BROCKLEHURST'S TEXTBOOK OF

Geriatric Medicine and Gerontology

6TH EDITION

Commissioning Editor: Miranda Bromage
Project Development Manager: Kim Benson
Project Manager: Hilary Hewitt/Keyword Publishing Services Ltd
Designer: Marie McNestry
Illustrations Manager: Mick Ruddy
Illustrators: Tim Loughhead, Marion Tasker
Cover Illustration: Rembrandt, follower of, an Old Man Seated in an
Armchair © National Gallery, London

BROCKLEHURST'S TEXTBOOK OF

Geriatric Medicine and Gerontology

6TH EDITION

Edited by

Raymond C Tallis MA FRCP FMedSci LittD DLitt
Professor of Geriatric Medicine
Division of Geriatric Medicine
University of Manchester Medical School;
Honorary Consultant Physician
Department of Care of the Elderly
Hope Hospital
Salford
UK

Howard M Fillit MD
Executive Director
The Institute for the Study of Aging;
Clinical Professor of Geriatrics and Medicine
Professor of Neurobiology
The Mount Sinai Medical Center
New York, NY
USA

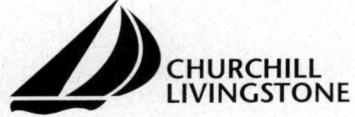
CHURCHILL
LIVINGSTONE

Churchill Livingstone
An imprint of Elsevier Science Limited

First edition 1973
Second edition 1978
Third edition 1985
Fourth edition 1992
Fifth edition 1998
Sixth edition 2003

ISBN 0-443-07087-3

British Library Cataloguing in Publication Data
A catalogue record for this book is available from the British Library

Library of Congress Cataloging in Publication Data
A catalog record for this book is available from the Library of Congress

Drug nomenclature
Directive 92/27/EEC requires use of the Recommended International Non-proprietary Name (rINN) for medicinal substances. In most cases the British Approved Name (BAN) and rINN are identical but where they differ the rINN has been used with the old BAN in parentheses.

There are two important exceptions: adrenaline and noradrenaline, where the BAN is used first followed by the new rINNS (epinephrine and norepinephrine) in parentheses.

Drug dosages
Medical knowledge is constantly changing. As new information becomes available, changes in treatment, procedures, equipment and the use of drugs become necessary. The authors and the publishers have taken care to ensure that the information given in this text is accurate and up to date. However, readers are strongly advised to confirm that the information, especially with regard to drug usage, complies with the latest legislation and standards of practice.

Printed in Spain

The
publisher's
policy is to use
**paper manufactured
from sustainable forests**

Table of Contents

Foreword

A textbook is "a manual of instruction in any science or branch of study, especially a work recognized as an authority"according to the Oxford English Dictionary. The Preface to the first edition of this textbook (1973) opened with the paragraph: "This Textbook of Geriatric Medicine and Gerontology is presented as an authoritative statement on research and current medical practice on all matters relating to aging and old age in man. While its main concern is with the medicine of old age, it is well recognized that this cannot be treated in isolation. Biological, psychological and social aspects of aging are all intertwined with geriatric medicine and all are interdependent." This philosophy continues to underlie this sixth edition.

While geriatrics as a medical specialty may have been born in the United Kingdom with the inception of the National Health Service in 1948, the advent of this first major textbook in 1973 was particularly relevant as a contribution to the struggle for the recognition among its peers as a legitimate medical specialty. Emerging medical specialties have traditionally faced a hostile reception from some members of the profession—for varying reasons. In the case of geriatrics, criticism centered on the notion that "it has no particular scientific basis," nor did it focus on one body system. And it had no endoscope or other special item of equipment.

The 44 contributors to the first edition of this textbook in 760 pages defined the scientific basis of geriatric medicine and reviewed the widespread research on which this rested.

The Textbook is now presented in its sixth edition with 180 contributors and over 1500 pages. This growth reflects the huge amount of research undertaken world wide in the biology, psychology, sociology and medicine of old age in the last 29 years. It reflects also the considerable change in life expectancy during that time and the consequent increased proportion of populations aged 70 and over world wide.

The first edition had an entirely British authorship with three exceptions, namely Bouliere from France, Munnichs from the Netherlands and Sourander from Finland. Since then the balance of readership and authorship has changed, most particularly with the emergence of specialization in geriatrics in the United States and Canada in the 1980s. The certificate of Added Qualification in Geriatric Medicine instituted by the joint American Boards of Internal Medicine and Family Practice in 1988 was a major contributor to this development.

In response to these changes—and the growing field of research—two distinguished geriatricians, one British and one American joined the editorial team of this Textbook for the fourth edition in 1992. Raymond Tallis, Professor of Geriatric Medicine at the University of Manchester is now one of the leaders of British geriatrics. While his particular medical interest is the neurology of old age, he is also widely recognized and respected as a philosopher (with five books in this field) as well as a writer of fiction and poetry. Howard Fillit, MD is a clinical professor of geriatrics, medicine and a professor of neurobiology in the pioneering department of geriatrics at the Mount Sinai Medical Center in New York City. He is also the founding executive director of the Institute for the Study of Aging, a biomedical venture philanthropy dedicated to catalyzing and funding research on cognitive aging and Alzheimer's disease. The total authorship of this sixth edition now reflects an equal balance between Britain and America, with a small number of contributors from other countries.

The Dutch artist Rembrandt van Rijn is one of the world's greatest portraitists of old age—both men and women. His last two self portraits were painted in the 63rd (and last) year of his life. His portrait of "An old man seated on armchair" (1652) was chosen as an appropriate adornment for the cover of the first edition of this textbook, and appears on the cover of all subsequent editions (by permission of the British National Gallery).

Now that the time has come for my withdrawal from the editorship of this textbook it is with confidence and gratitude that I hand over complete responsibility for this sixth edition to professors Tallis and Fillit. In their capable and scholarly hands its continuing authority is ensured.

JOHN C. BROCKLEHURST
Professor Emeritus
Geriatric Medicine
University of Manchester
2002

Contributors

HARITHA R ALLA MD
Fellow of Cardiovascular Medicine
Division of Cardiovascular Medicine
Medical College of Wisconsin
Milwaukee
WI
USA

REBECCA S ALLEN PhD
Assistant Professor of Psychology;
Associate Director, Applied Gerontology
Program
The University of Alabama
Tuscaloosa
AL
USA

WILBERT S ARONOW MD FACC AGSF
FGSA
Clinical Professor of Medicine
Divisions of Cardiology and Geriatrics;
Chief, Cardiology Clinic
New York Medical School;
Adjunct Professor of Geriatrics and Adult
Development
Mount Sinai School of Medicine
New York
NY
USA

MARGARET B ARTZ PhD RPh
Research Scientist
Institute for the Study of Geriatric
Pharmacotherapy
College of Pharmacy
University of Minneapolis
MN
USA

FRÉDÉRIC ASSAL MD
International Scholar
Clinique de Neurologie
Geneva
Switzerland

WILLIAM H BARKER MD FRCPEdin
Professor, Preventive Medicine and
Gerontology
University of Rochester
Rochester
NY
USA

PAUL BELCHETZ BA BChir MA MB MRCP
MSc FRCP
Consultant Physician/Endocrinologist
Department of Endocrinology
Leeds General Infirmary
Leeds
UK

GERALD CJ BENNETT MB BCh FRCP
Professor, Health Care of the Older People
Barts and The London Queen Mary's School
of Medicine and Dentistry
The Royal London Hospital (Mile End)
London
UK

STEVEN L BERK MD
Regional Dean and Mirick-Myers Chair of
Geriatric Medicine
Texas Tech School of Medicine
Amarillo
TX
USA

ARNAB BHOWMICK MB ChB FRCS
Specialist Registrar in Surgery
South Manchester University Hospital Trust
Wythenshawe Hospital
Manchester
UK

ITALO BIAGGIONI MD
Professor of Medicine and Pharmacology
Vanderbilt University
Nashville
TN
USA

DAVID A BLACK MA MBA FRCP
Medical Director and Consultant Geriatrician
Queen Mary's Hospital
Sidcup
Kent
UK

GERALD BLANDFORD MBBS MRCP
(Lond) FRCP(C) FACP
Medical Director
Division of Geriatrics
Montefiore Medical Center
Bronx
NY
USA

MARY R BLISS MBBS FRCP(UK)
Consultant Geriatrician Emeritus
St Bartholomew's and Hackney Hospitals
London
UK

CLIVE E BOWMAN BSc FRCPEdin & Lond
Medical Director
BUPA Care Services
Horsforth
Leeds
UK

LAWRENCE J BRANDT MD MACG FACP
FAAPP
Professor of Medicine and Surgery
Albert Einstein College of Medicine
Chief of Gastroenterology
Montefiore Medical Center and
Albert Einstein College of Medicine
New York
NY
USA

JOHN C BROCKLEHURST CBE MD
MSc FRCP (Lond)
Professor Emeritus
Geriatric Medicine
University of Manchester
Manchester
UK

SCOTT E BRODIE MD
Associate Professor
Department of Ophthalmology
Mount Sinai Medical Center
New York
NY
USA

REBECCA CC BROOKE BSc MB ChB
MRCP
Research Fellow
The Dermatology Centre
University of Manchester School of Medicine
Hope Hospital
Salford
UK

ALAN DG BROWN MB ChB FRCOG
FRCSEd
Consultant Obstetrician and Gynaecologist
Simpson Centre for Reproductive Health
Royal Infirmary
Edinburgh
UK

JOHN BRUNS, JR MD
Clinical Assistant Professor
Department of Emergency Medicine
Mount Sinai School of Medicine
New York
NY
USA

ALASTAIR BURNS MD FRCP FRCPsych
Professor of Old Age Psychiatry
School of Psychiatry and Behavioural Sciences
Wythenshawe Hospital
Manchester
UK

ANDREW BURROUGHS MB ChB Hons
FRCP
Professor of Hepatology
Liver Transplantation & Hepatobiliary Medicine
Royal Free Hospital
London
UK

ROBERT N BUTLER MD
Professor of Geriatrics
Mount Sinai School of Medicine;
President & CEO
International Longevity Center
New York
NY
USA

CHRIS CLOUGH FRCP
Consultant Neurologist
King's College Hospital
Department of Clinical Neurosciences
London
UK

MARTIN J CONNOLLY MD FRCP
Senior Lecturer in Medicine and Geriatrics
University of Manchester
Platt Rehabilitation Unit 2
Manchester Royal Infirmary
Manchester
UK

TARA K COOPER MRCOG
Consultant Gynaecologist & Obstetrician
St Johns Hospital at Howden
West Lothian Healthcare NHS Trust
Livingston
UK

RICHARD A COWIE BSc MB ChB FRCSE
FRCSE (SN)
Consultant Neurosurgeon
Hope Hospital
Salford
UK

SIMON CM CROXSON BM MD FRCP
Consultant Physician
Department of Medicine for the Elderly
Bristol General Hospital
Bristol
UK

JEFFREY L CUMMINGS MD
Augustus S Rose Professor of Neurology;
Professor of Psychiatry and
Behavioral Sciences;
Director, UCLA Alzheimer's Disease Center
Los Angeles
CA
USA

IOAN DAVIES PhD
Lecturer in Biological Gerontology
Department of Pathological Sciences
Schools of Medicine and Biological Sciences
University of Manchester
Manchester
UK

MARTIN S DENNIS MD FRCP(Ed)
Professor of Stroke Medicine
Department of Clinical Neurosciences
Western General Hospital
Edinburgh
UK

HUGH DEVLIN BDS BSc MSc PhD
Senior Lecturer in Restorative Dentistry
University Dental Hospital of Manchester
Prosthodontics Unit
Manchester
UK

A BALLAV DEY MD
Department of Medicine
All India Institute of Medical Sciences
New Delhi
India

SUSIE DINAN BEd PostgradDip
Senior Clinical Excercise Practitioner and
Research Fellow
Department of Primary Care and Population
Sciences
Royal Free and University College
School of Medicine
London
UK

REBECCA B DUNN FRCP
Consultant Geriatrician
Royal United Hospital NHS Trust
Bath
UK

SIJMEN A DUURSMA
Professor of Geriatric Medicine
University Medical Centre
Ultrecht University Hospital
Bunnik
The Netherlands

SHAH EBRAHIM DM MSc FRCP FFPHM
Professor in Epidemiology of Ageing
Department of Social Medicine
University of Bristol
Bristol
UK

JESSE EISLER MD
Department of Orthopaedics
Mount Sinai Medical Center
New York
NY
USA

TIMO ERKINJUNTTI MD PhD
Chief, Memory Research Unit
Department of Neurology
University of Helsinki
Finland

WILLIAM B ERSHLER MD
Director
Institute for Advanced Studies in Aging
Washington, DC
USA

JUDITH ESTRINE
Senior Science Writer
International Longevity Center
New York
NY
USA

WILLIAM EVANS PhD
Director, Nutrition, Metabolism, and
Excercise Laboratory;
Professor of Geriatrics, Physiology and
Nutrition
Donald W Reynolds Department of Geriatrics
University of Arkansas for Medical Sciences
Little Rock
AR
USA

MARIE FALLON MB ChB MD FRCP
MRCGP
Senior Lecturer in Palliative Care
Department of Oncology
Western General Hospital
Edinburgh
UK

MARK W J FERGUSON BSc BDS PhD
FFD FDS FMedSci CBE
Professor, School of Biological Sciences
University of Manchester
Manchester
UK

HOWARD M FILLIT MD
Executive Director
The Institute for the Study of Aging;
Clinical Professor of Geriatrics
Mount Sinai Medical Center
New York
NY
USA

HOWARD A FINK MD MPH
Assistant Professor of Medicine
VA Medical Center
Minneapolis
MN
USA

ROGER M FRANCIS MB ChB FRCP
Reader in Medicine (Geriatrics)
University of Newcastle upon Tyne
Bone Clinic
Freeman Hospital
Newcastle upon Tyne
UK

MICHAEL L FREEDMAN MD FACP
The Diane and Arthur Belfer Professor of
Geriatric Medicine;
Professor of Medicine;
Director of the Diane and Arthur Belfer
Geriatric Center
New York University
School of Medicine and the New York
University Medical Center
New York
NY
USA

ANTHONY J FREEMONT BSc MD FRCP
FRCPath
Professor of Osteoarticular Pathology
Musculoskeletal Research Group
School of Medicine
University of Manchester
Manchester
UK

JESSICA GALLINA MD
Department of Orthopaedics
Mount Sinai Medical Center
New York
NY
USA

NICHOLAS J R GEORGE MBBS MD
FRCS
Senior Lecturer / Consultant Urologist
Deparment of Urology
Withington Hospital
Manchester
UK

GARY GERSTENBLITH MD
Professor of Medicine
Cardiology Division
Johns Hopkins University School of Medicine
Baltimore
MD
USA

BARBARA A GILCHREST MD
Professor & Chairman of Dermatology
Boston University School of Medicine
Department of Dermatology
Boston
MA
USA

MARIA H GILLEECE MD BSc (Hons)
MRCP MRCPath
Consultant Haematologist
Department of Haematology
Ysbyty Gwynedd
Bangor
Gwynedd
UK

NEIL D GILLESPIE BSc(Hons) MB ChB
MD MRCP(UK)
Senior Lecturer in Ageing and Health
Department of Medicine (Ageing and Health)
Ninewells Hospital and Medical School
Dundee
UK

THOMAS A GLASS PhD
Associate Professor of Epidemiology
Johns Hopkins Bloomberg School of
Public Health
Department of Epidemiology
Baltimore
MD
USA

MARGOT GOSNEY MD FRCP
Senior Lecturer in Geriatric Medicine
University Clinical Departments
University of Liverpool
Liverpool
UK

STEFAN GRAVENSTEIN MD MPH FACP
Professor of Medicine
John Franklin Chair of Geriatrics
Chief, Division of Geriatrics
Director, Glennan Center for
Geriatrics and Gerontology
Eastern Virginia Medical School
USA

DAVID GREENWALD MD
Associate Professor of Medicine
Albert Einstein College of Medicine
Gastroentrology Fellowship Director
Montefiore Medical Center
Bronx
NY
USA

CHRISTOPHER E M GRIFFITHS BSc
MD FRCP
Professor of Dermatology
The Dermatology Centre
University of Manchester
Salford
UK

EMILY M D GRUNDY MA MSc PhD
Reader in Social Gerontology
Centre for Population Studies
London School of Hygiene & Tropical Medicine
London
UK

DAVID R P GUAY PharmD FCP FCCP
FASCP CGP
Professor and Head
Experimental and Clinical Pharmacology;
Director of Education
Institute for the Study of Geriatric
Pharmacotherapy
College of Pharmacy
University of Minnesota
Minneapolis
MN
USA

PETER HAMMOND MA BM BCh MD FRCP
Consultant Physician/Endocrinologist
Harrogate District Hospital
Harrogate
UK

JOSEPH T HANLON PharmD
Professor of Pharmacy
College of Pharmacy
University of Minnesota
Minneapolis
MN
USA

DANIELLE HARARI FRCP
Clinical Senior Lecturer and Consultant in
Geriatric Medicine
Elderly Care Unit
St Thomas' Hospital
London
UK

S MITCHELL HARMAN MD PhD
Director
Kronos Longevity Research Institute
Phoenix
AZ
USA

JOHN HARRIS FMedSci BA DPhil
Sir David Alliance Professor of Bioethics
School of Law
University of Manchester
Manchester
UK

ROBERT D HELME MBBS PhD FRACP
FFPMANZCA
St Vincent's Hospital
Barbara Walker Pain Management Centre
Fitzroy
Victoria
Australia

KENNETH W HEPBURN PhD
Associate Professor
Department of Family Practice &
Community Health;
Director, Aging and Geriatric Medicine
Program
Medical School
University of Minnesota
Minneapolis
MN
USA

CHRISTOPHER HEWARD PhD
Vice President of Research and Development
The Kronos Group
Phoenix
AZ
USA

JERROLD HILL PhD
Director of Outcomes Research
Institute for the Study of Aging
New York
NY
USA

CHRISTINE H HIMES MD
Director of Geriatirics
Group Health Cooperative
Seattle
USA

MICHAEL A HORAN MB PhD FRCP
Consultant in Care of the Elderly
Hope Hospital
Salford
UK

OLIVER F W JAMES FRCP FMedSci
Head of School Clinical Medical Sciences
Medical School
University of Newcastle
Newcastle upon Tyne
UK

SARBJIT VANITA JASSAL MB BCh MD
MRCP(UK) MSc FRCP(C)
Assistant Professor, University of Toronto;
Staff Nephrologist, University Health Network
Toronto
Ontario
Canada

NICOLE L JENKINS PhD
Post Doctoral Fellow
The Buck Institute for Age Research
Novato
CA
USA

ERIK JOHNSON MD
Department of Orthopaedics
Mount Sinai Medical Center
New York
NY
USA

RAJENDRA JUTAGIR PhD
Assistant Clinical Professor
Mount Sinai School of Medicine
New York
NY
USA

ALEXANDRE KALACHE MD PhD
Coordinator
Ageing and Life Course Programme
World Health Organisation
Geneva
Switzerland

LALIT KALRA MD PhD FRCP(Lond)
Professor of Stroke Medicine
Department of Internal Medicine
Guy's, King's and St Thomas' Medical School
London
UK

ROSALIE A KANE PhD
Professor, Health Services Research and Policy
School of Public Health
University of Minnesota
Minneapolis
MN
USA

CORNELIUS L E KATONA MD FRCPsych
Dean
Institute of Medicine and Health Sciences
University of Kent at Canterbury
Canterbury
Kent
UK

BENNY KATZ MBBS FRACP FFPMANZCA
Director, Pain Management Clinic
Melbourne Extended Care and
Rehabilitation Service
Parkville
Victoria
Australia

SEYMOUR KATZ MD FACP FACG
Clinical Professor of Medicine (New York
University School of Medicine)
Nassau Gastroenterology Associates, P.C.
Great Neck
NY
USA

LESLIE I KATZEL MD PhD
Associate Professor
University of Maryland School of Medicine
Department of Medicine
Division of Gerontology
Baltimore VA Medical Center GRECC
Baltimore
MD
USA

HORACIO KAUFMANN MD
Associate Professor of Neurology
Mount Sinai School of Medicine;
Director, Autonomic Disorders Research and
Treatment Program
Mount Sinai Medical center
Department of Neurology
New York
NY
USA

VISHAL Y KAUSHIK MBBS MRCP
Consultant Physician
Department of Gastroenterology
The Royal Infirmary
Blackburn
UK

PAUL W KEELEY MB ChB MRCGP
Department of Palliative Medicine
Beatson Oncology Centre
Western Infirmary
Glasgow
UK

NICHOLAS A KEFALIDES MD PhD
Professor
Departments of Medicine and Biochemistry
and Biophysics
University of Pennsylvania School of Medicine
Philadelphia
PA
USA

CATHERINE L KELLEHER MD
Assistant Professor of Medicine
Nephrology Division
Denver Health Medical Center
University of Colorado Medical Center
Denver
CO
USA

INGRID KELLER MSc MPH
Associate Professional Officer
Ageing and Life Course Programme
World Health Organisation
Geneva
Switzerland

DAVID C KENNIE MB ChB FRCP DCH
DRCOG
Consultant Physician
Department of Ageing and Health
The Royal Infirmary
Stirling
UK

ROSE ANNE KENNY MD FRCPI FRCP
Professor of Cardiovascular Research
Falls and Syncope Service
Care of the Elderly Offices
Royal Victoria Infirmary
Newcastle upon Tyne
UK

THOMAS B L KIRKWOOD MA MSc PhD
FMedSci
Professor of Medicine
University of Newcastle upon Tyne
Department of Gerontology
Institute for Ageing and Health
Newcastle General Hospital
Newcastle upon Tyne
UK

BRANDON KORETZ MD
Assistant Clinical Professor of
Geriatric Medicine
University of California at Los Angeles
School of Medicine
Division of Geriatrics
Los Angeles
CA
USA

MARK A KOSINSKI DPM
Professor
Division of Medical Sciences
New York College of Podiatric Medicine
New York
NY
USA

ALISTAIR LAMMIE MA MB BChir PhD
MRCPath
Consultant Neuropathologist
Department of Pathology
University of Wales College of Medicine
Cardiff
UK

ALAN LAZAROFF MD
Director of Geriatric Medicine
Centura Senior Care;
President
Geriatric Medicine Associates
Denver
CO
USA

MYRNA I LEWIS PhD
Assistant Professor
Mount Sinai School of Medicine
New York
NY
USA

CATHERINE LINDBLAD PharmD
University of Minnesota
College of Pharmacy
Minneapolis
MN
USA

GORDON J LITHGOW PhD
Associate Professor
The Buck Institute for Age Research
Novato
CA
USA

GILL LIVINGSTON MD FRCPsych
Reader in Psychiatry/Hon. Consultant in
Mental Health Care of the Elderly
UCL Department of Psychiatry and
Behavioural Sciences
London
UK

ROBERT L MAHER Jr PharmD
Assistant Professor of Clinical Pharamacy
Duquesne University School of Pharmacy
Pittsburgh
PA
USA

ALASTAIR MAKIN FRCP
Consultant Gastroenterologist
Manchester Royal Infirmary
Manchester
UK

JAMES MALONE-LEE MD FRCP
Professor of Medicine
Departmental of Medicine
Whittington Hospital Campus
University College London
London
UK

ROBERT E MANSEL MB MS FRCS
Professor of Surgery
University Hospital of Wales
Cardiff
UK

KENNETH G MANTON PhD
Research Professor and Scientific Director
Demographic Studies
Center for Demographics Studies
Duke University
Durham
NC
USA

BRYAN C MARKINSON DPM
Assistant Professor of Orthopedics
Mount Sinai School of Medicine;
Adjunct Professor, Medical Sciences
NY College of Podiatric Medicine
New York
NY
USA

EDWARD J MASORO PhD
Charleston
SC
USA

GAWAIN McCOLL PhD
Post Doctoral Fellow
The Buck Institute for Age Research
Novato
CA
USA

CHARLES N McCOLLUM MD FRCS
Professor of Surgery
Education and Research Centre
South Manchester University Hospital Trust
Wythenshawe Hospital
Manchester
UK

CLAUDINE McCREADIE MA(Cantab)
DipSocAdmin (LSE)
Research Fellow
Institute of Gerontology
King's College London
London
UK

JOLYON MEARA MD FRCP
Senior Lecturer in Geriatric Medicine
University of Wales College of Medicine
(North Wales)
Glan Clwyd Hospital
Rhyl
Clwyd
UK

MYRON MILLER MD FACP
Professor of Medicine,
Department of Medicine
Johns Hopkins University School of Medicine;
Academic Director
Division of Geriatric Medicine
Sinai Hospital of Baltimore
Baltimore
MD
USA

CHARLES VERNON MOBBS PhD
Associate Professor
Neurobiology and Geriatrics
Mount Sinai School of Medicine
Kastor Neurobiology of
Aging Laboratories
New York
NY
USA

KEVIN MORGAN BSc PhD
Professor of Gerontology
Department of Human Sciences
Loughborough University
Leicestershire
UK

CHARLOTTE MULLER PhD
Co-director of Research
International Longevity Center-USA;
Professor Emerita
Doctoral Economics Program
City University of New York
New York
NY
USA

JAMES W MYERS MD
Associate Professor of Medicine
Department of Internal Medicine
East Tennessee State University
Johnson City
TN
USA

DAVID NEARY MD FRCP
Professor of Neurology and Consultant
Neurologist
Great Manchester Neuroscience Centre
Hope Hospital
Salford
UK

MARY LYNN R NIERODZIK
MD FACP
Clinical Associate Professor
of Medicine
New York University School
of Medicine
New York
NY
USA

DIMITRIOS G OREOPOULOS MD PhD
FACP FRCP(Glasgow)
Professor of Medicine
University of Toronto
Toronto Western Hospital
University Health Network
Toronto
Ontario
Canada

JOSEPH G OUSLANDER MD
Professor of Medicine and Nursing
Director, Division of Geriatric Medicine and
Gerontology;
Chief Medical Officer, Wesley Woods Center
of Emory University;
Director, Emory Center of Health in Aging;
Investigator, Geriatric Research, Education,
and Clinical Center;
Atlanta VA Medical Center
Atlanta
GA
USA

JAMES T PACALA MD MS
Associate Professor
Vice-Chair for Medical Student Affairs
University of Minnesota Medical School
Department of Family Practice and
Community Health
Minneapolis
MN
USA

VALERIE M POMEROY PhD FCSP BA
GradDipPhys
Professor of Rehabilitation for Older People
St George's Hospital Medical School
London
UK

PETER POMPEI MD
Associate Professor of Medicine
Stanford University School of Medicine
Department of Medicine and VA Palo Alto
Health Care System
Palo Alto
CA
USA

JOHN F POTTER DM FRCP
Professor of Medicine for the Elderly
Glenfield Hospital
Leicester
UK

MARIA LUISA RAIMONDO MD
Clinical Fellow
Royal Free Hospital
Liver Transplantation & Hepatobiliary
Medicine
London
UK

LAKSHMI RAMANATHAN PhD
Assistant Professor of Pathology
Mount Sinai School of Medicine;
Assistant Director
Henry Dazian Department of Chemistry
The Mount Sinai Hospital
New York
NY
USA

BRION D REICHLER MD
Associate Professor
Department of Neurology
The Mount Sinai School of Medicine
New York
NY
USA

DAVID B REUBEN MD
Professor of Medicine;
Chief of the Division of Geriatrics;
Director, Multicampus Program in Geriatric
Medicine and Gerontology
University of California at Los Angeles School
of Medicine
Division of Geriatrics
Los Angeles
CA
USA

MARK E ROBERTS MB ChB BSc MRCP MD
Consultant Neurologist
Department of Neurology
Withington and Hope Hospitals
Manchester
UK

KENNETH ROCKWOOD MD MPA
FRCPC
Professor of Medicine (Geriatric Medicine and
Neurology) & Kathryn Allen Weldon Professor
of Alzheimer Research
Geriatric Medicine Research Unit
Dalhousie University
Halifax
Nova Scotia
Canada

CHRISTOPHER A RODRIGUES PhD
FRCP
Consultant Physician
Medical Unit
Kingston Hospital
Kingston-upon-Thames
Surrey
UK

DAVID H ROSENBAUM MD
Associate Clinical Professor of Neurology
Mount Sinai School of Medicine
New York
NY
USA

LAURENCE Z RUBENSTEIN MD MPH
FACP
Professor of Geriatric Medicine
VA Medical Center
Sepulveda
CA
USA

LISA V RUBENSTEIN MD MSPH FACP
Professor of General Internal Medicine
VA Medical Center
Sepulveda
CA
USA

EVELYN M RUSSELL MD MRCPsych
Consultant in Old Age Psychiatry
Withington Hospital
Manchester
UK

GERRY J F SALDANHA MA(Oxon)Hons
MRCP
Consultant Neurologist
Department of Neurology
Pembury Hospital
Kent
UK

LASZLO SARKOZI PhD FACB
Professor of Pathology
Mount Sinai School of Medicine;
Director, Henry Dazian Department of
Chemistry
The Mount Sinai Hospital
New York
NY
USA

K WARNER SCHAIE PhD
Evan Pugh Professor of Human Development
and Psychology;
Director, Gerontology Center
Pennsylvania State University
PA
USA

KENNETH SCHMADER MD
Associate Professor of Medicine – Geriatrics
Durham VA Medical Center
Durham
NC
USA

DAVID L SCOTT BSc MD FRCP
Professor of Clinical Rheumatology
King's College Hospital
London
UK

D GWYN SEYMOUR MB ChB BSc MD
FRCP
Professor of Medicine (Care of the Elderly)
Medicine for the Elderly
Foresterhill Health Centre
Aberdeen
UK

ASIT SHAH MD
Department of Orthopaedics
Mount Sinai Medical Center
New York
NY
USA

MO SHARIF PhD
Lecturer
Department of Anatomy
University of Bristol
Bristol
UK

ALAN J SINCLAIR MSc(Syd) MD FRCP(Edin)
FRCP(Lond)
Professor of Medicine and Consultant
Diabetologist
Diabetes Research Unit
Section of Geriatric Medicine and
Gerontology
The University of Warwick
Coventry
UK

JULIE S SNOWDEN PhD AFBPsS
CPsychol
Senior Neuropsychologist
General Function Unit
Greater Manchester Neuroscience Centre
Hope Hospital
Salford
UK

JOHN D SORKIN MD PhD
Assistant Professor
University of Maryland School of Medicine
Department of Medicine, Division of
Gerontology;
Chief, Biostatistics and Informatics
Baltimore VA Medical Center GRECC
and University of Maryland Claude D Pepper
Older Americans Independence
Baltimore
MD
USA

RANDALL K SPOERI PhD
Vice President
Medical and Quality Informatics
HIP Health Plans
New York
NY
USA

W ZOE D STITT MD
Assistant Professor of Dermatology
Boston University School of Medicine
Boston
MA
USA

ROBERT W STOUT MD DSc FRCP
FMedSci
Professor of Geriatric Medicine
Department of Geriatric Medicine
Queens University Belfast
Belfast
UK

ELTON STRAUSS MD FACS
Associate Clinical Professor
Chief of Orthopaedic Traruma and Adult
Reconstruction
Chief of Orthopaedic Geriatrics
Mount Sinai Medical Center
New York
NY
USA

IAN A STUART-HAMILTON MA(Oxon)
PhD AFBPS CPsychol ILTM
Professor of Psychology
University College Worcester
Department of Psychology
Worcester
UK

ALLAN D STRUTHERS BSc MD FRCP
FESC
Professor of Cardiovascular Medicine and
Therapeutics
Department of Clinical Pharmacology
Ninewells Hospital
Dundee
UK

DAVID SUTIN MD
Clinical Assistant Professor of Medicine
New York University
New York
NY
USA

DAVID A TABERNER BA BM BCh FRCP
FRC Path
Honorary Consultant Haematologist
University Hospital of South Manchester
Manchester
UK

RAYMOND C TALLIS MA FRCP FMedSci
LittD DLitt
Professor of Geriatric Medicine; Honorary
Consultant Physician
Hope Hospital, University of Manchester
Medical School
Division of Geriatric Medicine
Salford
UK

ROBERT E TEPPER MD FACP FACG
Teaching Assistant in Medicine (New York
University School of Medicine)
Nassau Gastroenterology Associates, P.C.
Great Neck
NY
USA

ANITA J THOMAS PhD FRCP
Consultant Physician Geriatric and General
Internal Medicine;
Associate Medical Director
Plymouth Hospitals NHS Trust;
Clinical Sub Dean, Peninsula Medical School
Derriford Hospital
Plymouth
UK

ANTHEA TINKER PhD FKC AcSS CBE
Professor of Social Gerontology
Institute of Gerontology
King's College London
London
UK

JONATHAN H TOBIAS MD PhD FRCP
Consultant Senior Lecturer in Rheumatology
Rheumatology Unit
Bristol Royal Infirmary
Bristol
UK

DONALD D TRESCH† MD
Formerly Professor of Medicine
Medical College of Wisconsin
Division of Cardiology and Geriatrics
Milwaukee
WI
USA

ARNOLD WALD MD FACG
Professor of Medicine
The University of Pittsburgh Medical Center
Division of Gastroenterology, Hepatology
and Nutrition
Pittsburgh
PA
USA

MARION F WALKER PhD PPhil SROT
Lecturer in Stroke Rehabilitation
Division of Stroke Medicine
Nottingham City Hospital
Nottingham
UK

SAMUEL W WARBURTON Jr MD
National Medical Director, Quality
Management
Aetna Health Plans
Blue Bell
PA
USA

KATHERINE WARD DPM
Assistant Professor
Division of Medical Sciences
New York College of Podiatric Medicine
New York
NY
USA

HUBER R WARNER PhD
Associate Director
Biology of Aging Program
National Institute on Aging
Bethesda
MD
USA

VIVIENNE WATKIN MB ChB BSc Med
Hons MRCPsych
Consultant in Psychiatry
Colindale Hospital
London
UK

† Deceased

ANDREW D WEINBERG MD FACP
Associate Professor of Medicine and Medical
Director for Long-Term Care
Wesley Woods Center of Emory University
Atlanta
GA
USA

CYRIL WEINKOVE BSc MB ChB FCP(SA)
PhD
Consultant Chemical Pathologist
Hope Hospital
Salford
UK

BARBARA E WEINSTEIN PhD
Professor of Audiology
Lehman College
The City University of New York
Gradnote School and University Center
New York
NY
USA

DOUGLAS L WELSH MA
Doctoral Student
Clinical Psychology
University of Alabama
Northport
AL
USA

JOHN WELSH FRCP MRCP MB ChB
BSc(Hons)
Consultant in Palliative Medicine
University of Glasgow
Beatson Oncology Center
Western Infirmary
Glasgow
UK

GORDON K WILCOCK DM (Oxon)
FRCP
Professor in Care of the Elderly
University of Bristol
Department of Care of the Elderly
Frenchay Hospital
Bristol
UK

SHERRY L WILLIS PhD
Professor of Human Development
Gerontology Center
Pennsylvania State University
PA
USA

KAREN WU MD
Department of Orthopaedics
Mount Sinai Medical Center
New York
NY
USA

JEAN F WYMAN PhD RN
Professor of Nursing
School of Nursing
University of Minnesota
Minneapolis
MN
USA

ARCHIE YOUNG BSc MB ChB FRCP
(Lond, Glasg, Edin)
Professor of Geriatric Medicine
The University of Edinburgh
Geriatric Medicine
Edinburgh
UK

JOHN YOUNG MB(Hons) MSc MBA FRCP
Consultant Geriatrician
Department of Elderly Care
St Luke's Hospital
Bradford
UK

SUSAN J ZIEMAN MD
Assistant Professor of Medicine
Johns Hopkins University School of Medicine
Cardiology Division, Department of Medicine
Baltimore
MD
USA

Acknowledgements

The massive effort of putting together this textbook would not have been possible without tremendous support from others. Professor Tallis would particularly like to thank Mrs Penny Essex and Mrs Barbara Jones for their fantastic secretarial support and, in particular, keeping a very close eye on the commissioning process and the flow of chapters. Dr Howard Fillit would like to acknowledge Ms Carren Gordon for her assistance in the administrative aspects of coordinating the editing of the book and Ms Gloria Picariello, an excellent geriatric nurse practitioner, who assisted in reviewing the chapters for content.

Both Dr Fillit and Professor Tallis would wish to pay special tribute to the outstanding editorial support from Dr Kim Benson at Elsevier Science. Kim has proved to be a peerless chaser of contributors, collator of contributions and overall a faultless organizer of the textbook and has moreover remained exceptionally cheerful throughout what was often a difficult process.

The earlier contribution of Miranda Bromage in the planning of the book and the more recent contribution of Maureen Allen in dealing with the proofs are also gratefully acknowledged.

R.C. Tallis
H.M. Fillit

Chapter 1

Introduction

Raymond C. Tallis and Howard M. Fillit

In the developed world, most people can now expect to live to old age. In developing countries, although the average life expectancy is less, the absolute numbers of older people are far greater than in the developed world, and most of the increase in older persons worldwide during the next century will, in fact, come from the developing world. The impact of these dramatic demographic changes has been reflected in medicine and science, with increasing research and knowledge; in society, in a constant endeavor to improve services, making them more sensitive to the specific needs of older people; and among older people themselves, with appropriately increased expectations of good health, and excellent care when health fails. Biological, social, and psychological gerontology and the clinical discipline of geriatric medicine are now firmly established throughout much of the world. The health and social care needs of older people, for so long regarded as being of relatively marginal importance, are now an important concern to both developed and developing societies.

In the last edition we noted that the field of gerontology—the application of fundamental science to understanding the complex biopsychosocial processes of aging—was advancing rapidly. Indeed, there have been dramatic developments in our understanding of the molecular genetics of aging and cellular physiology, so that gerontology is even more interesting and relevant now than it was 5 years ago. For scientists, gerontology remains an exciting scientific field of the present and future. For clinicians, in dealing with elderly people, knowledge of gerontology is necessary in order that they should incorporate an understanding of the physiology of aging into their approach to clinical problems. Advances in gerontology and geriatric medicine, which have played a major part in our understanding of phenomena such as frailty, must also inform the medical, nursing, and social care systems provided for old people. This is why *Brocklehurst's Textbook of Geriatric Medicine and Gerontology* has retained a major section on basic gerontology with a focus on clinically relevant issues.

All of those engaged professionally in caring for elderly people must have ready access to reliable information over a dauntingly wide range of topics—from the cellular biology of aging to the management of hepatic failure in an older person; from the multidisciplinary approach to stroke to best practice in the institutional care of frail older people; from demographic trends to attitudes in society toward older people. The question then arises as to what form this source of information should take. The world of medical informatics, and the scope of basic and clinical gerontology, have both changed dramatically since the first edition of the textbook in 1973, and the pace over the last few years has quickened.

In preparing this sixth edition of what, since its first edition, has been recognized as the leading international textbook in the field, we have been acutely aware of these changes and the questions they pose. Our first consideration has been to ensure that the text is as up-to-date as possible. The reader will note the large number of post-2000 articles in the references cited by authors. Even so, given the time they take to produce, major textbooks cannot compete with electronic sources of information that can be more rapidly updated and so they must offer something in addition. We believe that the present textbook does.

First of all, we provide readers with a "one-stop shop." Our coverage is comprehensive. Even so, we have deliberately kept the text within the confines of a single volume. Multivolume texts are often frustrating; somehow the volume in one's hand is never the one that contains the information one requires. The initial section on gerontology encompasses age-related changes at every level from demography to cell biology, from genetic mechanism to life chances, from physiology to social consequences. Although gerontology has a section of its own, the clinical implications of the basic sciences are emphasized. Moreover, in the very extensive second section on geriatric medicine, the systemic and organ-specific changes relevant to aging are addressed with respect to each of the clinical areas of interest. Because the impact even of focal organ-based illness may be global in the biologically aged person, and management likewise needs to be whole-person, the clinical section is preceded by 11 chapters on "general issues" and there is a third major section devoted to problem-based geriatric medicine, which integrates much of the material provided in the preceding sections. Furthermore, it is essential to look beyond the whole body to the whole person, and beyond that, to the older person in society. This is therefore addressed in the fourth section devoted to health systems and geriatric medicine.

The core of the textbook comprises the 71 chapters devoted to individual diseases. While we have aimed at comprehensive coverage and an "internal stitching" and cross-referencing that ensures integration of the elements of the textbook, there are other attractive characteristics of this latest edition. Most importantly, there is the quality of the contributions. Each chapter has been commissioned from an authority in the field—roughly equal numbers from either side of the Atlantic—and what is offered is not merely information but clinical wisdom. While we have expected (and received) chapters committed to evidence-based practice, we have expected (and received) something more: authoritative accounts of the topic in question informed with practical understanding of the real challenges of medical care which, especially in the case of the management of older people, may require decisions that go beyond currently available evidence. (There is a difference between evidence-based practice, which is to be welcomed, and evidence-biased, or evidence-imprisoned, practice, which is not.) The extensive references at the end of each chapter are meant not only to justify the assertions made in them but also to guide readers to further exploration of the topic. The intention to be user-friendly as well as authoritative is reflected in the provision, where appropriate, of Key Points lists and Summary of Management Algorithms (SOMAs). (These are examples of how, when planning the latest edition of this classic textbook, the editors took note of helpful suggestions made in reviews of the previous edition.) In pursuit of excellence, we have taken on many new authors and added new chapters which has resulted in significant changes to the overall organization of the book.

We believe, therefore, that the present edition of the textbook, like its predecessors, will make a major contribution to fostering good practice in the care of older people by equipping practitioners with the knowledge they need.

SECTION 1
Gerontology

Chapter 2

The epidemiology of aging

Emily M. D. Grundy

Epidemiology is commonly defined as "the study of the distribution of a disease or a physiological condition in human populations and of the factors that influence this distribution,"[1] and it is this emphasis on populations rather than individuals that most clearly distinguishes epidemiology from other health-related sciences. The study of the epidemiology of aging presents greater challenges than applying epidemiological methods to the study of a particular disease and, as Greenhouse[2] noted, arriving at a satisfactory definition of what is meant by the epidemiology of aging is itself problematic. However, four elements which together constitute the core of the subject may be identified. These are:

1. studies concerned with the identification of risk factors which may elucidate the etiology of specific conditions primarily affecting elderly people;
2. studies in which epidemiological methods are used in the evaluation of preventive or therapeutic interventions in elderly populations;
3. studies of the general health status of older populations, either descriptive or concerned with the identification of factors associated with variations in general indicators of health;
4. studies of age-related change in indicators of health status, both general and disease-specific.

In this chapter the chief focus will be on the more general studies included in the third and fourth categories listed above. The epidemiology of specific conditions, and the evaluation of therapeutic interventions, are of course important areas of activity, and references to these kinds of studies are included in other chapters in this volume. However, a more general inventory of the health status of older populations is essential for public health planning, and comparisons between populations and population subgroups may provide insights into factors associated with health problems in later life. Planning for the future requires an assessment of age-related changes in health status, which may also further our understanding of basic aging processes.

Major conceptual and methodological problems make the compilation and interpretation of population-based statistics on aging and health particularly difficult. Health is an elusive concept, hard to measure or define at either the individual or population level. The World Health Organization definition of health is "a complete state of physical mental and social well-being,"[3] which, while admirable in emphasizing the multifactorial nature of health, is hard to operationalize and, if applied rigorously, would probably consign most individuals in most populations to the ranks of the unhealthy. Research on "positive health" has recently attracted growing attention; but in practice negative measures of morbidity—rather than health—predominate. While perhaps simpler to conceptualize, defining morbidity is also problematic. Should someone with occult or subclinical disease, for example, be considered healthy or unhealthy? Recent developments in genetics raise further complexities in this area. The consequences of particular pathological processes for health more broadly defined may vary considerably as a result of psychosocial factors and host–environment interactions, with the result that the same level of morbidity may have differing effects on function and quality of life depending on, for example, availability of assistive devices, appropriate housing and social support.

For all these reasons it is now largely accepted that the distinction between health and ill-health is a quantitative rather than a qualitative one and that both the causes and consequences of particular pathological processes may be multifactorial.[4]

POPULATION HEALTH

The measurement of health at the population level represents more than aggregation of individual-level data and represents particular challenges. In some respects population-level indicators should be simpler to devise than individual ones, if only because the degree of error associated with generalizing from large distributions is less than that associated with the prediction of particular observations. To take one example, chronological age is an unreliable predictor of performance or health in an individual,[5] but at the population level it is quite

Table 2-1 **Deaths at ages 0–4 and 75+ in England and Wales**		
Percentage of all deaths at ages		
Year	**0–4 years**	**75+ years**
1901	37	12
1999	0.8	64

Sources: UN (1988),[8] ONS (2001).[9]

a sensitive discriminator between groups.[6] However, in many other respects the measurement of health is more complex at the population than at the individual level. This is not simply a function of the problems associated with reliable ascertainment of health status in large groups, but also reflects the differing dynamics of health at the population and individual levels. Healthcare interventions—environmental or behavioral changes which reduce the risk of disability from, for example, hypertension—may represent a health gain at the individual level but result in a higher prevalence of morbidity from this cause in the population. Selective survival effects may mean that the health trajectories of individuals differ from those in populations.[7] Cohort effects represent a further major factor complicating elucidation of trends over time or between age groups.

These issues, and the basic questions of how to define and measure health, have become particularly pressing in contemporary developed populations with old age structures in which most deaths occur at advanced ages from degenerative diseases. As shown in Table 2-1, in England and Wales in 1999 nearly two-thirds of all deaths occurred among those aged 75 and over and only a tiny proportion among infants and young children. In 1901, by contrast, well over a third of all deaths occurred among infants under 5 years. This enormous change reflects not just the welcome reduction in the risk of death early in life, but also age structure changes in the population. One important consequence of the shift of most mortality and much associated morbidity to later ages is that in many populations addressing age-associated disease now represents the biggest public health challenge.

POPULATION AGING

The demographic determinants of a population's size and age structure are fertility, mortality, and migration. It has long been recognized that fertility is potentially the most important of these parameters in all but the highest of high-mortality populations.[10–12]

Children, if they survive to maturity, will in most cases become the parents of children who themselves may reproduce. Each birth thus represents not just an addition to the current generation of children, but a potentially exponentially increasing contribution to the size of subsequent generations of children. Historically, and apparently paradoxically, improvements in mortality in the now developed world served to partially offset the trend toward population aging, as they chiefly benefited the young—and led to increases in the proportion surviving to have children themselves. Primary population aging—a once and for all shift to an older age structure—is a consequence of long-term downward trends in fertility. In much of the now developed Western world this shift, termed the "demographic transition," occurred in the late nineteenth or early twentieth century. As a consequence in countries like England and Wales, the proportion of people aged 65 and over had already reached 10 percent by the mid-twentieth century, as illustrated in Figure 2-1. In Japan and the USA, also shown in the figure, the proportion of elderly people was lower than in England and Wales until very recently when Japan "overtook" England and Wales, and many other European countries, on this indicator of population aging. The USA continues to have a slightly lower proportion of elderly people than England and Wales and many other European countries, largely because fertility rates are higher and also because of the rejuvenating effects of continuing immigration. Japan was the first country outside the West to undergo the demographic transition from high to low fertility, and the speed of its decline in fertility was unprecedented. During the period 1947 to 1957 the total fertility rate (average number of children that would be born to a woman experiencing the age-specific fertility rates of the period throughout the childbearing years) fell by more than half from 4.5 to 2.0 children per woman.[17] Largely as a consequence of this, the pace of population aging in Japan has also been very fast and has been amplified by recent trends in mortality considered in more detail below. Subsequently other countries, notably China, have experienced even more rapid declines in fertility and in these the pace of age structure change will be faster still.

Declines in death rates at older ages and a further shift to very low fertility (total fertility rates of 1.5 or lower) in some regions, particularly southern and eastern Europe, has resulted in the further aging of many populations which had already experienced an initial shift to an older structure. As illustrated in Figure 2-2, population projections suggest that in several European countries close to a quarter of the population will be aged 65, and over and 3 percent aged 85 or over (Figure 2-3) by 2020. By 2050, the most recent United Nations projections indicate that there will be 19 countries, including France, Germany, Italy, Japan, Spain, and the UK, in which at least 10 percent of the population is aged 80 or more. By then Europeans aged 60 or more will constitute one in three of the population and outnumber children aged under 15 by a ratio of 2.6 to 1.[18]

In poorer parts of the world the proportion of elderly people is lower but in many it is rapidly increasing. The transition to lower, deliberately controlled fertility—the precursor of population aging—is now close to being a global phenomenon. In 1990, only 17 percent of the world's population lived in countries where no appreciable downturn in fertility was then evident[19] (although in many there are now signs that this is occurring). In these populations, predominantly in sub-Saharan Africa, the proportion of elderly people aged 65 and over is very small and is not projected to increase significantly in the short term. It is important to remember, however, that these populations are growing rapidly and this includes enormous growth in the *absolute* number of elderly people.

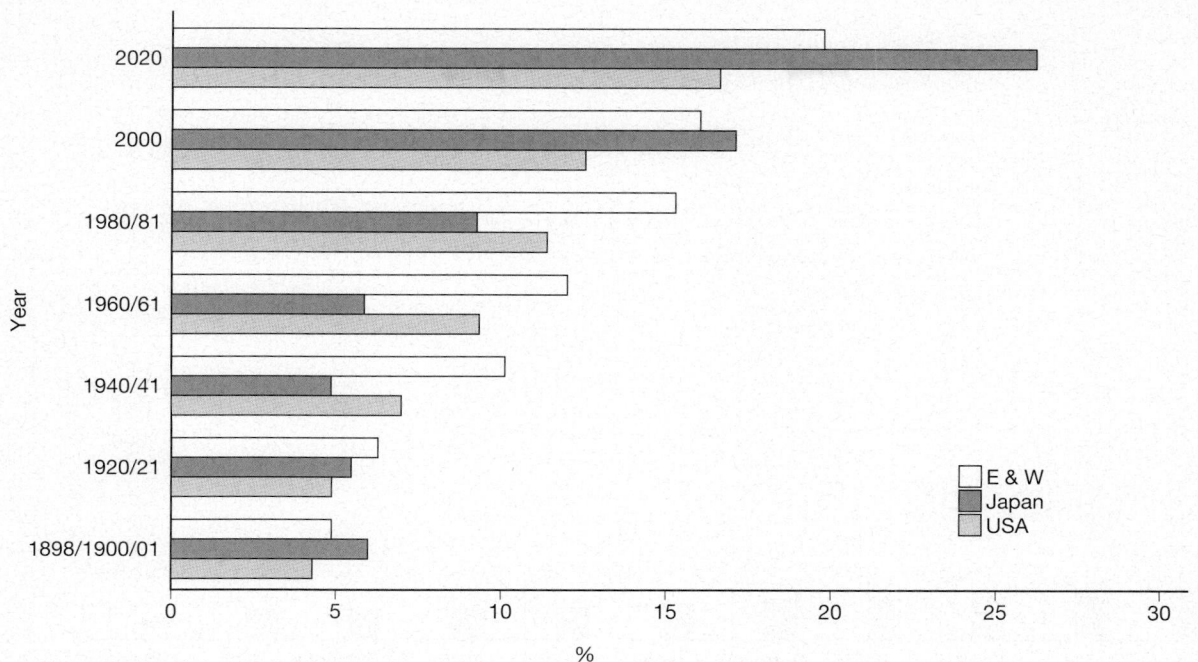

Figure 2-1 Percentage of the population aged 65 and over in England and Wales, the USA, and Japan, 1900 to 2020. Historical data: census data and estimates in Grundy[13] (England and Wales); Treas[14] (USA); Kono[15] (Japan). Projections from United Nations.[16]

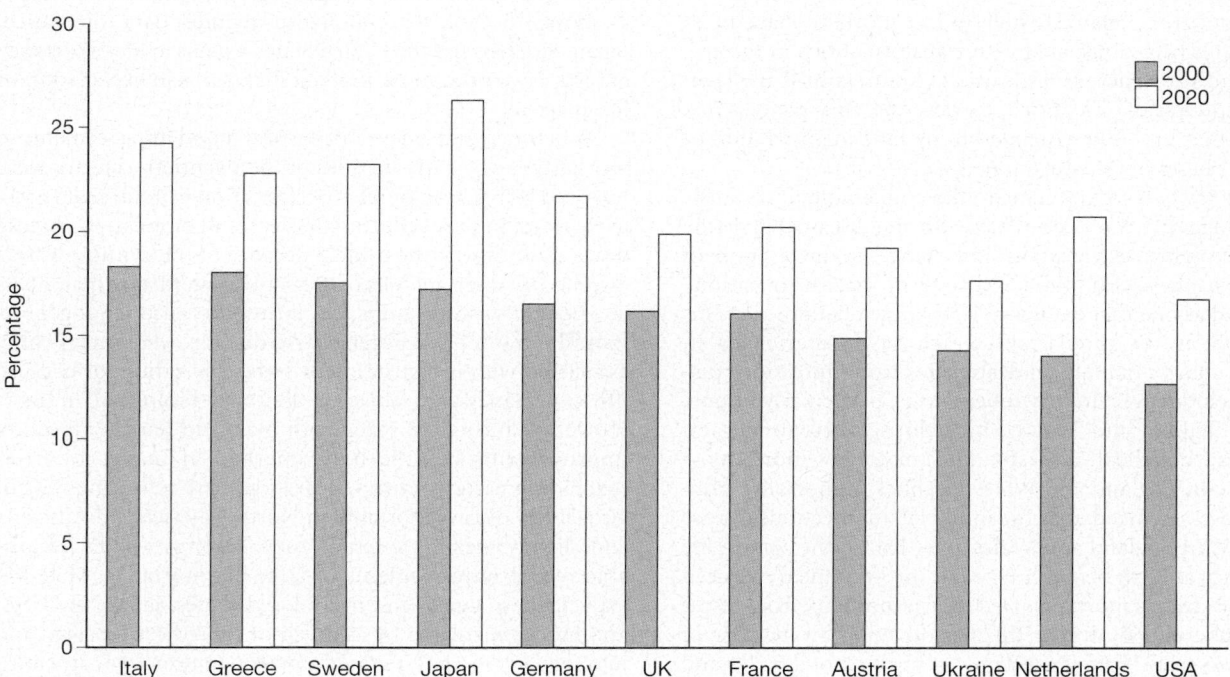

Figure 2-2 Percentage of the population aged 65 and over in selected industrialized countries, 2000 and 2020. Source: United Nations.[16]

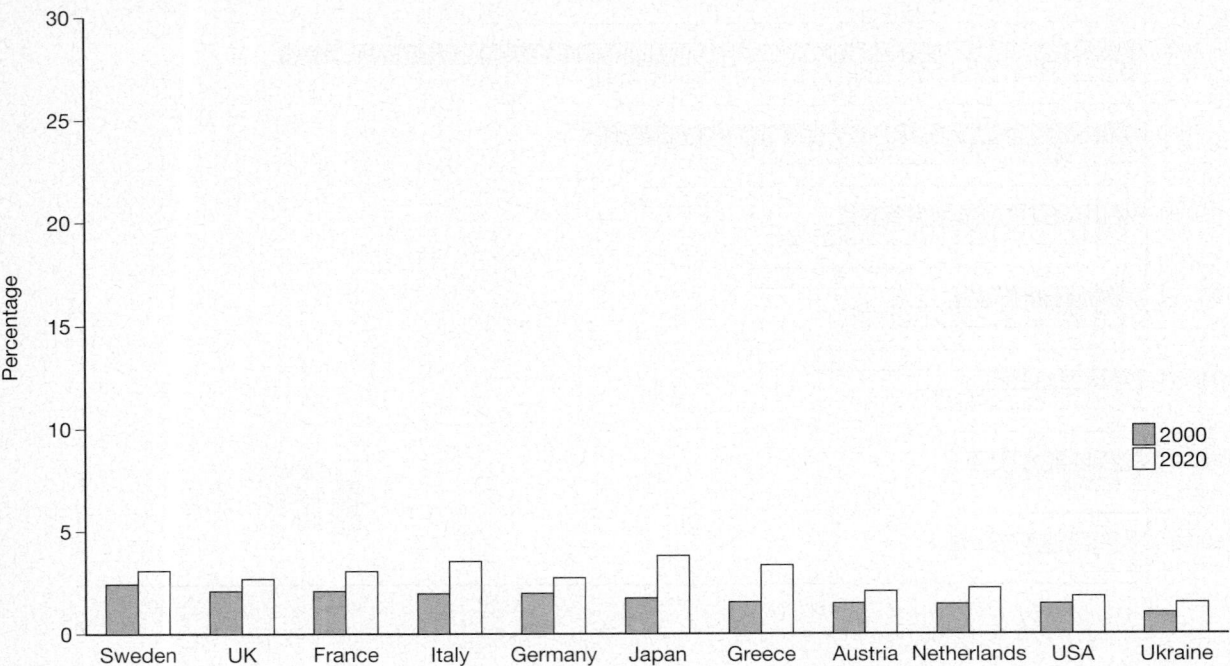

Figure 2-3 Percentage of the population aged 85 and over in selected industrialized countries, 2000 and 2020. Source: United Nations.[16]

MORTALITY, MORBIDITY, AND THE HEALTH TRANSITION

Transitions from relatively high to low mortality have in all populations been associated with transformations in the age, cause, and sex structure of death.[20] Omran coined the term "epidemiological transition" to describe this process,[21] a concept that has been expanded to include identification of separate phases of the transition.[22]

There are two components to the epidemiological transition: changes in the processes of health and disease that define the epidemiological transition, and changes in the response of societies to these conditions.[23] The term "health transition" was posed as one that embraced both these phenomena. This transition, in all populations which have experienced it, involves substantial falls in death rates from: infectious diseases (including respiratory tuberculosis, particularly important in England and Wales); bronchitis, pneumonia, and influenza; diarrheal diseases; and maternal mortality—although, in England and Wales, declines in mortality from these causes occurred after the initial fall in infectious disease mortality. In England and Wales, over half of the gain in life expectancy at birth between 1871 and 1911 was due to reduced infectious disease mortality. Declines in mortality from respiratory tuberculosis during this period led to an increase of nearly two years in life expectancy at birth among males and nearly two and a half years for females—some 20 percent of the total gain.[24]

Long-term trends in mortality by age in England and Wales are shown for men and women, respectively, in Figures 2-4 and 2-5. It can be seen that in all periods there is a strong relationship between age and mortality, with the risk of dying being lowest before puberty and then rising with age. Improvements in mortality over the whole of this period have been greatest in younger age groups. As a result— as shown in Table 2-2 which also includes data for France, Japan, Sweden, and the United States—gains in life expectancy at birth have been more marked than gains in expectation of life at age 65.

As in much of the developed world, rapid improvements in mortality in the early decades of the twentieth century were followed by a period of relative stagnation in adult male mortality rates, in part reflecting increases in circulatory-disease death rates during the middle decades of the century. It was assumed by some analysts of the period that further major falls in mortality were unlikely, either because endogenous mortality rates from degenerative diseases were inextricably associated with urbanization or industrialization, or because life expectancy was close to assumed biological limits.[25] However, during the 1970s both male and female mortality improvements became more marked in many countries (excluding eastern Europe), in large part reflecting falls in circulatory disease mortality in North America and Australia and, slightly later, in western Europe. Table 2-2 reveals remarkable recent improvements in later life mortality. Male life expectancy at age 65 in England and Wales, Japan, the USA, and France increased by as much or more between 1970 and 1995 than in the whole period from 1900 to 1970. In many countries death rates at the very highest ages have also fallen markedly, leading to large increases in the (admittedly still small) numbers reaching extreme ages of 100 or more.[26,27] An exception in western Europe seems to be the Netherlands where death rates among those aged 85 or over have stagnated or increased since the mid-1980s.[28]

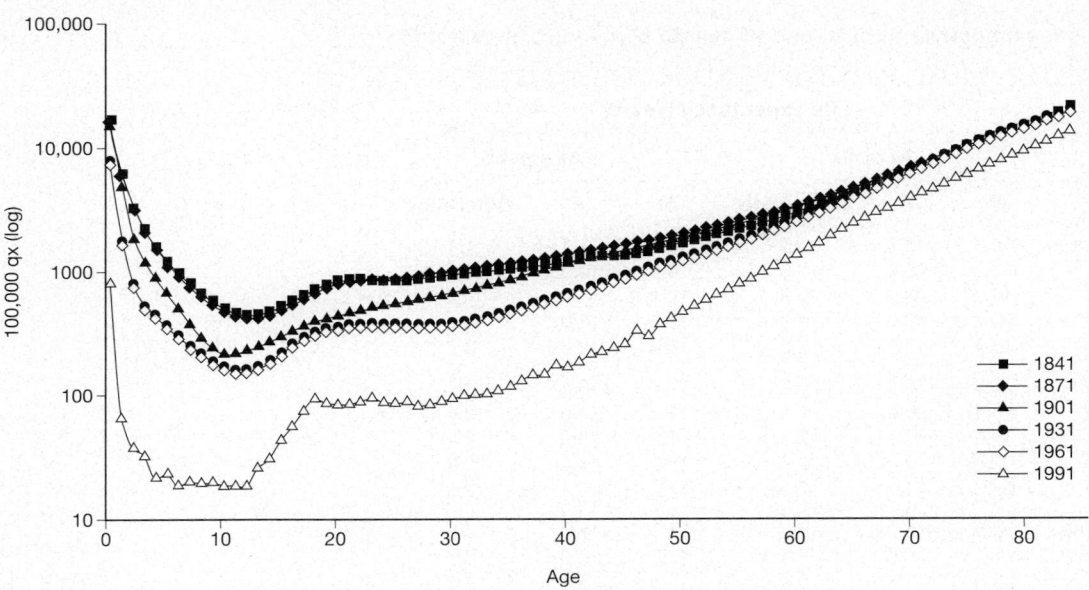

Figure 2-4 Male mortality by age in England and Wales, 1841 to 1991. Source: Government Actuary's Department, analyzed in Grundy,[31] with permission. (qx denotes probability of death from one age to the next.)

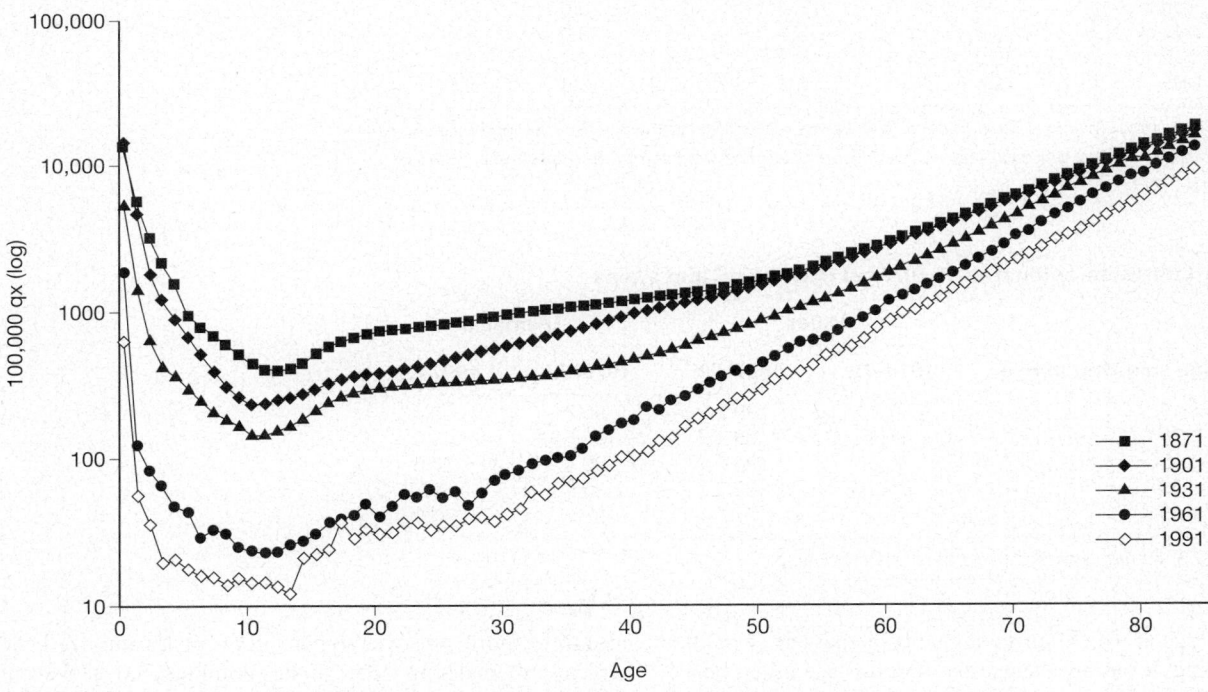

Figure 2-5 Female mortality by age in England and Wales, 1871 to 1991. Source: Government Actuary's Department, analyzed in Grundy,[31] with permission.

The effect of recent changes in mortality on the chances of survival to high ages is illustrated in Table 2-3, which shows period life-table estimates of survivorship based on the age-specific mortality schedules for England and Wales in 1970–72 and 1997–99. Already by 1970–72 current mortality rates implied almost universal survival to age 45 and survival to age 65 for a substantial majority. By 1997–99 the chance of survival to extreme old age had increased dramatically. Changes in survivorship from age 65 to age 85 were proportionately much greater than the changes between 1970–72 and 1997–99 in survivorship to specified younger ages. This is now a society in which current death rates imply that over 40 percent of females can expect to celebrate their 85th birthday.

Consequences of mortality changes

One consequence of these mortality changes—and a useful way of summarizing overall mortality trends—has been a marked

Table 2-2 Trends in life expectancy at birth and at age 65 by gender, in selected developed countries

| | | Life expectancy (years) | | | | | |
| | | At birth | | | At age 65 | | |
		M	F	Difference	M	F	Difference
1900/01	England & Wales	44.8	48.7	3.9	10.1	11.1	1.1
	France	43.2	46.9	3.8	10.0	10.9	0.9
	Japan	44.0	44.9	0.9	10.1	11.4	1.2
	Sweden	50.8	53.6	2.9	12.1	13.0	0.9
	USA	46.4	49.0	2.6	11.4	12.0	0.7
1950/1	England & Wales	65.3	70.3	5.0	10.8	13.4	2.6
	France	63.4	69.2	5.8	12.2	14.6	2.4
	Japan	57.6	60.9	3.3	10.9	13.0	2.1
	Sweden	69.8	72.4	2.6	13.5	14.3	0.8
	USA	65.6	71.1	5.5	12.8	15.1	2.3
1970/1	England & Wales	68.8	75.0	6.2	11.9	15.8	3.9
	France	68.4	75.8	7.4	13.0	16.8	3.7
	Japan	69.3	74.7	5.4	12.5	15.4	2.8
	Sweden	72.2	77.2	5.0	14.3	16.9	2.6
	USA	67.2	74.9	7.7	13.1	17.1	4.0
1995	England & Wales	74.4	79.6	5.2	14.8	18.4	3.6
	France	73.9	81.9	8.0	16.1	20.6	4.5
	Japan	76.4	82.8	6.4	16.5	20.9	4.4
	Sweden	76.2	81.5	5.3	16.0	19.7	3.7
	USA	72.4	79.3	6.9	15.3	19.2	3.8

Sources: Government Actuary's Department (E&W); Berkeley Mortality database (http://demog.berkeley.edu/ wilmoth/mortality); Ministry of Health and Welfare (Japan), Statistics and Information Department, 18th life-tables, Tokyo, 1998.

Table 2-3 Life-table estimates of survival in England and Wales

| | Males | | Females | |
Percentage surviving to age	1970–72	1997–99	1970–72	1997–99
5	97.7	99.2	98.2	99.4
25	96.4	98.4	97.6	99.0
45	93.3	96.0	95.4	97.6
65	70.4	82.3	82.4	88.7
85	11.4	24.2	27.2	40.9

Source: OPCS mortality statistics;[29,30] based on period data.

shift in the age at which, on average, people have 15 years of life remaining. It has been suggested that this age might be a more sensible indicator of passage to elder status than the rather arbitrary ages enshrined in social security legislation.[6] As can be seen in Figure 2-6, between 1901 and 1991 this age increased by ten years from 58 to 68 for women and from 55 to 63 for men. A further consequence of recent trends is that, because improvements in mortality have been greatest in absolute terms in adult, including elderly adult, age groups where the scope for further improvement was greatest, changes in death rates at older ages have come to play an increasingly important role in overall mortality change. Myers,[32] in a detailed examination of changes in six developed countries, found that in five of them the proportion of overall life expectancy increase in the 1980s, due to gains among those

aged 65 or more, was over 40 percent for males and nearly 60 percent for females. In Japan, in the period 1985–90, 48 percent of the female and 31 percent of the male gain in life expectancy at birth was due to falls in mortality among those aged 75 or over. In the period 1955–60, by contrast, half of female and two-thirds of male gains were due to falls in mortality, while changes among those aged 65 or over had no or a negative effect on life expectancy.[33] These changes have been evident even at the very highest ages.

Not only have changes in late-life mortality come to play a much more dominant role in determining the *overall* level and pace of change in mortality, but in a low-fertility, low-mortality population with already relatively high proportions of elderly people, mortality changes are now the major determinant of *further* population aging. It has been estimated that

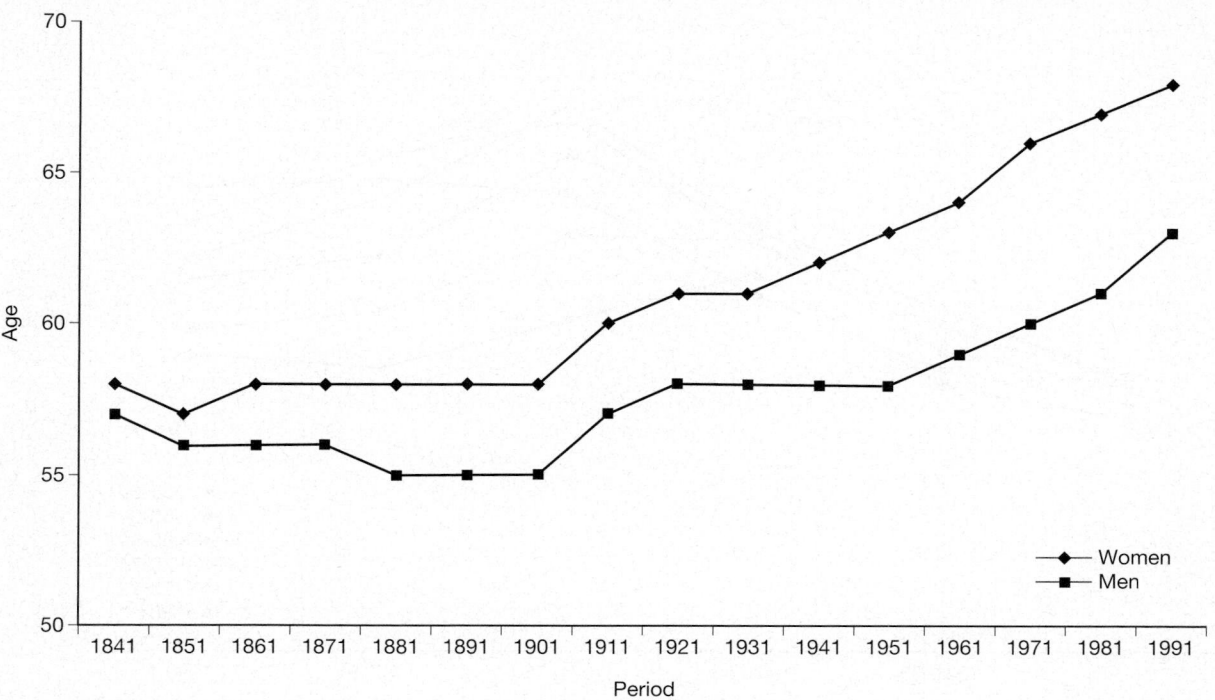

Figure 2-6 Age at which further life expectancy equals 15 years in England and Wales, 1841 to 1991. Source: GAD data analyzed in Grundy,[31] with permission.

38 percent of the increase in the proportion of elderly people in the UK between 1951 and 1981 was due to mortality change;[34] and it has been demonstrated that in Sweden, Japan, and the USA falls in mortality at older ages are now a major determinant of continued population aging.[35]

Sex differentials in mortality

Apart from age variations in the extent of mortality decline experienced during the transition period from relatively high to relatively low rates, a notable feature is the widening of sex differentials in death rates and so life expectancy which is a general feature observed in populations experiencing mortality decline. Waldron[36] reviewed the literature on reasons for this shift, and pointed to:

- declines in causes of death specifically or primarily affecting women (such as maternal mortality and tuberculosis);
- gender differences in health-related behavior and exposure to occupational hazards;
- the possibly greater susceptibility of men to stresses associated with socio-economic change;
- changes in the intrahousehold allocation of resources

as factors which resulted in greater mortality benefits for women than men during the period of mortality transition.

As can be seen from Table 2-2, there are signs that the sex differential in mortality in England and Wales and the USA (and a number of other developed countries)[8] is beginning to narrow again. Changes in the relative propensity of men and women to smoke are undoubtedly an important factor in this. Figure 2-7 hows the ratio of male to female death rates from neoplasms tor periods during the twentieth century for groups

aged 55–59 to 80 and over. This ratio rose until the mid century in younger groups, until 1971–75 in the 70–74 age group and until the late 1980s in the 75–79 age group, but then began to fall as cohorts with less sex-divergent smoking exposures reach the relevant age group. This is an example of a cohort effect.

Current gender differentials in further life expectancy at birth and at age 65 for a larger number of developed countries are shown in Figures 2-8 and 2-9. The gap between men and women is smallest in southern European countries where nutritional and lifestyle factors may protect men from some risks which their counterparts in other countries are exposed to, and largest in eastern Europe where excess alcohol consumption plays a large part in determining risk.[38] An important result of these sex differentials in mortality is the high proportion of widows in elderly populations.

Cohort effects

All the indicators of mortality presented above pertain to defined periods. Thus the (period) life-table measures are derived from age-specific mortality rates current at the specified time and show what would be the experience of a hypothetical group who throughout their lives experienced current rates of mortality. These hypothetical measures will diverge considerably from the actual experiences of particular cohorts if mortality rates change; and the past experience of those cohorts who today make up the elderly population is of course different from that of current groups of younger people. The oldest old alive today comprise only a very small proportion of their original birth cohort and so are more "selected" than their later born successors. In England and Wales, for example, only 24 percent of men and 36 percent of

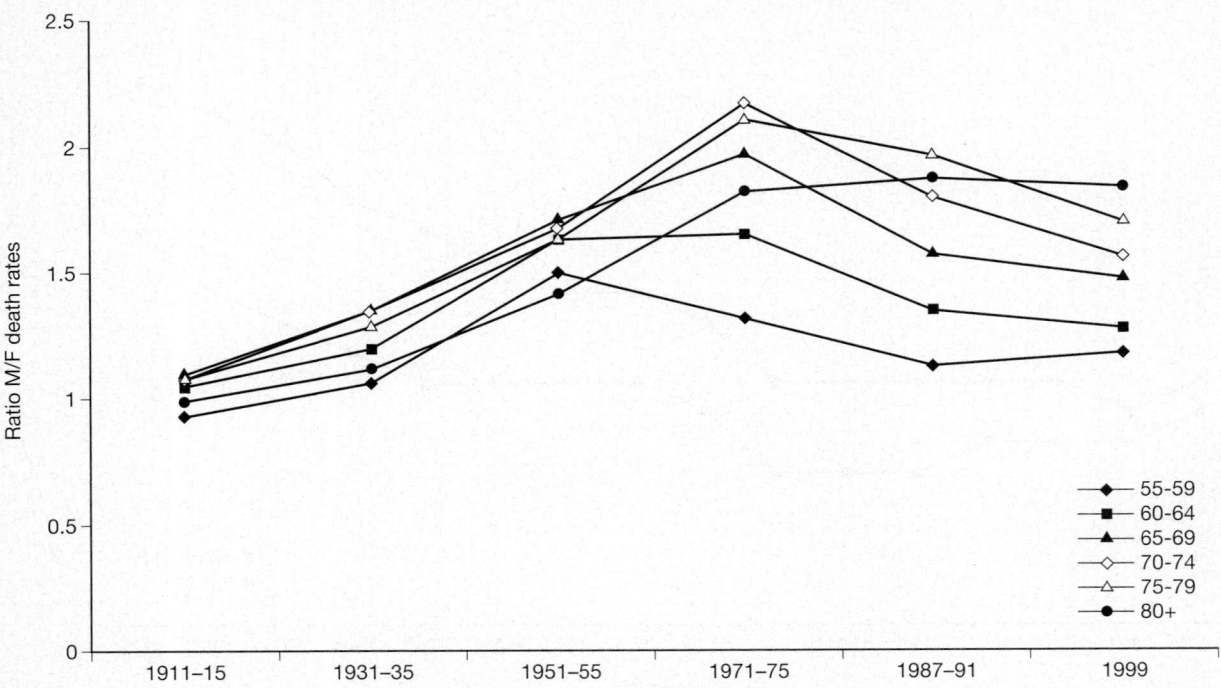

Figure 2-7 Sex ratios in death rates from neoplasms, for England and Wales. Source: OPCS historical data and ONS.[37]

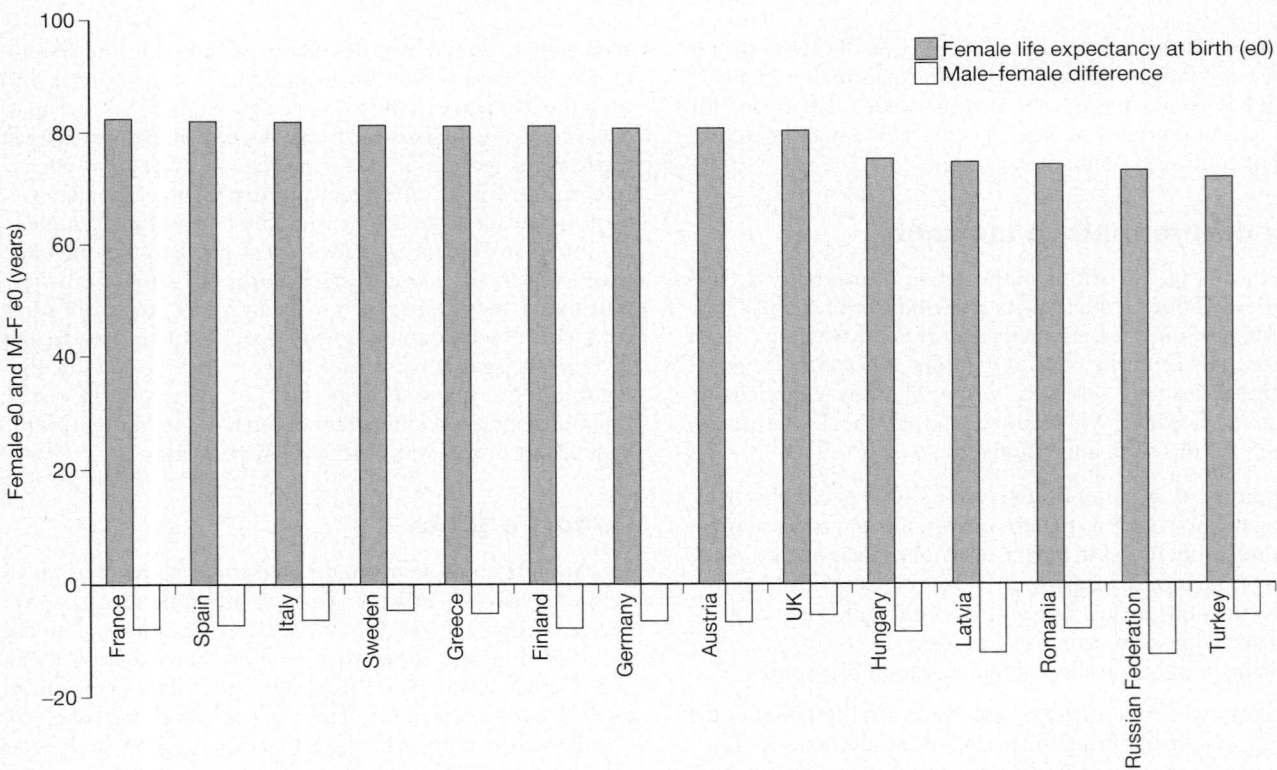

Figure 2-8 Female life expectancy at birth and the male–female difference, for selected European countries, 1995 to 2000. Source: United Nations.[16]

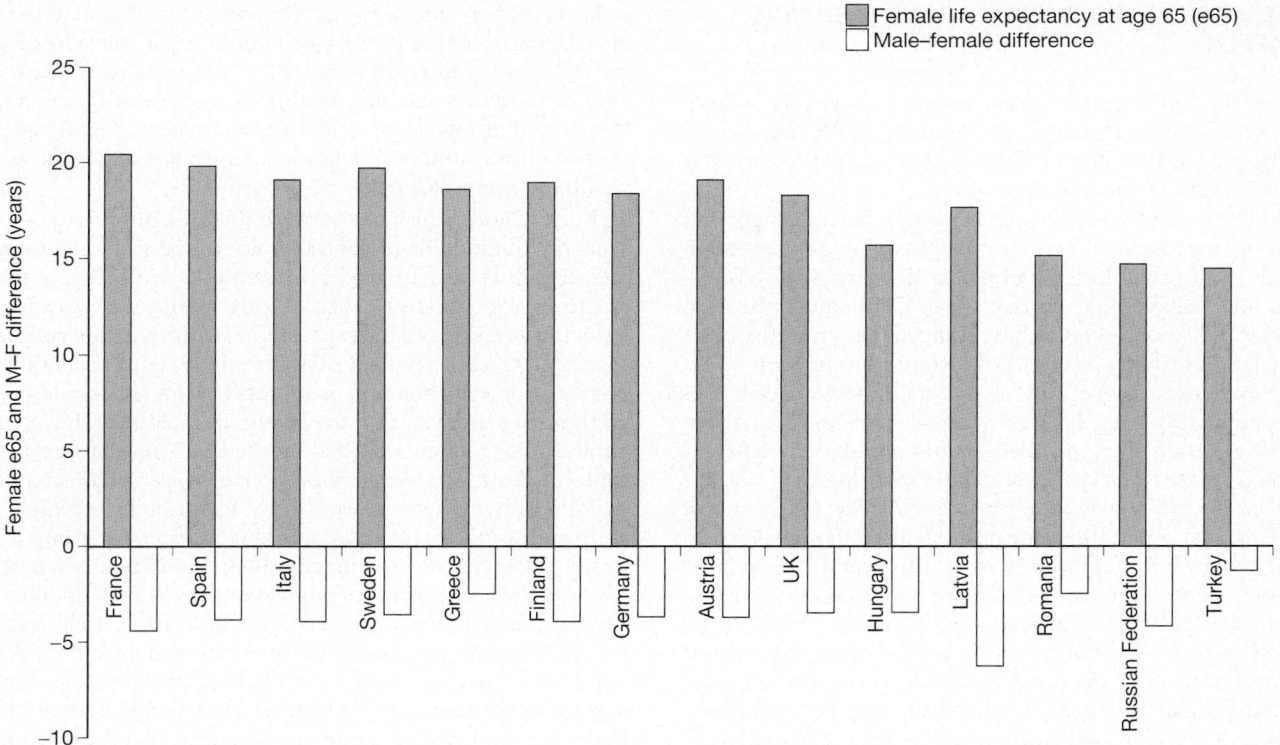

Figure 2-9 Female life expectancy at age 65 and the male–female difference, for selected European countries, 1995 to 2000. Source: United Nations.[16]

women born in 1881 survived to celebrate their 75th birthday in 1956. Among those born 40 years later, the proportions surviving to age 75 (in 1996) were 41 percent and 58 percent, respectively.[31] The past experience of these cohorts includes exposure to various environmental challenges that may have a continuing influence on health even in old ages.

The importance of cohort influences on health has long been recognized,[39] and cohort differences in, for example, mortality from smoking-related diseases have been extensively documented.[40] Other causes of death, such as suicide, also show marked variations by birth cohort.[41] More recently there has been growing interest in the effects of wartime experiences on the subsequent health of the cohorts affected,[42,43] and a renewed emphasis on early life influences on adult mortality.[44] Much of this research has focused on early (including in utero) nutritional influences on health in later life and the possible adverse consequences of early nutritional deprivation followed by relative affluence.[45,46] Although the methods employed in some of these studies, particularly those based on ecological data, have been criticized,[47] clearly this issue is an important one and links between circumstances, including health, in early and later life have been demonstrated in a range of studies. Kaplan et al.,[48] for example, have shown significant and graded associations between parental socio-economic position and cognitive function in a population-based study of Finnish men aged 58 and 64. Childhood mental ability, which may partly reflect early life factors, has itself been shown to be associated

with survival to age 76.[49] Birthweight and early growth have been found to be associated with mortality and with other markers of aging such as increased lens opacity score, reduced grip strength, and thinner skin 60–70 years later.[50]

Apart from the effect of childhood environmental legacies, genetic factors are also important. Some genetic characteristics, such as having the ApoE2 gene, are associated with greater longevity,[51] and studies of twins and other close relatives suggest that perhaps 25 percent of the variation in adult lifespans is due to genetic variation.[52,53] Genetic factors also seem to be associated with variations in the functional ability of women aged 80 and over.[54]

Prior exposures and experiences in adulthood, as well as in childhood, of course also influence health in old age and the social and economic resources available to older people, which may themselves be associated with health.[55,56] However, there are also a number of studies which suggest that current circumstances may have as great, or indeed a greater, effect on mortality in late life. Kannisto's work on mortality rates among those aged over 80 indicated that period rates were more important than cohort ones.[26] He and coworkers also found that children born or conceived during the Finnish famine of 1866–68 suffered higher mortality in childhood than did immediately preceding or succeeding cohorts, but similar mortality in later life.[57] Similarly twins, who tend to have lower birthweights than singletons, have been found to suffer from excess mortality only up to the age of six.[58]

SELECTIVE SURVIVAL AND HEALTH STATUS

Identifying and understanding trends in the relationship between mortality and morbidity at older ages is complicated by the need to allow for these differences between cohorts and for the effects of selective survival.

Individuals are endowed at birth with different genetic and early environmental inheritances, and further differentiation occurs throughout the lifespan as a result of exposure to favorable and unfavorable environmental influences. Because weaker individuals tend to have a shorter survival, the older population includes a larger proportion of those with favorable health characteristics and the age trajectories of death rates for a population may differ substantially from the age pattern of risk for individual members of that population.[7] There is some evidence that the relationship between mortality and age weakens in extreme old age,[59] which may reflect the status of centenarians as a healthy elite of survivors; although it is possible that this apparent pattern is artefactual.[60] Similarly, prospective studies often show a pattern of "unhealthy" groups becoming "healthier" with length of follow-up.[61] Manton and his colleagues,[62] who have contributed extensively to the development and specifications of this thesis, have also suggested that selective survival may account for the apparent "crossover" in the mortality risks of blacks and whites in the USA, although again there is countervailing evidence that this may be an artefact.[63]

One problem in trying to assess the impact of increased survivorship on the health status of populations is that environmental changes or medical interventions are often likely to both increase survivorship among the frail (thus increasing population morbidity) and improve the health of those who would have survived even in the absence of any intervention (so decreasing ill-health in the population, at least in the short term).

MORTALITY AS AN INDICATOR OF POPULATION HEALTH

Mortality patterns in populations are of interest not just because of their effect on age structure, but also because of the inferences about health status, and about the process of aging itself, which may be drawn from them. Aging in the individual is associated with decrements in homeostatic mechanisms that bring about adaptive response to environmental challenges. The end result of this process is death, and increases in mortality with age are commonly used as an indicator of senescence.[4]

However, even the use of this most basic indicator poses a number of problems common to all areas of gerontological research. Firstly there is the issue of measurement. Incomplete death registration, age misreporting and numerator denominator biases in the registration and census data from which mortality rates are derived, may all produce biases which distort the true pattern of mortality trends and differentials. While these problems are particularly serious in less-developed countries, they may also influence the validity of mortality statistics in developed countries. Age misreporting by the very

old is a problem in both the USA[64] and Britain,[59] and numerator denominator biases mean that uncorrected mortality data for these age groups are unreliable. Comparisons of cause-specific mortality data may be further complicated by variations in coding practices.[65] These measurement problems aside, the usefulness of mortality data as an indicator of population health has been challenged.

Ruzicka and Kane[23] have argued that one important consequence of the epidemiological or health transition has been a decline in the usefulness of conventional indicators of the health of a population, such as case fatality rates, cause-specific mortality, and life expectation. While it is appropriate to calculate case fatality rates for many acute infectious diseases, this is not possible, or appropriate, for chronic degenerative diseases given that the person affected may die from another cause, often after a long interval. The usefulness of cause-of-death data (unless multiply coded) as an indicator of major health problems is also limited by the high, and apparently increasing, extent of comorbidity in older age groups.[66] Considerable controversy surrounds the issue of trends in indicators of the health status of populations, including disability. To a large extent this controversy, and its lack of certain resolution, arises from measurement problems and the difficulties involved in making comparisons between health indicators derived in different ways.[67] However, there is also an underlying theoretical debate about the implications of declining mortality rates for the health status of the population. Criticisms of the unquestioning use of life expectancy as a measure of population health arises from the concerns expressed by some that recent reductions in mortality may be due partly to the prolongation of the process of dying rather than to an extension of healthy life.[68–71]

Adherents of this interpretation of recent trends in mortality and morbidity have argued that reductions in mortality at older ages have been achieved partly through medical interventions that postpone the lethal sequelae of chronic diseases, rather than by reducing the incidence or rate of progression of degenerative conditions. In short, the relationship between morbidity and mortality has changed, but with the unfavorable consequence of an increase in the prevalence of morbidity and disability.

A diametrically opposed view of morbidity trends has been advanced by Fries[72] and rests on the concept of a fixed biological limit to the lifespan. Fries argued that the limit to the lifespan was about 115, and that in any population average life expectancy was unlikely to exceed 85. Improvements in health, brought about by the acceptance of personal responsibility for health and appropriate lifestyle changes, would result not in further mortality decline, but in a "compression of morbidity" at the end of the lifespan. Those who adopted the appropriate responsible behaviors could hope to enjoy a vigorous life followed by a short period of ill-health and then a "natural death" resulting from biological senescence rather than a specific disease process.

Fries' argument (largely unmodified in his more recent work) has been challenged on methodological, theoretical, and empirical grounds.[73–75] Even if there is a fixed biological limit to the lifespan, which many dispute,[76] far from reaching a mortality "ceiling" many countries are experiencing continuing falls in mortality at advanced ages, and it has been argued that recent mortality data show a wider dispersion by age rather than signs of increasing concentration.[77] Recent analysis of data from Sweden, Japan, and the USA[78] indicates that mortality has been compressed and survival curves become more rectangular, but that this process has now slowed or been reversed.

Although the arguments of Fries on the one hand and Gruenberg on the other seem irreconcilable, adherents of both interpretations share an assumption that the relationship between morbidity and mortality is changing. Manton[79] proposed a third hypothesis of "dynamic equilibrium." He used US multicause coded mortality data to examine the frequency with which certain chronic diseases were mentioned at all compared with the frequency with which they featured as the underlying cause of death—in effect a kind of chronic-disease case fatality rate. This analysis led him to conclude that the prevalence of chronic diseases was increasing, but not as a result of the postponement of lethal sequelae. Rather, Manton suggested, the rate of progression of certain degenerative diseases had slowed down, partly as a result of medical interventions, resulting in a "dynamic equilibrium" between mortality and morbidity.

There is some empirical evidence to support both positive and negative interpretations. On the pessimistic side, the survival of old people with dementia seems to have increased.[80,81] However, this may reflect this group sharing the improvements in life expectancy experienced by the general population rather than any "excess" increase in survival.[82] Observed increases in the incidence of fractured neck of femur have also been associated with decreases in mortality,[83] possibly suggesting that the increased survival of frailer groups may be partly responsible. There are also some trend data which show an increase in some indicators of poor health in several populations. Results from the British General Household Survey, for example, show increases over time in reported limiting longstanding illness.[84] US data from the National Health Interview Survey also indicate increased reported disability between the mid-1960s and mid-1970s,[85] as do several other US studies.[70,71] Results from many developed countries also show large increases in claims for disability-related benefits, although factors other than disability may be a strong influence on these.[86]

More optimistically, more recent analysis of trends in the health of older Americans suggests some improvement in disability status.[87] Even more encouraging are results from a trend study of very old people in the USA based on longitudinal data and including those in institutions, which showed a marked decline in disability between the early 1980s and the mid-1990s.[88] Hayward et al.[89] suggest a noticeable shift in the USA from initial declines in late-age mortality being associated with increased morbidity to a more recent pattern of longer life foretelling better rather than worse health. Additionally, although the British GHS data suggest an increase in limiting longstanding illness, the more detailed information on the functional abilities of elderly people collected in some rounds of the GHS show a marked improvement.[90] Results from a number of other European countries also suggest declines in more serious disability, but possibly some increase in milder disability.[91] Overall this is the picture that emerges most clearly from the literature: that is, a scenario of declines in serious disability but increases in reported limiting longstanding illness, reported prevalence of some conditions,[92] and mild disability.

It should be noted that prospective studies of elderly people have shown that the best predictors of mortality are the markers of established disease or degree of functional capacity.[93–95] It is also clear that population subgroups with the highest mortality suffer more morbidity and the longest periods of disability.[96,97] This suggests a continuing strong link between morbidity and mortality.

MEASURING HEALTH

Part of the confusion about trends in morbidity and disability arises because of the difficulty of measuring these in population surveys, especially surveys relying on self-reported data, and the wide range of measures and concepts used in studies of health status. The simplest type of measure used in many surveys, and in some national population censuses, is based on questions about general health status. Two types of questions on self-assessments of general health status are commonly used. The first asks respondents for a general assessment of their health, sometimes in relation to others of the same age. The second focuses on whether respondents in surveys have longstanding illnesses and sometimes whether or not these affect their activities.

Self-perceptions of health have been shown in a number of studies to be fairly well correlated with other indicators, such as consultation rates and mortality.[98,99] While this measure may therefore be useful for investigations into the health status of a defined population, unfortunately it seems to be less helpful in making comparisons between populations which might throw light on factors influencing the health status of older people. The examination of trends over time, an extremely important issue, is also seriously complicated by possible changes in health expectations. Responses to questions on longstanding illness may be influenced by health expectations and, crucially in the older population, the extent to which older people attribute limitations to old age rather than illness. As shown in Figure 2-10, which is derived from the 2000 round of the Health Survey for England,[100] the prevalence of longstanding illness is high. Some 70 percent of both 65–79 year olds and people aged 80 and over report longstanding illness, and of these about half have two or more longstanding conditions. As would be expected, prevalence rates are higher among those living in care homes than in the private household population (community), but variation by age is relatively slight. This is because this measure is not sensitive to differences in the extent of health problems; other measures based on functional ability show much greater variation with age. The types of longstanding illness which are most common in later life are illustrated in Figure 2-11 using data from the USA. Arthritis is the most common, particularly among women, followed by circulatory diseases which are more common among men than women.

Disorders such as arthritis may be indirectly associated with mortality (by, for example, increasing the risk of falls and other accidents) and are a major predictor of the development of functional limitations,[102] but they are rarely recorded as causes of death. Reliance on mortality data alone would tell us little

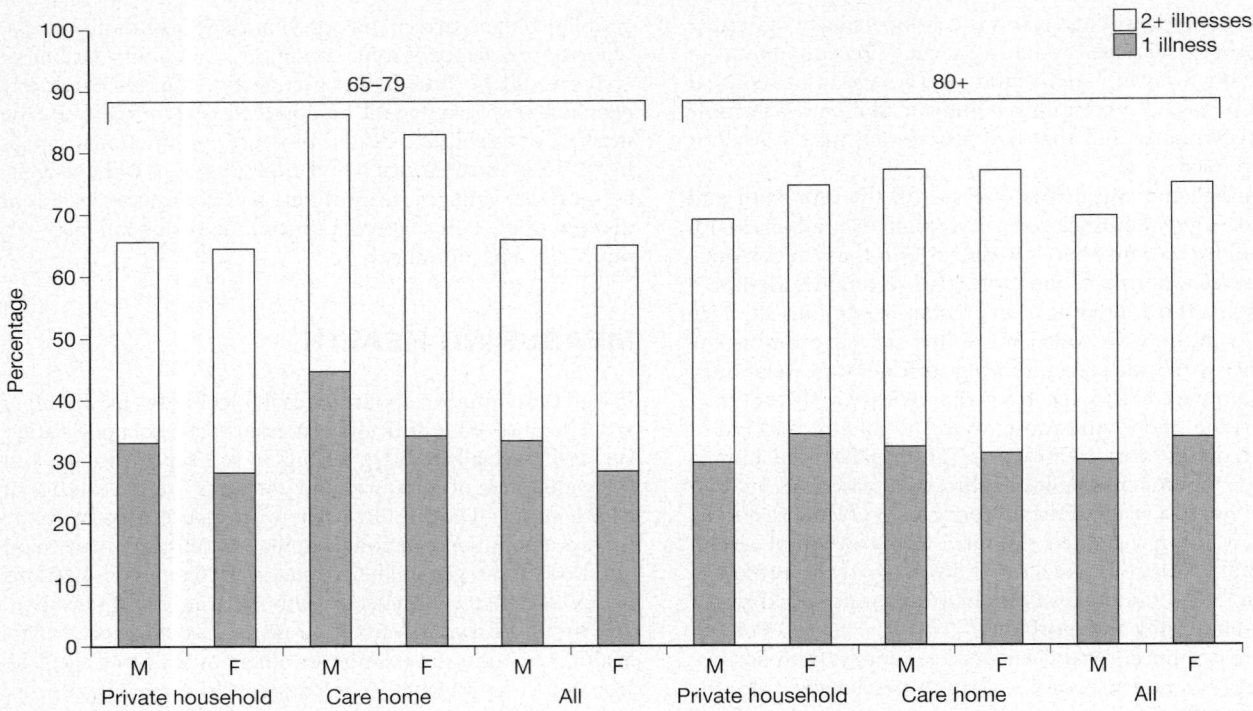

Figure 2-10 Percentage of people in England aged 65 and over reporting longstanding illnesses in 2000. Source: Health Survey for England.[100]

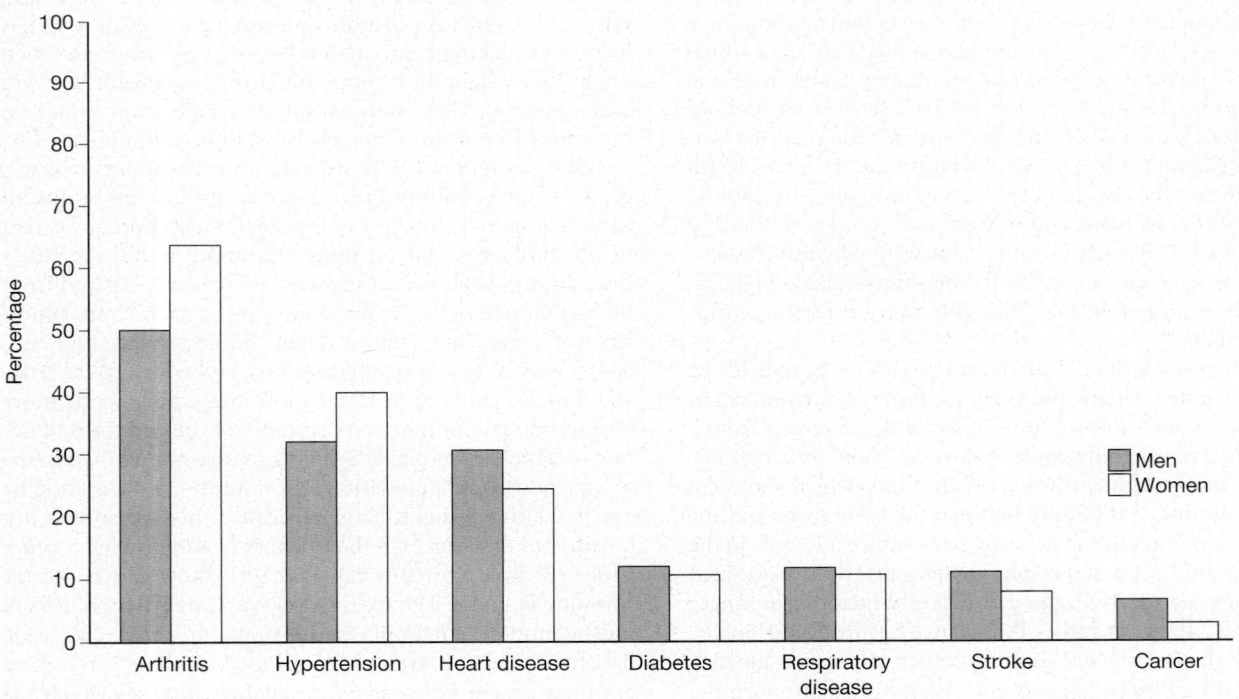

Figure 2-11 Percentage of people in the USA aged 70 and over reporting selected chronic conditions in 1995. Source: US National Health Interview Survey data, reported in Kramarow et al.[101]

Table 2-4 Percentage of people aged 70 and over who have difficulty performing, or are unable to perform, one or more activities of daily living (ADLs) and instrumental activities of daily living (IADLs), USA 1995

Age group	Gender	At least one ADL		At least one IADL	
		Performs with difficulty	Unable to perform	Performs with difficulty	Unable to perform
70–74	M	14	4	6	8
	F	20	5	13	16
75–79	M	17	6	8	11
	F	19	9	12	21
80–84	M	20	10	8	20
	F	24	12	14	27
85+	M	23	19	8	27
	F	33	23	13	44
70+	M	17	7	7	13
	F	22	10	13	23

Source: US National Health Interview Survey data, reported in Kramarow et al.[101]

about the problems arising from these common conditions. Heart and other circulatory diseases, by contrast, are associated with common causes of death among the elderly. Current age- and cause-specific mortality statistics imply that over half of all older Americans (and a similar proportion of the UK population aged 65 and over) will eventually die from circulatory diseases.[103] Even so, morbidity as well as mortality data are needed in any assessment of the health impact of these diseases, as changes in case fatality rates, rather than in incidence, may account for changes in mortality.

Data on morbidity from specific conditions are therefore subject to measurement biases, cohort and selective survival effects which may distort true relationships between aging and disease processes. Changes in case fatality rates and in awareness and reporting of conditions further complicate the comparison of prevalence rates. For these reasons, incidence data are to be preferred to prevalence data in epidemiological studies concerned with the etiology of particular diseases. However, such data are difficult and expensive to collect and for service planning purposes both incidence and prevalence data are needed, particularly if changes in the duration or severity of the disease are suspected. For epidemiologists concerned with identifying possible risk factors, the incidence data are more revealing, but public health and other service planners need also to know about trends in prevalence. Even more importantly, information on the implications of morbidity for general health status, in the WHO sense of well-being, is needed. Elderly people vary enormously in the extent to which their activities are affected by disease processes; thus the same degree of arthritis may not result in the same level of disability. This is particularly true given the multiple pathology common at older ages. In the Alameda County Study, for example, 41 percent of those aged 60 and over reported three or more diseases or health problems.[66] Social and environmental factors, as well as host differences, are also important influences on the general health implications of particular pathological processes. For these reasons we need to consider general indicators of health, particularly functional health.

Functional health status

As noted above, knowing whether or not someone reports a longstanding illness gives little indication of the effects of that illness on function or assistance needs; for this, more detailed information is needed which allows measurement of functional health or disability. Measures based on indicators of functional ability, such as activities of daily living (ADL) and instrumental activities of daily living (IADL) scores, are now very widely used both as an indicator of the health of elderly populations and population subgroups, and in clinical assessments. ADL scales usually include items on basic activities, such as eating and bathing, while IADL scales include questions about activities such as preparing food and shopping.

Theoretically these measures might appear preferable to self-reports of perceived health, since although they are influenced by environmental factors, a more standardized form of calibration may be possible. ADL and IADL measures have the advantage of being directly related to needs for services. Within populations, ADL measures also seem to correlate well with other indicators, such as mortality and indeed self-assessed health. Table 2-4, derived from data from the USA collected in 1994–96, shows that inability to undertake, or difficulty in undertaking, one or more ADLs or IADLs was strongly associated with age. In this survey the ADLs considered were bathing or showering; dressing; eating; getting in or out of bed or chair; walking; getting outside and getting to and using the toilet. A third of women aged 85 and over had difficulty performing at least one of these activities and a third were unable to perform at least one at all. Moreover this survey excluded those in institutions (nearly a quarter of the US 85+ population) among whom ADL limitations would be far more prevalent, and so underestimates the true extent of functional health limitations in the total population.

The higher prevalence of disability among women when compared with men partly reflects their greater risk of musculoskeletal disorders such as osteoporosis and arthritis. In the USA, for example, half of all women aged 85 and over have bone densities low enough to meet the WHO definition of osteoporosis.[101] Although the incidence of disability among older men and women is similar, women survive longer with disabilities than do men, with the result that prevalence rates are higher. This partly reflects sex differences in the most common causes of disability discussed above.

Questions about mobility or ability to undertake tasks such as bathing certainly show much stronger associations with age than more general questions about perceived health status or limiting longstanding illness. This suggests greater specificity in questions relating to particular activities (as would be expected). On the other hand, questions about serious disabilities are obviously not designed to be sensitive to more prevalent mild or moderate limitations on health or activity.

Data on activities of daily living are widely used to derive indices of functional health.[104] These provide a useful summary measure well correlated with other health indicators. However, major differences between studies in estimates of functional disability have been reported,[105] suggesting that local environmental factors, methods of data collection, and other variables affect the results obtained.

An alternative approach to ADL and IADL measures is derivation and use of indicators based on the WHO International Classification of Impairments, Diseases and Handicaps (ICIDH).[106] The ICIDH, currently being revised, involves distinguishing between impairments resulting from morbidity and trauma, disabilities or limitations resulting from these, and handicaps or limits to participation which result from lack of socially inclusive policies (for example, design of housing, streets, and public facilities which limits access for those with disabilities). ICIDH-based scales have been used in a number of national surveys and have the advantage of providing greater sensitivity for detecting less serious disabilities than ADL measures and of providing more detail, including in many cases information on impairments or the type of functional limitation (such as difficulty in reaching and stretching) which may result in functional disability (for example, inability to dress unaided). However, considerably more information must be collected, which increases costs. Results from the 1996/97 British survey of disability,[86] which used scales conceptually based on the ICIDH, for the population aged 75 and over are shown in Figure 2-12. Seventy percent of those in the survey, which included only those in private households, had some degree of disability on the scales used. Disabilities of locomotion, hearing, seeing, dexterity, and personal care were the most prevalent. Of those with some degree of disability, this survey also found that a quite high proportion—20 percent of those aged 80 or over—needed regular daily assistance with an essential task.

LIFE-TABLE ESTIMATES OF ACTIVE/DISABLED LIFE EXPECTANCY

A growing number of researchers have used life-table methods to analyze data on mortality and on various estimates of disability, to produce estimates of expectation of life divided into "active" or "disability-free" years and years with some form of impairment.[67,89,91,92,107–110] "Health expectancy" is the generic term used to describe these and other conceptually similar indications, such as the World Bank's estimation of disability-adjusted life years (DALYs) lost.[111]

Health expectancy measures are useful summary indicators which may be readily interpreted. Largely under the auspices of the REVES group,[67] great advances have been made in standardizing terminology and methodology. Nevertheless the

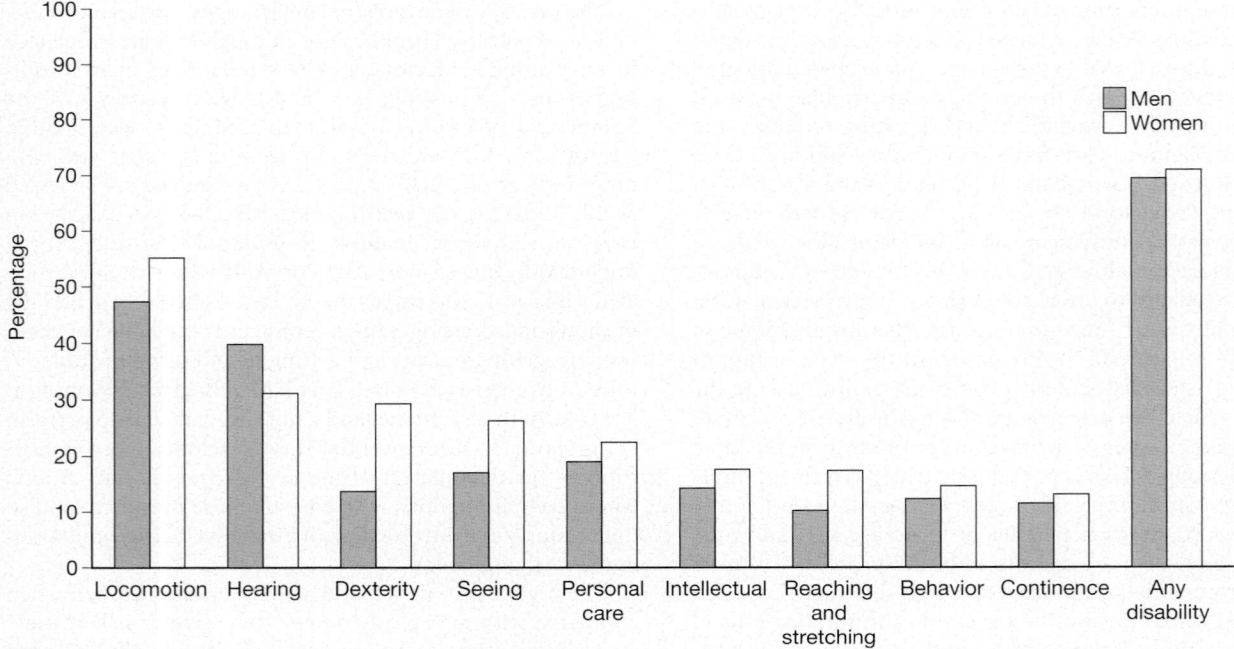

Figure 2-12 Prevalence of specified types of disability among the population aged 75 and over in Britain in 1996/97. Source: 1996/97 Disability Survey of Great Britain, data reported in Grundy et al,[86] with permission.

estimates of health expectancy which have now been prepared for some 40 countries are not directly comparable because of the substantial differences in the methods and data used to derive them.

Measures of health expectancy represent a major conceptual advance and a potentially valuable way for governments, healthcare providers, and individuals to assess health prospects and possibly the effects of interventions. However, the utility of any output measure depends crucially on the validity of the input data; and in many cases, as discussed in preceding sections of this chapter, these are deficient. Despite the problems, some general conclusions can be drawn about differentials in health expectancy. In nearly all countries, for example, women have a longer life expectancy than men but also spend proportionately longer in a state of impaired health. An example of this type of measure used in the 1998 Chinese longevity study[112] is shown in Figure 2-13. This study showed that, although there were differences between the further life expectancy of men and women, there were no differences between urban and rural dwellers. Most of the further life expectancy of those aged 80 was "active"—that is, free of disability; and even at age 90 the proportion of further life expectancy with any degree of disability was less than in the "active" population. In common with other studies, women suffered proportionately more disability than men, and this survey also shows an advantage for rural elders in comparison with urban dwellers. The authors suggested this might reflect both the difficulties elderly people with more serious disabili-

ties might have in remaining in rural areas (perhaps leading to migration to cities), and perhaps the beneficial effects of a physically active life on health status in old age. The short- and long-term benefits of physical activity have been highlighted in many other studies.[113] (See also Chapter 19.)

For a few countries, estimates of health expectancy are available for different time periods, based on input measures which, at least in design, are consistent. Potentially these results may hold the answer to the very important question of whether falls in mortality in older age groups are associated with reductions or increases in the extent of health limitations. Not surprisingly the results of these calculations are in line with assessments of trends in morbidity, from which they are partly derived, and suggest that much of the gain in life expectancy in the 1960s and 1970s was a gain in life with an impairment or disability. In the USA, for example, calculations based on NHIS data indicate that male life expectancy in good health increased by only 0.3 years between 1962 and 1976, while life expectancy with an activity restriction increased by 1.5 years. However, work including more recent periods suggests a much more favorable trend since the 1970s.[88,89] Results from Great Britain similarly appear at first sight to suggest an unfavorable trend as far as life expectancy free of longstanding illness is concerned. Between 1976 and 1991, male life expectancy in longterm ill-health increased by 1.6 years, while life expectancy free of long-term ill-health increased by 1.4 years.[107] However, these results are based on responses to general questions in the General Household Survey, which may well reflect changes in

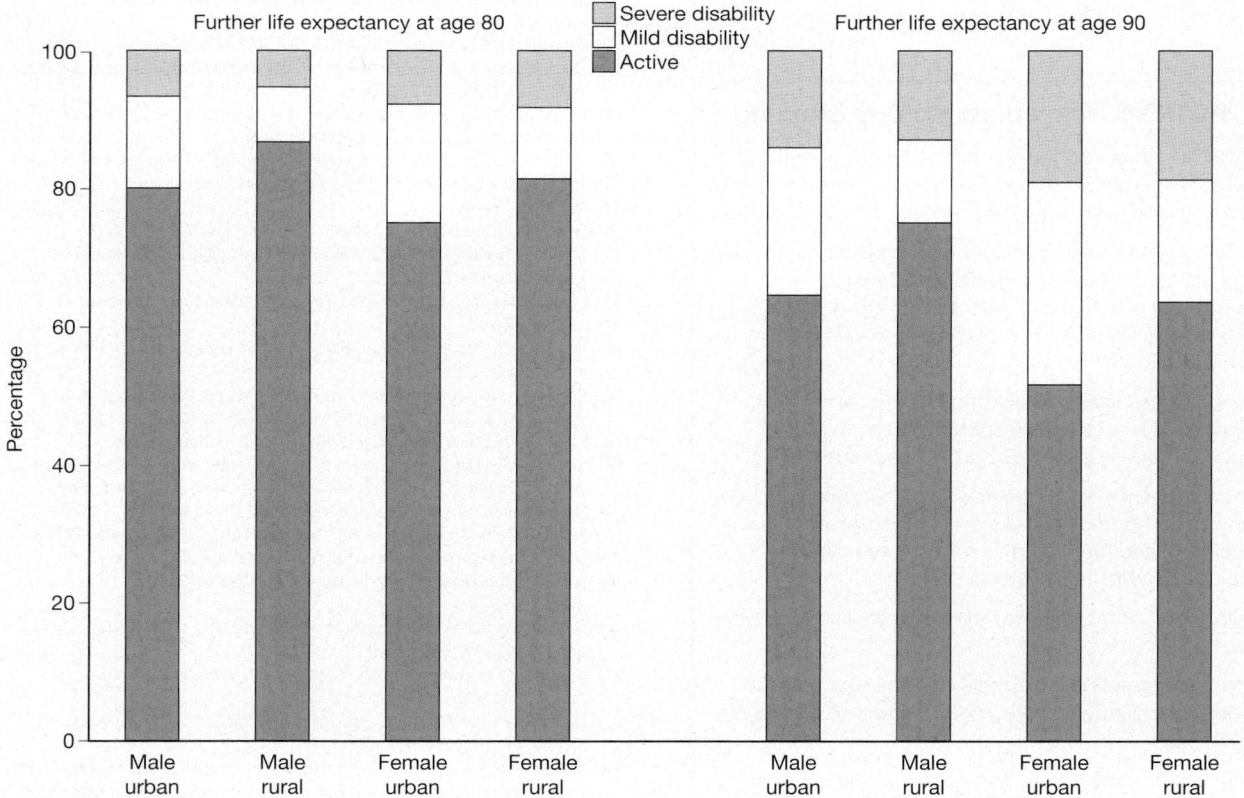

Figure 2-13 Proportion of further life expectancy at age 80 and age 90 spent in different states of health, China 1998.
Source: Chinese Health Longevity Survey data, reported in Zeng et al.[112]

health *expectations* rather than health *expectancy*. Analyses based on the more detailed ADL questions suggest some reduction in at least the proportion of life lived with a more severe disability.[75]

AGING AND USE OF SERVICES

As the elderly are far more likely than the young to experience health problems, it is not surprising that their use of medical and other services is high, and this of course is one of the reasons why policy-makers are concerned about the economic implications of increases in the size of the very old population. In the UK the average annual cost to the National Health Service of a person aged 85 and over is approximately six times the cost for a 16–44 year old and four times the cost for a 45–64 year old. Moreover, costs might be higher still if elderly people received clinically indicated treatments to the same extent as younger ones.[114] However, much of this cost is associated with care in the year before death and so perhaps should be regarded as associated with proximity to death rather than with age.[115] Most older people with disabilities live in the community and relatives provide much of the help they may need. Even so, one recent British study found that over a third of elderly people living in private households who had limitations to daily activity were wholly or partly dependent on formal services for help.[116]

DISCUSSION

Aging is associated with biological changes which increase the risk of morbidity, disability, and death. Later life is also marked by changes in economic status, in family and household composition (resulting from, for example, widowhood) and in other relationships, all of which may be associated with changes in health status. Social aspects of aging are considered in detail in Chapter 17, but we should note here the evidence showing links between social networks and mortality and other indicators of health, including cognitive function,[117] the important role played by family and friends in supporting elderly people with disabilities,[116] and the increasing evidence that economic and other social disadvantages compound the effects of aging in some groups of the population.[55,118] Elderly populations are heterogeneous and their characteristics are influenced by historical events and the effects of selective survival. Health is an elusive concept, difficult to define and measure. It is not surprising, therefore, that studies of aging and health present major difficulties. Further methodological work on overcoming these difficulties, and on collecting data which allow valid comparisons between and within populations at different points in time, is urgently needed to further our knowledge of the epidemiology of aging.

REFERENCES

1. Lilienfeld DE: Definitions of epidemiology. Am J Epidemiol 1978;107:87–90
2. Greenhouse SW: Definitions of ageing. In Haynes SG, Feinleib M (eds): Proceedings of the Second Conference on the Epidemiology of Aging. US Dept of Health and Human Services, Bethesda, MA, 1980
3. World Health Organization: Text of the constitution of the World Health Organization. Off Rec World Health Organ 1948;2:100
4. Evans JG: Ageing and disease. In Evered D, Whelan J (eds): Research and the Ageing Population (Ciba Foundation Symposium 124). John Wiley, Chichester, 1988
5. Brouwer A: The nature of ageing. In Horan MA and Brouwer A (eds): Gerontology: Approaches to Biomedical and Clinical Research. Edward Arnold, London, 1990:1–10
6. Seigel JS: A Generation of Change: A Profile of America's Older Population. Russell Sage Foundation, New York, 1992
7. Vaupel JW, Manton KG, Stallard E: The impact of heterogeneity in individual frailty on the dynamics of mortality. Demography 1979;16:439–454
8. United Nations: Population Bulletin 25. UN, New York, 1988
9. Office for National Statistics (ONS): Health Statistics Quarterly, no. 9. HMSO, London, 2001
10. Lotka A: Relation between birth rates and death rates. Science 1907;26:21–22
11. Notestein F: Some demographic aspects of aging. Proc Am Philosoph Soc 1954;98:229–233
12. Carrier N: Demographic aspects of the ageing of the population. In Welford AT, Argyle M, Glass DV, Morris JW (eds): Society, Problems and Methods of Study. Routledge & Kegan Paul, London, 1962
13. Grundy E: Health, health care and death among older adults in England and Wales: a hundred years' perspective. In Zaba B, Blacker J (eds): Brass Tacks. Athlone Press, London, 2001:270–291
14. Treas J: Older Americans in the 1990s and beyond (Population Bulletin 50.2). Population Reference Bureau, Washington, DC, 1995
15. Kono S: Population ageing in Japan. Rev Clinical Gerontol 1996;6:205–211
16. United Nations: World Population Prospects: The 1998 Revision, vols I and II. UN, New York, 1999
17. Kuroda T: Population ageing in Japan, with reference to China. Asia–Pacific Pop J 1987;2:3–22
18. United Nations: World Population Prospects: The 2000 Revision, Highlights. UN, New York, 2001
19. United Nations Economic Commission for Europe/United Nations Fund for Population: Changing Age Structures: Demographic and Economic Consequences and Implications. UN, Geneva, 1992
20. Preston SH: Mortality Patterns in National Populations. Academic Press, New York, 1976

KEY POINTS The epidemiology of aging

- By 2050 it is expected that one in three Europeans will be aged 60 or over and in several countries 10 percent or more of the population will be aged 80 or over.

- Survival to and through older ages has increased enormously. At current mortality rates in England and Wales, 40 percent of girls born now will reach the age of 85; likely future improvements suggest this proportion will in fact be much larger.

- In developed countries, deaths and ill-health are now concentrated in older age groups and addressing age-associated disease is the major public health challenge.

- One consequence of the epidemiological transition from high to low mortality is that mortality data no longer suffice as indicators of population health—we also need data on morbidity, disability, and quality of life.

- Health in later life is associated with earlier life events as well as current circumstances.

- Aging is associated with biological changes, and also with economic and family changes, which themselves have health implications.

- Much remains to be learned about the epidemiology of aging. Further progress requires both methodological work and expanded sources of population-based data.

21. Omram A: The epidemiological transition: a theory of the epidemiology of population change. Millbank Mem Fund Qtly 1971;64:355–391

22. Olshansky SJ, Ault AB: The fourth stage of the epidemiologic transition: the age of delayed degenerative diseases. Millbank Mem Fund Qtly 1986;64:355–391

23. Ruzicka L, Kane P: Health transition: the course of morbidity and mortality. In Caldwell J, Findley S, Caldwell P et al (eds): What We Know About Health Transition: The Cultural, Social and Behavioural Determinants of Health, vol. I. Australian National University, Canberra, 1990

24. Casselli G: Health transition and cause-specific mortality. In Schofield R, Reher D, Bideau A (eds): The Decline of Mortality in Europe. Clarendon Press, Oxford, 1991:68–96

25. Bourgeois-Pichat J: Essai sur la mortalité "biologique" de l'homme. Population 1952;3:381–394

26. Kannisto V: Development of oldest-old mortality 1950–1990. Odense University Press, Odense, 1994

27. Kannisto V: The advancing frontier of survival: life-tables for old age. Odense University Press, Odense, 1996

28. Nusselder W, Mackenbach J: Lack of improvement of life expectancy at advanced ages in the Netherlands. Int J Epidemiol 2000;29:140–148

29. OPCS: Mortality Statistics Serial Tables 1841–1985 (Series DHI, no. 19). HMSO, London, 1989

30. OPCS: Life Tables 1970–72 (Series DS, no. 2). HMSO, London, 1979

31. Grundy E: The health and health care of older adults in England and Wales 1841–1991. In Charlton JC, Murphy M (eds): The Health of Adult Britain 1841–1991. Stationery Office, London, 1997:183–204

32. Myers G: Comparative study of mortality trends among older persons in developed countries. In Casselli G, Lopez A (eds): Health and Mortality Among Elderly Populations. Clarendon Press, Oxford, 1996

33. Kono S: Demography and population ageing in Japan. In Ageing in Japan. JARC, Tokyo, 1994

34. Benjamin B: The demographic outlook. In Benjamin B, Haberman S, Helowicz G, Kay G, Wilkie D (eds): Pensions: The Problems of Today and Tomorrow. Allen & Unwin, London, 1987

35. Preston SH, Himes C, Eggers M: Demographic conditions responsible for population aging. Demography 1989;26:691–704

36. Waldron I: What do we know about sex differences in mortality? (Population Bulletin no. 18). United Nations, New York, 1986

37. Office for National Statistics: Mortality Statistics, Cause, England and Wales, 1999 (Series DH2, no. 26). Stationery Office, London, 2000

38. McKee M, Shkolnikov V, Leon DA: Alcohol is implicated in the fluctuations in cardiovascular disease in Russia since the 1980s. Ann Epidemiol 2001;11(1):1–6

39. Kermack W, McKendrick A, McKinlay P: Death rates in Great Britain and Sweden: some general regularities and their significance. Lancet 1934;226:698–703

40. Alderson MR, Ashwood F: Projection of mortality rates for the elderly. Pop Trends 1985;42:22–29

41. Murphy E, Lindesay J, Grundy E: Sixty years of suicide in England and Wales: a cohort study. Arch Gen Psych 1986;43:969–976

42. Horiuchi S: The long term impact of war on mortality: old age mortality of First World War survivors in the Federal Republic of Germany. United Nations Population Bulletin 1983:5

43. Caselli G: The influence of cohort effects on differentials and trends in mortality. In Vallin J, D'Souza S, Palloni A (eds): Measurement and Analysis of Mortality: New Approaches. Clarendon Press, Oxford, 1990

44. Barker DJP (ed): Fetal and infant origins of adult disease. BMJ Publishing Group, London, 1992

45. Forsdahl A: Are poor living conditions in childhood and adolescence an important risk factor for arteriosclerotic heart disease? Br J Prevent Soc Med 1977;31:91–95

46. Forsdahl A: Living conditions in childhood and subsequent development of risk factors for arteriosclerotic heart disease. J Epidemiol Commun Health 1978;32:34–37

47. Elo IT, Preston SH: Effects of early life conditions on adult mortality: a review. Popul Index 1992;58:186–212

48. Kaplan G, Turrell G, Lynch J et al: Childhood socio-economic position and cognitive function in adulthood. Int J Epidemiol 2001;30:256–263

49. Whalley L, Deary J: Longitudinal cohort study of childhood IQ and survival up to age 76. BMJ 2001;322:819

50. Sayer A, Cooper C, Evans J et al: Are rates of ageing determined in utero? Age Ageing 1998:579–583

51. Tilvis R, Strandberg T, Juva K: Apolipoprotein E phenotypes, dementia and mortality in a prospective population sample. J Am Ger Soc 1998;46:712–715

52. McGue M, Vaupel J, Holm B, Harvald B: Longevity is moderately heritable in a sample of Danish twins born 1870–1880. J Gerontol A 1993;48:B237–B244

53. Herskind A, McGue M, Holm N et al: The heritability of human longevity. Hum Genet 1996;97:319–323

54. Christensen K, McGue M, Yashin A et al: Genetic and environmental influences on functional abilities in Danish twins aged 75 years and older. J Gerontol A 2000;55:M446–M452

55. Grundy E, Holt G: Adult life experiences and health in early old age in Great Britain. Soc Sci Med 2000;51:1061–1074

56. Blane D, Berney L, Smith GD, Gunnell DJ, Holland P: Reconstructing the life course: health during early old age in a follow-up study based on the Boyd Orr cohort. Pub Health 1999;113(3):117–124

57. Kannisto V, Christensen J, Vaupel J: No increased mortality in later life for cohorts born during famine. Am J Epidemiol 1997;145:987–994

58. Christensen K, Vaupel J, Holm N et al: Mortality among twins after age 6: fetal origins hypothesis versus twin method. BMJ 1995;18:432–436

59. Thatcher AR: Trends and prospects at very high ages. In Charlton JC, Murphy M (eds): The Health of Adult Britain 1841–1991. HMSO, London, 1997

60. Coale AJ, Kisker EE: Defects in data on old age mortality in the United States: new procedures for calculating mortality schedules and life tables at the highest ages. Asian Pacific Pop For 1990;4:1–31

61. Fox AJ, Goldblatt PO, Adelstein AM: Selection and mortality differentials. J Epidemiol Commun Health 1982;36:69–79

62. Manton K, Stallard E: Recent Trends in Mortality Analysis. Academic Press, New York, 1984

63. Elo I, Preston S: Examining African–American mortality from incomplete data. Demography 1994;31:427–458

64. Kestenbaum B: A description of the extreme aged population based on improved Medicare enrolment data. Demography 1992;29:411–426

65. Alderson M: International mortality statistics. Macmillan Press, London, 1981

66. Seeman TE, Guralnik JM, Kaplan GA, Knudsen L, Cohen R: The health consequences of multiple morbidity in the elderly. J Aging Health 1989;1:55–66

67. Robine JM, Blanchet M, Dowd JE: Health expectancy; 1st workshop of the International Health Life Expectancy Network (REVES). Studies on Medical and Population Subjects no. 54. HMSO, London, 1992

68. Gruenberg EM: The failures of success. Millbank Mem Fund Qtly 1977;55:3–24

69. Kramer M: The rising pandemic of mental disorders and associated chronic diseases and disabilities. Acta Psych Scand 1980;62(suppl):285

70. Verbrugge L: Longer life but worsening health? Trends in health and mortality in middle-aged and older persons. Millbank Mem Fund Qtly 1984;62:475–519

71. Rogers A, Rogers RG, Belanger A: Longer life but worse health? Measurement and dynamics. Gerontologist 1990;30:640–647

72. Fries J: Aging, natural death and the compression of morbidity. N Engl J Med 1980;303:130–135

73. Bromley D, Isaacs B, Bytheway B: Review symposium: ageing and the rectangular curve. Ageing Society 1982;2:383–392

74. Schneider E, Brody J: Aging, natural death and the compression of morbidity: another view. N Engl J Med 1983;309:854–856

75. Grundy E: Mortality and morbidity among the old. BMJ 1984;288:663–664

76. Gavrilov LA, Gavrilova NS: The biology of lifespan: a quantitative approach. Harwood Academic, London, 1991

77. Rothenberg R, Lentzner H, Parker R: Population aging patterns: the expansion of mortality. J Gerontol 1991;46:S66–S70

78. Wilmoth JR, Horiuchi S: Rectangularization revisited: variability of age at death within human populations. Demography 1999;36:475–495

79. Manton KG: Changing concepts of morbidity and mortality in the elderly population. Millbank Mem Fund Qtly 1982;60:183–224

80. Blessed G, Wilson I: The contemporary natural history of mental disorder in old age. Br J Psychiat 1982;141:59–67

81. Christie A: Changing patterns in mental illness in the elderly. Br J Psychiat 1982;140:154–159

82. Wood E, Chitfield E, Christie A: Changes in survival in demented hospital inpatients 1957–1987. Int J Geriat Psychiatry 1991;6:523–528

83. Finsen V: Improvements in general health among the elderly: a factor in the rising incidence of hip fractures? J Epidemiol Commun Health 1988;42:200–203

84. Dunnell K: Population review: (2) Are we healthier? Popul Trends 1995;82:12–18

85. Colvez A, Blanchet M: Disability trends in the United States population 1966–76: analysis of reported causes. Am J Pub Health 1981;71:464–471

86. Grundy E, Ahlburg D, Ali M, Breeze E, Sloggett A: Disability in Great Britain: results from the 1996/97 Disability Survey (Department of Social Security Research Report). Stationery Office, London, 1999.

87. Crimmins E, Saito Y, Reynolds S: Further evidence on recent trends in the prevalence and incidence of disability among older Americans from two sources: the LSOA and the NHIS. J Gerontol 1997;52:S59–S71

88. Manton KG, Stallard E, Corder LS: The dynamics of dimensions of age-related disability 1982 to 1994 in the US elderly population. J Gerontol A 1998;53:B59–B70

89. Hayward M, Crimmins E, Saito Y: Cause of death and active life expectancy in the older population of the United States. J Aging Health 1998;10:192–213

90. Grundy E: Population review: people aged 60 and over. Popul Trends 1996;84:14–20

91. Boshiuzen HC, Van de Water HPA: An international comparison of health expectancies. TNO Health Research, Leiden, 1994

92. Crimmins E, Saito Y: Change in the prevalence of diseases among older Americans: 1984–1994. Demog Res 2000;3:9 [www.demographic-research.org]

93. Campbell J, Diep C, Reinken J, McCosh L: Factors predicting mortality in a total population sample of the elderly. J Epidemiol Commun Health 1985;39:337–342

94. Warren MD, Knight R: Mortality in relation to the functional capacities of people with disabilities living at home. J Epidemiol Commun Health 1985;36:220–223

95. Ruigómez A, Alonso J, Auto JM: Functional capacity and five year mortality in a sample of urban community elderly. Eur J Pub Health 1993;3:165–171

96. Manton KG, Stallard E, Corder L: Education-specific estimates of life expectancy and age-specific disability in the US elderly population: 1982 to 1991. J Aging Health 1997;9:419–450

97. Preston SH, Taubman P: Socio economic differences in adult mortality and health status. In Martin LG, Preston JH (eds): Demography of Aging. National Academic Press, Washington, DC, 1994:279–318

98. Blaxter M: Self definition of health status and consultation rates in primary care. Qtly J Soc Affairs 1985;1:131–171

99. Idler EL, Kasl S: Health perceptions and survival: do global evaluations of health status really predict mortality? J Gerontol 1991;46:S55–S65

100. Health Survey for England. Analysis of tables available on www.doh.gov.uk/public/healtholderpeople2000.htm

101. Kramarow E, Lentzner H, Rooks R et al: Health and Aging Chartbook: Health United States 1999. National Center for Health Statistics, Hyattsville, MA, 1999

102. Boult C, Kane R, Thomas A et al: Chronic conditions that lead to functional limitation in the elderly. J Gerontol A 1994;49:M28–M36

103. World Health Statistics Annual. WHO, Geneva, 1998

104. Katz S, Branch LG, Branson MH, Papsidero JA, Beck JC, Greer DS: Active life expectancy. N Engl J Med 1983;309:1218–1224

105. Weiner JM, Hanley RJ, Clark R, Van Nostrand JF: Measuring the activities of daily living: comparisons across national surveys. J Gerontol 1990;45:S229–S237

106. World Health Organization: International Classification of Impairments, Disabilities and Handicaps. WHO, Geneva, 1980

107. Bone MR, Bebbington AC, Jagger C, Morgan K, Nicolaas G: Health expectancy and its uses. HMSO, London, 1996

108. Crimmins E, Saito Y, Ingegneri D: Changes in life expectancy and disability-free life expectancy in the United States. Pop Devel Rev 1989;15:235–267

109. Robine JM: Health expectancies in current research. Rev Clin Gerontol 1997;7:73–81

110. Robine JM, Mormiche P, Sermet C: Examination of the causes and of the mechanisms of the increase in disability-free life expectancy. J Aging Health 1998;10:171–191

111. World Bank: World Development Report 1993: Investing in Health, World Development Indicators. Oxford University Press, Oxford, 1983

112. Zeng Y, Vaupel J, Xiao Z et al: The healthy longevity survey and the active life expectancy of the oldest old in China. Population (an English selection) 2001;13:95–116

113. Bowling A, Bond M, McKee D et al: Equity in access to exercise tolerance testing, coronary angiography, and coronary artery bypass grafting by age, sex and clinical indications. Heart 2001;85:680–686

114. McMurdo, Marion: A healthy old age: realistic or futile goal? BMJ 2000;321:1149–1151

115. Hanlon P, Walsh D, Whyte B et al: Hospital use by an ageing cohort: an investigation into the association between biological, behavioural and social risk markers and subsequent hospital utilization. J Pub Health Med 1998;20:467–476

116. Medical Research Council: Cognitive Function and Ageing Study and Resource Implications Study. Profiles of disability in elderly people: estimates from a longitudinal population study. BMJ 2001;318:1108–1111

117. Fratiglioni L, Wang H, Ericsson K et al: Influence of social networks on occurrence of dementia: a community-based longitudinal study. Lancet 2000;355:1315–1319

118. Medical Research Council: Topic Review: The Health of the UK's Elderly Population. Medical Research Council, London, 1994

Chapter 3

The future of old age

Kenneth G. Manton

The future of old age in the twenty-first century in the USA and other economically developed countries will be dynamic and will generate historically unprecedented demographic, social, and medical conditions. This will be due to quantitative and qualitative population, social, and health factors. Some quantitative demographic factors are well known—although details of their operation are not fully appreciated.

First, in the USA, there were rapid declines in mortality at young ages from at least 1900 due to reductions in infectious disease risks and infant and maternal mortality. Responsible for these declines were improved nutrition, new antibiotic therapies, immunization and vaccination programs for childhood diseases, and improved public hygiene (e.g. improved sanitation, drinking water, and, recently, air quality). The likelihood of surviving to age 65 for US males in 1900 was 37.3 percent; for females it was 41.0 percent.[1] By 1950 the figures had reached 61.8 percent for males and 74.3 percent for females; and in 2000 they were 75.9% for males and 86.4% for females. From 1954 to 1968, US mortality was viewed as static—male mortality rates increased 0.2 percent per year; female mortality rates, in contrast, declined 0.8 percent per year. Federal agencies began to plan, and operate, as if the upper limit to population life expectancy had been reached.[2] Projections of the Social Security beneficiary population in the mid-1970s assumed that mortality would decline no further.[3] This view was also expressed by epidemiologists who suggested that the third phase of the epidemiological transition would have increased the prevalence of chronic degenerative diseases[4] caused by adverse social[5] and public health conditions intrinsic to industrial society.[6]

Second, the size of birth cohorts increased. Post-WWII baby boom cohorts reached a maximum in 1963 in the USA. The first of those cohorts reaches age 65 in 2012, and age 85 in 2032. The largest cohorts reach age 65 in 2029 and 85 in 2049. The larger size of recent cohorts, and improved mortality up to age 65, will produce large future increases in the elderly population in the USA. Similar population dynamics operate in other developed, and some developing, countries. This will produce severe strains on economic and medical programs for elderly populations.

Third, after being static from 1954 to 1968, US mortality above age 65 began to decline, in part due to the start of national research programs on chronic diseases. The National Heart Institute was created in 1949. The Framingham Heart Study began in 1950. Actually, although reductions in chronic disease mortality were identified as starting in 1968, a more comprehensive examination suggests that mortality declines for chronic diseases began earlier. From 1950 to 1998, age-standardized heart disease mortality rates declined 58.8 percent; stroke mortality declined 71.7 percent. Declines in stroke mortality can be traced back to at least 1925.[7] Declines in male heart disease prevalence became evident after examining data on US Civil War veterans aged 65 and over who were assessed for pensions in 1910. A comparison of heart disease prevalence in Civil War veterans in 1910 with that in WWII veterans aged 65 and over in 1985 showed a decline of 66 percent in the intervening 75 years.[8]

Reductions in chronic disease mortality raised concern about society's "carrying" capacity for a growing elderly population, because it suggested that the number of years individuals live after age 65 would be significantly extended. Although Social Security finances benefit from an increasing number of persons living through their labor force years to age 65, living beyond 65 increases the financial burden on Social Security—and Medicare and Medicaid—programs. Recognition of the declines after 1968 in chronic disease mortality, and life expectancy increases above age 65, raised concerns about the long-term fiscal stability of the US Social Security system. In 1982, in addition to payroll tax increases, increases in the Social Security normal retirement age from 65 to 67 were scheduled for early in the twenty-first century. Increases in the retirement age to age 70, or even 72, are currently being debated. Similar problems are faced in other developed countries. A Japanese study suggested that future economic growth could be compromised by population aging. That study anticipated that one-quarter of Japan's population will be over 65 by 2025—using estimates of life expectancy limits that were exceeded by three years by Japanese females in 1992.[9,10]

Policy and social responses to population aging depends upon a fourth dynamic—changes in the average health of the elderly. Was the health of a person age 70 in 1995 better, on average, than the health of a 70-year-old in 1970? Will the health of an 80-year-old in 2020 be better than the health of an 80-year-old in 1995? US data suggest that the answers to these questions are yes. Significant declines in the prevalence of chronic disability and morbidity in the elderly population were observed from 1982 to 1999—and appear likely to continue to 2001 and beyond.[11–14]

Such health changes have profound effects on the social and economic institutions of a country—as well as on its healthcare delivery and financing system.[15] There are already popular responses in the perceived lower limit to "old age" in the USA. A recent survey suggested that persons aged 50 thought a person has to reach age 80 before being "elderly." This was due to changing social perceptions, and economic realities due to the growing proportion of the total US population over age 65, and the effects on housing, insurance, and other private markets as well as to physical changes in younger old persons. Fundamental research issues involve determining parameters of the population health dynamics underlying changing social perceptions and economics. Whether or not improvements in health and functioning continue at late ages, and can be accelerated by judicious public health and medical innovations and investments, will affect how the USA's and other developed countries' social and economic institutions respond to a growing elderly population.

A difficulty in anticipating future improvements in health at, for example, ages 85 and 95 is that changes depend, in part, upon both historical and future conditions. Historical factors are important because the individuals who will be the elderly and oldest-old cohorts in the next 65 years are already alive and have accumulated significant early exposures that partly determine the age trajectories of health parameters. Historical factors determine both the number of elderly persons (by reducing early mortality), and the mix of health problems they present (i.e. parameters of individual health changes with age vary due to differences in the prior risk factor experiences of birth cohorts). That is, depending both upon the cohort an elderly person is in, and the individual's life experiences, the principal health manifestations of aging may vary considerably. For example, very elderly cohorts may have little early smoking experience, and hence little chronic pulmonary disease. Recent cohorts of postmenopausal females, due to the early use of exogenous estrogens, may have reduced osteoporosis and coronary heart disease (CHD) risks. An analysis of future conditions is necessary because we are in a historically unique period where many biomedical technologies, and their clinical application, are maturing so that many conditions once palliatively managed are now subject to disease-modifying treatments (e.g. rheumatoid arthritis,[16] more recently osteoarthritis using glucosamine[17]).

The remainder of this chapter will briefly review historical and future inputs to the health dynamics of the elderly population, and then forecast what "old age" will signify in the future.

HISTORICAL DETERMINANTS OF THE FUTURE HEALTH OF THE ELDERLY

The realized human lifespan is increasing. The first well-documented case of a centenarian was reported in 1800.[18] The first well-documented achievement of the age of 110 years was in 1932. The first well-documented achievement of the age of 120 years (Jean Marie Calment; who lived to 122) was in 1995. There are partly documented reports of ages of 125 years being achieved for a Brazilian female; and 127 years for a US Hispanic female. Thus, the maximum documented human lifespan increased 10 years from 1800 to 1932, and over 12 years from 1932 to 1997; that is, at over twice the earlier rate. The number of centenarians in the USA increased 7 percent per year from 1960 to 1987—that growth continues with 54,000 centenarians estimated to be alive in 1995 and centenarians estimated to be alive in 2000.[19] Similar annual rates of increase in the number of centenarians are found in other developed countries.[20] Thus, centenarians are no longer a rarity—although studies of their current, and past, health characteristics are.[21] The age range of new elderly, and extreme elderly, cohorts is now broad enough (e.g. 65 to 115 years of age) that the parameters of the health consequences of aging will differ significantly across the cohorts represented by that range (i.e. aging health changes are partly determined by historical processes).

Evidence suggests that the health of the extreme elderly is improving and that interventions can be successful at late ages. One factor in health improvements is the effect of early mortality on the health of very elderly populations; "high" early mortality in a cohort "selects out" its genetically less fit members between ages 50 and 85. In a Swedish study, the relative risk of CHD mortality in monozygotic twin pairs was roughly 15 to 1 in middle age. Above age 85, the relative risk was 1.0.[22] Selection caused thyroid autoantibodies in Italian centenarians to be only as prevalent as they were at 50—even though their prevalence increased from ages 50 to 85.[23] Genetically determined lung cancer (due to defects in the cytochrome P-450 enzyme system) peak at 70 percent at age 50; by age 70 the genetic form of the disease is 20 percent of cases.[24] ApoE4, (apolipoprotein E4), associated with heart disease and dementia risk, declines with age from a prevalence of over 20 percent at age 80 to about 5 percent at age 100.[25] The null allele C4B*Qo is associated with heart attack risk in middle-aged males, with such risks (and selection against the genotype) occurring at later ages for females.[26,27]

If mortality selection were the only factor determining the health of extreme elderly populations, their average health would decline as the percentage surviving from birth to late ages in a cohort increased. However, many other factors affect the health of the extreme elderly.

A study of surgery performed on patients aged 90 to 103 showed that intraoperative mortality declined from 29 percent in the 1960s to 8 percent by 1985.[28] The study was performed because surgery rates over age 90 increased five-fold from 1979 to 1989. The 5-year survival of this group (mean age 93.5 years), was better than in the general population (i.e. a 5-year survival of 21 percent versus 16 percent in regional life-tables). A factor in the success of surgical interventions was the small number of "ever smokers" in the cohort and the low prevalence of chronic pulmonary disease.

Nutritional factors were thought to cause the reductions in chronic morbidity in Fogel's study of Civil War veterans.[8] One theory suggests that prenatal nutrition affects the risk of chronic disease at late ages[29–31] because the prenatal development of major organ systems is affected by maternal nutrition. In US Civil War veterans born 1825 to 1844, the high prevalence of chronic disease was thought to be due to poor maternal and early nutrition differentially affecting the development of major organ systems. Improvements between 1910 and 1985 in physiological status at late ages was argued to be due to improved early nutrition between the experience of the 1825 to 1844, and 1900 to 1920, cohorts. This Fogel traced to temporal increases in stature and body mass index (BMI) on Waaler surfaces.[32]

Another theory suggests that improved food hygiene reduced exposures to viral and other chronic "slow" infections (e.g. cytomegalovirus, herpesvirus, *Chlamydia pneumoniae*[33,34]) in animal food sources causing later reductions in atherosclerosis in adults.[35] They suggest that thermal food processing and tighter regulations on livestock production reduced the risk of chronic circulatory diseases and certain cancers[36] by reducing the risk of chronic viral and other infections.[35,37] That is, recent declines in heart disease mortality were traced to the ingestion of atherogenic viruses in pre-WWII, and postwar declines in infection rates as food hygiene improved. A number of events shaped these trends; vesicular exanthema, a viral disease of swine, was discovered in 1932. Controls for this and other livestock infections began in California between 1945 and 1949, a state showing early (1950) declines in heart disease. An outbreak of vesicular exanthema in 1952 mandated national regulations requiring thermal processing of livestock feed. Hog cholera eradication programs began in 1962. The Swine Health Protection Act was passed in 1980 to prevent another virus from entering the food chain. Thermal processing of prepared foods, although existing as a technology at the turn of the century, expanded rapidly after WWII. Some early models of atherosclerosis[38,39] suggested that infectious agents were involved—in addition to inflammatory processes, homeostatic factors, and blood lipids.[40] However, the technical ability (e.g. polymerase chain reaction [PCR] or fluorescence in-situ hybridization [FISH]) to detect the presence of agents, their genetic effects, or persistent immunological responses is recent.[41]

Another model suggests that chronic circulatory disease change was, in part, due to changes in the dietary levels of micronutrients such as vitamins A, B, C, E, and D. A, C, and E are antioxidants and may reduce the rate of oxidation of low-density lipoprotein (LDL) cholesterol in macrophages (producing "foam cells")—a factor in atherogenesis.[40] Vitamins A and E are cellular redifferentiating agents reducing the risk of some cancers.[42] The dietary levels of vitamins A (and other retinoids) and C depends upon the availability of fresh fruits and vegetables—foodstuffs difficult to preserve before refrigeration and transportation technologies allowed people in northern temperate climates to continue to consume such foodstuffs through the winter. This also could affect hypertension and stroke in that refrigeration reduced the use of salt as a food preservative. Increased consumption of fruits may have increased potassium intake and lowered hypertension.

Vitamin D has long been a supplement. Moon et al.[43] noted that the curative effects of cod liver oil on rickets were documented in 1917. By 1923, the USA imported half a million gallons of fish liver oil; nearly three million gallons in 1930. Ultraviolet radiation of milk began in the USA in 1924. Production of vitamin D rose from 35 pounds in 1948 to 14,000 pounds in 1972. Supplementation became problematic in that vitamin D is a potent hormonal agent with a narrow therapeutic trough. Reductions in supplementation were mandated by the Food and Drug Administration (FDA) in 1972.

Vitamin D metabolism is complex, including effects on cellular calcium metabolism and parathyroid hormone production, possibly leading to hypertension.[44] Vitamin D interferes with the uptake of magnesium. Concomitant with increased vitamin D supplementation were declines in magnesium in the US diet due to the use of nitrogen-based fertilizers. Vitamin D also increases the absorption of iron, so oversupplementation could affect heart disease by reducing magnesium (which could increase production of aldosterone[45]) and by increasing iron absorption-increasing LDL oxidation (also by causing increases in serum calcium and calcification of plaques), stroke (by affecting hypertension), and osteoporosis (by direct effects on osteoclasts and bone resorption).

A fourth model involves elevated homocysteine due to increased meat consumption and genetic or dietary deficiencies of vitamins B_6 and B_{12}. Decreasing renal function with age may adversely affect physiological vitamin B levels, as may age changes in liver metabolism through the eighth decade of life. The homocysteine model suggests that atherosclerosis is, in part, a disease of protein toxicity whereby failure to detoxify certain sulfur-based amino acid products of protein metabolism leads to damage in arterial endothelium.[46] The homocysteine model may not only explain initiating events in circulatory disease,[47] but also possibly osteo- and rheumatoid arthritic changes (by affecting cartilage matrix formation) and increases in dementia.[48] Vitamin B_6 also has a wide range of physiological effects (e.g. DNA binding and nuclear localization) on a superfamily of ligand-activated transcription factors that exert biological effects by regulating target gene expression.[49,50]

CURRENT AND FUTURE BIOMEDICAL INPUTS TO AGING

The factors described above determined health parameters of persons now entering advanced age ranges. To respond to this heterogeneity of aging parameters, and recent changes in the physiological manifestation of aging changes, are treatment modalities made possible by recent biomedical research. Research focused on aging per se began in the USA with the creation of National Institute on Aging (NIA) in 1974. In the 1960s, biological senescence was often viewed as a genetically determined cellular process operating universally in all tissue types, and chronic diseases were believed to be manifestations of its effects. Hayflick[51] suggested such a model after observing that human fibroblasts could reproduce only 50 to 60 times. An experiment[52] challenging this view examined the number of cell replications remaining for fibroblasts drawn from persons aged 30 to 80 years. Cells lost one replication for every five years of life. Thus, if this is the basic mechanism of senescence, it would not limit lifespans near current levels. Recently it has been suggested that defects in mitochondrial DNA may be a more likely biological limitation to the maximum human lifespan, suggesting a limit of 129 years.

In the 1970s it became clear that many aging studies had design flaws (i.e. the rate of loss of physiological function was tracked in "representative" populations). This confounded the intrinsic physiological rate of aging with the age-dependent prevalence of chronic disease determined by the history of environmental exposures. Studies of populations screened for existing chronic disease lowered estimates of the age rate of loss of physiological functions (e.g. the age rate of loss of cardiac function in an active elderly population was one-half that in earlier studies[53]). Age-related disease processes were found to be physiologically more complex, with much wider variation in expression than previously thought.[54,55]

In the 1980s, medical science began to demonstrate potential for modifying chronic disease processes. Atherosclerosis was once thought to be a product of an aging circulatory system. Now it appears to be reversible by nutritional modification (e.g. cholesterol reduction) and other interventions,[56,57] with functional responses evident before anatomical changes[58,59] and facilitated by antioxidant therapy.[60] Left ventricular hypertrophy (LVH) was thought to be due to age-related remodeling of cardiomyocytes. However, angiotensin-converting enzyme (ACE)-II inhibitors, as well as controlling hypertension, can also cause regression of LVH,[61] possibly by blocking the effects of aldosterone in remodeling myocytes as fibrotic tissue.[62] Many classic signs of senescence, or old age, are now well-defined pathological processes (e.g. frailty and osteoporosis, cognitive impairment, and Alzheimer's disease). With the pathological mechanisms identified, it is possible to develop disease-modifying interventions and, thus, to re-mold the aging process.

Some early chronic disease and aging interventions were initiated serendipitously. Exogenous estrogens were used by three million US women in 1985 for postmenopausal symptoms. By 1994 this had grown to 10 million women. Now it appears that exogenous estrogen reduces the risk of osteoporosis and CHD[63] in postmenopausal women.[64] Research[65] also suggests that estrogen supplementation could reduce the risk of dementia by 50 percent. Evidence is beginning to suggest that testosterone supplementation may have benefits for males in terms of reduced dementia risk. Data from the 1999 NLTCS suggests there were large declines in dementia risk from 1982 to 1999.[14]

Aspirin has long been used as an analgesic and to control fever. Recently, its potential in secondary prevention of stroke and heart attack by affecting platelet adhesion has been realized.[66] An association of aspirin consumption with reduced risk of colorectal cancer was found, as has an association of up to 80 percent reduction in Alzheimer's disease risks.[67] Nonsteroidal anti-inflammatory drugs (NSAIDs), by blocking inflammatory tissue responses, may affect other cancers by affecting the ability of tumor cells to metastasize and clonally organize.

Modeling senescence as the genetic control of the number of cell replications was given impetus by investigations of the end-segment of the human chromosome, the telomere, and an enzyme, telomerase, that induces its lengthening.[68] The evidence for the telomere controlling senescence is mixed. The telomere does decrease in length as the cell replicates. However, when a given length is reached, although the cell ceases to divide, it exhibits stable metabolism and function. Bone marrow and blood cells express low levels of telomerase, with that activity distributed across different cell types. Thus, there may not be an absolute shutoff of telomerase in somatic cells but continuing production at low levels. This is consistent with templates of telomerase ribonucleic acid (RNA) existing in somatic cells and the ability of tumor cells to express telomerase after a crisis phase.[69]

Evidence of the role of telomerase in neoplastic growth is clear. Normally, cells stop replicating while the telomere is still long. It may be that the p53 mediated pathway to apoptosis[70] is activated when the telomere drops below a functionally suboptimal length. Then, the cell enters a crisis phase that leads either to cell death or a reactivation of telomerase, a stabilized telomere length, and an immortal cell line.[71] Confirmation was found that telomerase activity was present in 68 percent of stage I tumors, and in 95 percent of advanced-stage breast tumors, but not in normal tissue. Telomerase was expressed in 45 percent of fibroadenomas, benign breast lesions.[72]

The search for mechanisms of senescence is difficult.[73] Many physiological mechanisms associated with aging and cell growth have proved to be more mutable by environmental factors, even at the genetic and molecular level, than once thought.[41,74,75] Some authors[76] have argued that human life expectancy is limited to 85 years, unless medical science develops interventions at the molecular level to modify parameters of aging. The problem with these arguments is defining

molecular interventions; many existing interventions operate at a molecular level. Nutritional factors (e.g. vitamins A and B) may affect receptor structure in the cell membrane, the message to DNA, and the transcription of genetic code to specific proteins. Some interventions have been used for a long time, even though their mechanisms were initially not understood. The anthracycline, doxorubicin, is a potent chemotherapeutic agent disrupting cell replication by affecting nuclear proteins, topoisomerase II α and β.[74] Early chemotherapeutic techniques were based on relatively simple principles where cell death was a function of drug concentration. Now the ways (e.g. interactions of c-*myc*, *bcl*-2 and *p53* genes[41]) in which apoptosis is induced, and interventions in ancillary processes such as angiogenesis, growth factor dependency, metastatic invasion, and cellular redifferentiation, are all therapeutic avenues being investigated at the molecular level.

To illustrate, an agent in use a long time, for which the mechanisms of molecular action are still being elaborated, is the antiestrogen, tamoxifen. This compound was given to older women with advanced, estrogen-receptor-positive breast cancer, to control its growth.[77] At first, growth inhibition was attributed to competitive binding with estrogen in a tumor cell's estrogen receptors. This initially raised concern that tamoxifen would exacerbate osteoporosis and heart disease. However, tamoxifen's interaction with the receptor was more complex—sometimes being an agonist (i.e. it was protective against bone loss and circulatory disease). It appears that tamoxifen affects the ability to induce transcriptional activity in the carboxy-terminal ligand binding domain.[78] Of further interest was that tamoxifen affected estrogen-receptor-negative tumor cells, and in interaction with chemotherapeutic agents (e.g. cisplatin[79]), by synergistically interacting in inducing apoptosis with other agents (e.g. vitamin D[80]); possibly by increasing the expression of estrogen receptors; or by blocking the action of drug-resistant genes by affecting the calcium channel membrane transport of the drug.[81,82] The effects on estrogen-receptor-negative breast cancer cells may be due to the induction of apoptosis by overexpression of c-*myc*, mRNA, and protein.[83] These effects may be enhanced by retinoic acid and vitamin D_3 analogs.[84,85] Interventions into the transcriptional expression of genotypes by known agents is interesting, given growing insights into the relation of carcinogenesis and senescence.[71,86,87]

THE FUTURE OF AGING

The above suggest (1) that the physiological expression of aging changes will vary in the future owing to major changes in nutrition, infectious disease risks, and hygiene, some exposures inducing stable genetic aberrations;[41,75] and (2) that we already have many agents and therapies affecting the molecular transcriptional expression of genotype, although our knowledge of the details of those mechanisms, and how to intervene, are not complete. It can be argued, however, that we have only recently developed the scientific tools (e.g. PCR; restriction fragment length polymorphism [RFLP]; chromosome painting[41,75]) to accelerate our understanding of these mechanisms, and of the techniques and agents for intervening (e.g. rational drug design; nonimmunosuppressive cyclosporin, PSC833[88]).

Techniques intervening at a molecular level are not restricted to cancer treatments but are used also in many other disorders.[89] A promising area is the improved regulation of the aging immune system.[90] A promising recent development was the observation that interleukin-10 (IL-10) suppressed tumor growth and inhibited spontaneous metastasis.[91,92] This was a surprise because IL-10 suppressed macrophage and helper T-cell function, and delayed hypersensitivity reactions. In suppressing macrophage activity, IL-10 suppressed release of proinflammatory cytokines, nitric oxide, and reactive oxygen intermediaries. It, however, stimulated natural killer (NK) cells, and chemoattraction of CD8+ cells and neutrophils. Inhibition of macrophage activity may have a tumor suppressive effect by reducing the local production of multiple growth or angiogenesis factors. Alterations of immune function (e.g. by vitamin A, C, or E supplementation[93,94]), and inflammatory responses and angiogenesis may be important in autoimmune disorders[95] and in certain stages of atherogenesis.[96,97] As in other cases, nutritional factors hold promise for modifying abnormal immunoresponse (e.g. the role of fish oil supplementation on MHC-II molecules and the membranes of human white blood cells affecting autoimmune disorders[98]). Omega-3 fatty acids may protect against chronic obstructive lung disease in "ever" smokers.[99]

Thus, there is a matrix of interrelations of physiological processes that underly the major chronic diseases expressed in old age. For example, the expression of Lp(a), a factor in circulatory disease risks, also has a strong association with breast cancer risk and its ability to metastasize.[100] The role of inflammatory response, and of the local production of growth factors, is likely crucial to both tumor growth and the development of atherosclerotic plaques.[92,96,97] There are likely associations of osteoporosis and atherosclerosis due to altered calcium metabolism.[101] Osteoporosis may be linked to hypertension and renal function by vitamin D metabolism.[89,102]

Because of this rapidly increasing understanding of disease processes and therapeutic interventions at the molecular level, it is reasonable to anticipate future and accelerating changes in disease and mortality risks at late ages. One of the crucial factors is to develop therapeutics with positive effect profiles. This is possible because of the above-mentioned matrix of physiological functions that interrelate many age-dependent pathologies at the molecular level. For example, ACE-II inhibitors have positive effects on lipid and glucose metabolism, reduce LVH, and possibly increase β-receptor density as well as control hypertension.[103–105] Certain β-blockers may improve β-receptor activity in the myocardium by down-regulating both response to norepinephrine and activity as an antioxidant.[106] The reason that IL-10 is promising is because it does not produce the serious side-effects found with many other cytokines.[107]

One argument may be that this increased understanding of disease mechanisms may produce medical interventions too expensive to provide en masse to a rapidly growing elderly population (e.g. the prescription of human growth hormone). This may, however, be due to a misunderstanding of the economics of scientific innovation, in that the initial development of new technologies is expensive; the evolution of subsidiary production technologies reduces unit costs and more of the population is treated (i.e. development costs are amortized over larger numbers of patients and the full benefits for the population are realized). For example, ACE-II inhibitors reduce the number of days of hospitalization required for congestive heart failure (CHF).[108] As a result, the cost–benefit ratio of ACE-II inhibitors, appropriately applied, can be quite high.[61] *Helicobacter pylori* was characterized in 1984. The role of *H. pylori* in the mechanism for most ulcers and gastric cancers[109] identified new treatment modalities that are very cost-effective. Antibiotic treatment for *H. pylori* costs about $200, compared to about $100 per month for the use of histamine blockers, which do not cure the disease. Given that there may be 4.5 million ulcer cases in the USA, the savings would be significant. Technologies also prove cost-effective, such as day surgery and plastic lens implants for cataracts;[110] newer forms of pacemakers more appropriate for cardiac functional decline at late ages, dual-chamber pacemakers, can respond to the increasing role of arterial pulse in cardiac output with age.[111] Thus, the correct understanding of a disease mechanism and linkages may produce synergistic interventions that eventually prove economic, especially if disease control is also accompanied by functional increases at late ages. Estimates of the savings to Medicare of reductions in functional disability prevalence from 1982 to 1995 could be over 7 percent of costs; or $180 to $200 billion (in 1995 dollars[11]).

If costs are not a limiting factor to advancement of health at late ages, what might aging in the mid-twenty-first century look like? Projections for the USA suggest that control of major circulatory disease risk factors, over a long enough time for their regulation to affect existing disease, could significantly increase the mean age at which CHD and stroke deaths occur.[112] The predominant forms of CHD would involve interactions of hypertension, atherosclerotic change, and age-related declines in cardiac function (e.g. age-related loss of β-receptor binding efficiency) that would become further dominated by the age-related changes in cardiac function. Cancer mortality, especially for solid tumors, in the next 10–15 years will begin to show significant declines due to treatments now in clinical trials. Evidence suggests that significant breast cancer mortality reductions have occurred owing to the use of tamoxifen in estrogen-receptor-positive disease, and adjuvant therapy in early node-negative disease.[113,114] Greenspan[115] suggests current chemotherapy, rigorously applied, could reduce the number of US breast cancer deaths by one-third. The aging of the population could promote this trend, as recent studies indicate that very young women with breast cancer may respond less favorably than older women to chemotherapy.[116,117] This is due to the generally less aggressive nature of disease in older women and probably to better management of the adverse effects of more aggressive treatments at later ages (e.g. use of granulocyte-colony stimulating factor [G-CSF]). The mix of cancers affecting an older population will change significantly. This will be related to the nature of the host tissue in which the tumor arises. For example, cancer related to infectious processes (liver cancer, gastric cancer) or food spoilage may decline. Other neoplasia related to biological aging processes (e.g. prostate cancer, multiple myeloma, certain types of lymphoma, late-onset breast cancer) will increase in importance—although the mean age of death from those cancers will also increase. The effects of viral diseases on cancer risks and possibly on atherogenesis and general immunological dysfunction (e.g. plasma cell dyscrasia of unknown significance, which often progress to multiple myeloma[90]) will become more treatable as antiviral agents improve and as our understanding of the chronic effects of viruses on the immune system advances.

Thus, there are a number of areas where therapeutic advances could occur, affecting multiple stages of very lengthy chronic disease processes. In addition, therapeutic advances could be supported by behavioral and lifestyle changes among middle-aged and elderly people. This can be anticipated in that:

- the proportion of elderly cohorts who are better educated is increasing—that is, better educated populations tend to be more amenable to public health messages;[118]
- physical activity has been shown to have benefits to extreme ages.[119–121]

It has now also been documented that biomedical advances began to significantly reduce total cancer mortality in the USA in 1991,[122] in contrast to the arguments put forward in Bailar and Smith[123] and Bailar and Gornik.[124]

These changes could increase life expectancy in the next 50–60 years (i.e. by 2050 to 2060) to 95 to 100 years.[125,126] This compares to US Census Bureau high life expectancy projections for 2050 of 86.4 years for males and 92.3 years for females.[19] Census Bureau life expectancy estimates are based on extrapolations of mortality trends. Our higher estimates are based on using multiple risk factor data, their dynamics, and assumptions about the ability to jointly control those factors.[125,126] Our projections do not assume that heart disease, stroke, and cancer are eliminated. They do assume that the mean age at death for each is increased due to preventative and disease-modifying interventions on risk factor profiles. Those changes will also affect the proportion of deaths due to specific causes. Male cancer mortality could increase from about 20 to 40 percent of deaths at all ages. The largest changes would come from increased proportions of cancer deaths above age 85. For females, cancer mortality would increase relatively more (to about 60 percent of all deaths), because the adverse effects of menopausal changes in multiple cardiovascular disease (CVD) risk factors are assumed controlled in the projections. CVD risks would decline moderately (from 65 to 50 percent) for males as a proportion of all deaths, but those deaths would occur at later ages. For females, the projected declines in CVD deaths are much larger.

The two sets of projections imply different things for US society's carrying capacity for the elderly. In census projections, the high life expectancy series project a US population of 416 million by 2050. In this projection, 1 percent would be over age 100 (4.1 million), 7.2 percent would be over age 85 (30 million), and 23.3 percent would be over age 65 (97 million). The proportion of the population above a given age in the census projections is strongly affected by fertility assumptions. For example, Social Security Administration (SSA) cohort life-tables for people born in 1950 (which use less favorable mortality assumptions) imply that 5.6 percent of females and 1.5 percent of males live to age 100. Assuming a 3 to 1 survival advantage for females to age 100, this suggests that 4.6 percent of the 1950 cohort survives to age 100. For the 1990 cohort, survival to age 100 is 10.2 percent for females and 3.3 percent for

males, or 8.4 percent combined. Thus, in a stable population, a large proportion of people reach age 100 even in less optimistic SSA 1990 life-tables. In our risk factor-based projections, the US population is projected to be 456 million in 2050, with 14 percent over age 85, and 33 percent over age 65. Although these proportions are larger than in the census projections, they are not grossly different from the 25 percent of the Japanese population expected to be over age 65 in 2025. If fertility and immigration is lower than assumed in Japanese census projections, then the proportion of the population over age 65 and over 85 would be higher. Even the extreme projections made from risk factor data do not take into account recent studies suggesting that human mortality never exceeds 50 percent at any age (i.e. 50 percent is the maximum mortality rate). This assumption has, for example, been built into the US Society of Actuaries' 1994 group annuity tables.[127] Such estimates are consistent with estimates from multiple studies showing that the annual increase in mortality rates slows to very low values (2–3 percent) at about age 100.[21] These slow increases in mortality are apparently due to the high mortality rates of very elderly persons with high levels of disability. Thus, the average level of disability at about age 95 tends to stabilize owing to the equilibrium with mortality rates at those ages.[112]

The question emerges of how a society can cope with a population with such a high proportion of elderly people. This is a problem only if there is not a commensurate change in the age-specific health status of the population. The health–mortality factors discussed above suggest that their natural dynamics enforce this in part. There is also evidence of such changes in current health expenditures. Lubitz et al.[128] found that the average Medicare expenditure for those who died at age 70 was $35,511, compared with $65,633 for those who survived to age 101. Thus, the average Medicare expense per year for centenarians from ages 65 to 101 was $1823, compared with $7100 per year for those who died at age 70. Thus, the pattern of a declining rate of Medicare expenditures with age contrasts with the accumulated liability of increased life expectancy for Social Security.

If disability declines, as observed from 1982 to 1999, health costs will decrease even more rapidly at later ages. This pattern

---

KEY POINTS **The future of old age**

- Population aging
- Morbid conditions prevalent at advanced ages
- Centenarians and growth of extreme elderly
- Barker's hypothesis
- Nutritional supplementation and exercise as modifiers of aging
- Biological inputs to aging and drug therapies
- Regenerative medicine: hormonal modulation
- Epidemiological transition
- Disability prevalence declines
- Mortality declined in the second half of the twentieth century

also seems consistent with the different patterns of medical problems that may be faced at late ages in the future. Disability will not only be prevented; in the future, functional loss will be reversed by "regenerative medicine." Thus, the primary response to the social costs of such large elderly populations would be increased in the normal retirement age for Social Security. Each year of increase in the normal retirement age for Social Security has a large fiscal impact. Thus, if the normal retirement age could be increased to age 70 or 72—because the physiological status now at those ages is equivalent to the physiological status at age 65 in, say, 1982—then a large portion of the fiscal burden of population aging could be addressed.

REFERENCES

1. Social Security Administration: Life Tables for the United States Social Security Area 1900–2080 (Actuarial Study 107). Social Security Administration (SSA pub no. 11–11536), Baltimore, 1992
2. National Center for Health Statistics: The change in mortality trends in the United States (Series 3, no. 1). Public Health Service, Washington, DC, 1964
3. Myers GC: Future age projections and society. In Gilmore AG (ed): Aging: A Challenge to Science and Social Policy. Oxford University Press, New York, 1981
4. Omran AR: The epidemiologic transition: a theory of the epidemiology of population change. Milbank Mem Qtly 1971;49:509–538
5. Antonovsky A: Social class and the major cardiovascular diseases. J Chron Dis 1968;21:65–106
6. Dubos R: Man adapting. Yale University Press, New Haven, 1965
7. Lanska DJ, Mi X: Decline in US stroke mortality in the era before antihypertensive therapy. Stroke 1993;24:1382–1388
8. Fogel RW: Economic growth, population theory, and physiology: the bearing of long-term processes on the making of economic policy. Am Econ Rev 1994;84:369–395
9. Nihon University: Population aging in Japan: problems and policy issues in the 21st century. In Kuroda T (ed): International Conference on an Aging Society: Strategies for the 21st Century Japan. Nihon University Population Research Institute, Tokyo, 1982
10. World Health Organization: World health statistics annual. WHO, Geneva, 1994
11. Manton KG: Future trends and perspectives in long-term care. In Jolt H, Leibovici MM (eds): Health Care Management: State of the Art Review Series. Hanley & Befus, Philadelphia, 1997
12. Manton KG, Corder LS, Stallard E: Estimates of change in chronic disability and institutional incidence and prevalence rates in the US elderly population from the 1982, 1984, and 1989 National Long Term Care Survey. J Gerontol B 1993;47:S153–S166
13. Manton KG, Stallard E, Corder LS: Changes in morbidity and chronic disability in the US elderly population: evidence from the 1982, 1984, and 1989 National Long Term Care Surveys. J Gerontol 1995;50B:S194–S204
14. Manton KG, XiLiang Gu: Changes in the prevalence of chronic disability in the United States black and nonblack population above age 65 from 1982 to 1999. Proc Natl Acad Sci USA 2001;98:6354–6359
15. Ikegami N, Campbell J: Medical care in Japan. N Engl J Med 1995;333:1295–1299
16. Tugwell P, Pincus T, Yocum D et al: Combination therapy with cyclosporine and methotrexate in severe rheumatoid arthritis. N Engl J Med 1995;333:137–141
17. Reginster J, Deroisy R et al: Long-term effects of glucosamine sulphate on osteoarthritis progression: a randomised, placebo-controlled clinical trial. Lancet 2001;357:251–256
18. Thoms WS: Human longevity, its facts and its fictions. John Murray, London, 1873
19. Day JC: Population projections of the United States, by age, sex, race, and Hispanic origin: 1995 to 2050, Series P25–1130. US Government Printing Office, Washington, DC, 1996
20. Vaupel JW, Jeune B: The emergence and proliferation of centenarians. Aging Research Unit, Odense University Medical School, Odense, Denmark, 1994
21. Manton KG, Stallard E: Longevity in the US: age and sex specific evidence on life span limits from mortality patterns: 1962–1990. J Gerontol A 1996;B362–B375
22. Marenberg ME, Risch N, Berkman LF et al: Genetic susceptibility to death from coronary heart disease in a study of twins. N Engl J Med 1994;330:1041–1046
23. Marriotti S, Sansoni P, Barbesino G et al: Thyroid and other organ-specific auto-antibodies in healthy centenarians. Lancet 1992;339:1506–1508
24. Sellers TA, Bailey-Wilson JE, Elston RC et al: Evidence for Mendelian inheritance in the pathogenesis of lung cancer. J Natl Cancer Inst 1990;82:1272–1279
25. Louhija J, Miettinen HE, Kontula K et al: Aging and genetic variation of plasma apolipoproteins: relative loss of the apolipoprotein E4 phenotype in centenarians. Arterioscler Thromb 1994;14:1084–1089
26. Kramer J, Fulop T, Rajczy K et al: A marked drop in the incidence of the null allele of the B gene of the fourth component of complement (C4B*Q0) in elderly subjects: C4B*Q0 as a probable negative selection factor for survival. Hum Genet 1991;86:595–598
27. Kramer J, Rajczy K, Hegyi L et al: C4B*Q0 allotype as risk factor for myocardial infarction. BMJ 1994;309:313–314
28. Hosking MP, Warner MA, Lodbell CM et al: Outcomes of surgery in patients 90 years of age and older. JAMA 1989;261:1909–1915
29. Barker D, Meade T, Fall C et al: Relation of fetal and infant growth to plasma fibrinogen and factor VII concentrations in adult life. BMJ 1992;304:148–152
30. Hale C, Barker D, Clark P et al: Fetal and infant growth impaired glucose tolerances at age 64. BMJ 1991;303:1019–1022
31. Barker DJP, Martyn CN: The maternal and fetal origins of cardiovascular disease. J Epidemiol Commun Health 1992;46:8–11
32. Waaler H: Height, weight, and mortality, the Norwegian experience. Acta Med Scand 1983;679(suppl 1):1–56
33. Grayston JT: Chlamydia in atherosclerosis. Circulation 1993;87:1408–1409
34. Linnanmäki E, Leinonen M, Mattila K et al: *Chlamydia pneumoniae*—specific circulating immune complexes in patients with chronic coronary heart disease. Circulation 1993;87:1130–1134
35. Mozar HN, Bal DG, Farag SA: The natural history of atherosclerosis: an ecologic perspective. Atherosclerosis 1990;82:157–164
36. Mozar HN, Bal DG, Farag SA: Human cancer and the food chain: an alternative etiologic perspective. Nutr Cancer 1989;12:29
37. Melnick JL, Schattner A: Viruses and atherosclerosis. Isr J Med Sci 1992;28:463–465
38. Klotz O, Manning MF: Fatty streaks in the intima of arteries. J Pathol Bacteriol 1912;16:211
39. Frothingham C: The relation between acute infectious diseases and arterial lesions. Arch Intern Med 1911;8:153
40. Ross R: The pathogenesis of atherosclerosis—an update. N Engl J Med 1986;314:488–500
41. Sheer D, Squire J: Clinical applications of genetic rearrangements in cancer. Cancer Biol 1996;7:25–32
42. Prasad KN, Edwards-Prasad J: Vitamin E and cancer prevention: recent advances and future potentials. J Am Coll Nutr 1992;11:487–500
43. Moon RC, Rao KVN, Detrisac CJ, Kelloff GJ: Animal models for chemoprevention of respiratory cancer. J Natl Cancer Inst Monogr 1992;13:45–49
44. Eastell R, Yergery A, Vieira N et al: Interrelationship among vitamin D metabolism, true calcium absorption, parathyroid function, and age in women: evidence of an age-related intestinal resistance to 1,25 dihydroxyvitamin A action. J Bone Mineral Res 1991;6:125
45. Ichihara A, Suzuki H, Saruta T: Effects of magnesium on the renin–angiotensin–aldosterone system in human subjects. J Lab Clin Med 1993;122:432–440
46. McCully KS: Homocystein theory of arteriosclerosis: development and current status. Arteriosclerosis 1983;2:157–246
47. von Eckardstein A, Malinow R, Upson B et al: Effects of age, lipoproteins, and hemostatic parameters on the role of homocyst(e)inemia as a cardiovascular risk factor in men. Arterioscler Thromb 1994;14:460–464
48. Riggs KM, Spiro A, Tucker K, Rush D: Relations of vitamin B-12, vitamin B-6, folate, and homocysteine to cognitive performance in the normative aging study. Am J Clin Nutr 1996;63:306–314
49. Tully DB, Allgood VE, Cidlowski JA et al: The steroid hormone receptors and their mechanism of action. In Nutrition and Gene Expression. CRC Press, Boca Raton, 1993:549–567

50. Allgood VE, Powell-Oliver FE, Cidlowski JA: Vitamin B_6 influences glucocorticoid receptor-mediated gene expression. J Biol Chem 1990;265:12424

51. Hayflick L: The limited in vitro lifetime of human diploid cell strains. Exp Cell Res 1965;37:614–636

52. Martin GM, Spaque CA, Epstein CJ: Replicative life-span of cultivated human cells: effects of donor's age, tissue and genotype. Lab Invest 1970;23:86–92

53. Kasch FW, Boyer JL, Van Camp SP et al: Effect of exercise on cardiovascular aging. Age Ageing 1993;22:5–10

54. Lakatta E: Health, disease, and cardiovascular aging. In America's Aging: Health in an Older Society. National Academy Press, Washington, DC, 1985

55. Lakatta EG: Deficient neuroendocrine regulation of the cardiovascular system with advancing age in healthy humans. Circulation 1993;87:631–636

56. Ornish D, Brown SE, Scherwitz LW et al: Can lifestyle changes reverse coronary heart disease? The Lifestyle Heart Trial. Lancet 1990;336:129–133

57. Brown BG, Zhao XQ, Sacco DE, Alberts JJ: Lipid lowering and plaque disruption and clinical events in coronary disease. Circulation 1993;87:1781–1791

58. Treasure C, Klein J, Weintraub W et al: Beneficial effects of cholesterol-lowering therapy on the coronary endothelium in patients with coronary artery disease. N Engl J Med 1995;332:481–487

59. Benzuly K, Padgett R, Kaul S et al: Functional improvement precedes structural regression of atherosclerosis. Circulation 1994;89:1810–1818

60. Anderson T, Meredith I, Yeung A et al: The effect of cholesterol-lowering and antioxidant therapy on endothelium-dependent coronary vasomotion. N Engl J Med 1995;332:488–493

61. Paul SD, Kuntz KM, Eagle KA, Weinstein MC: Costs and effectiveness of angiotensin converting enzyme inhibition in patients with congestive heart failure. Arch Intern Med 1994;154:1143–1149

62. Weber K, Brilla C: Pathological hypertrophy and cardiac interstitium. Circulation 1991;83:1849–1865

63. Nabulsi A, Folsom A, White A et al: Association of hormone-replacement therapy with various cardiovascular risk factors in postmenopausal women. N Engl J Med 1993;328:1069–1075

64. Belchetz P: Hormonal treatment of postmenopausal women. N Engl J Med 1994;330:1062–1071

65. Tang M, Jacobs D et al: Effect of oestrogen during menopause on risk and age at onset of Alzheimer's disease. Lancet 1996;348:429–432

66. Antiplatelet Trialists' Collaboration: Collaborative overview of randomized trials of antiplatelet therapy. I: Prevention of death, myocardial infarction, and stroke by prolonged antiplatelet therapy in various categories of patients. BMJ 1994;308:81–106

67. in't Veld BA, Ruitenberg A, Hofman A et al: Nonsteroidal antiinflammatory drugs and the risk of Alzheimer's disease. N Engl J Med 2001;345:1515–1521

68. Morin GB: The structure and properties of mammalian telomerase and their potential impact on human disease. Semin Cell Devel Biol 1996;7:5–13

69. Villeponteau B: The RNA components of human and mouse telomerases. Semin Cell Devel Biol 1996;7:15–21

70. Carson D, Ribeiro J: Apoptosis and disease. Lancet 1993;341:1251–1254

71. Bacchetti S: Telomere dynamics and telomerase activity in cell senescence and cancer. Semin Cell Devel Biol 1996;7:31–39

72. Hiyama E, Gollahon L, Kataoka T et al: Telomerase activity in human breast tumors. J Natl Cancer Inst 1996;88:116–122

73. Rowe J: Aging and geriatric medicine. In Wyngaarden W, Smith L (eds): Cecil, Textbook of Medicine. Harcourt, Brace Jovanovich, Philadelphia, 1988

74. Alton P, Harris A: Annotation: the role of DNA topoisomerases II in drug resistance. Br J Haematol 1993;85:241–245

75. Ramsey MJ, Moore DH, Briner JF et al: The effects of age and lifestyle factors on the accumulation of cytogenetic damage as measured by chromosome painting. Mutat Res 1995;338:95–106

76. Olshansky SJ, Rudberg MA, Carnes BA et al: Trading off longer life for worsening health: expansion of morbidity hypotheses. J Aging Health 1991;3:194–216

77. McDonald C, Stewart H: Fatal myocardial infarction in the Scottish adjuvant tamoxifen trial. BMJ 1991;303:435–437

78. Wolf DM, Fuqua AW: Mechanisms of action of antiestrogens. Cancer Treat Rev 1995;21:247–271

79. McClay EF, McClay ME, Albright KD et al: Tamoxifen modulation of cisplatin resistance in patients with metastatic melanoma: a biologically important observation. Cancer 1993;72:1914–1918

80. Welsh J: Induction of apoptosis in breast cancer cells in response to vitamin D and antiestrogens. Biochem Cell Biol 1994;82:537–545

81. Rowlands MG, Budworth J, Jarman M et al: Comparison between inhibitions of protein kinase C and antagonism of calmodulin by tamoxifen analogues. Biochem Pharmacol 1995;50:723–726

82. Lam HY: Tamoxifen is a calmodulin antagonist in the activation of cAMP phosphodiesterase. Biochem Biophys Res Commun 1984;118:27–32

83. Kang Y, Cortina R, Perry RR: Role of c-*myc* in tamoxifen-induced apoptosis in estrogen-independent breast cancer cells. J Natl Cancer Inst 1996;88:279–284

84. Vink-van Wijngaarden T, Pols HA, Buurman CJ et al: Inhibition of breast cancer cell growth by combined treatment with vitamin D_3 analogues and tamoxifen treatment. Cancer Res 1994;54:5711–5717

85. Anzano MA, Byers SW, Smith JM et al: Prevention of breast cancer in the rat with 9-*cis*-retinoic acid as a single agent and in combination with tamoxifen, Cancer Res 1994;54:4614–4617

86. Cutler RG, Semsei I: Development, cancer and aging: possible common mechanisms of action and regulation. J Gerontol 1989;44:25–34

87. Warner HR, Fernandes G, Wange E: A unifying hypothesis to explain the retardation of aging and tumorigenesis by caloric restriction. J Gerontol A 1995;50:B107–B109

88. Sikic BI: Reversing multidrug resistance with the nonimmuno-suppressive cyclosporin PSC 833. Cancer Invest: Abstracts 1996;14(suppl 1):55

89. Armbrecht H, Nemani R, Wongsurawat N: Protein phosphorylation: changes with age and age-related diseases. J Am Geriatr Soc 1993;41:873–879

90. Bowden M, Crawford J, Cohen H, Noyama O: A comparative study of monoclonal gammopathies and immunoglobulin levels in Japanese and United States elderly. J Am Geriatr Soc 1993;41:11–14

91. Kundu N, Beaty TL, Jackson MJ, Fulton AM: Antimetastatic and anti-tumor activities of interleukin 10 in a murine model of breast cancer. J Natl Cancer Inst 1996;88:536–541

92. Allione A, Consalvo M, Nanni P et al: Immunizing and curative potential of replicating and non-replicating murine mammary adenocarcinoma cells engineered with interleukin (IL)-2, IL-4, IL-6, IL-7, IL-10, tumor necrosis factor α, granulocyte-macrophage colony-stimulating factor, and γ-interferon gene or admixed with conventional adjuvants. Cancer Res 1994;54:6022–6026

93. Penn N, Purkins L, Kelleher J et al: The effect of dietary supplementation with vitamins A, C and E on cell-mediated immune function in elderly long-stay patients: a randomized controlled trial. Age Ageing 1991;20:169–174

94. Penn N, Purkins L, Kelleher J et al: Ageing and duodenal mucosal immunity. Age Ageing 1991;20:33–36

95. Carlquist J, Anderson J: HLA, autoimmunity, and rheumatic heart disease: apparent or real association. Circulation 1993;87:2060–2062

96. Buja L, Willerson J: Role of inflammation in coronary plaque disruption. Circulation 1994;89:503–505

97. van der Wal A, Becker A, van der Loos C, Das P: Site of intimal rupture or erosion of thrombosed coronary atherosclerotic plaques is characterized by an inflammatory process irrespective of the dominant plaque morphology. Circulation 1994;89:36–44

98. Hughes DA, Pinder AC, Piper Z et al: Fish oil supplementation inhibits the expression of major histocompatibility complex class II molecules and adhesion molecules on human monocytes. Am J Clin Nutr 1996;63:267–272

99. Shahar E, Folsom A, Melnick S et al: Dietary n-3 polyunsaturated fatty acids and smoking-related chronic obstructive pulmonary disease. N Engl J Med 1994;31:228–233

100. Kokoglu E, Karaarslan I, Karaarslan HM, Baloglu H: Elevated serum Lp(a) levels in the early and advanced stages of breast cancer. Cancer Biochem Biophys 1996;14:133–136

101. Moon J, Bandy B, Davison A: Hypothesis—etiology of atherosclerosis and osteoporosis: are imbalances in the calciferol endocrine system implicated? J Am Coll Nutr 1992;11:567–583

102. MacGregor GA, Cappuccio FP: The kidney and essential hypertension: a link to osteoporosis? J Hypertens 1993;11:781–785

103. Pollare T, Lithell H, Berne C: A comparison of the effects of hydroclorothiazide and captopril on glucose and lipid metabolism in patients with hypertension. N Engl J Med 1989;321:868–873

104. Pouleur H, Rousseau M, van Eyll C et al: Effects of long-term enalapril therapy on left ventricular diastolic properties in patients with depressed ejection fraction. Circulation 1993;88:481–491

105. Gilbert E, Sandoval A, Larrabee P et al: Lisinopril lowers cardiac adrenergic drive and increases b-receptor density in the failing heart. Circulation 1993;88:472–480

106. Packer M, Bristow MR, Cohn JN: The effect of carvedilol on morbidity and mortality in patients with chronic heart failure. N Engl J Med 1996;334:1349–1355

107. Nicolson GL: Bioregulators come of age in the control of tumor growth and metastasis. J Natl Cancer Inst 1996;88:479–480

108. SOLVD Investigators: Effect of enalapril on survival in patients with reduced left ventricular ejection fractions and congestive heart failure. N Engl J Med 1991;325:293–302

109. Fennerty M: *Helicobacter pylori*. Arch Intern Med 1994;154:721–727

110. Taylor A: Cataract: relationships between nutrition and oxidation. J Am Coll Nutr 1993;12:138–146

111. Bush D, Finucane T: Permanent cardiac pacemakers in the elderly. J Am Geriatr Soc 1994;42:326–334

112. Manton KG, Stallard E, Woodbury MA, Dowd JE: Time-varying covariates in models of human mortality and aging: multidimensional generalization of the Gompertz. J Gerontol A 1994;49:B169–B190

113. Nab H, Hop W, Crommelin M et al: Changes in long-term prognosis for breast cancer in a Dutch cancer registry. BMJ 1994;309:83–86

114. Olivotto I, Bajdik C, Plenderleith I et al: Adjuvant systemic therapy and survival after breast cancer. N Engl J Med 1994;330:805–810

115. Greenspan EM: The cure of breast cancer by combination chemotherapy. Cancer Invest 1996;14(suppl 1):70

116. Fowble BL: Section IV: Treatment. J Natl Cancer Inst Monogr 1994;16:67–68

117. Antman K, Ayash L, Elias A et al: High-dose cyclophosphamide, thiotepa, and carboplatin with autologous marrow support in women with measurable advanced breast cancer responding to standard-dose therapy: analysis by age. J Natl Cancer Inst Monogr 1994;16:91–94

118. Preston S: Demographic change in the United States, 1970–2050. In Manton K, Singer B, Suzman R (eds): Forecasting the Health of Elderly Population. Springer-Verlag, New York, 1992

119. Fiatarone M, Marks E, Ryan N et al: High-intensity strength training in nonagenarians. JAMA 1990;263:3029–3034

120. Fiatarone M, O'Neill E, Doyle N et al: The Boston FICSIT study: the effects of resistance training and nutritional supplementation on physical frailty in the oldest old. J Am Geriatr Soc 1993;41:333–337

121. Fiatarone M, O'Neill E, Ryan N et al: Exercise training and nutritional supplementation for physical frailty in very elderly people. N Engl J Med 1994;330:1769–1775

122. Hoeksema M, Law C: Cancer mortality rates fall: a turning point for the nation. J Natl Cancer Inst 1996;88:1706–1708

123. Bailar J, Smith E: Progress against cancer? N Engl J Med 1986;314:1226–1232

124. Bailar J, Gornik H: Cancer undefeated. N Engl J Med 1997;336:1569–1574

125. Manton KG, Stallard E, Singer BH: Projecting the future size and health status of the US elderly population. Int J Forecast 1992;8:433–458

126. Manton KG, Stallard E, Singer BH: Methods for projecting the future size and health status of the US elderly population. In Wise D (ed): Studies of the Economics of Aging. University of Chicago Press, Chicago, 1994

127. Society of Actuaries: 1994 Group Annuity Mortality Table and 1994 Group Annuity Reserving Table. Society of Actuaries, Exposure Draft, Schaumburg, IL, 1994

128. Lubitz J, Beebe J, Baker C: Longevity and Medicare expenditures. N Engl J Med 1995;332:999–1003

Chapter 4

Evolution theory and the mechanisms of aging

Thomas B. L. Kirkwood

The question "Why does aging occur?" calls for answers both at the level of proximate, physiological mechanisms and also at the level of ultimate, evolutionary origins. This chapter provides an understanding of why aging has evolved and examines what evolution theory can tell us about the kinds of mechanisms we might regard as prime candidates to explain senescence.

Evolution theory is well recognized as a powerful tool with which to inquire about the generic basis of the aging process.[1–4] Although human aging has its roots long ago in our past, the study of its evolution can throw important light on key present-day challenges. For example, a range of population-based studies, including one based on genealogical analysis of the entire population of Iceland, has shown consistent evidence for a generic contribution to human longevity.[5] Impelled in part by the human genome project, there is interest in knowing how many and what kinds of genes are likely to be involved in this heritability.[6] There is also interest in human genetic disorders such as Werner's syndrome that are characterized by acceleration of many aspects of the senescent phenotype. The identification by positional cloning of the gene responsible for Werner's syndrome[7] has raised interesting questions about its relation to other genes responsible for aging and age-associated diseases.

Before addressing questions about the evolutionary origin of aging it is important to be precise about how the term "aging" is to be understood. In this chapter, aging is defined as "a progressive, generalized impairment of function, resulting in a loss of adaptive response to stress and in a growing risk of age-related disease." The overall effect of these changes is summed up in the increase in the probability of dying, or age-specific death rate, in the population.

This definition of aging—in terms of a mortality pattern showing progressive increase in age-specific mortality—allows comparisons to be made even among species where the detailed features of the aging process may differ markedly. In phylogenetic terms, aging is widespread but by no means universal.[8–11] The fact that not all species show an increase in age-specific mortality indicates that aging is not an inevitable consequence of wear-and-tear. On the other hand, the fact that very many species do show such an increase is evidence that the evolution of aging has occurred under rather general circumstances.

EVOLUTION OF AGING

Theories on the evolution of aging seek to explain why aging occurs through the action of natural selection. The decline in survivorship, which is often also accompanied by a decline in fertility, means that there is an age-associated loss of Darwinian fitness that is clearly deleterious to the organism in which it occurs. Natural selection acts to increase fitness, so it is at once clear that selection should be expected, other things being equal, to oppose aging. The challenge to evolution theory is thus to explain why aging occurs in spite of its drawbacks.

Programmed or "adaptive" aging

It is sometimes suggested that in spite of its disadvantages to the individual, aging is beneficial and even necessary at the species level, for example, to prevent overcrowding.[12,13] In this case, genes that actively cause aging might have evolved specifically to program the end of life, in the same way as genes program development.

The difficulty with this view is that there is little evidence that aging serves as a major contributor to mortality in natural populations,[14] which means that aging apparently does not play the adaptive role suggested for it. The theory also embodies the questionable supposition that selection for advantage at the species level will be more effective than selection among individuals for the advantages of a longer life. Aging is clearly a disadvantage to the individual, so any mutation that inactivated the hypothetical adaptive aging genes would confer a fitness advantage, and therefore, the nonaging mutation should spread through the population unless countered by selection at the species or group level. Conditions under which "group selection" can work successfully are highly restrictive,[15] especially when there is selection in the opposite direction acting at the level of the individual. Briefly, it is necessary that the population be divided among fairly isolated groups, and that the introduction of a nonaging genotype into a group should rapidly lead to the group's extinction. The latter condition is necessary to provide the selection between groups that might, in principle, counter the tendency for selection at the level of individuals to favor the spread of nonaging mutants. It appears unlikely that these conditions will be met with sufficient generality to explain the evolution of aging.

Selection weakens with age

An observation of central importance to the evolution of aging is that the force of natural selection—that is, its ability to discriminate between alternative genotypes—weakens with age.[14,16–19] Because natural selection operates through the differential effects of genes on fitness, its discriminatory power must decline with age in proportion to the decline in remaining fraction of the organism's lifetime expectation of reproduction. This is true whether or not the species exhibits aging.

The attenuation in the force of natural selection with age means inevitably that there is only loose genetic control over the later portions of the lifespan. For this reason it has been suggested that aging might be due to an accumulation in the germ-line of mutations, which potentially are deleterious but are not expressed, or which produce no phenotypic effect until late in life.[14]

The idea is that if deleterious mutations are expressed so late that most individuals will already have died from some other cause, such as predation, even though the genes involved have the potential to cause harm they will be subject to very little selection against them. Over the generations a large number of such genes might accumulate. These would cause aging and death only when an individual is removed to a protected environment, away from the hazards of the wild, and so lives long enough to experience their negative effects.

A stronger version of this theory was proposed by Williams,[17] who suggested that because of the declining force of natural selection with age, any gene that conferred an advantage early in life would be favored by selection even if the same gene had deleterious effects at older ages. Such pleiotropic genes could explain aging. The decline in the force of natural selection with age would ensure that even quite modest early benefits would outweigh severe harmful side-effects, provided the latter occurred late enough.

Disposable soma theory

The disposable soma theory[1,4,20-22] explains aging through asking how best an organism should allocate its metabolic resources, primarily energy—between, on the one hand, keeping itself going from one day to the next, and on the other hand producing progeny to secure the continuance of its genes when it has itself died. No species is immune to hazards such as predation, starvation, and disease. All that is necessary by way of maintenance is that the body remains in sound condition until an age after which most individuals will have died from accidental causes. In fact, a greater investment in maintenance is a disadvantage, because it eats into resources that, in terms of natural selection, are better used for reproduction. The theory concludes that the optimum course is to invest fewer resources in the maintenance of somatic tissues than are necessary for indefinite survival (Fig. 4-1). The result is that aging occurs through the gradual accumulation of unrepaired somatic defects, but the level of maintenance will be set so that the deleterious effects do not become apparent until an age when survivorship in the wild environment would be extremely unlikely.

Comparison of the evolutionary theories

The adaptive program theory is in a category of its own and support for this theory is weak; it will not be considered further in this chapter.

The disposable soma and pleiotropic genes theories are adaptive in the sense that aging is the result of positive selection for aspects of the organism's life history, but the essential difference is that aging itself is not adaptive but is a negative trait that arises only as a by-product or tradeoff of some other benefit. The late-acting deleterious mutations theory assumes an essentially neutral evolutionary process, the accumulation

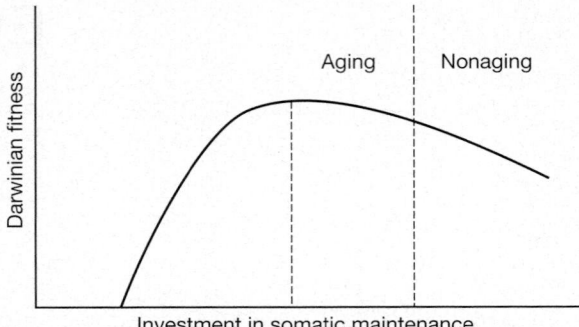

Figure 4-1 Relation between Darwinian fitness and investment in somatic maintenance predicted by the disposable soma theory of aging. Fitness is maximized at a level that is less than that which would be required for indefinite longevity (nonaging).

of mutations reflecting the inability of natural selection to maintain tight control over the later portions of the lifespan.

Among the nonadaptive theories there is a common strand, namely that old organisms count less. This is not due to any implicit assumption of frailty or obsolescence (this would render the theories circular), but to the simple mathematics of mortality. Even if old organisms retain exactly the same vigor as young ones, to the extent that old and young are physiologically indistinguishable, the fact that each cohort becomes numerically attenuated with age means that the selection force weakens. The nonadaptive theories are not mutually exclusive. Thus, aging might in principle be due to a combination of any of them.

As regards the nature of gene action, the disposable soma theory is the most specific of the evolutionary theories, for it suggests not only why aging occurs but also predicts that the genetic basis of aging is to be found in the genes that regulate levels of somatic maintenance functions. Neither the pleiotropic genes theory nor the late-acting deleterious mutations theory is specific about the nature of the genes involved.

GENETICS OF LIFESPAN

This section looks at the genetics of lifespan, first from the point of view of interspecies comparisons. That is, it will ask the question why do species have the lifespans they do? It will then look at intraspecies variation and heritability of lifespan. Finally, there is a brief discussion of Werner's syndrome as a model of genetically accelerated senescence.

Species differences in longevity

In addition to explaining why aging occurs, evolution theory also must account for differences in species lifespans. This raises basic questions about the genetic control of aging: specifically, how many genes are involved and how are these modified by selection to produce changes in lifespan?

For each of the nonadaptive theories, the generality of the selection forces that are involved suggests that multiple genes will be implicated. If there is a very large number of independent genes causing aging, however, the lifespan may be slow to change, because modifying a single gene may have little effect by itself and the probability of simultaneous independent modifications will be low. This suggests that either a reasonably small number of primary genes are responsible for aging, or that there exists some mechanism for coordinate regulation.

The evolution of increased lifespan is most readily explained if it is assumed that an adaptation occurs that results in a general lowering of the accidental (age-independent) death rate. In the late-acting deleterious mutations theory, this may result in new pressure to eliminate or postpone the deleterious gene effects. In the pleiotropic genes theory, the balance between early benefit and late cost may be shifted in favor of reducing the harmful effects on late survival. In the disposable soma theory, there may be selection to tune the optimum investment in maintenance to a higher level.

Variation within species

The variability in lifespan observed within a species or population clearly owes much to chance, but there is a significant heritable component as well.[5] Martin et al.[3] have applied the terms "public" and "private" to denote genetic factors related to aging that may either be specific to individuals or shared across a population (perhaps even across species). Late-acting deleterious mutations are strong candidates for private genes, because the fate of such alleles is determined largely by random genetic drift. Public genes are more likely to be those that arise through tradeoffs. In particular, the genes involved in regulating mechanisms of somatic maintenance are likely to be public genes of considerable importance. While these genes are "public" in the sense that all individuals have them, there may nevertheless be variations within a population in the precise levels at which these functions are set. These variations in setting may in turn be the cause of genetic variation in life expectancy.

As predicted by the disposable soma theory, the level of individual somatic maintenance systems should be set high enough so that the organism remains in sound condition through its natural expectation of life in the wild environment, but not much higher than this, or resources will be wasted. Numerous maintenance systems operate in parallel to preserve viability (Fig. 4-2). Depending on the levels at which they are set, each maintenance system can be thought of as "assuring" a given span of life (see also Cutler[23] and Sacher[24] for earlier discussion of the concept of "longevity assurance"). When any one of these critical mechanisms has exhausted its potential for assuring longevity, which happens because the accumulated defects threaten survival, the organism is liable to die.

If we now recall the shape of the fitness curve in Figure 4-1, we see that its peak—the point towards which natural selection is expected to exert evolutionary pressure—is rounded instead of sharp, and so we can expect a fair amount of intrapopulation variance in the precise settings of maintenance processes. Selection is expected to direct these settings toward the peak, but once within the region of the peak, the fitness differences on which selection can operate become quite small.

Putting these ideas together generates the prediction summarized in Figure 4-2. On the average, we expect the longevity assured by individual maintenance systems to be similar. This is because if the setting of any one mechanism is so low that it consistently fails before any of the others, then selection will tend to increase the level at which it is set. Conversely, if any mechanism tends always to fail after the others, then to the extent that this mechanism involves a metabolic cost, there will be selection to tune down the level at which it is set. In individuals, however, the genetic variance within the population is expected to result in variation in the extent to which the organism is predisposed to age from specific causes. For example, some individuals are likely to be less well protected against oxygen radicals than others, and these individuals will therefore experience greater oxidative damage.

Instances of extreme longevity, such as human centenarians, are of special interest for they are likely to be endowed with unusually high levels of each of the important ingredients of the cellular defense network.[6] Such individuals may also be distinguished by their freedom from alleles that predispose toward diseases that otherwise might shorten life expectancy. Schächter et al.[26] have performed a genetic study comparing centenarians with younger adult controls, which indicates the potential of this approach.

Werner's syndrome

Werner's syndrome is a rare autosomal recessive disorder affecting around 10 in one million people, who prematurely develop a variety of major age-related diseases, including arteriosclerosis, ocular cataracts, osteoporosis, malignant neoplasms, and type II diabetes. Cells grown from Werner-syndrome patients show reduced division potential and increased chromosomal instability compared with age-matched controls, and there is evidence that the pathology associated with Werner's syndrome may be related rather generally to impaired cell proliferation.

Yu et al.[7] identified the gene responsible for Werner's syndrome as a DNA helicase, an enzyme responsible for

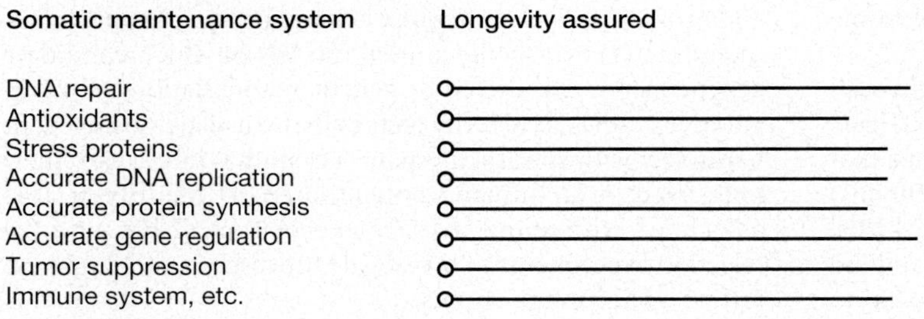

Somatic maintenance system	Longevity assured
DNA repair	
Antioxidants	
Stress proteins	
Accurate DNA replication	
Accurate protein synthesis	
Accurate gene regulation	
Tumor suppression	
Immune system, etc.	

Figure 4-2 Polygenic control of longevity predicted by the disposable soma theory of aging. On average, the period of longevity assured by individual somatic maintenance systems is predicted to be similar, but some genetic variance about the average is also expected, as shown.

unwinding DNA for purposes of replication, repair, and expression of the genetic material. This discovery strongly supports the concept that accumulation of somatic defects is important in aging, and it well illustrates the predicted involvement of longevity-assurance genes in determining the rate of aging. A defective helicase increases the rate of accumulation of DNA defects in actively dividing cell populations. A defect in this gene leads to accelerated aging particularly in tissues in which cell division continues throughout life. In terms of the scheme shown in Figure 4-2, the mutation responsible for Werner's syndrome can be considered equivalent to shortening the line for longevity assurance through DNA repair. However, as Figure 4-2 illustrates, DNA repair is but part of the network of longevity assurance mechanisms that determine overall rate of aging. It is striking that Werner's syndrome is not associated with accelerated aging in post-mitotic tissues such as brain and muscle, which is consistent with the fact that these tissues, by virtue of having little or no cell division during adult life, are relatively unaffected by having a defective DNA helicase.

TESTS OF THE EVOLUTIONARY THEORIES

A key prediction of the evolutionary theories is that altering the rate of decline in the force of natural selection will lead to the evolution of a concomitantly altered rate of aging. This has been tested by applying artificial selection on life history variables or by making comparisons within and between species on the effects of different levels of extrinsic mortality. For practical reasons, most studies have focused on short-lived species, in particular the fruit fly *Drosophila melanogaster* and the nematode worm *Caenorhabditis elegans*.

Evidence for tradeoffs between early and late fitness components, as predicted by both the disposable soma and pleiotropic genes theories, comes from the success of artificial selection for increased longevity in *Drosophila*.[27–32] A general correlate of delayed senescence has been reduced fecundity in the long-lived flies. A similar tradeoff has also been reported for a human population, based on analysis of birth-and-death records of British aristocrats.[33]

The nematode *Caenorhabditis elegans* has yielded a growing number of long-lived mutants in which increased longevity has been consistently associated with increased resistance to biochemical and other stresses. Many of the affected genes are linked to pathways that control a switch between the normal developmental process of the worm and an alternative long-lived form called the *dauer* larva, which is invoked during times of food shortage. The emerging picture points to a fundamental link between metabolic control, growth and reproduction, and somatic maintenance,[34–37] as predicted by the disposable soma theory.

From the comparative perspective, the evolutionary theories predict that in safe environments (those with low extrinsic mortality) aging will evolve to be retarded. Adaptations that reduce extrinsic mortality (wings, protective shells, large brains) are generally linked with increased longevity (bats, birds, turtles, humans). Field observations comparing a mainland population of opossums subject to significant predation by mammals, with an island population not subject to mammalian predation, found the predicted slower aging in the island population.[38]

At the molecular and cellular levels, the disposable soma theory predicts that the effort devoted to cellular maintenance and repair processes will vary directly with longevity. Numerous studies support this idea. A direct relation between species longevity and rate of mitochondrial ROS production in captive mammals has been found,[39,40] as has a similar relationship between mammals and similar-sized but much longer-lived birds.[41] DNA repair capacity has been shown to correlate with mammalian lifespan in numerous comparative studies,[42] as has the level of poly(ADP-ribose) polymerase,[43] an enzyme that plays an important role in the maintenance of genomic integrity. The quality of maintenance and repair mechanisms may be revealed by the capacity to cope with external stress. Comparisons of the functional capacity of cultured cells to withstand a variety of imposed stressors have shown that cells taken from long-lived species have superior stress resistance to that of cells from shorter-lived species.[44,45]

Tests of the evolutionary theories support the idea that it is the evolved capacity of somatic cells to carry out effective maintenance and repair that mainly governs the time taken for damage to accumulate to levels where it interferes with the organism's viability, and hence regulates longevity.

CONCLUSIONS

Our answers to the question "Why does aging occur?" have broad implications for how we perceive the likely genetic basis of aging. Firstly, evolution theory can illuminate a long-running debate about whether programmed or stochastic events, such as DNA damage, drive the aging process. The weakness of evolutionary support for the adaptive aging genes hypothesis calls the program theory into question. Any notion of an aging "clock" needs to be qualified by recognition of this fact. The existence of temporal controls in development and in cyclic processes such as diurnal and reproductive cycles does not provide a sufficient basis to suggest the existence of a clock that regulates aging. Nor does the broad reproducibility of many features of aging provide any real evidence for an underlying active program. This is not to say, however, that the nature and rate of aging are not genetically determined. The issue that distinguishes programmed from stochastic theories of aging is not whether the factors that determine longevity are specified within the genome, but rather, how this is arranged.[46]

Secondly, evolution theory clearly indicates a polygenic basis for aging. Different mechanisms and even different kinds of genes may operate together. This presents a major challenge, and progress is likely to require a combination of approaches, including (1) transgenic animal models in which candidate genetic factors are altered by genetic manipulation, (2) comparative studies to identify factors that correlate positively or negatively with species' lifespans, (3) studies of the extremely long-lived (e.g. human centenarians) to identify factors associated with above-average expectation of life, and (4) selection experiments to investigate the response of lifespan to artificial selection pressures.

KEY POINTS Aging

- We are not programmed to die.

- Aging occurs because, in our evolutionary past, when life expectancy was much shorter, natural selection placed limited priority on long-term maintenance of the body.

- Aging is caused by gradual accumulation of cell and tissue damage. Much of the damage arises as a side-effect of essential biochemical processes, like the utilization of oxygen to generate chemical energy through oxidative phosphorylation.

- Accumulation of damage begins early and continues progressively throughout life, resulting after several decades in the overt frailty, disability, and disease associated with aging.

- Multiple processes cause the damage that contributes to aging, and multiple genes regulate the efficacy of "longevity-assurance" processes, such as DNA repair, that together influence the rate of aging.

- Nongenetic factors, such as nutrition and exercise, can have important effects in modulating the rate of build-up of damage within the body.

REFERENCES

1. Kirkwood TBL, Rose MR: Evolution of senescence: late survival sacrificed for reproduction. Phil Trans R Soc Lond B 1991;332:15–24
2. Partridge L, Barton NH: Optimality, mutation and the evolution of ageing. Nature 1993;362:305–311
3. Martin GM, Austad SN, Johnson TE: Genetic analysis of ageing: role of oxidative damage and environmental stresses. Nature Genet 1996;13:25–34
4. Kirkwood TBL, Austad SN: Why do we age? Nature 2000;408:233–238
5. Cournil A, Kirkwood TBL: If you would live long, choose your parents well. Trends Genet 2001;17:233–235
6. Schächter F, Cohen D, Kirkwood TBL: Prospects for the genetics of human longevity. Hum Genet 1993;91:51
7. Yu C-E, Oshima J, Fu Y-H et al: Positional cloning of the Werner's syndrome gene. Science 1996;272:258–262
8. Comfort A: The Biology of Senescence, 3rd edn. Churchill Livingstone, Edinburgh, 1979
9. Kirkwood TBL: Comparative and evolutionary aspects of longevity. In Finch CE, Schneider EL (eds): Handbook of the Biology of Aging, 3rd edn. Van Nostrand Reinhold, New York, 1985:45–66.
10. Finch CE: Longevity, Senescence and the Genome. Chicago University Press, Chicago, 1990
11. Martinez DE: Mortality patterns suggest lack of senescence in hydra. Exp Gerontol 1997;33:217–225
12. Weismann A: Essays Upon Heredity and Kindred Biological Problems, vol. 1. Clarendon Press, Oxford, 1891
13. Wynne-Edwards VC: Animal Dispersion in Relation to Social Behaviour. Oliver & Boyd. Edinburgh, 1962
14. Medawar PB: An Unsolved Problem of Biology. H.K. Lewis, London, 1952
15. Maynard Smith J: Group selection. Qtly Rev Biol 1976;51:277–283
16. Haldane JBS: New Paths in Genetics. George Allen & Unwin, London, 1941
17. Williams GC: Pleiotropy, natural selection and the evolution of senescence. Evolution 1957;11:398–411
18. Hamilton WD: The moulding of senescence by natural selection. J Theor Biol 1966;12:12–45
19. Charlesworth B: Evolution in Age-structured Populations, 2nd edn. Cambridge University Press, Cambridge, 1994
20. Kirkwood TBL: Evolution of ageing. Nature 1977;270:301–304
21. Kirkwood TBL, Holliday R: The evolution of ageing and longevity. Proc R Soc Lond B, 1979;205:531–546
22. Kirkwood TBL: Repair and its evolution: survival versus reproduction. In Townsend CR, Calow P (eds): Physiological Ecology: An Evolutionary Approach to Resource Use. Blackwell Scientific Publications, Oxford, 1981:165–181.
23. Cutler RG: Evaluating biology of senescence. In Behare JA, Finch CE, Moment GB (eds): The Biology of Aging. Plenum Press, New York, 1978:311–360.
24. Sacher GA: Evolution of longevity and survival characteristics in mammals. In Schneider E (ed): The Genetics of Aging. Plenum Press, New York, 1978:151–167.
25. Kirkwood TBL, Franceschi C: Is ageing as complex as it would appear? Ann NY Acad Sci 1992;663:412–417
26. Schächter F, FaureDelanef L, Guenot F, Rouger H, Froguel P, Lesueurginot L, Cohen D: Genetic associations with human longevity at the APOE and ACE loci. Nature Genet 1994;6:29–32
27. Rose MR: Laboratory evolution of postponed senescence in Drosophila melanogaster. Evolution 1984;38:1004–1010
28. Luckinbill LS, Arking R, Clare, MJ et al: Selection for delayed senescence in Drosophila melanogaster. Evolution 1984;38:996–1003
29. Partridge L, Prowse N, Pignatelli P: Another set of responses and correlated responses to selection on age of reproduction in Drosophila melanogaster. Proc R Soc Lond B 1999;266:255–261
30. Buck S, Vettraino J, Force AG, Arking R: Extended longevity in Drosophila is consistently associated with a decrease in larval viability. J Gerontol A 2000;55:292–301
31. Zwaan B, Bijlmstra R, Hoekstra RF: Direct selection on life span in Drosophila melanogaster. Evolution 1995;49:646–659
32. Stearns SC, Ackermann M, Doebeli M, Kaiser M: Experimental evolution of aging, growth, and reproduction in fruitflies. Proc Natl Acad Sci USA 2000;97:3309–3313
33. Westendorp RGJ, Kirkwood TBL: Human longevity at the cost of reproductive success. Nature 1998;396:743–746
34. Lithgow GJ: Invertebrate gerontology: the age mutations of Caenorhabditis elegans. Bioessays 1996;18:809–815
35. Johnson TE: Genetic influences on aging. Exp Gerontol 1997;32:11–22
36. Hsin H, Kenyon C: Signals from the reproductive system regulate the lifespan of C. elegans. Nature 1999;399:362–366
37. Van Voorheis WA, Ward S: Genetic and environmental conditions that increase longevity in Caenorhabditis elegans decrease metabolic rate. Proc Natl Acad Sci USA 1999;95:11399–11403
38. Austad SN: Retarded senescence in an insular population of opossums. J Zool 1993;229:695–708
39. Ku H-H, Brunk UT, Sohal RS: Relationship between mitochondrial superoxide and hydrogen-peroxide production and longevity of mammalian species. Free Rad Biol Med 1993;15:621–627
40. Barja G, Herrero A: Oxidative damage to mitochondrial DNA is inversely related to maximum life span in the heart and brain of mammals. FASEB J 2000;14:312–318
41. Herrero A, Barja G: 8-oxo-deoxyguanosine levels in heart and brain mitochondrial and nuclear DNA of two mammals and three birds in relation to their different rates of aging. Aging Clin Exp Res 1999;11:294–300
42. Kirkwood TBL: DNA, mutations and aging. Mutat Res 1989;219:1–7
43. Grube K, Bürkle A: Poly(ADP-ribose) polymerase activity in mononuclear leukocytes of 13 mammalian species correlates with species-specific life span. Proc Natl Acad Sci USA 1992;89:11759–11763
44. Ogburn CE et al: Cultured renal epithelial cells from birds and mice: enhanced resistance of avian cells to oxidative stress and DNA damage. J Gerontol B 1998;53:287–292
45. Kapahi P, Boulton ME, Kirkwood TBL: Positive correlation between mammalian life span and cellular resistance to stress. Free Rad Biol Med 1999;26:495–500
46. Kirkwood TBL, Cremer T: Cytogerontology since 1881: a reappraisal of August Weismann and a review of modern progress. Hum Genet 1982;60:101–121

Chapter 5

Methodological problems in research on aging

John D. Sorkin and Leslie I. Katzel

The principal aims of gerontology are to identify changes that occur during aging, to quantify the rate at which the changes occur, and to understand the mechanisms behind the changes. Aging is the result of (1) intrinsic biological processes that are genetically determined (biological aging), (2) age-associated lifestyle changes (e.g. decreased physical activity, increased obesity), and (3) age-associated increased incidence and prevalence of disease. This chapter will describe five study designs—cross-sectional, time-series, longitudinal, case–control, and cohort—that can be used to identify change, to quantify the rate at which change occurs at different ages, and to separate biological aging from the effects of lifestyle and disease. Additionally, problems and limitations associated with the designs will be described.

CROSS-SECTIONAL, TIME-SERIES, AND LONGITUDINAL DESIGNS
Cross-sectional design

The cross-sectional design is the type most commonly used to study the relation between a variable of interest and age. A cross-sectional study is performed by assembling and

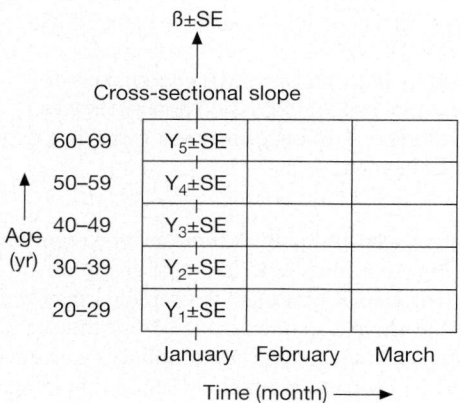

Figure 5-1 The design of a cross-sectional study. Over a short time period, 1 month in this example, a group of subjects 20–69 years of age is enrolled in a study. The subjects are divided into age decades. For each age decade, a mean and a standard error are calculated for the variable being studied ($Y_1 \pm SE$ through $Y_5 \pm SE$). Additionally, a cross-sectional slope, $\beta \pm SE$, is computed by entering all the data (ignoring the division into age decades) into a regression analysis in which the variable being studied, Y, is the dependent variable and age is the independent variable, X.

studying a group of subjects of different ages at a fixed point in time, or over a short period of time. Each subject is examined only once (Fig. 5-1).

When a subject is examined, his or her age is recorded, and the variable of interest is measured. Subjects are placed into age groups, often decades of life, and the data are reported by presenting the mean value of the variable of interest for each age group. Alternatively, the data can be entered into a regression analysis that relates the parameter studied (the dependent variable Y) to the independent variable age (the X variable). If height were being studied, the equation obtained from the linear regression would be

$$height = \beta_0 + \beta_1 \times age$$

The coefficient of the age term (β_1, the slope of age) gives the average difference in height between subjects who differ in age by 1 year.

Cross-sectional studies are relatively easy to perform, inexpensive, and can be completed quickly. Unfortunately, inferences from cross-sectional studies are subject to two errors, either of which can lead to incorrect conclusions about the relation between age and the variable studied.

The first type of error, bias due to birth cohort effects, is a difference between subjects caused solely by the era in which the subjects were born (Fig. 5-2), not by any age difference between subjects. Progressive improvements in nutrition, for example, may allow more recently born subjects to achieve a greater adult height than subjects born years earlier. A cross-sectional study of height in a hypothetical population where there is no change in height with aging will indicate that height decreases with age—not because height is lost as people get older, but because people born in the past did not grow to be as tall as people born recently.

The second type of error, bias due to selective mortality, occurs when the variable studied, Y, affects the survival of study subjects. If, for example, low values of Y are associated with an increased probability of survival to old age, and high values of Y with decreased probability of survival, the majority of old subjects will have low values of Y. Younger subjects, who are too young to have suffered significant mortality, will demonstrate the full range of values of Y. Even if Y does not change with age, a cross-sectional study of Y will lead to the conclusion that Y decreases with age (Fig. 5-3). Owing to the high mortality rate in the oldest old, selective mortality can be a major confounder of studies in this population.

Because of the problems inherent in the cross-sectional design (the potential for bias due to selective mortality and birth cohort effects), findings from cross-sectional studies should, whenever possible, be tested in longitudinal studies.

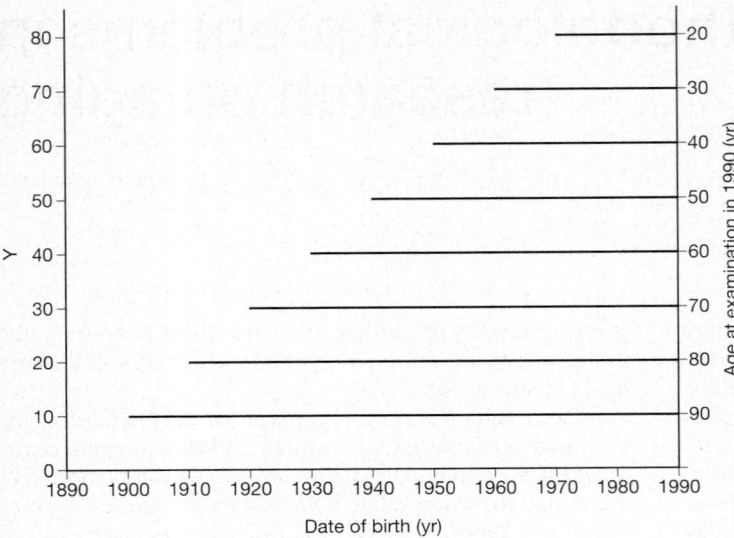

Figure 5-2 Differences related to a subject's birth cohort can bias the cross-sectional relation between a variable Y and age. There is no change in Y with age in any individual subject. Each subject's value of Y is determined solely by his date of birth. Subjects born in 1970 are 20 years old when examined in 1990. They were born with a Y value of 80, and maintain this value throughout their lives. This is indicated by the shortest horizontal line. (The next line is for subjects who are 30 years old when examined in 1990; they were born in 1960, and have a lifetime Y value of 70.) Recently-born subjects have higher Y values than subjects born years earlier. In 1990, 40-year-old subjects have a Y value of 60, 60-year-old subjects 40, and 90-year-old subjects a Y value of 10. As a result of the birth cohort effect, a cross-sectional study performed in 1990 will lead to the incorrect conclusion that Y decreases with age.

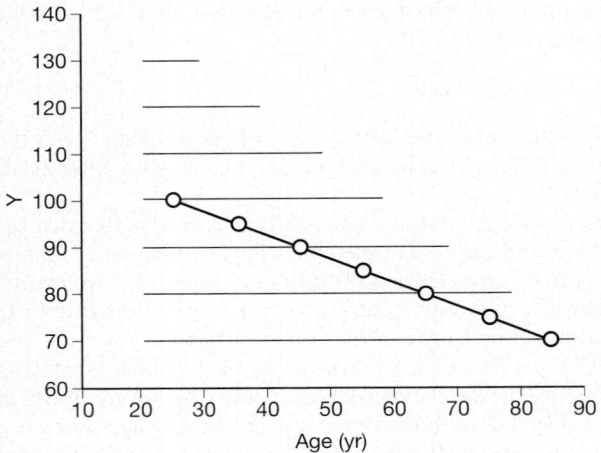

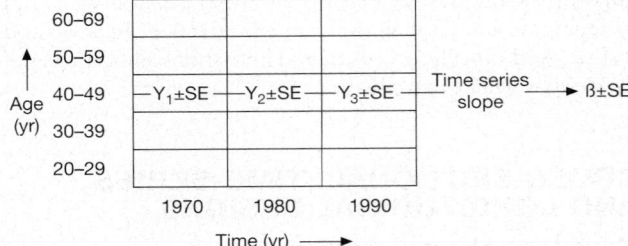

Figure 5-4 The design of a time-series study. At three distinct periods of time, 1970, 1980, and 1990, three distinct groups of subjects are recruited and studied once. The three groups are selected to have the same mean age at the time they are examined. For each of the three groups, a mean and a standard error are calculated for the variable being studied ($Y_1 \pm SE$ through $Y_3 \pm SE$). Additionally a time-series slope, $\beta \pm SE$, is computed by entering all the data (ignoring the division into time periods) into a regression analysis in which the variable being studied, Y, is the dependent variable and age is the independent variable, X.

Figure 5-3 Selective mortality can bias cross-sectional studies. In this example, Y does not change with age in any individual subject (the horizontal lines), and high levels of Y are associated with early mortality. If a random cross-section of the population is recruited, all possible values of Y will be seen in young subjects. Thus, in subjects 20–29 years of age, the mean value of Y will be 100. Because all subjects with a Y value above 120 die before they reach 30 years of age, the mean value of Y in subjects 30–39 years of age is 95. Because only those subjects with the lowest value of Y survive beyond age 80, the only value of Y in subjects 80–89 years of age is 70. (The diagonal line in the figure indicates the cross-sectional mean values of Y seen at different ages.) Thus, although Y does not change with age in any subject, a cross-sectional study of Y would indicate that Y decreases with age.

Time-series design

Gerontologists are often interested in examining differences that occur in a population over the course of time. For example, it may be of interest to know if the average cholesterol concentration in 45-year-old men in 1970 was the same as that seen in 45-year-old men in 1980 and 1990. A time-series design can answer this question. In a time-series study, a group of subjects of a given age (or a small age range) is assembled at a fixed point in time, and the group is examined once. Some time later, usually after several years, a second group of subjects is assembled and examined. The second group is chosen so that its age distribution, and mean age, are the same as were the age distribution and mean age of the first group when the first group was examined (Fig. 5-4). When a subject is examined, the age at which he or she is examined is noted, as is the value of the parameter being studied.

Any difference between the groups can be ascribed to the time at which the groups were examined and not to the age of the groups; the groups have the same mean age when they are examined. Data from a time-series study are reported by presenting the mean value of the parameter of interest by time period. Alternatively, the data obtained from all subjects can be entered into a regression analysis, which relates the variable studied (the dependent variable *Y*) to the independent variable, *X*, the date of examination. The slope obtained from the regression gives the average difference in the variable of interest between two different subjects of the same age who were examined at two different periods of time.

Time-series studies are subject to two errors that can lead to incorrect conclusions about the association between the factor being studied and time. The first type of error occurs when there is a differential selection of study subjects in the two periods that leads to a biased sample of the variable being studied. An example would be a study of height in which 40-year-old hypothyroid dwarfs are studied in 1980 and 40-year-old acromegalic giants are studied in 1990. The conclusion that 40-year-old people are taller in 1990 than were 40-year-old people in 1980 would be the result of studying subjects having different disease determined heights, rather than a temporal change in height from 1980 to 1990. The second type of error occurs as a result of methodological change or drift over time. For example, assume that cholesterol concentration is studied in 1980 and 1990. In 1980 one cholesterol assay is used and in 1990 a second assay that reads 5 mg/dL higher than the first. If the difference is not recognized, a time-series analysis of cholesterol concentration will suggest that cholesterol concentration has increased from 1980 to 1990.

Longitudinal design

Subjects who participate in a longitudinal study are followed for an extended period to determine the rate at which a variable changes. In order to conduct a longitudinal study, a group of subjects is assembled, examined, and then re-examined once, or several times, as the subjects are aging (Fig. 5-5). If each subject is examined exactly twice, the study is sometimes referred to as a cohort study. (This is not to be confused with birth cohort effects previously discussed.) If subjects are examined more than two times, the study is sometimes referred to as a longitudinal study. Each time a subject is examined, his or her age is noted and the variable of interest is measured.

Proper analysis of longitudinal data requires special techniques. If an analysis of longitudinal data is attempted using standard regression techniques (i.e. entering all the data into a single regression analysis), incorrect inferences may result (Fig. 5-6).

Several techniques have been used to analyze data obtained from a longitudinal study. The easiest to understand is the two-stage random-effects model (Fig. 5-7). In the first stage of the model a separate linear regression is performed for each subject. Each regression quantifies the rate (through the slope) at which the variable of interest (the dependent variable *Y*) changes with age (the independent variable *X*) for a single subject. If 100 subjects were enrolled in the study, 100 regressions would be performed resulting in 100 slopes. Each of the 100 slopes gives the average annual rate of change in the variable of interest for a different subject. In the second stage of the model, subjects are placed into age groups based on their age at entry to the study (or their mean age during the course of the study). A mean slope is calculated for each age group (Fig. 5-8).

Frequently some subjects in a longitudinal study will be examined more times than others. Subjects may die, drop out of the study, or be lost to follow-up prior to the end of the follow-up period. This leads to an important question about the method used to compute the mean slope for the age groups. Should the slopes of subjects who were studied more times than other subjects (and thus are computed from more points) be weighted by the number of data points used to compute the slope? If this is done, subjects who were examined many times will contribute more to the mean slope of their age group than

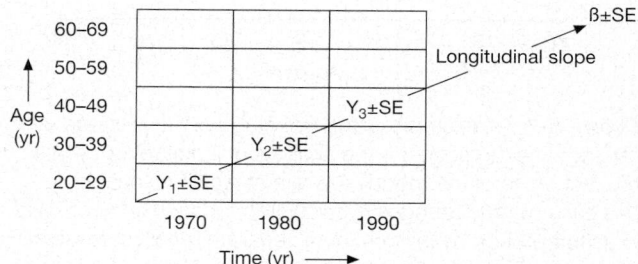

Figure 5-5 The design of a longitudinal study. In 1970, a group of subjects, 20–29 years old, is recruited and studied. In 1980, these subjects are studied again. At this time they are 30–39 years old. In 1990, the subjects are 40–49 years old and they are studied one last time. For each of the three time periods, a mean and a standard error are calculated for the variable being studied ($Y_1 \pm$ SE through $Y_3 \pm$ SE). A longitudinal slope, $\beta \pm$ SE, is computed using a two-stage random-effects model. The slope characterizes the rate at which Y changes as subjects are aging from age 20–29 to age 40–49. See text for details.

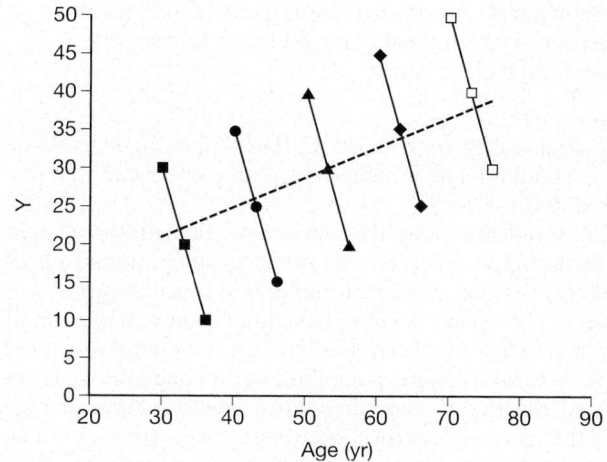

Figure 5-6 Standard regression techniques (i.e. entering all data into a single regression analysis) can result in an incorrect conclusion about the relation between a variable and age. In this example, data are plotted for five subjects (the five solid lines). For each subject Y decreases as the subject gets older. The regression line obtained by entering all the data into a single regression analysis is depicted by the dashed line. The dashed line incorrectly indicates that Y increases with age.

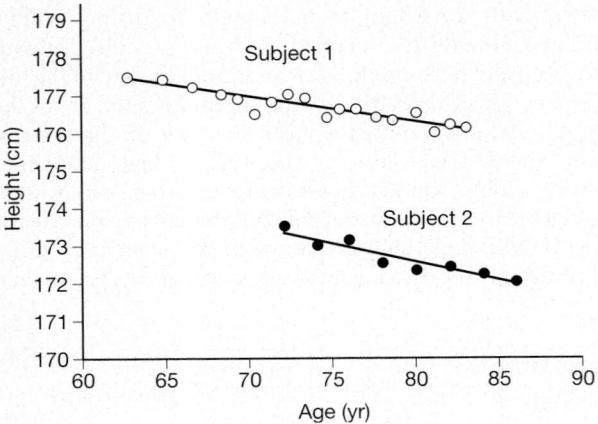

Figure 5-7 An example of the first stage of a two-stage random effects model for the analysis of longitudinal data. In the first stage of the model, the rate at which a variable, in this case height, changes is calculated for each subject. This is accomplished by performing a separate linear regression for each subject in which the dependent variable, *Y*, is height and the independent variable is age, *X*. For subject 1, the regression is performed using data from 18 observations (the open circles); for subject 2, eight (the closed circles). In the second stage, each subject is placed into an age group (often an age decade) based on age at entry to the study. In this example, subject 1 would be placed into the 60–69 year age decade, subject 2 into the 70–79 year age decade. (Alternatively, each subject could be placed into an age decade based upon his mean age during the time he was studied. In this case, subject 1 would be placed into the 70–79 year age decade, subject 2 would also be placed into the 70–79 year age decade.) In the second stage of the model (Fig. 5-8), each age group is characterized by the mean of the ages (either mean of the ages at entry or mean of each subject's mean age) and the mean of the slopes of the subjects assigned to the age group.

will subjects who were examined fewer times. In general, the slopes should not be weighted; weighting slopes can lead to a biased mean slope.

The problem produced by averaging weighted slopes is best understood by way of an example. Consider a longitudinal study of the change in serum cholesterol concentration. Each subject's cholesterol is measured annually for a maximum of 20 years. (Any subject can thus have his cholesterol measured up to 21 times.) High serum cholesterol concentrations are associated with early mortality. If two subjects of the same age have the same cholesterol concentration at entry to the study, the subject whose cholesterol concentration increases most rapidly will achieve higher levels at a younger age than will the subject whose concentration increases more slowly. Because high concentrations are associated with a high probability of death, the subject with the faster rate of increase will in all likelihood die at an earlier age than the subject whose rate of increase was slower. The subject with the faster rate of increase will therefore be less likely to remain in the study for 20 years than will the subject with the slower rate of increase. The slope for the subject with the faster rate of increase will be computed

from fewer points than will the slope for the subject with the slower rate of increase. If the individual slopes are weighted by the number of points used to calculate the slope, the slope from the subject with the faster rate of increase will have a smaller weight than the slope from the subject with the slower rate of increase. The average slope will thus be more heavily influenced by subjects with a slower rate of increase than by subjects with a faster rate of increase. The average slope will be biased; the longitudinal analyses will suffer from selective mortality. (The same bias occurs if the individual slopes are weighted by the inverse of their variance.) In general, if the rate of change of the variable studied is related to survival (i.e. the length of time a subject remains in the study), weighted slopes will result in a biased estimate of the rate at which the variable changes with aging.

Unlike cross-sectional studies, longitudinal studies are not subject to bias due to selective mortality and are relatively immune from incorrect inferences due to birth cohort effects. If unweighted slopes are used, each subject will contribute equally to the average slope in his age group, regardless of the time at which the subject leaves the study, the number of data points the subject contributes to the analysis, or the time at which the subject is lost to follow-up or dies. Thus the age-specific slopes are not unduly influenced by data from those subjects who are followed for the longest time. Thus there is no selective mortality, which, as described above, can lead to a biased estimate of the age-specific slopes if the value of the variable being studied affects the time a subject remains in the study.

Birth cohort effects generally are not important confounders of longitudinal studies because all of the subjects within a given age group were born within a relatively short period. Thus the average slope by which each age group is characterized comes from a "single" birth cohort, and for each age group there should be little influence of date of birth on factors influencing interutero growth and subsequent development. (There could be other factors influencing growth and development such as the subjects' socio-economic status during childhood, but these factors generally will vary randomly among subjects in a single age group. The factors generally will not be related to date of birth within the narrow range of dates of birth within a given age group.) Between age groups—for example, age groups defined by age decades—there may be birth cohort effects because the difference in dates of birth between younger and older age groups may be large. Fortunately, these effects are generally easily identified in a longitudinal study. A plot of the line segments representing the rates of change within age groups will not show a smooth pattern of change with one line segment starting where the previous segment ended (Fig. 5-8A), but rather a series of unconnected line segments, similar to that seen when there is a secular change during the course of the study (Fig. 5-8B).

Longitudinal studies can be very sensitive to small changes in assay methodology. The changes can result from changing to a new measuring instrument, from use of a new reagent lot, or from a change in the personnel measuring the variable of interest. A small change in methodology can make a variable that does not change with age appear to change (Fig. 5-9).

Several steps can be taken to lessen the probability of methodological change during the course of longitudinal study,

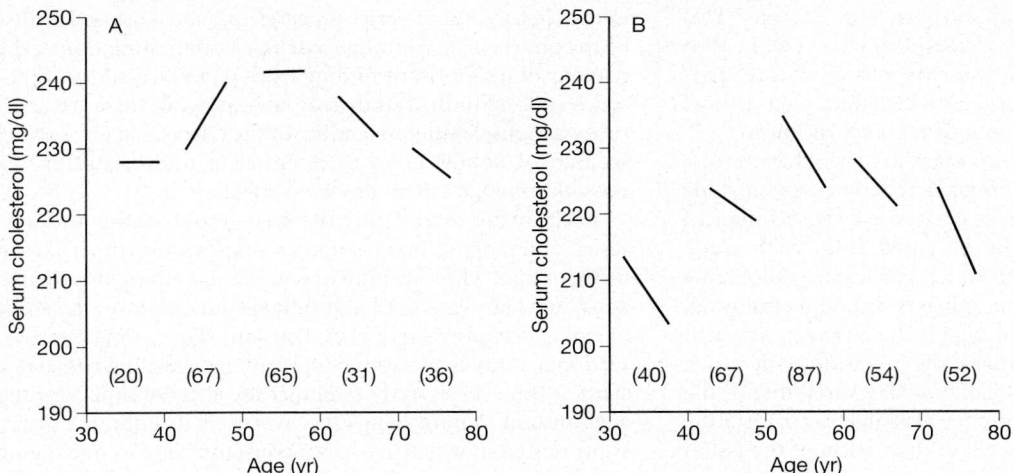

Figure 5-8 Longitudinal change in serum cholesterol in men from the Baltimore Longitudinal Study of Aging. The longitudinal change in each decade of life is represented by a line segment whose slope is the mean rate of change in cholesterol concentration for men whose mean age during longitudinal follow-up fell within the age decade. The midpoint of each line segment is plotted at the cross-sectional mean cholesterol concentration and cross-sectional mean age for the age decade. The horizontal length of each line (i.e. the difference between the age at the end and beginning of each line) represents the mean follow-up. The number of subjects included in each age decade is indicated by the numbers in parentheses. Panel A depicts the change from 1963 through 1971. During this period cholesterol increased from young adulthood to middle age. Longitudinal analyses and cross-sectional analyses (represented by the midpoint of each line) show similar results. This pattern is consistent with a pure aging effect. Panel B depicts the change from 1969 to 1977. In this period, cholesterol concentration drops in all five age decades; cross-sectional and longitudinal analyses disagree. In the youngest three age decades, the cross-sectional mean for each age decade, represented by the middle of each line segment, is at a progressively higher value as the mean age of the subjects increases; there is a cross-sectional increase in cholesterol with increasing age. During this period, the longitudinal slope in each of the age decades indicates that within each age decade cholesterol falls as subjects are aging. This pattern is consistent with a secular drop in cholesterol, which the authors felt was the result of "environmental factors." Source: Hershcopf et al,[14] with permission.

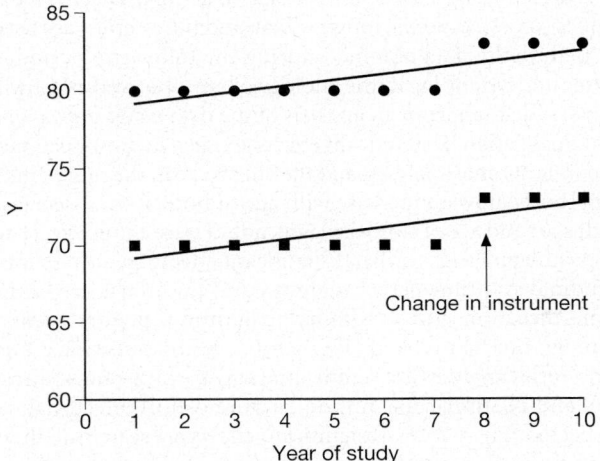

Figure 5-9 A small change in assay methodology can have a profound effect on a longitudinal study. In this example, a new instrument is used to measure Y in the eighth year of a longitudinal study. The new instrument reads three units higher than the old instrument. Although there is no increase in Y with aging, the effect of the introduction of the new instrument is to change the slope for each subject from zero to a positive value. The average of the two slopes will be a positive number rather than the correct value of zero.

including thorough training of study personnel (with periodic refresher courses), periodic measurement of a known standard throughout the course of the study, and a cross-over period when switching from an old to a new instrument. In the cross-over period, duplicate samples are run on the new and old instruments, and a correction factor is generated that converts values from the new machine to values that would have been obtained on the old machine.

Even if great care has been taken to ensure assay stability, it remains important to look for methodological error prior to data analysis. This is one of the most important steps in the analysis of longitudinal data; it is also one of the least frequently discussed. A review of techniques that can be used to test for methodological error is beyond the scope of this chapter. A brief review of two techniques is presented in Elahi et al.[1]

The average lifespan of the subjects of longitudinal studies is usually longer than the period during which any individual subject is studied. As a result, if the aim of a study is to understand the change in a variable that occurs over the course of adult life, the age range studied is generally broken into shorter intervals, often age decades. Each subject is placed into an age decade, based either upon age at entry to the study, or mean age during the period he or she participated in the study, and a mean slope is calculated for each age decade. If the average rate of change for each age decade is plotted (or tabulated) by the natural order of the age decades, a sense of the change of a variable over the entire adult lifespan will emerge. This methodology allows a pattern of nonlinear change to be seen (Fig. 5-8A). (Even if the lifetime trajectory of a variable is curvilinear, the change in most biological variables over a short period, such as a decade, can be approximated as linear.)

A longitudinal study is more complex to design than a cross-sectional or time-series study. Important design issues include the size of the group that must be studied, the number of measurements that should be obtained from each study participant, the frequency with which participants should be studied, and the length of time subjects should be followed. Factors that will influence the design include the rate at which the parameter of interest changes, the precision with which the parameter is measured, the day-to-day variability in the parameter, and the time and money available to perform the longitudinal study. For an excellent discussion of the issues involved in planning a longitudinal study, see Schlesselman.[2,3]

CAUTIONS ABOUT INFERENCES DERIVED FROM CROSS-SECTIONAL, TIME-SERIES, AND LONGITUDINAL STUDIES

A statistically significant longitudinal change in a variable (a longitudinal slope that is significantly different from zero) does not ensure that the change is the result of aging. A secular trend in lifestyle could account for the change. A secular trend (sometimes referred to as a "temporal trend") is a change occurring over a long time period, generally years or decades. Examples of secular trends include the decrease in cardiovascular disease mortality and infant mortality that occurred in the USA over 45 years.[4] As an example of the effect of a secular trend, consider a longitudinal study of cholesterol concentration that finds a decrease in serum cholesterol with aging. The decrease might be due to biological aging (i.e. the genetics of aging), but it might be due to a secular decrease in the consumption of fat over the course of the study, which in turn leads to the decrease in serum cholesterol concentration.

Just as a significant change in a variable seen in a longitudinal study does not ensure that the change is due to aging, a significant difference in a cross-sectional study does not ensure that the difference is due to age. Consider a cross-sectional study that finds a cross-sectional decrease in height with age. Older subjects may be shorter than younger subjects because of biological aging (e.g. an age-determined progressive loss of bone calcium leading to an increased incidence of compression fractures of the spinal vertebral bodies leading to loss of height), or the cross-sectional height differences may be due to birth cohort effects (Fig. 5-2).

As used above, a birth cohort effect (also known as a "generation effect") is "a variation in health status that arises from the different factors to which each birth cohort in the population is exposed to as the environment and society changes."[5] A cohort effect that might affect height would be the progressively better nutrition in utero, in infancy, and in childhood that occurred in the USA over the last century. The progressive improvement in nutrition during growth and development may allow more recently born subjects to achieve a greater fraction of their genetic height potential than was possible for subjects born earlier. Similarly, an apparent secular (temporal)

effect seen in a time-series analyses may be confused with a birth cohort effect. Although a definitive determination of the etiology of a significant finding from a cross-sectional, time-series, or longitudinal study may be impossible from the usual study designs, an understanding of the effects of a pure aging, secular, or cohort effect is essential to understanding the possible etiologies of an observed effect.

Each of the three study designs—cross-sectional, time-series, and longitudinal—studies a single factor (time, date of birth, or age) while keeping one of the remaining two factors constant (Fig. 5-10A). A longitudinal study explores the effect of aging, keeping date of birth constant (Fig. 5-10A). A cross-sectional study explores the effect of age, keeping time constant. A time-series study examines the effect of time, keeping age constant. A pure aging effect will exert its influence in any study design in which age is not constant. Thus, a pure aging effect will induce significant differences in cross-sectional and significant changes in longitudinal studies (Fig. 5-10B). A pure secular effect will exert its influence in any dimension in which time is not constant. A pure secular effect will induce significant change in longitudinal studies and significant differences in time-series studies (Fig. 5-10C). Finally, a pure cohort effect will be seen in those study designs in which date of birth is not constant. A pure cohort effect will therefore affect cross-sectional and time-series analyses (Fig. 5-10D).

If the subjects of a longitudinal study are recruited from a wide age range (e.g. 30 to 84 years), and are followed for a reasonable time period (perhaps 15 years), the longitudinal study will have embedded within itself a series of cross-sectional studies. (The first five years of the study might be combined into one cross-sectional study, the second five years into another cross-sectional study, etc.) If the first five years, the second five years, and the last five years of longitudinal follow-up are divided into age groups, perhaps by 5 years of age, the data can be analyzed using a time-series design. If all three analytic techniques (cross-sectional, longitudinal, and time-series) are used to analyze the data obtained during the follow-up period, a better understanding of the etiology of any observed effect will be possible than from an analysis of the data using only a longitudinal design. If significant effects are seen in cross-sectional and longitudinal analyses, and the effects are in the same direction (both show an increase with age or both show a decrease with age) and are of similar magnitude, a pure aging effect can be postulated (Fig. 5-10B). If significant effects are seen in longitudinal and time-series analyses (and the effects are in the same direction and of similar magnitude) a pure secular etiology can be invoked (Fig. 5-10C). If cross-sectional and time-series analyses are significant (and are in the same direction and of similar magnitude), a pure cohort effect may be suspected (Fig. 5-10D). If significant effects are seen in all three analytic methodologies, a mixed effect is probably responsible. Conversely, a pure aging effect should be postulated only if consistent significant effects are seen in cross-sectional and longitudinal analyses and not in time-series analyses (Fig. 5-10B); a pure secular effect only if consistent significant effects are seen in longitudinal and time-series analyses but not in cross-sectional analyses; and a pure cohort effect only if consistent significant effects are seen in time-series and cross-sectional analyses but not in longitudinal analyses. An excellent description of a study in which longitudinal data were analyzed

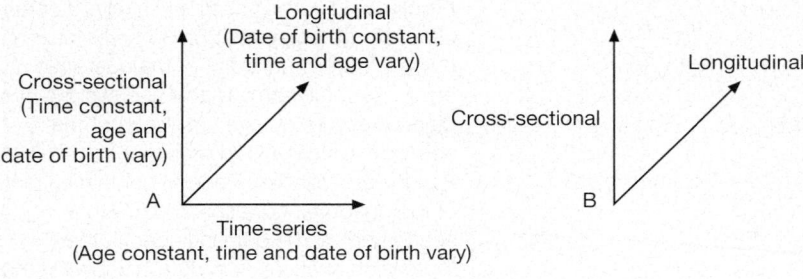

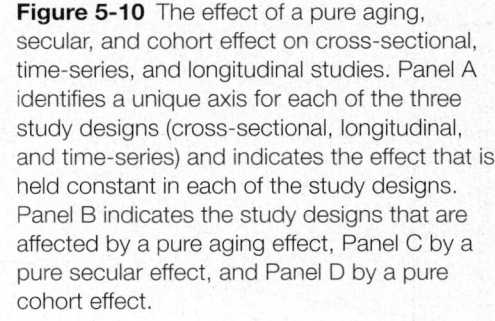

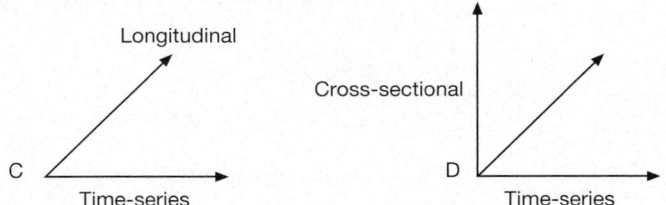

Figure 5-10 The effect of a pure aging, secular, and cohort effect on cross-sectional, time-series, and longitudinal studies. Panel A identifies a unique axis for each of the three study designs (cross-sectional, longitudinal, and time-series) and indicates the effect that is held constant in each of the study designs. Panel B indicates the study designs that are affected by a pure aging effect, Panel C by a pure secular effect, and Panel D by a pure cohort effect.

using longitudinal, cross-sectional, and time-series methodologies is presented in Elahi et al.[6]

Although the three study designs provide helpful summaries of the effects of age, time, and aging on a variable, they can hide important information. For example, a cross-sectional analysis of the relation between age and systolic blood pressure, summarized by a plot of the equation obtained by regressing age on systolic blood pressure (Fig. 5-11A), demonstrates that systolic blood pressure increases with age. The simple to understand plot, unlike a scattergram of the data, "hides" the fact that at all ages there is substantial variability in the relation between age and blood pressure. A large fraction of the oldest subjects and a larger fraction of young adults (subjects in their twenties and thirties) have blood pressures in the range 100–150 mmHg (Fig. 5-11B). Similarly a number of the oldest subjects have blood pressures that are higher than those seen in all but one or two young adults. Finally, at any age a wide range of blood pressures is seen. In young adult subjects the range is approximately 70 mmHg (i.e. approximately 80–150 mmHg); the range increases as the age of the subjects increases and is approximately 100 mmHg in the oldest subjects. In addition to the summary provided by a cross-sectional, time-series, or longitudinal analysis, a full understanding of the effect age, time, and aging have on a variable requires an examination of the data that were included in the analysis.

CASE–CONTROL AND COHORT DESIGNS

The methodologies discussed up to this point are applicable to continuous data that can take on a wide range of values (e.g. serum cholesterol concentration, or height). If the data can have only one of two values (i.e. the presence or absence of a characteristic such as being diabetic versus not being diabetic), other methods must be used. Two widely used methods for the analysis of data that can be classified as "o versus 1" or "yes versus no" are the case–control and cohort designs. (The use of the term "cohort" in this context is unfortunate as it can be confused with a longitudinal study in which every subject is examined exactly twice. Hopefully, the context in which the word is used will make its intended meaning clear.) A case–control study is related to a cross-sectional study in that each subject in the former is examined only once. A cohort study is related to a longitudinal study in that every subject is examined at least twice. Case–control studies are also referred to as "retrospective" and "case-referent" studies. Cohort studies are sometimes called "longitudinal studies."

Case–control design

Type II diabetes, defined as 2-hour plasma glucose concentration greater than or equal to 200 mg/dL on an oral glucose tolerance test, is a common finding in elderly people. It has been postulated that diabetes (an exposure) predisposes the elderly to myocardial infarction (a disease). A quick test of this hypothesis could be provided by a case–control study.[7–9] A case–control study begins by enrolling subjects tested and shown to have the disease of interest, and a group of controls, subjects who are tested and shown not to have the disease. At the time they are enrolled, cases and controls are examined for the presence of (or are asked if they were exposed to) a putative risk factor for the condition being studied. Although the history of exposure often comes from the subject's self-report or an examination of the subject, the history of exposure will at times be obtained from records (e.g. occupational, military, or medical). In the diabetes example, exposure status might be determined by a 2-hour glucose concentration greater than or equal to 200 mg/dL on an oral glucose tolerance test performed at the time subjects are enrolled in the study. On the basis of the presence or absence of the condition being studied and subjects' exposure history, a 2 × 2 table is produced that cross-tabulates disease status by exposure history (Table 5-1). The measure of the association between disease and exposure in a case–control study is the *odds ratio*. Using the symbols from Table 5-1, the odds ratio is defined as follows:

$$(a/c)/(b/d) = ad/bc$$

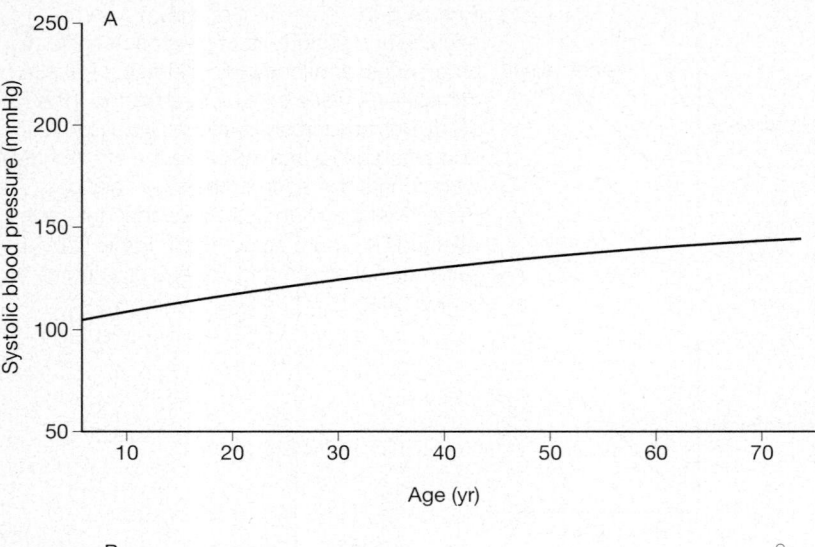

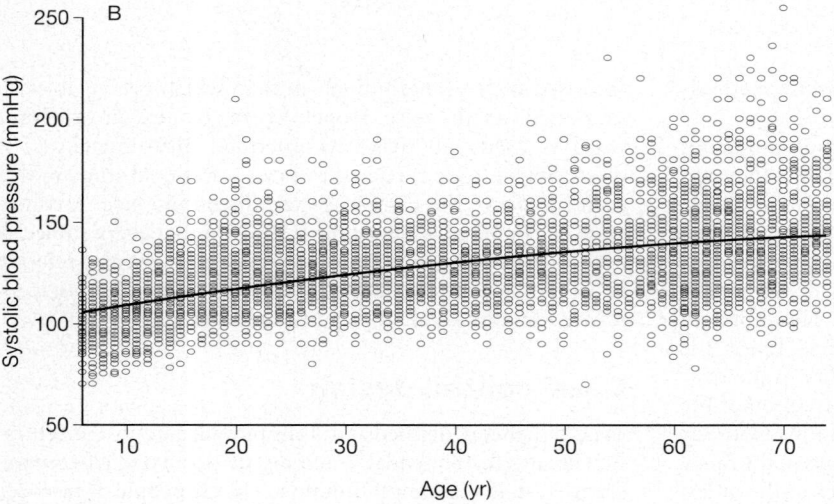

Figure 5-11 Cross-sectional analysis of the effect of age on systolic blood pressure. The curve in panel A is a plot of the quadratic equation obtained by regressing systolic blood pressure on age; i.e. a plot of the equation systolic blood pressure = $\beta_0 + \beta_1 age + \beta_2 age^2$. Panel B contains a plot of the quadratic equation along with a scatter plot of the data included in the regression analysis. The data included in the analysis are from white males who participated in the NHANES II survey.[15]

Table 5-1 **Cross-tabulation of disease by history of exposure to a putative risk factor**		
History of exposure	Diagnosed as having disease	
	Yes	No
Yes	a	b
No	c	d

An odds ratio greater than 1 indicates that exposure is associated with disease. An odds ratio less than 1 indicates that exposure is associated with protection from disease. The rationale for using the odds ratio as the measure of association; its relation to the probability of disease in exposed subjects compared with unexposed subjects; and the methods used to determine the statistical significance of an odds ratio—are beyond the scope of this chapter. Interested readers are referred to Kahn and Sempos.[7]

Case–control studies are open to several types of bias. The first is *recall bias*. In an effort to understand why they have a disease, subjects who have the disease may be more fastidious in "searching their memory" for a history of exposure than are subjects who are disease-free. This bias can be avoided if exposure status is determined from existing records rather than the subject's memory, or by measuring exposure status at entry with an objective test such as an oral glucose tolerance test. A test for the presence of recall bias can be performed by asking subjects to indicate their past exposure to a series of factors, only one of which is a putative risk factor. A significant association between the putative risk factor (as well as several of the "dummy" risk factors) and outcome suggests the presence of recall bias.

Another potential source of bias is *assignment bias*. If the researcher is aware of the subject's exposure status, he or she may be predisposed to interpret questionable signs or symptoms of disease as indicating that the disease is present (or absent). Knowing disease status may induce the investigator to probe the subject's history more vigorously for evidence of prior exposure. Assignment bias can be avoided if subjects are assigned to disease status without knowledge of exposure status, and if exposure status is determined without knowledge of disease status. It is essential to follow an established protocol when determining disease and exposure status (e.g. asking a standard set of questions or performing a standard series of laboratory techniques).

Case–control studies have an important weakness: the inability to determine whether there is a temporal association between exposure and the presence of disease. If the risk factor being studied causes disease, exposure to the risk factor must precede the appearance of disease. Because exposure and disease status are determined at the same time, at entry to the case–control study, it is not possible to determine whether the putative risk factor resulted in the disease or whether the disease process resulted in the observed status of the risk factor. A case–control study may indicate that elevated cholesterol concentration (defined as a serum cholesterol greater than or equal to 240 mg/dL) is associated with a history of myocardial infarction. Although this may be true, an alternative hypothesis would be that elevated cholesterol concentration promotes survival in those people who suffer an infarction. If this hypothesis is true, people with low cholesterol concentrations will not survive their myocardial infarction. The pool of subjects who have had a myocardial infarction will be enriched with subjects whose cholesterol concentration is high (*a* from Table 5-1) and will have few subjects whose cholesterol is low (*c* from Table 5-1). The pool of subjects who did not have a heart attack will not be affected by this selection pressure. Increasing *a* and decreasing *c* without affecting *b* and *d* will bias the odds ratio, *ad/bc*, toward values greater than 1. Thus case–control studies, much like cross-sectional studies, are subject to selective mortality.

Case–control studies are often used to study rare diseases where many thousands of unaffected subjects would have to be followed in order to obtain a single subject who develops the disease. In this situation, cases are often obtained by accessing a disease registry, or by enrolling patients followed at a referral center specializing in the disease.

The problems inherent in the case–control design will often require a case–control study to be confirmed by a study conducted according to a cohort design.

Cohort design

Disability is an important problem for elderly people. It has been suggested that obesity in young adulthood (an exposure), defined as a BMI (body mass index, an index of weight adjusted for height) greater than 27 kg/m^2, may lead to disability in old age (a disease). A cohort study could explore this question. A cohort study begins by screening a group of subjects to see whether they have the condition being studied. The screening can be accomplished by examination, laboratory testing, or questioning the subject. Only those subjects who are free of the disease or condition of interest are enrolled into the study. At the time subjects are enrolled, a risk factor is measured and subjects are placed into an exposed or unexposed group. Some time in the future, at the time of follow-up, subjects are again screened to see whether they have the disease or condition. On the bases of the results of the second screening, and the exposure status determined at entry to the study, a 2 × 2 table is created (Table 5-2).

The measure of the association between disease and exposure in a cohort study is the *relative risk*, defined (using the symbols from Table 5-2) as follows:

$$[a/(a+b)]/[c/(c+d)]$$

Table 5-2 Cross-tabulation of disease incidence during follow-up by exposure status at entry to a cohort study

Exposure at entry	Diagnosed as having disease during follow-up		Totals
	Yes	No	
Yes	*a*	*b*	*a + b*
No	*c*	*d*	*c + d*

The relative risk, unlike the odds ratio, is a direct comparison of the rate at which disease develops in exposed subjects compared with unexposed subjects. A relative risk greater than 1 indicates that subjects who are exposed to the risk factor have a higher probability of developing the disease or condition than do subjects who are not exposed. Thus, a relative risk greater than 1 indicates that exposure is associated with disease. A relative risk less than 1 indicates that exposure is associated with protection from disease. The method used to determine the statistical significance of a relative risk is beyond the scope of this chapter. Interested readers are referred to Kahn and Sempos.[7]

Because exposure status for each subject is determined at the time of enrollment into the study, before the disease or condition being studied develops, cohort studies, unlike case–control studies, are free from recall bias. Assignment bias can, however, occur if the person who evaluates subjects for the presence of disease at the end of the follow-up knows the subjects' exposure status. Cohort studies, in contrast to case–control studies, can establish a temporal relation between exposure and disease incidence. Unfortunately, cohort studies take longer to complete and are more expensive to perform than case–control studies.

Cohort studies can suffer from confounding as a consequence of loss to follow-up. If some subjects who were enrolled in the study never return for follow-up examination, they will not be included in the 2 × 2 table and hence will not be included in the computation of the relative risk. The computation of relative risk will be biased if the relation between exposure and disease is different in subjects lost to follow-up than it is in subjects who remain in the study. This survival bias is a form of selective mortality. As having no loss to follow-up is the only way to avoid survival bias, every attempt possible should be made to locate subjects who do not return for follow-up examination and convince them to return. Because some loss to follow-up is almost inevitable (subjects die, get sick, move, etc.), an important step in the analysis of a cohort study is to determine the potential effect of the loss to follow-up. Two methods have been used to accomplish this goal.

The first method is to assume that every subject who was lost to follow-up developed the condition being studied at the time they were lost to follow-up, add the subjects to the 2 × 2 table, and then re-analyze the data. This analysis is followed by one in which it is assumed that subjects who were lost to follow-up did not develop the condition being studied. If both analyses come to the same qualitative conclusion about the putative risk factor (i.e. both indicate that exposure increases risk, or both indicate that exposure is protective), and these results are qualitatively the same as those obtained from an analysis that excludes subjects who were lost to follow-up, then loss to follow-up might change the magnitude of the association between exposure and disease, but it will not change a protective factor into a risk factor for disease nor will it change a risk factor into a protective factor. If the two analyses come to different qualitative conclusions, the potential effect of loss to follow-up is uncertain, and any conclusion derived from the study is weakened.

The second method of assessing the potential of effect of loss to follow-up is to compare baseline characteristics of subjects lost to baseline characteristics of subjects who were followed to the end of the study. A typical comparison might include age, sex, race, exposure status, and socio-economic status. If there are no systematic differences between subjects who were lost to follow-up and those who were not, it is unlikely that the lost subjects had a different relation between exposure and outcome than did subjects who were not lost. In this case, loss to follow-up is unlikely to have a substantial effect on the inferences derived from the study.

Extensions to the case–control and cohort designs

Case–control and cohort designs are important tools in the analysis of the relation between an outcome variable that can be in one of two states, diseased or not diseased, and a single independent variable, exposure status, which can take on two states, exposed or nonexposed. Rather straightforward modifications of the designs permit exposure status to have more than two discrete values.[7] These modifications, however, do not allow the exposure variable to be expressed as a continuous variable, and the modifications are limited in their ability to allow additional covariates to be added to the model. (In a study of the relation between diabetes and mortality, it might be of interest to include the subject's age as an additional covariate.) Logistic regression,[7] which is closely related to case–control methodology, and Cox proportional hazards regression,[10] which is closely related to cohort methodology, allow the exposure to be expressed as a continuous variable rather than as "yes" or "no" (e.g. actual cholesterol concentration can be used rather than hypercholesterolemia versus a normal concentration). Although logistic regression and the Cox model are more "sophisticated" than are the case–control and cohort methodologies, they are subject to the same biases as are their respective simpler models.

COMPARISON OF RATES: DIRECT ADJUSTMENT

Disease incidence and mortality rates are of general medical interest; but because death and the incidence of many diseases such as cancer and heart are more common in older than younger people, the rates are of particular interest to gerontologists. Rather than give disease incidence or mortality rates for a series of age groups (e.g. by age decade), a single rate is often given for the entire population. For example, in the USA in 1998 there were 865 deaths per 100,000 population.[16] (A single rate is given because it is "easier" to remember a single mortality or disease incidence rate than it is to remember a series

of age-specific rates.) The health of the nation, and in some sense the success (or failure) of the medicine establishment, can be judged by comparing mortality rates across time.

Because mortality rates (and incidence rates of many diseases) vary by age, a comparison of rates across time can be confounded by changes in the age distribution of the population. This can best be understood by considering two populations consisting of 200 people. The first population contains 150 young and 50 old people. The second population, studied some years later, contains 50 young and 150 old people. Assume that 1 percent (1 out of 100) of the young people and 5 percent (5 out of 100) of the old people will die during a one-year period. The annual mortality rate is calculated as the number of deaths in the young group (calculated as the mortality rate in the young multiplied by the number of young people in the population) plus the number of deaths in the old group (calculated as the mortality rate in the old multiplied by the number of old people in the population) divided by the total number of people in the population. The annual mortality rate in the first population is $[(0.01 \times 150) + (0.05 \times 50)]/(150 + 50) = 0.02$, or 2000 per 100,000 population. The annual mortality rate in the second population is $[(0.01 \times 50) + (0.05 \times 150)]/(50 + 150) = 0.04$, or 4000 per 100,000 population. The difference in the age distributions of the two populations results in two different mortality rates despite the fact that the age-specific mortality rates are the same in the populations and makes it difficult to compare the mortality rates in the two populations.

In order to allow rates to be compared without the confounding caused by differences in the age distributions of the populations, the age-specific rates from different populations (or time periods) are used to compute disease rates in a standard population. The same standard population is used for all computations, regardless of whether the rates come from the first or second population, and regardless of the time at which the rates were obtained. For example, to allow us to compare the rates from our two populations, we can choose a standard population containing 100 young and 100 old subjects. We will compute an adjusted annual mortality rate for the first population using the age-specific mortality rates from the first population and the age distribution of the standard population. The adjusted annual mortality rate in the first population is $[(0.01 \times 100) + (0.05 \times 100)]/(100 + 100) = 0.03$, or 3000 per 100,000 population. Similarly we use the standard population when we compute an adjusted annual mortality rate in the second population. The adjusted rate in the second population is $[(0.01 \times 100) + (0.05 \times 100)]/(100 + 100) = 0.03$, or 3000 per 100,000 population. The adjusted rates in the two populations are thus the same. This technique of adjustment is often referred to as *direct adjustment*.[11]

Care must be taken when comparing directly adjusted rates. Until recently the population distribution of the USA in 1940 was widely used as the standard population. Directly adjusted rates have now been computed using the population distribution of the USA in 2000.[12] Thus older directly adjusted rates may not be comparable to recently computed directly adjusted rates.

A comparison of the unadjusted mortality rates (often referred to as "crude death rates") and the rates adjusted (using direct adjustment) to the age distribution of the USA in 1940 (Fig. 5-12) shows that the annual mortality rate has generally

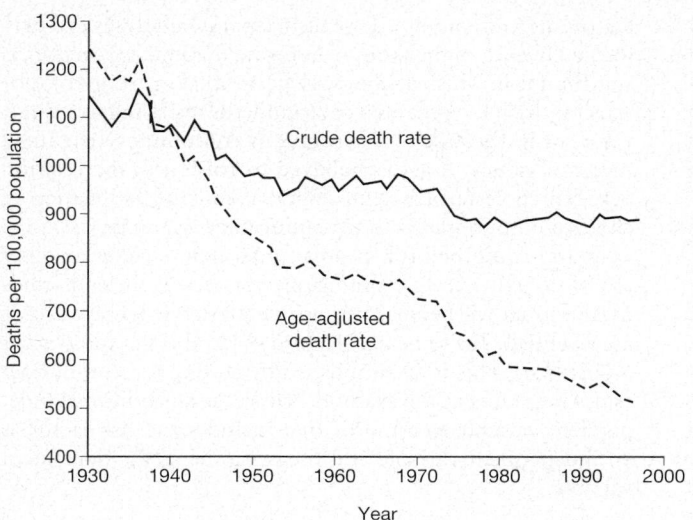

Figure 5-12 A comparison of the crude (solid line) and age-adjusted (dashed line) mortality rates in the USA from 1930 to 1998. Adjustment rates were computed using the direct method. The standard population used in the direct adjustment was the age distribution of the USA in 1940. See text for details. Adapted from Murphy.[16]

improved from 1930 to 1998 and that the age-adjusted rate has fallen faster than the crude death rate. The crude death rate has fallen more slowly than the age-adjusted death rate because from 1930 to 1998 the USA population became older. For example, over this period the percentage of Americans aged 65 and older almost doubled, from 7 to 13 percent. The increasing age of the population tends to increase the death rate. Improvements in medical care and access to medical care, public health measures, lifestyle changes, etc. during this period increased the average lifespan, decreasing the death rate. The crude death rate is influenced by factors that increase and factors that decrease the rate: (1) the age distribution of the population used to compute the crude rate became progressively older from 1930 to 1998 increasing the rate and (2) medical care, etc. improved from 1930 to 1998 decreasing the rate. The age-adjusted death rate is influenced only by the improvements in medical care, etc. from 1930 to 1998 because the same standard population is used to compute the age-adjusted death rate regardless of the year for which the computation is performed.

CAUTIONS ABOUT THE INTERPRETATION OF STUDIES

A statistically significant relation between a risk factor and outcome, regardless of study design, does not guarantee that the association is "true." False associations can be produced by chance, bias, or confounding. A chance association is an association that is due to the random variation seen in a sample of a larger population. The paradigm followed in almost every study of the association between a risk factor and an outcome is to select a sample of subjects from the total population and then perform a test to see whether there is an association between the risk factor and outcome in the sample. Based upon the association (or lack of one) in the sample, an inference is made about the association of the risk factor and outcome in the entire population. The major problem with this paradigm is that the findings in the sample may not be generalizable to the total population. It is unlikely that the exact same relation between risk factor and outcome would be seen in two distinct

samples of the population. There will always be some variation in the characteristics of the subjects that make up different samples. Additionally there will be variation in the way in which a study is performed in the samples, such as the time of day the studies are performed, etc. This variation will introduce variability in the observed relation between risk factor and outcome. If the variation is large enough, it is possible that one sample will indicate that the risk factor is associated with disease and a second sample will indicate that the risk factor protects subjects from disease.

Chance variation between samples, or between a sample and the population, can be minimized by studying as large a random sample of the population as possible. Additionally, mathematical techniques are available to estimate the magnitude of the inter-sample variation that might be expected due to chance alone. Statistical tests and the probability values (P values) obtained from the tests have been used to quantify the degree to which chance variability may account for the observed association. In medical research, a probability less than 5 percent ($P < 0.05$) is considered sufficient evidence to conclude that an association is unlikely to be due to chance variation and to reject the null hypothesis that there is no association between exposure and outcome. A probability greater than or equal to 5 percent ($P \geq 0.05$), is considered insufficient evidence to exclude the possibility that chance variation is the source of the observed association. More recently, interest has focused on the computation of a "confidence interval," which gives the range within which the true magnitude of an association lies with a certain degree of assurance. A discussion of the relative utility of P values versus confidence intervals is provided by Rothman.[8]

Bias refers to any error in the planning, execution, or evaluation of a study that leads to a systematic error in the estimation of the association between a putative risk factor and outcome. Several, but not all, sources of bias, and techniques for dealing with them, have been discussed earlier in this chapter.

Confounding refers to a condition in which the association between a putative risk factor and outcome is distorted by the effect of a third factor. Figure 5-13 depicts a hypothetical relation between a risk factor (BMI) and outcome—mortality in two groups of subjects, smokers and nonsmokers.

The percentage of subjects who are smokers is inversely related to BMI throughout the range of BMIs seen in the population. At low BMI values, 90 percent of the subjects studied are smokers and the remaining 10 percent are nonsmokers. In the middle of the BMI range, 50 percent of all subjects are smokers and 50 percent are nonsmokers. At the highest BMIs, 10 percent of the subjects are smokers and 90 percent are nonsmokers.

The relation between BMI and mortality in smokers is shown by the upper dashed line; mortality increases with both high and low BMI. Minimal mortality occurs in the middle of the BMI range. The relation between BMI and mortality in nonsmokers (the lower dashed line) is the same as that seen in smokers; mortality increases with both high and low BMI. At any given BMI, however, the mortality rate is higher in smokers than it is in nonsmokers. If the relation between BMI and mortality is studied separately in smokers and nonsmokers (i.e. the analysis is "stratified by smoking status") the true U-shaped relation between BMI and mortality is seen. If, however, the relation between BMI and mortality is studied without regard to smoking status (the subjects are analyzed as a single group), the relation between BMI and mortality seen is depicted by the solid line. At low BMI values, the mortality rate of the subjects will be close to that seen in smokers, since essentially all subjects are smokers. At high BMI values, the mortality rate will be close to that of nonsmokers, since almost all subjects are nonsmokers. For subjects whose BMI is close to the middle of the BMI range, the overall mortality rate will be close to midway between that seen in smokers and nonsmokers, because approximately half of the subjects are smokers and the remaining half are nonsmokers. Thus, smoking confounds the relation between BMI and mortality. If the confounding is not recognized and eliminated, the true U-shaped relation between smoking and mortality will not be seen.

Several steps can be taken to minimize the detrimental effects of confounding. (Attempting to eliminate the detrimental effects of confounding is often referred to as "adjusting" an analysis.) *Stratification* into groups based upon the value of a suspected confounder—for example, into smokers and nonsmokers—will often allow the true relation between a risk factor and outcome to be seen if separate analyses are performed in each of the groups. A second method, *restriction*, is a technique in which analyses are performed in groups of subjects in which the potential confounder is restricted to a single value, or in the case of a continuous confounder, to a small range of values. If age is believed to confound the relation between cholesterol and mortality, a study of the relation of cholesterol to mortality in the entire adult age range (i.e. 20 to 99 years) could be broken down into eight smaller analyses (20 to 29, 30 to 39, etc.). Within any age decade, the confounding due to age will be small because the subjects in any age decade are essentially the same age. A third method is the *multvariate adjustment*. This is accomplished by adding the confounder (smoking status in the example below), as an additional independent variable to a model that includes the risk factor as an independent variable and the outcome as the dependent variable:

- unadjusted model:
  mortality rate $= \beta_0 + \beta_1 \times$ BMI
- adjusted model:
  mortality rate $= \beta_0 + \beta_1 \times$ BMI $+ \beta_2 \times$ smoking status

where β_0 is the intercept, β_1 is the slope for BMI, and β_2 is the slope for smoking status.

A fourth technique is *matching*. In case–control analysis, subjects, at the time they are recruited, can be chosen so that cases and controls are "matched" on a potential confounder. If race is believed to be a confounder, for each of the cases selected, a control could be selected that is the same race as its respective control. Several races could participate in the study (as long as each case is matched with a control of the same race). Matching removes the racial difference between a case and its respective control. The case–control methodology previously described assumes that cases and controls were not matched. The analysis of a matched case–control study is slightly more complex.[7–9,13] Matching can also be performed in cohort studies.[8]

Regardless of the technique used to adjust for a potential confounder, if the relation between a putative risk factor and

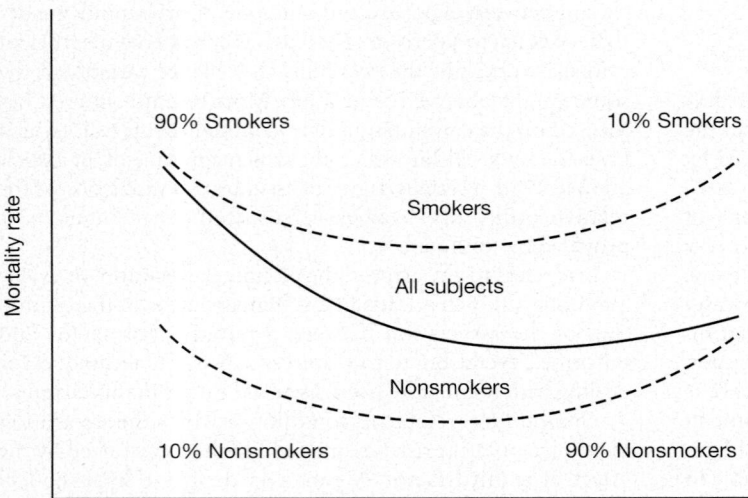

Figure 5-13 The hypothetical relation between a risk factor, BMI, is confounded by smoking status. See text for details.

outcome is the same before and after adjustment, there is no confounding and the "confounder" can be ignored. If the results are different, the potential confounder is a true confounder, and the true relation between risk factor and outcome can be determined only after adjustment is performed. A complete discussion of chance, bias, and confounding, and the methods that can be used to avoid them, is beyond the scope of this chapter. Interested readers are referred to any epidemiology textbook, including Rothman,[8] Hennekens et al.,[9] and Kahn et al.[7]

The final methodological problem in research on aging is to determine the generalizability of the results of a study. Regardless of the care taken in the planning, execution, and evaluation of a study, unrecognized bias, confounding, and chance variation may be present. Thus, the results of a study may not be generalizable to the entire population. Many of the techniques used to lessen the probability of bias and confounding result in restricting the population studied.

Unfortunately, the more restrictive the conditions are under which a study is performed, the more difficult it is to assume that the results can be generalized to the entire population. It is only through a comparison of the results of several studies, performed at different times, in different populations, under different conditions, that we can begin to address the question of the generalizability of an association. It is, therefore, of utmost importance that every study be conducted in a manner that will ensure, to as great an extent possible, that the results are correct. This means that great care must be taken to assure that the study design, execution, and interpretation are as free of bias, confounding, and chance as possible.

KEY POINTS   Methodological issues

■ The cross-sectional design is the most commonly used in studies of the relation between a variable of interest and age. Cross-sectional studies are relatively easy and inexpensive to perform and can be completed quickly, but are subject to two errors: bias due to birth cohort effects and bias due to selective mortality.

■ The time-series design is used to look for changes that occur in a population over the course of time. Time-series studies are subject to two errors: biased selection of subjects in the time periods and methodological change.

■ Subjects in a longitudinal study are followed over an extended period to determine the rate at which a variable changes as the subjects get older. Special techniques are required for proper analysis of longitudinal data. Longitudinal studies are subject to error due to methodological change, but they do not suffer from birth cohort effects or selective mortality.

■ Case–control and cohort designs are similar to cross-sectional and longitudinal studies, but they are used to study data that can have only one of two values. Several types of bias can affect case–control studies: recall bias, assignment bias, and selective mortality bias. Cohort studies, unlike case–control studies, can establish a temporal relation between exposure and disease incidence, but they take longer to complete and are more expensive to perform. They are subject also to bias due to loss to follow-up.

REFERENCES

1. Elahi D, Muller DC, Rowe JW: Design, conduct, and analysis of human aging research. In Schneider EL, Rowe JW (eds): Handbook of the Biology of Aging, 4th edn. Academic Press, San Diego, 1996
2. Schlesselman JJ: Planning a longitudinal study. I: Sample size determination. J Chronic Dis 1973;26:553–560
3. Schlesselman JJ: Planning a longitudinal study. II: Frequency of measurement and study duration. J Chronic Dis 1973;26:561–570
4. Kochanek KD, Hudson BL: Advance Report of Final Mortality Statistics. National Center for Health Statistics, Hyattsville, MA, 1995
5. Last J: A Dictionary of Epidemiology, 2nd edn. Oxford University Press, New York, 1988
6. Elahi VK, Elahi D, Andres R, Tobin JD, Butler MG, Norris AH: A longitudinal study of nutritional intake in men. J Gerontol 1983;38(2):162–180
7. Kahn HA, Sempos CT: Statistical Methods in Epidemiology. Oxford University Press, New York, 1989
8. Rothman KJ: Modern Epidemiology. Little Brown, Boston, 1986
9. Hennekens CH, Buring JE, Mayrent SL: Epidemiology in Medicine, 1st edn. Little Brown, Boston, 1987
10. Lee ET: Multivariate analysis: Cox proportional hazards model for survival data. In Statistical Methods for Survival Data Analysis. John Wiley, New York, 1992:250–263
11. Curtin LR, Klein RJ: Healthy People 2000: Statistical Notes no. 6, Direct Standardization (Age-adjusted Death Rates). National Center for Health Statistics, Hyattsville, MA, 1995
12. Klein RJ, Schoenborn CA: Healthy People: Statistical Notes no. 20, Age Adjustment Using the 2000 Projected US Population. National Center for Health Statistics, Hyattsville, MA, 2001
13. Armitage P, Berry G: Statistical Methods in Medical Research, 2nd edn. Blackwell Scientific, Oxford, 1987:282–295
14. Hershcopf RJ, Elahi D, Andres R, Baldwin HL, Raizes GS, Schocken DD et al: Longitudinal changes in serum cholesterol in man: an epidemiologic search for an etiology. J Chronic Dis 1982;35(2):101–114
15. US Public Health Service: Plan and Operation of the Second Health and Nutrition Examination Survey, 1976–1980 (DHHS Pub no. PHS 81–1317, Series 1, no. 15. US Government Printing Office, Washington, DC, 1981
16. Murphy SL: Deaths: Final Data for 1998. National Center for Health Statistics, Hyattsville, MA, 2000

Chapter 6

Biology of aging

Huber R. Warner

A discussion about the biology of aging demands that one first define what is meant by aging and the aging process. There are many definitions proposed, but the one provided by Richard Miller of the University of Michigan seems particularly useful for this chapter in a textbook on geriatric medicine.[1] He defines aging as the "process that progressively converts physiologically and cognitively fit healthy adults into less fit individuals with increasing vulnerability to injury, illness and death." The study of the biology of aging began with discovery research which mostly focused on describing and cataloging aging changes. To understand how these age-related changes relate to Miller's definition, the challenge then becomes to distinguish among:

- pathologically neutral age-related changes, such as the graying of hair;
- changes which may contribute to the development of one or more age-related pathologies, such as the accumulation of oxidatively damaged molecules;
- changes which may cause or indicate overt pathology, such as the development of plaques and tangles in the brain as risk factors for Alzheimer's disease.

Over the years a large number of theories of aging has been proposed,[2] but the complexity of the process diminishes the possibility that any one theory would completely explain aging. The concept that some age-related changes may be programmed, whereas others are stochastic and unpredictable, is now generally accepted. However, some theories include both kinds of changes and are impossible to classify uniquely as one or the other. A further complication is the need to distinguish between the process of aging itself, and the effects due to age-related phenomena such as diseases. The discussion in this chapter will mostly focus on the stochastic aspects of age-related changes, as Chapter 7 covers genetically programmed age-related change.

The most viable components of the stochastic biological theories include free radical damage,[3] DNA damage and repair,[4] nonenzymatic glycation,[5] and protein cross-linking. Beckman and Ames have written an excellent review of the free radical theory of aging,[6] which includes a discussion of many aspects of these overlapping phenomena.

MODEL SYSTEMS

Two important factors in aging research are the choice and appropriate use of a suitable animal model.[7] The choice of model is driven by a variety of considerations, including length of lifespan, quality of the genetic system, availability of genome sequence, ease of husbandry, and relevance to human biology. The most commonly used models are rats, mice, fruit flies (*Drosophila melanogaster*), nematodes (*Caenorhabditis elegans*), and yeast (*Saccharomyces cerevisiae*). Various characteristics of these model systems are provided in Table 6-1. In practice, mice and rats have been widely used for physiological studies,[7] whereas the shorter-lived invertebrate species have been particularly useful for studies on the genetic basis of longevity.[8]

Another animal model of more recent use is the nonhuman primate. This model is obviously desirable because it most closely resembles humans, but less desirable because of its substantially longer lifespan than rodents. Rhesus monkeys are currently being used for testing whether an intervention known as caloric restriction extends the lifespan of primates,[9,10] as it does for rodents,[11] and for studying the biology of the menopause.[12]

The human fibroblast grown in culture has been used as a possible model for aging at the cellular level, following the discovery by Leonard Hayflick that fibroblasts do not continue

Table 6-1 Animal models used in aging research

Organism	Lifespan	Genetic system	Genome sequence	Ease of husbandry
Yeast	20 doublings	Excellent	Known[81] 6000 genes	Excellent
Nematode (*C. elegans*)	20 days	Excellent	Known[82] 20,000 genes	Excellent
Fruit fly (*D. melanogaster*)	50 days	Excellent	Known[83] 14,000 genes	Excellent
Mouse	3 years	Excellent	Known 2001?[84] (about 30,000 genes)	Good
Rat	3 years	Poor	Known 2003?[84] (about 30,000 genes?)	Good
Rhesus monkey	30 years	None	Not known (about 30,000 genes?)	Expensive

to replicate indefinitely.[13] This growth cessation is now referred to as "replicative senescence"; the potential importance of this model has been heightened by the identification of senescent cells in human tissue.[14] This model is discussed in detail in Chapter 8.

DAMAGE AND REPAIR: A CENTRAL ROLE FOR MITOCHONDRIA

Denham Harman first proposed that oxygen free radical production is a major risk factor for aging.[3] The major source of these reactive oxygen species (ROS) is leakage from the electron transport system in mitochondria during the synthesis of adenosine triphosphate (ATP) by the process known as "oxidative phosphorylation." It has been estimated that 1–5 percent of the oxygen metabolized during this process is converted to a reactive oxygen specie in the form of superoxide anion[15] (see Figure 6-1). Mitochondria contain superoxide dismutase activity which converts the superoxide anion to hydrogen peroxide, which then either leaks out of the mitochondrion or damages mitochondrial components. The release of hydrogen peroxide by mitochondria increases with age.[16] Hydrogen peroxide can directly damage membrane lipids by peroxidation of their double bonds; or, in the presence of iron, it may be converted into the very damaging hydroxyl radical. The high protein-bound iron content of mitochondria due to the presence of the many cytochromes involved in the electron transport system increases the likelihood that this reaction will occur inside the mitochondria, thus damaging these same electron transport proteins and other proteins found there. Any hydrogen peroxide leaking out of the mitochondrion will either be inactivated by cytoplasmic catalase or glutathione peroxidase, converted to hydroxyl radical by cytoplasmic protein-bound iron,[17] or leak into the nucleus and oxidatively damage the genome.

The importance of maintaining mitochondrial structure and function cannot be overestimated. Not only are the mitochondria the primary source of the adenosine triphosphate (ATP) needed for nearly all cellular processes requiring energy, but if cytochrome c leaks out of damaged mitochondria, this may trigger apoptosis.[18] Apoptosis is a genetically programmed form of cell death, which occurs during development to remove unwanted cells, or in response to excessive and irreparable cellular damage, such as occurs during a stroke or heart attack. The roles of apoptosis in aging processes will be discussed below, and have been summarized by Warner et al.[19]

Proteins are susceptible to oxidative damage, and such damage increases with age.[20] There is also evidence that the ability to degrade damaged proteins decreases with increasing age, thus leading to accumulation of damaged protein,[21] often in the form of aggregates. Two mitochondrial enzymes involved in production of ATP appear to be particularly vulnerable to oxidation. These are the mitochondrial form of *cis*-aconitase,[22] which is an essential enzyme involved in the citric acid cycle, and adenine nucleotide translocase,[23] which is essential for transport of ATP from inside the mitochondrion where it is made, to the cytoplasm where it will be used. The oxidation of both of these enzymes increases with increasing age, which could compromise ATP production. Oxidative damage in general, and mitochondrial oxidative damage in particular, may be a major risk factor for a variety of degenerative diseases.[24]

Oxidative damage to DNA is another potential source of problems for the aging organism. Bruce Ames of the University of California in Berkeley has estimated that as many as 10,000 oxidized bases may be generated per human cell per day,[24] but newer techniques for isolating DNA indicate that this estimate is probably about 100-fold too high owing to oxidation during isolation of the DNA.[25] Nevertheless, oxidized bases are produced in living cells, leading to point mutations due to mispairing during subsequent DNA replication, if replication occurs before repair is complete. Levels of oxidized bases in mitochondrial DNA are 5–20 times higher than in nuclear DNA,[25] presumably because more oxidative damage occurs in mitochondria. While numerous studies report that mutations do increase with age in mice, a causal link between mutations and aging has not been established. In general, point mutations tend to be greater in replicating tissues than in nonproliferating tissues, because DNA replication "sets" the mutation in place.[26,27]

DNA deletions also occur with increasing frequency with age in both mice and humans, particularly in the mitochondrial DNA.[28] In this case, deletion frequencies are higher in nonreplicating tissues such as muscle, heart, and brain, but different brain regions exhibit widely varying deletion frequencies.[29] Mitochondrial DNA deletions colocalize with electron

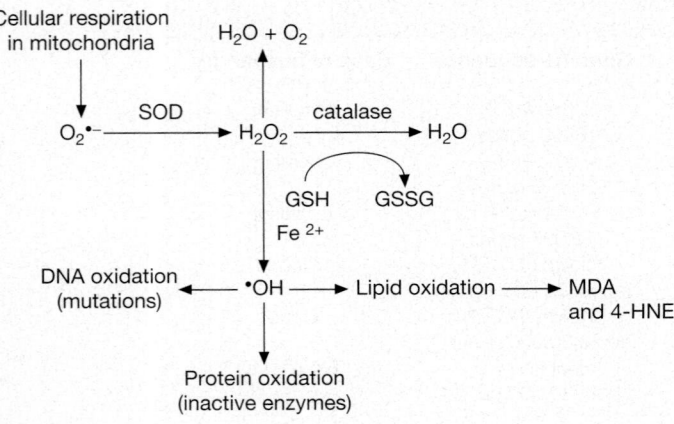

Cellular respiration in mitochondria

$H_2O + O_2$

$O_2^{\bullet -} \xrightarrow{\text{SOD}} H_2O_2 \xrightarrow{\text{catalase}} H_2O$

GSH   GSSG

Fe^{2+}

DNA oxidation (mutations) ← $^{\bullet}OH$ → Lipid oxidation → MDA and 4-HNE

Protein oxidation (inactive enzymes)

Figure 6-1 Production and metabolism of reactive oxygen species in vivo. $O_2^{\bullet-}$, superoxide anion; H_2O_2, hydrogen peroxide; SOD, superoxide dismutase; GSH, glutathione; $^{\bullet}OH$, hydroxyl radical; MDA, malondialdehyde; 4-HNE, 4-hydroxy-2-nonenal.

transport system dysfunction, muscle fiber atrophy, and oxidative damage in fiber sections.[30] Thus, these deletions may be a risk factor for age-related sarcopenia. The impact of these deletions on aging per se is not yet clear, as most results suggest that the percentage of mitochondria per cell containing any particular deletion is less than 2 percent. However, this value is an average, and the real value in any given cell can be much higher if many cells have mostly deletion-free mitochondrial DNA molecules.[31] Because a muscle fiber functions as a linear unit, a localized defect may compromise the function of the entire fiber. It has been reported that the mutation spectrum in mitochondrial DNA in human fibroblasts does change with age, with some point mutations occurring in as many as 50 percent of the mitochondrial genomes in fibroblasts from individuals above 65 years of age.[32]

The hypothesis that DNA damage and its repair may be important factors in aging[4] is supported by the discovery that the protein produced by the gene implicated in Werner's syndrome, a human syndrome that resembles premature aging, possesses both DNA helicase[33] and exonuclease[34] activities. It is likely that one or both of these activities could play an important role in DNA repair, with the obvious inference that this DNA repair deficiency may be a cause of the premature aging. Cells from Werner-syndrome patients do show an increase in mutations and chromosome alterations,[35] but this does not prove that they cause the premature aging per se.

Oxidative stress may be involved in aging in several more subtle ways as well. Two of these ways lead to protein cross-linking, which in itself may contribute to aging. One process is called nonenzymatic glycosylation, or glycation.[5] This process begins with a reaction between the aldehyde group of glucose and an amino group, often one found in protein, such as the ε-amino group of lysine. A Schiff's base is formed from this nonenzymatic reaction between glucose and a protein, and this structure undergoes multiple rearrangements and oxidative reactions to produce a variety of intermediates, eventually leading to reaction of these intermediates with the amino group of a lysine molecule in a second protein, thus linking the two protein molecules together. Cross-linked proteins may not be efficiently degraded by the cell's proteolytic systems, and in fact may act as an inhibitor of the proteolytic complex,[36] thus leading to an accumulation of cross-linked, nonfunctional protein in the cell. When an individual is hyperglycemic this process is exacerbated, leading to increased production of reaction oxygen species in aortic endothelial cells, and increased glycation.[37]

Another adverse process, from the standpoint of cellular homeostasis, begins with the peroxidation of double bonds in unsaturated fatty acids (those typically found in large abundance in membranes), leading to the eventual formation of malondialdehyde (MDA) and 4-hydroxy-2-nonenal (4-HNE).[38] Both of these aldehydic compounds can cross-link proteins which also act as inhibitors of the usual protein degradation systems, producing the same result as discussed above.[36] The mitochondrial protein α-ketoglutarate dehydrogenase appears to be particularly vulnerable to inactivation by 4-HNE, especially with increasing age.[39] Whether, or how, this accumulation of altered, nonfunctional protein in cells is a factor in aging remains controversial, but the amount of cross-linked collagen present in connective tissue[40] has been proposed as a biomarker of aging of an individual organism.

THE CALORIC RESTRICTION PARADIGM

The one intervention which has been shown to reliably, and possibly universally, extend both average and maximum lifespan is an intervention known as "caloric restriction." Discovered first in research by McCay using rodents,[41] the procedure involves first determining how much a cohort of rats or mice will eat if given free access to food. A second cohort is provided with all the essential nutrients, but the calories made available are reduced by 30–50 percent. The restricted cohort not only lives 30–40 percent longer, but the "restricted" rats or mice are also more active, and appear to be healthier for longer. The onset of many age-related pathologies is delayed by caloric restriction, including cancer, kidney disease, and autoimmune disease.[11] In terms of lifespan extension, this intervention appears to work in every species in which it has been adequately tested so far.[42] Three major questions about this intervention are:

- How does it work?
- Will it work in humans?
- Can the effect be induced without actually subjecting an individual to caloric restriction?

In spite of considerable research, the answer to none of these questions is known.

One consistent finding has been that caloric restriction reduces oxidative stress.[43,44] Oxygen consumption is lowered by caloric restriction and this reduction is accompanied by a lowered proton leak[45] and less production of superoxide anion from the mitochondria. As would be expected, calorically restricted rodents have lower circulating glucose levels, so levels of glycosylated serum proteins are also lower in these animals. The level of circulating glycosylated hemoglobin is used as an indicator of diabetes, although it is not known whether glycosylated hemoglobin presents any particular problem in either the diabetic or the older individual. It can be assumed that such hemoglobin molecules will have an altered ability to pick up oxygen in the lungs and release it to other tissues. Caloric restriction has recently been shown to reduce oxidative damage in skeletal muscle in mammals,[46] and might thereby delay age-related sarcopenia.

There are many age-related changes in gene expression,[47] and many of these are reversed by caloric restriction. It is not known which, if any, of the reversals induced by caloric restriction are critical to the lifespan extension. Other interventions that cause extension of lifespan in rodents and other animal model systems have provided some clues about what are some critical factors regulating the rate of aging. Genetic interventions that extend lifespan in yeast, nematodes, fruit flies, and mice have been identified, and some of these are summarized in Table 6-2. Several of these appear to show similarities to changes induced by caloric restriction; for example, caloric restriction extends lifespan and reduces oxidative stress, while many of these mutations both extend lifespan and increase resistance to various forms of stress. The two most interesting possibilities are modulation of growth hormone levels[48] and the activity of the insulin/IGF-1 signaling pathway.[49,50]

Levels of circulating growth hormone decrease with age, so growth hormone replacement has been suggested as a

Table 6-2 Genetic interventions to extend lifespan in animal models

Gene	Organism	Biochemical function	Comments	References
v-Ha-RAS	Yeast	Oncogene	Lifespan varies with level of expression	85
sir2	Yeast	NAD-dependent histone deacetylase	Activity required for normal lifespan; overexpression increases lifespan	86, 87
Sch9	Yeast	Akt/protein kinase B	Operates in insulin signaling pathway; mutations extend lifespan and increase resistance to oxidative stress	55
age1/daf23	Nematode	PI-3-kinase	Operates in insulin signaling pathway; mutations extend lifespan	49,88
daf16	Nematode	Transcription factor	Expression required for lifespan extension by daf2 or daf23 mutations	89
tkr1	Nematode	Tyrosine kinase	Overexpression extends lifespan and increases stress resistance	90
daf2	Nematode	Insulin/IGF-1 like receptor	First step in insulin signaling pathway; mutations extend lifespan	50,91
InR, CHICO	Fruit fly	Insulin/IGF-1 like receptor	First step in insulin signaling pathway; mutations extend lifespan	53,54
mth	Fruit fly	Transmembrane protein	Partial loss-of-function mutations extend lifespan and increases stress resistance	92
indy	Fruit fly	Dicarboxylic acid transport protein	Partial loss-of-function extends lifespan	56
SOD-1	Fruit fly	Cu/Zn-superoxide dismutase	Overexpression extends lifespan	93
p66shc	Mouse	Signal transduction response to oxidative stress	Mutations extend lifespan and increase resistance to apoptosis	94
pit1/prop1	Mouse	Required for pituitary development	Mutant mice are deficient in GH, prolactin, and TSH, and grow slowly, and have extended lifespan	48,95

possible intervention to prevent age-related loss of muscle mass in humans. An early trial by Rudman et al.[51] using subcutaneous injection of biosynthetic human growth hormone three times per week for 6 months into men over 60 years of age elevated circulating levels of IGF-1 into the youthful range, increased lean body mass by about 9 percent, and decreased adipose tissue by about 14 percent. However, there are some concerns about adverse side-effects such as diabetes, so larger studies were begun in the mid-1990s to test this intervention more completely. The results of these studies are not yet available, but it is now known that mice deficient in growth hormone production (dwarf mice) live substantially longer than normal mice.[48] Mice lacking the ability to make the growth hormone receptor are also longer-lived.[52] These results suggest that, even if growth hormone replacement therapy has short-term benefits, it could be harmful if continued for a long time.

Experiments with nematodes have implicated the insulin signaling pathway in regulating the rate of aging. Several classes of mutants already known to be defective in their ability to form a special larval state (known as a dauer larva) have subsequently been found to be long-lived. One class of these mutants codes for an insulin-like growth factor receptor,[50] indicating that shutting off the insulin signaling pathway lengthens lifespan in nematodes. Very similar results have been found in fruit flies.[53,54] These results suggest that a role for IGF-1 signaling in regulating longevity may be a general phenomenon in the animal kingdom. Another class of mutants interferes with this pathway by knocking out the downstream signal transduction enzyme, phosphatidylinositol 3 kinase, and these mutants are also long-lived.[49] Although the molecule recognized by the insulin-like growth factor receptor in nematodes has not yet been identified, it is clear that this signaling pathway in some unknown way regulates longevity. Knocking out the Akt/protein kinase B gene in yeast, another gene involved in the insulin signaling pathway, extends lifespan up to three-fold and increases resistance to oxidative stress.[55]

Another possible insight into how caloric restriction works was provided by the observation that mutations partially knocking out a dicarboxylic acid transport enzyme in fruit flies also extends lifespan.[56] This enzyme facilitates the transport of dicarboxylic acids, which are citric acid cycle intermediates, across membranes. This suggests that failure to maintain high levels of these acids in the mitochondria could slow down the cycle, thereby reducing the rate of both oxygen consumption and superoxide anion production, thus reducing oxidative stress.

Another piece of evidence suggesting that oxidative stress is an important factor in aging is the observation that a pharmacological compound known as EUK-134 also extends the lifespan of nematodes.[57] EUK-134 possesses both superoxide dismutase and catalase activities, so it can neutralize both the superoxide anion and hydrogen peroxide. Although oxidative stress has been implicated as a factor in a variety of age-related diseases, and dietary supplementation with vitamin E has been associated with reducing the risk for these diseases in some epidemiological studies, vitamin E supplementation has not been shown to extend the lifespan of any animal model. EUK-134 may be a more powerful alternative because it neutralizes the reactive oxygen species close to the source of their production.

APOPTOSIS AND AGING

It would be easy to assume that cell death in the adult is necessarily bad, but this is not so.[58] It has been known for a long time that death of certain cells is necessary during development to create the appropriate biological structures for adult life, and that failure to remove damaged cells can lead to cancer.[59] It is now known that well-regulated cell death is necessary to maintain homeostasis in certain tissues. One example of this with implications for aging is the delicate balance between osteoblasts and osteoclasts during bone remodeling.[60] If there are too many osteoclasts then bone resorption will exceed bone synthesis and osteoporosis will be the ultimate result. Although all the factors modulating this balance are not known, it is known that estrogen stimulates osteoclast apoptosis, at least partially explaining why osteoporosis often occurs in post-menopausal women.

Apoptosis is also essential for proper regulation of the immune system.[61] Lymphocytes which are reactive to "self" proteins must be destroyed, or autoimmune disease will result. It has been estimated that more than 90 percent of the lymphocytes produced are destroyed before leaving the thymus to prevent autoimmune disease. Genetically induced autoimmune disease in mice can be reduced by caloric restriction, suggesting the possibility that one of the effects of caloric restriction may be to stimulate apoptosis.[62] Experimental support for this idea has been published.[63,64] There is also evidence that senescent fibroblasts are resistant to apoptosis,[65] suggesting that one problem in maintaining tissue homeostasis with increasing age is an inability to rid a tissue of senescent, and possibly dysfunctional, cells. This is a speculative, but unproven idea, although senescent cells have been identified in human tissues.[14]

Of particular importance is the role of apoptosis in neurodegenerative diseases. These are characterized by the loss of specific neurons: Alzheimer's disease (hippocampus, cortex), amyotrophic lateral sclerosis (motor neurons), Huntington's disease (striatum), and Parkinson's disease (substantia nigra). Both genetic and environmental factors are risk factors for these diseases, but the onset of each is age-dependent, suggesting that some slow but chronic process is involved. A possibility is that oxidative damage is involved leading to apoptosis in each of these cases.[19]

BIOLOGICAL INTERVENTIONS

The levels of several circulating hormones decrease with age in humans, so the question arises whether hormone replacement therapy will maintain or restore youthful function. Besides growth hormone and estrogen which have been mentioned above, levels of circulating melatonin and dehydroepiandrosterone (DHEA) also decline with age, and have been proposed as dietary supplements to retard aging. Despite the existence of a large body of research on DHEA,[66] support for DHEA supplementation remains weak. This may be because most studies have been done in rodents, which have little if any circulating DHEA. However, further research using carefully designed and rigorously controlled studies might eventually lead to a therapeutic role for DHEA.[67]

The case for melatonin is even weaker. The seminal paper in the field reporting the extension of mouse lifespan by melatonin is compromised by the use of too few mice, and the failure to control for the effects of possible caloric restriction.[68] Although melatonin may be useful for regulating the sleep cycle in humans, it is not recommended as a supplement to promote healthy aging.

Insulin-like growth factor 1 (IGF-1) is a mediator of anabolic pathways in skeletal muscle cells, and therefore might be useful in place of growth hormone in repair and maintenance of muscle tissue with increasing age. In a mouse model where IGF-1 is transgenically overexpressed only in skeletal muscle, age-related muscle atrophy is delayed and the proliferative response to muscle injury characteristic of younger animals is retained.[69] This suggests a possible clinical strategy for treatment of age- or disease-related muscle frailty, provided undesirable pathological changes can be avoided.

An area of current intense interest is the potential of cell replacement therapy to restore function to dysfunctional tissues compromised by the apoptotic loss of critical cells, as in the case of neurodegenerative diseases. A major question is whether to attempt such therapeutic approaches with embryonic stem cells obtained from fetal tissue, or with adult stem cells found in a patient's own tissues. This choice is affected by both ethical and practical issues. Whereas embryonic stem cells may possess greater potential to develop into any cell type required, its development may also be more difficult to regulate. The finding that bone marrow can be introduced into a mouse and become central nervous system neurons indicates that adult stem cells may retain sufficient pluripotency to be useful for a wide range of therapeutic targets.[70] Bone marrow stem cells have also been successfully used to repair damage from an artificially induced heart attack in mice.[71] This potential should alleviate the problem of immune rejection if the stem cells can be isolated from the patient. An early trial using cells from aborted fetuses injected into the putamen to treat Parkinson's disease has resulted in adverse side-effects in 15 percent of the patients.[72] Thus, it is far from clear that embryonic stem cells will ultimately be the best choice for cell replacement therapies.

NEW APPROACHES FOR STUDYING AGING MECHANISMS

Aging is accompanied by changes in the expression of many genes, some going up and some going down. Early research on aging has been characterized by numerous attempts to document such changes in humans and animal models gene by gene using relatively laborious techniques.[47] In most cases it is not known which changes may be causal factors in aging, and which are secondary effects caused by aging. Nevertheless, it is clear that the pattern of age-related changes in gene expression must be determined in a variety of tissues under a variety of conditions to fully understand aging and age-related pathology.

This task promises to be made considerably easier by the use of gene expression microarray technology. In this technology, small DNA probes are attached to a solid support such as a glass slide or nylon membrane in arrays of thousands.

These arrays are then exposed to the solution to be tested—usually a preparation of messenger RNA molecules labeled with either radioactivity or dyes—and the amount of RNA binding to each spot is measured to determine the amount of mRNA in the solution complementary to each DNA probe.

Although absolute values are difficult to determine, relative values can be obtained. Thus, this technology is particularly useful for comparing two different but comparable preparations with each other; e.g., young vs old, normal vs pathological tissue, induced vs noninduced, etc. The technique has already been used to compare gene expression in young vs old and old vs old calorically restricted mouse skeletal muscle,[73] brain,[74] and liver,[75] and dividing vs senescent human fibroblasts.[76] Although data management and interpretation using this technique remains a problem because of the relatively minor changes associated with aging, this DNA-based microarray is potentially very powerful; and as the reliability and sensitivity of the technology improves, it should become very useful in evaluating the physiological status of aging animals and/or humans.

Another important question is why aging is so different among different individuals within a population. The sequencing of the human genome[77,78] provides a new approach to this problem. Once genes have been sequenced, re-sequencing of the same gene from different individuals in the population will uncover the single nucleotide polymorphisms (SNPs) in each gene, which are expected at a frequency of about one every thousand base pairs.[79] Over 80 percent of these SNPs are present in more than 10 percent of the population. Thus, almost all human genes will contain SNPs, and associations between SNPs in specific genes and age-related pathology will implicate these genes in aging and age-related disease. The best example of this so far is the role of the apoE gene. The frequency of the E4 allele of this gene found within the human population decreases with increasing age,[80] and the apoE4 allele is associated with increased risk for Alzheimer's disease and vascular disease.

KEY POINTS   Biology of aging

- Aging is defined here as the process that progressively converts physiologically and cognitively fit healthy adults into less fit individuals with increasing vulnerability to injury, illness, and death.

- Theories of aging are of three types: genetically programmed aging changes (if any?); stochastic biological aging changes—free radical damage (DNA, proteins, lipids) or nonoxidative changes in protein structure and function; and declines in function of physiological systems—immune system, endocrine systems, muscle function, neurodegenerative changes.

- Mitochondria are a major in vivo source of oxygen free radicals and cellular ATP, and play a role in initiating apoptosis of damaged cells.

- Interventions in aging in mammals have included: caloric restriction—demonstrated in rodents (and nonhuman primates?); reduced production of growth hormone—demonstrated in mice; and cell replacement therapy—unproven potential of stem cells?

REFERENCES

1. Miller RA: Kleemeier Award Lecture: Are there genes for aging? J. Gerontol 1999;54A:B297–B307
2. Warner HR, Butler RN, Sprott RL, Schneider EL (eds): Modern biological theories of aging. Raven Press, New York, 1987
3. Harman D: Aging: a theory based on free radical and radiation chemistry. J Gerontol 1956;2:298–300
4. Hart RW, Setlow RB: Correlation between deoxyribonucleic acid excision repair and life-span in a number of mammalian species. Proc Natl Acad Sci USA 1974;71:2169–2173
5. Monnier VM: Nonenzymatic glycosylation, the Maillard reaction and the aging process. J Gerontol 1990;45:B105–B111
6. Beckman KB, Ames BN: The free radical theory of aging matures. Physiol Rev 1998;78:547–581
7. Miller RA, Nadon NL: Principles of animals use for gerontological research. J Gerontol 2000;55:B117–B123
8. Guarente L, Kenyon C: Genetic pathways that regulate ageing in model organisms. Nature 2000;408:255–262
9. Lane MA, Ingram DK, Roth GR: Beyond the rodent model: calorie restriction in rhesus monkeys. Age 1997;20:45–56
10. Wanagat J, Allison DB, Weindruch R: Caloric intake and aging: mechanisms in rodents and a study in non-human primates. Toxicol Sci 1999;52:35–40
11. Weindruch R, Walford RL (eds): The retardation of aging and disease by dietary restriction. Charles C. Thomas, Springfield, IL, 1988
12. Gilardi KVK, Shideler SE, Valverde CR et al: Characterization of the onset of menopause in the rhesus macaque. Biol Reprod 1997;57:335–340
13. Hayflick L: The limited in vitro lifetime of human diploid cell strains. Exp Cell Res 1965;37:614–636
14. Dimri GP, Lee X, Basile G et al: A novel biomarker identifies senescent human cells in culture and aging skin in vivo. Proc Natl Acad Sci USA 1995;92:9363–9367
15. Boveris A, Chance B: The mitochondrial generation of hydrogen peroxide: General properties and effect of hyperbaric oxygen. Biochem J 1973;134:707–716
16. Sohal RS, Sohal BH: Hydrogen peroxide release by mitochondria increases during aging. Mech Ageing Dev 1991;57:187–202
17. Stadtman ER, Oliver CN: Metal-catalysed oxidation of proteins. Science 1991;266:2005–2008
18. Green DR, Reed JC: Mitochondria and apoptosis. Science 1998;281:1309–1312
19. Warner HR, Hodes RJ, Pocinki K: What does cell death have to do with aging? J Am Geriat Soc 1997;45:1140–1146
20. Stadtman ER: Protein oxidation and aging. Science 1992;257:1220–1224
21. Conconi M, Szweda LI, Levine RL et al: Age-related protein oxidation and proteolysis during aging and decline of rat liver multicatalytic proteinase activity and protection from oxidative inactivation by heat shock protein 90. Arch Biochem Biophys 1996;331:232–240
22. Yan L-J, Levine RL, Sohal RS: Oxidative damage during aging targets mitochondrial aconitase. Proc Natl Acad Sci USA 1997;94:11168–11172
23. Yan L-J, Sohal RS: Mitochondrial adenine nucleotide translocase is modified oxidatively during aging. Proc Natl Acad Sci USA 1998;95:12896–12901
24. Ames BN, Shigenaga M, Hagen T: Oxidants, antioxidants, and the degenerative diseases of aging. Proc Natl Acad Sci USA 1993;90:7915–7922
25. Hamilton ML, Gus ZM, Fuller CD et al: A reliable assessment of 8-oxo-2-deoxyguanosine levels in nuclear and mitochondrial DNA using the sodium iodide method to isolate DNA. Nucl Acids Res 2001;29:2117–2126
26. Dolle MET, Giese H, Hopkins CL et al: Rapid accumulation of genome rearrangements in liver but not brain of old mice. Nature Genet 1997;17:431–434
27. Dolle MET, Snyder WK, Gossen JA et al: Distinct spectra of somatic mutations accumulated with age in mouse heart and small intestine. Proc Natl Acad Sci USA 2000;97:8403–8408
28. Cortopassi GA, Wong A: Mitochondria in organismal aging and degeneration. Biochem Biophys Acta 1999;1410:183–193
29. Cortopassi GA, Shibata D, Soong N-W, Arnheim N: A pattern of accumulation of a somatic deletion of mitochondrial DNA in aging human tissues. Proc Natl Acad Sci USA 1992;89:7370–7374

30. Wanagat J, Cao Z, Pathare P, Aiken JM: Mitochondrial DNA deletion mutations colocalize with segmental electron transport system abnormalities, muscle fiber atrophy, fiber splitting and oxidative damage in sarcopenia. FASEB J 2001;15:322–332

31. Khrapko K, Bodyak N, Thilly WG et al: Cell-by-cell scanning of whole mitochondrial genomes in aged human heart reveals a significant fraction of myocytes with clonally expanded deletions. Nucl Acid Res 1999;27:2434–2441

32. Michigawa Y, Mazzucchelli F, Bresolin N et al: Aging-dependent large accumulation of point mutations in the human mtDNA control region for replication. Science 1999;286:774–779

33. Gray MD, Shen JC, Kamath-Loeb AS et al: The Werner syndrome protein is a DNA helicase. Nature Genet 1997;17:100–103

34. Huang S, Li B, Gray MD et al: The premature aging syndrome protein WRN is a 3′ to 5′ exonuclease. Nature Genet 1998;20:114–116

35. Fukuchi K, Martin GM, Monnat RJ: Mutator phenotype of Werner syndrome is characterized by extensive deletions. Proc Natl Acad Sci USA 1989;86:5893–5897

36. Friguet B, Stadtman ER, Szweda LI: Modification of glucose-6-phosphate dehydrogenase by 4-hydroxy-2-nonenal: formation of cross-linked protein that inhibits the multicatalytic protease. J Biol Chem 1994;269:21639–21643

37. Nishikawa T, Edelstein D, Brownlee M: The missing link: a single unifying mechanism for diabetic complications. Kidney Int 2000;58(suppl 77):26–30

38. Lucas DT, Szweda LI: Cardiac perfusion injury: aging, lipid peroxidation and mitochondrial dysfunction. Proc Natl Acad Sci USA 1998;95:510–514

39. Lucas DT, Szweda LI: Declines in mitochondrial respiration during cardiac reperfusion: age-dependent inactivation of α-ketoglutarate dehydrogenase. Proc Natl Acad Sci USA 1999;96:6689–6693

40. Elgawish A, Glomb M, Friedlander M, Monnier VM: Involvement of hydrogen peroxide in collagen cross-linking by high glucose *in vitro* and *in vivo*. J Biol Chem 1996;271:12964–12971

41. McCay CM, Crowell MP, Maynard LA: The effect of retarded growth upon the length of the life span and upon the ultimate body size. J Nutr 1935;10:63–79

42. Masoro EJ: Caloric restriction and aging: an update. Exp Gerontol 2000;35:299–305

43. Sohal RS, Weindruch R: Oxidative stress, caloric restriction, and aging. Science 1996;273:59–63

44. Yu BP: Aging and oxidative stress: modulation by dietary restriction. Free Rad Biol Med 1996;5:651–668

45. Lal SB, Ramsey JJ, Monemdjou S et al: Effects of caloric restriction on skeletal muscle mitochondrial proton leak in aging rats. J Gerontol 2001;56A:B116–B122

46. Zainal TA, Oberley TD, Allison DB et al: Caloric restriction of rhesus monkeys lowers oxidative damage in skeletal muscle. FASEB J 2000;14:1825–1836

47. Van Remmen H, Ward WF, Sabia RV, Richardson A: Gene expression and protein degradation. In: Masoro EJ (ed): Handbook of Physiology—Aging. Oxford University Press, New York, 1995:171–234

48. Bartke A, Brown-Borg H, Mattison J et al: Prolonged longevity of hypopituitary dwarf mice. Exp Gerontol 2001;36:21–28

49. Morris JZ, Tissenbaum HA, Ruvkun GA: A phosphatidyl inositol-3-OH kinase family member regulating longevity and diapause in *Caenorhabditis elegans*. Nature 1996;382:536–539

50. Kimura KD, Tissenbaum HA, Liu Y, Ruvkun G: daf-2, an insulin receptor-like gene that regulates longevity and diapause in *Caenorhabditis elegans*. Science 1997;277:942–946

51. Rudman D, Feller AG, Nagraj HS et al: Effects of growth hormone in men over 60 years old. N Engl J Med 1990;323:1–6

52. Coschigano KT, Clemmons D, Bellush LL, Kopchick JJ: Assessment of growth parameters and life span of GHR/BP gene disrupted mice. Endocrinology 2000;141:2608–2613

53. Tatar M, Kopelman A, Epstein D et al: A mutant *Drosophila* insulin receptor homolog that extends life-span and impairs neuroendocrine function. Science 2001;292:107–109

54. Clancy DJ, Gems D, Harshman LG et al: Extension of life-span by loss of CHICO, a *Drosophila* insulin receptor substrate protein. Science 2001;292:104–106

55. Fabrizzio P, Pozza F, Pletcher SD et al: Regulation of longevity and stress resistance by *Sch9* in yeast. Science 2001;292:288–290

56. Rogina B, Reenan RA, Nilsen SP, Helfand S: Extended life-span conferred by cotransporter gene mutations in *Drosophila*. Science 2000;290:2137–2140

57. Melov S, Ravenscroft J, Malik S et al: Extension of life-span with superoxide dismutase/catalase mimetics. Science 2000;289:1567–1569

58. Raff M: Cell suicide for beginners. Nature 1998;396:119–122

59. Williams GT: Programmed cell death: apoptosis and oncogenesis. Cell 1991;65:1097–1098

60. Manolagas SC: Birth and death of bone cells: basic regulatory mechanisms and implications for the pathogenesis and treatment of osteoporosis. Endocrine Rev 2000;21:115–137

61. Ogawa N, Dang H, Talal N: Apoptosis and autoimmunity. J Autoimmun 1995;8:1–19

62. Warner HR, Fernandes G, Wang E: A unifying hypothesis to explain the retardation of aging and tumorigenesis by caloric restriction. J Gerontol 1995;50A:B107–B109

63. Grasl-Kraupp B, Bursh W, Ruttkay-Nedecky B et al: Food restriction eliminates pre-neoplastic cells through apoptosis and antagonizes carcinogenesis in rat liver. Proc Natl Acad Sci USA 1994;91:9995–9999

64. James SJ, Muskhelishvili L: Rates of apoptosis and proliferation vary with caloric intake and may influence incidence of spontaneous hepatoma in C57BL/6 × C3HF1 mice. Cancer Res 1994;54:5508–5510

65. Wang E, Lee MJ, Pandey S: Control of fibroblast senescence and activation of programmed cell death. J Cell Biochem 1994;54:432–439

66. Bellino FL, Daynes RA, Hornsby PJ et al (eds): Dehydroepiandrosterone (DHEA) and aging. Ann NY Acad Sci 1995;774

67. Nestler JE: DHEA: a coming of age. Ann NY Acad Sci 1995;774:ix–xi.

68. Pierpaoli W, Regelson W: The pineal control of aging, the effect of melatonin and pineal grafting on aging mice. Proc Natl Acad Sci USA 1994;91:787–791

69. Musaro A, McCullagh K, Paul A et al: Localized IGF-I transgene expression in senescent skeletal muscle. Nature Genet 2001;27:195–200

70. Brazelton TR, Rossi FMV, Keshet GI, Blau HM: From marrow to brain: expression of neuronal phenotypes in adult mice. Science 2000;290:1775–1779

71. Orlic D, Kajstura J, Chimenti S et al: Bone marrow cells regenerate infracted myocardium. Nature 2001;410:701–705

72. Freed CR, Greene PE, Breeze RE et al: Transplantation of embryonic dopamine neurons for severe Parkinson's disease. N Engl J Med 2001;344:710–719

73. Lee C-K, Klopp RG, Weindruch R, Prolla TA: Gene expression profile of aging and its retardation by caloric restriction. Science 1999;285:1390–1393

74. Lee C-K, Weindruch R, Prolla TA: Gene-expression profile of the ageing brain in mice. Nature Genet 2000;25:294–297

75. Han E-S, Hilsenbeck SG, Richardson A, Nelson JF: cDNA expression arrays reveal incomplete reversal of age-related changes in gene expression by caloric restriction. Mech Ageing Devel 2000;115:157–174

76. Ly DH, Lockhard DJ, Lerner RA, Schultz PG: Mitotic misregulation and human aging. Science 2000;287:2486–2492

77. Venter JC, Adams MD, Myers EW et al: The sequence of the human genome. Science 2001;291:1304–1351

78. International Human Genome Sequencing Consortium: Initial sequencing and analysis of the human genome. Nature 2001;409:860–921

79. Chakravarti A: To a future of genetic medicine. Nature 2001;409:822–823

80. Schächter F, Faure-Delanef L, Guenot F et al: Genetic associations with human longevity at the APOE and ACE loci. Nature Genet 1994;6:29–32

81. The yeast genome directory. Nature 1997;387 (May special issue)

82. The *C. elegans* Sequencing Consortium: Genome sequence of the nematode *C. elegans*: a platform for investigating biology. Science 1998;282:2012–2018

83. Adams MD, Celniker SE, Holt RA et al: The genome sequence of *Drosophila melanogaster*. Science 2000;287:2185–2195

84. Marshal E: Rat genome spurs an unusual partnership. Science 2001;291:1872

85. Chen JB, Sun J, Jazwinski SM: Prolongation of yeast life span by the *V-Ha-RAS* oncogene. Molec Microbiol 1990;4:2081–2086

86. Kim S, Benguria A, Lai CY, Jazwinski SM: Modulation of life-span by histone deacetylase genes in *Saccharomyces cerevisiae*. Mol Biol Cell 1999;10:3125–3136

87. Kaeberlein M, McVey M, Guarente L: The SIR 2/3/4 complex and SIR2 alone promote longevity in *Saccharomyces cerevisiae* by two different mechanisms. Genes Dev 1999;13:2570–2580

88. Johnson T: Increased life span of age-1 mutants in *Caenorhabditis elegans* and lower Gompertz rate of aging. Science 1990;249:908–912

89. Lin K, Dorman JB, Rodan A, Kenyon C: daf-16: an HNF-3/forkhead family member that can function to double the life span of *Caenorhabditis elegans*. Science 1997;278:1319–1322

90. Murakami S, Johnson TE: Life extension and stress resistance in *Caenorhabditis elegans* modulated by the *tkr-1* gene. Curr Biol 1999;24:1091–1094

91. Larsen PL, Albert PS, Riddle DL: Genes that regulate both development and longevity in *Caenorhabditis elegans*. Genetics 1995;139:1567–1583

92. Lin Y-J, Seroude L, Benzer S: Extended life-span and stress resistance in the *Drosophila* mutant *Methuselah*. Science 1998;282:943–946

93. Sun J, Tower J: FLP recombinase-mediated induction of Cu/Zn superoxide dismutase transgene expression can extend life span of adult *Drosophila melanogaster* flies. Mol Cell Biol 1999;19:216–228

94. Migliaccio E, Giorgio M, Mele S et al: The p66[shc] adaptor protein controls oxidative stress response and life span in mammals. Nature 1999;402:309–313

95. Brown-Borg HM, Borg KE, Meliska CJ, Bartke A: Dwarf mice and the ageing process. Nature 1996;384:33

Chapter 7

Genetic mechanisms of aging

Nicole L. Jenkins, Gawain McColl and Gordon J. Lithgow

Whilst the mechanistic and physiological causes of aging remain essentially unknown, it is clear that genes determine the rate of aging and influence the etiology of age-related disease. Consequently, genetic experimentation is key to unraveling the physiological causes of aging. Molecular genetics often provides powerful insights into complex biological processes, and mutations that radically alter the processes provide a rapid way to find major effect genes. The availability of the full sequence of the human genome has considerably increased the influence of genetic approaches. This, together with extensive transgenic analysis and functional genomic technologies, will make possible significant progress in our understanding of lifespan determination.

For the consideration of genetic mechanisms, aging is best defined by its effect on a population of animals rather than on changes within an individual animal.[1] The most reliable endpoint measured experimentally is death. Death is simultaneously straightforward to determine and generally avoids experimenter bias associated with the choice of a marker for aging.

Hence, aging is best defined as an increase in age-specific mortality rate with age. The rate of increase in mortality can be thought of as a rate of aging. Although this rate tends to be characteristic of animal species, the rate of aging is known to change radically with increasing age. For example, in late life, mortality rates do not always increase, as was once thought to be the case.[2,3] Such a demographic definition is not based on any aging theory but rather on the observation that animals that exhibit senescent changes tend to exhibit an increased probability of death with increasing age.

THE ORIGINS OF AGING GENES

Genes do determine the rate at which animals age, but it is unlikely that animals are genetically "programmed" to die. An understanding of the evolutionary origins of aging is vital for the interpretation of genetic alterations in lifespan and when contemplating interventions in aging. As mentioned elsewhere in this volume, evolutionary theories of aging suggest that aging is nonadaptive.[4–6] Under natural selection, the effect of a gene has greater consequences for fitness if it acts early in life than if it acts late in life. Genes that influence aging may exist because an allele of a gene can affect more than one process (pleiotropic effects).[7] Alleles may be selected early in life because of a beneficial effect but then have a detrimental effect later in life, and thus such genes may cause or contribute to aging. Also, as genomes move through evolutionary time, it is likely that they accumulate mutations that do not affect fitness. Some of these mutations may be detrimental in late life and may also cause aging.[8]

Based on this we can see that the effect of genes on aging is distinct from the "effect" of genes on development. Genes driving development have evolved roles that clearly define highly ordered sequential events. In contrast, major effect "aging genes" are likely to be important for processes other than aging and influence aging only indirectly.

THE GENETICS OF HUMAN LONGEVITY

Certain allelic forms of human genes are clearly the cause of specific age-related diseases or are major risk factors. These genetic effects are dealt with elsewhere in this volume. The identities of genes that effect human longevity are unclear, although efforts have been made to estimate heritability and measure the effects of candidate genes.

Twin studies indicate that up to 35 percent of longevity is heritable,[9] although estimates vary from zero to 89 percent.[10–12] The most common method of identifying individual genes responsible for the heritable component has been association studies. For example, the epsilon4 allele of Apolioprotein E (ApoE) has been reported to be associated with increased human cardiovascular disease and increased risk of Alzheimer's disease, whilst the epsilon2 allele is associated with increased longevity in French centenarians.[13] The frequency of the epsilon2 allele was also found to be significantly increased in Finnish centenarians relative to the general population.[14] However, the difficulties inherent in correlation studies are highlighted by the fact that such results are not obtained from every population studied.[15]

In contrast to a candidate gene association study, linkage analysis is an unbiased approach to finding aging genes. A study of families exhibiting exceptional longevity (131 sibships) examined markers across the entire human genome. One marker (D4S1564) exhibited linkage with longevity and indicates a major longevity effect gene located on chromosome 4.[16] Such studies are likely, in the long term, to provide novel insights into physiological determinates of the human lifespan.

Another clue to genetic influences on human aging comes from the study of the progeroid diseases. These are rare, deleterious, heritable conditions that are characterized by a short lifespan and the accelerated appearance of a range of features associated with normal aging. The gene (*WRN*) associated with the adult progeria, Werner's syndrome, encodes a member of the RecQ family of DNA helicases.[17,18] *WRN* also exhibits exonuclease activity[19–21] and interacts with the heterodimeric factor of 70 and 80 kDa implicated in the repair of double-strand DNA breaks.[22,23] Overall, it appears *WRN* is involved in recombination and transcription processes and in the DNA damage response during replication.[24] It is not yet clear how such molecular processes lead to the complex pathologies of Werner's syndrome. These complexities include heart valve calcification, intense atherosclerosis, premature hair graying, skeletal muscle atrophy, and hypogonadism. In addition, carriers of this autosomal recessive mutation also exhibit neoplasms of connective tissues. The phenotypes of mutation of homologous genes in other animals may aid these investigations.[25]

MODEL GENETIC SYSTEMS FOR AGING STUDIES

Considerable information now exists on some of the main determinates of lifespan in a range of microbial organisms and simple animal models. This is a direct consequence of genetic interventions and transgenic technology, but other factors contributing to this success include the short lifespan exhibited by many of the model systems, and the ability to maintain large populations at relatively low cost (Table 7-1). The availability of complete genome sequences and the ability to determine the levels of expression of all known genes through transcript profiling and proteomic techniques allow for a great degree of sophistication in the analysis of aging in these systems. Aging research on these organisms has developed beyond genetics to the physiology and endocrinology of aging.

Genetic mechanisms in yeast and other fungi

In the budding yeast, *Saccharomyces cerevisiae*, lifespan can be measured as the number of divisions made by mother cells.[26,27] *S. cerevisiae* divides by asymmetric budding of a small daughter cell from a larger mother cell. The mother cell continues to divide but the number of divisions is limited and the mother cell granulates and death occurs. This number defines the yeast cell's replicative lifespan and is directly related to the chronological lifespan. A second system that has been described as an aging model is the long-term survival of yeast cells in a non-growth media. In this instance, long-term survival is taken as an indication of lifespan.

At least 19 genes influence yeast replicative lifespan. The range and diversity of proteins encoded by these genes supports the existence of multiple pathways and physiological processes influencing aging.[28] Overall, however, a body of studies support the general theme that metabolic control is a key modulator of yeast aging.[29]

For example, genes encoding components of the retrograde response (RR) have been shown to influence the number of daughter cells produced. RR is a compensatory mechanism, whereby mitochondrial dysfunction signals numerous changes in nuclear gene expression, including stress-response genes.[30] Another metabolic regulator, the Ras protein, also influences yeast replicative lifespan. Yeast has two forms of Ras, each encoded by a different gene (*Ras1* and *Ras2*). If extra copies of the *Ras2* are introduced by recombinant DNA techniques, a 30 percent increase in replicative lifespan results. In contrast, *deletion* of *Ras1* is associated with lifespan extension.[28]

Other genes that influence replicative lifespan suggest that chromatin structure and wide-ranging alterations in gene expression play a role. Loss of transcriptional silencing during aging has been demonstrated in yeast.[31] As aging progresses, it is thought that there is acceleration towards inappropriate expression of genes, which may ultimately lead to loss of homeostasis. Histone deacetylases assist in maintenance of an equilibrium between transcriptionally active and silent regions of chromatin. The *sir2* gene encodes a histone deacetylase that mediates chromatin silencing in a NAD (nicotinamide adenine dinucleotide)-dependent manner.[32] Modulation of *sir2* gene activity can affect mother cell lifespan.[33] Mutations in *sir2* result in the loss of transcriptional silencing, and exhibit a decrease in lifespan, whereas expressing extra copies of *sir2* extends life span. It has been hypothesized that *sir2* may act to coordinate lifespan with nutrient availability and hence its effects may be linked with other metabolic processes.

Table 7-1 Major genetic systems for aging studies

Species	Genetic techniques	Advantages	Lifespan extension
Human	Association studies Lineage analysis	Direct relevance to human disease	
Rodent	Generation of mutants Quantitative trait mapping Transgenesis	Good recombinant DNA tools Close relationship to humans	Three single gene mutations extend lifespan
Drosophila (fruit-fly)	Generation of mutants Quantitative trait mapping Transgenesis	Short lifespan Low cost of maintenance Excellent genetic tools Good recombinant DNA tools	Selective breeding Four single gene mutations extend lifespan Transgenesis
C. elegans (nematode roundworm)	Generation of mutants Genetic mosaic analysis Quantitative trait mapping Transgenesis	Short lifespan Low cost of maintenance Excellent genetic tools Good recombinant DNA tools	Approx 100 single gene mutations extend lifespan Transgenesis
Saccharomyces cerevisiae (budding yeast)	Generation of mutants Recombinant DNA technology	Short lifespan Very low cost of maintenance Excellent genetic tools Excellent recombinant DNA tools	Single gene mutations Recombinant strains with extended lifespan

Filamentous fungi have also been utilized as an aging model as measured by limited vegetative growth. Although less frequently studied, these fungi are providing insights into the influence of mitochondrial function and aging, a theme that is also prevalent in vertebrate aging genetics.[34]

Invertebrate aging systems

The potential of using invertebrate model systems to study the genetics of aging was realized with three important experimental approaches. The first was the demonstration by Rose,[35,36] and independently by Luckinbill and coworkers, of laboratory selection experiments for longevity in the fruit-fly *Drosophila melanogaster*. Large populations of flies were subjected to selection over many generations for late-life fertility resulting in longer-lived stocks. These initial observations prompted many additional studies in which investigators looked for correlated responses as a result of such selection.[6,37] For example, some investigators reported that flies with "postponed senescence" exhibited a deficit in early fertility. In addition, longer development times and higher larval viability accompanied longevity. However, these findings were not universal and characters observed associated with longevity are dependent on the environment in which they are measured. For some selected lines the differences in mortality rate between longevity-selected and control lines are abolished when fertility is prevented.[38] This suggests that the lifespan differences derived by the laboratory selection scheme is acting on genes involved with fertility, and consequently is strong evidence for the idea that many genes determining aging also act early in life—an important prediction of evolutionary theory of aging.

The second important indicator that aging was a tractable genetic problem was the construction of recombinant inbred (RI) strains with differing lifespans of the soil nematode *Caenorhabditis elegans*.[39,40] *C. elegans* has been a major system for the study of development and a range of complex biological traits.[41] It has a simple, defined anatomy with 959 cells in the hermaphrodite. It is straightforward to grow and maintain and was the first multicellular organism to have its genome entirely sequenced. The RI strains were produced by crossing two strains followed by self-fertilization over many generations. The result is effectively a series of strains with different assortments of the contributing parental genes. The lifespan of these strains varied from 10 to 31 days and quantitative genetic strategies have been proposed for the identification of the genes that account for this variability (quantitative trait loci—QTLs).[42] Such approaches have also been undertaken in rodents where QTLs affecting age-associated immune function characters have been identified. Although these experiments spectacularly demonstrated the genetic determination of lifespan, they have not directly lead to the identification of individual genes.

The third important experimental approach has been the most successful precisely because it leads to the cloning of individual genes. In 1988, Friedman and Johnson, working with strains of *C. elegans* isolated by Mike Klass,[43] demonstrated that a single gene mutation could greatly extend lifespan.[44,45] The mutation was in a gene which Johnson called *age-1* and increased mean lifespan by 65 percent and maximum lifespan by 110 percent. The lifespan increase was a result of a slowed acceleration of the age-specific mortality rate (Gompertz rate).[46]

Single-gene age mutations in C. elegans

C. elegans normally develops through four larval stages before moulting into a reproducing adult. However, when nutrition is low at the first larval stage, the animal bypasses normal development and undergoes "dauer" formation.[47] The dauer larvae is a diapause stage that does not feed or reproduce and is also long-lived (a mean lifespan of 60 days)[48] and stress-resistant.[49] Many of the genes that influence this early life, developmental checkpoint also influence lifespan. In fact, it is generally the case that many mutants that were initially identified because of their effects on other phenotypes have subsequently been found to affect nematode lifespan. Examples of these phenotypes not only include dauer formation (e.g. *daf-2*[50]), but also fertility (e.g. *spe-10*), growth (e.g. *gro-1*[51]), chemosensory perception (e.g. *osm-1*[52]), and neurosecretory control (e.g. *unc-64*[53]). In all cases there are single gene mutations that affect both lifespan and these phenotypes, but, importantly, some single gene mutations of these classes that have no affect on lifespan. For example, mutations in either *daf-2* or *daf-4* genes affect dauer formation in *C. elegans*, but many *daf-2* mutants have increased lifespan whereas *daf-4* mutants do not.[54]

Insulin-like signaling in C. elegans

Identification of the molecular nature of mutations that extend lifespan in nematodes, coupled with genetic analysis, has lead to the discovery of a major pathway that regulates lifespan in this organism. The *age-1* gene has been shown to encode a nematode homologue of the p110 subunit of phosphatidylinositol 3-kinase (PI 3-kinase),[55] that is part of an insulin-like signaling pathway. Many other genes encoding components of this pathway have been identified. Much work has been done on *daf-2*, which is upstream of *age-1* in the insulin-like signaling pathway and encodes an insulin/IGF-1 receptor.[56] A number of mutations in the *daf-2* gene have been characterized into classes based on their observed phenotypes.[57] With strong alleles, larvae develop into dauers rather than reproductive adults. Weaker alleles develop into adults but have a variety of altered phenotypes, including formation of dauers at high temperatures, reduced fertility, stress resistance, fat accumulation, and increased longevity.

The lifespan extension of *daf-2* and *age-1* mutants are suppressed by mutations in *daf- 16*,[50,54] which places the action of this gene downstream in the insulin-like signaling pathway. *daf-16* has been identified as a forkhead/winged helix family transcription factor.[58,59] Longevity mutations of *daf-2* and *age-1* are loss-of-function mutations. In wild-type worms, under conditions of abundant food, DAF-2 and AGE-1 proteins act to indirectly suppress the activity of *daf-16*.[60] Lack of signaling in the mutants causes increased activity of *daf-16*, which leads to the observed phenotypes, including increased lifespan. The DAF-2 protein exerts its effects through functioning in neurones.[61,62]

Mutations in *daf-18* also suppress lifespan extension of *daf-2* and *age-1*.[54,63] *daf-18* is a homologue of the PTEN phosphatase, which is a negative regulator of signaling.[64–66] Comparison of this signaling pathway in *C. elegans* to insulin signaling in mammals has lead to the identification of further genes in this pathway, such as *akt-1* and *akt-2*[67] and *pdk-1*.[68]

Analysis of these single gene mutants, their molecular characterization, and their phenotypic effects indicates that aging is controlled hormonally in *C. elegans*. Lifespan extension has been postulated to occur in a number of ways, including a decrease in the overall metabolic rate[69] or a metabolic shift to fat production.[70] However, other studies are not consistent with these interpretations. For example, some potential indicators of metabolic rate has also been reported to be higher in long-lived mutants.[71]

Mutants in the insulin-like signaling pathway that increase lifespan are generally loss-of-function mutations. Not surprisingly, overexpression of some genes also leads to an extension in lifespan. For example, when transgenic worms were constructed that maintained extra copies of a tyrosine kinase-like gene, *tkr-1*, lifespan was extended.[72] This lifespan extension also required a wild-type copy of *daf-16*, indicating that *tkr-1* determines lifespan in an insulin-like signaling-dependent manner.[73]

Other C. elegans *aging mutants*

Another class of mutant that affects lifespan in *C. elegans* has a very different series of associated phenotypes. These are known as clocks (clk), a term that refers to the altered developmental and behavioral timing exhibited by these mutants.[74] Four maternal effect genes have been found that affect lifespan, embryonic and post-embryonic development, rate of egg production, fecundity, and feeding/defecation cycles.[51,75] One of these genes, *clk-1*, has also been cloned and found to have a high similarity to a yeast gene involved in mitochondrial respiration.[76] The yeast homologue encodes the protein Coq7p, a mitochondrial protein required for biosynthesis of coenzyme Q.[77] It was thought that the nematode function had diverged from that of yeast, as nematodes lacking in Q would not be expected to be viable.[76] However, it is clear that *clk-1* mutant worms do have a defect in Q synthesis and actually rely upon a dietary source for normal respiratory function, growth, and extended lifespan. However, it is not yet clear why altered regulation of Q biosynthesis leads to an extended lifespan.[78]

Together, mutations in *daf-2* and *clk-1* are associated with a synergistic increase in longevity,[75] suggesting that insulin signaling and *clk* mutations operate in separate pathways. It has been suggested that *clk* mutations may increase lifespan in a manner similar to caloric restriction (CR).[79] Mutations that affect the rate of feeding may also mimic CR. For example, a mutation in a gene called *eat-2* reduces feeding and also increases longevity. When *eat-2* was combined with *daf-2*, lifespan increased more than for each mutant alone; however, when *eat-2* was combined with *clk-1* no further increase was seen, suggesting that *eat-2* and *clk-1* act through a similar mechanism.[79]

A class of Age mutants that are involved in sensory perception have been identified and are associated with a variety of defects including cilia defects (*daf-10, daf-19, osm-1, osm-5, osm-6, che-2, che-3, che-11, che-13*), support cell defects (*daf-6, mec-8, osm-3*), and signal transduction defects (*tax-2, tax-4*).[52] As with mutants in the insulin-like signaling pathway, the lifespan extension of these mutants is suppressed by *daf-16*.

However, in this case suppression is not complete, suggesting a *daf-16* independent pathway may exist downstream of some of these functions.

Single gene mutations in the fruit-fly Drosophila melanogaster

Recent work in *D. melanogaster* provides evidence that the role of an insulin/IGF signaling pathway in aging has been conserved across large evolutionary distances and that it is not just a peculiarity of *C. elegans* physiology. In *Drosophila*, reduced insulin/IGF signaling has been shown to mediate lifespan extensions. The *InR* gene encodes the insulin-like receptor, where specific heteroallelic combinations of mutations can increase lifespan by up to 85 percent.[80] However, these effects do differ with sex, with high early then reduced late adult mortality seen in males. Tatar and coworkers suggest that *InR* affects the neurosecretory regulation of juvenile hormone, the regulator of insect reproductive diapause. Adult *D. melanogaster* have reduced aging rates during diapause. Thus, lifespan extension phenotypes of *InR* mutants may represent ectopic expression of physiological strategies characteristic of diapause.[81]

Mutation of the gene encoding the insulin receptor substrate, Chico, also increases adult lifespan.[82] Again the greatest effects are seen in females, where homozygous mutants exhibit up to 41 percent increase in maximum lifespan. However, in *Drosophila*, the correspondence between lifespan effects and stress resistance characteristic of *C. elegans* insulin/IGF signaling mutants is not as clear. Heat resistance is not altered but resistance to oxidative stress is slightly increased, with elevated levels of the antioxidant enzyme superoxide dismutase.

Other single gene mutations that extend lifespan have been uncovered in *Drosophila*. Mutation of a gene called *Indy* ("I'm not dead yet") was found to extend heterozygote lifespan by 15–80 percent (depending on the genetic background).[83] *Indy* encodes a protein homologous to a mammalian sodium dicarboxyate cotransporter, a membrane transporter of Krebs cycle intermediates. The adult localization of the INDY protein includes the fat body, mid-gut, and oenocytes, the key sites of metabolite absorption, storage, and intermediary metabolism. The mutant phenotype may mimic the metabolic state seen in caloric-restricted individuals. With respect to other life history traits, no decrease was observed in fertility and fecundity across lifespan or developmental timing.

Mutation of another *Drosophila* gene, *methuselah*, has been found to give a 35 percent increase in lifespan.[84] This mutation also confers resistance to a variety of stressors, including heat, starvation, and paraquat (a generator of oxygen free radicals). The process by which *methuselah* regulates lifespan and stress resistance remains unclear. The *methuselah* gene encodes a novel G-protein coupled receptor. This large family of membrane-bound receptors are typically involved in mediating signals into the cell, which suggests the *methuselah*-encoded protein may be a component of a novel stress signaling pathway.[84]

The mouse lifespan mutants

Genetic studies in lifespan determination in complex eukaryotic systems have not progressed to match the studies exploiting simple eukaryotic model systems. However, a number of examples of single gene mutations that prolong lifespan have been observed.

Two highly compelling examples are the Snell and Ames dwarf mouse strains. These strains carry mutations in the pituitary-1 (*Pit-1*) gene and profit of pit-1 (*Prop-1*) gene, respectively.[85] *Pit-1* is a homeotic gene required for the differentiation of somatotrophs, lactotrophs, and thyrotrophs; hence mutant animals display a serve pituitary deficiency.[86] *Prop-1* is required for the normal development of cells that express *Pit-1*. Animals homozygous for either of the mutant genes are generally infertile. Brown-Borg and coworkers demonstrated that the homozygous *Prop-1* genotype was also leading to at least a 40 percent increase in mean lifespan.[85] The Snell mouse is also long-lived.[87] Although these mutations lead to longevity, they are clearly highly detrimental. As to the reasons for longevity, they do exhibit elevated antioxidant enzyme activities and a lowered metabolic rate, consistent with oxygen radical theory discussed below.[88] It seems likely that a growth hormone (GH) deficiency may contribute to longevity as suggested by the discovery that a GH receptor mutant mouse exhibits a 55 percent increase in lifespan.

Migliaccio et al.[89] have provided another example of a gene that appears to limit lifespan in a vertebrate system, this being mammalian proto-oncogene SHC locus (*p66^{shc}*). A single targeted mutation in the gene encoding the p66^{shc} was found to confer an increase of 30 percent in the lifespan of homozygous mutant mice. p66^{shc} is a cytoplasmic signal transducer with roles in mitogenic signaling from activated receptors to Ras. In addition, embryo fibroblasts (MEFs) from these p66^{shc−/−} mice exhibit heightened resistance to agents that cause oxidative damage (hydrogen peroxide and UV light).[89]

Conservation of aging mechanisms from yeast to mammals

Although there are many genes reported to increase lifespan in model systems, what does this mean for other organisms? Some of these genes are likely to be organism-specific, but most of those identified also have orthologues in other organisms. The existence of aging genes and maintenance of co- phenotypes suggests underlying and conserved regulatory mechanisms. In particular, it seems that genes involved in repair of oxidative damage and general stress resistance mechanisms are likely to be commonly involved in many species. Genetics provides a direct route to assess commonality of aging mechanisms in diverse species.

A very good example of such conservation of gene influence in aging comes from studies that indicate that *sir-2* gene silencing may affect lifespan of both the nematode and yeast.[90,91] *C. elegans* has four genes with similarity to the yeast *sir2*, the most homologous being *sir2.1*. A number of strains with duplications of various chromosomal regions were used to assess whether any of the *sir2* homologues affected nematode lifespan. Comparison of strains with a duplication of chromosome IV containing the gene *sir2.1* and those with a duplication of chromosome IV that had 90 percent similarity but lacked *sir2.1* indicated that extra copies of *sir2.1* increased both mean and maximum lifespan. These results were confirmed using transgenic lines overexpressing just *sir2.1*. The lifespan

extension in the transgenic lines was suppressed by mutation of *daf-16*, indicating that *sir2.1* is likely to be involved in silencing genes upstream of the insulin-like signaling pathway.[91] Assuming the same mode of action of *sir2* in both systems, these results suggest that some genetic mechanisms of aging are indeed conserved across species.

THE OXYGEN RADICAL THEORY OF AGING

Aging research has been strongly influenced by a number of theories but none more so than the free radical theory of aging. Genetic variants with extended lifespan have been used to test the oxygen radical theory of aging and there is mounting evidence that oxygen radicals do indeed play a role in determining lifespan.

Evidence that oxidative damage may be important in aging in *C. elegans* comes from the increased resistance to oxidative stress found in both *age-1*[92] and *daf-2*[93] mutants. Age mutants have higher levels of superoxide dismutase (SOD) and catalase and *daf-2* has elevated Mn-SOD mRNA and accumulates oxidative damage slowly. *daf-2* also has elevated Mtl-1 mRNA[94] which encodes the metal regulating protein, metallothionin. Similarly, *Drosophila* InR and Chico mutants both express elevated levels of SOD.[80,82] It has also been found that *C. elegans* mutants that exhibit an accelerated increase in oxidative damage, such as *mev-1* and *ctl-1*, have shortened lifespans. *mev-1* mutants have a defect in the mitochondrial electron transport chain; the *mev-1* gene encodes a subunit of succinate dehydrogenase cytochrome b.[95] This leads to increased oxidative damage, evident by the accumulation of lipofuscin granules. Similarly, increased oxidative damage is found in *ctl-1* mutants which lack a cytosolic catalase that is thought to be a general defense against oxygen radicals. Mutants in *Drosophila* that lack catalase[96] and SOD[97] also exhibit decreased lifespan, and a correlated increase in sensitivity to oxidative stress. Mice that are lacking the mitochondrial enzyme MnSOD also have multiple pathologies and drastically reduced lifespan.[98] In addition, it has been demonstrated that treating *mev-1* mutants with antioxidant compounds rescues their lifespan deficit.[99] Treating wild-type worms with these compounds also increases longevity by an average of 44 percent. In flies, simultaneous overexpression of catalase and Cu/Zn-SOD in adults has been reported to extend lifespan by up to 34 percent.[100] More recently, overexpression of Cu/Zn-SOD alone extended lifespan by up to 48 percent, and overexpression of catalase alone was found to increase stress resistance, but not lifespan.[101] Overexpression of human SOD1 in *Drosophila* motorneurons alone also increases both stress resistance and lifespan.[102]

GENETICS, STRESS RESISTANCE, AND AGING

Oxidative damage may not be the only stress to influence aging. Mutations that increase longevity in *C. elegans* are not just resistant to oxidative stress, but also have increased resistance to a range of stressors, including heat[103,104] and UV radiation.[105] As alluded to previously, the *methuselah* mutant in fruit-flies is also resistant to multiple stressors.[84] It is possible that general repair mechanisms are important in increasing longevity in such mutants.

Mild or nonlethal stress pretreatments have been shown to increase longevity in *C. elegans*[104] and *Drosophila*.[106] These experiments are consistent with the idea that increased levels of stress response proteins can confer increased lifespan. In addition, increased levels of hsp22 RNA levels have been reported in *Drosophila* lines that have been genetically selected for increased longevity.[107] Tatar and coworkers demonstrated directly that increasing levels of a stress response protein, HSP-70, conferred extended lifespan.[108] As it is thought that HSP-70 protects cells during stress by preventing protein aggregation, this work points to the possibility that maintaining protein conformation is an important factor determining lifespan.[109]

THE NEW BIOLOGY OF AGING

The genetic manipulation of model organisms has provided a key breakthrough in the biology of aging. Critically, it is now known that some genetic mechanisms have a large influence on the rate of aging. This is apparent in the identification of signaling pathways affecting the lifespan of nematodes and fruit-flies, and in the discovery of large effect loci in human longevity facilitated by the human genome project. In model systems the studies of lifespan have moved well beyond genetic analysis to experimentation on the endocrine and physiological mechanisms. As a result some commonality in lifespan determination is emerging. For example, there appears to be a strong correlation between stress resistance and lifespan extension and this may be due to oxidative stress being a major cause of aging. In addition, there are many instances of aging being influenced by processes that are also involved in nutrition sensing and metabolism. It is expected that studies on such processes will be informative in the long-standing question of why caloric restriction extends mammalian lifespan. Whilst the molecular and physiological causes of aging are still not fully understood, genetic experimentation has proved essential for identifying such processes.

KEY POINTS Genetic mechanisms of aging

- Genetic techniques are key to determining the nature and causes of aging.

- Aging is a nonadaptive process such that genes influencing aging rate generally affect other life history processes.

- Mutations in single genes can have large positive affects on lifespan.

- Genetic interventions in aging demonstrate that invertebrate lifespan is influenced by a range of neuroendocrine signaling and metabolic processes.

- Some commonality in aging mechanisms between diverse species is apparent.

- Genetic variability is likely to account for a significant fraction of human lifespan variability, and genes with major effects can be identified.

REFERENCES

1. Finch CE: Longevity, Senescence and the Genome. University of Chicago Press, Chicago, 1990
2. Carey JR, Liedo P, Orozco D, Vaupel JW: Slowing of mortality rates at older ages in large medfly cohorts. Science 1992;258:457–461
3. Fukui HH, Xiu L, Curtsinger JW: Slowing of age-specific mortality rates in *Drosophila melanogaster*. Exp Gerontol 1993;28:585–599
4. Medawar PB: An Unsolved Problem of Biology. H. K. Lewis, London, 1952
5. Kirkwood TBL, Holliday R: The evolution of ageing and longevity. Proc R Soc Lond B 1979;205:531–546
6. Rose MR: Evolutionary Biology of Aging. Oxford University Press, New York, 1991
7. Williams GC: Pleiotropy, natural selection, and the evolution of senescence. Evolution 1957;11:398–411
8. Hamilton WD: The moulding of senescence by natural selection. J Theor Biol 1966;12:12–45
9. McGue M, Vaupel JW, Holm N, Harvald B: Longevity is moderately heritable in a sample of Danish twins born 1870–1880. J Gerontol A 1993;48:B237–B244
10. Korpelainen H: Variation in the heritability and evolvability of human lifespan. Naturwissenschaften 2000;87:566–568
11. Korpelainen H: Genetic maternal effects on human life span through the inheritance of mitochondrial DNA. Hum Hered 1999;49:183–185
12. Herskind AM et al: The heritability of human longevity: a population-based study of 2872 Danish twin pairs born 1870–1900. Hum Genet 1996;97:319–323
13. Schachter F et al: Genetic associations with human longevity at the APOE and ACE loci. Nat Genet 1994;6:29–32
14. Frisoni GB, Louhija J, Geroldi C, Trabucchi M: Longevity and the epsilon2 allele of apolipoprotein E: the Finnish Centenarians Study. J Gerontol A 2001;56:M75–M78
15. Galinsky D et al: Analysis of the apo E/apo C-I, angiotensin converting enzyme and methylenetetrahydrofolate reductase genes as candidates affecting human longevity. Atherosclerosis 1997;129:177–183
16. Puca AA et al: A genome-wide scan for linkage to human exceptional longevity identifies a locus on chromosome 4. Proc Natl Acad Sci USA 2001;98:10505–10508
17. Gray MD et al: The Werner syndrome protein is a DNA helicase. Nat Genet 1997;17:100–103
18. Martin GM: The Werner mutation: does it lead to a "public" or "private" mechanism of aging? Mol Med 1997;3:356–358
19. Huang S et al: The premature ageing syndrome protein, WRN, is a 3'→5' exonuclease. Nat Genet 1998;20:114–116
20. Kamath-Loeb AS, Shen JC, Loeb LA, Fry M: Werner syndrome protein. II: Characterization of the integral 3'→5' DNA exonuclease. J Biol Chem 1998;273:34145–34150
21. Shen JC et al: Werner syndrome protein. I: DNA helicase and dna exonuclease reside on the same polypeptide. J Biol Chem 1998;273:34139–34144
22. Orren DK et al: A functional interaction of Ku with Werner exonuclease facilitates digestion of damaged DNA. Nucleic Acids Res 2001;29:1926–1934
23. Li B, Comai L: Requirements for the nucleolytic processing of DNA ends by the Werner syndrome protein–Ku70/80 complex. J Biol Chem 2001;276:9896–9902
24. Oshima J: The Werner syndrome protein: an update. Bioessays 2000;22:894–901
25. Kusano K, Berres ME, Engels WR: Evolution of the RECQ family of helicases: a drosophila homolog, Dmblm, is similar to the human bloom syndrome gene. Genetics 1999;151:1027–1039
26. Sinclair D, Mills K, Guarente L: Aging in *Saccharomyces cerevisiae*. Annu Rev Microbiol 1998;52:533–560
27. Jazwinski SM: Coordination of metabolic activity and stress resistance in yeast longevity. Results Probl Cell Differ 2000;29:21–44
28. Jazwinski SM: Longevity, genes, and aging: a view provided by a genetic model system. Exp Gerontol 1999;34:1–6
29. Jazwinski SM: Metabolic control and gene dysregulation in yeast aging. Ann NY Acad Sci 2000;908:21–30
30. Kirchman PA, Kim S, Lai CY, Jazwinski SM: Interorganelle signaling is a determinant of longevity in *Saccharomyces cerevisiae*. Genetics 1999;152:179–190

31. Defossez PA, Lin SJ, McNabb DS: Sound silencing: the Sir2 protein and cellular senescence. Bioessays 2001;23:327–332

32. Imai S, Armstrong CM, Kaeberlein M, Guarente L: Transcriptional silencing and longevity protein Sir2 is an NAD-dependent histone deacetylase. Nature 2000;403:795–800

33. Kaeberlein M, McVey M, Guarente L: The SIR2/3/4 complex and SIR2 alone promote longevity in Saccharomyces cerevisiae by two different mechanisms. Genes Dev 1999;13:2570–2580

34. Borghouts C, Osiewacz HD: Nuclear–mitochondrial interactions involved in aging in Podospora anserina. Ann NY Acad Sci 2000;908:291–294

35. Hutchinson EW, Rose MR: Quantitative genetics of postponed aging in Drosophila melanogaster. I: Analysis of outbred populations. Genetics 1991;127:719–727

36. Hutchinson EW, Shaw AJ, Rose MR: Quantitative genetics of postponed aging in Drosophila melanogaster. II: Analysis of selected lines. Genetics 1991;127:729–737

37. Partridge L: Evolutionary theories of ageing applied to long-lived organisms. Exp Gerontol 2001;36:641–650

38. Sgro CM, Partridge L: A delayed wave of death from reproduction in Drosophila. Science 1999;286:2521–2524

39. Johnson TE, Wood WB: Genetic analysis of life-span in Caenorhabditis elegans. Proc Natl Acad Sci USA 1982;79:6603–6607

40. Brooks A, Johnson TE: Genetic specification of life span and self-fertility in recombinant-inbred strains of Caenorhabditis elegans. Heredity 1991;67:19–28

41. Riddle et al. In Riddle DR, Blumenthal T, Meyer BJ, Priess JR (eds): C. elegans II. CSHL, New York, 1997:1–22

42. Shook DR, Brooks A, Johnson TE: Mapping quantitative trait loci affecting life history traits in the nematode Caenorhabditis elegans. Genetics 1996;142:801–817

43. Klass MR: A method for the isolation of longevity mutants in the nematode Caenorhabditis elegans and initial results. Mech Ageing Dev 1983;22:279–286

44. Friedman DB, Johnson TE: A mutation in the age-1 gene in Caenorhabditis elegans lengthens life and reduces hermaphrodite fertility. Genetics 1988;118:75–86

45. Friedman DB, Johnson TE: Three mutants that extend both mean and maximum life span of the nematode, Caenorhabditis elegans, define the age-1 gene. J Gerontol A 1988;43:B102–B109

46. Johnson TE: Increased life-span of age-1 mutants in Caenorhabditis elegans and lower Gompertz rate of aging. Science 1990;249:908–912

47. Riddle DL, Albert PS. In Riddle DL, Blumenthal T, Meyer BJ, Priess JR (eds): C. elegans II. CSHP, New York, 1997:739–768

48. Klass M, Hirsh D: Non-ageing developmental variant of Caenorhabditis elegans. Nature 1976;260:523–525

49. Anderson GL: Responses of dauer larvae of Caenorhabditis elegans (Nematoda: Rhabditidae) to thermal stress and oxygen deprivation. Can J Zool 1978;56:1786–1791

50. Kenyon C, Chang J, Gensch E, Rudner A, Tabtiang R: A C. elegans mutant that lives twice as long as wild type. Nature 1993;366:461–464

51. Hekimi S, Boutis P, Lakowski B: Viable maternal-effect mutations that affect the development of the nematode Caenorhabditis elegans. Genetics 1995;141:1351–1364

52. Apfeld J, Kenyon C: Regulation of lifespan by sensory perception in Caenorhabditis elegans. Nature 1999;402:804–809

53. Ailion M, Inoue T, Weaver CI, Holdcraft RW, Thomas JH: Neurosecretory control of aging in Caenorhabditis elegans. Proc Natl Acad Sci USA 1999;96:7394–7397

54. Larsen PL, Albert PS, Riddle DL: Genes that regulate development and longevity in Caenorhabditis elegans. Genetics 1995;139:1567–1583

55. Morris JZ, Tissenbaum HA, Ruvkun G: A phosphatidylinositol-3-OH kinase family member regulating longevity and diapause in Caenorhabditis elegans. Nature 1996;382:536–539

56. Kimura KD, Tissenbaum HA, Liu Y, Ruvkun G: daf-2, an insulin receptor-like gene that regulates longevity and diapause in Caenorhabditis elegans. Science 1997;277:942–946

57. Gems D et al: Two pleiotropic classes of daf-2 mutation affect larval arrest, adult behavior, reproduction and longevity in Caenorhabditis elegans. Genetics 1998;150:129–155

58. Ogg S et al: The Fork head transcription factor DAF-16 transduces insulin-like metabolic and longevity signals in C. elegans. Nature 1997;389:994–999

59. Lin K, Dorman JB, Rodan A, Kenyon C: daf-16: an HNF-3/forkhead family member that can function to double the life-span of Caenorhabditis elegans. Science 1997;278:1319–1322

60. Gottlieb S, Ruvkun G: daf-2, daf-16 and daf-23: genetically interacting genes controlling dauer formation in Caenorhabditis elegans. Genetics 1994;137:107–120

61. Apfeld J, Kenyon C: Cell nonautonomy of C. elegans daf-2 function in the regulation of diapause and life span. Cell 1998;95:199–210

62. Wolkow CA, Kimura KD, Lee MS, Ruvkun G: Regulation of C. elegans life-span by insulin-like signaling in the nervous system. Science 2000;290:147–150

63. Dorman JB, Albinder B, Shroyer T, Kenyon C: The age-1 and daf-2 genes function in a common pathway to control the lifespan of Caenorhabditis elegans. Genetics 1995;141:1399–1406

64. Ogg S, Ruvkun G: The C. elegans PTEN homolog, DAF-18, acts in the insulin receptor-like metabolic signaling pathway. Mol Cell 1998;2:887–893

65. Rouault JP et al: Regulation of dauer larva development in Caenorhabditis elegans by daf-18, a homologue of the tumour suppressor PTEN. Curr Biol 1999;9:329–332

66. Kokel M, Borland CZ, DeLong L, Horvitz HR, Stern MJ: clr-1 encodes a receptor tyrosine phosphatase that negatively regulates an FGF receptor signaling pathway in Caenorhabditis elegans. Genes Dev 1998;12:1425–1437

67. Paradis S, Ruvkun G: Caenorhabditis elegans Akt/PKB transduces insulin receptor-like signals from AGE-1 PI3 kinase to the DAF-16 transcription factor. Genes Dev 1998;12:2488–2498

68. Paradis S, Ailion M, Toker A, Thomas JH, Ruvkun G: A PDK1 homolog is necessary and sufficient to transduce AGE-1 PI3 kinase signals that regulate diapause in Caenorhabditis elegans. Genes Dev 1999;13:1438–1452

69. Van Voorhies WA, Ward S: Genetic and environmental conditions that increase longevity in Caenorhabditis elegans decrease metabolic rate. Proc Natl Acad Sci USA 1999;96:11399–11403

70. Kimura KD, Tissenbaum HA, Liu Y, Ruvkun G: daf-2, an insulin receptor-like gene that regulates longevity and diapause in Caenorhabditis elegans. Science 1997;277:942–946

71. Vanfleteren JR, De Vreese A: The gerontogenes age-1 and daf-2 determine metabolic rate potential in aging Caenorhabditis elegans. FASEB J 1995;9:1355–1361

72. Murakami S, Johnson TE: Life extension and stress resistance in Caenorhabditis elegans modulated by the tkr-1 gene. Curr Biol 1998;8:1091–1094

73. Murakami S, Tedesco PM, Cypser JR, Johnson TE: Molecular genetic mechanisms of life span manipulation in Caenorhabditis elegans. Ann NY Acad Sci 2000;908:40–49

74. Wong A, Boutis P, Hekimi S: Mutations in the clk-1 gene of Caenorhabditis elegans affect developmental and behavioral timing. Genetics 1995;139:1247–1259

75. Lakowski B, Hekimi S: Determination of life-span in Caenorhabditis elegans by four clock genes. Science 1996;272:1010–1013

76. Felkai S et al: CLK-1 controls respiration, behavior and aging in the nematode Caenorhabditis elegans. EMBO J 1999;18:1783–1792

77. Jonassen T et al: Yeast Clk-1 homologue (Coq7/Cat5) is a mitochondrial protein in coenzyme Q synthesis. J Biol Chem 1998;273:3351–3357

78. Jonassen T, Larsen PL, Clarke CF: A dietary source of coenzyme Q is essential for growth of long-lived Caenorhabditis elegans clk-1 mutants. Proc Natl Acad Sci USA 2001;98:421–426

79. Lakowski B, Hekimi S: The genetics of caloric restriction in Caenorhabditis elegans. Proc Natl Acad Sci USA 1998;95:13091–13096

80. Tatar M et al: A mutant Drosophila insulin receptor homolog that extends life-span and impairs neuroendocrine function. Science 2001;292:107–110

81. Tatar M, Yin C: Slow aging during insect reproductive diapause: why butterflies, grasshoppers and flies are like worms. Exp Gerontol 2001;36:723–738

82. Clancy DJ et al: Extension of life-span by loss of CHICO, a Drosophila insulin receptor substrate protein. Science 2001;292:104–106

83. Rogina B, Benzer S, Helfand SL: Drosophila drop-dead mutations accelerate the time course of age-related markers. Proc Natl Acad Sci USA 1997;94:6303–6306

84. Lin YJ, Seroude L, Benzer S: Extended life-span and stress resistance in the Drosophila mutant methuselah. Science 1998;282:943–946

85. Brown-Borg HM, Borg KE, Meliska CJ, Bartke A: Dwarf mice and the ageing process. Nature 1996;384:33

86. Bartke A et al: Prolonged longevity of hypopituitary dwarf mice. Exp Gerontol 2001;36:21–28

87. Flurkey K, Papaconstantinou J, Miller RA, Harrison DE: Lifespan extension and delayed immune and collagen aging in mutant mice with defects in growth hormone production. Proc Natl Acad Sci USA 2001;98:6736–6741

88. Hauck SJ, Bartke A: Effects of growth hormone on hypothalamic catalase and Cu/Zn superoxide dismutase. Free Radic Biol Med 2000;28:970–978

89. Migliaccio E et al: The p66shc adaptor protein controls oxidative stress response and life span in mammals. Nature 1999;402:309–313

90. Guarente L: SIR2 and aging. Trends Genet 2001;17:391–392

91. Tissenbaum HA, Guarente L: Increased dosage of *a sir-2* gene extends lifespan in *Caenorhabditis elegans*. Nature 2001;410:227–230

92. Larsen PL: Aging and resistance to oxidative damage in *Caenorhabditis elegans*. Proc Natl Acad Sci USA 1993;90:8905–8909

93. Honda Y, Honda S: The *daf-2* gene network for longevity regulates oxidative stress resistance and Mn-superoxide dismutase gene expression in *Caenorhabditis elegans*. FASEB J 1999;13:1385–1393

94. Barsyte D, Lovejoy DA, Lithgow GJ: Longevity and heavy metal resistance in *daf-2* and *age-1* long-lived mutants of *Caenorhabditis elegans*. FASEB J 2001;15:627–634

95. Ishii N et al: A mutation in succinate dehydrogenase cytochrome b causes oxidative stress and ageing in nematodes. Nature 1998;394:694–697

96. Mackay WJ, Bewley GC: The genetics of catalase in *Drosophila melanogaster*: isolation and characterization of acatalasemic mutants. Genetics 1989;122:643–652

97. Phillips JP, Campbell SD, Michaud D, Charbonneau M, Hilliker AJ: Null mutation of copper/zinc superoxide dismutase in *Drosophila* confers hypersensitivity to paraquat and reduced longevity. Proc Natl Acad Sci USA 1989;86:2761–2765

98. Melov S et al: A novel neurological phenotype in mice lacking mitochondrial manganese superoxide dismutase. Natl Genet 1998;18:159–163

99. Melov S et al: Extension of life-span with superoxide dismutase/catalase mimetics. Science 2000;289:1567–1569

100. Orr WC, Sohal RS: Extension of life-span by overexpression of superoxide dismutase and catalase in *Drosophila melanogaster*. Science 1994;263:1128–1130

101. Sun J, Tower J: FLP recombinase-mediated induction of Cu/Zn-superoxide dismutase transgene expression can extend the life span of adult *Drosophila melanogaster* flies. Mol Cell Biol 1999;19:216–228

102. Parkes TL et al: Extension of *Drosophila* lifespan by overexpression of human SOD1 in motorneurons. Nat Genet 1998;19:171–174

103. Lithgow GJ, White TM, Hinerfeld DA, Johnson TE: Thermotolerance of a long-lived mutant of *Caenorhabditis elegans*. J Gerontol A 1994;49:B270–B276

104. Lithgow GJ, White TM, Melov S, Johnson TE: Thermotolerance and extended life span conferred by single-gene mutations and induced by thermal stress. Proc Natl Acad Sci USA 1995;92:7540–7544

105. Murakami S, Johnson TE: A genetic pathway conferring life extension and resistance to UV stress in *Caenorhabditis elegans*. Genetics 1996;143:1207–1218

106. Maynard Smith J: Prolongation of the life of *Drosophila subobscura* by brief exposure of adults to a high temperature. Nature 1958;181:496–497

107. Kurapati R, Passananti HB, Rose MR, Tower J: Increased hsp22 RNA levels in *Drosophila* lines genetically selected for increased longevity. J Gerontol A 2000;55:B552–B559

108. Tatar M, Khazaeli AA, Curtsinger JW: Chaperoning extended life. Nature 1997;390:30

109. Lithgow GJ. In Schneider EL, Rowe JW (eds): Handbook of the Biology of Aging. Academic Press, San Diego, 1996:55–73

Chapter 8

Cellular mechanisms of aging

Ioan Davies

All multicellular organisms undergo changes with time through a progression of development, reproductive maturity, aging, and death, although age changes are not easily recognized until the post-reproductive stages of the lifespan. In mammals, the expression of the aging phenotype takes place progressively over a long time-scale, but even so attributing an accurate chronological age to an organism is often difficult. Some of the crude markers of aging in humans include loss of height, a reduction in lean body mass, graying of hair, wrinkling of skin, changes in eyesight, and to some extent reduced coordination of movement. However, all these changes are not necessarily present in an elderly individual, although they are described as features of "normal" aging.

This chapter sets out to (1) define aging and discuss some of the issues involved in identifying aging changes; and (2) evaluate critically some of the recent progress in investigating cellular and molecular aging, including:

- age changes in vitro and in vivo
- genomic stability
- gene expression.

Of necessity the material is highly selected. The chapter covers the major growth areas rather than trying to cover the whole field. However, an historical perspective is given for each area since experience shows that readers consulting a textbook have slightly different requirements from those reading in-depth scientific reviews.

A common definition of aging is presented in the box.[1] Aging occurs at many different levels: social, psychological (behavioral), physiological, morphological, cellular, and molecular. A definition encompassing all of these strata does

Definition of aging

Aging is characterized by a failure to maintain homeostasis under conditions of physiological stress. This failure is associated with a decrease in viability, and an increase in vulnerability, of the individual.

not exist, and may be impossible. Strehler[2] introduced four criteria to help separate aging from other time-related changes of development, maturation, and age-associated disease; these criteria included the concept of changes being universal to a species, degenerative, progressive, and intrinsic. However, no specific biological event features in the definition, or the limiting criteria, so they remain unsatisfactory.

Our problems become greater when we try to extend the definition to aging cells. No one disputes that cells undergo age changes, but how do we know if a cell is young or old? Indeed, is aging the same in mitotic and terminally differentiated cells, or is cellular aging the same in vitro and in vivo? Since this is a chapter in a textbook of geriatric medicine, the links between the physiological functioning of the whole organism and its cells and molecules will be maintained as much as possible. Biological gerontologists generally believe that age changes in cells lead to tissue and organ deficiencies and ultimately the expression of aging, and/or disease. Most gerontology textbooks show plots of physiological function against time. The graphs of nerve conduction velocity, cardiac index, maximum breathing capacity, and glomerular filtration rate show a considerable decline with age (Fig. 8-1). These findings are usually from cross-sectional studies and show a decrease

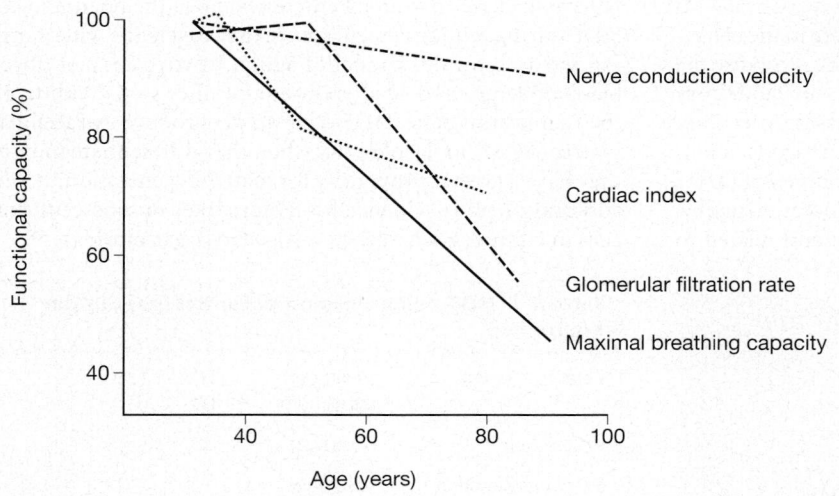

Figure 8-1 Changes in the effectiveness of several human physiological functions with age.

Nerve conduction velocity

Cardiac index

Glomerular filtration rate

Maximal breathing capacity

in physiological effectiveness from about the age of 35 years onwards. While these data have limitations, they generally support our "definition" of aging showing a potential increase in the vulnerability of multicellular organisms with time. Measuring complex physiological functions shows the degenerative change found in older animals and underscores the loss of integration of finely tuned regulatory mechanisms. The central thesis of cellular and molecular gerontology is that the breakdown of this complex system has an explanation based in altered cellular and molecular function.

Clearly, it is impossible to derive detailed explanations of the aging process simply by studying humans, and much of the information in this chapter is collected from a variety of sources. Laboratory rodents, frequently "specific pathogen free" and usually inbred, form the backbone of material for researching tissue, and cellular, age changes in vivo.[3,4] Recent papers have challenged this approach. Data from genetically homogeneous rodents may not be ideal for many investigations, and the use of heterogeneous mice and rats would allow researchers to reach more robust conclusions, less likely to reflect strain-specific peculiarities.[5] Invertebrates have always figured in gerontological research;[1,6] *Drosophila melanogaster* has had an illustrious career,[6] and the nematode *Caenorhabditis elegans* has been at the forefront of recent genetic approaches.[7] These metazoan invertebrates are useful because their genetics are well understood; they have a mainly nonmitotic cell population and a short lifespan, and they are easily manipulated in strictly controlled environments. However, they do have significant drawbacks; little is known about the physiology and pathology of aging in these animals, and the relative simplicity of their organization, particularly the number of different cell types contributing to tissue and organ structure, makes it difficult to extrapolate from invertebrates to vertebrates. Studies on human cells are also important since changes seen here more likely pertain to alterations in patients. To many this focus on human material is the raison d'être for aging research, and in vitro techniques offer the option of studying human mitotic cells directly.[8]

Gerontological research has a number of confounding factors. Research into mechanisms of aging using a particular species is a relatively straightforward matter; the problem comes when we try to extrapolate from one species to another. This is a major issue particularly when extrapolating from invertebrates to mammals, or from studies of single cells in culture to the behavior of cells in vivo. However, many studies fail to recognize the primary importance of pathological changes in laboratory animals. Early research detected marked increases in albumin synthesis by the liver in rodents during the lifespan.[9] Explanations for this increase in protein synthesis included compensation for genomic damage from somatic mutations or other errors;[9,10] however, the reason was more commonplace and related to the development of kidney pathology in old rodents. The result of age-associated kidney disease in rodents is proteinuria leading to a compensatory increase in plasma protein, particularly albumin, synthesis by the liver. Similarly, healthy donors should supply the cells used in basic gerontological research; otherwise significant errors of interpretation can be made (see later). This topic is discussed elsewhere,[11] but the study of changes in cellular function with age present many challenges (confounding factors are listed in the box).

CELL AGING

There are numerous manifestations of cell aging. Histological studies of tissues and organs from aged individuals reveal evidence for atrophy, cell death, and neoplasia.[11] However, the explanation of functional changes in tissues and organs with increasing age is a difficult problem, particularly when they are composed of several different cell types. Since the early twentieth century, researchers have been developing culture techniques to investigate the functional behavior of individual cells.[12] Eventually it was shown that cells from a variety of normal human tissues proliferate in culture only for a defined period before degenerating and apparently dying.[13] These cultured cells are known as human diploid, fibroblast-like (HDF) cells, and they divide only a certain number of times before the rate of division slows and eventually ceases. The cells are said to have undergone replicative senescence (the "Hayflick" limit), and it was argued that this process was equivalent to the cellular expression of aging in vivo.[14]

The phenotype of HDF in vitro

Accumulated population doublings are the principal measure of the age of a cell in culture (Table 8-1). The cells display different growth characteristics at different stages of the culture cycle. In the early stages of growth, cells proliferate rapidly and the sub-cultivation intervals are short; but in the senescent phase of the culture, the cells become larger and divide more slowly. The average number of population doublings of fetal lung and skin fibroblasts, before the senescent phase, is approximately 50, and the total number of doublings is 63 (Fig. 8-2).[14] Norwood et al.[8] give an extensive review of the phenotype of HDF during replicative senescence that covers the wide-ranging research on this model of aging. In vitro dermal fibroblasts undergo marked alterations after they stop dividing. In their replicating state, HDF cells rapidly produce extracellular matrix (ECM) molecules, but when they differentiate in vitro they have a greater propensity for matrix degeneration.[15–17] In addition, there is evidence for a biomarker of senescent skin cells in culture, a senescence-associated β-galactosidase.[18]

Factors affecting studies of cellular and molecular aging

- Age of subject/donor
- Genetic background
- Pathological status of subject/donor
- Composition of diet/nutritional factors

Table 8-1 HDF cells: division potential (population doublings)

Fetal (lung/skin)	Average:	50
	Maximum:	63
Adult (skin)	Average:	30
Progeria (Werner's)	Average:	10

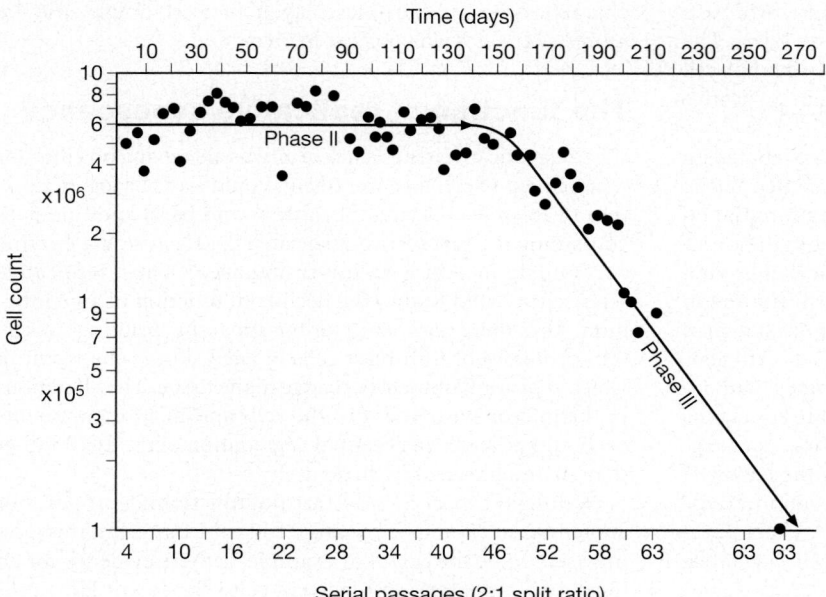

Figure 8-2 The lifecycle of human diploid fibroblast-like (HDF) cells in vitro. From Hayflick,[14] with permission.

Although the major feature of HDF cells in vitro is replicative senescence, these cells survive for a long time. Cultures can remain in the post-replicative state for periods of more than 12 months, a situation more akin to terminal cell differentiation.[19,20] The cells continue to support many biosynthetic functions, and they appear to differ from cells of earlier passage number only in their ability to initiate DNA synthesis before cell division.[21–23] Senescent HDF cells, when stimulated by mitogens, begin the process of DNA synthesis by expanding nucleotide pools and inducing certain enzymes,[24] but the genes needed for the progression of the cell cycle are repressed. It has been suggested that replicative senescence and differentiation may be the same thing,[20,25] although this is disputed.

Replicative senescence

Several investigators argue that multiple dominant-acting genes control replicative senescence.[25] The roles of cytoplasmic factors during in vitro senescence have been investigated by hybridization experiments.[26] Hybrids between anucleate cytoplasm (cytoplasts) and "inactivated" normal HDF cells showed that the enzymes of untreated cytoplasts replaced inactivated enzymes of whole cells and permitted hybrid cell survival. The hybrids formed by old cytoplasts plus old cells and young cytoplasts plus old cells had a low doubling potential, whereas those hybrids involving young cells had similar doublings to controls.[26] Thus, senescent HDF cells may synthesize some specific repressor molecule(s) that inhibits the initiation of DNA synthesis.[27] Subsequent work showed that in heterokaryons between old HDF and either SV80 transformed HDF, or HeLa cells, DNA synthesis was initiated in the old nuclei.[28] These results strongly implicate positive control of DNA synthesis by the HeLa and SV80-transformed cells overcoming the putative repressor. If young HDF cells were in the S-phase of the cell cycle when they were fused to senescent cells, then DNA synthesis continued.[29] On the other hand, entry into the

S-phase was inhibited because young HDF cells in the G1-phase of the cell cycle (when fused with senescent HDF) did not synthesize DNA.[29] These results were consistent with the hypothesis that senescence involves a block preventing cells in G1 entering the S-phase.[30]

Fusion of different immortal human cells can produce the senescent phenotype and this approach has enabled the isolation of four distinct complementation groups.[31] Three of the complementation groups have been assigned to chromosomes 1, 4, and 7, although other chromosomes have induced replicative senescence in immortal cell lines.[32–34] Despite the discovery of the chromosomes involved in senescence, the genes have not been identified. There is some controversy here: the number of chromosomes that induce senescence is greater than the number of complementation groups, and although attempts have been made to explain the situation, it is difficult to understand the failure to characterize the genes. It has been suggested that the complementation phenomenon is due to delayed toxicity of the drugs used to select the hybrids,[35] but this has been refuted.[25]

Greater progress has been made in discovering the way that cultured cells may count the number of divisions they undergo. In HDF cells, telomeres, which are "tails" of nucleotide repeats at the ends of chromosomes, progressively shorten during replicative senescence. On the other hand, immortalized tumor cells have stable telomeres that retain a constant length. In addition, the telomere length in stem cells is greater than that found in somatic cells, and the length of the telomeres in germ-line cells is constant, despite the age of the donor. Out of these observations came the telomere hypothesis of aging and immortalization.[36,37] Germ-line cells maintain the length of their chromosomes by the activity of an enzyme, telomerase, which extends one strand of the chromosome without a DNA template. At some stage during embryogenesis the telomerase is repressed, and telomere shortening takes place in somatic cells during cell division. When HDF cells reach the Hayflick limit, one or more telomeres will have lost most telomeric repeats, and the cells stop dividing. The telomerase hypothesis suggests a way in which the dividing cell may count its number of divisions, and may explain replicative senescence in vitro.

A telomerase knockout mouse has been constructed to examine the role of telomerase in normal and neoplastic growth.[38] The mice remained viable for six generations but no telomerase activity could be detected. The cells from these animals could be made immortal in vitro or transformed by viral oncogenes, and the transformed cells could form tumors in nude mice. As may be predicted, the telomeres shortened progressively through each generation, and from the fourth generation onward the ends of their chromosomes had no detectable telomeres. The cells from the telomerase knockouts had a variety of chromosomal abnormalities. These data suggest that telomerase is essential for maintaining the length of telomeres but not for the processes of immortalization, transformation, or tumor formation in these animals.[38] A later paper showed that these knockout mice were genetically unstable, which led to shortening of the lifespan and an increased incidence of spontaneous malignancy.[39] Other investigators transfected human retinal pigment epithelial cells and foreskin fibroblasts with the human telomerase catalytic subunit.[40] The telomerase-expressing clones exceeded their normal in-vitro lifespan by 20 population doublings, had long telomeres, divided normally, and showed a reduction in staining for β-galactosidase. The nontransfected control cells were senescent and had shortened telomeres.[40]

These studies could simply be viewed as contradictory, but that would be an oversimplification.[41] The telomerase knockout mice should not have survived, and the dire predictions of spontaneous transformations in the telomerase-transfected somatic cells were not borne out. However, telomerase and telomeres are important components for normal cellular function. Recent studies have highlighted a potential mechanism for the modification of gene expression during the replicative lifespan of cells in vitro, in a report of a telomere position effect in HeLa cells.[42] Clones of HeLa cells containing a luciferase reporter adjacent to a newly formed telomere express 10 times less luciferase than control clones generated by random integration. Overexpression of complementary DNA coding for human telomerase reverse transcriptase (hTRT) resulted in telomere elongation and a further decrease in luciferase expression if the reporter was close to the telomere, but not if the hTRT was randomly integrated into the genome.[42] More recently the mean length of the terminal restriction fragments (TRFs) from primary cultures of HDF cells from four healthy centenarians was compared with those from 11 individuals of different ages.[43] There was no correlation between mean TRF length and donor age. However, telomere shortening was detected during in-vitro propagation of centenarian fibroblasts, suggesting that for fibroblasts aged in vivo the telomeres had not reached a critical, minimum length. In blood cells from the various subjects, the expected inverse correlation between mean TRF length and donor age was found. In particular, a substantial difference (about 2 kb) between telomere length in fibroblasts and blood cells was observed in the same centenarians. These data suggest that telomere shortening could play different roles in different cell types, and that the characteristics of fibroblasts aged in vitro might not be representative of what occurs in vivo.[43]

The function of replicative senescence

Clearly, replicative senescence in any tissue relying on constant replacement of certain components could lead to a loss of function (Table 8-2). Dermal fibroblasts and basal keratinocytes containing the senescence-associated β-galactosidase enzyme accumulate in skin with increasing age.[25] Thus, replicative senescence could lead to the decline in function of an epithelium. Also, there is evidence for the apparent "priming" of certain proteases of fibroblast cells in aged skin,[44] the result of which is pro-inflammatory change in the tissue. The alterations in the microenvironment of the cells and ECM components of this tissue lead to a potential degradation of the ECM rather than maintenance of its structure.

We might expect cells that are not functioning properly, or are senescent, would be removed from the tissue but this does not seem to be the case. For example, is there evidence for an increase in apoptosis in senescent cells? Senescent HDF cells in vitro are resistant to apoptosis,[25,45] and if fibroblasts are similarly resistant to programmed cell death in vivo there is potential for the accumulation of nonfunctioning cells in tissues. As usual the data are complicated, and one has to examine each paper carefully to understand exactly what the investigators are reporting. Current evidence seems to suggest an age-related decrease in the potential for apoptosis in HDF and in thymocytes, although the molecular mechanisms may differ depending on the cell type[46] (see also Chapter 6).

Replicative senescence may also be important in the process of tumor suppression. Many tumors contain cells that have passed the limits of replicative senescence, and it is known that mutations leading to neoplasia allow mitotic cells to escape replicative control.[25] Cell division is regulated by proto-oncogenes acting as "accelerators," and tumor-suppressor genes acting as "brakes." In senescent HDF cells, several proto-oncogenes can be activated by mitogens, but two tumor-suppressor

Table 8-2 **Summary of the phenotypes of young and senescent HDF cells**	
Young	**Senescent**
Small spindle-shaped cell	Large "spread" cell
Cell division rapid	Cell division stopped
ECM: net synthesis	ECM: degradation
Mitogens stimulate division	Mitogens initiate process but genes for progression of cell cycle are repressed
Telomeres intact	Telomeres short
Telomerase: negative	Telomerase: negative Tumor suppressor genes: *p53* and *Rb* activated *p21* overexpression Apoptosis resistant Senescent form of β-galactosidase

genes, *p53* and *Rb* (retinoblastoma), remain strongly activated.[25] Both *p53* and *Rb* must be inactivated in order to extend the lifespan of pre-senescent cells and to reactivate DNA synthesis in senescent HDF cells.[25] Finally, there is strong evidence that the dominant arrest of growth observed in senescent HDF cells is related to a small group of candidate proteins, of which the overexpression of *p21* is the best studied.[25,47]

Numerous interesting avenues of research can be explored by studying the senescence of cells in culture. Fibroblast-like cells from different species respond to culture conditions in different ways. Chick fibroblast-like cells have a stable, limited lifespan and never appear to produce "immortal" cell lines. Similar cells from mice and rats have a different growth pattern that comprises rapid proliferation of the cells followed by a reduced rate of division, and then typically spontaneous transformation into an immortal cell line. Human cells, in contrast, need to be "transformed" into immortal cells by some treatment, such as exposure to the SV40 virus.[48] Early studies suggested that the growth potential of cells in culture decreases with the age of the donor.[49] However, recent research does not confirm these early findings, and suggests that earlier studies did not control carefully for the health status of the donors.[50] The outgrowth of cells from human skin explants increases linearly with age, although this phenomenon is subject to a great deal of individual variation that also depends on donor age.[51]

Mitotic cells in vivo and in vitro

Attempts have been made to test whether the division potential of mitotic cells in vivo limits the lifespan of an organism. Early studies used transplantation techniques to focus on the ability of cells, tissues, and organs to function in hosts of differing ages. Transplants of ovaries and skin between young and old animals suggested that young tissues functioned less well in old compared with young recipients, although the experiments were generally equivocal.[52] In particular, skin grafting data were difficult to interpret. In some cases the grafts from old animals grew as well as those from younger mice; however, during successive transplants, the grafts became progressively smaller and many were lost, but this was common to samples from both young and old animals. A major problem was that cells from the host tissue migrated into the transplant during wound repair. Subsequently, transplants of bone marrow stem cells were used to reduce the problem of identifying the donor and host cells. Whole-body irradiation was used to kill the intrinsic stem-cell population, and then the animal was inoculated with donor cells. One elegant study used a chromosomal abnormality to identify donor tissue in a test of the division capacity of marrow stem cells in mice.[53] Every year, for four years, marrow cells were serially transplanted into recipients, but after this the stem cells had a reduced capacity to repopulate the host's marrow. It was concluded that the maximum lifespan of the mouse was very close to that of the functional division capacity of the marrow cells and that they were programmed in some way to age and die at the same time.[53]

Subsequently it was shown that successive transplants caused nonspecific damage to stem cells, and the stem-cell pool could be "exhausted" when under the stress of constant division.[54] Definitive studies were carried out on mice with a genetic defect that causes hereditary anemia due to stem-cell abnormalities.[55] In this case the mice did not require lethal irradiation and if a transplant was successful the anemia was cured. Red cell production was measured in the recipients after transplantation, so a direct measure of stem-cell function was obtained. Since the cure of the hereditary anemia never occurred spontaneously, the donor cells were identified unambiguously, and the effects of cells from both young and old donor cells could be compared in the recipients. Thus, there was no evidence for intrinsic aging of the red cell producing stem cells in these mice.[55]

Genetic models of aging

HDF cells have been used extensively in the study of progeroid syndromes. Progeroid syndromes are human genetic conditions with accelerated pathobiological changes resembling the phenotype of old age. The three classical progerias are Hutchinson–Gilford, Werner's, and Cockayne syndromes,[56,57] which are characterized by young individuals having a senile appearance. HDF cells isolated from such individuals have been used to study age-associated changes in functional ability. Each of these conditions is autosomal recessive in its mode of inheritance.[57] HDF cells from individuals with these syndromes have a shorter in-vitro lifespan than cells from normal adults of the same age. The HDF cells from Hutchinson–Gilford and Werner patients undergo 10 doublings when compared with the average of 30 doublings in cells derived from normal adults. Decreases in mitotic activity, DNA synthesis, DNA repair efficiency, and cloning efficiency have been reported in cells isolated from people with progeria. Werner's syndrome has been studied extensively in terms of the clinical and biochemical features of the disorder, and in the last decade a genetic linkage study identified proximity of the mutation to a group of markers on chromosome 8.[58] One line of evidence implicated the structural gene for DNA polymerase β as a likely source of defective DNA metabolism in Werner's syndrome cells. Subsequently, positional cloning enabled the localization of the Werner's syndrome gene (*WRN*).[59,60] The predicted protein is 1432 amino acids in length and is very similar to a DNA helicase. Four mutations were identified in Werner's patients. Two of the mutations are splice-junction mutations, with the predicted result being the exclusion of exons from the final messenger RNA (mRNA). One of these mutations, causing a frameshift and a predicted truncated protein, was found in the homozygous state in 60 percent of the Japanese Werner's patients examined. The other two mutations are nonsense mutations.

The identification of a mutated putative helicase as the gene product of the Werner's syndrome gene suggests that defective DNA metabolism is involved in the complex process of aging in these patients.[60] An analysis of the replicative ability of HDF cells from Werner's syndrome patients shows that these cells exit, apparently irreversibly, from the cell cycle at a faster rate than do normal HDF cells. It has been proposed that the *WRN* gene controls the number of times cells can divide before terminal differentiation.[61] A recent study of telomere length, telomeric DNA damage and repair, in relation to the progression of aging, showed telomeres are shorter in HDF cells from old donors compared with those from young donors, shortest in cells from a patient with Werner's syndrome, and relatively long in HDF cells from a patient with Alzheimer's disease. Telomeric DNA repair efficiency was lower in cells from old donors than from young donors, normal in Alzheimer cells, and lower in Werner cells. It is possible that this decline in telomeric repair with aging is of functional significance to an age-related decline in genomic stability.[62] However, a study of the kinetics of the loss of telomeric repeats in Werner syndrome cells showed that the mean length of telomere restriction fragments from the earliest passages of Werner syndrome cells were similar to those of controls.[63] Thus, while accelerated loss of telomeric repeats may explain the rapid decline in proliferation of Werner syndrome cells, it is possible that the cells exit the cell cycle through different mechanisms to senescent cells from normal subjects.

Clearly, the analysis of genetic markers offers a powerful approach to unraveling the mechanisms underlying specific components of the senescent phenotype in any species, but isolated HDF cells from the progerias are a unique resource for the study of aging in humans. Martin[64] argues that, while the *WRN* helicase locus could be important in this regard, several lines of evidence suggest that mutation at that locus leads to a "private" mechanism of aging (as opposed to a universally expressed "public" mechanism). Recent studies have focused on a number of important issues relating to *WRN* gene expression and the function of the WRN protein. In general, progeroid features, and age-associated diseases, do not become apparent until after puberty. This may be because *WRN* expression is induced at the time of puberty; alternatively it may be that it is expressed at all ages, but the phenotype of deficiency becomes apparent only after puberty.[65] *WRN* is expressed as early as at 49 days of gestation and there was no significant reduction in adult tissues;[65] thus, the Werner syndrome phenotype is not manifest because of peripubertal induction of *WRN* expression. It is thought that the deficit in Werner's syndrome cells is impaired global or regional transcription that may be the primary molecular defect responsible for the clinical phenotype.[66] The purified WRN protein is now confirmed as a helicase and an exonuclease, and has associated adenosine triphosphatase activity. It interacts physically and functionally with replication protein A, which stimulates the helicase action.[67] The WRN exonuclease activity can be blocked by certain DNA lesions and not by others; thus, while WRN does not bind to DNA damage per se, it may have properties that allow it to sense the presence of damage in DNA.[67]

Despite the obvious "physiological" drawbacks of an in vitro cellular model, it is an extremely powerful tool in the study of aging mitotic cells, particularly in humans. Indeed, the study of aging in vitro has led to the proposal of theories to explain senescence in culture, such as the "commitment theory"[68] and the model of "clonal attenuation."[69] These ideas are reviewed elsewhere.[8,12,25]

Cell aging in vivo

One of the challenges facing researchers studying aging using the in vitro model is persuading investigators working "in vivo" that their model means anything at the level of the whole organism. Observations used to marshal support for the in vitro model include:

- the age-associated reduction in proliferative ability of cells from old donors;
- the shorter lifespan of cells from short-lived species;
- the shorter replicative lifespan of progeroid subjects;
- altered control of gene regulation in senescent cells.

The main area of joint interest is typically the escape of cells into unrestrained growth and neoplasia.[70] However, there are other important body constituents comprising a large proportion of nondividing, terminally differentiated cells. What happens to this population of cells throughout the lifespan? Post-mitotic cell populations in skeletal muscle and the central nervous system appear to survive intact until late in the lifespan. Until recently it was thought that neurons were lost in large numbers from the cerebral cortex of the brain, although in the evolutionary older parts of the brain—the hypothalamus and the brainstem—neuronal populations stay intact.[71–73] Research on the morphology of the aged brain now suggests that in healthy individuals atrophic change is more a feature of neuronal aging than cell death.[74–79] Clearly, neurons and skeletal muscle cells do undergo senescent changes, but they occur late in the lifespan and are subject to complex alterations that take place in the environment of the body, whether this is related to maintained blood flow, levels of growth factors, or even chronic stimulation with adrenal[80] or ovarian[81] hormones.

Unfortunately, the study of cells in vivo is complicated. Although we can show changes in physiological regulation with age, the identification of a cellular, or molecular, lesion as the cause of the disruption is not a simple matter. In physiological systems we rarely know all of the steps in a chain of reactions. The difficulties of pinpointing defects in organs are not trivial owing to the diverse cell populations involved. The deterioration of the vascular system (whether due to pathological changes or what has been termed "physiological aging") is frequently a confounding factor in aging studies. Changes in blood circulation may produce effects in cells and tissues that are incorrectly attributed to intrinsic alterations. The ultimate causes of aging will be due to molecular changes, probably because certain molecules cannot be replaced or repaired. Precisely how, or why, these molecular changes take place is another matter. The passage of time may lead to a molecular defect, or defects, which will influence the ability of a cell to maintain its structural integrity. Furthermore, the process of differentiation early in life may limit the potential a cell has for the repair of constituent tissues later in the lifespan. The result for the intact organism is a failure to maintain homeostasis, and investigation of in vivo systems is essential to identify age-associated changes and their precise location. However, the application of molecular biological methods to the study of aging in vivo is fundamental, because these techniques enable us to improve the precision of our questions about cellular function in tissues and organs.

MOLECULAR MECHANISMS IN AGING

Most investigators agree that we need satisfactory biomarkers of aging at the cellular level.[18,82–85] However, the most obvious change—the presence of the age-pigment, lipofuscin, in aged, terminally differentiated post-mitotic cells—is not a reliable indicator. At present a simple marker is elusive; no consistent structural alteration can be used to identify the nucleus of an aging cell, for example, as seen in cells undergoing programmed cell death.[86] What we do have is a series of general indicators of compromised function in aged cells. In the early days of aging research, many of these indicators were pathological, and related to human age-related diseases. To a great extent age-related pathology is still the driving force for much of current research, a fact that is lamented by some who believe that too much effort is placed on understanding aging diseases rather than the biological process of aging itself.[87] However, there is a considerable literature describing the age-related biochemical, molecular, and structural changes in cells and tissues. With hindsight, it is noteworthy that many of the theories and mechanisms about aging followed rapidly in the wake of current advances in cell biology and biochemistry. It was not long after the publication of the structure of DNA and the genetic code that those theories on mutations as a cause of aging, and errors in protein synthesis, were proposed. A very early hypothesis argued a role for free radicals in aging,[88] and this theory has outlasted others as a likely fundamental mechanism of aging.

REACTIVE OXYGEN SPECIES AND FREE RADICALS IN AGING

It is appropriate at this point to discuss the potential role of reactive oxygen species (ROS) and free radicals in aging. The splitting of a covalent bond in a molecule, so that each atom joined by the bond retains an electron from the shared pair, produces free radicals. These reactions are common in normal cell physiology, producing free radicals which are short-lived (survival time measured in femtoseconds) by-products of electron transport.[89] Research has uncovered a potential role for certain free radicals in cell signaling.[90,91] With respect to aging, it is proposed that uncontrolled free radical reactions may be an important source of pathological cellular damage.[91] Free radical damage probably takes place throughout the lifespan, causing a progressive deterioration of both nuclear and cytoplasmic components.

The respiring organism faces a dilemma: it respires and obtains energy from the metabolism of oxygen, but oxygen itself can be extremely toxic. Most of the oxygen in an aerobic organism is reduced to water by the cytochrome oxidase enzyme complex of the inner mitochondrial membrane. However, some oxidases within the cell can generate hydrogen peroxide, an extremely toxic ROS:

$$O_2 + 2H^+ + 2e^- \rightarrow H_2O_2$$

In the presence of transition metal ions such as iron, hydrogen peroxide can decompose to form the hydroxyl radical:

$$Fe^{2+} + H_2O_2 \rightarrow {}^\bullet OH + Fe^{3+} + H_2O$$

Other enzymes catalyze oxidation reactions in which a single electron is transferred from a substrate onto oxygen, which produces the superoxide radical:

$$O_2 + e^- = O^\bullet_2$$

Superoxide is a by-product of various enzyme reactions (particularly in the mitochondrial and chloroplast electron transport systems), and can be caused by environmental agents such as UV light, ultrasound, X- and γ-rays, toxic chemicals, and metal ions.

Free radicals can also cause lipid peroxidation.[92] Membrane lipids contain polyunsaturated fatty-acid side-chains that undergo lipid peroxidation involving the generation of carbon radicals and finally lipid hydroperoxides. Lipid hydroperoxides decompose into cytotoxic aldehydes (e.g. malondialdehyde) and other products, causing damage to both enzymes and membranes. The various radicals react with, and damage, all molecules found within cells. However, the most vulnerable targets seem to be the lipid and protein components of membranes and mitochondrial DNA (mtDNA).

Clearly, cells do not continuously disintegrate because of free radical damage. Several protective molecular mechanisms have evolved to protect cells from free radical damage (see the box). The thiol peptide molecules seem to be implicated in a cellular signaling system based on intracellular oxidation/reduction (redox) status. The redox-sensitive signaling circuitry comprises metal- and thiol-containing proteins such as glutathione and thioredoxin. Changes in the redox status of the cell are thought to be communicated by these signaling molecules and serve as common mechanisms linking environmental stressors to adaptive cellular responses.[93] Thus, while it is known that at one extreme reactive oxygen species cause damage to biological structures, low, physiologically relevant concentrations can regulate some aspects of gene expression through thiol-containing proteins.[94] Electron flow through the functional CH_2-SH groups in the side-chains of these proteins accounts for the redox-sensing properties and protein thiol groups with high thiol-disulphide oxidation potentials are likely to be redox-sensitive. Signal transduction from the cell surface to the nucleus is through phosphorylation and dephosphorylation chain reactions of cellular proteins, and protein phosphorylation, one of the most fundamental mediators of cell signaling, is redox-sensitive. Studies have also shown that certain transcription factors are also redox-regulated. Intracellular calcium homeostasis is regulated by the redox status of cellular thiols, and calcium ions are intimately involved in protein phosphorylation and proteolytic processing of proteins, two major intracellular events that are implicated in signal transduction from the cell surface to the nucleus. Thus, these "protective" molecules provide a potentially important link between the redox potential of a cell and gene expression; it may not simply be a matter of damage.

Natural protection against reactive oxygen species

- "Scavenging" systems such as vitamin E (α-tocopherol)
- Thiol peptides such as glutathione, a tripeptide containing "free" sulphydryl groups
- Catalases and peroxidases, removing of hydrogen peroxide
- Superoxide dismutase (SOD), removing superoxide radical

Age-associated reductions in glutathione, glutathione reductase, and superoxide dismutase from blood cells,[95,96] liver,[96] and the eyes[97] have been reported. However, no correlation has been found between the maximum lifespan potential and levels of SOD in primates.[98] The fact that an increase in the oxygen to nitrogen ratio shortens the lifespan of *Drosophila*, and leads to an increase in the concentration of lipofuscin, has been used as evidence of the toxic effects of oxygen.[99] Lipofuscin (or age-pigment granule) accumulation with age is well described (Fig. 8-3). The pigment emits a yellow–green to orange fluorescence when excited by UV-light and this is thought to be related to the malondialdehyde content of lipofuscin (Fig. 8-4). The lipofuscin granule is extremely heterogeneous; it contains proteins, carbohydrates, lipids, and various enzymes associated with lysosomal activity and oxidative metabolism. Under the electron microscope, lipofuscin is highly irregular in shape and the variation in structure is dependent on the cell type.

There are two schools of thought about what lipofuscin does: firstly, that the pigment causes intracellular malfunction; and secondly, that it is an indicator of age-associated cellular damage. The levels of lipofuscin and cytoplasmic RNA in tissue sections from autopsy samples of human central nervous system are negatively correlated,[100] but there is little other quantitative evidence to support the idea that lipofuscin may suppress protein synthesis. The high concentration of lipofuscin found in tissues from aging animals (and, incidentally, from those with a vitamin E deficiency) suggests that age-pigment may be associated with damage to subcellular components, possibly by way of free-radical reactions and lipid peroxidation.[101,102] This view is supported by various studies. However, an investigation of the effects of age on the structure and function of neuroendocrine cells (the antidiuretic hormone- and oxytocin-producing cells) of the mouse hypothalamus showed an age-associated increase in the concentration of lipofuscin, although the volumes of other subcellular organelles measured

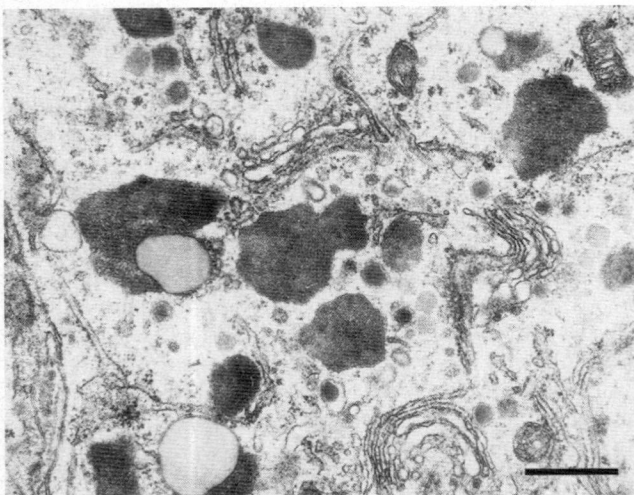

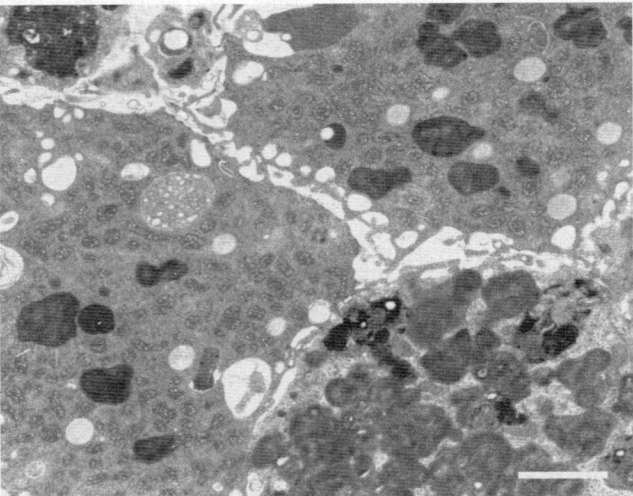

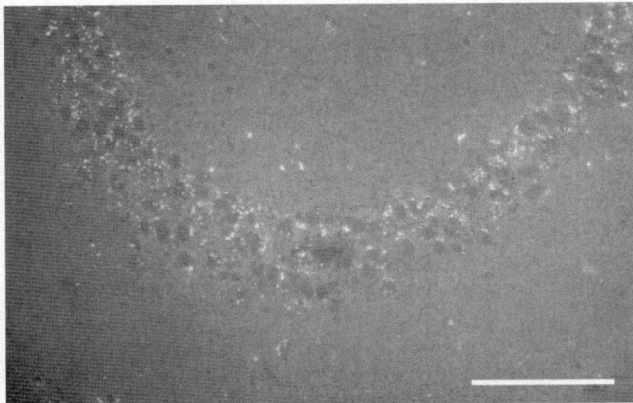

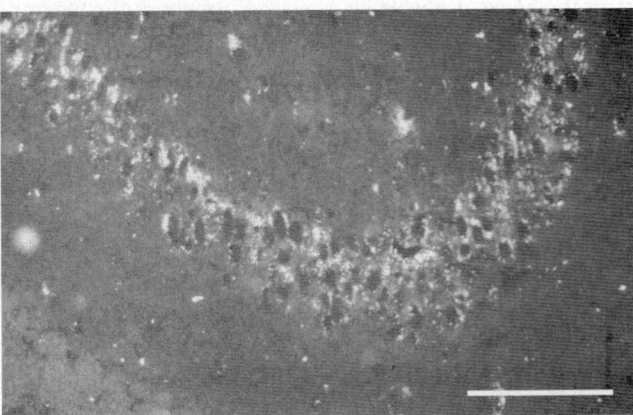

Figure 8-3 The upper panel is an electron micrograph of lipofuscin from a neuron in the supraoptic nucleus of a 28-month-old male mouse. Note the granular electron-dense structures with electron-lucent inclusions. Scale bar = 0.5 μm. The lower panel is an electron micrograph of lipofuscin in adrenal cortical cells of a 28-month-old male mouse. Note the appearance of the electron-dense granules and the lack of electron-lucent inclusions. Scale bar = 1 μm.

Figure 8-4 Photomicrographs showing the increase in levels of the autofluorescent age-pigment, lipofuscin, in hippocampal neurons of mice. At the top is a preparation from a 6-month-old animal, and below is one from a 28-month-old mouse. Scale bar = 100 μm.

in a quantitative morphological study were not significantly different from those found in young mice.[103,104]

Early experiments tried to extend rodent survival by feeding antioxidants such as cysteine hydrochloride, ethoxyquin, 2-mercaptoethylamine hydrochloride, 2,2′-diaminodiethyl-disulphide dihydroxide, and vitamin E through the lifespan.[105–107] The data were inconclusive. Mean lifespan increased by 10–15 percent depending on the strain of animal, but the maximum lifespan remained unaltered. These dosing experiments are difficult to interpret. Firstly, the studies were conducted with small numbers of animals and could not provide statistically reliable results. Secondly, no assessments were made of the physiological or pathological state of the control and treated animals to ensure that increased survival was in fact due to delayed aging and not to an effect on pathology. Thirdly, most of the treatments resulted in a decrease in body-weight.[105,106,108] It was suggested that these animals might have been restricting their food intake, which in itself can lead to an extension of life.[106] More recently, the maximum lifespan of *C. elegans* has been successfully extended using small synthetic superoxide dismutase/catalase mimetics. The treatment of wild-type worms increased their mean lifespan by 44 percent, and treatment of prematurely aging worms resulted in a 67 percent increase in lifespan.[109]

Transgenic *Drosophila*, overexpressing the gene for CuZn-SOD, showed a small but statistically significant increase in the mean lifespan for several strains of this insect,[110] although maximum lifespan was not improved. Other transgenics, overexpressing both catalase and CuZn-SOD, showed significant extensions of lifespan in *Drosophila*.[111] However, other attempts to genetically manipulate the enzymes involved in the metabolism of reactive oxygen species have been made, although they have not been successful in extending lifespan.[91] The transgenic studies require further work before we can be satisfied that increasing the expression of antioxidant defense mechanisms is beneficial.[91] However, there is correlative evidence suggesting that the feeding of antioxidants reduced the levels of fluorescent pigments in animal tissues.[112,113] Diets inadequate in vitamin E were generally successful in accelerating the deposition of the age-pigment, lipofuscin, in both the nervous system and the adrenal glands of rats and mice.[104,114] Lipofuscin has been associated with free-radical damage within cells and is considered to be a marker of increased autophagic activity in injured cells. Damage to the cell by free radicals or reactive oxygen species is now considered to be fact, and issues relating to the oxidation of different molecules will be raised elsewhere in this discussion on the mechanisms of cellular aging. Clearly, it is possible to augment the cells' protective mechanisms against ROS damage, but with varying degrees of success.

GENE EXPRESSION IN AGED CELLS

Age-associated changes take place in the number, and range, of genes transcribed by cells. Age can be associated with a complete loss of function, with an alteration in the rate of a particular process, or with some change in sensitivity to intra- and extracellular communication. The expression of genes and the production of macromolecules late in the lifespan are of critical importance when trying to understand aging at the cellular level. The key question is the extent to which somatic cells retain the ability to produce the correct synthetic responses to the demands of the body as a whole and local functional demand. The sources of age-related changes in gene expression are, therefore, many and various. Chromosomes and DNA may be damaged with age, or genes may be modified as they undergo, for example, methylation (epigenetic changes), or transcription rates may be changed due to altered availability of transcription factors.

In this author's view, it is naive to imagine that we will find a universal alteration in gene expression with age. What we usually mean when we discuss age-associated changes in gene expression is that there are alterations in the stability of function in a particular tissue. For this reason, numbers of studies that examine whole organs, such as the brain or liver, without fractionating them into specific cell types reveal little of value about the source of changes in functional stability. The data available suggest that qualitatively there is very little difference in cell and tissue-specific gene expression with advancing age. Exceptions to this finding are the involution of organs like the thymus, and the ovary in the post-reproductive stage of the lifespan.[11] The following subsections examine some of the components involved in gene expression and their alterations with increasing age (see Table 8-3).

Genomic alterations

Chromosomes and chromatin

The age-related decline in cell function, whether in terms of replicative potential or the production of new protein, implies some alteration in the genome. Ultimately, we must think of gene expression, and this can involve the transcriptional regulation of single genes or modifications to the state of the DNA that can influence gene expression, particularly transcriptional competence.

It is known that the topology (superhelicity) of DNA can influence transcription dramatically. At another level the state of the chromatin in which the gene is embedded, specifically the higher-order packing of nucleosomes, is another important component. Changes in chromosomes and chromatin in aged cells were discovered many years ago. Polyploidy leads to an increase in the DNA content of hepatocytes,[115,116] and some neurons.[117] The thermal stability of chromatin increases, and chromatin template activity may decrease with age. However, these observations are more due to changes in chromatin proteins rather than DNA, since the removal of proteins from

---

Table 8-3 Genomic alterations and DNA metabolism with age

- Chromosome rearrangements and aberrations: increased
- Epigenetics: DNA demethylation/reversal of gene silencing
- DNA oxidation: increased
- DNA strand breaks: double and single increased
- mtDNA: oxidation and deletion
- DNA repair: evidence disputed, changes in HDF cells in terminal stages of senescence
- DNA synthesis: DNA polymerase data suggest changes late in the lifespan

the chromatin eliminates many age-associated differences.[118] The physiological, chemical modification of chromosomal proteins (phosphorylation and acetylation) generally decreases with age, but the major drop in the acetylation of histone proteins, for example, is during the developmental period of the lifespan, rather than in the post-reproductive stages. Some conclude that no reliable age-associated changes in histones have been shown and that quantitative changes are small; others argue that detailed changes do take place. The differences between the various studies may be more to do with methodology. Overall, no change has been identified in the degradation of either histones or nucleotides with age in cell nuclei isolated from heart or brain. The nucleosome core size remains stable (approximately 140 base-pairs) for all tissues investigated, and the nuclease, DNAse I, does not cleave DNA at different sites for the respective sets of young, mature, and old nuclei.[118]

Recently, this subject area has reopened with studies of senescence in the budding yeast *Saccharomyces cerevisiae*. In *S. cerevisiae*, a suite of silent information regulator (*sir*) proteins are involved in "silencing" or inactivating entire regions of chromosomes. In this budding yeast, the number of cell divisions in a mother cell lineage measures the lifespan. In some ways this process is analogous to the "Hayflick" limit in HDF cells, but has also been equated to organism aging by yeast cell biologists, since the renewal process of budding of daughter cells occurs from an ultimately senescent, soma-like, lineage of mother cells.[119] In the mother cells that have undergone several divisions there is a breakdown in genomic silencing at certain loci, leading to the expression of the **a** and α mating-type genes; this leads to the simultaneous expression of genes of both mating types, resulting in sterility.[119] The identification of the SIR4-42 "longevity mutation" suggested a link between senescence and chromosomal silencing. In this mutation the *Sir2/3/4* proteins are directed from the telomeres where they normally act, to the ribosomal DNA (rDNA) region of the yeast genome. Under normal conditions *Sir2* mediates silencing of the rDNA region without the assistance of other *Sir* proteins; mutations that lead to the deletion of *Sir2* show a short lifespan, and extra copies of this gene lead to extended lifespans.[119]

Environmental and developmental factors also can influence the expression of genes.[120] The structure of chromatin at the site of a gene governs the way a gene is expressed. DNA methylation is a major factor in gene control. The expression of certain genes is correlated strongly with demethylation, particularly in embryonic and fetal tissues (e.g. globin genes in a variety of species, and genes from certain viruses).[21] This group of genes is demethylated in tissues where they are expressed, and methylated where they are not. In another group of genes demethylation is not apparently correlated with expression in tissues, and in at least one case methylation is associated with actual expression.[121] DNA methylation may decrease with age, although this is not the case for all genes.[122] The level of 5′-methylcytosine in the DNA of human, mouse, and hamster diploid fibroblasts declines during serial subculture. The rate of decline is greatest in mouse fibroblasts and slowest in human cells, suggesting that the maintenance of methylation may be a prerequisite of long-term survival in vitro.[123] Since diploid fibroblasts are connective tissue cells, it is possible that

demethylation may activate genes that are normally repressed, so leading to their aging and death. This idea has some support from studies using the demethylating agents azacytidine or azadeoxycytidine. A single treatment of young cells with a low dose of either of these compounds is followed by recovery, with a completely normal morphology and growth rate, but the cells die prematurely.[124] These studies are indirect evidence for the view that the maintenance of methylation is important for long-term survival of HDF cells.[125] There are other age-associated alterations in DNA methylation; for example, the genomes of certain endogenous viruses are demethylated in specific tissues with advancing age.[126] Thus, this epigenetic phenomenon may influence the aging of cells and tissues, and may prove to be a link between aging and cancer.[121]

The idea of aging being due to the loss of the differentiated state has been discussed.[127] The early experiments, although interesting, were not conclusive. It was shown that there was an increased expression of globin by the DNA of old "brain" when compared with young, and the ratio of globin RNA to total RNA in the cytoplasm was increased with age for each age group.[128] However, no attempt was made to differentiate between the diverse cells found in "brain" tissue, thus negating the impact of the findings. Other observations were more persuasive. There is a random inactivation of one of the two X-chromosomes in each cell of female placental animals during early development. This inactivation is stable through mitosis so that all descendants have the same active X-chromosome and the same inactive one.[129] Each adult female is a mosaic with regard to X-chromosome activity.[129] An experiment conducted several years ago showed that the gene responsible for coat color in mice could be inactivated by inserting it into an X-chromosome. The gene involved is wild-type tyrosinase, which on inactivation produces an albino coat. However, as these mice grew older they became progressively more pigmented, indicating that the tyrosinase gene was reactivated.[130] A similar observation was made on the expression of sex-linked ornithine carbamoyl transferase gene in the liver.[131] Since methylation has a role in maintaining the stability of the inactive X-chromosome, demethylation may be the cause of the reactivation process. Other studies have shown that, in heterozygous women with a severe deficiency of the enzyme hypoxanthine phosphoribosyltransferase, there is rare, age-associated reactivation of this X-linked gene. However, demethylation with 5-azacytidine induced activity in white cells from old donors but not young ones.[132] These findings are not necessarily incompatible with the notion that imperfect inheritance of gene methylation patterns causes gene reactivation with increasing age.[133] Evolutionary reasons might mean that the control of X-inactivation is likely to be far tighter in long-lived than short-lived species. The fact that the gene was reactivated more easily in white cells from old donors suggests that some demethylation had taken place, even though there was no detectable reactivation of the gene.

DNA methylation is one way of regulating gene expression but there are many others. There are processes that mediate both gene activation and repression. The idea of differential gene expression goes with the process of cell differentiation. Transcriptional control involves the transfer of genetic information from DNA to RNA, with specific interaction of transcription regulatory proteins and specific regulatory DNA sequences. These processes occur in the promoter and enhancer regions of the gene. The regulatory DNA sequences are the *cis*-acting sequences usually at the 5' end of the coding region, although this is not always the case. The *cis*-acting sequences serve as recognition sites for the binding of specific *trans*-acting, or transcription, factors that serve to activate or repress gene expression. Some investigators have focused on the signaling pathways associated with the expression of the so-called "stress response genes" that include the early immediate genes (*c-fos* and *c-jun*) and the heat shock proteins. Many of these genes undergo age-associated changes.[134] The AP-1 *cis*-acting site binds *fos–jun* dimers that are members of a superfamily of transcription factors induced by polypeptide hormones, growth factors, cytokines, and neurotransmitters. These transcriptional factors undergo post-translational modifications that determine their level of activity. In rat hepatocytes, there is a rise in constitutive levels of both *c-fos* and *c-jun* in the absence of known stress factors, suggesting chronic stress or constant stimulation of these genes.[135] In addition, AP-1 binding activity is more strongly induced in the hippocampus of aged rats.[136]

Recently it has been discovered that intracellular redox status, a tightly regulated variable, can influence gene expression. The mechanism by which the transcription of specific eukaryotic genes is regulated by the redox state is complex but involves redox-sensitive transcription factors.[137] It is thought that the redox-sensitive signaling circuitry comprises metal- and thiol-containing proteins such as glutathione and thioredoxin. Changes in the redox status of the cell are thought to be communicated by these signaling molecules and serve as common mechanisms linking environmental stressors to adaptive cellular responses.[93] NF-κB and AP-1 are transcription factors that are induced by a wide variety of exogenous and endogenous stimuli and have important roles in cell growth and differentiation, immunity, inflammation, and other cellular processes; they also respond to environmental stressors— chemicals, drugs, or other agents that appear to alter the redox status of the cell.[93] In addition, age-associated changes in heat shock protein have been detected in senescent HDF cells, hepatocytes, and hippocampus.[134] Induction of heat shock proteins by various stimuli in senescent HDF cells is significantly reduced, and is attributed to a reduction in the transcription of the HSP70.[138] The reduced transcription observed correlated with the loss of heat shock factor binding activity that activates the HSP70 gene.[139] Numbers of different lines of research are now converging with connections being made between heat shock gene expression, oxidative stress, and factors that may determine lifespan of animals. Mutant strains of the nematode *C. elegans* show a 70 percent increase in mean and maximum lifespan. The Age mutations show an increased thermal tolerance to temperature stress and overexpression of a nematode heat shock protein.[9] This is a rapidly developing field that is bringing together several different lines of research. Clearly, from the data described here the interconnections between oxidative stress, stress proteins, and lifespan determination are closely interwoven.

Expression profiling techniques using differential display[140] and DNA microarrays[141–143] to analyze age-related changes in gene expression have been appearing in the literature. Initial studies have tended to look at the expression of many genes simultaneously, but hopefully more appropriate experimental designs and improved data analysis techniques will refine the experimental approaches.

Differential display was used to survey gene expression in the brain, heart, and liver of aged rats.[140] Only about 2 percent of the genes expressed in these organs showed significant changes during aging. The data confirm the increased expression of glial fibrillary acidic protein in the aged brain. A decrease in fos, a component of the AP-1 transcription factor, was also identified.[140] Although this topic has not been dealt with directly in this chapter, there is evidence that certain strains of mice (e.g. Ames dwarf mice) live 40–70 percent longer than normal nonmutant siblings. These animals are homozygous for the dwarf (df) allele at the Prop1 locus and have a hereditary growth hormone, prolactin, and thyrotropin deficiency. This mutation has been linked with the single gene mutations in *C. elegans* where insulin/insulin-like growth factor-1 (IGF-1) signaling appears to be involved in the regulation of lifespan. A gene expression profile of these mice at different ages was assembled for 265 liver genes in df/df and age- and sex-matched controls. The analysis was complex but the proportion of genes showing relatively large changes between 5 and 13 months, or from 13 to 22 months of age, was not diminished by the df/df genotype. The data do not support the idea that the dwarf mutation leads to a global delay, or deceleration of the pace of age-dependent changes in gene expression. This is a complex area of investigation that needs more research.

It must be remembered that while the genetic pathways regulating lifespan in *C. elegans* are well established, and the homology of the nematode genes with mammalian genes is accepted, the functional status of the pathway is largely unknown. The indications from the study of these dwarf mice is that the growth hormone (GH)/IGF-1 axis may accelerate aging; but in humans, some physiological changes in elderly people resemble symptoms of GH deficiency that can be corrected by GH replacement.[144] Messenger RNA levels were measured in actively dividing fibroblasts isolated from normal young, middle-aged and old-age humans and individuals with Hutchinson–Gilford syndrome. It was found that 61 genes (approximately 1 percent of the genes monitored) showed consistent changes of more than 2-fold in the level of expression between young and middle age in normal subjects. Over half of these genes could be grouped into those whose products are involved in the cell cycle, while others were involved in maintenance and remodeling of the extracellular matrix (ECM). The data suggest that an underlying mechanism of aging involves increasing numbers of errors in the mitotic machinery of mitotic cells in the post-reproductive stage of life, which may lead to chromosomal pathologies.[143]

Chromosomal aberrations

Chromosomal aberrations are found with increasing frequency in aged cells.[145] The aberrations consist of chromosomal bridges and fragments seen in dividing cells, particularly the liver. In long-lived strains of mice, the aberrations increase from an incidence of approximately 10 percent in 2-month-old animals to about 35 percent in 24-month-olds. In short-lived mice, they develop much more rapidly, from 20 percent at 2 months to

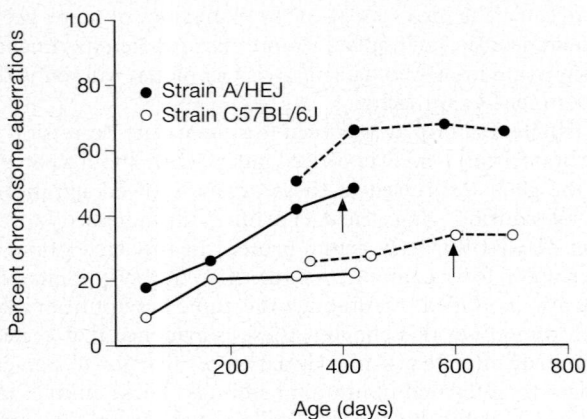

Figure 8-5 Incidence of chromosome aberrations in regenerating liver cells of two inbred strains of female mice, plotted as a function of age. The median lifespan of each strain is indicated by the arrows. From Crowley and Curtis.[242]

80 percent at 20 months (Fig. 8-5). There appears to be a correlation between lifespan and the rate of development of chromosome aberrations.[145]

However, there are anomalies: some mice with a very short lifespan have a rate of accumulation of aberrations similar to that found in mice with a long lifespan.[145] These short-lived animals develop severe terminal pathology, such as leukemia or mammary carcinomas, and do not live to a lifespan achieved by other strains. A more serious problem is that F_1 hybrids derived from parents with different lifespans develop chromosomal aberrations at a rate intermediate between that of the parents but live longer.[145] However, lymphocytes from aged individuals showed higher chromosomal aberration frequencies and longer duration of G2 than cells from young individuals.[146] In *S. cerevisiae*, incompletely silenced chromatin and the accumulation of extra-chromosomal rDNA circles has been implicated in causing senescence in these cells.[147] Chromosomal damage may be related to the action of reactive oxygen species, and some aberrations may be the result of errors in DNA replication as a function of use. Of particular interest is the peculiarly mammalian property of the escape of cells from normal proliferative homeostasis into neoplasia[70] midway through the lifespan.

DNA damage

General issues

DNA is considered a prime target for age changes. DNA is unique: it has to replicate and maintain itself, to preserve the primary genetic message of the cell through division and ongoing accidental events that may damage it. The functional integrity of DNA has to be maintained throughout the lifespan of the cell, although the nuclear DNA of some mammalian somatic cells undergoes a series of alterations that change it from the structure inherited through the germ-line—for example, the genomic rearrangements and mutations of immunoglobulin genes during the differentiation of B-lymphocytes.

However, endogenous or exogenous physical, chemical, or biological agents damage DNA.[148] DNA molecules exist at 37°C, which contributes to the loss of bases from the DNA polymer, and the subsequent development of "single-strand" breaks.[149] Mutations can arise from errors in DNA replication during the process of mitosis, by the mispairing of bases at a site of damage in the DNA molecule, or because of errors generated during the synthesis of DNA. At the end of World War II, evidence rapidly accumulated in survivors of the atomic bomb detonations in Japan, that ionizing radiation appeared to accelerate aging.[145] Superficially, irradiated survivors showed pathological changes similar to those seen in old humans.[11] Controlled studies on mice irradiated with a single dose of X-rays showed a shortening of the lifespan proportional to the dose. UV-radiation, γ- and X-rays cause specific types of damage ranging from the distortion of the helix by UV, and either base removal or damage from free radicals generated by γ- or X-rays. Chemical mutagens and carcinogens also cause damage to DNA, as does viral-DNA, which can be inserted into the genome of the host cell and alter the information content.

The effect of DNA damage depends on several factors (Fig. 8-6). The physiological consequences of a mutation depend on whether the organism is a homo- or heterozygote, and whether the gene affected is dominant or recessive. Most mutations are probably not lethal, especially since in a differentiated cell much of the DNA is not expressed. Therefore, it is highly likely that a mutation would be in a nontranscribed or repressed region. A mutation in a repressed zone would be "silent." However, this situation might change if the cell had to either undergo division, or respond to some unusual stimulus, involving the utilization of a previously unused region of the genome. Mutations in gene-control regions could cause inappropriate gene repression or activation. If the mutation involved genes controlling cell division, then abnormal cell proliferation might lead to tumor production. A mutation in the transcribed region of the DNA would be expressed in terms of altered RNA and hence protein.

Two theories have argued that aging is due to somatic mutations.[10,150] One proposal was that dominant mutations were the cause of cell damage or death,[150] while the other considered that aging in diploid cells was due to recessive mutations.[10] The calculated rate of mutation in germ cells failed to account for the lifespan of most species, so it was unlikely that recessive mutations could affect the survival of somatic cells. One prediction of the recessive mutation theory was that inbred organisms should live longer than outbred ones. Inbred animals are homozygous at most loci, whereas outbred are heterozygous at many positions. Inbred organisms cannot be homozygous for genetic defects because this is often lethal; and since they will be heterozygous for very few "faults," it follows that they will express close to the species-specific lifespan. However, the evidence obtained on inbreeding effects point to a reduction in lifespan. Other observations are inconsistent with the notion of recessive mutations causing aging. Diploid organisms should have a longer lifespan than haploids, and haploids should be more vulnerable to life-shortening effects such as ionizing radiation. Studies on the haploid and diploid males of the wasp *Habrobracon* have shown that such predictions are not true. The haploid males have the same lifespan as the diploid, which is inconsistent with the theory, although haploids are more

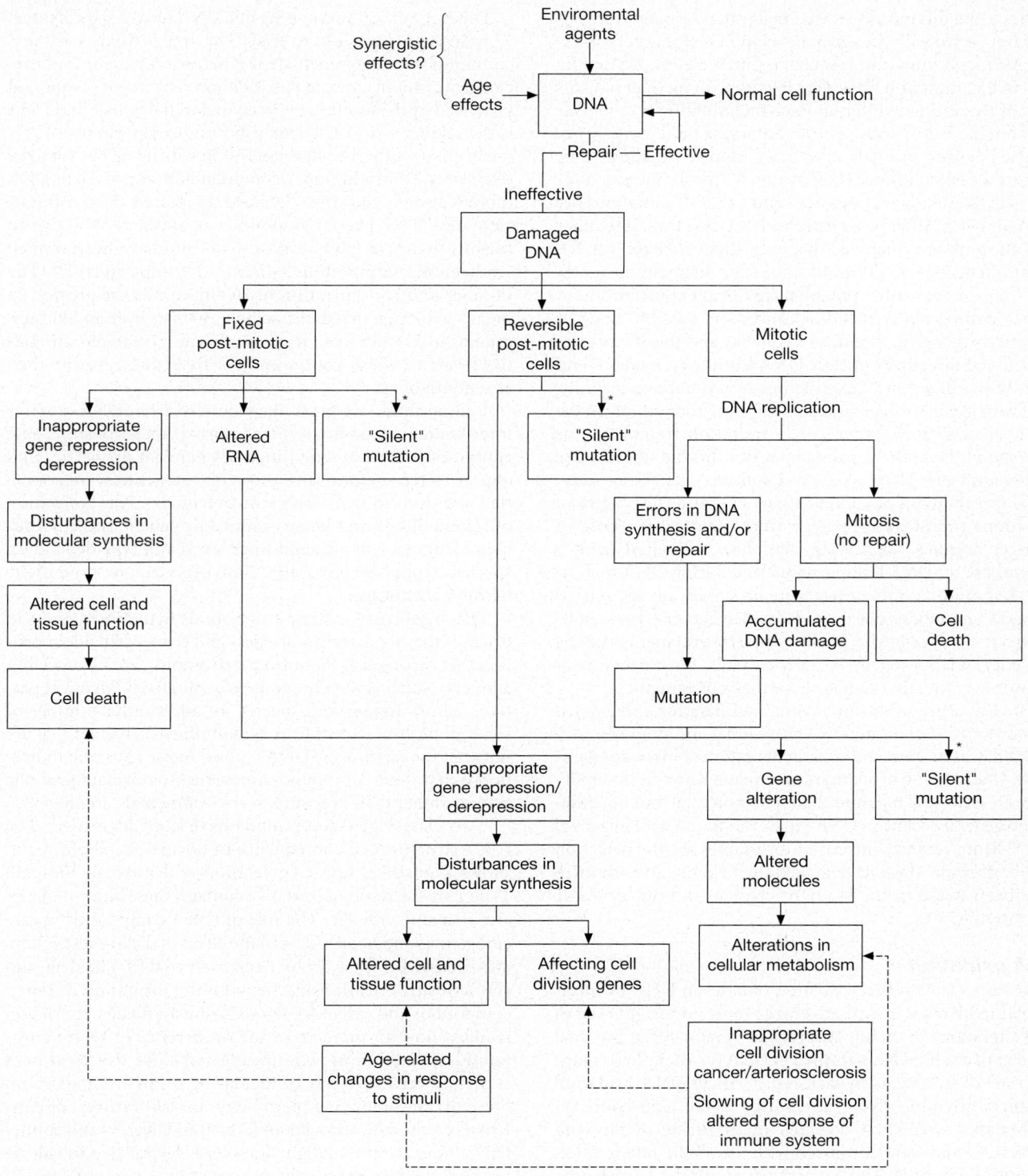

Figure 8-6 Diagrammatic view of the possible forms of damage to DNA and subsequent cellular responses. *These changes are of consequence only during redifferentiation and/or stimulation of further mitoses.

susceptible to the effects of ionizing radiation. Studies of rodents subjected to radiation damage showed signs of acceleration of both malignant and nonmalignant causes of death. However, the onset of age-associated conditions, both benign and malignant neoplasms, and senile cataracts, was different between normal aging and radiation-induced life-shortening.[151–153]

The recent development of the Big Blue lacI transgenic mouse enables the study of mutational frequency and specificity, and mutation rates in different tissues in vivo.

Studies using this mouse showed that mutation rates were not fixed but varied with the age or developmental stage of the tissue. Although mutation frequencies increased more rapidly early in life, mutation rates were lower in young than old animals. It was estimated that in mice the mutation rate in liver fell from 4.9×10^{-8} to 1.1×10^{-8} mutations per base pair per month between animals aged <1.5 months to those ≥ 1.5 months, a 4-fold decrease.[154] Mutation frequency increased 30-fold over the same ages (3.9×10^{-9} and 1.3×10^{-7} mutations per base pair per cell division, respectively). Using these and other data, the authors concluded that even slight changes in DNA repair efficiency could lead to significant increases in mutation frequencies, with a potential significant contribution to human pathogenesis, including cancer and possibly aging.[154] The effects of age on mutation frequency and specificity were determined directly in nuclear DNA from liver, bladder, and brain of Big Blue lacI transgenic mice.[155] Mutations accumulated with age in the liver and bladder, but more rapidly in the latter. A small initial increase in mutation frequency was observed in the brain of young mice but this did not increase further with age. There were no significant changes in mutational specificity in any tissue at any age, and the spectra of mutations found in aged mice were identical to those in younger animals, suggesting that they originated from a common set of DNA lesions manifested during DNA replication. It is of interest that there were no significant age-related changes in mutations due to oxidative damage, or errors resulting from changes in the fidelity of DNA polymerase or the efficiency of DNA repair.[155] Coincidentally, these data do not support the oxidative damage hypothesis of aging.

The literature up to 1990 contained data for and against chromosomal alterations, DNA cross-links, and strand-breaks, but there was no clear and consistent pattern of increased damage to DNA.[156,157] Correlations were made between the ability to repair DNA and maximum lifespan potential, but nonetheless no general decline in DNA repair was found with increased age.[156] More recently improved techniques for the detection of alterations in DNA have moved the field on, and advances have been made in the study of changes in both genomic and mtDNA.

DNA oxidation
It has been claimed that oxidation of bases in DNA by intracellular oxidants is quantitatively the most important class of base alterations in mammalian cells.[158] Estimates of the total number of oxidized bases formed in DNA on a daily basis range from 10^4 to 10^6 events in each cell.[159] Small DNA oxidation products, thymine glycol, thymidine glycol, and hydroxymethyuracil, were first detected in the urine of rats and humans,[160] and were correlated with metabolic rate in mice, rats, and humans.[161] The concentration of 8-hydroxydeoxyguanosine (8-OHdG) was found to increase with age in rat DNA.[162] In addition, DNA repair enzymes (glycosylases) that remove oxidized bases from DNA are positively correlated with lifespan in many mammals.[148] The mutagenic potential of oxidized bases in DNA is emphasized by the finding that the loss of the glycolase specific for the repair of 8-OHdG leads to an increase in the spontaneous mutation rate.[158] However, recent data directly measuring age-related increase in mutations due to oxidative damage have failed to support this hypothesis.[155]

Other modifications to genomic DNA by free radical intervention have been discovered. The highly toxic carbonyl compound malondialdehyde is a major mutagenic and carcinogenic product of lipid peroxidation. The major compound produced by the reaction between malondialdehyde and DNA is the adduct 3-β-D-2′- deoxyribofuranosylpyrimidol [1,2]-purin-10(3H)-one, but its relationship with aging has yet to be established.[163] In addition, I-compounds, bulky covalent DNA modifications, could be detected as altered deoxyribonucleotides.[163,164] These compounds accumulate with age in various tissues of laboratory rodents and have been termed "indigenous compounds" (hence I-compounds).[165] The number and concentration of I-compounds are greatest in organs with high metabolic activity, such as liver and kidney. Studies of Fischer 344 rats show that in 2-year-old animals the levels of these compounds is five times greater than at 1 month of age.[166]

I-compounds are most likely derived from DNA-reactive intermediates generated during normal metabolism. These compounds have a wide range of chemical properties and appear to represent diverse molecular structures, suggesting they are derived from different precursors. The formation of I-compounds may be determined by genetic and environmental factors and age; and their levels and type depend on species, strain, gender, diet, and exposure to potentially harmful chemicals.

The argument for these compounds being indigenous in origin is the characteristic species- and tissue-dependent profiles that distinguish them from exogenous carcinogen-DNA adducts, which generally produce qualitatively identical patterns across tissues and species. In addition, a number of I-compounds in rodent liver exhibit diurnal changes that are not seen for carcinogen-DNA type adducts. Thus, the indication is that these compounds are related to normal metabolic activity rather than exposure to environmental carcinogens.

Two classes of I-compounds have been identified. The type 1 structure is a consequence of normal metabolism and shows a positive, linear correlation with median lifespan. Type 2 are the result of oxidative damage; these bulky moieties also increase with age. The role of type 1 compounds in carcinogenesis and neoplasia, and the effect of dietary restriction, are discussed extensively by Randerath et al.[167] The data suggest a positive relationship between the formation of type 1 compounds and carcinogenesis. Curiously, dietary restriction studies show an increase in the occurrence of type 1 compounds. This finding was unexpected since this treatment is the only effective way of increasing mean and maximum lifespan and reducing pathology in laboratory rodents. However, the data are cited for kidney and liver,[163] and epithelial tumors are the malignancies least responsive to calorie restriction.[168] It may simply mean that the increased concentrations of type 1 compounds with age and malignancy is a spurious correlation.

This field is in an early stage of development. The assays are extremely sensitive and the number of changes detected is small.[11] The ability to measure this small level of DNA damage is a major advance in the field; but the low levels of damage, even though the percentage increase through the lifespan is quite large, suggests that genomic DNA damage may not be a major factor in aging without accompanying disease.

Mitochondrial DNA (mtDNA)

Mitochondrial DNA is a circular molecule and contains genes for two ribosomal RNAs (rRNAs), 22 transfer RNAs (tRNAs), and 13 peptides. These peptides are components of five multi-subunit enzymes of the oxidative–phosphorylation machinery of the inner mitochondrial membrane. Mitochondrial DNA is "naked" and attached to the inner mitochondrial membrane; and since about 2 percent of the oxygen reduced by the mitochondrion escapes as superoxide from the electron transport chain in the inner mitochondrial membrane, the DNA is potentially very vulnerable to oxidative damage. Large deletions have been detected in mtDNA with increasing age in human, rats, mice, and nematodes,[163] and have been implicated as a factor in, or even the cause of, cellular aging.[169] The deletions detected usually involve large segments of the genome located between the origins of replication, and often involve directly repeated sequences that facilitate some form of intramolecular recombination. In addition, in some human myopathies, and in diabetes, large sections of the mitochondrial genome have undergone rearrangements[170] (see also Chapter 6).

Mitochondria are the most important intracellular source of reactive oxygen species. The mtDNA is subject to severe oxidative damage to a much higher degree than genomic DNA. The oxidative damage is detected by the presence of oxidized bases, particularly 8-OHdG. This base modification can lead to point mutations because of mispairing. The level of 8-OHdG in mitochondrial DNA increases with age in rat and human liver, muscle, and brain tissues. It also increases in the mitochondrial genome of the housefly.[163,171] The latter findings are interesting in that a decrease in the physical activity of the housefly prolongs lifespan and reduces the level of 8-OHdG in both nuclear and mitochondrial DNA.[171] These observations are discussed in detail elsewhere.[167] Mitochondrial DNA is also partially fragmented in aged cells, possibly because of some of the deletions taking place.

For many years it was considered that mtDNA did not have the facility to repair damage. However, this is now known to be incorrect and it seems that DNA repair processes in mitochondria resemble those seen in the nontranscribing DNA of the nucleus.[172] This finding alters our view of how mtDNA might be affected by damage, but it does not preclude the possibility that mutations can accumulate in mitochondrial genomes, leading eventually to dysfunction of the cell. In addition, mtDNA can be inserted into nuclear DNA. This occurs continuously in yeast, and isolated sequences have been identified in human cells.[170,173] However, no evidence for the transfer of mtDNA sequences to the nucleus was found in aged human fibroblasts, suggesting that such transfers are rare in humans.[173]

Damage to mitochondria and the potential importance in cellular aging is an exciting and growing field, and is already proving extremely productive in the study of human disease. However, despite the very large increases in the alterations seen in mtDNA over the lifespan, particularly in post-mitotic tissues, the overall level of mitochondrial genomes containing deletions is less than 0.1 percent of the total mtDNA in a given tissue. This rather general statement of damage may be misleading because histochemical studies suggest that the mutant genomes are unevenly distributed, and highly concentrated in cells where energy metabolism may be impaired. The photomicrographs of muscle tissue taken from human myopathies indicate that the changes in muscle fibers are extremely complex.

DNA repair

Under conditions of normal homeostasis, and particularly under conditions of physiological stress, the integrity of the genome and consequently of gene expression depends on the ability to repair DNA damage. This mechanism is crucial to survival.[149] Calculations suggest that if endogenous changes in DNA accumulated unchecked, 10 percent of the bases in the DNA of the average cell of an old human would be altered, and this is not compatible with life.[149] In general, the repair of DNA damage is very effective, although the rate of damage caused by UV radiation in full sunlight is close to swamping the repair system.[149]

Damage to DNA may or may not be random in nature since the structure of the chromatin may make certain areas more susceptible to attack by outside agents. Repair of chromatin may also be restricted because of limited accessibility.[118,148] Animals with long maximum lifespan potentials generally have a more efficient DNA repair system.[174] Evidence for this has been obtained from studies on fibroblast cultures exposed to high doses of UV-radiation. Both the initial rate, and maximum incorporation, of radioactively labeled DNA precursors into DNA increases with the lifespan potential of the species, as shown in Figure 8-7. Subsequent work showed a strong correlation between DNA repair and longevity among

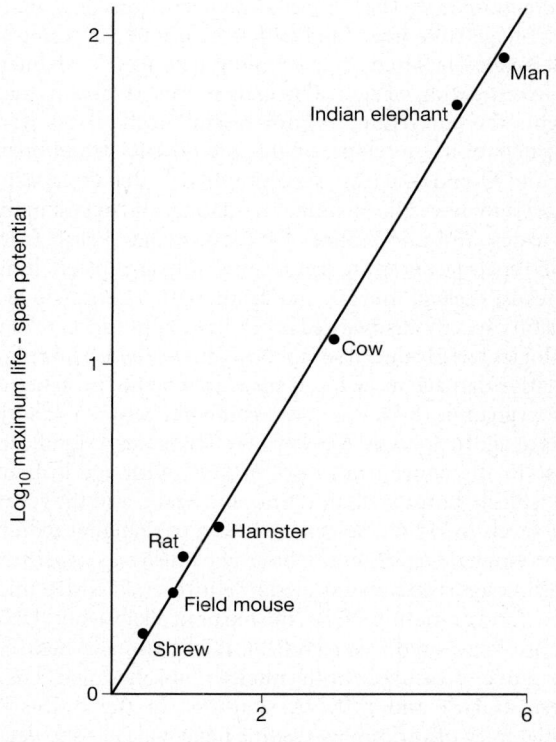

Figure 8-7 Diagrammatic representation of the correlation between the logarithm of the maximum lifespan potential of several species and the efficiency of repair of UV-damaged DNA in fibroblast cultures. From Hart and Setlow.[174]

mice,[175,176] and primates.[177] Late-passage cultures of HDF cells showed less DNA repair activity than did young cells after exposure to UV radiation.[178,179] These results indicate a decrease in the ability of senescent cells to integrate the various operations needed for DNA repair. However, the decline in UV-induced repair with culture age occurs only in the passage prior to cessation of cell division, prompting the conclusion that this deficiency in repair is not the basis of in vitro aging.[180]

It has been suggested that the reduced capacity to repair double-strand breaks in human DNA appears to be more pronounced in elderly women than in elderly men (and may begin after age 65 years). Moreover, the reported age-related decline in double-strand break induction occurs more rapidly in women than in men. This analysis revealed a gender-specific pattern in the correlation between the percentage of double-strand breaks induced, and the percentage of double-strand breaks rejoined. At comparable levels of induced double-strand breaks, cells from men rejoin a higher percentage than cells from women.[181] The repair of apurinic/apyrimidinic (AP) sites in DNA has been investigated in young and old IMR90 cells and human leucocytes. The number of AP sites in the aged IMR90 cells was two to three times higher than that in young cells, and in human leucocytes from old donors was seven times greater than that in young donors. Furthermore, the repair of AP sites was slower in senescent compared with young IMR90 cells owing to an age-related decline in the activity of the 3-methyladenine DNA glycosylase that removes methylated bases in IMR90 cells and in human leucocytes.[182]

Early studies of age-related DNA-repair in nonmitotic tissues were quite rare. The cerebellar neurons from dogs up to 13 years of age were irradiated with X-rays and the resulting "strand-breaks" repaired equally rapidly at all ages.[183] An interesting investigation of several organs in rats of various ages highlights the confusion.[184] Four repair mechanisms were investigated: excision repair, single- and double-strand break repair, and Q-endonuclease susceptibility.[184] Repair capacity was highest in liver, spleen, kidney, and lung, and lowest in the brain, testes, and duodenum. An age-associated shift from excision repair to rejoining strands was noted in spleen, lung, heart, testis, skeletal muscle, and brain, with a complete loss of excision capacity at advanced age .[184] The application of new technologies has produced some clarity in the field. The repair of oxidative damage in DNA, as measured by the presence of 8-hydroxyguanine (8-OHG), was no different between 5 and 30 months of age in Sprague–Dawley rats. There was a significant increase in the concentration of 8-OHG with age in liver, kidney, spleen, lung, small intestine, and brain, and the repair activity levels in kidney, spleen, and lung were higher than in the liver, small intestine, brain, but the pattern was consistent for the three age stages investigated.[185] However, in NMRI mice between 3 and 27 months of age, the repair of alkali-labile, DNA strand breaks was reduced significantly in brain and heart.[186] Others have measured both nuclear unscheduled DNA synthesis (UDS) and mtDNA synthesis in the brains of untreated mice of various ages. Some neuronal cells showed a decline of both UDS and mtDNA synthesis with age, whereas endothelial cells and the majority of glial cells showed no age-related alterations of UDS.[187] Another investigation used the polymerase chain reaction (PCR) to amplify fragments of transcribed (β-actin, p53) and non-transcribed (IgE, heavy-chain) genes in brain and spleen DNA from γ-irradiated and control 2- and 28-month-old rats.[188] The β-actin and IgE gene fragments of spleen DNA from old rats showed a higher level of lesions inhibiting the thermostable DNA polymerase derived from *Thermus thermophilus* (Tth polymerase) compared to analogous fragments of brain DNA from the same animals. After γ-irradiation, there was no preferential fast repair of lesions in the actively transcribed gene (β-actin) compared to the nontranscribed gene (IgE, heavy-chain) in the brain and spleen of the young and old rats. The data suggest that equal amounts of DNA lesions were repaired in the brains of both young and old rats during the fast-repair phase (0–30 minutes post-irradiation). However, in the slow-repair phase (>5 hours post-irradiation) there was a decrease in the efficiency of DNA repair in the brains of the old rats.[188]

DNA polymerases

Reduced function in the DNA polymerase enzymes with age in either activity or lowered fidelity might lead to a failure to synthesize new functional DNA. Early studies measuring the activity of DNA polymerases showed some variability. For example, the activities of polymerases differed between different tissues. Studies on the activity and fidelity of chromatin-associated DNA polymerase β from aging mice of different lifespans showed that the DNA synthetic activity of liver chromatin remained constant in both species throughout their lifespan.[189] Chromatin-directed, and non-chromatin-directed, copying of a dinucleotide polymer was similar in both *Mus musculus* (relatively short-lived), and *Peromyscus leucopus* (relatively long-lived), and was unaltered in older animals.[189]

More recent studies have examined DNA synthesis and associated polymerase activity. In primary hepatocyte cultures, the effect of epidermal growth factor (EGF) on the stimulation of replication of specific genes (dihydrofolate reductase: DHFR) and *c-myc*, and total mtDNA was examined.[190] Primary hepatocyte cultures were established from young adult (6 months) and senescent (24 months) rats; and basal and EGF-stimulated tritiated thymidine ([3H]-thymidine) incorporation, DNA polymerase α activity, and total cellular DNA, were assessed. It was found that EGF-stimulated [3H]-thymidine incorporation, DNA polymerase α activity, total cellular DNA, DHFR, and *c-myc* gene-specific DNA replication were reduced with age, but mtDNA replication was not affected by either EGF or age. Since mainly DNA polymerase α mediates chromosomal DNA replication, and mtDNA replication is mediated by DNA polymerase γ, the age-related decline in stimulated DNA replication appears to be associated mainly with the DNA polymerase α activation pathway. DNA synthesis has been compared in isolated nuclei from the livers of young and old rats.[191] In addition, normal liver was compared with regenerating tissue at each age. DNA synthesis in nuclei from normal liver was lower than in regenerating liver, and in regenerating liver synthetic activity was lower in nuclear preparations from aged rats. These data suggest that changes in DNA polymerase β are closely related to abnormal replication when DNA polymerases α and δ are inhibited, and that the effect of cytosol on DNA synthesis, as well as the DNA synthetic capacity of isolated nuclei, becomes lower in regenerating rat liver during aging.[191] Recent studies of DNA polymerases in isolated neurons suggest that the activity of polymerase β is reduced with age.[192]

On the other hand, the fidelity of DNA polymerase enzymes is claimed to be reduced in extracts from aged HDF cells maintained in tissue culture, with error frequencies 2–3.4 times greater than for enzymes prepared from young cultures. The main mispairing that seems to take place is between guanine and thymine, but great care must be taken in the interpretation of these results, because the error frequency of DNA polymerase in vitro is much greater than when DNA is synthesized in vivo.[193] Studies of DNA excision repair in human cells showed a decline in efficiency as an apparent function of decreased DNA polymerase α specific activity with increased age of the cell donor.[194] More recently, the DNA polymerase α and an exonuclease involved in the proofreading of DNA synthesis have been isolated from lung-derived HDF (TIG-1) cells at various population doublings.[195] The fidelity of the DNA polymerase α remained high until late passage and fell suddenly just before the end of the lifespan at between 65 and 69 doublings (maximum 70 population doublings). The activity of the exonuclease remained unchanged from 21 to 61 doublings, but decreased rapidly at later stages. The exonuclease activity at 69 population doublings was about 50 percent of that in TIG-1 cells at 21 population doublings. Late-passage (69 population doublings) TIG-1 cells showed an increased incorporation of noncomplementary nucleotides into DNA; in addition, many of the errors were not removed by the proofreading process, suggesting an increase in the mutation frequency in TIG-1 cells just before the end of the lifespan.[195]

Protein synthesis

Age-associated changes in gene expression would have a major impact on protein metabolism, which in turn would have far-reaching effects on the physiology of cell, and ultimately organ, homeostasis. Inadequate or faulty replacement of protein components, particularly under conditions of maximum demand, could explain the lower physiological capabilities of senescent animals.

Alterations in RNA levels may be brought about by a reduction in gene expression or by changes in the activity of RNA polymerases. There is no experimental evidence to suggest that RNA synthesis is reduced to the extent that there is a damaging lack of protein synthesis, nor is there any undisputed evidence for loss of RNA polymerase activity with age. A careful study of specific mRNA species found in hepatocytes from animals of various ages showed that there was no general trend in the synthesis of mRNA with age.[196] Age did not seem to affect the size of the mRNA molecules, nor was there a change in the post-transcriptional processing of five mRNA species studied. The age-associated alterations in mRNA species were similar to the changes in the levels of the proteins coded for by these mRNAs. Thus, age-associated changes in the transcription of mRNA are the primary site of the regulation of protein concentrations at advanced ages.[196] Furthermore, the fidelity of transcriptional processes in nonmitotic cells is not affected by aging.[118,197]

In a review of this length, it is difficult to provide enough background data to present a comprehensive picture of protein synthesis, but other reviews deal with this issue.[11,118,197–199] In many cellular studies there is a lack of important information, such as the pool sizes of the constituents involved in protein

synthesis, including the appropriate amino acids, tRNA, and tRNA synthetase concentrations, which are appropriately controlled in only a few definitive studies. However, it is generally accepted that aging is accompanied by a reduction in RNA and protein synthesis in rodents.

Studies on humans are complicated to interpret, although new technologies are improving the process of measurement.[200] Human research suggests that aging is associated with reduced tissue energy metabolism,[201] and this implies a change in protein metabolism. Elderly people are more likely to be affected by various biological, environmental, and social factors that would generally increase protein needs above those for younger adults. The decline in energy intake in old people, together with its possible consequences for reducing the efficiency of dietary protein utilization, also will tend to increase the protein requirement for elderly subjects, relative to that for more physically active young adults. It has been advocated that an appropriate protein allowance would be 12–14 percent of the total energy intake.[202] However, the data obtained on the measurement of any variable will reflect the population under study: gender, health status, and so on.[200] Studies completed in roughly the past twenty years have failed to demonstrate age changes in total protein synthesis in healthy, nonobese elderly men. Sophisticated techniques using radiolabeled glycine and leucine showed that total body protein metabolism did not alter when normalized for bodyweight.[203–206] However, there are clear changes in body composition and mass even in healthy elderly people, particularly in the 85+ age group. Age-related changes in bodyweight fall into three categories: wasting, cachexia, and sarcopenia.[207] The issue of definition is very important here; for example, cachexia is usually associated with cancer and other chronic diseases, and does not readily fit into the concept of a "healthy" old person.

While the data on total body protein metabolism are interesting, they are still not particularly helpful when trying to assess the functional status of individual cells and organs. The effect of age on the synthesis of specific proteins has been investigated. An example is the liver protein α_{2u}-globulin. Marked age-related decreases in the transcription of the mRNA for this protein have been described.[208–210] Subsequent studies have shown that the subpopulation of hepatocytes that synthesize α_{2u}-globulin is reduced in the liver late in the lifespan.[211] Rats on a calorie-restricted diet show no age-associated change in α_{2u}-globulin transcription, and this has been related to hormone changes brought about by this treatment.[209] Perhaps the major differences described in the literature are not necessarily associated with aging but, more likely, with methods of investigation and shortcomings in techniques.[212] This makes extrapolation from in-vitro to in-vivo situations more hazardous than usual.

Protein structural changes with age

Studies of age-associated changes in enzyme activities have shown increases, decreases, or no change, almost at random. The lack of pattern and consistency suggest that little can be concluded from an investigation of crude tissue extracts, and the reader is directed to extensive reviews on this topic.[11,118,198,199] Research on structural changes in protein with age has a long history, with many studies focusing on the effect of age on collagen cross-linking. In 1963, Leslie Orgel[213,214] proposed one of the first testable theories about aging, suggesting that errors in protein synthesis led to the production of abnormal proteins and was the cause of cellular aging. The suggestion was that incorrect amino acids were more likely to be incorporated into proteins in aged cells; preliminary estimates of the error rate ranged from a low value of 3 in 10^8 correct insertions, and a high one of 1 in 10^4 insertions. Incorrect amino acid insertions would have various effects depending on where they were within a protein. If the "errors" were at the catalytically active site of an enzyme, for example, this could alter its activity (or specificity) for a substrate. An alteration at an allosteric site might result in a loosening of control over its activity, while a change at an amino acid residue involved in the maintenance of the three-dimensional structure of a protein might affect its biophysical characteristics.

In many proteins (e.g. those undergoing rapid turnover) these changes may have little effect. However, errors in enzymes like the DNA and RNA polymerases might be potentially more damaging. These polymerases have long half-lives and catalyze a large number of reactions before they are degraded. Any alteration in their function could lead to the introduction of a large number of error-containing proteins that would accumulate within a cell. Orgel suggested that a critical level of such proteins may occur in a cell, and this would be followed by an "error catastrophe" and cell death. Orgel subsequently withdrew his support for the idea[215] and the theory is no longer considered a primary mechanism of aging, although it cannot be completely discounted.[216] However, some predictions of the hypothesis have been confirmed. Some enzyme proteins do accumulate in the cells and tissues of aging organisms in forms that are enzymically inactive, but the fact that not all proteins are affected suggests this is no universal phenomenon in cells in vitro or in vivo.

Post-translational protein modifications

One factor consistently ignored by many of the investigators testing the "error" theory was the possibility of post-synthetic modifications in protein structure.[217–219] For example, it was known that as human and rabbit erythrocytes age in vivo, several enzymes accumulate in inactive, or abnormally heat-labile, forms.[220] Since protein synthesis does not occur in erythrocytes at the time of this change, the production of these abnormal proteins must be due to post-synthetic modifications. Altered proteins also accumulate in the fiber cells of the lens during aging even though protein synthesis has ceased, indicating that post-synthetic modifications must be occurring.[221] Various post-synthetic modifications to proteins have been recorded including deamidation at asparagine or glutamine residues,[221] cleavage of peptide bonds,[221] acetylation of amino-terminal residues,[222] and glycation of free amino groups.[223] Other reactions include phosphorylation at serine residues, sulphydryl–disulphide bond interchange, changes involving cross-linking,[224] and oxidation.[225,226]

The oxidation of amino acid residues in proteins can occur by direct or indirect mechanisms. Carbonyl groups are formed after free radical damage to amino acid side-chains. The carbonyl content of proteins increased exponentially with age in cultured HDF cells.[227] It was speculated that the oxidized protein in an aged animal may be as much as 30–50 percent of the total cellular protein, a value consistent with the reduced catalytic activity of many enzymes found in old animals.[228] If proteins are exposed to reactive oxygen species in vitro, they undergo marked oxidative damage. Interactions between proteins and reducing sugars or reactive aldehydes in the cellular environment also cause the formation of carbonyl groups. Glycation of proteins involves the interaction of the carbonyl group of a reducing sugar with lysine residues of a protein to form Schiff base derivatives, which lead ultimately to fluorescent end-products (Maillard products).[229] The contribution of glycation and other oxidative reactions to the total carbonyl content of tissues is not fully understood, but there are clearly a number of common pathways, through the ubiquitous Schiff base reaction. Interestingly when aged animals are fed compounds that prevent free radical damage, such as the spin-trap compound phenylbutylnitrone (PBN or N-tert-butyl-α-phenylnitrone), the carbonyl content of tissues decreases, and when treatment is withdrawn the carbonyl groups reappear.[228]

Glycation, the process of nonenzymic addition of sugars to amino acid residues in proteins, is considered a major feature of the pathophysiology of aging.[230] We know that adult-onset diabetes with increased blood glucose raises the extent of the glycation of hemoglobin[231,232] and collagen.[233–235] The progressive glycation of collagen from human skin[233,234] and basement membranes[235] with age is well described, although the change is not universal in long-lived proteins (e.g. lens crystallins from normal human subjects[236]). The end-product of a glycation process is known as an "advanced glycation end-product" (AGE).[237] This area has been thoroughly reviewed elsewhere but is increasing in importance at the interface between biological aging processes and age-related disease.[230,238]

Much of the early literature on aging included detailed analyses of the cross-linkage of macromolecules, particularly the connective tissue proteins collagen and elastin, although the cross-linkage of strands of DNA and DNA-protein within the chromosome also fell into this general area. Collagen undergoes very low turnover rates in adult animals,[239] and is a very strong candidate for post-translational changes. The formation of glycation products suggests that collagen can undergo modification unrelated to its normal maturation after synthesis. Research has examined some of the complex collagen cross-links, and this is reviewed by Finch.[11]

The presence of altered protein molecules in old cells may be a direct result of a decrease in the degradation of intracellular protein. It is now clear that several pathways exist for the removal of proteins within the cell. Short-lived proteins, in either normal or abnormal form, are degraded in a proteolytic pathway in the cytosol. One pathway involves ubiquitin as a marker that identifies proteins for rapid degradation. A substrate protein for degradation is "tagged" with ubiquitin in a covalent linkage that is ATP-dependent. The protease, which degrades the ubiquitin-labeled proteins, is also ATP-dependent; although it is thought that other proteases must exist. The cytosolic proteases, the calpains, which are calcium-activated, may also have a role in protein degradation.[240] The balance of evidence suggests that protein degradation in the intact animal decreases with age.[198] Some of the pitfalls involved in the study of intracellular proteolysis have been discussed above, but it is intriguing to speculate on the possible effects of age-associated changes in the removal of damaged molecules,[241] and the effect this may have on cellular function and the process of cellular senescence.

CONCLUSION

The literature on aging has expanded dramatically. Cell and molecular biological studies are increasing our knowledge of the steps involved in cellular regulation and enabling us to ask new and more detailed questions. We have made real progress in our understanding of aging and age-associated changes. The challenge, as always, is to pinpoint mechanisms, and this is still the most difficult task. We rely too heavily on correlative data, and extrapolate too readily from factors that affect lifespan, when studying the mechanisms of aging. Much of the genetic research is to do with survival of organisms and does not seem to have produced a mechanism; many of the impressive lists of gene pathways are poorly defined in terms of physiological function.

The interface between biological aging processes and age-related diseases also is a major challenge, in terms of both definition and distinction. The separation of these two components seems to be a perennial issue; disease in mammals is a problem when designing studies to understand aging and it is difficult to interpret some investigations, human or rodent, because of a failure to control for sickness in the sample population. Similar, criticisms can be levelled at genetically modified organisms where the survival and health profile of the organism has not been described.

The cellular mechanism that is considered the "hottest" area, the effect of reactive oxygen species, has been around for at least forty years, and the evidence for it is still only correlative. Perhaps we should expect little more; after all, we are dealing with one of the final frontiers in biology. The ability to investigate gene expression more effectively is a major step forward, but in this author's view the temptation will be to use this technology as a data-gathering exercise. That may be no bad thing; biological gerontology has always been rich in theory but starved of data. However, researchers ought perhaps to focus on individual cells when investigating complex tissues like the brain, especially when there are known age-related alterations within the component cell populations.

KEY POINTS Cellular mechanisms of aging

- High-quality research into aging requires high-quality material; from humans with defined health status, to genetically defined model systems, whether mammalian or invertebrate animals.

- Studies of replicative senescence have focused on the role of telomeres and telomerase, using both telomerase knockout mice and human cells transfected with additional copies of the human telomerase catalytic subunit. Clearly, telomerase and telomeres are important components for normal cellular function, but telomere shortening may play different roles in different cell types.

- It is becoming clear that the characteristics of fibroblasts aged in vitro may not represent the situation in vivo.

- Recent studies on the molecular biology of aging have focused on gene expression and aspects of metabolic regulation. Epigenetics and gene silencing by methylation has been revisited, and studies on the yeast *S. cerevisiae* have identified the *Sir* gene as crucial in the regulation of this process.

- Macromolecular damage to DNA (genomic and mitochondrial), and post-translational modifications to proteins, have been explored in more detail.

- The linking of molecular and subcellular organelle damage, to the uncontrolled actions of reactive oxygen species and free radical reactions, has continued, although the data are primarily correlative.

- Interventions with a new generation of antioxidant drugs have been successful in extending lifespan in *C. elegans*, raising hopes for potential drug treatments in mammals.

- Gerontologists still rely too heavily on correlative data rather than cause and effect.

REFERENCES

1. Comfort A: The Biology of Senescence, 3rd edn. Elsevier, New York, 1979
2. Strehler BL: Time, Cells and Aging. Academic Press, New York, 1962
3. Gibson DC, Adelman RC, Finch C: Development of the Rodent as a Model System of Aging. US Department of Health, Education and Welfare, Bethesda, 1978
4. Miller RA, Nadon NL: Principles of animal use for gerontological research. J Gerontol A 2000;55:B117–B123
5. Miller RA, Austad S, Burke D et al: Exotic mice as models for aging research: polemic and prospectus. Neurobiol Aging 1999;20:217–231
6. Lints FA: Non-mammalian Models for Research on Aging. Karger, Basel, 1985
7. Johnson TE, Lithgow GJ: The search for the genetic basis of aging: the identification of gerontogenes in the nematode *Caenorhabditis elegans*. J Am Geriatr Soc, 1992;40:936–945
8. Norwood TH, Smith JR, Stein G: Aging at the cellular level: the human fibroblast-like cell model. In Schneider EL, Rowe JW (eds): Handbook of the Biology of Aging. Academic Press, San Diego, 1990:131–154
9. Lithgow GJ: Temperature, stress response and aging. Rev Clin Geront 1996;6:119–128
10. Szilard L: A theory of ageing. Nature (Lond) 1959;184:957
11. Finch CE: Longevity, Senescence and the Genome. University of Chicago Press, Chicago, 1990
12. Kirkwood TBL, Cremer T: Cytogerontology since 1891: a reappraisal of August Weismann and a review of modern progress. Hum Genet 1982;60:101–121
13. Hayflick L, Moorhead PS: The serial cultivation of human diploid cell strains. Exp Cell Res 1961;25:585–621
14. Hayflick L: The limited in-vitro lifetime of human diploid cell strains. Exp Cell Res 1965;37:614–636
15. West MD, Pereira-Smith OM, Smith JR: Replicative senescence of human skin fibroblasts correlates with a loss of regulation and overexpression of collagenase activity. Exp Cell Res 1989;184:138–147
16. Wick M, Burger C, Brusselbach S et al: A novel member of human tissue inhibitor of metalloproteinases (TIMP) gene family is regulated during G1 expression, mitogenic stimulation, differentiation and senescence. J Biol Chem 1994;269:18953–18960
17. Millis AJ, Hoyle M, McCue HM et al: Differential expression of metalloproteinase and tissue inhibitor of metalloproteinase genes in aged human fibroblasts. Exp Cell Res 1992;201:373–379
18. Dimri GP, Lee X, Basile G et al: A biomarker that identifies senescent human cells in culture and aging skin in vivo. Proc Natl Acad Sci USA 1995;92:9363–9367
19. Hornsby PJ, Gill GN, Bell E: Loss of division potential in culture; aging or differentiation. Science 1980;208:1482

20. Bayreuther K, Rodemann HP, Hommel R et al: Human skin fibroblasts in vitro differentiate along a terminal cell lineage. Proc Natl Acad Sci USA 1988;85:5112–5116

21. Olashaw NE, Kress ED, Cristofalo VJ: Thymidine triphosphate synthesis in senescent WI-38 cells: relationship to loss of replicative activity. Exp Cell Res 1983;149:547–554

22. Pendergrass WR, Saulewicz AC, Salk D et al: Induction of DNA polymerase alpha in senescent cultures of normal and Werner's syndrome cultured skin fibroblasts. J Cell Physiol 1985;124:331–336

23. Rittling SR, Brooks KM, Cristofalo VJ et al: Expression of cell cycle-dependent genes in young and senescent WI38 fibroblasts. Proc Natl Acad Sci USA 1986;83:3316–3320

24. Goldstein S: Replicative senescence: the human fibroblast comes of age. Science 1990;249:1129–1133

25. Campisi J, Dimri G, Hara E: Control of replicative senescence. In Schneider EL, Rowe JW (eds): Handbook of the Biology of Aging. Academic Press, San Diego, 1996:121–149

26. Wright WE, Hayflick L: Nuclear control of cellular ageing demonstrated by hybridization of anucleate and whole cultured normal human fibroblasts. Exp Cell Res 1975;96:113–122

27. Norwood TH, Pendergrass WR, Sprague CA et al: Dominance of the senescent phenotype in heterokaryons between replicative and post-replicative human fibroblast-like cells. Proc Natl Acad Sci USA, 1974;71:2231–2234

28. Norwood TH, Pendergrass WR, Martin GM: Reinitiation of DNA synthesis in senescent human fibroblasts upon fusion with cells of unlimited growth potential. J Cell Biol 1975;64:551–557

29. Yanishevsky RM, Stein GH: Ongoing DNA synthesis continues in young human diploid cells (HDC) fused to senescent HDC, but entry into S-phase is inhibited. Exp Cell Res 1980;126:469–472

30. Stein GH, Yanishevsky RM: Entry into S-phase is inhibited in two immortal cell lines fused to senescent human diploid cells. Exp Cell Res 1979;120:155–166

31. Pereira-Smith OM, Smith JR: Genetic analysis of indefinite division in human cells: identification of four complementation groups. Proc Natl Acad Sci USA 1988;85:6042–6046

32. Hensler P, Annab LA, Barrett JC et al: A gene involved in control of human cellular senescence on human chromosome 1q. Mol Cell Biol 1994;14:2292–2297

33. Ning Y, Weber JL, Killary AM et al: Genetic analysis of indefinite division in human cells: evidence for a senescence-related gene(s) on human chromosome 4. Proc Natl Acad Sci USA 1991;88:5635–5639

34. Ogata T, Ayusawa D, Namba M et al: Chromosome 7 suppresses indefinite division of nontumorogenic immortalized human fibroblast cell lines KMST-6 and SUSM-1. Mol Cell Biol 1993;13:6036–6043

35. Ryan PA, Maher VM, McCormick JJ: Failure of infinite lifespan human cells from different immortality complementation groups to yield finite lifespan hybrids. J Cell Physiol 1994;159:151–160

36. Harley CA, Flutcher AB, Greider CW: Telomeres shorten during ageing of human fibroblasts. Nature (Lond) 1990;345:458–460

37. Harley CB, Vaziri H, Counter CM et al: The telomere hypothesis of aging. Exp Gerontol 1992;27:375–382

38. Blasco MA, Lee HW, Hande MP et al: Telomere shortening and tumor formation by mouse cells lacking telomerase RNA. Cell 1997;91:25–34

39. Rudolph KL, Chang S, Lee HW et al: Longevity, stress response, and cancer in aging telomerase-deficient mice. Cell 1999;96:701–712

40. Bodnar AG, Ouellette M, Frolkis M et al: Extension of life-span by introduction of telomerase into normal human cells. Science 1998;279:349–352

41. Sedivy JM: Can ends justify the means? Telomeres and the mechanisms of replicative senescence and immortalization in mammalian cells. Proc Natl Acad Sci USA 1998;95:9078–9081

42. Baur JA, Zou Y, Shay JW et al: Telomere position effect in human cells. Science 2001;292:2075–2077

43. Mondello C, Petropoulou C, Monti D et al: Telomere length in fibroblasts and blood cells from healthy centenarians. Exp Cell Res 1999;248:234–242

44. Ashcroft GS, Horan MA, Ferguson MWJ: The effects of ageing on cutaneous wound healing in mammals. J Anat 1995;187:1–26

45. Wang E, Lee MJ, Pandey S: Control of fibroblast senescence and activation of programmed cell death. J Cell Biochem 1994;54:432–439

46. Warner HR, Hodes RJ, Pocinki K: What does cell death have to do with aging? J Am Geriatr Soc 1997;45:1140–1146

47. Chang BD, Watanabe K, Broude EV et al: Effects of p21 Waf1/Cip1/Sdi1 on cellular gene expression: implications for carcinogenesis, senescence, and age-related diseases, Proc Natl Acad Sci USA 2000;97:4291–4296

48. Cristofalo VJ, Stanulis BM: Cell aging: a model system. In Behnke JA, Finch CE, Moment GB (eds): The Biology of Aging. Plenum Press, New York, 1978

49. Martin GM, Sprague CA, Epstein CJ: Replicative lifespan of cultivated human cells: effects of donor's age, tissue and genotype. Lab Invest 1970;23:86–92

50. Cristofalo VJ, Allen RG, Pignolo RJ et al: Relationship between donor age and the replicative lifespan of human cells in culture: a reevaluation. Proc Natl Acad Sci USA 1998;95:10614–10619

51. Waters H, Walford RL: Latent period for outgrowth of human skin explants as a function of age. J Gerontol 1970;25:381–383

52. Krohn PL: Review lectures on senescence. II: Heterochromic transplantation in the study of ageing. Proc R Soc Lond Series B 1962;157:128–147

53. Ogden DA, Micklem HS: The fate of serially transplanted bone marrow cell populations from young and old donors. Transplantation 1976;22:287–298

54. Ross EAM, Anderson N, Micklem HS: Serial depletion and regeneration of the murine haematopoietic system: implications for haematopoietic organisation and the study of cellular aging. J Exp Med 1982;155:432–444

55. Harrison DE, Astle CM, Delaittre JA: Loss of proliferative capacity in immunohemopoietic stem cells caused by serial transplantation rather than aging. J Exp Med 1978;147:1526

56. Epstein CJ, Martin GM, Schultz AL et al: Werner's syndrome: a review of its symptomatology, natural history, pathological features, genetics and relationship to the natural aging process. Medicine 1966;45:177–186

57. Martin GM: Genetic syndromes in man with potential relevance to the pathobiology of ageing. In Bergsma D, Harrison DE (eds): Genetic Effects of Aging. Alan R Liss, New York, 1978:5–39

58. Goto M, Rubenstein M, Weber J et al: Genetic linkage of Werner's syndrome to five markers on chromosome 8. Nature (Lond) 1992;355:735–738

59. Goddard KA, Yu CE, Oshima J et al: Toward localization of the Werner syndrome gene by linkage disequilibrium and ancestral haplotyping: lessons learned from analysis of 35 chromosome 8p11.1–21.1 markers. Am J Hum Genet 1996;58:1286–1302

60. Yu CE, Oshima J, Fu YH et al: Positional cloning of the Werner's syndrome gene. Science 1996;272:258–262

61. Faragher RG, Kill IR, Hunter JA et al: The gene responsible for Werner syndrome may be a cell division "counting" gene. Proc Natl Acad Sci USA 1993;90:12030–12034

62. Kruk PA, Rampino NJ, Bohr VA: DNA damage and repair in telomeres; relation to aging. Proc Natl Acad Sci USA 1995;92:258–262

63. Schulz VP, Zakian VA, Ogburn CE et al: Accelerated loss of telomeric repeats may not explain accelerated replicative decline of Werner syndrome cells. Hum Genet 1996;97:750–754

64. Martin GM: Genetics and the pathobiology of ageing. Phil Trans R Soc Lond Series B 1997;352:1773–1780

65. Wang L, Evans AE, Ogburn CE et al: Werner helicase expression in human fetal and adult aortas. Exp Gerontol 1999;34:935–941

66. Balajee AS, Machwe A, May A et al: The Werner syndrome protein is involved in RNA polymerase II transcription. Mol Biol Cell 1999;10:2655–2668

67. Bohr VA, Cooper M, Orren D et al: Werner syndrome protein: biochemical properties and functional interactions. Exp Gerontol 2000;35:695–702

68. Kirkwood TBL, Holliday R: Commitment to senescence: a model for the finite and infinite growth of diploid and transformed human fibroblasts in culture. J Theor Biol 1975;53:481–497

69. Prothero J, Gallant JA: A model of clonal attenuation. Proc Natl Acad Sci USA 1981;78:333–337

70. Martin GM, Fry M, Loeb LA: Somatic mutation and aging in mammalian cells. In Sohal RS, Birnbaum LS, Cutler RG (eds): Molecular Biology of Aging: Gene Stability and Gene Expression. Raven Press, New York, 1985:7–22

71. Vijayashankar N, Brody H: A study of aging in the human abducens nucleus. J Comp Neurol 1977;173:433–439

72. Vijayashankar N, Brody H: Aging in the human brain stem: a study of the nucleus of the trochlear nerve. Acta Anat 1977;99:169–173

73. Vijayashankar N, Brody H: Quantitative study of the pigmented neurons in the nuclei locus coeruleus and subcoeruleus in man as related to aging. J Neuropathol Exp Neurol 1979;38:490–497

74. Haug H, Barmwater U, Eggers R et al: Anatomical changes in aging brain: morphometric analysis of the human prosencephalon. In Cervos-Navarro J, Sarkander H-I (eds): Brain Aging: Neuropathology & Neuropharmacology. Raven Press, New York, 1983:1–12

75. Haug H: Macroscopic and microscopic morphometry of the human brain and cortex: a survey in the light of new results. Brain Pathol 1984;1:123–149

76. Terry RD, Deteresa R, Hansen LA: Neocortical cell counts in normal human adult aging. Ann Neurol 1987;21:530–539

77. Finch CE: Neuron atrophy during aging: programmed or sporadic? TINS 1993;16:104–110

78. Wickelgren I: The aging brain: for the cortex, neuron loss may be less than thought. Science 1996;273:48–50

79. Wickelgren I: Is hippocampal cell death a myth? Science 1996;271:1229–1230

80. Landfield PW, Eldridge JC: Evolving aspects of the glucocorticoid hypothesis of brain aging: hormonal modulation of neuronal calcium homeostasis. Neurobiol Aging 1994;15:579–588

81. Johnson SA, Finch CA: Changes in gene expression during brain aging: a survey. In Schneider EL, Rowe JW (eds): Handbook of the Biology of Aging. Academic Press, San Diego, 1996:300–327

82. Hochschild R: Improving the precision of biological age determinations. 1: A new approach to calculating biological age. Exp Gerontol 1989;24:289–300

83. Meites J: Neuroendocrine biomarkers of aging in the rat. Exp Gerontol 1988;23:349–358

84. Skalicky M, Viidik A: The collagen biomarker of aging can be influenced by physical exercise also in senescent rats. Exp Gerontol 2000;35:595–603

85. Ingram DK, Nakamura E, Smucny D et al: Strategy for identifying biomarkers of aging in long-lived species. Exp Gerontol 2001;36:1025–1034

86. Wyllie AH, Duvall E, Blow JJ: Intracellular mechanisms in cell death in normal and pathological tissues. In Davies I, Sigee DC (eds): Cell Ageing and Cell Death. Cambridge University Press, Cambridge, 1984:269–294

87. Hayflick L: New approaches to old age. Nature 2000;403:365

88. Harman D: Ageing: a theory based on free radical and radiation chemistry. J Gerontol 1956;11:298–300

89. Gutteridge JMC: Free radicals and aging. Rev Clin Geront 1994;4:279–288

90. Butler AR, Flitney FW, Williams DL: NO, nitrosonium ions, nitroxide ions, nitrosothiols and iron-nitrosyls in biology: a chemist's perspective. TIPS 1995;16:18–22

91. Finkel T, Holbrook NJ: Oxidants, oxidative stress and the biology of ageing. Nature (Lond) 2000;408:239–247

92. Halliwell B: Free radicals, oxygen toxicity and ageing. In Sohal RS (ed): Age Pigments. Elsevier/North-Holland Biomedical Press, Amsterdam, 1981:1–62

93. Gius D, Botero A, Shah S et al: Intracellular oxidation/reduction status in the regulation of transcription factors NF-kappaB and AP-1. Toxicol Lett 1999;106:93–106

94. Sen CK: Cellular thiols and redox-regulated signal transduction. Curr Top Cell Regul 2000;36:1–30

95. Glass GA, Gershon D: Enzymatic changes in rat erythrocytes with increasing cell and donor age: loss of superoxide-dismutase activity associated with increases in catalytically defective forms. Biochem Biophys Res Commun 1981;103:1245–1253

96. Stohs SJ, Al-Turk WA, Angle CR: Glutathione S-transferase and glutathione-reductase activities in hepatic and extra-hepatic tissues of the female mice as a function of age. Bioch Pharm 1982;31:2113–2116

97. Dovart A, Gershon D: Rat lens superoxide-dismutase and glucose-6-phosphate-dehydrogenase: studies on the catalytic activity and the fate of enzyme antigen as a function of age. Exp Eye Res 1981;33:651–661

98. Tolmasoff JM, Ono T, Cutler RG: Superoxide dismutase: correlation with life-span and specific metabolic rate in primate species. Proc Natl Acad Sci USA 1980;77:2777–2781

99. Miquel J, Lundgren PR, Bensch KG: Effects of oxygen-nitrogen (1:1) at 760 Torr on the life span and fine structure of Drosophila melanogaster. Mech Age Devel 1975;4:41–59

100. Mann DMA, Yates PO: Lipoprotein pigments: their relationship to ageing in the human nervous system. I: The lipofuscin content of nerve cells. Brain 1974;97:481–488

101. Sohal RS: Age Pigments. Elsevier/North-Holland Biomedical Press, Amsterdam, 1981

102. Aloj Totaro E, Glees P, Pisanti FA: Advances in Age Pigments Research. Pergamon Press, Oxford, 1987

103. Davies I, Fotheringham AP: Lipofuscin: does it affect cellular performance? Exp Gerontol 1981;16:119–125

104. Davies I, Davidson YS, Fotheringham AP: The effect of vitamin E deficiency on the induction of age pigment in various tissues of the mouse. Exp Gerontol 1987;22:127–137

105. Harman D: Prolongation of the normal life-span and inhibition of spontaneous cancer by antioxidants. J Gerontol 1961;16:247–255

106. Comfort A, Youhotsky-Gore I, Pathmanathan K: Effect of ethoxyquin on the longevity of C3H mice. Nature (Lond) 1971;229:254–255

107. Pryor WA: The free-radical theory of aging revisited: a critique and a suggested disease-specific theory. In Warner HR, Butler RN, Sprott RL et al (eds): Modern Biological Theories of Aging. Raven Press, New York, 1987:89–112

108. Kohn RR: Effect of antioxidants on lifespan of C57BL mice. J Gerontol 1971;26:378–380

109. Melov S, Ravenscroft J, Malik S et al: Extension of life-span with superoxide dismutase/catalase mimetics. Science 2000;289:1567–1569

110. Reveillaud J, Niedzwiecki A, Bensch KG et al: Expression of bovine superoxide dismutase in Drosophila melanogaster augments resistance to oxidative stress. Mol Cell Biol 1991;11:632–640

111. Orr WC, Sohal RS: Extension of life-span by overexpression of superoxide dismutase and catalase in Drosophila melanogaster. Science 1994;263:1128–1130

112. Epstein J, Gershon D: Studies on ageing in nematodes. IV: The effect of anti-oxidants on cellular damage and life-span. Mech Age Devel 1972;1:257–264

113. Freund G: Effects of chronic alcohol and vitamin E consumption on ageing pigments and learning performance in mice. Life Sci 1979;24:145–152

114. Tappel AL, Fletcher B, Deamer D: Effect of antioxidants and nutrients on lipid peroxidation fluorescent products and aging parameters in the mouse. J Gerontol 1973;28:415–424

115. Middleton J, Gahan PB: A quantitative cytochemical study of acid phosphatases in rat liver parenchymal cells of different ploidy values. Histochem J 1979;11:649–659

116. Enesco HE, Shimokawa I, Yu BP: Effect of dietary restriction and aging on polyploidy in rat liver. Mech Age Devel 1991;59:69–78

117. Mann DM, Yates PO: Polyploidy in the human nervous system. I: The DNA content of neurones and glia of the cerebellum. J Neurol Sci 1973;18:183–196

118. Rothstein M: Biochemical Approaches to Aging. Academic Press, New York, 1982

119. Guarente L, Kenyon C: Genetic pathways that regulate ageing in model organisms. Nature 2000;408:255–262

120. Lamb MJ: Epigenetic inheritance and aging. Rev Clin Geront 1994;4:97–105

121. Mays-Hoopes LL: DNA methylation: a possible correlation between aging and cancer. In Sohal RS, Birnbaum LS, Cutler RG (eds): Molecular Biology of Aging: Gene Stability and Gene Expression. Raven Press, New York, 1985:49–65

122. Vijg J, Uitterlinden AG, Mullaart E, et al: Processing of DNA damage during aging: induction of genetic alteration. In Sohal RS, Birnbaum LS, Cutler RG (eds): Molecular Biology of Aging: Gene Stability and Gene Expression. Raven Press, New York, 1985:155–171

123. Wilson VL, Jones PA: DNA methylation decreases in aging but not in immortal cells. Science (Washington) 1983;220:1054–1057

124. Holliday R: Strong effects of 5-azacytidine on the in-vitro lifespan of human diploid fibroblasts. Exp Cell Res 1986;166:543–552

125. Holliday R: Toward a biological understanding of the aging process. Pers Biol 1988;32:109–123

126. Ono T, Shinya K, Uehara Y et al: Endogenous virus genomes become hypomethylated tissue—specifically during aging process of C57BL mice. Mech Age Devel, 1989;50:27–36

127. Cutler RG: Dysdifferentiative hypothesis of aging: a review. In Sohal RS, Birnbaum LS, Cutler RG (eds): Molecular Biology of Aging: Gene Stability and Gene Expression. Raven Press, New York, 1985:307–340

128. Ono T, Cutler RG: Age-dependent relaxation of gene expression: increase of endogenous murine leukaemia virus-related and globin-related RNA in brain and liver of mice. Proc Natl Acad Sci USA 1978;75:1431–1435

129. Holliday R: Ageing: X-chromosome reactivation. Nature (Lond) 1987;327:661–662

130. Deol MS, Truslove GM, McLaren A: Genetic activity at the albino locus in Cattanach's insertion in the mouse. J Embryol Exp Morphol 1986;96:295–302

131. Wareham KA, Lyon MF, Glenister PH et al: Age-related reactivation of an X-linked gene. Nature (Lond) 1987;327:725–727

132. Migeon BR, Axelman J, Beggs AH: Effect of ageing on reactivation of the human X-linked HRPT locus. Nature (Lond) 1988;335:93–96

133. Holliday R: X-chromosome reactivation and ageing. Nature (Lond) 1989;337:311

134. Papaconstantinou J, Reisner PD, Liu L et al: Mechanisms of altered gene expression with aging. In Schneider EL, Rowe JW (eds): Handbook of the Biology of Aging. Academic Press, San Diego, 1996:150–183

135. Fujita T, Maruyama N: Elevated levels of c-jun and c-fos transcripts in the aged rat liver. Biochem Biophys Res Comm 1991;178:1485–1491

136. Kaminska B, Kaczmarek L: Robust induction of AP-1 transcription factor DNA binding activity in the hippocampus of aged rats. Neurosci Lett 1993;153:189–191

137. Arrigo AP: Gene expression and the thiol redox state. Free Radic Biol Med 1999;27:936–944

138. Liu AY-C, Lin Z, Choi HS et al: Attenuated induction of heat shock gene expression in aging diploid fibroblasts. J Biol Chem 1989;264:12037–12045

139. Liu AY-C, Choi HS, Lu Y-K et al: Molecular events involved in transcriptional activation of heat shock genes become progressively refractory to heat stimulation during aging of human diploid fibroblasts. J Cell Physiol 1991;149:560–566

140. Goyns MH, Charlton MA, Dunford JE et al: Differential display analysis of gene expression indicates that age-related changes are restricted to a small cohort of genes. Mech Age Devel 1998;101:73–90

141. Dozmorov I, Bartke A, Miller RA: Array-based expression analysis of mouse liver genes: effect of age and of the longevity mutant Prop1df. J Gerontol A 2001;56:B72–B80

142. Kayo T, Allison DB, Weindruch R et al: Influences of aging and caloric restriction on the transcriptional profile of skeletal muscle from rhesus monkeys. Proc Natl Acad Sci USA 2001;98:5093–5098

143. Ly DH, Lockhart DJ, Lerner RA et al: Mitotic misregulation and human aging. Science 2000;287:2486–2492

144. Bartke A: Growth hormone and aging. Endocrine 1998;8:103–108

145. Curtis HJ: Genetic factors in aging. Adv Genet 1971;16:305–324

146. Pincheira J, Gallo C, Bravo M et al: G2 repair and aging: influence of donor age on chromosomal aberrations in human lymphocytes. Mutation Res 1993;295:55–62

147. Sinclair DA, Guarente L: Extrachromosomal rDNA circles: a cause of aging in yeast. Cell 1997;91:1033–1042

148. Bernstein H, Gensler HL: DNA damage and aging. In Yu BP (ed): Free Radicals in Aging. CRC Press, Boca Raton, 1993:89–122

149. Setlow RB: Theory presentation and background summary. In Warner HR, Butler RN, Sprott RL et al (eds): Modern Biological Theories of Aging. Raven Press, New York, 1987:177–182

150. Failla G: The ageing process and carcinogenesis. Ann NY Acad Sci 1958;71:1124–1135

151. Alexander P: The relationship between ageing and cancer: somatic mutations or breakdown of host defence mechanisms. Bull Schweiz Akad Med Wiss 1969;24:258–271

152. Yuhas JM: Age and susceptibility to reduction in life expectancy: an analysis of proposed mechanisms. Exp Gerontol 1971;6:335–344

153. Price GB, Makinodan T: Ageing: alteration of DNA-protein information. Gerontologia 1973;19:58–70

154. Stuart GR, Glickman BW: Through a glass, darkly: reflections of mutation from lacI transgenic mice. Genetics 2000;155:1359–1367

155. Stuart GR, Oda Y, de Boer JG et al: Mutation frequency and specificity with age in liver, bladder and brain of lacI transgenic mice. Genetics 2000;154:1291–1300

156. Tice RR, Setlow RB: DNA repair and replication in aging organisms and cells. In Finch CE, Schneider EL (eds): Handbook of the Biology of Aging. Van Nostrand Reinhold, New York, 1985:173–224

157. Rattan SIS: DNA damage and repair during cellular aging. Int Rev Cytol 1989;116:47–88

158. Marnett LJ, Burcham PC: Endogenous DNA adducts: potential and paradox. Chem Res Toxicol 1993;6:771–785

159. Ames BN, Gold LS: Endogenous mutagens and the causes of aging and cancer. Mutation Res 1991;250:3–16

160. Ames BN, Saul RL, Schwiers E et al: Oxidative DNA damage as related to cancer and aging: assay of thymine glycol, thymidine glycol and hydroxymethyuracil in human and rat urine. In Sohal RS, Cutler RG (eds): Molecular Biology of Aging: Gene Stability and Gene Expression. Raven Press, New York, 1985:137–144

161. Adelman R, Saul RL, Ames BN: Oxidative damage to DNA: relation to species metabolic rate and lifespan. Proc Natl Acad Sci USA 1988;85:2706–2707

162. Fraga CG, Shigenaga MK, Park JW et al: Oxidative damage to DNA during aging: 8-hydroxydeoxy-guanosine in rat organ DNA and urine. Proc Natl Acad Sci USA 1990;87:4533–4537

163. Randerath K, Randerath E, Filburn C: Genomic and mitochondrial DNA alterations with aging. In Schneider EL, Rowe JW (eds): Handbook of the Biology of Aging. Academic Press, San Diego, 1995:198–214

164. Randerath K, Reddy MV, Gupta RC: 32P-labeling test for DNA damage. Proc Natl Acad Sci USA 1981;78:6126–6129

165. Randerath K, Li D, Nath R et al: Exogenous and endogenous DNA modifications as monitored by 32P-postlabeling: relationships to cancer and aging. Exp Gerontol 1992;27:533–549

166. Randerath K, Hart RW, Zhou G-D et al: Enhancement of age-related increases in DNA I-compound levels by caloric restriction: comparison of male B-N and F-344 rats. Mutation Res 1993;295:31–46

167. Randerath K, Randerath E, Zhou GD et al: Bulky endogenous DNA modifications (I-compounds): possible structural origins and functional implications. Mutation Res 1999;424:183–194

168. Holehan AM, Merry BJ: The experimental manipulation of ageing by diet. Biol Rev 1986;61:329–368

169. Richter C: Oxidative damage to mitochondrial DNA and its relationship to ageing. In Esser K, Martin GM (eds): Molecular Aspects of Aging. John Wiley, Chichester, 1995:99–108

170. Wallace DC: Mitochondrial DNA mutations in human disease and aging. In Esser K, Martin GM (eds): Molecular Aspects of Aging. John Wiley, Chichester, 1995:163–177

171. Agarwal S, Sohal RS: DNA oxidative damage and life expectancy in house-flies. Proc Natl Acad Sci USA 1994;91:12332–12335

172. Linn S: DNA repair in mitochondria: How is it limited? What is its function? In Esser K, Martin GM (eds): Molecular Aspects of Aging. John Wiley, Chichester, 1995:191–196

173. Shay JW, Werbin H, Piatyszek MA: Does aging favour translation of mito-chondrial DNA fragments to the nuclear genome? In Esser K, Martin GM (eds): Molecular Aspects of Aging. John Wiley, Chichester, 1995:179–189

174. Hart RW, Setlow RB: Correlation between deoxyribonucleic acid excision repair and life-span in a number of mammalian species. Proc Natl Acad Sci USA 1974;71:2169–2173

175. Hart RW, D'Ambrosio SM, Ng KG et al: Longevity, stability and DNA repair. Mech Age Devel 1979;9:203–224

176. Sacher GA, Hart RW: Longevity, aging and comparative cellular and molecular biology of the house mouse, *Mus musculus*, and the white-footed mouse, *Peromyscus leucopus*. In Bergsma D, Harrison DE (eds): Genetic Effects on Aging. Alan R Liss, New York, 1978:71–96

177. Hart RW, Daniel FB: Genetic stability in vitro and in vivo. Adv Pathobiol 1980;7:123–141

178. Mattern MR, Cerutti PA: Age-dependent excision repair of damaged thymine from gamma-irradiated DNA by isolated nuclei from human fibroblasts. Nature (Lond) 1975;254:450–452

179. Hart RW, Setlow RB: DNA repair in late-passage human cells. Mech Age Devel 1976;5:67–77

180. Painter RB, Clarkson JM, Young BR: Ultra-violet induced repair replication in aging diploid human cells (WI-38). Radiat Res 1973;56:560–564

181. Mayer PJ, Lange CS, Bradley MO et al: Gender differences in age-related decline in DNA double-strand break damage and repair in lymphocytes. Ann Hum Biol 1991;18:405–415

182. Atamna H, Cheung I, Ames BN: A method for detecting abasic sites in living cells: age-dependent changes in base excision repair. Proc Natl Acad Sci USA 2000;97:686–691

183. Wheeler KT, Lett JT: On the possibility that DNA repair is related to age in non-dividing cells. Proc Natl Acad Sci USA 1974;71:1862–1865

184. Niedermuller H: DNA repair during aging. In Sohal RS, Birnbaum LS, Cutler RG (eds): Molecular Biology of Aging: Gene Stability and Gene Expression. Raven Press, New York, 1985:173–193

185. Hirano T, Yamaguchi R, Asami S et al: 8-hydroxyguanine levels in nuclear DNA and its repair activity in rat organs associated with age. J Gerontol A 1996;51: B303–B307

186. Zahn RK, Jaud S, Schroder HC et al: DNA status in brain and heart as prominent co-determinant for life span? Assessing the different degrees of DNA damage, damage susceptibility, and repair capability in different organs of young and old mice. Mech Age Devel 1996;89:79–94

187. Schmitz C, Axmacher B, Zunker U et al: Age-related changes of DNA repair and mitochondrial DNA synthesis in the mouse brain. Acta Neuropathol (Berl) 1999;97:71–81

188. Ploskonosova II, Baranov VI, Gaziev AI: PCR assay of DNA damage and repair at the gene level in brain and spleen of gamma-irradiated young and old rats. Mutation Res 1999;434:109–117

189. Fry M, Loeb LA, Martin GM: Nuclease digestion studies of mouse chromatin as a function of age. J Gerontol 1981;34:672–679

190. Kitano S, Bohr VA, Reed TD et al: Effect of aging on EGF-stimulated replication of specific genes in rat hepatocytes. J Cell Physiol 1998;176:32–39

191. Taguchi T, Fukuda M, Ohashi M: Differences in DNA synthesis in vitro using isolated nuclei from regenerating livers of young and aged rats. Mech Age Devel 2001;122:141–155

192. Rao KS, Annapurna VV, Raji NS et al: Loss of base excision repair in aging rat neurons and its restoration by DNA polymerase beta. Brain Res Mol Brain Res 2000;85:251–259

193. Murray V, Holliday R: Increased error frequency of DNA-polymerases from sensescent human fibroblasts. J Mol Biol 1981;146:55–76

194. Busbee D, Sylvia V, Stec J et al: Lability of DNA polymerase alpha correlated with decreased DNA synthesis and increased age in human cells. J Nat Cancer Inst 1987;79:1231–1239

195. Fukuda M, Taguchi T, Ohashi M: Age-dependent changes in DNA polymerase fidelity and proofreading activity during cellular aging. Mech Age Devel 1999;109:141–151

196. Richardson A, Rutherford MS, Birchenall-Sparks MC et al: Levels of specific messenger RNA species as a function of age. In Sohal RS, Birnbaum LS, Cutler RG (eds): Molecular Biology of Aging: Gene Stability and Gene Expression. Raven Press, New York, 1985:229–241

197. Reff ME: RNA and protein metabolism. In Finch CE, Schneider EL (eds): Handbook of the Biology of Aging. Van Nostrand Reinhold, New York, 1985:225–254

198. Makrides SC: Protein synthesis and degradation during ageing and senescence. Biol Rev 1983;58:343–422

199. Richardson A, Roberts MS, Rutherford MS: Aging and gene expression. Rev Biol Res Aging 1985;2:395–419

200. Heymsfield SB, Nunez C, Testolin C et al: Anthropometry and methods of body composition measurement for research and field application in the elderly. Eur J Clin Nutr 2000;54(Suppl 3):S26–S32

201. Fukagawa NK, Bandini LG, Young JB: Effect of age on body composition and resting metabolic rate. Am J Physiol 1990;259:E233–E238

202. Fukagawa NK, Young VR: Protein and amino acid metabolism and requirements in older persons. Clin Geriatr Med 1987;3:329–341

203. Fukagawa NK, Minaker KL, Young VR et al: Glucose and amino acid metabolism in aging man: differential effects of insulin. Metabolism 1988;37:371–377

204. Fukagawa NK, Minaker KL, Young VR et al: Leucine metabolism in aging humans: effect of insulin and substrate availability. Am J Physiol 1989;256:E288–E294

205. Gersovitz M, Bier D, Matthews D et al: Dynamic aspects of whole body glycine metabolism: influence of protein intake in young adult and elderly males. Metabolism 1980;29:1087–1094

206. Gersovitz M, Munro HN, Udall J et al: Albumin synthesis in young and elderly subjects using a new stable isotope methodology: response to level of protein intake. Metabolism 1980;29:1075–1086

207. Roubenoff R: The pathophysiology of wasting in the elderly. J Nutr 1999;129:256S–259S

208. Roy AK, Nath TS, Motwani NM et al: Age-dependent regulation of the polymorphic forms of α_{2u}-globulin. J Biol Chem 1983;258:10123–10127

209. Richardson A, Butler JA, Rutherford MS et al: Effect of age and dietary restriction on the expression of α_{2u}-globulin. J Biol Chem 1987;262:12821–12825

210. Murty CVR, Mancini MA, Chatterjee B et al: Changes in transcriptional activity and matrix association in α_{2u}-globulin gene family in the rat liver during maturation and aging. Biochim Biophys Acta 1988;949:27–34

211. Motwani NM, Caron D, Demyan WF et al: Monoclonal antibodies to α_{2u}-globulin synthesizing hepatocytes during androgenic induction and aging. J Biol Chem 1984;259:3653–3657

212. Filion A-M, Laughrea M: Translation fidelity in the brain, liver, and hippocampus of the aging Fischer 344 rat. In Sohal RS, Birnbaum LS, Cutler RG (eds): Molecular Biology of Aging: Gene Stability and Gene Expression. Raven Press, New York, 1985:257–261

213. Orgel LE: The maintenance of the accuracy of protein synthesis and its relevance to ageing. Proc Natl Acad Sci USA 1963;49:517–521

214. Orgel LE: The maintenance of the accuracy of protein synthesis and its relevance to ageing—a correction. Proc Natl Acad Sci USA 1970;67:1476

215. Orgel LE: Ageing of clones of mammalian cells. Nature (Lond) 1973;243:441

216. Rothstein M: Evidence for and against the error catastrophe hypothesis. In Warner HR, Butler RN, Sprott RL et al (eds): Modern Biological Theories of Aging. Raven Press, New York. 1987:139–154

217. Gershon D: Current status of age altered enzymes: alternative mechanisms. Mech Age Devel 1979;9:189–196

218. McKerrow JH: Non-enzymatic post-translational amino acid modifications in ageing: a brief review. Mech Age Devel 1979;10:371–377

219. Sharma HK, Rothstein M: Altered enolase in aged Turbatrix aceti results from conformational changes in the enzyme. Proc Natl Acad Sci USA 1980;77:5865–5868

220. Fornaini G, Leoncini G, Segni P et al: Relationship between age and properties of human and rabbit glucose-6-phosphate dehydrogenase. Eur J Biochem 1969;7:214–232

221. VanKleef FSM, DeJong WW, Hoenders HJ: Stepwise degradations and deamidation of the eye lens protein crystallin in ageing. Nature (Lond) 1975;258:264–267

222. Hoenders HJ, Schoenmakers JGG, Garding JJJ et al: The N-terminus of lens protein alpha-crystallin. Exp Eye Res 1968;7:291–297

223. Bailey AJ, Robbins SP: Development and maturation of the crosslinks in the collagen fibres of the skin. Front Matrix Biol 1973;1:130–156

224. Zs-Nagy I, Nagy K: On the role of cross-linking of cellular proteins in ageing. Mech Age Devel 1980;14:245–251

225. Kay MMB: Age effects on colony-forming human peripheral blood T and B cells. Gerontology 1985;31:278–284

226. Kay MMB, Bosman G, Notter M et al: Life and death of neurons: the senescent cell antigen. Ann NY Acad Sci 1988;521:155–169

227. Oliver CN, Ahn BW, Moerman EJ et al: Age-related changes in oxidised proteins. J Biol Chem 1987;262:5488–5491

228. Stadtman ER: Protein oxidation and aging. Science 1992;257:1220–1224

229. Gutteridge JMC: Oxygen radicals, transition metals and aging. In Aloj Totaro E, Glees P, Pisanti FA (eds): Advances in Age Pigments Research. Pergamon Press, Oxford, 1987:1–22

230. Harding JJ, Beswick HT, Ajiboye R et al: Non-enzymatic post-translational modification of proteins in aging: a review. Mech Age Devel 1989;50:7–16

231. Koenig RJ, Peterson CM, Jones RL et al: Correlation of glucose regulation and hemoglobin A1c in diabetes mellitus. N Engl J Med 1976;295:417–420

232. Bunn HF: Nonenzymatic glycosylation of protein: relevance to diabetes. Am J Med 1981;70:325–330

233. Schnider SL, Kohn RR: Glucosylation of human collagen in aging and diabetes mellitus. J Clin Invest 1980;66:1179–1181

234. Schnider SL, Kohn RR: Effects of age and diabetes mellitus on the solubility and nonenzymatic glucosylation of human skin collagen. J Clin Invest 1981;67:1630–1635

235. Garlick RL, Bunn HF, Spiro RG: Nonenzymatic glycation of basement membranes from human glomeruli and bovine sources: effect of diabetes and age. Diabetes 1988;37:1144–1155

236. Patrick JS, Thorpe SR, Baynes JW: Nonenzymatic glycosylation of protein does not increase with age in normal human lenses. J Gerontol 1990;45:B18–B23

237. Lee AT, Cerami A: Modifications of proteins and nucleic acids by reducing sugars: possible role in aging. In Schneider EL, Rowe JW (eds): Handbook of the Biology of Aging. Academic Press, San Diego, 1990:116–130

238. Levine RL, Stadtman ER: Protein modifications with aging. In Schneider EL, Rowe JW (eds): Handbook of the Biology of Aging. Academic Press, San Diego, 1996:184–197

239. Molnar JA, Alpert N, Burke JF et al: Synthesis and degradation rates of collagens in vivo in whole skin of rats, studied with $^{18}O_2$ labelling. Biochem J 1986;240:431–435

240. Zeman R, Kameyama T, Matsumoto K et al: Regulation of protein degradation in muscle by calcium: evidence for enhanced nonlysosomal proteolysis associated with elevated cytosolic calcium. J Biol Chem 1985;260:13619–13624

241. Dice JF, Goff SA: Error catastrophe and aging: future directions of research. In Warner HR, Butler RN, Sprott RL et al (eds): Modern Biological Theories of Aging. Raven Press, New York, 1987:155–168

242. Crowley C, Curtis HJ: The development of somatic mutations in mice with age. Proc Natl Acad Sci USA 1963;49:626–628

Chapter 9

Physiology of aging

Edward J. Masoro

When broadly defined, aging refers to all time-associated events that occur during the lifespan of an organism. During this time, many changes occur in the physiological processes. These changes may be beneficial, neutral, or deteriorative. During the developmental period of life most changes are due to the maturation of the physiological processes and tend to be beneficial. However, during the post-maturation period of life most of the changes are detrimental, although some may be neutral, such as the graying of the hair. Indeed, the term "senescence" is used to denote this post-maturation deterioration. Senescence is defined as the deteriorative changes with time during post-maturation life that underlie an increasing vulnerability to challenges, thereby decreasing the ability of the organism to survive. Although senescence is a subset of aging, in common usage, aging is often used to mean senescence. Unfortunately, this meaning is usually not explicitly stated. In this chapter, aging and senescence will be used as synonyms. This usage is particularly appropriate in a textbook of geriatric medicine.

This brief chapter can cover only concepts and provide a limited number of examples. Section 11 of the *Handbook of Physiology* series published by the American Physiological Society is dedicated to the physiology of aging.[1] That volume provides in-depth coverage of most age changes in the physiological systems and should be consulted by readers who desire further information in a particular subject area.

PHYSIOLOGICAL DETERIORATION AND THE AGING PHENOTYPE

A major characteristic of the aging phenotype is the difference in physiological processes in elderly people compared to young adults. Indeed, physiological deterioration plays an important role in the age-associated increase in the age-specific mortality rate. Thus, knowledge of the age changes in the physiological systems is invaluable for both the geriatric physician tending elderly patients and the biological gerontologist in the quest for an understanding of the biological nature of aging.

Causes of age-associated physiological deterioration

The progressive deterioration with age of the physiological systems that starts during young adulthood is caused by the many damaging processes and agents that organisms encounter during life. Apparently, repair systems during post-maturational life are not able to fully eliminate the damage. The result is a progressive functional inadequacy of the physiological systems due to the accumulation of damage. The extent of this functional inadequacy and its rate of occurrence varies among species and among individuals within a species, as well as among the physiological systems of an individual. It is convenient to classify the damaging processes responsible for the age-associated physiological deterioration in the following three categories: (1) damage resulting from intrinsic living processes, (2) damage caused by extrinsic factors, and (3) damage resulting from age-associated diseases.

Damage resulting from intrinsic living processes

Many of the processes essential to life also have damaging aspects. For example, aerobic metabolism, which enables organisms to readily generate metabolic energy from ingested nutrients, has the negative aspect of the generation of highly reactive compounds such as superoxide radicals, hydroxyl radicals, and hydrogen peroxide due to the univalent reduction of oxygen. These oxygen-containing compounds are potentially highly damaging. Protection from, and repair of, damage from these substances has evolved, but is not totally effective. Therefore, an accumulation of oxidative damage with increasing age occurs.[2] The extent of protection and the ability to repair the damage varies among species. Thus, it is not surprising that there is interspecies variation in the rate of accumulation of oxidatively damaged macromolecules. Another example involves glucose, a most important fuel for most organisms. However, in addition to serving as an energy source, glucose also participates in the glycoxidation of proteins and nucleic acids and, in this way, alters their biological functions.[3] Again, there are protective mechanisms, as well as processes that eliminate the damaged macromolecules, which vary in efficacy among species. Probably there is no intrinsic living process that does not also have the ability to cause damage.

Damage caused by extrinsic factors

There is general agreement that extrinsic factors contribute to the aging phenotype. In spite of this, many do not subscribe to the view that these extrinsic factors are part of the aging process. This view is based on long-held criteria for aging processes enumerated by Strehler[4] in 1977. One of the criteria is "intrinsicality," the view that aging is entirely an intrinsic phenomenon. Busse[5] recognized the conceptual difficulty that this criterion caused and tried to resolve the problem by proposing the concept of primary and secondary aging. Primary aging was defined as universal changes occurring with age within a species or population, changes not caused by disease or environment. Secondary aging was defined as changes due to the interactions of primary aging with disease processes and environmental factors. This concept may be faulty for two reasons. First, if aging is the result of the progressive accumulation of unrepaired damage, it is irrelevant whether that damage originates from intrinsic living processes or is caused by extrinsic agents. Second, extrinsic agents cause damage only because of interactions with biological materials and processes. For example, it has recently been shown that the effect of genes on the lifespan and aging of *Drosophila melanogaster* is dependent on environmental interactions.[6] In a sense, all damage is intrinsic whether it originates as a result of basic living processes or from reactions to extrinsic factors. However, this view downplays the importance of environmental factors which is not desirable because such factors can be modified and thus should be the focus of research on aging interventions.

Indeed, the marked effect that environmental factors can have on the aging process is particularly well illustrated by the effects of long-term restriction of food intake by laboratory mice and rats.[7] Restricting the food intake by 30–50 percent of that eaten by ad-libitum fed animals markedly increases longevity (see Figure 9-1 for its typical effect on population survival characteristics[8]), prevents or delays age-associated disease, and maintains a broad array of physiological processes in a youthful state until very advanced ages. Examples of the scope of these beneficial effects on physiological systems include: immune function,[9] cardiac function,[10] female reproductive function,[11] and gene expression.[12] Indeed, reduction of food intake retards most, but not all, age-associated changes in physiological processes of rats and mice that have been studied. It has been established that the reduction in energy (calorie) intake is the dietary factor responsible for this retardation of age changes in the physiological systems.[7] While there is no evidence that restricting energy intake of humans during adult life would globally retard age-associated physiological deterioration, it has been shown to influence the physiological systems of nonhuman primates in a fashion similar to its effects on rats and mice.[13] Moreover, there is evidence that diet can influence the occurrence or progression of age-associated human disease.[14] For example, high-fat, high-calorie diets are believed to promote age-associated human pathology such as atherosclerosis,[15] hypertension,[15] and insulin resistance and impaired glucose tolerance.[16]

The lifestyle factor that has received the most attention relates to the fact that with increasing age many people become increasingly sedentary.[17] Studies on the effect of exercise

training in old human subjects indicate that much of the decline in cardiovascular function with advancing age in sedentary people is due to the effects of exercise deficiency and, therefore, probably can at least in part be reversed by physical activity even at advanced ages.[18] Skeletal muscle mass and strength decrease with increasing age,[19] and both the mass and the strength of skeletal muscle can be increased by resistance training even at very advanced ages.[20] It is likely that the frequently occurring increase in body weight in people between the ages of 20 and 70 years is primarily the result of a sedentary lifestyle.[21] Exercise has also been found to attenuate the age-associated increase in body fat content.[22] Most importantly, exercise improves the distribution pattern of body fat in elderly men and women.[23] There is also evidence that exercise can attenuate the increase in insulin resistance and the reduction in glucose tolerance that occurs in many people with advancing age.[24] There can be little doubt that the increasingly sedentary lifestyle with advancing age contributes greatly to the deterioration of physiological functions of old people.

There is no clear demarcation between lifestyle factors and personal habits. For example, excessive exposure to the sun results in changes in skin structure and function that are generally considered to be part of the aging phenotype.[25] Such exposure may be an inevitable consequence of the occupation of individuals and/or the climatic conditions of the geographic region in which they reside. If so, excessive sun exposure probably should be in the lifestyle category. However, recreational choice leading to excessive exposure such as sunbathing can be viewed either as lifestyle or as personal habit. The personal habit that has received the most attention in regard to aging is cigarette smoking. It is established that wrinkling of the skin, a hallmark of aging, is promoted by smoking.[26] Also, many age-associated diseases that cause marked physiological deterioration are promoted by smoking. Examples are chronic obstructive lung disease[27] and atherosclerosis.[28]

Although yet to be intensively studied, there is suggestive evidence that psychosocial factors markedly influence age changes in physiological function.[29,30] For example, it has been established that social network emotional support enhances the maintenance of physical performance.[29] Elderly people commonly encounter reductions in autonomy and control because of many factors, such as a reduction in economic resources and institutional living facilities,[14] which lead to the deterioration of physiological functions. Also, both bereavement and residential relocation have been found to increase mortality and morbidity in elderly people and, therefore, it is likely that they negatively impact the physiological systems. It has been proposed that a reduction in social support plays a causative role[14] in the physiological deterioration of elderly people. The epidemiological research associating low educational level with an increased risk of a decline in mental function with increasing age focuses on another psychosocial factor capable of influencing age changes in the physiological systems.[14] Clearly, the subject of the influence of psychosocial factors on human aging is in the very preliminary stages of study and requires much further investigation. In particular, the pathways linking the psychosocial factors to the physiological systems must be delineated.

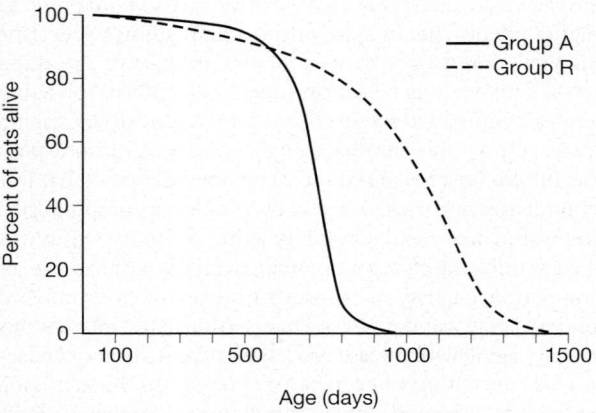

Figure 9-1 Survival curves for ad-libitum fed male F344 rats (group A, *n* = 115) and rats restricted to 60 percent of the mean ad-libitum intake (group R, *n* = 115). From Yu et al.[8]

Damage resulting from age-associated diseases

There is general agreement that much of the physiological deterioration of elderly people is secondary to age-associated disease. It is also recognized that the occurrence and progression of age-associated disease is strongly influenced by age-associated physiological deterioration. However, there is disagreement as to whether age-associated disease is part of the normal aging process. Indeed, the concept of "normal aging" has emerged[31] and is widely used by those conducting physiological studies on aging humans. It is defined as senescence in the absence of disease and more appropriately should be called "atypical aging" rather than "normal aging." Most elderly people have one or more age-associated disease and it is to be expected that the fraction of elderly free of age-associated disease will become vanishingly small as advances in technology increasingly uncover occult disease, as Lakatta[32] has done by using the thallium-stress test to determine occult coronary heart disease in elderly people. Indeed, in order to study what many investigators call "normal aging," great effort is made to exclude from the population to be studied subjects with age-associated disease.[33] These studies are invaluable because such a reductionist approach is a powerful tool in dissecting the details of the aging processes.

However, the view that "normal aging" does not involve the occurrence of age-associated disease is not conceptually sound in terms of basic biology. Evolutionary biologists propose that aging (senescence) occurs because of the decline in the force of natural selection with advancing age.[34] Because of this, biological processes that result in detrimental effects expressed late in life cannot be selected against. It is for this reason that physiological deterioration increases with increasing age, and it is for the same reason that age-associated disease increasingly expresses with advancing age. It is true that some people (a very small subset) may age without evidence of discernible age-associated disease, but this may relate to the fact that the distinction between age-associated disease and age-associated physiological deterioration is arbitrary. For example, loss of bone mass is a well-recognized age-associated physiological deterioration and osteoporosis is a major age-associated disease; the boundary in this case of when to label a physiological change as a disease is not obvious.

For all of the above reasons, in this chapter, deterioration of physiological systems secondary to age-associated disease will be considered to be an integral part of aging. Of course, it is always important to know the specific reason for the altered physiology, and when an age-associated disease is the major immediate cause, it should certainly be identified.

INTERSPECIES AND INTRASPECIES VARIATION IN AGE-ASSOCIATED PHYSIOLOGICAL DETERIORATION

In general terms, mammalian species are remarkably similar in that a progressive, but usually not linear, deterioration in the physiological systems occurs with advancing post-maturational age.[35] However, there is considerable interspecies variation in the details of these physiological changes.

There is also great intraspecies heterogeneity in age changes in the physiological systems, a phenomenon that has been well

characterized in humans. Rowe and Kahn[14] have developed the concept of "usual aging" and "successful aging" for considering the differences among individuals in age changes in physiological functions. "Usual aging" refers to elderly who are functioning well but are at risk for disease, disability, and premature death. They may exhibit modest increases in systolic blood pressure and abdominal fat, and deterioration of one or more physiological processes. "Successful aging" refers to a small group of disease-free elderly people who exhibit the following characteristics:

- low risk of disease or disability;
- high level of mental and physiological function;
- active engagement in life.

Rowe and Kahn focus on environment and lifestyle as the major determinants for achieving "successful aging" and point to adequate physical exercise, good diet, good personal habits (not smoking or abusing drugs and using alcohol in moderation), and good psychosocial environment as being particularly important. Surprisingly, they barely mention the role of genetics in achieving "successful aging."

Although the concept of "successful aging" is provocative, there are questions regarding its value and usefulness. One question is how common is "successful aging" now or is it likely to become if most people were to live in a good environment and adhere to an appropriate lifestyle. As of now, only a small fraction of those in the eighth decade of life would meet the criterion of being free of a chronic disease; i.e. almost all suffer from one or more of the following diseases: osteoarthritis, osteoporosis, coronary heart disease, cerebrovascular disease, congestive heart failure, dementia, type II diabetes, Parkinson's disease, cancer, benign prostatic hyperplasia, and cataracts. And this does not fully cover the list of such diseases.

A related question is what fraction of those who meet the criteria of "successful aging" in the eighth decade of life will continue to when in the ninth and tenth decades of life or when they are centenarians. If most of them undergo marked physiological deterioration before death, what does the concept of "successful aging" provide in addition to the well-known fact that individuals age at different rates? The concept of biological age as distinct from chronological age was proposed long ago.[36]

Thus the question arises as to whether the concept of "successful aging" is useful or misleading. It is likely that most centenarians were in the "successful aging" category when in the eighth decade of their lives. However, most centenarians exhibit marked physiological deterioration[37] which must have occurred during the ninth and tenth decades of life and/or after they became centenarians. Thus it would be more appropriate to say that these centenarians undergo a slow rate of aging rather than "successful aging." This is not merely an academic issue but one with societal implications because "successful aging" implies that physiological deterioration due to aging can be avoided rather than merely delayed. Such a view can lead to misguided public policy decisions based on the view that an appropriate lifestyle and environment will enable people to reach very old age without the disabilities that are so costly in societal resources. Indeed, it is possible that such an environment and lifestyle may have just the opposite effect.

Jeune and Kanisto[38] believe that centenarians will become commonplace during the twenty-first century; and in so far as the environment and lifestyle advocated for the achievement of "successful aging" contributes to this, it could result in an increase in the fraction of the population requiring much in the way of societal resources because of marked physiological deterioration.

AGE CHANGES IN THE PHYSIOLOGY OF SPECIFIC ORGANS AND ORGAN SYSTEMS

All organs and organ systems exhibit age-associated physiological deterioration, if not in all individuals, at least in a significant fraction of the population. This subject area is so vast that it cannot begin to be covered in this brief chapter. The volume on aging[1] of the *Handbook of Physiology* series of the American Physiological Society provides a systematic and extensive coverage for those needing in-depth information about a particular organ or organ system. Also, the other chapters of this textbook provide a substantial discussion of age changes on the physiology of specific organs and organ systems relevant to the subject matter of the chapter. In this chapter a few specific examples have been selected for discussion solely for the purpose of illustrating the general concepts presented above.

Before starting this discussion it is important to point out that most of the studies on age changes in the physiology of organs and organ systems have used the cross-sectional study design. The interpretation of cross-sectional studies is often confounded by factors not related to aging.[39] What are called "cohort effects" or "generational effects" is a major type of confounder.[40] For example, during the twentieth century, the number of years of education progressively increased in the developed nations.[41] Therefore when comparing cognitive abilities of 30-year-olds and 80-year-olds in a cross-sectional study, the difference in educational levels confounds any conclusions about the effects of aging. What is referred to as "selective mortality" is the other major type of confounder of cross-sectional studies.[42] The older the age group being studied, the smaller is the fraction of its birth cohort still alive. Members of the birth cohort with risk factors for fatal diseases tend to die at younger ages than others in the birth cohort. Thus, for example, a difference in the blood level of HDL-cholesterol between those in the age range of 80–90 years compared to those in the age range of 50–60 years may relate more to "selective mortality" than to aging.

The age changes in the physiology of the heart illustrate several concepts particularly well. The early studies on the effect of age on human cardiac function noted marked changes with advancing age. The results of recent studies have shown much less dramatic age changes. The major reason for the differences between the older and the more recent studies resides in the selection of the human subjects for study. The investigators in the early studies did not recognize the need (or often did not have the tools) to carefully screen for physical fitness or age-associated disease, particularly occult coronary artery disease. For example, left ventricular wall thickness increases with increasing age in humans, but in some individuals, the increase

is moderate. Indeed, the extent of this age change is markedly increased in individuals with coronary artery disease, in those with hypertension, and in individuals with a sedentary lifestyle.[43] Resting cardiac output normalized to body surface area (i.e. cardiac index) has been reported to be markedly decreased with age,[44] mildy decreased,[45] and unchanged.[46] The reasons for these discrepancies in the literature is that resting cardiac index is influenced by hypertension, body composition, and undoubtedly other factors, and each of the populations studied probably differed in regard to these factors. In some studies, a reduced stroke volume index during vigorous exercise at advanced ages has been reported,[47] while in other studies, either no change[48] or an increase[49] has been observed. The heterogeneity in these results is probably due to differences in the populations studied in regard to occult coronary artery disease, physical fitness, and body composition. However, not all changes in cardiac function with age have been related to age-associated disease, lifestyle, or body composition. For example, the reduced increase in heart rate in response to exercise has been observed in all subjects with advancing age, including those who are physically fit and free of occult coronary artery disease.[43] Another example is the decreased ability with advancing age of β-adrenergic agonists to increase heart rate;[50] it appears that aging blunts this response because of multiple changes in the molecular system coupling β-receptors and postreceptor mechanisms in all people with advancing age. Those age changes in cardiac physiology that have not been related to disease, lifestyle, or environmental factors are felt to be due to intrinsic aging processes and inevitable. However, one cannot be certain that they do not arise from a yet to be recognized extrinsic factor or disease. Moreover, it is important to note that those age changes in cardiac function that are secondary to lifestyle and other environmental factors are not inevitable and may be modifiable even at advanced ages, at least to some extent. Indeed, advances in medicine and public health have already made modifiable some age changes in cardiac function due to disease.

It has long been believed that a decrease in the glomerular filtration rate is an inevitable occurrence with advancing age.[51] This belief was based on cross-sectional studies. However, a longitudinal study[52] conducted on subjects of the Baltimore Longitudinal Study of Aging has revealed that not all people exhibit a decline in glomerular filtration rate (Fig. 9-2). The mean decrease in creatinine clearance in 446 male subjects followed over a 23-year period was 0.87 mL per minute per year. However, one-third of the subjects showed no decline in creatinine clearance, as illustrated by the data of six subjects in the bottom panel of Figure 9-2. In contrast, the subjects recorded in the top panel exhibited a marked decline, and those recorded in the middle panel, a small but statistically significant decline. Unlike the heart, reasons for the differences among people in changes with age in kidney function have not been established. Lindeman[51] has suggested that the decline in renal function noted in cross-sectional studies may be due to the fact that many in the population suffered from intervening pathology such as undetected glomerulonephritis or interstitial nephritis secondary to infections, immunological insults, drugs and other toxic exposures, vascular occlusions resulting in ischemic injury, urinary tract obstruction, and infection.

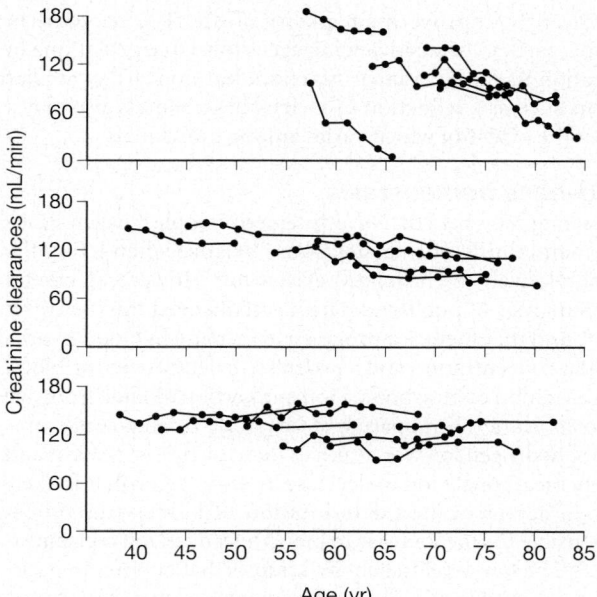

Figure 9-2 Age changes in creatinine clearance of male subjects studied serially in the Baltimore Longitudinal Study of Aging. The top panel presents the findings of six subjects from the group who exhibited marked decreases in creatinine clearance with increasing age; the middle panel presents the findings of six subjects from the group who exhibited a small but significant decrease in creatinine clearance with increasing age; the bottom panel presents the findings of six subjects from the group who exhibited no decrease in creatinine clearance with increasing age. From Lindeman et al.,[52] with permission of Blackwell Science Inc.

Indeed, it has been shown that hypertensive subjects have a more rapid age-associated decline in renal function than normotensive subjects.[53] It is also possible that lifetime dietary preferences play a role, since excessive dietary protein is believed to promote renal functional deterioration. Indeed, if the deterioration of renal function with age is primarily due to disease and/or environmental factors, then it is potentially modifiable by various public health measures.

The appearance of the skin is widely used as an indicator of the age of a person. The changes in skin underlying the altered appearance with increasing age are fine wrinkling, dryness, laxity, and proliferative lesions such as age spots, cherry angiomas, and seborrheic keratoses. However, most of these changes are not intrinsic but result from cumulative sun damage, since their extent is much reduced in skin areas protected from the sun.[54] Cigarette smoking is the other major factor that promotes skin wrinkling. Indeed, sun exposure and cigarette smoking appear to act synergistically to promote skin aging.[26] Thus, a commonly used marker of aging has little relation to intrinsic processes but primarily relates to environmental factors and can be readily modified by altering lifestyle. In addition to the change in appearance, many other skin functions deteriorate with age, including the barrier function, immune function, inflammatory response, wound healing, and vitamin D production;[25] the extent to which the age changes in these

functions may be secondary to sun exposure and cigarette smoking has yet to be carefully examined.

These three examples make clear that many age changes are not primarily due to intrinsic aging processes but, to varying degrees, are secondary to (or are at least promoted by) age-associated disease or extrinsic factors or both. To view them as not part of the aging process removes from consideration major problems that confront individuals as they age, nor is there any biological basis for such a view. It is true that deterioration due to disease or extrinsic factors may be preventable and, in some cases, reversible, but that hardly lessens their involvement in aging. Indeed, much of what we currently consider to be intrinsic may ultimately be found to be of extrinsic origin or at least influenced by extrinsic factors. And what is considered to be extrinsic has its actions by interacting with intrinsic processes. Indeed, what is considered to be lifestyle may have a strong intrinsic base. For example, the sedentary lifestyle adopted by many people as they age also occurs in laboratory rats,[55] which in the case of the rodent is probably better viewed to be intrinsic rather than a lifestyle choice. Moreover, as discussed above, there are strong reasons to believe that most age-associated diseases are part of the aging process, making their separation from other aspects of aging arbitrary. Nevertheless, identification of age-associated diseases is obviously essential in the practice of geriatric medicine and is also invaluable in experimental biogerontology by providing the detailed information needed for interpretation of the findings of human and animal studies.

AGE CHANGES IN ORGANISMIC FUNCTION

Given the many deteriorative changes that occur in the physiology of organs and organ systems, it is to be expected that the functional competence of the organism is compromised with advancing age. Indeed, organismic functional deficits occur that can be classified in the following way: (1) compromised ability to cope with challenges, (2) reduced functional capacity, and (3) altered homeostasis. A few examples of these organismic functional deficits are presented below.

Ability to cope with challenges
The reduced ability to cope with challenges, or what are often referred to as stressors, is a hallmark of the aging phenotype.[56] It is well known that secretion of glucocorticoids by the hypothalamic–adenohypophyseal–adrenocortical system and an increase in the activity of the adrenal medullary–sympathetic nervous system are responses common to all stressors, and that they play an important role in enabling mammalian organisms to cope with all stressors.[56] Also, induction of the heat shock protein system is a common response, enabling organisms of almost all species to withstand many different cellular stressors.[57] Of course, in addition to these general responses, there are defenses that are specific for particular stressors or challenges. However, because the loss with advancing age in ability of organisms to cope appears to occur with all types of stressors, it might be expected that there is deterioration of one or more of the general mechanisms. The currently available evidence does not indicate that the ability of the

hypothalamic–adenohypophyseal–adrenocortical system to respond to challenges by increasing the secretion of glucocorticoid hormone is compromised by aging.[58] Of course, that does not rule out the possibility of a reduced ability of the glucocorticoid target site to respond to the hormone, but studies designed to address this possibility have yet to be done. There is some indication that the response of the adrenal medullary–sympathetic nervous system to challenges may be attenuated with advancing age,[56] but these findings are hard to interpret because basal levels of catecholamines are elevated with increasing age. There is also evidence that there is a blunting with increasing age of at least some adrenergic responses in target tissues. Nevertheless, based on current information, it does not seem that an inadequate response of the adrenal medullary–sympathetic nervous system plays a major role in the age-associated reduction in the ability of the organism to meet challenges. In contrast to these neuroendocrine responses, the evidence is clear that the ability to induce heat shock proteins in response to cellular stressors markedly decreases with increasing age of mammals,[59] and this may play a major role in the loss in ability to cope with stressors. However, because the deterioration in physiological systems occurs with advancing age in most organs and organ systems, functional deficits in specific responses may underly the reduced ability of the aged to deal with a broad scope of challenges. A case in point is the decrease in the ability of the immune system to protect the organism from damage due to infectious agents.[60] Thus, although it has long been known that successfully meeting challenges is compromised with advancing age, the basis of this deficit remains to be fully elucidated.

Aerobic capacity

The ability of the cardiopulmonary system to supply oxygen to exercising muscles and the ability of these muscles to use this oxygen in energy metabolism is referred to as the "aerobic capacity." It is a measure of the maximum ability to carry out exercise and is determined by measuring the maximum rate of oxygen consumption attainable when performing an exercise test of increasing intensity that requires a large proportion of the total skeletal muscle mass. Aerobic capacity decreases in healthy sedentary men and women at the rate of about 10 percent per decade.[61] Since physical fitness markedly influences aerobic capacity, some of this decrease may be due to the fall in physical activity with advancing age. Of course, the decline in aerobic capacity is much greater in elderly people suffering from chronic disease, particularly atherosclerotic disease. Well-trained endurance athletes at all ages have a higher aerobic capacity than untrained people of the same age. However, it is striking that the trained athlete also exhibits an age-associated decline in aerobic capacity, making it evident that a decrease in physical fitness is not the only factor underlying this age-related decline. Nevertheless, there is suggestive but not unequivocal evidence that the rate of decline in aerobic capacity with age is less in trained athletes than in the untrained.[62] The aerobic capacity of sedentary men and women in the age range of 60–80 years can be increased by physical training,[63] but even if the training is maintained, age-associated decline occurs. Nevertheless, elderly people who continue the physical training maintain an aerobic capacity greater than that of their sedentary peers, which under certain circumstances can significantly improve their quality of life. The decrease in aerobic capacity with advancing age is to a large extent due to alteration in cardiovascular function, but noncardiovascular factors such as a reduction in skeletal muscle mass also play a role,[17] the extent of which varies among individuals.

Acid–base homeostasis

It has long been held that healthy elderly people have no problem maintaining normal acid–base balance when living the usual relatively unchallenged existence.[51] However, a careful meta-analysis of published data has challenged this view.[64] It was found that there is a progressive increase in blood hydrogen ion concentration and a progressive decrease in the blood concentration of bicarbonate ion and carbon dioxide from age 20 to 80 years. The apparent steady-state plasma concentration of hydrogen ion was found to increase by 6–7 percent and that of bicarbonate ion to decrease by 12–16 percent. It is likely that an age-associated deterioration of kidney function is responsible for the increase in blood hydrogen ion concentration.[65] The low-level metabolic acidosis that appears to occur in many people with advancing age may play a role in age-associated bone loss, a factor that has received little attention from those who study bone loss and aging.

Lean body mass

Lean body mass, or probably better called "fat-free mass," is fairly stable in men and women through about 40 years of age, and then decreases with advancing age with the rate of loss accelerating.[62] Clearly, the homeostatic system regulating fat-free mass is deranged at advanced age. Although an increasingly sedentary lifestyle is undoubtedly involved, physical fitness does not fully prevent the age-associated loss of fat-free mass, because it also occurs in trained athletes.[22] The principal component in this fall of fat-free mass is the loss of skeletal muscle mass with advancing age.[66] It is this loss of muscle mass that is the primary reason for the decrease in muscle strength with age.[67] Although muscle mass is lost with age in sedentary people and in athletes alike, exercise can improve the functional capacity of elderly people. High-intensity resistance training has been found to increase muscle size and strength,[20] which can be invaluable in enabling an elderly individual to maintain an independent existence of reasonable quality.

Fat mass

Cross-sectional studies indicate that body fat mass increases with age in both men and women.[62] In women, a linear increase in percentage body fat with age occurs through the eighth decade of life, with the average value being 25 percent and 41 percent at 25 and 75 years of age, respectively. In men the increase in body fat with age is similar to that of women through 50 years of age, but slows at more advanced ages. Even in those people whose body weight does not increase with age, body fat increases as lean body mass decreases. The homeostatic regulation of fat mass clearly becomes faulty with advancing age. Indeed, Pollack et al.[22] found that even in athletes who remain competitive, there is a small increase in fat content with advancing age. Apparently, therefore, exercise can attenuate but not totally prevent the age-associated increase in body fat. In men, the increase in fat mass with age occurs primarily in the abdominal region, while such is not the case for women until after the age of 54 years.[68,69] Exercise not only decreases the age-associated increase in body fat but, most importantly, it also attenuates the disproportionate increase in abdominal fat.[70] The great concern about abdominal fat is due to the extensive evidence indicating that it is a risk factor for several age-associated pathologic problems including hypertension, type II diabetes, cardiovascular disease, as well as some types of cancer.[71] Thus, interventions aimed at preventing the abdominal accumulation of fat with advancing age are most important to develop.

Bone mass

Every population that has been studied shows age-associated bone loss,[72] which suggests that it is an inevitable consequence of aging. Much progress is currently being made in regard to the molecular basis of this bone loss but, as of now, a clear understanding of the biological basis has not emerged. Nearly all bones are affected to varying degrees. The age of onset of bone loss depends on gender and type of bone. Vertebral bone loss in women may start as early as the third decade of life, while the loss of appendicular bone occurs at a much older age.[72] Bone loss accelerates following menopause, with the inevitable occurrence of estrogen deficiency being the major responsible factor.[73] Bone loss in men begins at an older age than in women, and for some the extent of loss is trivial. Although all people lose bone, the extent of bone loss and its clinical consequences vary among individuals. Black women have a higher bone mass as young adults and, as a consequence, are less prone to bone fractures with advancing age than are white women.[74] There is evidence that exercise attenuates age-associated bone loss[75] and that an adequate intake of dietary calcium is needed to minimize loss.[76] Cigarette smoking and the consumption of alcohol and caffeine have been implicated as factors promoting age-associated bone loss.[77,78]

Although the homeostatic ability to maintain bone mass becomes faulty in all people with advancing age, interventions are possible that will enable many to avoid much of the negative consequences during their lifetime. Estrogen replacement therapy markedly blunts the accelerated postmenopausal loss of bone, but its use must be evaluated in relation to the possible negative aspects of such therapy. Dietary supplements and exercise programs are also potential avenues of intervention. Moreover, giving up cigarette smoking, and moderation in other personal habits such as in the consumption of alcohol- and caffeine-containing beverages, should be helpful.

Body temperature

The homeostatic regulation of body temperature and the ability to adapt to different thermal environments deteriorates with advancing age.[79] The extent of this deterioration varies among individuals and is influenced by health status, physical fitness, and personal habits such as cigarette smoking and alcohol consumption.[80] Part of the loss in ability to cope with extremes in environmental temperature stems from the reduction in the perception of the thermal environment. Because of this, individuals fail to make appropriate behavioral responses.[80] However, physiological homeostatic failure also underlies the impaired ability to maintain body temperature. In response to a hot environment, the elderly are not able to increase cutaneous blood flow as effectively as young people.[81] Sweating is also impaired,[82] and this may be due to the decrease in physical fitness with increasing age.[83] The response to a cold environment is also compromised,[84] with both the cutaneous vasoconstrictor response and the shivering response being less effective; in many cases, this can at least in part be traced to medications used to treat chronic age-associated diseases. To a great extent, the physiological deficits can be compensated by appropriate conscious behavioral responses, but even this avenue becomes less trustworthy because of the perception deficit. The rise in body temperature in response to pyrogens is blunted with increasing age.[85] This deficit deprives elderly people of the possible benefits of fever in coping with infections.

Glucose homeostasis

A diminished homeostatic regulation of plasma glucose concentration is a common characteristic of the aging phenotype.[16] When this regulatory ability declines sufficiently, a diagnosis of type II diabetes is made—a common age-associated disease. The major tool for examining glucose homeostasis has been the oral glucose tolerance test. Typical of the findings are those reported by Chen et al.,[86] shown in Figure 9-3. They administered orally 100 g of glucose to groups of healthy old and young subjects; plasma glucose rose to higher levels and remained elevated longer in the old than in the young, while the rise in plasma insulin level was delayed in the old but with time reached that of the young. A reduced ability to secrete insulin does not appear to be a major reason for this alteration in glucose homeostasis with age.[87] There is strong evidence that an increased resistance to insulin action is a major factor in the diminished homeostatic glucose regulation in old people.[88] With advancing age, people become increasingly sedentary and show an increase in body fat, particularly in the abdominal region—factors that are known to increase insulin resistance and to blunt the glucose homeostatic responses. Indeed, Zavaroni et al.[89] have reported that the effect of aging on glucose tolerance is essentially eliminated after correcting for the effects of physical inactivity and adiposity. This view is consistent with the finding that there are old people who are similar to young people in regard to glucose tolerance and insulin sensitivity.[90] However, there is evidence that a small component of glucose intolerance and insulin resistance with advancing age is independent of physical inactivity and adiposity.[91] Nevertheless, most people of middle-age and older can greatly improve their homeostatic regulation of glucose by modifying their lifestyle to reduce adiposity and increase physical fitness.

SUMMARY AND CONCLUSIONS

Physiological deterioration is a hallmark of the aging phenotype. This deterioration is caused by (1) damage resulting from intrinsic living processes, (2) damage due to extrinsic factors such as diet, lifestyle, personal habits, and psychosocial factors, and (3) age-associated diseases. Although mammalian species are similar in that all show a progressive deterioration of physiological processes with advancing age, the details of this deterioration vary among species. Thus, the detailed characteristics of the deterioration probably has a strong genetic component. There is also a considerable intraspecies variation in the rate

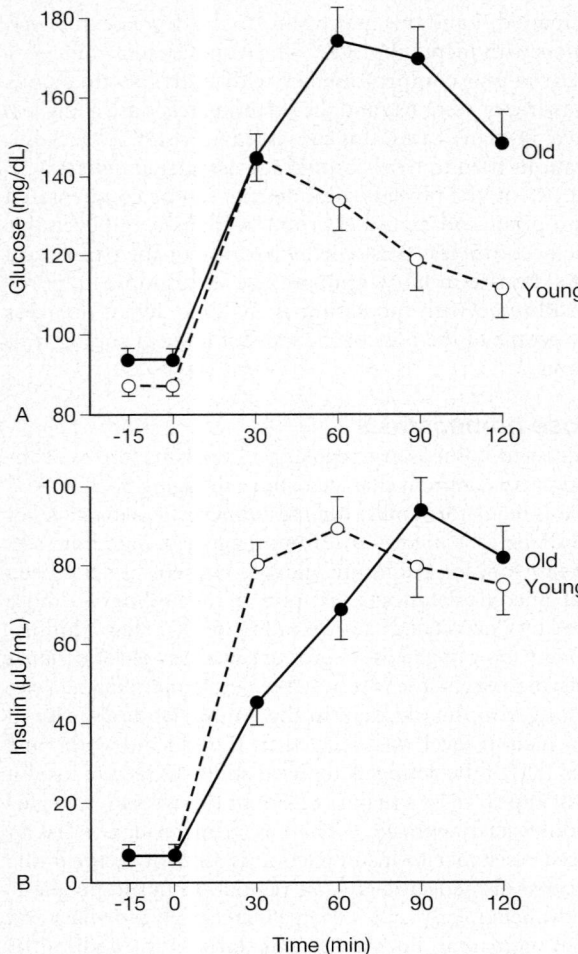

Figure 9-3 Influence of age on the response of plasma glucose and insulin concentration to an oral load of glucose. Young and old healthy human subjects were given 100 g of glucose orally. From Chen et al.,[86] with permission of Blackwell Science Inc.

KEY POINTS Physiology of aging

- Physiological deterioration of organisms occurs with advancing adult age and is manifested by decreased ability to cope with challenges, reduced functional capacity, and compromised homeostasis.

- Age-associated physiological deterioration results from three sources of damage: intrinsic living processes, environmental factors, and age-associated diseases.

- There is marked heterogeneity among individuals of the same chronological age in the extent of physiological deterioration. Those who have undergone little deterioration are said to have undergone "successful aging" from a physiological standpoint. Although "successful aging" is a popular concept, this author finds it to be a misleading rather than useful concept.

- Most of the research on the effects of aging on human physiology has utilized a cross-sectional design. Findings of studies using this design are often confounded by factors not related to aging, and the possibility of such confounders must be carefully evaluated when interpreting the results of these studies.

REFERENCES

1. Masoro EJ (ed): Handbook of Physiology. Section 11: Aging. Oxford University Press, New York, 1995
2. Sohal, RS, Weindruch, R: Oxidative stress, caloric restriction, and aging. Science 1996;273:59–63
3. Sell DR, Lane MA, Johnson WA et al: Longevity and the genetic determination of collagen glycoxidation kinetics in mammalian senescence. Proc Natl Acad USA 1996;93:485–490
4. Strehler BL: Time, cells, and aging, 2nd edn. Academic Press, New York, 1977
5. Busse, EW: Theories of aging. In Busse EW, Pfeiffer E (eds): Behavior and adaptation in adult life. Little Brown, Boston, 1969:11
6. Vieira C, Pasyukova EG, Zeng ZB et al: Genotype–environment interaction for quantitative trait loci affecting life span in *Drosophila melanogaster*. Genetics 2000;154:213–227
7. Masoro EJ: Caloric restriction and aging: an update. Exp Gerontol 2000;35:299–305
8. Yu BP, Masoro EJ, Murata I et al: Life span study of SPF Fischer 344 male rats fed ad libitum or restricted diets: longevity, growth, lean body mass and disease. J Gerontol 1982;37:130–141
9. Pahlavani MA: Intervention in the aging immune system: influence of dietary restriction, dehydroepiandrosterone, melatonin, and exercise. Age 1998;21:153–155
10. Kelley GR, Herlihy JR: Food restriction alters the age-related decline in cardiac β-adrenergic responsiveness. Mech Aging Dev 1998;103:1–12
11. McShane T, Wise PM: Life-long caloric restriction prolongs reproductive life span in rats without interrupting estrous cyclicity: effects on the gonadotrophin-releasing hormone/luteinizing hormone axis. Biol Reprod 1996;54:70–75
12. Lee C-K, Klopp RG, Weindruch R, Prolla TA: Gene expression profile of aging and its retardation by caloric restriction. Science 1999;285:1390–1393
13. Roth GS, Ingram DK, Lane MA: Caloric restriction in primates: Will it work and how will we know? J Am Geriat Soc 1999;47:896–903
14. Rowe JW, Kahn RL: Successful Aging. Pantheon Books, New York, 1998
15. Lipschitz DA: Nutrition and ageing. In Evans JG, Williams TF (eds): Oxford Textbook of Geriatric Medicine. Oxford University Press, Oxford, 1992:119
16. Halter JB: Carbohydrate metabolism. In Masoro EJ (ed): Handbook of Physiology. Section 11: Aging. Oxford University Press, New York, 1995:119

and character of physiological deterioration with advancing age. Much of the difference among individuals of the same species appears to relate to extrinsic factors. Age-associated deterioration occurs in all organs and organ systems. The extent to which extrinsic factors and age-associated disease play a role varies among organ systems and among individuals but, in most cases, they play a major role. These age changes in the physiology of organs and organ systems compromise the functional abilities of the organism and underly the decreasing ability to survive with advancing age. The physiological deficits of the aging organism can be summarized as (1) a reduced functional capacity, (2) a decreased ability to cope with challenges, and (3) an altered homeostasis. Because much of the physiological deterioration with advancing age is caused by extrinsic factors, organismic aging can be modified by altering lifestyle and environmental factors. Also, the large role that age-associated disease plays in the physiological deterioration can be modulated by presently available medical and public health measures and undoubtedly much more by those that will be developed in the future.

17. Spirduso WW: Physical Dimensions of Aging. Human Kinetics, Champaign, IL, 1995

18. Ehsani AA, Ogawa T, Miller TR et al: Exercise training improves left ventricular systolic function in older men. Circulation 1991;83:96–103

19. Grimby G: Muscle performance and structure in the elderly as studied cross-sectionally and longitudinally. J Gerontol A 1995;50(Special Issue):17–22

20. Evans WJ: Effects of exercise on body composition and functional capacity of the elderly. J Gerontol A 1995;50(Special Issue):147–150

21. Hallfrisch J, Muller D, Drinkwater D et al: Continuing diet trends in men: the Baltimore Longitudinal Study of Aging (1961–1987). J Gerontol A 1990;45:M186–M191

22. Pollock ML, Foster C, Knapp D et al: Effect of age and training on aerobic capacity and body composition of master athletes. J Appl Physiol 1987;62:725–731

23. Kohrt WM, Obert KA, Holloszy JO: Exercise training improves fat distribution patterns in 60- and 70-year-old men and women. J Gerontol A 1992;47:M99–M105

24. Goldberg AP, Dengel DR, Hagberg JM: Exercise physiology and aging. In Schneider EL, Rowe RW (eds): Handbook of the Biology of Aging, 4th edn. Academic Press, San Diego, 1996:331

25. Chuttani A, Gilchrest BA: Skin. In Masoro EJ (ed): Handbook of Physiology. Section 11: Aging. Oxford University Press, New York, 1995:309

26. Kadence DP, Burr R, Gress R et al: Cigarette smoking: a significant risk factor for premature facial wrinkling. Ann Intern Med 1991;114:840–844

27. Sparrow D, Weiss ST: Respiratory system. In Masoro EJ (ed): Handbook of Physiology. Section 11: Aging. Oxford University Press, New York, 1995:475

28. Crow MT, Bilato C, Lakatta EG: Atherosclerosis. In Birren JE (ed): Encyclopedia of Gerontology, vol 1. Academic Press, San Diego, 1996:123

29. Seeman TE, Berkman LF, Charpentier PA et al: Behavioral and psychosocial predictors of physical performance: MacArthur studies of successful aging. J Gerontol A 1995;50:M177–M183

30. Berkman LF, Seeman TE, Albert M et al: High, usual, and impaired functioning in community-dwelling older men and women: findings from the MacArthur Foundation research network on successful aging. J Clin Epidemiol 1993;46:1129–1140

31. Shock NW (ed): Normal Human Aging: The Baltimore Longitudinal Study of Aging (NIH Pub 84–2450). US Government Printing Office, Washington, DC, 1982

32. Lakatta EG: Health, disease, and cardiovascular aging. In Committee on an Aging Society, Institute of Medicine and National Research Council: America's Aging-Health in an Older Society. National Academy Press, Washington, DC, 1985:73

33. Rowe JW, Wang SY, Elahi D: Design, conduct, and analysis of human aging research. In Schneider EL, Rowe JW (eds): Handbook of the Biology of Aging, 3rd edn. Academic Press, San Diego, 1990:63

34. Rose MR: Evolutionary Biology of Aging. Oxford University Press, New York, 1991

35. Finch CE: Longevity, senescence, and the genome. University of Chicago Press, Chicago, 1990

36. Borkan GA, Norris AH: Assessment of biological age using a profile of physical parameters. J Gerontol 1980;35:177–184

37. Forette B: Centenarians: health and frailty. In Robine J-M, Vaupel JW, Jeune B, Allard M (eds): Longevity: To the Limits and Beyond. Springer Verlag, Berlin, 1997:105

38. Jeune B, Kannisto V: Emergence of centenarians and supercentenarians. In Robine J-M, Vaupel JW, Jeune B, Allard M (eds): Longevity: To the Limits and Beyond. Springer Verlag, Berlin, 1997:77

39. Costa PT Jr, McCrae RR: Design and analysis of aging studies. In Masoro EJ (ed): Handbook of Physiology. Section 11: Aging. Oxford University Press, New York, 1995:25

40. Evans DA: Human studies. In Masoro EJ (ed): Handbook of Physiology. Section 11: Aging. Oxford University Press, New York, 1995:83

41. Katzman R: Human nervous system. In Masoro EJ (ed): Handbook of Physiology. Section 11: Aging. Oxford University Press, New York, 1995:325

42. Elahi D, Muller DC, Rowe JW: Design, conduct, and analysis of human aging research. In Schneider EL, Rowe JW (eds): Handbook of the Biology of Aging, 4th edn. Academic Press, San Diego, 1996:24

43. Lakatta EG: Cardiovascular system. In Masoro EJ (ed): Handbook of Physiology. Section 11: Aging. Oxford University Press, New York, 1995:413

44. Brandonfbrener M, Landowne M, Shock NW: Changes in cardiac output with age. Circulation 1955;12:557–566

45. Coggan AR, Spina RJ, Rogers MA et al: Histochemical and enzymatic characteristics of skeletal muscle in master athletes. J Appl Physiol 1990;68:1896–1901

46. Fleg JL, Gerstenblith G, Zonderman AB et al: Prevalence and diagnostic significance of exercise-induced silent myocardial ischemia detected by thallium scintigraphy and electrocardiography in asymptomatic volunteers. Circulation 1990;81:423–436

47. Kuickka JT, Lansimies E: Effect of age on cardiac index, stroke index and left ventricular ejection fraction at rest and during exercise as studied by radiocardiography. Acta Physiol Scand 1982;114:339–343

48. Fleg JL, Gerstenblith G, Schulman SP et al: Gender differences in exercise hemodynamics of older subjects: effects of conditioning status. Circulation 1990;82:III-239 (abstract)

49. Mann DL, Dennenberg BS, Gash AK et al: Effects of age on ventricular performance during graded supine exercise. Am Heart J 1986;111:108–115

50. Stratton JR, Cerqueira MD, Schwartz RS et al: Differences in cardiovascular responses to isoproterenol in relation to age and exercise training in healthy men. Circulation 1992;86:504–512

51. Lindeman RD: Renal and urinary tract function. In Masoro EJ (ed): Handbook of Physiology. Section 11: Aging. Oxford University Press, New York, 1995:485

52. Lindeman RD, Tobin JD, Shock NW: Longitudinal studies on the rate of decline in renal function with age. J Am Geriatr Soc 1985;33:278–285

53. Lindeman RD, Tobin JD, Shock NW: Association between blood pressure and the rate of decline in renal function with age. Kidney Int 1984;26:861–868

54. Gilchrest BA: Physiology and pathophysiology of aging skin. In Goldsmith L (ed): Physiology, Biochemistry and Molecular Biology of the Skin, 2nd edn. Oxford University Press, New York, 1991:1425

55. McCarter RJM: Caloric restriction, exercise and aging. In Sen CK, Packer L, Hanninen O (eds): Handbook of Oxidants and Antioxidants in Exercise. Elsevier Science, Amsterdam, 2000:797

56. Mobbs CV: Neuroendocrinology of aging. In Schneider EL, Rowe JW (eds): Handbook of Biology of Aging, 4th edn. Academic Press, San Diego, 1996:234

57. Lindquist S: The heat shock response. Ann Rev Biochem 1986;55:1151–1191

58. Masoro EJ: Glucocorticoids and aging. Aging: Clin Exper Res 1995;7:407–413

59. Heydari AR, Gutsmann A, You S et al: Effect of dietary restriction on the genome function of cells: alterations in the transcriptional apparatus of cells. In: Hart RW, Neumann DA, Robertson RT (eds): Dietary Restriction: Implications for the Interpretation of Toxicity and Carcinogenicity Studies. ILSI Press, Washington, DC, 1995:213

60. Miller RA: Aging and the immune response. In Schneider EL, Rowe JL (eds): Handbook of the Biology of Aging, 4th edn. Academic Press, San Diego, 1996:355

61. Buskirk ER, Hodgson JL: Age and aerobic power: the rate of change in men and women. Federation Proc 1987;46:1824–1829

62. Holloszy JO, Kohrt WM: Exercise. In Masoro EJ (ed): Handbook of Physiology. Section 11: Aging. Oxford University Press, New York, 1994:633

63. Kohrt WM, Malley MT, Coggan AR et al: Effects of gender, age, and fitness level on response of $\dot{V}O_{2max}$ to training in 60 to 71 year-olds. J Appl Physiol 1991;71:2004–2011

64. Frassetto L, Sebastian A: Age and systemic acid–base equilibrium: analysis of published data. J Gerontol A 1996;51:B91–B99

65. Lubran MM: Renal function in the elderly. Ann Clin Lab Sci 1995;25:122–133

66. Cohn SH, Vartsky D, Yasumura S et al: Compartmental body composition based on total-body potassium and calcium. Am J Physiol 1980;239:E524–E530

67. Evans WJ: What is sarcopenia? J Gerontol A 1995;50(Special Issue):5–8

68. Ley CJ, Lees B, Stevenson JC: Sex- and menopause-associated changes in body fat distribution. Am J Clin Nutr 1992;55:950–954

69. Shimokata H, Tobin JD, Muller DC et al: Studies in the distribution of body fat: I. Effects of age, sex, and obesity. J Gerontol A 1989;44:M66–M73

70. Kohrt WM, Malley MT, Dalsky DP, Holloszy JO: Body composition of healthy sedentary and trained, young and older men and women. Med Sci Sports Exerc 1992;24:832–837

71. Elahi D, Dyke MM, Andres R: Aging, fat metabolism, and obesity. In Masoro EJ (ed): Handbook of Physiology. Section 11: Aging. Oxford University Press, New York, 1995:147

72. Kalu DN: Bone. In Masoro EJ (ed): Handbook of Physiology. Section 11: Aging. Oxford University Press, New York, 1995:395

73. Slemenda C, Hui SL, Longcope C, Johnston CC: Sex steroids and bone mass: a study of changes about the time of menopause. J Clin Invest 1987;80:1261–1269

74. Garn SM: Bone loss and aging. In Goldman R, Rockstein M (eds): Physiology and Pathology of Human Aging. Academic Press, New York, 1975:39

75. Sandler RB, La Porte R, Sashin D et al: The epidemiology of physical activity and postmenopausal bone loss. First year of a clinical trial. In Christiansen C, Arnaud CD, Nordin BEC et al (eds): Osteoporosis I. Aalborg Stiftsbogtrykkeri, Glostrup, 1984:317

76. Cuming RG: Calcium intake and bone mass: a quantitative review of the evidence. Calcif Tissue Int 1990;47:194–210

77. Heaney RP: Calcium intake, bone health and aging. In Young EL (ed): Nutrition, Aging and Health. Alan R. Liss, New York, 1986:165

78. Seeman E, Melton LJ, O'Fallon WM, Riggs BL: Risk factors of spinal osteoporosis in men. Am J Med 1983;75:977–983

79. Collins KJ, Exton-Smith AN: Thermal homeostasis in old age. J Am Geriatr Soc 1983;31:519–524

80. Lybarger JA, Kilbourne EH: Hyperthermia and hypothermia in the elderly: an epidemiologic view. In Davis BB, Wood WC (eds): Homeostatic Function and Aging. Raven Press, New York, 1985:149

81. Kenney WL: Control of heat-induced cutaneous vasodilation in relation to age. Eur J Appl Physiol 1988;57:120–125

82. Inoue Y, Nakao M, Araki T, Murakami H: Regional differences in the sweating responses of older and younger men. J Appl Physiol 1991;71:2453–2459

83. Tankersly CG, Smolander J, Kenney WL, Fortney SM: Sweating and skin blood flow during exercise: effects of age and maximum oxygen uptake. J Appl Physiol 1991;71:236–242

84. McCarter RJM: Energy utilization. In Masoro EJ (ed): Handbook of Physiology. Section 11: Aging. Oxford University Press, New York, 1995:95

85. Norman DC, Grahn D, Yoshikawa TT: Fever and aging. J Am Geriatr Soc 1985;33:859–863

86. Chen M, Halter JB, Porte D: The role of dietary carbohydrate in the decreased glucose tolerance of the elderly. J Am Geriatr Soc 1987;35:417–424

87. Muller DC, Elahi D, Tobin JD, Andres R: The effect of aging on insulin resistance and secretion. Sem Neurobiol 1996;16:289–298

88. Supiano MA, Hogikyan RV, Morrow LA et al: Aging and insulin resistance: role of blood pressure and sympathetic nervous system. J Gerontol A 1993;48:M237–M243

89. Zavaroni I, Dall'Aglio E, Bruschi F et al: Effect of age and environmental factors on glucose tolerance and insulin secretion in a worker population. J Am Geriatr Soc 1986;34:271–275

90. Broughton DL, James OWF, Alberti KGMM, Taylor R: Peripheral and hepatic insulin sensitivity in healthy elderly human subjects. Eur J Clin Invest 1991;21:13–21

91. Shimokata H, Muller DC, Fleg JL et al: Age as an independent determinant of glucose tolerance. Diabetes 1991;40:44–51

Chapter 10   Connective tissues and aging

Nicholas A. Kefalides

Aging is a continuous process which constitutes a cycle studded with events that affect all systems in the body, including the connective tissues. The interrelationship between the aging process and connective tissues is complex, involving a variety of factors and interactions acting in a reciprocal fashion. One could inquire into the effects of aging on connective tissues and, conversely, one may ask how the components of connective tissue contribute to the aging process. To answer these questions, it is important to have some understanding of the structural biochemistry of connective tissues, some knowledge of the processes involved in their biosynthesis, modification, extracellular organization, and molecular genetics, as well as of the factors affecting the properties of connective tissue cells and the extracellular matrix (ECM). Armed with this knowledge, it becomes apparent that there can be a huge number of events in the development of connective tissues that may be associated, directly or indirectly, with the processes or effects of aging. These have been and continue to be areas of intensive research.

This chapter presents an abbreviated discussion of the various components of the ECM, their structure, molecular organization, biosynthesis, modification, turnover, and molecular genetics. It discusses some concepts on the effects of aging on the ECM and the effects of aging on the properties of various connective tissues, as well as the involvement of connective tissue physiology on diseases associated with aging.

THE PROPERTIES OF CONNECTIVE TISSUES

The properties of connective tissues are derived primarily from the properties of the components of the ECM surrounding, and secreted by, the cells of those tissues. Some connective tissues such as cartilage or tendons may be comprised primarily of a single cell type (e.g. chondrocytes or fibroblasts) whose synthesis and secretion of ECM and other factors largely determine the properties of the tissue. Some tissues, such as bone and blood vessels, contain a number of different connective tissue cell types (e.g. osteoblasts and osteoclasts in bone and endothelial and smooth muscle cells in blood vessels) which contribute to both their structural and functional properties. Other tissues, such as cardiac muscle and kidney, may have properties dependent upon connective tissue components whose biological roles are separate from the major physiological function of the tissue and which may have influence over the properties of that tissue during the process of aging. Different cell types will exhibit different phenotypic patterns of ECM production which, in turn, will influence the structural properties of a given connective tissue.

The major components of the ECM fall into three general classes of molecules: (1) the structural proteins, which include the collagens (of which there are now 19 types recognized) and elastin; (2) the proteoglycans, which contain several structurally distinct molecular classes; and (3) the structural glycoproteins, whose contribution to the properties of connective tissues has been recognized only within the past 20–25 years. The interactions between these materials determine the development and properties of the connective tissues.

The collagens

STRUCTURE   The collagens are a family of connective tissue proteins having a triple-stranded organization and containing molecular domains within which the strands are coiled around one another in a triple helix. The reader is referred to two recent reviews on collagen biochemistry.[1,2]

The genes of at least 19 distinct collagen types have been characterized.[1] The interstitial collagens, types I, II, III, and V, exist as large, extended molecules which tend to organize into fibrils.[1] There may be more than one collagen type within these fibrils.[3] Type IV collagen, also known as *basement membrane collagen*, does not exist in fibrillar form, but rather in a complex network of collagen molecules linked by disulfide and other cross-linkages and associated with noncollagenous molecules, such as laminin, entactin, and proteoglycans, to form an amorphous matrix.[4,5] Although at least 19 collagen types are recognized, the protein of only the first 11 collagens has been isolated from tissues.

Table 10-1 contains a summary of the collagen gene family. There are 33 genes corresponding to the α chains of 19 collagen types. The most abundant collagen and the most abundant protein in the body is type I. The table classifies the various collagens into seven groups, depending on the nature of the fibrils they form. The basic unit of the type I collagen fibril is a triple helical heterotrimer, tropocollagen, consisting of two identical chains, termed $\alpha1(I)$, and a third chain, $\alpha2(I)$.[1] The other collagen types have been given similar designations; however, some of the types are homotrimers containing three identical chains, and some contain three genetically distinct α chains as indicated in Table 10-2.

The collagen α chain has a unique amino acid composition with glycine occupying every third position in the sequence. Thus the collagenous domains consist of a repeating peptide triplet, -Gly-X-Y-, in which X and Y are amino acids other than glycine. A large percentage of amino acids in the Y position is occupied by proline. In addition, collagen contains two unique amino acids derived from post-translational modifications of the protein, 4- and 3-hydroxyproline and hydroxylysine. The presence of 4-hydroxyproline provides additional sites along the α chain capable of forming hydrogen bonds with adjacent α chains, which are important in stabilizing the triple helix so that it maintains its structure at body temperatures.

Table 10-1 **Collagen gene family**		
Fibrillar collagen genes	I, II, III, V, XI	9 genes
Fibril-associated collagens (FACIT)	IX, XII, XIV	5 genes
Network-forming collagen genes	IV	6 genes
Short-chain collagen genes	VIII, X	3 genes
Collagens forming filamentous beads	VI	3 genes
Anchoring fibers	VII	1 gene
Multiple domain collagens	XIII, XV, XVI, XVII, XVIII, XIX	6 genes
Total		33 genes

Table 10-2 **Types of collagens**		
Type	**Chain composition**	**Tissue distribution**
I	$[\alpha1(I)]_2\alpha2(I)$	Skin, tendon, bone, cornea, blood vessels
II	$[\alpha1(II)]_3$	Cartilage, intervertebral disc, vitreous body
III	$[\alpha1(III)]_3$	Skin, blood vessels
IV	$[\alpha1(IV)]_2\alpha2(IV)$ $[\alpha3(IV)]_2\alpha5(IV)[\alpha4(IV)]_2\alpha6(IV)$	Basement membranes
V	$[\alpha1(V)]_2\alpha2(V)$	Placenta, skin, cardiovascular system
VI	$\alpha1(VI),\alpha2(VI)\alpha3(VI)$	Cornea, blood vessels
VII	$\alpha1(VII)$	Skin, cornea, GI tract
VIII	$\alpha1(VIII)$	Cardiovascular system, placenta, cornea
IX	$\alpha1(IX),\alpha2(IX)\alpha3(IX)$	Cartilage, cornea
X	$\alpha1(X)$	Cartilage
XI	$\alpha1(XI),\alpha2(XI)\alpha3(XI)$	Cartilage
XII	$\alpha1(XII)$	Tendons, periosteum
XIII	$\alpha1(XIII)$	Many tissues
XIV	$\alpha1(XIV)$	Skin, bone, cornea, blood vessels
XV	$\alpha1(XV)$	Placenta, heart, colon
XVI	$\alpha1(XVI)$	Placenta, heart, colon
XVII	$\alpha1(XVII)$	Skin hemidesmosomes
XVIII	$\alpha1(XVIII)$	Several tissues, particularly kidney and liver
XIX	$\alpha1(XIX)$	Rhabdomyosarcoma cells

If hydroxy-proline formation is inhibited, the triple helix dissociates into its component α chains at $37°C$.

The presence of glycine in every third position, along with the extensive hydrogen bonding, provides the triple helix with a compact protected structure resistant to the action of most proteases. The structures of collagens can be stabilized further through the formation of covalent cross-linkages derived from modification and condensation of certain lysine and hydroxylysine residues on adjacent α chains.[2,6] Cross-linkage formation is important in stabilizing collagen fibrils and contributes to their high tensile strength.

BIOSYNTHESIS[1,7] Type I collagen α chains are synthesized as a larger precursor, procollagen, containing noncollagenous sequences at their C and N termini. As each pro-α chain is synthesized, intracellular prolyl and lysyl hydroxylases act to form hydroxyproline and hydroxylysine. The triple helix is formed intracellularly and stabilized by the formation of interchain disulfide bonds near the carboxyl termini of the component pro-α chains. After secretion of the triple helical collagen, procollagen peptidases remove most of the noncollagenous portions at each end of the procollagen. Extracellular lysine and hydroxylysine oxidases oxidize the amino groups of lysine or hydroxylysine to form aldehyde derivatives, which can go on to form Schiff base adducts, the first cross-linkages. These can rearrange and become reduced to form the various other cross-linkages. The subject of collagen cross-linking is elegantly discussed in three reviews.[2,8,9] Increased number of collagen cross-linkages has been reported in a pathological state known as scleroderma.

COLLAGENOLYSIS Extracellular degradation of collagen is accomplished by enzymes known as tissue collagenases. These enzymes cleave triple helical collagen at a site three-quarters from the amino terminus, resulting in the formation of two triple helical fragments which denature at temperatures above $32°C$ to form nonhelical peptides which can now be degraded by tissue proteinases. Cleavage by tissue collagenase is considered to be the rate-limiting step in collagenolysis of triple helical collagen. Collagenolysis is the subject of reviews by Harris et al.,[10] Seiki,[11] and Kleiner and Stetler-Stevenson.[12]

Collagenolysis is an important physiological process responsible to a large extent for the repair of wounds and processes of tissue remodeling in which undesired accumulations are removed as new connective tissue is laid down. However, in conditions such as rheumatoid arthritis and osteoporosis, as well as aging, the production of collagenases may be stimulated, resulting in an elevated degradation of synovial tissue or bone.

Tissue collagenases are secreted by connective tissue cells as a precursor, procollagenase, which must be activated to become enzymatically active. This can be achieved in vitro by the action of trypsin on the latent enzyme. Other proteinases, including lysosomal cathepsin B, plasmin, mast cell proteinase, and plasma kallikrein, also can activate latent collagenases.[10,12] Thus inflammatory cells can secrete factors which lead to collagenase activation, accounting for the inflammatory sequelae of the arthritides. Collagenases are also under the influence of plasma inhibitors, of which α_2 macroglobulin accounts for most of the inhibitory process. In addition, inhibitors of plasminogen activation can indirectly prevent the activation of procollagenases by plasmin. Fibroblasts and other connective tissue cells also secrete inhibitors of collagenases, suggesting a complex system of extracellular control of collagenolysis.[10,12]

Elastin

The biochemistry and molecular biology of elastin have been subjects of some excellent reviews.[13,14] Like the interstitial collagens, glycine makes up about one-third of the amino acid content of elastin. Unlike collagen, however, glycine is not present in every third position. In addition, elastin is an exceedingly hydrophobic protein, with a large content of valine, leucine, and isoleucine.

Elastin is synthesized as a precursor molecule, tropoelastin, with a molecular weight of about 70 kDa. However, in tissues, elastin is found as an amorphous, macromolecular network. This is due to the condensation of tropoelastin molecules through the formation of covalent cross-linkages unique to elastin. These cross-linkages arise through the condensation of four lysine residues on different tropoelastin molecules to form the cross-linking amino acids, desmosine and isodesmosine, characteristic of tissue elastin. The reader is referred to reviews by Bailey et al.[2] and Eyre et al.[6] for discussions of the details of collagen and elastin cross-linking.

The hydrophobicity together with the formation of cross-linkages endow elastin with its elastic properties as well as an extreme insolubility and amorphous structure. Elastin accounts for most of the elastic properties of skin, arteries, ligaments, and the lungs. The presence of elastin has been demonstrated in other tissues such as the eye and the kidney. In most tissues, elastin is found in association with microfibrils which contain several glycoproteins, including fibrillin. Microfibrils have been identified in many tissues, and the importance of their assemblies as determinants of connective tissue architecture has been brought into focus by the identification of mutations in fibrillin in the heritable connective tissue disorder, Marfan syndrome.[15]

An elegant review summarizes the current knowledge of the structure of the elastin gene, including consideration of the heterogeneity observed in mature mRNA due to alternative splicing in the primary transcript.[16] Analysis of the bovine and human elastin genes revealed the separation of those exons coding for distinct hydrophobic and cross-linking domains. Comparison of the cDNA and genomic sequences, as well as S1 analyses, demonstrated that the primary transcript of both species is subject to considerable alternative splicing. It is likely that this accounts for the presence of multiple tropoelastins found in several species. It is suggested that the differences in alternative splicing may be correlated with aging.[16]

The proteoglycans

Proteoglycans are characterized by the presence of highly negatively charged, polymeric chains (glycosaminoglycans or "GAGs") of repeating disaccharide units covalently attached to a "core" protein. The disaccharide units comprise an N-conjugated amino sugar, either glucosamine or galactosamine, and a uronic acid, usually D-glucuronic acid or, in the instances of dermatan sulfate, heparan sulfate and heparin, L-iduronic acid. In cartilage and in the cornea, another GAG, keratan sulfate, containing D-glucose instead of a uronic acid has been demonstrated. The amino group of the hexosamine component is usually acetylated and the GAGs are usually O-sulfated in hexosamine residues with some N-sulfation, instead of acetylation, in the instances of heparan sulfate and heparin. Depending on the source and type of proteoglycan, the number of GAGs attached to the core protein can vary from three or four all the way up into the twenties, with each GAG having a molecular size in the tens of thousands of daltons. In addition, as in the case of the cartilage proteoglycans, there may be more than one type of GAG attached to the core protein. In cartilage, several proteoglycan molecules may be associated with another very large GAG, hyaluronic acid, consisting of disaccharide units of glucuronyl N-acetylglucosamine. The compositional structure of the glycosaminoglycans is summarized in Table 10-3.

The overall effect of these structures is the creation of huge, negatively charged highly hydrophilic complexes. The hydration and charge properties of these complexes causes them to become highly extended, occupying a hydrodynamic volume in the tissue much larger than would be predicted from their chemical composition. In the instance of synovial cartilage, it is suggested that the hydration endows the tissue with shock absorbing properties in which applied pressure to the joint is counteracted by the extrusion of water from the complex, forcing a compression of the negative charges within the molecule. Upon the release of pressure, the electronegative repulsive forces drive the charges apart with a concomitant influx of water to restore the initial hydrated state. The metachromatic staining properties of connective tissues is due mainly to their proteoglycan content.

Some excellent reviews of proteoglycan biochemistry have been written.[17–19]

In recent years, several proteoglycans have been identified in the pericellular environment, either associated with cell

Table 10-3 Properties and tissue distribution of glycosaminoglycans

Glycosaminoglycans	Composition	Distribution
Hyaluronic acid	N-acetylglucosamine D-glucuronic acid	Blood vessels, heart, synovial fluid, umbilical cord, vitreous
Chondroitin sulfate	N-acetylgalactosamine D-glucuronic acid 4- or 6- O-sulfate	Cartilage, cornea, tendon, heart valves, skin, etc.
Dermatan sulfate	N-acetylgalactosamine L-iduronic acid 4- or 6- O-sulfate	Skin, lungs, cartilage
Keratan sulfate	N-acetyglucosamine D-galactose O-sulfate	Cornea, cartilage, nucleus pulposus
Heparan sulfate	N-acetylglucosamine	Blood vessels, basement membranes, lung, spleen, kidneys
Heparin	N-sulfamino-glucosamine D-glucuronic acid L-iduronic acid O-sulfates	Mast cells, lung, Glisson's membranes

surfaces or interacting with ECM components, such as interstitial collagens, fibronectin, and TGF-β. In recent reviews, Groffen et al.[18] and Iozzo and Murdoch[20] described the structures of the protein cores, their gene organization, their functional characteristics, and tissue distribution. Table 10-4, which is a modification of the one published by Iozzo and Murdoch, lists the structure and biological characteristics of pericellular proteoglycans. The first five on the list constitute a group of small leucine-rich proteoglycans (SLRP). They are multidomain assemblies of protein motifs with a relatively elongated and highly glycosylated structure having several protein domains shared with other proteins. In their review, Groffen and colleagues discuss the role of perlecan as a crucial determinant of glomerular basement membrane permselectivity and suggest that the additional presence of agrin, another heparan sulfate proteoglycan species, makes the latter important contributors to glomerular function.

The presence of lumican, one of the leucine-rich proteoglycans, in articular cartilage was demonstrated in a study by Grover et al.[21] They showed that the relative abundance and size of lumican varied with age. Lumican was most abundant in adult cartilage extracts, where it exhibited a molecular size in the range 55–80 kDa. Extracts from juvenile cartilage had a more restricted size variation corresponding to the higher molecular size range present in the adult. In the neonate the sizes were in the range 70–80 kDa.

The biosynthesis of proteoglycans begins with the synthesis of the core protein. The sugars of the GAG chain then are sequentially added to serine residues of the protein (in most instances), utilizing uridine diphosphate (UDP) conjugates of the component sugars, with sulfation following as the chain elongates. (The mechanism of sulfation is beyond the scope of this discussion.) Most of the chain elongation and sulfation is associated with the Golgi apparatus. The degradation of proteoglycans is mediated through the action of lysosomal glycosidases and sulfatases specific for the hydrolysis of the various structural sites within the GAG chain.

Genetic abnormalities in the production or synthesis of these enzymes have been shown to be the main causes of the "mucopolysaccharidoses" whose victims may exhibit severe tissue deformities and a high incidence of mental retardation.

The structural glycoproteins

In addition to the collagen and elastin components of connective tissues, there are groups of glycoproteins, the structural glycoproteins, that have important roles in the physiology and structural properties of connective and other types of tissues. These proteins, which include fibronectin, laminin, entactin, thrombospondin, and others, are involved during development, in cell attachment and spreading, and in tissue growth and turnover.

Fibronectin
One of the best characterized of the structural glycoproteins is fibronectin. It was originally isolated from serum where it was referred to as "cold-insoluble globulin" (CIG). As it became recognized that fibronectin was an important secretory product of fibroblasts and other types of cells, and was involved in cell adhesion, the term "fibronectin" replaced CIG. Comprehensive reviews on the structure and function of fibronectin have been published by Lafrenie and Yamada[22] and Ruoslahti.[23]

Fibronectin exists as a disulfide-linked dimer with a molecular weight of about 450 kDa, each monomer having a molecular size of 250 kDa. Fibronectin exists in at least two forms, a tissue form and plasma fibronectin. Plasma fibronectin is somewhat smaller and is more soluble at physiological pH than the cellular form. Spectrophotometric and ultracentrifugal studies indicate that both forms are elongated molecules composed of structured domains separated by flexible, extensible regions. Limited proteolytic digestion has

Table 10-4 **Structure and properties of secreted pericellular proteoglycans**

Designation (gene product)	Protein core size (kDa)	Glycosamino-glycan type	Chromosomal location (human)	Tissue distribution
Decorin	36	CS/DS	12q21.3–q23	Ubiquitous, collagenous matrices, bone, teeth, mesothelia, floor plate
Biglycan	38	CS/DS	Xq28	Interstitium, and cell surfaces
Fibromodulin	42	KS	1q32	Collagenous matrices
Lumican	38	KS	12q21.3–q22	Cornea, intestine, liver, muscle, cartilage
Epiphycan	36	CS/DS		Epiphyseal cartilage
Versican	265–370	CS/DS	5q13.2	Blood vessels, brain, skin, cartilage
Aggrecan	220	CS	15q26	Cartilage, brain, blood vessels
Neurocan	136	CS		Brain, cartilage
Brevican	100	CS		Brain
Perlecan	400–467	HS/CS	1p36	Basement membranes, cell surfaces, sinusoidal spaces, cartilage
Agrin	200	HS	1p32-pter	Synaptic sites of neuromuscular junctions, renal basement membranes
Testican	44	HS/CS	21	Seminal fluid

revealed the presence of specific binding sites for a number of ligands, including collagen, fibrin, cell surfaces, heparin (heparan sulfate proteoglycan), factor XIIIa, and actin.

Fibronectin plays a role in blood clotting by becoming cross-linked to fibrin through the action of factor XIIIa transamidase that catalyses the final step in the clotting cascade. Fibroblasts and other cell types involved in the repair of injury adhere to the clot by interacting with the cell-binding domain of fibronectin. Fibronectin also enables cells to migrate in developing embryos. Fibronectin contains a unique peptide sequence, arginylglycylaspartylserine (RGDS or RGD) which binds to specific cell surface proteins (integrins) which span the plasma membrane.[23] Purified RGD can inhibit fibronectin from binding the cells, and can even displace bound fibronectin. The integrins have a complex molecular organization and appear to interact with certain intracellular proteins, thereby providing a mechanism for the control of a number of events by components of the extracellular environment.

Fibronectin is encoded by a single gene and its complete primary structure has been determined by the DNA sequencing of overlapping cDNA clones.[24] From such studies, it became recognized that there are peptide segments derived from alternative splicing of fibronectin mRNA at three distinct regions, termed extra domain A (ED-A), ED-B, and connecting segment (III CS). A middle region of the polypeptide containing homologous repeating segments of about 90 amino acids, called type III homologies, has been identified.[25] Using immunological techniques with monoclonal antibodies, it was shown that the ED-A exon is omitted during splicing of

fibronectin mRNA precursor in arterial medial cells, while the expression of fibronectin containing ED-A is characteristic of modulated smooth muscle cells such as those in culture or those involved in intimal thickening and atherosclerotic lesions. It would appear that this process of alternative splicing is used during embryonic development or tissue repair as a mechanism to generate different forms of fibronectin in the extracellular matrix by the inclusion or exclusion of specific segments.[26] This could be the source of differences between the plasma and cellular forms of fibronectin. This phenomenon of alternative splicing may also be involved in the synthesis of collagens and elastin, and may well be implicated in processes of aging.

Laminin

Laminin is the major structural glycoprotein of basement membranes. In addition to its association with the molecular components of basement membranes (e.g. type IV collagen, entactin/nidogen, and heparan sulfate proteoglycan), it plays some important roles in cell attachment and neurite growth.[27–30] Laminin is difficult to isolate from whole tissues or from basement membranes owing to its poor solubility, and so most of our knowledge of it is derived from extracts of tumor matrices.

Laminin is a very large complex composed of at least three protein chains associated by disulfide linkages. The largest of these, the $\alpha1$, has a molecular weight of about 440 kDa, whereas the smaller units, $\beta1$ and $\gamma1$ chains, have molecular weights of about 200–250 kDa. Several laminin isoforms have been described in recent years,[30] necessitating a new nomenclature of its component chains.[31] The first new chain ($\alpha2$) has been found in preparations from normal tissues but is absent from those from neoplastic tissues.[32,33] Table 10-5 lists the various laminin isoforms and their tissue distribution. Laminin has been shown to have a twisted cruciform shape consisting of three short arms and a single long arm with globular domains at the extremities of each arm. In several of the newer isoforms of laminin, the $\alpha1$ chain has a smaller molecular size, lacking a portion of its amino terminus.

Laminin can influence processes of differentiation, cell growth, migration, morphology, adhesion, and agglutination, as well as being involved in the structural organization of basement membranes. Laminin exhibits a preferential binding to type IV collagen compared with other collagen types. Laminin contains domains similar to those of fibronectin that bind to different proteins, and cell surface components containing a RGD sequence on the $\alpha1$ chain and a YIGSR sequence on the $\beta1$ chain, both of which bind to different integrins on the cell surface and which are involved in cellular attachment and migratory behaviors.

Entactin

Entactin, a novel sulfated glycoprotein, is an intrinsic component of basement membranes. Entactin was first identified in the extracellular matrix synthesized by mouse endodermal cells in culture.[34] Subsequently, a degraded form, termed nidogen, was isolated from the Englebreth–Holm–Swarm sarcoma and mistakenly identified as a new basement membrane component.[35] Both terms, entactin and nidogen, are used interchangeably in the modern literature.

Entactin forms a tight stoichiometric complex with laminin. Rotary shadowing electron microscopy has revealed its association with the γ1 chain of laminin. Entactin has been shown to promote cell attachment via an RGD sequence, and calcium ions have been implicated in its properties.[36] Its role in basement membrane assembly and in epithelial morphogenesis has already been noted in the previous section.

Thrombospondin

Thrombospondins are a family of extracellular, adhesive proteins that are widely expressed in vertebrates. Five distinct gene products—designated thrombospondin 1–4 and cartilage oligomeric matrix protein (COMP)—have been identified. Thrombospondin-1 and -2 have similar primary structures. The molecule (450 kDa) is composed of three identical disulfide-linked protein chains. It is one of the major peptide products secreted during platelet activation, and it is also secreted by a diversity of growing cells. Thrombospondin has 12 binding sites for calcium ion and depends upon it for its confirmational stability. It binds to heparin (and heparan sulfate proteoglycan) and to cell surfaces, and appears to modulate a number of cell functions, including platelet aggregation, progression through the cell cycle, and cell adhesion and migration.[37,38]

Integrins and cell attachment proteins

As indicated above, cell surfaces contain groups of proteins, the integrins, that mediate cell-matrix interactions. The integrins behave as receptors for components of the extracellular matrix and interact, as well, with components of the cytoskeleton.[39] This provides a mechanism for the mediation by components of the ECM of intracellular processes, including control of cell shape and metabolic activity. The integrins exist as paired molecules containing α and β subunits. They appear to have a significant degree of specificity for ECM proteins which apparently is conferred by combinations of different α and β subunits.

In addition to the integrins, cell attachment proteins (CAMs) are present on the cell surface. These confer specific cell–cell recognition properties. For reviews on integrins and CAMs, see Albelda and Buck,[39] Buck and Horwitz,[40] and Danen and Yamada.[41]

Table 10-5 Isoforms of laminin

New name	New composition	Descriptive name	Localization
Laminin 1	$\alpha1\beta1\gamma1$	EHS laminin	All basement membrane except skeletal muscle
Laminin 2	$\alpha2\beta1\gamma1$	Merosin	Striated muscle, peripheral nerve, placenta
Laminin 3	$\alpha1\beta2\gamma1$	S-laminin	Synapse, glomerus, arterial blood vessel walls
Laminin 4	$\alpha2\beta2\gamma1$	S-merosin	Myotendinous junction, trophoblast
Laminin 5	$\alpha3\beta3\gamma2$	Kalinin/nicein/epiligrin	Dermal–epidermal junction, stromal–epidermal junction
Laminin 6	$\alpha3\beta1\gamma1$	K-laminin	Dermal–epidermal junction, stromal–epidermal junction
Laminin 7	$\alpha3\beta2\gamma1$	KS-laminin	Amnion, fetal skin
Laminin 8	$\alpha4\beta1\gamma1$		Lung, heart, blood vessels, smooth muscle, endothelial cells, placenta
Laminin 9	$\alpha4\beta2\gamma1$		Heart, blood vessels, placenta, lung
Laminin 10	$\alpha5\beta1\gamma1$	*Drosophila* laminin	Heart, blood vessels, placenta, lung, kidney

AGING AND THE PROPERTIES OF CONNECTIVE TISSUES

From the foregoing discussion, it becomes apparent that there can be a multitude of possible loci in the development, structural organization, metabolism, and molecular biology of connective tissues for the introduction of alterations in the properties of these tissues. For a given tissue, changes in the composition of the ECM or changes in the factors that control the production of ECM can feed back through complex mechanisms to induce changes in the properties of the tissue. The process of aging may well involve some of these factors. It is probable that, during the aging process, the phenotypical expression of ECM—i.e. the patterns of ECM composition—will change. It is also probable that many of the components of the ECM may evolve with time as a function of their long biological half-lives and the enzymatic and nonenzymatic modifications that take place. These can include processes of maintenance and repair, responses to inflammation, nonenzymatic glycosylation, cross-linkage formation, etc.

In a sense, it may be important to differentiate between those processes of senescence that are genetically programmed (i.e. innate senescence), and the contributions to aging induced by "environmental" factors. However, it becomes difficult to distinguish whether a given alteration is an effect or a cause of aging.

In this section an attempt is made to discuss some of the factors and conditions involving connective tissues that may be involved in the aging process. This includes aspects of cellular senescence, inflammatory and growth factors, photoaging of the skin, diabetes mellitus, nonenzymatic glycosylation, the etiology of osteoporosis, osteoarthritis, collagen cross-linking, and the arthritides.

Cellular senescence

A large body of research has established conclusively that normal diploid cells have a limited replicative lifespan and that cells from older animals have shorter lifespans than those from younger animals.[42] Thus, the process of aging could be attributed to cellular senescence. A number of observations suggest that connective tissue proteins may be affected during cellular senescence. In an extensive study on the properties of murine skin fibroblasts, van Gansen and van Lerberghe[43] concluded that among the main effects of cellular mitotic age were a depression of chromatin plasticity, changes in the organization of cytoplasmic filaments, and changes in the organization of the ECM. They implicated an involvement of collagen fibers in the intracellular events both in vivo and in vitro. Although senescent fibroblasts may not be dividing, they are biosynthetically active, showing an increased synthesis of fibronectin[44] and increased levels of fibronectin mRNA.[45] However, both senescent and progeroid cells demonstrated a decreased chemotactic response to fibronectin and developed a much thicker extracellular fibronectin network than did young fibroblasts.[44] There is some indication that, with increasing age, cells become less able to respond to mitogens—which may have a bearing on age-related differences in wound healing. It was also shown that senescent human skin fibroblasts in culture show a loss of collagenase regulation with a 20-fold

elevation in trypsin-activated collagenolytic activity.[46] Thus it would appear that there is some correlation between cellular senescence and changes in the regulation of connective tissue metabolism and cellular interactions.

Inflammatory and growth factors

One of the active areas of contemporary connective tissue biology is the study of the influences of inflammatory and growth factors on the properties of connective tissues. It is well recognized that inflammatory cells accumulate in damaged and infected tissues as part of the inflammatory response. These cells secrete lymphokines, such as the interleukins, and other factors which may influence connective tissue metabolism. In addition, a number of growth factors, including epidermal growth factor (EGF), platelet-derived growth factor (PDGF), fibroblast growth factors (FGFs), and transforming growth factors (TGFs), can have extensive control over connective tissue metabolism. As indicated above, senescent cells may not respond to these factors as do young cells. In addition, it is possible that stimulation of cell replication by certain of these factors may accelerate the progression of cells toward senescence. To add to the complexity are the findings that many cells can synthesize certain of these factors, including interleukin I, PDGF, FGFs, and TGFs, endowing the cellular components of tissues with autocrine and paracrine properties.

In studies reported by Boonen et al.,[47] age-related bone resorption is probably associated with, in addition to lack of vitamin D-related mechanisms, a decline in skeletal content of anabolic growth factors, such as insulin-like growth factor-I. In their review of the properties of TGF-β, Roberts and Sporn[48] emphasize this complexity. They indicate that this factor has profound effects on all vascular cell types—including endothelial, smooth muscle, and adventitial cells. TGF-β plays a role in the vasculogenesis and angiogenesis characteristic of embryogenesis and inflammation, and also in the arterial thickening associated with hypertension. These actions of TGF-β are very complex, inhibiting vascular cell proliferation in vitro but enhancing the organization of endothelial cells into tubular structures indicative of angiogenesis. TGF-β also increases fibronectin synthesis but decreases protease secretion by both endothelial cells and fibroblasts, both of which can influence the phenotypical patterns of extracellular matrix formation and structure and thereby contributing to the development of fibrosis. TGF-β can also regulate PDGF synthesis by these cells, adding another degree of complexity to these systems. In vivo, TGF-β is a chemoattractant for macrophages and stimulates expression of mRNAs for several growth factors. PDGF, FGFs, and EGF are powerful mitogens for smooth muscle cells, fibroblasts, and keratinocytes.

The extent of involvement of these interacting factors in the aging process is not clear, but it is probable that they contribute to the process.

Mechanisms of cutaneous aging

Cutaneous aging is a complex biological activity consisting of two distinct components: (a) intrinsic, genetically determined degeneration; and (b) extrinsic aging, due to exposure to the environment, also known as "photoaging." These two processes are superimposed in the sun-exposed areas of skin, with their profound effects on the biology of cellular and structural elements of the skin.[49] The symptoms of photoaging are different from those of intrinsic aging, and evidence suggests that these two processes have different mechanisms.

A variety of theories have been advanced to explain aging phenomena and some of them may be applicable to innate skin aging as well. Hayflick postulated in 1979 that diploid cells, such as dermal fibroblasts, have a finite lifespan in culture.[50] This observation, when extrapolated to the tissue level, could be expected to result in cellular senescence and degenerative changes in the dermis. Another theory suggests that free radicals may damage collagen in the dermis,[51] and a third theory implicates nonenzymatic glycosylation of proteins, such as collagen, leading to increased cross-linking of collagen fibrils. It is postulated that this process is the major cause of dysfunction of collagenous tissues in old age.[2,52] Finally, cutaneous aging may be attributed to differential gene expression of extracellular matrix of connective tissue. It has been demonstrated that the rate of collagen biosynthesis is markedly reduced in the skin of elderly people.[49] Collectively, the observations on dermal connective tissue components in innate aging suggest an imbalance between biosynthesis and degradation, with less repair capacity in the presence of ongoing degradation.

Additional changes in the aged dermis concern the architecture of the collagen and elastin networks. The spaces between fibrous components are more compact owing to a loss of ground substance. Collagen bundles appear to unravel and there are signs of elastolysis. Scanning electron microscopic studies of the three-dimensional arrangement of rat skin from animals ranging in age from 2 weeks to 24 months showed that, during postnatal growth, there was a "dynamic rearrangement" of the collagen and elastic fibers, with an ordered arrangement of mature collagen bundles being attained by producing distortions of relatively straight elastic fibers. During adulthood, there is a tortuosity of these elastic fibers coupled with an incomplete restructuring of the elastic network that was deposited to interlock with the collagen bundles.

The effects of photodamage on dermal connective tissue are exemplified in the histopathological pictures of photoaging. The hallmark of photoaging is the massive accumulation of the so-called "elastotic" material in the upper and mid-dermis. This phenomenon, known as "solar elastosis," has been attributed to changes in elastin.[49] Solar elastotic material is composed of elastin, fibrillin, versican, a large proteoglycan, and hyaluronic acid. Even though the elastotic material contains the normal constituents of elastic fibers, the supramolecular organization of solar elastotic material and its functionality are severely perturbed.[53] It was also known that elastin gene expression is markedly activated in cells within the sun-damaged dermis. In addition, it has been shown that accumulation of elastotic material is accompanied by degeneration of the surrounding collagen meshwork.[53] Parallel studies provide evidence implicating matrix metalloproteinases (MMPs) as mediators of collagen damage in photoaging.[53]

In a review, Kligman[54] corroborated the manifestations of the effects of photoaging noted earlier. She stated that elastosis to the degree found in photoaging never occurs in normal protected skin, even of very old individuals. The main culprit

appears to be the UV-B portion of the ultraviolet spectrum, although UV-A and infrared radiation also contribute to the damage. In UV-A irradiated hairless mice, there appears to be alteration in the ratio of type III to type I collagen in addition to the elastosis. It has been shown that UV irradiation of fibroblasts in culture enhances expression of MMPs. UV exposure of skin was shown to induce tissue inhibitors of MMPs.[49] There is also an increase in the levels of the components of the ground substance in photoaged skin (predominantly dermatan sulfate, heparan sulfate, and hyaluronic acid). In human aged skin, mast cells are numerous and appear to be degranulated. These cells are known to produce a variety of inflammatory mediators so that photoaged skin is chronically inflamed. In innate aging, the skin tends to be hypocellular. The microcirculation of the skin is also affected, becoming sparse, with the horizontal superficial plexus almost destroyed. While atrophy may be presented in end-stage photoaging in the elderly population, ongoing photoaging is characterized by more, not less.

The effects of photoaging could be totally prevented by broad-spectrum sunscreens. While severe photoaging in the human is considered to be irreversible, in hairless mice it was found that repair could take place after the cessation of irradiation, with the newly deposited collagen appearing totally normal. A similar repair was observed in biopsies of severely photodamaged human skin after several years of avoidance of exposure to the sun. It has been found that the administration of retinoic acid accelerated the repair in irradiated mice, with the deposition of a repair zone of normal-appearing collagen and with the appearance of numerous, metabolically active fibroblasts.[54] This provides a potential opportunity for the development of a therapeutic approach to the connective tissue damage of photoaged skin.

Diabetes mellitus

Diabetics often show signs of accelerated aging, primarily as a result of the complications of vascular disease and impaired wound healing so common in this disease. It is well documented that diabetics will exhibit a thickening of vascular basement membranes which, at least in part, is believed to be related to the observed susceptibilities.[55]

The biological basis for this thickening is as yet obscure but could well be related to abnormalities in cell attachment or the response to factors affecting basement membrane formation, to excessive nonenzymatic glycosylation of proteins, or to an abnormal turnover of basement membrane components. Fibroblasts from diabetic individuals exhibit a premature senescence in culture.[56] The role of inhibitors of aldose reductase was investigated by Sibbett et al.[57] They showed that, in normal human fibroblasts, the mean population doubling times, population doublings to senescence, saturation density at confluence, tritiated thymidine incorporation, and response to PDGF were inhibited with increasing glucose concentrations in the media. They found that inhibitors of aldose reductase, sorbinil and tolrestat, completely prevented these inhibitions. Myoinositol had similar effects. However, no data were presented to indicate that aldose reductase inhibitors would reverse the premature senescence in fibroblasts from diabetic individuals. Thus it is not clear whether prevention of the formation of reduced sugars can have a therapeutic effect, nor is it clear that all of the aging effects of diabetes are mediated by reduced sugars.

Eaton et al.[58] examined the clinical response to long-term treatment of limited joint mobility in diabetes mellitus using an aldose reductase inhibitor. After treating two patients with IDDM for more than ten years with Sorceinil, an aldose reductase inhibitor, these investigators found a sustained correction of limited joint movement. They also observed that both subjects were homozygous for the Z-2 allele (A-C) 23 that has been linked to microvascular complications of diabetes mellitus.

Fleischli et al.[59] compared the material properties of connective tissue in human metatarsal bones from young diabetic donors and older nondiabetic donors. There were no significant differences between the two groups, suggesting that the effects of aging are comparable to the effects of diabetes on the structural integrity of human metatarsal bones.

Nonenzymatic glycosylation and collagen cross-linking

When enzymes attach sugars to proteins, they usually do so at sites on the protein molecule dictated by the specificity of the enzyme for the regional sequence to be glycosylated. On the other hand, nonenzymatic glycosylation, a process long known to cause food discoloration and toughness, proceeds nonspecifically at any site sterically available.[60] The longer a protein is in contact with a reducing sugar, the greater the chance for nonenzymatic glycosylation to occur. In uncontrolled diabetics, elevated circulating levels of glucosylated hemoglobin and albumin are found. Since erythrocytes turn over every 120 days, the levels of hemoglobin A_{1c} are an index of the degree of control of hyperglycemia over a 120-day period. The same is true for glucosylated albumin over a shorter period. Proteins such as collagen, which is extremely long-lived, have also been shown to undergo nonenzymatic glucosylation. Sell and Monnier[61] demonstrated an accelerated age-related browning of human collagen in diabetes.

The nonenzymatic reactions between glucose and proteins are collectively known as the Maillard or browning reaction. The initial reaction is the formation of a Schiff base between glucose and an amino group on the protein. This is an unstable structure and can spontaneously undergo an Amadori rearrangement in which a new ketone group is generated on the adduct. This can condense with a similar product on another peptide sequence to produce a covalent cross-linkage.[60] Initially, glycation affects the interaction of collagen with cells and other matrix components, but the most damaging effects are caused by the formation of glucose-mediated intermolecular cross-linkages. These cross-linkages decrease the critical flexibility and permeability of the tissues and reduce turnover. Another fibrous protein that is similarly modified by glycation is elastin.[62] Verzijl et al.[63] have shown that, during aging, nonenzymatic glycation results in the accumulation of the advanced glycation end-product pentosidine in articular cartilage aggrecan.

The arthritides

The development of rheumatoid diseases, particularly osteoarthritis, is a common event in aging individuals. Early assertions that chondrocytes are terminally differentiated cells, incapable of replication, have come under challenge.[64] Studies have confirmed that articular chondrocytes from aged animals can proliferate both in vivo and in vitro, and furthermore can synthesize macromolecules as is seen in younger animals. It has been reported that osteoarthritis is not the result of diminished metabolic activity, but rather that metabolic activity is elevated.[65] ECM synthesis and cell replication proceed at elevated rates in damaged tissue, but so do the levels of degradative lysosomal enzymes. Hollander et al.[66] have reported that in aging and osteoarthritis there is increased denaturation of type II collagen in cartilage. The damage starts at the articular surface and spreads into the deeper zones, involving articular chondrocytes. Thus proteoglycan content of articular cartilage decreases in proportion to the severity of the disease because of a greater rate of matrix degradation over synthesis.

In inflammatory arthritis, degradative enzymes including tissue collagenases are present in the rheumatoid lesion, leading to degradation of both cartilage and bone. It is believed that inflammatory factors stimulate abnormal levels of these enzymes.[67] Bunning et al.[68] demonstrated that interleukin-1 (IL-1), originally believed to be produced by monocytes and macrophages, can also be produced by synovial cells. IL-1 is also mitogenic for synovial cells and can stimulate the production of collagenases, proteoglycanases, plasminogen activator, and prostaglandins. These investigators suggest that IL-1 plays an important role in the pathogenesis of rheumatoid arthritis. It has also been shown that injections of type II collagen can lead to synovitis coupled to the appearance of antibodies against type II collagen. However, in spontaneously arthritic mice, synovitis appeared earlier than the peak levels of antibodies to type II collagen. It was suggested that, in these mice, induction of antibodies to type II collagen is triggered by joint cartilage destruction with subsequent type II collagen release.

Osteoporosis

Bone mass loss associated with aging can lead to osteoporosis, which is associated with multiple bone fractures with impaired healing. Ferris et al.,[69] in a study of biopsy material from osteoporotic fractures of the iliac crest, demonstrated an altered orientation of the proteoglycan components of the noncollagenous bone matrix, although the amounts of the material seemed unchanged. This implied that the quality as well as the quantity of bone is affected in osteoporosis. In a study of human trabecular bone taken at autopsy, Oxlund et al.[70] examined bone collagen and reducible and nonreducible collagen cross-linkages in relation to age and osteoporosis. The extractability of collagen from vertebral bone of control individuals was increased with age. Bone collagen of osteoporotic individuals showed increased extractability and a marked decrease in the concentration of the divalent reducible collagen cross-linkages compared with sex- and age-matched controls. No alterations were observed in the concentration of trivalent pyridinium cross-linkages. These changes would be expected to reduce the strength of the bone trabeculae and could explain why the osteoporotic individuals had bone fractures although the collagen density did not differ from that of the sex- and age-matched controls.

A marked increase in reducible collagen type I cross-linkages was reported in chronically immobilized monkeys with osteoporosis, by Yamauchi et al.[71] The low values returned to control levels after 40 months of ambulatory recovery. Mature, stable cross-linkage concentrations remained constant throughout immobilization and recovery. These studies strongly suggest that, during the osteoporotic state, rapid new collagen synthesis took place. With long-term recovery, this returned to normal values. Thus it appears that progressive bone loss in osteoporosis may result from bone resorption in excess of bone deposition. Croucher et al.[72] have quantitatively assessed cancellous structure in 35 patients with primary osteoporosis. Their data demonstrate that, for a given cancellous area, structural changes in primary osteoporosis are similar to those observed during age-related bone loss in normal subjects. These findings strongly implicate an abnormal increase in the activity(ies) of osteoclast-derived resorption enzymes, acting on the degradation of the ECM, in the etiology of osteoporosis.

Werner's syndrome

Werner's syndrome (WS) is a rare autosomal recessive condition with multiple progeroid features. It is caused by mutations of RecQ type DNA helicase. Clinical and biological manifestations in four major body systems—the nervous, immune, connective tissue, and endocrine systems—similar to normal aging, appear at an early stage of the patient's life.[73] WS may cause abnormalities in connective tissue metabolism that are rarely seen in normal aging, such as scleroderma-like skin.[74] Arakawa et al.[75] reported increased collagen synthesis in fibroblasts from two WS patients. This was accompanied by a near doubling of the levels of procollagen mRNA over normal controls. Similarly, studies by Hatamochi et al.[76] demonstrated that WS fibroblast-conditioned medium brought about activation of normal fibroblast proliferation but failed to alter the relative rates of collagen and noncollagenous protein synthesis by such fibroblasts. In a recent review, Shen and Loeb[77] presented evidence that the WS gene product (SRN), a DNA helicase, also contains an exonuclease activity and is involved in resolving aberrant DNA structures that may arise during the process of DNA replication and transcription. Such processes generate regions of single-stranded DNA that may provide a substrate for the initiation of recombination.

Alzheimer's disease

It is known that β-amyloid fibrils are deposited at the basement membrane of the cerebromicrovasculature in the brains of patients with Alzheimer's disease, and the assembly of the fibrils may be in continuation with the core of senile plaques.[78] Clinical and experimental studies have shown that cerebral perfusion is progressively decreased during increased aging, and this decrease in brain blood flow is significantly greater in Alzheimer's disease.

In a recent review, de la Torre[79] proposes that advanced aging, in association with vascular risk factors, promotes a critically attained threshold of cerebral hypoperfusion (CATCH). With time, CATCH induces brain capillary degeneration characterized by abnormal protein synthesis and neurotransmission failure.

Evidence that brain vascular basement membrane is implicated in Alzheimer's disease was presented by Zarow et al.[80] This microangiopathy is characterized by the immunocytochemical localization of heparan sulfate proteoglycan, collagen type IV, and laminin. In Alzheimer's patients, capillaries appeared ragged and irregular, with diameters of varying thickness and considerable variations from one region to another: in some areas they were sparse while in others they were tightly packed. All capillary beds stained with antibodies against type IV collagen, but heparan sulfate proteoglycans (HSGP) were disrupted at the endothelial surfaces, with a significant colocalization of HSGP with amyloid deposits. It was suggested that the vascular basement membrane may serve as a nidus for senile plaque, playing a role in the development of both amyloid and neuritic elements in Alzheimer's disease.[81]

Stevens and Kisilevsky[82] have reviewed current data on the relationship between immunoglobulin light chain-related fibrils of amyloid and glycosaminoglycans. They state that invariably the fibrils are associated with glycosaminoglycans, predominantly heparan sulfate. Primary structures of immunoglobulin light chains involved in amyloid fibril formation exhibit extensive mutation and diversity, rendering some proteins lightly amyloidogenic and others nonpathological. The interactions between light chains and glycosaminoglycans are also affected by amino acid variation, and may influence the clinical course of disease by enhancing fibril stability and by contributing to resistance to protease degradation.

In a recent editorial, Fillit[83] reviewed the current knowledge concerning the role of amyloidogenesis and proteoglycans in the pathogenesis of Alzheimer's disease. It appears that with aging and senile dementia of the Alzheimer's type, morphological changes of the synaptic terminal, and presumably of the synaptic extracellular matrix, occur. It is hypothesized that dysregulated synaptic plasticity or neuronal response to injury contributes to the evolution of amyloid deposition and senile plaque formation.

SUMMARY

This chapter has reviewed some aspects of connective tissue biochemistry and molecular biology, and the involvement of connective tissue in processes of aging. There is a complexity inherent in the control of connective tissue structure, metabolism, and molecular biology, and aging might contribute to alterations in these and vice versa. Among the phenomena that may prove central to the aging process are the processes of collagen cross-linking and nonenzymatic glycosylation, alternative gene splicing, effects of solar radiation, the interplay of cytokines and growth factors on the control of connective tissue phenotype, production of degradative enzymes, factors that affect cell replication, connective tissue diseases and intracellular factors that control senescence. The causes and effects of aging are an active area of contemporary research in which the involvement of connective tissue is an important segment.

KEY POINTS Connective tissues and aging

- Changes in the structural integrity and production of connective tissue macromolecules are associated with the process of aging.

- Loss of tissue function in aging is associated with increased cross-linking of collagen and elastin fibrils and subsequent decrease in their turnover.

- Alternative splicing in the mRNA of connective tissue macromolecules has been implicated in the process of aging.

- There is a correlation between cellular senescence and changes in the regulation of connective tissue metabolism.

- Nonenzymatic glycation of collagen and elastin is accelerated with aging and may be associated with changes in diabetes.

- In age-related osteoporosis, a decrease in divalent reducible collagen cross-linkages may lead to reduced bone strength and may explain increased bone fractures.

- In aging and in senile dementia of the Alzheimer's type, there is colocalization of heparan sulfate proteoglycan and amyloid plaques.

Acknowledgment

I wish to thank Ms Zahra Ziaie for her enormous help with the preparation of the manuscript.

REFERENCES

1. Prockop DJ, Kivirikko, KI: Collagens: molecular biology, diseases and potentials for therapy. Annu Rev Biochem 1995;64:403–430
2. Bailey AJ, Paul RG, Knott L: Mechanisms of maturation and aging of collagen. Mech Aging Devel 1998;106:1–56
3. Linsenmayer TF, Fitch JM, Birk DE: Heterotypic collagen fibrils and stabilizing collagens. Ann NY Acad Sci 1990;580:143–160
4. Yurchenko PD, O'Rear J: Supramolecular organization of basement membranes. In Rohrbach DH, Timpl R (eds): Molecular and Cellular Aspects of Basement Membranes. Academic Press, London, 1993:19
5. Kefalides NA, Alper R: Structure and organization of macromolecules in basement membranes. In Nimni ME (ed): Collagen: Chemistry, Biology and Biotechnology. CRC Press, Boca Raton, FL, 1988:73–94
6. Eyre DR, Paz MA, Gallop PM: Crosslinking in collagen and elastin. Ann Rev Biochem 1984;53:717–748
7. Mazzorana M, Gruffat H, Sergeant A, van der Rest M: Mechanisms of collagen trimer formation: construction and expression of a recombinant mini gene in HeLa cells reveals a direct affect of prolyl hydroxylation on chain assembly of type XII collagen. J Biol Chem 1993;268:3029–3032
8. Richard-Blum S, Ville G: Collagen crosslinking. Cell Mol Biol 1989;34:581–590
9. Tanzer ML: Collagens and elastin: structure and interactions. Curr Opin Cell Biol 1989;1:968–973
10. Harris ED, Welgus GA, Krane SM: Regulation of mammalian collagenases. Collagen Rel Res 1984;4:493–512
11. Seiki M: Membrane-type matrix metalloproteinases. APMIS 1999;107:137–143.
12. Kleiner DE, Stetler-Stevenson WG: Matrix metalloproteinases and metastasis. Cancer Chemother Pharmacol 1999;43(Suppl):S42–S51
13. Sandberg LB. Elastin structure in health and disease. Int Rev Connect Tissue Res 1976;7:159–210
14. Rosenbloom J, Abrams WR, Mecham R: Extracellular matrix 4: the elastic fiber. FASEB J 1993;7:1208–1218
15. Tiecke F, Katzke S, Booms P et al: Classic, atypically severe and neonatal Marfan syndrome: twelve mutations and genotype–phenotype correlations in FBN1 exons 24–40. Eur J Human Genet 2001;9:13–21
16. Bashir M, Indik Z, Yeh H et al: Elastin gene structure and mRNA alternate splicing. In Davidson J, Tamburro A (eds): Elastin: Chemical and Biological Aspects. Galatina Congedo Editore, Italy, 1990:48–70
17. Bernfield M, Kokenyesi, R, Kato, M et al: Biology of the syndecans: a family of transmembrane heparan sulfate proteoglycans. Annu Rev Cell Biol 1992;8:365–393
18. Groffen AJ, Veerkamp JH, Monnens LA: Recent insights into the structure and functions of heparan sulfate proteoglycans in the human glomerular basement membrane. Nephrol Dial Transplant 1999;14:2119–2129
19. Scott JE: Structure and function in extracellular matrices depend on interactions between anionic glycosaminoglycans. Pathol Biol (Paris) 2001;49:284–289
20. Iozzo RV, Murdoch AD: Proteoglycans of the extracellular environment: clues from the gene and protein side offer novel perspectives in molecular diversity and function. FASEB J 1996;10:598–614
21. Grover J, Chen X-N, Korenberg JR, Roughley, PJ: The human lumican gene: organization, chromosomal location, and expression in articular cartilage. J Biol Chem 1995;270:21942–21949
22. Lafrenie RM, Yamada KM: Integrins and matrix molecules in salivary gland cell adhesion, signaling, and gene expression. Ann NY Acad Sci 1998;842:42–48
23. Ruoslahti E: Fibronectin and its receptors. Annu Rev Biochem 1988;57:375–413
24. Kornblihtt AR, Umezawa K, Vibe-Pedersen K, Baralle FE: Primary structure of human fibronectin: different splicing may generate at least 10 polypeptides from a single gene. EMBO J 1985;4:1755–1759
25. Oldberg A, Ruoslahti E: Evolution of the fibronectin gene: exon structure of the cell attachment domain. J Biol Chem 1986;261:2113–2116
26. French-Constant C, Hynes RO: Alternate splicing of fibronectin is temporally and spatially regulated in the chicken embryo. Development 1989;106:375
27. Kleinman HK, Sephel GC, Tashiro K-I et al: Laminin in neural development. Ann NY Acad Sci 1990;580:311–323
28. Mayer U, Kohfeldt E, Timpl R: Structural and genetic analysis of laminin–nidogen interaction. Ann NY Acad Sci 1998;857:130–142
29. Rao CN, Kefalides NA: Identification and characterization of a 43-kilodalton laminin fragment from the "A" chain (long arm) with high-affinity heparin binding and mammary epithelial cell adhesion-spreading activities. Biochemistry 1990;29:6769–6777
30. Engvall E: Laminin variants: why, where and when. Kidney Int 1993;43:2–6
31. Burgeson RE, Chiquet M, Deutzmann R et al: A new nomenclature for the laminins. Matrix Biol 1994;14:209–211
32. Ohno M, Martinez-Hernandez A, Ohno N, Kefalides NA: Laminin M is found in placental basement membranes but not in basement membranes of neoplastic origin. Connect Tiss Res 1986;15:199–207
33. Ohno M, Martinez-Hernandez A, Ohno N, Kefalides NA: Comparative study of laminin found in normal placental membranes with laminin of neoplastic origin. In Shibata S (ed): Basement Membranes. Elsevier Science, Amsterdam, 1985:3–11
34. Chung AE, Freeman IL, Braginski JE: A novel extracellular membrane elaborated by a mouse embryonal carcinoma cell line. Biochem Biophys Res Commun 1977;79:859–868
35. Timpl R, Dziadek M, Fujiwara S, Nowack H. Wick G: Nidogen: a new self-aggregating basement membrane protein. Eur J Biochem 1983;137:455–465
36. Chakravarti S, Tam M, Chung AE: The basement membrane glycoprotein entactin promotes cell attachment and binds calcium ions. J Biol Chem 1990;265:10597–10603
37. Mosher DF: Physiology of thrombospondin. Annu Rev Med 1990;41:85–97
38. Newton G, Weremowicz S, Morton CC et al: The thrombospondin-4 gene. Mammal Genome 1999;10:1010–1016
39. Albelda SM, Buck CA: Integrins and other cell adhesion molecules. FASEB J 1990;4:2868–2880
40. Buck CA, Horwitz AF: Integrin, a transmembrane glycoprotein complex mediating cell-substratum adhesion. J Cell Sci Suppl 1987;8:231–250
41. Danen EH, Yamada KM: Fibronectin, integrins, and growth control. J Cell Physiol 2001;189:1–13
42. Cristofalo VJ, Stanulis-Paeger BM: Cellular senescence in vitro. Adv Cell Culture 1982;2:1–68
43. van Gansen P, van Lerberghe N: Potential and limitations of cultivated fibroblasts in the study of senescence in animals: a review of the murine skin fibroblast system. Arch Gerontol Geriatr 1988;7:31–74

44. Shevitz J, Jenkins CS, Hatcher VB: Fibronectin synthesis and degradation in human fibroblasts with aging. Mech Aging Develop 1986;35:221–232

45. Smith JR, Pereira-Smith OM: Altered gene expression during cellular aging. Genome 1989;31:386–389

46. West MD, Pereira-Smith OM, Smith JR: Replicative senescence of human skin fibroblasts correlates with a loss of regulation and over-expression of collagenase activity. Exp Cell Res 1989;184:138–147

47. Boonen S, Aerssens J, Broos P et al: Age-related bone loss and senile osteoporosis: evidence for both secondary hyperparathyroidism and skeletal growth factor deficiency in the elderly. Aging 1995;7:414–422

48. Roberts AB, Sporn MB: Regulation of endothelial cell growth architecture and matrix synthesis by TGF-beta. Am Rev Resp Dis 1989;140:1126–1128

49. Uitto J, Bernstein EF: Molecular mechanisms of cutaneous aging: connective tissue alterations in the dermis. J Invest Derm Symp Proc 1998;3:41–44

50. Hayflick L: The cell biology of aging. J Invest Dermatol 1979;73:8–14

51. Dale Carbonate M, Pathak, MA: Skin photosensitizing agents and the role of reactive oxygen species in photoaging. J Photochem Photobiol 1994;14:105–124

52. Bucala R, Cerami A: Advanced glycation: chemistry, biology and implications for diabetes and aging. Adv Pharmacol 1992;23:1–34

53. Bernstein EF, Chen YQ, Kopp JB et al: Long-term sun exposure alters the collagen of the papillary dermis: comparison of sun-protected and photoaged skin by Northern analysis, immunohistochemical staining and confocal laser scanning microscopy. J. Am Acad Dermatol 1996;34:209–218

54. Kligman LH: Photoaging: manifestations, prevention and treatment. Clin Geriatr Med 1989;5:235–251

55. Reddi AS: Diabetic microangiopathy. I: Current concepts of the chemistry and metabolism of the glomular basement membrane. Metabolism 1978;27:107–124

56. Archer FJ, Kaye R: Aging of diabetic and non-diabetic skin fibroblasts in vitro: life span and sequential growth curves. J Gerontol A 1989;44:M93–M99

57. Sibbitt WL, Mills RG, Digler CF et al: Glucose inhibition of human fibroblast proliferation and response to growth factors is prevented by inhibitors of aldose reductase. Mech Aging Dev 1989;47:265–270

58. Eaton RP, Sibbitt WL, Shah VO et al: A commentary on 10 years of aldose reductase inhibition for limited joint mobility in diabetes. J Diabetes Complications 1998;12:34–38

59. Fleischli JG, Laughlin TJ, Lavery LA et al: The effects of diabetes mellitus on the material properties of human metatarsal bones. J Foot Ankle Surg 1998;37:195–198

60. Cerami A, Vlassara H, Brownlee M: Glucose and aging. Sci Am 1987;256:90–96

61. Sell DR, Monnier VM: Isolation, purification and partial characterization of novel fluorophores from aging human insoluble collagen-rich tissue. Connect Tiss Res 1989;19:77–92

62. Paul RG, Bailey AJ: Glycation of collagen: the basis of its central role in the late complications of ageing and diabetes. Int J Biochem Cell Biol 1996;28:1297–1310

63. Verzijl N, Degroot, J, Bank RA et al: Age-related accumulation of the advanced glycation endproduct pentosidine in human articular cartilage aggrecan: the use of pentosidine levels as a quantitative measure of protein turnover. Matrix Biol 2001;20:409–417

64. Hough AJ, Webber RJ: Aging phenomena and osteoarthritis: cause or coincidence? Ann Clin Lab Sci 1986;16:501–510

65. Bora FW, Miller G: Joint physiology, cartilage metabolism and the etiology of osteoarthritis. Hand Clin 1987;3:325–336

66. Hollander AP, Pidoux I, Reiner A et al: Damage to type II collagen in aging and osteoarthritis starts at the articular surface, originates around chondrocytes and extends into the cartilage with progressive degeneration. J Clin Invest 1995;96:2859–2869

67. Mainardi CL: Biochemical mechanisms of articular destruction. Rheum Dis Clin N Am 1987;13:215–233

68. Bunning RA, Richardson HJ, Crawford A et al: The effects of interleukin-1 on connective tissue metabolism and its relevance to arthritis. Agents Actions 1986(Suppl);18:131–152

69. Ferris BD, Klenerman L, Didds RA et al: Altered organization of non-collagenous bone matrix in osteoporosis. Bone 1987;8:2285–2288

70. Oxlund H, Mosekilde L, Ortoft G: Reduced concentration of collagen reducible cross-links in human trabecular bone with respect to age and osteoporosis. Bone 1996;19:479–484

71. Yamauchi M, Young DR, Chandler GS, Mechanic GL: Crosslinking and new bone collagen synthesis in immobilized and recovering primate osteoporosis. Bone 1988;9:415–418

72. Coucher PI, Garrahan NJ, Compston JE: Structural mechanisms of trabecular bone loss in primary osteoporosis: specific disease mechanism or early aging? Bone Miner 1995;25:111–121

73. Lebel M: Werner syndrome: genetic and molecular basis of a premature aging disorder. Cell Mol Life Sci 2001;58:857–867

74. Goto SM: Hierarchical deterioration of body systems in Werner's syndrome: implications for normal aging. Mech Ageing Dev 1997;98:239–254

75. Arakawa M, Hatamochi A, Takeda K, Ueki H: Increased collagen synthesis accompanying elevated mRNA levels in cultured Werner's syndrome fibroblasts. J Invest Dermatol 1990;94:187–190

76. Hatamochi A, Arakawa M, Takeda K, Ueki H: Activation of fibroblast proliferation by Werner's syndrome fibroblast-conditioned medium. J Dermatol Sci 1994;7:210–216

77. Shen J, Loeb LA: Unwinding the molecular basis of the Werner syndrome. Mech Ageing Dev 2001;122:921–944

78. Inoue S, Kuroiwa M, Kisilevsky R: Basement membranes, microfibrils and beta amyloid fibrilogenesis in Alzheimer's disease: high resolution ultrastructural findings. Brain Res Brain Res Rev 1999;29:218–231

79. de la Torre JC: Cerebral hypoperfusion, capillary degeneration, and development of Alzheimer disease. Alzheimer Dis Assoc Dis 2000;14(Suppl 1):S72–S81

80. Zarow C, Barron E, Chui HC, Perlmutter LS: Vascular basement membrane pathology and Alzheimer's disease. Ann NY Acad Sci 1997;826:147–160

81. Perlmutter LS, Chui HC, Saperia D, Athanikar J: Microangiopathy and the colocalization of heparan sulfate proteoglycan with amyloid in senile plaques of Alzheimer's disease. Brain Res 1990;508:13–19

82. Stevens FJ, Kisilevsky R: Immunoglobulin light chains, glycosaminoglycans, and amyloid. Cell Mol Life Sci 2000;57:441–449

83. Fillit H: Disorders of the extracellular matrix and pathogenesis of senile dementia of the Alzheimer's type. Lab Invest 1995;72:249–253

Chapter 11

Clinical immunology of aging

Stefan Gravenstein, Howard M. Fillit, and William B. Ershler

As a fundamental organ necessary for the maintenance of life, the immune system first appeared in primitive organisms about 480 million years ago.[1] The intimate relation between acquired immunity and infection was apparent early in recorded history. Observing an epidemic of plague in 430 B.C., Thucydides reported that anyone who had recovered from the disease was never attacked again. The era of modern immunology was probably initiated by Jenner's report in 1798 on an effective vaccine employing cowpox pustules to prevent smallpox in humans. The linkage of advances in infectious disease and in immunology continued throughout the nineteenth and twentieth centuries. For example, identification of bacterial organisms ultimately resulted in the discovery of antibodies that could neutralize the toxins produced by these organisms, leading to modern methods for the development of vaccines. The discovery of antibody structure during the 1960s finally began the era of modern immunochemistry. With regard to cellular immunity, despite the early work of Metchnikoff and his followers, the role of cells in acquired immunity was not truly appreciated until the 1950s. Finally, although concepts of "recognition of self," and "autoimmunity" as a mechanism of disease appeared early in the twentieth century, the causes of autoimmune disease remain poorly understood.

Immunogerontology is a relatively new field, probably introduced by Walford in 1969.[2] Walford proposed that immune mechanisms play an important role in the pathogenesis, but not the etiology of the aging process. The immunological theory of aging linked life span with the genetic repertoire of the individual via the major histocompatibility genes. Walford proposed that disorders in the immune system that occur with aging account for three major causes of disease in old age: increased autoimmunity causing organ-specific disease, including vascular disease; failing surveillance allowing the expression of cancers; and the increased susceptibility to infectious diseases. Current evidence supports the notion that the decline in immune function with aging may be viewed as a form of idiopathic acquired immunodeficiency in old age, which is generally mild in nature. More recent complexity has been added to our understanding of immune dysfunction in malignancies, including a component of immune dysregulation. Elderly people may also suffer secondary, potentially reversible causes of acquired immunodeficiency that may be clinically significant.[3] Among these are cancer, malnutrition, and the acquired immune deficiency syndrome (AIDS).

CHANGES IN THE HUMAN IMMUNE SYSTEM WITH AGING
Nonspecific host defense

Primary immunity is the first line of defense against invading pathogens. It differs from secondary immunity in that it does not require sensitization, or prior exposure, to offer protection. Examples of primary immunity include the mucocutaneous barriers, cellular barriers that perform the function of phagocytosis, and cellular (natural killer cells) and noncellular (complement) systems that mediate nonspecific lysis of foreign cells.

Phagocytosis

Phagocytosis involves the engulfment and usually lysis and/or digestion of foreign substances. The capacity of neutrophils, macrophages, and monocytes for phagocytosis is determined by their number and ability to reach the relevant site. Thus, absolute number, endothelial adherence and chemotaxis, and phagocytosis itself with subsequent digestion of the organism are critical factors determining the efficiency of this mechanism in primary immunity.[4] The study of alterations in phagocytosis with age must then involve examinations of each of these steps, and are inherently more difficult in human populations than in disease-free inbred animals.

Extrapolation of studies of senescent mice to humans would suggest that age itself does not attenuate response to bacterial capsular antigens in a well-vascularized area such as the lung; the pulmonary inflammatory reaction is similar between young adult and old animals.[5,6] Niwa and colleagues[7] reported a deterioration in neutrophil chemotaxis and increase in serum lipid peroxidase in the nonsurviving cohort of a 7-year longitudinal study, suggesting a preterminal but not necessarily "normal" aging alteration in these factors. However, age-related effectiveness in chemotaxis may be reduced in less vascular areas in vivo, such as in the skin, which also has a host of other changes that may impair the ability of cells in the vascular compartment to reach a site of infection.[8] Although in-vitro neutrophil function (including endothelial adherence, migration, granule secretory behavior, etc.) is insignificantly affected by age,[9] significantly fewer neutrophils arrive at the skin abrasion sites studied in older people.[10] How this translates to immune response and immune-mediated repair in infected or otherwise physiologically stressed older people remains unknown.

Macrophage activation also appears to change with age; this may be partially attributable to a reduced gamma interferon signal from T lymphocytes.[11–13] Less signal at the site of infection could be a consequence of reduced numbers of activated T cells locally. Fewer T cells and the defective expression of homing markers to attract T cells from peripheral blood into inflamed tissues[14] suggests that increased susceptibility of old mice to, for example, tuberculosis, reflects an impaired capacity to focus mediator cells and the additional cytokine they may express at sites of infection[13] (more on T-cell changes with age, below). These observations may help explain why late-life tuberculosis, or, for that matter, reactivation tuberculosis occurs and remains clinically important.

Cell lysis

Cell lysis is mediated via a variety of pathways, including the complement system, natural killer (NK) cell activity, and neutrophil activity. Complement activity does not appear to decline significantly with age, and neutrophil function changes only arguably as noted above. However, kinetics of NK activity—lytic activity by cells that do not require prior exposure to the offending infected or malignant cells in order to lyse them—may be another factor that participates in infections such as tuberculosis. In longitudinal studies of nonhuman primates, NK activity does appear to be affected by age[15] and acute stressors such as illness.[16]

Specific host defense

Aging is accompanied by changes in the immune system, which are evidenced by alterations in both cellular and humoral immunity. Animal models have been used extensively to investigate these changes, but will not be discussed here in detail as more definitive reviews are available.[17–19]

Human aging is associated with decreased thymic function, an important factor for age-related changes in thymic dependent immunity.[20] Declines in serum thymic hormones precede the decline in thymic tissue. By the age of 60, few of the thymic peptides are measurable in human peripheral blood,[21] and most of the thymic epithelial tissue is replaced by fibrotic scar. Thymic hormone replacement may improve immune function in old age,[22,23] but there are no current clinical indications for the use of thymic hormones in practice.

In the cellular immune system, most studies show no significant changes with human aging in the total number of peripheral blood cells, including total lymphocytes, monocytes, NK cells, or polymorphonuclear leukocytes.[24–30] The appearance of lymphocytopenia is associated with mortality in elderly people, but is not an age-related finding.[25,31,32] Most studies show no changes in the percentages of B- and T-lymphocyte populations in the peripheral blood,[24,27,29,33,34] although chronically ill elderly people may particularly have a decline in total T-cell numbers.[34] Equivocal changes in the ratio of helper cells to suppressor cells (T4/T8) occur in normal aging.[26,27,34–36] These findings are in contrast to human immunodeficiency virus (HIV)-induced acquired immunodeficiency syndrome (AIDS) associated with a decreased T4/T8 ratio.[37] Finally, there is a specific age-related increase in memory cells, cells that express the CD45 surface marker.[38–42]

The function of lymphocytes is altered with aging. There is a robust decline in the proliferative capacity of T lymphocytes to nonspecific mitogens.[30,33,36,43,44] In addition, antigen-specific declines in the proliferative potential of T cells to specific viruses have been demonstrated.[45,46] The number and the affinity of mitogen receptors on T lymphocytes do not change with age.[47] However, the number of T lymphocytes capable of dividing in response to mitogens is reduced, and the activated T cells do not undergo as many divisions.[48]

Superimposed upon the accumulation of a relatively inert naïve T-cell fraction observed with advancing age, there appears also to be a shift in predominance of helper T-cell responses from type 1 (TH1) to type 2 (TH2). Cells of the TH1 type produce IL-2, interferon-γ, TNF-α, and predominantly

Table 11-1 **Inducers, products, and inhibitors of TH subsets**		
	TH1	**TH2**
Inducers	IL-12	IL-1
Products	IFN-g, IL-2	IL-4, IL-5, IL-6, IL-9, IL-10, IL-13
Consequences	CMI, IgG2a	IgG1, IgE
Inhibitors	IL-4, IL-10	IFN-g

mediate cell-mediated immune and inflammatory responses, whereas cells of the TH2 type produce IL-4, IL-5, IL-6, and IL-10, factors that enhance humoral immunity (Table 11-1).[49]

The abnormality in T-cell proliferative capacity is not related to an abnormality in accessory cell function.[43] Changes in the fluidity of the cell membrane occur with aging in most cells, including lymphocytes,[50] which may impair the proliferative response by preventing cross-linking and capping of receptors, a process necessary for cell activation. Cell activation is also dependent on cellular shifts of calcium (Ca). Lymphocytes from old humans may have abnormalities in Ca signaling cascades that ultimately lead to deoxyribonucleic acid (DNA) synthesis.[51] There may be intrinsic T-cell defects in DNA mechanisms of proliferation that may be involved in this decline in proliferative capacity.[52] Fewer activated T cells from old humans progress through the cell cycle after activation, and fewer old human T cells re-enter the cell cycle and continue to proliferate.[53]

The decline in proliferation may also be caused by decreased T-cell lymphokine production and regulation, particularly interleukin 2 (IL-2), during the proliferative response to mitogens.[25,36,54,55] Decreases in the percentage of IL-2 receptor positive cells, IL-2 receptor density, and in the expression of IL-2 and IL-2 receptor specific mRNA in old humans have been reported.[36,56] IL-2 production in response to specific antigens also declines. Vaccination with influenza results in increased IL-2 secretion in response to viral antigen in vitro.[57,58] In addition, the number of influenza-specific cytotoxic T cells declines with age, with no increase after vaccination.[59] The sensitivity of T cells to prostaglandins is also altered in aging.[60,61] However, little decline has been noted in the serum levels or secretion of inflammatory cytokines; although chronically ill, frail patients may have elevated serum levels, which predict mortality,[62,63] and there is an age-related increase in IL-6 which is both age-related and appears to be inhibited by estrogen. IL-6 is of interest because it can be linked to other age-associated disorders (such as multiple myeloma and benign monoclonal gammopathy—see below) that are or have been suggested to be immune related (Alzheimer's disease[64,65] and osteoporosis[66]).[67]

There is a decline in delayed-type skin hypersensitivity (DTH),[45] which may reflect the decline in in-vitro lymphocyte proliferation.[45,46] Anergy, the lack of DTH to a battery of injected antigens, indicates incompetence of cell-mediated immunity.[68] Generally, a battery of skin test antigens (usually four to six antigens) is necessary to adequately assess DTH in elderly people. Anergy to both mitogens and specific antigens increases with age.[44,45,69,70] The number of skin test positive reactions declines with age from over 80 percent in young individuals to less than 20 percent in older individuals.[44]

Variations in populations studied are important factors in determining rates of anergy in elderly people. In one study,[70] 17.9 percent of subjects over age 66 years and living at home were anergic; 41 percent of subjects living in a nursing home but able to care for themselves were anergic; and 60 percent of subjects who were functionally impaired and living in a nursing home were anergic. In addition, a number of acute and chronic illnesses may impair the DTH response, suggesting the need for longitudinal studies of DTH to determine the nature of the defect in DTH present in an individual patient or in various populations.[68] Concomitant in-vitro testing suggests that not all anergic patients have impaired in-vitro measures of lymphocyte function such as proliferative capacity,[24,71] suggesting that both in-vivo cutaneous DTH testing and in-vitro lymphocyte testing may be necessary to identify individuals who are truly anergic and presumably immunodeficient.[72] Associations between anergy and mortality have been repeatedly demonstrated.[32,44,70,73–75] These changes in cellular immunity may be responsible for reactivation infections such as tuberculosis and varicella (shingles—more on this below) in aged individuals.

The issue of DTH testing in tuberculosis has also received particular interest because of the clinical implications of tuberculin skin reactivity for the diagnosis and treatment of tuberculosis in elderly people.[48,53,76–78] In this regard, the size of the skin test reaction appears to have some significance in the clinical interpretation of results. Positive skin tests are often found after repeated testing, suggesting the presence of a "booster" effect, requiring additional interpretation and analysis.[78]

In the humoral immune system, there are no changes in the number of peripheral blood B cells in old age.[79] Most studies indicate an increase in total serum immunoglobulin (IgG) and IgA levels, and no change in IgM.[80,81] Declines in antibody titers to specific foreign antigens have been noted, including naturally occurring antibodies to the isoagglutinins,[82] and titers of antibody to foreign antigens such as microbial antigens.[83–87] Both the primary[88] and secondary immune responses to vaccination are impaired. Elderly patients tend to have lower peak titers of antibody and more rapid declines in titers after immunization,[89,90] as well as the peak titer occurring slightly later (2–6 weeks rather than 2–3 weeks post-vaccination) than in younger people.[91] In contrast, serum autoantibodies may have organ specificity, such as antiparietal cell, antithyroglobulin, and antineuronal antibodies.[92–99] Organ nonspecific autoantibodies, such as antibodies to DNA and rheumatoid factors, also increase with age. Circulating immune complexes may also increase with advancing age.[96,100] The reason why autoantibodies increase with age is not known. Several explanations are possible, including alterations in immune regulation and an increase in stimulation of B-cell clones due to recurrent or chronic infections or increased tissue degradation. Intrinsic B-cell abnormalities may be important in defective Ig production.[83,101–103] Changes in the human B-cell proliferative response, similar to the defect found in human T cells, have been investigated with varying findings.[30,104] Abnormalities in a specific B-cell subtype, the CD5 B cell, may be responsible for the abnormal production of autoantibodies, particularly rheumatoid factors, and the occurrence of certain myeloproliferative disorders in old age.[105] Changes in

Table 11-2 Cytokines and aging		
Decreased level or function	Unchanged, mixed reports, or not studied	Increased level or function
IL-2	IL-1	IL-6
IL-3	TNF-α	IL-10
GM-CSF	Interferon-γ	
IL-12	IL-4	

T-cell function may contribute to the B-cell dysfunction with age.[84,102,103,106]

Cytokine dysregulation and aging

There has been an increased awareness of alterations in the production and degradation of cytokines with age (Table 11-2). Whereas the decline in IL-2 and IL-12 may contribute to the observed decline in cellular immune function, the increase in proinflammatory cytokines (particularly IL-6) may contribute to the metabolic changes associated with frailty. Normally, IL-6 is typically a tightly controlled mediator of acute inflammatory responses, and levels in the serum are typically below the level of detection. Among the regulators of IL-6 are the sex steroids (estrogen and testosterone), and at menopause, detectable IL-6 levels appear in the blood in apparently healthy individuals. It has been proposed that a chronic exposure to such proinflammatory signals contributes to the phenotype of frailty.[107] In fact, elevated IL-6 levels have been shown to correlate well with functional decline and mortality in a population of community dwelling elderly people.[108,109]

AUTOIMMUNITY AND AGING

Walford[2] speculated that autoimmunity plays an important role in the aging process. Kay[110] and others[111] have alternatively proposed that autoimmunity may play an important physiological role in the regenerative and reparative process that is ongoing during aging. Certain autoimmune diseases have their highest incidence in old age, such as pernicious anemia,[112] thyroiditis,[113–115] bullous pemphigoid,[116] rheumatoid arthritis,[117,118] and temporal arteritis,[119] suggesting that the age-related increase in autoantibodies may have clinical significance.

Autoimmunity may also play a role in vascular disease in old age.[120] Giant cell arteritis is a common disease in old age.[119,121] Of interest, giant cell arteritis is associated with degenerative vascular disease.[119] Indeed, immune mechanisms may result in atherosclerosis, a final common pathway of pathology secondary to a variety of vascular insults.[122,123] A number of antivascular antibodies have been described in man[124–127] that are associated with diseases of the vasculature. Antiphospholipid antibodies are associated with a variety of pathological states of the vasculature, including stroke and vascular dementia,[128,129] temporal arteritis,[130] and ischemic heart disease.[131] However, the exact mechanism by which antiphospholipid antibodies cause vascular injury remains unknown.[132] The increased occurrence of antiphospholipid antibodies with age[133–135] and the association of these autoantibodies with vascular disease may represent a predisposing immunological factor for immune-mediated vascular disease in elderly people. Autoantibodies to vascular heparan sulfate proteoglycans (vHSPG) may also be important in vascular injury in old age,[126] since vHSPG plays an important role in normal anticoagulation and cholesterol metabolism.[136]

Immunosenescence and cancer in old age

Age is the single greatest risk for cancer.[137] Since immune mechanisms play an important role in the elimination of malignant clones via cytotoxic mechanisms, the decline of the immune system in old age could be related to the increased rate of cancer in old age. Nevertheless, the exact relation between immunosenescence and the increased incidence of cancer is unknown. Among explanations of why tumors increase in frequency with age is the observation that tumors may go undetected for decades; thus, the reason for increased frequency in late life relates to easier detection when they finally achieve sufficient size, and the host has had sufficient time for the tumor to progress through each of the necessary promoting events. An alternative explanation suggests that the host and host factors change over time, favoring progression and expression in later life. These two hypotheses to explain the increase in late-life malignancy have aptly been described as "seed vs soil."[138]

From an immunological and "soil" standpoint, there are two principal observations that relate to malignancies and age. There is both evidence of dysregulation of proliferation of cells directly controlled by the immune system, and evidence of increased malignancies in late life that could be hypothetically restrained by nonsenescent immunity. These will be discussed sequentially.

Proliferative disorders of the lymphocyte are common in old age. Although bimodal in incidence, the peak in late-life lymphoma includes a disproportionate incidence of nodular B-cell types.[139] Both old humans and mice have commonly exhibited a monoclonal gammopathy (paraprotein) in the last quartile of the life span.[140-144] Monoclonal gammopathies increase with age and may occur in 79 percent of sera from subjects over the age of 95 years.[145,146] Radl[145] has defined four categories of age-associated monoclonal gammopathy: (1) myeloma or related disorders; (2) benign B-cell neoplasia; (3) immune deficiency, with T-cell greater than B-cell loss, and (4) chronic antigenic stimulation. He speculates that the third category is by far the most common, and that this is what occurs with immune senescence. It is possible that age-associated immune dysfunction is initially associated with markers of aberrant immune regulation such as paraproteinemia and/or autoantibody, and later contributes to the pathogenesis of lymphoma (Fig. 11-1).

Monoclonal gammopathies may cause morbidity, particularly renal disease in the absence of overt multiple myeloma.[147] In a minority of cases of monoclonal gammopathies, a malignant evolution may occur.[148-150] Multiple myeloma also has an age-related increase in incidence.[151] Although treatment is not generally indicated for monoclonal gammopathies,[150] treatment of myeloma is often useful. Another common malignant transformation of the lymphocyte in old age is chronic lymphocytic leukemia.[152] Non-Hodgkin's lymphoma increases in incidence with age, while Hodgkin's lymphoma has a bimodal distribution.[153] The increased prevalence of solid tumors[154] in old age may be related to defective immune surveillance, although this is now being disputed (more on immune surveillance below). An alternative theory holds that there is a natural balance where the immune system has both immune restraining as well as growth-enhancing effects on the tumor, related in part to the cascade of cytokines released by the cells that infiltrate the tumor. With advancing age there may be an imbalance in these two factors that is more permissive or potentially can promote tumor growth (such as with multiple myeloma).[138]

Finally, a discussion of cancer development and aging would not be complete without considering the importance of the decline in immunity and associated failure of "immune surveillance." It has long been proposed that the decline in immune function contributes to the increased incidence of malignancy. However, despite the appeal of such an hypothesis, scientific support has been limited and the topic remains controversial.[155,156] Proponents of an immune explanation point to experiments in which outbred strains of mice with heterogeneous immune functions were followed for their lifespan.[157] Those who demonstrated better functions early in

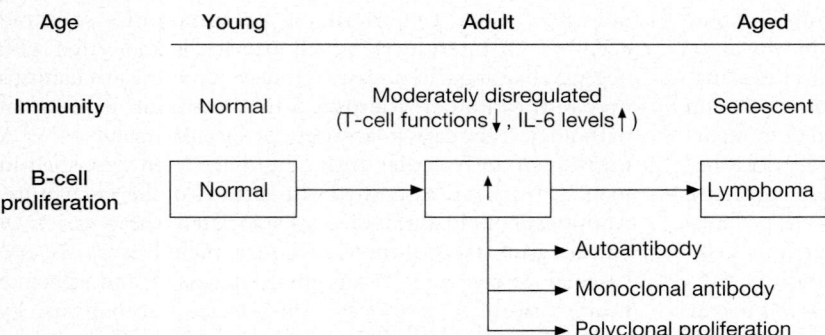

Figure 11-1 The relationship of immune changes with age and B-cell proliferation. A required second trigger, such as *H ras* expression, is necessary for the development of lymphoma.

life (as determined by a limited panel of assays available at the time on a small sample of blood) were found to have fewer spontaneous malignancies and a longer life than those estimated to be less immunologically competent. Furthermore, it is difficult to deny that profoundly immunodeficient animals or humans are subject to a more frequent occurrence of malignant disease, and it would stand to reason that others with less severe immunodeficiency would also be subject to more malignancy, perhaps less dramatically so. However, the malignancies associated with profound immunodeficiency (e.g., with AIDS or after organ transplantation) are usually lymphomas, Kaposi's sarcoma, or leukemia, and not the more common malignancies of geriatric populations (lung, breast, colon, and prostate cancers). Accordingly, it is fair to say that the question of the influence of age-acquired immunodeficiency on the incidence of cancer in elderly people is unresolved. However, there is much greater consensus on the importance of the immunodeficiency of aging in the clinical management of cancer, eluding the problems associated with infection and disease progression.

Immunosenescence and infections in old age

The most profound result of immunosenescence is the increased morbidity and mortality from infections. The rates of a number of infections and their morbidity and mortality increase with age,[158] particularly influenza, pneumonia, urinary tract infections, skin infections, recrudescent latent infections (herpes zoster), *Clostridium difficile* diarrhea, and tetanus. There is also an increase in hospital-acquired and nursing home infections in elderly people. These susceptibilities to infection are due to both immune senescence and other changes more common among older individuals—such as a reduced ciliary escalator efficiency and cough reflex predisposing to aspiration pneumonia; urinary and fecal incontinence predisposing to urinary tract and perineal skin infections; and immobility predisposing to pressure sores and wound infections. Immunosenescence also results in the atypical presentation of infections in old age.[159] Infections are more frequent and prolonged in elderly people.[160]

Old individuals, particularly the oldest old, may not respond as well to therapy for infection and present with infections by unusual organisms, recurrent infections with the same pathogen, or reactivation of quiescent diseases such as those caused by tuberculosis and herpes zoster virus. The impaired immune and inflammatory response in old age changes the clinical expression of infections.[161] Typical signs of infection can be absent, and a higher index of suspicion may be necessary to diagnose infection in elderly patients. Old individuals may not present with typical "hard" signs of infection such as spiking fever, leukocytosis, prominent inflammatory infiltrates on chest X-ray in patients with pneumonia, or rebound tenderness in patients with an acute abdomen. Lower baseline temperatures may require the need for monitoring the change in temperature, rather than the absolute temperature, in old age.[162]

Influenza

Most of the significant morbidity and excess mortality during influenza epidemics occurs in older adults.[163] Age itself, in addition to and separate from the many comorbid conditions

of older people, is a significant risk factor for severe complications of influenza.[164] It is widely held that much of the increased susceptibility of elderly people to influenza and its complications is attributable to immunological factors, including reduced antibody responsiveness and influenza-specific cell-mediated immunity. The role of humoral immunity, especially in the form of neutralizing antibody, is perhaps most important for preventing and limiting the initial infection[165] rather than promoting recovery. T-cell-mediated responses appear to be more important and primarily involved in post-infection viral clearance and recovery; influenza specific cytotoxic T lymphocyte (CTL) activity correlates with rapid clearance of virus in infected human volunteers, even in the absence of detectable serum antibody,[166] and has been experimentally confirmed in adoptive transfer of influenza-specific CTL experiments using the mouse model.[167,168] No doubt influenza-specific antibody declines with age, whether due to natural infection or vaccination,[169–171] and this presumably translates to an increased risk of influenza infection. However, and perhaps equally importantly, CTL,[59,172] human leukocyte antigens (HLA) restriction by influenza-specific T-cell clones, and lymphocyte proliferative responses[173] also decline with age. T-cell-mediated cytokine responses, such as IL-2, which mediate the humoral response to influenza may also decrease with age, although this has not been as clearly established for healthy elderly people[58] as it has been for frail elderly people.[57] Together these observations can account for much of the age-related increase in influenza susceptibility and morbidity. It is important to note that, despite all of the changes occurring with age and comorbid conditions of age, influenza vaccine still is highly cost-effective in reducing influenza-related infections and complications.[174,175] Furthermore, although influenza in otherwise healthy unvaccinated elderly people leads to an illness that lasts nearly twice as long as their younger counterparts—a clinical consequence of immune senescence—influenza illness duration in those elderly people previously vaccinated (i.e., vaccine failures) is comparable to the illness duration in vaccinated healthy young adults.[175a] This observation remains true when the vaccine-to-circulating strain match is poor, negating poor vaccine match as a reason not to vaccinate seniors annually.

Pneumococcal disease

Reduced immunocompetence due to age, disease, or drug therapy introduces risk for complications from pneumococcal disease. One study found the incidence of pneumococcal disease to be 70 cases per 100,000 in individuals over the age of 70 compared to 5 cases per 100,000 in younger adults.[176] *Streptococcus pneumoniae* is a Gram-positive lancet-shaped coccus that normally colonizes the nasopharynx, and was present in up to 70 percent of individuals before the antibiotic era. The pathogenic form is encapsulated diplococci, and the capsule carries the antigenic determinants in currently available pneumococcal vaccines. The rising prevalence of penicillin-resistant pneumococcus[177] poses interesting implications for future antimicrobial treatment of these infections in older adults and for long-term care settings, and reinforces the need for prevention as a primary management strategy for pneumococcal disease.

Pneumonia is the most prevalent expression of infection with *S. pneumoniae*. Other infections associated with pneumococcus include otitis media, sinusitis, meningitis, septic arthritis, pericarditis, endocarditis, peritonitis, cellulitis, glomerulonephritis, and sepsis (especially post-splenectomy). Chronic obstructive pulmonary disease is an independent risk factor for complications from pneumococcal pneumonitis, and this might relate to the altered mechanics of clearing secretions as well as altered immunity within the lung itself. Risk factors for pneumococcal infections also include conditions which predispose an individual to aspiration of pneumococci into the lung. Most conditions affecting swallowing function and mechanics increase in prevalence with age such as dementia, stupor, stroke, alcoholism, seizure disorders, and foreign bodies in the esophagus. Many of these conditions also affect immunity, potentially contributing to the underlying risks from immune senescence.

Prevention is the best form of defense, and the polysaccharide antigens of the pneumococcal vaccine are considered largely to generate a T-cell independent response, a theoretical advantage for older adults because immune senescence is thought to primarily perturb T-cell more so than B-cell responses (see discussion, above). Yet, studies on pneumococcal vaccine efficacy in disease prevention often have been disappointing or inconclusive,[178] with more recent studies suggesting efficacy and cost-effectiveness.[179,180] Consequently, underutilization of pneumococcal vaccine has been held accountable for the development of outbreaks in nursing facilities, underscoring the need for appropriate utilization of the vaccine.[181-183] Currently, revaccination is recommended for persons aged 65 and older if they received vaccine 5 or more years previously and were less than 65 years of age at time of vaccination. Meanwhile, new vaccine designs aim to better stimulate the immune response in older adults by recruiting T-cell help through polysaccharide conjugation with a peptide combined with cytokine[184] or by using a peptide target.[185] Whether these approaches are superior for an immune senescent patient remains to be seen.

Varicella zoster virus

Herpes zoster (shingles) is caused by varicella zoster virus (VZV) and is increasingly prevalent with advancing age, as are its severity and complications.[186-193] Incidence doubles to an annual attack rate of 0.8 percent from the age of 50 to 80 years,[188,189,192] and the majority of cases occurring after the age of 60. Two major complications of herpes zoster, post-herpetic neuralgia and cranial nerve zoster (often of the ophthalmic nerve, and not infrequently resulting in lower motor neuron paresis), are the most disabling. Post-herpetic neuralgia occurs in over 25 percent of patients at least 60 years old and is strongly associated with sleep disturbance and depression.[186,187,191,192,194-199] Bell's palsy[200] and Ménière's [201] disease, both conditions associated with advanced age, have also been linked to herpes zoster. VZV-specific cell-mediated immunity correlates closely with susceptibility to herpes zoster in large populations, such as patients with lymphomas, bone marrow transplant recipients, and immunocompetent elderly persons.[202-215] It is less clear whether boosting currently available measures of humoral or cellular immunity to VZV antigens will specifically reduce risk from developing herpes zoster,[207,211-218] but it is hoped that this will indeed be the case, making herpes zoster a vaccine preventable disease.[219]

SECONDARY CAUSES OF ACQUIRED IMMUNODEFICIENCY IN OLD AGE

In contrast to the normative changes that may result in a mild idiopathic acquired immunodeficiency with aging, a variety of secondary causes of acquired immunodeficiency occur in elderly people that may be severe, yet reversible. The distinction between secondary causes of immunodeficiency from "normal" age-related changes is an important clinical distinction. The clinician needs a high index of suspicion for acquired immunodeficiency in old age, since many causes are reversible and can be the primary reason for the infection risk, altered presentation of infection, or inadequate response to usual therapy.

The effects of malnutrition on the immune system may be profound, and clearly increase the risk of infection in elderly people.[220,221] Immune deficits in undernourished ambulatory elderly people may be reversed by nutritional supplementation.[222] Malnutrition affects up to 50 percent of hospitalized elderly people and is highly associated with poor acute care outcomes, including death among hospitalized elderly people.[223-226] Severe protein, calorie, vitamin, and elemental deficiencies such as zinc (a cofactor for the function of thymic hormone) may cause immunodeficiency and poor outcomes in response to infection.[227,228] An absolute lymphocyte count below 1,500 cells/mm^3 generally indicates some degree of malnutrition, and a count below 900 cells/mm^3 indicates severe malnutrition and immunodeficiency.[229] Chronic illnesses such as congestive heart failure[230] and Alzheimer's disease[231,232] may be associated with progressive cachexia despite adequate food intake, and may be mediated via tumor necrosis factor or other inflammatory mediators. In patients with dementia, despite adequate nutritional intake, malnutrition affected 50 percent of patients and was associated with a four-fold increase in infections.[232]

Since elderly people are frequently at iatrogenic risk of polypharmacy, drug-induced acquired immunodeficiency is probably far more common than is generally clinically recognized. Numerous commonly used drugs cause neutropenia and lymphocytopenia.[233,234] Analgesics, nonsteroidal anti-inflammatory agents, steroids, antithyroids, antibiotics, antipsychotics, antidepressants, hypnotics/sedatives, anticonvulsants, antihypertensives, diuretics, (H$_2$) blockers, hypoglycemics, and other medications (such as allopurinol) commonly prescribed in old age may suppress the inflammatory immune responses. T lymphocytes also have calcium channels, and cholinergic, histaminic, and adrenergic receptors—all of which may have effects on immune function.[235] Hypogammaglobulinemia may also be induced by medications.[236] Recent studies have also demonstrated that medications may also be associated with an impaired[237] or enhanced response to vaccination.[238]

HIV infection may be a cause of acquired immunodeficiency in elderly people, and should always be considered part of the differential diagnosis of acquired immunodeficiency in elderly patients with lymphopenia and appropriate risk factors.[239-243] The most common source of AIDS in elderly people was via transfusion before the blood screening methods were changed,[244] and now again is through sexual activity.[245] Dementia is often a common presenting feature of AIDS,[246] and AIDS should be considered part of the differential diagnosis of dementia in aged patients with appropriate risk factors. The possibility that many cases of AIDS may go undetected in elderly people has considerable implications for geriatric-healthcare workers.

Psychosocial isolation, depression, and stress are probable causes of immune dysfunction in old age.[247,248] There is an increased incidence of cancer during periods of psychosocial stress and depression related to bereavement.[249,250] Social isolation and marital discord may impair immune function.[251,252] Chronic stress in the form of caregiving for a demented spouse also reduces influenza vaccine response.[253] Interventions to enhance social contact improve immune function, as measured by a variety of laboratory measures.[254] Immobility may also cause immune dysfunction, and exercise may maintain function in old age in both animals and humans.[255,256] These aspects of psychoneuroimmunology obviously have particular relevance in the interdisciplinary practice of geriatrics, given the high prevalence of psychosocial problems in elderly people.

The tests necessary to perform an immunological evaluation to establish the diagnosis of acquired immunodeficiency in old age are readily available to the clinician.[257] The humoral immune system is readily tested by measuring the serum protein electrophoresis, immunoelectrophoresis, and other methods for quantitation of Ig levels, as well as the measurement of specific antibody titers, such as isoagglutinins. The cellular immune system is tested by blood leukocyte counts, including absolute lymphocyte counts, delayed skin test hypersensitivity employing a panel of at least six antigens, and in-vitro testing such as measurements of suppressor and helper lymphocyte ratios (T4/T8), and the ability of lymphocytes to proliferate in response to mitogens and specific antigens. The latter tests are often performed in a standard clinical immunology laboratory. Other more sophisticated immune tests are also available from the clinical immunology consultant and laboratory.

Specific potentially reversible causes of acquired immunodeficiency, such as malnutrition or medications, should be sought in aged patients with recurrent or unusual infections, particularly those with lymphocytopenia and/or anergy. At a minimum, a medication review and a nutritional assessment should be performed, with monitoring of neutrophil or lymphocyte counts during nutritional supplementation or mediation withdrawal. HIV infections should always be considered in high-risk patients, including the very old, particularly because of the risks for spread of HIV among healthcare workers and family members caring for frail elderly persons.[240,241]

Numerous interventions have been employed in an attempt to enhance immune function in old age. Thymic hormones, other hormones, mediations, and cytokines have been proposed as immunoenhancing agents, but none of these has gained clinical acceptance.[258,259] In animals, calorie restriction without undernutrition clearly prolongs life and is associated with immune competence into late life, but the benefits of calorie restriction in man remain unknown.[260] Zinc and other trace metals may have benefit in some older patients in restoring lymphocyte proliferation in vitro, and in enhancing delayed-type skin hypersensitivity reactions, but their effects in preventing or reducing the morbidity of infections or other problems potentially related to immunodeficiency in old age have not been demonstrated.[261,262] Vitamin C and other antioxidants may have beneficial effects on immune function.[259, 264] Megadose dietary supplementation does not significantly improve immune function in the normal aged animal.[265]

Vaccinations are critically important in maintaining the health of elderly people in the face of declining immunity, and are effective in preventing pneumococcal pneumonia, influenza and tetanus and reduce mortality from these illnesses.[256,266–268] Although elderly people achieve lower peak titers and more rapid declines of serum antibody levels, the majority of healthy elderly people achieve titers that are generally presumed protective.[87,90] However, chronically ill, frail elderly people—particularly institutionalized, malnourished individuals—may not achieve adequate protective peak antibody titers against pneumococcal pneumonia or influenza when immunized with a single dose of vaccine, and supplemental doses are recommended by some experts.[269–272] Older persons may require revaccination with tetanus toxoid more frequently than every 10 years (as currently recommended) to maintain protective levels of antibodies in the serum.[84] The use of new protein conjugate[273] and immunoconjugate[274] vaccines may improve the response in older people.

CONCLUSIONS

The immune system changes with apparently normal aging in ways that affect clinical presentation. These changes contribute to morbidity and mortality primarily by increasing susceptibility to infection, but also through other mechanisms. Reversible causes of acquired immunodeficiency in old age result in morbidity and mortality, particularly in high risk, chronically ill elderly people and need to be considered when developing a treatment plan. Maintenance of adequate nutrition, the prevention of polypharmacy, the reduction of psychosocial stress, and other preventive measures such as the effective use of vaccines may minimize the morbid effects of immune dysfunction in old age. Newer therapeutic approaches may ultimately be useful in the treatment of acquired immunodeficiency in elderly people, particularly in high-risk individuals who are substantially impaired by the effects of aging and diseases of old age on the immune system.

KEY POINTS Clinical immunology of aging

- The immune system changes with age, primarily affecting T-cell function.
- Changes in the immune system are relevant to the changing clinical presentation and expression of disease.
- Immune senescence affects vaccine effectiveness.

REFERENCES

1. Silverstein AM: History of immunology. In Paul WE (ed): Fundamental Immunology. Raven Press, New York, 1984:23
2. Walford RL: The Immunologic Theory of Aging. Williams and Wilkins, Baltimore, 1969
3. Fillit H: Reversible acquired immunodeficiency in the elderly: a review. Age 1991;14:83–89

4. Lehrer RI, Ganz T, Selsted ME et al: Neutrophils and host defense. Ann Intern Med 1988;109:127–142

5. Esposito AL, Poirer WJ, Clark CA: In vitro assessment of chemotaxis by peripheral blood neutrophils from adult and senescent C57BL/6 mice: correlation with in vivo responses to pulmonary infection with Type 3 Streptococcus pneumoniae. Gerontology 1990;36:2–11

6. Mancuso P, McNish RW, Peters-Golden M, Brock TG: Evaluation of phagocytosis and arachidonate metabolism by alveolar macrophages and recruited neutrophils from F344×BN rats of different ages. Mech Aging Dev 2001;1899–1913

7. Niwa Y, Kasama T, Miyachi Y et al: Neutrophil chemotaxis, phagocytosis and parameters of reactive oxygen species in human aging: cross-sectional and longitudinal studies. Life Sci 1989;44:1655–1664

8. Branchet MC, Boisnic S, Frances C et al: Skin thickness changes in normal aging skin. Gerontology 1990;36:28–35

9. Lord JM, Butcher S, Killampali V, Lascelles D, Salmon M: Neutrophil aging and immunesenescence. Mech Aging Dev 2001;122:1521–1535

10. MacGregor RR, Shalit M: Neutrophil function in healthy elderly subjects. J Gerontol 1990;45:M55–M60

11. Orme IM, Miller ES, Roberts AD et al: T lymphocytes mediating protection and cellular cytolysis during the course of Mycobacterium tuberculosis infection. J Immunol 1992;148:189–196

12. Murray HW: Interferon-gamma, the activated macrophage, and host defense against microbial challenge. Ann Intern Med 1988;108:595–608

13. Orme IM: Senescence of cellular immunity to tuberculosis infection in the mouse: some radical departures from previous thinking. In Powers DC, Morley JE, Coe RM (eds): Aging, Immunity and Infection. Springer Publishing, New York, 1994:27–40

14. Schimizu Y, Newman W, Tanaka Y, Shaw S: Lymphocyte interactions with endothelial cells. Immunology Today 1992;13:106–112

15. Ershler WB, Coe CL, Gravenstein S et al: Aging and immunity in nonhuman primates: I. Effects of age and gender on cellular immune function in rhesus monkeys (Macacca mulatta). Am J Primatol 1988;15:181–188

16. Proust JJ, Bender BS, Nagel JE et al: Developmental biology and senescence. Natural Immun 1989;392–439

17. Goidl EA: Aging and the Immune Response. Marcel Dekker, New York, 1987:1–364

18. Doria G, Adorini L, Sabbadini E et al: Immunoregulation in aging. Ann NY Acad Sci 1988;521:182–188

19. Miller RA: Aging and the immune response. In Schneider EL, Rowe JW (eds): Handbook of the Biology of Aging. Academic Press, San Diego, 1990:157–180

20. Boyd E: The weight of the thymus gland in health and disease. Am J Dis Child 1932;43:1162–1214

21. Lewis VM, Twomey JJ, Bealmear P et al: Age, thymic involution and circulating thymic hormone activity. J Clin Endocrinol Metab 1978;47:145–150

22. Weksler ME, Innes JB, Goldstein G: Immunological studies of aging. IV. The contribution of thymic involution to the immune deficiencies of aging mice and reversal with thymopoietin. J Exp Med 1978;148:996–1006

23. Gravenstein S, Duthie EH, Miller BA et al: Augmentation of influenza antibody response in elderly men by thymosin alpha one: a double-blind placebo-controlled study. J Am Geriatr Soc 1989;37:1–8

24. Barcellini W, Borghi MO, Sguotti C et al: Heterogeneity of immune responsiveness in healthy elderly subjects. Clin Immunol Immunopath 1988;47:142–151

25. Thompson JS, Wekstein DR, Rhoades JL et al: The immune status of healthy centenarians. J Am Geriatr Soc 1984;32:274–281

26. Nagel JE, Chrest FJ, Adler WH: Enumeration of T lymphocyte subsets by monoclonal antibodies in young and aged humans. J Immunol 1981;127:2086–2088

27. Schwab R, Staiano-Coico L, Weksler ME: Immunological studies of aging. IX. Quantitative differences in T lymphocyte subsets in young and old individuals. Diagn Immunol 1983;1:185–201

28. Weksler ME, Hutteroth TH: Impaired lymphocyte function in aged humans. J Clin Invest 1974;53:99

29. Gupta S, Good RA: Subpopulations of human T lymphocytes. X Alterations in T, B, third population cells, and T cells with receptors for immunoglobulin M or G in aging humans. J Immunol 1979;122:1214–1219

30. Murasko DM, Nelson BJ, Silver R et al: Immunologic response in an elderly population with a mean age of 85. Am J Med 1986;81:612–618

31. Bender BS, Nagel JE, Adler WH, Andres R: Absolute peripheral blood lymphocyte count and subsequent mortality of elderly men. J Am Geriatr Soc 1986;34:649–654

32. Proust J, Rosenzweig P, Debouzy C, Moulias R: Lymphopenia induced by acute bacterial infections in the elderly: a sign of age-related immune dysfunction of major prognostic significance. Gerontology 1985;31:178–185

33. Hallgren HM, Kersey JH, Dubey DP, Yunis EJ: Lymphocyte subsets and integrated immune function in aging humans. Cell Immunol 1978;10:65–78

34. Hallgren HM, Bergh N, Rodysill KJ, O'Leary JJ: Lymphocyte proliferative response to PHA and anti-CD3/Ti monoclonal antibodies, T cell surface marker expression, and serum IL-2 receptor levels as biomarkers of age and health. Mech Ageing Dev 1988;43:175–185

35. De Paoli P, Battistin S, Santini GF: Age-related changes in human lymphocyte subsets: progressive reduction of the CD4 CD45R (suppressor inducer) population. Cell Immunol 1988;48:290–296

36. Nagel JE, Chopra RK, Chrest FJ et al: Decreased proliferation, interleukin-2 synthesis, and interleukin-2 receptor expression are accompanied by decreased mRNA expression in phytohemagglutinin-cells from elderly donors. J Clin Invest 1988;81:1096–1102

37. Fauci AS, Masur H, Gelmann EP et al: The acquired immunodeficiency syndrome: an update. Ann Intern Med 1985;102:800–823

38. Okumura M, Fujii Y, Takeuchi Y et al: Age-related accumulation of LFA-1[high] cells in a CD8+CD45RA[high] T cell population. Eur J Immunol 1993;23:1057–1063

39. Cossarizza A, Ortolani C, Paganelli R et al: CD45 isoforms expression on CD4+ and CD8+ T cells throughout life, from newborns to centenarians: implications for T cell memory. Mech Ageing Dev 1996;86:173–195

40. Utsuyama M, Hirokawa K, Kurashima C et al: Differential age-change in the numbers of CD4+CD45RA+ and CD4+CD29+ T cell subsets in human peripheral blood. Mech Ageing Dev 1992;63:57–68

41. Miller RA: Short analytical review: accumulation of hyporesponsive, calcium extruding memory T cells as a key feature of age-dependent immune dysfunction. Clin Immunol Immunopathol 1991;58:305–317

42. Xu X, Beckman I, Ahern M, Bradley J: A comprehensive analysis of peripheral blood lymphocytes in healthy aged humans by flow cytometry. Immunol Cell Biol 1993;71:549–557

43. Schwab R, Hausman PB, Rinnooy-Kan E, Weksler ME: Immunological studies of aging. X. Impaired T lymphocytes and normal monocyte response from elderly humans to the mitogenic antibodies OKT3 and Leu 4. Immunology 1985;55:677–684

44. Roberts-Thompson IC, Whittingham S, Youngchaiyud U, Mackay IR: Ageing, immune response, and mortality. Lancet 1974;ii:368–370

45. Burke BL, Steele RW, Beard OW et al: Immune response to varicella-zoster in the aged. Arch Intern Med 1982;142:291–293

46. Miller AE: Selective decline in cellular immune response to varicella-zoster in the elderly. Neurology 1980;30:582–587

47. Antel J, Oger JJF, Dropcho E et al: Reduced T lymphocyte cell reactivity as a function of human aging. Cell Immunol 1980;54:184–192

48. Hefton JM, Darlington GJ, Casazza BA, Weksler ME: Immunologic studies of aging. V. Impaired proliferation of PHA-responsive human lymphocytes in culture. J Immunol 1980;125:1007–1010

49. Swain SL, Bradley LM, Croft M et al: Helper T-cell subsets: phenotype, function and the role of lymphokines in regulating their development. Immunol Rev 1991;123:115–144

50. Rivnay B, Bergman S, Shinitzky M, Globerson A: Correlations between membrane viscosity, serum cholesterol, lymphocyte activation and aging in man. Mech Ageing Dev 1980;125:1007–1010

51. Kennes B, Hubert C, Brohee D, Neve P: Early biochemical events associated with lymphocyte activation in aging. I. Evidence that Ca^{2+}-dependent processes induced by PHA are impaired. Immunology 1981;42:119–126

52. Gutkowski JK, Innes J, Weksler ME, Cohen S: Induction of DNA synthesis in isolated nuclei by cytoplasmic factors. II. Normal generation of cytoplasmic stimulatory factors by lymphocytes from aged human with depressed proliferative responses: J Immunol 1984;132:559–562

53. Staiano-Coico L, Darsynkiewicz Z, Melamed MR, Weksler ME: Immunological studies of aging. IX. Impaired proliferation of T lymphocytes detected in elderly humans by flow cytometry. J Immunol 1984;132:1788–1792

54. Gillis S, Kozak R, Durante M, Weksler ME: Immunological studies of aging. Decreased production of and response to T cell growth factor by lymphocytes from aged humans. J Clin Invest 1981;67:937–942

55. Rabinowich H, Gosis Y, Reshef T, Klajman A: Interleukin-2 production and activity in aged humans. Mech Ageing Dev 1985;32:213–226

56. Orson FM, Saadeh CK, Lewis DE, Nelson DL: Interleukin-2 receptor expression by T cells in human aging. Cell Immunol 1989;124:278–291

57. McElhaney JE, Beattie BL, Devine R et al: Age-related decline in interleukin-2 production in response to influenza vaccine. J Am Geriatr Soc 1990;38:652–658

58. McElhaney JE, Meneilly GS, Beattie BL et al: The effect of influenza vaccination on IL2 production in healthy elderly: implications for current vaccination procedures. J Gerontol 1992;47:M3–M8

59. Powers DC: Influenza A virus-specific cytotoxic T lymphocyte activity declines with advancing age. J Am Geriatr Soc 1993;41:1–5

60. Goodwin JS: Changes in lymphocyte sensitivity to prostaglandin E, histamine, hydrocortisone and x-irradation with age: studies in a healthy elderly population. Clin Immunol Immunopath 1982;25:243–251

61. Goodwin JS, Messner RP: Sensitivity of lymphocytes to prostaglandin E2 increases in subjects over age 70. J Clin Invest 1979;64:434–439

62. Mooradian AD, Reed RL, Osterweil D, Scuderi P: Detectable serum levels of tumor necrosis factor alpha may predict early mortality in elderly institutionalized patients. J Am Geriatr Soc 1991;39:891–894

63. Mooradian AD, Reed RL, Scuderi P: Serum levels of tumor necrosis factor alpha, interleukin-1 alpha and beta in healthy elderly subjects. Age 1991;14:61–64

64. Huberman M, Sredni B, Stern L et al: IL-2 and IL-6 secretion in dementia: correlation with type and severity of disease. J Neurol Sci 1995;130:161–164

65. Hüll M, Berger M, Volk B, Bauer J: Occurrence of interleukin-6 in cortical plaques of Alzheimer's disease patients may precede transformation of diffuse into neuritic plaques. Ann NY Acad Sci 1996;777:205–212

66. Manolagas SC, Bellido T, Jilka RL: New insights into cellular, biochemical, and molecular basis of postmenopausal and senile osteoporosis: roles of IL-6 and gp 130. Int J Immunopharmacol 1995;17:109–116

67. Ershler WB, Sun WH, Binkley N: The role of interleukin-6 in certain age-related diseases. Drugs Aging 1994;5:358–365

68. Zweiman B, Levinson AI: Cell-mediated immunity. In Middleton E, Reed CE, Ellis EF (eds): Allergy: Principles and Practice. Mosby, St. Louis, 1983:75

69. Dorken E, Grzybowski S, Allen EA: Significance of the tuberculin test in the elderly. Chest 1987;92:237–240

70. Marrie TJ, Johnson S, Durant H: Cell-mediated immunity of healthy adult Nova Scotians in various age groups compared with nursing home and hospitalized senior citizens. J Allergy Clin Immunol 1988;81:836–844

71. Castle S, Peris T, Chang M et al: Correlation of delayed type hypersensitivity (DTH) with in vitro test of cell-mediated immunity in elderly nursing home patients. Gerontology 1989;29:195A

72. Murasko DM, Wener P, Kaye D: Association of lack of mitogen-induced lymphocyte proliferation with increased mortality in the elderly. Aging: Immunol Infect Dis 1988;1:1–6

73. Cohn JR, Hohl CA, Buckley CE: The relationship between cutaneous cellular immune responsiveness and mortality in a nursing home population. J Am Geriatr Soc 1983;32:808–809

74. Stead WW, To T: The significance of the tuberculin skin test in elderly persons. Ann Intern Med 1987;107:837–842

75. Wayne SJ, Rhyne RL, Garry PJ, Goodwin JS: Cell-mediated immunity as a predictor of morbidity and mortality in subjects over 60. J Gerontol A 1990;45:M45–M48

76. Creditor MC, Smith EC, Gallai JB, Baumann M, Nelson KE: Tuberculosis, tuberculin reactivity, and delayed cutaneous hypersensitivity in nursing home residents. J Gerontol A 1988;43:M97–M100

77. Barry MA, Regan AM, Kunches LM et al: Two-stage tuberculin testing with control antigens in patients residing in two chronic disease hospitals. J Am Geriatr Soc 1987;35:147–153

78. van den Brande P, Demedts M: Four-stage tuberculin testing in elderly subjects induces age-dependent progressive boosting. Chest 1992;101:447–450

79. Nagel JE, Adler WH: Immunology. In Kent B, Butler RN (eds): Human Aging Research: Concepts and Techniques. Lippincott-Raven, Philadelphia, 1988:299–309

80. Buckley CEI, Buckley EG, Dorsey FC: Longitudinal changes in serum immunoglobulin levels in older humans. Fed Proc 1974;33:2036–2039

81. Phair JP, Kauffman CA, Bjornson A et al: Host defenses in the aged: evaluation of components of the inflammatory and immune responses. J Infect Dis 1978;138:67–73

82. Makinodan T, Adler W: The effects of aging on the differentiation and proliferation potentials of cells of the immune system. Fed Proc 1975;34:153–158

83. Antel JP, Oger JJF, Wrabetz LG et al: Mechanisms responsible for reduced in vitro immunoglobulin secretion in aged humans. Mech Ageing Dev 1983;23:11–19

84. Kishimoto S, Tomino S, Mitsuya H et al: Age-related decline in the in vitro and in vivo synthesis of anti-tetanus toxoid antibody in humans. J Immunol 1980;125:2347–2352

85. Antonaci S, Jirillo E, Lucivero G et al: Humoral immune response in aged humans: suppressor effect of monocytes on spontaneous plaque forming cell generation. Clin Exp Immunol 1983;52:387–392

86. Pahwa SG, Pahwa RN, Good RA: Decreased in vitro humoral immune responses in aged humans. J Clin Invest 1981;67:1094–1102

87. Kjeldsen K, Simonsen O, Heron I: Immunity against diphtheria and tetanus in the age group 30–70 years. Scand J Infect Dis 1988;20:177–185

88. Waldorf DS, Wilkens RF, Decker JL: Impaired delayed hypersensitivity in an aging population: association with antinuclear reactivity and rheumatoid factor. JAMA 1968;203:111–114

89. Shapiro ED, Berg AT, Austrian R et al: The protective effect of polyvalent pneumococcal polysaccharide vaccine. N Engl J Med 1991;325:1453–1460

90. Huang Y, Gauthey L, Martine M et al: The relationship between influenza vaccine-induced specific antibody responses and vaccine-induced nonspecific autoantibody responses in healthy older women. J Gerontol A 1992;47:M50–M55

91. Levine M, Beattie BL, McLean DM, Corman D: Characterization of the immune response to trivalent influenza vaccine in elderly men. J Am Geriatr Soc 1987;35:609–657

92. Hooper B, Whittingham S, Mathews JD et al: Autoimmunity in a rural community. Clin Exp Immunol 1972;12:79–87

93. Rosenthal M: Age and immunity: III. Circulating immune complexes in different age groups. Blut 1978;37:271–274

94. Hijmans W, Radl J, Bottazzo GF, Donlach D: Autoantibodies in highly aged humans. Mech Ageing Dev 1984;26:83–89

95. Pandey JP, Fudenberg JJ, Ainsworth SK, Loadholt CB: Autoantibodies in healthy subjects of different age groups. Mech Ageing Dev 1979;10:399–404

96. Goodwin JS, Searles RP, Tung KSK: Immunological responses of a healthy elderly population. Clin Exp Immunol 1982;48:403–410

97. Hallgren HM, Buckley CE, Gilberstein VA, Yunis EJ: Lymphocyte phytohemagglutinin responsiveness, immunoglobulins, and autoantibodies in aging humans. J Immunol 1973;111:1101–1105

98. Manousskakis MN, Tziosfas AG, Sills MP et al: High prevalence of anti-cardiolipin and other autoantibodies in a healthy elderly population. Clin Exp Immunol 1987;69:557–565

99. Siskind GW, Weksler ME: The effect of aging on the immune response. Ann Rev Geriatr Geront 1982;3:3–26

100. Delespesse G, Gausset PH, Sarfati M et al: Circulating immune complexes in old people and in diabetics: correlation with autoantibodies. Clin Exp Immunol 1980;40:96–101

101. Hollingsworth JW, Otte RG: B lymphocyte maturation in cultures from blood of elderly men: a comparison of plaque-forming cells, cells containing intracytoplasmic immunoglobulin and cell proliferation. Mech Ageing Dev 1981;15:9–18

102. Ceuppens JL, Goodwin JS: Regulation of immunoglobulin production in pokeweed mitogen-stimulated cultures of lymphocytes from young and old adults. J Immunol 1982;128:2429–2434

103. Rodriquez MA, Ceuppens JL, Goodwin JS: Regulation of IgM rheumatoid factor production in lymphocyte cultures from young and old subjects. J Immunol 1982;128:2422–2428

104. Whisler RL, Williams JW Jr., Newhouse YG: Human B cell proliferative responses during aging. Reduced RNA synthesis and DNA replication after signal transduction by surface immunoglobulins compared to B cell antigenic determinants CD20 and CD40. Mech Ageing Dev 1991;61:209–222

105. Kipps TJ: The CD5+ B cell. Adv Immunol 1989;47:117–186

106. Delfraissy JF, Galanaud P, Dormont J, Wallon C: Age related impairment of the in vitro antibody response in the human. Clin Exp Immunol 1980;39:208–214

107. Ershler WB, Keller ET: Age-associated increased IL-6 gene expression, late-life diseases and frailty. Ann Rev Med 2000;51:245–270

108. Cohen HJ, Pieper CF, Harris T, Rao KM, Currie MS: The association of plasma IL-6 levels with functional disability in community-dwelling elderly. J Gerontol A 1997;52:M201–M208

109. Cohen HJ, Piper CS, Harris T: Markers of inflammation and coagulation predict decline in function and mortality in community dwelling elderly. J Am Geriatr Soc 2001;S1:A3
110. Kay MMB: Immunological aspects of aging. In Makinodan T (ed): Aging, Immunity and Arthritic Disease. Raven Press, New York, 1980:33–78
111. Cohen IR: Autoimmunity: physiologic and pernicious. Adv Intern Med 1984;29:147–165
112. MacLennan WJ, Andrews GR, Macleod C, Caird FI: Anemia in the elderly. Quart J Med 1973;42:1–13
113. Blumenthal HT, Perlstein IB: The aging thyroid. II. An immuncytochemical analysis of the age-associated lesions. J Am Geriatr Soc 1987;35:855–863
114. Blumenthal HT, Perlstein IB: The aging thyroid. I. A description of lesions and an analysis of their age and sex distribution. J Am Geriatr Soc 1987;35:843–854
115. Tunbridge WMG, Evered DC, Hall R et al: The spectrum of thyroid disease in a community: the Whickham survey. Clin Endocrinol 1977;7:481–493
116. Rook AJ, Waddington E: Pemphigous and pemphigoid. Br J Dermatol 1953;65:425–431
117. Pope RM, Talal N: Autoimmunity in rheumatoid arthritis. Concepts Immunopathol 1985;1:219–250
118. Trentham DE, Dynesius RA, Rocklin RE, David JR: Cellular sensitivity to collagen in rheumatoid arthritis. N Engl J Med 1978;299:327–332
119. Machado EBV, Gabriel SE, Beard CM et al: A population-based case-control study of temporal arteritis: evidence for an association between temporal arteritis and degenerative vascular disease? Int J Epidemiol 1989;18:836–841
120. Mathews JD, Whittingham S, Mackay IR: Autoimmune mechanisms in human vascular disease. Lancet 1974;ii:1423–1427
121. Boesen P, Sorensen SF: Giant cell arteritis, temporal arteritis, and polymyalgia rheumatica in a Danish county. Arth Rheum 1987;30:294–299
122. Minick CR, Alonso DR, Rankin L: Role of immunologic arterial injury in atherogenesis. Thromb Haemostas 1978;39:304–311
123. Beaumont JL: Immunologic factors in atherosclerosis. In Blumenthal HT (ed): Handbook of Diseases of Aging. Van Nostrand, New York, 1982:317–325
124. Fillit HM, Kemeny E, Luine V et al: Antivascular antibodies in the sera of patients with senile dementia—Alzheimer's type. J Gerontol 1987;42:180–184
125. Faaber P, Rijke TPM, van de Putte LBA et al: Cross-reactivity of human and murine anti-DNA antibodies with heparan sulfate. The major glycosoaminoglycan in glomerular basement membrane. J Clin Invest 1986;77:1824–1830
126. Fillit HM, Mulvihill M: Association of autoimmunity to vascular heparan sulfate proteoglycan and vascular disease in the aged. Gerontology 1993;39:177–182
127. Cines DB: Disorders associated with antibodies to endothelial cells. Rev Infect Dis 1989;11:s705–711
128. Briley DP, Coull BM, Goodnight SH: Neurological disease associated with antiphospholipid antibodies. Ann Neurol 1989;25:221–227
129. Asherson RA, Mercey D, Phillips G et al: Recurrent stroke and multi-infarct dementia in systemic lupus erythematous: association with antiphospholipid antibodies. Ann Rheum Dis 1987;46:605–611
130. McHugh NJ, James ID, Plant GT: Anticardiolipin and antineutrophil antibodies in giant cell arteritis. J Rheumatol 1990;17:916–922
131. Klemp P, Cooper RC, Strauss FJ et al: Anticardiolipin antibodies in ischemic heart disease. Clin Exp Immunol 1988;74:254–257
132. Lockshin MD: Antiphospholipid antibody and antiphospholipid syndrome. Curr Opin Rthem 1991;3:797–802
133. Mannoussakis MN, Tziousfas AG, Silis MP et al: High prevalence of anti-cardiolipin and other autoantibodies in a healthy elderly population. Clin Exp Immunol 1987;69:557–565
134. Ruffati A, Rossi L, Callgaro A et al: Autoantibodies of systemic rheumatic diseases in the elderly. Gerontol 1990;36:104–111
135. Alving CR: Antibodies to liposomes, phospholipids, and cholesterol: implications for autoimmunity, atherosclerosis, and aging. Prog Clin Biol Res 1990;343:41–51
136. Wight TN: Cell biology of arterial proteoglycans. Arteriosclerosis 1989;9:1–20
137. Newell GR, Boutwell WB, Morris DL: Epidemiology of cancer. In De Vita VTJ, Hellman S, Rosenberg SA (eds): Cancer: Principles and Practice of Oncology. Lippincott, Philadelphia, 1982:3–32
138. Ershler WB: Guest Editorial: Why tumors grow more slowly in old people. J Natl Cancer Inst 1986;77:837–839
139. Cantor KP, Fraumeni JF Jr: Distribution of nonHodgkin's lymphoma in the United States between 1950 and 1975. Cancer Res 1980;40:2645–2652
140. Radl J, Sepers JM, Skvaril F et al: Immunoglobulin patterns in humans over 95 years of age. Clin Exp Immunol 1975;22:84–90
141. Radl J, Hollander CF, van den Berg P, de Glopper E: Idiopathic paraproteinaemia. I. Studies in an animal model—the ageing C57BL/KaLwRij mouse. Clin Exp Immunol 1978;33:395–402
142. Radl J: Idiopathic paraproteinemia—a consequence of an age-related deficiency in the T immune system. Three-stage development—a hypothesis. Clin Immunol Immunopathol 1979;14:251–255
143. Radl J, De Glopper ED, Schuit HR, Zurcher C: Idiopathic paraproteinemia. II. Transplantation of the paraprotein-producing clone from old to young C57BL/KaLwRij mice. J Immunol 1979;122:609–613
144. Ligthart GJ, Radl J, Corberand JX et al: Monoclonal gammopathies in human aging: increased occurrence with age and correlation with health status. Mech Ageing Dev 1990;52:235–243
145. Radl J, Weis J, Hoogeveen CM: Immunoblotting with (sub) class-specific antibodies reveals a high frequency of monoclonal gammopathies in persons thought to be immunodeficient. Clin Chem 1988;34:1839–1842
146. Kyle RA, Robinson RA, Katzmann JA: Clinical aspects of biclonal gammopathies. Am J Med 1981;71:999–1008
147. Buxbaum JN, Chuba JV, Hellman GC et al: Monoclonal immunoglobulin deposition disease: light chain and light and heavy chain deposition diseases and their relation to light chain amyloidosis. Ann Intern Med 1990;112:455–464
148. Fine JM, Lambin P, Muller JY: The evolution of asymptomatic monoclonal gammopathies. Acta Med Scand 1979;205:339–341
149. Crawford J, Eye MK, Cohen HJ: Evaluation of monoclonal gammopathies in the "well" elderly. Am J Med 1987;82:39–45
150. Kyle RA: Benign monoclonal gammopathy—after 20 to 35 years of follow-up. Mayo Clin Proc 1993;68:26–36
151. Cohen HJ: Multiple myeloma in the elderly. Clin Geriatr Med 1985;827–855
152. Stahl RL, Silber R: Chronic lymphocytic leukemia. Clin Geriatr Med 1985;1:857–867
153. Antin JH, Rosenthal DS: Acute leukemias, myelodysplasia and lymphomas. Clin Geriatr Med 1985;1:795–826
154. Dorn HF, Cutler SJ: Morbidity from cancer in the United States. Public Health Monographs 1956;56
155. Ershler WB: The influence of an aging immune system on cancer incidence and progression. J Gerontol A 1993;48:B3–B7
156. Miller RA: Aging and cancer: another perspective. J Gerontol A 1993;48:B8–B10
157. Covelli V, Mouton D, Mojo V et al: Inheritance of immune responsiveness, life span and disease incidence in interline crosses of mice selected for high or low multispecific antibody production. J Immunol 1989;142:1224–1234
158. Smith PW, Roccaforte JS, Caly PB: Infection and immune response in the elderly. Ann Epidemiol 1992;2:813–822
159. Berman P, Hogan DB, Fox RA: The atypical presentation of infection in old age. Age Ageing 1987;16:201–207
160. Kohn P: Cause of death in very old people. JAMA 1982;247:2793–2797
161. Castle SC: Clinical relevance of age-related immune dysfunction. Clin Infect Dis 2000;31(2):578–585
162. Castle SC, Norman DC, Yeh M et al: Fever response in elderly nursing home residents: are the older truly colder? J Am Geriatr Soc 1991;39:853–857
163. Glezen WP: Serious morbidity and mortality associated with influenza epidemics. Epidemiol Rev 1982;4:25–44
164. Barker WH, Mullooly JP: Impact of epidemic type A influenza in a defined adult population. Am J Epidemiol 1980;112:798–813
165. Clements ML, Betts RF, Tierney EL et al: Serum and nasal wash antibodies associated with resistance to experimental challenge with influenza A wild-type virus. J Clin Microbiol 1986;24:157–160
166. McMichael AJ, Gotch FM, Noble GR et al: Cytotoxic T-cell immunity to influenza. N Engl J Med 1983;309:13–17
167. Taylor PM, Askonas BA: Influenza nucleoprotein specific cytotoxic T cell clones are protective in vivo. Immunol 1986;58:417–420
168. Yap KL, Ada GL, McKenzie IFC: Transfer of specific cytotoxic T lymphocytes protects mice inoculated with influenza virus. Nature 1978;273:238–239
169. Davenport FM, Hennessey AV, Francis T Jr: Epidemiological and immunological significance of age distribution of antibody to antigenic variants of influenza virus. J Exp Med 1953;98:641–656

170. Noble GR, Kaye HS, Kendal AP et al: Age-related heterologous antibody responses to influenza virus vaccination. J Infect Dis 1977;136:S686–692

171. Beyer WEP, Palache AM, Bljet M et al: Antibody induction by influenza vaccines in the elderly: a review of the literature. Vaccine 1989;7:385–394

172. Powers DC, Belshe RB: Effect of age on memory cytotoxic T lymphocyte responses to inactivated influenza virus vaccine. J Infect Dis 1993;167:584–592

173. Schwab R, Russo C, Weksler ME: Loss of MHC-restricted T cell recognition of influenza antigens in aging. Aging Immunol Infect Dis 1990;2:111–116

174. Nichol KL, Margolis KL, Wuorenma J, Von Sternberg T: The efficacy and cost effectiveness of vaccination against influenza among elderly persons living in the community. N Engl J Med 1994;331:778–784

175. Patriarca PA, Arden NH, Koplan JP, Goodman RA: Prevention and control of type A influenza in nursing homes: benefits and costs with four approaches using vaccination and amantadine. Ann Intern Med 1987;107:732–740

175a. Gravenstein S, McElhaney JE, Vij S et al: The effect of zanamivir treatment and vaccination on naturally acquired influenza with advancing age in outpatients. Presented at the GSA, Chicago, IL, 11/30/00. (Unpublished.)

176. Breiman RF, Spika JS, Navarro VJ, Darden PM, Darby CP: Pneumococcal bacteremia in Charleston County, South Carolina. A decade later. Arch Intern Med 1990;150:1401–1405

177. Breiman RF, Butler JC, Tenover FC, Elliott JA, Facklam RR: Emergence of drug-resistant pneumococcal infections in the United States. JAMA 1994;271:1831–1835

178. Simberkoff MS, Cross AP, Al-Ibrahim M et al: Efficacy of pneumococcal vaccine in high-risk patients: results of a Veterans Administration Cooperative Study. N Engl J Med 1986;315:1318–1327

179. Sims RV, Steinmann WC, McConville JH et al: The clinical effectiveness of pneumococcal vaccine in the elderly. Ann Intern Med 1988;108:653–657

180. Gable CB, Holzer SS, Engelhart L et al: Pneumococcal vaccine; efficacy and associated cost savings. JAMA 1990;264:2910–2915

181. Quick RE, Hoge CW, Hamilton DJ et al: Underutilization of pneumococcal vaccine in nursing home in Washington State: report of a serotype-specific outbreak and a survey. Am J Med 1993;94:149–152

182. Centers for Disease Control and Prevention. Outbreaks of pneumococcal pneumonia among unvaccinated residents in chronic-care facilities—Massachusetts, October 1995, Oklahoma, February 1996, and Maryland, May–June 1996. MMWR 1997;46:60–62

183. Nuorti JP, Butler JC, Crutcher JM et al: An outbreak of multidrug-resistant pneumococcal pneumonia and bacteremia among unvaccinated nursing home residents. N Engl J Med 1998;338:1861–1868

184. Buchanan RM, Briles DE, Arulanandam BP et al: IL-12-mediated increases in protection elicited by pneumococcal and meningococcal conjugate vaccines. Vaccine 2001;19:2020–2028

185. Nabors GS, Braun PA, Herrmann DJ et al: Immunization of healthy adults with a single recombinant pneumococcal surface protein A (PspA) variant stimulates broadly cross-reactive antibodies to heterologous PspA molecules. Vaccine 2000;18(17):1743–1754

186. de Moragas JM, Kierland RR: The outcome of patients with herpes zoster. Am Arch Dermatol 1957;75:193–196

187. Burgoon CF Jr, Burgoon JS, Baldridge GD: The natural history of herpes zoster. JAMA 1957;164:265–270

188. McGregor RM: Herpes zoster, chicken-pox, and cancer in general practice. Br Med J 1957;i:84–87

189. Hope-Simonson RE: The nature of herpes zoster: a long-term study and new hypothesis. Proc R Soc Med 1965;58:9

190. Molin L: Aspects of the natural history of herpes zoster. Acta Derm Venereol 1969;49:569–583

191. Rogers RS III, Tindall JP: Geriatric herpes zoster. J Am Geriatr Soc 1971;19:495–504

192. Ragozzino MW, Melton LJ III, Kurland LT et al: Population-based study of herpes zoster and its sequelae. Medicine 1982;61:310–316

193. Weksler ME: Immune senescence. Ann Neurol 1994;35(suppl):S35–7

194. Hope-Simpson RE: Postherpetic neuralgia. J Roy Coll Gen Pract 1975;25:571

195. Huff JC, Bean B, Balfour HH et al: Therapy of herpes zoster with oral acyclovir. Am J Med 1988;85:84–89

196. Wood MJ, Ogan PH, McKendrick MW et al: Efficacy of oral acyclovir treatment of acute herpes zoster. Am J Med 1988;85:79–83

197. Harding SP, Lipton JR, Wells JCD: Natural history of herpes zoster ophthalmicus: predictors of postherpetic neuralgia and ocular involvement. Br J Ophthalmol 1987;71:353–358

198. Loeser JD: Herpes zoster and postherpetic neuralgia. Pain 1986;25:149–164

199. Watson CPN: Postherpetic neuralgia. Neurol Clin 1989;7:231–248

200. Moffat MM, Ritchie L, Collacott I, Brown T: Is Bell's palsy a reactivation of varicella zoster virus? J Infect 1995;30:29–36

201. Welling DB, Daniels RL, Brainard J et al: Detection of viral DNA in endolymphatic sac tissue from Meniere's disease patients. Am J Otol 1996;15:639–643

202. Straus SE, Ostrove JE, Inchauspe G et al: Varicella-zoster virus infections; biology, natural history, treatment, and prevention. Ann Intern Med 1988;108:221–237

203. Arvin AM: Cell-mediated immunity to varicella-zoster virus. J Infect Dis 1992;166(suppl 1):S35–41

204. Dolin R, Reichman RC, Mazur MH, Whitley RJ: Herpes zoster-varicella infections in immunosuppressed patients. Ann Intern Med 1978;89:375–388

205. Goffinet DR, Glatstein EJ, Merigan TC: Herpes zoster-varicella infections and lymphoma. Ann Intern Med 1972;76:235–240

206. Guinee VF, Guido JJ, Pfalzgraf KA et al: The incidence of herpes zoster in patients with Hodgkin's disease; an analysis of prognostic factors. Cancer 1985;56:642–648

207. Arvin AM, Pollard AM, Gamberg P et al: Cellular and humoral immunity in the pathogenesis of recurrent herpes viral infections in patients with lymphoma. J Clin Invest 1980;65:869

208. Meyers JD, Flournoy N, Thomas ED: Cell-mediated immunity to varicella-zoster infection after allogenic marrow transplant. J Infect Dis 1980;141:479

209. Schuchter LM, Wingard JR, Piantadosi S et al: Herpes zoster infection after autologous bone marrow transplantation. Blood 1989;74:1424–1427

210. Wilson A, Sharp M, Koropchak CM et al: Subclinical varicella-zoster virus viremia, herpes zoster, and T lymphocyte immunity to varicella-zoster viral antigens after bone marrow transplantation. J Infect Dis 1992;165:119–126

211. Miller AE: Selective decline in cellular immune response to varicella-zoster in the elderly. Neurology 1980;30:582–587

212. Berger R, Florent G, Just M: Decrease of the lymphoproliferative response to varicella-zoster virus antigen in the aged. Infect Immun 1981;32:24–27

213. Burke BL, Steele RW, Beard OW et al: Immune responses to varicella-zoster in the aged. Arch Int Med 1982;142:291–293

214. Hayward AR, Herberger M: Lymphocyte responses to varicella zoster virus in the elderly. J Clin Immunol 1987;7:174–178

215. Hayward A, Levin M, Wolf W et al: Varicella-zoster virus-specific immunity after herpes zoster. J Infect Dis 1991;163:873–875

216. Brunell PA, Novelli VM, Keller PM, Ellis RW: Antibodies to the three major glycoproteins of varicella-zoster virus: search for the relevant host immune response. J Infect Dis 1987;156:430–435

217. Giller RH, Winistorfer S, Grose C: Cellular and humoral immunity to varicella zoster virus glycoproteins in immune and susceptible human subjects. J Infect Dis 1989;160:919–928

218. Levin MJ, Murray M, Rotbart HA et al: Immune response of elderly individuals to a live attenuated varicella vaccine. J Infect Dis 1992;166:253–259

219. Trannoy E, Berger R, Hollander G et al: Vaccination of immunocompetent elderly subjects with a live attenuated Oka strain of varicella zoster virus: a randomized, controlled, dose-response trial. Vaccine 2000;18(16):1700–1706

220. Chandra RK: Nutritional regulation of immunity and the risk of infection in old age. Immunology 1989;67:141–147

221. Lesourd B: Immune response during disease and recovery in the elderly. Proc Nutr Soc 1999;58(1):85–98

222. Chandra RK: The relation between immunology, nutrition and disease in elderly people. Age Ageing 1990;19:s25–s31

223. Epstein AM, Leighton JR, Hoefer M: The relation of body weight to length of stay and charges for hospital services for patients undergoing elective surgery: a study of two procedures. Am J Public Health 1987;77:993–997

224. Agarwahl M, Acevedo F, Leighton LS et al: Predictive ability of various nutritional variables for mortality in elderly people. Am J Clin Nutr 1988;48:1173–1178

225. Weinsier RL, Hunker EM, Krumdieck CL, Butterworth CE: Hospital malnutrition: a prospective evaluation of general medical patients during the course of hospitalization. Am J Clin Nutr 1979;32:418–426

226. Lansey S, Waslien C, Mulvihill M, Fillit H: The role of anthropometry in the assessment of malnutrition in the hospitalized frail elderly. Gerontology 1993;39:346–353

227. Corman LC: The relationship between nutrition, infection and immunity. Med Clin North Am 1985;69:519–531

228. Lesourd BM: Nutrition and immunity in the elderly: modification of immune responses with nutritional treatments. Am J Clin Nutr 1997;66(2):478S–484S

229. Lewis EF, Bell SJ: Nutritional assessment of the elderly. In Morley JE, Glick Z, Rubinstein LZ (eds): Geriatric Nutrition. Raven Press, New York, 1990:73

230. Levine B, Kalman J, Mayer L et al: Elevated circulating levels of tumor necrosis factor in severe chronic heart failure. N Engl J Med 1990;323:236–241

231. Singh S, Mulley GP, Losowsky MS: Why are Alzheimer's patients thin? Age Ageing 1988;17:21–28

232. Sandman P, Adolfsson R, Nygren C et al: Nutritional status and dietary intake in institutionalized patients with Alzheimer's disease and multiinfarct dementia. J Am Geriatr Soc 1987;35:31–38

233. Dale DC: Neutropenia. In Williams WJ, Beutler E, Erslev AJ, Lichtman MA (eds): Hematology. McGraw-Hill, New York, 1989:807–816

234. Williams WJ: Lymphocytopenia. In Williams WJ, Beutler E, Erslev AJ, Lichtman MA (eds): Hematology. McGraw-Hill, New York, 1989:964–966

235. Plaut M: Lymphocyte hormone receptors. Ann Rev Immunol 1987;5:621–669

236. Travin M, Macris NT, Block HM, Schwimmer D: Reversible common variable immunodeficiency syndrome induced by phenytoin. Arch Int Med 1989;149:1421–1422

237. Gross PA, Quinnan GV, Weksler ME et al: Relation of chronic disease and immune response to influenza vaccine in the elderly. Vaccine 1989;7:303–308

238. Ershler WB, Hacker MP, Burroughs BJ et al: Cimetidine and the immune response: I. In vivo augmentation of nonspecific and specific immune response. Clin Immunol Immunopathol 1983;26:10–17

239. Moss RJ, Miles SH: AIDS and the geriatrician. J Am Geriatr Soc 1987;35:460–464

240. Fillit HM, Fruchtman S, Sell L, Rosen N: AIDS in the elderly: a case and its implications. Geriatrics 1989;44:65–70

241. Rosenzweig R, Fillit H: Probable heterosexual transmission of AIDS in an aged woman. J Am Geriatr Soc 1992;40:1261–1264

242. Bestilny LJ, Gill MJ, Mody CH, Riabowol KT: Accelerated replicative senescence of the peripheral immune system induced by HIV infection. AIDS 2000;14(7):771–780

243. Al-Harthi L, Marchetti G, Steffens CM et al: Detection of T cell receptor circles (TRECs) as biomarkers for de novo T cell synthesis using a quantitative polymerase chain reaction-enzyme linked immunosorbent assay (PCR-ELISA). J Immunol Methods 2000;237(1–2):187–197

244. Peterman TA, Jaffe HW, Feorino PM: Transfusion acquired immunodeficiency syndrome in the United States. JAMA 1985;254:2913–2917

245. Woolery WA. Occult HIV infection: diagnosis and treatment of older patients. Geriatrics 1997;52(11):51,55–58,61

246. Weiler PG, Mungas D, Pomerantz S: AIDS as a cause of dementia in the elderly. J Am Geriatr Soc 1988;36:139–141

247. Guidi L, Bartolini C, Frasca D et al: Impairment of lymphocyte activities in depressed aged subjects. Mech Ageing Dev 1991;60:13–24

248. Glaser R, MacCallum RC, Laskowski BF et al: Evidence for a shift in the Th-1 to Th-2 cytokine response associated with chronic stress and aging. J Gerontol A 2001;56(8):M477–M482

249. Bartrop RW, Lazarus L, Lockhurst E et al: Depressed lymphocyte function after bereavement. Lancet 1977;i:834–836

250. Schleifer SJ, Keller SE, Camerino M et al: Suppression of lymphocyte stimulation following bereavement. JAMA 1983;250:374–377

251. Thomas RD, Goodwin JM, Goodwin JS: Effect of social support on stress-related changes in cholesterol level, uric acid level, and immune function in an elderly sample. Am J Psychiatry 1985;142:735–737

252. Kiecolt-Glaser JK, Fisher P, Ogrocki P et al: Marital quality, marital disruption and immune function. Psychosom Med 1987;49:13–34

253. Kiecolt-Glaser JK, Glaser R, Gravenstein S, Malarkey WB, Sheridan J: Chronic stress alters the immune response to influenza virus vaccine in older adults. Proc Natl Acad Sci USA 1996;93:3043–3047

254. Kiecolt-Glaser JK, Glaser R, Willinger D et al: Psychosocial enhancement of immunocompetence in a geriatric population. Health Psychol 1985;4:25–41

255. Pahlavani MA, Cheung TH, Chesky JA, Richardson A: Influence of exercise on the immune function of rats of various ages. J Appl Physiol 1988;64:2997–3001

256. Soppi E, Varijo P, Eskola J: Effect of strenuous physical stress on circulating lymphocyte number and function before and after training. J Clin Lab Immunol 1982;8:43–46

257. Grieco MH, Meriney DK: Immunodiagnosis for Clinicans. Chicago, Year Book, 1983

258. Daynes RA, Araneo BA: Prevention and reversal of some age-associated changes in immunologic responses by supplemental dehydroepiandrosterone sulfate therapy. Aging Immunol Infect Dis 1992;3:135–155

259. Delafuente JC: Immunosenescence: clinical and pharmacologic considerations. Med Clin N Am 1985;69:465–486

260. Masoro EJ: Dietary restriction and aging. J Am Geriatr Soc 1993;41:994–999

261. Gershwin ME, Beach R, Hurley L: Trace metals, aging and immunity. J Am Geriatr Soc 1983;31:374–378

262. Bodey B, Bodey B, Jr, Siegel SE, Kaiser HE: The role of zinc in pre- and postnatal mammalian thymic immunohistogenesis. In Vivo, 1998;12(6):695–722

263. Penn ND, Purkines L, Kelleher J et al: The effect of dietary supplementation with vitamins A, C and E on cell-mediated immune function in elderly long-stay patients: a randomized controlled trial. Age Ageing 1991;20:169–174

264. Buzina-Suboticanec K, Buzina R, Stavljenic A et al: Ageing, nutritional status and immune response. Int J Vitam Nutr Res 1998;68(2):133–141

265. Goodwin JS, Garry PJ: Relationship between megadose vitamin supplementation and immunologic function in a healthy elderly population. Clin Exp Immunol 1983;51:647–653

266. Busby J, Caranasos GJ: Immune function, autoimmunity and selective immunoprophylaxis in the aged. Med Clin N Am 1985;69:465–474

267. Bentley DW: Pneumococcal vaccine in the institutionalized elderly: a review of past and recent studies. Rev Infect Dis 1981;3s:s61–70

268. Gross PA, Quinnan GV, Rodstein M et al: Association of influenza immunization with reduction in mortality in an elderly population. Arch Intern Med 1988;148:562–565

269. Ammann AJ Schiffman G, Austrian R: The antibody responses to pneumococcal capsular polysaccharides in aged individuals. Proc Soc Exp Biol Med 1980;164:312–316

270. Forrester HL, Jahnigen DW, LaForce FM: Inefficiency of pneumococcal vaccine in a high-risk population. Am J Med 1987;83:425–430

271. Peters NJ, Meiklejohn G, Jahnigen DW: Antibody response of an elderly population to a supplemental dose of influenza B vaccine. J Am Geriatr Soc 1988;36:593–599

272. Simberkoff MS, Cross AP, Al-Ibrahim M et al: Efficacy of pneumococcal vaccine in high-risk patients. N Engl J Med 1986;315:1318–1327

273. Gravenstein S, Drinka P, Duthie EH et al: Efficacy of an influenza hemagglutinin-diphtherian toxoid conjugate vaccine in elderly nursing home subjects during an influenza outbreak. J Am Geriatr Soc 1994;42:245–251

274. Hibberd PL, Rubin RH: Immunization strategies for the immunocompromised host: the need for immunoadjuvants. Ann Intern Med 1989;110:955–956

Chapter 12

Normal cognitive aging

Ian A. Stuart-Hamilton

Material in this chapter contains contributions from the previous edition, and we are grateful to the previous author for the work done.

This chapter provides an overview of the principal features of cognitive change in normal older adults. It considers changes in intelligence (i.e. the skill measured by standardized intelligence tests) and, more broadly, intellectual skills (i.e. skills with a discernible cognitive component which are not simply direct synonyms of memory or IQ tests) and memory. Each topic will be discussed in turn, before a final section, considering some of the problems inherent in testing older adults' cognitive skills. Following standard practice, it is assumed that "normal" in this context refers to older people with no discernible mental illness, and whose physical health is typical of their age group.

INTELLIGENCE
The nature of age-related change in intelligence

Early research on the effects of aging on intelligence produced a basic and often-replicated finding. Namely, scores on intelligence tests rise through childhood and peak in the late teens; thereafter there is a plateau of performance at more or less the same level before a decline in later life. This pattern of rise–level–drop is known as the *classic aging curve*. Early research, based on cross-sectional studies (see below), argued that the length of the plateau was relatively short, and that the onset of decline began in the late twenties or early thirties.[1] However, as will be seen below, this was due to measurement artefacts, and modern researchers place the decline for most skills in the sixties.[2,3] However, the shape (if not the relative proportions) of the classic aging curve was and generally is not disputed (i.e. lifespan cognitive change is seen as growth–retention–decline). It would be comforting for researchers if the matter could rest here, but unfortunately behind this simple façade lies a web of caveats, and the description is at best a gloss of a complex and at times contradictory set of findings. To examine this issue, it is necessary to approach the measurement of intelligence change from several angles. Before doing this, some parameters must be established.

First, it is important to note that the aging curve applies only to *raw* scores (quite simply, the number of questions correctly answered). If the intelligence quotient (IQ) is considered, then this remains relatively stable throughout life. This is because a person's IQ is a derived score, measuring an individual's cognitive status relative to the rest of his or her age group *only*, and not to the population as a whole. An individual tends to retain approximately the same IQ throughout life. In other words, a person remains at roughly the same intellectual status *relative to his or her age peers*. Thus, a person who performs better than 90 percent of age peers when aged 20 will still be likely to perform better than about 90 percent of age peers when aged 80. It follows from this that different raw scores are required to produce a particular IQ at different ages. Thus, to obtain a particular IQ score will require a bigger raw score in early than in late adulthood. This point needs to be stressed because many commentators use "IQ" as a shorthand for "intelligence," leading to fundamental misconceptions in the unwary reader.

A second caveat is derived from the fact that the core literature on cognitive aging is based on studies of performance on standardized intelligence tests. It may at first appear obvious to note that intelligence tests are designed to identify individual *differences* in test scores. However, this carries the implication that it is the end-result of cognitive functioning which is being measured and not cognitive functioning itself. Conversely, studies of change in aging cognitive processes (which ultimately produce the individual differences) have deliberately ignored individual differences in performance; instead, the goal has been to identify a common model of functioning. This creates potential disparities between studies of the nature of aging change and studies of its causes, since they are often derived from different disciplines with contrary goals.

A third caveat is that the waters are muddied further by the fact that most intelligence tests (and certainly the bulk of those used in psychogerontological research) are designed to assess aptitude rather than knowledge; in other words, ability divorced from skills learnt from experience and education. Whether any psychometric test can be totally divorced from prior knowledge is debatable,[4] but arguably emphasizing aptitude at the expense of experience is making a statement about what intelligence "truly" is which may be to the benefit of some age groups and types of people at the expense of others. To take one (rather obvious) example: older adults by definition will have had greater experience than younger adults; therefore, if an intelligence test sets out to ignore experience, this excludes a larger component of an older than a younger person's mental life and abilities. This would be seen by many researchers as being perfectly reasonable: there appears to be an explicit or at least tacit assumption in much of the literature that experience should be seen as either a contaminant or at best as something which will allow an older adult to prop up a failing of "pure" intelligence by recourse to tried and trusted mental ploys acquired through experience. This may be an entirely reasonable step to take—perhaps prior experience has no part in "true" intelligence—but there are times when an observer may get an uneasy feeling of foreclosure. This, and the previous considerations, should be borne in mind when considering the research literature.

In approaching the study of psychological change in later life, perhaps the biggest single problem is that any comparison of older and younger adults is not just a comparison of age differences. It is a commonplace that society has changed rapidly in the last hundred years. Thus, the upbringing of a typical older person was arguably impoverished relative to a younger adult. Examples of the better living conditions of today's youth compared with those of earlier generations are legion. For example, a person growing up in the 1930s and 40s (i.e. at the time of writing, today's 60- and 70-year-olds) will have experienced rationing and the stress of warfare, either as a civilian or as a member of the armed forces. Such delights have escaped today's teenagers, who, inter alia, have arguably been provided with more educational opportunities, better healthcare, ready access to more information through television and the Internet, greater freedom of expression, greater abundance of consumer goods, and more personal disposable income. It is thus perfectly reasonable to argue that today's youth have experienced a far more privileged upbringing than that of cohorts of 40 or more years ago. It follows that the size of the difference between older and younger adults may in part be the result of radically different early experiences and lifestyles rather than age per se; a phenomenon known as the "cohort effect." Controlling for this is problematic. Some academic journals have a wise policy of barring publication of age-difference studies which do not control for educational background and similar easily quantifiable measures. However, the simple and regrettable truth is that there are a great many other potentially influential variables which have not and cannot be plausibly measured and controlled for. A considerable handicap in researching the formative influences on adults is that many cohort effects would have been difficult to quantify at the time (e.g. quality of life in childhood) and now are rendered impossible because there is no method of verifying them. In other words, demonstrating that an age difference exists after controlling for cohort effects a, b, and c does not mean that the unmeasured influences of d through to z might not have had an effect.[5] This may appear a piece of armchair criticism which can be easily directed at hard-working researchers doing the best they can to control a plethora of confounding variables. However, the fact remains that when cohort effects are even partly controlled for in a reasonably effective manner, age differences are severely curtailed.

Most studies of age differences adopt a *cross-sectional design*. In other words, two age groups are tested at the same point in historical time. This is quick and easy to do, but it is prone to cohort effects. The alternative (known as the *longitudinal study*) measures the same group of people at different ages. This is logistically acceptable in testing an organism with the life expectancy of a fruit fly, but is a major undertaking in human aging research. Because significant age group differences are not usually seen in under a decade, participants must be followed for a great number of years. This raises many problems including those of maintaining compliance, gambling that the tests used in the original study will still be valid upon retesting, and the thorny issue of losing participants (through both death and the more mundane matter of changing addresses without notifying the experimenters). Not surprisingly longitudinal studies are expensive to run, and it is therefore small wonder that they are relatively rare. However, the longitudinal method carries a major advantage which at times outweighs its practical limitations. If the same people are compared at different ages, then any age difference between their scores cannot be due to differences in upbringing, since the older and younger groups are composed of the same people. This means that the cohort effects discussed above are eliminated. Longitudinal studies have traditionally found significantly smaller age differences and a later age of onset of decline in the aging curve.[6,7]

However, the longitudinal method is not ideal, and in effect, one cohort effect is removed only to be replaced by another. Following the same group of people over time measures how aging affects that particular cohort; it does not mean that other cohorts would necessarily show the same pattern of age change. To escape this problem requires the use of a more sophisticated version of the longitudinal study, called the *overlapping longitudinal study*,[8,9] in which several age groups are compared in a cross-sectional manner and then are retested at regular intervals. This enables researchers to follow each age group longitudinally; and, by comparing the longitudinal changes of the different groups, it is possible to estimate what are genuine aging changes and what are due to peculiarities of individual cohorts. Such a study is complex and expensive to run, but results are arguably the most reliable available. The findings indicate that an appreciable decline in general intelligence does not typically occur until after the mid-sixties.[9]

Notwithstanding their usefulness, the expense and impracticality of the longitudinal study and related methods means that, for almost all purposes, studies of aging change must rely on cross-sectional methods, and with them the problem that age differences demonstrated in most studies are almost inevitably exaggerated by a cohort effect. This is important because it is necessary that we know what is truly due to aging (what might be termed "pure aging") rather than method of upbringing. Arguably any future treatments for aging will affect pure aging but are unlikely to change cohort effects. It is therefore very important to know the proportion of the "aging decline" which can be feasibly altered by therapeutic means. However, in another sense knowing how much of an age difference is due to "pure aging" and how much is due to cohort effects is a matter of academic interest. The fact remains that whatever the cause of the decline, a decline still exists. To take an analogy: if a man is attacked and robbed by a mugger, the man's missing wallet and sore head are the same whether the mugger's actions were primarily caused by an innate psychopathy or poor socialization. In other words, the problem exists whatever its real cause.

Thus, the test method chosen will exaggerate or diminish the extent of age differences. It would be comforting if this were the only methodological problem besetting the subject; but regardless of the longitudinal versus cross-sectional debate, the findings on age-related change also vary according to the type of intelligence test employed. An "intelligence test" is almost inevitably a measure of *general intelligence*. Although researchers are sometimes divided on the precise construction of this ability,[10,11] the generally accepted definition is that general intelligence or g is a measure of overall ability at all types of intellectual tasks. General intelligence can be broken down into more specialized component skills, such as visuospatial intelligence (ability to process information about shapes and other visual images), verbal intelligence, and so forth. Each is strongly correlated with g, but also has some independence of its own. This means that most people have roughly the same level of ability at most tasks, but not an identical ability at everything—thus they may have relative strengths and weaknesses in specific skills. That is why schoolchildren who are good at one subject tend to be good at others, but will generally show a relative strength for either the arts or sciences.

Another commonly used method of breaking down g is to divide it into *fluid intelligence* and *crystallized intelligence*.[12–15] Fluid intelligence is the principal ingredient of most intelligence tests, and measures the degree to which a person can solve novel problems for which prior training has no effect (very loosely, it is a measure of "native wit"). Measures of fluid intelligence typically involve familiar "brain teasers" such as "Which is the next number in the series?", "Which is the odd one out?" etc. Participants usually must answer these questions against the clock (typically tests require people to answer as many questions as they can within a time limit) so speed as well as accuracy of thought are important. Crystallized intelligence, in contrast, is a gauge of the knowledge a person has acquired. Tests thus usually require participants to answer general knowledge questions and/or provide definitions of obscure words. There is typically an implicit value judgment in crystallized intelligence tests that only certain kinds of knowledge are of value, so measures of the skill concentrate on the sort of information acquired by a fairly traditional education (e.g. knowing what the *Apocrypha* are or what *adumbrate* means). Be that as it may, a cardinal feature of crystallized tests is that, unless the participant knows the answers before the test, they have no means of working them out from first principles. To this extent they are the opposite of fluid tests, where prior knowledge should have no influence, and the answers can be worked out only from first principles. Crystallized intelligence tests are usually not timed (i.e. people can take as long as they like to answer the questions).

The general finding is that fluid intelligence declines (often spectacularly) in older adults[16] whilst crystallized intelligence is preserved or even slightly improves.[17] Various explanations have been offered for this. One often cited in one format or another is that, given fluid intelligence is known to be positively correlated with physical health and status whilst crystallized intelligence is not,[15,18] it is tempting to explain the relative decline and preservation of the skills as a symptom of a general physical aging change. As will be seen in the section below on causes of change, this argument has considerable support, but it is also worth noting that to some extent the age difference on fluid and crystallized tests is a product of measurement artefacts. An ingenious demonstration of this was made by Storandt,[19] who observed that many fluid intelligence tests require considerable manual dexterity and speed of fine motor movements (e.g. in writing down answers in the spaces provided quickly and neatly). Older people may be disadvantaged, not because of mental failings, but through physical weakness and the effects of aging-associated illnesses such as rheumatism and arthritis. Thus, part of the age difference in test scores may not reflect intellectual differences, but rather, differences in handwriting speed. When Storandt controlled for this,

then age differences were significantly lowered (though not totally removed). It was subsequently demonstrated that compensating for other physical limitations (e.g. increasing the print size of the test to allow for poorer eyesight[20]) also diminished the age difference.

Not all measurement artefacts are necessarily acting against older adults: although some may be magnifying age differences in fluid skills, others are probably masking a real decline in crystallized intelligence. As has already been noted, crystallized tests are not against the clock. However, if a time limit is imposed, then a significant age difference arises.[21] Likewise, marking criteria are often quite lax on crystallized tests. If stricter rules are imposed, then, once again, older people are significantly worse.[22] The conclusion that crystallized skills are inviolate to normal aging change is thus probably incorrect, just as the "true" size of the difference in fluid skills is exaggerated. However, it would be wrong to assume that real differences in the two skills do not exist. First, they represent radically different cognitive processes. Second, for all the distortion introduced by measurement error, crystallized skills are much more effectively preserved relative to fluid skills, and appear to be based on different physiological mechanisms; a notable instance of this is that crystallized skills tend to be preserved for longer in many patients suffering from dementia.[23] It should also be noted that whatever the cause of the age difference, the fact remains that once again a large difference exists, and like the mugging analogy made above, the uncertainty as to the true cause of age difference does not disprove the existence of a problem.

Discussion of age changes in intelligence test performance have so far largely concentrated on group performance. However, there is also considerable individual variation; certainly it is far from true that the pattern of change for an individual is a close copy of the age group average. This was illustrated by the concept of *terminal drop*.[24] It is known that age group mean scores decline gently over time. However, observations of participants in longitudinal studies have found that not all individuals imitate this pattern. Instead, some show a relatively abrupt decline in abilities, and this typically predicts death within a few months of the last test session they attended. The terminal drop theory in its strongest form argued that everybody displays this pattern, and that the sudden decline in intellectual abilities reflects the onset of a fatal decline in physical functioning (the reason why group means decline gently is due to simple averaging out of the individual test scores). More recent research has demonstrated that the phenomenon applies only to the relatively young elderly (i.e. those under 75) and that it probably reflects the effects of onset of a comparatively sudden fatal illness. Older adults are less likely to show a sudden drop.[25]

Another interpretation of individual differences is the variability in preservation of skills. Although there is an average decline in the aging population, this is not mirrored in every individual: at its most simplistic, some adults decline more than others, and the population change is the average of this. In fact, variability in individual test scores is bigger in older adults than in any other adult age group,[26,27] and thus, contrary to stereotypes, older adults are less likely to fit their cohort average than any other adult age group. It should also be noted that a minority (perhaps up to 15 percent[26]) of older adults maintain their youthful intelligence test scores throughout life.[25]

Intellectual skills

Some cognitive skills are not directly reducible to psychometric measures of intelligence or memory (although they may both be major components and statistically be good predictors).

A skill often confounded with intelligence is *wisdom*. The term has a variety of meanings, but generally refers to a pragmatic sense of how a problem might be resolved rather than pure logical skill. For example, several Roman emperors are credited with resolving the problem of starvation amongst the wild beasts of the Roman circuses by feeding them with human prisoners (thereby simultaneously solving a problem of prison overcrowding). The solution is *logical* but it is hardly *wise*. A wise solution to a problem may not necessarily adopt the optimal working method, but it is the one which is likely to satisfy the greatest number of people. A high level of wisdom is not a preserve of older adults, contrary to stereotypes, and is found in adults of all ages.[28] The skill correlates strongly with intelligence and some psychometric personality measures, but there is still a significant quantity of unexplained variance,[29,30] indicating that wisdom is more than just intelligence in another guise.

Another skill sometimes confused with intelligence is *creativity*. The term refers to the ability to produce novel and appropriate solutions to a given problem. A typical creativity test requires a person to produce novel uses for a mundane household object, such as a brick (e.g. scraping the surface to produce powder paint). This is a measure of *divergent thinking*: the person must produce ideas which diverge or spread out from a single source (conversely, intelligence tests are measures of *convergent thinking*: the person must use a set of information to converge onto a single solution). Studies of divergent thinking typically demonstrate an age-related decline, even if older and younger participants are matched for intelligence and education levels.[31,32] However, two caveats must be raised. The first is that the findings might reflect a cohort effect: educational methods have arguably shifted from stressing convergent to divergent skills over the past few decades, so older adults may simply not have been encouraged to be creative when growing up. Second, there is evidence that divergent thinking tests are poor predictors of real life creativity,[33,34] partly because the source of creative inspiration may shift towards personal experience in later life,[35] thereby lessening the need for divergent thinking skills. Studies of real life creativity are in turn potentially error-prone. It can be demonstrated that output of creative work dries up for most individuals who have ever been considered to be creative by the time they reach their sixties.[36] However, this does not mean that aging automatically destroys creativity. That some individuals have continued to be creative into extreme old age (Titian being a notable example) indicates that aging does not automatically block creativity. A more prosaic answer is that older creative adults either get tired of their work, they are made to retire, or the public tires of their work (e.g. it is very rare for a fashionable artist to remain fashionable for decade

after decade) thereby removing the drive to continue producing work.

A final skill to be considered is that of *attention*. The term refers to the ability to concentrate and/or remember items in spite of distracting stimuli (which may also require processing). The skill is used in several contexts. *Sustained attention* is the ability to respond to a particular stimulus only (the *target*) which appears sporadically in a presentation of a sequence of targets and *distractors*. The task is akin to a radar operator surveying a largely unchanging screen for the rare sighting of a target. Older adults show little or no change in this skill.[37] *Selective attention* tasks require a response when a target is present amongst an array of distractors (the task is not unlike looking for a familiar face in a crowd). Older adults are usually disadvantaged at this task,[38] though the majority of findings indicate that, if the target appears with reasonable consistency at a particular location in a display, older people become faster at identifying targets in that position.[39] In effect this implies that older adults have some free processing space available to monitor what they are doing in the task. Although the age difference in selective attention is partly attributable to general slowing (see below), there is sufficient unexplained variance to indicate other as yet unexplained factors may play a role.[40] It should also be noted that because selective attention is in part dependent upon good sensory acuity, altering the physical parameters of the test (e.g. the colors and size of the targets) can appreciably alter the performance of older people.[41] There is also evidence that older people's performance on auditory selective attention tasks (e.g. trying to detect messages played against a background of distracting noise) is appreciably worse than younger people's.[42] However, other research[43] has demonstrated that this may be due at least in part to failure to compensate for hearing loss. When volume levels are adjusted to account for auditory acuity, age differences are largely eliminated.

The final form of attention to be considered is *divided attention*. This is the ability to attend to and process more than one source of information simultaneously. A common measure of this skill is the *dichotic listening task* in which participants must attend to messages played to the right and left ears simultaneously; typically, participants must then repeat back the messages to the left and right ears separately. As might be imagined, the task is difficult, and older adults are especially disadvantaged.[44] The pattern and nature of the responses older people make are very similar to those of younger adults, so it is unlikely that there is a notable change in the types of mental processes used.[44] This implies that the phenomenon may be explained in general terms of a lowering of cognitive capacity (see below). The root cause of this is in part attributable to neurological changes, both in failure adequately to screen out neural noise[45] and, at a grosser anatomical level, by a decline in frontal lobe function.[46]

The causes of age-related change in intelligence

As has been seen, studies of aging intelligence and intellectual skills have revealed an extensive catalog of decline, notwithstanding methodological considerations. We shall now examine some possible causes of this. Reduced to its simplest level, a decline in intelligence test score can be attributed to two basic factors. First, older people's skills may worsen because they no longer have the ability or "basic processes" to support intellectual activity at the levels they previously enjoyed. This can be principally attributed to a decline in physical health— slower neural transmission; poorer metabolism and so forth will all help to create a brain which can no longer conduct mental activity with the efficiency of yore. This is most notably expressed in the *general slowing hypothesis* and its derivatives, which argue that aging decline is attributable to slower and less efficient neural processing, and in studies of the varied effects of decline in different regions of the brain. The second factor is that older adults simply neglect intellectual skills so that they decline through lack of practice. This is in effect the old adage of "use it or lose it," more prosaically known as the *disuse theory*. The two models encapsulate much of the major research on aging change and we shall consider each in turn.

The general slowing hypothesis has its roots in a well-established observation; namely, that older adults tend to have slower reaction times (the time taken to respond to a stimulus).[47] Reaction times are assessed by presenting the participant with a stimulus and measuring how long it takes him or her to provide a prearranged response. The simplest version (called not surprisingly the "simple reaction time") involves the presentation of a single stimulus (typically a light or a sound) and a single response (typically pressing a button). This provides a basic measure of how quickly a person can respond to stimulation. A more sophisticated version (the "complex reaction time") presents the participant with one of a set of stimuli to which the participant responds with a different action for each stimulus. A common version of this involves several distinct visual stimuli (e.g. *A*, *B*, *C*, and *D*) and a different button to be pressed for each stimulus (e.g. button 1 for *A*, button 2 for *B*, etc.). Because the complex reaction time task requires participants to make a decision about which button to press, responses are slower than for simple reaction times, where less thought needs be given to what type of response has to be made. By measuring the extra time taken in a complex reaction time task, it is possible to gain at least a rudimentary insight into how long it takes to make a decision between choices.

The reaction time is thus a simple "ready reckoner" of the speed at which a person's nervous system can transmit information. The slower the reaction time, the slower the processing speed and the slower the mental processes involved. Older adults generally display relatively little slowing in simple reaction time tasks, but a much bigger worsening in complex reaction time performance.[48] This has key implications for intellectual functioning. The first is that, prosaically enough, if neurons take longer to send signals, then it will take a person longer to process information and hence longer to answer questions, solve problems, etc. As has been noted above, measures of fluid intelligence are against the clock, and accordingly, a slowing in processing speed will be reflected in a lowering of test scores. Indeed, there is a robust correlation between reaction time and intelligence test score.[49] Furthermore, if reaction time differences between older and younger adults are statistically controlled for, all or most of their differences in fluid intelligence are removed;[50] and

conversely, controlling for fluid intelligence removes all or most of the age differences in reaction times.[51]

However, the situation is more complex and far-reaching than just a simple slowing of neural transmission (though this in itself is a serious enough problem). Reaction times are a gauge not only of speed but of the general health and efficiency of the nervous system. Declining reaction times may be indicative of neural degeneration, increased neural noise (leading to less accurate storage and processing of information), loss of storage integrity, etc. Thus, reaction times may be a useful guide to the general physical status of the older person's brain. However, although reaction times are a useful gauge of this, they are not necessarily the most accurate. Some researchers have criticized the reaction time measurement as being too crude to give a reliable insight into the components of neural activity involved in a mental process.[52] Furthermore, relatively recent research has found that a better indicator than the reaction time are other indices of neural status, such as sensory acuity, and impressive claims have been made for the amount of variance in older adults' test scores which can be accounted for by this. For example, in one key study by Baltes and Lindenberger,[53] having controlled for vision and hearing, age-related variance in the cognitive skills being assessed was reduced to a trifling 3 percent.

If the decline in intelligence in older adults is due to a general slowing, then a simple prediction is that decline on similar intellectual tasks should be explicable in terms of a common factor of reduced processing speed. Initial evidence seemed to contradict this, however. If adults are given a set of tasks with a common core but differing levels of difficulty (e.g. sorting cards into red and black versus into diamonds, hearts, clubs, and spades) then they get slower the more complex the task. Furthermore, the older adults are slower than the younger adults. However, older adults get disproportionately worse the more complex the task: in other words, the gap between older and younger adults grows relatively bigger the harder the task they have been set. This is known as the *age times complexity effect*,[54] and at first sight appears to contradict the idea that a simple rule governs both complex and simple versions of the same task. However, if the older and younger adults' scores are plotted against each other (i.e. older groups' mean time on task 1 plotted against younger groups' time on task 1, older groups' time on task 2 plotted against younger groups' task 2 time, etc.) then the relationship is found to be linear (the *Brinley plot*).[55–57] This indicates that the age differences in performance may be governed by a simple rule of a difference in speed of processing. The model is an attractive one, since it apparently indicates that much of the aging change in intelligence can be explained by a simple drop in processing speed. This in turn implies that improving intellectual performance could largely be a matter of tweaking basic neural functioning, thereby putting the preservation of normal intelligence within the bounds of medical intervention.

Unfortunately, there is some evidence that Brinley plots may be an oversimplification. The criticisms revolve around the statistical regression technique used to demonstrate it, which may artificially exaggerate a linear relationship and in effect mask a high proportion of variability in the more complex tasks scores.[58] Other researchers have argued that Brinley plots measure a relationship between the relative standard deviations of younger and older people's scores, and not general slowing as such.[59] Again, it has been argued that other statistical techniques (such as curvilinear regression) give a better explanation of the data, but do not demonstrate a simple linear relationship.[60]

More generally, associating aging intelligence with reaction times and other neural and sensory changes is not as simple a connection as may first appear. First, although reaction times decline in later life, this is a decline in *mean* reaction times, not their *range*. In other words, at top speed, older adults are capable of responding as quickly as younger adults; the difference lies in the *typical* reaction time, which is slower in older adults.[61–63] This indicates that the change in processing is in average, not absolute, performance. Second, measures of reaction times, sensory acuity and similar are often taken as "pure" measures of "basic" ability. However, having good eyesight, sharp reactions, good hearing, etc. must to some extent be indicative of a lifetime of sensible healthcare. In short, a good sensory system may be as much a product of intelligent behavior as a cause of it.[64]

Third, it should be noted that measures of, say, reaction time and acuity are relatively crude measures of neural processing. Although they are arguably more "basic" than cognitive skills measured by test solving abilities (though Rabbitt[64] makes an intriguing case that in measuring speed one is measuring the product, not the root of the system), they are not necessarily the true "cognitive primitives."[65] Fourth, several studies have reported that senses and speed are at best indifferent predictors of the specific cognitive skills which were studied,[66] whilst in some broader assessments of batteries of cognitive skills, a significant proportion of age-related variability may be left unexplained.[67] A fifth and final consideration is that a distorted view may have been obtained because researchers have taken an inappropriate measure of "speed," for example by failing to gauge it against an appropriate baseline of performance.[68,69]

Armed with the current evidence, all that can be said is that measures of slowing are plausible indicators. In other words, they are guides to the general state of neural efficiency, not necessarily precise measures. Thus, explaining aging intelligence in terms of general slowing is an attractive goal, if only because it affords such a simple, easily quantifiable model.[70] However, for the reasons outlined, support for the model must be qualified.

Studies of the effects of decline in different regions of the brain indicate that links between neural status and mental functioning may also exist at grosser levels of anatomy. Studies of brain-damaged patients have long established that different anatomical regions specialize in specific mental operations. Since it is known that aging is associated with a depletion in brain cell numbers and extent of neural interconnections,[71] it is an intuitively obvious prediction that the loss will be reflected in a commensurate decline in mental functioning; and in addition to studies of general "neural efficiency" through the general slowing hypothesis, a considerable body of research has concentrated on declines in specific regions of the brain and their effects. For example, Schaie and Schaie[72] observed that the pattern of aging decline on subtests of the WAIS (Wechsler Adult Intelligence Scale IQ test battery) closely resembled the performance of patients with right hemisphere damage. Thus,

the authors argued, aging cognitive decline may be attributable at least in part to an imbalance in the rate of decline in the two hemispheres. The concept is an interesting one and not without some empirical support. However, as Kaszniak and Newman[73] observe in an excellent review of the subject, there are problems. First, there is no supporting evidence from neurological studies for differential hemispheric decline.[74] Second, psychological tests which assess right hemispheric skills tend to be more cognitively demanding, and therefore any age differences may be because in effect right hemisphere tests are "harder" rather than because the right hemisphere is being tested per se. Indeed, this is a problem which bedevils the psychogerontological literature. Disproportionate age differences on tasks linked to a specific region of the brain may indicate an especially concentrated decline in functioning in that region, or it may mean that the cognitive load of those tasks is greater than realized by researchers. The issue is extraordinarily difficult to resolve and easily slips into teleological reasoning. Caution in interpreting reports is accordingly advised.

In recent years, the right hemisphere hypothesis has been supplanted by the frontal lobe hypothesis. It is known that the frontal lobes show higher levels of decay than many other areas. Since the frontal lobes are known to be involved in, inter alia, planning and memory of sequences of actions, it might be assumed that cognitive tasks which are based on such skills will be especially badly affected by aging, and indeed, many researchers have found evidence supporting this.[75–77] However, others have noted that, although frontal lobe decline is linked to cognitive changes, the size of the effect is ameliorated if measures of function in other cortical regions are taken into account.[78,79] Indeed, Salthouse et al.[80] noted that many supposedly localized cortical effects share a high proportion (58 percent) of aging-related variance with other variables. Such findings indicate that aging change in cognitive skills is associated with general neural decline as much as with specific regions of the brain (and thus might more properly be seen as part of general slowing). Nonetheless, at least part of age-related variance is attributable to region-specific decline.[73] It should be noted that, in a permutation of the "mugging" analogy made above, whether a deficit in a particular region is part of a general decline or is unique does not remove the very practical problem that there is a problem.

Some caveats need to be added to these statements. The first is that, although there is a correlation between brain and mental state, the direction of the relationship is not always clear. Although it might be intuitively thought that brain will determine cognitive state, there is reasonable evidence that a more "intellectual" lifestyle is reflected in greater brain volume, neuronal interconnectivity and resistance to dementia.[71] However, the issue immediately begs the question of whether people would have "intellectual" lifestyles without the neurological framework to support it. Indeed, the issue can rapidly turn into a tedious chicken and egg debate. Notwithstanding this, it is tempting to perceive every cognitive process as grounded in a neural explanation. Whilst it is intuitively obvious that (Cartesian doubts aside) all mental processes must be performed using neurons, it is possible to become too slavishly dedicated to "proving" that mental processes are an inevitable product of a physical activity. This is best explained by analogy. A television program can be seen and heard properly only if the television set, the aerial, and the transmitting apparatus are all working effectively. In a similar way, mental functioning can occur efficiently only when the brain is working effectively. However, which television program a person chooses to watch has nothing to do with the physical state of the apparatus transmitting and receiving it. In a similar way, the physical state of the brain does not force a person to think about specific topics to the exclusion of others. The analogy is not total, because arguably a less efficient brain will limit the range and efficiency with which a topic can be mentally processed, whereas poor TV reception does not mean a person can only watch soap operas. But the essential point is that the status of the brain does not in itself determine which thought processes are adopted, only how well they will be performed. The evidence for a physical causation for aging intellectual decline is thus strong, but not overwhelming. This leads to consideration of whether the mental processes themselves play a causal role in their own preservation.

Disuse theory, like general slowing, can produce some strong arguments in its favor, but there are a number of caveats which have to be made. It is intuitively clear that nearly all skills must be practised if they are to be maintained. It follows from this that the decline in intelligence test scores might be partly explained as a failure to practise intellectual skills at the level necessary to maintain a youthful level of performance. This may initially sound fanciful, especially given the general slowing argument that decline is inevitable, but there is some evidence to support it. First, it can be established that if older adults are trained on certain types of intelligence test performance, they can usually recover all or most of their youthful level.[81] Second, it is apparent that older adults who have practised a skill as part of their daily lives also match younger adults in performance of it. Two strands of evidence may be produced to support this argument. The first is that there is no or little relationship between a person's performance of their everyday occupation and their age.[82] The second is a series of ingenious experiments by Charness[83–86] who demonstrated that (with the possible exception of world-class players at the absolute peak of form) older chess and bridge players could match younger opponents for ability. Of interest is that the older adults had poorer "basic" skills, such as memory, but compensated for this by having a greater store of tactics and experience of similar games played in the past (a phenomenon known unsurprisingly as *compensation*). Other researchers have demonstrated a similar phenomenon in older typists. Compared with younger colleagues, they had slower finger movements, but were more adept at other skills, such as planning sequences of finger movements over the keys more proficiently.[87,88] It is important to note that practice is not necessarily "preserving" skills: it is true that older adults are maintaining a youthful or near-youthful level of overall performance, but the manner in which the tasks are performed to obtain this end-result may have changed considerably.

Practise can thus make older adults more adept and may help preserve skills. However, the disuse theory, like the general slowing model, has problems in explaining some phenomena. For example, although practice will lessen many age differences, it will not remove all of them. Salthouse and colleagues[89,90] demonstrated that older architects and pilots, although proficient at visuospatial tasks (as might logically be expected), were slightly but significantly worse than younger architects and pilots on the same tasks. (It should be noted, however, that Salthouse et al. were measuring a relatively basic skill, and this did not take account of compensatory skills such as experience in other aspects of the participants' occupations.) Again, practise tends to be very specific in its effects. Practice at cognitive skill *A* will not necessarily improve cognitive skill *B* or *C* unless they are very similar tasks.[91] This implies that aging brings with it a general decline, which practice can only offset on a piecemeal basis by tackling specific symptoms rather than the root cause.

Evidence for the slowing and disuse theories is thus equivocal and it is improbable that decline is due to either factor alone; almost certainly both play a role and may also interact with each other. This is a pragmatic and not entirely unsurprising conclusion: few if any commentators would hazard a statement that aging change is entirely a product of either neural decay or practise. The statement also unfairly trivializes the research, which has not sought such grandiose claims as "explaining" the whole of cognitive aging. Instead, it has concentrated on the detailed examination of specific processes with the practical advantage that findings may aid therapeutic regimes, give practitioners and designers a clearer understanding of the capabilities of older people as patients and consumers, and so forth.

However, searching for causes of decline carries with it a tacit assumption which is rarely commented upon in the research literature. There is little reason for studying a phenomenon unless it has some practical relevance. However, what is the practical relevance of aging intellectual skills? There are clear reasons for being alarmed at a decline which reaches the extent of dementia, but normal intellectual aging does not leave a person enfeebled and incapable of leading an independent life. To play Devil's Advocate for a moment, we might ask what purpose is served by wanting older people to maintain a youthful level of intelligence. The majority of human activities are designed so that people from widely different educational and intellectual backgrounds can participate. A decline within this broad band of ability is not going to exclude anyone from participating, and as we have seen, practise at a particularly loved pastime is in any case likely to maintain the level of performance. The one group of people whose lives may be affected by senescent change is that of academics and other members of the self-proclaimed intelligentsia. In everyday life, decline may only be glaringly obvious in skills where accomplishment is possible only for those working at the extremes of ability. However, most people in the population would not consider it worrying if one day the *The Times* crossword took more than ten minutes to complete or they no longer had the mental stamina to cope with an Iris Murdoch novel. However, few people stretch themselves this far in everyday life.

This is of course a deliberate overstatement. Older adults of all intellectual abilities *do* comment on intellectual changes (whether real or imaginary) and they are often the cause for negative affect.[92] Furthermore, there are some routine activities which usually require a mundane level of ability, but periodically demand a limit-stretching level of performance. A key example of this is driving, in which an older motorist may be capable of routine driving but may find certain situations (e.g. very busy junctions) beyond their processing capacity.

The higher incidence of potentially lethal driving behavior in older adults indicates that, under certain specialized circumstances, cognitive aging decline will impinge on everyday activities. However, this does not alter the fact that, although some everyday mental skills may become harder to perform, the majority of activities are rarely made impossible in normal senescence, and it is only if one has very high expectations of intellectual status that a decline may genuinely not just mar but actually block a significant proportion of everyday functioning.

Thus, changes in intellectual status may have less relevance for many older people than might be supposed from a first reading of the situation. Furthermore, the changes may be less severe in their impact than the evidence presented so far suggests. The research outlined above has largely been built upon the findings of psychometric intelligence tests. However, raw scores on these measures are not necessarily the fairest representations of aging cognitive ability. The intelligence test was designed primarily for distinguishing between the aptitude levels of different schoolchildren. It was later used (not totally successfully) for identifying adults of different abilities, principally in connection with job selection. Generally, the further the behavior in question is divorced from the classroom or education, the poorer its correlation with intelligence test scores.[93] The use of the psychometric intelligence test as a measure of intellectual changes in later life is thus not automatically justified. Again, it has already been noted that most tests of intelligence (particularly those with a high weighting towards fluid intelligence) assume that the best measure of intellectual skills is aptitude rather than experience. However, it has also been noted that a cardinal feature of the aging intellect is compensation. This is traditionally viewed as a prop to hold up skills weakened by a decline in fluid intelligence. But by precisely the same argument, fluid intelligence is arguably a less appropriate gauge of later-life cognitive skills.

To take an analogy: suppose that as people age they lose leg strength to such an extent that a wheelchair is the only pragmatic solution; this means that practically everybody aged over 50 uses a wheelchair. Suppose it is decided to compare the mobility of younger and older adults. Because younger adults use their legs, it is decided that everyone will be compared on their walking ability. Of course the older adults will perform badly on this comparison, and although there will be some exceptions (i.e. a minority of adults who still have some leg strength), it will be concluded that older people have little or no means of movement. Of course this is wrong—the older adults *do* have a means of movement, which is perfectly efficient. But by applying a too-narrow criterion for measuring ability, this fact has been overlooked. In a similar manner, deciding that because fluid intelligence has always been accepted as the definitive measure of "pure" intellectual functioning, it must continue to be the prime benchmark test, leads to some potentially misleading conclusions.

This can be seen in the following example. Salthouse[90] demonstrated that, across a wide range of intelligence tests and measures of subskills, the mean test scores of older adults fall considerably below younger adults' means on the same tests. In some instances, older adults' means, placed on the younger adults' distribution curves, were approaching two standard deviations below the younger adults' mean. This is a considerable decline, but it should be put in perspective. Two standard deviations below the mean is taken by many authorities to indicate severe educational problems (what was once termed "educationally subnormal"). This means one of two things. First, it could mean that the results are a fair reflection of everyday life, and that the average older adult really is behaving at a cognitive level which at school would attract the close attention of remedial teachers and educational psychologists. This is, however, unrealistic. The alternative, borne out by everyday experience, is that quite palpably older adults are not behaving at such a level in everyday life. Hence, the psychometric measures of intelligence are not a fair gauge of older adults' cognitive status.[5,66]

Such arguments indicate that we should be cautious about using psychometric data (and particularly those weighted towards measures of fluid intelligence) too slavishly in measuring later life changes. However, the argument can be pushed too far. If older adults are misrepresented by psychometric measures, this is a relative, not an absolute problem. Intelligence test scores correlate reliably, if not always highly, with most everyday intellectual skills, so it is fair to assume that performance on intelligence tests indicates the general *trends* in cognitive ability. Assuming that test scores are a heuristic measure of cognitive status is not unreasonable. But it would be unwise to go further and assume that intelligence test performance in its own right is an indicator of all that is happening to cognitive skills in later life—as the confounding effects of compensation, problems in measurement, and design flaws in the tests themselves all too readily demonstrate.

Before leaving the topic of intelligence testing, a further argument will be considered. So far we have analyzed intellectual change with the assumption that older and younger adults are using essentially the same set of cognitive mechanisms, and that the primary difference lies in the efficiency with which these operate and also the skill with which they are used. Thus, faced with a particular cognitive task, older and younger adults would use the same set of mental processes (for the sake of argument, labeled *A*, *B*, and *C*) to attempt to solve it. *A*, *B*, and *C* might be operating faster and more accurately in younger than older adults, but it is assumed that nonetheless, the same set of skills are used in both cases. In many instances, research seems to indicate that just such a thing occurs.[66] However, on some occasions, older adults may adopt ways of thinking radically different from younger people. In other words, instead of using *A*, *B*, and *C*, older adults might be using *A*, *D*, and *F* to perform the same task.

Research by the child psychologist Jean Piaget (1896–1980) found that children under the age of 7 or 8 years were capable of making what to adult eyes appear remarkably illogical errors when faced with specific types of problems. For example, judgments of whether objects are alive or not tend to be based on whether the object moves (e.g. a bicycle might be "alive");[94] and in his most famous study of *conservation*, children would judge that the quantity of clay in a ball had changed when it was rolled out into a sausage shape.[95] Piaget explained the children's errors as being due to an immature logic system. His theories have been heavily criticized,[96] but nobody disputes that by the teenage years at the very latest, unhandicapped children will be capable of performing the tasks he devised. It has been tacitly assumed by most researchers that people then perform Piagetian tasks correctly for the rest of their lives. However, the available evidence indicates that adults, and especially older adults (who are not, it must be stressed, suffering from dementia), have difficulty with some of the apparently "obvious" and "simple" problems. For example, there is evidence of a rise in animism,[94] a decline in conservation skills,[97] and a shift in the manner in which moral dilemma problems are solved.[98]

The results are surprising, not least because of the strong tacit assumption that the tasks are so "obvious" to an adult that they should not be failed except by an individual with severe intellectual disadvantages. However, the failure is very real and furthermore is not particularly well correlated with level of fluid or crystallized intelligence.[99] If the change is not due to a loss of ability, then this implies that the change is a product of a shift in logical processes (i.e. how people chose to view events in intellectual terms). To take a deliberately extreme analogy: suppose that a man decides that, having learnt the basics of astronomy, he prefers the idea that the waning of the moon is due to its being made of cheese which gets nibbled away every month by galactic mice. Adopting this whimsical thought may in scientific terms be fundamentally wrong; but the man does not have to have suffered a decline in intelligence to move from logic to whimsy. Perhaps he prefers to live his life that way because it is more enjoyable; and provided he is not employed in an astrophysics department, it is hard to see what harm this belief might cause. This echoes the argument made above that declines in intelligence test scores may often be of interest only to academics. Because an apparent loss of logic appears serious to one group does not mean that it impinges on the lives of other people.

Ability to succeed in Piagetian tasks is very important for academics because they (the tasks) measure the basic skills felt to underpin many higher cognitive skills. Doing well at cognitive tasks matters to academics, but not necessarily to everybody else. If older adults who fail the Piagetian tasks are doing so because they are deliberately adopting a different way of looking at things, then a simple prediction can be made. Namely, Piagetian task performance should be closely associated with a measure of choice of intellectual lifestyle. This is what has been found: level of ability at Piagetian tasks in later life is strongly positively correlated with *need for cognition*,[99] a measure of drive to pursue cognitively demanding activities. Thus, a person with a high need for cognition is more likely to pursue intellectual activities, be interested in intellectual and other "high brow" matters, etc. It is unsurprising that this should be related to Piagetian task performance: doing well at Piagetian tasks indicates that a person is still immersed in the assumptions and beliefs of an intellectually active person. However, a person who is uninterested in such a lifestyle is not necessarily lacking in aptitude. Indeed, need for cognition is a better predictor of Piagetian skills than is intelligence test performance.[99] Furthermore, it has been demonstrated that people who fail Piagetian tasks can easily be retrained, indicating that there is no fundamental block to retaining the necessary skills.[100] This implies that people who pursue an intellectually active life into old age may not only maintain a relatively youthful level of cognitive skill, as disuse theory already has indicated, but also will maintain a particular mindset of ways of thinking which is in tune with intellectually active younger adults. Those

who have a relatively low drive for pursuing cognitively demanding activities may well "regress" to a set of cognitive viewpoints which are less sophisticated. This indicates that changes in the aging intellect may not be solely a matter of neural decay and practise, but also of lifestyle choice. Thus, cutting across issues of differences in size of scores is the consideration that a significant subgroup of older adults may be employing radically different methods of reasoning.

MEMORY

The nature of age-related change in memory

Memory changes in later life may be described in the same general terms as changes in intelligence: overall there is a decline, but with considerable differences in patterns of change between the types of memory and also the individuals concerned. A comprehensive taxonomy of types of memory is beyond the confines of this chapter, though there are excellent texts available for those interested in pursuing the issue further.[101] However, it is important to recognize the principal categories into which memory skills are grouped. First, memory can be divided up into the length of time the items have been mentally stored (this provides the distinctions between *short-term*, *long-term*, and *prospective* and *remote* memory listed below). It can also be divided into the types of materials being stored (i.e. whether they are visual or verbal, whether they are facts or events peculiar to an individual's life, etc.). Again, memory can be seen in terms of the processes involved, and researchers distinguish between the mental stages of encoding materials for storage, the storage itself, and the retrieval from storage. Overarching this is *metamemory*; namely, the understanding of the processes involved and an awareness of the most effective ways of memorizing particular types of material. Thus, memory involves rather more than the lay concept of "remembering things in the past," encompassing such skills as remembering when to do things in the future (e.g. keeping appointments), remembering details of one's autobiographical past, and keeping track of information in an ongoing cognitive process (e.g. remembering what has been said in a paragraph of prose so that what is currently being read can both be made sense of and be placed in the correct semantic context). In describing the effects of aging on this, we shall examine each of the principal types of memory in turn.

Short term memory

Memory for information which is presented to a person and must be recalled immediately or after a short delay (of up to about 30 seconds) is called short-term memory (STM). The traditional measure of this skill is to present the participant with a sequence of letters, words, or numbers and request that they are repeated back. Sequences are varied in length until the maximum length a participant can reliably (experimenters vary in their definition of this term) repeat back is discovered. Using this method, it has been found that there is a small but statistically significant decline in STM in older adults.[102] The age difference is typically increased, or perhaps more accurately, exaggerated, if the cognitive workload of the task is raised. For example, if participants are required to repeat the list in reverse order of presentation,[103] or to remember the list whilst performing another task simultaneously,[104] then span decreases for everyone, but the decline is disproportionately greater in older adults. Such findings indicate that memory is maximally effective when the mind can give its full attention to it: once a person must not only memorize items but also perform other tasks simultaneously, memory will suffer.

This phenomenon is another manifestation of the "age times complexity" argument described in the intelligence section above: namely, the more complex the task, the disproportionately greater the age difference becomes. Another way of approaching this issue is through a model common in psychology in which a cognitive process is seen as occupying a particular quantity of "mental space": the more complex the task, the more space is occupied. Since the total amount of space available for all mental processes is finite, it follows that the more space is occupied by a specific task, the less is available for performing other tasks which need to be conducted simultaneously. This is why, it is argued, memory span declines when a concurrent task must be performed. Older adults will be especially disadvantaged, however, because as part of the general cognitive decline of later life (see above), processing space has shrunk, so "space demanding" tasks (such as memory) will be especially disadvantaged. The concept of mental space is of course a metaphor: the limits on the quantity of information and tasks which can be processed simultaneously are determined by the efficiency of the neural networks, but their parameters of speed, maximum processing load, etc. must at some level be analogous to the concept of storage space.

Early studies of STM tended to concentrate on (frankly rather dull) studies of how many items a person would remember and what interfered with this. However, later researchers promoted the concept of STM as a more dynamic process, and one with active involvement in many types of cognitive processing. This is best expressed by Baddeley and Hitch's *working-memory model*.[105] In its basic form, it has the simple premise that STM is organized by a controller (the *central executive*) which allocates incoming items to be remembered to a set of slave systems: the *visuospatial sketchpad* (for memory of visual and spatial information) and the *phonological loop* (for verbal materials). Copies of the material being processed in working memory are sent for long-term storage, and if these items are sufficiently memorable (e.g. through being rehearsed—mentally practised) then a permanent memory trace will be formed.

The working-memory model makes various predictions about how people will perform given particular memory tasks, and the model has proven sufficiently accurate for it to be widely accepted. Of interest here is the degree to which aging affects the operations of working memory. The general consensus is that, in qualitative terms, older and younger adults' working memories are very similar. In both cases, if a younger group find working memory task *X* harder than task *Y*, then so will the older group. For example, the working-memory model creates a prediction that similar sounding letters (B, D, E, G) will be harder to remember than dissimilar sounding ones (G, W, S, H): the *phonemic similarity effect*. This is because the phonological loop is felt to be very sensitive to phonological structure. It thus gets easily "confused" by similar sounding letters (akin to a tongue twister marring pronunciation).

Research has demonstrated that older and younger adults are both prone to the phonemic similarity effect to the same relative extent, indicating that their phonological loops are operating in an analogous manner.[106] However, for all the similarities in operation, it is also clear that older adults are disproportionately disadvantaged when the cognitive workload of a working memory task is raised.[104] In other words, increase the demands of a distracting task, and older adults are disproportionately disadvantaged.

Baddeley[101,106] has argued that the problem may principally be with the central executive, which cannot organize items to be remembered with sufficient efficiency. For example, it has been argued that in a working-memory task, younger adults may be capable of sending a copy of to-be-remembered material to a longer-term store which can be used as a back-up if the original memory trace is lost; older adults may simply lack the processing space to do this.[107] The argument that problems with STM may be principally with cognitive skills involved in organizing it rather than in memory per se is a plausible one, since as has already been seen, there are no or few age differences on very "simple" STM tasks (i.e. just remembering items without having to perform other tasks simultaneously). If the principal problem with STM is the cognitive skills necessary to process information involved in memory tasks, it follows that older people's performance on STM tasks should correlate well with other cognitive measures and gauges of neurological status, such as intelligence test scores and sensory acuity. Indeed, this is the case, and studies have generally found that the higher the intelligence test score, the lower the STM problems.[108,109] To this extent, a worsening of memory in later life can be seen as part and parcel of the general cognitive decline, and to be caused by much the same reasons. This argument is further reinforced by the identification of STM deficits with decay in areas of the brain heavily involved in memory and cognition, such as the hippocampus[110] and the frontal lobes.[111]

However, as with explanations of changes in intelligence, ascribing everything to a single causal factor is attractive but impractical. Two principal caveats must be raised. The first is that, although there may be a decline associated with loss of processing capacity, older adults may also be changing strategies for remembering items which may contribute to their memory loss. An example of this is *chunking*: a process of grouping a list of items to be remembered into convenient "chunks" rather than one long list. The presentation of telephone and credit card numbers are a case in point: rather than present a single row of digits, the numbers are often presented as sequences of groups, each containing three or four digits. Chunking items to be remembered enhances memory, yet it is something which older adults do less frequently than younger adults. Older adults who do chunk have little or no decline in memory span.[112] If the age difference in memory is in part due to a difference in choice of strategies rather than a product of unavoidable decay, then this implies that older adults' memories might be improved by encouraging them to adopt better memorization techniques. Researchers have found that training does seem to improve memory span. For example, one popular method is the *method of loci* technique. This requires a person to imagine a very familiar scene, then create mental images of the items to be remembered and place them at prominent positions in the scene. When the person needs to retrieve the items, he or she mentally scans the scene and detects where the items have been placed. The technique works well for nearly all people, and can revive older adults' memories for some lists. However, it should be noted that the efficacy of such treatments is limited, and although they improve memory scores, do not necessarily completely restore them to a youthful level.[113] In addition, improvements are restricted to the specific type of memory task used in training: they do not have a widespread "knock-on" effect to other types of memory.[91] Therefore, improving older adults' memories through training would involve separate and painstakingly specific regimes for every type of material to be remembered.

Another caveat is that memory decline is not restricted solely to the encoding of information prior to being placed in a memory store. There is good evidence that older adults' memories of items are "weaker" than those of younger adults. For example, compared with younger adults, older adults typically are disproportionately better on recognition than on recall tasks. A recall task requires participants to report the items just presented; in a recognition task, they are presented with the items (the *targets*), along with items which did not appear (the *distractors*) and decide which have been encountered before and which have not. A recall task requires, in effect, a person to bring an item out from memory, and to be able to do this accurately the storage and retrieval must be effective. An old analogy in psychology is to compare memory to storing books in a library. For storage to work effectively, the librarian must first correctly catalog the book and put it on the right shelf; the book must then stay on the shelf and not be pushed off or allowed to rot with mildew; finally, the book must be correctly retrieved by identifying the right catalog number and finding the right shelf. Similarly, a recalled item must have been stored properly, have been kept in a memory store, and then brought out of storage intact. Recognition requires less cognitive effort. Targets and distractors must be compared against items in storage to judge if there is a sufficiently close resemblance for a judgment of recognition to be made. However, the cognitive effort required to do this is less than for recall. To return to the library analogy, instead of having to identify the precise book, it is sufficient to find one which looks similar to one being sought. The disproportionate advantage older adults experience on recognition tasks indicates that their memory storage and retrieval may be markedly less efficient than younger adults'. This argument is supported by Parkin and Walter,[114] who found that older adults are far less confident about the subjective "strength" or "sharpness" of their memories, even when they can produce the correct response in a memory task. This further indicates that storage of memories may become less efficient with age.

Although STM declines in later life, it should be noted that normal changes do not approach the catastrophic loss experienced in dementia, and can to some extent be compensated for by means of *aides-mémoires* such as a notepad or mnemonic strategies such as the method of loci. However, the decline in working memory can potentially have more pervasive effects. Working memory's principal role is in the storage and retrieval of ongoing information needed during cognitive tasks.[109] An example commonly given is of remembering a phone number one has been told whilst writing it down, but there are many others, such as remembering a section of prose just read in order to make sense of what is now being read, or keeping a set of directions in mind whilst driving a car. Because working memory is involved in so many commonplace tasks with a strong cognitive content, its influence is considerable. For example, Kemper[115] has demonstrated that older adults' ability to process syntax and use syntactically complex phrases in speech and writing declines. She plausibly ascribes this to memory loss: if older adults cannot hold complex linguistic constructions in working memory whilst composing a statement, then syntax is likely to become simplified. An elegant demonstration of this is the "simplification" of language in diary entries by older adults who have kept diaries for most of their lives.[116,117] Leaving aside questions of whether some of this simplification is a matter of changing fashions in writing styles rather than a response to loss,[66] the evidence does seem to indicate that memory is affecting linguistic skills.

Thus, STM in either its "traditional" form or when regarded as working memory shows an aging decline which gets more pronounced the more complex the interference from competing tasks becomes. Although some of the decline may be offset by compensatory tactics, nonetheless, the changes are still considerable.

Long-term memory

Long-term memory (LTM) is memory for items or events which occurred at a time more distant than that covered by STM. Since this in effect encompasses the whole of a person's life, the span of time covered by LTM is dictated by a person's age. LTM is not treated as a single entity, however, but is used as a collective term for a set of disparate skills, each concerned with a different subject matter. The effects of aging on LTM are mixed, with decline varying from considerable to practically nonexistent. To relieve the monotony of discussing aging skills in terms of decline, this section begins with a survey of some aspects of LTM which are relatively unaffected by aging.

The type of LTM which corresponds most closely to a layperson's idea of "memory" is probably *autobiographical memory*, which is memory of events specific to an individual's life. Measuring the extent of autobiographical memory is fraught with difficulties. For example, perhaps the most obvious problem is that it is practically impossible to judge if a person is producing an accurate memory. Suppose that a person says that they can remember going for a picnic with their parents when they were 7 years old, and as supporting evidence they describe in great detail where they went, what they ate, and so forth. How can one know whether it is true or false? Faced with either rejecting every memory which cannot be backed up by documentary evidence (and having no research materials as a result), or accepting a pragmatic view that it is perhaps best to place some trust in participants, researchers sensibly adopt the latter approach (fortunately, the majority of recollections are so banal that it is unlikely that they are fabricated). However, this is not the end of the researcher's problems. A further consideration is the method used to elicit memories, which can have a surprisingly strong effect. For example, asking people to produce a list of their most "vivid" memories produces a high proportion from childhood and adolescence. So does giving a person a cue word (e.g. "elephant") and asking for a memory associated with it (e.g. "I remember seeing an elephant on a visit to the zoo when

I was eight"), provided the memory has to be dated at the same time. However, if a person must provide memories associated with a set of cue words and only date when the memories occurred after completing the whole set, then the majority of memories tend to be from the recent past.[118] Choice of test technique is thus very important.

Notwithstanding these considerations, most adults (younger and older) tend to produce most memories from the past 10 years, and older memories tend to be concentrated in the period when the person was between 10 and 30 years of age,[119] a time period known as the *reminiscence peak*. Arguably this is because this is the period of personal development when the majority of key events are likely to occur for the first time: moving home, employment, sex, marriage, parenthood, etc.; at least some of these events become less memorable the more times they are experienced. Autobiographical memories are not necessarily dipped in a honeyed glow of nostalgia; the majority of recollections in at least one study were described as predominantly unpleasant.[120] It is also clear that the vividness of memories declines with age;[121] older adults tend to produce recollections lacking in details and which at times verge on the generic (e.g. "I remember going to the zoo with my parents when I was a child" as opposed to "When I was seven we went to London Zoo during a holiday in the capital with my parents; I particularly remember seeing Gus the gorilla"). Thus, although it was stated that there is not necessarily a decline in autobiographical memory, the quality of the recall may suffer. This is strongly associated with intelligence levels,[122] implying that level of cognitive skills may influence the fidelity and detail of memories; in addition, it is possible that people with greater cognitive skills are also more likely to observe and retain details in memory across their lifespans.

Alongside autobiographical memory is memory for events which have occurred during a person's lifetime but which were not part of that person's personal experience; what is often called *remote memory*. This is typically tested by giving people lists of names or events which were famous at some point during their lives and asking if they recognize them. The test would be very simple and inaccurate if all the items were so famous that they were part of general knowledge. For example, asking people in their eighties if they recognize the name "Adolf Hitler" or if the "Second World War" was a real event is not testing their remote memory. Such names and events are so famous that practically anybody of any age will recognize them, even if they were too young to have known them as contemporary figures or events. Therefore, remote memory tests are limited to items and events which were briefly famous but which have not been discussed in the media since. An example (with no disrespect implied) might be the boxer John Conteh, who was famous in Britain in the 1970s, but who has now largely disappeared from public view. Remote memory tests of this kind typically reveal that older adults outperform younger adults on more temporally remote names and events (not surprisingly perhaps), and that names and events which fall within the lifetimes of all age groups tend to be equally well remembered by all ages.[123] It is important to note that for even the oldest participants, recent events are remembered better than distant events. This contradicts the popular assumption that older people's memories are better for the past than the present (an opinion which once found support in the now-outmoded *Ribot's hypothesis*[124]). It should also be noted that remote memory tests are not necessarily measures of remote memory alone. Studies have found that young adults are often capable of recognizing a higher than chance proportion of names and events which occurred a long time before they were born. Furthermore, the probability of a particular name or event being recognized relative to the other names or events in the same test does not significantly differ across the ages of the participants (e.g. if "Ian Smith" was twentieth most-recognized name by 70-years-old participants, then Ian Smith would be at or near twentieth position for 50- or 20-years-old participants).[125] This indicates that at least some of the responses in remote memory tests may be the product of recognizing the name from general knowledge rather than from a genuine remote memory. That the hierarchy of recognition is the same for nearly all groups indicates the remarkable consistency with which names are highlighted by the media to which all age groups are exposed.

Not all items in memory are tied to specific events or periods of time. Most facts and items of knowledge are stored independent of experience (e.g. people know that the Second World War occurred between 1939 and 1945 without knowing when or how they learnt this information) and are known collectively as *semantic memory*. At a broad level of judging the quantity of facts a person knows, there is little or no age difference.[126] Furthermore, older and younger adults are equally accurate in *feeling of knowing*; that is, judging whether the answer they give is correct (i.e. the less certain they are that they are correct, the lower the probability that they are correct).[127] These findings are what would be expected from research on crystallized intelligence cited earlier in the chapter. Since older adults lose little or no general knowledge required for crystallized intelligence, so memory for facts should be expected to follow the same pattern. However, just as crystallized intelligence is less well preserved than might first appear (see above), so is semantic memory. Whilst knowledge of previously learnt material is on a par with younger adults, the storage of newly learnt facts is less secure,[102] and for all semantic memories, retrieval of information may be slower and less detailed.[128] Thus, as for crystallized intelligence, semantic memory is only aging-immune if one adopts fairly lax marking criteria.

Older adults are also often unimpaired (at least at a surface level) in *implicit memory* tasks.[129] These measure the ability of a person to recall information which has been previously encountered but which was not explicitly indicated at the time as material to be remembered. Implicit memory is commonly tested by giving people a cognitive task and later testing memory of items which at the time appeared incidental to the task at hand (e.g. the initial task might be to judge a selection of words for level of pleasant feelings evoked; later, recall of these words might be tested). There are no or relatively low age differences when the implicit memory task has a low cognitive load, but age differences tend to increase when the tasks used are made more difficult.[66] In other instances, aging effects have been reported which may be due to differences in the approaches older and younger adults take to psychological tests. In some implicit memory studies, younger participants may realize that the first experiment they are asked to do is in effect a "front" for the real test which will follow, and thus they will try harder to memorize the items they encounter, creating an age difference in implicit memory.[130]

Examples of superiority of older adults' recall in some types of remote, implicit, and semantic memory tasks are, however, exceptions rather than the rule. When presented with new information to memorize, older adults are significantly worse than younger people, whether on standard controlled laboratory studies[109] or in eyewitness testimony of "real life" events.[131] However, this failure of recall is not necessarily as grave as it may first appear. If asked to recall a story or other events with a strong narrative content, then there is typically little difference in memory for the key points of the narrative. In other words, older and younger adults recall the central plot of what they were exposed to with an accuracy roughly equal to that of a younger person. Aging deficits are more likely to occur in relatively peripheral details (e.g. color of the clothes a person was wearing rather than the part the person played in the story). The most plausible explanation for this is once again one of processing space. Older and younger adults both recognize recall of the plot as the prime goal, and relatively peripheral information is picked up if there is sufficient "free" processing space after the plot has been stored in memory. Because younger adults have greater free space, they can store more of the peripheral information and thus have a better overall memory for narrative.[132]

Although LTM is often thought of in terms of memory for the past, it also encompasses memory to perform a particular action in the future (*prospective memory*), because a person must maintain a memory of what has to be done over a considerable period of time before the action can be completed. This also is affected by aging under certain circumstances. When a prospective memory experiment requires a person to remember to phone or otherwise contact an experimenter at a prearranged time and date in the future, there is usually no age difference and indeed older adults may even be better than younger people.[133] The same applies when remembering to adhere to a simulated medication regime requiring people to take their "medicine" at specific times of the day over two periods of seven days each.[134] This may be due to cohort effects. First, there is a potential difference in upbringing: many older adults were raised to be punctual for appointments, a piece of etiquette not quite so rigidly implanted in many people in their teens and twenties (the typical ages of the comparison groups used). Second, there is a potential difference in lifestyle: older adults generally have less busy lives, and accordingly are less likely to be distracted into forgetting appointments.

However, the direction of the age difference is reversed when another method of assessing prospective memory is used. In this instance, the task requires a participant to remember to do something minutes rather than days or weeks in the future. For example, a person is engaged in doing a series of psychological tasks, but must remember at a particular point in the proceedings (e.g. upon leaving, or when a bell sounds) to perform a particular action (e.g. return a small item such as a pen to the experimenter). In such circumstances, a strong age difference is found.[135] It might be thought that this is another example of the "make the task more complex, and the elderly will suffer" phenomenon, and certainly age differences increase the more complex the task is made;[136] but it must be stressed

that the rise in workload need only be very slight for the age difference to appear (indeed, intelligence test score—a reasonable guide to processing ability—is a relatively poor predictor[137]). For example, Maylor[138] found an aging decline in a task where she asked participants to make judgments on a set of pictures of famous people and included a prospective memory component of asking people to indicate every time a picture of a person wearing spectacles appeared. Another study simply required people to remember to sign a paper at the end of the test session. This implies that prospective memory may be seriously affected by aging once it moves out of the confines of a very well-rehearsed skill of remembering social appointments. However, it can be argued that this is because many of the tests of prospective memory which find age differences are not really tests of prospective memory. Instead, they measure the ability to coordinate a set of different tasks which must be run simultaneously. Thus, in Maylor's task, people are not treating the "indicate people wearing glasses" instruction as a "remember to do this" type of instruction, but more as another component of the ongoing task of judging faces. This is a moot point, and in any case does not remove the practical problem that whatever the proper term for the skill is, older adults are especially disadvantaged at remembering to do something as part of a set of ongoing cognitive tasks.

LTM in later life is thus a curious mixture of the preserved and the decaying. As with STM, not all of this decay is necessarily serious if older people make use of memory aids. Thus, writing down key items to remember (be they new pieces of information or a prompt to do something important in the near future) may remove many of the obstacles created by age-related decline. However, the relative failure to retain new information indicates that, as with STM, there may be situations in which memory decline can have potentially serious consequences (e.g. in learning new skills). This argument must not be overplayed, however, and cannot be used as "proof" that older people are incapable of learning new information. Studies of the acquisition of real-life cognitive skills indicate that older adults will reach criterion levels of learning, even if the training time is slightly longer.[86,139] Also, as for intelligence, there are considerable individual differences in memory skills, and thus some individual older people will show no decline.

So far the memory of older people has been studied from the viewpoint of objective measures of memory skills. However, what do older people know about their own memories? The issue is an important one not least because the state of one's memory is often seen as an indicator of how successfully aging is occurring, which in turn plays upon fears of the severe amnesia of the dementias. The accuracy of older people's self-awareness of their memory skills depends to some extent upon the type of memory skill being considered. It has already been noted that given the task of judging if the answer to a semantic memory question is correct, older people are reasonably accurate and certainly are no worse than younger comparison groups. In other situations, an age difference has been found, but arguably this may be a product of the test methods used. For example, if older people are asked to rate the quality of their memories, then some studies have found that older people report a decline relative to younger people[140,141] whilst others have found the reverse: in other words, the younger adults are the ones who complain more about poor memories.[142] This is probably due to the types of questions given and the choice of test participants. For example, if a study makes older people more aware of the image of later life as a time of decay, then they may present themselves as in a period of decline. Conversely, if people are made to concentrate on the range of activities they undertake, then younger people may report a higher number of incidents of memory failure, because they have busier lives and thus in absolute terms have more memory lapses (even though these may form a smaller proportion of their total mental activity than do the memory lapses in older people's lives). Since self-reports of memory have a generally poor correlation with objective measures of memory,[140,143] the whole issue may be too flawed to merit further consideration. However, it is worth noting that memory self-rating correlates robustly with level of depression.[92]

Causes of memory change

A final aspect of memory to be considered concerns the causes of memory change in later life. It is clear that older adults process, store, and encode information less efficiently than younger people. This has been noted above on several occasions and can be seen encapsulated in the *tip of the tongue* (TOT) phenomenon. This describes the situation familiar to everyone of having a word on the "tip of the tongue" without being able to enunciate it. Typically the number of syllables, the word's general sound (e.g. what rhymes with it) and other features can be identified, but the word itself remains obstinately hidden from the mind's eye. The phenomenon is interesting in its own right, since it indicates that memories for items are stored as a set of components which must be reassembled before they enter conscious awareness. Since TOT states are relatively rare, experimenters must either try to generate them artificially in the laboratory (typically by giving people definitions of rare words and asking them to provide the word) or give participants diaries and hope that over several weeks they: (a) will have some TOT states and (b) will remember to write them down in the diary. Studies have usually found that older adults have more TOTs than younger people.[144] Furthermore, when in the TOT state, older adults can produce fewer features of the word they are trying to retrieve. This implies that memory stores are less robust in older adults. Items can be retrieved less easily from memory; and when only partial information is available, the memory traces may in effect be too faint for the person to interpret them sensibly. Such findings provide more support for the argument that a principal problem with memory in later life is that it operates at a much lower level of fidelity. This in turn points the finger of blame once more at the aging nervous system.

There are several grounds for implying that neurological changes will cause aging deficits in memory. The first, derived from the general slowing hypothesis (see above), is that a decline in processing speed means that information cannot be processed quickly enough before the memory trace fades. This leads to the prediction that memory decline should be associated with a fall in performance on measures known to be heavily reliant on processing speed, such as fluid intelligence and reaction times, and this has been found to be the case.[145] Again, declining processing speed is associated

with a general worsening of neurological functioning. For example, the increase in neural noise created by a thinning of the myelin sheath will in itself cause a considerable loss in the fidelity of signals and storage.[146] Likewise, the decline may be associated with a failure to inhibit earlier memories and/or irrelevant information from intruding into current memory processes (the *inhibition deficit hypothesis*). Although there is some support for this,[109] recent evidence suggests it may be a product of the research methodologies used.[147] A further consideration is the general loss in numbers of neurons. The resulting impoverishment of neural nets means that memory traces cannot be stored as clearly and unambiguously. It should thus once again not be surprising to find a correlation between memory and neurological status, and has already been noted above, researchers have indeed demonstrated this.[73,109]

Furthermore, brain imaging studies have found that patterns of activity in older and younger adults engaged in memory tasks differ significantly.[111] For example, auditory cortical activity (principally, the pattern of N100 responses) differs markedly between young and old adults engaged in an STM task.[148] It has already been noted that age-related loss centered on "memory-sensitive" areas of the brain such as the hippocampus[110] and the frontal lobes[111] is also linked with a decline in memory test scores. Baddeley[106] has plausibly argued that central executive functioning is centered in the frontal lobes. Using a PET scan, Reuter-Lorenx et al.[149] have recently demonstrated that the pattern of frontal lobe activity differs between younger and older adults when performing working-memory tasks. (Specifically, younger adults show left lateralization for verbal tasks and right lateralization for spatial tasks, whilst older adults show bilateral activation on both tasks.) It can thus be reasonably concluded that aging memory is strongly associated with neurological changes.

However, whilst neurological changes are undoubtedly a key factor, they are not the only cause. First, it is apparent that changes in one type of memory are not necessarily predictive of changes in other types.[91] Thus, neurological change does not act uniformly across all kinds of memory, either because the anatomical mechanisms upon which they are preserved are not uniformly affected, or because different memory skills are subject to different levels of compensation. Second, several studies have indicated that a significant proportion of memory changes may be attributable to chronological age rather than a specific measure. Third, even relatively mild sensory changes, such as slight hearing loss, can act as a significant handicap in verbal memory tasks.[150] This indicates that the predictive strength of a neural explanation may be less than originally presumed. A possible solution to this is that there is a more accurate measure of memory waiting to be discovered, or that a proportion of aging change is attributable to a myriad of minor causes which in tandem are best explained as "general aging."

PROBLEMS IN TESTING OLDER ADULTS' COGNITIVE SKILLS

The evidence surveyed so far has presented a picture of wholesale decline, interspersed with an occasional preservation of a skill (often relatively minor). However, these studies of aging cognitive change are predicated on assumptions which are at times questionable. First, there is the issue of what should be classified as "normal" aging. Throughout this chapter, it has been assumed that, following standard practice, "normal" refers to older people with no discernible mental illness, and whose physical health is typical of their age group. This creates potential distortions. In younger age groups, excluding people with mental illnesses likely to interfere with cognitive function, removes a small proportion of the population. However, excluding older adults with dementia, severe depression, etc., removes much larger proportions and these increase the older the sample considered (e.g. about a quarter of people aged over eighty[151]). Thus, "normal" aging can under certain circumstances be a misnomer, since the term usually carries the implicit meaning of "typical of the overwhelming majority." However, the older the sample considered, the more this definition is stretched.

Problems with overselectivity of who is tested do not end with the barring of the mentally ill, and just as there are problems of exclusion, so there are also problems of inclusion. Older adults are usually accepted as participants if their physical health is reasonably typical of their age. This means that probabilistically, the older the group, the higher the proportion of, inter alia, cardiovascular complaints, rheumatism, arthritis, cancers, etc. Since it has already been established that physical health is strongly correlated with preservation of intelligence, it follows from this that older groups will be automatically carrying a greater handicap and that in effect a cohort effect is built in to the research being conducted. This is very difficult to control for. Attempting statistically to remove effects presupposes that the full effect of illness can be gauged objectively. The alternative of choosing only participants who are A1 fit is perhaps more unsatisfactory because they are highly unlikely to be representative of a typical older person, not only in health but also in lifestyle, behavior, and so forth. Electing to exclude participants suffering from some illnesses but not others smacks of indecision and implies a prejudgment that only certain kinds of illness can have a major effect. In short, the researcher is presented with a paradox: exclude participants and the sample is unrepresentative, but include participants and there are almost certainly uncontrollable cohort effects.[5,66]

Problems also exist in the general assumptions about the function of aging. Research in cognitive aging has often been remarkably unconcerned about how the observed changes might fit in to a general framework of lifespan development. Models such as general slowing or age times complexity have been concerned with explaining change in terms of decline from a youthful level which by default is considered the optimal state. Even "successful aging" is often seen in terms of maintaining a youthful level of performance, not in the creation of an identity specific to later life. Our view of normal aging is thus shaped by several key questions:

- What is the extent and nature of the decline?
- Can the decline be ameliorated?
- What are the causes of the decline?
- Can the decline be explained in terms of a model?

Few would dispute these as a rather bland description of the field's key aims. However, underlying this is a deeper supposition that the decline in normal cognition is automatically a cause for concern and something which older people are trying to fight, or if not, should be trying to fight. If the decline in cognitive skills in later life were felt to be of little or no consequence, then quite simply the vast scholarly activity which has been devoted to the subject would never have occurred. However, *why* should the whole issue of decline be given the importance it has? First, it is apparent that normal cognitive decline is just that: it is not the inevitable precursor of dementia. Second, although it is apparent that older adults are concerned about cognitive changes as they age,[152] it is often unclear whether they are concerned about relatively minor senescent changes per se, or whether they are fearful they are harbingers of dementia. Third, changes on laboratory tasks are not necessarily sound predictors of real-life change. Certainly there have been studies which have demonstrated that level of self-esteem and self-rating of memory skills are related.[92] However, at least part of the connection between self-esteem and perceived worsening of performance may be attributable to other factors, such as belief in stereotypes about aging.[152] Again, it has been noted that laboratory test performances of two standard deviations below the mean of younger adults do not appear to be translated into a decline in "real life" skills of commensurate importance. Older adults who perform "badly" on laboratory tasks can leave the test center, do their weekly shopping without being defrauded by unscrupulous shopkeepers, and return home without spending several hours wandering the streets aimlessly before finding their house.

The discrepancy between severe decline on basic skills and relatively slight decline in everyday functioning can be readily explained by two factors: first, compensation, and second, the fact that most everyday tasks are relatively simple and designed so that they can be accomplished by people with a wide variety of cognitive abilities. Perhaps because of these, the decline in cognitive skills may be of less concern to older people than it is to some geropsychologists. To pursue this argument: for most people, a relatively small drop in scores on psychometric tests may be of small concern. As was noted above, people with a low need for cognition tend to lose intellectual skills faster. If this is so, then perhaps the "decline" in normal cognition is less a "failure" than an abnegation of skills which no longer need to be maintained to the same degree. The physical changes associated with normal cognitive aging, such as declining reaction times and sensory acuity, will also contribute to these changes, perhaps acting as an accelerant. However, this hypothesis cannot be sustained given the current evidence. Aging changes may be guided by lifestyle, but it is hard to prove or disprove that lifestyle is not in turn shaped by more basic cognitive skills.

As stated at the beginning of this chapter, normal cognitive aging provides a simple overall picture (to paraphrase, "on the whole, things get worse") but this hides a plethora of explanations. This should not be surprising. Since it is difficult enough to identify the causes of intellectual attainment in teenagers,[4] why should we expect simple answers in considering people with a further 50 or more years' exposure to environmental influences, changes in physiology, etc.? Current research has identified a plausible collection of factors which probably in tandem account for a great deal of aging change. But to claim that any alone is the prime mover is, based on present evidence, probably untenable.

KEY POINTS   Normal cognitive aging

- The classic aging curve consists of rise, plateau, and fall.

- Aging studies are prone to the cohort effect.

- Longitudinal studies have established that the fall begins in the mid-sixties for most skills.

- There is increased individual variability in later life.

- Some aspects of intelligence (notably crystallized skills) are better preserved than others.

- Wisdom is not a prerogative of later life.

- Creativity typically declines in later life; there may be strong cohort effects.

- Attention declines on most forms of the skill, probably for a group of reasons.

- Causes of intellectual decline are largely polarized around disuse and general slowing models.

- Proof for general slowing includes the Brinley plot, but there is evidence that it oversimplifies.

- Cognitive changes are strongly *associated* with general changes in brain anatomy and function.

- Proof for disuse theory includes compensation and effects of training, but still some age effects.

- Caveats include: problems with choice of tests; possibility of alternative methods of thinking.

- STM shows stronger aging effects the more complex the task.

- Working memory decline indicates potentially severe "real life" consequences.

- Generally, LTM skills decline the more the task requires the use of new or ongoing information.

- Causes of memory decline are strongly associated with general neurological changes.

- Findings are shaped by inclusion/exclusion of "normal" aging participants.

- What constitutes "normal" aging is not clear-cut.

- Aging cognitive change may be a product of changing needs rather than a "decline."

REFERENCES

1. Thompson DN: Contributions to the history of psychology: CVIII. On aging and intelligence: history teaches a different lesson. Percept Motor Skills 1997;85:28–30

2. Bayley N: Behavioral correlates of mental growth: birth to thirty-six years. Am Psychol 1968;23:1–17

3. Schaie KW, Hertzog C: Toward a comprehensive model of adult intellectual development: contributions of the Seattle Longitudinal Study. In Sternberg RJ (ed): Advances in Human Intelligence, vol. 3. Erlbaum, Hillsdale, NJ, 1986:79–118

4. Sternberg RJ, Wagner RK, Williams WM, Horvath JA: Testing common sense. Am Psychol 1995;50:912–927

5. Stuart-Hamilton I: Intellectual changes in late life. In Woods RT (ed): Psychological Problems of Ageing. John Wiley, Chichester, 1999:27–47

6. Owens WA: Is age kinder to the initially more able? J Gerontol 1959;14:334–337

7. Purdue U: Age and mental abilities: a second adult follow-up. J Educ Psychol 1966;57:311–325

8. Schaie KW: The Seattle Longitudinal Study: a 21-year exploration of psychometric intelligence in adulthood. In Schaie KW (ed): Longitudinal Studies of Adult Psychological Development. Guilford Press, NY, 1983:64–135

9. Schaie KW: The course of adult intellectual development. Am Psychol 1994;49:304–313

10. Eysenck HJ, Kamin L: The Intelligence Controversy. John Wiley, New York, 1981

11. Kail R, Pelligrino JW: Human Intelligence: Perspectives and Prospects. Freeman, San Francisco, 1985

12. Cattell RB: Abilities: Their Structure, Growth and Action. Houghton Mifflin, Boston, 1971

13. Horn JL: Human ability systems. In Baltes PB (ed): Life-span Development and Behavior, vol. 1. Academic Press, New York, 1978:211–256

14. Horn JL: The theory of fluid and crystallised intelligence in relation to concepts of cognitive psychology and aging in adulthood. In Craik FIM, Trehub S (eds): Aging and Cognitive Processes. Plenum, New York, 1982

15. Horn JL, Cattell RB: Age differences in fluid and crystallised intelligence. Acta Psychol 1967;26:107–129

16. Cunningham WR, Clayton V, Overton W: Fluid and crystallised intelligence in young adulthood and old age. J Gerontol 1975;30:53–55

17. Hayslip B, Sterns HL: Age differences in relationships between crystallised and fluid intelligence and problem solving. J Gerontol 1979;34:404–414

18. Emery CF, Pedersen NL, Svartengren M, McClearn GE: Longitudinal and genetic effects in the relationship between pulmonary function and cognitive performance. J Gerontol B 1998;53:311–317

19. Storandt M: Speed and coding effects in relation to age and ability level. Develop Psychol 1976;2:177–178

20. Storandt M, Futterman A: Stimulus size and performance on two subtests of the Wechsler Adult Intelligence Scale by younger and older adults. J Gerontol 1982;37:602–603

21. Rabbitt PMA: Memory impairment in the elderly. In Bebbington PE, Jacoby R (eds): Psychiatric Disorders in the Elderly. Mental Health Foundation, London, 1984;101–119

22. Botwinick J, Storandt M: Vocabulary ability in later life. J Geriatr Psychol 1974;125:303–308

23. Carswell LM, Graves RE, Snow WG, Tierney MC: Postdicting verbal IQ of elderly individuals. J Clin Exper Neuropsychol 1997;19:914–921

24. Kleemeier RW: Intellectual changes in the senium. Proc Soc Stat Sect Am Stat Assoc 1962;1:290–295

25. White N, Cunningham WR: Is terminal drop pervasive or specific? J Gerontol 1988;43:141–144

26. Rabbitt PMA: Does it all go together when it goes? Qtly J Exper Psychol 1993;46A:385–434

27. Morse CK: Does variability increase with age? An archival study of cognitive measures. Psychol Aging 1993;8:156–164

28. Sternberg RJ: Cognitive Psychology. Harcourt Brace, Fort Worth, 1996

29. Staudinger UM, Lopez DF, Baltes PB: The psychometric location of wisdom-related performance: Intelligence, personality and more? Personal Soc Psychol Bull 1997;23:1200–1214

30. Staudinger UM, Maciel AG, Smith J, Baltes PB: What predicts wisdom-related performance? A first look at personality, intelligence and facilitative experiential contexts. Eur J Personal 1998;12:1–17

31. Alpaugh PK, Birren JR: Variables affecting creative contributions across the adult life span. Hum Devel 1977;20:240–248

32. McCrae RR, Arneberg D, Costa PT: Declines in divergent thinking with age: cross-sectional, longitudinal, and cross-sequential analyses. Psychol Aging 1987;2:130–137

33. Simonton DK: Creativity and wisdom in aging. In Birren JW, Schaie KW (eds): Handbook of the Psychology of Aging, 3rd edn. Academic Press, San Diego, 1990

34. Hendricks J: Creativity over the life course: a call for a rational perspective. Int J Aging Hum Devel 1999;48:85–111

35. Sasser-Coen JR: Qualitative changes in creativity in the second half of life: a life-span developmental perspective. J Creat Behav 1993;27:18–27

36. Rebok GW: Life-span Cognitive Development. Holt, Rinehart & Winston, New York, 1987

37. Salthouse TA: Adult Cognition. Springer, New York, 1982

38. Rabbitt PMA: Some experiments and a model for changes in attentional selectivity with old age. In Hoffmeister F, Muller C (eds): Bayer Symposium VII: Evaluation of Change. Springer, Bonn, 1979

39. Nissen NJ, Corkin S: Effectiveness of attentional cueing in older and younger adults. J Gerontol 1985;40:185–191

40. Walsh DA: The development of visual information processes in adulthood and old age. In Craik FIM, and Trehub S (eds): Aging and Cognitive Processes. Plenum, New York, 1982

41. Albert MS: Cognitive function. In Alvert MS, Moss MB (eds): Geriatric Neuropsychology. Guilford, New York, 1988

42. Dubno JR, Dirk DD, Morgan DE: Effects of age and mild hearing loss on speech recognition in noise. J Acoust Soc Am 1984;76:87–96

43. Murphy DR, McDowd JM, Wilcox KA: Inhibition and aging: similarities between younger and older adults as revealed by the processing of unattended auditory information. Psychol Aging 1999;14:44–59

44. Salthouse TA: Adult Cognition. Springer, New York, 1985

45. Woodruff-Pak DS: The Neuropsychology of Aging. Blackwell, Oxford, 1997

46. Lowe C, Rabbitt P: Cognitive models of ageing and frontal lobe deficits. In Rabbitt P (ed): Methodology of Frontal and Executive Function. Taylor & Francis, Hove, 1997:39–59

47. Birren JE, Fisher LM: Aging and speed of behavior: possible consequences for psychological functioning. Ann Rev Psychol 1995;46:329–353

48. Kermis MD: The Psychology of Human Aging: Theory, Research and Practice. Allyn & Bacon, Boston, 1983

49. Ferraro FR, Moody J: Consistent and inconsistent performance in young and elderly adults. Develop Neuropsychol 1996;12:429–441

50. Hertzog C: Aging, information processing speed, and intelligence. In Schaie KW, Lawton P (eds): Annu Rev Gerontol Geriatr 1991;11:55–79

51. Rabbitt PMA, Goward L: Effects of age and raw IQ test scores on mean correct and mean error reaction times in serial choice tasks: a reply to Smith and Brewer. Br J Psychol 1986;77:69–73

52. Bashore TR, Ridderinkhof KR, van der Molen MW: The decline of cognitive processing speed in old age. Curr Direct Psychol Sci 1997;6:163–169

53. Baltes PB, Lindenberger U: Emergence of a powerful connection between sensory and cognitive functions across the adult life span: a new window to the study of cognitive aging? Psychol Aging 1997;12:12–21

54. Botwinick J: Cognitive Processes in Maturity and Old Age. Springer, New York, 1967

55. Brinley JF: Cognitive sets, speed and accuracy in the elderly. In Welford AT, Birren JE (eds): Behavior, Aging and the Nervous System. Springer, New York, 1965

56. Cerella J: Information processing rate in the elderly. Psychol Bull 1985;98:67–83

57. Cerella J: Aging and information processing rate. In Birren JE, Schaie KW (eds): Handbook of the Psychology of Aging, 3rd edn. Academic Press, San Diego, 1990

58. Rabbitt PMA: Speed of processing and ageing. In Woods R (ed) Handbook of the Clinical Psychology of Ageing. John Wiley, Chichester, 1996;59–72

59. Ratcliff R, Spieler D, McKoon G: Explicitly modelling the effects of aging on response time. Psychonom Bull Rev 2000;7:1–25

60. Sliwinsky M, Hall CB: Constraints on general slowing: a meta-analysis using hierarchical linear models with random coefficients. Psychol Aging 1998;13:164–175

61. Rabbitt PMA: A fresh look at reaction times in old age. In Stein DG (ed): The Psychology of Ageing: Problems and Perspectives. Elsevier, New York, 1980

62. Rabbitt PMA: The faster the better? Some comments on the use of information processing rate as an index of change in individual differences in performance. In Hindmarch I, Aufdembrinke B, and Ott H (eds): Psychopharmacology and Reaction Time. John Wiley, London, 1988

63. Rabbitt PMA: Does fast last? Is speed a basic factor determining individual differences in memory? In Gruneberg MM, Morris PE, Sykes RN (eds): Practical Aspects of Memory, vol. 2. John Wiley, Chichester, 1988

64. Rabbitt PMA: Measurement indices, functional characteristics, and psychometric constructs in cognitive aging. In Perfect TJ, Maylor EA (eds): Models of Cognitive Aging. Oxford University Press, Oxford, 2000:160–187

65. Perfect TJ, Maylor EA: Rejecting the dull hypothesis: the relation between method and theory in cognitive aging research. In Perfect TJ, Maylor EA (eds): Models of Cognitive Aging. Oxford University Press, Oxford, 2000:1–18

66. Stuart-Hamilton I: The Psychology of Ageing: An Introduction, 3rd edn. Jessica Kingsley Publishers, London, 2000

67. Ansley KJ, Luszcz MA, Sanchez L: A reevaluation of the common factor theory of shared variance among age, sensory function, and cognitive function in older adults. J Gerontol B 2001;56:3–11

68. Verhaeghen P: The parallels in beauty's brow: time–accuracy functions and their implications for cognitive aging theories. In Perfect TJ, Maylor EA (eds): Models of Cognitive Aging. Oxford University Press, Oxford, 2000:50–86

69. Fisher DL, Duffy SA, Katsikopoulos KV: Cognitive slowing among older adults: what kind and how much? Perfect TJ, Maylor EA (eds): Models of Cognitive Aging. Oxford University Press, Oxford, 2000:87–124

70. Salthouse TA: Aging and measures of processing speed. Biol Psychol 2000;54:35–54

71. Coffey CE, Saxton JA, Ratcliff G, Bryan RN, Lucke JF: Relation of education to brain size in normal aging: implications for the reserve hypothesis. Neurology 1999;53:189–196

72. Schaie KW, Schaie JP: Clinical assessment and aging. In Birren JE, Schaie KW (eds): Handbook of the Psychology of Aging. Van Nostrand Reinhold, New York, 1977:692–723

73. Kaszniak AW, Newman MC: Toward a neuropsychology of cognitive aging. In Qualls SH, Abeles N (eds): Psychology and the Aging Revolution. American Psychological Association, Washington, DC, 2000:43–67

74. Mttenberg W, Seidenberg M, O'Leary DS, DiGiulio DV: Changes in cerebral functioning associated with normal aging. J Clin Exper Neuropsychol 1989;11:918–932

75. Chao LL, Knight RT: Prefrontal deficits in attention and inhibitory control with aging. Cerebral Cortex 1997;7:63–69

76. Isingrini M, Vazou F: Relation between fluid intelligence and frontal lobe functioning in older adults. Int J Aging Hum Develop 1997;45:99–109

77. Duncan J, Emslie H, Williams P, Johnson R, Freer C: Intelligence and the frontal lobe: the organization of goal-directed behavior. Cognit Psychol 1996;30:257–303

78. Robbins TW, James M, Owen AM, Sahakian BJ, Lawrence AD, Mcinnes L, Rabbitt PMA: A study of performance on tests from the CANTAB battery sensitive to frontal lobe dysfunction in a large sample of normal volunteers: implications for theories of executive functioning and cognitive aging. J Int Neuropsychol Soc 1998;4:474–490

79. Foster JK, Black SE, Buck BH, Bronskill MJ: Ageing and executive functions: a neuroimaging perspective. In Rabbitt P (ed): Methodology of Frontal and Executive Function. Taylor & Francis, Hove, 1997:117–134

80. Salthouse T, Fristoe N, Rhee SH: How localized are age-related effects on neuropsychological measures? Neuropsychology 1996;10:272–285

81. Plemons JK, Willis SL, Baltes PB: Modifiability of fluid intelligence in aging: a short-term longitudinal training approach. J Gerontol 1978;33:224–231

82. McEvoy GM, Cascio WF: Cumulative evidence of the relationship between employee age and job performance. J Appl Psychol 1989;74:11–17

83. Charness N: Memory for chess positions: resistance to interference. J Exper Psychol Hum Learn Mem 1976;2:641–653

84. Charness N: Components of skill in bridge. Can J Psychol 1979;33:1–16

85. Charness N: Aging and skilled problem solving. J Exper Psychol: General 1981;110:21–38

86. Charness N: Can acquired knowledge compensate for age-related declines in cognitive efficiency? In Qualls SH, Abeles N (eds): Psychology and the Aging Revolution. American Psychological Association, Washington, DC, 2000:99–117

87. Salthouse TA: Effects of age and skill in typing. J Exper Psychol: General 1984;13:345–371

88. Bosman EA: Age-related differences in motoric aspects of transcription typing skill. Psychol Aging 1993;8:87–102

89. Salthouse TA, Babcock RL, Skovronek E, Mitchell DR, Palmon R: Age and experience effects in spatial visualization. Develop Psychol 1990;26:128–136

90. Salthouse TA: Reasoning and spatial abilities. In Craik FIM, Salthouse TA (eds): The Handbook of Aging and Cognition. Lawrence Erlbaum, Hillsdale, NJ, 1992

91. Herman DJ, Rea A, Andrzejewski S: The need for a new approach to memory training. In Gruneberg MM, Morris PE, Sykes RN (eds): Practical Aspects of Memory: Current Research and Issues. John Wiley, Chichester, 1988

92. Collins MW, Abeles N: Subjective memory complaints and depression in the able elderly. Clin Gerontol 1996;16:29–54

93. Sternberg RJ, Wagner RK, Williams WM, Horvath JA: Testing common sense. Am Psychol 1995;50:912–927

94. McDonald L, Stuart-Hamilton I: The meaning of life: animism in the classificatory skills of older adults. Int J Aging Hum Develop 2000;51:1–12

95. Piaget J: The Origins of Intelligence in Children. International Universities Press, New York, 1952

96. Smith L: Jean Piaget: Critical Assessments. Routledge, London, 1992

97. Papalia DE: The status of several conservation abilities across the life-span. Hum Develop 1972;15:229–243

98. McDonald L, Stuart-Hamilton I: Older and more moral? Age related changes in performance on Piagetian moral reasoning tasks. Age Ageing 1996;25:402–404

99. Stuart-Hamilton I, McDonald L: Do we need intelligence? Some reflections on the importance of g. Educ Gerontol 2001;27:399–407

100. Blackburn JA, Papalia DE: The study of adult cognition from a Piagetian perspective. In Sternberg RJ, Berg C (eds): Intellectual Development. Cambridge University Press, Cambridge, 1992

101. Baddeley AD: Memory. Lawrence Erlbaum, London, 1995

102. Craik FIM, Anderson ND, Kerr SA, Li KZH: Memory changes in normal ageing. In Baddeley AD, Wilson BA, Watts FN (eds): Handbook of Memory Disorders. John Wiley, Chichester, 1995:211–242

103. Bromley DB: Some effects of age on short-term learning and memory. J Gerontol 1958;13:398–406

104. Morris RG, Gick ML, Craik FIM: Processing resources and age differences in working memory. Mem Cognit 1988;16:362–366

105. Baddeley AD, Hitch G: Working memory. In Bower GH (ed): Attention and Performance, vol. 6. Academic Press, New York, 1974.

106. Baddeley AD: Working Memory. Oxford Science, Oxford, 1986

107. Morris RG, Craik FIM, Gick ML: Age differences in working memory tasks: the role of secondary memory and the central executive system. Qtly J Exper Psychol 1990;42A:67–86

108. Salthouse TA: Theoretical Perspectives on Cognitive Aging. Lawrence Erlbaum, Hillsdale, NJ, 1991

109. Light LL: Memory changes in adulthood. In Qualls SH, Abeles N (eds): Psychology and the Aging Revolution. American Psychological Association, Washington, DC, 2000:73–98

110. West RL: An application of prefrontal cortex function theory to cognitive aging. Psychol Bull 1996;120:272–292

111. Cabeza R, Anderson ND, Houle S, Mangels JA, Nyberg L: Age-related differences in neural activity during item and temporal-order memory retrieval: a positron emission tomography study. J Cognit Neurosci 2000;12:197–206

112. Belmont JM, Freeseman LJ, Mitchell DW: Memory and problem solving: the cases of young and elderly adults. In Gruneberg MM, Morris PE, Sykes RN (eds): Practical Aspects of Memory, vol. 2. John Wiley, Chichester, 1988

113. Lindenberger U, Kliel R, Baltes PB: Professional expertise does not eliminate age differences in imagery-based memory performance during adulthood. Psychol Aging 1992;7:585–593

114. Parkin A, Walter BM: Recollective experience, normal aging, and frontal dysfunction. Psychol Aging 1992;7:290–298

115. Kemper S: Life-span changes in syntactic complexity. J Gerontol 1987;42:323–328

116. Kemper S: Adults' diaries: changes to written narratives across the life span. Presented at a Conference on Social Psychology and Language, 20–24 July, 1987

117. Kemper S: Geriatric psycholinguistics: syntactic limitations of oral and written language. In Light LL, Burke DM (eds): Language, Memory and Aging. Cambridge University Press, New York, 1988

118. Cohen G: Memory and the Real World. Lawrence Erlbaum, Hove, 1989

119. Rubin DC, Rahhal TA, Poon LW: Things learned in early adulthood are remembered best. Mem Cognit 1998;26:3019

120. Rabbitt PMA, Winthorpe C: What do old people remember? The Galton paradigm reconsidered. In Gruneberg MM, Morris PE, Sykes RN (eds): Practical Aspects of Memory, vol. 2. John Wiley, Chichester, 1988

121. Nigro G, Neisser U: Point of view in personal memories. Cognit Psychol 1983;15:465–482

122. Winthorpe C, Rabbitt PMA: Working memory capacity, IQ, age and the ability to recount autobiographical events. In Gruneberg MM, Morris PE, Sykes RN (eds): Practical Aspects of Memory, vol. 2. John Wiley, Chichester, 1988

123. Craik FIM: Age differences in human memory. In Birren JE, Schaie KW (eds): Handbook of the Psychology of Aging. Van Nostrand Reinhold, New York, 1977

124. Ribot T: Disorders of Memory. Kegan, Paul, Tench and Co., London, 1882

125. Stuart-Hamilton I, Perfect T, Rabbitt P: Remembering who was who. In Gruneberg MM, Morris PE, Sykes RN (eds): Practical Aspects of Memory, vol. 2. John Wiley, Chichester, 1988

126. Sharps MJ: Age-related change in visual information processing: toward a unified theory of aging and visual memory. Curr Psychol 1998;16:284–307

127. Fozard JL: The time for remembering. In Poon LC (ed): Aging in the 1980s: Psychological Issues. American Psychological Association, Washington, DC, 1980

128. Kozora E, Cullum CM: Generative naming in normal aging: total output and qualitative changes using phonemic and semantic constraints. Clin Neuropsychol 1995;9:313–320

129. Gaudreau D, Peretz I: Implicit and explicit memory for music in old and young adults. Brain Cognit 1999;40:126–129

130. Park DC, Shaw RJ: Effect of environmental support on implicit and explicit memory in younger and older adults. Psychol Aging 1992;7:632–642

131. Yarmey AD, Yarmey MJ: Eyewitness recall and duration estimates in field settings. J Appl Soc Psychol 1997;27:330–344

132. Meyer BJF: Reading comprehension and aging. In Schaie KW (ed): Annual Review of Gerontology and Geriatrics, vol. 7. Springer, New York, 1987

133. Maylor EA: Age and prospective memory. Qtly J Exper Psychol 1990; 42A:471–493

134. Rendell PG, Thomson DM: The effect of ageing on remembering to remember: an investigation of simulated medication regimes. Austr J Ageing 1993;12:11–18

135. Cockburn J, Smith PT: Effects of age and intelligence on everyday memory tasks. In Gruneberg MM, Morris PE, Sykes RN (eds): Practical Aspects of Memory, vol. 2. John Wiley, Chichester, 1988

136. Einstein GO, McDaniel MA, Guynn MJ: Age-related deficits in prospective memory: the influence of task complexity. Psychol Aging 1992;7:471–478

137. Maylor EA: Aging and forgetting in prospective and retrospective memory tasks. Psychol Aging 1993;8:410–428

138. Maylor EA: Changes in event-based prospective memory across adulthood. Aging Neuropsychol Cognit 1998;5:107–128

139. McDonald L: Learning aptitude in later life. In Glendenning F, Stuart-Hamilton I (eds): Learning and Cognition in Later Life. Arena, Aldershot, 1995:95–113

140. Perlmutter M: What is memory aging the aging of? Develop Psychol 1978;14:330–345

141. Ponds RW, Van Boxtel MP, Jolles J: Age-related changes in subjective cognitive functioning. Educ Gerontol 2000;26:67–81

142. Rabbitt PMA, Abson V: "Lost and found": some logical and methodological limitations of self-report questionnaires as tools to study cognitive ageing. Br J Psychol 1990;81:1–16

143. Herrman DJ: Questionnaires about memory. In Harris JE, Morris PE (eds): Everyday Memory, Actions and Absentmindedness. Academic Press, London, 1984

144. Cohen G, Faulkner D: Memory for proper names: age differences in retrieval. Br J Develop Psychol 1986;4:187–197

145. Salthouse TA: The processing-speed theory of adult age differences in cognition. Psychol Rev 1996;103:403–428

146. Myerson J, Ferraro FR, Hale S, Lima SD: General slowing in semantic priming and word recognition. Psychol Aging, 1992;7:257–270

147. Grant JD, Dagenbach D: Further considerations regarding inhibitory processes, working memory, and cognitive aging. Am J Psychol 2000;113:69–94

148. Golob EJ, Starr A: Age-related qualitative differences in auditory cortical responses during short-term memory. Clin Neurophysiol 2000;111:2234–2244

149. Reuter-Lorenz PA, Jonides J, Smith EE, Hartley A, Miller A, Marshuetz C, Koeppe RA: Age differences in the frontal lateralization of verbal and spatial working memory revealed by PET. J Cognit Neurosci 2000;12:174–187

150. Van Boxtel MPJ, Van Beijsterveldt CEM, Houx PJ, Anteunis LJC, Metsemakers JFM, Jolles J: Mild hearing impairment can reduce verbal memory performance in a healthy adult population. J Clin Exper Neuropsychol 2000;22:47–154

151. White LR, Cartwright WS, Cornoni-Huntley J, Brock DB: Geriatric epidemiology. In Einsdorfer C (ed): Annual Review of Gerontology and Geriatrics, vol. 6. Springer, New York, 1986

152. Ward R: The impact of subjective age and stigma on older persons. J Gerontol 1977; 32:227–232

Chapter 13

The aging personality and self: diversity and health issues

Rebecca S. Allen, Douglas L. Welsh,
Sherry L. Willis, and K. Warner Schaie

Personality may be defined as the pattern of thoughts, feelings, and behaviors that shape an individual's interface with the world, distinguish one person from another, and manifest across time and situations.[1–3] Personality is impacted by biological, cognitive, and environmental determinants, including the impact of culture and cohort. Theoretical approaches to personality are as varied as the breadth of the construct they attempt to describe and explain. Yet each approach, to varying degrees, emphasizes stability and change within individuals across time and situations.

The impact of personality across the adult lifespan touches every domain: personal, professional, spiritual, and physical. Some current theories of the regulation of interpersonal relations allude to the possibility that perception of the time remaining to live may have direct influence on behavior. Certainly, personality characteristics have direct and indirect influences on health status, health behaviors, and behavioral interactions with healthcare professionals. Although no single chapter can adequately condense such rich, empirical study, we will attempt to provide a concise overview of stage models, trait theory, and social–cognitive approaches to personality. We will focus on aspects of personality development among cognitively intact older adults, not personality changes that may ensue as the result of dementia. For an overview of social relations research, including social networks, social support, and sense of control, we refer the reader to Antonucci.[4]

In each section of this chapter we provide an overview of classic as well as the most current research on stability and maturational and environmental change within adult personality. The focus is on longitudinal data. Second, we include cross-cultural comparisons of adult personality where available. This focus provides a unique contribution to recent reviews of adult personality and aging.[4,5] Third, we examine the health correlates of adult personality, focusing on morbidity and mortality, well-being, life satisfaction, positive and negative affect, anxiety, and depression. Finally, we discuss measurement issues and provide examples of current assessment instruments.

PERSONALITY STAGES AND EGO DEVELOPMENT

Freudian theory

The psychoanalytic approach to adult personality development has its roots in the theories of Sigmund Freud. His theories encompass four domains: level of consciousness, personality structure, defense mechanisms, and stages of psychosexual

development.[6,7] Freudian theory postulates that adult personality is made up of three aspects: (a) the id, operating on the pleasure principle generally within the unconscious; (b) the ego, operating on the reality principle within the conscious realm; and (c) the superego, operating on the morality principle at all levels of consciousness. The interplay of these personality structures generates anxiety that must be reduced through various defense mechanisms (Table 13-1). These mechanisms act to obscure the true, anxiety-laden reasons for one's behavior. Freud's theory of psychosexual development begins in infancy with the oral stage and progresses through the toddler years and the anal stage, with toilet training being the primary developmental challenge. Children then enter the phallic stage of development from age 4 to age 7 or 8. During this stage, boys must resolve the Oedipal complex and girls must resolve the Electra complex, erotic attachment to the

---

Table 13-1 The most common defense mechanisms postulated by Freud

- *Denial.* Refusing to perceive an unacceptable reality
- *Intellectualization.* Avoiding negative affect by focusing on logic and reason
- *Overcompensation.* Emphasizing desirable characteristics as a means to hide perceived weaknesses
- *Acting out.* Engaging in excessive, socially undesirable behavior as a means of garnering attention
- *Splitting.* Reacting to others in an "all good" or "all bad" manner without taking their full character into consideration
- *Repression.* Preventing undesirable or dangerous thoughts from entering consciousness
- *Projection.* Attributing one's own unacceptable behavior, emotions, or motives to others
- *Reaction formation.* Exaggerated behavior seemingly opposite to one's true feelings
- *Displacement.* Releasing hostile feelings on safe objects other than the threatening objects arousing the hostile feelings
- *Rationalization.* Developing reasonable excuses for one's unworthy behaviors
- *Regression.* Retreating to an earlier developmental stage involving less responsibility and mature behavior
- *Sublimation.* Using frustrated sexual energy in the service of substitute, socially acceptable activities
- *Identification.* Raising one's self-esteem by affiliating with a prestigious person or institution
- *Fixation.* Arresting emotional development by attaching oneself in a dependent way to another person

Source: Adapted from Phares and Chaplin.[3]

opposite-sex parent and resulting jealousy of the same-sex parent. Freud believed personality development to be essentially complete by adolescence, when individuals progress from the latency to the genital stage of psychosexual development.

Although seminal in the expansion of our understanding of the human psyche, Freud's specific theories receive little attention in the scientific study of personality today.[6] Freud proposed his theories of development based on an extremely limited sample of affluent, verbal Viennese women presenting to him for psychotherapy. His theories are resistant to scientific inquiry in that they frequently lead to nonspecific hypotheses, wherein failure to find expected effects may simply be due to unknown defense mechanisms. Feminist theorists from Karen Horney to Carol Gilligan have taken issue with Freud's ideas about women and penis envy.[3,8,9] Additionally, having postulated that personality development essentially ends in adolescence, Freud's theories have limited applicability to the fields of gerontology and geriatric medicine.

Post-Freudian theorists

In contrast, some post-Freudian theorists have conceptualized personality development as a continuing process focused on current interpersonal and/or family-of-origin issues as the source of individual distress and coping patterns. Carl Jung was one of the first to propose that, as individuals age, they achieve a balance between the expression of their masculine characteristics (animus) and feminine characteristics (anima).[10,11] Findings regarding increased balance of gender roles with age have emerged in different cultures around the world, lending some support to Jung's hypothesis.[2]

In a series of studies validating a projective sentence-completion test, Jane Loevinger identified six stages of adult personality development: conformist, conscientious-conformist, conscientious, individualistic, autonomous, and integrated.[12,13] Cross-sectional and longitudinal work shows that these stages have modest correlations with chronological age.[2] Loevinger proposed that adult development depends on changes in four areas: character (i.e. goals and values), interpersonal style, conscious preoccupation, and cognitive style. Her ego development score has been found to be associated with measures of openness in coping style and resolving social dilemmas.[14,15]

Erik Erikson's stages of psychosocial development are perhaps the best known of the stage theories of adult personality. The sequence of Erikson's eight stages of development is based on the epigenetic principle, which means that the growing personality moves through these stages in an ordered fashion at an appropriate rate.[3,16] Two of the eight stages describe personality change during the adult years. From age 25 to 65 the individual is focused on *generativity versus stagnation*. In this stage, individuals seek ways to give of their talents and experiences to the next generation, moving beyond the self-concerns of identity and the interpersonal concerns of intimacy.[5] Successful resolution of this stage results in the development of a sense of trust and care for the next generation and the assurance that society will continue. Unsuccessful resolution of this stage results in self-absorption.

Ego integrity versus despair is Erikson's final stage of ego development, beginning around age 65 and continuing until death. In this stage, individuals become increasingly internally focused and more aware of the nearness of death. Successful resolution of this stage results in being able to look back on one's life and find meaning, developing a sense of wisdom before death. Alternatively, meaninglessness and despair can ensue if the process of life review results in focus on primarily negative outcomes.

Erikson, Erikson, and Kivnick interviewed 29 adults aged 75–95 and found evidence of generativity in a focus on "the future well-being of the world as a whole" (p. 66).[17] In a qualitative review of research concerning religion, personality, and aging, McFadden used the lifespan perspective to argue that most of the world's religions facilitate the development of generativity later in life.[18] McFadden posited that Judaism, Christianity, and Islamic traditions motivate concern for creating a world of justice and mercy for future generations. McFadden also proposed that religion promotes the development of ego integrity by fostering an inward turn via meditative practices and symbolic expressions of the connections between humanity and the sacred.

Difficulties arising from attempts to empirically investigate Erikson's theory include the lack of specification regarding how developmental crises are resolved so that an individual may move from one stage to the next. The insistence that these stages are encountered in an orderly, prespecified sequence by all individuals is also problematic. One 22-year empirical investigation of three cohorts found significant age changes supportive of Erikson's theory.[19] Middle-aged adults expressed emotions and cognitions consistent with successful completion of more psychosocial developmental crises than younger adults. The environmental influences of culture and cohort on adult personality, however, have been minimized. Thus, relatively little empirical research has addressed Erikson's psychosocial stages.[11] More recent theorists postulate that the ego integrity versus despair period initiates a process of life review.[20]

Life review

The exception to this lack of empirical investigation regarding stage theories of adult personality is the research attention given to the concept of life review.[20,21] *Life review* can be thought of as a systematic cognitive–emotional process occurring late in life in which an individual thinks back across his or her life experiences and integrates disparate events into general themes. Although this approach to adult personality development can be conceptualized as a cognitive process in which identity emerges from the story, we have chosen to include it with stage models because it is most frequently described as occurring near the completion of one's life. Nevertheless, it should be acknowledged that individuals likely undergo a process of life review periodically throughout the adult years.

Analytic techniques used to assess the impact and correlates of life review vary from case studies to large, longitudinal investigations of aging.[22,23] Some investigators have found life review to be associated with themes of generativity and ego integrity as ongoing components of self-identity.[21,24] Others have failed to find this association, but have found life review to be negatively associated with death anxiety.[25] Although Coleman and colleagues revealed maintenance of life story themes,[22] there were no differences in tendency to engage in life review between young-old (aged 65–75) and old-old (aged 75+) adults.

In responding to the question "Who am I?," 516 participants of the Berlin Aging Study aged 70–103 revealed central themes of life review, health, and family.[23] Individuals throughout this age range were likely to engage in life review. The focus of self-defining statements was present-oriented; relatively few statements referred to the past or the future. Contrary to expectations, thoughts about death and dying were rare. However, there were some age-related differences in the content of self-definitions. Very old individuals (aged 85+) were more likely to mention daily living routines and sociodemographic variables but less likely to mention family/relatives, interests and hobbies outdoors, social participation, or interpersonal style. They were more likely than individuals aged 70–84 to make statements about the past. Although individuals across the entire age range generated more positive than negative evaluations of their self-definition, the ratio of positive to negative evaluations declined with age.

The life review process has also revealed spirituality themes.[21,26] Melia conducted life review interviews with 39 older Catholic women religious.[21] These interviews revealed continuous themes throughout individual lives, but no sequential pattern of late life development. Themes included faith, family, education, friends, community, caring, and prayer. Meddin found that among ten prominent older Australians, acquiring knowledge throughout life, engaging in altruistic behavior and experiencing transcendence were frequent.[26] These individuals reported that life review and the sense of developing wisdom were associated with a personal sense of coherence and continuity and an optimistic view of human nature.

Haight and colleagues have conducted a series of interventions incorporating life review in an attempt to improve quality of life among nursing home residents.[27–29] Haight and Dias found that 8 weeks of structured, evaluative life review performed on an individual basis was most effective in producing positive outcomes in life satisfaction, psychological well-being, and self-esteem.[27] Comparing life review to friendly visit comparison conditions, Haight and colleagues have found significant improvement immediately on measures of clinical depression and after 3 years on measures of depression, life satisfaction, and self-esteem.[28,29]

Stage theories and diversity

Hardly any of the studies investigating stage theories of personality have focused on diverse cultural or racial/ethnic groups. Most of the stage models, like Freud's original theories, were based on highly select samples. Only some investigations of life review have succeeded in recruiting participants reflecting the general population of interest.[23,28,29] Without such data, the universality of life review and the generalizability of the basic assumptions must be questioned.[30]

Stage theories and health

There has been limited investigation of the relation between stage approaches to adult personality and health. Once again, the exception to this is the investigation of life review processes. The intervention studies conducted by Haight and colleagues among nursing home residents support the contention that life review, in comparison with nonspecific but supportive interventions, has a positive impact on health, life satisfaction, well-being, and depression. These effects have been shown to be immediate and maintained up to three years post-intervention.

In the Freund and Smith study, health was a frequently mentioned theme of self-definition for individuals aged 70–103.[23] Forty-one percent of individuals in this age range mentioned hobbies and interests away from home, suggesting that their self-concepts are more active than anticipated. The number of positively evaluated self-definitions was related to experience of positive emotions, whereas the number of negatively evaluated self-definitions was related to the experience of both positive and negative emotions. These relations held even when physical health factors were controlled. Low functional capacity had a negative impact on well-being regardless of the number of domains of self-definition eliciting positive evaluations.

Measurement issues

The primary methodological problem plaguing empirical research involving stage theory approaches to adult personality development is the lack of specification of change mechanisms. Stating precise, testable hypotheses based on these models has proven difficult. Consequently, with the exception of Loevinger's projective sentence-completion test,[12,13] few standardized assessment instruments have been developed.

The most current stage approach to adult personality in our organizational scheme involves the concept of life review near the end of life. Although recent empirical research and intervention studies have embraced this concept, not every investigation of life review has yielded positive results. Fuchs notes the lack of a standardized approach to life review as a therapeutic technique in the delivery of interventions.[31] Additionally, methods of measurement vary widely.[31] A classic methodological limitation in much of this research is the problem of making causal inferences of age-related personality change from cross-sectional studies. In these studies, age-related differences could be observed due to the impact of aging or due to cohort differences. Without cohort-sequential data, it is impossible to tease apart these influences. Yet another issue in need of further study is the potential positive impact negative life events may play in initiating the process of life review and serving as a catalyst for continued development.[32] Thus, although stage theories of adult personality have intuitive appeal, their contribution is limited by fuzzy delineation of constructs and methodology.

THE BIG FIVE PERSONALITY TRAITS

In contrast to stage approaches to adult personality development, empirical research regarding trait approaches has experienced a great boon in recent years. In fact, it is safe to say that this is the standard, if not uncontested, method of personality assessment today, with multiple instruments available (see the measurement subsection). The "Big 5 Model" of personality description is intended to provide a broad framework for organizing the hundreds of traits, or individual differences, that characterize people.[33] This approach to personality description is based on the lexical hypothesis—that the most important individual differences in human transactions will be incorporated into many or most of the world's languages as single descriptors.[33] These five broad domains are obtained from factor analysis of self-report and peer/observer ratings, although some minor variations occur between specific measures.[33] Personality characteristics have been related to behaviors as diverse as handshaking.[34] A description of the most commonly identified five factors can be found in Table 13-2.

Early studies suggested that maturational changes in personality continue through the adult years, with age 30 serving as an identifiable cutoff indicative of relative intra-individual stability in traits.[35-39] Costa and McCrae have shown, via cross-sectional methods, small age-related declines in Neuroticism, Extraversion, and Openness to Experience, with age-related increases in Agreeableness and Conscientiousness from age 18 to 21 to adults at midlife.[40] Depending on how stability is measured, however, the idea that traits remain stable after age 30 has not received uniform support. For example, Field and Milsap found increases in mean-level agreeableness in a 14-year longitudinal study of adults aged 69–83.[41]

A recent meta-analysis of data from 152 longitudinal studies revealed that test–retest correlation coefficients of rank-order stability in trait consistency increased from 0.31 in childhood to 0.54 during college and 0.64 at the conventional cutoff age of 30.[42] However, trait consistency measured with the time interval held constant at 6.7 years plateaued around 0.74 between ages 50 and 70. It is important to note that this method of evaluating stability measures whether individuals maintain the same rank-order in traits across time. In this review, the majority of test–retest coefficients (77 percent) were coded into one of the Big 5 categories. As one would expect, longer longitudinal time intervals were associated with lower levels of trait consistency. In other words, assessment intervals longer than 6.7 years were more likely to be associated with change in personality traits.

Roberts and DelVecchio observed no gender differences in trait consistency.[42] Among the Big 5, measures of extraversion and agreeableness were most consistent ($M = 0.55$), although all Big 5 traits exhibited considerable consistency across time (from 0.50 to 0.52). The authors concluded that trait consistency increases at three points during the life course: from infancy and toddlerhood to the preschool period, from the college years to the early stages of young adulthood, and then from early middle age (age 40–49) to later middle age (age 50–59+). Since the peak level of consistency was well below unity, the authors also concluded that personality traits do not stop changing at some specific point in the life course. Hence, there is movement in the research literature toward process-oriented studies integrating concepts such as generativity and the Big 5 personality traits.[5]

Trait theories and diversity

Cross-cultural studies have most frequently compared non-Hispanic whites in the USA with individuals living in other countries.[43-45] Using the California Psychological Inventory (CPI), two studies compared factor structures similar to the Big 5 among adults in the USA and the People's Republic of China.[43,45] Such studies seek to estimate the effects of environment on different age cohorts by comparing adults in cultures with different recent histories. To the extent that cross-sectional studies in multiple countries reveal age-related differences that really reflect cohort effects (i.e. are due to different cultural experiences), then the pattern of age-related trait differences should be different across countries.[45]

Comparisons of adults in the USA and the People's Republic of China, however, reveal very similar patterns of age correlations.[43,45] In the Yang study, the Chinese sample was an average of 25 years younger than the US sample, and age effects were smaller in the US sample. The results were generalizable across gender, however, in both countries. Likewise, Labouvie-Vief and colleagues found high congruence on all four personality factors derived from the CPI: extraversion, control/norm orientation, flexibility, and femininity/masculinity.[43] Older cohorts across cultures had lower scores on extraversion and flexibility and higher scores on control/norm orientation. Once again, age differences were more pronounced among Chinese than US adults. Smaller cultural differences were found among the youngest age groups than among the oldest groups.

Using the NEO PI-R, McCrae and colleagues studied parallels in adult personality traits across five cultures: Germany, Italy, Portugal, Croatia, and South Korea.[44] Once again, these authors argued that different cultures would be likely to produce different patterns of age changes if environmental factors play a major role in adult personality development. In contrast, intrinsic maturational perspectives would suggest that even widely different cultures should show similar age trends. Results showed that, across cultures, midlife adults scored higher on measures of Agreeableness and Conscientiousness and lower on Neuroticism, Extraversion, and Openness than 18- to 21-year-olds. Congruence was strongest for Openness and weakest for Neuroticism, for which only two cultures (Germany, South Korea) replicated the American pattern.

In general, the results of these cross-cultural studies are consistent with the hypothesis that there are universal intrinsic maturational changes in personality.[43-45] Yang and colleagues reported, however, that across the span from 18 to 65 years, age never accounted for more than 20 percent of the variance in

---

Table 13-2 The Big 5 personality traits

- *Emotional stability vs neuroticism.* Anxiety, depression, emotional instability, self-consciousness, hostility, and impulsiveness vs relaxation, poise, and steadiness
- *Extraversion or surgency.* Gregariousness, assertiveness, activity level, and positive emotions vs silence, passivity, and reserve
- *Culture/intellect or openness to experience.* Imagination, curiosity, and creativity vs shallowness, imperceptiveness, and stupidity
- *Agreeableness or pleasantness.* Attributes such as kindness, trust and warmth that are considered pleasant and attractive to others vs hostility, selfishness, and distrust
- *Conscientiousness or dependability.* Encompasses organization, responsibility, ambition, perseverance, and hard work vs carelessness, negligence, and unreliability

Source: Adapted from Goldberg.[33]

CPI scale scores.[45] Gender did not influence the pattern of results in any of these cross-cultural studies. The authors differed in their interpretation of the influence of environmental factors. In the Yang and McCrae studies, the authors maintained that the results offered little support for historical cohort effects being major determinants of cross-sectional age differences in adult personality traits. Although noting the high degree of similarity in personality traits across cultures, Labouvie-Vief and colleagues also noted that cultural climate and cultural change do impact the relation between age and personality.[43] Such effects may best be observed at more precise levels of measurement; the aggregated Big 5 factors, being general descriptors, seem most influenced by maturational processes.

One of the most intriguing theories relevant to personality traits, diversity, and health is the "John Henryism hypothesis."[46] The term connotes a strong personality predisposition toward prolonged, high-effort coping with difficult psychological stressors in one's environment and refers to the strong African American man of legend who out-worked a steam engine but then died from the strain.[47] Using the 12-item John Henryism Scale for Active Coping, James and colleagues proposed that John Henryism (JH) traits among lower socio-economic groups without the resources to successfully cope with difficult psychological stressors are primarily responsible for the increased prevalence of hypertension among these groups.[46] Thus, individuals who are low in socio-economic status but have high JH scores are most at risk for hypertension and elevated blood pressure. Among those low in JH, the prevalence of hypertension and elevated blood pressure does not differ by socio-economic status.[46,47]

James and colleagues found that JH was significantly associated with life satisfaction and perceived health among blacks and whites.[47] Race was found to be a highly significant predictor of JH, with blacks scoring higher than whites even after controlling for sociodemographic and perceptual variables. However, these investigators failed to replicate the association between JH and negative health effects among rural white southerners. Black men and women did not differ on their JH scores in James' 1987 study,[47] but white women scored significantly lower than white men. Similarly, Dressler and colleagues found that, among African Americans, the relation between John Henryism and blood pressure was dependent on gender.[48] For black men, blood pressure and the risk for hypertension increased as scores on the John Henryism Scale for Active Coping increased. For black women, blood pressure and the risk for hypertension decreased as JH scores increased.

The association between JH and negative health correlates including incidence of hypertension and increased blood pressure has proven illusive in some studies.[49] For example, the impact of high JH on blood pressure has not been found among well-educated African Americans.[49,50] Wiist and Flack failed to find the relation with blood pressure, but did find that high JH and low SES were related to higher cholesterol levels.[51] In an age-restricted sample from the CARDIA study (aged 18–30), no association between JH, education, and blood pressure was found.[52]

In one of the only investigations of the John Henryism hypothesis among African American and white adults aged 50 and older, Weinrich and colleagues found two underlying factors for the John Henryism Scale for Active Coping: tenacity/hard work and personal efficacy.[53] An internal consistency estimate for the measure across age and race groups was $\alpha = 0.71$. Reliability was slightly but nonsignificantly higher among older than middle-aged adults ($\alpha = 0.73$ versus 0.67, respectively). There were differences due to race, gender, and education level: African Americans had higher JH scores than whites, men had higher JH scores than women, and those with lower levels of education had higher JH scores than those with more education.

Thus, although more research is needed, the "John Henryism hypothesis" seems to be confined to low-educated, low-occupational-status African American men in the rural southeastern USA. Limitations of the research noted to date include the restricted adult age range, with most studies including individuals aged 20–50. James and colleagues cited the limited variability in SES among blacks in their sample.[47] Additionally, almost all studies of the John Henryism hypothesis have been cross-sectional. Prospective studies are needed to investigate socio-economic status, race/ethnicity, and the incidence of hypertension among high JH individuals over time. Additional studies of the impact of high JH on job-related stress, particularly in low-status healthcare professions such as Certified Nursing Assistants, are also needed.

Trait theories and health

Numerous investigations using data from the VA Normative Aging Study of adult men have provided data on the relation of adult personality and health. Siegman and colleagues found that the dominance factor derived from the Minnesota Multiphasic Personality Inventory (MMPI-2) is an independent risk factor for incidence of fatal coronary heart disease and nonfatal myocardial infarction among older men with an average age of sixty-one.[54] Using the three Cook–Medley subscales of hostility from the MMPI, Kubzansky and colleagues found that lower levels of education and greater hostility were associated with greater "wear and tear" on the body in cross-sectional analyses of 818 men.[55] Niaura and colleagues found that, among such older men, greater hostility may be associated with a pattern of obesity, central adiposity, and insulin resistance, which can exert effects on blood pressure and serum lipids.[56] In this study, the effects of hostility on the metabolic syndrome appeared to be mediated by body mass index and waist/hip ratio. LoCastro and colleagues found that Neuroticism as measured by the Eyesenck Personality Inventory partially mediated the effects of having a family history of alcoholism on number of drinks per day and the number of alcohol problems.[57]

Measurement issues

Multiple measurement instruments of adult personality traits that in some way contribute to the Big 5 are available.[58–60] Regardless of the specific measurement instrument used, however, these measures prove remarkably consistent in the derivation of five dimensions of personality via factor analysis.[33]

Multiple methodological issues are yet to be resolved within the trait approach to adult personality research. For example, there is a dearth of research examining stability and change in personality traits among the old-old (aged 75–84) and the very old (aged 85+). Also, some investigations of the relation between personality traits, diversity, and health (i.e. John Henryism hypothesis) are hampered by restriction of research to cross-sectional samples. Trait approaches to the study of personality development overlap considerably with social–cognitive constructs such as the self.[5] One major complication of stability estimates in adult personality research involves what kind of stability is under consideration: intra-individual stability,[61] mean-level stability, or rank-order stability across time.[42]

The impact of cohort and time of measurement on trait consistency within the longitudinal studies conducted to date has not been fully considered.[42] Longitudinal studies of gender role differences have shown that age is not as good a predictor as the life experiences of different cohorts on personality traits of men and women across time.[62,63] Thus, it may be that earlier-born cohorts have developed more consistent personality traits earlier in life as the result of numerous social/historical and lifespan-related influences.

On a broader scale, the relative impact of biological and environmental variables on stability and change in adult personality has yet to be evaluated. Although the influence of genetic factors has been investigated in the development of personality among monozygotic and dyzygotic twins over a 10-year period, no such investigations have addressed the contribution of genetics to the maintenance of personality across the adult age range. Regarding the impact of environmental influences, with time and age individuals may encounter fewer novel experiences.[42] Thus, the stability of personality factors may be causally related to the decreasing novelty of the environment in which individuals live rather than genetic factors. Sophisticated research designs (i.e. perhaps monozygotic versus dyzygotic cohort-sequential twin studies) are needed to parse apart the relative contributions of genetics and the environment to adult personality development. Expansion of theory-driven research in adult personality would also assist in this endeavor. Although research regarding the Big 5 personality traits has been mostly descriptive, social–cognitive approaches to adult personality development have embraced theory-driven research.

SOCIAL–COGNITIVE APPROACHES TO PERSONALITY

The social–cognitive approach to the study of adult personality and self lends itself well to process-oriented investigation. This approach focuses on the processes underlying stability and change in one's perception of the self, and emphasizes the impact of necessary, adaptive adjustments in one's personality. Within this framework, an individual's sense of self is proposed to develop through the interaction of internal and environmental factors. Although the content of the developing self may change, this model proposes that the mechanisms by which changes are integrated into the concept of self are stable. The cohesion of internal and environmental factors in the development of the self is influenced by maturational changes and cohort differences. Thus, the development of the self as a dynamic construct reflects one's identity, perception of

possible selves, need for affiliation, and perceived remaining lifespan.

Identity and the self

Whitbourne describes a lifespan approach to one's core identity development. She refers to *identity* as an individual's developing sense of self, an organizing schema through which internal and external life experiences are interpreted.[64] Identity includes physical functioning, cognition, social relationships, and environmental experiences.[65] Two constructs underlie identity: the scenario and the life story. The scenario represents an individual's expectations for a future life path. The life story, in contrast, describes the personal history constructed after significant events occur. Thus, adults must differentiate and resolve the incompatibility between their scenario and life story, societal norms and expectations.[2] In this model, the impact of context on identity development assumes great importance. This context includes family relationships, work experiences, and life/cohort experiences in the social and historical world.

The scenario and life story provide key frameworks from which life success and the achievement of personal life goals can be evaluated. Assessment of goal achievements occurs through assimilation and accommodation.[64] Identity assimilation refers to the process through which one interprets life events according to acquired cognitive and affective schemes of identity.[64] An individual's reaction to medical illness and decisions regarding specific medical treatments, for example, may be dependent on the interpretation of the illness and how it impacts identity.[66] In contrast, when experience cannot easily be assimilated into the individual's existing framework of the self, the process of identity accommodation modifies both cognitive and affective schemas of self so that these life experiences may be included.[64] Successful aging consists of integrating information about the self via assimilation and accommodation, providing an organized framework by which experiences are interpreted. Note, once again, that negative life events and acute or chronic stressors such as care-giving may serve as catalysts for positive self-development.[32]

Whitbourne and Collins examined the self-report of 242 adults aged 40–95 years regarding the relation between identity and changes in physical functioning.[67] They found that 40-year-olds were sensitive to age-related changes. Individuals aged 65 and older reported paying particular attention to perceived changes in competence. These individuals were more likely to use identity assimilation (i.e. reinterpretation of experiences to coincide with the self) in the area of cognitive functioning than were other age groups. Across the adult age range, identity assimilation was shown to positively associate with self-esteem. The authors concluded that, by making behavioral changes in one's identity, individuals adapt to the aging process in healthy ways.

In addition to cognitive reinterpretation of events at odds with identity, older adults are believed to closely regulate their emotions on the basis of their thoughts about self and others. The self is linked to emotion through its ability to generate goals;[68] these goal-oriented aspects of the aging self provide a framework for understanding motivation to engage in social relationships. Researchers interested in understanding the self from a lifespan perspective often utilize the theoretical framework provided by the "possible selves" model.[69] The construct of "possible selves" postulates that individuals are guided in their actions by aspects of the self that represent what the individual could become, would like to become, and is afraid of becoming. Possible selves serve as psychological resources that may motivate an individual and direct future behavior. Indeed, there has been a growing literature documenting the positive relationship between achievement of identity-relevant goals and well-being.[70]

Ryff found empirical support for the concept of possible selves.[71] Young, middle-aged, and older adults were asked to judge their past, present, future, and ideal selves on dimensions related to self-acceptance, positive relations with others, autonomy, environmental mastery, purpose in life and personal growth. Ryff found that older people are more likely than younger adults to downwardly adjust their ideal self and to view their past more positively.[71] Cross and Markus found that, in comparison with younger adults, older adults report fewer possible selves that are more closely tied to their current selves.[72] Thus, older adults may use cognitive reappraisal more frequently than younger adults and may be more facile in doing so.[73]

Not every social–cognitive approach to adult personality development, however, emphasizes the integration of internal and external information into a cohesive sense of self. Lomranz defined the concept of "aintegration": the notion that there are intra-individual differences in the need for personal consistency.[74] Some individuals are able to feel well without having integrated all their various biopsychosocial levels into an overriding whole. The concept of "aintegration" has also been related to resiliency, wherein the ability to hold multiple diverse perspectives simultaneously without anxiety is conceptualized as a strength of aging.[42]

Socio-emotional selectivity theory

Another social–cognitive approach to the study of adult personality development is Carstensen's socio-emotional selectivity theory.[75–77] This theory focuses on the agentic choices made by adults in their social world for the purpose of regulating knowledge-oriented and emotion goals. Carstensen proposes that purposeful selective reduction in social interaction begins in early adulthood, and that emotional closeness remains stable or increases within selected relationships as one ages.[75–77] The theory postulates two general categories of social motives: those related to the acquisition of knowledge and those related to the regulation of affect. When time is perceived as open-ended, acquisition of knowledge is prioritized. When time is perceived as limited, however, emotional goals assume primacy. Older adults select social relationships in which they want to invest their resources and in which they expect reciprocity and positive affect, thereby optimizing their social networks. Thus, older adults' social networks reduce by choice, as individuals decrease contact with acquaintances but seek to maintain contact with certain relatives and close friends into their eighties and beyond, as a function of increased saliency of emotional attachment to one's life goals.[75–77]

Carstensen and colleagues suggest that the perception of time left in life is fundamental to motivation and that age is correlated with time perspective.[78] They postulate that perceiving an ending plays an important role in identity processes, such that endings promote greater self-acceptance and less striving toward an abstract ideal.[71,72] Thus, older adults have been shown to be more present-oriented than concerned about the past and less concerned than young adults about the future.[79] This is not due to maturational changes per se, but due to changes in the perceived time left to live. Rather than age being the causal factor in shifts in self-perception and social goals, it is the inverse association of chronological age with number of years left to live that produces observed relations.

In an effort to decouple chronological age from number of years left to live, Carstensen and Fredrickson examined the salience of affect in preferences for social partners among young gay men similar in age but disparate in health status (i.e. HIV-negative, HIV-positive with symptoms, or HIV-positive without symptoms).[80] Their findings were supportive of socio-emotional selectivity theory. They found that increasing closeness to death, rather than chronological age, was associated with increasing importance of the emotional connection one has with social partners.

Social–cognitive theories and diversity

There are few empirical investigations incorporating diverse cultural or racial/ethnic groups in the study of social–cognitive approaches to adult personality development, outside the topical arena of social relations.[4] Hypothetical and empirical research in this area has focused on socio-emotional selectivity theory. For example, Carstensen and colleagues proposed that, since African culture and African American subcultures encourage a temporal focus on the present,[81] the social networks within these cultures may be populated with emotionally close social partners owing to the optimization of emotion goals inherent in a present-time orientation.[78]

Gross and colleagues found consistent age differences in the subjective report of emotional experience and control across diverse cultures: Norwegians, Chinese Americans, African Americans, European Americans, and Catholic nuns.[82] Across all groups, older adults reported fewer negative emotional experiences and greater emotional control. Likewise, Fung et al. found support for the notion that socio-emotional selectivity is due to perceived limitations in time among adults in the USA and Hong Kong.[83] In both countries, older individuals displayed a preference for familiar social partners in comparison with younger adults within usual circumstances. When older adults were asked for their social preferences given an unlimited lifespan, the preference for familiar social partners disappeared.

Moreover, the handover of Hong Kong to the People's Republic of China in 1997 was shown to impact individuals' social preferences. This sociopolitical event appeared to impact the evaluation of time limitations. Specifically, one year before the transition, only older adults showed a preference for familiar social partners. Two months prior to the handover, however, both younger and older adults showed such preferences. This similarity across age in preference for social partners disappeared again one year after the handover, when the typical pattern of relation returned. Thus, perceived limitations in time impacting agentic preferences for social partners are not restricted to perceived time until death but also include sociocultural endings.

Social–cognitive theories and health

In general, empirical research regarding identity and the self has explored relations with physical health outcomes whereas research regarding socio-emotional selectivity theory has focused on relations with emotional outcomes. Age-related changes in physical functioning have been examined in relation to an individual's sense of self. As one advances in age, people define themselves increasingly in terms of health and physical functioning.[23] It appears that people cognitively manage their expectations and social comparison processes so that they are, in general, no less satisfied with their health status despite increasing physical limitations.

Using her multiple threshold model of aging,[84] Whitbourne investigated changes in a person's sense of self that coincide with changes in physical functioning.[65] According to her model, individuals are particularly vigilant to age-related physical changes within areas of functioning that are central to the self-concept. The concept of physical identity refers to the individual's self-perception of the body's appearance, competence, or the body's ability to perform tasks as needed in daily activities, and limitations.[85] Physical identity is theorized to follow the assimilation and accommodation processes referred to previously; individuals view changes in one's body in terms of current conceptualizations of the self. These self-perceptions often serve to protect one's sense of self, since the physical aging process is a constant challenge to the maintenance of a stable sense of identity by serving as a constant reminder of mortality. A particularly salient example of this for women is the onset of menopause.

The content of possible selves and self-regulatory processes associated with specific possible selves have been examined in relation to subjective well-being, health, and health behaviors. Hooker and Kaus found that having a possible self in the realm of health was more strongly related to reported health behaviors than was a global measure of health values.[86] Examination of possible selves in older adults living with a chronic illness will provide for a better understanding of how the self handles long-term care management and future outlook.

In socio-emotional selectivity theory, individuals alter their environmental interactions such that optimization of emotional experience is prioritized in later life.[87] As one ages, there is greater emotional attachment invested in each close relationship.[88] Lang and colleagues found that average emotional closeness to social network members serves an important adaptive function in late life.[89] This idea is supported by the finding that older adults reduce the amount of social support they provide to others, while the amount of perceived support received from others does not change.[4,90] Older adults with limited social contact may still perceive their social networks as supportive. Part of this perceived satisfaction may result from continuity in the quality of social interactions.

Measurement issues

Diverse measurement approaches are associated with social–cognitive investigations of adult personality. The "possible selves" construct is measured using a questionnaire inventory,[72] whereby respondents describe hoped-for and feared possible selves and evaluate their ability to achieve or avoid these manifestations of self in their anticipation of their own aging processes. After listing all of their possible selves, participants are asked to identify the three most important hoped-for selves (and the three most feared selves) and explain why each is important (or feared). A series of self-regulatory questions (e.g. "How capable do you feel of achieving this possible self?") are rated on 7-point Likert scales for each possible self. Socio-emotional selectivity theory, in contrast, has relied on self-report, observation of marital interactions, and card sorting of potential social partners on the basis of similarity judgments, with the resulting categories submitted to multidimensional scaling analysis.[78]

The strength of social–cognitive approaches lies in the positing of explanatory processes for personality development. Unlike stage or trait approaches, the identification of specific, testable processes such as identity assimilation, identity accommodation, possible selves, or socio-emotional selectivity promote theoretical advance via empirical hypotheses testing. Much more work is needed regarding identity development within diverse racial/ethnic groups. Likewise, more work relating socio-emotional selectivity theories to health outcomes is needed.

Social–cognitive researchers interested in personality and self in later life investigate domains where, albeit time-limited, growth and development in old age are possible, and contribute to an individual's perception of possible selves, need for affiliation, and content of life review. Today, we are living longer and want our last years to be as enjoyable and productive as our younger years. Research examining the effects of psychosocial and health variables on well-being and quality of life in old age needs to be at the forefront of this research perspective.

SYNTHESIS AND FUTURE DIRECTIONS

This chapter has reviewed several issues central to the conceptualization of adult personality. The issue of stability versus maturational change or cohort differences in personality development is highly dependent on the theory and measurement approach used. For example, the review of trait approaches highlighted the fact that the Big 5 personality variables, being large aggregates of more specific characteristics, may be relatively stable. Thus, the Big 5 may be largely dependent on genetic or biological factors. In contrast, measurement of more precise traits may be more influenced by cognitive and environmental (i.e. cohort) influences. Thus, specific individual traits would be expected to be less stable across time than the Big 5 personality aggregates. As stated in the section on trait theory, clarity in the definition of stability (i.e. intra-individual, mean-level, or ordinal) is critical to ensure that conclusions drawn from differing research methodologies are interpreted uniformly.

In the effort to tease apart environmental and biological influences on stability and change, cross-cultural comparisons of adult personality have been particularly useful. Comparison of adults of the same age who have experienced different environments across the lifespan provide evidence regarding the extent of environmental influence on personality. More research is needed, however, addressing personality development of very old individuals in diverse cultures. Additionally, investigation of health effects of adult personality in diverse cultures provides invaluable information for health service provision and the development of preventive interventions. Specifically, prospective studies of theories like the John Henryism hypothesis could influence the design of interventions for cardiovascular health and improve the dramatic and alarming health disparities between whites and African Americans in the USA.

Finally, it is time to apply the wealth of accumulated information regarding personality across adulthood to the provision of services designed to enhance quality of life.

KEY POINTS The aging personality and self

- Personality is the pattern of thoughts, feelings, and behaviors that shape an individual's interface with the world, distinguish one person from another, and manifest across time and situations. It is impacted by biological, cognitive, and environmental determinants.

- Stage theorists include Freud, Jung, and Erikson (eight stages of development are based on the idea that the growing personality moves through stages in an ordered fashion). The psychoanalytic approach to adult personality encompasses four domains: level of consciousness, personality structure, defense mechanisms, and stages of psychosexual development. Few studies investigating stage theories of personality have focused on diverse cultures, racial/ethnic groups, or health.

- Trait approaches are the standard method of personality assessment today with multiple instruments available. The Big 5 personality traits include: Neuroticism. Extraversion, Openness to Experience, Agreeableness, and Conscientiousness. In general, the results of cross-cultural studies are consistent with the hypothesis that there are universal intrinsic maturational changes in personality.

- The John Henryism (JH) hypothesis describes the strong personality predisposition toward prolonged, high-effort coping with difficult psychological stressors in one's environment. Race was found to be a highly significant predictor of JH, with African Americans scoring higher than whites.

- The social–cognitive approach focuses on the individual's sense of self, developing through the interaction of internal and environmental factors.

- The socio-emotional selectivity theory focuses on the agentic choices made by adults in their social world for the purpose of regulating knowledge-oriented emotion goals. In socio-emotional selectivity theory, individuals alter their environmental interactions such that optimization of emotional experience is prioritized later in life. There are few empirical investigations incorporating diverse cultural or racial/ethnic groups in the study of social–cognitive approaches to adult personality development, outside the topical arena of social relations.

Identification of personality processes that drive specific behaviors (i.e. handshaking) and choices (i.e. medical treatments) is needed. There is powerful evidence that personality characteristics can affect health status and health behaviors. For example, interventions such as life review have successfully enhanced quality of life in the nursing home. Similarly, a knowledge of John Henryism characteristics among certified nursing assistants and other economically disadvantaged but essential healthcare providers could guide the development of interventions to reduce caregiving burnout and job stress. Using social–cognitive approaches to adult personality development and the processes of identity assimilation, identity accommodation, and socio-emotional selectivity could inform interventions designed to improve the process of advance care planning for the implementation of life-sustaining or palliative treatments at the end of life.

Furthermore, applied intervention research will not only enhance service provision but also drive theoretical advances in the concept of the self in old age. For example, palliative care and/or hospice interventions designed to provide services targeting personal, physical, and spiritual needs can inform aspects of socio-emotional selectivity theory involving present-time orientation and time remaining to live. Incorporating aspects of life review could also provide advances in theories driving therapeutic approaches to depression. Interventions for bereaved personal and professional caregivers as well as interventions for the terminally or chronically ill older adult are desperately needed. It is the authors' contention that the time to apply our knowledge of adult personality across the lifespan is now, thereby deriving benefit from accumulated knowledge as well as driving advances in theory.

Acknowledgments
Preparation of this chapter was supported by funding from the National Institute on Aging to R. Allen-Burge (1K01AG00943–01A1). Special thanks are extended to Karen Quarles and Adriana Coates for assistance in manuscript preparation.

REFERENCES

1. Allport GW: Personality. Holt, Rinehart & Winston, New York, 1937
2. Schaie KW, Willis SL: Adult Development and Aging, 5th edn. Prentice-Hall, New York, 2002
3. Phares EJ, Chaplin WF: Introduction to Personality, 4th edn. Addison Wesley, New York, 1997
4. Antonucci TC: Social relations: an examination of social networks, social support, and sense of control. In Birren JE, Schaie KW (eds): Handbook of the Psychology of Aging, 5th edn. Academic Press, New York, 2001:427–453
5. Ryff CD, Kwan CML, Singer BH: Personality and aging: flourishing agendas and future challenges. In Birren JE, Schaie KW (eds): Handbook of the Psychology of Aging, 5th edn. Academic Press, New York, 2001:477–498
6. Baron RA: Psychology, 4th edn. Allyn & Bacon, Needham Heights, MA, 1997
7. Freud S: Three essays on the theory of sexuality. In Freud S (ed): The Standard Edition, vol. VII. Hogarth, London, 1953
8. Horney K: Feminine Psychology, 1st edn. W.W. Norton, New York, 1967
9. Gilligan C: In a Different Voice: Psychological Theory and Women's Development. Harvard University Press, Cambridge, MA, 1982
10. Jung CG: Analytical Psychology: Its Theory and Practice. Vintage, New York, 1968
11. Allen-Burge R, Willis SL, Schaie KW: The aging personality and self. In Tallis R, Fillit H, Brocklehurst JC (eds): Brocklehurst's Textbook of

Geriatric Medicine and Gerontology, 5th edn. Churchill Livingstone, London, 1998

12. Loevinger J, Wessler R: Measuring Ego Development. 1: Construction and Use of a Sentence Completion Test. Jossey-Bass, San Francisco, 1970

13. Loevinger J: Ego Development: Conception and Theory. Jossey-Bass, San Francisco, 1976

14. Blanchard-Fields F: Reasoning on social dilemmas varying in emotional saliency: an adult developmental study. Psychol Aging 1986;1:325–333

15. Labouvie-Vief G, Hakim-Larson J, Hobart CJ: Age, ego level and the life-span development of coping and defense processes. Psychol Aging 1987;2:286–283

16. Erikson E. Childhood and Society, 2nd edn. Norton, New York, 1963

17. Erikson EH, Erikson JM, Kivnick HQ: Vital Involvement in Old Age. W.W. Norton, New York, 1986.

18. McFadden SH: Religion, personality and aging: a life span perspective. J Pers 1999;67:1081–1104

19. Whitbourne SK, Zuschlag MK, Elliot LB et al: Psychosocial development in adulthood: a 22-year sequential study. J Pers Soc Psychol 1992;63:260–271

20. Butler RN, Lewis MI: Aging and Mental Health, 3rd edn. C.V. Mosby, St Louis, 1982

21. Melia SP: Continuity in the lives of elder Catholic women religious. Int J Aging Hum Dev 1999;48(3):175–189

22. Coleman PG, Ivani-Chalian C, Robinson M: Self and identity in advanced old age: validation of theory through longitudinal case analysis. J Pers 1999; 67:819–849

23. Freund AM, Smith J: Content and function of the self-definition in old and very old age. J Gerontol B 1999;54:P55–P67

24. Taft LB, Nehrke MF: Reminiscence, life review, and ego integrity in nursing home residents. Int J Aging Hum Dev 1990;30(3):189–196

25. Fishman S: Relationships among an older adult's life review, ego integrity, and death anxiety. Int Psychogeriatr 1992;4(suppl 2):267–277

26. Meddin JR: Dimensions of spiritual meaning and well-being in the lives of ten older Australians. Int J Aging Hum Dev 1998;47(3):163–175

27. Haight BK, Dias JK: Examining key variables in selected reminiscing modalities. Int Psychogeriatr 1992;4(suppl 2):279–290

28. Haight BK, Michel Y, Hendrix S: Life review: preventing despair in newly relocated nursing home residents short- and long-term effects. Int J Aging Hum Dev 1998;47(2):119–142

29. Haight BK, Michel Y, Hendrix S: The extended effects of the life review in nursing home residents. Int J Aging Hum Dev 2000;50(2):151–168

30. Merriam SB: Butler's life review: how universal is it? Int J Aging Hum Dev 1993;37(3):163–175

31. Fuchs T: Reminiscence therapy with the elderly. Psychother Psychom Med Psychol 1992;49(9–10):308–314

32. Diehl M: Self-development in adulthood and aging: the role of critical life events. In Ryff CD, Marshall VW (eds): The Self and Society in Aging Processes. Springer, New York, 1999;150–183

33. Goldberg LR: The structure of phenotypic personality traits. Am Psychol 1993; 48:26–34

34. Chaplin WF, Phillips JB, Brown JD et al: Handshaking, gender, personality, and first impressions. J Pers Soc Psychol 2000;79(1):110–117

35. Costa PT, McCrae RR: Personality in adulthood: a six-year longitudinal study of self-reports and spouse ratings on the NEO Personality Inventory. J Pers Soc Psychol 1988;54:853–863

36. Costa PT, McCrae RR: Personality continuity and the changes of adult life. In Storandt M, VandenBos GR (eds): The Adult Years: Continuity and Change. American Psychological Association, 1989;45–77

37. Costa PT, McCrae RR: Longitudinal stability of adult personality. In Hogan R, Johnson J, Briggs S (eds): Handbook of Personality Psychology. Academic Press, San Diego, 1997:269–292

38. McCrae RR, Costa PT: Personality in Adulthood. Guilford Press, New York, 1990

39. McCrae RR, Costa PT: The stability of personality: observation and evaluations. Curr Direct Psychol Sci 1994;3:173–175

40. Costa PT, McCrae RR: Professional Manual: Revised NEO Personality Inventory (NEO PI-R) and NEO Five-Factor Inventory (NEO-FFI). Psychological Assessment Resources, Odessa, FL, 1992

41. Field D, Milsap RE: Personality in advanced old age: continuity or change? J Gerontol B 1991;46:P299–P308.

42. Roberts BW, DelVecchio WF: The rank-order consistency of personality traits from childhood to old age: a quantitative review of longitudinal studies. Psychol Bull 2000;126:3–25

43. Labouvie-Vief G, Diehl M, Tarnowski A et al: Age differences in adult personality: findings from the United States and China. J Gerontol B 2000;55:P4–P17.

44. McCrae RR, Costa PT, Pedroso de Lima M et al: Age differences in personality across the adult life span: parallels in five countries. Dev Psychol 1999;35:466–477

45. Yang J, McCrae RR, Costa PT: Adult age differences in personality traits in the United States and the People's Republic of China. J Gerontol B 1998;53:P372–P383

46. James SA, Hartnett SA, Kalsbeek WD: John Henryism and blood pressure differences among black men. J Behav Med 1983;6(3):259–278

47. James SA, Strogatz DS, Wing SB et al: Socioeconomic status, John Henryism, and hypertension in blacks and whites. Am J Epidemiol 1987;126:664–673

48. Dressler WW, Bindon JR, Neggers YH: John Henryism, gender, and arterial blood pressure in an African American community. Psychosom Med 1998; 60:620–624

49. Adams JH, Aubert RE, Clark VR: The relationship among John Henryism, hostility, perceived stress, social support, and blood pressure in African American college students. Ethn Dis 1999;9:359–368

50. Jackson LA, Adams-Campbell LL: John Henryism and blood pressure in black college students. J Behav Med 1994;17(1):69–79

51. Wiist WH, Flack JM: A test of the John Henryism hypothesis: cholestorol and blood pressure. J Behav Med 1992;15(1):15–29

52. McKetney EC, Ragland DR: John Henryism, education, and blood pressure in young adults. The Coronary Artery Risk Development in Young Adults (CARDIA) study. Am J Epidemiol 1996;143:787–791

53. Weinrich SP, Weinrich MC, Keil JE et al: The John Henryism and Framingham type A scales: Measurement properties in elderly blacks and whites. Am J Epidemiol 1988;128:165–178

54. Siegman AW, Kubzansky LD, Kawachi I et al: A prospective study of dominance and coronary heart disease in the Normative Aging Study. Am J Cardiol 2000;86:145–149

55. Kubzansky LD, Kawachi I, Sparrow D: Socioeconomic status, hostility, and risk factor clustering in the Normative Aging Study: any help from the concept of allostatic load? Ann Behav Med 1999;21:330–338

56. Niaura R, Banks SM, Ward KD et al: Hostility and the metabolic syndrome in older males: the Normative Aging Study. Psychosom Med 2000;62(1):7–16

57. LoCastro J, Spiro A, Monnelly E et al: Personality, family history, and alcohol use among older men: the VA Normative Aging Study. Alcohol Clin Exp Res 2000;24:501–511

58. Gough HG, Bradley P: California Psychological Inventory Manual, 3rd edn. Consulting Psychologists Press, Palo Alto, 1996

59. Costa PT, McCrae RR: The NEO Personality Inventory Manual. Psychological Assessment Resources, Odessa, FL, 1985

60. Costa PT, McCrae RR: Revised NEO Personality Inventory (NEO-PI-R) and NEO Five-Factor Inventory (NEO-FFI) Professional Manual. Psychological Assessment Resources, Odessa, Fl, 1992

61. Costa PT, McCrae RR: Stability and change in personality from adolescence through adulthood. In Halverson CF, Kohnstamm GA, Martin RP (eds): The Developing Structure of Temperament and Personality from Infancy to Adulthood. Erlbaum, Hillsdale, NJ, 1994:139–150

62. Lynott PP, McCandless NJ: The impact of age vs. life experience on the gender role attitudes of women in different cohorts. J Women Aging 2000;12(1–2):5–21

63. Schaie KW: Intellectual development in adulthood: the second longitudinal study. Cambridge University Press, New York, 1996

64. Whitbourne SK, Connolly LA: The developing self in midlife. In Willis SL, Reid JK (eds): Life in the Middle: Psychological and Social Development in Middle Age. Academic Press, San Diego, 1999:25–45

65. Whitbourne SK: Physical changes in the aging individual: clinical implications. In Nordhus IH, VandenBos GR (eds): Clinical Geropsychology. American Psychological Association, Washington, DC, 1998:79–108

66. Zwahr MD, Park DC, Shifren K: Judgements about estrogen replacement therapy: the role of age, cognitive abilities, and beliefs. Psychol Aging 1999;14(2):179–191

67. Whitbourne SK, Collins KJ: Identity processes and perceptions of physical functioning in adults: theoretical and clinical implications. Psychotherapy 1998; 35:519–530

68. Heckhausen J, Schultz R: Selectivity in life-span development: biological and societal canalizations and individuals' development goals. In

Brandstadter J, Lerner RM (eds). Action and self-development: theory and research through the life-span. Sage, Thousand Oaks, CA, 1999:67–103

69. Markus H, Nurius P: Possible selves. Am Psychol 1986;41:954–969

70. McGregor I, Little BR: Personal projects, happiness, and meaning: on doing well and being yourself. J Pers Soc Psychol 1998;74:494–512

71. Ryff CD: Possible selves in adulthood and old age: a tale of shifting horizons. Psychol Aging 1991;6:286–295

72. Cross S, Markus H: Possible selves across the life span. Hum Dev 1991;34:230–255

73. Carstensen LL, Gross J, Fung H: The social context of emotion. Annu Rev Geriatr Gerontol 1997;17:325–352

74. Lomranz J: An image of aging and the concept of integration: coping and mental health implications. In Lomranz J (ed): Handbook of Aging and Mental Health: An Integrative Approach. Plenum Press, New York, 1998:217–250

75. Carstensen LL: Age-related changes in social activity. In Carstensen LL, Edelstein BA (eds): Handbook of Clinical Gerontology. Pergamon, New York, 1987:222–237

76. Carstensen LL: Selectivity theory: social activity in life-span context. In Schaie KW, Lawton MP (eds): Annual Review of Gerontology and Geriatrics. Springer, New York, 1991:195–215

77. Carstensen LL: Social and emotional patterns in adulthood: support for socioemotional selectivity theory. Psychol Aging 1992;7:331–338

78. Carstensen LL, Isaacowitz DM, Charles ST: Taking time seriously: a theory of socioemotional selectivity. Am Psychol 1999;54(3):165–181

79. Fingerman K, Perlmutter M: Future time perspective and life events across adulthood. J Gen Psychol 1995;122:95–111

80. Carstensen LL, Fredrickson BL: Influence of HIV status and age on cognitive representations of others. Health Psychol 1998;17:494–503

81. Jones JM: Cultural differences in temporal perspectives: instrumental and expressive behaviors in time. In McGrath JE (ed): The Social Psychology of Time: New Perspectives. Sage, Newbury, CA, 1988:21–38

82. Gross JJ, Carstensen LL, Pasupathi M et al: Emotion and aging: experience, expression, and control. Psychol Aging 1997;12:590–599

83. Fung HH, Carstensen LL, Lutz AM: Influence of time on social preferences: implications for life-span development. Psychol Aging 1999;14:595–604

84. Whitbourne SK: The Aging Individual: Physical and Psychological Perspectives. Springer, New York, 1996

85. Whitbourne SK: Physical changes. In Cavanaugh JC, Whitbourne SK (eds): Gerontology: An Interdisciplinary Perspective. Oxford University Press, New York, 1999:91–122

86. Hooker K, Kaus CR: Health-related possible selves in young and middle adulthood. Psychol Aging 1994;9(1):126–133

87. Carstensen LL, Charles ST: Emotion in the second half of life. Curr Direct Psychol Sci 1998;7(5):144–149

88. Carstensen LL, Gross JJ, Fung HH: The social context of emotional experience. In Schaie KW, Lawton MP (eds): Annual Review of Gerontology and Geriatrics. Springer, New York, 1998:325–352

89. Lang FR, Staudinger UM, Carstensen LL: Perspectives on socioemotional selectivity in late life: how personality and social context do (and do not) make a difference. J Gerontol B 1998;53:P21–P29

90. Krause N: Satisfaction with social support and self-rated health in older adults. Gerontologist 1987;27:301–308

Chapter 14

The pharmacology of aging

David R. P. Guay, Margaret B. Artz, Joseph T. Hanlon, and

Kenneth Schmader

Each day worldwide, elderly people consume millions of doses of medications. This remarkable amount of medication use benefits many elderly people greatly by preventing and treating disease, preserving functional status, prolonging life, and improving or maintaining good quality of life. However, this level of medication exposure may also harm elderly people via adverse drug reactions and is associated with problems such as drug interactions. The harmful and beneficial responses of elderly individuals to drugs are, in part, dependent upon age-related physiological changes that influence how the body handles a given drug (i.e. pharmacokinetics) and what a drug does to the body (i.e. pharmacodynamics). To obtain the desired therapeutic response and avoid drug-related problems, it is also useful to have an understanding of drug use patterns in the elderly. Therefore, this chapter first examines the epidemiology of drug use in elderly populations around the world, followed by age-related alterations in drug pharmacokinetics and pharmacodynamics, and finally drug interactions.

EPIDEMIOLOGY OF DRUG USE

In general, the number of medications (prescription and nonprescription) used by older individuals is greater than the number used by younger persons.[1] The number and type of medications used by elders are based, in part, on living situations and access to medications, as detailed below.

In the community

More than 75 percent of community-dwelling elderly people use one or more medications, with percentages varying by country: Sweden (93), Netherlands (90), USA (88), Italy (93), Canada (75), and Ireland (75).[2–7] The average number of medications being used at a given time is higher for US elders compared to elders elsewhere. The US average ranges between three and eight, whereas Sweden's average is 4.2, Taiwan's is 4.7, and Italy's is 3.5.[2,4,5,8–10] The most common types of medications are cardiovascular, gastrointestinal, central nervous system, analgesic, and vitamin agents.[1,2,5,6,10–13] The most common factor associated with medication use is gender, with females using more medications than males.[1,5,12–16] Increasing age has also been associated with increased medication use in the USA, Canada, and the UK.[11,12,14,16] In the USA, race has been associated with differences in medication use, with African Americans and Hispanic Americans demonstrating less use than Caucasians.[9,17]

In hospitals

Medication use by elderly people at the time of hospital discharge is slightly higher than that of community-dwelling elders; it ranges, on average, from about three medications in Germany to five in the USA, Australia, and the Netherlands.[18–21] There is a paucity of information with regard to the types of medications used by elders in this setting. However, in small studies conducted in the Netherlands, the USA, and Australia, the most common types of medications are cardiovascular, gastrointestinal, central nervous system, and analgesic agents, with noticeably high use of antimicrobials and laxatives.[18–20] There are conflicting studies regarding whether gender, increasing age, and number of medical conditions are factors enhancing medication use in this setting.[1,7,18–21]

In long-term-care facilities

The level of medication use of elderly people in long-term-care facilities (LTCFs) is generally higher than that of elders living at home.[22] For example, more than 75 percent of US LTCF residents receive four or more medications compared to 51 percent of Italian residents, 41 percent of Japanese residents, and 27 percent of Irish residents.[7,8,23] There is also disparity worldwide in the percentages of LTCF residents taking large numbers of medications. In the USA and Iceland, 33 percent of LTCF residents take 7–10 medications, whereas only 5 percent of residents have this high degree of use in Denmark, Italy, Japan, and Sweden.[23] The average number of routinely scheduled medications in most LTCF populations ranges from four to five, except in the USA and Sweden where the average is six to seven.[2,7,8,22,24–26]

The most common types of medications used are cardiovascular, central nervous system, laxative, and analgesic agents.[7,8,27] Overuse of certain centrally active medications, namely psychotropics, can be a particular problem in the LTCF setting.[28] Factors that have been associated with increased psychotropic use include dementia or mental illness and lack of drug monitoring.[29] Prior to 1987, there was a higher rate of usage of these agents in US LTCFs.[28] Federal legislation was then enacted which defined clear indications for appropriate prescribing of these agents and mandated close monitoring of them (Omnibus Budget Reconciliation Act or OBRA), resulting in a dramatic reduction in use.[29] Psychotropic medication usage rates are much higher in LTCFs in countries where there is no such monitoring.[29]

Access to medications

Universal public health insurance programs for elderly people in Australia, Sweden, Canada, France, Germany, Japan, New Zealand, and the UK provide some level of drug benefit coverage, with the drug benefits differing in the amount of cost sharing, the maximum amount of coverage, and the specific pharmaceuticals covered.[30] The US health insurance program for the elderly, Medicare, does not cover outpatient prescription drugs, but poor elders can receive drug benefit coverage through public assistance programs. While elderly Americans may purchase drug benefit coverage through retiree or individual insurance plans, 35 percent of elders are still without any drug benefit coverage, with the greatest impact likely on those who are near poverty and ineligible for public assistance programs.[31,32] Additionally, in developing countries, the supply of medications may be inadequate or too expensive for elders to purchase.[33]

ALTERED PHARMACOKINETICS

Table 14-1 illustrates an overview of age-related changes in drug pharmacokinetics.[34–36] The text herein details these changes in drug absorption, distribution, metabolism, and elimination.

Absorption

Numerous changes occur in the physiology of the gastrointestinal tract as a function of advancing age that might be expected to affect the absorption of drugs administered orally.[37] Gastric pH rises owing to the development of atrophic gastritis (as well as the use of acid-suppressive medications to treat age-related GI disorders such as peptic ulcer and gastroesophageal reflux). Gastric emptying is somewhat delayed and decreases are seen in intestinal blood flow (30–40 percent from age 20 to 70 years), intestinal motility, and number of functional absorptive cells.

Most drugs administered orally are absorbed via the process of passive diffusion, a process minimally affected by aging. A few agents require active transport for GI absorption and

their bioavailability may be reduced as a function of aging (e.g. calcium in the setting of hypochlorhydria). Of more significance is the decrease in first-pass intestinal wall and/or hepatic extraction that occurs with aging, resulting in an enhancement in systemic bioavailability for drugs like propranolol, morphine, and meperidine after oral administration.[37]

The effect of aging on drug absorption from other sites of administration such as rectum, muscle, and skin is poorly understood. For example, conflicting results have been published regarding the effect of aging on the pharmacokinetics of transdermal fentanyl.[38]

Distribution

A number of changes in physiology occur with aging that may impact drug distribution.[39,40] Body fat as a proportion of body weight rises from 18 to 36 percent in males and from 33 to 45 percent in females from age 20 to 70 years, while lean body mass decreases by 19 percent in males and by 12 percent in females, and plasma volume decreases by 8 percent from age 20 to 80 years. Total body water decreases by 17 percent from age 20 to 80 years and extracellular fluid volume decreases by 40 percent from 20 to 65 years of age. In addition, cardiac output declines approximately 1 percent per year from age 30 years, and brain and cardiac vessel blood flow rates decline 0.35 to 0.5 and 0.5 percent per year, respectively, beyond age 25 years. Additionally, frailty and concurrent disease may result in substantial changes in the serum concentrations of the two major drug-binding plasma proteins (albumin, which binds acidic drugs, decreases while alpha-1 acid glycoprotein, which binds basic drugs, remains the same or rises).[41]

As a result of the above factors, the volume of distribution of water-soluble (hydrophilic) drugs is decreased and that of fat-soluble (lipophilic) drugs is increased. Moreover, changes in volume of distribution can directly affect the loading doses of medications. For example, the loading dose of digoxin should be reduced in the presence of renal dysfunction (by 65 percent when the creatinine clearance is less than or equal to 10 mL/min).[34] Decreases in serum albumin concentration can lead to a reduction in the degree of plasma protein binding of acidic drugs such as naproxen, phenytoin, tolbutamide, and warfarin, thus increasing the drug-free fraction. Increases in alpha-1 acid glycoprotein due to inflammatory disease, burns, or cancer can lead to enhancement in the degree of plasma protein binding of basic drugs such as lidocaine, β-blockers, quinidine, and tricyclic antidepressants, thus reducing the drug-free fraction. Provided there is no compromise in excretory pathways, these potential changes are unlikely to be clinically significant. However, plasma protein binding changes can alter the relationship of unbound (free) and total (unbound + bound) plasma drug concentrations, making drug concentration interpretation more difficult. In these cases, the measurement of free plasma drug concentrations may be preferable to the usual use of total plasma drug concentrations.

Metabolism

Although drug metabolism can occur in numerous organs, most of the available data concern the effects of aging on

---

Table 14-1 Age-related changes in drug pharmacokinetics

Pharmacokinetic phase	Pharmacokinetic parameters
Gastrointestinal absorption	Unchanged passive diffusion and no change in bioavailability for most drugs ↓ active transport and ↓ bioavailability for some drugs ↓ first-pass effect and ↑ bioavailability for some drugs
Distribution	↓ volume of distribution and ↑ plasma concentrations of water-soluble drugs ↑ volume of distribution and ↑ terminal disposition half-life (t½) for fat-soluble drugs ↑ or ↓ decreased free fraction of highly plasma protein bound drugs
Hepatic metabolism	↓ clearance and ↑ t½ for some oxidatively metabolized drugs ↓ clearance and ↑ t½ of drugs with high hepatic extraction ratio
Renal excretion	↓ clearance and ↑ t½ of renally eliminated drugs

↑ = increased; ↓ = decreased.

Table 14-2 Selected cytochrome P450 substrates by isozyme

CYP1A2	CYP2C9	CYP2C19	CYP2D6	CYP3A4
Caffeine	Diclofenac	Diazepam	Codeine	Alprazolam
Clozapine	Phenytoin	S-mephenytoin	Desipramine	Astemizole
Olanzapine	Tolbutamine	Omeprazole	Dextromethorphan	Ciclosporin
Theophylline	S-warfarin	Phenytoin	Encainide	Midazolam
			Haloperidol	Nifedipine
			Metoprolol	Quetiapine
			Paroxetine	Terfenodine
			Risperidone	Triazolam
			Thioridazine	Verapamil

the liver. Over the age of 30 years, there is an approximate 1 percent per year decline in liver blood flow and liver mass.[42]

Drugs are metabolized by two types of reactions: phase I (oxidative reactions) and phase II (conjugative/synthetic reactions wherein an acetyl group or a sugar is conjugated to the drug to enhance its polarity, water-solubility, and hence, excretion via the kidneys). Most phase I reactions are mediated by cytochrome P450 (CYP 450) mono-oxygenase enzymes. Table 14-2 illustrates five CYP 450 isozymes of clinical importance and selected substrates. Age-related declines in drug oxidation (which are substrate-specific in their extent) are thought to more closely relate to reductions in liver volume (i.e. hepatocyte mass) than reductions in hepatic enzymatic activity.[43] Age-related decreased phase I metabolism, resulting in reduced total body clearance and increased terminal disposition half-life, has been reported for diazepam, chlordiazepoxide, piroxicam, theophylline, and quinidine (Table 14-3). The effect of aging on polymorphic drug metabolism has not been well-studied, although available data suggest that advancing age has no significant effect on drug acetylation or cytochrome P450 2D6 polymorphism.[44,45] Differences in enantiomeric disposition as a function of age are substrate-specific. For example, age-dependent changes in enantiomeric disposition have been reported for hexobarbital, propranolol, mephobarbital, and warfarin.[46–48] Phase II reactions appear to be generally spared from any adverse effect of aging.

Age-associated reductions in hepatic blood flow can reduce the clearance of high hepatic extraction ratio drugs such as tricyclic antidepressants, lidocaine, several opioids, and propranolol (Table 14-3).[42] Numerous confounders such as race, gender, frailty, smoking, diet, and drug interactions can significantly enhance or inhibit hepatic drug metabolism in the elderly.[49]

Elimination

Few data are available regarding the effect of aging on the biliary system. However, aging is associated with a significant reduction in renal mass and number and size of nephrons. In addition, glomerular filtration rate, tubular secretion, and renal blood flow decrease approximately 0.5, 0.5, and 1 percent per year, respectively, over the age of 20 years.[50,51] However, elderly people are a heterogeneous group, with up to one-third of healthy elders having no decrement in renal function as measured by creatinine clearance, a surrogate for glomerular filtration. In addition, tubular secretion and glomerular

filtration may not decline in parallel.[52] The estimation of creatinine clearance (CrCl), using any of a number of equations, serves as a useful screen for renal impairment in lieu of the use of serum creatinine (SCr), which is an imperfect marker of renal function in the elderly due to the reduction of muscle mass with advancing age (i.e. a "normal" serum creatinine does not equate with "normal" renal function in the elderly).[53] One useful estimation equation is that of Cockcroft and Gault:[54]

$$CrCl \, (males) = \frac{(140 - age \, in \, years) \times (total \, body \, weight \, in \, kg)}{72 \times SCr \, in \, mg/dL}$$

For females, multiply the result by 0.85.

Numerous medications are primarily renally-excreted and/or have renally-excreted active metabolites. Evidence exists of age-related reduction in the total body clearances of drugs which are primarily renally-cleared (Table 14-4). The risk

Table 14-3 Drugs whose hepatic metabolism is impaired with advancing age

Amlodipine	Nifedipine
Chlordiazepoxide	Nortriptyline
Diazepam	Phenytoin
Enalapril	Piroxicam
Erythromycin	Propranolol
Fosinopril	Quinidine
Imipramine	Theophylline
Levodopa	Triazolam
Lidocaine	Verapamil
Morphine	

Table 14-4 Drugs whose renal elimination is impaired with advancing age

ACEI	Furosemide
Acetazolamide	Lithium
Amantadine	Metformin
Aminoglycosides	Procainamide/NAPA
Chlorpropamide	Ranitidine
Cimetidine	Vancomycin
Digoxin	

ACEI, angiotensin-converting enzyme inhibitor; NAPA, N-acetylprocainamide.

of adverse clinical consequences are likely increased for those drugs with narrow therapeutic margins (e.g. digoxin, aminoglycosides).

ALTERED PHARMACODYNAMICS

In contrast to the relationship of aging to altered pharmacokinetics, fewer data are available investigating the effect of aging on pharmacodynamics (drug response). Theoretically, altered pharmacodynamics could be due to two mechanisms: (1) altered sensitivity owing to changes in receptor number or affinity and changes in post-receptor response, and (2) age-related impairment of physiological and homeostatic mechanisms.[55] This section reviews altered responses of elderly people to medications mediated by these two mechanisms.

Altered sensitivity

Table 14-5 lists those medications for which there are reasonable data documenting altered drug sensitivity in elderly people. Firm evidence exists that elders are less responsive to β-blockers and β-agonists.[56,57] There is a diminished maximal response to furosemide.[55] Firm evidence also exists that elders are more sensitive to the effects of benzodiazepines. Using psychomotor testing, this has been established for nitrazepam, temazepam, midazolam, loprazolam, and diazepam.[55,58] Enhanced sensitivity has also been demonstrated for opioids, metoclopramide, dopamine agonists, levodopa, and traditional neuroleptics.[55] It is well-established that elderly people have enhanced sensitivity to the effects of oral anticoagulants. The underlying mechanism of this effect is unknown.[55] There is evidence for both enhanced and reduced sensitivity to calcium-channel blockers in elders measured as blood pressure response or electrocardiographic (P–R interval) response.[55,58]

Alterations in physiological and homeostatic mechanisms

Physiological and homeostatic impairments in elderly people that may affect drug response include autonomic nervous system dysfunction (orthostasis, bowel/bladder dysfunction), impaired thermoregulation, reduced cognitive function reserve, impaired postural stability, glucose intolerance, and immunosenescence.[59–63] The loss of efficiency of homeostatic mechanisms puts elders at risk of symptomatic orthostasis/falls (with antihypertensives, traditional neuroleptics, tricyclic antidepressants), urinary retention and constipation (with drugs with anticholinergic properties), falls and delirium (with virtually every sedating drug), and accidental hypothermia or heatstroke (with neuroleptics) (Table 14-5).

DRUG INTERACTIONS

Drug interactions can be defined as the effect that the administration of one medication has on another drug.[64] The two major types of drug interactions include pharmacokinetic interactions, wherein drug absorption, distribution, metabolism, and excretion are affected; and pharmacodynamic interactions, wherein pharmacological effect is altered. Drugs may also interact with food or exacerbate pre-existing diseases.

Pharmacokinetic interactions

Increased drug bioavailability may be seen with the concurrent ingestion of grapefruit juice owing to its inhibitory effect on cytochrome P450 isozyme 3A4-mediated first-pass metabolism in the gut wall and liver. This may result in exaggerated pharmacological effects.[65] Decreased bioavailability can be seen when phenytoin is administered with enteral feedings.[66] Multivalent cations (e.g. antacids, sucralfate, iron, calcium supplements) can reduce the bioavailability of tetracycline and quinolone antimicrobials.[67]

Drug interactions involving drug distribution are primarily related to altered plasma protein binding. Although a number of drugs may displace other drugs from plasma protein binding sites, especially acids such as salicylate, valproic acid and phenytoin, this type of drug interaction is rarely clinically significant.

Drug interactions most likely to be clinically significant are those that involve the inhibition or induction of metabolism of narrow therapeutic margin drugs.[68] Table 14-2 provides examples of selected cytochrome P450 substrates whereas Table 14-6 illustrates selected cytochrome P450 enzyme inducers and inhibitors. It does not appear that young and elderly individuals differ in the magnitude of hepatic enzyme inhibition after exposure to drugs like cimetidine, macrolide antimicrobials (e.g. erythromycin, clarithromycin), quinidine, and

---

Table 14-5 Drugs whose sensitivity is altered with advancing age

β-Agonists (↓)	H₁-antihistamines (↑)
β-Blockers (↓)	Metoclopramide (↑)
Benzodiazepines (↑)	Neuroleptics (↑)
Calcium antagonists (↓ ↑)	Opioids (↑)
Dopaminergic agents (↑)	Warfarin (↑)
Furosemide (↓)	Vaccines (↓)

↑ = increased; ↓ = decreased.

Table 14-6 Selected cytochrome P450 inducers and inhibitors by isozyme

CYP1A2	CYP2C	CYP2D6	CYP3A4
Inducers	*Inducers*	*Inducers*	*Inducers*
Char-broiled beef	Rifampin	None known	Carbamazepine
Cruciferous			Phenytoin
vegetables	*Inhibitors*	*Inhibitors*	Rifampin
Omeprazole	Amiodarone	Fluoxetine	St John's Wort
Smoking	Fluconazole	Paroxetine	
	Fluvastatin	Quinidine	*Inhibitors*
Inhibitors		Ritonavir	Erythromycin
Cimetidine			Ketoconazole
Ciprofloxacin			Nefazodone
Fluvoxamine			

ciprofloxacin.[67,69] However, there is controversy regarding the effect of hepatic enzyme inducers in young versus elderly individuals, with some studies demonstrating no difference between the age groups while others suggest that elders do not respond as well to enzyme induction.[46,70–72] It may be that these effects are substrate- and/or inducer-specific.

Inhibition of renal clearance of one drug by another drug can also result in clinically significant effects.[73] Many of these drug interactions involve competitive inhibition of tubular secretion of anionic or cationic drugs. Table 14-7 provides a list of selected anionic or cationic drugs actively secreted via the renal tubules. For example, a nonsteroidal anti-inflammatory drug such as indometacin can inhibit the renal clearance of methotrexate. Another important interaction is the effect of quinidine on the renal clearance of digoxin.

Pharmacodynamic interactions

Some drugs may alter the response of another drug and produce adverse effects. A good example of this is the synergistic effect of taking more than one anticholinergic agent concurrently which can result in delirium, urinary retention, constipation, and other problems.[64] Other examples include additive bradycardia when β-blockers are administered concurrently with verapamil or diltiazem, additive hypotension when several antihypertensives are administered concurrently, and sedation/falls when several CNS depressants (e.g. benzodiazepines, sedative-hypnotics, antidepressants, neuroleptics) are administered concurrently.

Drug–disease interactions

Drug interactions can also be considered in a broader sense when they involve medications that can affect and can be affected by disease states. Elderly people are at higher risk for adverse outcomes with drug–disease state interactions owing to alterations in homeostatic mechanisms, diminished physiological reserve, and multiple comorbidities. Recently, a national expert panel from Canada and another from the USA developed a list of clinically important drug–disease state interactions (Table 14-8).[74,75] For example, nonsteroidal anti-inflammatory drugs can exacerbate hypertension and heart failure.[38]

Table 14-7 Selected drugs actively secreted by renal tubules

Basic (cationic) agents	Acidic (anionic) agents
Amiodarone	Cephalosporins
Cimetidine	Indometacin
Digoxin	Methotrexate
Procainamide	Penicillins
Quinidine	Probenecid
Ranitidine	Salicylates
Trimethoprim	Thiazides
Verapamil	

Table 14-8 Drug–disease interactions to avoid in the elderly as defined by explicit criteria by Canadian and US consensus panels[74,75]

Drug or drug class	Disease
α-Blockers	Urinary incontinence
Anticholinergic antihistamines	Benign prostatic hypertrophy
	Constipation
Anticholinergic antispasmodics	Benign prostatic hypertrophy
	Constipation
Anticholinergic tricyclic antidepressants	Benign prostatic hypertrophy
	Constipation
	Glaucoma
Amphetamines	Hypertension
Aspirin (>325 mg/day)	Peptic ulcer
Benzodiazepines, long half-life	Dementia
	Syncope/falls
β-Agonists	Insomnia
β-Blockers	Asthma/chronic obstructive pulmonary disease
	Diabetes
	Heart failure[a]
	Peripheral vascular disease, Raynaud's disease, Syncope/falls
Bethanechol	Benign prostatic hypertrophy
Calcium-channel blockers	Heart failure
Chlorpromazine	Postural hypotension
	Seizures
Clozapine	Seizures
Corticosteroids (systemic)	Diabetes
Decongestants	Insomnia
Desipramine	Insomnia
Disopyramide	Heart failure
Genitourinary antispasmodics	Benign prostatic hypertrophy
	Constipation
Methylphenidate	Insomnia
Metoclopramide	Seizures
Monoamine oxidase inhibitors	Insomnia
Narcotics	Benign prostatic hypertrophy
	Constipation
Nonsteroidal anti-inflammatory drugs	Chronic renal failure
	Heart failure
	Hypertension
	Peptic ulcer
Phenylpropanolamine	Hypertension
Potassium supplements	Peptic ulcer
Sedative/hypnotics	Chronic obstructive pulmonary disease
Skeletal muscle relaxants	Benign prostatic hypertrophy
Selective serotonin reuptake inhibitors	Insomnia
Theophylline	Insomnia
Thiazide diuretics	Gout
Thioridazine	Seizures
Tricyclic antidepressants	Arrhythmia
	Heart block
	Postural hypotension

[a]This combination may be beneficial in some patients.

SUMMARY

Elderly people consume a disproportionate share of medications. Factors enhancing medication utilization include the concurrent presence of multiple diseases, female gender, increasing level of care, and increasing age. Other factors that probably influence drug use in elderly people include provider prescribing behaviors, cultural milieu, psychosocial issues (i.e. living alone, anxiety, depression) and direct-to-consumer advertising by the pharmaceutical industry.

The most common classes of medications in the elderly include cardiovascular, gastrointestinal, central nervous system, and analgesic agents. Many studies have documented that the aging process alters drug disposition and response. Changes in body composition with aging result in an altered volume of distribution for many drugs. Age-related changes in plasma protein binding may alter the relationship of unbound and total plasma drug concentrations. Phase I hepatic metabolism is often reduced in older patients, resulting in reduced clearance and increased elimination half-life of many commonly used drugs. Age-related decline in renal function decreases clearance and increases the elimination half-life of renally-eliminated drugs. Pharmacodynamic studies indicate that elderly individuals tend to be more sensitive to the effects of benzodiazepines, opioids, dopamine-receptor antagonists, and warfarin. Drug–drug and drug–disease interactions may also impact elders' well-being.

Knowledge of this information is important for achieving the maximal benefits of medications in the elderly while avoiding drug-related problems.

KEY POINTS   Pharmacology of aging

- The elderly are avid consumers of medications.

- Age-related alterations in drug pharmacokinetics are most pronounced for decline in the hepatic metabolism and renal elimination of certain drugs.

- Age-related alterations in drug pharmacodynamics are under-studied, but elderly people seem to be more sensitive to the effects of benzodiazepines, opioids, dopamine-receptor antagonists, and warfarin.

- Potential drug–drug and drug–disease interactions are common in elderly people and may have an impact on health-related quality of life.

REFERENCES

1. Nolan L, O'Malley K: Prescribing for the elderly. II: Prescribing patterns: differences due to age. J Am Geriatr Soc 1988;36:245–254
2. Giron MST, Claesson C, Thorslund M et al: Drug use patterns in a very elderly population: a seven-year review. Clin Drug Invest 1999;17:389–398
3. Veehof LJG, Stewart RE, Meyboom-de Jong B et al: Adverse drug reactions and polypharmacy in the elderly in general practice. Eur J Clin Pharmacol 1999;55:533–536
4. Helling DK, Lemke JH, Semla TP et al: Medication use characteristics in the elderly: the Iowa 65+ rural health study. J Am Geriatr Soc 1987;35:4–12
5. Nobili A, Tettamanti M, Frattura L et al: Drug use by the elderly in Italy. Ann Pharmacother 1997;31:416–422
6. Millar WJ: Multiple medication use among seniors. Health Rep 1998;9:11–17
7. Passmore AP, Crawford VLS, Beringer TRO et al: Determinants of drug utilization in an elderly population in North and West Belfast. Pharmacoepidemiol Drug Safety 1995;4:147–160
8. Stewart RB, Cooper JW: Polypharmacy in the aged: practical solutions. Drugs Aging 1994;4:449–461
9. Hanlon JT, Fillenbaum GG, Burchette B et al: Drug-use patterns among black and nonblack community-dwelling elderly. Ann Pharmacother 1992;26:679–685
10. Hsu RY, Lin MS, Chou MH et al: Medication use characteristics in an ambulatory elderly population in Taiwan. Ann Pharmacother 1997;31:309–314
11. Rathore SS, Mehta SS, Boyko WL et al: Prescription medication use in older Americans: a national report card on prescribing. Fam Med 1998;30:733–739
12. Rumble RH, Morgan K: Longitudinal trends in prescribing for elderly patients: two surveys four years apart. Br J Gen Pract 1994;44:571–575
13. Stoehr GP, Ganguli M, Seaberg EC et al: Over-the-counter medication use in an older rural community: the MoVIES Project. J Am Geriatr Soc 1997;45:158–165
14. Chrischilles EA, Foley DJ, Wallace RB et al: Use of medications by persons 65 and over: data from the Established Populations for Epidemiologic Studies of the Elderly. J Gerontol A 1992;47:M137–M144
15. Laukkanen P, Heikkinen E, Kauppinen M et al: Use of drugs by non-institutionalized urban Finns born in 1904–1923 and the association of drug use with mood and self-rated health. Age Ageing 1992;21:343–352
16. Tamblyn R: Medication use in seniors: challenges and solutions. Thérapie 1996;51:269–282
17. Espino DV, Lichtenstein MJ, Hazuda HP et al: Correlates of prescription and over-the-counter medication usage among older Mexican Americans: the Hispanic EPESE study. J Am Geriatr Soc 1998;46:1228–1234
18. Beers M, Dang J, Hasegawa J et al: Influence of hospitalization on drug therapy in the elderly. J Am Geriatr Soc 1989;37:679–683
19. Gonski PN, Stathers GM, Freiman JS et al: A critical review of admission and discharge medications in an elderly Australian population. Drugs Aging 1993;3:358–362
20. van Kraaij DJW, Haagsma CJ, Go IH et al: Drug use and adverse drug reactions in 105 elderly patients admitted to a general medical ward. Neth J Med 1994;66:166–173
21. Nikolaus T, Kruse W, Bach M et al: Elderly patients' problems with medication: an in-hospital and follow-up study. Eur J Clin Pharmacol 1996;49:255–259
22. Furniss L, Craig SKL, Burns A: Medication use in nursing homes for elderly people. Int J Geriatr Psychiat 1998;13:433–439
23. Hughes CM, Lapane KL, Mor V et al: The impact of legislation on psychotropic drug use in nursing homes: a cross-national perspective. J Am Geriatr Soc 2000;48:931–937
24. Stichele RHV, Mestdagh J, Van Haecht CH et al: Medication utilization and patient information in homes for the aged. Eur J Clin Pharmacol 1992;43:319–321
25. Butler R, Fonseka S, Barclay L et al: The health of elderly residents in long-term care institutions in New Zealand. NZ Med J 1999;112:427–429
26. Tobias DE, Sey M: General and psychotherapeutic medication use in 328 nursing facilities: a year 2000 national survey. Consult Pharm 2001;16:54–64
27. Lunn J, Chan K, Donoghue J et al: Study of the appropriateness of prescribing in nursing homes. Int J Pharm Prac 1997;5:6–10
28. Beardsley RS, Larson DB, Burns BJ et al: Prescribing of psychotropics in elderly nursing home patients. J Am Geriatr Soc 1989;37:327–330
29. Hughes CM, Lapane KL, Mor V: Influence of facility characteristics on use of antipsychotic medications in nursing homes. Med Care 2000;38:1164–1173
30. Freund DA, Willison D, Reeher G et al: Outpatient pharmaceuticals and the elderly: policies in seven nations. Health Aff 2000;19:259–266
31. Anderson GF, Hussey PS: Population aging: a comparison among industrialized countries. Health Aff 2000;19:191–203
32. Donelan K, Blendon RJ, Schoen C et al: The elderly in five nations: the importance of universal coverage. Health Aff 2000;19:226–235
33. Magrath I, Litvak J: Cancer in developing countries: opportunity and challenge. J Natl Cancer Inst 1993;85:862–874
34. Chapron DJ: Drug disposition and response in the elderly. In Delafuente JC, Stewart RB (eds): Therapeutics in the Elderly, 3rd edn. Harvey Whitney, Cincinnati, 2000:257–288
35. Kiniross MT, Crome P: Clinical pharmacokinetic considerations in the elderly: an update. Clin Pharmacokinet 1997;33:302–312
36. Hammerlein A, Derendorf H, Lowenthal DT: Pharmacokinetic and pharmacodynamic changes in the elderly: clinical implications. Clin Pharmacokinet 1998;35:49–64

37. Iber FL, Murphy PA, Connor ES: Age-related changes in the gastrointestinal system: effects on drug therapy. Drugs Aging 1994;5:34–48

38. Guay D, Lackner T, Hanlon JT: Pharmacologic management: non-invasive modalities. In Weiner DK, Herr K, Rudy TE (eds): Improving the lives of older adults with persistent pain: an interdisciplinary guide. Springer, New York, 2002 (in press)

39. Edelman IS, Leibman J: Anatomy of body water and electrolytes. Am J Med 1959;27:256–277

40. Forbes GB, Reina JC: Adult lean body mass declines with age: some longitudinal observations. Metabolism 1970;19:653–663

41. Grandison MK, Boudinot FD: Age-related changes in protein binding of drugs: implications for therapy. Clin Pharmacokinet 2000;38:271–290

42. Woodhouse K, Wynne HA: Age-related changes in hepatic function. Drugs Aging 1992;2:243–255

43. Sotaniemi EA, Arranto AJ, Pelkonen O et al: Age and cytochrome P450-linked drug metabolism in humans: an analysis of 226 subjects with equal histopathologic conditions. Clin Pharmacol Ther 1997;61:331–339

44. Korrapati MR, Sorkin JD, Andres R et al: Acetylator phenotype in relation to age and gender in the Baltimore Longitudinal Study of Aging. J Clin Pharmacol 1997;37:83–91

45. Agundey JA, Rodriguez I, Olivera M et al: CYP206, NAT2 and CYP2E1 genetic polymorphisms in nonagenarians. Age Ageing 1997;26:147–151

46. Smith DA, Chandler MH, Shedlofsky SI et al: Age-dependent stereoselective increase in the oral clearance of hexobarbitone isomers caused by rifampicin. Br J Clin Pharmacol 1991;32:735–739

47. Zhou HA, Whelan E, Wood AJ: The effect of aging on the stereochemical disposition of propranolol. Br J Clin Pharmacol 1992;33:121–123

48. Lalonde RL, Tenero DM, Buelow BS et al: Effects of age on the protein binding and disposition of propranolol stereoisomers. Clin Pharmacol Ther 1990;47:447–455

49. O'Mahony MS, Woodhouse KW: Age, environmental factors and drug metabolism. Pharmacol Ther 1994;61:279–284

50. Davies DF, Shock NW: Age changes in glomerular filtration rate, effective renal plasma flow and tubular excretory capacity in adult males. J Clin Invest 1950;29:496–507

51. Miller JH, McDonald RK, Shock NW: Age changes in the maximal rate of tubular reabsorption of glucose. J Gerontol 1952;7:196–200

52. Ujhelyi MR, Bottorff MB, Schur M et al: Aging effects on the organic base transporter and stereoselective renal clearance. Clin Pharmacol Ther 1997;62:117–128

53. Malmrose LC, Gray SL, Pieper CF et al: Measured versus estimated creatinine clearance in a high-functioning elderly sample: MacArthur Foundation Study of Successful Aging. J Am Geriatr Soc 1993;41:715–721

54. Cockroft DW, Gault MH: Prediction of creatinine clearance from serum creatinine. Nephron 1976;16:31–41

55. Feely J, Coakley D: Altered pharmacodynamics in the elderly. Clin Geriatr Med 1990;6:269–283

56. Vestal RE, Wood AJJ, Shand DG: Reduced beta adrenoceptor sensitivity in the elderly. Clin Pharmacol Ther 1979;26:181–186

57. Turner MJ, Mier CM, Spina RJ et al: Effects of age and gender on the cardiovascular responses to isoproterenol. J Gerontol A 1999;54:B393–B400

58. Klotz U: Effect of age on pharmacokinetics and pharmacodynamics in man. Int J Clin Pharmacol Ther 1998;36:581–585

59. Johnson RH, Smith AC, Spalding JMK: The effect of posture on blood pressure in elderly patients. Lancet 1965;1:731–733

60. Collins KJ, Exton-Smith AN, James MH: Functional changes in autonomic nervous responses with aging. Age Ageing 1980;9:17–24

61. Sheldon JH: The effect of age on the control of sway. Geront Clin 1963;5:129–138

62. Swift CA: Postural instability as a measure of sedative drug response. Br J Clin Pharmacol 1984;18:87S–90S

63. Collins KJ, Dove C, Exton-Smith AN: Accidental hypothermia and impaired temperature regulation in the elderly. BMJ 1977;1:353–356

64. Seymour RM, Routledge PA: Important drug–drug interactions in the elderly. Drugs Aging 1998;12:485–494

65. Dresser GK, Bailey DG, Carruthers SG: Grapefruit juice–felodipine interaction in the elderly. Clin Pharmacol Ther 2000;68:28–34

66. Yeung Au SCS, Ensom MHH: Phenytoin and enteral feedings: does evidence support an interaction. Ann Pharmacother 2000;34:896–905

67. Guay DG: Quinolones. In Piscitelli SC, Rodvold KA (eds): Drug interactions in infectious diseases. Humana Press, Totowa, 2000:121–150

68. Michalets EL: Update: clinically significant cytochrome P-450 drug interactions. Pharmacotherapy 1998;18:84–112

69. Loi CM, Parker BM, Cusack BJ et al: Aging and drug interactions. III: Individual and combined effects of cimetidine and cimetidine and ciprofloxacin on theophylline metabolism in healthy male and female nonsmokers. J Pharmacol Exp Ther 1997;280:627–637

70. Crowley JJ, Cusack BJ, Jue SG et al: Aging and drug interactions. II: Effect of phenytoin and smoking on the oxidation of theophylline and cortisol in healthy men. J Pharmacol Exp Ther 1988;245:513–523

71. Dilger K, Hofmann U, Klotz U: Enzyme induction in the elderly: effect of rifampin on the pharmacokinetics and pharmacodynamics of propafenone. Clin Pharmacol Ther 2000;67:512–520

72. Hamman MA, Bruce MA, Haehner-Daniels BD et al: The effect of rifampin administration on the disposition of fexofenadine. Clin Pharmacol Ther 2001;69:114–121

73. Hansten PD, Horn JR, Koda-Kimble MA et al: Drug interactions: a clinical perspective and analysis of current developments. Applied Therapeutics, Vancouver, WA, 2000

74. McLeod PJ, Huang AR, Tamblyn RM et al: Defining inappropriate practices in prescribing for elderly people: a national consensus panel. Can Med Assoc J 1997;156:385–391

75. Beers MH: Explicit criteria for determining potentially inappropriate medication by the elderly. Arch Int Med 1997;157:1531–1536

Chapter 15

Anti-aging interventions

S. Mitchell Harman and Christopher Heward

Material in this chapter contains contributions from the previous edition, and we are grateful to the previous authors for the work done.

During the twentieth century, an unprecedented increase in human life expectancy (mean lifespan) occurred in the USA and most developed countries.[1] The reasons for this increase are not completely understood, but it is likely that modern sanitation, improved public health programs, better personal hygiene, reduced environmental hazards, and more effective medical interventions, such as antibiotics, all contributed. This increase in life expectancy has led, in turn, to an alteration in population demography such that a greatly increased proportion of the residents of developed nations are now over the age of 65. Moreover, persons over age 85 are now the fastest growing segment of the population in the developed nations.[2] The societal and economic implications of an aging world population are impossible to predict, but recent analyses concluded that increased life expectancy might constitute the single largest source of gains in our standard of living over the past 100 years.[1,3] It is still a matter of controversy as to whether this trend will continue.[4,5]

The answer to the question as to whether the trend for increasing human life expectancy will continue or plateau depends upon our ability to impact the fundamental aging process and extend the maximum human lifespan. Most experts agree that, unless we can address the fundamental process of biological aging, the trend toward increased life expectancy will slow dramatically in the near future.[4] There is considerable optimism that anticipated advances in medical science, based in part on the recent revolution in molecular biology and genetics, may soon lead to interventions that will retard or reverse the process of aging, but it is important to state, at the outset of this discussion, that no such interventions currently exist.

In spite of the existence of a "professional society" in the USA with the name "Anti-aging Medicine," anti-aging medicine remains a dream. There is, as yet, no convincing evidence that administration of any medicinal compound, natural or artificial, can slow, let alone reverse, human aging. Effective pharmacological interventions have yet to be demonstrated even in mice or rats. Claims to the contrary are both blatantly false and misleading to consumers. By misrepresenting what is currently possible, such claims understate the need for a greater understanding of the biology of aging and undermine the eventual development of authentic anti-aging interventions. It should be noted at this juncture that even the question whether it would be desirable or ethical to develop effective interventions to slow aging and extend the maximum human lifespan is controversial.[6]

In contrast to anti-aging medicine, the practice of geriatric medicine is a critically important specialty in all developed countries where population aging is a demographic certainty. Geriatric medicine focuses upon combating the degenerative diseases associated with aging (heart disease, cancer, stroke, type 2 diabetes, arthritis, Alzheimer's, osteoporosis, etc.). It is not the purpose of geriatric medicine to influence the aging process itself, but rather to prevent, treat, or ameliorate the consequent morbidity of known age-related diseases. It is interesting to note that, even in the absence of all fatal diseases, humans would not become immortal. Under such conditions, life expectancy would be determined entirely by environmental risks. The result would be an average lifespan on the order of 600 years, according to currently estimated risk levels.[7]

For many years, some scientists have questioned whether interventions to slow the aging process are desirable, but the more important issue is whether such interventions are even possible. Recently, however, investigations into the biological basis for the longevity of various nonhuman organisms have produced a number of promising targets for further research by biogerontologists. For example, caloric restriction (restricting caloric intake without causing malnutrition) seems to slow the rate of aging.[8,9] It is important to note that, in this model of extended lifespan, the result is not a prolonged period of frailty and senescence. Rather, the onset of a wide range of age-related diseases and disabilities, including cancers, immune senescence, cognitive decline, loss of muscle mass and strength, cataracts, and many others appears to be delayed and the period of relatively vital middle age appears to be prolonged.[10–15] Alterations of certain biochemical pathways in invertebrate animals have also been shown to extend lifespan.[16] In some species, lifespan extension has been achieved by genetic manipulation. Modification of certain single genes in various species can lead to a 20–50 percent increase in longevity, producing changes both in average, and in maximum, lifespan.[17–19] Analysis of the survival curves of animals produced using these methods suggests that these mutations may be increasing lifespan by an effect on the rate of aging itself. Several of these life-extending mutations share a common characteristic: they block the production of, the effects of, or the response to growth hormone, or its second messenger, insulin-like growth factor I (IGF-I). This is particularly ironic because it is common practice among many so-called anti-aging doctors to prescribe human growth hormone to combat aging.

In spite of the exciting results obtained in nonhuman laboratory animals, none of the approaches that slows aging in animals to date is a practical model for slowing or reversing aging in humans. In the opinion of the present authors, neither genetic modification nor voluntary caloric restriction deserves serious consideration as an anti-aging therapy in humans.

The importance of these research findings is that they demonstrate that (a) aging can be slowed down dramatically through simple means, and (b) practical pharmacological approaches to effective deceleration of the aging process are theoretically possible. Furthermore, it is the authors' contention that pharmacological interventions in humans which could extend lifespan similarly to the experimental models would make possible the prevention or treatment of a wide range of late-life ailments now considered to be incurable chronic diseases. Such interventions will require substantial basic and translational research before they become part of the armamentariums of practitioners of preventive and geriatric medicine. Thus, at least for the foreseeable future, ethical healthcare practitioners must be content to help patients cope with the problems of aging using traditional medical technologies for the prevention, diagnosis, and treatment of age-related diseases.

A GENETIC AND EVOLUTIONARY PERSPECTIVE

It is likely that, at the finest level, aging is the process of progressive and cumulative unrepaired damage to biomolecules due to endogenous and exogenous energetic processes. Because repair processes are neither 100 percent efficient nor 100 percent accurate, molecular damage occurs at a rate greater than molecular repair. This leads to what the prominent gerontologist, Dr Leonard Hayflick, has referred to as "molecular disorder."[20] The end-result is declining functionality and increasing vulnerability to environmental hazards and disease (i.e. aging).

Modern understanding of evolutionary biology has shed considerable light on the likely nature of biological aging and senescence.[21,22] It has been clear since Darwin's description of the process that natural selection favors the preservation of traits (i.e. genes) in a population that lead to reproductive success. Such traits are usually those which lead to greater capacity in vital systems that enable individuals to obtain sustenance, avoid premature death (escape predation, disease, accidents, and environmental extremes), and compete for mates, in the particular niches they inhabit. In the absence of premature death from predation, accident, etc., longevity is determined by the level of physiological reserve that remains after reproductive maturity. There is, *a priori*, no selective pressure, and perhaps even a disadvantage in terms of wasted resources, to evolving greater physiological reserve capacity than that required for maximal reproductive success in a particular environment. To restate, *there is no procreative advantage to greater longevity than that required for reproductive success.* Excess physiological reserve capacity must therefore evolve as a secondary consequence of a natural selection process based upon reproductive competence, not longevity. Longevity can evolve only in circumstances in which high physiological reserve favors reproductive success.

These considerations inevitably lead to the conclusion that genes and genetic interactions that tend to favor longevity may exist, in any species, but there are no "clock" genes that have been systematically selected to age the individual or limit the species lifespan. The existence of genes that shorten individual lifespan (and there are many which have been identified—i.e. "genetic diseases") must therefore be "accidental." Moreover, no gene whose sole or major effect is to shorten the lifespan to the point of reducing reproductive potential can become very widely distributed in a population (e.g. be present in a majority of individuals). The implication of the above is that a detailed understanding of the actions of those genes which have been selected because they increase longevity, especially in species such as our own, in which long life favors successful reproduction, could lead to interventions which extend lifespan still further.

AGING: A CLINICAL DEFINITION

Physicians, scientists, and bureaucrats have long debated the distinction between aging and disease.[23] Part of the difficulty in reaching a consensus stems from our ignorance of the fundamental mechanisms of these processes, particularly of aging. Although there is no consensus about the fundamental mechanisms responsible for aging, most scientists share the practical view that it is a universal, intrinsic, and deleterious biological process that manifests itself as a decline in functional capacity and an increased risk of mortality over time.[24] This definition refers to what many gerontologists think of as "primary aging"; whereas, "secondary aging" refers to those diseases that tend to accompany primary aging and their sequelae. While it may not be appropriate to consider aging itself to be a disease, it is abundantly clear that it is not healthy.

It is important, at this point, also to make a distinction between aging and the aged. Aging is a negative biological process that happens, as people grow chronologically older. It is not the people themselves. One can be against aging without being against elderly people, just as one can be against cancer without being against people who have cancer. It is equally important not to confuse some of the desirable concomitants of old age with aging itself. Aging *per se* is not experience. Aging is not knowledge. Aging is not growth. Aging is not wisdom. Aging is associated with these things only because time is required for us to acquire them (although their acquisition is by no means guaranteed) and aging also happens with the passage of time. The connection, however, is coincidental. In fact, it is probably more accurate to say that the desirable consequences of old age happen in spite of aging, not because of it. This brings us to the question of coping with and, more important, preventing the health consequences of aging in a clinical environment. Among gerontologists, this is now being referred to as "longevity medicine."

LONGEVITY MEDICINE

The Baltimore Longitudinal Study of Aging (BLSA), initiated in 1958, is America's oldest continuing scientific examination of human aging.[25] Its purpose is to describe and understand those age-associated changes and processes that can be attributed to primary aging and to document the onset of secondary aging. To accomplish this, BLSA participants are thoroughly tested at regular intervals in order to reveal changes in the functioning of a variety of important biochemical and physiological systems. These include various vital organs, the immune system, metabolism, the endocrine system (hormone levels), mental abilities, etc. As a result of this sustained effort, the BLSA database has become nothing less than a national treasure. It has made in the past, and will continue to make in the future, an invaluable contribution to our understanding of human aging.

Perhaps the most important conclusion emerging from the BLSA data is that there is no single, chronological timetable of human aging.[26] People do not all age at the same rate. Even within one individual, different tissues and organs appear to age at different rates. This suggests that aging involves a variety of distinct processes or determining factors. These factors can be grouped into two general categories—genetic (hereditary) and environmental. The variety in the pattern of expression of these factors in different individuals is enormous.

The most straightforward way to gauge the decline in physiological function associated with biological aging is to measure the functional reserves of the cells, tissues, organ systems, or organisms under study. This is the approach taken by the BLSA, monitoring each test subject's functional capacity for a variety of measures of physiological function over their lifetime. Although there is considerable heterogeneity in the rate of decline for the many measures of physiological function as we age, the general trend can be expressed as a total body average that reflects an individual's lifespan potential. This is useful in expressing graphically an idealized pattern of functional capacity throughout a typical human lifespan. (Fig. 15-1). The graph, of course, incorporates periods of both development and aging.

The first phase of life is characterized by development or maturation. It begins at birth and ends when the individual becomes fully mature (i.e. completely functional, both mentally and physically). Depending upon the individual, this usually happens between the ages of 15 and 25 years and is characterized by a general peak in functional capacity.

This peak in functional capacity marks the beginning of the second phase of life. It is characterized by degeneration and functional decline (aging). The early years of this phase are associated with a high degree of sexual (reproductive) activity,

excellent health, intellectual prowess, physical strength, and general vigor. This is followed by "middle age," more obviously associated with a progressive, degenerative decline in function. Libido wanes and sexual activity becomes less frequent. Women go through the menopause and men begin to experience the first signs of a gradual and constant decline of testosterone. There is a general loss of physical strength and activity owing to a loss of muscle mass. Insulin sensitivity declines and blood glucose creeps up. Flexibility and mobility wane. Wrinkled skin, aching joints, graying hair, slower reflexes, and reading glasses all declare to the world that "the bloom is off the rose." In addition, insomnia often becomes a problem—minor at first, but increasing with age.

As time goes by, minor health problems begin to occur more frequently and last longer. There is increasing physiological stress, complete with hormone imbalances and deficiencies, resulting in a negative nitrogen balance, loss of lean muscle mass, and increasing fat mass. General health, functional capacity, and vitality are all in decline. The rate of decline is highly variable from person to person, but nobody escapes it.

Finally, for everyone, as the progressive degeneration continues, the symptoms of bodily imbalance reach clinical thresholds and one or more diseases are diagnosed. Immune function continues to decline and susceptibility to infections increases. Medical intervention at this point is usually aimed at relieving the symptoms and lessening the consequences of disease rather than eliminating their causes. Youthful health and vitality become faint memories and, finally, the battle for life itself is lost. This is the inexorable pattern of human aging.

Remedial medicine: diagnose and treat

The relationship between health and functional capacity is undeniable—loss of one is loss of the other. This fact alone belies the notion of a healthy 80-year-old man. Every 80-year-old man has health problems, most of which are age-related. Even so, many people would be happy if they made it to the age of 80. The majority of us die at a much younger age, usually from one of the many age-related diseases described elsewhere in this book.

One of the reasons for this stems from the fact that individuals do not age uniformly. Some organs and tissues often seem to age more rapidly than others. Different people age differently as a direct result of the interaction between their genetics and environment. Figure 15-2 shows an example of uneven aging—in this case the person's cardiovascular system is declining prematurely (perhaps due, in part, to environmental factors, such as a poor diet). This decline in functional capacity threatens to end the person's life well before the age of 100.

Cardiovascular disease is a common cause of death in the USA. The conventional approach is to wait until symptoms of actual disease develop before taking action. Only then is the problem diagnosed and only when treatment becomes "medically necessary" is intervention begun. If treatment is successful, then life is briefly prolonged, albeit at a relatively low level of functional capacity. This is the nature of remedial medicine. Perhaps the greatest shortcoming of current healthcare delivery systems is that they focus almost exclusively upon treating existing disease, rather than preventing its onset.

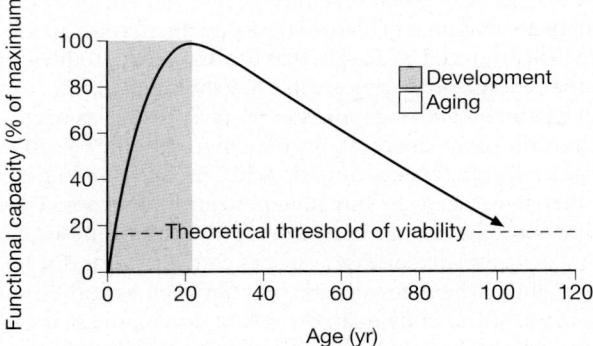

Figure 15-1 Normal (idealized) pattern of uniform development and aging. Note that aging begins as a young adult and is a more or less linear decline in functional capacity, occurring simultaneously (uniformly) in all systems, ending in death when the functional capacity of one or more systems reaches the threshold of viability.

Preventive medicine: assess and intervene

Unlike remedial medicine, preventive medicine is directed at preventing the natural consequences of aging. As depicted in Figure 15-3, the goal is to identify those processes and organ systems that are declining prematurely and, where possible, intervene in ways designed either to return them to a more youthful (healthy) state or to slow the progression from preclinical pathology to clinical disease. If successful, this will result not only in prolongation of the patient's life, but prolongation of the period of his or her lifespan associated with a high level of physiological function, free of age-related diseases and symptoms. See Chapter 20 for further coverage of this topic.

General clinical guidelines

The clinical guidelines described below are designed to preserve, for as long as possible, the patient's health and functional capacity. Each patient's intervention program

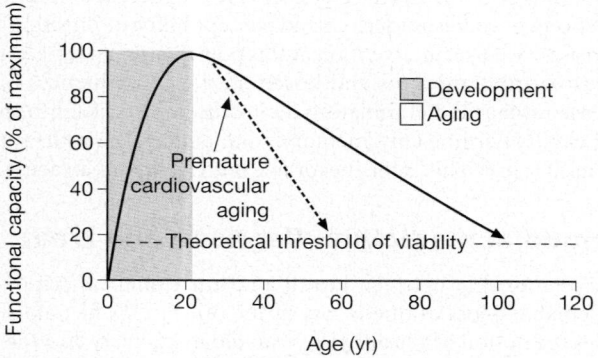

Figure 15-2 Nonuniform aging. In this example, it is the cardiovascular system that is aging prematurely. Such premature aging can occur in any of the major organ systems of the body and, usually, in more than one at a time.

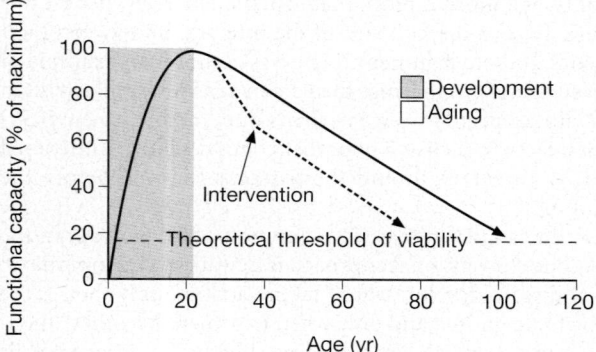

Figure 15-3 Nonuniform aging with successful early intervention. Accelerated decline in cardiovascular function is successfully countered by early intervention and the normal (much lower) rate of age-related functional decline is restored. Thus, an extremely premature death is avoided.

should be unique and customized specifically to meet his or her individual needs.

Interventions that can prevent or delay specific age-related diseases and disabilities include nutritional recommendations (such as increases in fiber, certain supplements, fruits and vegetables), alterations in behavior (such as weight loss, use of seat belts and sunscreens, adoption of regular exercise programs, and avoidance of tobacco products), and drug treatments (such as the use of antibiotics to prevent peptic ulcers and stomach cancer or cholesterol lowering agents to prevent heart disease). Patient adherence to such recommendations deserves strong encouragement and follow-up by the physician.

For patient convenience, customized compounding is often useful for the development of individualized patient treatment protocols. This also provides the highest possible level of control over the quality of the products prescribed to the patient. The ability to produce virtually any preparation that a physician can prescribe is the stock-in-trade of the compounding pharmacy. This affords the physician great flexibility in designing each patient's custom intervention program.

Dietary supplementation

Some scientists maintain that most people in developed countries get enough nutrients from a typical "well-balanced" diet and that additional supplementation is an unnecessary waste of money. Others do not share this view. For example, the US government's recommended daily allowance (RDA) is not designed for optimum health and longevity. It more closely represents a minimum daily requirement and is clearly not optimum for many vitamins (e.g. B complex, C, D, and E) and minerals (e.g. zinc, selenium). It also ignores other important nutrients entirely (e.g. phytochemicals, co-enzyme Q-10, beta-carotene).[27,28] Therefore, it is likely that a customized regimen of dietary supplementation provided to patients based upon their biochemical test results will result in better health outcomes in the long term. Supplementation regimens may include vitamins, minerals, herbs, and other nutrients. It should be stressed that the efficiency and cost-effectiveness of the procedures described above have not been demonstrated, but rather represent the authors' estimate of the best that can be done at this point in time to optimize age-related health outcomes and lifespan.

One of the most common targets of intervention addressed by supplementation is oxidative stress. Reactive oxygen species (ROS) are produced by all cells that use oxygen as products of essential, energy-producing aerobic metabolism and, also, to a lesser extent, by ionizing radiation (X-rays, cosmic rays, etc.) and certain toxic chemicals in the environment.[29–31] ROS damage cell components (nucleic acids, proteins, and lipids) and thereby weaken the functional integrity of tissues. They are known to have important roles in the pathogenesis of a variety of age-related diseases, such as cardiovascular disease, cancer, and Alzheimer's disease.[32] It has been hypothesized that, in any given individual, the risk of developing many of the age-related diseases is a function of, among other factors, the steady-state level of ROS-mediated damage ("oxidative stress").[33] The lower the rate of damage, the higher the probability of a long and healthy life.

Thus, by measuring various markers of oxidative damage together with known protection factors (endogenous and exogenous antioxidants), it may now be possible to gauge an individual's level of oxidative stress. Individuals under high oxidative stress should be ideal candidates for antioxidant interventions. However, there is still considerable controversy on this issue. Hucksters and charlatans have touted antioxidants as anti-aging "miracle treatments" for many years. The proponents of antioxidants claim that ingesting these substances (primarily vitamins such as C and E) will quench excess free radicals and therefore help prevent the damage they cause. Such claims inappropriately extend and exaggerate the anticipated health and longevity benefits of ingesting free radical scavengers. Although antioxidant supplements have many well-known health benefits, which include reducing the risk of certain age-related diseases, there is no scientific evidence to suggest that they can significantly extend lifespan in mammalian species.

Hormone replacement

One of the most promising interventions designed to achieve significant longevity and youthful function involves maintaining optimum homeostatic balance using hormone replacement (or supplementation) therapy. In theory, the best outcomes should be obtained if the hormone regimen is "bioidentical"; that is, the hormonal agents have the same chemical identity and are supplied in a dose and pattern that reproduces the blood levels observed in healthy younger persons of the same sex. In fact, there are no good data demonstrating that this is the case in all situations or for all hormones. Rather, there are limited data (e.g. for estrogen or progesterone replacement) suggesting that the bioidentical approach may yield better results with regard to biochemical changes with potential for producing adverse effects.

In principle, the approach is simple. The hormones in which one is deficient are determined and these hormones are replaced using bio-identical hormones in amounts sufficient to return blood levels to youthful norms. Hormone replacement therapy is a long-term proposition, possibly continuing for many years or even for the rest of a patient's life. Thus, great care must be taken to insure that optimum blood levels of the hormones are achieved and maintained.

A number of hormones, including growth hormone, testosterone, estrogens, progesterone, and others, have been shown in clinical trials to modify some of the physiological attributes associated with human aging. However, controlled long-term prospective studies of the health effects of the use of hormones in adult humans have not been conducted. Furthermore, negative side-effects have been associated with the use of many of these hormones.

A notable exception to the above statement is estrogen replacement therapy, both with (HRT) and without (ERT) opposing progesterone. Estrogen replacement in postmenopausal women has been demonstrated to be beneficial in various studies for preventing progression of osteoporosis and fractures,[34–36] improving lipid profiles and reducing risk of cardiovascular events,[37–40] and decreasing the risk or early onset of Alzheimer's disease.[41,42] Finally, in post-menopausal women, long-term HRT and ERT have been shown to significantly reduce the risk of death from all causes, in spite of increasing the risks of certain types of cancer.[43–46]

Nonetheless, there have been relatively few, randomized prospective trials of HRT. In one recently completed randomized, double-blind, placebo-controlled trial studying 222 postmenopausal women 45 years of age or older,[47] the average rate of progression of subclinical atherosclerosis was slower in healthy post-menopausal women taking unopposed ERT with 17beta-estradiol than in women taking placebo. In another controlled study of HRT in hypertensive women, transdermal HRT associated with an antihypertensive helped reduce cardiovascular risk as assessed by ventricular wall thickness.[48] However, in a randomized trial of secondary coronary heart disease (CHD) prevention, using HRT in women with pre-existing CHD (HERS trial),[49] there was a pattern of early increase in risk of cardiac events followed by a favorable pattern after several years of therapy, but no overall cardiovascular benefit. Consistent with the above trial are findings in a randomized study, using angiography to assess coronary narrowing, that HRT failed to prevent progression of existing atherosclerotic lesions;[50] and another study showing that, in older post-menopausal women, favorable effects of estrogen on brachial artery flow-mediated vasodilation may be limited to those who have not yet developed atherosclerotic vascular disease.[50] Thus, HRT does not appear appropriate for secondary prevention of CHD, but is likely to be effective if initiated early, before significant plaques develop. Final determination of benefits and risks has, thus, yet to be completed, even for HRT. For all other hormones, more research is needed even to begin to determine their proper application within a clinical environment.

Despite the above caveat, it is common practice among "anti-aging" practitioners to "replace" testosterone, dehydroepiandrosterone (DHEA), and growth hormone (GH) in middle-aged and older adults. These interventions are frequently "sold" to patients as a method of rejuvenation, with the promise that not only will function and appearance be improved, but also that lifespan will be extended. This is essentially an empty promise.

Testosterone has the capacity, in individuals actually deficient in testosterone (serum levels <250–300 ng/dL), to improve bone mineral density.[51] Testosterone may also increase lean body and skeletal muscle mass; although, in the absence of concomitant resistance exercise, the effects on muscle strength are uncertain, and improvements in actual capacity to perform activities of daily living have yet to be demonstrated.[52,53] The precise prevalence of testosterone deficiency in normal aging men is also uncertain, but clearly increases during the sixth to eighth decades to substantial levels (30 percent and more in most studies).[54,55]

DHEA is not a hormone. No specific receptor or action of DHEA has been identified in humans. Rather it is a hormone precursor, secreted in large quantities by the adrenal glands at puberty, which circulates conjugated mainly to sulfate, and is converted peripherally to active androgen and, to a lesser extent, estrogen. Because DHEA declines precipitously and monotonically with age, it remains a perennial favorite of anti-aging doctors as a recommended "youth hormone." In fact, no large controlled human study has ever demonstrated a beneficial effect of DHEA administration in normal aging. Several small studies have shown one or another effect, such as improved quality of life, or slightly increased IGF-I, but none of these findings has been replicated from one investigation to the next.[56–58] Moreover, the observed actions, such as they are, are almost certainly attributable to DHEA's weak and variable androgenic and estrogenic effects. Because DHEA is available over the counter, it continues to be consumed in large quantities for its putative anti-aging effects. It may have some limited benefit with regard to bone, muscle, and libido in post-menopausal women who are androgen-deficient due to the loss of ovarian androgen and the normal decrement in adrenal DHEA production. The role for androgen replacement by any modality in older women is, as yet, poorly defined, but some data suggest that selected women may benefit, so long as androgens are administered in appropriate female doses and along with estrogen-based HRT. Oral androgens in general should be avoided because of their deleterious effects to lower plasma HDL and raise LDL cholesterol.

Growth hormone is a potent anabolic agent with actions in many tissues, mediated in part directly and in part via stimulation of its "second messenger," insulin-like growth factor-I (IGF-I). Under normal circumstances, GH is secreted in 8–10 discrete pulses lasting less than an hour, with very low levels in the circulation in between. The amplitude of these pulses is higher at night during slow-wave sleep, producing a pronounced diurnal variation in GH secretion rates. While replacement by injection with recombinant human GH has been shown to be beneficial in, and has now been FDA approved for, adults with GH deficiency due to pituitary pathology, there are no long-term studies demonstrating benefits of GH administration in healthy elderly people whose serum IGF-I levels are consistent with a "somatopause." In fact, studies to date of GH effects on bone density in menopausal women have been disappointing. GH has been shown to increase lean body mass, reduce body fat, and cause small improvements in lipid profiles in older men and women, but effects on muscle strength have been equivocal and no benefits in terms of function or quality of life have been demonstrated.

Furthermore, GH administration in older men and women has been associated with a plethora of adverse effects, including carpal tunnel symptoms, arthralgias, and fluid retention with edema.[59] Of greater concern is the production of hyperinsulinemia and glucose intolerance,[59] occasionally reaching diabetic levels, and the potential for accelerated growth of malignancies. Risks of both prostate and breast cancer have been shown, in epidemiological studies, to increase with increasing circulating IGF-I.[60–62] These findings, while not conclusive as to causality, should inject a note of caution with regard to GH supplementation in older patients. Finally, it is clear that patients with acromegaly (excessive GH levels due to a secretory tumor of the pituitary gland) die prematurely of cardiovascular and cerebrovascular disease, cancer, and pulmonary disease, suggesting that GH excess is a form of premature aging. This impression is further supported by animal models in which genetic GH excess shortens, and deficiency of GH secretion or action lengthens, lifespan.

It is possible that new methods of replacing GH, in which pituitary secretion of endogenous GH in the physiological pulsatile pattern is augmented to resemble that of youth, may have a better risk/benefit profile than that achieved with GH injections, but this too remains to be demonstrated.

Optimum nutrition

Dietary intervention is notoriously difficult to control in an outpatient environment. Thus, the physician can do little more than inform patients about foods that are not consistent with optimum health. Dietary guidelines should include what specific foods to eat and not to eat, how to prepare them, and a simple explanation of the role of calories in health and aging. The physician should encourage consumption of the minimum number of calories required to obtain all of the vital nutrients that are necessary for optimum health. The goal is to build an understanding of how nutrition and energy intake affect aging in order to help make better nutrition a daily habit of each patient.

Dietary guidelines for optimum aging should strongly discourage the consumption of "empty calories"—energy-dense foods with little or no nutritional content. The physician should promote a diet that contains a wide variety of nutritious fruits, green and colorful vegetables, nuts, and other nutrient-dense foods, including lean meat, fish, and poultry. Such foods are rich in complete protein, good-quality essential fats, and natural antioxidants. Limiting the intake of saturated fats and "trans-" fatty acids should be strongly encouraged. Another good way to reduce total caloric intake is to restrict the intake of refined carbohydrates such as grains, sugars, and concentrated starches. Such a diet will produce better nutrition with fewer calories, almost certainly leading to improved health and longevity.

This emphasis upon calories is not arbitrary. Reducing caloric intake has been shown to increase longevity in virtually every species in which it has been studied.[63] The underlying mechanism by which this occurs is not yet fully understood. Although caloric restriction has not yet been scientifically demonstrated to prolong lifespan in humans, there is little reason to think that it will not do so. Also, there is little doubt about the detrimental health effects of obesity even in the absence of any longevity benefits of reduced caloric intake. Thus, even if they are not obese, most people would probably benefit from some degree of caloric restriction, assuming they do so without becoming nutritionally deficient.

Exercise

The benefits of exercise in achieving optimum health, longevity, and a better "quality of life" are well documented.[64–66] Guidelines should emphasize that no new exercise program should be undertaken by persons over 40 years of age until medical evaluation has shown that there is no occult heart, skeletal, or other disease, which could be exacerbated by too-vigorous physical activity. In the presence of such problems, exercise may still be an attractive option, but intensity and type should be adjusted to account for individual limitations. In general a well-balanced exercise program should include the elements of: aerobic exercise to condition the cardiovascular system and improve endurance; resistance exercise to maintain lean body mass, preserve performance of day-to-day tasks requiring muscle power, help prevent bone loss, and reduce the risk of falls; and stretching to limit the loss of flexibility that accompanies aging. Each patient should be encouraged to seek the advice of a certified personal trainer or other exercise professional, as needed, to prevent injury and help ensure adherence.

Pharmaceuticals

The role of pharmaceuticals in delaying the onset of age-related disease is a limited but important one. As a general rule, natural interventions to correct homeostatic imbalances are preferable to pharmaceuticals, if at all possible. This is because interventions designed to prevent the onset of age-related diseases are likely to be required for the remainder of the patient's life. Patients are often less likely to resist chronic interventions when they are natural. In addition, natural substances are often (but not always) less expensive, less toxic, and better tolerated than drugs. In the absence of a natural therapy, pharmaceuticals may be useful in treating early symptoms of age-related diseases not otherwise subject to control. Certain age-related degenerative processes cannot be addressed using supplements and/or natural hormones. Thus, pharmaceutical therapy may be appropriate for correcting and/or preventing age-related changes in these instances. For example, pharmaceutical agents (statins, niacin, fibrates) may be required, and have been demonstrated to be effective for correcting an abnormally high-risk blood lipid profile in patients for whom other interventions have failed. Other examples of effective pharmaceutical intervention include antihypertensive therapy, especially with angiotensin-converting enzyme (ACE) inhibitors, for prevention of cardiovascular disease and preservation of renal function,[67,68] and bis-phosphonate therapy for treatment of osteoporosis.

Ongoing monitoring

Once admitted into a long-term preventive health program, patients should be continually monitored for physiological and biochemical health status. First and foremost, it must be verified that the initial intervention protocol is working. When appropriate, a trend line should be established for each parameter that is changing significantly. This will provide an indication of how well the patient is doing, so that the person won't have to wait for years to observe the results of his or her efforts. Timely feedback on the efficacy of a patient's intervention program is extremely helpful in maintaining the motivation necessary for long-term adherence. Information from follow-up testing is used to improve and refine the intervention program.

ANTI-AGING MEDICINE: FUTURE PROSPECTS

Since 1889, when Brown-Sequard unsuccessfully attempted to rejuvenate failing testicular function in human subjects,[69] scientists have sought interventions designed to combat the aging process. In recent years, with a better understanding of the biochemical and neuroendocrine determinants of aging, anti-aging research is on a more solid foundation.[70,71] Although most studies are concerned with elucidating basic mechanisms of aging, many also have practical implications with respect to combating the diseases of aging.[72] Today, by carefully applying technology developed since the 1980s, it may be possible to significantly delay the onset of many age-related diseases. For the first time in history, there is now strong evidence that the aging process itself may be manageable. Moreover, evidence suggests that reducing the aging rate could decrease the risks of many serious age-related diseases, and that so doing would greatly extend both longevity and the healthy robust portion of the lifespan.[73] Credible scientists are now seriously discussing

well-defined research pathways that could produce a rational, testable strategy for developing interventions to slow aging in human beings.

The rationale for seeking anti-aging interventions ("anti-aging medicines") is that they would dramatically increase the number of years of active, healthy, productive lifespan for many people. In rodents, interventions that retard aging extend longevity by as much as 40–50 percent. In addition to lifespan, such interventions also increase healthspan, the time period over which the animals stay active and free of diseases and disabilities. In contrast, a successful intervention to cure cancer or heart disease would extend human lifespan by a relatively small percentage.

In the future, better methods for measuring the consequences of aging will be developed, including immune function testing, cognitive function testing, cancer screening tests, and genetic testing. These tests will, in turn, lead to improved techniques for maintaining youthful function in all areas. Studies of long-lived animal models, as well as basic laboratory investigations, have generated a list of promising avenues for future research in longevity extension, and thus to prevention of multiple late-life diseases.

TRANSLATIONAL RESEARCH

"Translational research" is a relatively new term that has gained popularity over the last few years. Most experts agree about the need for more translational research. However, as with "clinical research," different people mean different things when they use the term.

The call for more translational research, and perhaps the very creation of the concept, probably came as a reaction to the broadening of the scope of the meaning of "clinical research" to include investigations not clearly linked to human health benefits. It would be beneficial, in the long term, if the concept of translational research can be restricted to research activities in which intact human subjects, patients and/or normal volunteers, are employed in studies investigating the potential of new information and insights gained in basic research laboratories (i.e. investigations utilizing genes, cells, tissues, or living animals) for application to the treatment or prevention of human disease, or the improvement of human life. Research studies should be considered translational to the extent that they are designed to explore potential applications of novel insights from the realm of basic research, which have not yet been proven useful in living human beings.

There are very serious obstacles to translational research on anti-aging medicines, and it is time to give these obstacles serious consideration. These obstacles include (a) the very long time period that would be needed to test, in humans, drugs or other interventions that are thought likely to diminish late-life illnesses by their effects on the aging process; (b) the possibility that promising interventions might have undesirable side-effects not detectable in short-term trials; (c) the current lack of well-validated surrogate tests ("biomarkers") by which one could monitor the progress of clinical trials at intermediate stages; and (d) the understandable reluctance of for-profit corporations to commit their resources to testing agents that cannot begin to generate revenues for many years. Strategies for surmounting some of these problems—such as seeking approval for use of putative anti-aging medicines for short-term treatment of specific illnesses in the hope that they will then become widely used for "off-label" preventive therapies—raise new problems, both scientific and legal.

CONCLUSION

The dramatic changes in life expectancy in the last 100 years, attributable to improved nutrition, vaccination, and antisepsis, as well as to progress in medicine, surgery, and pharmacology, have brought with them equally striking adjustments in related social and economic arrangements, including shifts in housing, job choice, pension planning, and allocations of resources to healthcare. Effective anti-aging interventions, if they were indeed able to add decades of healthy and productive lifespan for the typical adult, would bring with them changes in economic and social structures of similar magnitude to those already seen within the lifetime of our oldest citizens, and these consequences merit careful forethought. Issues of this sort are too new, and too complicated, for easy resolution, and deserve wide discussion among economists, public figures, health providers and laypersons, as well as among research scientists.

In research laboratories around the world, great progress is being made toward a better understanding of aging. As a result, many promising technologies are on the horizon that may soon enable us to provide clinical interventions to combat some of the fundamental causes of aging. Interventions that affect the fundamental mechanisms of aging may enable us to significantly increase late-life functional capacity, life expectancy, and maximum lifespan all at the same time. Only when this is possible will we truly be using "anti-aging interventions."

KEY POINTS Anti-aging interventions

- Currently, authentic anti-aging medicine does not exist. Until anti-aging medicine becomes a reality, ethical healthcare practitioners must be content to help patients cope with the problems of aging using traditional medical technologies for the prevention, diagnosis, and treatment of age-related diseases.

- Anti-aging medicine is not anti-elderly patients any more than anti-cancer medicine is anti-cancer patients.

- Medical practitioners have historically taken a remedial (diagnose and treat) approach to healthcare. The future promises a more preventive (assess and intervene) approach.

- Currently, preventive healthcare technology is limited to clinical and laboratory assessment of disease risk factors followed by targeted preventive interventions including certain pharmaceuticals, supplementation, hormone replacement therapy, diet, and exercise.

- Future advances in anti-aging medicine will require both basic research, to discover new, safe and effective ways to combat aging, and translational research, to rapidly move such new discoveries from the laboratory to the clinic.

REFERENCES

1. Wilmoth JR: The future of human longevity: a demographer's perspective. Science 1998;280:395–397
2. Myers GC: Comparative mortality trends among older persons in developed countries. In Casselli G, Lopez AD (eds): Health and Mortality Among Elderly Populations. Oxford: Clarendon Press, 1996:87–111
3. Passell P: Exceptional Returns: The Economic Value of America's Investment in Medical Research. Santa Monica: Milliken Institute, 2000
4. Olshansky SJ, Carnes BA, Desesquelles A: Demography—prospects for human longevity. Science 2001;291:1491–1492
5. Olshansky SJ, Carnes BA, Cassel C: The future of long life. Science 1998;281:1612–1613; discussion 1613–1615
6. Hayflick L: The future of ageing. Nature 2000;408:267–269
7. Walford R: Maximum Lifespan. New York: WW Norton, 1983
8. McCay CM, Crowell MF, Maynard LA: The effect of retarded growth on the lifespan and upon the ultimate body size. J Nutr 1935;10:63–79
9. Masoro EJ: Life span extension and food restriction. Compr Ther 1988;14(6):9–13
10. Iwasaki K, Gleiser CA, Masoro EJ et al: Influence of the restriction of individual dietary components on longevity and age-related disease of Fischer rats: the fat component and the mineral component. J Gerontol A 1988;43:B13–B21
11. Effros RB, Walford RL, Weindruch R, Mitcheltree C: Influences of dietary restriction on immunity to influenza in aged mice. J Gerontol A 1991;46:B142–B147
12. Kritchevsky D: Caloric restriction and cancer. J Nutr Sci Vitaminol (Tokyo) 2001;47(1):13–19
13. Mayhew M, Renganathan M, Delbono O: Effectiveness of caloric restriction in preventing age-related changes in rat skeletal muscle. Biochem Biophys Res Commun 1998;251:95–99
14. Colman RJ, Roecker EB, Ramsey JJ, Kemnitz JW: The effect of dietary restriction on body composition in adult male and female rhesus macaques. Aging Milano 1998;10(2):83–92
15. Pariza MW: Dietary fat, calorie restriction, ad libitum feeding, and cancer risk. Nutr Rev 1987;45(1):1–7
16. Weindruch R, Keenan KP, Carney JM et al: Caloric restriction mimetics: metabolic interventions. J Gerontol 2001;56a(Special Issue 1):20–33
17. Orr WC, Sohal RS: Extension of life-span by overexpression of superoxide dismutase and catalase in *Drosophila melanogaster*. Science 1994;263:1128–1130
18. Brown-Borg HM, Rakoczy SG: Catalase expression in delayed and premature aging mouse models. Exp Gerontol 2000;35:199–212
19. Kimura KD, Tissenbaum HA, Liu Y, Ruvkun G: *daf-2*, an insulin receptor-like gene that regulates longevity and diapause in *Caenorhabditis elegans*. Science 1997;277:942–946
20. Hayflick L: Aging and the genome. Science 1999;283:2019
21. Masoro EJ: The biological mechanism of aging: is it still an enigma? Age 1996;19:141–145
22. Bowles J. Shattered: Medawar's test tubes and their enduring legacy of chaos. Med Hypotheses 2000;54:326–339
23. Johnson HA (ed): Relations Between Normal Aging and Disease. New York: Raven Press, 1985
24. Strehler B: Time, Cells, and Aging. New York: Academic Press, 1982
25. Shock NW, Greulich RC, Andres RA et al: Normal human aging: the Baltimore Longitudinal Study of Aging. Washington, DC: National Institute on Aging, 1984
26. Hayflick L: How and Why We Age. New York: Balleantine Books, 1994
27. Murry MT: Encyclopedia of Nutritional Supplements. Rockland, CA: Prima Health, 1996
28. Saltman P, Gurin J, Mothner I: University of California, San Diego, Nutrition Book. New York: Little Brown, 1993
29. Cutler RG: Evolution of human longevity: a critical overview. Mech Ageing Dev 1979;9(3–4):337–354
30. Harman D: Aging and oxidative stress. J Int Fed Clin Chem 1998;10(1):24–27
31. Niki E: Free radicals in the 1900s: from in vitro to in vivo. Free Radic Res 2001;33:693–704
32. Forsberg L, de Faire U, Morgenstern R: Oxidative stress, human genetic variation, and disease. Arch Biochem Biophys 2001;389(1):84–93
33. Floyd RA, West M, Hensley K: Oxidative biochemical markers: clues to understanding aging in long-lived species. Exp Gerontol 2001;36(4–6):619–640

34. Ettinger B, Genant HK, Cann CE: Long-term estrogen replacement therapy prevents bone loss and fractures. Ann Intern Med 1985;102:319–324

35. Weiss NS, Ure CL, Ballard JH et al: Decreased risk of fractures of the hip and lower forearm with postmenopausal use of estrogen. N Engl J Med 1980;303:1195–1198

36. Cauley JA, Seeley DG, Ensrud K et al: Estrogen replacement therapy and fractures in older women. Ann Intern Med 1995;122:9–16

37. Nabulsi AA, Folsom AR, White A et al: Association of hormone replacement therapy with various cardiovascular risk factors in postmenopausal women. N Engl J Med 1993;328:1069–1075

38. Sherwin BB, Gelfand MM, Schucher R, Gabor J: Postmenopausal estrogen and androgen replacement and lipoprotein lipid concentrations. Am J Obst Gyne 1987;156:414–419

39. Herrington DM, Werbel BL, Riley WA, Pusser BE, Morgan TM: Individual and combined effects of estrogen/progestin therapy and lovastatin on lipids and flow-mediated vasodilation in postmenopausal women with coronary artery disease. J Am Coll Cardiol 1999;33:2030–2037

40. Bush TL, Fried LP, Barrett-Connor E: Cholesterol, lipoproteins, and coronary heart disease in women. Clin Chem 1988;34(8B):60–70

41. Birge SJ: The role of estrogen in the treatment of Alzheimer's disease. Neurology 1997;48(5 suppl 7):S36–S41

42. Slooter AJ, Bronzova J, Witteman JC et al: Estrogen use and early onset Alzheimer's disease: a population-based study. J Neurol Neurosurg Psychiat 1999;67:779–781

43. Bush TL, Barrett-Conner E, Cowan LD: Cardiovascular mortality and noncontraceptive use of estrogen in women: results from the Lipid Research Clinics Program follow-up study. Circulation 1987;75:1102–1109

44. Bush TL, Cowan LD, Barrett-Connor E et al: Estrogen use and all-cause mortality: preliminary results from the Lipid Research Clinics Program follow-up study. JAMA 1983;249:903–906

45. Col NF, Eckman MH, Karas RH et al: Patient-specific decisions about hormone replacement therapy in postmenopausal women. JAMA 1997;277:1140–1147

46. Rodriguez C, Calle EE, Patel AV et al: Effect of body mass on the association between estrogen replacement therapy and mortality among elderly US women. Am J Epidemiol 2001;153:145–152

47. Hodis HN, Mack WJ, Lobo RA et al: Estrogen in the prevention of atherosclerosis: a randomized, double-blind, placebo-controlled trial. Ann Intern Med 2001;135:939–953

48. Modena MG, Molinari R, Muia N: Double-blind randomized placebo-controlled study of transdermal estrogen replacement therapy on hypertensive postmenopausal women. Am J Hypertens 1999;12(10 Pt 1):1000–1008

49. Hulley S, Grady D, Bush T et al: Randomized trial of estrogen plus progestin for secondary prevention of coronary heart disease in postmenopausal women. Heart and Estrogen/Progestin Replacement Study (HERS) research group. JAMA 1998;280:605–613

50. Herrington DM, Espeland MA, Crouse JR et al: Estrogen replacement and brachial artery flow-mediated vasodilation in older women. Arterioscler Thromb Vasc Biol 2001;21:1955–1961

51. Snyder PJ, Peachey H, Hannoush P et al: Effect of testosterone treatment on bone mineral density in men over 65 years of age. J Clin Endocrinol Metab 1999;84:1966–1972

52. Snyder PJ, Peachey H, Hannoush P et al: Effect of testosterone treatment on body composition and muscle strength in men over 65 years of age. J Clin Endocrinol Metab 1999;84:2647–2653

53. Bhasin S, Bagatell CJ, Bremner WJ et al: Issues in testosterone replacement in older men. J Clin Endocrinol Metab 1998;83:3435–3448

54. Harman SM, Metter EJ, Tobin JD, Pearson J, Blackman MR: Longitudinal effects of aging on serum total and free testosterone levels in healthy men. Baltimore Longitudinal Study of Aging. J Clin Endocrinol Metab 2001;86:724–731

55. Kaufman JM, Vermeulen A: Declining gonadal function in elderly men. Baillière's Clin Endocrinol Metab 1997;11:289–309

56. Hornsby PJ: DHEA: a biologist's perspective. J Am Geriatr Soc 1997;45:1395–1401

57. Yen SS, Morales AJ, Khorram O et al: Replacement of DHEA in aging men and women. Potential remedial effects: dehydroepiandrosterone (DHEA) treatment reverses the impaired immune response of old mice to influenza vaccination and protects from influenza infection. Ann NY Acad Sci 1995;774(15):128–142

58. Morales AJ, Haubrich RH, Hwang JY, Asakura H, Yen SS: The effect of six months' treatment with a 100 mg daily dose of dehydroepiandrosterone (DHEA) on circulating sex steroids, body composition and muscle strength in age-advanced men and women. Clin Endocrinol (Oxf) 1998;49:421–432

59. Rudman D, Feller AG, Cohn L et al: Effects of human growth hormone on body composition in elderly men. Horm Res 1991;36(suppl 1):73–81

60. Chan JM, Stampfer MJ, Giovannucci E, Gann PH, Ma J, Wilkinson P, et al: Plasma insulin like growth factor-I and prostate cancer risk: a prospective study [see comments]. Science 1998;279(5350):563–566

61. Harman SM, Metter EJ, Blackman MR, Landis PK, Carter HB: Serum levels of insulin-like growth factor I (IGF-I), IGF-II, IGF-binding protein-3, and prostate-specific antigen as predictors of clinical prostate cancer. J Clin Endocrinol Metab 2000;85(11):4258–4265

62. Hankinson SE, Willett WC, Colditz GA, Hunter DJ, Michaud DS, Deroo B, et al: Circulating concentrations of insulin-like growth factor-I and risk of breast cancer [see comments]. Lancet 1998;351(9113):1393–1396

63. Weindruch R, Walford R: The Retardation of Aging and Disease by Dietary Restriction. Springfield, IL: Charles C Thomas, 1988

64. Coll R, Izquierdo J, Salto G: Benefit of physical exercise in medicine. An Med Interna 1991;8(2):101 (in Spanish)

65. The American College of Sports Medicine Physicians Stand: Exercise and physical activity for older adults. Med Sci Sports Exerc 1998;30:992–1008

66. Schilke JM: Slowing the aging process with physical activity. J Gerontol Nurs 1991;17(6):4–8

67. Hoogwerf BJ, Young JB: The HOPE study: ramipril lowered cardiovascular risk, but vitamin E did not. Cleve Clin J Med 2000;67(4):287–293

68. Kshirsagar AV, Joy MS, Hogan SL, Falk RJ, Colindres RE: Effect of ACE inhibitors in diabetic and nondiabetic chronic renal disease: a systematic overview of randomized placebo-controlled trials. Am J Kidney Dis 2000;35:695–707

69. Brown-Sequard CE: Des effects produits chez la homme ardes injections sus-cutanees d'um liquide retire des testicules frais de cobayes et de dheins. Comptes Rend Soc Biol 1889;41:414–422

70. Butler RN: "Anti-aging" elixirs. Geriatrics 2000;55(6):3–4

71. Yu BP: Approaches to anti-aging intervention: the promises and the uncertainties. Mech Ageing Dev 1999;111(2–3):73–87

72. Rattan SI: Is gene therapy for aging possible? Indian J Exp Biol 1998;36(3):233–236

73. Holloszy JO: The biology of aging. Mayo Clin Proc 2000;75(suppl):S3–S8; discussion S8–S9

Chapter 16

Successful aging

Thomas A. Glass

"One of the major aims of gerontology is to provide society and individuals with advice on the making of societal and individual choices about such things as retirement policy, social security policy, housing, where and with whom to live, how to relate oneself to one's family, what to do in free time. In order to provide good advice, it is essential to have a theory of successful aging."[1]

Interest in the virtues of old age dates back to antiquity in both Eastern and Western philosophical traditions (for example, see reference 2 on Plato). While "successful aging" is regarded by some as a new area of investigation, the modern use of the term dates back more than 50 years to work done by social scientists of the "Chicago School" to better understand the process of social adjustment to old age.[3,4] In the postwar period, papers including the term "successful aging" were published at a brisk pace by Havighurst,[1] Rupp et al.,[5] Schonfield,[6] and Palmore.[7] An interest in understanding the correlates of successful aging was an aim of several longitudinal cohort studies of elderly people, including the Duke Longitudinal Studies of Aging, the Established Populations for the Epidemiologic Studies of the Elderly (EPESE), the MacArthur Studies of Successful Aging, the Gothenburg Study in Sweden, and the Bonn Longitudinal Study of Aging (BOLSA).

More recent interest in the concept was catalyzed by an article appearing in *Science* more than 25 years after Havighurst by Rowe and Kahn,[8] who introduced a distinction between "usual" and "successful" aging as two subclasses of "normal aging," asserting that "a major component of many age-associated declines can be explained in terms of lifestyle, habits, diet, and an array of psychosocial factors extrinsic to the aging process" (p. 143). The impact of this paper was not that it yielded a clear solution to the problem of how to define successful aging, but was due to the forcefulness with which these authors reframed the focus of gerontological research on the possibility that age-associated losses in function may not be inevitable, but may be the consequences of modifiable factors. The high visibility of this paper has overshadowed earlier ground-breaking publications by Capsi and Elder,[9] Ryff,[10] and Butler.[11] Additionally, the study of successful aging had an early start in European gerontology[12–14] and has persisted for 20 years through the pioneering work of Paul and Margaret Baltes and colleagues.

A recent search of Medline produced 881 articles containing the term "successful aging." The number of meanings and measures may be nearly as large. The term has become a conceptual ink-blot onto which a wide variety of ideas have been projected. The term has spawned more discussion and theorizing than empirical research. Despite the widespread use of the term, relatively few empirical studies have been conducted. As Carol Ryff[10] has said: "Like goodness, truth, and other human ideals, successful aging may appeal more than in illuminates" (p. 209). This chapter seeks to ascertain the degree to which the concept has been illuminating.

Two distinct approaches to the study of successful aging will be described: the *psychosocial approach* (that characterized much of the earlier work described above) and the *biomedical approach* that has dominated more recent work. These are rough categories. However, if the concept of successful aging is to play a fruitful role in gerontology, some synthesis of these approaches is required that recognizes the inherent multidimensionality of the concept as well as the need for multidisciplinary approaches to its study. In the final analysis, successful aging must be more than psychological adjustment, just as it must be something other than the avoidance of illness and functional loss. This chapter aims to be a potentially useful synthesis.

DEFINITIONS AND CONCEPTUALIZATIONS OF SUCCESSFUL AGING

The core concept underlying the literature on successful aging is heterogeneity. In its simplest form, successful aging extends the range of possible pathways in old age beyond what is either *pathological* or *normal*. Normal aging is inadequate to describe the magnitude of variability that can be observed in a variety of parameters in old age.[15] The evidence from cohort studies including the Kansas City Studies of Adult Life, the Duke Longitudinal studies, the Baltimore Longitudinal Study on Aging, and the Seattle Longitudinal study of Intellectual Aging have converged on the notion that aging is an exceedingly variable phenomenon, impacted by many factors embedded in the genetic, social, and historical context of human development. Normal patterns of aging fail also to account for a subset of individuals who exceed normative expectations—sometimes substantially. As observed by Baltes and Baltes,[16] what is normal does not tell us what is possible.

Along with heterogeneity, a closely related concept underlying much of the literature on successful aging is *plasticity*, which might be defined as the modifiability of functional systems through the mobilization of reserve capacity. In part, interest in plasticity arises from neurological studies showing that training or differential experience can induce neurochemical changes in the mammalian cerebral cortex in various parameters, including weight of cortex, cortical thickness, size of synaptic contacts, number of dendritic spines, and dendritic branching.[17] The discovery of reserve capacity in the brain has stimulated an interest in the possibility of reserve capacity in other functional systems. This research has demonstrated that among other things, with cognitive training, elderly people exhibit considerable capacity for learning and that the magnitude of improvements after cognitive training is equivalent to the declines seen in observational studies.[18]

Most people agree that successful agers exhibit a pattern of aging that is relatively free of significant mental or physical pathology, and characterized by a relative (or complete) absence of the age-related incapacities so exhaustively detailed in this volume. That having been said, a clear set of criteria for successful aging is difficult to identify. How do we define the term with sufficient precision that it might be measured in the conduct of research? Can a person exhibit signs of pathology in one area and still be "successful"? How should successful aging be differentiated from related concepts such as "productive aging," "optimal aging," or "positive aging"? These are questions that have not as yet been answered.

A wide range of conceptual definitions of successful aging have appeared, including: continued growth and development in late life,[10] avoidance of ill-health,[19] the successful adaptation to stress,[20] maintenance of personal control,[21] continued patterns of midlife activity,[1] as well as successful disengagement from those patterns of activity.[22] Across this vast literature, two primary approaches can be discerned: the *psychosocial* and *biomedical* approaches. Each is described briefly below.

The psychosocial approach

Most of the earliest literature on successful aging was done by social scientists, predominantly in psychology and human development. This early literature treated the term as a near synonym for life-satisfaction.[9,23–25] Life-satisfaction was defined broadly to include self-concept, mood, vitality, and the degree to which desired goals had been either achieved or accommodated. In the mid-1970s, Maddox and Wiley[26] argued that life-satisfaction was the most frequently studied variable in American gerontology. This may reflect the American preoccupation with personal happiness. The study of life-satisfaction in older persons succeeded in dispelling the myth that old age is a time of unhappiness and low morale.[27–29] Interestingly, the preoccupation with absence of disease or functional loss that can be seen in the literature today is almost entirely absent from these early studies.

Within the psychosocial tradition (as well as a more biomedical approach) the term "successful aging" has been assumed to be multidimensional. Ryff[27] outlines six criteria for successful aging, which are self-acceptance, positive relations with others, autonomy, environmental mastery, purpose in life, and personal growth. The first Duke Longitudinal Study of Aging defined successful aging as a combination of survival to age 75, a physical function rating indicating less than 20 percent disability, and a self-report of happiness.[7] In a classic paper, Havighurst[1] specified four criteria: an age-appropriate way of life, maintenance of middle-age activity, a feeling of satisfaction with one's present status and activities, and life-satisfaction.

Although the psychosocial tradition has been criticized repeatedly for weak theory, there are two important examples that have moved the field forward theoretically: *lifespan developmental theory* and the theory of *selective optimization with compensation* (SOC). The lifespan developmental perspective is grounded (to some extent) in Erikson's psychosocial stage model of ego development.[30,31] Of particular importance are his ideas about the primary ego challenge of late-adulthood: ego integrity versus despair. Although the definition of ego integrity is not entirely clear, a reasonable set of characteristics might include emotional integration, acceptance of the reality of death without fear, adaptation to changes in one's capacities, a balanced perspective on one's accomplishments in life, and a series of ongoing and meaningful connections to others.

A core assumption of the lifespan developmental model is that success in late life is defined in terms of developmental goals unique to this life stage. These developmental challenges go well beyond physical health, and absence of disease, but are instead theoretically grounded in a lifespan developmental formulation. Erikson's concept of ego integrity has influenced many investigators in the psychosocial tradition (although the concept does not appear in the biomedical literature). A few researchers have attempted to operationalize and study features of ego integrity.[32,33] Further attempts to frame successful aging in terms of a broader life-course developmental context can be found in Schulz and Heckhausen[34] and Ryff and Essex.[35]

A considerable body of literature makes clear that a core feature of the successful ager is adaptation to late-life changes, elaborated most thoroughly by Paul Baltes and colleagues[36] in their theory of selective optimization with compensation (SOC). These authors describe SOC as a "prototypical strategy of successful aging" (p. 21), designed to serve as a "guideline for an individual's thoughts and actions and for social policy." The theory emphasizes the need to maintain a sense of control over one's environment in the face of the dynamic interplay between gains and losses in late life.[36,37] The three main elements of this theory begin with *selection*, referring to conscious restriction of the range of functional activities in response to age-related losses of capacity and reserve. Secondly, *optimization* is the strategy of engaging in actions and behaviors that enhance or augment remaining strengths and capacities. Finally, *compensation* involves the use of psychological strategies (such as the use of mnemonic devices) or compensatory technology (e.g. hearing aids) to replace lost functional abilities. The emphasis on optimization and selective reframing of goals found in the SOC model serves to remind the field that happiness itself may not be a satisfactory cornerstone to successful aging—a point made decades earlier in the classic study by Angus Campbell, *The Quality of American Life*.[38]

The theory of SOC has been increasingly subject to empirical scrutiny in various populations, including nursing homes,[39,40] working seniors,[40] and low socio-economic groups.[41] Freund[42] measured self-reports of selection, optimization, and compensation in the Berlin Aging Study and found that these factors predicted several measures of well-being independent of other psychological predictors of successful aging, including neuroticism, extraversion, openness, control beliefs, and intelligence.

The biomedical approach

Although interest in successful aging first emerged from the social sciences, a trend can be seen toward the biomedicalization of the field. A more recent group of authors have emphasized physiological and cognitive function in biomedical terms without explicit connection to underlying theories of human development or psychological well-being. This approach tends to define successful aging as the absence of disease or disability (and sometimes as longevity or related ideas such as the compression of morbidity[43]). Despite the efforts of Rowe and Kahn to emphasize factors other than physical health, some subsequent studies have been narrow in focus.

This includes the MacArthur foundation studies of successful aging, a subset of the larger EPESE cohort studies.[44–47] In that study, successful aging was operationalized as performance in the top third of functional ability in both physical and cognitive function. Owing in part to the absence of available measures, no attempt was made to include indicators of ego integrity, life satisfaction, or other psychosocial dimensions. Concern about the tendency to define successful aging as absence of disease and disability, rather than in terms of presence of positive aspects of late-life growth, can be found in numerous critiques.[27,48,49]

The biomedical approach has focused on variability and its correlates in age-related biophysiological parameters, including glucose metabolism, bone density, and memory loss.[8] The existence of this heterogeneity itself calls attention to the possibility of a tail of high performing individuals, but it does not solve the problem of how successful aging should be defined. Substantial heterogeneity is likely to be observed within any group defined using any criteria for successful aging. As Gold et al.[47] have shown, for example, racial differences in blood pressure continue to be observed even among "successful agers."

While it seems clear that gerontologists remain unclear about the definition of successful aging, the term appears to have face validity for elderly people. When asked about the meaning of the term "successful aging," their answers reflect an emphasis on existential and interpersonal factors rather than biological or medical ones. In a study by Abrams, only 2 percent of older persons could not define successful aging. Fisher[50] content-analyzed responses to questions about successful aging from people aged 60–90 and found five content areas: interactions with others, a sense of purpose, self-acceptance, personal growth, and autonomy. In similar work, Ryff[51] found that while middle-aged respondents stressed self-confidence, self-acceptance, and self-knowledge, older persons emphasized an "others orientation" (being a caring, compassionate person, and having good relationships) as well as accepting change as important qualities of positive aging.

The study of successful aging extends from an understanding of the heterogeneity across multiple dimensions of function in late life. This heterogeneity can be observed across a wide range of biological, psychological, and social parameters. While genetic determination of the trajectory of development in early life is well accepted, genetics appears to determine a smaller proportion of variability in late life.[52] There is evidence that ancestral longevity is an even weaker predictor of psychosocial vitality. For example, Vaillant[53] studied a cohort of 184 men from socio-economically advantaged ancestors who were carefully followed from ages 18 to 65; while ancestral longevity predicted chronic illness until age 60, and mortality until age 68, no significant advantage of long-lived parents was seen at age 65 for measures of psychosocial vigor and mental health. In what follows, existing literature of the psychosocial correlates of successful aging are described with particular attention to both the individual and contextual factors.

PSYCHOSOCIAL CORRELATES OF SUCCESSFUL AGING: INDIVIDUAL CHARACTERISTICS

A number of psychological characteristics are associated with positive well-being or disease resistance. Barefoot et al.[54] showed that Rotter's trust scale predicted functional health 8 years later as well as mortality differences after 14 years of follow-up. Perceptions of personal control, mastery, and self-efficacy also appear to be robust predictors of successful aging. Self-efficacy beliefs have been perhaps the strongest and most consistent predictors of a variety of indicators of successful aging, including cognitive function[55] and physical function.[56,57] Seeman et al.[58] found that instrumental efficacy predicted maintenance over time in verbal but not nonverbal memory. Others have focused on perceived control.[21,59] Personal mastery has also been shown to be associated with remaining productive[46] and with optimism.[60] Personal mastery also appears to be a robust predictor of the maintenance of physical activity and exercise.[61] The degree to which perceived competence and control fluctuates over time may be important in its own right. Intraindividual variability in perceived control appears to predict mortality.[62] Some of the individual characteristics associated with optimal function (such as self-efficacy beliefs) appear to be anchored in features of the social atmosphere. Lang et al.[63] found that self-efficacy beliefs fluctuate in persons who believe that social relationships are unstable.

Numerous authors within both the psychosocial[17,36,64–66] and biomedical[67,68] traditions have focused on resilience (or the rate and extent of recovery from challenge). While some evidence suggests that old age may be associated with decreased resilience in the face of challenge, the picture is mixed. Kudielka et al.[69] found that older men had lower cardiovascular responses and comparable endocrine response patterns compared with young men exposed to a standardized stress test. Paradoxically, what may be most adaptive for low-status groups is a stubborn unwillingness to except societal definitions of self. Barusch[70] studied low-income older women who defined themselves as "fortunate" or "blessed" despite objective evidence to the contrary. A strategy of self-definition that insulates the self from negative influences may be an important feature of resilience.

Resilience may also represent the capacity to absorb the shock of physical illness without having it negatively effect morale or mental well-being. Some evidence suggests that declines in health do not lead to declines in morale and emotional health to the extent seen in younger adults.[71] Foster argues that "an abundance of evidence suggests that mental health diverges from physical health in that coping, adaptation and resilience (CAR) functions are surprisingly well-preserved throughout most of the lifespan.[66]

Several other habits of mind have been shown to correlate with successful aging variously defined. For example, a tendency toward more integrative and instrumental reminiscence but less obsessive reminiscence was observed in "successful agers" in a study by Wong and Watt.[72] Other personality factors that have been hinted at in the literature include androgeny,[73] stamina,[74] and intelligence.[75]

Among the more interesting points to make about individual predictors of successful aging is that several otherwise robust predictors of health status in younger populations are weak predictors of successful aging. For example, while an association between socio-economic status and several indicators of successful aging was seen in the MacArthur studies of successful aging,[56] other cohort studies have failed to observe this well-established association.[76]

PSYCHOSOCIAL CORRELATES OF SUCCESSFUL AGING: CHARACTERISTICS OF THE SOCIAL ENVIRONMENT

In addition to the individual characteristics reviewed briefly above, several psychosocial factors external to the individual appear also to impact patterns of aging. In broad terms, the increasing heterogeneity seen in older groups can be partially accounted for by social processes that sort and constrain individuals to be increasingly different from each other over time.[15]

Various indicators of social network integration and social support have been shown to predict survival in at least nine longitudinal studies.[77] While the precise mechanisms through which social integration and support may be related to well-being are not known, one study suggests that social support may operate through lowering the risk of alcohol abuse, smoking, and depressive disorder.[78] Although social support and social network ties may be important predictors of successful aging to the extent that they facilitate adaptation, it is crucial that social integration not be confused with successful aging as an outcome. This is particularly important given findings from the MacArthur studies of successful aging, showing that among men, greater use of instrumental social support is associated with an increased risk of ADL (activities of daily living) disability.[79]

Other studies have begun to show more clearly that continued social engagement, particularly with friends and distant relatives, is protective against the risk of disability.[80,81] The Duke Longitudinal Study found that frequency of activities with secondary networks (social groups and more distant friends) but not primary groups predicted who would show successful aging at follow-up.[7] This places the emphasis on actual performance of social roles as distinct from the receipt of support or the existence of ties.

Ageist attitudes in society appear to shape the self-perceptions of elderly people.[82,83] There is some evidence that cultural beliefs about aging may impact performance on memory tests.[84] Older people have differing attitudes in general toward the desirability and controllability of age-related personality and cognitive changes.[85] Ageist attitudes also appear to negatively impact access to medical care and other societal assets.[86,87] Some process of social comparison seems to be at play; that is, persons tend to compare themselves favorably to others who are worse off when they themselves feel stressed or ill, as a way of feeling better about themselves.[88] The social comparison phenomenon helps explain the paradoxical finding that, among schizophrenics for example, those who have lived in restricted or deprived social circumstances the longest have the highest life-satisfaction.[89] Despite a rich tradition of examining social comparison processes in children and adults, little work has been done to examine patterns of social comparison in seniors (see Heidrich and Ryff[90] for a notable exception).

STRESS AND ALLOSTATIC LOAD

Recent work has established the link between environmental stress and well-being in late life. Extending earlier work on stress and adaptation, McEwen and Stellar[91] introduced the concept of "allostatic load" defined as the cumulative strain on the body produced by repeated physiological responses across multiple systems. Seeman and colleagues[92] developed measures of allostatic load based on levels of physiological activity across a range of regulatory systems pertinent to disease risk. Those measures were found to be associated with poorer cognitive and physical function and predicted larger decrements in cognitive and physical functioning among participants of the MacArthur studies of successful aging. That group later showed that allostatic load was associated with 7-year survival and (marginally) with incident cardiovascular disease events, independent of standard sociodemographic characteristics and baseline health status.[93] Measures of allostatic load (particularly urinary cortisol excretion) have also been shown to predict memory function.[94] The study of environmental stress and the resulting allostatic load has shown considerable promise; although it is not clear whether biomarkers of stress are attributable to environmental or more endogenous stressors such as depression or attribution.

SUCCESSFUL AGING AND INTERVENTION

Relatively little work has been done to translate theories of successful aging into specific intervention strategies (excluding specific interventions aimed at improving one of the components of successful aging such as physical activity). A notable exception is the work of Fozard and colleagues, who tested a complex multifactorial intervention designed to optimize adaptation by intervening both at the level of individuals and environmental design.[95,96] The model was designed to improve cognitive function and memory but serves as an example of how a broad, multidisciplinary intervention program might look. A variety of other intervention models have been developed to improve cognitive performance.[97–99]

Another important example is the Intervention of Elderly in Göteborg study (IVEG) in Sweden, an interdisciplinary intervention in a representative population sample of 1206 70-year-olds designed to improve physical, mental, and social functioning through activity promotion.[100] The study hypothesized that significant age-related loss of function and disability could be postponed by providing four factors: adequate medical services, adequate levels of physical and social activity, an optimal lifestyle, and an emphasis on productivity. Although the intervention was underpowered to detect differences in disability risk, preliminary results suggest that the program was well-tolerated and that significant increases in participant activity and social engagement levels were achieved.[101] The work done in Sweden shows the utility of the "use-it-or-lose-it" model to intervention design.

TOWARD A SYNTHESIS

Having reviewed the existing literature on definitions and correlates of successful aging, the remainder of this chapter will outline a possible synthesis between what has been described above as two divergent approaches. It may be asked: "Why is a synthesis needed?" It may not be needed in all cases. It would be counterproductive for biological scientists interested in the study of glucose metabolism in late life to be required to interject psychosocial elements on principle alone. On the other hand, both research traditions stand to benefit from an expanded set of criteria from which to view successful aging. From a policy standpoint, it is important that, to borrow once again from Havighurst, our theory of successful aging recognize the need to encompass medical and nonmedical aspects of the "good life." To ignore either side of the equation is to be left with an impoverished view of what the research and policy objectives of gerontology should be. Qualitative research has taught us that, when asked, elderly people clearly tell us that health, social functioning, existential concerns, and functional independence are all important.

Let the reader not be lulled into a false sense of comfort. The synthesis of biological and psychosocial views of successful aging is a difficult enterprise. This is due in part to the insight provided by Dannefer,[15] who argued that a biomedical orientation to the study of aging is anchored in an "ontogenic" conception of human development, in which the lifespan is viewed as the natural unfolding of a pre-programmed algorithm inherent within the organism. This approach, he argues, results in an emphasis on normality and central tendency and a propensity to ignore heterogeneity. A psychosocial orientation, on the other hand (e.g. the lifespan developmental theory), questions the idea that development is universal, sequential, irreversible, and pre-programmed. Instead, patterns of variation are the products of social forces external to the individual. The difficulty of synthesizing these approaches should not be underestimated.

The basic idea that successful late-life development should involve multiple dimensions—physical, social, and psychological—is by no means new. Vaillant[102] described successful aging as a combination of physical health, mental health, psychosocial adjustment, and life satisfaction. There seems to be little doubt that any fruitful attempt to define successful aging, either conceptually or operationally, must include multiple dimensions, including at least the physical, cognitive, social, and psychological ones. Other features of obvious relevance to the definition of successful aging have been ignored—including sexuality[103] and spiritual or existential well-being.[104]

Figure 16-1 presents one approach to synthesizing these two perspectives, each of which has been productive although to

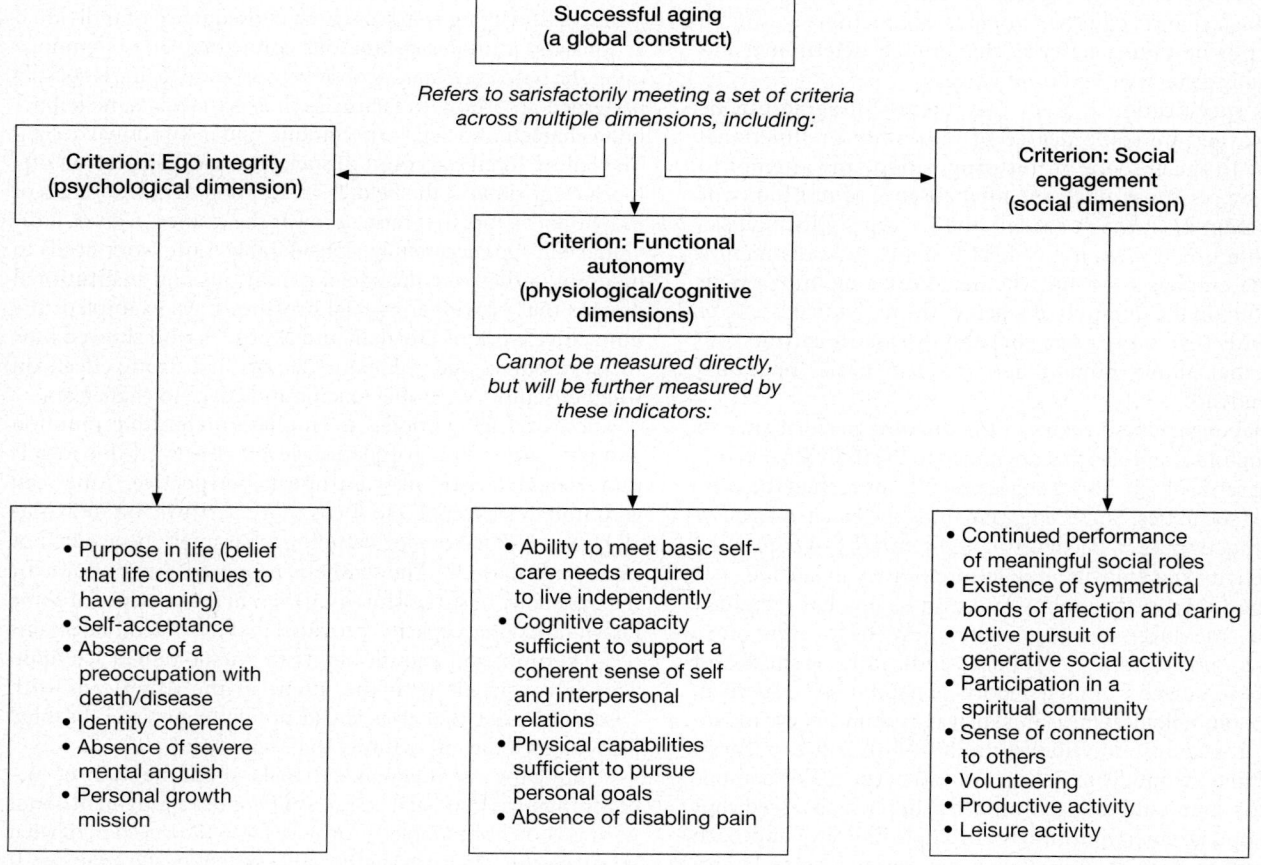

Figure 16-1 Conceptual model of successful aging, with emphasis on multiple subdimensions as well as potential empirical indicators.

some extent perhaps less than complete. The model depicted falls short of a formal theory, but is intended instead to propose a set of criteria for more clearly defining and operationalizing successful aging. The model is conceptual and not causal, meaning that the multitude of factors that give rise to, or are modifiers of, successful aging are not depicted. The model is meant to tell a story when read vertically (beginning at the top). The model is motivated by three hypotheses:

- Successful aging is a global construct of theoretical and empirical interest that bridges the full spectrum of domains of function in late life.
- There are four relevant core functional domains: the psychological, the physiological, the cognitive, and the social.
- The model posits three core criteria for successful aging, including (a) ego integrity, (b) functional autonomy, and (c) social engagement. Successful aging can therefore be defined as meeting all three of these criteria at some minimal level. The choice of these criteria reflects what Baltes and Baltes[36] call the "multicriteria approach" in an attempt to unify the key insights from both the psychosocial and the biomedical traditions.

Ego-integrity is a psychological construct referring to the extent to which an individual perceives himself to have a consistent and coherent sense of self, despite (and potentially because of) the challenges and pitfalls of late life. Functional autonomy refers to the capacity to remain independent in physiological and cognitive domains of function so as to be free to pursue valued activities that are self-determined and potentially generative and productive.

This specification implies that successful aging can be achieved despite some degree of morbidity or functional decline. In the absence of this proposition, any attempt to define successful aging as the total absence of morbidity or impairment of function renders the concept indistinguishable from broad measures of health status. This distinction puts the emphasis not on whether disease or impairment exists, but on the question of whether the individual is able to cope with (or compensate for) the disease/impairment in a way that allows him or her to retain basic functional independence.

Social engagement refers to the ongoing performance of meaningful social roles that are linked to the individual's continuing sense of self. Social engagement is more than the existence of social ties. Social engagement is the enacted tense of social functioning,[105] recognizing the centrality of continued productivity and enjoyment of leisure activity in late life.

If the conceptualization of successful aging has remained unclear, measurement approaches have been even more scattered and primitive. Proposed indicators of successful aging have ranged from self-reports of happiness, to survival, to more physiological measures such as exploratory eye movements in response to visual stimuli.[106] A fourth hypothesis underlying the model in Figure 16-1 is that the major components of successful aging cannot be directly observed, but can be operationalized through a multiple indicator approach that seeks to identify pools of common variance underlying a set of empirical items that might be caused by the latent construct of interest. Several potential empirical indicators of each of the three main criteria are specified in the figure. Conceptual overlap with more circumscribed concepts such as self-efficacy, productivity, and social networks are minimized so that these factors can be studied as potential correlates of successful aging.

POLICY IMPLICATIONS AND CONSIDERATIONS

By the year 2030, the size of the elderly population in the USA will have doubled to more than 70 million; one in five Americans will be 65 or older. One third of the human lifespan will be lived after the milestone of retirement, giving rise to what has been referred to as the "third age." However, while society has articulated a number of individual rights that obtain in older age, it has not agreed on a commensurate set of obligations, roles, and responsibilities that could help define what constitutes a good third age. Among the most important potential contributions of the concept of successful aging may be increased attention to the need to address the structural lag that has created a vacuum of opportunity for meaningful social engagement. A vision of the post-retirement years as an extended vacation in a sun-drenched paradise is not a sustainable vision of successful aging. What is needed most are social policy initiatives that aim to create structures of opportunity that sustain social and productive role performance for seniors.

Successful aging is not only the consequence of individual actions and attitudes. Numerous contextual factors impinge upon the outcomes that we observe. Successful aging is socially patterned according to factors such as social class, neighborhood character, societal expectations, and institutional design. The failure to take account of social context has been an oft-repeated critique of the field.[107] In addition to more studies of individual factors that raise or lower the chances a given individual will age successfully, considerably more work needs to be done to discover the social conditions and institutional designs that provide for social prosthesis. An example is the innovative work of Holahan and Moos,[108] who showed how social resources and contextual factors had strong effects on whether seniors were able to cope and adapt to challenges.

Successful aging implies an emphasis on health promotion and prevention at a population-level. However, this idea is more characteristic of a European perspective. American gerontology has tended to focus more narrowly on individually based risk factors for pathology that might be avoided or intervened upon.[109] The synthesis proposed above allows for the possibility of successful aging even in the presence of some loss of functional capacity, provided that the individual retains self-determination and the ability to pursue valued activities. This is consistent with the intent of the Americans with Disabilities Act that uses social policy to provide disabled persons with the opportunity to be successful.

Among the essential points to make about the study of successful aging is that what is *successful* implies a judgment about what is good or desirable.[34] Any answer to the question of what is "successful" depends on the value system of the enquirer. It is not surprising, given American cultural values, oriented as they are to individualism, and material success and achievement, that a preoccupation with successful aging has flourished in the USA. It is essential to remain skeptical of attempts to treat successful aging in purely scientific terms without recognition of the inherently value-laden nature of the term.[110] Any inquiry into successful aging will be as much about culture and values as about scientific truth. This should not paralyze the empirical study of successful aging or its determinants; however, it is important to remain aware of the cultural context of this work.

CONCLUSION

The main objective of this chapter was to review the state of the art of conceptualization and research into the concept of successful aging in an attempt to better define the term and to synthesize the psychosocial and biomedical approaches. The core conclusions of this chapter are shown in the Key Points box.

Considerable effort remains to further explicate the concept of successful aging to the point that it illuminates more than it obscures. While work has begun to understand the biology of plasticity and resilience across physiological systems, much more work needs to be done to understand the social and cultural factors that shape the phenotype of the aging person. A fuller integration of biomedical and psychosocial approaches will require significant attention to the development of more refined criteria and measures. In addition, there is a need for more qualitative studies of both the processes of adaptation and the meanings attached to aging.[111]

KEY POINTS Successful aging

- Although successful aging is a core concept in gerontology, it remains a vague and general construct that is not yet clearly defined and operationalized.

- Two distinct traditions or approaches can be seen, one older (the psychosocial approach) and another (the biomedical approach) focusing on physiological and cognitive function. To date, these two perspectives have not been integrated well.

- A synthesis of these approaches is proposed whereby successful aging is defined as meeting three criteria representing multiple dimensions. Proposed criteria include ego integrity, functional independence, and social engagement.

- A satisfactory definition of successful aging places the emphasis on adaptation and compensation for age-related losses, and not merely the presence or absence of those losses. Age-related functional loss does not necessarily preclude successful aging.

- The study of successful aging must pay greater attention to the role played by social context, including social class, neighborhood features, societal attitudes toward elderly people, and institutional design.

- The study of successful aging is inherently culture-bound and value-laden.

REFERENCES

1. Havighurst RJ: Successful aging. Gerontologist 1961;1:8–13
2. Griffin JJ: Plato's philosophy of old age. Geriatrics 1949;4:242–255
3. Lawton G: Aging Successfully. Columbia University Press, New York, 1946
4. Pollak O: Social Adjustment in Old Age: A Research Planning Report. US Social Science Research Council, Bulletin 59, 1948
5. Rupp C, Duffy EL, Danish MM: Successful adaptation to aging. I: Psychologic, social, and psychiatric aspects. J Am Geriatr Soc 1967;15:1137–1143
6. Schonfield D: Geronting: reflections on successful aging. Gerontologist 1967;7:270–273
7. Palmore E: Predictors of successful aging. Gerontologist 1979;19(5 Pt 1):427–431
8. Rowe JW, Kahn RL: Human aging: usual and successful. Science 1987;237:143–149
9. Capsi A, Elder GH: Life satisfaction in old age: linking social psychology and history. Psychol Aging 1986;1:18–26
10. Ryff CD: Successful aging: a developmental approach. Gerontologist 1982;22:209–214
11. Butler RN: Successful aging. MH 1974;58(3):6–12
12. Lehr U: ["Successful aging" requires "proper" living: a social challenge through trends in population development]. Fortschr Med 1984;102(33):70–71
13. Blucher VG: [Determinants of successful aging in Switzerland]. Aktuelle Gerontol 1982;12(5):180–183
14. Tempelman JJ: ["Successful aging," een leetheoretische visie]. Neder Tijdsch Geneesk 1977;121:1662–1665
15. Dannefer D: What's in a name? An account of the neglect of variability in the study of aging. In Birren JE, Bengston VL (eds): Emergent Theories of Aging. Springer, New York, 1988:356–384
16. Baltes PB, Baltes MM (eds): Successful Aging: Perspectives from the Behavioral Sciences. Cambridge University Press, Cambridge, 1990
17. Rosenzweig MR, Bennett EL: Psychobiology of plasticity: effects of training and experience on brain and behavior. Behav Brain Res 1996;78:57–65
18. Schaie KW, Willis SL, Hertzog C et al: Effects of cognitive training on primary mental ability structure. Psychol Aging 1987;2:233–242
19. Carson PJ, Nichol KL, O'Brien J et al: Immune function and vaccine responses in healthy advanced elderly patients. Arch Intern Med 2000;160:2017–2024
20. Smyer M, Reid J, Zarit S: Successful aging as adaptation to stress. Exper Aging Res 1991;17:93–94
21. Brandtstädter J, Baltes-Götz B: Personal control over development and quality of life perspectives in adulthood. In Baltes PB, Baltes MM (eds): Successful Aging: Perspectives from the Behavioral Sciences. Cambridge University Press, Cambridge, 1990:197–224
22. Henry WE, Cummings E: Personality development in adulthood and old age. J Proj Tech 1959;23:383–390
23. Havighurst RJ: Successful aging. In Williams RH, Tibbits C, Dohahue W (eds): Processes of Aging. Atherton Press, New York, 1963:299–320
24. McClelland KA: Self-conception and life satisfaction: integrating aged subculture and activity theory. J Gerontol 1982;37:723–732
25. Leonard WM: Successful aging: an elaboration of social and psychological factors. Int J Aging Hum Dev 1981;14:223–232
26. Maddox GL, Wiley J: Scope, concepts and methods in the study of aging. In Binstock RH, Shanas E (eds): Handbook of Aging and the Social Sciences. Academic Press, San Diego, 1976
27. Ryff CD: Beyond Ponce de Leon and life satisfaction: new directions in quest of successful aging. Int J Behav Dev 1989;12:35–55
28. Maddox GL: Activity and morale: a longitudinal study of selected elderly subjects. Soc Forces 1963;42:195–204
29. Herzog AR, Rodgers W, Woodworth J: Subjective Well-being Among Different Age Groups. University of Michigan Institute for Social Research, Ann Arbor, MI, 1982
30. Erikson EH: The Life Cycle Completed: A Review. W.W. Norton, New York, 1982
31. Erikson EH: Childhood and Society. 1950
32. Taft LB, Nehrke MF: Reminiscence, life review, and ego integrity in nursing home residents. Int J Aging Hum Dev 1990;30:189–196
33. Whitbourne SK: Psychological adaptation in old age. Long Term Care Health Serv Adm Qtly 1977;1(2):145–151
34. Schulz R, Heckhausen J: A life span model of successful aging. Am Psychol 1996;51:702–714

35. Ryff CD, Essex MJ: The interpretation of life experience and well-being: the sample case of relocation. Psychol Aging 1992;7:507–517

36. Baltes PB, Baltes MM: Psychological perspectives on successful aging: the model of selective optimization with compensation. In Baltes PB, Baltes MM (eds): Successful Aging: Perspectives from the Behavioral Sciences. Cambridge University Press, New York, 1990:1–34

37. Atchley RC: Continuity theory and the evolution of activity in later adulthood. In Kelly JR (ed): Activity and Aging: Staying Involved in Later Life. Sage, Newbury Park, 1993:5–16

38. Campbell A, Converse PE, Rodgers WL: The Quality of American Life. Russell Sage, New York, 1976

39. Baltes MM, Reisenzein R: The social world in long-term care institutions: psychological control toward dependency. In Baltes MM, Baltes PM (eds): The Psychology of Control and Aging. Lawrence Erlbaum, Hillsdale, NJ, 1986:315–343

40. Abraham JD, Hansson RO: Successful aging at work: an applied study of selection, optimization, and compensation through impression management. J Gerontol B 1995;50:94–103

41. Baltes MM, Lang FR: Everyday functioning and successful aging: the impact of resources. Psychol Aging 1997;12:433–443

42. Freund AM, Baltes PB: Selection, optimization, and compensation as strategies of life management: correlations with subjective indicators of successful aging. Psychol Aging 1998;13:531–543

43. Fries JF: Medical perspectives on successful aging. In Baltes PM, Baltes MM (eds): Successful Aging: Perspectives from the Behavioral Sciences. Cambridge University Press, New York, 1990:35–49

44. Schoenfeld DE, Malmrose LC, Blazer DG et al: Self-rated health and mortality in high-functioning elderly—a closer look at healthy individuals. MacArthur Field Study of Successful Aging. J Gerontol A 1994;49:M109–M115

45. Seeman TE, Robbins RJ: Aging and hypothalamic–pituitary–adrenal response to challenge in humans. Endo Rev 1994;15:233–260

46. Glass TA, Seeman TE, Herzog AR et al: Change in productive activity in late adulthood. MacArthur Studies of Successful Aging. J Gerontol B 1995;50:S65–S76

47. Gold DT, Pieper CF, Westlund RE et al: Do racial differences in hypertension persist in successful agers? Findings from the MacArthur Study of Successful Aging. J Aging Health 1996;8:207–219

48. Friedan B: The Fountain of Age. Simon & Schuster, New York, 1993

49. Lawton MP: The varieties of wellbeing. In Malatesta CZ, Izard CE (eds): Emotion in Adult Development. Sage, Beverly Hills, CA, 1984:67–84

50. Fisher BJ: Successful aging, life satisfaction, and generativity in later life. Int J Aging Human Dev 1995;41:239–250

51. Ryff CD: In the eye of the beholder: views of psychological well-being among middle-aged and older adults. Psychol Aging 1989;4:195–201

52. Vaupel JW, Carey JR, Christensen K et al: Biodemographic trajectories of longevity. Science 1998;280:855–860

53. Vaillant GE: The association of ancestral longevity with successful aging. J Gerontol 1991;46:292–298

54. Barefoot JC, Maynard KE, Beckham JC et al: Trust, health, and longevity. J Behav Med 1998;21:517–526

55. Albert MS, Jones K, Savage CR et al: Predictors of cognitive change in older persons. MacArthur Studies of Successful Aging. Psychol Aging 1995;10:578–589

56. Berkman LF, Seeman TE, Albert M et al: High, usual and impaired functioning in community-dwelling older men and women: findings from the MacArthur Foundation Research Network on Successful Aging. J Clin Epidem 1993;46:1129–1140

57. Rodin J: Aging and health: effects of the sense of control. Science 1986;233:1271–1276

58. Seeman T, McAvay G, Merrill S et al: Self-efficacy beliefs and change in cognitive performance. MacArthur Studies of Successful Aging. Psychol Aging 1996;11:538–551

59. Brandtstädter J, Rothermund K: Self-percepts of control in middle and later adulthood: buffering losses by rescaling goals. Psychol Aging 1994;9:265–273

60. Seeman M, Seeman TE: Health behavior and personal autonomy: a longitudinal study of the sense of control in illness. J Health Soc Behav 1983;24(June):144–160

61. Simonsick EM, Guralnik JM, Fried LP: Who walks? Factors associated with walking behavior in disabled older women with and without self-reported walking difficulty. J Am Geriatr Soc 1999;47:672–680

62. Eizenman DR, Nesselroade JR, Featherman DL et al: Intraindividual variability in perceived control in an older sample. MacArthur Successful Aging Studies. Psychol Aging 1997;12:489–502

63. Lang FR, Featherman DL, Nesselroade JR: Social self-efficacy and short-term variability in social relationships. MacArthur Successful Aging Studies. Psychol Aging 1997;12:657–666

64. Kahn RL: Retention, resilience, and enhancement: components of vitality throughout the life course. In The MacArthur Foundation Successful Aging Program. San Francisco, 1991

65. Rudinger G, Thomae H: The Bonn Longitudinal Study of Aging: Coping, life adjustment, and life satisfaction. In Baltes PB, Baltes MM (eds): Successful Aging: Perspectives from the Behavioral Sciences. Cambridge University Press, Cambridge, 1990:265–295

66. Foster JR: Successful coping, adaptation and resilience in the elderly: an interpretation of epidemiologic data. Psychiatr Qtly 1997;68:189–219

67. Minaker KL, Meneilly GS, Rowe JW. In Finch CE, Scheider EL (eds): Handbook of the Biology of Human Aging: Academic Press, London, 1985:433–456

68. Seals DR, Hagberg JM, Allen WK et al: Glucose tolerance in young and older athletes and sedentary men. J Appl Physiol 1984;56:1521–1525

69. Kudielka BM, Schmidt-Reinwald AK, Hellhammer DH et al: Psychosocial stress and HPA functioning: no evidence for a reduced resilience in healthy elderly men. Stress 2000;3:229–240

70. Barusch AS. Self-concepts of low-income older women: not old or poor, but fortunate and blessed. Int J Aging Hum Dev 1997;44:269–282

71. Sullivan MD: Maintaining good morale in old age. West J Med 1997;167:276–284

72. Wong PT, Watt LM: What types of reminiscence are associated with successful aging? Psychol Aging 1991;6:272–279

73. Shimonaka Y, Nakazato K, Homma A: Personality, longevity, and successful aging among Tokyo metropolitan centenarians. Int J Aging Hum Dev 1996;42:173–187

74. Colerick EJ: Stamina in later life. Soc Sci Med 1985;21:997–1006

75. Poon LW, Martin P, Clayton GM et al: The influences of cognitive resources on adaptation and old age. Int J Aging Hum Dev 1992;34:31–46

76. Roos NP, Havens B: Predictors of successful aging: a twelve-year study of Manitoba elderly. Am J Pub Health 1991;81:63–68

77. House JS, Landis KR, Umberson D: Social relationships and health. Science 1988;241:540–545

78. Vaillant GE, Meyer SE, Mukamal K et al: Are social supports in late midlife a cause or a result of successful physical aging? Psychol Med 1998;28:1159–1168

79. Seeman TE, Bruce ML, McAvay GJ: Social network characteristics and onset of ADL disability. MacArthur Studies of Successful Aging. J Gerontol B 1996;51:S191–S200

80. Mendes de Leon CF, Glass TA, Beckett LA et al: Social networks and disability transitions across eight intervals of yearly data in the New Haven EPESE. J Gerontol B 1999;54:S162–S172

81. Mendes de Leon CF, Gold DT, Glass TA et al: Disability as a function of social networks and support in elderly African Americans and whites. The Duke EPESE 1986–1992. J Gerontol B 2001;56:S179–S190

82. Bondevik M: Historical, cross-cultural, biological and psychosocial perspectives of aging and the aged person. Scand J Caring Sci 1994;8(2):67–74

83. Brown R, Middendorf J: The underestimated role of temporal comparison: a test of the life-span model. J Soc Psychol 1996;136:325–331

84. Levy B, Langer E: Aging free from negative stereotypes: successful memory in China and among the American deaf. J Pers Soc Psychol 1994;66:989–997

85. Heckhausen J, Baltes PB: Perceived controllability of expected psychological change across adulthood and old age. J Gerontol B 1991;46:P165–P173

86. Bowling A: Ageism in cardiology. BMJ 1999;319:1353–1355

87. Bates MS, Rankin-Hill L, Sanchez-Ayendez M: The effects of the cultural context of health care on treatment of and response to chronic pain and illness. Soc Sci Med 1997;45:1433–1447

88. Wilson SR, Benner LA: The effects of self-esteem and situation upon comparison choices during ability evaluation. Sociometry 1971;34:381–397

89. Franz M, Meyer T, Reber T et al: The importance of social comparisons for high levels of subjective quality of life in chronic schizophrenic patients. Qual Life Res 2000;9:481–489

90. Heidrich SM, Ryff CD: The role of social comparisons processes in the psychological adaptation of elderly adults. J Gerontol B 1993;48:P127–P136

91. McEwen BS, Stellar E: Stress and the individual: mechanisms leading to disease. Arch Int Med 1993;153:2093–2101

92. Seeman TE, Singer BH, Rowe JW et al: Price of adaptation—allostatic load and its health consequences. MacArthur Studies of Successful Aging. Arch Intern Med 1997;157:2259–2268

93. Seeman TE, McEwen BS, Rowe JW et al: Allostatic load as a marker of cumulative biological risk. MacArthur Studies of Successful Aging. Proc Natl Acad Sci USA 2001;98:4770–4775

94. Seeman TE, McEwen BS, Singer BH et al: Increase in urinary cortisol excretion and memory declines. MacArthur Studies of Successful Aging. J Clin Endocrin Metab 1997;82:2458–2465

95. Fozard JL, Popkin SJ: Optimizing adult development: ends and means of an applied psychology of aging. Am Psychol 1978;33:975–989

96. Treat NJ, Poon LW, Fozard JL et al: Toward applying cognitive skill training to memory problems. Exp Aging Res 1978;4:305–319

97. Lachman ME: Improving the sense of control over memory. Exp Aging Res 1991;17:81–82

98. Lachman ME, Weaver SL, Bandura M et al: Improving memory and control beliefs through cognitive restructuring and self-generated strategies. J Gerontol B 1992;47:P293–P299

99. Baltes PM, Lindenberger U: On the range of cognitive plasticity in old age as a function of experience: 15 years of intervention research. Behav Ther 1988;19:720–725

100. Eriksson BG, Mellstrom D, Svanborg A: Medical–social intervention in a 70-year-old Swedish population: a general presentation of methodological experience. Compr Gerontol C 1987;1:49–56

101. Svanborg A: A medical–social intervention in a 70-year-old Swedish population: is it possible to postpone functional decline in aging? J Gerontol 1993;48(spec no.):84–88

102. Vaillant GE: Avoiding negative outcomes: evidence from a forty-five year study. In Baltes PB, Baltes MM (eds): Successful Aging: Perspectives from the Behavioral Sciences. Cambridge University Press, New York, 1990:332–358

103. Wiley D, Bortz WM: Sexuality and aging—usual and successful. J Gerontol A 1996;51:M142–M146

104. Reker GT, Peacock EJ, Wong PT: Meaning and purpose in life and well-being: a life-span perspective. J Gerontol 1987;42:44–49

105. Glass TA: Conjugating the "tenses" of function: discordance among hypothetical, experimental, and enacted function in older adults. Gerontologist 1998;38:101–112

106. Daffner KR, Scinto LF, Weintraub S et al: The impact of aging on curiosity as measured by exploratory eye movements. Arch Neurol 1994;51:368–376

107. Riley MW: Successful aging. Gerontologist 1998;38:151

108. Holahan CJ, Moos RH: Personal and contextual determinants of coping strategies. J Personal Soc Psychol 1987;52:946–955

109. Bowling A: The concepts of successful and positive aging. Fam Pract 1993;10:449–453

110. Coan RW: Hero, Artist, Sage, or Saint? A Survey of Views on What is Variously Called Mental Health, Normality, Maturity, Self-actualization, and Human Fulfillment. Columbia University Press, New York, 1977

111. Clark F, Carlson M, Zemke R et al: Life domains and adaptive strategies of a group of low-income, well older adults. Am J Occup Ther 1996;50:99–108

Chapter 17

Social gerontology

Kenneth W. Hepburn

Social gerontology is a field of inquiry that examines how individuals age in a social setting. It may, perhaps, be more correct to speak of social gerontology as a collection of subsets of various academic fields than to construe it as a discrete academic enterprise. Economics, anthropology, sociology, psychology, family social science, and numerous other fields, including the arts and humanities, all contribute to social gerontology. Geriatrics is clearly one of these intersecting disciplines.

This chapter will not provide an overview of the history of social gerontology. That history was well represented in the last edition of this textbook and the reader interested in an overview is encouraged to review Malcolm Johnson's chapter there.

There is an underlying recognition in the social gerontology literature that social and physical well-being exert reciprocal effects, and that both, together, can interact to promote well-being or to hasten a downward cycle of frailty. For example, an extensive and effective social network of family and friends may provide important support to a person who has experienced an acute medical event (e.g. stroke or the onset of a chronic disabling disease).[1] Members of the network might provide transportation to an outpatient rehabilitation setting, restructure the home environment to a more therapeutic configuration, and in general promote a positive psychosocial environment for rehabilitation efforts that, in turn, promote optimum physical functioning. Conversely, psychosocial states like loneliness (social isolation) or depression can contribute to poor health. Such states can promote or reinforce negative behaviors (in areas like diet, alcohol consumption, etc.) which may contribute to bad health outcomes (e.g. hypertension, the development of cardiac disease or diabetes), ultimately leading to decreased functioning and increased utilization of healthcare resources.[2,3]

As the field of social gerontology has developed, particular emphasis has been placed on examining the ways in which social institutions and processes intersect with intrapersonal processes and characteristics to affect a broad target outcome, "successful aging."[4] The literature is replete with terms that stand as cognates for aging well—such as life satisfaction, quality of life, happiness, and integration. For purposes of this chapter, the term "social functioning" will be used to indicate an optimum condition in aging.

Figure 17-1 provides a conceptual map for the chapter. At the center is *social functioning*, the vivifying metaphor of social gerontology and the animating force of the field's inquiry to increase understanding about ways to improve life in aging. Arrayed in close proximity to this target are the three main social factors that contribute to (or detract from) social functioning. First is *status*, the place that people hold (or to which they are assigned or relegated) in the larger society. Second is *connections*, the way in which people fit within their own self-defined social networks—as well as what those social networks look like and do. Third is *personal resources*, the way in which persons construe themselves—both individually, within their social networks, and *vis-à-vis* the larger social fabric—along with the capacities they bring to bear on their social reality. A fourth factor—*health conditions and behaviors*—draws geriatrics into the scheme.

The figure is drawn to represent the interconnectedness of the factors. The four are postulated to affect social functioning directly, but also to affect one another and thus have an indirect effect on social functioning as well. For example, a person's income very likely affects health behavior, access to health services, and his or her opportunities for participation in the social world. The figure also incorporates two background factors that contribute to social functioning: *occupations* (the nature and kind of social involvement) and *life events* (things that happen close to the person that may have a profound effect on social functioning). Neither of these is represented as having a direct or indirect effect on social functioning. The effort rather is to portray them as being integral to the fabric of a person's world, thus affecting, in a pervasive or general way, that person's social functioning.

Each of the three social factors and the two background conditions are discussed separately in the chapter. For each, the discussion describes the factor and delineates how it contributes to social functioning. Research literature is cited to indicate key concepts associated with each factor/condition and the main ways it interacts with the other social and health factors. The chapter ends with a brief discussion of the clinical implications of social gerontology for the fourth factor, geriatrics.

STATUS

One of the earliest and most enduring concepts in sociology is that status plays an important part in social functioning.

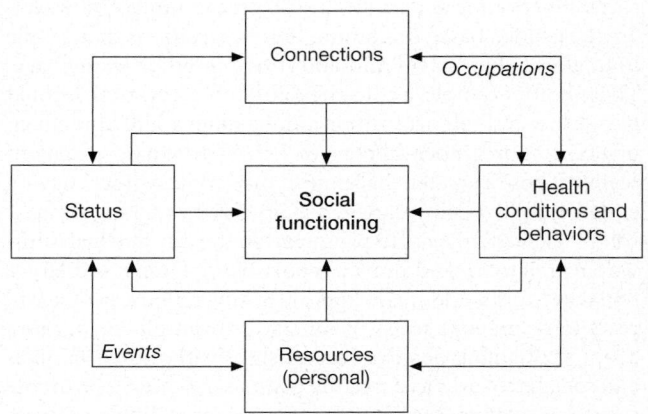

Figure 17-1 Interrelated factors affecting social functioning.

Discussion of social status typically includes four elements: income and education, gender, race and ethnicity, and geographical location. In this discussion, age—usually not considered, in itself, as a status element—will also be included as an important component of status. As with the other major factors contributing to social functioning, status serves as an indicator of a person's capacities and vulnerabilities—identifying the advantages a person may have or the challenges he or she may face in optimizing social functioning.

Income and education

Income and education are usually very highly correlated. People who are better educated typically have higher incomes, and so the two often stand as surrogates for one another. Both income and education have a direct effect on a person's access to and use of resources, opportunities, institutions, or structures that directly bear on social functioning such as community health or social services. This has both to do with knowing about the services as well as knowing how to use them.[5-9] Income and education seem to produce a greater sense of entitlement which facilitates and destigmatizes the use of services. For example, a person of very low means economically is less likely than a person of wealth to have access to, or to take advantage of, organizations that foster social interaction, intellectual or creative activities, or physical activity. Persons of lower means may be less likely to engage in elder hostel or health club activities or to participate in a wide range of volunteer organizations than are more affluent elders. The relationship to access is not hard and fast. Importantly, income and education don't bear all that significantly on participation in religious organizations or on volunteering in these organizations, both of which are positively associated with social functioning.[10]

Gender

Gender relates to social functioning in many ways, but it is important to recognize that many of these relationships are bound, in part, to age cohorts. For the near future, gender is likely to predict marital status. In the current and impending generations of elderly people, women are more likely than men to spend the last years of their lives alone. If ever married, their older and shorter-lived husbands will have died, and, given the diminished number of marriage-eligible males in their age cohort, there is only a slim likelihood of remarriage. As discussed below, this deficit in connection can bear adversely on social functioning and health.[11,12] Of greater impact, however, are the gender-based limitations and expectations that people hold about themselves and about one another as they age. There is, for example, a considerable body of research devoted to role loss and role acquisition among older adults, and much of it centers on gender differences.[13,14] In particular, retirement seems to pose a greater challenge to men while women, having ended a child-raising career, are involved in taking on new roles.[15] Gender appears to play a part in the way in which individuals relate to, and draw support from, family and larger social networks, and it also appears to suggest how people will react to or manage stress. Women, for example, seem more adept at retaining positive relationships within their families and social networks and making good use of those to promote social functioning. Men appear to have a more difficult time of this. Women, on the other hand, appear to manifest greater distress in situations such as caregiving.[16-19] Even in the area of health behavior, gender enters in. While both men and women appear to benefit from concerted physical activity and designed exercise programs, women seem to experience barriers to participation that are based, at least in part, on their own internalized sense of what kind of physical activities are proper or possible for a woman to do.[20]

Race and ethnicity

Especially over the last decade, race and ethnicity have received considerable attention in the social gerontology literature. The particular issues are much the same as those with income. There appears to be differential access to, and use and outcomes of, services by people depending on their membership in various racial or ethnic groups.[21-23] For people in minority groups, access to and use of health and social services appears to be part of a larger pattern of there being a distance between these individuals and those organizations. In the USA, the organizations are often predicated on service to a non-Hispanic white population, and the culture and expectations within the service are set by this orientation. This often produces a disconnection between the organization and persons of other races or cultures which may, in some cases, create disinclination for use or disinclination to serve.[24-26]

Of equal interest, the literature has begun to identify the unique ways in which various cultural, racial, and ethnic groups conceive of old age within their broader social reality. These fundamental conceptualizations bear on the way these groups organize around critical life events and also on the way in which they link with social structures such as helping organizations in times of these events.[27,28] For example, how one thinks about Alzheimer's disease will partly determine how openly help will be sought or how carefully guarded the family's "shameful secret" will be kept.[29,30] Culture-linked beliefs about health, death, and the afterlife profoundly affect the very different ways that people approach conversations about disease, the discussion of advance directives, or the performance of autopsy.[31-33] Similarly, generational differences and culture-linked expectations about the role of women in family caregiving will produce widely different conversations, tensions, and care arrangements in various cultural and ethnic groups.[34]

Geographical location

The fourth status concept—where a person lives (an inner city, a suburb, or a rural area)—is often a function (as well as an indicator) of income and education, but can also have independent bearing on health outcomes and social functioning.[35,36] Social functioning is reliant to a certain degree on opportunity, and location affects opportunity for being a member of and taking part in a larger social reality as well as access to types of care. For example, it is well documented that rural elderly people have difficulty accessing health and social services.[37-39] Access to other mechanisms affecting social function may be limited as well. The growing proportion of the aged who occupy rural counties is largely a function of out-migration by children and grandchildren. For the rural elderly, family networks, while possibly robust through distance communication (phone, e-mail, etc.), are likely to be weaker than those of the urban elderly whose children are less likely to have moved away, granting them the opportunity for frequent unstructured and informal interaction with family. While some structures in the rural area—in particular, churches—may focus effectively on the social needs of elderly people, there are fewer such structures in rural, compared with urban, settings.[40,41] People living in inner cities in large metropolitan areas have constraints of a different sort, but which lead to the same outcome—less opportunity for social interaction and reduced participation in family networks (although the opportunities for religious participation are present).[42,43]

Age

How old a person is can serve as an epidemiological indicator of a number of important facets of function. Thus, age (in conjunction with gender) can provide a working estimate of life expectancy and active life expectancy; it can also allow a person to be placed into risk categories for numerous diseases as well as overall functional decline or well-being.[44,45] But age—as an indicator of an age-cohort—is a status component of a more subtle sort. It can, for example, suggest something about the likely density or attenuation of a person's social network (the very old are likely to have fewer surviving friends or family members than the young old).[46,47] Age also offers clues about the cultural grounding and social experience of individuals. A member of the cohort that was in its childhood during the First World War and spent its early adulthood in the depression may hold very different values and expectations from one born 30 years later on the leading edge of the baby boom. Taken in conjunction with race and gender, age may suggest very different patterns of response to hardships or opportunity, beliefs about self-care, or other significant intrapersonal resources that affect positive social functioning.[48]

CONNECTIONS

Central to social gerontology is the notion that there is a larger social world in which the aged are embedded, in one fashion or another. The composition of this social world and the ways in which elders are connected to, contribute to, and/or draw support from it frame key lines of inquiry for the field. Investigation of ways to promote social interaction, to facilitate access to social networks, and to strengthen these networks' capacities to provide support for elders form important auxiliary lines of inquiry. Typically the social world of elders is conceptualized to include family, friends, and, at a greater distance, various kinds of voluntary or social organization.

In general, isolation is seen as the antithesis of social integration and is strongly associated with impaired health and social functioning.[49–51] In an earlier era, disengagement was considered a normative process of aging. Disengagement theory postulated that, cut off from the gender-based roles and responsibilities of work (for men) and marriage and childbearing (for women), older people would, in effect, quit the field to find their own meaning in the face of impending death. Failure to disengage—a form of denial of the role loss that was occurring—would result in decreased morale.[52,53] Disengagement theory has faded from vogue. Gender role changes of the last 40 years have undercut its premises, as has an appreciation that class and ethnic differences produce very different patterns of experiences and expectations as people

age. Nevertheless, the spectre of disengagement remains. The emergence of the pre-retirement counseling industry confirms the power of the concern people have with role loss and change with aging. More positively, disengagement theory has prompted substantial inquiry into what constitutes continued development and productivity in aging and the part social networks play in those processes.[54–56]

The health-based literature focusing on successful aging strongly endorses the importance of social connectedness to overall well-being in old age.[57,58] Robust social networks are associated with many of the key outcomes in geriatrics, including reduced risk for mortality and better physical and mental health outcomes.[59–64] At the level of function, participation in social networks is associated with reduced risk of decline or disability in activities of daily living (ADLs).[65] Similarly, robust social networks are associated with a greater likelihood of recovery of ADL function in the event of illness or trauma that produces a decline in that function.[66]

A running debate has focused on whether social networks serve to replace or reinforce self-care and promote dependency. It appears, on balance, that social networks serve to reinforce rather than preclude self-care behaviors and do not (except possibly in the case of older men) increase the risk for new or recurrent ADL disability. In the purely psychosocial realm, robust social networks tend to promote stronger self-efficacy beliefs (see the personal resources section below) and also serve to buffer the impact of major negative life events on the person.[67,68]

Four concepts have ongoing importance in the literature on social connectedness: (1) appraisal of the network, (2) history and quality of network relationships, (3) intimacy of the relationships, and (4) size of the social network.

APPRAISAL   A sense of belonging—a person's appraisal of his or her place in a social network—seems to trump all other considerations. The extent to which a person feels he or she belongs to a network (i.e. is or is not an integral part of a social group) profoundly affects the ability of that network to produce the kinds of positive outcomes of which they seem capable.[69–72] Appraisal, a subjective evaluation, can be influenced and might be considered the object of intervention in cases where a social network appears not to be playing as strong a role in the well-being of an older person as might be anticipated. The other factors surrounding a social network (see below) may enter into the appraisal but also may be affected by it, which needs to be considered in any potential intervention.

HISTORY AND QUALITY   A considerable body of work has pointed to the need to examine the historical quality of relationships within social networks. The presence of a discernible number of family and friends with apparent connections to an older person can give the impression of a supportive social network. However, it is essential to discover how those relationships have played over time and whether relations—in particular those between an older person and his or her spouse and children—have been historically positive and of good quality or conflictual, disappointing, or difficult.[73–76]

INTIMACY   Even in the context of a large and positive social network, the literature further points to the importance of the older person's having one or more confidants within the network. An older person might rely on various members of a network to assist with normal tasks of living, assistance that is important to day-to-day social functioning. However, the person is also experiencing more profound changes and facing more serious questions as he or she experiences losses, faces mortality, and engages in a continued search for meaning. It is at this level that the need to be intimately connected—to have a confidant—is seen as particularly important. The person who is without a confidant, even though surrounded by a network that supports function, is seen as being disadvantaged.[77–80]

SIZE The size of a social network—the number of people who are defined by an individual to be part of his or her network—is an insufficient measure of its ability to affect social functioning. Other important elements of size include: frequency and quality of contact (whether contacts are superficial, instrumental, or of a more personal nature), the kind and intensity of commitment of network members, the kinds of tasks the network performs, and the adequacy (or completeness) with which the network addresses an individual's needs.[81,82]

Overall, there is no simple measure of a social network, but these four domains have to be taken into account in assessing the degree to which a person's social network can promote or support optimal social function. Thus, for example, a person with only three members of a network but who sees these people on a regular basis, and is in intense contact with them, may be considerably better supported by that network than a person with dozens of more distant relatives and friends with whom the individual has infrequent contact and with whom personal matters are discussed almost not at all. On the other hand, if the network fails to provide some of the instrumental supports needed by the person, even though it may meet the person's more deep-seated needs for contact, the network might be ineffective. A large network might, for example, be able to buffer the loss of a person's spouse but be unable, by virtue of distance and lack of resources, to provide needed material assistance in the event of a health crisis requiring intensive rehabilitation.

PERSONAL RESOURCES

No other factor of social functioning has received more attention in the research literature than personal or inner resources. This area is broad and encompasses many facets, but the concept fundamentally comes down to two main capacities: (1) the ability to be effective or to act effectively in the world, and (2) the ability to respond effectively to the world. Taken together, the two capacities (being effective and reacting effectively) constitute a presentation of the self in the world that affects connectedness, is influential in the choice of occupations in aging, and shapes the responses to common events of aging.

The first capacity—being effective—speaks to the base from which a person acts in the social world. This base includes some apparently fundamental, fixed qualities such as personality and character. While persons may be more or less aware of their

personality and how it intersects with the social world, they are unlikely (or unable) to change personality.[83–85]

The second capacity—reacting effectively—speaks to a set of acquired characteristics such as skill and knowledge. The most salient finding for this subset of personal resources is that they appear to be malleable across the lifespan. They can be developed and strengthened, and when they are, they contribute positively to the realm of social functioning.[86,87] Coping style, for example, is frequently discussed in relation to older persons' reactions to stressful situations. Strategies such as cognitive behavioral therapy have demonstrated the ability of older persons to modify their coping behaviors or to adopt new coping behaviors that are more effective within the situation.[88–91] By buffering stress, these behaviors can help to prevent negative outcomes such as depression or burden. Outlook or attitude—a mediating factor in the stressful situation—also appears to be a modifiable trait. Programs targeted to outlook have demonstrated not only the ability to change outlook in desired ways, but also to affect outcomes within a broader stress situation.[92–94] The literature extensively discusses the concept of "resilience" or "hardiness." This is more of a pattern of the individual in terms of his or her response to the challenges presented over a lifetime. The concept suggests that resilience can be both strengthened through intervention and eroded by the cumulative effects of repeated stress.[95–98]

A particularly important form of personal resource is encompassed in the concept of self-efficacy belief or mastery.[99] There is a strong association between positive self-efficacy belief and physical function. Strong self-efficacy beliefs appear to contribute to overall physical performance and to the maintenance of good physical function. Weak self-efficacy beliefs are associated with declines in functional status.[100–102] In the more psychosocial realms, strong self-efficacy beliefs appear to buffer the effects of stress on mental health as well as physical health and to contribute to increased productivity (an important component of occupation).[103] In women, strong self-efficacy beliefs are associated with good choice-making, good performance, and persistence of effort.[104] Notably, self-efficacy is more often applied to specific situations than across the entire personality. Thus, a person may be said to have good self-efficacy beliefs about falls prevention or about handling difficult family situations. Especially important is that, as noted above for other personal resources, self-efficacy can be strengthened or improved. Reflection on self-efficacy in one area of living can be supportive of the development and strengthening of self-efficacy in another. Self-efficacy can be modeled as well as reinforced by role models or people who are trusted.

OCCUPATIONS

As noted above, the field has responded to disengagement theory by emphasizing the need for, and value of, continued engagement and productivity in later life.[105] The broadest general expression of this is in the work of Erik and Joan Erickson who added an eighth developmental stage to their theory of adult development. This stage, that of old age, pits Integration against Despair as the dynamic developmental activity of aging.[106] The basic task for the individual is to offer back—to whatever social context he or she defines—the fruits of wisdom. It is especially important that this creative activity is understood to be more than intrapsychic in nature. That is, it is an activity that occurs in the social realm and may therefore be seen as an integral part of social functioning,[107–110] even when age-associated declines in activity occur.[111] Retirement, a tangible life course event, represents an opportunity to change occupation. This is most usually a positive change, but may be negative if it is mandated by bad health or is the result of a substantial fall-off of income.[112,113]

Aside from connectedness with a social network, at least three kinds of other occupations have been studied extensively as a form of engagement. These include leisure-time activities, volunteerism (as well as continued paid post-retirement work), and membership in religious organizations.

LEISURE ACTIVITIES   The nature of the leisure-time activity is less important (from a social gerontological perspective) than is the individual's willingness and ability to pursue leisure-time activity in the face of changing health or other social conditions. Occupation in a leisure activity may be viewed as the continued orientation of the person to engage in play of one form or another. At root this constitutes a form of self-affirmation; the person is asserting that the capacity for and interest in play remains intact throughout the lifespan regardless of rate-limiting factors associated with physical or social condition.[114–116] At a less profound level, it is of particular note that, over the last decade, we have seen greatly increased numbers of opportunities for elderly people to pursue a wide variety of leisure-time activities. Evidence of this is the continued expansion of the elder hostel movement, the emergence of a subset of the travel industry directed toward older adults, and a growing number of community-based opportunities offered through senior centers and the public school community education system.

VOLUNTEER ACTIVITIES   Older people have been and continue to be the backbone of the US volunteer network. The literature indicates that volunteerism increases across the lifespan from young adulthood through middle age. Of particular note, the level of volunteerism remains relatively constant from middle age through older adulthood.[117] The underlying theory is that as persons reach middle age, their skills for volunteerism and the motives and rewards for it are most fully developed. As the person ages, his or her interests and special skills for volunteerism are honed. Finally as the person leaves the workforce either gradually or definitively, he or she is freer to maintain, in a selective fashion, commitments to voluntary organizations. Equally, the expanded free time provides elderly people with the opportunity to change or extend their volunteer commitments.

A subset of older persons remain in the workforce.[118] Some do so for financial reasons, and others do so for other forms of reward and/or to retain either commitment to or influence in their chosen field. Whether it is continued work, continued volunteerism, or some combination of the two, the growing reality for older persons is that there are multiple vehicles by which to remain occupied in the important structures of their community, and a growing number of older adults are exercising these options. From the perspective of social functioning, this is a positive trend.

RELIGIOUS PARTICIPATION   Older adults continue to be the cohort that is most involved with organized religion. This occupation with religion is important for two reasons. First, there is a body of research that suggests a positive association between involvement in religion and overall well-being in old age.[119,120] Second, involvement in organized religion is, in itself, an opportunity for volunteerism. Churches frequently offer their members (or expect) the opportunity to contribute to the community—whether it be the church community or the larger community. Thus, religion can be an important occupation for older people.[121,122]

LIFE EVENTS

Life events are included in the schema of social functioning as an ongoing backdrop for the life of elderly people. These are externalities that can have a significant impact on social functioning. In the case of elders, the archetypal life events involve losses, especially losses that lead to grief, a change in or loss of social roles, and an acquisition of the family caregiving role.

ONSET OF GRIEF   Grief produced by the death or illness of someone within the social network has a number of ramifications.[123] At the simplest level it affects connections by altering or reducing the number and kind of connections available to the person. The grief event creates a demand on personal resources. People experiencing grief employ coping mechanisms to manage it.[124] They draw down on their reserves of resilience to recover from the loss. Their outlook on life in general and on their own personal life may be challenged by the grief event. Particularly in the death of a spouse or confidant, the person may be called upon to re-engineer his or her social networks and to acquire new skills for negotiating not only the network but also the social world (for example, a widowed spouse may need to learn housekeeping skills he had not been called upon to use before). A grief event may also affect status, especially in women.[125] A woman dependent upon her husband's pension and social security may suffer a loss of income as a result of the death of that husband. She will also find herself in a different (and less advantaged) social stratum—namely that of a single older woman. Equally, a grief event may affect occupation in that opportunities to participate in voluntary organizations and volunteerism may be affected by the loss of a close relative or friend upon whom one depended for psychological support and encouragement or for more instrumental help such as transportation.[126]

CHANGING SOCIAL ROLES   A less specific kind of loss event typically entails the loss of social roles. This frequently occurs in retirement, but also might occur through the cessation of voluntary or membership activities—possibly produced by health-related events.[127,128] One key loss, the cessation of driving, can have substantial effects on social functioning.[129]

In the course of development, a person may find that he or she is making less of a contribution (or has a perception of making less of a contribution), having left the workforce or having been forced to leave occupations that the individual defined as contributing to the greater social good. Role losses have implications for social connectedness. Well-established patterns of friendship can be rapidly and irreversibly severed, causing an overall deterioration in the network and/or forcing a redefinition and recreation of a network.

Losses affect personal resources in a number of ways. A person's self-appraisal is affected by how the individual sees himself or herself in terms of various occupations. Because of the readjustment a person is often called upon to make, the reserves of resilience are drawn upon. Depending on the nature of the loss, a person's overall outlook on life can be challenged even to the point where his or her evaluation of life itself is diminished.

ACQUISITION OF THE CAREGIVING ROLE   More than 24 million Americans are involved in providing care to relatives who are affected with chronic diseases.[130] A substantial proportion of these carers are older adults. Such caregiving is not only prevalent, but is also often a longlasting occupation. As such, caregiving is well understood to affect the other domains of social functioning and to affect social functioning directly. The nature of the illness affecting the care recipient (and, accordingly, the nature and extent of caregiving) can jeopardize social connectedness, often disrupting normal patterns of friendship and weakening connections to acquaintances. Interaction closer inside the social network, particularly with family members, is often complicated by the illness and the attendant caregiving, producing new or exacerbating existing tensions. Caregiving can occupy many hours of the day, and there are frequent reports of caregivers withdrawing from voluntary and membership activities as a result. The impact on family caregivers themselves has been exceptionally well documented. Such persons are at multiple jeopardy for physical, psychological, social, economic, and familial problems.[131–134]

SUMMARY ON SOCIAL GERONTOLOGY

The effort of this chapter has been to portray and discuss major factors in the social reality of elderly people that affect their functioning in the world. The effort has been two-fold. First, there has been an effort to point out the power of individual factors or elements in promoting or deterring maximal social functioning. Whether one focuses on the presence of a confidant, the accumulated effects of race or poverty, or the acquisition or strengthening of self-efficacy, individual aspects of psychosocial functioning can be seen to operate powerfully to affect social functioning. At the same time the chapter draws attention to the interrelatedness, not only of the main factors of social gerontology, but also of these factors to domains more typically associated with geriatrics. Thus, whether one focuses on the reinforcement for positive health behaviors that can be provided by social networks, or the barriers to healthy lifestyle opportunities created by rural life, or the benefits to health of continued sense of creativity, one is continually reminded of the interplay of social and health factors affecting overall functioning of the aging individual.

CLINICAL NUANCES OF SOCIAL GERONTOLOGY

Geriatricians and other practicing clinicians seldom have time or opportunity to assess the social functioning of those who come under their care. As even this brief chapter indicates, the issues affecting social functioning are multifactorial, interrelated, and complex. However, as also indicated in the chapter, social functioning and physical functioning impinge upon one another. In consequence, clinicians will want to have at least a broad sense of the way in which psychosocial factors might come into play in the overall well-being of patients. Table 17-1 is offered as a mechanism for clinicians to quickly scan the social situation of a patient in order to generate an impression about the degree to which the person has psychosocial assets or liabilities. The table is structured by the mnemonic SCORE. The first column of the table recalls the major subheadings of this chapter. The second column recapitulates the main points of each of these subheadings. The assessment is not meant to yield a single "score." Rather, it is meant to provide clinicians with a checklist they may use to tally factors that may be working on behalf of, or contrary to, the overall well-being of the person. Some of the elements are immutable—this is true to virtually all of the status variables. In this case, the physician can at least get a sense of whether the direction of status is a benefit or a deficit for the individual. For example, a very old

Table 17-1 Factors to assess in the area of social functioning

Domain	Key areas of interest
Status	Age Economic condition: income/education Gender Race/ethnicity Living situation (access to services; housing situation)
Connections	Kind (spouse, kin, friends) Quality of relationship(s) Presence of a confidant Network size Connectedness (sense of belonging vs sense of isolation)
Occupations	Activities (work, volunteering, religion, other) Appraisal (how engaged/disengaged?)
Resources (personal)	Mastery (self-appraisal for managing life events) Coping style (how manages current situations) Outlook (how values life) Resilience/hardiness (how affected by life events) Personality (confident, dependent, neurotic)
Events	Caregiving (taking care of a member of the family?) Grief (recent experience of grief related to member of network) Loss (loss of social role or capability)

woman from a minority racial group living in poverty in an inner city will present a different set of challenges from that facing a recently retired well-to-do non-Hispanic Caucasian male living in the suburbs. The two situations are not equal. The older woman does face more challenges, and promoting well-being for her will be at least a more complicated if not more difficult task. The clinician should be aware of this.

Other of the factors are more mutable. Knowing about the kind and quality of connections and whether or not a person has a confidant can lead the clinician to make suggestions, and more importantly make referrals. A family or marriage therapist might be considered for older couples or older individuals who are having difficulty in their relationships or find themselves without a confidant. As noted above, a number of the personal resource factors are malleable. The sense of mastery and the choice of coping styles can be improved through various types of therapy, including psychoeducation and cognitive behavioral therapy. Thus the clinician noting an ineffective coping style or observing a person being overwhelmed by a situation ought to consider referral to a patient educator, a psychologist, a social worker, or other mental health specialist. Certainly the category of occupation lends itself to change. Recognizing the value of engagement, a clinician can offer advice or suggestions to become even more engaged and can refer patients who seem disengaged or isolated to a social worker or even a senior center and certainly to a religious figure (where religion enters the picture). Finally, life events clearly have a major impact on older persons and ought to be assessed. Each of the kinds of life events may require different types of care and different sorts of referrals, but a clinician ought to be aware of these and keep them in mind.

In sum, the SCORE sheet is meant to provide clinicians with an easy way to recall the many factors of social gerontology that affect the overall well-being of elderly people. It is not meant to be used in a quantified way. There is a sense that even a cursory examination of the factors can indicate whether a person has either a profound deficit or an accumulation of deficits that should be attended to, or conversely whether a person has assets that can be used in the development and implementation of a longer treatment plan.

KEY POINTS   Social gerontology

■ Physical and social factors interact in complex ways to affect overall functioning in elderly people.

■ Social status (including race, gender, income, education, and location), social connectedness, psychological characteristics, life events, and social involvement interact in complex ways to contribute to—or detract from—optimal social functioning.

■ Clinicians can keep the importance of such factors in mind, incorporate these factors in their overall assessment of older patients, and, as appropriate, make referrals to other clinicians for attention to psychosocial issues.

REFERENCES

1. Kincade-Norburn JE, Bernard SL, Konrad TR et al: Self-care and assistance from others in coping with functional status limitations among a national sample of older adults. J Gerontol B 1995;50:S101–S109

2. Mendes de Leon CF, Seeman TE, Baker DI et al: Self-efficacy, physical decline, and change in functioning in community-living elders: a prospective study. J Gerontol B 1996;51:S183–S190

3. Penninx BWJH, van Tilburg T, Boeke AJP et al: Effects of social support and personal coping resources on depressive symptoms: different for various chronic diseases? Health Psychol 1998;17:551–558

4. Rowe JW, Kahn RL: Successful aging. Gerontologist 1997;37:433–440

5. Kubansky LD, Berkman LF, Glass TA et al: Is educational attainment associated with shared determinants of health in the elderly? Findings from the MacArthur Studies of Successful Aging. Psychosom Med 1998;60:578–585

6. House JS, Lepkowski JM, Kinney Am et al: The social stratification of aging and health. J Health Soc Behav 1994;35:213–234

7. Crimmins EM, Hayward MD, Saito Y: Differentials in active life expectancy in the older population of the United States. J Gerontol B 1996;51:S111–S120.

8. Cairney J, Arnold R: Social class, health and aging: socio-economic determinants of self-reported morbidity among the noninstitutionalized elderly in Canada. Can J Pub Health 1996;87:199–203

9. Ross CE, Mirowsky J: Refining the association between education and health: the effects of quantity, credential, and selectivity. Demography 1999;36:445–460

10. Zorn CR, Johnson MT: Religious well-being in noninstitutionalized elderly women. Health Care Wom Int 1997;18:209–219

11. Hungerford TL: The economic consequences of widowhood on elderly women in the United States and Germany. Gerontologist 2001;41:103–110

12. Klesges LM, Pahor M, Shorr RI et al: Financial difficulty in acquiring food among elderly disabled women: results from the women's health and aging study. Am J Pub Health 2001;91:68–75

13. Richardson VE: Women and retirement. J Wom Aging 1999;11(2–3):49–66

14. Lee GR, DeMaris A, Bavin S et al: Gender differences in the depressive effect of widowhood in later life. J Gerontol B 2001;56:S56–S61

15. Achenbaum WA, Bengtson VL: Re-engaging the disengagement theory of aging: on the history and assessment of theory development in gerontology. Gerontologist 1994;34:756–763

16. Fitting M, Rabins P, Lucas MJ et al: Caregivers for dementia patients: a comparison of husbands and wives. Gerontologist 1986;26:248–252

17. Pruchno RA, Resch NL: Husbands and wives as caregivers: antecedents of depression and burden. Gerontologist 1989;29:159–165

18. Palo Stoller E, Cutler SJ: The impact of gender on configurations of care among married elderly couples. Res Aging 1992;14:313–330

19. Sparks MB, Farran CJ, Donner E et al: Wives, husbands, and daughters of dementia patients: predictors of caregivers' mental and physical health. Sch Inq Nurs Pract 1998;12:221–234

20. O'Brien Cousins S: "My heart couldn't take it": older women's beliefs about exercise benefits and risks. J Gerontol B 2000;55:P283–P294

21. Johnson FL, Foxall MJ, Kelleher E et al: Comparison of mental health and life satisfaction of five elderly ethnic groups. West J Nurs Res 1988;10:613–628

22. Hopper SV: The influence of ethnicity on the health of older women. Clin Geriatr Med 1993;9:231–259

23. Bassford TL: Health status of Hispanic elders [review]. Clin Geriatr Med 1995;11:25–38

24. Blackhall LJ, Murphy ST, Frank G et al: Ethnicity and attitudes toward patient autonomy. JAMA 1995;274:820–825

25. Ventres W, Nichter M, Reed R et al: Limitation of medical care: an ethnographic analysis. J Clin Ethics 1993;4:134–142

26. Espino DV, Lichtenstein MJ, Hazuda HP et al: Correlates of prescription and over-the-counter medication usage among older Mexican Americans: the Hispanic EPESE study. J Am Geriatr Soc 1998;46:1228–1234

27. Hopp FP, Duffy SA: Racial variations in end-of-life care. J Am Geriatr Soc 2000;48:658–663

28. Miller B, Campbell RT, Farran CJ et al: Race, control, mastery, and caregiver distress. J Gerontol B 1995;50:S374–S382

29. Cox C, Monk A. Strain among caregivers: comparing the experiences of African American and Hispanic caregivers of Alzheimer's relatives. Int J Aging Hum Dev 1996;43:93–105

30. Segall M, Wykle M: The black family's experience with dementia. J Appl Soc Sci 1988;13:170–191

31. Caralis PV, Davis B, Wright K, Marcial E: The influence of ethnicity and race on attitudes toward advance directives, life-prolonging treatments, and euthanasia. J Clin Ethics 1993;4:155–165

32. Perkins HS, Supik JD, Hazuda HP: Autopsy decisions: the possibility of conflicting cultural attitudes. J Clin Ethics 1993;4:145–154

33. Carrese JA, Rhodes LA: Western bioethics on the Navajo reservation. JAMA 1998;274:826–829

34. Versen GR: Native American elderly formal and informal support systems. J Soc Work Soc Welf 1981;8:513–528

35. McLaughlin DK: Rural women's economic realities [review]. J Wom Aging 1998;10(4):41–65

36. Elreedy S, Krieger N, Ryan PB et al: Relations between individual and neighborhood-based measures of socio-economic position and bone lead concentrations among community-exposed men: the normative aging study. Am J Epidemiol 1999;150:129–141

37. Snustad DG, Thompson-Heisterman AA, Neese JB et al: Mental Health Outreach to Rural Elderly: Service Delivery to a Forgotten Risk Group. Clin Gerontol 1993:95–111

38. Silveira JM, Winstead-Fry P: The needs of patients with cancer and their caregivers in rural areas. Oncol Nurs For 1997;24:71–76

39. Glasser M: Alzheimer's disease and dementing disorders: practices and experiences of rural physicians. Am J Alzheimer's Care Rel Dis Res 1993;July/August:28–35

40. Sonnenberg FA: Health information on the Internet. Arch Intern Med 1997;157:151–152

41. Wright LK, Bennet G, Gramling L: Telecommunication interventions for caregivers of elders with dementia. Adv Nurs Sci 1998;20(3):76–88

42. Mookherjee HN: Perceptions of well-being among the older metropolitan and nonmetropolitan populations in the United States. J Soc Psychol 1998;138:72–82

43. Brown V: The effects of poverty environments on elders' subjective well-being: a conceptual model [review]. Gerontologist 1995;35:541–548

44. Lev EL, Paul D, Owen SV: Age, self-efficacy, and change in patients' adjustment to cancer. Cancer Pract 1999;7(4):170–176

45. King KM, Koop PM: The influence of the cardiac surgery patient's sex and age on caregiving received. Soc Sci Med 1999;48:1735–1742

46. Martire LM, Schulz R, Mittelmark MB et al: Stability and change in older adults' social contact and social support: the Cardiovascular Health Study. J Gerontol B 1999;54:S302–S311

47. Ajrouch KJ, Antonucci TC, Janevic MR: Social networks among blacks and whites: the interaction between race and age. J Gerontol B 2001;56:S112–S118

48. Shaw BA, Krause N: Exploring race variations in aging and personal control. J Gerontol B 2001;56:S119–S124

49. Wenger GC: Social networks and the prediction of elderly people at risk. Aging Ment Health 1997;1:311–320

50. Page RM, Cole GE: Demoralization and living alone: outcome from an urban community study. Psychol Rep 1992;70:275–280

51. LaVeist TA, Sellers RM, Brown KA et al: Extreme social isolation, use of community-based senior support services, and mortality among African American elderly women. Am J Commun Psychol 1997;25:721–732

52. Cumming E, Henry WE: Growing Old. Basic Books, New York, 1961

53. Maddox GL: Disengagement theory. Gerontologist 1964;4:80–82,103

54. O'Reilly P, Caro FG: Productive aging: an overview of the literature [review]. J Aging Soc Policy 1994;6(3):39–71

55. Moen P: A life course perspective on retirement, gender, and well-being [review]. J Occup Health Psychol 1996;1(2):131–144

56. Stevens ES: Making sense of usefulness: an avenue toward satisfaction in later life. Int J Aging Hum Dev 1993;37:313–325

57. Seeman TE: Social ties and health. Ann Epidemiol 1996;6:442–451

58. Newsom TT, Schulz R: Social support as a mediator in the relation between functional status and quality of life in older adults. Psychol Aging 1996;11(1):34–44

59. Strawbridge WJ, Cohen RD, Shema SJ et al: Successful aging: predictors and associated activities. Am J Epidemiol 1996;144:135–141

60. Guralnik JM, Kaplan GA. Predictors of healthy aging: prospective evidence from the Alameda County Study. Am J Pub Health 1989;79:703–708

61. Mendes de Leon CF, Glass TA, Beckett LA et al: Social networks and disability transitions across eight intervals of yearly data in the New Haven EPESE. J Gerontol B 1999;54:S162–S172

62. Fisher L, Lieberman MA: The effects of family context on adult offspring of patients with Alzheimer's disease: a longitudinal study. J Fam Psychol 1996;10:180–191

63. Davies B, Reimer JC, Martens N: Family functioning and its implications for palliative care. J Palliat Care 1994;10(1):29–36

64. Blanchard CG, Albrecht TL, Ruckdeschel JC et al: The role of social support in adaptation to cancer and to survival. J Psychosoc Oncol 1995;13:7–95

65. Unger JB, McAvay G, Bruce ML et al: Variation in the impact of social network characteristics on physical functioning in elderly persons: MacArthur Studies of Successful Aging. J Gerontol B 1999;54:S245–S251

66. Bloom JR: The relationship of social support and health. Soc Sci Med 1990;30:635–637

67. Seeman TE, Charpentier PA, Berkman LF et al: Predicting changes in physical performance in a high-functioning elderly cohort: MacArthur Studies of Successful Aging. J Gerontol A 1994;49:M97–M108

68. Kincade-Norburn JE, Bernard SL, Konrad TR et al: Self-care and assistance from others in coping with functional status limitations among a national sample of older adults. J Gerontol B 1995;50:S101–S109

69. Hagerty BM, Williams RA: The effects of sense of belonging, social support, conflict, and loneliness on depression. Nurs Res 1999;48:215–219

70. Thompson MG, Heller K: Facets of support related to well-being: quantitative social isolation and perceived family support in a sample of elderly women. Psychol Aging 1990;5:535–544

71. Berkman LF: The role of social relations in health promotion. Psychosom Med 1995;57:245–254

72. Doeglas D, Suurmeijer T, Krol B et al: Social support, social disability, and psychological well-being in rheumatoid arthritis. Arthritis Care Res 1994;7(1):10–15

73. Lawrence RH, Tennstedt SL, Assmann SF: Quality of the caregiver–care recipient relationship: does it offset negative consequences of caregiving for family caregivers? Psychol Aging 1998;13:150–158

74. Kramer BJ: Marital history and the prior relationship as predictors of positive and negative outcomes among wife caregivers. Fam Relat 1993;42:367–375

75. Giese-Davis J, Hermanson K, Koopman C et al: Quality of couples' relationship and adjustment to metastatic breast cancer. J Fam Psychol 2000;14:251–266

76. Williamson GM, Schulz R: Relationship orientation, quality of prior relationship, and distress among caregivers of Alzheimer's patients. Psychol Aging 1990;5:502–509

77. Mullins LC, Mushel M, Cook C et al: The complexity of interpersonal relationships among older persons: an examination of selected emotionally close relationships. J Gerontol Soc Work 1994;22(1–2):109–130

78. Wu Z, Pollard MS: Social support among unmarried childless elderly persons. J Gerontol B 1998;53:S324–S335

79. Tijhuis MAR, DeJong-Gierveld J, Feskens EJM et al: Changes in and factors related to loneliness in older men: the Zutphen elderly study. Age Ageing 1999;28:491–495

80. Reinhardt JP: The importance of friendship and family support in adaptation to chronic vision impairment. J Gerontol B 1996;51:P268–P278

81. Potts MK: Social support and depression among older adults living alone: the importance of friends within and outside of a retirement community. Soc Work 1997;42:348–362

82. Hanson BS, Isacsson SO, Janzon L, Lindell SE: Social network and social support influence mortality in elderly men. The prospective population study of "Men born in 1914" Malmo, Sweden. Am J Epidemiol 1989;130:100–111

83. McCrae RR, Costa PT: Personality, coping, and coping effectiveness in an adult sample. J Pers 1986;54:385–405

84. Hooker K, Monahan DJ, Bowman SR et al: Personality counts for a lot: predictors of mental and physical health of spouse caregivers in two disease groups. J Gerontol B 1998;53:P73–P85

85. Reis MF, Andres D, Gold DP et al: Personality traits as determinants of burden and health complaints in caregiving. Int J Aging Hum Dev 1994;39:257–271

86. Pearlin LI, Schooler C: The structure of coping. J Health Soc Behav 1978;19:2–21

87. Lucke KT: Knowledge acquisition and decision-making: spinal cord injured individuals' perceptions of caring during rehabilitation. Sci Nurs 1997;14(3):87–95

88. Halford WK, Harrison C, Kalyansundaram et al: Preliminary results from a psychoeducational program to rehabilitate chronic patients. Psychiatr Serv 1995;46:1189–1191

89. Whitlatch CJ, Zarit SH, Goodwin PE et al: Influence of the success of psychoeducational interventions on the course of family care. Clin Gerontol 1995;16(1):17–30

90. Lazarus RS, Folkman S: Coping and adaptation. In Gentry WD (ed): The Handbook of Behavioral Medicine. Guilford, New York, 1984:282–325

91. Billings AG, Moos RH: The role of coping responses and social resources in attenuating the stress of life events. J Behav Med 1981;4:139–157

92. Hepburn K, Tornatore J, Center B et al: Dementia family care training: affecting beliefs about caregiving and caregiver outcomes. J Am Geriatr Soc 2001;49:450–457

93. Mittelman MS, Ferris SH, Shulman E et al: Family intervention to delay nursing home placement of patients with Alzheimer's disease. JAMA 1996;276:1725–1756

94. Shifren K, Hooker K: Stability and change in optimism: a study among spouse caregivers. Exp Aging Res 1995;21:59–76

95. Gallagher TJ, Wagenfeld MO, Baro F et al: Sense of coherence, coping and caregiver role overload. Soc Sci Med 1994;39:1615–1622

96. Intrieri RC, Rapp SR: Self-control skillfulness and caregiver burden among help seeking elders. J Gerontol B 1994;49:P19–P23

97. Lutzky SM, Knight BG: Explaining gender differences in caregiver distress: the roles of emotional attentiveness and coping styles. Psychol Aging 1994;9:513–519

98. Johansson I, Larsson G, Hamrin E: Sense of coherence, quality of life, and function among elderly hip fracture patients. Aging (Milano) 1998;10:377–384

99. Bandura A: Self-efficacy mechanism in human agency. Am Psychol 1982;37:122–147

100. Seeman TE, Unger JB, McAvay G et al: Self-efficacy beliefs and perceived declines in functional ability: MacArthur studies of successful aging. J Gerontol B 1999;54:P214–P222

101. Clark NM, Dodge JA: Exploring self-efficacy as a predictor of disease management. Health Educ Behav 1999;26:72–89

102. Smarr KL, Parker JC, Wright GE et al: The importance of enhancing self-efficacy in rheumatoid arthritis. Arthritis Care Res 1997;10(1):18–25

103. Gignac MAM, Gottlieb BH: Caregivers' appraisals of efficacy in coping with dementia. Psychol Aging 1996;11:214–225

104. Toobert DJ, Glasgow RE, Nettekoven LA, Brown JE: Behavioral and psychosocial effects of intensive lifestyle management for women with coronary heart disease. Patient Educ Couns 1998;35:177–188

105. Fisher BJ: Successful aging, life satisfaction, and generativity in later life. Int J Aging Hum Dev 1995;41:239–250

106. Erikson EH, Erikson JM, Kivnick HQ: Vital involvement in old age. W.W. Norton, New York, 1986

107. Lawton MP, Moss M, Hoffman C et al: Health, valuation of life, and the wish to live. Gerontologist 1999;39:409–416

108. Harlow RE, Cantor N: Still participating after all these years: a study of life task participation in later life. J Pers Soc Psychol 1996;71:1235–1249

109. Ardelt M: Wisdom and life satisfaction in old age. J Gerontol B 1997;52:P15–P27

110. Clark F, Azen SP, Zemke R et al: Occupational therapy for independent-living older adults: a randomized controlled trial. JAMA 1997;278:1321–1326

111. Herzog AR, Kahn RL, Morgan JN et al: Age differences in productive activities. J Gerontol B 1989;44:S129–S138

112. Mutchler JE, Burr JA, Massagli MP et al: Work transitions and health in later life. J Gerontol 1999;54:S252–S261

113. Quick HE, Moen P: Gender, employment, and retirement quality: a life course approach to the differential experiences of men and women. J Occup Health Psychol 1998;3:44–64

114. McGuinn KK, Mosher-Ashley PM: Participation in recreational activities and its effect on perception of life satisfaction in residential settings. Activ Adapt Aging 2000;25(1):77–86

115. Everard KM, Lach HW, Fisher EB et al: Relationship of activity and social support to the functional health of older adults. J Gerontol B 2000;55:S208–S212

116. Hugman R: Ageing, occupation and social engagement: towards a lively later life. J Occup Sci 1999;6(2):61–67

117. Cutler SJ, Hendricks J: Age differences in voluntary association memberships: fact or artifact. J Gerontol B 2000;55:S98–S107

118. Parnes HS, Sommers DG: Shunning retirement: work experience of men in their seventies and early eighties. J Gerontol B 1994;49:S117–S124

119. Krause N, Ingersoll-Dayton B, Ellison CG et al: Aging, religious doubt, and psychological well-being. Gerontologist 1999;39:525–533

120. Krause N: Neighborhood deterioration, religious coping, and changes in health during late life. Gerontologist 1998;38:653–664

121. Fry PS: Religious involvement, spirituality and personal meaning for life: existential predictors of psychological wellbeing in community-residing and institutional care elders. Aging Ment Health 2000;4:375–387

122. Ayele H, Mulligan T, Gheorghiu S et al: Religious activity improves life satisfaction for some physicians and older patients. J Am Geriatr Soc 1999;47:453–455

123. Thompson LW, Gallagher-Thompson D, Futterman A et al: The effects of late-life spousal bereavement over a 30-month interval. Psychol Aging 1991;6:434–441

124. Lee GR, DeMaris A, Bavin S et al: Gender differences in the depressive effect of widowhood in later life. J Gerontol B 2001;56:S56–S61

125. Gonyea JG: The paradox of the advantaged elder and the feminization of poverty [review]. Soc Work 1994;39:35–41

126. Zautra AJ, Reich JW, Guarnaccia CA: Some everyday life consequences of disability and bereavement for older adults. J Pers Soc Psychol 1990;59:550–561

127. Ross CE, Drentea P: Consequences of retirement activities for distress and the sense of personal control. J Health Soc Behav 1998;39:317–334

128. Adelmann PK: Multiple roles and psychological well-being in a national sample of older adults. J Gerontol B 1994;49:S277–S285

129. Marottoli RA, de Leon CFM, Glass TA et al: Consequences of driving cessation: decreased out-of-home activity levels. J Gerontol B 2000;55:S334–S340

130. National Alliance for Caregiving, American Association of Retired Persons: Family Caregiving in the United States: Findings from a National Survey—Final Report. National Alliance for Caregiving, Bethesda, MA, 1997 (abstract).

131. Schulz R, Beach SR: Caregiving as a risk factor for mortality: The caregiver health effects study. JAMA 1999;282:2215–2219

132. Mui AC: Perceived health and functional status among spouse caregivers of frail older persons. J Aging Health 1995;7:283–300

133. Ory MG, Hoffman RR, Yee JL et al: Prevalence and impact of caregiving: a detailed comparison between dementia and nondementia caregivers. Gerontologist 1999;39:177–185

134. Schulz R, Newsom J, Mittelmark M et al: Health effects of caregiving: the caregiver health effects study: an ancillary study of the cardiovascular health study. Ann Behav Med 1997;19:110–116

Chapter 18

Productive aging

Robert N. Butler, Charlotte Muller, and Judith Estrine

Productive aging is defined as the capacity of an individual or population to serve in the paid workforce and in volunteer activities, to assist in the family, and to maintain, to varying degrees, autonomy and independence for as long as possible. The concept was created primarily in response to stereotyped depictions of older persons as dependent and a burden to society. It served to draw attention to the fact that productivity does not stop when a person grows older, and that the older population is being underutilized by society. It reflected both the need for older persons to work longer in an older society, and the persistence and universality of prejudice against them in the workplace.[1] The concept of productive aging was also a reaction to the tendency of economists to omit the voluntary activities and informal contributions made by older adults when measuring a nation's gross domestic product (GDP).

The extent to which an older person can remain productive is determined by a variety of personal factors, including physical and emotional well-being, motivation, attitude, education, and experience, as well as by changing technologies and societal attitudes and structures. The interplay between personal issues and societal norms has an important influence on both paid and unpaid productive activities. Confirming the landmark study by the National Institute of Mental Health of healthy community-resident aged men conducted in the 1950s and 60s, the MacArthur Study of Successful Aging in America found that engagement in meaningful activities contributes to good health, satisfaction with life, and longevity, as well as providing a potentially effective means of reducing costs of physical and emotional illness in later life. Older persons who have goals and structure are more likely to live longer than people who lack motivation and purpose.

Paid work includes remunerative self-employment as well as work for others. For older employees, the central issue regarding participation in paid work is retirement. Many factors influence an individual's decision to retire, including health, economic status, the quality of the work environment, the structure of social security and private pension plans, the availability of part-time work and/or flexibility of work hours, and age discrimination. Other significant factors are education, marital status, and a spouse's labor force participation. Race and gender may also influence a person's decision to retire.[2]

DEMOGRAPHY

Infant mortality has declined dramatically, and at the same time as the birth rate drops, there is also an unprecedented reduction in maternal, childhood, and late-life mortality and morbidity rates. Population projections from the Social Security Administration show a decline in the working-age population (20–64) per capita after 2010.[3] In 1950, the ratio of US citizens aged 20–64 to those aged 65 and above was 16.5 to 1. In 2001, it was 3.3 to 1. By 2030, it will decline further to 2 to 1.[4]

Viewed another way, the world's population is growing at an annual rate of 1.7 percent, but the population over 65 increases by 2.5 percent per year.[5] In the USA, workers aged 55–64 have become the fastest-growing segment of the workforce.[6] Most developing countries as well are aging rapidly. In Latin America and most of Asia, the number of people over 60 will double by 2030, to 14 percent of the population. In China, that number will rise to 22 percent.

In Europe, projections indicate that by 2050 retirees will outnumber workers, and some fear that nations will be unable to finance their public pension systems. There is concern that if older workers retire in large numbers, sometime after 2010 there will be fewer workers to support more retirees, with the consequent reduction of growth in material standards of living among many European nations. These fears stem, in part, from the inappropriate interpretation of the dependency ratio, which, broadly applied, compares the number of dependents in a population (children plus persons 65 and older) to the population of younger adults. Moreover, the cost of raising a child to age 18 is estimated conservatively at $200,000 ($300,000 if the child goes on to college). Furthermore, given that not everyone between the ages of 18 and 64 is working, that fewer children are being born, and that many people over 65 are economically independent through continuing employment, savings, private pensions and social security based on contributions they have made to society over the course of many years, a more accurate measure of dependency would compare the economically dependent population with the population that is economically active.[7] The social and household cost of maintaining nonworkers is clearly not only due to retirees.

Thanks to the technology revolution, productivity is a more important measure of a nation's economic well-being than the size of its workforce. For example, food is far more plentiful now than it was a century ago, even though 37 percent of Americans in 1900 were engaged in agriculture compared with 2 percent today. As productivity grows in a variety of industries there will be less need for workers of any age to maintain present output, and the continuing low birth rates in the industrialized world will not pose significant problems.

It has been suggested that if it were possible to maintain a constant number of years in retirement, rather than automatically leaving the workforce after completing a constant number of years in paid employment, labor-force participation rates of older workers would increase. Thus, the reduced growth in labor supply would not by itself cause living standards to be lower than they were in 1997.

RETIREMENT

Juanita M. Kreps noted in 1977 that retirement was a relatively new life stage, and that it was quickly becoming a device for balancing the numbers of job seekers with the demand for workers.[8] And in the 1950s, social gerontologists Eugene Friedmann and Robert Havighurst wrote: "retirement is not a rich man's luxury or an ill man's misfortune. It is increasingly the common lot of all kinds of people. Some find it a blessing; others, a curse. But it comes anyway, whether blessing or curse, and it comes often in an arbitrary manner, at a set age, without direct reference to the productivity or the interest of the individual in his work."[9]

Prior to the industrial revolution, people worked until they died and retirement was virtually unknown. Following industrialization, in 1889, Germany's Chancellor Otto Von Bismarck established the first national contributory pension program in the modern era. At the turn of the twentieth century, the rise of labor unions in industrialized countries created worker protection that included retirement benefits. During most of the twentieth century, early retirement was an important labor market tool, serving to balance the number of people looking for jobs with the demand for workers and, in particular, supporting the careers of younger workers. Between 1910 and 1998/99, there was a drop of 1.2 years per decade in the age at which men retired from paid employment, so that the average male retirement age fell from 74 years to 63. Since male life expectancy has increased about 0.8 years per decade in the same period as the retirement age fell, late twentieth-century workers have spent an increasingly significant portion of their lives in retirement. It is estimated that, for many, retirement will last longer than their lives from birth until their entrance into the workforce.[10] Having said that, it must be noted that a trend toward later retirement appears to be developing, with baby-boomers indicating their intention to work beyond the age of 65.

In today's labor market, demographic trends that include a longer life expectancy and fewer younger people entering the workforce are at odds with benefit programs inherited from an era that provided incentives for early retirement for older workers. Traditional defined benefit pensions still in force include provisions that often discourage people from working past a certain age. For example, pensions are denied some workers who wish to remain on their jobs in a part-time capacity after formal retirement, and employers' concerns about legal or tax ramifications can also work against flexible work options. There is a shift away from defined benefit pensions to defined contributions, and therefore this problem is diminishing. This can favor staying on the job with less expense to the employer. It also permits workers to take pensions with them if they move from job to job, which contributes to continuing productive aging.

Retirement trends vary between nations owing to differences in the overall job markets; and in countries with higher unemployment, financial disincentives are still used to discourage the continued employment of older workers.[11] A 1998 study of 24 OPEC countries showed that in 1950 the average retirement age was 65 or higher, but by 1995 there was a drop to age 62 in many of these nations. The decrease in the average retirement age of women has been even faster.[12]

In the 1950s, the USA was placed in the middle of countries surveyed for retirement ages, but by 1995 it had one of the highest, with only Iceland, Japan, Norway, and Switzerland having a higher male retirement age, and Iceland, Japan, Norway, Sweden, and Turkey having a higher female retirement age (Table 18-1).

In the USA, social security is the main source of cash income of households headed by an individual aged 65 or older. It provides slightly more than 40 percent of the total cash income received by this population. Social security replaces about 42 percent of the final wages earned by a fully employed single worker who earns the average wage and begins collecting at 65, and 63 percent of the final wages of a worker with a nonworking dependent spouse. Until recently, a retirement means test was used to prevent older workers who collected social

Table 18-1 Statutory age for normal retirement and workforce participation rates for selected countries, 2000

Country	Women aged 65+ as % of all women	Statutory age of normal retirement		Workforce participation rate (%) by age group					
		Men	Women	Men			Women		
				55–59	60–64	65+	55–59	60–64	65+
Developed countries									
Italy	20.9	64	59	64.5	31.9	6.6	21.1	9.3	1.8
Germany	19.8	63	63	74.5	29.8	3.9	42.8	8.9	1.3
Sweden	19.8	65	65	85.6	60.0	6.6	80.4	52.9	2.5
Belgium	19.5	65	61	46.3	15.7	1.7	17.1	3.3	0.4
Japan	19.4	60	60	93.6	72.1	33.4	55.2	38.0	14.4
Developing countries[a]									
Latvia	18.0	60	57	85.3	52.7	20.4	49.9	33.2	11.1
Hungary	17.7	60	57	59.1	3.3	0.9	4.8	1.5	0.2
Ukraine	17.7	60	55	76.8	27.9	9.3	28.2	13.2	3.4
Estonia	17.3	62.5	57.5	85.2	48.6	23.8	52.4	34.0	14.1
Belarus	17.1	60	55	84.7	37.7	11.6	33.2	18.3	4.3

[a]*The five developed countries were selected because they have the highest percent of women aged 65+ of all women. The same criterion was used for the developing countries.*

Sources: (1) Social Security Programs Throughout the World. Social Security Administration, Office of Policy, Office of Research, Evaluation and Statistics. Washington, DC, 1999. (2) World Population Prospects: The 1998 Revision. United Nations, New York, 1999. (3) Year Book of Labour Statistics, various issues, 1990–2000. International Labour Office, Geneva.

security from continuing to earn more than a certain amount annually in paid employment. Workers aged between 65 and 69 lost $1 in benefits for every $3 they earned in excess of $17,000. In 2000, the Senior Citizens' Freedom to Work Act eliminated earnings penalties of social security recipients aged 65 and older, allowing potential retirees to receive full benefits regardless of earnings. As a result, the number of older persons who rejoin the workforce on a part-time, seasonal, or full-time basis is expected to rise, adding substantially to the gross domestic product by 2008. However, the new law does not apply to workers aged 62–65. Furthermore, for every $2 in annual earnings in excess of the designated limit ($10,800), a worker between 62 and 65 loses $1 in annual benefits.

Another step which might promote productive aging was passed by the US Congress in 1983, with implementation beginning in 2003. The age at which retirees can claim full social security benefits in the USA will gradually increase from 65, reaching 67 by 2027. Recommendations have been made to raise the retirement age to 70 by 2029 and as needed after that, in accordance with further increases in life expectancy. Many OECD nations are also gradually increasing the age at which workers become eligible for retirement benefits. Incentives are being considered to encourage people to delay retirement benefits or continue working while they receive benefits. For example, the UK has equalized retirement ages for men and women by raising the retirement age for women.

Increasing the average age of full pension entitlement and removing pension earnings rules and penalties for working past a certain age would allow healthy people to continue paid employment while increasing the length of time during which contributions are made to pension funds. However, it must be noted that at the same time as these changes extend years of salaried employment, they represent a cut in benefits to the beneficiary. Protection must also be made available to those unable to work for health reasons.

PAID EMPLOYMENT

Complete retirement is much less prevalent among older US citizens than is commonly believed. At least 50 percent of all workers "partially retire" by taking part-time jobs toward the end of their working lives, and the chance that an individual will re-enter the labor force after initial retirement is about one in four. Older workers employed in nontraditional paid work arrangements include independent contractors, on-call and temporary workers, and those engaged in home-based work, part-time work, and post-career bridge jobs. In 2000, only about 13 percent of older Americans worked; but a recent survey conducted by the AARP (formerly the American Association for Retired Persons) found that about 80 percent of baby-boomers plan to continue working after retirement, 35 percent at least part-time.[13]

With the drop in fertility in most industrialized nations, their future labor force will grow slowly, requiring them to invest in physical capital that will reduce labor needs, establish continuous education programs, liberalize immigration policies, train physicians to care appropriately for people as they grow older so they can continue to be productive, and encourage more women with children and older workers to remain in the workforce. Removing disincentives and creating positive incentives for older workers to stay employed can contribute to sustaining growth in industrialized nations. Policies that encourage phased retirement would include changing federal tax and pension laws to allow for the collection of partial benefits. Such laws would stimulate valued employees to remain on the job in flexible work situations, while eliminating some of the costs associated with their employment. Flexible employment options include job sharing, which allows two workers to split the responsibilities of one position, part-time work, and temporary employment. Another option is work from home. Large companies report that from 1995 to the turn of the twenty-first century, the percentage of employees who shared jobs overall rose by 70 percent, and the number who worked from home climbed 81 percent. A 1999 survey of more than 500 large corporations found that 16 percent are experimenting with flexible hours for older workers, and early quantitative data indicate a positive impact on productivity.[14] Finally, long-time employees could serve as consultants or mentors.

A German flexible retirement proposal offers employees incentives higher than those already established by law. Unions and employers in Baden Wuertenberg established a plan that allowed 55-year-old workers to work half-time and receive 82 percent of their salary. If the employer did not wish to participate, at age 61 the worker could opt to work half-time on 70 percent of full salary. Whatever the decision, the pension contribution would continue at 95 percent of the full-time rate.

AGEISM IN THE WORKPLACE

Ageism is discrimination based on age, and it creates official and societal acceptance of limits on the employment of older persons, contributing to later-life displacement. Financial disincentives, workplace discrimination, and inadequate retraining are factors which must be considered when discussing the continued paid employment of older persons. National surveys conducted in the USA in the 1980s suggest that 80 percent of Americans in general and 61 percent of employers in particular believe that most employers discriminate against older people and make it difficult for them to find work.[15] Until 1967, when the Age Discrimination in Employment Act was passed, approximately one-half of private-sector job openings were advertised as closed to applicants over 55, and one-quarter were barred to workers over 45. Age discrimination is the complaint most often lodged against employers, according to the Equal Employment Opportunity Commission, and a study in 1994 for the AARP showed that discrimination against older workers was about the same as that against African Americans and Hispanics of all ages.[16]

Although the relationship between age and job performance is exceedingly weak, misconceptions are common. They include the belief that most older workers are limited by health conditions, are less flexible on the job, are less educated, possess skills that are technologically obsolete, and are difficult to retrain. In a research study to determine whether worker performance declines with age, the literature showed that the only jobs for which performance appeared to decline with age were those requiring manual labor. No correlation was found between age and work quality for supervisors and professionals, and job performance in sales was shown to improve with age.

British economist Richard Disney notes that although a younger workforce may be more adaptable and quicker to learn, it is also true that they have less training and experience. Although some individuals in an older workforce may experience a degree of depreciation in skills and difficulty in retraining during periods of rapid technological change, overall they have greater experience and maturity, are more dependable, and embody high productivity and less absenteeism.[17] Of course, continuing educational opportunities would further increase the value of continuing employment of older workers.

The proportion of chronically disabled older Americans has fallen steadily in the past decades, and fewer older people are unable to work because of disability. According to the results of the *National Long-Term Care Survey*, the proportion of US citizens aged 65 and older who were chronically disabled declined to 21 percent in 1994 from 24 percent in 1982.[4] There can be some decline in mental and physical functioning; but in general older workers remain productive in spite of these limitations by finding ways to compensate for both functional conditions and chronic diseases. In fact, disabilities are more likely to involve hearing or eyesight problems than a complete inability to function. Employer accommodation can be relatively easy—for example, adjusting font sizes on computer monitors or being sensitive to an employee's need to take medications while at work.

Historically, a large number of the lifetime contributions to scholarship, the arts, and sciences were made by men and women in their later years. In fact, the period of life after age 50 accounts for the major portion of output in most scholarly and scientific fields. Ages 70–79 alone account for 20 percent of the output in the fields of scholarship and 15 percent in the sciences.[18] Today, employers report that their older workers are as creative as younger employees, more dependable, and far more experienced. According to a Harris poll of 774 corporate human resource directors, 80 percent agree that older workers had less turnover, and 71 percent said they had as much ability as younger workers to acquire new skills.

Industrialized nations are just beginning to take action against persistent ageism. For example, Australia's Council on Ageing (COTA) has begun to urge employers, businesses, trade unions, academics, and workers themselves to look for solutions to age-based discrimination.

Effective laws are needed to ensure that older workers receive equal opportunities for training to keep up with changing technology and to encourage lifelong learning. Reforms must be passed to ensure that job opportunities are available for older workers, and that they are equipped with the necessary skills and level of competence. Restructuring the job environment to accommodate older workers and developing innovative ways to reorganize work for long-tenure employees can increase productivity and help skilled older employees remain competitive. For example, in Norway, the government has undertaken a major national lifelong-learning initiative, which is known as Competence Reform. Employees who have been working at least three years and employed by the same employer for the last two years have the right to full-time or part-time study leave for up to three years. The purpose is to raise the level of competence and provide the country with a highly skilled and flexible workforce, and one of its benefits will be to help older workers stay abreast of new technologies and remain competitive in the workplace.

It has become increasingly important that computer-related training, like training in general, be customized to physically accommodate older trainees (e.g. offering larger monitors, screen displays, and a keyboard and mouse that can accommodate a limited range of motion), in addition to research into new technology (e.g. perfecting a voice-activated computer that eliminates the need for keyboard and mouse).[19] In a collaborative effort between the private and public sectors, computer learning centers in the USA that accommodate older students, computer software companies and aging organizations, have begun to work together to promote computer literacy among older adults.

UNPAID WORK

Free time was once the exclusive province of the well-to-do, especially women; but now millions of older persons have the time that younger people lack. A 1999 survey[20] reports that nearly half of all US citizens aged 55 or older engage in some form of unpaid work.

Unpaid work includes volunteer work performed through formal organizations such as hospitals, churches, and schools; informal help to relatives and friends, including caregiving and home maintenance; and unpaid help in a family business.[21] Formal volunteering in a community can be a substitute for paid labor, either producing services at a pre-existing level, expanding the product of a community's public and private organizations, or creating a new service, such as volunteer service organizations. Examples include mentoring programs for inner-city children, foster grandparent programs, and the recruitment of retired medical professionals in the development of free health clinics for the delivery of healthcare to the medically underserved.

Domestic activities include home maintenance and production of goods or services for home consumption. Older members add significantly to the nation's welfare in activities that include care of young, sick, or functionally limited family members and the transmission of values to younger generations.

Older people fill an important role as informal parent-surrogates to grandchildren. In 1998 this cohort was responsible for the care of nearly 4 million children, or 5.6 percent of all US children under the age of 18. Over 2.5 million maintained families with or without legal parents also in residence, and in more than 888,000 households they raised the children alone. Among families with preschoolers and employed mothers, 17 percent received primary child care from the child's grandparents.[22] Family dynamics and financial constraints mitigate against adoption; and often lacking legal status as guardians, grandparents can experience financial difficulties maintaining themselves and their grandchildren.

Unpaid labor by family members, which reduces labor costs of a family enterprise, is predominantly the purview of older persons. Beyond economic considerations, their participation may have the positive effect of enriching family relationships as well as enhancing the older person's sense of self-worth.

THE CASE OF JAPAN

Japan's population is aging much faster than in any other industrialized country. It has one of the lowest birthrates of any developed nation and the longest-living population. Employment opportunities for elderly people in Japan are limited, and the unemployment rate has increased. In the mid-1970s, twice as many workers entered the job market as were retiring, and the legal minimum age at which employees could retire and receive a pension was 55. But, as the twenty-first century unfolds, two workers will retire for every worker entering the job market. Sooner or later, industries will find it impossible to recruit enough young workers to the labor market to replace workers who have left.

In 1998, the legal minimum age of retirement in Japan was raised to 60, and it will gradually be raised to age 65 by 2013 for men, and by 2018 for women. Thirty-seven percent of Japanese men work after age 60, in contrast to 10 percent of American men. Japanese employers retain some of their older workers at lower wages, and transfer some others to subsidiaries or related firms. Workers also can find jobs with their old firm's suppliers or customers.[23]

With a view to expanding even further the employment of older workers, the Japanese government is beginning to offer companies a variety of incentives to encourage their older workers to remain in the workforce. Incentives include subsidies to businesses whose total workforce has more than 10 percent older workers and to employers who have eliminated mandatory retirement. Other incentives include partial coverage of expenses for employers who have adapted facilities and equipment in the workplace to make them better suited for older workers.

DEVELOPING NATIONS

The United Nations estimates that, by 2025, more than 75 percent of the over-60 population will live in developing nations, including 70 percent of the world's 604 million women over age 60. Forty percent of older people in developing nations will live in the countryside, but very few studies of this population have been undertaken.

Traditionally, old people who lived in rural poverty could depend upon their adult children to care for them as they aged. Today, modern industries and opportunities for advancement draw the young to the cities, leaving the elders in the community to cope as best they can with limited resources. Since rural economies depend predominantly on heavy manual labor, frail older persons are often left without visible means of support. Women especially lack the resources, skills, and social independence to cope with the changing social conditions. International nonprofit organizations, such as the United Nations Subcommittee on Ageing, the International Women's Movement, and Help Age International, are in the early stages of addressing the problems of impoverished older women in developing countries.

Small-loan programs in developing nations limit credit availability to older people, but there are notable exceptions Since 1976, a Bangladeshi nonprofit organization, Grameen Bank, has made small, unsecured loans available to people of all ages to begin small businesses, which are known as "microenterprises." Older women are particularly encouraged to participate in these entrepreneurial endeavors. Action for Welfare and Awakening in Rural Environment (AWARE), in Hyderabad, India, is one of several agencies that enable older workers to buy materials for individual work projects. In Colombia, Pro Vida, a nongovernmental agency, has developed programs to redirect or retrain the skills of older people (e.g. one town's innovative program gives impoverished older persons a monopoly on employment in a recycling program). In Ecuador, bakeries employ older people, and in the Philippines, they are trained in car repair and encouraged to open their own businesses. Laundries, home repair services, general merchandise shops, equipment rentals, industrial sewing, childcare, and hand-made crafts are other types of enterprises that have provided work for older persons in developing nations.[24]

CONCLUSION

In the twenty-first century, declining mortality and disability rates in early old age measure the improved health of older people. In some ways, retirement has been a twentieth-century phenomenon. It was required when the majority of people labored in mines, factories, and foundries, and it continues to be humane and necessary for individuals who have reasons to stop working after a lifetime of toil. Analyses of a variety of occupations and their physical requirements show that today a much smaller proportion of jobs require strenuous physical effort, and a large percentage require only moderate or light physical exertion. They suggest that the physical demands of work are easier to meet than they were in the past.[25]

A social norm that is appropriate to the new longevity and to a world trend toward human rights would be one in which all people are considered individually and collectively as a resource to meet their own and society's needs; one in which retirement remains a desired goal, as indeed it is, after a lifetime of work. At the same time, the new added life expectancy necessitates a commensurate increase in work expectancy, as long as there are jobs and people can work without age discrimination.

The responsibility for preserving one's human capital ultimately rests with the individual. If older individuals can continue to develop their productive potential, whether in paid employment, by service to family and community, or by sharing artistic and avocational abilities, their lives will be enriched, at the same time as they continue to benefit society. Late-life productivity is multifaceted, encompassing altruism, citizenship, stewardship, creativity, and the search for faith. A study found that while elderly people think that older workers should not stand in the way of younger workers, they also believe that "life is not worth living if you cannot contribute to the well-being of others."[26]

KEY POINTS   Productive aging

■ Productive aging is the capacity of an individual or population to engage in paid work and in non-remunerative activities, such as volunteer service to the family and community. It is affected by both internal and external factors. Internal factors include physical and emotional health, motivation, attitude, and experience. External factors involve society's willingness and ability to accommodate the special needs of elderly people.

■ Factors that encourage paid employment in later years include worker demand, educational level, changing technologies that may require retraining, and societal attitudes and structures. The age at which a country mandates or encourages its workers to retire influences the productive aging of its citizens.

■ Ageism is discrimination based on age, and it creates official and societal acceptance of limits on the employment of elderly people. Financial disincentives, workplace discrimination, and inadequate retraining are factors that have an impact on their continued employment.

■ Some benefit programs discourage workers from remaining on their jobs and provide incentives for early retirement. This is at odds with the projected demographics of greater life expectancy and fewer younger people entering the workforce. Removing disincentives to retirement and creating incentives for older workers to stay employed and employers to retain them can contribute to sustained growth in industrialized nations. Incentives include retraining older workers in new technologies, making accommodations for disabilities that do not impact on their ability to do the job, and developing options for job-sharing and part-time employment.

■ Means tests penalize older workers who receive pension benefits from earning more than a specified amount. For example, in 2000 the USA eliminated earnings penalties of social security recipients aged 65 and above. Many OECD nations are also gradually increasing the age at which workers become eligible for retirement benefits.

■ Older persons contribute significantly to a nation's benefit in activities that contribute to the care of young, sick, or functionally limited family members and the transmission of values to younger generations. Unpaid labor by older family members can significantly reduce labor costs of a family enterprise.

REFERENCES

1. Butler RN: Health, productivity, and aging. In Butler RN, Gleason HP (eds): Productive Aging: Enhancing Vitality in Later Life. Springer, New York, 1985:1–13

2. Knapp K, Muller C: Productive lives: paid and unpaid activities of older Americans. Working paper, International Longevity Center, New York, 2000:3–4

3. Toder E, Sandeep S: Effects of demographic trends on labor supply and living standards. The Retirement Project. Occasional Paper 2, Urban Institute, 1999:5–6

4. Martin D: Work first, invest later? Not these days. New York Times, 14 January 2001

5. Anonymous: The scope of the challenge. Online, available at www.who.int/ageing/scope.html

6. Toder E, Sandeep S: Effects of demographic trends on labor supply and living standards. The Retirement Project. Occasional Paper 2, Urban Institute, 1999:10,26

7. Muller C, Honig, M: Charting the productivity and independence of older persons. International Longevity Center, New York, 2000:11–12

8. Kreps JM: Age, work, and income. Southern Econ J 1977;43:1423–1437

9. Freidmann EA, Havighurst R: The Meaning of Work and Retirement. University of Chicago Press, Chicago, 1954:2

10. Burtless G, Quinn J: Retirement trends and policies to encourage work among older Americans. Presented at the Annual Conference of the National Academy of Social Insurance, Washington, DC, 26–27 January 2000:3

11. Smeeding T, Butler RN, Schaber G: The consequences of population aging for society. Workshop report, International Longevity Center, New York, 1999:10–12

12. Blondal, S, Scarpetta S: The retirement decision in OECD countries. Economics Department Working Paper 202, OECD, Paris, 1998

13. American Association of Retired Persons: Baby boomers envision their retirement: an AARP segmentation analysis. Roper Starch Worldwide and AARP, 1998

14. Anonymous: Phased retirement—reshaping the end of work, 1999. Online, available at www.watsonwyatt.com

15. Atchley R: Social Forces and Aging, 5th edn. Wadsworth, Belmont, CA, 2000

16. Lavelle M: On the edge of age discrimination. New York Times Magazine, 9 March 1997:66–69

17. Disney R: Can we afford to grow older? MIT Press, Cambridge, MA, 1996:187

18. Dennis W: Creative productivity between the ages of 20 and 80 years. J Gerontology 1966;21:1–8

19. Research and Policy Committee of the Committee for Economic Development: New opportunities for older workers. New York, 1999:43

20. Wang P: Is this retirement? Money 2000 (November):101–108

21. Knapp K, Muller C: Productive lives: paid and unpaid activities of older Americans. Working paper, International Longevity Center, New York, 2000:9

22. Casper LM: Who's minding our preschoolers? US Bureau of the Census—Current Population Reports: Household Economic Studies P70–53. US Department of Commerce, Economics and Statistics Administration, March 1996

23. Muller C, Huh MS: International Leadership Center on Longevity and Society: Almanac on Longevity and Society: Japan and the United States Compared. Mount Sinai School of Medicine, 1993:40

24. United Nations: Ageing: guide to achieving of national targets. Online, available at www.un.org/esa/socdev/ageing/agetarg7.htm

25. Burtless G: Living longer, living better: the policy challenge of an aging workforce. Presentation for the Special Committee on Aging, United States Senate, 21 November 2000:5

26. Rowe JW, Kahn RL: Successful Aging. Random House, New York, 2000:178

SECTION 2
Geriatric medicine

Chapter 19

Health promotion and physical activity

David C. Kennie, Susie Dinan, and Archie Young

HEALTH PROMOTION AND PREVENTIVE CARE

Many people (whatever their age) neither wish for, nor have the discipline to attain, the "perfect health" defined by the World Health Organization (WHO) as a "state of complete physical, mental and social well-being."[1] Instead, most prefer a tradeoff, aiming for optimal health where the cost of any further improvement outweighs the value attached to that improvement.[2] Such optimal health in old age is the product of a matrix of factors:

- freedom from illness;
- optimal functional status;
- an adequate system of social support;
- continuing personal development.

The traditional biomedical model of preventive care operating within health services has focused—through primary and secondary prevention—on freedom from disease. It has come in for much criticism for narrowly focusing "downstream," for at times being inappropriate, for causing iatrogenic problems, and for drawing attention and resources away from the other spheres of activity that maintain and promote the health of elderly people.

Health promotion has had a wider remit, aiming not only at avoiding disease but also at assisting the personal development of elderly people toward a better understanding and control of their own health and toward positive well-being. Its strategies have focused on society and the environment[3] and have therefore demanded a societal, multiagency, and intersectoral approach with much activity taking place outside the traditional health arena.

Nevertheless, elderly people need *both* preventive care and health promotion, so it is essential that health professionals become fully engaged in all areas of activity. A unified, multi-dimensional strategy is required (Fig. 19-1). For this holistic model of preventive care and health promotion to be effective for older people, many tasks need to be performed by many sectors of society (Table 19-1).

The range of strategies

Minimizing illness

Considerable progress has been made in the prevention of vascular damage in old age. Evidence for the benefit of treating hypertension continues to mount with at least some of that evidence pointing to benefit even in the very old. A clearer understanding has emerged on the respective benefit of various medications, and guidelines are now available for the management of this condition in older people.[4] The use of statin drugs in reducing vascular end-point damage in elderly people shows particular promise, with studies indicating their cost effectiveness for high-risk groups in old age.[5] The fact that statin medications are of benefit in those with and without elevated cholesterol levels suggests the benefits extend to an impact on the vascular endothelium that holds promise for secondary prevention in old age. The relative contributions of different approaches to preventing the complications of type II diabetes have recently been clarified,[6] with emphasis on blood pressure control and treatment of the vascular component of the disease probably being at least as effective as strict glycemic control.[7]

Whilst scientific evidence for the effectiveness of pneumococcal vaccination in frail elderly populations remains in doubt, the benefits of influenzal vaccination are now based on more substantial evidence. Moreover, evidence is emerging that for those in institutions, vaccination of *staff* may be more beneficial in reducing resident mortality than vaccination of the residents themselves.[8]

Several new drugs are available to combat the progress of Alzheimer's disease, randomized trials showing less deterioration in cognition, less functional decline, and less behavioral

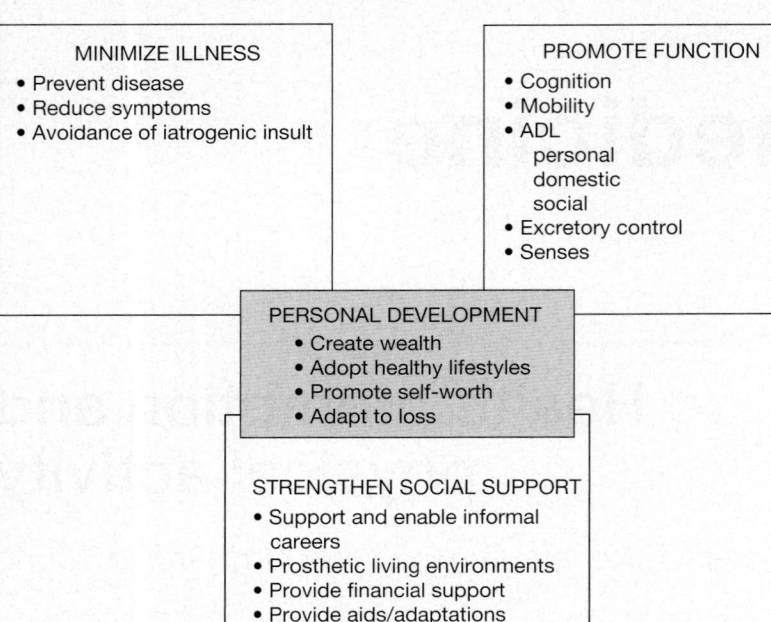

Figure 19-1 A multidimensional strategy for ensuring health and well-being in old age.

Table 19-1 **The tasks of health promotion**

Target group	Task
Elderly individuals	Generate wealth for and into old age Continue self-development Adopt a healthy lifestyle Adapt to loss
Families and carers	Provide informal support Respect the older person's autonomy Avoid overprotection
Healthcare providers	Educate, adopt, and document healthcare in a multidimensional fashion that promotes function and maintains social support systems as well as reducing illness Multiskill nursing and therapy support staff Validate preventive strategies scientifically Tailor preventive strategies to individual needs Reduce iatrogenic insult Recognize the needs of family carers
Public health	Guide organizations that purchase health services in buying appropriate preventive strategies Assist in the appropriate reorientation of funding between traditional health-service and non-health-service organizations Assess and catalyze the development of local community health strategies (see Table 19-2) Promote health education for the older population
Social services	Agree a protocol for health promotion measures to be adopted upon referral for complex home support services, social daycare or on admission to long-term care
Government	Provide a nurturing environment for the generation of wealth Ensure financial manipulation of "risk goods" to modify health behavior Provide legislation to modify health behavior
Collective	Educate to dispel agism Minimize costs

disturbance over time. There is also emerging evidence that these medications may be beneficial in patients with more severe cognitive impairment than in those who were originally enrolled in trials as well as in other types of dementia.

The value, or otherwise, of cancer screening in old age remains unclear. A fundamental reason is the failure to include elderly people in such trials, despite the increasing prevalence of cancer with increasing age. Nevertheless, future studies must also take account of the possibility that the identification of cancer may be of limited relevance in a very old person with significant comorbidity, and that the resulting therapeutic intervention may carry a high risk of iatrogenic morbidity.

Promoting function

MAINTAINING MOBILITY AND AVOIDING FALLS Safe mobility is the cornerstone of independent physical functioning, and strategies to promote this are essential components of health promotion for elderly people. There is good evidence that multifaceted prevention programs are effective for community populations. Randomized controlled trials also suggest that specific activities to train posture and balance may be of additional benefit. Fall prevention is discussed in Chapters 20 and 106, and the contribution of physical activity to the prevention of falls is considered in more detail later in this chapter.

It is now appreciated that even a short illness can result in deconditioning that can reduce mobility. Several trials of inpatient geriatric assessment units have shown improved functional outcomes by time of discharge.

MAINTAINING INDEPENDENCE IN THE ACTIVITIES OF DAILY LIVING Functional decline is common in very old people, with around 80 percent of those aged 80 and older requiring help with both their personal and domestic care.[9] Hart and workers have shown the benefits of a screening program for the provision of aids to daily living; those identified by screening and given aids showed significant reduction in disability.[10]

When discharged from hospital after acute medical illness, around 30 percent of those over 70 years have not regained their ability (often permanently) to feed or toilet or dress themselves.[11] It is encouraging that multifaceted inpatient strategies based on the principles of good geriatric medical practice prevent a significant proportion of this disability.[12] The functional benefits of physical activity are considered in more detail later in this chapter.

Maintaining and strengthening social supports

AVOIDING SOCIAL MARGINALIZATION Many elderly people experience a reduction in their level of social functioning. This occurs as a result of bereavement, weakness, fatigue, and the "ecological gap"[13] (i.e. the demands made by urban environments on a relatively disabled population, who may have difficulty walking distances, may no longer own a car, and may feel unsafe on the streets after dark). Local governments should, therefore, support and promulgate models of urban planning that take into account the needs of elderly people and facilitate social integration (Table 19-2).

Table 19-2 **The promotion of social function**	
Objectives	**Actions**
Supportive environment	Provide convenient and accessible public toilets Provide regularly spaced sitting areas Ensure good street lighting Ensure effective community policing Provide home security and alarm provision Provide personal attack alarms Develop victim support schemes
Transport and access	Manage traffic according to the needs of older drivers and pedestrians Ensure ease of access to public buildings Ramp kerbs Provide convenient and adapted public transport Provide dial-a-lift services
Leisure	Provide mobile library services to the housebound Provide library services to those in long-term care homes Provide audio and large-print books Inform about services and interests relevant to older people Encourage sport and activity before retirement Ensure dedicated sessions for elderly people (e.g. at public swimming pools) Increase attention paid to privacy in changing rooms
Continuing education	Provide pre-retirement education courses Provide self-education groups Ensure curricula relevant to the personal development and interests of retired people Develop educational models such as the "University of the Third Age"

Social marginalization is caused in part by the relative poverty of the older population. It is also caused by geographic, cultural, and linguistic barriers and by agism, which is pervasive within society. Health promotion measures to counteract agism within the health services include: professional education on the opportunities in caring for older people, legal action on age-related discrimination in the provision of healthcare, and greater participation by elderly people in service planning and policy-making. Initiatives outside the health sector include: positive media stereotypes of old people, a greater political voice for elderly people, and intergenerational projects. Health promotion must strive to eliminate the marginalization of elderly people and foster their inclusion in the wider concept of "community."

APPROPRIATE HOUSING Housing is a key element in providing for health, well-being, and independence, yet nearly one-half of all unfit properties are occupied by elderly people.[3]

Substandard housing leads to: illness from dampness, hypothermia from inadequate heating and drafts, problems of access and being housebound from inadequate design, falls and accidents from problems of layout, and frustration and anxiety from the need for repair.

Effective health promotion strategies include: home care and repair schemes, gardening chore workers, heating and insulation strategies, and the installation of aids and adaptations. Strategies aimed at allowing the elderly inhabitant to stay put and avoid unnecessary moves are also effective; they include the provision of personal and domestic care services and community alarm systems.

MINIMIZING CARER STRESS AND BURDEN   The impact of the caring role on the health of the family and other informal caregivers can be considerable. Several studies attest to a significant degree of physical and psychological ill-health. Caregiving also involves a degree of financial penalty and may place intolerable strains on family relationships.

Regrettably, identification of the impact of the caring role on caregivers is a skill rarely taught to healthcare professionals. Most rely on open-ended and unstructured interviews. Identification can, however, be enhanced through the use of validated measurement instruments for burden and stress.[14]

Health promotion strategies such as daycare and respite care, counseling, and skill training improve informal caregivers' well-being[15] and prolong the time for which they are willing to undertake that role.

Promoting personal development

GENERATING WEALTH   Financial security is not only important in itself, it is also a prerequisite for access to healthy choices in lifestyle. Elderly people make up the largest low-income group in the UK, with one-half of all pensioner households depending on their state pension for 75 percent of their income.[16] This has serious implications for their health. Poverty (or more precisely, relative poverty) shows a clear association not just with mortality in old age, but with increased morbidity in terms of chronic conditions and deteriorating functional status (Fig. 19-2).[17]

The traditional response has been to lobby government to ensure that elderly people are given an adequate basic pension and, if necessary, additional welfare benefits. This safety net is vital, but the scale of the issue makes adequate public subsidy unreliable in future years. For example, figures from the US Department of Health Education and Welfare indicate that, of the 64 percent of people who survive to 65 years of age, 54 percent have to rely on family or government for financial support, 5 percent continue working because of financial necessity, and only 5 percent are well-off or wealthy with the choices such financial independence brings to them. The magnitude of the reliance on governmental support threatens the fiscal integrity of most nations with an aging society.

A task of health promotion may, therefore, be to educate middle-aged and elderly people into the techniques of once again generating their own income, probably not through employment, but perhaps through home-based business, made possible through technological improvements in communication and through the Internet. For this to be effective,

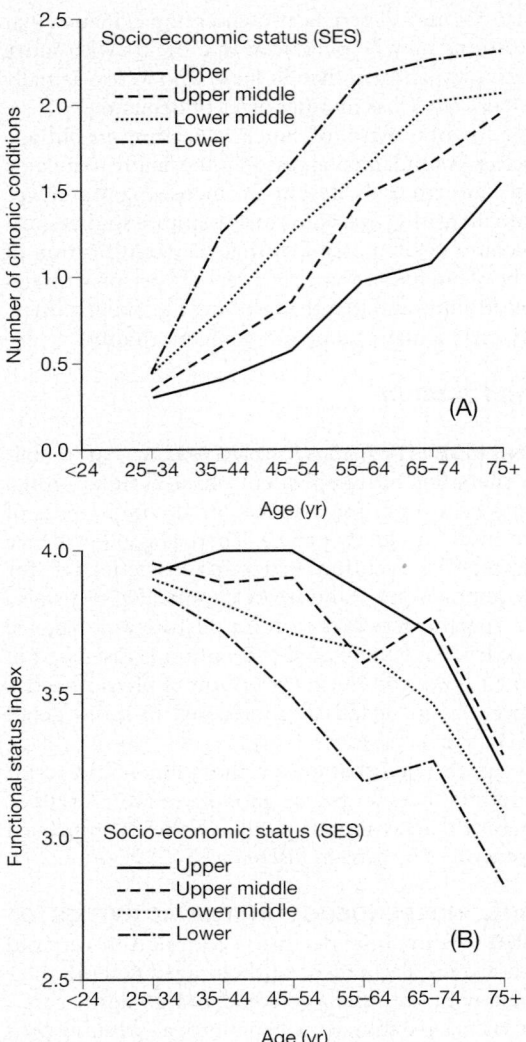

Figure 19-2 Relationship between socio-economic status and health at different ages. (A) Chronic conditions; (B) functional status. From House et al.,[17] with permission of Blackwell Publishers, Oxford

however, some disincentives must be removed from the income tax structure. Alternatively, governments might consider a greater financial acknowledgment of the role of older people as caregivers.

PROMOTING HEALTHY LIFESTYLE PRACTICES   In younger adults, there is a correlation between lifestyle and morbidity. In cross-sectional studies, this association is sometimes less clear for elderly people. Nevertheless, considerable scientific evidence, including some prospective studies, suggests scope for promoting health by addressing key lifestyle practices in older people.

Quitting smoking   Smoking has a well-documented correlation with vascular, respiratory, and neoplastic disease and for elderly people has the additional concerns of osteoporosis, cataract, macular degeneration, accentuated skin wrinkling, decline in functional performance, and fire risk in those with dementia.

Contrary to popular opinion there is much evidence to suggest it is still worthwhile for people to quit smoking, even in old age. The reduction in risk of lung cancer[18] and coronary artery disease[19] in quitters appears to be much the same for older and younger populations. Older adults who quit show improved lung function, a reduction in respiratory symptoms, and a reduction in hospitalization from influenza and pneumonia. Quitting smoking has been shown to result also in a significant and reasonably rapid reduction in risk of stroke.

At least two studies in older populations have shown significant benefit from implementing quit-smoking strategies. One British randomized controlled trial in smokers aged over 60 showed that a single input of counseling from their general practitioner, followed with support from the practice nurse, achieved a 14 percent 6-month quit rate.[20] In Pennsylvania, USA, the use of free nicotine patches for elderly smokers achieved a 29 percent 6-month quit rate.[21] Against this scientific background there appears to be significant agism amongst medical staff. Hospital doctors were less likely to advise older patients on the hazards of smoking, irrespective of their physical or mental health.[22] This is regrettable for, even in financial terms, the cost-effectiveness of brief counseling on stopping smoking appears to be a "good buy." When made during routine doctor–patient contact it has been estimated to be $950 and $1411 per life-year saved for men and women, respectively, aged 65–69 years.[23]

Ensuring good nutrition Enhanced nutrition for older people continues to hold out much promise for improved health, though much of the evidence base is still evolving. At its most gross, weight loss and protein-energy undernutrition are endemic in nursing homes[24] and in acute hospitals.[25] Increased staff awareness of feeding dependence, regular weighing, and biochemical and anthropometric measurements can all assist in the identification of the at-risk patient. Several studies have suggested improved outcomes for patients in whom enteral support has been given early in the rehabilitation process, though a Cochrane review of such measures after surgery for hip fracture suggests more cautious interpretation of benefit.

There is little doubt that high fruit and vegetable diets are correlated with lower risks of cancers and, although attempts at reducing cancer risk with β-carotene antioxidant supplementation have so far been unimpressive, there is a suggestion that increased folate in elderly people may protect against colorectal cancer.[26]

The Recommended Dietary Allowances (RDAs) for various nutritional substances for the older population is now mostly based on their impact on health rather than just the level that will prevent a deficiency state. Thus, often they may be achieved only by overt nutritional supplementation rather than relying solely on dietary content. Examples include the older person's increased need for vitamin D (because of less opportunity for sunlight exposure and less effective skin synthesis of this vitamin, and also the decreased ability of the kidney to convert it to active form), their increased need for vitamin B_{12} (due to atrophic gastritis and bacterial colonization of the upper gastrointestinal tract), their increased need for calcium, and their increased need for folate (to depress homocysteine levels with their accompanying cardiac risk[27]).

Increasing habitual physical activity A physically active lifestyle contributes to a lower risk of several important diseases, enhanced physical and mental function, richer opportunities for social interaction, and a greater sense of control over one's own health and well-being.[28] These will be discussed in more detail later in the chapter.

IMPROVING HEALTH LITERACY Elderly people may lack the skills necessary to gain access to, or to understand and use, information in ways that promote good health. This might impair motivation to adopt healthy lifestyle practices, or might impede the safe and effective use of medications. Improved esteem and self-worth can empower the elderly person to have the necessary confidence to become more health literate. Specific health education programs may also be employed, tailoring their messages for greatest impact. The promotion of health literacy also requires the development of personal and state resources for self-care.

AVOIDING AGISM AND PROMOTING SELF WORTH Many elderly people have a relatively low opinion of their value to society. Perhaps more than any, they hold agist attitudes. These perceptions arise from many factors: their cultural inheritance, low income, social marginalization, boredom, and loneliness. These negative perceptions of self-worth delay self-referral for illness and disability, diminish advocacy and control, and reduce motivation to seek positive resources for health.

Many, very varied, factors can maintain self-esteem. They range from gainful and income-generating activity, through socialization, to a rewarding sex life. Participation on health planning and implementation groups can improve the sense of control. Elderly people also need more positive images of old age, providing a vision of what might be possible. Unless as a society we allow older people a dream of what old age can be like at its most favorable, we will continue with agist stereotypes and with old people themselves assuming little responsibility or drive for their own future. Perhaps most of all, elderly people need positive affirmation by all sectors of society, from government to loved ones, of a belief in their value as human beings.

ADAPTING TO LOSS AND IMMINENT DEATH In the final analysis, every elderly person has to adapt to various sorts of loss and to the imminence of death. The ability to do this successfully and with dignity is the final life goal.[29] It largely depends on intrinsic coping skills acquired through life, but may be enhanced by open communication with loved ones and society at large and by freedom from pain and distress in the dying trajectory.

Tailoring strategies to individuals

The potential number of health promotion and preventive care strategies for elderly people are legion yet they must be tailored to suit individuals according to the scheme outlined in Figure 19-3. Certain steps should be taken to ascertain whether a potential preventive care strategy (particularly if this involves screening) is relevant to the older patient. This depends both on the strength of the scientific argument and on several characteristics of the individual

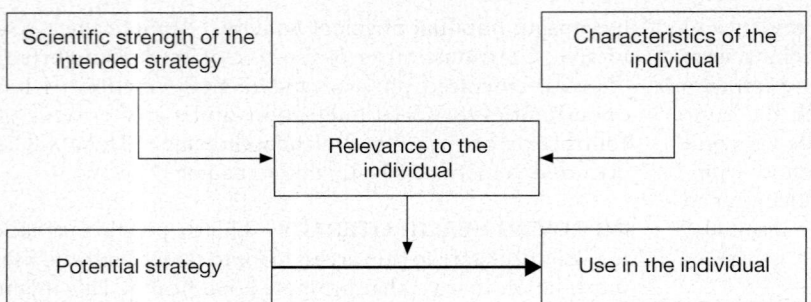

Figure 19-3 Tailoring strategies to individuals.

concerned (Fig. 19-3). These, in turn, depend principally on the following.

The importance of the health problem under consideration
This should relate to the elderly person's suffering, disability, morbidity, and mortality. The degree of burden that the problem imposes on caregivers and its impact on society in general are also important.

The problem's ability to be easily and accurately detected
In primary and secondary prevention, the priority issue is to refine the accuracy of identification of those individuals at risk of, or with, the particular health problem. For tertiary prevention, improved detection depends first on increasing the awareness of healthcare professionals that there might be a problem at all.

The proven effectiveness of an intervention once the problem has been identified   The Canadian Task Force on the Periodic Health Examination, the US Preventive Services Task Force, and the various Cochrane Reviews have done much to summarize the scientific evidence upon which many strategies are based. However, for strategies to be effective they must be transportable from the randomized controlled trial to the "real world," with the individuals under consideration being sufficiently similar to those in the trial, with adequate resources being available, with adequate compliance being likely, and with due respect for ethical considerations in care.

The cost of the intervention   Despite popular misconception, the scientific evidence suggests that the majority of health promotion strategies add to costs rather than create savings.[2,30] Wherever possible, therefore, the assessment of any health promotion strategy should include scrutiny of cost-effectiveness.

The individual's degree of risk   The person's degree of risk for the condition in question should be quantified.

The individual's expected survival   This should be estimated from tables showing survival against physiological age (the latter converted from chronological age according to self-reported health status).[31] If the patient's anticipated survival time, perhaps because of comorbidity, is likely to be less than the lag between implementing the preventive care strategy and evidence of improvement in morbidity or mortality, the preventive care strategy would appear to have little benefit to that older individual. For example, in many cancer screening programs the time between screening and reduced disease-specific mortality is in the region of 3–5 years.

An extreme example of this issue comes with the end-stage of irremediable disease. The sensitive physician will recognize that death is a legitimate end-point and that the patient's health promotion needs are for symptom control and a dignified death rather than for life extension.

The individual's predisposition to dependence   Certain preventive care strategies, particularly those offering additional home support, can at times foster increased dependence. The physician should appreciate that there is a critical intervention time or "window" when it is appropriate to prescribe such supportive measures but be aware that their premature implementation may be to the elderly person's ultimate detriment in terms of functional autonomy.

The individual's expressed wish to be left with an "unhealthy" lifestyle   It is agist not to discuss the potential benefits of a particular health promotion strategy fully and openly with an elderly individual. Nevertheless, many frail older people are a captive audience at particular risk of inappropriate or overzealous application of preventive care strategies. The physician should listen to the person's wishes, respect his or her autonomy, and be prepared to withhold the intended strategy.

PHYSICAL FUNCTION AND AGING

Physical activity as a health promotion strategy

The health benefits of habitual physical activity are at least as great in later life. The special importance of habitual physical activity as we age is its ability to preserve functional independence in activities of daily living by counteracting some of the age-related decline in physical performance. The ability to perform everyday activities comfortably and safely is central to well-being. This reflects the importance of physical function for autonomous and wide-ranging social function, and perhaps also the esthetic satisfaction of optimal physical function. The promotion of a physically active lifestyle, therefore, is potentially a very important strategy.[32] The justification and requirements of such a strategy are now considered, along the lines suggested above.

Age-related changes in physical function

STRENGTH   From middle age onward, there is a steady loss of muscle mass. This results in a progressive and substantial loss of strength. Even in the absence of symptomatic or diagnosed disease, people aged 65–89 years show differences in strength consistent with the loss of strength at some 1–2 percent per year[33] (see also Chapters 53 and 68).

The muscular cachexia (or "sarcopenia") of aging has sometimes been attributed to a reducing level of habitual physical activity. This explanation is unconvincing, however, as it leaves unexplained the similar age-related decline in performance seen in elite, veteran sportsmen competing in strength events.

The loss of muscle is principally a reduction in the number of muscle fibers. This, in turn, is associated with a reduced number of motoneurones. It seems likely that the sarcopenia of aging is due to a slowly progressive denervation, incompletely compensated by an increase in the size of the remaining motor units. In addition to the reduction in the number of muscle fibers, there may also be a reduction in the size of the remaining fibers, especially in the presence of pathology, following immobilization, and in advanced old age. Unlike the reduction in the number of muscle fibers, this may be amenable to improvement by increased activity.[34,35]

POWER   "Strength" and "power" are not synonymous. "Strength" refers to the maximum force (or torque) that can be exerted. "Power," the rate of performing work, is calculated as the product of force and speed. Age-related differences in explosive power observed in healthy elderly subjects are even more severe than the differences in strength.[33] Similarly, differences in power between healthy elderly people and patients of the same age are much greater than the differences in strength.

The weaker a muscle, the slower the contraction it must make to overcome an unchanged external resistance. As a result, power is reduced not only to the same degree as strength, but also as a result of an enforced shift to a less favorable point on the power–velocity relationship. The greater the required force in relation to the muscle's maximal strength, the more pronounced is this "extra" deficit in power.[36]

ENDURANCE   The ability to perform prolonged dynamic exercise without fatigue or discomfort depends on the percentage of the individual's maximum aerobic power (maximal oxygen uptake, or $\dot{V}O_2$ max) required for the activity. $\dot{V}O_2$max declines with increasing age at approximately the same rate as, and perhaps because of, the loss of muscle mass.[37,38] The contribution of the gradual age-related reduction in maximal heart rate is still a matter for debate. The age-related decline in performances of elite veteran endurance athletes indicates that the age-related decline in $\dot{V}O_2$ max cannot be explained as merely the result of habitual inactivity.

Functional consequences

STRENGTH AND POWER   A young person's strength includes a generous safety margin, but even healthy elderly people have strength (and power) below, or near to, functionally important thresholds and so have lost, or are in danger of losing, the ability to perform some important everyday tasks.[39–41] Women are weaker than men, both in absolute terms and also in relation to body weight. Data from the English National Fitness Survey (a representative sample of noninstitutionalized people) suggest that their lower power to weight ratios mean that women are functionally vulnerable about 20 years earlier than men.[41] This helps explain the greater prevalence of disability and of falls among elderly women than among elderly men, and the age-related decline in the percentage of elderly women using public transport on their own. There is a strong case, therefore, for ensuring that any interventions to improve muscle function are directed at least as strongly to women as to men.

The adverse effect of cooling on muscle power may be especially important in those elderly people who are immobile, thin, and living in poorly heated accommodation, perhaps contributing to the increased incidence of indoor falls and fractures in cold weather.

ENDURANCE   The age-related decline in $\dot{V}O_2$ max, especially when combined with the effects of disease, means that many elderly people need only a small further decline to render some everyday activities either impossible or so dependent on anaerobic metabolism as to be unpleasant to perform.[39]

For aerobic power, as for explosive power, a woman is functionally disadvantaged in weight-bearing activities (compared to a man of the same age) by her lower power to weight ratio. This happens at least 15 years earlier for women than for men.[41] For example, in the English National Fitness Survey, 80 percent of women (but only 35 percent of men) aged 70–74 recorded a $\dot{V}O_2$ max so low as to imply that they had lost the ability comfortably to sustain a walking speed of just 3 miles per hour. By age 80, even just 2 miles per hour (in comfort) is probably impossible for most women. Indeed, for a detrained, 80-year-old female patient, even just sitting still may demand such a high proportion of $\dot{V}O_2$ max that this apparently trivial activity cannot be sustained for more than 2–3 hours at a time.[42]

SUPPLENESS   In patients with arthritis, more than 120 degrees of shoulder abduction are necessary to wash hair without difficulty.[43] In the English National Fitness Survey,[41] there was a gradual reduction in the mean range of shoulder abduction with increasing age, which was somewhat more pronounced in the women. More than a quarter of the men aged 75 and over, and more than one-third of the women aged 75 and over, had a range of shoulder abduction below this functional threshold.

Detecting the need for intervention

Although the benefits of physical training for the performance of everyday tasks do not become prominent until late middle age, increased physical activity brings other health benefits throughout life. The promotion of physical activity is therefore a population-based intervention, from which elderly people must not be excluded. Population data on the strength, power, endurance, and suppleness of older people are invaluable, not so much to detect those who need the intervention, but to identify those who are likely to be most receptive to a promotional message based on the preservation of functional abilities.

Effectiveness of physical training

PROMOTING PSYCHOSOCIAL FUNCTION AND WELL-BEING   There is a growing body of evidence for a therapeutically useful effect of physical activity in the treatment of depression, chronic pain, and poor sleep in elderly people.[28,44] Physical activity can also improve short-term alertness[45,46] and perhaps even longer-term cognitive function.[47,48] Recreational exercise certainly offers important opportunities for socially acceptable, nonclinical, physical contact, for socialization, and for renewal of a contracting social network.

PREVENTING DISEASE Habitual physical activity protects against conditions important in old age, notably osteoporosis, noninsulin-dependent diabetes mellitus (NIDDM), hypertension, ischemic heart disease, stroke, and probably also colonic cancer.[49–51] This protection appears still to apply in those who are physically active in later life.[28] More data are required, however, before one can be confident about the effect on cardiovascular and cerebrovascular mortality of the new adoption of physical activity in later life.[28]

IMPROVING PHYSICAL FUNCTION Physical function depends on strength, power, endurance, coordination (including balance), and suppleness. Even in the absence of disease, these attributes are all eroded with increasing age, but all can be improved by appropriate physical training. Disability can even be ameliorated in the presence of established disease (e.g. in angina, claudication, chronic heart failure, airflow limitation).[52]

Strength, power, and related functional ability   Training by maximal or near maximal muscle contractions produces improvements in strength and power. Typically, strength training might comprise one, two, or three sets of 8–15 muscle contractions at perhaps greater than 70 percent of maximal strength, for each muscle group.[53] The weakness of old age, however, means that this can be achieved with very little in the way of specialized equipment.[54] Indeed, just body weight can be used to good effect.[55]

Randomized controlled trials have confirmed that elderly people (mean age 80 and over) respond to strength training with improvements at least as great (in percentage terms) to those seen in much younger subjects. This is true for elderly people who are healthy,[54] who are living in institutional care,[56,57] and who are recovering after hip fracture[58,59] and/or after an injurious fall.[60] Unfortunately, there is no evidence that strength training halts the underlying loss of muscle fibers. Nevertheless, even if strength continues to be lost at some 1–2 percent per year, an improvement in isometric strength of, say, 20–25 percent is still equivalent to a substantial "rejuvenation" of strength.

Training-induced improvements in strength and power may result in improvement in selected functional abilities,[54,59] but functional gains are more likely if the performance of strengthening exercises is accompanied by practice of the specific functional skills.[61]

Endurance and related functional ability   Endurance training in old age has received less attention than strength training. Nevertheless, it is apparent that, even into their eighties, women can expect endurance training to result in a 10–20 percent improvement in $\dot{V}o_2$ max, associated with a meaningful reduction in the strain of submaximal exercise.[62] Functional benefit in everyday life, however, cannot be assumed, no matter how likely it seems. This is an important area for further research.

Balance and falls   A growing body of evidence supports the value of exercise for fall prevention. It is clear from the best summaries of the evidence[63,64] that elderly people who are liable to fall should be offered a program of exercise incorporating muscle strengthening and balance training (e.g. adapted Tai Chi), preferably individually prescribed and preferably as part of a multifactorial intervention which also addresses other risk factors for falling.

Tailoring strategies to individuals
Program content
The content of an exercise program for older people includes all the elements common to any general fitness program but with an emphasis on particular areas and with appropriate adjustment of speed, intensity, and selection of exercises. A combination of regular recreational brisk walking and swimming, plus specific exercises to improve strength, flexibility, and balance, and participation in everyday activities such as gardening, general housework, and shopping, would benefit most elderly people. But this rather general advice takes no account of the fluctuating health and functional limitations of older people. Individually tailored, evidence-based physical activity programs that incorporate specific advice, education, and a variety of opportunities are preferable.

Principal components of an exercise program for elderly people

As for any age group...

- Safe
- Progressive
- Regular
- Balanced
- Strength
- Endurance
- Flexibility
- Coordination
- All major muscle groups
- Full ranges of movement
- Enjoyable

Also, specifically for older people...

- Load the bones
- Target postural, pelvic floor, and functional muscles
- Target functional movements
- Develop body awareness and dynamic balance
- Cater for a wider range of
  - initial activity levels
  - disabilities and pathologies
  - personal goals
- Injury prevention an even higher priority

Even very vulnerable older patients can exercise safely and effectively provided that the exercise program is appropriately designed and adapted, optimal functional gains are the priority, and heterogeneity is respected. The poorer the health and the greater the frailty of the participant, the greater the need for individualized advice, supervision, encouragement, and reassurance.[65] The shorter the remaining life expectancy, the greater the emphasis on maintaining independent mobility and functional abilities rather on disease prevention. Similarly, bone protection will be by hip protectors rather than by bone-loading exercises.

There is published guidance for exercise referral[66] and for the supervision of exercise by healthy older people and by older patients,[52,67,68] but the design and supervision of an exercise group for older participants are specialized skills. Efforts to improve the range and number of seniors' exercise groups should include insistence that instructors hold an appropriate specialist qualification to ensure increased enjoyment, effectiveness, and safety.

Safety

The health benefits of suitably adapted physical activity greatly outweigh any potential hazards. Nevertheless it is essential that everything possible be done to ensure the optimal balance between benefit and hazard for each individual. This is especially important for those participants most at risk of adverse events. This requires accurate identification of those for whom the standard exercise advice for older participants requires further modification or who warrant some other precaution. For example, is there a history of recurrent falls? Or, is the participant taking medication that might increase the risk of a fall?

Safety also requires that the intensity of the activity can be accurately judged and controlled, to ensure an intensity high enough to produce benefit but not so high as to be unduly hazardous. Again, frailer older participants will require more preparation and closer monitoring especially in the initial stages. Assessment is the key to meeting the safety requirements, in order to take account of the considerable diversity in age, initial fitness level, and coincidental chronic disease found in an unselected group of elderly people.

ASSESSMENT OF POTENTIAL PARTICIPANTS Healthy older people who plan just to increase their daily walking or undertake other light or moderate intensity activities may need no special evaluation or advice and are recommended simply to discuss their plans with their primary care physician. Referral to an exercise professional is appropriate if the person is likely to need help with current exercise practice, motivation, supervision, monitoring, choice of duration, frequency, time, type, and intensity of physical activity directed at specific health and functional outcomes.[66] The frailest and most vulnerable older patients routinely require referral to specialist exercise professionals. Programs should be individually tailored and based on a pre-exercise medical review that is "enabling"—i.e. one that emphasizes benefits rather than risks and actively facilitates safer, more effective participation.

Those at greatest risk of an adverse event during exercise are often people with most to gain from increasing their habitual level of physical activity. The purpose of assessment,

therefore, is not the exclusion of those at increased risk but, instead, to identify the characteristics of each individual that determine how he or she may enjoy effective exercise with the greatest safety. Pre-exercise assessment should be widely promoted as a positive, nonmedicalized, common-sense process in which the person, and if appropriate the medical adviser and exercise instructor, all participate.

Effective referral (i.e. the reliable transfer of relevant information) is a crucial part of the assessment process. This should be done in accordance with authoritative guidance[69] and recommended quality standards.[66] A suitable referral instrument may be helpful to guide the referring health professional in the sort of information likely to be important (Fig. 19-4).

RESPONSIBILITIES The referring doctor, practice nurse, or therapist has four key responsibilities:

- To identify and accurately communicate the patient's current pathologies and medications to the exercise professional.
- To indicate ways these may influence the individual's safety or comfort during physical activity. Any specifically contraindicated exercises or activities and other advice given to the patient should be included.
- To educate the patient in the early recognition of symptoms indicating that the exercise program may be in some way unsuitable. For example, the patient with osteoarthritic knees should be taught to respect and report an increase in pain, stiffness, or swelling.
- To monitor and review the patient's progress, encouraging; feedback from the patient and a productive dialogue with the exercise practitioner. These clinical responsibilities rest with the referrer.

The responsibility for applying the clinical information to the administration, design, delivery, and ongoing evaluation of the patient's exercise program and communication with the referrer rests with the exercise professional or exercise service. Responsibility for consenting to take part in the exercise program and observing its design and advice rests with the participant.

Health professionals should also acquire some understanding of the specific health benefits of exercise in old age, the components of an effective program for older people, and the professional requirements for those supervising the activities, and local knowledge of appropriate opportunities, settings, and professionals. They should also forge partnerships with local recreation providers, jointly to create opportunities for the independent use of recreational sports facilities by elderly people and for a range of supervised sessions catering for their diverse health, functional, social, and personal needs. To take their share of the overall responsibility, exercise professionals must be able to demonstrate that they are properly trained and that they respect confidentiality and professional boundaries.

ASSESSMENT OF EXERCISE INTENSITY There is a "window" of exercise intensity for the optimal balance between benefit and hazard. As a result of the decline in maximal oxygen uptake with increasing age, the older the participant, the smaller the window and the more accurate the control of exercise intensity must be.

REFERRAL FOR EXERCISE
(Exercise Practitioner Service)

DETAILS OF PATIENT

Surname.. D.O.B. ....

Forename .... Tel no: ....

Address ....

....

G.P. Dr .... Tel no: .... Fax no: ....

G.P's Address ....

Referrer's signature .... Date ....

REASON FOR EXERCISE REFERRAL: ....

CLINICAL DIAGNOSES AND/OR CURRENT PROBLEMS

1... Supine BP ....

2... Standing BP ....

3...

4...

MEDICATION:

1................................... 4................................... 7...................................

2................................... 5................................... 8...................................

3................................... 6................................... 9...................................

Possible effects of current medication and/or diagnoses on patient's safe/comfortable conduct of exercise

☐ Heart rate not an indicator of exercise intensity

☐ Suppression of pain

Susceptible to:

☐ Arrhythmia   ☐ Dizziness, falls

☐ Hypotension   ☐ Skin irritation/rashes/infection

☐ Hypoglycemia   ☐ Asthma

☐ Angina   ☐ Infection

☐ Osteoporosis   ☐ Joint pain

☐ Abnormal muscle tone   ☐ Urinary frequency

☐ Impaired alertness   ☐ Impaired cognition

Other precautions to be taken or what patient has been told:

Specific exercises/approaches to be included (if known):

Stage of health behavior change- (tick Activity Status)

☐ PRECONTEMPLATION   ☐ CONTEMPLATION   ☐ PREPARATION
(not considering exercise)   (considering)   (beginning)

☐ MAINTENANCE   ☐ RELAPSE   ☐ UNKNOWN

☐ ACTION:
(regularly active < 6 months)

Figure 19-4 Exercise referral form used by health professionals to transfer clinical information meaningfully to the exercise practitioner. Reproduced with permission of its authors, S. Dinan, A. Young, S. Iliffe, and P. Wallace.

Pulse counting is still widely used in an attempt to monitor, and so control, the intensity of self-paced exercise. There are several reasons why this is usually futile. It is rarely accurate, and the relationship between the "immediate" post-exercise heart rate and the exercising heart rate is inconsistent.[70] Furthermore, even if pulse rate could be reliably monitored, the intensity rating still depends on knowing the individual's maximal heart rate. However, there is considerable interindividual variation in maximal heart rate among subjects of the same age. (For example, it ranged from 110 to 180 beats per minute in a small group of healthy 80-year-old men.[71]) A useful age-based prediction of maximal heart rate is not possible for an individual, and direct measurement in the laboratory for every potential participant would be completely impracticable. Finally, there is a further problem in the use of the heart rate if the participant is taking digoxin or a β-blocker.

The "talk test" has been suggested as an alternative. This ruled that the ability to converse during exercise indicated that the intensity was not excessive and was based on the supposition that speech during exercise would impose a concurrent additional demand for ventilation.[72] This is now known to be incorrect; speech during exercise is achieved by a temporary *reduction* in ventilation, in order to permit phonation.[73] Moreover, young subjects could still read a test passage even at nearly 90 percent of their predicted maximal heart rate.[73] The degree of respiratory embarrassment during simultaneous speech and exercise may yet provide an aid to the subjective assessment of exercise intensity, but the original concept of the "talk test" cannot be relied upon.

In the end, one must still rely on reasoned, sensible guidelines and on exercise teachers' observational and communication skills. Most important of all are the participants' subjective judgments and their ability to "listen to their body." This skill is taught during a very gradual increase in exercise intensity from a very low starting level over the first few months of an exercise program. It uses a scale for the Rating of Perceived Exertion to help the person measure and describe the intensity of his or her effort during both endurance and strength activities.[74] Equivalent scales are also useful for assessing changes in chronic pain[74] or breathlessness[75] during exercise.

INJURY AVOIDANCE   To maintain enjoyment and adherence, the avoidance of even minor soft-tissue injuries and the recommendation of adequate rest between activity sessions should have high priority. "Too much too soon" greatly increases the risk of injury, possibly as a result of fatigue or through the precipitation of delayed-onset muscle soreness.

TEACHERS' COMPETENCE AND KNOWLEDGE   An approach, such as that outlined above, which aims to exclude virtually no one and which depends primarily on the use of the participant's own judgment for the assessment of exercise intensity, demands excellent communication between participants and their exercise advisers. It also demands that those working with elderly participants be aware of the features of conditions likely to be present and of how to adapt their exercise advice accordingly. The coaching, teaching, and programming skills required to work effectively and safely with elderly participants are, in many ways, as specialized as those required to work with elite athletes.

The need for specialized skills when designing and supervising exercise programs for elderly people has been widely recognized in recent years, most notably by the World Health Organization, the American College of Sports Medicine, the International Society for Aging and Physical Activity, and by government. This need, and the level of skill, increase with frailer participants and multiple pathology. Opportunities for health professionals and fitness professionals to acquire these specialist skills and to have them recognized by the award of academically validated qualifications are increasing.[66,76] Referrers, employers, and participants alike must insist on them.

Recommendations for safe, successful exercise sessions for elderly people

For teachers

- Emphasize posture and technique
- Give more coaching points and repeat more often
- Give earlier warning of directional and step changes
- Break moves and instructions down into step-by-step stages
- Allow longer times for transitions
- Improve own demonstration and communication skills
- Improve own observation, analytical, and correction skills
- Improve own monitoring skills and self-monitoring skills of participants
- Have adaptations/alternatives for all exercises to cater for all functional levels
- Ensure variety
- Integrate information to educate and motivate
- Be polished, patient, punctual, and persistent

For programming

- Include older people in planning, staffing, evaluation, and promotional material
- Ensure effective pre-exercise assessment prior to participation
- Aim to include an individual functional assessment
- Offer progressive, multilevel, multiactivity programs
- Ensure facilities meet health and safety and comfort requirements
- Keep registers, follow up absence, and offer telephone support
- Schedule socialization and individual feedback
- Provide and monitor a home exercise program
- Encourage an education program

On the other hand, the necessary change in elderly people's exercise habits will not be achieved if it depends on exercise supervision by a relatively small group of specialist teachers. There just cannot be enough of them. Instead, the specialist teachers' role is evolving into the conduct of "introduction to exercise" groups and the supervision of very highly specialized groups for people with particularly severe disability or disease. Most older people are going to have to take responsibility for *maintaining* their increased level of habitual physical activity. An important development to support them has been the collaboration of professional physical training bodies with age agencies to train lay seniors as "peer mentors" and "exercise buddies."

Changing exercise behavior

In an experimental setting, even a deeply engrained, multifactorial habit, such as customary physical activity, can be changed.[77] It is less clear whether this holds true for elderly people in more realistic settings. There are a few promising early indications.[78,79] Older people once engaged have particularly good adherence rates.[80,81] Telephone support may be helpful in maintaining adherence.[82]

Despite legitimate concerns about over-medicalizing recreational activities, situating the initial induction sessions in a familiar and convenient healthcare setting, such as a primary care waiting room, assists confidence in exercise participation for some frail older patients with poor self-efficacy.[83] The frailer the individual, the greater the attention given to the transition to a more recreational, community setting.[65,84]

Measuring changes in habitual physical activity Adequate evaluation of strategies to promote physical activity requires a suitable method for the objective measurement of the duration and intensity of episodes of increased activity. Diaries and recall are insufficient. Movement monitors have been used, but may be insensitive to changes in the intensity of exercise. Twenty-four-hour recordings of heart rate have also been used, as a proxy for oxygen consumption; but it is not possible to identify which episodes of tachycardia are due to emotion or to intensive use of small muscle groups and which (the important ones) are due to the intensive use of large muscle groups. Perhaps a combination of the two approaches will prove suitable, although applicable only to small numbers of people.

Cost

A demedicalized, population-based strategy for the promotion of physical activity, perhaps with an emphasis on walking as the core activity, will avoid excessive costs. There need be no equipment or clothing costs. Nevertheless, adherence will depend on the individual participant finding the activity enjoyable. For many this will mean the use of leisure center facilities, at a cost. Those who wish to join an exercise group with a skilled teacher will have to pay. There may be medical costs associated with the management of soft-tissue injuries.

On the benefit side of the balance, it is hard to know what value to put on subjective well-being, but reasoned estimates can be made of the savings to be expected from reductions in disease, disability, and dependence. Although the estimates are rather vague, exercise promotion among those below retirement age is clearly a "good buy."[85-87] The economic "bottom line" for promoting physical activity among older people also seems encouraging.[88] For example, individualized, home-based exercise programs for people aged 75+ or 80+ cost a mere £500 per fall prevented (1998 prices), even before taking account of hospital costs averted.[82,89]

The optimal time for implementation

All the evidence to date is that the fitness of elderly people is just as trainable, in relative terms, as that of younger people. The message is simple: it's never too late for potentially beneficial physiological adaptations in response to increased physical activity.

The crucial question is: At what stage in life are people most open to advice about changes in exercise behavior? We still need to know a great deal more about the factors (such as beliefs, attitudes, expected benefits, self-efficacy, educational level) that might influence receptiveness of elderly people to such advice.[81] Nevertheless, it is appealing to suppose that future generations of seniors will find it easier to become, or remain, physically active in later life if they have been equipped with a suitably broad-based, multiactivity, physical "literacy" during childhood. Real change requires recognition that, throughout life, physical activity is normal and physical inactivity is abnormal.

Acknowledgments

Ms Dinan gratefully acknowledges valuable discussions and experience with her colleagues in the Royal Free & University College Medical School (Primary Care for Older People project), the Royal Free Hospital ("Bone Wise" and "Balance Wise" programmes, and Old Age Psychiatry Exercise Practitioner service), Merton, Sutton & Wandsworth Health Authority (Falls Prevention Programme), the Department of Health, the British Heart Foundation Centre for Physical Activity and Health, Leicester College, and Age Concern.

Summary management algorithm

Exercise promotion with an elderly person

- If the person is healthy and experienced—recommend a gradual increase in daily walking or other light/moderate intensity activities.

- If the person is likely to need guidance, supervision, instruction, or motivation—refer to an exercise professional.

- If the person is frail or otherwise vulnerable—refer to a specialist exercise professional.

- *If not referring*, the health professional should educate the person to recognize promptly any adverse symptoms, and should monitor and review.

- *If referring*, the health professional should additionally identify and transfer all relevant clinical information, and maintain dialogue with the exercise professional.

- The exercise professional should combine the clinical information with a personal professional assessment to ensure safe, effective exercise.

- The exercise professional should continue to evaluate the person's progress and changing needs and maintain dialogue with the referrer.

- The participant should agree to participate, to follow advice, and to maintain communication with referrer and exercise professional.

KEY POINTS   Physical activity to promote health

- Physical activity is normal, physical inactivity is abnormal.

- The health benefits of suitably adapted physical activity greatly outweigh potential hazards. Those at greatest risk of an adverse event are often those with most to gain.

- A quality-assured exercise referral system offers access to appropriate specialist exercise skills. This requires a unified, multidimensional, intersectoral strategy.

- The reliable transfer of relevant information is essential for effective referral and pre-exercise assessment. The purpose of pre-exercise assessment is to enable, not to exclude.

- The health professional can be a powerful motivating influence.

- It's never too late.

REFERENCES

1. World Health Organization: Constitution of the World Health Organization: Annexe 1. The First Ten Years. WHO, Geneva, 1958

2. Cohen DR, Henderson JB (eds): Health, Prevention and Economics. Oxford University Press, Oxford, 1988

3. Kennie DC: Preventive Care for Elderly People. Cambridge University Press, Cambridge, 1993

4. Scottish Intercollegiate Guidelines Network: Hypertension in Older People. Royal College of Physicians, Edinburgh, 2001

5. Hamilton VH, Racicot FE, Zowall H, Coupal L, Grover SA: The cost effectiveness of HMG-CoA reductase inhibitors to prevent coronary heart disease: estimating the benefits of decreasing HDL-C. JAMA 1995;273:1032–1038

6. McCormack J, Greenhalgh T: Seeing what you want to see in randomised controlled trials: versions and perversions of UKPDS data. United Kingdom Prospective Diabetes Study. BMJ 2000;320:1720–1723

7. Adler AI, Stratton IM, Neil HA: Association of systolic blood pressure with macrovascular and microvascular complications of type 2 diabetes (UKPDS36): prospective observational study. BMJ 2000;321:412–419

8. Carman WF, Elder AG, Wallace LA et al: Effects of influenza vaccination of health-care workers on mortality of elderly people in long-term care: a randomised controlled trial. Lancet 2000;355:93–97

9. Cohen RA, Van Nostrand JF: Trends in the health of older Americans: US National Center for Health Statistics 1994. Vital Health Stat 1995;3(30)

10. Hart D, Bowling A, Ellis M, Silman A: Locomotor disability in very elderly people: value of a programme for screening and provision of aids for daily living. BMJ 1990;301:216–220

11. Sager MA, Franke T, Inouye SK et al: Functional outcomes of acute medical illness and hospitalization in older persons. Arch Intern Med 1996;156:645–652

12. Landefeld CS, Palmer RM, Kresevic DM, Fortinsky RH, Kowal J: A randomized trial of care in a hospital medical unit especially designed to improve the functional outcomes of acutely ill older patients. N Engl J Med 1995;332:1338–1344

13. Evans JG: A framework for promoting mobility and independence. In Towards a Framework for Promoting the Health of Older People. Four Perspectives of the Multiperspective Framework: Workshop Papers. Health Education Authority, London, 1996:1–9

14. Vitaliano PP, Young HM, Russo J: Burden: a review of measures used among caregivers of individuals with dementia. Gerontologist 1991;31:67–75

15. Knight BG, Lutzky SM, Macofsky-Urban F: A meta-analytic review of interventions for caregiver distress: recommendations for future research. Gerontologist 1993;33:240–248

16. Teale C: Caring for older people: money problems and financial help. BMJ 1996;313:288–290

17. House JS, Kessler RC, Herzog AR: Age, socioeconomic status and health. Milbank Q 1990;68:383–411

18. Pathak DR, Samet JM, Humble CG, Skipper BJ: Determinants of lung cancer risk in cigarette smokers in New Mexico. J Natl Cancer Inst 1986;76:597–604

19. Colsher PL, Wallace RB, Pomrehn PR et al: Demographic and health characteristics of elderly smokers: results from established populations for epidemiologic studies of the elderly. Am J Prev Med 1990;6:61–70

20. Vetter NJ, Ford D: Smoking prevention among people aged 60 and over: a randomized controlled trial. Age Ageing 1990;19:164–168

21. Orleans CT, Resch N, Noll E et al: Use of transdermal nicotine in a state-level prescription plan for the elderly: a first look at "real-world" patch users. JAMA 1994;271:601–607

22. Maguire CP, Ryan J, Kelly A, O'Neill D, Coakley D, Walsh JB: Do patient age and medical condition influence medical advice to stop smoking? Age Ageing 2000;29:264–266

23. Cummings SR, Rubin SM, Oster G: The cost-effectiveness of counseling smokers to quit. JAMA 1989;261:75–79

24. Morley JE, Silver AJ: Nutritional issues in nursing home care. Ann Intern Med 1995;123:850–859

25. Anonymous: Malnourished inpatients: overlooked and undertreated. Drug Therapeut Bull 1996;34:57–60

26. Mason JB, Levesque T: Folate: effects on carcinogenesis and the potential for cancer chemoprevention. Oncology 1996;10:1727–1736, 1742–1743

27. Selhub J, Jacques PF, Wilson PW, Rush D, Rosenberg IH: Vitamin status and intake as primary determinants of homocysteinemia in an elderly population. JAMA 1993;270:2693–2698

28. Young A: The health benefits of physical activity for a healthier old age. In Young A, Harries M (eds): Physical Activity for Patients: An Exercise Prescription. Royal College of Physicians of London, 2001:31–42

29. Christiansen D: Dignity in ageing: notes on geriatric ethics. J Humanist Psych 1978;18:41–54

30. Russell LB: Is Prevention Better than Cure? Brookings Institution, Washington, DC, 1986

31. Welch HG, Albertsen PC, Nease RF, Bubolz TA, Wasson JH: Estimating treatment benefits for the elderly: the effect of competing risks. Ann Intern Med 1996;124:577–584

32. Casperson CJ, Powell KE, Merritt RK: Measurement of health status and well-being. In Bouchard C, Shephard RJ, Stephens T (eds): Physical Activity, Fitness, and Health: International Proceedings and Consensus Statement. Human Kinetics, Champaign, IL, 1994:180–202

33. Skelton DA, Greig CA, Davies JM, Young A: Strength, power and related functional ability of healthy people aged 65–89 years. Age Ageing 1994;23:371–377

34. Aniansson A, Grimby G, Hedberg M: Compensatory muscle fibre hypertrophy in elderly men. J Appl Physiol 1992;73:812–816

35. Klitgaard H, Mantoni M, Schiafino S et al: Function, morphology and protein expression of ageing skeletal muscle: a cross-sectional study of elderly men with different training backgrounds. Acta Physiol Scand 1990;140:41–54

36. Harridge SDR, Young A: Skeletal muscle. In Pathy MSJ (ed): Principles and Practice of Geriatric Medicine, 3rd edn. John Wiley, London, 1997

37. Asmussen E: Ageing and exercise. In Horvath SM, Yousef MK (eds): Environmental Physiology: Ageing, Heat and Altitude. Elsevier North-Holland, Amsterdam, 1980:419–428

38. Lakatta EG: Hemodynamic adaptations to stress with advancing age. Acta Med Scand 1986;(suppl 711):39–52

39. Young A: Exercise physiology in geriatric practice. Acta Med Scand 1986;(suppl 711):227–232

40. Buchner DM, Larson EB, Wagner EH et al: Evidence for a non-linear relationship between leg strength and gait speed. Age Ageing 1996;25:386–391

41. Skelton D, Young A, Walker A, Hoinville E: Physical Activity in Later Life: Further Analysis of the Allied Dunbar National Fitness Survey and the Health Education Authority National Survey of Activity and Health. Health Education Authority, London, 1999

42. Young A: Exercise, fitness and recovery from surgery, disease, or infection. In Bouchard C, Shephard RJ, Stephens T et al (eds): Exercise, Fitness and Health: A Consensus of Current Knowledge. Human Kinetics, Champaign, IL, 1990:589–600

43. Badley EM, Wagstaff S, Wood PHN: Measures of functional ability (disability) in arthritis in relation to impairment of range of joint movement. Ann Rheum Dis 1984;43:563–569

44. Mockett S, Doherty M: The health benefits of physical activity for patients with osteoarthritis. In Young A, Harries M (eds): Physical Activity for Patients: An Exercise Prescription. Royal College of Physicians of London, 2001:7–16

45. Chodzko-Zajko W, Moore KA: Physical fitness and cognitive functioning in ageing. Exerc Sport Sci Rev 1994;22:195–220

46. Netz Y, Jacob T: Exercise and the psychological state of institutionalized elderly: a review. Percept Motor Skills 1994;79:1107–1118

47. Williams P, Lord SR: Effects of group exercise on cognitive functioning and mood in older women. Austr NZ J Pub Health 1997;21:45–52

48. Kramer AF, Hahn S, Cohen NJ et al: Ageing, fitness and neurocognitive function. Nature 1999;400:418–419

49. Powell KE, Blair SN: The public health burdens of sedentary living habits: theoretical but realistic estimates. Med Sci Sports Exerc 1994;26:851–856

50. Pate RR, Pratt M, Blair SN et al: Physical activity and public health: a recommendation from the Centers for Disease Control and Prevention and the American College of Sports Medicine. JAMA 1995;273:402–407

51. Blair SN, Franks AL, Shelton et al (eds): Physical Activity and Health: A Report of the Surgeon General. US Department of Health and Human Services, Centers for Disease Control and Prevention, National Center for Chronic Disease Prevention and Health Promotion, Atlanta, 1996

52. Young A, Harries M. (eds): Physical Activity for Patients: An Exercise Prescription. Royal College of Physicians of London, 2001

53. Feigenbaum MS, Pollock ML: Prescription of resistance training for health and disease. Med Sci Sports Exerc 1998;31:38–45

54. Skelton DA, Young A, Greig CA, Malbut KE: Effects of resistance training on strength, power, and selected functional abilities of women aged 75 and older. J Am Geriatr Soc 1995;43:1081–1087

55. Aniansson A, Gustafsson E: Physical training in elderly men with special reference to quadriceps muscle strength and morphology. Clin Physiol 1981;1:87–98

56. Fiatarone MA, O'Neill EF, Ryan ND et al: Exercise training and nutritional supplementation for physical frailty in very elderly people. N Engl J Med 1994;330:1769–1775

57. McMurdo MET, Rennie LM: Improvements in quadriceps strength with regular seated exercise in the institutionalised elderly. Arch Phys Med Rehabil 1994;75:600–603

58. Sherrington C, Lord SR: Home exercise to improve strength and walking velocity after hip fracture: a randomized controlled trial. Arch Phys Med Rehabil 1999;78:208–212

59. Mitchell SL, Stott DJ, Martin BJ, Grant SJ: Randomized controlled trial of quadriceps training after proximal femoral fracture. Clin Rehabil 2001;15:282–290

60. Hauer K, Rost B, Rutschle K et al: Exercise training for rehabilitation and secondary prevention of falls in geriatric patients with a history of injurious falls. J Am Geriatr Soc 2001;49:10–20

61. Skelton DA, McLaughlin AW: Training functional ability in old age. Physiotherapy 1996;82:159–167

62. Malbut KE, Dinan S, Young A: Aerobic training in the "oldest old": the effect of 24 weeks of training. Age Ageing 2002;31:255–260

63. American Geriatrics Society, British Geriatrics Society and American Academy of Orthopaedic Surgeons Panel on Falls Prevention: Guideline for the prevention of falls in older persons. J Am Geriatr Soc 2001;49:664–672

64. Gillespie LD, Gillespie WJ, Robertson MC, Lamb SE, Cumming RG, Rowe BH: Interventions for preventing falls in elderly people. Cochrane Database Syst Rev 2001;3:1–129

65. Dinan S: Delivering an exercise prescription for vulnerable older patients. In Young A, Harries M (eds): Physical Activity for Patients: An Exercise Prescription. Royal College of Physicians of London, 2001:53–70

66. UK Department of Health: Exercise Referral Systems—A National Quality Assurance Framework. Stationery Office, London, 2001

67. Durstine JL, Bloomquist LE, Figoni SF, Moore GE, Painter P, Pitetti KH, Pope CJ, Roberts SO (eds): ACSM's Exercise Management for Persons with Chronic Diseases and Disabilities. Human Kinetics, Champaign, IL, 1997

68. American Geriatrics Society Panel on Exercise and Osteoarthritis: Exercise prescription for older adults with osteoarthritis pain: consensus practice recommendations. J Am Geriatr Soc 2001;49:808–823

69. Haskell WL: Medical clearance for exercise program participation by older persons: the clinical versus the public health approach. In Huber G (ed): Healthy Ageing, Activity and Sports. Health Promotion Publications, Gamburg. 1997:192–204

70. Bell JM, Bassey EJ: Postexercise heart rates and pulse palpation as a means of determining exercising intensity in an aerobic dance class. Br J Sports Med 1996;30:48–52

71. Malbut KE, Dinan SM, Verhaar H, Young A: Maximal oxygen uptake in 80-year-old men. Clin Sci 1995;89(suppl 33):31P (abstract)

72. Cotes JE: The ventilatory cost of activity. Br J Ind Med 1975;32:220–223

73. Doust JH, Patrick JM: The limitation of exercise ventilation during speech. Resp Physiol 1981;46:137–147

74. Borg GAV: Borg's Perceived Exertion and Pain Scales. Champaign, IL, Blackwell Science, 1995

75. Burdon JGW, Juniper EF, Killian KJ et al: The perception of breathlessness in asthma. Am Rev Resp Dis 1982;126:825–828

76. Laventure B: The future: the clinical exercise practitioner. In Young A, Harries M (eds): Physical Activity for Patients: An Exercise Prescription. Royal College of Physicians of London, 2001:119–127

77. Dishman RK, Buckworth J: Increasing physical activity: a quantitative synthesis. Med Sci Sports Exerc 1996;28:706–719

78. Frändin K, Johannesson K, Grimby G: Physical activity as part of an intervention program for elderly persons in Göteborg. Scand J Med Sci Sports 1992;2:218–224

79. Hillsdon M, Thorogood M: A systematic review of physical activity promotion strategies. Br J Sports Med 1996;30:84–89

80. Iliffe S, See Tai S, Gould M, Smith P: Delivering an exercise prescription for patients in primary care. In Young A, Harries M (eds): Physical Activity for Patients: An Exercise Prescription. College of Physicians of London, 2001:43–51

81. Martin KA, Sinden AR: Who will stay and who will go? A review of older adults' adherence to randomized controlled trials of exercise. J Aging Phys Activ 2001;9:91–114

82. Robertson MC, Devlin N, Gardner MM, Campbell AJ: Effectiveness and economic evaluation of a nurse-delivered home exercise programme to prevent falls. 1: Randomised controlled trial. BMJ 2001;322:697–701

83. Gargaro G, Lenihan P, Iliffe S: Targetting at-risk elderly groups in an inner-city general practice. Commun Pract 2000;73:757–759

84. Clark CJ, Sword D, Cochrane LM: Delivering an exercise prescription for patients with chronic obstructive pulmonary disease. In Young A, Harries M (eds): Physical Activity for Patients: An Exercise Prescription. Royal College of Physicians of London, 2001:83–89

85. Morris JN: Exercise in the prevention of coronary heart disease: today's best buy in public health. Med Sci Sports Exerc 1994;26:807–814

86. Kaman RL, Patton RW: Costs and benefits of an active versus an inactive society. In Bouchard C, Shephard RJ, Stephens T (eds): Physical Activity, Fitness, and Health. Human Kinetics, Champaign, IL, 1994:134–144

87. Shephard RJ: Costs and benefits of an exercising versus a nonexercising society. In Bouchard C, Shephard RJ, Stephens T (eds): Exercise, Fitness, and Health. Human Kinetics, Champaign, IL, 1990:49–60

88. Shephard RJ: Ageing, Physical Activity, and Health. Human Kinetics, Champaign, IL, 1997:370–373

89. Robertson MC, Gardner MM, Devlin N, McGee R, Campbell AJ: Effectiveness and economic evaluation of a nurse-delivered home exercise programme to prevent falls. 2: Controlled trial in multiple centres. BMJ 2001;322:701–704

Chapter 20

Preventive and anticipatory care

James T. Pacala

As illnesses and adverse conditions become more prevalent with advancing age, the opportunity for prevention becomes increasingly important in elderly people. Preventive activities can be divided into five broad categories: prevention of diseases, prevention of frailty, prevention of accidents, prevention of iatrogenic problems, and prevention of psychosocial illnesses. Disease prevention practices are designed to:

- prevent illnesses from occurring in the first place (primary prevention);
- detect and treat disease at an early stage, thereby minimizing the morbidity and mortality caused by that disease (secondary prevention);
- optimize treatment of existing conditions, usually chronic illnesses, to prevent adverse sequelae from these diseases (tertiary prevention).

The accumulation of chronic diseases and adverse conditions with aging often leads to severely threatened or outright loss of function, widely known as "frailty"; efforts to prevent this often common end-point are particularly pertinent in the older adult population. Elderly people are particularly prone to injuries from accidents, constituting another area of opportunity for preventive efforts. It is well established that medical care itself has a propensity to cause harm which is increased with aging, indicating a need for prevention of iatrogenic problems, particularly among those who are frail. Finally, psychosocial illnesses also commonly pose a threat to functioning in older adults, and prevention of these illnesses is gaining increasing attention.

Not all elderly people stand to benefit equally from each type of preventive activity. They exhibit a great range of health and functional status, from highly functioning persons who are free of disease and injury to those who are frail and totally functionally dependent. Different types of preventive activities will have different yields, depending in part on the baseline health and functioning of the person. To maximize efficiency and patient benefit, individualizing prevention by devoting time and resources towards those activities which are most likely to prevent morbidity and mortality given the status of the older adult patient seems warranted.

This chapter describes strategies for each type of preventive activity. Then, a scheme for prioritizing those activities by patient status is presented.

DISEASE PREVENTION
Primary and secondary disease prevention

Primary and secondary disease prevention encompasses several activities. *Screening* refers to activities that detect a previously unknown condition in asymptomatic individuals. Detected risk factors are then altered, and through lowering of risk, the target disease is primarily prevented. Diseases discovered in their early stages are treated, thereby secondarily preventing more severe manifestation of advanced disease. *Immunoprophylaxis* prevents significant illnesses through vaccination. *Counseling* promotes lowering of disease risk through behavioral change. Improving disease risk by administering medications is known as *chemoprophylaxis*.

Both the US Preventive Services Task Force (USPSTF)[1] and the Canadian Task Force on the Periodic Health Examination (CTFPHE)[2] have rigorously reviewed a wide variety of primary and secondary prevention practices. Preventive services for elderly people that are recommended by the organizations, with selected additions based on recent evidence, are shown in Table 20-1. Table 20-2 lists activities currently not recommended by either USPSTF or CTFPHE, but which have been endorsed by other specialty organizations. The preventive efficacy of the procedures in Table 20-2 is not well established; as such, they might be considered more selectively in elderly people.

Tertiary disease prevention

As some elderly people age, they accumulate chronic illnesses that pose a threat to their functioning and quality of life. Although chronic illnesses by definition cannot be cured, proper management of these diseases can prevent further disease-induced functional loss. Chronic diseases which commonly lead to morbidity and mortality in the older population include the following.

- *Arthritis.* Osteoarthritis and rheumatoid arthritis affect about a half of all people aged 65 and over, and lead to mobility impairment, which in turn increases the risk for numerous other conditions—osteoporosis, deconditioning, and bedsores to name a few.[3] Therefore, aggressive management of arthritis through medication and exercise is indicated. (See Chapter 71 on arthritis.)

Table 20-1 Recommended disease prevention activities[a]

Type of activity	Disease to be prevented/detected	Activity	Frequency
Screening	Hypertension	Blood pressure measurement	At least yearly
	Obesity, malnutrition	Height and weight measurement	At least yearly
	Breast cancer	Mammography	Every 1–2 years[b]
	Cervical, uterine cancer	Pap smear	At least every 3 years[c]
	Colon cancer	Fecal occult blood testing (FOBT); sigmoidoscopy; colonoscopy	FOBT; yearly Sigmoidoscopy: every 3–5 years Colonoscopy: once
	Coronary artery disease	Serum lipid measurement yearly for persons with prior myocardial infarction, angina, or diabetes mellitus	every 5 years for primary prevention
	Hearing deficit	Hearing test	Yearly
	Visual deficit	Vision test	Yearly
	Alcoholism	Alcoholism screening questionnaire	At initial visit and when problem drinking is suspected
Immunoprophylaxis	Influenza	'Flu shot	Yearly
	Pneumococcal disease	Pneumovax vaccination	Once at age 65
	Tetanus	Tetanus booster	Every 10 years
Counseling	Cardiopulmonary disease, several cancers	Smoking cessation	At every visit of patients who smoke
	Obesity, coronary artery disease	Low fat diet	Yearly
	Osteoporosis	Adequate calcium intake; hormone replacement discussion	At menopause; at least once thereafter
	Coronary artery disease, osteoporosis	Exercise counseling	Yearly
	Malnutrition, tooth decay, oral cancers	Encourage visits to the dentist	Yearly

[a]As endorsed by the US Preventive Services Task Force and/or the Canadian Task Force on the Periodic Health Examination, with selected modifications based on recent evidence.

[b]Should be continued past age 70 in women who have a reasonable life expectancy.

[c]Stop at age 65 if regularly tested throughout adult life and there were no positive results; if never tested, can stop after two normal pap smears one year apart.

- *Diabetes.* Older adults exhibit significantly increased risk of retinopathy, nephropathy, and coronary disease when glycohemoglobin (HgbA1C) fractions exceed 7.9 percent.[4] Clinicians should attempt to achieve HgbA1C concentrations at least below 8 percent in diabetic patients, and even lower in those who are not frail. Aggressive prevention of foot ulcers should also be undertaken through patient education and foot exams at each visit. (See Chapter 96 on diabetes.)

- *Vascular disease.* Patients with prior history of coronary, cerebral, or peripheral arterial disease are at markedly increased risk of a disabling event. There is good evidence that treatment of vascular risk factors in older adults with prior myocardial infarction (MI), angina, prior stroke, or claudication significantly reduces the risk of a subsequent MI, stroke, or limb loss.[5] The risk factors include hypertension, smoking, diabetes, atrial fibrillation, and dyslipidemia. (See Chapters 34, 49, and 38 on coronary, cerebral, and peripheral vascular disease.)

- *Congestive heart failure* (CHF). CHF accounts for a great deal of suffering in elderly people and has a higher mortality than many forms of cancer. Proper and aggressive treatment of CHF, especially systolic dysfunction, has been shown to reduce hospitalization rates, functional decline, and even mortality.[6,7] (See Chapter 33 on CHF.)

- *Osteoporosis.* With the availability (and Medicare coverage in the USA) of bone density measurement, osteoporosis can now be detected before a disabling fracture. Treatment of osteoporosis, both in patients with and without prior fracture, has been shown to prevent new fractures. (See Chapter 70 on osteoporosis.)[8,9]

Tertiary prevention is accomplished through disease management. Aiding chronic disease management is the development of expert guidelines and practice-based protocols for specific illnesses, such as the series published by the Agency For Health Care Policy and Research. A disease-specific case management program can also be a powerful intervention for tertiary prevention, frequently employing a specially trained nurse to coordinate protocol-driven care, arrange support services, and provide patient education. The Cooperative Health Care Clinic model, in which groups of patients with the

Table 20-2 **Additional disease prevention activities which may be applicable to selected elderly people**

Type of activity	Disease to be prevented/detected	Activity and frequency	Comment
Screening	Diabetic complications	Blood glucose testing Every 1–3 years	Some experts recommend screening obese persons
	Prostate cancer	Digital rectal exam and/or prostate specific antigen testing Yearly	Effective for early detection, but efficacy for preventing prostate cancer death is unknown (randomized trials in progress)
	Dementia, delirium	Mental status testing Yearly	May grow in importance if early treatment of dementia is shown to change outcomes
	Osteoporosis	Bone density measurement Once after age 65; serial measurements may be useful for determining future risk	Expensive; commonly recommended in asymptomatic women with several osteoporosis risk factors, or in women and men with chronic glucocorticoid use
	Skin cancer	Skin exam Yearly	Treatment of false positives has low morbidity
	Hypothyroidism	Thyrotropin measurement Yearly	Some experts recommend screening women
Chemoprophylaxis	Coronary artery disease, stroke, colon cancer	Aspirin therapy 81–325 mg q.d. p.o.	Inexpensive; few side-effects

same chronic illness receive group teaching coupled with nurse and physician visits, has shown promise as an effective method of managing chronic illness.[10] Finally, specialty referral for management of patients whose chronic illness is particularly difficult to stabilize can accomplish better outcomes, especially when the specialist and primary care physician work collaboratively. See Chapter 120 for more information regarding implementation of disease management programs in health systems.

PREVENTION OF FRAILTY

Aside from preventing individual diseases, the larger question remains of whether or not their frequent end-point—frailty—can be prevented. Frailty refers to a condition where loss of physiological reserve makes the afflicted individual particularly susceptible to disability from minor stresses.[11] Frail individuals commonly exhibit significant functional deficits, weakness, muscle wasting, deconditioning, frequent falls, and incontinence. Control of a chronic condition becomes labile, resulting in frequent functional decompensation and hospitalization.

Can frailty be prevented? Data from long-term cohort studies are beginning to accumulate which suggest that it can, primarily through exercise and proper nutrition. Healthy adults who exercise are at lower risk of becoming frail, and functionally impaired older adults who exercise are less likely to experience further functional loss. To be most effective, an exercise program should include the following components.[12]

- *Aerobic conditioning*—at least 20 minutes of activity at 50–75 percent of maximum heart rate three times per week. Brisk walking is an activity which many older adults can perform for aerobic conditioning.

- *Weight (resistance) training*—three sets of 8–15 repetitions at least twice a week.
- *Flexibility*—at least 15 seconds of static stretching per muscle group daily.
- *Balance*—activities such as dance and Tai Chi which have shown promise in helping older adults maintain good balance.

Proper nutrition is important for prevention of many conditions contributing to frailty, including certain forms of cancer, osteoporosis, obesity, and malnutrition. Studies have consistently shown less morbidity and mortality in those who eat diets featuring:

- *Low fat*—less than 30 percent of total calories, with no more than 10 percent coming from saturated fats.[13]
- *Low sodium*—a 3 gram sodium diet is recommended but difficult to maintain; a 4–5 gram sodium diet is a more reasonable goal in most older adults.[14,15]
- *High calcium*—older adults need 1200 mg of calcium per day; most American diets contain only 500–700 mg per day. Calcium supplementation should be provided if the diet contains less than 1200 mg per day.[16]
- *Adequate vitamins and minerals*—ensured largely through eating fruits and vegetables. Some experts recommend supplementation with vitamin D (400–700 IU/day) for bone health, folate (at least 200 μg/d) to keep homocysteine levels low, and the use of vitamin E (200–400 IU/d) and selenium (200 μg/d) for their antioxidant effects.[13,16]
- *High fiber*—best obtained from eating fruits, vegetables, and grains.[13]
- *Moderate alcohol intake*—about 1–2 ounces of alcohol per day can actually promote health; more can be harmful.[17]

PREVENTION OF ACCIDENTS

Falls constitute a significant risk in older adults. Falls prevention programs (see Chapter 105 on falls) can be implemented for those who are at high risk of a fall or who have already fallen.

Slowed reaction time, sensory deficits, dementia, and a host of other age-associated conditions place elderly people at higher risk of injuring themselves and others while driving. Correction of these conditions whenever possible and routine driving tests can minimize risks. All older adults should be reminded to use seat belts when traveling in an automobile. Cessation of driving poses a great threat to the autonomy of older persons, so addressing the driving ability of the geriatric patient should be undertaken with great care and sensitivity.

Household environments can also present a variety of accident hazards. For example, persons with peripheral neuro-pathy are at increased risk of burns from excessively hot water; setting the hot water temperature at less than 120–130°F can obviate this problem. Harm from fires can be reduced by the use of smoke detectors. Demented persons face many accident risks in the home, especially when operating electrical and gas appliances; the use of alarms and automatic shutoff features can be effective in these instances. A *home safety checklist* can be completed by patients or their caregivers to assess environmental hazards which could lead to an injurious fall. Many physical and occupational therapy (PT/OT) departments perform home visits for accident risk assessment. For elderly people who are particularly vulnerable to injury, PT/OT consultation can be extremely helpful in reducing their accident risk.

PREVENTION OF IATROGENIC PROBLEMS

Several age-associated factors place elderly people at increased risk of iatrogenic problems. As physiological reserve progressively decreases, the margin for clinical error gets smaller, thereby increasing the risk of an adverse effect of a medical intervention. Older adults who accumulate chronic diseases also accumulate medical providers, often resulting in a lack of care coordination. Having multiple providers frequently leads to polypharmacy. Elderly people are hospitalized more than younger persons; hospitalization presents a host of iatrogenic risks, such as nosocomial infection, polypharmacy, transfusion reactions, and so on.[18]

In addition to the above factors, the explosion of advances in medical technology has presented further opportunity for iatrogenic illness. Technological interventions such as cardiopulmonary resuscitation (CPR), valvular replacement surgery, carotid endarterectomy, combination intravenous antibiotics, and artificial feeding tubes have dramatically increased the therapeutic options during life-threatening illnesses. While their positive effects are often lifesaving, the potential adverse effects of these interventions are usually severe, such as brain damage from CPR, sudden death or MI from valvular replacement surgery, stroke from carotid endarterectomy, fluid overload from combination IV antibiotics, and unwanted prolonged life from feeding tubes.

Compared with younger persons, older adults more often experience these untoward outcomes. When elderly people confront critical illnesses, the decision of whether or not to undergo high-risk, potentially lifesaving interventions must be faced. Unfortunately, research has shown that physicians are frequently unaware of patients' preferences for aggressive care and often do not discuss these issues with patients.[19,20] The morbidity experienced from a medical or surgical procedure that was not wanted in the first place is thus iatrogenic.

The first step in preventing iatrogenic problems is to recognize which patients are the most vulnerable to adverse effects of medical care. Patients most susceptible to iatrogenic problems are those who have *multiple chronic illnesses*, see *multiple physicians*, and take *multiple medications*. There is a direct correlation between the number of chronic illnesses and the chances that treatment of one illness will adversely affect the other. Persons with multiple chronic illnesses frequently see multiple physicians. It is very difficult for numerous providers to consult with each other every time they see a common patient. As a result, changes in a patient's therapeutic regimen are frequently made without the input of other providers, often increasing the risk of iatrogenesis. Chronically ill and frail people also take numerous medications. The average elderly person takes two to three times the prescription and over-the-counter medicines than a younger person. Higher rates of drug use and chronic illness lead to a markedly increased risk of drug–drug or drug–disease adverse interactions. This risk of polypharmacy is particularly increased in patients who are malnourished or who have renal failure.

One other significant risk factor for iatrogenic problems is hospitalization. Acutely ill older adults are at increased risk of treatment-related delirium, adverse drug reactions, pressure sores, and nosocomial infections. Patients with dementia and/or conditions causing immobility are at particular risk of hospital-induced iatrogenic problems, especially when undergoing surgery.

Once high-risk patients are identified, several interventions can be implemented to prevent iatrogenic complications.

CASE MANAGEMENT   The primary function of a case manager is care coordination. Case managers can be employed by physician groups, parent health plans, and community or governmental organizations. Research has shown that case management is most effective of achieving beneficial outcomes in elderly people who are frail.[21,22] Case managers facilitate communication between providers, ensure that needed services are provided, and avoid duplication of services.

GERIATRIC EVALUATION AND MANAGEMENT   A GEM team can be called upon to evaluate all of the patient's problems simultaneously and formulate a coordinated care plan. This intervention is resource-intensive and should be applied to only the most complex of patients.[23]

PHARMACIST CONSULTATION   A consulting pharmacist can be particularly helpful to prevent complications from polypharmacy.[24]

ACUTE CARE FOR THE ELDERLY UNITS   ACE units are specific wards of a hospital with dedicated staff, all designed to address the special needs of elderly inpatients. As such, these units are in tune with the iatrogenic risks of hospitalization and take specific measures to avoid these complications.[25]

ADVANCED DIRECTIVES Advanced directives, including designation of proxies for medical decision-making, can be helpful in avoiding administration of undesired medical treatments during periods of critical illness when patients are unable to speak for themselves. Research on the effectiveness of advanced directives has been somewhat disappointing, showing that they are rarely completed by patients, occasionally not obeyed by providers, and frequently changed when patients' conditions become dire; interventions designed to increase their effectiveness have been largely unsuccessful.[26] However, designation by the patient of a proxy for medical decision-making can often circumvent many of these limitations.

PREVENTION OF PSYCHOSOCIAL ILLNESSES

Aging is frequently accompanied by loss and isolation. Spouses and close friends become disabled or die; children often move far away from home. Retirement not only brings stoppage of work but also distancing from one's peers. Immobility and other conditions make travel much more difficult. Increasing disability and functional dependence leads to loss of autonomy. Depression, loneliness, family discord, and other psychosocially derived illnesses and conditions can result from these challenges of aging.

Research has shown that older adults with psychosocial illness suffer higher rates of functional dependence and mortality.[27,28] Less well established is whether or not these illnesses can be prevented. The major challenge in psychosocial illness prevention is the fact that the usual major antecedents—death or relocation of loved ones—are essentially not modifiable. Despite this challenge, the preponderance of psychosocial illness and its strong association to morbidity and mortality in older adults warrants concerted preventive efforts.

Depression is common in elderly people. Although major depression leading to suicide attempts and/or hospitalization appears to be less common than in younger persons, depressive symptoms (sometimes called minor or situational depression) can be quite prevalent—over 10 percent.[29] Unfortunately, depression is often unrecognized in primary care practice,[30] prompting the question of whether screening for depression in older adults is indicated. Screening would have a higher yield in patients with depressive risk factors: female, single, positive family history, financial problems, and lack of social supports. Several simple screening instruments have been developed and do not require a physician for administration. Coupling the ease of screening with the availability of effective and safe antidepressants, many clinicians have incorporated depression screening into their practices for older patients.

It is well established that elders with increased social contact experience better health.[31] Clinicians should take a social history from their patients, inquiring about situations of loneliness and isolation. In those who are isolated, efforts to increase social contact can theoretically prevent morbidity and mortality. Senior centers, social clubs, and increased family involvement are potentially effective interventions.

A sense of self-worth has also been linked to health in older adults.[32] Healthy seniors often speak of the importance of feeling needed by someone else. Remaining productive at work or leisure activities is also often cited as a correlate of successful aging. Again, though supporting research has not been performed, interventions such as obtaining a pet, performing volunteer work, contributing to household chores, or any other activity which confirms a sense of social connectedness are potentially effective in preventing psychosocial (and even physical) disability.

INDIVIDUALIZING PREVENTION

Since the elderly population exhibits marked heterogeneity of health status, tailoring preventive efforts to match the condition of the patient would seem indicated. Although a continuum in reality, the health and functional status of elderly people divides the population into three basic groups as shown in Figure 20-1. *Healthy* older adults, comprising the majority of this population, have minimal or no chronic disease and are functionally independent. Those who are *chronically ill* have an accumulation of incurable conditions; these persons usually have no or mild functional impairment, frequently take several prescription medications, and occasionally are hospitalized from exacerbations of chronic illness. *Frail* older adults, the smallest group, typically have numerous and severe chronic illnesses, marked functional dependence, and loss of functional reserve. These persons are frequently hospitalized and institutionalized. Each of these three groups is presented with different threats to its health and functioning, calling for different preventive emphases.

Table 20-3 provides an overview of prevention in the elderly population, matching preventive priorities with patient condition. In healthy older adults, who have yet to experience disease and functional decline, primary and secondary disease prevention as well as frailty prevention should be the focus of health maintenance efforts. In those who are chronically ill, it is most likely that complications from their longstanding

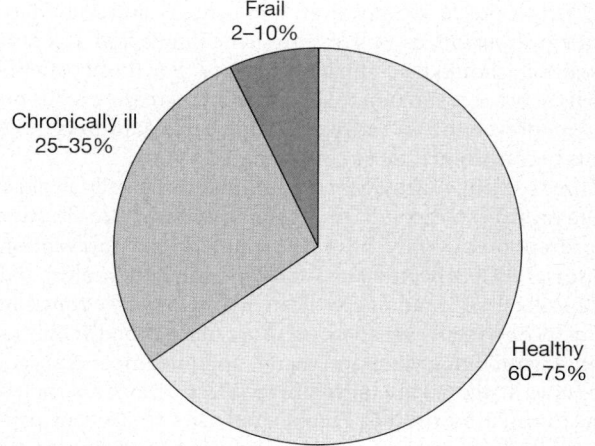

Figure 20-1 A population of elderly people.

Table 20-3 Overview of preventive strategies for elderly people

Activity	Methods	Priority target population
Primary and secondary disease prevention	Screening Immunoprophylaxis Counseling Chemoprophylaxis (see Tables 20-1 and 20-2)	Healthy and functionally independent

Tertiary disease prevention	Disease management of chronic illness:
	    Practice guidelines and protocols
	    Formal disease management programs
	    Cooperative Health Care Clinics
	    Specialty referral
		Chronically ill

Prevention of frailty	Exercise:
	    Aerobic
	    Weight training
	    Flexibility
	    Balance
	Diet
		Healthy and chronically ill who are functionally independent

Prevention of accidents	Falls prevention Driving tests Seat belts Home safety checklist PT/OT referral for environmental assessment	Chronically ill and frail
Prevention of iatrogenic illness	Case management GEM Pharmacist consultation ACE units Advance directives	Chronically ill and frail

Prevention of psychosocial illness	Depression screening
	Increased social contact
	    Senior centers
	    Social clubs
	Increased self-worth
	    Volunteer work
	    Caregiving
	    Pets
		All older adults

illnesses will be the cause of future morbidity and functional decline. Thus, the highest preventive priority for these patients should center around tertiary prevention and frailty prevention. This is not to say, however, that primary and secondary disease prevention, as well as iatrogenic illness and accident prevention, should be completely ignored. For those patients who have become frail, there should be an increasing focus on accident prevention and iatrogenic illness prevention, as these events become much more common.

Three preventive activities are applicable to virtually all older adults regardless of condition. First, exercise can be effective for prevention of frailty, has a role in the primary prevention of diseases such as heart disease and cancer in both healthy and chronically ill older adults, and can help to preserve function and reduce accidents in patients who are frail. Secondly, immunization with influenza shots (yearly) and pneumococcal vaccine (once at age 65) are inexpensive, effective, and associated with minimal morbidity. Finally, activities to prevent psychosocial illness as described in the above section can be applied uniformly across all older adults.

PREVENTIVE PRACTICE SYSTEMS

Provider knowledge of which preventive activities are indicated for the aging population is not sufficient for the appropriate delivery of preventive care. Implementation of an efficient disease prevention and health promotion system in a geriatric practice can be quite challenging. Older patients tend to have more acute care needs, manifested frequently as flare-ups of chronic conditions, the management of which occupies the majority of contact time with providers. Owing to the diverse nature of primary care practices, a "one size fits all" approach to implementing a disease prevention and health promotion program is not advisable. However, research has demonstrated that the following strategies result in greater degrees of successful preventive activities.

USE OF NONPHYSICIAN PERSONNEL Implementation of screening, immunoprophylactic, and counseling prevention activities are all essentially guideline driven and can be very well managed by nurses or other personnel. Research has consistently shown that nonphysicians do a better job of achieving greater compliance with cancer and other disease screening guidelines.[33,34] Nonphysicians can be successfully used for worthwhile but time-consuming counseling and behavioral change activities such as those involved in smoking cessation and dietary weight reduction.[35–37]

USE OF INFORMATION SYSTEMS   Computer reminders to prompt physicians and patients regarding periodic prevention activities have been extremely successful in enhancing preventive care.[38,39] Written checklists and hard-copy flow sheets have limited effectiveness since they are often not filled out.[39,40]

PATIENT AND PROVIDER EDUCATION   Increasing the knowledge and awareness of patients and providers about preventive activities serves to promote such activities in clinical practice. Evidence-based guidelines aid medical personnel in the design of preventive systems.[41,42] Pamphlets, posters, and other education materials can increase the awareness of and demand for preventive activities among patients.

COMMUNITY-WIDE PROMOTION   Healthcare organizations can promote preventive activities through mass mailings, public information, and advertisements such as through billboards and over the Internet to affect a more population-wide increase in prevention interest.[37,43]

CREATION OF INCENTIVES FOR PREVENTION   Reimbursement structures often favor acute care services over preventive services. Realignment of incentives to reward achievement of preventive guidelines can be a powerful intervention to increase disease prevention activities.[44] Changing reimbursement to cover preventive services can also be a strong motivator of change.[45–47] Finally, audit-and-feedback programs to physicians can serve to increase subsequent preventive behaviors.[48,49]

Designing practice-based disease prevention programs necessitates the direct involvement of the practitioners and staff. Working together, physicians and staff should review appropriate prevention literature, decide which disease prevention activities will be emphasized, define barriers to practicing prevention, and design systems which will overcome those barriers.[50]

KEY POINTS   Prevention

- Five categories of conditions can be addressed for prevention: diseases (primary, secondary, and tertiary), frailty, psychosocial illness, injuries, and iatrogenic problems.

- Disease prevention and health promotion must be individually tailored to the elderly person's health status and functional level.

- Successful disease prevention and health promotion care systems usually feature extensive use of nonphysician personnel, computer reminders for periodic preventive activities, educational interventions for both providers and patients, and alignment of incentives to promote preventive activities.

- See also Table 20-3.

REFERENCES

1. US Preventive Services Task Force: Guide to Clinical Preventive Services, 2nd edn. Williams & Wilkins, Baltimore, 1996
2. Canadian Task Force on the Periodic Health Examination: Canadian Guide to Clinical Preventive Health Care. Canadian Communication Group, Ottawa, 1994
3. Ettinger WH, Fried LP, Harris T, et al for the CHS Collaborative Research Group: Self-reported causes of physical disability in older people: the Cardiovascular Health Study. J Am Geriatr Soc 1994;42:1035–1044
4. Gasper B, Hirsch IB: The effects of improved glycemic control on complications in type 2 diabetes. Arch Intern Med 1998;158:134–140
5. Corti MC, Guralnik JM, Bilato C: Coronary heart disease risk factors in older persons. Aging (Milano) 1996;8(2):75–89
6. Rich MW, Beckham V, Wittenberg C et al: A multidisciplinary intervention to prevent the readmission of elderly patients with congestive heart failure. N Engl J Med 1995;333:1190–1195
7. Naylor MD, Brooten D, Campbell R et al: Comprehensive discharge planning and home follow-up of hospitalized elders: a randomized clinical trial. JAMA 1999;281:613–620
8. Ettinger B, Black DM, Mitlak BH et al: Reduction of vertebral fracture risk in postmenopausal women with osteoporosis treated with raloxifene: results from a 3-year randomized clinical trial. JAMA 1999;282:637–645
9. Harris ST, Watts BN, Genant HK et al: Effects of risedronate treatment on vertebral and nonvertebral fractures in women with postmenopausal osteoporosis. JAMA 1999;282:1344–1352
10. Beck A, Scott J, Williams P et al: A randomized trial of group outpatient visits for chronologically ill older HMO members: the Cooperative Health Care Clinic. J Am Geriatr Soc 1997;45:543–549
11. Campbell AJ, Buchner DM: Unstable disability and the fluctuations of frailty. Age Ageing 1997;26:315–318
12. Trajano D, Pacala JT: Prescribing exercise for older adults. Clin Fam Pract 1999;1:321–331
13. Expert Panel on Detection, Evaluation, and Treatment of High Blood Cholesterol in Adults: Executive Summary of the Third Report of the National Cholesterol Education Program (NCEP) Expert Panel on Detection, Evaluation, and Treatment of High Blood cholesterol in Adults (Adult Treatment Panel III). JAMA 2001;285:2486–2497
14. Whelton PK, Appel LJ, Espeland MA et al: Sodium reduction and weight loss in the treatment of hypertension in older persons: a randomized controlled trial of nonpharmacologic interventions in the elderly (TONE). TONE Collaborative Research Group. JAMA 1998;279:839–846
15. Hajjar IM, Grim CE, George V, Kotchen RA: Impact of diet on blood pressure and age-related changes in blood pressure in the US population: analysis of NHANES III. Arch Intern Med 2001;161:589–593
16. NOF: Physicians' Guide to Prevention and Treatment of Osteoporosis. National Osteoporosis Foundation, Washington, DC, 1999
17. Rimm EB, Klatsky A, Grobbee D, Stampfer MJ: Review of moderate alcohol consumption and reduced risk of coronary heart disease: is the effect due to beer, wine or spirits? BMJ 1996;312:731–736
18. Rothschild JM, Bates DW, Leape L: Preventable medical injuries in older patients. Arch Intern Med 2000;160:2717–2728
19. Teno JM, Hakim RB, Knaus WA et al: Preferences for cardiopulmonary resuscitation: physician–patient agreement and hospital resource use. J Gen Intern Med 1995;10:179–186
20. Bedell SE, Delbanco TL: Choices about cardiopulmonary resuscitation in the hospital: when do physicians talk with patients? N Engl J Med 1984;310:1089–1993
21. Burns LR, Lamb GS, Wholey DR: Impact of integrated community nursing services on hospital utilization and costs in a Medicare risk plan. Inquiry 1996;33:30–41
22. Leveille SG, Wagner EH, Davis C et al: Preventing disability and managing chronic illness in frail older adults: a randomized trial of a community-based partnership with primary care. J Am Geriatr Soc 1998;46:1191–1198
23. Boult C, Boult L, Morishita L et al: A randomized clinical trial of outpatient geriatric evaluation and management. J Am Geriatr Soc 2001;49:351–359

24. Follin SL, Kwong NM: Enhancement of a pharmacy consultation program on a transitional care unit. Am J Health Syst Pharm 2000;57:1990–1993

25. Landefeld CS, Palmer RM, Kresevic DM et al: A randomized trial of care in a hospital medical unit especially designed to improve functional outcomes of acutely ill older patients. N Engl J Med 1995;332:1338–1344

26. Hanson LC, Tulsky JA, Danis M: Can clinical interventions change care at the end of life? Ann Intern Med 1997;126:381–388

27. Wells KB, Stewart A, Hays RD et al: The functioning and well-being of depressed patients: results from the Medical Outcome Study. JAMA 1989;262:914–919

28. Spitzer RL, Kroenke K, Linzer M et al: Health-related quality of life in primary care patients with mental disorders: results from the PRIME-MD 1000 Study. JAMA 1995;274:1511–1517

29. Harwood DG, Barker WW, Ownby RL et al: Factors associated with depressive symptoms in non-demented community-dwelling elderly. Int J Geriatr Psychiatry 1999;14:331–337

30. Simon GE, Vonkorff M: Recognition, management, and outcomes of depression in primary care. Arch Fam Med 1995;4:99–105

31. Bosworth HB, Schaie KW: The relationship of social environment, social networks, and health outcomes in the Seattle Longitudinal Study: two analytical approaches. J Gerontol B 1997;52:P197–P205

32. McAnley E, Blissner B, Katula J et al: Physical activity, self-esteem, and self-efficacy relationships in older adults: a randomized controlled trial. Ann Behav Med 2000;22:131–139

33. Cargill VA, Conti M, Neuhauser D et al: Improving the effectiveness of screening for colorectal cancer by involving nurse clinicians. Med Care 1991;29:1–5

34. Imperial Cancer Research Fund OXCHECK Study Group: Effectiveness of health checks conducted by nurses in primary care: final results of the OXCHECK study. BMJ 1995;310:1099–1104

35. Fries JF, Bloch DA, Harrington H et al: Two-year results of a randomized controlled trial of a health promotion program in a retiree population: the Bank of America study. Am J Med 1993;94:455–462

36. Mayer JA, Jermanovich A, Wright BL et al: Changes in health behaviors of older adults: the San Diego Medicare Preventive Health Project. Prev Med 1994;23:127–133

37. Thompson RS, Taplin SH, McAfee TA et al: Primary and secondary prevention services in clinical practice: twenty year' experience in development, implementation, and evaluation. JAMA 1995;273:1130–1135

38. McPhee SJ, Bird JA, Fordham D et al: Promoting cancer prevention activities by primary care physicians: results of a randomized, controlled trial. JAMA 1991;266:538–544

39. Frame PS, Dowulich BA, Llewellyn AM: Improving physician compliance with a health maintenance protocol. J Fam Pract 1984;19:341–344

40. Madlon-Kay DJ: Improving the periodic health examination: use of a screening flow check for patients and physicians. J Fam Pract 1987;25:470–473

41. Karuza J, Calkins E, Feather J et al: Enhancing physician adoption of practice guidelines. Arch Intern Med 1995;155:625–632

42. Grimshaw JM, Russell IT: Effect of clinical guidelines on medical practice: a systematic review of rigorous evaluations. Lancet 1993;342:1317–1322

43. Curry SJ, McBride C, Grothaus LC et al: A randomized trial of self-help materials, personalized feedback, and telephone counseling with nonvolunteer smokers. J Consult Clin Psychol 1995;63:1005–1014

44. Morrow RW, Gooding AD, Clark C: Improving physicians' preventive health care behavior through peer review and financial incentives. Arch Fam Med 1995;4:165–169

45. Burton LC, Paglia MJ, German PS et al: The effect among older persons of a general preventive visit on three health behaviors: smoking, excessive alcohol drinking, and sedentary lifestyle. Prev Med 1995;24:492–497

46. Burton LC, Steinwachs DM, German PS et al: Preventive services for the elderly: would coverage affect utilization and costs under Medicare? Am J Pub Health 1995;85:387–391

47. Lave JR, Ives DG, Traven ND et al: Evaluation of a health promotion demonstration program for the rural elderly. Health Serv Res 1996;31:261–281

48. McPhee SJ, Bird JA, Jenkins CNH et al: Promoting cancer screening: a randomized controlled trial of three interventions. Arch Intern Med 1989;149:1866–1872

49. Shank JC, Powell T, Llewelyn J: A five-year demonstration project associated with improvement in physician health maintenance behavior. Fam Med 1989;21:273–278

50. Dietrich AJ, Woodruff CB, Carney PA: Changing office routines to enhance preventive care: The preventive GAPS approach. Arch Fam Med 1994;3:176–183

Chapter 21

Rehabilitation: general principles

John Young

Material in this chapter contains contributions from the previous edition, and we are grateful to the previous author for the work done.

Rehabilitation, always at the heart of geriatric medicine, has a rich heritage that dates back in the United Kingdom to early pioneers such as Sheldon, Warren, and Adams. Their contributions were based on systematic observations, on common sense, and on simple principles which we would still recognize today as central to the process of rehabilitation. In our modern health services, practitioners are nervous when challenged to justify the effectiveness of rehabilitation. Early evidence of the potential of rehabilitation in the UK was provided by Warren with the unblocking of chronic sick beds to such an extent that whole wards could be permanently closed. In one of her several inspiring papers, Warren described the factors that had led to her success.[1] They included taking a positive approach, the importance of individual patient assessment and patient involvement, team-working, and the concept of promoting independence by optimizing the patient's environment and by special and general therapeutic techniques. Contemporary evidence of the continued success of these core processes of rehabilitation comes from a recent meta-analysis,[2] demonstrating the superior effectiveness of "comprehensive geriatric assessment"—clearly a reassuring finding in the current climate of evidence-based practice. A more consistent application of the "Marjorie Warren" process across our contemporary medical and surgical wards, and in the community, would make a major contribution to the health of older patients. Indeed, it seems frustrating and perplexing that there has been a resistance to applying established rehabilitation concepts beyond elderly care departments. This has now been recognized in the UK and has stimulated the National Service Framework for Older People.[3]

This chapter describes the core principles of rehabilitation practice, and their underlying evidence-base. Additional detail for the specific rehabilitation techniques is provided in Chapter 22. Although the core principles of rehabilitation are generalizable to various healthcare settings in different countries, this chapter adopts a largely UK perspective. Chapter 114 provides a description of the rehabilitation services in the USA.

DEFINITIONS OF REHABILITATION

Several definitions and explanations of rehabilitation have been proposed. Although the similarities between the definitions are considerable, the perceived diversity of view has contributed to a confusion over the purpose and process of rehabilitation. This apparent ambiguity, and the intangible qualities of rehabilitation, have been in contrast to the concrete "ologies" of contemporary organ-based medicine and has contributed to the vulnerability of rehabilitation in some hospital-based services. Some general definitions of rehabilitation include:

- "Rehabilitation comprises re-ablement—the acquisition of skills needed for independent life—and re-settlement, the restoration of the person to his (or her) own or to another environment."[4]
- "[Rehabilitation is the] restoration of the individual to his (or her) fullest physical, mental and social capability."[5]
- "[Rehabilitation is the] combined and co-ordinated use of medical, social, education and vocation measures for training and retraining the individual to the highest level of functional ability."[6]
- "The primary objective of rehabilitation involves restoration (to the maximum degree possible) of either a function (physical or mental) or a role (within the family, social network or workforce)."[7]
- "Rehabilitation is a problem-solving and educational process aimed at reducing the disability and handicap experienced by someone as a result of disease, always within the limitations imposed both by the available resources and by the underlying disease."[8]
- "The primary objective of rehabilitation is to seek a role which is appropriate to the personality, functional ability and social position of the patient in the light of a realistic assessment of his (or her) functional prognosis; and to seek his (or her) co-operation and that of the professionals complementary to medicine in achieving this aim."[9]

Isaacs is one of the few authors to suggest what rehabilitation is *not*: "The aim of rehabilitation is not (although it is often assumed to be) the attainment of an objective appropriate to the needs of the service; i.e. an early discharge of the patient from hospital."[9]

One common thread within these definitions appears to be a focus on *restoration* of function. However, frequently used terminology in elderly care distinguishes between *active* and *maintenance* rehabilitation. The former implies an expectation of improvement in function; and the latter, an expectation of prevention of deterioration where restoration does not readily apply.

The concept of *frailty* is a further complexity for an understanding of rehabilitation in respect of elderly people. Frailty is regarded as a disease- or age-related loss of physiological reserve such that minor stress events result in disproportionate functional consequences. This has led to the notion of *unstable disability*,[10] characterized by the marked fluctuations in functional abilities that are familiar to professionals working with "old-elderly" people.

In these definitions of rehabilitation, value judgment words such as "fullest" or "optimal" are used. This begs the question of whether results are being judged from the perspective of the doctor, the nurse, the therapist, or perhaps the patient or carer. In stroke, for example, a "good recovery" as far as the therapy team is concerned relates to the maximum impairment at stroke onset as the baseline against which recovery is judged. For the patient, however, the baseline is the pre-stroke lifestyle.[11] A patient with a fractured neck of femur may not share the notion of a "successful" home discharge when returning to the prospect of a living-room commode. Such ambiguities of perspective, commonly unvoiced, can smoulder and lie at the heart of disability adjustment difficulties.

As with many complex issues, it is often rewarding to return to the beginning. Rehabilitation in the UK, at least for older people, emerged as a remedy for aged incurables: the bedridden chronic sick who languished in the Poor Law workhouses. The process was a holistic one in which the central theme was careful individual assessment "both for the establishment of a correct diagnosis and for full treatment" which was to be "undertaken by a (rehabilitation) team."[1] The novelty lay in its emphasis on *function*—not of a body part (for example, surgical revascularization to preserve a limb), but at the level of the whole person set in the context of his or her personal circumstances: family, social, and home environment.

A further important distinction between rehabilitation and other health interventions is that patients are not the passive recipients of a treatment. Rather, rehabilitation is a highly energetic process in which the patient struggles against his or her disability with guidance from a rehabilitation team. The process is characterized by active, positive, and planned actions taken with the patient working at the extremes of physical and functional capabilities.

OLDER AGE AND REHABILITATION NEED

Between 7 and 10 percent of the world population are significantly affected by disablement, defined as the limiting consequences of chronic health conditions.[12] Disablement affects persons of all ages but there is a strong association between older age and disablement so that most disability occurs in later life. The Office of Population Censuses and Surveys (OPCS) in the UK reported a near doubling of disability prevalence rates with each ten-year increment in age, from 7 percent of those aged 40–49, to 68 percent to those aged 80 and above.[13] This most recent OPCS report caused a considerable upward revision in the estimated numbers of disabled people living in the UK. The figure now stands at over 6 million and represents a substantial increase from the previous estimate of just over 3 million. The recent survey used a more realistic and broader operational definition of disability which took better account of restriction of function, and was therefore more reliable in the assessment of disability consequences for conditions such as arthritis and cardiorespiratory disease which commonly affect locomotor function. For people in private households, arthritis is the commonest cause of disability, accounting for 48 percent of disability. It is second only to cognitive impairment in the disabling disorders seen in institutional care residents.

As far as older people in the UK are concerned, an estimated 4.3 million people over 60 years are disabled—this represents 70 percent of all disabled people and 46 percent of all older people. Most (over 90 percent) older disabled people live in their own homes, and most (over 80 percent) have only "mild" disability, but many have several types of disability. Indeed, these self-reported disability categories are more diverse than often appreciated (Table 21-1) and have resource implications across nearly all health and social service departments. In the UK, people aged over 65 years constitute 14 percent of the population but consume nearly half of health[14] and social service[15] expenditure, and this is expected to rise by 3 percent a year.[16]

General disability surveys, and disease-specific epidemiological surveys, provide quantitative information which is important for indicating the scale of disablement, and are valuable for service planning purposes. However, they provide little insight into the experience of disablement for the sufferer. This more human dimension to disablement requires qualitative research methods. Mildred Blaxter's work remains exemplary because of its rigor and clarity, and because it was a longitudinal observation of patients at several points through what Blaxter termed their "career in disability."[17] The study followed 194 people after discharge from hospital with new-onset disability. What emerged was a fairly universal feeling of intense frustration and unnecessary hardship experienced by these people. Blaxter demonstrated how the disabled person could be surrounded by a bewildering array of potentially helpful professions and agencies who lacked visibility, coordination, or an identifiable structure. This resulted in confusion for patients and carers and a consequent failure to access services. Blaxter demonstrated how interventions (for example, equipment provision) often occurred more by chance or as a result of the ruthless determination by a patient or carer than by the consequence of service engagement. In the succeeding quarter century, despite frequent

Table 21-1 Estimates of prevalence of disability types, in rate per thousand population, for people over 75 years

Locomotion	464
Reaching and stretching	129
Dexterity	180
Seeing	225
Hearing	307
Personal care	263
Continence	120
Communication	112
Behavior	88
Intellectual functioning	107

Source: Office of Population Censuses and Surveys (1989).[13]

changes and reorganizations, the experience of being old and disabled all too often remains one of frustration. A recent King's Fund review described the pressing requirements for an effective rehabilitation system most of which would be judged as disappointingly basic.[18] The consequence of disability continues to be that of multiple waiting lists with poorly coordinated services.[19] A person may wait separately and sequentially for a wheelchair assessment, and for wheelchair delivery, and then experience more waiting for an access ramp.[20] There is no reason to expect that matters are better organized in many other countries.

PREVENTION OF DISABLEMENT

"Prevention is better than cure" is a familiar adage. But can disability be prevented in older people? This is an attractive notion to currently independent middle-aged and older people and to service funders (largely taxpayers) struggling to meet the steadily rising health and social care expenditure for age-related disability. Almost certainly much more could be done to minimize the disabling consequences of disease in elderly people: firstly, by better disease prevention, much of which could be quite simple (e.g. improved hypertension management to reduce stroke incidence);[21] and secondly, by more widespread implementation of rehabilitation procedures and systems of proven effectiveness.[22] Beyond the wider implementation of best clinical practices lies the issue of primary disability prevention.

The first step in tackling primary disability prevention/limitation is a more profound understanding of proximal factors, particularly teasing out directional relationships (e.g. does depression predispose the physical disability, or does physical disability generate sufficient misery to trigger depression?). Cross-sectional studies are cheap (and therefore plentiful) but are limited by cohort effects and by ambiguous directional inferences. Longitudinal studies are complex and expensive (and therefore scarce) but allow baseline factors to be examined against future events, thereby more precisely locating cause and effect.

A recent systematic review brought together several longitudinal observational studies in which functional decline was the main outcome measure.[23] The synthesis was carried out carefully, with transparent solutions to the testing problems of quality assessment and results formulation across diverse studies. The findings are interesting. Firstly, a big surprise was the number of studies identified (78). The big disappointment was the meager contribution from Europe (UK, 2 studies; other European countries, 10 studies). The lion's share came from the USA (62, and hugely larger sample sizes). The review findings are largely comfortable in that they support rather than contest established thinking. The baseline risk factors associated with subsequent functional status decline in older people were: cognitive impairment; depression; disease burden (comorbidity); increased and decreased body mass index; lower-extremity functional limitation; low frequency of social contacts; low level of physical activity; no alcohol use compared to moderate use; poor self-perceived health; smoking; and vision impairment. Such observational relationships do not necessarily imply that risk factor modification will translate

into desired disability reduction; only randomized controlled intervention trials can reliably establish this. Falls prevention/exercise programs have progressed to this level of evidence, even for frail older people,[24] and the solid paradigm relating exercise to disability prevention/limitation should encourage action from practitioners and service providers.

On a wider, population scale, is there evidence of a reducing burden of disability? One aspect is the thesis of compression of morbidity: people living longer but with a shorter phase of late-life physical and/or mental decline.[25] Some evidence is now available to support this thesis, with reports that older people have improved health reflecting a legacy of better childhood nutrition, less exposure to infection, and more education.[26] However, the evidence is far from substantial, and the relative contributions of genetic factors, environmental lifestyle, and socio-economic factors remain to be unraveled.

POLICY FRAMEWORK FOR REHABILITATION SERVICES FOR ELDERLY PEOPLE IN THE UK

Healthcare policy is the mechanism by which local and national authorities can encourage a desired outcome from a service or services. It has been a crude and clumsy tool for rehabilitation. Rehabilitation relies heavily on culture ("the way we do things around here") and interprofessional and interagency relationships as key organizational attributes; none of which is easily orchestrated. Moreover, squabbles have broken out concerning cost-shifting (for example, faster hospital discharges have represented a cost burden to social services). And distracting, mundane arguments have occurred (for example, the differentiation of a "health" from a "social" bath). A special difficulty has been the entanglement of rehabilitation with long-term care.

The bedrock of evidence-based medicine as a foundation of clinical practice has led to demands for a similar standard of evidence-based healthcare policy.[27] Unfortunately, much policy remains opinion-driven, largely because of the short time scale of the political cycle that imposes a demand for visible changes. There is therefore a temptation for large-scale reforms rather than incremental learning from restricted pilot schemes. Moreover, there is a further temptation to avoid commissioning research for the fear that the findings might prove an embarrassment.[28] Much of recent healthcare strategy for rehabilitation of older people is opinion-driven.

The NHS and Community Care Act

The 1980s witnessed a rapid expansion in private institutional care, fueled by the easy availability of social security payments which were related to expressed rather than to assessed need.[29] This represented an easy option for hard-pressed hospitals that readily grasped an exit solution for "bed blockers" and with it an associated loss of impetus to maintain, let alone improve, the rehabilitation component of acute care. Expenditure increased dramatically and prompted the NHS and Community Care Act (1990) which was implemented in 1993. The Act required systematic needs assessment and case management, and made long-term care funding cost-limited. Local Authority social services departments became the lead agency, resulting in fundamental changes to the traditional social worker role: it changed from that of adviser and counselor to one of a resource manager. However, the die was cast and insidious rehabilitation decline continued within acute hospitals.

The strategic shift of continuing care for elderly people from (free) NHS to (means-tested) social services was not to change. Rather too late it was recognized that this strategic shift had been too extreme and a readjustment was attempted in the form of a "guidance" document from the Department of Health to health authorities.[30] Somewhat ambitiously, the "guidance" set out a clarification of continuing care in the much wider context of a respecification of all the services expected from the NHS for older people. The range of services was to embrace rehabilitation, continuing, palliative and respite care, community services and even special transport. However, no new money accompanied the initiative and implementation required dis-investment from elsewhere.[31] In terms of political priorities in the NHS, little could compete with the obsession with the surgical waiting list, and, as a result, little changed.

"The coming of age: Improving care services for older people"

In this influential report, the Audit Commission took stock and emphasized the accumulated damage to rehabilitation services.[32] It was estimated that, in the five years 1989/90 to 1994/95, the average length of stay in elderly care in hospital fell by 45 percent—from 36 to 20 days. Opportunities for recovery and rehabilitation therefore had probably diminished and there was a recognition that hospital provision of rehabilitation for older people was foundering.[22] Moreover, there had been no compensatory increase in community-based rehabilitation. Rather, the notion of a "vicious cycle of care" was promoted in which lack of community rehabilitation services stimulated increasing demand for hospital admission. There was an associated earlier discharge of incompletely recovered people; and this drove higher requirements for expensive residential and nursing home care. It was clear that the "magic remedy"—rehabilitation—had withered in the hospital sector and had atrophied in the community.

"Not because they are old"

This was a critical report from the Health Advisory Service concerning the care of elderly people in 16 randomly selected acute hospitals across the UK (sample size: 71 patients; 59 relatives; 305 staff).[33] Although the methods used were far from robust, the report was influential because it drew upon the prevailing concerns about hospital services and was a further stimulus to the urgent formulation of the National Service Framework for Older People. The survey identified that basic deficiencies in care were jeopardizing effective recovery and rehabilitation of elderly people. The physical environment of the wards was often poor, access to basic rehabilitation equipment such as chairs was chaotic, privacy and dignity for the patients was not sufficiently respected, and staff training was a low priority.

National Beds Enquiry

A succession of politically embarrassing winter NHS bed crises prompted the Department of Health to commission the National Beds Enquiry.[34] This laid out facts that were already well known.[35] Pressures caused by year-on-year rising emergency admissions[36] and cost-driven bed closures had necessitated steadily reducing lengths of stay;[32] and rehabilitation, as a less visible component of care, had tended to become squeezed out.[22]

The National Beds Enquiry offered three possible scenarios to improve future service provision. The first option was essentially a status quo with a slight rise in bed capacity in the acute sector and moderate expansion of the primary and community care services. The second option was a larger expansion of the hospital sector with rehabilitation being predominantly provided in hospital settings. The third option, "care closer to home," was an active expansion and development of community health and social services into a new critical mass sufficient to address avoidable hospital admissions.

Although this was a consultative report, the Health Secretary signaled his preference strongly in favor of the third scenario and it has become accepted as the current healthcare policy for rehabilitation.[37]

A primary care-led NHS

The current strategic policy framework for older people, including rehabilitation, is located within a primary care-led NHS reflected in the new structure of the Primary Care Group/Trust (PCG/T).[38] The PCG/T is expected to have a strategic role in the planning, purchasing, and commissioning of a broad range of services. General practitioners, therefore, will be increasingly held responsible for local health services. Each PCG/T is intended to serve up to 100,000 patients, many of whom will be elderly and disabled and using resources disproportionately. A potential weakness is that most general practitioners have never worked in an elderly care department,[39] and so their perceptions of service need may be influenced by the considerable demands made upon primary care from the private nursing and residential care home sector.[40] Moreover, and encouraged by the limited public appeal of low technology health interventions,[41] rehabilitation may again become a tempting target for financial cuts.

On the other hand, there are genuine opportunities for rehabilitation contained within the PCG/T and a primary care-led NHS. One obvious possibility is the development of locality-based rehabilitation teams working within the PCG. Such an approach would maximize the opportunities for rehabilitation at various points in the overall system of health and social care, and at various times in the "career" of older people with disability. Such an initiative would need careful coordination and implementation strategy by health authorities as part of their Health Improvement Programmes (HImPs).

Intermediate care services

Clarity for a fresh strategic approach to rehabilitation for older people has consequently gradually emerged. It has been summarized using the umbrella term "intermediate care." The concept of intermediate care is therefore the final product of a policy cycle encompassing the last one to two decades.

Definitions of intermediate care have moved from the conceptual[42] to the prescriptive[43] (see box), the shift reflecting genuine experience and learning.[44] Examples of intermediate care (Table 21-2) are, at first glance, comfortably familiar.

Table 21-2 Examples of intermediate care services

Geriatric day-hospital
Home-at-home schemes
Hospital-based rehabilitation
Nursing home-based rehabilitation
Community hospitals
Rapid-response teams
Community assessment and rehabilitation teams (CARTs)
Nurse-led wards
Social service schemes:
    day-centre rehabilitation
    residential-care rehabilitation

Conceptual definition of intermediate care

That range of services designed to facilitate transition from hospital, and from medical independence to functional independence, where the objects of care are not primarily medical, the patient's discharge destination is anticipated, and a clinical outcome of recovery (or restoration of health) is desired. (King's Fund, 1997)[42]

Prescriptive definition of intermediate care

Intermediate care should be regarded as describing services that meet *all* the following criteria:

- targeted at people who would otherwise face unnecessarily prolonged hospital stays or inappropriate admission to acute inpatient care, long-term residential care, or continuing NHS inpatient care;

- provided on the basis of a comprehensive assessment, resulting in a structured individual care plan that involves active therapy, treatment and opportunity for recovery;

- having a planned outcome of maximizing independence and typically enabling patients/users to resume living at home;

- time-limited, normally no longer than 6 weeks, and frequently as little as 1–2 weeks or less.

- involving cross-professional working, with a single assessment framework, single professional records and shared protocols. (Based on Health Service Circular, 2001)[43]

For example, both the geriatric day hospital and the community hospital have long pedigrees. Rehabilitation in social settings such as residential care homes, however, is less familiar and is a recent development. This form of intermediate care was introduced partly as a response to the irritation felt by some social service departments forced into the position of taking older people discharged prematurely from acute wards. It was considered necessary to fill the rehabilitation gap created by inadequate health service provision. However, these social service solutions to unmet rehabilitation need have now been put on a more collaborative and consultative footing within the framework of Joint Investment Plans (JIPs).[38] Indeed, JIPs provide insight into the real novelty of intermediate care services. They are *not* about the relaunching of old style services. There is an expectation that intermediate care services will become a platform to incorporate new patterns of working and new professional relationships both between disciplines and

between agencies. It is an attempt to impose a strategic structure in the hitherto chaotic area of community care characterized by competing demands, conflicting pressures, and resource rationing. Unlike earlier community care initiatives, this one comes with a promised injection of resources, and on a large scale: £900 million by 2003/04.[37] At present, however, the UK-wide implementation of intermediate care is a political initiative. The involvement of geriatricians is ambiguous and the PCG/T, as the lead agency to develop intermediate care services, is still relatively immature.

The concept of intermediate care has not been universally well received by UK elderly care specialists.[45] However, the British Geriatrics Society has recommended that geriatricians should become involved with the planning and delivery of these services.[46] This implies a greater commitment from geriatricians to community working in the future.[47] In some areas, the medical input to intermediate care services will be discharged by a community geriatrician,[48] but at present there is no training program for such a post. There is a wider issue of training as one practical implication of this service reconfiguration will be appropriate preparation of future consultant geriatricians to contribute to intermediate care services.[49]

The program of intermediate care service implementation now has a massive momentum.[32,38] It is consistent with a primary care-led NHS and the imperative of joint working between health and social services. It has a self-evident role in post-acute care for elderly people to complement the scaled-down district general hospital by re-installing a time-space for rehabilitation and functional recovery. The main concern has been the additional proposed function of intermediate care for admission avoidance: to bypass, or delay access to, specialist district general hospital assessment and investigation facilities. Acute ill-health in elderly people typically presents in an ill-defined way. For example, an older person "found lying on the floor" might have simply rolled out of bed but, alternatively, may have a fractured neck of femur, pneumonia, or heart failure. Admission avoidance could easily become an institutional barrier in the expeditious assessment of sick older people. This worrying aspect of intermediate care has been reflected in its being referred to as "indeterminate care."[46]

UNDERSTANDING DISABILITY
The disablement process

The medical model concerns itself with diseases and their effects on the body. An abnormality of insulin production, release, or receptor binding causes varying degrees of hyperglycemia: the disease of diabetes. During the early stages, this may have no impact on well-being (no symptoms), and indeed the disease may be diagnosed only unexpectedly after a routine screening blood test. Diabetes is, however, an example of a progressive disease and eventually the chronic hyperglycemia will produce symptoms—sometimes, for example, nerve damage resulting in a peripheral neuropathy. At this stage, the person (in medical terminology now a patient) will find some previously routine everyday activities, such as walking to the shops, more difficult. The disease has now impacted on the person's daily life—a process of disablement has occurred, or the person has become disabled.

On this simple level disability is straightforward. However, a precise definition is elusive. Consider the different impact of the disease when the patient lives near to shops; or a similar diabetic patient already restricted by severe knee arthritis. In both cases the new disease of diabetes may have no noticeable additional impact. The disablement process needs therefore to describe how chronic and acute conditions affect specific physical and mental functions, and daily living activities, but also to account for the personal and environmental factors that have the potential to mediate the disablement process.[50] Thus, the wider context of disability requires us to understand the process as a gap between personal capability and environmental demand. It would appear, therefore, that disability is a relative phenomenon and difficult to capture unequivocally in a simple description.

Consider another patient, a bilateral amputee living in a nursing home. He enjoys socializing, trips out, singing, and placing racing bets by telephone. He is clearly content and has a fulfilled life. Is there a process of disablement here? A further difficulty lies in the origins of the disease process. Disability tends to conjure up an image of physical insult. So how should we regard the restricted life of a person with agoraphobia? And how should we accommodate the degree or quantity of disability? Presumably there is a continuum from "mild" to "severe." This implies that some form of objective measure should apply, but should this be based upon an external judgment, or upon the patient's perception? Obvious inconsistencies arise, when, for example, a patient who is "slightly" disabled from an external "objective" assessment perceives a "severe" disability. Moreover, disability definition may take several forms: legal/administrative; medical; cultural; self-definition. Administrative disability is particularly confusing. A person may be administratively disabled and qualify for a special parking permit, but administratively not disabled and ineligible for the attendance allowance benefit, and disabled by virtue of age (over 75) and eligible for a free television license. The fog surrounding an adequate and agreed definition for disability has been summarized aptly by Townsend:

"Although society may have been sufficiently influenced in the past to seek to adopt scientific measures of disability, so as to admit people to institutions, or regard them as eligible for social security or occupational and social services, these measures may be applied in a distorted way, or may not be applied at all, or may be replaced by more subjective criteria by hard pressed administrators, doctors and others. At the least, there may be important variations between 'social' and 'objective' assessments of severity of handicap."[51]

The WHO classification

The complexities of disability demand some form of classification map capable of providing a systematic method to describe the disablement process at the level of an individual. This has been the purpose of the International Classification of Impairments, Diseases and Handicap (ICIDH), first published by the World Health Organization in 1980. It is generally regarded as a useful classification framework within which to consider the rehabilitation process. The framework relates illness to four levels: pathology, impairment, disability, and handicap:

- *pathology:* the process of damage in an organ or organ system that results in disease;
- *impairment:* any loss or abnormality of psychological, physiological, or anatomical structure or function;
- *disability:* any restriction or lack of ability (resulting from an impairment) to perform an activity in a manner or within a range considered normal;
- *handicap:* a disadvantage for a certain individual, resulting from an impairment or disability, that limits or prevents his or her fulfillment of a role that would be normal for that individual.

The value of this classification in relation to older people is that it prompts the need to uncover a cause (pathology and impairment) for the disability when the person presents with, for example, a mobility problem; whilst also prompting examination of the consequences of the disease in functional terms (disability) and in relation to the lifestyle and environment of the individual patient (handicap). Thus a balanced approach is achieved between disease modification (usually drugs or surgery) and maximizing independence (physical treatments, aids, and adaptations). A common misunderstanding is to assume a progressive and proportional relationship between the four levels. The relationships are often discontinuous. For example, cerebral infarcts (pathology) are commonly found on head CT scans without associated impairments; severe knee osteoarthritis (pathology) may restrict a person to a wheelchair (mobility disability), and necessitate institutional care, but the individual may adjust, develop a new and contented lifestyle and have a strong sense of purpose and well-being (minimal handicap). The variable relationship between the levels emphasizes the need for individual patient assessments that respect fully the perspective of the patient and close supporters.

Illness or role rehabilitation

To some, the ICIDH classification has represented an over-medicalized model of disability in which disablement is seen as located primarily within the individual.[52] In the social model of disability, disablement is perceived less as an attribute of a person and more as a set of circumstances, many of which arise from the external environment.[53] Handicap is caused by having steps into buildings and not just by difficulty in walking. Within this paradigm, "the disabled elderly" can be considered as a disadvantaged minority group, an argument that forms a component of a larger thesis concerning the social construction of old age.[54] A continuation of this perspective is to discuss disablement in the language of social discrimination and oppression.[55] Here, problems are located at the level of an individual but caused through a prevailing unhelpful attitude towards disablement by society as a whole. This underpins arguments for a more inclusive research agenda which acknowledges more fully that disablement is a personal experience created as much by wider society as by the individual.[55] The debate over the relative merits of the different models of disability continues,[52,53,55,56] and it is the intention that both models will be encapsulated in the forthcoming revised version of the ICIDH (see below).

The two competing rehabilitation paradigms—medical and social—translate to an illness (sickness) model and role (person) model. Illness rehabilitation is most apparent when it is tacked on to various medical specialties. Examples are cardiac or pulmonary rehabilitation programs. Although these programs have extended the spectrum of care available to patients, they have not usually been integral to the medical specialty concerned but generally require a purposeful secondary referral. However, it has become increasingly recognized that these disease-specific rehabilitation programs have tangible benefits.[57–59] The lack of medical enthusiasm engendered by these programs can be located within our contemporary curative medical approach with its emphasis on brief interventions. Unfortunately, complexity appears integral to the effectiveness of rehabilitation programs,[60] and it is far easier to introduce a novel drug than a novel rehabilitation program.

The revised ICIDH model (ICIDH-2)

The ICIDH has been criticized for its unwieldiness, and for the consequent unreliability of the codes arising from it.[49,61–63] The original ICIDH included 1009 impairment items, 338 disability items, and 72 handicap items. However, it was designed as a comprehensive classification scheme, not as a measurement instrument in its own right. After two decades of use, the ICIDH is undergoing a major revision. The revision is prompted partly by the need for a more profound recognition of the social determinants of disability, and partly to reflect a positive description of health rather than the negative description of illness.

The new version, known as ICIDH-2, is described as a multipurpose classification designed to provide a common framework for understanding the dimensions of disablement and function at three different levels: body, person, and society. The wider application is its integration with the International Classification of Disease and it therefore uses a standardized common language permitting communication about health and healthcare across the world in various disciplines and sciences. Its use therefore goes beyond that of a practical clinical tool—for example, for service planning, policy development, and to progress human rights issues. As such, it attempts much and therefore can be criticized as being too all-embracing and unwieldy for the clinician. The general scheme of ICIDH-2 is given in Figure 21-1. The definitions of the components of the framework model comprise:

- *impairment*: a loss or abnormality of body structure or a physiological or psychological function;
- *activity*: the nature and extent of functioning at the level of the person;
- *participation*: the nature and extent of a person's involvement in a life situation in relation to impairment, activities, health condition, and contextual factors.

Activities may be limited in nature, duration, and quality (e.g. taking care of oneself, maintaining a job). Participation may be restricted in nature, duration, and quality (e.g. participation in community activities, obtaining a driving license).

Thus, as with ICIDH-1, there are four dimensions (with the inclusion of pathology), but with outcomes expressed as negative or positive levels of function. In effect, a continuum has been created between the expression of problems (e.g. impairment,

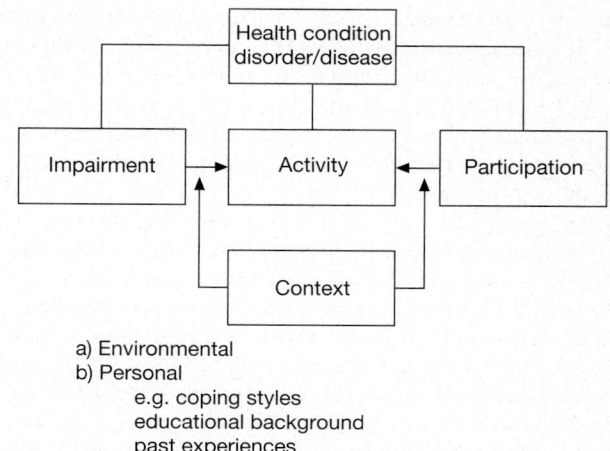

Figure 21-1 The revised World Health Organization ICIDH model of illness.

activity limitation, or participation restrictions), summarized under the umbrella term *disability*; and, at the opposite end, non-problematic (neutral) aspects of health and health-related states, summarized under the umbrella term *function*. However, the negative levels comprise impairments, activity *limitation* and participation *restriction*, and in this respect ICIDH-2 appears no different from its deriving parent, other than the substitution of one word for another: disability becomes activity while handicap becomes participation. The disablement process is again illuminated by the consequence of the dynamics between the four levels. However, the changes implicit in the proposed new model is more profound than simple substitutions of more politically correct words. The emphasis is on contextual factors which act as mediators between the levels of the model, thereby changing the process from one of general disablement to one which becomes highly individualized. The contextual mediators are subdivided into environmental and personal factors. Important examples of personal context factors are goals (what the person aspires to) and beliefs (the person's own explanation and understanding of his or her illness).[64] These aspects are, in turn, influenced by personal educational and life experiences, by family and supporters, and by wider prevailing societal values.

How, and to what extent, the ICIDH-2 will impact on rehabilitation thinking—and indeed how clinical practice might change—is speculative. It will depend on whether the opportunities perceived are sufficiently attractive to overcome resistance to a more complex classification model. One view is that considerable change in rehabilitation practice may occur.[64] The current version, ICIDH-2 beta-1, is undergoing field-testing. The situation is clearly fluid with constant incremental change which is best followed on the WHO website (www.who.ch/icidh).

ASSESSMENT AND REHABILITATION POTENTIAL

Many elderly people have several conditions of varying severity, and it can be challenging to unravel and identify the components and then to develop a personalized intervention plan. This process is called *assessment* and has been central to good practice since the inception of special services for older people.[1] The process aims to determine impairments, disabilities, and handicap, and then to trigger selective interventions at one or more of these levels, followed by observation and evaluation of response.

There is reliable evidence that the process is effective in improving outcomes for elderly people, but with the common sense proviso that the assessment process is closely linked to interventions.[65] The effectiveness studies have been summarized in a systematic review and meta-analysis.[2] The studies included (15 in North America, 8 in the UK, and 5 others) are heterogeneous but have as a common thread an evaluation of "comprehensive geriatric assessment": a core process characterized by multidisciplinary assessment and treatment. The pooled estimates of effectiveness across a range of outcome measures were encouragingly positive (Table 21-3). The best effects were obtained for comprehensive geriatric assessment delivered by hospital-based elderly care departments, in which the assessment process and subsequent interventions were integrated and when organized post-discharge follow-up was arranged. In a review of the literature, Wade concluded that successful assessment is more likely if the assessor is experienced and if multiple aspects are covered by the assessor(s), but that, at present, there is little evidence to guide the most appropriate or efficient methods of assessment.[66]

The process of assessment is self-evidently complex—generally more so than determining a drug prescription or planning an elective operation. Part of the complexity arises from the nature of the clinical problems: their diversity, varying severity, and multiplicity. Moreover, the problems interact at the level of personhood, so that disentangling physical and psychological factors is challenging. In addition, there may be a close association with social and environmental factors, and the interventions used are themselves complex (see Chapter 22). Interventions are based on human skills and therefore subject to variation, and they rely considerably on active patient participation which is also subject to variation.

Standardized assessment measures or professional assessment?

The scientific basis of rehabilitation demands objective measurement.[66] One problem has been the multitude and diversity of standardized measurement tools available[67]—described aptly as "a tower of Babel."[68] The most important consideration in selecting a particular measure is whether it is appropriate to the task in hand.[67] Additionally, measurement tools require research studies involving different patient groups in different settings and using advanced statistical methods to demonstrate various properties[69]:

- *Validity:* Does the instrument actually measure what it purports to measure?
- *Reliability:* Does the instrument give similar scores when used on the same patient by two observers, or when repeated on stable patients?
- *Sensitivity:* Does the instrument detect clinically important changes?
- *Acceptability:* Is the instrument simple and quick to apply, easy to understand, and easy for patients to complete (so that there is a high response rate)?

These instrument measurement properties are not independent and perfect scales do not exist. Compromises have to be achieved between, for example, sensitivity and reliability—a scale sensitive to small changes has low reliability.

In the USA, a task force established a Uniform Data System for Medical Rehabilitation which incorporated the use of the Functional Independence Measure.[70] In the UK, the Royal College of Physicians and the British Geriatrics Society have jointly recommended six standardized assessment instruments for routine use when assessing older people (Table 21-4).[71] However, few of these instruments have been adopted in routine practice.

Indeed, in clinical rehabilitation practice, as opposed to research, debate continues over the balance between professional assessment and the use of objective standardized measures. Compared to professional assessment, standardized measures have the advantage of being less subject to bias, more systematic, more communicable, and able to provide a numerical result. Further, they open up the possibility for postal or telephone disability assessment, or assessment by support staff rather than senior staff. On the other hand, a disadvantage is that the result from a measurement instrument is not easily related to an intervention. This is not surprising because rehabilitation measures have not been designed to do this. For example, a Barthel score of 16, although providing a useful disability profile summary, does not equate to a patient treatment strategy. To determine a treatment strategy

Table 21-3 Outcomes of "comprehensive geriatric assessment"—hospital geriatric unit versus alternative care	
	Odds ratio (and 95 percent confidence limits) at 6 months
Living at home	1.8 (1.28–2.53)
Reduced mortality	0.68 (0.45–0.91)
Improved physical function	1.63 (1.00–2.65)
Improved cognitive function	2.0 (1.13–3.55)
Source: Stuck et al. (1993).[3]	

Table 21-4 Standardized assessment instruments jointly recommended by the Royal College of Physicians of London and the British Geriatrics Society for routine use when assessing elderly people	
Domain of interest	**Recommended scale**
ADL disability	Barthel Index
Vision and hearing	Lambeth Disability Screening Score
Mental impairment	Hodgkinson Abbreviated Mental Test
Depression	Geriatric Depression Score
Quality of life	Philadelphia Geriatric Center Morale Scale
Social circumstances	Social Indicators Checklist
Source: RCP London (1992).[71]	

requires an exploratory, discursive process that seeks to identify patient-related problems and their context. This is the antithesis of the pervasive reductionalism characterizing the conventional biomedical model. Rather, it is the bio-psycho-social model propounded by Engel,[72] summarized as: "Do my doctors/therapists know who I am, who I have been, who I still want to be? Do they understand what I am going through, my suffering, my pain, my distress? Do they understand my hopes and aspirations, my fears and shames, my vulnerability and strengths, my needs and obligations and my values? Above all do they sense my personhood and my individuality?" It is impossible to achieve this level of understanding through standardized assessment instruments.

Isaacs[9] has argued for a discursive approach to the assessment of elderly people, with a list of open questions designed to identify problems but located in the context of the patient's personal attributes, daily life, family and friends. This type of semistructured format is a part of what has been described as narrative-based medicine.[73–75] There is a concern that narrative-based medicine is becoming a lost tradition and should be revived in mainstream medical practice.[75] Its special relevance lies in the series of unfolding events told, importantly, from the viewpoint of the patient. These events provide meaning, context, and perspective for the patient's predicaments. The attraction of the narrative approach is that it is both diagnostic and therapeutic. The telling of the story helps the patient make sense of events and, from the rehabilitation professional point of view, one outcome includes the possibility that novel and specific treatment options can be identified, or that a specific and especially valued element of information can be provided. One problem in practice is the difficulty in capturing adequately the richness of a narrative within the usual healthcare case records. This is one important reason why each multidisciplinary team member will wish to listen first-hand to a patient's account. This can appear frustratingly inefficient to healthcare managers, but it is in the small details that the special events and circumstances surrounding, for example, a fractured neck of femur emerge and change the commonplace (another admission with fractured neck of femur) to the particular narrative of an individual person with a fractured neck of femur.

DETECTION OF DEPRESSION AND DEMENTIA   It has been long recognized that depression and cognitive impairment can be significant barriers to successful rehabilitation.[76] There is therefore a good argument for routinely assessing patients on these domains using standardized instruments. Depression is common in elderly people,[77] but it can be difficult to detect because of overlap between the physical symptoms of organic disease, the vegetative symptoms of depression, and somatization of psychological distress.[78] The short version of the self-report Geriatric Depression Scale[79] can be used to screen for depression in medically ill older people and has a sensitivity and specificity of over 70 percent when compared with formal psychiatric diagnosis.[80] However, some of the questions (e.g. "Have you dropped many of your activities or interests?") have questionable face validity in the presence of a new condition, such as a fractured neck of femur or stroke. The Hospital Anxiety Depression Score[81] is another commonly used mood scale. It is easy to use and encompasses both depression and anxiety in separate subscales. However, the validity and reliability of this instrument for frail elderly people remains to be established. Several brief cognitive screening tools are available, such as the Abbreviated Mental Test[82] and the Mini Mental State Examination Score,[83] and their routine use in rehabilitation involving older people has been recommended.

Significant aphasia and severe deafness may make formal assessment of mood and cognitive impairment difficult. Also, these screening tools are not diagnostic instruments: they merely indicate that cognitive impairment or depression may be present. For example, the Abbreviated Mental Test score has a false positive rate of up to 25 percent.[84] Careful patient observation and information from supporters remain fundamental. This approach has been reinforced by the recently described observation-based rating scale for use by nurses or care staff in daily contact with the patient.[85] It comprises six questions and has acceptable sensitivity and specificity for the identification of depression.

Rehabilitation potential

Part of the initial assessment process is to determine the rehabilitation potential of a patient. Although this is a nebulous concept, it is a common and challenging clinical task with an inherent self-fulfillment risk for the patient who is classified as possessing "limited rehabilitation potential." Caution is needed with a one-off, snapshot assessment, as there is evidence that agreement on rehabilitation potential even within a multidisciplinary team is unreliable.[86] Repeated assessments or a "trial of rehabilitation" may be the preferred clinical approaches, but are not yet adequately researched.

Assessment of mobility

Restriction of mobility is one of the most serious health-related problems. If an elderly person has insufficient mobility to be able easily to leave home, it follows that the person must be dependent on others for basic activities such as shopping, and there is also the important loss of social opportunities. Objective assessment of gait and mobility is therefore important.[87]

A gait laboratory is capable of describing and reporting many of the components of a gait cycle and is considered the gold standard in gait analysis—though it is too expensive, cumbersome, and time-consuming for use as a routine clinical tool.[88] It is therefore gratifying to note that simple clinical observation of gait *can* be rewarding: in a study of frail elderly people at high risk of falls, those who were observed to "stop walking when talking" were at the highest risk of falling during the next 6 months.[89] Unfortunately, though, gait assessment based on observation alone can be unreliable.[90,91] There is no shortage of standardized approaches to assessment: a recent review identified 42 measures of balance and gait.[92]

The timed walking test

The timed walking test is quick, needs little equipment (only a stopwatch and tape measure), and can be done easily in the clinic or at home. It has been described as "remarkably simple, reliable, valid, sensitive, communicable, useful, and relevant—almost the perfect measure."[67] It involves timing patients using a stopwatch as they walk a measured 10-meter distance, or walk 5 meters and return (more applicable for home assessment). It has been found to correlate with recovery after stroke,[93] and with other aspects of gait—such as a functional walking test and number of steps taken,[94] balance,[95] use of walking aids,[96,97] falls,[98] and extent of personal mobility.[99] Gait speed measurement is suitable for routine use in geriatric day-hospital practice.[100] A practical point is that the first walk is often significantly slower than subsequent walks and should be regarded as a warm-up/practice measurement and excluded from gait speed measurement results.[101]

Selection of a walking aid

An appropriate walking aid can lessen many gait impairments and reduce disability. The commonest aids are walking sticks[102] and various types of walking frame. The introduction of the walking frame is ascribed to a 12-year-old Cincinnati boy who designed and constructed a frame for his aunt who had sustained a fractured neck of femur.[103]

There are now over 40 types of frame available in the UK,[104] including the Zimmer and various wheeled frames (e.g. the delta rollator). There are several disadvantages to the Zimmer frame because it promotes a slow and abnormal gait characterized by an intermittent stop/start or nonphysiological stepping pattern. Wheeled walking frames, on the other hand, encourage a smooth, physiological, striding type of gait pattern.

Comparison studies favor wheeled frames,[105] but the clinical issue is to select the most helpful walking aid for an individual patient. The "S test" has been designed to fulfill this practical clinical task.[106] It comprises a series of assessments in which the patient is asked to complete set maneuvers with different mobility aids. Patients are tested in their normal clothing and footwear in a carpeted area. Initially the therapist adjusts the aids usually to a height of the wrist crease and gives basic instruction. Subjects start the test seated in a chair and are then required to stand and walk a measured 5 meters which is timed by a stopwatch. They then make a 180-degree turn before walking a further 5 meters. Finally they make a 180-degree left turn before reversing into the chair. The test is repeated with different walking aids and the preferred aid is determined by considering five factors: safety, stability, stance, step/stride pattern, and speed. It is surprising how often this test selects a wheeled frame as the preferred walking aid.

Mobility handicap

One system which readily depicts mobility handicap is based on the concept of "life spaces."[99] Life spaces are divided into five concentric zones into which the individual can be placed: the bedroom, the rest of the dwelling, grounds surrounding the dwelling, the block, and the area across a traffic-bearing street. The system facilitates a better understanding of the relationship of the individual to his or her surroundings and stimulates an examination of barriers—i.e. why a person cannot move from one circle to the next.

In a community survey of arthritis sufferers, the availability of a car, the type of housing, and the distance to local shops emerged as the most restrictive barriers.[107] Ease of access to shops is important for elderly people as it fosters independence and re-enforces ties with friends and neighbors. It is an activity that might well be curtailed even in the face of modest mobility restriction if the environmental factors are hostile.

It is not just external environmental factors that are important. The internal architecture and distances between rooms are other important factors that can elevate a modest disability into a severe handicap. For example, in a survey of 15 "typical homes" in East Cumbria, 80 percent of the houses had their main living room separated from the nearest toilet by a distance of more than 20 meters.[91] For some elderly people, this might represent a handicapping distance. This may be one reason why accommodation that is more sympathetic to the needs of disabled older people, such as sheltered housing schemes, is associated with a reduction in mobility handicap.[108]

Assessment of disability

Activities of daily living

"Activities of daily living" (ADLs) is a term commonly used by rehabilitation professionals. It reflects the disability level of disease consequence in the WHO classification model. ADLs include tasks such as washing, dressing, transferring, toileting, and mobility. These may initially appear as a disparate collection of activities that have been force-fitted together. However, ADLs can be considered as a unified construct and, importantly, performance is critical for elderly people struggling to maintain independent living.[109] The systematic assessment of ADLs, therefore, is an important aspect of the overall assessment of elderly people. Once again, a multitude of standardized instruments has been developed—a testament both to the perceived importance of this area in rehabilitation practice, and to the difficulty in producing the optimal instrument. Fortunately, most ADL measures are remarkably similar, at least in item content.[8,109]

The Barthel Index

The Barthel Index has become widely adopted in routine clinical practice in British geriatric medicine and elsewhere. The popularity of the Barthel Index against the backdrop of numerous other rival ADL standardized instruments supports its clinical utility. The Barthel Index originated as an empirically derived measure for younger disabled adults.[110] Its widespread adoption into routine practice owes much to Wade and colleagues[111] who were the first to demonstrate its reliability and validity.[112]

The Barthel Index is an ordinal scale (as are most rehabilitation measures). Consequently, an improvement in score from, say, 5 to 6 does not represent the same clinical improvement as a score of 10 moving to 11. It assesses levels of independence or dependence for ten ADL tasks with a score range of 0 (dependent) to 20 (independent):

- Dressing
- Feeding
- Grooming
- Toilet
- Bathing
- Bed/chair transfers
- Walking
- Stairs
- Bladder
- Bowels

The Barthel Index score correlates well with mortality,[113] length of hospital stay,[114] and requirement for institutional care.[115] It is a simple measure that is easy to interpret in clinical practice, and it can both aid systematic disability assessment and also monitor rehabilitation progress if repeated at intervals.[116] It is an independent indicator of nursing dependency levels.[117]

One disadvantage of the Barthel Index is that the steps on the scale are fairly large, so it is not very sensitive to small changes. Also, especially for disabled people living at home, there is a marked "ceiling" effect—patients can score the maximum 20 points and be "independent" according to the index, but still have daily living restrictions. This low ceiling effect limits its applicability for outpatient rehabilitation settings such as the day-hospital.[118]

Extended activities of daily living

One limitation of the ADL scales is the restricted range of the content items. Living independently at home requires a more extensive repertoire of skills—including kitchen, domestic, transport use, and leisure activities. These types of activity are referred to variously as "instrumental," "extended," social," or "advanced" activities of daily living. Although there is a conceptual understanding of instrumental activities of daily living, there is no agreement on the exact categories to be included in such measures.[119] Examples of these measures include the Frenchay Activities Index[120] and the Nottingham Extended Activities of Daily Living scale.[121] These measures are less reliable both in total scores and individual items than ADL scores, probably because they rely on recall of activities undertaken during the preceding weeks.[122]

Assessment of handicap

Handicap, the disadvantage to the individual as a result of ill-health, is from the patient's point of view the critical level at which to effect change. There is an increasing recognition that the ultimate goal of rehabilitation for older people should be reintegration into normal patterns of life.[123] This involves placing the individual in the context of his or her home, local environment, and facilities, and the person's relationships, motivation, mood, and expectations. Unsurprisingly, the uniqueness of this context makes the development of a generic standardized assessment tool difficult. The development of robust measures of handicap has proved difficult,[67] and has only recently been described for stroke. Even here it remains a research tool for assessing the outcome of services rather than assisting rehabilitation assessment.[124]

The World Health Organization's ICIDH contains six basic "survival roles" in the handicap section: orientation (including sight, hearing, and cognition); physical independence; mobility; occupation (including employment, domestic work, and recreation); social integration; and economic self-sufficiency. Its main limitation is that it is a classification system rather than an assessment tool. Alternatively, the Rankin scale is often cited as a handicap measure but is, in fact, a crude disability scale and moreover heavily biased towards mobility.[125]

Social activity is an important domain of handicap and an important aspect of the reintegration process.[126] As there has been greater success in the development of measures of social activity, referred to above as "extended activities of daily living," these measures are the best current clinical compromise for a standardized approach to handicap assessment.

Location of assessment

Assessment was originally conceived as a hospital-based process, and the evidence for effectiveness is strongest for multidisciplinary teams working in the setting of hospitals. Emergency day-hospital assessment has been described as an alternative.[127]

Much less information is available on successful assessment of disabled elderly people at home. Here, the primary healthcare team is the main health contact for disabled older people working in collaboration with social service staff. The effectiveness of assessment of primary healthcare teams, and community rehabilitation teams, has become a more pressing concern following the introduction in the UK of intermediate care services. The first healthcare contact for elderly people struggling to cope at home is frequently the community nurse. Each year about half the population aged over 85 years is seen by a community nurse.[128] Such nurses work closely with general practitioners to coordinate the care with social service staff and therapists, and to organize services such as respite care and day-center attendance. A recent comprehensive review conducted by the Audit Commission concluded that there was considerable scope to improve the service, with a specific recommendation for the introduction of improved standardized assessment methods accompanied by an associated training program.[128]

The Easycare assessment

Easycare was developed on behalf of the European Regional Office of the World Health Organization for use in Europe as a first-stage assessment of elderly people in primary or community-care settings. It is designed as a system for rapid assessment of an older person's physical, mental, and social well-being, and provides a broad picture of the person's needs. It focuses on quality of life rather than disease, and recognizes the roles of family and carers. It comprises a structured assessment of hearing, vision and chewing; self-care and mobility; social functioning; and mood and cognition.

Provisional evaluation of Easycare has confirmed its usefulness as a combined medical and social assessment of elderly people in domiciliary settings.[129] Completion time is between 14 and 40 minutes.[130] However, the extent to which the Easycare system leads to improved outcomes for elderly people living at home has not yet been researched.

Home assessment

Home assessment shifts the rehabilitation orientation from disability to handicap. The UK College of Occupational Therapists defines a home visit as "a visit to the home of a hospital in-patient which involves an occupational therapist in accompanying the consumer to assess his/her ability to function independently within the home environment or to assess the potential for the consumer to be as independent as possible with the support of carers."[131] This is an overly narrow definition that ignores home assessment visits for elderly people who are not in hospital. Also, a home assessment should allow the patient and the rehabilitation team to obtain first-hand experience of the challenges faced in coping at home and thereby trigger new interventions and rehabilitation goals.

Like much in rehabilitation practice, the home assessment visit has become absorbed into mainstream practice in an uncritical way and its effectiveness is uncertain. Moreover, the function of the pre-discharge assessment visit has insidiously changed from a handicap assessment to inform the rehabilitation process, to an administrative component of the hospital discharge process. A systematic review of pre-discharge home assessment visits identified only five reports—of which two described retrospective surveys, and three were descriptive surveys of current clinical practice.[132] One randomized controlled trial involving 50 cases has since been published.[133] It investigated the important but relatively specific issue of falls. Pre-discharge home assessment visits and subsequent environmental modifications resulted in a significant reduction in the fall rate during the 12 months of follow-up, but the treatment effect was confined to those high-risk patients with a history of falls in the preceding year. Another systematic review (15 studies) has examined the effectiveness of preventative home assessment visits and reported inconclusive findings for relatively low-risk elderly people at home.[134]

TEAMWORK IN REHABILITATION

The concept of teamwork, arguably formalized first in rehabilitation,[1] is now familiar in most areas of healthcare: primary healthcare teams, surgical teams, cancer teams, palliative care teams, etc.[135] However, teamworking in rehabilitation has two distinctive features. Firstly, the team is built around the patient rather than a condition (such as a cancer or a surgical treatment). Secondly, the range of professional staff involved is exceptionally diverse in terms of professional backgrounds, and this necessitates careful coordination of each member's contribution.

Multidisciplinary team care

More has been written about successful and unsuccessful teamwork in the context of general management. A consistent finding has been that successful teams are made up of people with different styles and backgrounds who bring different angles to the issues at hand, rather than "clones" who are likely to adopt similar approaches.[136] Creativity and successful problem-solving therefore require a mix of character styles and skills, albeit at the expense of some tension when inevitable differences arise. The multidisciplinary rehabilitation team structure for rehabilitation, therefore, may be ideally suited for the complex problem-solving required for elderly people with disabilities.

Rehabilitation staff generally endorse the team approach and it is regarded as established practice. There is evidence of its importance as up to 75 percent of disabilities may go unrecognized by hospital doctors;[137] and although general practitioners are probably more aware, they still fail to recognize 40 percent of disabilities.[138] Successful impairment and disability assessment requires separate assessments by each member of the multidisciplinary team if problems are not to be overlooked.[86] However, there is little consensus and few empirical studies provide insight into the best methods to promote effective teamwork. Measurement of important aspects of team care, such as clinical and interpersonal skills, interprofessional relationships, and group dynamics are poorly developed. It has been suggested that effective teamwork requires at least three components: agreed and explicit aims; recognition of the contribution of different team members; and structures to facilitate collaborative working.[139]

Issues of role overlap are rarely addressed openly,[140] and professional "tribalism" can occur with recurring conflicts caused by the failure to understand and value the contribution of other team members,[141] resulting in arguments over professional boundary issues.[141,142] There are both inter- and intra-professional tensions. For example, one view is that physiotherapy has veered too far toward a biomedical reductionist approach with an emphasis on physical symptoms and the level of impairment, and too far from a more behavior/educational holistic approach.[143] Also, status problems can develop,[144] frequently resulting in jealousy and lack of cooperation.[145] Autonomy of rehabilitation staff within a team structure is required to realize the full potential of the team, but needs careful nurturing.[146] An effective team should be prepared to modify its approach in the light of emerging research, but relating practice to an evolving evidence base remains poor owing to insufficient time to read and discuss research literature.[147]

Interdisciplinary team care

Professional and clinical overlap inevitably occurs between members of a multidisciplinary rehabilitation team. Arguments have been advanced for a "generic therapist,"[148] but separate therapy disciplines remain the norm in the UK and elsewhere. Some progress has been made with generic therapy assistants within vocational training programs, but complex professional regulations have presented daunting practical obstacles. Team overlap and areas of duplication have led to a greater emphasis on interdisciplinary working.[141,149] This approach has been further promoted by limited resources and national shortfalls in trained rehabilitation staff, resulting in some rehabilitation disciplines being severely rationed or unevenly available—particularly clinical psychologists and speech and language therapists.

Interdisciplinary working is a higher order of team functioning than the traditional multidisciplinary approach. It involves acknowledging the overlap between disciplines, with greater sharing of duties and responsibilities. Formal strategies to promote interdisciplinary working are largely untested but include collaborative clinical records, shared goal-setting, and closer working practices. Interdisciplinary training programs may be one practical way of promoting this style of working. Such programs can be developed and implemented without additional resources and are associated with improvements in rehabilitation process, patient outcome, and a more positive attitude amongst nurses toward rehabilitation work.[150–152]

The role of the nurse in rehabilitation

Literature reviews of stroke and elderly care nursing suggest there is a lack of clarity over the role of the nurse in multidisciplinary teams, of sufficient degree to impede the effective functioning of those teams.[140,153–155] It has been argued that nurses lack the confidence, knowledge, or skills to assume an appropriate role in rehabilitation,[156] and findings from action research seem to confirm this.[157]

Previous work has drawn attention to competing models of care between the traditional caring/doing role of nurses and the encouraging/facilitating role more appropriate to rehabilitation.[154,158,159] These competing models of nursing care are not simply of theoretical interest: they exist as observed practice.[153,154,160] Addressing deficiencies in nurses' knowledge is believed to increase motivation to work with rehabilitation patients and improve team communication, coordination, and collaboration.[157,159]

It is clear, therefore, that nurses working in elderly care should receive additional training to enable them to incorporate some of the treatment concepts used by therapists as an integral component of their work. Training programs are now proposed in the UK by the Royal College of Nursing to underpin the new post of the gerontological nurse specialist.[161]

Promoting teamwork

One strategy to promote coordination of rehabilitation teams is based on shared documentation. This has been considered as expected practice in the UK for new intermediate care services.[43] One study involving the implementation of such an approach reported that patients made faster progress, with an associated increased rate of home discharge.[162] The system under study was a relatively simple one—of shared documentation for assessment and progress. There were weekly summary sheets on which treatment goals and patient expected progress were recorded. A particular difficulty with the generalizability of such documentation is disentangling the effects attributable to the documentation from the process undertaken by the local team in arriving at the documentation. The exercise inevitably involves team-building and shared ownership of the final product, either of which may independently improve patient outcomes.

Teamwork can also be promoted by multidisciplinary ward rounds. In a trial ($n = 1102$) investigating multidisciplinary ward rounds (physician, nurse, pharmacist, nutritionist, and social worker), clinical outcomes were unchanged but there were useful resource benefits, including decreased length of hospital stay and associated lower hospital costs.[163]

AN INTEGRATED CARE PATHWAY (ICP)   This is a technique that uses a proforma template to describe explicitly the content and timing of complex multidisciplinary care. It is overseen by a delegated professional, usually a nurse. Intuitively, ICPs should be of greatest value if the starting position is one of disorganization, and of least value in well-ordered settings. Thus, they have been shown to reduce hospital length of stay when introduced for fractured neck of femur,[164] but had no additional advantage in an established stroke unit where the care was already well organized.[165]

THE CONTENT OF REHABILITATION

The content of rehabilitation is of great concern to patients. It is, after all, what the patient and carer actually experience. In this sense, assessment, teamwork, goals, and rehabilitation professionals are collectively the vehicle to deliver the treatment elements that have the potential to improve functional abilities and health status. The vehicle has a daunting task, for the repertoire of rehabilitation treatments is enormous. Selecting the right interventions, in the right order, for the right patient, in the right circumstance, requires fine judgment. Moreover, negative experiences, or critical incidents, have lingering effects and impede disability adjustment.[166]

A recent report identified a staggering 35 systematic reviews for rehabilitation topics of relevance to older people.[60] Reviews were available for back pain, neck pain, diabetes, fractured neck of femur, occupational therapy in nursing homes, chronic pulmonary disease, cardiac rehabilitation, falls, and stroke. However, these reviews disguise an important general deficiency in our knowledge. They largely describe the effects of complex interventions—sometimes called *packages* of care. The content of rehabilitation packages can appear chaotic and the relative contribution of an item, or items, is speculative. The term "black box" has become a fashionable concept to indicate our imprecise understanding of these rehabilitation packages. Some light has now been let in to the black box and, as anticipated, it contains individualized, dynamic, and multicomponent interventions.[166–168]

One approach that can be helpful in understanding and clarifying the components is to consider rehabilitation in terms of "hard" and "soft" elements (Figure 21-2).[169] Traditionally, rehabilitation has been described in terms of hard components. Many of these are described in Chapter 22. These are the tangible entities—aids, physical treatments, environmental adaptations—that can be observed, counted, and costed. However, patient descriptions of the experience of rehabilitation emphasize the importance and value of soft rehabilitation: talking to, listening, understanding, encouraging, and counseling.[166–168] These are less visible components, harder to quantify and record, and easily neglected in hard-pressed services. Successful rehabilitation requires an appropriate and unique balance between the hard and soft components for each patient and his or her family.

Rehabilitation goals

Rehabilitation goals are highly focused statements of intent which result from a distillation of the assessment process.[169]

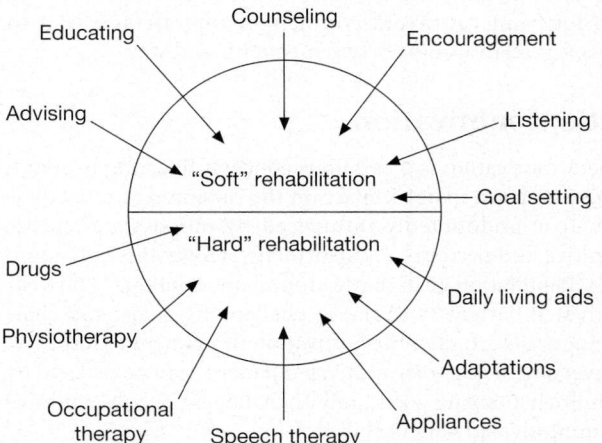

Figure 21-2 The concept of "hard" and "soft" rehabilitation. From Young,[169] with permission.

A helpful definition of a rehabilitation goal is "a future state that is desired and/or expected. The state might refer to relative changes or to an absolute achievement. It might refer to matters affecting the patient, the patient's environment, the family or any other party."[170] Goal-setting is "the process of agreeing on goals, this agreement usually being between the patient and all other interested parties. The process might include setting goals at various levels and in various time frames."[170] A goal is not a vague statement (for example: "to improve mobility"), but is a clear, unambiguous, and measurable statement (for example: "Mrs Brown will walk with her Zimmer frame without assistance six times each day").

The literature on goal-setting covers conceptual approaches,[172] consideration of their applicability,[171,172] direct practical advice on the use of goals,[173] and the use of goal-setting as an outcome tool.[174] Good descriptions of the importance and construction of rehabilitation goals are available.[174] Research evidence has demonstrated that using goals improves rehabilitation outcome provided that there is significant patient involvement, that both short-term and long-term goals are developed, and that the planning of goals is supported with specific interventions.[170] However, the research base is derived almost exclusively from studies of stable disability, generally in the context of outpatient work. The extent to which these studies generalize to the "frail" elderly population is speculative. Moreover, there is little consensus about how goal-setting should take place. Its implementation in practice varies considerably, and there appears to be no widely accepted method to promote patient and carer ownership of rehabilitation goals.[175]

Within the concept of goal-setting, there is often tension between idealized and actual practice, between negotiated/patient-centered and more externally imposed goals, and between explicit (written) and implicit goals. The goal-setting process itself may highlight differences in expectations of patients and therapists.[176] In essence, a delicate balance needs to be struck in order to present a meaningful challenge and thereby to promote recovery. Importantly, while goal-setting may be a recognized and established part of the rehabilitation process, an understanding of the term is not always shared by patients and carers.[11] The process of negotiation and renegotiation of goals with patients and carers can be laborious but can avoid conflicts of interest and lead to improved relationships between patients and staff.[177]

Patient motivation

Patient motivation is a nebulous concept, referring to something that has a major impact on the outcome of rehabilitation. It is undoubtedly influenced by mood-state and by cognitive and perceptual impairments. However, motivation and rehabilitation goals dance around one another. "The well-motivated patient" will rise to challenging goals, and challenging goals can raise the motivation of a patient to improve. Conversely, "the poorly motivated patient" can be deflated by even unchallenging goals, and unchallenging goals can leave the unmotivated patient stalled.

Although rehabilitation professionals commonly believe that motivation of patients has an important role in determining outcome, there is a lack of shared understanding about

the term "motivation."[178] In an important qualitative study, Maclean et al.[179] investigated the factors affecting motivation for rehabilitation in stroke patients. Information about rehabilitation, favorable comparisons with other stroke patients, and the desire to leave hospital were positive determinants of motivation; whereas overprotection by family members and professionals, lack of information and the provision of mixed messages about rehabilitation, and unfavorable comparisons with other patients were negative determinants of motivation. It seems, therefore, that the wider context of motivation lies in the nature of the relationship between patient and professional. Indeed, Blaxter observed that problems in adjustment and rehabilitation were very likely when the patient's own view of his or her condition differed from that of the rehabilitation team.[17]

Patient education programs

A natural extension of patient involvement in the planning of goals is patient participation in chronic-disease educational programs. These should not be confused with the largely passive provision of information more commonly undertaken in rehabilitation. Simple provision of information to patients and carers may not influence outcome.[180] With the emergence of chronic disease as the largest threat to health status and the largest reason for healthcare expenditure, the potential scope for patient self-management has assumed increased importance.

Much of the work on chronic-disease patient self-management programs has been conducted in the USA, where there are many examples of education programs for specific chronic conditions which have increased helpful behaviors, improved health status and/or decreased healthcare costs of their participants. A bibliography of more than 400 such patient educational studies has been published.[181] The components incorporated into such programs are diverse: cognitive symptom management; exercise; nutrition; fatigue and sleep management; use of community resources; use of medication; dealing with the emotions of fear, anger, and depression; communication with others, including health professionals; problem-solving; and decision-making. These components can be specific to different chronic diseases. One study provided a self-management program for patients with heart disease, lung disease, stroke, or arthritis: improved outcomes in terms of health behaviors, health status, and health resource use resulted.[182]

The carers

Despite the wider recognition that a large component of support for disabled elderly people is provided by informal carers,[183] the needs of carers are still frequently overlooked.[184] The stated intention of the UK government as expressed in the National Strategy for Carers is to "support people who choose to be carers."[185] The reality, however, is that exercising such choice can be extremely difficult. Many carers either drift insidiously into their role or take up their duties in a state of "initial innocence."[186] Carers who take on their role suddenly, or who feel poorly prepared, often experience higher levels of burden.[187] It is therefore important to consider the preparation for care-giving.[188]

Since 1996, Local Authorities in the UK have had a statutory duty to recognize the needs of carers independently during a community-care assessment of a client.[189] A focused approach with attention to four main areas is recommended: practical training for the physical aspects of care; preparing for the emotional aspects of care; learning how to deal with stress; and negotiating access to services.[190] A systematic review of 31 studies addressing the issue of stroke and informal carers concluded that carers' ability to cope with stroke was enhanced both by the use of positive coping strategies (for example, self-control skills) and by more concrete measures (such as stroke information).[191] Overall, the literature indicates that time should be allocated specifically to carers for separate needs assessment and appropriate supportive and practical interventions. Providing support routinely to carers of stroke patients appears well received and is effective.[192,193]

Undetected psychological and physical health problems in carers,[194,195] and deficiencies in training in safe handling skills with consequent risk of injury,[196] are particular concerns. The underprovision of aids and equipment leads some carers to improvise with potentially dangerous home-made gadgets designed to assist with transfers, toileting, and self-care.[197]

Daily living aids and adaptations

The use of aids and adaptations is an important component of rehabilitation content.[198,199] When carefully and correctly identified, they have potential to close "the ecological gap" between what the patient is able to do and what he or she is required to do. Unfortunately, inappropriate prescribing is common,[200] and there is no substitute for individual assessment so that equipment meets a clearly defined objective within a wider rehabilitation program.

Walking aids,[104] bath and toilet aids,[201] chairs,[202] and special kitchen equipment are commonly needed by elderly people with disabilities. Bathing difficulties are common, so it seems perverse that painful joints should be denied the helpful soothing of hot water because of the ergonomics of a "standard" bath. A home assessment visit by an occupational therapist to select and order the appropriate bathing aid, followed by a second visit after delivery for patient instruction, significantly improved the number of arthritic sufferers who were able to bath independently.[203] This finding has special relevance in the light of a study reviewing the frequency with which elderly people get stuck in the bath—an unnerving and undignified situation.[204]

A range of simple aids (raised toilet seat, teapot tipper, tap turner, shoe-horn, elastic laces, and double-handed saucepans) made a major impact in maintaining the independence of elderly people.[205] For patients with rheumatoid arthritis, home-based occupational therapy advice, treatment, and aids provision resulted in a significant improvement in daily living skills.[206]

The provision and organization of even simple aids and adaptations is poor in the UK. The mean delay between requesting and fitting an access ramp for wheelchair users in one study was 14 weeks, with the longest delay reported of 11 months.[20] Many patients experience multiple waiting lists for essential equipment and adaptations. Such waiting lists are less visible than the more politically sensitive surgical waiting lists.

A global indicator that incorporates waiting times for aids and adaptations has been proposed as a mechanism to promote a more user-focused service.[19] The current situation for the provision of aids and adaptations is clearly unsatisfactory, and a recent Audit Commission report was highly critical.[207] It investigated the five equipment services that are the largest in terms of user numbers and cost: orthotics, prosthetics, wheelchair services, community equipment, and audiology. In some sites, and some services, the situation was well-organized; but for most it was shambolic and the main findings of the audit were: lack of involvement of users; low priority afforded by senior managers; underinvestment; and geographic variations in people eligible to receive services, in the range and quantity of equipment provided, in the time spent waiting for its delivery, and in the number of staff trained.[207]

REHABILITATION SERVICES

Rehabilitation is the most complex of all health interventions. There is no other type of service that is required to provide such highly individualized treatments on a scale dictated by the highly prevalent conditions that underlie disability. The complexity appears intrinsic to effectiveness—on the whole, single or simple standardized rehabilitation interventions are unsuccessful.[60] In the face of this process complexity, the structure of services becomes a critical issue. Structure is the cement that binds the process elements and prevents dissipation of effectiveness. The term "packages of care" can be misleading as it can give the impression of production-line sameness. It is the variability that needs to be stressed: each package should have a different content dictated by the needs of the individual elderly person. Structures that have facilitated the complexity and variability of the rehabilitation process for older people include day-hospitals, stroke units, rehabilitation wards, and orthogeriatric units. In these examples the structure is explicit in as much as patients are geographically brought together. For community rehabilitation teams, the structure is more virtual and arises through a common team purpose and shared service objectives.

Location of rehabilitation

Arguments between service providers or professionals about location of rehabilitation tend to be emotionally charged. The currently available research evidence (a systematic review of 45 trials) strongly favors hospital-based rehabilitation.[208] Improved outcomes are reported for hospital stroke-unit care compared with general medical wards (19 trials), and for geriatric assessment units compared with nonspecialist care (11 trials). Early-discharge schemes provide similar outcomes to extended hospital stay but have associated hospital bed-releasing potential. The former group of trials (12 trials) include early discharge for surgical, orthopedic, and medical elderly patients, but the predominant evidence is for stroke (7 trials). Orthogeriatric units—where improved coordination between surgical, geriatric, and rehabilitation staff is the aim—have been widely promoted[209] and are accepted as good practice.[210] However, the overview evidence for effectiveness is inconclusive (7 studies).[164] One reason may be the considerable variation in need of elderly patients with fractures. "Old age" spans three decades and patients range from relatively fit elders with single pathology (osteoporosis) to frail older people with multiple pathology. A systematic review demonstrated that depression, delirium, and dementia are common comorbidities in patients with a fractured neck of femur and have a detrimental effect on outcome.[211] A single trial has reported that patients with dementia are a particular subgroup who may obtain improved outcomes from an orthogeriatric unit.[212]

One argument against hospital care for elderly people is the complexity of hospital healthcare pathways and systems. These fail routinely and regularly and constitute a greater hazard than we commonly acknowledge. Much of the evidence comes from North America and Australia, but a recent report in the UK by the Chief Medical Officer has openly accepted that similar circumstances apply to UK hospitals.[213] The report estimates there could be 85,000 serious adverse healthcare events per year, at a cost of over £2 billion. Half of these adverse events are considered preventable—this represents a genuine challenge for clinical governance. A rationale for services designed to avoid hospital admission for elderly people has been demonstrated[214] but are not yet adequately investigated (3 trials).[208] There is only one randomized trial comparing the effectiveness of stroke unit against domiciliary care for early stroke rehabilitation.[215] Stroke unit care was more effective in reducing mortality, the need for institutional care, and dependence. Thus, best evidence continues to support the stroke unit to optimize outcomes following early stroke rehabilitation.[216]

Although the evidence base is stronger for hospital-based rehabilitation for elderly people, this is to simplify and polarize a complex service situation. The location of rehabilitation is not an either/or situation. The requirement is for the provision of rehabilitation opportunities for elderly people at whatever point they contact health and social care services.[18] The best hospital-based rehabilitation should be multidisciplinary and intensive, and should offer 24-hour supportive care; but it is short-term, disability-orientated, and expensive. Home-based rehabilitation, on the other hand, is less intensive and more likely to be uniprofessional, but has the potential to be more handicap-orientated, involve carers more, take a longer-term perspective, and is cheaper. In a qualitative comparison study of patients treated at home or in hospital, the major difference was that patients at home took the initiative and were more able to express and determine their own goals.[217]

Home-based rehabilitation

The general concept of home-based rehabilitation has attracted widespread support for many years, but it has remained a vague intent rather than a clearly developed set of services. There has recently been an important shift in emphasis from a begrudging alternative to hospital care to a greater recognition of the primacy of home rehabilitation within the wider context of community care. Thus, the perception of home-based rehabilitation as a subsidiary, supporting role (for example, to allow patients to leave hospital more quickly) is changing. It seems common sense that enabling disabled people to do more for themselves in their own homes is eminently more desirable than simply supplying ever-more supportive care: that a therapeutic approach is preferable to a prosthetic one.

Joseph Sheldon was arguably the first to recognize the potential of home-based rehabilitation.[218] His insights were the product of the first systematic survey of disabled older people living in their own homes in which he observed their practical struggles and difficulties. Against this background he reflected on the most appropriate help and services and came to recognize the special relevance and applicability of home-based rehabilitation to address these problems. The UK has needed a full half-century of the National Health Service to endorse Sheldon's conclusions. Even 15 years ago, little home-based physiotherapy was available.[219] Home-based rehabilitation could be relevant to most of the common disabling conditions facing older people.

A systematic review identified 36 randomized controlled trials which evaluated interventions designed to reduce falls.[24] These included short-term exercise programs and home environmental assessments. Clear conclusions were hampered by variability in the interventions and in the outcomes studied. However, there was "reasonable evidence" that exercise programs offer benefit in reducing risk of falls. How such programs should be implemented in routine practice requires more study; but given the recipient patient group, the coverage needed, and the nature of the exercise programs, locality-based services would be a practical way forward. Indeed, the review identified several trials in which the initial falls risk assessment was undertaken in the elderly person's home as this allowed an environmental appraisal and resulted in risk-reduction measures such as home safety modification. In general, the higher the risk of falling, and the more multifaceted the interventions, the greater the benefit.[24]

Osteoarthrosis of hip and knee is a major public health problem affecting elderly people in the UK, with many patients being referred to outpatient physiotherapy departments. However, it is clear from the literature that the main treatment emphasis should be on exercise programs that can readily be delivered in the patient's own home.[220,221] These programs are easy, cheap, and effective; and there is no evidence that routinely used electrotherapies have additional advantages.[222] The principal practical task is to encourage patients to comply with their exercise programs, as those who persevere do best.[220]

Given that hospital stroke-unit care confers proven benefits,[217] this model of care should be seen as the gold standard by service commissioners. Nevertheless, the need to continue the rehabilitation process beyond the hospital period has been recognized for many years.[223] This important area has been considerably under-researched,[224] but recent studies have shown that community rehabilitation does have an important role to play. Several studies[225–230] have selected patients after discharge from a stroke unit where rehabilitation care is optimized and where it might be considered that additional function and improvements improbable. The natural phase of intrinsic, neuroplastic recovery should have long past. Yet, improvements in dressing ability,[227] daily living skills,[225,226] leisure activities,[228] mobility,[229] and reduced readmission[225] have all been reported. However, one trial, the largest occupational therapy trial, reported no benefit.[230]

Perhaps the most surprising finding has been the modest levels of therapy input required. For example, between 15 and 20 home physiotherapy visits to a patient over the 6 months following discharge from hospital appears to be a level of treatment associated with benefit.[231] This modest intervention intensity supports the special relevance of home-based rehabilitation where individual patient and carer problems are more readily identified and addressed. The therapy team operates to minimize handicap and can maximally involve carers (formal and informal). This is in contrast to outpatient therapy when carer involvement is minimal (left at home) and the interventions are at the lower level of disability rather than handicap. Moreover, outpatient attendance for stroke patients has low acceptability.[232]

The geriatric day-hospital

The first geriatric day-hospital was opened in the UK in 1952.[233] Day-hospitals then developed rapidly during the 1960s as an important component of elderly care provision designed to complement inpatient services.[234,235] The model has since been widely applied in New Zealand, Australia, Canada, the USA, and several European countries.

The objective of day-hospital attendance has been succinctly summarized as "to facilitate prolonged independent living for the elderly in the community."[236] There is a strong emphasis on rehabilitation, reflected in the multidisciplinary staffing structure. Reasonable amounts of therapy input can be achieved during a day-hospital attendance and provided in repeated short sessions—a form of delivery particularly suitable to older people with decreased stamina and exercise tolerance.[237,238] The service is sufficiently flexible to respond to a wide range of conditions and associated varying disabilities[237] and needs[239] of the attenders. Patients enjoy attending,[240] and carers find the day-hospital helpful.[241] Indirect supportive evidence for the day-hospital concept comes from instances of sudden day-hospital closure precipitated by industrial action: a short-term closure produced only marginal effects,[242] but a 16-week closure produced an appreciable increase in acute hospital admissions and deaths.[243] A retrospective review estimated that day-hospital attendance had shortened inpatient treatment in 8 percent of patients but had delayed or prevented admission in 42 percent.[244]

Day-hospitals are an expensive form of patient care,[244–247] and the National Audit Office has raised concerns about their cost-effectiveness.[248] More than twice-weekly attendance may be more costly than inpatient care.[249] Patients therefore need to be selected carefully so that only those with potential benefit are asked to attend. One study showed that up to 50 percent of general practitioner referrals to day-hospital could be managed by alternative and cheaper services.[250] Another study showed that nearly half the day-hospital attenders failed to complete their planned course of treatment.[251] Up to 20 percent may be unable to attend owing to motion sickness.[252]

The day-hospital trials have now been synthesized in a systematic review of 12 trials.[253] It was concluded that day-hospital care was an effective outpatient service for older people but was no more effective, and possibly more expensive, than other forms of well-organized elderly care. It appears to be less cost-effective than home-based physiotherapy for stroke after-care.[254] Attempts have been made to re-focus the day-hospital concept and use the multidisciplinary team structure to provide rapid assessment of elderly people and so avoid hospital admission.[127] A continuing role for the day-hospital is likely to depend on the development of more flexible operational policies to encompass rehabilitation outreach, brief outpatient attendance, and problem-based assessment clinics (e.g. falls, continence, movement disorders).[255]

CONCLUSION

Despite the impressive unraveling of the genetic and molecular pathophysiological bases for disease, a simple fact remains that a large proportion of the ill-health faced by elderly people is not amenable to a "cure." Worse, these chronic and (usually) progressive conditions adversely impact on, and limit, personal independence. The role of rehabilitation is to use a diverse collection of interventions to reduce this impact and maximize independence.

KEY POINTS Rehabilitation

- The burden of disability is considerable for elderly people, with an estimated 4.3 million people over 60 years in the UK reporting disability, which represents 46 percent of all older people.

- Rehabilitation is concerned with maximizing functional independence at the level of the whole person set in the context of his or her personal circumstances: family, social, and home environment.

- The World Health Organization's International Classification of Impairments, Disability and Handicap (ICIDH) is a useful model of disease consequence upon which to base the rehabilitation process.

- The practice of rehabilitation requires multidisciplinary assessment and teamwork with a mixture of "hard" approaches (e.g. physical treatments, daily living aids) and "soft" approaches (e.g. educational programs, counseling).

Acknowledgments

Part of this chapter is based on: Young, Brown, Forster, and Clare, "An overview of rehabilitation for older people," Reviews in Clinical Gerontology 1999;9:183–96—with permission from the coauthors, editor, and publisher.

REFERENCES

1. Warren M: Care of the chronic aged sick. Lancet 1946;(i):841–843
2. Department of Health: National Service Framework for Older People. DoH, London, 2001. Available at www.doh.gov.uk/nsf/olderpeople.htm
3. Stuck AE, Siu AL, Wieland GD, Adams J, Rubenstein LZ: Comprehensive geriatric assessment: a meta-analysis of controlled trials. Lancet 1993;342:1032–1036
4. Gompertz P, Ebrahim S: Organisation of rehabilitation services. Rev Clin Gerontol 1992;2:329–343
5. Mair A: Report of Sub-committee of the Standing Medical Advisory Committee, Scottish Health Service Council on Medical Rehabilitation. HMSO, Edinburgh, 1972
6. Aho K, Harmsen S, Marrquardsen J: Cerebrovascular diseases in the community: results of a WHO collaborative study. Bull World Health Org 1980;58:113–130
7. Nocan A, Baldwin S: Trends in Rehabilitation Policy. Audit Commission, London, 1998
8. Wade DT: Measurement in Neurological Rehabilitation. Oxford University Press, Oxford, 1992

9. Isaacs B: Rehabilitation for the elderly. Int Rehabil Med 1984;6:v–viii

10. Campbell AJ, Buchner DM: Unstable disability and the fluctuations of frailty. Age Ageing 1997;26:315–318

11. Lawler J, Dowswell G, Hearn J, Forster A, Young J: Recovering from stroke: a qualitative investigation of the role of goal setting in late stroke recovery. J Adv Nurs 1999;30:401–419

12. Thuriaux MC: Consequences of disease and their measurement: introduction. World Health Stat Quart 1989;42:110–114

13. Martin J, Meltzer H, Eliot D for the Office of Population Censuses and Surveys: The Prevalence of Disability Among Adults. HMSO, London, 1989

14. Wistow G: The changing scene in Britain. In Harding T, Meredith B, Wistow G (eds): Options for Long-Term Care. HMSO, London, 1996

15. Wistow G: Increasing private provision of social care: implications of policy. In Lewis B (ed): Care and Control: Personal Social Services and the Private Sector (Discussion Paper 15). London, Policy Studies Institute, 1987

16. Robins A, Wittenberg R: The Health of Elderly people: Economic Aspects. HMSO, London, 1996

17. Blaxter M: The Meaning of Disability. Heinemann, London, 1976

18. Robinson J, Batstone G: Rehabilitation: A Development Challenge. King's Fund, London, 1996

19. Young J, Turnock S: Community care waiting lists and older people. BMJ 2001;322:254

20. Wanklyn P, Kearney M, Hart A, Mulley GP: The provision of ramps for wheelchair users. Clin Rehab 1996;10:81–82

21. Mulrow C, Lau J, Cornell J, Brand M: Antihypertensive Treatment in the Elderly. The Cochrane Library, Oxford (update software)

22. Young J, Robinson J, Dickinson E: Rehabilitation for older people. BMJ 1998;316:1108–1109

23. Stuck AE, Walthert JM, Nikolaus T, Bula CJ, Hohmann C, Beck JC: Risk factors for functional status decline in community-living elderly people: a systematic literature review. Social Sci Med 1999;48:445–469

24. Effective Health Care: Preventing Falls and Subsequent Injury in Older People. NHS Centre for Reviews and Dissemination, University of York, UK, 1996

25. Fries JF: Ageing, natural death, and a compression of morbidity. N Engl J Med 1980;303:130–135

26. Grundy P: Ageing, ill-health and disability. In Tallis R (ed): Increasing Longevity: Medical, Social and Political Implications. Royal College of Physicians of London, 1998

27. Ham C, Hunter DJ, Robinson R: Evidence-based policy making. BMJ 1995;310:71–72

28. Smith R: Scientific basis of health services. BMJ 1995;311:961–962

29. Audit Commission: Making a Reality of Community Care. HMSO, London, 1986

30. Department of Health: NHS Responsibilities for Meeting Continuing Health Care Needs—HSG (98)8. DoH, London, 1995

31. Pearson M, Wistow G: The boundary between health care and social care. BMJ 1995;311:208–209

32. Audit Commission: The Coming of Age: Improving Care Services for Older People. HMSO, London, 1998

33. Health Advisory Service: Not Because They Are Old: An Independent Enquiry into the Care of Older People on Acute Wards at General Hospitals. Health Advisory Service, 2000

34. Department of Health: Shaping the Future NHS: Long Term Planning for Hospital Services. DoH, London, 2000

35. Vetter NJ: Hospitals, Jim, but not as we know them. Rev Clin Gerontol 1997;7:195–197

36. Capewell S: The continuing rise in emergency admissions. BMJ 1996;313:991–992

37. Department of Health: The NHS Plan: A Plan for Investment; a plan for reform. DoH, London, 2000

38. Secretary of State for Health: The New NHS. HMSO, London, 1998

39. British Geriatrics Society: General Practitioner Vocational Training in Geriatric Medicine (compendium document F5). BGS, London, 1997

40. Kavanagh S, Knapp M: The impact on general practitioners of the changing balance of care for elderly people living in institutions. BMJ 1998;317:322–327

41. Dowling A: What People Say about Prioritising Health Services. King's Fund, London, 1993

42. Steiner A: Intermediate Care: A Conceptual Framework and Review of the Literature. King's Fund, London, 1997

43. Health Service Circular 2001/01: LAC 2001/01

44. Vaughan B, Lathlean J: Intermediate Care: Models in Practice. King's Fund, London, 1999

45. Grimley Evans J, Tallis R: A new beginning for care for elderly people? BMJ 2001;322:807–808

46. British Geriatrics Society: Intermediate Care: Medical Guidance for Purchasers and Providers (compendium document D4). BGS, London, 1998

47. Young J, Philp I: Future directions for geriatric medicine. BMJ 2000;320:133–134

48. Morris J: The case for a community geriatrician. BMJ 1994;308:1184

49. Bansal A, Young J: A survey of community training experience for specialist registrars in elderly-care medicine. Age Ageing 2001;30:533–534

50. Verbrugge LM, Jette AM: The disablement process. Soc Sci Med 1994;38(1):1–14

51. Townsend P: Poverty in the United Kingdom. Penguin, Harmondsworth, 1979:688

52. Tennant A: Models of disability: a critical perspective. Disabil Rehabil 1997;19:478–479

53. Marks D: Models of disability. Disabil Rehabil 1997;19:85–91

54. Philipson C: Capitalism and the Construction of Old Age. Macmillan, London, 1982

55. Swain J, Finkelstein V, French S, Oliver M (eds): Disabling Barriers—Enabling Environments. Sage, London, 1993

56. Oliver M: The Politics of Disablement. Macmillan, London, 1990

57. Sridhar MK: Pulmonary rehabilitation: improves quality of life in chronic lung disease, but evaluation must continue. BMJ 1997;314:1361

58. Griffiths TL, Burr ML, Campbell IA et al: Results at 1 year of outpatient multidisciplinary pulmonary rehabilitation: a randomised controlled trial. Lancet 2000;355:362–368

59. de Bono DP: Models of cardiac rehabilitation. BMJ 1998;316:1329–1330

60. Sinclair A, Dickinson E: Effective Practice in Rehabilitation: The Evidence of Systematic Reviews. King's Fund, London, 1998

61. Prince M: The classification and measurement of disablement, with emphasis on depression, and its applications for clinical gerontology. Rev Clin Gerontol 1998;8:227–240

62. Behrens E, Brambring M: Inter-rater reliability of the ICIDH of the World Health Organization. Int J Rehabil Res 1987;10:391–404

63. Lankhorst GJ, Hoppener MG, van der Kaaij JE: Preliminary experiences with WHO's ICIDH; a user's report. Int Rehabil Med 1985;7:70–72

64. Wade DT: Personal context as a focus for rehabilitation. Clin Rehabil 2000;14:115–118

65. Tallis R: Measurement and the future of rehabilitation: the Marjorie Warren lecture 1988. Geriatr Med 1989;19:31–40

66. Wade DT: Evidence relating to assessment in rehabilitation. Clin Rehabil 1998;12:183–186

67. Wade DT: Measurement in Neurological Rehabilitation. Oxford University Press, Oxford, 1995

68. Barer D: Assessment in rehabilitation. Rev Clin Gerontol 1993;3:169–186

69. Jones L: The standardised test. Clin Rehabil 1991;5:177–180

70. Granger C, Brownscheidle C: Outcome measurement in medical rehabilitation. Tech Assess Health Care 1995;11:262–268

71. Royal College of Physicians and British Geriatrics Society Joint Workshops: Standard Assessment Scales for Elderly People. Royal College of Physicians, London, 1992

72. Engel GL: How much longer must medicine's science be bounded by a seventeenth century world view? Psychother Psychosom 1992;57:3–16

73. Greenhalgh T, Hurwitz B: Narrative based medicine: why study narrative? BMJ 1999;318:48–50

74. Launer J: Narrative based medicine: a narrative approach to mental health in general practice. BMJ 1999;318:117–119

75. Elwyn G, Gwyn R: Narrative based medicine: stories we hear and stories we tell—analysing talk in clinical practice. BMJ 1999;318:186–188

76. Adams GF, Hurwitz LJ: Mental barriers to the recovery from stroke. Lancet 1963;(ii):533–537

77. Burn WK, Davis KM, McKensie FR, Rothwell JA, Wattis JP: The prevalence of psychiatric illness in acute geriatric admissions. Int J Geriatr Psychiat 1993;8:171–174

78. House A: Mood disorders in the physically ill: problems of definition and measurement. J Psychomat Res 1988;32:345–353

79. D'Ath P, Cattonia P, Mullan P, Evans S, Cattonia C: Screening, detection and management of depression in primary care attenders. 1: The acceptability and performance of the fifteen item geriatric depression scale and the development of shorter versions. Fam Pract 1994;11:260–266

80. Shah A, Herbert R, Lewis, Mabendran R, Platt J, Bhattacharyya B: Screening for depression among acutely ill geriatric in-patients with a short geriatric depression scale. Age Ageing 1997;26:217–221

81. Zigmond AS, Snaith RP: The hospital and anxiety depression scale. Acta Psychiatr Scand 1983;67:361–370

82. Hodkinson HM: Evaluation of a mental test score for assessment of mental impairment in the elderly. Age Ageing 1992;1:233–238

83. Folstein MF, Folstein SE, McHugh PR: "Mini Mental State"—a practical method for grading the cognitive state of patients for the clinician. J Psychiatr Res 1975;12:89–98

84. Harwood D, Hope T, Jacaby R: Cognitive impairment in medical inpatients. 1: Screening for dementia. Is history better than mental state? Age Ageing 1997;26:31–35

85. Hammond MF, O'Keefe ST, Barer DH: Development and validation of a brief observer-rated screening scale for depression in elderly medical patients. Age Ageing 2000;29:511–515

86. Cunningham C, Horgan F, O'Neill D: Clinical assessment of rehabilitation potential of the older patient: a pilot study. Clin Rehabil 2000;14:205–207

87. Berman P, O'Reily SC: Gait disturbance in the elderly. Rev Clin Gerontol 1995;5:83–88

88. Young JB, Perkins P, Chamberlain MA: Initial experience with a telemeterised gait analysis system. Clin Rehabil 1989;3:205–209

89. Lundin-Olsson L, Nyberg L, Gustafson Y: "Stops walking when talking" as a predictor of falls in elderly people. Lancet 1997;349:617

90. Goodkin R, Driller L: Reliability among physical therapists in diagnosis and treatment of gait deviations in hemiplegics. Percept Motor Skills 1973;37:727–734

91. Chin PL, Rosie A, Irving M, Smith R: Studies in hemiplegic gait. In Rose C (ed): Advances in Stroke Therapy. Raven Press, New York, 1982:197–211

92. MacKnight C, Rockwood K: Assessing mobility in elderly people: a review of performance-based measures of balance, gait and mobility for bedside use. Rev Clin Gerontol 1995;5:464–486

93. Brandstater ME, de Bruin H, Gowland C, Clark BM: Hemiplegic gait: analysis of temporal variables. Arch Phys Med Rehabil 1983;64:583–587

94. Witte US, Carlsson JY: Self-selected walking speed in patients with hemiparesis after stroke. Scand J Rehabil Med 1997;29:161–165

95. Bohannon RW: Correlation of lower limb strengths and other variables with standing performance in stroke patients. Physiother Can 1989;41:198–202

96. Holden MK, Gill KM, Maglizzi MR: Gait assessment for neurologically impaired patients. Phys Ther 1986;66:1530–1539

97. Wade DT, Wood VA, Heller A, Maggs J, Langton-Hewer R: Walking after stroke: measurement and recovery over the first three months. Scand J Rehabil Med 1987;19:25–30

98. Wolfson L, Whipple R, Amerman P, Tobin JN: Gait assessment in the elderly: a gait abnormality rating scale and its relation to falls. J Gerontol A 1990;11:M12–M19

99. May D, Nayak USL, Isaacs B: The life-space diary: a measure of mobility in old people at home. Int Rehabil Med 1985;7(4):182–186

100. Martin BJ, Cameron M: Evaluation of walking speed and functional ambulation categories in geriatric day hospital patients. Clin Rehabil 1996;10:44–46

101. Green J, Forster A, Young J: Reliability of gait speed measured by a timed walking test in patients one year after stroke. Clin Rehabil 2002;16:306–314

102. Mulley GP: Walking sticks. In Everyday Aids and Appliances. BMJ, London, 1989

103. Dobrin L: Origin and evolution of the walkerette. Mount Sinai J Med 1980;47:172–174

104. Mulley GP: Walking frames. In More Everyday Aids and Appliances. BMJ, London, 1991

105. Malloney J, Euhardy RPT, Carnes M: A comparison of a two-wheeled walker and a three-wheeled walker in a geriatric population. J Am Geriatr Soc 1992;40:208–212

106. Prajapati C, Watkins C, Cullen H, Orugun O, King D, Rowe J: The "S" test—a preliminary study of an instrument for selecting the most appropriate mobility aid. Clin Rehabil 1996;10:314–318

107. Chamberlain MA: Mobility of the elderly arthritic. In Wright V (ed): Bone and Joint Disease in the Elderly. Churchill Livingstone, Edinburgh, 1983

108. Young JB: Sheltered housing for the elderly: too many unanswered questions. Arch Geriatr Gerontol 1991;12:13–23

109. Liang MH, Larson MG, Cullen KE, Schwartz JA: Comparative measurement efficiency and sensitivity of five health status instruments for arthritis research. Arthritis Rheum 1985;28:542–547

110. Mahoney FI, Barthel DW: Functional evaluation: the Barthel Index. Maryland State Med J 1965;14:61–65

111. Wade DT, Collin C: The Barthel ADL Index: a standard measure of physical disability. Int Disabil Stud 1988;10:64–67

112. Collin C, Wade DT, Davies S, Horne V: The Barthel ADL Index: a reliability study. Int Disabil Stud 1988;10:61–63

113. Wade DT, Hewer RL: Functional disabilities after stroke: measurement, natural history and prognosis. J Neurol Neurosurg Psychiat 1987;50:172–182

114. Wylie CM: Gauging the response of stroke patients to rehabilitation. J Am Geriatr Soc 1967;15:797–805

115. Wade DT, Wood VA, Hewer RL: Hospital admission for acute stroke: who, for how long, and to what effect? J Epidemiol Commun Health 1985;39:347–352

116. Stone SP, Ali B, Auberleek I, Thompsell A, Young A: The Barthel Index in clinical practice: use on a rehabilitation ward for elderly people. J R Coll Physicians Lond 1994;28:419–423

117. Al-Khawaja I, Wade DT, Turner F: The Barthel Index and its relationship to nursing dependency in rehabilitation. Clin Rehabil 1997;11:335–337

118. Harwood RH, Ebrahim S: Measuring the outcomes of day hospital attendance: a comparison of the Barthel Index and London Handicap Scale. Clin Rehabil 2000;14:527–531

119. Chong DK: Measurement of instrumental activities of daily living in stroke. Stroke 1995;26:1119–1122

120. Holbrook M, Skilbeck CE: An activities index for use with stroke patients. Age Ageing 1983;12:166–170

121. Nouri FM, Lincoln NB: An extended activities of daily living scale for stroke patients. Clin Rehabil 1987;1:301–305

122. Green J, Forster A, Young J: A test–retest reliability study of the Barthel Index, the Rivermead Mobility Index, the Nottingham Extended Activities of Daily Living Scale, and the Frenchay Activities Index in stroke patients. Disabil Rehabil 2001;15:670–676

123. Wood-Dauphine SL, Opzoomer MA, Williams JI, Marchard B, Spitzer WO: Assessment of global function: the reintegration to normal living index. Arch Phys Med Rehabil 1988;69:583–590

124. Harwood RH, Ebrahim S: Manual of the London Handicap Scale. Dept of Health Care of the Elderly, University of Nottingham, Nottingham, UK, 1998

125. Van Swieten JC, Koudstaal PJ, Visser MC, Schouten HJA, Van Gijn J: Inter-observer agreement for the assessment of handicap in stroke patients. Stroke 1988;19:604–607

126. Trigg R, Wood VA, Langton-Hewer R: Social reintegration after stroke: the first stages in the development of the Subjective Index of Physical and Social Outcome (SIPSO). Clin Rehabil 1999;13:341–353

127. Black DA: Emergency day hospital assessments. Clin Rehabil 1997;11:344–346

128. Audit Commission: First Assessment: A Review of District Nursing Service in England and Wales. HMSO, London, 1999

129. Philp I: Can a medical and social assessment be combined? J R Soc Med 1997;90:11–13

130. Philp I, Newton P, Rowse G, McKee KJ, Bath PA, Dixon S: Feasibility, cost and benefits of a standardised approach to the over-75 health checks in primary care. Final report of the SCOPE project, University of Sheffield, UK, 1999

131. UK College of Occupational Therapists: Statement on Home Visiting with Hospital In-patients (SPP 170), 1990

132. Patterson CJ, Mulley GP: The effectiveness of predischarge home assessment visits: a systematic review. Clin Rehabil 1999;13:101–104

133. Cumming RG, Thomas M, Szonyi G, Salkeld G, O'Neill E, Westbury C, Frampton G: Home visits by an occupational therapist for assessment and modification of environmental hazards: a randomised trial of falls prevention. J Am Geriatr Soc 1999;47:1397–1402

134. van Haastregt JCM, Diederiks JPM, van Rossum E, de Witte LP, Crebolder HFJM: Effects of preventative home visits to elderly people living in the community: a systematic review. BMJ 2000;320:754–758

135. UK General Medical Council. Working in Teams. Available at www.gmc.org.uk

136. Belbin M: Management Teams: Why They Succeed or Fail. Heinemann, Oxford, 1981

137. Calkins DR, Rubenstein LV, Cleary PD: Failure of physicians to recognise functional disability in ambulatory patients. Ann Intern Med 1991;114:451–454

138. Patrick DL, Peach H, Gregg I: Disablement and care: a comparison of patient views and general practitioner knowledge. J R Coll Gen Pract 1982;32:429–434

139. McGrath JR, Davis AM: Rehabilitation: where are we going and how do we get there? Clin Rehabil 1992;6:225–235

140. Waters KR, Luker KA: Staff perspectives on the role of the nurse in rehabilitation wards for elderly people. J Clin Nurs 1996;5:103–114

141. Barnitt R, Pomery V: A holistic approach to rehabilitation. Br J Ther Rehabil 1995;2:87–92

142. Strasser DC, Falconer JA, Martino-Saltzmann D: The rehabilitation team: staff perceptions of the hospital environment, the interdisciplinary team environment and interprofessional relations. Arch Phys Med Rehabil 1994;75:177–181

143. Stachura K: Professional dilemmas facing physiotherapists. Physiotherapy 1994;80:357–360

144. Neal LJ: The rehabilitation nursing team in the home health care setting. Rehabil Nurs 1995;20:32–36

145. Benson L, Ducanies A: Nurses' perceptions of their role and role conflicts. Rehabil Nurs 1995;20:204–211

146. Bergman B: Professional role and autonomy in physiotherapy: a study of Swedish physiotherapists. Scand J Rehabil Med 1990;22:79–84

147. Pollock AS, Legg L, Langhorne P, Sellars C: Barriers to achieving evidence-based stroke rehabilitation. Clin Rehabil 2000;14:611–617

148. Andrews K, Brocklehurst JC: Provision of remedial therapists in geriatric medicine. BMJ 1984;289:661–663

149. Davis A, Davis S, Moss N: First steps toward an interdisciplinary approach to rehabilitation. Clin Rehabil 1992;6:237–244

150. Dowswell G, Forster A, Young J, Sheard J, Wright P, Bagley P: The development of a physiotherapist-led stroke training programme for nurses. J Clin Nurs 1999;8:743–752

151. Forster A, Dowswell G, Young J, Bagley P, Sheard J, Wright P: Effect of a physiotherapist-led training programme on attitudes of nurses caring for patients after stroke. Clin Rehabil 1999;13:113–122

152. Forster A, Dowswell G, Young J, Sheard J, Wright P, Bagley P: Effects of a physiotherapist-led stroke training programme for nurses. Age Ageing 1999;28:567–574

153. O'Connor S: Nursing and rehabilitation: the interventions of nurses in stroke patient care. J Clin Nurs 1993;2:29–34

154. Costello J: The role of the nurse in the multidisciplinary team. Rev Clin Gerontol 1994;4:169–176

155. Nolan M, Nolan J: Nursing and rehabilitation: towards new horizons. Rev Clin Gerontol 1998;8:319–329

156. Myco F: Stroke and its rehabilitation: the perceived role of the nurse in the medical and nursing literature. J Adv Nurs 1984;9:429–439

157. Gibbon B, Little V: Improving stroke care through action research. J Clin Nurs 1995;4:93–100

158. Wilden Holmqvist L, Wrethagen N: Education programmes for those involved in the total care of the stroke patient. In Banks MA (ed): International Perspectives in Physical Therapy. Churchill Livingstone, Edinburgh, 1986

159. Passarella PM: Integration of nursing and therapy: an educational approach. Rehabil Nurs 1983;8:32–35

160. Booth J, Davidson I, Winstanley J, Waters K: Observing washing and dressing stroke patients: nursing intervention compared with occupational therapists. What is the difference? J Adv Nurs 2001;33(1):98–105

161. Ford P, McCormack B: Future directions for gerontology: a nursing perspective. Nurse Educ Today 2000;20:389–394

162. Rosenberg W, Parkes J, Jenkins A et al: Making a rehabilitation hospital for the elderly work. Health Trends 1986;18:66–72

163. Curley C, McEachern JE, Speroff T: A firm trial of interdisciplinary rounds on the inpatient medical wards: an intervention designed using continuous quality improvement. Med Care 1998;36:AS4–AS12

164. Cameron I, Crotty M, Currie C: Geriatric rehabilitation following fractures in older people: a systematic review. Health Technol Assess 2000;4:no. 2

165. Sulch D, Perez I, Melbourne A, Kalra L: Randomised controlled trial of integrated care pathway for stroke rehabilitation. Stroke 2000;31:1929–1934

166. Pound P, Gompertz P: A patient-centred study of the consequences of stroke. Clin Rehabil 1998;12:338–347

167. Dowswell G, Lawler J, Young J: Unpacking the "black box" of a nurse-led stroke support service. Clin Rehabil 2000;14:160–171

168. Pound P, Bury M, Gompertz P, Ebrahim S: Views of survivors of stroke on benefits of physiotherapy. Qual Health Care 1994;3:69–74

169. Young J: Rehabilitation and older people. BMJ 1996;313:677–681

170. Wade DT: Evidence related to goal planning in rehabilitation. Clin Rehabil 1998;12:273–275

171. King I: The theory of goal attainment. In Frey MA, Sieloff CL (eds): Advancing King's Systems Framework and Theory of Nursing. Sage, London, 1995

172. Roy C, Andrews HA: The Roy Adaptive Model: the Definitive Statement. Appleton & Lange, Norwalk, CT, 1991

173. Kemp N, Richardson E: The Nursing Process and Quality Care. Arnold, London, 1994

174. Rockwood K: Setting goals in geriatric rehabilitation and measuring their attainment. Rev Clin Gerontol 1994;4:141–149

175. Playford ED, Dawson L, Limbert V, Smith M, Ward CD, Wells R: Goal-setting in rehabilitation: report of a workshop to explore professionals' perceptions of goal-setting. Clin Rehabil 2000;14:491–496

176. Reid A, Chesson R: Goal attainment scaling. Physiotherapy 1998;84:136–144

177. Becker MC, Abrams KS, Onder J: Goal setting: a joint patient staff method. Arch Phys Med Rehabil 1974;55:87–89

178. Maclean N, Pound P: A critical review of the concept of patient motivation in the literature on physical rehabilitation. Soc Sci Med 2000;50:495–506

179. Maclean N, Pound P, Wolfe C, Rudd A: Qualitative analysis of stroke patients' motivation for rehabilitation. BMJ 2000;321:1051–1054

180. Forster A, Smith J, Young J, House A, Knapp P, Wright J: A Systematic Review of Information Provision to Stroke Patients and Carers. The Cochrane Library, Oxford (update software)

181. Center for the Advancement of Health, Center for Health Studies of Group Health Cooperative of Puget Sound: An Indexed Bibliography on Self-management for People with Chronic Disease, 1st edn. Washington, DC: CA Health, 1996

182. Lorig KR, Sobel DS, Stewart AL: Evidence suggesting that a chronic disease self-management program can improve health status while reducing hospitalisation: a randomised trial. Med Care 1999;37(1):5–14

183. Robins A, Wittenberg W: The Health of Elderly People: Economic Aspects in the Health of Elderly People—An Epidemiological Overview. HMSO, London, 1992

184. Carers National Association: Listen to Carers. London, 1992

185. Department of Health: Caring about Carers: A National Strategy for Carers. DoH, London, 1999

186. Taraborrelli P: Exemplar A—becoming a carer. In Gilbert N (ed): Researching Social Life. Sage, London, 1993

187. Archbold PG, Stewert BJ, Greenlick MR, Harvarth TA: The clinical assessment of mutuality and preparedness in family caregivers of frail older people. In Funk SG, Tornquist EMT, Champagne MT, Wiese RA (eds): Key Aspects of Elder Care: Managing Falls, Incontinence and Cognitive Impairment. Springer, New York, 1992:328–339

188. Brereton L, Nolan M: "You do know he's had a stroke, don't you?" Preparation for family care-giving—the neglected dimension. J Clin Nurs 2000;9:498–506

189. Carers (Recognition and Services) Act 1995. HMSO, London

190. Stewert BJ, Archbold PG, Harvath TA, Nkongho NO: Role acquisition in family caregivers of older people who have been discharged from hospital. In Funk SG, Tornquist EH, Champagne MT, Weise RA (eds): Key Aspects of Caring for the Chronically Ill: Hospital and Home. Springer, New York, 1993:219–231

191. Low JTS, Payne S, Roderick P: The impact of stroke on informal carers: a literature review. Soc Sci Med 1999;49:711–725

192. Dowswell G, Lawler J, Young J, Forster A, Hearn J: A qualitative study of specialist nurse support for stroke patients and care-givers at home. Clin Rehabil 1997;11:293–301

193. Mant J, Wade D, Winner S: Family support for stroke: a randomised controlled trial. Lancet 2000;356:808–813

194. Canwath TCM, Johnson DAW: Psychiatric morbidity among spouses of stroke. BMJ 1987;294:409–411

195. Wade DT, Leigh-Smith J, Hewer RL: Effects of living with and looking after survivors of stroke. BMJ 1986;293:418–420

196. Brown AR, Muley GP: Injuries sustained by caregivers of disabled elderly people. Age Ageing 1997;26:21–23

197. Brown AR, Mulley GP: Do it yourself: home made aids for disabled elderly people. Disabil Rehabil 1997;19:20–25

198. Chamberlain MA: Aids and the equipment for the arthritic. Practitioner 1980;224:65–71

199. Cochrane G: Aids in the home. Br J Hosp Med 1983;29:121–126

200. George J, Binns VE, Clayton AD, Mulley GP: Aids and adaptations for the elderly at home. BMJ 1988;296:1365–1366

201. Chamberlain MA, Thornley G, Wright V: Evaluation of aids and equipment for the bath and toilet. Rheumatol Rehabil 1978;17:187–194

202. Ellis MI, Minston JS, Chamberlaine MA: Seating for the Elderly and Arthritic. DHSS, London, 1983

203. Chamberlain MA, Thornley G, Stowe J, Wright V: Evaluation of aid and equipment for the bath. II: A possible solution to the problem. Rheumatol Rehabil 1981;20:38–43

204. Gooptu C, Mulley GP: Survey of elderly people who get stuck in the bath. BMJ 1994;308:762

205. Hart D, Bowling A, Ellis M, Silman A: Locomotor disability in very elderly people: value of a programme for screening and provision of aids for daily living. BMJ 1990;301:216–217

206. Helewa A, Goldsmith CH, Lee P: Effects of occupational therapy home service on patients with rheumatoid arthritis. Lancet 1991;337:1453–1456

207. Audit Commission: Fully Equipped. HMSO, London, 2000

208. Parker G, Bhakta P, Katbamna S et al: Best place of care for older people after acute and during subacute illness: a systematic review. J Health Serv Res Policy 2000;5(3):176–189

209. Audit Commission: United They Stand. HMSO, London, 1995

210. Pearse M, Woolf A: Care of elderly people with fractured neck of femur. Health Trends 1992;24:134–136

211. Holmes JD, House AO: Psychiatric illness in hip fracture. Age Ageing 2000;29:537–546

212. Huusko TM, Karppi P, Avikainen V, Kautianen H, Sulkava R: Randomised, clinically controlled trial of intensive geriatric rehabilitation in patients with hip fracture: subgroup analysis of patients with dementia. BMJ 2000;321:1107–1111

213. Expert Group on Learning from Adverse Events in the NHS: An Organisation with a Memory. Stationery Office, London, 2000. Available at www.doh.gov.uk/orgmemreport/index.htm

214. Coast J, Inglis A, Morgan K, Gray S, Kammerling M, Frankel S: The hospital admissions study in England: are there alternatives to emergency hospital admission? J Epidemiol Commun Health 1995;49:194–199

215. Kalra L, Evans A, Perez I, Knapp M, Donaldson N, Swift CG: Alternative strategies for stroke care: a prospective randomised controlled trial. Lancet 2000;356:894–899

216. Collaborative systematic review of randomised trials of organised inpatient (stroke unit) care after stroke. The Stroke Trialists' Collaboration. BMJ 1997;314:1151–1159

217. von Koch L, Wottrich AW, Holmqvist LW: Rehabilitation in the home versus the hospital: the importance of context. Disabil Rehabil 1998;10:367–372

218. Sheldon JH: The Social Medicine of Old Age. Oxford University Press, Oxford, 1948

219. Partridge CJ: Physiotherapy in the community. J R Coll Gen Pract 1987;37:194–195

220. Chamberlain MA, Gore G, Hartfield B: Physiotherapy in OA knees. Int J Rehabil Med 1982;4:101–106

221. Callaghan MJ, Oldham JA, Hunt J: An evaluation of exercise regimes for patients with osteoarthritis of the knee: a single blind randomised trial. Clin Rehabil 1995;9:213–218

222. Young J: Rheumatological rehabilitation. Rev Clin Gerontol 1991;1:283–296

223. Garraway WM, Akhtar AJ, Hockey L, Prescott RJ: Management of acute stroke in the elderly: follow-up of a controlled trial. BMJ 1980;281:827–829

224. Young JB: Is stroke better managed in the community? BMJ 1994;309:1356–1358

225. Corr S, Bayer A: Occupational therapy for stroke patients after hospital discharge. Clin Rehabil 1995;9:291–296

226. Logan PA, Gladman JRF, Lincoln NB: A randomised controlled trial of enhanced social service occupational therapy for stroke patients. Clin Rehabil 1997;11:107–113

227. Walker MF, Drummond AER, Lincoln NB: Evaluation of dressing practice for stroke patients after discharge from hospital: a crossover design study. Clin Rehabil 1996;10:23–31

228. Drummond AER, Walker MF: A randomised controlled trial of leisure rehabilitation after stroke. Clin Rehabil 1995;9:283–290

229. Wade DT, Collen FM, Robb GF, Warlow CP: Physiotherapy intervention late after stroke. BMJ 1992;304:609–613

230. Parker CJ, Gladman JRF, Drummond AER et al: A multicentre randomised controlled trial of leisure therapy and conventional occupational therapy after stroke. Clin Rehabil 2001;15:42–52

231. Gladman J, Forster A, Young J: Hospital and home based rehabilitation after discharge from hospital for stroke patients: analysis of two trials. Age Ageing 1995;24:49–53

232. Smith DS, Goldenburg E, Ashburn A: Remedial therapy after stroke: a randomised controlled trial. BMJ 1981;282:517–520

233. Farndale J: The Day Hospital Movement in Great Britain. Pergamon Press, Oxford, 1961

234. Irvine RE: Geriatric day hospitals: present trends. Health Trends 1980;12:68–71

235. Brocklehurst JC, Tucker JS: Progress in Geriatric Day Care. King Edward's Hospital Fund, London, 1980

236. Donaldson C, Wright KG, Maynard AK, Hamil JD, Sutcliffe E: Day hospital for the elderly: utilisation and performance. Commun Med 1987;9:55–61

237. Forster A, Young JB: Day hospital and stroke patients. Int Disabil Stud 1989;11:181–183

238. Nolan MR: The future role of day hospitals for the elderly: the case for a nursing initiative. J Adv Nurs 1987;12:683–690

239. McNicoll M, Comben S: Geriatric day hospital, remedial or social centre? Physiotherapy 1979;65:210–211

240. Peach H, Pathy MS: Evaluation of patients' assessment of day hospital care. Br J Prevent Soc Med 1977;31:209–210

241. Anard KB, Thomas JH, Osbourne KL, Osmolski R: Cost effectiveness of a geriatric day hospital. J R Coll Physicians Lond 1982;16:53–56

242. Bhattacharyya BK, Isherwood J, Sutcliffe RLG: Survey of elderly day hospital patients during a period of industrial action. Age Ageing 1980;9:106–111

243. Berrey PNE: Increase in acute admissions and deaths after closing a geriatric day hospital. BMJ 1986;292:176–178

244. MacFarlane JPR, Collings T, Graham K, MacIntosh JC: Day hospitals in modern clinical practice: cost benefit. Age Ageing 1979;8(suppl):80–86

245. Ross DN: Geriatric day hospitals: counting the cost compared to other methods of support. Age Ageing 1976;5:171–175

246. Donaldson C, Wright KG, Maynard AK: Determining value for money in day hospital care for the elderly. Age Ageing 1986;15:1–7

247. Forster A, Young JB: Cost analysis of geriatric day hospital care. J Clin Exper Gerontol 1991;13:247–262

248. UK National Audit Office: National Health Service Day Hospitals for Elderly People in England. HMSO, London, 1994

249. Hildick-Smith M: Geriatric day hospitals: changing emphasis in costs. Age Ageing 1984;13:95–100

250. George J, Young JB: General practitioners and the geriatric day hospital. Health Trends 1989;21:24–25

251. Zeeli D, Isaacs B: The efficiency and effectiveness of geriatric day hospitals. Postgrad Med J 1988;64:683–686

252. Stokoe D, Zuccollo G: Travel sickness in patients attending a geriatric day hospital. Age Ageing 1985;14:308–311

253. Forster A, Langhorn P, Young J: Systematic review and meta-analysis of day hospital care for older people. BMJ 1999;318:837–841

254. Young J, Forster A: Day hospital and home physiotherapy for stroke patients: a comparative cost effectiveness study. JR Coll Physicians Lond 1993;27:252–257

255. Young J, Forster A: What should we do with our day hospitals? Geriatric Med 1992;Sept:15–16

Chapter 22

Rehabilitation: therapy techniques

Valerie M. Pomeroy and Marion F. Walker

Geriatric rehabilitation has a major impact on length of hospital stay and unnecessary admissions to institutionalized care, burden on carers, and numbers of crisis "social" admissions.[1] In recognition of the contribution of rehabilitation, the recent National Service Framework for Older People in the UK emphasizes the importance of promoting elderly people's health and independence.[2] Therapy is an important component of this service. Specific techniques are used to prevent the onset of disability and to restore, maintain, and control the deterioration of functional ability.

Loss of functional ability can take many different forms. These include the loss of the ability to communicate, remember, walk, perform personal care tasks, and/or perform social roles which are perceived as the norm. Indeed, loss of functional ability can itself lead to secondary difficulties such as depression, muscle wasting, and withdrawal from social interaction and activity.

Rehabilitation is therefore a multifaceted service with therapy provided by a multiprofessional team. For example, speech and language therapists provide interventions targeted at communication difficulties and swallowing problems; psychologists provide interventions targeted at emotional function and cognitive function (e.g. memory and perception); and nurses provide interventions targeted at personal care, mobility, and psychosocial interactions. Effective teamwork is central to the success of rehabilitation. Multiprofessional assessment is followed by treatment and goal-setting with individual patients who are also recognized as being members of the rehabilitation team. Most treatment packages are therefore complex and require continued teamwork to ensure integrated delivery and adjustment.

The complexity of the rehabilitation package is widely recognized and it is frequently perceived as a "black box," particularly by medical members of the team. The aim of this chapter is to describe for doctors *some* of the techniques that are used by therapists to help elderly people maintain or regain optimal independence. To make this task more manageable, the techniques described in this chapter are restricted to those provided by occupational therapists and physiotherapists. Of course, the therapy component of rehabilitation services for elderly people consists of much more than is outlined here, with many other professional groups making key contributions. The techniques outlined in this chapter are therefore presented as *examples* of therapy, illustrating how these are combined for specific patients and groups of patients. The findings of narrative and systematic reviews are used where these are available, but this chapter does not seek to provide a thorough review of the effectiveness of the interventions described.

Descriptions of therapy techniques would be meaningless without placing them in the context of professional expertise and clinical application. Therefore the next section outlines the core skills of occupational therapists and physiotherapists, the therapy research culture, and the process of therapy. Therapy techniques are then connected with the specific conditions of stroke, fractured neck of femur following a fall, Parkinson's disease, and frailty.

OCCUPATIONAL THERAPY AND PHYSIOTHERAPY

Occupational therapy

Occupational therapy has been defined as "the treatment of physical and psychiatric conditions through specific activities in order to help people reach their maximum level of function and independence in all aspects of daily life."[3] An earlier definition by Turner[4] captures the more holistic approach, still favored by many occupational therapists today: "Occupational therapy is the treatment of the whole person by their active participation in purposeful living."

The roots of occupational therapy were first established in the eighteenth century with the work of the French physician and psychiatrist Phillipe Pinel, and the Englishman William Tuke, who—in founding an asylum, "The Retreat at York"—made early attempts to rehabilitate the mentally ill.[5] By the twentieth century a group of professionals evolved the concept of occupation as a restorative agent and of the person as an active participant in promoting personal health.

George Burton coined the term "occupational therapy" in 1914 and the first school of occupational therapy in Great Britain was founded in Bristol in 1930.[6] The main impetus came to occupational therapy during World War II with the first curative workshop set up at Shepherd's Bush Military Hospital by Sir Robert Jones, an eminent British surgeon of the day. He enthused about the value of occupational therapy and urged the War Office to set up other centers. Unfortunately at this time treatment activities were limited to the field of crafts, as the more realistic occupations were not possible because of trade prejudice.[6] This liaison with crafts is where the erroneous concept of the occupational therapist as "diversional therapist" originated.

Reed and Sanderson[7] list some basic concepts that do *not* belong to occupational therapy:

- Occupational therapy should not be used as a means of keeping a person busy.

- Occupational therapy does not provide employment.
- Occupational therapy should not be unplanned or a haphazard program of activities.

Since the early 1900s, occupational therapists have recognized the importance of having a strong theory of occupation to support their practice. Several authors have contributed to this theoretical base in the last 30 years, generating and expanding many models and approaches to be used in treatment.[5] The actual techniques used in day-to-day practice by occupational therapists are both numerous and diverse; and as clinicians primarily use a pragmatic eclectic approach to treat individual patients, it would be inappropriate simply to list them in a book of this nature. However, the main techniques used with elderly people are set out in this chapter.

The skills of the occupational therapist

Joice and Coia[8] describe the core skills of the occupational therapist as follows.

1. The use of selected activity which must be purposeful and meaningful to the individual. For example, in preparation for discharge from hospital to home the occupational therapist would encourage the patient to practise making a hot snack. The task would be purposeful and meaningful either because the patient lives alone or the main carer is out at work all day.
2. Activity analysis to break activities down into physical, cognitive, interpersonal, social, behavioral, and emotional components. To use the example given above: Can the patient manage both the physical and the cognitive components of making a hot snack? Can the person stand for long periods at the sink and cooker unaided, or does he or she require the use of a seat or perching stool? Can the person remember putting toast under the grill? Is the person aware of the sequencing of the tasks involved in making a hot drink? Does the person need to use any specialized equipment to achieve the task independently? If the individual's visual field has been affected by a stroke, can he or she see all the ingredients on the worktop and use them appropriately? Does the person have sufficient concentration and motivation to achieve the task?
3. Assessment and treatment of functional capabilities. The therapist must have the knowledge and ability competently to assess the functional, cognitive, and emotional capabilities of the individual and apply the appropriate treatment. A thorough knowledge of pre-hospital ability is essential for setting appropriate goals. "Competent assessment" in the current climate of evidence-based practice should, where possible, include the use of standardized, valid, and reliable measures. These will permit objective measurement of patients' progress.

The occupational therapist therefore strives to promote recovery through purposeful activity, and encourages the patient to retrain, to practise, and to become independent in some chosen activities of everyday life. These activities may incorporate personal care tasks such as washing, dressing, feeding, toileting, and bathing (known as activities of daily living, ADLs) or more demanding tasks such as outdoor mobility, using public transport, household tasks, and leisure interests (known as extended activities of daily living, EADLs; or instrumental activities of daily living, IADLs).

Occupational therapy training

In the UK, training in occupational therapy involves a four-year course culminating in an honors degree. Topics covered during training include anatomy and physiology, behavioral science, psychology, clinical sciences medicine and psychiatry, research methods, management and social policy, profession-related practice, fieldwork education, theoretical frameworks, therapeutic activity, and core professional skills.

Occupational therapy settings

In the UK, occupational therapists work in a variety of settings: hospitals (ward-based), day-hospitals, day-centers, outpatient departments, social service departments, and health centers. In parts of the UK, and in response to government initiatives (see Chapter 21), new community occupational therapy posts are developing within primary care settings, such as in general practitioner surgeries or within healthcare centers. These posts mainly come under the jurisdiction of the Primary Care Groups, or more recently, Primary Care Trusts.

The social services occupational therapist (SSOT) can provide occupational therapy also in the patient's own home. Local Health Authorities currently fund these posts. This specialist group of occupational therapists is concerned mainly with clients who have permanent and substantial disability, with the aim of helping these people to live independently in the community. They can provide equipment to help a client function more independently, or may supply equipment simply to ease the burden on the carer—such as by the provision of a hoist for bathing. Another remit of the SSOT is to give advice and facilitate structural changes within the disabled person's environment. This may range from outside ramps to enable wheelchair access, to major adaptations such as building a ground-floor bathroom. Social services occupational therapists also provide advice on financial benefits when appropriate.

Surveys indicate that, although social services occupational therapists are highly valued specialists, staffing levels and limited resources mean that their individual case contribution is often very limited.[9]

Physiotherapy

Since its inception in 1895, the profession of physiotherapy has been concerned with movement. Physiotherapists use many techniques to prevent the onset of movement problems, to facilitate recovery in the acute phase following injury, and to rehabilitate people who have a longer-term movement problem. These therapies can be broadly classified as: exercise; manipulation and mobilization of joints and soft tissues; electrotherapy; acupuncture; and hydrotherapy. Physiotherapists also advise on the suitability of various types of devices (e.g. walking aids and orthoses) to assist movement and mobility. Problems with movement occur as the result of many processes, including fractures, arthritis, whiplash injuries, back pain, stress incontinence, repetitive strain injuries, cystic fibrosis, sports injuries, stroke, and stress disorders. Physiotherapists work in many healthcare, social care, and community settings.

The skills of the physiotherapist

Understanding how and why people move as they do underpins the core skill of physiotherapy. Physiotherapists have extensive knowledge and experience of "normal" movement throughout the lifespan and how this is altered by various pathologies and lifestyle processes. An initial assessment identifies what the person can do, what he or she cannot do, where movement becomes difficult, and why. From this a treatment plan is drawn up, in partnership with the patient if possible. Assessment and treatment are therefore based on theoretical knowledge and clinical experience of neural and musculo-skeletal mechanisms involved in movement control and how these are affected by pathology, age, gender, lifestyle, and treatment modality.

Specialization is important to ensure that patients receive high-quality treatment. Physiotherapists specialize in a number of areas of healthcare, including orthopedics, intensive care, pediatrics, musculoskeletal injury, elderly care, sports injuries, psychiatry, neurology, and rheumatology. Consequently physiotherapists have additional core skills pertinent to their particular area of specialization. In addition to specialist knowledge and experience of particular conditions, specialist skills also include those relevant to the theory and practice of specific physical therapy techniques which are gained through postgraduate education and training. This chapter, which outlines only the physical therapy techniques used with elderly people, testifies to the range of skills deployed by physiotherapists.

Development of a research culture

In the UK, physiotherapy became an all-degree profession in 1992. Since then the number of physiotherapists with research skills has risen considerably. In the early 1980s only a few physiotherapists in the UK had been awarded a PhD. In 1997 there were 70 physiotherapists with doctorates and eight professors.[10] At the beginning of 2001 there were 100 physiotherapists with doctorates and 23 professors (nine without doctorates; T. Bury, personal communication). This is a dramatic increase, but still only a small proportion of the 35,000 physiotherapists in the UK.

Occupational therapy is also relatively new to the world of research, with many training schools introducing research modules into the curriculum only in the mid-1990s. The British College of Occupational Therapists has developed a research strategy to meet the research needs of occupational therapists.[11] Occupational therapists are required by the Code of Ethics and Professional Conduct to have: "A duty to ensure that wherever possible their professional practice is based upon established research findings."[12]

The increase in research-aware and research-active therapists is resulting in a more critical approach and a better evidence base for clinical practice. Despite these advances and the recommendations made in a Position Statement to the Department of Health in 1994,[13] standard career paths which include research activity have not yet been established.

However, with the increase in the number of research-active therapists and the publication of high-quality research in peer-reviewed journals, this situation is likely to change.

THE THERAPY PROCESS

Rehabilitation is an active participatory process, so the first contact with the patient is crucial in establishing a good rapport and therapeutic relationship. Assessment—which is essential to determine subsequent interventions and should be an ongoing activity throughout the rehabilitation process—begins at the first meeting.[14] Assessment ascertains what the patient can do, what he or she cannot do, where activities become difficult, and importantly *why* difficulties are experienced.

For example, the Rivermead Perceptual Assessment Battery[15] can be used to assess individual components of perceptual competence. One subtest examines the ability of the individual to discern specific objects in the foreground of a complex picture (figure/ground). Any difficulty experienced with this subtest could explain why a patient cannot simply select trousers from a group of clothes lying on a bed. When a specific problem has been identified, the therapist can suggest the most appropriate therapy.

It is also important at this early stage to ascertain the pre-hospital history of functional ability. Was a patient who has suffered a stroke, for example, able to walk before the stroke, or is the deficit only part of a history of progressive disability? Specific information is needed about the type of activities the patient participated in before referral to therapy, such as how active the person was, what help is presently available at home, and what the person wishes to attain through the therapist's intervention. On interpreting a detailed assessment, movement and functional diagnoses can be made and both are considered with the pathology and medical prognosis.

Goal-setting and treatment planning[16] are based on levels of existing functional and cognitive ability, discussion with the patient (and if appropriate the carer), and clinical judgment. Goals must always be realistic and attainable. As the patient progresses, they need to be reassessed and updated where necessary.

Therapists will also describe, to the patient and carer, their role within the multidisciplinary team and how they would hope to be able to contribute to the restoration of functional ability and social activity.

The framework for assessment, goal-setting, and intervention can be described by the bio-psycho-social approach of healthcare.[17] This holistic approach considers all elements of health: what is happening to parts of the body (pathology, impairment); what processes are happening at the level of the person's experience (disability); and what is happening in the person's wider social context (handicap). This framework is therefore complementary to the commonly used one proposed by the International Classification of Impairments, Disabilities and Handicaps (ICIDH),[18] which was recently updated with important terminological changes—see Chapter 21. As each framework is closely linked with the other, it is immaterial which is used by therapists.[19]

Once intervention has started, continued involvement and education of the main carer is essential if that person is to be able to use the techniques taught to best effect. This is particularly important when the patient is discharged from hospital, at a time when therapeutic interventions are often minimal. Patients, carers, therapists, social services personnel, and home-care services are essential collaborators when planning a successful discharge back into the community.

It is also prudent for the therapist to listen to the patient and carer, as much can be learned from their experiences and suggestions for solutions to individual problems. Therapists also help and support carers throughout the rehabilitation process by providing an ear and an environment where they can express their feelings of frustration, anger, depression, and possibly guilt.[20]

SOME SPECIFIC THERAPY TECHNIQUES

The context for the description of therapy techniques is provided here by four of the most common conditions presenting to therapists: stroke; fractured neck of femur following a fall; Parkinson's disease; and frailty. However, it should be appreciated that a patient may have more than one problem. For example, an elderly person having recently sustained a cardiovascular insult may also demonstrate longer-term frailty with deconditioning and/or permanent impairment of the cardiovascular and musculoskeletal systems. In such circumstances, a therapist addressing each of a patient's difficulties may adopt a "mix and match" approach in devising a treatment program. *Adaptability* and *flexibility* are key therapy skills. This might explain why therapists report using a large number of different interventions for defined clinical presentations—for example, 31 interventions for gait apraxia[21] and 175 interventions for post-stroke shoulder pain.[22] Such detailed description of techniques is important, especially if interventions are being tested in clinical trials; but as the aim of this chapter is to give an overview, techniques will be described here in rather less detail.

Although research into the effectiveness of specific therapy interventions for elderly people is limited at present, there are several therapy topics which are now the subject of Cochrane reviews. However, caution needs to be used when interpreting the results of these reviews. For example, it is difficult to collate the findings from different primary trials because of variation in aims, interventions, and outcomes,[23,24] and the identification of small numbers of compatible trials for meta-analysis.[25,26] Where adequate numbers of compatible trials are available, positive effects of some therapy interventions have been reported—for example, behavioral interventions and targeting environmental hazards to prevent elderly people sustaining a fall.[25] On the other hand, the optimum amount of therapy—its intensity, duration, and timing in the course of treatment[27]—is also uncertain. The descriptions that follow are therefore a snapshot of a changing science of therapy interventions for elderly people.

Stroke

Stroke is the commonest cause of permanent disability in elderly people and is an important area in rehabilitation as evidenced by its use as a "tracer" condition in the Audit Commission's report "The Way to Go Home: Rehabilitation and Remedial Services for Older People."[28] Therapy forms an important part of the multidisciplinary stroke care package which has been shown to prolong life and reduce disability,[29] an effect that is maintained 10 years after stroke.[30] The UK National Clinical Stroke Guidelines recommend that patients in the early phase should see a therapist each working day if possible and that they should be given as much therapy as they find tolerable.[31]

Before looking at some specific therapy techniques, it is important to touch on an issue of particular relevance to physical therapy—the use of "labels" to describe groups of techniques. Physical therapy given after stroke has historically been described by named approaches, and there have been a succession of these (Partridge[32] describes nine). Narrative reviews and trials, however, have not found any one "approach" to be better than any other at reducing disability.[33–35] Currently in the UK, the majority of physiotherapists and 50% of occupational therapists probably use the Bobath approach,[36–38] which emphasizes the facilitation of normal muscle tone and normal, good-quality movement[39] in preference to the direct training of movement tasks. Outside of the UK, the Bobath approach is not as predominant and other approaches are more favored—for example, the "movement science" approach which emphasizes the importance of training everyday activities.[40] However, describing therapy by using these labels probably does not allow any inferences to be made about which specific techniques are used.[41] For example, a recent survey (already alluded to) of nurses, occupational therapists, and physiotherapists in England found that 175 different types of interventions were reported as used for post-stroke shoulder pain, and suggested that there was intraprofessional variation.[22] These data support the clinical impression that the same label can be applied to different collections of therapy techniques, and so this chapter will not describe specific named approaches. Instead we want to give a flavor of the type of techniques that have been described in the stroke rehabilitation literature.

Initial steps

During the early period after stroke in patients with major motor impairment, *positioning*—the use of specific body postures—is advised in the UK National Clinical Stroke Guidelines.[31] A recent survey of physiotherapists found that the most common positions recommended during the first week after stroke were sitting in an armchair, side-lying on the hemiplegic side, and side-lying on the opposite side, with particular importance given to the position of the proximal joints of the limbs. For example, in side-lying on the hemiplegic side, the five most important components were found to be: head in neutral; scapular protraction; glenohumeral external rotation; hip extension; and knee flexion.[42]

During this early rehabilitation period, occupational therapists undertake a comprehensive ADL assessment and screen for perceptual and cognitive difficulties (e.g. the Rey figure screening tool[43]). Perceptual problems are common in both right and left hemiplegic stroke patients.[44] Perceptual screening involves asking the patient to copy a drawing of a complex figure made up of 18 components. This assessment is particularly important if the patient has the physical ability to complete a specified task but still remains dependent on assistance. If ADL difficulties are persistent and unexplained, the occupational therapist will then carry out a more detailed perceptual assessment, using perhaps the Rivermead Perceptual Assessment Battery.[15] This may clarify the type and nature of the perceptual problem and act as a pointer to the specific strategies to be used.

It is also important, early after stroke and throughout the rehabilitation process, to provide information to patients and carers on the nature of stroke, the difficulties they are experiencing, and the therapy interventions they are receiving. This will ensure that patients and carers are totally involved and knowledgeable about the therapeutic aims and objectives of the rehabilitation sessions. Compliance with the treatment regime will therefore be greater. Stroke Family Support Workers also provide much practical, psychological, and emotional support. This support is especially valuable when discharge from hospital is imminent.

Also from the very beginning of the rehabilitation process, therapists emphasize the importance of integration of interventions, and teach other members of the team (including informal carers) specific techniques for individual patients. For example, the occupational therapist may teach techniques to help with dressing, toileting, and/or feeding. These specifics may be directed at improving patients' ability to dress themselves. Some examples are:

- Cross the paretic leg over the the non-paretic one to be able to reach the paretic foot.
- Use a footstool to reach the feet.
- Adopt clothes that are easier to put on and take off, such as elastic-waisted jogging trousers (this can be modified as function returns).
- Use visual cues—such as red thread around armholes, or red thread next to one button and one hole for correct alignment of buttons.
- Practise backwards chaining. Start with the last step in a functional task and then, when this is achieved, work backwards to the first step, so that eventually the person is able to complete the whole task.
- Encourage and exploit progression of ability by, for example, reducing the support provided by a firm chair with arms, to sitting on a bed whilst getting dressed.

The physiotherapist may place a description/diagram of recommended positions above the patient's bed and/or run study days on the principles of normal movement.[22]

Re-education of movement

Therapists are often concerned with the re-education of movement, and many techniques have been used or are being developed.[41]

Active movement   The patient can be asked to produce, or attempt to produce, a voluntary contraction of paretic muscle.[45,46]

Biofeedback   Biofeedback has been used to provide patients with information about muscle activity during movement.[47,48] The technique involves placing EMG electrodes over the belly of the target muscle and producing a visual display of the electrical activity during a movement or functional task.

Constraint-induced therapy   This is based on experimental evidence of the benefits of "forced" use in monkeys (reviewed by Morris et al.[49]). Essentially the technique involves using a sling or a bulky mitten to restrict the nonparetic upper limb. During the period of restriction the patient is provided with an intensive functional exercise program and is encouraged to use the paretic upper limb during everyday activity.[50–56] This technique has not yet been the subject of evaluation in definitive clinical trials and is not in widespread clinical use. Research is ongoing.

Electrostimulation   Electrodes are placed on motor points of wrist and finger extensor muscles to produce full wrist and finger extension with 10 seconds on and 10 seconds off, one hour a day for 15 sessions.[57,58] Francisco and colleagues[59] placed electrodes on extensor carpi radialis and gradually increased the stimulus threshold with each session as voluntary recruitment increased. Functional electrical stimulation is also used particularly to improve ankle dorsiflexion during walking.[60] The technique involves stimulating the common peroneal nerve or tibialis anterior muscle, with the stimulation triggered during the swing phase of gait by a force-sensitive switch placed in the patient's shoe.

Facilitated muscle activity and movement   An example is weight-bearing through the heel of the hand with an extended elbow.[45,46,61] A particular example relating to postural adjustment was described by Pomeroy and colleagues.[22] The therapist sits behind the patient and the therapist's hands are placed each side of the patient's thorax whilst the therapist mobilizes the patient's trunk to produce lateral movement of the thorax on the pelvis.

Gross movement can also be facilitated. For example, stepping is effected by the therapist facilitating a patient to displace his or her weight diagonally forwards and outwards, so that balance reactions produce a forward stepping movement with the opposite lower limb. In effect the therapist is facilitating the accentuation of normal posture changes during movement. This technique can also be used to facilitate sit-to-stand. This activity requires an accentuation of the forward and downward movement of the head and shoulders which occurs during normal standing from a chair.

These techniques require a detailed knowledge of the mechanisms of both normal and disrupted movement (see the section on fracture neck of femur following a fall).

Aerobic exercise   An example is cardiorespiratory and musculoskeletal fitness training, typically over a period of about 10 weeks, using a cycle ergometer.[62] Over the first 4 weeks the initial workload of 30–50 percent of maximal effort is gradually increased to the highest level subjects could attain, and this level is then maintained for the last 6 weeks of the training period.

Functional activities   These include leg and arm training.[63] Training techniques for improving sitting balance include that described by Dean and Shepherd.[64] Patients are seated and undertake reaching tasks to retrieve different objects placed beyond arm's length. Distance and direction are varied, as are seat height, movement speed, object weight, and extent of thigh support on the seat. During reaching, patients are trained to give attention to placing weight through their paretic lower limb.[64]

Walking is a functional activity that is re-educated using numerous therapy techniques depending on the approach being used. A recent development has been to train walking as a whole activity using partial (< 40 percent) body weight support whilst walking on a treadmill.[65–69] Essentially patients receive partial body weight support from a "parachute harness" which allows them to walk at a low velocity on a treadmill with or without manual guidance from a therapist to ensure that the gait pattern is as normal as possible.

Massage and self-stroking An example of this is tapping and rubbing the skin overlying the paretic muscle.[46]

Orthotic assistance Orthoses might be provided to improve control of the ankle during walking. A variety of orthoses is available. Some, such as the Air-Stirrup brace, limit ankle eversion and inversion;[70] others "control" ankle dorsiflexion and plantarflexion.[70–73]

Positional feedback Specific interventions include feeding information back to patients: about weight distribution recorded by devices to measure force,[74–76] and about posture or joint angle recorded by devices to measure deviation from a set position.[77–80]

Resistive exercises Resistive exercise training can be given for grasp, hand extension, and ballistic extension including flicking a table-tennis ball at a paper cup target.[81] Other techniques include training grip strength by squeezing two bars separated by springs, and performing wrist extension with weights attached to the dorsum of the hand.[82] Yet other interventions have involved the use of a dynamometer to produce the resistance.[83]

Robot-aided therapy This is a novel therapy which is currently being developed and tested. The technique uses a robotic arm which is programmed to guide the patient's hand to a target if the patient cannot produce the required movement unaided.[84]

Secondary complications

Prevention and management of secondary complications, such as pain and contractures, is important. Specific interventions include pain assessment and management, and passive movements and stretching.[45] Other specific techniques include providing information about the structure and function of the shoulder, giving frequent feedback to the patient about the position of the arm, and reminding the patient to support the arm all the time.[22]

Training of ADLs

Training of ADLs is another area for specific therapy interventions. For example, in teaching dressing techniques the therapist can place the armhole of a garment between the patient's legs. The patient puts the paretic upper limb into the armhole with the paretic elbow resting on the paretic knee. The therapist then takes the sleeve over the patient's elbow and

shoulder before the person puts his or her non-paretic upper limb into the garment.[22]

Attention is given to the supply of assistive equipment. Examples are a stocking aid, and special cutlery and kitchen equipment (such as belly clamp, one-handed tin-opener, Dycem matting, etc.).[85]

Prior to discharge

As hospital discharge approaches, therapists give particular attention to preparing patients for living with a disability outside the protected hospital environment. A pre-discharge home visit is essential to assess safety (see later in the fractured neck of femur section) and to provide the opportunity for patients to test how they will manage essential personal care and move around their home after stroke. Important activities are practised, such as getting out of bed, bathing, getting dressed, moving between rooms, and getting in and out of the house.

A home visit is an encounter with the real world and it is often the first time that patients and carers fully appreciate the impact of the stroke on their everyday life. The realization that "at a stroke" they have become disabled and that everything is not going to be fine when they go home can be devastating. Aspects of the home environment which were not even noticed before the stroke—such as a step down into the kitchen—are now seen to threaten a severe restriction on independence. For this reason the home visit and the days following it can be emotionally charged. Counseling is often required. Following these visits it may be necessary to refer the client on to a social services occupational therapist, particularly if larger pieces of equipment such as bath aids and ramps or structural changes to accommodation are required.

After discharge

After hospital discharge, therapy may continue and improvements continue to be made.[86–89] Specific interventions include problem-solving, repetitive practice of ADL activities, advice about self-management and re-education of abnormal components of gait by providing practice and provision of appropriate walking aids.[86] Re-integration of social activity is promoted, and information is given on such facilities as Dial-a-Ride, shopmobility, and suitable swimming classes, where they are available. Leisure activities are promoted; and where previous leisure interests are no longer possible, alternative activities are explored. Where possible, every effort is made to regain the independence in every aspect of the patient's pre-stroke life. Unfortunately, rehabilitation in nursing or residential homes to date has been sparse, haphazard, and poorly defined;[90] this area is currently being researched.

Fractured neck of femur following a fall

During the acute postoperative period, therapists are most concerned with enabling patients to regain mobility and independence in personal self-care tasks. Of course all therapy interventions are influenced by the particular surgical procedure undertaken, so information given here can only be general in nature. Very early mobilization techniques frequently require patients to be assisted by one or two members of the therapy team so that they can practice fundamental skills such as moving around in bed and standing. Assistive devices such as tilt tables, wheelchairs,[91] raised toilet seats, and dressing aids (e.g. long-handled shoe-horn and stocking aids) might also be used. At this stage in rehabilitation it is also important to establish the patients' pre-injury level of independence so that appropriate goals, both formal and informal, can be set with patients and carers. As patients become more independent in everyday tasks, more emphasis is given to the prevention of further falls.

Mobility training is often based on an understanding of "normal" biomechanical models of performing particular tasks. Deficient or missing biomechanical components are identified and individualized exercises are given to each patient to remedy the deficient component. Exercises to increase flexibility, strength, and movement control are given in the context of the task being trained. If patients are unable to complete the whole task, then components of the task are practiced in isolation before being incorporated into the desired activity.[92]

For example, sit to stand has two major phases of initial forward trunk lean (first 35 percent of rising) and upward movement.[93] This division of the task can be further divided into four phases[94]:

1. *Flexion momentum* is initiation of movement to just before buttocks "lift off." The trunk and pelvis rotate anteriorly whilst femurs, shanks, and feet remain stationary.
2. *Momentum transfer* is "lift off" to maximum ankle dorsiflexion. The center of mass moves anteriorly and upward.
3. *Extension* begins just after maximum ankle dorsiflexion and ends when the hips cease to extend.
4. *Stabilization* begins when the hips cease to extend and finishes when all motion associated with rising is complete—although the end-point is not easy to define.

Some patients have difficulty with the momentum transfer phase because of lack of explosive power in the knee extensors. In this case, strength training of knee extensors combined with practicing "sit to stand" from an initial hip flexion angle of 120 degrees, and gradually reducing this to 90 degrees, is frequently used. Other aspects of functional mobility, such as transfers, gait and stair-climbing, are addressed through movement analysis.

In combination with specific techniques, opportunities are taken throughout the day to ensure that a conducive rehabilitation environment surrounds the patient. For example, the use of a perching stool (a high stool with slight downward slope to the seat) whilst shaving has the advantage over a standard chair of encouraging weight-bearing through the lower limbs.

A pre-discharge home visit identifies the potential risks that may cause the patient to fall. Such environmental hazards might include inappropriate heights of beds and chairs, loose or ill-fitting footwear, loose rugs, and slippery floor surfaces.[95] Of course it is not always possible to eliminate such hazards, so therapists need to respect the autonomy of patients and carers in making their own decisions—and remove, replace or modify any environmental hazards only with the person's consent.[96] At the very least, the therapist's role is to raise awareness of potential hazards and to teach patients and their carers the appropriate strategies to avoid them.

Other therapies designed to prevent further falls include[96–98]:

- balance retraining—e.g. standing balance exercises in front of a mirror progressing through different feet positions, correction of a tendency to fall backwards (by applying pressure to the front of the body), and ADL practice;
- strengthening lower limb muscles;
- increasing flexibility of the trunk and lower limbs;
- providing mobility aids and appliances;
- raising awareness of unhelpful strategies adopted to avoid a fall—e.g. fixation on the target and therefore being unaware of environmental changes on the way, and tensing muscles to avoid falling (the "walking on ice" strategy) which does not allow for subtle postural adjustments.

Further falls do happen, nevertheless, so it is useful to teach methods of rising from the floor. The conventional method is to help the person on to the floor and then teach him or her how to get on to the knees, so that the person is in a position to rise by pulling on available furniture. An alternative method is to use backward chaining of the task—i.e. first teach the ability to achieve the last component of the task successfully, and then to work successively backwards through the preceding components so that eventually the person is able to stand up independently when placed on the floor.[99,100] It is also possible to teach methods of summoning help, moving about, and keeping warm whilst on the floor.

Fear of falling is a problem for elderly people—they perceive themselves to be at risk of falling, and then they anticipate adverse consequences of doing so.[101] Fear of falling may negate any gains made through rehabilitation[102] and therefore is a major focus of therapy intervention. This may be resolved by graded exposure to a hierarchy of anxiety-provoking situations agreed by the patient and therapist—starting with the situation least feared until fear is reduced and confidence increased, then moving on to the next situation in the hierarchy. Relaxation techniques may be used as an adjunct to therapy.[98]

Parkinson's disease

As Parkinson's disease is a progressive condition, it is clear that therapy techniques will alter as a patient's disability changes. For example, patients with mild disability might receive a preventative exercise program and counseling, whilst those with severe disability might receive respiratory exercises and assistive devices.[103] A range of specific techniques suitable for people with Parkinson's disease is described in this section, but it is important to appreciate that these will be modified for individual patients depending on factors such as cognitive impairment, medication, and secondary changes in musculoskeletal and cardiovascular systems.[104]

Early in the disease, interventions might be aimed at maximizing trunk and pelvic range of movement and strength. Interventions are focused on stretching and strengthening the trunk and pelvic muscles,[102,103,106] rhythmic walking, turning, and maintaining the length of flexor muscle groups. Particular techniques may include the therapist resisting the patient walking forward by placing hands on the patient's pelvis at the anterior superior iliac spines.[105] Group exercise to music is frequently encouraged with warm-up, aerobic conditioning, and cool-down sections to each session. One paper describing such exercise groups reported that participants exercised initially at 65 percent of their maximum heart rate and this was increased by 5 percent every 4 weeks over a 12-week exercise period. Participants were actively discouraged from exceeding 85 percent of their maximum heart rate.[107]

Functional mobility

As disability becomes more pronounced, other therapy techniques are incorporated into treatment. Techniques to improve functional mobility "are based on the assumption that normal movement can be obtained by teaching strategies to avoid the basal ganglia pathology."[103]

External cues can be visual, auditory, or sensory.[108] An example of the use of visual cues to aid mobility exercises would be placement of colored objects in boxes positioned at different levels on the side opposite to the active upper limb, to encourage trunk rotation.[109] Auditory cues include a metronome and music with a steady beat to increase temporal spatial parameters of gait, such as stride length and velocity.[108] Sensory cues might include repetitive movement alternatively to left and right, to initiate walking in those with gait initiation difficulty.[110]

Internally generated cues have also been given, such as training patients to concentrate on heel strike so that the foot is lifted from the ground and bigger steps are taken,[111,112] and counting whilst walking.[112] Interventions can increase awareness of abnormal posture and how to correct it by using a mirror and feedback from the therapist during gait training.[103]

Attentional strategies can be taught. For example, when turning consciously think of a clock and place feet at specific points on the clock face to ensure larger steps and turning circle. Other attentional strategies include asking the patient to focus on the point in the movement where difficulty begins and then beginning re-training activity. Specific re-training strategies are teaching people to walk with larger steps, encouraging them to lean forward when standing up, and promoting participation in everyday physical activity.

Cognitive strategies include mental rehearsal and visualization, and patients can be advised to concentrate on one task at a time so that available cognitive resources are used to "control" the required task, rather than relying on subcortical movement control mechanisms. Mental rehearsal involves patients thinking through the steps of a task before performing it. This may also include prior visualization, so that patients imagine themselves performing the activity before they physically attempt it.

One can change the form of the task. For example, patients can be taught to turn in a larger circle to avoid smaller and smaller steps and falls, and break down complex sequences of movement tasks into simpler components.

A recent therapy approach is based on the principle of improving functional mobility directly by *repetitive practice*. One example is treadmill training with partial body weight support[113] (as outlined above in the section on techniques used with people who have had a stroke). Another is practising the components of walking on one spot.[103] It has been proposed that the current approach to therapy might change if further evidence emerges to support the finding that older people with Parkinson's disease (Hoehn and Yahr stages II and III) can

improve the performance of movement following repetitive practice.[114]

In addition to the techniques used to improve the movement required for functional mobility, therapists also apply techniques to improve *facial mobility*. Techniques include brushing muscles, applying ice to muscles, and asking patients to blow through a straw.[115]

Therapists also use specific techniques aimed at limiting the *effects* of immobility, social isolation, and psychological withdrawal—so-called "secondary disability."[20] Depression is frequently encountered especially as mobility and communication skills decline. Group therapy provides a safe supportive environment in which to practise several types of skills.[20] For example, an integrated physical and occupational therapy rehabilitation program has been described which consists of 69 repetitive exercises to improve range of motion, endurance, balance and gait, and fine motor dexterity. These exercises were provided for one hour, three times a week, for four consecutive weeks.[116] Such a group activity has clear opportunities for communication practice and enables therapists to identify difficulties that might be alleviated by the provision of a word chart or communication device. A speech and language therapist should ideally be involved in such group activities.

Of course there are times when *compensatory strategies* are appropriate. Compensatory strategies to enable "sit to stand" include: training the patient to stand up by placing hands on the armrests of the chair and by edging to the front of the seat before beginning to rise; and raising the seat height of the chair. Changes to the environment might also be needed[104] similar to those outlined already. Assistive devices can be supplied, such as elastic shoelaces and the replacement of small fasteners with Velcro.

Environmental changes

Eating is often a particular problem and therapists advise the use of plate warmers to keep food hot. Other useful devices include enlarged handles on utensils (weighted to dampen tremor), and use of a Dycem mat under the plate to improve stability. Sometimes raising the table to a height at which the patient can use one elbow as a pivot can enhance control during eating.

Other simple changes can be made to the environment to ensure that the patient is able to continue with desired activities. For example, place all of the most frequently used kitchen ingredients on one shelf to avoid unnecessary stretching and bending, and/or use a kitchen trolley which improves the walking pattern and increases stability, as well as reducing energy expenditure. There are a number of devices available to help, such as an electric tin-opener and teapot tipper.

Educating the carers

As in many other areas of geriatric rehabilitation, an important focus of therapy is educating the carer. Carers need to be advised that, although it may appear easier to carry out the task for the person, it is in fact kinder and indeed more therapeutic to let him or her struggle (within reason) with the task. This helps avoid inactivity and reduced self-esteem. Therapists work with carers and patients to set a hierarchy of tasks that should be done for the patient and those that the patients should do themselves. As the disease progresses, carers require training on positioning, moving, and handling. Specialist equipment might be needed such as a hospital bed, hoist, and/or wheelchair. Therapists work closely with patients and carers to ensure a best match of therapeutic interventions to abilities, needs, and the environment.

Frailty

In this chapter we shall use the definition of frailty proposed by Campbell and Buchner: "a condition or syndrome which results from a multi-system reduction in reserve capacity to the extent that a number of physiological systems are close to, or past, the threshold of symptomatic clinical failure."[117] The components of frailty appropriate for restorative therapy techniques are musculoskeletal function and aerobic capacity which might interact with an adverse environment to result in difficulty with mobility, personal care, and social interaction.[118] Therapists are also involved in the prevention of decline in the mobility and daily activities of elderly people, and consider it important to maintain function at the highest level possible, especially during periods of acute inpatient hospital care.[119] The detrimental effects of immobility are well recognized and even a relatively brief period of nonuse of a limb or a limb segment can lead to muscle atrophy and shortening.[120]

People who are frail are clearly at risk from falls, immobility, and social isolation. The specific therapy techniques to address these problems have been outlined in previous sections. This present section will therefore concentrate on techniques to improve the mobility and daily activity of frail elderly people. Many of these techniques are contained within exercise programs to improve mobility of joints and body segments, stability in weight-bearing postures, and control of functional movement.[118,121–129]

Exercise programs *(see also Chapter 19)*

Knee contracture might be helped by therapist-provided low-load prolonged stretch to increase knee extension while the patient lies supine, and then maintaining the extended position using foam roll or wedges under the knee before strapping the knee into the position on the supporting surface.[129]

Exercises can be designed to move each joint passively through its full range of movement.[122] Progression is effected through a program of active exercises by patients to produce voluntary movement through a full range of joint movement,[122,124,125] and when appropriate resistance to movement is provided.[122,125] Resistance can come from the patient's own body weight,[127] arm pulleys,[130] external weights,[128,130] and Thera-band (a color-coded series of different resistive strength latex rubber which can be cut to the required length for individual patients).[122,125,127,130] Resistive exercises are often provided for muscle groups such as knee extensors, hip flexors, deltoid and biceps brachii concentrically and eccentrically.[130,131] Some therapists also promote the use of resistance to movement which is required for functional ability.[127,128] An isokinetic exercise system might be used to provide progressive resistance to the lower limb movement required during walking,[126] as might an exercise bike.[130]

An appropriate sized gymnastic ball[132–134] can be used by frail elderly people in sitting or standing, and the automatic responses stimulated by the ball's inherent stability can be used to improve dynamic balance. The attending therapist provides stability or instability as appropriate. To increase stability

of the ball to enable elderly people to gain confidence in its use, it can be placed inside a cuff positioned on the floor to encircle the ball.[133]

There may be a need for functional training of tasks such as transfers, walking, wheelchair propulsion, and personal care.[122] The biomechanical approach to analysis and remediation is usually followed as set out in the section above on fractured neck of femur. The current trend seems to be towards use of assistive devices such as treadmill retraining of gait with partial body weight support.[135]

The techniques mentioned above are not applied in isolation and delivery is often in the form of group exercise to music. Schedules for these groups vary but include a selection of warm-up exercises, conditioning exercises (aerobic, balance, hand–eye coordination, hand–foot coordination, strengthening), a stretching period, functional exercises (walking, seated exercise to stretch trunk, chair rising, stair ascent and descent) and a relaxation/cool-down period.[136–138] Although exercise programs are frequently recommended, it is important to appreciate that frail elderly people may lack confidence in their ability to undertake exercise. Therapists therefore have to balance this lack of confidence with providing an exercise program which is sufficiently challenging to produce functional improvements quickly in order to motivate continuation.[139]

Exercise programs frequently provide a forum for the provision of information on exercise, safety in the home (set out in the earlier section on fractured neck of femur), and footcare. Footwear has been shown to affect performance of functional activities[140,141] and is addressed specifically in treatment programs.[124,142] Finlay[142] gives examples of dangerous footwear, including a shoe with excessive wear on the medial border thus "forcing" the foot into an everted position. Therapists provide information to patients and carers about the preferred shoe, avoiding in particular excessive heel height and using nonslip soles. It is sometimes necessary to refer to an orthotist for special footwear and/or to a podiatrist for special footcare; this is particularly important in diabetic patients. In addition the exercise classes allow the therapist to assess the need for, and current condition of, assistive devices such as walking aids, wheelchairs, dressing aids, and hoists.[143] It is not uncommon for therapists to find patients using unsafe equipment or equipment in need of repair. Other areas of daily life may also benefit from a technology assessment and subsequent provision of appropriate assistive devices.

Cognitive impairment does not preclude the provision of therapy. However, the therapist must be adaptable and flexible.[144,145] Exercise programs involving treadmills, bicycles, and weight-lifting have all been used with frail elderly people with cognitive impairment.[146]

The environment

Good seating is important for elderly people. It helps to maintain mobility if it is easy to get in and out of the chair. It facilitates communication and social interaction if the chair is orientated in a room appropriately. A good chair can prevent or reduce postural pain and promote comfort and security—and thus reduce agitation. The chair can enable adequate nutrition and hydration, and maximize respiratory function through adequate postural support. Therapists consider the following important features of chairs.[147]

- The seat depth should be adequate to support the thighs whilst leaving about 5 cm behind the knees to avoid compression of the popliteal fossae, which would impair circulation and the nervous system.
- The seat should be wide enough to avoid compression of tissues but allow the sitter to use the armrests for support.
- The seat height should be at least equal to the floor-to-knee height of the user, to make it easier to stand up and sit down.
- The back rest should support the whole of the back, preferably with contoured spinal curve support.
- The seat-to-back angle should be 95 degrees ideally.
- The armrests should be level with the patient's elbow and as long as the seat depth.

Therapists can provide individualized cushioning to adapt chairs,[147,148] including pressure-relief cushions. It is very important for each patient to have more than one chair in which to sit, as it is not normal to sit in one position or in one chair for long periods.

Also important for frail elderly people is the promotion of *personal energy conservation*. Organization of the environment can make best use of a person's abilities. For example, gather all garments before attempting to dress, dress all the lower half at once, reduce the difficulty of fastenings by applying Velcro, and reduce the burden of full weight-bearing by using a perching stool during kitchen activities.

FUTURE DIRECTIONS

The rapid expansion of rehabilitation doctorates, academic posts, and research output[10,149] is indicative of the increasing commitment of the therapy professions to base their practice on evidence. Therapists are now more critical of the methodology and rationale that governs their practice. As the research culture grows, therapists will test conventional techniques for their purported effects and implement those found to be most effective. Future innovations in therapy should therefore be based on research evidence in addition to clinical impressions.[150]

A recent UK Medical Research Council document[151] provides an excellent basis for a research strategy in geriatric rehabilitation, highlighting the need for systematic investigation of techniques, and combinations of techniques, in both exploratory and definitive clinical trials. However, in the present climate of a rapidly developing rehabilitation research base, it remains essential to remember that clinical evidence outside of formal research studies can also be an important source of information. Moreover, not all experimental evidence reaches peer-reviewed journals. Trials with positive results are still deemed to be more attractive by publishers and the inconclusive or negative trials are less likely to be published. Therefore the evidence base might actually be evidenced-biased.[152]

Expert opinion in the absence of scientific evidence has an important part to play in the rehabilitation process. Indeed, it is imperative that we do not throw away years of clinical judgment, especially in an area of rehabilitation as complex as elderly care. Specialist multidisciplinary groups such as SRR (Society for Research in Rehabilitation) and profession-specific bodies including OCTEP (Occupational Therapy for Elderly People) and AGILE (chartered physiotherapists working with older people) are essential networks from which future developments in elderly rehabilitation will flourish.

KEY POINTS   Rehabilitation techniques

- Rehabilitation consists of a complex package of techniques delivered by a multiprofessional team and involving the active participation of patients and carers. It makes an important contribution to maintaining independence and quality of life of elderly people.

- To reduce the complexity of description, this chapter uses some of the techniques used by occupational therapists and physiotherapists as exemplars to illustrate the range of possibilities within the package.

- Although techniques are described here within sections of stroke, fractured neck of femur following a fall, Parkinson's disease, and frailty, these techniques are often used in different combinations to meet the complex needs of elderly people.

- The research culture in the therapy professions is growing fast as more therapists obtain doctorates and pursue research into the most effective techniques to maintain the independence of elderly people.

REFERENCES

1. Mulley GP: In rehabilitation. Age Ageing 1994;23:S28–S30
2. Department of Health: National Service Framework for Older People. DoH, London, 2001
3. World Federation of Occupational Therapists: British Journal of Occupational Therapy, May OT News Supplement, 1989
4. Turner A: Occupational Therapy and Physical Dysfunction: Principles, Skills and Practice. Churchill Livingstone, Edinburgh, 1981
5. Hagedorn R: Occupational Therapy: Foundations for Practice, 2nd edn. Churchill Livingstone, Edinburgh, 1997
6. McDonald EM: Occupational Therapy in Rehabilitation, 2nd edn. Baillière Tindall, London, 1964
7. Reed KL, Sanderson SR: Concepts of occupational therapy. Williams & Wilkins, Baltimore, 1983
8. Joice A, Coia D: A discussion on the skills of the occupational therapist working in a multidisciplinary team. Br J Occup Ther 1989;52:466–468
9. Social Services Inspectorate: Occupational Therapy—The Community Contribution. DoH, London, 1994
10. Bury T: The status and development of physiotherapy research in the United Kingdom. Phys Ther Rev 1997;2:165–171
11. Eakin P, Ballinger C, Nicol M, Walker MF, Alsop A, Ilott I: College of Occupational Therapists: research and development strategy. Br J Occup Ther 1997;60:484–486
12. UK College of Occupational Therapists: Code of Ethics and Professional Conduct. COT, London, 1995
13. College of Occupational Therapists, College of Speech and Language Therapists, and the Chartered Society of Physiotherapy: Research and Development in Occupational Therapy, Physiotherapy and Speech and Language Therapy: A Position Statement. London, 1994
14. Wade DT: Measurement in Neurological Rehabilitation. Oxford Medical Publications, Oxford, 1992
15. Whiting SE, Lincoln NB, Cockburn J, Bhavnani G: The Rivermead Perceptual Assessment Battery. NFER-Nelson, Windsor, 1985
16. Wade DT: Evidence relating to goal planning in rehabilitation. Clin Rehabil 1998;12:273–275
17. Engel G: The clinical application of the biopsychosocial model. Am J Psychiat 1980;137:535–544

18. World Health Organization: The International Classification of Impairments, Disabilities and Handicaps. WHO, Geneva, 1980

19. Barnitt R, Pomeroy V: An holistic approach to rehabilitation: fact or fiction? Br J Ther Rehabil 1995;2:87–92

20. Szekely BC, Kosanovich NN, Sheppard W: Adjunctive treatment in Parkinson's disease: physical therapy and comprehensive group therapy. Rehabil Liter 1982;43:72–76

21. Mickelborough J, Liston R, Harris B, Pomeroy VM, Tallis RC: Physiotherapy for higher-level gait disorders associated with cerebral multi-infarcts. Physiother Theory Pract 1997;13:127–138

22. Pomeroy VM, Niven DS, Barrow S, Faragher EB, Tallis RC: Unpacking the black box of nursing and therapy practice for post-stroke shoulder pain: a precursor to evaluation. Clin Rehabil 2001;15:67–83

23. Cameron ID, Handoll HHG, Finnegan TP, Madhok R, Langhorne P: Co-ordinated multidisciplinary approaches for inpatient rehabilitation of older patients with proximal femoral fractures. Cochrane Database Syst Rev 2000;(4)

24. Parker MJ, Handoll HHG, Dynan Y: Mobilisation strategies after hip fracture surgery in adults. Cochrane Database Syst Rev 2000;(4)

25. Gillespie LD, Gillespie WJ, Cumming R, Lamb SE, Rowe BH: Interventions for preventing falls in the elderly. Cochrane Database Syst Rev 2000;(4)

26. Price CIM, Pandyan AD: Electrical stimulation for preventing and treating post-stroke shoulder pain. Cochrane Database Syst Rev 2000;(4)

27. Keith RA: Treatment strength in rehabilitation. Arch Phys Med Rehabil 1997;78:1298–1304

28. Audit Commission: The Way to Go Home: Rehabilitation and Remedial Services for Older People. Audit Commission, London, 2000

29. Stroke Unit Trialists' Collaboration: Collaborative systematic review of the randomized trials of organized inpatient (stroke unit) care after stroke. BMJ 1997;314:1151–1159

30. Indredavik B, Bakke R, Slordahl SA, Rokseth R, Haheim LL: Stroke unit treatment: 10 year follow-up. Stroke 1999;8:1524–1527

31. Intercollegiate Working Party for Stroke: National Clinical Guidelines for Stroke. Royal College of Physicians of London, 2000

32. Partridge CJ: Different approaches to physiotherapy in stroke. Rev Clin Gerontol 1995;5:199–209

33. Ernst E: A review of stroke rehabilitation and physiotherapy. Stroke 1990;21:1081–1085

34. Ashburn A, Partridge C, de Souza L: Physiotherapy in the rehabilitation of stroke: a review. Clin Rehabil 1993;7:337–345

35. Langhammer B, Stanghelle JK: Bobath or Motor Relearning Programme? A comparison of two different approaches of physiotherapy in stroke rehabilitation: a randomized controlled study. Clin Rehabil 2000;14:361–369

36. Sackley CM, Lincoln NB: Physiotherapy treatment for stroke patients: a survey of current practice. Physiother Theory Pract 1996;12:87–96

37. Davidson I, Waters K: Physiotherapists working with stroke patients: a national survey. Physiotherapy 2000;86:69–80

38. Walker MF, Drummond AER, Gatt J, Sackley CM: Occupational therapy for stroke patients: a survey of current practice. Br J Occup Ther 2000;63:367–372

39. Lennon S: The Bobath concept: a critical review of the theoretical assumptions that guide physiotherapy practice in stroke rehabilitation. Phys Ther Rev 1996;1:35–45

40. Carr J, Shepherd R: Neurological Rehabilitation: Optimizing Motor Performance. Butterworth–Heinemann, Oxford, 1998

41. Pomeroy VM, Tallis RC: Physical therapy to improve movement performance and functional ability post stroke. 1: Existing evidence. Rev Clin Gerontol 2000;10:261–290

42. Chatterton HJ, Pomeroy VM, Cratton J: Positioning for stroke patients: a survey of physiotherapists' aims and practices. Disabil Rehabil 2001;23:413–421

43. Lincoln NB, Drummond AER, Edmans JA, Yeo D, Willis D: The Rey Figure copy as a screening instrument for perceptual deficits after stroke. Br J Occup Ther 1998;61:33–35

44. Edmans J, Lincoln NB: The frequency of perceptual deficits after stroke. Clin Rehabil 1987;1:273–281

45. Parry RH, Lincoln NB, Appleyard MA: Physiotherapy for the arm and hand after stroke. Physiotherapy 1999;85:417–425

46. Hummelsheim H, Hauptmann B, Neumann S: Influence of physiotherapeutic facilitation techniques on motor evoked potentials in centrally paretic hand extensor muscles. Electroencephalogr Clin Neurophysiol 1995;97:18–28

47. Schleebaker RE, Mainous AG: Electromyographic biofeedback for neuromuscular re-education in the hemiplegic stroke patient: a meta-analysis. Arch Phys Med Rehabil 1993;74:1301–1304

48. Moreland J, Thompson MA: Efficacy of Electromyographic biofeedback compared with conventional physical therapy for upper extremity function in patients following stroke: a research overview and meta-analysis. Phys Ther 1994;74:534–547

49. Morris DM, Crago JE, DeLuca SC, Pidikiti RD, Taub E: Constraint-induced movement therapy for motor recovery after stroke. Neuro Rehabil 1997;9:29–43

50. Ostendorf CG, Wolf SF: Effect of forced use of the upper extremity of a hemiplegic patient on changes in function. Phys Ther 1981;61:1022–1028

51. Taub E, Miller NE, Novack TA et al: Technique to improve chronic motor deficit after stroke. Arch Phys Med Rehabil 1993;74:347–354

52. Blanton S, Wolf SL: An application of upper-extremity constraint-induced movement therapy in a patient with subacute stroke. Phys Ther 1999;79:847–853

53. Kunkel A, Kopp B, Muller G et al: Constraint-induced movement therapy for motor recovery in chronic stroke patients. Arch Phys Med Rehabil 1999;80:624–628

54. Miltner WR, Bauder H, Somer M, Dettmers C, Taub E: Effects of constraint-induced movement therapy on patients with chronic motor deficits after stroke: a replication. Stroke 1999;30:586–592

55. van der Lee JH, Wagenaar RC, Lankhorst GJ, Vogelaar TW, Deville WL, Bouter LM: Forced use of the upper extremity in chronic stroke patients: results from a single-blind randomised clinical trial. Stroke 1999;30:2369–2375

56. Dromerick AW, Edwards DF, Hahn M: Does the application of constraint-induced movement therapy during acute rehabilitation reduce arm impairment after ischaemic stroke? Stroke 2000;31:2984–2988

57. Glanz M, Klawansky S, Stason W et al: Functional electrostimulation in poststroke rehabilitation: a meta-analysis of the randomized controlled trials. Arch Phys Med Rehabil 1996;77:549–553

58. Chae J, Bethoux F, Bohinc T, Dobbos L, Davis T, Friedl A: Neuromuscular stimulation for upper extremity motor and functional recovery in acute hemiplegia. Stroke 1998;29:975–979

59. Francisco G, Chae J, Chawla H et al: EMG-triggered neuromuscular stimulation for improving the arm function of acute stroke survivors: a randomized pilot study. Arch Phys Med Rehabil 1998;79:570–575

60. Burridge JH, Taylor PN, Hagan SA et al: The effects of common peroneal stimulation on the effort and speed of walking: a randomised controlled trial with chronic hemiplegic patients. Clin Rehabil 1997;11:201–210

61. Brouwer BJ, Ambury P: Upper extremity weight-bearing effect on corticospinal excitability following stroke. Arch Phys Med Rehabil 1994;75:861–866

62. Potempa K, Lopez M, Braun LT, Szidon P, Fogg L, Tincknell T: Physiological outcomes of aerobic exercise training in hemiparetic stroke patients. Stroke 1995;26:101–105

63. Kwakkel G, Wagenaar RC, Twisk JWR, Lankhorst JC: Intensity of leg and arm training after primary middle-cerebral-artery stroke: a randomized trial. Lancet 1999;354:191–196

64. Dean CM, Shepherd RB: Task-related training improves performance of seated reaching tasks after stroke: a randomized controlled trial. Stroke 1997;28:722–728

65. Hesse S, Berelt C, Schaffrin A, Malezic M, Mauritz KH: Restoration of gait in nonambulatory hemiparetic patients by treadmill training with partial body-weight support. Arch Phys Med Rehabil 1994;75:1087–1093

66. Hesse S, Bertelt C, Jahnke MT, Schaffrin A, Baake P, Malezic M, Mauritz KH: Treadmill training with partial body weight support compared with physiotherapy in nonambulatory hemiparetic patients. Stroke 1995;26:976–981

67. Hesse S, Konrad M, Uhlenbrock D: Treadmill walking with partial body weight support versus floor walking in hemiparetic subjects. Arch Phys Med Rehabil 1999;80:421–427

68. Mackro RF, DeSouza CA, Tretter LD et al: Treadmill aerobic exercise training reduces the energy expenditure and cardiovascular demands of hemiparetic gait in chronic stroke patients: a preliminary report. Stroke 1997;28:326–330

69. Visintin M, Barbeau H, Korner-Bitensky N, Mayo NE: A new approach to retrain gait in stroke patients through body weight support and treadmill stimulation. Stroke 1998;29:1122–1128

70. Burdett RG, Borello-France D, Blatchley C, Potter C: Gait comparison of subjects with hemiplegia walking unbraced, with ankle-foot orthosis and with Air-Stirrup brace. Phys Ther 1988;68:1197–1203

71. Diamond MF, Ottenbacher KJ: Effect of a tone-inhibiting dynamic ankle-foot orthosis on stride characteristics of an adult with hemiparesis. Phys Ther 1990;70:423–430

72. Lehmann JF, Condon SM, Price R, Delateur BJ: Gait abnormalities in hemiplegia: their correction by ankle–foot orthosis. Arch Phys Med Rehabil 1987;68:763–771

73. Tyson S, Thornton H, Downes A: The effect of a hinged ankle–foot orthosis on hemiplegic gait: four single case studies. Physiother Theory Pract 1998;14:75–85

74. Engardt M: Rising and sitting down in stroke patients: Auditory feedback and dynamic strength training to enhance symmetrical body weight distribution. Scan J Rehabil Med 1994; (Suppl 31):1–57

75. Sackley CM, Lincoln NB: Single blind randomized controlled trial of visual feedback after stroke: effects on stance symmetry and function. Disabil Rehabil 1997;19:536–546

76. Shumway-Cook A, Anson D, Haller S: Postural sway biofeedback: its effect on re-establishing stance stability in hemiplegic patients. Arch Phys Med Rehabil 1988;69:395–400

77. Colborne GR, Olney SJ, Griffen MP: Feedback of ankle joint angle and soleus electromyography in the rehabilitation of hemiplegic gait. Arch Phys Med Rehabil 1993;74:1100–1106

78. De Weerdt W, Crossley SM, Lincoln NB: Restoration of balance in stroke patients: a single case study design study. Clin Rehabil 1989;3:139–147

79. Dursun E, Hamamci N, Donmez S, Tuzunalp O, Cakci A: Angular biofeedback device for sitting balance of stroke patients. Stroke 1996;27:1354–1357

80. Koheil R, Reg PT, Mandel AR: Joint position biofeedback facilitation of physical therapy in gait training. Am J Phys Med 1980;59:288–297

81. Trombly CA, Thayer-Nason L, Bliss G, Girard CA, Lyrist LA, Brexa-Hooson A: The effectiveness of therapy in improving finger extension in stroke patients. Am J Occup Ther 1986;40:612–617

82. Butefisch C, Hummelsheim H, Denzler P, Mauritz KH: Repetitive training of isolated movements improves the outcome of motor rehabilitation of the centrally paretic hand. J Neurol Sci 1995;130:59–68

83. Mercier C, Bourbonnais D, Bilodeau S, Lemay JF, Cross P: Description of a new motor re-education programme for the paretic lower limb aimed at improving the mobility of stroke patients. Clin Rehabil 1999;13:199–206

84. Volpe BT, Krebs HI, Hogan N, Edelstein L, Diels C, Aisen M: A novel approach to stroke rehabilitation: robot-aided sensorimotor stimulation. Neurology 2000;54:1938–1944

85. Mann WC, Ottenbacher KJ, Fraas L, Tomita M, Granger CV: Effectiveness of assistive technology and environmental interventions in maintaining independence and reducing home care costs for the frail elderly: a randomized controlled trial. Arch Fam Med 1995;8:210–217

86. Wade DT, Collen FM, Robb GF, Warlow CP: Physiotherapy intervention late after stroke and mobility. BMJ 1992;304:609–613

87. Drummond AER, Walker MF: A randomized controlled trial of leisure rehabilitation after stroke. Clin Rehabil 1995;9:283–290

88. Walker MF, Drummond AER, Lincoln NB: Evaluation of dressing practice for stroke patients after discharge from hospital: a cross-over design study. Clin Rehabil 1996;10:23–31

89. Walker MF, Gladman JRF, Lincoln NB, Siemonsma P, Whiteley T: Occupational therapy for stroke patients not admitted to hospital: a randomized controlled trial. Lancet 1999;354:278–280

90. Sackley CM, Gatt J, Walker MF: The use of rehabilitation services by private nursing homes: a census and interview study. Clin Rehabil 2000;14:455

91. Liss SE, Wylie WJ: Practical aspects of mobilizing the elderly patient following hip fracture. Texas Med 1978;74:69–73

92. Drabsch T, Lovenfosse J, Fowler V, Adams R, Drabsch P: Effects of task-specific training on walking and sit-to-stand after total hip replacement. Aust J Physiother 1998;44:193–198

93. Nuzik S, Lamb R, VanSant A, Hirt S: Sit-to-stand movement pattern: a kinematic study. Phys Ther 1986;66:1708–1713

94. Schenkman M, Berger RA, Riley PO, Mann RW, Hodge WA: Whole-body movements during rising to standing from sitting. Phys Ther 1990;70:638–651

95. Obonyo T, Drummond M, Isaacs B: Domiciliary physiotherapy for old people who have fallen. Int Rehabil Med 1983;5:157–160

96. Simpson JM, Harrington R, Marsh N: Guidelines for managing falls among elderly people. Physiotherapy 1998;84:173–177

97. Tinetti ME, Baker DI, Gottschalk M, Garrett P, McGeary S, Pollack D, Charpentier P: Systematic home-based physical and functional therapy for older persons after hip fracture. Arch Phys Med Rehabil 1997;78:1237–1247

98. Riley G, Holding D: Tackling a fear of falling using graded exposure: case report. Physiotherapy 2000;86:143–145

99. Reece AC, Simpson JM: Preparing older people to cope after a fall. Physiotherapy 1996;82:227–235

100. Adams JMG, Tyson S: The effectiveness of physiotherapy to enable an elderly person to get up from the floor: a single case study. Physiotherapy 2000;86:185–189

101. Simpson JM: Addressing older peoples' anxiety about falling. Physiother Theory Pract 1999;15:57

102. Petrella RJ, Payne M, Myers A, Overend T, Chesworth B: Physical function and fear of falling after hip fracture rehabilitation in the elderly. Am J Phys Med Rehabil 2000;79:154–160

103. Viliani T, Pasquetti P, Magnolfi S, Lunnardelli ML, Giorgi C, Serra P, Taiti G: Effects of physical training on straightening-up processes in patients with Parkinson's disease. Disabil Rehabil 1999;21:68–73

104. Morris ME: Movement disorders in people with Parkinson disease: a model for physical therapy. Phys Ther 2000;80:578–595

105. Chan J, Lee J, Neubert C: Physiotherapy intervention in parkinsonian gait. NZJ Physiother 1993;April:23–28

106. Bridgewater KJ, Sharpe MH: Trunk muscle training and early Parkinson's disease. Physiother Theory Pract 1997;13:139–153

107. Bridgewater KJ, Sharpe MH: Aerobic exercise and early Parkinson's disease. J Neuro Rehabil 1996;10:233–241

108. Dibble LE, Nicholson DE: Sensory cueing improves motor performance and rehabilitation in persons with Parkinson's disease. Neurol Report 1997;21:11–124

109. Dam M, Tonin P, Casson S, Bracco F et al: Effects of conventional and sensory-enhanced physiotherapy on disability of Parkinson's disease patients. Adv Neurol 1996;69:551–555

110. Schenkman M, Donovan J, Tsubota J et al: Management of individuals with Parkinson's disease: rationale and case studies. Phys Ther 1989;69:944–955

111. Kamsma YPT, Brouwer WH, Lakke JPWF: Training of compensational strategies for impaired gross motor skills in Parkinson's disease. Physiother Theory Pract 1995;11:209–229

112. Nieubower A, Feys P, de Weerdt W, Dom R: Is using a cue the clue to the treatment of freezing in Parkinson's disease? Physiother Res Int 1997;2:125–134

113. Miyai I, Fujimoto Y, Ueda Y, Yamamoto H, Nozaki S, Saito T, Kang J: Treadmill training with body weight support: its effect on Parkinson's disease. Arch Phys Med Rehabil 2000;81:849–852

114. Behraman AL, Cauraugh JH, Light KE: Practice as an intervention to improve speeded motor performance and motor learning in Parkinson's disease. J Neurol Sci 2000;174:127–136

115. Katsikitis M, Pilowsky I: A controlled study of facial mobility treatment in Parkinson's disease. J Psychosom Res 1996;40:387–396

116. Comella CL, Stebbins GT, Brown-Toms N, Goetz CG: Physical therapy and Parkinson's disease: a controlled clinical trial. Neurology 1994;44:376–378

117. Campbell AJ, Buchner DM: Unstable disability and the fluctuations of fraility. Age Ageing 1997;26:315–318

118. Harada N, Chiu V, Fowler E, Lee M, Reuben DB: Physical therapy to improve functioning of older people in residential care facilities. Phys Ther 1995;75:830–838

119. Palmer RM: Acute hospital care of the elderly: minimizing the risk of functional decline. Cleve Clin J Med 1995;62:117–128

120. Hachisuka K, Umexu Y, Ogata H: Disuse muscle atrophy of lower limbs in hemiplegic patients. Arch Phys Med Rehabil 1997;78:13–18

121. Lonnerblad L: Exercises to promote independent living in older patients. Geriatrics 1984;39:93–101

122. Mulrow CD et al: Effects of physical therapy on functional status of nursing home residents. J Am Geriatr Soc 1993;41:326–328

123. Mulrow CD, Gerety MB et al: A randomised trial of physical rehabilitation for very frail nursing home residents. JAMA 1994;271:519–526

124. Koch M, Gottschalk M, Baker DI, Palumbo S, Tinetti ME: An impairment and disability assessment and treatment protocol for community-living elderly persons. Phys Ther 1994;74:286–294

125. McMurdo MET, Johnstone R: A randomized controlled trial of a home exercise programme for elderly people with poor mobility. Age Ageing 1995;24:425–428

126. Smith S, Simpson JM, Hastie I: Elderly in-patients need more exercise: a functional exercise system. Physiotherapy 1995;81:605–610

127. Skelton DA, McLaughlin AW: Training functional ability in old age. Physiotherapy 1996;82:159–167

128. Brill P, Probst J, Greenhouse DL, Schell B, Macera C: Clinical feasibility of a free-weight strength-training program for older adults. J Am Board Fam Pract 1998;11:445–451

129. Fox P, Richardson J, McInnes B, Tait D, Bedard M: Effectiveness of a bed positioning program for treating older adults with knee contractures who are institutionalized. Phys Ther 2000;80:363–372

130. Carpenter C, Ewart LJ: Implementation and evaluation of a weight training program for the elderly in a long-term care facility. Physiother Can 1997;Fall:302–310

131. McCool JF, Schneider JK: Home-based leg strengthening for older adults initiated through private practice. Prevent Med 1999;28:105–110

132. Carriere B: The "Swiss Ball": An effective tool in physiotherapy for patients, families and physiotherapists. Physiotherapy 1999;85:552–561

133. Oddy R: Taming the gymnastic ball. Physiotherapy 1996;82:477–479

134. LaPier TL, Bain C, Moses S, Dunkle SE: Balance training through ball throwing activities: a research-based rationale. Phys Occup Ther Geriatr 1996;14:23–40

135. Cherniack EP, Caprio D, Fischer AA, Tuckman J: A novel device for walking training in elderly patients. Physiotherapy 1999;85:144–153

136. Lord SR, Ward JA, Williams P: Exercise effect on dynamic stability in older women: a randomized controlled trial. Arch Phys Med Rehabil 1996;77:232–236

137. Cochrane T, Davey R, Munro J, Nicholl J: Exercise, physical function and health perceptions of older people. Physiotherapy 1998;84:598–602

138. Gillies E, Aitchison T, MacDonald J, Grant S: Outcomes of a 12-week functional exercise programme for institutionalized elderly people. Physiotherapy 1999;85:349–357

139. Blyth J: Exercise prescription to improve function in the elderly: a case report. NZ J Physiother 1999;27:35–38

140. Finlay O, van der Meer DC, Beringer TRO: Use of gait analysis to demonstrate benefits of footwear assessment in elderly people. Physiotherapy 1999;85:451–456

141. Arnadottir SA, Mercer VS: Effects of footwear on measurements of balance and gait in women between the ages of 65 and 93 years. Phys Ther 2000;80:17–27

142. Finlay OE: Footwear management in the elderly care programme. Physiotherapy 1986;72:172–178

143. Cooper BA, Stewart D: The effect of a transfer device in the homes of elderly women. Phys Occup Ther Geriatr 1997;15:61–77

144. Pomeroy VM: The effect of physiotherapy input on mobility skills of elderly people with severe dementing illness: a pilot study. Clin Rehabil 1993;7:163–170

145. Pomeroy VM, Warren CM, Honeycombe C et al: Mobility and dementia: is physiotherapy treatment during respite care effective? Int J Geriatr Psychiat 1999;14:389–397

146. Arkin SM: Elder rehab: a student-supervised exercise program for Alzheimer's patients. Gerontologist 1999;39:729–735

147. Nitz JC: The seating dilemma in aged care. Aust J Physiother 2000;46:53–58

148. Pope PM: Postural management and special seating. In Edwards S (ed): Neurological Physiotherapy: A Problem-Solving Approach. Churchill Livingstone, London, 135–160

149. Walker MF: Stroke rehabilitation: a multi-disciplinary challenge. Targeting Stroke, Cerebro-vascular series 2001;2:13–14

150. Pomeroy VM, Tallis RC: Need to focus stroke rehabilitation. Lancet 2000;355:836–837

151. UK Medical Research Council: A Framework for Development and Evaluation of RCTs for Complex Interventions to Improve Health. MRC, London, 2000

152. Grimley Evans J: Evidence-based and evidence-biased medicine. Age Ageing 1995;24:461–463

Chapter 23

Palliative care

John Welsh, Marie Fallon, and Paul W. Keeley

"No moral impulse seems more deeply embedded than the need to relieve suffering ... it has become a foundation-stone for the practice of medicine and it is at the core of the social and welfare programmes of all civilised nations."[1]

Palliative care is defined as "the active total care of patients whose disease is not responsive to curative treatment. Control of pain, of other symptoms and of psychological, social and spiritual problems is paramount. The goal of palliative care is achievement of the best possible quality of life for patients and their families."[2]

BACKGROUND

Palliative care is not new but its re-emergence to a position of prominence owes much to the efforts of the pioneers of the modern hospice movement. Dame C. Saunders, who founded St Christopher's Hospice, London, in 1967 is the mother figure of this modern focus. The stimulus and motivation for this phenomenon was largely due to a reaction to change in the mainstream medical thrust occurring during the first half of the twentieth century. Medicine's traditional emphasis on relief of symptoms was obfuscated by a healthy scientific quest to find the cause of illnesses. This change in emphasis, coinciding with major technological and investigational advances, unconsciously produced a focus on the etiology of disease. The endpoint became cure, and person-centered medicine suffered. By the late 1950s and early 1960s the pioneers of hospice care were forced to move out of the National Health Service into the charitable sector to provide for, and to meet, needs that had become subordinated in the quest to understand and conquer all.

The underpinning tenet of the modern hospice movement is the philosophy of the importance of care for the whole person, and features of palliative care philosophy are listed in Table 23-1. Whole-person care comprises attention to physical, psychological, social, and spiritual needs, all of which are affected to varying degrees by chronic progressive incurable illness. The needs of the family are also assessed and met by relevant team members. The term "unit of care" was coined

Table 23-1 Palliative care philosophy

- Affirms life and regards dying as a normal process
- Neither hastens nor postpones death
- Provides relief from pain and other distressing physical symptoms
- Supplies integrative psychosomatic and spiritual care for patients
- Offers a system to help patients live as actively as possible until their death
- Offers a support system for the family to enable them to cope during the patient's illness and subsequently in their bereavement

by Dame C. Saunders to signify the patient and family who are the focus of care.

The first hospice for dying people is said to have been founded in Lyons, France, by Mademoiselle Garnier in 1842.[3] There has been a rapid growth in the number of hospice services in the UK and there are now 202 inpatient units providing a total of 3069 beds,[4] compared with 106 units in 1987.[5]

Palliative medicine became a specialty in the UK in 1987, recognized by the Royal College of Physicians, and there is now a recognized training pathway for future consultants.

"Palliative care" is an all-embracing phrase, but in reality it is divided into levels of specialism. The following definitions of the different forms or levels of palliative care are adapted from Findlay and Jones.[6]

- *Basic palliative care.* Care delivery with a palliative approach is a core skill that every health professional in whatever setting dealing with chronic incurable disease should possess.
- *Specialist palliative care.* This is care provided by a multidisciplinary team, led by clinicians with recognized specialist palliative medicine training. The team works collaboratively with those providing a palliative approach and deals with the more complex problems.
- *Specialist palliative intervention.* This is noncurative treatment aimed specifically at modifying the illness. The treatment is performed by specialists in medicine, clinical and medical oncology, or surgery.

Modern developments

The term "hospice" is tending to be replaced by the term "specialist palliative care service" (SPCS). A SPCS may be based within a specialist palliative care unit (SPCU) sited in a hospital or in the grounds of a hospital, or may be free standing, as the traditional hospice. The traditional hospice provides specialist palliative care and ideally comprises:

- inpatient facilities;
- day hospice/units;
- home care service;
- educational service;
- domiciliary and hospital medical/nursing advisory service;
- bereavement service;
- 24-hour telephone advisory service.[7]

The above bears remarkable similarities to the geriatric model. The analogy can be taken further as the modern SPCU acts as an assessment and rehabilitation facility with a full multidisciplinary team and liaises closely with the community. A more recent development has been the concept of Hospice at Home services in which hospice staff will provide a 24-hour service for a limited period to allow patients to die at home or for crisis intervention to prevent inpatient admission. The rigorous assessment of the effectiveness of such services has proved difficult and has so far been inconclusive.[8]

A SPCS responds to referrals from primary healthcare and from secondary and tertiary centers. The involvement of a SPCS may lead to inpatient care in the SPCU; attendance at the day unit; involvement of the SPCS's home care team; an advisory, liaison, and supportive input to the patient and family; or support and advice to those health professionals already involved.

The patients

The three chief categories admitted to inpatient units are patients with the potential for rehabilitation after symptom control; those admitted for respite, which in effect includes reassessment; and those admitted who are in the terminal stage of their illness and will not live long. The average length of stay in UK hospices is 14 days, and the average discharge rate is 50 percent.[9] Traditionally the vast majority of patients admitted to palliative care programs have cancer,[10] the remainder chiefly comprising motor neuron disease and human immunodeficiency virus or acquired immunodeficiency syndrome.

Quality of care

Most healthcare professionals feel adept at providing palliative care, but how good are their efforts? There is evidence of poor knowledge of pain control.[11] A survey of 145 physicians, of whom 73 percent were primary care physicians, identified knowledge about 14 fundamental cancer pain principles. It found that there were deficits in 9 out of 14 of these principles. Inappropriate attitudes to managing cancer pain were found in only two of nine cancer pain management concepts.[12] Similarly a Cancer Relief Macmillan Fund survey[13] found that 50 percent of a sample of general practitioners (GPs) rated themselves as inadequate or worse in dealing with terminally ill patients. The study demonstrated that the appointment of a GP facilitator in palliative care improved peer knowledge. Complaints about care in the National Health Service are increasing,[14] the majority concerning poor communication between professionals and relatives especially around the time of death.

EDUCATION AND TRAINING This is the major area in which substantial improvement in quality of care can be made in a cost-efficient manner. Critical-mass experience is often lacking for individual general practitioners. Ongoing interactive problem-based educational programs should therefore be widely available. Postgraduate and basic educational needs must be assessed locally and learning programs established. Curricula exist for medical students, for GPs, for palliative medicine specialist registrars,[15] and for nurses.[16,17] The UK General Medical Council[18,19] has recommended that medical graduates should be better equipped to meet the demands of this sensitive area. Major revision of the traditional medical curriculum is under way and one of the innovations in many British medical schools is a more prolonged and intensive period of training in communication skills. Thus it appears that some of the educational deficiencies are being recognized and remedied.

SYMPTOMATOLOGY

Tolerance to illness may be reduced in the elderly by preexisting, usually progressive, alterations in normal physiology. Declining physiological reserves can result in an exaggerated response to illness and associated symptoms. In addition, reduced tolerance to treatment and slower recovery may be apparent.[20]

Cancer is predominantly a disease of the elderly, with the incidence increasing with age.[21] In Europe, 22 percent of all deaths are due to cancer and 150,000 cancer deaths per annum occur in Great Britain.[22] Fifty percent of cancers occur in only 15 percent of the population (i.e. those over 65 years of age).[21] Likewise, in the USA 50 percent of all cancers occur in those over 65 years of age.[21] Therefore, the geriatrician will see a large number of cancer patients, many of whom will have pain.[23]

There is an increasing tendency to site-specialization in medicine. However, palliative care is an exception as there is a remarkable similarity of symptoms experienced by patients with a wide spectrum of different progressive incurable conditions. Research is lacking on symptoms suffered by those with nonmalignant, progressive incurable conditions, but studies in this area show considerable distress in noncancer patients. Cartwright and Seale[24] found similarities in symptoms between cancer and noncancer patients. In 639 adults over 75 years of age, the incidence of pain was 75 percent in those with cancer, compared with an incidence in noncancer patients of 68 percent. Pain intensity in patients with cancer was more severe but the duration of pain in noncancer cases was longer. In particular, chronic pain—in this case defined as pain present for more than 1 year—was not infrequent after stroke. Nausea, vomiting, anorexia, and constipation were significantly more common in cancer patients.

In a study of 1000 patients with different cancer types, the most common symptoms reported were pain, easy fatigue, weakness, anorexia and weight loss, xerostomia, constipation, and dyspnea.[25]

Palliative care focuses on relief of symptoms caused by an illness, not primarily on an attempt to modify the underlying incurable disease. As with any medical problem, the approach to symptom control is one of taking a careful history; listening attentively; careful examination; appropriate investigations (avoiding the unnecessary); and analysis and diagnosis of the pathogenesis of the symptom.

Appropriate treatment should be instigated with as much information given as the patient desires. The information should be presented at the patient's pace, free of jargon, and given in an understandable and empathic manner. With the patient's consent, the family should be included in this information exchange. Control of cancer-related symptoms is generally achieved by drugs, the average number of medications being six per day.[26] Control of symptoms in patients with preexisting disease will inevitably lead to polypharmacy. Care must be taken to review drug regimens regularly and to be aware of potential interactions. Prescribing principles for the elderly are described in Chapter 14 and will not be considered here.

Many of the symptoms and principles of management described below are shared in both malignant and nonmalignant conditions. Symptoms will be illustrated mainly by the use of cancer cases. Various important symptoms are now considered.

PAIN CONTROL

The problem

Chronic pain affects the person functionally, physically, and psychosocially.[27] The influence of pain on these components of the whole person must be accurately assessed. The study of pain and pain control in the elderly is a neglected area. Less than 1 percent of approximately 4000 articles on pain published per annum concern pain in the elderly.[28] Ferrell[29] reviewed eight textbooks of geriatric nursing, finding that of 5000 pages only 18 pages were devoted to pain and its management.

This is further put in perspective when it is considered that the incidence of pain in the elderly is probably higher than in younger age groups. However, there is conflicting evidence. Some evidence exists to support the view that there is no difference in incidence of pain in patients below 65 years of age and those above 65.[30,31] Epidemiological studies in the UK on this topic are lacking, but Bowling and Browne[32] reported a survey of 662 persons over the age of 85 years showing that 70 percent complained of pain. In an American study[33] the prevalence of pain in patients aged 60 years and above was found to be 25 percent, being double that of younger patients who had a prevalence of 12 percent. Other studies have estimated the prevalence of pain in elderly patients to vary between 45 and 80 percent.[34–37]

Despite the high incidence of pain in all ages, it appears from several hospital studies that, in general, control of this symptom is suboptimal.[38–43] The findings do not appear to have altered over time. Closs et al.[44] showed a similar lack of pain control in the elderly. There is evidence of a number of deficiencies in the knowledge of physicians in relation to cancer pain treatment.[45–47] These deficits relate to both knowledge and attitudes.

Control of pain requires accurate assessment. Assessment of pain in the elderly may sometimes be difficult for several reasons.[48] First, the elderly may report pain differently from younger age groups; this may be because they perceive aging and pain as inevitable. Second, cultural differences and differences in the perception of suffering add to the problem. Third, cognitive impairment, dysphasia, or dementia may make pain assessment difficult.[49,50] Fourth, there may be a reluctance to administer analgesia out of an exaggerated fear of side-effects, especially respiratory depression. Finally, there may be a perception that the elderly do not experience the same intensity of pain.[51] It is well known that elderly patients may have painless abdominal catastrophes[52,53] or "silent" myocardial infarction.[54] However, the mechanism of this phenomenon is not known and may not be related to aging as such.

Aide-mémoire when assessing pain

P = provoking or palliating factors

Q = quality of pain (e.g. dull, burning, stabbing)

R = radiation or referral of pain

S = severity of pain

T = timing of pain (e.g. constant, intermittent)

Age-related reduction in pain intensity has not been shown experimentally.[55–58] Clinical experience supports this, and a study by Wendy et al.[59] found that 75 percent of 239 cancer patients over 65 years of age had pain on admission to hospice care. This figure correlates well with the incidence of pain in the general hospice population.[31] There was no statistically significant difference between the intensity of pain in the study sample and a younger comparison group with advanced cancer.[59] However, discrepancies exist between patients', caregivers' and professionals' perception of pain intensity. Grossman et al.[60] found that correlation between the physicians' and caregivers' ratings of pain and that of the patient were close when the patient reported mild pain, with a concordance of 78 percent. When pain intensity increased to a moderate or severe level, the concordance level fell to 27 percent.

It has been shown in a large prospective study[61] of over 2000 patients with cancer that 88 percent of pain problems can be adequately controlled by adherence to the World Health Organization (WHO) guidelines for pain control.[62] Other studies have confirmed these results using the WHO guidelines.[63–65] Despite this, the public has a perception that if cancer develops a painful death is inevitable. In addition to *chronic pain*, which is defined as background pain present for more than 3 months, breakthrough and incident pain arise.[66] *Breakthrough pain* occurs without warning and is perceived above background pain. *Incident pain* is predictable pain associated with a particular function, such as standing, walking, or inspiration.

For diagnostic and therapeutic purposes, pain types can be divided into the following:

- nociceptive pain;
- visceral pain;
- neuropathic pain;
- sympathetically mediated pain;
- pain of mixed etiology;
- emotional pain or anguish.

Pains are commonly of mixed etiology, further complicating their management.

Pain management

The approach to successful pain management involves obtaining a careful history from which the type and severity of pain and its influence on function and psyche can be ascertained. This must be followed by a thorough examination to establish a diagnosis or differential diagnoses. Relevant investigations should be carried out, provided the patient is fit enough and a positive or negative result is likely to influence treatment. Pain relief should not be withheld until all investigations have been completed.

Depending on the severity of the pain, appropriate analgesia should be prescribed. The WHO analgesic ladder[62] (Fig. 23-1) is the "gold standard." Step one of the ladder is for mild pain and involves the use of basic analgesics such as paracetamol. Step two requires the use of opioids for moderate pain (e.g. codeine). Step three, for severe pain, employs strong opioids, commonly morphine. At all stages adjuvant analgesics, such as nonsteroidal anti-inflammatory drugs, should be prescribed as appropriate. An adjuvant analgesic is defined

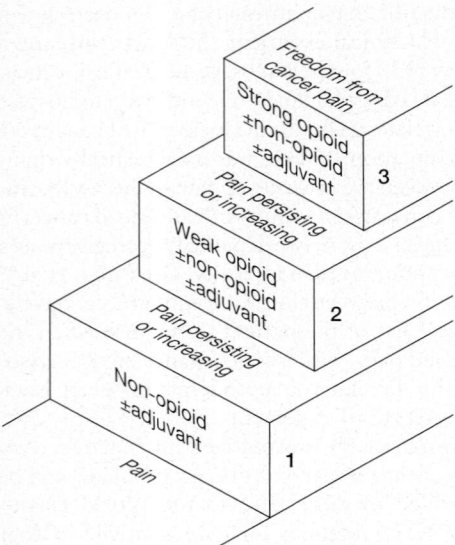

Figure 23-1 The three-step analgesic ladder. From World Health Organization.[2]

Table 23-2 **Adjuvant analgesics**

Drug	Indication	Dose per 24 hours
Dexamethasone	Soft tissue infiltration Hepatic capsular pain Nerve compression pain Nerve infiltration pain Spinal cord compression Raised intracranial pressure	12–16 mg
Amitriptyline	Neuropathic pain (especially if altered sensation and constant)	10–150 mg
Gabapentin	Neuropathic pain (especially if lancinating)	900–2700 mg
Nonsteroidal anti-inflammatory drugs	Bone pain Any inflammatory pain	Depends on choice of drug
Bisphosphonates	Bone pain	

as a drug that has a primary indication other than pain, but is analgesic in some painful conditions.[67,68] Table 23-2 lists examples of adjuvant analgesics and their indications. The patient should be introduced to the ladder at whichever level is appropriate to the degree of pain experienced. Before moving up a step, the maximum tolerated dose of analgesia together with an adjuvant analgesic should have been tried. There is no gain in moving laterally on the ladder (unless one equipotent analgesic is better tolerated). An accompanying summary box contains the basic guidelines for the use of analgesia in chronic pain.

The use of opioids

The strong opioid most commonly used on a worldwide basis is morphine. The reader is referred to two reviews describing morphine's clinical use.[70,71]

Morphine

There are numerous formulations. In uncontrolled severe pain, use of an immediate-release morphine gives greater flexibility for dosage change than do sustained-release preparations.[72] Morphine has a half-life of about 3 hours,[73,74] and for effective analgesia the immediate-release formulation should be given regularly every 4 hours. Provision for relief of breakthrough pain must be made. The dose of opioid required for breakthrough pain is one-sixth of the total 24-hour oral morphine dose. An immediate-release morphine formulation should be used to determine a patient's morphine requirement. Thereafter a sustained-release morphine preparation can be substituted.

In comparisons of the pharmacokinetic parameters of morphine in young and elderly patients, the elderly study group had a decreased morphine clearance with a trend to a smaller volume of distribution. Also the elderly group had a greater area under the plasma concentration–time curve. The time to reach maximum concentration was the same in both groups.[75,76] In clinical practice this means that the starting dose will generally be reduced to prevent undue adverse reactions. Successful pain management in the elderly is often complicated because of renal, hepatic, or gastrointestinal impairment. Elderly patients generally require a lower dose of morphine than younger patients,[77] but each patient's morphine dose should be titrated individually to achieve the best therapeutic outcome. Clinical prescribing guidelines are suggested in the the accompanying box.

The oral route should be used if possible. Morphine is a safe drug when used according to accepted guidelines.[78,79] The only ceiling to morphine dose escalation is the adverse-effect profile. If appropriately titrated, doses of several grams have been used safely.[80] If the patient cannot tolerate the oral route, the opioid should be given subcutaneously. Diamorphine is more soluble in water than morphine and is the opioid of

A morphine regimen

- Start with immediate-release morphine 4-hourly orally.
- Generally the starting dose will be 2.5 or 5 mg every 4 hours.
- Prescribe morphine at one-sixth of the total 24-hour dose for breakthrough or incident pain.
- Titrate the dose against the individual's level of pain and side-effect profile.
- Increase the dose by 20–50 percent or by the amount of breakthrough morphine used in the previous 24 hours.
- When pain is controlled, convert to a sustained-release formulation in an equivalent dosage.
- Prescribe a regular laxative, unless contraindicated.
- **Conversion of oral morphine dose to subcutaneous diamorphine dose**:

  Total 24-hour dose of oral morphine (mg) divided by 2 or 3. For example, if the oral morphine dose were to be 60 mg in 24 hours, the "equivalent" diamorphine dose should be 20–30 mg in 24 hours.

Misconceptions about opioids among physicians

- Poor pain assessment
- Reluctance to follow pain guidelines
- Reluctance to prescribe analgesia regularly
- Reluctance to prescribe maximally tolerated analgesia with respect to the severity of pain
- Belief that opioid side-effects are unpreventable
- Belief that oral opioids are ineffective
- Belief that use of opioids for analgesia will induce psychological dependence
- Belief that tolerance to opioid analgesia will develop
- Belief that tolerance to certain side-effects will not develop
- Belief that complete pain relief in patients with cancer is unattainable

choice for injection in the UK.[81–83] The oral morphine to subcutaneous diamorphine dose conversion factor is shown in the box. In emaciated patients it is less painful to administer appropriate drugs subcutaneously than intramuscularly.

Table 23-3 shows some of the side-effects of morphine.[84] Tolerance to some of the adverse effects such as nausea, vomiting, and sedation occurs. Tolerance to constipation, xerostomia,[85] and the analgesic effect does not occur. Nausea and vomiting will occur in approximately 40 percent of opioid-naive patients.[86] The antiemetic of choice is haloperidol in a dose of 1.5 mg orally twice a day. Normally this can be discontinued after 3 or 4 days.

Constipation requires a dual-action laxative, such as codanthramer, with dose titration as indicated. Prescription of laxatives should be proactive, not reactive. Drowsiness will

Table 23-3 Some side-effects of opioids

Common	Less common
Nausea/vomiting	Urinary retention
Xerostomia	Itch (uncommon in adults)
Constipation	Hypotension
Drowsiness	Bronchospasm
Loss of concentration	Myoclonus
	Respiratory depression
	Gastric stasis
	Sweating

usually resolve after a few days, but care should be taken to avoid concurrent sedating medicines. Dry mouth requires regular mouth care and prompt and effective treatment of any infection.

Other opioids

The majority of patients tolerate morphine well, but a small minority have side-effects which limit the dose of morphine which can be given and thus the control of pain.[87] In these patients, the notion of opioid rotation has been used to describe the conversion to an equianalgesic dose of an alternative opioid with the intention of attenuating dose-limiting side-effects.[88]

While morphine remains the opioid of first choice in severe cancer pain, other strong opioids have become available in recent years. Two opioids for severe pain which have been licensed in the UK in recent years are hydromorphone and oxycodone. Both are available in sustained-release and immediate-release preparations which are prescribed 12-hourly and 4-hourly in much the same way as morphine. There is good evidence for the effective treatment of pain in cancer patients with both agents.[89,90] Hydromorphone is approximately 7.5 times as potent as morphine,[89] while oxycodone has a potency ratio of 2:1.[91]

A transdermal therapeutic system (TTS) with fentanyl is available in the UK, having been available in the USA for some time. Fentanyl is a potent μ-agonist, hence its action can be reversed by naloxone. Fentanyl is a step 3 analgesic used for severe pain. The first fentanyl patch applied has a slow onset of action, reaching therapeutic plasma levels after 8–16 hours.[92] Owing to the slow onset of action, TTS fentanyl should be reserved for patients whose pain has been previously stabilized on immediate-release morphine. Breakthrough pain should be treated using immediate-release morphine.

Oral transmucosal fentanyl citrate (OTFC) became available in the UK in 2000. This is a sugar-free matrix containing fentanyl which is rubbed over the buccal mucosa, dissolves in saliva and is absorbed there and in the upper gut. About 25% of the dose is absorbed by the buccal mucosa and due to the rapid absorption, onset of analgesia usually occurs within 5 minutes. The remainder of the drug is swallowed and a further 25% is absorbed more slowly in the duodenum. Oral bioavailability is therefore about 50%. The rapid onset of analgesia makes this preparation particularly useful in selected patients—for example those with incident pain or patients having painful procedures performed.[93] Fentanyl has an important role in controlling pain, although its use currently requires careful surveillance. Pharmacokinetic parameters after TTS fentanyl are not significantly altered in elderly patients,[94] but when given intravenously in elderly patients fentanyl has a reduced clearance and prolonged half-life.[95]

Finally, there have been reports of the successful use of topical diamorphine in painful skin ulcers and other conditions.[96]

Rectal administration

The rectal route may be chosen for administration of analgesia. Morphine, dextromoramide, and oxycodone suppositories are available. The dose and frequency of administration of morphine rectally is identical to the oral route.[97,98]

Morphine-induced confusion

Patients who are morphine-toxic generally exhibit signs of somnolence, pseudo-hallucinations, confusion and myoclonus,[99] hypotension and respiratory depression.[100] However, more subtle signs, such as mild agitation or restlessness, can occur. In this situation the dose of morphine should be reduced. Adjuvant drugs should be prescribed in a morphine-sparing attempt. A careful reappraisal of the patient's drug regimen and level of anxiety should be made. If the patient is unable to tolerate morphine, changing to oxycodone, hydromorphone or transdermal fentanyl (if pain is stable) may allow upward dose titration with fewer side effects than morphine. Hallucinations can be controlled by a small dose of haloperidol. Morphine toxicity is usually a result of inappropriate dose escalation, poor pain assessment, deteriorating renal function, and failure to appreciate and treat underlying and associated psychological factors.

Difficult pain

Some pains prove more difficult to control. Generally these pains are classified as "opioid poorly responsive." However, opioids should be titrated to their maximally tolerated dose before arriving at this conclusion. Careful reappraisal of the etiology of the pain and use of appropriate adjuvant agents and nondrug interventions should be considered.

There has been a major interest in pain research in the past 20 years and knowledge of the nociceptive and antinociceptive pathways has increased greatly. The etiology of pains (often neuropathic) that are less opioid-responsive is clearer following recognition of the role of AMPA (RS-α-amino-3-hydroxy-5-methylisoxazole-4-proprionic acid) and NMDA (N-methyl-D-aspartate) receptors.[101] If the NMDA receptor pathway is activated, central sensitization develops, frequently accompanied by a clinical triad of signs and symptoms. This triad, comprising allodynia, hyperesthesia, and hyperpathia, is indicative of central sensitization. Morphine acts as an analgesic by its pure agonist effect on μ-receptors but is inactive at the NMDA receptor. Ketamine, an anesthetic agent, has analgesic properties at low doses and is an NMDA receptor antagonist. Its use as an analgesic in this situation has been evaluated in a number of situations and research continues into its therapeutic potential.[102] It has been shown to be effective in chronic neuropathic pain of malignant[103] and non-malignant[104] origin, phantom limb pain,[105] and fibromyalgia.[106] There are encouraging trials of its use in ischemic limb pain. The drug has been used orally,[107] parenterally,[108] and via the epidural route.[109] The dissociative symptoms associated with ketamine mean that its use should be limited to specialists with experience of the drug.

Pain due to nerve compression or infiltration may respond to high-dose dexamethasone added to the analgesic regimen.[110]

NAUSEA AND VOMITING

Nausea and/or vomiting occur in 60 percent of patients with advanced cancer.[111,112] It is distressing and if persistent can rapidly result in symptoms of dehydration and hypovolemia in elderly patients. Vomiting and retching is a complex reflex process. Nausea is mediated via autonomic stimulation of somatic nerves. The vomiting center coordinates the process, receiving input and integrating this from several sources. Figure 23-2 is a diagrammatic representation of the mechanisms of vomiting.

It is important to determine the etiology in each patient as the treatment selected depends on the cause. Examination will include fundoscopy and usually rectal exam. Blood analysis is

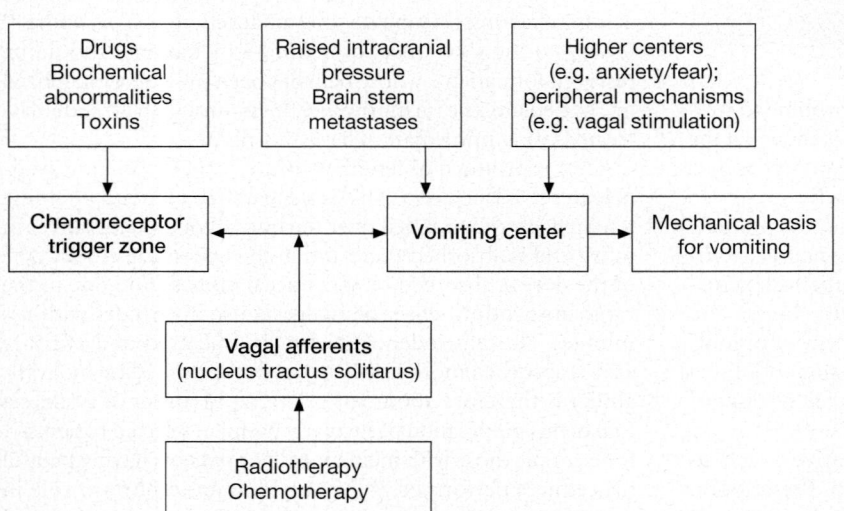

Figure 23-2 Coordination of nausea and vomiting.

Table 23-4 Causes of nausea and vomiting in advanced cancer

Caused by cancer	Caused by cancer and/or debility	Caused by treatment	Concurrent causes
Metabolic	Cough	Radiotherapy	Peptic ulcer
Gastroparesis (paraneoplastic visceral neuropathy)	Infection	Chemotherapy	Functional dyspepsia
Hepatomegaly		Surgery	Hiatal hernia
Tense ascites		Drugs	
Bowel obstruction			
Functional			
Partial or complete			
Constipation			
Cough			
Raised intracranial pressure			
Pain			
Anxiety			

often necessary and may reveal a reversible cause (e.g. hypercalcemia or digoxin toxicity). A review of all drugs is important, especially opioids. Sometimes patients find it difficult to differentiate among expectoration, regurgitation, and vomiting. A specific question about cough may be helpful as cough-induced retching resulting in vomiting requires treatment of the cause of the cough. Causes of nausea and vomiting in advanced cancer are listed in Table 23-4.

Management of nausea and vomiting

Management hinges on correction of the reversible, employing nondrug measures as appropriate and prescribing the correct antiemetic. Nondrug measures may include avoiding the smell or even the sight of food, avoiding exposure to foods that precipitate nausea, and presenting food in small, attractive quantities.

The choice of antiemetic depends on (1) knowledge of the emetic receptor(s) through which the cause of the vomiting is mediated, and (2) the receptor specificity of the antiemetic. Unless the cause can be removed, drug therapy must be administered regularly. The formulation of the antiemetic will depend on the pervasiveness and severity of the symptom. Oral, rectal, and parenteral preparations are available.

If a persistent pattern of vomiting is established, parenteral administration may be necessary. In the palliative care setting the subcutaneous route with a continuous infusion using a Graseby or similar lightweight portable pump is frequently used. This pump has the advantage of being small, suitable for use at home, and allowing a mixture of antiemetic and analgesia as indicated.[113] For patients wishing to avoid needles, the rectal route is an alternative (cyclizine, prochlorperazine, chlorpromazine, and domperidone are available in suppository form). Table 23-5 offers a systematic approach to antiemetic prescribing.

INTESTINAL OBSTRUCTION

Until the advent of the modern palliative care approach to malignant gastrointestinal obstruction, such patients had only two treatment options: palliative surgery, which carried high morbidity and mortality rates,[114] or conservative management with intravenous fluids, nothing by mouth, and a nasogastric tube. The latter has obvious physical and psychological drawbacks. The use of appropriate analgesics and antiemetic drugs by continuous subcutaneous infusion has been shown to control symptoms.[115] Malignant gastrointestinal obstruction is encountered most commonly in patients with advanced abdominal or pelvic cancers. It occurs in 10–28 percent of primary bowel cancer, in 5 percent of primary ovarian cancer, and in over 40 percent of patients with advanced ovarian cancer.[116]

The following recommendations apply to those patients who have no tumoricidal options open to them or who are awaiting tumoricidal treatment to take effect.

Table 23-5 Choice of antiemetic

Cause of nausea and vomiting	Antiemetic of choice
Drug-induced	Haloperidol 1.5–3 mg nocte
	Prochlorperazine 5–10 mg
Radiotherapy	Haloperidol 1.5–5 mg b.i.d.
Chemotherapy	5-HT$_3$ receptor antagonist (e.g. ondansetron)
	Metoclopramide (high dose)
	Dexamethasone
Metabolic	Haloperidol 5–20 mg/24 hr
Raised intracranial pressure	Cyclizine 50–100 mg t.d.s.
Middle-ear pressure/irritation	Hyoscine (Kwells) 0.3 mg SL t.d.s. or q.d.s.
Bowel obstruction[a]	Hyoscine butylbromide 60–120 mg SC/24 hr
	Octreotide 300–600 µg SC/24 hr
Delayed gastric emptying	Metoclopramide 10–20 mg q.d.s.
	Domperidone 10–20 mg q.d.s.
Drug-related gastric irritation	Treat gastritis; change medication as necessary

[a]See section on intestinal obstruction. Haloperidol, cyclizine metoclopramide, hyoscine butylbromide, octreotide, and dexamethasone can all be given by continuous subcutaneous infusion. Mixing dexamethasone with other drugs in a syringe driver is not recommended, but it can be given with diamorphine. Cyclizine is not compatible with octreotide.

The etiology of bowel obstruction in advanced malignancy can be complicated and should not automatically be assumed to be due to tumor alone. Adhesions, constipation, drugs, unrelated benign conditions, or a combination of factors should be considered. Obstruction may be functional, complete or partial, persistent or transient, high or low, single or at multiple sites.

There is almost always an element of continuous abdominal pain from the underlying cancer. Vomiting and intestinal colic occurs in about 80 percent of patients.[117] Distention varies with the level of obstruction, and bowel habit may vary from absolute constipation to diarrhea. Bowel sounds may be hyperactive but may also be absent.

Plain abdominal X-rays may confirm constipation. Computed tomography or magnetic resonance imaging can demonstrate obstruction at more than one level and are of use in deciding the technical feasibility of palliative surgery. Surgical intervention is unlikely to be successful in the following situations:

- radiological or previous surgical evidence that technically a surgical procedure will not be successful;
- diffuse intra-abdominal carcinomatosis (diffuse palpable intra-abdominal tumors);
- massive ascites that reaccumulates rapidly after paracentesis;[118]
- poor general physical status.

Management of intestinal obstruction

Medical management of malignant gastrointestinal obstruction hinges on an accurate assessment with attempts to reverse the reversible (e.g. constipation), and to palliate the irreversible. A nasogastric tube and intravenous fluids are rarely necessary. The principles of pharmacological management are shown in an accompanying box.

Persistent large-volume vomiting despite the pharmacological interventions mentioned may respond to the somatostatin analog, octreotide. This drug is antisecretory and proabsorptive with the resultant net effect of decreasing the volume of fluid in the gut lumen.[120,121] This has the effect of eliminating vomiting completely or reducing volume and frequency of vomiting. Octreotide has also been shown to decrease forward peristalsis and may have direct analgesic activity.[121] Octreotide does not have a direct antiemetic action, and if background nausea still exists, it can be combined with haloperidol in a syringe for continuous SC infusion.[122] A starting dose of 300 µg/24 hr is recommended as this is the mean dose required to control vomiting.[123] Titration beyond 600 µg/24 hr is usually unhelpful, but this has also to be judged on a clinical basis. Clinical impression and a recent study[124] suggest that the higher the obstruction, the higher the dose of octreotide required. Octreotide, although expensive, is undoubtedly cost effective in many patients. A small-scale trial has compared this with hyoscine butylbromide and concluded it is more effective than hyoscine.[125]

Diamorphine, octreotide, and haloperidol can be mixed in the same syringe and infused using a portable syringe driver. Octreotide does not appear compatible with cyclizine, levomepromazine, or dexamethasone in the same syringe.[123]

Steroids can be useful in some cases of malignant obstruction. The postulated mechanism is a reduction of peritumor

Intestinal obstruction

Pharmacological management

- Adequate analgesia should be given for background pain using a continuous subcutaneous infusion of diamorphine. Dose depends on current dose. If opioid-naive, start at diamorphine 10 mg SC in 24 hours.

- If colic is present avoid all prokinetics, bulk-forming, osmotic, and stimulant laxatives. If colic persists add subcutaneous hyoscine butylbromide, starting at 60 mg/24 hr and increasing up to 200 mg/24 hr. Some reports suggest increasing to 380 mg/24 hr,[119] but this is rarely necessary.

- Nausea and vomiting should be controlled. The choice of antiemetic depends on whether the patient is experiencing colic. If the symptoms are suggestive of an incomplete obstruction and colic is not a feature, a trial of the prokinetic, metoclopramide 60 mg SC/24 hr, is worthwhile. If the obstruction is more functional than mechanical this may resolve the problem.

- For other patients with nausea and vomiting, haloperidol 5–20 mg/24 hr or cyclizine 100–150 mg/24 hr are used as first-line treatment. Haloperidol is a dopamine antagonist with its main effect at the chemoreceptor trigger zone, whereas cyclizine acts on histamine and muscarinic cholinergic receptors, its main site of action being the vomiting center.

- A general principle in palliative medicine is to use the least number of drugs possible, thus avoiding unnecessary side-effects. If control with the first antiemetic is not achieved, the second should be added, and if successful, a trial without the first advocated.

inflammatory edema. The dose used is dexamethasone 8–16 mg/24 hr by intravenous or subcutaneous route. Trials of steroids in malignant bowel obstruction have been inconclusive.[126]

The role of laxatives in obstruction depends on the analysis of the situation. If a single colonic or rectal obstruction is suspected, then a fecal softening laxative is justified (e.g. docusate). In the more usual situation of small bowel obstruction, laxatives have no role. Where obstruction is due to a combination of tumor compressing the bowel and hard impacted stool in the bowel lumen, both rectal and stoma suppositories and enemas can tip the balance in favor of the bowel opening.

Dietary advice in obstruction depends on the symptoms present. Many patients even with complete obstruction can eat and drink in modest amounts when symptoms are controlled. Diet is often liquid and low residue.

The symptom of dry mouth is usually best dealt with by frequent sips of cool fluids and ice to suck, along with regular mouth care. Administration of intravenous fluid is less helpful in dealing with the symptom of dry mouth per se, largely because this symptom is a complex physical and emotional phenomenon that depends on many factors. It may, however, be entirely appropriate to administer intravenous or subcutaneous fluids to some patients,[127] and this has to be judged on an individual basis. The majority of patients with malignant obstruction who are unsuitable for surgery can be managed by appropriate drug regimens. A few patients, usually with a high obstruction, may require a venting gastrostomy. The patient benefits of this procedure need to be properly evaluated in clinical trials.

CACHEXIA AND ANOREXIA

Nausea and vomiting may exacerbate anorexia and, if they are controlled, appetite may improve. However, cachexia occurs in 90 percent of patients with advanced cancer and will further reduce mobility and exacerbate weakness due to depletion of muscle mass.[128] Enteral and parenteral feeding does not reverse this syndrome;[129] but in a double-blind placebo-controlled study, Downer[130] showed that the use of megesterol acetate improved appetite and general well-being. There may be a dose–response curve to megesterol acetate as shown by Tchekmedyian.[131] Megesterol acetate is generally well tolerated but fluid retention may be problematic.[132] Early studies in the use of megesterol acetate and nonsteroidal inflammatory drugs is encouraging in cachexia associated with some tumors.[133] In a double-blind placebo-controlled study of patients attending an oncology clinic, prednisolone 15 mg/d was shown to be statistically superior to placebo in improving appetite.[134]

CONSTIPATION

Constipation is one of the most troublesome and persistent symptoms in patients with advanced cancer. Forty-five percent of patients complain of constipation on admission to a hospice.[135] The etiology is usually multifactorial but the common causes are listed in Table 23-6. Prevention is the mainstay of management. Good general symptom control, attention to toileting arrangements, mobility, diet, fluid intake, and prescription of an appropriate laxative in a therapeutic dose, are all essential elements in the prevention and management of constipation.

The choice of laxative will depend on the bowel history but there frequently needs to be a combination of a stimulant and a softener (e.g. codanthramer or codanthrusate alone, or senna and lactulose given together). The dose should be titrated until the desired effect is achieved. Rectal laxatives are overprescribed, often because an inadequate dose of an oral laxative is used. However, some conditions such as spinal cord compression necessitate the use of regular rectal laxatives. In these situations a careful balance between oral and rectal laxatives gives pseudocontrol of the bowel.

Fecal impaction leading to overflow diarrhea, urinary incontinence, or urinary retention is not uncommon in a patient with cancer who has become bedbound and is taking constipating medication. Diarrhea secondary to impaction is frequently mistreated by antidiarrheal drugs.

The sequence of undiagnosed constipation leading to abdominal pain, which then is treated inappropriately by opioids, is unfortunately common in advanced cancer. This vicious circle causes much distress for patients.

The prevention and management of constipation is multifactorial; however, there is definite evidence that immobility can be a greater causal component in constipation than opioids.[136] Aggressive titration of laxatives in immobile patients is advised.

TERMINAL RESTLESSNESS

It is a fundamental right of humanity that, when natural death approaches, the passage from life to death should be dignified and peaceful with no undue distress. Moreover, it has also been shown that the quality of care, manner of dying, and support given to relatives influences the bereavement outcome of survivors. Pain or restlessness prior to death are unacceptable and distressing for all, not least the dying. The underlying principle of continuing attention to the whole person care is vital. The patient may be fearful and anxious about what is happening. As the patient enters the terminal phase, the approach to care must continue to be diligent, and attention to psychological, spiritual, and physical needs should continue. Careful positioning, ensuring an optimum environment, and attention to the remaining basic needs of the person may alone settle distress.

A study by Wilson et al.[137] showed that 32 percent of elderly patients in a long-stay ward and 41 percent in an assessment ward were distressed in the last week of life. Agitation was the most common manifestation of distress. Restlessness was especially prominent if there were respiratory symptoms or cardiac decompensation. Fifty-six percent of the 150 patients studied were taking opioids. However, the average dose was low at 2.5–5 mg immediate-release morphine 4-hourly orally. This dose range, if compared with the average dose in a SPCU, is low. The median dose of oral morphine in 955 inpatients at St Christopher's Hospice was 10 mg 4-hourly.[138] In a terminally restless patient there should be an attempt to determine the etiology of the distress (see Table 23-7).

If a cause for terminal restlessness is diagnosed, a decision must be made as to whether to treat the cause or palliate the

---

Table 23-6 **Causes of constipation**

Inactivity/poor mobility	Cancer-related
Poor diet	Tumor in bowel wall
Poor fluid intake	Tumor causing extrinsic
Drugs	compression of bowel
Opioids	Hypercalcemia
Anticholinergics	Cord compression
Antacids	Other illnesses
Anticonvulsants	Unsatisfactory toileting
Iron	arrangement
Vincristine	

Table 23-7 **Some causes of terminal restlessness**

Unrelieved pain	Cerebral metastases
Psychosocial factors:	Hiccoughs
anxiety, fear, unfinished business	Dyspnea
Retention of urine	Cough
Full rectum, impaction	Drugs
Dry mouth	Dehydration
Infection: chest, urine, wound	
Metabolic (e.g. hypercalcemia,	
hypoglycemia)	

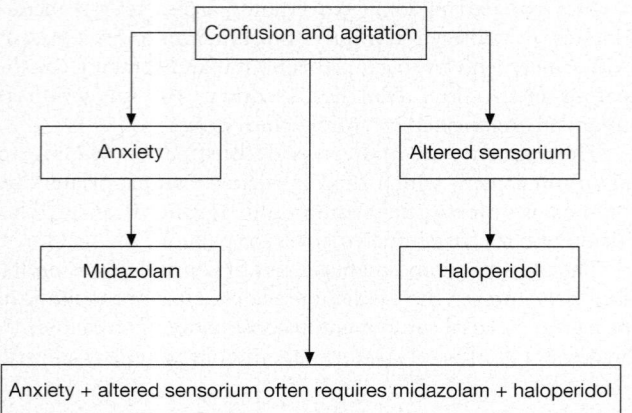

Figure 23-3 Treatment of terminal restlessness.

symptom. If the decision is taken to palliate the cause of the distress, various drugs are available.

Analgesia must be continued and if swallowing becomes difficult an alternative route, usually subcutaneously, should be used. Additional analgesia should be available for breakthrough pain, calculated as described earlier in this chapter.

The level of sedation required and nature of the distress will usually dictate which medication is used. Midazolam, haloperidol, levomepromazine, and indirectly hyoscine hydrobromide are commonly used. Midazolam is used subcutaneously in a syringe driver in doses ranging from 5 to 80 mg/24 hr.[139] The dose varies and for anxiety that cannot be alleviated by counseling and personal support a low dose of 5–20 mg/24 hr is normally sufficient, especially in patients elderly . If pain is present, diamorphine is compatible with midazolam and can be mixed in the same syringe driver. Midazolam also raises the seizure threshold. Dosage increase, if necessary, may be made in increments of 10 to 15 mg in 24 hours. Haloperidol is indicated in cases of agitation with altered sensorium. This drug can be administered via a syringe driver subcutaneously in doses between 2.5 and 25 mg/24 hr.

Levomepromazine, a phenothiazine, has antiemetic, antipsychotic, and sedative properties and is claimed to have analgesic properties.[140] It can be administered subcutaneously via a syringe driver and is a potent sedating agent. In the elderly patient, haloperidol is safer than levomepromazine. Figure 23-3 summarizes the approach.

If oropharyngeal secretions accumulate and produce a "rattle or gurgle," usually the patient is unconscious and unaware. The noise is distressing for relatives and other patients. Excessive secretions may be eased by using hyoscine hydrobromide if sedation is also desired. Hyoscine butylbromide is an alternative if sedation is not required. Diazepam (5–10 mg) or chlorpromazine (50–100 mg) can be administered rectally.

DYSPNEA

Dyspnea is an unpleasant awareness of difficulty in breathing. Dyspnea, like pain, is subjective and involves both the perception of the symptom by the patient and his or her reaction to that sensation. The symptom can be very variable even in the same patient not only because its severity is usually directly related to activity, but also because the speed of onset, more than the severity, may influence the patient's perception of breathlessness. In addition, patient's previous experience of a symptom, whether suffered by themselves or witnessed in others, undoubtedly colors their reaction.

There is frequently considerable disparity between doctors' and patients' assessments of symptoms, and indeed patients and their close relatives may well have differing points of view.[141] The tumors most commonly associated with dyspnea are lung, colorectal, breast, and prostate cancers.[142,143] Dyspnea in patients with cancer may be caused by the tumor itself, the treatment of the tumor, pre-existing cardiorespiratory disease, infection, or any combination of these factors. Anemia, pulmonary emboli, or congestive heart failure may arise as a manifestation of debility caused by both the disease and its treatment. Dyspnea has been noted as the most common severe symptom in the last days of life.[144] In a longitudinal survey of 1700 inpatient hospice patients in the USA, 70 percent of patients with a wide range of malignancies had dyspnea in the last weeks of life.[142] The same rate was reported in patients with lung cancer.[145] In one study neither lung nor heart disease could be identified as the cause of this symptom in one-quarter of patients.[143] The explanation given by the authors in this case was debility of terminal cancer, while an alternative explanation could be functional dyspnea.[146]

The pathogenesis of dyspnea is poorly understood and like pain is likely to be much more complex than previously thought. Factors as diverse as chemical stimulation of the respiratory center in the medulla and the tone of bronchial, diaphragmatic, and intercostal muscles are important. The innervation of the lung is complex and includes excitatory cholinergic parasympathetic and inhibitory adrenergic sympathetic neurons. More recently a nonadrenergic–noncholinergic network has been described. These latter are opioid receptors and, together with endogenous opioids, have been demonstrated in the lung.[147–149] There is growing evidence that they have an important role in the pathophysiology of breathlessness.[150,151]

The multiple aspects of the physiology of respiration are summarized in Figure 23-4.

Symptomatic treatment of dyspnea

The fundamental principles are a comprehensive clinical assessment, analysis of symptomatology, and reversal of the reversible and symptomatic relief of the irreversible based on the underlying cause(s). It is important to remember that a dyspneic patient is often an anxious patient (Fig. 23-5).

In cases where a reversible cause is identified, symptomatic relief should not be withheld while more definitive treatment is being applied, such as aspiration of pleural or ascitic fluid, radiotherapy, chemotherapy, treatment of infection, or laser therapy. The approaches to symptomatic treatment are, broadly, nonpharmacological and pharmacological. The former include the following:

- explanation and reassurance;
- calm presence;
- comfortable position;
- walking aid;

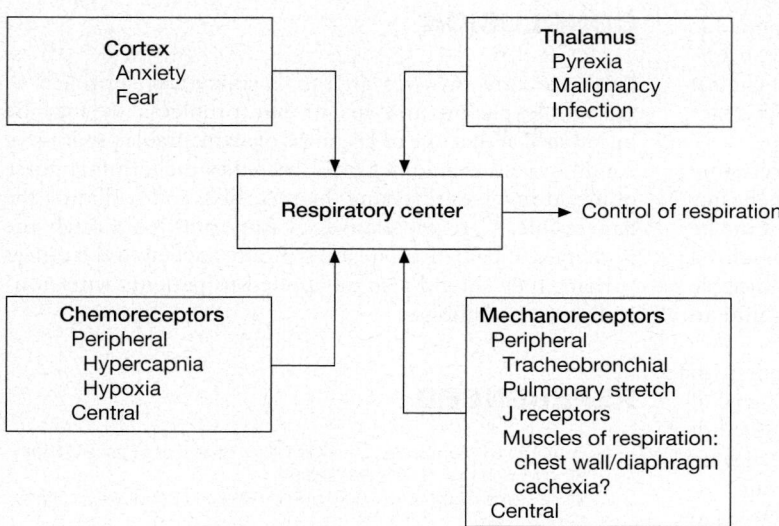

Figure 23-4 The physiology of respiration.

- bed rest;
- bed downstairs;
- cool air use of a fan;
- wheelchair;
- help with activities of daily living;
- breathing exercises;
- relaxation therapy.

Pharmacological intervention should be integrated with the above as follows. A low-dose systemic opioid, usually morphine, is the treatment of choice of most palliative medicine physicians for dyspnea in malignant disease.[152,153] Although many physicians worry about the respiratory depressant effect of opioids, this is not normally a problem if care is given to the choice of dose and dose titration. There is clinical evidence that patients with chronic obstructive pulmonary disease (COPD) and high arterial carbon dioxide levels tolerate opioids well.[154,155]

Several factors must be considered before choosing the route and dose of opioid. Among these factors are (1) history of exposure to opioids (whether or not opioid-naive); (2) current opioid dose and side-effect profile; (3) renal function; (4) coexisting COPD. A typical starting dose for oral morphine would be 5 mg 4-hourly (but see below). For a patient already on morphine, the dose should be gently titrated against dyspnea and adverse effects, using the same principles as in pain control.

Titration is always better achieved by using a 4-hourly immediate-release morphine preparation. This allows specific questions, such as time to onset of action, degree of relief, and duration of action, to be answered more accurately by the patient. Subsequently a more efficient titration to reach the desired balance between control of dyspnea and adverse effects is achieved. A dose equal to the individual 4-hourly dose should be prescribed for breakthrough dyspnea at any time.

Often in elderly opioid-naive patients a smaller starting dose of immediate-release morphine such as 2.5 mg 4-hourly may be sufficient. In renal dysfunction as little as 2.5 mg immediate-release morphine 6-hourly or less can reach a better balance between control of dyspnea and adverse effects. There is no evidence that sustained-release morphine compounds are less effective than immediate-release morphine preparations in control of dyspnea. If a stable immediate-release morphine dose is reached this can be converted to sustained-release morphine compound for ease of administration for the patient.

The mechanism of action of opioids in the control of dyspnea is not fully understood and is certainly complex, probably involving several areas. Morphine acts on (1) the cerebral cortex; (2) the respiratory center; (3) stretch (J) receptors in the lungs; (4) peripheral opioid receptors in the lungs; and (5) the cardiovascular system.

Morphine can also be given by nebulizer.[156] Clinical experience suggests nebulized morphine may help to control dyspnea in patients with interstitial lung disease, rather than in patients with encasing lung disease. In a randomized controlled trial in dyspneic patients with cancer, no difference in efficacy was found between nebulized morphine and nebulized saline.[157]

There is no evidence that diazepam has any central or peripheral effect on dyspnea per se. However, in the patient who becomes anxious, with resultant worsening of dyspnea, it has an obvious role. The dose of diazepam will vary with the individual patient, from 2 mg nocte to 10 mg t.d.s. and 20 mg nocte. In patients unable to swallow medication, midazolam is the anxiolytic of choice by continuous subcutaneous infusion. A starting dose of midazolam would be 10 mg over 24 hours.

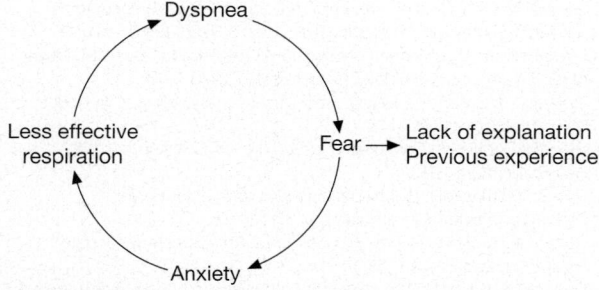

Figure 23-5 The interplay between dyspnea and anxiety.

Nebulized salbutamol has an interesting role in dyspnea due to malignancy. It seems to have much more than a bronchodilator effect and is often of use in the absence of clinical bronchospasm. Salbutamol has been shown to increase voluntary muscle strength.[158]

Nebulized 0.9 percent saline (2–5 mL) is also an interesting drug with much more than a mucolytic action. Although clinical research is lacking, the general impression is that it can be an effective treatment for the relief of dyspnea.[141] Nebulized lignocaine is disappointing in both the treatment of intractable cough and of dyspnea, performing poorly against saline in one study.[159]

In patients with cancer-related dyspnea, the benefit of oxygen is not dependent on correction of hypoxia; a trial of oxygen therapy is the only way to determine benefit, not improvement in blood gases. This has only been investigated superficially,[160] and needs to be looked at in more detail.

In summary, dyspnea is a common symptom that needs to be analyzed in the individual patient. All reversible factors should be dealt with and steps taken to give symptomatic relief. A combined approach is necessary to deal with the physical symptomatology and accompanying anxiety. A stepwise approach using simple methods such as nebulized saline and salbutamol, progressing to systemic opioid therapy, is advised. A combination of treatments is often required.

KEY POINTS   Palliative care

- The philosophy of palliative care is generic and can be applied to all patients with progressive, incurable disease.

- The education of medical students, doctors caring for patients with incurable, progressive disease, and all health workers in relevant sectors is an important part of the work of palliative physicians.

- Cancer is predominantly a disease of older people. Physicians caring for the elderly are likely to see large numbers of patients with symptoms related to their cancer and its treatment.

- The incidence of pain and other symptoms in the elderly is higher than in younger groups of patients.

- Good pain control is achievable in 80–90 percent of patients with cancer using the WHO three-step analgesic ladder.

- Pain requires careful assessment to be managed successfully.

- New step-3 synthetic opioids are available which will allow a more tailored approach to the management of severe cancer pain.

- New agents are available for use in the management of neuropathic pain.

- Services are becoming available in hospitals (the provision of palliative care support teams) and in the community (hospice at home projects) in addition to traditional, freestanding inpatient units.

- The evidence-base of palliative care is expanding, but progress is slow against the background of a new specialty with a small academic and research base.

CONCLUSION

Palliative care involves an active, analytical approach to the whole person and his or her problems. It may be introduced at the time of diagnosis of an incurable progressive condition and should not be restricted to the terminal phase of life. It involves reversing the reversible and palliating the irreversible. Care of relatives is important. Although the principles of palliative care are typically applied to the cancer patient, they should also be applied to patients with nonmalignant conditions.

REFERENCES

1. Callaghan D: The Troubled Dream of Life: In Search of a Peaceful Death. Simon & Schuster, New York, 1993:94
2. World Health Organization: Cancer Pain Relief and Palliative Care. WHO, Geneva, 1990
3. Doyle D, Hanks G, MacDonald N (eds): Oxford Textbook of Palliative Medicine. Oxford University Press, Oxford, 1993:3
4. Directory of Hospice and Palliative Care Services in the United Kingdom and Republic of Ireland. St Christopher's Hospice Information Service, London, 2000:xiii
5. Lunt B, Hillier R: St Christopher's Hospice Information Service, London, 1987
6. Findlay IG, Jones RVH: Outreach palliative care services: definitions in palliative care. BMJ 1995;311:754
7. National Council for Hospice and Specialist Palliative Care Services: Specialist palliative care: a statement of definitions, Occasional paper 8. London, 1995
8. McWhinney IR, Bass MJ, Donner A: Evaluation of a palliative care service: problems and pitfalls. BMJ 1994;309:1340–1342
9. Eve A, Higginson IJ: Minimum dataset activity for hospice and hospital palliative care services in the UK 1997/98. Palliat Med 2000;14(5):395–404
10. Directory of Hospice and Palliative Care Services in the United Kingdom and Republic of Ireland. St Christopher's Hospice Information Service, London, 1996:x
11. Hamilton J, Edgar L: A survey examining nurses' knowledge of pain control. J Pain Sympt Manage 1992;7:18–26
12. Elliot TE, Murray DM, Elliot BA et al: Physician knowledge and attitudes about cancer pain management: a survey from the Minnesota Cancer Pain Project. J Pain Sympt Manage 1995;10:494–504
13. Cancer Relief Macmillan Fund: In GP Facilitators Project. Section B: Project Activities 1992–94:x
14. Reid W: Just for the Record. Department of Health. Redhouse Lane Communications, 1995
15. Association of Palliative Medicine of Great Britain and Ireland: Palliative Medicine Curriculum, 1992
16. WHO: A core Curriculum for a Post Basic Course in Palliative Nursing. The International Society for Nurses in Cancer Care approved by the Cancer and Palliative Care Unit. WHO, Geneva, 1991
17. Commission of the European Communities and the European Oncology Nursing Society: A Core Curriculum for Post-Basic Nursing. Brussels, 1991
18. General Medical Council: Recommendations on General Clinical Training. Kiek & Read, London, 1992
19. General Medical Council: Tomorrow's Doctors—Recommendations on Undergraduate Medical Education. Kiek & Read, London 1993
20. Leventhal EA: The dilemma of cancer in the elderly. In Veeth JM, Meyer J (eds): Cancer and the Elderly. Karger, Basel, 1986:1–13
21. Crawford J, Cohen HJ: Relationship of cancer and aging. Clin Geriatr Med 1987;3:419–431
22. Office of Population Censuses and Surveys (OPCS): Monitor 1992. HMSO, London, 1993
23. Roy R, Thomas MR: Elderly persons with and without pain: a comparative study. Clin J Pain 1987;3:102–106
24. Cartwright A, Seale C: The Year Before Death. Aldershot, Ashgate Publishing, 1994:113–116
25. Donnelly S, Walsh D: The symptoms of advanced cancer. Semin Oncol 1995;22:67–72

26. Leishman JG, McGovern EM, McKay S et al: An Audit of the Pharmaceutical Care Provided to Terminally Ill Patients in the Hospice and Community. Clinical Resource and Audit Group, Scottish Office Home and Health Department, Edinburgh, 1995

27. Portenoy RK, Miransky J, Thaler HT: Pain in ambulatory patients with lung or colon cancer, prevalence, characteristics and impact. Cancer 1992;70:1616–1624

28. Melding PS: Is there such a thing as geriatric pain? Pain 1991;46:119–121

29. Ferrell BA: Pain management in elderly people. J Am Geriatr Soc 1991;39:64–73

30. Stein WM, Mieck RP: Cancer pain in the elderly hospice patient. J Pain Sympt Manage 1993;8:474–482

31. Twycross RG: Incidence of pain. Clin Oncol 1984;3:5–15

32. Bowling A, Browne PD: Social networks, health and emotional well-being among the oldest old in London. J Gerontol 1991;46:20–32

33. Kane RL, Ouslander JG, Abrass IB: Essentials of Clinical Geriatrics, 2nd edn. McGraw-Hill, New York, 1989

34. Roy R: A psychological perspective on chronic pain and depression in the elderly. Social Work Healthcare 1986;12:27–36

35. Lau-Ting C, Poon WO: Aches and pains among Singapore elderly. Singapore Med J 1988;29:164–167

36. Ferrell BA, Ferrell BR, Osterweil D: Pain in the nursing home. J Am Geriatr Soc 1990;39:64–73

37. Davis MA: Epidemiology of osteoarthritis. Clin Geriatr Med 1988;4:241–255

38. Marks RM, Sachar EJ: Undertreatment of medical inpatients with narcotic analgesics. Ann Intern Med 1973;78:173–181

39. Sriwatanakul K, Weis OF, Alloza JL et al: Analysis of narcotic usage in the treatment of postoperative pain. JAMA 1983;250:926–929

40. Melzack R, Abbott FV, Zackon W et al: Pain on a surgical ward: a survey of the duration and intensity of pain and the effectiveness of medication. Pain 1987;29:67–72

41. Seers CJ: Pain, Anxiety and Recovery in Patients Undergoing Surgery. Unpublished PhD thesis, Department of Nursing Studies, University of London, London, 1987

42. Carr ECJ: Post operative pain: patient's expectations and experiences. J Adv Nurs 1990;15:89–100

43. Kuhn S, Cook K, Collins M et al: Perception of pain after surgery. BMJ 1990;300:1687–1690

44. Closs SJ, Fairtlough HL, Tierney AJ, Currie CT: Pain in elderly orthopaedic patients. J Clin Nurs 1993;2:41–45

45. Cleeland CS, Cleeland LM, Dar R, Rinchardt LC: Factors influencing physicians' management of cancer pain. Cancer 1986;58:796–800

46. Elliot TE, Elliot BA: Physician attitudes and beliefs about use of morphine for cancer pain. J Pain Sympt Manage 1992;7:141–148

47. Rife BL, Inik N, Painter JD: A comparative study of the attitudes of physicians and nurses toward the management of cancer pain. J Pain Sympt Manage 1993;8:132–139

48. Closs SJ: Pain in elderly patients: a neglected phenomenon? J Adv Nurs 1994;19:1072–1081

49. Reid W, Stott DJ: Pain relief in elderly patients. Ther Update 1993;Sept:309–316

50. Hayes R: Pain assessment in the elderly. Br J Nurs 1995;4:1199–1204

51. Fordyce WE: Evaluating and managing chronic pain. Geriatrics 1978;33:59–62

52. Bender JS: Approach to the acute abdomen. Med Clin North Am 1989;73:1413–1422

53. Clinch D: Absence of abdominal pain in elderly patients with peptic ulcer. Age Ageing 1984;13:120–123

54. Bayer AJ, Chada JS, Farag RR, Pathy MS: Changing presentation of myocardial infarctions with increasing old age. J Am Geriatr Soc 1986;34:263–266

55. Collins G, Stone LA: Pain sensitivity, age and activity level in chronic schizophrenics and in normals. Br J Psychiatry 1965;112:33

56. Harkins SW, Chapman CR: Detection and decision factors in pain perception in young and elderly men. Pain 1976;2:253

57. Harkins SW, Chapman CR: The perception of induced dental pain in young and elderly women. J Gerontol 1977;428–435

58. Tucker MA, Andrew MF, Ogle SJ, Davison JG: Age associated change in pain threshold measured by transcutaneous neuronal electrical stimulation. Age Ageing 1989;18:241–246

59. Wendy M, Stein MD, Ralph P, Miech MD: Cancer pain in the elderly hospice patient. J Pain Sympt Manage 1993;8:474–482

60. Grossman SA, Shiedler VR, Sweden K et al: Correlation of patient and care giver rating of cancer pain. J Pain Sympt Manage 1991;6:53–57

61. Zech DFJ, Grond S, Lynch J et al: Validation of World Health Organization guidelines for cancer pain relief: a ten year prospective study. Pain 1995;63:65–76

62. World Health Organization: Cancer Pain Relief and Palliative Care. Report of a World Health Organization Expert Committee. Technical Report Series 804. WHO, Geneva, 1990

63. Takeda F: Results of field testing in Japan of the WHO draft interim guidelines on relief of cancer pain. Pain Clin 1986;1:83–89

64. Ventafridda V, Tamburini M, Carceni A et al: A validation study of the WHO method for cancer pain relief. Cancer 1987;59:851–856

65. Walker VA, Hoskin PJ, Hanks GW, White ID: Evaluation of WHO analgesic guidelines for cancer pain in a hospital-based palliative care unit. J Pain Sympt Manage 1988;3:145–149

66. Portenoy RK, Hagen NA: Breakthrough pain: definition, prevalence and characteristics. Pain 1990;41:273–281

67. Portenoy RK: Adjuvant analgesics in pain management. In Doyle D, Hanks G, MacDonald N (eds): Oxford Textbook of Palliative Medicine. Oxford University Press, Oxford, 1993:187–203

68. Russell K, Portenoy MD, Steven D, Waldman MD: Adjuvant analgesics in pain management: 2. J Pain Sympt Manage 1994;9:390–391

69. McCaffery M: Nursing Management of the Patient With Pain. Lippincott-Raven, Philadelphia, 1972

70. Gorman DJ: Opioid analgesics in the management of pain in patients with cancer: an update. Palliat Med 1991;5:277–294

71. Report of an Expert Working Group of the European Association for Palliative Care: Morphine in cancer pain: modes of administration. BMJ 1996;312:823–826

72. Hanks GW: Controlled release morphine in advanced cancer: the European experience. Cancer 1989;63:2378–2382

73. Sawe J: High dose morphine and methadone in cancer patients. Clinical pharmacokinetics: considerations of oral treatment. Clin Pharmacokinet 1986;11:87–106

74. Portenoy RK, Foley KM, Stulman J et al: Plasma morphine and morphine-6-glucuronide during morphine therapy for cancer pain: plasma profiles, steady state concentrations and the consequences of renal failure. Pain 1991;47:13–19

75. Owen JA, Sitar DS, Barger L et al: Age related morphine kinetics. Clin Pharmacol Ther 1983;34:364–368

76. Baille SP, Bateman ON, Coates PE, Woodhouse KW: Age and the pharmacokinetics of morphine. Age Ageing 1989;18:258–262

77. Rees WD: Opioid needs of terminal care patients: variations with age and primary site. Clin Oncol 1990;2:79–83

78. Scottish Intercollegiate Guidelines Network. Control of Pain in Patients with Cancer. SIGN: Edinburgh, 2000 (SIGN publication no.44)

79. Hanks GW et al. Morphine and alternative opioids in cancer pain: the EPAC recommendations. Br J Cancer 2001;84(5):587–593.

80. Smith KJ, Miller AJ, McKellar J, Court M: Morphine at gramme doses: kinetics, dynamics and clinical need. Postgrad Med 1991;67:55–59

81. Diamorphine hydrochloride. In Dollery C (ed): Therapeutic Drugs, vol. 1. Churchill Livingstone, London, 1991

82. Reynolds J (ed): Martindale: The Extra Pharmacopoeia, 31st edn. Royal Pharmaceutical Society, London, 1996:63

83. The Pharmaceutical Codex, 12th edn. In Lus W (ed): Morphine. Pharmaceutical Press, London. 1994

84. Portenoy RK: Management of common opioid side effects during long-term therapy of cancer pain. Ann Acad Med Singapore 1994;23:160–170

85. White ID, Hoskin PJ, Hanks GW, Bliss JM: Morphine and dryness of the mouth. BMJ 1989;298:1222–1223

86. Inturrisi CE, Hanks G: Opioid analgesic therapy. In Doyle D, Hanks G, MacDonald N (eds): Oxford Textbook of Palliative Medicine. Oxford University Press, Oxford, 1993:166–181

87. Fallon M: Opioid rotation: does it have a role? Palliat Med 1997;11(3):177–178

88. Mercadante S: Opioid rotation for cancer pain: rationale and clinical aspects. Cancer 1999;86:1856–1866

89. Moriarty M, McDonald IJ, Miller AJ: Randomised crossover comparison of controlled release morphine tablets in patients with cancer pain. J Clin Res 1999;2:1–8

90. Bruera E, Belzile M, Pituskin E, Fainsinger R, Darke A, Harsanyi Z et al: Randomized, double-blind, cross-over trial comparing safety and efficacy

of oral controlled-release oxycodone with controlled-release morphine in patients with cancer pain. J Clin Oncol 1998;16:3222–3229

91. Kaiko R, Lacouture P, Hopf K, Brown J, Goldenheim P: Analgesic onset and potency of oral controlled-release (CR) and CR morphine. Clin Pharmacol Ther 1996;59:130

92. Plezia PM, Kramer TH, Linford J: Transdermal fentanyl: pharmacokinetics and preliminary clinical evaluation. Pharmacotherapy 1989;9:2–9

93. Mercadante S, Fulfaro F: Alternatives to oral opioids for cancer pain. Oncology (Huntington) 1999;13:215–220

94. Data on file Janssen Pharmaceutical, Rowbotham, N91173, 1992

95. Bentley JB, Borel JD, Gillespie TJ et al: Fentanyl pharmacokinetics in obese and non-obese patients. Anesthesiology 1981;55:A177

96. Krajnik M, Zylicz Z, Finlay I, Uczak J, van Sorge AA: Potential uses of topical opioids in palliative care – report of 6 cases. Pain 1999;80:121–125

97. Pannueti I, Rossi AP, Lafelice G: Control of chronic pain in very advanced cancer patients with morphine hydrochloride administered by oral, rectal and sublingual route. Clinical report and preliminary results on morphine pharmokinetics. Pharmacol Res Commun 1982;14:369–380

98. Raiko RF, Healy N, Pav J et al: The comparative bio-availability of M.S. Contin tablets following rectal and oral administration. In Twycross RG (ed): The Edinburgh Symposium on Pain Control and Medical Education. Royal Society of Medicine, London, 1989:235–241

99. Snodgrass SR: Myoclonus: analysis of monoamine, GABA and other systems. FASEB 1990;4:2775–2788

100. Schug SA, Zech D, Grond S et al: A long-term survey of morphine in cancer pain patients. J Pain Sympt Manage 1992;7:259–265

101. Woolf CJ, Thompson SWN: The induction and maintenance of central sensitization is dependent on N-methyl-D-aspartic acid receptor activation; implications for the treatment of post-injury pain hypersensitivity states. Pain 1991;44:293–299

102. Fallon MT, Welsh J: What is the role of ketamine in pain control? Eur J Palliat Care 1996;3:143–146

103. Mercadante S: Ketamine in cancer pain: an update. Palliat Med 1996;10(3):225–230

104. Mathisen LC, Skjelbred P, Skoglund LA, Oye I: Effect of ketamine, an NMDA receptor inhibitor, in acute and chronic orofacial pain. Pain 1995;61:215–220

105. Stannard CF, Porter GE: Ketamine hydrochloride in the treatment of phantom limb pain. Pain 1993;54:227–230

106. Sorensen J, Bengtsson A, Ahlner J, Henriksson KG, Ekselius L: Bengtsson fibromyalgia—are there different mechanisms in the processing of pain? A double blind crossover comparison of analgesic drugs. J Rheumatol 1997;24:1615–1621

107. Enarson MC, Hays H, Woodroffe MA: Clinical experience with oral ketamine. J Pain Sympt Manage 1999;17:384–386

108. Grant IS, Nimmo WS, Clements JA: Pharmacokinetics and analgesic effects of i.m. and oral ketamine. Br J Anaesth 1981;53:805–810

109. Takahashi H, Miyazaki M, Nanbu T, Yanagida H, Morita S: The NMDA-receptor antagonist ketamine abolishes neuropathic pain after epidural administration in a clinical case. Pain 1998;75:391–394

110. Vecht ChJ, Haaxma-Reiche H, van Putten WLJ et al: Initial bolus of conventional versus high dose dexamethasone in metastatic spinal cord compression. Neurology 1989;39:1255–1257

111. Curtis EB, Krech R, Walsh TD: Common symptoms in patients with advanced cancer. J Palliat Care 1991;7:25–29

112. Dunlop DM: A study of the relative frequency and importance of gastrointestinal symptoms and weakness in patients with far advanced cancer: student paper. Palliat Med 1989;4:37–43

113. Johnson I, Paterson S: Drugs used in combination in the syringe driver: a survey of hospice practice. Palliat Med 1992;6:125–130

114. Chan A, Woodruff K: Intestinal obstruction in patients with widespread intra-abdominal malignancy. J Pain Sympt Manage 1992;7:339–342

115. Baines MJ, Oliver DJ, Carter RL: Medical management of intestinal obstruction in patients with advanced malignant disease: a clinical and pathological study. Lancet 1985;2:990–993

116. Ripamonti C: Malignant bowel obstruction in advanced and terminal cancer patients. Eur J Palliat Care 1994;1:16–19

117. Twycross R: Symptom management in advanced cancer. Radcliffe Medical Press, Oxford, 1995:175

118. Krebs H, Goplerud DR: Surgical management of bowel obstruction in advanced ovarian cancer. Obstet Gynecol 1983;61:327–330

119. Ventafridda V, Ripamonti C, Catraceni A et al: The management of inoperable gastrointestinal obstruction in terminal cancer patients. Tumori 1990;76:389–393

120. Mercadante S: The role of octreotide in palliative care. J Pain Sympt Manage 1994;9:406–411

121. Fallon MT: Physiology of somatostatin and its synthetic analogue octreotide. Eur J Palliat Care 1994;1:20–22

122. Mercadante S, Spoldi E, Caraceni A et al: Octreotide in relieving gastrointestinal symptoms due to bowel obstruction. Palliat Med 1993;7:42–46

123. Riley J, Fallon MT: The use of octreotide in malignant intestinal obstruction. Eur J Palliat Care 1994;1:23–25

124. Riley J, Khoo D, Waxman J: Randomised and controlled trial of octreotide versus placebo in malignant gastrointestinal obstruction. (in press)

125. Mercadante S, Ripamonti C, Casuccio A, Zecca E, Groff L: Comparison of octreotide and hyoscine butylbromide in controlling gastrointestinal symptoms due to malignant inoperable bowel obstruction. Support Care Cancer 2000;8(3):188–191

126. Laval G, Girardier J, Lassaunière JM, Leduc J, Haond C, Schaerer R: The use of steroids in the management of inoperable intestinal obstruction in terminal cancer patients: do they remove the obstruction? Palliat Med 2000;14:3–10

127. Fainsinger RL, MacEachern T, Miller MJ et al: The use of hypodermoclysis for rehydration in terminally ill cancer patients. J Pain Sympt Manage 1994;9:298–302

128. Erick RE: Current concepts in anorexia and cachexia. Am J Hospice Care 1987;4:13–15

129. Bruera E: Clinical management of anorexia and cachexia in patients with advanced cancer. Oncology 1992;2:35–42

130. Downer S: Double blind placebo controlled trial of response to medroxyprogestron in cancer cachexia. Br J Cancer 1993;67:1102–1105

131. Tchekmedyian NS: High dose megesterol acetate—a possible treatment for cachexia. JAMA 1987;257:1195–1198

132. Schmall J: Megesterol acetate in cancer cachexia. Semin Oncol 1991;18:32–34

133. MacMillan DC, O'Gorman P, Fearon KC, McArdle CS: A pilot study of megestrol acetate and ibuprofen in the treatment of cachexia in gastrointestinal cancer patients. Br J Cancer 1997;79:788–790

134. Willox JC, Corr J, Shaw J et al: Prednisolone as an appetite stimulant in patients with advanced cancer. BMJ 1984;288:27

135. St Christopher's Hospice. Annual Statistics. St Christopher's Hospice, London, 1986

136. Fallon MT, Hanks GW: Morphine, constipation and performance status in advanced cancer patients. Palliat Med 1999;13:159–160

137. Wilson JA, Lawson PM, Smith RG: The treatment of terminally ill geriatric patients. Palliat Med 1987;1:149–153

138. Twycross R: Pain Relief in Advanced Cancer. Churchill Livingstone, Singapore, 1994:313

139. McNamara P, Minton M, Twycross RG: Use of midazolam in palliative care. Palliat Med 1991;5:244–249

140. Beaver WT, Wallenstein S, Houde RW, Rogers A: A comparison of the analgesic effects of methotrimeprazine and morphine in patients with cancer. Clin Pharmacol Ther 1966;7:436–446

141. Higginson I, Wade A, McCarthy M: Palliative care: views of patients and their families. BMJ 1990;301:277–281

142. Ruben DB, Mor V: Dyspnoea in terminally ill cancer patients. Chest 1986;89:234–236

143. Heyse-Moore LH, Ross V, Mullee MA: How much of a problem is dyspnoea in advanced cancer? Palliat Med 1991;5:20–26

144. Higginson I, McCarthy M: Measuring symptoms in terminal cancer: are pain and dyspnoea controlled? J R Soc Med 1989;82:264–267

145. Krech RL, Davis J, Dedan W, Curtis EB: Symptoms of lung cancer. Palliat Med 1992;6:309–315

146. Davis CL: The therapeutics of dyspnea. In Cancer Surveys, Vol. 21: Palliative Medicine: Problem Areas in Pain and Symptom Management. Cold Spring Harbor Laboratory Press, New York, 1994:85–98

147. Hughes J, Kosterlitz HW, Smith TW: The distribution of methionine-enkephalin and leucine–enkephalin in the brain and peripheral tissues. Br J Pharmacol 1977;61:639–647

148. Miedle A, Manigalt I, Wajda IJ: Distribution of opiate-like substances in rat tissues. Neurochem Res 1979;4:399–410

149. Hedner T, Cassuto J: Opioids and opioid receptors in peripheral tissues. Scand J Gastroenterol 1987;130(suppl):27–40

150. Frossard M, Barnes PJ: MU opioid receptors modulate non-cholinergic constrictor nerves in guinea-pig airways. Eur J Pharmacol 1987;141:519–522

151. Belvisi MG, Rogers DF, Barnes PJ: Neurogenic plasma extravasation: inhibition by morphine in guinea-pig airways in vivo. J Appl Physiol 1989;60:268–272

152. Hoskin PJ, Hanks GW: The management of symptoms in advanced cancer: experience in a hospital-based continuing care unit. J R Soc Med 1988;81:341–344

153. Ahmedzai S: Palliation of respiratory symptoms. In Doyle D, Hanks GW, MacDonald N (eds): Oxford Textbook of Palliative Medicine. Oxford University Press, Oxford, 1993:362–365

154. Gray JMB, Henry DA, Paice B et al: Acute respiratory failure and CNS-depressing drugs. Postgrad Med J 1981;57:279–282

155. Walsh TD: Opiates and respiratory function in advanced cancer. Recent Results. Cancer Res 1984;89:115–117

156. Davis CL: The pharmacokinetics of nebulised morphine. Abstract 995 presented at the 7th World Congress on Pain. IASP Publications, Seattle, 1993

157. Davis CL, Penn K, Daniels J, Slevin M: Single dose randomised wcontrolled trial of nebulised morphine in patients with cancer related breathlessness. Palliat Med 1996;10:64–65

158. Matineau L: Salbutamol, a β-adrenoceptor agonist, increases skeletal muscle strength in young men. Clin Sci 1992;83:615–621

159. Wilcock A, Corcoran R, Tattersfield AE: Safety and efficacy of nebulised lignocaine in patients with cancer and breathlessness. Palliat Med 1994;8:35–38

160. Bruera E, de Stoutz N, Velasco-Leiva A et al: Effects of oxygen on dyspnoea in hypoxaemic terminal cancer patients. Lancet 1993;342:13–14

Chapter 24

Ethical issues in geriatric medicine

John Harris

An individual's entitlement to the concern, respect, and protection of the community does not diminish with age. We might call this the first principle of gerontology and it is one that would surely command wide respect both as a general moral principle and as an appropriate one for geriatric medicine. Clearly this principle is itself the application of a more general principle. That more general principle is sometimes called "the equality principle," which states that *each person is entitled to the same concern, respect, and protection of society as is accorded to any other person in the community*. The equality principle has the advantage of being generally accepted and versions of it are enshrined in many national constitutions throughout the world (the USA and France, for example). The first principle of gerontology simply reminds us that the equality principle applies as much in the face of discrimination on the basis of chronological age or life expectancy as it does to discrimination on the basis of gender, race, and other arbitrary features.[1,2] Below we will explore the consequences of accepting such a principle for geriatric medicine and gerontology; this will help to show just how plausible a principle this is and also will allow us to review some of the most important ethical dilemmas that arise within gerontology. But why start with such a principle? Where do such principles come from?

Moral principles are not just plucked from the air, but neither are they derived from unassailable premises or immutable absolutes. They articulate central elements of a shared morality. Like the "Ten Commandments" they remind us of that morality and our commitment to it, and like the famous commandments they require interpretation. Does the proscription on killing include animals and plants? Are some commandments more important than others? Is the prohibition against coveting neighbors' oxen more or less important than that against coveting neighbors' wives?

However, moral principles also differ from commandments in important ways. Unlike commandments they do not attempt self-justification; they do not purport to explain *why* they ought to be accepted. So, when we articulate a moral principle we are reminding ourselves of what we believe to be an important part of the morality we accept. We should follow the principle *because* we accept the morality, but the principle cannot give us *reasons for* accepting the morality. When we encounter a principle we need first to reflect on our morality to see whether and how the principle fits with it. We then need to explore the consequences of accepting the principle to see whether we can adhere to it consistently with other moral beliefs we share and wish to retain. If the principle can be applied consistently with our general morality, well and good; if not, we have to choose whether to abandon the principle or abandon the elements of our morality that are not consistent with it.

ETHICS-BASED MEDICINE

Let us now attempt this process with our principle and see what working through this process tells us about ethics-based medicine.

The principle with which we began, that an individual's entitlement to the concern, respect, and protection of the community does not diminish with age, is clearly part of a bigger idea, an idea that deals with entitlements or rights and in particular with entitlements to concern, respect, and protection. This group of entitlements is often termed *respect for persons*, and we will need to analyze this idea into its constituent parts. But before doing so we must examine another assumption that has been made.

This assumption is that medical ethics, or "healthcare ethics" as it is now more usually termed, is part of ethics more generally and that what it is ethical to do to and for people within a healthcare system, or "clinically," is constrained by our general morality. The assumption being made, then, is that the delivery of healthcare, both individually and within a healthcare system, is a dimension of our more general obligations to one another—and, in particular, that it is entailed by those commitments we have to honor other people's entitlements to concern, respect, and protection. In short, the duties of healthcare professionals, insofar as they are ethical duties, are derived from general morality and are not part of a particular ethics of healthcare. The ethical *dilemmas* that arise within a health service may be different from those arising within a prison service, for example, but the principles that inform the *resolution* of those dilemmas are drawn from our general morality.

Resistance to this idea often comes from a confusion about the different sorts of normative systems that operate within any society. Our general morality is just one of the normative systems that operate within society, albeit the one to which all others are answerable. Other general normative systems include the rules governing good manners or etiquette, and, of course, the legal system. Then there are the rules of particular professions, occupations, corporations, or clubs that are often rather misleading, referred to as "codes of professional ethics" or "corporate ethics." All or any of these normative systems may enjoin or forbid things in the name of morality, and the operation of these normative systems may generate ethical dilemmas. But the breach or observance of the requirements of any of these systems is not of itself an ethical issue except insofar as it *also* involves our general morality. For example, although it is always wrong (incorrect) to break the law, it is not always morally wrong. The law requires us to drive on the left in the United Kingdom. There is nothing unethical about driving on the right except insofar as it is dangerous to do so where others are conforming to the law. If it is morally wrong to commit murder it is so not because law forbids it; rather the law forbids it because it is morally wrong.

Medical or healthcare ethics may then be construed as the ethical code of a particular profession or professions or of the healthcare system. So construed it has limited force and will appeal, at most, only to members of those professions, or perhaps, more pessimistically, to those who wish to continue to be members of those professions. As we shall construe it, however, it is the application of our general morality to the dilemmas of healthcare.[3–5] Thus construed, healthcare ethics applies as much to patients and their friends and relatives as it does to doctors and nurses, and it is as concerned with the general obligations of society to provide healthcare as it is with doctors' duties to deliver it.

RESPECT FOR PERSONS

Respect for persons, which is the basis of any ethics of care, and of which our first principle of gerontology is an expression, involves four crucial elements. They are: (1) concern for the welfare of others; (2) respect for their wishes; (3) respect for the intrinsic value of their lives; and (4) respect for their interests.

When I suggest that these four elements are crucial to any respectable conception of respect for persons, I mean simply that no one could claim to respect persons if their attitude to others failed to take account of these four elements. This, of course, does not take us very far because we need to know both how to *understand* each of these elements, and also, of course, how to *prioritize* them. Obviously people can have self-harming preferences, and where they do we need to decide whether it is more important to respect their wishes or demonstrate concern for their welfare.

However, these four dimensions of what it is to respect persons provide a useful framework for considering the ethics of geriatric medicine and gerontology because they remind us of the particular ethical dilemmas facing all those involved in patient care.

Achieving the right balance between concern for welfare and respect for wishes not only serves to remind us that welfare is not an end in itself but an instrumental good that, at a certain level, frees individuals to create their own lives, but also invites us to consider whether and to what extent individuals are in fact capable of authentic choices. Thinking about the intrinsic value of lives reminds us that many people think that the intrinsic value of lives differs between individuals and that this provides a basis for prioritization not only between individuals but between groups of individuals, young and old, for example. Finally, thinking about just what is involved in respecting people's interests reminds us that it is not always in someone's interests to remain alive or to have their life prolonged and that we may have a legitimate interest both in the manner and the timing of our own death.

The agenda we have set for ourselves can thus be seen to embrace some of the more traditional "headings" of medical ethics in the context of geriatric medicine: euthanasia, informed consent (especially in the mentally incompetent patient), equity

and rationing, and limiting treatment (do-not-resuscitate orders and withholding aggressive treatments). We can now work through this agenda and see where and to what extent the first principle of gerontology can be of use in resolving the dilemmas we will encounter.

EUTHANASIA

Euthanasia is in a sense the ultimate issue for any ethic of respect for persons, and advocacy of any form of euthanasia is sometimes thought to be inconsistent with such an ethic. I shall be concerned with two types of euthanasia:

- voluntary, where the individual wishes to die and has clearly expressed such a wish;
- nonvoluntary, where the individual is no longer competent, but it is believed euthanasia is in the individual's best interests or where it is believed the individual would have wished to die in these circumstances.

We will start by trying to clarify the ethics of voluntary euthanasia. Where respect for the intrinsic value of life, and indeed concern for another's welfare, seem to conflict with respect for that person's wishes, what should we do? We must consider these two possible conflicts separately.

Welfare versus wishes

To resolve the apparent conflict between concern for welfare and respect for wishes, we need to remind ourselves of the point of valuing liberty—freedom of choice. The point of autonomy, the point of choosing and having the freedom to choose between competing conceptions of how, and indeed why, to live is simply that it is only thus that our lives become in any real sense our own. The value of our lives is the value we give to our lives. And we do this, so far as this is possible at all, by shaping our lives for ourselves. Our own choices, decisions, and preferences help to make us what we are, for each helps us to confirm and modify our own character and enables us to develop and to understand ourselves. So autonomy, as the ability and the freedom to make the choices that shape our lives, is quite crucial in giving to each life its own special and peculiar value.

Concern for welfare, and the paternalist control it is so often used to justify, ceases to be legitimate at the point at which, so far from being productive of autonomy, so far from enabling the individual to create his or her own life, it operates to frustrate the individual's own attempts to create his or her own life. And of course this also applies in the limiting case of suicide or, of course, to voluntary euthanasia, where the individual's attempts to create his or her own life involve creating its ending also.

Welfare thus conceived has a point, as does concern for the welfare of others; it is not simply a good in itself. We need welfare, broadly conceived in terms of health, freedom from pain, mobility, shelter, nourishment, and so on, precisely because welfare is *liberating*. It is what we need to be able to pursue our lives to best advantage. So where concern for welfare and respect for wishes are incompatible one with another, concern for welfare must give way to respect for autonomy.

Does voluntary euthanasia conflict with an ethic of valuing life?

This question has been much illuminated by recent debates surrounding the issue of permanent vegetative state (PVS) and we will try to resolve it by considering the issues raised by PVS. This is the condition that was at issue in two crucial cases of highest jurisdiction in the USA and in the UK, those of Nancy Cruzan and Tony Bland. We will take the Bland case as our exemplar.[6,7] Both Nancy Cruzan and Tony Bland had been left in a PVS following accidents. This is an unconscious state that, after 6 months' to a year's duration, is accepted as permanent and irreversible. People in PVS do not require life support as this is usually understood, although they do require tube feeding and hydration. They are not, nor without assistance will they become, "dead" according to any of the current criteria or accepted definitions of death.

Tony Bland's parents asked the courts to rule that his death could be brought about by withdrawal of feeding and withholding of other life-sustaining measures including antibiotics. After withdrawal of feeding he was expected to succumb to infections from which he would die without antibiotics. In advance of the various hearings, it had been expected that the issue in court would turn on whether it was lawful to withdraw feeding and starve someone to death. There were legal precedents for decisions to withdraw life-sustaining *medical* treatment, but few considered feeding to be a "treatment" and hence something that doctors could withdraw on the basis of their judgments as to whether the measure at issue was in the patient's best interests or could be afforded by the healthcare system. To their credit the courts did not attempt to stretch the meaning of "medical treatment" to cover feeding, thus attempting to give the doctors clinical discretion in the matter, but squarely faced the issue of whether or not Tony Bland should continue alive.

The three judges of the Court of Appeal and the five judges in the House of Lords were unanimous in concluding, albeit for very different and sometimes inconsistent reasons, that it was lawful to withdraw feeding in order to end Tony Bland's life. Their decision was in effect one permitting nonvoluntary euthanasia. Because Tony Bland was not dead, and would not die unless the Law Lords permitted a definite course of action that would result in his death, their decision effectively brought his life to an end. And indeed, such a decision was sought by Tony Bland's parents for precisely that reason. Because the Law Lords knew that Bland's parents fully intended to halt tube feeding if they permitted it, they knew Tony Bland's life or death hung on their decision.

If we ask what justified the nonvoluntary euthanasia of Tony Bland, I believe none of the reasons given by the various judges is satisfactory. If it is believed that there is a sanctity that attaches to the lives of humans then, as a live human, Tony Bland does not relevantly differ from others whom it is wrong to kill. If, however, it is the lives of *persons* that are sacred in this sense and if the value of their lives is expressed in terms of the respect due to persons in virtue of their personhood, we get a different answer. For although a live human being, Tony Bland, at the time of the courts' deliberations, was no longer a person. Respect for persons no longer applied to him.

It is always helpful in ethics to try to present a clear and positive account, if only to provide those who disagree with all

they require for effective refutation. We should, however, note two obvious sorts of objection to the above account. The first would be, and was indeed, presented by the Law Lords who rejected the idea that end-of-life decisions such as those taken in the case of Tony Bland amount to euthanasia. The Lords held that even decisions such as theirs, which effectively brought about the death of an individual, did not in law amount to euthanasia.

Of course, opponents of euthanasia also differ from the position defended above, although they can, and often do, agree with accounts such as this in all its essentials. The point of difference between those who reject euthansia and those who defend it usually turns, as I have indicated, on whether or not the sanctity of existence applies to humans or rather to persons. If to the former, then euthansia must be rejected; if to the latter a different conclusion follows.[8] To be clearer about why this is so we must look more closely at the idea of personhood.

Personhood

We have so far avoided addressing specifically the question of just what it is that makes individuals persons, but we must now say something about this absolutely crucial idea. Personhood is that set of characteristics that distinguishes persons from other creatures, such as most animals and all plants, and that accounts for the special importance we attach to individuals. It is the sense of self, the characteristics that enable us to have a life in which we can take an interest and which enables us to have interests that we wish to see protected. When personhood has permanently disappeared, as in PVS, we are inclined to use language that suggests that the individual we once knew is no longer there although the living human body they once animated is still present. I do not have space here to do justice to the concept of personhood. I have tried to do so elsewhere.[3,4] However, I do not believe that any sense can be made, for example, of the various legal judgments in the Bland case without resort to such a concept. In the words of Lord Keith of Kinkel in his judgment in that case: "It is, however, perhaps permissible to say that to an individual with no cognitive capacity whatever, and no prospect of ever recovering any such capacity in this world, it must be a matter of complete indifference whether he lives or dies."[7] Lord Keith's, perhaps unconscious, use of the term "individual" rather than that of "person" in this part of his judgment makes the point I am trying to express, namely that not all human beings, not all individuals, are persons.

The idea of respect for persons

Respect for persons requires that it is persons who will be respected and hence their interests. Where, however, the person no longer exists, the interests of the former person, although still worthy of our respect, must of necessity give way to the significant interests or preferences of actual people. Thus John's interest, if he can be said to have one, in a further 30 years of life in a PVS would give way to the significant interests or preferences of any actual persons, persons to whom the satisfaction, or not, of their desires can continue to matter. And this would surely accord with our intuitions here. We would not, I imagine, think that someone who could no longer benefit from, or appreciate the life he was leading, should have that life sustained, when to do so would cost the lives of others who could appreciate, and benefit from, their continued existence.[3]

If euthanasia is to be permitted, this will not be because everyone should accept that it is right, nor because to fail to do so violates a defensible conception of the sanctity of life, but simply because to deny a person control of what, on any analysis, must be one of the most important decisions of life, is a form of tyranny, which like all acts of tyranny is an ultimate denial of respect for persons.[9]

We have looked at some of the arguments that would sustain approval of voluntary euthanasia and euthanasia where an individual has permanently ceased to be a person, as in the case of PVS. The most problematic cases of euthanasia, however, are those where consent is itself problematic, and before drawing any conclusions about these we must look at the issue of consent more generally.

CONSENT

The centrality of consent in healthcare ethics is a function of the importance accorded to autonomy; and autonomy itself, as I have suggested, is part of our concept of the person. It is because we accept that the meaning and purpose of an individual's life are largely acts of self-creation that we are concerned to protect those attempts at self-creation even where we are convinced that they are misguided or even self-harming. However, although the importance of consent derives from our concept of the person, its procedural primacy in healthcare is owed to the common law tradition that protects individuals from assaults, that is, from unlawful touchings. It is consent that makes laying your hands on someone else lawful—hence the importance of obtaining valid consents to all medical procedures that involve interventions that compromise the bodily integrity of patients.

Just as forcing someone to go on living when they find life intolerable is a terrible form of tyranny and constitutes a denial of the ethic of respect for persons, so also does treating someone who has not consented and who is capable of choosing whether or not he or she wants treatment. This principle is a cornerstone of medical ethics and is endorsed by the law in most jurisdictions. Both ethics and prudence therefore combine to support it. However, there are many cases where consent is problematic or cannot be obtained prior to treatment, and these raise not only special problems of justification, but also special problems of explaining why interventions are justified.

Problematic consent

Because there are so many cases in healthcare practice that necessitate touching patients in circumstances where their consent cannot be obtained and where knowledge of their wishes is absent, the law has contrived various fictional consents to protect well-intentioned practitioners from the guilt of unlawful conduct. The moral necessity of obtaining a valid consent where this can be obtained does not require further discussion. To violate the bodily integrity of persons who reject such violation is a form of tyranny and should be accepted and treated as such. We must, however, look more closely at those cases where consent or its refusal is problematic, and at the fictionalized consents that are often manufactured in these circumstances.

There are a number of instances in healthcare where the patient's consent is appealed to and used, where his or her actual consent is unobtainable. These are circumstances in which the patient is either unconscious or unable to process the information required to give a valid consent, or is temporarily or permanently lacking the relevant capacity to consent. In such cases terms like "proxy consent," "substituted judgment," "presumed consent," or even "retrospective consent" are used to justify treating a patient. However, not only are these all fictions, but they totally fail to be justifications for treating the patient in particular ways.

Here I shall be advancing a thesis that runs counter to much contemporary thinking on consent that seems at home with attributing consent to individuals who are totally unaware that they are supposed to be consenting or are unaware at the time the consent is operative (as in the case of retrospective consent).

The reason why it is right to do what presumed consent or substituted judgment seems to suggest in these cases, is simply because treating the patient in the proposed ways is in his or her best interests and to fail to treat would be deliberately to harm the person. It is the principle that we should do no harm that justifies treating the patient in particular ways. The justification for treatment is not that the patient consented, nor that he or she would have, nor that it is safe to presume that the person would have, nor that the person will when he or she regains consciousness or competence, but simply that it is the right thing to do, and it is right precisely *because* it is in the patient's best interests. That it is the "best interests" test that is operative is shown by the fact that we do not presume consent to things that are not in the patient's best interests, even where it is clear that he or she would have consented. We do not, except where we believe it to be in the patients' best interests, amputate healthy limbs of patients suffering body dysmorphic disorder, and patients are often denied access to alcoholic beverages or cigarettes, even when they specifically request them.

Of course, we do not give beneficial treatment to patients who have refused them, say by advanced directive, because to do so would constitute an assault and a violation of their will. But it is not a violation of someone's will, nor is it an assault, to give a treatment they have not refused, the withholding of which would constitute an injury. And the reason it is not a violation is not because they have consented in some notional or fictional sense, but because it is the right thing to do. And the reason it is the right thing to do is that to fail or omit to do it would injure the patient. It is the infliction of that injury, by act or omission,[10,11] that would constitute the violation or assault. In short, if someone has not indicated clearly that it would be a violation of his or her will to refrain from causing injury, then we should not injure that person.

It is widely held that not only should we not harm people who do not want to be harmed, we also should not harm even those who do want to be harmed, and that this is sufficient reason not to withhold treatment the absence of which would harm. This raises the question of the right to harm oneself. What of the responsibilities of the shopkeeper who sells cigarettes? Two points need to be made here. The first is that the shopkeeper, as we have here suggested, has sufficient moral reason not to sell cigarettes and would not be wrong to refuse to do so regardless of the preferences of his customers. Second, the delivery of healthcare is not straightforwardly like the marketplace, and health professionals have often refused to give "treatments," for example, those they regard as mutilating, regardless of the expressed preferences of patients for such treatments.

Not only do we not need the concept of implied or assumed or proxy consent, because it literally does not work; we do not need it because it misleads us as to the character and meaning of our actions. The nineteenth century philosopher Jeremy Benthan was rightly scathing of fictional consents, and he remarked:[12]

> "In English law, fiction is a syphilis, which runs in every vein, and carries into every part of the system the principle of rottenness. Fiction of use to justice? Exactly as swindling is to trade. It affords presumptive and conclusive evidence of moral turpitude in those by whom it was invented and first employed."

So where, in medical contexts, we act in the best interests of patients who cannot consent, we do so, I suggest, because we rightly believe we should not harm those in our care and not because some irrelevant person or the law has constructed a consent. This does not help with the vexed problem of who is and who is not competent to consent, but it does explain the justification for intervening in the lives of those we are satisfied are not able to give the consents that would otherwise be required.

If the treatment of those whose consent is impaired is problematic, and decisions to discharge them from care equally so, what of research?

Research on cognitively impaired elderly subjects

There is nothing special about research on cognitively impaired elderly subjects. Cognitive impairment is only significant in this context insofar as it also involves impairment of autonomy and the elderly are not importantly different from other age groups from the point of view of consent.[13]

First we should note the difficulty of distinguishing between research and therapy. Many definitions have been provided and most rely at some point on making the distinction by reference to the intentions of those carrying out the work.[14–16] However, any distinctions based on intent are at best suspect and at worst susceptible to manipulation. The intentions of people are usually mixed and confused. Medical staff may, and doubtless often do, simultaneously intend to do many things when they treat their patients. They may intend to care for patients, offer relief of symptoms, identify and eradicate causes of disease, hone their medical skills, further their careers, satisfy their curiosity, generate research data, carry out instructions, and so on. Identifying *primary* intent is hardly more helpful because it either relies on a degree of self-awareness that few can achieve, or it simply stipulates one of many possible or actual intentions as paramount for the purposes of bringing the activity into an appropriate or permitted category.

This does not mean that there is no distinction to be drawn between research and therapy, but rather that the distinction cannot be drawn sufficiently clearly to sustain claims that therapy is justified whereas research is not. This is perhaps less worrying than might at first appear. The work supposedly done by the distinction between research and therapy might as easily be accomplished by concentrating on the degree of advantage to the patient. We could say that interventions, whether motivated by research or therapeutic imperatives, are permissible if either the patient accepts and consents to the interventions, or, where consent is unobtainable, that the interventions are the best available treatment for the patient, whether or not they also constitute research.

However, it is worth pursuing the distinction between therapeutic and nontherapeutic research a bit further, because, insofar as it is coherent, it relies on a suspiciously narrow view about the definition of "therapeutic" and also about what is, in fact, in every patient's best interests.

The following two claims are often made in this context:

1. The patient's interests are paramount.
2. Research on patients who cannot consent for themselves must be either (i) therapeutic *or* (ii) in the patient's own interests *or* of potential benefit for the patient herself, *or* (iii) if not directly for the benefit of the particular patient in question, at least for the benefit of the category of patients to which the subject belongs, so that for example, if the patient has Alzheimer's disease, then research will be justified only if the research will be of benefit if not to the patient, at least to other patients with Alzheimer's disease.

Neither claim seems sustainable, and since the claims are often repeated, it is worth taking a moment to see why this is so.

The patient's interests cannot be paramount for the simple and sufficient reason that being or becoming a patient is not the sort of thing that could conceivably increase either your rights or your moral claims. All people are morally important and with respect to one another each has a claim to equal consideration. No one has a claim to overriding consideration. To say that the patient's interests are paramount, if it means anything, must be seen as a way of reasserting that health professionals are concerned primarily for the patients in their care and may have special contractual duties to them. However, as a general remark about the obligations of the healthcare system, or of society, it is not sustainable.

The second claim is equally problematic. To assert that research must be therapeutic or in the patient's own interests is not plausible when interpreted as confining research to work that will benefit particular patients directly, in the sense that they will themselves, so to speak, "feel the benefit" or that it will serve their continuing interests.

Let us first look at the idea of what is or is not in someone's interests. We must be wary of being too conservative about what does or does not benefit someone or of defining someone's interests too narrowly. We all benefit from living in a society in which medical research is carried out and which utilizes the benefits of past research. It is both of benefit to patients and it is in their interests to be patients in a society that pursues and actively accepts the benefits of research and where research and its fruits are given a high priority. We all have benefited and continue to benefit from research that was not targeted on us, indeed most of us will have benefited from research undertaken before we were born. We all also benefit from the knowledge that research is ongoing, into diseases or conditions from which we do not currently suffer but to which we may succumb. It makes us feel more secure and gives us hope for the future, for ourselves and our descendants, and others for whom we care. If this is right, then I have a strong general interest that there be research, and in all well-founded research; not excluding but not exclusively, research on me and on my condition. All such research is also of clear benefit to me. A narrow interpretation of the requirement that research be of benefit to the subject of the research is, I believe, perverse.

The third suggestion, that research that is not directly beneficial to the patient be confined to research that will benefit the category of patients to which the subject belongs is also untenable. What arguments sustain the idea that the most appropriate reference group is that of fellow sufferers from a particular disease, Alzheimer's, for example? Surely any moral obligation I have to accept risk or harm for the benefit of others is not plausibly confined to others who are narrowly like me. This is surely close to claiming that research should be confined to others who are "black like me" or "English like me" or "God-fearing like me." The most appropriate category is surely "a person like me."

Justice

Where I benefit from research but refuse to participate in it I am clearly acting unfairly in some sense. I am free-riding on the back of the contribution of others. Although we may conclude that people are ultimately entitled to act unfairly in this way if they choose, that they should not normally be compelled to contribute or participate, there is no reason to presume that those who cannot consent would have wished to be free-riders. Indeed, as I have argued, there is no justification for any presumptions about their willingness to consent, in the absence of clear indications about their preferences. What is clear, I believe, is that there is no basis for any presumption that those who cannot consent should be excluded from research, whether that research be targeted on their condition or not. Nor, of course, is there any basis for the presumption that those who cannot consent should be, so to speak, "professional research subjects." They should neither be automatically included in research perhaps because they happen to be readily available in institutions or under continuing care, nor should they be automatically excluded.

We have been talking very generally and assuming a favorable risk/benefit balance for the research subjects—namely that the risks and pain, discomfort, or inconvenience of the research are minimal, and the projected benefits clear. There is clearly a tradeoff between risks and benefits and a fairly steep upward curve where we demand that the benefits be clear and urgent before we will accept significant risks or pain inconvenience and so on for ourselves. We should surely apply the same standards to those who cannot consent. I cannot say anything useful or original about this balance. Clearly I will only accept significant risk of death for myself if without accepting such risk there is an almost certainly and substantially worse

outcome for myself or those I care about. However, even here the risks are not plausibly undertaken only to benefit oneself. Live kidney donors, for example, clearly accept significant risks for others and we usually applaud their decision to do so.

We should note also that while generally we judge the decision whether or not to participate in research, as one for individuals to make for themselves, whether or not we reserve the right to criticize their decision, we do not accept that there is no obligation to take risks in the public interest nor that compulsion is always ruled out in such cases. There clearly is an obligation (sometimes) to make sacrifices for the community or an entitlement of the community to deny autonomy in the public interest, and this obligation is recognized in a number of ways. For example: control of dangerous drugs, control of road traffic, vaccination, quarantine for communicable disease, compulsory military service, detention under mental health acts, restriction on sexual and professional activities with the human immunodeficiency virus.

An example that seems to illustrate, and to an extent explain, our attitude to the imposition of risk in the public interest involves the following story. Imagine an ocean liner on a cruise. The captain receives a radio message that there is another ship in distress some miles to the north. There are 200 people aboard this other ship and his liner has 1000 aboard. His is the only ship that can effect the rescue before the stricken ship will founder. He knows that if he diverts into the storm he will impose some risk on his passengers and crew. There will be a small but significant risk of death for all. The storm is a bad one but the modern liner should be able to cope. There is a greater, but still small, risk of death for a few of his passengers and crew in the rough and tumble of the rescue. Finally, because the storm is severe, he will almost certainly be subjecting his many elderly passengers to risk of minor injuries in the rough seas and certainly to discomfort, fear, and inconvenience. Significantly, we don't have to ask what he should do. The captain knows he must attempt the rescue and subject his passengers and crew to the attendant risks and few would disagree. He also knows that he can and must do so without asking for the consent of his passengers and crew, for they would be wrong to withhold their consent and the captain would be wrong to act on it.

The list of areas in which, I believe, similar decisions are made in our society shows that the principles involved are not unfamiliar or indeed unacceptable. Why then should we assume, when considering the ethics of research involving say, cognitively impaired elderly subjects, that different principles should apply?

First, let us just remind ourselves what these principles are, and then go on to see if they are constrained in any way by the situation of patients whose consent is problematic. The principles involved are all dimensions of the principle of equality from which our first principle of gerontology was derived. That principle is, it will be remembered, *that each person is entitled to the same concern, respect, and protection of society as is accorded to any other person in the community.* This principle reminds us that the passengers on the stricken liner have as good a claim to our protection as any other persons (although they may not be fellow citizens); and that although we are not obliged to afford that protection at all costs, we are obliged to act morally when the costs of so doing are reasonable given the importance of what is at stake. I hope it is obvious that if acting morally were only obligatory when doing so was cost free to the agent, morality would not exist. It is not plausible to believe that the costs of acting morally fall only on those competent to consent. So long as we ensure that such costs do not fall *more heavily* on those not competent to consent than on others, I can see no sound argument for exempting them from the demands of morality. They may not be *accountable* in law, if they do wrong, but there is no reason to ensure that they do wrong, by exempting them from their moral obligations. The fact that the moral obligations in question are not mandatory, in that competent individuals may not, usually, be coerced into fulfilling them, does not seem to be a reason for exempting those not competent to consent. We do not allow children (or we should not) to do wrong because some adults may freely do so. However, we constrain children not only because we are, in part, morally responsible for their actions, but also because this is part of an education process. The right parallel with adults who lack competence might be to include them in research when, although not competent to consent or refuse, they make no overt objection to inclusion or complaint about it. Where they do object or complain, we should perhaps respect that, albeit incompetent, rejection of this particular moral obligation.

Doubtless this defense of the idea that there can be an obligation to participate in research in certain circumstances, whether those who participate are capable of consenting or not, will strike some as controversial. The prohibition of research on those incapable of consent except where the research is in their own therapeutic interest is a principle founded on the highest of motives, that of the need to protect the vulnerable. However, the same motive animates the position defended here. It is not only the incompetent who are vulnerable in the requisite sense. We are all vulnerable unless research is pursued. The issue is one of balance. If research can be pursued without recourse to those whose consent is dubious, then so much the better. This should be our first choice. However, if such a prohibition jeopardizes our capacity to pursue well-founded research then perhaps we should remember that free-riding is not an attractive principle, nor is it a moral principle. We should not, as I have indicated, assume that those incompetent to consent would wish to be free-riders, nor that they be excluded from discharging an obligation of good citizenship that we all share.

We must now turn to the vexed question of the application of constraints on resources to the treatment of older people.

EQUITY AND RESOURCES

In discussing the problem of what an equitable distribution of resources for gerontology and geriatric medicine would look like I want to try to do two modest things. The first is to outline what I believe a principled approach to care of the elderly would look like, and the second is to say why at least one, and by implication most, of the alternatives are far from equitable. We must begin by returning to the equality principle, which we identified as the "parent" of the first principle of gerontology.[17]

The equality principle revisited

I shall again assume that it is accepted that no allocation of public resources should discriminate unfairly between rival claimants or groups of claimants and that this happens when each person's claim to the equal concern, respect, and protection of the community, of the society in which they live, is not respected.

The principle of equality involves the idea that people's lives and fundamental interests are of equal importance and that they must in consequence be given equal weight and be equally protected. This principle has powerful intellectual appeal and intuitive force. It is often enough to discredit a proposal or a theory simply to show that it violates this principle. When measures are said to be discriminatory or unfair it is this principle that is in play.

If people's lives and fundamental interests are of equal value, then it is unjust to treat people differently in ways that effectively accord different values to their lives or fundamental interests. Deliberately to give one person a better chance of remaining healthy and of having as long a life as possible than another is to value their life and their fundamental interest in health more than the person not so benefited. It is to discriminate in their favor. Where literally all cannot be benefited, equality requires that the method of selecting who will benefit and who will not is fair. This is why scarce resources that bear upon the value of life or the fundamental interests of persons must be allocated justly.

No dogs in mangers

One method of allocation of a scarce resource that apparently satisfies the requirements of justice is not to allocate that resource to anyone! All are then treated equally, in the sense that they are all left equally without benefit of the resource in question.

Another superficially distinct but in fact morally similar procedure might be to go on redistributing resources until a distribution was achieved that satisfies the "envy test"—that is, one in which no one envies anyone else's life chances as provided by those resources.

This is often thought to be a viable application of the requirements of justice and indeed to constitute a just allocation of resources. The fallacy of such a supposition is easily illustrated. The principle of justice, and indeed the principle of equality, are *moral* principles; that is, they are principles with some moral content, principles that are designed to be more than impartial, that are designed among other things to respect and to do justice to persons. In some sense this must involve some benevolent attitude to persons that is often abbreviated as "respect for person." Such an attitude to others is as different as it is possible to be from simply showing *an equality of lack of respect or an equal indifference to the fate of others.*

The failure to allocate resources that would save lives or protect individuals could not then be part of a claim to satisfy the requirements of equality because this principle has at its heart the claim that people's lives and fundamental interests *are of value, that they matter.* Anyone who denied life-saving resources, or resources that would protect life and other fundamental interests, is not valuing the lives of those to whom he or she denies these protections. Although the person is treating them all equally in the sense of treating them all *the same*, he or she is not treating them *as equals*, as people who matter and hence matter equally.[18] The alternative dog-in-the-manger approach treats all people as *equally unimportant* and hence as equally without value.

It is an integral part of the equality principle that people's moral claims are not diminished by who they are, or how old they are, or by how rich or poor, or powerful or weak they are or by the quality of their lives. The equality principle covers young and old, healthy and sick, weak and strong, regardless of race, creed, color and gender, quality of life, or life expectancy.

The anti-agist argument

Implicit in this discussion has been an argument against agism in the distribution of resources for healthcare. This argument can be stated thus:[3]

> "*All of us who wish to go on living have something that each of us values equally although for each it is different in character, for some a much richer prize than for others, and none of us know its true extent. This thing is of course 'the rest of our lives.' So long as we do not know the date of our deaths then for each of us the 'rest of our lives' is of indefinite duration. Whether we are 17 or 70, in perfect health or suffering from a terminal disease we each have the rest of our lives to lead. So long as we each wish to live out the rest of our lives, however long that turns out to be, then if we do not deserve to die, we each suffer the same injustice if our wishes are deliberately frustrated and we are "cut off prematurely."*

An important element of anti-agism expressed in this way is that it links opposition to discrimination on the basis of chronological age to discrimination on the basis of life expectancy. These are not necessarily linked. Some people have defended what might be termed a "fair-innings argument."[3,19] This suggests that people are entitled to every opportunity to live a fair lifespan—perhaps the traditional three score years and ten. Up to that point they have equal entitlement to health-care, but beyond the fair innings they are given very low priority. This argument is tempting because it explains the strong intuition people have that there is something wrong with treating the claims of an octogenarian and those of a 20-year-old as equal. However, the fair-innings argument has a number of defects. It assumes that the value of a life is to be measured in units of lifetime, the more the better up to a certain point but thereafter extreme discounting begins. The problem is that people value particular events within their life disproportionately to the time required to experience those events. Although the fair-innings argument gives great impor-tance to a life having shape and structure, these things are again not necessarily achieved only within a particular time span. On the fair-innings argument, Nelson Mandela's entitlement to life-saving care from the community was over before he left Victor Verster prison; the long road to freedom would have ended before (personal) freedom was achieved. And it is not only for such as Mandela that the most important part of their life might well begin after a so-called fair innings had been achieved.

Without the vast detail of each person's life, and the person's hopes and aspirations within that detail, we cannot hope to do justice between lives. I believe the only sensible alternative is to count each life for one and none for more than

one, whatever the differences in age and in other quality considerations.

It is this outlook that explains why murder is always wrong and wrong to the same degree. When you rob someone of life you take from them not only all they have but all they will ever have; it is a difference in degree so radical that it makes for a difference in the quality of the act. However, the wrongness consists in taking from them something that they want. That is why, as has been suggested, voluntary euthanasia is not wrong and murder is.

Those who believe in discriminating in favor of the young or against the old must believe that, insofar as murder is an injustice, it is less of an injustice to murder the old than the young; and because they also believe that life years are a commodity like any other,[20] it is clear that in robbing people of life you take less from them the less life expectancy they have.

Fairness and quality of life

The same ideas that underpin discrimination against the old on the grounds of fairness would also entail trying to equalize quality as well as quantity of life. The argument here would be that resources required for survival should be distributed not only so as to favor the young but also so as to favor those whose quality of life has been relatively poor. Consider this:[20]

> "*Two patients...both about 40 years old...need a liver transplant but only one suitable liver is available. One of the patients [the first] has had a much worse life than the other. In this case it seems most fair to give the liver to the first person. This supports the life time view.*"

Again, such a view has some appeal but it has two major problems, one practical and the other theoretical.

The practical problem is that we could never make decisions as to how to allocate life-saving or indeed other scarce resources between people until we had their whole (and very complete and detailed) life history. Without it all sorts of injustices would be compounded. This problem is related to that we noted attendant upon the fair-innings approach. Better again to treat each person as counting for one and none for more than one than even to embark on the massively invasive (of privacy) data collection that it would be necessary to hold and have instantly available on each and every citizen and that could never be complete, accurate, or proof against abuse. This incidentally is also the reason why it is wrong to discriminate against smokers, for example in the provision of coronary artery bypass grafts.

The theoretical problem is that if it is right to attempt to even out quality of life as between people then we should do so as a matter of public policy throughout society, not simply in the rare cases where resource allocation decisions in health-care arise. This might have to include making sure that no one lived longer than the person who has the shortest lifespan and no one was happier than the most miserable. This might be dysfunctional in terms of species survival unless a different principle can support leveling up rather than leveling down.

Ultimately we will be comparing different moral priorities. However, there is much to be said for taking individual persons and their wishes and fundamental interests as what matters from the point of view of morality. This means that we must recognize that, although their lives will all differ in length, happiness, and success—in short, in the degree to which their fundamental interests are satisfied—people matter morally despite these differences not because of them.

I have defended an argument that shows why we should decline to discriminate against the old. Many think that this is precisely what we *should* do.[20–22] Their arguments either support a fair innings or suggest that an evidence-based medicine requires the maximization of life years to be gained from treatment. If health gain is defined in terms of life years gained, then the old will very often lose out. There is no doubt that it is highly attractive to healthcare providers to measure health gain in terms of life years per treatment and that this accords with our intuitions or our commonsense morality on some occasions. It seems fairer to rescue the 30-year-old rather than the 90-year-old, other things being equal. However, it seems less obvious that we ought always to prefer the 30-year-old to the 32-year-old. If we generalize the ethic of preferring to maximize life years gained from treatment or care, then geriatric medicine will always be a low priority and palliative care will not rank at all! The two approaches we have examined not only reflect different interpretation of an ethics of healthcare delivery but also of different conceptions of morality. I have here defended one such conception, the defense of the alternative must be left to others.[20–22]

DECISIONS TO LIMIT TREATMENT

We are now in a position to turn to our final topic, which concerns decisions to limit treatment. When may these legitimately be taken and by whom? Here again it is useful to remind ourselves of the first principle of gerontology and of the purpose of this branch of medicine. If the healthcare system is rightly seen as a dimension of the community's commitment to the protection of the individual, then so long as the delivery of that care does in fact protect, and no more important values are compromised by the delivery of that protection, then clearly it should continue.

A classic case

One dilemma in geriatric medicine always seems to be a priority for practitioners. It concerns the dilemmas surrounding the decision to discharge home a frail patient where it is feared that this may involve some risk to the person's health or life, and it is unclear how aware of this risk the patient may be, and perhaps where caregivers who may be family members or even neighbors are worried by this risk. Among the questions that arise are the following: How much risk can or should we allow a person to take with his or her own health? Is it reasonable to think the level of risk varies with the level of competence? What consideration should be given to the wishes of caregivers in view of their very real concerns?

The difficulty of these dilemmas arises not so much from any problems about answering questions such as these, but rather from the difficulty of knowing enough about the terms used in the questions. It is clear from the present discussion of issues such as "euthanasia" and "informed consent" that people are permitted to take risks, within the law, with their own health. The wishes of caregivers are important, but such wishes

cannot be permitted to imprison a competent individual within a context from which he or she has elected to be removed. The problem of this classic case is simply that it is often unclear just how competent the patient is to make a decision to leave a protected environment, and equally unclear just how competently he or she will be able to function at home. However, what ethics can contribute here is perhaps the reflection that we are talking of the liberty of the individual. That liberty should not be constrained lightly, and the presumption must be that the individual is competent to make decisions unless there is clear evidence to the contrary.

We have seen that to attempt to treat a competent patient against his or her own wishes is not only unethical but also, in most jurisdictions, a criminal act. Where the patient is not competent and the treatment is in the patient's interests, then again as we have seen, the ethics are simple: we should not injure the patient by withholding beneficial treatment.

Advance directives or "living wills"

Much discussion has arisen about the ethics of advance directives. However they are, I believe, both straightforward and unproblematic. All decisions we take bind us to a certain extent for the future. If I now consent to the administration of an anesthetic, I cannot revoke that consent until I wake up. If I decide to bind myself in the event of my losing competence in the future the principle is the same. So long as my instructions are clear, then any treatment of me contrary to those instructions is unethical and probably unlawful.

We should note two features of advance directives. The first is that I can direct people only to forbear; I have no power to command others to do things to me. Although this must be so it does not follow that health professionals or others can disregard my positive wishes. If health professionals would normally act on a patient request for treatment, the fact that the request is expressed in advance should make no difference to the willingness to act. Second, the directive, while it may be written or oral, must be clear and unequivocally the patient's own authentic request. Health professionals should be wary of hearsay. To give a concrete example, if an unconscious patient is admitted needing treatment and the person accompanying him, ostensibly his wife, says "he wouldn't have wanted that" or "he always said never to let that happen to him," this of itself is not adequate evidence of the existence of an advance directive. The accompanying person may not be related to the patient; nor, if she is, may she be a reliable guide either to his wishes or his best interests. Relatives often have vested interests, inheritance prospects for example. Certainly nothing that might harm the patient should be done on the basis of uncorroborated claims about the patient's wishes from unauthenticated sources.

Do-not-resuscitate

When might it be legitimate to decide in advance not to resuscitate a patient? What does such an instruction mean? It means that a relatively simple and inexpensive procedure, albeit one that may be painful and undignified for the patient, that offers a chance of reversing an immediately life-threatening event, will not be attempted. It is an instruction to take the earliest opportunity to ensure that a particular life comes to an end. Such an instruction could be ethical only in two sets of circumstances. The first is where the patient has expressly directed that no such treatment be given. The second is where the patient's life has deteriorated to such an extent that continued life as a person is no longer possible. This latter was in essence the nature of the decision taken by the House of Lords in the case of Tony Bland which we examined above.[7]

Certainly, wherever a patient can be consulted about whether or not he or she wants to go on living then this should be done, and a DNR decision should be taken only if the patient understands the effects of such a decision and explicitly rejects resuscitation. A DNR decision is not a matter of clinical judgment, because the question of whether a life is worth living, or whether or not it is better that it should end, is not a clinical question; these are moral and mortal questions. Moreover they are questions the answer to which is a matter of life or death to the patient; and wherever patients have a life as a person in which they continue to be interested, then any decision to end that life (when it could continue) that is not requested by the patient is a gross and emphatic violation.[10,23,24]

Against the position I have just articulated it might be claimed that decisions not to resuscitate have traditionally been regarded as clinical matters, and for good reason. Only a clinician is in a position to know when resuscitation will be futile and when the individual concerned is too frail to benefit from attempts at resuscitation. However, both these objections involve a misunderstanding or at least an equivocation over the meaning of the word "futile." If a procedure is genuinely futile, in that nothing that the patient wants or could possibly want can thereby be achieved, then this is a sufficient reason for not attempting it. Or, if the patient is so frail that attempts at resuscitation are simply not possible, then again this is a sufficient reason for not attempting them, and judgments of clinicians in either case are not in dispute. The crucial idea here is that of the patient having a life *in which he continues to be interested* and which *could continue*. What must be capable of continuance is the sort of life the patient wants to continue to lead (if such a life is the only alternative) and that might possibly be restored by resuscitation. If resuscitation could not restore such a life then it will indeed be futile. The decision as to whether resuscitation could restore such a life *is* a clinical decision. However, the decision as to whether or not a life is worth living to a particular individual is not a clinical matter. It is and *could only be* a matter for the individual.

Immortality?

We are all "designed" to age and die, but is this simply a design fault?[3,25] If our bodies could repair damage due to disease and aging "from within," we would certainly live much longer and healthier lives. New research is being reported which would not only constitute major contributions to the treatment of disease but which could in principle lead to the indefinite extension of life, to the extent perhaps that we would begin to think of people who had received such life-extending treatment as immortals.

We should note that immortality is not the same as invulnerability, and even these "immortals" could die or be killed. Increased longevity and its logical extension, some would say its *reductio ad absurdum*, immortality, have a long history. Certainly the human imagination is familiar with the idea of immortals and mortals living alongside one another, interacting and interbreeding. *The Iliad*, *The Odyssey*, *The Ramayama*, and Shakespeare have all made such ideas familiar. What imaginative sources have largely ignored are the ethical and political consequences of such possibilities.

A vital ethical and social question is how we should view the prospect of the indefinite extension of individual lives, and whether we can legitimately do anything to stop it.

If life extension proves possible, we will face the prospect of parallel populations, of "mortals" and of "immortals" existing alongside one another. This of course is precisely the destiny for which the poetic imagination has prepared us, literally from "time immemorial." While such parallel populations seem inherently undesirable, it is not clear that we could, or even that we should, do anything about preventing such a prospect for reasons of justice or morality. For if immortality or increased life expectancy is a good, it is doubtful ethics to deny palpable goods to some people because we cannot provide them for all. We don't refuse kidney transplants to some patients unless and until we can provide them for all with renal failure. We don't usually regard ourselves as wicked in Europe because we perform many such transplants while low-income countries perform few or none at all.

Whatever we feel about the prospect of enabling some to live longer, perhaps indefinitely longer, it is not clear what ethically could be done to prevent such developments. Remember that immortality is not unconnected with preventing or curing a whole range of serious diseases. It is one thing to ask the question "Should we make people immortal?" and answer in the negative; quite another to ask whether we should make people immune to heart disease, cancer, dementia, and many other diseases and decide that we shouldn't.

> ### KEY POINTS   Ethics
>
> - Chronological age does not diminish entitlement to healthcare.
>
> - Life expectancy does not diminish entitlement to healthcare.
>
> - All persons have an equal claim to the care of the healthcare system.
>
> - Where all claims to care cannot be met, some fair method of prioritization must be used. No such method will be fair if it accords low priority on the basis of either life expectancy or chronological age.

Acknowledgments
I would like to thank Ray Tallis and Sarah Hobson for very helpful comments on an earlier version of this chapter.

REFERENCES

1. Harris J: What is the good of health care? Bioethics 1996;10
2. Harris J (ed): Introduction. In *Bioethics*. Oxford University Press, Oxford, 2001
3. Harris J: The Value of Life. Routledge & Kegan Paul, London, 1985
4. Harris J: The concept of the person and the value of life. Kennedy Inst Ethic J 1999;9:293–308
5. Harris J: Intimations of immortality. Science 2000;288(5463):59
6. Cruzan v Director, Missouri Department of Health, 497, US 261 (1990)
7. Airdale NHS Trust v Bland [1993] 1 All ER 858 (H.L.)

8. Keown J (ed): Euthanasia Examined: Ethical Clinical and Legal Perspectives. Cambridge University Press, Cambridge, 1995:6–71

9. Dworkin R: Life's Dominion. HarperCollins, London, 1993

10. Harris J: Violence & Responsibility. Routledge & Kegan Paul, London, 1980

11. Lord Mustil: Judgment in Airedale NH Trust v Bland [1993] 1 All ER 821 (H.L.)

12. Steiner H: A Theory of Rights. Blackwell, Oxford, 1994:258

13. Hirsch S, Harris J (eds): Consent and the Incompetent Patient. Royal College of Psychiatrists, London, 1988

14. British Medical Association: Medical Ethics Today: Its Practice and Philosophy. BMA, London, 1993:219–229

15. Freeman M, Lewis A (eds): Law and Medicine. Oxford University Press, Oxford, 2000

16. Ciba Foundation Study Group: Medical research: civil liability and compensation for personal injury—a discussion paper. BMJ 1980;280:1172–1175

17. Harris J: More and better justice. In Mendus M, Bell M (eds): Philosophy and Medical Welfare. Cambridge University Press, Cambridge, 1988:75–97

18. Dworkin R: Taking Rights Seriously. Duckworth, London, 1977

19. Callahan C: What Kind of Life: The Limits of Medical Progress. Georgetown University Press, 1995

20. Kappel K, Sandoe P: QALYs, age and fairness. Bioethics 1992;6:297–316

21. Singer P, McKie J, Kuhse H, Richardson J: Double jeopardy and the use of QALYs in health care allocation (review). Med Ethics 1995;21:144–150

22. McKie J, Richardson J, Singer P, Kuhse K. The Allocation of Health Care Resources. Ashgate, Dartmouth, 1998

23. Glover J: Causing Death and Saving Lives. Penguin, Harmondsworth, 1977

24. British Medical Association: Consent Rights and Choices in Health Care For Children and Young People. BMJ Books, 2001

25. Kirkwood T: Time of Our Lives. Phoenix Books, 1999

Chapter 25

Presentation of disease in old age

Brandon Koretz and David B. Reuben

Not only are diseases more common in elderly people, they may be more difficult to diagnose accurately. Classic presenting symptoms of common diseases may be absent. For example, older persons presenting with myocardial infarction may not report having chest pain. Conversely, nonspecific or unusual symptoms may be the earliest or only manifestations in this age group. For example, many infections (e.g. pneumonia, urinary tract infection) may present with a change in mental status and lethargy but few or no organ-specific symptoms.

A number of possible explanations may account for such atypical presentations: multiple comorbid conditions may alter the presentation of disease, age-related physiological changes may alter the perception of stimulus, and cognitive impairment may prevent the patient from providing an accurate history. As a result, these atypical presentations may be more common than classical presentations, as illustrated in Table 25-1. Moreover, an atypical presentation may predict a poor outcome for hospitalized elderly patients,[1] perhaps as a result of delays in diagnosis and initiation of appropriate therapy.

This chapter examines a variety of common diseases, discussed by organ system, in order to explore the differences in disease presentation between younger and older patients.

GASTROINTESTINAL DISEASES

Gastrointestinal complaints are common in elderly people. This section discusses several gastrointestinal diseases, organizing them according to the organ that they primarily affect.

Achalasia

Although idiopathic achalasia usually occurs in young adults, it may present in late life. In one study, older persons with this disorder had a significantly lower incidence of chest pain than younger persons; similar percentages of patients in each age group presented with complaints of dysphagia and regurgitation.[2] Nevertheless, the two age groups appear to respond equally well to pneumatic dilation.[2]

Gastroesophageal reflux disease

Symptoms of gastroesophageal reflux disease (GERD) are common among elderly patients. Approximately 8 percent of older men and 15 percent of older women experience symptoms of GERD on a daily basis.[3] The typical symptom is post-prandial substernal burning exacerbated by reclining. However, among older persons referred for endoscopy, almost 20 percent have erosive or complicated esophagitis.[4] People in this subgroup are more likely to complain of dysphagia, respiratory

Table 25-1 **Common and uncommon symptoms in elderly people**			
Disorder	**Most common presenting symptom(s) in the elderly**	**Symptoms that are less frequent in the elderly**	**Symptoms that are more frequent in the elderly**
Achalasia	Dysphagia	Chest pain	
Peptic ulcer		Abdominal pain	Bleeding, nausea, vomiting, anorexia
Appendicitis	Abdominal pain		
Cholecystitis	Abdominal pain	Abdominal pain	
Colitis	Abdominal pain, diarrhea	Abdominal pain	
Myocardial infarction	Chest pain, dyspnea		Delirium, syncope, stroke
Pneumonia	Fever, cough	Fever, pleuritic chest pain, rigors	Delirium
Bacteremia	Fever	Chills, sweats, malaise, headaches, arthralgias	
Gout			Indolent course, polyarticular, tophaceous deposits
Rheumatoid arthritis			Fever, weight loss, fatigue
Urinary tract infection		Dysuria	Confusion

symptoms (chronic cough, hoarseness, or wheezing), and vomiting than patients without severe esophagitis. However, this atypical presentation may relate more to the extent of disease rather than age per se. A study of 476 veterans referred for endoscopy found no age-related difference in symptoms of GERD.[5]

Peptic ulcer disease

Among patients with endoscopically diagnosed ulcers, elderly people are less likely to have presented with abdominal pain.[6] Conversely, they are more likely to have presented with bleeding, a shorter duration of symptoms, and other symptoms not typically considered to be associated with peptic ulcer disease (nausea, vomiting, anorexia, or abdominal pain not relieved by eating or drinking).[7]

In part, these differences may reflect age-related differences in the pathophysiology of ulcers. Older patients are more likely to have used nonsteroidal anti-inflammatory drugs (NSAIDs). But even after adjusting for this variable, other differences remain—older patients have more gastric ulcers and are less likely to have *Helicobacter pylori* found in association with their ulcers.[7] It is not clear, however, whether these differences alone are sufficient to explain the variability in clinical presentation.

Intra-abdominal infections

This is a broad category of diseases that includes appendicitis, cholecystitis, and pyogenic liver abscesses, all of which are associated with significant morbidity and mortality in elderly patients.[8] When these infectious processes are considered together as a whole, it appears that older and younger patients present differently. The elderly are less likely to present with nausea, vomiting, or fever and are more likely to be hypothermic and relatively neutropenic (polymorphonuclear leukocyte count $<2000/mm^3$).[9] All of these characteristics are consistent with an atypical presentation. One important difference between these two groups is the relative frequency of the sites of these infections—elderly patients are more likely than younger patients to have biliary or pancreatic sources.[9] We will now consider these different infections separately.

APPENDICITIS While appendicitis is more common in younger patients, its mortality is substantially higher among older persons.[10] The classical presentation is periumbilical pain that rapidly localizes to the right lower abdominal quadrant in association with peritoneal signs. While this pattern may not be as common in elderly persons, most older patients will develop right lower quadrant pain at some time during the illness.[10] Though variable, the frequency of nausea, vomiting, leukocytosis, and fever do not appear to be significantly different between older and younger patients.[10] In contrast, abdominal rigidity, decreased bowel sounds, and the presence of a mass appear to be more common in older patients.[11]

CHOLECYSTITIS The typical presentation of cholecystitis is right upper quadrant pain, fever, nausea, vomiting, and leukocytosis. These findings may not be present in elderly patients. Although most present with abdominal pain, in one study of 39 cholecystitis patients who were older than 60 years, only three-quarters had abdominal tenderness and only half had peritoneal signs.[12]

PYOGENIC LIVER ABSCESSES Pyogenic liver abscesses are associated with a high mortality rate in the elderly population. Patients typically present with fevers, chills, nonlocalizing gastrointestinal symptoms, and liver tenderness or enlargement. It is not clear whether these symptoms and signs are less common in affected elderly patients.[10]

Colitis

Inflammatory bowel disease has a bimodal distribution. There is an initial peak in the third and fourth decades of life followed by a second peak in the sixth and seventh decades.[13] When considering patients who have had the diagnosis of Crohn's disease made after the age of 50, the most common signs and symptoms are abdominal pain (82 percent), diarrhea (70 percent), and weight loss (56 percent).[14] A quarter of patients present with gastrointestinal bleeding. Whether this represents a difference relative to younger patients is controversial. Some believe that there is no age-related difference in clinical presentation,[15] whereas others have described significant differences.[16] In one study, patients between the ages of 64 and 85 were less likely to have reported abdominal pain or have abdominal masses on examination.[16] They also had a longer duration of symptoms before the definitive diagnosis was made (6.4 versus 2.4 years).

CARDIOVASCULAR DISEASE
Myocardial infarction

The classical presentation of myocardial infarction (MI) is usually described as sudden, severe, crushing precordial chest pain that radiates to the left arm or jaw. However, presenting symptoms of cardiac ischemia vary considerably from patient to patient. While many studies have noted the classical symptom complex is the most common presentation among older persons,[17–20] others have found that dyspnea or congestive heart failure are more common presenting symptoms.[21–23] A third category of presenting symptoms is neurological. In one series, delirium was the presenting symptom in 13 percent of patients with MI, while syncope and stroke were the presenting symptoms in 7 percent each.[23] Some of these differences may be due to different patient populations and differing definitions of chest pain.[20] Since patients with impaired cognition may be more likely to present with atypical symptoms of MI,[24] variable inclusion of these patients in studies could also be a factor.

Some studies have directly compared the presenting symptoms of MI in younger and older patients. In a Finnish study, typical presentations occurred more commonly in younger patients while older patients more commonly presented with dyspnea, vertigo, and loss of consciousness.[18] A second study found that chest pain became less common as a presenting symptom of MI as patients aged; however, most patients of all ages had chest pain accompanying their MI.[25] The presence of syncope, stroke, and delirium as initial symptoms was significantly associated with increased age.[25]

PULMONARY DISEASE

Pneumonia

Pneumonia is the fifth leading cause of death among elderly people.[26] The typical presentation of pneumonia consists of fever, cough, chills, and pleuritic chest pain. However, atypical presentations occur more frequently.[26] These atypical presentations tend to fall into one of two patterns. The first is a nonspecific deterioration in a patient's health status—decreased oral intake, falling, or confusion. The second is an abrupt worsening of an underlying chronic medical condition (e.g. hemiplegia from a prior stroke).

The presence of symptoms commonly associated with pneumonia is variable in elderly people. Fever has been reported in 27–80 percent of older patients with pneumonia.[27–30] A cough has been noted in 54–82 percent of elderly patients admitted to the hospital with community-acquired pneumonia,[27,31,32] though it may occur less frequently in a nursing-home population.[32,33] Chills or rigors are noted in about one-quarter of patients and a similar percentage present with falls.[31] Chest pain may be present in one-third.[31]

The signs of pneumonia are similarly variable. Fever is found in 33–80 percent of older patients with pneumonia.[27–29] Tachypnea is common—three-quarters or more of elderly patients with pneumonia may present with respiratory rates greater than 20/min.[30,34] Tachypnea may be one of the earliest signs of pneumonia and can be noted 24–48 hours prior to the clinical diagnosis.[35] Delirium occurs in 15–47 percent of patients with pneumonia and seems to be more common among nursing-home patients (approximately 48 percent) than those who live independently.[27,28,30,32] Signs of consolidation (bronchial breath sounds, egophony, and whispered pectoriloquy) are variable—some have noted rates of almost 50 percent,[36] while others have found them substantially less often.[27,31]

Several studies have compared the presenting symptoms of pneumonia in younger patients with those of older patients. In general, it appears that older patients are less likely to mount fevers, experience pleurisy, or have rigors.[37,38] They are, however, more likely to die as a result of their pneumonia.[38,39] The largest study to examine the effect of age on symptoms and signs of pneumonia included over 1800 patients.[40] Older age was associated with a lower incidence of both respiratory and nonrespiratory symptoms. Increasing age was also associated with increasing respiratory rates. It is controversial whether age per se is responsible for these atypical presentations. Others have noted that when demented patients are excluded, the incidence of nonspecific presentations become equal in older and younger age groups.[41]

INFECTIOUS DISEASES

The age-dependent differences between the clinical presentations of intra-abdominal infections and pneumonia have been described. There are additional differences with other infections that are worth mentioning.

Fever

While not a disease itself, fever is the prototypical symptom of many infections. Its presence serves as a warning sign for potentially life-threatening diseases.[42] But, as already mentioned, the febrile response may be absent in infected older patients. While errors in measurement may account for some of this variability,[43] older patients, on average, have a lower basal temperature than younger persons.[44] To compensate for this, some have suggested that the use of change from basal temperature might be more sensitive for the presence of infection than absolute temperature.[44]

Bacteremia

One of the most serious complications of bacterial infections is bacteremia. Its presence is associated with significantly higher mortality rates.[45,46] In elderly people the three most commonly identified sources are the urinary tract, the lungs, and the gastrointestinal tract.[45–47] Classically, the symptoms associated with bacteremia are fevers, rigors, and chills. In clinical practice, however, the symptoms are often nonspecific. In a retrospective study of 50 consecutive patients with bacteremia admitted to a geriatric unit, 60 percent were febrile, 36 percent were delirious, and 30 percent complained of weakness or falls.[46] The author did not comment on the frequency of rigors or chills. However, others have noted that older patients with bacteremia may be less likely to chills, sweats, or malaise than younger patients.[48,49] Nonspecific symptoms of bacteremia (headache, abdominal pain, and arthralgias) also seem to be less common in older patients.[49] One physical examination sign of bacteremia, tachycardia, also appears to be less common in older patients.[48,49]

RHEUMATOLOGICAL DISEASES

Gout

The classic presentation of gout is an acute monoarticular arthritis affecting the first metatarsophalangeal joint of a middle-aged man who is fond of rich food and alcohol. In the elderly population, the clinical features may be different. The male predominance noted in younger patients does not seem to be present among older persons.[50] The disease may follow a more indolent course and be more likely to be polyarticular.[51] There is a strong association with long-term diuretic use; renal excretion of uric acid is inhibited due to volume contraction.[52,53] For the same reason, tophaceous deposits are more likely to be present in elderly people.

Rheumatoid arthritis

Typically, patients who are affected by rheumatoid arthritis (RA) are women aged 20–40 years. Affected patients most commonly note the insidious onset of symmetric polyarthritis which may be accompanied by systemic complaints. Older patients who develop RA seem to demonstrate several differences in their clinical presentation. The gender difference in disease incidence noted in younger patients seems to be less pronounced in patients who develop RA after the age of 60.[54–57] Older patients also tend to have more constitutional symptoms (fever, weight loss, and fatigue), are more likely to present with an acute onset of arthritis, have more shoulder involvement, and have a negative assay for rheumatoid factor.[54-57] However, there are some concerns about the methodological rigor of the studies on which these conclusions are based.[58]

URINARY TRACT INFECTION AND UROSEPSIS

Bacteriuria becomes increasingly common with advancing age. In the absence of symptoms, its association with increased mortality is controversial.[59] It is clear, however, that the urinary tract is the most common source for bacteremia in elderly patients admitted to a hospital.[45]

The clinical picture of urinary tract infections is variable. The typical symptoms associated with lower tract infections—dysuria, urgency, and suprapubic pain—are commonly absent in older patients with bacteriuria.[60] Similarly, the flank pain, fevers, and chills that typically accompany upper urinary tract infections may be absent. In one series of elderly patients with bacteremia from urinary sources, 30 percent presented with confusion, 29 percent with a cough, and 27 percent with dyspnea.[61] Other studies suggest that the febrile response to urinary tract infection remains intact, but also suggest that confusion is a common presenting sign.[62] Finally, the presence of costovertebral angle tenderness in elderly patients with pyelonephritis is inconsistent.[63]

CONCLUSION

Many studies support the notion that common diseases present differently in the elderly population. What is less clear is whether it is appropriate to call these presentations atypical. In fact, when the atypical presentation is more common than the classic presentation described for younger persons, perhaps it should be termed the typical presentation in the older age group. If it is unreasonable to expect a physical performance of a 75-year-old person to be equivalent to that of a 25-year-old person, it may not be reasonable to expect pneumonia to behave similarly in these two individuals. Rather than using the 25-year-old as the reference standard for all age groups, perhaps a better course would be for practitioners to remain aware that diseases have different clinical features depending upon the age of the affected patient.

KEY POINTS Presentation of disease

- Nonspecific presentations of disease are more common among elderly patients.

- Because they have lower basal body temperatures, infected elderly people may have a fever despite temperature readings that would be normal for younger people.

- Practitioners should remember that many common diseases may present differently in younger and older patients.

REFERENCES

1. Jarrett PG, Rockwood K, Carver D et al: Illness presentation in elderly patients. Arch Int Med 1995;155:1060–1064
2. Clouse RE, Abramson BK, Todorczuk JR: Achalasia in the elderly: effects of aging on clinical presentation and outcome. Digest Dis Sci 1991;36:225–228
3. Raiha IJ, Imipivaara O, Seppala M et al: Prevalence and characteristics of symptomatic gastroesophageal reflux disease in the elderly. J Am Geriatr Soc 1992;40:1209–1211
4. Raiha I, Hietanen E, Sourander L: Symptoms of gastro-oesophageal reflux disease in elderly people. Age Ageing 1991;20:365–370
5. Triadafilopoulos G, Sharma R: Features of symptomatic gastroesophageal reflux disease in elderly patients. Am J Gastrol 1997;92:2007–2011
6. Clinch D, Banerjee AK, Ostick G: Absence of abdominal pain in elderly patients with peptic ulcer disease. Age Ageing 1984;13:120–123
7. Kemppainen H, Raiha I, Sourander L: Clinical presentation of peptic ulcer disease in the elderly. Gerontology 1997;43:283–288
8. Fenyo G: Acute abdominal disease in the elderly. Am J Surg 1982;143:751–754
9. Cooper GS, Shlaes DM, Salata RA: Intraabdominal infection: differences in presentation and outcome between younger patients and the elderly. Clin Infect Dis 1994;19:146–148
10. Norman D, Yoshikawa TT: Intraabdominal infections in the elderly. J Am Geriatr Soc 1983;31:677–683
11. Telfer S, Fenyo G, Holt PR et al: Acute abdominal pain in patients over 50 years of age. Scand J Gastroenterol 1988;23:47–50
12. Morrow DJ, Thompson J, Wilson SE: Acute cholecystitis in the elderly. Arch Surg 1978;113:1149–1152
13. Rogers BHD, Clark IM, Kirsner JB: The epidemiologic and demographic characteristics of inflammatory bowel disease: an analysis of a computerized file of 1400 patients. J Chron Dis 1971;24:743–773
14. Roberts PL, Schoetz DJ, Pricolo R et al: Clinical course of Crohn's disease in older patients. Dis Col Rect 1990;33:458–462
15. Eisen GM, Schutz SM, Washington MK et al: Atypical presentation of inflammatory bowel disease in the elderly. Am J Gastroenterol 1993;88:2098–2101
16. Harper PC, McAuliffe TL, Beeken WL: Crohn's disease in the elderly: a statistical comparison with younger patients matched for sex and duration of disease. Arch Intern Med 1986;146:753–755
17. Tinker GM: Clinical presentation of myocardial infarction in the elderly. Age Ageing 1981;10:237–240
18. Acta Med Scand 1977;604(suppl):9–68
19. Bayer AJ: Presentation and management of myocardial infarction in the elderly. Br J Hosp Med 1998;40:300–301, 304–306
20. MacDonald JB: Presentation of acute myocardial infarction in the elderly—a review. Age Ageing 1984;13:196–200
21. Rodstein M: The characteristics of nonfatal myocardial infarction in the aged. Arch Intern Med 1956;98:84–90
22. Aronow W: Prevalence of presenting symptoms of recognized acute myocardial infarction and of unrecognized healed myocardial infarction in elderly patients. Am J Cardiol 1987;60:1182
23. Pathy MS: Clinical presentation of myocardial infarction in the elderly. Br Heart J 1967;29:190–199
24. Black DA: Mental state and presentation of myocardial infarction in the elderly. Age Ageing 1987;16:125–127
25. Bayer AJ, Chadha JS, Farag RR et al: Changing presentation of myocardial infarction with increasing old age. J Am Geriatr Soc 1986;34:263–266
26. Fein AM: Pneumonia in the elderly. Med Clin North Am 1994;78:1015–1033
27. Musgrave T, Verghese A: Clinical features of pneumonia in the elderly. Semin Respir Infect 1990;5:269–275
28. Harper C, Newton P: Clinical aspects of pneumonia in the elderly veteran. J Am Geriatr Soc 1989;37:867–872
29. Andrews J, Chandrasekaran P, McSwiggan D: Lower respiratory tract infections in an acute geriatric male ward: a one-year prospective surveillance. Gerontology 1984;30:290–296
30. Venkatesan P, Gladman J, Macfarlane JT: A hospital study of community acquired pneumonia in the elderly. Thorax 1990;45:254–258
31. Starczewski AR, Allen SC, Vargas E et al: Clinical prognostic indices of fatality in elderly patients admitted to hospital with acute pneumonia. Age Ageing 1988;17:181–186

32. Marrie TJ, Durant H, Yates L: Community-acquired pneumonia requiring hospitalization: 5-year prospective study. Rev Infect Dis 1989;11:586–599

33. Marrie TJ: Pneumonia. Infect Dis 1992;8:721–734

34. Peterson PK, Stein D, Guay DRP et al: Prospective study of lower respiratory tract infections in an extended-care nursing home program: potential role of oral ciprofloxacin. Am J Med 1988;85:164–171

35. McFadden JP, Price RC, Eastwood HD et al: Raised respiratory rate in elderly patients: a valuable physical sign. BMJ 1982;284:626–627

36. Marrie TJ, Durant H, Kwan K: Nursing home-acquired pneumonia. J Am Geriatr Soc 1986;34:697–702

37. Esposito AL: Community-acquired bacteremic pneumococcal pneumonia effect of age on manifestations and outcome. Arch Intern Med 1984;144:945–948

38. Finkelstein MS, Petkun WM, Freedman ML et al: Pneumococcal bacteremia in adults: age-dependent differences in presentation and outcome. J Am Geriatr Soc 1983;31:19–27

39. Marrie TJ, Haldane EV, Faulkner RS: Community-acquired pneumonia requiring hospitalization: is it different in the elderly? J Am Geriatr Soc 1985;33:671–680

40. Metlay JP, Schulz R, Li Y et al: Influence of age on symptoms at presentation in patient with community-acquired pneumonia. Arch Intern Med 1997;157:1453–1459

41. Johnson JC, Jayadevappa R, Baccash PD et al: Nonspecific presentation of pneumonia in hospitalized older people: age effect or dementia? J Am Geriatr Soc 2000;48:1316–1320

42. Keating HJ, Klimek JJ, Levine DS et al: Effect of aging on the clinical significance of fever in ambulatory adult patients. J Am Geriatr Soc 1984;32:282–287

43. Darowski A, Najim Z, Weinberg J et al: The febrile response to mild infections in elderly hospital inpatients. Age Ageing 1991;20:193–198

44. Castle SC, Norman DC, Yeh M et al: Fever response in elderly nursing home residents: are the older truly colder? J Am Geriatr Soc 1991;39:853–857

45. Esposito AL, Gleckman RA, Cram S et al: Community-acquired bacteremia in the elderly: analysis of one hundred consecutive episodes. J Am Geriatr Soc 1980;28:315–319

46. Windsor ACM: Bacteraemia in a geriatric unit. Gerontology 1983;29:125–130

47. Meyers BR, Sherman E, Mendelson MH et al: Bloodstream infections in the elderly. Am J Med 1989;86:379–384

48. Chassagne P, Perol MB, Doucet J et al: Is presentation of bacteremia in the elderly the same as in younger patients? Am J Med 1996;100:65–70

49. Terpenning MS, Buggy BP, Kauffman CA: Infective endocarditis: clinical features in young and elderly patients. Am J Med 1987;83:626–634

50. Meyers OL, Monteagudo FSE: A comparison of gout in men and women. South African Med J 1986;70:721–723

51. Fam A: Gout in the elderly clinical presentation and treatment. Drugs Aging 1998;13:229–243

52. Michet CJ, Evans JM, Fleming KC: Common rheumatologic diseases in elderly patients. Mayo Clin Proc 1995;70:1205–1214

53. Platt PN, Dick WC: Diuretic-induced gout: the beginnings of an epidemic? Practitioner 1985;229:281–284

54. Bajocchi G, La Corte R, Locaputo A et al: Early onset of rheumatoid arthritis: clinical aspects. Clin Exper Rheumatol 2000;18(suppl 20):S49–S50

55. Deal CL, Meenan RF, Goldenberg DL et al: The clinical features of elderly-onset rheumatoid arthritis. Arthr Rheum 1985;28:987–994

56. Terkeltaub R, Esdaile J, Decary F et al: A clinical study of older age rheumatoid arthritis with comparison to a younger onset group. J Rheumatol 1983;10:418–424

57. Yazici Y, Paget SA: Geriatric rheumatology: elderly-onset rheumatoid arthritis. Rheum Dis Clin North Am 2000;26:517–526

58. Kavanaugh AF: Rheumatoid arthritis in the elderly: is it a different disease? Am J Med 1997;103:40S–48S

59. Nordenstam GR, Brandeberg A, Oden AS et al: Bacteriuria and mortality in an elderly population. N Engl J Med 1986;314:1152–1156

60. Boscia JA, Kobasa WD, Abrutyn E et al: Lack of association between bacteriuria and symptoms in the elderly. Am J Med 1986;81:979–982

61. Barkham TMS, Martin FC, Eykyn SJ: Delay in the diagnosis of bacteraemic urinary tract infection in elderly. Age Ageing 1996;25:130–132

62. Berman P, Hogan DB, Fox RA: The atypical presentation of infection in old age. Age Ageing 1987;16:201–207

63. Gleckman R, Blagg N, Hibert D et al: Community-acquired bacteremic urosepsis in elderly patients: a prospective study of 34 consecutive episodes. J Urol 1982;128:79–81

Chapter 26

Multidimensional geriatric assessment

Laurence Z. Rubenstein and Lisa V. Rubenstein

Geriatric assessment is a multidimensional, usually interdisciplinary, diagnostic process intended to determine a frail elderly person's medical, psychosocial, and functional capabilities and problems with the objective of developing an overall plan for treatment and long-term follow-up. It differs from the standard medical evaluation in its concentration on frail elderly people with their complex problems, its emphasis on functional status and quality of life, and its frequent use of interdisciplinary teams and quantitative assessment scales.

The process of geriatric assessment can range in intensity from a limited assessment by primary care physicians or community health workers focused on identifying an older person's functional problems and disabilities (screening assessment), to more thorough evaluation of these problems by a geriatrician or multidisciplinary team (comprehensive geriatric assessment), often coupled with initiation of a therapeutic plan. This chapter discusses both limited geriatric assessment, such as can be performed by a single practitioner in an office setting, and comprehensive geriatric assessment, usually requiring a specialized geriatric setting.

Because the ultimate goal of geriatric assessment is to improve quality of life for elderly people, readers may find Figure 26-1 helpful.[1] As diagrammed, quality of life includes health status and socio-economic and environmental factors. Health status can be quantified both by measures of disease, such as signs, symptoms, and laboratory tests, and by measures of functional status. By functional status, we mean the individual's ability to participate fully in the physical, mental, and social activities of daily life. The ability to function fully in these

arenas is strongly affected by an individual's physiological health, and can often be used as a measure of the seriousness of a patient's multiple diseases. A comprehensive geriatric assessment should be able to evaluate and plan care for all these areas.

BRIEF HISTORY OF GERIATRIC ASSESSMENT

The basic concepts of geriatric assessment have evolved over the past 70 years by combining elements of the traditional medical history and physical examination, the social worker assessment, functional evaluation, and treatment methods derived from rehabilitation medicine, and psychometric methods derived from the social sciences. By incorporating the perspectives of many disciplines, geriatricians have created a practical means of viewing the "whole patient."

The first published reports of geriatric assessment programs came from the British geriatrician Marjory Warren, who initiated the concept of specialized geriatric assessment units during the late 1930s while in charge of a large London infirmary. This infirmary was filled primarily with chronically ill, bedfast, and largely neglected elderly patients who had not received proper medical diagnosis or rehabilitation and who were thought to be in need of lifelong institutionalization. Good nursing care kept the patients alive, but the lack of diagnostic assessment and rehabilitation kept them disabled. Through evaluation, mobilization, and rehabilitation, Warren was able to get most of the long bedfast patients out of bed and often discharged home. As a result of her experiences, Warren advocated that every elderly patient receive comprehensive assessment and an attempt at rehabilitation before being admitted to a long-term care hospital or nursing home.[2]

Since Warren's work, geriatric assessment has evolved. As geriatric care systems have been developed throughout the world, geriatric assessment programs have been assigned central roles, usually as focal points for entry into the care systems.[3] Geared to differing local needs and populations, geriatric assessment programs vary in intensity, structure, and function. They can be located in different settings, including acute hospital inpatient units and consultation teams, chronic and rehabilitation hospital units, outpatient and office-based programs, and home visit outreach programs. Despite diversity, they share many characteristics. Virtually all programs provide multidimensional assessment, utilizing specific measurement instruments to quantify functional, psychological, and social parameters. Most use interdisciplinary teams to pool expertise and enthusiasm in working toward common goals. Additionally, most programs attempt to couple their

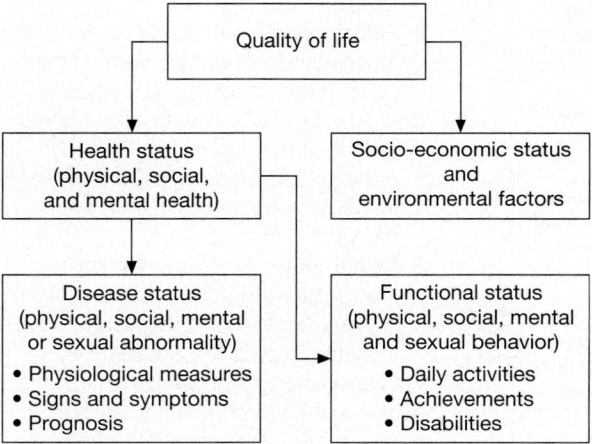

Figure 26-1 Conceptual components of quality of life—relationship to health and functional status. Adapted from Rubenstein et al.,[1] with permission of Blackwell Science, Inc.

assessments with an intervention, such as rehabilitation, counseling, or placement.

Today, geriatric assessment continues to evolve in response to increased pressures for cost-containment, avoidance of institutional stays, and consumer demands for better care. Geriatric assessment can help achieve improved quality of care and plan cost-effective care. This has generally meant more emphasis on noninstitutional programs and shorter hospital stays. Geriatric assessment teams are well positioned to deliver effective care for elderly persons with limited resources. Geriatricians have long emphasized judicious use of technology, systematic preventive medicine activities, and less institutionalization and hospitalization.

STRUCTURE AND PROCESS OF GERIATRIC ASSESSMENT

Geriatric assessment begins with the identification of deteriorations in health status or the presence of risk factors for deterioration. These deteriorations include both worsening of disease and worsening of functional status. If disease alone has worsened, without affecting function, the patient should be able to be cared for in usual primary care settings. In addition, when functional status problems are mild and are not rapidly progressive, it is appropriate for a primary care practitioner to proceed with the assessment. However, because families and patients identify functional status problems early, and because internists and family practitioners often are unfamiliar with the concept of "treating" functional status impairment as a problem in its own right, patients often self-refer to geriatric care settings for these functional status problems when such settings are available. Patients who have new severe or progressive deficits should ideally receive comprehensive multidisciplinary geriatric assessment. Figure 26-2 outlines an approach for evaluating elderly outpatients with health status deterioration and deciding who should be referred to multidimensional geriatric assessment settings.

Using this approach, an elderly patient presenting with a deterioration in health status of any kind, be it a markedly elevated blood glucose, a vertebral collapse, or a new inability to perform errands, should be evaluated briefly to determine the full extent of functional disabilities. Many experts believe that frail elderly people, defined generally as people over the

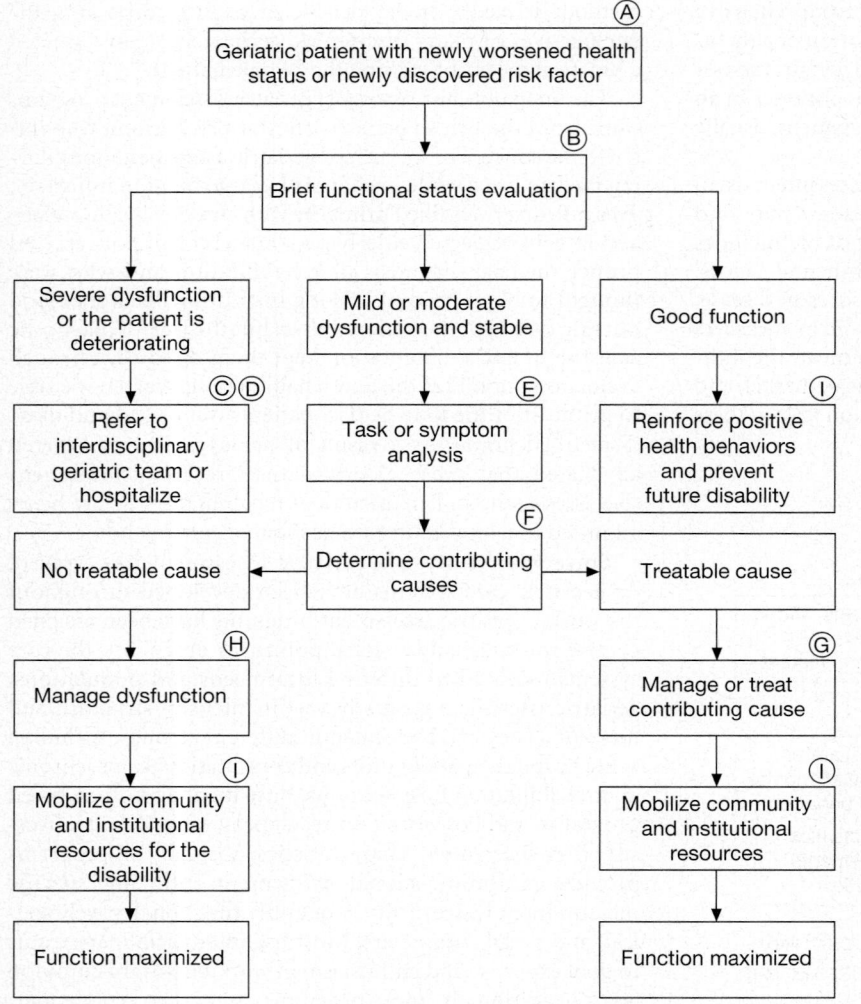

Figure 26-2 Evaluating and treating health status deterioration among geriatric outpatients.

A. Elderly patients with a new deterioration in health status or newly discovered risk factor(s) may need geriatric assessment. Examples of patients needing assessment include the following:
   1. Frail elderly people with a new functional disability or risk factor for deterioration detected on routine screening
   2. Elderly people with a new or worsened medical complaint or laboratory finding (e.g. "I fell last week" or the X-ray shows a new vertebral compression fracture)
   3. Elderly people with a new or worsened functional disability complaint ("I can't go to church because of my health")
B. Brief functional status evaluation should include the following:
   1. Activities of daily living (ADL)[13–16,23,24]
   2. Instrumental activities of daily living (IADL)[14,23,24]
   3. Mental status (e.g. Folstein Mini-Mental State)[20]
   4. Affective status (e.g. Yesavage Geriatric Depression Scale)[21,23]
C. Full multidimensional geriatric assessment and/or hospitalization is necessary for elderly patients with new severe or progressive functional disability

age of 75, or over age 65 with chronic disease, should also be screened for functional disability or risk factors at regular intervals such as once a year, even when no known acute health insults have occurred.[1,4–7] When a new disability or high-risk state is detected through screening, such patients may also be appropriate for a full geriatric assessment.

A typical geriatric assessment begins with a functional status "review of systems" that inventories the major domains of functioning. The major elements of this review of systems are captured in two commonly used functional status measures—basic activities of daily living (ADL) and instrumental activities of daily living (IADL). Several reliable and valid versions of these measures have been developed,[8–12] perhaps the most widely used being those by Katz et al.,[13] Lawton and Brody,[14] and Barthel.[15,16] These scales are used by clinicians to detect whether the patient has problems performing activities that people must be able to accomplish to survive without help in the community. Basic ADL include self-care activities such as eating, dressing, bathing, transferring, and toileting. Patients unable to perform these activities will generally require 12- to 24-hour support by caregivers. Instrumental activities of daily living include heavier housework, going on errands, managing finances, and telephoning—activities that are required if the individual is to remain independent in a house or apartment.

To interpret the results of impairments in ADL and IADL, physicians will usually need additional information about the patient's environment and social situation. For example, the amount and type of caregiver support available, the strength of the patient's social network, and the level of social activities in which the patient participates will all influence the clinical approach taken in managing deficits detected. This information could be obtained by an experienced nurse or social worker. A screen for mobility and fall risk is also extremely helpful in quantifying function and disability, and several observational scales are available.[17,18] An assessment of nutritional status and risk for undernutrition is also important in understanding the

extent of impairment and for planning care.[19] Likewise, a screening assessment of vision and hearing will often detect crucial deficits that need to be treated or compensated for.

Two other key pieces of information must always be gathered in the face of functional disability in an elderly person. These are a screen for mental status (cognitive) impairment and a screen for depression.[8,9,12] Of the several validated screening tests for cognitive function, the Folstein Mini-Mental State is one of the best because it efficiently tests the major aspects of cognitive functioning.[20] Of the various screening tests for geriatric depression, the Yesavage Geriatric Depression Scale[21] and the Zung Self-Rating Depression Scale[22] are in wide use, and even shorter screening versions are available without significant loss of accuracy.[23]

The major measurable dimensions of geriatric assessment, together with examples of commonly used health status screening scales, are listed in Table 26-1.[7–37] The instruments listed are short, have been carefully tested for reliability and validity, and can be easily administered by virtually any staff person involved with the assessment process. Both observational instruments (e.g. physical examination) and self-report (completed by patient or proxy) are available. Components of them—such as watching a patient walk, turn around, and sit down—are routine parts of the geriatric physical examination. Many other kinds of assessment measures exist and can be useful in certain situations. For example, there are several disease-specific measures for stages and levels of dysfunction for patients with specific diseases such as arthritis,[31] dementia,[32] and parkinsonism.[33] There are also several brief global assessment instruments that attempt to quantify all dimensions of the assessment in a single form.[34–37] These latter instruments can be useful in community surveys and some research settings but are not detailed enough to be useful in most clinical settings. More comprehensive lists of available instruments can be found by consulting published reviews of health status assessment.[7–11,38]

D. Targeted assessment for patients in office practice is appropriate for the following:
   1. Patients whose functional disabilities or medical problems are mild enough to make multiple appointment feasible
   2. Patients whose disability is stable enough to permit assessment over weeks to months
E. To perform task or symptom analysis, select the patient's major symptom or disability or chief complaint (the one that bothers him/her the most, the disability upon which resolution of other health problems depends, or the one that is the most treatable). Then, determine the exact maneuvers necessary to complete the task, or the exact components of the symptom (e.g. "difficulty getting dressed" due to difficulty putting on shoes because of inability to bend; or "difficulty with housework" because of failure to complete tasks despite adequate physical ability to perform them)
F. To determine contributing causes:
   1. Perform a targeted history, guided by the functional disabilities detected and by the known common occult causes of disability in the elderly (see text)

   2. Perform a targeted physical examination, always including postural blood pressure changes, vision and hearing screening, observations of gait (at least get up, walk 25 feet, turn around, sit down). Determine all specific physical disabilities such as hip flexor weakness, or poor hand mobility, that explain the observed functional disability
G. Manage or treat contributing cause(s). Begin appropriate medical treatments and evaluations. Mobilize community and institutional resources as appropriate (low-vision resources for blindness; Alcoholics Anonymous for alcoholics, etc.). Identify key members of the multidisciplinary team and refer as needed (e.g. social worker for social isolation, physical therapist for gait disorder, or psychiatrist for depression)
H. When the disability cannot be reversed, maximize function using available services and behavioral or physical adaptation. For example, rearranging schedule to maximize activity, providing adaptive devices, or arranging for home support services might be indicated
I. Always reinforce positive health behaviors.

Table 26-1 Measurable dimensions of geriatric assessment with examples of specific measures

Dimension	Basic context	Specific examples
Basic ADL[23,24]	Strengths and limitations in self-care, basic mobility, and incontinence	Katz (ADL);[13] Lawton Personal Self-Maintenance Scale;[14] Barthel Index[15,16]
IADL[24]	Strengths and limitations in shopping, cooking, household activities, and finances	Lawton (IADL);[14] Older Americans Resources and Services, IADL Section[28]
Social activities and supports[25]	Strengths and limitations in social network and community activities	Lubben Social Network Scale;[29] Older Americans Resources and Services, Social Resources Section[28]
Mental health— affective[27]	The degree to which the person feels anxious, depressed, or generally happy	Yesavage Geriatric Depression Scale;[21,23] Zung Self-Rating Depression Scale[22]
Mental health— cognitive[27]	The degree to which the person is alert, oriented, and able to concentrate, and perform complex mental tasks	Folstein Mini-Mental State;[20] Kahn Mental Status Questionnaire[30]
Mobility—gait and balance[9,11]	Quantitative scale of gait, balance, and risk of falls	Tinetti Performance Oriented Mobility Assessment;[17] Get up and go test[18]
Nutritional adequacy[19]	Current nutritional status and risk of malnutrition	Nutrition Screening Initiative Checklist;[19] Mini-Nutritional Assessment[26]

Abbreviations: ADL, activities of daily living; IADL, instrumental activities of daily living.

Table 26-2 Determining the intensity and location of the geriatric assessment

	Office setting	Outpatient unit/team	Inpatient unit/team
Level of disability	Low	Intermediate	High
Cognitive dysfunction	Mild	Mild to severe	Moderate to severe
Family support	Good	Good to fair	Good to poor
Acuity of illness	Mild	Mild to moderate	Moderate to severe
Complexity	Low	Intermediate	High
Transportation access	Good	Good	Good to poor

A number of factors must be taken into account in deciding where an assessment should take place. These are outlined in Table 26-2. Mental and physical impairment make it difficult for patients to comply with recommendations and to navigate multiple appointments in multiple locations. Functionally impaired elders must depend on families and friends, who risk losing their jobs because of chronic and relentless demands on time and energy and in their roles as caregivers, and who may be elderly themselves. Each separate medical appointment or intervention has a high time-cost to these caregivers. Patient fatigue during periods of increased illness may require the availability of a bed during the assessment process. Finally, enough physician time and expertise must be available to complete the assessment within the constraints of the setting.

Most geriatric assessments do not require the full range of technology nor the intense monitoring found in the acute-care inpatient setting. Yet hospitalization becomes unavoidable if no outpatient setting provides sufficient resources to accomplish the assessment fast enough. A specialized geriatric setting outside an acute hospital ward, such as a day hospital or subacute inpatient geriatric evaluation unit, will provide the easy availability of an interdisciplinary team with the time and expertise to provide needed services efficiently, an adequate level of monitoring, and beds for patients unable to sit or stand for prolonged periods. Inpatient and day-hospital assessment programs have the advantages of intensity, rapidity, and ability to care for particularly frail or acutely ill patients. Outpatient programs are generally cheaper and avoid the necessity of an inpatient stay.

Assessment in the office practice setting

A streamlined approach is usually necessary in the office setting. An important first step is setting priorities among problems for initial evaluation and treatment. The "best" problem to work on first might be the problem that most bothers a patient or, alternatively, the problem upon which resolution of other problems depends (alcoholism or depression often fall into this category).

The second step in performing a geriatric assessment is to understand the exact nature of the disability through performing a task or symptom analysis. In a nonspecialized setting, or when the disability is mild or clear-cut, this may involve only taking a careful history. When the disability is more severe, more detailed assessments by a multidisciplinary or interdisciplinary team may be necessary. For example, a patient may present with difficulty dressing. There are multiple tasks associated with dressing, any one of which might be the stumbling block (e.g. buying clothes, choosing appropriate clothes to put on, remembering to complete the task, buttoning, stretching to put on shirts, or reaching downward to put on shoes). By identifying the exact areas of difficulty, further evaluation can be targeted toward solving the problem.

Once the history has revealed the nature of the disability, a systematic physical examination and ancillary laboratory tests are needed to clarify the cause of the problem. For example, difficulty dressing could be caused by mental status impairment, poor finger mobility, or dysfunction of shoulders, back, or hips. Evaluation by a physical or occupational therapist may be necessary to pinpoint the problem adequately, and evaluation by a social worker may be required to determine the extent of family dysfunction engendered by or contributing to the dependency. Radiological and other laboratory testing may be necessary.

Each abnormality that could cause difficulty dressing suggests different treatments. By understanding the abnormalities that contribute most to the functional disability, the best treatment strategy can be undertaken. Often one disability leads to another—impaired gait may lead to depression or decreased social functioning; and immobility of any cause, even after the cause has been removed, can lead to secondary impairments in performance of daily activities due to deconditioning and loss of musculoskeletal flexibility.

Almost any acute or chronic disease can reduce functioning. Common but easily overlooked causes of dysfunction in elderly people include impaired cognition, impaired special senses (vision, hearing, balance), unstable gait and mobility, poor health habits (alcohol, smoking, lack of exercise), poor nutrition, polypharmacy, incontinence, psychosocial stress, and depression. To identify contributing causes of the disability, the physician must thus look for worsening of the patient's chronic diseases, occurrence of a new acute disease, or appearance of one of the common occult diseases listed above. The physician does this through a refocused history guided by the functional disabilities detected and their differential diagnoses, and a focused physical examination. The physical examination always includes, in addition to usual evaluations of the heart, lungs, extremities, and neurological function, postural blood pressure, vision and hearing screening, and careful observation of the patient's gait. The mini-mental state examination, already recommended as part of the initial functional status screen, may also determine what parts of the physical examination require particular attention as part of the evaluation of dementia or acute confusion. Finally, basic laboratory testing including a complete blood count and a blood chemistry panel, as well as tests indicated on the basis of specific findings from the history and physical examination, will generally be necessary.

Once the disability and its causes are understood, the best treatments or management strategies for it are often clear. When a reversible cause for the impairment is found, a simple treatment may eliminate or ameliorate the functional disability. When the disability is complex, the physician may need the support of a variety of community or hospital-based resources.

In most cases, a strategy for long-term follow-up and often, formal case management should be developed to ensure that needs and services are appropriately matched up and followed through.

Multidimensional geriatric assessment

If referral to a specialized geriatric setting has been chosen, the process of assessment will probably be similar to that described above, except that the greater intensity of resources and the special training of all members of the multidisciplinary team in dealing with geriatric patients and their problems will facilitate carrying out the proposed assessment and plan more quickly, and in greater breadth and detail. In the usual geriatric assessment setting, key disciplines involved include, at a minimum, physicians, social workers, nurses, and physical and occupational therapists, and optimally may include other disciplines such as dieticians, pharmacists, ethicists, and home-care specialists. Special geriatric expertise among the multidisciplinary team members is crucial.

The interdisciplinary team conference, which takes place after most team members have completed their individual assessments, is critical. Most successful trials of geriatric assessment have included such a team conference. By bringing the perspectives of all disciplines together, the team conference generates new ideas, sets priorities, disseminates the full results of the assessment to all those involved in treating the patient, and avoids duplication or incongruity. Development of fully effective teams requires commitment, skill, and time as the interdisciplinary team evolves through the "forming, storming, and norming" phases to reach the fully developed "performing" stage.[39] Involvement of the patient (and carer if appropriate) at some stage is important in maintaining the principle of choice.[39,40]

EFFECTIVENESS OF GERIATRIC ASSESSMENT PROGRAMS

A large and still growing literature supports the effectiveness of geriatric assessment programs (GAPs) in a variety of settings. Early descriptive studies indicated a number of benefits from GAPs such as improved diagnostic accuracy, reduced discharges to nursing homes, increased functional status, and more appropriate medication prescribing. Because they were descriptive studies, without concurrent control patients, they were not able to distinguish the effects of the programs from simple improvement over time. Nor did these studies look at long-term, or many short-term, outcome benefits. Nonetheless, many of these early studies provided promising results.[41–45]

Improved diagnostic accuracy was the most widely described effect of geriatric assessment, most often indicated by substantial numbers of important problems uncovered. Frequencies of new diagnoses found ranged from almost one to more than four per patient. Factors contributing to the improvement of diagnosis in GAPs include the validity of the assessment itself (the capability of a structured search for "geriatric problems" to find them), the extra measure of time and care taken in the evaluation of the patient (independent of the formal elements of "the assessment"), and a probable lack of diagnostic attention on the part of referring professionals.

Improved living location on discharge from a healthcare setting was demonstrated in several early studies, beginning with T. F. Williams' classic descriptive pre–post study of an outpatient assessment program in New York.[46] Of patients referred for nursing home placement in the county, the assessment program found that only 38 percent actually needed skilled nursing care, while 23 percent could return home, and 39 percent were appropriate for board and care or retirement facilities. Numerous subsequent studies have shown similar improvements in living location.[47–62] Several studies that examined mental or physical functional status of patients before and after comprehensive geriatric assessment coupled with treatment and rehabilitation showed patient improvement on measures of function.[47–51,55,59]

Beginning in the 1980s, controlled studies appeared that corroborated some of the earlier studies and documented additional benefits such as improved survival, reduced hospital and nursing home utilization, and in some cases, reduced costs.[47–71] These studies were by no means uniform in their results. Some showed a whole series of dramatic positive effects on function, survival, living location, and costs, while others showed relatively few if any benefits. However, the GAPs being studied were also very different from each other in terms of process of care offered and patient populations accepted. To this day, controlled trials of GAPs continue, and as results accumulate, we are able to understand which aspects contribute to their effectiveness and which do not.

One striking effect confirmed for many GAPs has been a positive impact on survival. Several controlled studies of different basic GAP models demonstrated significantly increased survival, reported in different ways and with varying periods of follow-up. Mortality was reduced for Sepulveda geriatric evaluation unit patients by 50 percent at 1 year, and the survival curves of the experimental and control groups still significantly favored the assessed group at 2 years.[47,63,64] Survival was improved by 21 percent at 1 year in a Scottish trial of geriatric rehabilitation consultation.[59] Two Canadian consultation trials demonstrated significantly improved 6-month survival.[55,56] Two Danish community-based trials of in-home geriatric assessment and follow-up demonstrated reduction in mortality,[48,61] and two Welsh studies of in-home GAPs had beneficial survival effects among patients assessed at home and followed for 2 years.[50,51] On the other hand, several other studies of geriatric assessment found no statistically significant survival benefits.[52,54,58,59]

Multiple studies followed patients longitudinally after the initial assessment and thus were able to examine the longer-term utilization and cost impacts of assessment and treatment. Some studies found an overall reduction in nursing home days.[47,59,65,66] Hospital utilization was examined in several reports. For hospital-based GAPs, the length of hospitalization was obviously affected by the length of the assessment itself. Thus, some programs appear to prolong initial length of stay[45,67,68] while others reduce initial stay.[53,59–61,69] However, studies following patients for at least 1 year have usually shown reduction in use of acute-care hospital services, even in those programs with initially prolonged hospital stays.[41,48,57]

Compensatory increases in use of community-based services or home-care agencies might be expected with declines in nursing home placements and use of other institutional services. These increases have been detected in several studies[48,50,55,70] but not in others.[47,57,62] Although increased use of formal community services may not always be indicated, it usually is a desirable goal. The fact that several studies did not detect increases in use of home and community services probably reflects the unavailability of community service or referral networks rather than that more of such services were not needed.

The effects of these programs on costs and utilization parameters have only seldom been examined comprehensively, owing to methodological difficulties in gathering comprehensive utilization and cost data, as well as statistical limitations in comparing highly skewed distributions. The Sepulveda study found that total first-year direct healthcare costs had been reduced owing to overall reductions in nursing home and rehospitalization days, despite significantly longer initial hospital stays on the geriatric unit.[47] These savings continued through 3 years of follow-up.[63] Hendriksen's program[48] reduced the costs of medical care, apparently through successful early case-finding and referral for preventive intervention. Williams' outpatient GAP[57] detected reductions in medical care costs owing primarily to reductions in hospitalization. Although it would be reasonable to worry that prolonged survival of frail patients would lead to increased service use and charges—or, of perhaps greater concern, to worry about the quality of the prolonged life—these concerns may be without substance. Indeed, the Sepulveda study demonstrated that a GAP could improve not only survival but prolong high-function survival,[47,63] while at the same time reducing use of institutional services and costs.

A 1993 meta-analysis attempted to resolve some of the discrepancies between study results, and to try to identify whether particular program elements were associated with particular benefits.[72,73] This meta-analysis included published data from the 28 controlled trials completed as of that date, involving nearly 10,000 patients, and was also able to include substantial amounts of unpublished data systematically retrieved from many of the studies. The meta-analysis identified five GAP types: hospital units (six studies), hospital consultation teams (eight studies), in-home assessment services (seven studies), outpatient assessment services (four studies), and "hospital–home assessment services" (three studies), the latter of which performed in-home assessments on patients recently discharged from hospitals. The meta-analysis confirmed many of the major reported benefits for many of the individual program types. These statistically and clinically significant benefits included reduced risk of mortality (by 22 percent for hospital-based programs at 12 months, and by 14 percent for all programs combined at 12 months), improved likelihood of living at home (by 47 percent for hospital-based programs and by 26 percent for all programs combined at 12 months), reduced risk of hospital (re)admissions (by 12 percent for all programs at study end), greater chance of cognitive improvement (by 47 percent for all programs at study end), and greater chance of physical function improvement for patients on hospital units (by 72 percent for hospital units).

Clearly not all studies showed equivalent effects, and the meta-analysis was able to indicate a number of variables at both the program and patient levels that tended to distinguish trials with large effects from ones with more limited ones.

When examined on the program level, hospital units and home-visit assessment teams produced the most dramatic benefits, while no major significant benefits in office-based programs could be confirmed. Programs that provided hands-on clinical care and/or long-term follow-up were generally able to produce greater positive effects than purely consultative programs or ones that lacked follow-up. Another factor associated with greater demonstrated benefits, at least in hospital-based programs, was patient targeting; programs that selected patients who were at high risk for deterioration yet still had "rehabilitation potential" generally had stronger results than less selective programs.

The meta-analysis confirmed the importance of targeting criteria in producing beneficial outcomes. In particular, when use of explicit targeting criteria for patient selection was included as a covariate, increases in some program benefits were often found. For example, among the hospital-based GAPs studies, positive effects on physical function and likelihood of living at home at 12 months were associated with studies that excluded patients who were relatively "too healthy." A similar effect on physical function was seen in the institutional studies that excluded persons with relatively poor prognoses. The reason for this effect of targeting on effect size no doubt lies in the ability of careful targeting to concentrate the intervention on patients who can benefit, without diluting the effect with persons too ill or too well to show a measurable improvement.

Studies performed after the meta-analysis have been largely corroborative. However, with principles of geriatric medicine becoming more diffused into usual care, particularly at places where controlled trials are being undertaken, differences between GAPs and control groups seem to be narrowing.[74–79] For cost reasons, growth of inpatient units has been slow, despite their proven effectiveness, while outpatient programs have increased, despite their less impressive effect size in controlled trials. However, some newer trials of outpatient programs have shown significant benefits in areas not found in earlier outpatient studies, such as functional status, psychological parameters, and well-being, which may indicate improvement in the outpatient-care models being tested.[75–79]

A continuing challenge has been obtaining adequate financing to support adding geriatric assessment services to existing medical care. Despite GAPs' many proven benefits, and their ability to reduce costs documented in controlled trials, health-care financiers have been reluctant to fund geriatric assessment programs—presumably out of concern that the programs might be expanded too fast and that costs for extra diagnostic and therapeutic services might increase out of control. Many practitioners have found ways to "unbundle" the GA process into component services and receive adequate support to fund the entire process. In this continuing time of fiscal restraint, geriatric practitioners must remain constantly creative in order to reach the goal of optimal patient care.

CONCLUSION

Published studies of comprehensive geriatric assessment have confirmed its efficacy in many settings. While there is no single optimal blueprint for geriatric assessment, the participation of the multidisciplinary team and the focus on functional status and quality of life as major clinical goals are common to all settings. Although the greatest benefits have been found in programs targeted to the frail subgroup of elderly people, a strong case can be made for a continuum of GAPs—screening assessments performed periodically for all older persons and comprehensive assessment targeted to frail and high-risk patients. Clinicians interested in developing these services will do well to heed the experiences of the programs reviewed here in adapting the principles of geriatric assessment to local resources. Future research is still needed to determine the most effective and efficient methods for performing geriatric assessment and on developing strategies for best matching needs with services.

KEY POINTS Geriatric assessment

- Geriatric assessment is a systematic multidimensional approach to improving diagnostic accuracy and planning care for frail elderly people.

- Controlled trials have documented many benefits from geriatric assessment, including, improved functional status and survival and reduced hospital and nursing-home admissions.

REFERENCES

1. Rubenstein LV, Calkins DR, Greenfield S et al: Health status assessment for elderly patients: reports of the society of general internal medicine task force on health assessment. J Am Geriatr Soc 1989;37:562–569
2. Matthews DA: Dr Marjory Warren and the origin of British geriatrics. J Am Geriatr Soc 1984;32:253–258
3. Brocklehurst JC: Geriatric care in advanced societies. MTP, Lancaster University Park Press, Baltimore, 1975
4. Canadian Task Force on the Periodic Health Examination: Can Med Assoc J 1979;121:1193–1254
5. Rubenstein LZ, Josephson KR, Nichol-Seamons M, Robbins AS: Comprehensive health screening of well elderly adults. J Gerontol 1986;41:343–352
6. US Congress, Office of Technology Assessment: Preventive Health Services for Medicare Beneficiaries: Policy and Research Issues (OTA-H-416). US Government Printing Office, Washington, DC, 1990
7. Rubenstein LV: Using quality of life tests for patient diagnosis or screening. In Spilker B (ed): Quality of Life and Pharmacoeconomics in Clinical Trials, 2nd edn. JB Lippincott, Philadelphia, 1996
8. Rubenstein LZ, Campbell LJ, Kane RL: Geriatric Assessment. WB Saunders, Philadelphia, 1987
9. Rubenstein LZ, Wieland D, Bernabei R: Geriatric Assessment Technology: The State of the Art. Kurtis Publishers, Milan, 1995
10. Kane RL, Kane RA: Assessing Older Persons. Oxford University Press, New York, 2000
11. Osterweil D, Brummel-Smith K, Beck JC: Comprehensive Geriatric Assessment. McGraw-Hill, New York, 2000
12. Gallo JJ, Fulmer T, Paveza GJ, Reichel W: Handbook of geriatric assessment, 3rd edn. Aspen Publishers, Rockville, MD, 2000
13. Katz S, Ford AB, Moskowitz RW et al: Studies of illness in the aged. The index of ADL: a standardized measure of biological psychosocial function. JAMA 1963;185:914–919
14. Lawton MP, Brody EM: Assessment of older people: self-maintaining and instrumental activities of daily living. Gerontologist 1969;9:179–186
15. Mahoney FI, Barthel DW: Functional evaluation—the Barthel Index. Maryland State Med J 1965;14:61–65
16. Wade DT, Colin C: The Barthel ADL Index—a standard measure of physical disability. Int Disabil Studies 1988;10:64–67
17. Tinetti ME: Performance oriented assessment of mobility problems in elderly patients. J Am Geriatr Soc 1986;34:119–126
18. Mathias S, Nayak USL, Isaacs B: Balance in elderly patients: the "get up and go" test. Arch Phys Med Rehab 1986;67:387–389

19. Vellas B, Guigoz Y: Nutritional assessment as part of the geriatric evaluation. In Geriatric Assessment Technology: The State of the Art. Kurtis Publishers, Milan, 1995

20. Folstein M, Folstein S, McHugh P: Mini-mental state: a practical method for grading the cognitive state of patients for the clinician. J Psychiatr Res 1975;12:189–198

21. Yesavage J, Brink T, Rose T et al: Development and validation of a geriatric screening scale: a preliminary report. J Psychiatr Res 1983;17:37–49

22. Zung WWK: A self rating depression scale. Arch Gen Psychiatr 1965;12:63–70

23. Hoyl T, Alessi CA, Harker JO et al. Development and testing of a 5-item version of the geriatric depression scale. J Am Geriatr Soc 1999;47:873–878

24. Hedrick SC: Assessment of functional status: activities of daily living. In Rubenstein LZ, Wieland D, Bernabei R (eds): Geriatric Assessment Technology: The State of the Art. Kurtis Publishers, Milan, 1995

25. Kane RA: Assessment of social function: recommendations for comprehensive geriatric assessment. In Rubenstein LZ, Wieland D, Bernabei R (eds): Geriatric Assessment Technology: The State of the Art. Kurtis Publishers, Milan, 1995

26. Rubenstein LZ, Harker JO, Salva A, Guigoz Y, Vellas B: Screening for undernutrition in geriatric practice: developing the short-form Mini-nutritional Assessment (MNA-SF). J Gerontol A 2001;56:M366–M372

27. Gurland BH, Wilder D: Detection and assessment of cognitive impairment and depressed mood in older adults. In Rubenstein LZ, Wieland D, Bernabei R (eds): Geriatric Assessment Technology: The State of the Art. Kurtis Publishers, Milan, 1995

28. Duke University Center for the Study of Aging and Human Development: The OARS Methodology. Duke University Press, Durham, NC, 1978

29. Lubben JE: Assessing social networks among elderly populations. Fam Commun Health 1988;8:42–52

30. Kahn R, Goldfarb A, Pollack M et al: Brief objective measures of mental status in the aged. Am J Psychiatr 1960;117:326–328

31. Chambers LW, MacDonald LA, Tugwell P et al: The McMaster Health Index Questionnaire as a measure of quality of life for patients with rheumatoid disease. J Rheumatol 1982;9:780–784

32. Reisberg B, Ferris SH, DeLeon MJ et al: The global deterioration scale for assessment of primary degenerative dementia. Am J Psychiatr 1982;139:1136–1139

33. Hoehn MM, Yahr MD: Parkinsonism: onset, progression, and mortality. Neurology 1967;17:427–442

34. Stewart AL, Hays RD, Ware JE: Communication: the MOS short-form general health survey: reliability and validity in a patient population. Med Care 1988;26:724–735

35. Nelson E, Wasson J, Kirk J et al: Assessment of function in routine clinical practice: description of the Coop chart method and preliminary findings. J Chron Dis 1987;40:55S

36. Bergner M, Bobbit R, Carter WB: The sickness impact profile: validation of a health status measure. Med Care 1981;19:787–805

37. Jette AM, Davies AR, Calkins DR et al: The functional status questionnaire: reliability and validity when used in primary care. J Gen Intern Med 1986;1:143

38. Van Swearington JM, Brach JS: Making geriatric assessment work: selecting useful measures. Phys Ther 2001;81:1233–1252

39. Campbell LJ, Cole KD: Geriatric assessment teams. Clin Geriatr Med 1987;3:99–110

40. Wieland D, Kramer BJ, Waite MS, Rubenstein LZ: The interdisciplinary team in geriatric care. Am Behav Sci 1996;39:655–664

41. William J, Stokoe IH, Gray S et al: Old people at home: their unreported needs. Lancet 1964;i:1117–1120

42. Lowther CP, MacLeod RDM, Williamson J: Evaluation of early diagnostic services for the elderly. BMJ 1970;3:275–277

43. Brocklehurst JC, Carty MH, Leeming JT, Robinson JH: Medical screening of old people accepted for residential care. Lancet 1978;ii:141–143

44. Applegate WB, Akins D, Vander Zwaag R et al: A geriatric rehabilitation and assessment unit in a community hospital. J Am Geriatr Soc 1983;31:206–210

45. Rubenstein LZ, Josephson KR, Wieland GD et al: Geriatric assessment on a subacute hospital ward. Clin Geriatr Med 1987;3:131–143

46. Williams TF, Hill JH, Fairbank ME, Knox KG: Appropriate placement of the chronically ill and aged: a successful approach by evaluation. JAMA 1973;266:1332–1335

47. Rubenstein LZ, Josephson KR, Wieland GD et al: Effectiveness of a geriatric evaluation unit: a randomized clinical trial. N Engl J Med 1984;311:1664–1670

48. Hendriksen C, Lund E, Stromgard E: Consequences of assessment and intervention among elderly people: three-year randomized controlled trial. BMJ 1984;289:1522–1524

49. Thomas DR, Brahan R, Haywood BP: Inpatient community-based geriatric assessment reduces subsequent mortality. J Am Geriatr Soc 1993;41:101–104

50. Vetter NJ, Jones DA, Victor CR: Effects of health visitors working with elderly patients in general practice: a randomized controlled trial. BMJ 1984;288:369–372

51. Vetter NJ, Lewis PA, Ford D: Can health visitors prevent fractures in elderly people? BMJ 1992;304:888–890

52. Winograd CH, Gerety M, Lai N: A negative trial of inpatient geriatric consultation: lessons learned. Arch Intern Med 1993;153:2017–2023

53. Collard AF, Bachman SS, Beatrice DF: Acute care delivery for the geriatric patient: an innovative approach. Qual Rev Bull 1985;(June):180–185

54. Allen CC, Becker PM, McVey LJ et al: A randomized controlled clinical trial of a geriatric consultation team: compliance with recommendations. JAMA 1986;255:2617–2621

55. Hogan DB, Fox RA, Badley BWD, Mann OE: Effect of a geriatric consultation service on management of patients in an acute care hospital. Can Med Assoc J 1987;136:713–717

56. Hogan DB, Fox RA: A prospective controlled trial of a geriatric consultation team in an acute care hospital. Age Ageing 1990;19:107–113

57. Williams ME, Williams TF, Zimmer JG et al: How does the team approach to outpatient geriatric evaluation compare with traditional care: a report of a randomized controlled trial. J Am Geriatr Soc 1987;35:1071–1078

58. Gilchrist WJ, Newman RH, Hamblen DL, Williams BO: Prospective randomized study of an orthopaedic geriatric inpatient service. BMJ 1988;297:1116–1118

59. Reid J, Kennie DC: Geriatric rehabilitative care after fractures of the proximal femur: one-year follow-up of a randomized clinical trial. BMJ 1989;299:25–26

60. Pathy MSJ, Bayer A, Harding K, Dibble A: Randomized trial of case finding and surveillance of elderly people at home. Lancet 1992;340:890–893

61. Hansen FR, Spedtsberg K, Schroll M: Geriatric follow-up by home visits after discharge from hospital: a randomized controlled trial. Age Ageing 1992;21:445–450

62. Gayton D, Wood-Dauphine S, de Lorimer M et al: Trial of a geriatric consultation team in an acute care hospital. J Am Geriatr Soc 1987;35:726–736

63. Rubenstein LZ, Josephson KR, Harker JO, Wieland D: The Sepulveda GEU study revisited: long-term outcomes, use of services, and costs. Aging: Clin Exp Res 1995;7:212–217

64. Rubenstein LZ, Wieland D, Josephson KR et al: Improved survival for frail elderly inpatients on a geriatric evaluation unit (GEU): who benefits? J Clin Epidemiol 1988;41:441–449

65. Schuman JE, Beattie EJ, Steed DA et al: The impact of a new geriatric program in a hospital for the chronically ill. Can Med Assoc J 1978;118:639–645

66. Lefton E, Bonstelle S, Frengley JD: Success with an inpatient geriatric unit: a controlled study. J Am Geriatr Soc 1983;31:149–155

67. Berkman B, Campion E, Swagerty E, Goldman M: Geriatric consultation teams: alternative approach to social work discharge planning. J Gerontol Soc Work 1983;5:77–88

68. Lichtenstein H, Winograd CH: Geriatric consultation: a functional approach. J Am Geriatr Soc 1984;32:356–361

69. Burley LE, Currie CT, Smith RG, Williamson J: Contribution from geriatric medicine within acute medical wards. BMJ 1979;263:90–92

70. Tulloch AH, Moore V: A randomized controlled trial of geriatric screening and surveillance in general practice. J R Col General Pract 1979;29:733–742

71. Rubenstein LZ, Wieland D, Bernabei R: Geriatric assessment: international research prospective. Aging: Clin Exp Res 1995;7:157–260

72. Stuck AE, Siu AL, Wieland GD et al: Comprehensive geriatric assessment: a meta-analysis of controlled trials. Lancet 1993;342:1032–1036

73. Stuck AE, Wieland D, Rubenstein LZ et al: Comprehensive geriatric assessment: meta-analysis of main effects and elements enhancing effectiveness. In Rubenstein LZ, Wieland D, Bernabei R (eds): Geriatric Assessment Technology: The State of the Art. Kurtis Publishers, Milan, 1995

74. Reuben DB, Borok GM, Wolde GT et al: A randomized clinical trial of comprehensive geriatric assessment consultation for hospitalized HMO patients. N Engl J Med 1995;332:1345–1350

75. Burns R, Nichols LO, Martindale-Adams J et al: Interdisciplinary geriatric primary care evaluation and management: two-year outcomes. J Am Geriatr Soc 2000;48:8–13

76. Stuck AE, Minder CE, Peter-Wuest I et al: A randomized trial of in-home visits for disability prevention in community-dwelling older people at low and high risk for nursing home admission. Arch Intern Med 2000;160:977–986

77. Boult C, Boult LB, Morishita L et al: A randomized clinical trial of outpatient geriatric evaluation and management. J Am Geriatr Soc 2001;49:351–359

78. Elkan R, Kendrick D, Dewey M et al: Effectiveness of home-based support for older people: systematic review and meta-analysis. BMJ 2000;323:1–9

79. Rubenstein LZ, Stuck AE: Preventive home visits for older people: defining criteria for success. Age Ageing 2001;30:107–109

Chapter 27

Biochemical tests

Laszlo Sarkozi and Lakshmi Ramanathan

Biochemical tests are performed on various body fluids, for several purposes. They are useful in physiological assessment, diagnosis and treatment of diseases, and for monitoring therapeutic drug levels. A measured or observed laboratory test result from an individual is compared with a reference value.[1] Previously used terms, such as "normal value" and "normal range," are based on assumptions. Statistical distribution of biological data most often does not fall into the gaussian symmetric "normal" bell-shaped distribution curve. In addition, by definition of the "95th percentile range," 5 percent of healthy individuals fall outside the normal range. Reference intervals (a range of values obtained from the reference value set) are based on the recommendations of the Expert Panel on Theory of Reference Values of the International Federation of Clinical Chemistry, and the published guidelines of the National Committee for Clinical Laboratory Standards, C28-P.[2]

Gradual physiological changes that occur over time as part of the aging process affect several analytes. With the introduction of clinical laboratory automation and large-scale multiphasic screening programs during the 1960s, it became possible to collect a sufficient database to document age- and sex-dependent changes and reference intervals for most biochemical diagnostic tests.[3–5]

PREANALYTIC AND ANALYTIC VARIABLES

Biochemical test results are collected from reference populations under controlled preanalytic and analytic variables. Similarly, specimens from a patient population must be obtained and processed under controlled circumstances. Several of the preanalytic variables to be considered are listed in Table 27-1.[2,6] Some of the variables might be more characteristic in the elderly population.

Drug regimen

The most commonly ignored preanalytic variable is the fact that elderly subjects are often on a drug regimen. Law and Chalmers[7] found in 1976 that, in Great Britain, 87 percent of people over 75 years old living at home were on medication and 34 percent were on at least three different drugs daily. Drugs may have in-vivo and/or in-vitro effects on biochemical tests. Young[8] provides an updated list of these effects with very extensive references.

Multiple disease and severe illness

Reference values are helpful in ruling out certain diagnoses. Values outside the reference may not be as valuable owing to their lack of specificity. Several analytes, especially some

Table 27-1 **Selected preanalytic variables**		
Subject preparation	**Specimen collection**	**Specimen handling**
Prior diet	Environmental conditions	Clotting
Fasting or nonfasting	Time	Transport
Drug regimen	Body posture	Centrifugation
Biological rhythms	Specimen type	Storage
Physical activity	Collection site	Preparation for analysis
Stress	Technique	

From National Committee for Clinical Laboratory Standards,[2] with permission of Blackwell Science, Inc.

elevated enzyme activities, may be the result of a chronic condition, eliminating their diagnostic utility.[9] Dehydration is a frequent condition in elderly people, with concurrent effect on renal function and homeostasis.

Recent hospitalization or prolonged bed rest

Calcium, sodium, potassium, and phosphate excretions are decreased, presumably owing to decreased metabolism of skeletal muscle.[10] Fluid retention may result in decreased serum protein and albumin concentrations and, correspondingly, reduction of protein-bound constituents.

GERIATRIC REFERENCE VALUES

A comprehensive book (86 contributors) on geriatric clinical chemistry presented data on 134 analytes.[11] Tietz et al.[12] determined 15,000 laboratory values in 236 individuals between the ages of 60 and 90 years, 22 individuals between 90 and 99 years, and 69 individuals at 100 years and above—an unprecedented wealth of information. They avoided the use of the term "reference ranges" in the group of nonagenarians and centenarians. It is difficult to distinguish between symptoms of a disease and normal manifestation of aging. The selected individuals 90 years old or younger appeared to be mentally and physically fit and mobile; 72 of them had some health problems or some diseases that were controlled by medication. Although the number of observations in the groups aged over 90 years may not satisfy statistical requirements,[13] nevertheless, this is the first published data on these groups and presents valuable information. The reports are compiled into a simplified format in Table 27-2. This chapter discusses only the tests whose mean values significantly differ from the young adult population.

Table 27-2 Laboratory ranges (95th percentile) and mean values of young adults, 60- to 90-year-olds, and those 90 years and older

Analyte	Method	Sex	Young adults Range	Young adults Mean	60–90 Range	60–90 Mean	>90 Range	>90 Mean
Albumin, g/L	Rate nephelometry	M + F	34–48	41	32–46	40	29–45	36
Albumin, urine, mg/L	Rate nephelometry	M + F	2–24	6.7			1–100	21
Albumin/creatinine, urine, g/mol		M + F	0.22–1.48	0.57			0.3–12.2	3.0
α_1-Antitrypsin, g/L	Rate nephelometry	M	0.40–2.05	1.41			1.22–2.50	1.78
		F	0.64–2.53	1.53			1.30–2.36	1.80
ALP, U/L	PNPP substrate AMP buffer, 37°C	M	53–128	85	56–119	81	56–155	97
		F	42–98M	67	53–141	82	43–160	92
Amylase, U/L	Maltotetraose, 37°C	M + F	27–131	65	24–151	71		
	PNP-α-MP, PNP-α-MH, 37°C	M + F	20–104	55			25–147	73
ALT, U/L	Oxidation of NADH P-5'-P, 37°C	M	10–40	20			6–38	14
		F	7–35	12			5–24	13
	Oxidation of NADH 30°C	M	6–16	11	7–24	11.2		
		F	6–16	9	7–16	8.7		
Amylase P-type, U/L	PNP-α-MP, PNP-α-MH, and wheat germ inhibitor 37°C	M + F	27–70	48			<10–82	39
Andostenedione, ng/L	RIA after selective solvent extraction	M	750–2050				270–1160	681
		F	850–2750				30–2250	566
nmol/L		M	2.6–7.2				0.9–4.1	2.4
		F	3.0–9.6				0.1–7.9	2.0
AST, U/L	Oxidation of NADH P-5'-P, 37°C	M	16–42	24.6			11–38	25
		F	14–29	19			18–30	24
	Oxidation of NADH, 30°C	M	10–20	14	11–26	14.7		
		F	9–20	13	10–20	14.2		
Bilirubin, total mg/L	Modified Jendrassik–Grof	M + F	3–12	6	2–11	5	2–9	4.2
μmol/L			15–21	10	3–19	9	3–15	7
Bilirubin, conjugated mg/L	Jendrassik–Grof	M + F	1–3	2	<1–1	1	<1–2	1.1
μmol/L			2–5	3	<2	2	<2–3	2
C3 activator, mg/L	Rate nephelometry	M + F	200–470	320	220–440	330	220–480	325
Calcium, total mmol/L	o-Cresolphtalein complexone	M + F	2.15–2.50	2.30	2.20–2.55	2.35	2.05–2.40	2.25
Calcium, ionized, mmol/L	Ion-selective electrode	M + F	1.15–1.27	1.21	1.16–1.29	1.22	1.12–1.32	1.22
CEA, μg/L	Solid-phase immunoenzymatic assay	M + F	Nonsmoker 0–3 Smoker 0–5				0.4–9.2	3.8
Ceruloplasmin, mg/L	Rate nephelometry	M	180–480	280			160–450	320
		F	200–560	340			240–460	350
Cholesterol, total, mg/L	Cholesterol oxidase	M	1290–2780 (recommended <2000)	1920	1670–3360	2270	1110–2560	1790
		F	1260–2800 (recommended <2000)	1750	1680–3480	2460	1480–2690	2010
Cholesterol, total, mmol/L		M	3.34–7.19 (recommended <5.17)	4.97	4.32–8.69	5.87	2.87–6.62	4.63
		F	3.26–6.83 (recommended <5.17)	4.53	4.34–9.00	6.36	3.83–6.96	5.20

Table 27-2 (Continued)

Analyte	Method	Sex	Young adults Range	Young adults Mean	60–90 Range	60–90 Mean	>90 Range	>90 Mean
Cl, mmol/L	Mercuric thiocyan.	M + F	98–107	103	98–107	103	98–111	104
CK, U/L	Reduction of	M	52–200	112			21–203	50
	NADP, 37°C	F	35–165	85			22–99	40
	Reduction of	M	25–80	53	20–110			
	NADP, 30°C	F	20–75	38	16–81			
CO_2, mmol/L	Cresol red	M + F	23–29	26	23–31	27		
	Enzymatic oxidation	M + F	20–29	25			20–29	26
Complement C_3, g/L	Rate nephelometry	M + F	0.78–1.75	1.16	0.82–1.70	1.19	0.82–1.58	1.05
Complement C_4, mg/L	Rate nephelometry	M	120–540	260			120–350	210
		F	110–340	220			140–420	240
Copper, µg/L	AAS	M	700–1400		860–1730	1330	50–1840	1390
		F	800–1550		1070–1890	1500	1000–1970	1490
µmol/L		M	11.0–22.0		13.5–27.2	20.9	11.8–29.0	21.9
		F	12.6–24.4		16.8–29.7	23.6	15.7–31.0	23.5
Corticobinding globulin (transcortin), µg/L	RIA in dilute serum	M + F	23–39				12–29	
Corticotropin, ng/L	RIA	M + F	0–100				10–106	40
pmol/L			0–22				2–23	9
Cortisol, µg/L	RIA, competitive binding	M + F	50–230	150	78–225	140	56–230	140
nmol/L			138–635	414	215–621	386	154–635	386
C-peptide, µg/L	RIA, competitive binding	M + F	1.4–4.3	2.3	1.5–4.9	2.7	0.6–4.4	2.1
Creatinine serum mg/L	Jaffe, rate	M	9–13	11	8–13	10	10–17	12
		F	6–11	9	6–12	8	6–13	9
µmol/L		M	80–115	97	71–115	88	188–150	106
		F	53–97	80	53–106	71	53–115	80
DHEA, µg/L	RIA after column chromatography	M + F	1.60–8.00				0.17–1.69	0.79
nmol/L			5.5–27.8				0.6–5.9	2.7
DHEAS, µg/L	RIA in dilute serum after hydrolysis	M	1800–4500				40–750	287
		F	1200–3150				20–600	231
µmol/L		M	4.9–12.2				0.1–2.0	0.8
		F	3.3–8.5				0.1–1.6	0.6
Estradiol, ng/L	RIA after column chromatography	F	Follicular: 30–100				<5–20	6
			Luteal: 70–300					
pmol/L			Follicular: 110–367					
			Luteal: 257–1,101				<18–73	22
Estrone, ng/L	RIA after column chromatography	F	Follicular: 30–100				<5–58	29
			Luteal: 90–160					
pmol/L			Follicular: 110–370					
			Luteal: 333–592				<18–215107	
Folate, serum µg/L	RIA, competitive binding	M	3.2–12.4	7.0	1.6–10.8	5.2	3.3–16.0	7.8
		F	3.2–15.9	7.7	1.8–12.2	5.7	3.0–16.0	8.8
nmol/L		M	7–28	16	4–24	12	8–36	18
		F	7–36	17	4–28	13	7–36	20
FSH, milli-int. units/L	RIA	M	2.2–14.0	6.5			8–112	53
		F	(Midcycle: 12–33)				66–168	111
γ-Globulin, g/L	Electrophoresis	M + F	6.0–14	9	6.0–16.0	10.0	5.0–16.0	10.0
Gastrin, ng/L	RIA, competitive binding	M + F	0–100	171	100–800		40–150	80
GGT, U/L	g-Glutamyl p-nitroanilide and glycylglycerine, 37°C	M	10–34	19	11–42	25		
		F	7–30	13	9–55	23		
	g-Glutamyl p-nitroanilide and glycylglycerine, 30°C	M	7–47	17			3–47	15
		F	4–25	11			4–44	15

Table 27-2 (Continued)

Analyte	Method	Sex	Young adults		60–90		>90	
			Range	Mean	Range	Mean	Range	Mean
Glucose, mg/L	Hexokinase	M + F	780–1050	920	820–1150	950		
mmol/L			4.3–5.8	5.1	4.6–6.4	5.3		
mg/L	Glucose oxidase	M + F	740–1060	890			750–1210	960
mmol/L			4.1–5.9	4.9			4.2–6.7	5.3
HDL cholesterol, mg/L	Cholesterol oxidase after PEG precipitation	M	200–690 (recommended 280–700)	420	280–1060	480	280–820	450
		F	270–850 (recommended 370–910)	530	280–1040	630	320–830	525
mmol/L		M	0.52–1.78 (recommended 0.72–1.81)	1.09	0.72–2.53	1.24	0.72–2.12	1.16
		F	0.70–2.20 (recommended 0.96–2.35)	1.37	0.72–2.69	1.63	0.83–2.15	1.36
HDL cholesterol, %	Calculated	M	9–43 (Low risk: >37)	23	11–40	22	13–45	25.5
		F	14–54 (Low risk: >40)	31	12–45	26	14–43	26
Hemoglobin, g/L	Coulter counter	M	140–180				121–171	140
		F	120–160				107–151	131
Hematocrit, %	Coulter counter	M	40–54				36–51	42
		F	37–47				32–46	39
Heptaglobulin, g/L	Rate nephelometry	M + F	0.28–1.78	0.94	0.36–1.73	1.08	0.22–1.97	1.15
Iron, µg/L	Colorimetric, ICSH method	M	600–1700	920			400–1290	870
		F	450–1600	970			350–1330	860
µmol/L		M	11–30	16			7–23	16
		F	8–29	17			6–30	15
IgA, g/L	Rate nephelometry	M	0.76–5.46	2.31			0.94–9.56	3.28
		F	0.74–4.20	1.99			0.98–8.18	2.95
IgD, mg/L	Radial immunodiffusion	M + F	0–80				0–60	10
IgE, Roto-int. units/L	Two-site sandwich immunoassay	M + F	0.7–463	71.5			1.2–352	69
IgG, g/L	Rate nephelometry	M	7.36–13.86	10.32			1.56–17.50	12.06
		F	6.95–16.70	11.00			3.88–18.85	12.00
IgG, urine mg/L	Fixed-time nephelometry	M + F	<8.0				5.0–38	8.0
IgM, g/L	Rate nephelometry	M	0.52–2.99	1.48			0.28–1.98	0.91
		F	0.46–3.90	1.69			0.42–2.90	1.05
Insulin, mU/L	RIA, competitive binding	M + F	6–23	11.8	6.6–36.7	16.4	2.4–19.0	7.2
pmol/L		M + F	43–165	85	47–263	118	17–136	52
K, mmol/L	Flame emission	M + F	3.8–4.9	4.3	3.9–5.3	4.5		
	Ion select. electrode	M + F	3.7–4.8	4.3			3.6–5.5	4.4
LD, U/L	L → P, colorimetric (AM Blue 610), 37°C	M + F	93–184	138			99–284	163
	Reduction of NADP, 30°C	M + F	48–102	69	55–104	76		
Lead, µg/L	AAS	M + F	<250				<150	
µmol/L			<1.21				<0.72	
LH, milli-int. units/L	RIA	M	2.5–19.7	8.9			19–115	53
		F	3.5–31.0 (midcycle: 48–175)	8			35–154	82
Lipase, U/L	Turbidimetric, 30°C	M + F	13–141	63	0–302			
	Modified turbidimetric 30°C	M + F	31–186	82			26–267	104
Magnesium, mg/L	AAS	M + F	16–25		16–24	20	17–23	20
mmol/L			0.66–1.03		0.66–0.79	0.82	0.70–0.95	0.82

Table 27-2 (Continued)

Analyte	Method	Sex	Young adults Range	Mean	60–90 Range	Mean	>90 Range	Mean
Microsomal antibodies	Hemagglutination	M + F	Negative				6.9% positive	
Na, mmol/L	Flame emission	M + F	137–143	140			137–144	140
	Ion select. electrode	M + F	138–144	141			132–146	141
Osmolality, serum mOsm/kg	Freezing-point depression	M + F	278–299	286	280–301	290	277–301	290
pH	Potentiometric	M + F	7.35–7.45		7.31–7.42	7.37	7.26–7.43	7.35
Phosphorus, mmol/L	Molybdenum blue	M	0.87–1.32	1.07	0.74–1.20	0.97	0.71–1.26	0.97
		F	0.84–1.29	1.07	0.90–1.29	1.10	0.81–1.36	1.10
Prealbumin, mg/L	Rate nephelometry	M	200–400	280			150–300	220
		F	150–290	220			140–360	230
Progesterone, ng/L	RIA after selective solvent extraction	M	130–970				<200–480	
		F	Follicular: 150–700 Luteal: 2000–25,000				<200–540<	
nmol/L		M	0.4–3.1				<0.6–1.5	
		F	Follicular: 0.5–2.2 Luteal: 6.4–79.5				<0.6–1.7	
Prolactin, µg/L	IRMA	M	3.9–22.1	9.5			8–25	15.5
		F	3.5–27.0	11.5			7–53	18
Prostatic acid phosphatase, mg/L	Solid-phase enzyme immunoassay	M + F	<2.0				0–3.2	0.7
PTH, pmol/ng midmolecule	RIA, competitive binding	M + F	36–86	54			49–118	71
RBP, mg/L	Radial immunodiffusion	M	34–88	58			26–96	56
		F	25–81	45			31–91	52
Sex hormone-binding globulin, µg/L	Competitive binding assay	M	9–19				11–45	23
		F	10–30				11–60	26
T₃, µg/L	RIA	M + F	1.12–2.12	1.56	1.00–2.00	1.43		
nmol/L			1.7–3.3	2.4	1.5–3.1	2.2		
µg/L		M + F	1.02–2.05	1.52			0.70–1.66	1.13
nmol/L			1.6–3.1	2.3			1.1–2.5	1.7
T₄, µg/L	RIA	M + F	50–120	81	50–107	78		
nmol/L			64–154	104	64–138	100		
µg/L		M	46–105	74				
		F	55–110	78				
nmol/L		M	59–135	95			53–100	74
		F	71–142	100			68–129	95
TBG, mg/L	Two-site IRMA	M + F	16–34	22.6			18–29	22
Testosterone, free, ng/L	Equilibrium dialysis	M	52–280				11.8–74.6	26.7
pmol/L			180.3–971.8				40.9–258.8	92.6
Testosterone, % free	Calculated	M	1.5–3.2				0.4–1.3	0.8
Testosterone, bioactive, µg/L	Competitive binding assay of non-SHBG bound fraction	M	1.28–4.30				0.27–1.76	0.67
nmol/L			4.4–14.9				0.9–6.1	2.3
Testosterone, % bioactive	Calculated	M	36.6–41.7				10.0–33.7	20.2
		F	11.0–26.0				8.2–28.2	16.5
Testosterone, total, µg/L	RIA after column chromatography	M	3.50–10.30				2.15–6.71	3.40
nmol/L			12.1–35.7				7.5–23.3	11.9
Thyroglobulin antibodies	Hemagglutination	M + F	Negative				17.2% positive	
Total protein, g/L	Biuret	M + F	63–78	70	62–77		60–80	
Transferrin, g/L	Rate nephelometry	M + F	2.57–4.29	3.22	1.91–3.75	2.73	1.86–3.47	2.64
Triglycerides, mg/L	GPO Trinder	M	410–1930 (recommended 400–1600)	1010	310–3500	1250	770–1110	940
		F	300–1850 (recommended 350–1350)	820	350–3380	1090	430–1440	1090

Table 27-2 (Continued)

Analyte	Method	Sex	Young adults		60–90		>90	
			Range	Mean	Range	Mean	Range	Mean
mmol/L		M	0.46–2.18 (recommended 0.45–1.81)	1.14	0.18–4.20	1.41	0.87–1.25	1.06
		F	0.23–2.15 (recommended 0.40–1.52)	0.93	0.40–3.82	1.23	0.49–1.63	1.23
Trypsin, μg/L	RIA	M + F	11–55	28	16–76	38		
nmol/L		M + F	0.5–2.3	1.2	0.8–3.2	1.5		
TSH, milli-int. units/L	RIA	M + F	1.8–8.8	4.7	2.1–15.5	5.2		
	Two-site IRMA	M + F	0.7–7.0	2.8			0.4–7.2	2.8
Urea nitrogen, serum mg/L	o-Phthalaldehyde reaction	M + F	60–210	122	80–230	150	100–310	197
nmol/L			2.1–7.1	4.4	2.9–8.2	5.4	3.6–11.1	7.0
Uric acid, mg/L	Reduction of phosphotungstate	M	44–76	62	42–80	61	35–83	60.5
		F	23–66	43	35–73	51	22–77	50
μmol/L		M	262–452	369	250–476	363	208–494	357
		F	137–393	256	208–434	303	131–458	297
Vitamin B$_{12}$, ng/L	RIA, competitive binding	M + F	128–701	399	110–769	380	58–872	318
pmol/L			94–517	294	81–567	280	43–644	235
Zinc, μg/L	AAS	M + F	700–1500		630–1070	850	520–990	750
μmol/L			10.7–23.0		9.6–16.4	13.0	8.0–15.1	11.5

ALT, alanine transaminase; AST, aspartate transaminase; CEA, carcinoembryonic antigen; AMP, adenosine monophosphate; Cl, chloride; CK, creatinine kinase; DHEA, dehydroepiandrosterone; NADP, nicotinamide adenine nucleotide phosphate; subluxation; RIA, radioimmunoassay; FSH, follicle-stimulating hormone; CGT, cortisol glucose tolerance; HDL, high-density lipoprotein; PEG, polyethylene glycol; ICSH, interstitial cell-stimulating hormone; PTH, parathyroid hormone; RBP, retinol-binding protein; TBG, thyrone-binding globulin; IRMA, immunoradiometric assay.

From Tietz et al.,[12] with permission.

SELECTED ANALYTES

Albumin

In both males and females, serum albumin concentration decreases gradually with age but generally remains within the "normal" range.[14] This may not be the result of the aging process alone, but also of the decreased state of health of those individuals.[15] Significantly increased albumin concentration in urine was reported in one study,[16] and correspondingly there is a significantly increased urinary albumin/creatinine ratio in the oldest group.

Alkaline phosphatase

The 60- to 90-year-old group of females has 20–25 percent elevated alkaline phosphatase activity, compared with young adults. This may be the result of postmenopause hormonal changes,[17] while in the same age group of males it remains constant. In the 90-years-and-older group, alkaline phosphate activities are equally elevated in both sexes. Elevated activities may not be only age-related, they may be the result of subclinical osteomalacia associated with secondary hyperparathyroidism[18] or therapeutic drug administration,[19] or Paget's disease with high bone turnover.[20]

Cholesterol, triglycerides and other markers for cardiovascular disease

CHOLESTEROL Total cholesterol levels are increased in the 60- to 90-year-old group, especially in females. In the oldest group the cholesterol level decreased more in the male group than in the female group.[21,22] HDL cholesterol is increased with age in men with a decrease in total cholesterol and LDL cholesterol.[23] The use of "desirable level," derived from prospective epidemiological studies directly relating to coronary heart disease, is recommended instead of reference limits.

TRIGLYCERIDES Levels in the 60- to 90-year-old age group are considerably higher than in the young adult group, followed by a decrease, especially in males.[24] Factors influencing the triglyceride levels in the elderly group include adiposity, use of diuretics, weight loss, and genetic differences. Changes may relate to changes in lifestyle as individuals grow older.[25] Exercise levels tend to fall through adult life, and total energy expenditure falls appreciably as a consequence. Food consumption tends to fall[26] in parallel with the fall in energy expenditure, but body fat tends to increase with age up to a peak in late middle life, while muscle mass falls progressively in response to a lower exercise level.

OTHER MARKERS Several markers of lipid status and inflammation are being used to assess an individual's risk of progressing to cardiovascular disease (CVD). Among these are highly sensitive C-reactive protein (CRP), homocysteine and lipoprotein(a).[27,28] It appears that high-sensitivity CRP is the strongest univariate predictor of risk of CAD events compared with homocysteine, lipoprotein(a), total cholesterol, fibrinogen, and tPA antigen in postmenopausal women.[29]

Insulin

Early detection and effective management of diabetes is necessary in the elderly population.[30] In the 60- to 90-year-old group, insulin is sharply elevated, then it drops below the young adult mean. The increase is related to various metabolic and homeostatic disorders[31] and has been attributed to progressively lessened sensitivity of muscular tissue to insulin,[32,33] insulin resistance,[34] and decreased number of insulin receptors in fat cells.[35] It has been suggested that obesity and glucose intolerance are more important determinants of insulin levels in elderly people than is age per se.[36]

Luteinizing hormone

Mean values of luteinizing hormone (LH) increase six- to ten-fold in the 90-years-and-older age group compared with values of young adults. In males it is probably due to the reduction of testosterone concentration.[37] The LH increase in females is attributed to the lack of negative feedback of ovarian steroids.[38]

Prostate-specific antigen

Prostate cancer occurs in 50 percent of the male population over the age of 70 years. As with other cancers, effective treatment of prostate cancer is more successful with early diagnosis.[39] Prostate-specific antigen (PSA) also is useful in monitoring treatment of patients with prostatic cancer. PSA screening is recommended by the American Urological Association and the American Cancer Society for all men 50 years or older.[40] Studies on African American[41] and Asian populations,[42,43] though not totally conclusive, demonstrate the distribution of serum PSA levels along ethnic lines. Age-specific PSA reference ranges are reported to improve the sensitivity for prostate cancer detection in younger men and the specificity in older men. Elevated PSA values may be seen in nonmalignant diseases of the prostate and other adjacent genitourinary tissues. Patients with confirmed prostatic carcinoma frequently have serum PSA concentrations within the range of those observed in healthy subjects. Serum PSA concentrations should be used only along with information from other diagnostic procedures and clinical evaluation of the patient.[44] PSA concentrations of 4 ng/mL or less are considered normal. Percentage of free PSA is used to determine whether a patient with a normal digital rectal exam and a total serum PSA level between 4.0 and 10.0 ng/mL would benefit from an initial or repeat biopsy having had at least one negative biopsy.[40]

Urea nitrogen

There is an age-related, steady increase of urea nitrogen, parallel with declining renal function.[45] The decrease in renal function is assumed to be due to the decrease in number of glomeruli, which are estimated to decrease by 33–50 percent in the population older than 70 years. Decreased renal function in this age group may also be due to decreased renal blood flow, as a result of decreased cardiac output, anatomical narrowing of blood vessels, and a persistent vasoconstriction.[46]

THERAPEUTIC DRUG MONITORING

Elderly people have a relatively high risk of developing adverse drug reactions. When an elderly patient is being evaluated, a major part of that evaluation should be a thorough medication history. Elderly patients frequently have four to five simultaneous prescriptions, and they may also be self-medicating with over-the-counter drugs, or taking drugs offered by friends.[47] Pharmacodynamics (what a drug does to the body) and pharmacokinetics (what the body does to the drug) in the elderly have been explored, but no clear answers are available.

Because of changes in protein and lipid metabolism, failure of blood circulation and renal function in old age, rational pharmacotherapy of geriatric patients is suggested.[48] The elderly have an increased sensitivity to some drugs and decreased or unchanged response to others. Because of decreased functioning of organs, elderly people are considered less able to maintain homeostasis than are younger patients. Pharmacokinetics (drug liberation, absorption, distribution, metabolism, excretion) in the elderly requires therapeutic drug monitoring more frequently than in younger adults.[49] Lithium is administered in lower doses owing to a combination of a reduced volume of distribution and reduced renal clearance.[50] Phenytoin is administered in much lower doses than to younger adults and the blood concentration is monitored.[51] Decisions to maintain, decrease, or increase dosage depend upon whether there is evidence of adequate response to therapy as well as evidence of possible toxic effects.

Laboratory markers for Alzheimer's disease

Along with increased understanding of the events that lead to Alzheimer's disease (AD), much work is being done on the identification of biochemical markers in the preclinical phase. The most promising is beta-amyloid (BA), which is increased in the blood and cerebrospinal fluid (CSF) of AD patients. Tau protein, a microtubule-associated protein that functions within the axons and the neurons, is also elevated in other neurological diseases other than AD, limiting its usefulness as a clinical marker.[52] Though glutamine synthetase is increased in the lumbar CSF of AD patients, it is not specific owing to the strong astrogliosis in brain.[53] It is suggested that cholesterol fractions could be involved in both Alzheimer's disease and vascular dementia.[54] The expert panel of the Ronald Reagan Institute of the US Alzheimer's Association has suggested that an appropriate marker of AD should have a specificity and a sensitivity of greater than 80 percent relative to other dementias and be noninvasive and inexpensive.[55]

Laboratory markers for osteoporosis

Osteoporosis is a major health problem in the elderly population. Bone loss is attributed to several factors, including calcium, vitamin D, PTH status, insulin-like growth factor (IGF-1), growth hormone, dehydroepiandrosterone (DHEA), and changes in the sex hormones.[56,57] Hormone replacement therapy in older men and women have benefical effects on bone mass as well as decreasing cardiovascular risk.[58,59] Biochemical markers of bone turnover—rather than total alkaline phosphatase and hydroxyproline—are being used.[60] Urinary cross-linked N-teleopeptide of type I collagen is considered to be the most sensitive predictor of bone loss. Serum vitamin D metabolites (25 hydroxy and 1,25 dihydroxy vitamin D) are lowered in the elderly, increasing the risk of potential fractures.[61] Bone loss can be partly stopped and hip fractures prevented with calcium and vitamin D supplements.[62]

DECISION LEVELS

"Some people see things as they are, and say 'Why?' I dream of things that never were, and say, 'Why not?'"   R. F. Kennedy

Reference ranges are what they are, not what should be achieved by intervention. The Report of the National Cholesterol Education Program (NCEP) Expert Panel[63] of the National Heart, Lung and Blood Institute established the following criteria for interpreting serum total cholesterol values: Levels below 200 mg/dL are classified as "desirable," those 200–239 mg/dL as "borderline high," and those 240 mg/dL and above as "high blood cholesterol." The report of the NCEP noted that 240 mg/dL corresponds to the 75th percentile of the adult US population; but clearly, it was the change in risk of coronary heart disease (CHD), not the distribution of the cholesterol in the total population (nor the reference range derived from that distribution), that determined the selection of 240 mg/dL as a critical point. However, other factors also have to be considered, such as the selective effect of survival (survival of the fittest). Characteristics that confer poorer prognosis may be eliminated by earlier death and so be seen less often in old age. An evaluation of the relationship between serum cholesterol level and all-cause CHD, and non-CHD mortality as a function of age, found that—contrary to clinical expectations—the 5-year survival rate of 73 percent for 80-year-old men in the highest two subgroups of cholesterol level (cholesterol level greater than 6.21 mmol/L or greater than 240 mg/dL) was better than the 49 percent for those in the two lower subgroups (cholesterol level ≤ 6.21 mmol/L).[64] They concluded that there is no definitive basis for recommending lipid-lowering treatment in men and women above 65–70 years of age.

A decision level is a threshold value above which or below which a particular management action is recommended.[65] Reference intervals are insufficient for this task. One cannot necessarily deduce a clinical decision simply on the basis of whether a lab result is outside a particular reference interval.[66] Recent directions in laboratory medicine,[67] such as patient-specific predictive values to guide in interpreting serial results, outcome-based reference end-points (such as 200 mg/dL cholesterol level), and dynamic interpretation of biochemical laboratory results, will add greatly to the clinician's ability to make appropriate decisions.

KEY POINTS   Biochemical tests

■ Pre- and postanalytical variables must be considered when evaluating reference values for the geriatric population. Drug regimen, multiple disease, chronic condition, dehydration, recent hospitalization, and prolonged bed rest are some of the major factors that affect laboratory values.

■ Analytes that show the greatest variation with age are albumin, alkaline phosphatase, cholesterol, triglycerides, insulin and luteinizing hormone. Age-specific PSA reference ranges are reported to improve sensitivity in younger men and specificity in older men.

■ High sensitive C-reactive protein may add to the predictive value of other markers, such as homocysteine, lipoprotein(a), LDL-cholesterol, fibrinogen, and tPA antigen in postmenopausal women, to assess the risk of cardiovascular and peripheral vascular disease.

■ Beta-amyloid shows promise as one of the biochemical markers for Alzheimer's disease.

■ Urinary cross-linked N-teleopeptide of type I collagen is considered to be the most sensitive predictor of bone loss in osteoporosis.

REFERENCES

1. Solberg HE: Establishment and use of reference values. In Burtis CA, Ashwood ER (eds): Tietz's Fundamentals of Clinical Chemistry, 4th edn. Saunders, Philadelphia, 1996:182–191

2. NCCLS: How to define, determine, and utilize reference intervals in the clinical laboratory; proposed guideline. NCCLS document C28P (ISBN 1-56238-143-1). NCCLS, 940 West Valley Road, Suite 1400, Wayne, Pennsylvania 19087, USA, 1992

3. Ratliff RR, Casey AE, Thrasher GS: Automatic instrumentation for mass screening procedures in metabolic profile studies. In Automation in Analytical Chemistry (Technicon Symposia 1966). Mediad, New York, 1967:321–325

4. Allerhand J, McCarrick L, Eisler L: The biochemical profile of blood-donors and healthy employees by AutoAnalyzer. In Automation in Analytical Chemistry (Technicon Symposia 1967). Mediad, New York, 1968:61–65

5. Tolls RE, Werner M, Hultin JV: Sex and age dependence of seven serum constituents in a large ambulatory population. In Advances in Automated Analysis (Technicon International Congress 1969), Vol. 111. Mediad, New York, 1970:9–14

6. Statland BE, Winkel P: Selected preanalytical sources of variations in reference values. In Grasbeck R, Alstrom T (eds): Reference Values in Laboratory Medicine. John Wiley, New York, 1981:127–137

7. Law R, Chalmers C: Medicines and elderly people: a general practice survey. BMJ 1976;i:565–568

8. Young DS: Effects of Preanalytical Variables on Clinical Laboratory Tests. AACC Press, Washington, 1993

9. Friedman RB, Young DS: Effects of Disease on Clinical Laboratory Tests, 2nd edn. AACC Press, Washington, 1993

10. Deitrick JE, Whedom GD, Shorr E: Effect of immobilization upon various metabolic and physiologic functions of normal men. Am J Med 1948;4:3–36

11. Faulkner WR, Meites S (eds): Geriatric Clinical Chemistry. AACC Press, Washington, 1994

12. Tietz NW, Shuey DF, Wekstein DR: Laboratory values in fit aging individuals—sexagenerians through centenarians. Clin Chem 1992;38:1167–1185

13. Lott JA, Mitchell LC, Moeschberger ML, Sutherland DE: Effects of reference ranges: how many subjects are needed? Clin Chem 1992;38:648–650

14. Greenblatt DJ: Reduced serum albumin concentration in the elderly: a report from the Boston collaborative drug surveillance program. J Am Geriatr Soc 1979;27:20–22

15. Campion EW, deLabry LO, Glynn RJ: The effect of age on serum albumin in healthy males: report from the normative aging study. J Gerontol A 1988;43:M18–M20

16. Rowe DJF, Dawnay A, Watts GGF: Microalbuminuria in diabetes mellitus: review and recommendation for the measurement of albumin in urine. Ann Clin Biochem 1990;27:297–312

17. Fülöp T, Vórum I, Varga P et al: Blood laboratory parameters of carefully selected healthy elderly people. Arch Gerontol 1989;8:151–163

18. Kelly A, Munan L, PetitClerc C: Patterns of change in selected serum chemical parameters of middle and later years. J Gerontol 1979;34:37–40

19. Chen FWK, Millard PH: The effect of aging on certain biochemical values. Mod Geriatr 1972;March:92–106

20. Siris ES: Paget's disease of bone. J Clin Endocrinol Metab 1995;80:335–338

21. Garry PJ, Hunt WC, VanderJagt DJ, Rhyne RL: Clinical chemistry reference intervals for healthy elderly subjects. Am J Clin Nutr 1989;50:1219–1230

22. Garry PJ, Hunt WC, Koehler KM et al: Longitudinal study of dietary intakes and plasma lipids in healthy elderly men and women. Am J Clin Nutr 1992;55:682–688

23. Ferrara A, Barrett-Connor E, Shan J: Total LDL and HDL cholesterol decrease with age in older men and women: the Rancho Bernado Study, 1984–1994. Circulation 1997;96:37–43

24. Alvarez C, Orejas A, Gonzales S et al: Reference intervals for serum lipids, lipoproteins, and apolipoproteins in the elderly. Clin Chem 1984;30:404–406

25. Hodkinson HM: Reference values for biological data in older persons. In Evans JG, Williams TF (eds): Oxford Textbook of Geriatric Medicine. Oxford University Press, Oxford, 1992:725–727

26. Garry PJ, Hunt WC, VanderJagt DJ, Rhyne RL: Clinical chemistry reference intervals for healthy elderly subjects. Am J Clin Nutr 1989;50:1219–1230

27. Herrmann W, Quast S, Ullrich M, Scultze H, Bodis M, Giesel J: Hyperhomocysteinemia in high aged subjects; relation to B vitamins, folic acid, renal function and the methylene tetrahydrofolate reductase mutation. Atherosclerosis 1999;144:91–101

28. Shlipak MG, Simon JA, Vittinghoff E, Lin F, Barrett-Connor E, Knopp RH, Levy RI, Hulley SB: Estrogen and progestin, lipoprotein(a) and the risk of recurrent coronary heart disease events after menopause. JAMA 2000;283:1845–1852

29. Ridker PM, Hennekens CH, Buring JE, Rifai N: C reactive protein and other markers of inflammation in the prediction of cardiovascular disease in women. N Engl J Med 2000;342:836–843

30. Bent N, Rabbitt P, Metcalfe D: Diabetes mellitus and the rate of cognitive aging. Br J Clin Psychol 2000;39:349–362

31. Carantoni M, Zuliani G, Volpato S, Palmieri E, Mezzetti A, Vergnani L, Fellin R: Relationships between fasting plasma insulin, anthropometrics, and metabolic parameters in a very old healthy population. Associazione Medica Sabin. Metabolism 1998;47:535–540

32. Dilman VM: Age-associated elevation of hypothalmic threshold to feedback control, and its role in development, aging, and disease. Lancet 1971;i:1211–1219

33. Schrier RW (ed): Clinical Internal Medicine in the Aged. WB Saunders, Philadelphia, 1982

34. Barzilai N, Stessman J, Cohen P et al: Glucoregulatory hormone influence on hepatic glucose production in the elderly. Age 1989;12:13–17

35. Modan M, Karasik A, Halkin H et al: Effect of past and concurrent body mass on prevalence of glucose intolerance and type 2 (non-insulin-dependent) diabetes and on insulin response. Diabetologia 1986;29:82–89

36. Bjorntop P, Berchtold P, Tibblin G: Insulin secretion in relation to adipose tissue in man. Diabetes 1971;20:65–70

37. Harman SM, Tsitouras PD: Reproductive hormones in aging men. 1: Measurement of sex steroids, basal luteinizing hormone and Leydig cell response to human chorionic gonadotropin. J Clin Endocr Metab 1980;51:35–40

38. Sowers JR, Felicetta JV (eds): Endocrinology of Aging. Raven Press, New York, 1988

39. Oesterling JE, Jacobsen SJ, Chute CG et al: Serum prostate-specific antigen in community-based population of healthy men. JAMA 1993;270:860–864

40. Polascik TJ, Oesterling JE, Partin AW: Prostate specific antigen. A decade of discovery—what we have learned and where we are going. J Urol 1999;162:293–306

41. Cooney KA, Strawderman MS, Wojno KJ et al: Age-specific distribution of serum prostate-specific antigen in a community-based study of African-American men. Urology 2001;57:91–96

42. Saw S, Aw TC: Age-related intervals for free and total prostate-specific antigen in a Singaporean population. Pathology 2000;32:245–249

43. Lee SE, Kwak C, Park MS, Lee CH, Kang W, Oh SJ: Ethnic differences in the age-related distribution of serum prostate-specific antigen values: a study in a healthy Korean male population. Urology 2000;56:1007–1010

44. Catalona WJ, Smith DS, Ratliff TL et al: Measurement of prostate specific antigen in serum as a screening test for prostate cancer. N Engl J Med 1991;324:1156–1161

45. Landahl S, Aurell M, Jagenburg R: Glomerular filtration rate at the age of 70 and 75. J Clin Exp Gerontol 1981;3:29–45

46. Chen FWK, Millard PH: The effect of aging on certain biochemical values. Mod Geriatr 1972;March:92–106

47. Warner A: Therapeutic drug monitoring in the elderly. In Faulkner WR, Meites S (eds): Geriatric Clinical Chemistry. AACC Press, Washington, 1994:134–144

48. Dyderski S: Pharmacokinetic aspects of geriatric therapy. Pol Merkuriusz Lek 1999;7(37):29–32

49. Cooper JW: Reviewing geriatric concerns with commonly used drugs. Geriatrics 1989;44:79–86

50. Sproule BA, Hardy BG, Schulman KI: Differential pharmacokinetics of lithium in elderly patients. Drugs Aging 2000;3:165–177

51. Bachman KA, Belloto RJ: Differential kinetics of phenytoin in elderly patients. Drugs Aging 1999;3:235–250

52. Sainato D: Laboratory testing for Alzheimer's disease. Clin Lab News 2000;26:10

53. Shen TH, Peter JB, Bruck W: Glutamine synthetase in cerebrospinal fluid, serum and brain: a diagnostic marker for Alzheimer's disease. Arch Neurol 1999;56:1241–1246

54. Bonarek M, Barberger-Gateau P, Letenner L, Deschamps V, Iron A, Dubroca B, Dartigues JF: Relationship between cholesterol, apolipoprotein E, polymorphism and dementia: a cross-sectional analysis from the PAQUID study. Neuroepidemiology 2000;19(3):141–148

55. Working Group on Molecular and Biochemical Markers of Alzheimer's Disease: Consensus report. Neurobiol Aging 1998;19:109–116

56. Sahota O: Osteoporosis and the role of vitamin D and calcium–vitamin D deficiency, vitamin D insufficiency and vitamin D sufficiency. Age Ageing 2000;29:301–304

57. Fassbender WJ, Balli M, Gortz B, Hinrichs B, Kaiser HE, Tracker HS: Sex steroids, biochemical markers, bone mineral density and histomorphometry in male osteoporosis patients. In Vivo 2000;14:611–618

58. Villareal DT, Holloszy JO, Kohrt WM: Effects of DHEA replacement on bone mineral density and body composition in elderly women and men. Clin Endocrinol (Oxf) 2000;53:561–568

59. Zanger D, Yang BK, Ardans J, Waclawiw MA, Csako G, Wanl LM, Cannon RO: Divergent effects of hormone therapy on serum markers of inflammation in postmenopausal women with coronary artery disease on appropriate medical management. J Am Coll Cardiol 2000;36:1797–1802

60. Garnero P, Binachi F, Carlier MC, Gentry V, Jacob N, Kamel S, Kindermans C, Plouvier E, Pressac M, Souberbielle JC: Biochemical markers of bone remodeling: preanalytical variations and guidelines for their use. SFBC (Societe Francaise de Biologic Clinique) Work Group. Ann Biol Clin (Paris) 2000;58:683–704

61. Theiler R, Stahelin HB, Kranzlin M, Tyndall A, Bischoff HA: High bone turnover in the elderly. Arch Phys Med Rehabil 1999;80:485–489

62. Maunier P: Prevention of hip fractures by correcting calcium and vitamin D insufficiencies in elderly people. Scand J Rheumatol Suppl 1996;103:75–78

63. National Cholesterol Education Program: Report of the NCEP Expert Panel on Detection, Evaluation, and Treatment of High Blood Cholesterol in Adults. Arch Intern Med 1988;148:36–39

64. Kronmal RA, Cain KC, Zhan Y, Omenn GS: Total cholesterol levels and mortality risk as a function of age. Arch Intern Med 1993;153:1063–1073

65. Barnett R: Medical significance of laboratory results. Am J Clin Pathol 1968;50:671–676

66. Statland BE: Clinical Decision Levels for Lab Tests. Medical Economics, Oradell, NJ, 1983

67. Harris KE, Boyd JC: Statistical Bases of Reference Values in Laboratory Medicine. Marcel Dekker, New York, 1995

Chapter 28

Social assessment of geriatric patients

Rosalie A. Kane

Social functioning is a broad concept, embracing all human relationships and activities. Social functioning, therefore, is multidimensional and cannot be measured meaningfully in a single scale. Physicians caring for older people will need routinely to assess at least some aspects of the social functioning of their patients. In some instances, physicians will also need to understand and use assessments done by the social worker on their own hospital teams, by local authority social workers (in the UK), or by case managers in community long-term care programs (in the USA). For these purposes, it is useful to consider the nature of available assessment technology, the particular aspects of social functioning that should be assessed, and the usefulness of the information derived for the actual planning of care.

SOCIAL ASSESSMENT AS PART OF COMPREHENSIVE ASSESSMENT

Particularly in the USA, but also in other developed countries, frail elderly persons often receive their first general, multidimensional assessment from a social worker or nurse who is defined as a case manager or care coordinator.[1–2] Such assessments are typically performed in the patient's own home, but they may also be performed in the hospital prior to the patient's discharge. The assessor uses a structured information-gathering schedule (often contained in a rather long booklet) to pose questions directly to the older person or (if the older person is incapable of participating) to a surrogate informant. Such assessments can take an hour or more to complete. They do not involve a physical examination or laboratory tests.

Multidimensional assessment used by case managers will typically include the following components:

- Factual information about the older person's marital status, household composition, housing situation, and income.
- Assessment of physical health based on some combination of the following checklist: symptoms; diseases the respondent believes he or she has; reports of overall utilization of hospitals, physicians, and other healthcare; reports of days sick; reports of medications used; summary of deficits in hearing, vision, speech, and dentition; and self-reported estimate of one's own health.
- Assessment of the ability to perform basic activities of daily living using a standardized scale. Such scales, at a minimum, measure independence in bathing, dressing, toileting, transferring out of bed or chair, and feeding, but may also include information about mobility, hand control, continence, and endurance.
- Ability to perform more complex social skills associated with independent living, sometimes called IADL (instrumental activities of daily living). Items that may or may not be scored on such a scale include cooking, cleaning, doing laundry, shopping, using transportation, communicating by telephone, managing money, and taking medications.
- Direct screening for cognitive impairment (to determine whether the respondent is reliable).
- Direct assessment of depressive affect and other possible psychological disturbances.
- Assessment of the social functioning of the older person in terms of the range of activities and relationships that the person pursues, the help available to or used by him or her, the presence of a confidante, and, perhaps, the subjective satisfaction of the older person with social interactions.
- Enumeration of the help the older person is receiving from family members and friends, from social programs, and from privately paid helpers directly employed by the older person and family.

Such batteries of questions are common in the USA, where they are in wide use in public programs. Many are derived from an assessment protocol developed at the Older Americans Research and Service (OARS) program at Duke University and commonly called the OARS methodology,[3] which has had extensive work done on its psychometric properties[4] and which has been extensively adapted. Another multidimensional tool that has had substantial work is the CARE (Comprehensive Assessment and Referral Evaluation) interview, developed by Gurland and colleagues[5] for a collaborative study done in the USA and the UK and later refined by the development of scales.[5–9] But the protocols in actual use for case management programs vary enormously in the way they combine questions and scales.

Some general points can be made about these multidimensional assessment tools and their use by social workers and case managers with geriatric patients.

DESCRIPTIVE OVERVIEW The batteries usually attempt a descriptive overview of physical and psychiatric functioning, but make no claims to diagnostic capability. Rather, in the context of an overall social assessment, the questions on physical and psychological health are designed to point out when fuller geriatric or psychogeriatric assessments should be sought. Thus, the presence of questions about health status, health utilization, and medications are designed not to encroach on physicians' diagnostic prerogatives, but to identify persons needing medical attention as well as to take medical conditions into account in planning care.

SCORES Scores may be derived for various subsections of the assessment, but the assessments seldom can generate an overall well-being score that has clinical significance.

COMPREHENSIVE ASSESSMENT PROTOCOLS These vary in the extent to which the information is based on queries made directly to the older person versus judgments of the assessor on the enumerated items. Unless careful instruction and training accompanies the assessment instrument, it is likely that the resultant information will not distinguish well between the older person's responses and the assessor's judgments.

FUNCTIONAL ABILITIES These are at the heart of the assessment, but are difficult to standardize and interpret. Although substantial agreement has been achieved on items for inclusion on ADL and IADL scales, variations occur in detail and approach to measurement. Sometimes, for example, the information about functioning is based on observation and sometimes on the older person's report. Sometimes the individuals are queried about what activities they are able to perform, and sometimes about activities they actually do perform. Sometimes the score is based on demonstration under test conditions, and sometimes professionals rate performance based on their observations. Widely varying time frames may be used (e.g. the last few weeks, the last few months, right now). There is also variation in the standard for adequate performance and the extent to which pain and discomfort of the older person, or elapsed time to complete a task, are taken into account. Recent work has been done to combine ADL and IADL items in a general scale. Rather than using the conventional but arbitrary system of according equal points for each item, Finch et al.[10] did empirical work to develop a scale where items are weighted according to their overall importance in functional capacity.

SERVICE PROVISION When used by case managers or social workers, the assessment protocol is meant to inform decisions about the services that should be arranged and the priority the particular older person's needs should get. However, there is seldom a clear set of rules to guide the assessor in translating the information from the assessment into guidelines for a service plan. Glass shows the intimate relationship between social factors and ADL functioning.[11] Taking advantage of a data set where respondents were asked about functioning in terms both of what they thought they could do and what they did do, he identified "underachievers" who failed to perform to their perceived capacity and, oddly enough, "overachievers" who claimed to do what they believed they were incapable of doing. Further inspection showed remarkable resourcefulness and creativity among the overachievers, and a variety of social and psychological factors (lack of wish to do the function, lack of transportation, lack of opportunity, lack of money, family factors) among the underachievers.[11]

ASPECTS OF SOCIAL FUNCTIONING

The multidimensional, comprehensive batteries described above are composed of constituent parts, designed to measure various aspects of functioning. The groundwork for measuring those dimensions is often laid in earlier research with the particular set of questions or scales. Let us now consider what aspects of social functioning should be measured.

All behavior of human beings might be termed social. But many aspects of social functioning hardly need be measured in detail for geriatric care. In a multivolume review of measures pertaining to old people, Mangen and Peterson[12] devote chapters to measurement of dimensions such as religiosity, interspousal relationships, and filial relationships. Relevant social dimensions for geriatric care constitute a shorter list, which has been summarized in a number of review works.[13,14] Suggested below is the information on social functioning that is needed, excluding health utilization and basic performance of ADL, which are important components but are covered elsewhere in this volume. Note, however, that ADL and IADL performance will be enhanced or impeded by social factors, and, conversely, social factors can influence the repercussions of ADL or IADL impairment. To deal with the latter, Allen and Mor[15] elaborated on functional measures by incorporating follow-up questions designed to assess any deleterious consequences of insufficient help (e.g. "Have there been times in the past month when you were not able to bathe as often as you would have liked because no one was available to help you?" or "Have there been times in the past month when you were unable to eat when you were hungry because no one was available to help you?"). They refer to these as indices of unmet need.

First, the *ability to perform social roles*, sometimes called social skills, is relevant. For younger people, such measures usually encompass their performance as employees, family members, and citizens.[16] For older people, perhaps shortsightedly, the measurement of role performance is usually limited to ability to perform the so-called instrumental ADL (cooking, cleaning, laundry), which are, in turn, related to household management and independent living.

Second, information about *social relationships* (their frequency, context, and quality), *social activities* (again their frequency, nature, and quality), *social resources* (including income, housing, and environmental conditions) is useful to geriatric providers. Third, *social support* is a salient concept to examine; it may include the help the patient is receiving and can expect to continue to receive from others in the environment, and the degree to which this help is perceived as supportive. Fourth, *subjective social well-being* can be measured more generally.

A fifth area of social function—*family burden* or family stress—has come into prominence in the last decade.[17] Although highly relevant to geriatric care, this measure pertains to family caregivers rather than to the older person receiving the care. The idea is that an understanding of the type and degree of burden that caregiving creates for the relative primarily responsible will help determine whether the arrangement is realistic, humane, and fair, and the extent to which relief for the family member is necessary.

A sixth emerging area concerns personal autonomy, values, and preferences. In recent years, there has been much interest in *personal autonomy and values* of older persons receiving long-term care.[18] This is fueled by growing social science literature that suggests that older people who perceive that they have lost control and choice over their lives experience adverse health outcomes, including depression, increased morbidity, and even increased mortality.[19–21] Some attempts have been made to estimate a measure of autonomy, although these measures are not ordinarily incorporated into everyday clinical practice. A related effort entails assessing the values and preferences that may be important to geriatric patients.[22]

Finally, substantial work has been done to seek a satisfactory approach to assessing the older person's *satisfaction* with the care and help received. Before briefly discussing each of these areas, some general comments about the problems of measuring social functioning are warranted.

Problems in assessing social functioning

First, social concepts such as social isolation, social support, or social well-being are value-laden abstract constructs, subject to interpretation. Thus, several scales containing different items may purport to measure the same thing, whereas scales that seem to be similar in content carry different labels.[12] It is important not to be deceived by the name of the scale, but to examine its contents.

Second, most social variables have both an objective and a subjective component. For example, one can measure social support by quantifying the support network and its activities, or by asking whether the older people view themselves as supported in various ways. Similarly, one can examine the burden of caregivers by quantifying their objective tasks with the patient and their other obligations, or one can measure the extent to which they feel burdened. Both approaches may be important.

Third, adequate social functioning can be achieved through diverse patterns. One seldom finds clear norms for interpreting the results of social information. A person who states that he or she has 10 friends is not necessarily twice as well befriended as a person with five, nor can one say that a person who spends much time playing cards is better off than one who spends the same amount of time fishing. Growing out of this observation are two important points in interpreting social information: (1) a change in social functioning may be as important as the actual value on a scale; and (2) information about adequate thresholds of functioning is needed. Regarding the latter, the objective of social measurements for geriatric caregivers is not to achieve a perfectly scaled measure of a social property such as isolation or social support; rather, it is to determine whether these dimensions have fallen below some threshold that means that the patient is at risk.

Fourth, social role expectations for the elderly are unclear at best and vary according to ethnic groups as well as over time. Nobody seems to know what constitutes adequate role performance for a retiree, a grandparent, or an elderly widow or widower, and establishing these norms is more complicated because of their likely sensitivity to cultural differences.

Finally, much social functioning involves people in interaction with others. They fill social roles, cope with stress, receive help from family members, and so on. How well a particular older person functions socially is, in part, dependent on the behavior of others, which complicates the assessment process. Glass and colleagues[23] have pioneered in expanding the range of social functioning examined in older people. In studies underway at Yale and later at Harvard, the team has attempted to develop better measures of social functioning related to productive aging in social and economic roles, incorporating housework, yardwork, childcare, and other family roles, paid work, and volunteer work.

Social relationships, activities, and resources

The aggregated social relationships of a client, viewed descriptively, are sometimes called the *social network*. "Social network" refers to the web of social relationships and contacts that an individual may have. Although difficult because of the amount of data collection needed, objective properties of social networks can be described using terms such as size (how many people are in the network), density (the number of people who know each other in the network), homogeneity (similarity of network members on various characteristics), multiplexity (the number of different types of interactions exchanged), and reciprocity (the balance or imbalance between perception of giving and receiving support).[24] Researchers point out that "social network" is a static concept referring to relationships across the lifespan; the term "social convoy" has been suggested as a more dynamic concept.[25] Measures in this area have been extensively reviewed by Levin.[26]

Although social networks have properties—such as size, density, frequency and intensity of contact, permeability, and directionality[24–29]—from the viewpoint of geriatric care, the large number of properties that can be elaborated upon for social research can be reduced to an interest in the frequency and nature of the patient's human contacts in the course of a day, week, or month. One approach, often incorporated into assessment, involves querying the patient about the frequency of contacts in person, by telephone, or by mail by categories of people (adult children, other relatives, friends, others), using a metric such as "frequently, occasionally, seldom, or never," or attempting more exact quantification (less than once a week, and so on). Such questions are sometimes followed up by asking the person whether he or she has contact with these people more than desired, about the right amount, or less than desired. The OARS methodology, a multidimensional assessment tool described above,[5] contains an often-used measure of social contacts.

Some efforts have been made to combine social contacts and social activities in brief social network scales, designed to predict the individual's well-being and need for service. The Berkman Social Network Scale,[30] developed in a general population, and the Lubben Social Network Scale,[31] developed for the elderly, are examples. Typically, marital status, membership in formal groups, and religious participation are included with other brief measures of social contact to form a short scale.

To assess social resources, well-planned, consistently asked questions are better than scales. Each assessment of social functioning does well to contain straightforward questions about household income and assets, and income and assets of the older person with the disability. It is also important to determine the composition of the household and the nature and adequacy of the housing. In some social contexts, access to a car and transportation is also an important social resource. Depending on the political context, information about insurance coverage, veteran status, and specific disability status may provide a key to resources that could be available for the person. Other information that is important in developing a plan and coming to know the individual includes information about the individual's occupation or former occupation, and interests; typically such items are overlooked.

Social support

A description of the social network does not automatically translate into an understanding of how well the patient's needs are met, nor does it permit a prediction of how well the needs may continue to be met in the future. Being enmeshed in a large network of family and friends may, depending on the network, be reassuring or stressful, helpful or harmful, informative or misleading. Social support is the positive tangible and intangible assistance drawn from the social network.[32] A social network or convoy has multiple functions, which also can be measured.[26,27] These include giving informational support, such as facts and advice; affective support, such as comfort, encouragement, and love; social support and stimulation, such as companionship; and tangible help, such as money or physical assistance. It is obvious that the geriatric team has an interest in knowing whether a given patient has a network that can or does provide such support. The social network is the potential vehicle for social support, but may be associated with negative as well as positive effects. Social scientists have studied the complex stress process that involves interaction of life events, chronic life strains, self-concepts, coping skills, and social supporters.[33]

If the geriatric patient already has tangible needs for physical help from others, one measure of social support is a straightforward tabulation of the kinds of help received and their frequency. Assessment tools usually attempt, however, to go beyond this simple count to an estimation of the likelihood that the help can continue into the future, and the prospects for a replacement, if the person giving most of the help cannot continue. Research suggests that often the patient's social support in terms of physical help depends on one person whose own health may be fragile, or who cannot continue indefinitely because of competing demands.[34] In such cases, planning can begin to broaden the base of social support. In other instances, additional relatives and friends are available to help, but the primary family caregiver assumes that nobody else is capable or willing. If the patient has not previously needed physical help, then an estimation of the likelihood of this help is needed. A few key questions can assist in making this prediction; for example: "If necessary, is there someone who could come and help you during the day?" or "Is there someone who could stay overnight with you if necessary?" Social support measures are also summarized in Levin's recent review.[26]

Subjective well-being

An overall measure of the patient's well-being is sometimes sought in a comprehensive assessment tool. Such measures are also often used to evaluate the worth of long-term care programs.[35,36] The two most frequently used measures in this regard are Lawton's Philadelphia Geriatric Center Morale Scale[37] and the Life Satisfaction Index (LSI-A) of Neugarten, Havighurst, and Tobin.[38,39] Both these scales are relatively brief and simple to administer, both have developed an extensive use history, and both measure elements of life satisfaction by asking clients to consider the extent to which their expectations in life were met. At the same time, both also measure aspects of existential well-being or happiness.

Although these two scales are often used for program evaluation, it is unclear how much these measures should change as a result of a worthwhile program. For example, a meal program may be performing an important and appreciated function, and yet the answer to the question "Overall, have I achieved most of my goals in life?" would remain the same. In general, it seems best to measure satisfaction with a program directly, through questions that specifically ask about satisfaction with various elements of the program itself.[13]

Caregiver burden

In both the USA and in Europe, social services authorities for the elderly recognize that their programs would be inadequate to meet the needs for care were it not for the volunteered efforts of family members. Indeed, unpaid family members give most of the personal care and housekeeping help that is received by community-dwelling older people. In the USA, almost 80 percent of in-home services for elderly people are given by family members. It has become a widespread program principle that social services should supplement and enhance family care, when appropriate, but should not replace it.

Given this situation, it becomes important to assess the well-being of family caregivers to estimate (1) how long such care may be expected to continue, and (2) legitimate needs for relief. Somewhat unfortunately because of its negative connotations, this area of measurement is often called measurement of "family burden." Many scales have been developed in the last decade to assess family caregiver burden.[40–45] These scales are often themselves multidimensional (including, for example, physical burden, emotional burden, social burden, and financial burden), and they may concentrate on subjective burden or objective burden, or both. Other scales designed especially to examine the stress-engendering aspects of family care for persons with dementia specifically measure the presence and frequency of a range of troublesome behavior. Pearlin and colleagues[46] have contributed a careful conceptual model of the stress process related to family caregiving, complete with brief measures of the relevant aspects of the phenomenon (including problematic behavior, overload, relational deprivation, family conflict, job-caregiving conflict, economic strain, role captivity, loss of self, caregiving competence, personal gain, management of situation, management of meaning, and management of distress). This series of measures is designed for research rather than clinical practice, yet it reminds us that the concept of caregiver burden is by no means straightforward. In general, it has been well documented that objective needs of the older person and objectively defined tasks occasion varying degrees of burden. The Caregiving Hassles Scale[47] can be used to measure the extent to which care of an elderly relative causes small daily tribulations or, in the vernacular, "hassles." Some authorities believe that the daily hassles produce more stress than dramatic life crises. Less attention has been given to the positive aspects of caregiving, sometimes called "uplifts," though these, too, have been measured and studied.[48]

The stress or burden of family caregivers, balanced against positive aspects of the role, should be part of a comprehensive assessment of an older person. However, the social worker or case manager must then be prepared to interpret and use the information to decide when and how much relief should be offered to family members. It is important also to understand the information collected according to the relationship of the family caregiver to the patient (spouse, adult offspring, other relative) and the competing obligations of that family caregiver (which could include employment, care of younger children, care of another disabled or elderly relative, or even dealing with their own failing strength).

In addition to applying specific measures that generate scores, clinical teams can benefit by consulting a practical reference work by Lustbader and Hooyman,[49] which lists sets of assessment questions that are useful for specific caregiving situations. For example, when a spouse is a caregiver, they suggest that one ask about the length of the marriage prior to the illness; the health of the caregiving spouse; the predisability marital patterns; the timing of onset relative to the couple's retirement plans; the impact of the illness on the couple's financial resources; the impact on their sexual functioning; and the availability of backup help from other family and friends. If siblings are sharing caregiving, the assessment might include these questions: Is concern about a potential inheritance straining sibling relationships? Is there financial disparity among siblings? Is there a natural leader, a parental favorite? Is there a healthcare professional among them? Are there step-siblings among them? What have been the adult siblings relationships to each other? And what obligations must each sibling meet in addition to parental care?

Personal autonomy, preferences, and values

In the last decade in the USA, there has been an attempt to record older people's preferences regarding life-sustaining medical treatment.[50–53] Such information is desired partly for legal reasons, to prevent liability, and partly to guide clinicians in giving good care. If taken seriously, however, assessment of such preferences is notoriously difficult. The validity of the data depends on whether accurate information has been adequately disclosed to the respondent and has been understood by the respondent. Some work has been undertaken to construct and study such measures, though in practice many assessment batteries merely contain a notation of the older person's preference for such services as cardiopulmonary resuscitation, artificial hydration, or respirators, and their preferences about who they want to act in their stead if they become temporarily or permanently unable to make decisions—without any assurance that the questions were asked or comprehended in any consistent way.

Others have sought to assess values of geriatric patients directly, a pursuit that is fraught with conceptual and methodological difficulties.[54] Using a tool that is meant to be an exercise in self-discovery rather than precise measurement, Gibson, a philosopher, and her colleagues[55,56] developed a Values History, which they recommend for distribution to clients to complete at leisure and with discussion among families. At the other extreme, Doukas and McCullough[57] have developed an approach that uses a few true–false questions to tap into values about risk, life and death, and spirituality.

Work has been done to assess systematically the ordinary values and preferences of older people that might be related to their care. Although not amenable to generating an overall scale, it is feasible to incorporate a list of topics that the patient rates in terms of importance, providing descriptive detail. Using a stem that relates the topic to care that they might need now or in the future, the instrument developed asks the person to rate the importance of the following: performing everyday routines in a particular way; participating in certain activities at home or away from home; personal privacy; specific events or milestones being anticipated or projects being completed; freedom from pain; taking risks as opposed to being protected but less free; involving or not involving family in their care; qualities desired in a helper; and qualities desired in a place to live. Older clients were willing to respond to such questions, revealing differences in the importance these issues hold and in the content of what they deemed important. However, clinicians were often somewhat reluctant to enter into such discussions, partly because of the time involved (about 20 minutes) and partly because of a sense of being intrusive or being unable to act on the preferences expressed.[22,58]

Although considerable hubris is involved in attempting to assess values and preferences, and assessors doing so must guard against believing that they have encapsulated the essence of another human being in a few simple items, it seems equally improper to ignore this arena. In fact, systematic efforts to assess the patient's values and preference are likely to restructure the encounter between social workers and geriatric patients in important ways. Moreover, insights into the values and preferences of the older persons served may be the best safeguard against inappropriate or paternalistic decision-making about their lives.

Satisfaction

Although the technical quality of care procedures may be assessed by professionals using objective criteria, increasing emphasis has been given to seeking a reliable way to elicit the patient's perspective, particularly with reference to home help and personal assistance. It is argued that the intimacy of care and its close connections to daily life requires that professionals have a way of determining how patients view that care. Indeed, evidence suggests that older people are often reluctant to accept the help suggested, and speculation has been that this reaction is related to dislike of the way services are offered. Geron[59,60] conducted focus groups with older home care clientele from varying ethnic backgrounds to identify the elements of quality important to consumers. With great consistency across ethnicity, older people identified the following elements of good care: humaneness (helpers who were likable, pleasant, courteous, caring), competence, dependability, continuity (i.e. if the previous two criteria were met, consumers preferred consistency rather than change, adequacy in terms of amount of help, and choice in the type and timing of help received). They then developed and tested a satisfaction tool. It is noteworthy, however, that such tools are quite specific to the service context.

Satisfaction has come to be seen as a measure of experience mediated by expectations. As such, it is bedeviled by the propensity of people to adjust their expectations downwards or to hold low expectations in the first place. Measurement of satisfaction is also rendered technically difficult if those whose reports are sought are dependent on the services or, worse, feel intimidated—the latter being a possibility for those living in group residential settings. Nonetheless, substantial progress has been made in measuring satisfaction.[61]

Social functioning of people with dementia

A large number of scales have been developed for rating or assessing the social functioning of persons with dementia in terms of presence of appropriate behavior and absence of behaviors considered disruptive.[62,63] Initially these instruments relied on ratings by professional caregivers or family carers. More recently, observational and even physiological tools have been used to measure social stress and social well-being on the part of those who cannot communicate.[64] In the late 1990s, several tools were developed and tested that depend on self-report from the person with dementia. Notably Brod et al.[65] developed a short set of Likert-type quality of life ratings called the DqoL, and Logsdon et al.[66] developed an even shorter set of 13 dichotomous questions for self-report of quality of life. Both these tools have reported good reliability. Teri and Logsdon[67] developed the Pleasant Events Schedule-AD, which is used either with the person with dementia or a proxy observer, to zero in on the existential experience of the person with dementia.

An emerging concern is the discordance found between the rating of the older person and that of a family or staff proxy when paired ratings are available. This has called proxy rating into question without presenting any substitute to measure social well-being in those persons whose dementia is too advanced for self-report. It would seem prudent to use proxies most when highly objective information about social functioning is sought, and to provide clear definitions of the behavior being observed, an approach taken in the multidimensional observational scale for older adults (MOSES).[68]

Social assessment within congregate group settings

Assessments of social functioning and social well-being within the context of a nursing home or board-and-care home need to take into account the nature of the setting. Although elaborate approaches to examine how the individual fits into the community have been made for research purposes,[69] this area of assessment is in its infancy in terms of scale development to be applied to residents. Sometimes this work is lumped with satisfaction measures that are tailored to specific residential programs. A large ongoing project funded by the US Department of Health and Human Services concentrates on measuring quality-of-life outcomes for nursing home residents and has developed short scales to tap 11 dimensions of quality of life: meaningful activity, individuality, dignity, privacy, enjoyment, relationships, comfort, functional competence, spiritual well-being, sense of security and order, and

autonomy.[70] These measures largely deal with social as opposed to physical functioning, and choice or systematic attention, although elaborate measures of environmental climates have been made for research purposes.

EMERGING AREAS OF SOCIAL ASSESSMENT

Other areas of social assessment are amenable to measurement and may be important in specific situations, but measurement approaches are just evolving. Also some new themes are getting attention. The following are some examples.

Measures of housing environments and housing satisfaction This is an underdeveloped arena.[71] Some work has recently been done to separate factors related to assisted living environments (often called "housing with services"). One such study identified personal care services, general services, apartment, control/choice and housekeeping/dining as separate constructs.[72]

Assessment of formal support in the form of help from personnel from healthcare and social service organizations Such a measure of assistance may or may not be thought of as part of the social assessment; but, however classified, it is necessary. It is often helpful to divide "formal care" into types of tasks: nursing tasks, such as help with medicines or procedures; personal care, such as help with bathing, toileting, eating, and transferring; housekeeping tasks, such as laundry, cooking, cleaning; help with transportation; help with business matters; and help with arranging for services, such as case management. Assessments usually develop indicators of frequency (days/visits per month, week, or day) and intensity (total hours of help of each type in a given period).

Assessment of the specific tasks performed by family carers Some assessment tools develop parallel questions to use in inquiring about the type of tasks and the frequency and intensity provided by both formal and informal sources. It is only by comparing formal and informal help received with needs for assistance that an estimation of unmet need is developed. Typically, care plans developed by social workers are designed to meet unmet needs.

Assessing social well-being across cultures Attention is now being given in general to the extent to which assessments of elderly people cross cultural lines. Cultural relativity would be particularly important for making normative judgments about social well-being. This topic was flagged in an issue of the *Journal of Mental Health and Aging*, where both methodological and content considerations are reviewed.[72]

ASSEMBLING THE ASSESSMENT PROTOCOL

As this chapter has suggested, assessment of social functioning can be as detailed as the geriatric team desires, touching on many or few dimensions of social functioning. The assessment may also vary in its mix of scales, single items, clinical ratings, and reliance on open-ended, unstructured approaches. This chapter recommends a consistent and standardized approach to assessing aspects of social functioning. Commitment to consistency and routine approaches is probably more important than which particular instrument is selected. Initial parsimony is also suggested, followed by more detailed assessment as necessary. It is highly likely that there will be an inverse relationship between the amount of information collected and the reliability and validity of the assessment interview.

A social worker is highly accepted as a member of a geriatric team. However, the importance of social information—whether collected specifically by a social worker or collected by a generalist who is gathering information to be used by all professionals on the team—has been insufficiently appreciated.

KEY POINTS Social assessment

■ Social functioning is a multidimensional construct that cannot be well measured in a single scale.

■ Relevant domains of social functioning with available measures include: ability to perform social roles; social relationships; social support; family carer well-being; autonomy; values and preferences; and satisfaction.

■ Measurement strategies for social functioning must take into account that most domains have an objective and subjective component; that normative social role definitions in old age are lacking; that there appear to be multiple ways to achieve satisfactory social functioning; and that research is needed to establish thresholds with clinical significance.

■ Advances have been made in conceptualizing quality of life for persons with dementia and for eliciting reliable direct responses from those with substantial cognitive impairment. Observational approaches have been developed for those who cannot be interviewed.

■ Measures of social well-being need to be modified or augmented for people who live in congregate group settings in order to receive care.

■ Topics highlighted for developmental work include: housing environments and housing satisfaction; assessment of help from paid individuals and organizations; the type and intensity of care activities performed by family carers; and cross-cultural measures of social functioning.

REFERENCES

1. Davis D, Challis D: Matching Resources to Need in Community Care: An Evaluated Demonstration of a Long-Term Care Model. Gower Publishing, Aldershot, Hampshire, 1987
2. Kane RA: Long-term case management for older adults. In Kane RL, Kane RA (eds): Assessing Older Persons: Measures, Meaning, and Practical Applications. Oxford University Press, New York, 2000
3. Fillenbaum GL: Multidimensional Functional Assessment of Older Adults: The Duke Older Americans Resources and Services Procedures. Lawrence Erlbaum, Hillsdale, NJ, 1988
4. George LK, Fillenbaum GG: OARS methodology: a decade of experience in geriatric assessment. Geriatr Soc 1985;33:607–615
5. Gurland BJ, Kuriansky L, Sharpe L et al: The Comprehensive Assessment and Referral Evaluation (CARE): rationale, development and reliability. Int J Ageing Dev 1978;8:9–42
6. Gurland BJ, Wilder DE: The CARE interview revisited: development of an efficient, systematic, clinical assessment. J Gerontol 1984;29:129–137
7. Golden RR, Teresi JA, Gurland BJ: Development of indicator scales for the Comprehensive Assessment and Referral Evaluation (CARE) Interview Schedule. J Gerontol 1984;29:138–146
8. Teresi JA, Golden RR, Gurland BJ et al: Construct validity of indicator scales developed for the Comprehensive Assessment and Referral Evaluation Interview Schedule. J Gerontol 1984;29:147–157
9. Teresi JA, Golden RR, Gurland BJ: Concurrent and predictor validity of indicator scales developed for the Comprehensive Assessment and Referral Evaluation Interview Schedule. J Gerontol 1984;29:158–167
10. Finch M, Kane RL, Philp I: Developing a new metric for ADLs. Am Geriatr Soc 1995;43:877–884
11. Glass, TA: Hypothetical vs enacted. Conjugating the tenses of function: discordance among hypothetical, experimental, and enacted function in older adults. Gerontologist 1998;38:101–112
12. Mangen D, Peterson W (eds): Research instruments in social gerontology, vols I–III. University of Minnesota Press, Minneapolis, 1982
13. Kane RL, Kane RA (eds): Assessing Older Persons: Measures, Meaning, and Practical Applications. Oxford University Press, New York, 2000
14. Kane RA: Assessment of social functioning: recommendations for comprehensive geriatric assessment. In Rubenstein LZ, Wieland D, Bernebei R (eds): Geriatric Assessment Technology: The State of the Art. Editrice Kurtis, Milan, 1995
15. Allen SM, Mor V: The prevalence and consequences of unmet needs: contrast between older and younger adults with disability. Med Care 1997;35:1132–1148
16. Kane R, Kane RL, Arnold S: Measuring social functioning in mental health studies: concepts and instruments. US Department of Health and Human Services, National Institute of Mental Health, Rockville, MD, 1985
17. Gaugler JE, Kane RA, Langlois J: Assessment of family caregivers of older adults. In Kane RL, Kane RA (eds): Assessing Older Persons: Measures, Meaning, and Practical Applications. Oxford University Press, New York, 2000
18. Kane RA: Values and preferences. In Kane RL, Kane RA (eds): Assessing Older Persons: Measures, Meaning, and Practical Applications. Oxford University Press, New York, 2000
19. Avorn J, Langer E: Induced disability in nursing home patients: a controlled trial. J Am Geriatr Soc 1982;30:397–400
20. Langer E, Avorn J: Impact of psychosocial environment of the elderly on behavior and health outcomes. In Hess B, Markson E (eds): Growing Old in America, 3rd edn. Transition Books, New Brunswick, NJ, 1985
21. Rodin J: Aging and health: effects of the sense of control. Science 1986;233:1271–1276
22. Degenholtz HD, Kane RA, Kivnick, HQ: Care-related preferences and values of elderly community-based LTC consumers: can case managers learn what's important to clients. Gerontologist 1997;37:767–777
23. Glass TA, Seeman TE, Herzog AR et al: Change in productive activity in late adulthood: MacArthur studies of successful aging. J Gerontol B 1995;50:S65–S76
24. Sauer W, Coward R (eds): Social Support Networks and the Care of the Elderly: Theory, Research, Practice, and Policy. Springer, New York, 1985
25. Antonucci TC: Social supports and social relationships. In Binstock RH, George LK (eds): Handbook of Social Science and Aging, 3rd edn. Academic Press, San Diego, 1990
26. Levin C: Social functioning. In Kane RL, Kane RA (eds): Assessing Older Persons: Measures, Meaning, and Practical Applications. Oxford University Press, New York, 2000
27. Kahn R: Aging and social support. In Riley MW (ed): Aging From Birth to Death. Westview, Boulder, Co, 1979
28. Antonucci TC, Depner CE: Social support and informal helping relationships. In Wills T (ed): Basic Processes in Helping Relationships. Academic Press, New York, 1982
29. Mitchell R, Trickett E: Task force reports: social networks as mediators of social support. J Commun Ment Health 1980;16:274
30. Berkman LF: The assessment of social networks and social supports in the elderly. J Am Geriatr Soc 1983;31:743–749
31. Lubben JE: Assessing social networks among elderly populations. Commun Health 1988;11:42–52
32. Hirsch BF: Psychological dimensions of social networks: a multimethod analysis. Am J Commun Psychol 1979;7:263–277

33. Pearlin LI, Menaghan EG, Lieberman MA et al: The stress process. J Health Soc Behav 1981;22:337–356

34. Kane RA, Reinardy J, Penrod JD, Huck S: After the hospitalization is over: a different perspective on family care of older people. J Gerontol Soc Wk 1999;31(1/2):119–142

35. Stock WA, Okun MA, Benin M: Structure of subjective well-being among the elderly. Psychol Aging 1986;1:91–102

36. Larsen RJ, Diener E, Emmons RA: An evaluation of subjective well-being measures. Soc Indicators Res 1985;17:1–17

37. Lawton MP: The Philadelphia Geriatric Center Morale Scale: a revision. J Gerontol 1975;30:85–89

38. Neugarten BL, Havighurst RJ, Tobin SS: The measurement of life satisfaction. J Gerontol 1961;16:141–143

39. Liang J: Dimensions of the Life Satisfaction Index A: a structural formulation. J Gerontol 1984;39:613–622

40. Kosberg JI, Cairl RE, Keller DM: Components of burden: interventive implications. Gerontologist 1990;30:236–242

41. Montgomery RV, Stull DE, Borgatta EF: Measurement and the analysis of burden. Res Aging 1985;7:137–152

42. Robinson B: Validation of a caregiver strain index. J Gerontol 1983;38:344–348

43. Zarit SH, Reever KE, Bach-Peterson J: Relatives of the impaired elderly: correlates of feelings of burden. Gerontologist 1980;20:649–655

44. Zarit SH, Zarit JM: The memory and behavior problem checklist and burden interview. Pennsylvania State University, Technical Report, 1983

45. Vitaliano PP, Young HM, Russo H: Burden: a review of measures used among caregivers of individuals with dementia. Gerontologist 1995;31:67–75

46. Pearlin LI, Mullan JT, Semple SJ et al: Caregiving and the stress process: an overview of concepts and their measures. Gerontologist 1990;30:583–584

47. Kinney J, Stephens MAAP: Caregiving Hassles Scale: assessing the daily hassles of caring for a family member with dementia. Gerontologist 1989;29:328–332

48. Brody EM, Hoffman C, Kleban MH et al: Caregiving daughters and their local siblings: perceptions, strains, and interactions. Gerontologist 1989;29:529–538

49. Lustbader W, Hooyman N: Taking Care of Aging Family Members. Free Press, New York, 1994

50. Diamond EL, Jemigan JA, Moseley RA et al: Decision-making ability and advance directive preferences in nursing home patients and proxies. Gerontologist 1989;29:622–626

51. Henderson M: Beyond the living will. Gerontologist 1990;30:480–485

52. Wetle T, Levkoff S, Cwikel J et al: Nursing home resident participation in medical decisions: perceptions and preferences. Gerontologist 1988;28(Suppl):53–58

53. Zweibel NR, Cassel CK: Treatment choices at the end of life: a comparison of decisions by older patients and their physician-selected proxies. Gerontologist 1989;29:615–621

54. Froberg D, Kane RL: Methodology for measuring health state preferences, I–IV. J Clin Epidemiol 1989;42:345–354, 459–471, 485–592, 675–685

55. Gibson JM: Values history focusses on life and death decisions. Med Ethics 1990;5:1–2,17

56. Gibson JM: Continuity of care and ethics. Continuing Care 1990;11–32

57. Doukas DJ, McCullough LB: The values history: the evaluation of the patient's values and advance directives. J Fam Pract 1991;32:145–153

58. Kane RA, Degenholtz HD, Kane RL: Adding values: an experiment in systematic attention to values and preferences of community long-term care clients. J Gerontol B 1999;54:S109–S119

59. Geron SM: Using measures of subjective well-being and client satisfaction in health assessments of older persons. Health Care in Later Life 1(6):185–196

60. Geron SM, Smith K, Tennstedt S, Jette J, Chassler D, Kasten L: The home care satisfaction measure: a client-centered approach to assessing the satisfaction of frail older adults with home care services. J Gerontol B 2000;55:S259–S270

61. Smith MA: Satisfaction. In Kane RL, Kane RA (eds): Assessing Older Persons: Measures, Meaning, and Practical Applications. Oxford University Press, New York, 2000

62. Teresi JA, Lawton MP, Ory M, Holmes D: Measurement issues in chronic care populations: dementia special care. Alzheimer Dis Assoc Disord 1994;8(Suppl):S144–S183

63. Cohen-Mansfield J: Reflections on the assessment of behavior in nursing home residents. Alzheimer Dis Assoc Disord 1994;8(Suppl):S217–S222

64. Harper, GJ: Assessing older adults who cannot communicate. In Kane RL, Kane RA (eds): Assessing Older Persons: Measures, Meaning, and Practical Applications. Oxford University Press, New York, 2000

65. Brod M, Stewart AL, Sands L, Walton P: Conceptualization and measurement of quality of life in dementia: the Dementia Quality of Life Instrument (DQoL). Gerontologist 1999;39:25–35

66. Logsdon RG, Gibbons L, McCurry S, Teri L: Quality of life in Alzheimer's disease: patient and caregiver reports, J Men Health Aging 1999;5:60–74

67. Teri L, Logsdon RG: Identifying pleasant activities for Alzheimer's disease patients: the pleasant events schedule-AD. Gerontologist 1991;31:124–127

68. Helmes E, Csapo K, Short GA: Standardization and validation of the multidimensional observational scale for elderly subjects (MOSES). J Gerontol 1987;42:395–405

69. Moos RL, Lemke S: Evaluating Residential Facilities. Sage, Thousand Oaks, CA, 1996

70. Kane RA: Long-term care and a good quality of life: bringing them closer together. Gerontologist 2001;41:293–304

71. Cutler L: Physical environments of older adults. In Kane RL, Kane RA (eds): Assessing Older Persons: Measures, Meaning, and Practical Applications. Oxford University Press, New York, 2000

72. Skinner JH, Terese JA, Homes D, Stahl SM, Stewart AL (eds): Measurement in old ethnically diverse populations. J Men Health Aging 2001;7:1–181

Chapter 29

Surgery and anesthesia in old age

D. Gwyn Seymour

This chapter provides a general overview of surgery and anesthesia in old age, but lays particular stress on those areas of the subject that are changing most rapidly and/or are attracting most clinical and research interest. After a brief introduction dealing with epidemiological trends, the elderly surgical patient is evaluated from a predominantly medical viewpoint. It is not possible to go into details of anesthetic or surgical technique here, but these have been considered at length elsewhere.[1–4]

Rehabilitation of the elderly orthopedic patient, important though it is, is also not dealt with here, as it is discussed elsewhere in this textbook.

TRENDS IN SURGERY AND ANESTHESIA IN OLD AGE

The surgical treatment of elderly patients is not a late twentieth century invention. Of 100 cases of strangulated hernia operated on by van Assen in Amsterdam between 1903 and 1906, 18 were between 50 and 70 years of age, 17 were between 70 and 80 years, and three were over 80.[5] Inhalational anesthesia was used in one-third of the cases, with local anesthesia in the others. There were only two deaths, but one of those was of a patient aged 81.

In the last 25 years, however, the increase in surgical activity in patients aged 65 and over has been much greater than would have been expected from demographic trends alone.[6,7] This increase has not just been in life-saving procedures, but has also been seen in procedures such as cataract surgery or total hip replacement, which are predominantly aimed at increasing quality of life. Figures 29-1 and 29-2 look at Scottish trends in hospital admission rates to the specialties of general surgery and ophthalmology over the last 20 years. In both specialties, but particularly in ophthalmology, there has been a dramatic increase in admission rates in the older age groups, while admission rates in younger groups have been static or have increased much more slowly. Note that the rising admission rates in the old, and particularly the very old, are not due to demographic changes, as these have already been allowed for by expressing referral rates relative to 100,000 patients of comparable age in the general population.

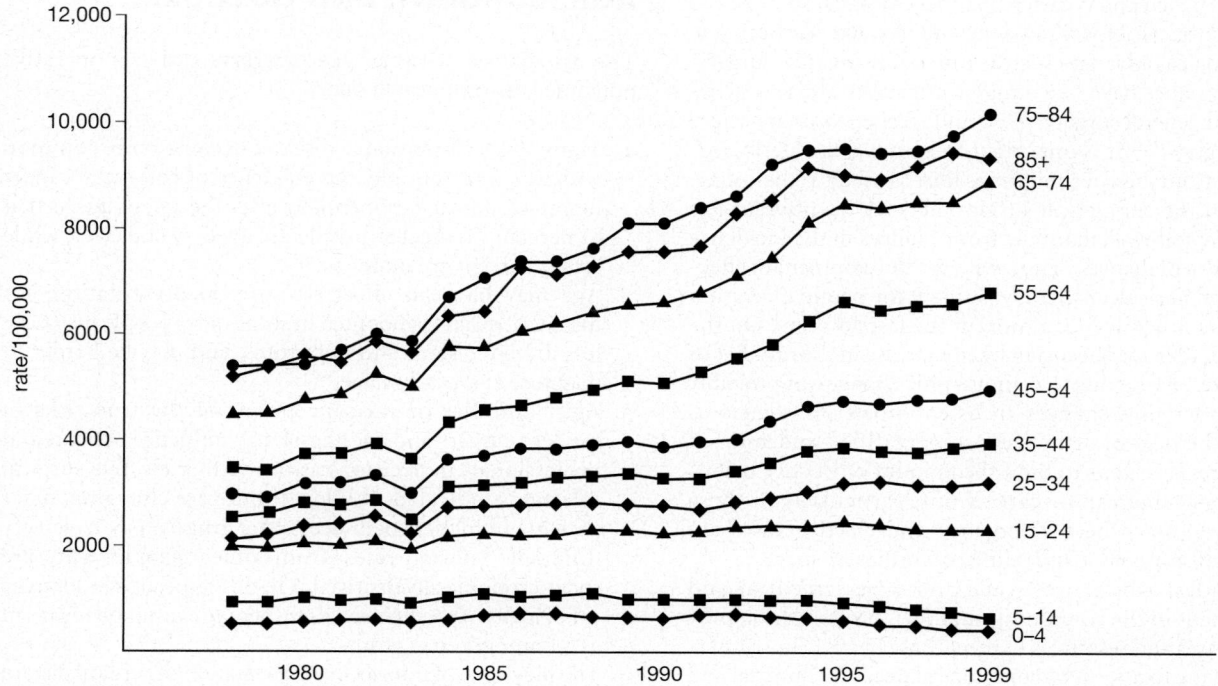

Figure 29-1 General surgery admissions to Scottish hospitals, according to age group. Data courtesy of the Information and Statistics Division, Edinburgh, Scotland.

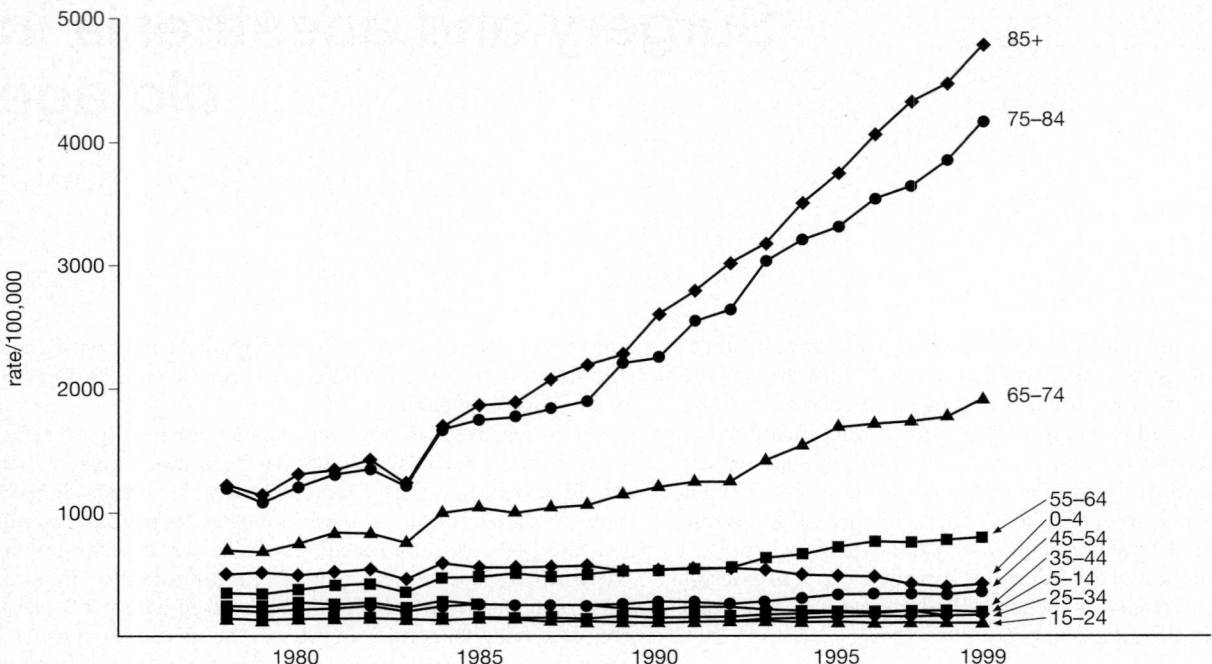

Figure 29-2 Ophthalmology admissions to Scottish hospitals, according to age group. Data courtesy of the Information and Statistics Division, Edinburgh, Scotland.

Surgery for cataract and total hip replacement for osteoarthritis are two prime examples of high-technology approaches to a surgical problem that have had a major impact on the quality of life of elderly patients. They neatly refute the simplistic assumption that high-technology "cures" are for the young, and low-technology "care" is for the old. As Grimley Evans puts it: "curing is caring."[8] In recent years, some of the increased surgical activity in young and old alike has been due to technological advances such as minimally invasive surgery. These techniques have had a major impact in urology, gynecology, and general surgery[1,4,6,7,9] and even in coronary artery bypass surgery.[10,11] It is important to ensure that elderly people benefit from these techniques as least as much as the young.

Some of the changes in surgical activity in different age groups have followed naturally from changes in the incidence or prevalence of disease.[7] Thus, with the development of effective medical anti-ulcer therapy, surgery for peptic ulceration has become much less common in the last 20 years. On the other hand, there has been a marked increase in the number of hip fractures, partly due to demographic change but probably due to underlying changes in osteoporosis prevalence as well.[12] In the field of orthopedic surgery, this "epidemic" of hip fractures threatens to limit the amount of elective orthopedic surgery that can be carried out, particularly in those orthopedic units where emergency and elective cases are competing for the same operating room/theater space.

In an ideal world, we would first assess medical and surgical needs in the community and then provide the appropriate services and resources to meet those needs. Those interested in trying to assess epidemiological needs for surgical and medical services, as a stimulus to more rational planning, are recommended to read a series of reviews edited by Stephens and Raftery.[13] In the context of the elderly surgical patient, the chapters on colorectal cancer, total hip replacement, total knee replacement, cataract surgery, hernia repair, varicose vein treatment, and prostatectomy are particularly relevant.

AGE, SURGERY, AND OUTCOME

The association between age, surgery, and postoperative outcome is a complicated one.

1. Many surgically treatable diseases become more common with age. For example, the incidence of colorectal cancer increases almost exponentially after the age of 40, so that 41 percent of affected people are aged 75 and over, while only 5 percent are under 50.[14]
2. Age may have an effect on surgical presentation; for instance, an acute abdomen in some older people may have less dramatic signs and symptoms, and may be harder to diagnose at an early stage.[15]
3. Agist attitudes or misconceptions of the true risks of modern surgery and anesthesia may influence patients and professionals in decisions as to whether elective surgical referral is indicated. While attitudes are changing, older patients in higher socio-economic groups may have very different referral rates from older people who are socio-economically deprived.[16] In this respect, as in so many other areas of medicine, elderly people cannot be regarded as a homogeneous group.
4. The incidence of nonelective presentation of surgical disease tends to rise sharply with age,[17] probably from a mixture of the above factors.

5. Nonelective surgical procedures have much higher rates of morbidity and mortality than elective procedures.[17–19]

6. Elderly surgical patients often have one or more coexisting medical conditions.[20] When these involve major organs such as the heart or lungs, then the risks of surgery and anesthesia tend to increase.[17,21]

7. Even in the absence of coexisting medical disease, gerontological studies point to a diminution in homeostatic reserve with age. Under conditions of extreme stress it might therefore be expected that the fit elderly patient would have less chances of survival than the fit young patient. This does indeed appear to be the case for multiple trauma or extensive burns,[22–24] but it is important that this does not lead to nihilism, as vigorous intensive therapy in elderly patients with burns and multiple trauma has led to improved survival rates.[24,25]

8. The increasingly common "league table" approach, by which the surgical mortality rates of individual institutions are widely publicized, may have a detrimental effect on the care of elderly surgical patients with multiple medical problems. Even when the patient, surgeon, and anesthetist are in agreement that the potential benefits of surgery outweigh the risks in an individual case, there may be managerial pressures to avoid surgery in high-risk patients because of the "detrimental" effect that a postoperative death would have on the league table. Case-mix stratification is a theoretical way around this problem, but is very difficult to achieve in practice.[26]

How can all these effects be disentangled? A fair summary of the available evidence is that it appears to be age-associated illness rather than the aging process itself that is the main reason for the increase in morbidity and mortality following surgery and anesthesia in old age.[6,27] Lines of evidence to support this assertion include:

- The APACHE III system, which looks at risk factors predicting mortality in intensive-care unit patients, has indicated that almost 50 percent of the variability in mortality is due to the intensity of the acute illness, whereas only 3 percent is due to chronological age.[28]

- In general surgical patients studied by the author in Dundee (Scotland) and Cardiff (Wales), the rate of postoperative complications for those aged 65 to 74 was almost the same as that for those aged 75 and over, provided that no preoperative medical problems were present (Fig. 29-3).[29] Similar conclusions have been reached by Dunlop and colleagues[30] in a group of general surgical patients, where medical status was stratified using the Medisgroups system, and by Shabot and Johnson[25] in a group of trauma patients, stratified by the Simplified Acute Physiology Score and the Injury Severity Score.

- Multivariate analyses relating several preoperative risk factors to postoperative outcome in elderly general surgical patients have not usually shown age to be a major *independent* predictor of postoperative outcome. Once major clinical factors (such as improved cardiovascular function or the presence of malignancy or sepsis) are entered into multivariate analyses, the predictive effect of age becomes less or disappears altogether.[31] At first sight, the logistic regression analyses of Pedersen et al.[32,33] relating preoperative status to postoperative outcome appear to contradict this statement, as the variable "age 70 and over" is associated with an odds ratios of 7.1 for postoperative cardiovascular complications, 5.6 for respiratory complications, and 9.0 for in-hospital mortality. However, this variable is expressed relative to patients aged between 20 and 49 years who are likely to have very little concomitant disease, and expressing the odds ratio relative to the age group 50–69 yields values of 2.0, 1.3, and 2.1. These are much lower than the odds ratios associated with major preoperative medical problems such as heart failure, ischemic heart disease, chronic lung disease, and renal failure.

Thus, attempts to set upper age limits for certain operations are suspect not simply from an ethical point of view, but are technically incompetent, because age by itself is such a poor predictor of adverse postoperative outcome in an individual elderly person.[16,28,34] Each person with a surgical problem—whatever his or her age—needs and deserves an individual assessment. The aim of a preoperative assessment of an elderly person is identical to the aim of a preoperative assessment of a young person. In each case there is a need to estimate, on an individual basis, whether the potential benefits of a surgical operation outweigh the potential risks.

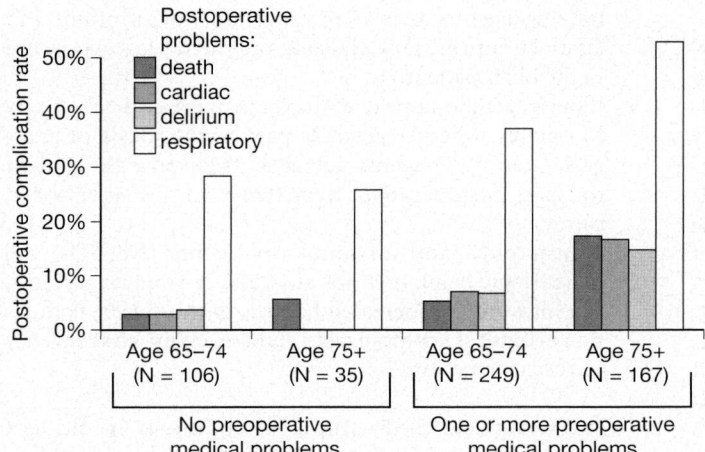

Figure 29-3 Age, preoperative medical status, and postoperative outcome in general surgical patients aged 65 and over. From Seymour,[29] with permission.

ANESTHETIC FACTORS

Morbidity and mortality following anesthesia

In some elderly individuals, factors such as the extent and type of surgical pathology and the presence of serious coexistent medical disease may suggest that the potential risks of surgical intervention outweigh the potential benefits. Under such circumstances, in discussions with patient and relatives it is tempting to resort to the phrase that the patient is "not fit for an anesthetic." However, in fairness to our anesthetic colleagues and the published evidence, this temptation should be resisted, as postoperative deaths occurring *solely* because of anesthesia are very rare at any age. Reviewing a number of retrospective surveys, Pedersen[17,38] came up with an estimate of one death in 10,000 anesthetics. In his own prospective study of 7306 consecutive anesthetics in patients of all ages studied between 1986 and 1987, one death in 2500 was thought to be attributable to anesthesia, with about one-third of these being potentially preventable.[17]

The total in-hospital postoperative mortality in Pedersen's series was 1.2 percent, but it was difficult to judge whether or not anesthesia had contributed to individual deaths, many of which occurred in elderly patients having major surgery for malignant disease. Difficulties in attributing the relative contribution to postoperative mortality of multiple factors such as urgency of presentation, extent of medical and surgical pathology, age-changes, type of surgical procedure, and anesthetic technique is a constant problem in surgical audit, as the excellent reports from the National Confidential Enquiry into Post-operative Deaths (NCEPOD)[35,36] and the Scottish Society for Surgical Mortality (SASM)[37] continue to show.

In Pedersen's[17] series of patients of all ages, nonfatal complications directly attributable to anesthesia occurred in one patient in 170, whereas the overall rate of postoperative cardiopulmonary complications was as high as 1 in 11. For complications directly attributable to anesthesia, there was no correlation with age. For problems not directly attributable to anesthesia, in-hospital mortality and cardiorespiratory complications were rare below the age of 50, but there was a steady increase in incidence of these postoperative problems for age groups 50–69, 70–79, and 80 and over.

Anesthetic drugs in elderly patients

Dodds[39] has described anesthesia as "applied clinical pharmacology with enough pathophysiology to confuse the picture." As both drug handling and pathophysiology are particularly variable in old age, the scope for confusion of the picture is greatly increased, particularly if pre-existing polypharmacy is present.

The recent review of anesthetic drugs in the elderly population by Dodds[39] is recommended in its entirety as a concise guide to an enormous subject. However, nine key points from that review are highlighted here, with the permission of the author.

1. The minimum alveolar concentration (MAC) is that concentration of an anesthetic gas that suppresses movement in response to a surgical stimulus in 50 percent of subjects. MACs tend to fall with age: in one study, halothane had a MAC of 1.08 percent in children but 0.64 percent at age 81.

2. With increasing age, there is a tendency to increased shunting in the lungs and decreased cardiac output. These pathophysiological changes have complex effects on the uptake of volatile gases, as a low cardiac output favors rapid uptake, while a decreased lung function produces the opposite effect. Such effects are less with the more insoluble gases, which therefore tend to produce a more stable rate of induction.

3. Where there is pre-existing ischemic heart disease, the patient may be vulnerable to the cardiac depressant effects of some anesthetics and there is also theoretical risk that isoflurane, enflurane, sevoflurane, and desflurane might "steal" blood from ischemic myocardium by increasing vasodilatation in normal vessels.

4. Hepatic metabolism and/or clearance of drugs tends to be affected by age, but there is considerable variability. Insoluble anesthetic agents that require no hepatic metabolism should be safer than soluble agents. Some agents such as halothane also have potentially hepatoxic metabolites, and this agent may also produce a fall in protein synthesis.

5. Hepatic metabolism releases inorganic fluoride from some hydrocarbon anesthetics such as sevoflurane, and where blood fluoride levels become elevated, nephrotoxicity can theoretically occur.

6. Because of reduced neuronal density and a reduced metabolic rate, the elderly may be more sensitive to a given amount of anesthetic drug. This raises the danger of overdosage. In patients with a delayed circulation time, there is increased potential for overdosage when intravenous agents are given too fast, as a delayed response may be mistaken for a lack of therapeutic effect, so that when the drug eventually reaches the brain, too much drug has been given. Smaller doses, slower rates of infusion, or repeated small boluses are recommended in elderly people.

7. Neuromuscular blocking agents can be classified into depolarizing types (of which suxamethonium is the only drug in common use), and nondepolarizing types. The nondepolarizing agents are usually favored in old age. Atracurium, vecuronium, and pancuronium are the nondepolarizing agents that have been most commonly used in general anesthetic practice, but atracurium has often been favored in elderly patients because it is not dependent on renal and hepatic metabolism for its clearance.[40] Newer nondepolarizing agents such as mivacurium, rocuronium, and cisatracurium are now available, but there is less experience in the older patient.

8. Elderly people appear to have an increased sensitivity to opiates, whether given as part of anesthesia or analgesia, and these agents may also predispose the patient to late postoperative hypoxemia, as is mentioned below.

9. Nonsteroidal anti-inflammatory agents (NSAIDs) are increasingly being used for analgesia in younger patients, but may present increased hazards in the elderly population because of nephrotoxicity, fluid retention, and tendency to gastric irritation.

For a more detailed account of anesthesia in old age, specialist texts should be consulted.[1–3]

RESPIRATORY PROBLEMS IN THE OLDER SURGICAL PATIENT

Incidence of postoperative respiratory complications

Respiratory complications are common after surgery in elderly patients, and while the majority of such patients survive, deaths from respiratory causes still rank alongside cardiac and thromboembolic deaths as major potentially preventable causes of postoperative mortality.[17,21]

The reported incidence of postoperative respiratory problems depends on the definitions used in individual research studies and on whether studies were prospective or retrospective. In general surgical patients assessed prospectively in Cardiff (Wales) using predefined clinical criteria, postoperative respiratory problems were found in 33 percent of those aged 65–74, and 50 percent of those aged 75 and over, but these percentages became 20 percent and 24 percent, respectively, when uncomplicated atelectasis was disregarded.[41] The risk of postoperative respiratory complications in these patients, all of whom were 65 years and over, was increased in the presence of clinical factors such as pre-existing lung disease, smoking, volume depletion, and incisions near the diaphragm.[42] Using similar definitions of complications, Brooks-Brunn[43] found six risk factors to be independently associated with postoperative respiratory complications in adults aged 18 and over undergoing abdominal surgery. These were: age 60 or over; impaired preoperative cognitive function; smoking in the previous 8 weeks; body mass index 27 or more; history of cancer; and incision involving the upper abdomen (or upper and lower abdomen together). Similarly, in a logistic regression analysis of surgical patients of all ages, Pedersen et al.[44] found that age, major abdominal surgery, emergency operation, pre-existing chronic lung disease, prolonged anesthesia, and the presence of pancreatitis were all positively associated with an increased risk of postoperative respiratory problems.

Pathophysiology of respiratory problems in elderly surgical patients

Lung abnormalities are common in older people even in the absence of smoking or known lung disease, although it is difficult to be sure how much of the abnormality of function is due to aging and how much to other factors such as recurrent respiratory infections or pollution.[39] Pulford and Connolly[45] have pointed to an increased closing volume (i.e. the lung volume at which basal airways begin to collapse) as one of the most consistent abnormal respiratory findings in old age, and an increased closing volume appears to be important in the etiology of many postoperative respiratory complications.[46]

Postoperative respiratory complications most commonly begin with basal atelectasis. Simple atelectasis may produce only minor signs and a low-grade hypoxemia but becomes clinically important when the lungs are already compromised and/or where the atelectasis develops into frank pneumonia. It should be noted that in the majority of postoperative patients, atelectasis is thought to be initiated not by retained secretions but by basal airways collapse.[21,46] A rise in closing volume or a fall in functional residual capacity favors airways collapse. Age is a risk factor for increased closing volume; but in the surgical situation, incisions near the diaphragm, the supine posture, and postoperative sedation also play a part in causing the basal airways to collapse.[46] In addition, if anesthesia is given without periodic full inflation of the lungs (to mimic the spontaneous "sighs" that occur in the conscious patient about five to ten times an hour), atelectasis is more likely to occur.[46]

Implications of research into respiratory pathophysiology

Classic methods of physiotherapy (which emphasize expiratory maneuvers and percussion) are unlikely to produce benefit in a patient in whom airway collapse rather than retained respiratory secretions is the initial event, and newer methods employ inspiratory maneuvers both before and after surgery. Devices such as incentive spirometers may be useful for encouraging deep inspiration,[47] and a systematic review of trials carried out between 1966 and 1992 concluded that incentive spirometry, intermittent positive pressure breathing, and deep breathing exercises were all more effective than no physical therapy in the prevention of pulmonary complications after upper abdominal surgery.[48] Classic "expiratory" methods of percussion and encouragement of coughing may have a role in those minority of cases where the retained secretions are the primary cause of respiratory complications; but if these techniques do not produce significant amounts of sputum, say 30 mL, then they may do more harm than good.[49]

Estimation of respiratory risk

In thoracic surgery, there is a large literature on the role of preoperative respiratory function testing as an aid to decision-making.[50–52] In recent years, researchers have asked whether preoperative respiratory function testing could predict postoperative complications in patients undergoing nonthoracic surgery.[53–58] The main conclusions so far have been that, in nonthoracic surgery, such tests must be interpreted along with clinical history and examination.[57] Future research reports will probably provide more precise guidelines, but in the meantime a pragmatic approach is suggested based on the current incomplete evidence (see the Summary of Management Algorithm).

Late postoperative hypoxemia

In the early postoperative period, constant vigilance is needed to detect possible respiratory complications and/or hypoxemia, and the latter process has been greatly aided by the development of pulse oximeters (although the need for direct measurement of blood gases has not been removed entirely, as pulse oximeters indicate oxygen saturation rather than absolute oxygen tensions and give no indication as to carbon dioxide levels[59]). Pulse oximeters have also had a major role in identifying a phenomenon, well known in anesthetic and surgical circles, for episodes of profound hypoxemia to develop 2, 3, 4, or even more days following surgery. The earliest research reports of prolonged hypoxemia appeared in the 1980s,[60] and the basic underlying mechanisms are now reasonably well understood, although the conventional explanation offered here is probably an oversimplification.[46] The classic clinical situation is that a patient who has had little or no hypoxemia for the first 1 or 2 postoperative days starts to develop episodes of profound hypoxemia (perhaps going below 60 percent saturation of oxygen), many times during the second, third, or fourth postoperative night. These desaturations often coincide with the presence of rapid-eye-movement (REM) sleep, which causes a disturbance of the respiratory mechanism similar to obstructive sleep apnea. The stress of surgery and, in particular, the use of opiates at the time of operation appear to suppress REM sleep for 2–3 days after major surgery, and it is when the REM sleep reappears that the episodes of desaturation occur.[61] Initially, the suppression of REM sleep was blamed entirely on opiates, but the phenomenon also occurs in patients who have not been given opiates.

Hypoxemia would be expected to cause arrhythmias and myocardial ischemia, particularly in patients with pre-existing heart disease, and it is tempting to conclude that some of the previously unexplained postoperative deaths around the third postoperative day were due to unrecognized hypoxemia.[62–65] However, it has been difficult to show a one-to-one relationship between episodes of hypoxemia and cardiac disturbance,[66] and other factors such as previous levels of hypoxemia and current carbon dioxide levels might be important as well. Hypoxemia might also have a detrimental effect on wound healing and cerebral function,[67,68] but again, there is need for further research.

The episodes of late hypoxemia can be prevented almost entirely by giving continuous oxygen by nasal cannulae for several days after surgery.[69] Common regimens are "three days and five nights." However, there are practical difficulties in identifying the patients who will be at risk from hypoxemia, and there is a balance to be struck between trying to monitor large numbers of patients with pulse oximeters and the alternative strategy of giving oxygen to a high proportion of patients even though some may not need it. Older patients, patients having major procedures, and those with respiratory disease would seem to be at increased risk of postoperative hypoxemia, but research is still continuing in this interesting area.

CARDIAC PROBLEMS IN THE ELDERLY SURGICAL PATIENT

Incidence of postoperative cardiac complications

Clinical evidence of postoperative myocardial infarction has been reported after surgery in 1–4 percent of unselected general surgical patients aged 65 and over.[21] In unselected patients aged 75 and over, and in populations of patients with known ischemic heart disease, the incidence is at least twice as high. The association between increasing age and postoperative myocardial infarction is likely to be due in part to a secondary association between age and preoperative ischemic heart disease. Other risk factors that have been repeatedly reported to increase the chance of postoperative myocardial infarction include myocardial infarction within the last 6 months and active congestive cardiac failure.[70] A number of other factors have been highlighted by some studies, including age, angina, hypertension, diabetes, arrhythmias, peripheral vascular disease, valvular heart disease, smoking, and previous cardiac surgery.[70]

Most surveys report that cardiac failure occurs more often than myocardial infarction, but that it is associated with similar preoperative risk factors.[70] More extensive electrocardiographic monitoring in the perioperative period has also revealed that many elderly patients have repeated episodes of subclinical myocardial ischemia that might be amenable to treatment. As mentioned above, some of these episodes might be precipitated by episodes of profound hypoxemia that are respiratory rather than cardiac in origin. This might help to explain why even the most sophisticated preoperative cardiac assessment cannot predict all adverse postoperative cardiac outcomes.

Diagnosis of myocardial infarction in the postoperative period is particularly difficult because the symptoms may be masked by analgesia or anesthesia, and the expected cardiac enzyme changes (such as a rise in creatinine kinase) may be mimicked by surgical trauma to muscle. More specific enzyme tests are now available, such as troponin I and troponin C.[70–72] Once clear clinical signs and symptoms of postoperative myocardial infarction are present, the death rate has been reported to be as high as 50 percent.[17,21] However, in a recent study by Badner et al.[72] which used troponin estimations as part of the diagnostic process, there were only three deaths out of the 18 patients with a postoperative myocardial infarction.

Cardiac assessment of the noncardiac surgical patient

It has been estimated that for every patient with known heart disease undergoing cardiac surgery, there are about 10 patients with heart disease, recognized or unrecognized, undergoing noncardiac surgery.[70] Many such patients are elderly. A large literature has therefore grown up on the "cardiac assessment of the noncardiac surgical patient."[73,74] Even though extensive use of high-technology screening of cardiac and respiratory function might in theory be able to predict many postoperative complications,[75,76] the large number of patients involved would make such a policy impracticable. Apart from the practical and economic implications, there are also scientific objections to mass screening of patients with high-technology methods. Some of the cardiac tests are not without risk, and in addition, widespread preoperative cardiac screening in relatively low-risk patients would inevitably throw up large numbers of false positive results, which could result in the unnecessary postponement of much-needed surgery.

Are there "low-technology" strategies based on simple clinical assessment that would increase our chances of predicting postoperative cardiac complications? The earliest research using clinical findings to assess cardiac risk in patients undergoing noncardiac surgery looked at risk factors one at a time (univariate analysis).[70] Unfortunately, this type of data was difficult to apply clinically when more than one risk factor was present, and so Goldman and colleagues[77] in 1977 were pioneers in producing a multifactorial index of cardiac risk in general surgical patients aged 40 and over. The problem with any clinical risk index is that it tends to perform well on the dataset from which it was constructed (i.e. the training dataset) but usually performs less well on subsequent datasets (test datasets).[42] The original Goldman index was based on a training dataset only, and subsequent attempts to validate it in other datasets have given variable results, particularly when subsets of patients such as those undergoing vascular surgery have been considered.[21] A modification of the Goldman index by Detsky in 1986[78] attempted to increase the predictive power of the index by taking into account the nature of the underlying surgical illness, but Goldman[79] has recently acknowledged that these early risk indices have now been largely superseded by other approaches, as is described below.

The newer approaches have employed a more stepwise approach to risk prediction, with initial screening tests leading, where necessary, to more complicated investigations.[73,74] The guidelines described by the American College of Cardiology/ American Heart Association (ACC/AHA)[80] use this approach and deserve close reading, while the recent editorial by Goldman[79] looks at future prospects for risk reduction.

The ACC/AHA guidelines and the Goldman editorial are described in the two sections that follow. First, however, a more general point about risk prediction needs to be made, which has applications outside the field of cardiac assessment and also applies to medical as well as surgical situations. A major concept incorporated into the ACC/AHA guidelines is the principle that more complex evaluation of risk, by means of non-invasive or invasive investigations, is best applied in those patients whose risk has already been judged by normal clinical methods as being *neither very high nor very low*. The mathematical justification for this comes from Bayes' theorem and is related to the concept of prior probability. In essence this states that, because most medical tests are neither very good nor very bad but something in-between, they are most likely to influence decision-making when the prior estimation of risk is neither very high nor very low.[73,74] Where the prior probability of disease is very low then the available noninvasive tests do not usually have a sufficiently high sensitivity and specificity to "lift" the patient into the "moderate risk" group and so do not alter the clinical assessment. On the other hand, when the prior probability of heart disease is very high, say 90 percent, then even if the noninvasive tests are negative, this is not enough to "demote" the patient to a low risk category, and so the tests again do not alter management.

The American College of Cardiology/American Heart Association (ACC/AHA) Guidelines

The ACC/AHA guidelines were issued in 1996, but the task force that compiled them has undertaken to review them every two years. With the exception of patients whose surgical problems are so urgent that they need to go for surgery straight away, the guidelines recommend one of four courses of action depending on patient circumstances:

1. Proceed to surgery without further investigations.
2. Perform noninvasive cardiovascular investigations to define risk with more precision (further management depending on the results of these investigations).
3. Do invasive cardiovascular testing straight away.
4. Delay or cancel surgery, or perform a lesser procedure, because the estimated cardiac risk is very high.

The broad basis of classifying patients is shown in Table 29-1. It can be seen that three types of risk factor are considered:

- clinical predictors for increased perioperative cardiovascular risk (Table 29-2)
- functional capacity of the individual patient (Table 29-3)
- the type (and thus the extent) of surgery being considered (Table 29-4).

The method of estimating functional capacity of a patient (Table 29-3) is of general interest and deserves to be better

---

Table 29-1 ACC/AHA guidelines for perioperative cardiovascular evaluation prior to noncardiac surgery: basic concepts

Perioperative cardiovascular risk can be classified on the basis of:

1. Clinical predictors (Table 29-2): Major/intermediate/minor
2. Functional capacity (Table 29-3): <4 METs/> 4 METs (metabolic equivalents)
3. Type of surgery (Table 29-4): in the case of a surgical emergency, operate straight away; otherwise classify as high/intermediate/low risk

Source: After reference 80.

Table 29-2 Clinical predictors of increased perioperative cardiovascular risk

Major:
Unstable coronary syndromes
Decompensated congestive heart failure (CHF)
Significant arrhythmias

Intermediate:
Mild angina pectoris
Prior myocardial infarction (MI)
Compensated or prior CHF
Diabetes mellitus

Minor:
Advanced age
Abnormal electrocardiogram (ECG/EKG)
Rhythm other than sinus
Low functional capacity
History of stroke
Uncontrolled hypertension

Source: After reference 80.

Table 29-3 Classification of functional capacity (see also Hlatky et al.[81])

Estimated energy requirements in metabolic equivalents (METs) of various activities:

1–4 METS:
- Can take care of self—eat, dress, use the toilet
- Can walk indoors around the house
- Can walk a block or two on level ground at 2–3 miles/h
- Can do light housework like dusting or washing dishes

4–10 METS:
- Can climb a flight of stairs or walk up a hill
- Can walk on level ground at 4 miles/h
- Can run a short distance
- Can do heavy housework, e.g. scrubbing floors/lifting furniture
- Can play golf, go bowling, go dancing, play doubles tennis, throw a baseball

>10 METS:
- Can do strenuous sports (swimming, singles tennis, football, basketball, skiing)

Source: After reference 80.

Table 29-4 Cardiac risk stratification for noncardiac surgical procedures

High surgical risk (reported cardiac risk often over 5 percent):
Emergency major operation, particularly in the elderly
Aortic and other major vascular surgery
Peripheral vascular surgery
Anticipated prolonged surgical procedures associated with large fluid shifts and/or blood loss

Intermediate surgical risk (reported cardiac risk generally < 5 percent):
Carotid endarterectomy
Head and neck surgery
Intraperitoneal and intrathoracic surgery
Orthopedic surgery
Prostate surgery

Low surgical risk (reported cardiac risk generally <1 percent):
Endoscopic procedures
Superficial procedures
Cataract surgery
Breast surgery

Source: After reference 80.

---

known in both surgical and medical circles. The maximal capacity of a patient is defined in terms of metabolic equivalents (METs), with 1 MET being the basal energy expenditure of a person at rest.[81] The ACC/AHA recommendation is that patients with a maximal functional capacity of 4 METs or less should be considered at high risk.

At the center of the ACC/AHA document is an algorithm which, on the basis of the three risk factors, recommends which of the four courses of action should be pursued. The original papers or website[80] should be consulted by those intending to use the algorithm in clinical practice, but Table 29-5, gives a broad summary of the principles of the algorithm, and also corrects a minor typographical error that appeared in the algorithm published in 1996.

While the ACC/AHA guidelines draw on a growing body of research evidence, many of their recommendations are not fully "evidence-based," with expert opinion being used where necessary to fill shortfalls in the published literature. It is therefore to be expected that refinements and alterations will be required as more research information becomes available, and as actual experience in applying the guidelines is published. Ali et al.[82] have recently presented data about the sensitivity and specificity of the guidelines when applied retrospectively to 119 cardiology and anesthesia consultations in Toronto. Two broad types of adverse postoperative outcome were defined, with "outcome 1" encompassing myocardial ischemia/infarction, heart failure, arrhythmia, and death; and "outcome 2" also including cancellation of surgery due to cardiac risk. The overall conclusion of Ali and colleagues, which might well be of importance in other areas of surgical risk prediction, was that the "medical" predictors listed in the guidelines had high sensitivity while the "surgical" predictors had high specificity. Thus, for Outcomes 1 and 2, the ACC/AHA medical predictors had a sensitivity of 87–89 percent, with the surgical predictors showing a specificity of 89 percent. When medical and surgical predictors were considered simultaneously, sensitivity was 93 percent but specificity fell to around

Clinical predictor (Table 29-2)	Functional status (Table 29-3)	Surgical classification (Table 29-4)	Recommended course of action
Major	Any	Any	Consider coronary angiography or modify surgery
Intermediate	<4 METs	Any	Noninvasive testing
Intermediate	>4 METs	High	Noninvasive testing
Intermediate	>4 METs	Intermediate or low	Proceed to surgery
Minor	<4 METs	High	Noninvasive testing
Minor	<4 METs	Intermediate or low	Proceed to surgery
Minor	>4 METs	Any	Proceed to surgery

Table 29-5 Basic strategy of algorithm used to determine next action

Source: After reference 80 (see for full details).

46–51 percent. However, as Ali and coworkers point out, prospective studies are now required to confirm these early findings.

It should also be recognized that, as currently formulated, the ACC/AHA guidelines would lead to practical problems for many clinicians and healthcare administrators. For example, as peripheral vascular disease is classified as having a "high" surgical risk, the guidelines would indicate that all such patients should routinely undergo noninvasive cardiac testing before surgery. In most UK centers this is not current common practice and would present considerable logistical problems.

A final point to make about *all* predictive systems is that they are only part of the process of risk reduction. While a broad stratification of preoperative risk is a reasonable aim (not least as a means of allowing the patient an informed choice as to whether he or she wants surgery), risk reduction also demands that a major effort should be directed into peri- and postoperative care. Such care would require careful monitoring at a level appropriate to the patient's condition, with adequate provision of high-dependency units and intensive-therapy units if clinically indicated. Within a UK setting, there is concern that existing facilities are not always sufficient to provide optimal levels of postoperative care, with the result that older frailer patients who are being monitored extremely closely during the period of their operation may rapidly find themselves back on a general surgical ward soon afterwards, where little specialized monitoring is available.[35–37]

Future trends in the detection and reduction of cardiac risk

The 1977 multivariate index of cardiac risk published by Lee Goldman and colleagues[77] has had a major influence on risk assessment prior to noncardiac surgery, and Goldman's contribution to the research literature since that time has been considerable. The recent editorial by Goldman therefore deserves our attention as an authoritative view of the last quarter century of research, and as a guide to the developments that can be anticipated in the near future.[79] In regard to the assessment of high-risk patients, Goldman broadly endorses the approach of the ACC/AHA guidelines. In reviewing multivariate risk indices carried out at a single point of time,

Goldman concludes that older approaches—including the American Society of Anesthesiologists' classification,[83] the Canadian Cardiovascular Society classification,[84] the original Goldman Index,[77] the Detsky Index,[78] and a clinical approach derived from vascular surgery patients who were selected for noninvasive testing[85]—may not perform as well as reported in the past.[86]

As a possible improvement on earlier multifactorial indices, Goldman draws attention to a recently derived index published by Lee et al.[87] which may stratify cardiac risk with more efficiency than the earlier risk indices. This index incorporates six risk factors: high-risk surgery; presence of ischemic heart disease; history of congestive cardiac failure; history of cerebrovascular disease; insulin therapy for diabetes; and preoperative elevation of creatinine. It remains to be seen, however, whether the new index will perform as well when it is applied to older patients in other geographical areas.

An important new development in the field of cardiac management is the possibility of effective medical intervention to reduce cardiac risk. The most promising approaches so far have used β-blockade, and Goldman highlights studies by Mangano et al.[88] and Poldermans et al.[89] which demonstrated benefit from perioperative β-blockers in reducing the risk of adverse outcomes at one year and in-hospital major cardiac complications in high-risk patients identified by stress echocardiography. Another report looked at the effects of mivazerol, an α-II agonist, in a study of patients with coronary heart disease who underwent noncardiac surgery.[90] This randomized controlled trial demonstrated a significant reduction in cardiac deaths, although all-cause death rate and myocardial infarction rate were not significantly reduced. However, in a pre-planned subgroup analysis of patients undergoing vascular surgery, myocardial infarction and all-cause death rate was reduced as well as cardiac death rate.

At the end of his editorial, Goldman suggests three research priorities for the near future:

- more precise criteria to determine which patients should have preoperative noninvasive testing;
- clearer guidelines on which patients should receive perioperative beta-blockers;
- clarification of the role of coronary revascularization prior to noncardiac surgery.

As Goldman states: "the bad news is that we still do not have all the answers. The good news is that approaches to the treatment of a cardiac patient undergoing noncardiac surgery are increasingly being driven by data, including data from randomized control trials."

Cardiac surgery

Paradoxically, the prediction of risk in patients who are undergoing cardiac as opposed to noncardiac surgery is less of a problem, as most cardiac patients will have had sophisticated and invasive preoperative cardiac testing. Even more importantly, such patients are closely monitored postoperatively, usually in an intensive-therapy unit. Under favorable circumstances, the mortality rate following cardiac surgery in patients aged 70 and over is of the order of 5 percent, compared with a rate of about 2.5 percent in patients under 69.[91] Reports from Washington, DC,[91] and from St George's Hospital, London,[92] have indicated that about one-quarter of cardiac surgical patients in both centers are currently over the age of 70. However, these are both specialist teaching centers and there has been concern that in many parts of Britain referral practices and cardiac surgical rates in older patients are suboptimal.[93-95] Recent research has shown that the quality of life and functional improvement after cardiac surgery is at least as good for patients who are 70 or over as it is for those under 70.[96-97] Such studies add weight to the argument that procedures such as angioplasty, and operations such as coronary artery bypass grafting and aortic valve replacement, should be more widely available in elderly people.

Another growth area of potential benefit to older surgical patients is "minimally invasive cardiac surgery." To those outside the field, minimally invasive cardiac surgery appears to be a contradiction in terms, but there is a growing interest in techniques such as "beating heart anastomoses" which can avoid the problems of cardiac bypass.[10,98] For anatomical reasons, minimally invasive techniques cannot replace all conventional coronary artery bypass procedures; but where facilities are available, they could take their place alongside more conventional surgery and percutaneous coronary angioplasty as one of a basket of techniques that could benefit elderly people with ischemic heart disease.

NUTRITION

Undernutrition in middle-aged and elderly surgical patients is at long last attracting significant research interest. There are a number of theoretical reasons why nutritional problems might be of particular relevance in older surgical patients. These include altered immune response, impaired wound healing, risk of infection, and anatomical and physiological effects on gastrointestinal, cardiovascular, and respiratory systems.[99,100] It would therefore seem good practice for nutritional assessment to be part of the routine evaluation of older patients who are being considered for surgical treatment. At a practical clinical level, however, there remains concern in the UK that many medical students, doctors, and health workers are insufficiently trained in the field of nutritional assessment and therapy,[99,101] and similar concerns exist elsewhere. Corish[100] has recently reviewed the literature on preoperative nutritional assessment in adults, paying particular attention to those aspects of the subject that are relevant to elderly people. His review shows that the nutrition of older patients coming into medical and surgical wards is often suboptimal and that this is clinically relevant to their management. Even within hospital the older patient may not be nutritionally safe. Corish points to studies which indicate that elderly hospital inpatients who are "eating normally" have a dietary intake well below their estimated energy requirements, and observations of food wastage indicate that as little as 60 percent of the food that is served to older patients is actually consumed. A deterioration in nutritional status following admission is therefore quite common.

Nutritional assessment

Much of the recent research interest in undernutrition in adult hospital patients was prompted by studies in the 1970s. Since the pioneering work of Bistrian et al.[102] in 1974, a popular study design in the field of surgical nutrition has been to take nutritional assessment methods that have been used in general population surveys and apply them to surgical patients in hospital. Using this approach, Bistrian concluded that one-half of all surgical patients were malnourished. Although this statement had a stimulating effect on some clinicians, it caused a backlash among many others who simply could not believe that one-half of all their patients, of all ages and all surgical problems, were suffering from clinically important malnutrition.[103] More recent reviews have tended to emphasize that severe (as opposed to moderate or mild) malnutrition is found in much less than 50 percent of the surgical population, and that it is on this severely malnourished group that our main diagnostic and therapeutic efforts should be concentrated.[104,105] The evidence that led to this major re-evaluation of previous attitudes to surgical nutrition will now be briefly described.

Criticisms of Bistrian's 1974 estimates[102] of the prevalence of surgical malnutrition appeared as early as 1979. Gray and Gray[106] pointed out that the anthropometric norms used by Bistrian were not based on contemporaneous age- and sex-matched data from a comparable population. Even more importantly, the cutoff points were set as a simple percentage of the mean value rather than as a percentile or as a fixed number of standard deviations. This had bizarre effects, depending on the distribution and/or skewness of the parameter being considered. Another criticism of Bistrian's nutritional criteria, albeit one that can be leveled at the majority of subsequent studies of surgical nutrition, is that the serum albumin was included as one of the nutritional parameters. In recent years, it has become clear that there are so many non-nutritional factors that can affect the serum albumin of an ill patient, that it is safer to regard it as a general index of illness severity rather than as an indicator of nutritional status.[103,107] For instance, in a surgical patient with a low serum albumin and an intra-abdominal abscess, it is as likely that the sepsis is causing the low albumin as it is that malnutrition is causing the sepsis.

Nutritional supplementation

While we can argue about precise definitions of malnutrition, there is ample evidence that malnutrition is associated with a range of problems in medical and surgical patients.[99] However, a research study that shows a statistical association between markers of malnutrition and poor postoperative outcome does not necessarily prove that the relationship is one of cause and effect. Still less does it prove that nutritional enhancement will improve postoperative outcome. The only way to assess the benefits or otherwise of nutritional supplementation on undernourished elderly patients is to carry out randomized controlled trials.[99,100] Such trials are not easy to do, and three recent reviews of nutritional supplementation in the elderly population have commented on the poor quality of many of the trials and have recommended that methodologies need to be more standardized.[99,108,109]

In the earliest of these reports, Potter et al.[108] carried out a systematic review of the 1966–1996 literature concerning protein-energy supplementation in adults with medical and surgical problems. Of the 30 papers selected, two looked at postoperative supplementation in elderly hip fracture patients and are included in the Avenell review discussed below. Seven of the remaining studies involved adult surgical patients; but in six of these, all patients had malignant disease. The main conclusion of the review was that further research was needed. While Potter and colleagues agreed that supplementation appeared to improve nutritional indices, they concluded that "there are insufficient data in trials which meet strict methodological criteria to be certain if mortality is reduced."[108]

The Cochrane review of Avenell and Handoll[109] confined its attention to postoperative nutritional supplementation in elderly patients with hip fractures. Fifteen randomized trials published between 1982 and 2000 involving 1054 participants were selected. Again, the review commented that many of the studies were of poor quality, and advocated caution in drawing any firm conclusions from the results. It was, however, suggested that the strongest evidence for the effectiveness of nutritional supplementation existed for oral protein and energy feeds. In the five studies using oral multinutrient feeds, the combined end-point of "death plus complications" appeared to be significantly reduced, but there was no statistically significant evidence for an effect on mortality as a single end-point (relative risk 0.85, but 95 percent confidence interval 0.42 to 1.70). The three studies using nasogastric multinutrient feeding that provided enough data for meta-analysis[110–112] similarly showed no statistically significant effect on mortality (relative risk 0.99, 95 percent confidence interval 0.50 to 1.97); but they had very different case-mix patterns, and apart from the pioneering early study by Bastow et al.,[110] they did not draw a distinction between very malnourished and other patients. This might well have been an important omission as, following nasogastric feeding, the hospital mortality in Bastow's "very thin" category of patients was reduced relative to the "thin" group (relative risk 0.37 vs 1.12). However, the confidence intervals were very wide owing to small patient numbers, and so the results were not statistically significant. Similarly, when morbidity was the outcome measured, it was the "very thin" group who appeared to benefit most.

If the evidence that nutritional support is most likely to be of benefit when targeted on very malnourished patients is borne out by future research, this will be good news for both patients and health service managers. For instance, the study by McWhirter and Pennington[113] indicated that 27 percent of general surgical patients, 39 percent of orthopedic surgery patients, and 43 percent of medical elderly patients were "undernourished." However, when only severe malnutrition was considered, the figures became 1 percent, 6 percent, and 19 percent, respectively, with moderate malnutrition being identified in 16 percent, 5 percent, and 20 percent.

In fairness to the many dedicated investigators who have pioneered research in the area of nutritional supplementation, it should be appreciated that performing nutritional intervention studies, particularly in surgical patients, is far from easy. Patients with the highest rates of preoperative malnutrition and postoperative morbidity tend to be elderly and/or to present as emergencies. The bedside nutritional evaluation of such patients is technically difficult, as is described below. In addition, postoperative problems such as sepsis may have many causes, only some of which are likely to be preventable by nutritional intervention. While, in theory, 2 weeks' nutritional support would be advisable before surgery (see below), this is rarely practicable in emergency cases. In an attempt to reduce heterogeneity, a popular experimental design has been to simplify data-gathering by excluding nonelective admissions, and by focusing on conditions such as gastrointestinal malignancy, where there is a strong likelihood of preoperative malnutrition.[105,114–119]

A comprehensive review on the "existence, causes and consequences of disease-related malnutrition in the hospital and the community, and the clinical and financial benefits of nutritional intervention" has been produced by Green[99] on behalf of the British Association of Parenteral and Enteral Nutrition (BAPEN) and deserves a wide readership. A section of the review deals with nutritional supplementation of general surgical patients, and Green concludes that the overall evidence points to "clinically significant benefits" of preoperative supplementation in patients undergoing moderate to major gastrointestinal surgery, particularly if they are malnourished, and if it is possible to give 10–14 days of preoperative therapy.[103–105,116] The statistically significant benefits demonstrated to date have been related to morbidity and length of stay rather than to mortality, but this probably indicates that bigger studies are needed. The costs and benefits of intervention will also need to be explored in future studies, although the encouraging message is that, where it can be given, enteral nutrition appears to be as least as effective as parenteral nutrition, so that the very high costs (as well as the procedure-associated complications) of the latter can often be avoided.[99]

At a practical clinical level, how should we assess nutritional status in elderly patients on a busy surgical ward? The review by Corish[100] contains a useful practical discussion about screening techniques that might be used. However, the comment is made that most techniques include a combination of objective and subjective variables and that none has been developed specifically for the elderly surgical patient. As broad indicators of nutritional risk, Corish draws attention to the American Society for Parenteral and Enteral Nutrition (ASPEN) guidelines. Risk factors listed by ASPEN include: involuntary loss or gain before hospital admission of more than 10 percent of usual body weight within 6 months (or 5 percent in one month); a weight of 20 percent over or under ideal body-weight; the presence of chronic disease; increased metabolic requirements; alterations to the normal diet as a result of recent surgery, illness, or trauma; and an inadequate nutritional intake for greater than 7 days.

In regard to individual measurements that have been claimed to reflect nutritional status, Corish[100] makes the important point that "all the traditional markers in nutrition lose their specificity in the sick adult." However, some of the methods that can be used include pre-admission weight loss, anthropometry, various serum proteins, creatinine/height index, functional status, immunological competence, and bio-electrical impedance. The strengths and weaknesses of these methods are discussed in detail by Corish. Pre-admission weight loss is important to record provided that accurate weights prior to admission are available. As well as the ASPEN criteria listed above, different "rules of thumb" have been suggested as being clinically significant weight losses in the elderly population. These include 4.5 kg over two years, 2 kg per year, 4 or 5 percent over one year and 7.5 percent over 6 months. While there is thus some dispute about exact criteria, Corish points out that a weight loss of 20 percent of body weight is almost invariably associated with physiological impairment, and that older people may well be less tolerant of weight loss than the young.

Anthropometric methods of assessing nutrition may appear to be more "scientific" than other methods, but there are considerable problems in applying them to elderly people in general and old surgical patients in particular. Anthropometric measurements that can potentially be used in routine clinical practice are weight, height, body mass index (BMI) (weight in kilograms divided by the square of the height in meters), triceps skinfold thickness, mid-arm circumference, mid-arm muscle circumference, hand-grip strength, a history of weight loss, and measured weight change. McWhirter and Pennington[113] remind us that the BMI by itself is not a sensitive indicator of protein-energy malnutrition in adults, as it does not distinguish between depletion of fat or muscle. There are added problems in assessing BMI in older people, as some of them lose height as the result of osteoporosis. Some researchers substitute knee height or arm demi-span for body height, but then, as for all the other anthropometric measurements, it is necessary to establish age- and sex-matched norms in a comparable general population.[113] Furthermore, in acutely ill surgical patients, even the measurement of body weight presents practical problems.

A number of multi-item nutrition risk indices are also reviewed by Corish,[100] including the Nutritional Risk Index, Nutritional Risk Score, Subjective Global Assessment, Mini Nutritional Assessment, Prognostic Nutritional Index, Likelihood of Malnutrition Index, and the Instant Nutritional Assessment. All of these have strengths and weaknesses with the usual tradeoff between sensitivity and specificity and varying usage of specialized laboratory tests. Details are given by Corish, although he refers to two recent studies in which the Mini Nutritional Assessment was incorporated into an anesthetic consultation in general surgical patients and orthopedic patients.

From an academic standpoint, we might conclude that randomized control trials do not as yet permit the construction of detailed guidelines for nutritional assessment and support in elderly surgical patients. However, in the meantime, we need to do the best we can for our patients, and several lines of advice are available. Allison,[104] in a wide-ranging review of nutritional support in medical and surgical practice, points out that it is much easier to maintain physical and mental function by early feeding than it is to regain function once it has been lost. His broad criteria for nutritional support are (1) weight loss of more than 10 percent and continuing, (2) continuing inadequate oral intake, and (3) the presence of disease whose known natural history is associated with likely accelerated weight loss and poor intake for 10 days or more. Guidelines from BAPEN and ASPEN are published periodically and give detailed guidance on individual medical and surgical conditions.[101,120] On the organizational level, it is widely accepted that each major hospital needs a defined nutritional team to give advice and guidance on all aspects of nutritional support, but particularly where parenteral nutrition is contemplated.[101]

While further research evidence is awaited, a practical strategy for the bedside assessment of surgical patients has been devised by Windsor and Hill,[103,121,122] who are surgeons with an extensive experience in nutritional research. They have attempted to target nutritional therapy in surgical patients, by a structured clinical assessment together with basic anthropometric and laboratory tests. A summary of the methods that they advocate is shown in Table 29-6. The points to note from this table are that recent weight loss is probably of more

---

Table 29-6 Hill and Windsor's approach to nutritional assessment of surgical patients

Basic concepts:
- Recent weight loss (in past 3 months) more important than earlier weight loss
- Evidence of undernutrition together with significant impairment of function more important than undernutrition alone

Patients classified into three groups:
- I: weight loss (in past 3 months) less than 10 percent of body weight
- II: weight loss of more than 10 percent of body weight, but no impairment of function
- III: weight loss of more than 10 percent of body weight, and with impairment of function

Impairment of function:
A significant impairment in function is recorded when two or more of the following have coincided with the period of weight loss.

- Reduction in activity level
- Reduction in skeletal muscle function (such as hand grip strength)
- Respiratory impairment (check respiratory effort and sound of coughing and dyspnea)
- Impaired wound healing (unhealed wounds, sores or scratches, and/or skin sepsis)
- Serum albumin < 32 g/L
- Impaired psychological status (impaired mood, alertness, ability to concentrate, irritability)

Hill and Windsor found that only in group III patients were there statistically significant increases in postoperative pneumonia, septic complications, other major complications, and hospital stay. They recommend that nutritional support be concentrated on this group.

Sources: Windsor,[103] Hill,[121] and Windsor and Hill.[122]

importance than absolute body weight, and that where nutritional depletion appears to be affecting physiological function (see the table for definition), then there is more likely to be significant need for nutritional support than when physiological function is not affected. The technique of Windsor and Hill is open to a degree of interobserver variation, and there may also be interpretational problems in older patients where physiological impairment could well be due to coexistent disease rather than nutritional deficiencies. However, until these questions are settled by further research, the practical benefits of the system appear to outweigh the disadvantages.

Future trends in nutritional support and therapy

More fundamental laboratory-based research in the field of nutrition is also having an impact on clinical practice. At the cellular and molecular levels, knowledge about the interactions of nutrition, immune function, stress response, and gene activation is growing rapidly.[123–126] This type of information has already led to clinical interest in the selective use of particular nutritional agents (such as glutamine, branched-chain amino acids, arginine, and omega-3 fatty acids) both as supplements and as pharmacological agents to alter immune response.[104,124,125] Heys and Gardner[127] have provided a useful update on the potential of "nutritional pharmacology" in surgical patients particularly in respect to L-arginine and L-glutamine.

OBESITY

The pathophysiology of obesity has been discussed by Bray,[128] who divides patients into five categories based on their BMI. Individuals who are not obese (class 0) have BMIs of 20–25 kg/m², while the BMIs of individuals in class I (low risk from obesity), II (moderate risk), III (high risk), and IV (very high risk) are 25–30, 30–35, 35–40, and greater than 40 kg/m², respectively. In reviewing the anesthetic risks of obesity, Wilson and Reilly[58] take 35 kg/m² or over as their definition, and have discussed the physiological and anatomical changes that make the tasks of the anesthetist and surgeon more difficult. However, even in patients with severe obesity it has been difficult to demonstrate an increase in postoperative mortality; the main excess risk appears to be postoperative wound infections, with some studies also reporting an increase in thromboembolic complications.[58]

As Wilson and Reilly's review shows,[58] studies of postoperative outcome in mild or moderately obese patients are surprisingly uncommon in the literature. Garrow et al.[129] prospectively studied 469 patients undergoing abdominal surgery of whom 73 were classified as obese (taking a BMI of 27 or more in men and 30 or more in women so as to embrace the top 15 percent of BMIs in the population). The obese group had significantly more postoperative wound infections, but no differences were found in respect of deep venous thrombosis, pulmonary embolism, chest infections, urinary infections, and unexplained fever. Postoperative deaths (one in the obese group and six in the nonobese group) were too few for statistical analysis.

Garrow's series[129] was not confined to elderly people, but in an earlier survey of general surgical patients aged 65 and over, patients above the 75th percentile of triceps thickness had twice the rate of postoperative wound infections, but no increase in postoperative chest infections or in-hospital mortality.[130] In a more recent study of elderly general surgical patients,[19] patients were classed as being underweight or overweight by simple visual inspection. It was the underweight patients who had the worst in-hospital mortality and 5-year mortality; patients classified as being overweight had a survival pattern that was identical with that of patients who were classified as normal (Seymour et al., unpublished observations). This is of interest, as there is evidence from a number of medical and population studies that, once a patient has achieved old age, it is being underweight rather than being overweight that is associated with the worse long-term survival.[131–133] There would seem to be a need for further research studies in older surgical patients, correlating both low and high body weight with postoperative outcome.

A retrospective study of perioperative morbidity following primary knee and hip replacement defined obesity as being 20 percent above ideal weight for height, based on life insurance tables. On this criterion, 103 out of 154 patients were classified as obese (joint replacement patients with osteoarthritis tend to be overweight, in contrast to hip fracture patients who tend to be underweight). While the obese patients had longer operative times, their stay in hospital, number of days with a fever, number of transfusions, and analgesic use were no different from the nonobese.[134]

In a retrospective study of 924 North American coronary artery bypass graft patients who were aged between 60 and 86, obesity was significantly related to a prolonged length of hospital stay, but was less important as a predictor than congestive cardiac failure, renal impairment, and being aged 75 years and over.[135]

FLUID AND ELECTROLYTE IMBALANCE

The 1991–1992 National Confidential Enquiry Into Perioperative Deaths[35] stressed the critical importance of fluid balance in elderly surgical patients. In the 1999 review,[36] which concentrated on patients aged 90 and over, examples of over- and under-administration of fluid were encountered although particular attention was drawn to the former. In regard to postoperative fluid management, the following six key points were made.

1. Fluid imbalance can contribute to serious postoperative morbidity and mortality.
2. Fluid imbalance is more likely in elderly people as they tend to have renal impairment or other comorbidity.
3. Accurate monitoring, early recognition, and appropriate treatment of fluid balance are essential.
4. Fluid balance should be accorded the same status as drug prescription.
5. Training in fluid management, for medical and nursing staff, is required to increase awareness and spread good practice.

6. There is a fundamental need for improved postoperative care facilities.

However, the assessment and treatment of fluid and electrolyte disturbance in surgical patients is difficult, particularly for emergency patients where the deficits are likely to be most severe. There is no simple "cookbook" approach that will guarantee perfect fluid balance every time, and the sad news for the busy junior hospital doctor is that the best that can usually be hoped for is to make an initial broad assessment of fluid and electrolyte needs, to start treatment on that basis, and to monitor progress constantly thereafter. If cookbook rules are difficult to formulate for young surgical patients, then they are even more difficult to draw up for older patients; here, the increased prevalence of pre-existing renal disease and homeostatic impairment in the cardiovascular system and renal system[136] produces a need for tighter control, while at the same time the signs and symptoms of salt and/or water depletion are more difficult to interpret.[21,137]

Assessment of fluid and electrolyte status

The standard surgical strategy when assessing perioperative fluid and electrolyte requirements in patients of any age is (1) to assess pre-existing deficits, (2) to estimate maintenance needs, and (3) to allow for continuing losses.[21,138]

The assessment of pre-existing fluid and electrolyte deficits is more difficult in elderly patients because many of the classical signs of water and salt depletion such as reduced skin turgor and postural hypotension are neither sensitive nor specific in old age. For example, postural hypotension or lax skin tone may exist in elderly patients who are not volume-depleted, whereas a compensatory tachycardia may fail to develop in elderly people who are.[21,137,139] There is a need not just to examine the patient but to look at the whole clinical context over the previous few days. For instance, a patient who has been vomiting for 2 days is likely to be depleted of both salt and water even if the clinical signs are equivocal.

Water depletion

Another of the basic principles of assessing electrolyte and fluid balance is to try to estimate the type of fluid that has been lost and to identify the main body compartment that has been affected. It is helpful to remember that losses predominantly of water have very different effects from losses of salt and water together.[21,138,139] When pure water depletion occurs, then the intracellular compartment is primarily affected, and the initial symptoms and signs are nonspecific, being drowsiness, irritability, and perhaps low grade fever.[21,137] In healthy younger patients, thirst is a reliable indicator of water depletion, but this may not be true in a proportion of healthy older patients,[136,139] and the symptom may in any case be impossible to elicit in acutely ill surgical patients. The main fact to remember about water depletion is that hypernatremia tends to develop, and Lye[140] has estimated that 90 percent of cases of hypernatremia in geriatric clinical practice are due to water depletion.

Salt and saline depletion

Loss of salt (or saline, as salt loss is usually associated with water loss as well) has its predominant effect on the extracellular compartment, which includes the vascular compartment.[21,138,139] Middle-aged patients with this type of depletion classically develop postural hypotension and tachycardia, but the presence or absence of these signs may be difficult to interpret in older patients where postural hypotension from other causes may occur in one-quarter of patients, and where autonomic reflexes are often blunted.[139]

The patient with severe salt (or saline) depletion will eventually develop circulatory collapse and poor peripheral circulation, but these are late signs. A low jugular venous pressure (obtained by lying the patient flat and observing the neck) is a test of volume depletion that is underused.[21] In severe cases, more invasive methods such as central venous pressure monitoring or the estimation of pulmonary artery pressure may be needed. Although noninvasive means of estimating pulmonary artery wedge pressure are being developed,[141,142] none has yet entered into routine medical practice. Whereas a high serum sodium can be used to diagnose water depletion, a low serum sodium is unfortunately not a good sign of salt depletion, as hyponatremia can occur in a variety of clinical conditions, including congestive cardiac failure, where total body stores of sodium tend to be high, and where intravenous administration of saline might lead to clinical disaster.

In a younger patient with salt and water depletion, the appropriate kidney response is to produce a urine that is concentrated and low in salt. If a young patient develops oliguria, and the urine has these features, then a "prerenal" deficit can be presumed and fluid challenge can be given. Where oliguria is not associated with such features, then permanent renal impairment is often inferred and caution is usually advised with fluids. In the elderly patient, where a degree of coincidental renal impairment is common, oliguria may develop primarily as a result of prerenal causes, but the urine may be misleading because the pre-existing renal damage does not allow for salt and water conservation. Again, there is the need to take into account the whole clinical situation and not one set of biochemical results. If the clinical signs and history point to a likely volume depletion, then the correct course of action is to treat cautiously and monitor closely.

Defining dehydration

In the discussion so far, the word "dehydration" has deliberately been avoided. Strictly this word should apply to water depletion on its own, and this is the way it is used by Levinsky.[143] However, in general usage, dehydration is often taken to mean a deficit of water or salt or both, and the classical signs of dehydration under this usage are actually signs of salt depletion such as postural hypotension. A recent useful review of salt and water depletion in elderly medical patients[139] appears to use the term "dehydration" in this more general sense. As has been argued above, the signs, symptoms, and treatment of salt depletion on the one hand, and water depletion on the other, are different. It is therefore unfortunate that the word "dehydration" is often used in a nonspecific sense to smudge both of these together. However, as the usage is so widespread, the best course of action is probably to avoid the word "dehydration" altogether and to try to specify the nature and amount of the fluid that has been lost, and which body compartment is primarily affected.

Practical aspects of fluid and electrolyte therapy

Some broad "rules of thumb" that may be useful in assessing and treating fluid/electrolyte disturbance in elderly surgical patients are as follows:

1. A water loss of 2 kg or more is probably significant in an elderly patient.[140]
2. In regard to younger adults, Shires and Canizaro[144] suggest that a saline loss of 4 percent of the body weight is "mild," 6–8 percent is "moderate," and 10 percent is "severe." Elderly patients are not specifically mentioned, but are probably at more risk from a given percentage of saline depletion because of their more limited homeostatic reserve.
3. It has been estimated that, in the younger surgical patient, 4 L of saline are lost before signs of depletion appear, and 4 L of saline are gained before edema develops.[145] There appear to be no comparable estimates for older patients.
4. The recommended rate of fluid administration depends on the type of fluid that has been lost.

- In cases of water depletion, rapid replacement may be hazardous, as cerebral edema can result. Van Zee and Lowry[138] recommended that only one-half of the calculated water deficit should be administered over the first day, with the remainder being replaced over the next 1–2 days. Water repletion can be achieved by 5 percent dextrose infusions intravenously or subcutaneously. Water by the oral or nasogastric route is an alternative.
- In cases of volume depletion, rapid replacement is usually desirable. In young patients with severe volume depletion, Shires and Canizaro[144] recommend an initial infusion rate of 2 L per hour, but state that this rate should be halved as soon as signs of improvement appear. Even then, when rates of infusion are above 1 L per hour, they recommend that a physician be in constant attendance. For older patients with severe volume depletion, Shires and Canizaro point out that the benefits of rapid repletion may be partly offset by the risks of fluid overload, and they state that monitoring by central venous line or a pulmonary artery catheter is desirable.

CENTRAL NERVOUS SYSTEM
Postoperative stroke

Postoperative stroke is a relatively rare complication following general surgery, although the incidence rises with age, being around 1 percent in the over-65 and 3 percent in the over-80 age group. However, as is discussed below, procedures on the carotid arteries, and coronary artery bypass procedures, carry a higher stroke risk than general surgical procedures. In the case of carotid endarterectomy for symptomatic stenosis, the balance of risks and benefits has been worked out in two recent controlled clinical trials, but the place of surgery in asymptomatic stenosis is still a matter for debate.[146–148]

The risk of stroke after open heart surgery appears to be falling but still remains higher than that for general surgery.[149] The improvement in outcome in cardiac bypass patients has usually been attributed to better techniques of extracorporeal circulation, but two recent studies of postoperative cardiac patients have claimed that the main risk of postoperative stroke is to be found in a small subset of patients with pre-existing cerebrovascular or carotid disease.[150,151] If these findings are confirmed, preventive strategies targeted on this subset of patients might show clinical benefit.

Postoperative delirium

Postoperative mental impairment following surgery has been a topic of interest for many years. A proportion of patients develop postoperative delirium. This has an incidence of 10–40 percent depending on the type of operation, on the exact definition of delirium employed, and on whether the study was prospective or retrospective.[41,152] Many of the precipitants of delirium in the postoperative situation are the same as those causing delirium in the medical patient;[153] they include acute illness (particularly infection), the effects of drugs, and withdrawal from alcohol or psychoactive drugs such as tranquillizers. However, delirium following surgery may also be due to premedication (especially with anticholinergics), anesthetic drugs, associated surgical complications, and episodes of late hypoxemia. Diagnosis of the cause of delirium may also be more difficult postoperatively. For instance, delirium tremens developing postoperatively in an emergency surgical patient who has been unwilling or unable to give a history of heavy alcohol intake prior to admission, may be attributed to "surgical" causes.

A painstaking prospective study of the risk factors for postoperative delirium has been carried out.[154] Independent predictors of delirium were: an age of 70 or over; self-reported alcohol abuse; poor cognitive status; poor functional status; markedly abnormal preoperative sodium, potassium, or glucose; noncardiac thoracic surgery; and aortic aneurysm surgery. While it is sometimes stated that delirium is less common after regional as opposed to general anesthesia, in a large randomized controlled study of patients undergoing elective total knee replacement, Williams-Russo et al.[155] found no statistical difference between the incidence of postoperative delirium in patients following general anesthesia (12/128 or 9.4 percent) and that following epidural anesthesia (16/134 or 12 percent).

Although it is good practice to try to minimize risk factors that might cause delirium in elderly surgical patients, and minimal use of premedication in older surgical patients is one way of doing this, the main clinical requirement is probably to recognize delirium when it occurs and to treat the cause vigorously. However, trials of strategies aimed at reducing the incidence of delirium in older people in a variety of clinical situations are now being reported.[156] In a recent randomized controlled study of hip fracture patients it was reported that daily visits from a geriatrician reduced the overall incidence of postoperative delirium.[157] Another recent study of hip fracture patients used a nurse-led intervention program, and while the incidence of delirium was not reduced, the duration of delirium episodes was shortened.[158]

Postoperative dementia

The more difficult question involving postoperative mental status is whether dementia ever occurs as a primary event following surgery and anesthesia. There has been argument about this in the literature for many years following two pioneering studies that attempted to identify patients who had "never been the same since their operation."[159,160] Since that time the search has been out for patients who had an apparently uneventful surgery and anesthesia but who suffered mental impairment thereafter. Many of the early studies in this area were uncontrolled and did not have a baseline mental assessment measurement.[161] Some were also associated with emergency surgical procedures where a number of factors such as hypotension or sepsis might have had a permanent effect on cerebral function that was not directly due to surgery or the anesthetic process.[161]

In recent years there have been attempts to carry out properly controlled trials, with detailed psychological testing before and after surgery.[161] The problem with such trials is that the need to make precise preoperative psychological assessments tends to limit them to elective patients who are undergoing anesthesia under carefully controlled conditions and so the risk of postoperative complications of any type is likely to be small. Such formal trials have not demonstrated objectively that anesthesia, whether general or regional, has a permanent effect on mental functioning. For instance, in the study of Jones et al.,[162] objective tests of cognitive function were not statistically significantly different before surgery and 3 months afterward, although there was a group of 21 out of the 129 patients who reported some subjective changes. It is not clear whether these patients had real but subtle changes in cognitive function that could not be picked up by the standard tests, or whether they had other conditions such as depression or postoperative fatigue that were not primary dementing processes. A subsequent prospective randomized study of local versus general anesthesia for cataract surgery in patients aged 65–98 years found no cognitive decline at 3 months after surgery, and no difference between the two anesthetic groups.[163]

Subsequently, Williams-Russo and colleagues found no long-term (6-month) difference in mental functioning between elderly patients undergoing elective orthopedic surgery under regional anesthesia and those undergoing general anesthesia.[155] However, the cognitive function of 12 out of the 231 patients (7/114 of those having an epidural anesthetic and 5/117 having a general anesthetic) was worse at 6 months than it had been preoperatively. In the absence of long-term follow-up information of nonoperative patients using the same cognitive assessment protocols, it is difficult to assess whether a decline of this amount would have occurred even in the absence of surgery.

Many of the earliest studies could be criticized because they had no controls and/or because preoperative psychological testing was limited or absent. However, the first ISPOCD (International Study of Post-Operative Cognitive Dysfunction) study was specifically designed with these criticisms in mind,

and still came to the worrying conclusion that 25.8 percent patients had POCD (postoperative cognitive dysfunction) 7 days after surgery and that 9.9 percent of all patients still had evidence of POCD on the repeat neuropsychological tests carried out at 3 months (with corresponding values for controls being 3.4 percent and 2.8 percent).[164] Contrary to expectations, no correlation was found between perioperative hypoxemia and/or hypotension and the subsequent development of early or late POCD. Indeed, despite analyses of the effects of more than 25 other clinical parameters, only age showed a statistically significant correlation with late POCD.

Because the first ISPOCD study did not provide definitive guidance with regard to the prevention or treatment of POCD, ISPOCD2 was designed to look at a variety of other factors that might be related to cognitive impairment, although this study is yet to report. However, in the meantime, a cautious note of optimism is possible, because a subset of the ISPOCD1 patients has now been followed for 1–2 years.[165] While about one postoperative patient in ten in this longer follow-up study still had cognitive impairment, this prevalence was now similar to the rate of cognitive impairment found in nonoperated controls. This might indicate that some of the cognitive deficits noted 3 months after surgery were reversible. While numbers are small, and confidence intervals correspondingly wide, Abildstrom and coworkers suggest that POCD is a reversible condition in the majority of older patients undergoing noncardiac surgery, and their best current estimate for the long-term persistence of POCD is 1 percent.

This research area is still being explored but, on current evidence, it is fair to advise elderly surgical patients that elective surgery under controlled conditions is unlikely to lead to a permanent memory problem, although a transient delirium is relatively common.

Postoperative sepsis

Wound sepsis is a common cause of postoperative morbidity, and large-scale studies involving elderly patients have suggested that the incidence goes up with age. This might be due to subtle changes in immune function; but prosaic explanations, such as the tendency for older people to undergo more operations on the gastrointestinal tract and to present with more advanced surgical disease, are probably more important. More serious sepsis such as intra-abdominal sepsis or widespread septicemia with multiorgan failure, remains a major cause of postoperative mortality at all ages but particularly in the elderly population. The pathophysiology of such states is complex,[166] and mortality rates remain high despite intensive therapy.[167]

The concept of giving single doses of antibiotics to prevent postoperative sepsis has developed in recent years and is mentioned briefly here as it appears to run counter to normal antibiotic practice. Animal work over two decades ago[168,169] showed that sepsis in a wound or operative site was often initiated at the time of the first incision, and that this could be prevented if high levels of antibiotics were in the blood at that precise time. A single dose of an intravenous antibiotic given one-half hour before surgery is often sufficient to achieve this benefit, although subsequent doses are sometimes given during prolonged procedures. Antibiotic prophylaxis of this type is indicated where the risk of infection is high (such as in operations involving the gastrointestinal tract) or in situations where the risk of infection is low but the consequences of infection would be disastrous (such as in joint replacement surgery).[169] Where there is an established infection prior to surgery, such as in the case of a ruptured abscess, then full antibiotic courses need to be given and this should be distinguished from prophylactic antibiotic use. In practical terms, the administration of prophylactic antibiotics is usually in the hands of the surgical team, and there is a need to comply with local guidelines, particularly as antibiotic sensitivities can differ from place to place. The Scottish Intercollegiate Guidelines Network guidelines issued in July 2000 are, however, a very useful source of advice, and will be updated on a regular basis.[170]

The area of antibiotic prophylaxis more familiar to the physician is that needed to prevent the development of bacterial endocarditis when a patient with a pre-existing heart valve lesion undergoes a procedure such as dental therapy, which might cause a transient bacteremia. The scope of this type of therapy has recently been extended to encompass surgical procedures on the urinary and biliary tract and also some procedures on the upper and lower bowel.[169,170]

Postoperative thromboembolism

Pulmonary embolism is difficult to diagnose clinically, particularly in the postoperative period, and its true incidence is almost certainly underestimated in elderly patients. In 1979, before prophylaxis was widely used, Palmberg and Hirsjarvi[171] reported that the postoperative death rate from pulmonary embolism in general patients aged 70 and over was 3 percent, accounting for one-third of the total postoperative mortality in their series.

The risk factors for thromboembolism in surgical patients are similar to those in medical patients and include presence of malignancy, age, and prolonged periods of immobility. The additional factor in surgical patients is that the surgical procedure itself may initiate the process of venous thrombosis.[21] For example, in general surgical patients, the period of calf flaccidity during general anesthesia may be enough to start off a process of thrombosis that can then spread proximally. In surgical operations involving the hip or pelvis there is danger of direct trauma to pelvic veins, which can cause thrombosis and subsequent pulmonary embolism. In the former situation, a dose of heparin, which would be insufficient to treat thrombosis once it develops, appears effective in preventing a large proportion of venous thrombosis.[21] This is the rationale for low-dose prophylactic subcutaneous heparin use prior to many general surgical procedures, the typical dose being 5000 U twice a day until the patient is mobile.

More difficult decisions arise in the case of pelvic surgery or orthopedic surgery. Here the risk of thrombosis is higher and may be more than subcutaneous heparin can deal with; but the risk of hemorrhage is also increased. Various regimens have attempted to either supplement a low dose of heparin with other physical interventions, or to look at higher doses of anticoagulants, or to look at alternative antithrombotic methods.[172] As in the case of antibiotic prophylaxis, it is highly desirable to comply with local guidelines when prescribing prophylaxis for thromboembolism in surgical patients.

SURGICAL AND ANESTHETIC AUDIT

Audit is a process that has been well established for many years among surgeons and anesthetists, and physicians have much to learn from their colleagues in these specialties. A major advance in Britain has been the establishment of a National Confidential Enquiry into Perioperative Deaths (NCEPOD) for the UK excluding Scotland, and the corresponding Scottish Audit of Surgical Mortality (SASM)—the regular reports arising from these sources are well worth reading.[35-37] These reports give illustrative case reports of situations where deaths of individual surgical patients might have been avoided; and as around two-thirds of all the deaths reported occur in patients over the age of 70, they are particularly relevant to the present discussion. Recurrent themes over the years have been the necessity for nonelective patients to be treated in units with appropriate facilities and by staff with the appropriate levels of experience. In some of the individual case reports, potentially preventable factors have included a lack of medical stabilization of patients prior to surgery. It must be acknowledged, however, that this is a difficult judgment to make, as excessive delay before surgery is also associated with increased complication rates in many conditions, including hip fractures.

As well as looking at the medical circumstances of individual cases, audits such as NCEPOD and SASM have stressed the importance of having appropriate organizational structures in place to deal with high-risk groups such as the elderly emergency surgical patient. These structures involve the availability of adequate numbers of trained staff, the provision of high-dependency units and intensive-care beds, and the ready availability of operating rooms/theaters.[35-37] Less easy to define, but probably as important, is the whole style and atmosphere of an individual surgical service. This is likely to involve its degree of cooperation with medical specialists including geriatricians in the preoperative period, the postoperative period, and during any rehabilitation that is necessary.

The establishment of audit, the general acceptance of well-designed guidelines for patient management, and thinking of an "evidence-based" type are examples of general measures that are likely to improve postoperative outcome of all elderly surgical patients, but it may be difficult to prove the benefit of any individual intervention. This approach is complementary to the more usually discussed method of reducing risk in operative patients, which is to target high-risk patients prior to surgery and to put in maximal effort at this point. It is becoming clear, however, that perfect targeting of patients is unlikely ever to be achieved and that a combined approach involving selective targeting, peri- and postoperative monitoring, and close attention to the general environment, structure, and interprofessional links of the surgical service are all important.[25] A wider look at the subject might also consider the process of referral in the first place, and would also examine the attitudes of society to high-technology treatment in old age.[8,16,173] It is arguable, for instance, that if more elderly patients were referred at an earlier stage for surgery, then some emergencies could be avoided with a likely reduction in morbidity and mortality. While such approaches might have benefit, they need to be proven by controlled trials before they are introduced.

MEASUREMENT OF QUALITY OF LIFE

Surgeons and anesthetists have traditionally recorded deaths and surgical complications in the postoperative period as their only outcome measures. In so doing, they have given the lead to their physician colleagues, who have usually collected no outcome measures of any type. However, all groups of clinicians have realized in recent years that there is a need to look at the wider impact of treatment on a patient's ability to pursue those activities in life that are important to him or her. The exact definition of "health-related quality of life" is difficult, and, as McDowell and Newell[174] have pointed out, it is common for the terms "general health status measures" and "measures of health-related quality of life" to be used interchangeably. However, the aspects usually included in quality-of-life assessments are physical function and mobility, cognitive function, self-care, emotional status, sensory function, and pain.[175]

There is increasing interest in measuring health-related quality of life in surgical patients,[176,177] and studies are starting to have an impact on attitudes to surgery in old age. The measurement of quality of life after cardiac surgery[96,97] has supported the argument that more cardiac operations should be carried out in elderly people. Similarly, the decision whether or not to have a total hip replacement depends crucially on the ability of the surgery to reduce pain and increase activity, and thus to allow patients to pursue those activities in life that are most important to them.[178] Follow-up studies from intensive-care units have started to consider qualitative aspects of outcome as well as simple survival.[175] Again, these studies seem to favor the more widespread use of intensive care for treatment of elderly people, as well as showing that age by itself has very little to do with the survival process.[175]

Questionnaires designed to measure health-related quality of life fall into three categories, considered below.

DISEASE-SPECIFIC MEASURES These are designed to look at one particular surgical or medical problem. Thus, a questionnaire to look at patients following varicose vein surgery would be very different from that used to evaluate patients being treated for osteoarthritis.[179]

GENERIC MEASURES The second approach is to use more generic questionnaires such as the Sickness Impact Profile, the Short-Form-36 Health Survey, or the Nottingham Health Profile, which include questions about a wide range of physical, social, and mental function.[174] The advantages of generic questionnaires are that they allow different conditions to be compared in different populations, and that they are likely to have been well validated. The main disadvantage is that many of the questions may be of limited relevance for a specific clinical problem. For instance, questions on mobility are more relevant after hip replacement than after breast surgery. In practice, it is common for both disease-specific and generic scales to be used in individual surgical studies, as they tend to give complementary information.[178,180]

PATIENT-SPECIFIC MEASURES A third approach to measuring quality of life in an individual patient is to allow that person to nominate those areas of life that are most important to him or her and then to devise a tailor-made scale

to see how these areas change after therapy. These type of techniques are only in their infancy but include the MACTAR (McMaster-Toronto Arthritis Patient Preference Disability Questionnaire),[181] the SEIQoL (Schedule for the Evaluation of Individual Quality of Life),[182] and the PGI (Patient Generated Index).[183] To date, patient-specific scales have mainly been applied in the fields of orthopedics and rheumatology, but they could easily be extended to other surgical situations.

FUTURE TRENDS

Factors increasing the number of surgical procedures in old age

It is highly likely that the technical developments in surgery and anesthesia that have occurred recently will continue in the future and will allow potentially beneficial surgery to be extended to ever older and frailer patients. Such developments are also likely to lead to more favorable attitudes to surgery in old age, so that more patients will be referred. Even if attitudes and techniques were not to change, demographic changes would lead to an increase in surgery in the old and the very old in the next two decades.

Factors decreasing surgical procedures in old age

It is to be hoped that preventive medicine or novel forms of medical therapy will reduce the need for surgical intervention in some conditions in the future. This has already been seen in regard to modern medical therapy for peptic ulceration. An increase in minimally invasive techniques might also lead to a reduction in the number of major surgical operations being performed. For instance, gall bladder surgery is increasingly being performed by laparoscopic techniques rather than via a laparotomy.[9]

A reduction in surgical activity in some conditions because of better medical therapies or the substitution of less invasive procedures is obviously to be applauded. Much more sinister, however, is the tendency for politicians and health planners to contemplate that some forms of potentially beneficial surgery should be rationed on the basis of age, even though there is very poor evidence that age has any significant effect on the ability of a patient to benefit from a given surgical procedure.

If elderly patients are denied surgery simply on the basis of their age, this is by definition agist and such practices need to be challenged vigorously.[16,34] However, more subtle forms of discrimination may occur because of reduced equity of access of older people to medical and surgical services, and a UK Medical Research Council review has concluded that "research is needed to examine the extent of differences in access to the NHS according to age group."[184] While detection of inequity of access is difficult for both medical and surgical conditions, the research is technically simpler in the surgical situation, as interventions and end-points tend to be more clearly defined. Preliminary investigations by Seymour and Garthwaite[16] suggest that inequity of access for surgical patients on the basis of age does exist, but that this interacts with inequity based on patient deprivation.[13] Age-related inequity is probably decreasing with time, but inequity on the basis of deprivation may be more resistant to change.[16]

KEY POINTS   Surgery and anesthesia

- In the last 25 years the increase in surgical activity involving patients aged 65 and over has been much greater than that which would have been expected from demographic trends alone. This change has been seen not only for life-saving procedures, but also in procedures predominantly aimed at increasing quality of life.

- The association between age, surgery, and postoperative outcome is a complex one. However, there are scientific and ethical reasons to argue that age by itself should not be a barrier to surgery. Each patient, whatever his/her age, needs an individual assessment so that the potential benefits and risk of surgery and anesthesia can be identified.

- Anesthetic techniques are becoming more and more sophisticated and are allowing surgical procedures to be performed in patients who have advanced medical problems. The concern of many anesthetists in the UK lies not so much with the patient at the time of anesthesia, but with the intensity of care that is available in the hours and days immediately after.

- Respiratory problems are a common cause of postoperative morbidity, and a smaller but important cause of postoperative mortality. Research into the mechanism of postoperative respiratory complications has allowed a more logical approach to prevention and treatment, but further research is required to define an optimal set of strategies.

- Postoperative hypoxemia can occur for a variety of reasons and is not confined to the immediate hours following surgery. Pulse oximetry has made it easier to monitor and treat hypoxemia, but research is still going on into the underlying mechanisms.

- "Cardiac assessment of the noncardiac surgical patient" has been an area of research activity for many years. Guidelines issued by the American College of Cardiology and the American Heart Association (ACC/AHA) provide a coherent approach to the management of surgical patients who have coincidental cardiac disease. However, while there is a considerable evidence base supporting these guidelines, further research is needed and ACC/AHA have undertaken to update these guidelines on a regular basis.

- Undernutrition in middle-aged and elderly surgical patients has only recently attracted the research attention that it deserves. Broad guidelines for identifying older surgical patients at risk and for designing nutritional interventions are available, but the evidence base is still patchy.

- A greater risk of postoperative fluid and electrolyte imbalance in the elderly patient with impaired homeostasis is to be expected on theoretical grounds and is often observed clinically, not least in death audits. Unfortunately, examples of severe fluid overload and severe fluid underload both feature in audits, and there is no simple strategy that will suit all clinical situations. In the chapter a variety of strategies are offered to try to assess fluid–electrolyte status with more accuracy in elderly surgical patients, but this is an area where repeated assessment, cautious trials of therapy, and close clinical observation are likely to be needed for a considerable time.

- The causes of acute delirium in surgical patients are similar to the causes in elderly nonsurgical patients. A major and continuing concern over the years, however, has been whether permanent cognitive dysfunction can occur simply as a result of an uneventful anesthetic. The first International Study of Postoperative Cognitive Dysfunction (ISPOCD1) was designed to answer these questions once and for all, but some doubts have still remained and a series of investigations under the ISPOCD2 banner have been launched.

- Surgeons and anesthetists have led the way in showing the value of clinical audit in looking for potentially modifiable factors for morbidity and mortality. However, it is increasingly being realized that other outcomes such as quality-of-life measurements need to be considered, particularly in the case of operations such as hip replacement or cataract surgery where the primary aim is not to save life but to alleviate symptoms, improve function, and enhance well-being. This is a complex field, and it is important that medical and surgical researchers take advantage of theoretical advances made in fields such as psychology, psychometrics, and sociology in regard to the definition and measurement of "quality of life."

REFERENCES

1. Crosby DL, Rees GAD, Seymour DG (eds): The Ageing Surgical Patient: Anesthetic, Operative and Medical Management. John Wiley, Chichester, 1992
2. McLeskey CH: Geriatric Anesthesiology. Williams & Wilkins, Baltimore, 1997
3. Muravchick S: Geroanesthesia: Principles for Management of the Elderly Patient. Mosby Yearbook, St Louis, 1997
4. Rosenthal RA, Zenilman ME, Katlic MR (eds): Principles and Practice of Geriatric Surgery. Springer-Verlag, New York, 2001
5. Van Assen, quoted by Coley WB: Hernia. In Keen WW (ed): Surgery: Its Principles and Practice. W.B. Saunders, Philadelphia, 1913:587
6. Seymour DG: The aging surgical patient—an update. Rev Clin Gerontol 1999;9:221–233
7. Seymour DG: Future trends. In Crosby DL, Rees GAD, Seymour DG (eds): The Ageing Surgical Patient: Anesthetic, Operative and Medical Management. John Wiley, London, 1992:417–427
8. Evans JG: Curing is caring. Age Ageing 1989;18:217–218
9. Efron DT, Bender JS: Laparoscopic surgery in older adults. J Am Gerontol Soc 2001;49:658–663
10. Duhaylongsod FG: Minimally invasive cardiac surgery defined. Arch Surg 2000;135:296–301
11. Mack MJ: Is there a future for minimally invasive cardiac surgery? Eur J Cardiothor Surg 1999;16(suppl 2):S119–S125
12. Royal College of Physicians: Fractured neck of femur, prevention and management. J R Coll Physicians Lond 1989;23:8–12
13. Stevens A, Raftery J (eds): Health Care Needs Assessment. The Epidemiologically Based Needs Assessment Reviews, Vols 1 and 2. Radcliffe Medical Press, Oxford, 1994
14. Mountney L, Sanderson H, Harris J: Colorectal cancer. In Stevens A, Raftery J (eds): Health Care Needs Assessment. The Epidemiologically Based Needs Assessment Review. Radcliffe Medical Press, Oxford, 1994:379–410
15. De Dombal FT: Acute abdominal pain in the elderly patient. In Diagnosis of Acute Abdominal Pain, 2nd edn. Churchill Livingstone, Edinburgh, 1991:161–171
16. Seymour DG, Garthwaite PH: Age, deprivation category and rates of inguinal hernia surgery in men: is there evidence of inequity of access to health care? Age Ageing 1999;28:485–490
17. Pedersen T: Complications and death following anesthesia: a prospective study with special reference to the influence of patient-, anesthesia-, and surgery-related risk factors. Danish Med Bull 1994;41:319–331

18. Le Néel J-C, Guiberteau B, Borde L et al: Prise en charge des patients âgés de plus de 75 ans presentant une pathologie digestive ou abdominale: a propos de 660 observations. Chirurgie 1993–94;119:143–147

19. Edwards AE, Seymour DG, McCarthy JM, Crumplin MKH: A five-year survival study of general surgical patients aged 65 years and over. Anaesthesia 1996;51:3–10

20. Arvidsson S, Ouchterlony J, Nilsson S et al: The Gothenburg study of perioperative risk. I: Pre-operative findings, post-operative complications. Acta Anesth Scand 1994;38:679–690

21. Seymour DG, Rees GAD, Crosby DL: Introduction and general principles. In Crosby DL, Rees GAD, Seymour DG (eds): The Ageing Surgical Patient: Anesthetic, Operative and Medical Management. John Wiley, Chichester, 1992:1–90

22. Day RJ, Vinen J, Hewitt-Falls E: Major trauma outcomes in the elderly. Med J Aust 1994;160:675–678

23. Smith DL, Cairns BA, Ramadan F et al: Effect of inhalation injury, burn size, and age on mortality: a study of 1447 consecutive burn patients. Trauma 1994;37:655–659

24. Herruzo-Cabrera R, Fernandez-Arjona M, Garcia-Torres V et al: Mortality evolution study of burn patients in a critical care burn unit between 1971 and 1991. Burns 1995;21:106–109

25. Shabot MM, Johnson CL: Outcome from critical care in the "oldest old" trauma patients. J Trauma 1995;39:254–260

26. Parsonnet V: Risk stratification in cardiac surgery: is it worthwhile? J Cardiac Surg 1995;10:690–698

27. Lubin MF: Is age a risk factor for surgery? Med Clin North Am 1993;77:327–335

28. Knaus WA, Wagner DP, Draper EA et al: The APACHE III prognostic system: risk prediction of hospital mortality for critically ill hospitalized adults. Chest 1991;100:1619–1636

29. Seymour DG: Ageing and ageism: a medical and surgical perspective. Aberdeen Univ Rev 1996;3:344–359

30. Dunlop WE, Rosenblood L, Lawrason L et al: Effects of age and severity of illness on outcome and length of stay in geriatric surgical patients. Am J Surg 1993;165:577–580

31. Seymour DG: Prediction of Risk in the Elderly Surgical Patient. MD thesis, University of Birmingham, England, 1988

32. Pedersen T, Eliasen K, Henriksen E: A prospective study of risk factors and cardiopulmonary complications associated with anesthesia and surgery: risk indicators of cardiopulmonary morbidity. Acta Anesthesiol Scand 1990;34:144–155

33. Pedersen T, Eliasen K, Henriksen E: A prospective study of mortality associated with anesthesia and surgery: risk indicators of mortality in hospital. Acta Anesthesiol Scand 1990;34:176–182

34. Grimley Evans J: The rationing debate: rationing health care by age: the case against. BMJ 1997;314:822–825

35. NCEPOD reports: Available from the Administrator, National Confidential Enquiry into Peri-Operative Deaths, 35–43 Lincoln's Inn Fields, London WC2A 3PN, UK. Website:www.ncepod.org.uk

36. NCEPOD: Extremes of Age—The 1999 Report of the National Confidential Enquiry into Peri-Operative Deaths. See reference 35

37. Scottish Audit of Surgical Mortality (SASM): Annual reports available at www.show.scot.nhs.uk/sasm; or from SASM, Royal College of Physicians and Surgeons of Glasgow, 232–242 St Vincent Street, Glasgow G2 5RJ, UK. Email:surg.audit@rcpsglasg.ac.uk

38. Pedersen T, Johansen SH: Serious morbidity attributable to anesthesia: considerations for prevention. Anaesthesia 1989;44:504–508

39. Dodds C: Anesthetic drugs in the elderly. Pharmacol Ther 1995;66:369–386

40. Slavov V, Khalil M, Merle JC et al: Comparison of duration of neuromuscular blocking effect of atracurium and vecuronium in young and elderly patients. Br J Anaesthesia 1995;74:709–711

41. Seymour DG, Vaz FG: A prospective study of elderly general surgical patients. II: Post-operative complications. Age Ageing 1989;18:315–326

42. Seymour DG, Green M, Vaz FG: Making better decisions: the construction of clinical scoring systems using the Spiegelhalter and Knill-Jones approach. BMJ 1990;300:223–226

43. Brooks-Brunn JA: Predictors of postoperative pulmonary complications following abdominal surgery. Chest 1997;111:564–571

44. Pedersen T, Viby-Mogensen J, Ringsted C: Anesthetic practice and postoperative pulmonary complications. Acta Anesthesiol Scand 1992;36:812–818

45. Pulford EC, Connolly MJ: Respiratory disease in old age. Rev Clin Gerontol 1996;6:21–39

46. Jones JG, Sapsford DJ, Wheatley RG: Postoperative hypoxaemia: mechanisms and time course. Anaesthesia 1990;45:566–573

47. Hall JC, Tarala R, Harris J et al: Incentive spirometry versus routine chest physiotherapy for prevention of pulmonary complications after abdominal surgery. Lancet 1991;337:953–956

48. Thomas JA, McIntosh JM: Are incentive spirometry, intermittent positive pressure breathing, and deep breathing exercises effective in the prevention of pulmonary complications after upper abdominal surgery? A systematic overview and meta-analysis. Phys Ther 1994;74:3–16

49. Murray JF: The ketchup bottle method. N Engl J Med 1979;300:1155–1157

50. Epstein SK, Faling LJ, Daly BD, Celli BR: Predicting complications after pulmonary resection: preoperative exercise testing vs a multifactorial cardiopulmonary risk index. Chest 1993;104:694–700

51. Bolliger CT, Wyser C, Roser H et al: Lung scanning and exercise testing for the prediction of postoperative performance in lung resection candidates at increased risk from complications. Chest 1995;108:341–348

52. Ferguson MK, Reeder LB, Mick R: Optimizing selection of patients for major lung resection. J Thorac Cardiovasc Surg 1995;109:275–283

53. American College of Physicians: Preoperative pulmonary function testing. Ann Intern Med 1990;112:793–794

54. Zibrak JD, O'Donnell CR, Marton K: Indications for pulmonary function testing. Ann Intern Med 1990;112:763–771

55. Lawrence VA, Page CP, Harris GD: Preoperative spirometry before abdominal operations: a critical appraisal of its predictive value. Arch Intern Med 1989;149:280–285

56. Williams-Russo P, Charlson ME, MacKenzie R et al: Predicting postoperative pulmonary complications: is it a real problem? Arch Intern Med 1992;152:1209–1213

57. Celli BR: What is the value of preoperative pulmonary function testing? Med Clin North Am 1993;77:309–326

58. Wilson AT, Reilly CS: Anesthesia and the obese patient. J Obesity 1993;17:427–435

59. Hanning CD, Alexander-Williams JM: Pulse oximetry: a practical review. BMJ 1995;311:367–370

60. Catley DM, Thornton C, Jordan C et al: Pronounced, episodic oxygen desaturation in the postoperative period: its association with ventilatory pattern and analgesic regimen. Anesthesiology 1985;63:20–28

61. Knill RL, Moote CA, Skinner MI, Rose EA: Anesthesia with abdominal surgery lead to intense REM sleep during the first postoperative week. Anesthesiology 1990;73:52–61

62. Pateman JA, Hanning CD: Postoperative myocardial infarction and episodic hypoxaemia. Br J Anaesthesia 1989;63:648–650

63. Reeder MK, Muir AD, Foex P et al: Postoperative myocardial ischaemia: temporal association with nocturnal hypoxaemia. Br J Anaesthesia 1991;67:626–631

64. Gill NP, Wright B, Reilly CS: Relationship between hypoxaemic and cardiac ischaemic events in the perioperative period. Br J Anaesthesia 1992;68:471–473

65. Stausholm K, Kehlet H, Rosenberg J: Oxygen therapy reduces postoperative tachycardia. Anaesthesia 1995;50:737–739

66. Smith HL, Sapsford DJ, Delaney ME, Jones JG: The effect on the heart of hypoxaemia in patients with severe coronary artery disease. Anaesthesia 1996;51:211–218

67. Rosenberg J, Kehlet H: Postoperative mental confusion: association with postoperative hypoxemia. Surgery 1993;114:76–81

68. Rosenberg J: Hypoxaemia in the general surgical ward: a potential risk factor? Eur J Surg 1994;160:657–661

69. McBrien ME, Sellers WFS: A comparison of three variable performance devices for postoperative oxygen therapy. Anaesthesia 1995;50:136–138

70. Mangano DT: Perioperative cardiac morbidity. Anesthesiology 1990;72:153–184

71. Adams JE, Sicard GA, Allen BT et al: Diagnosis of perioperative myocardial infarction with measurement of cardiac troponin I. N Engl J Med 1994;330:670–674

72. Badner NH, Knill RL, Brown JE, Novick TV, Gelb AW: Myocardial infarction after noncardiac surgery. Anesthesiology 1998;88:572–578

73. Mangano DT, Goldman L: Preoperative assessment of the patient with known or suspected coronary disease. N Engl J Med 1995;333:1750–1756

74. Mangano DT: Preoperative risk assessment many studies, few solutions: is a cardiac risk assessment paradigm possible? Anesthesiology 1995;83:897–901

75. Gerson MC, Hurst JM, Hertzberg VS et al: Prediction of cardiac and pulmonary complications related to elective abdominal and noncardiac thoracic surgery in geriatric patients. Am J Med 1990;88:101–107

76. Older P, Smith R, Courtney P et al: Preoperative evaluation of cardiac failure and ischaemia in elderly patients by cardiopulmonary exercise testing. Chest 1993;104:701–704

77. Goldman L, Caldera DL, Nussbaum SR et al: Multifactorial index of cardiac risk in noncardiac surgical procedures. N Engl J Med 1977;297:845–850

78. Detsky AS, Abrams HB, McLaughlin JR et al: Predicting cardiac complications in patients undergoing non-cardiac surgery. J Gen Intern Med 1986;1:211–219

79. Goldman L. Assessing and reducing cardiac risks of noncardiac surgery. Am J Med 2001;110:320–323

80. American College of Cardiology/American Heart Association Task Force on Practice Guidelines: Guidelines for perioperative cardiovascular evaluation for noncardiac surgery. Circulation 1996;93:1278–1317. Published simultaneously in JACC 1996;27:910–948. For the original report and updates, see the American Heart Association website: www.americanheart.org

81. Hlatky MA, Boineau RE, Higginbotham MB et al: A brief self-administered questionnaire to determine functional capacity (Duke Activity Status Index). Am J Cardiol 1989;64:651–654

82. Ali MJ, Davison P, Pickett W, Ali NS: ACC/AHA guidelines as predictors of postoperative cardiac outcomes. Can J Anaesth 2000;47:10–19

83. American Society of Anesthesiologists: New classification of physical status. Anesthesiology 1963;24:111

84. Campau L: Grading of angina pectoris. Circulation 1976;54:522–523

85. L'Italien GJ, Paul DS, Hendel RC: Development and evaluation of Bayesian model for perioperative cardiac risk assessment in a cohort of 1081 vascular surgery patients. J Am Coll Cardiol 1996;27:779–786

86. Gilbert K, Larocque BJ, Patrick LT: Prospective evaluation of cardiac risk indices for patients undergoing non-cardiac surgery. Ann Intern Med 2000;133:356–359

87. Lee TH, Marcantonio ER, Mangione CM et al: Derivation and prospective validation of a simple index and prediction of cardiac risk of major non-cardiac surgery. Circulation 1999;100:1043–1049

88. Mangano DT, Layug AL, Wallace A, Tateo I: Effect of atenolol on mortality and cardiovascular morbidity after non-cardiac surgery. Multicenter Study of Perioperative Ischemia Research Group. N Engl J Med 1996;335:1713–1720

89. Poldermans D, Boersma E, Bax JJ: The effect of bisoprolol on peri-operative mortality and myocardial infarction in high-risk patients undergoing vascular surgery. Dutch Echocardiographic Risk Evaluation Study Group. N Engl J Med 1999;341:1789–1794

90. Oliver MF, Goldman L, Julian DG, Holme I: Effect of mivazerol on perioperative cardiac complications during noncardiac surgery in patients with coronary heart disease: the European Mivazerol Trial (EMIT). Anesthesiology 1999;91:951–961

91. Katz NM, Hannan RL, Hopkins RA, Wallace RB: Cardiac operations in patients aged 70 years and over: mortality, length of stay, and hospital charge. Ann Thorac Surg 1995;60:96–101

92. Unsworth-White MJ, Holmes L, Treasure T: Cardiac surgery in older people. Br J Hosp Med 1993;49:457

93. Elder AT, Shaw TRD, Turnbull CM, Starkey IF: Elderly and younger patients selected to undergo coronary angiography. BMJ 1991;303:950–953

94. Lawson-Matthew PJ, Channer KS: Reporting on reports: cardiological interventions in elderly people. J R Coll Phys Lond 1995;29:11–14

95. Northridge D, Hall RC: Cardiological services for the elderly. J R Coll Physicians Lond 1995;29:9–10

96. Jaeger AA, Hlatky MA, Paul SM, Gortner SR: Functional capacity after surgery in elderly patients. J Am Coll Cardiol 1994;24:104–108

97. Walter PJ, Mohan R: Coronary bypass surgery in the elderly: a multi-disciplinary opinion. Summary of proceedings of an international symposium held at Antwerp, Belgium, 9–11 March 1994. Qual Life Res 1995;4:279–287

98. Mack MJ: Is there a future for minimally invasive cardiac surgery? Eur J Cardiothor Surg 1999;16(Suppl 2):S119–S125. See also other articles in this supplement which is a report of a 1998 conference on minimally invasive cardiac surgery

99. Green CJ: Existence, causes and consequences of disease-related malnutrition in the hospital and the community, and clinical and financial benefits of nutritional intervention. Clin Nutr 1999;18(suppl 2):3–28

100. Corish CA: Pre-operative nutritional assessment in the elderly. J Nutr Health Aging 2001;5:49–59

101. Sizer T, Russell CA, Wood S et al: Standards and Guidelines for Nutritional Support of Patients in Hospital. British Association for Parenteral and Enteral Nutrition (BAPEN), Maidenhead, UK, 1996

102. Bistrian BR, Blackburn, Hallowell E, Heddle R: Protein status of general surgical patients. JAMA 1974;230:858–860

103. Windsor JA: Underweight patients and the risks of surgery. World J Surg 1993;17:165–172

104. Allison SP: The uses and limitations of nutritional support. Clin Nutr 1992;11:319–330

105. Campos ACL, Meguid MM: A critical appraisal of the usefulness of perioperative nutritional support. Am J Clin Nutr 1992;55:117–130

106. Gray GE, Gray LK: Validity of anthropometric norms used in the assessment of hospitalized patients. J Paren Enteral Nutr 1979;3:366–368

107. McLaren DS: A fresh look at protein-energy malnutrition in the hospitalized patient. Nutrition 1988;4:1–6

108. Potter J, Langhorne P, Roberts M: Routine protein energy supplementation in adults: systematic review. BMJ 1998;17:495–501

109. Avenell A, Handoll HH: Nutritional supplementation for hip fracture aftercare in the elderly. Cochrane Database Syst Rev 2000;2:CD001880

110. Bastow MD, Rawlings J, Allison SP: Benefits of supplementary tube feeding after fractured neck of femur: a randomised controlled trial. BMJ 1983;287:1589–1592

111. Hartgrink HH, Wille J, Konig P, Hermans J, Breslau PJ: Pressure sores and tube feeding in patients with a fracture of the hip: a randomized clinical trial. Clin Nutr 1998;17:287–292

112. Sullivan DH, Nelson CL, Bopp MM, Puskarich-May CL, Wallis RC: Nightly enteral nutrition support of elderly fracture patients: a phase I trial. J Am Coll Nutr 1998;17(1):155–161

113. McWhirter JP, Pennington CR: Incidence and recognition of malnutrition in hospital. BMJ 1994;308:945–948

114. Meguid MM, Campos AC, Hammond WG: Nutritional support in surgical practice: I. Am J Surg 1990;159:345–358

115. Meguid MM, Campos AC, Hammond WG: Nutritional support in surgical practice: II. Am J Surg 1990;159:427–443

116. Veterans Affairs Total Parenteral Nutrition Cooperative Study Group: Perioperative total parenteral nutrition in surgical patients. N Engl J Med 1991;325:525–532

117. Von Meyenfeldt MF, Meijerink WJHJ, Rouflart MMJ et al: Perioperative nutritional support: a randomised clinical trial. Clin Nutr 1992;11:180–186

118. Rana SK, Bray J, Menzies-Gow N et al: Short term benefits of post-operative oral dietary supplements in surgical patients. Clin Nutr 1992;11:337–344

119. Hessov I: Impact of sip therapy on postoperative surgical outcome. Nutrition 1995;11(suppl 2):221–223

120. American Society for Parenteral and Enteral Nutrition: Guidelines for the use of parenteral and enteral nutrition in adult and pediatric patients. J Parenteral Enteral Nutr 1993;17(suppl 4):1SA–52SA

121. Hill GL: Surgical nutrition: time for some clinical common sense. Br J Surg 1988;75:729–730

122. Windsor JA, Hill GL: Weight loss with physiological impairment: a basic indicator of surgical risk. Ann Surg 1988;207:290–296

123. Gallagher HJ, Daly JM: Malnutrition, injury, and the host immune response: nutrient substitution. Curr Opin Gen Surg 1993;92–104

124. Saunders C, Nishiwaka R, Wolfe B: Surgical nutrition: a review. J R Coll Surg Edinb 1993;38:195–204

125. Mainous MR, Deitch EA: Nutrition and infection. Surg Clin North Am 1994;74:659–676

126. Udelsman R, Holbrook NJ: Endocrine and molecular responses to surgical stress. Curr Prob Surg 1994;31:653–720

127. Heys SD, Gardner E: Nutrients and the surgical patients: current and potential therapeutic applications to clinical practice. J R Coll Surg Edinb 1999;44:283–293

128. Bray GA: Pathophysiology of obesity. Am J Clin Nutr 1992;55:488S–494S

129. Garrow JS, Hastings EJ, Cox AG et al: Obesity and postoperative complications of abdominal operation. BMJ 1988;297:181

130. Seymour DG: Medical Assessment of the Elderly Surgical Patient. Croom Helm, Beckenham, 1986

131. Campbell AJ, Spears GFS, Brown JS et al: Anthropometric measurements as predictors of mortality in a community population aged 70 years and over. Age Ageing 1990;19:131–135

132. Rajal SA, Haavisto HJ, Kaarela RH, Heikinheimo RJ: Body weight and the three year prognosis in very old people. Int J Obesity 1990;14:997–1003

133. Kushner RF: Body weight and mortality. Nutr Rev 1993;51:127–136

134. Jiganti JJ, Goldstein WM, Williams CS: A comparison of the perioperative morbidity in total joint arthroplasty in the obese and nonobese patient. Clin Orthopaed Rel Res 1993;289:175–179

135. Lahey SJ, Borlase BC, Lavin PT, Levitsky S: Preoperative risk factors that predict hospital length of stay in coronary artery bypass patients 60 years old. Circulation 1992;86(suppl 5):II181–185

136. Phillips PA, Johnston CI, Gray L: Disturbed fluid and electrolyte homeostasis following dehydration in elderly people. Age Ageing 1993;22:S26–S33

137. Gross CR, Lindquist RD, Woolley AC et al: Clinical indicators of dehydration severity in elderly patients. J Emerg Med 1992;10:267–274

138. Van Zee KJ, Lowry SF, and the American College of Surgeons: Emergency care. In Surgery. Scientific American, New York, 1995:1–16

139. Weinberg AD, Minaker KL, and the Council on Scientific Affairs, American Medical Association: Dehydration: evaluation and management in older adults. JAMA 1995;274:1552–1555

140. Lye M: Electrolyte disorders in the elderly. Clin Endocrinol Metab 1984;13:377–398

141. McIntyre KM, Vita JA, Lambrew CT et al: A noninvasive method of predicting pulmonary-capillary wedge pressure. N Engl J Med 1992;327:1715–1720

142. Vanoverschelde JL, Robert AR, Gerbaux A et al: Noninvasive estimation of pulmonary arterial wedge pressure with Doppler transmitral flow velocity pattern in patients with known heart disease. Am J Cardiol 1995;75:383–389

143. Levinsky NG: Fluids and electrolytes. In Isselbacher KJ, Braunwald E, Wilson JD et al. (eds): Harrison's Principles and Practice of Internal Medicine, 13th edn. McGraw-Hill, New York, 1994:242–253

144. Shires GT, Canizaro PC: Fluid and electrolyte management of the surgical patient. In Sabiston DC et al: Textbook of Surgery: The Biological Basis of Modern Surgical Practice, 13th edn. W.B. Saunders, Philadelphia, 1986:64–86

145. Tweedle DEF: Electrolyte disorders in the surgical patient. Clin Endocrinol Metab 1984;13:351–376

146. Rothwell PM, Slattery J, Warlow CP: A systematic review of the risks of stroke and death due to endarterectomy for symptomatic carotid stenosis. Stroke 1996;27:260–265

147. Rothwell PM, Slattery J, Warlow CP: A systematic comparison of the risks of stroke and death due to carotid endarterectomy for symptomatic and asymptomatic stenosis. Stroke 1996;27:266–269

148. Easton JD, Wilterdink JL: Carotid endarterectomy: trials and tribulations. Ann Neurol 1994;35:5–17

149. Sotaniemi KA: Long-term neurologic outcome after cardiac operation. Ann Thorac Surg 1995;59:1336–1339

150. Ricotta JJ, Faggioli GL, Castilone A, Hassett JM: Risk factors for stroke after cardiac surgery: Buffalo Cardiac-Cerebral Study Group. J Vasc Surg 1995;21:359–364

151. Redmond JM, Greene PS, Goldsborough MA et al: Neurologic injury in cardiac surgical patients with a history of stroke. Ann Thorac Surg 1996;61:42–47

152. Dyer CB, Ashton CM, Teasdale TA: Post-operative delirium: a review of 80 primary data-collection studies. Arch Inter Med 1995;155:461–465

153. Schor JD, Levkoff SE, Lipsitz LA et al: Risk factors for delirium in hospitalized elderly. JAMA 1992;267:827–831

154. Marcantonio ER, Goldman L, Mangione CM et al: A clinical prediction rule for delirium after elective noncardiac surgery. JAMA 1994;271:134–139

155. Williams Russo P, Sharrock NE, Mattis S et al: Cognitive effects after epidural vs general anesthesia in older adults: a randomized trial. JAMA 1995;274:44–50

156. Cole MG, Primeau FJ, Elie LM: Delirium prevention, treatment, and outcome studies. J Geriatr Psychiat Neurol 1998;11:126–237 and discussion 157–158

157. Marcantonio ER, Flacker JM, Wright RJ, Resnick NM: Reducing delirium after hip fracture: a randomized trial. J Am Geriatr Soc 2001;49:516–522

158. Milisen K, Foreman MD, Abraham IL et al: A nurse-led interdisciplinary intervention program for delirium in elderly hip-fracture patients. J Am Geriatr Soc 2001;49:523–532

159. Bedford PD: Adverse cerebral effects of anesthesia on old people. Lancet 1955;ii:256–263

160. Simpson BR, Williams M, Scott JF, Crampton Smith A: The effects of anaesthesia on old people. Lancet 1961;ii:887–893

161. Seymour DG: Anesthetics and the mental state. In Copeland JRM, Abou-Saleh MT, Balzer DG (eds): Principles and Practice of Geriatric Psychiatry. John Wiley, Chichester, 1994:995–1004

162. Jones MJT, Piggott SE, Vaughan RS et al: Cognitive and functional competence after anaesthesia in patients aged over 60: controlled trial of general and regional anaesthesia for elective hip or knee replacement. BMJ 1990;300:1683–1687

163. Campbell DNC, Lim M, Kerr Muir M et al: A prospective randomised study of local versus general anaesthesia for cataract surgery. Anaesthesia 1993;48:422–428

164. Moller JT, Cluitmans P, Rasmussen LS et al: Long-term postoperative cognitive dysfunction in the elderly: ISPOCD1 study. Lancet 1998;351:857–861

165. Abildstrom H, Rasmussen LS, Rentowl P et al, and the ISPOCD group: Cognitive dysfunction 1–2 years after non-cardiac surgery in the elderly. Acta Anesthesiol Scand 2000;44:1246–1251

166. Shaw JHF: Metabolic basis for management of the septic surgical patient. World J Surg 1993;17:154–164

167. Bender BS: Sepsis. Clin Geriatr Med 1992;8:913–924

168. Condon RE, Wittman DH: Surgical infections. In Morris PJ, Malt RA (eds): Oxford Textbook of Surgery. Oxford University Press, Oxford, 1994:27–44

169. Paluzzi RG: Antimicrobial prophylaxis for surgery. Med Clin North Am 1993;77:427–441

170. Scottish Inter-collegiate Guidelines Network 45: Antibiotic Prophylaxis in Surgery. Available at www.sign.ac.uk, July 2000

171. Palmberg GS, Hirsjarvi E: Mortality in geriatric surgery. Gerontology 1979;25:103–112

172. Merli GJ: Deep vein thrombosis and pulmonary embolism prophylaxis in orthopaedic surgery. Med Clin North Am 1993;77:397–411

173. Evans JG: This patient or that patient? In Rationing in Action. BMJ Publishing Group, London, 1993:118–124

174. McDowell I, Newell C: Measuring Health: A Guide to Rating Scales and Questionnaires, 2nd edn. Oxford University Press, New York, 1996

175. Chelluri L, Grenvik, Silverman M: Intensive care for critically ill elderly: mortality, costs, and quality of life. Arch Intern Med 1995;155:1013–1022

176. Wood-Dauphinee SL, Troidl H: Assessing quality of life in surgical studies. Theoret Surg 1989;4:35–44

177. Fraser SCA: Quality-of-life measurement in surgical practice. Br J Surg 1993;80:163–169

178. Laupacis A, Bourne R, Rorabeck C et al: The effect of total hip replacement on health-related quality of life. J Bone Joint Surg 1993;75A:1619–1626

179. Bellamy N, Buchanan WW, Goldsmith CH et al: Validation study of WOMAC: a health status instrument for measuring clinically important patient relative outcomes to antirheumatic drug therapy in patients with osteoarthritis of the hip or knee. J Rheumatol 1988;15:1833–1840

180. Bombardier C, Melfi CA, Paul J et al: Comparison of a generic and a disease-specific measure of pain and physical function after knee-replacement surgery. Med Care 1995;33(suppl):AS131–AS144

181. Tugwell P, Bombardier C, Buchanan WW et al: The MACTAR Patient Preference Disability Questionnaire—an individualized functional priority approach for assessing improvement in physical disability in clinical trials in rheumatoid arthritis. J Rheumatol 1987;14:446–451

182. O'Boyle CA, McGee H, Hickey A et al: Individual quality of life in patients undergoing hip replacement. Lancet 1992;339:1088–1091

183. Ruta DA, Garratt AM, Leng M et al: A new approach to the measurement of quality of life. The Patient-Generated Index. Med Care 1994;32:1109–1126

184. UK Medical Research Council: The Health of the UK's Elderly People—Topic Review. MRC, London, 1994

Chapter 30

Effects of aging on the heart

Wilbert S. Aronow

Age-related changes in the cardiovascular system, overt and occult cardiovascular disease, and reduced physical activity affect cardiovascular function in elderly people. With aging, there is a loss of myocytes in both the left and right ventricles, with a progressive increase in myocyte cell volume per nucleus in both ventricles.[1] With aging, there is also a progressive reduction in the number of pacemaker cells in the sinus node, with 10 percent of the number of cells present at age 20 remaining at age 75.[2]

AFTERLOAD

Afterload is the resistance to the ejection of blood by the left ventricle. Afterload is composed of two components: (1) peripheral vascular resistance, which is the steady-state component and the opposition to steady blood flow; and (2) characteristic aortic impedance, which is the dynamic component and the opposition to pulsatile blood flow. Peripheral vascular resistance is calculated by dividing the mean arterial pressure by the cardiac output and is inversely proportional to the cross-sectional area of the peripheral vascular beds. Characteristic aortic impedance is measured as the time variation in mean arterial pressure/flow through the aorta and is inversely proportional to the arterial compliance (the distensibility of the arterial wall). An indirect measurement of afterload is the pulse wave velocity, which measures the propagation speed of pressure waves traveling from proximal to distal arterial segments and which increases as arteries become less compliant.

With aging, the large elastic arteries become dilated with a reduction in compliance.[3] Progressive thickening of the aortic media and intima are associated with aortic enlargement.[4] There is an age-associated increase in arterial stiffness resulting from changes in the arterial media such as thickening of the smooth muscle layers, increased fragmentation of elastin, an increase in the amount and characteristics of collagen, and increased calcification.[5] These structural changes are associated with a reduction in aortic distensibility owing to increased aortic stiffness with an increase in pulse wave velocity.[6] These structural changes in the arterial wall are independent of coexisting atherosclerosis. Avolio et al.[6] demonstrated an increase in pulse wave velocity with age in farmers from Guanzhou Province in southern China despite a low prevalence of atherosclerosis in this population. The age-associated increase in stiffness and decrease in distensibility of large elastic arteries is not observed in distal arteries.[7]

Impedance spectral patterns have shown an age-related increase in characteristic aortic impedance and in peripheral vascular resistance.[8] The reduction in arterial compliance contributes more to the age-related increase in afterload than does the loss of peripheral vascular beds.[8] Peripheral vascular resistance was not age-related in healthy Baltimore Longitudinal Study of Aging participants screened for occult coronary artery disease,[9] but was increased with age in persons not screened for occult coronary artery disease.[10] Arterial stiffening appearing as an increase in pulse wave velocity is associated with degeneration of the vascular media independent of atherosclerosis. Arterial stiffening causes earlier occurrence of wave reflection from peripheral sites to the ascending aorta during left ventricular ejection. Therefore, aortic and carotid phasic pressures increase to a greater magnitude at a later time during left ventricular ejection, causing an increase in systolic and pulse pressures and a delayed peak in the aortic pressure pulse contour.

Circulating levels of catecholamines increase with age, especially with stress. However, β-adrenergic vasodilation of vascular smooth muscle decreases with aging.[11] α-adrenergic vasoconstriction of vascular smooth muscle does not change with aging.[12] The impaired vasodilator response to β-adrenergic stimulation with age is most important during exercise and contributes to the increased afterload associated with aging.

Increased afterload causes an increase in blood pressure. With aging, there is an increase in systolic blood pressure and a widening pulse pressure. A slight reduction in diastolic blood pressure occurs after the sixth decade.[13] The increase in systolic blood pressure is due to interactions of aging, cardiovascular disease, and lifestyle factors such as dietary sodium intake, level of physical activity, and body weight. An age-associated increase in the index of aortic stiffening was not found in normotensive persons on a low sodium chloride diet.[14] The increase in carotid augmentation index (which is an index of aortic stiffening) in highly trained elderly men was one-half of that expected on the basis of age alone.[15]

As aortic compliance decreases with aging, the transfer of kinetic energy from the blood ejected during left ventricular systole to potential energy stored in the elasticity of the aortic wall is decreased. Consequently, the return of the potential energy stored in the elasticity of the aortic wall back to the kinetic energy of blood flow during diastole also is decreased. Therefore, the left ventricle must eject its stroke volume into a less compliant aorta with greater pressure and force to achieve an adequate cardiac output. The increased pulse wave velocity also causes the pressure in the aorta to increase and peak later in systole, contributing to the increased systolic blood pressure and widened pulse pressure.

Posterior left ventricular wall thickness increased with increasing age in normotensive men and women in the Baltimore Longitudinal Study of Aging participants screened for occult coronary artery disease.[3] Data from the Baltimore study suggested that the increase in left ventricular wall thickness associated with aging is mediated by an increase in systolic blood pressure.[16] Aging is also associated with an increase in the prevalence of hypertension and cardiovascular disease. Therefore, the prevalence of echocardiographic left ventricular hypertrophy increases with age.

Age-associated left ventricular hypertrophy is caused by an increase in the volume but not in the number of cardiac myocytes. Fibroblasts undergo hyperplasia, and collagen is deposited in the myocardial interstitium. Increased afterload causes an increase in left ventricular systolic stress and the addition of sarcomeres in parallel. This results in increased left ventricular wall thickness with a normal or decreased left ventricular wall thickness.

In the Framingham Heart Study, echocardiographic left ventricular hypertrophy was demonstrated in 33 percent of men and 49 percent of women older than 70 years.[17] In our elderly population, echocardiographic left ventricular hypertrophy was observed in 44 percent of 1881 women, mean age 81 years, and in 43 percent of 924 men, mean age 80 years.[18] In our elderly population, hypertension was present in 108 of 215 blacks (50 percent), mean age 81 years; in 411 of 1140 whites (36 percent), mean age 82 years; and in 19 of 54 Hispanics (35 percent), mean age 81 years.[19] Echocardiographic left ventricular hypertrophy was present in 66 of 92 hypertensive blacks (72 percent), in 194 of 346 hypertensive whites (56 percent), and in 8 of 15 hypertensive Hispanics (53 percent).[19] However, echocardiographic left ventricular hypertrophy was present in only two of our 88 elderly persons (2 percent) without hypertension or overt cardiac disease.[20]

Regular aerobic endurance exercise attenuates age-related decreases in central arterial compliance and restores levels in previously sedentary healthy middle-aged and elderly men.[21] Regular aerobic endurance exercise also can prevent the age-associated loss in endothelium-dependent vasodilation and restore levels in previously sedentary middle-aged and elderly healthy men.[22] These are mechanisms by which regular aerobic endurance exercise contributes to a reduced risk of cardiovascular disease in the elderly population.[21,22]

PRELOAD

Preload is the filling volume of the left ventricle. Preload is determined by numerous factors that influence blood return to the heart and by the mechanical properties of the heart during diastolic filling of the left ventricle.

Resting left ventricular end-diastolic volume measured by echocardiography or by radionuclide ventriculography using multiple gated pool acquisition imaging is not age-related in healthy persons, indicating that resting preload does not change with age.[3,9,23] However, although resting preload does not change with age, left ventricular early diastolic filling is reduced with aging.

Passive filling of the left ventricle occurs during the rapid filling and diastasis phases of early diastole. With aging, left ventricular stiffness is increased, left ventricular compliance is decreased, left ventricular relaxation is impaired, and left ventricular early diastolic filling is decreased. This may result in hypotension if preload is decreased. An age-related increase in systolic blood pressure also impairs left ventricular early diastolic filling, leading to hypotension if preload is reduced. Left ventricular filling during early diastole decreases 50 percent from age 20 years to 80 years.[3,24,25]

Despite the reduction in early diastolic filling of the left ventricle with aging, preload is maintained because left atrial contraction becomes more vigorous to increase late diastolic filling of the left ventricle.[23–29] Augmentation of late diastolic filling of the left ventricle prevents a decrease in left ventricular end-diastolic volume with aging. The ratio of late diastolic Doppler peak transmitral velocity (peak atrial or A-wave velocity) to early diastolic Doppler peak transmitral velocity (peak rapid filling or E-wave velocity) increases from approximately 0.6 at 30 years of age to 1.2 at 70 years of age.[30] A decrease in E/A-wave ratio with aging reflects a reduction in left ventricular compliance. An age-related increase in left atrial size resulting from increased wall stress due to increased left atrial pressure counteracts the effects of decreased left ventricular compliance with aging. In our elderly population, 38 percent of 1881 women, mean age 81 years, and 30 percent of 924 men, mean age 80 years, had echocardiographic left atrial enlargement.[18]

In the Framingham Heart Study, age was the most powerful independent variable for left ventricular filling in healthy persons.[31] Age was inversely associated with the E wave (peak early diastolic filling velocity) and was directly associated with the A wave (peak late diastolic filling velocity). Other independent variables contributing to a lesser degree of left ventricular filling were heart rate, PR interval measured from the electrocardiogram, gender, systolic blood pressure, and left ventricular systolic function. Increasing heart rate reduces peak early diastolic filling and increases peak late diastolic filling velocity. The PR interval on the electrocardiogram is inversely associated with peak early diastolic filling velocity. Women have slightly higher peak early diastolic filling velocities than men. Left ventricular systolic function is directly associated with peak early diastolic filling velocity. Increasing systolic blood pressure increases the peak late diastolic filling velocity.[31,32]

A reduction of preload is not well tolerated in elderly people. Reduced intravascular volume, decreased venous return to the heart, vasodilation by drugs or disease states, and use of drugs such as nitrates or diuretics reduce preload and may cause a decreased cardiac output and hypotension in elderly people. Decreased compliance of the left ventricle and reduced cardiac and vascular responsiveness to β-adrenergic stimulation[33] cause elderly people to be greatly dependent on the Frank-Starling mechanism to increase cardiac output. They are more susceptible to develop orthostatic hypotension.[34–36] Impaired baroreceptor reflex sensitivity,[37] decreased cardiac responsiveness to β-adrenergic stimulation,[33] loss of arterial compliance, decreased venous return due to increased venous distensibility, impaired compensatory mechanisms for maintenance of fluid volume and electrolyte balance, increased incidence of common precipitating diseases and disorders, and the use of multiple drugs all contribute to orthostatic hypotension. Elderly people are also more susceptible to developing postprandial hypotension.[38–40]

Since left atrial contraction can contribute up to 50 percent of left ventricular filling in a poorly compliant left ventricle, development of atrial fibrillation may cause a marked reduction in cardiac output because of the loss of left atrial contribution to left ventricular late diastolic filling. A rapid ventricular rate associated with atrial fibrillation will also reduce the time for diastolic filling of the left ventricle.

The incidence of chronic atrial fibrillation also increases with age.[41,42] In 2101 elderly persons in a nursing home, the prevalence of chronic atrial fibrillation was 5 percent in persons aged 60–70 years, 13–14 percent in persons aged 71–90 years, and 22 percent in persons 91 years and older.[42]

Cardiac output is increased during exercise in healthy elderly persons by an increase in venous return to the heart, increasing diastolic filling of the left ventricle, and allowing an increased stroke volume to be ejected during exercise.[43] This is the Frank-Starling mechanism. In healthy persons in the Baltimore Longitudinal Study of Aging, the maximal heart rate response to exercise decreased with age.[9] However, exercise stroke volume increased with age to maintain the exercise cardiac output.[9] The increase in exercise stroke volume resulted from an increase in left ventricular end-diastolic volume (preload) by the Frank-Starling mechanism. In contrast, healthy nonelderly persons achieved an increase in exercise cardiac output primarily by an increase in heart rate. Exercise stroke volume increased in nonelderly healthy persons by a slight increase in left ventricular end-diastolic volume and by a large decrease in left ventricular end-systolic volume. The exercise-induced increase in heart rate and reduction in left ventricular end-systolic volume in nonelderly persons is probably mediated by β-adrenergic stimulation. The increase in left ventricular end-diastolic volume during exercise in healthy elderly persons suggests that the age-associated reduction in resting early diastolic filling of the left ventricle does not persist during exercise.

CONTRACTILITY

The intrinsic ability of the heart to generate force does not change with age in healthy people. However, the duration of contraction and relaxation is prolonged in senescent animals.[44,45] Prolongation of left ventricular ejection time[46] and of the pre-ejection period[47] with aging in healthy persons indicates that prolongation of contraction occurs with aging. Prolongation of the duration of contraction in senescent animals is associated with increased muscle stiffness and with prolongation of the action potential duration.[48] These age-related changes are associated with cellular changes in the excitation–contraction coupling mechanism,[49] and may be an adaptive response to preserve contractile function in response to an age-induced increase in afterload.

There is no reduction of resting left ventricular ejection fraction or circumferential fiber shortening in elderly persons with no evidence of heart disease.[3,9,23,50,51] Systolic function with exercise is impaired with aging. In the Baltimore Longitudinal Study of Aging, elderly persons showed less of an exercise-induced increase in left ventricular ejection fraction than did younger persons because of an age-related increase in left ventricular end-systolic volume.[9] However, absolute values of left ventricular ejection fraction at maximal exercise in healthy elderly persons rarely decreased from basal values.[9] Age-associated reductions in maximal heart rate and in left ventricular contractility during maximal exercise are manifestations of decreased β-adrenergic responsiveness with aging partially offset by exercise-induced dilatation of the left ventricle.[52]

DIASTOLIC FUNCTION

Aging is associated with prolongation of isovolumic relaxation time, a reduction in early diastolic filling of the left ventricle, and augmentation of late diastolic filling of the left ventricle.[24,27,30] Normal aging changes affecting left ventricular diastolic function include increase in systolic blood pressure, increase in left ventricular wall thickness, decrease in left ventricular early diastolic filling, prolongation of left ventricular diastolic relaxation, increase in left atrial size, and increase in left ventricular late diastolic filling.[53]

With aging occurs a slowing of the rate at which calcium is sequestered by the sarcoplasmic reticulum following myocardial excitation, which results in decreased relaxation of the left ventricule.[49,54,55] Accumulation of calcium at the onset of diastole may impair left ventricular diastolic relaxation and early diastolic filling.[54] Reduced oxidative phosphorylation and cumulative mitochondrial peroxidation occurring with aging may also impair left ventricular diastolic function.[56,57]

Increased left ventricular stiffness with aging due to increased interstitial fibrosis and cross-linking of collagen in the heart impairs left ventricular diastolic relaxation and filling.[1,58–60] Myocardial ischemia in the absence of coronary artery disease caused by reductions in capillary density and coronary reserve with aging may further impair left ventricular diastolic function in elderly people.[1,61]

In addition to a reduction in left ventricular diastolic relaxation and early diastolic filling caused by aging, elderly people are more likely to have left ventricular diastolic dysfunction because they have an increased prevalence of hypertension, myocardial ischemia due to coronary artery disease, and left ventricular hypertrophy due to hypertension, valvular aortic stenosis, coronary artery disease, hypertrophic cardiomyopathy, and other cardiac disorders. The increased stiffness of the left ventricle and prolonged left ventricular relaxation time impair left ventricular early diastolic filling and cause higher left ventricular end-diastolic pressures at rest and during exercise in elderly persons.[62,63]

In congestive heart failure (CHF) associated with left ventricular systolic dysfunction, the left ventricular ejection fraction is less than 50 percent. There is a decreased amount of myocardial fiber shortening, the stroke volume is reduced, the left ventricle is dilated, and the patient is symptomatic.

In CHF due to left ventricular diastolic dysfunction with normal left ventricular systolic function, the left ventricular ejection fraction is normal. Kitzman et al.[64] demonstrated during exercise that persons with CHF and normal left ventricular systolic function but abnormal left ventricular diastolic function were unable to normally increase stroke volume, even in the presence of increased left ventricular filling pressure. Myocardial hypertrophy, ischemia, or fibrosis causes slow or incomplete left ventricular filling at normal left atrial pressures. Left atrial pressure increases to augment left ventricular filling, resulting in pulmonary and systemic venous congestion. The development of atrial fibrillation may also cause a reduction in cardiac output and the development of pulmonary and systemic venous congestion, because of the loss of left atrial contribution to left ventricular late diastolic filling and decreased diastolic filling time due to a rapid ventricular rate.

The prevalence of CHF associated with left ventricular diastolic dysfunction with a normal left ventricular ejection fraction increases with age[65–71] and is higher in older women than in older men.[66–71] Table 30-1 shows the prevalence of a normal left ventricular ejection fraction in older persons with CHF.[65–71] Table 30-2 shows the association of CHF with a normal left ventricular ejection fraction with gender for different age groups.[69] A normal left ventricular ejection fraction was present in older persons with CHF in 44 percent of 55 African American men versus 58 percent of 110 African American women, in 46 percent of 24 Hispanic men versus 56 percent of 34 Hispanic women, in 35 percent of 148 white men versus 57 percent of 303 white women, and in 38 percent of 227 men versus 57 percent of 447 women.[70]

Left ventricular ejection fraction should be measured in all patients with CHF in order that appropriate therapy may be given.[72–76] For example, digoxin should not be used to treat persons with CHF and normal left ventricular ejection fraction if sinus rhythm is present.[53,77] By increasing contractility through increasing intracellular calcium ion concentration, digoxin may increase left ventricular stiffness, increasing left ventricular filling pressure, and adversely affecting CHF due to left ventricular diastolic dysfunction. Patients with CHF due to abnormal left ventricular ejection fraction tolerate higher doses of diuretics than do patients with CHF and normal left ventricular ejection fraction. Patients with CHF due to left ventricular diastolic dysfunction with normal left ventricular ejection fraction need high left ventricular filling pressures to maintain an adequate stroke volume and cardiac output and cannot tolerate intravascular depletion. These patients should be treated with a low-salt diet with cautious use of diuretics, rather than with large doses of diuretics.

CARDIOVASCULAR RESPONSE TO EXERCISE

The maximal oxygen consumption ($\dot{V}O_{2max}$) is the best overall measurement of cardiovascular fitness.[78] $\dot{V}O_{2max}$ is the product of cardiac output and systemic arteriovenous oxygen difference at peak exercise. Maximal cardiac output is the heart rate multiplied by the stroke volume at peak exercise, and is a more direct measurement of cardiovascular reserve than is $\dot{V}O_{2max}$.[78] $\dot{V}O_{2max}$ decreases with aging.[79,80] The degree of reduction of $\dot{V}O_{2max}$ with aging is affected by physical conditioning, subclinical coronary artery disease, smoking, and body weight. Table 30-3 summarizes the cardiovascular responses to exercise in healthy elderly people.

In the Baltimore Longitudinal Study of Aging, older male athletes had a higher peak exercise $\dot{V}O_{2max}$ than older sedentary men.[81] The greater peak exercise $\dot{V}O_{2max}$ in older male athletes than in older sedentary men was achieved by a higher cardiac index and a greater systemic arteriovenous oxygen difference. The higher peak exercise cardiac index in older male athletes than in older sedentary men was due to a higher stroke volume index with similar maximal heart rates.

Table 30-1 Prevalence of normal left ventricular ejection fraction in elderly people with congestive heart failure

Study	Normal left ventricular ejection fraction
Wong et al.[65]	41 percent of 54 patients, mean age 80 years, with CHF had normal LVEF
Aronow et al.[66]	47 percent of 247 patients, mean age 82 years, with CHF had normal LVEF
Cardiovascular Health Study[67]	59 percent of 186 patients, mean age 73 years, with CHF had normal LVEF
Pernenkil et al.[68]	34 percent of 501 patients aged ≥70 years with CHF had normal LVEF
Aronow et al.[69]	50 percent of 572 patients, mean age 82 years, with CHF had normal LVEF
Aronow et al.[70]	51 percent of 674 patients, mean age 81 years, with CHF had normal LVEF
Framingham Heart Study[71]	51 percent of 73 patients, mean age 73 years, with CHF had normal LVEF

Abbreviations: CHF, congestive heart failure; LVEF, left ventricular ejection fraction.

Table 30-2 Association of congestive heart failure and normal left ventricular ejection fraction with age and gender in 572 elderly people

Age (years)	Normal left ventricular ejection fraction
60–69	22 percent of 18 men and 37 percent of 38 women with congestive heart failure
70–79	33 percent of 54 men and 44 percent of 79 women with congestive heart failure
80–89	41 percent of 86 men and 59 percent of 219 women with congestive heart failure
≥90	47 percent of 19 men and 73 percent of 59 women with congestive heart failure
All ages	37 percent of 177 men and 56 percent of 395 women with congestive heart failure

Source: Adapted from Aronow et al.[69]

Table 30-3 Cardiovascular responses to exercise in healthy elderly people

- Maximal heart rate decreases with aging.
- Exercise stroke volume is increased with aging to maintain cardiac output.
- Increased exercise stroke volume with aging results primarily from increase in left ventricular end-diastolic volume by the Frank-Starling mechanism.
- Decrease in muscle mass with aging plays a role in age-associated reductions in systemic arteriovenous oxygen difference and in $\dot{V}O_{2max}$ at peak exercise.
- Left ventricular end-diastolic and end-systolic volumes increase during peak exercise with aging.
- Peak exercise left ventricular ejection fraction decreases with aging.
- Exercise-induced reduction in left ventricular end-systolic volume index and increases in cardiac index, stroke volume index, and left ventricular ejection fraction from rest were greater in older men than in older women.

A decrease in maximal systemic arteriovenous oxygen difference occurs with aging.[82] The reduction in muscle mass with aging may play a major role in the reduction in systemic arteriovenous oxygen difference at peak exercise and in $\dot{V}O_{2max}$ with aging.[83]

Fleg et al.[84] also investigated the effect of aging upon peak upright cycle exercise in healthy sedentary men and women aged 22–86 years in the Baltimore Longitudinal Study of Aging. Peak cycle work-rate decreased with aging in both men and women but was greater in men than in women at any age. Both men and women had, at peak exercise, decreases in heart rate, cardiac index, and left ventricular ejection fraction and increases in left ventricular end-diastolic volume index and end-systolic volume index with aging. Peak exercise stroke volume index did not vary with age in either men or women. The exercise-induced reduction in left ventricular end-systolic volume index and increases in cardiac index, stroke volume index, and left ventricular ejection fraction from rest were greater in older men than in older women.

CARDIOVASCULAR DISEASE

In addition to age-related changes in cardiovascular function and deconditioning due to a sedentary lifestyle in many elderly persons, this population also has a higher prevalence and incidence of cardiovascular disorders that impair cardiovascular performance than nonelderly persons. Table 30-4 lists the prevalence of some cardiovascular disorders in elderly men and in elderly women in a long-term healthcare facility.[18,40,70,85–89]

SUMMARY

Table 30-5 itemizes some age-related changes in cardiovascular function in healthy elderly people. Decrease in arterial compliance contributes more to the age-related increase in afterload than does the loss of peripheral vascular beds. The impaired vasodilator response to β-adrenergic stimulation with aging is most important during exercise and contributes to the increased afterload associated with aging. Resting preload does not change with age. Left ventricular early diastolic filling is decreased with aging. Augmentation of late diastolic filling of the left ventricle prevents a decrease in left ventricular end-diastolic volume with aging. The maximal heart rate response to exercise decreases with age. Exercise stroke volume is increased with age to maintain the exercise cardiac output. The increase in exercise stroke volume with age results from an increase in preload by the Frank-Starling mechanism. Contractility at rest does not change with age. However, the duration of left ventricular contraction and relaxation is prolonged with aging. Age-associated decreases in maximal heart rate and in left ventricular contractility during maximal exercise are manifestations of decreased β-adrenergic responsiveness with aging partially offset by exercise-induced dilation of the left ventricle. $\dot{V}O_{2max}$ and systemic arteriovenous oxygen difference at peak exercise decrease with aging. In addition to age-related changes in cardiovascular function and deconditioning due to a sedentary lifestyle in many elderly persons, this population also has a higher prevalence and incidence of cardiovascular disorders that impair cardiovascular performance than do nonelderly persons. Elderly persons, especially women, are more likely than nonelderly persons to develop CHF due to abnormal left ventricular diastolic dysfunction with normal left ventricular systolic function.

Table 30-4 Prevalence of some cardiovascular disorders in elderly men and women

Cardiovascular disorder	Mean age (years)		Prevalence			
	Men	Women	Men		Women	
			No.	%	No.	%
Coronary artery disease[85]	80	82	292/664	44	603/1488	41
Atherothrombotic brain infarction[86]	80	82	187/664	28	364/1488	24
Peripheral arterial disease[87]	80	82	158/559	28	291/1275	23
40–100 percent extracranial carotid arterial disease[88]	81	81	68/425	16	213/1421	15
Congestive heart failure[70]	80	81	260/922	28	534/1971	27
Hypertension[85,86]	80	82	255/664	38	651/1488	44
Aortic stenosis[18]	80	81	141/924	15	322/1881	17
Mitral annular calcium[18]	80	81	336/924	36	985/1881	52
≥1+ mitral regurgitation[18]	80	81	298/924	32	630/1881	33
≥1+ aortic regurgitation[18]	80	81	282/924	31	542/1881	29
Rheumatic mitral stenosis[18]	80	81	3/924	0.3	34/1881	2
Hypertrophic cardiomyopathy[18]	80	81	28/924	3	80/1881	4
Atrial fibrillation[40]	80	81	101/650	16	182/1451	13
Pacemaker rhythm[89]	81	82	16/326	5	34/827	4
Abnormal ejection fraction[18]	80	81	271/924	29	416/1881	22
Left ventricular hypertrophy[18]	80	81	393/924	43	831/1881	44
Left atrial enlargement[18]	80	81	278/924	30	709/1881	38
Idiopathic dilated cardiomyopathy[18]	80	81	10/924	1	19/1881	1

Table 30-5 Some age-related changes in cardiovascular function in healthy elderly people

- Decrease in arterial compliance contributes more to age-related increase in afterload than does loss of peripheral vascular beds.

- Resting preload does not change with age.

- Left ventricular early diastolic filling is decreased with aging.

- Augmentation of late diastolic filling of left ventricle prevents decrease in left ventricular end-diastolic volume with aging.

- Contractility at rest does not change with aging.

- Duration of left ventricular contraction and relaxation is prolonged with aging.

- Cardiovascular responses to exercise with aging are listed in Table 30-3.

- Age-associated decreases in maximal heart rate and in left ventricular contractility during maximal exercise are manifestations of decreased β-adrenergic responsiveness with aging partially offset by exercise-induced dilation of the left ventricle.

KEY POINTS   Effects of aging on the heart

- Care of the elderly patient with congestive failure is influenced by the physiological changes that accompany normal aging.

- Care of the elderly patient with cardiovascular disease is influenced by the physiological changes that accompany normal aging.

- Care of the elderly surgical patient is influenced by the physiological changes that accompany normal aging.

- Decision-making for the elderly surgical patient requires an assessment of treatment goals, therapeutic options, and their associated risks, as well as an understanding of the natural history of the disease.

REFERENCES

1. Olivetti G, Melissari M, Capasso JM, Anversa P: Cardiomyopathy of the aging human heart: myocyte loss and reactive cellular hypertrophy. Circ Res 1991;68:1560–1568
2. Davies MJ: The pathological basis of arrhythmias. Geriatr Cardiovasc Med 1988;1:181–183
3. Gerstenblith G, Fredericksen J, Yin FCP et al: Echocardiographic assessment of a normal adult aging population. Circulation 1977;56:273–278
4. Safar M: Aging and its effects on the cardiovascular system. Drugs 1990;39(suppl 1):1–8
5. Yin FCP: The aging vasculature and its effects on the heart. In Weisfeldt ML (ed): The aging heart: its function and response to stress. Vol 12: Aging. Raven Press, New York, 1980:137–214
6. Avolio AP, Fa-Quan D, Wei-Qiang L et al: Effects of aging on arterial distensibility in populations with high and low prevalence of hypertension: comparison between urban and rural communities in China. Circulation 1985;71:202–210

7. Boutouyrie P, Laurent S, Benetos A et al: Opposing effects of ageing on distal and proximal large arteries in hypertensives. J Hypertens 1992;10:587–591
8. Nichols WW, O'Rourke MF, Avolio AP et al: Effects of age on ventricular–vascular coupling. Am J Cardiol 1985;55:1179–1184
9. Rodeheffer RJ, Gerstenblith G, Becker LC et al: Exercise cardiac output is maintained with advancing age in healthy human subjects: cardiac dilatation and increased stroke volume compensate for a diminished heart rate. Circulation 1984;69:203–213
10. Brandfonbrener M, Landowne M, Shock NW: Changes in cardiac output with age. Circulation 1955;12:557–566
11. Pan HY, Hoffman BB, Pershe RA, Blaschke TF: Decline in beta-adrenergic receptor-mediated vascular relaxation with aging in man. J Pharmacol Exp Ther 1986;239:802–807
12. Buhler F, Kowski W, Van Brumeler P: Plasma catecholamines and cardiac, renal and peripheral vascular adrenoceptor mediated response in different age groups in normal and hypertensive subjects. Clin Exp Hypertens 1980;2:409–426
13. Landahl S, Bengtsson C, Sigurdsson JA et al: Age-related change in blood pressure. Hypertension 1986;8:1044–1049
14. Avolio AP, Clyde KM, Beard TC et al: Improved arterial distensibility in normotensive subjects on a low salt diet. Arteriosclerosis 1986;6:166–169
15. Vaitkevicius PV, Fleg JL, Engel JH et al: Effects of age and aerobic capacity on arterial stiffness in healthy adults. Circulation 1993;88:1456–1462
16. Lima JAC, Gerstenblith G, Weiss JL et al: Systolic blood pressure, not age mediates the age-related increase in left ventricular wall thickness within a normotensive population. J Am Coll Cardiol 1988;11:81A (abstract)
17. Levy D, Anderson KM, Savage DD et al: Echocardiographically detected left ventricular hypertrophy: prevalence and risk factors. The Framingham Heart Study. Ann Intern Med 1988;108:7–13
18. Aronow WS, Ahn C, Kronzon I: Prevalence of echocardiographic findings in 554 men and in 1243 women aged >60 years in a long-term healthcare facility. Am J Cardiol 1997;79:379–380
19. Aronow WS, Kronzon I: Prevalence of coronary risk factors in elderly blacks and whites. J Am Geriatr Soc 1991;39:567–570
20. Aronow WS, Koenigsberg M, Schwartz KS: Usefulness of echocardiographic left ventricular hypertrophy in predicting new coronary events and atherothrombotic brain infarction in patients over 62 years of age. Am J Cardiol 1988;61:1130–1132
21. Tanaka H, Dinenno FA, Monahan KD et al: Aging, habitual exercise, and dynamic arterial compliance. Circulation 2000;102:1270–1275
22. DeSouza CA, Shapiro LF, Clevenger CM et al: Regular aerobic exercise prevents and restores age-related declines in endothelium-dependent vasodilation in healthy men. Circulation 2000;102:1351–1357
23. Gardin JM, Henry WL, Savage DD et al: Echocardiographic measurements in normal subjects: evaluation of an adult population without clinically apparent heart disease. J Clin Ultrasound 1979;7:439–447
24. Bryg RJ, Williams GA, Labovitz AJ: Effect of aging on left ventricular diastolic filling in normal subjects. Am J Cardiol 1987;59:971–974
25. Iskandrian AS, Aakki A: Age-related changes in left ventricular diastolic performance. Am Heart J 1986;112:75–78
26. Spirito P, Maron BJ: Influence of aging on Doppler echocardiographic indices of left ventricular diastolic function. Br Heart J 1988;59:672–679
27. Miyatake K, Okamoto J, Kinoshita N et al: Augmentation of atrial contribution to left ventricular flow with aging as assessed by intracardiac Doppler flowmetry. Am J Cardiol 1984;53:587–589
28. Sartori MP, Quinones MA, Kuo LC: Relation of Doppler-derived left ventricular filling parameters to age and radius/thickness ratio in normal and pathologic states Am J Cardiol 1987;59:1179–1182
29. Fleg JL, Shapiro EP, O'Connor F et al: Left ventricular diastolic filling performance in older male athletes. JAMA 1995;273:1371–1375
30. Gardin JM, Rohan MK, Davidson DM et al: Doppler transmitral flow velocity parameters: relationship between age, body surface area, blood pressure and gender in normal subjects. Am J Noninvasive Cardiol 1987;1:3–10
31. Benjamin EG, Levy D, Anderson KM et al: Determination of Doppler indexes of left ventricular diastolic function in normal subjects (The Framingham Heart Study). Am J Cardiol 1992;70:508–515
32. Villari B, Hess OM, Kaufmann P et al: Effect of aortic valve stenosis (pressure overload) and regurgitation (volume overload) on left ventricular systolic and diastolic function. Am J Cardiol 1992;69:927–934

33. Lakatta EG: Age-related alterations in the cardiovascular response to adrenergic mediated stress. Fed Proc 1980;39:3173–3177

34. Robbins AS, Rubenstein LZ: Postural hypotension in the elderly. J Am Geriatr Soc 1984;82:769–774

35. Aronow WS, Lee NH, Sales FF, Etienne F: Prevalence of postural hypotension in elderly patients in a long-term health care facility. Am J Cardiol 1988;62:336

36. Lipsitz LA, Jonsson PV, Marks BL et al: Reduced supine cardiac volumes and diastolic filling rates in elderly patients with chronic medical conditions: implications for postural blood pressure homeostasis. J Am Geriatr Soc 1990;38:103–107

37. Gribbin B, Pickering TG, Sleight P, Peto R: Effect of age and high blood pressure on baroreflex sensitivity in man. Circ Res 1971;29:424–431

38. Lipsitz LA, Nyquist RP, Wei JY, Rowe JW: Postprandial reduction in blood pressure in the elderly. N Engl J Med 1983;309:81–83

39. Vaitkevicius PV, Esserwein DM, Maynard AK et al: Frequency and importance of postprandial blood pressure reduction in elderly nursing-home patients. Ann Intern Med 1991;115:865–870

40. Aronow WS, Ahn C: Postprandial hypotension in 499 elderly persons in a long-term health care facility. J Am Geriatr Soc 1994;42:930–932

41. Wolf PA, Abbott RD, Kannel WB: Atrial fibrillation as an independent risk factor for stroke: the Framingham Study. Stroke 1991;22:983–988

42. Aronow WS, Ahn C, Gutstein H: Prevalence of atrial fibrillation and association of atrial fibrillation with prior and new thromboembolic stroke in elderly patients. J Am Geriatr Soc 1996;44:521–523

43. Poliner LR, Dehmer GJ, Lewis SE et al: Left ventricular performance in normal subjects: a comparison of the responses to exercise in the upright and supine positions. Circulation 1980;62:528–534

44. Fraticelli A, Josephson R, Danziger R et al: Morphological and contractile characteristics of rat cardiac myocytes from maturation to senescence. Am J Physiol 1989;257:H259–H265

45. Capasso JM, Malhotra A, Remly RM: Effects of age on mechanical and electrical performance of rat myocardium. Am J Physiol 1983;245:H72–H81

46. Willems JL, Roelandt H, DeGeest H et al: The left ventricular ejection time in elderly subjects. Circulation 1970;42:37–42

47. Shaw DJ, Rothbaum DA, Angell CS, Shock NW: The effect of age and blood pressure upon the systolic time intervals in males aged 20–89 years. J Gerontol 1973;28:133–139

48. Lakatta EG: Do hypertension and aging have similar effects on the myocardium? Circulation 1987;75(suppl I):I69–I77

49. Lakatta EG, Yin FCP: Myocardial aging: functional alterations and related cellular mechanisms. Am J Physiol 1982;242:H927–H941

50. Port S, Cobb FR, Coleman RE, Jones RH: Effect of age on the response of the left ventricular ejection fraction to exercise. N Engl J Med 1980;303:1133–1137

51. Aronow WS, Stein PD, Sabbah HN, Koenigsberg M: Resting left ventricular ejection fraction in elderly patients without evidence of heart disease. Am J Cardiol 1989;63:368–369

52. Fleg JL, Schulman S, O'Connor F et al: Effect of acute β-adrenergic receptor blockade on age-associated changes in cardiovascular performance during dynamic exercise. Circulation 1994;90:2333–2341

53. Tresch DD, McGough MF: Heart failure with normal systolic function: a common disorder in older people. J Am Geriatr Soc 1995;43:1035–1042

54. Wei JY, Spurgeon HA, Lakatta EG: Excitation-contraction in rat myocardium: alterations with adult aging. Am J Physiol 1984;246:H784–H791

55. Morgan JP, Morgan KG: Calcium and cardiovascular function: intracellular calcium levels during contraction and relaxation of mammalian cardiac and vascular smooth muscle as detected with aequorin. Am J Med 1984;77(suppl 5A):33–46

56. Bandy B, Davison AJ: Mitochondrial mutations may increase oxidative stress: implications for carcinogenesis and aging? Free Radic Biol Med 1990;8:523–539

57. Corral-Debrinski M, Stepien G, Shoffner JM et al: Hypoxemia is associated with mitochondrial DNA damage and gene induction: implications for cardiac disease. JAMA 1991;266:1812–1816

58. Lie JT, Hammond PI: Pathology of the senescent heart: anatomic observation on 237 autopsy studies of patients 90 to 105 years old. Mayo Clin Proc 1988;63:552–564

59. Schaub MC: The aging of collagen in the heart muscle. Gerontologia 1964;10:38–41

60. Verzar F: The stages and consequences of aging collagen. Gerontologia 1969;15:233–239

61. Hachamovitch R, Wicker P, Capasso JM, Anversa P: Alterations of coronary blood flow and reserve with aging in Fischer 344 rats. Am J Physiol 1989;256:H66–H73

62. Ogawa T, Spina R, Martin WH et al: Effects of aging, sex and physical training on cardiovascular responses to exercise. Circulation 1992;86:494–503

63. Manning WJ, Shannon RP, Santinga JA et al: Reversal of changes in left ventricular diastolic filling associated with normal aging using diltiazem. Am J Cardiol 1989;67:894–896

64. Kitzman BW, Higginbotham MB, Cobb FR et al: Exercise intolerance in patients with heart failure and preserved left ventricular systolic function: failure of the Frank-Starling mechanism. J Am Coll Cardiol 1991;17:1065–1072

65. Wong WF, Gold S, Fukuyama O, Blanchette PL: Diastolic dysfunction in elderly patients with congestive heart failure. Am J Cardiol 1989;63:1526–1528

66. Aronow WS, Ahn C, Kronzon I: Prognosis of congestive heart failure in elderly patients with normal versus abnormal left ventricular systolic function associated with coronary artery disease. Am J Cardiol 1990;66:1257–1259

67. Kitzman DW, Gardin JM, Arnold A et al: Heart failure with preserved systolic LV function in the elderly: clinical and echocardiographic correlates from the Cardiovascular Health Study. Circulation 1996;94(Suppl I):I433 (abstract)

68. Pernenkil R, Vinson JM, Shah AS et al: Course and prognosis in patients ≥70 years of age with congestive heart failure and normal versus abnormal left ventricular ejection fraction. Am J Cardiol 1997;79:216–219

69. Aronow WS, Ahn C, Kronzon I: Normal left ventricular ejection fraction in older persons with congestive heart failure. Chest 1998;113:867–869

70. Aronow WS, Ahn C, Kronzon I: Comparison of incidences of congestive heart failure in older African Americans, Hispanics, and whites. Am J Cardiol 1999;84:611–612

71. Vasan RS, Larson MG, Benjamin EJ et al: Congestive heart failure in subjects with normal versus reduced left ventricular ejection fraction. J Am Coll Cardiol 1999;33:1948–1955

72. Konstam MA, Dracup K, Baker DW et al: Heart Failure: Management of Patients with Left-Ventricular Systolic Dysfunction. Quick Reference Guide for Clinicians, no. 11, AHCPR Publication 94–0613. Agency for Health Care Policy and Research, Rockville, MD, June 1994:1–21

73. Aronow WS: Echocardiography should be performed in all elderly patients with congestive heart failure. J Am Geriatr Soc 1994;42:1300–1302

74. Williams JF, Bristow MR, Fowler MB et al: Guidelines for the evaluation and management of heart failure. Report of the American College of Cardiology/American Heart Association Task Force on Practice Guidelines (Committee on Evaluation and Management of Heart Failure). J Am Coll Cardiol 1995;26:1376–1398

75. American Medical Directors Association: Heart failure. Clinical Practice Guideline. American Medical Directors Association, Columbia, MD. 1996:1–8

76. Aronow WS: Commentary on American Geriatrics Society Clinical Practice Guidelines from AHCPR Guidelines on Heart Failure: Evaluation and Treatment of Patients with Left Ventricular Systolic Dysfunction. J Am Geriatr Soc 1998;46:525–529

77. Aronow WS: Digoxin or angiotensin converting enzyme inhibitors for congestive heart failure in geriatric patients: which is the preferred treatment? Drugs Aging 1991;1:98–103

78. Fleg JL: Alterations in cardiovascular structure and function with advancing age. Am J Cardiol 1986;57:33C–44C

79. Dehn MM, Bruce RA: Longitudinal variations in maximal oxygen intake with age and activity. J Appl Physiol 1972;33:805–807

80. Heath GW, Hagberg JM, Ehsani AA, Holloszy JO: A physiological comparison of young and older endurance athletes. J Appl Physiol 1981;51:634–640

81. Fleg JL, Schulman SP, O'Connor FC et al: Cardiovascular responses to exhaustive upright cycle exercise in highly trained older men. J Appl Physiol 1994;77:1500–1506

82. Julius S, Amery A, Whitlock LS, Conway J: Influence of age on the hemodynamic response to exercise. Circulation 1967;36:222–230

83. Fleg JL, Lakatta EG: Role of muscle loss in the age-associated reduction in $VO2max$. J Appl Physiol 1988;65:1147–1151

84. Fleg JL, O'Connor F, Gerstenblith G et al: Impact of age on the cardiovascular response to dynamic upright exercise in healthy men and women. J Appl Physiol 1995;78:890–900

85. Aronow WS, Ahn C: Risk factors for new coronary events in a large cohort of very elderly patients with and without coronary artery disease. Am J Cardiol 1996;77:864–866

86. Aronow WS, Ahn C, Gutstein H: Risk factors for new atherothrombotic brain infarction in 664 older men and 1488 older women. Am J Cardiol 1996;77:1381–1383

87. Aronow WS, Ahn C: Correlation of serum lipids with the presence or absence of atherothrombotic brain infarction and peripheral arterial disease in 1834 men and women aged ≥62 years. Am J Cardiol 1994;73:995–997

88. Aronow WS, Ahn C, Schoenfeld MR, Gutstein H: Association of extracranial carotid arterial disease and chronic atrial fibrillation with the incidence of new thromboembolic stroke in 1846 older persons. Am J Cardiol 1999;83:1403–1404

89. Aronow WS: Correlation of arrhythmias and conduction defects on the resting electrocardiogram with new cardiac events in 1153 elderly patients. Am J Noninvas Cardiol 1991;5:88–90

Chapter 31

Atypical manifestations of cardiac disorders

Donald D. Tresch and Haritha R. Alla

Cardiac disorders are often misdiagnosed in elderly patients because clinical manifestations can be significantly different from those in younger patients with the same disorder. The failure to correctly diagnose these disorders has significant implications and may result in an unnecessary increase in morbidity and mortality.

The atypical manifestations may reflect a difference in the disease process between the age groups, or it may be related to the superimposition of normal physiological aging changes and the presence of concomitant diseases, which mask the usual clinical manifestations.

This chapter discusses four cardiac disorders which are common in elderly patients but which have different clinical manifestations from those usually associated with the disorders in younger patients: heart failure, aortic stenosis, mitral valve prolapse, and hyperthyroid heart disease. Atypical manifestations of ischemic heart disease in elderly patients are discussed in Chapter 34.

HEART FAILURE

Heart failure increases with age and is present in approximately 10 percent of persons over 80 years.[1] Heart failure is considered to be an emerging epidemic, with Medicare claims in the USA for the condition to be as high as 1.9 million in 1993 and estimated annual expenditures in excess of 40 billion dollars.[2]

Although the causes of heart failure in elderly patients are generally the same as those in younger patients, the clinical presentation can be different.[3] Frequently, the presentation is atypical and the diagnosis is delayed. This delay may cause the initial diagnosis of heart failure in elderly patients to be made at an advanced stage of the underlying disease process. The patient will be unstable and intensive-care monitoring will be necessary, and hospital stay will be prolonged.

Because of sedentary lifestyles, many elderly patients with heart failure do not experience progressive external dyspnea, which is usually considered the classical symptom of left ventricular failure in middle-aged and younger patients. Orthopnea and paroxysmal nocturnal dyspnea may not occur in elderly patients because of compensatory pulmonary vasculature changes in response to chronically elevated pulmonary pressure, or may reflect the common practice of the elderly person sleeping in a chair or recliner, and not assuming a supine position. Instead of dyspnea, many elderly patients with high pulmonary artery pressure complain of a dry cough as the initial symptom of heart failure.

When symptoms occur, nonspecific complaints of general weakness, impaired exercise tolerance, and fatigue often predominate. Mental disturbances such as insomnia, anxiety, or confusion may also be common symptoms of elderly patients with heart failure. Some studies have reported heart failure to be one of the most frequent precipitating causes of acute confusion in elderly patients.[4] In other elderly patients with heart failure, an increase in nocturia with daytime oliguria may be a major complaint, reflecting the low cardiac output with increased venous return and renal perfusion at night because of recumbence.

Some elderly patients will experience more typical symptoms of heart failure, but because of their nonspecificity and the presence of concomitant diseases the symptoms may be wrongly diagnosed. For example, a dry cough or mild shortness of breath may be mistakenly related to chronic pulmonary disease, which is common in elderly patients. Even more common, complaints of easy fatigability, generalized weakness, and impaired exercise tolerance are thought merely to reflect changes related to aging.

As with symptoms, the principal findings of heart failure in elderly patients can be difficult to interpret. The findings that are so impressive in younger patients may be subtler and even obscure in elderly patients. Some of the difficulty in interpreting the physical findings may be related to the superimposition of aging changes or the presence of other diseases, which mask or obscure the typical findings seen in younger patients. Resting tachycardia is uncommon in elderly people owing to the age-related decreased sympathetic responsiveness. Atherosclerotic changes in the vasculature make propagation of the pulse difficult, and stiffness of the arterial wall may obscure abnormality in the pulse contour. Because of the presence of pulmonary disease and increased chest diameter, cardiac auscultation may be difficult in elderly patients. The intensity of murmurs may be markedly diminished and gallops may be undetected. Even if detected, the S_4 gallop is not very helpful in diagnosing ventricular dysfunction, because the finding may be heard in many elderly without heart disease. Other physical findings, such as pulmonary rales or wheezes, may be present, although both are nonspecific and may be misinterpreted in being related to pulmonary disease, and not heart failure. Peripheral edema, a finding of right-sided heart failure, is usually a late manifestation if the right-sided failure is secondary to left ventricular failure. Moreover, peripheral edema is a common finding in elderly patients without heart failure, and not uncommonly is misdiagnosed as secondary venous insufficiency.

In certain elderly patients, heart failure will be sudden in onset and may be related to coronary artery disease.[5–7] Patients may be in their eighth or ninth decade and have no awareness of coronary artery disease until the development of acute pulmonary edema, commonly unaccompanied by chest pain. Signs of an acute myocardial infarction are typically not present, although the electrocardiogram may demonstrate myocardial ischemia, and angiographic studies will usually demonstrate three-vessel coronary disease. Only moderate left ventricular systolic dysfunction will be present. Most of these elderly patients have a long history of hypertension, and the etiology of left ventricular impairment will be acute myocardial ischemia superimposed on a hypertrophic left ventricle with resultant severe diastolic dysfunction.

Some elderly patients with acute left ventricular failure will demonstrate an acute ventricular overload, usually secondary to severe mitral regurgitation (see the later discussion of mitral valve prolapse). Acute aortic valvular regurgitation may be the etiology of acute volume overload in other elderly patients. Another possible etiology of the sudden onset of left ventricular failure in elderly patients will be accelerated hypertension with a resultant ventricular pressure overload.

After diagnosing heart failure in an elderly patient, it is mandatory to determine whether the person has primary systolic or diastolic ventricular dysfunction causing the heart failure.[8] Until recently, heart failure was usually attributed to an inadequate contraction of the ventricle (systolic dysfunction). It is now known that a subset of patients with clinical heart failure will have normally contracting hearts. The problem is not systolic, but ventricular diastolic dysfunction.[9,10] The prevalence of heart failure secondary to diastolic dysfunction varies from 30 to 40 percent, and the prevalence significantly increases with age.[11,12] Approximately 45 percent of patients 65 years or older with heart failure will demonstrate diastolic ventricular dysfunction, with the incidence higher in elderly women. The increased prevalence of heart failure secondary to diastolic dysfunction in elderly patients most likely reflects the concomitant effects of normal cardiovascular changes with aging and the high incidence of cardiac disorders in this age group that cause diastolic dysfunction, such as hypertension and myocardial ischemia.[8]

The clinical differentiation between diastolic and systolic dysfunction is difficult, and diastolic dysfunction is often unrecognized in elderly patients with heart failure. Although this differentiation is difficult, clues to the type of ventricular dysfunction may be discovered from the patient's history, physical examination, electrocardiogram, and chest X-ray (Table 31-1).[8]

In summary, heart failure in elderly patients may be difficult to diagnose because of lack of typical symptoms and physical findings that are so common in younger patients with this disorder. When the symptoms and signs are present, they may be mistakenly related to other disorders that are frequently present in elderly patients. In other elderly patients the symptoms and signs may be obscured by the presence of aging changes or the presence of other diseases. Therefore, it is mandatory that the physician be highly suspicious of heart failure in all elderly patients who have underlying heart disease, or who present with nonspecific symptoms that could represent heart failure.

AORTIC STENOSIS

Aortic valvular stenosis (AVS) is mainly a disease of the elderly. The disorder is 15 times more prevalent in persons over 60 years of age than in those younger than 30 years.[13] In the general population, the disorder is more common in males by a ratio of 4 to 1; however, with increasing age the ratio lessens and females may predominate among patients over 80 years of age.[14] People with AVS are usually asymptomatic and the first symptoms may not appear until the ninth decade. Once the symptoms appear the stenosis is usually severe, with rapid progression unless valve replacement is performed.[15]

Unfortunately, even though the disorder is common in elderly people, severe AVS is often misdiagnosed and proper treatment is delayed. Symptoms in elderly patients are similar to those experienced by younger patients with severe AVS,

---

Table 31-1 Clinical differentiation of diastolic versus systolic dysfunction in patients with heart failure

	Systolic dysfunction	Diastolic dysfunction
Past history	Hypertension	Hypertension
	Myocardial infarction	Renal disease
	Diabetes	Diabetes
	Chronic valvular insufficiency disorder	Aortic stenosis
Presentation	Younger than 65 years	65 years or older
	Progressive shortness of breath	Acute pulmonary edema
Physical examination	Displaced PMI	Sustained PMI
	S_3 gallop	S_4 gallop
Radiographic findings	Pulmonary congestion	Pulmonary congestion
	Cardiomegaly	Normal-sized heart
Electrocardiogram	Q waves	LVH
Echocardiogram	Decreased LVEF	Normal or increased LVEF

Abbreviations: LVEF, left ventricular ejection fraction; LVH, left ventricular hypertrophy; PMI, point of maximum impact.

Source: From Tresch and McGough,[8] with permission of Blackwell Science, Inc..

except that in the elderly patient the classical triad of angina, dyspnea, and dizziness or syncope may be misdiagnosed as caused by other disorders which are common in the age group. Angina may be misdiagnosed as being due to coronary artery disease; dyspnea is often considered to be related to pulmonary disease; and dizziness and syncope may be incorrectly ascribed to a neurological or vascular etiology.

The physical examination, which is usually considered to be the diagnostic hallmark of severe AVS, can be even more misleading than symptoms in elderly patients.[16] Studies have demonstrated a difference in the valvular pathological and auscultatory findings of severe AVS between younger and elderly patients.[17] Younger patients more commonly have congenital bicuspid or rheumatic valves with commissural fusion and heavy calcification, whereas older patients usually have tricuspid valves with severe stenosis and calcification but commissural fusion is unusual. The rigid, calcified valve with commissural fusion is thought to be responsible for the classical harsh, grunting systolic musical murmur, which is loudest at the right base with radiation upward to the right carotid. Commonly, the murmur is preceded by an ejection sound. In the elderly, by contrast, the calcified tricuspid valve lacks commissural fusion, resulting in a spray of blood rather than uniform ejection into the aorta. Consequently, in elderly patients the harsh murmur at the base may be less intense and comparatively inconspicuous, and an ejection sound is characteristically absent. Instead of the harsh murmur at the base, a more musical systolic murmur may be present which is transmitted across the entire precordium. This murmur is usually clearly audible at the apex, and due to its quality and location the murmur is easily confused with the murmur of mitral valve regurgitation.

In addition, elderly patients commonly have calcification of the mitral annulus, which can produce mitral valvular incompetence.[18] As a result, some elderly patients will have both AVS and mitral regurgitation, making the auscultatory findings even more confusing.

Besides the apical murmur, 25 percent of elderly patients with AVS will demonstrate atrial fibrillation, which is a rare finding in younger patients with AVS. The combination of atrial fibrillation with an apical systolic musical murmur may further lead to a mistaken diagnosis of mitral valvular regurgitation, instead of AVS, in elderly patients.

Other physical findings that may mislead the physician in evaluating elderly patients with severe AVS include the blood pressure reading and the carotid arterial pulse upstroke. Systemic hypertension is rarely present in younger patients with severe AVS, whereas a narrow pulse pressure and slowly rising carotid arterial pulse (parvus et tardus pulse) are usually present. Such findings may not be present in elderly patients. Systemic hypertension occurs in elderly patients with severe AVS, and the elevated pressure, combined with decreased arterial compliance, may result in the absence of a parvus et tardus arterial pulse.

Palpation of left ventricular hypertrophy and a systolic thrill, common findings in younger patients with severe AVS, may not be present in elderly patients owing to the presence of emphysema and an increase in chest diameter.

Electrocardiographic and chest X-ray findings may also be confusing. Younger patients with severe AVS will demonstrate an electrocardiographic finding of left ventricular hypertrophy with a strain pattern. Owing to emphysematous changes and an increase in chest diameter, the electrocardiographic voltage may not be impressive in elderly patients with severe AVS. In addition intraventricular conduction defects, common in elderly patients, can mask the hypertrophy. On chest X-ray, the heart is usually normal in size unless clinical heart failure is present. Aortic valvular calcification may be noted, but this is a nonspecific finding which may be seen in elderly patients with aortic valvular sclerosis (aortic valve thickening without stenosis).

In summary, AVS is a common disorder in elderly patients. With proper diagnosis and therapy, the prognosis is excellent. Owing to atypical physical findings, however, the disorder may be misdiagnosed in elderly patients and correct therapy will not be administered. It is mandatory that AVS be considered in any elderly patient with a systolic murmur, who has symptoms of angina, dyspnea, dizziness, or syncope.

MITRAL VALVE PROLAPSE

Mitral valve prolapse (MVP) is usually diagnosed in the third through fifth decade and is more common in women than men in this age group.[19,20] The gender difference has been reported by some investigators to decrease with age, although other studies have found an approximately 2 to 1 female to male ratio regardless of patient age.[21] In these patients with MVP, the typical auscultatory findings are usually a midsystolic click followed by mid-to-late systolic murmur. In other patients usually with more severe prolapse, the murmur will be holosystolic without a preceding click. A small percentage of patients will only demonstrate a click, without a murmur.

Many patients with MVP, regardless of age, will be asymptomatic and the diagnosis will be made on the basis of a heart murmur or echocardiographic findings. In other patients with MVP, symptoms will be nonspecific with palpitations and atypical chest pain not being unusual. Symptoms related to specific arrhythmias, including ventricular, do occur in some patients with MVP, although cardiac arrest is rare.

The main clinical feature that is different between older and younger patients with MVP is the presence of severe mitral regurgitation.[22] The increased severity of the valvular regurgitation in older patients not only results in heart failure, but also will change the auscultatory and echocardiographic findings in older patients. The frequency of isolated click or late systolic murmur, so commonly present in younger patients with MVP, decreases with age and holosystolic murmurs are more common in older patients. Differences in echo findings between age groups include a higher prevalence of pansystolic prolapse and flaccid valves in patients over 50 years of age. Furthermore, increased cardiac chamber dimensions are more common in older patients. In addition to differences in auscultatory and echo findings, older patients with MVP commonly demonstrate electrocardiographic findings of atrial fibrillation, plus left ventricular enlargement, which are less common in younger patients.

In younger patients with MVP, severe mitral regurgitation with resultant heart failure is rare, whereas in older patients the risk of developing severe mitral regurgitation that necessitates valvular surgery significantly increases. Some studies[23,24] have shown that at least 25 percent of patients over 60 with MVP develop heart failure. Besides age, numerous studies have found association between male gender and severity of mitral valvular regurgitation in patients with MVP, and as expected the risk of mitral valve surgery increases in males.[25,26]

In many elderly MVP patients, the development of severe mitral regurgitation will be abrupt with the sudden onset of heart failure.[27] Certain elderly patients will present with symptoms of acute pulmonary edema, whereas others will have a few weeks of progressive dyspnea. The typical history will be a 10–15 year history of an insignificant heart murmur in an asymptomatic male, then sudden onset of progressive symptoms of heart failure. At surgery, an enlarged, floppy mitral valve, plus commonly ruptured chordae tendinae,[27,28] are found. In many of these patients the valve can be repaired with excellent results, including symptomatic relief and long-term survival.

In other patients with MVP, there is a slow development of mild or moderate valve regurgitation progressing to severe regurgitation. Many of the patients are elderly and male, and will remain asymptomatic or have only mild symptoms for many years, even though the clinical findings of regurgitation are severe and cardiac chamber dimensions are increased. Patients who develop symptoms or who demonstrate significant cardiac chamber enlargement or decreased ventricular function require valvular surgery. Some investigators have found a high incidence of significant morbidity, including heart failure and atrial fibrillation, to occur in patients with flail mitral valves and severe regurgitation.[29,30] Early valvular surgery has been recommended in these patients. It is assumed that most patients with flail valves have underlying MVP and many will demonstrate ruptured chordae.[29,31]

In summary, severity of valvular regurgitation with resultant heart failure in patients with MVP is influenced by age and gender. Increasing age and male gender is associated with increasing regurgitation and heart failure. Recognition of this disorder and proper timing of valvular surgery is important since surgical intervention is associated with excellent results.

HYPERTHYROID HEART DISEASE

The peak incidence of hyperthyroidism occurs in the third to fourth decades, but 15–25 percent of all cases do not occur until after the seventh decade.[32] In younger patients, hyperthyroidism is four to eight times more common in women, whereas in older patients the disease occurs with equal frequency in men and women.

Clinically, hyperthyroidism may present in the activated (classical) or nonactivated (apathetic) forms.[33] While the activated form is easily recognized by its classical symptoms and physical findings of tremors, hyperactivity, exophalmos, tachycardia, and enlarged thyroid, the apathetic type is more difficult to recognize. It usually occurs in the elderly and is difficult to diagnose because of its insidious onset, meager symptoms, and lack of characteristic exophalmos and hyperkinetic appearance. Elderly apathetic hyperthyroid patients usually present with a prolonged period of generalized malaise and lethargy with progressive weight loss, and often the

symptoms are mistakenly diagnosed as related to major depression. Early in the course of the illness, the elderly patient may not demonstrate the typical findings of a rapid bounding pulse or hyperactive precordium, and the first heart sound may not be accelerated. Systolic ejection flow murmurs and a S_4 may be present, although these findings are nonspecific. Not until late in the course of illness, with progressive increase in cardiac output, will the elderly patient develop symptoms of heart failure due to volume overload with progressive dyspnea and ankle edema.[34] Associated with these symptoms, the patient may become aware of a rapid irregular pulse and hyperactive precordium. Not infrequently, new or accelerated angina will develop. At this time, the physical examination will demonstrate findings of left- and right-sided heart failure and an impressive heart murmur, which is suggestive of mitral valvular regurgitation. The electrocardiogram confirms the diagnosis of atrial fibrillation with a rapid ventricular rate and nonspecific ST–T wave changes. Because of these findings, the elderly hyperthyroid patient's heart failure and angina, plus the heart murmur, may be mistakenly diagnosed as caused by ischemic heart disease. The thyroid may not be enlarged and unless thyroid functions are obtained, hyperthyroidism will not be diagnosed.

Early reports of apathetic hyperthyroidism were referred to as "masked hyperthyroidism" and many investigators stressed the significant morbidity and mortality associated with the disorder.[35] They further warned that even though patients may not appear extremely ill, without proper therapy the course would be progressively downhill with devastating outcomes.

In summary, hyperthyroidism may have a different presentation in elderly patients compared to younger patients, so the diagnosis may be missed. Instead of an activated (classical) state, elderly patients with hyperthyroidism may present in a nonactivated (apathetic) state. When significant cardiac involvement occurs, the patient will usually present with findings of atrial fibrillation and heart failure. Recognition of hyperthyroidism is mandatory, because without proper therapy, mortality and morbidity are high.

KEY POINTS   Cardiac disorders

- Clinical manifestations of common cardiac disorders in elderly patients may be atypical, compared with younger patients. Typical symptoms may not be present.

- When symptoms are present they are commonly nonspecific and may be misdiagnosed, owing to the presence of other common disorders or the presence of aging changes.

- Physical findings may be absent, obscured, or masked by the presence of concomitant disorders or aging changes.

- A physician caring for an elderly patient has to have a high suspicion for the presence of cardiac disease.

REFERENCES

1. Kannel WB, Belanger AJ: Epidemiology of heart failure. Am Heart J 1991;121:951–957
2. O'Connell JB, Bristone MR: Economic impact of heart failure in the United States: time for a different approach. J Heart Lung Transplant 1994;13(suppl 10):S107–S112

3. Tresch, DD: The clinical diagnosis of heart failure in older patients. J Am Geriatr Soc 1997;45:1128–1133

4. Rockwood K: Acute confusion in elderly medical patients. J Am Geriatr Soc 1989;37:150–154

5. Siegel R, Clemens T, Wingo M et al: Acute heart failure in the elderly: another manifestation of unstable "angina." J Am Coll Cardiol 1991;17:149 (abstract)

6. Clark LT, Garfein OB, Dwyer EM: Acute pulmonary edema due to ischemic heart disease without accompanying myocardial infarction. Am J Med 1983;75:332–336

7. Kunis R, Greenberg H, Yeoh CB et al: Coronary revascularization for recurrent pulmonary edema in elderly patients with ischemic heart disease and preserved ventricular function. N Engl J Med 1985;313:1207–1209

8. Tresch DD, McGough MF: Heart failure with normal systolic function: a common disorder in older people. J Am Geriatr Soc 1995;43:1035–1042

9. Dougherty AH, Naccarelli GV, Gray EI et al: Congestive heart failure with normal systolic function. Am J Cardiol 1984;54:778–782

10. Soufer R, Wholgelernter D, Vita NA et al: Intact systolic left ventricular function in clinical congestive heart failure. Am J Cardiol 1985;55:1032–1036

11. Wong WF, Gold S, Fukuyama O et al: Diastolic dysfunction in elderly patients with congestive heart failure. Am J Cardiol 1989;63:1526–1528

12. Aronow WS, Ahn C, Kronszon I: Prognosis of congestive heart failure in elderly patients with normal versus abnormal left ventricular systolic function associated with coronary artery disease. Am J Cardiol 1990;66:1257–1259

13. Bloor CM: Valvular heart disease in the elderly. In Coodley EL (ed): Geriatric Heart Disease. PSG Publishing, 1985:295–303

14. Aronow WS, Schwartz KS, Koenigsberg M: Correlation of aortic cuspal and aortic root disease with aortic systolic ejection murmurs and with mitral annular calcium in persons older than 62 years in a long-term health care facility. Am J Cardiol 1986;58:651–652

15. Ross J, Braunwald E: Aortic stenosis. Circulation 1968;38(Suppl V):V61–V67

16. Tresch DD, Knickelbine T: Aortic valvular stenosis in the elderly: a disorder with a favorable outcome if correctly diagnosed and treated. Cardiovasc Rev Rep 1994;14:35–38

17. Roberts WC, Perloff JK, Constantino T: Severe valvular aortic stenosis in patients over 65 years of age. Am J Cardiol 1971;27:497–506

18. Fulkerson PK, Beaver BM, Auseon JC et al: Calcification of the mitral annulus: etiology, clinical associations, complications and therapy. Am J Med 1979;66:967–977

19. Fontana ME, Pence HL, Leighton RJ et al: The varying clinical spectrum of the systolic click–late systolic murmur. Circulation 1979;41:807–816

20. Barlow JB, Bosman CK, Pocock WA et al: Late systolic murmur and nonejection (mid-late) systolic clicks: an analysis of 90 patients. Br Heart J 1968;30:203–218

21. Savage DD, Garrison RJ, Devereaux RB et al: Mitral valve prolapse in the general population. I: Epidemiological features. The Framingham Study. Am Heart J 1983;106:571–576

22. Reddy G, Tresch DD: Mitral valve prolapse: not always a benign disorder in the older patient. Cardiovasc Rev Rep 1997;18:42–48

23. Tresch DD, Siegel R, Keelan MH et al: Mitral valve prolapse in the elderly. J Am Geriatr Soc 1979;27:421–424

24. Kolibash AJ, Bush CA, Fontana MB et al: Mitral valve prolapse syndrome: analysis of 62 patients aged 60 years and older. Am J Cardiol 1983;52:534–539

25. Zuppiroli A, Rinaldi M, Kramer-Fox R et al: Natural history of mitral valve prolapse. Am J Cardiol 1995;75:1028–1032

26. Wilcken DE, Hickey AJ: Lifetime risk for patients with mitral valve prolapse of developing severe valve regurgitation require surgery. Circulation 1988;78:10–14

27. Tresch DD, Doyle TP, Boncheck LI et al: Mitral valve prolapse requiring surgery. Am J Med 1985;78:245–250

28. Jeresaty RM, Edward JE, Chawla SK: Mitral valve prolapse and ruptured chordae tendinae. Am J Cardiol 1985;55:138–142

29. Ling LH, Enriquez-Sarano M, Seward JB et al: Clinical outcome of mitral regurgitation due to flail leaflet. N Engl J Med 1996;335:1417–1423

30. Enriquez-Sarano M, Orszulak TA, Schaff HV et al: Mitral regurgitation: a new clinical perspective. Mayo Clin Proc 1997;72:1034–1043

31. Ren FJ, Panidis IP, Kotler MN et al: Flail mitral valve syndrome: comparison with chronic mitral regurgitation of other etiologies. Am Heart J 1985;109:435–442

32. Davis PJ, Davis FB: Hyperthyroidism in patients over the age of 60 years: clinical features in 85 patients. Medicine 1974;53:161–181

33. Lahey FH: Non-activity (apathetic) type of hyperthyroidism. N Engl J Med 1931;204:747–748

34. Shimshek T, Tresch D: Heart failure, weight loss, and depression in an elderly woman. Hosp Phys 1987;23:43–48

35. Levine SA, Sturgis CC: Hyperthyroidism masked as heart disease. Boston Med Surg J 1924;190:233–237

Chapter 32

Atherosclerosis and lipid metabolism

Robert W. Stout

Atherosclerosis is the most important disease in old age. It is responsible for the majority of deaths in old people and is the most common cause of disability and dependency in the later years of life. The principal arteries affected by atherosclerosis are: the coronary arteries, leading to myocardial infarction and chronic ischemic heart disease, cardiac failure, and cardiac arrhythmias; the cerebral circulation, leading to stroke, transient ischemic attacks, and multi-infarct dementia; the aorta, leading to aneurysm; and the peripheral arterial system, leading to intermittent claudication, chronic ischemia, gangrene, and amputation. Atherosclerosis has the characteristics of a chronic degenerative disease; it takes decades to develop, the underlying cause is unknown, and it is irreversible by the time it becomes clinically apparent.

Atherosclerosis is a disease of multiple causes with several mechanisms operating at different times in any individual. The advanced lesion with its cellular proliferation, connective tissue deposition, calcification, necrosis, and thrombosis is the final common pathway of a number of different mechanisms. Although atherosclerosis becomes more prevalent with advancing age, it is becoming clearer that it can be prevented, or at least its progress delayed, and ischemic disease need not be an inevitable consequence of growing older.

PATHOGENESIS OF ATHEROSCLEROSIS

The normal artery

The arterial wall is divided into three layers: the intima, media, and adventitia.

The *intima* consists of a single layer of epithelial-like cells, the endothelium, which is separated from the internal elastic lamina by connective tissue containing a variable number of smooth muscle cells. The number of smooth muscle cells in the intima increases with advancing age to form diffuse intimal thickening. The endothelium acts as a barrier that protects the inner part of the artery from injurious substances in the circulation and as a blood compatible container. It is selectively permeable and allows the passage of nutrients to the inner part of the artery. The endothelium, which in total is a very large organ, is metabolically active and secretes a number of important substances, including: prostacyclin; factor VIII antigen; endothelium-derived vasoactive factors such as nitric oxide, prostacyclin, and endothelin; and cytokines and growth factors.[1]

The *media* consists of smooth muscle cells and is separated from the intima by the fenestrated internal elastic lamina. Smooth muscle cells, by their contraction and relaxation, modify the size of the lumen of the artery and maintain blood pressure. They also are the major synthetic cells of the artery,

manufacturing connective tissue, including collagen, fibrin, elastin, and proteoglycans, as well as cytokines and growth factors. Smooth muscle cells appear to exist in two phenotypic states—contractile or synthetic—and may change from one to the other depending on their environment.[1] In atheromatous lesions they appear to be in the synthetic state.

The *adventitia* consists of fibrous and fatty connective tissue and is the means by which the artery is linked to the surrounding tissues. The adventitia appears to play no part in the development of atherosclerosis.

Atherosclerosis

Atherosclerosis is a disease of the intima and inner part of the media of the artery. The term "atherosclerosis" or "atheroma" covers a number of lesions of which the most characteristic are the fatty streak and the fibrous plaque.[1,2] Fatty streaks are found in the lining of many arteries in children and younger adults. They are flat white or yellow longitudinal lesions on the intimal surface of the artery (Fig. 32-1) and consist of collections of lipid-engorged foam cells, overlain with an intact endothelium (Fig. 32-2). The foam cells originate from monocyte–macrophages and T-lymphocytes. The fibrous plaque is the advanced atheromatous lesion (Fig. 32-3). It consists of a fibrous cap made up of connective tissue containing elastic fibers, collagen, proteoglycans, and basement membrane, in which are embedded smooth muscle cells, and beneath which are variable amounts of intracellular and extracellular lipids, smooth muscle cells, macrophages, T-lymphocytes, connective tissue, and, in the depth of the lesion, necrotic debris, cholesterol crystals, and calcification (Fig. 32-4). The relative content of fibrous tissue and lipid within a plaque is variable, with lesions in the coronary arteries being largely fibrous. The surface of the fibrous plaque may be the site of thrombosis.

It is not known what determines whether a fatty streak evolves into a fibrous plaque, or what precipitates thrombus formation on the plaque. The distribution of the lesion within the arterial system remains unexplained, although hemodynamic factors such as shear stress may account for the sites of some of the lesions.[3]

The cells of the lesions

Atherosclerosis results from the interaction of four cells—two arterial cells (endothelial and smooth muscle cells), and two circulating cells (platelets and monocyte–macrophages).[1] These interact with each other and with lipoproteins, hormones, hemodynamic factors, and connective tissue in the arterial wall. Each of the cells is able to synthesize and secrete a wide variety of cytokines, growth factors, coagulation factors, and vasoactive substances.[1] These can act locally on adjacent cells

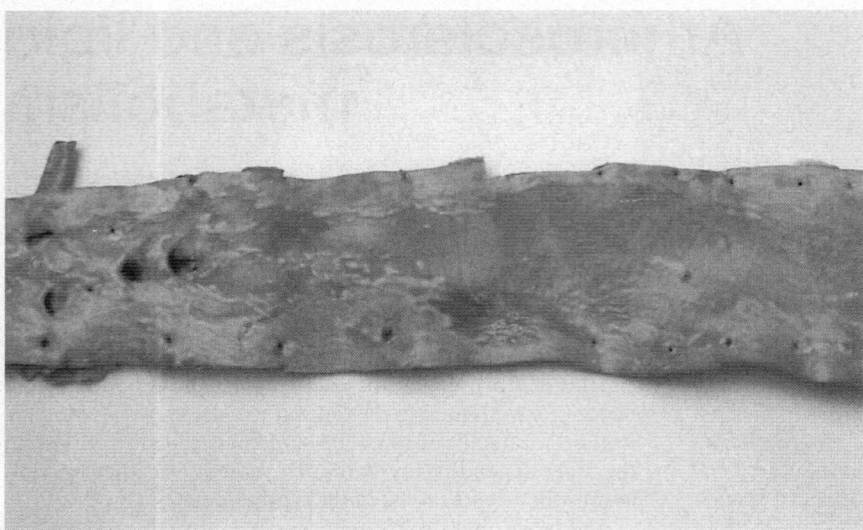

Figure 32-1 Surface of human aorta showing extensive involvement by fatty streaks. Courtesy of Dr J.D. Biggart, Department of Pathology, Queen's University of Belfast.

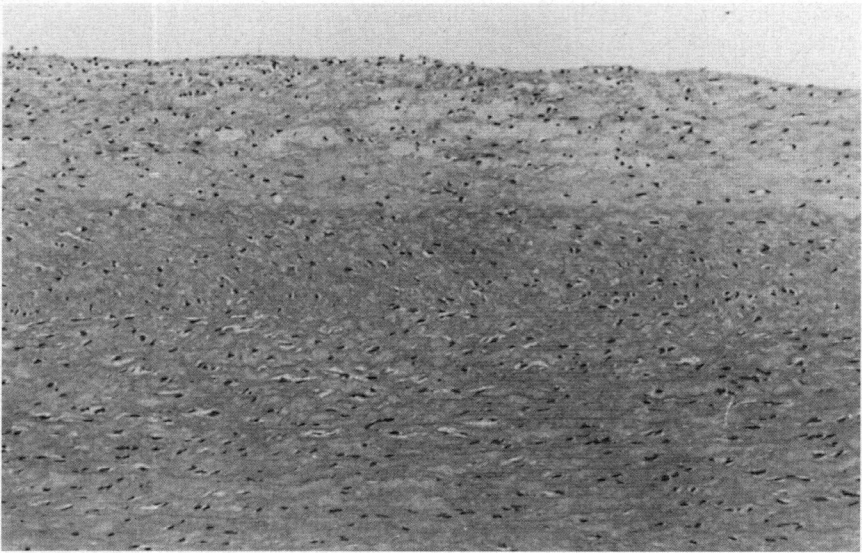

Figure 32-2 Photomicrograph of fatty streak showing foam cells in subintimal tissues. Courtesy of Dr J.D. Biggart, Department of Pathology, Queen's University of Belfast.

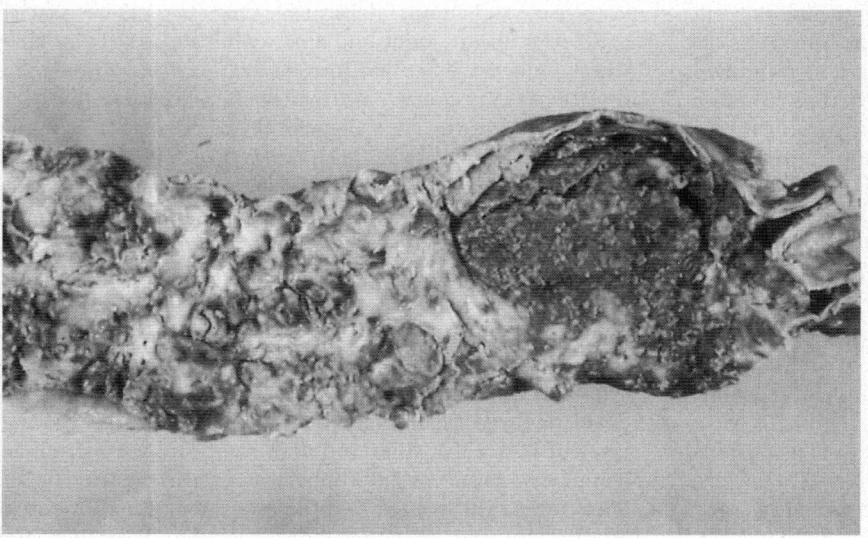

Figure 32-3 Surface of human aorta showing extensive involvement by fibrous plaques and a large thrombus. Courtesy of Dr J.D. Biggart, Department of Pathology, Queen's University of Belfast.

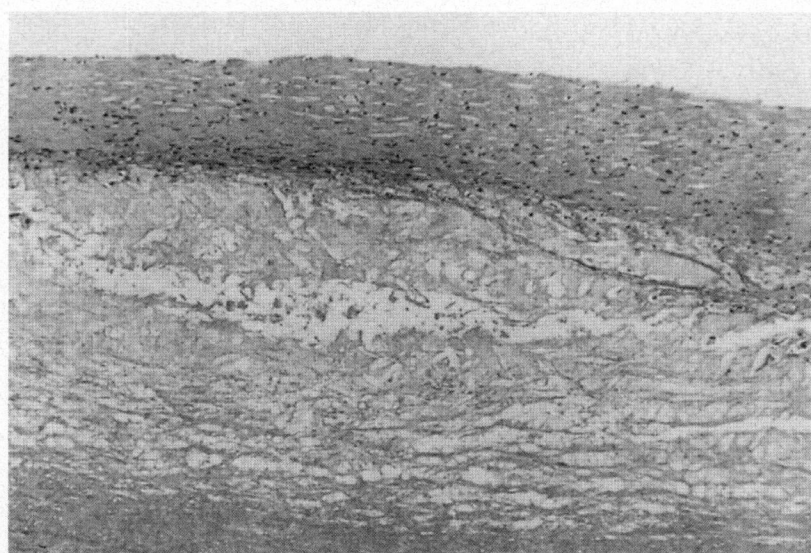

Figure 32-4 Photomicrograph of fibrous plaque showing fibrous cap with smooth muscle cells, foam cells and extracellular lipid, and necrotic debris. Courtesy of Dr J.D. Biggart, Department of Pathology, Queen's University of Belfast.

(paracrine function) and on the same cells (autocrine function). The interactions of these factors and circulating (endocrine) factors in the pathogenesis of atherosclerosis is complex and has not been completely elucidated.

ENDOTHELIAL CELLS   The endothelium consists of a single layer of epithelial cells which are normally quiescent but perform a number of essential functions. Endothelial cells regulate the transfer of metabolic substances between the plasma and the subendothelial space. They bind low-density lipoprotein (LDL) and "modify" it.[4–6] Modification by oxidation of LDL may be one of the most important early events in the development of atherosclerosis and may cause endothelial "injury."[5,6] They synthesize a number of biologically active molecules involved in hemostasis, in the regulation of vascular tone and in inflammation, and of particular relevance to atherosclerosis, a number of growth factors. In this way they may influence the growth and function of the other cells of the lesion and of themselves. Although the response-to-injury theory of atherogenesis presupposes an injury to the endothelial barrier, this "injury" may not result in loss of cells but may be a subtle alteration of endothelial function.[1]

SMOOTH MUSCLE CELLS   Proliferation of smooth muscle cells and their migration from the media to the intima is an important event in the development of the fibrous plaque. Smooth muscle cells synthesize connective tissue, and are the major components of the fibroproliferative lesion of atherosclerosis. They synthesize and secrete growth factors and cytokines and factors that attract monocytes into the artery.[7]

PLATELETS   These adhere to intimal surfaces that have been denuded of endothelium and release the contents of their granules, which include mitogens, platelet factor 4, β-thromboglobulin, and thromboxane A1. The platelet-derived growth factor (PDGF),[1] now known to be synthesized and secreted by many other cells as well as platelets, is particularly significant in atherogenesis, as it is a chemoattractant as well as

a mitogen to smooth muscle cells and also stimulates the interaction of low-density lipoproteins with their cell surface receptors.

MONOCYTES/MACROPHAGES   Circulating monocytes are the source of tissue macrophages and of many of the foam cells of the atheromatous lesion. In hypercholesterolemic animals, the earliest abnormality found in the arterial wall is attachment of monocytes to the surface of the endothelium. The monocytes then migrate between the endothelial cells into the subendothelium, where they accumulate lipid. Macrophages are considered to have a "scavenger" function in inflammatory reactions. They have scavenger receptors for modified LDL that are not subject to the normal regulation of LDL receptors, and hence there is unlimited uptake of modified LDL, with the formation of foam cells.[4] Macrophages secrete many growth factors and cytokines which act on the cells of the lesion. The mechanisms of the adherence and migration of monocytes in the artery wall are little understood.

Atherogenesis

One of the oldest ideas on the development of atherosclerosis suggests that it is a "response to injury,"[1] with modern emphasis being placed on an inflammatory process[8] (Fig. 32-5). The early stages of the development of atherosclerosis appear to be a disruption or alteration of the endothelium's barrier function (the "injury"). This may be caused by elevated or modified LDL, the effects of cigarette smoking, perhaps by means of free radicals, other risk factors such as hypertension or diabetes, elevated plasma homocysteine concentrations, genetic alterations, or perhaps infections. The altered endothelium becomes more adhesive to circulating cells, particularly leucocytes or platelets, and also increases its permeability. The dysfunctional endothelium tends to promote coagulation rather than preventing it. At a later stage, smooth muscle cells migrate and proliferate into the intima which also accumulates monocyte-derived macrophages and T-lymphocytes. Multiple enzymes, cytokines, and growth factors are released by the different cells and interact with the cells and with circulating

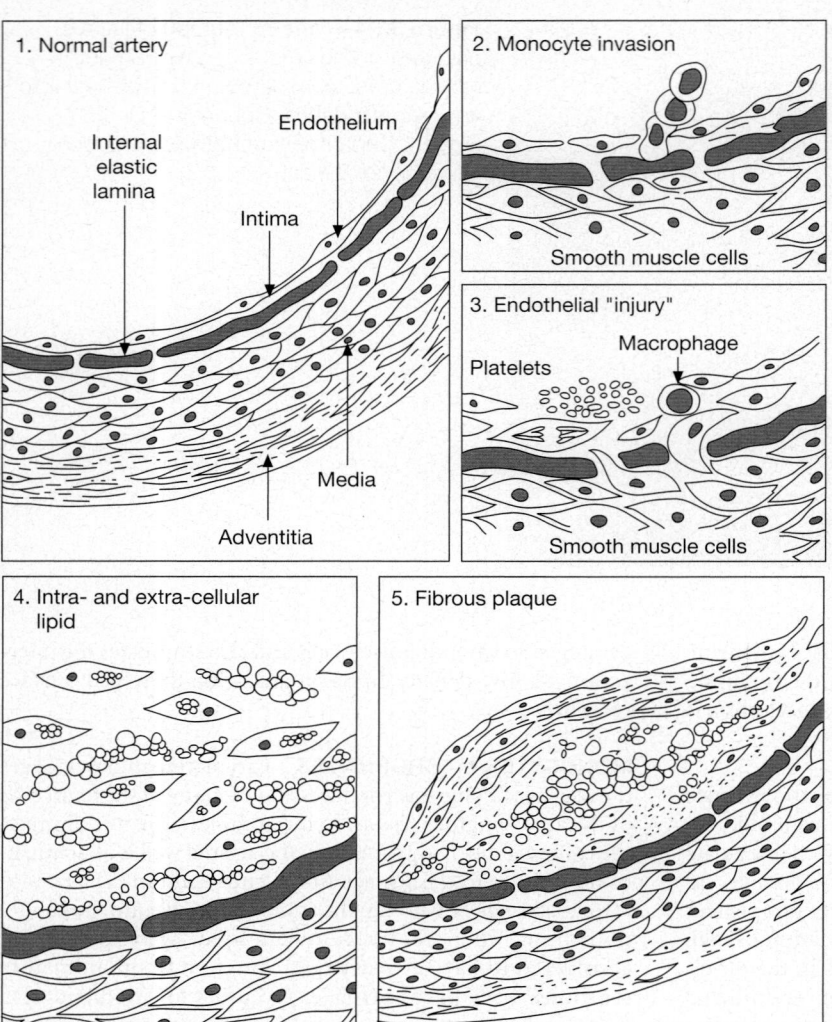

Figure 32-5 The pathogenesis of atherosclerosis; see text for details. Adapted from Stout.[111]

factors, including lipids and lipoproteins. The basic process is probably an inflammatory and repair mechanism and normally leads to reconstitution of the integrity of the artery, with the injury becoming covered by a continuous layer of endothelium, and the proliferating smooth muscle cells regressing.

In abnormal circumstances such as repeated injury or exposure to abnormal constituents of the circulation (e.g. hypercholesterolemia), the process changes from a repair to a proliferative process. This is characterized by an accumulation of smooth muscle cells in the arterial intima; the formation of extracellular connective tissue; the accumulation of foam cells, most of which are derived from monocyte macrophages that have engorged lipoproteins; calcification; ulceration; hemorrhage into the plaque; and superimposed thrombus formation. A small proportion of plaques are heavily engorged with lipid, both in foam cells and in the core of the lesion. These plaques appear to be unstable and at risk of fissuring, a process that predisposes to the formation of thrombus on the surface of the plaque.[2] It seems likely that there are a number of different stimuli that may be involved in the development of atherosclerosis, and that the advanced atherosclerotic lesion is the final common pathway of a number of pathogenic mechanisms.

Some of the evidence that atherosclerosis is an inflammatory disease comes from the presence of circulating inflammatory markers in patients who have had, or who are at high risk of, myocardial infarction. C-reactive protein and fibrinogen, both of which predict the outcome of myocardial infarction, are also associated with an increased risk of mortality from cardiac causes.[9,10] An elevated white cell has also been associated with coronary heart disease.[11] There is evidence of association between ischemic heart disease and infections with organisms such as herpes viruses and *Chlamydia pneumoniae*. Infection or inflammation may be a mechanism that links cardiovascular disease with risk factors such as dental disease, air pollution, and cold temperatures.[12,13]

Aging and atherosclerosis

Atherosclerosis and aging are intimately linked, and atherosclerosis is universally present in elderly people. The exact relationship between atherosclerosis and aging is difficult to define. On the one hand, the pathogenesis of atherosclerosis may be related to a biological aging process. On the other, the

Table 32-1 **Changes in the biological properties of arterial endothelial and smooth muscle cells in relation to in-vivo or in-vitro aging**	
Endothelial cells	**Smooth muscle cells**
Finite lifespan	Finite lifespan
Decreased population doublings	Decreased population doublings
Decreased binding and degradation of LDL	Longer latent period
No change in processing acetyl LDL	Reduced response to growth factors
Decreased angiotensin-converting enzyme activity	Decreased LDL degradation
	Decreased prostacyclin synthesis

Abbreviation: LDL, low density lipoprotein.

Source: Adapted from Stout (1987),[14] by permission of Oxford University Press.

Table 32-2 Risk factors for atherosclerosis

Intrinsic (irreversible)
- Age
- Male sex
- Genetic and familial factors

Extrinsic (reversible)
- Cigarette smoking
- Hypertension
- Dyslipoproteinemia
- Hyperglycemia and diabetes mellitus

Indirect (might be modified)
- Obesity
- Physical inactivity

Others
- Hyperfibrinogenemia
- Hyperhomocysteinemia
- Insulin resistance and hyperinsulinemia
- Hemostatic factors
- Hyperuricemia

relationship between age and atherosclerosis may simply be the time required for its development.

Aging and atherosclerosis may be related by age changes in the artery, or by age changes in cardiovascular risk factors. Changes occur in the cells of the artery during senescence, and these might contribute to the development of atherosclerosis[14] (Table 32-1). Endothelial cells lose their proliferative ability and hence their ability to repair an "injury" on the surface of the artery. The control of proliferation of smooth muscle cells and their interaction with lipoproteins is also altered with senescence. Hence, although atherosclerosis in old age is almost certainly the end point of a slow and prolonged process, it may be accelerated in older people because of changes in the cells that contribute to the development of the lesion.

Theories linking an aging process with atherosclerosis must take into account the evidence that nutrition in vitro or early infancy may profoundly influence the future development of cardiovascular disease.[15]

EPIDEMIOLOGY OF ATHEROSCLEROSIS

Atherosclerosis is a universal condition that is present in all elderly people. It first appears in the late teens or early twenties; autopsy studies in young men killed as a result of war or accidents have revealed extensive atherosclerosis in these relatively young age groups.[16] However, atherosclerosis can be detected in life only by sophisticated imaging techniques, and hence epidemiological studies usually measure other manifestations of cardiovascular disease, such as sudden death, cardiovascular death, or nonfatal myocardial infarction. Fewer epidemiological studies have looked at stroke or peripheral vascular disease, which are less common than coronary artery disease and, therefore, more difficult to investigate.

Risk factors

Studies of the epidemiology of atherosclerosis have concentrated on the identification of risk factors for the disease.[17] These are characteristics in asymptomatic people that

predispose to cardiovascular disease, and are identified by prospective epidemiological studies. Risk factors identify groups of people who are particularly susceptible to cardiovascular disease. They are not necessarily causal, but may be indirectly related to the disease or may even be early manifestations of the condition. As a result, alteration of a risk factor will not necessarily modify the course of the disease; intervention studies are required to test this. Risk factors that are associated with the clinical complications of atherosclerosis may or may not be related to the initiation of the disease in the vessel wall many years earlier, or to its progression to a stage where it causes clinical disease.

The risk factors for atherosclerosis may be divided into: intrinsic, which are currently not amenable to alteration; extrinsic, which to varying degrees can be altered; and indirect (Table 32-2).

Intrinsic risk factors

AGE   This is the most important risk factor for cardiovascular disease, which becomes progressively more common with advancing age in both men and women (Fig. 32-6). A reasonable hypothesis is that atherosclerosis is an age-related disease that is accelerated by the presence of other risk factors. Risk factors for atherosclerosis seem to continue to operate in old age.[19] With advancing age the chance of having significant atheromatous lesions increases and the presence of atheromatous plaques greatly increases the risk of a cardiovascular event.[17]

MALE SEX   This is another important risk factor for cardiovascular disease. Particularly in the younger age groups, men develop ischemic heart disease much more often than women[20] (Fig. 32-6). Beyond the age of menopause the incidence tends to equalize, becoming similar at about the age of 70. This is because atherosclerosis increases in women after the menopause.[21] The sex difference in incidence is less marked in stroke,[22] possibly because stroke tends to occur rather later in life than ischemic heart disease. The differences between

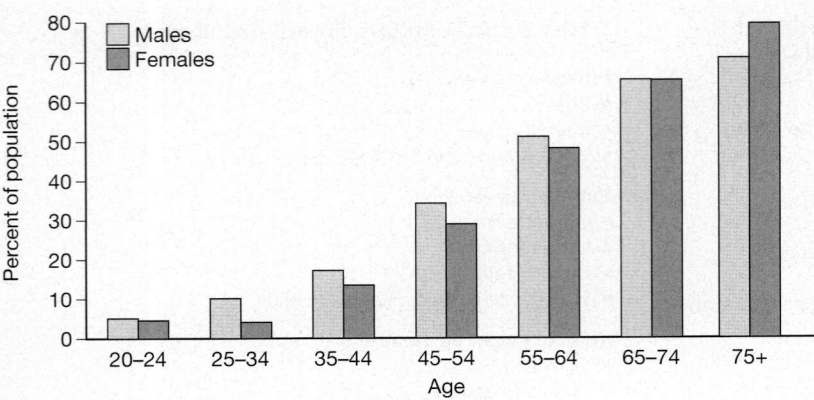

Figure 32-6 Prevalence of cardiovascular disease by age and sex in the USA, 1988–94. From American Heart Association.[18]

the epidemiology of coronary heart disease and stroke, two complications of atherosclerosis, indicate the need for caution in extrapolating the results of studies of clinical end-organ damage to disease of the arterial wall.

GENETIC FACTORS These are important and may operate in two ways. Many cardiovascular risk factors are, to a greater or lesser extent, under genetic influence (e.g. dyslipoproteinemia).[23] However, after taking account of this, there still appears to be a genetic and familial susceptibility to premature cardiovascular disease. In the Framingham study, death due to coronary artery disease in parents was associated with a 30 percent increase in risk of coronary artery disease in siblings.[24] This association was found in men and women and was independent of the effect of other cardiovascular risk factors. Although present in those who developed coronary artery disease later than age 60 years, the effect was stronger with earlier onset of the disease.

Extrinsic risk factors

CIGARETTE SMOKING This is totally extrinsic and the most completely preventable of all cardiovascular risk factors. Cigarette smoking is an important predisposing factor to premature cardiovascular disease, including ischemic heart disease[25] and stroke.[26] The risk increases with the number of cigarettes smoked. Cessation of smoking reduces the risk of myocardial infarction to that of those who never smoked in 2 or 3 years,[27] and also reduces the risk of stroke. The mechanism by which cigarette smoking increases cardiovascular disease is not known, although some of the toxic products of cigarette smoke may act on the cells of the arterial wall, causing changes in their biological functions.[28] The elimination of cigarette smoking would result in a considerable improvement in the health of the population.

HYPERTENSION Raised blood pressure has a number of effects on the cardiovascular system. Hypertension itself may cause specific problems in the renal and retinal arteriolar circulation and also predisposes to Charcot–Bouchard aneurysms and intracranial hemorrhage. However, hypertension is an important risk factor for atherosclerotic cardiovascular disease, including ischemic heart disease[29] and

stroke[30] (Fig. 32-7). Stroke is the most important cardiovascular complication of hypertension in terms of relative risk, although with respect to attributable risk, ischemic heart disease is numerically more important. Conversely, hypertension is the most important risk factor for stroke. Well-controlled therapeutic trials have shown that reduction of high blood pressure in people up to the age of 79 years prevents stroke but is less effective in preventing ischemic heart disease.[31]

DYSLIPOPROTEINEMIA This is a term that covers abnormal concentrations of plasma lipoproteins, including elevation of some lipoproteins (hyperlipoproteinemia) or decreased

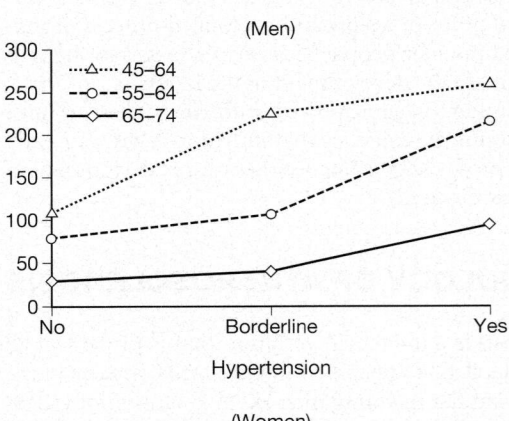

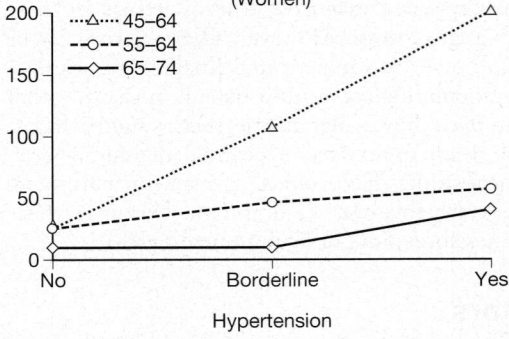

Figure 32-7 Cardiovascular mortality (per 10,000) in relation to hypertension in men and women. From Kannel et al.,[29] with permission.

high density lipoproteins. The closest relationship between lipids and cardiovascular disease is with plasma cholesterol[32,33] (Fig. 32-8). Cholesterol is carried in LDL, and both cholesterol and LDL are positively correlated with the incidence of ischemic heart disease throughout the lifespan,[34] and, to a somewhat lesser extent, with stroke[35] and peripheral vascular disease. There is an inverse relationship between the level of high-density lipoprotein cholesterol (HDL) and cardiovascular disease.[36] Plasma triglyceride levels are also a risk factor for ischemic heart disease[37] and, although there has been controversy as to whether this relationship is independent of the effects of cholesterol,[38] evidence favors such a relationship.[39] Dyslipoproteinemia is related to both genetic factors[23] and dietary factors.[40] Lipid metabolism is discussed in more detail later in this chapter.

DIABETES MELLITUS   This is associated with an increase in the incidence of cardiovascular disease, which is present in both insulin-dependent diabetes mellitus (IDDM) and non-insulin-dependent diabetes (NIDDM).[41,42] Cardiovascular disease is the leading cause of mortality and morbidity in diabetes. The absolute risk for major coronary events in otherwise healthy patients with NIDDM approaches that of nondiabetic patients with established coronary heart disease. The prognosis of coronary heart disease in patients with diabetes is also poor. The incidence of diabetes increases with advancing age and diabetes-related cardiovascular disease is a major health problem in elderly people. Diabetes confers a particularly high risk in women, so that in younger people with diabetes, the incidence of cardiovascular disease in women is equal to that in men (Fig. 32-9), while the excess risk associated with diabetes is present at least until age 75. Diabetes is the only condition in which the incidence of cardiovascular disease is the same in men and women at all ages.

The atherosclerosis that occurs in diabetes is morphologically and biochemically indistinguishable from atherosclerosis in the general population and is not related to diabetic microangiopathy.

Diabetes is associated with other cardiovascular risk factors including dyslipoproteinemia and hypertension. However, even when these risk factors are taken into account, diabetes doubles the risk of cardiovascular disease. The risk is not closely related to the blood sugar level, and currently available methods of treating diabetes do not prevent the excess frequency of cardiovascular disease. Increasing emphasis is being placed on identifying and treating other risk factors, such as hypertension,[43] in an attempt to prevent cardiovascular disease in people with diabetes.

These four risk factors account for about 50 percent of the variability in risk in high-risk populations. They can also explain up to 90 percent of the excess risk for coronary heart disease.[17]

Indirect risk factors

There are a number of risk factors for cardiovascular disease that probably act indirectly. Prominent among these are obesity[44,45] and a sedentary lifestyle.[46] Both of these are associated with disorders of lipid metabolism, hyperglycemia, and hypertension. Although the epidemiological relationship may be indirect, prevention or correction of obesity and increased physical activity may be effective ways of preventing cardiovascular disease.

Other risk factors

Other cardiovascular risk factors have been described but their place in the epidemiology of cardiovascular disease has been less well established than those mentioned above.

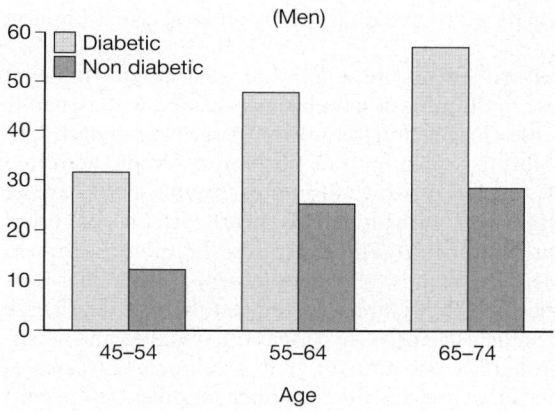

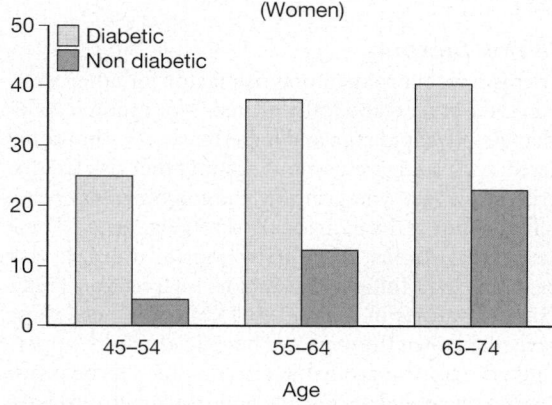

Figure 32-9 Annual incidence of cardiovascular disease in relation to the presence or absence of diabetes mellitus in men and women. From Kannel and McGee,[110] with permission.

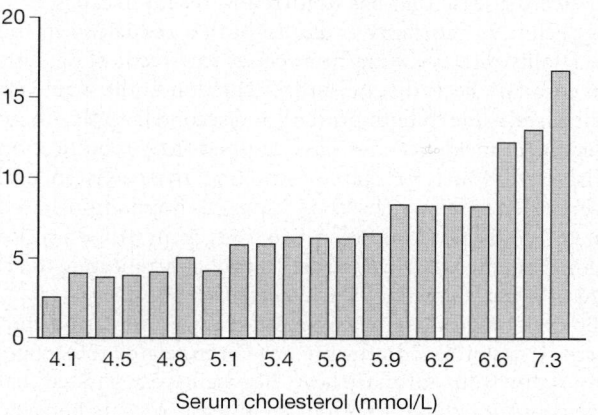

Figure 32-8 Six-year mortality from coronary heart disease (CHD) in relation to serum cholesterol. From Martin et al.,[32] with permission.

Raised serum *fibrinogen* is a risk factor for ischemic heart disease[47] and stroke.[48] Fibrinogen is involved in the coagulation process, and it seems likely that raised fibrinogen is related not only to the development of atherosclerosis but also to the thrombus, which often converts an atherosclerotic lesion into a complete occlusion of the artery.[2] In older people, fibrinogen levels are higher in winter than in summer.[49] This parallels the seasonal variation in the prevalence of both fatal and nonfatal ischemic heart disease. Fibrinogen levels are influenced by a number of other factors, including smoking, diet, and exercise; and being an acute-phase protein, fibrinogen is influenced by inflammatory processes and other body stress.[50]

Insulin resistance and hyperinsulinemia (sometimes called the "metabolic syndrome" or "syndrome X") are associated with cardiovascular disease and many of its risk factors.[51,52] The insulin-resistance syndrome[52] consists of a combination of high insulin levels, normal or mildly elevated glucose, high triglyceride and very-low-density lipoprotein (VLDL), low HDL, and hypertension. It occurs in relation to obesity and mild NIDDM, but may be present in the absence of either. Although many people with cardiovascular disease have several or all of the components of the insulin-resistance syndrome, prospective epidemiological studies have shown that high insulin levels are independently associated with the development of ischemic heart disease.[51] As well as its effects on other risk factors, insulin has direct effects on the arterial wall, promoting smooth muscle cell proliferation and lipid accumulation.[51] Hyperinsulinemia and insulin resistance may be corrected by avoiding obesity and by regular physical exercise.

As well as fibrinogen, a number of other factors that predispose to thrombosis have been associated with ischemic heart disease. Coagulation factor VII,[47] tissue plasminogen activator inhibitor (which inhibits fibrinolysis),[53] and activated protein C resistance (which promotes thrombosis)[54] have all been associated with ischemic heart disease or other thrombotic disorders. The exact role of these factors in atherosclerosis remains to be determined, as does their relation to aging.[55] They emphasize the fact that the classic risk factors for atherosclerosis—hypertension, smoking, and hypercholesterolemia—account for only a minority of cases of myocardial infarction and that the search for other factors must continue.

Multiple risk factors

Many patients have more than one risk factor for atherosclerosis. Often these are metabolically related—for example, obesity and diabetes, dyslipidemia and hypertension[52]—but some are unrelated, such as cigarette smoking and other risk factors. Multiple risk factors act synergistically, the combined risk being greater than the sum of the individual risks[56] (Fig. 32-10). There have been several studies of intervention on multiple risk factors, including the Multiple Risk Factors Intervention Trial[57] in the USA and studies in Finland.[58,59] Unfortunately, these studies have not shown the expected beneficial results, apparently because the control group has also modified its behavior and hence differences between study and control groups have not been apparent.

The predisposition to ischemic heart disease and stroke, and to many of their risk factors including changes in blood

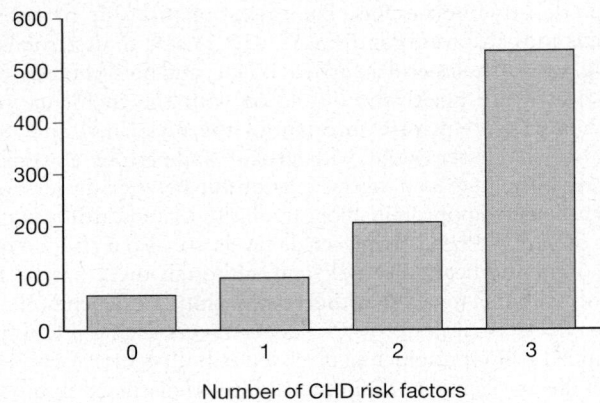

Figure 32-10 Twelve-year annual incidence of coronary heart disease in relation to number of risk factors present. The risk factors are cigarette smoking, hypertension, and hypercholesterolemia. From Kannel et al.[56]

pressure and circulating lipids, diabetes, and insulin resistance, seem to be determined in very early life—before, during, or soon after birth.[15] Fetal and neonatal nutrition seem to program the individual for the future development of serious and life-threatening conditions. The possibility that health in old age is influenced by events around the time of birth is a new challenge to preventive gerontology.

Other epidemiological findings

Geographical patterns of cardiovascular disease provide information on predisposing factors.[60] Migrant populations are very informative in this respect. Coronary heart disease is particularly common in people who have migrated from the Indian subcontinent to various parts of the world. The high rates cannot be explained by hypertension, smoking, or high serum cholesterol, but appear to be associated with low plasma HDL levels, high plasma triglyceride levels, and a high prevalence of NIDDM and hyperinsulinemia, suggesting a state of insulin resistance.[61]

One of the striking features of the epidemiology of atherosclerosis has been the decline in mortality rates from coronary heart disease that has occurred in recent decades.[62–64] The decline in mortality is due to both a reduction in the case-fatality rate, resulting from better treatment of patients with coronary heart disease, and a reduction in the incidence of the disease due to both primary and secondary prevention. A decline in incidence may have resulted from modification of risk factors such as cigarette smoking, hypertension, and hypercholesterolemia. If so, it supports population-based strategies for health promotion. Mortality from stroke has also declined but the fall started earlier,[65] probably reflecting treatment of hypertension or a decline in smoking.

Epidemiological studies in which changes in plasma cholesterol levels or blood pressure have been related to changes in mortality from coronary heart disease have suggested that there is an "incubation period" of at least 10 years between exposure to risk factors and the effects on mortality.[66] Studies in patients with diabetes have shown that atherosclerosis starts

KEY POINTS Atherosclerosis

- Atherosclerosis is the pathological process which is responsible for the majority of deaths and the greatest amount of disability and dependency in later life.

- There is increasing evidence that atherosclerosis is an inflammatory process.

- Atherosclerosis becomes more prevalent with advancing years, but the process is accelerated in the presence of certain risk factors, and may be delayed by reduction of those risk factors.

- Intrinsic risk factors for atherosclerosis are age, male sex, and genetic factors.

- The main extrinsic risk factors are cigarette smoking, hypertension, dyslipoproteinemia, and hyperglycemia/ diabetes mellitus. Other emerging risk factors include hyperfibrinogenemia, hyperhomocysteinemia, insulin resistance and hyperinsulinemia, and hemostatic changes.

- Multiple risk factors act synergistically. Hence, reduction of one of multiple risk factors may have disproportionate benefits.

- The most effective means of preventing or delaying atherosclerosis and cardiovascular disease are avoiding cigarette smoking, controlling blood pressure, and reducing cholesterol levels.

- Avoidance of obesity and regular physical exercise benefit several risk factors as well as general health.

at the same time in patients with and without diabetes but progresses more rapidly in those with diabetes.[67] This suggests that the initiation and progression of atherosclerosis may be influenced by different factors.

LIPIDS AND LIPOPROTEINS

Lipids

The major lipids of the circulation are cholesterol and fatty acids. Cholesterol is an essential structural component of cell membranes and a precursor of steroid hormones, bile acids, and other important molecules. It is derived both from dietary animal fat, and from synthesis in the liver, although most tissues have the capacity to synthesize cholesterol. Fatty acids are the major energy source of the body and circulate either unesterified (free fatty acids), or as components of triglycerides, phospholipids, or cholesteryl esters. Fatty acids may be ingested in the diet or synthesized in the liver.

As lipids are insoluble in water, they circulate in lipid–protein complexes. Free fatty acids are loosely complexed with albumin, while cholesterol, cholesteryl esters, triglycerides, and phospholipids circulate in association with specific peptides (apolipoproteins) as macromolecular complexes, the lipoproteins. These systems transport cholesterol and fatty acids to the peripheral tissues and return cholesterol to the liver, where it is converted to bile acids and excreted or repackaged into other lipoproteins.

Lipoproteins

The following lipoproteins occur in the circulation, in increasing order of density and decreasing order of size.

- *Chylomicrons* are the largest lipoproteins and consist of triglyceride and cholesterol of dietary origin, and apolipoproteins (Apo) B-48, E, and C-II. Normally, chylomicrons are cleared from the circulation within 4 hours of a meal by hydrolysis of triglyceride by the enzyme lipoprotein lipase. The resulting chylomicron remnants are present only transiently in the circulation and are taken up and metabolized by the liver.
- *Very-low-density lipoproteins* are the main carriers of endogenously synthesized triglyceride. They also contain cholesterol, cholesteryl ester, phospholipids, and apolipoproteins B-100, C-II, and E. The triglyceride is hydrolyzed in capillaries by the enzyme lipoprotein lipase to create intermediate-density lipoproteins (IDL), which are normally present only transiently in the circulation before being taken up by the liver.
- *Low-density lipoproteins* are the main carriers of cholesterol in the circulation. They also contain small amounts of triglyceride and phospholipids and apolipoprotein B-100.
- *High-density lipoproteins* contain nearly equal amounts of cholesterol and protein—apolipoproteins A-I and A-II. Two subclasses of HDL, HDL2 and HDL3, predominate in the circulation.

Lipid metabolism

Lipid metabolism may be conveniently considered as occurring in three pathways: the exogenous lipid pathway, the endogenous lipid pathway, and reverse cholesterol transport.[68]

Exogenous fat transport

The majority of lipid that is ingested in the diet is triglyceride, although cholesterol is also taken in. Triglyceride is broken down in the gastrointestinal tract by pancreatic lipase, reassembled in the intestinal epithelium, and absorbed into the lacteals, where it is complexed with cholesterol, also absorbed from the diet, cholesterol esters, and apoB-48, apoA-I, and apoA-IV to form chylomicrons.

In the circulation, chylomicrons acquire apoE, C-II, and C-III which is a cofactor for lipoprotein lipase and lose apoA-I and A-IV. After a meal, particularly one containing fat, the triglyceride level in the blood greatly increases, and blood that is allowed to stand has a creamy layer representing the absorbed lipid. It is usually cleared in about 4 hours by the activity of the enzyme lipoprotein lipase, which is secreted from endothelial cells in adipose tissue capillaries and which hydrolyzes chylomicron triglyceride to fatty acids that are taken up by adipose cells and stored to be used as energy. The chylomicron remnants are reprocessed in the liver, which has specific chylomicron remnant cell membrane receptors. Hepatic lipase has an important role in remodeling remnant particles.

Endogenous fat transport

Triglyceride is synthesized in the liver from glucose and fatty acid precursors and is secreted with cholesterol, apoB-100, C-II, C-III, and E as VLDL. VLDL triglyceride is hydrolyzed by the same lipoprotein lipase that hydrolyzes chylomicron triglyceride, and the released fatty acids are used by muscle as an energy source or stored in adipose tissue. The remnant particles (IDL) are reprocessed in the liver by way of receptors that bind apoE. Some are cleared from the plasma while others are reformed into LDL. LDL is the main cholesterol-carrying lipoprotein and is cleared predominantly by the liver by way of the LDL receptor, which recognizes apoB-100.[69] LDL receptors are also present in most of the cells of the body. Interaction of LDL with its receptor results in internalization of the lipoprotein receptor complex (Fig. 32-11). This triggers a number of intracellular biochemical processes, which include catabolism of the lipoprotein in the lysosomes, inhibition of the activity of the enzyme hydroxymethyl glutyryl coenzyme A (HMG-CoA) reductase, the rate-limiting enzyme in the cholesterol synthetic pathway, and inhibition of further LDL interaction with cell membrane receptors. In this way, cellular cholesterol synthesis is finely regulated.

Reverse cholesterol transport

High-density lipoprotein is responsible for reverse cholesterol transport, removing cholesterol from the tissues, and delivering it to the liver for reprocessing into other lipoproteins or for elimination by conversion to bile acids. Nascent HDL, secreted by the liver and the intestine, attracts material from the breakdown of chylomicrons and VLDL, and cholesterol from cells. The cholesterol is esterified by the enzyme lecithin cholesterol acyltransferase (LCAT), which uses apoA-I, present in nascent HDL, as a cofactor. With incorporation of cholesterol ester, HDL becomes larger and less dense, changing from HDL3 to HDL2. Some of the cholesterol of HDL2 is transferred to VLDL, IDL, and LDL by means of a cholesterol ester transfer protein (CETP). By this means, cholesterol is transported to the liver and can be eliminated from the body by excretion in the bile as bile acids or free cholesterol.

Control of lipid metabolism

Lipid metabolism is subject to many inherited and acquired disorders and to gene–environment interactions. Genetic disorders of most of the proteins involved in fat transport, the apolipoproteins, the cell membrane receptors, and the enzymes, have been described.[68] Many of the metabolic processes are influenced by hormones, particularly insulin but also thyroxine, corticosteroids, and catecholamines. Thus, conditions such as diabetes mellitus, obesity, hypothyroidism, and steroid therapy are associated with lipid abnormalities.

Lipid and lipoprotein levels vary throughout the lifespan[70] (Figs 32-12 and 32-13) in ways that parallel the incidence of atherosclerosis up to the age of about 50 years. The reduction in the rate of increase of lipids and lipoproteins after the age of 50 and the reduction in levels in old people[71] may be due to the phenomenon of exhaustion of susceptibles (i.e. those with high levels do not survive into old age), rather than a biological age change.

LIPIDS AND ATHEROSCLEROSIS

Cholesterol and low-density lipoproteins

The combined weight of evidence from epidemiology, experimental pathology, cell biology, and intervention studies[72] leaves no doubt that cholesterol has a role in the development of coronary heart disease. The strength, consistency, and graded nature of the relation between serum cholesterol and coronary heart disease mortality makes a causal link very likely.[73] There is inconsistent evidence that cholesterol is related to coronary heart disease in elderly people.[74–76] There is no association of total cholesterol levels with stroke;[77] it is possible, however, that studies of all strokes conceal different associations with ischemic strokes and hemorrhagic strokes.

Cholesterol-lowering trials show that the prevention of coronary heart disease depends on the magnitude and duration of cholesterol reduction, not on the way it is achieved. Overviews of clinical trials on cholesterol lowering, by diet or drugs, have shown a consistent relationship between the reduction in plasma cholesterol and the reduction in coronary heart disease risk, and the percentage reduction in coronary risk is similar to that predicted from epidemiological studies.

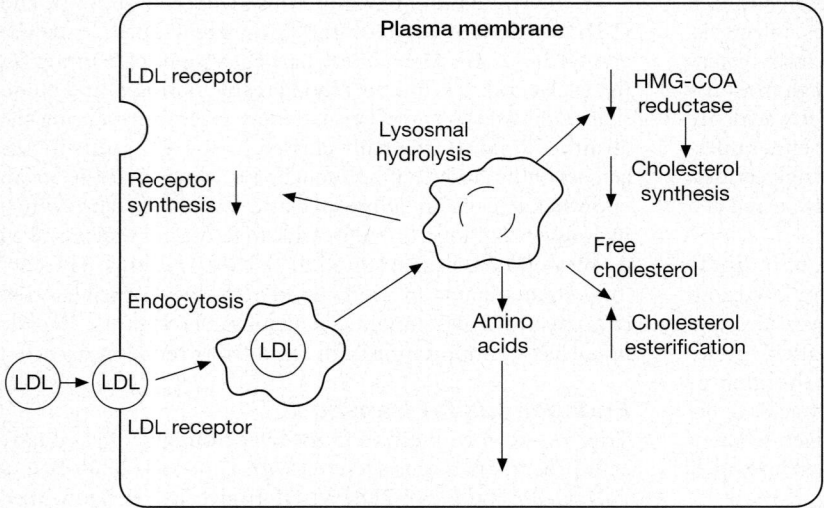

Figure 32-11 The low-density lipoprotein receptor pathway; see text for details. Adapted from Brown and Goldstein © The Nobel Foundation 1985.[69]

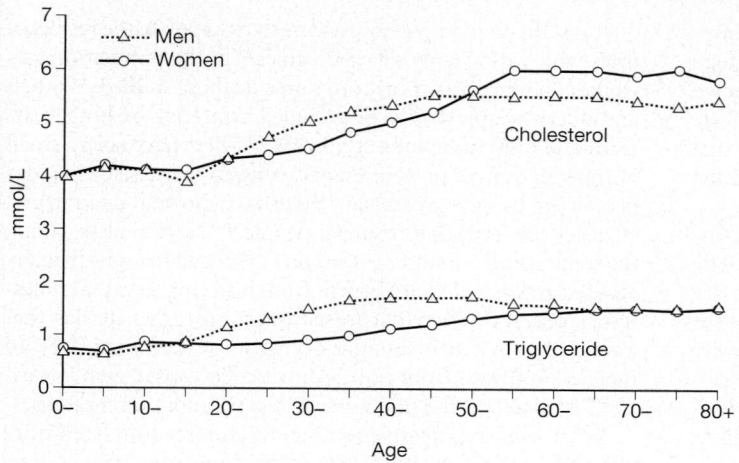

Figure 32-12 Plasma cholesterol and triglyceride levels in relation to age and sex. Data from Lipid Research Clinics Program Epidemiology Committee.[70]

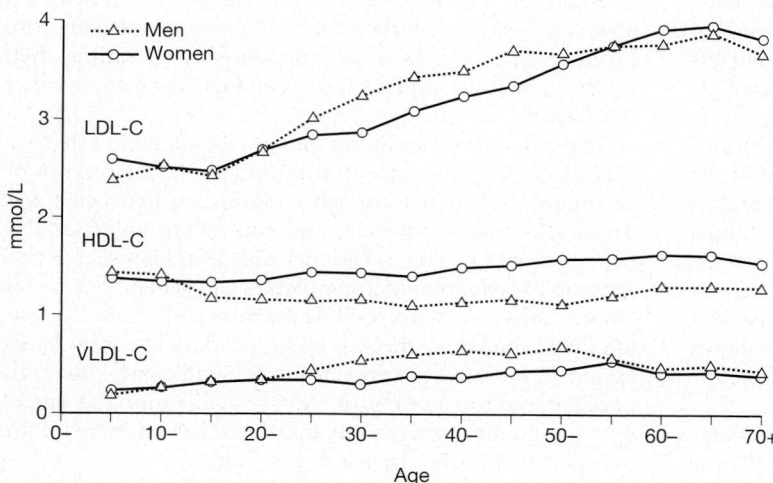

Figure 32-13 Plasma low-density lipoprotein cholesterol (LDL-C), high-density lipoprotein cholesterol (HDL-C), and very-low-density lipoprotein (VLDL-C) levels in relation to age and sex. Data from Lipid Research Clinics Program Epidemiology Committee.[70]

High-density lipoproteins

Clinical and epidemiological studies have shown an inverse relationship between HDL and coronary disease,[78,79] and it has been suggested that HDL has a protective role in atherogenesis.[80] The inverse relationship between HDL cholesterol and coronary heart disease mortality has been confirmed in elderly men[74,81] and women[80] but has also been refuted.[75] The mechanism by which HDL levels are inversely related to coronary heart disease remains unknown but presumably involves reverse cholesterol transport.

Reductions in the incidence of coronary heart disease and simultaneous rises in HDL levels have been found in some clinical trials, but there has been no clinical trial designed specifically to test the effect of raising HDL levels, nor are there any drugs that increase HDL levels without affecting other lipoproteins.

PREVENTION OF CARDIOVASCULAR DISEASE

General issues

Primary prevention aims to prevent the occurrence of cardiovascular disease in healthy asymptomatic people, while the objective of *secondary prevention* is to reduce the progression of atherosclerosis or the development of its complications and hence reduce the risk of further ischemic episodes in patients who have established cardiovascular disease. The latter are at the highest risk, and are priority targets for preventive measures.

Since atherosclerosis is a universal condition closely related to aging, it is unlikely that it can be totally prevented. Slowing the progression of atherosclerosis with prevention or delay in its effects on the cardiovascular system is, therefore, the aim. Regression of atherosclerosis may also be possible. Regression has been described in experimental atherosclerosis in animals[82] and in wasting diseases in humans,[83] and the results of angiographic studies in humans are consistent with regression of lesions in patients intensively treated with lipid-lowering drugs.[84,85]

There are two possible strategies for prevention by risk-factor reduction.[86,87] The *population strategy* is based on the realization that most cardiovascular disease results from the exposure of many people to moderately elevated levels of risk factors. This strategy, therefore, seeks to change people's behavior toward a healthier lifestyle by promoting, for example, healthy diets, exercise, and nonsmoking in the whole population. The *individual (or "high risk") strategy* seeks to identify the relatively small number of people within the population who are at particularly high risk of cardiovascular disease. Those at high risk include people with a family history of cardiovascular disease occurring at an early age and those who have cardiovascular risk factors. The individual strategy may target risk-factor assessment on people likely to have positive findings (selective screening); may use opportunistic screening by including an assessment of risk factors in the normal clinical consultation; or may perform general screening of the public.

The population and individual strategies are complementary, and each may enhance the effectiveness of the other. The population strategy is most useful for risk factors that are widespread and relatively mild, but would be inadequate for the minority of people with marked risk factors (e.g. severe hypertension or hyperlipidemia). Even when the high-risk strategy is used to target specific risk factors in individuals, it is essential that the general burden of risk be also addressed by changes in lifestyle.[88]

One of the problems of assigning targets for risk-factor modification is the fact that the relationship between most of the risk factors and cardiovascular disease is continuous and linear or curvilinear. Thus, the definition of any target or "normal" level is arbitrary. The synergistic effects of multiple risk factors must also be considered and any strategy must assess all risk factors, while assigning priority to the most important or the most readily modified. For example, in a cigarette smoker with diabetes, the importance of stopping smoking is overwhelming. The total level of risk for the individual must be assessed;[89] the higher the absolute risk, the greater the need for intervention. It is currently recommended that those with a risk of 30 percent or greater over 10 years should be treated.[88] Surveys have shown that there remains a considerable potential for prevention before everybody with this level of risk is being treated.

Trials aimed at preventing or delaying the progress of atherosclerosis by targeting lipids will be considered here. Those involving other risk factors are described elsewhere in the book.

Targeting lipid metabolism

Prevention studies using the most effective means of reducing serum cholesterol levels, the HMG-CoA reductase inhibitors (the statins), have clarified the role of cholesterol-lowering in the prevention of coronary heart disease.[90] They have finally removed any doubt that reducing cholesterol levels reduces the incidence of coronary heart disease. For every 1 percent reduction in cholesterol level, there is a 2–5 percent reduction in coronary heart disease incidence (the older the subjects, the lower the benefit),[91–93] and the full effect of the reduction in risk is achieved by 5 years.[94] It seems likely that the reduction in clinical coronary heart disease associated with lipid-lowering therapy results from depletion of cholesterol from the core of the atheromatous lesion and a decrease in the number of lipid-laden macrophage-derived foam cells.[85] In this way, the relatively small number of fatty lesions are stabilized, preventing fissuring and thrombosis. Cholesterol-lowering with statins also reduces the risk of stroke[95,96] and reduces early mortality following acute coronary disease.[97] The results of these trials, together with evidence that cholesterol-lowering slows the progression of atheromatous lesions or even results in their regression,[84,85,98] provide convincing evidence in favor of attempting to reduce serum cholesterol levels.

It is difficult to know how widely to extrapolate the results of trials which use highly selected subjects to the population as a whole and in particular to groups outside those studied. Women and elderly people tend to be excluded from trials on both treatment and prevention of heart disease.[99] There have been a small number of trials of prevention of cardiovascular disease in older people (up to age 75 years) and these have shown the same beneficial effects as trials in younger people.[100] Nevertheless, taking the results of all the studies, it would be difficult to argue that any age–sex group would not benefit from lowering elevated cholesterol levels. A concern that arose from some earlier studies, that a reduction in cardiovascular deaths was accompanied by an increase in deaths from noncardiovascular causes such as cancer[101] or violence, has not been a feature of more recent trials.

Because of the effectiveness, safety, and freedom from side-effects of statins, no other class of lipid-lowering drug is considered here. The benefits and convenience of these drugs, however, do not reduce the need for other measures to improve cardiovascular fitness, including smoking cessation, diet, weight reduction, regular exercise, and management of other risk factors.

The goal of lipid-lowering therapy should be to achieve a plasma cholesterol concentration of less than 5 mmol/L or 200 mg/dL.[87,102] For those whose levels are between 5 and 6 mmol/L, dietary advice[103] and counseling on other risk factors should be given. Patients with levels between 6 and 7 mmol/L need more intensive dietary and general risk-factor advice. If the cholesterol level is between 7 and 8 mmol/L, fasting lipids should be checked and secondary hyperlipidemia excluded. Intensive nutritional advice is indicated, and if this does not lead to a substantial reduction in plasma cholesterol over 3–6 months, drug treatment should be considered if the overall risk of cardiovascular disease is high.

For those with cholesterol levels more than 8 mmol/L, full investigation of the lipid abnormality, a search for causes of secondary hyperlipidemia, and consideration of familial hyperlipidemia are indicated. If intensive dietary advice does not reduce the plasma cholesterol to below 7 mmol/L (270 mg/dL) in 3–6 months, drug treatment should be considered. The most common causes of secondary hyperlipidemia are obesity, alcoholism, hypothyroidism, diabetes, and renal and hepatic disease. In considering the need for treatment, the presence of other risk factors, including existing cardiovascular disease, and the lipoprotein profile are taken into account.

The diet should have less than 30 percent of daily food energy intake from fat, with saturated fat contributing less than 10 percent of the total, less than 300 mg of cholesterol per day, and should contain foods rich in soluble fiber. Mild hypertriglyceridemia (3.0–6.0 mmol/L, 250–500 mg/dL) usually responds to weight reduction and decreased alcohol consumption; drugs may be used if this is not effective. Very high triglyceride levels (more than 6 mmol/L, 500 mg/dL) are associated with an increased risk of pancreatitis and should be vigorously treated with diet and drugs.

Treating elderly people

Should hypercholesterolemia be sought and treated in elderly people? The answer to this question is becoming clearer as the data on which a decision could be based become available.[104] Cholesterol remains a risk factor for cardiovascular disease in old age. Postponement of a myocardial infarction, stroke, or amputation for even a few years would have major benefits on the lives of elderly people. Lipid-lowering treatment by diet or drugs seems to be as effective in older as in younger people.[100,105,106]

A pragmatic approach should be taken. After a full assessment of the patient's physical, mental, and functional states and measurement of cardiovascular risk factors, a decision on the benefits and risks of treatment can be taken. An independent healthy person with significant hypercholesterolemia may be offered treatment. This should first consist of advice on weight, exercise, diet, and smoking. There is no contraindication to a low-fat, low-cholesterol diet in older people. If, after adherence to this advice, cholesterol levels remain high, drug treatment may be instituted. If this approach is used, the need for drug treatment of hypercholesterolemia in old age will be uncommon.

Despite the huge burden of cardiovascular disease, the high prevalence of cardiovascular risk factors, and the increasing evidence that prevention is possible, rates of use of lipid-lowering drugs remain very low,[107] especially in elderly people.[108]

OTHER RISK FACTORS

The beneficial effects of cessation of cigarette smoking are incontrovertible.

Hypertension is considered elsewhere in this book. Many studies, including some in elderly subjects,[31] have shown beneficial effects of treating hypertension on a number of fatal and nonfatal manifestations of cardiovascular disease.

There is no evidence that currently available methods of treating diabetes are effective in reducing the large-vessel complications.[41] There are, of course, other benefits from controlling hyperglycemia. More attention is now being paid to control of other risk factors such as cigarette smoking, hypertension, and hyperlipidemia in diabetes in an attempt to reduce the cardiovascular complications. There is good evidence that controlling blood pressure and lipid levels have beneficial effects in patients with diabetes.[43]

Avoidance of obesity[44] and regular physical exercise,[46] have beneficial effects on several risk factors and can be recommended as general health measures.

A different approach to prevention is to modify hemostatic function. Aspirin permanently inhibits cyclo-oxygenase-dependent platelet aggregation, and has been shown to be effective in the secondary prevention of cardiovascular disease.[109] Whether aspirin acts by reducing the progression of atheromatous lesions or by inhibiting thrombus formation on the lesions remains to be determined.

CONCLUSION

The burden of atherosclerosis in old age will increase as the aged population increases. Although there have been many advances in the treatment of cardiovascular disease, and many of these can be and are being used in elderly patients, they do not address the fundamental problem—atherosclerosis. Prevention of atherosclerosis requires a healthy lifestyle throughout the lifespan. Successful efforts at health promotion in younger people will result not only in increased survival but also a healthier old age.

Hypercholesterolemia

Summary of management algorithm

The goal is a plasma cholesterol of less than 5 mmol/L or 200 mg/dL.

- Cholesterol level 5–6 mmol/L—Dietary advice and attend to other risk factors

- Cholesterol level 6–7 mmol/L—Intensive dietary advice and attention to other risk factors

- Cholesterol level 7–8 mmol/L—Check fasting lipids; exclude secondary hyperlipidemia; try diet for 3–6 months; if not effective use a statin

- Cholesterol level more than 8 mmol/L—Search for secondary or familial hyperlipidemia; intensive dietary treatment followed by statin if diet ineffective

- Diet should provide less than 30 percent of daily energy intake from fat, less than 10 percent of which is saturated fat, and less than 300 mg cholesterol per day. It should contain foods rich in soluble fiber.

KEY POINTS Lipids

- Lipid metabolism is subject to genetic influences, to which environmental factors such as diet are added.

- In cross-sectional studies, lipid and lipoprotein levels increase to about age 50, and then decrease. The later decrease may be due to the exhaustion of susceptibles.

- High cholesterol and low-density lipoprotein (LDL) levels, and low high-density lipoprotein (HDL) levels, are associated with atherosclerosis.

- The statin class of drugs (HMG-CoA reductase inhibitors) are the most effective means of lowering cholesterol and have been shown to reduce the frequency of cardiovascular disease and delay the progression of atheromatous lesions.

- There is no evidence to support an age limit to the beneficial effects of treating hypercholesterolemia.

REFERENCES

1. Ross R: The pathogenesis of atherosclerosis: a perspective for the 1990s. Nature 1993;362:801–809
2. Fuster V, Badimon L, Badimon JJ, Chesebro JH: The pathogenesis of coronary artery disease and the acute coronary syndromes. N Engl J Med 1992;326:242–250, 310–318
3. Schwartz CJ, Kelley JL, Nerem RM et al: Pathophysiology of the atherogenic process. Am J Cardiol 1989;64:23G–30G

4. Steinberg D, Parthasarathy S, Carew TE et al: Beyond cholesterol: modifications of low-density lipoprotein that increase its atherogenicity. N Engl J Med 1989;320:915–924

5. Witztum JL: The oxidation hypothesis of atherosclerosis. Lancet 1994;344:793–795

6. Carew TE: Role of biologically modified low-density lipoprotein in atherosclerosis. Am J Cardiol 1989;64:18G–22G

7. Mazzone T, Jensen M, Chait A: Human arterial wall cells secrete factors that are chemotactic for monocytes. Proc Natl Acad Sci US 1983;80:5094–5097

8. Ross R: Atherosclerosis: an inflammatory disease. N Engl J Med 1999;340:115–126

9. Libby P, Ridker PM: Novel inflammatory markers of coronary risk: theory versus practice. Circulation 1999;100:1148–1150

10. Rader DJ: Inflammatory markers of coronary risk. N Engl J Med 2000;343:1179–1182

11. Kannel WB, Anderson K, Wilson PWF: White blood cell count and cardiovascular disease: insights from the Framingham Study. JAMA 1992;267:1253–1256

12. Woodhouse PR, Khaw KT, Plummer M et al: Seasonal variations of plasma fibrinogen and factor VII activity in the elderly: winter infections and death from cardiovascular disease. Lancet 1994;343:435–439

13. Crawford VLS, Sweeney O, Coyle PV, Halliday IM, Stout RW: The relationship between elevated fibrinogen and markers of infection: a comparison of seasonal cycles. QJM 2000;93:745–750

14. Stout RW: Ageing and atherosclerosis. Age Ageing 1987;16:65–72

15. Barker DJP (ed): Fetal and Infant Origins of Adult Disease. British Medical Association, London, 1992

16. Enos WF, Holmes RH, Beyer J: Coronary disease among United States soldiers killed in action in Korea. JAMA 1953;152:1090–1093

17. Grundy SM, Bazzarre T, Cleeman J et al: Prevention Conference V. Beyond secondary prevention: identifying the high-risk patient for primary prevention: Medical Office Assessment: Writing Group 1. Circulation 2000;101:e3–e11

18. American Heart Association: 2001 Heart and Stroke Statistical Update. AHA, Dallas, TX, 2000

19. Howard G, Manolio TA, Burke GL, Wolfson SK, O'Leary DH, for the Atherosclerosis Risk in Communities (ARIC) and Cardiovascular Health Study (CHS) investigators: Does the association of risk factors and atherosclerosis change with age? An analysis of the combined ARIC and CHS cohorts. Stroke 1997;28:1693–1701

20. Lerner DJ, Kannel WB: Patterns of coronary heart disease morbidity and mortality in the sexes: a 26-year follow-up of the Framingham population. Am Heart J 1986;111:383–390

21. Witteman JCM, Grobbee DE, Kok FJ et al: Increased risk of atherosclerosis in women after the menopause. BMJ 1989;298:642–644

22. Bamford J, Sandercock P, Dennis M et al: A prospective study of acute cerebrovascular disease in the community: the Oxfordshire Community Stroke Project 1981–86. I: Methodology, demography and incident cases of first-ever stroke. J Neurol Neurosurg Psychiatr 1988;51:1373–1380

23. Goldstein JL, Hazzard WR, Schrott HG et al: Hyperlipidemia in coronary heart disease. 2: Genetic analysis of lipid levels in 176 families and delineation of a new inherited disorder, combined hyperlipidemia. J Clin Invest 1973;52:1544–1568

24. Schildkraut JM, Myers RH, Cupples LA et al: Coronary risk associated with age and sex of parental heart disease in the Framingham Study. Am J Cardiol 1989;64:555–559

25. Fuller JH, Shipley MJ, Rose G et al: Mortality from coronary heart disease and stroke in relation to degree of glycaemia: the Whitehall study. BMJ 1983;287:867–870

26. Gill JS, Shipley MJ, Tsementzis SA et al: Cigarette smoking: a risk factor for hemorrhagic and nonhemorrhagic stroke. Arch Intern Med 1989;149:2053–2057

27. Rosenberg L, Palmer JR, Shapiro S: Decline in the risk of myocardial infarction among women who stop smoking. N Engl J Med 1990;322:213–217

28. Albers JJ, Bierman EL: The effect of hypoxia on uptake and degradation of low density lipoproteins by cultured human arterial smooth muscle cells. Biochem Biophys Acta 1976;424:422–429

29. Kannel WB, Gordon T, Schwartz MJ: Systolic versus diastolic blood pressure and risk of coronary heart disease: the Framingham study. Am J Cardiol 1971;27:345–355

30. Kannel WB, Dawber TR, Sorlie P, Wolf PA: Components of blood pressure and risk of atherothrombotic brain infarction: the Framingham study. Stroke 1976;7:327–331

31. Amery A, Birkenhager W, Brixko P et al: Mortality and morbidity results from the European Working Party on High Blood Pressure in the Elderly Trial. Lancet 1985;1:1349–1354

32. Martin MJ, Hulley SB, Browner WS et al: Serum cholesterol, blood pressure, and mortality: implications from a cohort of 361,662 men. Lancet 1986;ii:933–936

33. Stamler J, Wentworth D, Neaton JD, for the MRFIT Research Group: Is the relationship between serum cholesterol and risk of premature death from coronary heart disease continuous and graded? Findings in 356,222 primary screenees of the Multiple Risk Factor Intervention Trial (MRFIT). JAMA 1986;256:2823–2828

34. Castelli WP: Cholesterol and lipids in the risk of coronary artery disease: The Framingham Heart Study. Can J Cardiol 1988;4(suppl A):5A–10A

35. Iso H, Jacobs DR, Wentworth D et al: Serum cholesterol levels and six-year mortality from stroke in 350,977 men screened for the multiple risk factors intervention trial. N Engl J Med 1989;320:904–910

36. Gordon DJ, Rifkind BM: High-density-lipoprotein: the clinical implications of recent studies. N Engl J Med 1989;321:1311–1316

37. Carlson LA, Bottiger LE: Ischaemic heart-disease in relation to fasting values of plasma triglycerides and cholesterol: Stockholm prospective study. Lancet 1972;i:865–868

38. Castelli WP: The triglyceride issue: a view from Framingham. Am Heart J 1986;112:432–437

39. Cambien F, Jacqueson A, Richard JL et al: Is the level of serum triglyceride a significant predictor of coronary death in "normocholesterolemic" subjects? Am J Epidemiol 1986;124:624–632

40. Kushi LH, Lew RA, Stare FJ et al: Diet and 20-year mortality from coronary heart disease: the Ireland–Boston Diet–Heart Study. N Engl J Med 1985;312:811–818

41. Stout RW (ed): Diabetes and Atheroslerosis. Kluwer, Dordrecht, 1992

42. Grundy SM, Benjamin IJ, Burke GL et al: Diabetes and cardiovascular disease. Circulation 1999;100:1134–1136

43. UK Prospective Diabetes Study Group: Tight blood pressure control and risk of macrovascular and microvascular complications in type 2 diabetes: UKPDS 38. BMJ 1998;317:703–713

44. Eckel RH. Obesity and heart disease. Circulation 1997;96:3248–3250

45. Depres J-P, Lemieux I, Prud'homme D: Treatment of obesity: need to focus on high risk abdominally obese patients. BMJ 2001;322:716–720

46. Fletcher GF, Balady G, Blair SN et al: Statement on exercise: benefits and recommendations for physical activity programs for all Americans. Circulation 1996;94:857–862

47. Meade TW, Mellows S, Brozovic M et al: Haemostatic function and ischaemic heart disease: principal results of the Northwick Park Heart Study. Lancet 1986;ii:533–537

48. Kannel WB, Wolf PA, Castelli WP, D'Agostino RB: Fibrinogen and risk of cardiovascular disease: the Framingham study. JAMA 1987;258:1183–1186

49. Stout RW, Crawford V: Seasonal variations in fibrinogen concentrations among elderly people. Lancet 1991;338:9–13

50. Ernst E, Resch KL: Fibrinogen as a cardiovascular risk factor: a meta-analysis and review of the literature. Ann Intern Med 1993;118:956–963

51. Stout RW: Insulin and atheroma: 20-yr perspective. Diabetes Care 1990;13:631–655

52. Reaven GM: Role of insulin resistance in human disease. Diabetes 1988;37:1595–1607

53. Thompson SG, Kienast J, Pyke SDM et al, for the European Concerted Action on Thrombosis and Disabilities Angina Pectoris Study Group: Hemostatic factors and the risk of myocardial infarction or sudden death in patients with angina pectoris. N Engl J Med 1995;332:635–641

54. Ridker PM, Hennekens CH, Lindpaintner K et al: Mutation in the gene coding for coagulation factor V and the risk of myocardial infarction, stroke and venous thrombosis in apparently healthy men. N Engl J Med 1995;332:912–917

55. Stout RW, Crawford VLS, McDermott MJ et al: Seasonal changes in haemostatic factors in young and elderly subjects. Age Ageing 1996;25:256–258

56. Kannel WB, Doyle JT, Ostfeld AM et al, for the Atherosclerosis Study Group: Optimal resources for primary prevention of atherosclerotic disease. Circulation 1984;70:(suppl)157A–205A

57. Multiple Risk Factor Intervention Trial Research Group: Multiple Risk Factor Intervention Trial. Risk factor changes and mortality results. JAMA 1982;248:1465–1477

58. Puska P, Tuomilehto J, Salonen J et al: Changes in coronary risk factors during comprehensive five-year community programme to control cardiovascular disease (North Karelia project). BMJ 1979;2:1173–1178

59. Salonen JT, Puska P, Mustaniemi H: Changes in morbidity and mortality during comprehensive community programme to control cardiovascular disease during 1972–7 in North Karelia. BMJ 1979;2:1178–1183

60. Elford J, Phillips AN, Thomson AG, Shaper AG: Migration and geographic variations in ischaemic heart disease in Great Britain. Lancet 1989;i:343–346

61. McKeigue PM, Miller GJ, Marmot MG: Coronary heart disease in South Asians overseas: a review. J Clin Epidemiol 1989;42:597–609

62. Rosamond WD, Chambless LE, Folsom AR et al: Trends in the incidence of myocardial infarction and in mortality due to coronary heart disease, 1987 to 1994. N Engl J Med 1998;339:861–867

63. Levy D, Thom TJ: Death rates from coronary disease: progress and a puzzling paradox. N Engl J Med 1998;339:915–917

64. Hunink MG, Goldman L, Tosteson AN et al: The recent decline in mortality from coronary heart disease, 1980–1990: the effect of secular trends in risk factors and treatment. JAMA 1997;277:535–542

65. Haberman S, Capildeo R, Rose FC: Diverging trends in cerebro-vascular disease and ischaemic heart disease mortality. Stroke 1982;13:582–589

66. Rose G: Incubation period of coronary heart disease. BMJ 1982;284:1600–1601

67. Krolewski AS, Kosinski EJ, Warram JH et al: Magnitude and determinants of coronary artery disease in juvenile-onset, insulin-dependent diabetes mellitus. Am J Cardiol 1987;59:750–755

68. Breslow JL: Genetics of lipoprotein abnormalities associated with coronary heart disease susceptibility. Ann Rev Genet 2000;34:233–254

69. Brown MS, Goldstein JL: A receptor-mediated pathway for cholesterol homeostasis. Science 1986;232:34–47

70. Lipid Research Clinics Program Epidemiology Committee: Plasma lipid distributions in selected North American populations: the Lipid Research Clinics Program Prevalence Study. Circulation 1979;60:427–439

71. Ettinger WH, Wahl PW, Kuller LH et al: Lipoprotein lipids in older people: results from the Cardiovascular Health Study. Circulation 1992;86:858–869

72. Steinberg D: The cholesterol controversy is over. Why did it take so long? Circulation 1989;80:1070–1078

73. Marmot M: The cholesterol papers. Lowering population cholesterol concentrations probably isn't harmful. BMJ 1994;308:351–352

74. Weijenberg MP, Feskens JM, Kromhout D: Total and high density lipoprotein cholesterol as risk factors for coronary heart disease in elderly men during 5 years of follow-up. The Zutphen Elderly Study. Am J Epidemiol 1996;143:151–158

75. Krumholz HM, Seeman TE, Merrill SS et al: Lack of association between cholesterol and coronary heart disease mortality and morbidity and all-cause mortality in persons older than 70 years. JAMA 1994;272:1335–1340

76. Jacobsen SJ, Freedman DS, Hoffmann RG et al: Cholesterol and coronary artery disease: age as an effect modifier. J Clin Epidemiol 1992;45:1053–1059

77. Prospective Studies Collaboration: Cholesterol, diastolic blood pressure, and stroke: 13,000 stroke, in 450,000 people in 45 prospective cohorts. Lancet 1995;346:1647–1653

78. Gordon T, Castelli WP, Hjortland MC et al: High density lipoprotein as a protective factor against coronary heart disease: the Framingham study. Am J Med 1977;62:707–714

79. Gordon DJ, Probstfield JL, Garrison RJ et al: High-density lipoprotein cholesterol and cardiovascular disease: four prospective American studies. Circulation 1989;79:8–15

80. Miller GJ, Miller NE: Plasma-high-density-lipoprotein concentration and development of ischaemic heart-disease. Lancet 1975;i:16–19

81. Corti M-C, Guralnik JM, Salive ME et al: HDL cholesterol predicts coronary heart disease mortality in older persons. JAMA 1995;274:539–544

82. St Clair RW: Atherosclerosis regression in animal models: current concepts of cellular and biochemical mechanisms. Prog Cardiovasc Dis 1983;26:109–132

83. Wilens SL: The experimental production of lipid depositions in excised arteries. Science 1954;114:389–393

84. MAAS Investigators: Effect of simvastatin on coronary atheroma: the Multicentre Anti-Atheroma Study (MAAS). Lancet 1994;344:633–638

85. Brown BG, Zhao X-Q, Sacco DE, Albers JJ: Lipid lowering and plaque regression: new insights into prevention of plaque disruption and clinical events in coronary disease. Circulation 1993;87:1781–1791

86. Oliver MF: Strategies for preventing and screening for coronary heart disease. Br Heart J 1985;54:1–5

87. Pyorala K, De Backer G, Graham I et al, on behalf of the Task Force of the European Society of Cardiology, European Atherosclerosis Society and European Society of Hypertension: Prevention of coronary heart disease in clinical practice. Eur Heart J 1994;15:1300–1331

88. British Cardiac Society, British Hyperlipidaemia Association, British Hypertension Society, endorsed by the British Diabetic Association: Joint British recommendations on prevention of coronary heart disease in clinical practice. Heart 1998;80:1–29

89. Wilson PWF, D'Agostino RB, Levy D, Belanger AM, Silbersatz H, Kannel WB: Prediction of coronary heart disease using risk factor categories. Circulation 1998;97:1837–1847

90. Ross SD, Allen IE, Connelly JE et al: Clinical outcomes in statin treatment trials: a meta-analysis. Arch Intern Med 1999;159:1793–1802

91. Scandinavian Simvastatin Survival Study Group: Randomised trial of cholesterol lowering in 4444 patients with coronary heart disease: Scandinavian Simvastatin Survival Study (4S). Lancet 1994;344:1383–1389

92. Scandinavian Simvastatin Survival Study Group: Baseline serum cholesterol and treatment effect in the Scandinavian Simvastatin Survival Study (4S). Lancet 1995;345:1274–1275

93. Shepherd J, Cobbe SM, Ford I et al: Prevention of coronary heart disease with pravastatin in men with hypercholesterolemia. N Engl J Med 1995;333:1301–1307

94. Law MR, Wald NJ, Thompson SG: By how much and how quickly does reduction in serum cholesterol concentration lower risk of ischaemic heart disease? BMJ 1994;308:367–373

95. Hebert PR, Gaziano JM, Chan KS, Hennekens CH: Cholesterol lowering with statin drugs, risk of stroke, and total mortality. JAMA 1997;278:313–321

96. White HD, Simes RJ, Anderson NE et al: Pravastatin therapy and the risk of stroke. N Engl J Med 2000;343:317–326

97. Aronow HD, Topol EJ, Roe MT et al: Effect of lipid-lowering therapy on early mortality after acute coronary syndromes: an observational study. Lancet 2001;357:1063–1068

98. Furberg CD, Adams HP, Applegate WB et al: Effect of lovastatin on early carotid atherosclerosis and cardiovascular events. Circulation 1994;90:1679–1687

99. Bandyopadhyay S, Bayer AJ, O'Mahony MS: Age and gender bias in statin trials. QJM 2001;94:127–132

100. Lewis SJ, Moye LA, Sacks FM et al: Effect of pravastatin on cardiovascular events in older patients with myocardial infarction and cholesterol levels in the average range: results of the Cholesterol and Recurrent Events (CARE) trial. Ann Intern Med 1998;129:681–689

101. Lackner KJ, Schettler G, Kubler W: Plasma cholesterol, lipid lowering, and risk for cancer: an update of the results from epidemiologic studies and intervention trials. Klin Wochenschr 1989;67:957–962

102. Expert Panel: Summary of the second report of the National Cholesterol Education Program (NCEP) Expert Panel on Detection, Evaluation and Treatment of High Blood Cholesterol in Adults (Adult Treatment Panel II). JAMA 1993;269:3015–3023

103. Hooper L, Summerbell CD, Higgins JPT et al: Dietary fat intake and prevention of cardiovascular disease: systematic review. BMJ 2001;322:757–763

104. Grundy SM, Cleeman JI, Rifkind BM, Kuller LH, for the Coordinating Committee of the National Cholesterol Education Program: Cholesterol lowering in the elderly population. Arch Intern Med 1999;159:1670–1678

105. Bach LA, Cooper ME, O'Brien RC, Jerums G: The use of simvastatin, an HMG CoA reductase inhibitor, in older patients with hypercholesterolemia and atherosclerosis. J Am Geriatr Soc 1990;38:10–14

106. LaRosa JC, Applegate W, Crouse JR: Cholesterol lowering in the elderly: results of the Cholesterol Reduction in Seniors Program (CRISP) pilot study. Arch Intern Med 1994;154:529–539

107. Primatesta P, Poulter NR: Lipid concentrations and the use of lipid lowering drugs: evidence from a national cross sectional survey. BMJ 2000;321:1322–1325

108. Lemaitre RN, Furberg CD, Newman AB et al: Time trends in the use of cholesterol-lowering agents in older adults: the Cardiovascular Health Study. Arch Intern Med 1998;158:1761–1768

109. Hennekens CH, Buring JE, Sandercock P et al: Aspirin and other antiplatelet agents in the secondary and primary prevention of cardiovascular disease. Circulation 1989;80:749–756

110. Kannel WB, McGee DL: Diabetes and cardiovascular risk factors: the Framingham study. Circulation 1979;59:8–13

111. Stout RW: Hormones and atherosclerosis. MTP Press, Lancaster, 1982

Chapter 33

Chronic cardiac failure

Neil D. Gillespie and Allan D. Struthers

Cardiac failure increases in both prevalence and incidence with age.[1] It is a disease of middle and old age, although the underlying etiologies differ considerably as the patient becomes increasingly advanced in years.[2] In younger patients with cardiac failure the etiology is frequently coronary artery disease, whereas in the older patient valvular disease and hypertensive etiologies are more common. Most of the epidemiological studies are based on symptoms and signs of cardiac failure, but more recent data include objective assessments of ventricular function.[3]

The prevalence of heart failure is expected to continue to increase as more patients survive myocardial infarction as a result of fibrinolytic therapy. In addition, patients with hypertension are surviving longer as a result of continued improvements in the prevention of strokes.[4] Indeed, it appears that the effective treatment of hypertension merely delays the onset of heart failure.[5]

When considering the epidemiology of heart failure it is important to have a precise definition. In essence, heart failure is defined as the presence of symptoms and signs of cardiac decompensation, together with objective evidence of underlying structural heart disease. These are the definitions used by the European Society of Cardiology[6] and the American Heart Association[7] who have recently independently reached a consensus on the diagnosis of heart failure. This is an important step forward as it has resulted in a more focused approach when considering precisely what disease entity is being treated in individual patients. Heart failure is of major economic significance; in the UK it accounts for up to 5 percent of hospital admissions,[8] and in the rest of Europe hospitalization for heart failure is a significant financial burden for a number of countries.[9] Many elderly patients with heart failure also have multiple pathologies and coexistent disease which potentially make the diagnosis more difficult.[10]

EPIDEMIOLOGY

There are relatively few epidemiological data assessing the incidence and prevalence of heart failure in the older patient population. Much of the epidemiological data comes from Scandinavia[11] and the Framingham study,[12] although recently new data have come from the UK from a relatively young population.[3] The early data collected from studies were predominantly from medical record analysis and patient questionnaires, and this type of data collection has its limitations.

In a West London study,[13] the prevalence of heart failure in those aged under 65 was reported as 0.6 per thousand of the population, and 28 per thousand of the population in those over 65. It has been suggested that this study underestimated the severity of the problem as only patients who had been prescribed a diuretic were included; those patients with relatively mild disease may have been excluded as they did not require a diuretic for symptoms of fluid retention. Many of the earlier epidemiological studies were performed on populations which were inadequately described and give no information on the population at risk. The precise prevalence of left ventricular dysfunction in the whole population has been obscure until recent years. Studies in the late 1950s revealed a prevalence of 0.2 percent in the 45–64 year age group[14] and 1.9 percent in those over the age of 65. Another US study demonstrated prevalence rates of 1 percent and 6.5 percent in corresponding age groups.[15]

The criteria for heart failure used in the Framingham Heart Study population[12] were more strictly defined than in the previous two studies and the baseline prevalence was 0.3 percent of the population aged 62 or less. However, over a 34-year follow-up period the prevalence rate was 0.8 percent in ages 50–59 and 9.1 percent in the over-80s age group.[16] The most recent estimates of population prevalence come from a study in North Glasgow, Scotland, which estimated the prevalence of left ventricular systolic dysfunction based on echocardiographic criteria to be about 2.9 percent.[3] This figure was obtained from a population of 1640 patients between the ages of 25 and 74 and was based on an echocardiographic diagnosis. The systolic dysfunction was symptomatic in 1.5 percent of patients and asymptomatic in 1.4 percent. In this study it therefore appears that systolic dysfunction was at least twice as common as symptomatic heart failure defined by clinical criteria.

The longitudinal Framingham study suggested that prevalence rates doubled every decade and reached approximately 10 percent for people in their 80s.

Prescribing data also highlight the extent of the problem. In the USA, data suggest that up to 1 in 5 elderly patients were being treated for chronic cardiac failure.[17] In the UK, echocardiographic data in patients over 75 years of age suggest that prevalence may be around 10 percent of patients being managed in the community.[18]

Information on the incidence of heart failure also reveals a sharp increase over the age of 75 years. The best available incidence data are from the Framingham Heart Study[19] and the study of men born in 1913.[20] In the Framingham study, 5200 individuals have been followed since 1948 and the incidence rises markedly with age. The annual incidence was 2 percent per thousand in men and 1 percent per thousand in women under the age of 54, and 14 percent per thousand in men and 13 percent per thousand in women between the ages of 75 and 84. The Framingham study data probably underestimate the incidence, as the entry criteria did not include the milder forms of heart failure.

In the Scandinavian study of men born in 1913, the annual incidence for those in the 50–54 year age group was 1.5 per thousand per year, which increased to 10.2 at ages 61–67.

The Hillingdon Heart Failure Study[21] was a population-based surveillance system in which patients first developing heart failure were identified. Over a 20-month period, 220 patients fulfilled the criteria for heart failure and the incidence of the condition increased steeply with age and was higher in men than in women at all ages. Many of the studies performed before the advent of widespread echocardiography based the diagnosis of heart failure on clinical assessment, chest radiology, and electrocardiographic criteria. This approach, even accounting for prescribing patterns, is likely to underestimate the severity of heart failure, because many patients have asymptomatic left ventricular dysfunction, and heart failure with normal systolic function is increasingly recognized.[22]

Hospitalizations for chronic heart failure are frequent; but this may relate mainly to approaches to treatment and assessment, together with awareness of the condition, rather than be a reflection of the incidence or prevalence. The number of hospital discharges where a diagnosis of heart failure has been coded has increased in recent years both in Holland[23] and in Scotland.[24] In the USA in 1991, congestive heart failure was the primary discharge diagnosis in around 790,000 hospitalizations.[25]

As mentioned previously, the increased numbers of patients hospitalized for heart failure may reflect improved survival following myocardial infarction, but also an improvement in heart failure management. As a result patients with heart failure are living longer, with more episodes of decompensation requiring hospital admission. Data from North America suggest that there is a high rate of readmission in heart failure patients.[26] Emerging evidence suggests that a multidisciplinary approach to the treatment of heart failure may reduce the need for hospitalization in elderly patients with the condition.[27] Such an approach is crucial in the older patient where issues such as compliance, cognition, and continence figure prominently in the clinical decision-making process.

The prognosis for heart failure, although improved in recent years by drug treatment, is nevertheless still poor. The majority of patients with New York Heart Association Class IV disease (Table 33-1) will be unlikely to survive a year.

A study of elderly men admitted as inpatients with heart failure revealed that the 1-year mortality was in the region of 50 percent.[28] It is thus clear that heart failure is a relatively malignant condition and, although newer treatments have been shown to improve the prognosis for many patients, alleviation of symptoms and improved morbidity is as important as any potential mortality benefits in the older patient.[29]

PATHOPHYSIOLOGY

In the older patient with heart failure a number of issues are worth considering. There may be structural abnormalities within the heart together with overcompensatory mechanisms in the renin–angiotensin system, the sympathetic nervous system, and the peripheral vasculature. Although there are specific changes in the cardiovascular system with age, such as increased calcification, increased myocardial fibrosis, and reduced ventricular compliance,[30] most elderly patients with heart failure have additional pathology to explain their symptoms. In patients with an ischemic etiology for their heart failure, remodeling can result in alterations in the shape and morphology of the left ventricle with ultimate left ventricular dilatation and a large end-diastolic volume.[31] In addition to changes in the structure of the left ventricle, many elderly patients have associated calcific degeneration of both the aortic and mitral valves, with functional and hemodynamically significant consequences.[32] The cardiomyopathies[33] are also a small but significant cause of heart failure in older patients, although the widely seen asymmetrical septal hypertrophy itself is not of great significance.[34] In hypertensive patients with left ventricular hypertrophy, the increase in collagen content of the ventricular wall and associated myocardial fibrosis may lead to diastolic filling abnormalities,[35] which may contribute to the symptoms of heart failure. In addition, loss of atrial contraction can result in significant hemodynamic deteriorations as atrial systole has an increased importance in the older patients when left ventricular wall stiffness is increased.[36]

In a healthy person, cardiac output is influenced directly by stroke volume and heart rate. In the failing heart, stroke volume is maintained by increasing the left ventricular end-diastolic pressure and volume, which is the basis of Starling's Law of the heart. However, eventually at very high left ventricular end-diastolic volumes there will be no subsequent compensatory increase in cardiac output. One of the aims of heart failure treatment is to minimize increases in left ventricular end-diastolic pressure, so that cardiac output can be maintained and so that subsequent tissue oxygenation is adequate for perfusion of the vital organs.

The autonomic nervous system and the neuroendocrine systems initially support the failing heart, but ultimately the compensatory mechanisms may themselves prove harmful. Activation of the renin–angiotensin aldosterone system can result in increased levels of angiotensin in heart, kidney, brain, and vascular system, with undesirable consequences.[37] Furthermore, the associated high levels of plasma adrenaline and noradrenaline (epinephrine and norepinephrine) as well as reduced heart rate variability, are associated with a poor prognosis.[38]

Much of the fluid overload and edema in heart failure is as a result of the effects of the renin–angiotensin system on the kidney, and reduced bradykinin may be associated with increased vasoconstriction. Changes in the morphology of skeletal muscle may explain the fatiguability seen in heart failure patients over and above that expected with reduced tissue blood supply.[39] Disruption of the microvasculature is also seen with impaired endothelial function.[40] These changes are usually consequences of the disease process and not merely related to age—although in extremely old patients with mild symptoms of cardiac failure, true pathological processes and age-related processes may be difficult to differentiate.

Such age-related changes include a reduction of cardiac output on exercise, an increase in end-systolic volume, a decrease in ejection fraction with exercise, and a reduced heart rate with exercise.[41]

Table 33-1 **New York Heart Association classification of heart failure**	
Class I	No symptoms
Class II	Symptoms with ordinary activity
Class III	Symptoms with less than ordinary activity
Class IV	Symptoms at rest

Most of the established treatments for heart failure are in patients with systolic dysfunction. Even so, there are many elderly patients with normal systolic function who have symptoms and signs compatible with heart failure. Conversely, many elderly patients have these "diastolic abnormalities" on echocardiography but no symptoms of heart failure. The relative clinical significance of the diastolic abnormalities in these patients is unclear. They may go on to develop subsequent heart failure as a result of atrial fibrillation or systolic dysfunction, or may have intermittent episodes of mild cardiac decompensation possibly as a result of silent myocardial ischemia. Furthermore, echocardiographically determined measures of diastolic dysfunction are critically dependent on the degree of activation of the sympathetic nervous system. Such variables include transmitral flow velocities (the E to A ratio) and the isovolumic relaxation time.[42]

THE ETIOLOGY OF HEART FAILURE

Heart failure has been described as a syndrome rather than a diagnosis or disease, and the underlying etiology must always be sought in patients presenting with the syndrome. The most frequent cause of heart failure is left ventricular systolic dysfunction, usually as a consequence of ischemic heart disease, especially myocardial infarction. However in elderly patients, valvular heart disease frequently contributes to the symptoms. Figure 33-1 highlights the common etiologies of heart failure.

Less frequently, heart failure in the older patient may be caused by one of the cardiomyopathies, amyloidosis, storage diseases (e.g. hemochromatosis), secondary to chemotherapy or vitamin B deficiencies. In the over-80s, aortic or mitral valve disease frequently contributes to heart failure and many elderly patients in long-term care have background cardiac valvular disease.[43] Furthermore, as already noted, it is increasingly recognized that many patients have symptoms associated with heart failure in the presence of normal systolic function and no evident valvular disease. This is often called "diastolic heart failure" and may be responsible for as much as 30 percent of heart failure in the elderly population.[44] The etiology of this heart failure is unclear, but it is more likely to

Table 33-2 Factors which may precipitate heart failure in the elderly person

Anemia
Alcohol
Intercurrent infection, including endocarditis
Fluid overload (often postoperatively)
Thyrotoxicosis
Drugs (e.g. NSAIDs)
Atrial fibrillation
Altered drug compliance
Pulmonary emboli

be present in patients with hypertension and left ventricular hypertrophy. It is uncertain how these patients should be managed, as most of the major studies have addressed patients with left ventricular systolic dysfunction as a cause for their heart failure.[45–48]

Patients in heart failure with systolic dysfunction have a poorer prognosis than those with normal systolic function. It is also well established that patients with an increased left ventricular end-diastolic volume secondary to myocardial dilatation have a poor prognosis.[49] Not infrequently heart failure will be precipitated by anemia, alcohol, and a number of other factors[50] (Table 33-2).

DIAGNOSIS OF HEART FAILURE

Heart failure is a difficult disease to define. It is fairly easy to recognize heart failure in its more severe versions when the patient has pronounced symptoms and signs accompanied by echocardiographic evidence of left ventricular dysfunction.[51] However, diagnostic difficulties arise in its milder forms. The presence of atrial fibrillation or underlying valvular disease adds to the complexities.

The European Society of Cardiology (ESC) has developed guidelines for the diagnosis of heart failure[6] (Table 33-3). However, with any guidelines there is a degree of vagueness, and in particular there is no specific definition of precisely what is meant by cardiac dysfunction. An example to highlight some of the difficulties is the case of the elderly lady whose echocardiogram meets the criteria for "diastolic dysfunction" and who has swollen ankles with no breathlessness or fatigue. Does this type of patient really have heart failure? Nonetheless, the ESC guidelines have generally clarified the situation even if there are still a few areas of ambiguity.

For the clinician who is faced with an elderly patient with suspected heart failure, two questions should be considered before further assessment:

1. Are the patient's symptoms cardiac in origin?
2. If so, what kind of cardiac disease is producing these symptoms?[52]

Table 33-4 lists the typical and atypical symptoms in the elderly patient with suspected heart failure, as well as potential differential diagnoses.

The diagnosis of heart failure is especially difficult because it is not defined by an absolute level of any one parameter,

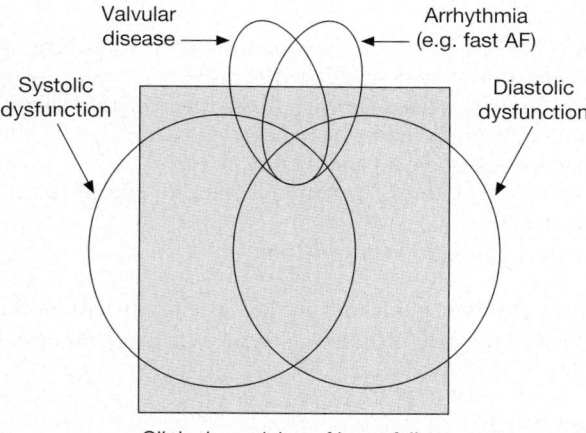

Figure 33-1 The common etiologies of heart failure.

> **Table 33-3 European Society of Cardiology guidelines for the diagnosis of heart failure**
>
> **Essential features**
> - Symptoms of heart failure (for example, breathlessness, fatigue, ankle-swelling).
> - Objective evidence of cardiac dysfunction (at rest).
>
> **Nonessential features**
> In cases where the diagnosis is in doubt, there is a response to treatment directed towards heart failure.

Table 33-4 Symptoms of heart failure in elderly patients, and differential diagnoses

Classical symptoms	Atypical features	Differential diagnoses
Dyspnea	Lethargy	Anemia
Orthopnea	Confusion	COPD
Peripheral edema	Falls	Depression or anxiety
	Dizziness	Hypothyroidism
	Syncope	Hypoalbuminemia
	Immobility	Malnutrition
		Renal disease
		Neoplasm

Abbreviation: COPD, chronic obstructive pulmonary disease.

as is the case with a number of other diseases. Consequently the diagnosis is a judgment based on a careful history and examination, chest radiology, electrocardiography, echocardiography, and other routine baseline investigations such as full blood count, serum biochemistry, and thyroid function.

Clinical history

The most classical symptom of heart failure is exertional breathlessness. However, this is a common symptom in the general population and in elderly people is often a result of chronic obstructive pulmonary disease (COPD).[53] Most people will experience some breathlessness with moderate exertion and, during exercise, the stage at which breathlessness is experienced depends on the overall level of fitness.

Anemia and obesity are confounding factors which make exertional dyspnea a very nonspecific symptom. Orthopnea is a more specific symptom which does not occur in normal patients, and is not usually a feature in respiratory disease. However, the disease process has to be relatively advanced before orthopnea occurs; and even if it is present, diuretics have often been instituted by the patient's general practitioner to relieve this symptom. Likewise, paroxysmal dyspnea (PND) is a more extreme version of dyspnea and is a result of fluid redistribution which increases the left ventricular end-diastolic pressure. Again, PND is specific but an insensitive symptom as it signifies fairly severe heart failure which should have been noted and previously treated.

Fatigue and lethargy are other common problems in heart failure, but they are probably even harder to define and assess than dyspnea, particularly in elderly patients. Fatigue is present in nearly every other disease.

Ankle edema is a common presenting feature, but again there are many alternative causes—such as cor pulmonale, recurrent pulmonary emboli, dependent edema, or hypoalbuminemia. Elderly women often have ankle edema which is not caused by heart failure: its precise cause is unknown, although venous insufficiency accompanied by pelvic obstruction to venous blood flow are commonly blamed. Indeed, it is elderly women with swollen ankles who most commonly cause false positives for heart failure when assessed subsequently by echocardiography.

Probably the best indication of underlying heart failure comes from the history, with a history of previous myocardial infarction or hypertension being useful indicators.[54] It should be remembered, however, that many elderly patients have silent myocardial ischemia or infarctions. In addition, many elderly patients are unsure whether a previous hospitalization for chest pain was for a myocardial infarction or angina. Additional features which may suggest the diagnosis of heart failure include excessive alcohol intake, a history of rheumatic fever, and the use of drugs such as nonsteroidals which might precipitate heart failure.

Physical signs

Many of the physical signs of heart failure are nonspecific and of relatively low predictive value. These include tachycardia, pulmonary crepitations, and peripheral edema. Equally, many of the physical signs which are specific to heart failure are insensitive because they occur only once the heart failure has become severe. These include elevation of the jugular venous pressure, a gallop rhythm, and displacement of the cardiac apex beat. The situation is further compounded by a variable ability of doctors to detect these clinical signs.[55] As a result, few of the symptoms and signs are of any value on their own. The probability of the diagnosis of heart failure is weighed up by the individual clinician making full use of clinical judgment together with the findings on examination and careful history taking.[56]

Investigations

The SIGN guidelines[57] for the diagnosis and treatment of heart failure due to left ventricular systolic dysfunction suggest that the purposes of clinical investigation in heart failure are:

1. to confirm or exclude the diagnosis of heart failure by demonstrating underlying cardiac disease;
2. to define the precise underlying cardiac cause of heart failure;
3. to identify precipitating or aggravating factors;
4. to guide management and treatment;
5. to provide baseline information to monitor effective treatment; and
6. to obtain prognostic information.

Even though these guidelines are not specifically written for the elderly patient, they provide a useful framework for investigations.

Chest X-ray

Chest X-ray is performed routinely and can produce useful information for patients with suspected heart failure. Cardiac enlargement (cardiothoracic ratio greater than 50 percent) implies cardiomegaly, and if present is a good guide to heart failure.[58] However, many heart failure patients do not exhibit cardiomegaly, so it tends to be a specific but insensitive test which identifies severe heart failure only. The other helpful findings of chest X-ray are pulmonary edema, upper lobe diversion, fluid in the horizontal fissure, and Kerly-B-lines in the costophrenic angles. In extreme cases, pleural effusions may be present, although clearly there are alternative explanations for pleural effusions such as bronchial carcinoma, pneumonia, or pulmonary emboli. In a recent meta-analysis of 29 studies,[59] Bayesian analysis found that chest radiography can only exclude heart failure (post-test probability less than 5 percent) and a decreased ejection fraction in patients who are asymptomatic can never confirm heart failure (post-test probability greater than 95 percent). However, it is likely that cardiomegaly represents underlying structural cardiac disease and in many patients heart failure will be present at some stage.

A chest X-ray can reveal other clues as to noncardiac disease which might be causing breathlessness. A lung tumor might be obvious, and emphysema may also be present. Nevertheless, the chest X-ray should be seen as a whole. For example, the finding of cardiomegaly plus bilateral pleural effusions with no other parenchymal lung disease makes heart failure extremely likely (although it should still be confirmed by echocardiography).

Electrocardiogram

The 12-lead electrocardiogram (ECG) should be performed routinely. Left ventricular systolic dysfunction is rare in the presence of a completely normal 12-lead ECG. Recent data[60] suggest that an abnormal resting ECG is sensitive (94 percent) with excellent negative predictive value (98 percent) but is much less specific (61 percent) and has poor positive predictive value (35 percent). Most studies suggest that this is the case, but where there is doubt an echocardiogram should be performed.

Other abnormalities on the ECG may be useful in the assessment of patients. For example, the presence of atrial fibrillation may be useful in concluding whether the patient should receive additional anticoagulation.

Echocardiography

The optimum investigation in the elderly patient with suspected heart failure is echocardiography.[61] Both qualitative and quantitative assessment can be useful. However, the degree of left ventricular systolic dysfunction can be assessed by a number of indices. Fractional shortening is usually sufficient in most instances.[62] Left ventricular ejection fraction,[63] and more recently a regional motion index,[64] have been shown to provide accurate assessments of left ventricular systolic function. Echocardiography can clearly distinguish whether the left ventricle is dilated or not; this approach to assessing left ventricular dimensions is preferable to chest X-ray. Left ventricular dilatation and left ventricular systolic dysfunction usually accompany each other, but occasionally the left ventricle is dilated despite the presence of normal systolic function. Nevertheless, left ventricular dilatation implies impending left ventricular systolic dysfunction and should probably be treated as such.

Echocardiography can also identify patients with mitral valve disease or aortic stenosis who may benefit from surgery. It can also assess diastolic dysfunction, although there is some controversy over this.[65] The problem relates to the fact that the left ventricle becomes stiffer as it ages, and it is difficult to define consistently when the stiff ventricle constitutes diastolic dysfunction. At the time of writing no echocardiographic criteria are fully accepted as measures of diastolic dysfunction.

However, there is one extreme version of diastolic dysfunction which can cause severe pulmonary edema. This occurs when the left ventricle is so stiff that left atrial pressure increases and leads to fast atrial fibrillation with profound breathlessness. In the short term, treatment is to reverse the abnormal rhythm, but longer-term strategies are required to prevent LV stiffness which leads to atrial fibrillation. Echocardiography also provides information about left ventricular hypertrophy if present, and this has treatment implications.[66]

Figure 33-2 suggests an approach for diagnosing heart failure in practice.

Natriuretic peptides

The natriuretic peptides (NPs) which are released from the atrium and ventricles have a variety of cellular effects, act as vasodilators, and cause a natriuresis. They have recently been shown to reflect left ventricular function, and levels correlate reasonably well with quantitative assessments of left ventricular function.[67] There is emerging evidence that the natriuretic peptides—and in particular BNP and ANP—have a role in identifying patients with left ventricular systolic dysfunction.[68,69] It is also becoming apparent that these agents may have a role in the preselection of patients for echocardiography when it is not always available. In patients following myocardial infarction, it appears that the levels of B-type natriuretic peptide closely relate to ejection fraction.[70] It has also been shown that in patients with acute dyspnea, plasma levels of BNP reflect left ventricular function.[71] Currently more easily performed assays are being developed, and testing is now possible with bedside Stix tests comparable to a BM Stix for blood sugar. In a recent community study, it was demonstrated

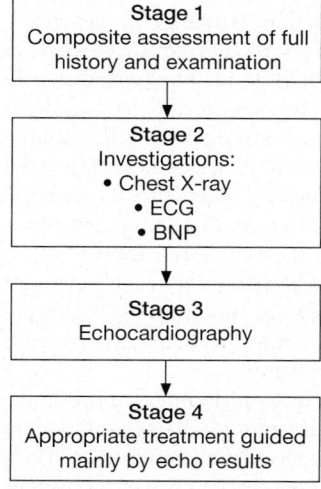

Figure 33-2 Diagnosing heart failure in practice.

that the natriuretic peptides are effective in detecting patients with left ventricular systolic dysfunction.[72]

In summary, the diagnosis of heart failure is a sequential one which relies on a clear clinical history and examination followed by either electrocardiography, chest radiology, or echocardiography. Echocardiography is desirable in all cases although it may not be always available, particularly in older patients.[73] Nevertheless, it is probably more important in the elderly patient to obtain an echocardiogram before instigating treatment, as structural abnormalities are more common and optimum treatment requires as accurate a diagnosis as possible so that adverse effects may be kept to a minimum.

When echocardiography proves to be technically difficult, objective assessments of left ventricular function may be made by radionuclide ventriculography. In the older patient, functional capacity can be assessed by performing a 6-minute walking test.[74] This can provide useful prognostic information.

TREATMENT OF HEART FAILURE
General issues

Since the 1960s, when the loop diuretics were introduced,[75] treatments for heart failure have diversified. As the pathophysiology of heart failure has become clearer, treatment options have broadened and a number of agents—including ACE inhibitors and β-blockers—have been shown to improve prognosis. It is now known that the negative influences of heart failure on left ventricular function and the peripheral circulation can be treated, with consequent hemodynamic improvement. Neurohumoral activation can be blocked and left ventricular remodeling can be reduced.[76] These adverse consequences of heart failure are the targets of drug treatment. As a result, patients may require multiple drug treatment and priorities need to be established. It is important that patients or their carers understand the implications of their treatment.

In the frail elderly patient, quality of life and alleviation of symptoms are as important as any prognostic benefit from treatment. The major clinical trials of heart failure have generally excluded older patients, and the majority of patients are in the age range 50–70 years. In such patients, the etiology of left ventricular systolic dysfunction is usually coronary artery disease and myocardial infarction, and in most clinical trials the compliance of patients is good. The typical elderly patient with heart failure, by contrast, often has multiple pathology and atypical presentation, together with variable compliance and often multiple etiologies, as well as associated comorbidity.[77] Consequently, when the older patient with heart failure is treated it is important to have as accurate a diagnosis as possible so that treatment can be tailored appropriately.

It is easy to forget that the older patient may have eyesight problems or impairment of cognitive function, so a multidisciplinary approach is the best method of managing patients both in hospital and in the community.

It is worth remembering and re-emphasizing that the different treatments are mediated by different mechanisms. Diuretics relieve the symptoms of fluid retention, but (apart from spironolactone[78]) there is little objective evidence to show any mortality benefit. While it would be unethical to perform a randomized controlled trial of diuretics today, the majority of such trials which earlier demonstrated a mortality benefit included patients who were receiving baseline diuretic treatment.

ACE inhibitors improve symptoms and exercise tolerance as well as prognosis in patients with heart failure.[45–47] This should be contrasted with β-blockers,[48,79–81] where symptomatic benefit may be mild and even deleterious in the early stages of treatment. So it is important to carefully guide a patient through treatment, making sure that he or she understands the process of the disease. The key point is that, in the long term, β-blockers slow progression and improve prognosis dramatically. More recently the angiotensin antagonists have been shown to be tolerated[82–84] and improve symptoms in patients with heart failure already taking diuretic treatment, but there is no strong evidence of prognostic benefit. In the last few years digoxin[85] has been shown convincingly to improve symptoms and reduce hospitalizations in patients with heart failure, although it appears that it does not alter mortality in patients who are in sinus rhythm with heart failure.

Nonpharmacological management of the patient is particularly important as mentioned previously, and compliance is a major issue. Where possible patients should be given advice about monitoring their weight, about the nature and relevance of their symptoms, and about the dosages of their drugs and the opportunity for flexible dosing dependent on symptoms. In general, patients should be advised to take moderate exercise and stop smoking. Patients who drink alcohol to excess should be advised to cut back. Often patient carers have a vital role to play in the nonpharmacological management.

In general, a drug should be started at a low dose and titrated in relation to the response, especially since patients may be taking over-the-counter preparations and the potential for drug interactions is considerable.[86] Each of the aforementioned drug classes will be considered in more detail; but in addition to the main therapeutic options, mention will be made of drugs which have less proven efficacy.

Diuretics

Diuretic treatment is fundamental to the treatment of chronic heart failure. The loop diuretics introduced in the 1960s were shown to be very effective in reducing symptoms associated with fluid retention and they had a clear hemodynamic benefit. Studies have shown deterioration in symptomatic heart failure when diuretics are withdrawn. This has added to the weight of evidence that diuretics are useful in the treatment of heart failure.[87]

The loop diuretics (which include frusemide and bumetanide) block the sodium–potassium–chloride transport exchange in the ascending limb of the loop of Henle.[88] Thiazides have a different site of action and work in the distal convoluted tubule.[89] Spironolactone has a yet different mode of action, antagonizing the aldosterone-mediated sodium exchange with potassium and hydrogen in the collecting ducts.[90] In older patients with heart failure, the rate of absorption of loop diuretics and time to peak plasma concentration are reduced as renal function is often impaired. High doses of diuretics may need to be used to produce a diuresis as the coexisting relative acidosis results in increased competition for the organic acid transport pathway at the proximal tubule. The bio-availability of frusemide can be very variable, from 20 to 80 percent, but is more consistent with bumetanide.[91] Most of the loop diuretics have a fairly short half-life, in the region of 1–2 hours. In contrast, the thiazide and potassium-sparing diuretics have longer half-lives which allow once-daily doses. Tolerance can occur to diuretics and this has a clinical relevance. The natriuretic response diminishes after the first dose but this can be reversed by restoring intravascular volume. Long-term administration of a loop diuretic can also result in tolerance, which can be combated by combining a loop and thiazide diuretic together.[92]

In patients with acute left ventricular failure, intravenous frusemide is effective, but prolonged use can result in a reduction in right-sided heart pressure with a consequent fall in cardiac output and increase in peripheral vascular resistance.[93] This can often be combated by treatment with a concomitant vasodilator such as a nitrate.[94] When frusemide is given to patients with severe acutely decompensating heart failure, high doses should be used until symptoms and signs of fluid overload have been controlled. An intravenous dose of 40–50 mg is often sufficient to control the symptoms; but when resistance to loop diuretics occurs, up to 250–500 mg per day may be required. In resistant cases, frusemide can be given by a continuous infusion of up to 4 g per day.

Metolazone[95] is a thiazide which can be used for resistant edema and heart failure. It blocks sodium reabsorption in the proximal convoluted tubule as well as having thiazide effects on the distal convoluted tubule. It is given orally at a dose between 1.25 mg and 10 mg per day. It can result in a profound diuresis and postural hypotension may be significant. Close monitoring of electrolytes is essential.

When patients with heart failure are being treated with a diuretic, it is essential to monitor plasma biochemistry regularly. Particular electrolyte disturbances include hypokalemia,[96] which may precipitate cardiac arrhythmias; hyponatremia,[97] which may cause drowsiness; and hypomagnesemia,[98] which may cause a number of cellular effects. Hypokalemia may be alleviated by the concomitant use of potassium-sparing diuretics such as spironolactone or an ACE inhibitor (see later). Diuretic treatment can also result in disturbances of lipid metabolism, glucose intolerance, and hyperuricemia.[99]

In addition to the above diuretic side-effects, older patients are prone to difficulties with urinary incontinence, immobility, postural hypotension, dehydration, and confusion. These problems should be prominent in the prescriber's mind when instigating treatment in an individual patient. It is also important not to administer intravenous frusemide rapidly as this may precipitate an irreversible hearing loss.[100]

A study in the Netherlands[101] of patients over the age of 65 assessed the impact of discontinuing diuretic therapy for relatively mild symptoms of heart failure (patients with severe symptoms and acute heart failure, and those requiring intravenous diuretics, were excluded). In the follow-up period, diuretic therapy had to be *reintroduced* in half of the patients in whom it had been withdrawn, owing to symptomatic deterioration. Even though the patients in whom diuretic therapy had to be restarted were relatively well, this study highlights the likelihood of a recurrence of symptoms if diuretics are discontinued in an elderly population.

Angiotensin-converting enzyme inhibitors

Angiotensin-converting enzyme (ACE) inhibitors have been available since the early 1980s, and evidence accumulated in the last 20 years confirms their considerable efficacy in the treatment of heart failure. ACE inhibitors block overactivity of the renin–angiotensin system and the sympathetic nervous system.[102] In addition to these effects, ACE inhibitors seem to enhance the bradykinin–nitric oxide system in the vascular endothelium.[103] They may also have an influence outside the circulation in various tissues.[104] In patients with mild to moderate heart failure and even asymptomatic left ventricular dysfunction, they reduce morbidity and mortality.[45–47] Mechanistically, ACE inhibitors are vasodilators with subsequent reduction in cardiac preload and afterload, resulting in hemodynamic and symptomatic improvement for patients with heart failure. In addition to reducing the overcompensatory activity of the renin–angiotensin system together with beneficial effects on the endothelium, ACE inhibitors may also have anti-ischemic effects[105] and have an influence on the deleterious effects of the remodeling of the left ventricle following myocardial infarction.

The first study which demonstrated a benefit was in patients with severe heart failure (New York Heart Association class IV). In the CONSENSUS Study,[45] patients were randomized to treatment with enalapril 2.5 mg titrated to 10 mg twice-daily if tolerated, or placebo. At 1-year follow-up, mortality was 52 percent in the placebo group and 36 percent in the enalapril group. There were also significant reductions in hospital admissions in the treatment group. In the SOLVD Study,[46] patients with mild to moderate heart failure treated with enalapril 10 mg twice-daily obtained a mortality benefit. This benefit also extended to patients in a prevention group of the SOLVD study as well as those in the treatment group. The trials not only demonstrated a mortality and symptomatic benefit, but also confirmed that, in general, treatment was well-tolerated. The patients in these studies were middle-aged, so it may not be possible to extrapolate the findings directly to frail elderly patients. Nonetheless, most physicians would probably treat the older patient who had systolic dysfunction with an ACE inhibitor. Treatment with an ACE inhibitor also reduces the likelihood of myocardial ischemic events. In the SAVE Study,[47] patients with asymptomatic left ventricular dysfunction (LVEF < 40 percent) following myocardial infarction were treated with titrated doses of captopril up to 50 mg three times daily. There was a risk reduction of 19 percent in mortality compared with patients treated by placebo.

Further evidence for the efficacy of ACE inhibitors in patients with heart failure following myocardial infarction was obtained by the AIRE study.[106] Patients were randomized to treatment with ramipril 2.5 mg twice daily, increased to 5 mg twice daily if tolerated. In the 15-month follow-up the mortality rate in those treated with ramipril was 17 percent, compared with 23 percent in the placebo group.

As a result of the findings of all these trials, the use of ACE inhibitors has become increasingly widespread in patients with left ventricular systolic dysfunction. However, concerns do remain about their use in the elderly population as some reports suggest there is a high prevalence of renovascular disease in the older patient with heart failure.[107]

The main contraindications to treatment with ACE inhibitors are obstructive valvular disease and renal impairment. Patients who are volume-depleted, particularly those with hyponatremia, are more likely to experience hypotension with initial dosage. However, this may be less marked with some ACE inhibitors than others.[108] Treatment should be gradually titrated in divided doses until the maximum achievable dose is obtained. In general terms the optimal benefit is obtained at the top end of the dose range. The recent ATLAS study[109] compared low and high doses of lisinopril in heart failure and patients with higher dosages fared better. Ideally, the diuretic dose should be reduced or curtailed to optimize intravascular volume at the time of initiation of therapy. This reduces the likelihood of hypotension. Renal function and electrolytes should be monitored at regular intervals, initially every few days or weekly and then every 3–6 months. It may be possible to reduce the dose of maintenance diuretic therapy once the patient has been established on ACE inhibition.

The effects of ACE inhibitors on heart failure appear to be a class effect. Individual drugs currently used include captopril, enalapril, lisinopril, perindopril, and quinapril. The main side-effects of ACE inhibitors include cough, hypotension, hyperkalemia and rarely angioneurotic edema. The ACE-inhibitor mediated cough may be partially alleviated by the use of sodium cromoglycate.[110]

The role of ACE inhibition in patients in heart failure with normal systolic function is unclear but is currently being addressed in a randomized trial.[111]

Beta-blockers

It has become increasingly clear in the last few years that β-blockade is beneficial for patients with left ventricular systolic dysfunction and heart failure. A role for β-blockers was suggested as far back as the early 1970s.[112] Part of the rationale behind their use relates to reducing the adverse consequences of overstimulation of the sympathetic nervous system in patients with heart failure.

The main historical concerns related to the relatively negative inotropic effects of β-blockers with the potential for hypotension and fatigue. However, the results of randomized trials now suggest that, after mild intolerance associated with starting treatment in some patients, the benefits of longer-term therapy are significant and worth pursuing. Improved understanding of the pathophysiology of heart failure has highlighted the potential role for β-blockers in reducing the effects of vasoconstriction and fluid retention associated with heart failure. Indeed it is the case that blockade of the sympathetic nervous system by β-blockers complements the beneficial effects of ACE inhibitors on the renin–angiotensin system. Beta-blockers also have an antiarrhythmic effect and additionally facilitate coronary blood flow by prolonging diastole. Blockade of the adrenergic system may reduce both adrenaline (epinephrine)-mediated myocyte cell loss and myocyte dysfunction, thus reducing associated left ventricular systolic dysfunction.[113] Furthermore, the promotion of cellular growth and ventricular remodeling which is mediated by noradrenaline (norepinephrine) is blocked by β-blockers. It also appears that β-blockade may reduce some of the uncoupling of the β-receptors from their G protein at a cellular level, preventing further deterioration in systolic function.[114]

In the last few years it has been confirmed that treatment with β-blockade initially in small dosages, with a number of agents, can result in significant mortality benefits for patients with heart failure.[79–81] It is important that the dose be carefully titrated, with a close evaluation following each up-titration in order to detect worsening heart failure or associated hypotension. Up-titration of the dose should occur only when the patient is stable. Although most patients will show some improvement in their clinical condition and the progression of heart failure is reduced, exercise capacity may be only partially improved by treatment. However, hospital admissions for decompensated heart failure are overall less frequent.

Although the evidence for the use of β-blockade in heart failure is strengthening, some earlier studies in the late 1980s and early 1990s showed only a mild benefit following treatment.[115] It is only with the MERIT Heart Failure study,[80] the CIBIS II,[81] and the US COPERNICUS Heart Failure study[48] that the evidence base for the use of β-blockers in heart failure has become robust.

- In the MERIT study, nearly 4000 patients with New York Heart Association class II–IV heart failure were treated with longacting metoprolol in divided and increasing doses. The treatment group started on a dose between 12.5 and 25 mg daily which was titrated to a target dose of 200 mg daily. Those patients treated had a reduced mortality rate of 34 percent in the 1-year follow-up period, the absolute mortality rate being reduced from 11 to 7.2 percent. Deaths from worsening heart failure and sudden deaths were both reduced significantly.
- In the CIBIS II study, the findings are similar with patients in New York Association class III–IV on standard treatment with diuretics and ACE inhibitors deriving additional benefit by treatment with bisoprolol, a β_1 selective adrenoceptor blocker. The dose of bisoprolol was titrated up to 10 mg daily, with the mortality rate being reduced from 13.2 to 8.8 percent in the treatment group. Carvedilol is a nonselective β-blocker with antioxidant, α-blocking, and vasodilator activity.[116] Following treatment with titrated doses of carvedilol,[79] patients with chronic heart failure, including those with severe heart failure, derived benefit following a 6.5-month follow-up period.
- In the COPERNICUS trial,[48] a 35 percent reduction in analyzed mortality was obtained in patients treated with carvedilol compared to placebo. The benefit was also significant in patients with NYHA class IV heart failure, with an annual mortality rate of 18.5 percent in the placebo group compared with 11.4 percent in the carvedilol group.

These landmark trials have convincingly demonstrated that β-blockers improve mortality in patients with chronic heart failure. The precise role of β-blockers in frailer older patients with associated cognitive impairment and more frequent postural hypotension and comorbidity is unclear. However, there is a compelling case for β-blockade in patients with no contraindications.

Contraindications include bradycardia, AV block, hypotension, asthma, or chronic obstructive pulmonary disease. Problems with tolerability may be accentuated if the patient is taking other cardioactive medications. Patients with peripheral vascular disease may also find β-blockers difficult to tolerate. Initiation of β-blockers is best undertaken in a supervised hospital setting.

Spironolactone

In the RALES study,[78] the effectiveness of spironolactone added to an ACE inhibitor and a loop diuretic for severe chronic heart failure was assessed. This was a randomized double-blind placebo-controlled trial in which 1633 patients with New York Heart Association class III–IV heart failure, and ejection fraction of less than 30 percent and established on full ACE inhibitor and diuretic therapy with or without digoxin, were included. Small doses of spironolactone (25–50 mg per day) were well tolerated and reduced total mortality by 30 percent in the treatment group. Deaths from progressive heart failure and sudden deaths were reduced equally, and the incidence of severe hyperkalemia was low.

Digoxin

Digoxin has been used in the treatment of heart failure for over 200 years. It is a positive inotrope and the effects of digoxin are mediated by inhibition of the Na^+/K^+ ATPase which influences intracellular sodium with resultant influences on sodium/calcium exchange across the sarcolemmal membrane.[117] It has a relatively narrow therapeutic window, with the result that side-effects are common, particularly in the elderly with renal impairment and hypokalemia.

In addition to its effects on the myocardium, digoxin is a weak diuretic and can cause gastric irritation[118] and has a mild estrogenic effect.[119] Digoxin improves the cardiac output and the stroke volume index with a resultant improvement in hemodynamic status in heart failure patients. The side-effects of digoxin are more pronounced in patients with hypokalemia as potassium competes for the binding site at the site of action.

Until recently there has been considerable controversy over the role of digoxin in patients with heart failure. Its role in patients with sinus rhythm was particularly unclear. In the DIG trial,[85] nearly 8000 patients were assessed in over 300 centers. Patients were randomized to digoxin or placebo and followed for an average of 3 years. The patients had clinical heart failure but were in sinus rhythm. In the majority of patients the cause of heart failure was ischemic heart disease and the average ejection fraction was 32 percent. Total mortality was no different between the digoxin and placebo groups. Heart failure deaths were reduced in the digoxin group but there was a trend towards an increase in deaths because of arrhythmias or myocardial infarction. Hospital admissions were significantly reduced. Thus digoxin can now be recommended to patients with heart failure and sinus rhythm who remain symptomatic despite the use of diuretics and ACE inhibitors, and β-blockers.

Clearly in older patients close monitoring of therapy is essential. Two relatively recent withdrawal studies[120,121] indicate that digoxin is a useful adjunct to treatment in patients on ACE inhibitors and diuretics. With impaired renal function and reduced clearance of the drug, symptomatic nausea and fatigue are probably the most frequent complication together with bradycardia. A number of therapeutically important drug interactions also exist with digoxin, particularly with quinidine and amiodarone.[122] It is also sometimes difficult to distinguish between digoxin toxicity and the underlying symptoms of cardiac failure.

Digoxin is particularly useful in controlling ventricular rate in patients with fast atrial fibrillation and heart failure. The recent Scottish Intercollegiate Guideline Network has suggested that patients with heart failure and atrial fibrillation who need control of their ventricular rate should be considered for treatment with digoxin.[57] Others to be considered include patients with moderately severe or severely symptomatic heart failure; those who remain symptomatic despite diuretic and ACE inhibitor therapy; those who have had more than one hospital admission for heart failure; and those who have had poor left ventricular systolic function and persisting cardiomegaly.

The maintenance dose of digoxin in heart failure should be in the region of 125 μg per day, but smaller doses may be necessary in some patients. Although additional therapeutic benefit may be obtained at higher doses, toxicity becomes increasingly likely.

Angiotensin antagonists

Attention recently has been directed towards angiotensin receptor blockade as a means of modifying the symptoms of heart failure.[123] It appears that there are at least two angiotensin receptors: AT I and AT II. Stimulation of the former results in vasoconstriction, while stimulation of the latter results in vasodilatation. Angiotensin I receptor antagonists are effective in hypertension and their use is becoming more widespread.

The effects of these agents in elderly patients with heart failure has been clarified recently in the ELITE[82,83] and Val HeFT[84] studies. In the former, where mortality was the primary endpoint, no mortality difference was seen between patients treated with losartan or captopril. In the Val HeFT study, (reporting at the time of writing) there appeared to be no improvement in mortality in patients with heart failure treated with valsartan on top of an ACE inhibitor. However, symptomatic improvement was demonstrated and the need for hospital admission was reduced by valsartan on top of an ACE inhibitor.

These agents are generally well tolerated and should certainly be used in patients who are intolerant of ACE inhibition because of cough. They are, however, licensed in the UK currently only as a treatment for hypertension.

Other pharmacology

Nitrates have a well-established role in the treatment of angina, but they also have a role in the management of cardiac failure. They act predominantly through stimulation of intracellular guanylate cyclase with subsequent sequestration of intracellular calcium and resultant vasodilatation. Beneficial hemodynamic effects include a reduction in blood pressure together with decreased pulmonary artery wedge pressure.[124]

These favor an increase in cardiac output by reducing the pre-load on the left ventricle.[125] Tolerance to nitrate therapy is well recognized but this can be reduced by nitrate-free periods.

A study of intravenous nitrate therapy showed that this treatment is effective in the treatment of acute pulmonary edema with reduction in symptoms of breathlessness and discomfort.[126] In the first Veterans Administration Cooperative Heart Failure trial (V-HeFT 1), isosorbide dinitrate and hydralazine[127] were compared with prazosin and placebo in patients with New York Heart Association class II–III heart failure. There was a mild improvement in mortality in the nitrate and hydralazine group and ejection fraction and exercise performance also improved. This highlights the potential value of nitrates, but their current role is probably as adjunctive treatment to agents with more proven long-term benefit. However, they are still commonly used in patients who have had an acute decompensation of their heart failure. In one trial of acute left ventricular failure, intravenous isosorbide dinitrate appeared better than intravenous frusemide.[128]

In addition to nitrates, other vasodilators such as calcium antagonists may have a role in heart failure. However, the PRAISE trial[129] showed that amlodipine has a neutral effect on mortality, which means that amlodipine can be used for its anti-ischemic effect in heart failure patients without worsening their heart failure.

Other agents have been evaluated in patients with cardiac failure but the abovementioned drugs are currently the conventional treatment. In general terms, positive inotropes have been largely unhelpful and phosphodiesterase inhibitors have merely increased mortality.[130,131] Flosequinan is also associated with increased mortality.[132] Short-term use of intravenous positive inotropes may be useful in occasional patients, but their overall benefit is limited. Other simple measures may be useful. In a patient with a mild anemia treatment of the anemia may improve tissue oxygenation and subsequent cardiac performance. This may require ferrous sulfate or even erythropoietin or both. In patients with nutritional deficiencies, vitamin B supplementation may also be useful. There has been some recent concern that treatment with aspirin may negate the beneficial effects of ACE inhibitors in patients with left ventricular systolic dysfunction.[133] The evidence for this is not strong and such patients with left ventricular systolic dysfunction should still be treated with an ACE inhibitor where possible. There is currently no strong evidence that anticoagulation for patients with heart failure in sinus rhythm is of any benefit. Patients with atrial fibrillation should receive treatment with warfarin if not contraindicated.[134]

Cardiac arrhythmias are relatively common in patients with heart failure. Patients with atrial fibrillation should be managed with anticoagulation where possible, although it should be remembered that the risks of hemorrhagic side-effects are likely to be greater in the older patient and tight control of the INR is mandatory. Anticoagulation should be avoided in patients who are frequent fallers. Rapid ventricular rates associated with fast atrial fibrillation can be controlled by digoxin and/or β-blockers. Conversion to sinus rhythm can prove difficult as often the atrial fibrillation is longstanding. However, as atrial systole has increased importance in the older patient,[36] attempts to maintain sinus rhythm should be made if possible, either electrically or pharmacologically with β-blockers or amiodarone.

Ventricular arrhythmias are also relatively common in patients with heart failure. These ventricular arrhythmias may cause considerable hypotension and may even be fatal. Amiodarone is often used in the context of symptomatic ventricular arrhythmias, but it has a number of noncardiac side-effects including pulmonary fibrosis, liver function abnormalities, thyroid dysfunction, and peripheral neuropathy. In a trial in South America,[135] 500 patients with heart failure were randomized to amiodarone or placebo at a relatively low dose and followed-up at 13 months. The mortality in the amiodarone group was 33.5 percent, compared with 41.4 percent in the placebo group—a risk reduction of 28 percent. In the CHF–STAT trial,[136] a higher dosage of amiodarone was used in a similar number of patients. At the higher dose, no mortality benefit was seen although there was a reduced mortality trend in patients with a nonischemic etiology. These studies would tend to suggest that amiodarone should be the antiarrhythmic of choice in patients with heart failure and symptomatic ventricular arrhythmias, but there is no role for widespread use of prophylactic amiodarone.

Drug interactions are frequently a problem in the elderly population and there are a number of significant interactions with amiodarone. The most significant of these is with warfarin and treatment should be carefully monitored. Patients with heart failure who have associated angina and myocardial ischemia should be treated for their ischemic heart disease by conventional means. Patients may require treatment with aspirin, β-blockade, statins, oral nitrates, calcium antagonists or other, nondrug, measures.

In patients with ischemic heart disease and mild to moderate impairment of left ventricular systolic functions, left ventricular performance may be improved by coronary bypass surgery. Such patients may have a hibernating area of myocardium which could potentially be salvaged following bypass surgery.

CONCLUSIONS

Chronic heart failure is a major cause of morbidity and mortality in older patients. Optimum treatment requires an accurate diagnosis. In the older patient the etiology of heart failure is often heterogeneous and the clinical and examination findings should be confirmed by more objective assessments including chest radiology, electrocardiography, and particularly echocardiography. Elderly patients often have limited access to echocardiography, but it is essential given the high prevalence of background valvular disease and structural heart disease.

Once an accurate diagnosis has been established, treatment of left ventricular systolic dysfunction should follow the recent guidelines of the European Society of Cardiology and the American Heart Association where possible, with consideration of the specific requirements of the individual patient. Close supervision of treatment is mandatory particularly with ACE inhibitors and β-blockers where the possibility of short-term side-effects is significant. Specific drug interventions should be tailored to individual patients, with cognitive impairment and additional pathology restricting the choice of agents available.

The prognosis for chronic heart failure is poor and at all times when treating the older patient emphasis should be on improving the patient's quality of life and symptom control.

Many of the major multicenter clinical trials have excluded older patients from analysis, but evidence should emerge about drug tolerability in patients over the age of 75. However, when there is evidence of fluid retention patients should be treated with a diuretic, and once evidence of left ventricular systolic dysfunction is confirmed they should be treated with an ACE inhibitor. Strong consideration should be given to treatment with a β-blocker. If the patient has severe heart failure, spironolactone (25 mg/day) should be added to the frusemide, ACE inhibitor, and β-blocker, but it is crucial to monitor the serum electrolytes carefully in the first month of therapy.

If the patient is in atrial fibrillation and control of the ventricular rate is an issue, digoxin should be used. Other agents should be chosen in the light of contraindications to these major treatments. Digoxin and nitrates improve symptoms, and spironolactone may improve mortality. As in any illness, the response to treatment should be carefully monitored by the physician.

KEY POINTS   Chronic cardiac failure

- Chronic heart failure is a major cause of morbidity and mortality in elderly patients.

- The optimum treatment requires an accurate diagnosis. In the older patient, the etiology of heart failure is often heterogeneous, so the clinical and examination findings should be confirmed by more objective assessments— including chest radiology, electrocardiography, and particularly echocardiography.

- Once an accurate diagnosis has been established, treatment of left ventricular systolic dysfunction should follow the recent guidelines of the European Society of Cardiology and the American Heart Association where possible, with consideration of the specific requirements of the individual patient.

- Close supervision of treatment is mandatory, particularly with ACE inhibitors and β-blockers where the possibility of short-term side-effects is significant.

- The prognosis for chronic heart failure is poor. Emphasis should be on improving the patient's quality of life and symptom control, although new treatments may also improve mortality.

- Many of the major multicenter clinical trials have excluded older patients from analysis, but evidence should emerge in the next few years about drug tolerability in patients over the age of 75.

- When there is evidence of fluid retention, patients should be treated with a diuretic. Once evidence of left ventricular systolic dysfunction is confirmed, they should be treated with an ACE inhibitor.

- Strong consideration should be given to treatment with a β-blocker. If the patient has severe heart failure, spironolactone (25 mg/day) should be added to the frusemide.

- If the patient is in atrial fibrillation and control of the ventricular rate is an issue, digoxin should be used.

- Other agents should be chosen in the light of contraindications to these major treatments. Digoxin and nitrates improve symptoms and spironolactone may improve mortality.

Summary of treatment options
Chronic heart failure

Diuretics	For symptoms of fluid overload and edema. Loop diuretic (frusemide or bumetanide) at appropriate dose. Also consider thiazide.
ACE inhibitor	Symptomatic and mortality benefit for systolic dysfunction following confirmation of diagnosis by echocardiography. Options include enalapril, lisinopril, captopril, perindopril, ramipril. Dose should be titrated.
β-blocker	Should be considered for symptomatic and mortality benefit in mild, moderate and even severe heart failure under close hospital supervision. Beneficial effects may not be immediate. Options include carvedilol, metoprolol, bisoprolol. Dose should be titrated
Spironolactone	Adjunctive treatment with a mortality benefit.
Digoxin	As adjunctive treatment for symptomatic benefit and control of atrial fibrillation. Also provides symptomatic improvement in sinus rhythm but no clear mortality benefit.
Nitrates	As adjunctive treatment for symptomatic benefit and control of associated angina.
Other options	Amlodipine, ferrous sulphate, erythropoietin, warfarin, amiodarone.
Nonpharmacological	Weight loss; low-salt diet; cessation of smoking; exercise; compliance aids. Multidisciplinary management.

REFERENCES

1. Dargie HJ, McMurray JJV: Diagnosis and management of heart failure. BMJ 1994;309:321–328
2. Sutton GC: Epidemiological aspects of heart failure. Am Heart J 1990;120:1538–1540

3. McDonagh TA, Morrison CE, Lawrence A et al: Symptomatic and asymptomatic left-ventricular systolic dysfunction in an urban population. Lancet 1997;50:829–833

4. Yusuf S, Thom T: Changes in hypertension treatment and in congestive heart failure mortality in the United States. Hypertension 1989;13(1):74–79

5. Kostis JB, Davis BR, Cutler J et al: Prevention of heart failure by antihypertensive drug treatment in older persons with isolated systolic hypertension. JAMA 1997;278:212–216

6. The Taskforce on Heart Failure of the European Society of Cardiology: Guidelines for the diagnosis of heart failure. Eur Heart J 1995;16:741–751

7. Report of the American College of Cardiology/American Heart Association Task Force on Practice Guidelines (committee on evaluation and management of heart failure): Guidelines for the evaluation and management of heart failure. Circulation 1995;92:2764–2784

8. Parameshwar J, Poole-Wilson PA, Sutton GC: Heart failure in a district general hospital. J R Coll Physicians Lond 1992;26:139–142

9. McMurray J, Hart W: The economic impact of heart failure on the National Health Service. Br Heart J 1993;69:19

10. Luchi RJ, Taffet GE, Teasdale TA: Congestive heart failure in the elderly. J Am Geriatr Soc 1991;39:810–825

11. Erikksson H, Svarsudd K, Larsson B et al: Risk factors for heart failure in the general population: the study of men born in 1913. Eur Heart J 1989;10:647–656

12. Kannel WB: Epidemiology and prevention of cardiac failure: Framingham study insights. Eur Heart J 1987;8(F):23–26

13. Parameshwar J, Shackell MM, Richardson A, Poole-Wilson PA, Sutton GC: Prevalence of heart failure in three general practices in north west London. Br J Gen Pract 1992;42:287–289

14. Logan WPD, Cushion AA: Morbidity Statistics from General Practice. HMSO, London, 1958

15. Gibson TC, White KL, Klainer LM: The prevalence of congestive heart failure in two rural communities. J Chronic Dis 1996;19:141–152

16. Ho KK, Pinsky JL, Kannel WB, Levy D: The epidemiology of heart failure: the Framingham study. J Am Coll Cardiol 1993;22:6–13

17. Aronow WS: Prevalence of the appropriate and inappropriate use of digoxin in elderly patients at the time of admission to a nursing home. J Am Geriatr Soc 1996;44:588–590

18. Morgan S, Smith H, Simpson I et al: Prevalence and clinical characteristics of left ventricular dysfunction among elderly patients in general practice setting: cross-sectional study. BMJ 1999;318:368–372

19. McKee PA, Castelli WP, McNamara M, Kannel WB: The natural history of congestive heart failure: the Framingham study. N Engl J Med 1971;285:1441–1446

20. Eriksson H, Svardsudd K, Caidahl K et al: Early heart failure in the population: the Study of Men Born in 1913. Acta Med Scand 1988;223:197–209

21. Parameshwar J, Poole-Wilson PA, Sutton GC: Heart failure in a district general hospital. J R Coll Physicians Lond 1992;26:139–142

22. Tresch DD, McGough MF: Heart failure with normal systolic function: a common disorder in older people. J Am Geriatr Soc 1995;43:1035–1042

23. Reitsma JB, Mosterd A, Koster RW et al: Increase in the number of admissions due to heart failure in Dutch hospitals in the period 1980–1992. Ned Tijdschr Geneeskd 1994;138:866–871

24. McMurray J, McDonagh T, Morrison CE, Dargie HJ: Trends in hospitalisation for heart failure in Scotland 1980–1990. Eur Heart J 1993;14:1158–1162

25. Haldeman GA, Croft JB, Giles WH et al: Hospitalisation of patients with heart failure: national hospital discharge survey 1985–95. Am Heart J 1999;137:352–360

26. Gooding J, Hetter AM: Hospital readmissions among the elderly. J Am Geriatr Soc 1985;33:595–601

27. Rich MW, Beckham V, Wittenberg C et al: A multidisciplinary intervention to prevent the readmission of elderly patients with congestive heart failure. N Engl Med J 1995;333:1190–1195

28. Taffet GE, Teasdale TA, Bleyler AZ, Kutka NJ, Luci RJ: Survival of elderly men with congestive heart failure. Age Ageing 1992;21:49–55

29. Gillespie N, Darbar D, Struthers A, McMurdo MET: Heart failure: a diagnostic and therapeutic dilemma in elderly patients. Age Ageing 1998;27:539–543

30. Lye M: Chronic heart failure: mechanisms and management. Scott Med J 1997;42(5):138–140 (review)

31. Pfeffer MA, Braunwald E: Ventricular remodelling after myocardial infarction. experimental observations and clinical implications. Circulation 1990;81:1161–1172

32. Otto CM: Valvular Heart Disease. W.B. Saunders, London, 1999

33. Report of the WHO/ISFC task force on the definition and the classification of the cardiomyopathies. Br Heart J 1980;44:672–673

34. Swinne CJ, Shapiro EP, Jamart JA et al: Age-associated changes in left ventricular outflow tract geometry in normal subjects. Am J Cardiol 1996;78:1070–1073

35. Sagie A, Benjamin E, Galderisi M: Reference values for Doppler indexes of left ventricular diastolic filling in the elderly. J Am Soc Echocardiogr 1993;6:570–576

36. Fleg JL: Alterations in cardiovascular structure and function with advancing age. Am J Cardiol 1986;57(C):33–44

37. Francis GS, Benedict C, Johnstone DE et al: Comparison of neuroendocrine activation in patient with left ventricular systolic dysfunction with and without congestive heart failure: a sub-study of the Studies of Left Ventricular Dysfunction (SOLVD). Circulation 1990;82:1724–1729

38. Periui R, Milesi S, Fisher NM: Heart rate variability during dynamic exercise in elderly males and females. Eur J Appl Physiol 200;82:8–15

39. Poole-Wilson PA, Ferrari R: Role of skeletal muscle in the syndrome of chronic heart failure. J Mol Cell Cardiol 1996;28:2275–2285

40. Lip GY, Lowe GD, Metcalfe MJ et al: Is diastolic function associated with thrombogenesis? A study of circulating markers of a prothrombotic state in patients with coronary artery disease. Int J Cardiol 1995;50:31–42

41. Sollott SJ, Lakatta EG: Normal ageing changes in the cardiovascular system. Cardiol Elderly 1993;1:349–358

42. Wong WF, Gold S, Fukuyama O et al: Diastolic dysfunction in elderly patients with congestive heart failure. Am J Cardiol 1989;63:1526–1528

43. Aronow WS, Ahn Chul, Kronzon I: Prevalence of echocardiographic findings in 554 men and 1243 women aged >60 years in a long-term-care health facility. Am J Cardiol 1997;79:379–380

44. Aronow WS, Ahn C, Kronzon I: Prognosis of congestive heart failure in elderly patients with normal versus abnormal left ventricular systolic function associated with coronary artery disease. Am J Cardiol 1990;66:1257–1259

45. The CONSENSUS Trial Study Group: Effects of enalapril on mortality in severe congestive heart failure. N Engl J Med 1987;316:1429–1435

46. The SOLVD Investigators: Effect of enalapril on survival in patients with reduced left ventricular ejection fractions and congestive heart failure. N Engl J Med 1991;325:293–302

47. Pfeffer MA, Braunwald E, Moye LA et al: Effect of captopril on mortality and morbidity in patients with left ventricular dysfunction after myocardial infarction: results of the Survival and Ventricular Enlargement Trial. N Engl J Med 1992;327:669–677

48. Carvedilol Randomised Prospective Cumulative Survival (COPERNICUS). European Society of Cardiology Congress 2000.

49. White H, Norris R, Brown M et al: Left ventricular end-systolic volume as the major determinant of survival after recovery from a myocardial infarction. Circulation 1987;76:44–51

50. Ghali JK, Kadakia S, Cooper R, Ferlinz J: Precipitating factors leading to decompensation of heart failure. Arch Intern Med 1988;148:2013–2016

51. Gillespie ND, McNeill G, Pringle T, Ogston S, Struthers AD, Pringle SD: Cross-sectional study of clinical assessment and simple cardiac investigations in diagnosis of left ventricular systolic dysfunction in patients admitted with acute dyspnoea. BMJ 1997;314:936–940

52. Struthers AD. The diagnosis of heart failure. Heart 2000;84:334–338

53. McNamara RM, Cionni DJ: Utility of the peak expiratory flow rate in the differentiation of acute dyspnoea; cardiac versus pulmonary origin. Chest 1992;101:129–132

54. Davie AP, Francis CM, Caruana L, Sutherland GR, McMurray JJ: Assessing diagnosis in heart failure: which features are any use? QJM 1997;90:335–339

55. Ishmail AA, Wings S, Ferguson J, Hutchison TA, Magder S, Flegel KM: Interobserver agreement by auscultation in the presence of a third heart sound in patients with congestive heart failure. Chest 1987;91:870–873

56. Poole-Wilson PA: Prediction of heart failure: an art aided by technology. N Engl J Med 1997;336:1381–1382

57. Scottish Intercollegiate Guidelines Network (SIGN). Issue 35—The Diagnosis and Treatment of Heart Failure due to Left Ventricular Systolic Dysfunction. Royal College of Physicians of Edinburgh, 1999

58. Madsen EB, Gilpin E, Slutsky RA, Ahnve S, Henning H, Ross J: Usefulness of the chest x-ray for predicting abnormal left ventricular

function after acute myocardial infarction. Am Heart J 1984;108:1431–1436

59. Badgett RG, Mulrow CD, Otto PM et al: How well can the chest radiograph diagnose left ventricular dysfunction? J Gen Intern Med 1996;11:625–634

60. Davie AP, Francis CM, Love MP et al: Value of the electrocardiogram in identifying heart failure due to left ventricular systolic dysfunction. BMJ 1996;12:222

61. Shah PM, Crawford M, De Maria A et al: Recommendations for quantitation of the left ventricle by two-dimensional echocardiography. J Am Soc Echocardiogr 1989;2:358–367

62. Francis CM, Caruana L, Kearney P et al: Open access echocardiography in management of heart failure in the community. BMJ 1995;310:634–636

63. Eagle KA, Quertermous T, Singer DE: Left ventricular ejection fraction: physician estimates compared with gated blood pool scan measurements. Arch Intern Med 1988;148:882–885

64. Berning J, Hoilund-Carlsen P, Nielson GG et al: Critical reappraisal of bedside echocardiographic parameters for estimation of left ventricular ejection fraction in acute myocardial infarction. Am J Noninv Cardiol 1992;6:269–278

65. Wong WF, Gold S, Fukuyama O, Blanchette PL: Diastolic dysfunction in elderly patients with congestive heart failure. Am J Cardiol 1989;63:1526–1528

66. Kannel W, Gordon T, Castelli W et al: Electrocardiographic left ventricular hypertrophy and risk of coronary heart disease: the Framingham Heart Study. Ann Intern Med 1970;72:813–822

67. Struthers AD: Prospects for using a blood sample in the diagnosis of heart failure. Q J Med 1995;88:303–306

68. Struthers AD: Ten years of natriuretic peptide research: a new dawn for their diagnostic and therapeutic use? BMJ 1994;308:1615–1619

69. Wilkins MR, Redondo J, Brown LA: The natriuretic-peptide family. Lancet 1997;349:1307–1310

70. Davidson NC, Naas AA, Hanson JK, Kennedy NS, Coutie WJ, Struthers AD: Comparison of atrial natriuretic peptide, B-type natriuretic peptide and N-terminal proatrial natriuretic peptide as indicators of left ventricular systolic dysfunction. Am J Cardiol 1996;77:828–831

71. Davis M, Espiner E, Richards G et al: Plasma brain natriuretic peptide in assessment of acute dyspnoea. Lancet 1994;343:440–444

72. Cowie MR, Struthers AD, Wood DA et al: Value of natriuretic peptides in assessment of patients with possible new heart failure in primary care. Lancet 1997;350:1347–1351

73. Clarke KW, Gray D, Hampton JR: Evidence of inadequate investigation and treatment of patients with heart failure. Br Heart J 1994;71:584–587

74. Bittner V, Weiner DH, Yusuf S, Rogers WJ, McIntyre KM, Bangdiwala SI et al: Prediction of mortality and morbidity with a 6-minute walk test in patients with left-ventricular dysfunction. JAMA 1993;270:1702–1707

75. Odlind B: Site and mechanism of action of the diuretics. Acta Pharmacol Toxicol 1984;54(1):5–15

76. Sharpe N: Management principles: much more to be gained. In Heart Failure Management. Martin Dunitz, London, 2000:15–28

77. Aronow WS: Treatment of congestive heart failure in older persons. J Am Geriatr Soc 1997;45:1252–1258

78. The RALES Investigators: Effectiveness of spironolactone added to an ACE inhibitor and a loop diuretic for severe chronic congestive heart failure. Am J Cardiol 1996;78:902–907

79. Packer M, Bristow MR, Cohn JN et al, for the US Carvedilol Heart Failure Study Group: The effect of carvedilol on morbidity and mortality in patients with chronic heart failure. N Engl J Med 1996;334:1349–1355

80. The MERIT-HF Study Group: Metoprolol CR/XL Randomised Intervention Trial in Congestive Heart Failure (MERIT-HF): mortality results. Lancet 1999;353:2001–2007

81. CIBIS-II investigators and committees: The Cardiac Insufficiency Bisoprolol Study II (CIBIS 2): a randomised trial. Lancet 1999;353:9–13

82. Pitt B, Martinez FA, Meures G et al, on behalf of the ELITE study investigators. Randomised trial of losartan versus captopril in patients over 65 with heart failure. Lancet 1997;349:747–752

83. Pitt B, Poole-Wilson PA, Sega R et al: Effect of losartan compared with captopril on mortality in patients with symptomatic heart failure: randomised trial. The Losartan Heart Failure Survival Study ELITE II. Lancet 2000;255:1582–1587

84. Cohn JN: Val-HeFT—Valsartan in Heart Failure Trial. Result presented at the American Heart Association Scientific Sessions, New Orleans, November 2000

85. The Digitalis Investigation Group: The effect of digoxin on mortality and morbidity in patients with heart failure. N Engl J Med 1997;336:525–533

86. McMurdo MET: Adverse drug reactions. Age Ageing 2000;29:5–6

87. Ginstead WC, Francis MJ, Marks GF: Discontinuation of chronic diuretic therapy in stable congestive heart failure secondary to coronary artery disease or idiopathic dilated cardiomyopathy. Am J Cardiol 1994;73:881–886

88. Olind B: Site and mechanism of action of the diuretics. Acta Pharmacol Toxicol 1984;54(1):5–15

89. Brater DC: Clinical pharmacokinetics of diuretics in cardiac insufficiency. Progr Pharmacol Clin Pharmacol 1992;9:363–370

90. Brater DC: Diuretic therapy. N Engl J Med 1998;339:387–395

91. Halstenson CE, Matzke GR: Bumetanide: a new loop diuretic. Drug Intell Clin Pharm 1983;17:786–797

92. Channer KS, McLean KA, Lawson-Matthew P: Combination diuretic treatment in severe heart failure: a randomised controlled trial. Br Heart J 1994;71:146–150

93. Gerlag PGG, van Meijel JJM: High-dose furosemide in the treatment of refractory congestive heart failure. Arch Intern Med 1988;148:286–291

94. Packer M: Are nitrates effective in the treatment of chronic heart failure? Antagonist's viewpoint. Am J Cardiol 1990;66:458–461

95. Kiyingi A, Field MJ, Pawsey CC et al: Metolazone in the treatment of severe refractory cardiac failure. Lancet 1990;335:29–31

96. Levy DW, Lye M: Diuretics and potassium in the elderly. J R Coll Physicians Lond 1987;21:148–152

97. Vermeulen A, Chadha DR: Slow-release frusemide and hydrochlorothiazide in congestive heart failure: a controlled trial. J Clin Pharmacol 1982;22:513–519

98. Dorup I, Sajaa K, Clausen T, Kjeldsen K: Reduced concentrations of potassium, magnesium and sodium-potassium pumps in human skeletal muscle during treatment with diuretics. BMJ 1988;296:455–458

99. McMurray J, McDevitt DG: Treatment of heart failure in the elderly. Br Med Bull 1990;46:202–229

100. David DS, Hitzig P: Diuretics and ototoxicity. N Engl J Med 1971;284:1328–1329

101. Walma EP, Hoes AW, van Dooren C et al: Withdrawal of long-term diuretic medication in elderly patients: a double blind randomised trial. BMJ 1997;315:464–468

102. Davis R, Ribner HS, Keung E et al: Treatment of chronic congestive heart failure with captopril, an oral inhibitor of angiotensin-converting enzyme. N Engl J Med 1979;301:117–121

103. Drexler H, Kurz S, Jeserich M et al: Effect of chronic ACE inhibition on endothelial function in patients with chronic heart failure. Am J Cardiol 1995;76(E):13–18

104. Dzau VJ, Re R: Tissue angiotensin system in cardiovascular medicine: a paradigm shift? Circulation 1994;89:493–498

105. Rump AFE, Rosen R, Korth A: Deleterious effect of exogenous angiotensin-I on the extent of regional ischaemia and its inhibition by captopril. Eur Heart J 1993;14:106–112

106. The Acute Infarction Ramipril Efficacy (AIRE) study investigators: Effect of ramipril on mortality and morbidity of survivors of acute myocardial infarction with clinical evidence of heart failure. Lancet 1993;342:821–888

107. MacDowall P, Kalra P, O'Donoghue DJ: Risk of morbidity from renovascular disease in elderly patients with congestive cardiac failure. Lancet 1998;352:13–16

108. Squire IB, MacFadyen RJ, Reid JL et al: Differing early blood pressure and renin–angiotensin system responses to the first dose of ACE inhibitors in congestive heart failure. Clin Cardiol 1996;19:1–15

109. The ATLAS investigators: Comparative effects of low-dose versus high-dose lisinopril on survival and major events in chronic heart failure: the Assessment of Treatment with Lisinopril and Survival (ATLAS) Study. Eur Heart J 1998;19:142 (abstract)

110. Hargreaves MR, Benson MK: Inhaled sodium cromoglycate in angiotensin-converting enzyme-inhibitor cough. Lancet 1995;345:13–16

111. Cleland JGF, Tendera M, Adamus J et al: Perindopril for elderly people with chronic heart failure: the PEP-CHF study. Eur J Heart Failure 1999;1:211–217

112. Waagstein F, Hjalmarson A, Varnauskas E: Effect of chronic beta-adrenergic receptor blockade in congestive cardiomyopathy. Br Heart J 1975;37:1022–1036

113. Paolisso G, Gambardella, Marrazo G: Metabolic and cardiovascular benefits derived from β-adrenergic blockade in chronic congestive heart failure. Am Heart J 1992;123:103–110

114. Bristow MR, Herschberger RE, Port JD et al: Beta-adrenergic pathways in non-failing and failing human ventricular myocardium. Circulation 1990;82(1):12–25

115. Waagstein F, Bristow M, Swedberg K et al: Beneficial effects of metoprolol in idiopathic dilated cardiomyopathy. Lancet 1993;342:1441–1446

116. Cleland JGF, Swedberg K: Carvedilol for heart failure, with care. Lancet 1996;347:1199–1200

117. Smith TW: Digitalis: mechanisms of action and clinical use. N Engl J Med 1988;318:358–365

118. Hayward R, Hammer J: Digitalis. Drugs for Heart Disease. Chapman & Hall, London, 1979

119. Stoffer SS, Hynes KM, Jiang NS et al: Digoxin and abnormal serum hormone levels. JAMA 1973;225:1643–1645

120. Uretsky BF, Young JB, Shahaidi FE et al: Randomised study assessing the effects of digoxin withdrawal in patients with mild to moderate chronic congestive heart failure. J Am Coll Cardiol 1993;22:955–962

121. Packer M, Gheorghiade M, Young JB et al: Withdrawal of digoxin from patients with chronic heart failure treated with angiotensin converting enzyme inhibitors. N Engl J Med 1993;329:1–7

122. Hughes SG: Prescribing for the elderly patient: why do we need to exercise caution? Br J Clin Pharmacol 1998;46:531–533

123. Sweet CS, Rucinska EJ: Losartan in heart failure: preclinical experiences and initial outcomes. Eur Heart J 1994;15:139–144

124. Ignarro LJ, Lippton H, Edwards JC et al: Mechanism of vascular smooth muscle relaxation by organic nitrates, nitrites, nitroprusside and nitric oxide: evidence for the involvement of S-nitrosothiols as active intermediates. J Pharmacol Exp Ther 1981;218:739–749

125. Swedberg K: Use of nitrates in acute and chronic congestive heart failure. Drugs 1987;33(4):147–149

126. Elkayam U, Roth A, Kumar A et al: Hemodynamic and volumetric effects of venodilation with nitroglycerin in chronic mitral regurgitation. Am J Cardiol 1987;60:1106–1111

127. Cohn JN, Archibald DG, Ziesche S et al: Effect of vasodilator therapy on mortality in chronic congestive heart failure: results of a Veterans Administration Cooperative Study. N Engl J Med 1986;314:1542–1547

128. Cotter G, Metzkor E, Kaluski E et al: Randomised trial of high-dose isosorbide dinitrate plus low-dose furosemide versus high-dose furosemide plus low-dose isosorbide dinitrate in severe pulmonary oedema. Lancet 1998;351:389–393

129. Packer M, O'Connor CM, Ghali JK et al: Effect of amlodipine on morbidity and mortality in severe chronic heart failure. N Engl J Med 1996;335:1107–1114

130. Dies FKM, Whitlow P, Liang CS et al: Intermittent dobutamine in ambulatory outpatients with chronic heart failure. Circulation 1986;74:138

131. Cowley AJ, Skene AM: Treatment of severe heart failure: quantity or quality of life? A trial of enoximone: enoximone investigators. Br Heart J 1994;72:226–230

132. Packer M, Rouleau JL, Swedberg K et al: Effect of flosequinan on survival in chronic heart failure: preliminary results of the profile study. Circulation 1993;88:301

133. Anon: Is aspirin safe for patients with heart failure? Br Heart J 1995;74:215–219

134. Raffaeli S, Paciaroni E: Stroke and atrial fibrillation: risks, prevention and therapy in the elderly. Arch Gerontol Geriatr 1995;20:23–28

135. Doval HC, Nul DR, Grancelli HO et al: Randomised trial of low dose amiodarone in severe congestive heart failure. Lancet 1994;344:493–498

136. Singh BN, Fletcher RD, Fisher SG et al: Amiodarone in patients with congestive heart failure and asymptomatic ventricular arrhythmia. N Engl J Med 1995;333:77–82

Chapter 34

Diagnosis and management of coronary artery disease

Susan J. Zieman, Donald D. Tresch, Haritha R. Alla, and

Gary Gerstenblith

The diagnosis and management of coronary artery disease in older individuals is an increasingly frequent and complex challenge. Although those aged over 65 years make up only about 13 percent of the total US population, they represent the majority of those with coronary disease. Approximately 60 percent of acute myocardial infarctions occur in persons 65 years or older, and 85 percent of all cardiovascular deaths occur in this age group.[1] Improvements in risk factor identification and reduction as well as advances in the diagnosis and treatment of ischemic heart disease in the young and middle-aged populations have led to increased numbers of older individuals with, or at increased risk for, coronary disease. Not only is coronary disease more common with increasing age, but it is also associated with increased morbidity and mortality. Nearly half of the deaths in this age group are due to cardiovascular causes and the vast majority of all cardiovascular deaths occur in the elderly.[2] In fact, age is now recognized as the most significant risk factor for ischemic heart disease. This chapter reviews how the aging process influences the incidence, presentation, and management of coronary artery disease.

PHYSIOLOGICAL CHANGES ASSOCIATED WITH CARDIAC AGING

There are several changes in cardiovascular parameters associated with the normal aging process which increase the likelihood for the development of cardiovascular disease, complicate its management, and increase the incidence of adverse consequences following an ischemic insult. These changes include an increase in central arterial stiffness, a decrease in β-adrenergic responsiveness, and a decrease in early left ventricular diastolic filling.[3]

Altered vascular properties

Age-associated alterations in both the structural and dynamic properties result in important physiological changes, including decreased compliance and increased afterload. The structural alterations in the large arteries which promote stiffness include a decrease and fraying of elastin fibers and an increase in collagen content. The former may be related to increased elastase activity with age[4] and the latter to increased transforming growth factor beta (TGF-β) expression.[5,6]

Age-associated changes in the dynamic properties of arterial compliance are manifest by diminished endothelial responsiveness. Nitric oxide, a mediator of local vasodilation, plays a major role in endothelial reactivity. With vascular aging, the response to acetylcholine,[7] and the brachial artery response to flow-mediated vasodilation,[8] are diminished. In aging animal models, endothelial dysfunction is probably not caused by diminished activity of nitric oxide synthase, the enzyme which produces nitric oxide.[9,10] Interestingly, the levels of plasma asymmetric dimethylarginine, a competitive inhibitor of nitric oxide synthase, rise with increasing age.[11] Other factors which limit, or result in defective, nitric oxide production may also contribute to the age-associated endothelial dysfunction. Manifestations of endothelial dysfunction in other settings include expression of adhesion molecules, loss of the permeability barrier, migration and proliferation of smooth muscle cells and fibroblasts, decreased lytic activity, and increased likelihood for vasoconstriction and resultant plaque disruption. Thus, endothelial dysfunction is involved in nearly every step in the development, progression, and manifestations of coronary atherosclerotic disease.

Increased central arterial stiffness has notable effects on cardiovascular hemodynamics. Decreased vascular compliance increases both the arterial systolic pressure load and the pulse wave velocity. Increased pulse wave velocity results in the reflected pulse wave returning to the central aorta in late systole, augmenting systolic pressure, rather than in early diastole, resulting in decreased diastolic pressure. The most common noninvasive index of increased stiffness is an age-associated rise in pulse pressure. In fact, pulse pressure is now recognized as one of the most important determinants of cardiovascular risk in the older population.[12–14] Increased pulse pressure is also a powerful and independent predictor of outcomes in the postinfarction setting,[15] and a significant predictor for the development of heart failure in elderly people.[16] Increased vascular stiffness also shifts the pressure–volume relationship such that, for any given alteration in intravascular volume, the resulting pressure change is greater in the older individual.[17] This alteration in the pressure–volume relationship manifests clinically as a reduction in the threshold for symptoms, including an increased likelihood for orthostatic changes in the setting of dehydration or over-diuresis, and for hypertension and pulmonary edema in the setting of volume overload. Interventions which decrease stiffness are associated with lower cardiac volumes for any given output and increased aerobic exercise capacity in older individuals,[18,19] and may represent an attractive therapeutic goal in older patients with, or at risk for, cardiovascular disease. Age-associated alterations in endothelial dysfunction can be improved with exercise in humans[20,21] and with angiotensin converting enzyme inhibition in animal models.[22]

Decreased responsiveness to β-adrenergic stimulation

Both animal and human data indicate that aging is associated with decreased cardiovascular β-adrenergic responsiveness. This is true for the inotropic,[23–25] chronotropic,[26] and vasodilating[27] effects of these agents. This diminished response is not due to decreased elaboration of catecholamines, but rather to age-associated changes in cardiac β-adrenergic receptor signaling. This is indicated by decreased L-type sarcolemmal calcium-channel availability and calcium influx in response to β-adrenergic receptor stimulation in aged animal models.[28,29] This change would be expected to decrease the cardiovascular reserve capacity in older individuals following an ischemic, as well as other, insults.

Delayed early left ventricular relaxation

Another important physiological change associated with cardiac aging is prolonged contraction and decreased early ventricular diastolic filling. There are several potential mechanisms, including alterations in intracellular calcium cycling due to slowed inactivation of the L-type calcium current,[30] reduced outwardly directed potassium current,[30] decreased sarcoplasmic reticulum pump activity[31] and site density,[32] and decreased percentage of myosin isozyme that has the most rapid adenosine triphosphate (ATP) hydrolytic rate.[33] Additional potential mechanisms include increased ventricular fibrosis, wall thickness, and heterogeneity during relaxation.[34] From a clinical standpoint, these changes would be expected to exacerbate abnormalities in ischemic-induced diastolic properties and to compromise diastolic filling during tachyarrhythmias. Older individuals, therefore, would be more likely than younger people to experience dyspneic symptoms for any given ischemic or tachycardiac insult.

STUDY OF ISCHEMIC HEART DISEASE IN ELDERLY PEOPLE

Before reviewing the data on ischemic heart disease in the elderly, it is important to evaluate their applicability. Although best practices are largely based on prospective randomized trials, the inclusion of older subjects in these studies continues to be limited. Explanations for their exclusion include increased comorbidities (including diabetes and vascular, renal, hepatic, and pulmonary diseases), alterations in drug metabolism, atypical presentation of conditions, cognitive and consent issues, frailty, the existence of another life-threatening condition, and social limitations. Many recommendations are derived from observational databases and carry with them the limits of such data. Because the incidence and severity of coronary disease increase with age, future work should focus on this age group.

RISK FACTORS FOR CORONARY ARTERY DISEASE

Recent studies indicate that elderly people benefit as much as younger individuals do from aggressive risk-factor reduction. In fact, since the absolute risk is so much greater in the older population, the absolute reduction in events for any given relative risk reduction resulting from these interventions is greater than it is in the younger population.

Hypertension/pulse pressure

Although studies have not specifically targeted reduced pulse pressure as a therapeutic goal, two large studies[35,36] indicate that treatment of isolated systolic hypertension (associated, by definition, with a widened pulse pressure) decreases myocardial infarction or death, as well as congestive heart failure, and dementia, in those 60 years or over. The benefit is particularly marked in older individuals with diabetes.[37]

Lipids

Elevated lipids are associated with increased risk in the older population and HMG Co-A reductase therapy provides both primary and secondary prevention benefits. In the Established Populations for Epidemiologic Studies of the Elderly report,[38] there was a 17 percent increase in the risk for coronary heart disease death for every one unit increase in the total cholesterol/HDL cholesterol ratio in nearly 5000 men and women 71 years and older. HDL cholesterol was also related to coronary outcomes in women and in those over 80 years. In the AFCAPS/TexCAPS[39] and West of Scotland Coronary Prevention[40] studies, there was significant reduction in the risks of nonfatal myocardial infarction and coronary heart disease death in the older age groups assigned to lovastatin and pravastatin, respectively; and in the CARE trial,[41] secondary prevention with pravastatin resulted in decreased cardiovascular events in 65–75 year old patients following myocardial infarction. In the "4S" trial,[42] simvastatin therapy was associated with a 0.73 relative risk of all-cause mortality and a 0.71 relative risk of a major coronary event, defined as coronary death, nonfatal myocardial infarction, or cardiac arrest in those 60 years of age or older.

Tobacco use

Another important remediable coronary risk factor in the elderly is cigarette smoking. The effects of smoking cessation were evaluated in a subset of participants in the CASS Registry.[43] The relative risk (and confidence limits) of myocardial infarction or death over a 6-year period for those who continued to smoke, as compared to those who stopped, was 2.9 (1.4, 5.9) for those men and women 70 years of age and older, and 1.5 (1.0, 2.3) for those aged 65–69 years. These were similar to, or greater than, the benefit in those under 65 years of age. Thus, there is strong suggestive evidence that older patients reduce cardiac risk when they stop smoking.

Estrogen status

As age increases, the ratio of women to men in the patient population with ischemic heart disease also increases. Although observational studies indicated that post-menopausal estrogen use was associated with a decrease in cardiovascular events,[44] and acute estrogen administration improves endothelial responsiveness in post-menopausal women,[45] a large prospective randomized secondary prevention trial demonstrated no overall benefit.[46] Thus, at the present time, estrogen cannot be recommended for primary or secondary cardiovascular prevention.

Other risk factors

There are other risk factors associated with coronary disease and mortality in the elderly population, although no prospective randomized trials indicate that changing these risk factors changes cardiovascular outcomes in this population. Obesity is one factor. In a study of over 41,000 elderly women, body fat distribution indexed by the waist to hip ratio (but not body mass index) was associated with a strong, monotonic increase in the risk of cardiovascular and total mortality.[47] The waist to hip ratio is also the best marker for the metabolic hazards of obesity, including insulin resistance, hypertension, and hyperlipidemia.[48]

Other factors associated with cardiovascular outcomes in older individuals are physical activity status,[49] dietary antioxidant flavonoid intake,[50] plasma fibrinogen and factor VIII activity,[51] depression,[52] insulin resistance syndrome,[53] polymorphisms for ACE and PAI-1,[54] and dietary, although not supplemental vitamin E, intake.[55]

DIAGNOSIS AND EVALUATION OF CORONARY DISEASE

The diagnosis of coronary disease in an older individual should be considered with the realization that although silent ischemia is undoubtedly present in individuals of all age groups, it is particularly likely in the aged. In patients referred to a medical center for stress testing, the prevalence of exercise-induced silent ischemia increased from 7 percent in those under 50 years of age to 36 percent in those 70 years or older.[56] In a report of 470 asymptomatic volunteers from the Baltimore Longitudinal Study of Aging, the prevalence of exercise-induced silent ischemia, defined by both electrocardiographic and thallium scintigraphic criteria, increased from 2 percent in the fifth decade to 15 percent in the ninth decade of life.[57] The true, or autopsy, prevalence of significant stenoses is several-fold higher than the clinical prevalence if the latter is judged by symptoms of exertional chest discomfort or history of a myocardial infarction. In an autopsy study reported by investigators from the Mayo Clinic, 72 percent of men and 54 percent of women 70 years or older had 75 percent or greater stenoses of at least one major coronary artery.[58] The high prevalence of silent, or unrecognized, ischemia may be due to a diminished sensation of chest discomfort, the increased likelihood that ischemia will be manifest as dyspnea rather than more typical pain symptoms, an age-associated decline in physical activity to a level at which symptoms are not present, and the fact that other, superimposed diseases may render the older individual less likely to exercise to the point at which anginal symptoms occur.

It is important, therefore, to go beyond just a negative history if a degree of certainty is required regarding the absence of significant ischemic disease in the elderly person. Often the most useful objective test is the exercise electrocardiogram. Although the specificity is somewhat less in the older age group,[59] it is generally useful with some known caveats. The first is that the predictive accuracy of a positive test is low in the setting of an abnormal baseline electrocardiogram. This is more likely in older individuals because of the increased prevalence of left bundle branch block, left ventricular hypertrophy, and digitalis ingestion. In these circumstances, an exercise imaging exam would be useful. It should also be noted that the predictive accuracy of a negative test is low in a population with a high prevalence of disease. Thus, a negative test in an older man with risk factors and some symptoms, who may have an 80 percent pretest likelihood of disease, may still be associated with a 50 percent post-test likelihood of significant disease. A third concern in the older population is an inability, because of other medical problems such as arthritis or pulmonary insufficiency, to exercise to 85–90 percent of the predicted maximum heart rate. In this setting, the predictive accuracy of a negative test is low, and pharmacological testing with dipyridamole, adenosine, or dobutamine in conjunction with electrocardiographic, isotope, or echocardiographic monitoring is useful.[60,61] For patients in whom good-quality echocardiograms can be obtained, this tool provides additional information that may be particularly useful in the older individual. These include the significance of aortic stenosis (which is often associated with anginal symptoms in the elderly), aortic sclerosis (an additional risk factor for coronary disease in the older population), the presence of left ventricular hypertrophy, and global and regional assessment of left ventricular function. The sensitivity and specificity of exercise echocardiography were 88 percent and 82 percent, respectively, and comparable to those with exercise thallium imaging. The sensitivities of dobutamine and dipyridamole echocardiography were 82 and 74 percent and specificities were 82 and 77 percent, respectively, for diagnosing the presence of coronary disease.[61]

Prognosis in patients with stable coronary disease is dependent upon coronary anatomy and left ventricular function. Although the severity of symptoms is one means of evaluating the severity of atherosclerosis, their absence, or the presence of only minimal symptoms, particularly in the older age groups, cannot be relied upon to indicate the presence of only minimal disease. In this situation as well, the noninvasive stress electrocardiogram is useful, not only in diagnosing disease, but also in assessing the likelihood of triple vessel or left main coronary stenoses.[62]

TREATMENT OF CORONARY DISEASE

It is often useful to consider whether noncardiac factors which increase demand determinants and/or decrease oxygen supply are present in the older individual with new-onset angina or a change in anginal pattern. Anemia, for example, frequently presents with ischemic symptoms in this age group. Hyperthyroidism in the elderly person often presents with cardiac manifestations, including arrhythmias and ischemia, rather than noncardiac symptoms, which are more common in the young. Emotional stress, weight gain, fever, supraventricular arrhythmias, hypertension, congestive heart failure, and medication noncompliance may also be responsible for new-onset or worsening angina. Identification and reversal of these precipitating factors, therefore, may return the older individual to the symptomatic status enjoyed previously.

Medical therapy

If medical therapy is needed, sublingual nitrates are the most effective agents for the relief of an acute ischemic episode. Continuous nitrates alone, however, are not capable of providing continuous prophylaxis because of tolerance, which is present for oral, topical, as well as continuous intravenous use. Therefore, a nitrate-free interval of 12–14 hours is generally recommended for patients using longacting nitrate preparations.

Tolerance is not an issue with β-blockers and these are excellent agents in patients with stable, exertional angina. The choice of an anti-ischemic β-blocker can be based on associated medical conditions and patient convenience. These can be used to decide whether to use a hydrophilic or lipophilic agent, as well as whether to use a relatively cardioselective agent. The latter, however, are cardioselective in only low doses and may lose their relative selectivity when moderate and high doses are employed. An additional consideration in the post-infarction patient is whether the β-blocker provides secondary prevention. Side-effects of β-blocker therapy in the older patient include mood changes, sleep disturbances, and fatigue. In patients who are intolerant of β-blocker, or who require additional medical therapy, calcium antagonists can be considered. The agents limiting heart rate may be more useful in patients not on β-blocker therapy, and the longacting dihydropyridine agents in those who are receiving β-blockers. For patients who continue to experience ischemic symptoms despite pharmacological therapy and who are not candidates for revascularization procedures, external counter-pulsation may be helpful. Aspirin, if not contraindicated, should also be considered in all patients with the diagnosis of coronary disease. ACE-inhibitor therapy may also provide secondary prevention in patients with coronary disease. In the HOPE trial, ramipril was shown to decrease cardiovascular events or death in older, as well as younger, high-risk individuals—defined as those with coronary disease or with diabetes and an additional risk factor.[63]

Age-associated changes in pharmacokinetics should also be considered. The decrease in lean body mass and increase in adipose tissue affects the volume of drug distribution, and the decreases in hepatic blood flow and renal glomerular filtration rate affect drug metabolism and excretion. In addition, concurrent comorbid conditions increase the potential for adverse drug reactions, as does polypharmacy.

Coronary angioplasty

Angioplasty is an increasingly attractive option in elderly individuals with continued symptoms despite medical therapy. This is particularly true in those who are at increased risk with bypass surgery because it avoids the thoracotomy, general anesthesia, and prolonged convalescence associated with surgery.

Although the National Heart, Lung, and Blood Institute (NHLBI) Percutaneous Transluminal Coronary Angioplasty (PTCA) registry initially reported a lower success rate and a higher complication rate, including death and need for subsequent bypass surgery, in patients over 65 years of age,[64] the development of new techniques, the introduction of stents, the use of IIB/IIIA inhibitors, and increased experience in the treatment of multivessel disease have increased the number of elderly people who are likely to experience significantly improved symptoms with angioplasty.

In a recent pooled analysis[65] comparing the results of coronary artery angioplasty and stenting in a total of 6186 patients, the 301 who were older than 80 years had a higher prevalence of moderate-to-severe target lesion calcification (30.4 vs 15.3 percent), and smaller reference vessel diameter (2.9 vs 2.98 mm), but a similar procedural success rate (97.4 vs 98.5 percent). However, in-hospital and 1-year mortality were higher (1.33 vs 0.1 percent and 5.65 vs 1.41 percent, respectively) as were bleeding complications (4.98 vs 1.00 percent). Clinical restenosis (11.19 and 11.93 percent) was similar in the two groups.

In another report[66] comparing results in those 70–79 years of age and those 80 years and above, angiographic success per lesion was 99 percent and 96 percent, respectively; and the incidences of in-hospital death (1.1 and 1.5 percent), myocardial infarction (2.9 and 6.2 percent), emergency CABG (1.3 and 0 percent), and local vascular complications (4.4 and 4.6 percent) were all comparable in the two groups, although the older group had a two-day longer hospital stay.

In a randomized trial of stent angioplasty versus bypass surgery for patients with multivessel coronary disease,[67] age older than 65 years was associated with a 2.22 odds ratio for death, myocardial infarction, stroke, and repeat procedure at 30 days in men, but was not associated with an increased risk for these events in women, or in the overall population.

It is important to note, however, that mortality in older individuals following angioplasty varies considerably and is strongly influenced by comorbidities, including acute myocardial infarction, ejection fraction, renal insufficiency, diabetes, and advanced age.[68]

Coronary bypass surgery

Consistent with the aging of the population and the age-associated increase in incidence and severity of coronary disease, the number of elderly—and the proportion which they represent of the total bypass population—is rapidly increasing.[69,70] In view of the fact that surgery is often reserved for older patients who have few other options, it is not surprising that perioperative survival is lower, and complications higher in this age group.

In 24,461 Medicare recipients 80 years of age or older who underwent bypass surgery,[69] in-hospital, 1-year, and 3-year mortality were 11.5, 19.3, and 28.8 percent, respectively. Although the perioperative risk is high, the long-term survival rate for these patients was actually similar to that of the general US octogenarian population.

The major predictors of operative mortality in the elderly population are left ventricular function, prior bypass surgery, female sex, the presence of peripheral vascular disease, and diabetes, whereas prior angioplasty is protective.[70]

The presence of comorbidities, including pulmonary and renal dysfunction, is also important. Advanced age is another important predictor of stroke, transient ischemic attack and cognitive decline following bypass operations. Among 2118 patients from 24 US centers undergoing the operation, age was an important predictor of both type 1 (focal injury, stupor, or coma) and type 2 (deterio-ration in intellectual function, memory deficit, or seizures) adverse cerebral outcomes.[71] Age is also a predictor of long-term, 5-year, cognitive decline following CABG.[72] It is possible that improved predictors of such outcomes and new operative techniques[73] may improve postoperative results in the elderly population.

ACUTE MYOCARDIAL INFARCTION

Symptoms of myocardial infarction (MI) in an elderly person are more likely to include dyspnea and those related to decreased cardiac output, including mental status changes, rather than typical chest pain.[74] Older individuals are also more likely to be female, experience a non-Q-wave myocardial infarction,[75,76] and have an enzyme pattern consisting of an elevated MB fraction in the presence of a normal total creatinine kinase (CK).[77]

Treatment of acute myocardial infarction in the elderly should be tempered by the knowledge that older individuals are several-fold more likely than their younger counterparts to suffer serious complications of the infarct, including death, congestive heart failure, recurrent infarction, and rupture.[78,79] The influence of age on mortality in patients with first myocardial infarction was reported by the Gruppo Italiano per lo Studio della Sopravvivenza mell'Infarto Miocardio (GISSI)-2 investigators.[78] In over 9700 patients receiving thrombolytic therapy for acute infarcts, mortality, congestive heart failure, and echocardiographic evidence of left ventricular dysfunction increased with age. There was no increase, however, in the investigators' measures of infarct size, including CK elevation and number of electrocardiographic leads involved with the infarct. The most striking finding on autopsy was a marked age-related increased finding of rupture. Rupture was present in over 80 percent of those older than 70 years of age who died and had autopsy examination. It is not clear why this was so high, particularly since there was no age-related increase in the extent of fixed coronary disease in these patients with first myocardial infarction. The rupture finding may relate to impaired healing in older individuals; to increased load on the infarcted regions because the noninfarcted territory cannot compensate as well for the myocardium lost as a result of the infarct; or to the fact that all of the patients received thrombolytic therapy.

The Thrombolysis in Myocardial Infarction (TIMI)-2 investigators also studied the impact of age on outcomes and the influence of postlytic management strategies in older infarction patients.[79] They reported an age associated increase in mortality, complications, and recurrent infarctions. This may have been linked to an age-related increase in delay in administration of the thrombolytic, perhaps due to the increased likelihood of atypical presentations in the older population, and to the fact that fewer older individuals were eligible to receive concomitant β-blocker therapy. There was no difference in

clinical outcomes between those 65–74 years of age who were randomized to an early intervention strategy with catheterization and revascularization, and patients who underwent an early conservative strategy in which revascularization was performed only if they had evidence of recurrent ischemia during the early post-infarction period.

There are several limitations of thrombolytic therapy, and some of these are particularly relevant in the older population. Older individuals are less likely to be eligible to receive thrombolytic therapy because of hypertension and/or a history of central nervous system disease or other major bleeding. Best results are probably achieved with TIMI-3 flow; this is present in only about 60 percent of patients who undergo lysis. In addition, the risks of thrombolytic therapy may be increased in the older population, particularly in women.[80] In a recent analysis of the Cooperative Cardiovascular Project database,[81] thrombolytic therapy was associated with a 30-day survival benefit for those 65–75 years of age, but with a 38 percent increased 30-day mortality for those 76–86 years of age. In the first PAMI trial, separate results were not reported for those over 70 years of age.[82] However, in a meta-analysis combining the Primary Angioplasty in Myocardial Infarction (PAMI) results with a Netherlands trial,[83] primary angioplasty was associated with a significant survival advantage and a decrease in stroke risk, as compared to thrombolytic therapy in those 70 years of age or older. More recent randomized reports,[84,85] as well as another analysis of the Cooperative Cardiovascular Project database comparing outcomes in Medicare beneficiaries who underwent primary angioplasty or thrombolytic therapy,[86] all suggest improved outcomes with angioplasty. In the latter study, the 30-day and 1-year adjusted hazard ratios of death were 0.74 and 0.88 for those who received primary angioplasty as compared with lytic therapy.

The benefits of post-infarction β-blocker and aspirin therapy are present in the older population, although significant numbers of Medicare patients are not prescribed these effective therapies.[87,88] Older post-infarction patients with congestive heart failure and left ventricular dysfunction benefit from ACE-inhibitor therapy as well,[89,90] although the survival advantage is less clear in lower-risk individuals and therapy should be individualized because of the increased risk of renal insufficiency in this population. As noted above, statin therapy decreases adverse events in older post-infarction patients; and in the Cholesterol and Recurrent Events Trial, lipid-lowering therapy decreased cardiac death or nonfatal myocardial infarction by 39 percent in those 65–75 years of age.[41]

Advanced age is also associated with increased adverse outcomes in patients with unstable angina or non-Q-wave myocardial infarctions and is, in fact, the most powerful risk factor in this patient population. Other markers include dynamic ST changes, evidence of associated left ventricular dysfunction, prior aspirin use, diabetes, multiple cardiac risk factors, and elevated biochemical markers.[91] The level of risk is important in determining the site of care as well as the need for therapies associated with increased risk themselves. Intensive medical therapy in a monitored setting is indicated for high-risk elderly patients. While thrombolysis is beneficial in patients with acute ST-elevation MI, it is of no value in the treatment of unstable angina or non-ST-elevation infarction.

Aspirin, β-blockers, and nitroglycerin are indicated, and unfractionated heparin or low-molecular-weight heparin also carry a class I indication.[92] Low-molecular-weight heparin is associated with broader activity, more predictable anticoagulant effect, and easier administration. The use of enoxaparin is associated with a reduction of MI, death, or recurrent ischemia, as compared with unfractionated heparin, in patients with acute coronary syndrome.[93] The addition of a glycoprotein IIb/IIIa inhibitor to aspirin and heparin improves short-term outcomes of death, myocardial infarction, and recurrent ischemia.[94] Although the risk of any hemorrhage is increased, there is no increase in major hemorrhage or intracerebral bleeding, and age should not be considered a contraindication for this therapy. A recent study has also indicated that early use of aggressive lipid lowering with statin therapy is beneficial in patients with acute coronary syndrome as well.[95]

The use of early coronary angiography and revascularization is indicated in patients with unstable angina or non-ST-elevation infarction whose symptoms are refractory to medical therapy. The role of routine catheterization and revascularization in these patients is more controversial, with studies comparing early invasive and early conservative strategies reporting different results. The VANQUISH study[96] found increased adverse outcomes with the early invasive approach. The more recent FRISC II study,[97] however, reported that patients treated with early catheterization and revascularization experienced fewer deaths or nonfatal infarctions, with a particular benefit in the older subgroup.

It is also important to note that cardiac rehabilitation is an important component of post-infarction care of an elderly person. Significant reductions in weight and lipid parameters as well as improvements in exercise capacity occur following cardiac rehabilitation programs in those over age 75 years.[98–100]

KEY POINTS   Coronary artery disease

- The incidence, prevalence, and adverse events associated with ischemic disease all increase dramatically with increasing age. This is related to altered physiology accompanying the normal aging process, an increased likelihood of co-existing disease, and altered response to many therapeutic interventions.

- Important physiologic changes likely include increased central vascular stiffness, decreased endothelial responsiveness, diminished response to beta adrenergic sympathetic stimulation, and slowed early diastolic filling.

- Identification and aggressive treatment of risk factors decreases cardiovascular risk in the older population. Non-traditional risk factors, including obesity, pulse pressure, physical activity status, depression, and insulin resistance, may be particularly important in the elderly.

- The diagnosis of coronary disease is often difficult because of the increased likelihood of atypical presentations, decreased activity status, and an abnormal baseline electrocardiogram.

- The goals of medical therapy for coronary artery disease are the same in the older and younger populations. These include reducing myocardial oxygen demand and increasing supply determinants. It is also important to identify any reversible precipitants in the older population, such as anemia, thyroid disease, and infection.

- Coronary interventions, including angioplasty and bypass surgery, are often safe and effective in the older population. However, in the presence of renal, peripheral vascular, and/or pulmonary disease, the risks are increased and in these settings, a careful weighing of the risks and benefits of aggressive therapy and patient preferences should be carefully considered.

- The mortality associated with acute myocardial infarction is markedly increased with age. Non-Q wave myocardial infarctions are more common. Primary angioplasty, if available, is usually preferred to thrombolytic therapy. Secondary prevention strategies are particularly useful in the older population and these should not be denied this age group because of a hypothetical concern for adverse effects. Cardiac rehabilitation is usually safe, preserves functional status, and improves outcomes.

ACKNOWLEDGMENTS

Dr. Zieman is an E. Cowles Adrus Scholar.

This work was supported in part by contract NOI-AG-82109 from the National Institute on Aging.

REFERENCES

1. American Heart Association: Heart and Stroke Statistical Update. AHA, Dallas, TX, 2000
2. Thom T, Epstein F: Heart disease, cancer, and stroke mortality trends and their interactions: an international perspective. Circulation 1994;90:574–582
3. Lakatta EG: Cardiovascular regulatory mechanisms in advanced age. Physiol Rev 1993;73:413
4. Robert L: Aging of the vascular wall and atherogenesis: Role of elastin–laminin receptor. Atherosclerosis 1996;123:169
5. Li Z, Froehlich J, Galis ZS et al: Increased expression of matrix metalloproteinase-2 in the thickened intima of aged rats. Hypertension 1999;33:116
6. Takasaki I, Chobanian AV, Sarzani R et al: Effect of hypertension on fibronectin expression in the rat aorta. J Biol Chem 1990;265:21:935
7. Egashira K, Inou T, Hirooka Y et al: Effects of age on endothelium-dependent vasodilation of resistance coronary artery by acetylcholine in humans. Circulation 1993;88:77–81
8. Celermajer DS, Sorensen KE, Spiegelhalter DJ et al: Aging is associated with endothelial dysfunction in healthy men years before the age-related decline in women. JACC 1994;24:471–476
9. Cernadas MR, de Miguel LS, Garcia-Duran M et al: Expression of constitutive and inducible nitric oxide synthases in the vascular wall of young and aging rats. Circ Res 1998;83:279–286
10. Zieman SJ, Gerstenblith G, Lakatta EG et al: Upregulation of the nitric oxide-cGMP pathway in aged myocardium: physiological response to L-arginine. Circ Res 2001;88:97–102
11. Miyazaki H, Matsuoka H, Cooke JP et al: Endogenous nitric oxide synthase inhibitor: a novel marker of atherosclerosis. Circulation 1999;99:1141–1146
12. Franklin SS, Larson MG, Khan SA et al: Does the relation of blood pressure to coronary heart disease risk change with aging? Circulation 2001;103:1245–1249
13. Franklin SS, Khan SA, Wong ND, Larson MG, Levy D: Is pulse pressure useful in predicting risk for coronary heart disease? The Framingham Heart Study. Circulation 1999;100:354–360
14. Lee M-LT, Rosner BA, Weiss ST: Relationship of blood pressure to cardiovascular death: the effects of pulse pressure in the elderly. Ann Epidemiol 1999;9:101–107

15. Mitchell GF, Moye LA, Braunwald E et al: Sphygmomanometrically determined pulse pressure is a powerful independent predictor of recurrent events after myocardial infarction in patients with impaired left ventricular function. Circulation 1997;96:4254–4260
16. Chae CU, Pfeffer MA, Glynn RJ et al: Increased pulse pressure and risk of heart failure in the elderly. JAMA 1999;33:951
17. Chen CH, Nakayama M, Nevo E et al: Coupled systolic-ventricular and vascular stiffening with age: implications for pressure regulation and cardiac reserve in the elderly. J Am Coll Cardiol 1998;32:1221
18. Nussbacher A, Gerstenblith G, O'Connor FC et al: Hemodynamic effects of unloading the old heart. Am J Physiol 1999;277:H1863–H1871
19. Chen FH, Nakayama M, Talbot M et al: Verapamil acutely reduces ventricular-vascular stiffening and improves aerobic exercise performance in elderly individuals. J Am Coll Cardiol 1999;33:1602–1609
20. Higashi Y, Sasaki S, Kurisu S et al: Regular aerobic exercise augments endothelium-dependent vascular relaxation in normotensive as well as hypertensive subjects: role of endothelium-derived nitric oxide. Circulation 1999;100:1194–1202
21. Rywik TM, Blackman MR, Zink RC et al: Endurance training improves endothelial function in older men. J Appl Physiol 1999;87:2136–2142
22. Michel JB, Heudes D, Michel O et al: Effect of chronic ANG I-converting enzyme inhibition on aging processes. II: Large arteries. Am J Physiol 1994;267:R124–R135
23. Lakatta EG, Gerstenblith G, Angell CS et al: Diminished inotropic response of aged myocardium to catecholamines. Circ Res 1975;36:262–269
24. Guarnieri T, Filburn CH, Zitnik G et al: Contractile and biochemical correlates of beta-adrenergic stimulation of the aged heart. Am J Physiol 1980;239:H501–H508
25. Jiang MT, Moffat MP, Narayanaan N: Age-related alterations in the phosphorylation of sarcoplasmic reticulum and myofibrillator proteins and diminished contractile response to isoproterenol in intact rat ventricle. Circ Res 1993;72:102–111
26. Yin FCP, Spurgeon HA, Greene HI et al: Age-associated decrease in heart rate response to isoproterenol in dogs. Mech Ageing Dev 1979;10:17–25
27. Pam HY, Hoffman RR, Perskin RA et al: Decline in beta adrenergic receptor-mediated vascular relaxation with aging in man. J Pharmacol Exp Ther 1986;239:802–807
28. Xiao R-P, Spurgeon HA, O'Connor F et al: Age-associated changes in beta-adrenergic modulation on rat cardiac excitation–contraction coupling. J Clin Invest 1994;94:2051
29. Xiao R-P, Tomhave ED, Xiangwu J et al: Age-associated reductions in cardiac beta one- and beta two-adrenoceptor responses without changes in inhibitory G proteins or receptor kinases. J Clin Invest 1998;101:1273
30. Walker KE, Lakatta EG, Houser SR: Age associated changes in membrane currents in rat ventricular myocytes. Cardiovasc Res 1993;27:1968
31. Froehlich JP, Lakatta EG, Beard E et al: Studies of sarcoplasmic reticulum function and contraction duration in young and aged rat myocardium. J Mol Cell Cardiol 1978;10:427–438
32. Tate CA, Taffet GE, Hudson EK et al: Enhanced calcium uptake of cardiac sarcoplasmic reticulum in exercise-trained old rats. Am J Physiol 1990;258:H431
33. Effron MB, Bhatnagar GM, Spurgeon HA et al: Changes in myosin isoenzymes, ATPase activity and contraction duration in rat cardiac muscle with aging can be modified by thyroxine. Circ Res 1987;60:238
34. Bonow RO, Vitale DF, Bacharach SL, Maron BJ, Green MV: Effects of aging on asynchronous left ventricular regional function and global ventricular filling in normal human subjects. J Am Coll Cardiol 1988;11:50–58
35. SHEP Cooperative Research Group: Prevention of stroke by antihypertensive drug treatment in older persons with isolated systolic hypertension. JAMA 1991;265:3255
36. Staessen JA, Fagard R, Thijs L et al: Randomized double-blind comparison of placebo and active treatment for older persons with isolated systolic hypertension. Lancet 1997;350:757
37. Tuomilehto J, Rastenyte D, Birkenhaber WH et al: Effects of calcium-channel blockade in older patients with diabetes and systolic hypertension. N Engl J Med 1999;340:677–684
38. Corti M-C, Guralnik JM, Salive ME et al: HDL cholesterol predicts coronary heart disease mortality in older persons. JAMA 1995;274:539–544
39. Downs JR, Clearfield M, Weis S et al: Primary prevention of acute coronary events with lovastatin in men and women with average cholesterol levels. JAMA 1998;279:1615–1622
40. Shepherd J, Cobbe SM, Ford I et al: Prevention of coronary heart disease with pravastatin in men with hypercholesterolemia. N Engl J Med 1995;333:1301–1307
41. Lewis SJ, Moye LA, Sacks FM et al: Effect of pravastatin on cardiovascular events in older patients with myocardial infarction and cholesterol levels in the average range. Ann Intern Med 1998;129:681–689
42. Scandinavian Simvastatin Survival Study Group: Randomized trial of cholesterol lowering in 4444 patients with coronary heart disease: the Scandinavian Simvastatin Survival Study (4S). Lancet 1994;344:1383–1389
43. Hermanson B, Omenn GS, Kronmal RA, Gersh BJ: Beneficial six-year outcome of smoking cessation in older men and women with coronary artery disease: results from the CASS registry. N Engl J Med 1988;319:1365–1369
44. Stampfer MJ, Colditz GA, Wilett WC et al: Postmenopausal estrogen therapy and cardiovascular disease: ten-year follow-up from the Nurses' Health Study. N Engl J Med 1991;325:756–762
45. Reis SE, Gloth ST, Blumenthal RS et al: Ethinyl estradiol acutely attenuates abnormal coronary vasomotor responses to acetylcholine in postmenopausal women. Circulation 1994;89:52
46. Hulley S, Grady D, Bush T et al, for the Heart and Estrogen/Progestin Replacement Study (HERS) Research Group: Randomized trial of estrogen plus progestin for secondary prevention of coronary artery disease in postmenopausal women. JAMA 1998;280:605–613
47. Folson AR, Kaye SA, Sellers TA et al: Body fat distribution and 5-year risk of death in older women. JAMA 1993;269:483–487
48. Bjorntorp P: The association between obesity, adipose tissue distribution and disease. Acta Med Scand 1988;723(suppl):121–134
49. Paffenbarger RS, Hyde RT, Wing AL, Hsieh C: Physical activity, all-cause mortality, and longevity of college alumni. N Engl J Med 1986;314:605–613
50. Hertog MGL, Feskens EJM, Holman PCH et al: Dietary antioxidant flavonoids and risk of coronary heart disease: the Zutphen Elderly Study. Lancet 1993;342:1007–1011
51. Woodhouse PR, Khaw KT, Plumer M et al: Seasonal variations of plasma fibrinogen and factor VII activity in the elderly: winter infections and death from cardiovascular disease. Lancet 1994;343:435–439
52. Ariyo AA, Haan M, Tangen CM et al: Depressive symptoms and risks of coronary heart disease and mortality in elderly Americans. Circulation 2000;102:1773–1779
53. Lempiainen P, Mykkanen L, Pyorala K, Laakso M, Kuusisto J: Insulin resistance syndrome predicts coronary heart disease events in elderly nondiabetic men. Circulation 1999;100:123–128
54. Heijmans BT, Westendorp RGJ, Knook DL, Kluft C, Slagboom PE: Angiotensin 1-converting enzyme and plasminogen activator inhibitor-1 gene variants: risk of mortality and fatal cardiovascular disease in an elderly population-based cohort. J Am Coll Cardiol 1999;34:1176–1183
55. Kushi LH, Folsom AR, Prineas RJ et al: Dietary antioxidant vitamins and death from coronary heart disease in postmenopausal women. N Engl J Med 1996;334:1156–1162
56. Callahan PR, Froelicher VG, Klein J et al: Exercise-induced silent ischemia: age, diabetes mellitus, previous myocardial infarction and prognosis. J Am Coll Cardiol 1989;14:1175–1180
57. Fleg JL, Gerstenblith G, Zonderman AB et al: Prevalence and prognostic significance of exercise-induced silent myocardial ischemia detected by thallium scintigraphy and electrocardiography in asymptomatic volunteers. Circulation 1990;81:428–436
58. Elveback L, Lie JT: Continued high incidence of coronary artery disease at autopsy in Olmstead County, Minnesota. Circulation 1979;70:345–349
59. Hlatky MA et al: Factors affecting sensitivity and specificity of exercise electrocardiography: multivariable analysis. Am J Med 1984;77:64–71
60. Bateman TM, O'Keefe JH. Pharmacological (stress) perfusion scintigraphy: methods, advantages, and applications. Am J Cardiac Imaging 1992;6:3–15

61. Beleslin BD, Ostojic M, Stepanovic J et al: Stress echocardiography in the detection of myocardial ischemia: head-to-head comparison of exercise, dobutamine, and dipyridamole tests. Circulation 1994;90:1168–1176

62. Blumenthal DS, Weiss JL, Mellits ED, Gerstenblith G: The predictive value of a strongly positive test in patients with minimal symptoms. Am J Med 1981;70:1005–1010

63. The Heart Outcomes Prevention Evaluation study investigators: Effects of an angiotensin-converting enzyme inhibitor, ramipril, on cardiovascular events in high-risk patients. N Engl J Med 2000;342:145–153

64. Mock MB, Holmes DR, Vliestra RE et al: Percutaneous transluminal coronary angioplasty (PTCA) in the elderly patient: experience in the National Heart, Lung, and Blood Institute PTCA registry. Am J Cardiol 1984;53:89C–91C

65. Chauhan MS, Kuntz RE, Ho KKL et al: Coronary artery stenting in the aged. J Am Coll Cardiol 2001;37:856–862

66. Ang PC, Farouque HM, Harper RW, Meredith IT: Percutaneous coronary intervention in the elderly: a comparison of procedural and clinical outcomes between the eighth and ninth decades. J Invas Cardiol 2000;12:488–494

67. Rodriguez A, Bernardi V, Navia J et al: Argentine randomized study: coronary angioplasty with stenting versus coronary bypass surgery in patients with multiple-vessel disease. J Am Coll Cardiol 2001;37:53–58

68. Batchelor WB, Anstron KJ, Muhlbaier LH et al: Contemporary outcome trends in the elderly undergoing percutaneous coronary interventions: results in 7472 octogenarians. J Am Coll Cardiol 2000;36:723–730

69. Peterson ED, Cowper PA, Jollis JG et al: Outcomes of coronary artery bypass graft surgery in 24,461 patients aged 80 years or older. Circulation 1995;92:85–91

70. Ivanov J, Weisel RD, David TE, Maylor CD: Fifteen-year trends in risk severity and operative mortality in elderly patients undergoing coronary artery bypass graft surgery. Circulation: 1998;97:673–680

71. Roach GW, Kanchbuger M, Mangano CM et al: Adverse cerebral outcomes after coronary bypass surgery. N Engl J Med 1996;335:1857–1863

72. Newman MF, Kirchner JL, Phillips-Bute B et al: Longitudinal assessment of neurocognitive function after coronary-artery bypass surgery. N Engl J Med 2001;344:395–402

73. Stamou SC, Corso PJ: Coronary revascularization without cardiopulmonary bypass in high-risk patients: a route to the future. Ann Thor Surg 2001;71:1056–1061

74. Solomon CG, Lee TH, Cook EF et al: Comparison of clinical presentation of acute myocardial infarction in patients older than 65 years of age to younger patients: the multicenter chest pain study experience. Am J Cardiol 1989;63:772–776

75. Nadelmann J, Frishman Wh, Ooi WL et al: Prevalence, incidence and prognosis of recognized and unrecognized myocardial infarction in persons aged 75 years or older: the Bronx Aging Study. Am J Cardiol 1990;66:533

76. Goldberg RJ, Gore JM, Gurwitz JH et al: The impact of age on the incidence and prognosis of initial acute myocardial infarction: the Worcester Heart Attack Study. Am Heart J 1989;117–543

77. Heller GV, Blaustein AS, Wei JY: Implications of increased myocardial isoenzyme level in the presence of normal serum creatine kinase activity. Am J Cardiol 1983;51:24–27

78. Maggioni AP, Maseri A, Fresco C et al: Age-related increase in mortality among patients with first myocardial infarction treated with thrombolysis. N Engl J Med 1993;329:1442–1448

79. Aguirre FV, McMahon RP, Hueler H et al: Impact of age on clinical outcomes and postlytic management strategies in patients treated with intravenous thrombolytic therapy: results from the TIMI II study. Circulation 1994;90:78–86

80. Gurwitz JH, Gore JM, Goldberg RJ, et al: Risk for intracranial hemorrhage after tissue plasminogen activator treatment for acute myocardial infarction. Ann Intern Med 1998;129:597–604

81. Thiemann DR, Coresh J, Schulman SP et al: Lack of benefit for intravenous thrombolysis in patients with myocardial infarction who are older than 75 years. Circulation 2000;101:2239–2246

82. Grines CL, Browne KF, Marco J et al: A comparison of immediate angioplasty with thrombolytic therapy for acute myocardial infarction. N Engl J Med 1993;328:673–679

83. O'Neill WW, Zijlstra F, Suryapranata H et al: Meta-analysis of the PAMI and Netherlands randomized trials of primary angioplasty versus thrombolytic therapy of acute myocardial infarction. Circulation 1993;88:I106

84. Stone GW, Grines CL, Browne KF et al: Predictors of in-hospital and 6-month outcome after acute myocardial infarction in the reperfusion era: the Primary Angioplasty in Myocardial Infarction (PAMI) trial. J Am Coll Cardiol 1995;25:370–377

85. The Global Use of Strategies to Open Occluded Coronary Arteries in Acute Coronary Syndromes (GUSTO IIb) Angioplasty substudy investigators: A clinical trial comparing primary coronary angioplasty with tissue plasminogen activator for acute myocardial infarction. N Engl J Med 1997;336:1621–1628

86. Berger AK, Schulman KA, Gersh BJ et al: Primary angioplasty vs thrombolysis for the management of acute myocardial infarction in elderly patients. JAMA 1999;282:341–348

87. Soumerai SB, McLaughlin TJ, Spiegelman D et al: Adverse outcomes of underuse of beta-blockers in elderly survivors of acute myocardial infarction. JAMA 1997;277:115–121

88. Krumholz HM, Radford MJ, Ellerbeck EF et al: Aspirin for secondary prevention after acute myocardial infarction in the elderly: prescribed use and outcomes. Ann Intern Med 1998;124:292–298

89. Pfeffer MA, Braunwald E, Moye LA et al: Effect of captopril on mortality and morbidity in patients with left ventricular dysfunction after myocardial infarction: results of the Survival and Ventricular Enlargement Trial. N Engl J Med 1992;327:669–677

90. Kober L, Torp-Pedersen C, Carlsen JE et al: A clinical trial of the angiotensin-converting-enzyme inhibitor trandolapril in patients with left ventricular dysfunction after myocardial infarction. N Engl J Med 1995;333:1670–1676

91. Antman EM, Cohen M, Bernink PF et al: The TIMI risk score for unstable angina/non-ST-elevation myocardial infarction: a method for prognostication and therapeutic decision making. JAMA 2000;284:835–842

92. Braunwald E, Antman EM, Beasley JW et al: ACC/AHA guidelines for the management of patients with unstable angina and non-ST-elevation myocardial infarction: executive summary and recommendations. Circulation 2000;102:1193–1209

93. Cohen M, Demers C, Gurfinkel EP et al, for the Efficacy and Safety of Subcutaneous Enoxaparin in Non-Q-Wave Coronary Events Study Group: A comparison of low-molecular-weight heparin with unfractionated heparin for unstable coronary artery disease. N Engl J Med 1997;337:447–452

94. Lincoff AM, Harrington RA, Califf RM et al: Management of patients with acute coronary syndromes in the United States by platelet glycoprotein IIb/IIIa inhibition. Circulation 2000;102:1093–1100

95. Schwartz GG, Olsson AG, Ezekowitz MD et al, for the Myocardial Ischemia Reduction with Aggressive Cholesterol Lowering (MIRACL) study investigators: Effects of atorvastatin on early recurrent ischemic events in acute coronary syndromes. JAMA 2001;285:681–689

96. Boden WE, O'Rourke RA, Crawford MH et al: Outcomes in patients with acute non-Q-wave myocardial infarction randomly assigned to an invasive as compared with a conservative management strategy. N Engl J Med 1998;338:1785–1792

97. FRISC II investigators: Invasive compared to non-invasive treatment in unstable coronary-artery disease: FRISC II prospective randomised multicentre study. Lancet 1999;354:708–715

98. Lavie CJ, Milani RV: Effects of cardiac rehabilitation and exercise training programs in patients ≥75 years of age. Am J Cardiol 1996;78:675–678

99. Stahle A, Mattsson E, Ryden L, Unden A, Nordlander R: Improved physical fitness and quality of life following training of elderly patients after acute coronary events. A 1-year follow-up randomized controlled study. Eur Heart J 1999;20:1475–1484

100. Stahle A, Nordlander R, Bergfeldt L: Aerobic group training improves exercise capacity and heart rate variability in elderly patients with a recent coronary event: a randomized controlled study. Eur Heart J 1999;20:1638–1646

Chapter 35

Hypertension

John F. Potter

Coronary heart disease and stroke remain the major causes of death in people aged over 65 years in westernized societies, with an elevated blood pressure (BP) level being the biggest treatable risk factor. With the ever-increasing number of elderly people in the population, hypertension is pre-eminent as a public health problem. It is perhaps surprising to realize that it was only in 1985 that the first large trial of blood pressure reduction in the elderly population was published, demonstrating the benefits of treatment in terms of reducing cardiovascular complications.[1] Prior to this, a general reluctance to treat hypertension in older people prevailed, based it would seem on a few case reports of the adverse effects of antihypertensive drugs. This chapter deals with some of the more important aspects of hypertension in elderly people, while highlighting areas where important questions remain unanswered.

EPIDEMIOLOGY

Blood pressure increases with age. This has been shown in both cross-sectional and longitudinal studies in nearly all industrialized cultures. The rise in systolic blood pressure (SBP) is almost linear up to age 80 years, values tending to plateau thereafter. Diastolic blood pressure (DBP) levels plateau earlier, at 50–60 years, and then fall.[2] These changes herald the important age-related changes that occur in pulse pressure (PP) and mean arterial pressure (MAP). PP tends to rise steeply after the age of 60 years irrespective of the SBP levels when young; whereas MAP shows a much greater increase with age in those with high values in their 30s and 40s and reaches a plateau after the age of 50–60 years.

There are many factors governing these changes, both environmental and genetic. For example, blacks tend to have a greater age-related rise than whites, especially in women. Important sex differences in the BP changes with age are also found when comparing the results from cross-sectional and longitudinal studies, with the former showing women to have higher SBP and DBP values than men after 50 years of age. Cohort studies show a different pattern, with SBP increasing to the same degree in both sexes with little difference in age-related values; whereas DBP levels for women are consistently lower than for men, of the order of 5 mmHg. It is possible that some of these differences in cross-sectional studies are due to selective mortality differences (such as death rates being higher in those with higher BP levels) resulting in an under-representation of those with initially high BP levels in the older age groups. Lifestyle differences probably account for some of these age-related alterations, little change in BP being seen with advancing years in some non-westernized cultures.

Prevalence and incidence

The prevalence of hypertension is dependent on the definition used. Classically the threshold is the BP levels at which treatment appears to offer benefit over nontreatment, but the actual BP levels taken for defining hypertension have changed considerably recently. Definite hypertension, as originally defined in the Framingham study (SBP ≥ 160 mmHg and/or DBP ≥ 95 mmHg or on antihypertensive treatment), was present in 39 percent of men and 48 percent of women in those aged 65–94 years.[2] Similar prevalence figures were recorded in NHANES,[3] being 35 and 37 percent for men and women aged 60–74, respectively, compared with 7.2 and 3.9 percent for those aged 30–39 years. However, if a more liberal definition of hypertension is taken ($> 140/90$ mmHg), prevalence rates markedly increase to 51 and 50 percent for 60–74 year old men and women, respectively.[4] These rates are based on two or three recordings at a single visit and, given the increased BP variability in older people, the estimates are probably too high and the rates based on repeated measurements are about 30 percent less than those quoted. For example, in a UK study of people aged 65+ years, 52.2 percent had hypertension at first screening compared with 10.3 percent at the third visit 6–12 weeks later.[5]

As the systolic BP tends to increase to a greater extent than the diastolic BP with advancing years, isolated systolic hypertension (ISH) is the commonest form of hypertension in older people. Prevalence rates for ISH in the BIRNH study were 9.9 percent in men and 11.7 percent in women aged 65–74 years, compared with rates for diastolic hypertension (DBP ≥ 95 mmHg) of 15.8 and 10.6 percent.[6] For those aged 75–89, ISH rates increased to 15.3 and 17.4 percent in men and women, whereas diastolic hypertension (DH) fell to 7.7 percent in men but increased slightly to 11.2 percent in women. Interestingly, 84 percent of all female hypertensives in the study were aware of their diagnosis, compared with less than 70 percent of men, highlighting the need for BP screening in this age group. Other studies using multiple BP recordings made on several visits have found prevalence rates for ISH of 4.2 percent, combined hypertension (CH) in 3.9 percent, and isolated DH of 1 percent in those aged 65–84 years.[5]

Favorable trends in terms of decreasing hypertension prevalence are being reported. In the USA, rates have declined progressively since 1971. For example, in the NHANES study, rates of hypertension in men aged 60–74 fell from 37.9 percent in 1971–74 to 35.4 percent in 1988–91, and for women from 64.7 percent in 1971–74 to 51.1 percent in 1988–91.[3] Incidence rates have changed little, being of the order of 9 percent and 6 percent per 2 years for men and women, respectively, in those aged 70–79 years.[7] However, reliable incidence data are relatively scarce, particularly in the very elderly population.

Blood pressure and risk

Framingham data have shown that elderly hypertensives have three times the risk of a cardiovascular (CV)-related death than age- and sex-matched normotensives.[8] There has been much discussion as to whether this relationship between BP and CV mortality is linear, U-shaped or J-shaped, giving rise to the opinion that there may be an optimum level to which elevated BP values should be reduced. Intervention studies have suggested that reducing BP levels too much may paradoxically increase cardiovascular and noncardiovascular risk. However, a U- or J-shaped relationship between BP and CV mortality has been reported in the placebo arms of these studies, so this could not be an effect of treatment per se.

Many of the studies suggesting an increased risk with lower BP levels were of relatively short duration and did not control for potentially confounding variables. In a large community study, Glynn et al[9] showed that, after adjustment for confounding factors such as frailty, presence of coronary heart disease (CHD), and excluding deaths within 3 years of follow-up, increasing levels of SBP and DBP were associated with a linear increase in CV mortality; those with SBP <130 mmHg had an adjusted relative risk of 0.89 (95 percent CI = 0.73–1.07) compared with the top quintile BP (>160 mmHg) who had a relative risk of 1.21 (1.01–1.44). For diastolic BP the linear trend was not as steep as for systolic, with only a 9 percent difference in relative risk of death between the lowest (<70 mmHg) and highest (90 mmHg) DBP quintile. The waters have been further muddied, however, by a recent reanalysis of the Framingham data which suggests that CV risk starts to increase only above an SBP >160 mmHg in those aged 65–74 years.[10]

The proportional risks of CV disease due to hypertension do decrease with age. In the Honolulu heart program, the attributable risk of stroke due to hypertension in men was 50.1 percent for those aged 45–54 years, compared with 18.2 percent for those aged 65–81 years.[11] Even though the age-adjusted risk ratio for CV events is lower in older hypertensives, the absolute risk remains greater because CV disease is so much more prevalent in this age group.

SBP, DBP, and risk

Systolic blood pressure is a bigger risk factor than DBP for cardiovascular disease in older people. In the Copenhagen heart study,[12] the risk ratio (RR) for stroke due to ISH (SBP ≥ 160 mmHg, DBP <90 mmHg) in men was 2.7, but for diastolic hypertension (DBP ≥ 90 mmHg irrespective of SBP) it was 1.7 compared with normotensives. For myocardial infarction no such difference was seen in the relative risk between ISH and diastolic hypertension. More importantly, borderline ISH (SBP 140–159, DBP < 90 mmHg) in the Physicians Health Study[13] was associated with a 32 percent increase in CV events compared with normotensives, and a 56 percent increase in CV deaths. If future studies show that treatment of borderline ISH reduces CV risk, this will have enormous implications because over 20 percent of those aged over 70 years fall into this BP category.

Pulse pressure and risk

Pulse pressure increases markedly after the age of 50 years, due to arterial wall stiffening with the associated increase in SBP and fall in DBP. In older age groups in the Framingham study,[14] coronary heart disease was found to be inversely related to DBP at any given level of SBP ≥ 120 mmHg, suggesting that higher pulse pressure is as important, if not more so, than any other component of BP in predicting CHD risk (Fig. 35-1). Pulse pressure was a better predictor than SBP, independent of DBP levels, for estimating the development of congestive heart failure (CHF); for each 10 mmHg increase in pulse pressure there was a 14 percent increased risk of CHF, compared with a 9 percent increase for the same change in SBP.

Although SBP and PP are the best predictors of coronary heart disease, the same is not necessarily true for stroke. Mean arterial pressure has been found, in some studies at least, to be a better predictor of stroke than either SBP or PP. In the Systolic Hypertension in the Elderly Programme,[15] a 10 mmHg increase in PP was associated with a relative risk of stroke of 1.11 (1.01–1.22) compared with 1.20 (1.02–1.42) for a similar MAP rise.

The finding that PP is as good a predictor of coronary heart disease as SBP has potential implications for treating hypertension, as there seems little point in lowering SBP and DBP to the same extent, (keeping PP unchanged) as this may contribute to maintaining some degree of CV risk. It would thus appear that, in elderly people, CHD events are more closely related to pulsatile load than steady-state components of blood pressure. This may explain why, overall, 30–60 percent of all

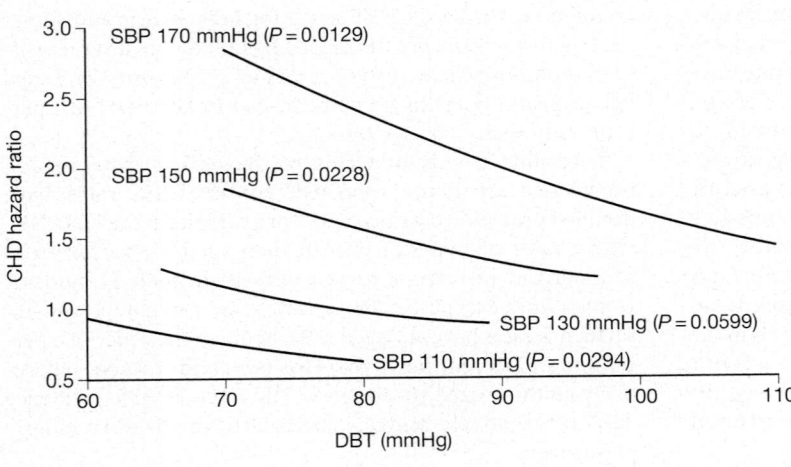

Figure 35-1 Influence of systolic and diastolic blood pressure on CHD risk in 50–79 year olds. CHD hazard ratios are determined from the level of DBP within SBP groups. Hazard ratios are set to a reference value of 1.0 for an SBP of 130 and a DBP of 80 mmHg. All estimates are adjusted for age, sex, body mass index, smoking, glucose tolerance, and total/HDL cholesterol. Data from the Framingham study, reprinted from Franklin et al. (1999).[14]

CV events in the elderly population are attributable to mild or moderate hypertension.

Blood pressure and risk in the very elderly

The effect of hypertension on CV mortality in those aged more than 75 years is unclear. Kannel et al.[8] demonstrated, in those aged 75–94 years, a U-shaped curve for CV mortality and increasing BP levels, with a marked rise in mortality rate in those with a systolic pressure above 120 mmHg, for both men and women. However, this excess mortality in the low-BP group probably reflects poor general cardiovascular health and not low SBP per se. Some studies have concluded that increasing BP levels at this age are in fact beneficial, being associated with a decrease in overall mortality; other studies have suggested the opposite. What to do about raised blood pressure in the very elderly population remains unclear.

PATHOGENESIS

Mean arterial pressure (MAP) is determined by cardiac output and peripheral vascular resistance (PVR) and is the steady-state component of blood pressure. The dynamic component, pulse pressure (PP), is the variation around the mean state and is influenced by large artery stiffness, early pulse-wave reflection, left ventricular ejection, and heart rate. A rise in PVR and large artery stiffness will increase the systolic BP component, while a decrease in PVR or an increase in large artery stiffness will result in a fall in diastolic BP, the latter being the dominant change in older hypertensives.

The main cardiovascular pathophysiological changes associated with aging are arterial dilation and a decrease in large artery compliance, especially in the aorta, due to loss of elastic fibers in the vessel wall and a concomitant increase in collagen. Arterial stiffening leads to enhanced pulse-wave velocity and early reflected waves augmenting the late systolic aortic pressure wave, resulting in a systolic increase and diastolic fall. The rise in mean aortic pressure is augmented by the rise in PVR, seen particularly in older women, enhanced by impaired endothelial release of nitric oxide, especially in older hypertensives. The increase in systolic load puts excess mechanical strain on the left ventricle, leading to concentric wall thickening. As coronary artery perfusion is primarily dependent on the diastolic pressure, any reduction in DBP can have adverse effects on coronary artery perfusion, especially as left ventricular myocardial demands are increased in hypertension. Intimal wall damage results in the development of atherosclerosis and an increased likelihood of thrombosis.

The other main features associated with hypertension in old age are a reduction in heart rate, cardiac output, intravascular volume, and glomerular filtration rate, and decreased cardiac baroreceptor sensitivity (BRS). This decrease in cardiac BRS accounts for the increase in BP variability found in older hypertensives, and it perhaps plays a role in the increased susceptibility to postural hypotension. Both renal plasma flow and plasma renin activity (PRA) levels decrease with age, the fall in PRA being more marked in elderly hypertensives than in normotensives. Plasma noradrenaline (norepinephrine) levels increase with age and are associated with a decrease in β-adrenoreceptor sensitivity. The effect of age and hypertension on α-adrenoreceptor sensitivity is still unclear.

OTHER CARDIOVASCULAR RISK FACTORS

Hypertension should not be considered in isolation. Irrespective of the age of the patient, it is important that overall cardiovascular risk be assessed, taking into account other important risk elements such as cholesterol levels, smoking habits, and the presence or absence of diabetes.

Lipid abnormalities

Around 25 percent of men and 40 percent of women aged over 65 years have raised serum total cholesterol (TC) levels, though controversy still abounds as to their predictive value in assessing coronary heart disease and cerebrovascular risk. Most studies suggest that serum TC levels increase with age and remain a significant independent predictor for CHD in men. The effect in women is less clear because the number studied has been too small to draw firm conclusions. The SHEP study[16] found that TC and LDL cholesterol remained significant indicators of risk in both sexes, such that a 1 mmol/L increase in TC was associated with a 30–35 percent higher CHD event rate.[16] For those aged 65–81 years in the Framingham study,[17] the risk of CHD comparing top and bottom quartiles of TC:HDL-cholesterol ratio was 2.3 for men and 3.3 for women, whereas for TC alone this was 1.2 (not significant) for men and 2.0 for women. This additional predictive power using HDL levels has been one of the reasons why recent guidelines have used the ratio rather than TC levels alone. Although the hazard ratio for TC:HDL-cholesterol decreases with age, this is somewhat offset by the higher incidence of CV disease in the older age groups resulting in a larger attributable risk. In those over 75 years a further paradox is found, with increasing TC concentrations being associated with increased longevity, due to fewer deaths from infections and cancer.

For all strokes, TC levels do not appear to be related to events, but increased HDL cholesterol levels may well protect against cerebral infarction. These divergent results probably arise from an inverse risk between TC and cerebral hemorrhage and a positive correlation with cerebral infarction.

Diabetes mellitus

Up to 10 percent of elderly people with hypertension will have impaired glucose tolerance, and diabetes doubles the risk of developing coronary heart disease and stroke in those aged 65–94 years. Like total cholesterol, however, its impact on CV events falls with age: women remain slightly more at risk than men, though the absolute risk from diabetes is greater in the elderly than the young.

Body mass index

Increasing body mass index (BMI) is associated with an elevation in blood pressure, but the risk of obesity-related hypertension declines with age, there being a 3-fold increase in hypertension in obese 20–45 year olds compared to a 1.5 increase in 65–94 year olds. For each unit of BMI increase (kg/m²), SBP can be expected to increase by 1.2 mmHg and DBP by 0.7 mmHg.

Interestingly, for elderly hypertensive men CV relative risk increases from 1.8 to 2.9 between the lowest and highest tertiles of BMI, whereas the reverse is true for women. Even so, hypertension still more than doubles the risk of developing CV disease in both sexes. In the European Working Party on Hypertension in the Elderly (EWPHE) study,[18] those with the lowest total mortality and CV terminating events were found in the moderately obese group with a BMI of 28–29 kg/m², while those with a BMI of 26–27 had the lowest cardiovascular mortality. Truncal obesity (reflected in an increased waist to hip ratio) is more strongly related to hypertension and is a better predictor for coronary heart disease and stroke than BMI alone.

Smoking

Although the number of smokers decreases with age, smoking remains a significant risk factor for CV mortality in older persons (the relative risk is 2.0 for males and 1.6 for females). The relative risk of stroke amongst older hypertensive smokers is five times that of normotensives but 20 times that of normotensive nonsmokers. The benefits of stopping smoking in terms of reducing coronary heart disease and stroke mortality are still present even in the 70+ age group, with the excess risk of mortality declining within 1–5 years of quitting. Older smokers should therefore be encouraged to stop. Hypertensive cigarette smokers have an increased relative risk of stroke nearly quadruple that of hypertensive nonsmokers (pipe/cigar use still increases the risk 3-fold). Encouragingly, hypertensive ex-smokers of <20 cigarettes/day have, after only a few years of quitting, a similar risk to that of hypertensive nonsmokers.

Atrial fibrillation and left ventricular hypertrophy

In patients with atrial fibrillation, hypertension doubles the stroke risk compared with normotensives. Electrocardiographically diagnosed left ventricular hypertrophy (LVH) increases with age, reported prevalence rates being 6 percent in men and 5 percent in women aged 65–74 years, compared with 9.4 and 10.8 percent, respectively, in those aged over 85. LVH has a significant effect on CV risk. Its presence in those aged 65–94 years nearly triples the risk for men and quadruples that in women, but this effect is less than that seen in younger age groups with a similar blood pressure.

Alcohol and diet

ALCOHOL The association between high alcohol consumption and blood pressure has been known for a very long time, although the relationship is not linear in most epidemiological studies. It takes on a J- or U-shaped form, with the lowest incidence of hypertension being seen in those consuming around 5–10 units of alcohol per week. Large falls in BP (19/10 mmHg) have been recorded with abstention in those aged 70–74 years who had a long history of heavy alcohol intake. Excessive alcohol intake has been directly related to stroke risk. It is unknown whether this is due to its direct pressor effect or to some other mechanisms, such as alcohol-induced cerebral vasoconstriction or cardiac dysrhythmia, particularly atrial fibrillation.

As there appears to be a mild protective effect of a small amount of alcohol in older people, two units per day would seem a reasonable upper limit to recommend.

DIET The relationship between dietary sodium intake and hypertension strengthens with age. For a 100 mmol per day increase, mean BP rises by 5 mmHg in those aged 20 years but this more than doubles in those aged 60–69 years. Conversely, increasing potassium intake by 60 mmol per day reduces BP in older people by as much as 10/6 mmHg. Increasing potassium dietary intake may also reduce stroke risk independently of its hypotensive effect. The average daily potassium intake in elderly people in the UK is around 60–70 mmol. This could be raised to over 100 mmol simply by increasing consumption of vegetables and fruit.

Physical exercise

Even mild-to-moderate physical exercise such as walking for 30 minutes 3–4 times a week has a hypotensive effect. Vigorous exercise in young to middle-aged persons prevents stroke in later life. Whether these effects are mediated solely through BP-lowering or are due to other mechanisms, such as exercise-induced decreases in fibrinogen levels or increase in HDL cholesterol, is unknown.

Hormone replacement

There has been considerable controversy over the benefits of hormone replacement therapy (HRT) in CV disease prevention, but a recent overview has suggested treatment reduces coronary heart disease by about 30 percent.[19] The effect of HRT on hypertension if present is small at best and, given the high risk of CHD in post-menopausal women, if BP is controlled, treatment will have a long-term benefit.

COMPLICATIONS OF HYPERTENSION

Stroke

Hypertension remains the major treatable risk factor for stroke, although the attributable risk for increasing BP levels decreases with age. For a 10 mmHg increase in usual diastolic BP, the risk of stroke is almost doubled. A reduction of 9/5 mmHg can be expected to produce about a 30 percent reduction in stroke incidence, while a fall of 18/10 mmHg halves the risk; these expectations are irrespective of baseline BP levels.

The relative risk of cerebral infarction varies depending on the hypertension type in older age groups.[20] Isolated systolic hypertension (ISH) is a bigger risk factor (ratio 2.3) than is combined systolic and diastolic hypertension (ratio 1.5). The population attributable risk for stroke in those aged 70–79 years with ISH is about 21 percent for women and 17 percent for men, while for those aged 50–59 years the figures are 5 percent for women and 4 percent for men. Although the relative risk of stroke from raised BP decreases with age, this is not because hypertension per se loses its effect as a risk factor, but that more strokes occur in those with "normal" blood pressure. Intracerebral hemorrhage is also closely related to hypertension, the relative risk varying from 2.0 to 9.0 between studies— being greater for combined hypertension than ISH, particularly in younger patients.

The effect of raised BP levels on outcome in the immediate post-stroke period is unclear. Hypertension is common in the first days to weeks after stroke, and BP levels tend to settle spontaneously. There is, however, increasing evidence that raised BP levels following acute stroke are associated with a poor outcome in terms of death and dependency.[21] There is a small but convincing body of evidence to suggest an almost linear relationship between increased BP values and stroke recurrence rate.

BP and asymptomatic cerebrovascular disease

Deep white matter lesions (leukoaraiosis) in asymptomatic hypertensive elderly patients are frequently found on magnetic resonance scanning. Whether these lesions account for the age-related cognitive impairment seen with hypertension that has been reported in many studies is unknown. It is also uncertain whether they increase the risk of subsequent cerebral infarction or hemorrhage. Isolated systolic hypertension, in particular, is associated with these subcortical lesions, and good BP control appears to have a protective effect. Large diurnal falls in BP are associated with silent subcortical white matter lesions and lacunar infarcts, but these are found also in those who have marked nocturnal rises in BP.

Cognitive impairment

The influence of blood pressure on cognitive decline and psychomotor function, over and above its association with vascular dementia, has been much debated. Some studies show no such relationship while others report a strong positive correlation. Recent controlled studies have emphasized a positive relationship between cognitive decline and hypertension. Cacciatore et al.[22] in a cross-sectional study, found that increasing diastolic BP, but not systolic, levels in 75–84 year olds resulted in impaired Mini-Mental State score (scoring <24) with an odds ratio of 1.6; but for those aged over 85 this rose to 5.2, independent of sex, educational level, geriatric depression score, and antihypertensive drug use. Similar results have been reported in large longitudinal studies.[23]

The pathogenesis of hypertension-related cognitive impairment is unclear. It could be linked to a decrease in cerebral blood flow with increasing BP levels and alteration in the cerebral metabolism over and above the changes associated with leukoaraiosis.

Cardiac disease

The relationship between coronary heart disease and hypertension is discussed in Chapter 34. Hypertension accelerates the development of coronary artery atheroma through many mechanisms, particularly in association with metabolic abnormalities as in the insulin-resistance syndrome. Increased blood glucose and insulin levels as well as changes in total cholesterol, HDL and LDL levels, and endothelial dysfunction result in impaired endothelial-dependent relaxation and increased leucocyte adherence, smooth muscle proliferation, intimal macrophagic accumulation, fibrosis, and arterial medial wall thickening. These changes, along with increased vascular oxidative stress and free radical production (see Chapter 32), result in inflammatory changes in the arterial wall, monocyte migration into the intima, and plaque formation.

DIAGNOSIS AND EVALUATION
General issues

Assessment of blood pressure levels in elderly people can pose particular problems, but it is essential that accurate measurements be made if patients are not to receive unnecessary or inadequate treatment. Minute-to-minute BP variations occur with respiratory and vasomotor changes. During the 24-hour period, BP fluctuations are related to mental and physical activity, sleep, and postprandial changes. Seasonal variations are also seen, with BP levels being higher during the winter months. Hypertensive patients have a greater absolute BP variability than normotensives, but when corrected for baseline values little difference exists. Clinically important differences are frequently found between individual readings at a single visit and between visits. Large falls in BP with repeated measurements in elderly hypertensives have been reported in nearly every placebo-controlled interventional trial, the effect increasing with age and amounting to as much as 10/5 mmHg decrease. The tendency for BP levels to decrease with time is related in part to regression to the mean as well as familiarity with the procedure of BP measurement. The British Hypertension Society (BHS) Guidelines recommend that in uncomplicated cases an average of two readings be taken sitting, on four occasions over a 2–3 month period during initial assessment.[24] It is particularly important to measure BP levels 1 and 3 minutes after standing to assess postural BP change in view of the frequency of orthostatic hypotension in this age group.

Measuring blood pressure

With the expected phasing out of mercury sphygmomanometers and their replacement by semiautomatic devices, it is important that manufacturers provide accurate equipment vali-dated in the elderly. A list of BP measuring devices that have been validated for use in young and elderly persons has recently been published in Europe.[25] Cuff size is important as under-cuffing gives falsely high BP values. Cuff width should be equal to two-thirds of the distance between axilla and antecubital fossa, and when the bladder is placed over the brachial artery it should cover at least 80 percent of the arm's circumference—which should be kept supported at heart level. Clinicians should obtain both standard and large cuffs and ensure they are used appropriately.

The measurement should be taken in both arms initially, as over 10 percent of elderly people have at least a 10 mmHg difference between arms. The arm with the highest reading should be used for subsequent measurements. All elderly people should have their BP measured every 5 years up to age 80 years at least, and in those with high normal BP (135–139/85–89 mmHg) it should be assessed annually.

Ambulatory blood pressure monitoring

The role of ambulatory monitoring (ABPM) in the assessment of elderly people with hypertension is still being defined.

24-hour monitoring reduces the variability and the alerting response to measurement, so that 75 percent of elderly hypertensives will have lower ABPM measurements than clinic values. Casual measurements tend to be in the order of 20/10 mmHg higher than 24-hour values. Daytime BP values are the best predictor of target organ damage.

The value of other information that the 24-hour ABPM profile can provide, such as day–night differences, is unknown. The Syst-Eur study[26] has emphasized that ABPM is a significantly better predictor of CV risk than are casual measurements. ABPM could be recommended in the following cases:

- to diagnose white-coat hypertension (persistently elevated clinic BP levels while normotensive on ABPM);
- when BP appears resistant to therapy (using three or more agents);
- in those with symptoms of postural hypotension and postprandial hypotension.

However, there is little justification as yet to use it routinely in all elderly hypertensive patients as it is expensive and time-consuming, though generally well tolerated.

Suggested normal values are: daytime ≤135/85 mmHg; night-time <120/70 mmHg; and 24-hour ≤130/80 mmHg. Abnormal values are: daytime >140/90 mmHg; night-time> 125/75 mmHg; and 24-hour >135/85 mmHg.[27]

Cuff measurements tend to underestimate intra-arterial levels of systolic BP by up to 5–10 mmHg, and to overestimate diastolic BP by about 5–15 mmHg. "Pseudohypertension" refers to falsely high noninvasive recordings caused by arterial rigidity which prevents the vessel collapsing during cuff inflation. The prevalence of this condition in an unselected elderly population is probably very low, of the order of 1–2 percent. Unfortunately there is no accurate way of predicting the condition. Osler's maneuver (said to be positive when the radial artery is still palpable following the occlusion of the brachial artery) is unreliable.

Clinical assessment and investigations

One common feature of hypertension in young and elderly people alike is that it is very often asymptomatic. Complaints often attributed to increased BP levels, such as headache, are in fact unrelated in most cases. History and examination should include assessment for the presence of important CV risk factors (such as diabetes), for symptoms and signs of secondary causes of hypertension, and for evidence of target organ damage. Other important factors to be considered are the presence of confusion, urinary incontinence, decreased mobility, other medication use (for possible drug interactions which will affect the need for and type of antihypertensive agent)—all of which will influence treatment decisions. Examination should focus on evidence of target organ damage, including peripheral pulses and bruits (renal or carotid), and cardiac murmurs. Ophthalmoscopy is used for possible malignant-phase as well as diabetic changes, and a neurological examination for signs of cerebrovascular disease and vascular dementia.

Initial investigations should include height, weight, blood samples for urea and electrolytes, creatinine and glucose estimations, and a 12-lead ECG (to exclude ischemic change, dysrhythmias, and left ventricular hypertrophy). In those aged ≤70 years for primary prevention, and in those ≤75 years for secondary prevention, total cholesterol and HDL cholesterol levels along with urine analysis for protein and blood should be included. Chest X-ray is of doubtful benefit, except in those who may have heart failure or chest disease. Plasma calcium and uric acid levels may also be useful, to look for primary hyperparathyroidism (which is more frequent in elderly people with hypertension) and to check for gout. Echocardiography is rarely needed.

Renal artery stenosis is the only major secondary cause of hypertension in this age group. It should be considered:

- when there is a sudden onset or rapid progression of hypertension;
- if BP control suddenly becomes difficult, particularly in those at greater risk of atherosclerotic renal artery stenosis—diabetics, smokers, and those with peripheral vascular disease;
- in those developing malignant phase hypertension;
- where there is rapid deterioration of renal function, particularly after starting angiotensin converting enzyme inhibitors.

Renal ultrasound is not reliable for making the diagnosis of renal artery stenosis, although a significant difference in renal size may be suggestive. Captopril renography is not always helpful, and imaging techniques—either duplex ultrasonography or MR angiography—are the mainstays of diagnosis.[28]

MANAGEMENT OF HYPERTENSION

This section summarizes briefly the results of the important trials of drug therapy on outcome in elderly people. Space does not allow a full description of each trial.

Several recent large intervention studies have assessed the effects of antihypertensive drug treatment on outcome in elderly people, all of which have shown a positive benefit for active treatment. This is perhaps surprising given the heterogeneity of the patients included in the trials (those with combined hypertension, combined and ISH, or ISH alone, the presence or absence of target organ damage, and varying CV risk factors), the differences in antihypertensive drugs used, and the varying length of follow-up.

Published trials

Trials in combined hypertension

The first large trial solely in elderly patients, which awoke widespread interest, was the European Working Party Hypertension in the Elderly (EWPHE) trial published in 1985.[1] The results suggested that, for every 1000 elderly patients treated for 1 year initially with a diuretic, 11 fatal cardiac events, 6 fatal and 11 nonfatal strokes, and 8 cases of congestive cardiac failure would be prevented. Other randomized controlled trials that have enrolled hypertensive patients over 70 years include: that reported by Kuramoto et al.[29] using thiazide diuretics as first-line therapy; the Hypertension in Elderly People trial,[30] using β-blockers; the MRC elderly study,[31] using thiazides or β-blockers; and the STOP-Hypertension trial,[32] again using thiazides or β-blockers as first-line agents. These have all shown

Table 35-1 Compelling and possible indications, contraindications, and cautions for use of the major classes of antihypertensive drugs in elderly people

Class of drug		Compelling indications	Possible indications	Compelling contraindications	Possible contraindications
A	ACE inhibitors	Heart failure Left ventricular dysfunction Type 1 diabetic neuropathy	Chronic renal disease Type 2 diabetic neuropathy	Renovascular disease	Renal impairment PVD
B	Beta-blockers	Myocardial infarction Angina	Heart failure	Asthma/COPD Heart block	Heart failure Dyslipidemia PVD
C	Calcium antagonists (dihydropyridine)	Elderly ISH	Elderly Angina	–	–
D	Thiazide diuretics	Elderly		Gout	Dyslipidemia
	Others				
	Alpha-blockers	Prostatism	Dyslipidemia	Urinary incontinence	Postural hypotension
	All antagonists	ACE-inhibitor-induced cough	Heart failure Intolerance of other antihypertensive drugs	Renovascular disease	PVD
	Calcium antagonists (rate-limiting)	Angina	Myocardial infarction	Heart block Heart failure	Combination with β-blockade

See text for explanation of ABCD classification. Abbreviations: ACE, angiotensin converting enzyme; ISH, isolated systolic hypertension; COPD, chronic obstructive pulmonary disease; PVD, peripheral vascular disease.

Source: Adapted from Ramsey et al. (1999),[24] with permission.

the benefits of treatment in reducing cardiovascular disease (Table 35-1).

MORTALITY   Of the five studies noted above, only the STOP-Hypertension trial reported a significant reduction in all-cause mortality following treatment (relative risk 0.57; 95% CI = 0.37–0.87). A meta-analysis of these five trials demonstrates an insignificant overall reduction in total mortality (odds ratio [OR] 0.90; 0.79–1.02), but overall cardiovascular deaths were significantly reduced (OR 0.78; 0.66–0.92), as were CHD deaths (OR 0.73; 0.59–0.91) and stroke deaths (OR 0.68; 0.50–0.94).

NONFATAL EVENTS   An overall picture of treatment effects on nonfatal events is difficult to formulate because different trials used different criteria for defining nonfatal events; for example, "cerebrovascular events" may have included or excluded transient ischemic attacks or minor strokes. With these provisos in mind, nonfatal stroke events were significantly reduced (OR 0.69; 0.54–0.87), as were CV events (OR 0.72; 0.60–0.88), but with considerable variation between trials. For example, nonfatal stroke events in the STOP-Hypertension trial were reduced by 38 percent and in the HEP trial by 27 percent, and nonfatal coronary events by 20 percent in HEP and by 9 percent in EWPHE.[33] The benefits of treatment in terms of proportional risk reduction were similar between studies (a 35–40 percent decrease in all stroke events), but the absolute benefit seen was related to the underlying patient risk. In the MRC study,[31] strokes prevented per 1000 patient–years of treatment were approximately 2.5, compared with around 14 in the STOP-Hypertension trial.[32] Drug therapy reduced the risk of hemorrhagic stroke within just 1 year of starting treatment, and within 2 years for ischemic stroke.

Trials in isolated systolic hypertension

Trials involving ISH patients only (SHEP,[34] Syst-Eur,[35] and Syst-China[36]) have shown similar reductions in stroke and, to a lesser extent, coronary heart disease. Syst-Eur and Syst-China were unique in their time as they were the first to use calcium-channel blockers (CCBs) as first-line antihypertensive treatment. Concerns had been raised about decreasing diastolic pressure further in patients with ISH, as low DBP levels in cross-sectional longitudinal studies have been shown to be associated with an adverse prognosis in this age group. However, these worries do not seem justified, as in the SHEP study treatment reduced DBP from 77.5 mmHg to 68 mmHg and yet significant reductions were seen in fatal and nonfatal stroke and myocardial infarct rates. Overall, for the ISH studies there were significant reductions in total mortality by 17 percent, in CV mortality by 25 percent, and in fatal and nonfatal stroke by 37 percent. These benefits are similar to those seen in non-ISH trials.

Combined results

The combined results of the CH and ISH trials are shown in Figure 35-2. They suggest that only 45 elderly people with hypertension would need to be treated for 5 years to prevent one CHD event, compared with 180 younger hypertensives. For stroke the benefits are even greater, with only 22 elderly patients needing treatment to prevent a cerebrovascular event, compared with 113 under 65 years. These benefits were achieved with relatively modest reductions in BP of about 20/10 mmHg. Drug compliance amongst elderly hypertensives is generally as good as that for younger patients despite numerous factors that can affect this, including poor eyesight and hearing, confusion, etc. Simple once-daily drug regimens, and perhaps increased use of combined preparations, will improve compliance and therefore blood pressure control.

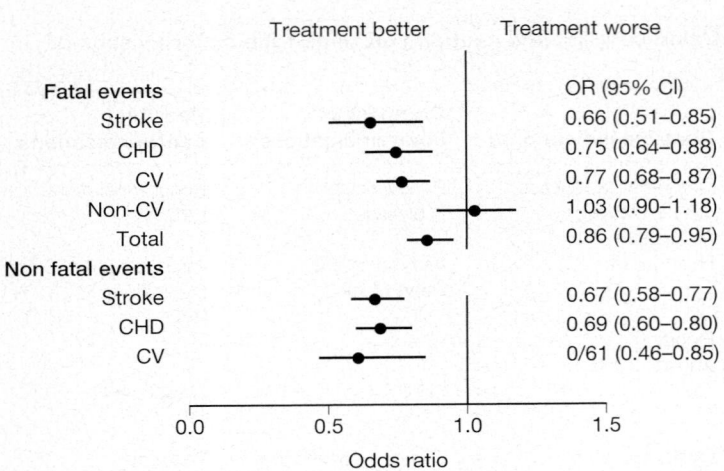

Figure 35-2 Effects of treatment on fatal and nonfatal events. Data from randomized outcome trials involving hypertensive patients aged 70 years and over.[1,29–36]

There is now convincing evidence that antihypertensive treatment should be introduced in nearly all patients up to the age of 80 years if they have a systolic BP ≥160 mmHg and/or a diastolic BP ≥100 mmHg despite nonpharmacological measures (see later). Treatment should also be introduced in those patients with an SBP of 140–159 mmHg and/or DBP ≥90–99 mmHg if target organ damage or other CV risk factors such as diabetes are present and their 10-year CHD risk is ≥15 percent (equivalent to a 20 percent CV risk). This risk can now be easily calculated using the Joint British Societies Coronary Risk Prediction Chart[24] or a similar computer program. This chart cannot be used to predict risk in those aged over 75 years or those on treatment, but it can be used for assessing the need for statin therapy based on the TC:HDL-cholesterol ratio and for the introduction of aspirin (see later).

Target BP levels for treatment

Target blood pressure levels in trials have varied considerably and have also fallen considerably with time; for instance, target levels in the HEP study were 170/105 mmHg, compared with <140 mmHg for systolic BP in SHEP. The fact that the degree of CV risk reduction was so similar between studies is even more remarkable. However, with the concern still present about a potential U- or J-shaped relationship between BP levels on treatment and outcome, it was unclear how far BP should be reduced as no trial had specifically looked at this aspect in elderly patients, or in those with ISH. Results from the EWPHE trial[1] suggested that all-cause mortality was lower in those with an SBP on treatment of 150 mmHg compared with those who achieved an SBP of 130 mmHg.

The HOT study has gone some way to answering questions.[37] This recruited 18,790 patients aged 50–80 years (mean 61.5 years) with a diastolic BP of 100–115 mmHg who were randomized to three target DBP groups: ≤80 mmHg; ≤85 mmHg; or ≤90 mmHg. All patients received initial therapy with the dihydropyridene calcium-channel blocker felodipine. In addition, patients were randomized to low-dose aspirin (75 mg daily) or no aspirin. Unfortunately it proved difficult to reach target BPs, particularly in the two lowest groups of DBP, despite triple therapy in the majority of patients. No differences were seen in outcome measures between the three target BP groups, apart from a borderline-significant reduction in myocardial infarctions in the <80 mmHg group compared with the <90 mmHg group. However, combining all patient groups showed that the lowest risk point for major cardiovascular events was a mean achieved SBP of 138.5 mmHg and a DBP of 82.6 mmHg, and CV mortality was lowest with a BP of 138.8/86.5 mmHg. For stroke, the lowest estimated incidence was with an SBP of 142 mmHg with no definite minimum DBP level. In a diabetic subgroup, however, major CV events were highly significantly reduced, the risk being halved for those in the ≤80 mmHg group compared with the ≤90 mmHg group. There seems to be little to be gained in reducing the diastolic BP below 80 mmHg except in diabetic patients.

Based on these results, the British Hypertension Society guidelines recommend that clinic BP levels for optimal control should be SBP <140 mmHg and DBP <85 mmHg, and in diabetics <140/80 mmHg, with minimum recommended levels for BP control of <150/90 mmHg and 140/85 mmHg, respectively.[24]

It is important to bear in mind that introducing antihypertensive treatment is only part of the risk-reduction process. It is the level of blood pressure while on treatment that is a much better predictor of subsequent events than baseline values—hence the need to achieve these target levels. This will mean three or more different antihypertensive agents in 20–30 percent of elderly hypertensives. It is also important that other CV risk factors be dealt with simultaneously, such as raised lipid levels and smoking.

Prophylaxis

Aspirin use

Although aspirin reduces deaths following myocardial infarction and stroke, its routine use in patients with uncomplicated hypertension has been unclear. In the HOT study,[37] those randomized to 75 mg of aspirin had a 15 percent (1–27 percent) reduction in major CV events, and MIs were reduced by 36 percent (15–51 percent); but stroke, total, and CV mortality rates were unaffected by treatment. Similar results were seen in a thrombosis prevention trial of men aged 45–69 years at high risk of CHD.[38] Both studies emphasized that if any benefit from aspirin were to be achieved, BP levels must be controlled;

that is, <150/90 mmHg before aspirin is started in patients with uncomplicated hypertension.

For elderly patients matters are less clear, as the benefits of prophylactic aspirin use appear to decrease with age. There was a 52 percent risk reduction with aspirin for CHD in those aged 45–49, compared with 29 percent increase in those aged 60–69 years. Those least likely to benefit were patients with a systolic BP >145 mmHg compared with those with SBP <130 mmHg.

Elderly hypertensive patients should receive low-dose aspirin (75 mg daily) only if BP levels are well controlled and their 10-year CV risk is ≥15%, unless there are other specific indications—i.e. after stroke or MI, with diabetes or other evidence of target organ damage. Even then, good BP control should be aimed at.

Statin use

No studies of statin use have specifically targeted people with hypertension, young or old. Conclusions drawn are therefore based on subgroup analysis of the large trials.

Insufficient data exist to support lipid-lowering therapy for primary prevention in patients aged over 70 years, and so routine lipid screening over this age is unnecessary. With regard to secondary prevention, there have been just two large studies of statin use in patients with CHD over the age of 65 years.[39,40] The results suggest that a much more proactive stance should be taken. Evidence indicates that 65–74 year olds with CHD (MI or angina) are as likely to benefit from statin therapy as much younger patients, in terms of reducing all major CHD events by about 25 percent and stroke by 30 percent over 5 years. We do not yet know whether stroke patients with raised total cholesterol (TC) will benefit from cholesterol reduction; but as most die from coronary heart disease if they survive the initial stroke, a case could be made for statin treatment. Ongoing studies will be able to answer the question as to whether those aged over 75 years should receive statin therapy, and whether those with a history of stroke, especially cerebral infarction, will also benefit.

There are no long-term studies of the effects of diet on lipid levels and CV events. Such measures are likely to reduce TC only by 10 percent. Effective reductions will therefore require potentially expensive statin treatment. Evidence suggests statin therapy could be justified in those with a 10-year CHD risk of 6 percent, which would mean that nearly two-thirds of the elderly population should be on treatment! This is unlikely to be possible, so guidelines recommend that patients up to the age of 75 years with CHD or overt atherosclerotic diseases should be considered for secondary prevention with a view to reducing TC to ≤5 mmol/L or by 25 percent, whichever is greater (or LDL cholesterol to ≤3 mmol/L or by 30 percent). For primary prevention, those up to the age of 70 years with TC ≥5 mmol/L and a 10-year CHD risk >30 percent should be considered for treatment.

Nonpharmacological methods

There is a general lack of enthusiasm for nondrug measures to reduce BP in elderly patients, despite the evidence of their efficacy (see later). Various guidelines have emphasized their importance as first-line treatment in trying to achieve normotension and in reducing other CV risk factors.

WEIGHT LOSS   A 2 kg weight loss over a 6-month period will reduce blood pressure by about 4/5 mmHg in elderly hypertensive subjects.[41] However, constant encouragement is needed to maintain this weight loss if the long-term benefit is to be seen. A body weight within 10 percent of ideal (or a BMI <26 kg/m²) should be encouraged, not just for its hypotensive effects but also to improve glycemic control and lipid profiles, and to improve mobility and respiratory and cardiac function.

SALT RESTRICTION   The hypotensive effect of reducing sodium intake increases with age. In elderly people with hypertension, an 80 mmol/day decrease in sodium intake will result in an 8 mmHg fall in SBP.[42] This level of sodium reduction can be achieved simply by avoiding salty foods and not adding salt whilst cooking or at the table. Reducing salt added to processed foods would make even greater reductions possible.

INCREASING POTASSIUM INTAKE   Increasing potassium intake by 40 mmol/day will have a significant hypotensive action, reducing clinic BP by 10/6 mmHg and 24-hour BP levels by 6/2 mmHg.[43] In addition, increasing dietary potassium intake may reduce stroke rates over and above any hypotensive action. The average intake of potassium in the UK is about 60–70 mmol/day, and an intake of 100–110 mmol/day can be achieved by encouraging greater consumption of fresh fruit and vegetables. Potassium supplements are not routinely recommended for their hypotensive action, and care must obviously be taken in those with renal impairment.

REDUCING ALCOHOL INTAKE   The alcohol–hypertension link has been firmly established, but the relationship is non-linear. Most epidemiological studies have shown a J-shaped curve, with the lowest incidence of hypertension in those drinking about 1 unit (10 g) alcohol per day.[44] Low levels of alcohol intake also appear to have a protective effect with regard to the development of coronary heart disease, even in older individuals, by raising HDL levels and having an antithrombotic effect.

OTHER MEASURES   Changing magnesium and calcium intake have not been found to have a significant effect on BP in the elderly population, although increasing vitamin C intake does have a mild hypotensive action as well as a positive effect on the lipid profile in older hypertensives.[45] Caffeine may have an acute pressor effect in caffeine-naive persons, but regular caffeine intake does not have a pressor effect (although some studies have shown increasing consumption is associated with an increased CHD risk). Mild aerobic exercise (walking 30 minutes a day 3–4 times a week) results in important reductions in BP (approximately 20/10 mmHg) in older hypertensives. It also decreases stroke risk independently of its hypotensive action, and improves glucose profiles, reduces weight, and improves general well-being.[46]

COMBINED EFFECTS   The combined effect of dietary interventions has been investigated in two important studies. The Dietary Approaches to Stop Hypertension (DASH) trial[47] studied the effects of a special diet rich in vegetables and fruit and low in diary products. It compared this to a standard diet, while varying levels of sodium intake in persons with and without hypertension. The DASH diet with a low sodium intake resulted in a BP fall of 7 mmHg in normotensives and 11.5 mmHg in hypertensives—similar effects to those that might be seen with a thiazide diuretic (see later). However, the duration of the trial was only 30 days.

The Trial Of Non-pharmacological intervention in the Elderly (TONE) study[41] randomized elderly hypertensives who were normotensive on monotherapy to drug treatment withdrawal and either sodium reduction (and, if obese, sodium reduction or weight loss or the combination) or usual care with a 30-month follow-up. End-points of restarting hypotensive drug treatment or developing a CV event were significantly reduced by all the interventions, with a 53 percent risk reduction in the obese on the combined sodium-restriction and weight-loss diet. The study was underpowered to find a significant decrease in CV events alone, but the nutritional interventions were well tolerated.

Approximately 25 percent of elderly people with mild hypertension could remain off drug treatment for 12 months or more using nonpharmacological measures. Predictors of those who will remain normotensive include the absence of ECG evidence of LVH, obesity, and patients with well-controlled SBP levels prior to withdrawal of treatment. In general, nonpharmacological methods should be tried initially in all patients and given time to work, though constant encouragement will be needed. In the majority of patients drug therapy will also be needed. Important synergistic effects between nonpharmacological and drug treatment are found, such as in sodium restriction with those patients treated with ACE inhibitors.

Drug treatments

Thiazides
Low-dose thiazide diuretics remain the first-choice antihypertensive agents in elderly patients for combined or isolated systolic hypertension.[24] Their mode of action has not been fully resolved, but is in part due to a reduction in peripheral vascular resistance. Although there are concerns that thiazides may induce postural hypotension this is not a significant side-effect. Mild hypokalemia, hyponatremia, and hyperuricemia can occur but are not normally clinically significant if low doses are used. Impotence can still be a problem with these agents, in all age groups. Serum electrolytes should be checked before and a few weeks after starting treatment to assess the need for additional potassium supplementation.

Beta-adrenoreceptor blockers
Beta-blockers, like thiazide diuretics, have been used as first-line therapy in several large intervention trials in the elderly. There are, however, theoretical reasons why they may not be the most obvious choice in elderly patients with hypertension as they reduce cardiac output and renin levels which are already reduced, and increase peripheral resistance. Although they can effectively reduce BP in this age group, they do not have a good side-effect profile. For instance, in the MRC study in the elderly,[31] 30 percent of the β-blocker group were withdrawn because of major side-effects, compared with 15 percent in the diuretic limb and 4 percent of those on placebo. There were also significant differences between treatment limbs in outcome measures in the trial. The β-blocker group showed

no significant reduction in coronary events, unlike the diuretic group.

A recent meta-analysis of all trials in elderly patients with hypertension using diuretics and/or β-blockers as first-line agents showed that, although β-blockers prevented all stroke events, they did not reduce stroke mortality; nor did they reduce CHD events, CV, or all-cause mortality, whereas diuretics showed a positive and significant advantage in all these outcome measures.[48]

In view of these findings, patient compliance and economic factors, thiazides are the drug of first choice for initial therapy. However, as over half of such patients will require two or more agents, β-blockers should still be considered as additional therapy. There are still those patients in whom β-blockers may be considered first-line agents, particularly those who have had a previous myocardial infarction or have angina.

Calcium-channel blockers
Recent intervention studies involving elderly people with hypertension—the Syst-Eur,[34] Syst-China,[35] and HOT[37] studies—have used members of the dihydropyridine CCB group as first-line therapy. There has been considerable debate about the safety of the dihydropyridines, and various meta-analyses have arrived at diametrically opposite conclusions. It is clear that the placebo-controlled intervention studies in the elderly using dihydropyridine CCBs as first-line treatment have shown significant benefits, particularly in terms of stroke and CV risk reduction. We still need the security of long-term safety data, but trial evidence indicates that these agents are generally well tolerated and effective, so are recommended as first-line agents in patients with isolated systolic hypertension in whom thiazide diuretics cannot be tolerated.[23] Short-acting calcium-channel blockers have no role in the treatment of hypertension.

Angiotensin converting enzyme inhibitors and AII antagonists
ACE inhibitors (ACEIs) are effective antihypertensive agents in young and old alike. First-dose hypotension may occur, especially in patients who are on large-dose diuretics, so it is usually recommended that these agents be stopped for a few days before initiating ACE inhibitor therapy. Hyperkalemia can be a problem, so potassium-sparing diuretics should be stopped with the introduction of these drugs. Problems with renal impairment have been reported in older patients taking NSAIDs and those with pre-existing renal impairment. Renal failure may be precipitated in those with occult renal artery stenosis, so it is recommended that urea and electrolytes be checked before and 1–2 weeks after starting treatment. Cough can be a problem in about 10 percent of patients, so an AII antagonist may be a suitable alternative. There are theoretical reasons to suggest that the combination of ACE and AII inhibitors could be potentially synergistic in their hypotensive actions, although it is too early to recommend this combination.

There are now several outcome studies using ACEIs as first-line therapy in the elderly. The recently published STOP-2 trial[49] compared the newer antihypertensive agents—a dihydropyridine CCB and an ACEI—against standard therapy with β-blockers and diuretics. Overall there was little difference in terms of outcome measures between the new and old agents.

A comparison of the ACEI and CCB groups showed a greater reduction in myocardial infarction and congestive heart failure in the ACEI group (by 23 and 22 percent, respectively) but a greater decrease in stroke mortality with CCBs. Overall CV mortality, total mortality, and all major CV events were similar in the ACEI and CCB groups, with CV mortality being 20.5 per 1000 patient–years in the ACEI group and 19.2 per 1000 patient–years in the CCB group. There have been no large outcome studies using ACEIs as first-line therapy in elderly people with hypertension. Further ongoing studies of new versus old agents may give more definitive answers as to whether one group is preferable to another as first-line therapy, but there is still no evidence that the newer drugs are any better than the older established antihypertensives—but they are more expensive!

Other agents

Alpha-blockers still have a minor role in treating elderly people with hypertension and are usually used as additional, rather than first-line, therapy. The withdrawal of doxazosin as initial therapy in the ALLHAT study[50] because of increased risks of heart failure and stroke compared with chlorthalidone supports this policy. Alpha-blockers may have a role in men with prostatic symptoms, and they can be used in renal failure though postural hypotension and urinary incontinence remain a drawback in a significant number of patients.

Methyldopa, hydralazine, and centrally acting agents are rarely used because of their adverse side-effect profiles. The former two agents need to be taken more than once a day, which does not aid compliance. There seems little reason to use agents that do not have a 24-hour hypotensive action when taken once-daily.

Combination therapy

Over 50 percent of these patients will need two or more agents if adequate blood pressure control is to be achieved.[37] Not all agents have a synergistic effect. For example, the addition of a calcium-channel blocker to a thiazide diuretic in most studies has a minimal additional hypotensive effect. Adoption of the "ABCD strategy" will help form logical combinations, such that antihypertensive combinations are likely to have an additional hypotensive effect if their mechanisms of action are complementary.[51]

The first-line agents in the elderly should be a thiazide diuretic (D) or, if that is not tolerated, a calcium-channel blocker (C). If control is not achieved, a first-line agent of the other group—i.e. ACEIs (A) or β-blockers (B)—could be tried. If good control is still not obtained, an additional agent from the other group is added along the following lines in the elderly: (C or D) → (A or B) → (A or B + C or D) → combination + third-line agent (Table 35-1).

SPECIAL CASES

The 80+ age group

Several trials have included patients over the age of 80, but it is still unclear whether they benefit from treatment. Longitudinal studies have shown that raised blood pressure in the very old (aged 75–80+ years) is not as big a risk factor as in younger people. However, the SHEP study[34] showed that only the 80+ age group had a significant reduction in CV risk with active treatment compared to placebo, though there were similar trends in the 60+ and 70+ age groups. A meta-analysis of these trials[52] that included all the patients aged 80+ years showed that treatment prevented 34 percent (18–52 percent) of strokes, with a reduction in major CV events (23 percent) and heart failure (42 percent). However, total mortality was increased by 15 percent in the actively treated group, leaving physicians with a considerable dilemma as what is best for very old hypertensive patients.

The currently ongoing HYpertension in the Very Elderly Trial (HYVET)[53] will, it is to be hoped, answer this important question. Firm recommendations for this age group cannot be given, but decisions should be based on biological rather than chronological age. Patients aged 80+ with newly diagnosed hypertension and who are generally fit with a reasonable life expectancy should be considered for treatment if they have evidence of target organ damage. Those who reach 80 years of age on treatment should probably continue therapy, though about 20 percent can probably have monotherapy withdrawn if blood pressure is controlled and they will remain normotensive.

Type II diabetes

Hypertension is common in elderly type II diabetics. Nearly two-thirds will have raised BP levels that require treatment. Elderly diabetics as much as their younger counterparts should be treated aggressively in terms of BP reduction. The UK Prospective Diabetes Study[54] showed that strict BP control reduces stroke by 44 percent (11–65 percent) and death related to diabetes by 32 percent (6–51 percent). A subgroup of elderly diabetics in the SHEP study[34] did similarly well, with a 5-year reduction of major CV events of 34 percent (6–54 percent) compared with placebo, and a reduction of nonfatal and fatal CHD events by 54 percent (12–76 percent). The HOT study[37] also included a group of diabetics and only this group showed a significantly better outcome in those in whom diastolic BP was reduced to <80 mmHg compared with <90 mmHg on treatment, with a 50 percent reduction in CV end-points in the lowest BP group. Diabetics in the STOP-2 study showed no difference in outcome between those on conventional therapy (low-dose thiazide diuretic or β-blocker) and those on the newer agents (ACE inhibitors and CCBs). This again highlights how it is the degree of BP reduction and not the agent used that predicts CV risk, and diabetics require lower target BP levels as evidenced by the HOT study. Hence, in diabetics, BP levels for the introduction of therapy should be ≥140/90 mmHg (lower starting BP levels than for nondiabetics) with optimum control levels set at <140/80 mmHg. No one group of antihypertensive agents appears more efficacious than another.

Cognitive function, dementia, and quality of life

Although increased blood pressure has been associated with impaired cognitive function, this does not mean that antihypertensive treatment will reduce this decline. Indeed, it has been suggested that antihypertensive treatment may actually hasten it. Reassuringly, the MRC study in the elderly found no difference in the changes in cognitive function between β-blocker- or diuretic-treated patients compared with placebo over a 54-month follow-up.[55]

Since hypertension is associated with both vascular dementia and Alzheimer's disease, it might be hoped that treatment could slow down or prevent cognitive decline. The Syst-Eur study,[35] encouragingly for a relatively short follow-up period of 2 years, found that active treatment reduced the incidence of dementia by 50 percent (though the numbers actually involved were very small) and improved the Mini-Mental State score slightly, whereas in the placebo group scores deteriorated significantly. However, the SHEP study[34] failed to find a decrease in the incidence of dementia with active treatment. It is to be hoped that current studies will guide us as to whether we can expect to prevent a decline in cognitive function with antihypertensive treatment.

Although there are relatively limited numbers of studies assessing the long-term effects of antihypertensives on quality-of-life measures, most have shown a long-term benefit. Quality of life should be an essential part of the overall patient assessment, but it does not necessarily require a lengthy or complex questionnaire. Simple clinical assessment of possible changes in physical function (e.g. mobility and balance, and ability for self-care), sexual function, energy levels and mood, cognitive function, life satisfaction, and social interaction is sufficient. Of particular importance are the effects of treatment on cognitive function, mood, and mobility. Thiazide diuretics appear to be the "cleanest" in terms of effects on quality-of-life factors, but there are at present too few data on the newer agents to assess whether some of the positive qualities of these agents (e.g. improved mood with ACEI use) are borne out in large clinical trials.

Stroke

Antihypertensive treatment helps to prevent primary stroke, but in the acute stroke and post-stroke situation the evidence for reducing an elevated BP is less clear. Acutely post-ictus, BP is frequently raised but the few antihypertensive intervention studies have been disappointing. Beta-blockers and calcium-channel blockers given orally or intravenously have been shown either to have no effect on prognosis or to be associated with an adverse outcome. The numbers of patients studied has been small and the study design often questionable, so there is a desperate need for a suitable trial to assess whether lowering of BP in the acute situation is of benefit. Until such evidence is available, in the majority of cases raised blood pressure is probably best left untreated, at least for the first 2 weeks.

Trials of BP reduction in the weeks and months following stroke have also been disappointing. There have been only two randomized intervention trials that have specifically recruited patients with raised BP levels following stroke, and only three others that have included both normotensive and hypertensive individuals. Overall these studies have shown that treatment does not reduce stroke recurrence or total mortality, but it does reduce the number of nonfatal strokes by 19 percent (5–32 percent) and all major CV events by 18 percent (5–28 percent). The recently published PROGRESS Trial taking patients with controlled BP levels several weeks to months after stroke has shown the benefits of the combination of perindopril and indapamide in reducing stroke recurrence by 43 percent and major vascular events by 40 percent.[56]

SUMMARY

Hypertension is the biggest single treatable risk factor for stroke and cardiovascular disease in those aged up to 80 years, and probably beyond, but it is becoming increasingly appreciated that other elements that dictate cardiovascular risk in older people—such as diabetes and abnormal lipid profiles—also require active management. Nonpharmacological methods of BP reduction should initially be tried in all patients. Thiazide diuretics are the first-choice antihypertensive in the vast majority of patients, there being no evidence to date that any of the newer antihypertensive agents is more efficacious. It is the level of BP reduction rather than any specific treatment that is important in reducing event rates, and the majority of patients will need two or more antihypertensive agents to obtain adequate BP control. Effective treatment leads to a substantial reduction in cerebrovascular and coronary heart disease events within a short time of starting treatment, without producing adverse side-effects or compromising quality of life. Statin therapy and prophylactic aspirin use (when BP levels are controlled) are warranted in patients at the appropriate level of cardiovascular risk.

Although we have come a long way in a short time in terms of evidenced-based management of the older hypertensive patient, there is still no room for complacency. Too many elderly patients remain undiagnosed or inadequately treated, in terms of BP reduction and management of other cardiovascular risk factors, for the full benefits of treatment to be realized.

KEY POINTS Hypertension

- Hypertension is the main treatable risk factor for cerebrovascular and coronary artery disease in elderly people, although significant numbers of elderly hypertensives remain inadequately treated.

- Hypertensives aged up to 80 years at least with sustained systolic BP ≥160 mmHg and/or diastolic BP ≥100 mmHg should be treated. Those with an SBP of 140–159 mmHg and/or a DBP of 90–99 mmHg, evidence of target organ damage (TOD), or a CHD risk of ≥15 percent over 10 years, should also receive antihypertensive treatment.

- For those aged over 80 years and newly diagnosed the benefits of treatment are unclear, but if TOD is present then therapy may be of value. For those aged 80+ years already on antihypertensive treatment, this should probably be continued particularly if TOD is present.

- Thiazide diuretics remain the preferred first-line therapy, although dihydropyridine calcium-channel blockers may be useful alternative agents in those with isolated systolic hypertension. Target clinic BP levels on treatment should be <140/85 mmHg in nondiabetics and <140/80 in diabetics. The majority of patients will require two or more antihypertensive drugs to achieve these levels.

REFERENCES

1. Amery A, Birkenhager W, Brixko R, Bulpitt C, Clement D et al: Mortality and morbidity results from the European working party on high blood pressure in the elderly trial. Lancet 1985;1:1349–1354
2. Volkonas PS, Kannel WB, Cupples LA: Epidemiology and risk of hypertension in the elderly: the Framingham study. J Hypertens 1988;6(Suppl 1):S3–S9
3. Burt VL, Cutler JA, Higgins M et al: Trends in the prevalence, awareness, treatment and control of hypertension in the adult US population: data from the Health Examination Surveys, 1960 to 1991. Hypertension 1995;26:60–69
4. Sagie A, Larson MG, Levy D: The natural history of borderline isolated systolic hypertension. N Engl J Med 1993;329:1912–1917
5. Ekpo EK, Ashworth IN, Fernando MU, White AD, Shah IU: Prevalence of mixed hypertension, isolated systolic hypertension and isolated diastolic hypertension in the elderly population in the community. J Hum Hypertens 1994;8:539–543
6. De Backer G, Myny K, De Henauw S et al: Prevalence, awareness, treatment and control of arterial hypertension in an elderly population in Belgium. J Hum Hypertens 1988;12:701–706
7. Dannenberg AL, Garrison RJ, Kannel WB: Incidence of hypertension in the Framingham study. Am J Pub Health 1988;78:676–679
8. Kannel WB, D'Agostino RB, Sibershatz H: Blood pressure and cardiovascular morbidity and mortality rates in the elderly. Am Heart J 1997;134:758–763
9. Glynn RJ, Field TS, Rosner B et al: Evidence for a positive linear relation between blood pressure and mortality in elderly people. Lancet 1995;345:825–829
10. Port S, Demer L, Jennrich R, Walter D, Garfinkel A: Systolic blood pressure and mortality. Lancet 2000;355:175–180
11. Curb JD, Abbot RD, MacLean CJ et al: Age-related changes in stroke risk in men with hypertension and normal blood pressure. Stroke 1996;27:819–824
12. Nielsen WB, Vestbo J, Jensen GB: Isolated systolic hypertension as a major risk factor for stroke and myocardial infarction and an unexploited source of cardiovascular prevention: a prospective population-based study. J Hum Hypertens 1995;9:175–180
13. O'Donnell CJ, Ridker PM, Glynn RJ et al: Hypertension and borderline isolated systolic hypertension increase risks of cardiovascular disease in mortality in male physicians. Circulation 1997;95:1132–1137
14. Franklin SS, Khan SA, Wong ND, Larson MG, Levy D: Is pulse pressure useful in predicting risk for coronary heart disease? The Framingham Heart Study. Circulation 1999;100:354–360
15. Domanski MJ, Davis BR, Pfeffer MA, Kastantin M, Mitchell GF: Isolated systolic hypertension: prognostic information provided by pulse pressure. Hypertension 1999;34:375–380
16. Frost PH, Davis BR, Burlando AJ et al, for the Systolic Hypertension in the Elderly Research Group: Serum lipids and incidence of coronary heart disease: findings from the Systolic Hypertension in the Elderly Program (SHEP). Circulation 1996;94:2381–2388
17. Kannel WB: Cardiovascular risk factors in the elderly. Coron Artery Dis 1997;8:565–575
18. Tuomilehto J: Body mass index and prognosis in elderly hypertensive patients: a report from the European working party on high blood pressure in the elderly. Am J Med 1991;90(3A):34S–41S
19. Barrrett-Connor E, Grady D: Hormone replacement therapy, heart disease and other considerations. Annu Rev Public Health 1998;19:55–72
20. Ueda K, Omae T, Hasuo Y et al: Prognosis and outcome of elderly hypertensives in a Japanese community: results from a long-term prospective study. J Hypertens 1988;6:991–997
21. Robinson TG, Waddington A, Ward-Close S, Taub N, Potter JF: The predictive role of 24-hour compared to casual blood pressure levels on outcome following acute stroke. Cerebrovasc Dis 1997;7:264–272
22. Cacciatore F, Abete P, Ferrara N et al, for the Osservatoria Geriatrico Campano Group: The role of blood pressure in cognitive impairment in an elderly population. J Hypertens 1997;15:135–142
23. Tzourio C, Dufouil C, Ducimetiere P, Alperovitch A, for the EVA Study Group: Cognitive decline in individuals with high blood pressure. Neurology 1999;53:1948–1952
24. Ramsey LE, Williams B, Johnston GD et al: Guidelines for the management of hypertension: report of the third working party of the British Hypertension Society. J Hum Hypertens 1999;9:569–592
25. O'Brien E, Waeber B, Parati G, Staessen J, Myers MG, on behalf of the European Society of Hypertension Working Group on Blood Pressure Monitoring: Blood pressure measuring devices: recommendations of the European Society of Hypertension. BMJ 2001;322:531–536
26. Staessen JA, Thijs L, Fagard R et al, for the Systolic Hypertension in Europe trial investigators: Predicting cardiovascular risk using conventional vs ambulatory blood pressure in older patients with systolic hypertension. JAMA 1999;282:539–546
27. O'Brien E, Coats A, Owens P et al: Use and interpretation of ambulatory blood pressure monitoring: recommendations of the British Hypertension Society. BMJ 2000;320:1128–1134
28. Safin RD, Textor SC: Renal artery stenosis. N Engl J Med 2001;344:431–441
29. Kuramoto K, Matsushita S, Kuwajima I, Murakami M: Prospective study on the treatment of mild hypertension in the aged. Jpn Heart J 1981;22:75–85
30. Coope J, Warrender TS: Randomised trial of treatment of hypertension in elderly patients in primary care. BMJ 1986;293:1145–1148
31. MRC Working Party: Medical Research Council trial of treatment of hypertension in older adults: principal results. BMJ 1992;304:405–412
32. Dahlof B, Lindholm LH, Hansson L et al: Morbidity and mortality in the Swedish Trial in Older Patients with Hypertension (STOP-Hypertension). Lancet 1991;338:1281–1285
33. Lever AF, Ramsey LE: Treatment of hypertension in the elderly. J Hypertens 1995;13:571–579
34. SHEP Cooperative Research Group: Prevention of stroke by antihypertensive drug treatment in older persons with isolated systolic hypertension: final results of the Systolic Hypertension in the Elderly Program (SHEP). JAMA 1991;265:3255–3264
35. Staessen JA, Fagard R, Thijs L et al, for the Systolic Hypertension in Europe (Syst-Eur) trial investigators: Randomised double blind comparison of placebo and active treatment for older patients with isolated systolic hypertension. Lancet 1997;350:757–764
36. Liu K, Wang JG, Gong L, Liu G, Staessen J, for the Systolic Hypertension in China (Syst-China) collaborative group: Comparison of active treatment and placebo in older Chinese patients with isolated systolic hypertension. J Hypertens 1988;16:1823–1829
37. Hansson L, Zanchetti A, Carruthers SG et al, for the HOT study group: Effects of intensive blood pressure lowering and lose dose aspirin in patients with hypertension: principal results of the Hypertension Optimal Treatment (HOT) randomised trial. Lancet 1998;351:1755–1762
38. Meade TW, Brennan PJ, on behalf of the MRC General Practice Research Framework: Determination of who may derive most benefit from aspirin in primary prevention: subgroup results from a randomised controlled trial. BMJ 2000;321:13–17
39. The Long-Term Intervention with Pravastatin in Ischaemic Heart Disease (LIPID) study group: Prevention of cardiovascular events and death with pravastatin in patients with coronary heart disease and a broad range of initial cholesterol levels. N Engl J Med 1998;339:1349–1357
40. Plehen JF, Davis BR, Sacks FM et al: Reduction of stroke incidence after myocardial infarction with pravastatin: the cholesterol and recurrent events (CARE) study. Circulation 1999;99:216–223
41. Whelton PK, Appel LJ, Espeland MA et al, for the TONE collaborative research group: Sodium reduction and weight loss in the treatment of hypertension in older persons: A randomised controlled trial of nonpharmacological interventions in the elderly. JAMA 1998;279:839–846
42. Fotherby MD, Potter JF: Effects of moderate sodium restriction on clinic and twenty-four hour ambulatory blood pressure in elderly hypertensive subjects. J Hypertens 1993;11:657–663
43. Fotherby MD, Potter JF: Potassium supplementation reduces clinic and ambulatory blood pressure in elderly hypertensive patients. J Hypertens 1992;20:1403–1408
44. Klatsky AL, Friedman GD, Siegelaub AB, Gerard MJ: Alcohol consumption and blood pressure: Kaiser-Permanente Multiphasic Health Examination Data. N Engl J Med 1977;296:1194–1199
45. Fotherby MD, Williams JC, Forster LA, Craner P, Ferns GA: Effect of vitamin C on ambulatory blood pressure and plasma lipids in older persons. J Hypertens 2000;18:411–415
46. Hagberg JM, Montain SJ, Martin WH, Ehsani AA: Effect of exercise training in 60- to 69-year old persons with essential hypertension. Am J Cardiol 1989;64:348–353
47. Appel LJ, Moore TJ, Obarzanek E et al, for the DASH collaborative research group: A clinical trial of the effects of dietary patterns on blood pressure. N Engl J Med 1997;336:1117–1124
48. Messerli F, Grossman E, Goldbourt U: Are β-blockers efficacious as first-line therapy for hypertension in the elderly? JAMA 1998;279:1903–1907

49. Hansson L, Kindholm LH, Ekbom T et al, for the STOP-Hypertension-2 study group: Randomised trial of old and new antihypertensive drugs in elderly patients: cardiovascular mortality and morbidity the Swedish Trial in Old Patients with Hypertension-2 study. Lancet 1999;354:1751–1754

50. The Officers and Coordinators for the ALLHAT collaborative research group: Major cardiovascular events in hypertensive patients randomised to doxazosin vs chlorthalidone: the Antihypertensive and Lipid Lowering Treatment to Prevent Heart Attack Trial. JAMA 2000;283:1967–1975

51. Dickerson JEC, Hingorani AD, Ashby MJ, Palmer CR, Brown MJ: Optimisation of antihypertensive treatment by crossover rotation of four major classes. Lancet 1999;353:2008–2013

52. Gueyffier F, Bulpitt C, Boissel J-P et al, for the INDANA group: Antihypertensive drugs in very old people: a subgroup meta-analysis of randomised controlled trials. Lancet 1999;353:793–796

53. Bulpitt C, Fletcher A, Beckett N et al: The Hypertension in the Very Elderly Trial (HYVET): protocol for the main trial. Drugs Ageing 2001;18:151–164

54. Adler AI, Stratton IM, Neil HAW et al, for the UK Prospective Diabetes study group: Association of systolic blood pressure with macrovascular and microvascular complications of type 2 diabetes (UKPDS 36): prospective observational study. BMJ 2000;321:412–419

55. Prince MJ, Bird AS, Blizard RA, Mann AH: Is the cognitive function of older patients affected by antihypertensive treatment? Results from 54 months of the Medical Research Council's treatment trial of hypertension in older adults. BMJ 1996;312:801–805

56. PROGRESS Collaborative Group: Randomised trial of a Perindopril based blood pressure lowering regimen among 6105 individuals with previous stroke or transient ischaemic attack. Lancet 2001;358:1033–1041

Chapter 36

Valvular heart disease

Wilbert S. Aronow

AORTIC STENOSIS

Etiology and prevalence of AS

Valvular aortic stenosis (AS) in elderly people is usually due to stiffening, scarring, and calcification of the aortic valve leaflets. The commissures are not fused as in rheumatic AS. Calcific deposits in the aortic valve are common in older persons and may lead to valvular AS.[1–7] Aortic cuspal calcium was present in 295 of 752 men (36 percent), mean age 80 years, and in 672 of 1663 women (40 percent), mean age 82 years.[6] Of 2358 persons, mean age 81 years, 378 (16 percent) had valvular AS, 981 (42 percent) had valvular aortic sclerosis (thickening of or calcific deposits on the aortic valve cusps with a peak flow velocity across the aortic valve ≤ 1.5 m/s), and 999 (42 percent) had no valvular AS or aortic sclerosis.[7] Calcific deposits in the aortic valve were present in 22 of 40 necropsy patients (55 percent) aged 90–103 years.[2] Calcium of the aortic valve and mitral annulus may coexist.[1–3,8,9]

In the Helsinki Aging Study, calcification of the aortic valve was diagnosed by Doppler echocardiography in 28 percent of 76 persons aged 55–71 years, in 48 percent of 197 persons aged 75–76 years, in 55 percent of 155 persons aged 80–81 years, and in 75 percent of 124 persons aged 85–86 years.[5] Aortic valve calcification, aortic sclerosis, and mitral annular calcium (MAC) are degenerative processes,[1,2,10–12] accounting for their high prevalence in an elderly population.

Otto et al.[11] showed that the early lesion of degenerative AS is an active inflammatory process with some similarities to atherosclerosis, including lipid deposition, macrophage and T-cell infiltration, and basement membrane disruption. In a study of 571 persons, mean age 82 years, 292 (51 percent) had calcified or thickened aortic cusps or root.[13] A serum total cholesterol ≥ 200 mg/dL, a history of hypertension, diabetes mellitus, and a serum high-density lipoprotein cholesterol < 35 mg/dL were more prevalent in older persons with calcified or thickened aortic cusps or root than in older persons with normal aortic cusps and root.[13]

In the Helsinki Aging Study, age, hypertension, and a low body mass index were independent predictors of aortic valve calcification.[14] In 5201 persons older than 65 years in the Cardiovascular Health Study, independent clinical factors associated with degenerative aortic valve disease included age, male gender, smoking, history of hypertension, height, and high lipoprotein (a) and low-density lipoprotein cholesterol levels.[12] In 1275 older persons, mean age 81 years, AS was present in 52 of 202 (26 percent) with 40–100 percent extracranial carotid arterial disease (ECAD) and in 162 of 1073 (15 percent) with 0–39 percent ECAD.[15] In 290 persons, mean age 79 years, with valvular AS who had follow-up Doppler echocardiograms, older persons with MAC had a greater reduction in aortic valve area/year than older persons without MAC.[16] Significant independent risk factors for progression of valvular AS in

102 persons, mean age 76 years, who had follow-up Doppler echocardiograms were cigarette smoking and hypercholesterolemia.[17] These and other data suggest that aortic valve calcium, MAC, and coronary atherosclerosis in older persons have similar predisposing factors.[11–19]

The frequency of AS increases with age. Valvular AS diagnosed by Doppler echocardiography was present in 141 of 924 men (15 percent), mean age 80 years, and in 322 of 1881 women (17 percent), mean age 81 years.[20] Severe valvular AS (peak gradient across aortic valve of ≥ 50 mmHg or aortic valve area <0.75 cm²) was diagnosed in 62 of 2805 older persons (2 percent).[20] Moderate valvular AS (peak gradient across aortic valve of 26–49 mmHg or aortic valve area of 0.75–1.49 cm²) was present in 149 of 2805 older persons (5 percent).[20] Mild valvular AS (peak gradient across aortic valve of 10–25 mmHg or aortic valve area ≥1.50 cm²) occurred in 25 of 2805 older persons (9 percent).[20] In 501 unselected persons aged 75–86 years in the Helsinki Aging Study, critical AS was present in 3 percent and moderate-to-severe AS in 5 percent of the 501 older persons.[5]

Pathophysiology of AS

In valvular AS, there is resistance to ejection of blood from the left ventricle (LV) into the aorta, with a pressure gradient across the aortic valve during systole and an increase in LV systolic pressure. The pressure overload on the LV leads to concentric LV hypertrophy, with an increase in LV wall thickness and mass, normalizing systolic wall stress, and maintenance of normal LV ejection fraction and cardiac output.[21,22] A compensated hyperdynamic response is common in older women.[23] Older persons with a comparable degree of AS have more impairment of LV diastolic function than do younger persons.[24]

The compensatory concentric LV hypertrophy leads to abnormal LV compliance, LV diastolic dysfunction with decreased LV diastolic filling, and increased LV end-diastolic pressure, further increased by left atrial systole. Left atrial enlargement develops. Atrial systole plays an important role in diastolic filling of the LV in persons with AS.[25] Loss of effective atrial contraction may cause immediate clinical deterioration in persons with severe AS.

Sustained LV hypertrophy eventually leads to LV chamber dilatation with reduced LV ejection fraction and, ultimately, congestive heart failure (CHF). The stroke volume and cardiac output decrease, the mean left atrial and pulmonary capillary pressures increase, and pulmonary hypertension occurs. Older persons with both obstructive and nonobstructive coronary artery disease have an increased incidence of LV enlargement and LV systolic dysfunction.[26] In a percentage of older persons with AS, the LV ejection fraction will remain normal and LV diastolic dysfunction will be the main problem.

In 48 older persons with CHF associated with unoperated severe valvular AS, the LV ejection fraction was normal in

30 (63 percent).[27] The prognosis of persons with AS and LV diastolic dysfunction is usually better than that of persons with AS and LV systolic dysfunction, but is worse than that of persons without LV diastolic dysfunction.[27,28]

Symptoms of AS

Angina pectoris, syncope or near syncope, and CHF are the three classic manifestations of severe AS. Angina pectoris is the most common symptom associated with AS in older persons. Coexistent coronary artery disease (CAD) is frequently present in these people. However, angina pectoris may occur in the absence of CAD as a result of an increase in myocardial oxygen demand with a decrease in myocardial oxygen supply at the subendocardial level. Myocardial ischemia in persons with severe AS and normal coronary arteries is due to inadequate LV hypertrophy with increased LV systolic and diastolic wall stresses causing reduced coronary flow reserve.[29]

Syncope in persons with AS may be caused by decreased cerebral perfusion following exertion when arterial pressure falls because of systemic vasodilatation in the presence of a fixed cardiac output. LV failure with a reduction in cardiac output may also cause syncope. In addition, syncope at rest may be caused by a marked decrease in cardiac output secondary to transient ventricular fibrillation or transient atrial fibrillation or transient atrioventricular block related to extension of the valve calcification into the conduction system. Coexistent cerebrovascular disease with transient cerebral ischemia may contribute to syncope in older persons with AS.

Exertional dyspnea, paroxysmal nocturnal dyspnea, orthopnea, and pulmonary edema may be caused by pulmonary venous hypertension associated with AS. Coexistent CAD and hypertension may contribute to CHF in older persons with AS. Atrial fibrillation may also precipitate CHF in these people.

CHF, syncope, or angina pectoris was present in 36 of 40 older persons (90 percent) with severe AS, in 66 of 96 older persons (69 percent) with moderate valvular AS, and in 45 of 165 older persons (27 percent) with mild valvular AS.[30]

Sudden death occurs mainly in symptomatic AS persons.[27,30–33] It may also occur in 3–5 percent of asymptomatic persons with AS.[31,33] Marked fatigue and peripheral cyanosis in persons with AS may be caused by a low cardiac output. Cerebral emboli causing stroke or transient cerebral ischemic attack, bacterial endocarditis, and gastrointestinal bleeding may also occur in older persons with AS.

Signs of AS

A systolic ejection murmur heard in the second right intercostal space, down the left sternal border toward the apex, or at the apex, is classified as an aortic systolic ejection murmur (ASEM).[3,4,34,35] An ASEM is commonly heard in older persons,[1,3,34] occurring in 265 of 565 unselected older persons (47 percent).[3] Of 220 older persons with an ASEM and technically adequate M-mode and two-dimensional echocardiograms of the aortic valve, 207 (94 percent) had aortic cuspal or root calcification or thickening.[3] Of 75 older persons with an ASEM, valvular AS was diagnosed by continuous-wave Doppler echocardiography in 42 (56 percent).[35]

Table 36-1 shows that an ASEM was heard in all 19 older persons with severe AS, in all 49 older persons with moderate

Table 36-1 Correlation of physical signs of aortic stenosis with severity in older persons (percentages)

	Severity of aortic stenosis		
	Mild ($n = 74$)	Moderate ($n = 49$)	Severe ($n = 19$)
Aortic systolic ejection murmur	95	100	100
Prolonged duration aortic systolic ejection murmur	3	63	84
Late-peaking aortic systolic ejection murmur	3	63	84
Prolonged carotid upstroke time	3	33	53
A_2 absent	0	10	16
A_2 reduced or absent	5	49	74

Abbreviation: A_2, aortic component of second heart sound.
Source: Adapted from Aronow et al. (1991),[4] with permission.

AS, and in 95 percent of 74 older persons with mild AS.[4] However, the ASEM may become softer or absent in persons with CHF associated with severe AS because of a low cardiac output. The intensity and maximal location of the ASEM and transmission of the ASEM to the right carotid artery do not differentiate among mild, moderate, and severe AS.[3,4,35] The ASEM may be heard only at the apex in some older persons with AS. The apical systolic ejection murmur may also be louder and more musical than the basal systolic ejection murmur in some older persons with AS. The intensity of the ASEM in valvular AS increases with squatting and by inhalation of amyl nitrite and decreases during the Valsalva maneuver.

Prolonged duration of the ASEM and late peaking of the ASEM best differentiate severe AS from mild AS.[3,4,35] However, the physical signs do not distinguish between severe and moderate AS (Table 36-1).[4,35]

A prolonged carotid upstroke time does not differentiate between severe and moderate AS in older persons.[4,35] A prolonged carotid upstroke time was palpable in 3 percent of older persons with mild AS, in 33 percent of older persons with moderate AS, and in 53 percent of older persons with severe AS (Table 36-1).[4] Stiff noncompliant arteries may mask a prolonged carotid upstroke time in older persons with severe AS. The pulse pressure may also be normal or wide rather than narrow in older persons with severe AS because of loss of vascular elasticity. An aortic ejection click is rare in older persons with severe AS because of loss of vascular elasticity. An aortic ejection click is rare in older persons with AS because the valve cusps are immobile.[4,35]

An absent or reduced A_2 occurs more frequently in older persons with severe or moderate AS than in persons with mild AS (Table 36-1). However, an absent or decreased A_2 does not differentiate between severe and moderate AS.[4,35] The presence of atrial fibrillation, reversed splitting of S_2, or an audible fourth heart sound at the apex also does not differentiate between severe and moderate AS in older persons.[35] The presence of a third heart sound in older persons with AS usually indicates the presence of LV systolic dysfunction and elevated LV filling pressure.[36]

Electrocardiography and chest roentgenography in AS

Echocardiography is more sensitive than electrocardiography in diagnosing LV hypertrophy in older person with AS.[4] Rounding of the LV border and apex may occur as a result of concentric LV hypertrophy. Poststenotic dilatation of the ascending aorta is commonly seen. Calcification of the aortic valve is best seen by echocardiography or fluoroscopy.

Involvement of the conduction system by calcific deposits may occur in older persons with AS. In a study of 51 older persons with AS who underwent aortic valve replacement, conduction defects occurred in 58 percent of 31 persons with MAC and in 25 percent of 20 persons without MAC.[9] In another study of 77 older persons with AS, first-degree atrioventricular block occurred in 18 percent of persons, left bundle branch block in 10 percent, intraventricular conduction defect in 6 percent, right bundle branch block in 4 percent, and left axis deviation in 17 percent.[37]

Complex ventricular arrhythmias may be detected by 24-hour ambulatory electrocardiograms in persons with AS. Older persons with complex ventricular arrhythmias associated with AS have a higher incidence of new coronary events than older persons with AS and no complex ventricular arrhythmias.[38]

Echocardiography and Doppler echocardiography in AS

M-mode and two-dimensional echocardiography and Doppler echocardiography are very useful in the diagnosis of AS. Of 83 persons with CHF or angina pectoris and a systolic precordial murmur in whom severe AS was diagnosed by Doppler echocardiography, AS was not clinically diagnosed in 28 (34 percent).[39] Echocardiography can detect thickening, calcification, and reduced excursion of aortic valve leaflets.[3] LV hypertrophy is best diagnosed by echocardiography.[4] Chamber dimensions and measurements of LV end-systolic and end-diastolic volumes, LV ejection fraction, and assessment of global and regional LV wall motion give important information on LV systolic function.

Doppler echocardiography is used to measure peak and mean transvalvular gradients across the aortic valve and to identify associated valve lesions. Aortic valve area can be calculated by the continuity equation using pulsed Doppler echocardiography to measure LV outflow tract velocity, continuous-wave Doppler echocardiography to measure transvalvular flow velocity, and two-dimensional long-axis view to measure LV outflow tract area.[40,41] Aortic valve area can be detected reliably by the continuity equation in older persons with AS.[41]

Shah and Graham[42] reported that the agreement in quantitation of the severity of AS between Doppler echocardiography and cardiac catheterization was greater than 95 percent. Persons with a peak jet velocity ≥ 4.5 m/s had critical AS, and those with a peak jet velocity <3.0 m/s had noncritical AS. Slater et al.[43] demonstrated a concordance between Doppler echocardiography and cardiac catheterization in the decision to operate or not to operate in 61 of 73 persons (84 percent) with valvular AS. In 75 persons, mean age 76 years, with valvular AS, the Bland–Altman plot showed that 4 of the 75 (5 percent) had disagreement between cardiac catheterization and Doppler

echocardiography that was outside the 95 percent confidence limits.[44]

Cardiac catheterization was performed in 105 persons in which Doppler echocardiography demonstrated an aortic valve area ≤ 0.75 cm^2 or a peak jet velocity ≥ 4.5 m/s, consistent with critical AS.[45] Doppler echocardiography was 97 percent accurate in this subgroup. Cardiac catheterization was performed in this study in 133 persons with noncritical AS. Doppler echocardiography was 95 percent accurate in this subgroup. Although most older persons do not require cardiac catheterization before aortic valve surgery, they require selective coronary arteriography before aortic valve surgery. Persons in whom Doppler echocardiography shows a peak jet velocity between 3.6 and 4.4 m/s and an aortic valve area >0.8 cm^2 should undergo cardiac catheterization if they have cardiac symptoms attributable to AS.[42] Persons with a peak jet velocity between 3.0 and 3.5 m/s and a LV ejection fraction <50 percent may have severe AS, requiring aortic valve replacement, and should undergo cardiac catheterization.[42] Persons with a peak jet velocity between 3.0 and 3.5 m/s and a LV ejection fraction >50 percent probably do not need aortic valve replacement but should undergo cardiac catheterization if they have symptoms of severe AS.[42]

Natural history of AS

Ross and Braunwald[31] demonstrated that the average survival rate was 3 years after the onset of angina pectoris in persons with severe AS. Ross and Braunwald also reported that the average survival rate after the onset of syncope in persons with severe AS was 3 years. They showed that the average survival rate after the onset of CHF in persons with severe AS was 1.5–2 years.

Persons with symptomatic severe valvular AS have a poor prognosis.[30–33,46] At the National Institutes of Health, 52 percent of persons with symptomatic severe valvular AS not operated on were dead at 5 years.[32,33] At 10-year follow-up, 90 percent of these people were dead.

At 4-year follow-up of patients aged 75–86 years in the Helsinki Aging Study, the incidence of cardiovascular mortality was 62 percent in persons with severe AS and 35 percent in persons with moderate AS.[47] At 4-year follow-up, the incidence of total mortality was 76 percent in persons with severe AS and 50 percent in persons with moderate AS.[47]

In a prospective study, at 19-month follow-up (range 2–36 months), 90 percent of 30 persons with CHF associated with unoperated severe AS and a normal LV ejection fraction were dead.[27] At 13-month follow-up (range 2–24 months), all 18 persons with CHF associated with unoperated severe AS and an abnormal LV ejection fraction were dead.[27]

Table 36-2 shows the incidence of new coronary events in older persons with no, mild, moderate, and severe AS. Independent risk factors for new coronary events in this study were prior myocardial infarction, AS, male gender, and increasing age.[30] In this prospective study, at 20-month follow-up of 40 older persons with severe AS, CHF, syncope, or angina pectoris was present in 36 of 37 (97 percent) who developed new coronary events and in none of 3 persons without new coronary events.[30] At 32-month follow-up of 96 older persons with moderate valvular AS, CHF, syncope, or angina pectoris was present in 65 of 77 (84 percent) who developed new

Table 36-2 **Incidence of new coronary events in older persons with no, mild, moderate, or severe aortic stenosis**				
	No AS (n = 1496)	Mild AS (n = 165)	Moderate AS (n = 96)	Severe AS (n = 40)
Age (years)	81	84	85	85
Follow-up (months)	49	52	32	20
New coronary events (percent)	41	62	80	93

Source: Adapted from Aronow et al. (1998),[30] with permission.

coronary events and in 1 of 19 (5 percent) without new coronary events.[30] At 52-month follow-up of 165 older persons with mild AS, CHF, syncope, or angina pectoris was present in 40 of 103 (39 percent) who developed new coronary events and in 5 of 62 (8 percent) without new coronary events.[30]

In a prospective study of 981 persons, mean age 82 years, with aortic sclerosis and of 999 persons, mean age 80 years, without valvular aortic sclerosis, older persons with aortic sclerosis had at 46-month follow-up a 1.8 times higher chance of developing a new coronary event than those without valvular aortic sclerosis.[7] Otto et al.[48] also reported in 5621 men and women ≥ 65 years of age that AS and aortic sclerosis increased cardiovascular morbidity and mortality.

Kennedy et al.[49] followed 66 persons with moderate AS diagnosed by cardiac catheterization (aortic valve area 0.7–1.2 cm^2). In 38 persons with symptomatic moderate AS and in 28 with minimally symptomatic moderate AS, the probabilities of avoiding death from AS were 0.86 for those with symptomatic AS and 1.0 for those with minimally symptomatic moderate AS at 1-year follow-up; 0.77 for those with symptomatic AS and 1.0 for those with minimally symptomatic AS at 2 years; 0.77 for those with symptomatic AS and 0.96 for those with minimally symptomatic AS at 3 years; and 0.70 for those with symptomatic AS and 0.90 for those with minimally symptomatic AS at 4 years.[49] During 35-month mean follow-up in this study, 21 persons underwent aortic valve replacement.

Hammermeister et al.[50] followed 106 persons with unoperated AS in the Veterans Administration Cooperative Study on Valvular Heart Disease for 5 years. During follow-up, 60 of 106 persons (57 percent) died. Multivariate analysis demonstrated that measures of the severity of the AS, the presence of CAD, and the presence of CHF were the important predictors of survival in unoperated cases.

Studies have shown that patients with asymptomatic severe AS are at low risk for death and can be followed until symptoms develop.[51–54] Turina et al.[51] followed 17 persons with asymptomatic or mildly symptomatic AS. During the first 2 years, none died or had aortic valve surgery. At 5-year follow-up, 94 percent were alive and 75 percent were free of cardiac events. Kelly et al.[52] followed 51 asymptomatic persons with severe AS. During 17-month follow-up, 21 (41 percent) of the persons became symptomatic. Only 2 of the 51 (4 percent) died of cardiac causes. In both these people, death was preceded by the development of angina pectoris or CHF. Pellikka et al.[53] showed that 113 of 143 persons (79 percent), mean age 72 years, with asymptomatic severe AS were not initially referred for aortic valve replacement or percutaneous aortic balloon valvuloplasty. During 20-month follow-up, 37 of 113 (33 percent) became

symptomatic. The actuarial probability of remaining free of cardiac events associated with AS, including cardiac death and aortic valve surgery, was 95 percent at 6 months, 93 percent at 1 year, and 74 percent at 2 years. No asymptomatic person with severe AS developed sudden death while asymptomatic.

Rosenheck et al.[54] followed 126 persons with asymptomatic severe AS for 22 months. Eight died and 59 developed symptoms necessitating aortic valve replacement. Event-free survival was 67 percent at 1 year, 56 percent at 2 years, and 33 percent at 4 years. Five of the six deaths from cardiac disease were preceded by symptoms. Of the persons with moderately or severely calcified aortic valves whose aortic jet velocity increased by 0.3 m/s or more within 1 year, 79 percent underwent aortic valve replacement or died within 2 years of the observed increase.

Medical management of AS

Prophylactic antibiotics should be used to prevent bacterial endocarditis in persons with AS regardless of severity, according to American Heart Association (AHA) guidelines.[55] Persons with CHF, exertional syncope, or angina pectoris associated with moderate or severe AS should undergo aortic valve replacement promptly. Valvular surgery is the only definitive therapy in these older persons.[56] Medical therapy does not relieve the mechanical obstruction to left ventricular outflow and does not relieve symptoms or progression of the disorder. Persons with asymptomatic AS should report the development of symptoms possibly related to AS immediately to the physician. If significant AS is present in asymptomatic older persons, clinical examination and an electrocardiogram and Doppler echocardiogram should be performed at 6-month intervals. Nitrates should be used with caution in persons with angina pectoris and AS to prevent the occurrence of orthostatic hypotension and syncope. Diuretics should be used with caution in persons with CHF to prevent a decrease in cardiac output and hypotension. Vasodilators should be avoided. Digitalis should not be used in persons with CHF and a normal LV ejection fraction unless needed to control a rapid ventricular rate associated with atrial fibrillation.

Aortic valve replacement

Aortic valve replacement is the procedure of choice for symptomatic older persons with severe AS (see the box). The bioprosthesis has less structural failure in older persons than in younger persons and may be preferable to the mechanical prosthetic valve for AS replacement in the elderly due to the anticoagulation issue.[57,58] Persons with mechanical prostheses need anticoagulant therapy indefinitely. Persons with porcine bioprostheses require anticoagulant therapy for 3 months after hospital discharge and then may be treated with antiplatelet therapy alone.[59]

Arom et al.[60] performed aortic valve replacement in 273 persons aged 70–89 years (mean age 75 years), 162 with aortic valve replacement alone, and 111 with aortic valve replacement plus coronary artery bypass graft surgery (CABGS). Operative mortality was 5 percent. Late mortality at 33-month follow-up was 18 percent. Actuarial analysis showed at 5-year follow-up that overall survival was 66 percent for those with aortic valve replacement alone, 76 percent for those with aortic valve replacement plus CABGS, and 74 percent for a similar age group in the general population.

Culliford et al.[59] performed aortic valve replacement in 71 persons aged ≥ 80 years, 35 with aortic valve replacement alone, and 36 with aortic valve replacement plus CABGS. Hospital mortality was 6 percent in those with aortic valve replacement alone and 19 percent in those with both aortic valve replacement plus CABGS. At 1-year follow-up, survival from late cardiac death was 100 percent for those who had aortic valve replacement alone and 96 percent for those who had aortic valve replacement plus CABGS. At 3-year follow-up, survival from late cardiac death was 100 percent for those who had aortic valve replacement alone and 91 percent for those who had aortic valve replacement plus CABGS. Freedom from all valve-related complications (thromboembolism, anticoagulant-related complications, endocarditis, and reoperation or prosthetic failure) was 93 percent at 1-year follow-up and 80 percent at 3-year follow-up. At follow-up, 65 percent of survivors were in New York Heart Association (NYHA) functional class I or II, 31 percent in class III, and 4 percent in class IV.

Levinson et al.[61] performed aortic valve replacement in 71 octogenarians, mean age 82 years; the operative mortality was 9 percent. At 28-month follow-up, all of the survivors were in NYHA functional class I or II. Actuarial 1-, 5-, and 10-year survival rates were 83, 67, and 49 percent, respectively. A UK heart valve registry showed in 1100 persons aged ≥ 80 years (56 percent women) who underwent aortic valve replacement that the 30-day mortality was 6.6 percent.[62] The actuarial survival was 89 percent at 1 year, 79 percent at 3 years, 69 percent at 5 years, and 46 percent at 8 years.

Aortic valve replacement is associated with a reduction in LV mass and in improvement of LV diastolic filling.[63,64] Hoffman and Burckhardt[65] performed a prospective study in 100 persons who had aortic valve replacement. At 41-month follow-up, the yearly cardiac mortality rate was 8 percent in persons with electrocardiographic LV hypertrophy and repetitive ventricular premature complexes ≥ 2 couplets per 24 hours

during 24-hour ambulatory monitoring, and 0.6 percent in persons without either of these findings.

If LV systolic dysfunction in persons with severe AS is associated with critical narrowing of the aortic valve rather than myocardial fibrosis, it often improves after successful aortic valve replacement.[66] In 154 persons, mean age 73 years, with AS and a LV ejection fraction ≤ 35 percent who underwent aortic valve replacement, the 30-day mortality was 9 percent. The 5-year survival was 69 percent in persons without significant CAD and 39 percent in persons with significant CAD. NYHA functional class III or IV was present in 58 percent of persons before surgery versus 7 percent of persons after surgery. Postoperative LV ejection fraction was measured in 76 percent of survivors at a mean of 14 months after surgery. Improvement in LV ejection fraction was found in 76 percent.[66]

Balloon aortic valvuloplasty

In a Mayo Clinic study, the actuarial survival of 50 older persons, mean age 77 years, with symptomatic severe AS in whom aortic valve replacement was refused (45 cases) or deferred (5 cases) was 57 percent at 1 year, 37 percent at 2 years, and 25 percent at 3 years.[67] Because of the poor survival in this group, balloon aortic valvuloplasty should be considered when operative intervention is refused or deferred.

Balloon aortic valvuloplasty is effective palliative therapy for some older persons with symptomatic AS, although restenosis with recurrence of symptoms is common.[68–77] On the basis of the available data, balloon aortic valvuloplasty should be considered for older persons with symptomatic severe AS who are not candidates for aortic valve surgery, and possibly for persons with severe LV dysfunction as a bridge to subsequent valve surgery.[75–77]

AORTIC REGURGITATION

Etiology and prevalence of AR

Acute aortic regurgitation (AR) in older persons may be due to infective endocarditis, rheumatic fever, aortic dissection, trauma following prosthetic valve surgery, or rupture of the sinus of Valsalva. It causes sudden and severe LV failure.

Chronic AR in older persons may be caused by valve leaflet disease (secondary to any cause of aortic stenosis, infective endocarditis, rheumatic fever, congenital heart disease, rheumatoid arthritis, ankylosing spondylitis, following prosthetic valve surgery, or myxomatous degeneration of the valve) or by aortic root disease. Examples of aortic root disease causing chronic AR in older persons include association with systemic hypertension, syphilitic aortitis, cystic medial necrosis of the aorta, ankylosing spondylitis, rheumatoid arthritis, Reiter's disease, systemic lupus erythematosus, Ehler–Danlos syndrome, and pseudoxanthoma elasticum. Mild or moderate AR was also diagnosed by Doppler echocardiography in 9 of 29 persons (31 percent) with hypertrophic cardiomyopathy.[78] Margonato et al.[79] linked the increased prevalence of AR with age to aortic valve thickening.

The prevalence of AR increases with age.[79–81] In a prospective study of 450 unselected persons, mean age 82 years, AR was diagnosed by pulsed Doppler echocardiography in 39 of 114 men (34 percent) and in 92 of 336 women (27 percent).[81]

Severe or moderate AR was diagnosed in 74 of 450 older persons (16 percent). Mild AR was diagnosed in 57 of 450 older persons (13 percent). In a prospective study of 924 men, mean age 80 years, and 1881 women, mean age 82 years, valvular AR was diagnosed by pulsed Doppler recordings of the aortic valve in 282 of 924 men (31 percent) and in 542 of 1881 women (29 percent).[20]

Pathophysiology of AR

The primary determinants of AR volume are the regurgitant orifice area, the transvalvular pressure gradient, and the duration of diastole.[82] Chronic AR increases LV ventricular end-diastolic volume. The largest LV end-diastolic volumes are seen in persons with chronic severe AR. LV stroke volume increases to maintain the forward stroke volume. The increased preload causes an increase in LV diastolic stress and the addition of sarcomeres in series. This results in an increase in the ratio of the LV chamber size to wall thickness. This pattern of LV hypertrophy is called "eccentric LV hypertrophy."

Primary myocardial abnormalities or ischemia due to coexistent CAD decrease the contractile state. LV diastolic compliance decreases, LV end-systolic volume increases, LV end-diastolic pressure rises, left atrial pressure increases, and pulmonary venous hypertension results. When the LV end-diastolic radius-to-wall thickness ratio rises, LV systolic wall stress increases abnormally because of the preload and afterload mismatch.[22,83] Additional stress then decreases the LV ejection fraction response to exercise.[84] Eventually, the LV ejection fraction, forward stroke volume, and effective cardiac output are decreased at rest. Aronow et al.[85] demonstrated that an abnormal resting LV ejection fraction occurred in 8 of 25 older persons (32 percent) with CHF associated with chronic severe AR.

In persons with acute severe AR, the LV cannot adapt to the increased volume overload. Forward stroke volume falls, LV end-diastolic pressure increases rapidly to high levels,[86] and pulmonary hypertension and pulmonary edema result. The rapid rise of the LV end-diastolic pressure to exceed the left atrial pressure in early diastole causes premature closure of the mitral valve.[87] This prevents backward transmission of the elevated LV end-diastolic pressure to the pulmonary venous bed.

Symptoms of AR

Persons with acute AR develop symptoms due to the sudden onset of CHF, with marked dyspnea and weakness. Persons with chronic AR may remain asymptomatic for many years. Mild dyspnea on exertion, and palpitations—especially on lying down—may occur. Exertional dyspnea, orthopnea, paroxysmal nocturnal dyspnea, fatigue, and edema are common clinical symptoms when LV failure occurs. Syncope is rare. Angina pectoris occurs less often in persons with AR than in persons with AS and may be due to coexistent CAD. However, nocturnal angina pectoris, often accompanied by flushing, diaphoresis, and palpitations, may develop when the heart rate slows and the arterial diastolic pressure falls to very low levels. Most persons with severe AR who do not have surgery die within 2 years after CHD develops.[88]

Signs of AR

The AR murmur is typically a high-pitched blowing diastolic murmur that begins immediately after A_2. When the AR is due

to valvular disease, the diastolic murmur is best heard along the left sternal border in the third and fourth intercostal spaces. When the AR is due to dilatation of the ascending aorta, the murmur is best heard along the right sternal border. The diastolic murmur is also best heard with the diaphragm of the stethoscope with the person sitting up, leaning forward, and holding the breath in deep expiration. The severity of AR correlates with the duration of the diastolic murmur, not with the intensity of the murmur.

Grayburn et al.[89] heard an AR murmur in 73 percent of 82 persons with AR and in 8 percent of 24 persons without AR. Saal et al.[90] heard an AR murmur in 80 percent of 35 persons with AR and in 10 percent of 10 persons without AR. Meyers et al.[91] heard an AR murmur in 73 percent of 66 persons with AR and in 22 percent of 9 persons without AR. An AR murmur was heard in 95 percent of 74 older persons with severe or moderate AR diagnosed by pulsed Doppler echocardiography, in 61 percent of 57 older persons with mild AR, and in 3 percent of 319 older persons with no AR.[81]

In persons with chronic severe AR, the LV apical impulse is diffuse, hyperdynamic, and displaced laterally and inferiorly. A rumbling diastolic murmur (Austin Flint) may be heard at the apex, with its intensity reduced by inhalation of amyl nitrite. A short basal systolic ejection murmur is heard. A palpable LV rapid filling wave and an audible S_3 at the apex are usually found. Physical findings due to a large LV stroke volume and a rapid diastolic runoff in persons with severe AR include a wide pulse pressure with an increased systolic arterial pressure and an abnormally low diastolic arterial pressure, an arterial pulse that abruptly rises and collapses, a bisferiens pulse, bobbing of the head with each heart beat, booming systolic and diastolic sounds heard over the femoral artery, capillary pulsations, and systolic and diastolic murmurs heard over the femoral artery when compressing it proximally and distally.

Electrocardiography and chest roentgenography in AR

The electrocardiogram may initially be normal in persons with acute severe AR. Roberts and Day[92] demonstrated in 30 necropsy cases of chronic severe AR that the electrocardiogram did not accurately predict the severity of AR or cardiac weight. Using various electrocardiographic criteria, the prevalence of LV hypertrophy varied from 30 percent ($RV_6 > RV_5$) to 90 percent (total 12-lead QRS voltage >175 mm). The P–R interval was prolonged in 28 percent of cases, and the QRS duration was ≥ 0.12 seconds in 20 percent of cases.[92]

The chest X-ray in persons with acute severe AR may show a normal heart size and pulmonary edema. The chest X-ray in those with chronic severe AR usually shows a dilated LV, with elongation of the apex inferiorly and posteriorly and a dilated aorta. Aneurysmal dilatation of the aorta suggests that aortic root disease is causing the AR. Linear calcifications in the wall of the ascending aorta are seen in syphilitic AR and in degenerative disease.

Echocardiography and Doppler echocardiography in AR

M-mode and two-dimensional echocardiography and Doppler echocardiography are very useful in the diagnosis of AR.

Two-dimensional echocardiography can provide information showing the etiology of the AR and measurements of LV function. Eccentric LV hypertrophy is diagnosed by echocardiography if the LV mass index is increased with a relative wall thickness <0.45.[93–95] Echocardiographic measurements reported to predict an unfavorable response to aortic valve replacement in persons with chronic AR include a LV end-systolic dimension >55 mm,[96] a LV shortening fraction < 25 percent,[96] a LV diastolic radius-to-wall thickness ratio >3.8,[97] a LV end-diastolic dimension index >38 mm/m²,[97] and a LV ventricular end-systolic dimension index >26 mm/m².[97]

Grayburn et al.[89] found that pulsed Doppler echocardiography correctly identified the presence of AR in all 57 persons with ≥2+ AR and in 22 of 25 (88 percent) with 1+ AR. Saal et al.[90] showed that pulsed Doppler echocardiography identified the presence of AR in 34 of 35 (97 percent) with documented AR. Continuous-wave Doppler echocardiography has also been demonstrated to be very useful in diagnosing and quantitating AR.[98,99] AR is best assessed by color flow Doppler imaging.[100]

Natural history of AR

The natural history of chronic AR is significantly different from that of acute AR. Persons with acute AR should have immediate aortic valve replacement because death may occur within hours to days. In one study of persons with hemodynamically significant chronic AR treated medically, 75 percent were alive at 5 years after diagnosis.[46,101] Of persons with moderate-to-severe chronic AR, 50 percent were alive at 10 years after diagnosis.[46,101] The 10-year survival rate for persons with mild-to-moderate chronic AR was 85–95 percent.[46,102]

During 8-year follow-up of 104 asymptomatic persons with chronic severe AR and normal LV ejection fraction, two persons (2 percent) died suddenly, and 23 (22 percent) had aortic valve replacement.[103] Of the 104 persons, 19 (18 percent) had aortic valve replacement because of cardiac symptoms and 4 (4 percent) had aortic valve replacement because of the development of LV systolic dysfunction in the absence of cardiac symptoms. Multivariate analysis showed that age, initial end-systolic dimension, and rate of change in end-systolic dimension and resting LV ejection fraction during serial studies predicted the outcome.

Medical and surgical management of AR

Asymptomatic persons with mild or moderate AR do not require therapy. However, prophylactic antibiotics should be used to prevent bacterial endocarditis in persons with AR, according to AHA guidelines.[55] Echocardiographic evaluation of LV end-systolic dimension should be performed yearly if the measurement is less than 50 mm but every 3–6 months if the LV end-systolic dimension is 50–54 mm. Aortic valve replacement should also be considered when the LV ejection fraction approaches 50 percent before the decompensated state.[82]

Persons with asymptomatic, chronic severe AR should be treated with hydralazine,[104] nifedipine,[105] or preferably angiotensin-converting-enzyme therapy[106] to decrease the LV volume overload. Infections should be treated promptly. Systemic hypertension increases the regurgitant flow and

should be treated. Drugs that reduce LV function should not be used. Arrhythmias should be treated. Persons with AR due to syphilitic aortitis should receive a course of penicillin therapy. Prophylactic resection should be considered in persons with Marfan's syndrome when the aortic root diameter exceeds 55 mm.[107]

Bacterial endocarditis should be treated with intravenous antibiotics. Indications for aortic valve replacement in persons with AR due to bacterial endocarditis are CHF, uncontrolled infection, myocardial or valvular ring abscess, prosthetic valve dysfunction or dehiscence, and multiple embolic episodes.[108–110]

CHF should be treated with sodium restriction, diuretics, digoxin if the LV ejection fraction is abnormal, vasodilator therapy, and aortic valve replacement. Angina pectoris should be treated with nitrates.

Persons with acute severe AR should undergo aortic valve replacement immediately. Those with chronic severe AR should have aortic valve replacement if they develop symptoms of CHF, angina pectoris, or syncope.[103] Aortic valve replacement should also be performed in asymptomatic persons with chronic severe AR if they develop LV systolic dysfunction.[103] Class I American College of Cardiology (ACC)/AHA indications for aortic valve replacement in persons with chronic severe AR include NYHA functional class III or IV symptoms and a LV ejection fraction ≥50 percent at rest; NYHA functional class II symptoms and a LV ejection fraction ≥50 percent at rest but with progressive LV dilatation or decreasing LV ejection fraction at rest on serial studies or decreasing effort tolerance on exercise testing; asymptomatic or symptomatic persons with a resting LV ejection fraction of 25–49 percent; and persons undergoing CABGS or surgery on the aorta or other valves.[111]

Elderly people undergoing aortic valve replacement for severe AR have an excellent postoperative survival if the preoperative LV ejection fraction is normal.[112–114] If LV systolic dysfunction was present for less than 1 year, persons also did well postoperatively. However, if the person with severe AR has an abnormal LV ejection fraction and impaired exercise tolerance and/or the presence of LV systolic dysfunction for longer than 1 year, the postoperative survival is poor.[112–114] After aortic valve replacement, women exhibit an excess late mortality, suggesting that surgical correction of severe chronic AR should be considered at an earlier stage in women.[115]

The operative mortality for aortic valve replacement in older persons with severe AR is similar to that in older persons with aortic valve replacement for valvular AS. The mortality rate is slightly increased in persons with infective endocarditis and in those needing replacement of the ascending aorta plus aortic valve replacement. The bioprosthesis is preferable to the mechanical prosthetic valve for aortic valve replacement in older persons, as in older persons with valvular AS.[58] Persons with porcine bioprostheses require anticoagulant therapy for 3 months after hospital discharge and then may be treated with antiplatelet therapy alone.[58]

In a prospective study, aortic valve replacement in 38 persons with severe AR normalized LV chamber size and mass in two-thirds of persons undergoing surgery.[116] At 9-month follow-up after AR replacement, 58 percent had a normal LV end-diastolic dimension and 50 percent had a normal LV mass. During further follow-up (18–56 months postoperatively),

66 percent had a normal LV end-diastolic dimension and 68 percent had a normal LV mass. The LV end-diastolic dimension normalized in 86 percent with a preoperative LV end-systolic dimension ≤55 mm. A preoperative LV end-systolic dimension >55 mm was present in 81 percent with postoperative persistent LV dilatation.

MITRAL ANNULAR CALCIUM

Mitral annular calcium (MAC) is a chronic degenerative process that is common in elderly people, especially women. The amount of calcium may vary from a few spicules to a large mass behind the posterior cusp, often extending to form a ridge or ring encircling the mitral leaflets, occasionally lifting the leaflets toward the left atrium. Sphincter function loss of the mitral annulus and mechanical stretching of the mitral leaflets can cause improper coaptation of the leaflets during systole, resulting in mitral regurgitation (MR).[8]

Although the calcific mass may immobilize the mitral valve, actual calcification of the leaflets is rare. In persons with severe MAC, the calcification may extend inward to involve the underside of the leaflets. Mitral stenosis (MS) may result from severe calcific deposits within the mitral annulus protruding into the orifice.[117,118] Calcific deposits may extend from the mitral annulus into the membranous portions of the ventricular septum, involving the conduction system and causing rhythm and conduction disturbances.[9,119,120] Although the annular calcium is covered with a layer of endothelium, ulceration of this lining can expose the underlying calcific deposits, which may serve as a nidus for platelet–fibrin aggregation and subsequent thromboembolic (TE) episodes.[121–123] In persons with endocarditis associated with MAC, the avascular nature of the mitral annulus predisposes to periannular and myocardial abscesses.[124–127]

Prevalence of MAC

MAC is a degenerative process that increases with age and occurs more frequently in women than in men.[2,3,10,18,20,121,128–133] MAC was present in 298 of 924 men (36 percent), mean age 80 years, and in 985 of 1881 women (52 percent), mean age 81 years.[20]

Predisposing factors for MAC

Because calcific deposits in the mitral annulus, in the aortic valve cusps, and in the epicardial coronary arteries are commonly associated in older persons and have similar predisposing factors, Roberts[18] suggested that MAC and aortic cuspal calcium are a form of atherosclerosis. MAC and aortic cuspal calcium may coexist.[2,8,18,19,121,130,134,135] The prevalence of CAD is higher in men and women with aortic valve calcium[6] and with MAC[6,136] than in men and women without aortic valve calcium and MAC.

Breakdown of lipid deposits on the ventricular surface of the posterior mitral leaflet at or below the mitral annulus and on the aortic surfaces of the aortic valve cusps is probably responsible for the calcification.[8] Increased LV systolic pressure due to AS increases stress on the mitral apparatus and may accelerate development of MAC.[2,3,8,121,135] Tricuspid annular

calcium and MAC may also coexist and have similar predisposing factors.[137]

Systemic hypertension increases with age and predisposes to MAC.[2,8,19,121,130,138] Persons with diabetes mellitus also have a higher prevalence of MAC than nondiabetic persons.[2,8,19,134] MAC occurs in the teens in persons with serum total cholesterol levels >500 mg/dL.[139] Waller and Roberts[2] suggested that hypercholesterolemia predisposes to MAC. The prevalence of hypercholesterolemia with a serum total cholesterol ≥200 mg/dL was higher in older persons with MAC than in older persons without MAC.[19]

Roberts and Waller[140] found that chronic hypercalcemia predisposes to MAC. Older persons with chronic renal insufficiency have a higher prevalence of MAC and aortic valve calcium than older persons with normal renal function.[141] Persons undergoing dialysis for chronic renal insufficiency have an increased prevalence of MAC.[140–147] MAC has also been found to be a marker of LV dilatation and reduced LV systolic function in persons with end-stage renal disease on peritoneal dialysis.[147] Cardiac calcium in persons with chronic renal failure has been attributed to secondary hyperparathyroidism.[143,146] Nair et al.[134] found a similar mean serum calcium, a higher mean serum phosphorus, and a higher mean product of serum calcium and phosphorus in persons younger than 60 years with MAC than in a control group. However, Aronow et al.[19] demonstrated no significant difference in mean serum calcium, serum phosphorus, or product of serum calcium and phosphorus between elderly persons with and without MAC.

By accelerating LV systolic pressure, hypertrophic cardiomyopathy predisposes to MAC.[8] Kronzon and Glassman[148] diagnosed MAC in 12 of 18 persons (67 percent) older than 55 years with hypertrophic cardiomyopathy and in 4 of 28 (14 percent) younger than 55 years with hypertrophic cardiomyopathy. Nair et al.[149] observed MAC in 12 of 42 persons (27 percent) with hypertrophic cardiomyopathy. Their patients with both MAC and hypertrophic cardiomyopathy were older than those with hypertrophic cardiomyopathy and no MAC. Motamed and Roberts[150] demonstrated MAC in 30 of 100 autopsy cases (30 percent) with hypertrophic cardiomyopathy older than 40 years and in none of 100 autopsy cases younger than 40 years with hypertrophic cardiomyopathy. Aronow and Kronzon[151] diagnosed MAC in 13 of 17 older persons (76 percent) with hypertrophic cardiomyopathy and in 176 of 362 older persons (49 percent) without hypertrophic cardiomyopathy.

Diagnosis of MAC

Calcific deposits in the mitral annulus are J, C, U, or O shaped and are seen in the posterior third of the heart shadow.[121,129,142,152–158] MAC may be diagnosed by chest X-ray or by fluoroscopy.[158] However, the procedures of choice for diagnosing MAC are M-mode and two-dimensional echocardiography.

Posterior MAC is diagnosed by M-mode echocardiography when a band of dense echoes is recorded anterior to the LV posterior wall and moving parallel with it.[159] These echoes end at the atrioventricular junction and merge with the LV posterior wall on echocardiographic sweep from the aortic root to the LV apex. Anterior MAC is diagnosed by M-mode echocardiography when a continuous band of dense echoes is observed at the level of the anterior mitral leaflet in both systole and diastole.[159] These echoes are contiguous with the posterior wall of the aortic root. Calcification may extend from the mitral annulus throughout the base of the heart and into the mitral and aortic valves.

Using multiple echocardiographic views, MAC may be classified as mild, moderate, or severe.[160] The echo densities in mild MAC involve less than one-third of the annular circumference (<3 mm in width) and are usually restricted to the angle between the posterior leaflet of the mitral valve and the LV posterior wall. The echo densities in moderate MAC involve less than two-thirds of the annular circumference (3–5 mm in width). The echo densities in severe MAC involve more than two-thirds of the annular circumference (>5 mm in width), usually extending beneath the entire posterior mitral leaflet with or without making a complete circle.

MAC was diagnosed in the original chest X-ray report in 3 of 8 persons (38 percent) with MAC diagnosed at autopsy.[129] Schott et al.[142] diagnosed MAC by chest X-ray in 2 of 41 persons (5 percent) with MAC diagnosed by echocardiography. Dashkoff et al.[161] detected MAC by chest X-ray in 5 of 8 persons (63 percent) with MAC diagnosed by echocardiography.

In a blinded prospective study, MAC was diagnosed by M-mode and two-dimensional echocardiography in 55 percent of 604 older persons.[158] The diagnosis of MAC by chest X-ray using a lateral view in addition to the posterior–anterior or anterior–posterior views had a sensitivity of 12 percent, a specificity of 99 percent, a positive predictive value of 95 percent, and a negative predictive value of 47 percent. Persons with radiographic MAC were more likely than those without radiographic MAC to have a more severe form of the disease, with significant MR, functional MS, or conduction defects. However, patients with echocardiographically severe MAC and significant MR, functional MS, or conduction defects may have no evidence of MAC on chest X-ray films.

Chamber size in MAC

Persons with MAC have a higher prevalence of left atrial enlargement[121,129–131,133,134,160,162] and LV enlargement[129,130,134,160,162] than those without MAC. In a prospective study of 976 older persons (526 with MAC and 450 without MAC), left atrial enlargement was 2.4 times more prevalent in those with MAC.[133]

Atrial fibrillation in MAC

Persons with MAC have a higher prevalence of atrial fibrillation than those without MAC.[121,129–131,133,160,163,164] The prevalence of atrial fibrillation was increased 12 times,[130] 5 times,[160] and 2.8 times[164] in persons with MAC.

Conduction defects in MAC

Because of the close proximity of the mitral annulus to the atrioventricular node and the bundle of His, persons with MAC have a higher prevalence of conduction defects, such as sinoatrial disease, atrioventricular block, bundle branch block, left anterior fascicular block, and intraventricular conduction defect, than those without MAC.[9,119–121,135,160] The calcific

deposits may also extend into the membranous portions of the interventricular septum involving the conduction system, or may even extend to the left atrium, interrupting interatrial and intra-atrial conduction. In addition, MAC may be associated with a sclerodegenerative process in the conduction system. Nair et al.[160] showed in their study that persons with MAC had a higher incidence of permanent pacemaker implantation because of both atrioventricular block and sinoatrial disease.

Mitral regurgitation in MAC

MAC is thought to generate systolic murmurs by the sphincter action loss of the annulus and the mechanical stretching of the mitral leaflets causing MR and from vibration of the calcified ring or vortex formation around the annulus. Table 36-3 shows that the prevalence of apical systolic murmurs of MR in persons with MAC ranged from 12 to 100 percent in different studies.[117,121,129,130,132,142,159,165] Table 36-4 states the prevalence of MR diagnosed by Doppler echocardiography in persons with MAC.[162,165,166] The prevalence of mitral regurgitation associated with MAC ranged from 54 to 97 percent in the Doppler echocardiographic studies.[162,165,166]

The greater the severity of MAC, the greater the severity of MR associated with it. Moderate to severe MR was diagnosed by Doppler echocardiography in 33 percent of 51 persons with MAC by Labovitz et al.[166] and in 22 percent of 1028 older persons with MAC by Aronow et al.[164] Kaul et al.[162] diagnosed severe MR in 7 percent of their 29 patients with MAC. Kaul and colleagues also concluded from their study that MR in persons with MAC is caused by a decreased sphincteric action of the mitral annulus, with MAC preventing the posterior annulus from contracting and assuming a flatter shape during systole.

Table 36-3 Prevalence of apical systolic murmurs of mitral regurgitation and of apical diastolic murmurs of mitral stenosis in persons with mitral annular calcium

Prevalence of MR murmur		Prevalence of MS murmur	
No.	%	No.	%
14/14	100[129]	3/14	21[129]
10/14	71[142]	2/14	14[142]
2/4	50[117]	1/4	25[117]
72/80	90[121]	5/59	8[154]
26/132	12[130]	2/132	2[130]
17/104	16[159]	7/104	7[159]
129/293	44[132]	28/293	10[132]
43/100	43[165]	6/100	6[165]

Table 36-4 Prevalence of mitral regurgitation and of mitral stenosis diagnosed by Doppler echocardiography in persons with mitral annular calcium

Prevalence of MR		Prevalence of MS	
No.	%	No.	%
28/51	55[166]	4/51	8[165]
54/100	54[165]	6/100	6[165]
28/29	97[162]	83/1028	8[164]

Mitral stenosis in MAC

An apical diastolic murmur may be heard in persons with MAC as a result of turbulent flow across the calcified and narrowed annulus (annular stenosis). Table 36-3 shows that the prevalence of apical diastolic murmurs of MS in persons with MAC ranged from zero to 25 percent in different studies.[117,129,130,132,142,154,159,165] Table 36-4 indicates that MS associated with MAC was diagnosed by Doppler echocardiography in 8 percent of 51 persons by Labovitz et al.,[166] in 6 percent of 100 persons by Aronow and Kronzon,[165] and in 8 percent of 1028 persons by Aronow et al.[164]

The decrease of mitral valve orifice in persons with MAC is due to the annular calcium and to decreased mitral excursion and mobility secondary to calcium at the base of the leaflets.[165] The commissures are fused in rheumatic MS but are not fused in MS associated with MAC. The mitral leaflet margins in MAC may be thin and mobile, and the posterior mitral leaflet may move normally during diastole. However, Doppler echocardiographic recordings show increased transvalvular flow velocity and prolonged pressure half-time and, therefore, smaller mitral valve orifice in persons with MS, regardless of the etiology.

Bacterial endocarditis in MAC

Bacterial endocarditis, with a high incidence of *Staphylococcus aureus* endocarditis, may complicate MAC.[121,124–127,133] Persons with MAC associated with chronic renal failure are especially at increased risk for developing bacterial endocarditis.[142] The calcific mass erodes the endothelium under the mitral valve, which is exposed to transient bacteremia. The avascular nature of the mitral annulus interferes with antibiotics reaching a nidus of bacteria, predisposing to periannular and myocardial abscesses and, consequently, to a poor prognosis.[124–127] Therefore, Burnside and DeSanctis[124] recommended prophylactic antibiotics to prevent bacterial endocarditis in persons with MAC.

Nair et al.[160] observed at 4.4-year follow-up no significant difference in incidence of bacterial endocarditis in 99 persons younger than 61 years with MAC compared to a control group of 101 persons. However, Aronow et al.[133] demonstrated at 39 months follow-up a 3 percent incidence of bacterial endocarditis in 526 older persons with MAC and a 1 percent incidence in 450 elderly persons without MAC. On the basis of these data, prophylactic antibiotics are recommended to prevent bacterial endocarditis in persons with MAC according to AHA guidelines.[55]

Cardiac events in MAC

In a prospective study of 107 persons (8 lost to follow-up) younger than 61 years with MAC and 107 (6 lost to follow-up) age- and sex-matched control subjects, Nair et al.[160] observed at 4.4-year follow-up that persons with MAC had a higher incidence of new cardiac events than control subjects (Table 36-5). In a prospective study of 526 older persons with MAC and 450 older persons without MAC, Aronow et al.[133] found at 39-month follow-up that the incidence of new cardiac events (myocardial infarction, primary ventricular fibrillation, or sudden cardiac death) was also higher in older persons with MAC than in older persons without MAC.

Table 36-5 Incidence of new cardiac events in persons with or without mitral annular calcium

	Cardiac events[a]		
	MAC %	No MAC %	Relative risk
Nair et al.[160] (99 with MAC, 101 without MAC)			
Total cardiac death	31	2	15.5
Sudden cardiac death	12	1	12.0
Congestive heart failure	41	6	6.8
Mitral or aortic valve replacement	9	0	–
Aronow et al.[133]			
Cardiac events, if atrial fibrillation (90 with MAC, 41 without MAC)	69	54	1.3
Sinus rhythm (436 with MAC, 409 without MAC)	36	26	1.4
All persons (526 with MAC, 450 without MAC)	42	28	1.5

[a]*Myocardial infarction, primary ventricular fibrillation, or sudden cardiac death.*

Mitral valve replacement

Nair et al.[167] reported that mitral valve replacement can be accomplished in persons with MAC with morbidity and mortality similar to those in persons without MAC. Following mitral valve replacement, subsequent morbidity and mortality during 4.4-year follow-up were also similar in persons with and without MAC.

Cerebrovascular events in MAC

Although the increased prevalence of atrial fibrillation, MS, MR, left atrial enlargement, and CHF predisposes persons with MAC to thromboembolic (TE) stroke, some investigators consider MAC a marker of other vascular disease causing stroke rather than the primary embolic source.[168] However, the prevalence of prior stroke was higher in 280 African American, Hispanic, and white men with MAC (40 percent) than in 484 without MAC (27 percent); and in 876 African American, Hispanic, and white women with MAC (36 percent) than in 799 without MAC (22 percent).[169] In addition, six prospective studies have demonstrated an increased incidence of new cerebrovascular events in persons with MAC than in persons without MAC.[133,160,164,170–172]

Nair et al.[160] showed at 4.4-year follow-up in 107 persons (8 lost to follow-up) younger than 61 years with MAC and 107 (6 lost to follow-up) age- and sex-matched control subjects that persons with MAC had a 5 times higher incidence of new thromboembolic cerebrovascular events than persons without MAC.

The Framingham study observed at 8-year follow-up in 160 persons with MAC and 999 persons without MAC that the incidence of stroke was increased 2.7 times in those with MAC compared with those without MAC.[170]

At 39-month follow-up of 526 older persons with MAC and 450 without MAC, Aronow et al.[133] observed a 1.5 times higher incidence of new TE stroke in persons with MAC than in persons without MAC if atrial fibrillation was present; a 1.6 times higher incidence if sinus rhythm was present; and a 1.7 times higher incidence overall.

The Boston Area Anticoagulation Trial for Atrial Fibrillation study demonstrated at 2.2-year follow-up in 129 persons with atrial fibrillation and MAC and 291 persons with atrial fibrillation without MAC a 4 times higher incidence of ischemic stroke in those with MAC.[171]

At 45-month follow-up, Aronow et al.[172] showed that the incidence of TE stroke was 1.5 times higher in 101 persons with 40–100 percent ECAD and MAC than in 49 persons with 40–100 percent ECAD and no MAC; and 2.2 times higher in 365 persons with MAC and 0–39 percent ECAD than in 413 persons with no MAC and 0–39 percent ECAD.

Table 36-6 shows the incidence of new TE stroke at 44-month follow-up in 310 older persons with chronic atrial fibrillation and in 1838 older persons with sinus rhythm, mean age 81 years.[164] MS and the severity of MR were diagnosed by Doppler echocardiography in this study. In older persons with chronic atrial fibrillation, MAC increased the incidence of new TE 2.1 times if MS was associated with MAC, 1.7 times if 2–4+ MR was associated with MAC, and 1.4 times if 0–1+MR was present. In older persons with sinus rhythm, MAC increased the incidence of new TE stroke 3.6 times if MS was associated with MAC, 3.1 times if 2–4+ MR was associated with MAC, and 2.7 times if 0–1 MR was present.

Aronow et al[172] found a higher prevalence of MAC in older persons with 40–100 percent ECAD (67 percent of 150 persons) than in older persons with 0–39 percent ECAD (47 percent of 778 persons). The increased prevalence of significant ECAD contributes to a higher incidence of TE stroke in older persons with MAC. Thrombi of the mitral annulus also contribute to TE stroke in this group.[173–175] In addition, MAC is associated with complex intra-aortic debris which could contribute to TE stroke.[176]

Since persons with MAC and atrial fibrillation or sinus rhythm have a higher incidence of TE stroke than those without MAC, antithrombotic therapy should be considered in those with MAC and no contraindications to antithrombotic therapy. In the Boston Area Anticoagulation Trial for Atrial Fibrillation study, warfarin significantly reduced the incidence of TE stroke in persons with MAC by about 90 percent.[177,178]

Until data from prospective, randomized studies evaluating the efficacy and risk of antithrombotic therapy in persons with MAC are available, the recommendation is to treat persons with MAC associated with either atrial fibrillation, MS, or moderate to severe MR with warfarin, if they have no contraindications to anticoagulant therapy. The INR should be maintained at between 2.0 and 3.0. The efficacy of antiplatelet treatment in persons with MAC is unknown.

MITRAL STENOSIS

Prevalence and etiology of MS

Mitral stenosis (MS) due to rheumatic heart disease was diagnosed by Doppler echocardiography in 3 of 924 men (0.3 percent), mean age 80 years, and in 34 of 1881 women (2 percent), mean age 81 years.[20] The most common cause of MS in older persons is MAC. The differentiation by echocardiography of MS due to rheumatic heart disease from that caused by MAC has been discussed in the section on MAC. In a study of 1699 persons, mean age 81 years, the prevalence of rheumatic MS was 6 percent in persons with atrial fibrillation versus 0.4 percent in those with sinus rhythm.[163]

Pathophysiology of MS

MS leads to an increase in left atrial pressure, pulmonary capillary pressure, and right ventricular and pulmonary artery systolic pressure, causing pulmonary hypertension. Atrial fibrillation predisposes persons with MS to develop stroke, peripheral arterial embolism, and CHF.

Symptoms and signs of MS

If MS is moderate or severe (especially if atrial fibrillation is present), exertional dyspnea, orthopnea, paroxysmal nocturnal dyspnea, and pulmonary edema may develop. Pulmonary hypertension leads to right-sided CHF. Hemoptysis may result from ruptured bronchial veins.

The loud first heart sound and opening snap heard in persons with MS may become softer or disappear if valvular calcification is present. An apical low-frequency diastolic murmur heard as a rumble with presystolic accentuation is heard at the point of maximum apical impulse. The low-frequency diastolic murmur begins after the opening snap, is prolonged with increasing severity of the MS, and increases in intensity after inhalation of amyl nitrite. The closer the opening snap is heard to A_2, the more severe the MS. If atrial fibrillation develops, the presystolic accentuation usually disappears.

Diagnostic tests in MS

The electrocardiogram and chest X-ray will often show left atrial enlargement. Electrocardiographic right ventricular hypertrophy (RVH) is usually present with severe MS. Documentation of MS and of the severity is made by Doppler echocardiography. Echocardiography will also rule out left atrial myxoma which can mimic mitral stenosis.

Table 36-6 **Incidence of new thromboembolic stroke at 44 months**	
	TE stroke %
Atrial fibrillation, no MAC (n = 85)	35
Atrial fibrillation with MS due to MAC (n = 42)	74
Atrial fibrillation with MAC and 2–4 + MR (n = 90)	59
Atrial fibrillation with MAC and 0–1 + MR (n = 93)	48
Sinus rhythm, no MAC (n = 1035)	9
Sinus rhythm with MS due to MAC (n = 41)	32
Sinus rhythm with MAC and 2–4 + MR (n = 134)	28
Sinus rhythm with MAC and 0–1 + MR (n = 625)	24

Abbreviations: MAC, mitral annular calcium; MS, mitral stenosis; MR, mitral regurgitation.

Source: Adapted from Aronow et al. (1998),[164] with permission.

Management of mitral stenosis

A rapid ventricular rate associated with atrial fibrillation is controlled by digoxin and/or β-blockers, verapamil, or diltiazem. Diuretics should be used to control congestive symptoms. Unloading therapy with vasodilators is not beneficial and may cause a significant reduction in cardiac output. Long-term anticoagulation with oral warfarin is indicated in persons with MS and atrial fibrillation (especially) or sinus rhythm to prevent systemic embolization. The INR should be maintained at between 2.0 and 3.0. Prophylactic antibiotics should be used to present bacterial endocarditis in persons with MS, according to AHA guidelines.[55]

Interventional therapy is indicated for symptomatic persons with severe MS. A mitral valve area of 1.0 cm² or less is considered severe MS. Mitral valve replacement is usually performed because the calcified mitral valve is usually not amenable to open mitral commissurotomy. For the few older persons who have an uncalcified mitral valve or mild calcific deposits, flexible mitral valve leaflets, and no or mild MR, percutaneous balloon valvuloplasty is the procedure of choice.[179]

MITRAL REGURGITATION

Acute mitral regurgitation

Acute severe mitral regurgitation (MR) in older persons may be caused by ruptured chordae tendineae or development of a flail mitral valve secondary to acute myocardial infarction, infective endocarditis, papillary muscle rupture, or mucoid degeneration of the mitral valve cusps. Acute severe MR usually results in severe CHF with pulmonary edema and right-sided CHF.

Signs of acute severe MR

The MR murmur associated with acute severe MR is characteristically a harsh systolic murmur (with an associated palpable thrill) heard at the apex which begins with the first heart sound but ends early when the noncompliant left atrium can no longer accept the large regurgitant volume. The first heart sound is soft, and the pulmonic component of the second heart sound is increased. A left ventricular third heart sound gallop and an atrial fourth heart sound gallop are heard at the apex.

Diagnosis and management of acute MR

Doppler echocardiography confirms the diagnosis of severe MR. Transesophageal echocardiography provides a highly accurate anatomic assessment of the etiology of the acute MR and assists in determining whether the mitral valve can be repaired or must be replaced.[180] CHF needs to be managed medically. Infective endocarditis should be treated with appropriate antibiotics. Mitral valve surgery should be performed urgently.

Chronic mitral regurgitation

Prevalence and etiology of chronic MR

Chronic MR was present in 298 of 924 men (32 percent), mean age 80 years, and in 630 of 1881 women (33 percent), mean age 81 years.[20] MR 2–4+ was present in 10 percent of 2148 persons, mean age 81 years.[164] The commonest cause of MR in older persons is MAC.[132] Other causes in older persons include papillary muscle dysfunction after myocardial infarction, rheumatic heart disease, myxomatous degeneration of the mitral valve leaflets and chordae tendineae with mitral valve prolapse (MVP), ruptured chordae tendineae, and following endocarditis. MR may also result from alteration in the geometry of the mitral annulus occurring with dilatation of the LV and CHF.

Pathophysiology of chronic MR

The regurgitant volume gradually increases in chronic MR, increasing the left atrial volume during systole and the LV volume during diastole. Eccentric LV hypertrophy occurs. Atrial fibrillation develops, and the LV cannot maintain an effective forward stroke volume because of depressed LV contractility. Left-sided CHF develops, resulting in increased pulmonary artery and right ventricular systolic pressure, and eventually right-sided CHF. Decreased LV systolic and diastolic function in persons with chronic MR contribute to the clinical manifestations of CHF.[181] Unrecognized MR may contribute to acute pulmonary edema in persons with normal or abnormal LV systolic function.[182]

Symptoms and signs of chronic MR

Older persons with chronic MR may be asymptomatic or have a reduction in exercise tolerance with easy fatigability. Dyspnea on exertion will develop with significant MR and progress to orthopnea, paroxysmal nocturnal dyspnea, and dyspnea at rest caused by left-sided CHF. Right-sided CHF will cause ankle swelling, anorexia, and right upper abdominal tenderness from hepatic congestion. Symptoms may also result from the development of atrial fibrillation. Atypical chest pain, palpitations, or syncope due to arrhythmias may be associated with mitral valve prolapse. In some persons, acute pulmonary edema may be the initial manifestation of severe mitral regurgitation from MVP.[183]

The heart murmur associated with chronic MR is heard as an apical holosystolic, late systolic, or early systolic murmur beginning with the first heart sound but ending in midsystole. The holosystolic murmur may radiate to the left axilla, to the back, and over the entire precordium. A nonejection systolic click may precede the mid-to-late systolic apical murmur associated with MVP. With severe MR, the first heart sound becomes decreased, and a LV third heart sound is heard at the apex.

Diagnosis of chronic MR

Doppler echocardiography can quantitate the severity of MR and assess LV size and function. Doppler echocardiography (especially transesophageal) can also determine the etiology of the MR. Vegetations are seen with infective endocarditis. Mitral valve prolapse and thickening of the mitral valve leaflets suggest myxomatous degeneration. MAC can be diagnosed. Thickened retracted leaflets and chordal fusion suggest rheumatic heart disease as the cause of MR. A flail mitral valve and ruptured chordae tendineae can be diagnosed. The sensitivity of transesophageal echocardiography in diagnosing specific causes of MR was 82 percent for vegetations, 99 percent for MVP, 100 percent for a flail mitral valve, and 84 percent for ruptured chordae tendineae.[180] In persons with severe chronic

MR, the electrocardiogram may show atrial fibrillation or left atrial enlargement, LV hypertrophy in about 50 percent of cases, and RVH in approximately 15 percent.

Management of chronic MR
Older persons with chronic MR should have Doppler echocardiograms every 6–12 months. There are no long-term studies supporting the use of vasodilator therapy in asymptomatic persons with chronic MR. Angiotensin-converting enzyme (ACE) inhibitors should be used in treating persons with symptomatic chronic MR.[184] Persons with atrial fibrillation should be treated with long-term oral warfarin to maintain the INR at between 2.0 and 3.0. CHF should be treated with standard medical therapy. Prophylactic antibiotics should be used to prevent bacterial endocarditis, according to AHA guidelines.[55]

Timing of surgery in chronic MR
Of 478 persons with nonischemic chronic severe MR undergoing surgery, the cause of MR was mitral valve prolapse in 79 percent, rheumatic in 8 percent, endocarditis in 8 percent, and miscellaneous in 4 percent.[185] Surgical repair of the mitral valve was performed in 68 percent of cases and mitral valve replacement in 32 percent. CABGS was performed in 27 percent of persons in association with mitral valve surgery.[185]

Tribouilloy et al.[185] reported no operative mortality for persons younger than 75 years. Above that age the operative mortality was 3.6 percent in those with NYHA class I or II symptoms, and 12.7 percent in those with severe symptoms. In persons with a LV ejection fraction ≥60 percent, the 10-year survival was 79 percent in those with class I or II symptoms versus 49 percent in those with class III or IV symptoms. In persons with a LV ejection fraction <60 percent, the 10-year survival was 75 percent in those with class I or II symptoms versus 41 percent in those with class III or IV symptoms.

Table 36-7 lists the ACC/AHA class indications for performing mitral valve surgery in persons with nonischemic severe MR.[111] Older persons with symptomatic severe MR and severely depressed LV function (LV ejection fraction <30 percent or LV end-systolic dimension >55 mm) should be treated medically. Older persons with chronic nonischemic MR who have NYHA class I symptoms and normal LV function should be followed at 3–6 month intervals. If LV dysfunction, atrial

fibrillation, or pulmonary hypertension develops, the person should be considered for cardiac catheterization and possible mitral valve surgery, especially if it is thought that the mitral valve can be repaired.

The prognosis for the person with ischemic MR is worse than that for MR from other causes. CABGS may improve LV function and decrease ischemic MR.[111] The best operation for ischemic MR is controversial.

TRICUSPID REGURGITATION

In older persons, tricuspid regurgitation (TR) is usually caused by dilatation of the right ventricle and tricuspid annulus associated with right-sided heart failure resulting from left-sided heart failure or pulmonary hypertension associated with pulmonary vascular disease.

The murmur of TR is usually high-pitched and holosystolic heard in the third or fourth intercostal space at the left sternal border and occasionally in the subxiphoid area, and increases with inspiration in 50 percent of persons. When TR is mild, the systolic murmur may be a short ejection murmur or absent. P_2 is increased with pulmonary hypertension. If TR is severe, a prominent large V wave is seen in the jugular venous pulse. Systolic pulsation of an enlarged tender liver is commonly present. Ascites and peripheral edema are frequent.

Diagnosis of TR is confirmed by Doppler echocardiography. Medical treatment of CHF is indicated. Surgery is rarely necessary.

TRICUSPID STENOSIS

Tricuspid stenosis (TS) in older persons is rare and due to multivalvular rheumatic heart disease or the carcinoid syndrome. Symptoms of right-sided heart failure occur. A low-frequency diastolic rumble is heard in the third or fourth intercostal space at the left sternal border which increases with intensity with inspiration. A prominent A wave with poor or absent Y descent is seen in the jugular venous pulse. The electrocardiogram shows tall right atrial probability waves and no RVH. The chest X-ray shows a dilated right atrium without an enlarged pulmonary artery segment. Diagnosis of TS is confirmed by Doppler echocardiography.

Medical therapy is indicated for mild TS. Balloon valvotomy is recommended for persons with TS with signs of right-sided heart failure or with a marked reduction in exercise tolerance due to an inability to increase cardiac output. If the tricuspid valve is calcified (rarely), tricuspid valve replacement is indicated. A porcine bioprosthetic heart valve is recommended in the tricuspid position.

PULMONIC REGURGITATION

In older persons, pulmonic regurgitation (PR) is almost always due to pulmonary hypertension resulting from left-sided heart failure or pulmonary vascular disease. A high-pitched, blowing decrescendo murmur beginning immediately after P_2 is heard in the second and third intercostal space to the left of the

---

Table 36-7 Class I indications for mitral valve surgery in persons with nonischemic severe mitral regurgitation

1. Acute symptomatic MR in which mitral valve repair is likely.
2. Persons with NYHA class II, III, or IV symptoms and normal LV function defined as LV ejection fraction >60 percent and LV end-systolic dimension <45 mm.
3. Symptomatic or asymptomatic persons with mild LV dysfunction defined as LV ejection fraction of 50–60 percent and LV end-systolic dimension of 45–50 mm.
4. Symptomatic or asymptomatic persons with moderate LV dysfunction defined as LV ejection fraction of 30–50 percent and/or LV end-systolic dimension of 50–55 mm.

Abbreviations: MR, mitral regurgitation; NYHA, New York Heart Association; LV, left ventricular.
Source: Adapted from Bonow et al. (1998),[111] with permission.

sternum. Diagnosis of PR is confined by Doppler echocardiography. Management of PR is directed at treating the underlying disorder and trying to reduce pulmonary artery pressure.

KEY POINTS Valvular heart disease

■ Persons with congestive heart failure, exertional syncope, or angina pectoris associated with moderate or severe aortic stenosis should undergo aortic valve replacement promptly.

■ Persons with chronic severe aortic regurgitation should undergo aortic valve replacement promptly if they develop symptoms of congestive heart failure, syncope, or angina pectoris.

■ Aortic valve replacement should be performed in asymptomatic persons with chronic severe aortic regurgitation if they develop left ventricular systolic dysfunction.

■ Persons with nonischemic chronic severe mitral regurgitation with New York Heart Association class II, III, or IV symptoms and normal left ventricular systolic function, or asymptomatic persons with mild or moderate left ventricular systolic dysfunction, should have mitral valve surgery performed promptly.

REFERENCES

1. Roberts WC, Perloff JK, Costantino T: Severe valvular aortic stenosis in patients over 65 years of age. Am J Cardiol 1971;27;497–506

2. Waller BF, Roberts WC: Cardiovascular disease in the very elderly: an analysis of 40 necropsy patients aged 90 years or over. Am J Cardiol 1983;51:403–421

3. Aronow WS, Schwartz KS, Koenigsberg M: Correlation of aortic cuspal and aortic root disease with aortic systolic ejection murmurs and with mitral annular calcium in persons older than 62 years in a long-term health care facility. Am J Cardiol 1986;58:651–652

4. Aronow WS, Kronzon I: Prevalence and severity of valvular aortic stenosis determined by Doppler echocardiography and its association with echocardiographic and electrocardiographic left ventricular hypertrophy and physical signs of aortic stenosis in elderly patients. Am J Cardiol 1991;67:776–777

5. Lindroos M, Kupari M, Heikkila J, Tilvis R: Prevalence of aortic valve abnormalities in the elderly: an echocardiographic study of a random population sample. J Am Coll Cardiol 1993;21:1220–1225

6. Aronow WS, Ahn C, Kronzon I: Association of mitral annular calcium and of aortic cuspal calcium with coronary artery disease in older patients. Am J Cardiol 1999;84:1084–1085

7. Aronow WS, Ahn Chul, Shirani J, Kronzon I: Comparison of frequency of new coronary events in older subjects with and without valvular aortic sclerosis. Am J Cardiol 1999;83:599–600

8. Roberts WC, Perloff JK: Mitral valvular disease: a clinicopathologic survey of the conditions causing the mitral valve to function normally. Ann Intern Med 1972;77:939–975

9. Nair CK, Aronow WS, Stokke K et al: Cardiac conduction defects in patients older than 60 years with aortic stenosis with and without mitral annular calcium. Am J Cardiol 1984;53:169–172

10. Sell S, Scully RE: Aging changes in the aortic and mitral valves. Am J Pathol 1965;46:345–365

11. Otto CM, Kuusisto J, Reichenbach DD et al: Characterization of the early lesion of "degenerative" valvular aortic stenosis. Circulation 1994;90:844–853

12. Stewart BF, Siscovick D, Lind BK et al: Clinical factors associated with calcific aortic valve disease. J Am Coll Cardiol 1997;29:630–634

13. Aronow WS, Schwartz KS, Koenigsberg M: Correlation of serum lipids, calcium, and phosphorus, diabetes mellitus and history of systemic hypertension with presence or absence of calcified or thickened aortic cusps or root in elderly patients. Am J Cardiol 1987;59:998–999

14. Lindroos M, Kupari M, Valvanne J et al: Factors associated with calcific aortic valve degeneration in the elderly. Eur Heart J 1994;15:865–870

15. Aronow WS, Kronzon I, Schoenfeld MR: Prevalence of extracranial carotid arterial disease and of valvular aortic stenosis and their association in the elderly. Am J Cardiol 1995;75:304–305

16. Nassimiha D, Aronow WS, Ahn C, Goldman ME: Rate of progression of valvular aortic stenosis in persons ≥60 years. Am J Cardiol 2001;87:807–809

17. Nassimiha D, Aronow WS, Ahn C, Goldman ME: Association of coronary risk factors with progression of valvular aortic stenosis in older persons. Am J Cardiol 2001;87:1313–1314

18. Roberts WC. The senile cardiac calcification syndrome. Am J Cardiol 1986;58:572–574

19. Aronow WS, Schwartz KS, Koenigsberg M: Correlation of serum lipids, calcium and phosphorus, diabetes mellitus, aortic valve stenosis and history of systemic hypertension with presence or absence of mitral annular calcium in persons older than 62 years in a long-term health care facility. Am J Cardiol 1987;59:381–382

20. Aronow WS, Ahn C, Kronzon I: Comparison of echocardiographic findings in African-American, Hispanic, and white men and women aged >60 years. Am J Cardiol 2001;87:1131–1133

21. Kennedy JW, Twiss RD, Blackmon JR, Dodge HT: Quantitative angiocardiography. III: Relationships of left ventricular pressure, volume and mass in aortic valve disease. Circulation 1968;38:838–845

22. Hood WP, Rackley CE, Rolett EL: Wall stress in the normal and hypertrophied human left ventricle. Am J Cardiol 1968;22:550–558

23. Carroll JD, Carroll EP, Feldman T et al: Sex-associated differences in left ventricular function in aortic stenosis of the elderly. Circulation 1992;86:1099–1107

24. Villari B, Vassalli G, Schneider J et al: Age dependency of left ventricular diastolic function in pressure overload hypertrophy. J Am Coll Cardiol 1997;29:181–186

25. Stott DK, Marpole DG, Bristow JD et al: The role of left atrial transport in aortic and mitral stenosis. Circulation 1970;41:1031–1041

26. Vekshtein VI, Alexander RW, Yeung AC et al: Coronary atherosclerosis is associated with left ventricular dysfunction and dilatation in aortic stenosis. Circulation 1990;82:2068–2074

27. Aronow WS, Ahn C, Kronzon I, Nanna M: Prognosis of congestive heart failure in patients aged ≥62 years with unoperated severe valvular aortic stenosis. Am J Cardiol 1993;72:846–848

28. Hess OM, Villari B, Krayenbuehl HP: Diastolic dysfunction in aortic stenosis. Circulation 1993;87(suppl IV):73–76

29. Julius BK, Spillmann M, Vassalli G et al: Angina pectoris in patients with aortic stenosis and normal coronary arteries: mechanisms and pathophysiological concepts. Circulation 1997;95:892–898

30. Aronow WS, Ahn C, Shirani J, Kronzon I: Comparison of frequency of new coronary events in older persons with mild, moderate, and severe valvular aortic stenosis with those without aortic stenosis. Am J Cardiol 1998;81:647–649

31. Ross J, Braunwald E. Aortic stenosis. Circulation 1968:37(suppl V):61–67

32. Frank S, Johnson A, Ross J: Natural history of valvular aortic stenosis. Br Heart J 1973;35:41–56

33. Braunwald E: On the natural history of severe aortic stenosis. J Am Coll Cardiol 1990;15:1018–1020

34. Bruns DL, Van Der Hauwaert LG: The aortic systolic murmur developing with increased age. Br Heart J 1958;20:370–378

35. Aronow WS, Kronzon I: Correlation of prevalence and severity of valvular aortic stenosis determined by continuous-wave Doppler echocardiography with physical signs of aortic stenosis in patients aged 62 to 100 years with aortic systolic ejection murmurs. Am J Cardiol 1987;60:399–401

36. Folland ED, Kriegel BJ, Henderson WG et al: Implications of third heart sounds in patients with valvular heart disease. N Engl J Med 1992;327:458–462

37. Finegan RE, Gianelly RE, Harrison DC: Aortic stenosis in the elderly: relevance of age to diagnosis and treatment. N Engl J Med 1969;281:1261–1264

38. Aronow WS, Epstein S, Koenigsberg M, Schwartz KS: Usefulness of echocardiographic abnormal left ventricular ejection fraction, paroxysmal ventricular tachycardia, and complex ventricular arrhythmias in predicting new coronary events in patients over 62 years of age. Am J Cardiol 1988;61:1349–1351

39. Rispler S, Rinkevich D, Markiewicz W, Reisner SA: Missed diagnosis of severe symptomatic aortic stenosis. Am J Cardiol 1995;76:728–730

40. Teirstein P, Yeager M, Yock PG, Popp RL: Doppler echocardiographic measurements of aortic valve area in aortic stenosis: a noninvasive application of the Gorlin formula. J Am Coll Cardiol 1986;8:1059–1065

41. Come PC, Riley MF, McKay RG, Safian R: Echocardiographic assessment of aortic valve area in elderly patients with aortic stenosis and of changes of valve area after percutaneous balloon valvuloplasty. J Am Coll Cardiol 1987;10:115–124

42. Shah PM, Graham BM: Management of aortic stenosis: is cardiac catheterization necessary? Am J Cardiol 1991;67:1031–1032

43. Slater J, Gindea AJ, Freedberg RS et al: Comparison of cardiac catheterization and Doppler echocardiography in the decision to operate in aortic and mitral valve disease. J Am Coll Cardiol 1991;67:1007–1012

44. Nassimiha D, Aronow WS, Ahn C, Goldman ME: Comparison of aortic valve area determined by Doppler echocardiography and cardiac catheterization in 75 older patients with valvular aortic stenosis. Cardiovasc Rev Rep 2000;21:507–509

45. Galan A, Zoghbi WA, Quinones MA: Determination of severity of valvular aortic stenosis by Doppler echocardiography and relation of findings to clinical outcome and agreement with hemodynamic measurements determined at cardiac catheterization. Am J Cardiol 1991;67:1007–1012

46. Rapaport E: Natural history of aortic and mitral valve disease. Am J Cardiol 1975;35:221–227

47. Livanainen AM, Lindroos M, Tilvis R et al: Natural history of aortic valve stenosis of varying severity in the elderly. Am J Cardiol 1996;78:97–101

48. Otto CM, Lind BK, Kitzman DW et al: Association of aortic-valve sclerosis with cardiovascular mortality and morbidity in the elderly. N Engl J Med 1999;341:142–147

49. Kennedy KD, Nishimura RA, Holmes DR, Bailey KR: Natural history of moderate aortic stenosis. J Am Coll Cardiol 1991;17:313–319

50. Hammermeister KE, Cantor AB, Burchfield CM et al: Clinical haemodynamic and angiographic predictors of survival in unoperated patients with aortic stenosis. Eur Heart J 1988;9(suppl E):65–69

51. Turina J, Hess O, Sepulcri F, Krayenbuehl HP: Spontaneous course of aortic valve disease. Eur Heart J 1987;8:471–483

52. Kelly TA, Rothbart RM, Cooper CM et al: Comparison of outcome of asymptomatic to symptomatic patients older than 20 years of age with valvular aortic stenosis. Am J Cardiol 1988;61:123–130

53. Pellikka PA, Nishimura RA, Bailey KR, Tajik AJ: The natural history of adults with asymptomatic hemodynamically significant aortic stenosis. J Am Coll Cardiol 1990;15:1012–1017

54. Rosenhek R, Binder T, Porenta G et al: Predictors of outcome in severe, asymptomatic aortic stenosis. N Engl J Med 2000;343:611–617

55. Dajani AS, Taubert KA, Wilson W et al: Prevention of bacterial endocarditis: recommendations by the American Heart Association. Circulation 1997;96:358–366

56. Tresch DD, Knickelbine T: Aortic valvular stenosis in the elderly: a disorder with a favorable outcome if correctly diagnosed and treated. Cardiovasc Rev Rep 1994;15(7):35–38

57. Hammermeister K, Sethi GK, Henderson WG et al: Outcomes 15 years after valve replacement with a mechanical versus a bioprosthetic valve: final report of the Veterans Affairs Randomized Trial. J Am Coll Cardiol 2000;36:1152–1158

58. Borkon AM, Soule LM, Baughman KL et al: Aortic valve selection in the elderly patient. Ann Thorac Surg 1988;46:270–277

59. Culliford AT, Galloway AC, Colvin SB et al: Aortic valve replacement for aortic stenosis in persons aged 80 years and older. Am J Cardiol 1991;67:1256–1260

60. Arom K, Nicoloff D, Lindsay W et al: Aortic valve replacement in the elderly: operative risks and long-term results. J Am Coll Cardiol 1990;15:96A (abstract)

61. Levinson JR, Akins CW, Buckley MJ et al: Octogenarians with aortic stenosis: outcome after aortic valve replacement. Circulation 1989;80(suppl I):49–56

62. Asimakopoulos G, Edwards M-B, Taylor KM: Aortic valve replacement in patients 80 years of age and older. Survival and cause of death based on 1100 cases: collective results from the UK Heart Valve Registry. Circulation 1997;96:3403–3408

63. Gilchrist IC, Waxman HL, Kurnik PB: Improvement in early diastolic filling dynamics after aortic valve replacement. Am J Cardiol 1990;66:1124–1129

64. Villari B, Vassalli G, Monrad ES et al: Normalization of diastolic dysfunction in aortic stenosis late after valve replacement. Circulation 1995;91:2353–2358

65. Hoffman A, Burckhardt D: Patients at risk for cardiac death late after aortic valve replacement. Am Heart J 1990;120:1142–1147

66. Connolly HM, Oh JK, Orszulak TA et al: Aortic valve replacement for aortic stenosis with severe left ventricular dysfunction: prognostic indicators. Circulation 1997;95:2395–2400

67. O'Keefe JH, Vlietstra RE, Bailey KR, Holmes DR: Natural history of candidates for balloon aortic valvuloplasty. Mayo Clin Proc 1987;62:986–991

68. Litvack F, Jakubowski AT, Buchbinder NA, Eigler N: Lack of sustained clinical improvement in an elderly population after percutaneous aortic valvuloplasty. Am J Cardiol 1988;62:270–275

69. Block PC, Palacios IF: Clinical and hemodynamic follow-up after percutaneous aortic valvuloplasty in the elderly. Am J Cardiol 1988;62:760–763

70. Safian RD, Berman AD, Diver DJ et al: Balloon aortic angioplasty in 170 consecutive patients. N Engl J Med 1988;319:125–130

71. Lewin RF, Dorros G, King JF, Mathiak L: Percutaneous transluminal aortic valvuloplasty: acute outcome and follow-up of 125 patients. J Am Coll Cardiol 1989;14:1210–1217

72. Brady ST, Davis CA, Kussmaul WG et al: Percutaneous aortic balloon valvuloplasty in octogenarians: morbidity and mortality. Ann Intern Med 1989;110:761–766

73. Letac B, Cribier A, Koning R, Lefebvre E: Aortic stenosis in elderly patients aged 80 or older: treatment by percutaneous balloon valvuloplasty in a series of 92 cases. Circulation 1989;80:1514–1520

74. Rodriguez AR, Kleiman NS, Minor ST et al: Factors influencing the outcome of balloon aortic valvuloplasty in the elderly. Am Heart J 1990;120:373–380

75. Kuntz RE, Tosteson ANA, Berman AD et al: Predictors of event-free survival after balloon aortic valvuloplasty. N Engl J Med 1991;325:17–23

76. Cheitlin MD: Severe aortic stenosis in the sick octogenarian: a clear indicator for balloon valvuloplasty as the initial procedure. Circulation 1989;80:1906–1908

77. Rahimtoola SH: Catheter balloon valvuloplasty for severe calcific aortic stenosis: a limited role. J Am Coll Cardiol 1994;23:1076–1078

78. Theard MA, Bhatia SJS, Plappert T, St John Sutton MG: Doppler echocardiographic study of the frequency and severity of aortic regurgitation in hypertrophic cardiomyopathy. Am J Cardiol 1987;60:1143–1147

79. Margonato A, Cianflone D, Carlino M et al: Frequency and significance of aortic valve thickening in older asymptomatic patients and its relation to aortic regurgitation. Am J Cardiol 1989;64:1061–1062

80. Akasaka T, Yoshikawa J, Yoshida K et al: Age-related valvular regurgitation: a study by pulsed Doppler echocardiography. Circulation 1987;76:262–265

81. Aronow WS, Kronzon I: Correlation of prevalence and severity of aortic regurgitation detected by pulsed Doppler echocardiography with the murmur of aortic regurgitation in elderly patients in a long-term health care facility. Am J Cardiol 1989;63:128–129

82. Gaasch WH, Sundaram M, Meyer TE: Managing asymptomatic patients with chronic aortic regurgitation. Chest 1997;111:1702–1709

83. Ross J: Afterload mismatch and preload reserve: a conceptual framework for the analysis of ventricular function. Prog Cardiovasc Dis 1976;18:256–264

84. Greenberg B, Massie B, Thomas D et al: Association between the exercise ejection fraction response and systolic wall stress in patients with chronic aortic insufficiency. Circulation 1985;71:458–465

85. Aronow WS, Ahn C, Kronzon I, Nanna M: Prognosis of patients with heart failure and unoperated severe aortic valvular regurgitation and relation to ejection fraction. Am J Cardiol 1994;74:286–288

86. Welch GH, Braunwald E, Sarnoff SJ: Hemodynamic effects of quantitatively varied experimental aortic regurgitation. Circ Res 1957;5:546–551

87. Mann T, McLaurin LP, Grossman W, Craige E: Assessing the hemodynamic severity of acute aortic regurgitation due to infective endocarditis. N Engl J Med 1975;293:108–113

88. Massell BF, Amezcua FJ, Czoniczer G: Prognosis of patients with pure or predominant aortic regurgitation in the absence of surgery. Circulation 1966;34(Suppl III):164 (abstract)

89. Grayburn PA, Smith MD, Handshoe R et al: Detection of aortic insufficiency by standard echocardiography, pulsed Doppler echocardiography, and auscultation: comparison of accuracies. Ann Intern Med 1986;104:599–605

90. Saal AK, Gross BW, Franklin DW, Pearlman AS: Noninvasive detection of aortic insufficiency in patients with mitral stenosis by pulsed Doppler echocardiography. J Am Coll Cardiol 1985;5:176–181

91. Meyers DG, Sagar KB, Ingram RF et al: Diagnosis of aortic insufficiency: comparison of auscultation and M-mode echocardiography to angiography. South Med J 1982;75:1192–1194

92. Roberts WC, Day PJ: Electrocardiographic observations in clinically isolated, pure, chronic, severe aortic regurgitation: analysis of 30 necropsy patients aged 19 to 65 years. Am J Cardiol 1985;55:431–438

93. Savage DD, Garrison RJ, Kannel WB et al: The spectrum of left ventricular hypertrophy in a general population sample: the Framingham study. Circulation 1987;75(suppl I):26–33

94. Aronow WS, Ahn C, Kronzon I, Koenigsberg M: Congestive heart failure, coronary events, and atherothrombotic brain infarction in elderly blacks and whites with systemic hypertension and with and without echocardiographic and electrocardiographic evidence of left ventricular hypertrophy. Am J Cardiol 1991;67:295–299

95. Koren MJ, Devereux RB, Casale PN et al: Relation of left ventricular mass and geometry to morbidity and mortality in uncomplicated essential hypertension. Ann Intern Med 1991;114:345–352

96. Henry WL, Bonow RO, Borer JS et al: Observations on the optimum time for operative intervention for aortic regurgitation. I: Evaluation of the results of aortic valve replacement in symptomatic patients. Circulation 1980;61:471–483

97. Gaasch WH, Carroll JD, Levine HJ, Criscitiello MG: Chronic aortic regurgitation: prognostic value of left ventricular end-systolic dimension and end-diastolic radius/thickness ratio. J Am Coll Cardiol 1983;1:775–782

98. Grayburn PA, Handshoe R, Smith MD et al: Quantitative assessment of the hemodynamic consequences of aortic regurgitation by means of continuous wave Doppler recordings. J Am Coll Cardiol 1987;10:135–141

99. Beyer RW, Ramirez M, Josephson MA, Shah PM: Correlation of continuous-wave assessment of chronic aortic regurgitation with hemodynamics and angiography. Am J Cardiol 1987;60:852–856

100. Perry GJ, Helmcke F, Nanda NC et al: Evaluation of aortic insufficiency by Doppler color flow mapping. J Am Coll Cardiol 1987;9:952–959

101. Dexter L: Evaluation of the results of cardiac surgery. In Jones AM (ed): Modern Trends in Cardiology, Vol 2. Appleton-Century-Croft, New York, 1969:311–333

102. Hegglin R, Scheu H, Rothlin M: Aortic insufficiency. Circulation 1968;38(suppl V):77–92

103. Bonow RO, Lakatos E, Maron BJ, Epstein SE: Serial long-term assessment of the natural history of asymptomatic patients with chronic aortic regurgitation and normal left ventricular systolic function. Circulation 1991;84:1625–1635

104. Greenberg B, Massie B, Bristow JD et al: Long-term vasodilator therapy of chronic aortic insufficiency: a randomized double-blind, placebo-controlled clinical trial. Circulation 1988;78:92–103

105. Scognamiglio R, Rahimtoola SH, Fasoli G et al: Nifedipine in asymptomatic patients with severe aortic regurgitation and normal left ventricular function. N Engl J Med 1994;331:689–694

106. Lin M, Chiang H-T, Lin S-L et al: Vasodilator therapy in chronic asymptomatic aortic regurgitation: enalapril versus hydralazine therapy. J Am Coll Cardiol 1994;24:1046–1053

107. McDonald GR, Schaff HV, Pyeritz RE et al: Surgical management of patients with the Marfan syndrome and dilatation of the ascending aorta. J Thorac Cardiovasc Surg 1981;81:180–186

108. Alsip SG, Blackstone EH, Kirklin JW, Cobbs CG: Indications for cardiac surgery in patients with active infective endocarditis. Am J Med 1985;78(suppl 6B):138–148

109. Karp RB: Role of surgery in infective endocarditis. Cardiovasc Clin 1987;17(3):141–162

110. Cobbs CG, Gnann JW: Indications for surgery. In Sande MA, Kaye D, Root RK (eds): Endocarditis. Churchill Livingstone, New York, 1984:201–212

111. Bonow RO, Carabello B, de Leon AC et al: Guidelines for the management of patients with valvular heart disease. Executive summary. A Report of the American College of Cardiology/American Heart Association Task Force on Practice Guidelines (committee on management of patients with valvular heart disease). Circulation 1998;98:1949–1984

112. Bonow RO, Picone AL, McIntosh CL et al: Survival and functional results after valve replacement for aortic regurgitation from 1976 to 1983: impact of preoperative left ventricular function. Circulation 1985;72:1244–1256

113. Bonow RO. Noninvasive evaluation: prognosis and timing of operation in symptomatic and asymptomatic patients with chronic aortic regurgitation. In Cohn LH, DiSesa VJ (eds): Aortic Regurgitation: Medical and Surgical Management. Marcel Dekker, New York, 1986:55–86

114. Turina J, Milincic J, Seifert B, Turina M: Valve replacement in chronic aortic regurgitation: true predictors of survival after extended follow-up. Circulation 1998;98:II100–II107

115. Klodas E, Enriquez-Sarano M, Tajik AJ et al: Surgery for aortic regurgitation in women: contrasting indications and outcomes compared with men. Circulation 1996;94:2472–2478

116. Roman MJ, Klein L, Devereux RB et al: Reversal of left ventricular dilatation, hypertrophy, and dysfunction by valve replacement in aortic regurgitation. Am Heart J 1989;118:553–563

117. Hammer WJ, Roberts WC, deLeon AC: "Mitral stenosis" secondary to combined "massive" mitral annular calcific deposits and small, hypertrophied left ventricles: hemodynamic documentation in four patients. Am J Med 1978;64:371–376

118. Osterberger LE, Goldstein S, Khaja F, Lakier J. Functional mitral stenosis in patients with massive annular calcification. Circulation 1981;64:472–476

119. Nair CK, Runco V, Everson GT et al: Conduction defects and mitral annulus calcification. Br Heart J 1980;44:162–167

120. Nair CK, Sketch MH, Desai R et al: High prevalence of symptomatic bradyarrhythmias due to atrioventricular node–fascicular and sinus node–atrial disease in patients with mitral annular calcification. Am Heart J 1982;103:226–229

121. Fulkerson PK, Beaver BM, Auseon JC, Graber HL: Calcification of the mitral annulus: etiology, clinical associations, complications and therapy. Am J Med 1979;66:967–977

122. Ridolfi RL, Hutchins GM: Spontaneous calcific emboli from calcific mitral annulus fibrosus. Arch Pathol Lab Med 1976;100:117–120

123. DeBono DP, Warlow CP: Mitral annulus calcification and cerebral or retinal ischaemia. Lancet 1979;2:383–385

124. Burnside JW, DeSanctis RW: Bacterial endocarditis on calcification of the mitral annulus fibrosus. Ann Intern Med 1972;76:615–618

125. Watanakunakorn C: Staphylococcus aureus endocarditis on the calcified mitral annulus fibrosus. Am J Med Sci 1973;266:219–223

126. Mambo NC, Silver MD, Brunsdon DFV: Bacterial endocarditis of the mitral valve associated with annular calcification. Can Med Assoc J 1978;119:323–326

127. D'Cruz IA, Collison HK, Gerrardo L, Hensel P: Two-dimensional echocardiographic detection of staphylococcal vegetation attached to calcified mitral annulus. Am Heart J 1982;103:295–298

128. Pomerance A, Darby AJ, Hodkinson HM: Valvular calcification in the elderly: possible pathogenic factors. J Gerontol 1978;33:672–676

129. Korn D, DeSanctis RW, Sell S: Massive calcification of the mitral annulus: a clinicopathologic study of fourteen cases. N Engl J Med 1962;267:900–909

130. Savage DD, Garrison RJ, Castelli WP et al: Prevalence of submitral (annular) calcium and its correlates in a general population-based sample (the Framingham Study). Am J Cardiol 1983;51:1375–1378

131. Aronow WS, Schwartz KS, Koenigsberg M: Correlation of atrial fibrillation with presence or absence of mitral annular calcium in 604 persons older than 60 years. Am J Cardiol 1987;59:1213–1214

132. Aronow WS, Schwartz KS, Koenigsberg M: Correlation of murmurs of mitral stenosis and mitral regurgitation with presence or absence of mitral annular calcium in persons older than 62 years in a long-term health care facility. Am J Cardiol 1987;59:181–182

133. Aronow WS, Koenigsberg M, Kronzon I, Gutstein H: Association of mitral annular calcium with new thromboembolic stroke and cardiac events at 39-month follow-up in elderly patients. Am J Cardiol 1990;65:1511–1512

134. Nair CK, Sudhakaran C, Aronow WS et al: Clinical characteristics of patients younger than 60 years with mitral annular calcium: comparison with age- and sex-matched control subjects. Am J Cardiol 1984;54:1286–1287

135. Nair CK, Sketch MH, Ahmed I et al: Calcific valvular aortic stenosis with and without mitral annular calcium. Am J Cardiol 1987;60:865–870

136. Adler Y, Herz I, Vaturi M et al: Mitral annular calcium detected by transthoracic echocardiography is a marker for high prevalence and severity of coronary artery disease in patients undergoing coronary angiography. Am J Cardiol 1998;82:1183–1186

137. Aronow WS, Schwartz KS, Koenigsberg M: Prevalence of tricuspid annular calcium diagnosed by echocardiography in elderly patients. Am J Noninvas Cardiol 1987;1:275–277

138. Roberts WC: Morphologic features of the normal and abnormal mitral valve. Am J Cardiol 1983;51:1005–1028

139. Sprecher DL, Schaefer EJ, Kent KM et al: Cardiovascular features of homozygous familial hypercholesterolemia: analysis of 16 patients. Am J Cardiol 1984;54:20–30

140. Roberts WC, Waller BF: Effect of chronic hypercalcemia on the heart: an analysis of 18 necropsy patients. Am J Med 1981;71:371–384

141. Aronow WS, Kronzon I: Prevalence of aortic valve calcium and of mitral annular calcium in older persons with and without chronic renal insufficiency. Cardiovasc Rev Rep 2000;21:623–624

142. Schott CR, Kotler MN, Parry WR, Segal BL: Mitral annular calcification: clinical and echocardiographic correlations. Arch Intern Med 1977;137:1143–1150

143. D'Cruz IA, Bhatt GR, Cohen HC, Glick G: Echocardiographic detection of cardiac involvement in patients with chronic renal failure. Arch Intern Med 1978;138:720–724

144. Nestico PF, DePace NL, Kotler MN et al: Calcium phosphorus metabolism in dialysis patients with and without mitral annular calcium. Am J Cardiol 1983;51:497–500

145. Forman MB, Virmani R, Robertson RM, Stone WJ: Mitral annular calcification in chronic renal failure. Chest 1987;85:367–371

146. Cohen JL, Barooah B, Segal KR, Batuman V: Two-dimensional echocardiographic findings in patients on hemodialysis for more than six months. Am J Cardiol 1987;60:743–745

147. Huting J: Mitral valve calcification as an index of left ventricular dysfunction in patients with end-stage renal disease on peritoneal dialysis. Chest 1994;105:383–388

148. Kronzon I, Glassman E: Mitral ring calcification in idiopathic hypertrophic subaortic stenosis. Am J Cardiol 1978;42:60–66

149. Nair CK, Kudesia V, Hansen D et al: Echocardiographic and electrocardiographic characteristics of patients with hypertrophic cardiomyopathy with and without mitral annular calcium. Am J Cardiol 1987;59:1428–1430

150. Motamed HE, Roberts WC: Frequency and significance of mitral annular calcium in hypertrophic cardiomyopathy: analysis of 200 necropsy patients. Am J Cardiol 1987;60:877–884

151. Aronow WS, Kronzon I: Prevalence of hypertrophic cardiomyopathy and its association with mitral annular calcium in elderly patients. Chest 1988;94:1295–1296

152. Roberts WC, Waller BF: Mitral valve "annular" calcium forming a complete circle or "O" configuration: clinical and necropsy observations. Am Heart J 1981;101:619–621

153. Sosman MC: The technique for locating and identifying pericardial and intracardiac calcifications. Am J Roentgenol 1943;50:461–468

154. Simon MA, Liu SF: Calcification of the mitral valve annulus and its relation to functional valvular disturbance. Am Heart J 1954;48:497–505

155. Windholz F, Grayson C: Roentgen demonstration of calcifications in the interventricular septum in cases of heart block. Am J Roentgenol 1947;58:411–421

156. Gabor GE, Mohr BD, Goel PC, Cohen B: Echocardiographic and clinical spectrum of mitral annular calcification. Am J Cardiol 1976;38:836–842

157. D'Cruz IA, Cohen HC, Prabhu R et al: Clinical manifestations of mitral annulus calcification, with emphasis on its echocardiographic features. Am Heart J 1977;94:367–377

158. Aronow WS, Schwartz KS, Koenigsberg M: Sensitivity, specificity, positive predictive value, and negative predictive value of mitral annular calcium detected by chest roentgenograms correlated with mitral annular calcium diagnosed by echocardiography in elderly patients. Am J Noninvas Cardiol 1987;1:252–253

159. Nair CK, Aronow WS, Sketch MH et al: Clinical and echocardiographic characteristics of patients with mitral annular calcification: comparison with age- and sex-matched control subjects. Am J Cardiol 1983;51:992–995

160. Nair CK, Thomson W, Ryschon K et al: Long-term follow-up of patients with echocardiographically detected mitral annular calcium and comparison with age- and sex-matched control subjects. Am J Cardiol 1989;63:465–470

161. Dashkoff N, Karakushensky M, Fortuin NJ: Echocardiographic features of mitral annulus calcification. Circulation 1975;52(suppl II):II34 (abstract)

162. Kaul S, Pearlman JD, Touchstone DA, Esquival L: Prevalence and mechanisms of mitral regurgitation in the absence of intrinsic abnormalities of the mitral leaflets. Am Heart J 1989;118:963–972

163. Aronow WS, Ahn C, Kronzon I: Echocardiographic findings associated with atrial fibrillation in 1699 patients aged >60 years. Am J Cardiol 1995;76:1191–1192

164. Aronow WS, Ahn C, Kronzon I, Gutstein H: Association of mitral annular calcium with new thromboembolic stroke at 44-month follow-up of 2148 persons, mean age 81 years. Am J Cardiol 1998;81:105–106

165. Aronow WS, Kronzon I: Correlation of prevalence and severity of mitral regurgitation and mitral stenosis determined by Doppler echocardiography with physical signs of mitral regurgitation and mitral stenosis in 100 patients aged 62 to 100 years with mitral annular calcium. Am J Cardiol 197;60:1189–1190

166. Labovitz AJ, Nelson JG, Windhorst DM et al: Frequency of mitral valve dysfunction from mitral annular calcium as detected by Doppler echocardiography. Am J Cardiol 1985;55:133–137

167. Nair CK, Biddle P, Kaneshige A et al: Mitral valve replacement in patients with mitral annular calcium. Chest 1991;100(Suppl):109S (abstract)

168. Sherman DG, Dyken ML, Fisher M et al: Cerebral embolism. Chest 1986;89:82S–98S

169. Aronow WS, Ahn C, Kronzon I, Gutstein H: Association of mitral annular calcium with prior thromboembolic stroke in older white, African-American, and Hispanic men and women. Am J Cardiol;85:672–673

170. Benjamin EJ, Plehn JF, D'Agostino RB et al: Mitral annular calcification and the risk of stroke in an elderly cohort. N Engl J Med 1992;327:374–379

171. Boston Area Anticoagulation Trial for Atrial Fibrillation Investigators: The effect of low-dose warfarin on the risk of stroke in patients with nonrheumatic atrial fibrillation. N Engl J Med 1990;323:1505–1511

172. Aronow WS, Schoenfeld MR, Gutstein H: Frequency of thrombo-embolic stroke in persons ≥60 years of age with extracranial carotid arterial disease and/or mitral annular calcium. Am J Cardiol 1992;70:123–124

173. Pomerance A: Pathological and clinical study of calcification of the mitral ring. J Clin Pathol 1970;23:354–361

174. Stein JH, Soble JS: Thrombus associated with mitral valve calcification: a possible mechanism for embolic stroke. Stroke 1995;26:1697–1699

175. Eicher J-C, Soto F-X, DeNadai L et al: Possible association of thrombotic, nonbacterial vegetations of the mitral ring: mitral annular calcium and stroke. Am J Cardiol 1997;79:1712–1715

176. Rubin DC, Hawke MW, Plotnick GD: Relation between mitral annular calcium and complex intraaortic debris. Am J Cardiol 1993;71:1251–1252

177. Aronow WS: The effect of low-dose warfarin on the risk of stroke in patients with nonrheumatic atrial fibrillation. N Engl J Med 1991;325:130 (letter)

178. Singer DE, Hughes RA, Gress DR et al: The effect of low-dose warfarin on the risk of stroke in patients with nonrheumatic atrial fibrillation. N Engl J Med 1991;325:131 (reply to letter)

179. Iung B, Garbarz E, Doutreland L et al: Late results of percutaneous mitral commissurotomy for calcific mitral stenosis. Am J Cardiol 2000;85:1308–1314

180. Enriquez-Sarano M, Freeman WK, Tribouilloy CM et al: Functional anatomy of mitral regurgitation: accuracy and outcome implications of transesophageal echocardiography. J Am Coll Cardiol 1999;34:1129–1136

181. Corin WJ, Murakami T, Monrad ES et al: Left ventricular passive diastolic properties in chronic mitral regurgitation. Circulation 1991;83:797–807

182. Stone GW, Griffin B, Shah PK et al: Prevalence of unsuspected mitral regurgitation and left ventricular diastolic dysfunction in patients with coronary artery disease and acute pulmonary edema associated with normal or depressed left ventricular systolic function. Am J Cardiol 1991;67:37–41

183. Tresch DD, Doyle TP, Boncheck LI et al: Mitral valve prolapse requiring surgery. Am J Med 1985;78:245–250

184. Levine HJ, Gaasch WH: Vasoactive drugs in chronic regurgitant lesions of the mitral and aortic valves. J Am Coll Cardiol 1996;28:1083–1091

185. Tribouilloy CM, Enriquez-Sarano M, Schaff HV et al: Impact of preoperative symptoms on survival after surgical correction of organic mitral regurgitation: rationale for optimizing surgical indications. Circulation 1999;99:400–405

Chapter 37

Cardiac arrhythmias

Wilbert S. Aronow

VENTRICULAR ARRHYTHMIAS

The presence of three or more consecutive ventricular premature complexes (VPCs) on an electrocardiogram (ECG) is diagnosed as ventricular tachycardia (VT).[1,2] VT is considered sustained if it lasts at least 30 seconds and nonsustained if it lasts less than 30 seconds.[2] Complex ventricular arrhythmias (VAs) include VT or paired, multiform, or frequent VPCs. This author considers frequent VPCs to be an average of at least 30/hour on a 24-hour ambulatory ECG or at least 6/minute on a 1-minute rhythm strip of an ECG.[2,3] Simple VAs include infrequent VPCs and no complex forms.

The prevalence of nonsustained VT diagnosed by 24-hour ambulatory ECGs in older persons without cardiovascular disease has been reported as 4 percent,[1,4,5] 2 percent,[6] and 4 percent in 729 elderly women and 13 percent in 643 elderly men in the Cardiovascular Health Study.[7] The prevalence was 9 percent in elderly persons with hypertension, valvular heart disease, or cardiomyopathies and 16 percent in elderly persons with coronary artery disease (CAD).[5]

The prevalence of complex VAs in elderly persons without cardiovascular disease has been reported as 50 percent,[1] 31 percent,[4] 30 percent,[5] 20 percent,[6] 16 percent in women and 28 percent in men,[7] and 33 percent.[3] The prevalence was 55 percent in elderly persons with hypertension, valvular heart disease, or cardiomyopathies,[5] 68 percent in elderly persons with CAD,[5] and 55 percent in 843 elderly persons with heart disease.[3] Complex VAs were present on a 1-minute strip of an ECG in 2 percent of 104 elderly persons without cardiovascular disease and in 4 percent of 843 elderly persons with cardiovascular disease.[3] In elderly persons with cardiovascular disease, there is a higher prevalence of VT and of complex VAs in those who have an abnormal left ventricular (LV) ejection fraction,[8] echocardiographic LV hypertrophy,[9] or silent myocardial ischemia.[10]

Prognosis of ventricular arrhythmias

Those with no heart disease Nonsustained VT or complex VAs diagnosed by 24-hour ambulatory ECGs[5,11,12] or by 12-lead ECGs with 1-minute rhythm strips[3] in elderly persons with no clinical evidence of heart disease were not associated with an increased incidence of new coronary events. Exercise-induced nonsustained VT[13] or complex VAs,[14] in elderly persons with no clinical evidence of heart disease, also were not associated with an increased incidence of new coronary events. Therefore, asymptomatic nonsustained VAs or complex VAs in elderly persons without heart disease should *not* be treated with antiarrhythmic drugs.

Those with heart disease In elderly persons with heart disease, nonsustained VT[5,10,12] or complex VAs[3,5,10,12] increased the incidence of new coronary events. At 2-year follow-up of 391 elderly persons with heart disease, the incidence of new coronary events was increased 6.8 times in elderly persons with VT plus an abnormal LV ejection fraction, and 7.6 times in elderly persons with complex VAs plus an abnormal LV ejection fraction.[5] At 27-month follow-up of 468 elderly persons with heart disease, the incidence of primary ventricular fibrillation or sudden cardiac death was increased 7.1 times in elderly persons with VT plus echocardiographic LV hypertrophy, and 7.3 times in persons with complex VAs plus echocardiographic LV hypertrophy.[12] At 37-month follow-up of 404 elderly persons with heart disease, the incidence of new coronary events was increased 2.5 times in elderly persons with VT plus silent ischemia, and 4.0 times in elderly persons with complex VAs plus silent ischemia.[10]

General therapy for ventricular arrhythmias

Underlying causes of complex VAs should be treated when possible. Treatment of congestive heart failure (CHF), LV dysfunction, digitalis toxicity, hypokalemia, hypomagnesemia, myocardial ischemia (by anti-ischemic drugs such as β-blockers or by coronary revascularization), hypertension, LV hypertrophy, hypoxia, and other conditions may abolish or reduce complex VAs. The person should not smoke or drink alcohol and should avoid drugs that may cause or increase a complex VA.

All elderly persons with CAD should be treated with aspirin[15–17] and with β-blockers[17–21] unless there are contraindications to these drugs. Elderly persons who have, after myocardial infarction (MI), congestive heart failure, an anterior MI, or an LV ejection fraction ≤40 percent should be treated with angiotensin-converting enzyme (ACE) inhibitors unless there are contraindications.[17,22–25] Elderly persons with CAD with serum low-density lipoprotein cholesterol levels ≥125 mg/dL should be treated with 3-hydroxy-3-methylglutaryl coenzyme A reductase inhibitors.[17,26–28]

Class I antiarrhythmic drugs are more proarrhythmic than class III. Except for β-blockers, all antiarrhythmic drugs can cause torsades de pointes VT (polymorphous appearance associated with prolonged QT interval).

CLASS I ANTIARRHYTHMIC DRUGS These are sodium-channel blockers. Class Ia have intermediate channel kinetics and prolong repolarization; these drugs include disopyramide, procainamide, and quinidine. Class Ib have rapid channel kinetics and shorten repolarization slightly; these drugs include lidocaine, mexiletine, phenytoin, and tocainide. Class Ic have slow channel kinetics and have little effect on repolarization; these drugs include encainide, flecainide, lorcainide,

Table 37-1 Effect of class I antiarrhythmic drugs on mortality in persons with heart disease and complex ventricular arrhythmias

Study	Results
International Mexiletine and Placebo Antiarrhythmic Coronary Trial[29]	At 1-year follow-up, mortality was 7.6% for mexiletine and 4.8% for placebo.
Cardiac Arrhythmia Suppression Trial I[30,31]	At 10-month follow-up, mortality for arrhythmia or cardiac arrest was 4.5% for encainide or flecainide versus 1.2% for placebo. Mortality was 7.7% for encainide or flecainide versus 3.0% for placebo. Adverse events including death were more frequent in elderly persons taking encainide or flecainide.
Cardiac Arrhythmia Suppression Trial II[31,32]	At 18-month follow-up, mortality for arrhythmia or cardiac arrest was 8.4% for moricizine versus 7.3% for placebo. Two-year survival rate was 81.7% for moricizine versus 85.6% for placebo. Adverse events including death were more frequent in elderly persons taking moricizine
Aronow et al.[33]	At 2-year follow-up, mortality was 65% for quinidine or procainamide versus 63% for no antiarrhythmic drug. Quinidine or procainamide did not reduce sudden death, total cardiac death, or total mortality in elderly persons with ischemic or nonischemic heart disease, abnormal or normal LV ejection fraction, and presence or absence of VT.
Moosvi et al.[34]	Two-year sudden death survival was 69% for quinidine, 69% for procainamide, and 89% for no antiarrhythmic drug. Two-year total survival was 61% for quinidine, 57% for procainamide, and 71% for no antiarrhythmic drug.
Hallstrom et al.[35]	At 108-month follow-up, the adjusted relative risk of death or recurrent cardiac arrest on quinidine or procainamide versus no antiarrhythmic drug was 1.17.

Abbreviations: LV, left ventricular; VT, ventricular tachycardia.

moricizine, and propafenone. None of the class I antiarrhythmic drugs has been demonstrated in controlled, clinical trials to decrease sudden cardiac death, total cardiac death, or total mortality.

Table 37-1 shows the effect of class I drugs on mortality in persons with heart disease and complex VA. A meta-analysis of six double-blind studies of persons with chronic atrial fibrillation (AF) who underwent direct-current cardioversion to sinus rhythm showed that the mortality at 1 year was higher in those treated with quinidine (2.9 percent) than in those treated with placebo (0.8 percent).[36]

Of 1330 patients in the Stroke Prevention in Atrial Fibrillation Study, 127 were treated with quinidine, 57 with procainamide, 34 with flecainide, 20 with encainide, and 7 with amiodarone.[37] The adjusted relative risk of cardiac mortality was 1.8 times increased and the adjusted relative risk of arrhythmic death was 2.1 times increased in persons receiving antiarrhythmic drugs versus no antiarrhythmic drugs. In persons with a history of CHF, the adjusted relative risk of cardiac death was 3.3 times increased and the adjusted relative risk of arrhythmic death was 5.8 times increased in those taking antiarrhythmic drugs versus no antiarrhythmic drugs.

An analysis was made of 59 randomized, controlled clinical trials including 23,229 patients that investigated the use of class I antiarrhythmic drugs after MI.[38] The drugs included aprindine, disopyramide, encainide, flecainide, imipramine, lidocaine, mexiletine, moricizine, phenytoin, procainamide, quinidine, and tocainide. Mortality was increased in persons receiving class I drugs compared with those not receiving an antiarrhythmic drug (odds ratio = 1.14). None of the 59 studies showed that the use of a class I antiarrhythmic drug decreased mortality in persons after MI.

On the basis of the available data, none of the class I antiarrhythmic drugs should be used to treat VT or complex VA in elderly or younger persons with heart disease.

CALCIUM-CHANNEL BLOCKERS These are not useful in the therapy of complex VAs. Although verapamil can terminate a left septal VT, hemodynamic collapse can occur if intravenous verapamil is given to persons with the more common forms of VT. An analysis was made of randomized, controlled clinical trials including 20,342 patients that investigated the use of calcium-channel blockers after MI.[38] Mortality was insignificantly increased in persons receiving calcium-channel blockers compared with those not receiving an antiarrhythmic drug (odds ratio = 1.04).

On the basis of the available data, none of the calcium-channel blockers should be used to treat VT or complex VAs in elderly or younger persons with heart disease.

BETA-BLOCKERS An analysis of 55 randomized, controlled clinical trials including 53,268 persons that investigated the use of β-blockers after MI showed that mortality was decreased in those receiving β-blockers versus placebo (odds ratio = 0.81).[38] Beta-blockers caused a greater decrease in mortality in older persons than in younger persons.[18–21,39] Table 37-2 indicates the effect of β-blockers on mortality in persons with heart disease and a complex VA.

The decrease in mortality by β-blockers in elderly persons with heart disease and a complex VA is due more to an anti-ischemic effect than to an antiarrhythmic effect.[45] Beta-blockers also abolish the circadian distribution of sudden cardiac death or fatal MI,[46] markedly decrease the circadian variation of complex VAs,[47] and abolish the circadian variation of myocardial ischemia.[48]

Table 37-2 Effect of β-blockers on mortality in persons with heart disease and complex ventricular arrhythmias

Study	Results
Hallstrom et al.[35]	At 108-month follow-up, the adjusted relative risk of death or recurrent cardiac arrest for β-blockers versus no antiarrhythmic drug was 0.62.
Beta Blocker Heart Attack Trial[39–41]	At 25-month follow-up, propranolol reduced sudden cardiac death by 28% in persons with complex VA and by 16% in persons without VA. Propranolol decreased total mortality by 34% in persons aged 60–69 years.
Norwegian Propranolol Study[42]	High-risk survivors of acute MI treated with propranolol for 1 year had a 52% decrease in sudden cardiac death.
Aronow et al.[43]	At 29-month follow-up, compared with no antiarrhythmic drug, propranolol caused a 47% reduction in sudden cardiac death, a 37% decrease in total cardiac death, and a 20% borderline significant decrease in total death.
Cardiac Arrhythmia Suppression Trial[44]	Persons on β-blockers had a reduction in all-cause mortality of 43% at 30 days, of 46% at 1 year, and of 33% at 2 years; and a decrease in arrhythmic death or cardiac arrest of 66% at 30 days, of 53% at 1 year, and of 36% at 2 years. Beta-blockers were an independent factor for reduced arrhythmic death or cardiac arrest by 40% and for decreased all-cause mortality by 33%.

Abbreviations: VA, ventricular arrhythmias; MI, myocardial infarction.

Table 37-3 Effect of class III antiarrhythmic drugs on mortality in persons with heart disease

Study	Results
Julien et al.[53]	At 1-year follow-up, mortality was not different in persons after MI on d,1-sotalol versus placebo.
Waldo et al.[54]	At 148-day follow-up, mortality in persons after MI was increased by d-sotalol (5.0%) versus placebo (3.1%).
Singh et al.[55]	At 2-year follow-up of persons with CHF and complex VA, survival was not different for amiodarone versus placebo.
Canadian Amiodarone MI Arrhythmia Trial[56]	At 1.8-year follow-up of persons after MI with complex VA, mortality was not different for amiodarone versus placebo.
European MI Amiodarone Trial[57]	At 21-month follow-up of persons after MI, mortality was not different for amiodarone (13.9%) versus placebo (13.7%).

Abbreviations: MI, myocardial infarction; CHF, congestive heart failure; VA, ventricular arrhythmias.

On the basis of the available data, β-blockers should be used to treat older and younger persons with heart disease and a complex VA if there are no contraindications.

ANGIOTENSIN-CONVERTING ENZYME INHIBITORS ACE inhibitors have been demonstrated to reduce sudden cardiac death in some studies of persons with CHF.[25,49] ACE inhibitors should be used to reduce total mortality in older and younger persons with CHF,[23,25,49,50] an anterior MI,[24] and a LV ejection fraction ≤40 percent after MI.[22,25] ACE inhibitors should be administered to treat elderly and younger persons with CHF with abnormal LV ejection fraction[23,25,49,50] or with normal LV ejection fraction.[51,52]

On the basis of the available data, ACE inhibitors should be used to treat older and younger persons with VT or a complex VA associated with CHF, an anterior MI, or a LV ejection fraction ≤40 percent after MI if there are no contraindications. Beta-blockers should be administered in addition to ACE inhibitors in treating these patients.

CLASS III ANTIARRHYTHMIC DRUGS These are potassium-channel blockers which prolong repolarization manifested by an increase in QT interval on the ECG. The drugs are effective in suppressing complex VAs, including nonsustained VT, by increasing the refractory period. However, antiarrhythmic aggravation can occur, especially torsades des pointes.

Table 37-3 shows the effect of class III antiarrhythmic drugs on mortality in persons with heart disease. None of the class III drugs has been found in a double-blind, randomized, placebo-controlled clinical trial to decrease mortality in persons with heart disease and a complex VA.

In 23 of 481 persons with VT (5 percent), oral sotalol caused torsades de pointes (12 cases) or an increase in VT episodes (11 cases).[58] On the basis of the available data, β-blockers are preferred to the use of d,1-sotalol in treating elderly and younger persons with heart disease and VT or a complex VA.

Amiodarone is very effective in suppressing VT and complex VAs associated with heart disease.[55,56,59] However, the incidence of adverse effects from amiodarone approaches 90 percent after 5 years of therapy.[60] In the Cardiac Arrest in Seattle study,[59] the incidence of pulmonary toxicity was 10 percent at 2 years in persons receiving 158 mg of amiodarone daily. Amiodarone can also cause hyperthyroidism or hypothyroidism, as well as cardiac, dermatological, gastrointestinal, hepatic, neurological, and ophthalmological adverse effects.

Because amiodarone has not been demonstrated to reduce mortality in elderly or younger persons with VT or a complex VA associated with prior MI or CHF, and has a very high incidence of toxicity, β-blockers are preferred in treating these persons. There are also data suggesting that persons receiving amiodarone plus a β-blocker had a better survival than persons receiving amiodarone.[61]

Invasive interventions

If a person has life-threatening VT or ventricular fibrillation resistant to antiarrhythmic drugs, invasive intervention should be performed. Persons with critical CAD and severe myocardial ischemia should undergo coronary artery bypass graft surgery to reduce mortality.[62]

Surgical ablation of the arrhythmogenic focus in a person with life-threatening ventricular tachyarrhythmias can be curative. This treatment includes aneurysmectomy or infarctectomy and endocardial resection with or without adjunctive cryoablation based on activation mapping in the operating room.[63–65] However, the perioperative mortality rate is high. Endoaneurysmorrhaphy with a pericardial patch combined with mapping-guided subendocardial resection frequently cures recurrent VT with a low operative mortality and improvement of LV systolic function.[66] Radiofrequency catheter ablation of VT has also been beneficial in the management of selected patients with arrhythmogenic foci of monomorphic VT.[67,68]

AUTOMATIC IMPLANTABLE CARDIOVERTER–DEFIBRILLATOR (AICD)
The AICD is the most effective treatment for persons with life-threatening VT or ventricular fibrillation. Table 37-4 indicates the effect of the AICD on mortality in persons with ventricular tachyarrhythmias. Tresch et al.[64,65] showed in retrospective studies that the AICD was very effective in treating life-threatening VT in elderly as well as in younger persons. The Canadian Implantable Defibrillator Study found that persons most likely to benefit from an AICD were those with at least two of the following factors: age at least 70 years, LV ejection fraction no more than 35 percent, and New York Heart Association function class III or IV.[75]

At 26-month follow-up, survival was 91 percent for persons treated with metoprolol plus an AICD versus 83 percent for those treated with sotalol plus an AICD.[76] These data favor using a β-blocker in persons with an AICD needing antiarrhythmic drug therapy. An observational study in 78 persons with CAD and life-threatening VA treated with an AICD showed at 490-day follow-up that the use of lipid-lowering drugs reduced recurrences of life-threatening VA.[77] These data require confirmation in a prospective randomized study.

The ACC/AHA guidelines recommend that class I indications for treatment with an AICD are (1) cardiac arrest due to VT or ventricular fibrillation not caused by a transient or reversible cause; (2) spontaneous sustained VT; (3) syncope of undetermined origin with clinically relevant, hemodynamically significant sustained VT or ventricular fibrillation induced at electrophysiological study when drug therapy is ineffective, not tolerated, or not preferred; and (4) nonsustained VT with CAD, prior MI, LV systolic dysfunction, and inducible ventricular fibrillation or sustained VT at electrophysiological study that is not suppressed by a class I antiarrhythmic drug.[78]

ATRIAL FIBRILLATION

Atrial fibrillation (AF) is the most common sustained cardiac arrhythmia. The prevalence of AF increases with age.[79–82] The prevalence of AF in 2101 persons, mean age 81 years, was 5 percent in persons aged 60–70 years, 13 percent in those aged 71–90 years, and 22 percent in those aged 91–103 years.[80] Chronic AF was present in 16 percent of elderly men and in 13 percent of elderly women.[80] The prevalence of chronic AF in a study of 1563 persons, mean age 80 years, living in the community and seen in an academic geriatrics practice was 9 percent.[82]

AF may be paroxysmal or chronic. Episodes of paroxysmal AF may last from a few seconds to several weeks. Spontaneous conversion of paroxysmal AF to sinus rhythm occurs in 68 percent of persons presenting with AF of less than 72 hours duration.[83]

Table 37-4 Effect of the automatic implantable cardioverter–defibrillator on mortality in persons with ventricular tachyarrhythmias

Study	Results
Multicenter Automatic Defibrillator Implantation Trial[69]	At 27-month follow-up, the AICD caused a 54% reduction in mortality.
Antiarrhythmics Versus Implantable Defibrillators Trial[70]	Compared with drug therapy, the AICD caused a 39% decrease in mortality at 1 year, a 27% reduction in mortality at 2 years, and a 31% decrease in mortality at 3 years.
Canadian Implantable Defibrillator Study[71]	Compared with amiodarone, at 3 years, total mortality rate was insignificantly decreased by 20% and the arrhythmic mortality was insignificantly reduced by 33%.
Hamburg Cardiac Arrest Study[72]	Propafenone was stopped at 11 months because mortality from sudden death and cardiac arrest recurrence was 23% for propafenone versus 0% for an AICD.
Hamburg Cardiac Arrest Study[73]	Compared with amiodarone or metoprolol, the 2-year mortality was decreased 37% by an AICD.
Multicenter Unsustained Tachycardia Trial[74]	Compared with electrophysiological guided antiarrhythmic drug therapy, the 5-year total mortality was borderline significantly decreased 20% by an AICD and the 5-year risk of cardiac arrest or death from arrhythmia was decreased 76% by an AICD.

Predisposing factors for AF

Factors predisposing to AF include alcohol, atrial myxoma, atrial septal defect, cardiomyopathies, chronic lung disease, conduction system disease, CHF, CAD, diabetes mellitus, drugs, emotional stress, excessive coffee, hypertension, hyperthyroidism, hypoglycemia, hypokalemia, hypovolemia, hypoxia, myocarditis, neoplastic disease, pericarditis, pneumonia, postoperative state, pulmonary embolism, systemic infection, and valvular heart disease. Table 37-5 lists the increased prevalence of echocardiographic findings in 254 older persons with chronic AF compared with 1445 older persons with sinus rhythm, mean age 81 years.[84] In the Framingham Heart Study, low serum thyrotropin levels were independently associated with a 3.1 times increase in the development of new AF in elderly persons.[85]

Associated risks of AF

The Framingham study showed that the incidence of death from cardiovascular causes was 2.0 times higher in men and 2.7 times higher in women with chronic AF than in men and women with sinus rhythm.[86] The study also demonstrated that after adjustment for pre-existing cardiovascular conditions, the odds ratio for mortality in persons with AF was 1.5 in men and 1.9 in women.[87] At 42-month follow-up of 1359 persons, mean age 81 years, with heart disease, persons with AF had a 2.2 times higher probability of developing new coronary events than those with sinus rhythm after controlling for other prognostic variables.[88]

In 106,780 Medicare beneficiaries at least 65 years of age from the Cooperative Cardiovascular Project treated for acute MI, AF was present in 22 percent.[89] Compared with sinus rhythm, elderly persons with AF had a higher in-hospital mortality (25 percent versus 16 percent), 30-day mortality (29 percent versus 19 percent), and 1-year mortality (48 percent versus 33 percent). AF was an independent predictor of in-hospital mortality (odds ratio = 1.2), 30-day mortality (odds ratio = 1.2), and 1-year mortality (odds ratio = 1.3). Elderly persons developing AF during hospitalization had a worse prognosis than those who presented with AF.

AF is an independent risk factor for thromboembolic (TE) stroke, especially in older persons.[79,80] In the Framingham study, the relative risk of stroke in persons with nonrheumatic AF compared with persons in sinus rhythm was 2.6 times higher in those aged 60–69 years, 3.3 times higher in those aged 70–79 years, and 4.5 times higher in those aged 80–89 years.[79]

AF was present in 313 of 2384 persons (13 percent), mean age 81 years.[90] AF was also present in 201 of 1024 persons (17 percent) with LV hypertrophy and in 112 of 1360 (8 percent) without LV hypertrophy. At 44-month follow-up, both AF (risk ratio = 3.2) and LV hypertrophy (risk ratio = 2.8) were independent risk factors for new TE stroke. The higher prevalence of LV hypertrophy in elderly persons with chronic AF contributes to the higher incidence of TE stroke.

At 45-month follow-up of 1846 persons, mean age 81 years, both AF (risk ratio = 3.3) and 40–100 percent extracranial carotid arterial disease (ECAD; risk ratio = 2.5) were independent risk factors for new TE stroke.[91] Elderly persons with both chronic AF and 40–100 percent ECAD had a 6.9 times higher probability of developing new TE stroke than those with sinus rhythm and no significant ECAD.[91]

Symptomatic cerebral infarctions were present in 22 percent of 54 autopsied patients aged 70 years or older with paroxysmal AF.[92] Symptomatic cerebral infarction was 2.4 times more common in older persons with paroxysmal AF than in older persons with sinus rhythm.[92] AF also causes silent cerebral infarction.[93]

AF is a predisposing factor for CHF in older persons. As much as 30–40 percent of LV end-diastolic volume may be attributable to left atrial contraction in older persons. Absence of a coordinated left atrial contraction decreases late diastolic filling of the LV because of loss of the atrial kick. A fast ventricular rate associated with AF also shortens the diastolic filling period, which further decreases LV filling.

A retrospective analysis of the Studies of Left Ventricular Dysfunction Prevention and Treatment Trials found that AF was an independent risk factor for all-cause mortality (risk ratio = 1.3), progressive pump failure death (risk ratio = 1.4), and death or hospitalization for CHF (risk ratio = 1.3).[94]

AF was present in 132 of 355 persons (37 percent), mean age 80 years, with prior MI, CHF, and an abnormal LV ejection fraction.[95] AF was also present in 98 of 296 (33 percent), mean age 82 years, with prior MI, CHF, and a normal LV ejection fraction. In this study, AF was an independent risk factor for mortality with a risk ratio of 1.5.

A fast ventricular rate associated with chronic or paroxysmal AF may cause a tachycardia-related cardiomyopathy, which may be an unrecognized curable cause of CHF.[96,97] Control of a fast ventricular rate by radiofrequency ablation of the atrioventricular (AV) node with permanent pacing caused an improvement in LV ejection fraction in persons with medically refractory AF.[98]

Clinical symptoms and diagnostic tests for AF

Elderly people with AF may be symptomatic or asymptomatic with their arrhythmia detected by physical examination or by an ECG. Examination of a person after a stroke may lead to the diagnosis of AF. Symptoms may include palpitations, skips in heartbeat, fatigue on exertion, exercise intolerance, cough, dizziness, chest pain, and syncope. A fast ventricular rate associated

---

Table 37-5 Echocardiographic findings in 254 persons with chronic atrial fibrillation and 1445 persons with sinus rhythm, mean age 81 years

Variable	Higher prevalence in atrial fibrillation
Rheumatic mitral stenosis	17.1 times
Left atrial enlargement	2.9 times
Abnormal LV ejection fraction	2.5 times
Aortic stenosis	2.3 times
≥1+ mitral regurgitation	2.2 times
≥1+ aortic regurgitation	2.1 times
LV hypertrophy	2.0 times
Mitral annular calcium	1.7 times

Abbreviation: LV, left ventricular.
Source: Adapted from Aronow et al. (1995),[84] with permission.

with loss of atrial contraction reduces cardiac output and may cause hypotension, angina pectoris, CHF, acute pulmonary edema, and syncope, especially in elderly persons with mitral stenosis, aortic stenosis, or hypertrophic cardiomyopathy.

When AF is suspected, a 12-lead ECG with a 1-minute rhythm strip should be obtained to confirm the diagnosis. If paroxysmal AF is suspected, a 24-hour ambulatory ECG should be obtained. All persons with AF should have an M-mode, two-dimensional, and Doppler echocardiogram to determine the presence and severity of cardiac abnormalities causing AF and to identify risk factors for stroke. Appropriate tests for non-cardiac causes of AF should be performed when clinically indicated. Thyroid function tests should be performed as AF or CHF may be the only clinical manifestations of apathetic hyperthyroidism in elderly people.

General treatment measures

Along with drug therapy, treatment of AF should include therapy of the underlying disorder (such as hyperthyroidism, pneumonia, or pulmonary embolism) when possible. Candidates for mitral valve replacement should undergo surgery if it is clinically indicated. If mitral valve replacement is not performed in those with significant mitral valve disease, elective cardioversion should not be performed in persons with AF. Precipitating factors such as CHF, hypoxia, hypokalemia, hypoglycemia, hypovolemia, and infection should be treated immediately. Alcohol, coffee, and drugs (especially sympathomimetics) that precipitate AF should be avoided. Paroxysmal AF associated with the tachycardia–bradycardia (sick-sinus) syndrome should be treated with permanent pacing in combination with the use of drugs to slow a fast ventricular rate associated with AF.[99]

Control of a very rapid ventricular rate

Immediate direct-current cardioversion should be performed in persons who have paroxysmal AF with a very fast ventricular rate associated with an acute MI, chest pain caused by myocardial ischemia, hypotension, severe CHF, or syncope. Intravenous verapamil,[100] diltiazem,[101] or β-blockers[102–105] may be used to immediately slow a very fast ventricular rate associated with AF.

> ### Indications for emergency cardioversion
>
> - Acute myocardial infarction.
> - Chest pain caused by myocardial ischemia.
> - Hypotension.
> - Severe congestive heart failure.
> - Syncope.

Control of a fast ventricular rate

Digitalis glycosides are ineffective in converting AF to sinus rhythm.[106] Digoxin is also ineffective in slowing a fast ventricular rate associated with AF if there is associated hyperthyroidism, fever, hypoxia, acute blood loss, or any condition involving increased sympathetic tone.[107] However, digoxin should be used for slowing a fast ventricular rate in AF unassociated with increased sympathetic tone, the Wolff–Parkinson–White syndrome, or hypertrophic obstructive cardiomyopathy, especially if there is LV systolic dysfunction. The usual maintenance oral dose of digoxin administered to persons with AF is 0.25–0.5 mg daily, with the dose decreased to 0.125–0.25 mg daily for elderly persons who are more susceptible to digitalis toxicity.[108]

Oral verapamil,[109] diltiazem,[110] or a β-blocker[111] should be added to the therapeutic regimen if a fast ventricular rate associated with AF occurs at rest or during exercise despite digoxin. These drugs act synergistically with digoxin to depress conduction through the AV junction. In a study of digoxin 0.25 mg daily, diltiazem-CD 240 mg daily, atenolol 50 mg daily, digoxin 0.25 mg plus diltiazem-CD 240 mg daily, and digoxin 0.25 mg plus atenolol 50 mg daily, digoxin and diltiazem as single drugs were least effective and digoxin plus atenolol was most effective in controlling ventricular rate in AF during daily activity.[112]

Amiodarone is the most effective drug for slowing a fast ventricular rate associated with AF.[113,114] However, its adverse effect profile limits its use in the treatment of AF. Oral doses of 200–400 mg daily may be administered to selected persons with symptomatic life-threatening AF refractory to other drug therapy.

Therapeutic concentrations of digoxin do not decrease the frequency of episodes of paroxysmal AF or the duration of episodes of paroxysmal AF detected by 24-hour ambulatory ECGs.[115,116] In fact, digoxin has been demonstrated to increase the duration of episodes of paroxysmal AF, a result consistent with its action in reducing the atrial refractory period.[115] Therapeutic concentrations of digoxin also do not prevent a rapid ventricular rate from developing in persons with paroxysmal AF.[115–117] Therefore, digoxin should be avoided in persons with sinus rhythm with a history of paroxysmal AF.

Nondrug therapies

Radiofrequency catheter modification of AV conduction should be performed in persons with symptomatic AF in whom a fast ventricular rate cannot be slowed by drug therapy.[118,119] If this procedure does not control the fast ventricular rate associated with AF, complete AV block produced by radiofrequency catheter ablation followed by permanent pacemaker implantation should be performed.[120] In persons with CHF and chronic AF, AV junction ablation with implantation of a VVIR pacemaker was superior to drug therapy in controlling symptoms in a randomized, controlled study of 66 persons.[121] Surgical techniques have also been developed for use in persons with AF in whom the rapid ventricular rate cannot be slowed by drug treatment.[122,123] Appropriate indications for using an implantable Atrioverter in the treatment of AF need further investigation.[124]

Tachycardia–bradycardia syndrome

Paroxysmal AF associated with the tachycardia–bradycardia (sick-sinus) syndrome should be treated with a permanent pacemaker in combination with drugs to decrease a rapid ventricular rate associated with AF.[99] Ventricular pacing is an independent risk factor for the development of chronic AF in persons with paroxysmal AF associated with the syndrome.[125] Persons with paroxysmal AF associated with the syndrome and no signs of AV conduction abnormalities should be treated with atrial pacing or dual-chamber pacing rather than with ventricular pacing, because atrial pacing is associated with less AF, fewer TE complications, and a lower risk of AV block than is ventricular pacing.[126]

Wolff–Parkinson–White syndrome

Direct-current cardioversion should be performed if a fast ventricular rate in paroxysmal AF associated with the Wolff–Parkinson–White syndrome is life-threatening or fails to respond to drugs. Drug treatment for paroxysmal AF associated with the syndrome includes propranolol plus procainamide, disopyramide, or quinidine.[127] Digoxin, verapamil, and diltiazem are contraindicated in persons with AF associated with the syndrome because these drugs shorten the refractory period of the accessory AV pathway, causing faster conduction down the accessory pathway. This results in a marked increase in ventricular rate. Radiofrequency catheter ablation or surgical ablation of the accessory pathway should be considered in persons with AF and fast AV conduction over the accessory pathway.[128]

Slow ventricular rate

Many elderly persons are able to tolerate AF without the need for treatment because the ventricular rate is slowed as a result of concomitant AV nodal disease. These persons should not be treated with a drug that depresses AV conduction. A permanent pacemaker should be implanted in those with AF who develop cerebral symptoms such as dizziness or syncope associated with ventricular pauses >3 seconds that are not drug-induced, as documented by a 24-hour ambulatory ECG. If persons with AF have drug-induced symptomatic bradycardia and the causative drug cannot be discontinued, a permanent pacemaker must be implanted.

Elective cardioversion

Elective direct-current cardioversion has a higher success rate of converting AF to sinus rhythm than does medical cardioversion.[129] Unfavorable conditions for this elective cardioversion include duration of AF >1 year, moderate-to-severe cardiomegaly, echocardiographic left atrial dimension >45 mm, digitalis toxicity (contraindication), slow ventricular rate (contraindication), sick-sinus syndrome (contraindication), mitral valve disease, CHF, chronic obstructive lung disease, recurrent AF despite antiarrhythmic drugs, and inability to tolerate antiarrhythmic drugs. Elective cardioversion of AF either by direct current or by antiarrhythmic drugs should not be performed in asymptomatic elderly persons with chronic AF.

Antiarrhythmic drugs that have been used to convert AF to sinus rhythm include amiodarone, disopyramide, dofetilide, encainide, flecainide, ibutilide, procainamide, propafenone, quinidine, and sotalol. None of these are as successful as direct-current cardioversion (which is 80–90 percent successful) in converting AF to sinus rhythm. All of these drugs are proarrhythmic and may aggravate or cause cardiac arrhythmias.

Encainide and flecainide caused atrial proarrhythmic effects in 6 of 60 persons (10 percent).[130] The proarrhythmic effects included conversion of AF to atrial flutter with a 1-to-1 AV conduction response and a very fast ventricular rate.[130]

Flecainide has induced VT and ventricular fibrillation in persons with chronic AF.[131] Antiarrhythmic drugs including amiodarone, disopyramide, flecainide, procainamide, propafenone, quinidine, and sotalol caused cardiac adverse effects in 73 of 417 patients (18 percent) hospitalized for AF.[132] Class Ic drugs such as encainide, flecainide, and propafenone should be avoided in persons with prior MI or LV systolic dysfunction because these drugs may cause life-threatening ventricular tachyarrhythmias.[30]

Ibutilide and dofetilide are class III antiarrhythmic drugs that have recently been used to try to convert AF to sinus rhythm. Twenty-three of 79 persons (29 percent) with AF treated with intravenous ibutilide converted to sinus rhythm.[133] Polymorphic ventricular tachycardia developed in 4 percent taking ibutilide in this study. All of these people had abnormal LV systolic function. Eleven of 75 persons (15 percent) with AF treated with intravenous dofetilide converted to sinus rhythm.[134] Torsades de pointes occurred in 3 percent treated with intravenous dofetilide.[135] After 1 month, 22 of 190 patients (12 percent) with CHF and AF had sinus rhythm restored with dofetilide compared with 3 of 201 patients (1 percent) treated with placebo.[135] Torsades de pointes developed in 25 patients (3 percent) treated with dofetilide and in none of the patients treated with placebo.[135] Although direct-current cardioversion of AF has a higher success rate in converting AF to sinus rhythm and a lower incidence of cardiac adverse effects than any antiarrhythmic drug, pretreatment with ibutilide has been shown to facilitate transthoracic cardioversion of AF.[136]

Unless transesophageal echocardiography has shown no thrombus in the left atrial appendage before cardioversion,[137] oral warfarin therapy should be administered for 3 weeks before elective direct-current cardioversion or drug cardioversion.[138] Anticoagulant therapy should be administered at the time of cardioversion and continued until sinus rhythm has been maintained for 4 weeks.[138] The left atrium becomes stunned and contracts poorly for 3–4 weeks, predisposing to TE stroke unless the patient is receiving oral warfarin.[139,140] The maintenance dose of oral warfarin should be titrated by serial prothrombin times so that the INR is 2.0–3.0.[138] A controlled, randomized, prospective clinical trial is needed to compare conventional anticoagulant treatment prior to cardioversion of AF with a transesophageal echocardiography-guided strategy.[141]

USE OF ANTIARRHYTHMIC DRUGS TO MAINTAIN SINUS RHYTHM The efficacy and safety of antiarrhythmic drugs after cardioversion has been questioned. It is unknown whether persons cardioverted from AF to sinus rhythm will have a decreased incidence of subsequent TE stroke. A meta-analysis of six double-blind, placebo-controlled studies of quinidine involving 808 persons who had direct-current cardioversion of chronic AF to sinus rhythm found that 50 percent receiving quinidine and 25 percent receiving placebo were in sinus rhythm at 1 year.[36] However, the mortality was higher in those treated with quinidine (2.9 percent) than in those receiving a placebo (0.8 percent).

In a study of 406 persons, mean age 82 years, with heart disease and complex VA, the incidence of adverse effects causing drug cessation was 48 percent for quinidine and 55 percent for procainamide.[142] The incidence of total mortality at 2-year follow-up was insignificantly higher in persons receiving quinidine or procainamide than in those not receiving an antiarrhythmic drug.

In another study, 98 persons were randomized to sotalol and 85 persons to quinidine after direct-current cardioversion of AF to sinus rhythm.[143] At 6-month follow-up, 52 percent of sotalol-treated persons and 48 percent of quinidine-treated persons were in sinus rhythm.

At 1-year follow-up of persons with AF cardioverted to sinus rhythm, 30 percent of 50 persons randomized to propafenone and 37 percent of 50 persons randomized to sotalol remained in sinus rhythm.[144]

Of 1330 persons in the Stroke Prevention in Atrial Fibrillation (SPAF) study, 127 persons were receiving quinidine, 57 procainamide, 34 flecainide, 20 encainide, 15 disopyramide, and 7 amiodarone.[37] Patients taking an antiarrhythmic drug had a 2.7 times increased adjusted relative risk of cardiac mortality and a 2.3 times increased adjusted relative risk of arrhythmic death compared with persons not taking an antiarrhythmic drug. Persons with a history of CHF taking an antiarrhythmic drug had a 4.7 times increased relative risk of cardiac death and a 3.7 times higher relative risk of arrhythmic death than persons with a history of CHF not taking an antiarrhythmic drug.

A meta-analysis of 59 randomized, controlled studies comprising 23,229 persons, including elderly persons, that investigated the use of aprindine, disopyramide, encainide, flecainide, imipramine, lidocaine, mexiletine, moricizine, phenytoin, procainamide, quinidine, and tocainide after MI showed that the mortality was higher in those receiving class I antiarrhythmic drugs (odds ratio = 1.14) than in those not receiving an antiarrhythmic drug.[38] None of the 59 studies demonstrated a decrease in mortality by class I antiarrhythmic drugs.

Ventricular rate control

Because maintenance of sinus rhythm with antiarrhythmic drugs may need serial cardioversions, exposes patients to the risks of proarrhythmia, sudden cardiac death, and other adverse effects, and requires anticoagulant treatment in those in sinus rhythm who have a high risk of recurrence of AF, many cardiologists (including the author) prefer the treatment strategy—especially in elderly persons—of ventricular rate control plus anticoagulant treatment. Beta-blockers such as propranolol 10–30 mg three to four times daily can be administered to control ventricular arrhythmias[43] and following conversion of AF to sinus rhythm. Should AF recur, β-blockers have the additional advantage of slowing the ventricular rate. Beta-blockers are also the most effective drugs in preventing and treating AF after coronary artery bypass graft surgery.[145] In a double-blind, randomized placebo-controlled study of 394 persons receiving metoprolol CR/XL or placebo after cardioversion of persistent AF, metoprolol was more effective than placebo in preventing recurrence of AF and in decreasing the ventricular heart rate if AF recurred.[146]

The Atrial Fibrillation Follow-Up Investigation of Rhythm Management (AFFIRM) study is currently randomizing persons with paroxysmal AF or chronic AF of up to 6 months duration at high risk for stroke to either maintenance of AF with ventricular rate control or to an attempt to maintain sinus rhythm with antiarrhythmic drugs after cardioversion.[147] Persons in both arms of this study will receive warfarin. The primary endpoint of the study is total mortality.

On March 18, 2002, preliminary data were presented at the Annual Scientific Meeting of the American College of Cardiology from the AFFIRM study in 3957 persons, mean age 70 years, with atrial fibrillation, who were at high risk for stroke.

Compared to persons randomized to the strategy of maintenance of sinus rhythm by antiarrhythmic drugs plus long-term warfarin to maintain an INR between 2.0–3.0, persons randomized to the strategy of ventricular rate control plus long-term warfarin had fewer deaths (306 vs 356, $p = 0.058$), had fewer strokes (5.7% vs 7.3%, p not significant), fewer hospitalizations (70% vs 78%, $p < 0.0001$), and no significant difference in quality of life or functional status.

RISK FACTORS FOR THROMBOEMBOLIC STROKE

Risk factors for TE stroke in persons with AF include:

- age;[79,148–151]
- diabetes mellitus;[149]
- echocardiographic left atrial enlargement;[152,153]
- echocardiographic LV systolic dysfunction;[151,153,154]
- echocardiographic LV hypertrophy;[151,152]
- ECAD;[91]
- history of CHF;[149,154,155]
- prior MI;[148,150,152,156]
- hypertension;[149,152,154,155]
- mitral annular calcium;[148,157]
- prior arterial thromboembolism;[80,91,149–151,154,155,158]
- rheumatic mitral stenosis;[151,152]
- and women older than 75 years.[154]

Table 37-6 lists independent risk factors for new TE stroke in 312 persons with chronic AF, mean age 84 years.

Table 37-6 Risk factors for new thromboembolic stroke in 312 elderly persons with chronic atrial fibrillation

Variable	Risk ratio
Age	1.03 per year increase
Prior stroke	1.6
Abnormal LV ejection fraction	1.8
Mitral stenosis	2.0
LV hypertrophy	2.8
Abnormal LV ejection fraction	1.8
Serum total cholesterol	1.01 per 1 mg/dL increase
Serum high-density lipoprotein cholesterol	1.04 per 1 mg/dL decrease

Abbreviation: LV, left ventricular.

Source: Adapted from Aronow et al. (1998),[151] with permission.

In the SPAF study[153,155] involving persons with non-rheumatic AF, mean age 67 years, recent CHF (within 3 months), a history of hypertension, prior arterial thrombo-embolism, echocardiographic LV systolic dysfunction, and echocardiographic left atrial enlargement were independently associated with new TE events. The incidence of new TE events was 18.6 percent per year if three or more risk factors were present, 6.0 percent per year if one or two risk factors were present, and 1.0 percent per year if none of these risk factors was present.[153] In the SPAF III study,[154] persons of mean age 72 years were considered to be at high risk for developing TE stroke if they had a previous thromboembolism, CHF or abnormal LV systolic function, or a systolic blood pressure higher than 160 mmHg, or if the person was a woman older than 75 years.

Antithrombotic therapy

Prospective, randomized studies have shown that warfarin was effective in reducing the incidence of TE stroke in persons with nonvalvular AF.[149,154,158–164] Analysis of pooled data from five randomized controlled trials demonstrated that warfarin decreased the incidence of new TE stroke by 68 percent and was more effective than aspirin in decreasing TE stroke.[149] Nonrandomized observational data from an elderly population, mean age 83 years, found that 141 persons with chronic AF treated with oral warfarin to achieve an INR between 2.0 and 3.0 (mean INR = 2.4) had a 67 percent decrease in new TE stroke compared with 209 persons with chronic AF treated with oral aspirin.[165] Compared with aspirin, warfarin caused a 40 percent decrease in new TE stroke in persons with prior stroke, a 31 percent reduction in those with no prior stroke, a 45 percent reduction in those with an abnormal LV ejection fraction, and a 36 percent reduction in those with a normal LV ejection fraction.

At 1.1-year follow-up in the SPAF III study, persons with nonvalvular AF considered to be at high risk for developing TE stroke randomized to therapy with oral warfarin to achieve an INR between 2.0 and 3.0 had a 72 percent decrease in ischemic stroke or systemic embolism compared with persons randomized to therapy with oral aspirin 325 mg daily plus oral warfarin to achieve an INR between 1.2 to 1.5. Adjusted-dose warfarin caused an absolute decrease in ischemic stroke or systemic embolism of 6.0 percent per year. In the second Copenhagen Atrial Fibrillation, Aspirin, and Anticoagulation (AFASK) study,[166] low-dose warfarin plus aspirin was also less effective in decreasing stroke or a systemic TE event in persons with AF (7.2 percent after 1 year) than was adjusted-dose warfarin to achieve an INR between 2.0 to 3.0 (2.8 percent after 1 year).

Analysis of pooled data from five randomized controlled trials showed that the annual rate of major hemorrhage was 1.0 percent for the control group, 1.0 percent for the aspirin group, and 1.3 percent for the warfarin group.[149] The incidence of major hemorrhage in persons taking adjusted-dose warfarin to achieve an INR of 2.0–3.0 in the SPAF III study (mean age 72 years) was 2.1 percent.[154] In the second Copenhagen AFASK study, the incidence of major hemorrhage in persons of mean age 73 years was 0.8 percent per year for those taking adjusted-dose warfarin to achieve an INR between 2.0 and 3.0, and 1.0 percent per year for those treated with aspirin 300 mg

daily.[167] The incidence of major hemorrhage in elderly persons, mean age 83 years, was 4.3 percent (1.4 percent per year) for those with chronic AF taking warfarin to maintain an INR between 2.0 and 3.0, and 2.9 percent (1.0 percent per year) for those with chronic AF treated with aspirin 325 mg daily.[165]

In the SPAF III study,[167] 892 persons of mean age 67 years at low risk for developing new TE stroke were treated with oral aspirin 325 mg daily. Mean follow-up was 2 years. The incidence of new ischemic stroke or systemic embolism (primary events) was 2.2 percent per year. The incidence of new ischemic stroke or systemic embolism was 3.6 percent in patients with a history of hypertension and 1.1 percent in those without a history of hypertension.

Recommendation

On the basis of the available data, elderly people with chronic or paroxysmal AF who are at high risk for developing TE stroke, or who have a history of hypertension and who have no contraindications to anticoagulation therapy, should receive long-term oral warfarin to achieve an INR of 2.0–3.0.[138] Hypertension must be controlled. Whenever the person has a prothrombin time taken, the blood pressure should also be checked. The physician prescribing the dose of oral warfarin should be aware of the numerous drugs which potentiate the effect of warfarin causing an increased prothrombin time and risk of bleeding.[168] Elderly people with AF who are at low risk for developing TE stroke or who have contraindications to therapy with long-term oral warfarin should be treated with aspirin 325 mg orally daily.

ATRIAL FLUTTER

Atrial flutter is usually paroxysmal and only rarely chronic. Untreated individuals with atrial flutter and no disease of the AV junction usually have a 2:1 AV conduction response with an atrial rate of about 300 beats per minute and a ventricular rate of 150 beats per minute. Over time, atrial flutter usually degenerates into AF.

Management of atrial flutter is similar to management of AF. Direct-current cardioversion is the treatment of choice for converting atrial flutter to sinus rhythm.[169] Thirty-eight percent of 78 persons with atrial flutter treated with intravenous ibutilide converted to sinus rhythm.[133] Fifty-four percent of 16 persons with atrial flutter treated with intravenous dofetilide converted to sinus rhythm.[134] Atrial pacing may also be used to try to convert atrial flutter to sinus rhythm.[170]

Intravenous verapamil,[100] diltiazem,[101] or β-blockers[102–105] may be used to immediately slow a very rapid ventricular rate associated with atrial flutter. Oral verapamil,[109] diltiazem,[110] or a β-blocker[111] should be added to the therapeutic regimen if a rapid ventricular rate associated with atrial flutter occurs at rest or during exercise despite digoxin use. Amiodarone is the most effective drug for slowing a rapid ventricular rate associated with atrial flutter.[114] Digoxin, verapamil, and diltiazem are contraindicated in persons with atrial flutter associated with the Wolff–Parkinson–White syndrome because these drugs shorten the refractory period of the accessory AV pathway, causing more rapid conduction down the accessory pathway. Drugs such as quinidine should never be used to treat persons with atrial flutter who are not being treated with digoxin, a β-blocker, verapamil, or diltiazem as a 1-to-1 AV conduction response may develop.

People with atrial flutter are at increased risk for developing new TE stroke.[171,172] Anticoagulant therapy should be administered prior to direct-current cardioversion or drug cardioversion of persons with atrial flutter to sinus rhythm using the same guidelines as for converting AF.[137–140] People with chronic atrial flutter should be treated with oral warfarin with the INR maintained between 2.0 and 3.0.[138]

OTHER CONDITIONS
Atrial premature complexes (APCs)

The prevalence of frequent APCs diagnosed by 24-hour ambulatory ECGs in elderly people was 18 percent in 729 women and 28 percent in 643 men in the Cardiovascular Health Study,[7] and 28 percent in 407 persons, mean age 82 years.[8] Although frequent APCs may trigger a paroxysm of AF, atrial flutter, or supraventricular tachycardia, they are of no clinical significance when found incidentally and should not be treated. If a supraventricular tachyarrhythmia is triggered by frequent APCs, a β-blocker should be administered.

Supraventricular tachycardia (SVT)

The ventricular rate in paroxysmal SVT usually ranges between 140 and 220 beats per minute and is extremely regular. The prevalence of short bursts of paroxysmal SVT diagnosed by 24-hour ambulatory ECGs in 1476 persons, mean age 81 years, with heart disease was 33 percent.[150] At 42-month follow-up of 1359 persons of mean age 81 years and with heart disease, paroxysmal SVT was not associated with an increased incidence of new coronary events.[88] At 43-month follow-up of 1476 persons of mean age 81 years, paroxysmal SVT was not associated with an increased incidence of new TE stroke.[150]

Sustained episodes of SVT should first be treated by increasing vagal tone by carotid sinus massage or the Valsalva maneuver. If vagal maneuvers are unsuccessful, intravenous adenosine is the drug of choice.[173] Intravenous verapamil, diltiazem, or β-blockers may also be used. If these measures do not convert SVT to sinus rhythm, direct-current cardioversion should be used.

Most people with paroxysmal SVT do not require long-term therapy. If long-term therapy is required because of symptoms due to frequent episodes of SVT, digoxin, propranolol, or verapamil may be administered.[174] These drugs are the initial choice for AV nodal re-entrant and AV re-entrant SVT—the commonest forms of SVT. For SVT associated with the Wolff–Parkinson–White syndrome, flecainide or propafenone may be used if there is no associated heart disease.[175] If heart disease is present, quinidine, procainamide, or disopyramide plus a β-blocker or verapamil should be used.[175] Radiofrequency catheter ablation should be used to treat older persons with symptomatic, drug-resistant SVT and should be considered an early treatment option.[176]

Nonparoxysmal atrioventricular junctional tachycardia (NPJT)

NPJT is a very rare cause of supraventricular tachycardia and is caused by enhanced impulse formation within the AV junction rather than by re-entry.[177] This arrhythmia is usually due to recent aortic or mitral valve surgery, acute MI, or digitalis toxicity. The ventricular rate usually ranges between 70 and 130 beats per minute. Treatment of NPJT is directed toward correction of the underlying disorder. Hypokalemia, if present, should be treated with potassium. Digitalis should be stopped if digitalis toxicity is present. Beta-blockers may be given cautiously if this is warranted by clinical circumstances.

Paroxysmal atrial tachycardia (PAT) with atrioventricular block

Digitalis toxicity causes 70 percent of cases of paroxysmal atrial tachycardia with AV block. Digoxin and diuretics causing hypokalemia should be stopped in these patients. If the serum potassium is low or low–normal, potassium chloride is the treatment of choice. Intravenous propranolol will cause conversion to sinus rhythm in about 85 percent of cases of digitalis-induced PAT with AV block, and in about 35 percent of cases of PAT with AV block not induced by digitalis.[178] By increasing AV block, propranolol may also be beneficial in slowing a rapid ventricular rate in PAT with AV block.

Multifocal atrial tachycardia (MAT)

MAT is usually associated with acute illness, especially in older persons with pulmonary disease. MAT is best managed by treatment of the underlying disorder. Intravenous verapamil has been reported to be effective in controlling the ventricular rate in MAT, with occasional conversion to sinus rhythm.[179] However, intravenous verapamil was not very effective in treating MAT.[180] The tendency of intravenous verapamil to aggravate pre-existing arterial hypoxemia also limits its use in the group of persons most likely to develop MAT.[179]

Bradyarrhythmias

With aging, there is a loss of specialized muscle cells (called P cells) within the sinus node which are responsible for initiating impulse formation. By age 75 years, the sinus node may consist of less than 10 percent P cells.[181] A progressive increase in the amount of collagen within the sinus node also occurs with aging.[182] There is an age-related reduction in conducting cells in the His bundle and both bundle branches, which are the distal parts of the cardiac conduction system. Diseases associated with aging such as CAD, hypertension, and valvular heart disease also adversely affect the cardiac conduction system.

Numerous drugs can cause bradyarrhythmias and conduction disturbances. Hypothyroidism, hyperkalemia, hypokalemia, and hypoxia can also depress cardiac impulse formation and conduction. Drugs and endocrine and metabolic disorders causing reversible cardiac impulse formation and conduction abnormalities must be considered before deciding to implant a permanent pacemaker.

A 12-lead ECG with a 1-minute strip may detect bradyarrhythmias caused by a sick-sinus syndrome, AV block, right and left bundle branch block, bifascicular block, and trifascicular block. ECG manifestations of sick-sinus syndrome include severe sinus bradycardia, sinus pause or arrest, sinus exit block, sinus node re-entrant rhythm, AF or atrial flutter with a slow ventricular rate not drug-induced, failure of restoration of sinus rhythm after cardioversion for tachyarrhythmias, a longer than 3-second pause after carotid sinus massage, and a tachycardia–bradycardia syndrome. The tachycardia–bradycardia syndrome is characterized by paroxysmal AF, atrial flutter, or SVT followed by periods of sinus bradycardia, sinus arrest, or sinoatrial block.

Dyspnea, weakness, fatigue, falls, angina pectoris, CHF, episodic pulmonary edema, dizziness, faintness, slurred speech, personality changes, paresis, and convulsions in older persons may be caused by bradyarrhythmias. Death may result from prolonged ventricular asystole. Older persons with symptoms that may be due to bradyarrhythmias should have a 12-lead ECG with a 1-minute rhythm strip. Since ECG abnormalities may be intermittent, a 24-hour ambulatory ECG may need to be performed.

In a prospective study of 148 persons, mean age 82 years, with unexplained syncope, 24-hour ambulatory ECGs diagnosed bradyarrhythmias with pauses greater than 3 seconds requiring permanent pacemaker implantation in 21 persons (14 percent).[2] Of these people, eight had sinus arrest, seven had advanced second-degree AV block, and six had AF with a slow ventricular rate not drug-induced. At 38-month follow-up after pacemaker implantation, recurrent syncope developed in only 3 of the 21 patients (14 percent).

In some elderly people without clinical evidence of heart disease and with recurrent episodes of unexplained syncope, a patient-activated memory loop event recorder may be used to capture the ECG tracings preceding and during syncope.[183] Elderly people with unexplained syncope and heart disease should undergo an electrophysiological study.[183]

The display box shows class I indications for permanent pacemaker implantation.[78] Modes of pacing, pacemaker codes, and pacemaker follow-up are discussed in detail elsewhere.[184]

Class I indications for permanent pacing

A. Third-degree atrioventricular (AV) block with:

1. Symptomatic bradycardia
2. Arrhythmias and other medical conditions that require drugs which cause symptomatic bradycardia
3. Pauses ≥3.0 seconds or any escape ventricular rate <40 beats per minute
4. After catheter ablation of AV junction
5. Postoperative AV block not expected to resolve
6. Neuromuscular diseases with AV block

B. Second-degree AV block with symptomatic bradycardia

C. Chronic bifascicular and trifascicular block with:

1. Intermittent third-degree AV block
2. Type II second-degree AV block

D. After acute myocardial infarction with:

1. Persistent second-degree AV block in His–Purkinje system with bilateral bundle branch block or third-degree AV block within or below His–Purkinje system
2. Transient second- or third-degree infranodal AV block and associated bundle branch block
3. Persistent and symptomatic second- or third-degree AV block

E. Sinus node dysfunction

1. Sinus node dysfunction with symptomatic bradycardia
2. Symptomatic chronotropic incompetence

F. Prevention and termination of tachyarrhythmias

1. Symptomatic recurrent supraventricular tachycardia terminated by pacing after drugs and catheter ablation fail to control arrhythmia or cause intolerable side-effects
2. Symptomatic recurrent sustained ventricular tachycardia as part of an automatic defibrillator system

G. Prevention of tachycardia

Sustained pause-dependent ventricular tachycardia, with or without prolonged QT, in which efficacy of pacing is documented

H. Hypersensitive carotid sinus and neurally mediated syncope

Recurrent syncope caused by carotid sinus stimulation; minimal carotid sinus pressure induces asystole >3 seconds in absence of any drug that depresses sinus node or AV conduction

Source: Adapted from Gregoratos et al. (1998),[78] with permission.

KEY POINTS   Cardiac arrhythmias

- Asymptomatic nonsustained ventricular tachycardia or complex ventricular arrhythmias in persons without heart disease should not be treated with antiarrhythmic drugs.

- Beta-blockers should be used to treat persons with heart disease and complex ventricular arrhythmias if there are no contraindications to β-blockers.

- The automatic implantable cardioverter–defibrillator is the most effective treatment for patients with life-threatening ventricular tachycardia or ventricular fibrillation.

- People with chronic or paroxysmal atrial fibrillation who are at high risk for developing stroke or who have a history of hypertension and who have no contraindications to anticoagulant therapy should receive long-term oral warfarin to maintain an INR (international normalized ratio) of 2.0–3.0.

REFERENCES

1. Fleg JL, Kennedy HL: Cardiac arrhythmia in a healthy elderly population: detection by 24-hour ambulatory electrocardiography. Chest 1982;81:302–307

2. Aronow WS, Mercando AD, Epstein S: Prevalence of arrhythmias detected by 24-hour ambulatory electrocardiography and the value of antiarrhythmic therapy in elderly patients with unexplained syncope. Am J Cardiol 1992;70:408–410

3. Aronow WS, Epstein S, Mercando AD: Usefulness of complex ventricular arrhythmias detected by 24-hour ambulatory ECG and by ECGs with one-minute rhythm strips in predicting new coronary events in elderly patients with and without heart disease. J Cardiovasc Technol 1991;10:21–25

4. Camm AJ, Evans KE, Ward DE, Martin A: The rhythm of the heart in active elderly subjects. Am Heart J 1980;99:598–603

5. Aronow WS, Epstein S, Koenigsberg M, Schwartz KS: Usefulness of echocardiographic abnormal left ventricular ejection fraction, paroxysmal ventricular tachycardia, and complex ventricular arrhythmias in predicting new coronary events in patients over 62 years of age. Am J Cardiol 1988;61:1349–1351

6. Kantelip JP, Sage E, Duchene-Marullaz P: Findings on ambulatory electrocardiographic monitoring in subjects older than 80 years. Am J Cardiol 1986;57:398–401

7. Manolio TA, Furberg CD, Rautaharju PM et al: Cardiac arrhythmias on 24-h ambulatory electrocardiography in older women and men: The Cardiovascular Health Study. J Am Coll Cardiol 1994;23:916–925

8. Aronow WS, Epstein S, Schwartz KS, Koenigsberg M: Prevalence of arrhythmias detected by ambulatory electrocardiographic monitoring and of abnormal left ventricular ejection fraction in persons older than 62 years in a long-term healthcare facility. Am J Cardiol 1987;59:368–369

9. Aronow WS, Epstein S, Schwartz KS, Koenigsberg M: Correlation of complex ventricular arrhythmias detected by ambulatory electrocardiographic monitoring with echocardiographic left ventricular hypertrophy in persons older than 62 years in a long-term healthcare facility. Am J Cardiol 1987;60:730–732

10. Aronow WS, Epstein S: Usefulness of silent ischemia, ventricular tachycardia, and complex ventricular arrhythmias in predicting new coronary events in elderly patients with coronary artery disease or systemic hypertension. Am J Cardiol 1990;65:511–522

11. Fleg JL, Kennedy HL: Long-term prognostic significance of ambulatory electrocardiographic findings in apparently healthy subjects ≥60 years of age. Am J Cardiol 1992;70:748–751

12. Aronow WS, Epstein S, Koenigsberg M, Schwartz KS: Usefulness of echocardiographic left ventricular hypertrophy, ventricular tachycardia and complex ventricular arrhythmias in predicting ventricular fibrillation or sudden cardiac death in elderly patients. Am J Cardiol 1988;62:1124–1125

13. Fleg JL, Lakatta EG: Prevalence and prognosis of exercise-induced nonsustained ventricular tachycardia in apparently healthy volunteers. Am J Cardiol 1984;54:762–764

14. Busby MJ, Shefrin EA, Fleg JL: Prevalence and long-term significance of exercise-induced frequent or repetitive ventricular ectopic beats in apparently healthy volunteers. J Am Coll Cardiol 1989;14:1659–1665

15. Antiplatelet Trialists' Collaboration: Collaborative overview of randomised trials of antiplatelet therapy. I: Prevention of death, myocardial infarction and stroke by prolonged antiplatelet therapy in various categories of patients. BMJ 1994;308:81–106

16. Goldstein RE, Andrews M, Hall WJ, Moss AJ, for the Multicenter Myocardial Ischemia research group: Marked reduction in long-term cardiac deaths with aspirin after a coronary event. J Am Coll Cardiol 1996;28:326–330

17. Ryan TJ, Antman EM, Brooks NH et al: 1999 update: ACC/AHA guidelines for the management of patients with acute myocardial infarction: executive summary and recommendations. A report of the American College of Cardiology/American Heart Association Task Force on Practice Guidelines (committee on management of acute myocardial infarction). Circulation 1999;100:1016–1030

18. Hjalmarson A, Herbiz J, Malek J et al: Effect on mortality of metoprolol in acute myocardial infarction. Lancet 1981;2:823–827

19. Gundersen T, Abrahamsen AM, Kjekshus J et al: Timolol-related reduction in mortality and reinfarction in patients ages 65–75 years surviving acute myocardial infarction. Circulation 1982;66:1179–1184

20. Pedersen TR, for the Norwegian Multicentre Study Group: Six-year follow-up of the Norwegian Multicentre Study on Timolol after acute myocardial infarction. N Engl J Med 1985;313:1055–1058

21. Beta-blocker Heart Attack Trial research group: A randomized trial of propranolol in patients with acute myocardial infarction. JAMA 1982;247:1707–1714

22. Pfeffer MA, Braunwald E, Moye LA et al: Effect of captopril on mortality and morbidity in patients with left ventricular dysfunction after myocardial infarction: results of the Survival and Ventricular Enlargement Trial. N Engl J Med 1992;327:669–677

23. The Acute Infarction Ramipril Efficacy (AIRE) study investigators: Effect of ramipril on mortality and morbidity of survivors of acute myocardial infarction with clinical evidence of heart failure. Lancet 1993;342:821–828

24. Ambrosioni E, Borghi C, Magnani B, for the Survival of Myocardial Infarction Long-term Evaluation (SMILE) study investigators: The effect of the angiotensin-converting-enzyme inhibitor zofenopril on mortality and morbidity after anterior myocardial infarction. N Engl J Med 1995;332:80–85

25. Kober L, Torp-Pedersen C, Carlsen JE et al: A clinical trial of the angiotensin-converting-enzyme inhibitor trandolapril in patients with left ventricular dysfunction after myocardial infarction. N Engl J Med 1995;333:1670–1676

26. Miettinen TA, Pyorala K, Olsson AG et al: Cholesterol-lowering therapy in women and elderly patients with myocardial infarction or angina pectoris: findings from the Scandinavian Simvastatin Survival Study (4S). Circulation 1997;96:4211–4218

27. Lewis SJ, Moye LA, Sacks FM et al: Effect of pravastatin on cardiovascular events in older patients with myocardial infarction and cholesterol levels in the average range: results of the Cholesterol and Recurrent Events (CARE) trial. Ann Intern Med 1998;129:681–689

28. The Long-term Intervention with Pravastatin in Ischaemic Disease (LIPID) study group: Prevention of cardiovascular events and death with pravastatin in patients with coronary heart disease and a broad range of initial cholesterol levels. N Engl J Med 1998;339:1349–1357

29. IMPACT research group: International Mexiletine and Placebo Antiarrhythmic Coronary Trial: I. Report on arrhythmia and other findings. J Am Coll Cardiol 1984;4:1148–1163

30. The Cardiac Arrhythmia Suppression Trial (CAST) investigators: Preliminary report—Effect of encainide and flecainide on mortality in a randomized trial of arrhythmia suppression after myocardial infarction. N Engl J Med 1989;321:406–412

31. Akiyama T, Pawitan Y, Campbell WB et al: Effects of advancing age on the efficacy and side-effects of antiarrhythmic drugs in post-myocardial infarction patients with ventricular arrhythmias. J Am Geriatr Soc 1992;40:666–672

32. The Cardiac Arrhythmia Suppression Trial II investigators: Effect of the antiarrhythmic agent moricizine on survival after myocardial infarction. N Engl J Med 1992;327:227–233

33. Aronow WS, Mercando AD, Epstein S, Kronzon I: Effect of quinidine or procainamide versus no antiarrhythmic drug on sudden cardiac death, total cardiac death, and total death in elderly patients with heart disease and complex ventricular arrhythmias. Am J Cardiol 1990;66:423–428

34. Moosvi AR, Goldstein S, VanderBrug Medendorp S et al: Effect of empiric antiarrhythmic therapy in resuscitated out-of-hospital cardiac arrest victims with coronary artery disease. Am J Cardiol 1990;65:1192–1197

35. Hallstrom AP, Cobb LA, Hui Yu B et al: An antiarrhythmic drug experience in 941 patients resuscitated from an initial cardiac arrest between 1970 and 1985. Am J Cardiol 1991;68:1025–1031

36. Coplen SE, Antmann EM, Berlin JA et al: Efficacy and safety of quinidine therapy for maintenance of sinus rhythm after cardioversion: a meta-analysis of randomized control trials. Circulation 1990;82:1106–1116

37. Flaker GC, Blackshear JL, McBride R et al: Antiarrhythmic drug therapy and cardiac mortality in atrial fibrillation. J Am Coll Cardiol 1992;20:527–532

38. Teo KK, Yusuf S, Furberg CD: Effects of prophylactic antiarrhythmic drug therapy in acute myocardial infarction: an overview of results from randomized controlled trials. JAMA 1993;270:1589–1595

39. Hawkins CM, Richardson DW, Vokonas PS, for the BHAT research group: Effect of propranolol in reducing mortality in older myocardial infarction patients. The Beta-Blocker Heart Attack Trial experience. Circulation 1983;67(suppl I):I94–I97

40. Friedman LM, Byington RP, Capone RJ et al: Effect of propranolol in patients with myocardial infarction and ventricular arrhythmia. J Am Coll Cardiol 1986;7:1–8

41. Lichstein E, Morganroth J, Harrist R, Hubble MS, for BHAT study group: Effect of propranolol on ventricular arrhythmia. The Beta-Blocker Heart Attack Trial experience. Circulation 1983;67(suppl I):I5–I10

42. Hansteen V: Beta blockade after myocardial infarction: The Norwegian Propranolol Study in high-risk patients. Circulation 1983;67(Suppl I):I57

43. Aronow WS, Ahn C, Mercando AD et al: Effect of propranolol versus no antiarrhythmic drug on sudden cardiac death, total cardiac death, and total death in patients ≥62 years of age with heart disease, complex ventricular arrhythmias, and left ventricular ejection fraction ≥40%. Am J Cardiol 1994;74:267–270

44. Kennedy HL, Brooks MM, Barker AH et al: Beta-blocker therapy in the Cardiac Arrhythmia Suppression Trial. Am J Cardiol 1994;74:674–680

45. Aronow WS, Ahn C, Mercando AD et al: Decrease of mortality by propranolol in patients with heart disease and complex ventricular arrhythmias is more an anti-ischemic than an antiarrhythmic effect. Am J Cardiol 1994;74:613–615

46. Aronow WS, Ahn C, Mercando AD, Epstein S: Circadian variation of sudden cardiac death or fatal myocardial infarction is abolished by propranolol in patients with heart disease and complex ventricular arrhythmias. Am J Cardiol 1994;74:819–821

47. Aronow WS, Ahn C, Mercando AD, Epstein S: Effect of propranolol on circadian variation of ventricular arrhythmias in elderly patients with heart disease and complex ventricular arrhythmias. Am J Cardiol 1995;75:514–516

48. Aronow WS, Ahn C, Mercando AD, Epstein S: Effect of propranolol on circadian variation of myocardial ischemia in elderly patients with heart disease and complex ventricular arrhythmias. Am J Cardiol 1995;75:837–839

49. Cohn JN, Johnson G, Ziesche S et al: A comparison of enalapril with hydralazine–isosorbide dinitrate in the treatment of chronic congestive heart failure. N Engl J Med 1991;325:303–310

50. Garg R, Yusuf S, for the Collaborative Group on ACE Inhibitor Trials: Overview of randomized trials of angiotensin-converting-enzyme inhibitors on mortality and morbidity in patients with heart failure. JAMA 1995;273:1450–1456

51. Aronow WS, Kronzon I: Effect of enalapril on congestive heart failure treated with diuretics in elderly patients with prior myocardial infarction and normal left ventricular ejection fraction. Am J Cardiol 1993;71:602–604

52. Philbin EF, Rocco TA: Use of angiotensin-converting-enzyme inhibitors in heart failure with preserved left ventricular systolic function. Am Heart J 1997;134:188–195

53. Julian DJ, Prescott RJ, Jackson FS, Szekely P: Controlled trial of sotalol for one year after myocardial infarction. Lancet 1982;i:1142–1147

54. Waldo AL, Camm AJ, deRuyter H et al: Effect of d-sotalol on mortality in patients with left ventricular dysfunction after recent and remote myocardial infarction. Lancet 1996;348:7–12

55. Singh SN, Fletcher RD, Fisher SG et al: Amiodarone in patients with congestive heart failure and asymptomatic ventricular arrhythmia. N Engl J Med 1995;333:77–82

56. Cairns JA, Connolly SJ, Roberts R, Gent M, for the Canadian Amiodarone Myocardial Infarction Arrhythmia Trial investigators: Randomised trial of outcome after myocardial infarction in patients with frequent or repetitive ventricular premature depolarisations: CAMIAT. Lancet 1997;349:675–682

57. Julian DG, Camm AJ, Frangin G et al: Randomised trial of effect of amiodarone on mortality in patients with left-ventricular dysfunction after recent myocardial infarction: EMIAT. Lancet 1997;349:667–674

58. Kehoe RF, MacNeil DJ, Zheutlin TA et al: Safety and efficacy of oral sotalol for sustained ventricular tachyarrhythmias refractory to other antiarrhythmic agents. Am J Cardiol 1993;72:56A–66A

59. Greene HL, for the CASCADE investigators. The CASCADE study: randomized antiarrhythmic drug therapy in survivors of cardiac arrest in Seattle. Am J Cardiol 1993;72:70F–74F

60. Herre J, Sauve M, Malone P et al: Long-term results of amiodarone therapy in patients with recurrent sustained ventricular tachycardia or ventricular fibrillation. J Am Coll Cardiol 1989;13:442–449

61. Boissel J-P, Boutitie F, Bernard C et al: Synergy between amiodarone and beta-blockers after myocardial infarction. Circulation 1998;98(suppl I):I–93 (abstract)

62. O'Rourke RA: Role of myocardial revascularization in sudden cardiac death. Circulation 1992;85(suppl I):I112–I117

63. Platia EV, Griffith LSC, Watkins L et al: Treatment of malignant ventricular arrhythmias with endocardial resection and implantation of the automatic cardioverter–defibrillator. N Engl J Med 1986;314:213–216

64. Tresch DD, Platia EV, Guarnieri T et al: Refractory symptomatic ventricular tachycardia and ventricular fibrillation in elderly patients. Am J Med 1987;83:399–404

65. Tresch DD, Troup PJ, Thakur RK et al: Comparison of efficacy of automatic implantable cardioverter–defibrillator in patients older and younger than 65 years of age. Am J Med 1991;90:717–724

66. Rastegar H, Link MS, Foote CB et al: Perioperative and long-term results with mapping-guided subendocardial resection and left ventricular endoaneurysmorrhaphy. Circulation 1996;94:1041–1048

67. Morady F, Harvey M, Kalbfleisch SJ et al: Radiofrequency catheter ablation of ventricular tachycardia in patients with coronary artery disease. Circulation 1993;87:363–372

68. Gonska B-D, Cao K, Schaumann A et al: Catheter ablation of ventricular tachycardia in 136 patients with coronary artery disease: results and long-term follow-up. J Am Coll Cardiol 1994;24:1506–1514

69. Moss AJ, Hall WJ, Cannom DS et al: Improved survival with an implanted defibrillator in patients with coronary disease at high risk for ventricular arrhythmia. N Engl J Med 1996;335:1933–1940

70. The Antiarrhythmics versus Implantable Defibrillators (AVID) investigators: A comparison of antiarrhythmic-drug therapy with implantable defibrillators in patients resuscitated from near-fatal ventricular arrhythmias. N Engl J Med 1997;337:1576–1583

71. Connolly SJ, Gent M, Roberts RS et al: Canadian Implantable Defibrillator Study (CIDS): a randomized trial of the implantable cardioverter–defibrillator against amiodarone. Circulation 2000;101:1297–1302

72. Siebels J, Cappato R, Ruppel R et al: Preliminary results of the Cardiac Arrest Study Hamburg (CASH). Am J Cardiol 1993;72:109F–113F

73. Cappato R, Siebels J, Kuck KH: Value of programmed electrical stimulation to predict clinical outcome in the Cardiac Arrest Study Hamburg (CASH). Circulation 1998;98(Suppl I):I495–I496 (abstract)

74. Buxton AE, Lee KL, Fisher JD et al: A randomized study of the prevention of sudden death in patients with coronary artery disease. N Engl J Med 1999;341:1882–1890

75. Sheldon R, Connolly S, Krahn A et al: Identification of patients most likely to benefit from implantable cardioverter–defibrillator therapy. The Canadian Implantable Defibrillator Study. Circulation 2000;101:1660–1664

76. Seidl K, Hauer B, Schwick NG et al: Comparison of metoprolol and sotalol in preventing ventricular tachyarrhythmias after the implantation of a cardioverter/defibrillator. Am J Cardiol 1998;82:744–748

77. De Sutter J, Tavernier R, De Buyzere M et al: Lipid lowering drugs and recurrences of life-threatening ventricular arrhythmias in high-risk patients. J Am Coll Cardiol 2000;36:766–772

78. Gregoratos G, Cheitlin MD, Conill A et al: ACC/AHA Guidelines for Implantation of Cardiac Pacemakers and Antiarrhythmia Devices: Executive Summary. A Report of the American College of Cardiology/American Heart Association Task Force on Practice Guidelines (committee on pacemaker implantation). Circulation 1998;97:1325–1335

79. Wolf PA, Abbott RD, Kannel WB: Atrial fibrillation as an independent risk factor for stroke: the Framingham Study. Stroke 1991;22:983–988

80. Aronow WS, Ahn C, Gutstein H: Prevalence of atrial fibrillation and association of atrial fibrillation with prior and new thromboembolic stroke in older patients. J Am Geriatr Soc 1996;44:521–523

81. Furberg CD, Psaty BM, Manolio TA et al: Prevalence of atrial fibrillation in elderly subjects (the Cardiovascular Health Study). Am J Cardiol 1994;74:236–241

82. Mendelson G, Aronow WS: Underutilization of warfarin in older persons with chronic nonvalvular atrial fibrillation at high risk for developing stroke. J Am Geriatr Soc 1998;46:1423–1424

83. Danias PG, Caulfield TA, Weigner MJ et al: Likelihood of spontaneous conversion of atrial fibrillation to sinus rhythm. J Am Coll Cardiol 1998;31:588–592

84. Aronow WS, Ahn C, Kronzon I: Echocardiographic findings associated with atrial fibrillation in 1,699 patients aged >60 years. Am J Cardiol 1995;76:1191–1192

85. Sawin CT, Geller A, Wolf PA et al: Low serum thyrotropin concentration as a risk factor for atrial fibrillation in older persons. N Engl J Med 1994;331:1249–1252

86. Kannel WB, Abbott RD, Savage DD, McNamara PM: Epidemiologic features of chronic atrial fibrillation: the Framingham Study. N Engl J Med 1982;306:1018–1022

87. Benjamin EJ, Wolf PA, D'Agostino RB et al: Impact of atrial fibrillation on the risk of death. The Framingham Heart Study. Circulation 1998;98:946–952

88. Aronow WS, Ahn C, Mercando AD, Epstein S: Correlation of atrial fibrillation, paroxysmal supraventricular tachycardia, and sinus rhythm

with incidences of new coronary events in 1359 patients, mean age 81 years, with heart disease. Am J Cardiol 1995;75:182–184

89. Rathore SS, Berger AK, Weinfurt KP et al: Acute myocardial infarction complicated by atrial fibrillation in the elderly: prevalence and outcomes. Circulation 2000;101:969–974

90. Aronow WS, Ahn C, Kronzon I, Gutstein H: Association of left ventricular hypertrophy and chronic atrial fibrillation with the incidence of new thromboembolic stroke in 2384 older persons. Am J Cardiol 1999;84:468–469

91. Aronow WS, Ahn C, Schoenfeld MR, Gutstein H: Association of extracranial carotid arterial disease and chronic atrial fibrillation with the incidence of new thromboembolic stroke in 1846 older persons. Am J Cardiol 1999;83:1403–1404

92. Yamanouchi H, Mizutani T, Matsushita S, Esaki Y: Paroxysmal atrial fibrillation: high frequency of embolic brain infarction in elderly autopsy patients. Neurology 1997;49:1691–1694

93. Ezekowitz MD, James KE, Nazarian SM et al: Silent cerebral infarction in patients with nonrheumatic atrial fibrillation. Circulation 1995;92:2178–2182

94. Dries DL, Exner DV, Gersh BJ et al: Atrial fibrillation is associated with an increased risk for mortality and heart failure progression in patients with asymptomatic and symptomatic left ventricular systolic dysfunction: a retrospective analysis of the SOLVD trials. J Am Coll Cardiol 1998;32:695–703

95. Aronow WS, Ahn C, Kronzon I: Prognosis of congestive heart failure after prior myocardial infarction in older persons with atrial fibrillation versus sinus rhythm. Am J Cardiol 2001;87:224–225

96. Shinbane JS, Wood MA, Jensen DN et al: Tachycardia-induced cardiomyopathy: a review of animal models and clinical studies. J Am Coll Cardiol 1997;29:709–715

97. Schumacher B, Luderitz B: Rate issues in atrial fibrillation: consequences of tachycardia and therapy for rate control. Am J Cardiol 1998;82:29N–36N

98. Wood MA, Brown-Mahoney C, Kay GN, Ellenbogen KA: Clinical outcomes after ablation and pacing therapy for atrial fibrillation: a meta-analysis. Circulation 2000;101:1138–1144

99. Pollak A, Falk RH: Pacemaker therapy in patients with atrial fibrillation. Am Heart J 1993;125:824–830

100. Aronow WS, Landa D, Plasencia G et al: Verapamil in atrial fibrillation and atrial flutter. Clin Pharmacol Therap 1979;26:578–583

101. Salerno DM, Dias VC, Kleiger RE et al: Efficacy and safety of intravenous diltiazem for treatment of atrial fibrillation and atrial flutter. Am J Cardiol 1989;63:1046–1051

102. Aronow WS, Uyeyama RR: Treatment of arrhythmias with pindolol. Clin Pharmacol Therap 1972;13:15–22

103. Aronow WS, Van Camp S, Turbow M et al: Acebutolol in supraventricular arrhythmias. Clin Pharmacol Therap 1979;25:149–153

104. Aronow WS. Use of beta-adrenergic blockers in antiarrhythmic therapy. Practical Cardiol 1986;12(6):75–89

105. Abrams J, Allen J, Allin D et al: Efficacy and safety of esmolol vs propranolol in the treatment of supraventricular tachycardia: a multicenter double-blind clinical trial. Am Heart J 1985;110:913–922

106. Falk RH, Knowlton AA, Bernard SA et al: Digoxin for converting recent onset atrial fibrillation to sinus rhythm: a randomized, double-blinded trial. Ann Intern Med 1987;106:503–506

107. Falk RH, Leavitt JI: Digoxin for atrial fibrillation: a drug whose time has gone? Ann Intern Med 1991;114:573–575

108. Aronow WS: Digoxin or angiotensin converting enzyme inhibitors for congestive heart failure in geriatric patients: which is the preferred treatment? Drugs Aging 1991;1:98–103

109. Lang R, Klein HD, Weiss E et al: Superiority of oral verapamil therapy to digoxin in treatment of chronic atrial fibrillation. Chest 1983;83:491–499

110. Roth A, Harrison E, Milani G et al: Efficacy and safety of medium- and high-dose diltiazem alone and in combination with digoxin for control of heart rate at rest and during exercise in patients with chronic atrial fibrillation. Circulation 1986;73:316–324

111. David D, Segni ED, Klein HO et al: Inefficacy of digitalis in the control of heart rate in patients with chronic atrial fibrillation: beneficial effect of an added beta adrenergic blocking agent. Am J Cardiol 1979;44:1378–1382

112. Farshi R, Kistner D, Sarma JSM et al: Ventricular rate control in chronic atrial fibrillation during daily activity and programmed exercise: a crossover open-label study of five drug regimens. J Am Coll Cardiol 1999;33:304–310

113. Gold RL, Haffajee CI, Charos G et al: Amiodarone for refractory atrial fibrillation. Am J Cardiol 1986;57:124–127

114. Chun SH, Sager PT, Stevenson WG et al: Long-term efficacy of amiodarone for the maintenance of normal sinus rhythm in patients with refractory atrial fibrillation or flutter. Am J Cardiol 1995;76:47–50

115. Rawles JM, Metcalfe MJ, Jennings K: Time of occurrence, duration, and ventricular rate of paroxysmal atrial fibrillation: the effect of digoxin. Br Heart J 1990;63:225–227

116. Murgatroyd FD, Gibson SM, Baiyan X et al: Double-blind placebo controlled trial of digoxin in symptomatic paroxysmal atrial fibrillation. Circulation 1999;99:2765–2770

117. Galun E, Flugelman MY, Glickson M, Eliakim M: Failure of long-term digitalization to prevent rapid ventricular response in patients with paroxysmal atrial fibrillation. Chest 1991;99:1038–1040

118. Morady F, Hasse C, Strickberger SA et al: Long-term follow-up after radiofrequency modification of the atrioventricular node in patients with atrial fibrillation. J Am Coll Cardiol 1997;27:113–121

119. Feld GK, Fleck P, Fujimura O et al: Control of rapid ventricular response by radiofrequency catheter modification of the atrioventricular node in patients with medically refractory atrial fibrillation. Circulation 1994;90:2299–2307

120. Fitzpatrick AP, Kourouyan HD, Siu A et al: Quality of life and outcomes after radiofrequency His-bundle catheter ablation and permanent pacemaker implantation: impact of treatment in paroxysmal and established atrial fibrillation. Am Heart J 1996;131:499–507

121. Brignole M, Menozzi C, Gianfranchi L et al: Assessment of atrioventricular junction ablation and VVIR pacemaker versus pharmacological treatment in patients with heart failure and chronic atrial fibrillation: a randomized, controlled study. Circulation 1998;98:953–960

122. Cox JL, Boineau JP, Schuessler RB et al: Successful surgical treatment of atrial fibrillation: review and clinical update. JAMA 1991;266:1976–1980

123. Leitch JW, Klein G, Yee R, Guiraudon G: Sinus node–atrioventricular node isolation: long-term results with the "Corridor" operation for atrial fibrillation. J Am Coll Cardiol 1991;17:970–975

124. Wellens HJJ, Lau C-P, Luderitz B et al: Atrioverter: an implantable device for the treatment of atrial fibrillation. Circulation 1998;98:1651–1656

125. Sgarbossa EB, Pinski SL, Maloney JD et al: Chronic atrial fibrillation and stroke in paced patients with sick sinus syndrome: relevance of clinical characteristics and pacing modalities. Circulation 1993;88:1045–1053

126. Andersen HR, Thuesen L, Bagger JP et al: Prospective randomised trial of atrial versus ventricular pacing in sick-sinus syndrome. Lancet 1994;344:1523–1528

127. Michelson EL: Clinical perspectives in management of Wolff–Parkinson–White syndrome. 2: Diagnostic evaluation and treatment strategies. Mod Concepts Cardiovasc Dis 1989;58:49–54

128. Jackman WM, Wang X, Friday KJ et al: Catheter ablation of accessory atrioventricular pathways (Wolff–Parkinson–White syndrome) by radiofrequency current. N Engl J Med 1991;324:1605–1611

129. Morris JJ, Peter RH, McIntosh HD: Electrical conversion of atrial fibrillation: immediate and long-term results and selection of patients. Ann Intern Med 1966;65:216–231

130. Feld GK, Chen P-S, Nicod P et al: Possible atrial proarrhythmic effects of class IC antiarrhythmic drugs. Am J Cardiol 1990;66:378–383

131. Falk RH. Proarrhythmia in patients treated for atrial fibrillation or flutter. Ann Intern Med 1992;117:141–150

132. Maisel WH, Kuntz KM, Reimold SC et al: Risk of initiating antiarrhythmic drug therapy for atrial fibrillation in patients admitted to a university hospital. Ann Intern Med 1997;127:281–284

133. Ellenbogen KA, Stambler BS, Wood MA et al: Efficacy of intravenous ibutilide for rapid termination of atrial fibrillation and atrial flutter: a dose–response study. J Am Coll Cardiol 1996;28:130–136

134. Falk RH, Pollak A, Singh SN, Friedrich T: Intravenous dofetilide, a class III antiarrhythmic agent, for the termination of sustained atrial fibrillation or flutter. J Am Coll Cardiol 1997;29:385–390

135. Torp-Pedersen C, Moller M, Bloch-Thomsen PE et al: Dofetilide in patients with congestive heart failure and left ventricular dysfunction. N Engl J Med 1999;341:857–865

136. Oral H, Souza JJ, Michaud GF et al: Facilitating transthoracic cardioversion of atrial fibrillation with ibutilide pretreatment. N Engl J Med 1999;340:1849–1854

137. Manning WJ, Silverman DI, Keighley CS et al: Transesophageal echocardiographically facilitated early cardioversion from atrial fibrillation using short-term anticoagulation: final results of a prospective 4.5-year study. J Am Coll Cardiol 1995;25:1354–1361

138. Laupacis A, Albers G, Dalen J et al: Antithrombotic therapy in atrial fibrillation. Chest 1998;114:579S–589S

139. Fatkin D, Kuchar DL, Thorburn CW, Feneley MP: Transesophageal echocardiography before and during direct current cardioversion of atrial fibrillation: evidence for "atrial stunning" as a mechanism of thromboembolic complications. J Am Coll Cardiol 1994;23:307–316

140. Black IW, Fatkin D, Sagar KB et al: Exclusion of atrial thrombus by transesophageal echocardiography does not preclude embolism after cardioversion of atrial fibrillation: a multicenter study. Circulation 1994;89:2509–2513

141. Grimm RA, Stewart WJ, Black IW et al: Should all patients undergo transesophageal echocardiography before electrical cardioversion of atrial fibrillation? J Am Coll Cardiol 1994;23:533–541

142. Aronow WS, Mercando AD, Epstein S, Kronzon I: Effect of quinidine or procainimide versus no antiarrhythmic drug on sudden cardiac death, total cardiac death, and total death in elderly patients with heart disease and complex ventricular arrhythmias. Am J Cardiol 1990;66:423–428

143. Juul-Moller S, Edvardsson N, Rehnqvist-Ahlberg N: Sotalol versus quinidine for the maintenance of sinus rhythm after direct current conversion of atrial fibrillation. Circulation 1990;82:1932–1939

144. Reimold SC, Cantillon CO, Friedman PL et al: Propafenone versus sotalol for suppression of recurrent symptomatic atrial fibrillation. Am J Cardiol 1993;71:558–563

145. Olshansky B: Management of atrial fibrillation after coronary artery bypass graft. Am J Cardiol 1996;78(suppl 8A):27–34

146. Kuhlkamp V, Schirdewan A, Stangl K et al: Use of metoprolol CR/XL to maintain sinus rhythm after conversion from persistent atrial fibrillation: a randomized, double-blind, placebo controlled study. J Am Coll Cardiol 2000;36:139–146

147. Planning and Steering Committees for AFFIRM Study: Atrial fibrillation follow-up investigation of rhythm management: the AFFIRM Study design. Am J Cardiol 1997;79:1198–1202

148. Boston Area Anticoagulation Trial for Atrial Fibrillation investigators: The effect of low-dose warfarin on the risk of stroke in patients with nonrheumatic atrial fibrillation. N Engl J Med 1990;323:1505–1511

149. Atrial Fibrillation investigators: Risk factors for stroke and efficacy of antithrombotic therapy in atrial fibrillation: analysis of pooled data from five randomized controlled trials. Arch Intern Med 1994;154:1449–1457

150. Aronow WS, Ahn C, Mercando AD et al: Correlation of paroxysmal supraventricular tachycardia, atrial fibrillation, and sinus rhythm with incidences of new thromboembolic stroke in 1476 old-old patients. Aging Clin Exp Res 1996;8:32–34

151. Aronow WS, Ahn C, Kronzon I, Gutstein H: Risk factors for new thromboembolic stroke in persons ≥62 years old with chronic atrial fibrillation. Am J Cardiol 1998;82:119–121

152. Aronow WS, Gutstein H, Hsieh FY: Risk factors for thromboembolic stroke in elderly patients with chronic atrial fibrillation. Am J Cardiol 1989;63:366–367

153. Stroke Prevention in Atrial Fibrillation investigators: Predictors of thromboembolism in atrial fibrillation. II: Echocardiographic features of patients at risk. Ann Intern Med 1992;116:6–12

154. Stroke Prevention in Atrial Fibrillation investigators: Adjusted-dose warfarin versus low-intensity, fixed-dose warfarin plus aspirin for high-risk patients with atrial fibrillation: Stroke Prevention in Atrial Fibrillation III randomised clinical trial. Lancet 1996;348:633–638

155. Stroke Prevention in Atrial Fibrillation investigators: Predictors of thromboembolism in atrial fibrillation. I: Clinical features of patients at risk. Ann Intern Med 1992;116:1–5

156. Peterson P, Kastrup J, Helweg-Larsen S et al: Risk factors for thromboembolic complications in chronic atrial fibrillation. Arch Intern Med 1990;150:819–821

157. Aronow WS, Ahn C, Kronzon I, Gutstein H: Association of mitral annular calcium with new thromboembolic stroke at 44-month follow-up of 2148 persons, mean age 81 years. Am J Cardiol 1998;81:105–106

158. EAFT (European Atrial Fibrillation Trial) study group: Secondary prevention in non-rheumatic atrial fibrillation after transient ischaemic attack or minor stroke. Lancet 1993;342:1255–1262

159. Peterson P, Boysen G, Godtfredsen J et al: Placebo-controlled, randomised trial of warfarin and aspirin for prevention of thromboembolic complications in chronic atrial fibrillation. Lancet 1989;1:175–179

160. Stroke Prevention in Atrial Fibrillation investigators: Preliminary report of the Stroke Prevention in Atrial Fibrillation Study. N Engl J Med 1990;322:863–868

161. Stroke Prevention in Atrial Fibrillation investigators: Stroke Prevention in Atrial Fibrillation Study: final results. Circulation 1991;84:527–539

162. Connolly SJ, Laupacis A, Gent M et al: Canadian Atrial Fibrillation Anticoagulation (CAFA) study. J Am Coll Cardiol 1991;18:345–355

163. Ezekowitz MD, Bridgers SL, James KE et al: Warfarin in the prevention of stroke associated with nonrheumatic atrial fibrillation. N Engl J Med 1992;327:1406–1412

164. Stroke Prevention in Atrial Fibrillation investigators: Warfarin versus aspirin for prevention of thromboembolism in atrial fibrillation: Stroke Prevention in Atrial Fibrillation II study. Lancet 1994;343:687–691

165. Aronow WS, Ahn C, Kronzon I, Gutstein H: Effect of warfarin versus aspirin on the incidence of new thromboembolic stroke in older persons with chronic atrial fibrillation and abnormal and normal left ventricular ejection fraction. Am J Cardiol 2000;85:1033–1035

166. Gullov AL, Koefoed BG, Petersen P et al: Fixed minidose warfarin and aspirin alone and in combination vs adjusted-dose warfarin for stroke prevention in atrial fibrillation. Second Copenhagen Atrial Fibrillation, Aspirin, and Anticoagulation Study. Arch Intern Med 1998;158:1513–1521

167. The SPAF III Writing Committee for the Stroke Prevention in Atrial Fibrillation investigators: Patients with nonvalvular atrial fibrillation at low risk of stroke during treatment with aspirin. Stroke Prevention in Atrial Fibrillation III Study. JAMA 1998;279:1273–1277

168. Frishman WH, Cheng A, Aronow WS: Cardiovascular drug therapy in the elderly. In Tresch DD, Aronow WS (eds): Cardiovascular Disease in the Elderly Patient, 2nd edn. Marcel Dekker, New York, 1999:739–768

169. Van Gelder IC, Tuinenburg AE, Schoonderwoerd BS et al: Pharmacologic versus direct-current cardioversion of atrial flutter and fibrillation. Am J Cardiol 1999;84:147R–151R

170. Orlando J, Del Vicario M, Aronow WS: High reversion of atrial flutter to sinus rhythm after atrial pacing in patients with pulmonary disease. Chest 1977;71:580–582

171. Mehta D, Baruch L: Thromboembolism following cardioversion of "common" atrial flutter: risk factors and limitations of transesophageal echocardiography. Chest 1996;110:1001–1003

172. Lanzarotti CJ, Olshansky B: Thromboembolism in chronic atrial flutter: is the risk underestimated? J Am Coll Cardiol 1997;30:1506–1511

173. Camm AJ, Garratt CJ: Adenosine and supraventricular tachycardia. N Engl J Med 1991;325:1621–1629

174. Winniford MD, Fulton KL, Hillis LD: Long-term therapy of paroxysmal supraventricular tachycardia: a randomized, double-blind comparison of digoxin, propranolol and verapamil. Am J Cardiol 1984;54:1138–1139

175. Ganz LI, Friedman PL: Supraventricular tachycardia. N Engl J Med 1995;332:162–173

176. Epstein LM, Chiesa N, Wong MN et al: Radiofrequency catheter ablation in the treatment of supraventricular tachycardia in the elderly. J Am Coll Cardiol 1994;23:1356–1362

177. Rosen KM: Junctional tachycardia: mechanisms, diagnosis, differential diagnosis, and management. Circulation 1973;47:654–664

178. Aronow WS: Management of supraventricular tachyarrhythmias. Compr Ther 1989;15(4):11–16

179. Hazard PB, Burnett CR: Verapamil in multifocal atrial tachycardia: hemodynamic and respiratory changes. Chest 1987;91:68–70

180. Aronow WS, Plascencia G, Wong R et al: Effect of verapamil versus placebo on PAT and MAT. Curr Ther Res 1980;27:823–829

181. Davies MJ, Pomerance A: Quantitative study of ageing changes in the human sinoatrial node and internodal tracts. Br Heart J 1972;34:150–152

182. Fujino M, Okada R, Arakawa K: The relationship of aging to histological changes in the conduction system of the normal heart. Jpn Heart J 1983;24:13–20

183. Aronow WS: Dizziness and syncope. In Hazzard WR, Blass JP, Ettinger WH, Halter JB, Ouslander JG (eds): Principles of Geriatric Medicine and Gerontology, 4th edn. McGraw-Hill, New York, 1998:1519–1534

184. Mercando AD: Bradyarrhythmias and cardiac pacemakers in the elderly. In Tresch DD, Aronow WS (eds): Cardiovascular Disease in the Elderly Patient, 2nd edn. Marcel Dekker, New York, 1999:599–615

Chapter 38

Syncope

Rose Anne Kenny and A. Ballav Dey

Syncope (from the Greek *syn*, "with" and the verb *koptein*, "to cut," or more appropriately in this case, "to interrupt") is a symptom defined as a transient, self-limited loss of consciousness, usually leading to falling. The onset of syncope is relatively rapid, and the subsequent recovery is spontaneous, complete, and usually prompt.[1–3]

The underlying mechanism is a transient global cerebral hypoperfusion. In some forms of syncope there may be a premonitory period in which various symptoms (e.g. light-headedness, nausea, sweating, weakness, and visual disturbances) offer warning of an impending syncopal event. Often, however, loss of consciousness occurs without warning. Recovery from syncope is usually accompanied by almost immediate restoration of appropriate behavior and orientation. Amnesia, although believed to be uncommon, may be more frequent than previously thought, particularly in older individuals. Sometimes the post-recovery period is marked by fatigue.

EPIDEMIOLOGY OF SYNCOPE

The epidemiology of syncope in old age has not been well studied. The greatest difficulty in assessing the magnitude of this problem is the overlap between syncope and falls. A substantial number of older subjects with syncope present with unexplained and recurrent falls. For example, nearly two-thirds of older patients with orthostatic hypotension,[4] and one-third of patients with carotid sinus syndrome,[5] present with falls and deny loss of consciousness. The reasons for this are amnesia for loss of consciousness[4,5] or falls caused by instability during hypotensive episodes. An accurate witness account of falls and syncope is not available in up to half of older patients.[6] A history from the patient may be unreliable, particularly if cognitive function is impaired or if the patient has amnesia for loss of consciousness. The problem is further complicated by the presence of multiple disorders that may synergistically cause syncope and by methodological difficulties in determining a relationship between circumstances, medications, and symptoms.

From available data, syncope accounts for 3 percent of emergency room attendances and 1 percent of medical admissions to a general hospital.[7] Syncope and collapse is the seventh-commonest reason for emergency admission of older patients.[8] Unexplained or nonaccidental falls (which include patients with syncope) were responsible for 15 percent of attendances to an A and E department of a total of almost 72,000 adults (over 50 years) screened.[6] In a study of 711 older subjects (mean age 87 years) living in a chronic care facility, the prevalence of syncope was reported to be 23 percent over a 10-year period with an annual incidence of 6 percent and recurrence rate of 30 percent, over a 2-year prospective follow-up.[9] This is undoubtedly an underestimate because falls were excluded.

In a study by Kapoor et al.[10] a cause of syncope could not be determined in 40 percent of patients among 210 community dwelling older subjects (mean age 71 years). Syncope due to a cardiac cause was associated with higher mortality rates irrespective of age. In patients with a noncardiac or unknown cause of syncope, older age, a history of congestive cardiac failure, and male sex were important prognostic factors of mortality. This study predated establishment of standardized tests for neurocardiogenic syncope and did not specifically investigate all patients for baroreflex abnormalities, namely carotid sinus syndrome, orthostatic hypotension, and vasovagal syncope. These conditions are responsible for a substantial proportion of unexplained syncope in older subjects. In more recent studies, syncope is unexplained in 10–20 percent.[11–13]

PATHOPHYSIOLOGY OF SYNCOPE IN ELDERLY PEOPLE

The temporary cessation of cerebral function that causes syncope results from transient and sudden reduction of blood flow to parts of the brain (brainstem reticular activating system) responsible for consciousness. Age related physiological impairments in heart rate, blood pressure, cerebral blood flow, in combination with comorbid conditions and concurrent medications account for the increased prevalence of syncope in the older person. Baroreflex sensitivity is blunted with aging, manifesting as a reduction in the heart rate response to hypotensive stimuli.[14,15] Older people are prone to reduced blood volume due to excessive salt wasting by the kidneys as a result of a decline in plasma renin and aldosterone,[16] a rise in atrial natriuretic peptide[17] and concurrent diuretic therapy. Low blood volume together with age-related diastolic dysfunction can lead to a low cardiac output which increases susceptibility to orthostatic hypotension and vasovagal syncope. Cerebral autoregulation which maintains a constant cerebral circulation over a wide range of blood pressure changes is altered in the presence of hypertension and possibly by aging.[14,15,18] Although a recent study has reported no age-related change in static or dynamic cerebral autoregulation in healthy elderly people and no differences in static or dynamic cerebral autoregulation in patients with recurrent vasovagal syncope.[19] In general it is agreed that sudden mild to moderate declines in blood pressure can affect cerebral blood flow markedly and render an older person particularly vulnerable to presyncope and syncope. Multiple age-related diseases and medications influencing circulation, together with age-related physiological alterations predispose as well as influence the outcome of syncope in older people.

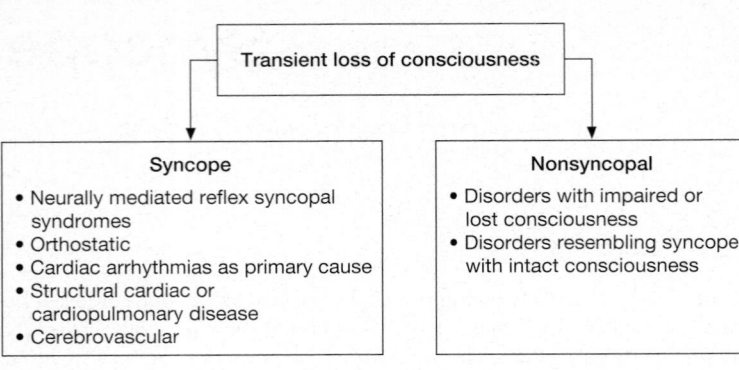

Figure 38-1 Initial investigation profile of patients with syncope (based on the recommendations from the European Cardiac Society Task Force on Syncope[180]).

ETIOLOGY

Syncope is a common symptom experienced by up to 30 percent of healthy adults at least once in their lifetime.[20,21] A wide variety of conditions, benign as well as life threatening, are causally related to syncope. An attributable cause of syncope can be identified by detailed history, examination, and specific laboratory investigations in most patients[22–24] (Fig. 38-1).

A subset of patients with recurrent syncope will remain undiagnosed despite extensive investigations, particularly older patients who have marginal cognitive impairment and for whom a witnessed account of events is often unavailable (40 percent).[5,12] Common causes of syncope are listed in Tables 38-1 to 38-3. Strict diagnostic criteria are essential for accurate diagnosis and management.

OVERLAP BETWEEN SYNCOPE AND FALLS

Syncope and falls are often considered as two separate entities with different etiologies. An overlap between syncope and falls has become increasingly evident.[4,12,25–27] In older adults, determining the cause of a fall may be difficult. Approximately 30 percent of cognitively normal older subjects fail to recall documented falls three months later[28] and up to half of syncopal episodes go unwitnessed.[12] Nearly 40 percent of patients with carotid sinus syndrome present with unexplained falls and deny loss of consciousness.[5] Amnesia for loss of consciousness has been observed in half of patients with carotid sinus syndrome who present with falls[27] and a quarter of all patients with carotid sinus syndrome, irrespective of presentation.[12] Amnesia for loss of consciousness in young adults has also been observed in syncope induced through a sequence of hyperventilation, orthostasis and Valsalva maneuver.[2] Falls are also associated with postprandial hypotension[29] and orthostatic hypotension,[4,12] suggesting that the phenomenon is generalized for cardiovascular syncope. More recent reports confirm a high incidence of falls in addition to traditional syncopal symptoms in older patients paced for sick sinus syndrome and atrioventricular conduction disorders.[30] Thus syncope and falls are often indistinguishable and in fact are manifestations of similar pathophysiological processes.

CAROTID SINUS SYNDROME

Carotid sinus syndrome (CSS) is an important but frequently overlooked cause of syncope and presyncope in older subjects.[31]

Episodic bradycardia and/or hypotension resulting from exaggerated baroreceptor-mediated reflexes or carotid sinus hypersensitivity (CSH) characterize the syndrome. The syndrome is diagnosed in subjects with unexplained symptoms, when 5–10 seconds of carotid sinus massage produces asystole exceeding 3 seconds (cardioinhibitory), or a fall in systolic blood pressure exceeding 50 mmHg in the absence of cardioinhibition (vasodepressor) or a combination of the two (mixed).[32,33] The first recognized case of carotid sinus syndrome was reported in 1930,[34] though slowing of the heart rate in response to carotid pressure was first published in 1799.[35] However, it was only in the 1920s that the anatomy and physiology of the carotid baroreflex were described in detail.[36]

Anatomy and physiology

The carotid sinus is the dilated portion of the internal carotid artery at the level of the carotid artery bifurcation.[37] The sinus wall is rich with elastic tissue. Sensory nerve endings emerge from the sinus as the carotid sinus nerve of Hering, before joining the glossopharyngeal nerve. Some of the fibers also join the vagus, hypoglossal, and cervical sympathetic nerves.[33] The afferent limb of the carotid sinus reflex terminates at the nucleus of the tractus solitarius in the medulla.[38] The efferent limb comprises the sympathetic nerves supplying the heart, vasculature, and the cardiac vagus nerve.[39] Sensory nerve endings in the walls of the carotid sinus respond to mechanical deformation with an increase in afferent traffic producing inhibition of sympathetic activity and stimulation of vagal activity. This results in hypotension and bradycardia.[39] Physiological rises in arterial blood pressure generate the stretch necessary to activate the reflex. In health, the carotid baroreceptors in conjunction with those of the aortic arch play a major role in the neural control of blood pressure.

Pathophysiology of carotid sinus syndrome

Baroreflex sensitivity, which normally declines with increasing age,[40] is enhanced in patients with carotid sinus syndrome compared with age-matched controls.[41] The exact site and mechanism for this hypersensitivity are not known. The lesion, theoretically, could lie within the carotid sinus itself, the afferent limb, central nucleus or efferent limbs of the reflex arc or even in the target organs, i.e., the heart and vasculature. Atherosclerotic change within the carotid sinus was considered as the cause of carotid sinus hypersensitivity[42] due to the

Table 38-1 Causes of syncope

Neurally mediated reflex syncopal syndromes
- Vasovagal faint (common faint)
- Carotid sinus syncope
- Situational faint
  - acute hemorrhage
  - cough, sneeze
  - gastrointestinal stimulation (swallow, defecation, visceral pain)
  - micturition (post-micturition)
  - post-exercise
  - others (e.g. brass instrument playing, weightlifting, postprandial)
  - Glossopharyngeal and trigeminal neuralgia

Orthostatic
- Autonomic failure
  - Primary autonomic failure syndromes (e.g. pure autonomic failure, multiple system atrophy, Parkinson's disease with autonomic failure)
  - Secondary autonomic failure syndromes (e.g. diabetic neuropathy, amyloid neuropathy)
  - Drugs and alcohol
- Volume depletion
  - Hemorrhage, diarrhea, Addison's disease

Cardiac arrhythmias as primary cause
- Sinus node dysfunction (including bradycardia/tachycardia syndrome)
- Atrioventricular conduction system disease
- Paroxysmal supraventricular and ventricular tachycardias
- Inherited syndromes (e.g. long QT syndrome, Brugada syndrome)
- Implanted device (pacemaker, ICD) malfunction, drug-induced proarrhythmias

Structural cardiac or cardiopulmonary disease
- Cardiac valvular disease
- Acute myocardial infarction/ischemia
- Obstructive cardiomyopathy
- Atrial myxoma
- Acute aortic dissection
- Pericardial disease/tamponade
- Pulmonary embolus/pulmonary hypertension

Cerebrovascular
- Vascular steal syndromes

Reproduced from Brignole et al.[180]

Table 38-2 Causes of nonsyncopal attacks

Disorders with impairment or loss of consciousness
- Metabolic disorders,[a] including hypoglycemia, hypoxia, hyperventilation with hypocapnia
- Epilepsy
- Intoxications
- Vertebrobasilar transient ischemic attack

Disorders resembling syncope without loss of consciousness
- Cataplexy
- Drop attacks
- Psychogenic "syncope" (somatization disorders)[b]

[a]*Syncope probably secondary to metabolic effects on cerebrovascular tone.*

[b]*May also include hysteria, conversion reaction.*

Reproduced from Brignole et al.[180]

Table 38-3 Disorders commonly misdiagnosed as syncope

- Transient ischemic attacks (TIA) of carotid origin
- Hypoglycemia
- Some forms of epilepsy
- Drop attacks
- Alcohol intoxication
- Drug-related cerebral states

Reproduced from Brignole et al.[180]

frequent association of the syndrome with cardiovascular disease. A higher incidence of bilateral atherosclerotic changes in the carotid arteries of patients with carotid sinus syndrome was observed using doppler ultrasonography, compared with controls matched for atherosclerotic risk factors.[43] The frequent occurrence of carotid sinus hypersensitivity in the presence of neck pathology supported this theory. However, the occurrence of symptoms which are not triggered by head movement,[44] the frequent overlap with vasovagal syncope, dissociation of cardioinhibition and vasodepression in many patients, and the normal release of arginine vasopressin during hypotension (for which intact afferent connections to the hypothalamus are essential) in patients with the syndrome[45] argue against this hypothesis. The efferent limb of the reflex arc, i.e., the vagus nerve, is responsible for the heart rate slowing response during carotid sinus massage.[46] Vagally mediated depression of sinoatrial automaticity and sinoatrial block lead to sinoatrial arrest and asystole.[47] Atropine in a dose of 400 µg can abolish bradycardia in 80 percent of subjects, whereas 700 µg will abolish the response in all patients.[48] Complete atrioventricular block may also occur and is reported to coexist with sinus arrest in up to 70 percent of patients.[31] Carotid sinus syndrome and sick sinus syndrome are two separate diagnostic entities, although up to 5 percent of patients with carotid sinus syndrome can have abnormal intrinsic sinus node function.[49] Conversely, a proportion of patients with sick sinus syndrome have altered autonomic tone.[50] It is possible that carotid sinus syndrome results from a central abnormality of baroreflex gain.[51] The frequent association of carotid sinus syndrome with atherosclerotic comorbidities has led to speculation that ischemia may play an important role in its pathogenesis.[52] Myocardial ischemia causing activation of vagal afferents capable of influencing central baroreflex pathways or ischemia at brainstem level may result in abnormalities of neurotransmitter function.[53] A recent hypothesis suggests upregulation of central post-synaptic alpha-2 adrenoceptors as the primary abnormality in carotid sinus hypersensitivity, but work from our group has shown that this is not the case[54] the pathophysiology remains elusive.

Prevalence of carotid sinus hypersensitivity and carotid sinus syndrome

The prevalence of carotid sinus reflex hypersensitivity in asymptomatic individuals is not known. However, it definitely increases with age and is rare in patients with syncope who are aged less than 50 years.[55] Early reports suggested that 10 percent of the healthy aged population have carotid sinus reflex hypersensitivity and that the prevalence was even higher in the presence of coronary artery disease or hypertension.[56–59] Such studies predated the standardization of diagnostic criteria for reflex hypersensitivity and involved long periods of carotid sinus massage, leading to skepticism regarding the existence of carotid sinus syndrome as a disease entity rather than an epiphenomenon for atherosclerotic vascular disease. However, recent studies suggest that it is not a feature of normal aging.[60] In a study of 25 healthy older subjects, none developed diagnostic or symptomatic cardioinhibition or vasodepression during carotid sinus massage.[60] In another series, abnormal cardioinhibition has been reported in 2 percent of 288 healthy subjects (age range 17–84 years).[61] Carotid sinus hypersensitivity was demonstrated in 19 percent of 538 patients (age > 50 years) who presented to an accident and emergency department of an inner city university hospital with unexplained falls, the prevalence increased to 21 percent among fallers aged more than 65 years. Abnormal responses to carotid sinus massage are more likely to be observed in asymptomatic individuals with coronary artery disease[52] and those on vasoactive drugs known to influence reflex sensitivity (digoxin, beta blockers, and alpha methyl dopa).[62–64] The prevalence of drug induced carotid sinus hypersensitivity among older fallers was 11 percent.[65] Though it was generally considered as a very rare condition (only 1 in a series of 204 syncopal patients),[66] referral centers which routinely perform carotid sinus massage in all older patients presenting with syncope diagnose carotid sinus syndrome in 20–45 percent.[13,67]

Carotid sinus massage

Carotid sinus reflex sensitivity is assessed by measuring heart rate and blood pressure responses to carotid sinus massage. In normal subjects, carotid sinus massage induces both cardioinhibition as well as vasodepression. In a study of 25 healthy older subjects, cardioinhibition of 1,038 ($\pm$195) milliseconds and vasodepression of 21 ($\pm$14) mmHg was observed following 5 seconds of carotid sinus massage.[60] No subject developed diagnostic cardioinhibition or vasodepression when supine, though 12 percent of subjects had asymptomatic vasodepression of more than 50 mmHg during upright carotid sinus massage. Cardioinhibition and vasodepression were more marked on right-sided carotid sinus massage and there was no fixed relationship between rate of heart rate slowing and fall in blood pressure. In patients with cardioinhibitory carotid sinus syndrome, over 70 percent have a positive response to right-sided carotid sinus massage either alone or in combination with left-sided carotid sinus massage.[44]

Carotid sinus massage is a crude and unquantifiable technique and is prone to intra- as well as interobserver variation. More scientific diagnostic methods using neck chamber suction[41] or drug-induced changes in blood pressure[40] can be used for carotid baroreceptor activation, but are not suitable for routine use. The recommended duration of carotid sinus massage is from 5 to 10 seconds.[68] The maximum fall in heart rate usually occurs within 5 seconds of the onset of massage.[33,51]

Complications resulting from carotid sinus massage include cardiac arrhythmias and neurological sequelae.[69–71] Fatal arrhythmias, both asystolic and ventricular, are extremely uncommon and have generally occurred in patients with underlying heart disease undergoing therapeutic rather than diagnostic massage.[69,72] Digoxin toxicity has been implicated in most cases of ventricular fibrillation.[73] Neurological complications are thought to result from either occlusion of or embolization from the carotid artery. Several authors have reported cases of hemiplegia following carotid sinus stimulation, often in the absence of hemodynamic changes.[71] Complications from carotid sinus massage, however, are extremely uncommon (0.14%).[74] Only 12 patients, in a retrospective analysis[75] of 16,000 instances of carotid sinus massage, developed neurological complications, which resolved within 24 hours in eight patients and within 1 week in two patients. Neurological deficits persisted in two patients. Serious ventricular arrhythmias were never encountered. Complications were immediate and in two-thirds of occasions followed a vasodepressor response to carotid sinus massage. Carotid doppler studies in these cases did not reveal significant carotid obstruction compared to age-matched controls. It was not possible to predict either from clinical characteristics or from doppler findings those who developed neurological sequelae.

It has been suggested that carotid sinus massage should not be performed in patients with known cerebrovascular disease or carotid bruits unless there is a strong indication. We do not use the presence of a carotid bruit as a contraindication and this practice has not adversely affected or complicated rates.[33] It should also be avoided immediately following myocardial infarction when reflex sensitivity may be increased.[51] It is prudent to rest patients for at least 10 minutes if there is a significant hypotensive response during the stimulus before standing them up for other tests.

In another prospective series of 1,000 consecutive cases, no patient had cardiac complications and 1 percent had possible neurological complications which resolved in most cases. Persistent neurological complications were uncommon, occurring in 0.4 percent.[76]

Diagnostic criteria for carotid sinus syndrome

Carotid sinus syndrome should be diagnosed when carotid sinus hypersensitivity is documented in a patient with otherwise unexplained syncope and in whom carotid sinus massage reproduces symptoms.[33] Three subtypes of carotid sinus hypersensitivity or of carotid sinus syndrome are currently recognized. The cardioinhibitory subtype is diagnosed if carotid sinus massage produces asystole exceeding 3 seconds, the vasodepressor subtype if there is a fall in systolic blood pressure exceeding 50 mmHg in the absence of significant cardioinhibition (or 30 mmHg in the presence of symptoms) and a mixed subtype if both responses are present.[32,33,46] The independent vasodepressor response can be confirmed by repeating carotid sinus massage after abolishing significant cardioinhibition using either atrio-ventricular sequential pacing or intravenous atropine.[46,77] Asystole exceeding 1.5 seconds should be regarded as "significant" in this regard. The frequency of each of the subtypes is similar. In a series of 64 consecutive cases with carotid sinus syndrome, a third each had cardioinhibitory, vasodepressor, and mixed responses.[43] A cerebral subtype has been described in which facial pallor and symptoms of cerebral hypoperfusion occurred during massage in the absence of any hemodynamic change.[78] These changes were attributed to reflex cerebral vasoconstriction. In our experience this subtype is rare if indeed it exists. Lown[72] showed that such symptoms develop as a result of carotid occlusion in the presence of contralateral carotid disease, and the existence of the cerebral subtype has since been largely discredited.

Symptom reproduction during carotid sinus massage was regarded by early investigators as essential in the diagnosis of carotid sinus syndrome,[33] but is not always justified in patients with reproducibly abnormal responses.[51,73] Spontaneous symptoms usually occur in the upright position.[33] So it is still worth repeating the procedure with the patient upright, even after demonstrating a positive response when supine. This aids in attributing a diagnosis with reproduction of symptoms, especially in patients with unexplained falls who deny loss of consciousness and have carotid sinus hypersensitivity.

Clinical characteristics

Carotid sinus syndrome is virtually unknown before the age of 50 and its incidence increases with age thereafter.[79] Males are more commonly affected and the majority have either coronary artery disease or hypertension.[80] The symptoms are usually precipitated by mechanical stimulation of the carotid sinus; i.e., by head turning, tight neckwear, neck pathology and by vagal stimuli such as prolonged standing.[33,44] Other recognized triggers for symptoms are postprandial state, straining, looking or stretching upwards, exertion, defecation, and micturition. In a significant number of patients no triggering event can be identified.[80] Abnormal response to carotid sinus massage may not always be reproducible necessitating repetition of the procedure if the diagnosis is strongly suspected.

Carotid sinus hypersensitivity is frequently associated with other hypotensive disorders such as vasovagal syncope and orthostatic hypotension,[44] indicating a common pathogenetic process. Overlap of hypotensive disorders can make attributable diagnosis more difficult. However, every attempt must be made to make an attributable diagnosis as interventions may vary and methods for assessment of response depend on the initial diagnosis. Carotid sinus syndrome is associated with appreciable morbidity. Approximately half of patients may sustain an injury during symptomatic episodes; fractures (especially of femoral neck) were sustained by 25 percent.[44] In a prospective study of falls in nursing home residents, a three-fold increase in the fracture rate in those with carotid sinus hypersensitivity was observed.[81] Indeed, carotid sinus hypersensitivity can be considered as a modifiable risk factor for fractures of the femoral neck.[82] Carotid sinus syndrome is not associated with an increased risk of death. The mortality rate in patients with the syndrome is similar to that of patients with unexplained syncope and the general population matched for age and sex.[83] Mortality rates are similar for the three subtypes of the syndrome.[83]

When the characteristics of patients with a cardioinhibitory response who presented with drop attacks and those who presented with syncope were compared, the drop attack group were more likely to be female, have more frequent episodes, and a shorter time period, and of those who lost consciousness during carotid massage, 95 percent of the drop attack group had amnesia for this compared with 20 percent of syncopal patients.[84]

Natural history

The natural history of CSH or CSS has not been well investigated. In one study, the majority (90 percent) of subjects with abnormal hemodynamic responses (CSH) but without syncopal symptoms, remained symptom free during a follow-up over 19 ± 16 months, while half of those who presented with syncope had symptom recurrence.[85] Similar observations were made in another study where 57 percent of patients with CSS were randomized to a nontreatment protocol during an average follow-up of 36 months.[86]

Treatment

No treatment is necessary in subjects with asymptomatic carotid sinus hypersensitivity. However, there is no consensus on the timing of therapeutic intervention in the presence of symptoms. Considering the high rate of injury in symptomatic episodes as well as low recurrence rate of symptoms, it is prudent to treat all patients with a history of two or more symptomatic episodes. The need for intervention in those with a solitary event should be assessed on an individual basis, taking into consideration the severity of the event and the patient's lifestyle.[79]

Treatment strategies in the past included carotid sinus denervation achieved either surgically or by radio-ablation.[87,88] Success rates with radio-ablation were variable and the procedure has largely been abandoned. Surgical denervation has been reported to relieve symptoms in approximately two-thirds of patients,[33] but is not without risk of postoperative orthostatic hypotension and hypertensive crises.[87,89] Denervation surgery is still occasionally considered in patients with coexisting neck pathology[90] or with vasodepression resistant to drug therapy.[91]

The treatment of patients with cardioinhibition has largely been superseded by newer treatment modalities. Cardioinhibition can be treated with anticholinergic agents such as atropine and propantheline bromide and some benefit has been reported.[92] However, frequent cholinergic adverse effects, particularly in older people, limit this treatment option.

Cardiac pacing, first used nearly a quarter of a century ago, is currently the treatment of choice in patients with symptomatic cardioinhibitory carotid sinus syndrome. Atrial pacing is contraindicated in view of the high prevalence of both sinoatrial and atrioventricular block in patients with carotid sinus hypersensitivity.[51] Ventricular pacing abolishes cardioinhibition but fails to alleviate symptoms in a significant number of patients. Such symptoms result from either aggravation of a coexisting vasodepressor response or the development of pacemaker-induced hypotension (pacemaker syndrome).[49] The latter occurs when ventriculoatrial conduction is intact and this is so for up to 80 percent of patients with the syndrome.[51] Atrioventricular sequential pacing is the treatment of choice for patients with symptomatic cardioinhibition.

Dual-chamber pacing has been shown to result in significantly less vasodepression than ventricular pacing during both supine and upright carotid sinus massage.[93] Moreover, with maintenance of atrioventricular synchrony, there is no risk of pacemaker syndrome. Randomized double-blind studies have demonstrated that a substantial number of patients prefer atrioventricular pacing.[94,95] Both dual sensing dual pacing inhibition (DDI) and dual sensing dual pacing inhibition and triggering (DDD) pacing modes have been widely used; DDD pacing carries a theoretical risk of inducing endless loop tachycardia but this has rarely been encountered.[79] With appropriate pacing, syncope is abolished in 85–90 percent of patients with cardioinhibition.[51,82]

In a recent report of cardiac pacing in older fallers (mean age 74 years) who had cardioinhibitory CSH (CICSH),[6] subsequent falls during 1 year of follow-up were reduced by two-thirds in patients who received dual chamber systems (Table 38-4). Subsequent syncopal episodes were much less frequent in participants overall but were also reduced by half.[6] It was concluded that patients with nonaccidental falls—either single or recurrent events—who have cardioinhibitory CSS, benefit from cardiac pacing. The series was too small to determine any benefit in fracture rates but injurious episodes were reduced by three-quarters. We postulate two explanations for this effect. The first is that older patients with CICSH have amnesia for loss of consciousness and only recall falling—this has been confirmed in up to a third of induced syncopal episodes during upright CSM. The second is that moderate hypotension, caused by significant reduction in heart rate, causes the older person to fall. Over half of the patients in the aforementioned series had gait abnormalities and three-quarters had balance abnormalities which would render individuals more susceptible to falls under such hemodynamic circumstances. The implications of this paper are far reaching in that falls and syncope are the commonest reason for adults to attend the emergency room—15 percent of falls are "nonaccidental," i.e., no apparent medical or accidental explanation for the event, and of these people almost 20 percent have CICSH, increasing to 30 percent in those over 70.

Treatment of vasodepressor carotid sinus syndrome is less successful due to poor understanding of its pathophysiology. Ephedrine has been reported to be useful,[96] but long-term use is limited by side-effects. Dihydroergotamine is effective but poorly tolerated.[97] Fludrocortisone, a mineralocorticoid widely used in the treatment of orthostatic hypotension, is used in the treatment of vasodepressor carotid sinus syndrome with good results but its use is limited in the longer term by adverse effects.[98] The medical treatment of vasodepressor carotid sinus syndrome remains unsatisfactory.

ORTHOSTATIC HYPOTENSION

Orthostatic or postural hypotension is arbitrarily defined as either a 20 mmHg fall in systolic blood pressure or a 10 mmHg fall in diastolic blood pressure on assuming an upright posture from a supine position.[99] Orthostatic hypotension implies abnormal blood pressure homeostasis and is a frequent observation with advancing age. Prevalence of postural hypotension varies between 4 percent[6] and 33 percent[100] among community-living older persons, depending on the methodology used. Higher prevalence and larger falls in systolic blood pressure have been reported with increasing age,[101] and often signify general physical frailty. Orthostatic hypotension is reported to be associated with excessive mortality.[102]

Physiology of orthostasis

Orthostasis is a physiological stress related to upright posture. On standing, the force of gravity in the vertical axis causes venous pooling in the lower limbs, a sharp decline in venous return and reduction in filling pressure of the heart which increase further on prolonged standing due to shifting of water to interstitial spaces and hemoconcentration.[103] These mechanical events can cause a marked reduction in cardiac output and consequent fall in arterial blood pressure. However, in normal people, cardiac output and blood pressure are maintained by powerful compensatory mechanisms involving a rise in heart rate.[104] Consequently the fall in stroke volume is compensated for and cardiac output declines only slightly. Blood pressure is maintained by a rise in peripheral resistance. These compensatory phenomena are initiated by the baroreceptors located at the aortic arch and carotid bifurcation. The baro-receptor input to brainstem centers leads to inhibition of cardiac vagal control, stimulation of sympathetic ganglia and release of noradrenaline from sympathetic nerve endings. Noradrenaline has a positive chronotropic and inotropic effect on the heart and also causes venous and arteriolar vasoconstriction.[105] Thus the compensatory response to orthostasis involves stimulation of the sympathetic nervous system and inhibition of the parasympathetic nervous system, and reflects the integrity of the total arterial baroreflex arc. Orthostatic hypotension results from failure of the arterial baroreflex, most commonly due to disorders of the autonomic nervous system.[106]

Aging and orthostasis

The heart rate and blood pressure responses to orthostasis occur in three phases: an initial heart rate and blood pressure response, an early phase of stabilization and a phase of prolonged standing; all are influenced by aging.[107–110] The maximum rise in heart rate and the ratio between the maximum and the minimum heart rate in the initial phase decline with age, implying a relatively fixed heart rate irrespective of

Table 38-4 Outcome during 1 year of follow-up in patients with carotid sinus syndrome who presented with falls

Outcome	Study participants	
	Control	Pacemaker
Falls	699	216
Syncope	47	22
Injury	198	58
Fracture	4	3
		(O.R. 0.42 CI 0.23–0.75)

Data from: Kenny and Richardson.[6]

posture.[108–110] Despite a blunted heart rate response, blood pressure and cardiac output are adequately maintained on standing in active, healthy, well hydrated, and normotensive older subjects.[109] The underlying mechanism involves decreased vasodilatation and reduced venous pooling during the initial phases and increased peripheral vascular resistance after prolonged standing. However, in older subjects with hypertension and cardiovascular disease receiving vaso-active drugs, these circulatory adjustments to orthostatic stress are disturbed, rendering them vulnerable to postural hypotension.[111]

Hypertension and orthostatic hypotension

Aging is associated with an increased risk for hypertension as well as hypotension. Hypertension itself increases the risk of hypotension by impairing baroreflex sensitivity and reducing ventricular compliance.[112,113] A strong relationship between supine hypertension and orthostatic hypotension has been reported amongst unmedicated institutionalized older subjects.[114] Hypertension increases the risk of cerebral ischemia from sudden declines in blood pressure. Older hypertensives are more vulnerable to cerebral ischemic symptoms even with modest and short-term postural hypotension, because the threshold for cerebral autoregulation is altered by prolonged elevation of blood pressure.[18] In addition, antihypertensive agents impair cardiovascular reflexes and further increase the risk of orthostatic hypotension.

Etiology of orthostatic hypotension

Several pathological conditions are associated with orthostatic hypotension. Autonomic failure[115] and drugs[116] are important causes of orthostatic hypotension. Ideally establishing a causal relationship between a drug and orthostatic hypotension requires identification of the culprit medicine, abolition of symptoms by withdrawal of the drug, and rechallenge of the drug to reproduce symptoms.[117] Rechallenge is an important step in the diagnosis but often omitted in clinical practice in view of the potential serious consequences. In the presence of polypharmacy, which is so common in older people, it becomes difficult to identify the culprit drug because of the synergistic effect of different drugs and drug interactions.[116] A number of non-neurogenic conditions are also associated with postural hypotension. They include myocarditis, atrial myxoma, aortic stenosis, constrictive pericarditis, hemorrhage, diarrhea, vomiting, ileostomy, burns, hemodialysis, salt-losing nephropathy, diabetes insipidus, adrenal insufficiency, fever, and extensive varicose veins.

Primary autonomic failure syndromes

These are three distinct clinical entities, namely: pure autonomic failure (PAF), multiple system atrophy (MSA) or Shy–Drager syndrome (SDS), and autonomic failure associated with idiopathic Parkinson's disease (IPD). PAF, the least common and a relatively benign entity, was previously known as idiopathic orthostatic hypotension. This condition presents with orthostatic hypotension, defective sweating, impotence, and bowel disturbances. No other neurological deficits are found, and resting plasma noradrenaline levels are low. MSA is the commonest of all and carries the poorest prognosis. Clinical manifestations include features of dysautonomia and motor disturbances due to striatonigral degeneration, cerebellar atrophy or pyramidal lesions. Additional neurological deficits include muscle atrophy, distal sensorimotor neuropathy, pupillary abnormalities, restriction of ocular movements, disturbances in rhythm and control of breathing, life-threatening laryngeal stridor and bladder disturbances. Psychiatric manifestations and cognitive defects are usually absent. Resting plasma noradrenaline levels are usually within the normal range but fail to rise on standing or tilting. The prevalence of autonomic failure in Parkinson's disease is not precisely known. Cerebellar and pyramidal signs are not seen. Orthostatic hypotension in Parkinson's disease can be due to factors other than dysautonomia, e.g., side-effects of anti-Parkinsonian drugs (levodopa, bromocriptine), accompanying effects of aging, autonomic neuropathy complicating coexisting diabetes mellitus, side-effects of drug therapy for other coexisting diseases (vasodilators for hypertension, alpha adrenergic antagonists for benign prostatic hypertrophy) and confusion with early MSA with predominant Parkinsonian features.[115]

Secondary autonomic dysfunction

Availability of sensitive tests of autonomic function has led to the identification of autonomic nervous system involvement in several systemic diseases. A large number of neurological disorders are also complicated by autonomic dysfunction which may involve several organs leading to a variety of symptoms in addition to orthostatic hypotension, namely: anhidrosis, constipation, diarrhea, impotence, retention of urine, urinary incontinence, stridor, apneic episodes, and Horner's syndrome. Important among them are multiple sclerosis, brainstem lesions, compressive and noncompressive spinal cord lesions, demyelinating polyneuropathies (Guillain–Barré syndrome), diabetic polyneuropathy, chronic renal failure, chronic liver disease, and connective tissue disorders.[115] In the absence of well-recognized conditions causing primary and secondary autonomic failure, aging can also be considered as a cause of autonomic failure.

Manifestations of orthostatic hypotension

The clinical manifestations of orthostatic hypotension are due to hypoperfusion of the brain and other organs. Depending on the degree of fall in blood pressure and cerebral hypoperfusion, symptoms can vary from dizziness to syncope associated with a variety of visual defects, from blurred vision to blackout.[118] Other reported ischemic symptoms of orthostatic hypotension are nonspecific lethargy and weakness, suboccipital and paravertebral muscle pain, low-back ache, calf claudication and angina.[118,119] Several precipitating factors for orthostatic hypotension have been identified; speed of positional change, prolonged recumbency, warm environment, raised intrathoracic pressure (coughing, defecation, micturition), physical exertion, and vasoactive drugs.

Orthostatic hypotension is an important cause of syncope accounting for 14 percent of all diagnosed cases in a large series on syncope. In a tertiary referral clinic dealing with unexplained syncope, dizziness, and falls, 32 percent of patients (age > 65 years) had orthostatic hypotension.[12] Irrespective of symptoms, orthostatic hypotension increases the risk of falls in older patients. Nineteen percent of older fallers attending an accident and emergency department had a diagnosis of orthostatic hypotension.[27] Orthostatic hypotension was the cause of "drop attacks" in 15 percent of 35 older patients (age > 50 years) and probably contributed to unexplained falls in a similar proportion of patients.[11] The diagnosis of orthostatic hypotension involves a demonstration of a postural fall in blood pressure after active standing. Reproducibility of orthostatic hypotension depends on the time of measurement and on autonomic function.[4] The diagnosis may be missed on casual measurement during the afternoon. The procedure should be repeated during the morning after maintaining supine posture for an adequate period (10 minutes). Sphygmomanometer measurement is as sensitive as sophisticated phasic blood pressure measurements and active standing is as diagnostic as head-up tilting.[4] In patients with unexplained syncope or falls, an attributable diagnosis of orthostatic hypotension depends on reproduction of symptoms.

Management of orthostatic hypotension

The goal of therapy for symptomatic orthostatic hypotension is to improve cerebral perfusion. There are several nonpharmacological interventions for orthostatic hypotension which include avoidance of precipitating factors for low blood pressure, elevation of the head of the bed at night[120] and application of graduated pressure from a support garment to the lower limbs to reduce venous pooling. There are reports to suggest benefit from implantation of cardiac pacemakers, in a small number of patients, by increasing heart rate during postural change.[121] However, the effects of tachypacing on improving cardiac output in patients with maximal vasodilatation remains conjectural. A large number of drugs have been used to raise blood pressure in orthostatic hypotension, including fludrocortisone, midodrine, ephedrine, desmopressin (DDAVP), octeotride, erythropoietin, nonsteroidal anti-inflammatory agents, and others. Fludrocortisone (9-alpha fluhydrocortisone) in a dose of 0.1–0.2 mg causes volume expansion, reduces natriuresis, and sensitizes alpha adrenoceptors to noradrenaline. In older people, the drug is poorly tolerated in larger doses and for long periods. Reported adverse effects in the older person include hypertension, cardiac failure, depression, edema, and hypokalemia.[122] Midodrine is a directly acting sympathomimetic vasoconstrictor of resistance vessels. Treatment is started at a dose of 2.5 mg three times daily and requires gradual titration to a maximum dose of 45 mg/day. The adverse effects include pilomotor erection, gastrointestinal symptoms, cardiovascular and central nervous system toxicity. Side-effects are usually controlled by dose reduction. Midodrine is comparable in its efficacy with other sympathomimetic agents but better tolerated. Midodrine is an effective and well-tolerated treatment for moderate to severe orthostatic hypotension.[123] It significantly increased standing blood pressure and improved symptoms of orthostatic hypotension. Side-effects were mostly mild and only 7 percent of patients discontinue treatment due to supine hypertension. DDAVP has potent antidiuretic and mild pressor effects. Intranasal doses of 5–40 μg at bedtime are useful. Side-effects include water retention. This agent can be combined with fludrocortisone with synergistic effect. The drug treatment for orthostatic hypotension requires frequent monitoring for supine hypertension, electrolyte imbalance, and congestive heart failure.

VASOVAGAL SYNCOPE
Clinical characteristics

The hallmark of vasovagal syncope is hypotension and/or bradycardia sufficiently profound to produce cerebral ischemia and loss of neural function. Vasovagal syncope has been classified into cardioinhibitory (bradycardia), vasodepressor (hypotension), and mixed (both) subtypes depending on the blood pressure and heart rate response.[124] In most patients, the manifestations occur in three distinct phases: a prodrome or aura, loss of consciousness and post-syncopal phase.[125] A precipitating factor or situation is identifiable in most patients which include extreme emotional stress, anxiety, mental anguish, trauma, physical pain, or anticipation of physical pain (e.g., anticipation of venesection), sight of blood, accident, warm environment, air travel, and prolonged standing. The commonest triggers in older individuals are prolonged standing and vasodilator medication.[12] In the authors' experience, drug-induced syncope in older adults is as often due to vasovagal syncope as orthostatic hypotension. Some patients experience symptoms in specific situations, namely micturition, defecation, and coughing. Prodromal symptoms include extreme fatigue, weakness, diaphoresis, nausea, visual defects, visual and auditory hallucinations, dizziness, vertigo, headache, abdominal discomfort, dysarthria, and paresthesias. The duration of prodrome varies greatly from seconds to several minutes, during which some patients take actions such as lying down to avoid an episode. The syncopal period is usually brief, during which some patients develop involuntary movements, usually myoclonic jerks, but tonic clonic movements also occur. Vasovagal syncope can masquerade as epilepsy.[126] Recovery is usually rapid but some patients can experience protracted symptoms such as confusion, disorientation, nausea, headache, dizziness, and a general sense of ill-health.

Pathophysiology of vasovagal syncope

The normal physiological responses to orthostasis, as described earlier, are an increase in heart rate, rise in peripheral vascular resistance (increase in diastolic blood pressure) and minimal decline in systolic blood pressure, to maintain an adequate cardiac output. In patients with vasovagal syncope, these responses to prolonged orthostasis are paradoxical. The precise sequence of events leading to vasovagal syncope are not fully understood. The possible mechanism involves a sudden fall in venous return to heart, rapid fall in ventricular volume and virtual collapse of the ventricle due to vigorous ventricular contraction.[127,128] The net result of these events is stimulation of ventricular mechanoreceptors and activation of Bezold–Jarisch reflex leading to peripheral vasodilatation (hypotension) and bradycardia.[128] Negative inotropic agents (beta blockers, disopyramide) can avert or diminish these responses in spontaneous or head-up tilt-induced vasovagal syncope.[128] Several neurotransmitters, namely serotonin, endorphins, and arginine vasopressin play an important role in the pathogenesis of vasovagal syncope, possibly by central sympathetic inhibition, although their exact role is not yet well understood.

Healthy older subjects are not particularly prone to vasovagal syncope compared to younger adults. Due to an age-related decline in baroreceptor sensitivity, the paradoxical responses to orthostasis (as in vasovagal syncope) are possibly less marked in older subjects. Thus situational syncope are less common in old age. However, in the presence of hypertension and atherosclerotic cerebrovascular disease, excessive loss of baroreflex sensitivity leads to dysautonomic responses during prolonged orthostasis (in which blood pressure and heart decline steadily over time) and patients become susceptible to vasovagal syncope. Diuretic or age-related contraction of blood volume further increases the risk of syncope.

Diagnosis

Several methods have evolved to determine an individual's susceptibility to vasovagal syncope such as Valsalva maneuvers, hyperventilation, ocular compression, and immersion of the face in cold water. However, these methods are poorly reproducible and lack correlation with clinical events. Using the strong orthostatic stimulus of head-upright tilting, maximal venous pooling and reflex vasovagal syncope can be reproduced in a susceptible individual. Head-up tilting as a diagnostic tool was first reported in 1986[129] and since then validity of this technique to identify susceptibility to neurocardiogenic syncope has been established.[31, 130–133] A classification of vasovagal responses to head-up tilting has been suggested by some investigators as follows:[124]

Type 1. *Mixed*: Heart rate rises on head-up tilting and later falls at the time of syncope with ventricular rate 40 beats per minute or less for less than 10 seconds with or without asystole for 3 seconds. Blood pressure may rise initially with tilting but then falls before the heart rate falls.

Type 2a. *Cardioinhibitory*: Heart rate rises on head-up tilting and then falls at the time of syncope with ventricular rate less than 40 beats per minute for more than 10 seconds or asystole occurs for more than 3 seconds. Blood pressure may rise initially with tilting but then falls before the heart rate falls.

Type 2b. *Cardioinhibitory*: Heart rate rises on head-up tilting and then falls at the time of syncope with ventricular rate less than 40 beats per minute for more than 10 seconds or asystole occurs for more than 3 seconds. Blood pressure may rise initially with tilting but only falls to hypotensive levels (less than 80 mmHg systolic) at or after the onset of rapid and severe heart rate fall as defined above.

Type 3. *Pure vasodepressor*: Heart rate rises progressively after adoption of the head-up position and does not fall more than 10 percent from its peak at the time of syncope. Blood pressure falls during tilt to cause syncope.

There are a few exceptions to these criteria:

1. Chronotropic incompetence: no heart rate rise during head-up tilting, possibly due to underlying sinoatrial disease.
2. Excessive heart rate rise, both at the onset and throughout the head-up tilt (>130 bpm), can be associated with types 1–3 due to different pathophysiology.
3. Association of carotid sinus hypersensitivity with any of the subtypes.

A modification of this classification has been proposed by Brignole's group who describe hemodynamic changes during classical vasovagal syncope (with passive tilt and glyceryl trinitrate (GTN) tilt) and dysautonomic responses which were more common in older persons, and orthostatic responses which occurred early during the tilt sequence.[134]

The sensitivity of head-up tilting can be further improved by provocative agents which accentuate the physiological events leading to vasovagal syncope. The most widely used agent is intravenous isoprenaline, which enhances myocardial contractility by stimulating beta adrenoreceptors. Isoprenaline is infused, prior to head-up tilting, at a dose of 1 µg per minute and gradually increased to a maximum dose of 3 µg per minute to achieve a heart rate increase of 25 percent.[135,136] Though the sensitivity of head-up tilt testing improves by about 15 percent,[137] the specificity is reduced.[138,139] In addition, as a result of the decline in beta receptor sensitivity with age, isoprenaline may be less useful as a provocative agent in elderly patients with a higher incidence of adverse effects.[50] The other agent which can be used as a provocative agent is nitroglycerin, which by reducing venous return due to vasodilatation can enhance the vasovagal reaction in susceptible individuals. The drug can be used by intravenous infusion[140] but more conveniently sublingually[141,142] with improved sensitivity and reduced period of tilting. The positivity of head-up tilting can also be improved by intravenous cannulation,[60] providing useful provocative stimulus without any adverse effects. GTN provocation during head-up tilt testing is preferable to other provocative tests in older patients: the event profile is less, the duration of testing less, and sensitivity and specificity are better than for isoprenaline.[143]

The precise sensitivity of head-up tilting is difficult to determine as no gold standard is available for comparison. However, the estimated sensitivity of head-up tilting in various reports is between 30 and 80 percent.[144–146] Vasovagal syncope can be produced by head-up tilting in less than 10 percent of healthy elderly subjects.[147,148] Healthy young subjects are more likely to experience syncope compared to older controls reflecting declining baroreflex sensitivity in old age.[146] Specificity of head-up tilting must be considered with the fact that vasovagal syncope results from a normal (though exaggerated) reflex response which can be induced in most individuals with proper conditioning. Therefore it must be recognized that in the absence of recurrent and unexplained syncopal symptoms, the value of positive head-up tilt is limited. Head-up tilt testing has a symptomatic reproducibility of 80–90 percent in patients with recurrent syncope.[148–151] Thus in symptomatic patients this test has extreme value in assessing the efficacy of intervention.

Treatment

Patient education involving avoidance of precipitating factors, vasodilator drugs and taking evasive action, e.g., lying down, during prodromal symptoms has great value in avoiding episodes of vasovagal syncope. However, many patients experience symptoms without warning necessitating drug therapy. A number of drugs are reported to be useful in alleviating symptoms. Beta blockers (atenolol 50 mg/day) by their negative inotropic actions decrease the force of ventricular contraction and thereby reduce the degree of mechanoreceptor discharge; and are useful in vasovagal syncope.[138] Disopyramide (200 mg twice daily) by its negative inotropic and anticholinergic effects,[152] has been recommended but efficacy is dubious.[153] Transdermal scopolamine (one patch every 3 days) works through its anticholinergic effects[133] and fludrocortisone (100–200 µg/day) by its volume expanding effect.[145] Recent reports suggest that serotonin antagonists such as fluoxetine (20 mg/day) and sertraline hydrochloride (25 mg/day) are effective in symptom relief.[154,155] The efficacy of midodrine in the management of vasovagal syncope has been recently observed in a double-blind randomized controlled trial.[156] More than 50 percent of patients experienced significant symptomatic improvement, delayed response to head-up tilting and improvement in quality of life. Midodrine presumably acts by reducing peripheral venous pooling and thereby improving cardiac output. Elastic support hose, relaxation techniques (biofeedback), and conditioning using repeated head-up tilt as therapy, are useful adjuvant therapies. Permanent cardiac pacing is beneficial in some patients, who have recurrent syncope and significant bradycardia,[157,158] dual chamber pacing being the preferred mode of pacing.[145] However, pacing influences the bradycardia component of the response and not vasodilatation and hypotension, which frequently dominates. Its utility is limited in some instances to prolongation of the prodrome in order to allow other evasive action.[159]

POSTPRANDIAL HYPOTENSION

The effect of meals on the cardiovascular system was appreciated from postprandial exaggeration of angina which was demonstrated objectively by deterioration of exercise tolerance following food.[160] Postprandial reductions in blood pressure manifesting as syncope and dizziness were subsequently reported,[161,162] leading to extensive investigation of this phenomenon. In healthy older subjects, systolic blood pressure falls by 11–16 mmHg,[163–165] and heart rate rises by 5–7 beats/minute[163,164] 60 minutes after meals of varying composition and energy content. However, the change in diastolic blood pressure is not as consistent. In older subjects with hypertension, orthostatic hypotension, and autonomic failure, the postprandial blood pressure fall is much greater with no corresponding rise in heart rate.[166] These responses are marked if the energy and simple carbohydrate content of the meal is high.[167] However, in the majority of fit as well as frail older subjects, most of these hypotensive episodes go unnoticed. Postprandial physiological changes include increased splanchnic and superior mesenteric artery blood flow at the expense of peripheral circulation[168] and a rise in plasma insulin levels[167,169,170] without corresponding rises in sympathetic nervous system activity. Vasodilator effects of insulin[171] and other gut peptides, namely neurotensin and vasointestinal peptide (VIP), are thought to be responsible for postprandial hypotension, although the precise mechanism remains uncertain. The clinical significance of a fall in blood pressure after meals is difficult to quantitate. However, postprandial hypotension is causally related to recurrent syncope and falls in older subjects.[12,172,173] In the authors' experience, postprandial symptoms occur in at most 20 percent of patients with symptomatic orthostatic hypotension. A reduction in simple carbohydrate content of food, its replacement with complex carbohydrates or high protein, high fat, and frequent small meals are effective interventions for postprandial hypotension. Drugs useful in the treatment are fludrocortisone and indomethacin,[174] octreotide,[175] and caffeine.[176,177] Given orally along with food, caffeine prevents hypotensive symptoms in fit as well as frail older subjects;[178,179] it should preferably be given in the mornings as tolerance develops if it is taken throughout the day.

GENERAL DIAGNOSTIC EVALUATION OF SYNCOPE

The diagnostic evaluation of syncope is that recommended by the European Cardiac Society Task Force on Syncope.[180] Figure 38-2 shows a flow diagram of an approach to the evaluation of syncope for all age groups.

Initial evaluation

The starting point for the evaluation of syncope is a careful history and physical examination including orthostatic blood pressure measurements.[180] In some young patients without heart disease a definite diagnosis of neurally mediated syncope can be made without any further examination. A 12-lead ECG should be usually part of the general evaluation of patients. This basic assessment will be defined as "initial evaluation."

Three key questions should be addressed during the initial evaluation:

- Is loss of consciousness attributable to syncope or not?
- Is heart disease present or absent?
- Are there important clinical features in the history that suggest the diagnosis?

Differentiating true syncope from other "nonsyncopal" conditions associated with real or apparent loss of consciousness is generally the first diagnostic challenge and influences the subsequent diagnostic strategy. Apart from the prognostic importance of the presence of heart disease, its absence excludes a cardiac cause of syncope with few exceptions. In a recent study,[181] heart disease was an independent predictor of a cardiac cause of syncope, with a sensitivity of 95 percent and a specificity of 45 percent; by contrast, the absence of heart disease allowed exclusion of a cardiac cause of syncope in 97 percent of the patients. Finally, accurate history taking alone may be diagnostic of the cause of syncope or may suggest the strategy of evaluation. It must be pointed out that syncope may be one of the accompanying symptoms which occur at the presentation of certain diseases, such as aortic dissection, pulmonary embolism, acute myocardial infarction, outflow

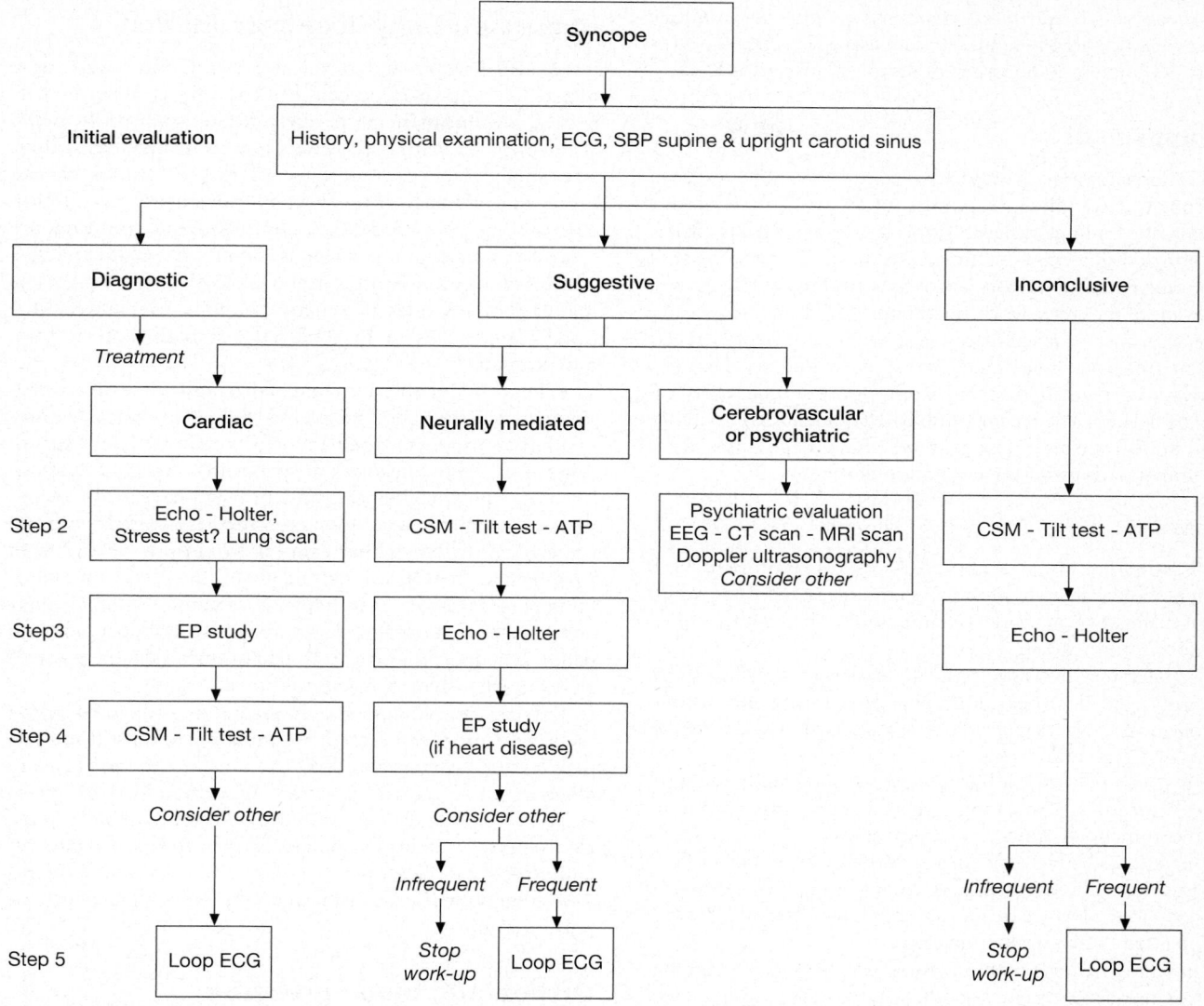

Figure 38-2 An approach to the evaluation of syncope for all age groups (based on the recommendations from the European Society Task Force on Syncope[180]).

tract obstruction, etc. In these cases, priority must be given to specific and immediate treatment of the underlying condition.

Certain or suspected diagnosis

Initial evaluation may lead to diagnosis based on symptoms, signs, or ECG findings. Under such circumstances, no further evaluation is needed, and treatment, if any, can be planned. More commonly, the initial evaluation leads to a suspected diagnosis, which needs to be confirmed by directed testing (Fig. 38-1). If a diagnosis is confirmed by specific testing, treatment may be initiated. On the other hand, if the diagnosis is not confirmed, then patients are considered to have unexplained syncope and are evaluated as follows.

Unexplained syncope

The most important issue in these patients is the presence of structural heart disease or an abnormal ECG. These findings

are associated with a higher risk of arrhythmias and a higher mortality at 1 year. In these patients, cardiac evaluation consisting of echocardiography, stress testing, and tests for arrhythmia detection such as prolonged electrocardiographic and loop monitoring or electrophysiological study are recommended. If cardiac evaluation does not show evidence of arrhythmia as a cause of syncope, evaluation for neurally mediated syndromes is recommended in those with recurrent or severe syncope.

In patients without structural heart disease and a normal ECG, evaluation for neurally mediated syncope is recommended for those with recurrent or severe syncope. The tests for neurally mediated syncope consist of tilt testing and carotid sinus massage. The majority of patients with single or rare episodes in this category probably have neurally mediated syncope. Additional consideration in patients without structural heart disease and a normal ECG is bradyarrhythmia or psychiatric illness. Loop monitoring is needed in patients with recurrent unexplained syncope whose symptoms are suggestive of arrhythmic syncope. Psychiatric assessment is recommended in patients with frequent recurrent syncope who have multiple other somatic complaints and initial evaluation raises concerns for stress, anxiety and possible other psychiatric disorders.

Reappraisal

Once the evaluation, as outlined, is completed and no cause of syncope is determined, reappraisal of the work-up is needed since subtle findings or new historical information may change the entire differential diagnosis. Reappraisal may consist of obtaining details of history and re-examining patients as well as review of the entire work-up. If unexplored clues to possible cardiac or neurological disease are apparent, further cardiac and neurological assessment is recommended. In these circumstances, consultation with appropriate specialty services may be needed. The recently published guidelines on syncope from the European Cardiac Society[180] have made a number of recommendations for the evaluation of syncope:

Class I:

- Routine use of basic laboratory tests is recommended if metabolic causes or blood loss are suggested by the results of the history or physical examination. Their routine use is not recommended.
- In patients with suspected heart disease, echocardiography, prolonged electrocardiographic monitoring and, if non-diagnostic, electrophysiological studies are recommended as first evaluation steps.
- In patients with palpitations associated with syncope, electrocardiographic monitoring and echocardiography are recommended as first evaluation steps.
- In patients with chest pain suggestive of ischemia before or after loss of consciousness, stress testing, echocardiography, and electrocardiographic monitoring are recommended as first evaluation steps.
- In young patients without suspicion of heart or neurological disease and recurrent syncope, tilt testing and, in older patients, carotid sinus massages are recommended as first evaluation steps.
- In patients with syncope occurring during neck turning, carotid sinus massage is recommended at the outset.
- In patients with syncope during or after effort, echocardiography and stress testing are recommended as first evaluation steps.
- In patients with signs of autonomic failure or neurological disease a specific diagnosis should be made.

Special features in older patients

Multiple illnesses are very common in older people: subjects over 65 years have an average of 3.5 illnesses.[182] It is thus important to carefully attribute a diagnosis, rather than assume that the presence of an abnormality known to produce syncope or hypotensive symptoms is the cause. In order to attribute a diagnosis, patients should have symptom reproduction during investigation and preferably alleviation of symptoms with specific intervention. In addition, more than one hypotensive disorder can coexist[12] in older patients, rendering a precise diagnosis difficult.

History and physical examination

A detailed history and physical examination results in a diagnosis in up to 40 percent of cases.[12,13] An accurate witness account can help to differentiate syncope from an accidental fall. Witnessed features of prodrome, e.g., pallor, sweating, presence or absence of loss of consciousness, presence or absence of involuntary movements, and clinical events after the episode, e.g., confusion and vomiting, are crucial in constructing a diagnostic picture. Nonetheless a witnessed account is often not available (40 percent). The majority of episodes of syncope or falls, even in institutional care, occur in the bedroom or bathroom and are unwitnessed.[183]

Patients frequently complain of dizziness alone or as a prodrome to syncope and unexplained falls. The clinical features of dizziness can further help to identify an underlying cause of symptoms. Four categories of symptoms—vertigo, dysequilibrium, light-headedness, and others—have been recognized.[184] Light-headedness is often associated with an underlying cardiovascular cause of symptoms, vertigo with peripheral or central lesions, and unsteadiness with an underlying central lesion.[185] In addition, dizziness is most likely attributable to a cardiovascular diagnosis if associated with pallor, syncope, prolonged standing or the need to lie down or sit down when symptoms occur.[185]

Physical examination should include morning orthostatic blood pressure measurement, examination of carotid and cardiac bruits, heart rate and rhythm and for the presence of atherosclerotic disease: e.g., peripheral vascular disease, hypertensive retinal changes etc. Assessment of gait, mobility, muscle strength, and use of walking aids are important in patients complaining of unexplained falls and possible syncope. Assessment of vision, hearing, and signs of Parkinson's disease are also important.

Orthostatic blood pressure measurement

Supine blood pressure measurements should be taken after a minimum of 10 minutes of rest. Blood pressure should then be recorded for up to 3 minutes while standing unaided.[186] In 90 percent of patients who have orthostatic hypotension, a significant reduction in standing blood pressure will have occurred by 1 minute during standing. Some studies have recorded blood pressure for up to 20 minutes[187] but prolonged standing leads to overlap of orthostatic symptoms and vasovagal symptoms.[127] A sustained 20 mmHg fall of systolic blood pressure or 10 mmHg fall in diastolic blood pressure or fall of systolic blood pressure to 90 mmHg or less is considered diagnostic for orthostatic hypotension.[186] However, in practice, patients can have symptom reproduction (dizziness) during transient falls in orthostatic blood pressure which are not sustained or which changes do not meet the standard criteria for orthostatic hypotension. This is particularly so in frailer old people in whom cerebral autoregulation is compromised. Digital photoplethysmography (Finapres) is a useful noninvasive technique for beat-to-beat blood pressure measurement during orthostasis. Alternatively, other systems for automated recording of blood pressure or repeated manual sphygmomanometry can be used but will miss transient hypotension. Reproducibility of orthostatic hypotension depends on the time of measurement and on autonomic nervous system function.[4] Where possible the procedure should be carried out in the morning. In patients with unexplained syncope, an attributable diagnosis of orthostatic hypotension depends on reproduction of symptoms or dramatic falls in orthostatic blood pressure.

Twelve-lead electrocardiogram

Causes of syncope such as acute myocardial infarction, bradyarrhythmias or tachyarrhythmias can be diagnosed from surface ECG. But an abnormal ECG is not necessarily the cause of symptoms—up to 32 percent of unselected older subjects have an abnormal surface ECG.[188] Ischemic changes, together with a history of palpitation, may indicate an underlying arrhythmogenic cause of syncope.

Echocardiography

Echocardiography is frequently used as a screening test to detect cardiac disease in patients with syncope. Although numerous published case reports have suggested an important role of echocardiography in disclosing the cause and/or mechanism of syncope, larger studies have shown that the diagnostic yield from echocardiography is low in the absence of clinical, physical, or electrocardiographic findings suggestive of a cardiac abnormality.[66,189,190]

In patients with syncope or presyncope and normal physical examination, the most frequent (from 4.6 to 18.5 percent of cases) finding is mitral valve prolapse.[190] This may be coincidental as both conditions are common. Other cardiac abnormalities include valvular diseases (most frequently aortic stenosis), myopathies, regional wall motion abnormalities suggestive of myocardial infarction, infiltrative heart diseases such as amyloidosis, cardiac tumors, aneurysms, atrial thromboembolism, and other abnormalities.[32–34,79] Even if echocardiography alone is only seldom diagnostic, this test provides information about the type and severity of underlying heart disease which may be useful for risk stratification. If moderate to severe structural heart disease is found, evaluation is directed toward a cardiac cause of syncope. On the other hand, in the presence of minor structural abnormalities the probability of a cardiac cause of syncope is not high, and the evaluation may proceed as in patients without structural heart disease.

Examples of heart disease in older persons in which cardiac syncope is likely include: cardiomyopathy with episodes of overt heart failure, systolic dysfunction (ejection fraction < 40 percent), ischemic cardiomyopathy following an acute myocardial infarction, hypertrophic cardiomyopathy, cardiac tumors, outflow tract obstruction, pulmonary embolism, and aortic dissection.

Electrocardiographic monitoring (noninvasive and invasive)

Holter monitoring

Most ECG monitoring in syncope is undertaken with external 24-hour cassette tape-recorders connected to the patient via external wiring and adhesive ECG patches. The advantages of this are that it is a noninvasive test, there is beat-to-beat acquisition, device costs are low, and there is relatively high fidelity over a short time-period. Conversely, limitations are many—patients may not tolerate adhesive electrodes, or electrodes may not remain adherent throughout monitoring or during an event. A recurrence of presenting symptoms may not occur during monitoring. The vast majority of patients have a syncope-free interval measured in weeks, months or years, but not days, and therefore, symptom ECG correlation can rarely be achieved with Holter monitoring. In an overview[191] of the results of eight studies of ambulatory monitoring in syncope, only 4 percent of patients (range between 6 and 20 percent) had correlation of symptoms with arrhythmia. Admittedly in 15 percent of patients, symptoms were not associated with arrhythmia. In these patients, a rhythm disturbance could potentially be excluded as a cause of syncope. The true yield of conventional ECG monitoring in syncope may be as low as 1–2 percent in an unselected population.[192–194]

External ECG event monitoring in syncope

Conventional event recorders are external devices equipped with fixed electrodes through which an ECG can be recorded by direct application to the chest wall. Recordings can be prospective or retrospective (loop recorders) or both. Prospective external event recorders have a limited value in syncope because the patient must be able to apply the recorder to the chest during the period of unconsciousness and activate recording. These recorders are more appropriate for the investigation of palpitations. In patients with frequent syncopal symptoms, external retrospective loop recorders show a relatively high diagnostic yield.[195] However, since patients usually do not comply for more than a few weeks with this instrument, symptom–ECG correlation cannot be achieved when the syncopal recurrence rate is infrequent.

Implantable ECG event monitoring in syncope

Recently an implantable ECG event monitor (implantable loop recorder) has become available. This device is placed subcutaneously under local anesthesia, and has a battery life of 18–24 months. The current version can store up to 42 minutes of continuous ECG. Retrospective ECG allows activation of the device after consciousness has been restored. Symptoms–ECG correlation is achieved in 59 to 88 percent of patients.[196,197]

One recent series supports the use of an implantable loop recorder (Reveal™: Medtronic) in a small series of older patients who had unexplained syncope despite investigation. The device yielded a diagnosis in half of patients[198] studied.

- Advantages of the implantable loop recorder include: continuous-loop high-fidelity ECG recording for up to 24 months; a loop memory which allows activation after consciousness is restored; removal of logistical factors which prevent good ECG recording during symptoms; and a potential for a high yield in terms of symptom–ECG correlation because of the high likelihood of recording during recurrence of presenting symptoms.
- Disadvantages include: the need for a minor surgical procedure; the lack of recording of any other concurrent physiological parameter, e.g., blood pressure; and the high cost of the implantable device.

The implantable loop recorder carries a high up-front cost. However, if symptom–ECG correlation can be achieved in a substantial number of patients within 12 months of implantation, then analysis of the cost per symptom–ECG yield could show that the implanted device may be more cost-effective than a strategy using conventional investigation. This remains to be confirmed.[196,197,199] Knowledge of what transpires during a spontaneous syncopal episode is the gold standard for syncope evaluation. For this reason it is likely that implantable monitors will become increasingly important in syncope. However, more information is required on the benefits of loop recorders for evaluation of falls and syncope in older patients.

Electrophysiological testing

Transesophageal electrophysiological study

The role of the noninvasive or transesophageal electrophysiological examination is limited to screening for fast supraventricular tachycardia due to atrioventricular nodal re-entrant tachycardia or atrioventricular re-entrant tachycardia in patients with normal resting ECG and a history of syncope associated with palpitations and to the evaluation of sinus node dysfunction in patients with syncope suspected to be due to bradycardia. It can also be used for risk evaluation in patients with pre-excitation, although a normal refractory period of the accessory pathway cannot rule out a risk of atrial fibrillation with a fast ventricular response.[200,201]

Invasive electrophysiological study

Electrophysiological studies use endocardial and (in the coronary sinus) epicardial electrical stimulation and recording to disclose abnormalities that suggest a primary arrhythmia as the cause of syncope. However, few studies have used Holter monitoring or implantable devices to confirm the results of the electrophysiological study. The true diagnostic yield of the electrophysiological study is therefore only partly known.[202–205]

Indeed, when neurally mediated syncope was excluded, Brignole et al.[202] showed that the presence of abnormal sinus node or His–Purkinje function (at baseline or after ajmaline provocation) disclosed the correct diagnosis in 86 percent of cases with spontaneous syncope due to sinus arrest or paroxysmal AV block, respectively. These results have been corroborated in subsequent reports on patients with either electrocardiographic monitoring performed before electrophysiological study or by a bradycardia-detecting pacemaker after an electrophysiological study.[206,207] Importantly, unrelated ventricular tachycardia and fibrillation and atrial tachyarrhythmias were induced in 22 percent of patients in the aforementioned studies, tachycardias that mistakenly might have been designated as the cause of syncope. Positive results at electrophysiological study occur predominantly in patients with evidence of organic heart disease.[208]

Suspected bradycardia

The pretest probability of a transient bradycardia is relatively high when syncope occurs suddenly, without premonitory symptoms, and is independent of posture and physical activity, is short-lasting, has no or subtle accompanying symptoms, and is followed by rapid recovery. Sinus node disease/sick sinus syndrome is present when symptoms and sinus bradycardia or pauses occur simultaneously as proven by ECG monitoring ("gold standard"). Sinus node dysfunction can be demonstrated by abnormal sinus cycle variations on resting ECG, chronotropic incompetence on exercise testing, and by prolonged sinus node recovery time (SRT or SNRT) or sinoatrial conduction time (SACT) on electrophysiological study.[209–211]

The major concern lies in limited sensitivity with all above mentioned methods, while specificity is high. There is no generally accepted protocol for evaluating sinus node function.[180]

Syncope in patients with bundle branch block (impending high-degree AV block)

The most alarming ECG sign in a patient with syncope is probably alternating complete left and right bundle branch block, or alternating right bundle branch block with left anterior or posterior fascicular block, suggesting trifascicular conduction system disease and intermittent or impending high-degree AV block.[212–215]

Patients with bifascicular block (right bundle branch block plus left anterior or left posterior fascicular block, or left bundle branch block) are at higher risk of developing high-degree AV block. A significant problem in the evaluation of syncope and bifascicular block is the transient nature of high-degree AV block and, therefore, the long periods required to document it by ECG.[215] Two factors were shown to increase the risk for AV block; a history of syncope and a prolonged HV interval. The risk of developing AV block increased from 2 percent in patients without syncope to 17 percent in patients with syncope.[216]

In order to increase the diagnostic yield of the electrophysiological evaluation incremental atrial pacing and pharmacological provocation were added. In five studies[215,217–220] evaluating the diagnostic value of pharmacological stress testing for a total of 333 patients, high-degree AV block was induced in 50 (15 percent) of the patients. During the follow-up ranging between 24 and 63 months, 68 percent (range 43–100) of these patients developed spontaneous AV block. Thus, the induction of AV block during atrial pacing and pharmacological testing is highly predictive of subsequent development of AV block. On the other hand, in patients with negative electrophysiological studies Link et al.[221] observed development of AV block in 18 percent (after 30 months) and Gaggioli et al.[222] in 19 percent (at 62 months). Finally, pacemaker therapy resulted in effective suppression of syncopal recurrences in almost all patients and was significantly better than no pacing, thus indirectly confirming the usefulness of the electrophysiological study.[219,223,224]

In conclusion, in patients with syncope and bifascicular block, an electrophysiological study is highly sensitive in identifying patients with intermittent or impending high-degree AV block. This block is the likely cause of syncope in most cases, but not of the high mortality rate observed in these patients. Indeed, the high total and sudden mortality seems mainly related to underlying structural heart disease and ventricular tachyarrhythmias. Unfortunately, ventricular programmed stimulation does not seem to be able correctly to identify these patients and the finding of inducible ventricular arrhythmia should therefore be interpreted with caution.

Suspected tachycardia

Supraventricular tachycardia presenting as syncope without accompanying palpitations is probably rare.[225] Both noninvasive (transesophageal) and invasive electrophysiological studies may be used to evaluate hemodynamic effects of an induced tachycardia, especially if combined with administration of isoprenaline or atropine. Ventricular tachycardia may present as syncope with or without palpitations or other accompanying symptoms. The major concern with programmed electrical stimulation as part of an electrophysiological study for inducing clinically significant ventricular arrhythmias is its varying sensitivity (and specificity) in different clinical settings[226] and the lack of a standard protocol.[227] Generally speaking, programmed electrical stimulation is thought to be a sensitive tool in patients with chronic ischemic heart disease (previous myocardial infarction) and susceptibility for a spontaneous monomorphic ventricular tachycardia. Applying the opposite perspective, the induction of a monomorphic ventricular tachycardia is thought to be a specific event that should guide therapy.[228]

Emerging diagnostic tests for bradyarrhythmias and tachyarrhythmias are the ATP test and ventricular signal-averaged electrocardiogram.

ATP test

Intravenous injection of adenosine triphosphate (ATP) has recently been proposed as a tool in the investigation of patients with unexplained syncope.[229,230] In predisposed patients with unexplained syncope, the stimulation of purinergic receptors, with a powerful dromotropic effect on the atrioventricular node, causes prolonged ventricular pauses due to atrioventricular block, which are considered as possibly responsible for spontaneous attacks. The action of ATP is due to its rapid catabolism to adenosine and the subsequent action of adenosine at purinoceptor sites. ATP and adenosine have similar effects in humans.[231] The test requires further evaluation before widespread use.

Ventricular signal-averaged electrocardiogram

Ventricular late potentials represent areas of slow conduction that can promote the occurrence of ventricular arrhythmias. These low-amplitude signals can be detected on the surface electrocardiogram using a signal averaging technique if the area of slow conduction is activated late during ventricular depolarization.[232]

Ambulatory blood pressure monitoring

Ambulatory blood pressure monitoring is predominantly used in the management of hypertensive disorders. It can, however, play a role in the diagnosis and management of hypotensive disorders. Information such as the pattern of diurnal blood pressure behavior, postprandial dips in blood pressure, and blood pressure changes after medication are useful in patients suffering from syncope and dizziness. A reversal of the diurnal blood pressure pattern is observed frequently in symptomatic orthostatic hypotension.[233]

Carotid sinus massage

Carotid sinus massage comprises measurement of heart rate and blood pressure responses during and after longitudinal massage over the point of maximum carotid impulse, usually located at the level of the upper border of the thyroid cartilage (Fig. 38-3). Heart rate responses are recorded using a continuous surface electrocardiogram (Fig. 38-4). Blood pressure is best measured by noninvasive phasic blood pressure monitoring equipment which allows accurate assessment of the blood pressure nadir (mean of 18 seconds after the onset of massage).[44,115,234] Massage should be carried out initially supine and then tilted head up to 70°. This is because up to one-third of patients with carotid sinus syndrome have an abnormal response only when upright.[84,234]

Head-up tilt testing

Prolonged head-up tilting tests the baroreflex response to prolonged standing. The optimal protocol for the test is as yet undefined. Thus a variety of methods are recommended concerning the angle of tilt, duration of tilt and use of additional provocation to induce syncope. A tilting angle within the range of 60°–80° provides the necessary orthostatic stress.[144] Duration of tilting in various studies has varied from 30 to 60 minutes. The test should be carried out during morning hours after an overnight fast and after withdrawal of all cardioactive drugs for at least five half-lives unless the role of culprit medication is of diagnostic relevance. The subject should be rested supine for a period of 15–30 minutes after which baseline blood pressure and heart rate is recorded. Blood pressure is ideally

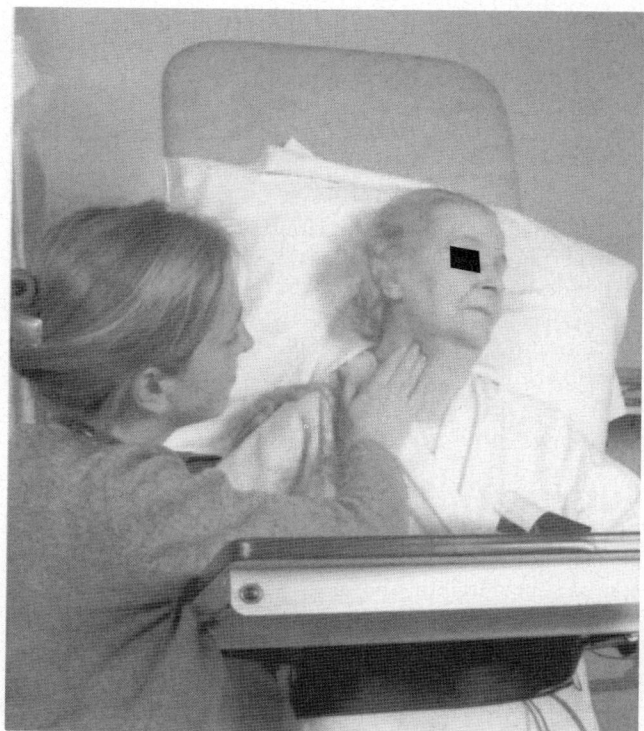

Figure 38-3 Procedure for carotid sinus massage while upright.

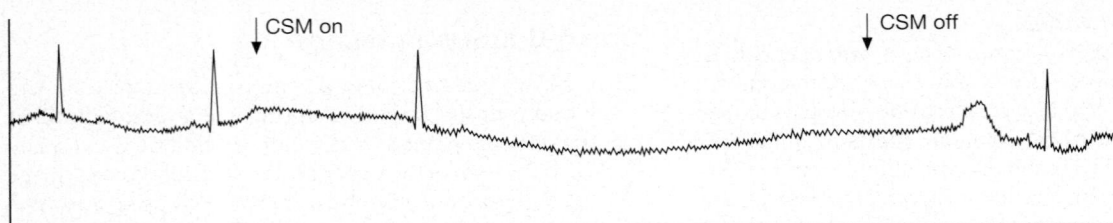

Figure 38-4 Cardioinhibitory carotid sinus response asystole of 5.2 seconds.

recorded by digital photoplethysmography (Finapres), which records beat-to-beat changes. Alternatively, other systems for automated blood pressure recording or repeated manual sphygmomanometer blood pressure recording and continuous surface ECG can be used for monitoring. The authors consider a tilting angle of 70° and duration of 40 minutes as adequate in most patients. The test is positive if the patient develops syncope and or presyncope together with hypotension and/or bradycardia during the upright period. The patient should be immediately lowered to supine position and the study terminated. Symptom reproduction during hemodynamic changes is preferable in order to attribute cause. Further shorter tilt tests are recommended if passive testing is not diagnostic and these include tests with GTN provocation and isoprenaline. Our group has recently published our preferred protocol for tilting.[136,236]

Head-up tilting is a useful investigation in the following instances:

1. The diagnosis of neurocardiogenic syncope. Additional provocative tests include intravenous isoprenaline,[139,237] sublingual or intravenous glyceryl trinitrate,[141,142] and intravenous cannulation.[143,238]
2. The diagnosis of orthostatic hypotension,[4] if patients have difficulty standing unaided.
3. The diagnosis of cardioinhibitory carotid sinus syndrome.[44,54]
4. It is a useful procedure (reproducing "syncope") in patients with psychiatric disorders without any change in blood pressure and heart rate.[44,148]
5. The diagnosis of hyperventilation syncope, where patients hyperventilate with reproduction of symptoms but without developing hypotension or bradyarrhythmia.
6. The diagnosis of central dizziness. Movement of the tilt bed can reproduce symptoms of dizziness without accompanying hemodynamic changes.[235]

SUMMARY

Syncope is a common symptom in older adults due to age-related neurohumoral and physiological changes. Common treatable causes of syncope encountered by the geriatrician are carotid sinus syndrome, orthostatic hypotension, vasovagal syncope, postprandial syncope, sinus node disease, and atrioventricular block. Algorithms for the assessment of syncope are similar to those for young adults, but the prevalence of carotid sinus syndrome and cardiac conduction disease is higher in older adults. A systematic approach to syncope will achieve a diagnosis in over 80 percent of cases. Cardiovascular syncope can present as falls and render an attributable diagnosis more difficult to make.

> **KEY POINTS** Syncope
>
> - Syncope is caused by a severe but reversible reduction in blood flow to the brainstem neurons responsible for supporting consciousness (reticular activating system).
>
> - Elderly people, especially those over 75 years, have the highest incidence of syncope of all age groups.
>
> - Syncope due to cardiac arrhythmias carries a poor prognosis, is usually associated with structural heart abnormalities, and should always be excluded first.
>
> - Syncope is most frequently caused by orthostatic hypotension either secondary to drugs, to chronic autonomic failure, or to neurally mediated syncope (i.e., vasovagal syncope).
>
> - Neurally mediated syncope is characterized by acute vasodilation and bradycardia. It is the most frequent cause of syncope in otherwise normal subjects.
>
> - Elderly people often take many medications that can cause syncope. Before undertaking aggressive evaluation, medications should be considered as a primary cause for syncope in elderly people, even in those patients who have cardiovascular disease.
>
> - Testing orthostatic tolerance during passive head-up tilt is the best available diagnostic procedure to evaluate patients with syncope in whom a cardiac cause has been excluded.

REFERENCES

1. Rossen R, Kabat H, Anderson JP: Acute arrest of cerebral circulation in man. Arch Neurol Psychiatr 1943;50:510–528
2. Lempert T, Bauer M, Schmidt D: Syncope: A videometric analysis of 56 episodes of transient cerebral hypoxia. Ann Neurol 1994;36:233–237
3. Hoefnagels WAJ, Padberg GW, Overweg J et al: Transient loss of consciousness: the value of the history for distinguishing seizure from syncope. J Neurol 1991;238:39–43
4. Ward C, Kenny RA: Reproducibility of orthostatic hypotension in symptomatic elderly. Am J Med 1996;100:418–422
5. Kenny RA, Traynor G: Carotid sinus syndrome—clinical characteristics in elderly patients. Age Ageing 1991;20:449–454
6. Kenny RA, Richardson DA et al: Carotid sinus syndrome: a modifiable risk factor for non-accidental falls in older adults. J Am Coll Cardiol 2001;38:1491–1496
7. Day SC, Cook EF, Funkenstein H, Goldman L: Evaluation and outcome of emergency room patients with transient loss of consciousness. Am J Med 1982;72:15–23

8. Kenny RA, Walker H: Impact of a dedicated syncope and falls facility for older adults on emergency bends. Age Ageing (in press)

9. Lipsitz LA, Wei JY, Rowe JW: Syncope in an elderly, institutionalised population: prevalence incidence and associated risk. Q J Med 1985;55:45–55

10. Kapoor W, Snustad D, Peterson J et al: Syncope in elderly. Am J Med 1986;80:419–428

11. Dey AB, Stout NR, Kenny RA: Cardiovascular syncope is the commonest cause of drop attacks in the older patient. Eur JCPE 1996;6(2):84–88

12. McIntosh SJ, DaCosta D, Kenny RA: Outcome of an integrated approach to the investigation of dizziness, falls and syncope in elderly patients referred to a syncope clinic. Age Ageing 1993;22:53–58

13. Allcock LM, O'Shea D: Diagnostic yield and development of a neurocardiovascular investigation unit for older adults in a district general hospital. J Gerontol A Biol Sci Med Sci 2000;55(8):M458–462

14. Lipsitz LA, Pluchino FC, Wei JY, Rowe JW: Syncope in institutionalised elderly: the impact of multiple pathological conditions and situational stress. J Chron Dis 1986;39:619–630

15. Lipsitz LA: Altered blood pressure homeostasis in advanced age: clinical and research implications. J Gerontol 1989;44:179–183

16. Crane MG, Harris JJ: Effect of ageing on renin activity and aldosterone secretion. J Lab Clin Med 1976;87:947–959

17. Epstein M, Hollenberg MK: Age a determinant of renal sodium conservation in normal man. J Lab Clin Med 1976;87:411–417

18. Strandgaard S: Autoregulation of cerebral blood flow in hypertensive patients: the modifying influence of prolonged antihypertensive treatment on the tolerance to acute drug induced hypotension. Circulation 1976;53:720–727

19. Carey BJ, Manktelow BN, Panerai RB, Potter JF: Cerebral autoregulatory responses to head-up tilt in normal subjects and patients with recurrent vasovagal syncope. Circulation 2001;104:898–902

20. Dermksian G, Lamb LE: Syncope in a population of healthy young adults: incidence mechanism and significance. J Am Coll Cardiol 1958;168:122–127

21. Murdoch BD: Loss of consciousness in healthy South African men: incidence, causes and relationship to ECG abnormality. S Afr Med J 1980;57:771–774

22. Schilinford JP: Syncope. Am J Cardiol 1970;26:609–612

23. Friedberg CK: Syncope: pathologic physiology, differential diagnosis and treatment. Mod Concepts Cardiovasc Dis 1971;40:54–63

24. Wright KE Jr, McIntosh HD: Syncope: a review of pathophysiologic mechanisms. Prog Cardiovasc Dis 1971;13:580–594

25. Rubenstein LZ, Robbins AS, Josephson KR, Schulman BL, Osterweil D: The value of assessing falls in an elderly population. Ann Intern Med 1990;113:308–316

26. Lipsitz LA: Abnormalities in blood pressure homeostasis that contribute to falls in the elderly. Clin Geriatr Med 1985;91:637–648

27. Davies AJ, Steen N, Kenny RA: Carotid sinus hypersensitivity is common in older patients presenting to an accident and emergency department with unexplained falls. Age Ageing 2001;30:289–293

28. Cummings SR, Nevitt MC, Kidd S: Forgetting falls: the limited accuracy of recall of falls in the elderly. J Am Geriatr Soc 1988;36:613–616

29. Aronow WS, Ahn C: Postprandial hypotension in 499 elderly persons in a long term health care facility. J Am Geriatr Soc 1994;42:930–932

30. Seifer C, Kenny RA: Atrioventricular block and sick sinus syndrome present with falls in addition to syncope. Am J Geriatr Cardiol (in press)

31. Strasberg B, Sagie A, Rechavie E et al: The non-invasive evaluation of syncope of suspected cardiovascular origin. Am Heart J 1989;117:160–163

32. Franke H: Uber das Karotissinus-Syndrom und den sogenannten hyperaktiven Karotissinus-Reflex. Friedrich-Karl Schattauer-Verlag, Stuttgart, 1963;149

33. Thomas JE: Diseases of the carotid sinus—syncope. In Vinken PJ, Bruyn GW (eds): Handbook of Clinical Neurology, Vol 11. North Holland Publishing, Amsterdam, 1972:532–551

34. Roskam J: Un syndrome nouveau. Syncopes cardiaques graves et syncopes repetees par hyperreflectivite sinocarotidienne. Presse Medical 1930;38:590–591

35. Parry CH: An Enquiry into Symptoms and Causes of Syncope Anginosa, Commonly Called Angina Pectoris. R Cruttwell, Bath, UK 1799

36. Hering HE: Der Sinus caroticus an der Ursprungsstelle der Carotis interna als Ausgangsort eines hemmenden Herzreflexes und eines depressorischen Gefassreflexes. Munch Med Wschr 1924;71:701–704

37. Binswanger O: Anatomische untersuchungen uber die ursprungsstelle und den anfongstheil der carotis interna. Arch Psychiatr Nervenkr 1879;9:351–368

38. Crill WE, Reis DJ: Distribution of carotid sinus and depressor nerves in cat brainstem. Am J Physiol 1968;214:269–276

39. Thomas JE: Hyperactive carotid sinus reflex and carotid sinus syncope. Mayo Clin Proc 1969;44:127–139

40. Bristow D, Honour J, Pickering GW, Sleight P, Smyth HS: Diminished baroreflex sensitivity in high blood pressure. Circulation 1969;39:48–54

41. Dehn TCB, Morley CA, Sutton R: A scientific evaluation of the carotid sinus syndrome. Cardiovasc Res 1984;18:746–751

42. Salomon S: The carotid sinus syndrome. Am J Cardiol 1958;2:342–350

43. Wiedermann G, Grotz J, Bewermeyer H, Hossmann V, Heiss WD: High-resolution real-time ultrasound of the carotid bifurcation in patients with hyperactive carotid sinus syndrome. J Neurol 1985;232:318–325

44. McIntosh SJ, Lawson J, Kenny RA: Clinical characteristics of vasodepressor, cardioinhibitory and mixed carotid sinus syndrome in the elderly. Am J Med 1993;95:203–208

45. Kenny RA, Lyon CC, Ingram AM et al: Enhanced vagal activity and normal arginine vasopressin response in carotid sinus syndrome: implications for a central abnormality in carotid sinus hypersensitivity. Cardiovasc Res 1987;21:545–550

46. Walter PF, Crawley IS, Dorney ER: Carotid sinus hypersensitivity and syncope. Am J Cardiol 1978;42:396–403

47. Gang ES, Oseran DS, Mandel WJ, Peter T: Sinus node electrogram in patients with the hypersensitive carotid sinus syndrome. J Am Coll Cardiol 1985;5: 1484–1490

48. Kenny, RA, McIntosh, S, Wynne, H: Pattern of inhibition of parasympathetic activity in response to incremental bolus doses of atropine in carotid sinus hypersensitivity. J Clin Auton Res 1994;4:63–66

49. Morley CA, Perrins EJ, Grant P, Chan SL, McBrien DJ, Sutton R: Carotid sinus syncope treated by pacing. Analysis of persistent symptoms and role of atrioventricular sequential pacing. Br Heart J 1982;47:411–418

50. Brignole M, Menozzi C, Gianfranchi L et al: Carotid sinus massage eyeball compression and head-up tilt test in patients with syncope of uncertain origin and in healthy control subjects. Am Heart J 1991;122:1651–1664

51. Morley CA, Sutton R: Carotid sinus syncope. Int J Cardiol 1984;6:287–293 (editorial)

52. Brown KA, Maloney JA, Smith HC et al: Carotid sinus reflex in patients undergoing coronary angiography: relationship of degree and location of coronary artery disease to response to carotid sinus massage. Circulation 1980;62:697–703

53. Wentink JRM, Jansen RWMM, Hoefnagels WHL: The influence of age on the response of blood pressure and heart rate to carotid sinus massage in healthy volunteers. Cardiol Elderly 1993;1:453–459

54. Parry SW, Baptist M, Gilroy JJ, Hutchinson M, Kenny RA: Central alpha-2 adrenoceptors have no role in the pathogenesis of the vasodepressor component of carotid sinus hypersensitivity. JACC 2000;35 (2, suppl 1): 261

55. Nathanson MH: Hyperactive cardioinhibitory carotid sinus reflex. Arch Intern Med 1946;77:491–502

56. Heidorn GH, McNamara AP: Effect of carotid sinus stimulation on the electrocardiograms of clinically normal individuals. Circulation 1956;14: 1104–1113

57. Sigler LH: The hyperactive cardioinhibitory carotid sinus reflex as an aid in the diagnosis of coronary disease. N Engl J Med 1942;226:46–51

58. Smiddy J, Lewis D, Dunn M: The effect of carotid sinus massage in older men. J Gerontol 1972;27:209–211

59. Sigler LH: Hyperactive vasodepressor carotid sinus reflex. Arch Intern Med 1942; 70:983–1001

60. McIntosh SJ, Lawson J, Kenny RA: Intravenous cannulation alters the specificity of head-up tilt testing for vasovagal syncope in elderly patients. Age Ageing 1994;23:317–319

61. Brignole M, Gigli G, Altomonte F et al: Cardioinhibitory reflex provoked by stimulation of carotid sinus in normal subjects and those with cardiovascular disease. G Ital Cardiol 1985;15:514–519

62. Quest JA, Gillis RA: Effect of digitalis on carotid sinus baroreceptor activity. Circ Res 1974;35:247–255

63. Reyes AJ: Propanolol and the hyperactive carotid sinus reflex syndrome. Br Med J 1973;2:662

64. Bauerfeind, Hall C, Denes P, Rosen KM: Carotid sinus hypersensitivity with alpha methyldopa. Ann Intern Med 1978;88:214–215

65. Richardson DA, Shaw FE, Bond J, Kenny RA: Prevalence of carotid sinus hypersensitivity among unexplained fallers presenting to accident and emergency department. (Communicated to PACE)

66. Kapoor W, Karp FM, Wieand S et al: A prospective evaluation and follow up of patients with syncope. N Engl J Med 1983;309:197–204

67. AGS, BTGS, AAOSP–Panel on Falls Prevention: Guideline for the prevention of falls in older persons. J Am Geriatr Soc 2001;49:664–672

68. O'Shea D, Parry SW, Kenny RA: The Newcastle protocol for carotid sinus massage. J Am Geriatr Soc 2001;49(2):236–237

69. Hilal H, Massumi R: Fatal ventricular fibrillation after carotid sinus stimulation. N Engl J Med 1966;275:157–158

70. Askey J: Hemiplegia following carotid sinus stimulation. Am Heart J 1946;31:131–137

71. Calverley JR, Millikan CH: Complications of carotid manipulation. Neurology 1961;11:185–189

72. Lown B, Levine SA: The carotid sinus: clinical value of its stimulation. Circulation 1961;23:766–789

73. Strasburg B, Rechavia E, Sagie A et al: Usefulness of head-up tilt table test in evaluating patients with syncope of unknown origin. Am Heart J 1989;118:923–927

74. Munro NC, McIntosh SJ, Lawson J et al: Incidence of complications after carotid sinus massage in older patients with syncope. J Am Geriatr Soc 1994;42:1248–1251

75. Davies AJ, Kenny RA: Frequency of neurological complications following carotid sinus massage. Am J Cardiol 1998;16:1434–1435

76. Richardson DA, Bexton R, Shaw FE et al: Complications of carotid sinus massage—a prospective series of older patients. Age Ageing 2000;29(5):413–417

77. Stryjer D, Friedensohn A, Schlesinger Z: Carotid sinus hypersensitivity: Diagnosis of vasodepressor type in the presence of cardioinhibitory type. PACE 1982;5:793–800

78. Weiss S, Baker JP: The carotid sinus reflex in health and disease: its role in the causation of fainting and convulsions. Medicine (Baltimore) 1933;12:297–354

79. Strasberg B, Sagie A, Erdman S et al: Carotid sinus hypersensitivity and the carotid sinus syndrome. Prog Cardiovasc Dis 1989;31:379–391

80. Draper AJ: The cardioinhibitory carotid sinus syndrome. Ann Intern Med 1950;32: 700–716

81. Murphy AL, Rowbotham BJ, Boyle RS et al: Carotid sinus hypersensitivity in elderly nursing home patients. Aust NZ Med 1986;16:24–27

82. Ward C, McIntosh S, Kenny RA: The prevalence of carotid sinus syndrome in elderly patients with fractured neck of femur. Age Ageing 1993;23 (suppl 1): A16 (abstract)

83. Brignole M, Oddone D, Cogorno S et al: Long-term outcome in symptomatic carotid sinus hypersensitivity. Am Heart J 1992;123:687–692

84. Parry SW, Kenny RA: The role of tilt table testing in neurocardiovascular instability in older adults. Eur Heart J 2001;22(5):370–372

85. Blanc JJ, Boshat J, Penther P: Hypersensibilite sino-carotidienne. Evolution a moyen terme en fonction du traitement et des symptomes. Arch Mal Coeur 1984;77:330–336

86. Brignole M, Menozzi C, Lolli G, Bottoni N, Gaggioli G: Long-term outcome of paced and nonpaced patients with severe carotid sinus syndrome. Am J Cardiol 1992;69:1039–1043.

87. Trout HH, Brown LL, Thompson JE: Carotid sinus syndrome treatment by carotid sinus denervation. Ann Surg 1979;189:575–580

88. Greeley HP, Smedal MI, Morset W: The treatment of the carotid sinus syndrome by irradiation. N Engl J Med 1955;252:91–94

89. Ford FR: Fatal hypertensive crisis following denervation of the carotid sinus for the relief of repeated attacks of syncope. Case history. Bull Johns Hopkins Hosp 1957;100:14–16

90. Frank JI, Ropper AH, Zuniga G: Vasodepressor carotid sinus syncope associated with a neck mass. Neurology 1992;42:1194–1197

91. Wenger TL, Dohrmann ML, Strauss HC: Hypersensitive carotid sinus syndrome manifested as cough syncope. PACE 1980;3:332–339

92. Sugrue DD, Gersh BJ, Holmes DR et al: Symptomatic 'isolated' carotid sinus hypersensitivity: natural history and results of treatment with anticholinergic drugs or pacemaker. J Am Coll Cardiol 1986;7:158–162

93. Madigan NP, Flaker GC, Curtis JJ et al: Carotid sinus hypersensitivity: beneficial effects of dual-chamber pacing. Am J Cardiol 1984;53:1034–1040

94. Brignole M, Sartore B, Barra M, Menozzi C, Lolli G: Is DDD superior to VVI pacing in mixed carotid sinus syndrome? An acute and medium-term study. PACE 1988;11:1902–1910

95. Morley CA, Perrins EJ, Chan SL, Sutton R: Longterm comparison of DVI and VVI pacing in carotid sinus syndrome. In Steinbach K, Gloggar D, Laszkowicz A, Scheibelhofer W, Weber H (eds): Proceedings of the VIIth World Symposium on Cardiac Pacing. Steinkopff-Verlag, Darmstadt 1983:929–935

96. Almquist A, Gornick C, Benson DW et al: Carotid sinus hypersensitivity: evaluation of the vasodepressor component. Circulation 1985;71:927–936

97. Morley CA, Perrins EJ, Sutton R: Pharmacological intervention in the carotid sinus syndrome. PACE 1983;6:A16

98. da Costa D, McIntosh S, Kenny RA: Benefits of fludrocortisone in the treatment of symptomatic vasodepressor carotid sinus syndrome. Br Heart J 1993;69:308–310

99. Mathias CJ, Bannister R: Investigation of autonomic disorders. In Bannister R, Mathias CJ (eds): Autonomic Failure: A Textbook of Clinical Disorders of the Autonomic Nervous System. Oxford Medical Publications, Oxford, 1992:255–290

100. Palmer KT: Studies into postural hypotension in elderly patients. NZ Med J 1983;96:43–45

101. Caird FI, Andrews GR, Kennedy RD: Effect of posture on blood pressure in the elderly. Br Heart J 1973;35:527–530

102. Schatz IJ, Masaki KH, Burchfiel CM, Curb JD, Chiu D: Orthostatic hypotension (OH) as a predictor of two year mortality in elderly men; the Honolulu heart program. Clin Autonom Res 1995;5:321

103. Sjostrand T: Regulation of the blood distribution in man. Acta Physiol Scand 1952;26:312

104. Ziegler MG: Postural hypotension. Ann Rev Med 1980;31:239–245

105. Rowe JW, Troen BR: Sympathetic nervous system and ageing in man. Endocrinol Rev 1980:1:167–179

106. Bannister R, Mathias CJ: Clinical features and manifestations and investigation of primary autonomic failure syndromes. In Bannister R, Mathias CJ (eds): Autonomic Failure: A Textbook of Clinical Disorders of the Autonomic Nervous System. Oxford Medical Publications, Oxford, 1992:531–547

107. Wieling W, van Brederode JFM, deRijk LG et al: Reflex control of heart rate in normal subjects in relation to age: a data base for cardiac vagal neuropathy. Diabetologia 1982;22:163–166

108. Wieling W: Laboratory assessment of disturbances in cardiovascular control. In Kenny RA (ed): Syncope in the Older Patient: Causes, Investigations and Consequences of Syncope and Falls. Chapman & Hall Medical, London, 1996:47–71

109. Imholz BPM, Dambrink JHA, Karemaker JM, Wieling W: Orthostatic circulatory control in the elderly evaluated by non-invasive continuous blood pressure measurement. Clin Sci 1990;79:73–79

110. Wieling W, Veerman DP, Dambrink JHA, Imholz BPM: Disparities in circulatory adjustment to standing between young and elderly subjects explained by pulse contour analysis. Clin Sci 1992;83:149–155

111. Van Dijk JG, Tjon-A-Tsien AML, Kamjoul BA et al: Effect of supine blood on interpretation of standing up test in 500 patients with diabetes mellitus. J Autonom Nerv Syst 1994;47:23–31

112. Gribbin B, Pickering TG, Sleight P, Peto R: Effect of age and blood pressure on baroreflex sensitivity in man. Circ Res 1971 29:424–431

113. Lakatta EG. Do hypertension and aging have a similar effect on myocardium. Circulation 1987;75:169–177

114. Lipsitz LA, Storch HA, Minaker KL, Rowe JW: Intra-individual variability in postural blood pressure in the elderly. Clin Sci 1985;69:337–341

115. Mathias CJ: The classification and nomenclature of autonomic disorders—ending chaos, resolving conflict and hopefully achieving clarity. Clin Autonom Res 1995;5:307–310

116. Wynne HA, Schofield S: Drug induced orthostatic hypotension. In Kenny, RA (ed): Syncope in the Older Patient: Causes, Investigations and Consequences of Syncope and Falls. Chapman & Hall Medical, London, 1996:137–154

117. Naranjo CA, Busto U, Sellers EM et al: A method of estimating the probability of adverse drug reactions. Clin Pharmacol Ther 1981;30:239–245

118. Mathias CJ: Primary autonomic failure in association with other neurological features—the syndromes of Shy–Drager and multiple system atrophy. In Kenny RA (ed): Syncope in the Older Patient: Causes, Investigations and Consequences of Syncope and Falls. Chapman & Hall Medical, London, 1996:237–248

119. Bleasdale-Barr K, Mathias CJ: Suboccipital (coat hanger) and other muscular pains—frequency in autonomic failure and other neurological problems, and association with postural hypotension. Clin Autonom Res 1994;4:82

120. Bannister R, Ardill L, Fentem P: An assessment of various methods of treatment of idiopathic orthostatic hypotension. Q J Med 1969;38:377–395

121. Moss AJ, Glaser W, Topol E: Atrial tachypacing in the treatment of a patient with primary orthostatic hypotension. New Engl J Med 1980;302:1456–1457

122. Hussain RM, McIntosh SJ, Lawson J, Kenny RA: Fludrocortisone in the treatment of hypotensive disorders in the elderly. Heart 1996;76:507–509

123. Jankovic J, Gilden JL, Hiner BC et al: Neurogenic orthostatic hypotension: a double blind placebo controlled study with midodrine. Am J Med 1993;95:38–48

124. Sutton R, Petersen M, Brignole M et al: Proposed classification for tilt induced vasovagal syncope. Eur J Card Pacing Electrophysiol 1992;2:180–183

125. Wayne HH: Syncope: physiologic considerations and an analysis of the clinical characteristics in 510 patients. Am J Med 1961;30:418–438

126. Parry SW, Kenny RA: Carotid sinus syndrome masquerading as treatment resistant epilepsy. Postgrad Med J 2000;76(900):656–658

127. Streeten DP, Andersen GH Jr, Richardson R, Deaver TF: Abnormal orthostatic changes in blood pressure and heart rate in subjects with intact sympathetic nervous function: evidence for excessive venous pooling. J Lab Clin Med 1988;111:326–335

128. Samoil D, Grubb BP, Brewster P et al: Comparison of single and dual chamber pacing techniques in prevention of head upright tilt induced vasovagal syncope. Eur J Pacing Electrophysiol 1993;1:36–41

129. Kenny RA, Ingram A, Bayliss J, Sutton R: Head-up tilt is a useful tool for investigating unexplained syncope. Lancet 1986;2:1352–1354

130. Fitzpatrick A, Sutton R: Tilting towards a diagnosis in unexplained recurrent syncope. Lancet 1989;1:658–660

131. Grubb BP, Temesy-Armos P, Hahn H, Elliot L: Utility of head upright tilt table testing in the evaluation and management of syncope of unknown origin. Am J Med 1991;90:6–10

132. Raviele A, Gasparini G, DePede F et al: Usefulness of head-up tilt table test in evaluating syncope of unknown origin and negative electrophysiologic study. Am J Cardiol 1989;65:1322–1327

133. Abi-Samara F, Maloney J, Fouad FM, Castle L: The usefulness of head-up tilt table testing and hemodynamic investigations in the workup of syncope of unknown origin. PACE 1987;10:406–410

134. Brignole M, Menozzi C, Del Rosso A et al: New classification of haemodynamics of vasovagal syncope: beyond the VASIS classification. Analysis of the pre-syncopal phase of the tilt test without and with nitroglycerin challenge, Vasovagal Syncope International Study. Europace 2000; 2:66–76

135. Kenny RA, Richardson DA: Carotid sinus syndrome and falls in older adults. Am J Geriatr Cardiol 2001;10(2):97–99 (review)

136. Kenny RA, O'Shea D, Parry SW: The Newcastle protocols for head-up tilt table testing in the diagnosis of vasovagal syncope, carotid sinus hypersensitivity, and related disorders. Heart 2000;83(5):564–569

137. Grubb BP, Samoil D: Neurocardiogenic syncope. In Kenny RA (ed): Syncope in the Older Patient: Causes, Investigations and Consequences of Syncope and Falls. Chapman & Hall Medical, London, 1996:91–106

138. Almquist A, Goldenberg I, Milstein S et al: Provocation of bradycardia and hypotension by isoproterenol and upright posture in patients with unexplained syncope. N Engl J Med 1989;320:346–351

139. Kapoor WN, Brant N: Evaluation of syncope by upright tilt testing with isoproterenol. A nonspecific test. Ann Intern Med 1992;116:358–368

140. Raviele A, Gasparini G, diPede F et al: Usefulness of nitroglycerin infusion during head-up tilt for the diagnosis of vasovagal syncope. J Am Coll Cardiol 1993;21:111A.

141. Kurbaan AS, Franzén A-C, Bowker TJ et al: Usefulness of tilt test-induced patterns of heart rate and blood pressure using a two-stage protocol with glyceryl trinitrate provocation in patients with syncope of unknown origin. Am J Cardiol 1999;84:665–670

142. Raviele A, Menozzi C, Brignole M et al: Value of head-up tilt testing with sublingual nitroglycerin to assess the origin of unexplained syncope. Am J Cardiol 1995;76:267–272

143. Graham LA, Gray JC, Kenny RA: Comparison of provocative tests for unexplained syncope: isoprenaline and glyceryl trinitrate for diagnosing vasovagal syncope. Eur Heart J 2001;22(6):497–503

144. Benditt D, Remole S, Bailin S et al: Tilt table testing for evaluation of neurally mediated syncope: rationale and proposed protocols. PACE 1991;14:1528–1537

145. Samoil D, Grubb BP: Vasovagal (neurally mediated) syncope: pathophysiology, diagnosis, and therapeutic approach. Eur J Card Pacing Electrophysiol 1992;2:234–241

146. Fish F, Benson DW: Tilt testing for unexplained syncope. Primary Cardiol 1992;18:87–97

147. Shvartz E: Reliability of quantifiable tilt table data. Aerospace Med 1968;39:1094–1096.

148. Fitzpatrick AP, Theodorakis G, Vardas P, Sutton R: Methodology of head upright tilt table testing in patients with unexplained syncope. J Am Coll Cardiol 1991;17:125–130

149. Chen XC, Chen MY, Remole S et al: Reproducibility of head upright tilt table testing for eliciting susceptibility to neurally mediated syncope in patients without structural heart disease. Am J Cardiol 1992;69:755–760

150. Sheldon R, Spelaniski J, Koestner J et al: Reproducibility of isoproterenol tilt tests in patients with syncope. Am J Cardiol 1992,69:1300–1305

151. Grubb BP, Wolfe D, Temesy Amos P et al: Reproducibility of tilt table test results in patients with syncope. PACE 1992,15:1477–1481

152. Milistein S, Buetikofer J, Lesser J et al: Usefulness of disopyramide for prevention of upright tilt induced hypotension and bradycardia. Am J Cardiol 1990;65:1339–1344

153. Morillo CA, Leitch JW, Yee R, Klein GJ: A placebo-controlled trial of intravenous and oral disopyramide for prevention of neurally mediated syncope induced by head-up tilt. J Am Coll Cardiol 1993;22(7):1843–1848

154. Di Girolamo E, Di Iorio C, Sabatini P et al: Effects of paroxetine hydrochloride, a selective serotonin reuptake inhibitor, on refractory vasovagal syncope: a randomised, double-blind, placebo-controlled study. J Am Coll Cardiol 1999;33(5):1227–1230

155. Grubb BP, Wolfe DA, Samoil D et al: Usefulness of fluoxetine hydrochloride for prevention of resistant upright tilt induced syncope. PACE 1993;16:458–464

156. Ward C, Gilroy J, Bishop J, Kenny RA: Midodrine in vasovagal syncope—a randomised controlled trial. (Communicated)

157. Connolly SJ, Sheldon RS, Roberts RS, Gent M: The North American vasovagal pacemaker study, a randomised trial of permanent cardiac pacing for the prevention of vasovagal syncope. J Am Coll Cardiol 1999;33:16–20

158. Raviele A, Brignole M, Sutton R et al: Effect of etilefrine in preventing syncopal recurrence in patients with vasovagal syncope: a double-blind, randomized, placebo-controlled trial. The Vasovagal Syncope International Study. Circulation. 1999;99(11):1452–1457

159. Grubb BP, Wolfe D, Samoil D et al: Adaptive rate pacing controlled by right ventricular pre-ejection interval for severe refractory orthostatic hypotension. PACE 1993;16:801–805

160. Goldstein RE, Redwood DR, Rosing DR et al: Alterations in the circulatory response to exercise following a meal and their relationship to post prandial angina pectoris. Circulation 1971;44:90–100

161. Seyer-Hansen K: Postprandial hypotension. Br Med J 1977;2:1262

162. Lipsitz LA, Nyquist RP, Wei JY, Rowe JW: Postprandial reduction in blood pressure in the elderly. N Engl J Med 1983;309:81–83

163. Lipsitz LA, Fullerton KJ: Postprandial blood pressure reduction in healthy elderly. J Am Geriatr Soc 1986;34:267–270

164. Westenend M, Lenders JWM, Thein T: The course of blood pressure after a meal: a difference between young and elderly subjects. J Hypertens 1985;3:S417–419

165. Peitzman SJ, Berger SR: Postprandial blood pressure decrease in well elderly persons. Arch Int Med 1989;149:286–288

166. Jansen RWMM, Penterman BJM, vanLier HJJ, Hoefnagels WHL: Blood pressure reduction after oral glucose loading and its relation to age, blood pressure and insulin. Am J Cardiol 1987;60:1087–1091

167. Potter JF, Heseltine D, Hartley G et al: Effects of meal composition on the postprandial blood pressure, catecholamine and insulin changes in elderly subjects. Clin Sci 1989;77:265–272

168. Sidery MB, Cowley AJ, Macdonald IA: Cardiovascular responses to a high fat and high carbohydrate meal in healthy elderly subjects. Clin Sci 1993;84:263–270

169. Jansen RWMM, Peeters TL, vanLier HJJ, Hoefnagles WHL: The effect of oral glucose, protein, fat and water loading on blood pressure and the gastrointestinal peptides VIP and somatostatin in hypertensive elderly subjects. Eur J Clin Invest 1990;20:192–198

170. Heseltine D, Dakak M, Macdonald IA et al: Effects of carbohydrate type on postprandial blood pressure, neuroendocrine and gastrointestinal hormone changes in the elderly. Clin Autonom Res 1991;1:219–224

171. Mathias CJ, daCosta DF, Fosbraey P et al: Hypotensive and sedative effects of insulin in autonomic failure. Br Med J 1987;295:161–163

172. Jonsson PV, Lipsitz LA, Kelly M, Koestner J: Hypotensive responses to common daily activities in institutionalized elderly. Arch Int Med 1990;150:1518–1524

173. Vaitkevicius PV, Esserwein DM, Maynard AK et al: Frequency and importance of postprandial blood pressure reduction in elderly nursing-home patients. Ann Int Med 1991;115:865–870

174. Robertson D, Wade D, Robertson RM: Postprandial alterations in cardiovascular hemodynamics in autonomic dysfunctional states. Am J Cardiol 1981;48:1048–1052

175. Raimbach SJ, Cortelli P, Kooner JS et al: Prevention of glucose induced hypotension by the somatostatin analogue octreotide (SMS 201–995) in chronic autonomic failure; hemodynamic and hormonal changes. Clin Sci 1989;77:623–628

176. Haigh R, Fotherby M, Harper G et al: Duration of caffeine abstention influences the acute blood pressure response to caffeine in elderly normotensives. Eur J Clin Pharmacol 1993;44:549–553

177. Potter JF, Haigh R, Harper G et al: Blood pressure, plasma catecholamine and renin response to caffeine in elderly hypertensives. J Hum Hypertens 1993;7: 273–278

178. Lenders JWM, Morre HLC, Smits P, Thien TH: The effect of caffeine on the postprandial fall in blood pressure in the elderly. Age Ageing 1988;17:236–240

179. Heseltine D, Dakak M, Woodhouse K et al: The effect of caffeine on postprandial hypotension in the elderly. J Am Geriatr Soc 1991;39:160–164

180. Brignole M, Alboni P, Benditt D et al: Guidelines on management (diagnosis and treatment) of syncope. Eur Heart J 2001;22(15):1256–1306

181. Alboni P, Brignole M, Menozzi C et al: The diagnostic value of history in patients with syncope with or without heart disease. J Am Coll Cardiol 2001;37:1921–1928

182. Besdine RW: Geriatric medicine—an over view. Annu Rev Gerontol 1980;1:135–153

183. Dimant T: Accidents in the skilled nursing facility. NY State J Med 1985;85:202

184. Drachman DA, Hart CW: An approach to the dizzy patient. Neurology 1972;22:323–324

185. Lawson J, Birchall JP, Fitzgerald J, Kenny RA: Benefits of an integrated diagnostic approach to the investigation of dizziness in the community. Br Med J (in press)

186. The Consensus Committee of the American Autonomic Society and the American Academy of Neurolepsy: Consensus statement on the defunction of orthostatic hypotension, pure autonomic failure and multiple system atrophy. Neurology 1996;46:1470–1479

187. Patel A, Maloney A, Damato AN: On the frequency and reproducibility of orthostatic blood pressure changes in healthy community dwelling elderly during 60 degrees head-up tilt. Am Heart J 1993;126:184–188

188. Camn AJ, Evans KE, Ward DE, Martin A: The rhythm of the heart in active elderly subjects. Am Heart J 1980;99:598–603

189. Surgue DD, Holmes DR, Gresh BJ et al: Impact of intracardiac electrophysiologic testing on the management of elderly patients with syncope or near syncope. J Am Geriatr Soc 1987;35:1079–1083

190. Denes P, Uretz E, Ezri MD, Borbola J: Clinical predictor of electrophysiologic findings in patients with syncope of unknown origin. Arch Intern Med 1988;146:1922–1928

191. Kapoor WN: Evaluation and management of the patient with syncope. JAMA 1992;268:2553–2560

192. Gibson TC, Heitzman MR: Diagnostic efficiency of 24 hour electrocardio-graphic monitoring for syncope. Am J Cardiol 1984;53:1013–1017

193. DiMarco JP, Philbrick JT: Use of electrocardiographic (Holter) monitoring. Ann Intern Med 1990;113:53–68

194. Bass EB, Curtis EI, Arena VC et al: The duration of Holter monitoring in patients with syncope: Is 24 hours enough? Arch Intern Med 1990;150:1073–1078

195. Linzer M, Pritchett ELC, Pontinen M, McCarthy E, Divine GW: Incremental diagnostic yield of loop electrocardiographic recorders in unexplained syncope. Am J Cardiol 1990;66:214–219

196. Krahn A, Klein GJ, Yee R, Norris C: Final results from a pilot study with an implantable loop recorder to determine the etiology of syncope in patients with negative noninvasive and invasive testing. Am J Cardiol 1998;82:117–119

197. Krahn AD, Klein GJ, Yee R, Takle-Newhouse T, Norris C: Use of an extended monitoring strategy in patients with problematic syncope. Reveal investigators. Circulation 1999;99:406–410

198. Armstrong VL, Lawson J, Kamper AM, Newton J, Kenny RA. Use of an implantable loop recorder in the investigation of unexplained syncope in older people. Age Aging 2002 (in press)

199. Zaidi A, Fitzpatrick AP: Single centre experience of 64 insertable loop recorders for investigation of unexplained syncope. PACE 1999;22:756 (abstract)

200. Oraii S, Maleki M, Minooii M, Kafai I: Comparing two different protocols for tilt table testing: sublingual glyceryl trinitrate versus isoprenaline infusion. Heart 1999;81:603–605

201. Raviele A, Giada F, Brignole M et al: Diagnostic accuracy of sublingual nitroglycerin test and low-dose isoproterenol test in patients with unexplained syncope. A comparative study. Am J Cardiol 2000;85:1194–1198

202. Brignole M, Menozzi C, Bottoni N et al: Mechanisms of syncope caused by transient bradycardia and the diagnostic value of electrophysiologic testing and cardiovascular reflexivity maneuvers. Am J Cardiol 1995;76:273–278

203. Fujimura O, Yee R, Klein G, Sharma A, Boahene A: The diagnostic sensitivity of electrophysiologic testing in patients with syncope caused by transient bradycardia. N Engl J Med 1989;321:1703–1707

204. Lacroix D, Dubuc M, Kus T et al: Evaluation of arrhythmic causes of syncope: correlation between Holter monitoring, electrophysiologic

205. Moazez F, Peter T, Simonson J et al: Syncope of unknown origin: clinical, noninvasive, and electrophysiologic determinants of arrhythmia induction and symptom recurrence during long-term follow-up. Am Heart J 1991;121:81–88

206. Bergfeldt L, Vallin H, Rosenqvist M et al: Sinus node recovery time assessment revisited: role of pharmacological blockade of the autonomic nervous system. J Cardiovasc Electrophysiol 1996;7:95–101

207. Englund A, Bergfeldt L, Rosenqvist M: Pharmacological stress testing of the His-Purkinje system in patients with bifascicular block. PACE 1998;21:1979–1987

208. Linzer M, Yang E, Estes M et al: Diagnosing syncope. Part II: Unexplained syncope. Ann Intern Med 1997;127:76–86

209. Bergfeldt L, Rosenqvist M, Vallin H, Nordlander R, Åström H: Screening for sinus node dysfunction by analysis of short-term sinus cycle variations on the surface electrocardiogram. Am Heart J 1995;130:141–147

210. Benditt DG, Gornick C, Dunbar D, Almquist A, Pool-Scheider S: Indications for electrophysiological testing in diagnosis and assessment of sinus node dysfunction. Circulation 1987;75 (suppl III):93–99

211. Freedman RA: Sinus node dysfunction. Cardiac Electrophysiol Rev 1999;3:74–79

212. Rosenbaum MB, Elizari MV, Lazzari JO: Los hemibloqueos. Buenos Aires, Parados, 1968

213. Demoulin JC, Kulbertus HE: Histopathological examination of concept of left hemiblock. Br Heart J 1972;34:807–814

214. Dhala A, Gonzalez-Zuelgaray J, Deshpande S et al: Unmasking the trifascicular left intraventricular conduction system by ablation of the right bundle branch. Am J Cardiol 1996;77:706–712

215. Bergfeldt L, Edvardsson N, Rosenqvist M, Vallin H, Edhag O: Atrioventricular block progression in patients with bifascicular block assessed by repeated electrocardiography and a bradycardia-detecting pacemaker. Am J Cardiol 1994;74:1129–1132

216. McAnulty JH, Rahimtoola SH, Murphy E et al: Natural history of "high risk" bundle branch block. Final report of a prospective study. N Engl J Med 1982;307(3):137–143

217. Gronda M, Magnani A, Occhetta E et al: Electrophysiologic study of atrio-ventricular block and ventricular conduction defects. G Ital Cardiol 1984;14:768–773

218. Dini P, Iaolongo D, Adinolfi E et al: Prognostic value of His-ventricular conduction after ajmaline administration. In Masoni A, Alboni P (eds): Cardiac Electrophysiology Today. Academic Press, London, 1982:515–522

219. Kaul U, Dev V, Narula J et al: Evaluation of patients with bundle branch block and "unexplained" syncope: a study based on comprehensive electrophysiologic testing and ajmaline stress. PACE 1988;11:289–297

220. Twidale N, Heddle W, Tonkin A: Procainamide administration during electrophysiologic study—utility as a provocative test for intermittent atrioventricular block. PACE 1988;11:1388–1397

221. Link M, Kim KM, Homoud M, Estes III M, Wang P: Long-term outcome of patients with syncope associated with coronary artery disease and a non diagnostic electrophysiological evaluation. Am J Cardiol 1999;83:1334–1337

222. Gaggioli G, Bottoni N, Brignole M et al: [Progression to 2d and 3d grade atrioventricular block in patients after electrostimulation for bundle-branch block and syncope: a long-term study]. [Italian] Giornale Italiano di Cardiologia 1994;24:409–416

223. Scheinman MM, Peters RW, Sauvé MJ et al: Value of the H-Q interval in patients with bundle branch block and the role of prophylactic permanent pacing. Am J Cardiol 1982;50:1316–1322

224. Rosen KM, Rahimtoola SH, Chquimia R, Loeb HS, Gunnar RM: Electrophysiological significance of first-degree atrioventricular block with intraventricular conduction disturbance. Circulation 1971;43:491–502

225. Goldreyer BN, Kastor JA, Kershbaum KL: The hemodynamic effects of induced supraventricular tachycardia in man. Circulation 1976;54:783–789

226. Bigger JT Jr, Reiffel JA, Livelli FD, Wang PJ: Sensitivity, specificity, and reproducibility of programmed ventricular stimulation. Circulation 1986;73(suppl II):73–78

227. Wellens HJJ, Brugada P, Stevenson WG: Programmed electrical stimulation of the heart in patients with life-threatening ventricular arrhythmias: what is the significance of induced arrhythmias and what is the correct stimulation protocol? Circulation 1986;72:1–7

228. Olshansky B, Hahn EA, Hartz VL, Prater SP, Mason JW: Clinical significance of syncope in the electrophysiologic study versus electrocardiographic monitoring (ESVEM) trial. Am Heart J 1999;137:878–886

229. Flammang D, Church T, Waynberger M, Chassing A, Antiel M: Can adenosine 5′ triphosphate be used to select treatment in severe vasovagal syndrome? Circulation 1997;96:1201–1208

230. Brignole M, Gaggioli G, Menozzi C et al: Adenosine-induced atrioventricular block in patients with unexplained syncope. The diagnostic value of ATP test. Circulation 1997;96:3921–3927

231. Belardinelli L, Linden J, Berne RM: The cardiac effects of adenosine. Prog Cardiovasc Dis 1989;22:73–97

232. Berbari EJ, Scherlag BJ, Hope RR, Lazzara R: Recording from the body surface of arrhythmogenic ventricular activity during the S-T segment. Am J Cardiol 1978;41:697–702

233. Senard JM, Charmontin B, Rascol A, Montastruc JL: Ambulatory blood pressure in patients with Parkinson's disease without and with orthostatic hypotension. Clin Autonomic Res 1992;2:99–104

234. O'Shea D, Parry SW, Kenny RA: The Newcastle protocol for carotid sinus massage. J Am Geriatr Soc 2001;49:236–237

235. Parry SW, Kenny RA: The management of vasovagal syncope. Q J Med 1999;92(12):697–705 (review)

236. Parry SW, Kenny RA: Tilt table testing in the diagnosis of unexplained syncope. Q J Med 1999;92(11):623–629 (review)

237. Kapoor WN, Smith MA, Miller NL: Upright tilt testing in evaluating syncope: A comprehensive literature review. Am J Med 1994;97:78–88

238. Parry SW, Bishop M, Kenny RA: Shortening the duration of the head up tilt—a randomized trial of passive versus GTN—prolonged tilt table testing. J Clin Coll Cardiol 2001 (in press)

Chapter 39

Vascular surgery

Arnab Bhowmick and Charles N. McCollum

The prevalence of atherosclerosis increases with advancing age, so it is hardly surprising that the majority of a vascular surgeon's patients are elderly and have a full range of concomitant diseases typical of such patients. Equally, specialists in geriatric medicine frequently find vascular disease in the patients they treat. Decisions regarding treatment need to be balanced against quality of life and cardiac and respiratory risk factors. In many patients neither invasive investigation by arteriography nor vascular surgery will be indicated. However, vascular surgery is now being performed with increasing safety in patients who have longer life expectancies. The principle of balancing benefit against risk of treatment is emphasized repeatedly throughout this chapter.

Elderly people suffer a range of vascular conditions, but this chapter covers the three most common problems presenting to vascular surgeons: (1) vascular disease of the limb, either acute or chronic; (2) carotid disease; and (3) abdominal aortic aneurysm. New techniques are rapidly changing our approach to the management of vascular conditions; for example, the use of percutaneous transluminal angioplasty as the sole treatment for lower-limb critical ischemia,[1] and the introduction of endovascular stent-grafts for the treatment of abdominal aortic aneurysms.[2]

ARTERIAL DISEASE OF THE LIMB

Most patients with peripheral vascular disease present with symptoms of chronic ischemia. This ranges from intermittent claudication with a benign prognosis, to critical ischemia presenting with rest pain, gangrene, ischemic ulceration, and the threat of amputation.

Acute ischemia of a limb may be due to emboli, but it is now more usually secondary to thrombosis in diseased arteries. The majority of emboli lodge at the bifurcation of a main vessel, giving rise to distal dysfunction. Acute ischemia may present with some or all of the classical symptoms such as pain, pallor, paresthesia, paralysis, and lack of pulse.

Chronic peripheral vascular disease

Prevalence

Atherosclerosis is the most common disease affecting peripheral arteries in the elderly population and may severely limit mobility and quality of life.[3] Amputation for peripheral vascular disease or gangrene is the second most common operation in patients aged over 90 years.[4] At least one-third of patients with arterial stenosis or arterial occlusion, particularly involving the superficial femoral artery at the adductor canal, are asymptomatic.[5] However, approximately 50 percent of patients presenting with intermittent claudication have a superficial femoral artery occlusion.[6] The prevalence of claudication is only 1.0–1.5 percent in men aged under 50 years, but it rises substantially thereafter—up to 20–25 percent in those over 85.[7,8]

Prognosis

Only 10 percent of individuals with intermittent claudication consult a doctor and only a minority of these will ever come to surgery.[9] The outlook for the legs in patients with claudication is good, but peripheral vascular disease is a strong predictor of subsequent mortality, which more than doubles that of non-claudicants.[10–12] The majority of claudicants die from associated cardiovascular events, in particular stroke and myocardial infarction, and this high mortality risk is only partly explained by the expected association of peripheral vascular disease with coronary artery disease owing to the generalized nature of atherosclerosis.[13–15] In the Speedwell prospective heart disease study,[15] men with intermittent claudication had a 30 percent 5-year mortality compared with 6 percent in men without intermittent claudication. The increased risk of cardiovascular death may stem from repeated ischemia/reperfusion injury in the leg muscle, leading to leucocyte and platelet activation and increased thrombogenicity.[16]

Investigations

Investigation of patients with intermittent claudication should concentrate on identifying risk factors for cardiac and cerebrovascular events. Smoking is strongly associated with intermittent claudication, as are diabetes, hypertension, and abnormal lipid levels.[10,15,17] In diabetic patients there is increased involvement of small vessels with distal artery occlusion, which carries a poor prognosis.[11]

The ankle brachial pressure index (ABPI) may be helpful in quantifying the severity of peripheral vascular disease, but only a minority of patients with abnormal APBIs are symptomatic.[18] As a general rule, patients with a mean ABPI of less than 0.6 who have symptoms or leg ulcers need vascular surgical assessment.[19]

Rest pain, ischemic ulceration, or gangrene is an absolute indication for investigation with a view to treatment. Duplex imaging or angiography may be used to identify the sites of stenotic or occlusive disease, but they are indicated only if surgery or angioplasty is being considered. Duplex imaging has become increasingly important in the diagnosis and follow-up of arterial lesions as it is noninvasive and can be repeated on many occasions to monitor disease progress, graft patency, and the need for intervention. It identifies arterial occlusions and hemodynamically significant stenoses with a sensitivity and specificity of 92 and 97 percent, respectively, and has the potential to replace angiography. The presence of multiple stenoses is the main limitation on diagnostic accuracy.[20–22]

Duplex imaging alone can be used to predict the indication for percutaneous transluminal angioplasty.[23]

Treatment

Treatment is directed at control of risk factors for cardiovascular and cerebrovascular mortality, such as hypertension, hyperlipidemia, and diabetes. Surgery or angioplasty for peripheral vascular disease is rarely indicated for intermittent claudication, but it may be offered to those whose symptoms are intolerable for their lifestyle despite a period of conservative care. The best advice for patients with claudication is to stop smoking, lose weight if appropriate, and keep walking. Exercise training can improve claudication distances significantly.[24]

The treatment for rest pain, ischemic ulceration, or gangrene depends on the state of the peripheral circulation. New treatment modalities have revolutionized the revascularization of lower-limb ischemia. Percutaneous transluminal angioplasty is becoming the most frequent option in the treatment of both claudication and revascularization for critical ischemia. If there is a lesion amenable to angioplasty, then this should be treated. Alternatively, whether reconstructive surgery is indicated depends on the level and length of arterial occlusions and the severity of disease distally in the limb.

Acute limb ischemia

The clinical distinction between arterial thrombosis or embolism can be difficult, but errors in diagnosis lead to a higher surgical failure rate and higher hospital mortality.[25,26] Acute ischemia of the lower limb may occur due to embolization into a previously patent arterial tree, but it is now more likely to be due to thrombosis in diseased arteries. The most frequent site of origin for an arterial embolus is the heart, resulting from poor atrial emptying in atrial fibrillation or from a mural thrombus following myocardial infarction. Alternatively, an embolus may originate from a previously undiscovered ventricular or aortic aneurysm.

Arterial emboli to the arm are infrequent and usually seen only in elderly patients. Approximately two-thirds of emboli are of cardiac origin, though peripheral aneurysm may account for up to 20 percent of cases.[27,28] Conservative management is appropriate for many of these patients if the hand is viable and the pressure index (relative to the opposite normal arm) is greater than 0.6.[29,30] Surgical embolectomy can be performed under local anesthesia and achieves excellent results. However, there is an associated mortality of greater than 10 percent, related predominantly to the underlying cardiac condition.[27]

Management of femoral embolism

Early femoral embolectomy is the standard for acute leg ischemia in patients with a strong clinical suspicion of an embolus, such as those with a short history of ischemia (less than 72 hours), an embolic source such as atrial fibrillation, and no past history of intermittent claudication.[31] Embolectomy using a Fogarty catheter will usually restore limb perfusion, but it has been associated with a 16–26 percent mortality due predominantly to coexisting cardiac disease.[31–33] Following embolectomy, the patient should be given long-term anticoagulant therapy, initially by heparin infusion and then with oral anticoagulants. Investigation by full blood count, echocardiography, and duplex imaging of the arterial supply to the leg is essential.

Management of acute thrombosis

In contrast, the management of acute critical ischemia due to arterial thrombosis is one of the more demanding surgical emergencies and should be dealt with only by an experienced vascular team. There is usually a little more time to make the diagnosis and arrange treatment as a collateral circulation offers some protection. Heparin should be given as soon as possible to reduce extension of the thrombus. If the limb is not completely anesthetic or paralyzed there should be sufficient time for adequate preoperative investigations by urgent duplex imaging and angiography if indicated to assess the distal arterial tree.

Intra-arterial thrombolysis achieves lysis of such thrombi (or emboli) in approximately two-thirds of cases.[34] Accelerated techniques of lysis such as clot suction and the pulse-spray method may be undertaken in as little as 30 minutes, but higher doses of thrombolytic agents tend to increase the risk of hemorrhagic complications.[35] Following lysis, the underlying arterial disease should be treated either by transluminal angioplasty or by arterial reconstruction. In patients requiring urgent surgery, "on table" operative angiography may be performed (Fig. 39-1) to assess the extent of the occlusion and the quality of the distal arteries. This should be repeated on completion of surgery to check the reconstruction and give an indication of prognosis.

Outcome of limb salvage for severe ischemia

An aggressive policy of revascularization achieves limb and patient survival rates of approximately 75 percent at 1 year, even in the elderly population.[36] Almost all patients with severe leg ischemia should be offered a limb salvage procedure as this is associated with a better quality of life (Fig. 39-2).[37] The availability of specialist vascular surgeons reduces the frequency of major lower limb amputations, with a concomitant increase in the number of distal reconstructions.[38] Arterial reconstruction to save the leg and alleviate pain is preferable to an amputation, particularly as few elderly patients regain mobility and independence after lower-limb amputation and most require institutional care or at least homes adapted for wheelchair use.[32] Although the initial operative costs of reconstructive surgery are higher than those of amputation, this cost is more than offset by the duration of inpatient stay and the high community costs of rehabilitating amputees.[33]

CAROTID DISEASE
Diagnosis and investigations
Diagnosis
Carotid disease may be asymptomatic or may present with stroke, transient ischemic attacks (TIAs), or possibly with vague symptoms such as dizziness. Carotid artery stenosis may cause

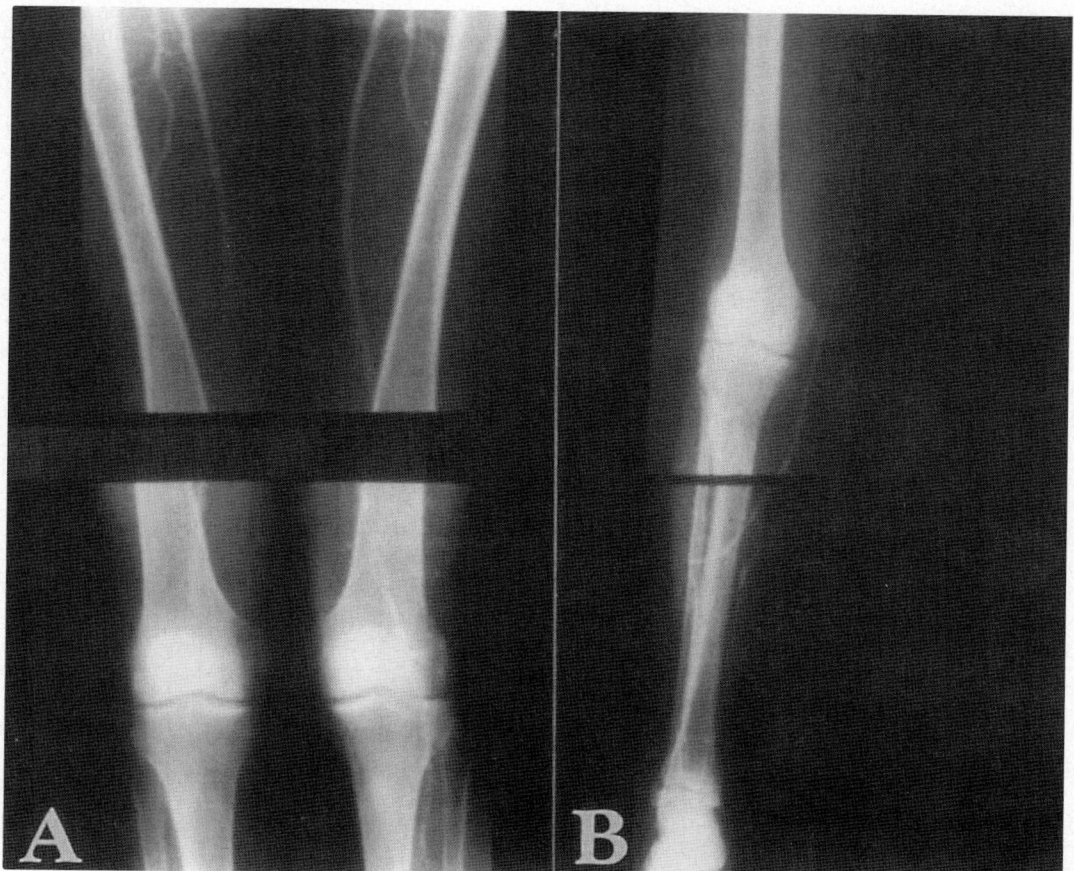

Figure 39-1 A sequence of arteriograms from a patient with acute right lower limb ischemia. In (A) there is no visualization of "run-off" below a recent occlusion in the proximal popliteal artery. Subsequent on-table angiogram using the distal popliteal artery revealed a patent anterior tibial artery. (B) Shows the completed bypass (with reversed saphenous vein).

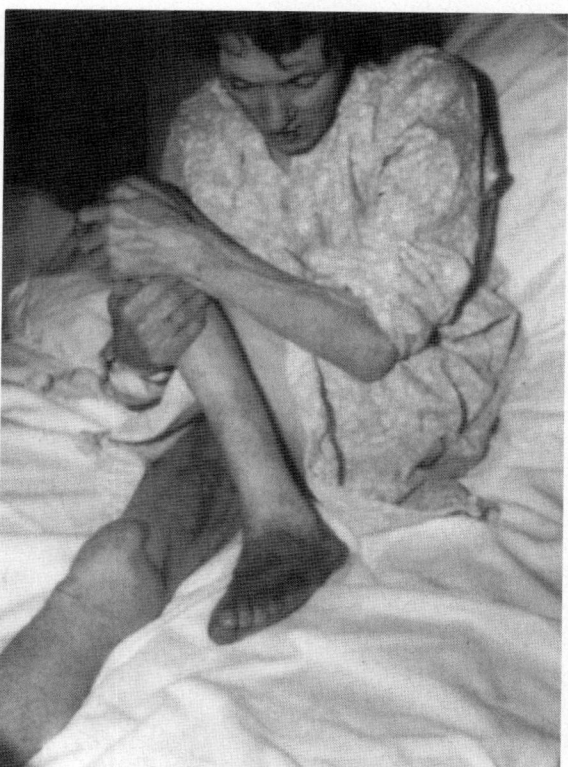

Figure 39-2 Prolonged rest ischemia, often requiring opiates, leads to distress, malaise, and general disability. Physiotherapy should be started immediately to release the flexion contracture of the knee.

stroke by hypoperfusion or by emboli; indeed many strokes are preceded by TIAs that are ignored by the patient and the doctor.

Carotid bruits can occur in the absence of significant internal carotid artery disease, and severe carotid disease may not produce a bruit. Thus, a bruit is not a reliable indicator of underlying carotid disease.[39,40] In a study examining the predisposing factors for acute cerebral infarction, only 14 percent had cervical bruits.[41] All patients presenting with either TIAs, or who recover from an appropriate stroke and are fit for surgery, should undergo carotid imaging; significant carotid artery disease is found in just over 30 percent of those with anterior circulation infarcts as classified by the Oxford Community Stroke Project Classification.[42,43]

Investigations

Noninvasive techniques to assess carotid disease include color duplex Doppler imaging, which incorporates continuous-wave Doppler to estimate blood velocity, and B-mode ultrasound to image the whole vessel. High-resolution B-mode scanning has also been shown to give prognostic information: echolucent (soft) plaques may have a greater propensity for embolization than echo-dense (hard) plaques.[44]

Portable continuous-wave Doppler (Fig. 39-3) can be used to assess the blood flow at the bifurcation and both the internal and external carotid arteries as far as the mandible. An experienced vascular technologist can readily distinguish the waveforms from each of these three vessels. Those from the internal carotid artery have a high diastolic component caused by low peripheral resistance from the cerebral circulation. In comparison, the external signal is more pulsatile with a sharp initial peak and usually a characteristic small second peak resembling the flow signals from the peripheral arteries. Increased blood velocity through a stenotic area is detected by increased frequency in the Doppler shift so that the grade of stenoses over 50 percent may be easily detected. As stenoses less than 50 percent have little or no hemodynamic significance, diagnostic accuracy and the value of the investigation improves as the degree of stenosis increases.

Although this method is simple, quick, and accurate for detecting stenoses of greater than 50 percent, mistakes can be made in heavily calcified vessels that may appear occluded if calcification prevents ultrasound penetration. In these circumstances, and where there are clinical symptoms relevant to carotid artery disease, duplex Doppler (Fig. 39-4) should be used to guide therapy. Occasionally, even duplex imaging may be difficult to interpret; in particular, total occlusion may be falsely diagnosed as trickles of blood flow through a very tight stenosis. In these cases digital subtraction angiography is indicated.

The most important risk of angiography is transient or permanent neurological deficits, with estimates in the ranges

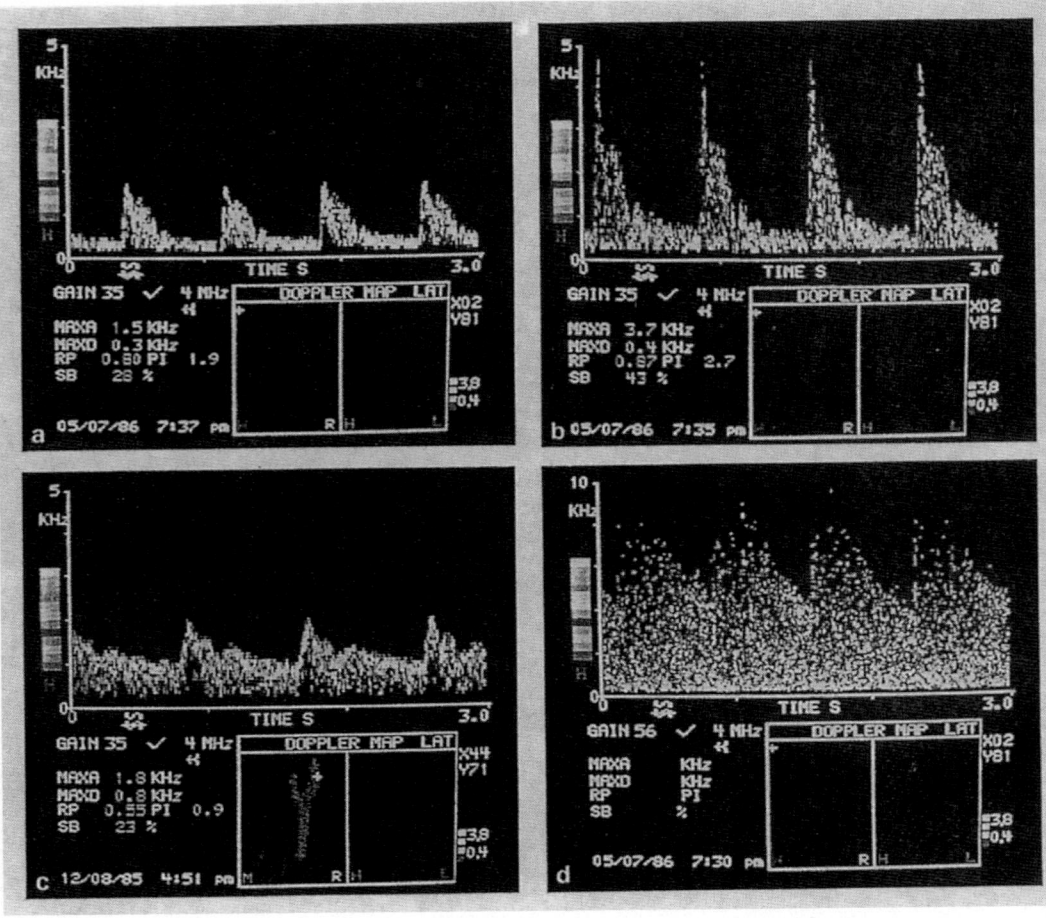

Figure 39-3 Doppler spectral analysis flow signals in normal (a) common carotid artery; (b) external carotid artery; (c) internal carotid artery; (d) a stenosed internal carotid artery demonstrating increased Doppler frequencies.

0.5–4 percent and 0.09–1.3 percent, respectively. Local complications include hematoma, dissection of the femoral artery, and embolism. Systemic complications such as allergic reactions and renal failure also occur. The overall complication rate is in the range 0.9–10 percent.[45,46]

In contrast, color duplex ultrasound is noninvasive and risk-free and has a positive predictive value of over 95 percent for significant stenosis.[47] The controversial issue of whether ultrasound alone is adequate as the definitive investigation prior to surgery is now resolving. Both magnetic resonance and digital subtraction angiography may well under- or overestimate the degree of carotid stenosis if a large plaque is situated asymmetrically within the vessel lumen.[48,49] It is also argued that angiography is necessary to exclude additional stenotic lesions elsewhere in the cerebral circulation, typically in the carotid siphon, or coincidental cerebral aneurysms, but the relevance of these so-called "tandem lesions" is uncertain.[50] Computed tomography (CT) angiography provides another noninvasive alternative in carotid assessment, but has yet to gain widespread acceptance.[51] In patients with a recent acute stroke, a cerebral CT scan (Fig. 39-5) should be performed to exclude intracerebral hemorrhage.

The risks and cost of angiography do not justify its routine use prior to carotid surgery. Exceptions to this policy are if the

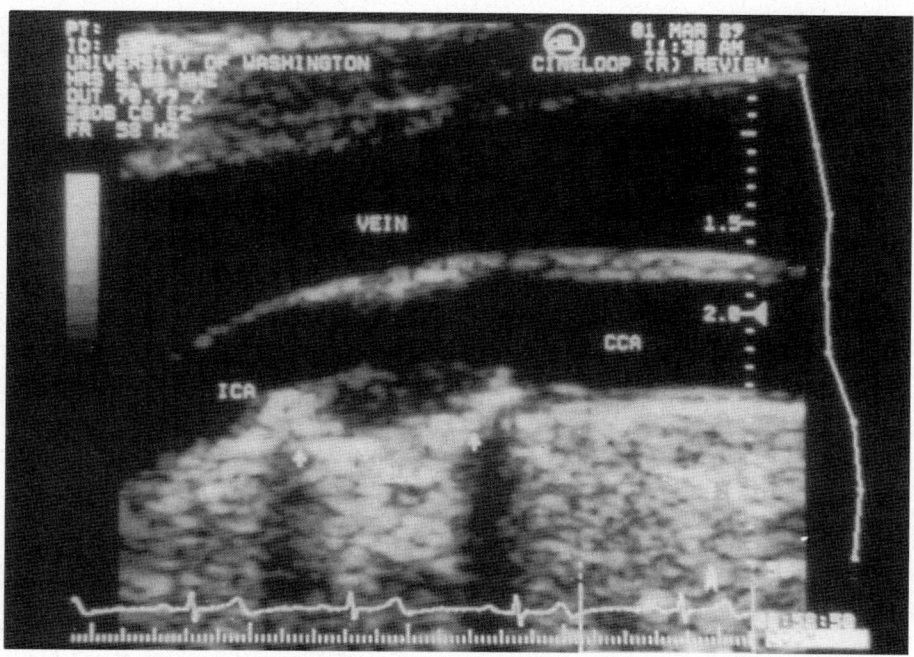

Figure 39-4 B-mode image of the carotid bifurcation demonstrating the jugular vein, common carotid (CCA), and internal carotid arteries (ICA). An ulcerated, calcified plaque is seen at the origin of the internal carotid.

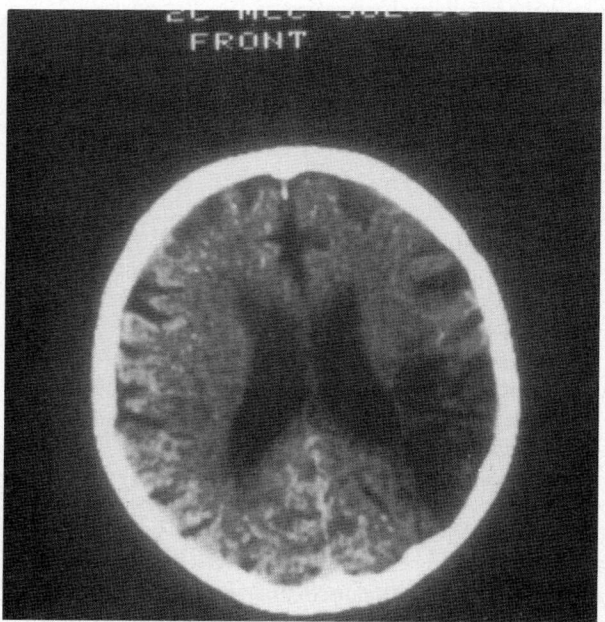

Figure 39-5 CT brain imaging of a large cerebral infarct in the left parietal region.

duplex imaging is inconclusive, or if the artery appears to be occluded on ultrasound when it is important to exclude the possibility of "trickle flow" through a very tight stenosis.

Carotid surgery

Benefits

The role of carotid surgery in the prevention of stroke in symptomatic patients with severe stenosis (70–99 percent) of the internal carotid artery is now well established. In the North American Carotid Surgery Trial[52] covering 50 clinical centers, patients with internal carotid stenosis and a history of a hemispheric or retinal transient ischemic attack or nondisabling stroke within 120 days of onset were randomized to surgery or best medical care. In patients with 70–99 percent stenosis (diameter reduction on angiography) of the symptomatic artery, the cumulative estimated risk at 2 years of an ipsilateral stroke was 26 percent in the 331 medical patients and 9 percent in the 328 surgical patients. For a major or fatal ipsilateral stroke, the corresponding rates were 13.1 and 2 percent. The perioperative stroke and death rate was 5.8 percent, but only 2.1 percent for major stroke and death.

In the European Carotid Surgery Trial,[53] patients with a stenosis of the relevant carotid artery who after a carotid territory nondisabling ischemic stroke, a transient ischemic attack, or amaurosis fugax were also randomized to surgery or best medical care. In patients with mild carotid stenosis (less than 69 percent), there was low 3-year risk of ipsilateral stroke, so any benefit from surgery was outweighed by the risks. In patients with severe carotid stenosis (greater than 70 percent), there was a 7.5 percent risk of stroke or death within 30 days of surgery. However, during the next 3 years the risks of ipsilateral stroke were only 2.8 percent for surgery patients and 16.8 percent for control patients. At 3 years, the total risk of death or any stroke was 12.3 percent for surgery and 21.9 percent for control patients.

Asymptomatic carotid artery stenosis

The role of carotid endarterectomy in patients with asymptomatic carotid artery disease remains unanswered. The Asymptomatic Carotid Atherosclerosis Study[54] suggested that endarterectomy halved the risk of stroke in patients with greater than 70 percent carotid stenosis. However, there were methodological anomalies and this is the first large randomized study to reach such a conclusion. This finding would also have massive cost implications as the rate of stroke was only 4–5 percent each year without surgery. The European equivalent, the asymptomatic Carotid Surgery Trial, is ongoing and so a conservative approach is recommended until the results of that study are known.

Mortality from carotid surgery

Current mortality and complication rates for carotid endarterectomy in the UK and Ireland are low: there is a 1.3 percent mortality and 2.1 percent stroke rate by 30 days postoperatively.[55] Over half of all perioperative strokes are caused by intraoperative or postoperative thrombosis and embolization.[56] Studies have confirmed that carotid endarterectomy can be performed safely in the elderly population, including nonagenarians, but outcome is dependent on the individual

surgeon.[57–60] Clearly, the key issues in the decision to offer carotid surgery are the risk of stroke, the quality of life enjoyed by the patient, and life expectancy.

Timing of carotid surgery after stroke

Traditionally, surgery is delayed for 2 months following acute stroke. In the 1960s, several studies of the role of urgent carotid surgery were published. The results were poor, and postmortem studies often demonstrated intracerebral hemorrhage.[61,62] It was concluded that urgent surgery precipitated hemorrhage within the infarct. However, CT was not available then to exclude a primary intracerebral hemorrhage, where surgery would be clearly inappropriate. Furthermore, many of the patients in those early studies had dense neurological deficits and were in "coma, semicoma or stupor."[63]

Interest in the role of urgent carotid surgery following acute stroke was renewed by reports of improvement in neurological deficits in patients with progressing stroke and limited deficit.[64] The rationale for carotid surgery in such patients is twofold: first to restore cerebral perfusion and limit neuronal death; and second, to reduce early recurrence or progression of stroke due to further emboli from the diseased carotid. Urgent surgery in patients with progressing strokes and acute stable strokes have shown better results than the natural history of acute stroke in small studies, but there has been no adequate trial on carotid surgery in acute stroke since CT scans were introduced.[65,66] A recent feasibility study concluded that trials of urgent carotid surgery should focus on partial anterior circulation infarcts and yet would still need large numbers of patients to be randomized.[67]

Carotid angioplasty and stenting

A future alternative in the treatment of carotid stenosis may lie in angioplasty and stenting. A recent multicenter randomized trial comparing these techniques with endarterectomy showed similar rates of disabling stroke or death in the two groups, at around 6 percent.[68] Concern has been raised, however, that lower complication rates than demonstrated in this study should be achievable by surgery.

ABDOMINAL AORTIC ANEURYSM
Prevalence and natural history

Prevalence

Abdominal aortic aneurysms are common. Mortality statistics from the UK Office of Population Censuses and Surveys show that each year approximately 10,000 deaths are due to aortic aneurysm in England and Wales. However, quoted statistics may vastly underestimate the number of deaths related to aortic aneurysms as most aneurysms remain undiagnosed and may be certified as myocardial infarction following sudden unexplained death in an elderly person. The true figure is estimated at nearer 25,000. Deaths from rupture are rare below the age of 50 years; deaths from rupture peak in men aged 75–79 years.[69]

The prevalence of aortic aneurysms is increasing, though some would argue that this finding merely reflects improved diagnosis, changing patterns of referral, and an increased awareness of the disease.[70,71] Difficulties arise in estimating the prevalence and mortality of aneurysms because of varying definitions of aneurysm and operative mortality, especially as aneurysm is still most frequently diagnosed on postmortem examination.

The Vascular Surgery Society proposed that an aneurysm was by definition 50 percent dilated above normal, "normal" being an estimate taken from the literature and adjusted for gender and radiological modality.[72] Collin[73] suggested that an abdominal aortic aneurysm was present by definition when the infrarenal aorta was at least 4 cm in diameter or exceeded the maximum diameter of the aorta between the origin of the superior mesenteric and left renal arteries by at least 0.5 cm. Sterpetti[74] has suggested that an abdominal aneurysm is present when the ratio of infrarenal to suprarenal measurements is 1.5 or greater. Screening of 4237 men and women aged 65–80 years around Chichester, UK, yielded aneurysms of 3 cm or more in 4.3 percent of cases and *aneurysmal changes* can be detected in 10.7 percent of men in the eighth decade of life.[75,76] The prevalence of aneurysms is higher in men over the age of 50, in first-degree male relatives of patients with proven aneurysms, and inpatients with hypertension or peripheral vascular disease.[77–79]

Natural history

Aneurysms less than 5 cm in diameter seldom rupture, but the outlook for larger aneurysms is grim without surgery; the 2-year mortality for aneurysms greater than 6 cm may be 72 percent, though this high mortality does reflect a bias against operating on patients who are unfit at diagnosis. However, the majority of deaths in patients with large aneurysms are due to rupture.[80,81] The expansion rate of aortic aneurysms depends on aneurysm size and in small aneurysms is approximately 2 mm per year, but growth is neither consistent, steady, or predictable.[82] Smoking may increase the rate of aneurysm growth.[83] Growth rates tend to accelerate as the aneurysm size increases, and the only reliable predictor of aneurysm rupture is aneurysm size and female sex.[74,80,84] Irrespective of size, symptomatic or tender aneurysms should be investigated with a view to surgery as soon as possible, as over 25 percent of these will rupture in the next year.

Clinical presentation and diagnosis

Presentation

Although most aortic aneurysms are asymptomatic or present with rupture, they may cause back or abdominal pain. This is not always classic lumbar back pain, and all abdominal or back pains in patients with an abdominal aortic aneurysm should be attributed to the aneurysm unless another diagnosis is obvious. Alternatively, the first presentation may be that of acute leg ischemia due to distal emboli from the aneurysm, although this is surprisingly rare considering the frequency of thrombus within the aneurysm sac.

When an aortic aneurysm ruptures, the vast majority of patients die immediately and without reaching hospital. The early survivors present with severe back or abdominal pain and hemorrhagic shock. Patients with retroperitoneal rupture, where the bleed is contained by the pressure of surrounding tissues, are more likely to reach hospital alive, but still the majority of patients die before reaching a hospital.[85] Less common presentations include rupture of the aneurysm into the vena cava (leading to a massive arteriovenous fistula and high-output cardiac failure) or into the gastrointestinal tract (hematemesis and melena) due to an aortoduodenal fistula.

Diagnosis

Most aneurysms are detected incidentally, usually either on physical examination or on abdominal ultrasound (Fig. 39-6). Physical examination tends to overestimate aneurysm size by about 20 percent owing to overlying retroperitoneal tissue and the thickness of the abdominal wall.[86] Although ultrasound is the most cost-effective imaging method for diagnosis and follow-up, further information should be obtained prior to elective repair. The relationship to the origin of the renal arteries should be defined, and patency and diameter of the iliac arteries confirmed. Most aortic aneurysms are infrarenal. If there

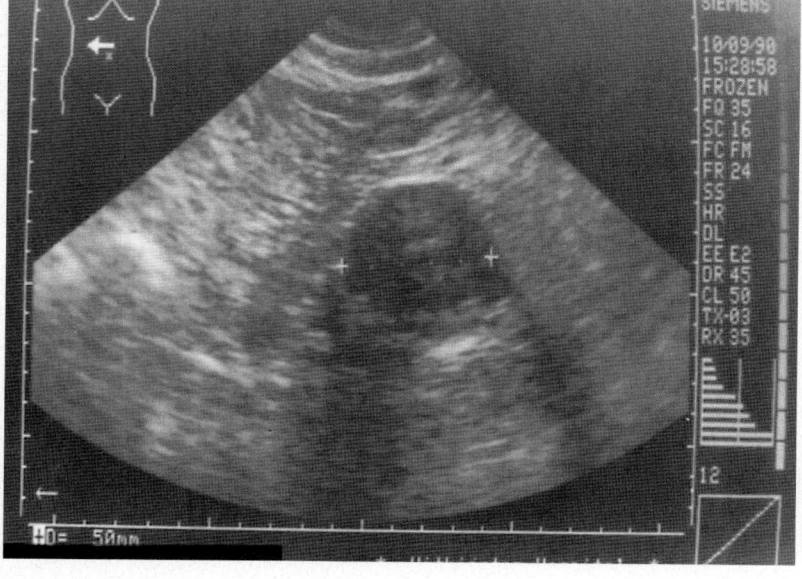

Figure 39-6 Abdominal ultrasound image demonstrating a large abdominal aortic aneurysm in transverse section.

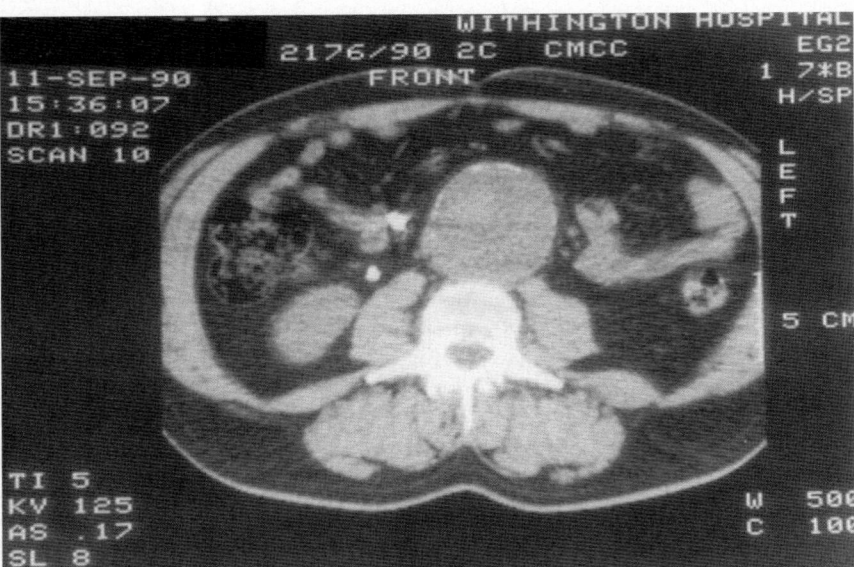

Figure 39-7 An 8 cm abdominal aortic aneurysm with calcified wall on CT imaging.

is suprarenal extension of the aneurysm, the operative difficulty increases, as does the operative mortality because of the need to cross-clamp above the renal arteries with subsequent increased risk of renal embolization and renal failure. Specialist centers favor either computed tomography (Fig. 39-7) or nuclear magnetic resonance imaging (MRI) for this assessment. Both are noninvasive and are sensitive to the level of the renal arteries.[87] Neither provides adequate information on occlusive arterial disease, either viscerally or peripherally, although MRI angiography is an option. Arteriography has been found to be unhelpful as it underestimates the size and extent of the aneurysm owing to luminal thrombus.

Complications of aneurysm surgery

Mortality from rupture

The operative mortality for a ruptured aneurysm varies between centers, from 31 percent to over 75 percent.[88,89] However, this represents only the tip of the iceberg, as the overall mortality is greater than 80 percent as only a minority of patients reach hospital alive.[85] Mortality rates for emergency surgery have improved very little over the years, with an overall rate in the UK of around 70 percent but with lower rates in specialized vascular centers.[90]

Operative mortality

The 30-day mortality for elective aneurysm surgery has been quoted from zero to 8.4 percent depending on the series of patients and the center.[91,92] However, independently assessed mortality in clinical trials is invariably much higher, at around 10–12 percent. Generally, in the UK mortality rates for elective surgery should be around 5 percent.

In a recent study of over 16,000 patients, operative mortality was increased by cerebral vascular occlusive arterial disease, chronic pulmonary disease, and impaired renal function.[93] Cardiac failure and diabetes have also been shown to adversely affect outcome.[94] Intraoperative hypotension, left renal vein ligation, and blood loss greater than 4 units are known to be associated with increased mortality,[95] and postoperative renal failure is the strongest predictor of death.[89] Following successful aneurysm repair, prognosis is excellent, with a life-expectancy comparable to that of an age- and sex-matched population.[93]

Cardiac complications

Aneurysm patients tend to have increased operative risk owing to concomitant cardiac and pulmonary disease. Just under half of these patients have electrocardiographic evidence of ischemic heart disease.[96] Myocardial infarction is the most frequent cause of death in patients undergoing elective aneurysm repair. If there is a history of significant angina, coronary angiography should be considered to define the coronary disease prior to elective surgery. An echocardiogram may be of some value in identifying segmental wall motion abnormalities indicative of underlying ventricular dysfunction, and in providing an estimate of the left ventricular ejection fraction. Patients with an ejection fraction greater than 60 percent are unlikely to experience significant cardiac problems postoperatively, but a low ejection fraction is a poor predictor of complications.

Respiratory complications

Severe pulmonary insufficiency with dyspnea at rest is a contraindication to surgery. A simple clinical assessment based on ability to walk or climb a flight of stairs without needing to rest identifies most "problem" patients, but arterial blood gases and pulmonary function tests may be useful in defining the severity of pulmonary insufficiency. Patients with obstructive lung disease require careful preoperative physiotherapy and bronchodilators to increase pulmonary capacity, thereby reducing postoperative morbidity and mortality.

Surgical approach may also influence outcome. Abdominal aortic aneurysm repair has traditionally been performed via a transperitoneal approach, but an extended retroperitoneal approach may be less stressful for elderly patients and those with limited pulmonary reserve.[97]

Renal complications

After cardiac causes, renal insufficiency is the next most frequent cause of death following aortic aneurysm repair. Elevated preoperative serum creatinine is significantly associated with postoperative mortality risk.[98] This pre-existing renal insufficiency may be caused by repeated embolization from an atheromatous aorta, coexisting atheroma of the renal arteries, or concomitant disease such as hypertension or diabetes. It is especially important to avoid perioperative hypovolemia in these patients.

Cerebrovascular complications

Stroke is an infrequent complication of aneurysm repair.[94] Noninvasive duplex Doppler investigation reliably identifies potentially treatable carotid artery stenosis, but carotid surgery is of proven benefit only in patients with appropriate symptoms in the relevant carotid territory.

Decreasing operative mortality

There are many ways to improve the outcome for patients undergoing elective abdominal aortic surgery. Patients should have the benefit of standard intensive monitoring including, electrocardiography (ECG), arterial pressure monitoring, and pulse oximetry. Intensive or high-dependency facilities must be available for postoperative care, ventilation, and monitoring as required. This type of monitoring has led to a progressive decrease in morbidity and mortality, as well as a decrease in the incidence of renal complications, by minimizing periods of hypotension.[99] Perioperative β-blockade reduces cardiovascular mortality significantly in patients with pre-existing cardiac disease.[100,101]

Modern vascular surgery should also include a strategy for managing blood transfusion. Techniques such as preoperative donation, perioperative hemodilution, and the use of salvage autotransfusion result in an appreciable saving of bank blood transfusion and a reduction in systemic inflammatory response. The many risks inherent in blood transfusions are obviated.[102]

The osmotic diuretic mannitol has been used sporadically in aortic surgery for the last 30 years to maintain urine output during aortic cross-clamping.[103] More recently, mannitol has been shown to scavenge oxygen free radicals produced by restoration of blood flow to ischemic tissues, and these are important in the development of ischemia/reperfusion injury. A prospective randomized clinical trial in elective aortic aneurysm repair has shown a significant benefit in postoperative pulmonary function in patients who received mannitol prior to cross-clamping.[104]

Aortic aneurysm repair in the elderly population

Aneurysm surgery can be well-tolerated in octogenarians, but mortality for aneurysm repair is undoubtedly increased in those aged over 75, mainly owing to comorbid conditions.[95] Regrettably, in a recent British survey nearly 50 percent of general practitioners would not refer to a specialist an 80-year-old with a palpable aneurysm.[105] Clearly, we should take advantage of the current enthusiasm for continued medical education to ensure that appropriately selected patients are offered elective repair before rupture occurs.

Endovascular techniques

Endovascular stent-grafts have been used successfully to exclude abdominal aortic aneurysms in selected patients. Currently, endovascular aneurysm repair (EVAR) is offered in the UK only as part of randomized controlled trials comparing this technique either to surgery or, in those unfit for surgery, to best medical care. The results of this study will not be available before 2003, but national audit data from the UK suggest a 1 percent 30-day mortality from EVAR if the patient is considered fit for surgery and a 17 percent mortality in those considered unfit.[106]

The stent-graft is assembled within the aorta via the femoral artery at operation. This avoids a laparotomy with its associated cardiac and respiratory morbidity in these high-risk patients. However, only a minority of patients are suitable for this technique, as a widely patent and not too tortuous iliac system is required through which the graft can reach its destination. A suitable length of nonaneurysmal aorta below the renal arteries is essential, as is a normal aorta above the bifurcation or acceptable iliac arteries for stent attachment.[2] These measurements are all taken during spiral CT or MRI imaging.

MANAGEMENT OF SMALL ANEURYSMS

For many years it remained unclear how to manage aortic aneurysms less than 5.5 cm in diameter. The UK Small Aneurysm Trial[107] randomized 1090 patients with aneurysms 4–5.5 cm in diameter to either surgery or regular surveillance by ultrasonography. No significant difference in survival was found between the two groups despite follow-up of up to 6 years. Hence surgery should now be reserved for aneurysms greater than 5.5 cm and smaller aneurysms monitored with regular ultrasound imaging. The cost-effectiveness of screening for aortic aneurysm compares favorably with breast and cervical cancer screening, provided surgery is offered only for asymptomatic aortic aneurysms greater than 5.5 cm in diameter.[108]

CONCLUSIONS

Informed consent for surgery in elderly people is especially important because of the concomitant risks but surgical intervention in selected patients is well-tolerated.

Carotid endarterectomy or revascularization for peripheral vascular disease are intended primarily to enhance quality of life. Without such treatments the elderly patient may lose independence through a stroke or limb amputation. The loss of independence and long-term care costs after limb amputation or stroke argue for the cost-effectiveness of an aggressive policy of early revascularization for limb salvage or carotid disease.

KEY POINTS Vascular surgery

- Intermittent claudication should be managed by lifestyle advice, exercise, and antiplatelet agents such as aspirin. Angioplasty/stenting and surgery are usually reserved for severe symptoms sufficient to impair quality of life or ischemic rest pain.

- Cardiorespiratory comorbidity indicates the risk of mortality after vascular surgery.

- Carotid endarterectomy is appropriate for symptomatic internal carotid artery stenosis of greater than 70 percent, provided the quality of life is good. Lesser symptomatic stenoses should be managed medically.

- Aortic aneurysms greater than 5.5 cm in diameter require open or endovascular repair. Below this diameter, regular ultrasonographic surveillance is indicated.

REFERENCES

1. London NJM, Varty K, Sayers RD et al: Percutaneous transluminal angioplasty for lower-limb critical ischaemia. Br J Surg 1995;82:1232–1235
2. Andrews SM, Cuming R, MacSweeney ST et al: Assessment of feasibility for endovascular prosthetic tube correction of aortic aneurysm. Br J Surg 1995;82:917–919
3. Pell JP, for the Scottish Vascular Audit Group: Impact of intermittent claudication on quality of life. Eur J Vasc Surg 1995;9:469–472
4. Adkins RB, Scott HW: Surgical procedures in patients aged ninety years and older. S Med J 1984;77:1357–1364
5. Widmer LK, Greensher A, Kannel WB: Occlusion of peripheral arteries: a study of 6400 working subjects. Circulation 1964;30:836–842
6. Wilson SE, Schwartz I, Williams RA, Owens ML: Occlusion of the superficial femoral artery. What happens without operation? Am J Surg 1980;140:112–117
7. Dormandy J, Mahir M, Ascady G et al: Fate of the patient with chronic leg ischaemia. J Cardiovasc Surg 1989;30:50–57
8. Hale WE, Marks RG, May FE et al: Epidemiology of intermittent claudication: evaluation of risk factors. Age Ageing 1988;17:57–60
9. Reid DD, Brett GZ, Hamilton PJ et al: Cardiorespiratory disease and diabetes among middle aged male civil servants. Lancet 1974;1:469–473
10. Kannel WB, McGee DL: Update on some epidemiologic features of intermittent claudication: the Framingham study. J Am Geriatr Soc 1985;33:13–18
11. Jonason T, Ringqvist I: Mortality and morbidity in patients with intermittent claudication in relation to the location of the occlusive atherosclerosis in the leg. Angiology 1985;36:310–314
12. Jelnes R, Gaardsting O, Hougard Jensen K: Fate in intermittent claudication: outcome and risk factors. BMJ 1986;293:1137–1140
13. O'Riordain DS, O'Donnell JA: Realistic expectations for the patient with intermittent claudication. Br J Surg 1991;78:861–863
14. Reunanen A, Takkunen H, Aromaa A: Prevalence of intermittent claudication and its effect on mortality. Acta Med Scand 1982;211:249–256
15. Bainton D, Sweetnam P, Baker I, Elwood P: Peripheral vascular disease: consequence for survival and association with risk factors in the Speedwell prospective heart disease study. Br Heart J 1994;72:128–132
16. Winn RK, Shara SR, Vedder NB et al: Leucocyte and endothelial adhesion molecules in ischaemia reperfusion injury. CIBA Foundation symposium 1995;189:63–78
17. Leng GC, Papacosta O, Whincup P et al: Femoral atherosclerosis in an older British population: prevalence and risk factors. Atherosclerosis 2000;152:167–174
18. Hooi JD, Kester AD, Stoffers HE et al: Incidence of and risk factors for asymptomatic peripheral arterial occlusive disease: a longitudinal study. Am J Epidemiol 2001;153:666–672
19. Yao ST: Haemodynamic studies in peripheral arterial disease. Br J Surg 1970;56:676–679
20. Whelan JF, Barry MH, Moir JD: Color flow Doppler ultrasonography: comparison with peripheral arteriography for the investigation of peripheral vascular disease. J Clin Ultrasound 1992;20:369–374
21. Legemate DA, Teeuwen C, Hoeneveld H et al: The potential of duplex scanning to replace aortoiliac and femoro-popliteal angiography. Eur J Vasc Surg 1989;3:49–54
22. Allard L, Cloutier G, Durand L-G et al: Limitations of ultrasonic duplex scanning for diagnosing lower limb arterial stenoses in the presence of adjacent segment disease. J Vasc Surg 1994;19:650–657
23. van der Heijden FHWM, Legemate DA, van Leeuwen MS et al: Value of duplex scanning in the selection of patients for percutaneous transluminal angioplasty. Eur J Vasc Surg 1993;7:71–76
24. Gardner AW, Katzel LI, Sorkin JD et al: Exercise rehabilitation improves functional outcomes and peripheral circulation in patients with intermittent claudication: a randomised controlled trial. J Am Geriatr Soc 2001;49:755–762
25. Jivegard L, Holm J, Schersten T: The outcome in arterial thrombosis misdiagnosed as arterial embolism. Acta Chir Scand 1986;152:251–256
26. Fogarty TJ: Management of arterial emboli. Surg Clin North Am 1979;59:749–753
27. Vohra R, Lieberman DP: Arterial emboli to the arm. J R Coll Surg Edinb 1991;36:83–85
28. Baguneid M, Dodd D, Fulford P et al: Management of acute non-traumatic upper limb ischaemia. Angiology 1999;50:715–720
29. Abbott WM, Maloney RD, McCabe CC et al: Arterial embolism: a 44 year perspective. Am J Surg 1982;143:460–464
30. Baird RJ, Lajos TZ: Emboli to the arm. Ann Surg 1964;160:905–909
31. Vohra R, Zahrani H, Lieberman DP: Factors affecting limb salvage and mortality in patients undergoing femoral embolectomy. J R Coll Surg Edinb 1991;36:213–215
32. Collin C, Collin J: Mobility after lower-limb amputation. Br J Surg 1995;82:1010–1011
33. Humphreys WV, Evans F, Watkin G, Williams T: Critical limb ischaemia in patients over 80 years of age: options in a district general hospital. Br J Surg 1995;82:1361–1363
34. Korn P, Khilnani NM, Fellers JC et al: Thrombolysis for native arterial occlusions of the lower extremities: clinical outcome and cost. J Vasc Surg 2001;33:1148–1157.
35. Braithwaite B, Birch P, Davies C et al: Accelerated high-dose bolus tissue plasminogen activator extends the role of peripheral thrombolysis but may increase risk. Br J Surg 1994;81:A619 (abstract)
36. Sayers RD, Thompson MM, Hartshorne T et al: Treatment and outcome of severe lower-limb ischaemia. Br J Surg 1994;81:521–523
37. Seabrook GR, Cambria RA, Freischlag JA et al: Health-related quality of life and functional outcome following arterial reconstruction for limb salvage. Cardiovasc Surg 1999;7:279–286
38. Lindholt JS, Bøvling S, Fasting H, Henneberg EW: Vascular surgery reduces the frequency of lower limb major amputations. Eur J Vasc Surg 1994;8:31–35
39. Chambers BR, Norris JW: Clinical significance of asymptomatic neck bruits. Neurology 1985;35:742–745
40. Crevasse LE, Logue RB: Carotid artery murmurs. Continuous murmur over carotid bulb—a new sign of carotid artery insufficiency. JAMA 1958;167:2177–2182
41. Sandercock PAG, Warlow CP, Jones LN, Starkey IR: Predisposing factors for cerebral infarction: the Oxfordshire Community Stroke Project. BMJ 1989;298:75–80
42. Bamford J, Sandercock P, Dennis M et al: Classification and natural history of clinically identifiable subtypes of cerebral infarction. Lancet 1991;337:1521–1526
43. Mead GE, Murray H, Farrell A et al: The potential role of carotid surgery in acute stroke. Br J Surg 1995;82:A1558 (abstract)
44. Feeley TM, Leen EJ, Colgan MP et al: Histologic characteristics of carotid artery plaque. J Vasc Surg 1991;13:719–724
45. Grzyska U, Freitag J, Zeumer H: Selective cerebral intraarterial DSA: complication rate and control of risk factors. Neuroradiology 1990;32:296–299
46. Waugh JR, Sacharias N: Arteriographic complications in the DSA era. Radiology 1992;182:243–246
47. Dinkel HP, Moll R, Debus S: Colour flow Doppler ultrasound of the carotid bifurcation: can it replace routine angiography before carotid endarterectomy? Br J Radiol 2001;74:590–594

48. Friese S, Krapf H, Fetter M et al: Ultrasonography and contrast-enhanced MRA in ICA-stenosis: is conventional angiography obsolete? J Neurol 2001;248:506–513

49. Spencer MP, Reid JM: Quantitation of carotid stenosis with continuous-wave Doppler ultrasound. Stroke 1979;10:326–330

50. Schuler JJ, Flanigan DP, Lim LT et al: The effect of carotid siphon stenosis on stroke rate, death and relief of symptoms following elective carotid endarterectomy. Surgery 1982;92:1058–1067

51. Goddard AJ, Mendelow AD, Birchall D: Computed tomography in the investigation of carotid stenosis. Clin Radiol 2001;56:523–534

52. North American Symptomatic Carotid Endarterectomy trial collaborators: Beneficial effects of carotid endarterectomy in symptomatic patients with high grade carotid stenosis. N Engl J Med 1991;325:445–453

53. European Carotid Surgery Trialists' Collaborative Group: MRC European Carotid Surgery Trial: interim results for symptomatic patients with severe (70–99%) or with mild (0–29%) carotid stenosis. Lancet 1991;337:1235–1243

54. Executive Committee for the Asymptomatic Carotid Atherosclerosis Study: Endarterectomy for asymptomatic carotid artery stenosis. JAMA 1995;273:1421–1428

55. McCollum PT, Da Silver A, De Cossart L: Carotid endarterectomy in the UK and Ireland. Eur J Vasc Endovasc Surg 1997;14:386–391

56. Jacobowitz GR, Rockman CB, Lamparello PJ et al: Causes of perioperative stroke after carotid endarterectomy: special considerations in symptomatic patients. Ann Vasc Surg 2001;15:19–24

57. Perler BA, Williams GM: Carotid endarterectomy in the very elderly: is it worthwhile? Surgery 1994;116:479–483

58. Ting AC, Taylor DC, Salvian AJ et al: Carotid endarterectomy in octogenerians. Cardiovasc Surg 2000;8:441–445

59. Schultz RD, Sterpetti AV, Feldhaus RJ: Carotid endarterctomy in octogenarians and nonagenarians. Surg Gynecol Obstet 1988;166:245–251

60. Maxwell JG, Taylor AJ, Maxwell BG et al: Carotid endarterectomy in the community hospital in patients age 80 and older. Ann Surg 2000;231:781–788

61. Wylie EJ, Hein MF, Adams JE: Intracranial haemorrhage following surgical revascularisation for treatment of acute strokes. J Neurosurg 1964;21:212–215

62. Hunter JA, Julian OC, Dye WS, Javid H: Emergency operation for acute cerebral ischemia due to carotid artery obstruction: review of 26 cases. Ann Surg 1965;162:901–904

63. Bauer RB, Meyer JS, Fields WS et al: Joint study of extracranial arterial occlusion. 3: Progress reports of controlled study of long term survival in patients with and without operation. JAMA 1969;208:509–518

64. Goldstone J, Moore WS, Moncure AC et al: Emergency carotid artery surgery in neurologically unstable patients. Arch Surg 1976;111:1284–1291

65. Gertler JP, Blankensteijn JD, Brewster DC et al: Carotid endarterectomy for unstable and compelling neurologic conditions: do the results justify an aggressive approach? J Vasc Surg 1994;19:32–40

66. Greenhalgh RM, Cuming R, Perkin GD, McCollum CN: Urgent carotid surgery for high risk patients. Eur J Vasc Surg 1993;7(suppl):25–32

67. Mead GE, Murray H, Farrell A et al: Pilot study of carotid surgery for acute stroke. Br J Surg 1997;84:990–992

68. CAVATAS investigators: Endovascular versus surgical treatment in patients with carotid stenosis in the Carotid and Vertebral Artery Transluminal Angioplasty Study: a randomised trial. Lancet 2001;357:1729–1737

69. UK Office of Population Censuses and Surveys (ed): Mortality Statistics Cause Series DH2, Vol 19: England and Wales. London, HMSO, 1992

70. Fowkes FGR, Macintyre CCA, Ruckley CV: Increasing incidence of aortic aneurysms in England and Wales. BMJ 1989;298:33–35

71. Collin J: The increasing incidence of aortic aneurysms. BMJ 1989;298:387–388

72. Johnston KW, Rutherford RB, Tilson MD et al: Suggested standards for reporting on arterial aneurysms. J Vasc Surg 1991;13:444–450

73. Collin J: A proposal for a precise definition of abdominal aortic aneurysm: a personal view. J Cardiovasc Surg 1990;31:168–169

74. Sterpetti AV, Schultz RD, Feldhaus RJ et al: Factors influencing enlargement rate of small abdominal aortic aneurysms. J Surg Res 1987;43:211–219

75. Scott RAP, Ashton HA, Kay DN: Abdominal aortic aneurysm in 4237 screened patients: prevalence, development and management over 6 years. Br J Surg 1991;78:1122–1125

76. Bengtsson H, Bergqvist D, Ekberg O et al: A population based screening of abdominal aortic aneurysms. Eur J Vasc Surg 1991;5:53–57

77. Twomey A, Twomey E, Wilkins RA, Lewis JD: Unrecognised aneurysmal disease in male hypertensive patients. Int Angio 1986;5:269–273

78. Collin J, Walton J: Is abdominal aortic aneurysm familial? BMJ 1989;299:49

79. Galland RB, Simmons MJ, Torrie EPH: Prevalence of abdominal aortic aneurysm in patients with occlusive peripheral vascular disease. Br J Surg 1991;78:1259–1260

80. Glimaker H, Holmberg L, Elvin A et al: Natural history of patients with abdominal aortic aneurysm. Eur J Vasc Surg 1991;5:125–130

81. Szilagyi DE, Elliott JP, Smith RF: Clinical fate of the patient with asymptomatic abdominal aortic aneurysm and unfit for surgical treatment. Arch Surg 1972;104:600–606

82. Cronenwett JL, Sargent SK, Wall MH et al: Variables that affect the expansion rate and outcome of small abdominal aortic aneurysms. J Vasc Surg 1990;11:260–269

83. MacSweeney STR, Ellis M, Worrell PC et al: Smoking and growth rate of small abdominal aortic aneurysms. Lancet 1994;344:651–652

84. Collin J, Heather B, Walton J: Growth rates of subclinical abdominal aortic aneurysms: implications for review and rescreening programmes. Eur J Vasc Surg 1991;5:141–144

85. Adam DJ, Mohan IV, Stuart WP et al: Community and hospital outcome from ruptured abdominal aortic aneurysm within the catchment area of a regional vascular surgical service. J Vasc Surg 1999;30:922–928

86. Brewster DC, Darling RC, Raines JK et al: Assessment of abdominal aortic aneurysm size. Circulation 1972;56(suppl 2):164

87. Salaman RA, Shandall A, Morgan RH et al: Intravenous digital subtraction angiography versus computed tomography in the assessment of abdominal aortic aneurysm. Br J Surg 1994;81:661–663

88. Kniemeyer HW, Kessler T, Reber PU et al: Treatment of ruptured abdominal aortic aneurysm, a permanent challenge or a waste of resources? Prediction of outcome using a multi-organ-dysfunction score. Eur J Vasc Endovasc Surg 2000;19:190–196

89. Harris LM, Faggioli GL, Fiedler R et al: Ruptured abdominal aortic aneurysms: factors affecting mortality rates. J Vasc Surg 1991;14:812–820

90. Berridge DC, Chamberlain J, Guy AJ et al: Prospective audit of abdominal aortic aneurysm surgery in the northern region from 1988 to 1992. Br J Surg 1995;82:906–910

91. Chalmers RTA, Stonebridge PA, John TG et al: Abdominal aortic aneurysm in the elderly. Br J Surg 1993;80:1122–1123

92. Lawrence PF, Gazak C, Bhirangi L et al: The epidemiology of surgically repaired aneurysms in the United States. J Vasc Surg 1999;30:632–640

93. Huber TS, Wang JG, Derrow AE et al: Experience in the United States with intact abdominal aortic aneurysm repair. J Vasc Surg 2001;33:304–311

94. Heller JA, Weinberg A, Arons R et al: Two decades of abdominal aortic aneurysm repair: have we made any progress? J Vasc Surg 2000;32:1091–1100

95. Amundsen S, Skjaerven R, Trippestad A, Sfreide O, members of the Norwegian Aortic Aneurysm Trial: Abdominal aortic aneurysms—a study of factors influencing postoperative mortality. Eur J Vasc Surg 1989;3:405–409

96. Bayly PJM, Matthews JNS, Dobson PM et al: In-hospital mortality from abdominal aortic surgery in Great Britain and Ireland: Vascular Anaesthesia Society audit. Br J Surg 2001;88:687–692

97. Leather RP, Shah DM, Kaufman JL et al: Comparative analysis of retroperitoneal and transperitoneal aortic replacement for aneurysm. Surg Gynecol Obstet 1989;168:387–393

98. Brady AR, Fowkes FG, Greenhalgh RM et al, for the UK Small Aneurysm Trial participants: Risk factors for post-operative death following elective surgical repair of abdominal aortic aneurysm: results of the UK Small Aneurysm Trial. Br J Surg 2000;87:742–749

99. Cohen JR, Mannick JA, Couch NP, Whittemore AD: Abdominal aortic aneurysm repair in patients with peri-operative renal failure. J Vasc Surg 1986;3:867

100. Mangano DT, Layug EL, Wallace A et al: Effect of atenolol on mortality and cardiovascular morbidity after noncardiac surgery: multicenter study of perioperative ischaemia research group. N Engl J Med 1996;335:1713–1720

101. Poldermans D, Boersma E, Bal D et al: The effect of bisoprolol on perioperative mortality and myocardial infarction in high-risk patients undergoing vascular surgery. N Engl J Med 1999;341:1789–1794

102. Haynes SL, Wong JC, Torella F et al: The influence of homologous blood transfusion on immunity and clinical outcome in aortic surgery. Eur J Vasc Endovasc Surg 2001;22:244–250

103. Barry KG, Cohen A, Kuchel JP et al: Mannitol infusion: the prevention of acute functional renal failure during resection of an aneurysm of the abdominal aorta. N Engl J Med 1961;264:967–971

104. Paterson IS, Klausner JM, Mannick JA et al: Pulmonary oedema after aneurysm surgery is modified by mannitol. Ann Surg 1990;210:796–801

105. Michaels JA, Galland RB: General practitioner referral of patients with symptoms of peripheral vascular disease. J R Coll Surg Edinb 1994;39:103–105

106. Sheffield Vascular Institute: The UK Registry for Endovascular Treatment of Aneurysms

107. UK Small Aneurysm Trial participants: Mortality results for randomised controlled trial of early elective surgery or ultrasonographic surveillance for small abdominal aortic aneurysms. Lancet 1998;352:1649–1655

108. St Leger AS, Spencely M, McCollum CN et al: Screening for abdominal aortic aneurysm: a computer assisted cost-utility analysis. Eur J Vasc Endovasc Surg 1996;11:183–190

Chapter 40

Thromboembolic disease

David A. Taberner

Venous and arterial thromboembolism are very common causes of death and morbidity in the elderly population. The risks increase with age[1-3] and are matched by the increased hazards of antithrombotic drugs.[4] For these reasons, the management of thromboembolic disease in elderly patients poses difficult questions concerning the risks and benefits of therapeutic interventions. The logistics of delivering effective and safe antithrombotic therapy are particularly challenging when patients cannot attend an anticoagulant clinic regularly or have difficulty in understanding and following treatment regimens, which may vary from week to week.

A thrombus is a mass of blood constituents found within the vascular tree during life. Its structure is quite different from a blood clot formed in a test tube. Indeed, its structure indicates the site of origin and mechanisms by which it formed.

Arterial thrombi are pale, reflecting a major platelet component, while venous thrombi are darker with more red cells and fibrin than platelets. Thrombi are laminated as a consequence of the sequential laying down of new thrombus and lysis of old. New thrombus often contains more platelets which generate multiple white lines, known as lines of Zahn.[5]

MECHANISMS OF THROMBUS FORMATION

As a natural repair process, damaged endothelium is sealed by adherent platelets. These are activated as they pass by in the blood stream, thereby sticking to the exposed subendothelium.

Subsequently there is repair with re-endothelialization, but fibrin formation may occur. Platelets, by providing an anionic phospholipid surface, bind clotting factors which may sequentially activate if initiated by tissue factor. Fibrin then formed may be lysed by the lytic system, but can propagate and lead to local thrombosis or embolism. There are many factors which interplay in these physiological and pathological processes. Broadly they can be categorized into disturbances of flow, disturbance within the vessel wall, and abnormalities of blood components. These three groups of factors make up the triad recognized by Virchow over 100 years ago.

Stasis is an important factor in the etiology of thrombosis, particularly in elderly people who may not be very mobile. In venous disease, failure to use the calf muscle pump, for example, encourages stasis. In arterial disease, low flow states may accompany poor cardiac output and narrowed vessels. Stasis promotes local accumulation of activated clotting factors and platelets. Lack of exercise is thought to discourage fibrinolysis. Factors within the blood contribute to stasis and may be of particular relevance to older patients. Increased hematocrit may occur following cardiorespiratory problems as well as in primary myeloproliferative disorders. Increased viscosity may occur in myeloma and other paraproteinemias, but more commonly may follow polyclonal increases in γ-globulins and fibrinogen which occur secondary to many inflammatory disease states or in malignancies.

Within the vessel wall the endothelium has a complex role (Fig. 40-1). It expresses anticoagulant, antiplatelet profibrinolytic and antifibrinolytic activities. The endothelium

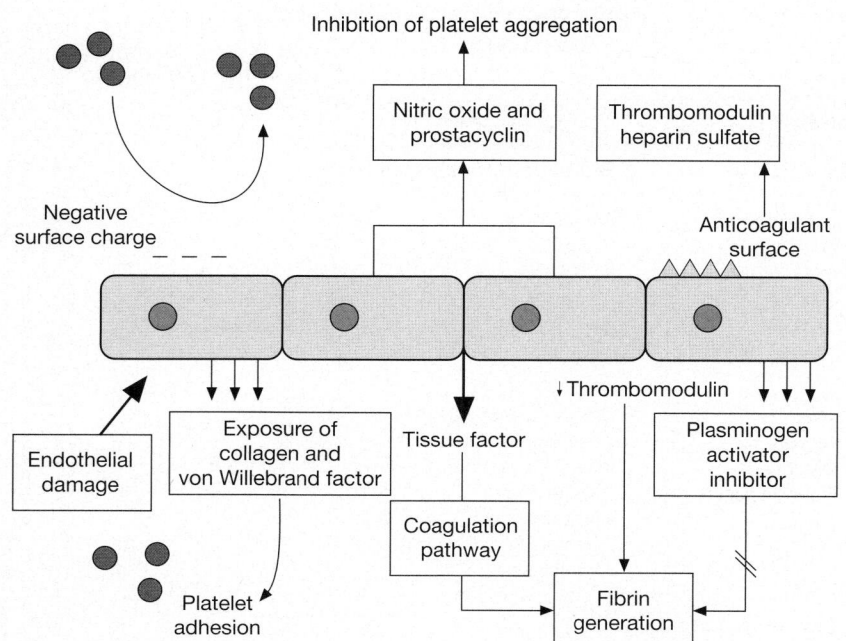

Figure 40-1 Endothelial hemostatic function. From Alford et al. (2000),[113] by kind permission of The Medicine Publishing Company.

interacts with the blood components to facilitate the two main natural anticoagulant mechanisms, namely capture of thrombin by antithrombin and proteolysis of activated forms of the two major procoagulant cofactors, factor VIIIc (hemophilic factor) and factor V by activated protein C. Quantitative and qualitative abnormalities of procoagulant and anticoagulant proteins may promote thrombosis. Decrease in activators of fibrinolysis and increase in the antifibrinolytic proteins, particularly plasminogen activator inhibitor I and α_2 antiplasmin, will discourage fibrinolysis and encourage fibrin propagation. The interplay of these factors is shown in Table 40-1. The important message is that thrombosis is consequent upon the interplay of these factors. It is rare that a single factor alone causes thrombosis. It is usually several factors working together which results in extension of fibrin with subsequent thrombotic occlusion or embolization.

Mechanisms and effects of arterial thrombosis

A major factor in arterial disease is damage to the vessel wall by atherosclerosis. Platelets and fibrin are thought to contribute to the growth of arterial plaques. Platelets release growth factors and mitogens after accumulation at sites of vessel injury or turbulent flow. Their release from platelets contributes to the accumulation of monocytes and the proliferation of smooth muscle cells that are the hallmarks of the early vascular lesion. As the plaque grows, it may ulcerate or disrupt and expose subendothelium and plaque material. High shear stresses beyond a tight stenosis may activate platelets, with the interaction with von Willebrand factor. Monocytes and endothelial expression of tissue factor may follow, initiating the coagulation cascade (Fig. 40-2). Platelet adhesion, aggregation, and release of vasoconstrictors may lead initially to a small platelet thrombus. This may embolize and is thought to contribute to transient cerebral ischemic attacks and unstable angina. Further extension of the fibrin formation may lead to vascular occlusion with retrograde extension and subsequent forward growth.

Mechanisms and effects of venous thrombosis

Stasis is recognized to be a major factor in the development of deep vein thrombosis (DVT). However, under experimental conditions, blood isolated in a ligated vein remains fluid for some time. If any activated factors are generated or added, fibrin formation rapidly follows.[6] Within deep veins, many thrombi begin within the valve pockets where there is local stasis.[7] Here the interplay of the many factors initiates thrombosis—see Table 40-2 and Figure 40-3. Within these cusps, shear forces are low and platelet incorporation is less evident, although some platelet deposition may occur as each new episode of fibrin formation is initiated.

Fibrinolytic activity is an important consideration. For example, most subclinical postoperative calf thrombi are thought to

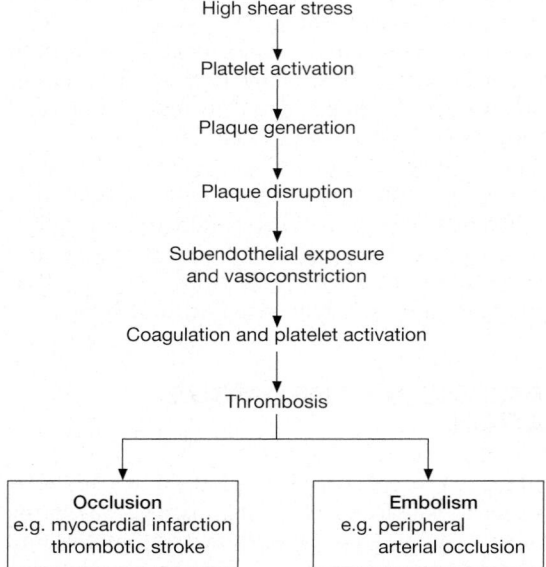

Figure 40-2 Mechanisms and effects of arterial thromboembolism.

Table 40-1 **Mechanisms of thrombus formation**			
Factors	**Vessel wall**	**Blood flow**	**Blood components**
Anticoagulant factors	Vasodilatation Antiplatelet activity Cofactor activity for anticoagulant pathways Profibrinolytic properties	Vasodilatation Hemodilution Good cardiac output Good calf muscle activity	Antithrombin Protein C/S Fibrinolytic factors (tPA uPA)
Procoagulant factors	Vasoconstriction Endothelial damage and exposure of subendothelium Generation of tissue factor and loss of anticoagulant cofactor activity	Stasis Stenosis Polycythemia Hyperviscosity	Procoagulant factor levels (e.g. VIIIc) Increased thrombi generation Antifibrinolytic factors (e.g. PAI and antiplasmin factor V Leiden)
tPA: tissue plasminogen activator; uPA: urokinase; PAI: plasminogen activator inhibitor.			

Table 40-2 Clinical risk factors for venous thromboembolism particularly relevant to elderly people

Immobility
Tissue trauma, particularly hip fracture and surgery
Myocardial infarction
Estrogen therapy
Obesity
Previous deep vein thrombosis
Congestive cardiac failure
Malignancy
Nephrosis
Advancing age
Collagen disorder, including antiphospholipid antibodies
Hyperviscosity
Myeloma and paraproteinemia
Myeloproliferative disorders
Some thrombophilic problems:
    factor V Leiden
    increasing factor VIII

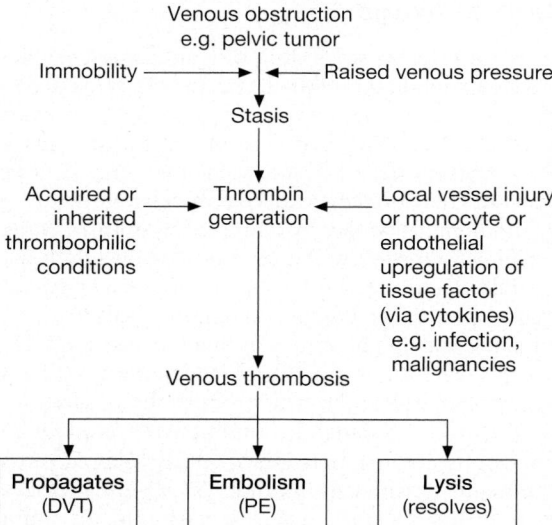

Figure 40-3 Mechanism and effects of venous thromboembolism.

lyse spontaneously.[8] However, at least 20 percent of untreated calf thrombi progress to proximal occlusion with a very high risk of pulmonary embolism (PE).[9] Post-phlebitic damage to the venous valvular system, and occlusion due to unresolved thrombi, contribute to subsequent symptoms. Swollen legs, with pigmentation and predisposition to venous ulceration, are common sequelae to iliofemoral deep vein thrombosis.[10] Even if there is not such severe damage, many patients suffering an episode of deep vein thrombosis will complain of slight swelling of legs after standing, restless legs at night, unusual sensations in the legs, and a tendency to nocturnal cramp.

HYPERCOAGULABLE STATES

Although changes in procoagulant, anticoagulant, and fibrinolytic factors may contribute to the development of thrombosis, it is only in certain circumstances that measurement of these factors influences the antithrombotic management of patients. Generally it is clinical events which determine the need for long-term anticoagulation and/or antiplatelet therapy.

For arterial disease, identifying inherited risk factors (other than metabolic defects such as diabetes mellitus, hyperlipidemias, and homocystemia) is not currently of value in assessing the likelihood of thrombosis in the individual patient. In epidemiological terms, genetic determinants of fibrinogen levels such as the G-455A β-fibrinogen gene promoter polymorphism are likely to be of biological importance in causing an elevated risk of thrombosis.[11] However, the magnitude of the effect is modulated by many environmental factors such as smoking. Plasminogen activator inhibitor I levels have also been proposed as a possible risk factor for arterial disease.[12] Higher levels have been associated with insulin resistance and obesity but, currently, its measurement is not of proven clinical value. Plasma fibrinogen levels and fibrin D-dimer have also been suggested as predictors of future arterial thrombotic events. Whether patients benefit from thromboprophylaxis remains to be established.[13]

For acquired hypercoaguable states in patients presenting with arterial events such as stroke, assessment of the presence of antiphospholipid antibodies is of value as their presence has been shown to indicate the likelihood of recurrent thrombosis.[14] These antibodies can be detected by solid-phase enzyme-linked immunoadsorbent assays (ELISA) for the presence of antibodies to phospholipid antigens such as cardiolipin, or by fluid-phase phospholipid-dependent coagulation tests, which detect the lupus anticoagulant. The continued presence of either or both of these antibodies associated with thrombosis constitutes the "antiphospholipid antibody syndrome" (APS). This syndrome identifies a cohort of patients in whom there may be particular risk of further thrombosis. APS may be primary, where patients do not have systemic lupus erythematosus (SLE), or secondary to lupus or lupus-like disorders. The presence of APS with arterial thrombosis indicates the need for thromboprophylaxis to prevent further arterial thrombotic events. Warfarin is the drug of first choice.[14] Although the antiphospholipid syndrome commonly presents in a young age group, increasingly these antibodies have been detected in older patients with thrombosis. Further research is required to assess their significance, particularly when the antibody titer is low.

In patients with established venous thrombotic disease, assessment of hypercoagulability may be more informative. The risk factors manifesting as inherited defects in the natural anticoagulant pathways characterized as deficiencies of antithrombin, protein C, and protein S are present in approximately 10 percent of patients presenting with deep vein thrombosis before the age of 45. Factor V Leiden and the G20210A prothrombin polymorphism are more common. These defects are therefore likely to be present with initial venous thrombosis in an older age group. Indeed, although current guidelines advise inherited thrombophilia screening only after venous events presenting in younger patients, more defects are detected when screening all age groups.

However, it is not the presence of thrombophilic defects but the number of clinical venous thrombotic events which, in most instances, determines the need for long-term anticoagulation.[15]

The presence of a severe life-threatening venous thromboembolism, with a familial thrombophilic defect, may indicate a need for lifelong warfarin,[16,17] but this would be the case regardless of the thrombophilic status. Patients with double defects such as homozygosity for factor V Leiden, or combined defects associated with a less severe clinical event, should be considered for long-term warfarin. In each case, the threat of severe morbidity or death due to recurrent venous thromboembolism should be evaluated against risks of life-threatening hemorrhage with long-term oral anticoagulation. Unusual affected sites, such as mesenteric vein or cerebral vein, may be indicative of a thrombophilic disorder. The antiphospholipid syndrome is also a recognized marker for recurrent venous thromboembolism.[14] However, although after a single venous thromboembolic event there is a high incidence of recurrence, long-term warfarin is not mandatory. Further recurrence usually is considered an indication for permanent warfarin.

ANTITHROMBOTIC TREATMENT

The most direct and logical approach to antithrombotic treatment is removal of the offending thrombus. This can be achieved by lysis or by physical means via catheter or surgery. Once the thrombus is removed it is important to inhibit further thrombus generation by antithrombotic and/or antiplatelet therapy. Anticoagulants are used for this purpose, primarily for venous disease where thrombi are rich in fibrin. Antiplatelet therapy is more appropriate for arterial disease where platelet-rich thrombi are found.

For the treatment of venous disease, anticoagulation alone will in most circumstances be sufficient. Here the strategy is to prevent any extension of established thrombus. The existing thrombus will be lysed by natural fibrinolysis. However, resolution may be slow or incomplete.

Fibrinolytic therapy

Although antithrombotic drugs remain the cornerstone of treatment of established thrombosis, lysis using plasminogen activation is widely used for myocardial infarction. It also has a role in some cases of severe venous thromboembolism and is being evaluated in acute stroke.

While fibrinolytic drugs generate plasmin, predominantly acting on the fibrin contained within the thrombus, they also induce a plasma proteolytic state.[18] The resulting plasminemia also destroys fibrinogen and some procoagulant clotting factors, and may therefore induce a widespread hemorrhagic state. Even with the newer agents where plasmin generation is mainly within fibrin and the action is not so systemic, lysis may not be confined to the thrombotic target. Hemostasis in other parts of the vascular tree may rely on the integrity of the fibrin plug. For this reason, fibrinolytic therapy can cause intracranial bleeding in the case of a cerebrovascular insult, an intracranial neoplasm, cranial surgery within 10 days, any form of major trauma to the head, or in controlled hypertension. After major surgery involving the thorax or abdomen, or with existing gastrointestinal lesions, fibrinolytic agents can cause massive hemorrhage. These clinical conditions are strong contraindications to fibrinolytic therapy.

The first-generation fibrinolytic drugs developed were urokinase and streptokinase. They have low fibrin specificity and streptokinase is antigenic. Second-generation agents are tissue plasminogen activator and streptokinase activator complex. There are now some third-generation agents derived from tissue plasminogen activator which may prove even more fibrin-specific. There are standard dosage regimens for established agents without the need for laboratory monitoring.[19]

These lytic agents can be given locally or systemically. For peripheral arterial conditions and some severe venous disorders, local delivery has the advantage of delivery to target and ability to improve resolution. For myocardial infarction, the number of patients requiring therapy and the degree of urgency makes intravenous therapy the more practical choice. For venous disease, for massive pulmonary embolism, fibrinolytic therapy may be life-saving and has a role in an incipient venous gangrene. Catheter-delivered fibrinolysis may be useful in occlusive deep vein thrombosis, but long-term results are still be to evaluated.[20]

Antiplatelet drugs

There are now several classes of drug with antiplatelet activity and these have an important role in the treatment of arterial disease. Aspirin, the irreversible cyclo-oxygenase inhibitor, remains the most widely used drug. For example, in the secondary prevention of myocardial infarction, aspirin not only reduces reinfarction rates but also reduces overall vascular mortality by one-sixth and nonfatal strokes by one-third.[21] At least 120 mg is required initially for effective therapy, but subsequently 75 mg daily may suffice. Gastrointestinal hemorrhage remains a potential problem even with low dosage and requires vigilance.

Dipyrimadole is an inhibitor of phosphodiesterase and occasionally is used as an additional antithrombotic agent to warfarin to prevent embolism with problematic prosthetic heart valves.[22,23]

Ticlopidine and clopidogrel[24] inhibit ADP binding to platelets and subsequent expression of GP IIb/IIIa receptors and subsequent fibrinogen binding. Ticlopidine causes reversible neutropenia and requires strict full blood count monitoring. It is sometimes used for a short time after coronary stenting. Clopidogrel may have a wider role in arterial disease, although there is still controversy regarding its additional benefit compared with aspirin.[25,26]

The platelet IIb/IIIa blockers are potent antiplatelet drugs. Abciximab is a Fab fragment of a humanized monoclonal antibody. Eptifabatide is a peptide specific for $\alpha IIb\beta_3$. Tirofiban is another agent with similar action.[25] These blockers need to be given intravenously and have a particular role in post-coronary angioplasty.

In addition to established use in coronary and cerebrovascular thrombotic disease, a recent meta-analysis has shown antiplatelet drugs to be of value in intermittent claudication.[27]

Anticoagulation

General issues

The well-established anticoagulants, heparin and warfarin, are still widely used for patients with thromboembolic disease. For rapid anticoagulation, heparin remains the drug of choice because, when given intravenously, its action is immediate.

In contrast, warfarin takes 4 days to become fully effective.[28] Newer anticoagulant drugs also have rapid action, but the full therapeutic potential of these antithrombin and anticlotting factor Xa agents has yet to be evaluated.

When the need for long-term anticoagulation is established, if immediate treatment is required, then it is usual to start heparin and warfarin together, continuing heparin until warfarin reaches an adequate therapeutic level.[29] Although for serious venous thromboembolism heparin alone may be used initially for several days prior to warfarinization, for submassive events warfarin may be safely started early to avoid prolonged heparinization.[30] Baseline prothrombin time, activated partial thromboplastin time, and platelet count are required to exclude any underlying hemostatic defect.[29] Subtherapeutic heparin levels early in treatment are associated with recurrent thromboembolism for both arterial and venous disease.[31] In the treatment of venous thrombosis, if oral anticoagulants are used alone, recurrence is more likely.[32]

Heparin

This heterogeneous drug preparation contains glycosaminoglycon chains[33] of varying molecular weight.[34] It is now formulated into two different drug types: unfractionated (standard) heparin, and low-molecular-weight (LMW) preparations. The anticoagulant effect depends on a unique pentasaccharide with a marked affinity for the endogenous coagulation inhibitor, antithrombin.[33] An allosteric effect following this binding induces subsequent conformational change to antithrombin.[35] This altered molecule has increased ability to capture the serine proteases of the coagulation pathway and thereby inactivate them. This inactivation is rapid and highly effective, particularly for thrombin and factor Xa. Thrombin is most sensitive to this interaction, during which a tertiary complex is formed with heparin binding to both antithrombin and thrombin. In contrast, factor Xa binds only to antithrombin without interacting with heparin. Low-molecular-weight heparin containing fewer than 18 saccharides cannot bind antithrombin and heparin simultaneously.[36] Low-molecular-weight heparin preparations, because the proportion of small saccharides is increased, show higher relative anti-Xa to antithrombin specificity compared with standard preparations. Potency and dosage comparisons between these various heparin types are difficult to assess.[37] Fortunately in most clinical circumstances for LMW heparins, fixed dose or bodyweight dosage gives adequate prophylactic or therapeutic levels. In contrast, with standard heparin, the dose–response relationship is more unpredictable and laboratory monitoring is usually required.[37]

The activated partial thromboplastin time (APTT) is the most commonly used method for monitoring standard unfractionated heparin,[38–40] which is usually given by continuous intravenous infusion. Guidelines usually indicate a therapeutic target of 1.5–2.5 times the average laboratory control value; but reagents vary in heparin sensitivity,[40] so local advice from the laboratory is recommended to determine the appropriate target. It is usual to give a loading dose of 5000 units of standard heparin as an intravenous bolus injection, with subsequent infusions of 24,000 to 30,000 units per 24 hours. Monitoring should be started 6 hours after induction and continued at least daily. Monitoring of the platelet count is recommended to exclude heparin-induced thrombocytopenia.[37] If thrombocytopenia is suspected, then heparin should be stopped immediately and an alternative immediate-acting anticoagulant used, as there is danger of arterial or venous heparin-induced thrombosis.[38]

Overdosage of heparin responds in a few hours to dose reduction or discontinuation. Intravenous protamine is prompt and effective if rapid reversal is required. If bleeding is severe, protamine sulfate should be given in a dose of 1 mg for every 100 international units of heparin infused over the previous hour.[41] Underdosage of heparin may require a further bolus as well as an increase in the infusion rate.

Subcutaneous standard heparin given 12-hourly has been used instead of intravenous heparin in some circumstances. However, low-molecular-weight preparations which are formulated specifically for the subcutaneous route give more sustained and predictable therapeutic levels. They can also be given once-daily for venous thromboembolic disease.[42–45] Bodyweight regimens with once-daily dosing have been shown to be satisfactory for the outpatient management of deep vein thrombosis[46] and pulmonary embolism.[47] Inpatient treatment can now be confined to the more serious occlusive venous thromboses where leg elevation may be required,[48] or serious pulmonary embolism where cardiac function needs assessment. Of course, outpatient management may not be appropriate in some domestic circumstances or where the patient has other medical or social problems.

Prophylactic subcutaneous heparin regimens are well established to prevent deep vein thrombosis and pulmonary embolism in hospitalized patients.[49] Standard heparin 5000 units twice-daily is effective, but low-molecular-weight regimens use once-daily dosing and are more effective in high-risk situations—such as after hip surgery where extended prophylaxis may be justified.[50] Adjusted-dose subcutaneous unfractionated heparin improves prophylaxis in hip surgery,[51,52] but the need for care with daily monitoring of dosage requirement makes it generally impracticable except in special circumstances.

Oral anticoagulants

These drugs are indicated when anticoagulation continues for more than 2 weeks. Low-molecular-weight heparin regimens have been used without warfarin for the full duration of treatment for venous thrombosis and found to be effective.[53] There may be circumstances where warfarin monitoring is difficult when this is a useful alternative. However, twice-weekly platelet counts are currently recommended during the early period of heparinization.[54]

Warfarin, nicoumalone, and phenprocoumon are in general use, with warfarin by far the most popular oral anticoagulant. They compete with vitamin K in the post-transcriptional carboxylation of glutamic acid residues of clotting factors II, IV, IX, and X and inhibiting proteins C and S. Warfarin has a plasma half-life of almost 1.5 days and takes up to a week for full effect. It is important to continue heparin until warfarin is fully effective,[29] which may take 5 days or more. Two days with adequate warfarin levels will usually indicate a full therapeutic effect.[28]

The therapeutic window for warfarin is narrow, and the danger of bleeding with overdose is high; therefore monitoring—using the prothrombin time (PT) test—has developed as the advised method for oral anticoagulation.[55] In order to standardize the prothrombin time method it is expressed in "international normalized ratios" (INRs). This takes into account the sensitivity of the local method which is expressed as the International Sensitivity Index (ISI). The index is the slope of the relationship between locally determined PT and international reference method PT, using a log scale; then INR = (PT ratio)^{ISI}.[56] The target varies for different clinical indications. The British Society of Haematology recommendations are given in tables which have been incorporated into a nationally recommended inpatient dosage chart[57] (Fig. 40-4).

During early days of warfarin induction, the dosage schedules are suitable for both inpatient[58] and outpatient[59] induction. Some induction schemes are slower in achieving therapeutic level, but require less frequent monitoring. Computerized assistance in determining dosage[60] is now widely used in outpatient clinics, and inpatient/induction/computer packages are available.

Long-term warfarin treatment requires regular INR assessment, and vigilance regarding dose compliance, drug interactions, and other medical problems. Blood specimens may be venous or capillary by thumb prick, collected at home, at local clinics or at hospital. Testing may be near-patient or within a central laboratory.[61] Dosage alteration may be immediate following direct dialog with the patient after the test, or later by post or direct communication. The dosage can be supervised by a hospital specialist, a general practitioner, a specialist nurse, a pharmacist, or a hematological scientist. Provided there is good communication with the patient or person supervising warfarin intake, and good protocols, then any of these configurations is satisfactory. Computer assistance is also of well established value in the quality of the dosage.[62] Good quality of control, however, depends on good communication. It is not infrequent for the patient to misunderstand written dosage instructions, in spite of verbal reinforcement. Gradual-onset cognitive impairment may be overlooked, so it is only by vigilance that life-threatening hemorrhagic complications are minimized. Annual rates of major bleeding of 2.4–8.1 percent have been reported, and although the risk is multifactorial, increasing age is often found to be associated with increased risk of major bleeding.[63,64] There is now an interest in self-management of oral anticoagulation with home monitors. Early studies indicate better control and increased patient satisfaction.[65] However, considerable effort is required in training patients and ensuring good quality control of testing methods. Older age would not contraindicate use of self-monitoring, but surveillance would still be required to ensure that all procedures continue to be performed satisfactorily as the patient becomes older.

Drug interactions continue to give major problems for patients in the warfarin clinic.[66] Ideally the clinic should be notified of any new or changed prescription, and the UK national anticoagulant booklet gives clear advice for the patient to notify doctor, dentist, or pharmacist about the use of warfarin. Such a booklet should always be used and be kept fully up to date with clinical and dosage information.

Clear guidelines have been formulated to deal with bleeding and for high INR readings.[29] If bleeding occurs with a therapeutic or low INR, a local cause must always be sought. Occult colonic neoplasms may bleed on warfarin and can therefore be detected early. This may aid successful surgery. Other side-effects are rare. Rashes and alopecia can occur.[67] Very rarely skin necrosis, involving microthrombosis of capillaries, can occur. This is associated with induction when there is an imbalance between warfarin effect of procoagulant and anticoagulant factors. If it occurs, inherited deficiency of protein C or S may also be present.[68]

Other anticoagulants

The newer anti-Xa and direct thrombin inhibitors are still under evaluation.[69,70] Recombinant hirudin has been used for venous thromboembolism prophylaxis and in patients with heparin-induced thrombocytopenia.[71] This drug, which is modeled on the leach anticoagulant, inhibits thrombin directly. It is a moderate-size peptide and therefore must be given by intravenous or subcutaneous injection. Other agents are not yet licensed in the UK but are likely to become available shortly.[69]

VENOUS THROMBOTIC DISEASE

Deep vein thrombosis (DVT) and pulmonary embolism (PE) are the main manifestations of venous thrombotic disease. Thromboembolism occurs with increasing frequency with age[1] and, although potentially treatable, surveys indicate that it is under-recognized and often misdiagnosed (Fig. 40-5). As many as two-thirds of patients with DVT may remain symptom-free,[72] and symptoms suggestive of DVT may be due to another condition in approximately 50 percent of patients.[72,73] Pulmonary embolism is estimated to be the cause of death in 3–6 percent of the general population in both the UK and the USA,[74,75] and postmortem studies show an incidence as high as 69 percent. Antemortem diagnosis is low: 90 percent of fatal PE may not be recognized in life,[76] and often the condition is not even considered.

The clinical diagnosis of DVT is based on the classical symptoms of pain and swelling of the calf, together with increased calf circumference, local warmth, induration of the soleus and gastrocnemius muscle bed, tenderness on palpation, and a positive Homans' sign (pain in the calf on dorsiflexing the foot). However, two-thirds of patients with venous thrombosis may not have any symptoms or signs,[72] and if the signs are present they may be due to another condition in at least 50 percent of patients (e.g. ruptured Baker's cyst or cellulitis).[72,73] In one study, signs were detected in only 9 of 53 legs with thrombosis, and these developed at least 2 days after a positive fibrinogen scan.

Nevertheless, the view that clinical signs are unreliable has been challenged.[78] Landfield et al.[79] found that swelling above or below the knee, recent immobility, cancer, and fever were independent predictors of acute proximal DVT. If venography had been carried out only in patients with one or more of these factors, it would have diagnosed 97 percent of cases and would have been avoided in 26 percent of patients with normal test results. By combining clinical findings with venous ultrasonography, Wells et al.[80] confirmed that it is possible to stratify patients into high, moderate, and low pretest probabilities,

Anticoagulant chart and referral form   *Hospital*

Guidelines for anticoagulation of adult patients

Patient ref no	:
Name	:
Address	:
	:
	:
	:
	:
Telephone	:
Date of birth	:

Lower doses may be required for
(i) the elderly, especially those with cardiac failure
(ii) patients with hepatic and/or severe renal failure

Unfractionated heparin infusion schedule

iv bolus   5000 units (in severe pulmonary embolism, 10 000 units may be used)
iv infusion   15 000 units/12 hours
Check APTT ratio after 2-6 hours
- acceptable range   1.5-2.5

Monitor platelets after 4 days heparin treatment

Adjust heparin as follows:-

> 5.0	stop for 1 hour		
	decrease by 6000 units/12 hours	- recheck APTT	in 2 - 6 hours
4.1 - 5.0	decrease by 3600 units/12 hours	- recheck APTT	in 2 - 6 hours
3.1 - 4.0	decrease by 1200 units/12 hours	- recheck APTT	in 2 - 6 hours
2.6 - 3.0	decrease by 600 units/12 hours	- recheck APTT	in 2 - 12 hours
1.5 - 2.5	no change	- recheck APTT within	24 hours
1.2 - 1.4	increase by 2400 units/12 hours	- recheck APTT	in 2 - 12 hours
< 1.2	increase by 4800 units/12 hours	- recheck APTT	in 2 - 6 hours

Check APTT 3-6 hours after starting heparin
Do not represcribe heparin for more than 24 hours
Checking APTT on a daily basis is the mandatory minimum for all patients receiving intravenous heparin
See overleaf for guidance on correction of over anticoagulation
For further information please contact consultant haematologist

Continue heparin until oral anticoagulation is established and the international normalized
ratio (INR) is stable in the appropriate therapeutic range

Subcutaneous low molecular weight heparin (LMWH) schedule

Name of LMWH=
Dose per kg body weight=

Treatment regimen for patients with confirmed DVT
And/or PE (where licensed)

Frequency of sc injection based on body weight once/twice* per day
(*delete as appropriate)

APTT monitoring is **not** routinely indicated

Treatment with LMWH should be for 5 days, and continued until the
INR is stable within the appropriate therapeutic range 2.0-3.0
(target INR 2.5) or 3.0-4.0 (target INR 3.5) - see page 3

Monitor platelets after 4 days heparin treatment

Weight _____ kg

Weight (kg)	dosage
130	
125	
120	
115	
110	
105	
100	
95	
90	
85	
80	
75	
70	
65	
60	
55	
50	
45	
40	

Figure 40-4 Anticoagulant chart and referral form. Reproduced from Hospital Medicine 2000; 61, no. 9, by kind permission of the Medicine Publishing Company.

Warfarin schedule

DVT	start warfarin same day as heparin (includes LMWH)
PE, DVT plus PE	start warfarin same day as heparin or when diagnosis is confirmed

Warfarin dosing

Day	INR	Dose mg
1	< 1.4	10.0
2	< 1.8	10.0
	= 1.8	1.0
	> 1.8	0.5
3	< 2.1	10.0
	2.0 - 2.1	5.0
	2.2 - 2.3	4.5
	2.4 - 2.5	4.0
	2.6 - 2.7	3.5
	2.8 - 2.9	3.0
	3.0 - 3.1	2.5
	3.2 - 3.3	2.0
	= 3.4	1.5
	= 3.5	1.0
	3.6 - 4.0	0.5
	>4.0	0.0

Warfarin dosing ... continued

Day	INR	Dose mg	
4	< 1.4		Refer to haematology department for advice
	= 1.4	8.0	
	= 1.5	7.5	
	1.6 - 1.7	7.0	
	= 1.8	6.5	
	= 1.9	6.0	
	2.0 - 2.1	5.5	
	2.2 - 2.3	5.0	
	2.4 - 2.6	4.5	
	2.7 - 3.0	4.0	
	3.1 - 3.5	3.5	
	3.6 - 4.0	3.0	
	4.1 - 4.5		Miss out one day's dose, then give 2.0 mg
	> 4.5		Miss out two day's dose, then give 1.0 mg
5 onward			Monitor INR daily until in range and stable (iv heparin can be stopped when two consecutive INR results in therapeutic range

BLEEDING WHILE ANTICOAGULATED (UNFRACTIONATED HEPARIN)

As heparin has a short half-life it is usually sufficient to stop infusion
If bleeding is severe reverse anticoagulation with iv protamine sulphate as follows
→ 1mg protamine for every 100 units of heparin given over previous hour
→ Halve protamine dose if heparin infusion has been stopped for 1 hour, quarter dose if stopped for 2 hours

Give protamine slowly (5mg/min), not more than 40mg at one time
Note: a further dose may be required as protamine has a short half-life

BLEEDING WHILE ANTICOAGULATED (LMWH)

If bleeding is severe reverse anticoagulation with iv protamine sulphate as follows
→ 40mg protamine sulphate

Give protamine slowly (5mg/min)
As LMWH is continuously absorbed, repeat treatment may be necessary

BLEEDING WHILE ANTICOAGULATED (WARFARIN)

Life-threatening haemorrhage
→ Stop warfarin
→ 5mg vitamin K by slow iv injection
→ Factor II, IX, X and VII concentrates at 50 iu/kg
→ If no concentrate use fresh frozen plasma (FFP) approx 1L in an adult (15ml/kg)

Less severe haemorrhage
→ Withhold warfarin for 1 or more days. Restart at reduced dose when INR < 5.0
→ Consider vitamin K 0.5 - 2.0 mg iv

Unexpected bleeding at therapeutic levels
→ Investigate for underlying cause

OVERANTICOAGULATION WITHOUT BLEEDING

INR>8.0 no bleeding
→ stop warfarin
→ give vitamin K 0.5mg iv or 5mg oral. Restart at reduced dose when INR<5.0

INR 5.0 - 8.0 without haemorrhage
→ Withhold warfarin for 1 or 2 days and review. Restart at reduced dose when INR<5.0

> **If in doubt contact consultant haematologist**

Figure 40-4 *Continued.*

Request for continuation of anticoagulant therapy as outpatient

An appointment for anticoagulant follow up *must* be made before the patient is discharged from hospital.

Telephone_____ . This form *must* be completed and sent to_____ .

Please tick one box	Venous thromboembolism	Target INR	range	Recommended duration
	Postoperative calf vein thrombosis without any risk factors	2.5	2-3	6 weeks
	Calf vein thrombosis in non-surgical patients without any risk factors	2.5	2-3	3 months
	Pulmonary embolus and proximal vein thrombosis	2.5	2-3	6 months
	DVT and/or PE with persistent risk factors	2.5	2-3	duration varies according to risk factor(s) - discuss with haematologist
	Recurrent DVT and/or PE	2.5	2-3	indefinite
	Recurrent DVT and/or PE while on warfarin (INR range 2-3)	3.5	3-4	indefinite

Atrial fibrillation (AF)

	Atrial fibrillation or other high risk arrhythmias	2.5	2-3	indefinite

Heart valve prostheses and other cardiac indications

	Mechanical prosthetic valves	3.5	3 - 4	indefinite
	Bioprosthetic heart valves (not aortic)	2.5	2 - 3	3 months*
	Cardiomyopathy, mural thrombus or akinetic segment	2.5	2 - 3	indefinite

* discontinue warfarin if there is no AF, intracardiac thrombus or history of systemic embolism
Patients not requiring warfarin should be considered for antiplatelet therapy, e.g. aspirin

Aspirin is first-line therapy for the following conditions:

If warfarin is considered appropriate:

	TIA/ischaemic stroke	3.5	3 - 4	indefinite
	Peripheral arterial thrombosis and grafts	3.5	3 - 4	indefinite
	Coronary artery thrombosis	3.5	3 - 4	indefinite
	Coronary artery graft thrombosis	3.5	3 - 4	indefinite
	Coronary angioplasty and coronary stents	3.5	3 - 4	indefinite

	Preferred treatment and date for anticoagulation		
	Other drug therapy:		
	If patient currently taking aspirin, should this continue?	YES / NO	
	Discharge home date/time		
	Date of follow-up as outpatient		
	Date of anticoagulant follow up		
	Yellow anticoagulant book issued to patient		
	Transport to anticoagulant clinic required	YES / NO	ambulance / car
	Signature of referring doctor / specialist nurse		

Figure 40-4 *Continued.*

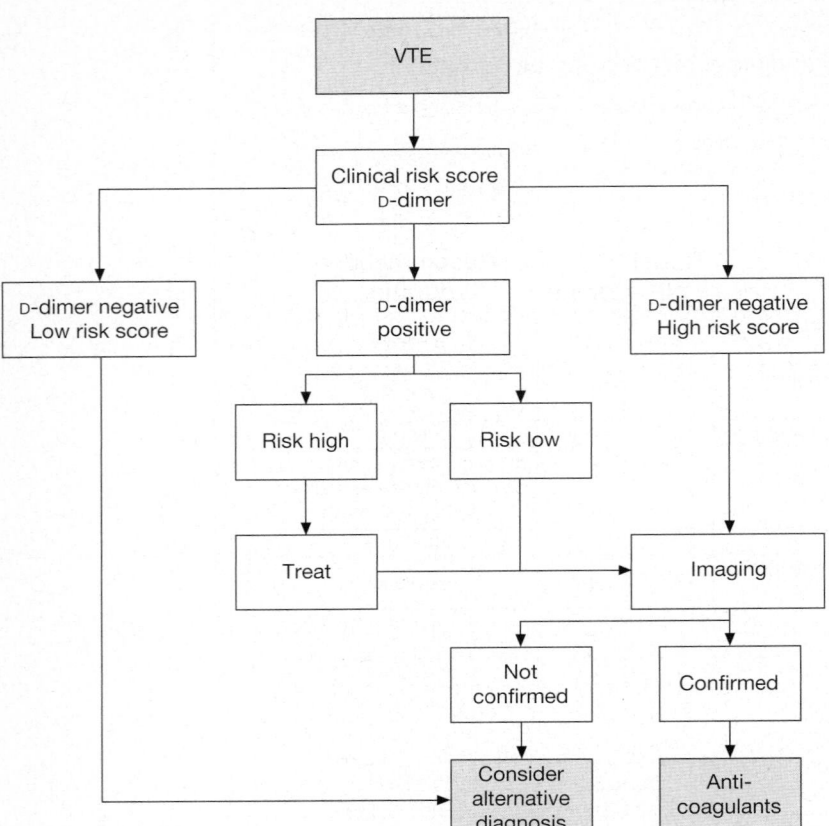

Figure 40-5 Algorithm outlining an approach to the investigation of a patient presenting with suspect venous thromboembolism (VTE).

limiting the need for invasive venography. The clinical signs can be used with measurement of the degradation product of cross-linked fibrin (D-dimer) to identify patients who are more likely to show a DVT when subsequent ultrasound and venography are performed.[81,82] Use of D-dimer as a screening method for DVT can reduce unnecessary duplex scanning or venography.[83–85] Patients with a positive D-dimer will still require imaging or sonography as the result is not specific for DVT.[82]

The symptoms and signs of pulmonary embolism may be absent, or the condition may give rise to shortness of breath and pleuritic pain or, in extreme cases, lead to life-threatening collapse. Hemoptysis is uncommon.[86] In massive PE, patients may be short of breath both upright and prone, with elevated jugular venous pressure. Chronic repeated PE may result in pulmonary hypertension. D-dimer estimation also may be helpful.[87]

The clinical diagnosis of venous thrombosis and PE require objective confirmation.[88,89] Generally first-line investigations are ultrasound for DVT and ventilation perfusion scanning for PE. Spiral computerized tomography is also useful for PE. Venography and pulmonary angiography remain the definitive investigations for venous thromboembolism.[86–88,90]

Initial treatment of venous thromboembolism is as previously described in this chapter—namely heparin, now usually LMW subcutaneous heparin given by bodyweight once-daily, and adjusted-dose warfarin. This can be given safely as an outpatient when the thrombosis is minor. Heparin continues until the INR is above 2.0 for at least 2 consecutive days.[91]

Warfarin is usually continued for several months. For postoperative venous thrombosis, 6 weeks is judged adequate.[92,93] Symptomatic calf vein thrombosis in nonsurgical patients without predisposing factors such as cancer or thrombophilia should be treated with warfarin for 3 months.[92–94] Longer periods of warfarin have been shown to reduce recurrence but not definitely reduce mortality.[95] Continued treatment should be considered where there are persistent risk factors, but the hazards of continued anticoagulation should be judged against the complications which may occur after recurrence of the thromboembolism.

Recurrence of venous thromboembolism may indicate a long-term requirement for warfarin. Recurrence while on warfarin indicates a need for high-intensity warfarin (INR 3.5), or alternative anticoagulant therapy such as the addition or alternative use of LMW heparin. It should also highlight the need to exclude malignancy or the antiphospholipid syndrome.[29]

Low-molecular-weight heparins prevent venous thrombosis more effectively than standard heparins, and the once-daily dosage is an advantage (though the risk of major bleeding is probably the same).[96] Prophylaxis is of value in some medical conditions. Four out of five studies showed a significant reduction in the incidence of DVT after myocardial infarction.[97] McCarthy et al[98,99] reported a large reduction in venous thrombosis following a stroke. However, there are potential hazards in the use of LMW heparins and heparinoids in acute ischemic stroke for the prevention of deep vein thrombosis and pulmonary embolism.[100]

There are clear benefits of prophylaxis for patients under-going general surgery. For patients following hip surgery, the rate for DVT was reduced from 50 to 20 percent.[97] The final end-point in prophylaxis must be to lower the incidence of fatal pulmonary embolus. In a large multicenter trial of over 4000 patients, only two of those treated with heparin died from PE, compared with 16 in the control group.[101] There are other methods for prophylaxis.[102,103] Hills et al.[77] reported that inter-mittent pneumatic calf compression was of value in general surgical patients, which was confirmed by Colditz et al.[104] Graduated elastic stockings alone were of less value.

In any strategy for prevention, patients should be stratified and treated according to the estimated risk of thrombo-embolism[102,103] (Table 40-3).

ARTERIAL THROMBOEMBOLISM

In general, except for specific conditions, the use of warfarin is not recommended for patients with arterial disease. Antiplatelet therapy, usually aspirin, is more appropriate.[29]

A particular exception is patients with atrial fibrillation (AF), both nonrheumatic and rheumatic.[105–107] It is the former who now comprise the major group of patients in warfarin clin-ics, many of whom are over the age of 60. There is still controversy in this area,[108] but the current recommendation is to give warfarin as first-line therapy in patients with AF and at least one risk factor (previous thromboembolism, age, hyper-tension, heart failure, abnormal left ventricular function, or echocardiography), to prevent thromboembolism. The recom-mendation is outlined in a North American consensus report:[109]

"Long-term [oral anticoagulant] with a target of 2.5 (range 2–3) is strongly recommended in AF patients at high risk of stroke such as patients with prior [transient ischemic attacks], stroke, or systemic embolism, patients aged >75 years, those with poor left ventricular function, hypertension, diabetes, coronary artery disease, and thyrotoxicosis. In the absence of these risk factors, aspirin is usually recommended under 65 years because of low stroke risk, and either aspirin or an anticoagulant can be given between 65 and 75 years."

This risk benefit may alter with age and additional illness. Aspirin is considered a less effective but safer alternative in patients when warfarin appears unusually hazardous.[29]

Other indications for warfarin include rheumatic mitral valve disease (even in the absence of AF), mural thrombosis, cardiomyopathy, and the use of a mechanical prosthetic heart valve.[29] For mechanical valve replacement the UK recom-mendation is an INR target of 3.5. Recommendations in the USA are to use an INR of 3.0–4.5 for caged-ball prostheses, 2.5–3.5 for a bileaflet mitral valve, 2.0–3.0 for a bileaflet aortic valve with sinus rhythm, and 2.5–3.5 for a bileaflet aortic valve with AF.[110] For bioprosthetic valves, warfarin is not required unless there is AF.[111,112] For ischemic stroke, peripheral arterial throm-bosis and grafts, coronary artery thrombosis, and coronary artery graft thrombosis, angioplasty and stents, aspirin is an appropriate prophylaxis.[29]

Table 40-3 Percentage incidence of venous thromboembolism[a] in hospitalized patients

	DVT	Proximal DVT	Fatal PE
Low risk	<10	<1	0.01
Moderate risk	10–40	1–10	0.1–1
High risk	40–80	10–30	1–10

In older patients—

Low risk: minor surgery less than 30 min with no other risk factors except age

Moderate risk:
• major surgery (except as below tabulated in high risk)
• major medical illness (heart or lung disease, cancer)
• inflammatory bowel disorder
• major trauma or burns
• minor surgery with previous venous thromboembolism (VTE)

High risk:
• fracture or major orthopedic surgery of pelvis, hip, or lower limb
• major pelvic or abdominal surgery for cancer
• major surgery with previous VTE
• lower-limb paralysis
• major limb amputation

[a]Meta-analysis suggests that the mean incidence of DVT after major surgery will be reduced from 25 to 9 percent by use of low-dose heparin prophylaxis.

KEY POINTS   Thromboembolic disease

■ The incidence of thromboembolism increases with age.

■ The hazards of antithrombotic drugs also increase with age.

■ Each decision to use antithrombin drugs should assess risks against benefits.

■ Long-term warfarin therapy is usually decided on clinical, not laboratory, grounds.

■ Drug interactions remain a common cause of warfarin overdosage.

■ Good communication is essential for safe antithrombotic therapy.

REFERENCES

1. Havig O: Deep vein thrombosis and pulmonary embolus. Acta Churg Scand 1977;478(Suppl):1–93
2. Nordstrom M, Lindblad B, Bergqvist et al: A prospective study of the incidence of deep vein thrombosis within a defined urban population. J Intern Med 1992;232:155–160
3. Anderson FA, Wheeler HB, Goldberg RJ et al: A population based perspective of the hospital incidence and case fatality rates of deep vein thrombosis and pulmonary embolism: the Worcester DVT study. Arch Intern Med 1991;151:933–938
4. Van der Meer FJM, Rosendaal FR, Vandenbroucke et al: Bleeding complications in oral anticoagulant therapy. Arch Intern Med 1993;153:1557–1562
5. French JE: Thrombosis. In Florey H (ed): General Pathology, 3rd edn. Lloyd-Luke, London, 1964:234

6. Wessler S: Thrombosis in the presence of vascular stasis. Am J Med 1962;33:648–666

7. Sevitt S, Gallagher NG: Venous thrombosis and pulmonary embolism: a clinicopathological study in injured and burned patients. Br J Surg 1961;48:475–489

8. Kakkar V, Flanc C, Howe C et al: Natural history of postoperative deep vein thrombosis. Lancet 1969;ii:230–233

9. Pellegrini V, Langhans M, Totterman S et al: Embolic complications of calf thrombosis following total hip arthroplasty. J Arthroplasty 1993;8:449–457

10. Young AE, Thomas ML, Browse NL: Comparison between sequelae of surgical and medical treatment of venous thrombosis. BMJ 1974;4:127–133

11. Humphreys SE, Luong L, Montgomery HE et al: Gene–environment interaction in the determination of levels of plasma fibrinogen. Thromb Haemost 1999;82:818–825

12. Juhan-Vague I, Alessi MC: Regulation of fibrinolysis in the development of atherothrombosis: role of adipose tissue. Thromb Haemost 1999;82:832–836

13. Lowe G, Rumley A, Norrie J et al: Blood rheology, cardiovascular risk factors and cardiovascular disease: the West of Scotland coronary prevention study. Thromb Haemost 2000;84:553–558

14. Greaves M, Cohen H, Machin SJ et al: Guidelines on the investigation and management of the antiphospholipid syndrome. Br J Haem 2000;109:704–715

15. Greaves M, Baglin T: Laboratory testing for inheritable thrombophilia: impact on clinical management. Br J Haem 2000;109:699–703

16. Marchetti M, Pistorio A, Barosi G: Extended anticoagulation for prevention of recurrent venous thromboembolism in carriers of factor V Leiden: cost-effectiveness analysis. Thromb Haemost 2000;84:752–757

17. Van der Belt AGM, Hutten BA, Prins MH et al: Duration of oral anticoagulant treatment in patients with venous thromboembolism and a deficiency of antithrombin protein C or protein S: a decision analysis. Thromb Haemost 2000;84:758–765

18. Weitz JI, Stewart RJ, Fredenburgh JC: Mechanism of action of plasminogen activators. Thromb Haemost 1999;82:974–982

19. British National Formulary: Fibrinolytic drugs. BNF 2000;40:120–121

20. Kandarpa K: Catheter directed thrombolysis of peripheral arterial occlusions and deep vein thrombosis. Thromb Haemost 1999;82:987–996

21. Greaves M, Taberner DA: Thrombotic disease. In Oxford Textbook of Medicine, 3rd edn. Oxford University Press, Oxford, 1999:3661–3676

22. Schafer AI: Antiplatelet therapy. Am J Med 1996;101:199–209

23. Savi P, Herbert JM: ADP receptors on platelets and ADP-selective antiaggregating agents. Med Res Rev 1996;16:159–179

24. Herbert JM, Frehel D, Vallee E et al: Clopidogrel, a novel antiplatelet and antithrombotic agent. Cardiovasc Drug Rev 1993;11:180–198

25. British National Formulary: Antiplatelet drugs. BNF 2000;40:117–119

26. CAPRIE Steering Committee: A randomised, blinded, trial of clopidogrel versus aspirin in patients at risk of ischaemic events. Lancet 1996;348:1329–1339

27. Girolami B, Bernadi E, Prins MH et al: Antithrombotic drugs in the primary medical management of intermittent claudication: a meta-analysis. Thromb Haemost 1999;81:715–722

28. Ginsberg J: Drug therapy: management of venous thromboembolism. N Engl J Med 1996;335:1816–1828

29. British Committee of Statistics in Haematology: Guidelines on oral anticoagulation, 3rd edn. Br J Haem 1998;101:374–387

30. Gallus A, Jackman J, Tillet J et al: Safety and efficacy of warfarin started early after submassive venous thrombosis or pulmonary embolism. Lancet 1986;2:1293–1296

31. Hull RD, Raskob CE, Hirsch J et al: Continuous intravenous heparin compared with intermittent subcutaneous heparin in the initial treatment of proximol vein thrombosis. N Engl J Med 1986;315:1109–1114

32. Brandjes DPM, Hejiboer H, Buller HR et al: Acenocoumarol and heparin compared with acenocoumarol alone in the initial treatment of proximal vein thrombosis. N Engl J Med 1986;327:1485–1489

33. Casu B. Heparin structure. Haemostasis 1990;20:62–73 (review)

34. Andersson LO, Barrowcliffe TW, Holmer E et al: Molecular weight dependency of the heparin potential inhibition of thrombin and activated factor X: effect of heparin neutralization in plasma. Thromb Res 1979;15:531–541

35. Rosenberg RD, Lam L: Correlation between structure and function of heparin. Proc Natl Acad Sci USA 1979;76:1218–1222

36. Casu B, Oreste P, Torri G et al: The structure of heparin oligosaccharide fragments with high antifactor Xa activity containing the minimal antithrombin III binding sequence: chemical and 13C nuclear magnetic resonance studies. Biochem J 1981;197:599–609

37. Kitchen S: Problems in laboratory monitoring of heparin dosage. Br J Haem 2000;111:397–406

38. Banez EI, Triplett DA, Koepke J: Laboratory monitoring of heparin therapy: the effect of different salts of heparin on the APTT. Am J Clin Path 1980;74:569–574

39. Van den Besselaar AMHP, Neuteboom J, Berhna RM: Monitoring heparin therapy: relationships between the APTT and heparin assays based on ex-vivo samples. Thromb Haemost 1990;63:16–23

40. Kitchen S, Jennings I, Woods TAL et al: Wide variation in the sensitivity of APTT reagents for monitoring heparin dosage. J Clin Path 1996;49:10–14

41. British Committee for Statistics in Haematology: Guidelines for the use and monitoring of heparin, 1992, 2nd edn. J Clin Path 1993;46:97–103

42. Leisorovicz A, Simonneau G, Decousous H et al: Comparison of efficacy and safety of low molecular weight heparins and unfractionated heparin in initial treatment of deep venous thrombosis: a meta-analysis. BMJ 1994;309:299–304

43. Lensing AWA, Prins MH, Davidson BL et al: Treatment of deep vein thrombosis with low-molecular weight heparins. Arch Intern Med 1995;155:601–607

44. Dolovich LR, Ginsber JS, Douketis JD et al: A meta-analysis comparing low-molecular weight heparins with unfractionated heparin in the treatment of venous thromboembolism. Arch Int Med 2000;160:181–188

45. Bijsterveld NR, Hettiarachchi R, Peters R et al: Low-molecular weight heparins in venous and arterial thrombotic disease. Thromb Haemost 1999;82(Suppl 1):139–147

46. Belcaro G, Nicolaides AN, Cesarone MR et al: Comparison of low-molecular-weight heparin, administered primarily at home, with unfractionated heparin, administered in hospital, and subcutaneous heparin, administered at home for deep vein thrombosis. Angiology 1999;50:781–787

47. Hull RD, Raskob GE, Brant RF et al: Low molecular weight heparin vs heparin in the treatment of patients with pulmonary embolism. American–Canadian Thrombosis Study Group. Arch Int Med 2000;160:229–236

48. Shetty HG: Management of deep vein thrombosis. Prescribers J 1997;37:167–172

49. Hirsch J: Heparin. N Engl J Med 1991;324:1565–1574

50. Thomas DP: Thromboprophylaxis after replacement arthroplasty. BMJ 2001;322:686–687

51. Levraz PF, Richard J, Bachmann F et al: Adjusted versus fixed dose subcutaneous heparin in the prevention of deep vein thrombosis after total hip replacement. N Engl J Med 1983;309:954–958

52. Taberner DA, Poller L, Thomson JM et al: Randomized study of adjusted versus fixed low dose heparin prophylaxis of deep vein thrombosis in hip surgery. Br J Surg 1989;76:933–935

53. Veiga F, Escriba A, Maluenda MP et al: Low molecular weight heparin (Enoxaparin) versus oral anticoagulant therapy (Acenocumarol) in the long-term treatment of deep vein thrombosis in the elderly: a randomized trial. Thromb Haemost 2000;84:559–565

54. Olson JD, Arkin CF, Brandt JT et al: Laboratory monitoring of unfractionated heparin. Arch Pathol Lab Med 1998;122:782–798 (review)

55. British Committee for Standards in Haematology: Guidelines on oral anticoagulation, 2nd edn. J Clin Path 1990;43:177–183

56. WHO Expert Committee on Biological Standardization: WHO technical report series no. 87, London. 1983;33:81–105

57. Rose P: Audit of anticoagulant therapy. J Clin Path 1996;49:5–9

58. Fennerty A, Dolben J, Thomas P et al: Flexible induction dose regimen for warfarin and prediction of maintenance dose. BMJ 1984;288:1268–1270

59. Tait RC, Sefcick A: A warfarin induction regimen for out-patient anticoagulation in patient with atrial fibrillation. Br J Haem 1998;101:450–454

60. Ryan P, Gilbert M, Rose P: Computer control of anticoagulant dose for therapeutic management. BMJ 1989;299:1207–1209

61. Machin S, Mackie I, Chitolie A et al: Near patient testing (NPT) in haemostasis: a synoptic review. Clin Lab Haem 1996;18:69–74

62. Poller L, Wright D, Rowlands M: Prospective comparative study of computer programs for management of warfarin. J Clin Path 1993;46:299–303

63. Landefeld CS, Beyth RJ: Anticoagulant related bleeding: clinical epidemiology, prediction and prevention. Am J Med 1993;95:315–328

64. Levine MN, Hirsh J, Landefeld CS et al: Haemorrhagic complications of anticoagulant treatment. Chest 1992;102(Suppl):352–363

65. Cromheecke ME, Levi M, Colly LP et al: Oral anticoagulant self-management by a specialist anticoagulant clinic: a randomized cross-over comparison. Lancet 2000;356:97–100
66. Routledge PA: Practical prescribing: warfarin. Prescribers J 1997;37:173–179
67. British National Formulary: Oral anticoagulants. BNF 2000;40:115–116
68. Craig A, Taberner DA, Foster D et al: Type 1 protein S deficiency and skin necrosis. Postgrad Med J 1990;66:389–391
69. Ahmed S, Yang LH, Atisan A et al: Pharmacokinetics of argatroban in primates: evidence of endogenous uptake. Int Angio 2000;19:126–134
70. Lewis BE, Ferguson IJ, Grossman ED et al: Successful coronary interventions performed with argatroban anticoagulation in patients with heparin-induced thrombocytopenia and thrombosis syndrome. J Invas Cardiol 1996;8:410–417
71. British National Formulary: Parenteral anticoagulants. BNF 2000;40:111–115
72. Salzman EW: Venous thrombosis made easy. N Engl J Med 1986;314:847–848
73. Cranlley JJ: Diagnosis of deep vein thrombosis: fallibility of clinical symptoms and signs. Arch Surg 1976;111:34–36
74. Dalen JE, Alpert JS: Natural history of pulmonary embolus. Prog Cardiovasc Dis 1975;17:259–270
75. Dismulie SE: Pulmonary embolus as a cause of death. JAMA 1986;255:2039–2042
76. Horrowitz PE, Tatter D: Lethal pulmonary embolism. In Sherry S, Brinkhouse KM, Stengle JM (eds): Thrombosis. National Academy of Science, Washington, DC, 1969
77. Hills NH, Pflug JJ, Jeyasingh K et al: Prevention of deep vein thrombosis by intermittent pneumatic compression of calf. BMJ 1972;1:131–135
78. Ramsey LE: Impact of venography on the diagnosis and management of deep vein thrombosis. BMJ 1983;286:698–699
79. Landfield CS, McGuire E, Cohen AM: Clinical findings associated with acute proximal deep vein thrombosis: a basis for quantifying clinical judgment. Am J Med 1990;88:382–388
80. Wells PS, Hirsch J, Anderson DR et al: Accuracy of clinical assessment of deep vein thrombosis. Lancet 1995;345:1326–1330
81. Bounameaux H, Moerloose P, Perrier A et al: D-dimer testing in suspected venous thromboembolism: an update. QJM 1997;90:437–442
82. Ginsberg JS, Kearon C, Douketis J et al: The use of D-dimer testing and impedance plethysmographic examination in patients with clinical indications of deep vein thrombosis. Arch Intern Med 1997;157:1077–1081
83. Van der Graaf F, van der Borne H, van der Kolk M et al: Exclusion of deep vein thrombosis with D-dimer testing: comparison of 13 D-dimer methods in 99 outpatients suspected of deep venous thrombosis using venography as reference standard. Thromb Haemost 2000;83:191–198
84. Bernardi E, Prandoni P, Lensing AWA et al: D-dimeer testing as an adjunct to ultrasonography in patients with clinically suspected deep vein thrombosis; prospective cohort study. BMJ 1998;317:1037–1040
85. Mauron T, Baumgartner I, Z'Brun A et al: SimpliRED D-dimer assay: comparability study of capillary and citrated venous whole blood, between assay variability and performance of the test for exclusion of deep vein thrombosis in symptomatic outpatients. Thromb Haemost 1998;79:1217–1219
86. Ledingham IGG, Weatherall DJ: Pulmonary embolism. In Oxford Textbook of Medicine. Oxford University Press, Oxford, 1996:2522–2527
87. Perrier A, Desmarais S, Miron M-J et al: Noninvasive diagnosis of pulmonary venous thromboembolism in outpatient including clinical probability, D-dimer and ultrasonography. Lancet 1999;353:190–195

88. Bell RB, Simon TL: Current status of pulmonary thromboembolic disease: pathophysiology, diagnosis, prevention and treatment. Am Heart J 1982;103:239–262
89. de Mooerloose P: D-dimer assays for the exclusion of venous thromboembolism: which test for which diagnostic strategy? Thromb Haemost 2000;83:180–181
90. Moser KM: Diagnosing pulmonary embolism. BMJ 1994;309:1525–1526
91. Anonymous: How to anticoagulate. Drugs Therapeut Bull 1992;30:77–80
92. Schuman S, Rhedin AS, Lindmarker P et al: A comparison of six weeks with six months of oral anticoagulant therapy after a first episode of venous thromboembolism. N Engl J Med 1995;332:1661–1665
93. Chesterman CN: After a first episode of venous thromboembolism. BMJ 1995;311:700–701
94. Hirsh J: The optimal duration of anticoagulant therapy for venous thrombosis. N Engl J Med 1995;332:1710–1711
95. Hutton BA, Prins MH: Duration of treatment with vitamin K antagonists in symptomatic venous thromboembolism. Cochrane Library 2000; issue 3.
96. Anonymous: Low molecular weight heparins in orthopaedic surgery. Drugs Ther Bull 1993;31:39–40
97. Kakkar VV: The prevention of venous thromboembolism. In McCarthy ST (ed): Peripheral Vascular Disease in the Elderly. 1983:150–164
98. McCarthy ST, Turner JJ, Robertson D et al: Low dose heparin as a prophylaxis against deep vein thrombosis after acute stroke. Lancet 1977;2:800–801
99. McCarthy ST, Turner JJ: Low dose subcutaneous heparin in the prevention of deep vein thrombosis and pulmonary embolus following acute stroke. Age Ageing 1986;15:84–88
100. Bath PMW, Iddenden R, Bath FJ: Low molecular weight heparins and heparinoids in acute ischaemic stroke. Stroke 2001;31:1770–1778
101. International Multicentre Trial: Prevention of post-operative pulmonary embolus by low doses of heparin. Lancet 1975;2:45–51
102. Thromboembolic risk factors (THRIFT) Consensus Group: Risk and prophylaxis for venous thromboembolism in hospital patients. BMJ 1992;305:567–574
103. Anonymous: Preventing and treating deep vein thrombosis. Drugs Ther Bull 1992;30:9–12
104. Colditz GA, Tuden RL, Oster G: Rates of venous thrombosis after general surgery: combined results of randomized clinical trials. Lancet 1986;2:143–146
105. Hart RG, Halperin JL: Atrial fibrillation and thromboembolism: a decade of progress in stroke prevention. Ann Intern Med 1999;131:688–695
106. Hart R, Benavente O, McBride R et al: Antithrombotic therapy to prevent stroke in patients with atrial fibrillation: a meta-analysis. Ann Intern Med 1999;131:492–501
107. Benavente O, Hart R, Koudstaal P et al: Antiplatelet therapy for preventing stroke in patient with non-valvular atrial fibrillation and no previous history of stroke or transient ischaemic attacks. Cochrane Library, issue 1, 2000
108. Taylor FC, Cohen H, Ebrahim S: Systematic review of long term anticoagulation or antiplatelet treatment in patients with non-rheumatic atrial fibrillation. BMJ 2001;322:321–325
109. Laupacis A, Albers G, Daker J et al: Antithrombotic therapy in atrial fibrillation. Chest 1998;114:5793–5795
110. Stein P, Alpert JS, Dalen JE et al: Antithrombotic therapy in patients with mechanical and biological prosthetic heart valves. Chest 1998;114:602S–610S
111. Turpie G, Canstensen J, Hirsch J et al: Randomized comparison of two intensities of oral anticoagulant therapy after tissue heart valve replacement. Lancet 1988;i:1242–1245
112. Turpie A: Valvular heart disease and heart valve prostheses. In Oral Anticoagulants. Arnold, London, 1996:143–149
113. Alford SI, Machin S: Haemostasis. Medicine 2000;28(2):10–14

Chapter 41

Age-related changes in the respiratory system

Martin J. Connolly

In common with all organ and control systems there are both structural and functional changes in the respiratory system associated with the aging process. An understanding of such changes is essential to the understanding of respiratory pathology. However, before such changes can themselves be understood it is necessary to have a grasp of normal respiratory function in younger adults.

RESPIRATORY FUNCTION TESTS

This section provides a brief introduction to the most commonly used nonradiological investigations in respiratory disease, together with the typical patterns seen in different classes of respiratory pathology in younger adults.

The most commonly used "breathing tests" are as follows:

- FEV_1: *forced expiratory volume in one second* (liters). This is the volume of air expired during the first second of a forced expiratory maneuver from vital capacity.
- FVC: *forced vital capacity* (liters). This is the total volume of air expired during forced expiration from vital capacity. It is usually identical to slow vital capacity (SVC) (i.e. that expired during an unforced maneuver). However, in severe emphysema with loss of elastic support, FVC may fall disproportionately more than SVC.
- PEFR (or PEF): *peak expiratory flow rate* (liters per minute). This is a simple measure of maximal expiratory flow rate.
- TL_{CO}: *transfer factor* (mmol/min). This is a measure of the ability of the lung to oxygenate hemoglobin. It is usually measured with a single-breath technique using carbon monoxide.
- K_{CO}: *transfer coefficient* (mmol/min/k/Pa/L_{BTPS}). This is essentially TL_{CO} corrected for lung volume.

In addition to the above, blood gas measurements are frequently performed in the investigation of patients with respiratory problems. Their purpose is to assess acid–base balance and oxygenation. The most important measures are therefore partial pressure of oxygen (Po_2), partial pressure of carbon monoxide (Pco_2), and pH.

An *acutely* rising Pco_2 (type 2 respiratory failure) will result in a fall in pH. This is most commonly seen in chronic obstructive pulmonary disease. A chronically high Pco_2 (also common in COPD) will be compensated for by renally mediated mechanisms and will thus be associated with a normal or near-normal pH. Hyperventilation (as in panic attacks, pulmonary embolism, Cheyne–Stokes respiration) will sometimes produce a high pH (alkalosis) due to "blowing off" of CO_2.

There are essentially two characteristic "patterns" of abnormal respiratory function. The *obstructive pattern* is most commonly found in asthma and chronic obstructive pulmonary disease and is characterized by the following:

- reduced FEV_1 and PEF;
- reduced FVC, though proportionately less so than FEV_1;
- reduced FEV_1/FVC ratio (normal approximately 70 percent);
- Po_2 usually normal in asthma (apart from severe exacerbation) but may be low in moderate to severe COPD (either chronically or more commonly during acute exacerbations);
- Pco_2 may be raised in chronic severe COPD or in acute exacerbations of COPD;
- pH may be low during acute exacerbations of COPD (respiratory acidosis).

Pco_2 is usually normal in asthma, though it often *falls* during acute episodes. A rising Pco_2 (due to patient exhaustion) in acute asthma (or a falling pH) is an adverse prognostic sign suggesting the need for assisted ventilation.

The *restrictive pattern* of abnormal respiratory function, as for example in interstitial fibrotic lung disease, is characterized by the following:

- reduced FVC;
- similarly reduced FEV_1;
- normal or sometimes high FEV_1/FVC ratio;
- reduced TL_{CO} and K_{CO};
- reduced Po_2;
- normal or low Pco_2 (secondary to hyperventilation);
- normal or high pH.

AGE-RELATED CHANGES IN THE RESPIRATORY SYSTEM

Basic issues

This section provides a summary of the relatively sparse data available on age-related changes in the respiratory system. It is theoretically important to distinguish between changes *due to* aging itself and those merely *associated with* old age—in other words, to distinguish between "aging" changes and "age-related" changes.

Age-related changes in structure and in function (excluding those in respiratory control and monitoring) may have an enormous number of potential causes. In Western populations the effects of disease far outweigh any effects due to aging itself. In particular, the effects of smoking (probably including passive smoking[1,2]) are of most importance. Much interest is currently focused upon reactive oxidants in the lung both in terms of smoking-related pathology and aging changes.[3] Reactive oxidants reduce the capacity of amino acid proteinase inhibitor (α-1-proteinase inhibitor) to prevent elastase damaging collagen elastin fibers. Smoking is thought to increase levels of reactive oxidants in the lung.[4] A variety of inconclusive studies have suggested a relationship between antioxidant status and preservation of respiratory function with aging. However, high antioxidant levels or a high antioxidant diet may be merely an epiphenomenon (possibly a socially related marker). This area has been reviewed fairly recently.[5]

Other theories of decline of respiratory function with age include previous respiratory infection (particularly in childhood), general nutritional status, environmental pollution, and increased bronchial responsiveness to irritants. It is difficult to distinguish here between "disease effects" and aging effects, and such mechanisms are discussed in more detail in Chapter 42.

There is, similarly, debate about the possibility that asthma in particular is an age-related disease. Age-related abnormalities in β_2-adrenoceptor status are recognized in a variety of bodily systems, including the lung, and are similar to those seen in young asthmatics. This is also discussed in more detail in Chapter 42, as is the possibility that atopic status may have implications for respiratory function even in the absence of clinically apparent atopic disease in the elderly population.

There is an absence of longitudinal studies (following patients into old age) in this area. Our information on the differences in the respiratory system of elderly and young people comes therefore from cross-sectional studies (comparing a group of young people to a group of elderly people). Because no other internal organ is so intimately exposed to external environmental influences as the lung, it is difficult even in the absence of disease to differentiate clearly between physical and physiological changes of aging itself and those brought about by a lifetime sum of diverse inspired "environmental" insults. These changes comprise physical (structural) changes and physiological (functional) changes, in the lung, in ventilatory control, and in oxygen exchange and uptake.

Age-related structural changes

The most important age-related change in the large airways is a reduction in the number of glandular epithelial cells. This results in reduced production of protective mucus and thus impaired defense against respiratory infection. There are few changes in the bronchi, but the area of the alveoli falls and the alveoli and alveoli ducts enlarge. Function residual capacity, residual volume, and compliance increase. There is deposition of amyloid in lung vasculature and alveolar septa, although the significance of this is unclear.

Small airways suffer qualitative[6] and quantitative changes in the supportive elastin and collagen, with coiling and rupture of fibers and consequent dilatation of alveolar ducts and airspaces (so-called "senile emphysema"),[7] and an increased tendency for small airways to collapse during expiration (see below). These changes may be exacerbated by reduced mobility (often consequent upon acute illness) with reduction in deep breaths, hypoventilation of dependent zones, failure to clear dependent sputum, and thus further risk of lower respiratory infection. There is up to a 20 percent reduction in alveolar surface area with consequent reduction in respiratory reserve, although this is of little or no significance in the healthy elderly.

The respiratory muscles comprise the diaphragm (responsible for perhaps 85 percent of respiratory muscle activity), the intercostals, the anterior abdominal muscles, and the accessory muscles of the neck, back, and upper chest. The accessory muscles can mainly only be brought into action by splinting of the arms (trapezius is an exception to this). In normal breathing, expansion of the chest (inspiration) is brought about by the action of these muscles whereas expiration is a passive phenomenon. Under increased demands the accessory muscles are brought into play for inspiration, and expiration becomes at least partially active. All respiratory muscles are made up of type I (slow), type IIA (fast-fatigue resistant) and type IIB (fast-fatiguable) fibers. This differentiation is based upon ATP activity in the myofibrils, and confers differing physiological properties.

The major age-related change in the respiratory muscles is a reduction in the proportion of type IIA fibers with consequent impairment of strength and (more importantly) endurance.[8] Reduced muscle strength has been suggested as an independent predictor of mortality (at least in women).[9]

In addition to age-related changes in muscle strength and endurance, the situation is complicated by changes brought about by systemic and respiratory pathologies common in the elderly population. Overall "lack of fitness" (deconditioning) will exacerbate age-related changes detailed above. Clearly musculoskeletal disorders can affect all striated muscles, but other common although less immediately obvious pathologies (e.g. osteomalacia) may also cause significant impairment of strength and endurance. Medications (particularly corticosteroids) may cause problems particularly in respiratory muscle strength. Acute infection—including but not exclusively respiratory infection—is often associated with muscle weakness due to toxemia.

Ossification of costal cartilages,[10] loss of vertebral disk space, increased anteroposterior diameter, and calcification of rib articulatory surfaces combine with muscle changes to produce impaired mobility of the thoracic cage. These "normal" changes may be compounded by osteoporotic vertebral collapse (leading to kyphosis) and/or rib or even sternal fracture. Atraumatic sternal fracture is indeed a recognized cause of "atypical" chest pain in the frail elderly population.

Age-related functional changes

Lung volumes (both static and expiratory) fall gradually with age and are an independent predictor of mortality.[9] Until recent years there have been no large studies of elderly patients in this regard, so apparent falls in FEV_1 and FVC have been extrapolated from data on younger patients. However, it is clear that this has produced an underestimate in rate of decline in these indices with age as hard data are now available for elderly populations.[11] Earlier studies by Milne[12] and Milne and Williamson[13] had also suggested this and in addition had produced longitudinal rather than cross-sectional data in support of the above. The FEV_1/FVC ratio falls by approximately 0.2 percent per year from 70 percent at the age of 40–45 years.[14]

There are sex differences in these age-related functional changes. The FEV_1/FVC ratio declines less rapidly in older men than in older women.[15] Maximal expiratory flow and maximum voluntary ventilation decline less rapidly in women.[15]

Flow in the small airways also declines with age.[16] However, the most clinically important functional changes in the aging respiratory system are:

- an increased tendency for small airways to collapse sooner (at higher lung volumes) during expiration (increased "closing volume");
- reduction in respiratory muscle strength and endurance;
- changes in the monitoring and control of breathing.

Increased closing volume results from degeneration of the collagen and elastin support structure of small airways. In the normal elderly airway, closure in the dependent zones takes place during tidal breathing,[17] with consequent impaired ventilation of the dependent areas, ventilation–perfusion mismatch, and reduced resting arterial oxygen tension.[18] Conversely, because of the sigmoid shape of the oxygen dissociation curve, percentage oxygen saturation is not significantly affected by normal aging at least until oxygen tension falls below 8 kPa (60 mmHg). Although small-airways closure and ventilation mismatch is the *main* reason for the fall in oxygen tension, minor structural alveolar changes also contribute to impaired gas transfer.

At least partially because of the rise in pulmonary artery pressure, blood flow in the healthy elderly lung is increased towards the apices.[19] This further enhances the tendency to mismatch, in that ventilation follows the pattern seen in young adults (i.e. greater ventilation at the bases than the apices).

Respiratory muscle strength and endurance fall, in major part a consequence of type IIA fiber atrophy. Such changes may again be of little or no functional significance in the healthy elderly person, but they lead to impaired reserve to combat respiratory challenges consequent upon acute respiratory disease. Although there is a wide range of normal, maximal, inspiratory mouth pressure (an indirect measure of inspiratory muscle strength), this falls by up to 35 percent in men from age 20 years to age 75 years.[20]

Interestingly, although the mechanisms underlying such changes are likely to be multiple and varied, and are to some extent unclear, the adoption of a sedentary "Western" lifestyle in Inuit communities has been shown to be associated with an acceleration in age-related lung function decline.[21]

A variety of age-related changes produce relative inefficiency in control monitoring and of ventilation. The much-quoted study of Kronenberg and Drage[22] suggested impaired ventilatory responses to both hypoxia and hypercapnia at rest in old age. More recent Anglo-Canadian work[23,24] has challenged some of the data by showing a normal response to resting eucapnic hypoxia, but an impaired response to hypoxia during sustained hypercapnia. Elderly people do show an *increased* ventilatory response to exercise-induced carbon-dioxide production,[25] an effect which may be more pronounced in males.[26] Conversely, episodes of sleep apnea are more common in the healthy elderly.[27,28] The significance of this latter observation is unclear. There has been a suggestion that

stroke disease may further interfere with respiratory control, producing posture-dependent hypoxia,[29] but this has not been confirmed by a recent study in the present author's own department.[30]

Elderly people are less able to objectively perceive acute bronchoconstriction;[31] indeed such perception falls progressively throughout adulthood. This may be due in part to the altered sensitivity of chemoreceptors to hypoxia as discussed above. Other possible mechanisms include the reduced ability to perceive elastic or resistive loads on inspiration or expiration,[33,34] impaired perception of tactile sensation and joint movement,[35–37] or age-associated abnormalities in central processing.[38–40] Such impaired perception of bronchoconstriction, whatever its cause, may have important clinical implications in terms of the awareness of respiratory symptoms, self-referral, and access to medical care and mortality from acute respiratory problems.[31,41,42]

Mucociliary clearance is reduced in old age.[43,44] However, what limited evidence is available suggests that the cough reflex is unaffected by the aging process.[45]

Maximal oxygen uptake ($\dot{V}O_{2max}$) declines with age (with a consequent decline in "reserve" and in exercise capacity). Whilst this is partly the result of cardiovascular changes (fall in maximum tachycardic response and cardiac output[18]), a fall in diffusing capacity[18] and alveolar capillary volume together with ventilation–perfusion mismatch are also implicated. The decline in maximal oxygen uptake with age can be attenuated by regular aerobic exercise,[46] and indeed well-conditioned ("fit") older adults have $\dot{V}O_2$ kinetics very similar to "fit" young subjects.[47]

In addition to "aging" changes specific to the respiratory system, there are significant changes in host defense which predispose elderly people to more frequent and severe bacterial viral and fungal infection. Many of these changes (especially local changes) are not specific to aging but occur in consequence of the pathologies seen more commonly in older subjects.

Colonization of the upper respiratory tract (pharynx) by potential pathogens is not uncommon in the elderly population, particularly those in institutions.[48,49] In particular, colonization may occur with Gram-negative enterobacteria. Colonization of the stomach may in fact precede airway colonization. Stomach colonization itself is facilitated by achlorhydria which is itself commoner in old age and may be further precipitated by antacids or H_2-blockers.[50–52] Concern has also been expressed that overuse of amoxycillin (and similar agents) may predispose to Gram-negative colonization and infection in old age.[53] Swallowing disorders, especially in association with stroke and other neurological diseases, together with tracheal intubation or the presence of nasogastric tubes may facilitate aspiration of pathogens. The mucus layer itself may be altered by smoking or chronic lung disease and the respiratory epithelium breached by the effects of chronic lung disease.[54]

Aging is characterized by increasing immune deficiency. The degree of change in immune function varies dramatically between individuals, and a large part of so-called aging changes may be the results of chronic disease, poor nutrition, and a variety of other factors not specific to aging itself. Defects occur in both cell-mediated immunity and humoral immunity, the latter probably secondary to T-cell dysfunction. Defects in humoral immunity predispose to bacterial infections and may partly explain the increased frequency of pneumonias, particularly pneumococcal pneumonia, in the elderly population. Humoral changes include both a reduction in the peak antibody response to immunization and a reduction in the duration of antibody response following immunization. These defects may in part explain why beneficial effects of pneumococcal and influenza immunization have historically been more difficult to prove in elderly populations.

Cell-mediated changes include reduction in the number of active peripheral T-cells with a corresponding increase in the proportion of circulating immature T-cells; a reduced thymic mass; a reduced T-cell response to interleukins; a reduced T-cell response to mitogens; and a reduction in the generation of cytotoxic T-cells.[5]

CONCLUSION

Data on aging or age-related changes in respiratory structure and function are surprisingly limited. The most clinically important changes so far recognized are functional rather than structural changes, the majority of the latter serving only to reduce the vast reserve capacity present in the young mature respiratory system. Further research work should therefore probably concentrate on functional changes, changes in control and monitoring of respiratory function and in the effects of depression of immune response (both local and systemic) on the predisposition to respiratory infection and neoplasia.

KEY POINTS Age-related changes in the respiratory system

- "Age-related" changes in the respiratory system (associated with diseases common in the elderly) have far greater importance than true aging changes.

- Most of the available information comes from cross-sectional studies rather than longitudinal studies, and is therefore potentially flawed.

- The most important structural change is reduction in the proportion of Type IIa fibres in respiratory muscles, leading to loss of endurance. The changes may assume functional importance in acute illness as they lead to impaired reserve.

- Fall in maximal oxygen uptake and a reduction in the subjective perception of bronchoconstriction are probably the most clinically important functional changes associated with aging.

REFERENCES

1. Sockrider M: The respiratory effects of passive tobacco smoking. Curr Opin Pulmon Med 1996;2(2):129–133
2. Law MR, Hackshaw AK: Environmental tobacco smoke. Br Med Bull 1996;52(1):22–34
3. Rahman I, MacNee W: Role of oxidants/antioxidants in smoking-induced lung diseases. Free Radic Biol Med 1996;21:669–681
4. Richards GA, Theron AJ, Van der Merwe CA et al: Spirometric abnormalities in young smokers correlate with increased chemiluminescence responses of activated blood phagocytes. Am Rev Respir Dis 1989;139:181–187
5. Smith HA, Grievink L, Taback C: Dietary influences on chronic obstructive lung disease and asthma: a review of the epidemiological evidence. Proc Nutr Soc 1999;58:309–319
6. Bellmont MJ, Portero M, Pamplona R et al: Evidence for the Maillard reaction in rat lung collagen and its relationship with solubility and age. Biochim Biophys Acta 1995;1272:53–60
7. Verbeken EK, Cauberghs M, Mertens I et al: The senile lung: comparison with normal and emphysematous lungs. 1: Structural aspects. Chest 1992;101:793–799
8. Brook MH, Kaiser KK: Muscle fiber-types: how many and what kind? Arch Neurol 1970;23:369–379
9. Schroll M, Avlund K, Davidsen M: Predictors of five-year functional ability in a longitudinal survey of men and women aged 75–80. The 1914-population of Glostrup, Denmark. Aging Milano 1997;2:143–152
10. Teale C, Romaniuk C, Mulley G: Calcification on chest radiographs: the association with age. Age Ageing 1989;18:333–336
11. Enright PL, Kraonma RA, Higgins M, Schenker M, Haponik EF: Spirometry reference values for men and women aged 65 to 85 years of age: cardiovascular health study. Am Rev Respir Dis 1993;147:125–133
12. Milne JS: Longitudinal respiratory studies in older people. Thorax 1978;33:547–554
13. Milne JS, Williamson J: Respiratory function tests in older people. Clin Sci 1972;42:371–381
14. Tager IB, Segal MR, Speizer FE, Weiss ST: The natural history of forced expiratory volumes: effect of cigarette smoking and respiratory symptoms. Am Rev Respir Dis 1988;138:837–849
15. Young RC, Borden DL, Rachel RE: Aging of the lung: pulmonary disease in the elderly. Age 1987;10:138–145
16. Knudson RJ, Slatin RC, Leibowitz MD, Burrows B: The maximal expiratory flow-volume curve, normal standards, variability and effects of age. Am Rev Respir Dis 1976;113:587–560
17. Anthoniesen NR, Danson J, Roberton PC et al: Airway closure as a function of age. Respir Physiol 1970;8:58–65
18. Young RC, Borden DL, Rachel RE: Aging of the lung: pulmonary disease in the elderly. Age 1987;10:138–145
19. Kronenberg RS, L'Heureux P, Ponto RA et al: The affect of ageing on lung perfusion. Ann Intern Med 1972;76:413–421
20. Dow L, Carroll M: The ageing lung: structural and functional aspects. In Connolly MJ (ed): Respiratory Disease in the Elderly Patient. London: Chapman & Hall, 1996:2–17
21. Rode A, Shepherd RJ: The ageing of lung function: cross-sectional and longitudinal studies of an Inuit community. Eur Respir J 1994;9:1653–1659
22. Kronenberg RS, Drage CW: Attenuation of the ventilatory and heart responses to hypoxia and hypercapnia with ageing in normal men. J Clin Invest 1973;52:1812–1819
23. Smith WDF, Cunningham DA, Paterson DH, Poulin MJ: Ventilatory responses to sustained isocapnic hypoxia in the eighth decade. Age Ageing 1995;24 (Suppl 2):P12
24. Poulin MJ, Cunningham DA, Paterson DH, Kowalchuk MJ, Smith WDF: Ventilatory sensitivity to CO_2 in hyperoxia and hypoxia in older aged humans. J Appl Physiol 1993;75:2209–2216
25. Brischetto MJ, Millman RP, Peterson DD et al: Effect of ageing on ventilatory response to exercise and CO_2. J Appl Physiol 1984;56:1143–1150
26. Poulin MJ, Cunningham DA, Paterson DH, Rechnitzer PA, Ecclestone NA, Koral JA: Ventilatory responses to exercise in men and women 55 to 86 years of age. Am J Resp Crit Care Med 1994;149(2 Pt 1):408–415
27. Hayward L, Mant A, Eyland A et al: Sleep disordered breathing and cognitive function in a retirement village population. Age Ageing 1992;21:121–128
28. Flamer HE: Sleep problems. Med J Aust 1995;162:603–607
29. Elizabeth J, Singarayar EJ, Bearer D, Lye M: Arterial oxygen saturation and posture in acute stroke. Age Ageing 1993;22:269–272
30. Chatterton HJ, Pomeroy VM, Connolly MJ et al: The effect of body position on arterial oxygen saturation in acute stroke. J Gerontol A 2000;55:M239–M244
31. Connolly MJ, Charan NB, Nielson CP, Vestal RE: Reduced subjective awareness of bronchoconstriction provoked by methacholine in elderly asthmatic and normal subjects as measured on a simple awareness scale. Thorax 1992;47:410–413

32. Marks GB, Yates DH, Sist M et al: Respiratory sensation during bronchial challenge testing with methacholine, sodium metabisulphite, and adenosine monophosphate. Thorax 1996;51:793–798

33. Rack M, Altose MD, Cherniack NS: Effects of ageing on respiratory sensations produced by elastic loads. J Appl Physiol 1981;50:844–850

34. Tack M, Altose MD, Cherniack NS: Effects of aging on the perception of resistive ventilatory loads. Am Rev Respir Dis 1982;126:463–467

35. Dyck PJ, Schultz PW, O'Brien PC: Quantitation of touch pressure sensation. Arch Neurol Chicago 1972;26:465–473

36. Kormen E, Bossemeyer RW, Williams WJ: Quantitative evaluation of joint motion in an ageing population. J Gerontol 1978;33:62–67

37. Levin HS, Benton AL: Age effects in proprioceptive feedback performance. Gerontol Clin 1973;15:161–169

38. Walsh DA: Age differences in central perceptual processing: a dichoptic backward masking investigation. J Gerontol 1976;31:178–185

39. Walsh DA, Williams MV, Hertzog CK: Age-related differences in two stages of central perceptual processes: the effects of short duration targets and criterion differences. J Gerontol 1979;34:234–241

40. Till RE, Franklin LD: On the locus of age differences in visual information processing. J Gerontol 1981;36:200–210

41. British Thoracic Society and others: The British Guidelines on Asthma Management—1995 review and position statement. Thorax 1997;52 (Suppl 1):S1–S21

42. The COPD Guidelines Group of the Standards of Care Committee of the British Thoracic Society: BTS guidelines for the management of chronic obstructive pulmonary disease. Thorax 1997;52 (Suppl 5):S1–S28

43. Goodman RM, Yergin BM, Landa JF, Golin Vaux MH, Sackner MA: Relationship of smoking history and pulmonary function tests to tracheal mucous velocity in non-smokers, young smokers, ex-smokers and patients with chronic bronchitis. Am Rev Respir Dis 1978;117:205–214

44. Joki S, Saano V: Influence of ageing on ciliary beat frequency and on ciliary response to leukotriene D4 in guinea-pig tracheal epithelium. Clin Exp Pharmacol Physiol 1997;24:166–169

45. Katsumata U, Tagasugi R, Kotaku K et al: Cough reflex does not decline with age. Am Rev Respir Dis 1991;143:A535

46. Bortz WM: Disuse and aging. JAMA 1982;248:1203–1208

47. Chilbeck PD, Paterson DH, Petrella RJ, Cunningham DA: The influence of age and cardiorespiratory fitness on kinetics of oxygen uptake. Can J Appl Physiol 1996;21:185–196

48. Valenti WM, Trudell RG, Bentley DW.: Factors predisposing to oropharyngeal colonisation with Gram-negative bacilli in the aged. N Engl J Med 1978;298:1108–1111

49. Crossley KB, Thurn JR: Nursing home-acquired pneumonia. Semin Respir Infect 1989;4:64–72

50. Du Moulin GC, Paterson DG, Hedley-Whyte J, Lisbon A: Aspiration of gastric bacteria in antacid-treated patients: a frequent cause of post-operative colonisation of the airway. Lancet 1982;1:242–245

51. Heyland D, Mandell LA: Gastric colonisation by Gram-negative bacilli and nosocomial pneumonia in the intensive care unit patient. Chest 1992;101:187–193

52. Inglis TJJ, Sherratt MJ, Sproat LJ et al: Gastroduodenal dysfunction and bacterial colonisation of the ventilated lung. Lancet 1993;341:911–913

53. Alzeer A, Mashlah A, Fakim N et al: Tuberculosis is the commonest cause of pneumonia requiring hospitalization during Hajj (pilgrimage to Makkah). J Infect 1998;36:303–306

54. Goodman RM, Yergin BM, Landa JF: Relationship of smoking history and pulmonary function tests to tracheal mucus velocity in non-smokers, young smokers, ex-smokers and patients with chronic bronchitis. Am Rev Respir Dis 1978;117:205–214

55. Schwalo R, Walters CA, Weksler ME: Host defense mechanisms and ageing. Semin Oncol 1989;16:20–27

Chapter 42

Asthma and chronic obstructive pulmonary disease

Martin J. Connolly

Respiratory diseases result in great morbidity and potentially avoidable mortality in elderly people. The burden of many respiratory diseases (asthma, COPD, pulmonary tuberculosis) is increasing in this age group. Elderly people themselves seem to regard respiratory conditions as second only to musculoskeletal disorders as a cause of severe disability; general practitioners can expect 700 respiratory consultations per year from every 1000 elderly patients on their list; and at least 8 percent of all hospital admissions among the elderly in England are attributable to respiratory conditions.[1-3]

In addition to the burden of respiratory problems in this age group, the likelihood of atypical and nonspecific presentation of respiratory problems is becoming increasingly recognized. The sensitivity and specificity of physical signs may be diminished. There is an age-related reduction in cardiovascular response to hypoxia, together with an age-related impairment of the subjective appreciation of bronchoconstriction and probably breathlessness in general.

The recognition of such differences has been relatively recent and has both occurred because of, and in turn stimulated interest and research into, the specific respiratory problems of elderly patients. Within the confines of the present work a comprehensive review is impossible, and reference will be made to both original research and recent more extensive reviews.

PATTERNS OF PHYSICAL SIGNS

Despite the fact that respiratory diseases in the elderly population may present nonspecifically in terms of both symptoms and physical signs, there remain classical features of the history and more particularly of examination which can be grouped into "patterns" suggestive of specific diagnoses or of more general diagnostic areas. Though elusive to define exactly, medical "experience" is in no small part based on pattern recognition, and so there follows a brief summary of patterns of examination features pointing towards asthma and/or chronic obstructive pulmonary disease (COPD).

The following refers to chronic obstruction, although many will also apply to acute obstruction (acute asthma or acute exacerbation of smoking-related airways obstruction):

- audible wheeze;
- use of accessory muscles (often with arms fixed on the hips, chair, or bed);
- high shoulders;
- increased anteroposterior diameter of chest;
- prolonged expiration time;
- inward movement of the costal margin;
- absent (or lowered) liver dullness;
- rhonchi and impaired air entry (in severe obstruction air entry may be so poor that rhonchi are absent).

"Patterns" similarly suggestive of other respiratory conditions are given in Chapter 43.

ASTHMA

Epidemiology of asthma

The true prevalence of asthma in elderly people is complicated by problems with diagnostic labeling. Epidemiological studies suggest a prevalence of between 6.5 and 17 percent.[4-9] Despite the fact that most subjects revealed in these studies to have asthma are symptomatic, the prevalence rate of *diagnosed* asthma in clinical practice falls after the age of 65 years, suggesting underdiagnosis and undertreatment.[8,10] This probably relates to a combination of reduced mobility (less exertion-related dyspnea), reduced expectation on the part of patient and physician, impaired subjective awareness of acute bronchoconstriction,[11] and the poor predictive value of "typical" respiratory symptoms in old age.[12,13] Whether screening tests in primary care (possibly as part of the "over-75 check" in the UK) or elsewhere is justified has not been studied.

Pathogenesis of asthma

Most elderly asthmatics have developed the disease as adults, not in childhood[5,14] (i.e. they have "late onset" asthma), although a history of childhood asthma is a significant predictor of late-onset disease.[15] In contrast to those with juvenile-onset asthma, those with late-onset disease are rarely atopic. The pathogenesis of such "intrinsic" disease is hotly debated. Absence of clinical atopy does not imply absence of the airway inflammation which is pathognomonic of asthma at all ages. The pathology underlying asthma in elderly patients is only recently becoming the subject of scrutiny, but intrinsic asthma in younger patients displays similar patterns of cellular immune response and eosinophil activation to those in atopic asthma.[16,17]

The search for the trigger for inflammation has produced several theories of pathogenesis which are not necessarily mutually exclusive. There is debate in the medical[18-23] and lay press about the relevance of atmospheric pollution in asthma *pathogenesis* (as opposed to exacerbating asthma in those with the condition). This debate is no less relevant to the elderly population, especially in view of their greater lifelong exposure to a greater variety of atmospheric pollutants. Agents hypothesized in this regard include smoke particulates (indoors from heating systems and outdoors from diesel engines), oxides of sulfur, nitrogen, and low-level ozone, and even "new" crops such as oilseed rape and soyabean. Most publicity has centered on outdoor pollution, with emphasis on the internal combustion engine; however, recent evidence suggests that nitrogen dioxide (from gas cookers) may reach significant levels indoors[24] and is associated with asthmatic symptoms and with other respiratory symptoms in children,[25,26] and even with IgE levels in infants.[27] A British epidemiological study has indicated that women (not men) who use a gas stove or have an open gas fire have significant impairment of lung function compared to women who do not,[28] and others have cited animal models linking nitrogen dioxide exposure with susceptibility to viral infection.[29] Elderly people have, by virtue of relative poverty, tended to live (historically) in well-ventilated ("draughty") homes. The otherwise laudable trends to home insulation and draught exclusion may have unwittingly increased indoor pollution levels, but the persistent relative poverty of elderly people may mean they are likely to use older, less well maintained cooking and heating appliances which might maximize any effect of nitrogen dioxide pollution.

Secondly, despite lack of obvious clinical atopic disease (including atopic-related exacerbations and elevated serum IgE levels), an atopic etiology cannot be dismissed. IgE levels are recognized to fall with age,[30] but remain a predictor of lung function in elderly populations independent of the presence or absence of asthma.[31] Although the possibility of a relationship between IgE levels and bronchial responsiveness (airway irritability, high levels of which characterize asthma) is not as clear in studies of older subjects as it is in the young, such a relationship may indeed exist.[15,30,32] There may also be interaction between cigarette consumption (and possibly environmental pollutants) and elevated IgE and serum eosinophil levels, in the pathogenesis of airways obstruction in old age.[31,33–35] This is consistent with the hypothesis of an overlap between chronic obstructive pulmonary disease and asthma in old age as mirrored in the experience of practising clinicians.

Possible imbalance between β-adrenergic, cholinergic, and α-adrenergic receptor pathways has also been suggested as possible causes. Most work in this area has concentrated on β-adrenergic receptors with evidence of exaggeration of the "normal" age-related changes in β-adrenoceptor activity being seen in elderly late-onset asthmatics,[36,37] and being directly associated not only with imbalance in autonomic regulation of airway smooth muscle[37] but also with the increased leucocyte activation necessary for airway inflammation.[28] Downregulation of glucocorticoid receptors in the elderly[39] may also be implicated as the β-adrenoceptor adenylyl cyclase pathway is modulated by corticosteroid activity.[40–43]

Genetic studies for atopy, bronchial hyperresponsiveness, and asthma in younger subjects have identified potential linkage markers on chromosomes 4, 6, 7, 11, 13, and 14, with particular interest centering on chromosome 6 (certain HLA genotypes and relations to IgE response, tumor necrosis factor), chromosome 5 (β-adrenoceptor, interleukin-4), chromosome 11 (FcεRI-beta) and chromosome 14 (high-affinity IgE receptor TCRα).[43–47] Particularly in the light of clinical observations on the linkage between even late-onset asthma and atopy, it is perhaps reasonable to suggest that late-onset asthma (and even

possibly reversible airways disease in general) in older individuals represents a delayed expression of the same phenotype as in younger asthmatics. Studies are currently in progress in this area, with preliminary results suggesting that this hypothesis may indeed be valid.[49]

Presentation of asthma

The classical presenting symptoms of asthma seen in young patients (intermittent cough, breathlessness, wheezing, tight-chestedness, often in association with viral infection, nonspecific respirable irritants, and exercise and emotion) are also seen in elderly asthmatics.[50–54] However, as well as the problems of diagnostic confusion (specificity) with other conditions common in this age group (e.g. COPD, cardiac failure, angina) and some rare ones (e.g. myasthenia gravis[55]), the sensitivity of symptoms is reduced in the elderly population. Perception of bronchoconstriction by asthmatics falls gradually throughout adulthood,[56] and acute bronchoconstriction is poorly perceived by elderly people whether asthmatic or not.[11] The same is true of other symptoms characteristic of asthma[53] and in particular the predictive value of the so-called "bronchial irritability syndrome" (wheeze, cough, and chest tightness on exposure to respirable irritants such as cold air and traffic fumes) is much less in the elderly than in the young.[12] Furthermore the intrinsic nature of asthma in old people together with reduced tendency to diurnal variation, "reversed" seasonal variation (elderly asthmatics tend to be worse in the winter), and the chronic nature of the condition (i.e. even with maximal treatment bronchoconstriction is rarely completely reversible) result in considerable diagnostic confusion with smoking-related COPD. Even the presence of right-sided cardiac failure (cor pulmonale), usually taken as evidence of COPD rather than asthma, does not exclude a diagnosis of the latter.[57] As discussed above, such apparent clinical "confusion" may in fact be explained by at least a moderate degree of continuity in etiology. As both COPD and asthma are common, they are not mutually exclusive,[54] but misdiagnosis and bias because of differences in age, sex, and social class is well recognized. Elderly men[58] and those of lower social class[59] seem more likely to receive a diagnosis of emphysema or COPD than one of asthma, irrespective of clinical features. There has recently been an interest in the literature in differentiation of asthma from COPD by the use of clinical algorithms, simple investigation, challenge testing, and examination of induced sputum, bronchoalveolar lavage (BAL), high resolution CT scanning, and transfer factor measurement.[60–63] However, although these may be of assistance in individual cases they are not widely applied in clinical practice.

Any misdiagnosis of asthma as COPD probably adversely influences treatment, as patients in general practice with a "label" of asthma are much more likely to receive inhaled bronchodilators than those with a "label" of COPD.[65] A survey in Northern Ireland recently revealed that over a quarter of all deaths in the 56–75 year age group registered as being due to COPD were in fact probably the result of asthma.[66] The same survey confirmed frequent misdiagnosis of sudden death from asthma being recorded as myocardial infarction or cardiac failure.

However, in contrast to a strong relationship between general-practice prescribing and hospital admission in young adults with asthma, there is some evidence that lack of appropriate GP prescribing in elderly patients with asthma does not increase the risk of hospital admission, although this in itself may reflect lack of diagnostic accuracy in elderly people.[67] Despite this, the hospital admission rate for asthma in old age is similar to that for asthma in young children.[68]

Management of asthma

The first step is clearly an accurate diagnosis and assessment of severity. Spirometry with reversibility assessment to inhaled or nebulized bronchodilators is essential. Although the reversibility detected may be less than in the young, it is usually in excess of 20 percent. For those without significant immediate reversibility, a course of inhaled or oral corticosteroid (for 6 weeks or 2 weeks, respectively) followed by repeat reversibility assessment may be helpful. It is possible that diurnal peak flow monitoring with reversibility assessment (at least four times daily[69]) may be useful; but as well as potential problems of unsupervised inhaler technique, the meters may prove difficult to read for elderly people with poor vision. Even if the figures on the meters themselves are readable, those on the peak flow graphs usually supplied with mini peak flow meters can be very difficult even for younger people to read and understand. It is a recommendation of this author that low-reading peak flow meters (peak flow ranging between 30 and 350 liters per minute) should be used as the scale is both appropriate and easier for elderly people to read. Patients should not be expected to chart a graph but should merely be asked to record their peak flow in simple tabular form.

A diurnal variability in peak flow of 15 percent or more suggests asthma, but (particularly in old age) lack of such variability does not exclude it. Measurement of peak flow less than four times daily significantly reduces the likelihood of detecting variability,[69] although the greatest variability is seen between measurements taken in the early morning and late afternoon.[70]

Assessment of bronchial responsiveness to methacholine may be helpful in a few cases (especially those in whom pulmonary function is normal or equivocal); but in addition to the lack of an accepted normal range of responsiveness in the elderly population, the test is not generally available and will probably remain chiefly a research tool. Chest radiography and electrocardiography should be performed to exclude pulmonary edema and help exclude ischemic heart disease. Allergy testing is usually unhelpful and rarely necessary, except (again) in a research setting.

MANAGEMENT OF THE CHRONIC CONDITION Guidelines[71] on asthma management have been published by the British Thoracic Society (BTS) and are widely accepted in the UK. They suggest stepwise increments in treatment depending on severity of the condition as judged chiefly (though not exclusively) by patient-reported symptoms. The principles of these guidelines are just as applicable to elderly asthmatics, but there are arguable differences in application. The first step in the BTS guidelines is "on demand" use of regular bronchodilators. This is probably inappropriate for elderly patients who are less able to appreciate acute bronchoconstriction,[11] and the prophylactic use of regular low-dose inhaled corticosteroids should be considered as a first step. Whether one should also give *prescribed* (as opposed to "on demand") regular inhaled bronchodilators is unclear (there is no available research to guide the decision). The possibility and likely clinical significance of downregulation (tachyphylaxis) of airway β-adrenoceptors due to regular use of inhaled β-agonists is discussed below under COPD.

The subsequent incremental steps—higher dose inhaled steroids (step 3), followed by additional regular β-agonists (step 4), followed finally by oral corticosteroids (step 5)—are appropriate. However, a recommended alternative to high-dose inhaled steroids for step 3 is low-dose inhaled steroids plus long-acting β-agonist bronchodilator. The latter may also be introduced in step 4, as may inhaled muscarinic antagonists (ipratropium or oxitropium). The evidence base for the use of long-acting bronchodilators before muscarinic antagonists in the elderly population is questionable. Age-related dysfunction in β-adrenoceptor-mediated responsiveness is recognized in respiratory, cardiac, and vasoregulatory systems.[36,72] Furthermore, there is known to be impaired bronchodilator response to salbutamol in elderly normals.[37] Ullah et al.[73] have shown similar impairment of response to salbutamol in older asthmatics. Also, although response to a muscarinic antagonist (ipratropium) was inversely related to age, reduction in ipratropium responsiveness was relatively less than that in salbutamol responsiveness, such that in older subjects ipratropium response was greater than that to salbutamol. Further studies in this area are in progress.

Leukotriene receptor antagonists have been shown to improve lung function and reduce inflammatory markers in chronic asthma. Studies have been invariably performed on younger subjects and none of the leukotriene antagonists has been specifically studied in elderly asthmatics. Thus their use in the management of asthma in elderly people has as yet no evidence base, although once again research is in progress in this area.

Emphasis should be placed on *objective* outcome measures (e.g. home peak flow measures) over subjective complaints (or more likely lack of these) in order to guide transitions between steps in management. Only a very small minority of elderly asthmatics should require regular oral corticosteroid steroid therapy for adequate control.

Asthmatic patients with psychotic illness have greater risk of asthma death.[74] This presumably relates to poor personal control of the condition among patients with psychiatric problems. It is likely that similar difficulties in control will be found in the chronically confused or those acutely confused for reasons other than their asthma, although surprisingly this seems to have been little studied. There is, however, evidence that the demented may *perceive* bronchoconstriction less well.[75] These factors may go part of the way to explaining the increased differential mortality from asthma in elderly people. Particular care must be taken over the chronic management of the condition in the elderly psychotic or chronically confused.

Inhaler management must be simplified as much as possible. This involves not just choosing the correct inhaler device for optimum technique (see below) but simplifying the inhaler *regimen*. Longer-acting inhaled β-agonists (salmeterol and eformoterol) may be administered twice instead of four times daily. They have been shown to be effective and safe in elderly patients.[76,77] Although twice the dose of inhaled steroid given once daily may not provide as tight control as the normal dose administered on a twice-daily basis, it can provide reasonable control in the more stable patients,[78] and may on occasion make home management with once-daily family support more feasible for the mildly demented elderly asthmatic.

There has been enormous amount of debate regarding inhaler technique in old people. The standard metered-dose inhaler (MDI) is probably obsolescent when used in isolation for elderly patients. Patients with reduced handgrip strength find difficulty coordinating inhalation and triggering of the device, and even the mildly confused elderly find MDI technique difficult to learn and retain.[79] The addition of a large-volume spacer device (Volumatic: Allen and Hanbury's Ltd; or Nebuhaler: Astra Pharmaceuticals Ltd) involves a technique which removes the problem of coordination, is easier for patients to learn and retain, and is preferred by elderly patients.[80] In addition, such devices ameliorate the problem of systemic absorption of significant quantities of inhaled corticosteroid when using high doses of such drugs.[81] Furthermore, large-volume spacers can be triggered by carers or relatives if the patients themselves find them difficult to use. Any consequent delay between triggering and inhalation in such circumstances is unlikely to have a major effect on deposition of the drug in the airways.[82]

A large number of breath-actuated devices are available. There is limited literature on inhaler technique with these devices, but the Turbohaler and the Autohaler seem relatively successful in the elderly, whereas the Rotahaler and the Diskhaler seem more difficult for the elderly to use.[83–86] Whichever inhaler is employed, it is important that where possible different drugs are given through the same type of device and that the patient has frequent demonstration and reinstruction on techniques. More tuition and reinstruction together with *inpatient* first prescription of inhalers and consequent opportunity for nurse-led reinforcement both improve inhaler technique in elderly people.[79,86,87] Allen[88] has demonstrated in a series of studies the type of inhaler device (categorized by number of "stages" needed to activate and inhale the device adequately) that patients with dementia are able to use adequately. Those patients with an abbreviated mental test score of 4 or less are unable to use any device, but the easiest device for the moderately demented seems to be a three-stage (inspiration triggered) inhaler.

ASSESSMENT AND MANAGEMENT OF THE ACUTE CONDITION Mortality rates for asthma are much higher in old age.[89] Most asthma mortality occurs during acute exacerbations and is frequently due to potentially avoidable factors.[90] Though asthma itself does not appear to increase overall mortality risk for the elderly,[91] most asthma deaths occur in elderly people.[92,93] There has, however, been speculation that some of this excess mortality from "asthma" in the elderly population may be due to inaccurate death certification.[94] Nonetheless, elderly asthmatics do underestimate the severity of acute bronchoconstriction[11] and take on average three times as long to get to hospital as their young counterparts during exacerbations.[95] Elderly people develop less tachycardia and pulsus paradoxus than the young with the same degree of bronchoconstriction,[95] and are thus more likely to be perceived by their medical attendants as having less severe exacerbations.

The BTS guidelines for the *management* of acute asthma[71] are generally applicable to the elderly asthmatic. However, in the light of the above, even more emphasis must be given to *objective* assessment rather than reliance on misleadingly "minor" symptoms and the "reassuring" absence of worrying physical signs. All patients should have peak flow estimated and compared with their predicted level or previous known best.[96] All those attending hospital should also have arterial blood gas estimations (preferably when breathing room air). Chest radiography should look for evidence of pneumothorax, pulmonary edema, and infections. Unsuspected abnormalities (often of immediate clinical significance) occur on the majority of chest radiographs in elderly acute asthmatics.[97]

Immediate treatment should include high-flow oxygen and nebulized β-agonists and ipratropium. Ipratropium should not be given in conjunction with β-agonists in those with diagnosed or suspected glaucoma. High doses of systemic corticosteroids (initially intravenously) are needed: 200 mg of hydrocortisone should be given followed by 30–40 mg of prednisolone daily.

Objective measurement of response should comprise regular peak flow monitoring (including response to nebulizers) and, if this is not clearly improving, repeat blood gas measurements. Blood gases should in any case be measured again at least once or if there is *any* suspicion of a clinical deterioration.

For those who do not respond to the above treatment, intravenous salbutamol and/or aminophylline should be considered. A rising $P\text{CO}_2$ (or even a normal $P\text{CO}_2$) may be an indication of impending patient exhaustion. Intermittent positive pressure ventilation (IPPV) via an endotracheal tube may be more often considered for the elderly asthmatic than for one with end-stage COPD. Advanced age is not a barrier to intensive care entry or to mechanical ventilation. The decision whether to ventilate an elderly patient is usually a difficult one and needs to be made in conjunction with the patient (if possible), relatives, the full multidisciplinary team, and the patient's own general practitioner if available. An enlightened discussion of this area is given in a review by Nielson.[98]

OTHER TREATMENT Respiratory infection may or may not be present in patients with severe asthma. If there is objective evidence of infection (raised white blood cell count, pyrexia, infiltration on the chest X-ray), then antibiotics should be chosen as discussed below for COPD. Many patients will need judicious intravenous rehydration.

CHRONIC OBSTRUCTIVE PULMONARY DISEASE (COPD)

Epidemiology of COPD

The British Thoracic Society (BTS) guidelines on COPD[99] define the condition as "a chronic slowly progressive disorder characterized by airways obstruction ... which does not change markedly over several months." COPD is almost always the result of cigarette smoking, and a smoking history of less than 10 pack-years (1 pack-year being 20 cigarettes per day for 1 year) strongly suggests the possibility of an alternative diagnosis (e.g. chronic asthma, bysinnosis). Following a long asymptomatic phase of decline in respiratory function, initial presentation of COPD usually occurs between the ages of 50 and 60 years. Epidemiological surveys reveal a high prevalence of COPD in elderly people, much of which is undetected clinically (probably for reasons similar to those discussed above for asthma) and thus untreated. Recent studies in the present author's institution suggest that nearly 30 percent of Caucasian inner-city community-dwellers over the age of 65 years have airways obstruction (COPD plus asthma), and that nearly two-thirds of these receive no treatment.[4] Other British, Canadian, European, and US epidemiological studies from less industrialized areas with lower rates of cigarette smoking report COPD prevalence of between 7 and 16 percent,[12,100–104] although a British survey of the more dependent elderly reported a prevalence (COPD plus asthma) of over 40 percent.[50]

COPD, for so long the disease of the Western world, no longer seems to be confined to developed populations. There is increasing and worrying evidence of the development of COPD in significant proportions of the populations of India and China, with one study in particular reporting a prevalence of nearly 3.5 percent among a population over the age of only 30 years in rural south India.[105,106]

Smoking rates appear to be falling, or at least leveling off, in Western men but are still increasing in women.[107] This is mirrored by a rise in the prevalence of COPD in women contrasted with a plateau in COPD prevalence in men in the UK.[108] The fall in smoking prevalence has been smaller in the less well educated, in ethnic minorities, and in those from poorer socioeconomic groups.[109] The cohort of people making up today's elderly have had the highest uptake of cigarette smoking and thus should be expected to have a higher prevalence of COPD than younger cohorts.[4] Indeed it is likely that the healthcare burden caused by COPD (particularly in women) in the Western world will continue to rise in absolute terms paralleling or exceeding the rise in the elderly population.[111] There is some evidence that this latter is in fact the case, and certainly COPD is no less common in elderly people than in the middle-aged,[4] with some evidence that it may in fact be more common in old age.[104] Although it is less frequently diagnosed and treated,[4,10] COPD produces major morbidity, disability, and impairment of quality of life in old age.[112–114]

Presentation of COPD

COPD is characterized by a variable phase (usually several years) of minimal symptoms (perhaps except "smokers cough") or physical signs before the onset of wheeze and/or breathlessness. Most of those who subsequently develop COPD will qualify for the "label" of chronic bronchitis (the production of sputum each day for at least 3 months on 2 consecutive years), but often do not regard sputum production as abnormal. The essential abnormality of lung function in COPD is obstructive (a reduced FEV_1 and FEV_1/FVC ratio), and it is only when FEV_1 fall below 60 percent of predicted (or even lower in elderly people) that breathlessness and wheeze on exertion become troublesome. Other presenting symptoms include general malaise, fatigue (often neglected), cough and sputum production (as for chronic bronchitis), and possibly sleep disturbance. As the condition progresses (FEV_1 below 40 percent of predicted), breathlessness and wheeze worsen and hyperinflation of the chest, cyanosis, and signs of right heart strain appear (due to pulmonary vasoconstriction from chronic hypoxia)—right ventricular heave, raised jugular venous pressure, and peripheral edema. Secondary polycythemia affects some sufferers. Sleep disturbance and daytime somnolence becomes more common. Nocturnal hyperventilation and hypoxia may interfere with sleep pattern.[115–117] It is usually only in this latter phase (FEV_1 below 40 percent of predicted) that sufferers become known to the hospital, generally because of emergency admission with intermittent exacerbations (see below). Gradual weight loss is common secondary to a combination of increased energy demands of breathing and in the latter stages reduced intake because of breathlessness on eating.[118]

Prognosis is inversely related to age and to lung function (particularly to post-bronchodilator lung function).[119] Preliminary results from work in the author's department indicate that the prognosis may also be independently inversely related to level of disability. The significance of this finding remains unclear.

Management of COPD

SMOKING CESSATION This is the cornerstone of management at all levels of severity. The argument that this is not possible in elderly patients is specious. Cessation is as successful in the motivated elderly[120] and possibly even more so,[121] with one year "quit rates" of 10–15 percent. However, research studies looking at "quit rates" by necessity have examined a subgroup of elderly patients (the motivated) which may not be representative of elderly smokers in general, and there is strong anecdotal evidence that elderly smokers overall are less motivated to join smoking cessation groups. This phenomenon needs further study. Unfortunately, there is some recent evidence that doctors are less likely to give antismoking advice to patients over the age of 65.[123] Nicotine replacement for the highly motivated including elderly people[121,122] may improve one-year quit rate to about 20 percent. Sudden cessation is more effective than gradual reduction.[124] The benefits of smoking cessation upon rate of loss in lung function decline with age but probably remain valuable up to the age of 80 years (particularly in women).[125] A more detailed review of smoking cessation in old age can be found in a recent editorial.[126]

Lung function testing (FEV_1 and FVC) is essential for diagnosis. PEFR measurement can be misleadingly high in COPD.[99] Bronchodilator reversibility testing should be carried out in all patients (FEV_1 before and 30 minutes after 2.5–5 mg nebulized salbutamol and 0.5 mg nebulized ipratropium). Classically a 15 percent improvement in FEV_1 was until recently considered significant; however, this can be misleading when baseline FEV_1 is very low, and current recommendations are that a significant improvement in FEV_1 comprises a 15 percent increase *and* an absolute improvement of 200 mL.[99] Response to oral steroids (30 mg of prednisolone daily for 2 weeks) or inhaled steroids (for 6 weeks) should be examined by repeating reversibility testing at the end of the steroid course. *Objective* response indicates the need for regular *inhaled* steroid prescription.

DRUG TREATMENT The use of "on demand" β-agonist treatment is not appropriate for elderly people in whom reduced appreciation of bronchoconstriction may impair "demand."[11] Such impaired demand with consequent failure to respond to worsening bronchoconstriction is recognized as contributory to increased mortality from asthma.[127] Some authorities argue that regular β-agonists are associated with an increased risk of mortality or near-death episodes from acute asthma. The mechanism for this is believed to be tachyphylaxis (downregulation) of lung β-receptors. The majority of the evidence for this comes from studies of fenoterol, a relatively nonselective (compared to salbutamol and terbutaline) β-agonist.[128–130] However, most of the excess mortality in these studies was in younger patients, and in the UK the Committee of Safety of Medicines and the Royal Society of Medicine have both concluded that the evidence against β-agonists is limited and not sufficient to recommend changes in their use.[131,132]

Inhaled medication usage (both technique and dosage compliance) is variable and probably worse in the elderly population. It is improved by regular follow-up visits and by the provision of feedback about inhaler use and technique.[133] In those with compliance problems, a safe and effective (though expensive) alternative may be the long-acting inhaled β$_2$-agonists salmeterol and eformoterol,[76,77] although there is some evidence that such long-acting agents may produce a small loss of bronchodilator effect with prolonged use together with a more rapid and significant decline in broncho-*protective* effect which is not prevented by concurrent use of inhaled corticosteroids.[134] Inhaled corticosteroids should be given only to those with a *documented* steroid response (i.e. objective improvement in lung function), although some would argue that there is limited value in a trial of oral steroids in those patients with COPD who gain clinical benefit from an inhaled steroid.[135] Conversely, data from the ISOLDE study suggests that abrupt withdrawal of inhaled corticosteroids should be monitored carefully even in patients who apparently have irreversible disease, because of the increased risk of exacerbation on withdrawal.[136] The results of large-scale trials (ISOLDE, Euroscop, and the Copenhagen City Lung Study) are awaited concerning the possible benefits of inhaled steroids on COPD *progression*, but at present there is only conflicting evidence of their value in those patients without documented objective response. Nonetheless, a meta-analysis of the effects of high-dose long-term inhaled corticosteroids in severe COPD did appear to show a reduced rate of decline in lung function over a 2-year period.[137]

An apparent response to steroids during an acute exacerbation does not necessarily imply response between exacerbations. There is little or no place for oral corticosteroids in the chronic management of COPD. Beta-blockers should be avoided as they may exacerbate bronchoconstriction. Even β-blocker eye-drops used for the treatment of glaucoma are recognized to produce bronchoconstriction which is reversible on stopping treatment. Where β-blocker eye-drops are essential, a "cardioselective" medication such as betaxolol should be used in preference to timolol or carteolol.[138,139] Spirometric screening before starting topical β-agonist therapy for glaucoma (with repeat spirometry after one month's treatment) can avoid the risk of respiratory impairment.[140]

Despite good evidence that elderly patients with COPD respond to inhaled anticholinergic drugs—in terms of improvement in spirometry and in breathlessness and exercise capacity[141]—the optimal dose of inhaled anticholinergic agent for the stable patient is not yet established with certainty. There is recent evidence, from a small study including patients up to the age of 76 years, that a dose of ipratropium of at least 160 μg (four times the standard dose) is necessary for maximal bronchodilation, and that such doses are needed before any improvement in exercise tolerance is seen.[142] This work needs confirmation in larger numbers of older subjects. Despite the theoretical effects of anticholinergics on cognition, inhaled cholinergics are essentially lipid-insoluble and thus should not cross the blood–brain barrier. In an elegantly designed study by Ramsdell et al.[143] there were no demonstrable effects over a 2-week period of ipratropium treatment on a battery of psychometric test scores.

Inhaler technique is discussed above under asthma. Whilst nebulizers do have a place for inhaled drug administration in COPD, they have too frequently been prescribed without objective evidence of benefit, and even more frequently are employed in an unsupervised way.[144] The elderly population in particular may find nebulizers difficult to manage, and often need the help of a carer for effective use.[145] This, among other things, implies that nebulizers should not be seen as the "simple" alternative to inhalers in the patient with inadequte inhaler technique. Hospital-based assessment of benefit from nebulizers is probably inadequate, and domiciliary assessment may be preferable.[146,147] Nebulizers need regular servicing and replacement of filters, and patients or carers should be aware of who to contact about this. There is evidence that compliance with nebulized therapy is surprisingly low (of the order of 50 percent), poor compliance being associated with low quality of life and with depression.[148,149] Also, the potential side-effects of such therapy have not been examined in the elderly population who may, at least theoretically, be more prone to cardiac side-effects of high-dose β-agonists and to β-agonist-related hypokalemia. Further trials are indicated.

Theophyllines are beneficial both as bronchodilators and in improving respiratory muscle strength. Unfortunately their side-effects are often prohibitive in elderly patients, particularly as clinically significant benefit is obtained only when plasma concentrations are at the upper end of the therapeutic range.[150] Sustained-release preparations reduce the incidence of side-effects. Both theophyllines and oral β-agonist preparations may be useful in the small number of patients (often the demented) who are unable to use any form of inhaled bronchodilator. In the USA where theophyllines are more widely used, it is interesting to note that they are among the commonest causes of self-poisoning in elderly people.[151]

LONG-TERM OXYGEN THERAPY LTOT is proven to prolong survival in COPD. The only other measure for which this claim can be made is smoking cessation. LTOT implies the delivery of oxygen (usually by oxygen concentrator) for at least 15 hours per day in order to alleviate or prevent right ventricular failure (cor pulmonale) which results from pulmonary hypertension precipitated by chronic hypoxia. It must be distinguished from giving intermittent oxygen for palliation of symptoms. The two studies which indicated a reduction in mortality on LTOT did not include large numbers of elderly people, and one, the MRC LTOT trial, *excluded* patients over 70 years of age.[152,153] Nonetheless, if assessment follows established criteria (as an inpatient at least overnight) there is little reason to suppose that elderly people are less likely to benefit; though preliminary data from the author's institution indicate (perhaps not surprisingly) that the mortality rate of the over-70s on LTOT is much higher than data on younger patients would suggest. The BTS guidelines on COPD management[99] recommend 6-month follow-up of all patients commenced on LTOT. In brief, criteria for selection for LTOT are:

- persistent irreversible airflow obstruction ($FEV_1 < 1.5$ L);
- nonsmoker;
- with or without hypercapnia;
- Po_2 less than 55 mmHg (7.3 kPa) on two sequential estimations at least one month apart, and not during an acute exacerbation;
- LTOT leads to increased Po_2 without a dangerous fall in pH or rise in Pco_2.

NONINVASIVE POSITIVE-PRESSURE VENTILATION NIPPV has been shown in studies including a few patients over the age of 70 years[115] to be of benefit, as an adjunct to LTOT, in selected patients with severe but stable COPD. In addition to patient compliance, motivation, and good cognitive function, criteria for possible benefit from NIPPV comprise documented nocturnal hypoventilation (hypoxia), reversible with NIPPV, together with daytime hypercapnia. Considerable improvement in quality of life in terms of reduced sleep disturbance, activity, and psychosocial factors may be possible.[115] Patients should have stable disease, and NIPPV should not be seen as a "last resort" in rapidly deteriorating end-stage disease.[116] This area is the subject of an excellent review,[117] and may provide further hope for elderly patients in the future. However, studies to date are small in scale, and further work needs to be done in larger numbers of elderly patients before the technique can be widely recommended in this age group.

NIPPV may also be used in acute exacerbation of COPD (AECOPD) as a less invasive alternative to positive-pressure ventilation via endotracheal tube. Clinical limitations in this situation are similar to those for the use of NIPPV in stable disease, with the additional factor that many patients cannot tolerate a mask because of extreme anxiety and panic caused by the "claustrophobic feeling of the mask." Furthermore, it is the recommendation of this author that NIPPV should be pursued in AECOPD only in an intensive-care or high-dependency setting, although in a recent review of the literature this was found not always to be the case.[154] Again there are few studies in the very elderly, but the available literature does suggest that age alone is not a significant prognostic factor for the success or failure of NIPPV; adverse prognostic indicators include a low body mass index, a higher Acute Physiology and Chronic Health Evaluation (APACHE) II score, and a low serum albumin level.[155]

Short-burst oxygen therapy may be symptomatically beneficial for relief of breathlessness. Opiates (including nebulized morphine) and diazepam are not of proven value in the alleviation of breathlessness.

Clinical depression and anxiety

Depression is extremely common in moderate or severe COPD, particularly in the elderly population[156–158] Studies at Manchester Royal Infirmary have indicated that approximately 40 percent of patients with disabling COPD suffer clinical depression which is difficult to detect without the use of specific questionnaires designed for this purpose. Most of the diagnostic assessment scales for depression take up to an hour to administer, but the BASDEC screening questionnaire (which takes 10 minutes for the patient to self-complete) has been shown in our hands to be highly predictive of clinical depression when compared to gold-standard diagnostic scales.[158]

The main predictors of depression appear to be level of disability and patient-perceived quality of life, with other pathophysiological variables including FEV_1, age, and body mass index not being predictive.[157] Clinical anxiety is common (again almost 40 percent) but only in those patients with clinical depression; its prevalence in the nondepressed may be as low as 5 percent.[158]

There have been few trials of the treatment of depression in this setting. Many elderly patients with depression-related COPD refuse to acknowledge that they have a depressive illness and decline treatment.[159] There is some evidence that treatment of depression in this situation produces a significant improvement in quality of life.[156]

Pulmonary rehabilitation

Pulmonary rehabilitation is the subject of an enormous amount of research, including some in elderly patients.[160–163] Pulmonary rehabilitation programs are a multidisciplinary effort comprising education, optimization of medical therapy, nutritional assessment and modification, psychological evaluation and support, relaxation techniques, smoking cessation support, and (essentially) exercise training and reconditioning.

Exercise reconditioning comprising aerobic training of both arms and legs, and expiratory and inspiratory resistive training ("respiratory muscle training"), are recognized to improve exercise tolerance in the short-term. Most frail elderly COPD patients *seem* able to perform the relatively intensive protocols needed to obtain improved exercise tolerance.[161,162,164,165] There is debate, however, even in younger patients, about the duration of benefit; some studies claim that improvement in exercise tolerance persists for up to a year in the absence of maintenance therapy, but others contradict this.[166,167] A Japanese study of fairly elderly patients with disabling COPD showed an improvement in 10-minute walking distance after 12 weeks of therapy, and the improvement was maintained at 16 weeks.[163]

Arguably of most importance is the question of whether improvement in exercise tolerance translates to improvement in quality of life. The data are scanty.[168] There is currently no evidence that respiratory rehabilitation reduces mortality or frequency of hospital admission in elderly patients, though there are some old data suggesting the latter in younger patients.[168] Recent experience at Manchester Royal Infirmary suggests that elderly patients who have completed a pulmonary rehabilitation program are less likely to be admitted to hospital in the subsequent 12 months, and that most of the improvement in exercise tolerance gained during the program is maintained at 12 months irrespective of whether the patient performs "maintenance" exercises.

Greater evaluation of respiratory rehabilitation is needed in elderly patients. Data from the USA have shown that only

5 percent of pulmonary rehabilitation programs include patients from a rehabilitation hospital setting.[169] In the UK, pulmonary rehabilitation is not a commonly offered service generally, and when it is offered it frequently does not include very elderly patients. Certainly, elderly patients with irreversible COPD and chronic asthma (provided they are able to exercise to a sufficient intensity to produce an aerobic training effect) should be considered for referral to existing respiratory rehabilitation programs. Home-based pulmonary rehabilitation may prove especially suitable for elderly subjects.[168,170]

All patients should be advised to remain as physically active as possible, and the obese given advice on weight reduction (which will reduce oxygen requirements of exercise). Conversely, malnutrition is common and correlates with mortality, but beneficial effects of nutritional supplements are unproven. Wheeled walking frames may improve exercise tolerance in the severely disabled.[171] In a recent study the use of wheeled frames did not improve distance walked but were associated with a major and significant reduction in breathlessness in patients (including elderly people) with severe COPD.[172] The high, wheeled gutter frame seems to improve exercise capacity and reduces exercise-associated oxygen desaturation in elderly COPD patients.[173]

Influenza vaccination is recommended for all those with COPD, not just elderly people,[174] and reduces mortality by over two-thirds.[175,176] However, the rate of uptake of vaccination in those in whom it is indicated is only around 50 percent,[177–179] with failure to offer the vaccine and refusal of the offer being almost equally common.[179] Failure of uptake of vaccine among elderly patients seems largely related to the absence of positive belief of its beneficial effects and the excess of erroneous negative beliefs regarding side-effects.[180] Thus a positive and enthusiastic approach from geriatricians to their patients regarding influenza vaccination should be encouraged. Simple clinic-based education measures are likely to have positive benefits on uptake, although currently the vast majority of influenza vaccination in the UK is provided by general practitioners. The *treatment* of influenza A and B with the antiviral agent zanamivir has recently been recommended by the National Institute of Clinical Excellence (NICE) for at-risk adults during influenza epidemics provided they are able to commence treatment within 24 hours of the onset of symptoms. Patients with COPD are recognized in this context as an at-risk group. Zanamivir reduces the onset and duration of symptoms by approximately 24 hours, but there is a paucity of data on hospitalization or mortality even in at-risk groups.

The value of polyvalent pneumococcal vaccine is not absolutely proven, though early studies in elderly people are encouraging with 45–80 percent protection over 3 years.[181] Its indications are similar to those for influenza vaccine.

Quality of life

In the context of what is an incurable disease, where the management aim should arguably shift towards enhancing quality of life, it is perhaps surprising that there remains considerable debate about the factors most affecting quality of life in COPD sufferers.[182–189] Most authors have concluded that the patient's emotional reaction to his or her condition is a significant (if not the most important) quality-of-life determinant, and that perhaps absolute level of respiratory function (spirometry) is of limited help in assessment. Whether age or socioeconomic status are independent variables continues to tax the minds of investigators. Epidemiological data from Manchester in middle-aged and elderly subjects suggest that airways obstruction has significant impact on quality of life, and that this is related to both baseline pulmonary function and to level of nonspecific bronchial responsiveness (airway irritability). In the population as a whole the impact of airways obstruction does not appear, in our studies, to decrease with advancing age.[190] In a more tightly defined group of elderly subjects (mean age 78 years) with severe disabling COPD, quality of life was mainly predicted by disability level and depressive ideation, with smaller contributions from exercise capacity and from advancing age—which appeared to be "protective" perhaps because of reduced subject expectation with aging.[191] In addition there may be a gender effect; similar levels of respiratory disability have a greater tendency to depression and impaired quality of life in elderly women than in elderly men.[192]

Management of AECOPD

Although most exacerbations are managed effectively in the community, it is during an acute exacerbation of COPD (AECOPD) that the patient is most likely to present to hospital. The peak age for hospital admissions for AECOPD is around 70 years.[193] Many, but not all, are the result of bacterial infection (acute infective bronchitis, pneumonia). Other causes include viral infection, pulmonary edema, peripheral edema, or pulmonary embolus. Symptoms may include fever, increased sputum volume and/or purulence, increased breathlessness and wheeze, fluid retention, confusion, and somnolence. The British Thoracic Society guidelines[99] detail the criteria to assess when deciding which AECOPD patients need hospital admission. Criteria suggesting need for admission include: severe breathlessness; poor or deteriorating general condition; cyanosis; increasing peripheral edema; confusion or impaired consciousness; inability to cope at home; and patients already receiving LTOT.

Immediate hospital investigations should include a chest radiograph and blood gas estimation (preferably when breathing room air). Further indications for admission are arterial pH less than 7.35, arterial P_{O_2} on air less than 7 kPa, or infiltration present on the chest radiograph.

The cause of death in AECOPD is usually hypoxia, so the aim is to achieve adequate oxygenation ($P_{O_2} \geq 6.6$ kPa) without a rise in P_{CO_2} or worsening acidosis. Oxygen delivery by nasal cannula is not controlled (i.e. the percentage of inspired oxygen is not predictable), so a Venturi mask should be used if at all possible. When the patient cannot tolerate a mask and nasal cannulas are employed, blood gas monitoring needs to be more frequently performed, and should be done within 30 minutes of commencement of supplemented oxygen. When delivery by a Venturi mask is possible, a 28 percent mask should be used initially and blood gases rechecked within an hour, adjusting the inspired oxygen delivery (different Venturi mask) as indicated by the results. Blood gases should be repeated if there is any change in consciousness level or other clinical deterioration.

Not all those with AECOPD need antibiotic treatment, but antibiotics are indicated if two or more of the following are present: increased sputum volume, increased sputum purulence, increased breathlessness. For the majority of infective episodes which develop in the community, amoxycillin, tetracycline, or co-amoyclav will be appropriate choices.[99] Episodes beginning in hospital may need different antibiotics depending on local sensitivities, and the choice(s) should cover Gram-negative bacilli (e.g. co-amoyclav, cefuroxime). Unfortunately such broad-spectrum antibiotics are prone to produce the potentially serious complication of pseudomembranous colitis in the elderly population. Any diarrhea in such circumstances, particularly if accompanied by abdominal pain and bloating, should be taken very seriously. The patient should be barrier-nursed and stool samples sent for culture—including that of *Clostridium difficile* (and toxin estimation)—and treatment with oral metronidazole and/or vancomycin commenced following local microbiological advice.

Bronchodilators should be given by nebulizer (driven by compressed air, not by oxygen) 4-hourly, beginning at 6–7am and continuing overnight if the patient is awake. Salbutamol 2.5–5 mg and ipratropium 0.5 mg are usually given together, but the latter should be omitted in patients with glaucoma because of the risk of an anticholinergic-precipitated acute episode.

For the severely bronchoconstricted who fail to respond to nebulized treatment, intravenous aminophylline (0.5 mg/kg/h) may be valuable, although research results are contradictory and mainly relate to acute asthma rather than AECOPD.[194–198] Intravenous aminophylline should be avoided in a patient already receiving methylxanthine, unless serum theophylline levels are available. Intravenous or subcutaneous β-agonists may be an alternative in the severely bronchoconstricted when nebulized drugs may penetrate poorly. Clinical experience suggests their usefulness, but controlled trials in the elderly population are lacking.

It is common practice to administer systemic corticosteroids to AECOPD patients, but their value in this condition is unclear.[99] The BTS guidelines suggest administration of a 1–2 week course if the patient has been previously shown to respond to steroids, is on maintenance steroid therapy, is presenting for the first time with AECOPD, or fails to respond to high-dose bronchodilators. It is important to recognize that steroid response in the acute episode does not necessarily justify maintenance inhaled steroid therapy.

In patients with severe respiratory acidosis (arterial pH < 7.25), intravenous doxapram may be useful. Close supervision with regular blood gas estimation is needed. Doxapram is contraindicated in the presence of coexisting ischemic heart disease (a common association).

If intermittent positive-pressure ventilation (IPPV) is available, it is valuable for some patients with respiratory acidosis. Old age is not a contraindication but the acutely confused respond less well.[199,200] Mechanical ventilation is similarly not precluded by age alone but is beyond the scope of this chapter. It has been reviewed recently elsewhere.[201]

Objective assessment of the severity of airways obstruction in AECOPD (by means of regular blood gas and peak flow estimation) is essential in all age groups but most particularly in elderly people. The absence of pulsus paradoxus and of tachycardia are common in severe airways obstruction in elderly people and is not reassuring.[95] Similarly the assertion by patients themselves that their dyspnea is not particularly troublesome or improving may be unreliable, as the elderly patient may have impaired perception of bronchoconstriction.[99]

Nebulized treatment should be changed to inhalers (unless the patient uses a home nebulizer) at least two days before discharge to allow time for monitoring of inhaler technique and exclusion of deterioration on dosage reduction. Inhaler technique should be demonstrated, checked repeatedly, and

Summary of management algorithm
Asthma and COPD

- The British Thoracic Society Guidelines on the Management of COPD and of asthma are generally applicable to the elderly patient

- Because of atypical presentation (particularly in terms of reduced appreciation of bronchoconstriction in old age) objective assessment (spirometry, blood gas estimation PEFR, etc.—dependent upon the clinical situation) is even more important in old age than in the young

- Smoking cessation is the only intervention proven to prolong life in most patients with COPD and is vital for the elderly patient

- LTOT prolongs life in the chronically hypoxic patient with COPD and needs careful assessment when the patient is medically stable

- It is arguable that (because of impaired awareness of bronchoconstriction) elderly patients with asthma or COPD should receive inhaled bronchodilators on a regular rather than an "on demand" basis

- Elderly patients with severe COPD or chronic asthma need careful assessment of disability and possible depression using validated screening tools

- Such patients may benefit for assessment for inclusion in pulmonary rehabilitation programs

- All patients with chronic lung disease should receive influenza and pneumococcal vaccination

KEY POINTS Asthma and COPD

- Respiratory diseases overall (most commonly COPD and asthma), are the second commonest cause of disability in old age.

- There are multiple (and potentially mutually inclusive) causes of late-onset asthma, with the possibility that it represents delayed phenotypic expression of the juvenile-onset (atopic) asthma genotype receiving the most current interest.

- Though cigarette smoking is by far the commonest cause of COPD, only 25% of moderate-heavy smokers will develop COPD. This may again reflect a different phenotypic expression of the *asthma* genotype (the "Dutch Hypothesis").

- Elderly patients with asthma and COPD are often undiagnosed or misdiagnosed and may present atypically, particularly in the acute situation.

- There is no room for nihilism in the management of the elderly smoker—an elderly smoker is in fact slightly more likely to be able to quit than a young smoker, provided he/she is motivated to do so.

documented as adequate prior to discharge. All patients should be seen by a respiratory nurse prior to discharge, and the opportunity for smoking-cessation counseling should be grasped enthusiastically by healthcare professionals.

REFERENCES

1. The Burden of Respiratory Disease. Factsheet 95/3, Lung and Asthma Information Agency, 1995
2. UK Department of Clinical Epidemiology, National Heart and Lung Institute: Respiratory Disease in England and Wales. Thorax 1988;43:949–954
3. Hunt A: The Elderly at Home: A Study of People Aged Sixty-five and Over Living in the Community in England in 1976. HMSO, London, 1976
4. Renwick DS, Connolly MJ: Prevalence and treatment of chronic airflow obstruction in adults over the age of 45. Thorax 1996;51:164–168
5. Burr ML, Charles TJ, Roy K, Seaton A: Asthma in the elderly: an epidemiological survey. BMJ 1979;1:1041–1044
6. Dodge RR, Burrows B: The prevalence and incidence of asthma and asthma-like symptoms in a general population sample. Am Rev Respir Dis 1980;122:567–575
7. Braman SS, Kaemmerlen JT, Davis SM: Asthma in the elderly: a comparison between patients with recently acquired and long-standing disease. Am Rev Respir Dis 1991;143:336–340
8. Parameswaran K, Hildreth AJ, Chadha D et al: Asthma in the elderly: underperceived, underdiagnosed and undertreated; a community survey. Respir Med 1998;92:573–577
9. Nejjari C, Tessier JF, Letenneur L et al: Prevalence of self-reported asthma symptoms in a French elderly sample. Respir Med 1996;90:401–408
10. Roberts SJ, Bateman DN: Which patients are prescribed inhaled anti-asthma drugs? Thorax 1994;49:1090–1095
11. Connolly MJ, Crowley JJ, Charan NB, Nielson CP, Vestal RE: Reduced subjective awareness of bronchoconstriction provoked by methacholine in elderly asthmatic and normal subjects as measured on a simple awareness scale. Thorax 1992;47:410–413
12. Dow L, Coggon D, Holgate ST: Respiratory symptoms as predictors of airways lability in an elderly population. Respir Med 1992;86:27–32
13. Renwick DS, Connolly MJ: Do respiratory symptoms predict chronic airflow obstruction and bronchial hyperresponsiveness in older adults? J Gerontol A 1999;54:M136–M139
14. Rackemann FM: Studies in asthma. 1: A clinical survey of 1074 patients with asthma followed for two years. J Lab Clin Med 1927;12:1185–1197
15. Parameswaran K, Hildreth AJ, Taylor IK, Keaney NP, Bansal SK: Predictors of asthma severity in the elderly: results of a community survey in northeast England. J Asthma 1999;36:613–618
16. Walker C, Bode E, Boer L et al: Allergic and nonallergic asthmatics have distinct patterns of T-cell activation and cytokine production in peripheral blood and bronchoalveolar lavage. Am Rev Respir Dis 1992;146:109–115
17. Bentley AM, Menz G, Storz CHR et al: Identification of T lymphocytes, macrophages and activated eosinophils in the bronchial mucosa in intrinsic asthma. Am Rev Respir Dis 1992;146:500–506
18. State of the art: health effects of outdoor air pollution. Am J Respir Crit Care Med 1996;153:3–50
19. Tattersfield AE: Altouyan Address. Air pollution: brown skies research. Thorax 1996;51:13–22
20. Aubier M, Lambrozo J: Atmospheric pollution linked to transportation. C R Acad Sci III 2000;323:641–649
21. Dutau H, Charpin D: Pollution and allergy: the epidemiological data. Allerg Immunol Paris 1998;30:329–336
22. Austin JB, Russel G, Adam MG et al: Prevalence of asthma and wheeze in the Highlands of Scotland. Arch Dis Child 1994;71:211–216
23. Barnes PJ: Air pollution and asthma. Postgrad Med J 1994;70:319–325
24. Coggon D: Air pollution in homes. BMJ 1996;312:1316 (editorial)
25. Burr ML: Indoor air pollution and the respiratory health of children. Paediatr Pulmonol Suppl 1999;18:3–5
26. Withers NJ, Low L, Holgate ST, Clough JB: The natural history of respiratory symptoms in a cohort of adolescents. Am J Respir Crit Care Med 1998;158:352–357
27. ETAC Study Group: Early treatment of the atopic child: determinants of total and specific IgE in infants with dermatitis. Pediatr Allergy Immunol 1997;8:177–184
28. Jarvis D, Chinn S, Luczynska C, Burney P: Association of respiratory symptoms and lung function in young adults with use of domestic gas appliances. Lancet 1996;347:426–431
29. Chauhan AJ, Krishna MT, Frew AJ, Holgate ST: Exposure to nitrogen dioxide and respiratory disease risk. Rev Environ Health 1998;13:73–90
30. Barbee RA, Halon M, Kaltenborn W et al: A longitudinal study of serum IgE in a community cohort: correlations with age, sex, smoking, and atopic status. J Allergy Clin Immunol 1987;79:919–927
31. Dow L, Coggon D, Campbell MJ et al: The interaction between immunoglobulin E and smoking in airflow obstruction in the elderly. Am Rev Respir Dis 1992;146:402–407
32. Burrows B, Martinez FD, Halonen M et al: Association of asthma with serum IgE levels and skin-test reactivity to allergens. N Engl J Med 1989;320:271–277
33. Pride N: Smoking, allergy and airways obstruction: revival of the "Dutch hypothesis." Clin Allergy 1986;16:3–6
34. Renwick DS, Connolly MJ: Persistence of atopic effects on airway calibre and bronchial responsiveness in older adults. Age Ageing 1997;26:435–440
35. Ariano R, Panzani RC, Augeri G: Late onset asthma clinical and immunological data: importance of allergy. J Investig Allergol Clin Immunol 1998;8:35–41
36. Connolly MJ, Crowley JJ, Charan N, Nielson CP, Vestal RE: Peripheral mononuclear leukocyte beta adrenoceptors and non-specific bronchial responsiveness to methacholine in young and elderly normal subjects and asthmatic patients. Thorax 1994;49:26–32
37. Connolly MJ, Crowley JJ, Charan NB, Nielson CP, Vestal RE: Impaired bronchodilator response to albuterol in healthy elderly men and women. Chest 1995;108:401–406
38. Nielson CP, Crowley JJ, Vestal RE, Connolly MJ: Impaired beta adrenoceptor function, increased leucocyte respiratory burst and bronchial hyperresponsiveness. J Allergy Clin Immunol 1992;90:825–832
39. Chang W, Roth G: In vitro biosynthesis of adipocyte proteins having the characteristics of glucocorticoid receptors. Biochim Biophys Acta 1980;632:58–72
40. Besse JC, Bass AD: Potentiation by hydrocortisone of responses to catecholamines in vascular smooth muscle. J Pharmacol Exp Ther 1966;154:224–238
41. Scarpace PJ, Abrass IB: Desensitization of adenylate cyclase and the downregulation of beta adrenergic receptors after in vivo administration of beta agonist. J Pharmacol Exp Ther 1982;223:327–331
42. Hui KK, Conolly MB, Tashkin DP: Reversal of the human lymphocyte beta-adrenoceptor desensitisation by glucocorticoids. Clin Pharmacol Ther 1982;32:566–571
43. Rimo G, Hanski E, Braun S, Levitski A: Mode of coupling between hormone receptors and adenylate cyclase elucidated by modulation of membrane fluidity. Nature 1978;276:394–396
44. Cookson WOCM, Sharp PA, Faux JA, Hopkin JM: Linkage between immunoglobulin E responses underlying asthma and rhinitis and chromosome 11q. Lancet 1989;i:1292–1295
45. Young RP, Dekker JW, Wordsworth BP et al: HLA-DR and HLA-DP genotypes and immunoglobulin E responses to common major allergens. Clin Exp Allergy 1994;24:431–439
46. Shirakawa TS, Li A, Dubowitz M et al: Association between atopy and variance of the beta subunit of the high affinity immunoglobulin E receptor. Nature Genet 1994;7:124–129
47. Moffatt MF, Hill MR, Cornelis F et al: Genetic linkage of the TCR-a/d complex to specific immunoglobulin E responses. Lancet 1994;343:1597–1600
48. Marsh DG, Neely JD, Breazeale DR et al: Linkage analysis of IL-4 and other chromosome 5q31.1 markers and total serum IgE concentrations. Science 1994;264:1152–1156
49. Ruse CE, Hill M, Parker SG et al: A lymphotoxin alpha promotor polymorphism is predictive of severity of disease in individuals with late onset airflow obstruction. Age Ageing 2001;30(suppl 1):29
50. Banergee DK, Lee GS, Malik SK, Daly S: Underdiagnosis of asthma in the elderly. Br J Dis Chest 1987;81:23–29
51. Lee HY, Stretton TB: Asthma in the elderly. BMJ 1972;4:93–95
52. Allen SC: Missed asthma: a study of 13 old people. Br J Clin Pract 1988;42:158–160
53. Bailey WC, Richards JM, Brooks CM et al: Features of asthma in older adults. J Asthma 1992;29:21–28
54. Burrows B, Barbee RA, Cline MG et al: Characteristics of asthma among elderly adults in a sample of the general population. Chest 1991;100:935–942

55. Putman MT, Wise RA: Myasthenia gravis and upper airway obstruction. Chest 1996;109:400–404

56. Martis GB, Yates DH, Sist M et al: Respiratory sensation during bronchial challenge testing with methacholine, sodium metabisulphite and adenosine monophosphate. Thorax 1996;51:793–798

57. Corris PA, Gibson GJ: Asthma presenting as cor pulmonale. BMJ 1984;288:389–390

58. Dodge R, Cline MG, Burrows B: Comparisons of asthma, emphysema and chronic bronchitis diagnoses in a general population sample. Am Rev Respir Dis 1986;133:981–986

59. Littlejohns P, Ebrahim S, Anderson R: Prevalence and diagnosis of chronic respiratory symptoms in adults. BMJ 1989;298:1556–1560

60. Dor A, Leibhart J, Malolepszy J: Specificity and sensitivity of some signs, symptoms and basic laboratory findings for differentiation between bronchial asthma and chronic obstructive pulmonary disease. Pneumonol Alergol Pol 1998;66:383–390

61. Liebhart J, Dor A: Diagnostic standard for differentiation between bronchial asthma and chronic obstructive pulmonary disease. Pneumonol Alergol Pol 1998;66:373–382

62. Thaidens HA, De-Bock GH, Dekker FW et al: Value of measuring diurnal peak flow variability in the recognition of asthma: a study in general practice. Eur Respir J 1998;12:842–847

63. Boulet LP, Turcotte H, Houdon C, Carrier G, Maltais F: Clinical, physiological and radiological features of asthma with incomplete reversibility of airflow obstruction compared to those of COPD. Can Respir J 1998;5:270–277

64. Hsu JY, Huang CM, King SL, Chaing CD: Important sputum differential cell counting in the diagnosis of airways disease. J Formos Med Assoc 1997;96:330–335

65. Littlejohns P, Ebrahim S, Anderson R: Treatment of adult asthma: is the diagnosis relevant? Thorax 1989;44:797–802

66. Smyth ET, Wright SC, Evans AE, Sinnamon DG, MacMahon J: Death from airways obstruction: accuracy of certification in Northern Ireland. Thorax 1996;51:293–297

67. Griffiths C, Naish J, Sturdy P, Pereira F: Prescribing in hospital admissions for asthma in East London. BMJ 1996;312:481–482

68. Harju T, Keistinen T, Tuuponen T, Kivela SL: Hospital admissions of asthmatics by age and sex. Allergy 1996;51:693–696

69. Gannon PFG, Newton DT, Pantin CFA, Burge PS: Effect of the number of peak expiratory flow readings a day on diurnal variation. Thorax 1992;48:845

70. Iwdshaki Y, Ueda M, Hashimoto S et al: Optimal time of the day for measuring peak expiratory flow rates in patients with asthma. Nihon Kyobu Shikkan Gakkai Zasshi 1996;34:885–889

71. British Thoracic Society et al: The British guidelines on asthma management: 1995 review and position statement. Thorax 1997;52(suppl 1):S1–S21

72. Connolly MJ: Asthma in old age: epidemiology and pathogenesis. In Connolly MJ (ed): Respiratory Disease in the Elderly Patient. Chapman & Hall, London, 1996

73. Ullah MI, Newman GB, Saunders KB: Influence of age on response to ipratropium and salbutamol in asthma. Thorax 1981; 36:523–529

74. Joseph KS, Blaisl Ernst P, Suissa S: Increased morbidity and mortality related to asthma among asthmatic patients who use major tranquillisers. BMJ 1996;312:79–82

75. Connolly MJ, Jarvis EH, Hendrick DJ: Late-onset asthma in a demented elderly patient: the value of methacholine challenge in diagnosis. J Geriatr Soc 1990;38:539–541

76. Starke ID, Luce P: The efficacy and safety of inhaled salmeterol 50 μg in older patients with reversible airflow obstruction. Age Ageing 1995;25:67–71

77. Cazola M, Matera MG, Santagelo G et al: Salmeterol and formoterol in partially reversible severe chronic obstructive pulmonary disease: a dose–response study. Respir Med 1995;89:357–362

78. Weiner P, Weiner M, Azgad Y: Long term clinical comparison of single versus twice daily administration of inhaled budesonide in moderate asthma. Thorax 1995;50:1270–1273

79. Allen SC, Prior A: What determines whether an elderly patient can use a metered-dose inhaler correctly? Br J Dis Chest 1986;80:45–49

80. Connolly MJ: Large volume spacer devices and inhaler technique in elderly patients. Age Ageing 1995;24:190–192

81. Selroos O, Halme M: Effect of a Volumatic spacer and mouth rinsing on systemic absorption of inhaled corticosteroids from a metered-dose inhaler and dry powder inhaler. Thorax 1991;46:891–894

82. Newman SP, Woodman G, Moren F, Clarke SW: Bronchodilator therapy with Nebuhaler: how important is the delay between firing the dose and inhaling. Br J Dis Chest 1988;82:262–267

83. Diggory P, Bailey R, Vallon A: Effectiveness of inhaled bronchodilator delivery systems for elderly patients. Age Ageing 1991;20:379–382

84. Harvey J, Williams JG: Randomised cross-over comparison of five inhaler systems for bronchodilator therapy. Br J Clin Pract 1992;46:249–251

85. Diggory P, Fernandez C, Humphrey A, Jones V, Murphy M: Comparison of elderly people's technique in using two dry powder inhalers to deliver zanamivir: randomised controlled trial. BMJ 2001;322:577–579

86. Armitage JM, Williams SJ: Inhaler technique in the elderly. Age Ageing 1988;17:275–278

87. Abbey C: Teaching elderly patients how to use inhalers: a study to evaluate an education programme on inhaler technique for elderly patients. J Adv Nurs 1997;25:699–708

88. Allen SC: Competence thresholds for the use of inhalers in people with dementia. Age Ageing 1997;26:83–86

89. Lung and Asthma Information Agency: Trends in Asthma Mortality in the Elderly. Factsheet 92/1, 1992

90. Model D: Preventable factors and death certification in death due to asthma. Respir Med 1995;21–25

91. Sherman CB: Late-onset asthma: making the diagnosis, choosing drug therapy. Geriatrics 1995;50:24–33

92. Jack CI, Lye M: Asthma in the elderly patient. Gerontology 1996;42:61–68

93. Renwick DS, Connolly MJ: Improving outcomes in elderly patients with asthma. Drugs and Aging 1999;14:1–9

94. Reid DW, Hendrick VJ, Aitken TC et al: Age-dependent inaccuracy of death certification in northern England, 1991–1992. Eur Respir J 1998;12:1079–1083

95. Petheram IS, Jones DA, Collins JV: Assessment and management of acute asthma in the elderly: a comparison with young asthmatics. Postgrad Med J 1982;58:149–151

96. Cook NR, Evans DA, Scherr PA et al: Peak expiratory flow rate and 5-year mortality in an elderly population. Am J Epidemiol 1991;133:785–794

97. Connolly MJ, Renwick DS, Gibson HN, Taylor PM: Admission chest radiograph in elderly patients admitted to hospital with acute severe asthma. Age Ageing 1995;24(suppl 2):13

98. Nielson C: Critical care. In Connolly MJ (ed): Respiratory Disease in the Elderly Patient. Chapman & Hall, London, 1996:209–230

99. The COPD Guidelines Group of the Standards of Care Committee of the BTS. The BTS guidelines for the management of chronic obstructive pulmonary disease. Thorax 1997;52(suppl 5):S1–S28

100. Horsley JR, Sterling IJ, Waters WE, Howell JB: Respiratory symptoms among elderly people in the New Forest area as assessed by postal questionnaire. Age Ageing 1991;20:325–331

101. Isoaho R, Puolijoki H, Huhti E et al: Prevalence of chronic obstructive pulmonary disease in elderly Finns. Respir Med 1994;88:571–580

102. Marco JL, Martin BJC, Corres IM, Luque DR, Zubillhea GG: Chronic obstructive lung disease in the general population: an epidemiologic study performed in Guipuzcoa. Arch Bronconeumol 1998;34:23–27

103. Sobradillo V, Miravitlles M, Jimenez CA: Epidemiological study of chronic obstructive pulmonary disease in Spain (IBERPOC): prevalence of chronic respiratory symptoms and airflow limitation. Arch Bronconeumol 1999;35:159–166

104. Whittemore AS, Perlin SA, DiCiccio Y: Chronic obstructive pulmonary disease in lifelong nonsmokers: results from NHANES. Am J Public Health 1995;85:702–706

105. Ray D, Abel R, Selvaraj KG: A 5-yr prospective epidemiological study of chronic obstructive pulmonary disease in rural south India. Indian J Med Res 1995;101:238–244

106. Rao X, Cai R, Huang Z: Effects of smoking on lung function in populations of Beijing and Guangzhou. Zhonghua Jie He He Hu Xi Za Zhi 1996;19:14–17 (in Chinese)

107. Lung and Asthma Information Agency: Trends in Lung Cancer and Smoking. Factsheet 93/1, 1993

108. Soriano JB, Maier WC, Egger P et al: Recent trends in physician diagnosed COPD in women and men in the UK. Thorax 2000;55:789–794

109. Davis RM, Novotny TE: The epidemiology of cigarette smoking and its impact on chronic obstructive pulmonary disease. Am Rev Respir Dis 1989;140:S82–S84

110. Lee PN, Fry JS, Forey BA: Trends in lung cancer, chronic obstructive lung disease, and emphysema death rates for England and Wales

1941–85 and their relation to trends in cigarette smoking. Thorax 1990;45:657–665

111. Feinleib M, Rosenberg HM, Collins JG: Trends in COPD morbidity and mortality in the United States. Am Rev Respir Dis 1989;140:9–18S

112. Renwick DS, Connolly MJ: Impact of obstructive airways disease on quality of life in older adults. Thorax 1996;51:520–525

113. Yohannes AM, Roomi J, Waters K, Connolly MJ: Quality of life in elderly patients with chronic obstructive pulmonary disease: measurement of predictive factors. Respir Med 1998;92:1231–1236

114. Connolly MJ: Obstructive airways disease: a hidden disability in the aged. Age Ageing 1996;25:265–267

115. Mecham Jones DJ, Paul EA, Jones PW, Wedzicha JA: Nasal pressure support ventilation plus oxygen compared to oxygen therapy alone in hypercapnic COPD. Am J Respir Crit Care Med 1995;152:538–544

116. Mecham Jones DJ, Wedzicha JA: Non-invasive positive pressure ventilation in advanced progressive chronic respiratory failure due to COPD. Am Rev Respir Dis 1993;147:A322

117. Wedzicha JA, Meecham Jones DJ: Domiciliary ventilation in advanced chronic obstructive pulmonary disease: where are we? Thorax 1996;51:455–457 (editorial)

118. Schols AMWJ, Soeters PB, Mostert R, Saris WHM, Woeters EFM: Energy balance in chronic obstructive pulmonary disease. Am Rev Respir Dis 1991;143:1248–1252

119. The Intermittent Positive Pressure Breathing Trial Group: Intermittent positive pressure therapy of chronic obstructive pulmonary disease. Ann Intern Med 1983;99:612–620

120. Vetter NJ, Ford D: Smoking prevention among people aged 60 and over: a randomized controlled trial. Age Ageing 1990;19:164–168

121. Campbell IA, Prescott RJ, Tjeder-Burton SM: Transdermal nicotine plus support in patients attending hospital with smoking-related diseases: a placebo-controlled study. Respir Med 1996;90:47–51

122. Russel MAH, Stapleton JA, Feyerbend C et al: Targeting heavy smokers in general practice: randomised controlled trial of transdermal nicotine patches. BMJ 1993;306:1308–1312

123. Maguire CP, Ryan J, Kelly A et al: Do patient age and medical condition influence medical advice to stop smoking? Age Ageing 2000;29:264–266

124. Flaxman J: Quitting smoking now or later: gradual, abrupt, immediate and delayed quitting. Behav Ther 1978;9:260–270

125. Burchfiel CM, Marcus EB, Curb D et al: Effects of smoking and smoking cessation on longitudinal decline in pulmonary function. Am J Respir Crit Care Med 1995;151:1778–1785

126. Connolly MJ: Smoking cessation in old age: closing the stable door? Age Ageing 2000;29:193–195 (editorial)

127. Stableforth DE: Asthma mortality and physician competence. J Allergy Clin Immunol 1987;80:463–466

128. Crane J, Pearce N, Flatt N et al: Prescribed fenoterol and death from asthma in New Zealand, 1981–83: case–control study. Lancet 1989;1:917–922

129. Grainger J, Woodman K, Pearce N et al: Prescribed fenoterol and death from asthma in New Zealand, 1981–7: a further case–control study. Thorax 1991;46:105–111

130. Sears MR, Taylor DR, Print CG et al: Regular inhaled beta-agonist treatment in bronchial asthma. Lancet 1990;336:1391–1396

131. Kuitert LM: Beta-agonists in asthma. State of the art: report on a Royal Society of Medicine seminar. Thorax 1992;47:568–569

132. Committee on Safety of Medicines: Report of the Beta-agonist Working Party. Medicines Control Agency, London, 1992

133. Simmons MS, Nides MA, Rand CS, Wise RA, Tashkin DP: Trends in compliance with bronchodilator use between follow-up visits in a clinical trial. Chest 1996;109:963–968

134. Sears MR: Long-acting beta-agonists, tachyphylaxis and corticosteroids. Chest 1996;109:862–864 (editorial)

135. Boothman-Burrell D, Delany SJ, Flannery EM, Hancox RJ, Taylor DR: The efficacy of inhaled corticosteroids in the management of non asthmatic chronic airflow obstruction. NZ Med J 1997;110:370–373

136. Jarad NA, Wedzicha JA, Burge PS, Calverley PM: An observational study of inhaled corticosteroid withdrawal in stable chronic obstructive pulmonary disease. Respir Med 1999;93:161–168

137. van Grunsven PM, van Schayck CP, Derenne JP et al: Long term effects of inhaled corticosteroids in chronic obstructive pulmonary disease: a meta-analysis. Thorax 1999;54:7–14

138. Diggory P, Cassels-Brown A, Vail A, Abbey LM, Hillman JS: Avoiding unsuspected respiratory side-effects of topical timolol with cardioselective or sympathomimetic agents. Lancet 1995;345:1604–1606

139. Diggory P, Cassels-Brown A, Fernandez C: Topical beta-blockade with intrinsic sympathomimetic activity offers no advantage for the respiratory in cardiovascular function of elderly people. Age Ageing 1996;25:424–428

140. Diggory P, Cassels-Brown A, Vail A, Hillman JS: Randomised, controlled trial of spirometric changes in elderly people receiving timolol or betaxolol as initial treatment for glaucoma. Br J Ophthalmol 1998;82:146–149

141. Teramoto S, Fukuchi Y: Improvements in exercise capacity and dyspnoea by inhaled anticholinergic drug in elderly patients with chronic obstructive pulmonary disease. Age Ageing 1995;24:278–282

142. Ikeda A, Nishimura K, Koama H et al: Dose response study of ipratropium bromide aerosol on maximum exercise performance in stable patients with chronic obstructive pulmonary disease. Thorax 1996;51:48–53

143. Ramsdell JW, Henderson S, Renvall MJ, Salmon DP, Ferguson P: Effects of theophylline and ipratropium on cognition in elderly patients with chronic obstructive pulmonary disease. Ann Allergy Asthma Immunol 1996;76:335–340

144. Anon: The nebuliser epidemic. Lancet 1984;2:789–790

145. Teale C, Jones A, Patterson CJ et al: Community survey of home nebulizer technique by elderly people. Age Ageing 1995;24:276–277

146. O'Driscoll BR, Kay EA, Taylor RJ, Bernstein A: Home nebulisers: can optimal therapy be predicted by laboratory studies? Respir Med 1990;84:471–477

147. Teale C, Morrison JFJ, Jones PC, Muers MF: Reversibility tests in chronic obstructive airways disease: their predictive value with reference to benefit from domiciliary nebuliser therapy. Respir Med 1991;85:281–284

148. Bosley CM, Corden ZM, Rees PJ, Cochrane GM: Psychological factors associated with the use of home nebulized therapy for COPD. Eur Respir J 1996;9:2346–2350

149. Pounsford JC: Nebulisers for the elderly. Thorax 1997;52 (suppl 2):S53–S55

150. McKay SE, Howie C, Thomson AH, Whiting B, Addis GJ: Value of theophylline treatment in patients handicapped by chronic obstructive lung disease. Thorax 1993;48:227–232

151. Haselberger MB, Kroner BA: Drug poisonings in older patients: preventative and management strategies. Drugs Aging 1995;7:292–297

152. Nocturnal Oxygen Therapy Trial Group: Continuous or nocturnal oxygen therapy in hypoxic chronic obstructive lung disease. Ann Intern Med 1980;93:391–398

153. Report of the Medical Research Council Oxygen Working Party: Long-term domiciliary oxygen therapy in chronic hypoxic cor pulmonale complicating chronic bronchitis and emphysema. Lancet 1981;1:681–685

154. Sinuff T, Cook D, Randall J, Allen C: Noninvasive positive-pressure ventilation: a utilization review of use in a teaching hospital. CMAJ 2000;163:969–973

155. Putinati S, Ballerin L, Piattella M, Panella GL, Potena A: Is it possible to predict the success of non-invasive positive pressure ventilation in acute respiratory failure due to COPD? Respir Med 2000;94:997–1001

156. Light RW, Merrill EJ, Despars JA et al: Prevalence of depression and anxiety in patients with COPD: relationship to functional capacity. Chest 1985;87:35–38

157. Yohannes AM, Roomi J, Baldwin RC, Connolly MJ: Depression in elderly outpatients with disabling chronic obstructive pulmonary disease. Age Ageing 1998;27:155–160

158. Yohannes AM, Baldwin RC, Connolly MJ: Depression and anxiety in elderly outpatients with chronic obstructive pulmonary disease: prevalence, and validation of the BASDEC screening questionnaire. Int J Geriatr Psych 2000;15:1090–1096

159. Yohannes AM, Connolly MJ, Baldwin RC: A feasibility study of antidepressant drug therapy in depressed elderly patients with chronic obstructive pulmonary disease. Int J Geriatr Psych 2001;16:451–454

160. Chauhan AJ, Leahy BC: Pulmonary rehabilitation in the elderly patient. In Connolly MJ (ed): Respiratory Disease in the Elderly Patient. London: Chapman & Hall, 1996:261–295

161. Couser JI, Guthmann R, Hameadeh MA, Kane CS: Pulmonary rehabilitation improves exercise capacity in older elderly patients with COPD. Chest 1995;107:730–734

162. Sudo E, Ohga E, Matsuse T et al: The effects of pulmonary rehabilitation combined with inspiratory muscle training on pulmonary function and inspiratory muscle strength in elderly patients with chronic obstructive pulmonary disease. Nippon Ronen Igakkai Zasshi 1997;34:929–934

163. Sudo E, Ohga E, Matsuse T et al: Duration of the effect of pulmonary rehabilitation in elderly patients with chronic obstructive pulmonary disease. Nippon Ronen Igakkai Zasshi 1997;34:739–742

164. Roomi J, Johnson MM, Waters K, Yohannes A, Connolly MJ: Respiratory rehabilitation, exercise capacity and quality of life in chronic airways disease in old age. Age Ageing 1996;25:2–16

165. Roomi J, Yohannes A, Connolly MJ: Respiratory rehabilitation improves exercise capacity in elderly patients with chronic airflow limitation. Thorax 1995;50(suppl 2):A56

166. Swerts PM, Kretzers LM, Terpstra-Windevan E, Verstappen FT, Woeters EF: Exercise reconditioning in the rehabilitation of patients with chronic obstructive pulmonary disease: a short and long-term analysis. Arch Phys Med Rehab 1990;71:570–573

167. Vale F, Reardon JZ, Zuwallack RL: The long-term benefits of out-patient pulmonary rehabilitation on exercise endurance and quality of life. Chest 1993;103:42–45

168. Ries AL: Position paper of the American Association of Cardiovascular and Pulmonary Rehabilitation. Scientific basis of pulmonary rehabilitation. J Cardiopulmon Rehab 1990;10:418–441

169. Glasman SJ: Pulmonary rehabilitation in the acute inpatient rehabilitation hospital. Respir Care Clin N Am 1998;4:47–57

170. Wijkstra PJ, van der Mark TW, Kraan J: Long-term effects of home rehabilitation on physical performance in chronic obstructive pulmonary disease. Am J Respir Crit Care Med 1996;153:1234–1241

171. Grant BJB, Capel H: Walking aid for pulmonary emphysema. Lancet 1972;ii:1125–1127

172. Dalton G, Ashley J, Rudkin ST, White RJ: The effect of walking aids on walking distance, breathlessness and oxygenation with patients with severe chronic obstructive pulmonary disease (COPD). Thorax 1995;50(suppl 2):A57

173. Roomi J, Yohannes AM, Connolly MJ: The effect of walking aids on exercise capacity and oxygenation in elderly patients with chronic obstructive pulmonary disease. Age Ageing 1998;27:703–706

174. Department of Health: Immunisation Against Infectious Disease. HMSO, London, 1992

175. Howells CHL, Vesselinova-Jenkins CK, Evans AD, James J: Influenza vaccination and mortality from bronchopneumonia in the elderly. Lancet 1985;1:381–383

176. Gross PA, Quinnan GV, Rodstein M et al: Association of influenza immunisation with reduction in mortality in an elderly population: a prospective study. Arch Intern Med 1988;148:562–565

177. Wulp CG van der, Perenboom RJM, Davidse W: Ontwikkelingen in de griepvaccinatie in Nederland. Maandbericht Gezondheid (CBS) 1995;2:4–9

178. Nicholson KG: Immunization against influenza among people aged over 65 living at home in Leicestershire during winter 1991–2. BMJ 1993;306:974–976

179. Frank JW, Henderson M, McMurray L: Influenza vaccination in the elderly. 1: Determinance of acceptance. Can Med Assoc J 1995;132:371–375

180. Honkanen PO, Keistinen T, Kivela SL: Factors associated with influenza vaccination coverage among the elderly: role of health care personnel. Public Health 1996;110:163–168

181. Shapiro ED, Berg AT, Austrian R et al: Protective efficacy of polyvalent pneumococcal polysaccharide vaccine. N Engl J Med 1991;325:1453–1456

182. Dudley DL, Glasser EM, Jorgenson Logan DL: Psychsocial and psychological concomitants to rehabilitation in COPD. 1: Psychosocial considerations. Chest 1980;77:413–420

183. Dudley DL: Coping with chronic obstructive pulmonary disease: therapeutic options. Geriatrics 1981;36:69–74

184. Cockcroft AE: Randomised controlled trial of rehabilitation in chronic respiratory disability. Thorax 1981;36:200–203

185. McSweeney AJ, Grant I, Heaton RK, Adams KM, Timms RM: Life quality of patients with chronic obstructive pulmonary disease. Arch Inten Med 1982;142:473–478

186. Prigatano GP, Wright EC, Levin D: Quality of life and its predictors in patients with mild hypoxemia and chronic obstructive pulmonary disease. Arch Intern Med 1984;144:1613–1619

187. Williams SJ: Chronic respiratory illness and disability: a critical review of the psychosocial literature. Soc Sci Med 1989;28:791–803

188. Cutris JR, Deyo RA, Hudson LD: Health-related quality of life among patients with chronic obstructive pulmonary disease. Thorax 1994;49:162–170

189. Okubadejo AA, Jones PW, Wedzicha JA: Quality of life in patients with chronic obstructive pulmonary disease and severe hypoxaemia. Thorax 1996;5144–5147

190. Renwick DS, Connolly MJ: Impact of obstructive airways disease on quality of life in older adults. Thorax 1996;51:520–525

191. Johannes AM, Roomi J, Waters K, Connolly MJ: Quality of life in elderly patients with chronic obstructive pulmonary disease: measurement and predictive factors. Respir Med 1998;92:1231–1236

192. Yohannes AM, Connolly MJ: Gender differences in prevalence of depression in elderly patients with chronic obstructive pulmonary disease. Age Ageing Abstract 2000;30(suppl 2):74

193. Vilkman S, Keistinen T, Tuuponen T, Kivela SL: Age distribution of patients treated in hospital for chronic obstructive pulmonary disease. Age Ageing 1996;25:109–112

194. Seigel D, Sheppard D, Gelb A, Weinberg PE: Aminophylline increases the toxicity but not the efficacy of an inhaled beta-adrenergic agonist in the treatment of acute exacerbations of asthma. Am Rev Respir Dis 1985;132:283–286

195. Self TH, Abou-Shala N, Burns R et al: Inhaler albuterol and oral prednisone in hospitalised adult asthmatics: does aminophylline add any benefit? Chest 1990;98:1317–1321

196. Wrenn K, Slovis CM, Murphy F, Greenberg RS: Aminophylline therapy for acute bronchospastic disease in the emergency room. Ann Intern Med 1991;115:241–247

197. Murphy DC, McDermott MJ, Rydman RJ et al: Aminophylline in the treatment of acute asthma when β_2-adrenergics and steroids are provided. Arch Intern Med 1993;153:1784–1788

198. Huang D, O'Brian RG, Harman E et al: Does aminophylline benefit adults admitted to hospital for an acute exacerbation of asthma? Ann Intern Med 1993;119:1155–1160

199. Bott J, Carroll MP, Conway J et al: Randomised controlled trial of nasal ventilation in acute ventilatory failure due to chronic obstructive airways disease. Lancet 1993;341:1555–1567

200. Brochard C, Mancebo J, Wysocki M et al: Noninvasive ventilation for acute exacerbations of chronic obstructive pulmonary disease. N Engl J Med 1995;338:817–822

201. Nielson C: Critical care. In Connolly MJ (ed): Respiratory Disease in the Elderly Patient. London: Chapman & Hall, 1996:209–230

Chapter 43

Nonobstructive lung disease and thoracic tumors

Martin J. Connolly and Margot Gosney

PRESENTATIONS

There are few or no age-related differences in the presentation and progression of fibrotic lung diseases, tuberculosis, pneumonia, and bronchogenic carcinomas. In simple terms, presentations fall into five pathological groups.

COLLAPSE
- Reduced movement of the affected side, tracheal deviation to the affected side, and displacement of the apex toward the collapse;
- Diminished breath sounds.

CONSOLIDATION
- Dullness to percussion;
- Reduced vocal fremitus;
- Increased vocal resonance (aegophony);
- Bronchial breathing;
- Signs of collapse often coexist;
- Crepitations.

PNEUMOTHORAX (air in the pleural space)
- Reduced or absent breath sounds;
- Pleural click (left-sided pneumothoraces only).

When a pneumothorax occurs with tension, other signs may occur in addition. "Tension" indicates increasing accumulation of air in the pleural space with each inspiration, due to a "flap" of pleura producing a one-way valve effect.

- Displacement of the apex and trachea *away* from the affected side;
- Hyper-resonance to percussion;
- Absent breath sounds;
- Tachycardia;
- Hypotension;
- Respiratory distress;
- Cyanosis;
- Sweating;
- Raised jugular venous pressure.

PLEURAL EFFUSION
- Reduced chest movement over the effusion;
- Profound dullness to percussion ("stony dullness");
- Reduced breath sounds;
- Reduced vocal fremitus and vocal resonance;
- Displacement of apex and trachea *away from* the effusion (if large).

DIFFUSE LUNG FIBROSIS (e.g. fibrosing alveolitis)
- Fine, late inspiratory or pan-inspiratory crepitations ("velcro-creps");
- Clubbing (often);
- Cyanosis.

NON-CANCEROUS DISEASES

NON-MYCOBACTERIAL RESPIRATORY INFECTIONS

Epidemiology and pathogenesis

Although death from respiratory infection is common in the elderly population, epidemiological studies of infection are patchy and many specifically exclude elderly people. The best estimate is that the death rate from respiratory infection for the over-65s approaches 500 per 10,000 population per year. This figure is 50 times higher than that in young adults.[1]

Factors which increase the risk of respiratory infection in old age are detailed in Chapter 42. Briefly these comprise: a depressed immune response; an increased closing volume; an increased prevalence of chronic lung disease (in turn producing impairment of the mucociliary escalator, impaired respiratory muscle strength and endurance, breaches of the respiratory epithelium, and alteration in the mucous layer); institutionalization leading to greater proximity to infected individuals; and colonization of the upper respiratory tract by pathogens (Gram-negative enterobacteria are particularly likely in some circumstances[2]). Other medical conditions common in elderly people also predispose to increased infection. For example, stroke and other neurological conditions increase the risk of aspiration, and impaired nutritional status further depresses immunity.

Influenza

The scale of the problem

Influenza is *not* more common in the elderly population. However, its complication rate, morbidity, and mortality are much greater. Hospitalization as a result of influenza is up to 20 times more common in elderly people, and even more so in those with other chronic illnesses.[3,4] Approximately a quarter of elderly patients suffer complications from influenza.[5] Acute infective bronchitis is up to 20 times more common after influenza in old people, and pneumonia nearly ten times more common.[6] The well recognized complication of staphylococcal pneumonia following influenza in fact accounts for only about a quarter of post-influenza pneumonias even during epidemic periods, and the most common bacterial pathogen following influenza is *Streptococcus pneumoniae.*[7] Pneumonia directly due to the influenza virus rather than bacterial superinfection is a frequent complication.

Influenza epidemics are associated with a peak of deaths from pneumonia and acute bronchitis in old people. However, there is also a large increase in deaths from cerebrovascular and cardiovascular disease which are precipitated by influenza infection.[8]

Vaccination

Influenza vaccination is recommended in the UK for residents of nursing or residential homes as well as those of all ages with diabetes, chronic renal failure, or chronic respiratory conditions.[9,10]

The UK Department of Health has recently changed its recommendations on influenza vaccine for the elderly population generally, reducing the recommended lower age limit from 75 years to 65 years[11] and thus moving into line with practice in North America and across most other European countries.[12–14] Vaccine is modified each year to cover serotype changes.

The main benefit of vaccination is in reducing the incidence of hospitalization (and other complications) and mortality: it is estimated that mortality is reduced by at least 60 percent.[4,15] Nevertheless, currently only a small minority of those elderly people eligible for influenza vaccination actually receive it in the UK and in other European countries.[16–19] Vaccine uptake rates are much higher in institutional care—although even in that setting the most common reason for failure to vaccinate is patient refusal.[20] In the community in the UK, the most common reason given by those unvaccinated is lack of information from the general practitioner, with fears about side-effects, concern about vaccine efficacy, and perception of personal good health.[18,21,22]

Simple strategies to increase vaccine uptake—computerized highlighting of high-risk patients and the sending of personal reminders—have been effective in the Netherlands[17] and in Ireland.[23] However, whilst agreeing with this general view, Siriwardena has shown that—for reasons that are unclear—of all the high-risk groups it is those with chronic lung disease who are particularly difficult to target and persuade to accept vaccination, with uptake rates of about 20 percent.[24] Other factors known to influence the uptake of influenza vaccination are personal income, marital status, and racial origin.[25,26]

In the hospital long-term care setting, vaccination of healthcare workers (as opposed to patients/residents) is associated with a major decrease in influenza-related mortality among patients, although with no reduction in nonfatal influenza infection.[27] Only recently has influenza vaccination been offered commonly to healthcare workers in the UK, and little is yet known about uptake.

Until recently the only effective antiviral drugs for influenza were the adamantane group (e.g. amantadine). These were effective only against influenza A, and although they did reduce illness severity they rapidly led to the production of drug-resistant strains and were poorly tolerated.

A new neuraminidase inhibitor, zanamivir, has been licensed recently in the UK. It is effective against all strains of influenza A and B and its tolerance is generally very good, although caution is recommended in patients with asthma or chronic obstructive pulmonary disease (COPD) because of the potential risk of bronchoconstriction. Zanamivir is given by inhalation and is estimated to reduce the time to alleviation of symptoms of illness by one or two days.[28,29] There has been controversy in the UK with regard to the use of zanamivir in the elderly population and in other high-risk groups, in terms of reduction in *mortality* from influenza, and further research is needed. Nonetheless, its efficacy in the reduction of duration and severity of symptoms *has* been demonstrated in elderly people.[29] There is some evidence that when given prophylactically it may have a protective effect, particularly when used to enhance protection given by influenza vaccine.[30,31] Again this requires confirmation in elderly patients; if it is confirmed, zanamivir may be useful, for example, during outbreaks in institutional care settings.

Pneumonia

The scale of the problem

Pneumonia is much more common in elderly than in younger adults. European studies suggest an incidence approaching 20 cases per 1000 population per year in the 70–79 age group, compared with one or two per 1000 in younger adults.[32,33] Over 90 percent of deaths from pneumonia in developed countries occur in the old.[34] UK national figures suggest that pneumonia is a primary cause in over 5 percent of deaths in the over-65s.[35] In the less developed world, pneumonia is the only major killer for which the mortality rate is not decreasing.[36,37]

In Britain and most developed countries, *Haemophilus influenzae* and pneumococcus are the most common causes of community-acquired pneumonia in the elderly population.[38–44] "Atypical" pneumonias in elderly people seem rare in the UK,[39] although less so in the USA. The exception to this is that mycoplasma infection is common in the UK during epidemics which tend to occur approximately every four years and peak between January and March.[38] Gram-negative enterobacteria have traditionally been thought to be uncommon as a cause of community-acquired pneumonia in Britain, although their role in nursing-home-acquired pneumonia elsewhere (particularly in the USA) has been the subject of investigation and speculation for some time.[43] It is probable that aspiration is underdiagnosed as a cause of pneumonia in elderly people,[45] and in this context it may be important that colonization of the mouth with Gram-negative bacilli is common in the institutionalized frail elderly.[46]

Risk factors for the development of pneumonia in old age include institutionalization, neurological disease (particularly when associated with swallowing difficulties), immobility, male sex, extreme old age, alcoholism, malnutrition, lack of receipt of influenza vaccine, and comorbidity—particularly chronic respiratory impairment or cardiac disease.[47–50] Many of these risk factors are also associated with poor prognosis and particularly with the development of bacteremic pneumonia.[48] Furthermore, the recurrence of pneumonia (again associated with high mortality) following hospitalization for previous pneumonia is predicted by the presence of chronic pulmonary disease and by advancing age.[51]

Presentation of pneumonia

The elderly person, particularly if cognitively impaired,[52] is likely to present with atypical (i.e. nonrespiratory) symptoms. The most common of these is confusion (up to 70 percent of cases versus 30 percent of younger adults[38,39,53,54]). Indeed, confusion is so common as a nonspecific presenting feature that a chest radiograph will reveal the diagnosis in nearly a quarter of cases of elderly patients presenting with acute confusion and no physical signs.[55] Tachypnea (>24/min) is a very early feature of pneumonia in elderly people,[56] though its specificity is poor. Signs of cardic failure are present in nearly a quarter of patients.[57] Pleuritic chest pain and rigors are uncommon.[58] Although oral or axillary temperature may not be raised, core temperature is almost always elevated in the first 24 hours after hospital admission[54]; in other words, the claim that elderly people do not develop a pyrexia is erroneous. However, it has also been suggested that *all* (both typical and atypical) symptoms in elderly patients with pneumonia are less commonly reported than in the young.[59]

Although most elderly patients with pneumonia will have localizing crackles on chest auscultation, the presence of isolated (especially bilateral) pulmonary basal crackles is a nonspecific finding in the ill elderly.[60] Similarly, dehydration—although much more common in older people than in younger people with pneumonia—may be difficult to detect clinically.[61] The present authors' own studies have shown that the presence of axillary sweating is highly suggestive that the patient is *not* dehydrated, although its absence is not as helpful a sign.[62]

Investigations and supportive measures

Investigations in hospital are not specific to elderly people. They should include urgent urea and electrolyte estimation, full blood count, chest X-ray, blood gas estimation, and (if possible) peak flow estimation. Measurement of ESR or C-reactive protein may give further evidence of infection in uncertain cases. However, this apparently simple and rational approach is not always applicable in old age where the investigations may be aimed at detecting the cause of an acute confusional state or other atypical presentation, and will initially therefore include more wide-ranging investigations. There is some evidence that the absence of a leucocytosis is more common in elderly people with pneumonia and may be an adverse prognostic factor.[34,63–65]

Blood cultures should be taken before institution of antibiotic therapy. However, antibiotic therapy should not be delayed by waiting for a sputum sample, as in the early stages fewer than 50 percent of patients are able to produce sputum. The bacterial etiology of pneumonia cannot be determined by means of analysis of clinical manifestation or radiological imaging alone, and in the acute setting bacteriological investigation is often unhelpful.[66] Microbiological identification is even more difficult in the elderly population,[57,67,68] in whom even in the situation of controlled clinical trials there is failure to identify a pathogenic organism in 30–60 percent of cases.[69–71] Failure to establish bacterial etiology does not apparently affect prognosis in the majority of patients. Gram staining is almost as valuable as culture of sputum[72] but is not available in all centers. Blood cultures should always be taken and will be positive in almost a third of patients with pneumococcal pneumonia.[38,39] Where bacteriological diagnosis is deemed essential, counter-current immune-electrophoresis (CIE) of sputum or urine is sensitive in the detection of pneumococcal capsular antigen.[38,39] However, it may give false positives in patients with chronic lung disease who are often colonized with pneumococcus.

General supportive measures include careful intravenous rehydration (necessary in the majority of patients) and oxygen treatment (often high-flow oxygen) as indicated by blood gases. Even if the patient is not initially dehydrated, intravenous fluids are often necessary to maintain hydration in a patient with reduced intake (secondary to anorexia and possibly confusion) and increased needs due to pyrexia and tachypnea.

Bacterial etiology and antibiotic treatment

Pneumococcus is the most common cause of community-acquired pneumonia in people, causing 30–60 percent of cases. It is less well recognized that viral pneumonia is the second most common cause (most particularly influenza viruses). Third comes *Haemophilus influenzae*.[39–44,73] The incidence of *Legionella* pneumonia in the elderly population is low, with fewer than 100 cases per year in England and Wales.[74] Similarly, mycoplasma pneumonia outside of epidemics is extremely rare in elderly people.[75] In contrast, staphylococcal pneumonia, though not common, affects elderly people as well as the young most particularly following influenza.[76] *Chlamydia* infection is not uncommon, with about 15 percent of all cases of psittacosis occurring in elderly people.[77]

Gram-negative enterobacteria are the most commonly identified cause of *nosocomial* pneumonia, accounting for over half of cases.[78,79] This probably relates to prior usage of antibiotics both in the individual patient and in the hospital. Staphylococcal infection is the second most common cause of nosocomial pneumonia in Britain, and there is now increased appreciation of the relevance of aspiration pneumonia, particularly in elderly people with neurological impairment. Whilst patients most commonly aspirate mouth and oropharyngeal commensal bacteria (including anaerobes), Gram-negative enterobacteria may also be important, particularly in patients who have been in hospital for a few days, as oropharyngeal colonization with Gram-negatives is common following hospitalization of elderly people.[46] There is some concern that *Pseudomonas aeruginosa* and methicillin-resistant *Staphylococcus aureus* (MRSA) may be becoming increasingly common causes of nosocomial pneumonia.[80]

Overall, nosocomial pneumonia is second only to urinary tract infection as a cause of hospital-acquired infection. Crude incidence rates are between 1.5 and 8 percent in the acute sector and about 8 percent in long-term care,[81,82] although there is a dearth of studies in this area. Pre-existing chest disease and recent antibiotics *do not* appear to increase the overall risk of nosocomial pneumonia.[81] Caution in diagnosis is needed here, as a preliminary report has suggested that in about one-third of cases urinary tract infection may be misdiagnosed as respiratory infection,[83] with implications for choice and duration of antibiotic therapy.

Recommendations for initial antibiotic therapy for pneumonia in elderly people differ greatly between community-acquired pneumonia and nosocomial pneumonia. For relatively mild community-acquired infection, ampicillin, amoxycillin, or erythromycin are the drugs of first choice. Clarithromycin may be substituted for erythromycin, the former being less likely to cause gastrointestinal upset, particularly nausea. The dose of erythromycin or clarithromycin will need to be reduced in patients with renal impairment. For the more severely ill patient with community-acquired pneumonia, a second- or third-generation cephalosporin (e.g. cefuroxime) plus erythromycin is the best first-line combination. For nosocomial pneumonia, a quinolone (e.g. ciprofloxacin) *plus* an aminoglycoside, *or* a second- or third-generation cephalosporin *plus* an aminoglycoside, should be employed. For patients with suspected aspiration, ampicillin or amoxycillin plus metronidazole is the most usual treatment. However, some authorities now recommend cefuroxime plus metronidazole in order to "cover" Gram-negative aspirates reliably. Ciprofloxacin should never be used alone in the primary treatment of pneumonia as it does not reliably kill pneumococcus.

Modification of antibiotic treatment may prove necessary once the results of sputum or blood culture are available.

The British Thoracic Society Guidelines on pneumonia have recently been published.[84]

Prognosis of pneumonia

Mortality from pneumonia is high in the elderly population. Most studies suggest mortality rates of 15–35 percent or even higher in the frailest elderly.[39,57,68,73,82,85] As well as deaths directly related to pneumonia, some (probably a minority) die of complications such as stroke and pulmonary embolus. Factors predicting death include tachopnea, dehydration, and hypotension.[86] Patients may spend prolonged periods in hospital and take many months to resume full activity.[39] The resolution of radiological abnormalities may be extremely slow, with nearly a third remaining abnormal 3 months after admission.[38] Thus a "slowly resolving" persistently abnormal chest X-ray should not necessarily prompt further investigations in the medium term, especially invasive investigations, unless there are accompanying persisting clinical features, or worsening signs on radiology (particularly progressive collapse).

Bronchiectasis

The true prevalence of bronchiectasis in the elderly population of the UK is unknown, but overall it is a relatively rare condition affecting 1–2 per 1,000 population. A recent Finnish study has suggested an overall prevalence of bronchiectasis in that country of 39 cases per million total population, rising to 104 cases per million in the over-65s.[87] For most patients the condition is merely a nuisance or a social embarrassment.

However, a minority (particularly those colonized by *Pseudomonas aeruginosa*) will have rapidly progressive disease with repeated severe exacerbations.

It is defined in terms of pathological changes: dilated bronchi and bronchioles and ciliary absence or dysfunction. Its causes are varied and include rare congenital causes (e.g. Kartagener's syndrome: bronchiectasis in association with dextrocardia) and cystic fibrosis (patients under 40 years). It can be post-infective (e.g. following tuberculosis or whooping cough) or obstructive (e.g. foreign body, carcinoma). It occurs rarely in association with pulmonary eosinophilia, *Aspergillus* infection, and allergic bronchopulmonary aspergillosis.[88]

There is replacement of the bronchial wall with squamous epithelium, often with ulceration; usually destruction of the bronchial walls and cartilage with significant infiltration of the lumen with inflammatory cells, particularly neutrophils; and hypertrophy of the bronchial arterial tree.

Typical clinical features are cough and the production of large amounts of purulent sputum (often deeply green). Hemoptysis is common (usually only streaks or small amounts but occasionally severe). Halitosis may produce profound social embarrassment in a minority. There is often associated airways obstruction, and severe bronchiectasis may produce a restrictive ventilatory deficit. In such cases the patient will complain of dyspnea and/or wheeze. Clubbing is common and there are usually coarse or mid-character crepitations chronically present in the affected region(s). For any patient with more than mild disease, early stages of infection may be difficult to identify as they involve only a slight qualitative or quantitative change in the production of already purulent sputum, perhaps with recurrence or exacerbation of hemoptysis.

The interpretation of microbiological results is difficult for several reasons. Most patients are chronically colonized by a variety of organisms (most commonly *Haemophilus influenzae*[89]). Secondly, different areas of the abnormal bronchial tree may harbor different bacterial pathogens, making sputum sampling somewhat patchy and possibly unrepresentative. Thirdly, some patients with bronchiectasis harbor forms of *Haemophilus* difficult to identify on sputum culture because of absence of a cell wall.[90] Finally, a small proportion of patients with bronchiectasis may develop mycobacterial colonization and infection in the bronchiectatic lung, often with atypical mycobacteria such as *Mycobacterium avium intracellulare*.[91]

THERAPY Preventative therapy essentially comprises regular postural drainage. Supportive treatment for established exacerbation is similar to that discussed above for pneumonia (or below for tuberculosis), with the addition of increased postural drainage (possibly using oxygen via a nasal cannula as postural changes may produce hypoxia). Even in the absence of *Pseudomonas* infection there is need for broad-spectrum antibiotics with β-lactamase activity. Supranormal doses may be needed to achieve sputum penetration with some evidence of increased efficacy and a longer exacerbation-free interval.[92,93]

Patients who have infective relapses frequently may respond to nebulized antibiotics as prophylaxis.[93] Recurrent infection with *Pseudomonas aeruginosa* is particularly problematic. Oral ciprofloxacin is a first-line treatment, but in most cases the organism develops early resistance to this agent.

TUBERCULOSIS (MYCOBACTERIAL INFECTION)

The prevalence of tuberculosis (TB) is once again increasing in the Western world and in less developed countries, with a disproportionate rise in prevalence in elderly people.[94–107] This may partly be due to increasing urban deprivation which disproportionately affects the elderly,[108,109] and to relative ease of transmission in nursing and residential homes.[99,110,111] Whatever the reason for the increase, tuberculosis is more common in elderly people, with notification rates approximately five times those in young adults, in the 65–75 age range (approximately 20 per 10,000 population) and up to 12 times those in young adults in the over-75s (approximately 60 per 10,000).[96,97]

Most cases of tuberculosis in the elderly population represent reactivation of previous (often unrecognized) disease. This may be precipitated by the depressed immunocompetence of normal aging, malnutrition (often in association with alcohol excess), HIV infection, diabetes mellitus, corticosteroid therapy, gastrectomy,[112] and even cigarette smoking.[113] Tuberculosis incidence is higher among those with relatively low serum vitamin D levels (perhaps owing to vitamin D's role in modulating macrophage function).[114] This has particular implications for the elderly and for Asian immigrants to the UK.

Presentation of tuberculosis

Very often the presenting features in old age are similar to those in younger patients and include weight loss, cough, hemoptysis, pyrexia, and night sweats. However, elderly patients with tuberculosis more often present atypically than the younger patients (especially in the presence of other chronic illnesses), often with pyrexia of unknown origin or other nonspecific features.[111] There is also some evidence that hemoptysis is a less common presenting feature in old age.[115] Elderly people are more likely to have lymphopenia, hypoalbuminemia, abnormal liver function tests, hypokalemia, and hyponatremia.[100,116] Miliary tuberculosis seems more common in the elderly, this presentation occurring in up to 1 in 20 cases.[95] The presence of miliary tuberculosis in the elderly population seems to be increasing[117] and it is probably underdiagnosed in this age group.[118] Presentation in such cases may again be atypical and subacute.

Renal and genitourinary tuberculosis may be *less* common in older people[95] but when present is often asymptomatic. However, nonpulmonary tuberculosis appears generally more common in children and in elderly people.[119] Bony and joint tuberculosis affects approximately 5 percent of elderly patients with the disease.[95] It most commonly involves the spine, often with paravertebral infection.[120,121] Such patients usually present with back pain and tenderness and up to two-thirds are febrile.[121] Bone tuberculosis can also present in the small bones of the hand or foot when it is often associated with painless fracture.[122,123] Other well-recognized nonpulmonary sites in elderly people include lymph nodes (commonly the neck),[119] the ileocecal area,[124] and other areas of colon[125] (which may present with fever, diarrhea, weight loss, and abdominal pain). Tuberculous meningitis may be particularly difficult to diagnose in the elderly person owing to a combination of lack of meningism and an acellular CSF aspirate.[126] Worryingly, a failure to diagnose the condition during life in elderly people is evidenced by an up to 20-fold disparity (versus the young) in the number of cases diagnosed at post mortem.[95,127]

Mortality is high in tuberculosis in old age and even in the developed world may reach 20–30 percent.[100,115,128,129] Whilst this may in part reflect the often atypical presentation and a reluctance on the part of elderly patients and their physicians to undergo invasive diagnostic procedures, such as bone marrow aspiration and bronchoscopy, it also suggests a low index of suspicion among physicians.

Investigations

The radiological features of tuberculosis in the elderly population are often similar to those in younger patients, but there is a greater prevalence of mid and lower zone shadowing.[95,101,115,120–132] Other radiological features which may be more common in old age include decreased frequency of cavitation,[130] diffuse infiltrates, atelectasis, and isolated hilar or mediastinal lymphadenopathy or even a normal chest X-ray,[132] mass lesions,[133] and extensive infiltration in both lungs.[134] Nonetheless, the most common radiological appearance is that of old healed disease with a peripheral calcified primary complex and calcified hilar nodes together with upper zone patchy calcification and possibly pleural thickening ("capping"). Cavitation is present in 20–30 percent of cases and pleural effusions in approximately 15 percent.[95,130] In such cases it may be difficult to differentiate tuberculosis from primary lung malignancy, especially in apical disease. The CT scan may be of use here when more invasive tests are thought inappropriate. A normal chest X-ray *almost* excludes pulmonary tuberculosis, though a very rare exception is endobronchial post-primary disease.[135] Endobronchial disease may also present with mass lesions.[136]

Other useful screening investigations include C-reactive protein or ESR estimation and tuberculin skin test, although the latter must be interpreted with caution in elderly patients with possible post-primary disease. Biochemical abnormalities (as discussed above) are common, as is a normochromic normocytic anemia and mildly raised peripheral white blood cell count.

A grade 3 or 4 positive Heaf skin test (a ring of six confluent papules filled-in at the center with induration and ulceration) or a >10 mm reaction on Mantoux skin testing is diagnostic of present *or past* tuberculous infection. Thus the emergence or "conversion" from skin test negativity to skin test positivity suggests active disease. However, repeated skin testing is known to produce a "booster" effect. This phenomena occurs in those who have suffered previous (often asymptomatic) infection but whose skin test reactivity has fallen over many years and is subsequently stimulated once again by skin testing—so that a first test is negative but a second or subsequent test may be positive.[137] More commonly a tuberculin skin test may be falsely negative in association with other infections (bacterial or viral), or with corticosteroid use, sarcoidosis, lymphoma, malnutrition, or even massive overwhelming tuberculous infection.

Isolation of *Mycobacterium tuberculosis* is the only *absolute* confirmation of active infection. The organism is isolated from approximately two-thirds of elderly patients treated for active disease, a slightly lower percentage than that in younger patients.[95] Smear positivity (identification of the organism by simple Ziehl–Neelsen or Kinyoun staining of sputum) in an untreated patient is very highly suggestive of infectivity. More commonly, sputum culture in a Lowenstein–Jensen medium is necessary and may require up to 8 weeks. Recommended practice is to send at least three good sputum samples for microscopy and culture before any antituberculous therapy is given.[138] This is important not only for confirmation of diagnosis but also to establish antimicrobial sensitivities.[138] Where sputum production is difficult this may be aided by physiotherapy and inhalation of ultrasonically nebulized saline. Bronchoscopy and washings of radiologically affected areas may occasionally be required, as may aspiration of pleural fluid together with pleural biopsy. Where renal or genitourinary infection is suspected, three samples of early-morning urine should be sent for microscopy and culture. Bone marrow aspiration, liver biopsy, synovial aspiration, or lymph node biopsy may be helpful in disseminated disease.

Treatment of tuberculosis

The British Thoracic Society (BTS) guidelines recommend that treatment of all patients should be supervised by physicians with full training in the management of tuberculosis and with direct working access to tuberculosis health visitors or nurse specialists.[138] In practice, this means that all elderly patients with tuberculosis should be referred to a department of respiratory medicine for supervision of their management.

For those with pulmonary disease, 6 months' treatment with rifampicin and isoniazid together with pyrazinamide and ethambutol for the first 2 months is advised. This is generally applicable to elderly people, with a possible reduction and dosage and monitoring of serum levels of ethambutol in patients with renal impairment. The same drugs may be appropriate to nonpulmonary disease, although the duration of chemotherapy may need to be longer (12 months for TB meningitis). Combined preparations are recognized to improve medication compliance, which may be particularly problematic.

Other agents may be helpful or even essential in a small minority of cases, depending on sensitivity results. These may include thiacetazone, para-aminosalicylic acid (PAS), capreomycin, kanomycin, cycloserine, prothionamide, and viomycin. Streptomycin is occasionally used but may produce vestibular damage and for this reason is usually avoided in the elderly patient.

Liver function tests should be checked before commencement of therapy. However, a transient hepatic enzyme rise is common and does not indicate the need for modification of treatment unless hepatitis or jaundice occur. If ethambutol is used, visual acuity should be checked by an ophthalmologist before and during treatment. Isoniazid-related peripheral neuropathy is preventable by pyridoxine 10 mg daily. Treatment side-effects seem to be more common in old people:[95,139] overall, almost 1 in 5 elderly people will experience treatment side-effects.

The BTS has also produced guidelines on the control and prevention of the spread of tuberculosis.[139] Patients with suspected pulmonary tuberculosis should be admitted to a single room *vented to the outside air* until their sputum status is known and risk assessments are made. Where there are other compromised patients on the ward, or where multiple drug-resistant tuberculosis is suspected or proven, patients

should remain in such a negative-pressure room. In other circumstances patients with pulmonary tuberculosis can be nursed in a normal single room on the ward. Patients with nonpulmonary tuberculosis can usually be nursed on a general ward. Patients whose bronchial washings are smear positive can usually be managed as noninfectious unless they have been in contact with compromised patients or they are known or suspected of having multiple drug-resistant tuberculosis.

The treatment of tuberculosis is not complete without contact tracing. The details of tracing procedures are beyond the scope of this article, so the reader is referred to BTS guidelines.[139] In contrast with data from the USA, there is little evidence that elderly residents of British nursing homes are at increased risk from tuberculosis.[140] If any recent resident of institutional care is diagnosed as having infectious tuberculosis, normal isolation and contact procedures should apply.[139]

ATYPICAL MYCOBACTERIAL INFECTION

This is relatively rare in Britain. There is no direct evidence that it is more common in elderly people, although some atypical mycobacteria seem to be more likely to cause infection in patients with pre-existing respiratory conditions which may be more common in elderly people.[141]

Clinical features of most atypical mycobacterial infections are similar to those of true tuberculosis, although upper lobe and pleural involvement appears to be more common.[142,143] Culture of nontuberculous mycobacteria may take longer than that of *Mycobacterium tuberculosis*, and sensitivity patterns are often unusual.

Clinical summaries and treatment guidelines have been published by the American Thoracic Society[142] and more recently by the British Thoracic Society.[143]

PULMONARY EMBOLIC DISEASE

Pulmonary embolic disease is common in elderly people population, particularly the ill elderly. It is estimated that over half of patients with pulmonary embolism are over the age of 65.[144] Indeed, the instance of pulmonary embolic disease increases exponentially with age.[145] Age-associated risk factors include immobility, malignancy, hemiplegia, cancer, surgery (especially orthopedic), hip fracture, and stroke.

Presentation

Clinical features of pulmonary embolism in elderly people differ little from those in the young.[146] They are usually acute and comprise breathlessness, severe central constricting chest pain (in large hemodynamically compromising emboli), pleuritic chest pain (in more peripheral emboli), and hemoptysis. Occasionally symptoms may be chronic or subacute due to multiple emboli and comprise gradual onset of breathlessness and right-sided cardiac failure. Only about one-fifth of elderly patients present atypically (usually with radiological abnormalities, most commonly linear atelectasis).[146] Presentation with atypical but consistent features in the context of known risks factors for pulmonary embolic disease or a clinical deep vein thrombosis should alert the physician to the strong possibility of pulmonary embolism.

Patients with very large emboli will present with chest pain, breathlessness, and severe hypotension, often with right ventricular heave and signs of right-sided cardiac strain. Physical signs as well as those of right-sided strain include tachypnea, cyanosis, tachycardia, localized crepitations, pleural rub, and (particularly in a patient with pre-existing asthma or COPD) wheeze.

Investigations

Unfortunately, diagnosis based on clinical features or on investigations short of pulmonary angiography is inaccurate, with high both false positive and false negative rates.[143,147] Diagnosis may be particularly difficult in patients (often elderly people) with previous respiratory disease. The accuracy of the ventilation–perfusion ($\dot{V}/\dot{Q}$) scan may be particularly compromised by this. Simple screening tests may do little other than enhance clinical suspicion. Electrocardiograms will show right-sided strain in a minority of cases. Abnormalities include right bundle branch block, P "pulmonale," S-wave in lead 1, Q-wave, and T-wave inversion in lead 3 ($S_1 Q_3 T_3$).[148–150] Pulmonary embolism may also precipitate atrial fibrillation. Blood gas estimation frequently reveals hypoxia in association with hypocapnia.[151] These findings are not specific. The chest X-ray may be normal (thus helping to exclude other pathologies) or occasionally may show effusions, basal atelectasis, or wedge-shaped areas of hypoperfusion.[150,152]

A ventilation–perfusion scan is the most widely used *diagnostic* test for pulmonary embolic disease. It is essentially non-invasive and can be performed rapidly in most patients. Unfortunately, many hospitals in the UK do not offer an "out-of-hours" service.[153] $\dot{V}/\dot{Q}$ scanning should be performed within 24 hours of clinical suspicion of pulmonary embolism.[154] Soon after this, scans may either normalize or show a matched defect. An entirely normal $\dot{V}/\dot{Q}$ scan performed within this time-frame essentially excludes pulmonary embolism. The presence of multiple perfusion defects with normal ventilation (a mis-matched scan) is highly suggestive of pulmonary embolic disease. In the context of clinical suspicion, up to a third of patients whose scans have been classified as having only low or intermediate probability for pulmonary embolism will in fact have pulmonary embolic disease.[143] Ventilation–perfusion scans should always be interpreted in the context of a chest radiograph performed on the same day.[154] The diagnostic value of ventilation–perfusion scanning is unaffected by age alone,[146] although many age-associated diseases (including COPD, cardiac failure, fibrotic lung disease, and bronchogenic carcinoma) may make interpretation difficult.

Arguably, the absolute diagnosis of minor or moderate pulmonary embolism is less critical in the presence of a proven diagnosis of deep venous thrombosis (DVT). Ultrasound and impedance plethysmography is the investigation of choice for potential DVT. It is as accurate as venography without the complications.[147]

The only absolutely definitive diagnostic investigation for pulmonary embolism is *pulmonary angiography*. This may be difficult or impossible in ill, frail, elderly patients and is not without risk—although the limited evidence available suggests the risks are no higher in elderly people.[146,147,155] Pulmonary angiography should be considered where other investigations have failed to establish a diagnosis or (urgently) when cardiovascular collapse or hypotension is present.[154]

For more details the reader is strongly referred to the British Thoracic Society guidelines on the management of pulmonary embolism.[154] These guidelines are particularly valuable for their discussion of spiral CT scanning, advances in lower limb ultrasound, the use of echocardiography, and the place of plasma D-dimer, detailed discussion of which is beyond the scope of this chapter.

Treatment of pulmonary embolism

Again the reader is referred to the British Thoracic Society guidelines.[154] Immediate supportive therapy comprises supplemental oxygen (usually a high inspired percentage as dictated by blood gas measurement) and analgesia in patients with pleuritic chest pain. Hypotensive patients should be resuscitated with colloid, and central venous pressure should be monitored with the aim of achieving a high pressure of 15–20 mmHg.[154] Anticoagulation, initially with intravenous or subcutaneous heparin, should aim to keep the activated partial thromboplastin time at about 1.5–2.5 times the control value. Low-molecular-weight heparin is as effective as standard heparin in the treatment of proximal deep vein thrombosis and non-life-threatening pulmonary embolism,[154] and needs no laboratory monitoring. Following 5–7 days of heparinization, maintenance therapy should be with oral anticoagulation, usually warfarin, aiming for an international normalized ratio (INR) of between 2 and 3. Recent evidence suggests that the traditional duration of anticoagulation was excessive, and that for pulmonary emboli 3 months of anticoagulation therapy is adequate, 1 month being adequate for DVT,[154,156] in the absence of a persisting underlying risk factor or thrombotic disorder.

Anticoagulation will need frequent hematological monitoring. Patients should receive written and verbal information regarding side-effects and what to do should these arise, as well as information on drug interactions and which drugs to avoid. Access to outpatient warfarin clinics may prove difficult for elderly patients, and domiciliary phlebotomy may need to be provided in some cases.

A small proportion of patients who suffer recurrent pulmonary emboli despite anticoagulation, or where anticoagulation is contraindicated, may benefit from the insertion of a filter device into the inferior vena cava.[154,157] These can now be inserted by a minimally invasive percutaneous procedure.

For patients with catastrophic acute pulmonary emboli associated with circulatory collapse the prognosis is dire, with a mortality rate of over 80 percent.[156] Thrombolysis is as successful as surgical embolectomy in such cases.[154] The British Thoracic Society guidelines therefore recommend thrombolysis in patients who are hemodynamically unstable and particularly those who have systemic hypotension.[154] The recommended dose is 250,000 units of streptokinase over 30 minutes followed by 100,000 units per hour for up to 24 hours. Hydrocortisone should be administered concurrently. Recombinant tissue plasminogen activator (rtPA) is an alternative. Thrombolysis is equally effective whether given through a pulmonary artery catheter or peripheral vein.

Great caution is needed with thrombolysis, especially in the early postoperative period.

Surgical embolectomy is rarely indicated but should be considered for a patient with massive pulmonary embolism who fails to respond to thrombolysis. It is clear that many frail elderly patients may not be suitable for such aggressive invasive measures. That is probably particularly true of those with medical conditions which put them at the highest risk of pulmonary embolic disease.

Prophylaxis of pulmonary embolism in the context of immobility, stroke, and surgery using pharmacological and physical measures (including compression hosiery) is recognized to dramatically reduce incidence, but there is widespread variation in practice [154] and need for more clinical trials particularly in stroke.

FIBROTIC (INTERSTITIAL) LUNG DISEASES

These conditions have a wide variety of pathologies and etiologies and are generally taken not to include carcinomas, lymphomas, other neoplasms, and infection. They have been the subject of recent guidelines published by the British Thoracic Society.[158]

The diagnosis and investigation of fibrotic interstitial lung disease is complex. Furthermore, even the less rare of the conditions described below is common. For both of these reasons, elderly patients with suspected interstitial lung disease who do not respond to the withdrawal of potential causative agents should be referred to a specialist respiratory physician for assessment, diagnosis, and management.

Epidemiology

Many fibrotic interstitial lung diseases have a higher incidence in elderly people. These include the relatively common conditions of fibrosing alveolitis in association with connective tissue disorders, cryptogenic fibrosing alveolitis (160 per 100,000 in the over-75s),[159] and the pneumoconioses associated with industrial dust exposure. Some of the rarer conditions are also more common in the elderly population. These include Wegener's granulomatosis, amyloidosis, and cryptogenic organizing pneumonia. Conversely, sarcoidosis is extremely rare as a primary presentation in elderly people, and chronic eosinophilic pneumonia is less common than in younger adults.

Mortality rate from all causes of pulmonary fibrosis is increasing in both men and women.[160] Deaths from all fibrotic causes (both absolute numbers of deaths and percentage of deaths per head of age-stratified population) peak in the 75–84 age group.[160] Over a near 20-year period (1979–96), the death rate from cryptogenic fibrosing alveolitis in England and Wales rose from 336 to 1035 cases,[161] with a much higher overall mortality with increasing age.[162]

Investigations

Fibrotic interstitial lung diseases classically produce a restrictive ventilatory defect on spirometry (relatively preserved forced expiratory flow with a reduced forced vital capacity and thus a normal or raised FEV_1/FVC ratio). Wegener's granulomatosis, however, usually produces an obstructive pattern (low FEV_1/FVC ratio). Total lung capacity is reduced, as is the transfer factor (TL_{CO}). The transfer coefficient (K_{CO}) which is essentially the transfer factor corrected for lung volumes is generally affected later than the TL_{CO}. Blood gas analysis commonly reveals hypoxia, often with hypocapnia (the latter secondary to hyperventilation).

Chest radiography may be normal in early disease, and even in some more advanced cases.[163] More commonly, characteristic parenchymal shadowing may be present, in the form of reticular, nodular, reticulonodular, linear, or ground-glass appearances. The distribution of such shadowing may be a clue to the diagnosis. For example, a "reversed bat's wing" appearance (peripheral shadowing) is commonly seen in chronic pulmonary eosinophilia and cryptogenic organizing pneumonia. The presence of nonparenchymal abnormalities on chest X-ray (e.g. eggshell calcification of hilar lymph nodes in silicosis, or pleural involvement in association with asbestosis) may be helpful. However, diagnosis based on the type of distribution of shadowing on chest radiographs is possible in fewer than 20 percent of cases.[164,165]

Conversely, CT or high-resolution CT scanning has a high diagnostic accuracy (approximately 95 percent).[164,166–168] Classification of CT scan abnormalities is based both upon the site of the abnormality and its nature. Abnormalities may be classified according to sites or compartments: the peripheral compartment (the pleura and interlobular sector); the middle compartment (most of the central areas of the lung); and the axial compartment (immediately surrounding the mediastinum and extending along the lymphatics, vascular and bronchial structures). A variety of characteristic abnormalities is seen, including a ground-glass appearance suggesting very active disease, a nodular appearance often associated with sarcoidosis and pneumoconiosis, or a cystic appearance of end-stage alveolitis.

CT patterns may be so helpful (both in diagnosis and estimation of disease activity and progression[166]) as sometimes to render other investigations such as lung biopsy redundant.[169] Occasionally bronchoalveolar lavage (BAL) may be indicated for differential diagnosis, and characteristic patterns of cellular abnormality have been described in different conditions.[170] Guidelines for the use of bronchial lavage are available.[171] Bronchial alveolar lavage can occasionally be diagnostic, particularly in suspected malignancy, infections, and some of the rarer forms of fibrotic lung disease. There is, however, as yet a poor evidence base on the value of this technique in diagnosis and assessment of prognosis of the more common forms of fibrotic lung disease. A more detailed description of this technique is beyond the scope of the present chapter, so the reader is referred to the European Respiratory Society and the British Thoracic Society guidelines.[158,172]

BIOPSY Lung biopsy may be by means of transbronchial technique, a percutaneous drill technique, or an open technique. All of these procedures involve morbidity and a small risk of mortality (see below) and so should not be undertaken lightly. Even if the patient is fit for biopsy, it is probably unnecessary in those with stable or mild disease or with a typical presentation.

When biopsy *is* necessary, transbronchial lung biopsy is least invasive and can be performed in patients who would be unfit for open biopsy. Multiple transbronchial biopsies are usually taken, with a high diagnostic rate,[173] especially in a disease with a characteristic histological pattern. The mortality rate of transbronchial biopsy in one very large series was 0.2 percent, the most common complications (overall rate less than 10 percent) being pneumothorax and bleeding.[174] Sampling error may pose diagnostic difficulties.

Percutaneous drill biopsy has been little studied and is not commonly used. This may reflect its slightly higher complication rate and lower diagnostic yield when compared with transbronchial biopsy.

Open lung biopsy is a surgical procedure, requiring a general anesthetic. It is most commonly employed when transbronchial biopsy has failed to achieve a diagnosis. As well as producing enough material for increased diagnostic certainty, the larger sample is usually able to produce a good estimate of disease activity. The mortality rate, however, is about 1 percent. Other complications include infection and persistent pneumothorax in approximately one in six patients.[175–177]

Specific conditions

Pneumoconiosis

This disease results from an abnormal lung parenchymal reaction to inspired *inorganic* dusts, usually in an occupational context. The most common dusts involved are coal (producing coal-workers' pneumoconiosis), silica (producing silicosis), and asbestos (producing asbestosis).

Coal-workers' pneumoconiosis is the result of fibrosis in alveoli and interlobular sectors with compensatory dilatation of other alveoli leading to centrilobular emphysema. This may progress (even after cessation of occupational exposure) to the insidious complicated pneumoconiosis or progressive massive fibrosis (PMF). PMF mainly affects the upper lobes which contain large fibrotic masses several centimeters across, often with necrotic centers. PMF is associated with the increased likelihood of autoimmune antibodies such as antinuclear antibody and rheumatoid factor.[178] Occasionally, in patients with rheumatoid arthritis, Caplan's syndrome may result. This takes the form of flitting radiological lesions in the lung which occasionally necrose or calcify. These may be associated with pleural effusion.

An obstructive ventilatory picture is common in patients with simple pneumoconiosis, especially where there is associated central alveolar emphysema. PMF produces both restrictive and obstructive defects, the restrictive defects in part being the result of reduced lung volume. Progression to cor pulmonale and respiratory failure is not uncommon.

Symptoms usually comprise those of chronic bronchitis together with the production of coal-stained black sputum (melanoptysis). Patients often erroneously feel that they have coughed up blood, although true hemoptysis is indeed common in PMF. Patients are not clubbed. General fatigue and loss of weight are common, particularly in severe end-stage disease.

There is no specific treatment other than supportive therapy and treatment of any reversibility of airways obstruction. Smoking cessation should be strongly encouraged and supported.

Silicosis

There is a high occupational risk for this disease in quarrying, sand blasting, mining (copper, tin, gold), boiler workers, and some forms of brick manufacture.

Acute silicosis may occur after intense brief exposure to silica dust, and such exposure is rare in old age. The condition is associated with extreme dyspnea and a chest X-ray appearance similar to that of pulmonary edema. It may be fatal within weeks or months. More commonly, chronic silicosis has similar pathological features to coal-workers' pneumoconiosis, with fibrosis of lymphatics, blood vessels, and bronchi, and some degree of secondary emphysema. Active chronic silicosis predisposes to pulmonary tuberculosis.

There are usually mixed obstructive and restrictive ventilatory defects, hypoxia, and cor pulmonale in the later stages. Typical radiological findings include miliary or nodular lesions throughout all the lung fields, especially in the middle and upper zones. There may in addition be larger (sometimes cavitated) shadowing. Eggshell calcification of the hilar lymph nodes is pathognomonic.

Symptoms are gradually progressive over several years. They are similar to those of chronic bronchitis and chronic obstructive pulmonary disease together with occasional hemoptysis, cachexia, and weight loss. In such circumstances tuberculosis needs to be actively excluded. Treatment is once again supportive (including smoking cessation).

Asbestosis

This is a fibrotic condition of the lungs due to usually prolonged occupational exposure to asbestos dust. Occupations at greatest risk include shipyard workers, asbestos factory workers, plumbers and gas fitters, insulation workers, rail workers, electricians, demolition workers, and builders. Asbestosis must be distinguished from asbestos-related pleural thickening and calcification, mesothelioma, and bronchogenic carcinoma—all of which can also be precipitated by asbestos exposure. Fibrosis originates in the alveoli and bronchioles. It is most marked in the lung bases but may spread to involve the whole of the lungs. Progressive massive fibrosis is not a common feature.

A recent survey has shown that there may be a nihilistic attitude towards fibrotic interstitial lung disease in those previously exposed to asbestos. This is inappropriate, especially as approximately 5 percent of such individuals in fact have another treatable interstitial lung disease.[179]

In common with mesothelioma and bronchial carcinoma, the latent period after exposure before the development of asbestosis may be in excess of 20 years and it is not unusual for symptoms to appear for the first time in an elderly person.

The major ventilatory defect is restrictive, with reduced transfer factor and reduced total lung compliance. Radiological appearances include fine mottling and patchy streaky fibrosis, often with associated pleural lesions (a diagnostic clue), most commonly on the diaphragm (coin lesions).

Symptoms initially comprise breathlessness on exertion and later cough, weight loss, and fatigue. Patients are usually clubbed with fine bilateral basal crepitations in nearly two-thirds of patients.[180] Treatment is supportive. Because of the recognized synergistic association of asbestos exposure and tobacco smoking in the etiology of bronchogenic carcinoma, smoking cessation should be encouraged and supported perhaps even more strongly in this condition than in other forms of fibrotic lung disease.

Extrinsic allergic alveolitis

This disease is essentially a type III immological reaction to organic dusts at the alveolar level. It follows chronic repeated exposure and is associated with the formation of systemic precipitating antibodies (precipitins). An acute form (type I reaction) can occur more rarely, with shivers, acute dyspnea, and cough. "Budgerigar-fanciers' lung" is probably the most common form.[181] There is some suggestion that the keeping of budgerigars as pets is most common in the elderly population, but that, independent of this, age is still an important prognostic indicator.[182] Other extrinsic alveolitides include "farmers' lung" (secondary to moulds in damp straw and hay), ventilation pneumonitis (due to thermophylic actinomycetes in air-conditioning systems), and "mushroom workers' lung" (from mushroom spores).

Symptoms include breathlessness on exertion, progressing to breathlessness at rest with production of sputum. Clubbing is uncommon but when present may be associated with a poorer prognosis.[183] Weight loss (often marked) is not unusual. Crackles on auscultation occur in only about one in four patients.[180] Diffuse ground-glass or micronodular patterns are the most common radiological abnormalities, and etiological diagnosis is by identification of the appropriate serum precipitins.

Treatment comprises removal of (or from) the offending antigen. This may prove difficult in a patient who is particularly attached to a pet. Furthermore, in some affected patients the disease is not progressive despite continued exposure to the offending antigen, whereas in others removal of the antigen does not prevent progression.[184] Some patients may require corticosteroid or immunosuppressive therapy, as discussed below for cryptogenic fibrosing alveolitis.

Cryptogenic fibrosing alveolitis

This is the most common interstitial lung disease in the elderly population. Estimates of the peak age at presentation have increased recently to a mean of about 60 years.[185] There may be a slight male excess in the prevalence.[186] Overall the estimated prevalence is about 5 cases per 100,000 population. There is a rare familial form of the disease but otherwise its etiology is unknown.

Histological appearances are many and varied. The two ends of the spectrum of histology are (a) a fibrotic pattern in which the alveoli are replaced by collagen and there is very little active inflammation, and (b) a cellular pattern with infiltration of lymphocytes, neutrophils, and eosinophils into the interstitium with the alveolar spaces containing larger numbers of macrophages. It is possible but not certain that the cellular form *progresses* to the fibrotic form. However, the cellular appearance is associated with an increased chance of steroid responsiveness and with a better prognosis.[186,187]

The typical presentation is breathlessness on exertion progressing to breathlessness at rest. There is some suspicion that elderly patients present later than younger patients, possibly because of reduced appreciation of breathlessness.[188] Many patients complain of a productive cough, and the volume of sputum produced relates negatively to prognosis.[189] Minor hemoptysis is fairly common. The vast majority of patients will have fine crepitations ("velcro-crep") at the bases, possibly extending to mid and even upper zones.[190,191] The majority

are clubbed[180] and hypertrophic pulmonary osteoarthropathy has been described.

In most patients the disease progresses slowly and insidiously, with an untreated 50 percent mortality at about 5 years.[185] In the rarer (though classically described) Hamman Rich syndrome, progression is more rapid (about 6 months to death if untreated). In such cases there may be pyrexia, cough, and purulent sputum.

There is a strong association with bronchial carcinoma. Advanced age seems to be associated with a poorer prognosis and with a recently recognized rise in overall mortality from the condition.[161,162,180,192]

Chest radiographs vary from normal to ground-glass appearance or miliary mottling. Abnormalities may be diffuse but are most common in the lower zones.

In addition to supportive treatment as for pneumoconiosis, specific treatment regimens are advocated for cryptogenic fibrosing alveolitis. It is perhaps surprising that there are no controlled trials comparing corticosteroid treatment with placebo for cryptogenic fibrosing alveolitis, the evidence being based on retrospective reviews.[158] There is, perhaps because of this, limited consensus on when to start treatment, even in younger patients, although in practice the decision is often based on clinical evidence of progressive disease. A relatively old survey suggested that elderly patients tend to receive less corticosteroid therapy than the young.[193] The objective response rate to high-dose corticosteroid therapy varies from 16–37 percent overall, but possibly less in elderly people (again based on retrospective reviews).[158] Clinical experience would suggest that the addition of azathioprine to high-dose corticosteroid therapy increases the response rate to perhaps as much as 50 percent. However, again there are no controlled trials which unequivocally show extra benefit from adding azathioprine to steroid therapy.[158] There is similar lack of controlled-trial evidence for the use of cyclophosphamide, which is commonly associated with the side-effects requiring a discontinuation of therapy. There seems to be little benefit in using immunosuppressives in a steroid-sparing role.[194,195]

The standard dose of prednisolone in high-dose regimens is up to 100 mg daily for up to 6–8 weeks, reducing by approximately 20 mg per day each month to a maintenance daily dose of 10 mg. However, as the British Thoracic Society guidelines point out,[158] there are no good comparative data on dose regimens or duration of therapy. Any response is usually seen within 3 months, and a response to corticosteroids is usually associated with improved survival—though it is unclear whether this is a causative relation.[158]

Fibrosing alveolitis in association with autoimmune disorders

Autoimmune disorders, particularly rheumatoid arthritis but also Sjorgren's syndrome, systemic sclerosis, and celiac disease, can lead to fibrotic lung disease in up to 5 percent of cases. Occasionally respiratory problems precede other manifestations of the disease. The association with rheumatoid arthritis and fibrotic lung disease seems stronger for elderly patients, and the condition is twice as common in men. Pathology and clinical features are very similar to those of cryptogenic fibrosing alveolitis, although pleural changes are more common on the chest radiograph.

Fibrosing alveolitis in association with systemic sclerosis probably has a better prognosis than cryptogenic fibrosing alveolitis.[196,197] The rate of progression of the disease appears slower. Corticosteroids, D-penicillamine, cyclophosphamide, and chlorambucil have been used in uncontrolled and/or retrospective trials with some evidence of benefit.[158]

In contrast to systemic sclerosis, fibrosing alveolitis in association with rheumatoid arthritis has a similar progression to cryptogenic fibrosing alveolitis.[190] Again there are very few controlled studies of corticosteroid and immunosuppressive therapy. The British Thoracic Society guidelines recommend that treatment should be similar to that for cryptogenic fibrosing alveolitis.[158]

Wegener's granulomatosis

This relatively rare condition is most common in the elderly population, with a peak age of onset at about 55 years. It is a granulomatous and vasculitic condition principally affecting the lung, upper respiratory tract, and kidneys. Patients present (either acutely, chronically, or following a relapsing and remitting course) with upper and lower respiratory symptoms including breathlessness, pleuritic chest pain, cough, hemoptysis, epistaxis, sinusitis, rhinitis, and otitis. However, upper respiratory problems are less common in elderly people, and renal involvement at initial diagnosis is more common in this age group.[198] Central nervous system involvement (vasculitis usually presenting with acute confusion or fits) is relatively common in old age.[198] Infective complications are not more prevalent in elderly people, although mortality from infection is significantly more common in this age group.[198]

Diagnosis is usually by biopsy of the upper and lower respiratory tract or kidneys.[199–201] Circulating antineutrophyl cytoplasmic antibodies (ANCA) are usually positive in the majority of patients.[198]

The usual treatment regimens comprise cyclophosphamide and high-dose steroids, with initially up to a 90 percent response rate at about 6–12 months. However, relapse rates are high (up to 50 percent).[202] There is no evidence that elderly patients with Wegener's granulomatosis show a less aggressive form of the disease, and intensive chemotherapy is usually indicated. Although infection is the cause of mortality in a large proportion of elderly patients, this does not seem to correlate with immune suppression due to chemotherapy.[200,203] Indeed there is no evidence that elderly people are more likely to suffer complications of treatment for this condition.

Drug-induced interstitial lung disease

Despite an overall incidence of adverse drug reactions of 10–25 percent in elderly people,[204] there is little evidence that elderly people are more prone to adverse drug reactions producing inflammatory lung disease.[205,206] However, such iatrogenic disease is more common in this age group probably by virtue of the increased exposure to multiple drugs. Perhaps the most commonly prescribed causes of iatrogenic lung disease are carbamazepine, phenytoin, nitrofurantoin, amiodarone, and aspirin. Others include the cytotoxic agents methotrexate, bleomycin, and busulphan, together with gold salts, penicillamine, sulphasalazine, and hydrallazine. Of particular relevance to elderly people is the occasional occurrence of lipoid pneumonia secondary to the chronic ingestion and aspiration of liquid paraffin. A careful drug history is essential, and it should be remembered that some drugs, particularly amiodarone and cyclophosphamide, may have been used without apparent problems by the patient for several years before the development of symptoms.[207,208]

Treatment comprises withdrawal of the offending drug with occasionally recourse to specific anti-inflammatory therapies.

Cryptogenic organizing pneumonia

This is a rare condition but is again slightly more common in the elderly population, with a peak age of onset of 50–60 years. It is characterized by the appearance of buds of connective tissue in the alveoli and small bronchioles. Presenting features are breathlessness on exertion, cough (a prominent symptom) and, in the majority of patients, pyrexia, weight loss, and general malaise. Clubbing is unusual. Radiological appearances are usually patchy and peripheral.

It shows a rapid (sometimes within days) and frequent (60 percent or more) response to high-dose corticosteroid therapy. Over half of the responders will relapse on stopping corticosteroids.

Chronic eosinophilic pneumonia

Once again this is a rare disease and is probably even rarer in the elderly population. Most patients have an atopic history, and thus wheeze is a common feature. Treatment with high dose corticosteroids (and occasionally other immunosuppressants) is usual.

Sarcoid lung disease

Over the whole population, sarcoidosis is the most common idiopathic interstitial lung disease. However, the appearance of sarcoidosis for the first time in an elderly patient is extremely unusual. There is limited evidence that when this does occur the prognosis is slightly worse. Serum angiotensin converting enzyme (ACE) does not have high sensitivity (approximately 60 percent) and has quite low specificity in the detection of sarcoidosis.[209,210] Its routine use is not recommended.[158]

The role of lung transplantation in fibrotic lung disease

Current guidelines suggest an upper age limit for lung transplantation of 65 years.[158] This is somewhat paradoxical as most fibrotic lung diseases are more common in the elderly population. However, there is no evidence base for lung transplantation in patients beyond their sixth decade. Indeed, the upper age limit of 65 years is 5 years higher than the usual upper limit for other organ transplantation.

KEY POINTS Nonobstructive lung disease

- British Thoracic Society Guidelines have recently been published in respect of pulmonary embolism, fibrotic lung disease, pneumonia and tuberculosis, and the reader is strongly advised to consult these.

- Tuberculosis is increasing in prevalence across the world, with a disproportionate rise in elderly people.

- Management of both tuberculosis and of fibrotic lung disease is a specialist domain and patients should be referred to respiratory physicians.

- Influenza vaccination is now recommended (in most western countries) for all people over the age of 65 years.

LUNG CANCERS

Lung cancer incidence rates are in general high and increase with age to a maximum at 80 years in men and 70 years in women. Above this, there is then a decline in incidence with increasing age. The high incidence of lung cancer with age probably reflects the highly carcinogenic nature of the by-products of cigarette smoking together with the lag period between the start of exposure to cigarette smoke and the development of lung cancer.[211]

Over time, the incidence of lung cancer has steadily fallen in males, especially during 1991–95. The decrease is probably due to the gradual decrease in the number of male smokers in the UK.[212,213] The increase in women smoking may also explain both the absolute and relative increase in lung cancer in females.

Pleural mesothelioma is the result of exposure to asbestos dust that may have occurred over a short or prolonged period. In the UK it primarily occurs as a result of occupational exposure. Owing to the long latent period (sometimes 20–40 years) between exposure to asbestos and development of the mesothelioma, it commonly occurs in older people.[214] Mesothelioma usually presents with a pleural effusion or pain due to invasion of the chest wall. In approximately 50 percent of patients pleural aspiration and conventional pleural biopsy will yield positive results.[215] If this fails to reveal either the diagnosis or positive histopathology, thoracoscopy with direct visualization of the pleura almost always provides the evidence required.[216] The treatment of mesothelioma is almost always palliative. Mean survival is less than 12 months and unfortunately the tumor is insensitive to chemotherapy or radiotherapy.

Unfortunately the true incidence of lung cancer in older people may be underestimated. As patients become older, the number who present to cancer registries as Death Certificate Only (DCO) cases increases. While 6 percent of men and 8 percent of women between the ages of 60 and 64 years present as DCO cases of lung cancer, these figures rise to 18 percent and 22 percent, respectively, for men and women aged 85 years or above.

Non-small-cell lung cancer (NSCLC) accounts for approximately 80 percent of all cases, with small-cell lung cancer (SCLC) accounting for the remaining 20 percent.[217]

INVESTIGATIONS OF SUSPECTED LUNG CANCER

A high index of suspicion is necessary. While the specific symptoms of cough, hemoptysis, and breathlessness may point towards pulmonary pathology, the coexistence of COPD or the patient attributing the symptoms to normal aging may delay diagnosis. Nonspecific symptoms such as weight loss, tiredness, or even the "giants of geriatric medicine" (confusion, falls, immobility, incontinence) make diagnosis even more difficult. Elderly patients present with more advanced disease and therefore investigations must be timely to ensure that both curative and palliative therapy are available.

It is imperative that patients be investigated fully before treatment decisions are made. Even if no active therapy is to be instigated, patients require a definitive diagnosis to ensure that they have access to palliative care services as well as practical and financial support. Bronchoscopy can be both diagnostic and therapeutic; and despite some concerns about its safety and efficacy, there is no evidence to support the exclusion of older people from such investigations.

In a study of 45 patients with a mean age of 65 years undergoing bronchoscopy, cardiovascular monitoring showed that the mean blood pressure rose initially with a further rise on intratracheal injection and remained high throughout the procedure.[218] The mean pulse rate rose from 93 to 134 bpm during the bronchoscopy, and in four patients an unexpected ST depression developed. A further three patients developed a bundle branch block; and when these seven patients were considered together they were older (72 versus 61 years), smoked more (63 versus 39 pack years) and had a greater tachycardia and higher blood pressure at commencement of the procedure. This and a study by Matot et al.[219] encourage the routine administration of atropine and ECG and oximetry monitoring. As many as 17 percent of the older subjects studied had myocardial ischemia which lasted 20 ± 8 minutes but had no permanent impairment.

Brown et al.[220] found that patients with suspected lung cancer who were reviewed by chest physicians were more likely to have a histological diagnosis which then increased the probability of their receiving active treatment ($P < 0.001$) than those patients seen by either a generalist or a geriatrician. Older people were significantly less likely to be reviewed by a chest physician ($P < 0.001$), and thereby less likely to have both histological verification and active treatment.

Although Kant et al.[221] found that presentation of lung cancer increased with advanced age, older people were more likely to have the stage of the cancer designated as unknown compared with younger people. In males this effect was significant ($P < 0.05$).

TREATMENT OF LUNG CANCER

Treatment principles

The treatment of choice for all lung cancer is surgery. This offers the main hope of cure for both NSCLC and SCLC. In addition, radiotherapy is suitable for either curative or palliative treatment of NSCLC, and either as palliative treatment of SCLC or as consolidation treatment either to the primary site or prophylactic cranial irradiation after definitive treatment of SCLC with chemotherapy. The main role for chemotherapy is in SCLC and in most cases it is palliative. There is increasing interest in the role of chemotherapeutic agents in the management of patients with NSCLC, although the data, particularly in older people, are still poor. Clearly, before major recommendations are made to elderly people the results of clinical trials are vital.

Trimble et al.[222] found that people aged 65 or above were under-represented in clinical cancer trials, given that cancer incidence and prevalence for this population. Men aged 65 years or older account for only 47.3 percent of patients in lung cancer trials and women only 43.6 percent of the trial population, despite over 50 percent of all lung cancer being in patients aged 75 years or above.

In order to promote evidence-based medicine within the National Health Service (NHS) in the UK, guidelines are playing an ever-expanding role in clinical practice.[223] The NHS Executive publishes cancer guidelines in two forms: Firstly the Manual and secondly the research evidence underpinning the guidance. The former provides the key recommendations for cancer care whereas the research document provides a summary of evidence that is relevant to the recommendations made in the manual. For lung cancer both documents were published in June 1998.[224,225]

Specific treatment of lung cancer includes surgery, radiotherapy, or chemotherapy commenced within 6–12 months of diagnosis. There is a marked decrease in the proportion of lung cancer patients who have specific treatment by age. Specific treatment decreases from more than 70 percent in younger age groups to under 10 percent in the older age groups. Males are significantly more likely than females to have specific treatment for lung cancer.

Surgery for lung cancer

For NSCLC, surgery offers the best hope of cure (Table 43-1). However, irrespective of the patient's age, 50 percent of tumors are obviously unresectable at initial presentation. Cardiovascular and respiratory diseases are common comorbid conditions that influence both morbidity and mortality.

Table 43-1 Surgical options for patients with NSCLC, by stage

Stage	Surgical option
I or IIa	Lobectomy or pneumonectomy
IIb or IIIa	Expert clinical judgment
IIIb or IV	No surgery

Preoperative staging is essential, and whilst CT and MRI scanning may detect the presence of lymphadenopathy this does not necessarily equate with metastatic disease, nor does the absence of lymphadenopathy confirm localized disease. Thus some tumors assessed as operable may be found to be inoperable at thoracotomy.

Age alone is not incompatible with curative resection, although a less radical resection may be advisable if the patient has existing comorbidity.[226] Unfortunately older patients are less likely to be referred for surgery despite having an operable tumor.[227–229]

Pneumonectomy is more commonly performed than lobectomy. In a group of 27 patients aged 70 years or above, operative mortality was 22 percent (compared with 3.2 percent in younger patients), and the 5-year survival was 11.5 percent (versus 30.5 percent). The apparent 19 percent difference in 5-year survival might suggest that pneumonectomy should be avoided in patients over 70 years of age. However, the study shows that two-thirds of patients in the older group survived up to 5 years following surgery after the initial postoperative mortality was accounted for, and this is similar to those patients under 70 years of age.[230]

It has been suggested that if patients can undergo lobectomy rather than pneumonectomy, survival is improved.[231] These authors also highlighted the need for preoperative digoxin, subcutaneous heparin, veno-occlusive stockings, and aggressive perioperative pulmonary toilet to reduce morbidity. They found that despite these measures the morbidity and mortality figures for older patients were worse than for the general group, but differed little from a further high-risk group studied.

Surgery should not be withheld even from octogenarians who may undergo surgery with an intention to cure. For 54 octogenarians undergoing either lobectomy or pneumonectomy, the mean postoperative stay was 6.3 days.[232] The overall 1-year survival was 86 percent and for stage I disease was 97 percent. The 5-year survival was 43 percent, with 57 percent for stage I disease.

Whilst most authors suggest that both morbidity and mortality are increased in those patients undergoing pneumonectomy when compared with those undergoing more limited resection, this was not the finding of Sioris et al.[233] In their series of 75 patients aged 75 years or above (of whom 13 were aged over 80), the overall perioperative mortality was 9 percent and morbidity was 29 percent, which included 21 percent of patients who had major complications. They found that mortality did not differ significantly between resection types but morbidity did, with an incidence of 13 percent in patients with limited resection, 21 percent after lobectomy, 50 percent after bilobectomy, and 60 percent after pneumonectomy.

Radiotherapy for lung cancer

Although the majority of radiotherapy is palliative in intent, some patients may be cured by aggressive therapy. It is therefore important that the side-effects of radiotherapy not be worse than the symptoms of the disease itself. Whilst conditions such as hypertension and diabetes may complicate the outcome of radiotherapy, it is important to separate the effects of normal aging from those of comorbidity. The safe delivery of radiotherapy requires immobilization and cooperation between patient and staff, and there is no evidence that older patients are less cooperative than younger ones. However, older patients with chronic arthritis, and/or respiratory or cardiac insufficiency, may find immobilization in the supine position difficult.[234]

Elderly patients with a tumor that is inoperable for medical reasons or simply because of age are often referred for radiotherapy,[235] and this may be the only therapy they receive.

Limited SCLC is best treated with a combination of chemotherapy and radiotherapy. In order to avoid toxicity, many patients are treated with palliative rather than curative intent. Additionally, it has been found that a combined approach using chemotherapy and radiotherapy does not result in unacceptable toxicity in this age group.[236]

In a study of over 1200 patients with primary bronchial or esophageal tumors from six prospective EORTC trials, Pignon et al.[237] found no association between age and the occurrence of acute toxicity. Indeed no difference was seen between acute or late toxicity, and the only important prognostic indicator was weight loss, which did show a trend with older people experiencing more loss of weight.

The clinical syndrome of *radiation pneumonitis* develops in 5–15 percent of all irradiated patients. There is no significant difference in the incidence of radiation pneumonitis between young and older subjects, however it does tend to be more severe if it occurs in older people.[238] There is no gross physiological change in the lung until 4–8 weeks after completion of irradiation, when clinical pneumonitis develops.

Whilst age, stage, and histology do not predict the development of symptomatic radiation pneumonitis, its prevalence is increased significantly in those patients with a low Karnofsky performance status, a history of smoking, comorbid lung disease, or poor pulmonary function tests—all conditions more likely to be seen in older patients.[239]

Larson et al.[240] prospectively studied patients with lung cancer over the age of 65 years undergoing radiotherapy to assess whether there were problems unique to elderly people. They found that the older group received a lower radiation dose, had more side-effects, more concurrent comorbidity, and less social support than the control group. However, they concluded that chronological age alone was not a sufficient criterion to determine whether therapy should be undertaken.

In a 1-year retrospective study of 149 patients aged over 75 years referred to a regional center with a diagnosis of lung cancer, Patterson et al.[241] reported that radiotherapy was well tolerated, with responses similar to those in younger patients. Whilst the majority of patients had palliative treatment, 90 percent were able to receive their therapy during a 1-week period and 81 percent had their treatment as an outpatient. They found that palliation was good, especially for hemoptysis, but less effective for dyspnea and cough. Side-effects were mild and reported in only 18 percent of patients. In keeping with this study, Zachariah et al.[242] found that patients over the age of 80 who received radiation therapy for various tumors (including 21 primary bronchial) tolerated the treatment well. Of particular interest is that 77 percent of this elderly study group were treated with curative intent.

While it was traditional teaching that postoperative radiotherapy may remove any malignant cells remaining in the tumor bed, at the resection margins, or in the adjacent lymph nodes—thus reducing local and regional recurrence and improving survival—there is now evidence that this may not be the case.[243] Data from nine randomized trials on 2128 patients who had undergone surgery found that postoperative radiotherapy was detrimental to patients with early-stage completely resected NSCLC, with a 21 percent relative increase in the risk of death and a reduced overall survival from 55 percent to 48 percent.[244] Thus caution must be exercised particularly in older patients when advising them about postoperative radiotherapy.

Radical radiation therapy is an effective treatment for small (T_1 or <3 cm) tumors and may provide an alternative to surgery in elderly or infirm patients.[235] In a study by Graham et al.[245] of radical radiotherapy for early NSCLC, most patients were elderly with squamous cell carcinoma of the lung, high comorbidity, and significant weight loss. The study found that the cause of death was not the patient's lung cancer in 28 percent of cases (cardiovascular 54 percent, respiratory 31 percent, and others 15 percent), and 77 percent of patients had no evidence of lung cancer at the time of death. Thus this may be an acceptable alternative with similar results to surgical resection in early-stage tumors.

The role of continuous hyperfractionated accelerated radiotherapy (CHART) is well-documented.[246] Significant improvement in survival of patients with NSCLC occurred following CHART; and while dysphagia was more common in the CHART group, there was no other difference in short- or long-term morbidity. In addition CHART was delivered over 12 consecutive days rather than 6 weeks, which may have been an advantage to older patients since inpatient stay was necessary because of the treatment schedule, thus avoiding repeated travel. Approximately one-quarter of the study group were aged 71 years or above and there was no evidence that age affected outcome. Whilst CHART included all patients from stage IA to IIIB, Bonner et al.[247] specifically studied patients with stage IIIA or IIIB treated by standard or accelerated hyperfractionated radiotherapy. Their study included patients up to the age of 86 years and found improved survival in those patients with hyperfractionated radiotherapy compared with standard radiotherapy, though they were unable to determine whether the addition of cisplatin improved survival further because of the mismatch in histological types between the treatment arms.

Chemotherapy for lung cancer

Balducci and Beghe[248] set out general guidelines on the administration of chemotherapeutic drugs for older people (defined as over 75 years).[248] These include the following recommendations:

- Agents that are renally excreted should be adjusted for dose according to the patient's glomerular filtration rate.
- Hemopoietic growth factors should be used in patients who are receiving moderately toxic chemotherapy, in order to reduce the duration and severity of neutropenia.
- High-dose chemotherapeutic regimens should be avoided because older people are more susceptible to complications as their functional reserves are decreased.
- Palliation for frail patients may include some form of chemotherapy.

It must be remembered that in many elderly patients, irrespective of their diagnosis, polypharmacy occurs[249] and this is important when considering the administration of chemotherapy.[250]

For some patients with NSCLC, chemotherapy may increase survival, but there is no consensus regarding the overall balance of benefits and costs at either the patient or health service level.[224] However, palliative chemotherapy may be offered to patients with advanced NSCLC and age should not be an adverse prognostic factor.[251]

Lung cancer guidelines recommend that all patients with SCLC be offered chemotherapy.[224] Small-cell lung cancer usually responds to cyclophosphamide, doxorubicin, vincristine, etoposide, and cisplatin. There is no evidence that response rate or survival is different in patients below or above the age of 70 years when administered CAV (cyclophosphamide, doxorubicin, and vincristine) versus EP (etoposide and cisplatin). However, once again it must be remembered that abbreviated treatment rather than dose reduction is an appropriate option.[252,253]

While intensive chemotherapy for older patients with limited SCLC is associated with both higher response rates and substantially more toxicity, some authors believe there is no major survival benefit.[254] Unfortunately 70 percent of patients when first diagnosed with small-cell lung cancer have extensive disease, so therapy is generally considered to be palliative rather than curative. Most tumors respond well to chemotherapy and this results in an increase in both quantity and quality of life. The 1998 guidelines *Improving Outcomes in Lung Cancer* recommend that all patients with small-cell lung cancer should be offered chemotherapy, and they do not recommend that older patients receive less than the standard six cycles of standard dose.[224] They do, however, suggest that patients who are less fit should be offered three to four cycles of a standard dose. Of note is that there is no recommendation to give lower dosage, even in elderly frail patients.

ETOPOSIDE The median survival for untreated elderly patients with SCLC remains between 6 and 12 weeks.[255] Etoposide is among the most active chemotherapeutic agents for small-cell lung cancer. It has a molecular weight of 588 Da, is poorly water-soluble, protein bound, with a mean half-life of 11.5 hours. Approximately 45 percent of the drug is excreted in the urine after 72 hours, of which 29 percent is as unchanged drug and 15 percent as metabolite.[256] Renal impairment, prior administration of cisplatin, and increasing age alter the pharmacokinetics of etoposide. Patients over the age of 60 years have an elevated volume of distribution at the steady state, an increased tendency for toxicity, but only minor influences on the systematic clearance of etoposide.[257] The optimal dose and schedule for etoposide is uncertain[258]; owing to etoposide's relatively rapid plasma clearance it has been suggested that it should be administered daily.[258]

Initial studies of etoposide demonstrated a significantly greater response rate and survival for patients receiving etoposide over 5 days than for patients receiving the same total dose over 24 hours.[259,260] Early data supporting the use of single-agent etoposide tended to concentrate on single outpatient treatment in combination with oral ifosfamide[261] or as a single-agent oral dose.[262] DeVore et al.[263] also found single-agent chronic oral etoposide to be the optimal treatment for extensive SCLC. Hainsworth et al.[264] administered oral etoposide daily in escalating doses for 21 consecutive days with good results, although the series was not exclusively older patients and therapy was frequently discontinued because of leucocyte counts of less than 2.0×10^9/L or platelet counts less than 75×10^9/L.

In a study of 94 patients with small-cell lung cancer (35 limited disease and 59 extensive disease), a 5-day regimen of etoposide was found to have equivalent activity to an 8-day regimen.[265] A pharmacokinetic association between concentrations of etoposide and response and toxicity was found, which supports the hypothesis that the schedule of etoposide administration may affect efficacy and toxicity and that prolonged exposure to low concentrations of etoposide may improve the therapeutic ratio of this drug. Whilst this study was not confined to elderly patients, the median age of the two groups was 64 and 65 years, respectively, and patients aged up to 77 years were included.

In a study by Carney and Bryne[255] of the 63 elderly patients treated with oral etoposide alone, 76 percent had an objective response—a complete response occurred in 20 patients and a median survival of 38 weeks was found.

Where administration of etoposide is prolonged, it is usually given orally. However, Thompson et al.[266] used a continuous infusion of etoposide for at least 21 days or until either the leucocyte count dropped to <2000/mm^3 or platelets dropped to <75,000/mm^3 or tumor progression occurred. While their study included only eight patients over the age of 60 years, and it is difficult to determine how many of them had SCLC, an objective response did occur in two of the three patients with previously untreated extensive SCLC.

Etoposide is often administered with other chemotherapeutic drugs. In one study, the co-administration of cisplatin did not result in an increase in leucocyte and platelet toxicities.[267] However, neither the response rate nor the median survival differed from those reported in studies employing oral etoposide as a single agent in previously untreated patients.

Loehrer et al.[268] found that the addition of cisplatin and ifosfamide to intravenous etoposide resulted in 37 percent complete remission, 34 percent partial remission, and an overall objective response rate of 71 percent. However, a disappointing median duration of response of 15 weeks (range 5–45) was seen.

TENIPOSIDE This drug, in common with etoposide, is a podophyllotoxin derivative that is active against small-cell lung cancer. Bork et al.[269] reported a 90 percent response rate with moderate toxicity when teniposide was administered intravenously. However, other authors have seen less convincing results. In a study of 26 patients aged 64–79 of whom 19 were aged more than 70 years, two cycles of teniposide resulted in two complete responses, twelve partial responses, five patients with stable disease, and only three with progressive disease.[270] The median duration of response was 7 months, and in this group of frail elderly patients the overall median survival was 9 months.

CARBOPLATIN   This drug is a relatively nontoxic cisplatin analogue active against SCLC in phase I/II trials.[271] Michel et al.[272] found that elderly patients with SCLC could be administered carboplatin and teniposide on an outpatient basis. After a median of 12 chemotherapy courses (range 2–31), the overall response rate was 67 percent, with five patients of the 24 studied in complete remission and 11 in partial remission. The median overall survival was 33 weeks and symptomatic improvement occurred in 86 percent of patients. Similar findings using carboplatin in combination with etoposide or etoposide, cyclophosphamide, and vincristine have also been described in elderly patients.[273]

VINORELBINE   There is little doubt that vinorelbine is a useful agent in elderly patients with inoperable NSCLC. Of 46 patients (median age 75 years, range 70–83 years) receiving 5-weekly infusions of vinorelbine, 27 had early discontinuation of treatment but 2 had partial response, 10 had some partial tumor regression, and 26 had tumor stabilization. The estimated median time to progression was 19 weeks and median survival 34 weeks.[274] A similar median survival of 9 months was found by Veronesi et al.[275] whose study of 83 patients included 23 over the age of 70 years. A median survival of 36 weeks was found by Gridelli et al.[276] although the doses administered were higher but for a shorter duration.

GEMCITABINE   The treatment of older patients with NSCLC is usually determined by their general condition. Unfortunately cisplatin treatment is often contraindicated and therefore agents such as gemcitabine in isolation or in combination are often considered. Patients ineligible for treatment with cisplatin on the grounds of their age or the presence of contraindications were studied following the administration of both gemcitabine and vinorelbine.[277] Of the study group, 35 percent achieved a partial remission for a median duration of 6 months, and 15 percent had stable disease for a median of 4 months. The median survival was 7 months with a 1-year actuarial survival rate of 31 percent. Of particular interest is that the treatment was well tolerated with only a third of patients having grade 3 or grade 4 granulocytopenia on day 14.

Similar results were found in a study of patients aged 70 years or over with advanced NSCLC who were randomly allocated to receive either vinorelbine on days 1 and 8 every 3 weeks or gemcitabine and vinorelbine on days 1 and 8 every 3 weeks.[278] The overall response rates were 22 and 15 percent in the combined and single-agent groups, respectively, and the median survival was 29 weeks compared with 18 weeks. In addition, combination therapy was associated with a clear delay in symptom and quality-of-life deterioration as assessed by a Modified Lung Cancer Symptom Scale Questionnaire.

DOCETAXEL   Hainsworth et al.[279] found that patients with advanced NSCLC tolerated a weekly dose of docetaxel. This agent provided an alternative treatment for older patients with advanced disease who could not tolerate combination chemotherapy.

CONCLUSION

Lung cancer continues to be a major cause of disability and death in elderly people. At present it is underinvestigated and undertreated. If the true extent of this disease is greater than that reflected in cancer registry statistics, the twenty-first century will look back on this as a prime example of agism. Treatments, both palliative and curative, are readily available and evidence suggests that in carefully selected patients they are safe. Geriatricians must work closely with their colleagues to ensure that patients have optimum therapy.

Summary of management algorithm
Lung cancer

- Investigate suspected lung cancer with bronchoscopy.
- Histopathology is mandatory.
- Depending on the extent of disease, decide whether palliative or curative treatment is the overall aim.
- Preoperative care must include a full functional assessment and antiembolic intervention.
- The most limited surgery must be undertaken.
- Radiotherapy is used for palliation of hemoptysis.
- Curative radiotherapy is used for those patients unable or unwilling to undergo curative surgery.
- Chemotherapy palliates small-cell lung cancer.
- Adjuvant chemotherapy for non-small-cell lung cancer may have a role in future management.
- Survival is short in most cases of lung cancer and early involvement with palliative care services is required.

KEY POINTS Lung cancers

- Investigation of lung cancer is mandatory even if curative therapy is not planned.
- There is no evidence that chemotherapy should be modified in elderly patients, but careful evaluation of clinical trials is essential.
- Limited resection is preferred over more radical surgery and provides the mainstay of curative therapy.
- Radiotherapy is well tolerated by all but the most frail patients, can be delivered in an outpatient setting, and is especially effective in reducing hemoptysis.

REFERENCES

1. Cockburn WC: The importance of infections of the respiratory tract. J Infect 1979;1(suppl 2):3–8

2. Valenti WM, Trudell RG, Bentley DW: Factors predisposing to oropharyngeal colonisation with Gram-negative bacilli in the aged. N Engl J Med 1978;298:1108–1111

3. Barker WH, Mullooly JP: Influenza vaccination of elderly persons: reduction in pneumonia and influenza hospitalizations and deaths. J Am Med Soc 1980;244:2547–2549

4. Glezen WP, Decca MD, Joseph SW, Mercready RG: Acute respiratory disease associated with influenza epidemics in Houston 1981–83. J Infect Dis 1987;155:1119–1126

5. Nicholson KG, Baker DJ, Farquhar A et al: Acute upper respiratory tract viral illness and influenza immunisation in homes for the elderly. Epidemiol Infect 1990;105:609–618

6. Connolly AM, Salmon RL, Lervy V, Williams DH: What are the complications of influenza and can they be prevented? Experience from the 1989 epidemic of H3N2 influenza A in general practice. BMJ 1993;306:1452–1454

7. Schwarzmann SW, Adler JL, Sullivan RJ, Marine WM: Bacterial influenza during the Hong Kong influenza epidemic 1968–69. Arch Intern Med 1971;127:1037–1041

8. Curwan M, Dunnell K, Ashley J: Hidden influenza deaths. BMJ 1990;300:896

9. UK Department of Health: Immunisation Against Infectious Disease. HMSO, London, 1992

10. UK Department of Health: Guideline on the Control of Infection in Residential and Nursing Homes. Public Health Medicine Environmental Group, Wetherby, 1996

11. UK Department of Health: Influenza Immunisation. HMSO, London, 2000

12. National Advisory Committee on Immunization (NACI): Statement on influenza vaccination for the 1991–1992 season. Can Dis Weekly Rep 1991;17–24:121–126

13. Centers for Disease and Control Prevention and Controls of Influenza: Recommendations of the immunization practices advisory committee (ACIP). MMWR 1992;40:1–17

14. Nicholson KG, Snacken R, Palache AM: Influenza immunization policies in Europe and the United States. Vaccine 1995;4:365–369

15. Howells CHL, Vesselinova-Jenkins CK, Evans AD, James J: Influenza vaccination and mortality from bronchopneumonia in the elderly. Lancet 1985;1:381–383

16. Nicholson KG, Wiselka MG, May A: Influenza vaccination of the elderly: perceptions and policies of general practitioners and outcome of the 1985–86 immunisation programme in Trent, UK. Vaccine 1985;5:302–306

17. Hak E, Hermens RP, Hoes AW et al: Effectiveness of a co-ordinated nationwide programme to improve influenza immunisation rates in the Netherlands. Scand J Prim Healthcare 2000;18:237–241

18. Gupta A, Makinde K, Morris G, Thomas P, Hasan M: Influenza immunization coverage in older hospitalized patients during winter 1998–99 in Carmarthenshire, UK. Age Ageing 2000;3:211–213

19. Nexoe J, Kragstrup J, Sogaard J: Decision on influenza vaccination among the elderly. A questionnaire study based on the Health, Belief, Moral and the Multi-dimensional and the Locus of Control Theory. Scand J Prim Healthcare 1999;17:105–110

20. Gupta A, Morris G, Thomas P, Hasan M: Influenza vaccination coverage in old people's home in Carmarthenshire, UK, during the winter of 1998/99. Vaccine 2000;18:2471–2475

21. Cornford CS, Morgan M: Elderly peoples' beliefs about influenza vaccination. Br J Gen Pract 1999;441:281–284

22. Findlay PF, Gibbons YM, Primrose WR, Ellis G, Downie G: Influenza and pneumococccal vaccination: patient perceptions. Postgrad Med J 2000;76:215–217

23. Igoe G, Bedford D, Howell F, Collins S: How to improve the uptake of influenza vaccination in older persons at risk. Ir J Med Sci 1999;168:107–108

24. Siriwardena AN: Targetting pneumococcal vaccination to high-risk groups: a feasibility study in one general practice. Postgrad Med J 1999;75:208–212

25. Pearson DC, Thompson RS: Evaluation of group health cooperative of Puget Sound's Senior influenza immunization program. Public Health Rep 1994;109:571–578

26. Wulp CG van der, Perenboom RJM, Davidse W: Ontwikkelingen in de griepvaccinatie in Nederland. Maandbericht Gezondheid (CBS) 1995;2:4–9

27. Carman WF, Elder AG, Wallace LA et al: Effects of influenza vaccination of healthcare workers on mortality of elderly people in long-term care: a randomised controlled trial. Lancet 2000;355:93–97

28. Calza L, Briganti E, Manfredi R, Chiodo F: Influenza. Recenti Progressi in Medicana 2000;91:657–666

29. Makela MJ, Pauksens K, Rostila T et al: Clinical efficacy and safety of the orally inhaled neuraminidase inhibitor zanamivir in the treatment of influenza: a randomized double-blind, placebo-controlled European study. J Infect 2000;40:42–48

30. Couch RB: Measures for control of influenza. Pharmacoeconomics 1999;16(suppl):141–145

31. Fenton RJ, Morley PJ, Owens IJ et al: Chemoprophylaxis of influenza A virus infections with single doses of zanamivir, demonstrates that zanamivir is cleared slowly from the respiratory tract. J Antimacrob Agents Chemother 1999;43:2642–2647

32. Ortquist A, Sterner G, Nilsson JA: Severe community-acquired pneumonia: factors influencing need of intensive care treatment and prognosis. Scand J Infect Dis 1985;17:377–386

33. Woodhead MA: Studies on pneumonia in the community and in hospital in Nottingham. DM thesis, University of Nottingham, 1988

34. Mouton CP, Bazaldua OV, Pierce B, Espino DV: Common infections in older adults. Am Fam Physician 2001;63:257–268

35. UK Office of Population Censuses and Surveys: Mortality Statistics. HMSO, London, 1990

36. Medina E, Kaempffer AM: Adult mortality in Chile. Revista Medica de Chile 2000;128:1144–1149

37. Leung KK, Tang LY, Chie WC, Lue BH, Lee LT: Mortality trends of elderly people in Taiwan from 1974 to 1994. Age Ageing 1999;28:199–203

38. The British Thoracic Society and the Public Health Laboratory Service: Community-acquired pneumonia in adults in British hospitals in 1982–1983: a survey of aetiology, mortality, prognostic factors and outcome. QJM 1987;62:195–230

39. Venkatesan P, Gladman J, MacFarlane JT: A hospital study of community acquired pneumonia in the elderly. Thorax 1990;45:254–258

40. Butler JC, Schuchat A: Epidemiology of pneumococcal infections in the elderly. Drugs Aging 1999;15(suppl):111–119

41. Anderson EC, Begg NT, Crawshaw SC et al: Epidemiology of invasive *Haemophilus influenzae* infections in England and Wales in the pre-vaccination era (1990–2). Epidemiol Infect 1995;115:89–100

42. Hedlund J: Community-acquired pneumonia requiring hospitalisation: factors of importance for the short- and long-term prognosis. Scand J Infect Dis Suppl 1995;971–976

43. Torres A, El-Ebirary M, Riquelme R, Ruiz M, Celis R: Community-acquired pneumonia in the elderly. Semin Respir Infect 1999;14:173–183

44. El-Solh AA, Sikka P, Ramadan F, Davies J: Etiology of severe pneumonia in the very elderly. Am J Respir Crit Care Med 2001;163:645–651

45. Marrie TJ: Pneumonia in the elderly. Curr Opin Pulm Med 1996;2:192–197

46. Preston AJ, Gosney MA, Noon S, Martin MV: Oral flora of elderly patients following acute medical admission. Gerontology 1999;45:49–52

47. Loeb M, McGeer A, McArthur M, Walter S, Simor AE: Risk factors for pneumonia and other lower respiratory tract infections in elderly residents of long-term care facilities. Arch Intern Med 1999;159:2058–2064

48. Garciea-Ordonez MA, Alvarez-Hurtado F, Cebrain-Gallardo JJ et al: Community-acquired bacteremic pneumonia in the elderly. An Med Interna 1999;16:345–348 (in Spanish)

49. Riquelme R, Torres A, El-Ebiary M et al: Community-acquired pneumonia in the elderly: clinical and nutritional aspects. Am J Respir Crit Care Med 1997;156:1908–1914

50. Riquelme R, Torres A, El-Ebiary M et al: Community-acquired pneumonia in the elderly: a multivariate analysis of risk and prognostic factors. Am J Respir Crit Care Med 1996;154:1450–1455

51. Hedlund J, Kalin M, Ortqvist A: Recurrence of pneumonia in middle-aged and elderly adults after hospital-treated pneumonia: aetiology and predisposing conditions. Scand J Infect Dis 1997;29:387–392

52. Harper C, Newton P: Clinical aspects of pneumonia in the elderly veteran. J Am Geriatr Soc 1989;37:867–872

53. Starczewski AR, Allen SC, Vargas E, Lye M: Clinical prognostic indices of fatality in elderly patients admitted to hospital with acute pneumonia. Age Ageing 1988;17:181–186

54. Esposito AL: Community-acquired bacteremic pneumococcal pneumonia: effect of age on manifestations and outcome. Arch Intern Med 1984;144:945–948

55. Puxty JAH, Andrews K: The role of chest radiography in the evaluation of "Geriatric Giants." Age Ageing 1986;15:174–176

56. McFadden JP, Price RC, Eastwood HD, Briggs RS: Raised respiratory rate in elderly patients: a valuable physical sign. BMJ 1982;284:626–627

57. Marrie TJ, Durant H, Yates L: Community-acquired pneumonia requiring hospitalization: 6-year prospective study. Rev Infect Dis 1989;11:586–599

58. La Croix AZ, Lipson S, Miles TP, White L: Prospective study of pneumonia hospitalizations and mortality of US older people: the role of chronic conditions, health behaviors and nutritional status. Public Health Rep 1989;104:350–360

59. Metlay JP, Schulz R, Li YH et al: Influence of age on symptoms at presentation in patients with community-acquired pneumonia. Arch Intern Med 1997;157:1453–1459

60. Connolly MJ, Crowley JJ, Vestal RE: Clinical significance of crepitations in elderly patients following acute hospital admission: a prospective survey. Age Ageing 1992;21:43–48

61. Weinberg AD, Minaker KL: Dehydration: evaluation and management in older adults. Counsel on Scientific Affairs, American Medical Association. JAMA 1995;274:1552–1556

62. Eaton D, Bannister P, Mulley GP, Connolly MJ: Axillary sweating in clinical assessment of dehydration in ill elderly patients. BMJ 1994;308:1271

63. Ahkee S, Srinheh L, Ramirez J: Community-acquired pneumonia in the elderly: association of mortality with lack of fever and leukocytosis. South Med J 1997;90:296–298

64. Werner H, Kuntsche J: Infection in the elderly: what is different? Z Gerontol Geriatr 2000;33:350–356

65. Dey AB, Nagarkar KM, Kumar V: Clinical presentation and predictors of outcome in adult patients with community-acquired pneumonia. Nat Med J India 1997;10:169–172

66. Leiberman D, Leiberman D: Community-acquired pneumonia in the elderly: a practical guide to treatment. Drugs Aging 2000;17:93–105

67. Garb JL, Brown RB, Garb JR, Tuthill RW: Differences in etiology of pneumonias in nursing homes and community patients. JAMA 1978;240:2169–2172

68. Marrie TJ, Haldane EV, Faulkner RS, Durant H, Kwan C: Community-acquired pneumonia requiring hospitalization: is it different in the elderly? J Am Geriatr Soc 1985;33:671–680

69. Rello J, Rodriguez R, Jubert P, Alvrez B: Severe community-acquired pneumonia in the elderly: epidemiology and prognosis. Study Group for Severe Community-Acquired Pneumonia. Clin Infect Dis 1996;23:723–728

70. Diaz-Fuenzalida A, Vera C, Santamarina J et al: Community-acquired pneumonia in the elderly requiring hospitalization: clinical features and prognosis. Medicina (B-Aires) 1999;59:731–738

71. El-Solh AA, Sikka P, Ramadan F, Davies J: Aetiology of severe pneumonia in the very elderly. Am J Respir Crit Care Med 2001;163:645–651

72. Levy M, Dromer F, Brion N, Leterdu F, Carbon C: Community-acquired pneumonia: importance of initial noninvasive bacteriologic and radiographic investigations. Chest 1988;93:43–48

73. Ausina V, Coll P, Sambeat M et al: Prospective study on the aetiology of community-acquired pneumonia in children and adults in Spain. Eur J Clin Microbiol Infect Dis 1988;7:343–347

74. Report from the PHLS Communicable Disease Surveillance Centre. BMJ 1988;296:778–779

75. Noah ND: *Mycoplasma pneumoniae* infection in the United Kingdom, 1967–73. BMJ 1974;2:554–556

76. Kaye MG, Fox MJ, Bartlett JG et al: The clinical spectrum of *Staphylococcus aureus* pulmonary infection. Chest 1990;97:788–792

77. Yung AP, Grayson ML: Psittacosis: a review of 135 cases. Med J Aust 1988;148:228–233

78. Horan TC, White JW, Jarvis WR et al: Nosocomial infection surveillance 1984. MMWR 1986;34:17ss–29ss

79. Diot P, Palmer LB, Uy LL et al: Technique for measurement of oropharyngeal clearance in the elderly. J Aerosol Med 1995;8:177–186

80. Kobashi Y, Fujita K, Karino T et al: Clinical analysis of pneumonia in the elderly in a community hospital: comparison of community-acquired pneumonia and nosocomial pneumonia. Kansenshogaku Zasshi 1999;73:884–892

81. Harkness GA, Bentley DW, Roghmann KJ: Risk factors for nosocomial pneumonia in the elderly. Am J Med 1990;89:457–463

82. Marrie TJ: Pneumonia in the elderly. Curr Opin Pulm Med 1996;2:192–197

83. Barkham TMS, Martin FC: The respiratory presentation of urinary tract infection in older patients. Age Ageing 1995;24(suppl 2):P18–P19

84. British Thoracic Society Standards of Care Committee et al: BTS Guidelines for the management of community acquired pneumonia in adults. Thorax 2001;56(suppl iv):iv1–iv63

85. Ebright JR, Rytel MW: Bacterial pneumonia in the elderly. J Am Geriatr Soc 1980;18:220–223

86. British Thoracic Society. Community-acquired pneumonia in adults in British hospitals in 1982–1983: a survey of aetiology, mortality, prognostic factors and outcome. QJM 1987;62:195–220.

87. Saynajakangas O, Keistinen T, Tuuponen T, Kivela SL: Evaluation of the incidence and age distribution of bronchiectasis from the Finnish hospital discharge register. Cent Eur J Public Health 1998;6:235–237

88. Vilar ME, Najib NM, Chowdhry I et al: Allergic bronchopulmonary aspergillosas as presenting sign of cystic fibrosis in an elderly man. Ann Allergy Asthma Immunol 2000;85:70–73

89. Roberts DE, Cole PJ: Use of selective media in bacteriological investigation of patients with chronic suppurative lung infection. Lancet 1980;1:796

90. Roberts D, Higgs E, Rutman A, Cole PJ: Isolation of sphero-plastic forms of *Haemophilus influenzae* from sputum in conventionally treated chronic bronchial sepsis using selective medium supplanted with *N*-acetyl-D-glucosamine: possible reservoir for re-emergence of infection. BMJ 1984;289:1409

91. Wallace RJ, Zhang Y, Brown BA et al: Polyclonal *Microbacterium avium* complex infections in patients with nudular bronchiectasis. Am J Respir Crit Care Med 1998;158:1235–1244

92. Cole PJ, Roberts DE: High dose antibiotic is logical, effective and economical in treatment of severe bronchial sepsis. Lancet 1983;1:248

93. Hill SL, Morrison HM, Burnett D, Stockley RA: Short term response of patients with bronchiectasis to treatment with amoxycillin given in standard or high doses orally or by inhalation. Thorax 1986;41:559–565

94. Powell KE, Farer LS: The rising age of the tuberculosis patient. J Infect Dis 1980;142:946–948

95. Teale C, Goldman JM, Pearson SB: The association of age with the presentation and outcome of tuberculosis: a 5 year survey. Age Ageing 1993;22:289–293

96. Duffield JS, Adams WH, Anderson M, Leitch AG: Increasing incidence of tuberculosis in the young and the elderly in Scotland. Thorax 1996;51:140–142

97. Leitch AG, Iubilar M, Kurnow J et al: Scottish national survey of tuberculosis notifications 1993 with special reference to the prevalence of HIV seropositivity. Thorax 1996;51:78–81

98. Iinuma Y: Tuberculosis. Rinsho byori 2000;48:1029–1035

99. Rajagopalan S, Yoshikawa TT: Tuberculosis in long-term-care facilities. Infect Control Hosp Epidemiol 2000;21:611–615

100. Al-Jahdali H, Al-Zahrani K, Amene P et al: Clinical aspects of miliary tuberculosis in Saudi adults. Int J Tuberc Lung Dis 2000;4:252–255

101. Janssens JP, Zellweger JP: Clinical epidemiology and treatment of tuberculosis in elderly patients. Schweiz Med Wochenschr 1999;129:80–89

102. Prikazsky V, Kubin M, Pikhartova J: Selected results of the tuberculosis control program in the Czech Republic. Sent Eur J Public Health 1999;7:116–121

103. Vachee A, Vincent P, Savage C et al: Molecular epidemiology of tuberculosis in the Nord Department of France during 1995. Tuber Lung Dis 1999;79:361–366

104. Tocque K, Bellis MA, Tam CM et al: Long-term trends in tuberculosis. Comparison of age-cohort data between Hong Kong and England and Wales. Am J Respir Crit Care Med 1998;158:484–488

105. Heath TC, Roberts C, Winks M, Capon AG: The epidemiology of tuberculosis in New South Wales 1975–1999: the effects of immigration in a low prevalence population. Int J Tuberc Lung Dis 1998;2:647–654

106. Baldo V, Menegon T, Zannoni F et al: Epidemiological aspects of tuberculosis in the Padua Health District 1985–1996. Eur J Epidemiol 1998;14:125–128

107. Banerji S, Bellomy AL, Uyu ES et al: Tuberculosis in San Diego county: a border community perspective. Public Health Rep 1996;111:431–436

108. Kearney HT, Wanklyn PD, Goldman JM, Pearson SB, Teale C: Urban deprivation and tuberculosis in the elderly. Respir Med 1994;88:703–704

109. Davies PD: The effects of poverty and ageing on the increase in tuberculosis. Monaldi Arch Chest Dis 1999;54:168–171

110. Morris CDW, Nell H: Epidemic of pulmonary tuberculosis in geriatric homes. S Afr Med J 1988;74:117–120

111. Rajagopalan S, Yoshikawa TT: Tuberculosis in the elderly. Z Gerontol Geriatr 2000;33:374–380

112. Snider DE: Tuberculosis after gastrectomy. Chest 1985;87:414–415

113. Dull R, Peto R: Mortality in relation to smoking: 20 years observations on male British doctors. BMJ 1976;2:215–225

114. Chan TY: Vitamin D deficiency and susceptibility to tuberculosis. Calcif Tissue Int 2000;66:476–478

115. Davies PD: Tuberculosis in the elderly: epidemiology and optimal management. Drugs Aging 1996;8:436–444

116. Morris CDW, Bird AR, Nell H: Haematological and biochemical changes in severe pulmonary tuberculosis. QJM 1989;73:1151–1159

117. McAdams JP, Erasmus J, Winter JA: Radiologic manifestations of pulmonary tuberculosis. Radiol Clin North Am 1995;33:655–678

118. Ormerod LP, Horsfield N: Miliary tuberculosis in a high prevalence area of the UK: Blackburn 1978–1993. Respir Med 1995;89:555–557

119. Daucourt V, Petit S, Pasquet S et al: Comparison of cases of isolated pulmonary tuberculosis with cases of other localizations of tuberculosis in the course of an active surveillance (Gironde, 1995–1996). Rev Med Intern 1998;19:792–798

120. Gorse GJ, Pais PJ, Kusske JA et al: Tubercular spondylitis: a report of six cases and review of the literature. Medicine 1983;62:1788–1784

121. Chelsom J, Solberg CO: Vertebral osteomyelitis at a Norwegian University Hospital 1987–97: clinical features, laboratory findings and outcome. Scand J Infect Dis 1998;30:147–151

122. Kali L, Lund F: Tuberculosis of the hand. Tidsskr Nor Laegeforen 2000;120:445–446

123. Reading AD, Stother IG: The painless fracture: could it be TB? J R Coll Surg Edinb 1998;43:410–411

124. Kelly J, Warren K, Coutts M, Jenkins A: An unusual case of ileocaecal tuberculosis in an 80-year-old Caucasion male. Int J Clin Pract 1999;53:77–79

125. Perez-Fernandez T, Moreira-Vicente V, Sanz-Villalobos E, Alvarez-Baleriola I: Isolated colonic tuberculosis. Gastro Enterol Hepatol 1997;20:490–493

126. Karstaedt AS, Valtchanova S, Barriere K, Crewe-Brown HH: Tuberculosis meningitis in South African urban adults. QJM 1998;91:743–747

127. Counsell S, Tan JS, Dittus RS: Unsuspected pulmonary tuberculosis in a community teaching hospital. Arch Intern Med 1989;149:1274–1278

128. Roblot F, Roblot P, Bourgoin A et al: Distinctive features of tuberculosis in the aged. Rev Med Intern 1998;19:629–634

129. Dahmash NS, Fayed DF, Chowdhury MN, Arora SC: Diagnostic challenge of tuberculosis in the elderly in hospital: experience at a university hospital in Saudi Arabia. J Infect 1995;31:93–97

130. Morris CDW, Nell H: Epidemic pulmonary tuberculosis in geriatric homes. S Afr Med J 1988;74:117–125

131. Perez-Guzman T, Torres-Cruz A, Villarreal-Velarde H, Vargas MH: Progressive age-related changes in pulmonary tuberculosis images and the effect of diabetes. Am J Respir Crit Care Med 2000;162:1738–1740

132. Van-den-Brande P, Dockx S, Valck B, Demedts M: Pulmonary tuberculosis in the adult in a low prevalence area: is the radiological presentation changing? Int J Tuberc Lung Dis 1998;2:904–908

133. Liaw YS, Yang BC, Yu CJ et al: A clinical spectrum of tuberculosis in older patients. J Am Geriatr Soc 1995;43:256–260

134. Chan CH, Woo J, Or KK, Chan RC, Chung W: The effect of age on the presentation of patients with tuberculosis. Tuber Lung Dis 1995;76:290–294

135. Ip MSM, Yo SY, Lam WK, Mok CK: Endo-bronchotuberculosis revisited. Chest 1986;89:727–729

136. Bour-Guichenez G, Guichenez P, Bonnamour C, Ruesch C, Gonthier R: Bronchial tuberculosis in the elderly: apropos of nine cases. Radioclinical, endoscopic and developmental aspects. Rev Med Intern 1997;18:26–29

137. Snider DE: The tuberculin skin test. Am Rev Respir Dis 1982;125:108–114

138. Joint Tuberculosis Committee of the British Thoracic Society. Chemotherapy and management of tuberculois in the United Kingdom: recommendations 1998. Thorax 1998;53:536–548

139. Joint Tuberculosis Commitee of the British Thoracic Society. Control and prevention of tuberculosis in the United Kingdom: Code of Practice 2000. Thorax 2000;55:887–901

140. Nisar M, Williams CSD, Ashby D, Davies PDO: Tuberculin testing in residential homes for the elderly. Thorax 1993;48:1257–1260

141. Connolly MJ, Magee JG, Hendrick DJ: *Mycobacterium malmoense* in the North-East of England. Tubercle 1985;66:211–217

142. American Thoracic Society: Diagnosis and treatment of disease caused by non tuberculous mycobacteria. Am Rev Respir Dis 1990;142:940–953

143. Sub-Committee of the Joint Tuberculosis Committee of the British Thoracic Society. Management of opportunist mycobaterial infections: Joint Tuberculosis Committee Guidelines 1999. Thorax 2000;55:210–218

144. PIOPED Investigators: Value of the ventilation/perfusion scan in acute pulmonary embolism: results of the prospective investigation of pulmonary embolism diagnosis (PIOPED). JAMA 1990;263:2753–2759

145. Anderson FA, Wheeler HB, Goldberg RJ et al: A population-based perspective of the hospital incidence and case-fatality rates of deep vein thrombosis and pulmonary embolism. Arch Intern Med 1991;151:933–938

146. Stein PD, Gottschalk A, Saltzman MA, Terrin ML: Diagnosis of acute pulmonary embolism in the elderly. J Am Coll Cardiol 1991;18:1452–1457

147. Dalen JE: Clinical diagnosis of acute pulmonary embolism: when should a V/Q scan be ordered? Chest 1991;100:1185–1186 (editorial)

148. Stein PD, Dalen JE, McIntyre KM et al: The electrocardiogram and acute pulmonary embolism. Prog Cardiovasc Dis 1975;17:247–257

149. Stein PD, Terrin ML, Hales CA et al: Clinical, laboratory, roentgenographic and electrocardiographic findings in patients with acute pulmonary embolism and no pre-existing cardiac or pulmonary disease. Chest 1991;100:598–603

150. Sutton GC, Honey M, Gibson RV: Clinical diagnosis of acute massive pulmonary embolism. Lancet 1969;I:271–273

151. Santolicandro A, Prediletto R, Fornai E et al: Mechanisms of hypoxaemia and hypocapnia in pulmonary embolism. Am J Respir Crit Care Med 1995;152:336–347

152. Stein PD, Goldhaber SZ, Henry JW: Alveolar-arterial oxygen gradient in the assessment of acute pulmonary embolism. Chest 1995;107:139–143

153. Bury RF, Smith AH: Out of hours scintigraphy: a survey of current practice. Nucl Med Comm 1993;14:126–129

154. British Thoracic Society, Standards of Care Committee: Suspected acute pulmonary embolism: a practical approach. Thorax 1997; 52 (suppl 4):S1–S24

155. Raskob GE, Hull RD: Diagnosis and management of pulmonary embolism. QJM 1990;76:787–789

156. Research Committee for the British Thoracic Society: Optimum duration of anticoagulation for deep vein thrombosis and pulmonary embolism. Lancet 1992;340:873–876

157. Magnant JG, Walsh DB, Juravsky LI, Cronenwett JL: Current use of inferior cava filters. J Vasc Surg 1992;16:701–706

158. British Thoracic Society, Standards of Care Committee: The diagnosis, assessment and treatment of diffused parenchymal lung disease in adults. British Thoracic Society recommendations. Thorax 1999;54(suppl 1):S1–S30

159. Coultas DB, Zumwalt RE, Black WC et al: The epidemiology of interstitial lung diseases. Am J Respir Crit Care Med 1994;150:967–972

160. Mannino DM, Etzel RA, Parrish RG: Pulmonary fibrosis deaths in the United States, 1979–1991: an analysis of multiple-cause mortality data. Am J Respir Crit Care Med 1996;153:1548–1552

161. UK Office of National Statistics: Mortality Statistics 1996. Stationery Office, London, 1998

162. Johnston I, Britton K, Kinnear W et al: Rising mortality from cryptogenic fibrosing alveolitis. BMJ 1990;301:1017–1021

163. Epler GR, McLoud TC, Gaensler AE et al: Normal chest roentgenograms in chronic infiltrative lung disease. N Engl J Med 1978;298:934–939

164. Mathiesom JR, Mayo JR, Staples CA, Muller ML: Chronic diffuse infiltrative lung disease: comparison of diagnostic accuracy of CT and chest radiography. Radiology 1989;181:111–116

165. McLoud TC, Carrington CB, Gaensler EA: Diffuse infiltrative lung disease: a new scheme for description. Radiology 1983;149:353–363

166. Padley SP, Adler B, Hansell DM et al: High-resolution computerised tomography of drug-induced lung disease. Clin Radiol 1992;46:232–236

167. Muller NL, Miller RR: Computed tomography of chronic diffuse infiltrative lung disease. Am Rev Respir Dis 1990;142:1206–1215

168. Padley SPG, Alder B, Muller NL: High resolution computed tomography of the chest: current indications. J Thoracic Imaging 1993;8:189–199

169. du Bois RM: Diffuse lung disease: an approach to management. BMJ 1994;309:175–179

170. Booth HL, Walters EH: Interstitial lung disease in the elderly patient. In: Connolly MJ (ed): Respiratory Disease in the Elderly Patient. Chapman & Hall, London, 1996:171–207

171. BAL Cooperative Group Steering Committee: Bronchoalveolar lavage constituents in healthy individuals, idiopathic pulmonary fribrosis, and selected comparison groups. Am Rev Respir Dis 1990;141:S169–S202

172. Klech H, Pohl W (eds): Technical recommendations and guidelines for broncho-alveolar lavage (BAL): report of European Society of Pneumonology Task Group on BAL. Eur Respir J 1989;2:561–585

173. Poe RH, Israel RH, Utell MJ, Hall WJ: Probability of positive transbroncheal lung biopsy result in sarcoidosis. Arch Intern Med 1979;139:761–763

174. Herf SM, Suratt PM: Complications of transbroncheal lung biopsies. Chest 1978;73:759–760

175. Bentzon N, Adamsen S, Jacobsen B et al: Video thoracoscopic lung biopsy by a stapling technique. Eur J Surg 1994;160:543–546

176. Nasim A, Akhtar RP, Spyt TJ et al: Video-thoracoscopic lung biopsy in diagnosis of interstitial lung disease. J R Coll Surg Edinb 1995;40:22–24

177. Krasna MJ, White CS, Aisner SC et al: The role of thoracoscopy in the diagnosis of interstitial lung disease. Ann Thorac Surg 1995;59:348–351

178. Soutar CA, Turner-Warwick M, Parkes WR: Circulating antinuclear antibody and rheumatoid factor in coal pneumoconiosis. BMJ 1974;3:145

179. Gaensler EA, Jedelinic PJ, Churg A: Idiopathic pulmonary fibrosis in absestos-exposed workers. Am Rev Respir Dis 1991;144:689–696

180. Epler GR, Carrington CB, Gaesler EA: Crackles (rales) in the interstitial pulmonary diseases. Chest 1978;73:333–339

181. Hendrick DJ, Faux JA, Marshall R: Budgerigar-fancier's lung: the commonest variety of allergic alveolitis in Britain. BMJ 1978;2:81–84

182. Allen DH, Williams GV, Woolcock AJ: Bird breeders' hypersensitivity pneumonitis: progress studies and lung function after cessation of exposure to the provoking antigen. Am Rev Respir Dis 1976;114:555–566

183. Sansores R, Salas J, Chapela R: Clubbing in hypersenstivity pneumonitis. Arch Intern Med 1990;150:1849–1851

184. Kokkarinen JL, Tukiainen HO, Terho EO: Effective corticosteroid treatment and the recovery of pulmonary function in farmer's lung. Am Rev Respir Dis 1992;145:3–5

185. Crystal RG, Bitterman PB, Rennard SI et al: Interstitial lung disease of unknown cause: disorders characterized by chronic inflammation of the lower respiratory tract. N Engl J Med 1984;310:154–166

186. Wright PH, Heard BE, Steel SJ, Turner-Warwick M: Cryptogenic fibrosing alveolitis: assessment by graded trephine lung biopsy: Histology compared with clinical radiographic and physical features. Br J Dis Chest 1981;75:61–70

187. Stack BHR, Choo-Kang YFJ, Heard BE: The prognosis of cryptogenic fibrosing alveolitis. Thorax 1972;27:535–542

188. Connolly MJ, Crowley JJ, Charan NB, Nielson CP, Vestal RE: Reduced subjective awareness of bronchoconstriction provoked by methacholine in elderly asthmatic and normal subjects as measured on a simple awareness scale. Thorax 1992;47:410–413

189. Hiwitari N, Shimura F, Sasaki T et al: Prognosis of idiopathic pulmonary fibrosis in patients with mucus hypersecretion. Am Rev Respir Dis 1991;143–145

190. Turner-Warwick M, Burrows B, Johnson A: Cryptogenic fibrosing alveolitis: clinical features and their influence on survival. Thorax 1980;35:171–180

191. Tukiainen P, Taskinen E, Holsti P et al: Prognosis of cryptogenic fibrosing alveolitis. Thorax 1983;38:349–355

192. Johnson I, Britton J, Kinnear W, Logan R: Rising mortality from cryptogenic fibrosing alveolitis. BMJ 1990;301:1017–1021

193. Turner-Warwick M, Burrows B, Johnson A: Cryptogenic fibrosing alveolitis: response to corticosteroid treatment and its effect on survival. Thorax 1980;35:593–599

194. Johnson MA, Kwan S, Snell NJC et al: Randomised control trial comparing prednisolone alone with cyclophosphamide and low dose prednisolone in combination in cryptogenic fibrosing alveolitis. Thorax 1989;44:280–288

195. Raghu G, Depaso WJ, Cain K et al: Azathioprine combined with prednisolone in the treatment of idiopathic pulmonary fibrosis: a prospective double-blind randomized placebo-controlled clinical trial. Am Rev Respir Dis 1991;144:291–296

196. Wells AU, Cullinan P, Hansell DM et al: Fibrosing alveolitis associated with systemic sclerosis has a better prognosis than lone cryptogenic fibrosing alveolitis. Am J Respir Crit Care Med 1994;149:583–590

197. Papiris SA, Vlachoyiannopoulos PG, Maniati MA et al: Idiopathic pulmonary fibrosis and pulmonary fibrosis in diffuse systemic sclerosis: two fibroses with different prognoses. Respiration 1995;64:81–85

198. Krafcik SS, Cobin RB, Lynch JP, Sitrin RG: Wegener's granulomatosis in the elderly. Chest 1996;109:430–437

199. Devaney KO, Travis WD, Hoffman GS et al: Interpretation of head and neck biopsies in Wegener's granulomatosis. Am J Surg Pathol 1990;14:555–564

200. Travis WD, Hoffma GS, Leavitt RY et al: Surgical pathology of the lung in Wegener's granulomatosis. Am J Surg Pathol 1991;15:315–333

201. Andrassy K, Erb A, Koderisch J et al: Wegener's granulomatosis with renal involvement: patient survival and correlations between initial renal function, renal histology, therapy and renal outcome. Clin Nephrol 1991;35:139–147

202. Fauci AS, Haynes BF, Katz P, Wolff SM: Wegener's granulomatosis: prospective clinical and therapeutic experience with 85 patients for 21 years. Ann Intern Med 1983;98:76–85

203. Bradley JD, Brandt KD, Katz BP: Infectious complications of cyclophosphamide for vasculitis. Arthritis Rheum 1989;32:415–453

204. Seidl LG, Thornton GF, Smith JW, Cluff LE: Studies on the epidemiology of adverse drug reactions. III: Reactions in patients on a general medical service. Bull Johns Hopkins Hosp 1966;119:299–315

205. Hurwitz N: Predisposing factors in adverse reactions to drugs. BMJ 1969;1:536–539

206. Levy M, Kewitz H, Altwein W et al: Hospital admissions due to adverse drug reactions: a comparative study from Jerusalem and Berlin. Eur J Clin Pharmacol 1980;17:25–31

207. Cooper JAD, White DA, Matthay RA: Drug-induced pulmonary disease. I: Cytotoxic drugs. Am Rev Respir Dis 1986;133:321–340

208. Cooper JAD, White DA, Matthay RA: Drug-induced pulmonary disease. II: Noncytotoxic drugs. Am Rev Respir Dis 1986;133:488–505

209. James DG: Clinical picture of sarcoidosis. In Schwrtz MI, King TE (eds): Interstitial Lung Disease. Mosby Year Book, St Louis, 1993

210. Newman LS, Rose CS, Maier LA: Sarcoidosis. N Engl J Med 1997;336:1224–1234

211. Williams C: Lung cancer In Morris D, Kearsley J, Williams C (eds): Cancer, a Comprehensive Guide. Harwood Academic, London, 1998:141–154

212. Doll R, Darcy S, Whitley E: Trends in mortality from smoking-related diseases. In Charlton J, Murphy M (eds): The Health of Adult Britain, 1841–1994, vol. 1. HMSO, London, 1997:128–155

213. Woll P, Thatcher N: Bronchus. In Price P, Sikora K (eds): Treatment of Cancer, 3rd edn. Chapman & Hall, London, 1995:437–472

214. Lung and Asthma Information Agency: Pleural mesothelioma. Factsheet 92/3, Department of Public Health Sciences, St George's Hospital Medical School, London, 1992

215. Boutin C, Rey F: Thoracoscopy in pleural malignant mesothelioma: a prospective study of 188 consecutive patients. Part 1: diagnosis. Cancer 1993;72:389–393

216. Boutin C, Rey F, Gouvernet J et al: Thoracoscopy in pleural malignant mesothelioma: a prospective study of 188 consecutive patients. Part 2: prognosis and staging. Cancer 1993;72:394–404

217. Ellis P, Smith I: Small cell lung cancer. In Horwich A (ed): Oncology: A Multidisciplinary Textbook. Chapman & Hall, London, 1995:585–598

218. Davies L, Mister R, Spence DP et al: Cardiovascular consequences of fibreoptic bronchoscopy. Eur Respir J 1997;10:695–698

219. Matot I, Kramer MR, Glantz L, Drenger B, Cotev S: Myocardial ischemia in sedated patients undergoing fiberoptic bronchoscopy. Chest 1997;112:1454–1458

220. Brown JS, Eraut D, Trask C, Davison AG: Age and the treatment of lung cancer. Thorax 1996;51:564–568

221. Kant AK, Glover C, Horm J, Schatzkin A, Harris TB: Does cancer survival differ for older patients? Cancer 1992;70:2734–2740

222. Trimble EL, Carter CL, Cain D et al: Representation of older patients in cancer treatment trials. Cancer 1994;74:2208–2214

223. Woolf SH, Grol R, Hutchinson A, Eccles M, Grimshaw J: Clinical guidelines: potential benefits, limitations, and harms of clinical guidelines. BMJ 1999;318:527–530

224. UK Department of Health: Improving Outcomes in Lung Cancer: The Manual. DoH, London, 1998

225. UK Department of Health: Improving Outcomes in Lung Cancer: The Research Evidence. DoH, London, 1998

226. Hasse J, Wertzel H, Kassa M, Burgard G: Thoracic cancer surgery in the elderly. Eur J Surg Oncol 1998;24:403–406

227. McKenna RJ: Clinical aspects of cancer in the elderly: treatment decisions, treatment choices and follow up. Cancer 1994;74:2107–2117

228. Zagonel V, Pinto A, Serraino D et al: Lung cancer in the elderly. Cancer Treat Rev 1994;20:315–329

229. Turner NJ, Hayward RA, Mulley GP, Selby PJ: Cancer in old age: is it inadequately investigated and treated? BMJ 1999;319:309–312

230. Mizushima Y, Noto H, Sugiyama S et al: Survival and prognosis after pneumonectomy for lung cancer in the elderly. Ann Thorac Surg 1997;64:193–198

231. Knott-Craig CJ, Howell CE, Parsons BD et al: Improved results in the management of surgical candidates with lung cancer. Ann Thorac Surg 1997;63:1405–1409

232. Pagni S, Federico JA, Ponn RB: Pulmonary resection for lung cancer in octogenarians. Ann Thorac Surg 1997;63:785–789

233. Sioris T, Salo J, Perhoniemi V, Mattila S: Surgery for lung cancer in the elderly. Scand Cardiovasc J 1999;33:222–227

234. Pignon T, Scalliet P: Radiotherapy in the elderly. Eur J Surg Oncol 1998;24:407–411

235. Dosoretz DE, Galmarini D, Rubenstein JH et al: Local control in medically inoperable lung cancer: an analysis of its importance in outcome and factors determining the probability of tumor eradication. Int J Radiat Oncol Biol Phys 1993;27:507–516

236. Jeremic B, Shibamoto Y, Acimovic L, Milisavljevic S: Carboplatin, etoposide, and accelerated hyperfractionated radiotherapy for elderly patients with limited small cell lung carcinoma: a phase II study. Cancer 1998;82:836–841

237. Pignon T, Gregor A, Schaake Koning C et al: Age has no impact on acute and late toxicity of curative thoracic radiotherapy. Radiother Oncol 1998;46:239–248

238. Koga K, Kusumoto S, Watanabe K et al: Age factor relevant to the development of radiation pneumonitis in radiotherapy of lung cancer. Int J Radiat Oncol Biol Phys 1988;14:367–371

239. Monson JM, Stark P, Reilly JJ et al: Clinical radiation pneumonitis and radiographic changes after thoracic radiation therapy for lung carcinoma. Cancer 1998;82:842–850

240. Larson PJ, Lindsey AM, Dodd MJ et al: Influence of age on problems experienced by patients with lung cancer undergoing radiation therapy. Oncol Nurs Forum 1993;20:473–480

241. Patterson CJ, Hocking M, Bond M, Teale C: Retrospective study of radiotherapy for lung cancer in patients aged 75 years and over. Age Ageing 1998;27:515–518

242. Zachariah B, Balducci L, Venkattaramanabalaji GV et al: Radiotherapy for cancer patients aged 80 and older: a study of effectiveness and side effects. Int J Radiat Oncol Biol Phys 1997;39:1125–1129

243. Munro AJ: What now for postoperative radiotherapy for lung cancer? Lancet 1998;352:250–251

244. PORT Meta-analysis Trialists Group: Postoperative radiotherapy in non-small-cell lung cancer: systematic review and meta-analysis of individual patient data from nine randomised controlled trials. Lancet 1998;352:257–263

245. Graham PH, Gebski VJ, Stat M, Langlands AO: Radical radiotherapy for early nonsmall cell lung cancer. Int J Radiat Oncol Biol Phys 1995;31:261–266

246. Saunders M, Dische S, Barrett A et al, on behalf of the CHART Steering Committee: Continuous hyperfractionated accelerated radiotherapy (CHART) versus conventional radiotherapy in non-small-cell lung cancer: a randomised multicentre trial. Lancet 1997;350:161–165

247. Bonner JA, McGinnis WL, Stella PJ et al: The possible advantage of hyperfractionated thoracic radiotherapy in the treatment of locally advanced nonsmall cell lung carcinoma. Cancer 1998;82:1037–1048

248. Balducci L, Beghe C: Pharmacology of chemotherapy in the older cancer patient. Cancer Control 1999;6:466–470

249. Boyle DM: Realities to guide novel and necessary nursing care in geriatric oncology. Cancer Nurs 1994;17:125–136

250. Gosney M Cancer. In Crome P, Ford G (eds): Drugs and the Older Population. Imperial College Press, London, 2000:601–651

251. Hickish TF, Smith IE, O'Brien ME, Ashley S, Middleton G: Clinical benefit from palliative chemotherapy in non small cell cancer extends to the elderly and those with poor prognostic factors. Br J Cancer 1998;78:28–33

252. Siu LL, Shepherd FA, Murray N et al: Influence of age on the treatment of limited-stage small cell lung cancer. J Clin Oncol 1996;14:821–828

253. Murray N, Grafton C, Shah A et al: Abbreviated treated for elderly, infirm, or noncompliant patients with limited-stage small cell lung cancer. J Clin Oncol 1998;16:3323–3328

254. Kelly P, O'Brien AA, Daly P, Clancy L: Small-cell lung cancer in elderly patients: the case for chemotherapy. Age Ageing 1991;20:19–22

255. Carney DN, Byrne A: Etoposide in the treatment of elderly/poor-prognosis patients with small-cell lung cancer. Cancer Chemother Pharmacol 1994;34(S):96–100

256. Carney DN, Keane M, Grogan L: Oral etoposide in small cell lung cancer. Semin Oncol 1992;19:40–44

257. Pflüger KH, Hahn M, Holz JB et al: Pharmacokinetics of etoposide: correlation of pharmacokinetic parameters with clinical conditions. Cancer Chemother Pharmacol 1993;31:350–356

258. Loehrer PJ: Chronic oral etoposide: trials at Indiana University and with the Hoosier Oncology Group. Semin Oncol 1992;19:48–52

259. Slevin ML, Clark PI, Joel SP et al: A randomized trial to evaluate the effect of schedule on the activity of etoposide in small-cell lung cancer. J Clin Oncol 1989;7:1333–1340

260. Abratt RP, Willcox PA, de Groot M et al: Prospective study of etoposide scheduling in combination chemotherapy for limited-disease small cell lung cancer. Eur J Cancer 1991;27:28–30

261. Cerny T, Lind M, Thatcher N, Swindell R, Stout R: A simple outpatient treatment with oral ifosfamide and oral etoposide for patients with small cell lung cancer (SCLC). Br J Cancer 1989;60:258–261

262. Carney DN, Grogan L, Smith EF et al: Single-agent oral etoposide for elderly small cell lung cancer patients. Semin Oncol 1990;17:49–53

263. DeVore R, Hainsworth J, Greco FA, Hande K, Johnson D: Chronic oral etoposide in the treatment of lung cancer. Semin Oncol 1992;19:28–35

264. Hainsworth JD, Johnson DH, Frazier SR, Greco FA: Chronic daily administration of oral etoposide: a phase 1 trial. J Clin Oncol 1989;7:396–401

265. Clark PI, Slevin ML, Joel SP et al: A randomized trial of two etoposide schedules in small-cell lung cancer: the influence of pharmacokinetics on efficacy and toxicity. J Clin Oncol 1994;12:1427–1435

266. Thompson DS, Hainsworth JD, Hande KR, Holzmer M, Greco FA: Prolonged administration of low dose infusional etoposide in patients with advanced malignancies. Cancer 1994;73:2824–2831

267. Johnson DH, Hainsworth JD, Hande KR, Greco FA: Combination chemotherapy with oral etoposide. Semin Oncol 1992;19:19–24

268. Loehrer PJ, Rynard S, Ansari R et al: Etoposide, ifosfamide, and cisplatin in extensive small cell lung cancer. Cancer 1992;69:669–673

269. Bork E, Hansen M, Dombernowsky P et al: Teniposide (VM-26), an overlooked highly active agent in small-cell lung cancer: results of a phase II trial in untreated patients. J Clin Oncol 1986;4:524–527

270. Tummarello D, Isidori P, Pasini F, Cetto G, Cellerino R: Teniposide as single drug therapy for elderly patients affected by small cell lung cancer. Eur J Cancer 1992;28A:1081–1084

271. Smith IE, Harland SJ, Robinson BA et al: Carboplatin: a very active new cisplatin analog in the treatment of small cell lung cancer. Cancer Treat Rep 1985;69:43–46

272. Michel G, Leyvraz S, Bauer J et al: Weekly carboplatin and VM-26 for elderly patients with small-cell lung cancer. Ann Oncol 1994;5:369–370

273. Raghavan D, Bishop JF, Stuart-Harris R et al: Carboplatin-containing regimens for small cell lung cancer: implications for management in the elderly. Semin Oncol 1992;19:12–16

274. Buccheri G, Ferrigno D: Vinorelbine in elderly patients with inoperable nonsmall cell lung carcinoma: a phase II study. Cancer 2000;88:2677–2685

275. Veronesi A, Crivellari D, Magri MD et al: Vinorelbine treatment of advanced non-small cell lung cancer with special emphasis on elderly patients. Eur J Cancer 1996;2A:1809–1811

276. Gridelli C, Perrone F, Gallo C et al: Vinorelbine is well tolerated and active in the treatment of elderly patients with advanced non-small cell lung cancer: a two-stage phase II study. Eur J Cancer 1997;33:392–397

277. Beretta GD, Michetti G, Belometti MO et al: Gemcitabine plus vinorelbine in elderly or unfit patients with non-small cell lung cancer. Br J Cancer 2000;83:573–576

278. Frasci G, Lorusso V, Panza N et al: Gemcitabine plus vinorelbine versus vinorelbine alone in elderly patients with advanced non-small-cell lung cancer. J Clin Oncol 2000;18:2529–2536

279. Hainsworth JD, Burris HA, Litchy S et al: Weekly docetaxel in the treatment of elderly patients with advanced non small cell lung carcinoma. Cancer 2000;89:328–333

Chapter 44

Neurobiology of aging

Charles Vernon Mobbs

Interest in brain functioning during aging arises from two general concerns: first, that brain functions deteriorate during aging; and second, that neuronal processes may drive some aspects of the process of senescence itself and ultimately determine lifespan. In comparison with the failure of other systems, such as the immune system, impairments in brain function (e.g. memory) may cause deterioration in the very sense of identity and what it means to be human. Similarly, impairments in brain functions, especially those involving sensory processing and memory, comprise among the most common complaints of the elderly population. The role of the brain in driving the aging process is less well-studied, but the concept that neuroendocrine failure may mediate at least some functional impairments during aging (especially those of the reproductive system) is almost as old as the systematic study of aging itself.

Given the broad purview of the neurobiology of aging, it is impossible to address the subject fully in a short survey. Indeed, a recent book on the subject[1] comprises almost 1000 pages but still cannot be considered comprehensive. Numerous recent reviews examining various specific aspects of brain aging have also been published.[2–7] In addition, several chapters in the present volume address key aspects of the aging of the nervous system, including reviews of stroke, cognitive disorders, movement disorders, sensory impairments, and neuroendocrine impairments. In the previous edition of the present volume, an excellent review by Michael and Mann[8] described a range of age-related changes in the central nervous system, and much of the essential descriptions in that review continue to be pertinent. However, three main general concepts have become clearer since that time, and therefore the present study will focus on these concepts.

First, and probably most important, whereas it was previously held that there was little utility in distinguishing between neurological pathologies and age-related changes in individuals apparently free of pathological symptoms, it is now appreciated that this distinction is critical both conceptually and practically, as discussed below. Second, new data have become available that demonstrate, contrary to previous expectations and possibly intuition, the contribution of heredity to age-related impairments actually increases with age, up until about the age of 70, after which the effect of environment becomes increasingly important. Finally, recent studies in animal models have demonstrated convincingly that the nervous system may play a definitive role in determining lifespan, consistent with correlative evidence in humans. The present review therefore focuses on these key recent conceptual advances in the neurobiology of aging. For detailed descriptions of specific neuropathological syndromes and age-correlated changes in the central nervous system, the reader is referred to the appropriate chapters in the present volume, the reviews cited above, or the text specifically concerned with the neurobiology of aging cited above.[1]

Since age-related impairments in cognitive, sensory, motor, and neuroendocrine functions are particularly associated with age-related neurobiological impairments, the key concepts examined in the present review will be developed with particular reference to these systems.

NEUROBIOLOGY OF AGING: NORMAL VERSUS PATHOLOGICAL

Use of diagnostic criteria

The neurobiology of aging is particularly compelling in the context of those extreme impairments associated with disease, especially Alzheimer's disease which is associated with profound loss of memory function and eventual loss of basic cognitive processes, even including a sense of identity. Nevertheless, as described below, the very fact that Alzheimer's disease can be diagnosed as a specific syndrome implies that the constellation of symptoms associated with Alzheimer's disease is not a universal concomitant of senescence. Thus, although Alzheimer's disease is an age-related disease, in that its incidence increases dramatically with age, not every individual eventually succumbs to Alzheimer's disease. On the other hand, mild cognitive impairments, relative to young individuals, also increase with age even in individuals who clearly do not exhibit the constellation of symptoms that characterize Alzheimer's disease.

These considerations led to the hypothesis that Alzheimer's disease is only an "exaggerated" form of aging, and the same hypothesis could be suggested for many other age-correlated pathologies, such as Parkinson's disease or glaucoma. In effect such a hypothesis implies that people with Alzheimer's disease are only at the extreme end of a normal distribution of symptoms, and that as people age they inexorably drift toward that set of symptoms.

However, careful analysis of the characteristics of both the behavioral symptoms of Alzheimer's disease, and histological assessment of brains from patients with Alzheimer's disease compared to age-matched controls, in contrast to the comparison of brains of older compared to younger individuals, indicates that in fact Alzheimer's disease comprises a characteristic set of pathologies that are quite distinct from those observed in age-matched, non-diseased brains.[9]

First, it must be recognized that Alzheimer's disease is defined by its histological characteristics, particularly the signature presence of amyloid plaques and neurofilament tangles especially in the neocortex.[10–14] Using a typical constellation of diagnostic criteria based on plaques and tangles, one study found the diagnostic accuracy to be 88 percent, the sensitivity to be 98 percent, and the specificity to be 69 percent.[11] On the other hand, the clinical interest in this histopathological diagnosis is the relationship between these markers and clinical impairments; thus although diagnosis based on plaque load has been applied at least since 1985,[10] at which time such a diagnosis was known to correlate well with functional impairments based on clinical diagnosis using a variety of psychological testing instruments,[10] work has continued on both histological and psychological criteria to improve the agreement between them.[11–14] Nevertheless it should be appreciated that on the whole both psychological[15] and histopathological diagnostic criteria are based on a bimodal distribution of outcome. Thus, by definition, individuals diagnosed with Alzheimer's disease by an experienced clinician are not simply at the extreme of a unimodal distribution, as would be the case if Alzheimer's disease were simply an "exaggerated" form of aging; rather, individuals diagnosed with the disease appear to constitute a qualitatively different population. Thus while various aspects of memory function may exhibit some impairments during nonpathological aging, the confusion, disorientation, and remarkable forgetting of specific experiences that characterize even the earliest stages of Alzheimer's disease are, taken together, qualitatively distinct from those observed even in quite elderly individuals who do not appear to exhibit the disease.[15] Similarly, while it is true that possibly during nonpathological aging some plaques and tangles may develop, in the significant majority of cases the qualitative distinction between Alzheimer's disease and nonpathological aging is immediately evident after routine silver-staining procedures.[16] Naturally the diagnosis of a few individuals, often in the early stage of the disease, will be ambiguous, since the diagnostic scores of these individuals may fall in between the modal distributions of nonpathological and pathological cases; but the existence of such individuals is inherent even when the pathological and the nonpathological states are qualitatively distinct.

Use of stereological cell counts

Even using standard criteria, the diagnosis of Alzheimer's disease may be ambiguous in a few individuals, but this ambiguity is largely eliminated if more laborious methodologies involving direct assessment of cell number are used. For example, at the earliest stages of Alzheimer's disease the entorhinal cortex invariably exhibits a substantial load of neurofibrillary tangles at levels never observed in young normal individuals, although nondiseased elderly individuals may exhibit a few such tangles.[17] Though based on tangles and other criteria there might be some overlap between diseased and nondiseased brains, much more laborious analysis of cell counts using modern stereological methods demonstrated that even very early Alzheimer's disease is characterized by significant loss of neurons in the entorhinal cortex, in contrast to no neuron loss at the same ages in individuals with no evidence of Alzheimer's disease.[18] Indeed, numerous studies using the now-standard stereological techniques have led to the consensus that neuropathological conditions can be qualitatively distinguished from nonpathological aging, in that the former, but not the latter, is invariably associated with neuron loss.[9] Such conclusions based on clinical data are consistent with the much more extensive data from animal models demonstrating that normal age-related impairments in memory function are not due to neuronal loss, and indeed that healthy aging animals rarely exhibit neuron loss.[19–21]

Incident rate analysis

An alternative analysis to distinguish between normal and pathological aging involves examination of rate-specific incidence rates of neurodegenerative diseases, based on the analysis of rate-specific mortality rates.[22] Mortality rates increase exponentially with age, although in both humans and other species[23,24] the slope of the linearized Gompertz equation begins to decrease at very old ages, and possibly the rate of mortality becomes constant (e.g. independent of age) in populations composed of very old individuals.

The Gompertz equation applies not only to mortality but also to diseases, and may be used to address the distinction, discussed above, between pathological and nonpathological age-related impairments. This distinction is not merely semantic but addresses fundamental questions of mechanism. As with mortality, the rate of onset of many neurological diseases increases exponentially with age.[25] (In the following analysis it is essential to keep in mind the difference between *incidence*, the rate at which new cases occur at a given age, and *prevalence*, which is the total number of extant cases in a population of that age. Rate equations such as the Gompertz curve describe only incidence, so incidence is the most informative from a mechanistic point of view.) The incidence rate of neurological diseases increases exponentially up to the age of maximum incidence, the age depending on the disease, but then the incidence of disease begins to decrease. For example, the age-specific incidence of Huntington's disease peaks at around 40 years of age,[26] the age-specific incidence of Parkinson's disease peaks at about 75 years of age,[27] and the age-specific incidence of Alzheimer's disease appears to peak at about 90 years of age.[28]

These examples also indicate the important mechanistic implications of incidence rate data. Typically, the incidence rate of familial forms of age-related diseases peaks at earlier ages than do the nonfamilial or sporadic forms. Thus mutations in the parkin gene lead to juvenile-onset Parkinson's disease, whose incidence peaks at around 20 years of age, and the incidence of Parkinson's disease due to mutations in α-synuclein peaks at around 50 years of age.[29] In contrast, the incidence rate of Parkinson's disease in the population as a whole peaks at around 70 years.[27] The mechanistic implications of the distinction between disease and senescence may be clarified by example. As described above, the incidence of Alzheimer's disease continues to increase until late in life. In addition, gradual impairments in memory functions also increase monotonically with age. As described above, these observations have suggested the hypothesis that Alzheimer's disease is an exaggerated form of nonpathological "normal" aging. This hypothesis implies that if one lives long enough, one would inevitably contract Alzheimer's disease, just as all women, if they live long enough, experience menopause. However, careful analysis of the incidence of Alzheimer's disease has demonstrated that, like all diseases, the incidence reaches a peak well before maximum lifespan. Thus, for example, centenarians exhibit a lower incidence of Alzheimer's disease than do individuals aged between 70 and 80.[28] This behavior indicates that Alzheimer's disease is not merely an accentuated form of "normal" age-related changes but is a distinct pathological process; conversely, the more universal (but milder) cognitive impairments observed during aging are not likely to be due to the same mechanism as that which causes Alzheimer's disease.

Relative contributions of heredity and environment to age-related impairments

From a clinical perspective, the degree to which age-related impairments in neurobiological function, whether pathological or nonpathological, are due to environment or heredity profoundly influences treatment options. Clearly in the case of age-related genetic diseases, the coupling between genotype and phenotype increases with age; for single-gene defects, this implies that genetic penetrance increases with age. For example, Huntington's disease is an autosomal-dominant disease with complete penetrance, since every individual bearing the disease-causing allele eventually develops the disease (if the individual lives long enough) and no individual without that allele develops the disease.[26] However, at birth there is no phenotypical difference between individuals bearing the mutation for Huntington's disease and normal individuals; the phenotype develops only during aging, and by age 70 there is almost 100 percent concordance between genotype and phenotype, the environment playing essentially no role. Thus penetrance of the Huntington's disease allele increases from zero to 100 percent during aging. Furthermore, cumulative environmental effects during aging may depend largely on genotype. For example, as described below, practice enhances skill, and a high-fat diet induces obesity, but the effect of these manipulations depends largely on genotype. Thus when individuals share a common environment, the effect of genotype may become more accentuated during aging even for environmentally induced phenotypes.

It has therefore become clear that assessing the coupling between genotype and phenotype during aging requires a careful analysis of the effect of age on genetic penetrance. As will be described below, such careful analysis in human twin studies has indicated that the relative contribution of genotype to neurobiological phenotype often increases with age to a peak at around 70 years of age, after which phenotype is increasingly determined by environment.

It is perhaps surprising that, at least until age 70, heredity is increasingly important in determining phenotype of, for example, cognitive function, since it might be hypothesized that effects of experience would dominate during aging. Since effects of environment, unique to each individual, must surely accumulate with age, it may seem counterintuitive that effects of genotype could increase with age at all. This apparent paradox can be more easily understood in the context of the following considerations. First, the effect of genes for age-related genetic diseases must, by definition, increase with age. Second, the incidence rate of familial forms of diseases peaks earlier than the incidence rate of sporadic or nonfamilial forms. As described below, the net effect of these two phenomena is that the concordance between genotype and phenotype increases with age, as the phenotype of genetic diseases develops, but then the relative contribution of genotype to phenotype decreases with age as the incidence rate of sporadic forms of diseases increases.

MOTOR SYSTEMS FUNCTIONALITY

As described in detail in other chapters of this book, motor system functionality is impaired with age. In humans, this decline is characterized by the development of several age-related diseases of motor systems (including Huntington's disease and Parkinson's disease) superimposed on universal but gradual impairments in neuromuscular functions, especially due largely to decrease in muscle mass. The incidence of each disease peaks at a characteristic age (for Huntington's disease around age 40, for Parkinson's disease around age 70), then begins to decline, but the relative contribution of the universal age-related declines in neuromuscular function continues to increase with age. As the incidence of disease increases, the contribution of disease to individual variation in motor function also increases; and to the extent that risk of disease is primarily genetic, genotype contributes substantially to phenotype during this time. However, as the incidence of motor diseases decreases (after about age 70) there is also a decline in the relative contribution of motor disease genes to age-related impairments in motor function.

Huntington's disease

Huntington's disease is an autosomal-dominant neurodegenerative condition associated with profound movement disorders, whose age-specific incidence peaks at around 40 years of age.[26] Monozygotic twins are essentially 100 percent concordant in the development of Huntington's disease, demonstrating the primary contribution of genotype to the risk.[30] More recent work has demonstrated that Huntington's disease is caused by a variable expansion of a CAG repeat producing a polyglutamine stretch in the gene product, huntingtin.[31] Characterization of the allele for Huntington's disease has made it possible to definitively test for the relationship between genotype and Huntington's phenotype. Thus Kremer et al.[32] studied 1007 late middle-aged patients who were clinically diagnosed with Huntington's disease from 565 families, and 113 controls with other age-related neurological diseases. Of the 1007 diagnosed patients, 995 were found to bear from 36 to 121 CAG repeats, whereas none of the patients with other neurological diseases was found to bear these repeats. Thus by late middle age the concordance between genotype and Huntington's phenotype is essentially 100 percent.

Nevertheless, at relatively young ages (under 20 years), there is little concordance between genotype and Huntington's phenotype, since at these ages only about 10 percent of individuals who express CAG repeats in the huntintin gene exhibit Huntington's phenotype. Therefore with respect to incidence, Huntington's disease represents an extreme form of the coupling between genotype and age-related phenotype, in which the coupling increases from very low below the age of 20 years (at which age the great majority of individuals bearing the CAG repeat do not exhibit the Huntington phenotype) to essentially 100 percent concordance by age 70 years (at which age almost every individual who bears the CAG repeat would have developed the disease). By the same token, however, the relative contribution of the CAG repeat to phenotypic variation in the whole population increases with age as the incidence of the disease peaks at about 40 years, but then begins to decline as the incidence of Huntington's disease decreases.

On the other hand, other aspects of the phenotype exhibit a more subtle relationship to genotype. For example, the number of CAG repeats can vary widely, from fewer than 30 to more than 100; the number of CAG repeats is highly (inversely) correlated with age of onset of Huntington's disease early in life, but the strength of this correlation decreases with age.[33,34] Therefore the coupling between genotype and the age of onset of Huntington's disease decreases with age.

Parkinson's disease

Parkinson's disease is about 10-fold more prevalent than Huntington's disease, and the incident rate of Parkinson's disease peaks later than that of Huntington's disease, at about 75 years of age, after which incidence rate begins to decline.[27] In stark contrast to the perfect concordance for Huntington's disease in identical twins, several studies have failed to observe any concordance for Parkinson's disease in identical twins.[35] This observation demonstrates a much lower overall contribution of genotype to Parkinson's phenotype than for Huntington's phenotype. On the other hand, several families have been studied in which the Parkinson's disease follows an autosomal-dominant pattern of inheritance,[36] and in several different families this led to the identification of an allele of α-synuclein as the genetic basis of the disease in these families.[37] In another group of families in which Parkinson's disease is inherited in an autosomal-recessive pattern, mutations in the gene coding for parkin account for the appearance of the Parkinson's phenotype.[38,39] Nevertheless, mutations in α-synuclein and parkin account for only a small subset of all cases of familial Parkinson's disease,[40] and thus of an even smaller subset of all cases of Parkinson's disease.

These observations demonstrate that the coupling of genotype to phenotype is much lower, and the genetic basis much more complex, in Parkinson's disease. On the other hand, Parkinson's disease is not only much more common than Huntington's disease, it is a much more heterogeneous syndrome, and thus plausibly involves a more heterogeneous set of pathophysiological processes. Thus for those forms of Parkinson's disease for which a single gene defect has been defined, the coupling between genotype and phenotype behaves as it does in Huntington's. Within kindreds in which α-synuclein mutations are common, at young ages there is no concordance between mutations in α-synuclein and Parkinson's phenotype, whereas by age 70 there is a very high concordance between genotype and phenotype. On the other hand, in the population as a whole this relationship is less evident since α-synuclein mutations account for only a small proportion of all cases of Parkinson's disease, in contrast to Huntington's disease, all of whose cases are accounted for by mutations in a single gene.

A key observation is that the incidence rate of familial forms of Parkinson's disease peaks earlier than in sporadic or nonfamilial forms. Thus mutations in parkin lead to juvenile-onset Parkinson's disease, whose incidence peaks at around 20 years of age, and the incidence of Parkinson's disease due to mutations in α-synuclein peaks at around 50 years of age. In contrast, the incidence rate of Parkinson's disease in the population as a whole peaks at around 70 years. Since twin studies indicated that genotype makes little contribution to the late-onset (and most common) form of the disease, taken together these data imply that the contribution of genotype to Parkinson's phenotype increases with age up until about age 50, then begins to decline such that, by age 70, there is little contribution of genotype to phenotype.[29]

Nonpathological age-related changes in motor function

For age-related diseases, the effect of genotype generally increases with age up until about age 70 (in humans), then begins to decline as the incidence of age-related diseases peaks and then declines. However, as the incidence of disease decreases in later life, the relative contribution of disease to the variance in age-related phenotype also begins to decline. Thus a major question is the extent to which genotype accounts for nondisease phenotype during aging. While it might be assumed that the effect of life-long environmental effects would increasingly dominate genetic effects, there is little evidence to support this as a general phenomenon. For example, twin studies have indicated that, although psychomotor speed declines with age, the effect of genotype and possibly early environment continues to dominate this phenotype during aging, at least up until age 67; in contrast, effects of exercise were minimal.[41] Nevertheless, the effect of age on the penetrance of genotype on psychomotor function has not been elucidated in detail.

COGNITIVE FUNCTION

Although genetic effects on motor diseases increase with age before they decrease, it might be hypothesized that cognitive functions are more likely to reflect cumulative experience during aging, and thus the contribution of genotype might be less for cognitive functions. However, as described below, effects of genotype are probably at least as great on cognitive functions during aging as for motor functions.

Alzheimer's disease

In contrast to Parkinson's disease, twin studies have demonstrated a much greater significant genetic contribution to the risk of developing Alzheimer's disease.[42–51] For example, in a study of Swedish twins, concordance between monozygotic twins was 67 percent, compared with only 22 percent for dizygotic twins.[45] Conclusions from twin studies have been corroborated in family studies. For example, offspring whose parents had both been diagnosed with Alzheimer's disease had a 47 percent chance of developing Alzheimer's disease by age 65, far higher than the risk of the general population at that age.[52] Similarly, analysis of 70 kindreds with evidence of hereditary forms of Alzheimer's disease indicated that offspring whose parents had Alzheimer's disease had a lifetime risk of developing the disease (by age 87) of 64 percent (compared with a risk of less than 10 percent in the general population by that age). Interestingly, the risk for offspring in families with early-onset Alzheimer's disease was only 53 percent, compared with a remarkable 86 percent for offspring in families with late-onset Alzheimer's disease.[53] Thus at least within these kindreds, there is evidence of increased penetrance of genotype during aging. On the other hand, the incidence rate of Alzheimer's disease appears to decrease after age 90.[28] Because of the relatively small number of individuals alive at these very advanced ages, it is not yet known whether the effect of genotype on the risk of Alzheimer's disease may decline after age 90.

As with Parkinson's disease, allelic variations in several specific genes (presenilin 1, presenilin 2, β-amyloid-precursor, and apolipoprotein E) have been implicated in the etiology of Alzheimer's disease.[54] Thus how aging influences the penetrance of these genes is of great interest. Campion et al.[55] addressed this question in a recent study which examined the genetic basis of early-onset autosomal-dominant Alzheimer's disease in the whole population of a single city in France. In this study early-onset autosomal-dominant disease was defined by the occurrence of Alzheimer's disease before the age of 61 years in three generations of a family. Thirty-four such families were observed in the city examined, with a population of almost 500,000. In 56 percent of the families, allelic variations in presenilin 1 were observed, and in 15 percent of the families allelic variations of the β-amyloid precursor were observed. In contrast, in nine families which did not exhibit an early-onset form of the disease, such allelic variations were not observed. These data suggest that the penetrance of presenilin 1 and β-amyloid precursor mutations reaches 100 percent at relatively young ages (around age 60). However, since the incidence of Alzheimer's disease before the age of 60 is less than 5 percent of the incidence at age 80–90, this demonstrates that the coupling between presenilin 1 (or β-amyloid precursor) and Alzheimer's disease phenotype peaks at around age 60, then returns to negligible by age 80. In contrast to the (eventual) complete penetrance of the presenilin and β-amyloid alleles, alleles of the ApoE gene are never completely penetrant, but nevertheless account for a much larger proportion (possibly 20 percent) of cases of Alzheimer's disease.[56] Nevertheless, the effect of ApoE genotype peaks at around age 70, then declines (but is significant even at 90 years of age).[56,57]

Taken together, the evidence indicates that the coupling between genotype and Alzheimer's disease phenotype peaks at about 70 years of age; then, as with other age-related diseases, the role of genotype begins to decline.

Nonpathological age-related impairments in cognitive function

Since the effect of genotype on performance in standardized intelligence tests has been examined in great detail in young populations, several studies have used similar methodologies to assess effects of aging on the contribution of genotype to performance on these tests.[58–63]

For example, Plomin et al.,[58] as part of the Swedish Adoption/Twin Study of Aging, examined cognitive functions in 112 pairs of twins (both monozygotic and dizygotic) reared apart and in 111 matched pairs of twins reared together. The age of the twins was 64.1 ± 7.5 (mean ± standard deviation) years. At this age, the average heritability of general cognitive function (a composite of spatial, verbal, memory, and speed of processing performances, after removal of effects of age and gender) was 80 percent. In a detailed review of studies from both the Swedish Adoption/Twin Study of Aging and the Minnesota Twin Study of Adult Development and Aging, Finkel et al.[59] concluded that both sets of studies suggested that heritability of general cognitive function is about 80 percent throughout adulthood (though this estimate is higher than has been observed in other studies), but evidence suggested a possible decrease in heritability after age 70 years. A further analysis of the Swedish Twin study appeared to corroborate this result, since in Swedish twins over the age of 80, heritability of general cognitive function was estimated to be about 62 percent.[60] Although direct comparisons are not conclusive, other studies have suggested that heritability of general cognitive function increases from about 50 percent in childhood and adolescence to about 80 percent in adulthood.[64,65]

It should be noted that although aging influences the heritability of general cognitive function, the effect of age on cognitive function itself is more specific to specific subsystems. In general, functions reflecting knowledge improve with age, whereas functions reflecting speed of processing and memory are impaired with age. Thus aspects of cognition reflected by the Wechsler subscales of Information, Vocabulary, and Comprehension are relatively unimpaired or even improve with age in nondemented individuals, whereas cognitive functions reflected by the subscales of Block Design, Picture Arrangement and Digit Symbol tend to deteriorate robustly with age.[66] Interestingly, the heritability of general cognitive function during aging is greater than the heritability of any of the functions reflected by subscales, which has been interpreted to indicate that the "nature of the genetic influence in the cognitive domain appears to be more general than specific."[58] Thus in contrast to the effect of age on the heritability of general cognitive function, heritability on memory function alone is reported to be stable with age.[67]

GENOTYPE INFLUENCES ON THE CUMULATIVE EFFECT OF ENVIRONMENT

Since cognitive function is defined by experience, it may seem surprising that heritability of cognitive function can increase with age at all (although decreasing after the age of 70). One resolution of this apparent paradox is that the influence of experience may greatly depend on genotype; that is, the effect of experience may be enhanced by genotype. For example, in a twin study examining the effect of genotype on the acquisition of a motor skill, Fox et al.[68] reported that, while genotype influenced the initial performance of the skill, the effect of genotype on the enhancement of the skill by practice was even greater. These investigators concluded that "the effect of practice is to decrease the effect of environmental variation (previous learning) and increase the relative strength of genetic influences on motor performance." Similarly, it seems plausible that genotype may influence the cumulative effect of experience on general cognitive functions. On the other hand, after the age of 70 it appears that these genetic effects have reached their peak, and the effects of unique experiences come to dominate.

A similar phenomenon may influence neuroendocrine functions during aging. For example, it has been reported that in males the heritability of body mass index is about

46 percent in those aged 46–59 years and 61 percent in those aged 60–76 years.[69] As with other phenotypes, the mechanism of this increasing penetrance on body mass index is unclear. However, work in rodents suggests a possible mechanism. Two strains of mice, C57BL/6J and A/J, have similar bodyweights throughout life if fed a standard laboratory chow, which is very low in fat. In contrast, when fed a diet high in fat, C57BL/6J gain a substantial amount of body weight and after several months develop diabetes; whereas A/J mice, while consuming the same amount of the diet, stay relatively thin and normoglycemic.[70] Thus in the presence of one environment (characterized by a low-fat diet), there is little effect of genotype on body weight or blood glucose, whereas in a different environment (characterized by a high-fat diet), the effect of genotype (which initially is very small) increases substantially as body weight and blood glucose increases over time in C57BL/6J mice, but not A/J mice. Furthermore, the increase of heritability of body weight over time on a high-fat diet appears to be mediated through a neuroendocrine mechanism, since the high-fat diet induces weight-reducing responses in the hypothalamus of A/J mice, but not in C57BL/6J mice.[71] Twin studies have also suggested that the heritability of age at menopause, which appears to entail neuroendocrine impairments, is about 60 percent.[72]

SENSORY FUNCTIONS

Age-related impairments in sensory functions may also involve genetic exacerbation of environmental insults. For example, C57BL/6J mice exhibit gradual age-related impairments in auditory function, leading to essentially complete loss of hearing by old age, whereas CBA and other strains of mice retain largely normal auditory function until old age; this effect of genotype is now known to be due to a recessive gene whose penetrance increases with age. Of particular interest, however, is that this recessive gene also greatly potentiates noise-induced hearing loss.[73] Thus, while the effect of genotype on hearing function clearly increases with age in mice, part of the mechanism by which this occurs may involve exacerbation of effects, as occurs in diet-induced obesity. Similarly, concordance of age-related macular degeneration was 100 percent in monozygotic twins but only 42 percent in dizygotic twins,[74] so again the effects of genotype on macular degeneration increase with age. Numerous environmental risk factors for macular degeneration have been observed (including smoking and diabetes), so it will be of interest to assess whether the genetic causes involve exacerbation of these deleterious events.

A NEURONAL PATHWAY MAY DRIVE SYSTEMIC AGING

In the discussions above, and in most of the chapters in the present volume, the focus is on impairments in neurobiological function that increase with advancing age. Generally, these impairments are thought of as "effects" of aging, though of course the impairments are effects of processes that continue over time.

In contrast, it is of interest to consider the role that neurobiological processes have in the development of more global age-related impairments, and in particular in the contribution of age-related neuronal impairments in causing mortality. In the case of some diseases, particularly Huntington's disease, this association is complete and clear: age-related mortality is completely accounted for by the neurobiological pathology. However, it has long been hypothesized that nonpathological neuronal processes, particularly neuroendocrine processes, may regulate more fundamental aspects of the aging process, and indeed may fundamentally regulate lifespan. For example, obesity and its associated metabolic syndrome including hypertension and other cardiovascular diseases are clearly associated with increased mortality. To the extent that obesity is due to impairments in the hypothalamic neurons that sense metabolic status and regulate bodyweight, the age-associated increase in obesity and its associated metabolic impairments may actually contribute to an age-related increase in mortality rate.[75] Recent results, reviewed below, have surprisingly supported such a hypothesis.

Since cellular functionality in many tissues is generally preserved during aging, age-related pathologies have long been hypothesized to be due to age-related impairments in the regulatory or hormonal milieu impinging upon these cells.[76] On the other hand, based in part on the precedent that lifespan is limited in spawning salmon by the activation of the hypothalamic–pituitary–adrenal axis,[77] several investigators have proposed that specific neuroendocrine systems may actively drive distinct senescent processes.[78–80] A more general hypothesis that neuroendocrine systems drive a fundamental process of senescence was supported by the observation that hypophysectomy may delay many aspects of senescence and extend lifespan.[81] Consistent with, and perhaps even more striking than, these observations, loss of function of single genes in two possibly related neuroendocrine pathways also increases maximum lifespan in mice. First, single gene defects that ablate hormone-producing pituitary cells[82] extend maximum lifespan of mice.[83] Similarly, ablation of the growth hormone receptor also increases lifespan in mice.[84] Furthermore, ablation of p66Shc, which appears to mediate some effects of growth factors including insulin,[85] also extends maximum lifespan in mice.[86] Similarly, loss of function of several individual genes in the insulin-like signaling pathway of *Caenorhabditis elegans* extends maximum lifespan in this species.[87] Finally, loss of function of a hormone/GTP-binding receptor-like protein also extends maximum lifespan in fruit-flies.[88] Taken together, these genetic studies suggest that the action of hormones may drive important processes in senescence, including the limitation of lifespan. However, the role of neuronal activity in driving these mechanisms has not been demonstrated definitively in mammals.

On the other hand, a recent series of investigations in the nematode has directly demonstrated a key role of the neuroendocrine system in regulating lifespan. In the nematode a group of genetic mutations has been established which lead to an extension of maximum lifespan.[89–91] Particularly striking was the discovery that a mutation in a single gene, termed age-1, reduces the Gompertz rate of mortality in *C. elegans*.[90] The existence of such a gene was largely unexpected, given evolutionary arguments implying that senescence is unlikely to be controlled by even a small number of genes.[92] When this gene was cloned it was discovered to code for a homologue of mammalian phosphatidylinositol-3-OH kinase.[93] While this clearly suggested a neuroendocrine mechanism, the ligand pathway mediated by this kinase was initially unclear. Subsequent to the discovery of age-1, however, other single genes were discovered that also extended lifespan in *C. elegans*; among these genes, DAF-2 was subsequently cloned and discovered to code for a homologue of the mammalian insulin receptor.[94] Further genetic analysis has now demonstrated conclusively that single gene defects extending lifespan act through an insulin signaling pathway remarkably similar to the mammalian insulin signaling pathway.[87] Furthermore, and most surprisingly, transgenic manipulation has now demonstrated that it is activity of the insulin-like pathway specifically in neurons, not muscle or other highly metabolically active tissue, that regulates lifespan in *C. elegans*.[95]

In essence, therefore, these studies indicate that sensescence (or at least a major component of senscence, since defects in this pathway reduce the Gompertz slope) arises from the activity of an insulin-like pathway acting through neurons regulated by this pathway (that is, presumably, neurons that are sensitive to an insulin-like ligand). As described below, considerable evidence has suggested that senescence may arise from metabolic activity. Therefore a logical hypothesis is that an insulin-like pathway drives senescence in *C. elegans* by enhancing metabolic activity. Furthermore, the life-extending effect of the insulin-like pathway appears to require activity of an unusual cytoplasmic catalase.[96] Taken together, these data suggest that reduction of senescence by attenuating the insulin-like pathway entails protection of neurons from free radical damage and that, conversely, integrity of neurons sensitive to this insulin-like pathway constitutes a limiting factor in lifespan of *C. elegans*.[95]

Whether insulin-sensitive neurons in the mammalian nervous system may play a similar role in regulating mammalian lifespan remains to be established. Several lines of evidence suggest a convergence of insulin and glucose signaling in glucose-sensitive neuroendocrine cells in mammals,[97–101] and indeed that many effects of insulin are mediated through glucose metabolism.[102] Another series of studies has indicated that an essential metabolic step mediating effects of caloric restriction on yeast lifespan is the conversion of NAD to NADH (and not, for example, ATP).[103] Several lines of evidence have now indicated that an essential metabolic step by which neuroendocrine cells sense glucose is also the conversion of NAD to NADH, rather than production of ATP.[104–106] Thus these data suggest that conversion of NAD+ to NADH in glucose-sensitive neuroendocrine cells may drive key aspects of the aging process.

Such observations are consistent with the hypothesis that glucose metabolism in glucose-sensitive neuroendocrine cells, especially in the mammalian hypothalamus, cumulatively compromises the function of these key neuroendocrine cells and leads to age-associated metabolic impairments.[75,107] This hypothesis has been supported by the evidence that a key subset of glucose-sensitive neurons in the hypothalamus produce proopiomelancortin (POMC),[108,109] impairments in which cause metabolic syndromes similar to those observed during aging,[110] and POMC-producing neurons are among the most vulnerable to early and robust age-related impairments in mice,[111] rats,[112] and humans.[113–115]

Thus it remains possible that not only are key neuronal functions impaired during senescence, but that in fact impairments in key neuronal functions may drive the process of senescence, and generally limit lifespan. Therapeutic interventions that reduce these age-related impairments in neuroendocrine function may therefore in some cases delay mortality in association with reduced functional pathologies, especially cardiovascular diseases associated with the metabolic syndrome.

KEY POINTS Neurobiology of aging

- Pathological and nonpathological age-related impairments are quantitatively and qualitatively distinct.

- Cognitive, motor, sensory, and neuroendocrine functions are all impaired with age, although the nonpathological age-related changes in the last three systems are more dependent on peripheral impairments than impairments in the central nervous system.

- The importance of heredity in determining age-related impairments increases with age up until about 70 years, after which environmental influences become increasingly important.

- Impairments in brain function may play a key role in determining lifespan.

REFERENCES

1. Hof PR, Mobbs CV (eds): Functional Neurobiology of Aging. Academic Press, San Diego, 2001
2. Barnes CA: Plasticity in the aging central nervous system. Int Rev Neurobiol 2001;45:339–354
3. Mattson MP, Duan W, Lee J, Guo Z: Suppression of brain aging and neurodegenerative disorders by dietary restriction and environmental enrichment: molecular mechanisms. Mech Ageing Dev 2001;122:757–778
4. Farkas E, Luiten PG: Cerebral microvascular pathology in aging and Alzheimer's disease. Prog Neurobiol 2001;64:575–611
5. Brandt J: Mild cognitive impairment in the elderly. Am Fam Physician 2001;63:620,622,625–626
6. Grady CL, Craik FI: Changes in memory processing with age. Curr Opin Neurobiol 2000;10(2):224–231
7. Toescu EC, Myronova N, Verkhratsky A: Age-related structural and functional changes of brain mitochondria. Cell Calcium 2000;28(5–6):329–338
8. Michael D, Mann A: Neurobiology of aging. In Tallis R, Fillit H (eds): Brocklehurst's Textbook of Geriatric Medicine and Gerontology. Harcourt, London, 1998:385–422
9. Morrison JH, Hof PR: Life and death of neurons in the aging brain. Science 1997;278:412–419
10. Khachaturian ZS: Diagnosis of Alzheimer's disease. Arch Neurol 1985;42:1097–1105
11. Kazee AM, Eskin TA, Lapham LW: Clinicopathologic correlates in Alzheimer disease: assessment of clinical and pathologic diagnostic criteria. Alzheimer Dis Assoc Disord 1993;7(3):152–164
12. National Institute on Aging, and Reagan Institute Working Group on Diagnostic Criteria for the Neuropathological Assessment of Alzheimer's Disease: Consensus recommendations for the postmortem diagnosis of Alzheimer's disease. Neurobiol Aging 1997;18(4 suppl):S1–S2
13. Newell KL, Hyman BT, Growdon JH, Hedley-Whyte ET: Application of the National Institute on Aging (NIA)–Reagan Institute criteria for the neuropathological diagnosis of Alzheimer disease. J Neuropathol Exp Neurol 1999;58:1147–1155

14. Wisniewski HM, Silverman W: Diagnostic criteria for the neuropathological assessment of Alzheimer's disease: current status and major issues. Neurobiol Aging 1997;18(4 suppl):S43–S50

15. Mohs RC, Knopman D, Petersen RC et al: Development of cognitive instruments for use in clinical trials of antidementia drugs: additions to the Alzheimer's Disease Assessment Scale that broaden its scope. The Alzheimer's Disease Cooperative Study. Alzheimer Dis Assoc Disord 1997;11(suppl 2):S13–S21

16. Powers JM: Diagnostic criteria for the neuropathologic assessment of Alzheimer's disease. Neurobiol Aging 1997;18(4 suppl):S53–S54

17. Hyman BT, Van Hoesen GW, Damasio AR: Memory-related neural systems in Alzheimer's disease: an anatomic study. Neurology 1990;40:1721–1730

18. Gomez-Isla T, Price JL, McKeel DW et al: Profound loss of layer II entorhinal cortex neurons occurs in very mild Alzheimer's disease. J Neurosci 1996;16:4491–4500

19. Gallagher M, Landfield PW, McEwen B et al: Hippocampal neurodegeneration in aging. Science 1996;274:484–485 (letter and comment)

20. Rapp PR, Gallagher M: Preserved neuron number in the hippocampus of aged rats with spatial learning deficits. Proc Natl Acad Sci USA 1996;93:9926–9930

21. Rapp PR, Stack EC, Gallagher M: Morphometric studies of the aged hippocampus. I: Volumetric analysis in behaviorally characterized rats. J Comp Neurol 1999;403:459–470

22. Riggs JE: The Gompertz function: distinguishing mathematical from biological limitations. Mech Ageing Dev 1993;69(1–2):33–36

23. Vaupel JW, Carey JR, Christensen K et al: Biodemographic trajectories of longevity. Science 1998;280:855–860

24. Curtsinger JW, Fukui HH, Townsend DR, Vaupel JW: Demography of genotypes: failure of the limited life-span paradigm in Drosophila melanogaster. Science 1992;258:461–463

25. Riggs JE: Age-specific rates of neurological disease. In Hof PR, Mobbs CV (eds): Functional Neurobiology of Aging. Academic Press, San Diego, 2001:3–12

26. Greenamyre JT, Shoulson I: Huntington's disease. In Calne DB (ed): Neurodegenerative Diseases. WB Saunders, Philadelphia, 1994:685–704

27. Martilla RJ: Epidemiology. In Koller W (ed): Handbook of Parkinson's disease. Marcel Dekker, New York, 1987:55–60

28. Lautenschlager NT, Cupples LA, Rao VS et al: Risk of dementia among relatives of Alzheimer's disease patients in the MIRAGE study: what is in store for the oldest old? Neurology 1996;46:641–650

29. Langston JW: Epidemiology versus genetics in Parkinson's disease: progress in resolving an age-old debate. Ann Neurol 1998;44(3 suppl 1):S45–S52

30. Sudarsky L, Myers RH, Walsh TM: Huntington's disease in monozygotic twins reared apart. J Med Genet 1983;20:408–411

31. Lunkes A, Trottier Y, Mandel JL: Pathological mechanisms in Huntington's disease and other polyglutamine expansion diseases. Essays Biochem 1998;33:149–163

32. Kremer B, Goldberg P, Andrew SE et al: A worldwide study of the Huntington's disease mutation: the sensitivity and specificity of measuring CAG repeats. N Engl J Med 1994;330:1401–1406

33. Crauford D, Dodge A: Mutation and age at onset in Huntington's disease. J Med Genet 1993;30:1008–1111

34. Kremer B, Squitieri F, Telenius H et al: Molecular analysis of late onset Huntington's disease. J Med Genet 1993;30:991–995

35. Lilienfeld DE: An epidemiological overview of amyotrophic lateral sclerosis, Parkinson's disease, and dementia of the Alzheimer's type. In Calne DB (ed): Neurodegenerative Diseases. WB Saunders, Philadelphia, 1994:399–425

36. Golbe LI, Di Iorio G, Sanges G et al: Clinical genetic analysis of Parkinson's disease in the Contursi kindred. Ann Neurol 1996;40:767–775

37. Polymeropoulos MH, Lavedan C, Leroy E et al: Mutation in the alpha-synuclein gene identified in families with Parkinson's disease. Science 1997;276:2045–2047

38. Kitada T, Asakawa S, Hattori N et al: Mutations in the parkin gene cause autosomal recessive juvenile parkinsonism. Nature 1998;392:605–608

39. Hattori N, Matsumine H, Asakawa S et al: Point mutations (Thr240Arg and Gln311Stop) in the Parkin gene. Biochem Biophys Res Commun 1998;249:754–758

40. Vaughan J, Durr A, Tassin J et al: The alpha-synuclein Ala53Thr mutation is not a common cause of familial Parkinson's disease: a study of 230 European cases. European Consortium on Genetic Susceptibility in Parkinson's Disease. Ann Neurol 1998;44(2):270–273

41. Simonen RL, Videman T, Battie MC, Gibbons LE: Determinants of psychomotor speed among 61 pairs of adult male monozygotic twins. J Gerontol A 1998;53:M228–M234

42. Rubinsztein DC: The genetics of Alzheimer's disease. Prog Neurobiol 1997;52:447–454

43. Plassman BL, Breitner JC: The genetics of dementia in late life. Psychiatr Clin North Am 1997;20(1):59–76

44. Bergem AL, Engedal K, Kringlen E: The role of heredity in late-onset Alzheimer disease and vascular dementia: a twin study. Arch Gen Psychiat 1997;54:264–270

45. Gatz M, Pedersen NL, Berg S et al: Heritability for Alzheimer's disease: the study of dementia in Swedish twins. J Gerontol A 1997;52:M117–M125

46. Raiha I, Kaprio J, Koskenvuo M, Rajala T, Sourander L: Alzheimer's disease in twins. Biomed Pharmacother 1997;51(3):101–104

47. Raiha I, Kaprio J, Koskenvuo M, Rajala T, Sourander L: Alzheimer's disease in Finnish twins. Lancet 1996;347:573–578

48. Gallo JJ, Breitner JC: Alzheimer's disease in the NAS–NRC Registry of aging twin veterans. IV: Performance characteristics of a two-stage telephone screening procedure for Alzheimer's dementia. Psychol Med 1995;25:1211–1219

49. Breitner JC, Welsh KA, Gau BA et al: Alzheimer's disease in the National Academy of Sciences–National Research Council Registry of Aging Twin Veterans. III: Detection of cases, longitudinal results, and observations on twin concordance. Arch Neurol 1995;52:763–771

50. Bergem AL: Heredity in dementia of the Alzheimer type. Clin Genet 1994;46(1 Spec No):144–149

51. Breitner JC, Gatz M, Bergem AL et al: Use of twin cohorts for research in Alzheimer's disease. Neurology 1993;43(2):261–267

52. Bird TD, Nemens EJ, Kukull WA: Conjugal Alzheimer's disease: is there an increased risk in offspring? Ann Neurol 1993;34:396–399

53. Farrer LA, Myers RH, Cupples LA et al: Transmission and age-at-onset patterns in familial Alzheimer's disease: evidence for heterogeneity. Neurology 1990;40 (3 Pt 1):395–403

54. Cruts M, Van Broeckhoven C: Molecular genetics of Alzheimer's disease. Ann Med 1998;30:560–565

55. Campion D, Dumanchin C, Hannequin D et al: Early-onset autosomal dominant Alzheimer disease: prevalence, genetic heterogeneity, and mutation spectrum. Am J Hum Genet 1999;65:664–670

56. Slooter AJ, Cruts M, Kalmijn S et al: Risk estimates of dementia by apolipoprotein E genotypes from a population-based incidence study: the Rotterdam Study. Arch Neurol 1998;55:964–968

57. Farrer LA, Cupples LA, Haines JL et al: Effects of age, sex, and ethnicity on the association between apolipoprotein E genotype and Alzheimer disease: a meta-analysis. ApoE and Alzheimer Disease Meta Analysis Consortium. JAMA 1997;278:1349–1356

58. Plomin R, Pedersen NL, Lichtenstein P, McClearn GE: Variability and stability in cognitive abilities are largely genetic later in life. Behav Genet 1994;24(3):207–215

59. Finkel D, Pedersen NL, McGue M, McClearn GE: Heritability of cognitive abilities in adult twins: comparison of Minnesota and Swedish data. Behav Genet 1995;25:421–431

60. McClearn GE, Johansson B, Berg S et al: Substantial genetic influence on cognitive abilities in twins 80 or more years old. Science 1997;276:1560–1563

61. Emery CF, Pedersen NL, Svartengren M, McClearn GE: Longitudinal and genetic effects in the relationship between pulmonary function and cognitive performance. J Gerontol B 1998;53:P311–P317

62. Finkel D, Pedersen NL, Plomin R, McClearn GE: Longitudinal and cross-sectional twin data on cognitive abilities in adulthood: the Swedish Adoption/Twin Study of Aging. Dev Psychol 1998;34:1400–1413

63. Swan GE, LaRue A, Carmelli D, Reed TE, Fabsitz RR: Decline in cognitive performance in aging twins: heritability and biobehavioral predictors from the National Heart, Lung, and Blood Institute Twin Study. Arch Neurol 1992;49:476–481

64. McCartney M, Harris MJ, Bernieri F: Growing up and growing apart: a developmental metanalysis of twin studies. Psychol Bull 1990;107:226–237

65. MaGue M, Bouchard TJ, Iaconon WG, Lykken DT: Behavioral genetics of cognitive ability: a life-span perspective. In Plomin R, McClearn GE (eds): Nature, Nurture, and Psychology. American Psychological Association, Washington, 1993:59–76

66. Botwinick J: Aging and Behavior. Springer, New York, 1978

67. Finkel D, McGue M: Age differences in the nature and origin of individual differences in memory: a behavior genetic analysis. Int J Aging Hum Dev 1998;47(3):217–239

68. Fox PW, Hershberger SL, Bouchard TJ: Genetic and environmental contributions to the acquisition of a motor skill. Nature 1996;384:356–358

69. Herskind AM, McGue M, Sorensen TI, Harvald B: Sex and age specific assessment of genetic and environmental influences on body mass index in twins. Int J Obes Relat Metab Disord 1996;20:106–113

70. Surwit RS, Kuhn CM, Cochrane C, McCubbin JA, Feinglos MN: Diet-induced type II diabetes in C57BL/6J mice. Diabetes 1988;37:1163–1167

71. Bergen HT, Mizuno T, Taylor J, Mobbs CV: Resistance to diet-induced obesity is associated with increased proopiomelanocortin mRNA and decreased neuropeptide Y mRNA in the hypothalamus. Brain Research 1999;850:198–203

72. Snieder H, MacGregor AJ, Spector TD: Genes control the cessation of a woman's reproductive life: a twin study of hysterectomy and age at menopause. J Clin Endocrinol Metab 1998;83:1875–1880

73. Erway LC, Shiau YW, Davis RR, Krieg EF: Genetics of age-related hearing loss in mice. III: Susceptibility of inbred and F1 hybrid strains to noise-induced hearing loss. Hearing Res 1996;93:181–187

74. Meyers SM, Greene T, Gutman FA: A twin study of age-related macular degeneration. Am J Ophthalmol 1995;120:757–766

75. Mobbs CV: Neurotoxic effects of estrogen, glucose, and glucocorticoids: neurohumoral hysteresis and its pathological consequences during aging. Rev Biol Res Aging 1990;4:201–228

76. Finch CE: The regulation of physiological changes during mammalian aging. Q Rev Biol 1976;51(1):49–83

77. Robertson OH: Prolongation of the lifespan of kokanee salmon (*O. nerka kennerlyi*) by castration before beginning development. Proc Natl Acad Sci USA 1961;47:609–621

78. Landfield PW: An endocrine hypothesis of brain aging and studies on brain–endocrine correlations and monosynaptic neurophysiology during aging. Adv Exp Med Biol 1978;113:179–199

79. Finch CE, Felicio LS, Mobbs CV, Nelson JF: Ovarian and steroidal influences on neuroendocrine aging processes in female rodents. Endocr Rev 1984;5:467–497

80. Sapolsky RM, Krey LC, McEwen BS: The neuroendocrinology of stress and aging: the glucocorticoid cascade hypothesis. Endocr Rev 1986;7(3):284–301

81. Everitt AV, Seedsman NJ, Jones F: The effects of hypophysectomy and continuous food restriction, begun at ages 70 and 400 days, on collagen aging, proteinuria, incidence of pathology and longevity in the male rat. Mech Ageing Dev 1980;12(2):161–172

82. Sornson MW, Wu W, Dasen JS et al: Pituitary lineage determination by the Prophet of Pit-1 homeodomain factor defective in Ames dwarfism. Nature 1996;384:327–333

83. Brown-Borg HM, Borg KE, Meliska CJ, Bartke A: Dwarf mice and the ageing process. Nature 1996;384:33

84. Coschigano KT, Clemmons D, Bellush LL, Kopchick JJ: Assessment of growth parameters and life span of GHR/BP gene-disrupted mice. Endocrinology 2000;141:2608–2613

85. Laurino C, Cordera R: Role of IRS-1 and SHC activation in 3T3-L1 fibroblasts differentiation. Growth Horm IGF Res 1998;8:363–367

86. Migliaccio E, Giorgio M, Mele S et al: The p66shc adaptor protein controls oxidative stress response and life span in mammals. Nature 1999;402:309–313

87. Guarente L, Ruvkun G, Amasino R: Aging, life span, and senescence. Proc Natl Acad Sci USA 1998;95:11034–11036

88. Lin YJ, Seroude L, Benzer S: Extended life-span and stress resistance in the *Drosophila* mutant methuselah. Science 1998;282:943–946

89. Friedman DB, Johnson TE: A mutation in the age-1 gene in *Caenorhabditis elegans* lengthens life and reduces hermaphrodite fertility. Genetics 1988;118(1):75–86

90. Johnson TE: Increased life-span of age-1 mutants in *Caenorhabditis elegans* and lower Gompertz rate of aging. Science 1990;249:908–912

91. Johnson TE, Lithgow GJ: The search for the genetic basis of aging: the identification of gerontogenes in the nematode *Caenorhabditis elegans*. J Am Geriatr Soc 1992;40:936–945

92. Rose MR: Can human aging be postponed? Sci Am 1999;281(6):106–111

93. Morris JZ, Tissenbaum HA, Ruvkun G: A phosphatidylinositol-3-OH kinase family member regulating longevity and diapause in *Caenorhabditis elegans*. Nature 1996;382:536–539

94. Kimura KD, Tissenbaum HA, Liu Y, Ruvkun G: daf-2, an insulin receptor-like gene that regulates longevity and diapause in *Caenorhabditis elegans*. Science 1997;277:942–946

95. Wolkow CA, Kimura KD, Lee MS, Ruvkun G: Regulation of *C. elegans* life-span by insulin-like signaling in the nervous system. Science 2000;290:147–150

96. Taub J, Lau JF, Ma C et al: A cytosolic catalase is needed to extend adult lifespan in *C. elegans* daf-C and clk-1 mutants. Nature 1999;399:162–166

97. Oomura Y: Significance of glucose, insulin, and free fatty acid on the hypothalamic feeding and satiety neurons. In Novin D et al (eds): Hunger: Basic Mechanisms and Clinical Implications. Raven Press, New York, 1975:145–157

98. Debons AF, Krimsky I, From A, Pattinian H: Diabetes-induced resistance of ventromedial hypothalamus to damage by gold thioglucose: reversal by adrenalectomy. Endocrinology 1974;95:1636–1641

99. Daniel JA, Thomas MG, Hale CS, Simmons JM, Keisler DH: Effect of cerebroventricular infusion of insulin and (or) glucose on hypothalamic expression of leptin receptor and pituitary secretion of LH in diet-restricted ewes. Domest Anim Endocrinol 2000;18(2):177–185

100. Bruning JC, Gautam D, Burks DJ et al: Role of brain insulin receptor in control of body weight and reproduction. Science 2000;289:2122–2125

101. Kulkarni RN, Bruning JC, Winnay JN et al: Tissue-specific knockout of the insulin receptor in pancreatic beta cells creates an insulin secretory defect similar to that in type 2 diabetes. Cell 1999;96:329–339

102. Kahn A: Transcriptional regulation by glucose in the liver. Biochimie 1997;79(2–3):113–118

103. Lin SJ, Defossez PA, Guarente L: Requirement of NAD and SIR2 for life-span extension by calorie restriction in *Saccharomyces cerevisiae*. Science 2000;289:2126–2128

104. Dukes ID, McIntyre MS, Mertz RJ et al: Dependence on NADH produced during glycolysis for beta-cell glucose signaling. J Biol Chem 1994;269:10979–10982

105. Yang XJ, Kow LM, Funabashi T, Mobbs CV: Hypothalamic glucose sensor: similarities and differences from pancreatic beta-cell mechanisms. Diabetes 1999;48:1763–1672

106. Eto K, Tsubamoto Y, Terauchi Y et al: Role of NADH shuttle system in glucose-induced activation of mitochondrial metabolism and insulin secretion. Science 1999;283:981–985

107. Mobbs CV: Genetic influences on glucose neurotoxicity, aging, and diabetes: a possible role for glucose hysteresis. Genetica 1993;91(1–3):239–253

108. Bergen HT, Mizuno TM, Taylor J, Mobbs CV: Hyperphagia and weight gain after gold-thioglucose: relation to hypothalamic neuropeptide Y and proopiomelanocortin. Endocrinology 1998;139:4483–4488

109. Mizuno TM, Makimura H, Silverstein J et al: Fasting regulates hypothalamic neuropeptide Y, agouti-related peptide, and proopiomelanocortin in diabetic mice independent of changes in leptin or insulin. Endocrinology 1999;140:4551–4557

110. Tritos NA, Maratos-Flier E: Two important systems in energy homeostasis: melanocortins and melanin-concentrating hormone. Neuropeptides 1999;33:339–349

111. Nelson JF, Bender M, Schachter BS: Age-related changes in proopiomelanocortin messenger ribonucleic acid levels in hypothalamus and pituitary of female C57B1/6J mice. Endocrinology 1988;123:340–344

112. Lloyd JM, Scarbrough K, Weiland NG, Wise PM. Age-related changes in proopiomelanocortin (POMC) gene expression in the periarcuate region of ovariectomized rats. Endocrinology 1991;129:1896–1902

113. Abel TW, Rance NE: Proopiomelanocortin gene expression is decreased in the infundibular nucleus of postmenopausal women. Brain Res Mol Brain Res 1999;69(2):202–208

114. Abel TW, Rance NE: Stereologic study of the hypothalamic infundibular nucleus in young and older women. J Comp Neurol 2000;424:679–688

115. Abel TW, Voytko ML, Rance NE: The effects of hormone replacement therapy on hypothalamic neuropeptide gene expression in a primate model of menopause. J Clin Endocrinol Metab 1999;84:2111–2118

Chapter 45

Neurological signs in old age

Frédéric Assal and Jeffrey L. Cummings

Material in this chapter contains contributions from the previous edition, and we are grateful to the previous author for the work done.

Neurological conditions are leading causes of morbidity and institutionalization in elderly people,[1] but geriatric neurology has not been recognized with disciplinary status as have geriatric medicine and geriatric psychiatry. The need for geriatric neurology is not only to cope with neurological diseases in elderly people but also to understand what alterations are due to normal aging of the central and peripheral nervous system. These changes have important diagnostic, therapeutic, and economical implications. In 1931, Critchley, a forerunner of contemporary geriatric neurology, described elderly people free of neurological diseases and suggested that many neurological signs were due to aging.[2] The question of the nature of aging is debated from the biological and clinical points of view (see Section 1). Commonly, neurologists look upon changes such as loss of muscle mass, and decreased balance as "normal" aging changes, whereas the increasing tendency to develop illnesses such as cerebral infarction or dementia with increasing chronological age is seen as disease. Clinically, the dividing line between normal aging and disease is somewhat arbitrary, for example for parkinsonism, gait disturbances, and many other signs reviewed here.

In clinical practice geriatric neurology is difficult. First, the basic concept of parsimony in neurology (one disease to explain signs and symptoms) is almost always challenged, since elderly people have many concurrent diseases. Second, neurological signs and symptoms (i.e., confusion, gait disturbances) frequently may announce non-neurological disorders (i.e., myocardial infarction, pulmonary embolism, urinary tract infection, fecal impaction). Third, hearing and vision losses as well as delirium and dementia tend to complicate the clinical examination. Finally, we have to integrate the fact that neurological signs may be influenced by other systems (e.g., motor function by joint diseases) (Table 45-1).

MENTAL STATUS

The mental status examination remains the first step of every neurological evaluation in geriatric neurology. It requires special emphasis and the reader is referred to other chapters of this book. In normal aging compared to younger adults, not all cognitive functions decline in parallel, and some may not decline at all (Ch. 12); speed of processing, attentional capacity, or visuospatial perception are impaired as well as certain aspects of memory (mainly episodic memory). Moreover, dementia (Chs. 62, 63, 64, 65, 66), delirium (Ch. 61), and depression (Ch. 67) all alter the mental status. Secondarily, these modifications or perturbations may alter the neurological

assessment of elderly people. For all these reasons the examiner must be prepared to consult other sources (e.g., family, friends, medical records) for relevant information and be aware that neurological examination in elderly people may be time consuming.

PRIMITIVE REFLEXES

These reflexes are termed "primitive," "archaic," or "developmental" reflexes, or cortical "disinhibition" or "release" signs because they are believed to represent release phenomena resulting from a diminution of cerebral inhibition on lower centers, permitting emergence of reflex associations that had existed at an earlier stage of ontogenetic development but were suppressed as the brain matured.

The palmomental reflex

A brief contraction of the mentalis muscle elicited by stroking the thenar eminence of the ipsilateral hand was first described in 1920 by Marinesco and Radovici.[3] Physiologically, it is considered as a polysynaptic and nociceptive reflex. Its afferent impulse travels through the median nerve, and also the ulnar nerve; the efferent fibers run with the facial nerve; the central pathways and connections, and the reflex center either in the pons, thalamus, or cortex remain unclear. A classical experimental study in human subjects using electrical stimulation showed the palmomental reflex was present in all normal subjects provided that the stimulus was of sufficient strength, and its presence or absence following palmar stroking merely reflected variations in the threshold for the response between individuals.[4]

Clinical studies testing the palmomental reflex at the bedside using subnoxious or slightly painful stimuli confirmed its presence before the age of 50 and showed an increased prevalence with increasing age,[5,6] although other authors did not replicate the latter finding.[7] In one of the biggest epidemiological surveys of palmomental reflex in normal elderly people, the increased prevalence with increasing age was confirmed with a frequency of 15.6 percent at 67 years of age, 15.9 percent at 72, 19.7 percent at 77, 30.7 percent at 82, and 36.4 percent at 87.[8] The frequency of the palmomental reflex in patients with parkinsonism did not differ significantly from the frequency in normal subjects of similar age.[9] Study differences may be due to different stimulation methods as mentioned above and various criteria in the assessment of a positive response.

The palmomental reflex lacks a clinical value. Some authors claimed that an asymmetrical reflex may mean an involvement

Table 45-1 Frequencies of most common neurological signs in normal aging (see text for references)

Neurological signs		Frequency[a] (%)	Remark
Primitive reflex	Palmomental	15.6–36.4	Frequent in isolation but considered pathological when combined
	Snout	33–73	
	Suck	4.7	
	Nuchocephalic	Up to 29	
	Corneomandibular	5.7	
	Grasp	Up to 67	
	Glabella	4–57.5	
Special senses	Decreased smell and taste	Common	Rule out secondary causes
	Decreased visual acuity	Common	Rule out ocular pathologies or irregularities
	Diminished or no pupillary response	5–19	
	Diminished upward gaze	Up to 64.7	Smooth pursuit and cogwheel tracking are common
	Loss of higher sound frequencies	Common	
Motor signs	Strength	21–45	Depend on the muscle examined
	Atrophy	Common	
	Speed or dexterity	20–23	
	Paratonia	4.2–21	
	Parkinsonism	14.9–52.4	Defined as two or more signs (bradykinesia, rigidity, tremor, gait disturbances)
	Orobuccofacial dyskinesias	1.5–38	Upper range overestimated
Sensory signs	Decreased vibration at the metatarsal or the medial malleolus of the ankle	11.8–67.7	
Myotatic reflex	Absent ankle reflex	7–55.9	
Gait and balance	Loss of balance on one foot	Common	
	Reduction in velocity and in length of stride	Common	

[a]Wide ranges reflect different inclusion and exclusion criteria, and different examination approaches.

of the central nervous system,[10] but this was on a small cohort of patients and before the modern imaging era. A nonfatiguing reflex occurring after repeated thenar stimulation may be suggestive of a cerebral cortical disinhibition process.[11]

The snout reflex

This reflex corresponds to the pouting or pursing of the lips elicited by pressing or gently tapping over the philtrum of the upper lip with the forefinger or the reflex hammer. As the palmomental reflex, the snout reflex is considered as a nociceptive reflex of the perioral musculature traveling through the trigeminal and facial nerves. In contrast to the palmomental reflex, it is not observed before the fifth decade,[6] and correlates with advanced age.[8,12] Studies of a community-dwelling population showed a prevalence of 33, 54, and 73 percent in the 65–74, 75–84, and 85 and over age groups respectively.[13] Its occurrence also correlates with impairment of cognition on psychometric testing,[14] and especially with advanced brain damage.[15] The snout reflex is twice as common in Alzheimer's disease than in age-matched controls.[16] The frequency of this reflex in parkinsonism patients did not differ significantly from the prevalence of normal subjects of similar ages in some studies,[9] and was increased in frequency in others.[17]

The suck reflex

Stroking the lips with the index finger or objects such as a reflex hammer handle elicits a response of the lips, which close around the finger or object; it is frequently associated with sucking movements of the lips, tongue, and jaw. Its frequency in normal aging is low (4.7 percent in an Italian cohort).[8] It occurs much more often in dementia,[14,16] and correlates with the severity of the cognitive impairment.[15] It has been labeled as a primitive release sign and because of its remarkable similarity with the oral type of behavior of the neonate, some authors have postulated a re-emergence of a lower level of integration related to the loss of cortical inhibitory function.[18]

The nuchocephalic reflex

This reflex is obtained by a rapid turning of the subject's shoulders in one direction, which is followed by turning of the head in the same direction after a lag of approximately one half second. In infants and children up to 4 years, the head remains central. Proprioceptive input from the trunk and neck, and possibly a vestibular input are presumed to play a role in the reflex. The inhibition of the response with the head turning in the same direction as the shoulder movement is assumed to be of cortical origin, similar to that of the mechanisms which inhibit the oculocephalic reflex. This reflex is absent before age 50. It reappears in old age where its frequency in normal volunteers can go up to 29 percent in the 80-year-old and older age group.[12] It is correlated with cognitive dysfunction.[19] Clinically, the examiner should be aware that movement of the head and shoulder en bloc, as may be seen with cervical spondylosis, common in the elderly, obscures the reflex and prevents assessments of the response.

The corneomandibular reflex

This reflex is positive when touching the lateral margin of the cornea with a rolled wisp of cotton wool elicits a contralateral deviation of the jaw due to the contraction of the ipsilateral lateral pterygoidus. Present in 50 percent of newborns,[20] the corneomandibular reflex subsequently disappears then reappears in diffuse brain disease or focal disease with corticobulbar damage.[21] With a different stimulation technique using a surgically gloved forefinger, its absence before the fifth decade was established. It was elicited bilaterally with an overall frequency of 5.7% of normal subjects from the fifth decade onward but unlike the snout and palmomental, there was no further increase with advancing age.[6] Another group found a relative increase in the very old compared to the younger old (8–25 percent).[5] There may be a $2\frac{1}{2}$ times greater frequency of corneomandibular reflex in patients with parkinsonism compared to normal controls.[9]

The grasp reflex

Three types of grasp reflex are recognized, suggesting an increased severity of disinhibition. The tactile grasp (grasp with palmar touch) appears first, followed by traction grasp (counter-pull when pulling away from the patient's grip) and magnetic grasp (following the examiner's hand to grasp it).[22]

The tactile grasp is elicited by firm pressure with the testing fingers across the palm from the ulnar to the radial side, with the patient's attention distracted. Usually, if first positive the examiner asks the subject to desist, then the test is repeated. The reflex is considered positive if the subject grasps the examiner's fingers in response to a palmar rubbing action. It has a tactile and a proprioceptive component. Cortical and especially medial frontal or basal ganglia lesions can elicit such a response. Lesions can be bilateral or unilateral and in the latter predict a contralateral response. Its prevalence is a matter of debate in normal aging and varies from 0.3 percent in an unselected sample of healthy elderly people[8] to 27–67 percent in another sample.[13] The latter authors also found an increase with increasing age. The grasp reflex is increased in Alzheimer's disease compared to controls,[16] and significantly correlated with the degree of cognitive impairment.[15]

The glabella reflex

Also called the glabella tap sign, the nasopalpebral reflex, the orbicularis oculi reflex, the blinking reflex and Myerson's sign, this reflex is a nociceptive trigeminofacial reflex. A normal response consists of up to 3–9 blinks following repeated tapping between the eyebrows with the finger avoiding a visual threat response, usually at a rate of two per second, further blinking

stopping at this point despite continuing tapping. First found in post-encephalic parkinsonism, the glabella reflex was first thought to be diagnostic of Parkinson's disease but since then numerous reports showed that it was not, although more common in Parkinson's disease.[23] It occurs in other neurodegenerative diseases, focal lesions and normal aging as well. Frequencies vary again in different studies ranging from 4 to 57.5 percent in normal aging, with and without significant increase with increasing age.[5,8,12,16] It is a sign of basal ganglia disinhibition and thus differs in physiology from cortical disinhibition reflexes.

Other reflexes

The root reflex is elicited by having the subject make a fist while the examiner gently strikes the most lateral portion of the upper lip. The reflex is considered present when the head turns in response to the examiner's action. The facial reflex is a facial twitch resulting from a stroke at the side of the subject's mouth. Data concerning these reflexes are scarce, with prevalence ranged from 5 to 37 percent in healthy elderly people.[13]

Comment on reflexes

All primitive reflexes were classically interpreted as signs of diffuse multifocal or frontal encephalic involvement. This wide generalization is often incorrect when applied in individual cases. First, the palmomental reflex can be elicited in all ages. Second, these signs have been reported in normal aging, even if the existing literature shows considerable variability in reported frequencies. Differences in eliciting and scoring, and different inclusion criteria for normal subjects and patients may explain the variability observed in the literature. Finally, we do not know with precision the structural correlates of these responses. Cerebral atrophy and ventricular enlargement on computed tomography, mainly in the frontal lobes, has been considered the most common anatomical substrate of these reflexes.[14,24] Patients with a positive snout reflex had a significantly lower count of large pyramidal cells in layers III through V of the frontal cortex, Brodman area 32.[25] These findings derive from studies in Alzheimer's disease patients. Taken in isolation, these reflexes are neither specific nor sensitive for any neurological disease. Although they are the most common noncognitive neurological abnormalities elicited in patients with dementia, the clinician should not gain the impression that these signs are actually characteristic or predictive of dementia. On the other hand, when they occur in combination, these reflexes (particularly the snout, the suck, and the grasp reflexes) are not present in normal aging, are more common in dementia, and correlate with severity of cognitive changes.[8,14,15,25–27]

CRANIAL NERVES AND SPECIAL SENSES
Smell and taste

Changes in the chemical senses of smell and taste are common aspects of Alzheimer's disease[28] and Parkinson's disease,[29] and normal aging as well, although their prevalence is not known. They may alter food choices and intake, and subsequently exacerbate disease states, impair nutritional status and immunity, and produce weight loss. Impairment of smell appears at both threshold and suprathreshold concentrations for most odors. The threshold in normal elderly people is higher than in young adults; elderly people have reduced capacity to discriminate the degree of differences between odors of different qualities, and performance on tasks that require identification of odors is impaired.[30] Medications, virus infection, exposure to toxic fumes, and head trauma may all alter olfaction in elderly people. In other cases, structural and functional changes in the upper airway, the olfactory epithelium, olfactory bulb, and nerves have been reported to alter these senses in normal aging.[30] Taste is also altered at threshold and suprathreshold perception: reduced sensitivity for sweet, sour, salty, bitter, as well as other tastes occurs in normal aging; however, some authors reported smaller differences, compared to young adults; normal elderly people perceive a broad range of tastes as being less intense than do young persons.[31,32] The causes of this taste loss are unclear. Some studies indicate that there is not a significant loss of taste buds in aging; neurophysiological recordings indicate there may be some decline in responses.[33] Practically, one must exclude secondary causes of impairment including medications (e.g., lipid-lowering drugs, antihistamines, antibiotics, anticonvulsants), surgical interventions, environmental exposure (e.g., smoking, alcohol), and also dentures which cover the soft palate, thereby diminishing the sensory input.[30]

Eyes and vision

Visual acuity is considerably worse in conditions of low contrast and luminance in elderly people.[34] This finding is consistent with previous anatomical and physiological studies, indicating a deterioration of photoreceptors after age 20.[35] There is also a general decline in sensitivity of the visual field and an increased rate of decline with eccentricity, which is less well understood.[36] Clinically, however, visual acuity in elderly people is affected primarily by presbyopia, cataract, glaucoma, and macular degeneration (see Ch. 59).

Pupillary modifications include sluggish reactions to light and loss of the near reflex in elderly subjects without known neurological disease.[37,38] Some authors found a significant difference between pupillary size between old and young subjects.[39] Pharmacological evaluation of the pupil permitted the same authors to conclude that these changes may be due to diminished preganglionic sympathetic tone. More recently Odenheimer confirmed absence of pupil reaction in 5–19 percent of healthy elderly people and reported that irregularities in pupil diameter were common with a rate of 10–22 percent.[13]

Eye movements change with gradual limitation of upward gaze with age.[40] Studies have also documented increased slowed smooth pursuit and cogwheel tracking with age; the reported frequency of these changes varies markedly (2–64 percent).[8,12,13,37,41,42] The anatomical substrate explaining these findings is not clarified. Practically, as in adult neurology, any limitation in downward gaze has to be considered as abnormal and investigated.

Hearing

Hearing loss, particularly of higher sound frequencies, is an almost invariable consequence of aging. Presbyacusis accounts for most of this age-related change. It is probably mostly due to the loss of cochlear hair cells in the organ of Corti and is discussed elsewhere (see Ch. 60). Speech discrimination also is affected. In a recent longitudinal study, there was a significant increase in pure tone threshold averages (about 1 dB per year) and speech reception threshold averages (about 2 dB per year), and a significant decrease in discrimination scores over the 5 years of follow-up in 57 normal older subjects.[43]

MOTOR SIGNS
Motor function

The examiner has to be aware of unique clinical difficulties associated with motor examination of elderly people. First, certain muscle groups, like the iliopsoas and glutei, are particularly difficult to test compared to younger adults so that functional testing (i.e., rising from a low chair with arms folded) may be more appropriate. Second, dexterity is a complex motor function related to pyramidal, extrapyramidal, proprioceptive, and cerebellar functions but also influenced by other medical conditions (i.e., rheumatoid arthritis).

Clinical data in elderly people regarding decrease in muscle strength show various results. Some authors found the strength of both upper and lower extremities gradually decreased (21–45 percent) with increasing age,[44] while others reported that these changes were infrequent,[37] or not significant when they were not attributable to major diseases.[13] In laboratory conditions, maximum voluntary contraction force and twitch tension in the quadriceps were 50% lower in old subjects compared to young ones.[45] These differences in study findings may be due to different evaluation techniques and differences in which muscle groups were examined.

Decrease of muscle power is often accompanied by loss of muscle bulk. A recent longitudinal study using computerized tomography showed a 12.5% reduction in the cross-sectional area of the thigh in a 12-year follow-up.[46] Atrophy of the intrinsic muscles of the hand, particularly the dorsal interossei and thenar muscles, without weakness or fasciculations is also frequently observed in clinical practice and present in over half of all elderly subjects in cross-sectional studies.[38] Muscle biopsy findings in longitudinal studies of aging subjects report conflicting loss of muscle fibers, predominantly type IIB, fast-twitch fibers,[47] reduction in percentage of type I fibers with no change in type I or II mean fiber area, and a decrease in the capillary-to-fiber ratio;[46] increase in the percentage of type I fibers.[48] In the latter study, the subjects were runners with a mean age at follow-up of 47–50 years. Functional improvement was achieved with high resistance weight training leading to significant gains in muscle strength, size, and functional mobility in a population of residents in a nursing home without any neurological diseases.[49]

Other motor functions may decline with aging. Speed of hand and tapping was reduced by 20–23 percent in one study.[44] There is a loss of coordination with increasing age.[50] Kaye showed some but nonsignificant dysmetric movements in the oldest old compared with younger old[42] and Kokmen found some terminal tremor or hesitation on finger-to-nose test but no actual dysmetria in neurologically normal subjects.[37]

Paratonia

Paratonia of Dupré or Gegenhalten of Kleist are similar terms. They correspond to an increase in tone with rapid passive movement of the limbs which disappears if passive movements are elicited slowly. Frequently the examiner can feel intermittent opposition to the passive movements despite instructions to relax. Paratonia also can be detected when the patient's arms, suspended 15 cm above the lap, remain elevated after being released, even after instructions to relax. It differs clinically from both spasticity and extrapyramidal rigidity. Its prevalence varies between 4.2–21%, increasing with advancing age.[8,12,41] Paratonia is more common in patients with Alzheimer's disease and is correlated with the severity of cognitive impairment.[51] Paratonia is sometimes regarded as a release sign and is probably a constituent of the postural reflexes. It may follow a prevalence pattern similar to the primitive release signs, which are prominent in the late stages of Alzheimer's disease.[51] Another hypothesis postulates that paratonia is a manifestation of age-related changes in the basal ganglia.[12]

Parkinsonism, tremor, and other movement disorders

Parkinson's disease and many other movement disorders occur more commonly in elderly people and are presented elsewhere (see Ch. 52) but various extrapyramidal signs have been described in healthy elderly people. Bradykinesia, rigidity, and even tremor have been shown to be frequent in isolation in normal aging with prevalence rates between 1.8 and 44 percent depending on the population, the parkinsonian sign, the limb examined, and the age of the patients studied.[13,38,41] The association of more than one parkinsonian sign is rarely discussed and the relationship with Parkinson's disease remains unclear, since all available studies are cross-sectional studies. Prevalence of parkinsonian signs defined as the presence of signs in two or more categories (bradykinesia, rigidity, tremor, gait disturbance) increased gradually from 14.9% for people aged 65–74 years of age to 52.4 percent for those 85 and older in a stratified random sample of 467 residents of East Boston.[52] Another important finding of this study was that parkinsonism was associated with a two-fold increase in the risk of death, which was strongly related to the presence of gait disturbance. Nevertheless this study design did not allow the authors to differentiate Parkinson's disease from other causes of parkinsonism, so some cases were probably mild subclinical Parkinson's disease. Rest tremor seems to be the most specific sign of Parkinson's disease in anatomical series.[53,54] Longitudinal studies of subjects with parkinsonism are still needed.

In a recent study, hyperechogenicity detected by transcranial sonography may be related to nigral injury in elderly people with parkinsonian signs without Parkinson's disease.[55] For the same reasons as previously mentioned, longitudinal follow-up data are needed. In human pathology, a linear decline of pigmented neurons within the substantia nigra has been described in advancing age, with a different cell loss pattern than in Parkinson's disease.[56] Lewy body formation in the brain stem and cell loss in the substantia nigra have been reported in Alzheimer's disease patients with parkinsonism.[57] The mechanisms of cell death may be due to apoptotic-like changes in substantia nigral neurons.[58]

Postural tremor is common in elderly people. When medications (i.e., amiodarone, valproate, bronchodilators, corticosteroids, antidepressants), alcohol, hyperthyroidism, hyperadrenergic states (e.g., anxiety) and dystonia are not potential etiologic factors, essential tremor may be considered, although there is still no absolute method for distinguishing it from other causes. Its prevalence varies between 1.7 and 23 percent in healthy elderly people aged 65 or older in different studies, reflecting an absence of standardization of diagnostic criteria.[59,60] In a recent community-based case-control study of subjects who did not meet strict criteria for essential tremor, a mild tremor was present in 98.7 percent of normal elderly people. An important clinical feature was that this so-called senile tremor was generally asymptomatic and did not require treatment. Its etiology remains uncertain, but this high prevalence led the authors to suggest that it was due to normal aging.[61] It remains unknown if severe forms of normal tremor and enhanced physiological tremor form a continuum with mild forms of essential tremor and the relative importance of genetic, aging, and environmental factors require further study.

Senile chorea is a rare entity, characterized by the presence of late onset, generalized chorea with no family history and no dementia.[2] Some may have late onset sporadic Huntington's disease confirmed with genetic testing and some may not.[62,63] One of the few pathological reports disclosed normal caudate nuclei but abnormal putamen, globus pallidum, and cerebellar nuclei.[64] Senile chorea is a syndrome, not a distinct disease.

The prevalence of idiopathic lingual–facial–buccal dyskinesias is elevated (6.8–38 percent) in people aged over 60 years but may be overestimated because studies were performed in hospital-based populations.[65] Some investigators found only 1.5% of idiopathic lingual–facial–buccal dyskinesias in two unselected samples of elderly people.[41,66] Neuroleptic-induced tardive dyskinesias should be considered in the differential diagnosis.

SENSORY SIGNS

In elderly people it is difficult to test sensation easily by clinical methods used in younger patients, but these modalities should not be neglected. As Critchley pointed out, findings on sensory system examination change with aging, mainly vibratory sense, which is mediated by the dorsal columns.[2] Since Critchley's original report, numerous authors have corroborated this observation at the bedside using a 128 Hz tuning fork placed at the metatarsal or the medial malleolus of the ankle.[37,38,44,67] Vibration sensation is impaired with a prevalence of 11.8–67.7 percent in subjects over 65 years old up to 85 and older,[13,41,42] and is increased with increasing age.[13,42] Using various stimulators and quantitative measurements, it has been shown that there is a progressive decrease in sensitivity with age at high frequencies but no change at low (25–40 Hz) frequencies;[68] vibration threshold progressively increased with age to a significant degree also in the finger,[69] or in both upper and lower extremities.[70] Some authors found a correlation between age and vibration perception, and between vibration perception and body sway standing on foam. This may suggest that increased body sway in elderly people may be due in part to reduced proprioception in the lower limbs.[71] Loss of proprioception or toe position sense was unchanged,[44] variously impaired with a 2 percent prevalence rate in one study,[8] 11.8–44.1 percent in another,[42] and 6–13 percent in a third one,[13] with an increase with increasing age for the latter two. Such discrepancies may imply a different mode of examination technique and subject recruitment. Diabetes, alcohol use, vitamin B12 deficiency, and neurotoxic drugs should be sought, since they can produce these abnormalities. Pathologically, these changes may be secondary to proliferation of connective tissue, arteriosclerotic changes of the nutritional arterioles, and degeneration of the nerve fibers with aging,[72] or loss of axons in the dorsal columns in the spinal cord.[73]

There have been less systematic investigations of changes in tactile sensitivity in elderly people. Skre showed a reduction in tactile sensation with increasing age in women but not in men;[67] Potvin found no change in touch or two-point discrimination in their quantitative examination.[44] Light touch thresholds increase with age,[74] but there is no significant loss in this modality on routine clinical examination.

Pain is a frequent complaint in geriatric neurology and geriatric medicine (see Chs. 47 and 109). Studies concerning normal aging of this sensory modality are less numerous and also controversial. Thermal sensitivity threshold showed a significant relationship with aging[75] or not[69] using different stimulators. The latter results parallel other observations that possible age-related decline in pinprick sensation is usually not detectable by routine clinical testing.[50]

A number of so-called cortical sensory changes have been reported in normal elderly people. Face–hand test,[16,37] stereognosis,[42] and double simultaneous stimulation[42] have all been found abnormal in some studies. Longitudinal studies with extensive neuropsychological testing should be performed in order to address their significance in normal aging.

MYOTATIC REFLEXES

Reflex testing is a very important objective measure of nervous system integrity in the adult neurological examination but is often very difficult in elderly people because of apprehension or musculoskeletal changes. Moreover, optimizing ankle position or reinforcement procedures are rarely performed. It is commonly accepted that reduction or loss of the ankle jerk is a normal variant in aging, although conditions such as diabetes or alcoholism were not exclusion criteria in some studies.[2,38,67,76] With these as exclusion criteria, the prevalence of absent ankle jerk varies in recent literature between 7 percent,[8] 21.3 percent,[41] and 55.9 percent.[42] Degenerative joint disease, and to a lesser extent visual impairment and obesity, have been correlated with absent ankle jerk.[41] These findings need longitudinal follow-up, since exclusion of incipient peripheral neuropathies was not assured. Babinski

sign or a positive extensor plantar response has been reported as rare by some authors.[2,37] In other series, a Babinski sign was seen in normal aging with a prevalence of 5.0 to 11.8 percent.[13,42] The meaning of these findings must be explored with modern neuroimaging and neuropathological studies.

GAIT AND BALANCE

Impaired locomotion is a significant source of disability in old age. Gait alterations of elderly people reflects changes in multiple systems, which if individually disrupted might not impair ambulation. Postural control is influenced by the visual, vestibular, motor, and proprioceptive systems. All these systems can be altered in normal aging as discussed earlier.

Loss of balance in elderly people is common. Healthy elderly people have greater difficulty to balance on one foot with eyes closed.[42,44] This has been confirmed with quantitative posturography; older people have greater body sway than younger individuals.[77,78] Kinematic studies reveal that elderly people exhibit a significant reduction in the velocity of gait and length of stride.[79,80]

Many older people develop a stooped posture with thoracolumbar kyphotic ankylosis, a posteriorly rotated immobile pelvis, excessive flexion at the hips and knees, a reduced toe–floor clearance, a slightly broad base, and a diminished arm swing.[2,38,80] These modifications have been referred to as the syndrome of cautious gait[81] or idiopathic senile gait.[82–84] However, the clinical picture of this senile gait disorder is variable, imprecisely defined and has not been studied with modern neuroimaging techniques. In an investigation on 153 healthy noninstitutionalized elderly people over 88 years of age, the authors showed that 61 percent had an abnormal gait due to a distinct disease, and 10 percent had a wide spectrum of gait abnormalities (mainly with ataxic features) without apparent cause, which could represent the idiopathic senile gait.[85] Some of these alterations may be secondary to non-neurological causes (i.e., degenerative joint disease). Nevertheless, clinicians recognize that there is substantial overlap with pathological conditions including normal pressure hydrocephalus, lower-body parkinsonism and lacunar state.[81] Prospective studies revealed that disequilibrium of unknown cause in elderly people was associated with frequent falls, concerns about falling, frontal atrophy, and subcortical white matter changes on magnetic resonance imaging.[86] Idiopathic senile gait disorders may be related to subclinical, cardiovascular disease; the risk of cardiovascular death was twofold higher than in subjects with normal gait.[87] So-called senile gait may be a preclinical or subclinical pathological condition.

CONCLUSION

Many abnormal signs and symptoms have been attributed to aging in the past. We reviewed the controversial data, some arguing that pathological signs are due to normal aging, others arguing they are disease-related signs. Many studies have used different inclusion criteria (inpatient, outpatient, or community-based populations), different exclusion criteria (diabetes, major medical illness) and different examination approaches. Even in the well-done community-based studies, various authors attribute many neurological signs to aging itself, particularly deficits in balance, vibration sense, smell, visual pursuit or upward gaze limitation, decreased pupillary reactivity, and the emergence of multiple primitive reflexes or mild postural tremor.[13,41,42] More studies with strict inclusion criteria and consensus for clinical diagnosis are needed. More longitudinal clinical data are required to interpretation of current observations. Finally, more clinical correlations with anatomical data and modern imaging techniques are warranted. These data will be useful not only for diagnostic criteria but also for the clinical decision-making processes. Information is needed to distinguish normal from pathological signs in elderly people, to know what to do and how far to go with diagnostic procedures, and to predict cost.

KEY POINTS   Neurological signs in old age

- Clinically, distinguishing normal aging from disease is challenging.

- Many older people have multiple concurrent diseases.

- Primitive reflexes are the most common noncognitive neurological findings in normal aging. Taken in isolation, they are neither specific nor sensitive for any neurological disease. When these reflexes occur in combination, they are more common in dementia.

- A limitation of upward gaze is common in normal aging but any limitation in downward gaze requires investigation.

- Isolated parkinsonian symptoms such as rigidity, bradykinesia, and tremor are frequent in normal aging and their relationship with Parkinson's disease remains unclear.

- Impairment of vibration sense or absent ankle jerks may be found in normal aging but may also reflect an incipient peripheral neuropathy. Diabetes, alcohol, and vitamin deficiencies should be excluded.

- So-called "idiopathic senile gait" is imprecisely defined. Normal pressure hydrocephalus, lower-body parkinsonism, lacunar state must be excluded. Signs of frontal atrophy and subcortical white matter changes are frequent on MRI in patients with gait changes.

Acknowledgments

This project was supported by an NIA Alzheimer's Disease grant (AG16570), and Alzheimer's Disease Research Center of California grant, the Sidell-Kagen Foundation (JLC), and a scholarship from the University Hospital, Geneva, Switzerland (FA).

REFERENCES

1. Kurtzke JF: The current neurologic burden of illness and injury in the United States. Neurology 1982;321:1207–1214
2. Critchley M: The neurology of old age. Lancet 1931;1:1221–1230
3. Marinesco G, Radovici A: Sur un réflexe cutané nouveau: le réflexe palmomentonnier. Rev Neurol 1920;27:237–240
4. Reis DJ: The palmomental reflex. Arch Neurol 1961;4:30–42
5. Orefice G, Modafferi N, Selvaggio M et al: Archaic reflexes in normal elderly people. Acta Neurol 1991;13:19–24
6. Jacobs L, Gossman MD: Three primitive reflexes in normal adults. Neurology 1980;30:184–188
7. Jensen JPA, Gron U, Pakkenberg H: Comparison of three primitive reflexes in neurological patients and in normal individuals. J Neurol Neurosurg Psychiatry 1983;46:162–167
8. Benassi G, D'Alessandro R, Gallassi R et al: Neurological examination in subjects over 65 years: an epidemiological survey. Neuroepidemiology 1990;9:27–38
9. Gossman MD, Jacobs L: Three primitive reflexes in parkinsonism patients. Neurology 1980;30:189–192
10. Marx P, Reschop J: The clinical value of the palmomental reflex. Neurosurg Rev 1980;3:173–177
11. Jenkyn LR, Walsh DB, Culver CM et al: Clinical signs in diffuse cerebral dysfunction. J Neurol Neurosurg Psychiatry 1977;40:956–966
12. Jenkyn LR, Reeves AG, Warren T et al: Neurologic signs in senescence. Arch Neurol 1985;42:1154–1157
13. Odenheimer G, Funkenstein HH, Beckett L et al: Comparison of neurologic changes in "successfully aging" persons vs the total aging population. Arch Neurol 1994;51:573–580
14. Tweedy J, Reding M, Garcia C et al: Significance of cortical disinhibition signs. Neurology 1982;32:169–173
15. Bakchine S, Lacomblez L, Palisson E et al: Relationship between primitive reflexes, extra-pyramidal signs, reflective apraxia and severity of cognitive impairment in dementia of the Alzheimer type. Acta Neurol Scand 1989;79:38–46
16. Galasko D, Kwo-on-Yuen PF, Klauber MR et al: Neurological findings in Alzheimer's disease and normal aging. Arch Neurol 1990;47:625–627
17. Vreeling FW, Verhey FRJ, Houx PJ et al: Primitive reflexes in Parkinson's disease. J Neurol Neurosurg Psychiatry 1993;56:1232–1236
18. Ajuriaguerra de J, Rego A, Tissot R: Le reflexé oral et quelques activités orales dans les syndromes démentiels du grand âge: leur signification dans la désintegration psycho-motrice. Encéphale 1963;52:179–219
19. Jenkyn LR, Walsh DB, Walsh BT et al: The nuchocephalic reflex. J Neurol Neurosurg Psychiatry 1975;38:561–566
20. Paulson GW, Bird MT: The corneomandibular reflex. Confin Neurol 1971;33:116–119
21. Gordon RM, Bender MB: The corneomandibular reflex. J Neurol Neurosurg Psychiatry 1971;34:236–242
22. Haerer AF: DeJong's The Neurologic Examination. Lippincott, Philadelphia, 1992
23. Pearce J, Aziz H, Gallagher JC: Primitive reflex activity in primary and symptomatic parkinsonism. J Neurol Neurosurg Psychiatry 1968;31:501–508
24. Burns A, Jacoby R, Levy R: Neurological signs in Alzheimer's disease. Age Ageing 1991;20:45–51
25. Foerstl H, Burns A, Levy R et al: Neurologic signs in Alzheimer's disease. Result of a prospective clinical and neuropathologic study. Arch Neurol 1992;49:1038–1042
26. Isakov E, Sazbon L, Costeff H et al: The diagnostic value of three common primitive reflexes. Eur Neurol 1984;23:17–21
27. Vreeling FW, Houx PJ, Jolles J et al: Primitive reflexes in Alzheimer's disease and vascular dementia. J Geriatr Psychiatry Neurol 1995;8:111–117
28. Serby M, Larson P, Kalkstein D: The nature and course of olfactory deficits in Alzheimer's disease. Am J Psychiatry 1991;148:357–360
29. Doty RL, Riklan M, Deems DA et al: The olfactory and cognitive deficits of Parkinson's disease: evidence for independence. Ann Neurol 1989;25:166–171
30. Schiffman SS: Taste and smell losses in normal aging and disease. JAMA 1997;278:1357–1362
31. Grzegorczyk PB, Jones SW, Mistretta CM: Age-related differences in salt taste acuity. J Gerontol 1979;34:834–840
32. Stevens JC, Cruz LA, Hoffman JM et al: Taste sensitivity and aging. Chem Senses 1995;20:451–459
33. Bradley RM: Effects of aging on the anatomy and neurophysiology of taste. Gerodontics 1988;4:244–248
34. Adams AJ, Wong LS, Wong L et al: Visual changes with age: some new perspectives. Am J Optom Physiol Opt 1988;65:403–406
35. Bagolini B, Porciatti V, Falsini B et al: Macular electroretinogram as a function of age of subjects. Doc Ophthalmol 1988;70:37–43
36. Jaffe GJ, Alvarado JA, Juster RP: Age-related changes of the normal visual field. Arch Ophthalmol 1986;104:1021–1025
37. Kokmen E, Bossemeyer RW Jr, Barney J et al: Neurological manifestations of aging. J Gerontol 1977;32:411–419

38. Prakash C, Stern G: Neurological signs in the elderly. Age Ageing 1973;2:24–27
39. Korczyn AD, Laor N, Nemet P: Sympathetic pupillary tone in old age. Arch Ophthalmol 1976;94:1905–1906
40. Chamberlain W: Restriction in upward gaze with advancing age. Am J Ophthalmol 1971;71:341–346
41. Waite LM, Broe GA, Creasey H et al: Neurologic signs, aging, and the neurodegenerative syndromes. Arch Neurol 1996;53:498–502
42. Kaye JA, Oken BS, Howieson DB et al: Neurologic evaluation of the optimally healthy oldest old. Arch Neurol 1994;51:1205–1211
43. Enrietto JA, Jacobson KM, Baloh RW: Aging effects on auditory and vestibular responses: a longitudinal study. Am J Otolaryngol 1999;20:371–378
44. Potvin AR, Syndulko K, Tourtellotte WW et al: Human neurologic function and the aging process. J Am Geriatr Soc 1980;28:1–9
45. Roos MR, Rice CL, Connelly DM et al: Quadriceps muscle strength, contractile properties, and motor unit firing rates in young and old men. Muscle Nerve 1999;22:1094–1103
46. Frontera WR, Hughes VA, Fielding RA et al: Aging of skeletal muscle: a 12-yr longitudinal study. J Appl Physiol 2000;88:1321–1326
47. Aniansson A, Hedberg M, Henning GB et al: Muscle morphology, enzymatic activity, and muscle strength in elderly men: a follow-up study. Muscle Nerve 1986;9:585–591
48. Trappe SW, Costill DL, Fink WJ et al: Skeletal muscle characteristics among distance runners: a 20-yr follow-up study. J Appl Physiol 1995;78:823–829
49. Fiatarone MA, Marks EC, Ryan ND et al: High-intensity strength training in nonagenarians. JAMA 1990;263:3029–3034
50. Nichols ME, Meador KJ, Loring DW et al: Age-related changes in the neurologic examination of healthy sexagenarians, octogenarians, and centenarians. J Geriatr Psychiatry Neurol 1994;7:1–7
51. Franssen EH, Reisberg B, Kluger A et al: Cognition-independent neurologic symptoms in normal aging and probable Alzheimer's disease. Arch Neurol 1991;48:148–154
52. Bennett DA, Beckett LA, Murray AM et al: Prevalence of parkinsonian signs and associated mortality in a community population of older people. N Engl J Med 1996;334:71–76
53. Rajput AH, Rozdilsky B, Ang L: Occurrence of resting tremor in Parkinson's disease. Neurology 1991;41:1298–1299
54. Hughes AJ, Daniel SE, Kilford L et al: Accuracy of clinical diagnosis of idiopathic Parkinson's disease: a clinico-pathological study of 100 cases. J Neurol Neurosurg Psychiatry 1992;55:181–184
55. Berg D, Siefker C, Ruprecht-Doerfler P et al: Relationship of substantia nigra echogenicity and motor function in elderly subjects. Neurology 2001;56:13–17
56. Fearnley JM, Lees AJ: Ageing and Parkinson's disease: substantia nigra regional selectivity. Brain 1991;114:2283–2301
57. Ditter SM, Mirra SS: Neuropathologic and clinical features of Parkinson's disease in Alzheimer's disease patients. Neurology 1987;37:754–760
58. Tompkins MM, Basgall EJ, Zamrini E et al: Apoptotic-like changes in Lewy-body-associated disorders and normal aging in substantia nigral neurons. Am J Pathol 1997;150:119–131
59. Louis ED, Ottman R, Hauser WA: How common is the most common adult movement disorder? Estimates of the prevalence of essential tremor throughout the world. Mov Disord 1998;13:5–10
60. Elble RJ: Tremor in ostensibly normal elderly people. Mov Disord 1998;13:457–464
61. Louis ED, Wendt KJ, Ford B: Senile tremor. Gerontology 2000;46:12–16.
62. Shinotoh H, Calne DB, Snow B et al: Normal CAG repeat length in the Huntington's disease gene in senile chorea. Neurology 1994;44:2183–2184
63. Garcia Ruiz PJ, Gomez-Tortosa E, del Barrio A et al: Senile chorea: a multicenter prospective study. Acta Neurol Scand 1997;95:180–183
64. Friedman JH, Ambler M: A case of senile chorea. Mov Disord 1990;5:251–253
65. Klawans HL, Barr A: Prevalence of spontaneous lingual-facial-buccal dyskinesias in the elderly. Neurology 1982;32:558–559
66. D'Alessandro R, Benassi G, Cristina E et al: The prevalence of lingual-facial-buccal dyskinesias in the elderly. Neurology 1986;36:1350–1351
67. Skre H: Neurological signs in a normal population. Acta Neurol Scand 1972;48:575–606
68. Verrillo RT: Age related changes in the sensitivity to vibration. J Gerontol 1980;35:185–193
69. Merchut MP, Toleikis SC: Aging and quantitative sensory thresholds. Electromyogr Clin Neurophysiol 1990;30:293–297
70. Goldberg JM, Lindblom U: Standardised method of determining vibratory perception thresholds for diagnosis and screening in neurological investigation. J Neurol Neurosurg Psychiatry 1979;42:793–803
71. Bergin PS, Bronstein AM, Murray NM et al: Body sway and vibration perception thresholds in normal aging and in patients with polyneuropathy. J Neurol Neurosurg Psychiatry 1995;58:335–340.
72. Takahashi K: A clinicopathologic study on the peripheral nervous system of the aged. Sciatic nerve and autonomic nervous system. Geriatrics 1966;21:123–133
73. Mufson EJ, Stein DG: Degeneration in the spinal cord of old rats. Exp Neurol 1980;70:179–186
74. Thornbury JM, Mistretta CM: Tactile sensitivity as a function of age. J Gerontol 1981;36:34–39
75. Doeland HJ, Nauta JJ, Van Zandbergen JB et al: The relationship of cold and warmth cutaneous sensation to age and gender. Muscle Nerve 1989;12:712–715
76. Bathia S, Irvine RE: Electrical recording of the ankle jerk in old age. Gerontol Clin 1973;15:357–360
77. Camicioli R, Panzer VP, Kaye J: Balance in the healthy elderly. Arch Neurol 1997;54:976–981
78. Baloh RW, Corona S, Jacobson KM et al: A prospective study of posturography in normal older people. J Am Geriatr Soc 1998;46:438–443
79. Murray MP, Kory RC, Clarkson BH: Walking patterns in healthy old men. J Gerontol 1969;24:169–174
80. Elble RJ, Thomas SS, Higgins C et al: Stride-dependent changes in gait of older people. J Neurol 1991;238:1–5
81. Nutt JG, Marsden CD, Thompson PD: Human walking and higher-level gait disorders, particularly in the elderly. Neurology 1993;43:268–279
82. Koller WC, Wilson RS, Glatt SL et al: Senile gait: correlation with computed tomographic scans. Ann Neurol 1983;13:343–344.
83. Sudarsky L, Ronthal M: Gait disorders among elderly patients: a survey study of 50 patients. Arch Neurol 1983;40:740–743
84. Koller WC, Glatt SL, Fox JH: Senile gait: a distinct neurological entity. Clin Geriatr Med 1985;1:661–669
85. Bloem BR, Haan J, Lagaay AM et al: Investigation of gait in elderly subjects over 88 years of age. J Geriatr Psychiatry Neurol 1992;5:79–84
86. Kerber KA, Enrietto JA, Jacobson KM et al: Disequilibrium in older people: a prospective study. Neurology 1998;51:574–580
87. Bloem BR, Gusseklo J, Lagaay AM et al: Idiopathic senile gait disorders are signs of subclinical disease. J Am Geriatr Soc 2000;48:1098–1101.

Chapter 46

Epilepsy

Raymond C. Tallis

There has been increasing interest in epilepsy in older adults over the last two decades. Until quite recently, only a tiny proportion of the huge epilepsy literature was specifically devoted to elderly patients. The growing awareness among epileptologists of geriatric patients is reflected in designated sessions at international meetings and in the recent publication of textbooks specifically on epilepsy of old age (e.g. Rowan and Ramsay;[1] Kramer[2]). The relative paucity of literature on seizures in old age might be due to several misconceptions: that epilepsy is rare in old age; that it matters less in an elderly person than in a younger one; and that it is the same as epilepsy in younger adults, so that whatever is learned about the latter can be applied directly to the former.

The importance of seizures in old age should not need to be spelled out. Even though epilepsy no longer carries the stigma it once did, the psychological impact of an epileptic fit may be profound. Elderly patients, in particular, may have childhood memories that go back to a time when epilepsy was poorly controlled, was often associated with serious brain damage, and was stigmatized. In many respects, the problem of epilepsy is comparable to that of recurrent falls: although the condition is episodic, the anxiety it causes may be constant. An elderly person may worry, and not without reason, that future fits may lead to injury—to road traffic accidents, fractures, burns, etc. The prolonged postictal states sometimes seen in old age[3] may add further hazards. Moreover, discontinuity of consciousness undermines self-confidence at the deepest level; to an elderly person, a fit may seem a harbinger of death. For these reasons, as will be discussed, reassurance—based upon information and education—is a crucial aspect of management.

DEFINITION

Seizures are defined pathophysiologically as being due to paroxysmal discharges of cerebral activity, in which a critical mass of neurons fires synchronously.

"Epilepsy" is not used to refer to a *single* seizure, but to a continuing *tendency* to epileptic seizures. In epidemiological studies, the term is usually used when a patient has suffered from more than one nonfebrile seizure of any type. It follows that a diagnosis of epilepsy cannot strictly be made on the basis of a single seizure, especially if the seizure has an external provocation. The distinction, however, is not as sharp as is sometimes implied; in old age at least, the majority of individuals who present with a single unprovoked seizure will go on to have further seizures.[4–6]

EPIDEMIOLOGY

As already noted, many doctors have the impression that seizures are comparatively rare in elderly people and that elderly-onset epilepsy is uncommon. Twenty-five percent of general practitioners[7] in one postal survey thought they had never seen epilepsy presenting for the first time in old age.

The belief that elderly-onset seizures are uncommon has no foundation in the recent literature. Twenty-five years ago, Hauser and Kurland[8] reported a rise in the prevalence of epilepsy above the age of 50 and an even steeper rise in incidence—from 12 per 100,000 in the 40–59 age range to 82 per 100,000 in those over 60. This rise has been confirmed in their more recent studies[9–10] and Luhdorf[11] reported a similar incidence of 77 per 100,000 in Denmark. This has also been confirmed by studies based in primary care. The United Kingdom National General Practice Survey of Epilepsy and Epileptic Seizures (NGPSE),[4] a prospective-based, community-based study, found that 24 percent of new cases of definite epilepsy were in subjects over the age of 60. A study of a primary care database covering 82 practices and nearly 370,000 subjects, 62,000 of whom were over the age of 60, revealed a continuing rise in the incidence of seizures in old age:[12] whereas the incidence for the overall population was 69 per 100,000, the incidence in the 65–69 age group was 87; in the 70s, 147 per 100,000; and in the 80s, 159 per 100,000. Over one-third of all incident cases placed on antiepileptic drugs (AEDs) were individuals over the age of 60. A more recent study of a much larger primary care database (see Fig. 46-1) has generated very similar findings.[13]

The high incidence is observed for both definite epilepsy and single seizures. Loiseau[14] found an annual incidence for all seizures (single and recurrent) of 127 in subjects over age 60 and that those over age 60 accounted for 28 percent of cases of confirmed epilepsy (two or more unprovoked seizures) and 52 percent of acute symptomatic seizures. The Rochester Minnesota survey[10] also found that both single unprovoked seizures and definite epilepsy increased sharply with age.

The dramatic rise of the incidence of seizures shown in Figure 46-1A may, in view of the predicted rise in the elderly population, be expected to continue. This rise is contrasted with the fall in incidence in younger people, so that the average incidence in the overall population is relatively unchanged. Older people are therefore emerging as the single most important part of the population with seizures.

Prevalence studies in epilepsy are less straightforward than studies of incidence because of the difficulty of arriving at an agreed definition of definite, active epilepsy. Nevertheless, the recent literature also shows a striking upsurge in prevalence of epilepsy in the older population compared with younger adults (see Fig. 45-1B). This is particularly true of the older elderly population, namely the over 75s. For example, in the Rochester study, Hauser[15] found a prevalence of 14.8 per 1,000 in subjects over 75, compared with an overall population average of 6.8 per 1,000. In the Rotterdam study[16] there was a rise in prevalence from 7 per 1,000 in those aged 55–64 to 12 per 1,000 in

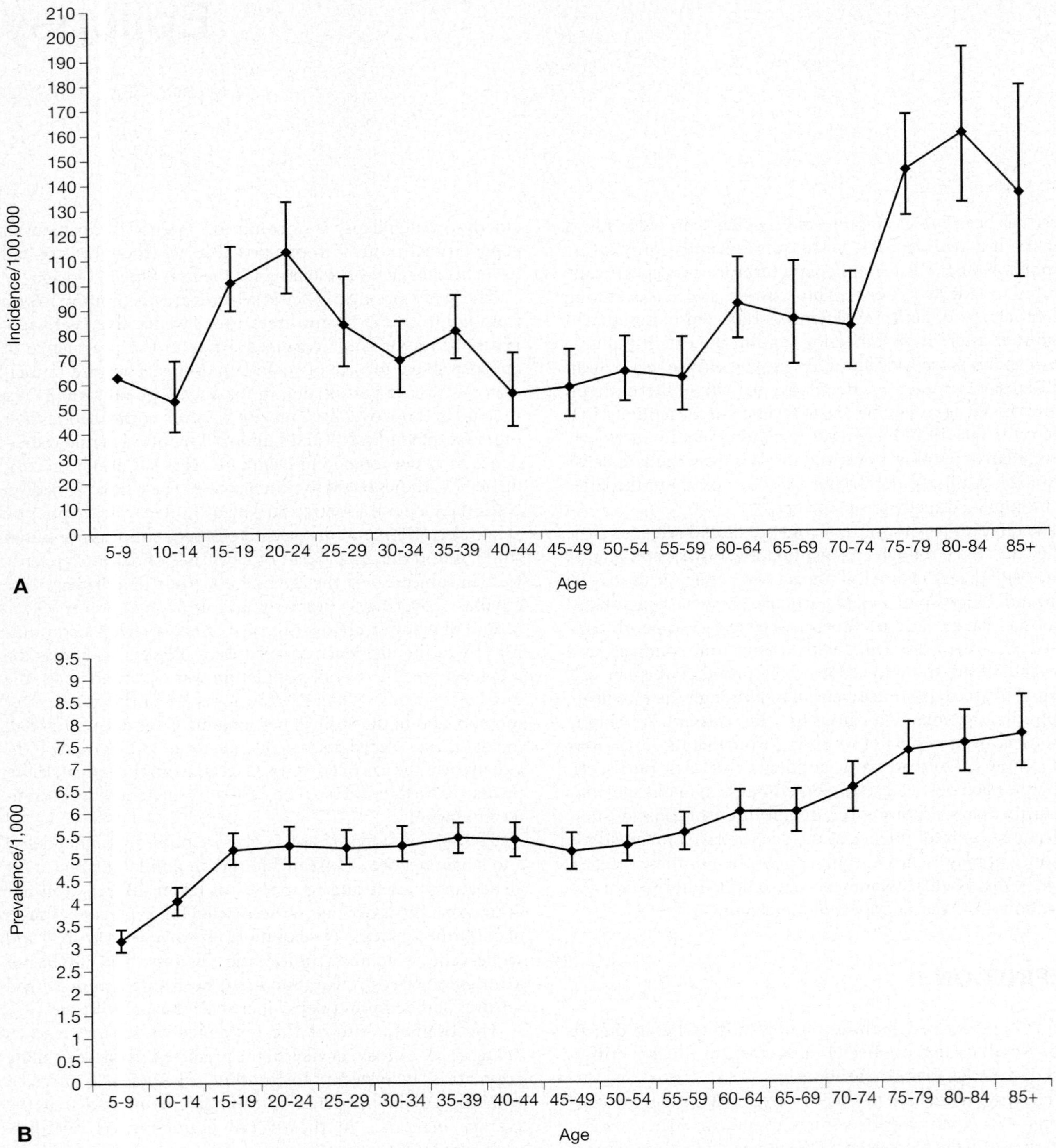

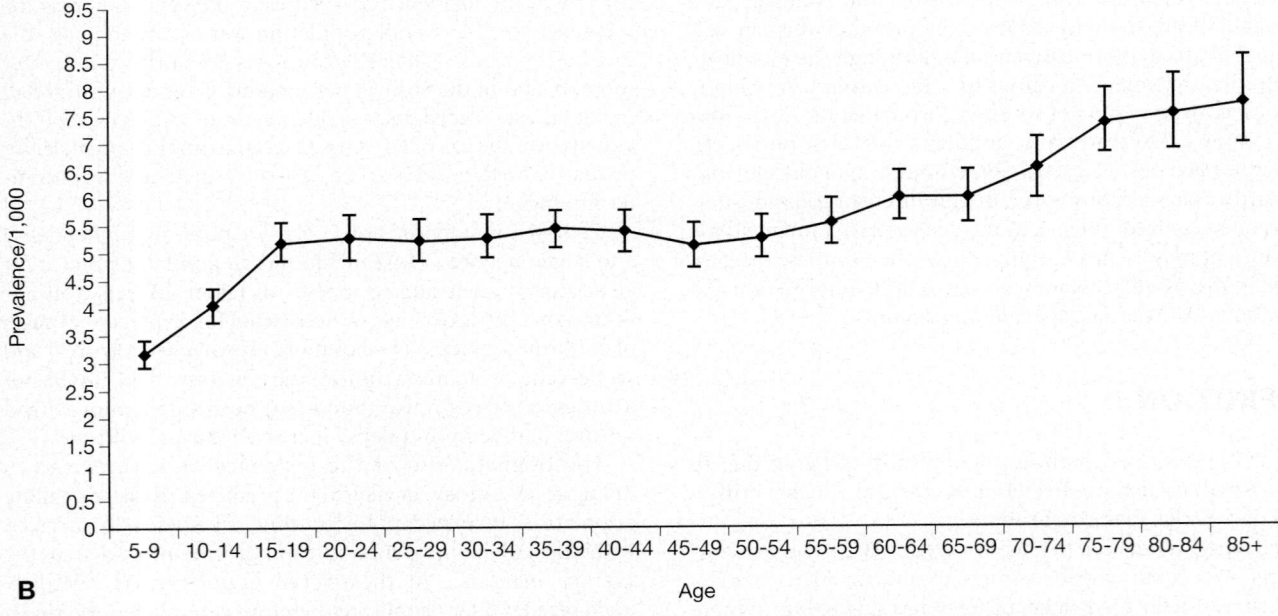

Figure 46-1 (A) Age-specific incidence of treated epilepsy per 100,000 persons. **(B)** Age-specific prevalence of treated epilepsy per 1,000 persons. (Source: Wallace, Shorvon, Tallis, Lancet: 1998;352:19–26 with permission.)

people aged between 85 and 94, with an overall prevalence in elderly people of 9. Hauser noted a dramatic increase in the prevalence in elderly people between the years 1940 and 1980—1.9 to 14.8 per 1,000 in the over 75s.[9] Of 45,000 patients in American long-term care facilities, at least 10% were on antiepileptic medication.[17]

This secular trend will have been in part due to improved case ascertainment, but this is clearly not the whole story.

Because cerebrovascular disease is the main cause of seizures in old age (see below) and there has been a decline in overt stroke during this period, the trend may seem paradoxical. However, it is possible that the increase in the prevalence of seizures may reflect an increase in the burden of "minor" or occult cerebrovascular disease that is sufficiently advanced to predispose to seizures, but not expressed as overt stroke or, where it is expressed in stroke, carries a lower mortality.

There are, that is to say, more people surviving with cerebrovascular disease.

Whatever the explanation, these data make epilepsy the third most common serious neurological disease of old age, following dementia and stroke. Why should its incidence and prevalence be so underestimated? Minor seizures may not be reported; they may not be recognized for what they are, getting lost in the pathologically rather busy situation of the biologically aged person; or, even if recognized, not referred to hospital and therefore excluded from hospital-based or hospital-biased series. In the NGPSE,[4] 20 percent of elderly patients with seizures were not referred to a hospital, compared with only 4 percent of younger patients. This is despite the fact that elderly people contributed a disproportionate number of additional cases of "possible" or "probable" epilepsy, confirming the increased diagnostic uncertainty in the aged.

TYPES OF SEIZURES

The manifestations of epilepsy are complex and varied and the methods of classifying seizures correspondingly complex. The revised 1981 International League against Epilepsy classification[18] correlates clinical seizure types with ictal and interictal electroencephalographic features. Table 46-1 gives those parts of the classification most relevant to elderly patients.

Primary generalized seizures are those in which the first clinical events suggest involvement of both hemispheres from the outset. This is confirmed by electroencephalogram (EEG) discharges during a fit that are bilateral from the outset. Such seizures may be convulsive or nonconvulsive. In the former case, motor manifestations are bilateral from the outset. In nonconvulsive seizures, there is impairment or interruption of consciousness without motor manifestations. Impairment of consciousness also may be the first event in a convulsive seizure. In partial seizures, the *first* changes suggest activation of neurons limited to part of one cerebral hemisphere. A partial seizure is classified as "simple" if consciousness is *not* impaired and as "complex" if it *is* impaired. Impairment of consciousness in a partial seizure usually implies bilateral spread of seizure activity affecting a large part of the cerebral cortex of both hemispheres. The clinical correlate of such generalized electrical activity may also include tonic–clonic features supervening on initially focal symptoms.

It may be helpful to map the current, more precise terminology onto the older terminology with which some readers may be more familiar. (For obvious reasons, the mapping cannot be exact and the older, more imprecise terminology should no longer be used.) Primary generalized convulsive seizures roughly correspond to the classical "grand mal" attack without a preceding aura. A grand mal attack preceded by an aura or other focal features corresponds to "partial seizures evolving to secondary generalized seizures." "Minor" or "focal" epilepsy covers simple and complex partial seizures. Most of the latter were previously classified as "temporal lobe epilepsy" as, among the focal seizures, it is those originating in the temporal lobes that are most likely to be associated with disturbances of consciousness. Some temporal lobe attacks may take the form of simple partial seizures with autonomic or psychic symptoms.

Table 46-1 Seizures occurring in elderly people
Generalized seizures: generalized from the onset
• Tonic–clonic seizures (including variations beginning with a clonic or myoclonic phase)
• Clonic seizures
• Tonic seizures
• Myoclonic seizures
• Atonic seizures
• Reflex seizures in generalized epilepsy syndromes
Partial or focal seizures
Simple focal seizures: consciousness unimpaired throughout
With motor symptoms:
• Focal motor with or without march
• Versive
• Postural
• Vocalization
With somatosensory or special-sensory symptoms:
• Somatosensory
• Visual
• Auditory
• Olfactory
• Gustatory
• Vertiginous
With autonomic symptoms or signs:
• Epigastric sensations
• Pallor
• Sweating
• Flushing
• Piloerection
• Pupillary dilatation
With disturbances of higher cerebral function:
• Dysphasic
• Dysmnestic
• Cognitive
• Affective
• Illusions (e.g., macropsia)
Secondarily generalized seizures: partial seizures progressing to convulsive or nonconvulsive generalized seizures[a]
Impairment of consciousness only[b]
Impairment of consciousness with automatism
Impairment of consciousness with tonic clonic feature

[a]Most generalized seizures in older people are secondarily generalized.

[b]Brief absences occurring in older people are most often due to complex partial seizures (they used to be called "temporal lobe absences"). Primary generalized seizures in older people are relatively rare.

(Modified from Commission on Classification and Terminology of the International League Against Epilepsy,[18] in two ways: amplification and simplification of some of the terms used; and removal of forms of seizures not occurring in older people.)

The *classification* of seizures in old age in epidemiological studies is rarely satisfactory. Large, population-based studies do not have full electrophysiological evaluation. This is a serious omission because seizures that appear clinically to be primarily generalized may actually be focal in origin (and symptomatic) though generalization occurs too fast for the initial focal features to be noted by an observer. Studies in which investigation has been adequate enough to ensure accurate classification are often derived from atypical populations attending neuromedical centers. The literature on the respective frequencies of different types of seizures has been usefully reviewed in Jallon and Loiseau.[19]

Current evidence suggests that up to 75 percent of elderly-onset seizures are focal, or focal in origin.[4,11,19] The actual figure may be higher as it seems unlikely that primary generalized seizures frequently occur spontaneously for the first time in old age. An individual with an idiopathic lowering of seizure threshold would have expressed this earlier in life. This said, a recent study[20] has suggested that idiopathic generalized epilepsy may, after all, occasionally occur for the first time in late middle or old age. The author even suggested a second peak in the incidence of these epilepsies (which typically present in childhood and adolescence) in older subjects. Interictal EEGs showed generalized spike-wave or polyspike abnormalities at about 3 Hz with no consistent asymmetrical discharges. Neuroimaging ruled out focal lesions. Occasionally a syndrome similar to juvenile myoclonic epilepsy may occur for the first time in later life[2] and myoclonic-type seizures may occur in Alzheimer's disease.[21] Identifying the small minority of elderly onset patients who have primary generalized seizures is important because it may influence the choice of medication.

Simple partial seizures have been reported as being more frequent than complex seizures.[19] This, however, may be because brief loss or impairment of consciousness may not be observed or reported. Moreover, Hauser[15] found that complex partial seizures accounted for nearly 50 percent of seizures in old age, while simple partial seizures accounted for only 13 percent. Among primary generalized seizures, over 90 percent are tonic–clonic. Epileptologists have increasingly drawn attention to absence status in elderly patients (see below). Finally, and not surprisingly, there is a high proportion of unclassifiable seizures in older people—in roughly 10 percent of cases.[4] The proportion of *misclassified*—as opposed to *unclassified*—seizures is probably even higher. Much still remains to be done in this area.

ETIOLOGY

An epileptic fit may be regarded as the result of an interaction between an individual predisposition, which is constitutional or hereditary, and a provoking cause that may be either an epileptogenic lesion in the brain or a systemic disturbance lowering the convulsive threshold. In elderly patients presenting with fits for the first time, it may be reasonably assumed that the contribution of the provoking cause usually outweighs that of the individual predisposition, because the latter would have already expressed itself earlier in life.

Cerebrovascular disease

Cerebrovascular disease is the main cause of epilepsy in older adults, accounting for between 30 and 50 percent of cases in different series.[4,14,19,22] It accounts for an even higher proportion—up to 75 percent[4]—of those cases in which an attributable cause is found.

Cerebrovascular disease and seizures may be linked in different ways: (1) in association with overt stroke, when there may be early (peristroke, onset) seizures or late (poststroke) seizures; and (2) in association with otherwise occult stroke disease, as evidenced by concurrent computerized tomography (CT) scan finding and/or subsequent development of stroke. There have been several important studies investigating the relationship between overt stroke and early and late seizures. Kilpatrick et al.[23] found that about 4 percent of patients had early seizures. Seizures occurred within 5 years of an ischemic stroke in about 10 percent of 675 patients with a first stroke (of whom 512 were at least 65 years old) in the Oxford Community Stroke Project.[24] The Oxford study found a much higher incidence of poststroke seizures in hemorrhagic stroke and this was also observed by Lancman.[25]

A population-based study of over 500 patients with ischemic stroke by So et al.[26] must be regarded as definitive. They divided seizures into early (within 1 week of the stroke) and late (after 1 week). Six percent of subjects developed early seizures, 78 percent of these within 24 hours. Late seizures developed in 5.5 percent of subjects. The cumulative probabilities of developing an initial late seizure were 3 percent at 1 year, nearly 5 percent at 2 years, and 7.5 percent at 5 years. Early seizure occurrence was a strong predictive factor for initial late seizures. Overall, ischemic stroke increased the chances of an individual developing epilepsy 17-fold. Poststroke seizures may occasionally proceed to status epilepticus. Velioğlu et al.[27] found poststroke seizures in 180 out of 1174 patients with first time strokes; of these, 9 percent went on to develop status epilepticus which was associated with a higher functional disability but not a higher mortality. Early onset of status epilepticus (within 7 days) was associated with a higher rise of recurrent status (nearly all patients) and a higher mortality rate. Later onset status did not appear to have this association.

The relationship between otherwise occult cerebrovascular disease and seizures is more problematic. It is true that the more carefully cerebrovascular disease is sought in epileptic patients, the more frequently it is found. Comparisons of CT scan appearances of patients with elderly-onset epilepsy and no evidence of cerebral tumor with those of age- and sex-matched controls may show an excess of ischemic lesions in epileptic patients despite normal clinical examination. This observation, however, may have to be treated with caution. The presence of areas of ischemia on a CT scan may not mean that they are the primary or even a contributory cause of the seizures. One study also showed an excess of previous seizures in patients admitted to the hospital with acute stroke compared with controls, suggesting that in a proportion of elderly patients, seizures may be the earliest manifestation of cerebrovascular disease.[28] This observation will need to be confirmed (the present author has ongoing studies) but in the meantime it may be prudent to assume that an elderly patient presenting with unexplained seizures should be fully screened for cardiovascular risk factors and treatment with low-dose aspirin or other preventative measures should be instituted where appropriate.

The strong relationship between age and the incidence and prevalence of cerebrovascular disease—as reflected in the almost exponential relationship between age and first-ever stroke—underlines the growing importance of this cause of elderly-onset seizures, particularly as the elderly population is itself aging.

Other cerebral disorders

Cerebral tumors

Clinicians are often concerned that elderly-onset epilepsy may indicate a cerebral tumor. Most series indicate that this is the underlying cause in only a minority of cases.[4,22,29] There is a large variation between studies in the incidence of tumors, presumably due to the different populations being surveyed (itself a reflection of different referral patterns), the different extent to which patients are investigated and, related to this, the different proportion of cases in which no cause is found. The most reliable figures so far suggest that about 10 to 15 percent of elderly-onset epilepsy may be due to neoplasm. In most cases, tumors are either metastatic or (inoperable) gliomas, though a few meningiomas are found. Until there is information on adequately documented, investigated, and sufficiently large population-based series, one cannot be certain what proportion of cases of very late-onset epilepsy are due to treatable and nontreatable tumors. Even less is known regarding the proportion of patients with seizures due to tumors in which there are no other pointers on history or examination to a space-occupying lesion. They certainly do occur from time to time (Fig. 46-2).

Nonvascular cerebral degenerative disease

A variable proportion of seizures is attributed to nonvascular cerebral degeneration. Again, the data are insufficient and will remain so until large series with uniform access to neuro-scanning facilities are reported. Mcareavey et al.[30] have suggested that Alzheimer dementia may cause seizures and this has been reiterated by Hesdorffer et al.[31] who reported a six-fold increased risk of unprovoked seizures. However, in neither study were "gold standard" criteria used for diagnosing Alzheimer's dementia and differentiating Alzheimer's from multi-infarct dementia or mixed Alzheimer's and multi-infarct dementia. However, a special form of myoclonic epilepsy associated with Alzheimer's disease has been described,[21] as has already been noted.

Subdural hematoma is a rare but important but remediable cause, especially as very elderly patients are prone to this condition because of cerebral atrophy. Because it may occur after a relatively trivial injury, the diagnosis may be missed.[32] Direct brain damage due to head injury is itself a relatively uncommon cause of elderly-onset epilepsy, except in one series,[33] where it accounted for over 20 percent of cases over the age of 60. This unusually high figure, however, derived from a tertiary referral hospital providing a head injury service.

Seizures may occur during the course of acute severe cerebral infections (meningitis, encephalitis), but under such circumstances should not strictly be called "epilepsy." Following recovery from such infections, however, epilepsy may arise due to scarring. This is a rare cause of epilepsy in elderly people.

Metabolic and toxic causes

Recent series[14] have underlined the importance of toxic and metabolic causes of seizures in old age. Alcohol is an important factor

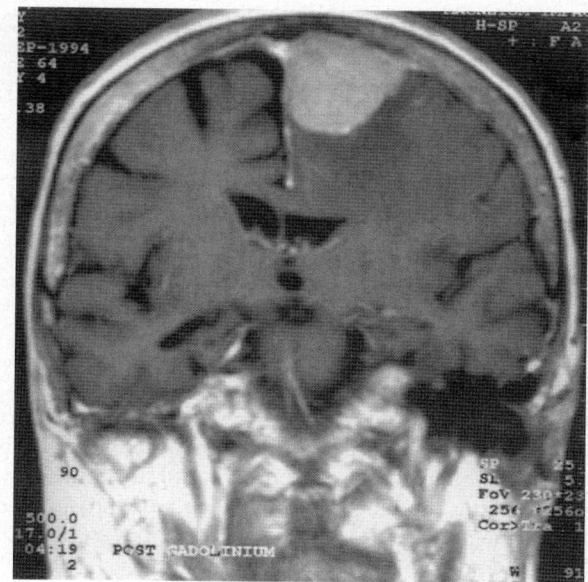

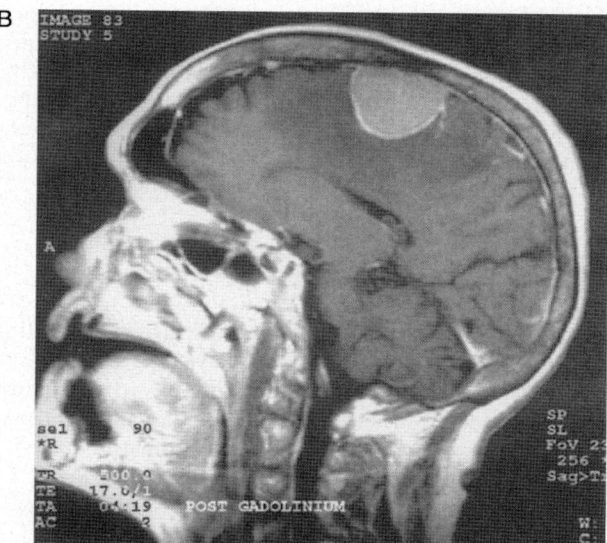

Figure 46-2 (A and B) MRI scans showing meningioma in an 82-year-old woman who presented with seizures commencing 2 years earlier. (Courtesy of the Department of Magnetic Resonance Imaging, Salford Royal Hospitals Trust.)

at any age.[34–35] Pyrexia and other acute conditions may precipitate seizures in older people[14] and pneumonia, which in the biologically aged may be more likely to cause hypoxia, may predispose to seizures, or precipitate them in an individual who has otherwise well-controlled epilepsy. Table 46-2 lists some important toxic and metabolic causes of seizures in elderly patients.

A wide range of drugs has been suspected of causing convulsions.[36] It is often difficult to prove that a given drug caused convulsions in a particular case, but in certain drugs the

<table>
<tr><td>

Table 46-2 Some toxic and metabolic causes of seizures in old age

- Pyrexia
- Hypoglycemia
- Electrolyte disturbance including water overload
- Pneumonia with or without respiratory failure
- Severe myxoedema
- Hepatic failure
- Renal failure
- Drugs and drug withdrawal
- Alcohol and alcohol withdrawal

</td></tr>
</table>

probability of a causal relationship seems to be high. Drug-induced seizures are particularly likely to occur when the drug is given in high dosage, parenterally, or to patients with impaired drug handling. Aminophylline, which has a narrow therapeutic index, and whose disposition may be altered by cigarette smoking, is especially prone to cause generalized seizures. Psychotrophic drugs, including tricyclic antidepressants and phenothiazines, are also particularly important. Benzodiazepine withdrawal may cause fits. Repeated hypoglycemic episodes due to excessive insulin or oral hypoglycemics may precipitate recurrent seizures. Drugs suspected of being epileptogenic are listed in Table 46-3. Strictly, seizures provoked by metabolic and toxic causes, even if they are recurrent, should not be called "epilepsy." Not infrequently, patients on antiepileptic drugs are on other medication with proconvulsant effects.[37]

Idiopathic

Occasionally, one encounters a patient whose seizures are apparently idiopathic, presenting for medical help for the first time in old age. Such patients may have had a lifetime of untreated epilepsy. As already noted, without such a long history, it is difficult to sustain a diagnosis of idiopathic epilepsy, though the possibility of elderly-onset idiopathic primary generalized seizures has already been discussed.

DIAGNOSIS AND INVESTIGATION

The diagnostic task when a patient presents with suspected seizures is complex. Figure 46-3 shows the questions that should be addressed. The most powerful tool for answering these questions is a detailed history from the patient or eye witness. In the context of a well-defined aura; clear progression from a tonic to a clonic phase; tongue-biting; incontinence or focal neurological features during an attack; and stupor or prolonged confusion, headache, muscle aching, neurological signs after the attack, diagnosis is straightforward. Post-event confusion and headache are particularly useful pointers to a fit. For obvious reasons, the history from the patient may be unsatisfactory and eyewitness reports must be sought. This may be difficult in a patient who lives alone and who has simply been "found on the floor." Even evidence from individuals who did not see the event itself but observed the patient's post-event state—neighbors, ambulance drivers,

Table 46-3 Drugs that may cause seizures in elderly people

Antibiotics
- Ampicillin
- Benzylpenicillin
- Oxacillin
- Carbenicillin
- Isoniazid
- Cycloserine
- Nalidixic acid
- Quinalones

Hormones
- Insulin
- Oral hypoglycemics
- Prednisone

Local anesthetics/antiarrhythmics
- Lignocaine
- Procaine
- Disopyramide
- Anticholinergics in overdose

Psychotropic drugs
- Chlorpromazine
- Other phenothiazines
- Tricyclic and other antidepressants
- Lithium

Analeptic drugs
- Aminophylline
- Doxapram
- Ephedrine
- Nikethamide

Anesthetic agents
- Ether
- Methohexitone
- Ketamine
- Halothane
- Althesin
- Propanadid

Anticonvulsants in overdosage
- Phenobarbitone
- Phenytoin

Miscellaneous
- D-Penicillamine
- Baclofen
- Hyperbaric oxygen
- Cyclosporin
- Interferon

Withdrawal fits
- Benzodiazepines
- Alcohol

casualty staff—may be helpful. In the case of an elderly person living alone, this may be the only source of useful history. The next most powerful tool is a wide-ranging, open-minded, physical examination. The third most powerful tool is time. It is better to wait and see than to initiate inappropriate treatment. Specialist investigations such as the EEG are only occasionally helpful in either positively diagnosing epilepsy or ruling it out. More useful, as we shall see, are tests of

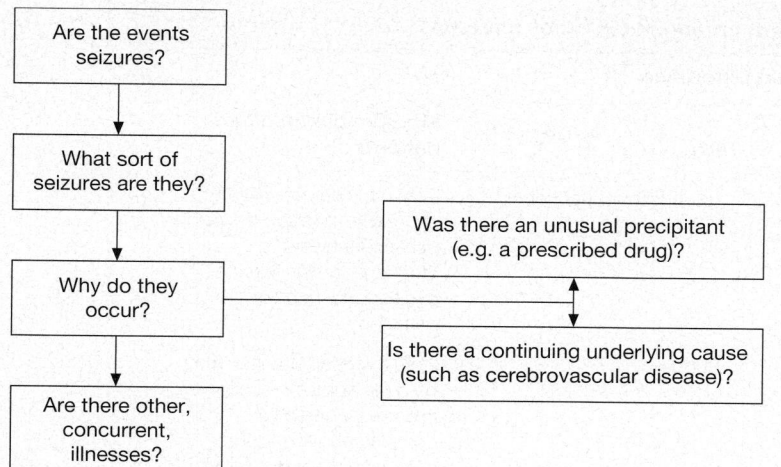

Figure 46-3 Epilepsy and suspected epilepsy in older people: a diagnostic algorithm.

cardiovascular function that may positively diagnose syncope as a cause of transient loss of consciousness.

Are the events seizures?

The most common feature of epilepsy in elderly people, as at any other age, is transient impairment or loss of consciousness. Sometimes disturbances of consciousness may be forgotten and the patient will report only a fall. The differential diagnosis will then encompass the numerous other causes of falls in elderly people. A fall occurring in the absence of any obvious environmental cause and which cannot be confidently attributed to orthopedic, cardiovascular, or nonepileptic neurological factors, should raise the suspicion of a fit.

In the case of a classic generalized or partial seizure, the diagnosis can be readily made on the basis of the history. Unfortunately, fits may be difficult to differentiate from a variety of nonepileptic paroxysmal events that also occur in old people. Some of these latter may, however, be relatively easily ruled out. Table 46-4 lists nonepileptic events that may be confused with epileptic fits.

Hypoglycemia is rare in a patient not on hypoglycemic medication. Where it does occur, however, it may not be associated in an old person with characteristic autonomic features (see Chapter 96). Nocturnal hypoglycemia due to longer-acting oral hypoglycemics such as chlorpropamide and glibenclamide may occasionally cause fits and present as early morning confusion and postictal headache. (Such oral hypoglycemics should be avoided in elderly people.)

Transient ischemic attacks do not typically cause disturbance of consciousness. They tend to have negative features, such as weakness and numbness, whereas focal seizures have positive features such as twitching and tingling or lancinating sensations.[38]

Recurrent paroxysmal behavioral disturbances are seen in dementias, in particular multi-infarct states. They may be confused with complex partial seizures (or vice versa, see below). Unlike the latter, they may have a predictable diurnal pattern (see Chapter 61).

Drop attacks[39] are associated with immediate (rather embarrassed) recovery, and do not cause loss of consciousness, though the patients may sustain nasty bruising—hence "genoux bleues." A patient might say, "My legs just gave way, doctor."

Table 46-4 **Nonepileptic events that may be confused with epilepsy**
• Syncope
• Hypoglycemia
• Transient ischemic attacks
• Recurrent paroxysmal behavioral disturbances secondary to organic brain disease
• Drop attacks and other nonepileptic causes of falls
• Transient global amnesia
• Psychogenic attacks
• Panic attacks
• Hypoventilation
• Pseudoseizures (nonepileptic attack disorder)

They tend to occur in a cluster and spontaneously remit. Other causes of recurrent falls may be inappropriately attributed to seizures. However, the reverse error is equally likely: fits may not be considered when the only available history is that of the patient repeatedly being found on the floor.

Transient global amnesia may be confused with complex partial seizures causing temporal lobe dysfunction and consequent memory disturbance. This, however, is less common, and has characteristic features (anguished disorientation and repeated asking of the same questions), typically lasts for 24 hours, and usually does not recur.[40]

Psychogenic attacks ("pseudo-seizures," "nonepileptic attack disorder")[41] do not usually occur for the first time in old age and there are usually other features of functional psychiatric illness and precipitating factors such as bereavement. However, the data on this are scanty. The differentiation from genuine seizure may be difficult without full videotelemetry recording to determine whether the attacks coincide with ictal activity on the electroencephalography. It is important to realize that some genuine epileptic fits—for example seizures of frontal lobe origin—may look like pseudo-seizures.

The most difficult differential diagnosis is *syncope*—transient loss of consciousness due to acute cerebral anoxia secondary to a fall in cerebral perfusion. Even when there is a reasonably good history, the features that characteristically differentiate fits from faints may not be as decisive as in younger adults, as is set out in Table 46-5. The diagnosis

Table 46-5 **The differences between faints and fits: problems in older patients**

	Usual Difference		
Features	**Faints**	**Fits**	**Modification in older patients**
Posture	Usually occur in the upright position	Not position-dependent	Faints in older people are not always position-dependent because they are often due to significant, position-independent, pathology
Onset	Gradual	Sudden	Loss of consciousness may be quite abrupt in syncope in an older person; complex partial seizures may have a gradual onset
Injury	Rare	More common	A syncopal attack may be associated with significant soft tissue or bony injury in an older person
Incontinence	Rare	Common	An individual prone to incontinence may be wet during a faint; partial seizures will not usually be associated with incontinence
Recovery	Rapid	Slow	A fit may take the form of a brief (temporal lobe) absence: a faint associated with a serious arrhythmia may be prolonged
Postevent confusion	Little	Marked	A prolonged hypoxic episode due to a faint may be associated with prolonged postevent confusion
Frequency	Usually infrequent with a clear precipitating cause	May be frequent and usually without precipitating cause	Faints associated with cardiac arrhythmias, low cardiac output, postural hypotension or carotid sinus sensitivity may be very frequent

and management of syncope in older adults is covered in Chapter 38 and comprehensively reviewed in Kenny's definitive textbook.[42] It will therefore be only briefly touched on here. Cardiogenic or neurocardiogenic syncope may be associated with brief myoclonic jerks, head turning, automatisms (lipsmacking, chewing), and upward deviation of the eyes and vocalizations may occur.[43] Differentiating fits from faints may be even more difficult when there are coexistent conditions predisposing to both syncope and seizures. It is well-known that transient cerebral anoxia, as for example in carotid sinus syncope—now recognized to be much more more common than before realized[44]—may itself cause convulsions. The convulsions of syncope are not usually followed by postictal stupor, or malaise. However, incontinence may occur and there may be transient throbbing headache.

Recurrent cardiac arrhythmias are particularly important: in one series of patients referred to a neurological department with a diagnosis of epilepsy, 20 percent were found to have cardiac arrhythmias that caused or significantly contributed to their symptoms.[45] The situation may be particularly confusing, as complex partial seizures affecting the temporal lobes may present with autonomic features, and attention has been drawn to the ictal bradycardia syndrome, in which episodic bradycardia or even asystole leading to syncope may itelf be an ictal event.[46]

It may, therefore, sometimes prove impossible to determine whether transient cerebral symptoms are cardiac or cerebral in origin. Even ambulatory 24-hour or even longer ECG, with or without other cardiovascular tests, and prolonged EEG monitoring may not permit a confident diagnosis. Nonspecific abnormalities on an EEG, or cardiac arrhythmias recorded on a 24-hour tape unrelated to the symptoms, may add to the confusion. Head-up tilt for up to 45 minutes with or without carotid sinus massage may induce bradycardia and/or hypotension and thus help differentiate convulsive syncope from epilepsy.[42] The golden rule is to avoid, as much as possible, approaching the patient with preconceptions: "As ye seek, so shall ye find." The correlative of this is that there are potential pitfalls in establishing isolated epilepsy clinics or syncope clinics for older people. Perhaps "paroxysmal disorder clinics" would be better. In the author's experience, the two-way traffic between his own epilepsy clinic and his colleague's syncope service is extremely heavy! Where there is continuing uncertainty my own practice is to investigate vigorously for causes of syncope in the first instance if only because undiagnosed cardiac arrhythmias are more likely to be life-threatening than undiagnosed epilepsy.

Some genuinely epileptic events may not be appreciated for what they are (Table 46-6). The temporal lobe is the terminus of the vestibular pathways; consequently, seizures originating in this area may present with episodic vertigo, often associated with nausea.[47] Sometimes these fits may evolve to full-blown tonic–clonic seizures, but until this happens they may be labeled as nonspecific dizziness, especially in an elderly person. Complex partial seizures, with or without automatisms, may be nonspecific confusional states or even, where there are affective[48] or cognitive features or hallucinations, as manifestations of functional psychiatric illnesses. Patients with nonconvulsive epileptic status may present with acute, behavioral changes—withdrawal, mutism, delusional ideas, paranoia, vivid hallucinations, and fugue states.[49] Fluctuating mental impairment may easily be attributed to other causes of recurrent confusional states or even misread as part of a dementing process.[50,51] Thomas[52] has recently reviewed epileptic confusional states in elderly people due to either absence status or partial complex status and noted how often they are triggered by psychotropic medication such as tricyclic antidepressants (usually in excessive doses), though there are often metabolic causes. Occasionally, patients present with abrupt loss of consciousness without tonic–clonic movements—so-called atonic seizures.[53] Perhaps because of age-related changes in the brain, but more likely because epilepsy in elderly people usually takes place against the background of cerebral damage, postictal states may be very prolonged, and this may be another source of diagnostic confusion. At least 14 percent of patients in one series suffered a confusional state lasting 24 hours or more and in some cases it could persist as long as a week.[3] A focal postictal paresis (Todd's palsy) is also more frequent in elderly patients. Todd's paresis after a fit may be misdiagnosed as stroke; in one series this was the most common nonstroke cause of referral to a stroke unit.[54] This is particularly likely where fits occur against a background of known cerebrovascular disease, and a recurrence of stroke may be incorrectly diagnosed.[55]

In the face of such difficulties, the clinician's primary duty is to acknowledge uncertainty where it exists and, if uncertainty remains after a careful history, examination, and appropriate investigations, simply to wait and see. A "therapeutic trial" of anticonvulsants as a diagnostic test is not generally recommended: it will rarely produce a clear answer unless

Table 46-6 Seizures that may be confused with other conditions

Epileptic event	Possible misdiagnosis
Epilepsia partialis continua (partial motor status)	Extrapyramidal movement disorder
Sensory epilepsy	Transient ischemic attack
Complex partial seizures	Organic or functional psychosis
Atonic seizures	Drop attacks/hysteria
Epileptic vertigo (due to temporal lobe attacks)	Brain stem/vestibular disease/nonspecific dizziness
Todd's palsy	Stroke/transient ischemic attack
Any kind of seizure	"Falls"

fits are very frequent and will add the burden of possibly unnecessary drug treatment to the patient's troubles.

INVESTIGATIONS

Investigations will be directed toward confirming the clinical diagnosis of epilepsy (and so differentiating this from other causes of "funny turns" and other transient impairments), defining the type of epilepsy (although the vast majority of cases of epilepsy in old age are focal in origin), and identifying remediable underlying causes.

General investigations

The choice of investigations will, of course, be determined by the history and by the findings on examination as well as by consideration of likely causes. Routine tests should include a full blood count, erythrocyte sedimentation rate, biochemical investigations (including urea, electrolytes, glucose, and liver function tests), electrocardiograph, and chest X-ray. It is important to rule out metabolic causes (see "Metabolic and Toxic Causes," above) as they will usually be amenable to treatment. An estimate of gamma-glutamyl transferase may be a useful marker of recent alcohol consumption. The threshold for carrying out thyroid function tests should be low, as myxoedema (which is occasionally associated with seizures) is common in older people and may present atypically. Diabetic control should be reviewed, especially where the presenting problem is that of nocturnal seizures in a patient on oral hypoglycemic agents. The choice of other investigations, such as serum tests for syphilis, will be influenced by history and findings on examination—and known prevalence of such conditions.

Specialist investigations

The hardest diagnostic challenge is often, as already indicated, to differentiate between fits and faints. If it decided that there is strong chance that the episodes are syncopal, then the patient should be carefully investigated along the lines suggested in Chapter 38.

In the absence of features suggesting acute infection of the nervous system, there is no indication for lumbar puncture which may, anyway, be dangerous if a space-occupying lesion has not been ruled out by neuroimaging. The remote possibility of neurosyphilis will be even more remote if blood testing does not show abnormal serology. A chest X-ray may reveal a relevant primary neoplasm. While a skull X-ray may show evidence of raised intracranial pressure, intracranial calcification, or other evidence of an intracerebral neoplasm, it is rarely helpful in the present era of neuroimaging.

A survey[56] of American neurologists' management of a single, unprovoked seizure showed a wide variation in the use of electroencephalography and neuroimaging. Some neurologists routinely ordered both investigations, some one but not the other, and some neither. There is clearly scope here for studies evaluating these different approaches to investigation.

Electroencephalography

Excessive reliance upon an EEG to make or to refute a diagnosis of epilepsy is potentially dangerous. A routine EEG may support the diagnosis of epilepsy, especially if clear-cut paroxysmal discharges are observed. The absence of such activity on a routine recording does not, however, rule out the diagnosis; after all, most recordings last for only 20 minutes and ictal or diagnostic interictal activity occurs only intermittently. The range of "normal" increases with age so that discriminating normal from abnormal is more difficult in an elderly patient. Nonspecific abnormalities are more common in old age. In summary, while the EEG may provide useful supporting evidence for the diagnosis of epilepsy, it should not overrule the clinical diagnosis nor, with rare exceptions such as nonconvulsive status, provide its sole basis. It should also be added that an EEG, in this age group as in any other, cannot alone determine the need for a treatment in a newly diagnosed case, establish the adequacy of treatment, or predict the safety of discontinuing therapy.

A focal abnormality on an EEG may support the clinical diagnosis of a focal origin for fits and suggest a local neurological cause. In those fits where there is an inadequate history or where the focal phase is too brief to be observed clinically, focal discharges may suggest a focal origin for the first time and guide further investigation. Persistent gross localized abnormalities on an EEG would strongly support a focal structural lesion. The EEG may be particularly useful in diagnosing nonconvulsive status or epilepsy presenting with recurrent behavioral disturbance or other neuropsychiatric manifestations (see above). Prolonged EEG recording via telemetry, sleep studies, and videotelemetry may help in the classification of difficult cases and may help differentiate epilepsy from syncope due to cardiac arrhythmias and ensure that patients with such problems are not treated with anticonvulsant drugs. Unfortunately, the access of elderly patients to such diagnostic facilities is often limited.

Neuroradiology

The older the age of presentation with epilepsy the greater the chance of a positive CT scan: as many as 60 percent of very late onset epilepsy patients may show a structural lesion.[57] This, however, would be an argument for routine scanning only if

identification of such lesions influenced management—as in the case of a space-occupying lesion amenable to neurosurgical removal (see Fig. 46-2). In only a minority of patients with elderly-onset epilepsy is a neoplasm or subdural hematoma the cause and in only a small proportion of tumor cases would neurosurgical intervention be appropriate. As already noted, in most series, tumors are more likely to be gliomas or metastases than meningiomas. Even where a meningioma is diagnosed, neurosurgical treatment may not be indicated.[58] There is an impression that some meningiomas in old age may be relatively inert and there is no doubt that craniotomy is often tolerated poorly by elderly patients. The discovery of an otherwise inert meningioma, especially if it is nonoperable because of its site or the patient's general condition, may not be of benefit to the patient. Even so, it is always useful to have a definitive diagnosis, as in, for example, established cerebrovascular disease, though definitive treatment for the underlying condition may not be available or considered inappropriate. Arguable indications for CT scanning are given in the accompanying box.

> ### Indications for computerized tomography in elderly-onset seizures
>
> - Unexplained focal neurological signs
> - Progressive or new neurological signs or symptoms
> - Poor control of seizures not attributable to poor compliance with antiepileptic drugs or continued exposure to precipitants such as alcohol.
> - Clear-cut, stereotyped focal seizures
> - Persistent marked slow-wave abnormality on the electroencephalogram

Magnetic resonance imaging (MRI) has been assessed in patients with seizures in whom there was no clear cause and CT scans have been normal. In some such cases, MRI has given diagnostically helpful information, confirming that it is a powerful and sensitive diagnostic tool; however, how often the information obtained using it would alter management in elderly-onset epilepsy still remains to be seen.[59]

It should not be forgotten that for many older people, an MRI scan is something of an ordeal, described by some as being "like burial at sea." Some have argued vigorously for cerebral imaging in all cases of elderly onset seizures.[2,60] In the absence of good data on the way the use of neuroradiological investigations influences the outcome for patients, personal opinion, the availability of resources, and patient expectation will shape investigative strategies. The more actively investigative approach to managing cerebrovascular disease (as we have noted, the commonest cause of seizures in old age) may, however, appropriately lower the threshold for cerebral imaging.

MANAGEMENT

Doctors tend to think of the care of patients with epilepsy predominantly in terms of drug treatment. Management, however, is much more than drug treatment. The problem of epilepsy for the patient, and the impact of seizures, goes far beyond their immediate consequences.[61]

General measures

Reassurance

Reassurance is of paramount importance: that, in the vast majority of cases, fits do not indicate serious brain damage; that epilepsy itself rarely causes brain damage; that fits are unrelated to psychiatric disturbance; and that they can be controlled by medication. Patients should be told that anyone's brain is capable of having seizures if the circumstances are right and that fits are the most commonest neurological problems after headache, with as many as 1 in 50 people having a fit at some time in their life. In epilepsy, almost more than in any other condition, giving patients the opportunity to air their beliefs, preconceptions, and worries about their condition is of paramount importance. This will not be achieved at a single interview. The patient will require "several bites of the cherry." In the management of epilepsy, as elsewhere, communication of a diagnosis is a process of education.

Education, information, and support

Patients will want to know whether their fits are brought on by any particular activity and whether, for this reason, they should lead restricted lives. The advice in this age group is the same as that given to any patients: avoid only those activities that would mean immediate danger if a fit occurred. The tendency of carers and supporters to discourage people with epilepsy from living a full and independent life should be anticipated and pre-empted.

Epileptic attacks are the most frequent cause of medical attacks at the wheel.[62] Driving regulations vary from country to country and even, as in the US, from state to state. In the UK, any driving licence holder diagnosed as having epilepsy must notify the Driver and Vehicle Licensing Authority and stop driving until further directed by the authority. The onus of responsibility to inform the Authority lies with the patient and not the doctor. The current regulations in the UK have been usefully summarized by Shorvon,[63] and the essence of his summary is contained in Appendix 46-1.

As so often in old-age medicine, management is multidisciplinary. A fit may cause severe loss of confidence and, in individuals who already have locomotor or other disability, this may lead not only to voluntary restriction of activities and a shrinkage of "life space," but may be also the beginning of a progressive descent into a vicious spiral of reduced mobility. In such patients, encouragement of mobility, assessment for walking or other aids, and a review of the home circumstances and need for social support services will require input from remedial therapists and social workers. A home visit by an occupational therapist to look for potential sources of dangers—unguarded fires, etc.—may be helpful. Where fits are frequent, especially when there is a warning aura, a body-worn personal alarm may be useful.

Factors that are known to precipitate fits, such as inadequate sleep or excess alcohol, should be avoided. The patient should be warned that alcohol will increase the side-effects of medication and that other drugs may trigger seizures or interact with antiepileptic drugs (AEDs). Patients should be encouraged to remind their doctors that they have epilepsy when they are seen about other conditions for which they may receive prescriptions. It should be made clear that AEDs are for life and not just "a course of treatment." In any patient presenting with seizures, existing medication should be reviewed, and drugs with a known epileptogenic potential[36] or liable to interfere with AEDs withdrawn if possible.

Contact numbers for local branches of the national epilepsy associations may be useful, though older patients may find the rest of the membership rather young. With the patient's permission, spouses, relatives, neighbors, and other caretakers should be advised as to how to manage seizures if they occur. Verbal information should be supplemented with clearly expressed, written information printed in a font of adequate size.

DRUG TREATMENT

Though the literature on AED therapy is enormous, it contains relatively little specific reference to elderly patients. In those few drug trials from which elderly patients are not actually excluded, they are seriously under-represented. Most of what we think we know about anticonvulsant therapy in the aging brain has therefore been extrapolated from studies on younger patients, many of whom do not have the focal lesions that are typical in elderly epileptic patients and all of whom lack the age-related changes seen in older people. The advice that follows, therefore, falls rather short of the ideals of evidence-based medicine.

When should antiepileptic drugs be started?

Epilepsy is defined as a tendency to recurring seizures and implicit in treatment with AEDs is the assumption that a patient does have such a tendency. A single seizure—especially if it has an obvious precipitating cause such as fever or alcohol—does not count as epilepsy, the assumption being that it does not imply an underlying tendency to recurrence. Here the correct approach is not AEDs, but removal of the cause. Where there is a single apparently unprovoked seizure, the decision whether or not to treat with AEDs is more difficult. It will be influenced by several considerations: the severity of the index seizure: the clinician's view as to the likelihood of recurrence (estimates range from 27 to 80 percent[64,65]), the estimate of the risks such as injury associated with a recurrent seizure; the conjectured hazards of AEDs; and the credibility one gives to the notion that "fits breed fits"[66] so that early treatment may prevent epilepsy becoming chronic or intractable. Ideally, there should be clear strategies for arresting epileptogenesis, either after a first seizure or after an event that predicts future seizures. At present, we have inadequate information upon which to base rational decisions as to whether a single unprovoked major seizure in an older person should be treated. Age itself is not a consistent predictor of recurrence, although the presence of a clear-cut etiological factor, such as a focal cerebral lesion, is. The relative dangers of nontreatment (e.g. injury due to further seizures) and of treatment (adverse effects of medication) have never been assessed in a systematic population-based, prospective manner. Until this has been done—and we have the results of the long-term outcome of trials such as the MESS[67,68] studies—the decision whether or not a single unprovoked fit should be treated is partly personal prejudice.[69]

At present, it seems reasonable to treat a single unprovoked major seizure only if it is prolonged or it has a clear-cut underlying cerebral cause such as a cerebral tumor which predicts recurrence. Where there is no such cause, and the fit has not been prolonged, the decision is more difficult. In the case of a short-duration generalized convulsive seizure or a partial or nonconvulsive seizure, it is probably best to wait. In a patient who has had a single fit, it is important to emphasize future prompt treatment of conditions such as chest infections that might lead to hypoxia and so precipitate further fits. Two or more unprovoked major seizures warrant AED treatment, for then the risk of recurrence is about 70 percent in the general adult population[65] and it will probably be higher in the older adult population, where there is more often a continuing underlying cause.

There is even less information regarding the prognosis of untreated minor seizures. Treatment of a single minor episode is probably overzealous and it would seem to be reasonable to wait and see how frequent and how upsetting the episodes are before embarking on drug therapy.

The choice of AED

Since the last edition of this textbook, there has been a significant increase in the information available to prescribers about AEDs and although not all of this can be extrapolated from the rather young population that tends to predominate in AED trials, some of it is highly relevant. Moreover, there has been a modest increase in the number of trials specifically looking at AEDs in older patients. More important than the increase in the total amount of information, however, has been the establishment of the Cochrane Collaboration which, over the last few years, has produced very high quality systematic reviews of the information made available in randomized controlled trials.[70] The problems of pooling the data have been addressed by extremely sophisticated methodologies including accessing, as far as possible, individual patient data made available by the trialists. Ironically, one of the messages that has come through most clearly from the conscientious labors of the Cochrane collaborationists has been the lack of information to support the therapeutic choices we make! There are, for example, no placebo-controlled randomized controlled trials evaluating the main AEDs as monotherapy in partial or generalized epilepsy and remarkably few adequately powered head-to-head comparisons. The third development since the last edition, has been a further proliferation of the new generation AEDs available to prescribers.

Perhaps not entirely unsurprisingly, the widening knowledge base and the increased range of therapeutic choices have made life more rather than less difficult for the thoughtful prescriber. Rational prescribing may become easier in future years particularly when the respective merits of the standard and new AEDs are clarified as a result of the SANAD (Standard and New Antiepileptic Drugs) trial to be published in 2005.[71] The recommendations that follow must be regarded as provisional, pending more robust information.

Standard antiepileptic drugs

The majority of cases with either primary or secondary generalized seizures or partial seizures can be controlled with a single, standard AED. Seventy percent of patients can expect a 5-year remission. For a long time, the evidence suggested that phenytoin, carbamazepine and sodium valproate were equally effective as first-line, broad-spectrum AEDs for unselected patients with seizures.[72] One of the first fruits of the Cochrane Collaboration has been to show that, at least in the case of elderly-onset seizures, the three standard broad-spectrum first-line AEDs are not equivalent. The strong clinical belief that carbamazepine appears to have an edge over sodium valproate in partial and secondarily generalized seizures, seems to be upheld. This is of particular relevance to older patients.[73] The Cochrane Overview was based on 1,265 patients derived from all trials that met the stringent entry criteria. The outcome measures used to evaluate the drugs were well chosen: time to treatment withdrawal (which would encompass both efficacy and adverse effects); 12-month remission; and time to first seizure. Carbmazepine was significantly superior to valproate in partial or secondary generalized seizures. It was also superior to valproate in elderly-onset seizures, which is what might be expected given that the latter are overwhelmingly partial or secondary generalized.[19] In the absence of further information, therefore, carbamazepine would seem to be the first-choice broad-spectrum AED in older people. A controlled-release preparation is probably preferable to a standard preparation.

It would probably be premature, however, to make carbamazepine the first-line choice in all cases. As we have noted, a small minority of seizures in older people are generalized in origin and these may benefit from sodium valproate rather than carbamazepine. These include myoclonic seizures in patients with Alzheimer's disease, and late-onset idiopathic primary generalized seizures. In such cases, and in our present state of uncertainty, valproate should be the first drug of choice.

If carbamazepine fails to control seizures or where it is poorly tolerated, monotherapy with one of the other first-line drugs should be tried. Whether one should switch to valproate or phenytoin is unclear because there have been no head-to-head Cochrane comparisons between these two drugs. Moreover, a multicenter comparative trial of efficacy in 150 elderly patients[74] showed both sodium valproate and phenytoin to be useful first-line, broad-spectrum AEDs in elderly onset seizures. There was no significant difference in efficacy nor, surprisingly, in adverse effects, between the two drugs. Interestingly, acturial analysis suggested that a 6-month remission by 12-month follow-up would be enjoyed by 78 percent of the patients on valproate and 76 percent of patients on phenytoin—very similar to the findings from monotherapy studies in the general adult population.

Many considerations, in addition to efficacy and adverse effects, may need to be taken into account in choosing a first-line AED. These include ease of use by both patient and physician. Phenytoin can be used once daily, which is an advantage in the case of patients requiring help from others with their medication. Though controlled release of sodium valproate (Epilim Chrono) has been used by some once daily, it is still usually given twice daily and the same is true of carbamazepine. Ease of use by the physician is also important. Phenytoin is unusual in exhibiting saturation kinetics near the therapeutic range so that a small change in the dose may be associated with a very large change in available drug creating the risk of a switch from subtherapeutic to toxic levels (see below). This makes the drug potentially problematic in inexperienced hands. There is also the question of drug–disease interactions. Finally, cost is an issue, though the difference in price between the three older-generation AEDs is small compared with the difference in price between the older and the newer AEDs.

Adverse effects are of paramount importance. AEDs may cause acute dose-related, acute idiosyncratic, and chronic toxic effects. These adverse effects are usefully summarized in Appleton et al.,[75] and the reader is strongly advised to be familiar with them when an AED is prescribed. It is important to appreciate that they may present rather subtly in an older patient who may have pre-existing pathology impairing either cognitive function or mobility.

The gross *neurological* side-effects include ataxia, dysarthria, nystagmus, dizziness, unsteadiness, blurring and doubling of vision, reversible dyskinesias, and asterixis. Although some neurotoxic effects may occur more frequently with certain drugs, there is so much overlap that most cannot be regarded as specific to any one drug; the effects are generally dose related, and in the general adult population, can usually be avoided or minimized by careful dosage titration.

Effects on cognitive function are of particular relevance. Earlier studies suggested that, of the commonly used broad-spectrum AEDs, maximum adverse impact was seen with phenytoin and lesser effects with sodium valproate and carbamazepine.[76] Interestingly, this difference has not been found in elderly patients. A detailed comparison of the impact of sodium valproate and phenytoin on various aspects of cognitive function, including attention, concentration, psychomotor speed, and memory[77] in elderly people failed to show major differences between the two drugs. This is in keeping with more recent literature which has also failed to demonstrate significant differences in the cognitive effects of AEDs in the general adult population.[78] It is probable, that if the dose of AEDs is kept to a minimum, adverse cognitive effects are less important.

Other neurological or neuropsychiatric side-effects—for example, subjective feelings of unsteadiness and tiredness (including falling asleep in front of one's favorite television program)—may, however, still be significant and there may be important differences in the frequency and severity of these. We know remarkably little about subtle adverse neurological and other effects of AEDs, even less in older people.

Of the many non-neurological side effects, osteomalacia[79] may be especially relevant, since this is more likely to occur in patients whose poor dietary intake of vitamin D and reduced exposure to sunlight already puts them at risk. Phenytoin, in particular, induces enzymes in the liver that accelerate the metabolism of vitamin D. There may, therefore, be a case for routine vitamin supplementation in patients on this AED. Sodium valproate, unlike phenytoin or carbamazepine, does not cause hypocalcemia or reduced vitamin D levels. Carbamazepine-induced hyponatremia increases significantly with age[80] and may occur at very low doses. The risk of hyponatremia may be even greater with oxcarbazepine (see below).[81] This will be important in patients on diuretics—especially potassium-sparing sodium-losing diuretics—or who are prone to hyponatremia from other causes such as recurrent chest infection. Skin rashes are an important problem especially with carbamazepine and a common reason for withdrawal from that drug. It may sometimes be severe and occasionally take the life-threatening form of toxic epidermal necrolysis.[82]

Monotherapy should be preferred to polytherapy, particularly in patients who are likely already to be on one or more medications. In younger subjects, where monotherapy is unsuccessful, this is very often due to poor compliance or sometimes associated with a serious underlying cerebral condition. Adding a second drug sometimes contributes only additional side-effects. In some patients who are on more than one drug, withdrawal of the second or third drug may actually improve control. The idea that epilepsy is better controlled with smaller doses of more than one drug makes even less sense in older people who are already on other medication. Though monotherapy should be the aim, there will be a proportion of patients who will require two AEDs—so-called "rational polypharmacy"—but before embarking on this course, the advice of an expert should be sought. When we have "cleaner" drugs whose actions are both more precise and better understood, it may be possible to tailor-make a "cocktail" of drugs with complementary actions, each given in relatively low doses. However, this approach lies in the future.

In summary, so far as standard AEDs are concerned, there is a case for carbamazepine as the first choice. However, there should be no blanket recommendation for elderly people. There may be individual drugs that are more suited to individual patients. Whatever drug is chosen, the prescribing physician should be familiar with its effects, kinetics, and its side-effects.

New antiepileptic drugs

When a patient is not satisfactorily controlled on one of the standard AEDs, the clinician is faced with a bewildering array of choices (see Summary of Management Algorithm). As may be expected, the evidence to guide the clinician through this maze of possible lines of action is scanty. Most importantly, we have little clear evidence about the comparative benefits and disadvantages of first- and second-line drugs. Information will be available when the UK study of the Standard and New Antiepileptic Drugs (SANAD) is published in 2005. There are some general characteristics of the new-generation AEDs that make them very attractive to physicians caring for older people with seizures. In trials of the general adult population, they may have equal efficacy, but fewer side-effects, than the older drugs. Their pharmacokinetics are often simpler. Perhaps most important of all, they have relatively few drug interactions.

There is certainly room for improvement on the performance of the standard AEDs. The multicenter comparative study in elderly-onset seizures referred to earlier[74] found a high rate of adverse effects (20 percent). Most of these were minor, but it might be anticipated that "minor" adverse effects in older patients who are often near to the threshold of failure may translate into a significant impact on function. Moreover, over 20 percent of patients were not satisfactorily controlled. Herein lies the potential significance of the new generation AEDs: to obtain the same, or better, levels of efficacy with fewer adverse effects. Against this, two important considerations should

Summary of management algorithm: antiepileptic drug treatment strategies when response is unsatisfactory

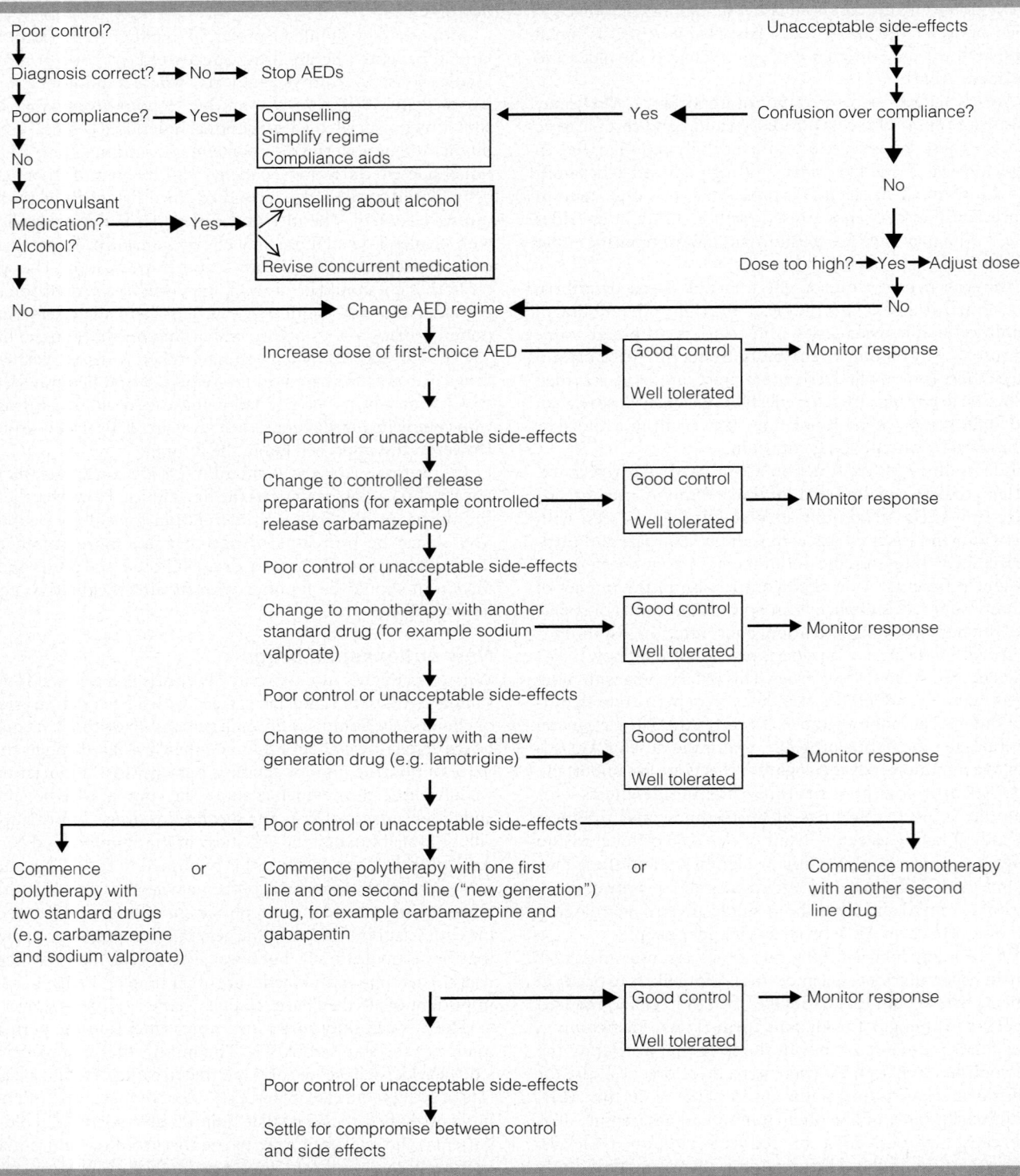

weigh against a wholesale switch in prescribing habits. First of all, the new-generation drugs are very much more expensive than the older ones and, since epilepsy is a chronic illness affecting large numbers of patients, this has huge implications for the national drug budget. Secondly, these drugs remain relatively little tried compared with the standard drugs and unexpected adverse effects may still emerge. This has been dramatically illustrated in the case of vigabatrin, the first tailor-made AED, which looked very promising indeed. However, it is no longer recommended because it is associated with serious irreversible visual field loss which might be difficult to pick up in older patients.[83] The following brief notes on new AEDs should therefore be seen as provisional reports from a rapidly changing situation.

Lamotrigine,[84] like phenytoin, acts by blockage of sodium-dependent channels. It exhibits linear kinetics and is not bound to plasma protein. It has been shown to be effective as add-on treatment in refractory partial seizures. More importantly, a recent multicenter, double-blind randomized comparison of monotherapy with lamotrigine with carbamazepine (which on the basis of the above discussion may be regarded as a reasonable first-choice standard AED in elderly patients with newly diagnosed seizures) has shown advantages for lamotrigine.[85] The main difference between the drugs was the rate of dropout due to adverse events (lamotrigine 18 percent vs carbamazepine 42 percent). This was partly due to a lower rash rate with lamotrigine. Lamotrigine patients also complained less frequently of somnolence. Although there was no difference between the drugs from time to first seizure, a greater percentage of lamotrigine-treated patients remained seizure free during the last 16 weeks of treatment. Overall, more patients continued on treatment with lamotrigine than carbamazepine (71 percent and 42 percent respectively) for the duration of study. The authors concluded that lamotrigine could be regarded as an acceptable choice of initial treatment for elderly patients with newly diagnosed epilepsy. Lamotrigine, in combination with other AEDs such as sodium valproate, can reduce seizures but the adverse effects of valproate may be increased.

Oxcarbazepine,[86] while only newly licensed in the UK, has been available in Scandinavian countries for over a decade. Since, however, experience elsewhere is relatively sparse this is still regarded as a "new-generation" drug. It is an analog of carbamazepine, developed in an effort to retain the therapeutic effects of the latter while offering improved tolerability. It is effectively a prodrug that is rapidly and completely metabolized and virtually all of its activity is due to its metabolites. Carbamazepine, by contrast, is converted to an active metabolite that accumulates and this is responsible for some of its side-effects. Unlike carbamazepine, oxcarbazepine does not induce its own metabolism, so that its half-life does not decrease with chronic administration which theoretically should make dosage titration easier. Finally, it has fewer drug interactions. Given these advantages and its equal efficacy to carbamazepine, there is a case for its being a drug of choice for older people. A comparative study[87] with carbamazepine in the general adult population with both primary generalization and partial and secondary generalized seizures showed similar efficacy and overall incidence of "severe" side-effects. There is, however, insufficient information in large numbers of elderly people and there is concern about

hyponatremia, though how important this is is still a matter of controversy.[88] Personal experience, moreover, indicates that one has to be as careful when introducing oxcarbazepine as carbamazepine despite the theoretical reason for thinking that it will be better tolerated in the early stages of titration.

Gabapentin acts via both sodium-channel blocking effects and potentiation of GABA receptor responses. Although it does not have linear kinetics (exhibiting saturability of gastrointestinal absorption), it is a relatively easy drug to use because it is excreted unchanged in the kidney, it is unbound to protein, and has a wide therapeutic window. Importantly, it has no interactions with other drugs. For these reasons, it is another potentially attractive first-line drug for older patients, particularly as it appears to be relatively free from side-effects.[89] There is, however, insufficient evidence to determine its place in monotherapy.[90] There is no doubt about its efficacy as add-on medication in resistant partial epilepsy.[91] As with other new drugs, research is needed into the effects of long-term use: studies have tended to focus on its short-term effects. There is certainly a case for more studies comparing gabapentin with carbamazepine and lamotrigine and oxcarbazepine as monotherapy in partial epilepsy and gabapentin and valproate as monotherapy in primary generalized epilepsy in older people.

Topiramate acts in at least four different ways and its use could justifiably be described "single-drug polypharmacy." Again, the kinetics are simple, with nonsaturability, mostly renal excretion, and lack of protein binding. There appear to be few significant interactions. There are no data for monotherapy in elderly patients. Topiramate is efficacious as add-on treatment in patients with drug-resistant partial epilepsy.[92] However, trials were of relatively short duration and provided no evidence for long-term efficacy. As with other add-on drugs, the results cannot be extrapolated to monotherapy or to patients with other types of epilepsy than partial epilepsy.

Tiagibine[93] is a GABA uptake inhibitor which is effective as add-on therapy in the management of patients with refractory partial epilepsy, producing sustained reduction in seizure frequency in studies of up to 12 months duration. Current information is insufficient to determine its usefulness when used as monotherapy. The possible disadvantage of tiagibine is its short half-life necessitating 2–4 times daily administration, which is a consideration in elderly patients.

Zonisamide[94] is as yet, a relatively little used drug. A recent Cochrane Review found that this was useful as add-on treatment in patients with drug-resistant partial epilepsy. Since the trials were of relatively short duration (12 weeks), the results are not able to confirm effectiveness in long-term seizure control; nor can the results be extrapolated to monotherapy or to patients with other seizure types or epilepsy syndrome. Add-on therapy is associated with increased adverse effects.

Leviteracetam is a novel AED which is structurally unrelated to other AEDs. A recent review found that leviteracetam reduced seizure frequency when used as add-on treatment for patients with drug-resistant epilepsy. Moreover, it is possibly better tolerated than other add-on therapy for partial seizures.[95]

In summary, the new AEDs still have promise of enhanced efficacy, either alone or in combination with other drugs in cases of intractable seizures; have simpler kinetics in some cases; exhibit fewer drug interactions and, in some cases, none; and have the possibility of less frequent or less marked adverse effects. In view of the fact that they are much more expensive, less widely tried and tested and few have been specifically evaluated in the elderly population, it would be premature to consider these as first-choice, first-line monotherapy for the generality of elderly patients with seizures with the possible exception of lamotrigine.

The physician who is looking for an alternative automatic choice first-line monotherapy for the broad range of seizures in old age must, therefore, wait a while. To quote a recent authoritative review:[96] "At present, the main use of the new agents is in patients refractory to first-line drugs … and further studies are required to characterize their activity spectrum as well as their potential value in monotherapy. In most patients, new drugs cannot be recommended for first-line use until evidence is obtained that potential advantages in tolerability or ease of use outweigh the drawback of their high cost."

On the basis of the present data, Marson and colleagues[97] suggest that, if add-on treatment is required with the drugs discussed above, gabapentin and lamotrigine offer the best option for patients with drug intolerance but adequate seizure control, while in patients with poor seizure control in whom potency is the main issue, topiramate might be an optimal choice. In either case, for the practicing geriatrician, these drugs should be used only in patients with seizures unresponsive to the conventional therapy and, hence, on the advice of a specialist. If the newest AEDs are to be used as initial monotherapy in older patients, this should usually be in the context of an ongoing drug trial in older people. At any rate, it is important that when the new drugs have demonstrated their efficacy in the younger adult population, they should be separately evaluated in older people; until such studies have been done, they should not be routinely recommended for people with elderly-onset seizures.

Prescribing strategies (see Summary of management algorithm on p. 562)

For the present, a sensible strategy is to use a conventional drug with which one is familiar, unless the considerations set out above dictate the choice of one of the other AEDs such as the newer AEDs. If this works, well and good; if, despite adequate dosage and good compliance, there is poor control, then one of the other first-line older-generation broad-spectrum AEDs should be tried. In a small minority of patients it may be necessary to use more than one AED at a time in either a combination of older AEDs or an older AED combined with a new one. Such patients should be referred to a physician with a special interest in seizures.

Some patients may not be fully controlled even with optimal AED treatment. This should not prompt ever-increasing, toxic doses of multiple drugs, but a more modest goal: to achieve a reduction in fit frequency to tolerable levels without unacceptable drug side-effects. Feeling continually wretched from the adverse effects of AEDs may be even worse than suffering the intermittent unpleasantness of a fit.

Dosages

The dosages recommended for the general adult population may be inappropriate for elderly patients. There is considerable evidence to support an age-related increase in pharmacodynamic sensitivity to certain AEDs.[98] For example, a study of carbamazepine found a greater effect on body sway with one 400 mg dose, despite the absence of pharmacokinetic differences. Even more important than age-related changes in pharmacodynamic sensitivity, are the altered pharmacokinetics of anticonvulsants in older patients.

The concentration of AEDs in the nervous system reflects the free or unbound concentration in the plasma rather than that bound to protein. Since albumin concentrations tend to be lower in elderly people—especially when ill—higher free concentrations of certain drugs are to be expected. This has been demonstrated in the case of phenytoin, sodium valproate, and certain benzodiazepines. The differences are particularly marked with valproate. There is also reduced clearance of certain AEDs. Single-dose studies have shown reduced clearance of valproate and in multiple-dose studies the maximum rate of phenytoin clearance and the clearance of unbound valproate are both reduced. In the case of phenytoin, there is an increased plasma half-time. This is due in part to reduced clearance, but also to the fact that the volume of distribution for lipid soluble drugs is increased in elderly people because of the increase of fatty tissue as a proportion of the total body mass. There is, therefore, a longer interval between initiation of a drug dosage and the attainment of a steady state. This does not appear to apply to valproate.

The information just given should not lead to an exaggerated estimate of present knowledge of age-related changes in pharmacodynamics or pharmacokinetics or its applicability to an individual patient. So-called age changes are often derived by comparing mean values for young and old groups. Differences within these groups may be at least as important as differences between them. In the case of phenytoin, for example, only 20 percent of the interindividual variation noted in one series was attributable to age alone.[99] In this context, as so often in clinical geriatrics, *age is more important as a source of unpredictable variability than of predictable change.*

Other sources of unpredictability arise from concurrent diseases, particularly those that affect pharmacokinetics through hepatic metabolism or that, for a variety of reasons, lead to a further reduction in albumin, and hence, protein binding; or those such as cerebral disease which affect pharmacodynamic sensitivity. The multiple pathology associated with old age will often mean multiple medication; many drugs interact with AEDs and they interact with one another. There are many sources of information about interactions. The British National Formulary[100] (updated three-monthly) is a good UK reference for clinically important interactions. Among these, interactions between AEDs such as phenytoin and anticoagulants are of particular importance in view of their potential seriousness and the escalating number of elderly patients who may benefit from anticoagulant prophylaxis against cardiovascular disease and this may direct the clinician towards those of the newer AEDs that do not interact with anticoagulants. Predicting plasma levels in a patient who is on more than two interacting drugs is especially more difficult.

All of this should make clear that to suggest specific doses "for elderly people" is misconceived. All that can be recommended is a general strategy: "start low and go slow" and be prepared to find that the response, either in terms of adverse effects or efficacy is not precisely what one had expected or hoped for. There is now sufficient evidence to suggest that the initial dose of phenytoin in an elderly person should not be more than 200 mg, possibly lower. Most patients will be controlled on 150 to 250 mg daily. It would seem reasonable to commence carbamazepine at 100 to 200 mg total daily dose, with a maintenance between about 400 mg and 1.2 g daily. Sodium valproate should be started at 400 mg total daily dose increasing to about 1 to 1.2 g total daily dose. Except where fits are frequent and control is a matter of urgency, dosage increases should be gradual. As for the newer drugs, the "start low, go slow" principle is even more relevant given the limited published information about their use in older people. At any rate, it is difficult, in view of the lack of clinical experience to make more specific dosage recommendations. Substituting one drug for another is even more complex, as is rationally determining the rate of addition of add-on drugs. In some cases, as in the replacement of sodium valproate by lamotrigine, there is useful guidance from the manufacturers. Caution in dosage alteration is particularly applicable to phenytoin where, as already noted, near the therapeutic range, an increment of as little as 25 mg may cause a marked rise in blood levels.

Anticonvulsant monitoring

The long-term management of patients with epilepsy was helped by the introduction in the 1970s of widely available AED monitoring.[101] This may be useful where: fits are not controlled by average doses of drugs; there are doubts about compliance, signs of intoxication, or odd neuropsychiatric syndromes; there is a sudden loss of control of fits; new interacting drugs are introduced; or where there are other diseases that may complicate treatment. The increased unpredictability between prescribed dose and blood levels in the patient makes AED monitoring particularly appropriate in the elderly.

It must be appreciated, however, that the most important part of *patient* monitoring is not measurement of AED levels, but the use of information derived from history and examination.[102] The patient or relative should keep a record of seizures; moreover, the patient should always be accompanied by a well-informed relative, neighbor, or caretaker to ensure that an accurate as possible account of events is obtained. Independent witnesses may also help the physician to pick up adverse effects that may be subtle in elderly people, and if not actively looked for, missed. Some attempt should be made to assess compliance and this should always be discussed with the patient. Increasing the dose because poor control due to variable compliance has been misinterpreted as implying insufficient dosage may lead to disaster. It is vital to emphasize the need to take medication consistently and indefinitely; some patients may have the erroneous notion that anticonvulsants need to be taken only when fits occur or as a "course." Finally, doctors should be aware that generic substitution may be associated with alteration in control and/or an increase in side-effects. This is particularly important with phenytoin, where different preparations have markedly different bioavailability.

Anticonvulsant levels are most helpful when they are used to answer a particular question or to resolve a particular uncertainty. Phenytoin is especially suitable for monitoring. First, its saturation kinetics mean a nonlinear relationship between dose and blood level: near the therapeutic range there will be a very steep dose–blood–level curve. Second, it has a propensity to produce adverse neuropsychiatric effects that may present nonspecifically or be lost in the noise of other neurological and other non-neurological pathology. Third, interindividual variation in kinetics is more marked than with the other two broad-spectrum AEDs. Fourth, there is a close correlation, at least at the population level, between blood values of this drug and, on the one hand, efficacy and, on the other, side-effects. Finally, because of the long half-life of phenytoin, single samples taken at random give a good approximation of the steady-state level.

The place of anticonvulsant monitoring is less well-defined for carbamazepine[103] and valproate.[104] The dosage of carbamazepine is a poor predictor of serum concentration (though after the initial period of enzyme induction the relationship between dose and plasma concentration in an individual is relatively linear) and many of the side-effects do appear concentration dependent. The relationship between carbamazepine concentration and clinical response is complicated by varying degrees of metabolism to its active metabolite and individual pharmacodynamic variability. The values given for the therapeutic range should be interpreted with caution: seizure control may be achieved throughout a very wide range of concentrations. Moreover, a single measurement may be meaningless because of great variations of concentration during a dosage interval. Both peak (3–4 hours after a dose) and trough (just after the next dose) levels need to be measured. In the case of sodium valproate, there is little correlation between blood levels and pharmacological effect and, because there may be diurnal variation in drug clearance, repeated levels on the same dose may show wide variation. Only a few of the side-effects, such as tremor, are concentration dependent. Monitoring, however, may help to rationalize treatment in patients on polypharmacy and to identify the cause for treatment failure when a patient is on an apparently adequate dose. Samples should be taken at a standard time in relation to doses.

Overdoing or overinterpreting anticonvulsant levels may lead to mismanagement.[102] As already indicated, levels are only a small part of the clinical assessment, and the results obtained from the laboratory must be interpreted in the light of the larger picture. Therapeutic ranges defined on general adult populations may not apply to the elderly population and certainly will not necessarily apply to any individual elderly patient. Doses should not be adjusted in fit-free nontoxic patients simply to bring the levels into the "therapeutic range." Conversely, a patient with symptoms suggestive of intoxication should not be required to continue on the same dose of an anticonvulsant simply because the values from the laboratory fall within the notional therapeutic range. It must be remembered that laboratory results may be incorrect for all sorts of technical reasons, ranging from the time the specimen was taken, through the labeling of the specimen, to the method used in the measurement.

Richens'[105] helpful review has set out the situations in which monitoring might be used: when seizure control is being established; if seizure control is lost; if adverse events occur; if the patient develops concomitant illnesses; if the patient's psychological state changes; and before withdrawing therapy. Limiting therapeutic monitoring to these patients Richens suggests, will strike the best cost-effective balance.

Improving compliance

People of all age groups with epilepsy tend to comply poorly with their medication—which is not surprising in view of the chronicity of treatment, the purely prophylactic nature of the benefit, and the frequency of side-effects. There is little evidence that noncognitively impaired elderly patients are much less compliant than younger people;[106] nevertheless, poor or variable compliance will be another reason for the lack of predictable relationship between prescribed dose and plasma level and between the doctor's action and the patient's response. Moreover, there are special problems for an older patient who may be on several drugs in addition to AEDs.

These are some of the ways in which compliance may be assisted:

* Simplifying regimes
* Giving clear instructions, both orally and written
* Making sure that medication is clearly labeled
* Making sure that medication is accessible (childproof bottles and blister packs may defeat the patient)
* Co-opting the help of caretakers, relatives, and others where appropriate
* Using compliance aids, such as dosette containers
* Adopting a nonadversarial approach to compliance
* Trying to determine the reason for noncompliance if it is detected
* Home visits or telephone contact by a specialist nurse (see below)

PROGNOSIS
Control of fits

There is little information on the proportion of elderly-onset patients who are satisfactorily controlled on AEDs. A report from the National General Practice Study of Epilepsy found that 9 years after the index seizure, 68 percent of subjects with definite epilepsy had had a 3–5 year remission and that age was not relevant.[107] In a comparative study of phenytoin with sodium valproate,[72] failure due to poor control was found in only 2 percent of patients on valproate and 4 percent of subjects on phenytoin (this difference was not significant), though 10 and 14 percent, respectively, had withdrawn due to adverse effects. We need larger numbers of subjects followed over a longer period of time to get a reliable picture. There is much work to be done to determine whether the newer AEDs will improve this picture. As already noted, lamotrigine seems to have the edge over carbamazepine in terms of patient acceptability.

Can drugs be withdrawn?

When should AEDs be withdrawn in patients with elderly-onset seizures? The literature[108,109] addresses much younger populations. A review of slow AED withdrawal in over 1,000 people who had been seizure free for at least 2 years found that while 78 percent of people on continuing treatment remained seizure free, this fell to 59 percent in patients taken off AEDs. Clinical predictors of relapse after drug withdrawal include age, seizure type, the number of AEDs being taken, whether seizures have occurred since AEDs were started and the period of remission before drug withdrawal. Because late-onset epilepsy, partial and secondarily generalized seizures (which are, of course, more common in the elderly), and the presence of known cerebral pathology (also more common in elderly epileptic patients) are associated with an increased rate of relapse, one may have to reluctantly concede that withdrawal of therapy should not be attempted in most elderly patients who have had a good reason to be placed on AEDs in the first place. However, this does not preclude attempted withdrawal in a patient who has a strong desire to be off AEDs after a full discussion of risks and benefits and the implications for driving if fits recur.

Mortality

Mortality is increased in people with epilepsy. However, the relative increase—the Standard Mortality Ratio—may be less marked in those diagnosed over 60 years of age than in those diagnosed in youth or middle age. Hauser et al.[110] found that the death rate from cardiac disease was increased in patients with elderly-onset epilepsy, but that the incidence of sudden cardiac death was increased only in patients with symptomatic epilepsy in whom cerebrovascular disease was the attributed cause. Luhdorf[111] followed 251 patients for a minimum period of 2 years. Survival at 6 years was 60 percent of what was expected. Most deaths were related to cerebrovascular disease or tumors and when patients with tumors or overt cerebrovascular disease were excluded, mortality was no higher than that of the age-matched population. It would appear that epilepsy per se does not increase mortality significantly.

In summary, what little evidence we have suggests that, in the absence of serious progressive disease, the prognosis both for control of seizures and for survival is good in elderly-onset cases. However, more prospective long-term studies are required, particularly because a report from Alabama[112] suggested a high death rate (4 percent) in elderly patients discharged from hospital with a primary diagnosis of convulsions.

SERVICES FOR PATIENTS WITH EPILEPSY

The challenge presented by a patient whose complaint suggests seizures is formidable. There is the diagnostic problem: are these events seizures and what is their underlying cause? Answering this question may require a good deal of clinical acumen and, sometimes, access to sophisticated investigative tools. Beyond this, there is the task of ensuring that patients are fully informed about their condition and its implications and that the necessary reassurance, education, and counseling is given. Finally, there is the difficulty of ensuring that the appropriate medication is prescribed, and taken, in the appropriate amounts over many years of a fluctuating condition affecting a patient who may have other illnesses that may influence the effects and adverse effects of the medication.

The nature of these challenges clearly argues for the development of specialist services. Perhaps these should not be addressed specifically to patients with epilepsy but should be open to patients who suffer from paroxysmal disorders of all kinds. Diagnosis-specific clinics—such as separate epilepsy clinics and separate syncope clinics—tend to prejudge diagnoses. Enthusiasts for the former may have a bias toward the diagnosis of epilepsy and for the latter toward syncope. We tend to find what we seek. My own epilepsy clinic operates in close partnership with a colleague's syncope clinic: there is only a "semipermeable membrane" between the two services. If such specialist services are developed, a crucial element is specific diagnostic facilities because the most difficult phase in management is confirming the diagnosis of seizures.

At present, there is little experience of such specialist services for older people. Elderly people with seizures may fall between two stools—between specialist geriatric services and specialist epilepsy services. It is important that the specialist clinics should not be regarded as sufficient in themselves. In an ideal world, they should be the hub of a population-based service crossing the divide between hospital and primary care services. At the least the clinic should be supported by, and reach out to, the wider geriatric medical services and to community services. There should be clear definition of the roles of general practitioners and specialists in what will, inevitably in a chronic disease, be "shared care."

Crucial to such services will be the specialist epilepsy nurse, which earlier research had suggested may be both effective[113] and cost-effective[114] in supporting patients with epilepsy in the long term, meeting their needs for information, education, counseling, and monitoring. A recent overview, however,[115] failed to find convincing evidence that specialist epilepsy nurses improve outcomes for people with epilepsy overall. Seizure frequency, psychosocial functioning, knowledge of epilepsy, general health status, work days lost, and depression and anxiety scores showed no significant improvement. It is important not to read too much into this finding. First of all, lack of evidence of benefit was not evidence of lack of benefit: the authors emphasize the need for further research. Moreover, nurses enable an overstretched service to reach out to more patients who would otherwise be overlooked and would not even be included in studies. Finally, these studies did not look at older patients whom one might expect to be more in need of support, for example over management of their medication. (Our ignorance of the benefits of specialist clinics is even more profound. To date there have been no controlled trials of suitable quality comparing them with nonspecialist clinics!)[116]

AREAS FOR RESEARCH

The observation made in previous editions of this textbook that geriatric epileptology is a relatively underdeveloped and under-researched field remains true. The outstanding research agenda is substantially the same.

Causes of seizures

Although it now seems clear that cerebrovascular disease is the most common cause of seizures in old age, the connection may be exaggerated because of the frequency of CT scan evidence of vascular disease in the general elderly population. More studies are needed to determine the frequency and type of cerebral tumors as a cause.

The physical impact of seizures

Seizures might be expected to have more adverse physical effects in old people. Is this the case? How frequent are fractures and other significant injuries?

The psychosocial impact of seizures

Jacoby and colleagues[117] have emphasized how "impact of a chronic illness is experienced not only through its physical symptoms, but also as a result of its effect on psychosocial

---

KEY POINTS Epilepsy

- Epileptic seizures occur more commonly in older people than in any other age group. Elderly people with seizures are now emerging as the most important single group of people with epilepsy.

- The vast majority of seizures in old age are either focal or focal in origin with secondary generalization.

- The most important cause of seizures in old age is cerebrovascular disease and otherwise unexplained epilepsy occurring for the first time in old age may be an early manifestation of cerebrovascular disease.

- Amongst the multitude of causes of provoked seizures, it is important not to forget iatrogenic drug-induced seizures and alcohol-related seizures.

- The most difficult step in the management of a person with suspected seizures is to determine whether or not the events are indeed epileptic fits. The most difficult differential diagnosis is between seizures and syncope. In many cases it is important to keep an open mind and where there is uncertainty aggressive pursuit of the diagnosis of syncope will often be more useful than repeated special investigations such as an EEG aimed at demonstrating epileptogenic activity.

- Electroencephalography has a smaller place in the diagnosis and classification of seizures than is generally appreciated by nonepileptologists. It may be useful if it can detect ictal activity in nonconvulsive status. Prolonged recordings with video telemetry may be helpful in difficult cases.

- The recent more active approach to diagnosis and management of cerebrovascular disease may lower the threshold for neuroimaging in patients with elderly onset seizures.

- The management of established epilepsy goes far beyond drug treatment. Key elements are reassurance, education, information, and support.

- There have been major developments in the drug treatment of epilepsy, some of which may be relevant to elderly people. Carbamazepine is probably the first choice of older generation drug for the majority of people with elderly onset seizures. The role of the very promising newer generation antiepileptic drugs is as yet uncertain.

(continued)

KEY POINTS (Continued)

- About 80 percent of people with elderly onset seizures will be controlled with the first choice drug or one of the other older generation antiepileptic drugs. Where these fail, expert advice should be sought and the strategy should be as set out in the Summary of Management Algorithm. In deciding when to start treatment and how hard to push treatment in cases that are difficult to control, it is important to weigh the benefits of seizure control, or improved seizure control, against the very real impact of adverse drug effects on quality of life.

- Interaction of antiepileptic drugs with medication for concurrent illness is a very important consideration in older people.

- Anticonvulsant monitoring may have a place in the management of some patients but monitoring the control of seizures and the overall clinical impact on the patient is even more important.

- Elderly patients with seizures require initial specialist assessment and should have access to continuing specialist services, in line with recommendations for younger people. The role of the multidisciplinary team including specialist epilepsy nurses, is central to managing this chronic condition and ensuring that it impacts as little as possible on the patient's life.

- Finally, there are many questions about the diagnosis and management of older people with epilepsy and the organization of services which remain unanswered. More targeted research is needed.

functioning. In the case of an illness such as epilepsy, where the physical manifestations are transient, the psychosocial consequences may, with time, come to be of greater concern." We know little or nothing about this in older people. What do they think about seizures? What misconceptions and/or fears do they have and how much do they contribute to inducing dependency and shrinking lifespace? What are their information needs? How should those needs be best met? A small start in trying to understand quality of life in older people has been made.[118]

When to use AEDs

Should one treat a single unprovoked tonic–clonic seizure in old age or wait for two or more seizures? The ongoing MESS study referred to earlier should help. What are the chances of recurrence where there is no overt cause? How easy are seizures to control in old age? More prospective studies are needed to answer these questions.

The role of the newer generation of AEDs

What is the place of monotherapy using the new generation of anticonvulsants in the de novo treatment of elderly onset seizures? Studies addressing these questions should focus not simply on the traditional endpoints such as seizure control. The importance of newer AEDs may lie more in reducing subtle adverse effects on gait and mobility than in improved seizure control, especially as "minor" effects of this sort may, in a frail elderly person, translate into significant dysfunction.

The organization of epilepsy services

How best should we provide a service for elderly people with seizures? What are the elements of an optimal overall comprehensive service? Who should provide it? How should we evaluate it? If we had answers to these questions our management of seizures in old age would be considerably better than it is now.

REFERENCES

1. Rowan AJ, Ramsay GR: Seizures and Epilepsy in The Elderly. Butterworth-Heinemann, Boston, 1997
2. Kramer G: Epilepsy in the Elderly: Clinical Aspects and Pharmacotherapy. Georg Thieme Verlag, Stuttgart, 1999
3. Godfrey JW, Roberts MA, Caird FI: Epileptic seizures in the elderly: 2. Diagnostic problems. Age Ageing 1982;11:29–34
4. Sander JWAS, Hart YM, Johnson AL, Shorvon SD: National General Practice Study of Epilepsy: newly diagnosed epileptic seizures in general population. Lancet 1990;336:1267–1270
5. Chadwick D: Epilepsy after first seizures: risks and implications. J Neurol Neurosurg Psychiatry 1991;54:385–387
6. Beghi E, Ciccione A: The First Seizure Trial Group: Recurrence after a first unprovoked seizure. Is it still a controversial issue? Seizure 1992;2:5–10
7. Craig I, Tallis RC: General practitioner knowledge and management of elderly-onset epilepsy. Care Elderly 1991;3:69–72
8. Hauser WA, Kurland LT: The epidemiology of epilepsy in Rochester, Minnesota, 1935 through 1967. Epilepsia 1975;16:1–66
9. Hauser WA et al: Prevalence of epilepsy in Rochester, Minnesota: 1940–1980. Epilepsia 1991;32:429–445
10. Hauser WA, Annegers JF, Kurland LT: Incidence of epilepsy and unprovoked seizures in Rochester, Minnesota: 1935–1984. Epilepsia 1993;34:453–468
11. Luhdorf K, Jensen LK, Plesner AM: Epilepsy in the elderly: incidence, social function, and disability. Epilepsia 1986;27:135–141
12. Tallis RC, Craig I, Hall G, Dean A: How common are epileptic seizures in old age? Age Ageing 1991;20:442–448
13. Wallace H, Shorvon S, Tallis RC: Age-specific incidence and prevalence rate of treated epilepsy in an unselected population of 2,052,922 and age-specific fertility rates of women with epilepsy. Lancet 1998;37;352:1970–1973
14. Loiseau J, Loiseau P, Duche B et al: A survey of epileptic disorders in Southwest France: seizures in elderly patients. Ann Neurol 1990;27:232–237
15. Hauser WA: Seizure disorders: the changes with age. Epilepsia 1992;33:S6–S14
16. de la Count A, Brezeler M, Meinardi H et al: A prevalence of epilepsy in the elderly: the Rotterdam study. Epilepsia 1996; 37:141–147
17. Cloyd JC, Lackner TE, Leppik IE: Antiepileptics in the elderly: Pharmacoepidemiology and pharmacokinetics. Arch Fam Med 1994;3:589–598
18. Commission on Classification and Terminology of the International League Against Epilepsy: Proposal for revised classification of epilepsies and epileptic syndromes. Epilepsia 1989;30:389–399
19. Jallon P, Loiseau P: Epileptic Seizures and Epilepsies in the Elderly. Sanofi Winthrop Scipp Vincennes, 1995
20. Luef G, Schauer R, Bauer G: Idiopathic generalised epilepsy of late onset: a new epileptic syndrome? Epilepsia 1996;37(suppl 4):4(abstract)
21. Hauser WA, Morris ML, Heston LL, Anderson VE: Seizures and myoclonus in patients with Alzheimer's disease. Neurology 1986;36:1226–1230
22. Luhdorf K, Jensen LK, Plesner A: Etiology of seizures in the elderly. Epilepsia 1986;27:458–463
23. Kilpatrick CJ, Davis SM, Tress BM et al: Epileptic seizures in acute stroke. Arch Neurol 1990;47:157–160
24. Burn JM, Dennis M, Bamford J, Sandercock P, Wade D, Warlow C: Epileptic seizures after a first stroke in the Oxford Community Stroke Project. Br Med J 1997;315:1582–1587
25. Lancman ME, Golimstok A, Norscini J, Granillo R: Risk factors for developing seizures after stroke. Epilepsia 1993;34:141–143
26. So EL, Annegers JF, Hauser WA et al: Population-based study of seizure disorders after cerebral infarction. Neurology 1996;46:350–355

27. Velioğlu SK, Özmenoğlu M, Boz C, Alioğlu Z: Status epilepticus after stroke. Stroke 2001;32:1169–1172

28. Shinton RA, Gill JS, Zezulk AV, Beevers DJ: The frequency of epilepsy preceding stroke. Lancet 1987;i:11–13

29. Ettinger AB: Structural causes of epilepsy. Tumor, cysts, stroke and vascular malformations. Neurol Clin 1994;12:41–57

30. Mcareavey BJ, Ballinger BR, Fenton GW: Epileptic seizures in elderly patients with dementia. Epilepsia 1992;33:657–660

31. Hesdorffer DC, Hauser WA, Annegers JF et al: Dementia and adult-onset unprovoked seizures. Neurology 1996;46:727–730

32. Jones SC, Bamford JM, Heath J, Heatley RV: Multiple forms of epileptic seizures secondary to a small chronic subdural haematoma. Br Med J 1989;299:439–441

33. Sung C-Y, Chu N-S: Epileptic seizures in elderly people: aetiology and seizure type. Age Ageing 1990;19:25–30

34. Heckmatt JA: Seizure induction by alcohol in patients with epilepsy. Experience in two hospitals. J R Soc Med 1990;83:6–9

35. Lechtenberg R, Worner TM: Total ethanol consumption as a seizure risk factor in alcoholics. Acta Neurol Scand 1992;85:90–94

36. Schackter SC: Iatrogenic seizures. Neurol Clin (N Am) 1998;16:157–170

37. Shorvon S, Tallis R, Wallace H: Antiepileptic drugs: co-prescription of proconvulsant drugs and oral contraceptives. A national study of antiepileptic drug prescribing practice. J Neurol Neurosurg Psychiatry 2002;72:114–115

38. Hankey GJ: Cerebrovascular disease: a clinical approach. Rev Clin Gerontol 1994;4:289–310

39. Overstall P: Drop attacks. In Kenny RA (ed): Syncope in the Older Patient. Causes, Investigations and Consequences of Syncope and Falls. Chapman & Hall, London, 1996

40. Hodges JR, Warlow CP: The aetiology of transient global amnesia: a case control study of 114 cases with prospective follow-up. Brain 1990;113:639–657

41. Betts T, Boden S: Diagnosis management and prognosis of a group of 128 patients with non-epileptic attach disorder. Part One. Seizure 1992;1:19–26

42. Kenny RA (ed): Syncope in the Older Patient. Causes, Investigations and Consequences of Syncope and Falls. Chapman & Hall, London, 1996

43. Lempert T, Bauser M, Schmidt D: Syncope: A videometric analysis of 56 episodes of transient cerebral hypoxia. Ann Neurol 1994;36:233–237

44. McIntosh S, DaCosta D, Kenny RA: Outcome of an integrated approach to the investigation of dizziness, falls and syncope in elderly patients referred to a "syncope" clinic. Age Ageing 1993;22:53–58

45. Schott GD, Macleod AA, Jewitt ED: Cardiac arrhythmias that masquerade as epilepsy. Br Med J 1977;i:1454–1457

46. Reeves AL, Nollet KE, Klass DW, Sharbrough FW: The ictal bradycardia syndrome. Epilepsia 1996;37(suppl 5):82(abstract)

47. Kogeorgos J, Scott DF, Swash M: Epileptic dizziness. Br Med J 1981;282:687–689

48. Blumer D: Epilepsy and disorders of mood. Adv Neurol 1991;55:185–195

49. Rowan AJ: Ictal amnesia and fugue states. Adv Neurol 1991;55:357–367

50. Ellis JM, Lee SI: Acute prolonged confusion in later life as an ictal state. Epilepsia 1978;19:119–128

51. Jamal GA, Fowler CJ, Leslie K et al: Non-convulsive status epilepticus as a cause of acute confusional state in the over-60 age group. J Neurol Neurosurg Psychiatry 1988;51:738

52. Thomas P: Epileptic confusional states in the elderly. Epilepsia 1996;37(suppl 4):36

53. Godfrey JW: Misleading presentation of epilepsy in elderly people. Age Ageing 1989;18:17–20

54. Norris JW, Hachinski VC: Mis-diagnosis of stroke. Lancet 1982;i:328–331

55. Fine W: Post hemiplegic epilepsy in the elderly. Br Med J 1967;1:199–201

56. Gifford DR, Vickrey BG: Neurologists vary in their test ordering and treatment decisions for a single, unprovoked seizure. Epilepsia 1995;36(suppl 4):95(abstract)

57. Ramirez-Lassepas M, Cipolle RJ, Morillo LR, Gumnit RJ: Value of computed tomography scan in the evaluation of adult patients after their first seizure. Ann Neurol 1984;15:436–443

58. Chadwick D: How far to investigate the elderly patient with epilepsy. In Tallis RC (ed): Epilepsy and the Elderly. Royal Society of Medicine Services, London, 1988:21–30

59. Kilpatrick CJ, Tress BM, O'Donnell C et al: Magnetic resonance imaging and late-onset epilepsy. Epilepsia 1991;32:358–364

60. Thomas RJ: Seizures and epilepsy in the elderly. Arch Intern Med 1997;157:605–617

61. Jacoby A, Baker GA: Quality of life in epilepsy beyond seizure counts in assessment and treatment. In Jacoby A, Baker GA (eds): The problems of Epilepsy. Harwood, Amsterdam, 2000

62. Driving and Vehicle Licensing Authority: At a Glance Guide to the Current Medical Standards of Fitness to Drive. March 2001

63. Shorvon S: Epilepsy and driving. Br Med J 1995;310:885–886

64. Chadwick D: Epilepsy after first seizures: risks and implications. J Neurol Neurosurg Psych 1991;54:385–387

65. Berg AT, Shinnar S: The risk of seizure recurrence following a first unprovoked seizure: A quantitative review. Neurology 1991;41:965–972

66. Sander JWAS, White SH: Disease modification in epilepsy. Prog Neurol Psychiatry, September 2001

67. Beghi E: First Seizure Trial Group. A randomised clinical trial of the efficacy and safety of the treatment of the first unprovoked epileptic seizure. Neuroepidemiology 1992;11:50–51

68. Medical Research Council: Multi-centre study of early epilepsy and single seizures (MESS)

69. Reynolds EH, Chadwick D: Controversies in treatment and management. Do anticonvulsants alter the natural course of epilepsy? Br Med J 1995;310:176–177

70. The Cochrane Library: Update Software, Oxford

71. NHS R&D Health Technology Assessment Programme: An RCT of longer-term clinical outcomes and cost-effectiveness of standard and new antiepileptic drugs. March 2000

72. Treiman DM: Efficacy and safety of antiepileptic drugs: a review of controlled trials. Epilepsia 1987;28(suppl 3):S1–S8

73. Marson AG, Williamson PR, Hutton JL, Clough ME, Chadwick DW: Carbamazepine versus valproate monotherapy for epilepsy (Cochrane review). In: The Cochrane Library, Issue 1, Update Software, Oxford, 2000

74. Tallis RC, Easter D, Craig I: Multicentre trial of sodium valproate and phenytoin in elderly patients with newly diagnosed epilepsy. Age Ageing 1994;23(suppl 2):5(abstract)

75. Appleton R, Baker G, Chadwick D, Smith D: Epilepsy, 3rd Ed. Martin Dunitz, London, 1993

76. Trimble MR: Anticonvulsant drugs and cognitive function: a review of the literature. Epilepsia 1987;28(suppl 3):S37–S45

77. Craig I, Tallis R: The impact of sodium valproate and phenytoin on cognitive function in elderly patients: results of a single-blind randomised comparative study. Epilepsia 1994;35:381–390

78. Meador KM, Loring DW, Huh K et al: Comparative cognitive effects of anticonvulsants. Neurology 1990;40:391–394

79. Gough H, Goggin T, Bissessar A et al: A comparative study of the relative influence of different anticonvulsants, UV exposure and diet on vitamin D and calcium metabolism in out-patients with epilepsy. Q J Med 1986;59:569–577

80. Lahr MB: Hyponatraemia during carbamazepine therapy. Clin Pharmacol Ther 1985;37:693–696

81. Houtkooper MA, Lammertsma A, Meyer JWA: Oxcarbazepine: a possible alternative to carbamazepine. Epilepsia 1987;28:693–698

82. Brodie MJ, Dichter MA. Established antiepileptic drugs. Seizure 1997;6:159–174

83. Kalviainen R, Nousiainen I, Mantyjarvi M et al: Vigabatrin, a gabaergic antiepileptic drug, causes concentric field defects. Neurology 1999;53:922–960

84. Richens A: Overview of the clinical efficacy of lamotrigine. Epilepsia 1991;32(suppl 2):S13–16

85. Brodie M, Overstall P, Giorgi L: The UK Lamotrigine Elderly Study Group. Multicentre, double blind, randomised comparison between lamotrigine and carbamazepine in elderly patients with newly diagnosed epilepsy. Epilepsy Res 1999;37:81–87

86. Lott RS, Helmboldt K: Oxcarbazepine. A carbamazepine analogue for partial seizures in adults and children with epilepsy. Formulary 2000;35:219–230

87. Dam M, Ekberh R, Loyninh Y et al: A double blind study comparing oxcarbazepine and carbamazepine in patients with newly diagnosed, previously untreated epilepsy. Epilepsy Res 1989;3:70–76

88. Van Amelsvoort T, Bakshi R, Devaux CB, Schwabe S: Hyponatraemia associated with carbamazepine and oxcarbazepine therapy: a review. Epilepsia 1994;35:181–188

89. Chadwick DW, Anhut H, Greuner MJ et al: A double blind trial of gabapentin monotherapy for newly diagnosed partial seizures. International Gabapentin Monotherapy Study Group 945–77. Neurology 1998;51:1282–1288

90. Marson AG, Chadwick DW: New drug treatment for epilepsy. J Neurol Neurosurg Psych 2001;70:143–148

91. Marson AG, Kadir ZA, Hutton JL, Chadwick DW: Gabapentin add-on for drug resistant partial epilepsy (Cochrane Review). In The Cochrane Library Issue 3, Update Software, Oxford, 2000

92. Jette NJ, Marson AG, Kadir ZA, Hutton JL: Topiramate add-on for drug resistant partial epilepsy (Cochrane Review). In: The Cochrane Library, Issue 1, Update Software, Oxford, 2001

93. Anking JC, Noble S: Tiagibine. A review of its pharmacodynamic and pharmacokinetic properties and therapeutic potential in the management of epilepsy Drugs 1998;55(3):437–460

94. Chadwick DW, Marson AG: Zonisamide add-on for drug resistant partial epilepsy (Cochrane Review). In The Cochrane Library, Issue 2, Update Software, Oxford, 2000

95. Dooley M, Plosker GI: Levetiracetam. A review of its adjunctive use in the management of partial onset seizures. Drugs 2000;60(4):871–930

96. Perucca E: The new generation of antiepileptic drugs: advantages and disadvantages. Br J Clin Pharm 1996;42:531–543

97. Marson AG, Kadir ZA, Chadwick DW: New antiepileptic drugs: a systematic review of their efficacy and tolerability. Br Med J 1996;313:1169–1174

98. Mawer G: Specific pharmacokinetic and pharmacodynamic problems of anticonvulsant drugs in the elderly. In Tallis RC (ed): Epilepsy and the Elderly. Royal Society of Medicine Services, London, 1988:21–30

99. Bauer LA, Blouin RA: Age and phenytoin kinetics in adult epileptics. Clin Pharmacol Ther 1982;31:301–304

100. British National Formulary: British Medical Association and the Royal Pharmaceutical Society of Great Britain, London, 19 June 2001

101. Rimmer EM, Richens A: Clinical pharmacology and medical treatment. In Laidlaw J, Richens A, Oxley J (eds): A Textbook of Epilepsy, 3rd Ed. Churchill Livingstone, Edinburgh, 1988

102. Chadwick DW: Overuse of monitoring of blood concentrations of anti-epileptic drugs. Br Med J 1987;294:723–724

103. Brodie MJ Hallworth MJ: Therapeutic monitoring of carbamazepine. Hosp Update 1987:57–63

104. Leading article: Sodium valproate. Lancet 1988;ii:1229–1231

105. Richens A: How valuable is therapeutic drug monitoring? Epidata Bull No. 8. British Epilepsy Association, London, 1996

106. Weintraub M: Compliance in the Elderly. Clinics in Geriatric Medicine. WB Saunders, Philadelphia, 1990

107. Cockerell OC, Johnson AL, Sander JWAS, Hart YM, Shorvon SD: Remission of epilepsy: results from the National General Practice Study of Epilepsy. Lancet 1995;346:140–144

108. Medical Research Council Antiepileptic Withdrawal Study Group: A randomised study of antiepileptic drug withdrawal in patients in remission of epilepsy. N Engl J Med 1991;337:1175–1180

109. Berg AT, Shinnar S: Relapse following discontinuation of antiepileptic drugs. Neurology 1994;44:601–608

110. Hauser WA, Annegers JF, Elveback LR: Mortality in patients with epilepsy. Epilepsia 1980;21:399–412

111. Luhdorf K, Jensen LK, Plessner AM: Epilepsy in the elderly: life expectancy and causes of death. Acta Neurol Scand 1987; 76:183–190

112. Geyer J, Kuzniecky R, Faught E: Admission and mortality rates for convulsive seizures in patients aged 65 years and older. Epilepsia 1995;36(suppl 4):148

113. Brown SW et al: An epilepsy needs document. Seizure 1993;2:91–103

114. Hartshorn JC: A nurse-managed clinic for individuals with epilepsy. Epilepsia 1995;36(suppl 4):99(abstract)

115. Bradley P, Lindsay B: Specialist epilepsy nurses for treating epilepsy (Cochrane Review). In The Cochrane Library Issue 1, Update Software, Oxford, 2001

116. Bradley P, Lindsay B: Epilepsy clinics versus general 'neurology or medical clinics' (Cochrane Review). In The Cochrane Library Issue 1, Update Software, Oxford, 2001

117. Jacoby A, Baker G, Smith D et al: Measuring the impact of epilepsy: the development of a novel scale. Epilepsy Res 1993;16:83–88

118. Baker GA, Jacoby A, Buck D, Brooks J, Potts P, Chadwick DW: The quality of life of older people with epilepsy: findings from a UK community study. Seizure 2001;10(2):92–99

APPENDIX 46-1

DRIVING AND EPILEPSY: UK REGULATIONS FOR ORDINARY LICENCE HOLDERS

- A patient may drive only if he or she is free of epileptic attacks during the year before the date when the licence is granted.
- If epileptic attacks occur only during sleep, the patient must have had a sleep-only pattern for 3 years or more.
- His or her driving must be unlikely to endanger the public where driving is compromised by drug treatment or associated neurological or neuropsychiatric disturbances.

SEIZURES
Single seizures

Single seizures are not regarded as epilepsy by the DVLA unless a continuing liability can be shown (usually by EEG or imaging). However, the DVLA usually prohibits driving for 12 months after a single seizure.

Provoked seizures

Provoked seizures are defined as seizures precipitated by exceptional nonrecurring circumstances in nonepileptic subjects. Driving is usually allowed once the provoking factor has been successfully treated or removed. The precipitating factor must be truly exceptional. Alcohol and illicit drugs do not qualify.

Mild seizures

Mild seizures are defined as, for example, myoclonic jerks and seizures not associated with loss of conciousness. These are treated the same as other attacks.

ATTACKS OCCURRING DURING CHANGES IN DRUG TREATMENT

Regulations apply to these attacks. Licence will be barred regardless of whether deliberate or accidental. Driving should be suspended during changes in drug treatment (advise not regulatory). When drugs are being totally withdrawn, driving should be suspended from the time withdrawal begins until 6 months after completion.

EEG CHANGES

Without overt seizures, these are not usually a bar to driving. The exception is unequivocal 3 Hz spike/wave in primary generalized seizures.

(From Shorvon S: Epilepsy and driving. Br Med J 1995; 310:885–886, with permission.)

Chapter 47

Headache and facial pain

Gerry J. F. Saldanha and Chris Clough

Wolff prefaced the first edition of his now famous *Handbook of Headache and Other Head Pain* with the pertinent observation that "Headache may be equally intense whether its implications are malignant or benign, and though there are few instances in human experience where so much pain may mean so little in terms of tissue injury, failure to separate the ominous from the trivial may cost life or create paralysing fear."

Few epidemiological studies have been carried out to estimate the size of the headache problem. In one year in the USA, 70 percent of the general population had a headache, 5 percent of whom sought medical attention.[1] Less is known about the frequency of headache in the elderly population, although in a large population-based study carried out in East Boston,[2] some 17 percent of patients over 65 years of age reported frequent headache, with 53 percent of women and 36 percent of men reporting headache in the previous year. Headache prevalence in the elderly age group ranged from 5 to 50 percent.[3,4] Overall, headache appears to be less frequently reported in the elderly population[5] and shows a decline with age.[2] Most studies agree that the prevalence of primary headache syndromes declines with increasing age.[6-9] One obvious limitation of these studies is that none is longitudinal and so may not differentiate an effect of aging from cohort or period effects. In addition, elderly patients may be less complaining, or the emergence of other more serious problems may have suppressed reporting of a benign symptom such as headache.

In elderly people headache is more likely to represent organic pathology.[10] A clinic-based retrospective case record study[11] concluded that, while it was less likely that elderly people would attend a hospital outpatients clinic for diagnosis of headache, there was a ten-fold increase in the likelihood of finding organic pathology. Recruitment bias is a problem in these studies. Nevertheless it is likely that headache is a more serious complaint from the elderly patient.

A large lifetime prevalence study[12] utilizing a population-based questionnaire found that, while migraine and tension-type headache appeared to decrease with increasing age, chronic tension headache has significantly higher prevalence rates in the elderly population.

The authors conclude that headache remains an extremely common condition of elderly people, much of it has benign origin, but more care needs to be taken with older patients to rule out underlying pathology especially when they present for the first time.

PRIMARY HEADACHE DISORDERS

Migraine

Migraine is an episodic disorder which is diagnosed from the history. Epidemiological studies are difficult to carry out and dogged by numerous problems.[13] There has been much controversy over whether migraine headache and tension headache are separate entities or different points on a continuum of headache disorder.[14] Only 5 percent of migraineurs consult specialists,[15] and so clinic-based studies will suffer from referral bias. Despite this limitation, a number of population-based studies has been carried out.[9,15-24] Criteria for the diagnosis of migraine have been developed by the International Headache Society[25] and there has been evaluation of these criteria.[26]

Rasmussen et al.[23] did not find a decrease in migraine prevalence with increasing age, in contrast to the findings of Stewart et al.[21] who also showed that it is uncommon for migraine to start in a person's later years.[9] The female preponderance of migraineurs persists in this age group.[15]

Symptoms and diagnosis of migraine

Migraine is classified into two main forms, migraine with aura (formerly "classical migraine") and migraine without aura (formerly "common migraine"), based on criteria of the International Headache Society.[25] Other varieties of migraine include ophthalmoplegic, retinal, basilar, and familial hemiplegic, complications of migraine such as migrainous infarction (a neurological deficit not reversible in 7 days), and status migrainosis (an attack of headache or aura lasting more than 72 hours). Migraine aura can exist without headache, and the same patient may at different times experience headache with aura, headache without aura, or aura without headache.[27,28]

To diagnose migraine without aura, five attacks are needed, each lasting 4–72 hours and having two of the following four characteristics: unilateral location, pulsating quality, moderate or severe intensity, and aggravation by routine physical activity. In addition, the attacks must have at least one of the following: nausea and/or vomiting and/or photophobia and phonophobia.

Migraine with aura is diagnosed when there have been at least two attacks with any three of the following features:

- one or more fully reversible aura symptoms;
- aura developing over more than four minutes;
- aura lasting less than 60 minutes;
- headache following aura with a free interval of less than 60 minutes.

A simpler working definition for the clinical diagnosis of migraine was proposed by Solomon and Lipton.[29] A positive diagnosis could be made on any two of the following four symptoms:

- unilateral headache;
- pulsating quality;
- nausea;
- photophobia and phonophobia.

A similar headache must have occurred in the past and structural disease excluded.

Migraine attacks may generally be divided into five phases: the prodrome (hours or days before the headache); the aura (migraine with aura); the headache; the headache termination; and the postdrome phase.[30] Symptoms of the prodrome may include mental, neurological and/or general (constitutional, autonomic) symptoms. The patients may experience depression, euphoria, irritability, restlessness, mental slowness, hyperactivity, and drowsiness. General symptoms may include a feeling of coldness, sluggishness, thirst, anorexia, diarrhea, constipation, fluid retention, and food cravings. Photophobia and phonophobia may also occur.

The aura is a group of neurological symptoms that precedes or accompanies the attack. They may be visual, sensory, or motor and may also cause language or brainstem disturbance. Headache usually occurs within 60 minutes of the end of the aura,[25] but may begin with the aura. Most patients may have more than one type of aura and progress from one type to another in subsequent attacks. Common visual symptoms are the positive phenomena such as hemianopic photopsia (flashes of light) and teichopsia or fortification spectra. Scotomota may follow. Complex visual distortions and hallucinations are reported but are more common in younger people.[27] Somatosensory phenomena, typically paresthesiae with anatomical march of symptoms, may occur and motor disturbance may result in hemiparesis. Aphasia has also been reported.[7,31]

Acephalgic migraine is an entity characterized by the neurological dysfunction of the aura but without headache. This is strictly a diagnosis of exclusion especially in elderly people. These so-called migraine accompaniments may occur for the first time in the older age group,[32] and can be easily confused with transient ischemic attacks (TIAs) except in the most classic of cases. Migraine with aura and acephalgic migraine can both be confused with TIAs, and vice versa. Headache occurred with 36 percent of TIAs in one series[33] and is more common in vertebrobasilar ischemia.[34,35] Migrainous aura in the elderly person presents a particularly difficult diagnostic dilemma. Transient hemiparetic or hemisensory symptoms occurring in elderly people for the first time should be assumed to be vascular (i.e. TIA) in etiology until proved otherwise. Alternating hemisensory/paretic symptoms are more likely to be migrainous but still could have an embolic cause. Investigation including carotid Doppler studies and echocardiography will be necessary to manage potentially treatable embolic sources. Visual disturbance is more likely to be helpful as fortification spectra and colored zigzag lines are unlikely to occur in straightforward TIAs and are almost always migrainous in origin. Migraine with aura can occur for the first time in the elderly person and may reflect the development of vascular change. It is often helpful in these cases to elicit a previous history of common migraine earlier in life.

The headache of migraine is typically throbbing in nature and exacerbated by exercise.[36] The pain may be unilateral in 60 percent of cases but bilateral at the outset in up to 40 percent.[7] Unilateral headache may later become bilateral during the attack. The intensity is moderate to severe and pain may radiate down the neck to the shoulder. Some 40 percent of migraineurs report short-lived jabs of pain lasting seconds and having a "needle"-like quality, the so called "ice-pick" pains.[37]

The common accompanying symptoms of nausea and vomiting may make it difficult for the patient to take oral medication. There is usually photophobia and phonophobia; many patients retire to a dark and quiet room for rest. Constitutional, mood, and mental changes are universal,[7] and the patient is usually left feeling lethargic for a period after the attack.

Basilar migraine is a variant characterized by brainstem dysfunction such as ataxia, dysarthria, diplopia, vertigo, nausea and vomiting, and alteration in cognition and consciousness. Headache is invariable. In the elderly person these symptoms should be assumed to be of vascular origin until proven otherwise.

Ophthalmoplegic migraine is rare and can be confused with the presentation of Berry aneurysm. Attacks of migraine-like pain occur around the eye with oculomotor nerve dysfunction and dilation of the pupil. The ophthalmoplegia may last from hours to months. The differential diagnosis includes orbital inflammatory disease and diabetic mononeuropathy.

Migraine attacks may vary in frequency from a few a year to several a week. Trigger factors include certain foods, red wine,[38] hormone replacement treatment in post-menopausal women,[39] irregular meals, and a change in sleep habit.[40] Environmental triggers include flickering lights, noise, and even certain types of weather. Head injury and stress may lead to migraine attacks.

Treatment of migraine

Once the diagnosis has been established, reassuring the patient may suffice. Any obvious precipitating cause such as diet, lack of sleep, or environmental factors should be discussed. Relaxation therapy may be helpful but special diets have little place in management.

Pharmacotherapy includes treatment of the acute attack and consideration of prophylactic therapy. Acute treatment should be started by the patient at the outset of an attack, and is best limited to simple soluble analgesics such as paracetamol or aspirin (Table 47-1). Combination analgesics such as co-proxamol should be avoided, if possible, because of side-effects and risk of addiction. For a more severe headache, nonsteroidal anti-inflammatory drugs are used.[41] Ibuprofen (200 mg t.d.s.) may be obtained in the UK without prescription, or naproxen (250 mg t.d.s.) by prescription, or diclofenac (75 mg twice-daily). This group of drugs should be administered with caution in the elderly population because of the increased risk

Table 47-1 Drugs of use in the treatment of migraine[a]

Migraine attack treatments	Migraine prophylaxsis
Soluble aspirin	Propranolol
Soluble paracetamol	Pizotifen
Antiemetics such as domperidone suppositories	Calcium antagonists
Nonsteroidal anti-inflammatory drugs	Methysergide
Sumatriptan (subcutaneous or oral)	Sodium valproate
Medihaler ergotamine and other ergotamine preparations	
Combination analgesia	

[a] Care must be taken with possible interactions with pre-existent treatments and conditions such as asthma (if β-blockers are to be prescribed). The table lists medication in order of preference.

of gastrointestinal hemorrhage, especially when there is a past history of peptic ulceration[42,43] or renal insufficiency.

For moderate to severe migraine not responding to simple analgesia, sumatriptan can be tried. The initial dose is 50 mg orally and can be increased to 100 mg if there is no response. Subcutaneous self-administration is the preferred route when there is significant nausea or vomiting. Sumatriptan is a $5HT_1$ agonist and is thought to act as a selective cerebral vasoconstrictor. Up to 80 percent of patients obtain relief from headache within 2 hours after an injection[44] and up to 65 percent after a tablet dose.[45] The advantage is that the drug may be administered at any point during an attack and repeated if necessary. Flushing, tingling in the neck and head, and chest tightness can occur in up to 5 percent of patients.[46] Since sumatriptan may cause coronary vasoconstriction, it is contraindicated in patients with ischemic heart disease or uncontrolled hypertension. Special care in the elderly person is required because the loss of subcutaneous fat may lead to intramuscular injection and more rapid absorption. Pharmacotherapy should be combined with rest and sleep. A number of newer triptans have been licensed for use in migraine treatment and may be selected for the individual patient.[47]

Ergotamine preparations are best reserved for occasional (>1 month interval) severe headaches. They are potent vasoconstrictors and are best avoided in patients with a history of vaso-occlusive disease, peripheral vascular disease, or hypertension, and those receiving β-blockers or with a history of Raynaud's phenomenon. Patients should be strongly encouraged to avoid overuse of these drugs, because this can lead to resistant medication-misuse headache. Admission for drug withdrawal may be required when this occurs.

The accompanying symptoms of nausea and vomiting are often as disabling as the headache and require treatment in their own right. Metoclopramide is the most commonly used antiemetic; and by promoting gastric emptying it aids absorption of coadministered medication. It can cause extrapyramidal side-effects, especially in the elderly person. Domperidone is less likely to cause this problem as it does not cross the blood–brain barrier but does not aid gastric emptying.

Prophylactic therapy is indicated when there is severe recurrent headache causing disruption to daily life—as a guide, more than two severe headaches per month. Various drugs are used including β-blockers, antidepressants, serotonin antagonists, calcium-channel blockers, and occasionally anticonvulsants. Treatment is started at a low dose and built to maintenance. Possible side-effects should be discussed and the regimen kept as simple as possible as many patients in this age group are likely to have coexistent medication. Patients should be weaned from therapy every 4–6 months.

Of the β-blockers, propranolol, metoprolol, and atenolol have all been shown to be effective in up to 60–80 percent of patients producing a greater than 50 percent reduction in attack frequency.[48,49] Atenolol (50–100 mg daily) has a better side-effect profile than propranolol (20–160 mg daily). Patients may complain of fatigue, dizziness, nightmares, and cold extremities. Care should be taken when there is peripheral vascular disease, and in combination with ergotamine.

The tricyclic antidepressants have been used in migraine prophylaxis, although the evidence for their efficacy is largely based on anecdotal reports or uncontrolled trials. Their effect in headache may be independent of their antidepressant effect.[48,50] Amitriptyline is most commonly used, although fluoxetine has fewer anticholinergic side-effects and causes less weight gain.[51] Paroxetine may be a suitable alternative where anxiety is a factor.[52] Because of their common side-effect of drowsiness, the tricyclics are administered at the lowest effective dose at bedtime and slowly increased as necessary. Elderly people are more vulnerable to the muscarinic side-effects. The typical starting dose for amitriptyline should be 10 mg, increasing to 150 mg if needed.

Sodium valproate (0.6–2.5 g daily) is well tolerated and there is clinical trial evidence of efficacy.[53] There is no current evidence to support the use of other antiepileptics.

Calcium-channel antagonists are not licensed for migraine prophylaxis in the UK but have been shown to be of benefit.[48] The mechanism of action of these compounds in migraine is uncertain and side-effects are common, including edema, flushing, dizziness, and not infrequently an initial increase in headache frequency. Improvement of headache may require several weeks of treatment.[54]

Of the serotonin antagonists, the two mostly commonly prescribed are pizotifen and methysergide. Pizotifen is a $5HT_2$ antagonist that is usually commenced in a dose of 0.5 mg at night and increased in stepwise manner to a dose of 4.5 mg. It has mild antidepressant activity but unfortunately stimulates appetite and leads to weight gain if diet is not controlled. It can produce beneficial effects in 40–79 percent of patients.[55] Methysergide is also a $5HT_2$ antagonist with some affinity for the $5HT_1$ receptor. It is effective prophylaxis in up to 60 percent of migraineurs, possibly with better results in those with migraine with aura.[56] Side-effects are common and include myalgia, weight gain, nausea, and hallucinations (especially after the first dose). The complication of retroperitoneal, endocardial, and pulmonary fibrosis is rare and prevented by stopping treatment for 3–4 weeks every 4–6 months. The starting dose is 1 mg at night but may be increased to 6 mg daily in divided dosage.

Feverfew (*Tenacetum parthenium*) is a herbal remedy long used for headache treatment. It has limited effect and the side-effects include mouth ulceration and loss of taste.[57,58]

Tension headache

Definition

The Classification Committee of the International Headache Society (IHS) in 1988 defined episodic tension headache as recurrent headaches lasting for 30 minutes to 7 days with fewer than 15 headache days per month and at least two of the following pain characteristics:

- pressing/tightening (non-pulsating) quality;
- mild or moderate intensity;
- bilateral location;
- no aggravation on walking up or down stairs or similar routine physical activity.

There should *not* be photophobia and phonophobia, although either alone is permitted within the definition. Patients should *not* experience nausea or vomiting (although the IHS criteria allow for nausea but not vomiting in the diagnosis of chronic tension-type headache).

Symptoms and diagnosis of tension headache

Chronic tension headache has the same pain characteristics as the episodic form but with a frequency of more than 15 headache days per month for more than 6 months. In both types of headache there may be pericranial muscle tenderness with or without increased electromyographic activity, although this does not assume that muscle tension is the cause of the headache.[59] In all age groups, tension-type headache is the most common form. However, only 5 percent of patients with chronic tension-type headache report onset after the age of 60 years.[60] Within all age groups, tension headache remains most common in females.[23]

The pain of tension-type headache is usually described as a constant ache which is infrequently pulsatile. Patients may describe a tight band about the head or a sensation of wearing a tight cap. There may be associated stiffness of the neck and upper back; in contrast to migraine, the pain is usually of lesser intensity. Scalp tenderness may lead to avoidance of hair brushing. This symptom is also recorded in migraineurs and it may persist for some days after the headache has subsided.[61]

The headache may be unilateral or bilateral, commonly occipital or frontal, but may involve any site. It can be relieved by changing position.

Patients with episodic tension headache may experience pericranial muscle tenderness with palpable nodules.[62] Depression, anxiety, and other psychological factors are important in the pathogenesis of tension headache, though not infrequently patients may initially deny any role.

Depression is common in the community at large, and in an average family practice in the UK is the fourth most commonly diagnosed disorder.[63] The headache associated with depression can have features described for tension-type headache, and the headaches are often present for years or even throughout the patient's life. The headache is typically diurnal, usually worse in the morning and in the evening. There may be identifiable emotional, physical, and psychic complaints. These problems merit attention in their own right, especially in the elderly person when organic pathology is more likely anyway. The presence of severe depression in elderly people may be easily overlooked. Other headache associated with depression can be described more bizarrely with almost a delusional tone. Such headaches may indicate a serious psychiatric disorder and should lead to urgent psychiatric referral.

Treatment of tension headache

Treatment includes reassurance, simple analgesia as abortive treatment for the acute attack, and treatment of any psychopathology that may be present. Paracetamol is the drug of choice and amitryptyline may be added as appropriate. The latter is especially useful when sleep disturbance is a prominent symptom. Fluoxitene (20 mg daily) is less sedating. Paroxetine (10 mg daily) may be helpful where there are additional anxiety symptoms. Monoamine oxidase inhibitors should be avoided if possible. Psychiatric help may be appropriate, although often initially rejected by patients. Relaxation therapy and biofeedback may also have a role.

The mixed headache syndrome—migraine and tension-type headache in the same patient—usually responds to treatment with tricyclic antidepressants with the addition of analgesia for acute episodes.

Chronic daily headache

The syndrome of chronic daily headache (CDH) accounts for 40 percent of patients seen in headache clinics.[64] The prevalence is 20 percent in the West, rising to 27 percent in those over 65 years.[65] Only 5 percent reported their headache as starting after 60 years of age.[60]

There are several subtypes of CDH (Table 47-2). The features of tension-type headache are discussed above. Analgesic overuse should be stopped with an appropriate explanation; the cycle of continuous headache may be broken with the use of sumatriptan and NSAIDs.[66] Once the cycle has been broken, prophylactic treatment may be required. Amitriptyline in an initial dose of 10 mg at night increased to 75 mg as tolerated is effective, with improvement seen at 2–14 days. The drug should be continued at an effective dose for 6 months and then withdrawn slowly over 3 months. Caution should be exercised in those with glaucoma and prostatism. Drugs commonly used in migraine prophylaxis may be effective, and sodium valproate has been used with favourable results.[67]

Episodic migraine may evolve into CDH. In one study, 489 of 630 patients (78 percent) with CDH had a clear preceding history of episodic migraine.[68] This so-called "transformed migraine" may be caused by excessive use of opioid and simple analgesics, barbiturates, ergot compounds, and caffeine, but not NSAIDS. Headaches are often more severe on waking owing to a drug-free withdrawal period overnight effectively causing rebound.

The differential diagnosis includes cervicogenic headache, temporal arteritis, mass lesions, and visual acuity problems. Since tension-type headache is often associated with depression, sleep disorder, and situational life events, especially in the elderly population, the treatment of CDH must include behavioral, psychological, and social aspects.

Cluster headache

This condition, although most common in young adults, may have its onset in the seventh decade.[69,70] The International Headache Society classification divides the condition into episodic and chronic cluster headache, the latter being more common in the elderly population.[71] The overall prevalence is 70 per 100,000 population, with a higher male preponderance in the young but more females over 60 years affected than males.[72]

Cluster headache is characterized by bouts of severe pain often described as "boring." The pain is constant, and patients walk around trying to find relief—in contrast to those with migraine who lie quietly. The pain is often centered on one eye and there may be ipsilateral watering of the eye with nasal stuffiness and a runny discharge. There is usually conjunctival

---

Table 47-2 Chronic daily headache subtypes

Chronic tension-type headache
Transformed migraine
    Drug-induced
    Nondrug-related
New daily persistent headache
Post-traumatic headache

injection and there may be an associated ptosis and miosis. The pain may spread to the whole side of the face. Bouts of pain occur 1–3 times per day with alarm-clock regularity, commonly an hour or so after going to sleep, and last from 15 minutes to a few hours. The cluster period typically lasts for 1–2 months and then subsides. During the cluster attacks alcohol is a potent precipitant, as are vasodilator drugs such as nitrates. The chronic form continues without remission often for many years.

Treatment is symptomatic. Oxygen at 100 percent is useful in the casualty department and can be given at home. More practically, sumatriptan by subcutaneous injection is the drug of choice for acute attacks.[73] Steroids (prednisolone 40 mg daily for a week and reducing by 10 mg a week) may abbreviate cluster attacks. No one thing works for everybody. Verapamil is superior to placebo[74] and compares favorably with lithium,[75] particularly in view of the plethora of potential neuropsychiatric side-effects of the latter. Sodium valproate may be tried in resistant cases.[76] Lithium carbonate given in standard psychiatric doses and monitored accordingly is useful in chronic cluster.

Rarely surgical intervention is attempted. Percutaneous radiofrequency trigeminal gangliorhizolysis or posterior fossa trigeminal sensory rhizolysis have been performed but are of unproven benefit. Operation can cause a reduction in facial sensation and corneal hypoesthesia with increased risk of corneal ulceration.[77]

Cluster headache is an underdiagnosed cause of recurrent paroxysmal cranial pain in the elderly population. It may not have the usual classical features in this age group. Treatment may need to be given empirically when there is doubt.

Chronic paroxysmal hemicrania (Sjaastad headache), a rare variant of cluster headache, differs in the brevity (3–45 minutes) and frequency (up to 40 times a day) of the attacks. The invariable response to indomethacin now forms part of the diagnostic criteria.[78]

FACIAL NEURALGIAS
Trigeminal neuralgia
Diagnosis

Trigeminal neuralgia is diagnosed clinically. It rarely begins before the age of 30 years.[79,80] The symptoms are pathognomonic. The pain is periodic, of high intensity and lancinating, lasting from 20–30 seconds followed by a period of relief lasting a few seconds to a minute and which may be followed by further paroxysms of pain. The pain usually commences in the maxillary and mandibular divisions of the trigeminal nerve and in fewer than 5 percent of cases begins in the ophthalmic division. In some 10–15 percent of cases all the divisions are involved and the symptoms may be bilateral in 3–5 percent.[81] Apart from the quality and characteristic site of pain, the patient can usually identify trigger factors such as brushing the teeth, washing the face, shaving, biting, chewing, or even a gust of cold wind on the face. Avoidance behavior is common. Slightly more females than males are affected and the prevalence is estimated to be 155 per million population.[82]

The pain may occur daily for weeks or months followed by remission of varying periods. Unfortunately there is a tendency for the disorder to deteriorate, with increased frequency of attacks increasingly resistant to treatment. Clinical examination should be normal, and any loss of facial sensation prompt investigation, preferably MRI of the brain, to rule out a compressive lesion of the trigeminal nerve.

Etiology

The etiology of trigeminal neuralgia is unexplained. The presence of chronic irritation of the roots of the trigeminal nerve has been demonstrated to cause neuralgia. This may also arise with more peripheral lesions. Animal laboratory data, however, are more consistent with a central mechanism mediated by the loss of segmental inhibition within the spinal trigeminal sensory nucleus. To reconcile these observations, Fromm et al.[83] proposed that spontaneous peripheral activity from the irritated nerve, in the presence of the failure of the normal central inhibitory mechanisms, may cause paroxysmal bursts of neuronal activity within the trigeminal nucleus and its thalamic relays, perceived as neuralgia by the patient. This has been likened to a form of "sensory reflex epilepsy".[84] Some evidence for the peripheral component of this hypothesis comes from the common finding of vascular loops in association with the nerve root in a majority of symptomatic patients.[85] Since vessels tend to become more ectatic with age, this may explain why the condition is more common in the elderly population.

Treatment

The treatment of this condition is firstly medical.[86–88] Occasionally the symptoms are so severe that hospital admission is required to control symptoms and prevent a downward spiral of increasing pain and depression.

The drugs of choice are anticonvulsants and it is usual to begin with carbamazepine; pain relief is usually obtained within 4–24 hours. Carbamazepine is commenced at 100 mg three times daily and increased every 48 hours in a stepwise manner until symptom relief or side-effects occur. Patients should be warned of the potential for drowsiness, rash, and unsteadiness. A baseline full blood count is recommended since leukopenia does occur commonly and agranulocytosis rarely; treatment should be stopped immediately if the latter occurs. Although carbamazepine is usually effective at blood levels of 25–50 mg/L, the dose can be titrated to the maximum tolerated in resistant cases. Therapy should be maintained until the patient has been free of pain for at least 4 weeks, after which slow reduction of dose by decrements of 100 mg of carbamazepine each week may allow for complete withdrawal of the drug.

If adequate pain relief is not obtained with standard doses of carbamazepine, a second drug such as baclofen (10 mg t.d.s. up to 1.03 mg/kg daily) can be administered. This may aggravate drowsiness. Alternatively phenytoin, clonazepam, or sodium valproate can be added. Polypharmacy should be avoided if possible because of additional side-effects and problems with compliance.

Surgical intervention should be considered if medical treatment fails. Up to 50 percent of patients may eventually require some form of surgical treatment. There are two main options, rhizotomy or microvascular decompression.

Radiofrequency rhizotomy or alternatively glycerol rhizolysis is relatively safe and simple. Patients require only light anesthesia and the procedure is carried out under radiographic screening control. Selective root lesioning is achieved if a stimulating electrode is employed, and this reduces the side-effects (see below). Acute pain relief can be accomplished in over 90 percent of patients, and this can be maintained in the long term with repeated treatments if necessary.[89] Glycerol injection into Meckel's cave acts as a neurotoxin.

The main side-effect is sensory loss (usually less with glycerol injection). Corneal hypoesthesia is a problem and may result in ulceration. Rarely there may be masseter weakness. Both forms of treatment have about 90 percent success and the patient can be discharged home within 24 hours. Unfortunately the reported recurrence rates are about 25 percent. In a study comparing glycerol rhizolysis and posterior fossa exploration, freedom from pain at 5 years was 59 and 68 percent, respectively.[90]

Microvascular decompression involves major neurosurgery with a posterior fossa approach. This procedure was pioneered by Janetta.[91] If a blood vessel is found in close association with the trigeminal root or deforming it, it is mobilized and a small sponge of polyvinyl chloride interposed between the nerve and the vessel. In elderly people this is a procedure of last resort because of a 1 percent mortality rate, additional morbidity, and the length of hospital stay.

Glossopharyngeal neuralgia

This syndrome has the same symptom characteristics as trigeminal neuralgia but the pain is felt in the region of the tonsil and ear. Trigger factors include swallowing, coughing, and talking, and the distribution of the pain is in the sensory territory of the glossopharyngeal nerve and the auricular and pharyngeal branches of the vagus nerve. Rarely the patient may become unconscious during an attack due to asystole.[92] Neurological examination is normal unless the syndrome is secondary to pathology such as neoplasm, infection, or inflammatory disease.

Treatment is the same as for trigeminal neuralgia with carbamazepine and other drugs. If there is no improvement, microvascular dissection of the intracranial section of the glossopharyngeal nerve and upper two rootlets of the vagus can be undertaken.

Post-herpetic neuralgia

Post-herpetic neuralgia occurs following 10 percent of attacks of shingles, but this figure rises to 50 percent in the over-60 age group.[93] The most common site is the ophthalmic division of the trigeminal nerve. The virus has a predilection for the trigeminal (23 percent of cases[94]) and upper cervical ganglia, and in the acute stages the herpetic eruption is seen in the appropriate distribution. The Ramsay Hunt syndrome is due to herpetic infection of the facial nerve. Excruciating pain may precede the eruption of vesicles by 1–3 days. The latter are seen over the external auditory meatus and mastoid process and may occur with edema and redness of the ear, making examination difficult. Occasionally other cranial nerves may be affected with involvement of the trigeminal nerve, leading to loss of sensation on the face and numbness of the palate occurring when the 9th nerve is affected. A careful search for vesicles around the ear and in the mouth will make the diagnosis clear. There may also be involvement of the 4th, 6th, and oculomotor nerves,[95] with the possibility of long-term paralysis.

The syndrome of post-herpetic neuralgia is characterized by a constant burning or aching pain with occasional stabbing components and occurs following healing of the rash. It may take several weeks or months to emerge. There is sensory loss over the affected area and invariably allodynia develops.

Treatment is symptomatic. In a recent review, acyclovir was shown to provide marginal evidence for reduction of pain incidence at 1–3 months following zoster onset. Famciclovir reduced the duration of the neuralgia but not its incidence, as did valacyclovir. Steroids had no effect on post-herpetic neuralgia.[96] Amitriptyline taken at the onset may reduce the incidence of post-herpetic neuralgia but more trials need to be undertaken.[96] Acyclovir (800 mg five times daily) may be prescribed if the rash is extensive or if there is a threat to eyesight. Opiate analgesia may be required. Once neuralgia is established, amitriptyline is of proven benefit[97,98] and carbamazepine may help to control the stabbing component of the pain. Relief of pain may be gained in up to 80 percent of cases. Nortriptyline and desimipramine may be better tolerated, causing less sedation; the former has been shown to be as effective as amitriptyline.[99] Transcutaneous electrical nerve stimulation (TENS) may sometimes be useful. Topical capsaisin cream has had variable success.[100,101] The drug gabapentin has been licensed for use in the USA following positive data in post-herpetic neuralgia.[102] The condition is notoriously difficult to treat and presently there is no role for surgery.

ATYPICAL FACIAL PAIN

This syndrome is rare in the elderly population. It is characterized by a continuous, chronic head or facial pain that does not follow dermatomal boundaries nor conform to any of the known patterns of headache or cranial neuralgia. The diagnosis can be made only after the exclusion of organic pathology, including dental and sinus disease. Many patients are believed to be depressed[33] and receive tricyclic antidepressants, generally with a good result. Lance[81] has proposed an organic basis to this syndrome. However, tricyclics remain the treatment of choice together with the judicious use of baclofen. Occasionally the pain may have a throbbing vascular nature, and when intermittent it is worth considering a diagnosis of facial or "lower half" migraine. In this case a trial of a β-blocker or sumatriptan may be useful.

HEADACHE ARISING FROM THE NECK

Cervical spondylosis, affecting the neck vertebrae, has a strong association with age.[103] Degenerative changes lead to a loss of intervertebral height with narrowing of the central canal and the intervertebral foramina. Spondylotic changes may compress cervical nerves and/or spinal cord. Symptomatic cervical spondylosis is more common in men than women and produces symptoms typically in the fifth and sixth decades. Neck pain and headache may result; and although most of the population over the age of 40 years has radiological changes consistent with cervical spondylosis without symptoms, in those with symptomatic disease (brachalgia or myelopathy) 40 percent reported headache as a chief symptom and

25 percent reported it as a major symptom.[104] Overall cervical spondylosis is an uncommon cause of headache.

The head pain resulting from cervical degenerative disease is frequently occipital in distribution but may radiate to the vertex or even the frontal area. The greater occipital nerve (C2) provides much of the sensory input from the back of the head, and irritation of this nerve typically causes occipital headache. The pain is usually described as constant, not throbbing, and of moderate intensity. Associated muscle tenderness, perhaps secondary to spasm, may be present and this may make differentiation from tension headache difficult. It is disputed whether the cervical spine itself gives rise to headache per se, but headache may arise as a secondary phenomenon due to muscle spasm in the neck.[103] Movements of the cervical spine may aggravate the headache, and examination will reveal reduced range of movement and suboccipital tenderness with muscle spasm.

Treatment is usually conservative with nonsteroidal drugs or simple analgesics. Cervical collars are of uncertain worth and anyway should be combined with referral to a physiotherapist for neck exercises. Surgery is considered when there is myelopathy or radiculopathy, especially when it is progressive.

Lesions of the bones of the upper cervical spine and base of skull can give rise to occipital ache by pressure on the cervical nerves. Myeloma, osteomyelitis, metastatic tumor, and erosive inflammatory disease such as rheumatoid arthritis may all cause headache and neurological deficit. Paget's disease can cause basilar invagination with traction on the upper cervical nerves and or hydrocephalus, both of which may result in headache.[104] A plain skull X-ray will usually rule out these possibilities if suspected.

SINUS DISEASE AND DENTAL DISEASE

Head and facial pain may be referred from the cranial sinuses. Experiments have shown that inflammation of the sinus lining is rarely painful, but that pain arises from inflammation of the ducts and ostia of the sinuses or inflammation of the nasal turbinates.[105] Disease of the frontal sinuses causes ache localized over these sinuses; that of the antrum is usually referred to the maxillary region and into the zygomatic or temporal areas. Headache associated with sphenoidal and ethmoidal disease is mainly felt behind the eyes and over the vertex of the skull.

The pain of sinus disease is usually deep-seated and dull, aching, and nonpulsatile. Adopting a recumbent position may relieve the headache of sinus disease, so these headaches are less prominent at night than during the day. Pain may be exacerbated by shaking the head or adopting a head-down position. Coughing or straining also exacerbates the pain by raising intracranial venous pressure.

The treatment of sinusitis is symptomatic with decongestants and analgesia, but unremitting pain may indicate a more sinister cause and merits further investigation.

Dental disease is referred to the distribution of the trigeminal nerve. In general, upper jaw disease is referred to the maxillary division and lower jaw disease to the mandibular division. The etiology of such pain is usually obvious, but continued facial pain may merit referral to a maxillofacial surgeon. Examination of the patient with facial pain includes assessment of the teeth and a search for tooth sensitivity with percussion.

VASCULAR DISORDERS AND HEADACHE

Giant cell arteritis

(See also Chapter 72)

This condition is rare below the age of 50 years, with incidence rising 10-fold between the sixth and ninth decades. The female to male ratio is approximately 4:1 and the prevalence varies from 7 per 100,000 in 50-year-olds to 70 per 100,000 in octogenarians.[106] Headache is the most common symptom (85 percent at some point in the disease). It is usually a severe, *persistent* ache and may have an additional throbbing component. Many patients also report an additional burning quality to the headache. The pain is usually bitemporal but may be unilateral, frontal, or generalized. Scalp tenderness is a common symptom and patients may avoid grooming the hair. The rare symptom of jaw claudication (facial pain when chewing) is virtually pathognomonic of this condition. Infarction of the tongue can follow this symptom. Although primarily a condition pathologically affecting the extracranial arteries, any vascular bed may be involved. Thus a plethora of symptoms can occur and there is an association with polymyalgia rheumatica. Patients may report a number of constitutional symptoms such as fatigue and malaise, lethargy, anorexia, and a low-grade fever. Weight loss and sweating are common.

Transient ischemic attacks can occur and sudden visual loss may affect up to 7 percent of cases.[107] This is a result of ischemia of the posterior ciliary arteries and secondary ischemic optic neuropathy, or infarction of the choroid.

The affected vessels become nodular, tortuous, and swollen. The superficial temporal artery may become palpable, tender, and pulseless. There is medial necrosis with formation of granulomatous tissue and invasion of lymphocytes and giant cells. Often there is thrombosis of the lumen.

Unfortunately the pathology is not continuous and "skip lesions" mean that there is a good chance that a temporal artery biopsy will be negative. The sedimentation rate is a vital diagnostic test but can be normal in up to 10 percent of cases.[108] One study found an ESR of less than 30 in 22.5 percent of cases.[109] Nonspecific abnormalities include a mild normochromic normocytic anemia, and leucocytosis. Plasma fibrinogen levels are elevated, as are other acute-phase proteins. Liver function tests are often abnormal, with an elevated alkaline phosphatase and elevated transaminases. An elevated creatine phosphokinase does not occur and should lead to a search for an alternative diagnosis.

If clinical suspicion is high the patient should be commenced on high-dose corticosteroids immediately since failure to act may cost the patient loss of vision. Prednisolone (60–80 mg) is given usually with rapid clinical effect. Failure of the symptoms to respond within 24–48 hours should lead to review of the diagnosis. This high dose is maintained for 1–2 weeks and then tapered gradually depending on the sedimentation rate and the patient's symptoms. The addition of NSAIDs can help to reduce minor recurrent symptoms.[110]

Patients will need treatment for many months and most for several years; relapse is most common in the first year after stopping steroids.[111] After stopping treatment the patient's sedimentation rate and symptoms should be monitored for at least 6 months to a year in case of relapse. Visual loss because of a relapse is unusual after a lengthy course of steroids. Osteoporosis prophylaxis may be necessary.

Temporal artery biopsy should be undertaken in all suspected cases to confirm the diagnosis, but this is not essential. It should not delay treatment if clinical suspicion is high. Biopsy can be undertaken after a few days of treatment and still be positive. The sample should be taken from the symptomatic side to try to maximize yield. Unfortunately this is a disorder that can be easily overlooked, with potential disastrous consequences. Any elderly person with malaise, arthralgia, depression, and vague headache should be considered a possible case until proven otherwise.

Cerebrovascular disease and hypertension

Headache is a common accompaniment to cerebrovascular disease,[112,113] and may occur before, during, or after transient ischemic attack or stroke. The pain is often throbbing in nature and exacerbated with effort. Usually it is lateralized to the side of ischemia. It occurs most frequently when there is parenchymal hemorrhage (57 percent), but also with TIAs (36 percent), thromboembolic infarct (29 percent), and lacunar infarction (17 percent).

Headache does not occur more frequently in the hypertensive than in the normotensive general population unless it is of extreme degree or associated with rapid rises of blood pressure, as in phaeochromocytoma.[114] Occasionally, however, migraine has undoubtedly been aggravated by the occurrence of hypertension.

Carotid and vertebral artery dissection

Carotid artery dissection and occlusion gives rise to ipsilateral pain involving the face and forehead and occasionally the neck. The pain is described as burning or throbbing but can be sudden and stabbing and may be mistaken for subarachnoid hemorrhage (see below). A Horner's syndrome may be present ipsilateral to the involved artery, with contralateral neurological signs.[108] Occasionally there are no associated neurological signs.

Vertebral artery dissection is associated with neck and occipital pain[115] and may occur more commonly than is thought in patients diagnosed with vertebrobasilar insufficiency. The occipital headache associated with this form of dissection is almost always associated with neurological deficits from the brainstem.

Subarachnoid hemorrhage

Intracerebral aneurysms are usually silent except when aneurysms cause compression of neural structures to produce focal signs and headache, or when they rupture. The sudden, severe catastrophic headache of subarachnoid hemorrhage is easily diagnosed and in the elderly patient the prognosis is usually poor.[116] Warning leaks are a concern and may presage fatal hemorrhage. Patients with sudden, severe headache may need screening urgently for the possibility of aneurysmal bleed.

Chronic subdural hemorrhage

This condition usually presents in an insidious manner and a history of head trauma may be absent or forgotten. Coagulopathy, particularly with a background of excessive alcohol consumption, is a well-recognized predisposing factor. Headache with fluctuating neurological signs, cognitive impairment, and a suggestive history should be investigated by means of a CT brain scan. Large symptomatic hematomas are usually evacuated, but smaller hematomas may be left and the patient's neurological state monitored clinically. The resolution of the hematoma is reviewed by serial CT scans.

Headache associated with trauma

Between 9 and 14 percent of those admitted to head injury units are over 65 years of age, and this group has the worst prognosis.[117] Headache after injury, sometimes apparently trivial, is a common complaint, but persistence of headache usually indicates a psychogenic component. CT brain scan should be reserved for those with focal signs or fluctuating consciousness. Simple analgesia should be used, but resistant headache may require psychological management and the use of psychotropic drugs.

INTRACRANIAL TUMORS

(See also Chapter 55)

While headache is present in 60 percent of those with an intracranial tumor, it is the presenting feature in only 20 percent,[118] and only 10 percent of elderly patients had headache in one series.[119] As in most age groups, the most common intracranial mass lesions in the elderly population are secondary tumors. Some tumors may grow to a large size in the elderly before symptoms and signs are evident; this is attributed to the increased space within the cranium secondary to cerebral atrophy.

The typical features of raised intracranial pressure are the same in the elderly population as in all age groups: morning headache, vomiting, and gradual visual loss. The headache may be exacerbated by coughing, straining, or bending forward. There may be incontinence, gait disturbance, and mental deterioration. Papilloedema is often absent. Mass lesions may cause less easily recognized types of headache. Stretching of dural structures by tumors may cause persistent focal headache. Occasionally tension headache and migraine may be mimicked. Thus further investigation including a brain scan may be indicated in an elderly patient whenever there is recent onset of head pain syndrome.[120] Headache persisting for more than 6 months is unlikely to have a structural cause. However, rarely, pituitary tumors which distort the sella turcica can cause long-term headache which is often deep-seated and retro-orbital.

The most common benign primary brain tumors are meningiomas, which are usually operable with good result in the otherwise fit elderly patient where there is headache. Asymptomatic meningiomas can be managed conservatively if monitored regularly.

LOW-PRESSURE HEADACHE SYNDROME

This is headache characterized by improvement on adopting a supine position and most commonly described in the context of lumbar puncture. It is less common in the elderly population[121–127] and may be associated with a variety of symptoms, including pain or stiffness of the neck, nausea, emesis, change in hearing, visual blurring, interscapular pain, and occasionally facial numbness or weakness and upper limb radicular symptoms. The most common site of the leak is in the spine around the point at which the spinal nerve roots pierce the dura, usually in the thoracic and cervicothoracic regions. Magnetic resonance imaging (MRI) may show typical diffuse meningeal enhancement; subdural and epidural collections may be seen. The management is conservative in the first instance; rarely blood patches may be required to provide relief.

DRUG-INDUCED HEADACHE

Drugs causing headache

A large number of the drugs prescribed for elderly people cause headache (Table 47-3). The pain is usually described as involving the whole head, but may be occipital or frontal.

Medication-misuse headache

It is estimated that 1 in 50 people suffer from this type of headache. The overuse of analgesics—particularly codeine-containing compounds and ergotamine—can lead to the development of chronic refractory headache, which then increases dependence on medication. Patients with initially intermittent migraine or tension-type headache may develop chronic daily headache because of analgesic abuse. These patients have higher depression scores, and attempted discontinuation leads to withdrawal symptoms and a refractoriness to prophylactic treatments.[128] Side-effects of the medication are also more likely— such as ergotism, analgesic nephropathy, and gastrointestinal problems.

The only option is to stop the analgesics, although this almost inevitably precipitates a temporary worsening of the headaches. Patients with severe headache should be admitted for drug withdrawal, and given temporary cover with opiates and steroids along with instigation of

Table 47-3 Drugs that can cause headache

Calcium-channel blockers	Nitrates
Indomethacin	Dipyridamole
Lithium	Corticosteroids
Hydralazine	Sympathomimetics
Monoamine oxidase inhibitors	Cimetidine
Ranitidine	Theophyllines

antidepressant therapy and consideration of migraine prophylaxis.[129]

HEADACHE AND THE EYE

The eye and orbit derive a rich innervation from the first division of the trigeminal nerve, and these structures are common causes of pain around the eye and of headache.

In the elderly population, glaucoma can be an important cause of eye pain and headache. Although the condition may be acute or chronic, it is the acute closed-angle glaucoma which causes sudden onset of severe constant pain, centered on the affected eye. This may spread to give a generalized headache and there are visual symptoms such as colored haloes in the visual field and misting of vision. There is photophobia and nausea or vomiting. Patients may be diagnosed as suffering from subarachnoid hemorrhage unless the history or signs of eye disease are discovered. Clinically there is limbic injection, corneal edema (hazy appearance), and the globe will be hard and tender to palpation. This condition represents an emergency that requires immediate referral to an ophthalmic casualty department for further treatment. Opiate analgesia will be necessary.

Proptosis, ophthalmoplegia, and pain can be caused by orbital pseudotumor.[130] Often there is an elevated sedimentation rate and a rapid response to high-dose corticosteroids. The differential diagnosis includes dysthyroid eye disease, or orbital neoplasia (secondary spread from, for example, melanoma). Superior orbital fissuritis (Tolosa–Hunt syndrome)[131] is one end of the spectrum of orbital inflammatory disease. MRI of the skull and/or CT of the skull should differentiate between these conditions, but often the response to steroids aids the diagnosis.[132,133]

Painful oculomotor paresis with retro-orbital pain is usually due to one of two main pathologies. If the pupil is fixed and dilated, then a surgical cause is likely, with aneurysm of the posterior communicating artery being the most common cause. If the pupil reacts to light, then the cause is likely to be nonsurgical and diabetes is the most likely. Angiography may still be necessary to rule out aneurysm even if the blood sugar is elevated.

Anterior and posterior uveitis are also causes of eye pain and visual disturbance. There may be evidence of coexistent systemic pathology to aid the diagnosis. Refractive disorders (so called "eye strain") rarely cause headache. Orbital pain may arise from entrapment of the greater occipital nerve as it emerges from between the occiput and first cervical vertebra. Pain usually starts in the occipital region and radiates forward to the eye, although it may be isolated to the orbit. Treatment is symptomatic, and a soft collar can be tried for a short period.

MISCELLANEOUS CAUSES OF HEAD PAIN

The hypnic headache syndrome was first described by Raskin[134] and reviewed by Newman et al.[135] It is an uncommon form of headache occurring only in the elderly population. Headaches wake the patient from sleep at a regular time each night. They are generalized and usually pulsating in quality. They may last up to half an hour and recur the same night. There are no associated autonomic symptoms. This disorder is believed to be a form of REM sleep disturbance. It is difficult to treat; lithium carbonate (300 mg nocte) may produce a remission but the limiting factor is side-effects, particularly tremor and gastrointestinal symptoms. The differential diagnosis includes mass lesions, temporal arteritis, and cluster headache, although the latter is characterized by additional autonomic features.

The "exploding head syndrome"[136] is another benign cause of disturbance experienced more commonly by elderly people. It is not a pain or headache but a loud noise occurring in the twilight of sleep and waking the patient. It may occur for a short period of weeks or months on an infrequent basis or recur irregularly but more frequently. The noise is deep in the center or back of the head and causes fear in the patient. Some may describe momentary difficulty in breathing, tachycardia, or sweating. There are no sequelae and usually patients do not have a preceding illness or history of neurological disease. The etiology of the condition is unknown and it is almost certainly underreported. Reassurance is usually all that is required.

About a third of patients with Parkinson's disease report occipital headache, usually dull in nature. The cause of this is not clear and it is not associated with nuchal rigidity.[137] Amitriptyline in low dose may be effective.[138]

Infections, whether bacterial or viral, may be associated with headache. Chronic meningitis may cause headache and be associated with gait disorder secondary to hydrocephalus. Multiple cranial nerve involvement may be associated with basal meningeal involvement as seen in carcinomatous meningitis and sarcoidosis. Other systemic causes of headache include: hypoxia and hypercapnia related to parenchymal lung disease or sleep apnea;[139] hypoglycemia of less than 2.2 mmol/L; hemodialysis; hypercalcemia; and severe anemia. Carbon monoxide poisoning from poorly ventilated gas appliances may be an insidious cause of chronic headache and nonspecific symptoms.[140]

THE DIAGNOSTIC APPROACH TO HEADACHE

As in any branch of medicine, the diagnosis rests heavily on the history of the complaint and use of appropriate investigations after a thorough physical examination. The duration of symptoms and their mode of onset together with the tempo of their development provide valuable diagnostic clues. Quality of headache is a less useful feature, but position and intensity together with radiation of the pain and the presence of exacerbating and relieving factors should be asked for. A complete drug history should be obtained; and appraisal of the patient's mood, sleep, and vegetative functions are helpful in discerning the impact of the illness and possible psychological background.

Although the vast majority of headaches in all age groups are benign, in the elderly population the risk of organic pathology is increased. The diversity of symptoms of temporal arteritis can often lead to a delay in diagnosis. Chronic malaise, myalgia, and arthralgia are frequently seen in giant cell arteritis but easily dismissed as nonspecific symptoms and resulting from the aging process. Severe pain of sudden onset, pain that is persistent and progressively worsening with time, early morning headache with vomiting, and exacerbation by coughing, straining and bending forward, all suggest underlying organic disease. Migraine can be identified when there is a long history or classical symptoms, but complicated migraine may be difficult to differentiate from TIAs[32] and complete investigation is warranted. The presence of other symptoms such as drowsiness, confusion, and memory loss will raise the index of suspicion. Other worrying symptoms include progressive visual disturbance, weakness, clumsiness, and loss of balance. It is important to realize that the cranial neuralgias are not associated in their simple form with neurological deficits and have a strict definition for a positive diagnosis. The description of bands of pain or a tight cap on the head is more likely to result from muscle tension as seen in tension-type headache or disease of the neck, but can be a symptom of a more serious disease. Injury to the head may precede the formation of a subdural hematoma which is more likely with coagulopathy or chronic alcohol abuse. Brachalgia together with myelopathy should point to the neck as the source of headache.

A normal neurological examination will often help rule out serious underlying disease and avoid unnecessary investigations.

Summary of management algorithm
Headache

○ **Indications for investigation**

New headache with:
- abnormal neurological signs
- a history suggesting raised intracranial pressure
- impairment of memory
- impairment of consciousness
- worsening pain which may disturb sleep
- headache on waking and associated with vomiting

Apparent "late-onset" migraine
Atypical facial pain

○ **Migraine**

Avoid easily identified triggers

Bedrest

Analgesia
- paracetamol or aspirin
- NSAIDs (beware peptic and renal side-effects)
- triptans for moderate to severe headache
- antiemetics if required

Prophylaxis
- β-blockers
- tricyclic antidepressants
- valproate sodium
- serotonin antagonists (e.g. pizotifen).

○ **Tension-type headache**
Reassurance after careful clinical assessment
Simple analgesia
Address possible psychological issues
Treat depression if identified (tricyclics useful)
? relaxation therapy and biofeedback
Avoid chronic analgesic abuse which can cause chronic daily headache

(continued)

Summary of management algorithm
(continued)

Trigeminal neuralgia
Diagnosed only on strict criteria
Carbamazepine is still first line
Alternatives include baclofen, phenytoin, sodium valproate, clonazepam, gabapentin, and lamotrigine
Up to 50 percent of patients may require surgical treatment

Post-herpetic neuralgia
Up to 50 percent of elderly patients may develop this syndrome
Amitriptyline and carbamazepine are both of proven benefit
Gabapentin has recently been shown to be of proven benefit

Giant cell arteritis
This medical emergency requires swift initiation of steroids
Jaw claudication is virtually pathognomonic
Constitutional symptoms are common
In up to 10 percent of cases the sedimentation rate may be normal

KEY POINTS   Headache

■ Headache is a common problem in the whole population. However, it is less reported by elderly people in whom there is a decline in prevalence, although the symptom is more likely to represent serious pathology.

■ Management of the common primary headache conditions is the same as for younger patients. Elderly people are more likely to have comorbidity that may limit their ability to tolerate medication, or side-effects resulting from drug interactions.

REFERENCES

1. Siberstein SD, Silberstein MM: New concepts in the pathogenesis of migraine headache. Pain Manag 1990;3:297–302
2. Cook NR, Evans DA, Funkenstein HH et al: Correlates of headache in a population-based cohort of elderly. Arch Neurol 1989;46:1338–1344
3. Newland CA, Illis LS, Robinson PK, Batchelor BG, Waters WE: A survey of headache in an English city. Res Clin Stud Headache 1978;5:1–20
4. Serratrice G, Serbanesco F, Sambuc R: Epidemiology of headache in elderly: correlations with life conditions and socio-professional environment. Headache 1985;25(2):85–89
5. Waters WE, O'Connor PJ: Epidemiology of headache and migraine in women. J Neurol Neurosurg Psychiat 1971;34(2):148–153
6. Nikiforow R: Headache in a random sample of 200 persons: a clinical study of a population in northern Finland. Cephalalgia 1981;1(2):99–107
7. Selby G, Lance JW: Observations on 500 cases of migraine and allied vascular headache. J Neurol Neurosurg Psychiat 1960;23(23):23–32
8. Rasmussen BK, Olesen J: Migraine epidemiology. Cephalalgia 1993;13(3):216–217 (letter/comment)
9. Stewart WF, Linet MS, Celentano DD, Van Natta M, Ziegler D: Age- and sex-specific incidence rates of migraine with and without visual aura. Am J Epidemiol 1991;134:1111–1120
10. Hale WE, May FE, Marks RG, Moore MT, Stewart RB: Headache in the elderly: an evaluation of risk factors. Headache 1987;27(5):272–276
11. Pascual J, Berciano J: Experience in the diagnosis of headaches that start in elderly people. J Neurol Neurosurg Psychiat 1994;57:1255–1257
12. Gobel H, Petersen-Braun M, Soyka D: The epidemiology of headache in Germany: a nationwide survey of a representative sample on the basis of the headache classification of the International Headache Society. Cephalalgia 1994;14(2):97–106
13. Linet MS, Stewart WF: Migraine headache: epidemiologic perspectives. Epidemiol Rev 1984;6:107–139 (review)
14. Featherstone HJ: Migraine and muscle contraction headaches: a continuum. Headache 1985;25(4):194–198
15. Silberstein SD, Lipton RB: Epidemiology of migraine. Neuroepidemiology 1993;12(3):179–194 (review)
16. Lipton RB, Stewart WF: The epidemiology of migraine. Eur Neurol 1994;34(suppl 2):6–11
17. Lipton RB, Stewart WF: Migraine in the United States: a review of epidemiology and health care use. Neurology 1993;43(6: suppl 3):S6–S10
18. Lipton RB, Silberstein SD, Stewart WF: An update on the epidemiology of migraine. Headache 1994;34(6):319–328 (review)
19. Rasmussen BK, Olesen J: Epidemiology of migraine and tension-type headache. Curr Opin Neurol 1994;7:264–271
20. Stang PE, Yanagihara T, Swanson JW, Beard CM, Melton LJ: A population-based study of migraine headaches in Olmsted County, Minnesota: case ascertainment and classification. Neuroepidemiology 1991;10(5–6):297–307
21. Stewart WF, Lipton RB, Celentano DD, Reed ML: Prevalence of migraine headache in the United States: relation to age, income, race, and other sociodemographic factors. JAMA 1992;267:64–69
22. Stewart WF, Shechter A, Rasmussen BK: Migraine prevalence: a review of population-based studies. Neurology 1994;44(6:suppl 4):S17–S23 (review)
23. Rasmussen BK, Jensen R, Schroll M, Olesen J: Epidemiology of headache in a general population: a prevalence study. J Clin Epidemiol 1991;44:1147–1157
24. Henry P, Michel P, Brochet B et al: A nationwide survey of migraine in France: prevalence and clinical features in adults: GRIM. Cephalalgia 1992;12(4):229–237
25. International Headache Society: Classification and diagnostic criteria for headache disorders, cranial neuralgia, and facial pain. Cephalalgia 1988;8(suppl 7):1–96
26. Rasmussen BK, Jensen R, Olesen J: A population-based analysis of the diagnostic criteria of the International Headache Society. Cephalalgia 1991;11(3):129–134
27. Silberstein SD, Saper JR: Wolff's Headache and Other Head Pain, 6th edn. Oxford University Press, Oxford, 1996
28. Ziegler DK, Hassanein RS: Specific headache phenomena: their frequency and coincidence. Headache 1990;30(3):152–156
29. Solomon S, Lipton RB: Criteria for the diagnosis of migraine in clinical practice. Headache 1991;31(6):384–387 (review)
30. Blau JN: Migraine prodromes separated from the aura: complete migraine. Br Med J 1980;281:658–660
31. Jensen K, Tfelt-Hansen P, Lauritzen M, Olesen J: Classic migraine: a prospective recording of symptoms. Acta Neurol Scand 1986;73:359–362
32. Fisher CM: Late-life migraine accompaniments: further experience. Stroke 1986;17:1033–1042 (review)
33. Lascelles RG: Atypical facial pain and depression. Br J Psychiat 1966;112:651–659
34. Loeb C, Gandolfo C, Dall'Agata D: Headache in transient ischemic attacks (TIA). Cephalalgia 1985;5(suppl 2):17–19
35. Andre C, Neves FF, Vincent MB: Headache in transient ischaemic attacks. Funct Neurol 1996;11(4):195–200
36. Iversen HK, Langemark M, Andersson PG, Hansen PE, Olesen J: Clinical characteristics of migraine and episodic tension-type headache in relation to old and new diagnostic criteria. Headache 1990;30:514–519
37. Raskin NH, Schwartz RK: Icepick-like pain. Neurology 1980;30(2):203–205
38. Littlewood JT, Gibb C, Glover V et al: Red wine as a cause of migraine. Lancet 1988;1:558–559
39. Kudrow L: The relationship of headache frequency to hormone use in migraine. Headache 1975;15(1):36–40
40. Baumel B, Eisner LS: Diagnosis and treatment of headache in the elderly. Med Clin N Am 1991;75:661–675
41. Pradalier A, Clapin A, Dry J: Treatment review: non-steroid anti-inflammatory drugs in the treatment and long-term prevention of migraine attacks. Headache 1988;28:550–557
42. Johnson AG, Day RO: The problems and pitfalls of NSAID therapy in the elderly: I. Drugs Aging 1991;1(2):130–143 (review)

43. Garcia Rodriguez LA, Jick H: Risk of upper gastrointestinal bleeding and perforation associated with individual non-steroidal anti-inflammatory drugs. Lancet 1994;343:769–772; erratum 343:1048

44. Subcutaneous Sumatriptan International Study Group: Treatment of migraine attacks with sumatriptan. N Engl J Med 1991;325:316–321

45. Oral Sumatriptan and Aspirin plus Metaclopramide Comparative Study Group: A study to compare oral sumatriptan with oral aspirin plus oral metaclopramide in the acute treatment of migraine. Eur Neurol 1992;32:177–184

46. Brown EG, Endersby CA, Smith RN, Talbot JC: The safety and tolerability of sumatriptan: an overview. Eur Neurol 1991;31:339–344

47. Goadsby PJ: A triptan too far? J Neurol Neurosurg Psychiat 1998;64(2):143–147

48. Andersson K, Vinge E: Beta-adrenoceptor blockers and calcium antagonists in the prophylaxis and treatment of migraine. Drugs 1990;39:355–373

49. Ramadan NM, Schultz LL, Gilkey SJ: Migraine prophylactic drugs: proof of efficacy, utilization and cost. Cephalalgia 1997;17:73–80

50. Ziegler DK, Hurwitz A, Hassanein RS et al: Migraine prophylaxis: a comparison of propranolol and amitriptyline. Arch Neurol 1987;44:486–489

51. Adly C, Straumanis J, Chesson A: Fluoxetine prophylaxis of migraine. Headache 1992;32(2):101–104

52. Hays P: Paroxetine prevents migraines. J Clin Psychiat 1997;58(1):30–31 (letter)

53. Rothrock JF: Clinical studies of valproate for migraine prophylaxsis. Cephalalgia 1997;17:81–83

54. Meyer JS, Hardenberg J: Clinical effectiveness of calcium entry blockers in prophylactic treatment of migraine and cluster headaches. Headache 1983;23:266–277

55. Peatfield R: Headache. In Conomy JP, Swash M (eds): Clinical Medicine and the Nervous System. Springer-Verlag, New York, 1986

56. Drummond PD: Effectiveness of methysergide in relation to clinical features of migraine. Headache 1985;25(3):145–146

57. Johnson ES, Kadam NP, Hylands DM, Hylands PJ: Efficacy of feverfew as prophylactic treatment of migraine. BMJ 1985;291:569–573

58. Murphy JJ, Heptinstall S, Mitchell JR: Randomised double-blind placebo-controlled trial of feverfew in migraine prevention. Lancet 1988;2:189–192

59. Silberstein SD: Tension-type and chronic daily headache. Neurology 1993;43:1644–1649 (review)

60. Langemark M, Olesen J, Poulsen DL, Bech P: Clinical characterization of patients with chronic tension headache. Headache 1988;28:590–596

61. Drummond PD: Scalp tenderness and sensitivity to pain in migraine and tension headache. Headache 1987;27(1):45–50

62. Hatch JP, Moore PJ, Cyr-Provost M: The use of electromyography and muscle palpation in the diagnosis of tension-type headache with and without pericranial muscle involvement. Pain 1992;49(2):175–178

63. Marsland DW, Wood M, Mayo F: Content of family practice. I: Rank order of diagnoses by frequency. II: Diagnoses by disease category and age/sex distribution. J Fam Pract 1976;3(1):37–68

64. Mathew NT: Chronic refractory headache. Neurology 1993;43(6:Suppl 3):S26–S33 (review)

65. Solomon GD, Kunkel RS, Frame J: Demographics of headache in elderly patients. Headache 1990;30(5):273–276

66. Diener HC, Haab J, Peters C et al: Subcutaneous sumatriptan in the treatment of headache during withdrawal from drug-induced headache. Headache 1991;31(4):205–209

67. Mathew NT, Ali S: Valproate in the treatment of persistent chronic daily headache: an open label study. Headache 1991;31(2):71–74

68. Mathew NT, Stubits E, Nigam MP: Transformation of episodic migraine into daily headache: analysis of factors. Headache 1982;22(2):66–68

69. Ekbom K: A clinical comparison of cluster headache and migraine. Acta Neurol Scand 1970:suppl 41:1

70. Ekbom K: Patterns of cluster headache with a note on the relations to angina pectoris and peptic ulcer. Acta Neurol Scand 1970;46(2):225–237

71. Kudrow L: Cluster Headache: Mechanisms and Management. Oxford University Press, London, 1980

72. Merikangas KR, Tierney C, Martin NG, Heath AC: Genetics of migraine in the Australian Twin Registry. In Rose FC (ed): New Advances in Headache Research, Vol. 27. Smith-Gordon, Cambridge, 1994

73. Ekbom K, Monstad I, Prusinski A: Subcutaneous sumatriptan in the acute treatment of cluster headache: a dose comparison study. The Sumatriptan Cluster Headache Study Group. Acta Neurol Scand 1993;88(1):63–69

74. Leone M, D'Amico D, Frediani et al: Verapamil in the prophylaxis of episodic cluster headache: a double-blind study versus placebo. Neurology 2000;54:1382–1385

75. Bussone G, Leone M, Peccarisi C et al: Double blind comparison of lithium and verapamil in cluster headache prophylaxis. Headache 1990;30:411–417

76. Hering R, Kuritzky A: Sodium valproate in the treatment of cluster headache: an open clinical trial. Cephalalgia 1989;9(3):195–198

77. Mathew NT, Hurt W: Percutaneous radiofrequency trigeminal gangliorhizolysis in intractable cluster headache. Headache 1988;28:328–331

78. Antonaci F, Sjaastad O: Chronic paroxysmal hemicrania (CPH): a review of the clinical manifestations. Headache 1989;29:648–656

79. Rothman KJ, Monson RR: Epidemiology of trigeminal neuralgia. J Chronic Dis 1973;26(1):3–12

80. Katusic S, Beard CM, Bergstralh E, Kurland LT: Incidence and clinical features of trigeminal neuralgia, Rochester, Minnesota, 1945–1984. Ann Neurol 1990;27(1):89–95

81. Lance JW: Mechanism and Management of Headache, 5th edn. Butterworth–Heinemann, Oxford, 1993

82. Selby G: Diseases of the fifth cranial nerve. In Dyck PH, Thomas PK, Lambert EH (eds): Peripheral Neuropathy. WB Saunders, Philadelphia, 1975:533–569

83. Fromm GH, Terrence CF, Maroon JC: Trigeminal neuralgia: current concepts regarding etiology and pathogenesis. Arch Neurol 1984;41:1204–1207

84. Pagni CA: The origin of tic douloureux: a unified view. J Neurosurg Sci 1993;37(4):185–194

85. Tash RR, Sze G, Leslie DR: Trigeminal neuralgia: MR imaging features. Radiology 1989;172:767–770

86. Zakrzewska JM, Patsalos PN: Drugs used in the management of trigeminal neuralgia. Oral Surg Oral Med Oral Pathol 1992;74:439–450 (review)

87. Sidebottom A, Maxwell S: The medical and surgical management of trigeminal neuralgia. J Clin Pharm Ther 1995;20(1):31–35 (review)

88. Green MW, Selman JE: The medical management of trigeminal neuralgia. Headache 1991;31:588–592 (review)

89. Kanpolat Y, Savas A, Bekar A, Berk C: Percutaneous controlled radio frequency trigeminal rhizotomy for the treatment of idiopathic trigeminal neuralgia: 25-year experience with 1600 patients. Neurosurgery 2001;48:524–532

90. Steiger HJ: Prognostic factors in the treatment of trigeminal neuralgia: analysis of a differential therapeutic approach. Acta Neurochir 1991;113(1–2):11–17

91. Jannetta PJ: Treatment of trigeminal neuralgia by suboccipital and transtentorial cranial operations. Clin Neurosurg 1977;24:538–549

92. Dalessio D: The major neuralgias, postinfectious neuritis, and atypical facial pain. In Delassio DJ, Silberstein SD (eds): Wolff's Headache and Other Head Pain, 6th edn. Oxford University Press, Oxford, 1993:345–364

93. Demoragas JM, Kierland RR: The outcome of patients with herpes zoster. Arch Dermatol 1957;75:193–196

94. Watson CPN: Postherpetic neuralgia: clinical features and treatment. In Fields HC (ed): Pain Syndromes in Neurology. Butterworth, London, 1990:223–238

95. Ragozzino MW, Melton LJ, Kurland LT, Chu CP, Perry HO: Population-based study of herpes zoster and its sequelae. Medicine (Balt) 1982;61:310–316

96. Alper BS, Lewis PR: Does treatment of acute herpes zoster prevent or shorten postherpetic neuralgia? J Fam Pract 2000;49:255–264

97. Max MB, Schafer SC, Culnane M et al: Amitriptyline, but not lorazepam, relieves postherpetic neuralgia. Neurology 1988;38:1427–1432

98. Watson CP, Evans RJ, Reed K et al: Amitriptyline versus placebo in postherpetic neuralgia. Neurology 1982;32:671–673

99. Kanazi GE, Johnson RW, Dworkin RH: Treatment of postherpetic neuralgia: an update. Drugs 2000;59:1113–1126

100. Jessell TM, Iversen LL: Capsaisin-induced depletion of substance P from sensory primary neurons. Brain Res 1979;152:132–188

101. Editorial: Post-herpetic neuralgia. Lancet 1990;336:537–538

102. Rowbotham MC, Harden N, Stacey B, Bernstein B, Magnus Miller L: Gabapentin for the treatment of postherpetic neuralgia: a randomised controlled trial. JAMA 1998;280:1837–1842

103. Iansek R, Heywood J, Karnaghan J, Balla JI: Cervical spondylosis and headaches. Clin Exp Neurol 1987;23:175–178

104. Edmeads J: The cervical spine and headache. Neurology 1988;38:1874–1878

105. Stevenson DD: Allergy, atopy, nasal disease, and headache. In Delassio DJ, Silberstein SD (eds): Wolff's Headache and Other Head Pain, 6th edn. Oxford University Press, Oxford, 1993:291–333

106. Bengtsson BA: Incidence of giant cell arteritis. Acta Med Scand 1982;58(suppl 6):15–17

107. Huston KA, Hunder GG, Lie JT, Kennedy RH, Elveback LR: Temporal arteritis: a 25-year epidemiologic, clinical, and pathologic study. Ann Intern Med 1978;88:162–167

108. Kansu T, Corbett JJ, Savino P, Schatz NJ: Giant cell arteritis with normal sedimentation rate. Arch Neurol 1977;34:624–625

109. Ellis ME, Ralston S: The ESR in the diagnosis and management of the polymyalgia rheumatica/giant cell arteritis syndrome. Ann Rheumatol Dis 1983;42(2):168–170

110. Kyle V, Hazelman BL: Stopping steroids in polymyalgia rheumatica and giant cell arteritis. BMJ 1990;300:344–345

111. Ayoub WT, Franklin CM, Torretti D: Polymyalgia rheumatica: duration of therapy and long-term outcome. Am J Med 1985;79:309–315

112. Edmeads J: The headache of ischemic cerebrovascular disease. Headache 1979;19:345–349

113. Portenoy RK, Abissi CJ, Lipton RB et al: Headache in cerebrovascular disease. Stroke 1984;15:1009–1012

114. Waters WE: Headache and blood pressure in the community. BMJ 1971;1:142–143

115. Caplan LR, Zarins CK, Hemmati M: Spontaneous dissection of the extracranial vertebral arteries. Stroke 1985;16:1030–1038

116. O'Sullivan MG, Dorward N, Whittle IR, Steers AJ, Miller JD: Management and long-term outcome following subarachnoid haemorrhage and intracranial aneurysm surgery in elderly patients: an audit of 199 consecutive cases. Br J Neurosurg 1994;8(1):23–30

117. O'Neill P: Cranio-cerebral trauma. In Tallis R (ed): The Clinical Neurology of Old Age. John Wiley, Chichester, 1989;285–296

118. Iversen MK, Strange P, Sommer W, Tjalve E: Brain tumour headache related to tumour size, histology and location. Cephalalgia 1987;7 (suppl 6):394–395

119. Godfrey JB, Caird FI: Intracranial tumours in the elderly: diagnosis and treatment. Age Ageing 1984;13:152–158

120. Forsyth PA, Posner JB: Headaches in patients with brain tumors: a study of 111 patients. Neurology 1993;43:1678–1683

121. Mokri B: Spontaneous intracranial hypotension. Curr Pain Headache Rep 2001;5(3):284–291

122. Mokri B: Spontaneous cerebrospinal fluid leaks: from intracranial hypotension to cerebrospinal fluid hypovolemia—evolution of a concept. Mayo Clin Proc 1999;74:1113–1123

123. Christoforidis GA, Mehta BA, Landi JL, Czarnecki EJ, Piaskowski RA: Spontaneous intracranial hypotension: report of four cases and review of the literature. Neuroradiology 1998;40:636–643

124. Kosmorsky GS: Spontaneous intracranial hypotension. J Neuro-Ophthalmol 1995;15(2):79–83

125. Moayeri NN, Henson JW, Schaefer PW, Zervas NT: Spinal dural enhancement on magnetic resonance imaging associated with spontaneous intracranial hypotension: report of three cases and review of the literature. J Neurosurg 1998;88:912–918

126. Jacobs MB, Wasserstein PH: Spontaneous intracranial hypotension: an uncommon and underrecognized cause of headache. West J Med 1991;155:178–180

127. Rando TA, Fishman RA: Spontaneous intracranial hypotension: report of two cases and review of the literature. Neurology 1992;43:(3 Pt 1):481–487

128. Mathew NT: Medication misuse headache. Cephalalgia 1998; 18(suppl 21):34–36

129. Clough C: Treating migraine. BMJ 1989;299:141–142 (review)

130. Min YG, Lee CH, Shin JS, Byun SW: Idiopathic orbital pseudotumours in adults. Rhinology 1996;34(1):60–63

131. Kline LB, Hoyt WF: The Tolosa–Hunt syndrome. J Neurol Neurosurg Psychiat 2001;71:577–582

132. Pascual J, Cerezal L, Canga A et al: Tolosa–Hunt syndrome: focus on MRI diagnosis. Cephalalgia 1999;19(suppl 25):36–38

133. Hunt WE, Brightman RP: The Tolosa–Hunt syndrome: a problem in differential diagnosis. Acta Neurochir Suppl 1988;42:248–252

134. Raskin NH: The hypnic headache syndrome. Headache 1988;88:534–536

135. Newman LC, Lipton RB, Solomon S: The hypnic headache syndrome: a benign headache disorder of the elderly. Neurology 1990;40:1904–1905

136. Pearce JM: Clinical features of the exploding head syndrome. J Neurol Neurosurg Psychiat 1989;52:907–910

137. Indo T, Naito A, Sobue I: Clinical characteristics of headache in Parkinson's disease. Headache 1983;83(5):211–212

138. Indaco A, Carrieri PB: Amitriptyline in the treatment of headache in patients with Parkinson's disease: a double-blind placebo-controlled study. Neurology 1988;38:1720–1722

139. Ulfberg J, Carter N, Talback M, Edling C: Headache, snoring and sleep apnoea. J Neurol 1996;243:621–625

140. Varon J, Marik PE, Fromm RE, Gueler A: Carbon monoxide poisoning: a review for clinicians. J Emerg Med 1999;17(1):87–93

Chapter 48

Stroke: pathology and epidemiology

Shah Ebrahim and Alistair Lammie

DEFINITIONS AND CRITERIA

Stroke is defined clinically rather than pathologically as "rapidly developing clinical signs of focal (or global) disturbance of cerebral function, with symptoms lasting 24 hours or longer or leading to death, with no apparent cause other than of vascular origin."[1] Events lasting less than 24 hours are classified as transient ischemic attacks (TIAs) and are excluded by the definition, whereas subarachnoid hemorrhages are included. In population surveys of stroke prevalence the simple question "Have you ever had a stroke?" performs well.[2]

The underlying vascular origins of stroke may be divided into two broad categories: ischemic (i.e., thrombosis or embolism) and hemorrhagic (see Fig. 48-1). Alternative classifications such as reversible ischemic neurological deficit (RIND)[3] and major and minor stroke are widely used terms but lack agreed operational criteria.[4] However, understanding of pathological processes is essential for the interpretation of secular and geographical trends and for the study of etiology.

Clinical diagnostic scales,[5,6] relying largely on symptoms and signs associated with raised intracranial pressure and meningism, can distinguish between large hemorrhagic and thrombotic stroke but are not sufficiently accurate for clinical management of patients. Computed tomography (CT) scanning is helpful in diagnosis, but in one-third to one-half of

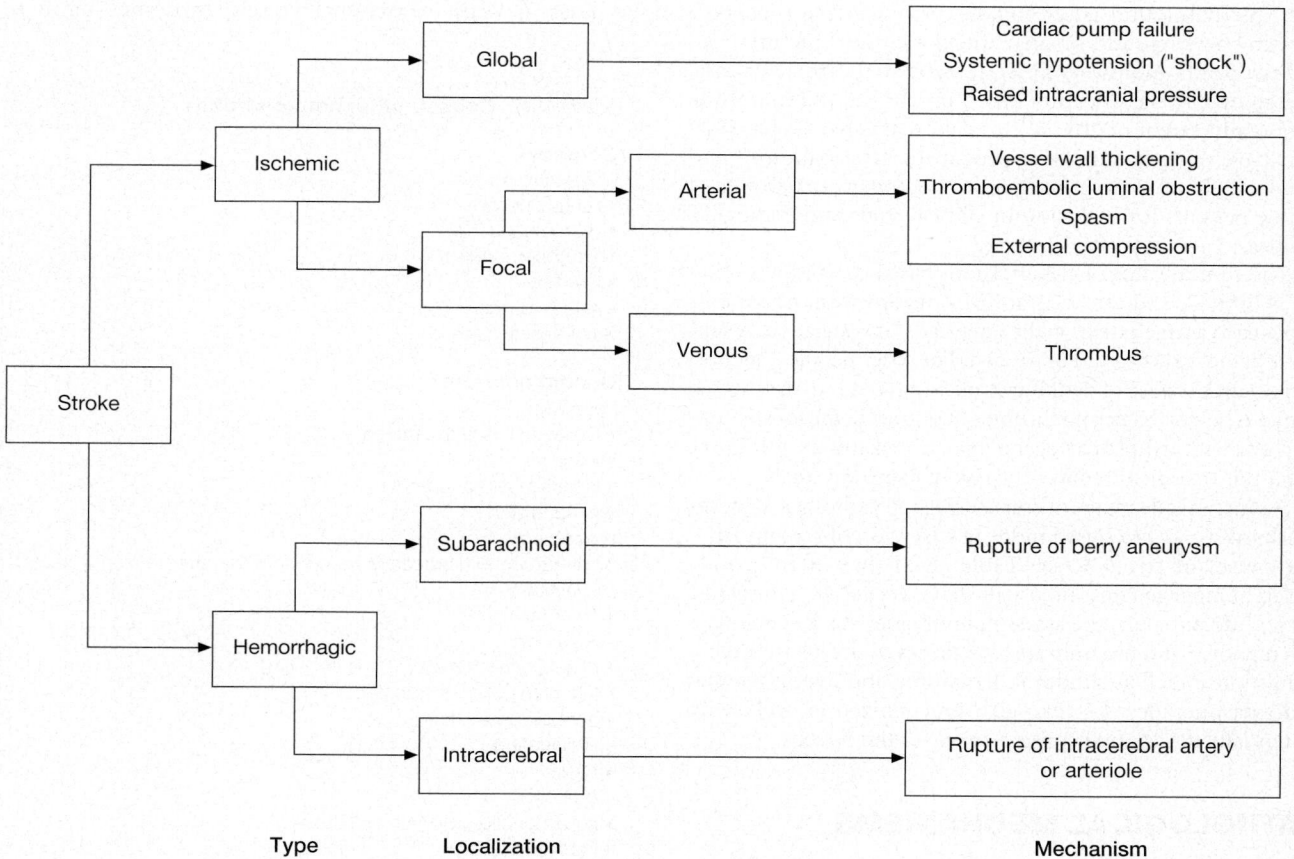

Figure 48-1 A simple pathological classification of stroke.

Table 48-1 A clinical classification of ischemic stroke subtypes and associated mortality

Stroke subtype	Proportion in community series (%)	Mortality at 6 months (%)
Anterior circulation infarct (ACI):		
Total anterior circulation infarct (TACI) (i.e., cortical and subcortical impairment)	17	56
Partial anterior circulation infarct (PACI) (i.e., only cortical impairment)	34	10
Lacunar anterior circulation infarct (LACI) (i.e., pure motor, pure sensory, motor-sensory, ataxic syndromes)	25	7
Posterior circulation infarct (POCI) vertebrobasilar circulation impairment	24	14

Data from Oxford Community Stroke Study, Bamford et al.[10]

patients no CT abnormality is found despite clinical evidence of stroke.[7,8]

An appraisal of stroke subtype requires information about the underlying pathogenesis or mechanism (i.e., thrombosis, embolus, hemorrhage, hemodynamic); the arterial site affected (i.e., internal carotid artery, middle cerebral artery, small perforating arteries, and so on); and the clinical picture (i.e., sudden death, motor hemiplegia, associated cardiac disease, and so on). A classification based on clinical criteria of the region and extent of arterial circulation affected (Table 48-1) may have value in improving prognostic information[9,10] and may be helpful in describing more homogeneous groups of stroke patients for inclusion in clinical trials and etiological studies.

The clinical value of classifications based on complex criteria is limited, and the accuracy of categorization of patients depends to a large extent on the intensity of investigation. A simple scheme is shown in Figure 48-1. For older people, the most important purpose of defining stroke subtypes is to distinguish between hemorrhagic and thrombotic stroke: in the former prophylaxis with antiplatelet agents may be hazardous, but in the latter this treatment reduces the risk of recurrent stroke.

A practical advantage of considering the pathological mechanism of stroke is a raised index of suspicion of rare underlying causes of stroke[11] (see Table 48-2) that often require different management and usually have a different natural history. Unfortunately, the assessment of older stroke patients is often poor,[12] and not only are rare causes of stroke missed but conditions (such as subdural hematoma and hypoglycemia) that masquerade as stroke go unrecognized as well, with potentially devastating consequences for the patient.

PATHOLOGICAL MECHANISMS

Ischemic stroke

Causes of vessel occlusion

The causes of occluded cerebral vessels are legion (Table 48-2), but in practice atherosclerosis is by far the most common cause

of cerebral infarction, mediated by thrombotic and embolic complications. Atherosclerosis is an almost universal feature of large and medium-sized arteries in elderly people and is most severe in the aortic arch, and at points of bifurcation (e.g. carotid bifurcation) and confluence (e.g. basilar artery). At least in large extracranial vessels, thrombus tends to

Table 48-2 Causes of ischemic stroke

Common
In-situ thrombosis:
• Atherosclerosis
• Hypercoaguability
Thromboembolism:
• Cardiac
• Artery-to-artery
Small vessel disease

Uncommon/rare
Vasculitis:
• Collagen vascular disease
• Infective
• Isolated CNS angiitis
• Drug related
Embolism:
• Fat, tumor, air, fibrocartilage, foreign body, atrial myxoma, septic
Dissection:
• Trauma
• Atheroma
• Infection/inflammation
• Inherited collagen disease
Traumatic neck injury:
• Penetrating
• Blunt
Metabolic:
• Mitochondrial cytopathy (MELAS)
• Fabry's disease
• Homocystinuria
Miscellaneous:
• Vasospasm
• CADASIL

complicate the ruptured or eroded "unstable" atherosclerotic plaque,[13] as in the coronary arteries. Such plaques are characterized by a large necrotic core covered by a thin, inflamed fibrous cap.[14] Exposure of the thrombogenic plaque core causes activation of platelets and triggering of the coagulation cascade. The resulting thrombus either occludes the vessel in situ, dislodges as embolus, or perhaps not uncommonly undergoes clinically silent lysis or healing and incorporation into the growing plaque. Rupture of unstable plaques appears to be less common in intracranial vessels, where atherosclerosis may more commonly mediate stroke by low-flow effects or by acting as luminal narrowings at which emboli impact.

The possible causes of small, deep (lacunar) infarcts are also many,[15] but in practice there are likely to be two important causes.[16] The first is small vessel atherosclerosis, and the second is a destructive lesion of small arteries ("lipohyalinosis") characterized in the acute phase by fibrinoid necrosis. The aetiopathogenesis of lipohyalinosis is uncertain, but may be linked to inherited and acquired disorders of small vessel tone.[17]

Cerebral veins and venous sinuses become thrombosed when a variety of constitutive and acquired factors, both local and systemic, promote hypercoaguability and/or venous stasis.[18]

Consequences of vessel occlusion

The size, shape, and location of occlusive arterial infarcts conform more or less to individual arterial supply zones, variations dependent upon interindividual differences in vascular anatomy, adequacy of collaterals, pre-existing vascular disease, and other factors. Hemorrhagic transformation of initially pale ischemic infarcts is relatively common following lysis, either spontaneous or therapeutic, of thromboemboli.[19] Bleeding may be severe enough to mimic a primary intracerebral hemorrhage.[20] The distribution of infarction in global cerebral circulatory insufficiency is diverse, but commonly involves spinal as well as cerebral arterial borderzones and selectively vulnerable brain regions such as the CA1 zone of the hippocampus, neocortical layers 3, 5, and 6, cerebellar Purkinje cells, and basal ganglia.[21,22] Venous infarcts characteristically do not conform to arterial supply zones, and are often accompanied by subarachnoid and intracerebral hemorrhage, and massive brain swelling.

Irrespective of size or location, brain infarcts are areas of ischemic coagulative necrosis of all cellular elements, ultimately becoming fluid-filled cavities.[23] Temporary or less severe ischemia may produce areas of so-called "incomplete infarction,"[24] characterized by death of only the most vulnerable cells, in particular neurons, representing perhaps a neuropathological substrate of transient ischemic attacks.[25] The ultimate fate of affected brain depends not only on the severity and duration of ischemia, but also on how selectively vulnerable is the region and its component neurons, and on the degree and duration of reperfusion ("delayed neuronal death").[26] In humans, cerebral blood flow must fall from an average normal value of about 50 ml $100 \text{ g}^{-1} \text{ min}^{-1}$ to 18–20 ml $100 \text{ g}^{-1} \text{ min}^{-1}$ before neurons become electrically silent and to 8–9 ml $100 \text{ g}^{-1} \text{ min}^{-1}$ before neuronal ion pumps fail.[27] The marginal zone of brain around the doomed ischemic core has cerebral blood flow levels between these thresholds of

synaptic transmission and membrane failure. This "penumbra," nonfunctional yet viable, remains the focus of potential therapeutic salvage.[28] Better understanding of the cascade of ischemic neuronal damage[29] may yet provide effective stroke therapy targets, and it is increasingly speculated that the future of stroke treatment lies in rapidly instituted combination therapy with thrombolytic, neuroprotective and ultimately perhaps regenerative/trophic agents.

Hemorrhagic stroke

Causes of vessel rupture

The causes of primary (i.e., nontraumatic) intracerebral hemorrhage are diverse (Table 48-3), although few are common. The commonest remains the classical spontaneous "hypertensive" hemorrhage, characteristically in basal ganglia, thalamus, lobar white matter, cerebellum, and pons, in approximate descending order of frequency.[30] Hypertension is the most important, but perhaps overemphasized and certainly not an invariable, risk factor. Their pathogenesis has been difficult to study, but circumstantial evidence points to the same, or closely related, lesion to that causing lacunar infarction,[31] with which it colocalizes and shares a common risk factor profile. Thus, a destructive lesion characterized by fibrinoid necrosis and associated with hypertension is considered by many to be the underlying vascular lesion in most cases.[32] In elderly people, an increasingly recognized form of spontaneous brain hemorrhage is due to cerebral amyloid angiopathy, in

---

Table 48-3 Causes of spontaneous intracerebral hemorrhage

Structural
Fibrinoid necrosis of small perforating vessels
Cerebral amyloid angiopathy
Vascular malformations:
• Arteriovenous malformations
• Cavernous angiomas
• Venous angiomas
Saccular ("berry") aneurysms
Arterial dissection
Moya moya syndrome
Vasculitis
Intracerebral tumors—primary and secondary

Hemodynamic
Hypertension
Acute increases in blood pressure/cerebral blood flow
Migraine

Hemostatic
Anticoagulants
Antiplatelet drugs
Thrombolysis
Leukemia
Thrombocytopenia
Hemophilia

Drug-related
Amphetamines
Cocaine
Alcohol

which bleeds are classically lobar, superficial, and multiple.[33] The mechanism of amyloid-related bleeds, their relation to classical "hypertensive" bleeds, and the contribution of amyloid angiopathy to cognitive decline in Alzheimer's disease are ill understood.

The most common cause of isolated, spontaneous subarachnoid hemorrhage is rupture of a berry aneurysm, about 85 percent of which in adults occur at proximal arterial bifurcations on the anterior circle of Willis.[34] Their aetiopathogenesis is disputed, but appears to involve acquired degenerative tunica media defects at arterial branch points, sometimes in genetically predisposed individuals.

Consequences of vessel rupture

Intracerebral hemorrhage is more often acutely fatal than ischemic stroke, due largely to its mass effect, and the consequent potential for raised intracranial pressure and reduced cerebral perfusion. Hematomas, however, tend to dissect and separate brain tissue, with relatively little direct parenchymal damage. Therefore, should the patient survive and the hematoma be cleared by phagocytic cells to leave a blood-stained slit-like cavity, the prognosis for recovery is potentially better than that for cerebral infarcts of similar size and location.

EPIDEMIOLOGY

An understanding of the distribution and determinants of stroke in populations is essential for health services planning and evaluation and for rational approaches to stroke prevention through risk factor reduction.

Since stroke comprises two major pathological mechanisms—hemorrhage and thrombosis—it is logical to examine the epidemiology of each type of stroke separately. However, it is not possible to distinguish accurately hemorrhagic from thrombotic stroke subtypes clinically or from routine sources of information,[5,35] although clinical diagnosis of specific subtypes of cerebral infarction may be reliable.[36] Consequently, most of the epidemiological information on stroke combines both hemorrhagic and thrombotic stroke, although the picture is dominated by the latter which predominates in most developed countries. With increased use of CT scanning in population-based stroke studies, it is becoming feasible to examine the distribution, risk factors, and natural history of subtypes of stroke.

Burden of stroke

Stroke is the third most common cause of death and the leading cause of severe disability in most of the developed world. In China there are about one million deaths per year attributed to stroke,[37] and worldwide each year approximately 44 million disability-adjusted life-years (DALYs) are lost because of stroke, of which only five million DALYs occur in countries with established market economies.[38] Given the rapid aging profile that is affecting most of the developing world, stroke will become an increasingly important cause of mortality and disability, and a high priority must be given to its prevention.[39]

In England and Wales, each year over 130,000 people suffer a first or recurrent stroke, and about 70,000 deaths are attributed to stroke, with the majority occurring in people over the age of 65. Although many people die rapidly from the stroke, there are about 300,000 stroke survivors living in the community, of whom one-half are unable to use public transport, one-quarter need help from a district nurse, and one-twentieth require long-term institutional care.[40]

Stroke is an expensive disease in terms of health services. In the United States it is estimated that $30 billion is spent each year,[41] and about 4–5 percent of total British National Health Service spending is on stroke.[42] However, direct health service costs (bed-days, investigations, treatments) account for only about half of total costs when loss of earnings and costs of family care-giving are considered.[43] Total lifetime costs are dominated by long-term care rather than acute hospital care costs,[44] although economic appraisals have tended to focus on the costs of acute care.

Projections of the future burden of stroke disability are difficult to make. While demographic trends will inevitably result in an increase in the number of strokes, it is possible that selective mortality of the most disabled and elderly survivors will lead to only modest increases in the number requiring institutional care.[45] However, case fatality is falling,[46] and possible increases in incidence, changes in the balance of care provided by public and private sources, and numbers of available family caregivers may make estimates of the future burden unreliable.

Variation in time, place, and person

Time trends

Stroke mortality rates have fallen over the twentieth century (Fig. 48-2), and the decline has been more rapid since the 1970s, with falls of 20–70 percent over two decades in many countries.[47] The abrupt rise in 1939/40 is probably due to coding changes associated with the introduction of the fourth revision of the International Classification of Diseases. However, the situation in central and eastern Europe and the former USSR shows an opposite trend, with mortality rates rising by 1–50 percent over the same time period.[48] The reason for the declining mortality trend in more affluent countries is not entirely clear,[49] as the study of secular variation in incidence is beset with problems of defining the population at risk, counting stroke events accurately, and variable presentation of data.[50]

The fall in mortality rates is thought to mirror a decline in stroke incidence,[51] although the decline in mortality might also be explained by a fall in case fatality and a stable incidence. During the 1980s the rates of decline in mortality and incidence appeared to be slowing, although case fatality was still declining.[46,52] The picture was complicated by differences in secular trends between countries, with some showing continued decline with a similar pattern for both hemorrhagic and thrombotic strokes.[53]

A recent Italian study reported continued declines in case fatality but no change in incidence rates between 1989 and 1997.[54] In Copenhagen, incidence has declined to 1993 but only among older (65+ years) men, whereas in other groups incidence has been unchanged since 1976.[55] In Finland, between 1986 and 1993 declines in incidence have been observed.[56]

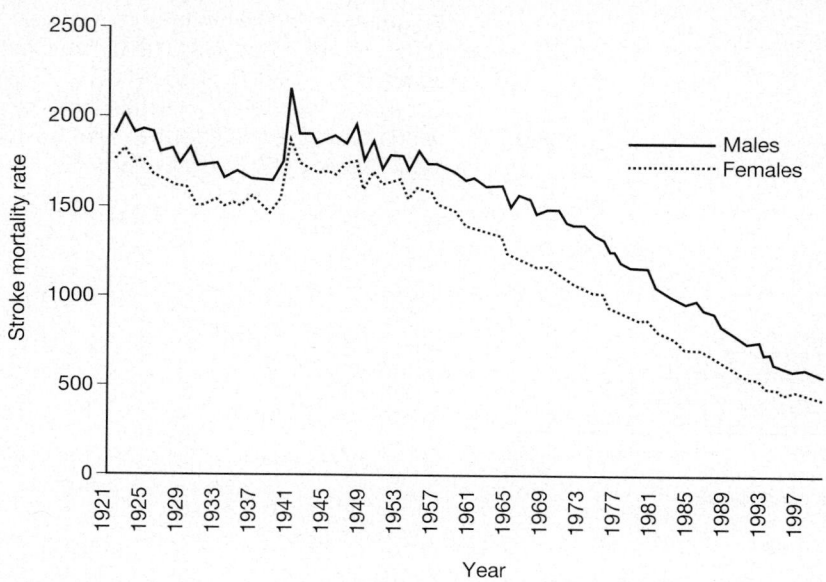

Figure 48-2 Secular trends in age standardized death rates per 100,000 from stroke for men and women 1921–1998, England and Wales. (Source: Health of Adult Britain, 1841–1994. London: Office of National Statistics, HMSO, 1997,[47] with permission.)

In Perth, Australia, repeated stroke incidence studies in 1985/6 and 1995/6 found a decline in incidence but no change in case fatality, suggesting that the decline in mortality was due to declining incidence only.[57]

Changes in major cardiovascular risk factors—blood pressure, smoking, and blood cholesterol—over the last few decades have occurred and may explain between one-third[58] and as much as two-thirds of the decline in stroke mortality.[59] In Japan, despite a rise in blood cholesterol levels from the 1960s to the 1980s, stroke rates have fallen dramatically.[60]

Better detection and treatment of high blood pressure is often put forward as an explanation for the declining risk of stroke.[61] However, in Australia and New Zealand, only marginal reductions in blood pressure have occurred, and it is estimated that only 10 percent of the decline in mortality among people younger than 70 years old can be attributed to treatment of high blood pressure.[62] In the United States better treatment does not seem to be the explanation.[63] Older people have also enjoyed a reduction in stroke mortality, despite less vigorous detection and treatment of high blood pressure than in younger people.

The divergent stroke mortality time trends in western and eastern European countries indicate that stroke risk is modifiable and therefore preventable. The higher prevalence of hypertension in Russia may be an explanation for the widening stroke risk in eastern and western Europe,[64] although alcohol consumption may also play a role.[65] The earlier concern that the era of declining mortality rates was coming to an end in affluent countries[52] may not be true for all countries. Mortality trends are determined both by incidence and by case fatality, and it is possible that changes in the ratio of hemorrhagic to thrombotic stroke, in addition to better medical care, and reductions in risk factors may play roles in influencing stroke incidence and case fatality to different degrees in different places and at different times.

Geographical trends

Stroke mortality varies by nine-fold among countries at ages 35–74 years, with the highest rates in the former USSR and Bulgaria and the lowest rates in the USA and Switzerland[48] (Fig. 48-3A and B). At older ages, variation between countries is not as marked, but the rank ordering of countries changes from that seen at ages 35–74 years, which may reflect diagnostic bias at older ages. Stroke incidence also shows considerable variation among countries, but there are major methodological problems in obtaining comparable data.[66] Mortality rates also vary within countries, with rates twice as high in the north of England as in the south,[67] higher in the north than the south of China,[68] and higher in the south of the USA.[69] Interestingly, people who migrate from areas of high mortality to low mortality acquire the low risk of the area to which they migrate,[70] suggesting that current environmental factors are more important determinants of risk than genetic or early-life factors.

Differences in stroke risk between and within countries demonstrate that stroke is preventable. Possible reasons for variation among populations include differences in the major risk factors (e.g. blood pressure, smoking), the underlying determinants of these risk factors or other unknown risk factors. One possible explanation is salt intake, which shows variations among countries[71] and accounts for some of the variation in population blood pressure distributions and may also contribute to secular trends in stroke risk. Vitamin C and potassium intake derived from fresh fruit and vegetables, which also varies between rich and poor countries and has changed over time, may also provide an explanation for differences in stroke risk both over time and from place to place.[72]

Individual risk factors

Variation in stroke risk between people is of major importance in guiding prevention policy and strategy. Risk factors can be classified as *inherent biological traits* such as genes, age, and gender, *physiological characteristics* such as blood pressure, *behaviors* such as smoking, *social characteristics* such as social class, and *environmental factors* such as temperature.[73] Prevention policy and practice vary depending on the strength of evidence implicating risk factors, their position in the causal chain, and the ease and cost with which they can be modified.

A

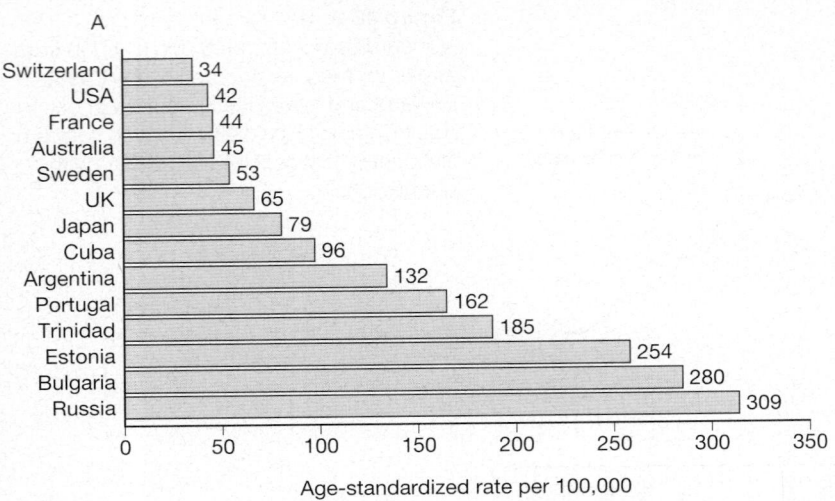

Figure 48-3 Stroke mortality in men aged (A) 35–74, (B) 75–84, circa 1990. (Source: adapted from Sarti C, Rastenyte D, Cepaitis Z, Tuomilehto J. International trends in mortality from stroke, 1968 to 1994. *Stroke* 2000;31:1588–1601.[48])

B

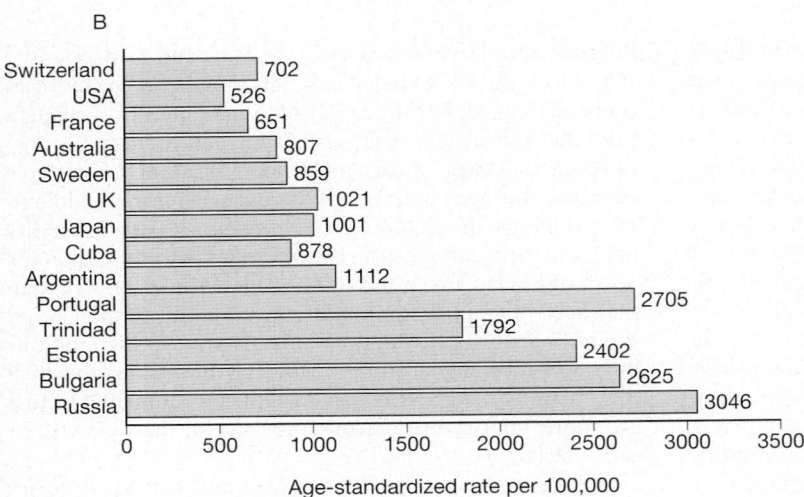

INHERENT BIOLOGICAL TRAITS

Age is the most important, but immutable, stroke risk factor, with an exponential increase in stroke mortality of 100-fold between the ages of 30–40 years and 80–90 years.[74] By the age of 85 years, one in four men and one in five women currently aged 45 can expect to suffer a stroke.[75] With increasing age the strength of association between some risk factors (e.g. blood pressure, smoking) and stroke tends to weaken, but because the absolute risk of stroke increases with age, the contribution of such risk factors remains important.[12,76]

People from different ethnic groups show variations in stroke mortality risk, with the highest rates in the UK among those born in the Caribbean.[77] The explanation for ethnic variation is not clear. In the United States, the excess risk of stroke among blacks compared with whites is associated with higher blood pressure levels, raised blood cholesterol, and diabetes mellitus.[78,79] In the UK, hypertension and diabetes are more prevalent among the black population but atrial fibrillation, excessive alcohol intake and smoking are less common.[80]

Stroke tends to run in families,[12,81] but with the exception of the cerebral autosomal dominant arteriopathy with subcortical infarcts and leucoencephalopathy (CADASIL) which is due to a mutation in the NOTCH:3 gene,[82] the genetic contribution to stroke is unclear. In a well-conducted Swedish twin registry with high levels of follow-up, similar concordance rates for stroke mortality in both monozygotic and dizygotic twins were found, suggesting that genetic factors are not important.[83] Greater concordance among monozygotic twins was found in a less well-designed US study.[84] Associations with apoE2 and apoE4,[85] with mitochondrial DNA mutations,[86] and with polymorphisms in the alpha(1)-antichymotrypsin gene[87] have been reported. Many such associations will represent type-I errors, therefore replication of such findings is required before they are accepted.

There is continued uncertainty about the relative contributions of genetic and environmental factors in stroke. Homocysteinemia is an interesting example of the way in which genetic inheritance can be modified by environmental factors. Homocysteinuria is an autosomal recessive inborn error of metabolism which, in addition to causing skeletal defects similar to those of Marfan's syndrome, is associated with increased risk of venous and arterial thrombosis. Heterozygous states are relatively common and may be associated with homocysteinemia, which is associated with increased risk of stroke.[88,89] Elevated homocysteine levels appear to be more strongly associated with large and small artery disease but not with embolic stroke.[90] As one of the common metabolic pathways affected in this condition is pyridoxine and folate dependent, dietary deficiency may lead to increased stroke risk,[91] possibly explaining the increased stroke risk with age. There is considerable interest in polymorphisms of the methyl-tetrahydrofolate reductase gene which regulates homocysteine levels.[92,93] Treatment with pyridoxine, B$_{12}$, and/or folate reduces homocysteinemia in heterozygotes,[91,94] but the effects on stroke risk are not yet known.

PHYSIOLOGICAL CHARACTERISTICS Raised blood pressure has been recognized for many years as an important stroke risk factor.[95] This observation has been confirmed in different parts of the world, and the association remains strong even at older ages.[76] Pharmacological reduction of blood pressure is associated with reduced risk of stroke even at ages up to 80 years.[96] The relationship between blood pressure and stroke is stronger for systolic than for diastolic blood pressure and is a graded response with no threshold of increased risk of stroke.[97,98] Consequently, clinical thresholds for diagnosis of hypertension are somewhat arbitrary, although there is a consensus that pressures over 160/95 require monitoring and treatment. More recent World Health Organization–International Hypertension Society guidelines[99] and British Hypertension Society guidelines[100] have proposed much lower levels of 140/90 which would have profound workload implications if implemented.

Blood cholesterol is not related to risk of stroke of undefined type in many populations.[76,101] However, it is most likely that this lack of association hides a positive relationship with ischemic stroke[102,103] and an inverse relationship with hemorrhagic stroke.[104] In trials of pharmacological cholesterol lowering with statins, reductions in stroke risk have been found, suggesting that the relationship with ischemic stroke is causal.[105]

SMOKING Smoking is of much greater importance than was initially thought,[106] and several studies have confirmed this.[107,108] Cessation of smoking is associated with a rapid reduction in stroke risk.[109] Although forced expiratory volume (FEV$_1$) is reduced by smoking, poorer lung function is associated with increased risk of stroke, independently of smoking habit.[110,111] Smoking interacts with high blood pressure, which is of great clinical importance in identifying those at high risk,[112] resulting in a 12-fold increased stroke risk among people who are both hypertensive and smoke.[113]

DIET Fruit and vegetable consumption,[114] vitamin C intake,[115] and dietary potassium[116] are associated with stroke, highlighting the possible role of antioxidant mechanisms. However, intervention trials of supplementation with antioxidant vitamins have failed to demonstrate clear reductions in stroke risk,[117] suggesting that associations found in observational studies represent the influence of uncontrolled confounding.[118] Fish consumption has also been reported to protect against stroke in observational studies,[119,120] although this has not been confirmed in all studies.[121,122] Eating whole grains has been reported to reduce risk of stroke,[123] but confirmation is awaited.

EARLY LIFE AND LIFE COURSE EXPOSURES Low birth weight, poor intrauterine growth and markers of maternal health are associated with increased risk of stroke and ischemic heart disease.[124–126] However, it has been postulated that these associations are due to confounding between socioeconomic status, health in early life, and risk of cardiovascular disease in adulthood. Evidence demonstrating relationships between intrauterine growth and cardiovascular risk factors—blood pressure and fibrinogen—suggests that the association between birthweight and stroke is biologically plausible.[127,128] However, a growing body of work has shown that intrauterine growth is only one factor operating early in life that has an influence on future risk of stroke. Growth in childhood and adult social class both modify the association between birthweight and stroke.[129] Adult height, a marker of childhood growth, is associated with ischemic stroke.[130] Surprisingly, a "reverse causality" has been demonstrated—birthweight of *offspring* is inversely associated with *parental* risk of cardiovascular death, suggesting that some factor, probably genetic, operating across generations is responsible for birthweight–cardiovascular disease associations.[131] Furthermore, it has been shown that social factors operating across the life course are associated with adult disease to different extents.[132] These new observations make it unlikely that the relationship between intrauterine growth and adult disease is simple or direct.

OTHER FACTORS Past history of ischemic heart disease and heart failure,[133] atrial fibrillation,[134,135] diabetes mellitus,[136] and intermittent claudication[137] are all associated with increased risk of stroke. Carotid artery intima-medial thickness is a marker of atherosclerosis and is associated with several cardiovascular risk factors,[138] and in prospective studies, is predictive of stroke events.[139]

Large-scale prospective studies have confirmed the importance of age, raised blood pressure, smoking, past cardiovascular disease, and diabetes mellitus as major determinants of stroke risk.[76,113,140,141] Risk factors for stroke are summarized in Table 48-4.

RISK FACTORS FOR STROKE SUBTYPES Several studies have examined the etiology of hemorrhagic and occlusive stroke subtypes. In general, raised blood pressure,[141,192–194] smoking,[163,165,193–196] and alcohol consumption[193,194,197–198] are associated with both hemorrhagic and occlusive stroke. Diabetes mellitus is not associated with hemorrhagic stroke.[137,199] Atrial fibrillation is associated with risk of cortical but not lacunar[200] or primary hemorrhagic stroke.[201] Minor ischemic stroke, lacunar stroke, and TIA have many risk factors in common.[200,202]

PREVENTION

The World Health Organization has promoted community-based stroke prevention and hypertension control for

Table 48-4 Stroke risk factors

Factor	Relative risk[a]
Inherent traits	
Genetic:	
Homocysteinemia	3–4[88,89]
Family history	2–3[142,143]
Monozygotic twin	1–5[83,84]
Age (55–64 vs 75)	5[113,144]
Race (black vs white American)	1.4[78,145,146]
Physiological characteristics	
High blood pressure	3[97,113]
Orthostatic hypotension (>20 mmHg systolic)	2[147]
Low forced expiratory volume	2[110]
Blood cholesterol (SD change)	1.12 ischemic, 0.76 hemorrhagic[148;149]
HDL-cholesterol	0.7[102,103]
Lp (a)	—[150]
Raised fibrinogen	—[151]
C-reactive protein	2[152]
Raised hematocrit	—[153]
Endogenous tissue plasminogenactivator	3.5[154,155]
Insulin resistance syndrome	1.6[156]
Obesity	1–2[157,158]
Snoring	2[159;160]
Behaviors	
Alcohol consumption (30 units/wk)	2.5–4[113, 80,161–164]
Smoking	2[107,113,165]
Low dietary vitamin C	1.5[115,166–168]
Low dietary potassium	2–5[116,169,170]
Exercise	0.3–0.5[171–173]
Life events (e.g., bereavement, loss of job)	2[174]
Hormone replacement therapy	0.5–2[175]
Oral contraceptive current use	2–3[175]
Environmental factors	
Low temperature	—[176–178]
Air pollution	—[179;180]
Social characteristics	
Lower social class	1.8[67,181,182]
Other factors	
Early-life environment and maternal nutrition	—[124–126,129,183]
Helicobacter infection	2[184]
Comorbid conditions:	
Heart failure	5[133]
Atrial fibrillation	5–7[134,135]
Carotid bruit	1–2[185,186]
TIA	7[187]
Diabetes mellitus	2–3[136,188,189]
Infection	5[184,190]
Warfarin treatment	7–10[191]

[a]Relative risk estimates for continuous variables are generally lowest compared with the highest quintiles of distributions. No estimate is given when the publication did not calculate a relative risk.

many years.[203] In England, a decade ago the Health of the Nation policy[204] set a goal of 40 percent reduction in mortality from stroke over 10 years. While this target was considered unambitious given the secular trends observed in the past, rather lower average annual declines have occurred, around 3.1 percent for men and 2.7 percent for women (see Fig. 48-2). More recent preventive health policy has again focused on stroke, emphasizing social inequalities in, and the control of, major risk factors.[205] Reducing disease and risk factor exposure is not solely the work of health services but requires much wider collaboration, both within central government and also at more local levels. Despite strong evidence that older people stand to benefit as much in relative terms, and more in absolute terms, from primary and secondary prevention, both the earlier and current Health of the Nation policies have failed to focus on those aged 75 years and over who are at greatest risk of stroke, reflecting the widespread agism in society.

High-risk approach

Identification of people at high risk of stroke is an essential step in primary prevention. An efficient stroke risk score has been developed[112] comprising age, systolic blood pressure, smoking, and presence of anginal symptoms. The score derived from these risk factors can be used to identify individuals who will subsequently suffer a stroke. Those in the highest quintile (fifth) of the score distribution suffer 80 percent of strokes occurring over a period of 5 years. Use of such a scoring system in primary care would reduce the amount of work required in identifying and targeting preventive strategies such as antihypertensive treatment, use of antiplatelet agents, and antismoking advice. The costs of primary prevention must also be considered, and vary markedly depending on the risk of the patients to be treated, the costs of treatment and discounting assumptions made. For example, cost-effectiveness of blood pressure detection and treatment may range from £500 (diuretic, woman aged 60 years, and undiscounted) to £21,000 (ACE inhibitor, woman aged 40, and discounted at 5 percent per year) per DALY gained.[206]

While use of aspirin for secondary prevention in those with established cardiovascular disease, smoking cessation advice, and cholesterol lowering with statins all fall within a cost per life-year gained considered reasonable (i.e., below £10,000 per life-year gained), carotid endarterectomy costs range from £16,000 to £86,000 per life-year gained depending on the assumptions made. Attempts to more accurately predict who among those with severe carotid stenosis are at greatest risk of suffering a stroke hold the promise of making endarterectomy a more cost-effective option.[207,208]

Population approach

Lowering the population distribution of a risk factor not only reduces the level of stroke but will also result in a reduction in the proportion of high-risk individuals.[209] Lowering a population's level of salt intake through reducing hidden salt in processed foods and alcohol consumption through increased taxation might be expected to result in lower blood pressure distributions,[71] although there is doubt about the size of the reduction that could be achieved.[210] Whether such changes can be achieved in practice depends largely on political will rather than scientific evidence. Repeated surveys show that, for example, the blood pressure distribution of the population is indeed falling,[211] but whether this can be claimed as a success for public health is not known.

Reduction in smoking and increase in physical activity are both measures that are of general importance in the control of stroke and other diseases. There is no doubt that population approaches through public health campaigns restricting smoking in the workplace, the sale of tobacco to children, and steady increases in tobacco taxation have had a population impact in shifting the levels of smoking in many countries downwards, and have strengthened the resolve of governments to review tobacco policy.[212] Similar public health campaigns focused on physical activity are urgently required. Evidence to support population approaches to prevention is sparse compared with that available to underpin pharmacological high-risk preventive treatments.[213,214]

KEY POINTS Stroke: pathology and epidemiology

■ Stroke is caused by two major pathological processes—hemorrhage and infarction—which have different causes and natural history.

■ Stroke is a common cause of death and the leading cause of severe disability, resulting in the loss of 44 million disability adjusted life-years worldwide and costs of 4–5 percent of National Health Service spending.

■ Stroke mortality, incidence and case-fatality have fallen dramatically over the course of the twentieth century in many developed countries, although rates have increased in central and eastern European countries.

■ Stroke mortality rates vary up to nine-fold between countries and some of this variation is due to differences in major risk factors.

■ Secular trends and geographical variation indicate that much of the burden of stroke can be prevented and is not genetically determined.

■ Individual susceptibility to stroke is largely explained by major risk factors—age, blood pressure, smoking, coexisting cardiovascular disease—but high dietary intake of fruit and vegetables and physical activity may be protective.

■ Prevention of stroke requires both modifying risk factors in those in the upper distribution of risk (i.e., the high risk strategy), and also attempts to lower the whole population distribution of risk factors (i.e., the population strategy).

REFERENCES

1. World Health Organization: Cerebrovascular disease: a clinical and research classification. Offset Series No 43. WHO, Geneva, 1978
2. O'Mahony PG, Dobson R, Rodgers H, James OF, Thomson RG: Validation of a population screening questionnaire to assess prevalence of stroke. Stroke 1995;26:1334–1337
3. National Institute of Neurological Disorders and Stroke: Classification of cerebrovascular disease III. Stroke 1990;21:637–676
4. Bamford J: Clinical examination in diagnosis and subclassification of stroke. Lancet 1992;339:400–402
5. Celani MG, Righetti E, Migliacci R et al: Comparability and validity of two clinical scores in the early differential diagnosis of acute stroke. Br Med J 1994;308:1674–1676
6. Poungvarin N, Viriyavejakul A, Komontri C: Siriraj stroke score and validation study to distinguish supratentorial intracerebral haemorrhage from infarction. Br Med J 1991;302:1565–1567
7. Sandercock P, Molyneux A, Warlow C: Value of computed tomography in patients with stroke: Oxfordshire Community Stroke Project. Br Med J 1985;290:193–197
8. Foulkes MA, Wolf PA, Price TR, Mohr JP, Hier DB: The Stroke Data Bank: design, methods, and baseline characteristics. Stroke 1988;19:547–554

9. Bamford J, Sandercock P, Jones L, Warlow C: The natural history of lacunar infarction: the Oxfordshire Community Stroke Project. Stroke 1987;18:545–551

10. Bamford J, Sandercock P, Dennis M, Burn J, Warlow C: Classification and natural history of clinically identifiable subtypes of cerebral infarction. Lancet 1991;337:1521–1526

11. Anonymous. Uncommon causes of stroke. Lancet 1989;1:26

12. Ebrahim S, Harwood RH: Stroke. Epidemiology, Evidence and Clinical Practice. OUP, Oxford, 1999

13. Lammie GA, Sandercock PA, Dennis MS: Recently occluded intracranial and extracranial carotid arteries. Relevance of the unstable atherosclerotic plaque. Stroke 1999;30:1319–1325

14. Davies MJ: Pathophysiology of acute coronary syndromes. Indian Heart J 2000;52:473–479

15. Pullicino PM: Pathogenesis of lacunar infarcts and small deep infarcts. In Pullicino PM, Caplan LR, Hommel M (eds): Advances in Neurology. Raven Press, New York, 1993:125–140

16. Fisher CM: Lacunar infarcts—a review. Cerebrovasc Dis 1991;1:311–320

17. Lammie GA: Pathology of small vessel stroke. Br Med Bull 2000;56:296–306

18. Mas JL, Meder JF: Cerebral venous thrombosis. In Ginsberg MD, Bogousslavsky J (eds): Cerebrovascular Disease. Blackwell Science, Oxford, 1998:1487–1501

19. Fisher CM, Adams RD: Observations on brain embolism with special reference to the mechanism of haemorrhagic infarction. J Neuropathol Exp Neurol 1951;10:92–94

20. Caplan LR: Intracerebral haemorrhage revisited. Neurology 1988;38:624–627

21. Adams JH, Brierley JB, Connor RC, Treip CS: The effects of systemic hypotension upon the human brain. Clinical and neuropathological observations in 11 cases. Brain 1966;89:235–268

22. Pulsinelli WA, Brierley JB, Plum F: Temporal profile of neuronal damage in a model of transient forebrain ischemia. Ann Neurol 1982;11:491–498

23. Garcia JH: The evolution of brain infarcts. A review. J Neuropathol Exp Neurol 1992;51:387–393

24. Garcia JH, Lassen NA, Weiller C, Sperling B, Nakagawara J: Ischemic stroke and incomplete infarction. Stroke 1996;27:761–765

25. Garcia JH, Mitchem HL, Briggs L et al: Transient focal ischemia in subhuman primates. Neuronal injury as a function of local cerebral blood flow. J Neuropathol Exp Neurol 1983;42:44–60

26. Kirino T, Tamura A, Sano K: Delayed neuronal death in the rat hippocampus following transient forebrain ischemia. Acta Neuropathol (Berl) 1984;64:139–147

27. Heiss WD, Rosner G: Functional recovery of cortical neurons as related to degree and duration of ischemia. Ann Neurol 1983;14:294–301

28. Heiss WD, Graf R: The ischemic penumbra. Curr Opin Neurol 1994;7:11–19

29. Lee JM, Zipfel GJ, Choi DW: The changing landscape of ischaemic brain injury mechanisms. Nature 1999;399:A7–14

30. MacKenzie JM: Intracerebral haemorrhage. J Clin Pathol 1996;49:360–364

31. Fisher CM: Pathological observations in hypertensive cerebral haemorrhage. J Neuropathol Exp Neurol 1971;30:536–550

32. Rosenblum WI: The importance of fibrinoid necrosis as the cause of cerebral hemorrhage in hypertension. Commentary. J Neuropathol Exp Neurol 1993;52:11–13

33. Vinters HV: Cerebral amyloid angiopathy. A critical review. Stroke 1987;18:311–324

34. Weller RO: Subarachnoid haemorrhage and myths about saccular aneurysms. J Clin Pathol 1995;48:1078–1081

35. Hawkins GC, Bonita R, Broad JB, Anderson NE: Inadequacy of clinical scoring systems to differentiate stroke subtypes in population-based studies. Stroke 1995;26:1338–1342

36. Lindley RI, Warlow CP, Wardlaw JM et al: Interobserver reliability of a clinical classification of acute cerebral infarction. Stroke 1993;24:1801–1804

37. Bonita R, Beaglehole R, Asplund K: The worldwide problem of stroke. Curr Opin Neurol 1994;7:5–10

38. World Bank: Investing in Health. World Development Report 1993. Oxford University Press, Oxford, 1993

39. Pearson TA, Jamison DT, Trejo-Gutierrez J: Cardiovascular disease. In Jamison DT, Mosley WH, Measham AR, Bobadilla JL (eds): Disease Control Priorities in Developing Countries. Oxford University Press, Oxford, 1993

40. Wade DT: Stroke (acute cerebrovascular disease). In Stevens A, Raftery J (eds): Health Care Needs Assessment, Volume 1. Ratcliffe Medical Press, Oxford, 1994

41. Gorelick PB: Stroke prevention. Arch Neurol 1995;52:347–355

42. Isard PA, Forbes JF: Cost of stroke to the National Health Service in Scotland. Cerebrovasc Dis 1992;2:47–50

43. Adelman SM: National Survey of Stroke. Economic impact. Stroke 1981;12 (suppl 1):I-69–I-87

44. Bergman L, van der Meulen JH, Limburg M, Habbema JD: Costs of medical care after first-ever stroke in The Netherlands. Stroke 1995;26:1830–1836

45. Malmgren R, Bamford J, Warlow C, Sandercock P, Slattery J: Projecting the number of patients with first ever strokes and patients newly handicapped by stroke in England and Wales. Br Med J 1989;298:656–660

46. Bonita R, Broad JB, Beaglehole R: Changes in stroke incidence and case-fatality in Auckland, New Zealand, 1981–91. Lancet 1993;342:1470–1473

47. Charlton J, Murphy M, Khaw KT, Ebrahim S, Davey Smith G: Cardiovascular diseases. In Murphy M, Charlton J (eds): Health of Adult Britain, 1841–1994. Office of National Statistics, HMSO, London, 1997:60–81

48. Sarti C, Rastenyte D, Cepaitis Z, Tuomilehto J: International trends in mortality from stroke, 1968 to 1994. Stroke 2000;31:1588–1601

49. Bonita R, Beaglehole R: Explaining stroke mortality trends. Lancet 1993;341:1510–1511

50. Malmgren R, Warlow C, Bamford J, Sandercock P: Geographical and secular trends in stroke incidence. Lancet 1987;2:1196–1200

51. Garraway WM, Whisnant JP, Furlan AJ, Phillips LH, Kurland LT, O'Fallon WM: The declining incidence of stroke. N Engl J Med 1979;300:449–452

52. Broderick JP, Phillips SJ, Whisnant JP, O'Fallon WM, Bergstralh EJ: Incidence rates of stroke in the eighties: the end of the decline in stroke? Stroke 1989;20:577–582

53. Kagan A, Popper J, Reed DM, Maclean CJ, Grove JS: Trends in stroke incidence and mortality in Hawaiian Japanese men. Stroke 1994;25:1170–1175

54. D'Alessandro G, Bottacchi E, Di Giovanni M et al: Temporal trends of stroke in Valle d'Aosta, Italy. Incidence and 30-day fatality rates. Neurol Sci 2000;21:13–18

55. Truelsen T, Prescott E, Gronbaek M, Schnohr P, Boysen G: Trends in stroke incidence. The Copenhagen City Heart Study. Stroke 1997;28:1903–1907

56. Fogelholm R, Murros K, Rissanen A, Ilmavirta M: Decreasing incidence of stroke in central Finland, 1985–1993. Acta Neurol Scand 1997;95:38–43

57. Jamrozik K, Broadhurst RJ, Lai N et al: Trends in the incidence, severity, and short-term outcome of stroke in Perth, Western Australia. Stroke 1999;30:2105–2111

58. Tuomilehto J, Bonita R, Stewart A, Nissinen A, Salonen JT: Hypertension, cigarette smoking, and the decline in stroke incidence in eastern Finland. Stroke 1991;22:7–11

59. Vartiainen E, Sarti C, Tuomilehto J, Kuulasmaa K: Do changes in cardio-vascular risk factors explain changes in mortality from stroke in Finland? Br Med J 1995;310:901–904

60. Shimamoto T, Komachi Y, Inada H et al: Trends for coronary heart disease and stroke and their risk factors in Japan. Circulation 1989;79:503–515

61. Garraway WM, Whisnant JP: The changing pattern of hypertension and the declining incidence of stroke. JAMA 1987;258:214–217

62. Bonita R, Beaglehole R: Does treatment of hypertension explain the decline in mortality from stroke? Br Med J 1986;292:191–192

63. Casper M, Wing S, Strogatz D, Davis CE, Tyroler HA: Antihypertensive treatment and US trends in stroke mortality, 1962 to 1980. Am J Pub Health 1992;82:1600–1606

64. Stegmayr B, Vinogradova T, Malyutina S et al: Widening gap of stroke between east and west. Eight-year trends in occurrence and risk factors in Russia and Sweden. Stroke 2000;31:2–8

65. Leon DA, Chenet L, Shkolnikov VM et al: Huge variation in Russian mortality rates 1984–94: artefact, alcohol, or what? Lancet 1997;350:383–388

66. Sudlow CL, Warlow CP: Comparable studies of the incidence of stroke and its pathological types: results from an international collaboration. International Stroke Incidence Collaboration. Stroke 1997;28:491–499

67. Acheson RM, Sanderson C: Strokes: social class and geography. Popul Trends 1978;12:13–17

68. Li SC, Schoenberg BS, Wang CC et al: Cerebrovascular disease in the People's Republic of China: epidemiologic and clinical features. Neurology 1985;35:1708–1713

69. Obisesan TO, Vargas CM, Gillum RF: Geographic variation in stroke risk in the United States. Region, urbanization, and hypertension in the Third National Health and Nutrition Examination Survey. Stroke 2000;31:19–25

70. Syme SL, Marmot MG, Kagan A, Rhoads G: Epidemiological studies of coronary heart disease and stroke in Japanese men living in Japan, Hawaii, and California. Introduction. Am J Epidemiol 1975;102:477–480

71. Elliott P, Stamler J, Nichols R et al: Intersalt revisited: further analyses of 24 hour sodium excretion and blood pressure within and across populations. Intersalt Cooperative Research Group. Br Med J 1996;312:1249–1253

72. Gillman MW, Cupples LA, Gagnon D et al: Protective effect of fruits and vegetables on development of stroke in men. JAMA 1995;273:1113–1117

73. Marmot MG, Poulter NR: Primary prevention of stroke. Lancet 1992;339:344–347

74. Bamford J, Sandercock P, Dennis M et al: A prospective study of acute cerebrovascular disease in the community: the Oxfordshire Community Stroke Project 1981–86. 1. Methodology, demography and incident cases of first-ever stroke. J Neurol Neurosurg Psych 1988;51:1373–1380

75. Bonita R: Epidemiology of stroke. Lancet 1992;339:342–344

76. Prospective Studies Collaboration. Cholesterol, diastolic blood pressure, and stroke: 13,000 strokes in 450,000 people in 45 prospective cohorts. Lancet 1995;346:1647–1653

77. Balarajan R: Ethnic differences in mortality from ischaemic heart disease and cerebrovascular disease in England and Wales. Br Med J 1991;302:560–564

78. Kittner SJ, White LR, Losonczy KG, Wolf PA, Hebel JR: Black-white differences in stroke incidence in a national sample. The contribution of hypertension and diabetes mellitus. JAMA 1990;264:1267–1270

79. Sacco RL, Kargman DE, Gu Q, Zamanillo MC: Race-ethnicity and determinants of intracranial atherosclerotic cerebral infarction. The Northern Manhattan Stroke Study. Stroke 1995;26:14–20

80. Hajat C, Dundas R, Stewart JA et al: Cerebrovascular risk factors and stroke subtypes: differences between ethnic groups. Stroke (Online) 2001;32:37–42

81. Wannamethee SG, Shaper AG, Ebrahim S: History of parental death from stroke or heart trouble and the risk of stroke in middle-aged men. Stroke 1996;27:1492–1498

82. Hassan A, Markus HS: Genetics and ischaemic stroke. Brain 2000;123:1784–1812

83. de Faire U, Friberg L, Lundman T: Concordance for mortality with special reference to ischaemic heart disease and cerebrovascular disease. Prevent Med 1975;4:509–517

84. Brass LM, Isaacsohn JL, Merikangas KR, Robinette CD: A study of twins and stroke. Stroke 1992;23:221–223

85. Kokubo Y, Chowdhury AH, Date C et al: Age-dependent association of apolipoprotein E genotypes with stroke subtypes in a Japanese rural population. Stroke 2000;31:1299–1306

86. Pulkes T, Sweeney MG, Hanna MG: Increased risk of stroke in patients with the A12308G polymorphism in mitochondria. Lancet 2000;356:2068–2069

87. Vila N, Obach V, Revilla M, Oliva R, Chamorro A: Alpha(1)-antichymotrypsin gene polymorphism in patients with stroke. Stroke (Online) 2000;31:2103–2105

88. Perry IJ, Refsum H, Morris RW et al: Prospective study of serum total homocysteine concentration and risk of stroke in middle-aged British men. Lancet 1995;346:1395–1398

89. Iler J, Nielsen GM, Tvedegaard KC et al: A meta-analysis of cerebrovascular disease and hyperhomocysteinaemia. Scand J Clin Lab Invest 2000;60:491–499

90. Eikelboom JW, Hankey GJ, Anand SS et al: Association between high homocyst(e)ine and ischemic stroke due to large- and small-artery disease but not other etiologic subtypes of ischemic stroke. Stroke 2000;31:1069–1075

91. Mason JB, Miller JW: The effects of vitamins B12, B6, and folate on blood homocysteine levels. Ann NY Acad Sci 1992;669:197–203

92. Markus HS, Ali N, Swaminathan R et al: A common polymorphism in the methylenetetrahydrofolate reductase gene, homocysteine, and ischemic cerebrovascular disease. Stroke 1997;28:1739–1743

93. Dekou V, Whincup P, Papacosta O et al: The effect of the C677T and A1298C polymorphisms in the methylenetetrahydrofolate reductase gene on homocysteine levels in elderly men and women from the British regional heart study. Atherosclerosis 2001;154:659–666

94. Homocysteine Lowering Trialists Collaboration: Lowering blood homocysteine with folic acid based supplements. Meta-analysis of randomised trials. Br Med J 1998;316:894–898

95. Kannel WB, Wolf PA, Verter J, McNamara PM: Epidemiologic assessment of the role of blood pressure in stroke. The Framingham study. JAMA 1970;214:301–310

96. Mulrow CD, Cornell JA, Herrera CR: Hypertension in the elderly: implications and generalisability of randomized trials. JAMA 1995;272:1932–1938

97. MacMahon S, Peto R, Cutler J et al: Blood pressure, stroke, and coronary heart disease. Part 1, Prolonged differences in blood pressure: prospective observational studies corrected for the regression dilution bias. Lancet 1990;335:765–774

98. Ni MC, Rodgers A, MacMahon S: The associations of diastolic blood pressure with the risk of stroke in Western and Eastern populations. Clin Exp Hypertens (NY) 1999;21:531–542

99. World Health Organization–International Society of Hypertension. Guidelines Subcommittee: World Health Organization–International Society of Hypertension guidelines for the management of hypertension. J Hypertens 1999;17:151–183

100. Ramsay LE, Williams B, Johnston GD et al: British Hypertension Society guidelines for hypertension management: summary. Br Med J 1999;319:630–635

101. Chen Z, Peto R, Collins R et al: Serum cholesterol concentration and coronary heart disease in population with low cholesterol concentrations. Br Med J 1991;303:276–282

102. Wannamethee SG, Shaper AG, Ebrahim S: HDL-Cholesterol, total cholesterol, and the risk of stroke in middle-aged British men. Stroke 2000;31:1882–1888

103. McCarron P, Greenwood R, Elwood P et al: The incidence and aetiology of stroke in the Caerphilly and Speedwell Collaborative Studies II: risk factors for ischaemic stroke. Pub Health 2001;115:12–20

104. Neaton JD, Blackburn H, Jacobs D et al: Serum cholesterol level and mortality findings for men screened in the Multiple Risk Factor Intervention Trial. Multiple Risk Factor Intervention Trial Research Group. Arch Int Med 1992;152:1490–1500

105. Ebrahim S, Smith GD, McCabe C et al: What role for statins? A review and economic model. Health Technol Assess 1999;3:i–91

106. Dawber, TR: The Framingham Study. Harvard University Press, London, 1980

107. Shinton R, Beevers G: Meta-analysis of relation between cigarette smoking and stroke. Br Med J 1989;298:789–794

108. Hart CL, Hole DJ, Smith GD: Risk factors and 20-year stroke mortality in men and women in the Renfrew/Paisley study in Scotland. Stroke 1999;30:1999–2007

109. Wannamethee SG, Shaper AG, Whincup PH, Walker M: Smoking cessation and the risk of stroke in middle-aged men. JAMA 1995;274:155–160

110. Wannamethee SG, Shaper AG, Ebrahim S: Respiratory function and risk of stroke. Stroke 1995;26:2004–2010

111. Dow L, Ebrahim S: Commentary: Lung function and risk of fatal and non-fatal stroke—The Copenhagen City Heart Study. Int J Epidemiol 2001;30:152–153

112. Coppola WG, Whincup PH, Papacosta O, Walker M, Ebrahim S: Scoring system to identify men at high risk of stroke: a strategy for general practice. Br J Gen Pract 1995;45:185–189

113. Shaper AG, Phillips AN, Pocock SJ, Walker M, Macfarlane PW: Risk factors for stroke in middle aged British men. Br Med J 1991;302:1111–1115

114. Ness AR, Powles JW: The role of diet, fruit and vegetables and antioxidants in the aetiology of stroke. J Cardiovasc Risk 1999;6:229–234

115. Daviglus ML, Orencia AJ, Dyer AR et al: Dietary vitamin C, beta-carotene and 30-year risk of stroke: results from the Western Electric Study. Neuroepidemiology 1997;16:69–77

116. Khaw KT, Barrett-Connor E: Dietary potassium and stroke-associated mortality. A 12-year prospective population study. N Engl J Med 1987;316:235–240

117. Leppala JM, Virtamo J, Fogelholm R et al: Controlled trial of alpha-tocopherol and beta-carotene supplements on stroke incidence and mortality in male smokers. Arterioscler Thromb Vasc Biol 2000;20:230–235

118. Egger M, Schneider M, Davey Smith G: Spurious precision? Meta-analysis of observational studies. Br Med J 1998;316:140–144

119. Keli SO, Feskens EJ, Kromhout D: Fish consumption and risk of stroke. The Zutphen Study. Stroke 1994;25:328–332

120. Morris MC, Manson JE, Rosner B et al: Fish consumption and cardiovascular disease in the physicians' health study: a prospective study. Am J Epidemiol 1995;142:166–175

121. Orencia AJ, Daviglus ML, Dyer AR, Shekelle RB, Stamler J: Fish consumption and stroke in men. 30-year findings of the Chicago Western Electric Study. Stroke 1996;27:204–209

122. Gillum RF, Mussolino ME, Madans JH: The relationship between fish consumption and stroke incidence. The NHANES 1 Epidemiologic Follow-up Study (National Health and Nutrition Examination Survey). Arch Int Med 1996;156:537–542

123. Liu S, Manson JE, Stampfer MJ et al: Whole grain consumption and risk of ischemic stroke in women: A prospective study. JAMA 2000;284:1534–1540

124. Barker DJ, Osmond C: Death rates from stroke in England and Wales predicted from past maternal mortality. Br Med J 1987;294:83–86

125. Rich-Edwards JW, Stampfer MJ, Manson JE et al: Birth weight and risk of cardiovascular disease in a cohort of women followed up since 1976. Br Med J 1997;315:396–400

126. Martyn CN, Barker DJ, Osmond C: Mothers' pelvic size, fetal growth, and death from stroke and coronary heart disease in men in the UK. Lancet 1996;348:1264–1268

127. Taylor SJ, Whincup PH, Cook DG, Papacosta O, Walker M: Size at birth and blood pressure: cross sectional study in 8–11 year old children. Br Med J 1997;314:475–480

128. Leon DA, Koupilova I, Lithell HO et al: Failure to realise growth potential in utero and adult obesity in relation to blood pressure in 50 year old Swedish men. Br Med J 1996;312:401–406

129. Eriksson JG, Forsen T, Tuomilehto J, Osmond C, Barker DJ: Early growth, adult income, and risk of stroke. Stroke 2000;31:869–874

130. McCarron P, Greenwood R, Davey Smith G, Ebrahim S, Elwood P: Adult height is inversely associated with ischaemic stroke. The Caerphilly and Speedwell Collaborative Studies. J Epidemiol Commun Health 2000;54:239

131. Davey Smith G, Hart C, Ferrell C et al: Birth weight of offspring and mortality in the Renfrew and Paisley study: prospective observational study. Br Med J 1997;315:1189–1193

132. Davey Smith G, Hart C, Blane D, Gillis C, Hawthorne V: Lifetime socioeconomic position and mortality: prospective observational study. Br Med J 1997;314:547–552

133. Kannel WB, Wolf PA, Verter J: Manifestations of coronary disease predisposing to stroke. The Framingham study. JAMA 1983;2942–2946

134. Flegel KM, Shipley MJ, Rose G: Risk of stroke in non-rheumatic atrial fibrillation. Lancet 1987;1:526–529

135. Wolf PA, Abbott RD, Kannel WB: Atrial fibrillation as an independent risk factor for stroke: the Framingham Study. Stroke 1991;22:983–988

136. Tuomilehto J, Rastenyte D, Jousilahti P, Sarti C, Vartiainen E: Diabetes mellitus as a risk factor for death from stroke. Prospective study of the middle-aged Finnish population. Stroke 1996;27:210–215

137. Jamrozik K, Broadhurst RJ, Anderson CS, Stewart-Wynne EG: The role of lifestyle factors in the etiology of stroke. A population-based case-control study in Perth, Western Australia. Stroke 1994;25:51–59

138. Ebrahim S, Papacosta O, Whincup P et al: Carotid plaque, intima media thickness, cardiovascular risk factors, and prevalent cardiovascular disease in men and women: the British Regional Heart Study. Stroke 1999;30:841–850

139. Chambless LE, Folsom AR, Clegg LX et al: Carotid wall thickness is predictive of incident clinical stroke: the Atherosclerosis Risk in Communities (ARIC) study. Am J Epidemiol 2000;151:478–487

140. Wolf PA, D'Agostino RB, Belanger AJ, Kannel WB: Probability of stroke: a risk profile from the Framingham Study. Stroke 1991;22:312–318

141. Harmsen P, Rosengren A, Tsipogianni A, Wilhelmsen L: Risk factors for stroke in middle-aged men in Goteborg, Sweden. Stroke 1990;21:223–229

142. Wannamethee G, Shaper AG, Ebrahim S: History of paternal death from stroke or heart trouble and risk of stroke in middle-aged men. Stroke 1996;27:1492–1498

143. Jousilahti P, Rastenyte D, Tuomilehto J, Sarti C, Vartiainen E: Parental history of cardiovascular disease and risk of stroke. A prospective follow-up of 14371 middle-aged men and women in Finland. Stroke 1997;28:1361–1366

144. Oxfordshire Community. Incidence of stroke in Oxfordshire: first year's experience of a community stroke register. Br Med J 1985;287:713–717

145. Davey Smith G, Wentworth D, Neaton JD, Stamler R, Stamler J: Socioeconomic differentials in mortality risk among men screened for the Multiple Risk Factor Intervention Trial: II. Black men. Am J Pub Health 1996;86:497–504

146. Gillum RF: Risk factors for stroke in blacks: a critical review. Am J Epidemiol 1999;150:1266–1274

147. Eigenbrodt ML, Rose KM, Couper DJ et al: Orthostatic hypotension as a risk factor for stroke: the atherosclerosis risk in communities (ARIC) study, 1987–1996. Stroke (Online) 2000;31:2307–2313

148. Hart CL, Hole DJ, Smith GD: The relation between cholesterol and haemorrhagic or ischaemic stroke in the Renfrew/Paisley study. J Epidemiol Commun Health 2000;54:874–875

149. Rogers A, MacMahon S: Blood pressure, cholesterol, and stroke in eastern Asia. Lancet 1998;352:1801–1807

150. Milionis HJ, Winder AF, Mikhailidis DP: Lipoprotein (a) and stroke. J Clin Pathol 2000;53:487–496

151. Kannel WB, Wolf PA, Castelli WP, D'Agostino RB: Fibrinogen and risk of cardiovascular disease. The Framingham Study. JAMA 1987;258:1183–1186

152. Gussekloo J, Schaap MC, Frolich M, Blauw GJ, Westendorp RG: C-reactive protein is a strong but nonspecific risk factor of fatal stroke in elderly persons. Arterioscler Thromb Vasc Biol 2000;20:1047–1051

153. Gagnon DR, Zhang TJ, Brand FN, Kannel WB: Hematocrit and the risk of cardiovascular disease—the Framingham study: a 34-year follow-up. Am Heart J 1994;127:674–682

154. Ridker PM, Hennekens CH, Stampfer MJ, Manson JE, Vaughan DE: Prospective study of endogenous tissue plasminogen activator and risk of stroke. Lancet 1994;343:940–943

155. Johansson L, Jansson JH, Boman K et al: Tissue plasminogen activator, plasminogen activator inhibitor-1, and tissue plasminogen activator/plasminogen activator inhibitor-1 complex as risk factors for the development of a first stroke. Stroke 2000;31:26–32

156. Pyorala M, Miettinen H, Halonen P, Laakso M, Pyorala K: Insulin resistance syndrome predicts the risk of coronary heart disease and stroke in healthy middle-aged men: the 22-year follow-up results of the Helsinki Policemen Study. Arterioscler Thromb Vasc Biol 2000;20:538–544

157. Walker SP, Rimm EB, Ascherio A et al: Body size and fat distribution as predictors of stroke among US men. Am J Epidemiol 1996;144:1143–1150

158. Shinton R, Sagar G, Beevers G: Body fat and stroke: unmasking the hazards of overweight and obesity. J Epidemiol Commun Health 1995;49:259–264

159. Harbison JA, Gibson GJ: Snoring, sleep apnoea and stroke: chicken or scrambled egg? Q J Med 2000;93:647–654

160. Koskenvuo M, Kaprio J, Telakivi T et al: Snoring as a risk factor for ischaemic heart disease and stroke in men. Br Med J 1987;294:16–19

161. Berger K, Ajani UA, Kase CS et al: Light-to-moderate alcohol consumption and risk of stroke among U.S. male physicians. N Engl J Med 1999;341:1557–1564

162. Wannamethee SG, Shaper AG: Patterns of alcohol intake and risk of stroke in middle-aged British men. Stroke 1996;27:1033–1039

163. Lee TK, Huang ZS, Ng SK et al: Impact of alcohol consumption and cigarette smoking on stroke among the elderly in Taiwan. Stroke 1995;26:790–794

164. Hansagi H, Romelsjo A, Gerhardsson de Verdier M, Andreasson S, Leifman A: Alcohol consumption and stroke mortality. 20-year follow-up of 15,077 men and women. Stroke 1995;26:1768–1773

165. Robbins AS, Manson JE, Lee IM, Satterfield S, Hennekens CH: Cigarette smoking and stroke in a cohort of U.S. male physicians. Ann Int Med 1994;120:458–462

166. Gey KF, Stahelin HB, Eichholzer M: Poor plasma status of carotene and vitamin C is associated with higher mortality from ischemic heart disease and stroke: Basel Prospective Study. Clin Invest 1993;71:3–6

167. Hirvonen T, Virtamo J, Korhonen P, Albanes D, Pietinen P: Intake of flavonoids, carotenoids, vitamins C and E, and risk of stroke in male smokers. Stroke (Online) 2000;31:2301–2306

168. Yochum LA, Folsom AR, Kushi LH: Intake of antioxidant vitamins and risk of death from stroke in postmenopausal women. Am J Clin Nutr 2000;72:476–483

169. Fang J, Madhavan S, Alderman MH: Dietary potassium intake and stroke mortality. Stroke 2000;31:1532–1537

170. Sasaki S, Zhang XH, Kesteloot H: Dietary sodium, potassium, saturated fat, alcohol, and stroke mortality. Stroke 1995;26:783–789

171. Hu FB, Stampfer MJ, Colditz GA et al: Physical activity and risk of stroke in women. JAMA 2000;283:2961–2967

172. Shinton R: Lifelong exposures and the potential for stroke prevention: the contribution of cigarette smoking, exercise, and body fat. J Epidemiol Commun Health 1997;51:138–143

173. Wannamethee G, Shaper AG: Physical activity and stroke in British middle aged men. Br Med J 1992;304:597–601

174. House A, Dennis M, Mogridge L, Hawton K, Warlow C: Life events and difficulties preceding stroke. J Neurol Neurosurg Psychiatry 1990;53:1024–1028

175. Gillum LA, Mamidipudi SK, Johnston SC: Ischemic stroke risk with oral contraceptives: A meta-analysis. JAMA 2000;284:72–78

176. Pan WH, Li LA, Tsai MJ: Temperature extremes and mortality from coronary heart disease and cerebral infarction in elderly Chinese. Lancet 1995;345:353–355

177. Feigin VL, Nikitin YP, Bots ML, Vinogradova TE, Grobbee DE: A population-based study of the associations of stroke occurrence with weather parameters in Siberia, Russia (1982–92). Eur J Neurol 2000;7:171–178

178. Rothwell PM, Wroe SJ, Slattery J, Warlow CP: Is stroke incidence related to season or temperature? The Oxfordshire Community Stroke Project. Lancet 1996;347:934–936

179. Knox EG: Meteorological associations of cerebrovascular disease mortality in England & Wales. J Epidemiol Commun Health 1981;35:220–223

180. Zhang ZF, Yu SZ, Zhou GD: Indoor air pollution of coal fumes as a risk factor of stroke, Shanghai. Am J Pub Health 1988;78:975–977

181. Hart CL, Hole DJ, Smith GD: The contribution of risk factors to stroke differentials, by socioeconomic position in adulthood: the Renfrew/Paisley Study. Am J Pub Health 2000;90:1788–1791

182. Hart CL, Hole DJ, Smith GD: Influence of socioeconomic circumstances in early and later life on stroke risk among men in a Scottish cohort study. Stroke (Online) 2000;31:2093–2097

183. Coggon D, Margetts B, Barker DJ et al: Childhood risk factors for ischaemic heart disease and stroke. Paed Perinat Epidemiol 1990;4:464–469

184. Markus HS, Mendall MA: Helicobacter pylori infection: a risk factor for ischaemic cerebrovascular disease and carotid atheroma. J Neurol Neurosurg Psych 1998;64:104–107

185. Van Ruiswyk J, Noble H, Sigmann P: The natural history of carotid bruits in elderly persons. Ann Intern Med 1990;112:340–343

186. Wolf PA, Kannel WB, Sorlie P, McNamara P: Asymptomatic carotid bruit and risk of stroke. The Framingham study. JAMA 1981;245:1442–1445

187. Koudstaal PJ, Algra A, Pop GA et al: Risk of cardiac events in atypical transient ischaemic attack or minor stroke. The Dutch TIA Study Group. Lancet 1992;340:630–633

188. Stegmayr B, Asplund K: Diabetes as a risk factor for stroke. A population perspective. Diabetologia 1995;38:1061–1068

189. Abbott RD, Donahue RP, MacMahon SW, Reed DM, Yano K: Diabetes and the risk of stroke. The Honolulu Heart Program. JAMA 1987;257:949–952

190. Grau AJ, Buggle F, Heindl S et al: Recent infection as a risk factor for cerebrovascular ischemia. Stroke 1995;26:373–379

191. Hart RG, Boop BS, Anderson DC: Oral anticoagulants and intracranial hemorrhage. Facts and hypotheses. Stroke 1995;26:1471–1477

192. Juvela S, Hillbom M, Palomaki H: Risk factors for spontaneous intracerebral hemorrhage. Stroke 1995;26:1558–1564

193. Stemmermann GN, Hayashi T, Resch JA et al: Risk factors related to ischemic and hemorrhagic cerebrovascular disease at autopsy: the Honolulu Heart Study. Stroke 1984;15:23–28

194. Tanaka H, Ueda Y, Hayashi M: Risk factors for cerebral haemorrhage and cerebral infarction in a Japanese rural community. Stroke 1982;13:62–73

195. Abbott RD, Yin Y, Reed DM, Yano K: Risk of stroke in male cigarette smokers. N Engl J Med 1986;315:717–720

196. Gill JS, Shipley MJ, Tsementzis SA et al: Cigarette smoking. A risk factor for hemorrhagic and nonhemorrhagic stroke. Arch Int Med 1989;149:2053–2057

197. Gill JS, Shipley MJ, Tsementzis SA et al: Alcohol consumption—a risk factor for hemorrhagic and non-hemorrhagic stroke. Am J Med 1991;90:489–497

198. Kiyohara Y, Kato I, Iwamoto H, Nakayama K, Fujishima M: The impact of alcohol and hypertension on stroke incidence in a general Japanese population. The Hisayama Study. Stroke 1995;26:368–372

199. Burchfiel CM, Curb JD, Rodriguez BL et al: Glucose intolerance and 22-year stroke incidence. The Honolulu Heart Program. Stroke 1994;25:951–957

200. Lodder J, Bamford JM, Sandercock PA, Jones LN, Warlow CP: Are hypertension or cardiac embolism likely causes of lacunar infarction? Stroke 1990;21:375–381

201. van Merwijk G, Lodder J, Bamford J, Kester AD: How often is non-valvular atrial fibrillation the cause of brain infarction? J Neurol 1990;237:205–207

202. Dennis MS, Bamford JM, Sandercock PA, Warlow CP: A comparison of risk factors and prognosis for transient ischemic attacks and minor ischemic strokes. The Oxfordshire Community Stroke Project. Stroke 1989;20:1494–1499

203. Hatano S, Shigematsu I, and Strasser T: Hypertension and Stroke Control in the Community. World Health Organization, Geneva, 1976

204. Secretary of State for Health. Health of the Nation. HMSO, London, 1992

205. Secretary of State for Health. Saving Lives. Our Healthier Nation. The Stationery Office, London, 1999

206. Ebrahim S: Cost-effectiveness of stroke prevention. Br Med Bull 2000;56:557–570

207. Rothwell PM, Warlow CP: Prediction of benefit from carotid endarterectomy in individual patients: a risk-modelling study. European Carotid Surgery Trialists' Collaborative Group. Lancet 1999;353:2105–2110

208. Rothwell PM: Who should have carotid surgery or angioplasty? Br Med Bull 2000;56:526–538

209. Rose G: Strategy of prevention: lessons from cardiovascular disease. Br Med J 1981;280:1847–1851

210. Davey Smith G, Phillips AN: Inflation in epidemiology: "the proof and measurement of association between two things" revisited. Br Med J 1996;312:1659–1661

211. McCarron P, Okasha M, McEwen J, Smith GD: Changes in blood pressure among students attending Glasgow University between 1948 and 1968: analyses of cross sectional surveys. Br Med J 2001;322:885–889

212. Secretary of State for Health. Smoking Kills. A White Paper on Tobacco. The Stationery Office, London, 1998

213. Gubitz G, Sandercock P: Prevention of ischaemic stroke. Br Med J 2000;321:1455–1459

214. Goldstein LB, Adams R, Becker K et al: Primary prevention of ischemic stroke: A statement for healthcare professionals from the Stroke Council of the American Heart Association. Stroke (Online) 2001;32:280–299

Chapter 49

Stroke: clinical presentation and management

Lalit Kalra

The term *cerebrovascular disease* refers to a broad group of disorders and includes any abnormality of the brain resulting from pathological processes involving blood vessels that leads to ischemia, infarction, or hemorrhage (Fig. 49-1). These disorders are classified into three main clinical categories: transient ischemic attacks (TIAs), stroke (occlusive or hemorrhagic), and cerebral multi-infarct states (cortical, subcortical, or diffuse).

Stroke is the cardinal manifestation of cerebrovascular disease and is defined as the acute onset of a neurological deficit lasting more than 24 hours or leading to death with no apparent cause other than vascular disease.[1] The neurological deficit is generally focal and is representative of the site and size of the anatomic lesion. Global presentations, associated with loss of consciousness, are occasionally seen. The abruptness of onset of the neurological deficit (minutes, hours, or days) is the characteristic feature of stroke. Another important characteristic is its clinical course: there is arrest of the neurological deficit followed by regression—depending on pathology to a greater or lesser extent—in all but fatal strokes.

Stroke ranks first in frequency, and probably urgency, among serious neurological disorders and accounts for nearly half of all neurological admissions seen in general hospitals.[2] It is a leading cause of death and disability in the western world. Nearly one-half of stroke patients die within 1 year of the acute episode,[3] with another 10 percent of survivors dying every year thereafter. Only a third of survivors make good recovery, and stroke is estimated to be responsible for 14–25 percent of cases of severe disability in the community.[4] The human cost of stroke to the individual, family, and society cannot be overestimated. The financial costs of managing stroke patients are high, irrespective of whether treatment takes place in a hospital or in the community. Overall, about 20 percent of the medical beds in a general hospital are occupied by stroke patients, and in western countries half of the survivors spend at least 4 weeks in the hospital.[5] There are concerns that these costs are likely to escalate as a consequence of demographic changes and the changing epidemiology of stroke.

In the past, stroke management has been dominated by negative and nihilistic attitudes, not only among physicians but also among patients and their families. Much of this pessimism has reflected the absence of effective medical treatment for acute stroke, ignorance about the benefits of nonpharmacological interventions, and a perception of universally poor outcome in this patient group. Fortunately, attitudes are changing, in part because of improved understanding of mechanisms underlying ischemic brain injury, advances in neuroimaging and vascular imaging techniques, as well as developments in therapeutics and changes in the philosophy of stroke management. The transition from a disease/organ-centered approach to a holistic patient-centered approach in recent years has been shown to be associated with a better outcome for patients at reduced service costs because of better organization of care.[6]

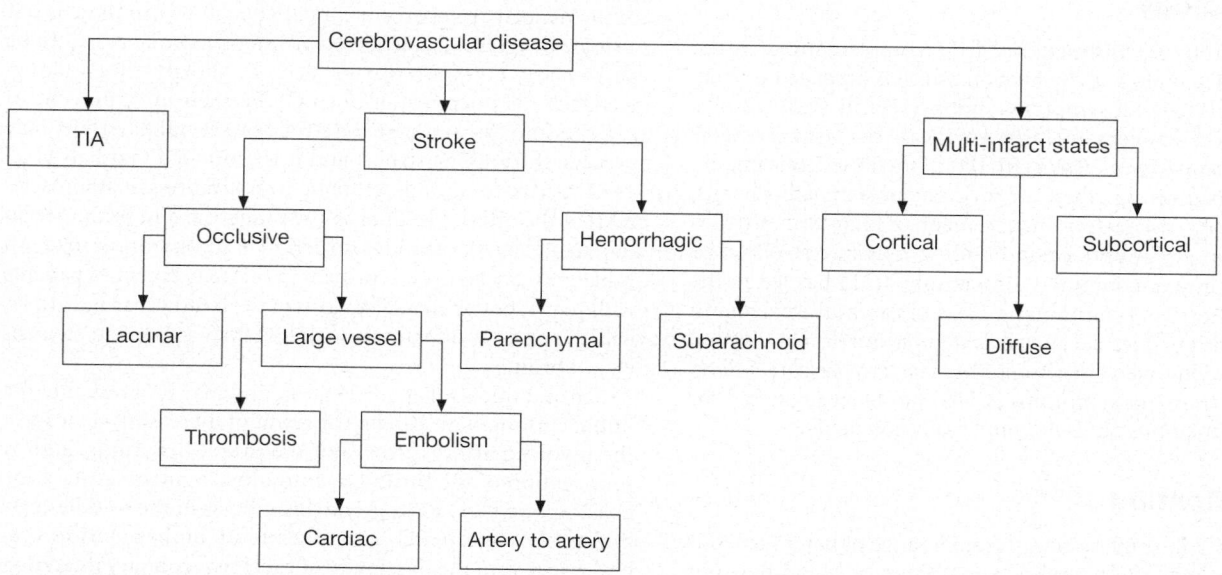

Figure 49-1 Classification of cerebrovascular diseases.

Awareness of the true costs of poor management of stroke patients and fears of spiraling costs in the future have provided further impetus to adopting a more positive attitude, with stroke prevention and treatment receiving high priority in most national health programs.

Stroke is primarily a disorder of the aging population and, in the United Kingdom at least, much of the care of stroke patients is undertaken by professionals with a special interest in care of elderly people. The association with aging has several important implications. Acute and late mortality are higher in this age group compared with that for younger stroke patients.[7,8] Older patients are more likely to be hospitalized because of severe loss of function and lack of adequate support mechanisms at home.[9] They are also more likely to have other pathology—notably ischemic heart disease, chronic heart failure, chronic pulmonary disease, arthritis, and visual or auditory impairment—which must be addressed as a part of overall stroke management. Background levels of chronic cognitive impairment increase with age and are likely to affect outcome, especially because much of rehabilitation involves learning and retention of new skills. Despite these considerations, there is no evidence suggesting that age, per se, affects neurological recovery or the duration of hospital stay in stroke patients.[10]

It is important to emphasize that stroke affects several domains of human performance and behavior, many of which lie outside traditional medical models of assessment and management. The whole philosophy of stroke assessment and management is based on multidisciplinary practice requiring the skills of many people including doctors, nurses, therapists, social workers, and other professionals who may be called on to help in the care of patients. Although this chapter concentrates mainly on the medical aspects of stroke presentation and management in an elderly population, emphasis is also placed on a holistic approach to assessment and treatment based on multidisciplinary practice.

CLINICAL ASPECTS

Terminology

TIAs are arbitrarily distinguished from complete stroke by the duration of neurological dysfunction, which is stipulated as being less than 24 hours. If symptoms (not necessarily signs) resolve within 1 week (3 weeks in North America)[11] the term *reversible ischemic neurological deficit* (RIND) is often used. It is important to remember that there are no differences in pathogenesis, epidemiology, risk factors, management, or long-term prognosis between a TIA and a nondisabling ischemic stroke. The increasing use of computed tomography (CT) has led to the identification of asymptomatic areas of cerebral ischemia in patients with first stroke as well as infarcts in relevant cerebral areas in patients who have had a TIA. The term *cerebral infarction with transient symptoms* (CITS) has been suggested for these presentations but is not universally accepted.[12]

Classification

Stroke is a syndrome resulting from a range of heterogeneous conditions that affect cerebral vasculature or blood flow but have a common clinical presentation. Strokes may be divided into those due to arterial occlusion and those due to hemorrhage (Fig. 49-1). Approximately 85 percent of strokes are occlusive and occur in the milieu of vascular risk characterized by advancing age and increased prevalence of hypertension, diabetes mellitus, and smoking.[3] Large vessel occlusion may affect extra- or intracranial arteries and may be due either to thrombotic changes on atheromatous plaques (local occlusion or artery to artery embolism) or due to emboli from a cardiac source. In addition, ischemic stroke may be a result of occlusion of small, penetrating arteries in the brain, causing damage to deep structures (lacunar stroke). Such strokes are seen in about one-fifth of ischemic stroke patients and exhibit significant differences in pathology, prognosis, recurrence, and natural history compared with large vessel disease. Hemorrhages account for 15 percent of stroke patients. These may be primary, due to microaneurysms (11–12 percent), or secondary, due to extracerebral rupture of intracranial vessels (3–4 percent).[3]

Thrombotic stroke

The most common cause of thrombotic stroke is atherosclerosis in the arteries of the brain which parallels, but is somewhat less severe than, atherosclerosis of the aorta, coronary, or renal arteries. The common sites of involvement are the internal carotid artery at the carotid sinus in the neck, the junction of the vertebral and basilar arteries, the main bifurcation of the middle cerebral artery, the posterior cerebral artery around the cerebral peduncle, and the anterior cerebral artery over the corpus callosum.[2] It is rare for cerebral arteries to be affected significantly beyond their first bifurcation. Degeneration, hemorrhage into atheroma, or rupture of atheromatous plaques damage the vascular endothelium and exposes subendothelial collagen. This, in association with other stimuli, activates platelets, leading to aggregation, adhesion, and thrombus formation. The thrombus may occlude the vessel at the site of formation or be carried downstream to lodge in a vessel with a smaller lumen (artery-to-artery embolism).

Thrombotic strokes are classically described as having "stuttering" intermittent progression over several hours or days after commencement. However, this intermittency is not seen in the majority (60 percent) of patients, in whom there is but a single progressive episode.[2] Thrombotic stroke is said to be particularly common during sleep or shortly after waking. Headache is uncommon but may be seen in 15 percent of patients and can antedate the stroke by several days. TIA may precede thrombotic stroke, and it is estimated that half of all TIAs are due to thromboembolic complications of atherosclerosis of the arteries leading to the brain. Carotid bruits are an unreliable sign of carotid obstruction in thrombotic stroke. An ipsilateral carotid bruit is present in only 64 percent of patients with 50 percent or greater stenosis of the internal carotid artery, while 11 percent of patients with less than 50 percent stenosis have a bruit.[14]

Thrombotic strokes are dynamic and may progress after the initial episode. This can be the result of increasing stenosis of the involved artery, growth of the mural thrombus, and/or propagation of the thrombus into other branches, hindering anastomotic flow. Retrograde thrombosis in the middle cerebral artery can extend back to the mouth of the anterior cerebral artery with the possibility of causing secondary infarction in the territory of that vessel. In addition, embolic particles traveling from the site of thrombosis to other vessels may precipitate abrupt changes in the neurological deficit after the main event.

Embolic stroke

The heart is the source of emboli in most cases of cerebral embolism, but artery-to-artery embolism may occur as mentioned previously. Although any region of the brain can be affected, the territory of the middle cerebral artery is most frequently involved. Cerebral embolization from the heart can be caused by atrial fibrillation; damaged, infected, or prosthetic valves; or damaged or dyskinetic myocardial segments. Cerebral emboli can be associated with severe neurological deficits because the rapidity of onset of complete occlusion prevents collateral perfusion from becoming established. Embolic stroke does not have any prodromal features and has been classically described as "a bolt out of the blue"; the full-blown neurological deficit develops within a few minutes of onset. Occasionally, in its passage along an artery, an embolus may produce significant neurological deficits which are transitory and resolve as the embolus breaks up or passes into a small branch supplying a relatively silent area of the brain. The clinical picture is then that of a TIA. Cardiogenic emboli are responsible for TIAs in 20 percent of patients presenting with transient weakness.[15] TIAs due to cardiogenic emboli are characterized by episodes in different vascular territories with differing patterns of neurological deficit, since it is unlikely that successive emboli will lodge at identical sites.

Hemorrhagic transformation

In many cases, the embolic clot subsequently breaks up into fragments which then enter smaller vessels before disappearing completely. Recanalization of the previously occluded vessel may then lead to bleeding in the necrotic area. Hemorrhagic transformation is estimated to occur in 30 percent of embolic infarcts.[16] Although hemorrhagic transformation is particularly linked to embolic stroke, this is not always the case. The extent of hemorrhagic transformation is dependent on the depth and duration of ischemia as well as on the intensity of reperfusion. Serial CT studies have shown that this is a dynamic process and can occur at any time during the first 2 weeks after stroke. Although hemorrhagic transformation is being more frequently recognized because of widespread use of CT scans in stroke, little is known about its clinical or therapeutic implications.

Hemorrhagic transformation is of particular significance in relation to early use of drugs that affect hemostatic mechanisms and is more likely to occur in patients already on such drugs at the time of their stroke.[16] The relationship with antithrombotic or antiplatelet drugs given after a cerebral infarct is less clear. Acute intervention studies have shown that the use of thrombolytic agents increases the risk of intraparenchymal bleeding three-fold, especially in patients with established infarcts or when thrombolysis is delayed beyond 3 hours.[17] The evidence on the early use of antiplatelet drugs or anticoagulants is not clear. The International Stroke Trial showed that although there was a small risk of increased hemorrhagic transformation with aspirin, this risk was not significant and did not outweigh the benefits of early aspirin use.[18] An overview of all trials on the early use of heparin or warfarin was inconclusive; the theoretical benefits of preventing clot propagation and early recurrence need to be balanced against the risks of hemorrhagic transformation in individual patients depending upon clinical assessment.[19]

Lacunar stroke

Lacunar lesions vary between 3–15 mm in diameter and include the residua of old small infarcts (Type I lacunes), small hemorrhages (Type II), or dilatation of the perivascular spaces (Type III).[20] The term is conventionally used to describe an area of infarction within the territory of a single perforating cerebral artery. Patients with such lesions may or may not present with clinical features of stroke, and recent CT evidence suggests that as many as 80 percent of lacunar infarcts may be clinically silent. Approximately 20 percent of occlusive strokes are lacunar, and their frequency increases with age.[21]

Lacunar strokes result from the occlusion of small perforating arteries which branch off from the major cerebral arteries and have few anastomotic branches. The areas most commonly affected are the caudate and lenticular nuclei, thalami, basis pontis, and cerebral or cerebellar white matter. The arteries are blocked not by platelet or fibrin thrombi (as would be expected in large vessel disease) but by a poorly understood process known as lipohyalinosis.[13] In some instances, lipohyalinosis results in false aneurysm formation resembling Charcot–Bouchard aneurysms of intracerebral hemorrhage. As lacunar strokes can affect any fibers descending from the cortex, they can cause a host of clinical syndromes. A small number of clinical syndromes appear to occur more commonly and have been correlated with relevant lacunae observed during subsequent autopsy. These are regarded as "classic" lacunar syndromes and include pure motor stroke, pure sensory stroke, dysarthria–clumsy hand syndrome, ataxic hemiparesis, and sensorimotor stroke.[22] The term *extended lacunar stroke* is used to describe cases in which lacunar strokes have been associated with additional features such as psychological disturbances or eye movement abnormalities. Little is known about this condition, which may have different pathophysiology and clinical implications compared with lacunar infarcts. A "corona radiata lacune," more commonly seen in elderly people, is not a true lacunar infarct but a partial watershed infarct between the area of supply of the medullary branches of the cortical middle cerebral artery and the lenticulostriate penetrating branches of the middle cerebral artery. It is usually larger, less distinct, and more superficial than a lacunar infarct.[22]

Pure motor stroke is the most common presentation of lacunar infarcts. The deficit is likely to evolve over hours and does not have any cortical features such as language problems, visual field defects, inattention, or visuospatial difficulties. Significant headaches, seizures, or impairment of consciousness are all uncommon in lacunar strokes. TIAs in 20 percent of patients may be due to the involvement of small perforating arteries and are a result of incipient occlusion rather than cardiogenic or artery-to-artery emboli (as in the case of large vessel disease). Incipient occlusion may also explain the crescendo of attacks (frequency and duration) sometimes seen immediately before the completion of deficit (capsular warning syndrome).[22]

Although lacunar strokes are more common in patients with hypertension, atherosclerosis, and diabetes, the underlying pathophysiology appears—as already described—to be different from that of large vessel occlusion. Significant ipsilateral carotid stenosis (resulting in artery-to-artery embolism) or potential cardiac sources of embolism (in particular atrial fibrillation) are less prevalent in lacunar stroke patients[21] and, where they are seen, their contribution to the disease process remains to be proven.[13] Consequently, there is debate about the choice of special investigations, antiplatelet therapy, and anticoagulation for these patients. A diagnosis of lacunar stroke should not preclude further investigation in elderly patients because these strokes develop in an atherogenic milieu similar to that of large vessel infarcts. The possibility that any proximal vascular lesions may be coincidental to the presenting stroke, however, should be borne in mind.[22]

Classification of cerebral infarcts

In almost all patients, classification of infarcts according to site and size can be achieved with considerable accuracy on the basis of clinical signs and symptoms alone. This approach has been favored by epidemiologists and clinical trialists because of its simplicity, lack of dependence on extensive investigations, and correlation with outcome and the uniformity of pathophysiological mechanisms within individual groups. A currently popular version, used in several clinical trials in Britain, classifies ischemic stroke into total anterior circulation infarction (TACI), partial anterior circulation infarction (PACI), posterior circulation infarction (POCI), and lacunar infarction.[23]

TACI is a result of occlusion of either the internal carotid artery or the proximal stem of the middle cerebral artery and involves almost all of the carotid territory. The grouping includes, but does not distinguish, patients who may have added anterior cerebral artery infarction. The proportion of TACIs caused by in-situ thrombosis, cardiogenic embolism, or artery-to-artery embolism from the internal carotid artery to the middle cerebral artery is not known. TACI is associated with high levels of mortality (more than 50 percent dead at 1 year) and dependence, suggesting that acute thrombolysis may

be most worthwhile in this group of patients. However, this needs to be tempered by the observation that patients with established CT scan changes at the time of thrombolysis or those with infarcts affecting more than a third of the cerebral hemisphere are more likely to have adverse outcomes.[17] PACI is generally due to involvement of smaller branches of the middle cerebral artery and is most frequently embolic in origin. There is a high risk of recurrence of stroke in these patients, especially within the first 3 months.[23] This suggests that patients with PACI need early investigation and institution of secondary preventive measures even—or especially—when there is relatively minor neurological deficit. Infarction in the border zones between two main arterial territories may occasionally present as PACI. This is usually caused by hemodynamic disturbance and if unilateral may indicate a tight stenosis of the ipsilateral internal carotid artery. The ratio of thrombotic to embolic events in POCI is 4:1. It is usually difficult to determine exact vascular involvement in this area because of the rich anastomoses in the posterior fossa. Lacunar anterior circulation infarction (LACI) is associated with less mortality and morbidity than other infarcts and does not have cortical features. Recurrence occurs at a steady rate subsequent to the initial event, suggesting that another perforating artery needs to be involved before further symptoms arise. Data from the Oxford Community Stroke Project suggest that 17 percent of cerebral infarcts are TACI, 34 percent are PACI, 24 percent are POCI, and 25 percent are LACI.

Improved understanding of stroke mechanisms and advances in secondary prevention have shifted the emphasis of stroke classification from clinical syndromes to etiological subtypes. The most commonly used classification is the TOAST (Trial of Org 10172 in Acute Stroke Treatment) system.[24] In this system, categorization as strokes due to large vessel atherosclerosis is based on clinical findings of cerebral cortical impairment with infarcts greater than 1.5 cm in diameter, history of hypertension, diabetes, hyperlipidemia or smoking, and evidence of atherosclerotic internal carotid artery disease (stenosis or heterogeneous plaque) on carotid duplex examination. The cardioembolic category includes patients with known cardiac disease, evidence of previous strokes or transient ischemic attacks in different vascular territories, valvular abnormalities, left atrial enlargement, or dyskinetic myocardial segments who have no other cause of stroke. Small artery occlusion is considered to be present in patients with lacunar syndromes who have no cortical signs, lesions less than 1.5 cm on CT or MRI scans, absence of carotid disease, and normal cardiac/ECG findings. Patients who do not fit into any of these categories are assigned to the "undetermined etiology" group. Patients in whom two different etiologies are equally likely are designated as having "mixed etiology."

Hemorrhagic stroke

The most common type of hemorrhagic stroke is primary intracerebral hemorrhage (PICH) and is associated with hypertension and increasing age. The nature of the vascular lesion that leads to arterial rupture is not fully known, but it is thought to be due to arterial wall changes leading to segmental lipohyalinosis or formation of microaneurysms from which bleeding occurs. These microaneurysms are usually located on small arteries, especially the lenticulostriate branches of the

---

Stroke subtypes according to site and size

Total anterior circulation infarction (TACI)
- Motor and sensory deficit
- Ipsilateral hemianopia
- Evidence of cortical dysfunction (dysphasia, visuospatial problems, and so on)

Partial anterior circulation infarction (PACI)
- Any two of the above, or
- Isolated disturbance of higher cerebral function

Posterior circulation infarction (POCI)
- Unequivocal signs of brain stem involvement, or
- Isolated hemianopia

Lacunar infarction (LACI)

Any one of the following:
- Pure motor stroke
- Pure sensory stroke
- Pure sensorimotor stroke
- Ataxic hemiparesis

middle cerebral artery and the cerebellar and pontine branches of the basilar artery. The extravasation forms a roughly oval or circular mass which disrupts the surrounding tissue and, depending on the size of the bleed, may cause a mass effect. The most common sites for PICH, in order of frequency, are the putamen and the adjacent internal capsule (50 percent of cases), various parts of the central white matter (frontal lobe, corona radiata, extension from the putamen), thalamus, cerebellar hemisphere, and pons. In some patients, intracerebral hemorrhages are superficial (lobar) and not associated with hypertension or other vascular risk factors. In such patients, an alternative cause such as arteriovenous malformation, neoplasm, amyloid angiopathy, or rarer vascular abnormalities, needs to be excluded.

Hemorrhagic stroke is said to have an abrupt onset, usually associated with activity, and a relentlessly progressive course dependent on the speed of bleeding. Hypertension is common, but there are no recognizable warning or prodromal symptoms. Moderate to large intracerebral bleeds (depending on hemorrhage volume and ventricular extension) are associated with a persistent and often severe neurological deficit from which rapid improvement is not to be expected. There is, however, increasing awareness that smaller bleeds, which are confined to cerebral parenchyma, may have a clinical course similar to that of cerebral infarction.[25] Severe headache occurs in only 50 percent of patients, and vomiting once or twice at the onset of hemorrhage may be an important feature. Epileptic fits occur in 10 percent of patients during the first few days of a stroke, especially in those with subcortical "slit hemorrhages" at the junction of white and gray matter. Once bleeding has stopped, early rebleeding is uncommon.

DIAGNOSTIC ISSUES

The clinical features of stroke are so distinctive that diagnosis is self-evident. The three major criteria underpinning a diagnosis of stroke are clinical setting, temporal profile, and evidence of focal brain damage. If this information is lacking, a diagnosis can still be established by undertaking CT scans of the brain. However, a significant proportion of acute CT scans in patients with clinically definite stroke do not show a relevant abnormality. In such circumstances, confirmation of diagnosis can be made by extending the period of observation and resorting to the golden rule that a physician's best diagnostic tool is the second and third examination. Factors that may contribute to difficulties in diagnosis in elderly patients include nonavailability of a reliable history because of the absence of a witness, dysphasia, dementia or confusion, unusual symptoms or signs due to pre-existing cerebrovascular disease, and multiple pathology which may mask or confound the clinical diagnosis of stroke.

The diagnosis of TIA depends almost entirely on clinical history, as signs are seldom present during examination and there are no objective investigations that can confirm or exclude the diagnosis. Approximately 15 percent of patients having their first stroke have a history of TIA, although in only half has this event been correctly identified.[15] Accuracy of diagnosis of TIA in elderly people is compromised by problems of obtaining a reliable history in some patients and nonspecificity

of symptoms (especially if they involve the vertebrobasilar territory), as well as a multiplicity of other conditions that may have a similar presentation (syncope, hypoglycemia, epilepsy).[26] In addition, there is considerable interobserver variability in the diagnosis of TIA between general physicians and neurologists and even between experienced neurologists. The difficulties in the diagnosis of TIA are due to lack of detail in the widely used definition and the absence of any precise, valid, reliable, generally acceptable criteria for diagnosis.[27] There have been attempts to develop and evaluate computer-assisted programs and clinical algorithms for evaluating patients with TIA. These programs take into account variables such as setting of symptoms (presence of risk factors), rapidity of onset and temporal profile (arrest and rapid resolution) of neurological symptoms, focal nature of the deficit, and the presence or absence of associated symptoms.[28] In patients with vague or uncharacteristic symptoms or in whom symptoms occur under unusual circumstances, a diagnosis of "possible TIA" should be made pending confirmation by witness accounts or reassessment over a period of time. The annual risk of stroke following a TIA is increased seven-fold over the first 5 years. It is hence imperative that patients with TIA or possible TIA be investigated as a matter of urgency, especially as the risk of stroke is highest during the first few weeks after the TIA.[15]

The clinical presentation of thrombotic and arterial occlusion depends on the occluded artery and varies according to the availability of collateral blood flow. There are countless variations in the size, shape, and completeness of infarcts depending on the speed of occlusion, cerebral autoregulation, and oxygenation variables. Focal ischemic lesions have traditionally provided one of the most instructive approaches in localizing function in the brain, with doctors learning neurology "stroke by stroke."[2] Although specific impairments may vary in different patients and according to the location and size of the infarct, there is sufficient uniformity to permit diagnosis within major vascular territories. In general, unilateral signs predominate in carotid system involvement (hemiplegia, hemianesthesia, hemianopia, dysphasia, and agnosia), whereas bilateral motor or sensory signs with cranial nerve or cerebellar involvement are more commonly found in vertebrobasilar disease. In general, hemorrhage within these vascular territories gives rise to effects similar to those observed with occlusive stroke. The overall clinical picture, however, is apt to differ from that for infarcts because of deep extension of the hemorrhage into other vascular territories and because of a mass effect giving rise to midline shift and raised intracranial pressure. Determination of the arterial territory involved in TIA is important because carotid endarterectomy may be a possible intervention for carotid circulation syndromes. It is usually possible to distinguish between carotid territory (80 percent) and vertebrobasilar territory (20 percent) involvement on the basis of clinical presentation and symptoms, especially if they are related to cortical function or include transient monocular blindness. The difficulty arises when the neurological symptoms are limited to pathways that receive their blood supply from the carotid or basilar circulation at different levels (e.g. corticospinal tracts, spinothalamic tracts, optic radiation). In such instances, localization of lesion on clinical criteria has limitations and ancillary investigations are needed to resolve diagnostic problems.

Differences between hemorrhage and infarction

The distinction between cerebral hemorrhage and infarction has become extremely important because of recent advances in the acute management and secondary prevention of stroke. It is particularly important to make this distinction before considering treatment with thrombolytics and in patients who may already be on drugs that modify hemostatic function. Accuracy of pathological diagnosis is also required in patients who may be candidates for invasive interventions aimed at secondary stroke prevention (anticoagulation, carotid angiography, carotid endarterectomy). It has been traditional to differentiate between hemorrhagic and ischemic strokes using clinical features derived retrospectively from autopsy series. These distinctions have been made on the basis of time of onset, temporal profile of symptoms, progression of deficit, and associated features of headache and vomiting. This method of clinical distinction, even when clinical scoring systems are used, is neither sensitive nor reliable because nearly 60 percent of stroke patients have a similar presentation regardless of pathology.[2] Differentiation based on clinical features alone is also not supported by CT scan data, which show considerable overlap in clinical presentation between primary intracerebral hemorrhage and cerebral infarction, especially in patients with smaller peripheral hemorrhages that have not ruptured into the ventricular system.[29] CT scanning soon after the initial episode is the only reliable way of distinguishing between an infarct and a hemorrhage as a cause of stroke. The radiological density of a hemorrhage changes with time, and delays beyond 2 weeks may necessitate magnetic resonance imaging (MRI) to distinguish reliably between hemorrhage and infarction (see below).

INVESTIGATIONS IN STROKE

Although the diagnosis of stroke or TIA is mainly clinical, investigations are needed to determine stroke pathology and etiology, which are essential for appropriate management of stroke patients. All patients need basic investigations to detect treatable vascular risk factors and other disorders that would alter management. Investigations may also be needed to identify possible treatable complications of stroke. The issue of appropriateness is important in determining the level of investigation in stroke patients. Although age in itself should never be a contraindication to undertaking further investigations, investigative zeal must be tempered by the clinical state of the patient and the potential for functional recovery, comorbidity (which may preclude aggressive management), risk–benefit appraisal of management options (some of which may actually favor elderly people), and suitability (as well as willingness) to undergo further investigation or intervention.

Baseline investigations in all stroke patients should include a CT scan, full blood count (polycythemia, thrombocyte disorders), erythrocyte sedimentation rate (hyperviscosity, vasculitis), blood glucose (glycemic status), urea and electrolytes (diuretics, renal function), serum cholesterol, electrocardiogram (atrial fibrillation, myocardial infarct), carotid/vertebral duplex studies, echocardiogram if in atrial fibrillation and a chest radiograph (metastatic disease, cardiomegaly, aspiration). Serum cholesterol

levels are representative only if a fasting specimen has been taken within 24 hours of stroke, otherwise they should be measured at least 6 weeks after the acute episode. Further investigations are indicated in younger patients (atherosclerosis being uncommon in this age group), and in those with no vascular risk factors or atypical features on presentation. These investigations may involve MRI scans, MR angiography, transoesophageal echocardiography, hemostatic profile, screening for dyslipoproteinemias, hemoglobinopathies, abnormal proteins (antithrombin III, proteins C and S), immunological profile, plasma electrophoresis, syphilis serology, and anticardiolipin antibodies. Conventional angiography, tests for inherited metabolic disorders, and tests for rare granulomatous diseases may also be needed.

CT scanning

CT scan studies are the cornerstone investigation in stroke and should be undertaken as early as possible in all suspected stroke patients. Although the Royal College of Physicians guidelines[30] recommend that CT scanning should be undertaken within 48 hours of stroke onset, many patients will benefit by earlier scanning. Indications for CT scanning on presentation include nonavailability of a clear history (unconscious or acutely confused patient), atypical symptoms or signs, rapid deterioration in clinical status, features of raised intracranial pressure, suspected cerebellar stroke, subarachnoid hemorrhage or history of anticoagulant use. Urgent CT scanning is also needed in patients within 3–6 hours of stroke onset who may be eligible for thrombolysis and in those with atrial fibrillation where the size of the cerebral lesion may determine the timing of anticoagulation. Early CT scanning may be necessary to establish a diagnosis in stroke patients with other pathology (e.g., malignant disorders) in whom progression of the pre-existing disease process is an alternative explanation for focal neurological deficits. Accuracy in diagnosis is important for prognosis, acute intervention (hemorrhage vs infarction), determining the need and nature of secondary prevention (large vs small vessel disease), and establishing specific rehabilitation needs (site and size of lesion), although the latter is influenced more by the level of impairments.

CT scanning is extremely useful for distinguishing hemorrhages from infarcts, especially in patients presenting early enough to contemplate thrombolysis. CT is highly sensitive in detecting intracerebral bleeding soon after the onset of stroke, which is seen as an area of high attenuation within the cerebral parenchyma. The sensitivity of CT scanning in detecting hemorrhages decreases with time because areas of high attenuation may become isodense or even hypodense with respect to surrounding brain tissue after 2 weeks of onset, making differentiation between hemorrhage and infarction difficult. CT scanning is less sensitive in detecting infarction in the acute phase and is negative in 25–30 percent of patients presenting with clinically established stroke.[31] This may be because the scan has been performed too early (CT scan infarction changes may take 1–2 days to appear) or because of the transitory "fogging effect" due to which infarcts may not be visible (infarcted areas become isodense within 1–3 weeks in 50 percent of cases). Other reasons for negative CT scans include infarcts less than 10 mm in size, or posterior fossa lesions. In-situ thrombosis may be seen occasionally as an area of high density in an artery on an ordinary CT scan, and follow-up scans may show a decrease in vessel density due to thrombus resolution. CT scanning has a sensitivity of 80 percent in detecting hemorrhagic infarcts, which are seen as areas of patchy high density, often in the territory of the middle cerebral artery. It can, however, be difficult to distinguish between a hemorrhagic infarct and PICH on a CT scan. Although this may not present significant problems in medical management (antihemostatic treatment being contraindicated in both conditions), it may make surgical decisions regarding possible endarterectomy (which may be required in some patients with hemorrhagic infarcts secondary to artery-to-artery embolization) more difficult.

MRI scanning

MRI is more sensitive than CT scanning in detecting infarcts, particularly if undertaken early or if the infarcts are small or occur in the posterior fossa.[31] The sensitivity of MRI in detecting hemorrhages or hemorrhagic infarcts in the acute phase is less than that of CT scanning, although its performance in detecting clinically relevant lesions in stroke can be increased by undertaking special studies.[32] In contrast to that of CT scanning, the sensitivity of MRI in detecting hemorrhage increases with time. This is because of the formation of methemoglobin in 3–5 days, which results in an increased signal on T_1 and T_2 images. At 2 weeks a low-intensity rim can be seen around the edge of a hematoma on T_2 images because of deposition of hemosiderin at the edge of the bleed. MRI does not have any significant advantages over CT scanning in differentiating between primary intracerebral hemorrhages and hemorrhagic transformation of infarcts.

MRI has particular value in patients with small vessel disease, in whom conventional CT scans seldom reveal the full extent of cerebrovascular disease. It is also of value in patients with multiple strokes: diffusion-weighted sequences can help distinguish new lesions from chronic or subacute lesions and help with diagnosis.[33] It is now possible to visualize the penumbra in acute stroke by combining MR perfusion imaging (which helps to quantitate the area of reduced blood flow) with diffusion sequences (which quantitate the areas of actual cellular damage).[34] Such imaging will allow a more informed and targeted approach to thrombolysis as thrombolysis can be specifically directed toward patients with significant mismatch, regardless of the duration since stroke onset (Fig. 49-2). It is also possible to perform MR angiography at the same time as undertaking MR imaging, which allows noninvasive visualization of intra- and extracranial vasculature and may help to identify the etiology of stroke.

It needs to be emphasized that MRI is still a second-level investigation for stroke in the UK and should be undertaken only where CT scanning does not provide relevant answers. MRI is expensive, not universally available, and contributes little toward resolving diagnostic issues important in stroke management over and above CT scanning. It is important to remember that nearly a fifth of patients with acute stroke are unable to undergo an MRI examination because of claustrophobia or contraindications, such as pacemakers.[35]

Other imaging techniques

The emphasis of imaging in the past has been on delineation of the anatomy and pathology of the lesion in stroke patients. In recent years, there has been considerable interest and developments in imaging techniques for studying the physiological aspects of stroke. Significant developments in this area include positron emission tomography (PET), single photon emission tomography (SPET), xenon CT, and magnetic resonance spectroscopy (MRS). Most of these techniques are research tools and are being used to study the pathophysiology (vascular and neurological) of acute stroke, the effect of acute interventions, and the changes associated with recovery, reactivation, and rehabilitation. Although these techniques have not been introduced in clinical practice, an overview is essential to facilitate better understanding of current research and its future implications.

Xenon CT and SPET have been used primarily to study cerebral blood flow in the acute phases of stroke. Xenon CT

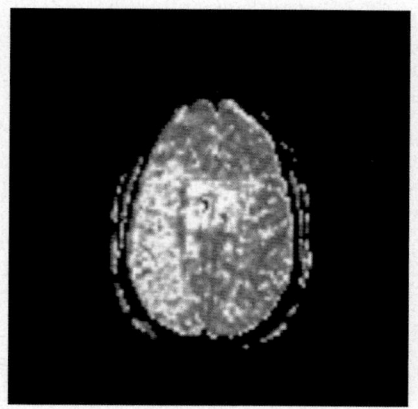
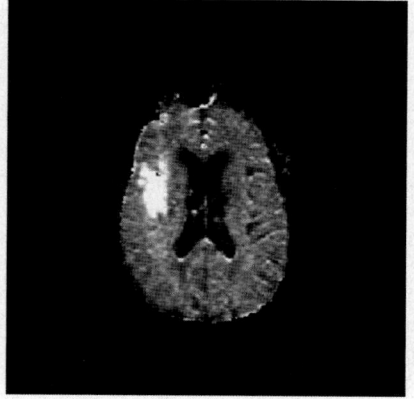
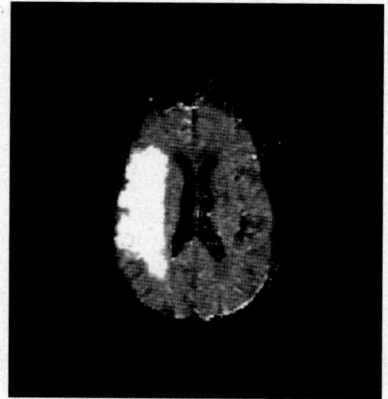

Perfusion deficit (MTT) at 12 hours

Neuronal injury (DWI) at 12 hours

Neuronal injury (DWI) at 4 days

Figure 49-2 Diffusion and perfusion scans at 12 hours after onset of symptoms to highlight the difference between the extent of the diffusion and perfusion abnormalities in the acute stage of the stroke. (Courtesy Dr David Lythgoe.)

can demonstrate the site and size of cerebral ischemic injury before any changes are seen on ordinary CT scans.[31] Xenon CT scanning can be performed immediately after conventional CT scanning and may have the potential of selecting patients for thrombolysis because of its ability to distinguish between patients with low cerebral blood flow (who are likely to benefit) and those with high cerebral blood flow (who are unlikely to benefit). SPET is essentially a research tool which provides high-resolution images of cerebral blood flow changes associated with acute stroke within 20 to 30 minutes of injection of a tracer isotope. SPET has been used for studying temporal changes in cerebral blood flow after acute stroke, monitoring the effects of acute treatment and predicting recovery.

PET, MRS, and functional MR imaging have been employed in the study of cerebral perfusion, oxygen consumption, and metabolic changes following stroke and their relationship to recovery.[37–39] It is now possible to examine the metabolic consequences of ischemia, the threshold between reversible and irreversible ischemia, and metabolic factors involved in neurological recovery. It may be possible to predict which patients are most likely to benefit from acute stroke intervention on the basis of perfusion and oxygen consumption patterns observed on PET scanning.[37] Studies using these modalities have suggested that there are changes in the metabolic activity of both the affected and the unaffected sides of the brain during recovery, with reactivation of previously silent areas.[39] This has considerable implications in the evaluation of recovery and therapy inputs in stroke. It may also be possible to identify biochemical markers of prognosis and response to therapy in acute stroke using PET or MRS techniques.

Vascular studies

Vascular studies are necessary in patients with recent carotid territory TIA or nondisabling stroke. They are most urgent in patients with nondisabling stroke because of the high risk of recurrence. Investigations include noninvasive procedures, such as carotid ultrasound and magnetic resonance angiography, and invasive tests such as conventional angiography, intra-arterial digital subtraction angiography (IA-DSA), and intravenous digital subtraction angiography (IV-DSA).

Ultrasound

Extracranial

Duplex carotid ultrasound, which combines the high reliability of Doppler studies in detecting hemodynamically significant internal carotid artery stenosis (more than 50 percent of diameter) with the high reliability of B-mode imaging in detecting mild to moderate lesions (25–50 percent of diameter), is the most effective noninvasive method of detecting extracranial carotid disease.[40] Doppler flow studies have high sensitivity (90–100 percent) and moderate specificity (55–90 percent in detecting moderate to severe stenosis but are less reliable in detecting milder disease that produces normal flow patterns. In contrast, B-mode imaging readily detects mild to moderate lesions with a high sensitivity (70–100 percent) but cannot reliably detect more advanced stenosis because of scattering of sound waves due to fibrosis or calcification. As

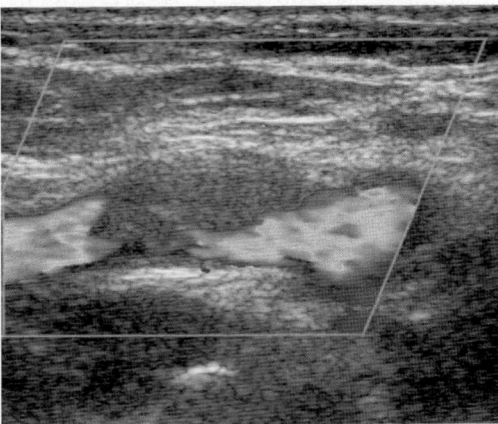

Figure 49-3 Carotid ultrasound showing carotid artery dissection.

advanced stenosis is usually accompanied by flow velocity changes, this limitation of B-mode echo is overcome by the Doppler flow element of the investigation.

Carotid duplex studies are widely used as a screening procedure for carotid artery disease (Fig. 49-3). However, their diagnostic utility may be restricted by a high carotid bifurcation, problems in distinguishing between internal and external carotid artery in some patients, incomplete plaque characterization because of the inability of sound waves to penetrate calcified atherosclerotic plaques and difficulties in distinguishing tight stenosis from occlusion because of markedly reduced blood flow. The reliability of carotid duplex studies is also dependent on the expertise of the examiner. In trained hands, this procedure can detect mild atherosclerotic disease in an extracranial artery with a sensitivity of 90 percent and a specificity of 85–95 percent.[40] The sensitivity of carotid duplex studies in detecting hemodynamically significant disease (more than 50 percent stenosis) is even higher (greater than 95 percent). The major problem encountered in such studies in mainstream practice is difficulty in differentiating between a tight but patent stenosis and complete occlusion. The positive predictive value of duplex in detecting occlusion is low (53–86 percent), suggesting that 14–37 percent of patients in whom a duplex study suggests an occlusion actually have a tight but patent internal cranial artery stenosis.[41] This has important implications because occlusion of the internal carotid artery precludes patients from carotid endarterectomy, whereas a tight symptomatic stenosis in the same territory is a definite indication for the procedure. It is hence appropriate that angiography be undertaken in all patients potentially suitable for endarterectomy suspected of having internal carotid artery occlusion on duplex studies because a significant proportion of them will be found to have treatable tight stenosis.[41]

Transcranial

Transcranial Doppler is a noninvasive procedure for measuring blood flow in the major intracranial arteries using a small, portable unit.[42] This method has been used to evaluate cerebral collateral flow in patients with extracranial carotid disease, monitor middle cerebral artery blood flow velocity during carotid endarterectomy, detect cerebral embolism during surgical procedures or in acute stroke, assess acute cerebral infarction and vessel recanalization, and detect posterior circulation flow disturbances in vertebrobasilar insufficiency. Transcranial Doppler is also used to evaluate the presence of hemodynamically significant intracranial stenosis of the major arteries.

Intracranial components of the cerebral circulation are difficult to investigate ultrasonically because they are surrounded by bone. The acoustic barrier of the brain has been overcome by using lower than conventional ultrasound frequencies and directing the beam through the natural foramina (foramen magnum) or the thinnest regions of the skull (temporal bone). Despite this, it is not possible to penetrate the acoustic barrier of the skull in 10 percent of patients, particularly elderly females and those of Afro-Caribbean or Asian origin (failure rate 30 percent).[43] The procedure is also highly operator dependent (more so than duplex scanning) and is further limited by patient cooperation, anatomic anomalies of the circle of Willis, inaccuracies in vessel identification, effect of pathological structural abnormalities, and abnormal collateral flow states. In addition, data provided by the procedure reflect blood velocity and not volume flow, which may be a more relevant measure.

Future developments

Carotid ultrasound is also being used in studying plaque morphology, early changes in the carotid arterial wall, and longitudinal progression of carotid disease. These applications are still being developed and are not a part of mainstream clinical practice. Technological advances include the development of color duplex sonography which combines real-time ultrasound imaging with semiquantitative color encoding of Doppler information, allowing turbulent flow to be more easily detected. This development has the potential of overcoming the most important current limitation of carotid duplex sonography because tight stenoses are likely to be associated with greatest turbulence in flow, whereas there should be no turbulence in cases of occlusion. Similar advances have been made in sonographic intracranial imaging with the development of low-frequency duplex color probes (transcranial color-coded sonography) for transcranial use. Although color-coded sonography requires a better acoustic window than conventional intracranial Doppler studies, it has the advantage of allowing more precise identification of vessels and structural abnormalities and more accurate measurement of blood flow velocities. It is likely that these developments in extra- and intracranial ultrasound imaging techniques will provide a noninvasive, safe, reliable alternative to angiography in stroke patients.

Angiography

Selective intra-arterial angiography, whether conventional or digitally subtracted, continues to be the gold standard for diagnosing vascular abnormality in stroke. An angiogram is indicated in stroke patients who are potential candidates for carotid endarterectomy. It may also be indicated in other patients with ischemic infarcts in whom carotid duplex studies have failed to demonstrate significant atheromatous disease. These patients include individuals with no risk factors, suspected subclavian steal syndrome, arteritis, and patients suspected to have carotid artery dissection. In addition, it may be necessary to undertake angiography in nondisabled survivors of cerebral hemorrhage, depending on the site of bleeding (e.g. lobar hematoma) and the lack of any obvious underlying cause (hypertension or bleeding diathesis). The objective is to exclude significant aneurysms or arteriovenous malformations which may be a treatable cause of the hemorrhage.

Eligibility for carotid endarterectomy is by far the most common indication for angiography in acute stroke. Carotid angiography should be undertaken if duplex studies show significant levels of stenosis (70–99 percent) in the extracranial section of the relevant internal carotid artery. The carotid artery on the symptomatic side is studied first, and if a potentially operable lesion is demonstrated (70–99 percent stenosis), the contralateral carotid is studied unless already well shown by duplex scanning. As the risk of recurrence or stroke after TIA is highest during the first few weeks after the initial event, it is logical that angiography and possibly carotid endarterctomy be performed as soon as the patient has recovered and is fit enough to undergo the procedure. In practice, this usually means surgery 4–6 weeks after the stroke, although it is being undertaken earlier at some facilities. Carotid angiography is a major procedure and has its own risks. The neurological complication rate of conventional angiography in patients suffering TIA or minor strokes is about 4 percent, with 1 percent of patients suffering disabling stroke resulting in permanent neurological deficit.[44] The risks are greatest for patients with tight stenosis of the external internal cerebral artery.

The risks of angiography must be balanced against the potential benefit of endarterectomy for the patient. There is no indication for undertaking angiography in stroke patients in whom carotid duplex studies have demonstrated mild to moderate stenosis. Even in those shown to have significant disease, it is important to ascertain that they are willing to proceed with carotid endarterctomy, if indicated, before being offered angiography. All patients should be told of the relative risk of stroke before and after endarterectomy, as well as the possibility of neurological complications caused by angiography and carotid endarterectomy, to help in the decision-making process. Although age in itself is not a criterion, there is no justification for proceeding with angiography in elderly patients who may not wish to undergo carotid endarterectomy for personal or cultural reasons or for fear of disabling consequences.

As mentioned previously, noninvasive MR angiography is safe and can be undertaken easily at the time of doing an MR scan. It is fast replacing conventional angiography in the assessment of intra- and extracranial vasculature in stroke patients.[45] However, MRA lacks the spatial resolution, selectivity, and dynamic character of conventional intra-arterial angiography, which remains essential for a more detailed assessment if surgery is contemplated.

Echocardiography

The role of routine echocardiography in the evaluation of stroke patients is controversial. Large series on echocardiography in stroke have shown low yields of clinically relevant lesions.[46] There is little evidence that management decisions, such as those regarding anticoagulation, are influenced by echocardiographic findings.[47] An abnormal echo does not prove that the ischemic lesion was caused by embolism or that the heart was the source of this embolism. Similarly, a normal echo does not exclude a cardiac source of embolism because the whole clot may have embolized, leaving no trace, or the clot may be less than 2 mm in diameter, too small to be detected by conventional echocardiography but not too small to lodge in a branch of the middle cerebral artery. The type of echocardiographic scan used is also important. The conventional two-dimensional transthoracic echo may occasionally detect intraventricular thrombi as small as 5 mm in diameter but cannot visualize the left atrium and appendage reliably. It is also of limited value in obese patients and those with emphysema, chest deformity, or prosthetic valves. Some of these limitations can be overcome by using transesophageal echocardiography, but this is expensive, has limited availability, and does not visualize the cardiac apex as well as the transthoracic procedure.[48]

The clinical value of echocardiography depends on appropriate patient selection and awareness of the relevance of the information it provides. Unrestricted use of echocardiography in stroke patients may be unjustified and unnecessary.[49] Echocardiography should be undertaken in stroke or TIA patients with no significant evidence of atheromatous disease or risk factors; those with evidence of relevant cardiac disease on clinical examination, chest radiograph, and electrocardiography (atrial fibrillation, aortic or mitral valve disease, vegetations, myocardial dyskinesia); and those with a family history of atrial myxoma or cardiomyopathy. Symptomatic patients with a high probability of atrial thrombus should be referred for transesophageal echocardiography if the two-dimensional echo is normal.

MANAGEMENT OF STROKE PATIENTS

Management of stroke patients is a complex process ranging from acute medical intervention to treatment of long-term disability and involves several specialities, disciplines, and settings. There is no single measure which in itself can overcome the burden of stroke to the patient, to health services, and to society. Management of stroke patients is based on a pragmatic strategy involving intervention at several levels. Effective management of stroke also requires true integration of services across different areas of interest (e.g., medical, rehabilitation, and social services) to ensure mechanisms for timely mobilization of appropriate resources and to achieve a seamless service from the onset of stroke to long-term care.[50]

Acute management

Several studies and guidelines for acute stroke management recommend immediate hospitalization of all stroke patients with access to specialist stroke care.[51,52] The "core" working practices of modern acute stroke units include rapid admission of patients within the first few hours of onset, comprehensive

> ### Summary of management algorithm
> ### Management of stroke patients
>
> Effective treatment
> - Medical intervention to minimize impairment
> - Prevention and early treatment of acute complications
> - Rehabilitation to minimize disability
> - Adaptations to minimize handicap
>
> Effective prevention (strokes and TIAs)
> - Modification of risk factors: e.g., hypertension, smoking, lifestyle
> - Medical treatment: antiplatelets, anticoagulants
> - Surgical treatment: carotid endarterectomy
>
> Effective support
> - Patient and family: counseling, education, training
> - Health services: community nursing, domiciliary rehabilitation
> - Statutory services: personal care, respite care
> - Voluntary agencies: clubs, information, day centers

investigations at the time of admission, and intensive medical, nursing, and therapy input.[53] The potential benefits of these units include an opportunity for early treatment with thrombolytic, neuroprotective, or anticoagulant drugs, maintenance of physiological homeostasis, prevention of stroke-related complications, secondary prevention, early mobilization and improved coordination within the stroke team. In addition, such units offer the opportunity to undertake trials of new interventions and novel investigations in acute stroke management, which have important implications for future practice. Despite the importance of specialist care in reducing morbidity and mortality in stroke, the proportion of stroke patients who are admitted to hospitals is as low as 50 percent in some areas, often due to exclusion of elderly people from specialist care.[54]

The benefits of hospital admission for stroke patients have not always been clear and it was long believed that most patients were admitted to hospital to meet nursing, rehabilitation, and social needs.[9] There was a view that a significant proportion of admissions to hospitals were unnecessary and led to inappropriate use of resources.[55] Several observational studies suggested that organized care at home could achieve similar outcomes to stroke unit care. A recent randomized controlled study did not support this assumption.[56] Nearly a third of the patients being managed at home had to be admitted to hospital despite well-defined criteria for patient selection, high levels of support from the specialist stroke team and community services operating in the most favorable configuration of health and social services. In addition, mortality and dependence were significantly higher at 3 and 12 months in patients managed at home or in general ward settings. The number of patients that were needed to be treated on the stroke unit for a favorable effect was 6 compared with other settings, which is much lower than required for many accepted interventions.

The predominant aim of management is to restore function. This can be achieved by reducing the size of the lesion (acute interventions aimed at the pathology of stroke), thereby reducing the severity of impairment, or alternatively, by treating impairment to prevent or reduce disability (acute rehabilitation). Acute medical treatment of stroke can be divided into:

1. General medical management in the acute phase
   - physiological homeostasis
   - prevention of complications
2. Measures to restore circulation and arrest the pathological process
   - thrombolysis
   - neuroprotection
3. Measures to prevent further strokes (secondary prevention)
4. Restoration of function
   - early mobilization
   - assessments for specialist rehabilitation

General medical measures

The management of patients with acute stroke requires the skills of a well-coordinated multidisciplinary team because of the number of problems associated with stroke (e.g. impaired consciousness, dysphagia), the high risk of stroke-related complications (e.g. aspiration pneumonia, venous thrombosis), and the specialized needs (e.g. communication problems, visuospatial impairment) of this patient group. Most of the treatment in acute stroke is supportive, allowing time for neurological injury to settle with minimization of further direct risk to the area of damage and indirect risk from complications that may arise. This includes maintaining stable respiratory and cardiovascular function, with particular attention to oxygenation and appropriate blood pressure; correction of fluid electrolyte imbalance and monitoring blood glucose levels; ensuring adequate nutrition; preventing hypo- or hyperthermia and complications such as aspiration pneumonitis, urinary retention or infection, venous thromboembolism, seizures, pressure sores, contractures, and dislocated or frozen shoulder. Areas that need special attention include the following.

1. Maintenance of airways and oxygenation: Despite its obvious importance in restricting the damage associated with stroke, this aspect of care is frequently poorly managed in clinical settings. It is particularly important in elderly patients, in whom alterations in consciousness level following stroke are common and who are more likely to suffer from chronic pulmonary disease or desensitization of central ventilatory mechanisms. Interventions include proper positioning, adequate nasopharyngeal suction, and oxygen administration. Aminophylline may be used in patients with Cheyne–Stokes breathing. Assisted ventilation and hyperbaric oxygen have been used in patients with acute stroke but their effectiveness remains to be demonstrated.[57]

2. Management of hypertension: High blood pressure is commonly seen in patients with acute stroke.[58,59] There is considerable controversy regarding optimal blood pressure control in acute stroke with opinions varying from no treatment at all to aggressive management of blood pressure. The only area of consensus is in the management of patients with intracerebral hemorrhage. Persistent marked elevation of blood pressure can promote further bleeding, increase cerebral blood flow, and raise intracranial pressure.[60] Markedly elevated blood pressure (higher than 125 mmHg diastolic) on admission and persistent inadequate blood pressure control have been shown to adversely affect the prognosis in intracerebral hemorrhage. There appears to be a case for controlling high blood pressure in patients with cerebral hemorrhage, although persistent hypotension (which may lead to secondary ischemia) should be avoided.

It is generally accepted at present that hypertension should not be treated soon after ischemic stroke.[61] Cerebral autoregulation is lost in the area around cerebral infarction, and perfusion is dependent on systemic blood pressure. Observational studies have shown that in the acute phase of ischemic stroke, elevation of blood pressure in the first few days helps to restore cerebral perfusion and activates collateral arterial supply.[62] SPET has shown that reducing blood pressure carries the risk of reducing the blood flow to the penumbra and increasing the area of infarct.[63] The effects of iatrogenic hypotension may be more significant in elderly hypertensives in whom age and hypertension may already have impaired cerebral autoregulatory mechanisms.[64]

Studies have shown a marked fall in systolic and diastolic blood pressure levels during the first 7 days after acute stroke in most patients,[65] and a wait-and-see policy is recommended. Antihypertensive treatment may be indicated in patients who continue to be hypertensive beyond the first week of stroke. The aim should then be to reduce blood pressure gradually into the high normal range. There may be benefits in using angiotensin-converting enzyme inhibitors, α-adrenergic blockers, or β-adrenergic blockers, which preserve cerebral blood flow, in preference to cerebral vasodilators such as nitroprusside and certain calcium channel blockers, which may result in cerebral edema or vascular steal from the ischemic area.

Early antihypertensive treatment may be necessary for ischemic stroke patients presenting with persistent high diastolic blood pressure levels greater than 130 mmHg, features of malignant hypertension, or complicating medical illness such as decompensated cardiac failure, persistent angina or aortic dissection.[61] Early control of hypertension may also be indicated in patients undergoing thrombolysis because of the increased risk of intracranial hemorrhage in patients with elevated blood pressure.[66] Systolic hypertension in acute stroke may be associated with early progression, but the causal relationship between systolic hypertension and early progression has not been established.[67] Confirmation of this relationship has the potential of altering future antihypertensive management in acute stroke, especially if shown to be amenable to therapeutic interventions.

Many stroke patients are admitted to hospital who were taking antihypertensive medication at the time of the stroke and there is no consensus whether these medications should be continued or withdrawn in the first few days after stroke onset. There is great variation in practice depending upon the views of treating physicians. Theoretically there are advantages in stopping antihypertensives in the acute phase because of the usual reasons of loss of cerebral autoregulation and the central blood pressure being the main driver for adequate cerebral perfusion. This needs to be balanced against specific patient needs, level of blood pressure, and comorbidity. The appropriateness of antihypertensive medication in the acute phase should be reviewed in individual patients keeping these parameters in mind. Patients who are normotensive on admission should be monitored regularly and antihypertensive medication reintroduced 1–2 weeks after stroke depending upon the level of blood pressure. We prefer not to stop antihypertensive medication if the patient is a known hypertensive with evidence of left ventricular hypertrophy or renal involvement and if the blood pressure is over 180 systolic and over 100 diastolic on several readings at the time of admission.

3. Glucose: Although 15–20 percent of patients with acute stroke are known to be diabetic, hyperglycemia has been reported in 25–50 percent of acute stroke patients on initial presentation.[68] Blood glucose levels of over 8 mmol/L in stroke patients have been associated with increased mortality and poor functional outcome, regardless of the cause of hyperglycemia or stroke subtype.[69] However, this is not accepted universally, as many studies have shown that blood glucose levels cease to have an independent effect when controlled for other variables in multivariate models.[70]

There is no consensus on the management of hyperglycemia in stroke patients. Clearly, diabetic patients and those with persistent blood glucose levels outside the normal range need to be treated. Practice is less clear in patients who are not diabetic and have blood glucose levels greater than 8 mmol/L. Despite the lack of any large trials, there is a trend toward treating these patients aggressively with insulin based on extrapolation of the findings of the DIGAMI study.[71] There is an ongoing study on the use of combined insulin, glucose and potassium infusions to reduce blood glucose levels in stroke patients with mild to moderate hyperglycemia, the results of which should be available in the near future.[72] Care should be taken in patients who require antihyperglycemia treatment because of the dangers of hypoglycemia.

4. Temperature: Hyperthermia (Temp. >37.5°C) is common in stroke and has been reported in 25–30 percent of patients.[73] Common causes of pyrexia include coexisting infection, infarct necrosis or disturbances of thermoregulatory mechanisms. Hyperthermia in stroke is associated with large infarcts, early neurological deterioration and increased mortality. This suggests that rises in temperature should be avoided in acute stroke patients by aggressive screening and prevention of infections as well as the use of antipyretics and cooling interventions. Although common sense and clinical experience support this strategy (followed on many stroke units), there are no large studies to support this intervention. If high temperatures increase infarct size and mortality in stroke, it can be argued that intentional hypothermia will have the opposite effect.[74] However, there are no controlled trials of hypothermia to support this practice, and large randomized trials are being proposed to test this intervention.

5. Hydration and biochemical imbalance: Stroke is often associated with disturbances of water, glucose, and salt mechanisms. These conditions may be due to impaired consciousness, inability to perceive or respond to hunger and thirst, or hypothalamic disturbances causing salt losing or retaining syndromes. Hydration should be maintained with care to reduce the risk of cerebral or pulmonary edema (chronic heart failure being common in the elderly) and hyponatremia.

6. Raised intracranial pressure: Cerebral edema due to a combination of vasogenic and cytotoxic mechanisms is a frequent complication of large middle cerebral artery territory or cerebellar infarcts and intracranial hemorrhages. The clinical picture is that of worsening consciousness levels and neurological deficits, 1–5 days after stroke onset. In addition to herniation, cerebral edma can compress and obstruct other intracranial arteries leading to secondary strokes in unrelated territories. Clinical symptoms suggestive of raised intracranial pressure are an important indication for repeating CT scans and undertaking transcranial Doppler studies to assess the level of intracranial tension and the evolution of secondary lesions. Several interventions have been suggested and include the use of mannitol, glycerol, steroids, diuretics and barbiturates.[75] None of these interventions is supported by robust clinical evidence. As the action of most osmotic agents is nonselective, there is a risk of worsening of neurological deficit because of their effect on the unaffected side. In clinical practice, mannitol has been used in selected patients, with apparently good results in some individuals. More recently, decompressive craniotomy has been used in patients with malignant middle cerebral artery territory infarction with good results.[76]

7. Nutrition: Malnutrition is common in acute stroke patients, especially if they have swallowing problems. Elderly patients are at greater risk than their younger counterparts because of the increased prevalence of background malnutrition in this age group.[77] Research has shown that the nutritional status of stroke patients (regardless of the presence of dysphagia) tends to decrease in the first few months after stroke.[78] This is compounded by low mood, anorexia, and starvation-induced weakness of the pharyngeal and respiratory muscles, leading to further malnutrition.[79] It is not known whether nutritional supplementation, over and above daily requirements, can influence recovery or outcome in stroke patients. Despite the awareness of nutritional depletion in such individuals, there are no universally accepted guidelines for feeding acute stroke patients. The decision to maintain nutrition depends on the clinical state of the patient, expected prognosis, and clinical practice at individual centers. In general, assisted nutrition (nasogastric or via a gastrostomy) may not be appropriate in deeply unconscious patients with poor prognosis. Swallowing problems in most other patients resolve rapidly in the first 2 weeks after stroke, and persistent problems are seen in only 10–15 percent of stroke survivors after this time. Adequate nutrition in these patients can be achieved through a nasogastric tube (with its inherent problems) or by undertaking a percutaneous endoscopic gastrostomy (PEG), which is a relatively simple and safe procedure for establishing nutrition in stroke patients. Although PEG has theoretical advantages over nasogastric feeding, there is no agreement on the timing of the procedure or its benefits over nasogastric feeding in patients who may recover rapidly in a few days.[80] Early PEG may be indicated in patients for whom clinical assessment by a speech and language therapist suggests that swallowing problems are unlikely to resolve in the near future.[81] The assessment and management of dysphagia is discussed in greater detail in a later section.

8. Prevention of complications: Prevention of complications is an important part of acute stroke management and should include general nursing measures and medical interventions aimed at preventing aspiration and chest infections, thromboprophylaxis using elasticated (TED) stockings or heparin, continence care, maintenance of skin integrity, and prevention of abnormal postures, contractures, or falls.

Specific therapies

RATIONALE FOR ACUTE INTERVENTION Specific therapies have been developed mainly for acute ischemic stroke due to large vessel disease and are aimed at re-establishing blood flow or limiting the neuronal consequences of hypoxia. Complete occlusion of the blood supply due to thrombosis or embolism leads to neuronal death within 5–10 minutes because of the high oxygen requirement of these cells. The effects of occlusion, however, are modified by the presence of collateral perfusion, leading to a small central area of infarct surrounded by an oligemic region between the infarcted area and healthy tissue. This area, called the ischemic penumbra, is defined as "the area of brain where blood flow is sufficient to prevent neuronal death, but not sufficient to sustain normal electrical activity."[82] It is characterized by impaired synaptic transmission but preserved ionic gradients and cell morphology. A flow rate just below the threshold necessary for electrical activity can be tolerated for several hours (Fig. 49-4). If the insult is sustained, cell death invariably occurs.

Neuronal death is a result of impaired energy metabolism in a cell due to disruption of oxidative phosphorylation and reduced adenosine triphosphate (ATP) production. This results in a loss of control over the transport of ions (particularly calcium) and neurotransmitters (particularly glutamate and aspartate) across the cell membrane.[83] The flux of these neurotransmitters overstimulates receptors such as the *N*-methyl-D-aspartate (NMDA) receptor, a subtype of glutamate receptor present on a large number of neurons, which initiates a massive influx of calcium ions in toxic doses into neurons and their mitochondria (Fig. 49-5). The massive influx of calcium against a background of homeostatic failure activates lipases, proteases, and endonucleases, resulting in cell destruction (ischemic cascade).[83] Calcium-activated phospholipases and intracellular metabolites also contribute to cell injury by stimulating nitric oxide synthase and the generation of highly reactive free radicals. These metabolites further compromise membrane and cellular processes, cause vascular vasospasm, increase local thrombogenesis, and release glutamate in huge quantities, fueling further calcium influx. The structural consequences of the ischemic cascade are swelling of the cells, which takes place between 24 and 48 hours after the acute injury and

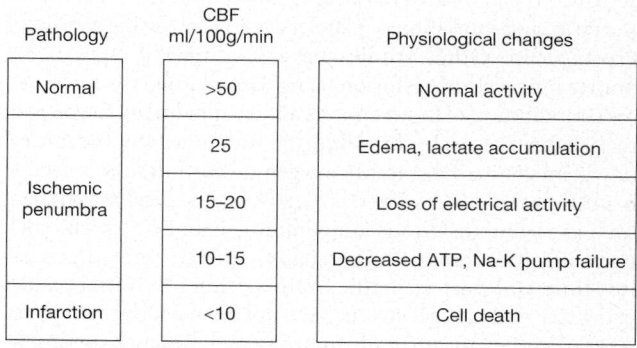

Pathology	CBF ml/100g/min	Physiological changes
Normal	>50	Normal activity
Ischemic penumbra	25	Edema, lactate accumulation
	15–20	Loss of electrical activity
	10–15	Decreased ATP, Na-K pump failure
Infarction	<10	Cell death

Figure 49-4 Pathophysiology of stroke.

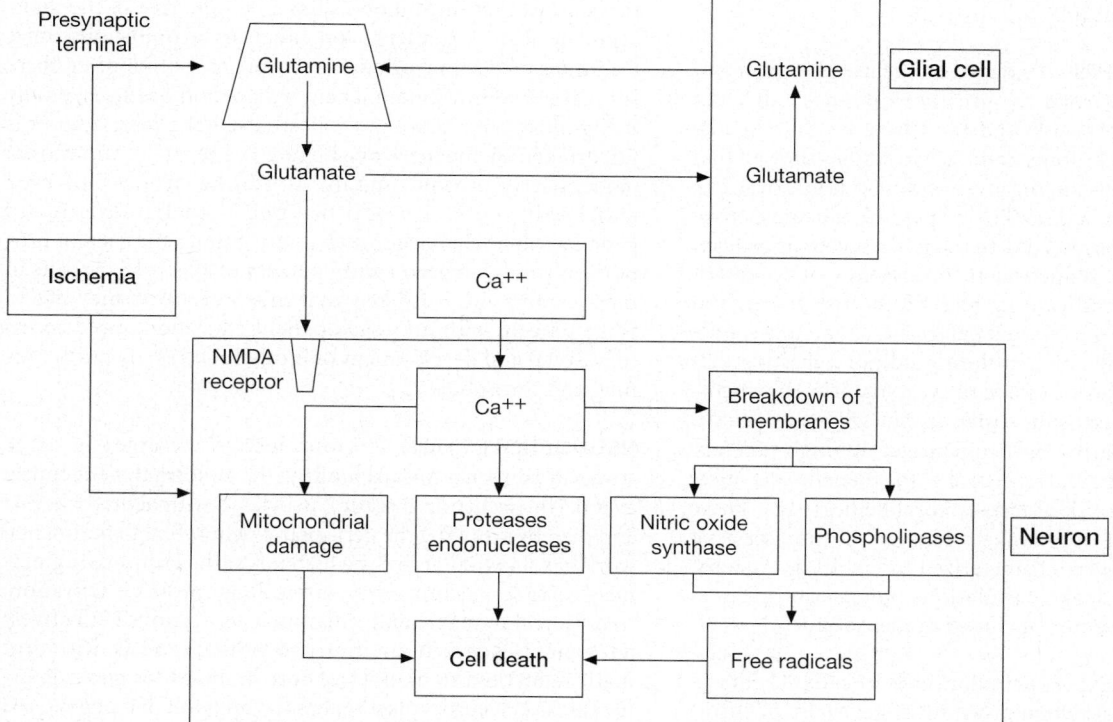

Figure 49-5 Simplified diagram of the ischemic cascade.

is followed by extracellular edema which occurs 3–5 days after stroke.[84] This may be seen clinically in association with large infarcts and causes deterioration after initial clinical improvement.

Therapeutic interventions have been targeted at these mechanisms and are specifically directed toward rescuing he ischemic penumbra. The favored strategies at present include:

- Early restoration of blood flow to ischemic tissue to prevent infarction or improve the ischemic penumbra and reduce the size of the infarct.
- Protection of ischemic neurons from consequences of the ischemic cascade by blocking excitatory pathways, inhibiting calcium influx, or scavenging free radicals.

Treatments aimed at restoration of blood flow and oxygenation include thrombolysis using tissue plasminogen activator (tPA) or urokinase, anticoagulation with heparin or warfarin, and inhibition of platelet aggregation using aspirin or prostacyclin. Other studies have investigated the role of improving cerebral perfusion using vasodilators, vasopressors, or hemodilution.[85] Interventions aimed at reducing the oxygen requirement of the brain include treatment with naftidrofuryl (an agent claimed to modify oxygen utilization) and selective hypothermia of the injured cortex.[85] Free-radical scavengers, such as 21-aminosteroids and vitamins E and C, which block peroxidization and lipoxygenase activity, may decrease ischemic and post-ischemic brain swelling.[86] Initial results using free-radical scavengers have not been encouraging, and further studies are currently in progress.[86] Recent experimental work in animal models has suggested that agents which block mediators of inflammatory response (e.g., ICAM) may be neuroprotective in acute stroke and offer treatment possibilities for the future.[87]

ASPIRIN AND HEPARIN Evidence on the use of aspirin and heparin in acute stroke is greatly influenced by the International Stroke Trial[18] and the Chinese Acute Stroke Trial.[88] The combined results of these two studies showed that aspirin in a dose of 150–300 mg given within 48 hours of stroke onset prevented death or disability in 1 percent of treated stroke patients at 4 weeks compared with those not receiving aspirin. There was a similar reduction in proportion of recurrent strokes without a significant increase in the risk of cerebral hemorrhage. Aspirin was started before a CT scan in a significant proportion of patients in these studies, suggesting that early use of aspirin may be safe in the vast majority of patients diagnosed to have an ischemic stroke on clinical grounds alone. The evidence on heparin was inconclusive; although early use of heparin decreased recurrent stroke, this benefit was offset by an increase in the risk of intracerebral hemorrhage. These data need to be interpreted in the context of the limitations of both studies, which were characterized by significant heterogeneity not only in stroke populations but also in practices within the different centers included in these studies.

THROMBOLYSIS Experimental models of cerebral infarction have shown that, when given intra-arterially or intravenously, thrombolytic agents such as streptokinase, tPA, and urokinase may lyse acute clots and reduce infarct size.[89]

These studies also showed that there was a narrow window for intervention, requiring that the drugs be given within 6 hours of the acute episode. Initial studies on stroke patients, which were mostly isolated and poorly controlled, showed mixed results but suggested potential benefits.[90] This has been confirmed in recent randomized controlled trials on thrombolysis, which include common design features such as mandatory CT scanning, defined time windows for intervention, use of standardized assessment techniques and a common endpoint (death or disability) measured at 3 months after stroke.

Streptokinase was used in three large trials, all of which were terminated prematurely because of an early increased risk of cerebral hemorrhage and death. Although no gains were demonstrated for any subgroup of patients at any time points, the studies had significant design flaws in terms of dose, timing of interventions and concommitant use of heparin and aspirin.[91] Alteplase (tPA) was used in four major trials with generally consistent results.[92] Only the NINDS trial in which tPA was used within a 3 hour time window showed clearly positive results. The proportion of patients with favorable outcome on both neurological and functional measures showed an absolute increase of 12 percent, without adversely affecting mortality. Supporting evidence comes from the European studies which had a longer time window (6 hours) and included more severe patients than the NINDS study. Although the European studies failed to show a significant effect on prespecified endpoints, post hoc analyses showed a significant effect if endpoints similar to those for the NINDS trial were used.[93] When subject to meta-analysis, the results unequivocally favor the use of thrombolysis in the first 3 and probably 6 hours after stroke onset.[92]

Thrombolysis for stroke has been in use in North America and Europe for over 5 years. The lessons learnt in clinical practice suggest that thrombolysis has a definite role in the management of stroke patients and enhances favorable outcomes if administered within 3 hours of stroke onset.[94] However, there is a real risk of intracerebral hemorrhage and death, especially if eligibility criteria are not followed strictly, intervention is undertaken by inexperienced teams, patients are monitored inadequately or concomitant aspirin/heparin is not used judiciously.[94] It is also clear that only a small proportion of patients will be eligible for such interventions; the current proportion varies between 1 and 3 percent of all stroke patients in most centers and it is likely that this proportion may rise to 15–20 percent with improved patient education, rapid access to hospital and development of infrastructures for early scanning and thrombolysis.

NEUROPROTECTION Cytoprotective therapies in acute stroke are directed toward limiting the abnormal biochemical events (the ischemic cascade) associated with acute ischemia and thereby salvaging the peri-infarct penumbra. Experimental work has shown that drugs which target the excitotoxic glutamate cascade, calcium entry, intracellular protease activation, free-radical damage, and inflammatory response effectively attenuate ischemic brain injury in animal models, with dramatic reductions in infarct size both in the cortex and subcortical areas.[95] Neuroprotection has the prospect of being offered universally, either alone or in combination with thrombolysis. Unlike thrombolysis, CT scanning may not be mandatory prior to commencing treatment, special monitoring facilities may not be needed and the treatment could be offered by family physicians or by the paramedical staff prior to transfer to a specialist facility. It is also possible that neuroprotection may extend the window for thrombolysis beyond 3 hours.

A large number of drugs are currently undergoing phase III clinical trials, and results available to date have been disappointing.[96] Many of the problems with previous studies have been attributed to poor design, and newer studies have been devised to overcome the problems identified with older studies. The results of ongoing trials are awaited, following which it will be important to assess the clinical implications of this strategy in future practice.

It is unlikely that any single pharmacological approach will be suitable for all stroke patients. It is more likely that future practice will be a combination of synergistic general and specific measures directed against different components of the ischemic process (e.g. combinations of thrombolysis, neuroprotection, free radical scavenging) aimed at restoring cerebral function after infarction.

Stroke prevention

The role of aggressive strategies aimed at stroke prevention cannot be overestimated. It is generally accepted that no intervention would have a greater impact on quality of life in old age than prevention of stroke.[97] A secondary prevention strategy which is not based on age but appropriateness makes good sense and is cost-effective because elderly people have a higher risk of stroke and will derive greater benefit from such interventions. There is overwhelming evidence to support active antihypertensive treatment in elderly patients with mild to moderate hypertension.[98] This has been facilitated by the availability of antihypertensive drugs which are effective, have minimal side-effects and can be administered once or twice a day. These properties make them ideal for use in elderly patients in whom compliance may be a problem. The role of lipid lowering agents in elderly patients with hypercholesterolemia is more controversial.[99] Extrapolation of data from high-profile studies in relatively young patients suggest that management with statins may be of benefit, especially if there is pre-existing vascular disease.[100] Lifestyle changes are an important aspect of stroke prevention. There is evidence that simple measures such as cessation of smoking,[101] and exercise[102] reduce the risk of stroke. Moderate alcohol consumption has been found to be protective, and the benefits are not limited to any particular type of alcoholic beverage.[103] The success of any preventative program based on lifestyle changes is dependent on adequate resources, targeting (individual risk approach), acceptance rate, and ability to provide effective continued intervention and follow-up.[104]

Antiplatelet drugs (e.g. aspirin 75–300 mg/day) in patients with TIA or minor stroke reduce the risk of recurrence by 15 percent.[105] There is also evidence that aspirin may decrease the risk of first-ever stroke in patients with vascular disease and recurrent stroke in patients with atrial fibrillation.[106] Despite the widespread use of aspirin in vascular disease, there are several questions that remain unanswered. It is not known whether inadvertent aspirin administration can worsen the condition of patients with primary intracerebral hemorrhage or whether patients on stroke prophylaxis with aspirin are more likely to have hemorrhagic infarcts. There is also considerable debate about when aspirin should be started after an ischemic stroke (risk of hemorrhagic transformation), what the effective dose should be (higher doses may not offer a greater benefit/risk ratio), and for what period of time it should be continued. The role of aspirin in the primary prevention of stroke in patients without established vascular disease remains equivocal. It is also possible that the benefits of aspirin are limited to large vessel occlusive disease and may not extend to patients with lacunar infarcts because of the difference in pathophysiology. Dipyridamole can be used as monotherapy in patients who cannot be given aspirin, although dipyridamole on its own is not as effective as aspirin in preventing stroke.[107] A combination of aspirin and dipyridamole has been shown to be significantly more effective than aspirin alone in the secondary prevention of stroke, but there is a high incidence of side-effects and subsequent discontinuation of treatment with the combination.[108] A large study using a new antiplatelet agent, clopidogrel, has shown a relative risk reduction of 8.7 percent over aspirin with no significant differences in safety.[109] Clopidogrel may be a suitable second-line intervention in patients who cannot tolerate aspirin or dipyridamole, continue to have recurrent TIAs on aspirin or have a history of ischemic heart disease. It is important to remember that the benefits of clopidrogel over aspirin are modest compared with the relative difference of costs between the drugs.[49]

Atrial fibrillation, common in elderly patients, is an important cause of thromboembolic stroke. Trials of anticoagulation in stroke have consistently shown two-thirds reduction in risk compared with 25 percent reduction in risk seen with aspirin.[106] The risks of stroke, and hence the benefits of anticoagulation, are greatest in patients with previous history of stroke or other embolic disease, structural valve lesions involving the mitral and aortic valves, prosthetic or infected valves, cardiomyopathy and chronic heart failure. Hypertension, diabetes, and increasing age are also associated with a higher risk of stroke in patients with atrial fibrillation. The benefits of anticoagulation need to be counterbalanced by the risks involved, especially in elderly patients who may be prone to falls, suffer from cognitive impairment compromising compliance and ability to monitor adverse events, take a large number of drugs (some of which may interfere with anticoagulation), or have significant comorbidity (recent bleed, peptic ulcer disease, malignancy, or alcoholism). However, recent studies have shown that anticoagulation is underused in a significant proportion of elderly people who meet eligibility criteria and do not have contraindications to warfarin use.[110] Research has also shown that anticoagulation for stroke prevention in clinical practice is feasible, safe and matches the effectiveness seen in randomized trials, even in older people.[111] Hence, long-term anticoagulation with adjusted-dose warfarin should be considered in all warfarin-eligible patients with atrial fibrillation who are at high thromboembolic risk, especially as studies have shown that aspirin or fixed, low-dose warfarin are not as effective.[112] In patients with atrial fibrillation for whom the risks of anticoagulation outweigh its benefits, treatment with aspirin may be a safe, although not as effective, alternative.

The increasing availability and proven efficacy of carotid endarterectomies (CEA) has been another important development in stroke prevention.[113] CEA is indicated in patients with a recent TIA or nondisabling stroke in whom the CT scan is compatible with a diagnosis of cerebral ischemia and duplex scanning has demonstrated a hemodynamically significant stenosis of the relevant extracranial internal carotid artery. Selective angiography is needed to demonstrate that the stenosis is amenable to surgery and that there are no other distal lesions that may preclude surgical intervention. The risks of surgery include minor neurological deficits which may be seen in 10–20 percent of patients and are usually transitory. Major neurological sequelae leading to permanent disability or death are seen in 1–5 percent of patients depending on the expertise available in the operating room and the skill of the surgeon. CEA is of proven effectiveness in patients with 70–99 percent extracranial internal carotid artery stenosis where the benefit for stroke reduction outweighs the risks of the procedure and angiography. Age per se should not be a contraindication to CEA because the risk of stroke increases with age, and elderly people with significant stenoses are likely to accrue greater health benefit than younger patients, provided that they are medically fit and willing to undergo the operation. CEA is of little benefit in patients with mild carotid stenosis (0–29 percent reduction in diameter), for whom the risks of the procedure are greater than the risk of stroke. The risk/benefit ratio in patients with moderate stenosis remains unclear. Progression in degree of stenosis occurs in about one-fourth of these patients, half of whom will develop a severe stenosis within 10 years. The cumulative risk of stroke in these cases has been estimated at 11 percent after 7 years. At present it is conventional not to offer surgery to patients with moderate stenosis except under specific circumstances. Recent advances in interventional neurovascular radiology have led to the development of cerebral percutaneous transluminal angioplasty as an alternative to surgical endarterectomy. This procedure is undergoing further evaluation, but preliminary data suggest a success rate of 90 percent with less than 10 percent morbidity. Despite their ability to prevent strokes in selected patients with tight carotid stenosis, carotid endarterectomy and angioplasty may not have a significant impact on stroke incidence. It is estimated that even if the availability of CEA were unrestricted, only one stroke per year would be prevented for every 20 procedures performed (estimated reduction in stroke incidence less than 1 percent), limiting its impact as a major stroke prevention strategy.[49]

RECOVERY AND REHABILITATION

Based on evidence from randomized trials and statistical overviews, there is little that medical treatment or surgery can do to alter eventual outcome in the vast majority of stroke patients. It is likely that this view will change as potentially effective treatments for acute stroke become available in the near future. However, it may be a few years before new interventions become routine practice in mainstream care. Until such time, early and planned multidisciplinary rehabilitation will remain the cornerstone of stroke management.

Recovery

Most patients who survive a stroke make some functional recovery. Recovery is of two types: intrinsic, which involves a degree of return of neural control, and adaptive, in which alternative strategies are used to overcome disability. The majority of patients show some degree of both intrinsic and adaptive recovery. Advances in neuroimaging techniques have shown that the adult brain has considerable potential for plasticity.[114] Recovery from brain injury occurs because of restoration of function of partially damaged pathways and strengthening of existing pathways (restitution), and by the development of new pathways in the unaffected areas of brain which take over the lost function (substitution).[115] Further studies have shown a number of cellular and histological changes, such as axonal sprouting and formation of new dendritic connections, in the unaffected hemisphere during recovery from stroke in experimental models.[115]

The process of reorganization of neural activity has been demonstrated in human subjects who have suffered a stroke.[116,117] Imaging studies have shown reorganization of activity in the peri-infarct cortex, supplementary areas and functionally similar areas in the ipsilateral hemisphere. The cerebellum, thalamus and prefrontal areas appear to play an important part in the restoration of function. It is now believed that there are multiple motor circuits in the brain which serve similar functions. Conventional pathways dominate in healthy subjects and inhibit the activity of alternative pathways in other areas of the brain. Disruption of traditional pathways in cerebral ischemia reduces or eliminates the inhibition normally exerted by these pathways and allows activation of alternate pathways in the premotor areas of the affected side and primary motor areas on the unaffected side. Hence, the paradigm for function has shifted from strict cerebral localization to that of interactive functioning of diverse cortical areas activated by the constantly changing balance of inhibitory and excitatory impulses.

An important question that remains unanswered is whether there are factors or processes which modify restoration of neural networks following ischemic damage. Early studies suggest that activation may be facilitated by sensory stimulation,[118] repetitive movement of the affected limbs[119] or the use of drugs which modify neurotransmitter release.[120] Their absence may also be important—loss of function will mean withdrawal of afferent stimulation arising out of voluntary activity and is supported by some experimental evidence in primates.[121] The timing and intensity of intervention, however, may be crucial: early movements in experimental models have shown an increase in the size of the cortical lesion.[122] This emerging picture fits in well with our knowledge about motor learning, which emphasizes the importance of repetition, attention, and goal-directed activity.[123] The concept of reorganization and its susceptibility to external influences is fundamental to the process of rehabilitation. Although most therapy regimens claim to modulate neuronal plasticity, there is little direct evidence that this is indeed the case.[124] More research is needed into the drivers which modulate restorative neuroplasticity before new therapies that are grounded firmly in the science of recovery can be developed.[123]

Recovery is the fastest in the first few weeks after stroke, with a further 5–10 percent occurring between 6 months and 1 year. About 30 percent of survivors are independent within 3 weeks, and by 6 months this proportion rises to 50 percent.[125] Measurable recovery seldom occurs after

12 months, although every clinician is aware of at least one patient who is an exception to this rule. Later neurophysiological recovery can continue for several years but is rarely significant in terms of improvement in overall functional ability.[126] Completeness of recovery depends largely on the severity of the initial deficit. The more severe the initial deficit, the less likely is it that complete recovery will occur. The pattern of recovery is not uniform and shows considerable variation between individuals and also between different deficits in the same individual. There is currently no validated method for predicting the precise mode or degree of recovery for a given individual. In addition, there can be considerable variation in day-to-day progress of individual patients, which may mask overall recovery or at times give rise to false optimism. This problem can be overcome by monitoring patients over time, as overall trends are more important than "one-off" assessments. Recovery may be affected adversely by the development of stroke-related complications. Although intensive and appropriate therapy may hasten recovery, it is debatable whether the ultimate overall extent of recovery is affected. Comorbidity in elderly patients is another variable that affects overall recovery and rehabilitation.

Rate of recovery varies for different impairments and disabilities. Some problems such as homonymous hemianopia, dysphagia, and sitting balance resolve very quickly in stroke survivors, whereas arm paralysis and language impairment recover more slowly and less completely. Perceptual problems may persist or take a very long time to recover.

HOMONYMOUS HEMIANOPIA   Improves within 4 weeks, usually within 10 days. Hemianopia present after 4 weeks usually persists.[127]

URINARY INCONTINENCE   This has been suggested as a prognostic measure in stroke,[128] although its clinical relevance may be limited by other variables such as consciousness, mobility, and nursing practices in different settings. About 60 percent of elderly stroke survivors are incontinent at 1 week, 42 percent at 4 weeks, 25 percent at 3 months, and 15 percent at 1 year. Persistence of urinary incontinence is associated with poor functional outcome, but it is not clear at what point in time this should be measured.

DYSPHAGIA   Swallowing problems are common in stroke and occur in up to 60 percent of patients within the first 24 hours of an acute episode.[129] Most swallowing difficulties in acute stroke, however, are transient and resolve in most patients within 2 weeks (mean 8.5 days) of the acute episode. Less than 15 percent of patients are symptomatic beyond 2 weeks, less than 2 percent beyond 3 months.

DYSPHASIA   This is normally slow to recover, maximum recovery occurring by 3 months. Some patients continue to recover up to 6 months.[126] The variability between the speed and degree of recovery among patients, compounded by lack of knowledge about predictors of recovery, has made prognostication difficult in this area. Spontaneous recovery is not influenced by the type of dysphasia or the age of the patient, which in turn does not influence functional recovery.[130,131]

SITTING BALANCE   Nearly 60 percent of stroke survivors recover sitting balance by 10 days, and 90 percent by 4 weeks.[132] Inability to maintain sitting balance at 3 months is associated with poor prognosis and is usually due to further strokes.

ARM WEAKNESS   Improvement in arm function is independent of overall stroke severity: 40 percent of patients gain full voluntary movement, and another 40 percent make partial recovery.[133] In general, if there is no recovery by 4 weeks, the prospects of full recovery are poor, although some patients may still show nonfunctional gains. The rate of arm recovery varies in different muscle groups. Wrist and finger flexors recover better than extensors, and shoulder movement is twice as likely to recover as hand movement.

WALKING   Leg function recovers quickly in patients who will finally walk: 45 percent of patients walk independently indoors by 4 weeks.[134] Walking outdoors presents greater problems, with only 25 percent of patients achieving this by 6 months.

PERCEPTUAL DISORDERS   The natural history of perceptual disorders is difficult to determine because of problems involving definition and measurement. Some perceptual problems, such as unilateral visual neglect and anosagnosia, tend to recover more quickly than other problems such as sensory inattention and sensory neglect. The presence of perceptual problems adversely influences speed of functional recovery, length of hospital stay, and destination of discharge even in the presence of good recovery in terms of other impairment.[135]

FUNCTIONAL RECOVERY   Functional recovery depends on the level of initial impairment and disability.[136] Mild to moderately disabled patients make measurable improvements up to 3 months following stroke, after which the recovery curve flattens.[137] There is evidence showing that the rate of functional recovery can be influenced by coordinated rehabilitation (Fig. 49-6). Patients with severe stroke may continue to show further functional improvement between 3 and 6 months.[138] The pattern of functional recovery often predicts the pattern of discharge from the hospital and the length of hospital stay (Fig. 49-6). If all stroke survivors are considered, 62 percent are independent in self-care at 3 months and 66 percent at the end of 1 year, despite persistence of neurological deficit in some patients.[139]

Rehabilitation (See also Chs 21–22)

Rehabilitation in stroke is not simply a matter of being treated by a therapist or a group of therapists but involves a whole range of approaches to managing disability provided by a coordinated multidisciplinary team and tailored to restore patients to their fullest possible physical, mental, and social capability.[140,141] The goals of rehabilitation are not always easy to define because it deals with many aspects of human performance. In general, rehabilitation should aim to maximize patients' role fulfillment and independence in their environment within the limitations imposed by underlying impairment and availability of resources.[142] It should help them to make the best adaptation possible to any difference between the roles desired and the roles achieved following stroke. Another important objective of the rehabilitation process is to

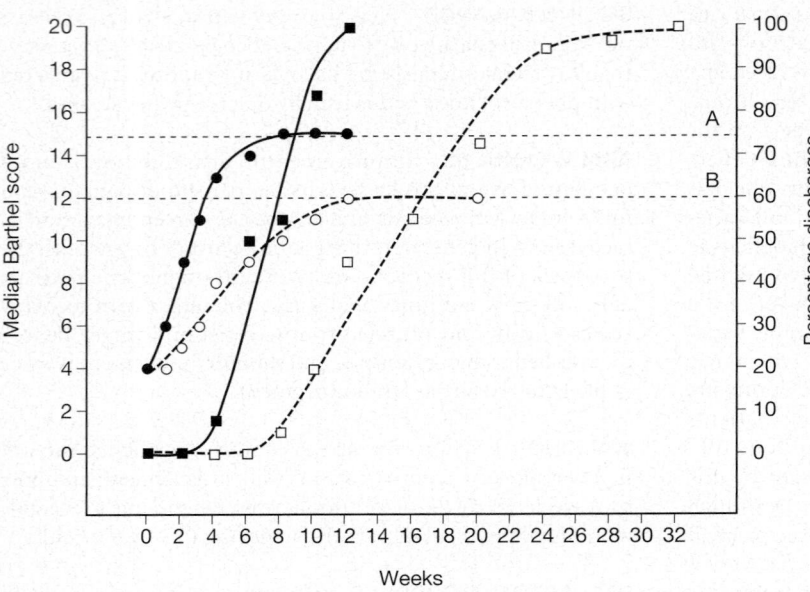

Figure 49-6 Weekly median Barthel scores and discharge rates of stroke survivors on stroke unit (*n* = 73) and general wards (*n* = 69) •, median Barthel score (stroke unit); ■, percentage discharges (stroke unit); ○, median Barthel score (general ward); □, percentage discharge (general ward). A, median discharge Barthel score of stroke unit group. B, median discharge Barthel score of general ward group.

monitor regularly the services provided to ensure that the best possible value is being obtained for the money and effort being expended.[141]

Progress in the development of rehabilitation techniques in stroke has been slow because of the lack of a conceptual model for stroke rehabilitation in the past.[143] The revised World Health Organization International Classification of Impairments, Disabilities, and Handicaps (ICIDH) is the most widely accepted model and allows measurement of outcomes in terms of body, person, and social function. The new revision has changed terminology; the terms disability and handicap have been replaced by limitations in activities and restriction in participation.[143] It is accepted that the focus of attention should pass from pathology to handicap and from patient to environment during the course of rehabilitation. The major areas of concern in rehabilitation are limitation of activity (disability) and restriction of participation (handicap).[144] Disability is defined as "restriction, or lack of ability, to perform an activity in the manner or within the range considered to be normal." Disability relates to function, and the ability to undertake basic activities of self-care is fundamental to any physical rehabilitation program. Handicap, the social consequence of disability, is defined as "limitations faced by stroke patients in fulfilling their normal role in the society." It is not always possible to differentiate handicap from disability, and most pragmatic approaches tend to combine these two dimensions, referring to them as social disability.

Process of rehabilitation

Rehabilitation in stroke is essentially a multidisciplinary activity which has been described as a problem-solving educational process focusing on disability and intended to reduce handicap.[145] The basic principles that should be applied throughout rehabilitation of stroke patients are the following:

- Documentation of impairments, disabilities, and handicaps and, where possible, measuring them using simple, valid scales

- Maximization of independence and minimization of learned dependency
- Holistic approach to patients, taking into account their physical and psychosocial background as well as their environment

The process of rehabilitation has four important components: assessment, planning, intervention, and evaluation.

ASSESSMENT This includes measurement of deficits, identification of problems, and analysis of underlying causes. Assessment is necessary to ascertain the precise nature and severity of deficits prior to commencement of a rehabilitation program. It provides a logical basis for treatment and management and enables monitoring of patients' progress. As rehabilitation deals with the ill-defined concept of human performance, there are many areas for potential assessment, but it may be pragmatic and productive to select a small group of scales relevant to the objectives of intervention rather than to use comprehensive assessments to evaluate the overall outcome of rehabilitation.[146] As all other processes of rehabilitation and the quality of overall management of stroke patients are dependent on performing appropriate, adequate assessments, this aspect of stroke management will be discussed in detail in a later section.

PLANNING This is the process of goal setting based on identification of aims, objectives, and targets.[147] Many difficulties arise in stroke rehabilitation because the goals of intervention are not set in advance or because these goals have not been discussed and agreed on by all relevant parties. The two major problems that arise in goal setting include failure to use a common language in communication between various professionals or between professionals and patients and, second, failure to agree on a time frame within which the rehabilitation process must be accomplished. There is often a discrepancy between the goals of patients and their families and those of professional staff members. An essential function of the whole rehabilitation team is to identify and modify unrealistically high (and sometimes unjustifiably low) expectations of patients and their families by making them more aware of the nature of residual deficit and expected prognosis as soon as these are reasonably clear. The areas of practical importance in goal setting are as follows:

- *Accommodation*: Where will the patient live and what physical adaptations will be needed?
- *Personal support*: What help will be essential for the patient?
- *Life satisfaction*: What roles will the patient be fulfilling within his or her social setting and how will they be occupying their time?

INTERVENTION The minimum requirement of any stroke intervention is to provide care necessary to maintain the status quo and prevent deterioration of the patient's condition or functional ability due to poor management or complications. Further intervention should be aimed at facilitating recovery and improving outcome by minimizing disability and preventing handicap. As mentioned previously, traditional therapy input lacks a proper physiological basis because little is known about the processes underlying the return of neurological function.[148] In addition, recent studies have suggested that many of the assumptions which underlie the most widely used physical therapy approach in the UK have a dubious foundation.[123] Hence, although rehabilitation packages improve outcome (often at great expense), stroke therapy is a long way from being rooted in science.[123]

Literature on therapeutic intervention in stroke is limited and deals largely with poorly designed studies undertaken with small groups of patients.[143,148,149] An overview of these studies suggests that, because of ethical considerations, it is virtually impossible to design trials comparing therapy with no therapy, despite the absence of proof of effectiveness. Of the few trials that compared different therapeutic techniques, none showed conclusively that one technique was superior to any other in the major areas of physical therapy[148] or in speech and language function.[150] Randomized studies on social services intervention and on counseling or education of patients and caregivers have proven generally more positive, but the effects are modest and vary between studies.[151,152]

The amount of formal therapy received by stroke patients is small and may be as little as 45 minutes each working day or 3–4 percent of a patient's waking time each week, even at specialized facilities.[56,153] The effects of intensive therapeutic input on recovery from stroke have been investigated in well-designed controlled studies.[154,155] These investigations have shown a small but definite relationship between the amount of therapy given and the amount of improvement in functional ability, which is independent of the nonspecific effects of changes in attention or adaptive mechanisms. There is increasing evidence from studies at stroke rehabilitation centers that early, intensive therapy has a beneficial effect on the speed of early recovery and discharge from the hospital, although the long-term benefits remain equivocal.[6]

EVALUATION Evaluation is the process of monitoring a patient's progress (or lack of it) and assessing the effectiveness of the rehabilitation process itself. Objective assessment of effectiveness of stroke rehabilitation has proved difficult for several reasons. These include the confounding effect of spontaneous recovery from stroke, difficulty in defining the extent of need, and perceptions of good outcome, which may vary with the perspective of different observers. Most patients who survive stroke exhibit varying degrees of spontaneous recovery due either to return of neural control mechanisms or to adaptive processes involving the use of alternative strategies. As recovery is fastest during the first 3 months and coincides with the period during which patients are likely to receive maximum rehabilitation input, it is difficult to disentangle the effects of rehabilitation from those of spontaneous recovery.

The extent of need is also difficult to define. Although most patients have some disabilities and problems related to the stroke, it is unlikely that the level of disability will always correlate with the scale of problems encountered by stroke patients. A severely disabled person who needs nursing home care seemingly has a lesser need for formal rehabilitation and does not seem to pose as serious a management problem. The rehabilitation needs of a moderately disabled person who chooses to live alone in inappropriate accommodation, on the other hand, are great and require an inordinately high level of resource input. Similarly, differences in expectations and, consequently, perceptions of what is considered good outcome, have resulted in considerable variability in evaluating the effectiveness of stroke rehabilitation programs. It is accepted that goals of rehabilitation vary according to the expectations of the parties involved. The goal of hospitals may be to discharge patients as soon as possible, whereas the goal of patients may be to return to their previous functional status even if this is unattainable. The goal of caregivers may be to minimize the level of input they need to provide even at the cost of institutionalization. Many of the difficulties ultimately faced in managing patients and in evaluating the effectiveness of interventions can be traced back to conflicts between the goals and objectives of different parties.

CONCLUSIONS There is consensus that well-organized, well-planned rehabilitation guided by well-defined goals based on adequate assessment and sensitive negotiation with patients and caregivers reduces disability and long-term institutionalization. There is, however, no evidence supporting any specific treatment technique for stroke patients. A pragmatic functional approach individualized for each patient's needs is recommended, and strict adherence to theories with little scientific basis or clinical evidence of effectiveness should be discouraged. There is also evidence suggesting that early, intensive intervention by therapists may speed recovery and hasten discharge from the hospital without increasing the total amount of therapeutic input.

ASSESSMENTS IN STROKE REHABILITATION

Assessment in rehabilitation is acquisition of the information needed to define rehabilitation goals. A large number of neurological, physical, and functional assessments are currently available and can be divided into global assessments (which determine the overall impact of stroke) and specific assessments (which deal with a single level or domain of impairment or disability). There are numerous scales for measuring global disease severity, which often use composite scoring systems.[156] Composite scores for global disease severity are unreliable because of the dominance of speech and language function over other indexes and because, when quite different disabilities are combined into one score, much specific information is lost. Most scores also mix a variety of impairments and disabilities without considering their interactions. A considerable amount of work has been undertaken in developing and validating simpler and more specific measures of stroke disability that are more appropriate in assessing and comparing stroke patients and their treatment.[157]

Ideally, all component items of an assessment at a given time should relate to the level being measured. Some overlap between assessments for different levels, however, is likely to occur in clinical settings because these levels are not discrete but form a continuum. The importance of knowing what information is wanted and why, that is the purpose of a measure, is central to choosing any measure in rehabilitation. It is also important to decide on the least amount of information necessary to achieve this purpose. The temptation to collect large amounts of data should be resisted because this practice is expensive in time and effort, and often results in reduced accuracy and completeness of the data collected. Assessment protocols based on a small selection of easy-to-use relevant measures have been recommended for wider use. The necessary characteristics of suitable measures are validity, reliability, sensitivity, simplicity, and communicability. It is best to use existing measures wherever possible provided that they are valid for the purpose in mind, reliable in the circumstances proposed, and appropriate to the needs and resources. Moreover, the use of established measures makes communication and interpretation of data easier.

The major reasons for undertaking assessments in stroke patients are (1) to define the type of patient and the potential for recovery and/or responding to intervention (prognostication); (2) to identify the main areas of difficulty and their underlying causes, the extent of disability, and the aims of the patient and the family; (3) to monitor the process of rehabilitation (evaluation); and (4) to assess the degree of recovery and residual disability at the end of the rehabilitation process (outcome).

Prognostication in stroke

Nature of stroke
PICH has traditionally been associated with high mortality and severe disability. Over two-thirds of patients with PICH die within 3 weeks of onset.[158] However, the increasing use of CT scanning has shown that some minor strokes are due to small hemorrhages deep within the parenchyma of the brain and are associated with good functional outcome. The functional outcome of patients with severe stroke who survive cerebral hemorrhage has also been improved considerably by the development of rehabilitation techniques, especially stroke rehabilitation units, in recent years.[159] The anatomical classification of stroke[23] is of prognostic significance in patients with cerebral infarction, as described earlier. The prognosis of patients with hemorrhagic transformation remains unknown. In general, CT scan

appearances of severe edema, midline shift, or herniation in association with a vascular lesion are indicative of poor outcome.

Stroke severity
Prognosis after stroke is directly related to the severity of initial impairments and disabilities, and there are several ways of predicting outcome.[160,161] These may utilize simple specific indicators or more complex assessment approaches including weighted formulas based on multivariate analysis. Simple indicators include urinary incontinence, changes in consciousness levels, and severity of individual motor, speech, or perceptual impairment. The more complex methods of determining prognosis include assessments of aggregated motor deficit, functional impairment scores, or a combination of motor and functional impairment scores incorporated into multivariate scores.

There has been considerable controversy over the relative merits of these different prognostic indicators and their applicability to stroke practice. Various studies have shown that prognostic indicators based on neurological examination can predict mortality or severe handicap but are of limited use in predicting functional outcome, destination of discharge, or care needs following discharge from hospital. Scores that include functional assessments are more predictive of functional outcome but often involve the use of multivariate formulas. There are some reservations about the use of multivariate formulas in predicting stroke outcome because of their perceived complexity and their lack of validity in data sets other than those from which they were derived. There is a trend toward promoting the use of simple single indicators, such as urinary incontinence, as predictors of outcome in clinical practice despite concerns about the sensitivity and reliability of any single indicator in predicting outcome. Although urinary continence has been demonstrated to be superior to five multivariate scales in predicting outcome,[128] it may not always be easy to assess incontinence in intensive care units.[162] In addition, urinary continence may continue to improve over several weeks, limiting its predictive value in the early phase of stroke management. Early in the course of their treatment, it is possible and clinically more relevant to group stroke survivors for expected outcome and resource use (health benefit grouping) using a simple validated bedside scoring system based on clinical assessment of power, balance, proprioception, and cognition.[163,164] Grouping of patients according to outcome and resource use has applications in monitoring the appropriateness of care for individual patients and in undertaking comparisons of the effectiveness of various therapy interventions or models of stroke care. It is important to remember that no prognostic criteria are applicable to all patients in all settings. These criteria must be used as part of overall clinical evaluation of individual patients when determining management strategies.

Monitoring rehabilitation

The wide variety of impairments and disabilities associated with stroke, as well as the large number of instruments available to measure each impairment and disability, have contributed significantly to the lack of a common assessment data set for stroke management. A sensible approach is to use simple assessments more frequently during the rehabilitation process to monitor and adjust the treatment program. A review of studies on stroke rehabilitation has shown the predominance of ADL scales in monitoring the rehabilitation process.[160] This may be because ADL scales measure independence (and, by implication, dependence on others) in undertaking basic daily activities, which is a fundamental goal of the rehabilitation process. The level of independence in ADL is not only the basis for more complete recovery but is also important in determining the care needs of, and resource use by, patients who continue to be dependent. Widespread use of ADL scales is further supported by the general agreement on the core ADL components (bladder and bowel function, feeding, cleanliness, dressing, and mobility), high inter-rater reliability in clinical settings which is not influenced by the method of data collection, and communicability within multidisciplinary teams.

The limitations of ADL scales should be acknowledged. The distinction between impairment and disability is often blurred, and ADL scales include items that could be considered impairments. Items on these scales may not be independent of each other or may be influenced by other aspects of disability (e.g. communication or orientation) that are not measured. ADL scales have a low ceiling effect and cannot identify the reasons why patients fail to achieve goals (e.g. incontinence may be due to immobility or bladder dysfunction) or how patients achieve independence (the quality of functional recovery).

Measurement of outcome

There is little consensus on the most relevant outcome, the method of measurement, or the most appropriate timing of such assessment in stroke patients.[143] The perception of a favorable outcome may vary depending upon professional, patient, or carer perspectives and how long after stroke it is assessed. It has been recommended that outcomes should be measured at different levels within the ICIDH framework but patients value their ability to undertake desired activities or to participate in social roles more than improvements in specific areas of performance. Specifying a favorable outcome is difficult because change may continue over months, and the rate and extent of change may vary between the different levels of the ICIDH model. Consequently, it is important to consider the timing of any assessments, the measurement of factors known to impact on the chosen outcomes and the likely statistical distribution of outcomes at the chosen end point.

Measures of impairment are the closest practical measures relating to the size of lesion and probably the best markers of prognosis. Impairment level measures help to assess case mix and act as surrogate measures of neurological outcome. Measures at the level of activities (disability) are the most important for outcome; measures of basic activities of daily living (e.g. the Barthel ADL Index) have significant weaknesses, and measures that assess higher level of activity and mobility need to be used (instrumental/extended ADL). These have the advantage of objectivity, reliability, and sensitivity, besides being simple and relevant to the patient. Measurement of participation and quality of life both appear attractive but may pose problems. There is great debate about the construct of "quality of life," and many of the measures said to assess the quality of life are also measuring activities or emotion. Measurement of emotion is important, given the frequency of depression and its relation to activities, participation, and quality of life. In any assessment of outcome in stroke, it needs to be accepted that some patients will be unable to complete the assessment because of impaired cognition or language. In such patients, proxy use of common measures of activity and participation has been shown to be a valid method of measuring outcome.

Appropriate timing of assessments is important and the natural history of recovery from stroke must be considered when selecting the time of assessment. The degree and timing of recovery also relate to the initial severity of stroke, and spontaneous recovery may not plateau until 6 months after a severe stroke. It follows that 6 months is the most appropriate time point at which to measure neurological and functional outcome. Wider interactions with environment and society become important after this stage, and measurement of participation, life satisfaction, and emotionality should preferably take place at a time when the patient's social condition has stabilized.

Mortality continues to be an important outcome because of its inclusion in several epidemiological and stroke outcome studies. Mortality in stroke can be divided into three phases: (1) early mortality due to brain damage, which is unlikely to be influenced by rehabilitation but may be affected by acute interventions; (2) delayed hospital mortality due to stroke-related complications, which is an indicator of quality of care; and (3) late mortality, which is multifactorial depending on the severity of stroke, rehabilitation, care requirements, community intervention, and comorbidity. The setting into which an individual is discharged after rehabilitation, when premorbid accommodation has been taken into account, has long been one of the most frequently used outcome indicators. Institutionalization implies unsuccessful rehabilitation, loss of freedom to live at home, and high costs to society. Destination of discharge, however, is not only dependent on the level of residual disability or success of rehabilitation but is also influenced by comorbidity, family support, and social variables which may be outside the control of the rehabilitation process. Despite these limitations, institutionalization has been used in several previous studies and is accepted as a useful outcome measure in stroke research.

SEQUELAE OF STROKE

Stroke patients may suffer a range of problems associated with primary pathology or due to secondary medical or neurological complications. Stroke-related disorders that are significant in patient management include visual problems (hemianopia or inattention), dysphagia with the risk of aspiration and infection, communication problems, venous thrombotic disease, urinary and bowel problems, spasticity and contractures, pressure sores, shoulder pain, associated reactions, cold hemiplegic arm, and edema of the limbs. The main neurological complications include depression, seizures, behavioral changes and, rarely, thalamic pain. Stroke patients are also at a higher risk of falls which, in association with osteoporotic bone changes in the hemiplegic limb, often result in fractures on the stroke side.

Various studies have shown that complications occur in about 60 percent of stroke patients undergoing rehabilitation and are more frequent in patients with severe disability.[165] The clinical aspects of some of the more important problems are discussed in the following sections.

Dysphagia

Swallowing problems are common after stroke and have been attributed in the past to brain stem or bilateral cerebral lesions. New research, however, suggests that this condition is also seen in a significant number of patients with unilateral hemispheric lesions.[166] Swallowing problems are associated with increased incidence of aspiration, chest infection, dehydration, and malnutrition.[79] The presence of dysphagia, in itself and in association with its complications, is linked with poor outcome following stroke.[167] Despite this, dysphagia is poorly recognized and poorly managed in most acute settings.

The diagnosis of dysphagia is conventionally dependent on clinical examination and a demonstrated absence of the gag reflex in stroke patients. The gag reflex is not a reliable sign of dysphagia, being present in some patients with significant swallowing problems and absent in others who may have no swallowing problems.[168] Several studies have shown that the bedside swallowing assessment is a simple, feasible, reliable method for screening patients for swallowing problems.[129] This assessment should be undertaken in patients with relevant neurological deficits (facial weakness, dysarthria, dysphonia), reasonable sitting balance, and ability to cooperate with the examination (appropriate sensorium). The patient is given a teaspoonful of water and observed for dribbling, cough, altered respiration, breathing problems, or wet dysphonia before being given more liquid and then a solid. Oral intake should be restricted in patients with definite or probable swallowing problems pending full assessment by a speech and language therapist.

The development of videofluoroscopic techniques has greatly facilitated objective assessment of swallowing problems.[169] Videofluoroscopy allows analysis of various phases of deglutition in great detail and can measure transit times for the bolus to complete the pharyngeal swallow accurately. It can demonstrate problems with initiating swallow (e.g. poor tongue control, inability to form bolus or move bolus to the pharynx), with swallowing itself (e.g. poor swallow reflex, inadequate laryngeal elevation, pooling, aspiration), or in the postpharyngeal phase of swallow (e.g. esophageal spasm). It also shows the presence of aspiration (entry of food or barium below the level of the true vocal cords) even when there are no clinical signs of a compromised airway or aspiration. Videofluoroscopy has made it possible to assess objectively and reliably the effectiveness of various interventions aimed at improving swallowing in stroke patients. It is important to remember that this procedure is not necessary in most stroke patients (who recover rapidly and spontaneously) and should be reserved for patients with atypical or persistent dysphagia or those with unexplained or recurrent pneumonia.

Most swallowing difficulties in acute stroke are transient and resolve in most patients within 2 weeks of the acute episode. The remainder respond well to compensatory techniques and dietary modifications under the supervision of speech and language therapists and dieticians, which remain the mainstay of treatment of dysphagia in stroke patients.[170] Treatment of patients with persistent dysphagia, however, presents problems. Most current strategies are directed toward establishing alternative means of nutrition (e.g. nasogastric tubes, PEG) until normal feeding can be established. Although stimulation of the pharynx by mechanical or thermal means is often used in patients with persistent swallowing problems, there are no proven interventions aimed directly at improving the swallowing process. Other measures under investigation include cortical stimulation with magnetic fields to stimulate the swallowing reflex and insertion of artificial electrical pacemakers to trigger laryngeal elevation.

Dysphasia

Dysphasia is a defect in language function manifesting as impairment in speech production, comprehension, reading, or writing in the absence of motor disturbances of voice production or writing, visual or auditory deficits, and intellectual or cognitive impairment. Although the left hemisphere is traditionally associated with speech in most people, there is evidence suggesting that the right hemisphere has some capacity for language, even in right-handed people.[171] In left-handed people, lesions of the left hemisphere can still result in speech problems because this is the dominant hemisphere in 70 percent of these individuals. In the remaining 30 percent, language functions are situated in the right hemisphere in 20 percent and equally distributed between the two hemispheres in 10 percent. Consequently, left-handed people are more likely to suffer from dysphasia as a group, regardless of which hemisphere is damaged. Dysphasia in left-handed patients, however, tends to be less severe and to recover more rapidly than that in right-handed patients, probably because of bilateral representation.[172] Evidence suggests that damage to subcortical nuclei may also result in dysphasia.[172] Structures mainly involved are the thalamus and the basal ganglia. Language deficits associated with lesions in these areas include alterations in fluency, nominal aphasia, hesitancy, word blocking, and impairment in reading and comprehension.

Patients may present with nonfluent dysphasia, which at its most severe consists of complete loss of speech and phonation. This is nearly always associated with an inability to comprehend anything but the most simple commands. Often there is buccofacial apraxia. Recovery is associated with the ability to phonate simple yes or no responses (or similar monosyllabic utterances) which are usually out of context and inappropriate. Less severe and more common forms present as agrammatic speech, although the information content may be adequate to convey appropriate meaning to a patient listener despite the hesitancy and distorted articulation. Fluent dysphasia is characterized by spontaneous speech which is abnormal and often incomprehensible because of the use of nonexistent words, wrong words (paraphasia), or inappropriately arranged words, which lose their meaning.

Impaired ability to understand speech is common in dysphasic patients. The difficulty in comprehension increases with increasing linguistic complexity of the speech presented and length of sentences used. The extent to which a dysphasic patient can understand what is being said is frequently overestimated, which can result in misunderstandings between patients and their families or professionals involved in patient care. It is important that speech and language problems be identified early in stroke patients because many therapy interventions are dependent on this function.

The more severe forms of dysphasia are often easy to diagnose on clinical examination in most stroke patients. The diagnosis of mild dysphasia may be more difficult, especially if the patient has a high-level language deficit.[173] It is also important to differentiate dysphasia from confusion secondary to cognitive impairment. Enquiries about the patient's language background (native language, profession, social and educational status), previous speech problems (e.g. stuttering) and hand dominance should be part of the examination. Problems in comprehension are particularly difficult to assess. A bedside measure can be obtained by assessing the patient's ability to respond to commands of increasing complexity, either in content or in linguistic structure. It should be remembered that in some patients, errors may occur because of dyspraxia or memory problems. Problems with expression usually present as difficulty in finding words, problems with naming objects, or inability to read or write during a bedside assessment. All patients suspected of having dysphasia should be assessed by speech and language therapists regardless of the severity of the impairment. Appropriate treatment of dysphasic patients consists of individualized therapy programs supervised by speech and language therapists, development of simple communication strategies to enable multidisciplinary rehabilitation, and educating caregivers in communication techniques appropriate to the patient's level of impairment.

Perception

Perception is an important but sadly neglected aspect of stroke management.[174] The outcome of rehabilitation frequently depends on effective management of perceptual problems rather than on motor recovery alone. Despite this, perceptual problems are poorly understood and difficult to assess objectively because of the paucity of valid assessment instruments. Their management is equally difficult and a subject of great controversy.

Perceptual problems after stroke can be divided into (1) neglect, which is the disregard of, and failure to attend to, one half of external space; (2) agnosias, which comprise problems with interpreting sensory data from the environment or the body (visual, tactile, autotopagnosia); and (3) apraxias, the collection of problems involving formulating, initiating, or sequencing motor activity. Although it is traditional to consider perceptual problems a consequence of nondominant (right) hemisphere lesions, there is increasing evidence that these difficulties may be equally common in both hemispheres but are hard to assess in patients with left hemisphere lesions because of dysphasia.

Total neglect of one side of the body is a result of extensive hemisphere damage and is usually combined with dense hemiplegia. Patients with visuospatial neglect tend to ignore objects on the affected side and classically leave food on one side of the plate or bump into objects on the affected side despite no obvious hemianopia. Common agnosias seen in stroke patients include visual agnosia (failure to recognize objects by sight alone) and problems with depth and movement perception. Visual problems are common and are present in about 25 percent of stroke survivors in the acute phase. Visuospatial dysfunction may significantly affect visual depth and movement perception and can be particularly disabling in stroke patients, as it affects their ability to judge distances and relationships between objects or between self and objects in a three-dimensional setting, causing severe restrictions in daily living activities.[135] Some patients with perceptual difficulties lose left–right discrimination, leading to inappropriate action, whereas others may suffer impairment of topographic awareness of the environment, causing them to become lost even in familiar surroundings. Some patients may be aware of their deficit but are unable to overcome it without paying extra attention to affected functional abilities.[175]

The simplest and perhaps most sensitive test for visuospatial impairments involves asking the patient to draw a clock face. Affected individuals fail to put numbers on the affected side. More formal tests include star or number cancellation tests and the Rivermead Perceptual Test Battery. It is not known whether these deficits respond to general stimulation or to specific remedial measures. Recent research suggests that neglect may be amenable to therapeutic interventions.[176,177] Electrical stimulation may also be of benefit in patients with neglect, but further studies are required to confirm this benefit.[178] Although visuospatial problems delay or compromise functional recovery in most patients, some individuals eventually make full recovery.

Other major agnosias affecting functional recovery are loss of body image, resulting in failure to identify parts of the body (autotopagnosia) and denial of the stroke or underestimation of its severity (anosoagnosia). Autotopagnosia is usually revealed when patients try to dress themselves and fail to dress completely, ignoring the affected part of the body. Some patients with right parietal lobe lesions complain about "phantom limbs" or other bizarre phenomena (e.g. having "withered" or "demonic" limbs), which can be very frightening for them. The clinical presentation of body agnosia is very characteristic, but further confirmation can be made by asking the patient to name body parts or draw a picture of a human body. More formal confirmation can be made by one of the many perceptual test batteries available (e.g. Rivermead Perceptual Assessment Battery). In patients with anosognosia the lack of awareness of any problem makes their rehabilitation difficult. Despite this, improvement is possible with specialist input provided by therapists trained in stroke management.

Apraxia is difficulty in performing purposive movements at will in the absence of sensation, comprehension, motor, or coordination deficits adequate to explain this inability. Learned skilled movements are performed incorrectly but may be performed spontaneously in response to subconscious stimuli. Several types of apraxia affect different activities (e.g. orofacial, gait, dress) and occur singly or in combination. In some patients apraxia is seen on the unaffected side (sympathetic apraxia). There is no effective treatment for apraxia. Management currently focuses on increasing the patient's awareness of the condition and its effects in the stroke setting, early recognition of the problem and its impact on the patient, education, and teaching of adaptive skills and coping strategies to patients and their relatives.

Tone and spasticity

Doctors and therapists have differing perceptions and definitions of tone and spasticity and different views regarding its clinical significance. Spasticity is a consequence of increased tone and is defined as the resistance to passive stretch of muscles. Tone is often reduced in the early days after a stroke, and return of tone is usually associated with good outcome. Physiotherapists emphasize that tone is a more dynamic, complex process that is part of an overall pattern of posture and movement. Appropriate management of tone is one of the fundamental principles of the Bobath method of facilitative physiotherapy in stroke patients, which gives priority to normalization of tone and improving symmetry even at the cost of postponing standing or walking. However, this preoccupation with normalization of tone is not supported by evidence and best practice remains open to question.[179]

The management of abnormal tone and spasticity is difficult, as it depends on achieving the right balance between hypo- and hypertonia between different muscle groups.[180] The problem is compounded by the fact that spasticity varies between different groups of muscles and times of day and with the emotional state of the patient, activity being undertaken, and posture of the limb. Inappropriate exercise can result in inappropriate tone patterns to the ultimate detriment of the patient. If not managed correctly, spasticity leads to bad gait patterns, contractures, and loss of function.

Management of spasticity should be undertaken jointly by doctors and physiotherapists.[181] It is important to consider spasticity in relation to other impairments and define functional goals of management in advance because interventions directed solely at reduction of spasticity are unlikely to result in significant gains. Treatment of abnormal tone is usually initiated by physiotherapists, who can offer a range of interventions including physical therapy, attention to posture and seating and conventional orthoses to reduce spasticity and its complications. Drug therapy should be initiated in consultation with therapists and adjusted to achieve optimal effects. Its main drawback is its lack of selectivity; since all muscle groups are affected equally, there may be undesirable hypotonia in some muscle groups (e.g. drugs for reducing spasticity in arm muscles may affect walking). Newer treatments such as botulinum toxin have been shown to be effective in reducing spasticity in short-term studies but this effect is short-lived (up to 3 months) and may not translate into functional improvements.[182] Electrical stimulation techniques are a useful adjunct to other treatments, particularly for treating spastic equinus deformities.[183] In some cases phenol nerve blocks can produce good results, especially when standard treatments fail or botulinum toxin produces beneficial or short-term effects. In patients refractory to medical treatments surgical interventions such as ablation of peripheral nerves, tenotomies or reconstruction of tendons and joints may be required.

The hemiplegic shoulder

Shoulder pain, restriction of movement, and subluxation of the shoulder joint are common problems in stroke patients. In hypotonic patients, the loss of muscle strength around the shoulder joint and the weight of the paralyzed arm may result in malalignment of the humeral head in the shallow glenoid cavity, predisposing to inferior subluxation of the shoulder. This can easily be detected clinically in the sitting or standing patient and confirmed on radiographs in the erect position. There is considerable variation in the reported incidence of subluxation in stroke patients, but it is estimated that one in every five patients is affected.[184] The clinical implications of subluxation and its effects on eventual recovery of function are not known.

Shoulder pain is more common and inconsistently related to subluxation, although its exact prevalence remains unknown. It is encountered in rehabilitation settings with disconcerting frequency and may be a result of spasticity in the shoulder muscles, glenohumeral subluxation, reflex sympathetic dystrophy (the shoulder–hand syndrome), or orthopedic causes such as rotator cuff injury, arthritis, or adhesive capsulitis made worse by immobility. Contributory factors include careless handling of patients and incorrect position of the hemiplegic arm. Management is empirical with no agreed-on guidelines. It should be undertaken in collaboration with physiotherapists and includes measures such as proper positioning of the arm during periods of inactivity, avoidance of abnormal arm movements causing excessive strain on the shoulder joint or inappropriate pulling of the hemiplegic arm during transfers, and early passive exercise to prevent joint stiffness and contractures. Patients should be advised to avoid overzealous, self-assisted arm movements. Treatment with analgesics, strapping and nonsteroidal anti-inflammatory drugs may help in some patients. Steroid injections in the shoulder may be helpful, but further studies are needed to confirm benefit.[185]

Edematous limbs

Swelling of the limbs on the affected side is common after stroke.[186] It causes considerable discomfort and concern to stroke survivors, especially because it may never resolve in some patients. Swelling of the leg is seen in about 25 percent of stroke survivors and in most cases is caused by underlying phlebothrombosis. This swelling is more common in elderly patients, increases with stroke severity, and predisposes to venous thrombosis. Management is conservative and includes measures such as early mobilization, avoidance of trauma, and leg elevation at rest. The role of stockings and long-term heparin prophylaxis remains to be determined. Anticoagulation may be necessary if there is proven deep vein thrombosis.

The precise etiology of edema of the hand of the paralyzed arm is not known, but it is thought to be due to reflex sympathetic dystrophy, posture, and lack of muscle activity. It is often unsightly and painful, especially on flexion of the fingers. Edema fluid has a high protein content and is unlikely to respond to diuretics. Treatment modalities include elevation of the hand, massage, and application of elastic bandages. Immersion of the hand in a tank of water cooled to 10°C has been shown to reduce the swelling considerably.[187]

Seizures

Cerebrovascular disease is the most common cause of late onset seizures (see also Chapter 46). Fits occurring at the onset of stroke are seen in about 2–6 percent of patients and are associated with lesions in carotid artery distribution.[188] These fits are most likely the result of acute local brain metabolic alteration induced by ischemia, and once these derangements are reversed, the seizures disappear. A single seizure after stroke does not need treatment unless prolonged or associated with complications and treatment with anticonvulsants hence may not be appropriate in these patients until further fits occur.[189] In acute stroke, seizures do not correlate with the size of the lesion, functional outcome, or mortality. In clinical practice, it is not always easy to distinguish between a stroke causing a seizure (anticonvulsants not indicated) or a seizure with a stroke-like presentation (possible treatment indicated), and it may be appropriate to undertake further investigations (including imaging) before making therapeutic decisions. It is important to remember that the risk of subsequent late seizures and post-stroke epilepsy is increased in patients with early seizures.[190]

Late-onset seizures (those appearing more than a week after the stroke is completed) can occur months to years after the stroke and are probably due to structural brain abnormalities leading to development of an epileptic focus. A longitudinal study has shown that the risk of developing epilepsy is about 10 percent at 5 years after stroke.[191] The risk of seizures is greatest with cortical lesions and least with subcortical or infratentorial lesions. The pathology of stroke is important: about 10 percent of patients with cerebral infarction, 25 percent of patients with primary intracranial hemorrhage, and over 30 percent of patients with subarachnoid hemorrhage developed epilepsy within 5 years of the original event in the Oxford Community Stroke Project. Late-onset seizures need to be treated and respond well to anticonvulsant treatment.

Depression

It is estimated that between 30 and 60 percent of stroke patients have clinically significant depression, the highest prevalence and severity occurring in the first 2 years after stroke.[192] Three different types of mood disorders have been recognized in stroke patients: (1) severe depression that meets the diagnostic criteria for major depression, (2) minor depressive illness fulfilling most of the criteria for a dysthymic disorder except the time frame, and (3) an indifferent, apathetic mental state often associated with false cheerfulness.[193] Diagnosis of mood disorders in patients with acute stroke is difficult because changes in appetite, sleep, or interest (all indicative of depression) may be a normal adjustment response to physical disability and changed roles. The diagnosis of depression in stroke is further hampered by the presence of dysphasia and impairments in attention or concentration which make assessment difficult. The presence of autonomic and psychological depressive symptoms (e.g. palpitations, anxiety, excessive sweating, loss of energy, concentration difficulties, pessimistic thoughts including suicide), however, strongly favors depression in the acute stroke period.

It is commonly accepted that depression in stroke is frequently associated with left hemisphere lesions despite some studies suggesting no laterality.[194] The frequency and severity of depression appears to be related to the proximity of the anterior boundary of the lesion to the left frontal pole. Anatomic work suggests that the deep nuclei of the forebrain and associated structures (mainly the head of the caudate and the anterior limb of the internal capsule) may play a special role in the pathogenesis of depression in stroke. There is no convincing evidence that the size of the lesion correlates with the severity of the depression observed. Depression is less frequent following right hemisphere lesions and is associated with posterior or retrorolandic pathology. Post-stroke depression appears to be more common in patients with a family or personal premorbid history of depression.

Post-stroke depression may last for 7–8 months or more without treatment and is highly correlated with failure to resume premorbid social and physical activities.[192] Depression also has a negative effect on functional and cognitive recovery, integration into the family environment, and caregiver stress in stroke patients.[195] There is growing evidence suggesting that early recognition of depression in stroke and early treatment with appropriate antidepressants can facilitate recovery, although most series are small.[196] Antidepressant therapy, however, needs to be used with caution and monitored carefully because of potential toxicity. It is also important to remember that the expectation of benefits from antidepressant therapy is based on extrapolation of existing data on depression in the general population to stroke patients. There are only a few well-designed prospective intervention studies in stroke patients with frontal lobe involvement and mood lability and evidence for the effectiveness of antidepressive treatment in the generality of stroke patients with depression is inconclusive. Equally importantly, the role of nonpharmacological interventions has not been properly evaluated. There is little information on which types of antidepressants are most effective in stroke patients, the time when antidepressants should be started, and the duration for which they should be continued. There is a prima facie case for preferring serotonin-specific reuptake inhibitor (SSRI)-type drugs over tricyclics because of the latter's side-effects, but this as well as their effectiveness is supported by only limited data in stroke patients.

Apathy

Apathy is a frequent sequel of stroke and is associated with older age, cognitive impairment, and premorbid deficits in activities of daily living.[197] Although it frequently coexists with depression, apathy can also present without marked depressive features. It appears to be more common in patients with lesions in the posterior limb of the internal capsule. The presence of this condition significantly affects functional recovery in stroke patients. It is not known whether apathy responds to drug intervention. It may be possible to improve motivation in these patients by adopting an enthusiastic approach, setting achievable goals, and praising achievements regardless of their magnitude.

PSYCHOSOCIAL ASPECTS AND SUPPORT

Stroke is a major life event which few, if any, are prepared for and presents major difficulties for patients, their spouses, and their families. It not only may result in physical dependency but also requires a wide range of emotional and social adjustments within families, often leading to role reversals and establishment of new hierarchies.[198] The post-stroke phase is a period of considerable turmoil during which patients and their families need to be supported in order to achieve good outcomes. The major areas of relevance are the following.

BEREAVEMENT The reaction to stroke is akin to bereavement. Initially, there is a phase of shock during which patients and caregivers have so much to cope with that they may not assimilate much of what is told to them about the illness. This is followed by a phase of realization of the enormity of the event and is usually associated with despondency. Then a period of positive thinking and optimism sets in as patients focus on the activities of the rehabilitation team, and many harbor unrealistic hopes of sudden recovery. It is important for the clinician to introduce the notion of gradual and perhaps incomplete recovery at this phase to prevent unrealistic expectations of outcome. This reduces the chances of ultimate disappointment, and it may pave the way to more successful adaptation to the reality of residual disability. As the recovery curve begins to reach a plateau, there may be a second phase of depression which may be aggravated when the patient leaves the hospital or is discharged from outpatient care. Stroke patients understandably feel rejected: they had expected to be cured yet remain disabled. They need counseling as well as practical support because they feel uncertain or gloomy about the future.

FEAR Another significant psychological problem faced by stroke patients is fear. They may be frightened of disfigurement, loss of physical function, falls, insanity, leaving the hospital, poverty, and even death. They worry about sexual impairment and wonder whether it will be safe to try to resume sexual activity. Fear of further stroke can be eased to some extent by explaining that 90 percent of survivors do not have a stroke in any given year, that drugs such as aspirin reduce the chances of further occlusive vascular disease, and that strokes are not caused by stress or exertion.

PERSONALITY CHANGES Alterations in personality may commonly occur after stroke and are a source of great distress to spouses and caregivers of stroke patients. One of the saddest comments made by spouses of stroke patients is "He (or she) is not the person I married." The changes noted are irritability, aggression, and anxiety; the patient may be described as "difficult." Some disabled stroke victims are models of good behavior in the hospital but become demanding tyrants after they go home. They may revert to childish behavior, eat messily, and be reluctant to cooperate.

LOSS OF SELF-ESTEEM People who were very active and independent feel distressed when they must rely on others to wash and shave them, cut their food, dress and bathe them, or wipe their bottom. The loss of esteem may lead to apathy and even depression if not addressed early during a patient's treatment. This is more likely to happen in the paternalistic environment of hospitals, and the attitude and approach of the medical team are crucial in enabling the patient to maintain

dignity. Esteem plummets when patients are not given much attention on hospital rounds or are depersonalized by staff who refer to them as "CVAs" or "hemis" rather than considering them unique individuals.

GUILT Even in secular societies, stroke may be seen as punishment for real or imaginary sins of omission or commission. The doctor must explain to the patient and family that no one is responsible for this illness; it was not caused by stress or overwork or nagging or anything else done by the victim or his or her relatives. The knowledge that a stroke is a reflection of the state of one's cardiovascular system and not of one's soul can be reassuring.

Care at home

Most stroke patients return home. Of these, a quarter are dependent on someone for feeding, dressing, and toileting.[199] In one survey, 65 percent of those relying on caregivers needed help with bathing, 54 percent with dressing, 38 percent with toileting, and 21 percent with feeding; 18 percent required attention every night.[200] Most stroke patients are cared for by their families with little outside support.[201] These informal caregivers who often shoulder a heavy burden, are mostly women and are often elderly themselves.

Caregivers, especially elderly people, may have their own health problems and suffer further physical ill health because of lifting (backache, hernias, injury) or accidents.[202] Depression is common (50 percent of caregivers are depressed at 3 years) and is frequently unrecognized. Depression is also common in caregivers of minimally disabled patients. In addition, they may have made significant changes in their lifestyle, such as giving up work (resulting in loss of income and self-esteem) or social pursuits. Being tied to the home is one of the most burdensome aspects of care-giving. There may be marital stress, especially if the patient is dysphasic, demanding, depressed, or irritable.

It is not uncommon for caregivers to feel exhausted, isolated, and depressed from time to time and to require support in their own right. Despite the heavy burden of care, most relatives who provide support have little respite: only one-third leave the patient unattended for all or part of the day. Those who provide the most care (because the patient is more severely disabled) are less likely to have frequent contact with neighbors. There is an increasing awareness that stroke families need continuing care and support which may be required for many years.[203] Support for stroke victims and their families is high on the agenda of many health and social service organizations. A large number of services supporting stroke patients and their caregivers are also being developed within the voluntary sector.[204]

There continues to be a medical role in the long-term management of stroke. This input should consist of monitoring of secondary preventive measures (e.g. lifestyle changes, cessation of smoking, and control of hypertension, hyperlipidemia, or diabetes); monitoring of disease progression (especially in patients with known moderate internal carotid artery stenosis); assessment of changes in disability or handicap and their potential for reversibility using therapy or environmental interventions; and identification of psychological and social support needs of patients and caregivers that may require referral to appropriate social or community care agencies. Long-term medical management goals can be achieved by regular review of stroke patients by their general practitioners, backed up with review by a specialist once or twice a year. Many disabled stroke patients survive for many years, and it is important that we ensure that their quality of life is as good as possible.[205]

CEREBRAL MULTI-INFARCT STATES

There is considerable heterogeneity of multi-infarct states associated with cerebrovascular disease. In general, cortical multi-infarct disease is characterized by clear-cut repeated atherothrombotic or cardioembolic strokes, obvious sensorimotor deficits, more severe aphasic disturbances, and abrupt onset of cognitive failure.[206] Subcortical multi-infarct states, on the other hand, are associated with pseudobulbar signs, isolated pyramidal deficits and depression or emotional lability, mildly impaired memory, disorientation, apathy, lack of concentration, preservation, and other behavioral problems attributable to frontal lobe dysfunction.[207] Cerebral multi-infarct states are classified into clinicoanatomic subtypes, although there is debate about classification and overlap between different subgroups.

CORTICAL MULTI-INFARCT DISEASE Cortical multi-infarct disease appears to be a result of multiple thromboembolic infarcts too small individually to produce a major clinical incident but synergistically causing impairment of cortical function. It is more common in elderly people, and the diagnosis is straightforward when a patient has repeated thromboembolic episodes (TIAs or physically nondisabling strokes) and brain imaging shows more than one cortical infarct. Depending on the location of infarcts, the clinical picture shows a combination of deficits in higher function (e.g. dysphasia, apraxia, neglect) with a significant memory disorder.[206] Not infrequently, apraxic gait disturbance becomes clinically significant before the onset of cognitive impairment.[208]

DISTAL FIELD INFARCTION This usually involves the anterior circulation and is thought to be due to disturbances of the frontal border zone perfusion secondary to internal carotid artery disease. The areas affected are distant from the centrosylvian structures with widespread or multifocal infarction (often bilateral) which includes the association areas of the anterior and posterior cerebrum.[209] A frontal syndrome predominates and is associated with aphasia, dyspraxia, or neglect rather than hemiparesis or hemianesthesia. Because the syndrome is related to a tight carotid artery stenosis, carotid endarterectomy theoretically may prove effective in slowing the progression of this form of dementia.

LACUNAR MULTI-INFARCT DISEASE This type of dementia is due to multiple deep infarcts and exhibits the classic features of subcortical multi-infarct disease—gait, continence, and emotional problems—which may be early markers for this syndrome.[210,211] Frontal lobe features often predominate and overshadow cognitive decline, which is usually subtle or mild.

In some patients, however, infarcts in the thalamus, caudate nucleus, or genu may have a disproportionate effect on cognitive function. These cases may be wrongly diagnosed as cortical multi-infarct disease.

BINSWANGER'S DISEASE This disease shares several of the features of, and is often clinically indistinguishable from, lacunar multi-infarct states. These features include pseudobulbar speech and abulic delay, prominent mood and behavior changes, bilateral pyramidal signs, and a mild memory disorder.[210,211] The clinical course features slow but relentless mental deterioration punctuated by transient focal symptoms. The most prominent pathological finding is severe white matter atrophy with sparing of the cortex. Imaging shows a high frequency of white matter lesions, although these may be seen in elderly patients not suffering from Binswanger's disease. The diagnosis is dependent on the demonstration of extensive deep white matter rarefaction with multiple deep infarcts on brain imaging in the clinical setting of dementia with frontal lobe and focal signs and evidence of cerebrovascular disease or risk factors.

AMYLOID ANGIOPATHY Two presentations of this rare condition are recognized: multiple lobar hemorrhages in an elderly nonhypertensive patient with preceding or supervening dementia, and diffuse white matter or focal cortical ischemic lesions with or without concomitant Alzheimer's disease.[212] A third, more recently described presentation is a syndrome of recurrent transient neurological symptoms, responding to anticonvulsants and suggestive of seizures provoked by microhemorrhages.[212] In all types, there is deposition of amyloid β protein in the cortical arterioles, replacing normal smooth muscles.

CADASIL (CEREBRAL AUTOSOMAL DOMINANT ARTERIOPATHY WITH SUBCORTICAL INFARCTS AND LEUKOENCEPHALOPATHY) This is a diffuse disease of small arteries predominantly affecting the brain. It starts during mid-adulthood and is characterized by recurrent ischemic events (transient or permanent), attacks of migraine with aura, severe mood disorders, subcortical dementia and widespread leukoencephalopathy on MRI scanning.[213] The disease was first reported in European families, but has also been reported in patients of African and Asiatic origin and is linked to single missense mutation in the NOTCH 3 gene locus on chromosome 19.

Dementia associated cerebral multi-infarct states

Cerebral multi-infarct disease is often associated with significant cognitive impairment and is the second most common cause of dementia after Alzheimer's disease.[214] The true incidence of dementia due to multi-infarct states is not known and, as stroke and Alzheimer's disease frequently coexist, it is often difficult to determine whether vascular disease is a cause of or is coincidental with the dementia. Despite this limitation, it is estimated that dementia secondary to multi-infarct states occurs in about 25 percent of stroke patients and in about 3 percent of patients without a history of stroke.[214] The diagnosis of dementia due to cerebral multi-infarct states requires that a patient have (1) evidence of cerebrovascular disease (history, examination, brain imaging); (2) memory impairment with at least two other cognitive deficits that interfere with ADL and are not explained by stroke-related physical deficits (e.g. dysphasia, agnosia, apraxia); (3) evidence of causality that includes a temporal relationship between dementia and stroke, stepwise deterioration with a fluctuating course, or specific brain image findings in relevant areas.[215] Supportive evidence includes a history of cerebrovascular risk factors, early appearance of gait disturbances or frequent falls, urinary incontinence not explained by urological disease, frontal lobe or extrapyramidal features, and pseudobulbar features with or without emotional liability. Cortical infarcts are seen in about 38 percent of patients with vascular dementia, subcortical in 46 percent, and combined lesions in the remaining 16 percent.[209] Multiple lesions predominate, although a small number of patients may have single lesions (strategic infarct dementia). These focal forms of dementia are due to damage to the temporal lobe and hippocampus (posterior type), basal ganglia or thalamus (basal type), or frontal lobes (frontal type). The clinical features depend on the specific location but are associated with confusion and significant memory loss.

Management of cerebral multi-infarct states

Interest in cerebral multi-infarct states has increased in recent years, not only because of the realization that they are more common than previously supposed but also because they may be more amenable to prevention and treatment at present than other forms of dementia. Generally speaking, the risk factors for most cerebral multi-infarct states are the same as those for stroke and include hypertension, diabetes mellitus, advanced age, male gender smoking, and cardiac disease.[216,217] In addition to the established association between hypertension and stroke, hypertension is an independent risk factor for Binswanger's disease.[218] Other rarer causes include lipohyalinosis, cerebral amyloid angiopathy, disruption of the blood–brain barrier, and altered regulation of cerebral blood flow.[219] Extracerebral causes include ischemic hypoxic dementia, vasculitis, hyperviscosity, and hemostasis abnormalities. This heterogeneity of causes of cerebral multi-infarct disease should be taken into account in developing a management approach for this group of disorders.

The evolving clinical approach to multi-infarct disease consists of several options aimed at preventing further cerebrovascular damage and managing related symptoms.[220] These include lifestyle changes (e.g. cessation of smoking, starting an exercise program, dietary changes) and treatment of hypertension, elevated cholesterol, and atrial fibrillation. In the presence of early signs of cerebrovascular disease, such as TIAs or subtle cognitive deficits supported by changes on brain imaging, a more aggressive approach may be warranted. This may include aspirin, anticoagulants, or even carotid endarterectomy. Recent research has shown that rehabilitation may also have a specific role to play in patients with gait disorders.[221] Most of the current management of cerebral multi-infarct disease is empirical and based on extrapolation of stroke data to this group of disorders. The effectiveness of any of the possible interventions in either preventing or slowing the progression of this condition has yet to be supported by appropriately designed prospective clinical trials.

KEY POINTS   Stroke: clinical presentation and management

- Stroke ranks first in frequency, and probably urgency, among serious neurological disorders and is a leading cause of death and disability in the western world.

- The nihilistic attitudes associated with stroke in the past have changed greatly because of improved understanding of stroke mechanisms, advances in imaging techniques, developments in therapeutics and changes in the philosophy of stroke management.

- Stroke affects several domains of human performance and behavior and the whole philosophy of stroke care is based on multidisciplinary practice requiring the skills of many people.

- Optimum acute care consists of early investigations for pathology and etiology, maintaining physiological homeostasis, thrombolysis, prevention of complications, early mobilization and secondary prevention.

- Early and planned multidisciplinary rehabilitation remains the cornerstone of stroke management. Rehabilitation should aim to maximize patients' role fulfillment and independence in their environment within the limitations imposed by underlying impairment and availability of resources.

- Stroke is a major life event, which not only results in physical dependency but also requires a wide range of emotional and social adjustments within families who need to be supported.

REFERENCES

1. World Health Organization: Special Report. Stroke: Recommendations on stroke prevention, diagnosis, and therapy. Stroke 1989;20:1407–1431

2. Adams RD, Victor M: Cerebrovascular diseases. In Adams RD, Victor M, Ropper AH (eds): Principles of Neurology, McGraw-Hill, New York, 1997:777–874

3. Bamford J, Sandercock P, Dennis M, Warlow C: A prospective study of acute cerebrovascular disease in the community: the Oxfordshire Community Stroke Project. II. Incidence, case fatality rates and overall outcome at one year of cerebral infarction, primary intracerebral and subarachnoid haemorrhage. J Neurol Neurosurg Psych 1990;53:16–22

4. Murray CL, Lopez AD (eds): The Global Burden of Disease: a comprehensive assessment of disability from disease, injuries and risk factors in 1990 and projected to 2020. Harvard University Press, Boston, 1996

5. Wade DT: Stroke. In Stevens A, Raferty J (eds): Health Care Needs Assessment. Radcliffe Medical Press, Oxford 1994

6. Stroke Unit Trialists Collaboration: Collaborative systemic review of the randomised trials of organised inpatient (Stroke Unit) care after stroke (Cochrane Review). In: The Cochrane Library, 1, 2001 Update Software, Oxford

7. Posner JD, Gorman KM, Woldow A: Stroke in the elderly: 1. Epidemiology. J Am Geriatr Soc 1984;32:95–102

8. Sheikh K, Bretinan PJ, Meade TW et al: Predictors of mortality and disability in stroke. J Epidemiol Community Health 1983;357:70–74

9. Bamford J, Sandercock P, Warlow C, Gray M: Why are patients with acute stroke admitted to hospital? Br Med J 1986;1:1369–1372

10. Kalra L: Does age affect benefits of stroke unit rehabilitation? Stroke 1994;25:346–351

11. National Institute of Neurological Disorders and Stroke: Classification of cerebrovascular diseases III. Stroke 1990;21:637–676

12. Bogousslavsky J, Regii F: Cerebral infarction with transient signs (CITS): do TIAs correspond to small deep infarcts in internal carotid artery occlusion? Stroke 1984;15:536–539

13. Lammie GA: Pathology of small vessel stroke. Br Med Bull 2000;56:296–306

14. Hankey GJ, Warlow CP: Symptomatic carotid ischaemic events: safest and most cost-effective way of selecting patients for angiography, before carotid endarterectomy. Br Med J 1990;300:1485–1491

15. Warlow CP, Davenport RJ: The management of transient ischaemic attacks. Prescrib J 1996;36:1–8

16. del Zoppo GJ: Thrombolytic therapy in the treatment of stroke. Drugs 1997;54(suppl 3):90–98

17. Hacke W, Brott T, Caplan L et al: Thrombolysis in acute ischemic stroke: controlled trials and clinical experience. Neurology 1999;53(7 suppl 4):S3–14

18. International Stroke Trial Collaborative Group: The International Stroke Trial (IST): a randomised controlled trial of aspirin, subcutaneous heparin, both or neither among 19,435 patients with acute ischaemic stroke. Lancet 1997;349:1569–1581

19. Berge E, Sandset PM: Heparin and aspirin in stroke. Lancet 2001;357:1044–1045

20. Poirier J, Derouesne C: Cerebral lacune: a proposed new classification. Clin Neuropathol 1984;3:266

21. Besson G, Hommel M, Perret J: Risk factors for lacunar infarcts. Cerebrovasc Dis 2000;10:387–390

22. Bamford J: Classic lacunar syndromes. In Bogousslavsky J, Caplan L (eds): Stroke Syndromes. Cambridge University Press, Cambridge, 1995:366–372

23. Bamford J, Sandercock P, Dennis M et al: Classification and natural history of clinically identifiable subtypes of cerebral infarction. Lancet 1991;337:1521–1526

24. Adams HP, Bendixen HB, Kappelle JL, Biller J, Love BB, Gordon DL, Marsh EE: Classification of subtype of acute ischemic stroke: definitions for use in a multicentre clinical trial. Stroke 1993;24:35–41

25. Jorgensen HS, Nakayama H, Raaschou HO, Olsen TS: Intracerebral haemorrhage versus infarction: stroke severity, risk factors and prognosis. Ann Neurol 1995;38:45–50

26. Hankey GJ: Recent advances in cerebrovascular disease. Rev Clin Gerontol 1992;2:187–206

27. Hankey GJ, Slattery JM, Warlow CP: Transient ischaemic attacks: which patients are at high (and low) risks of serious vascular events? J Neurol Neurosurg Psychiatry 1992;55:640–652

28. Hennessy MJ, Britton TC: Transient ischaemic attacks: evaluation and management. Int J Clin Pract 2000;54(7):432–436

29. Weir CJ, Murray GD, Adams FG et al: Poor accuracy of stroke scoring systems for differential clinical diagnosis of intracranial haemorrhage and infarction. Lancet 1994;344:999–1002

30. Intercollegiate Working Party on Stroke: National Clinical Guidelines on Stroke. Royal College of Physicians, London, 2000

31. Jager HR: Diagnosis of stroke with advanced CT and MR imaging. Br Med Bull 2000;56:318–333

32. Moseley I: Acute disturbances of cerebral function: stroke and cerebrovascular disease. In Magnetic Resonance Imaging in Diseases of the Nervous System: an Introduction. Blackwell, Oxford, 1988:20–34

33. Albers GW, Lansberg MG, Norbash AM et al: Yield of diffusion-weighted MRI for detection of potentially relevant findings in stroke patients. Neurology 2000;54:1562–1567

34. Latchaw R: The roles of diffusion and perfusion imaging in acute stroke management. Am J Neuroradiol 1999;20:957–959

35. Hommel M, Besson G, Le Bas JF et al: Prospective study of lacunar infarction using magnetic resonance imaging. Stroke 1990;21:546–554

36. Nuutinen J, Kuikka J, Roivainen E, Sivenius J: Early serial SPET in acute middle cerebral artery infarction. Nucl Med Commun 2000;21:425–429

37. Marchal G, Serrati C, Rioux P et al: PET imaging of cerebral perfusion and oxygen consumption in acute ischaemic stroke: relation to outcome. Lancet 1993;341:925–927

38. Saunders DE: MR spectroscopy in stroke. Br Med Bull 2000;56:334–345

39. Frackowiak R: Functional imaging of recovery from stroke: A review of personal experience. Cerebrovasc Dis 1999;9(suppl 5):23–28

40. Carroll BA: Carotid sonography. Radiology 1991;178:303–313

41. Humphrey P, Sandercock P, Siattery J: A simple method to improve the accuracy of noninvasive ultrasound in selecting TIA patients for cerebral angiography. J Neurol Neurosurg Psychiatry 1990;53:966–971

42. Markus HS: Transcranial Doppler ultrasound. Br Med Bull 2000;56:373–388

43. Martin PJ, Naylor AR: Transcranial sonography and its clinical applications. Hosp Update 1994;20:479–488

44. Hankey GJ, Warlow CP, Sellar RJ: Cerebral angiographic risk in mild cerebrovascular disease. Stroke 1990;21:209–222

45. Clifton AG: MR angiography. Br Med Bull 2000;56:367–372

46. Come PC, Riley MF, Bivas NK: Roles of echocardiography and arrhythmia monitoring in the evaluation of patients with suspected systemic embolism. Ann Neurol 1983;113:527–531

47. Sudlow M, Thomson R, Thwaites B, Rodgers H, Kenny RA: Prevalence of atrial fibrillation and eligibility for anticoagulants in the community. Lancet 1998;352:1167–1171

48. Pop G, Sutherland GR, Koudstaal PJ et al: Transesophageal echocardiography in the detection of intracardiac embolic sources in patients with transient ischaemic attacks. Stroke 1990;21:560–565

49. Hankey GJ, Warlow CP: Treatment and secondary prevention of stroke: evidence, costs and effects on individuals and populations. Lancet 1999;354:1457–1463

50. Wade DT: Evaluating outcome in stroke rehabilitation. Scand J Rehabil Med 1992;(suppl 26):97–104

51. Adams HP, Jr, Brott TG, Crowell RM et al: Guidelines for the management of patients with acute ischemic stroke. A statement for healthcare professionals from a special writing group of the Stroke Council, American Heart Association. Stroke 1994;25:1901–1914

52. Aboderin I, Venables G: Stroke management in Europe. Pan European Consensus Meeting on Stroke Management. J Intern Med 1996;240:173–180

53. Indredavik B, Bakke F, Slordahl SA, Rokseth R, Haheim LL: Treatment in a combined acute and rehabilitation stroke unit: which aspects are most important? Stroke 1999;30:917–923

54. Shah E, Harwood R: Acute management: admission to hospital. In Stroke: Epidemiology, Evidence and Clinical Practice, 2nd Ed. Oxford University Press, Oxford, 1999

55. Wade DT, Langton Hewer R: Hospital admission for acute stroke: who, for how long and to what effect? J Epidemiol Community Health 1985;39:347–352

56. Kalra L, Evans A, Perez I et al: Alternative strategies for stroke care: A prospective randomised controlled study of stroke unit, stroke team and domiciliary management of stroke. Lancet 2000;356:894–899

57. Ronnig OM, Guldvog B: Should stroke victims routinely receive supplemental oxygen? A quasi-randomised controlled trial. Stroke 1999;30:2033–2037

58. Phillips SJ: Pathophysiology and management of hypertension in acute ischaemic stroke. Hypertension 1994;23:131–136

59. Morfis L, Schwartz RS, Poulos R, Howes LG: Blood pressure changes in acute cerebral infarction and haemorrhage. Stroke 1997;28:1401–1405

60. Dandapani BK, Suzuki S, Kelley RE et al: Relation between blood pressure and outcome in intracerebral haemorrhage. Stroke 1995;26:21–24

61. The European Ad-Hoc Consensus Group: European strategies for early intervention in stroke. Cerebrovasc Dis 1996;6:315–324

62. Brainin M: Antihypertensive therapy in stroke: acute therapy, primary and secondary prevention. Acta Med Austriaca 1995;22:54–57

63. Lisk DR, Grotta JC, Lamki LM et al: Should hypertension be treated after acute stroke? A randomised controlled trial using SPECT. Arch Neurol 1993;50:855–862

64. Strandgaard S: Autoregulation of cerebral blood flow in hypertensive patients. Circulation 1976;53:720–727

65. Harper G, Castleden CM, Potter JF: Factors affecting changes in blood pressure after acute stroke. Stroke 1994;25:1726–1729

66. Brott T, Lu M, Kothari R et al: Hypertension and its treatment in the NINDS rt-PA stroke trial. Stroke 1998;29:1504–1509

67. Jorgensen HS, Nakayama H, Raaschou HO, Olsen TS: Effect of blood pressure and diabetes on stroke progression. Lancet 1994;344:156–159

68. Scott JF, Robinson GM, French JM et al: Prevalence of admission hyperglycaemia across clinical subtypes of acute stroke. Lancet 1999;353:376–377

69. Weir CJ, Murray GD, Dyker AG, Lees KR: Is hyperglycaemia an independent predictor of poor outcome after acute stroke? Results of a long-term follow-up study. Br Med J 1997;314:1303–1306

70. Tracey F, Crawford VLS, Lawson JT, Buchanan KD, Stout RW: Hyperglycaemia and mortality from acute stroke. Q J Med 1993;86:439–446

71. Scott JF, Gray CS, O'Connell JE, Alberti KGMM: Glucose and insulin therapy in acute stroke: why delay further? Q J Med 1998;91:511–515

72. Scott JF, Robinson GM, French JM et al: Glucose potassium infusions in the treatment of acute stroke in patients with mild to moderate hyperglycemia. Stroke 1999;30:793–799

73. Reith J, Jorgensen HS, Pedersen PM et al: Body temperature in acute stroke: relation to stroke severity, infarct size, mortality and outcome. Lancet 1996;347:422–425

74. Schwab S, Schwarz S, Spranger M et al: Moderate hypothermia in the treatment of patients with severe middle cerebral artery infarction. Stroke 1998;29:2461–2466

75. Bath PM: Optimising homeostasis. Br Med Bull 2000;56:422–435

76. Hacke W, Schwab S, Horn M et al: Malignant middle cerebral artery infarction. Arch Neurol 1996;53:309–315

77. Ek AC, Larsson J, von Schenck et al: The correlation between anergy, malnutrition and clinical outcome in an elderly population. Clin Nutr 1990;9:185–189

78. Axelsson K, Apslund K, Norberg A, Eriksson S: Eating problems and nutritional status during hospital stay of patients with severe stroke. J Am Diet Assoc 1989;89:1092–1096

79. Smithard DG, O'Neill MD, Park C et al: Complications and outcome following acute stroke: does dysphagia matter? Stroke 1996;27:1200–1204

80. Wanklyn P, Cox N, Belfield P: Outcome in patients who require a gastrostomy after stroke. Age Ageing 1995;24:510–514

81. Norton B, Homer-Ward M, Donnelly MT et al: A randomised prospective comparison of percutaneous endoscopic gastrostomy and nasogastric tube feeding after acute dysphagic stroke. Br Med J 1996;312:13–16

82. Astrup J, Symon L, Siejbo BK: Thresholds in cerebral ischaemia—the ischaemic penumbra. Stroke 1981;12:723–725

83. Castillo J, Davalos A, Noya M: Progression of ischaemic stroke and excitotoxic aminoacids. Lancet 1997;249:79–83

84. Randall JB, Hoff JT: In Weinstein PR, Faden AJ (eds): Protection of the Brain from Ischaemia. Williams and Wilkins, Baltimore, 1990

85. Harper G: Treatment of stroke in older patients: a state of the art review. Drugs Aging 1995;6:29–44

86. The RANTTAS Investigators: A randomised trial of trilizad mesylate in patients with acute stroke. Stroke 1996;27:1453–1458

87. Schneider D, Berrouschot J, Brandt T et al: Safety, pharmacokinetics and biological activity of enlimomab: an open label dose escalation study in patients hospitalised for acute stroke. Eur Neurol 1998;40:78–83

88. Chinese Acute Stroke Trial (CAST) Collaborative Group: Randomised placebo controlled trial of early aspirin use in 20,000 patients with acute ischaemic stroke. Lancet 1997;349:1641–1649

89. Small DL, Buchan AM: Animal models in stroke. Br Med Bull 2000;56:307–317

90. Levine SR, Brott TG: Thrombolytic therapy in cerebrovascular disorders. Prog Cardiovasc Dis 1992;34:235–262

91. Lees KR: Thrombolysis. Br Med Bull 2000;389–400

92. Wardlaw JM, del Zoppo G, Yamaguchi T: Thrombolysis for acute ischaemic stroke (Cochrane review). In The Cochrane Library, Issue 1, Update Software, Oxford, 2000

93. Hacke W, Bluhmki E, Steiner T et al: Dichotomized efficacy end points and global end-point analysis applied to the ECASS intention-to-treat data set: post hoc analysis of ECASS I. Stroke 1998;29:2073–2075

94. Mohr JP: Thrombolytic therapy for ischemic stroke: from clinical trials to clinical practice. JAMA 2000;283:1189–1191

95. Heiss WD, Theil A, Grond M, Graf R: Which targets are relevant for therapy of acute ischaemic stroke? Stroke 1999;30:1486–1489

96. Lees KR: Neuroprotection. Br Med Bull 2000;401–412

97. Wolf PA: Prevention of stroke. Lancet 1998;352(suppl III):15–18

98. Gubitz G, Sandercock P: Prevention of ischaemic stroke. Br Med J 2000;321:1455–1459

99. Prospective Studies Collaboration: Cholesterol, diastolic blood pressure and stroke. Lancet 1995;9:695–697

100. Scandinavian Simvastatin Survival Study Group: Randomised trial of cholesterol lowering in 4444 patients with coronary heart disease. Lancet 1994;344:1383–1389

101. Hankey GJ: Smoking and risk of stroke. J Cardiovasc Risk 1999;6:207–211

102. Shinton R, Sagar G: Lifelong exercise and stroke. Br Med J 1993;307:231–234

103. Hendriks HFJ, Veenstra J, Velthius-te Wierik EJ et al: Effect of moderate dose of alcohol with evening meal on fibrinolytic factors. Br Med J 1994;308:1003–1006

104. OXCHECK Study Group of the Imperial Cancer Research Fund: Effectiveness of health checks conducted by nurses in primary care: results of the OXCHECK study after one year. Br Med J 1994;308:308–312

105. Johnson ES, Lanes SF, Wentworth CE 3rd et al: A metaregression analysis of the dose-response effect of aspirin on stroke. Arch Intern Med 1999;159:1248–1253

106. Tong DC, Albers GW: Antithrombotic management of atrial fibrillation for stroke prevention in older people. Clin Geriatric Med 1999;15:645–662

107. Diener H-C: Antiplatelet drugs in the secondary prevention of stroke. Int J Clin Pract 1998;52:91–97

108. Wilterdink JL, Easton JD: Dipyridamole plus aspirin in cerebrovascular disease. Arch Neurol 1999;56:1087–1092

109. CAPRIE Steering Committee: A randomised, blinded trial of clopidogrel versus aspirin in patients at the risk of ischaemic events. Lancet 1996;348:1329–1339

110. Kalra L, Perez I, Melbourn A: Risk assessment and anticoagulation for primary stroke prevention in atrial fibrillation. Stroke 1999;30:1218–1222

111. Kalra L, Yu G, Perez I, Lakhani A, Donaldson N: Prospective cohort study to determine if trial efficacy of anticoagulation for stroke prevention in atrial fibrillation translates into clinical effectiveness. Br Med J 2000;320:1236–1239

112. Aronow WS, Ahn C, Kronzon I, Gutstein H: Incidence of new thromboembolic stroke in persons 62 years and older with chronic atrial fibrillation treated with warfarin versus aspirin. JAGS 1999;47:366–368

113. Rothwell PM: Who should have carotid surgery or angioplasty? Br Med Bull 2000;56:526–538

114. Weiller C, Ramsay S, Wise RJS, Friston KJ, Frackowiak RSJ: Individual patterns of functional reorganisation in the human cerebral cortex after capsular infarction. Ann Neurol 1993;33:181–189

115. Steinberg BA, Augustine JR: Behavioural, anatomical and physiological aspects of recovery of motor function following stroke. Brain Res Rev 1997;25:125–132

116. Dettmers C, Stephan KM, Lemon RN, Frackowiak RSJ: Reorganisation of the executive motor system after stroke. Cerebrovasc Dis 1997;7:187–200

117. Cramer SC, Nelles G, Benson RR et al: A functional MRI study of subjects recovered from hemiparetic stroke. Stroke 1997;28:2518–2587

118. Hamdy S, Rothwell JC, Aziz Q, Singh KD, Thompson DG: Long-term reorganization of human motor cortex driven by short-term sensory stimulation. Nat Neurosci 1998;1(1):64–68

119. Nudo RJ, Wise BM, SiFuentes F, Millken GW: Neural substrates for the effects of rehabilitative training on motor recovery after ischaemic infarct. Science 1996;272:1791–1794

120. Gledmacher DS: Enhancing recovery from ischaemic stroke. Neurosurg Clinics N Am 1997;8:245–251

121. Nudo RJ, Milliken GW, Jenkins WM, Merzenich MM: Use-dependent alterations of movement representations in primary motor cortex of squirrel monkeys. J Neurosci 1996;16:785–807

122. Kozlowski DA, James DC, Schallert T: Use-dependent exaggeration of neuronal injury after unilateral sensorimotor cortex lesions. J Neurosci 1996;16:4776–4786

123. Pomeroy VM, Tallis RC: Need to focus research in stroke rehabilitation. Lancet 2000;355:836–837

124. Wade D: Rehabilitation therapy after stroke. Lancet 1999;354:176–177

125. Wade DT, Langton Hewer R: Functional abilities after stroke: measurement, natural history and prognosis. J Neurol Neurosurg Psychiatry 1987;50:177–182

126. Skilbeck CE, Wade DT, Hewer RL, Wood VA: Recovery after stroke. J Neurol Neurosurg Psychiatry 1983;46:5–8

127. Gray CS, French JM, Bates D et al: Recovery of visual fields in acute stroke: homonymous hemianopia associated with adverse prognosis. Age Ageing 1989;18:419–421

128. Gladman JR, Harwood DM, Barer DH: Predicting the outcome of acute stroke: prospective evaluation of five multivariate models and comparison with simple methods. J Neurol Neurosurg Psychiatry 1992;55:347–351

129. Mann G, Hankey GJ, Cameron D: Swallowing disorders following acute stroke: Prevalence and diagnostic accuracy. Cerebrovasc Dis 2000;10:380–386

130. Undrum W, Lincoln NB: Spontaneous recovery of language in patients with aphasia between 4 and 34 weeks after stroke. J Neurol Neurosurg Psychiatry 1985;48:743–748

131. Oder W, Binder H, Baumgartner CH: Is aphasia an additional prognostic factor in ischemic stroke with regard to the severity of hemiparesis in the subacute phase? Acta Neurol Scand 1988;78:85–89

132. Partridge CJ, Johnston M, Edwards S: Recovery from physical disability after stroke: normal patterns as a basis for evaluation. Lancet 1987;1:373–375

133. Bard G, Hirschberg GG: Recovery of voluntary motion in upper extremity following hemiplegia. Arch Phys Med Rehabil 1965;46:567–572

134. Christie D: Aftermath of stroke: an epidemiological study in Melbourne, Australia. J Epidemiol Community Health 1982;36:123–126

135. Edmans JA, Lincoln NB: The relationship between perceptual deficits after stroke and independence in ADL. Br J Occup Ther 1990;53:139–142

136. Kalra L, Smith D, Crome P: Stroke in patients aged over 75 years: outcome and predictors. Postgrad Med J 1993;69:33–36

137. Kalra L: The influence of stroke unit rehabilitation on functional recovery from stroke. Stroke 1994;25:821–825

138. Andrews K, Brocklehurst JC, Richards B, Laycock PJ: The rate of recovery from stroke and its measurement. Int Rehabil Med 1981;3:155–161

139. Kotila M, Waltimo O, Niemi ML et al: The profile of recovery from stroke and factors influencing outcome. Stroke 1984;15:1039–1044

140. Langton-Hewer R: Rehabilitation after stroke. Q J Med 1990;279:659–674

141. Wade DT: Is stroke rehabilitation worthwhile? Curr Opin Neurol Neurosurg 1993;6:78–82

142. Harvey RL: Tailoring therapy to a stroke patient's potential. Postgrad Med 1998;104:78–88

143. Duncan PW, Jorgensen HS, Wade DT: Outcome measures in acute stroke trials: a systematic review and some recommendations to improve practice. Stroke 2000;31:1429–1438

144. Wade DT, de Jong BA: Recent advances in rehabilitation. Br Med J 2000;320:1385–1388

145. Wade DT: Stroke: rehabilitation and long-term care. Lancet 1992;339:791–793

146. Wade DT: Measurement in neurologic rehabilitation. Curr Opin Neurol 1993;6:778–784

147. Wade DT: Evidence relating to goal planning in rehabilitation. Clin Rehabil 1998;12:273–275

148. Wade DT: A framework for considering rehabilitation interventions. Clin Rehabil 1998;12:363–368

149. Hoenig H, Horner RD, Duncan PW, Clipp E, Hamilton B: New horizons in stroke rehabilitation research. J Rehabil Res Dev 1999;36:19–31

150. Pearson VA: Speech and language therapy: is it effective? Pub Health 1995;109:143–153

151. Mant J, Carter J, Wade DT, Winner S: Family support for stroke: a randomised controlled trial. Lancet 2000;356:808–813

152. Rodgers H, Atkinson C, Bond S et al: Randomized controlled trial of a comprehensive stroke education program for patients and caregivers. Stroke 1999;30:2585–2591

153. Wade DT, Skilbeck CE, Langton-Hewer R, Wood VA: Therapy after stroke: amounts, determinants and effects. Int Rehabil Med 1984;6:105–110

154. Sunderland A, Tinson DJ, Bradley EL et al: Enhanced physical therapy improves recovery of arm function after stroke: a randomised controlled trial. J Neurol Neurosurg Psych 1992;55:530–535

155. Kwakkel G, Wagenaar RC, Twisk JW, Lankhorst GJ, Koetsier JC: Intensity of leg and arm training after primary middle-cerebral-artery stroke: a randomised trial. Lancet 1999;354:191–196

156. Wade DT: Measurement in Neurological Rehabilitation. Oxford University Press, Oxford, 1992

157. Duncan PW, Lai SM, van Culin V et al: Development of a comprehensive assessment toolbox for stroke. Clin Geriatric Med 1999;15:885–915

158. Abu-Zeid HAH, Won Choi N, Hsu PH, Maini KK: Prognostic factors in the survival of 1484 stroke cases observed for 30 to 48 months. 1. Diagnostic types and descriptive variables. Arch Neurol 1978;35:121–125

159. Kalra L, Eade J: The role of stroke rehabilitation units in managing severe disability after stroke. Stroke 1995;26:2031–2034

160. Kwakkel G, Wagenaar RC, Kollen BJ, Lankhorst GJ: Predicting disability in stroke—a critical review of the literature. Age Ageing 1996;25:479–489

161. Stone SP, Allder SJ, Gladman JRF: Predicting outcome in acute stroke. Br Med Bull 2000;56:486–494

162. Kalra L, Dale P, Crome P: Evaluation of a clinical score for prognostic stratification of elderly stroke patients. Age Ageing 1994;23:492–499

163. Kalra L, Crome P: The role of prognostic scores in targeting stroke rehabilitation in elderly patients. J Am Geriatr Soc 1993;41:396–400

164. Lai SM, Duncan PW, Keighley J: Prediction of functional outcome after stroke: comparison of the Orpington Prognostic Scale and the NIH Stroke Scale. Stroke 1998;29:1838–1842

165. Langhorne P, Stott DJ, Robertson L et al: Medical complications after stroke: a multicenter study. Stroke 2000;31:1223–1239

166. Hamdy S, Aziz Q, Rothwell JC et al: The cortical topography of swallowing motor function in man. Nat Med 1996;2:1217–1224

167. Kidd D, Lawson J, Nesbitt R, MacMahon J: The natural history and clinical consequences of aspiration following acute stroke. Q J Med 1995;88:409–413

168. Davies AE, Kidd D, Stone SP, MacMahon J: Pharyngeal sensation and gag reflex in healthy subjects. Lancet 1995;345:487–488

169. Martino R, Pron G, Diamant N: Screening for oropharyngeal dysphagia in stroke: insufficient evidence for guidelines. Dysphagia 2000;15:19–30

170. Bath PM, Bath FJ, Smithard DG: Interventions for dysphagia in acute stroke. Cochrane Datab Systemat Rev 2000;(2):CD000323

171. Meador KJ, Loring DW, Lee K et al: Cerebral lateralization: relationship of language and ideomotor praxis. Neurology 1999;53(9):2028–2031

172. Oxbury J, Wyke MA: Disturbances of higher cerebral function. In Weatherall DJ, Leddingham JGG, Warrell DA (eds): Oxford Textbook of Medicine, 3rd ed. 1997

173. Gonzalez Rothi LJ, Nadeau SE, Ennis MR: Aphasia treatment: a key issue for research into the twenty-first century. Brain Lang 2000;71:78–81

174. Bowen A, McKenna K, Tallis RC: Reasons for variability in the reported rate of occurrence of unilateral spatial neglect after stroke. Stroke 1999;30:1196–1202

175. Lincoln NB, Drummond AE, Berman P: Perceptual impairment and its impact on rehabilitation outcome. SUE Study Group. Disabil Rehabil 1997;19:231–234

176. Robertson IH, Tegner R, Tham K et al: Sustained attention training for neglect: theoretical and rehabilitation implications. J Clin Exp Neuropsychol 1995;17:416–430

177. Kalra L, Perez I, Gupta S, Whittink M: The influence of visual neglect on stroke rehabilitation. Stroke 1997;28:1386–1391

178. Prada G, Tallis RC: Treatment of the neglect syndrome in stroke patients using a contingency electric stimulator. Clin Rehabil 1995;9:77–86

179. Pomeroy VM, Tallis RC: Physical therapy to improve movement performance and functional ability post-stroke. Part I. Existing evidence. Rev Clin Gerontol 2000;10:261–290

180. Pomeroy VM, Dean D, Sykes L et al: The unreliability of clinical measures of muscle tone: implications for stroke therapy. Age Ageing 2000;29:229–233

181. Bhakta BB: Management of spasticity in stroke. Br Med Bull 2000;56:476–485

182. Davis EC, Barnes MP: Botulinum toxin and spasticity. J Neurol Neurosurg Psych 2000;69:143–147 (editorial)

183. Wang RY, Chan RC, Tsai MW: Effects of thoraco-lumbar electric sensory stimulation on knee extensor spasticity of persons who survived cerebrovascular accident (CVA). J Rehabil Res Dev 2000;37:73–79

184. Roy CW: Shoulder pain in hemiplegia: a literature review. Clin Rehabil 1988;2:35–44

185. Snels IA, Beckerman H, Twisk JW et al: Effect of triamcinolone acetonide injections on hemiplegic shoulder pain: A randomized clinical trial. Stroke 2000;31(10):2396–2401

186. McGuire JR, Harvey RL: The prevention and management of complications after stroke. Phys Med Rehabil Clinics N Am 1999;10:857–874

187. Moon AH, Gragnani JA: Cold water immersion for the oedematous hand in stroke patients. Clin Rehabil 1989;3:97–101

188. So EL, Annegers JF, Hauser WA et al: Population-based study of seizure disorders after cerebral infarction. Neurology 1996;46:350–355

189. Bladin CF, Alexandrov AV, Bellavance A et al: Seizures after stroke: a prospective multicentre study. Arch Neurol 2000;57:1617–1622

190. Berges S, Moulin T, Berger E et al: Seizures and epilepsy following strokes: recurrence factors. Eur Neurol 2000;43:3–8

191. Viitanen M, Eriksson S, Asplund K: Risk of recurrent stroke, myocardial infarction and epilepsy during long-term follow up after stroke. Eur Neurol 1988;28:227–231

192. Rao R: Cerebrovascular disease and late life depression: an age old association revisited. Int J Geriatric Psychiatry 2000;15:419–433

193. Robinson RG, Lipsey JR, Pearlson CD: The occurrence and treatment of post-stroke mood disorder. Compr Ther 1984;10:19–24

194. Carson AJ, MacHale S, Allen K et al: Depression after stroke and lesion location: a systematic review. Lancet 2000;356:122–126

195. Robinson-Smith G, Johnston MV, Allen J: Self-care self-efficacy, quality of life, and depression after stroke. Arch Phys Med Rehabil 2000;81:460–464

196. Rigler SK: Management of poststroke depression in older people. Clinics Geriatric Med 1999;15:765–783
197. Maclean N, Pound P, Wolfe C. Rudd A: Qualitative analysis of stroke patients' motivation for rehabilitation. Br Med J 2000;321:1051–1054
198. Robinson RG, Murata Y, Shimoda K: Dimensions of social impairment and their effect on depression and recovery following stroke. Int Psychoger 1999;11:375–384
199. Tyson S, Turner G: Discharge and follow-up for people with stroke: what happens and why. Clin Rehabil 2000;14:381–392
200. Ebrahim S, Nouri F: Caring for stroke patients at home. Int Rehabil Med 1987;8:171–173
201. Weatherall M: Family support after stroke. Lancet 2000;356:2196
202. Blake H, Lincoln NB: Factors associated with strain in co-resident spouses of patients following stroke. Clin Rehabil 2000;14:307–314
203. Low JT, Payne S, Roderick P: The impact of stroke on informal carers: a literature review. Social Sci Med 1999;49:711–725
204. Harding J, Lincoln NB: An observational study of the Stroke Association family support organizer service. Clin Rehabil 2000;14:315–323
205. Knapp P, Young J, House A, Forster A: Non-drug strategies to resolve psycho-social difficulties after stroke. Age Ageing 2000;29:23–30
206. Erkinjuntti T: Types of multi-infarct dementia. Acta Neurol Scand 1987;75:391–393
207. Stuss DT, Cummings JL: Subcortical vascular dementia. In Cummings JL (ed): Subcortical Dementia. Oxford University Press, Oxford, 1990
208. Wilkieson C, Stott DJ, Wardlaw JM, Caird FI: Cerebral multi-infarct states: Rev Clin Gerontol 1994;4:29–42
209. Tatemichi TK: Dementia. In Bogousslavsky J, Caplan L (eds): Stroke Syndromes. Cambridge University Press, Cambridge, 1995
210. Roman GC: Vascular dementia today. Rev Neurol 1999;155(suppl 4):S64–72
211. Rockwood K, Bowler J, Erkinjuntti T, Hachinski V, Wallin A: Subtypes of vascular dementia. Alzheimer Dis Associat Disord 1991;13(suppl 3):S59–65
212. Yamada M: Cerebral amyloid angiopathy: an overview. Neuropathology 2000;20:8–22
213. Viitanen M, Kalimo H: CADASIL: hereditary arteriopathy leading to multiple brain infarcts and dementia. Ann NY Acad Sci 2000;903:273–284
214. Rocca WA, Kokmen E: Frequency and distribution of vascular dementia. Alzheimer Dis Associat Disord 1999;13(suppl 3):S9–14
215. Roman CG, Tatemichi TK, Erkinjuntti T et al: Vascular dementia: diagnostic criteria for research studies—report of the NINDS-AIREN International Workshop. Neurology 1993;43:250–260
216. Schmidt R, Schmidt H, Fazekas F: Vascular risk factors in dementia. J Neurol 2000;247:81–87
217. Gorelick PB, Erkinjuntti T, Hofman A et al: Prevention of vascular dementia. Alzheimer Dis Associat Disord 1999;13 Suppl 3: S131–139
218. Fujishima M, Tsuchihashi T: Hypertension and dementia. Clin Exp Hypertens 1999;21:927–935
219. Ogata J: Vascular dementia: the role of changes in the vessels. Alzheimer Dis Associat Disord 1999;13(suppl 3):S55–58
220. Galton CJ, Hodges JR: The spectrum of dementia and its treatment. J R Coll Physic Lond 1999;33:234–239
221. Liston R, Mickelborough J, Harris B, Wynn Hann A, Tallis RC: Conventional physiotherapy and treadmill retraining for higher-level gait disorders in cerebrovascular disease. Age Ageing 2000;29:311–318

Chapter 50

Stroke: organization of services

Martin S. Dennis

A few years ago no editor of a textbook on geriatric, general, or neurological medicine would have considered including a chapter on the organization of stroke services. However, things have changed, and after years of being largely ignored by doctors and health services managers, as well as by editors, the organization of stroke care has become an important issue. The frequency of stroke and its impact on patients' survival and function have led governments in many countries to identify stroke as a key area for improving health care. Several reports have suggested that stroke care is too often poorly organized and not tailored to the individual.[1,2] Perhaps this is not surprising, since in many countries no specialist group has taken stroke on as, for example, cardiologists have taken on myocardial infarction.

Until recently there was little reliable evidence that it mattered how services for stroke patients were organized. Since the 1960s, several randomized controlled trials (RCTs) had individually provided little to justify setting up stroke units. In 1991 a small RCT evaluating a stroke unit in Trondheim demonstrated that patients managed in the unit had reduced mortality and a better functional outcome than patients managed in a general medical setting.[3] This stimulated Langhorne and colleagues[4] to perform a systematic review of all RCTs, comparing the outcome of stroke unit care with that in a general medical setting. Despite the methodological problems associated with performing a meta-analysis of RCTs of relatively heterogeneous interventions and that measured different outcomes, this study provided fairly robust evidence that care in a stroke unit is associated with a significant reduction in mortality.[4] These data have focused attention on how stroke services should be organized, although they provide little direct evidence about the optimum type of general care and rehabilitation.

When considering the organization of stroke services, it is useful to list the components of care to ensure that each is adequately addressed to provide a comprehensive service so that particular groups of patients are not disadvantaged (see accompanying box). There has been little formal evaluation to establish the optimum method for delivering those components of stroke care not included within the functions of a stroke unit. However, one can make some commonsense recommendations based on what we know about patients' problems and needs and the clinical epidemiology of stroke. This chapter addresses some of the choices offered at different stages in a patient's treatment and discusses the rationale, or the evidence if any exists, for competing models of stroke service. It concludes with an outline of some of the issues surrounding the monitoring and integration of stroke services.

IMMEDIATE MANAGEMENT

Patients who recognize the initial symptoms of a stroke should be advised to (1) contact their family doctor, or (2) call an ambulance or (3) go straight to the nearest hospital.

The rationale for immediate self-referral to a hospital is that it reduces the delay in getting medical attention[5] and that if acute medical treatment for stroke is going to be successful it is likely to be most effective if initiated early. There is evidence supporting this. RCTs of thrombolytic therapy in acute ischemic stroke suggest that the benefits of treatment may be greater (and the risk of treatment, i.e., hemorrhagic transformation, less) if administered within the first 3 hours.[6] If these findings are confirmed, we will have to modify the preadmission care of stroke patients, perhaps including the kinds of arrangements currently made to ensure minimum delay between onset of myocardial infarction and thrombolysis therapy which have been used to facilitate the evaluation of early thrombolysis in acute stroke.[7] Currently, few medical centers use routine thrombolytic therapy, and therefore emergency admission of all patients is not easily justified and patients probably lose little by contacting their family doctor. Of course if acute medical treatments

Summary of service options

- Acute phase
  Home community team
  Rapid access neurovascular outpatient clinic
  Acclerated hospital admission to facilitate thrombolysis, etc.
  Routine hospital admission

- Acute hospital care
  Admission to a general ward
  Acute stroke unit
  - providing short-term care only
  - intensive care unit
  - "comprehensive" unit providing ongoing rehabilitation

- Rehabilitation
  Specialist stroke rehabilitation unit
  Generic rehabilitation unit

  Prolonged hospital-based rehabilitation
  Early supported discharge team

  Day hospital
  Community-based rehabilitation

- Long-term care
  Community
  Institution

that can be safely administered in the community without prior imaging are identified, the need for hospitalization will be reduced. However, it seems likely that the initial evaluation of such treatments would be hospital based.

HOSPITAL REFERRAL

Family doctors seeing patients with a stroke or transient ischemic attack (TIA) have two choices regarding referral to a hospital: (1) Managing patients in the community or referring them to a hospital, and (2) referring patients for outpatient (ambulatory) or inpatient care.

The proportion of stroke patients admitted to hospital varies widely from place to place, although some of this variation might be accounted for by different definitions of admissions.[8,9] For instance, in some healthcare systems attendance at an emergency department might be counted as an admission. Admission rates must reflect factors including the quality and confidence of family doctors; the population's perception of stroke and their expectations concerning acute treatment, general care, and rehabilitation; and the access to facilities in the community and in a hospital. Social factors, such as whether the patient lives alone, are often decisive.[8] One small trial randomized acute stroke patients to one of three care settings: an inpatient stroke unit; a general ward with advice from a visiting multidisciplinary stroke team; and management in the community. A third of the patients allocated management in the community were later admitted to the stroke unit and their mortality was higher and functional recovery less good than those managed in the stroke unit.[10]

There is an increasing consensus that all, or at least almost all, patients with stroke and TIA should be referred to a hospital for a detailed assessment.[11,12] Referral is usually justified on the basis that a specialist with hospital-based facilities can offer a more accurate and thorough assessment than a family doctor. Although the clinical diagnosis of stroke is usually reliable, the diagnosis of TIAs is prone to considerable interobserver variation.[13,14] However, a complete assessment includes a search for the underlying cause, which involves investigations to define the pathological type of stroke and in some patients with ischemic stroke to identify cardiac and extracranial vascular disease, and so the clinician needs ready access to appropriate imaging facilities.

Timing of referral

The history of an event and its neurological signs are most easily interpreted as soon as possible after the event. Computerized tomography (CT) scanning can reliably distinguish cerebral infarction from primary intracerebral hemorrhage only if it is performed within a week of onset.[15] This means that patients should see a specialist as soon as possible and has prompted the development of stroke or neurovascular clinics that provide early clinical assessment and fast-track investigation for patients who do not require hospital admission. The situation in many institutions where only inpatients have access to early investigation reflects a lack of organization and is bound to increase the service costs by encouraging unnecessary admissions to hospital.

Family doctors sometimes delay admission to see how the patient progresses, but this strategy has some inherent dangers. It can put undue pressure on the family who may later, even after a period of inpatient rehabilitation, be reticent about further involvement in the patient's long-term care. Also, inexpert handling at home may lead to injury to the patient or the care-giver.

Accessing the multidisciplinary team

Even after the diagnosis of stroke has been confirmed, the likely cause identified, and treatable underlying causes excluded, patients often require further detailed assessment. Thus, in all but the mildest or most transient cases, the patient should have prompt access to a team comprising at least a nurse, physiotherapist, speech and language therapist, and occupational therapist. In most places this usually requires referral to a hospital.

STROKE UNITS
Initial placement

Once the decision has been made to admit the patient to a hospital, the next choice is whether the patient should be admitted to (1) a general medical, geriatric, or neurological unit, or (2) a specialized acute stroke unit, that is, a unit that accepts direct, unselected admissions with stroke from the community.

There are few data from RCTs that help inform this choice. Several of the RCTs included in the stroke unit trialists collaboration admitted patients acutely and where appropriate offered several weeks of rehabilitation (so-called comprehensive stroke units).[16] Such units make some sense, since they facilitate:

- The introduction of guidelines and protocols to ensure consistently high standards of assessment and early treatment, perhaps including an assessment proforma[17,18]
- Research, especially to test the effectiveness of medical treatments for acute stroke
- Early involvement of specialists and members of a multidisciplinary team
- Monitoring of the performance of the unit since all cases are more easily identified at an early stage in their admission.

Stroke intensive care units

Some have suggested that acute stroke patients should initially be managed in high-tech stroke intensive care units where a range of physiological parameters, for example, intracranial pressure, can be monitored and attempts made to optimize them with for example hemicraniotomy, positive pressure ventilation, or mannitol.[19] However, little is known about the benefits, or indeed the risks, of either the monitoring itself or the interventions which follow. It seems unlikely that any improvement in outcome from such interventions would be dramatic, and thus we need to look for evidence of effectiveness from RCTs. Unfortunately little direct evidence is available. One small randomized trial of noninvasive monitoring and where appropriate, correction of abnormal physiological parameter (e.g. oxygen saturation, low blood pressure, and hyperglycemia) did show a reduction in early progression of stroke deficits but the monitoring took place in a normal ward environment.[20] The increased costs of intensive care units means that we should not set them up except to evaluate them or unless some acute intervention is shown to be effective and requires such close monitoring of patients.

The post-acute period—triage

Once the diagnosis has been made, investigations completed, and any early medical or surgical treatment given, the 90 percent of patients who survive the first few days can usually be divided into three groups depending on their condition. For each of these three groups of patients one must provide facilities that match their individual needs.

Mild strokes

Some patients, perhaps 20–30 percent, have minimal functional sequelae and are able to be discharged home within a few days. Their further treatment should primarily be directed at secondary prevention, although we should not underestimate their psychological needs. After all they may perceive their stroke as a major threat to their survival and independence. These patients should probably remain in the acute admission area or stroke unit until an early discharge. The period of inpatient care can be usefully employed in educating and informing the patient and relatives about stroke, although this process may need to be carried through into the post-discharge period. Once a strategy for secondary prevention has been developed, it should probably most sensibly be monitored in primary care, where this is well organized but, alternatively, the neurovascular clinic could fulfill this role.

The severest strokes

Some patients have been so badly damaged by the stroke itself or have coexistent pathologies, for example, dementia, that they are unable to participate actively in rehabilitation. Such patients may die, may remain in a severely dependent state, or may require time to improve to a level where they might benefit from a rehabilitation environment. For instance, those who remain in a coma or medically unwell might remain in the acute stroke unit where they can receive good nursing care and appropriate medical treatment. Obviously issues such as prevention of pressure sores, aspiration, deep venous thrombosis, dehydration, and malnutrition are important during this period. Where patients are likely to survive with an acceptable quality of life, they require active medical management of such problems. Such individuals often raise difficult ethical dilemmas, which makes good communication between professionals and with relatives particularly important. This may be an important reason for managing such patients in a designated area.

Strokes of intermediate severity

Many patients fall into an intermediate group who have neurological impairments and disabilities that make immediate discharge impossible. Such individuals need rehabilitation, and this can be provided in several different environments including (1) acute general medical, geriatric, or neurological units, (2) specialized stroke units (either part of a comprehensive unit or a separate stroke rehabilitation unit), and (3) generic rehabilitation units.

The systematic review of all RCTs of stroke units referred to in the introduction provides compelling evidence that patients, particularly those in the intermediate category, are better managed in a stroke unit. The care provided in a stroke unit compared with that offered in a general medical setting has been associated with about 17 percent reduction in the odds of death within the first year and a 23 percent reduction in the odds of death or long-term institutionalization.[16] Several characteristics may account for their effectiveness, including:

- Involvement of a multidisciplinary team whose members are interested in and have specialized in stroke care
- Regular (at least weekly) meetings of the multidisciplinary team to discuss progress and to plan treatment of patients
- In-service training for the staff
- Involvement and education of caregivers in the management of patients

Of course there are many different ways of delivering these services, and unfortunately there is little evidence supporting one particular model. There are, however, practical arguments for pursuing certain models of stroke unit care.

Combining or separating acute care and rehabilitation

Some of the more successful stroke units have combined both acute and rehabilitation functions, the so called comprehensive units.[3] The danger of this is that less acute patients compete unsuccessfully for nursing time, as occurs in an acute hospital setting where the needs of the acute patient (e.g., treatment of ischemic chest pain) may be perceived as more urgent and perhaps more important than those of the rehabilitating patient (e.g., regular toileting to maintain continence). Some splitting of the functions seems logical, but if this can be achieved in one unit, continuity of care and thus consistency of approach will be improved.

Stroke units vs mobile stroke teams

Most of the evidence from RCTs supported the concept of a geographically defined unit rather than one based in several locations that relies on the input from a roving multidisciplinary team. One of the main advantages of a geographically defined unit is that it facilitates full participation of the nurses in the multidisciplinary team. After all, the aim is for patients to receive consistent help toward regaining independence around the clock and not just during therapy sessions. Only two RCTs have evaluated a roving stroke team and neither provided evidence of benefit.[10,21]

Maintaining flexibility

One of the major disadvantages of a geographically defined unit is that unless one has extremely flexible staffing arrangements and use of beds, the number of patients who can be accommodated is limited. In most hospitals there are likely to be substantial fluctuations in the number of patients who might benefit from stroke unit care. Many of these fluctuations are due to random effects, although seasonal variation in stroke incidence and admission may play a part.[22] When the number of stroke admissions rises or the proportion of patients with severe stroke increases (so increasing mean length of stay), some patients cannot get into the unit. One partial solution is to operate a mobile stroke team which manages patients wherever they are as well as those in the stroke unit. An ideal solution is to have an expandable unit sized to match changing demands but this also requires enough trained staff.

Generic rehabilitation centers

In many countries patients are moved from acute care facilities, which may be stroke-specific or not, to generic rehabilitation facilities. The latter are often in separate departments or even at a different site than the acute facility. Such rehabilitation facilities may provide excellent multidisciplinary care but can lead to a loss of continuity of care. Also, if rehabilitation beds are scarce, patients may have to wait at an acute facility. Patients who are waiting for rehabilitation may become frustrated and may not receive the sort of care that will ensure their continued progress. There needs to be close integration of acute and rehabilitation facilities where these are geographically separated. It is still unclear whether generic rehabilitation services, which might include geriatric services, are as effective as stroke-specific ones.

Many other issues will need to be addressed in future RCTs, including questions regarding the optimum type of stroke unit and which features contribute most to their effectiveness.

Duration of hospitalization

Once a patient has been admitted to a hospital, it must be decided how long they should remain there. The length of stay varies greatly from place to place and depends on how much emphasis is placed on rehabilitation and what community facilities are available to provide care. For instance, in many developing countries the length of stay may be short because rehabilitation facilities are limited, and the extended family can provide a home environment in which a disabled patient can receive at least basic care. In some countries prolonged hospital care may be an option only for those who can afford to pay. In many countries there are considerable pressures to reduce length of hospital stay to limit the spiraling costs of medical care. Stroke accounts for a significant proportion of available bed days because of its high frequency and prolonged length of stay.[23] There is evidence that stroke unit care may be associated with reduced length of hospital stay.[16] Patients with disabling stroke require enough care to be able to live at home as well as to continue therapy to ensure that they reach their optimum outcome as regards function. "Early supported discharge" schemes that combine these two elements of care in the patient's own home are models that might reduce length of hospital stay. A systematic review of randomized trials suggests that an early supported discharge scheme can reduce length of stay for a selected minority (perhaps a third of hospitalized patients) by about a week, while achieving similar outcomes at no greater cost.[24]

OUTPATIENT REHABILITATION

Once patients have been discharged from an inpatient facility, whether the stay was prolonged or shortened by an early supported discharge scheme, some may benefit from further input from members of the team. Those responsible for organizing services may choose whether this input is provided (1) in the hospital, either in an outpatient or a day hospital environment, or (2) in the patient's own home.

In two randomized trials comparing the cost-effectiveness of hospital- and home-based continued therapy for stroke patients,[25–28] there were no convincing differences in patient outcome or in the cost of care.

LONG-TERM CARE

For patients with continuing disability one can choose to (1) provide enough continuing support in the community to allow them to return home, or (2) provide care in institutions (e.g. long-term hospital care or nursing home care).

Some patients may be so badly disabled by their stroke that a return to their previous accommodation is not possible given the resources in the community (family or social services). Of course, given unlimited resources it is possible to maintain anyone, whatever their functional status and care needs, at home. Those responsible for funding long-term care have to determine the balance between providing community and institutional care, a decision that should take account of patients' needs and wishes as well as the comparative costs.

After a stroke the timing of the decision to move a patient into long-term care is often difficult. Institutions may not provide the facilities or environment to ensure that the patient continues to improve or even maintain their level of independence. The patient may need to stay in the rehabilitation facility until everyone involved in their care, including the family and sometimes even the patient, is convinced that further rehabilitation is unlikely to make a long-term difference in their quality of life.

There is considerable uncertainty about the value of long-term maintenance therapy. One frequently sees patients who deteriorate after discharge from rehabilitation, perhaps because of an overly protective family and lack of practice, which can partly be avoided by properly instructing the caregiver. However, some patients seem to require long-term input, or at least intermittent input, from therapists to maintain their functional level. In such cases, this interaction may be essential to allow them to remain at home.

MONITORING STROKE SERVICES

A system of monitoring stroke services might demonstrate good or poor performance and identify particular problems that need to be addressed. Any system may depend on monitoring (1) structure, (2) process, and (3) outcome.[29]

There are few recommendations we can make about the structure of a service that are based on reliable evidence, but these include the recommendation that patients be managed in stroke units rather than in a general medical setting. Monitoring the process of care is more promising since several specific interventions have been shown to improve the outcome after stroke, most in the area of secondary prevention.[30–33] Therefore it seems sensible to monitor the use and appropriateness of well-defined interventions such as antiplatelet drugs, anticoagulants, and carotid surgery. The value of monitoring other aspects of process, such as use of imaging, quality of assessment, and access to a multidisciplinary team, is less certain since their effectiveness has not been demonstrated in RCTs. Also, it may be difficult to measure these aspects of care reliably.[34] The patient's survival and physical, social, or psychological outcome are perhaps the most relevant indications of the quality and effectiveness of stroke services. However, the outcome of patients managed by a particular service depends not only on the quality and effectiveness of care but also on the "case mix," the method of measuring outcome, and luck. The case mix is probably the most important determinant of outcome, its effect swamping any differences attributable to the treatment provided. Also, most stroke services do not manage sufficiently large numbers of patients to provide a precise enough estimate of, for example, the case fatality rate, to allow comparisons to be made between units or within the same unit in different periods.[35,36] Of course if a service has consistently poor outcomes, possible causes should be sought. Any differences or changes in the patients' outcomes must be interpreted in the light of detailed information about the case mix and with the utmost caution.

PROVIDING INTEGRATED STROKE SERVICES

In the preceding sections we have discussed some of the choices available to those planning stroke services. It is often not a matter of choosing one model or another but rather of finding a balance between them. For instance, how far does one strive to maintain disabled patients in their own home? In many cases there is little reliable evidence about how services are best organized. Thus choices often have to be based on local decisions taking into account existing resources, local geography, and funding arrangements. However, it seems clear that stroke services should be well organized and their structure based on some knowledge of patients' needs. Facilities need to ensure that all aspects of management can be provided, from acute care through long-term support for severely disabled survivors. Also, with rapid advances in our knowledge and treatment of patients with stroke, it is vital that services be flexible enough to incorporate changes dictated by developments. One example is the introduction of an acute drug treatment for stroke which might have a dramatic effect on the structure of stroke services. However, the precise structure of a stroke service is probably less important than having an individual or small group of people who are willing to take on the responsibility of organizing services for stroke patients. The latter should ensure that services are constructed to meet local needs and conditions.

> **KEY POINTS** Aspects of stroke management
>
> - Initial diagnosis (how can the patient access the appropriate services?)
> - Full assessment to identify the type, cause, and consequences of the stroke (crucial to the planning of all other aspects of care)
> - Specific acute medical and/or surgical treatment
> - General care in the acute period (although there may be little evidence supporting the use of specific acute treatments, a lot can be done to prevent and treat the complications and coexistent pathology in stroke patients)
> - Terminal care (an area bristling with ethical dilemmas)
> - Rehabilitation (often thought of as comprising simply physical therapies but should probably be thought of as a wider process which merges seamlessly with general care, i.e., rehabilitation should start immediately)
> - Long-term placement
> - Secondary prevention (an area where there are several interventions of proven effectiveness)
> - Management of long-term disability and handicap (some argue that stroke-specific services are most relevant in the first few months of a patient's stroke and that generic services for the disabled should become involved at this stage because of the complex inter-relationship of disabilities due to different pathologies)

REFERENCES

1. King's Fund Consensus Conference: Treatment of stroke. BMJ 1988;297:126–128
2. Rudd AG, Irwin P, Rutledge Z et al: The National Sentinel Audit for stroke: a tool for raising standards of care. Roy Coll Phys Lond J 1999;33:460–464
3. Indredavik B, Bakke F, Solberg R et al: Benefit of a stroke unit: a randomised controlled trial. Stroke 1991;22:1026–1031
4. Langhorne P, Williams BO, Gilchrist W, Howie K: Do stroke units save lives? Lancet 1993;342:395–398
5. Wester P, Radberg J, Lundgren B, Peltonen M, for the Seek-Medical-Attention-in-Time Study Group: Factors associated with delayed admission to hospital and in-hospital delays in acute stroke and TIA. A prospective, multicentre study. Stroke 1999;30:40–48
6. Wardlaw J, Yamaguchi T, del Zoppo G: Thrombolysis for acute ischaemic stroke. In the Cochrane Library. Update Software, Oxford, 2000
7. Alberts MJ, Perry A, Dawson DV, Bertels C: Effects of public and professional education on reducing the delay in presentation and referral of stroke patients. Stroke 1992;23:352–356
8. Bamford J, Sandercock P, Warlow C, Gray M: Why are patients with acute stroke admitted to hospital? BMJ 1986;292:1369–1372
9. Asplund K, Bonita R, Kuulasmaa K et al: Multinational comparisons of stroke epidemiology: evaluation of case ascertainment in the WHO MONICA Stroke Study. Stroke 1995;25:355–360
10. Kalra L, Evan A, Perez I et al: Alternative strategies for stroke care: a prospective randomised controlled trial. Lancet 2000;356:894–899
11. Adams HP Jr: The importance of the Helsingburg declaration on stroke management in Europe. J Intern Med 1996;240:169–180
12. RCP Consensus Statement 2000: Proceedings of the Royal College of Physicians of Edinburgh, 2001 Supplement
13. Koudstaal PJ, Van Gijn J, Staal A et al: Diagnosis of transient ischemic attacks: improvement of interobserver agreement by a check-list in ordinary language. Stroke; 1986;17:723–728

14. Quik-van Milligen MLT, Kuyvenhoven MM, de Melker RA et al: Transient ischemic attacks and the general practitioner: diagnosis and management. Cerebrovasc Dis 1992;2:102–106

15. Dennis MS, Bamford JM, Molyneux AJ, Warlow CP: Rapid resolution of signs of primary intracerebral haemorrhage in computed tomograms of the brain. BMJ 1987;295:379–381

16. Stroke Unit Trialists' Collaboration: Organised inpatient (stroke unit) care for stroke (Cochrane Review). In: The Cochrane Library, Issue 1. Update Software, Oxford, 2000

17. Davenport RJ, Dennis MS, Warlow CP: Improving the recording of the clinical assessment of stroke patients using a clerking proforma. Age Ageing 1995;24:43–48

18. Royal College of Physicians Research Unit and UK Stroke Audit Group: Stroke Audit Package. Royal College of Physicians, London, 1994

19. Hacke W, Schwab S, De Georgia M: Intensive care of acute ischaemic stroke. Cerebrovasc Dis 1994;4:385–392

20. Davis M, Hollymann C, McGiven M et al: Physiological monitoring in acute stroke. Age Ageing 1999;28(suppl 1):P45

21. Wood-Dauphinee S, Shapiro S, Bass E et al: A randomized trial of team care following stroke. Stroke 1984;15:864–872

22. Rothwell PM, Wroe SJ, Slattery J, Warlow CP: Is stroke incidence related to season or temperature? Lancet 1996;347:934–936

23. Caro JJ, Huybrachts KF, Duchesne I, for the Stroke economic analysis group: Management patterns and costs of acute ischaemic stroke. An international study. Stroke 2000;31:582–590

24. Early supported discharge trialists: Services for reducing duration of hospital care for acute stroke patients (Cochrane Review). In: The Cochrane Library, Issue 1. Update Software, Oxford, 2001

25. Young JB, Forster A: The Bradford Community Stroke Trial: results at six months. BMJ 1992;304:1085–1089

26. Young J, Forster A: Day hospital and home physiotherapy for stroke patients: a comparative cost-effectiveness study. J R Coll Physic Lond 1993;27:252–257

27. Gladman JRF, Lincoln NB: Follow-up of a controlled trial of domiciliary stroke rehabilitation (DOMINO Study). Age Ageing 1994;23:9–13

28. Gladman J, Forster A, Young J: Hospital- and home-based rehabilitation after discharge from hospital for stroke patients: analysis of two trials. Age Ageing 1995;24:49–53

29. Dennis M: Stroke services: the good, the bad, and the … J R Coll Physic Lond 2000;34:92–96

30. Antiplatelet Trialists' Collaboration: Collaborative overview of randomised trials of antiplatelet therapy. I. prevention of death, myocardial infarction, and stroke by prolonged antiplatelet therapy in various categories of patients. BMJ 1994;308:81–106

31. EAFT (European Atrial Fibrillation Trial) Study Group: Secondary prevention in non-rheumatic atrial fibrillation after transient ischaemic attack or minor stroke. Lancet 1993;342:1255–1262

32. North American Symptomatic Carotid Endarterectomy Trial Collaborators: Beneficial effect of carotid endarterectomy in symptomatic patients with high-grade carotid stenosis. N Engl J Med 1991;325:445–453

33. European Carotid Surgery Trialists' Collaborative Group: Randomised trial of endarterectomy for recently sympotmatic carotid stenosis: final results of the MRC European Carotid Surgery Trial (ECST): Lancet 1998;351:209–212

34. Gompertz P, Dennis M, Hopkins A, Ebrahim S: Development and reliability of the Royal College of Physicians stroke audit form. Age Ageing 1994;22:378–383

35. Davenport RJ, Dennis MS, Warlow CP: Effect of correcting outcome data for case mix following stroke. BMJ 1996;312:1503–1505

36. Scottish Stroke Outcome Group. Towards a national system for monitoring the quality of hospital-based stroke services. Stroke 2001;32:1415–1421

Chapter 51

Disorders of the autonomic nervous system

Horacio Kaufmann and Italo Biaggioni

Material in this chapter contains contributions from the previous edition, and we are grateful to the previous authors for the work done.

We will focus on the consequences of aging on autonomic cardiovascular control. The neurobiology of aging is dealt with in Chapter 44, and the effects of aging on gastrointestinal and urinary tract function are detailed in other sections in this book.

We will first provide a brief summary of autonomic pathways involved in cardiovascular control, and the methods used to assess their function. We will then review the effect of aging on the different components involved in autonomic cardiovascular control, namely, alterations in afferent and efferent function, and in end-organ responsiveness. We will then discuss the integrated effect of these changes on the response of elderly people to daily stresses of life, i.e., response to upright posture and to food ingestion. We conclude by discussing pathological disorders of the autonomic nervous system that are present clinically in elderly people, such as orthostatic hypotension, syncope, pure autonomic failure and multiple system atrophy.

BASIC CONCEPTS OF AUTONOMIC PHYSIOLOGY

Autonomic pathways

Autonomic regulation depends on three main components. Afferent fibers continuously sense changes in blood pressure (baroreceptors), blood content of oxygen and other chemical signals (chemoreceptors), pain (sensory afferents), and cortical stimulation. These signals are integrated in brainstem centers that ultimately modulate sympathetic and parasympathetic outflows, which are transmitted to target organs via efferent fibers. The baroreflex provides an example of these pathways (Fig. 51-1). This is a redundant system, with input from multiple independent afferent pathways that ensure maintenance of cardiovascular regulation even after partial damage.[1] The afferent limb of this reflex includes pressure-sensitive receptors located in the walls of cardiopulmonary veins, the right atrium and within almost every large artery of the neck and thorax but particularly within the carotid and aortic arteries. Stimulated by stretch, these low- and high-pressure baroreceptors monitor venous and arterial pressures, respectively, and relay that information to brainstem centers. Information both from the venous and the aortic arch baroreceptors is carried centrally via fibers that course within the vagus nerve (X cranial nerve). Carotid sinus baroreceptor nerve activity is relayed centrally by passage first through the carotid sinus (Hering's) nerve, then through the glossopharyngeal nerve (IX cranial nerve) before arriving at the same brainstem centers.

Afferent fibers from these multiple baroreceptors have their first synapse in the nucleus tractus solitarii (NTS) of the medulla oblongata.[2] This nucleus inhibits sympathetic tone and is crucial to baroreflex function. Its destruction, e.g., by experimental lesion[3] or neurological damage,[4] leads to loss of baroreflex function resulting in episodes of hypertension and tachycardia.[5] In addition to the afferent input arising from the baroreceptors, the NTS also receives modulating input from many other cardiovascular brain centers, such as the area postrema. The NTS provides excitatory inputs to the caudal ventrolateral medulla (CVLM), which in turn inhibits the rostral ventrolateral medulla (RVLM),[6,7] where the pacemaker neurons that originate sympathetic tone are believed to be located.[8] RVLM neurons project to the preganglionic sympathetic neurons in the intermediolateral column of the spinal cord that send fibers outside the CNS. Parasympathetic activity is also modulated by the NTS, through projections to preganglionic parasympathetic neurons in the nucleus ambiguus and the motor nucleus of the vagus (Fig. 51-1).

The importance of autonomic mechanisms in the regulation of blood pressure is most evident when they fail. Damage of baroreflex afferents, e.g., as consequence of radiation or surgery, leads to labile blood pressure that is very difficult to control.[5] At the other extreme, degeneration of central or efferent structures, as seen in patients with primary autonomic failure, leads to disabling orthostatic hypotension.[9] In the most severe cases, patients are unable to stand but for few seconds before profound orthostatic hypotension and loss of consciousness ensues. These disorders are described later in this chapter.

Methods used to test autonomic function

Posture (orthostatic) test

Perhaps the most informative and simplest autonomic evaluation is the posture test. The patient's blood pressure and heart rate are measured after 5–10 minutes in the supine position, and repeated after the subject stands motionless for 3–5 minutes. There is some value in repeating measurements at each of these time points, but just one measurement is informative. Virtually all patients with severe autonomic failure will have an immediate fall in blood pressure on standing. There are other

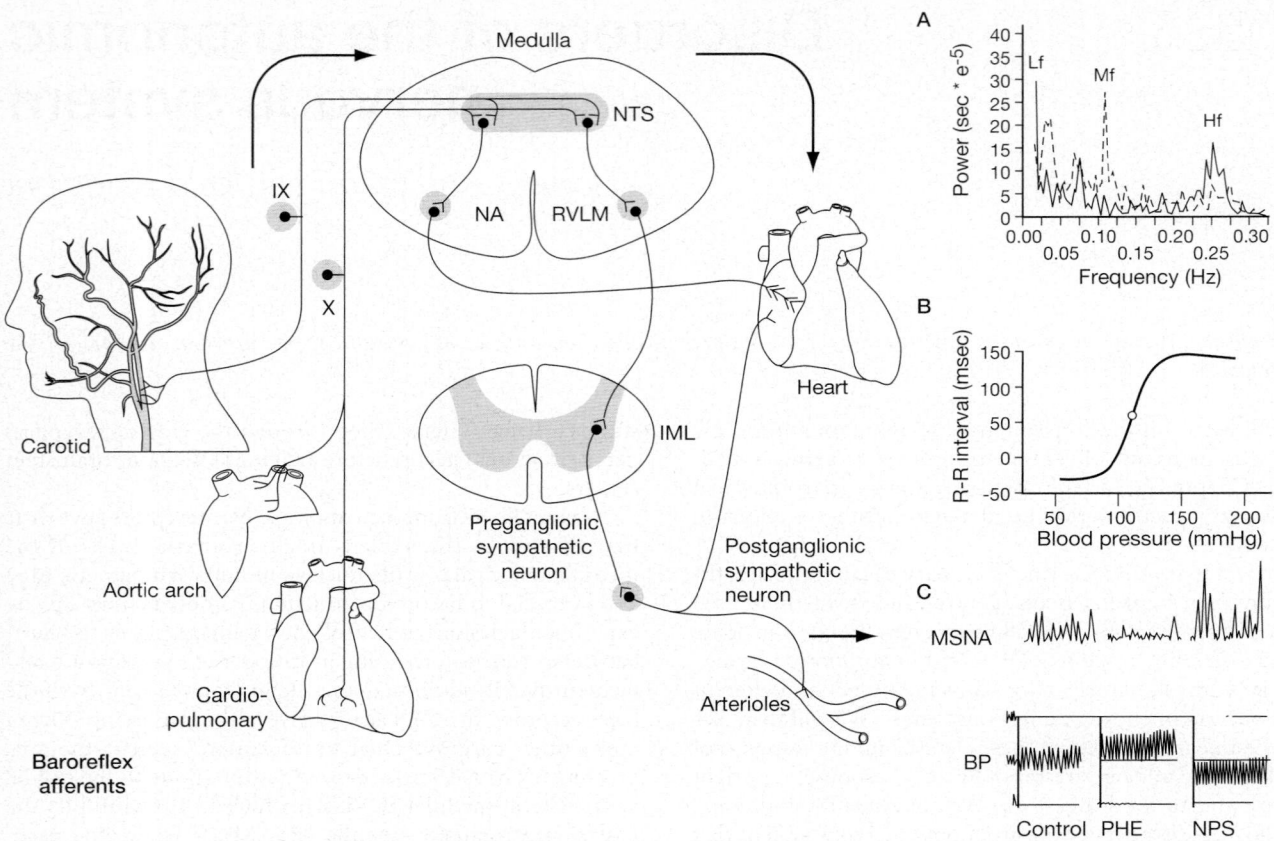

Figure 51-1 Simplified anatomical/functional scheme of baroreflex function. Afferent fibers located in the right atrium and in the cardiopulmonary veins (low-pressure baroreceptors), and in the aortic arch and carotid sinus (high-pressure baroreceptors) are activated by stretch and relay this information through the vagus (X) or glossopharyngeal (IX) nerves to the nucleus tractus solitarii (NTS) of the brainstem. The NTS provides excitatory inputs to the caudal ventrolateral medulla, which in turn inhibits the rostral ventrolateral medulla (RVLM)[6,7] (for simplicity the NTS is shown as projecting direct inhibitory pathways to the RVLM), where pacemaker neurons that originate sympathetic tone are believed to be located. These cell bodies send their efferent projections through the intermediolateral column of the spinal cord (IML). Baroreflex function can be simplified as follows: an increase in blood pressure is detected by arterial baroreceptors which increase their firing into the NTS; activation of the NTS leads to a greater inhibitory output to the RVLM; inhibition of pacemaker cells in the RVLM results in a compensatory reduction in sympathetic tone. Conversely, a decrease in blood pressure results in decreased firing in the NTS, withdrawal of the inhibitory influence of this nuclei on the RVLM, and a compensatory increase in sympathetic tone. Parasympathetic activity is also modulated by the NTS, through projections to the nucleus ambiguus (NA). An increase in blood pressure will lead to activation of the NTS and of the NA, with increased parasympathetic activity. Methods to assess baroreflex function include (A) spectral analysis, by correlating spontaneous changes in blood pressure and heart rate, and (B) by the neck barocuff method. Results obtained by these methods are influenced by afferent baroreceptor input, brainstem pathways, and end-organ responsiveness. Baroreflex modulation of sympathetic activity can be assessed with (C) microelectrode recording of postganglionic efferent sympathetic nerve activity (MSNA). In this example, blood pressure increment with phenylephrine (PHE) produced a baroreflex-mediated decrease in MSNA and blood pressure reduction with nitroprusside (NPS) produces a baroreflex-mediated increase in MSNA.

autonomic conditions associated with delayed orthostatic hypotension that require a 30-minute stand test for their diagnosis,[10] but these are usually not associated with widespread autonomic neuropathy. Heart rate is crucial in interpreting blood pressure changes. Patients with severe autonomic failure characteristically have no or little (about 10–15 bpm) increase in heart rate despite profound orthostatic hypotension. A greater increase in heart rate usually indicates that other conditions, e.g., volume depletion or medications, are contributing to orthostatic hypotension.

Noninvasive autonomic tests

The heart rate response to deep breathing (i.e., respiratory sinus arrhythmia) and to the Valsalva maneuver are simple yet informative autonomic tests. They require real-time monitoring of heart rate. Respiratory sinus arrhythmia is assessed during controlled breathing at a rate of six deep breaths per minute (Fig. 51-2). The sinus arrhythmia ratio is calculated by dividing the longest to the shortest R–R interval. This expiratory/inspiratory (E/I) ratio decreases progressively with age. Subjects younger than 40 usually have a ratio less

Normal   Autonomic failure

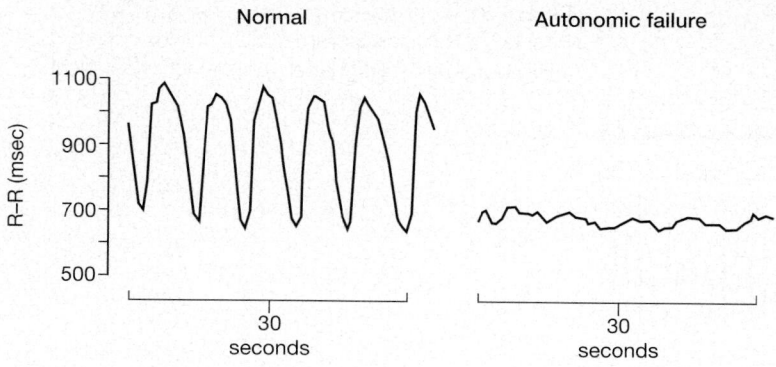

Figure 51-2 Successive electrocardiographic R–R intervals during paced breathing in a normal subject (left) and in a patient with autonomic failure (right).

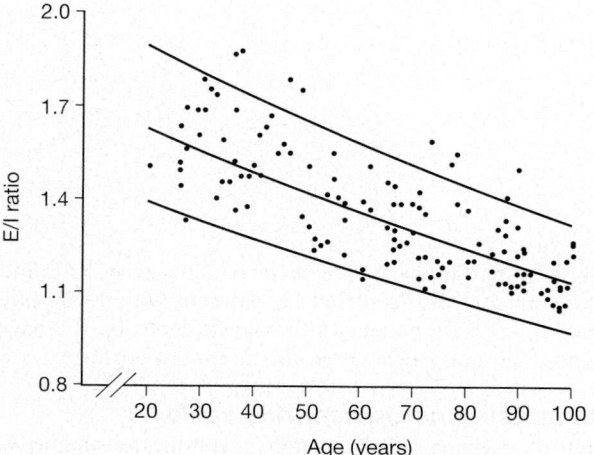

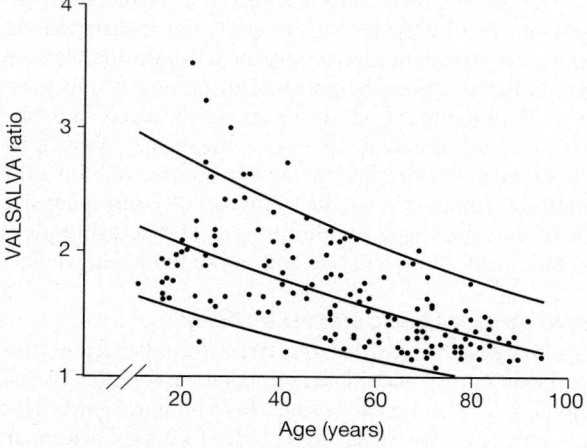

Figure 51-3 (Top) Expiratory/inspiratory (E/I) ratio during paced breathing in normal subjects according to age. Linear regression and confidence limits are shown. (Bottom) Valsalva ratio in normal subjects according to age. Linear regression and confidence limits are shown.

than 1.2 (Fig. 51-3). A Valsalva maneuver is induced by having the subject blow against a 40 mmHg pressure for 12 seconds. A 5–10 cc syringe can be used as a mouthpiece, and can be connected to a sphygmomanometer to monitor pressure. A small leak should be introduced into the system to ensure the subject uses thoracic effort. The increase in intrathoracic pressure

produces a transient fall in blood pressure with narrowing of pulse pressure during phase II (strain), whereas blood pressure overshoots above baseline values during phase IV (after release) (Fig. 51-4). In autonomic failure blood pressure continues to fall during phase II and the normal overshoot is absent during phase IV. Thus, appropriate evaluation of the Valsalva response requires continuous recording of blood pressure which can be accomplished noninvasively with finger plethysmography (Finapress, Portapress) or tonometry of the radial artery (Colin). Even if blood pressure cannot be monitored, however, heart rate responses are useful. The blood pressure changes described previously produce reciprocal baroreflex-mediated changes in heart rate; heart rate increases during the hypotensive phase II of the Valsalva maneuver, and decreases during the blood pressure overshoot of phase IV. The Valsalva ratio is calculated by dividing the fastest heart rate during phase II by the slowest heart rate during phase IV. As with the E/I ratio, Valsalva ratio decreases with age and results should be interpreted accordingly (Fig. 51-3).

Spectral analysis of heart rate and blood pressure

Blood pressure and heart rate are kept within a relatively narrow range because of autonomic baroreflex mechanisms. Within this narrow range, however, blood pressure shows substantial variability. Detailed analysis of this variability indicates that most of it is not random, but follows natural rhythmic patterns which can be studied using spectral analysis techniques. These patterns are importantly modulated by the respiratory frequency. In particular, respiration frequency influences heart rate variability, and this interaction is under baroreflex control via the vagus nerves. The "respiratory peak" of heart rate variability, therefore, can be used to assess cardiac parasympathetic function. Respirations also modulate blood pressure, but this is thought to be mediated through mechanical events and do not reflect autonomic mechanisms. In contrast, blood pressure shows a lower frequency rhythm (Mayer waves). This is mediated in part by sympathetic modulation of vascular tone. There is substantial interindividual variability in the spectral analysis of heart rate and blood pressure, making these methods less suitable for the diagnosis of individual patients with less than severe autonomic impairment. Nonetheless, population studies have shown that impaired heart rate variability as shown by spectral analysis of heart rate is a predictor of mortality in patients

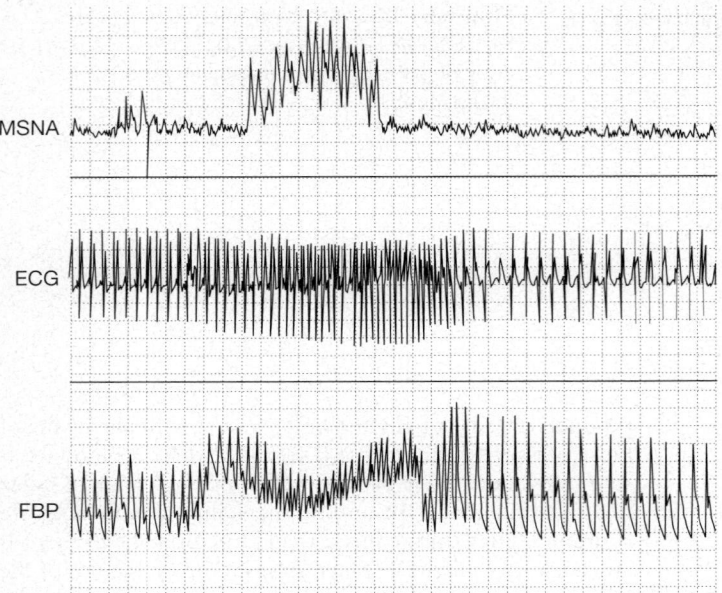

MSNA

ECG

FBP

Figure 51-4 Muscle sympathetic nerve activity (MSNA), electrocardiogram (ECG), and blood pressure (FBP) during Valsalva maneuver in a normal subject.

post myocardial infarction, and in patients with diabetes mellitus.

Assessment of baroreflex function

Several methods can be used to quantify the changes in heart rate (or R–R interval) produced by unit change of blood pressure. These methods require the simultaneous monitoring of blood pressure and heart rate. Baroreflex function can be assessed by measuring the reciprocal changes in blood pressure and heart rate that occur spontaneously, or during the phase IV of the Valsalva maneuver. Blood pressure can be increased with phenylephrine or decreased with nitroprusside and the gain of the baroreflex expressed as the change in R–R interval per unit blood pressure (expressed in msec/mmHg), during the linear portion of this relationship. Each of these methods provides slightly different normative values of baroreflex gain. It is important to note that changes in blood pressure affect all baroreflex afferents, including carotid sinus and aortic high-pressure receptors, and low-pressure receptors located in the venous circulation. The carotid sinus reflex can be selectively investigated by producing positive and negative pressure to the neck, to simulate decreases and increases in intracarotid pressure, respectively. All of the methods described above rely on instantaneous changes in heart rate, which depend exclusively on the parasympathetic limb of the baroreflex. The sympathetic limb of the baroreflex can be assessed by relating changes in blood pressure to reciprocal changes in muscle sympathetic nerve activity (see below).

Biochemical assessment of sympathetic function

Plasma norepinephrine provides a useful measure of sympathetic activity. It is particularly useful when measuring acute changes to standard stimuli. For example, upright posture induces a doubling of plasma norepinephrine. Patients with autonomic impairment have a blunted response. Basal norepinephrine, however, is different depending on the underlying pathology. It is low in patients with PAF and normal or slightly decreased in patients with MSA (see below). In contrast, patients with volume depletion will have enhanced norepinephrine response to upright posture.

Estimation of norepinephrine spillover

Despite the usefulness of plasma norepinephrine measurements, it is noteworthy that only a small percentage of the norepinephrine released by noradrenergic nerves actually reaches the circulation. Most of it is taken back into nerve terminals by the norepinephrine transporter (i.e., reuptake) or is metabolized. Norepinephrine clearance can be measured by infusing a known amount of titriated norepinephrine. During steady-state infusion it is assumed that clearance of titriated norepinephrine reflects clearance of endogenous norepinephrine. Once clearance is calculated, norepinephrine appearance rate into the circulation ("spillover") can be estimated. A comprehensive review of the advantages and limitations of this technique is beyond the scope of this chapter and can be found elsewhere.[11]

Muscle sympathetic nerve activity

Nerve activity can be recorded directly by introducing a recording electrode into an accessible peripheral nerve. Afferent and efferent fibers can be recorded using this technique. Sympathetic efferent activity can be selectively recorded by careful placement of the electrode. The peroneal nerve at the level of the knee is commonly used to measure postganglionic sympathetic nerve activity. While there is considerable interindividual variability in muscle sympathetic nerve activity, baseline recordings expressed as sympathetic bursts per minute are highly reproducible in a single individual between different recording sites, and when measured on different occasions. Muscle sympathetic nerve activity effectively monitors central sympathetic outflow and is tightly modulated by the baroreflex. Stimuli that increases blood pressure by activating central sympathetic outflow will be reflected as an increase in muscle sympathetic nerve activity. Conversely, stimuli that increases blood pressure directly (e.g. an injection of phenylephrine), will produce baroreflex-modulated suppression of muscle sympathetic nerve activity. This recording is also exquisitely sensitive to sympathetic withdrawal. For example, sympathetic activity disappears during neurogenic syncope.[12]

EFFECT OF AGING ON THE DIFFERENT COMPONENTS OF AUTONOMIC CARDIOVASCULAR CONTROL

Baroreflex function

There is a progressive decline in baroreflex sensitivity with aging, due to both vascular and neural deficits. Cardiovagal baroreflex gain, i.e., the reciprocal heart rate changes produced by changes in arterial pressure, declines with age but the ability of the cardiopulmonary baroreflex to inhibit sympathetic nerve traffic has been reported to be well preserved with age in healthy adults. Hence, vagal, but not sympathetic baroreflex gains vary inversely with subjects' ages and their baseline arterial pressures. There is no correlation between sympathetic and vagal baroreflex gains.[13]

Cardiac parasympathetic function

Cardiac vagal innervation decreases with age as clearly shown by a progressive reduction in respiratory sinus arrhythmia (Fig. 51-3). Experimental evidence suggests that long-term physical activity attenuates the decline in cardiovagal baroreflex gain by maintaining neural vagal control.[14] These findings may have important therapeutic implications.

Systemic sympathetic function

Muscle sympathetic nerve activity (MSNA) increases progressively with age likely due to increased central nervous system drive (Fig. 51-5). Sympathetic nerve traffic increases in a region-specific manner; however, outflow to skeletal muscle and the gut increases, but not to the kidney.[15] The increase in central sympathetic outflow result in higher levels of plasma norepinephrine with age, but reduced norepinephrine clearance appears to play a role as well.[16,17] It is suggested that age-related elevations in whole-body and abdominal adiposity can explain the increase in basal MSNA with age in healthy humans.[18] The relation between body fat and MSNA is observed in both young and older populations.[19] Tanaka et al.[18] showed that although body mass index (BMI) was similar in groups of young and older subjects, both total body fatness and abdominal adiposity were greater in the older subjects and were directly related to baseline levels of MSNA. Preliminary data[20] indicate that circulating concentrations of leptin are related to both adiposity and MSNA. Thus, age-associated elevations in total and abdominal adiposity may be linked to increases in MSNA, at least in part, via elevations in leptin levels.[18] In contrast to sympathetic neuronal activity, adrenaline secretion from the adrenal medulla is markedly reduced with age, and adrenaline release in response to acute stress is attenuated in older men. Plasma adrenaline concentrations remains normal, however, because of reduced plasma clearance.

End-organ responsiveness

Despite the number of beta-adrenergic receptors in lymphocytes being unaltered with age[21] and higher neurotransmitter levels,

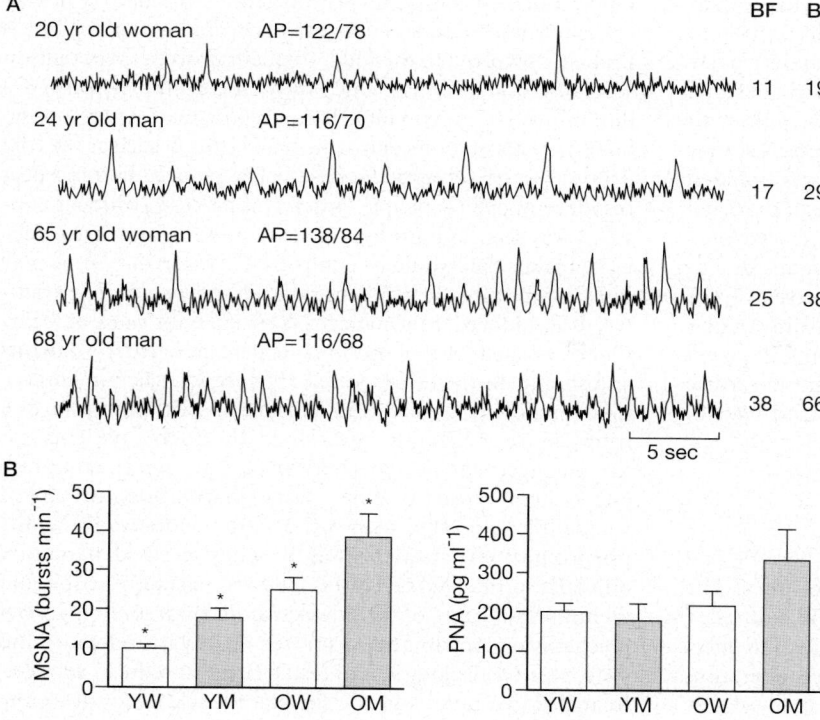

Figure 51-5 Age-associated increases in muscle sympathetic nerve activity. (A) muscle sympathetic nerve activity (MSNA) from four healthy adult humans under supine resting conditions (top to bottom): young female, young male, older female, older male. MSNA burst frequency (BF; bursts min^{-1}) and burst incidence (BI; bursts (100 heart beats)$^{-1}$) are higher in the neurograms of the older adults in both sexes. However, the female subjects demonstrate lower MSNA than the males at each age. AP, arterial blood pressure. (B) mean ± SEM; values for MSNA in four groups of subjects: young women (YW), young men (YM), older women (OW), and older men (OM). MSNA was at least twice as great in the older compared with the young subjects of the same sex. At each age, however, MSNA was significantly lower in the women. These age and sex differences in MSNA were not reflected in the corresponding antecubital venous plasma noradrenaline concentrations. PNA, plasma noradrenaline concentration; *$P < 0.05$ vs all other groups. Reproduced from Seals and Esler,[15] with permission.

beta-adrenergic responses to norepinephrine are blunted with progressive aging, probably due to beta-adrenergic receptor down-regulation in response to higher circulating levels of norepinephrine as well as a defect in G-protein receptor complexes and reduced adenyl cyclase activity.[22,23] Depressed beta$_1$ responses lead to impaired cardioacceleration and reduced cardiac contractility. Reduced beta$_2$ responses are manifested by increased vascular tone because alpha$_1$ vasoconstriction ability remains unchanged. The combination of age-related vascular stiffening and depressed beta-adrenergic function result in reduced arterial baroreflex sensitivity[24] in elderly subjects.[25–27] This reduces cardioacceleration during hypotension.[28] Reduced postural cardioacceleration, as well as decreased baroreceptor gain with age, increases the risk for orthostatic hypotension in elderly people.[29,30] Blood pressure in older subjects is sustained by increased peripheral vascular tone, in spite of depressed cardioacceleration. Due to a higher reliance on vascular resistance, dehydration, and vasodilator medications pose a high risk for hypotension and syncope in older subjects. On the other hand, vasovagal syncope is reportedly less frequent in elderly subjects.[31]

Vascular changes

Aging stiffens blood vessels[32] and alters vasomotor function. In elderly subjects, coronary vasodilatation capacity is reduced due to reduced nitric oxide release by the senescent endothelium. Conversely, endothelin release by the endothelium is increased in elderly people, promoting vasoconstriction.[33] These alterations increase susceptibility to myocardial ischemia, particularly during increased demand stresses such as tachyarrhythmias[34] and may also impair cerebral autoregulation, increasing susceptibility to syncope. Other age-dependent cardiovascular alterations that may increase predisposition to syncope are increased left ventricular afterload, and myocyte hypertrophy. These alterations lead to impaired diastolic filling and chronic ischemia that may predispose subjects to cardiac arrhythmias and decrease ventricular volume that may manifest as syncope. Decreased preload volume precipitated by vasodilators, dehydration, or blood pooling can dramatically reduce cardiac output and precipitate syncope. Susceptibility to atrial fibrillation increases with age due to reductions in pacemaker cells, progressive fibrosis of the cardiac conduction system and concomitant cardiovascular diseases that alter atrial morphology. In older patients, impaired diastolic filling and a reduction of up to 50 percent in cardiac output may develop during atrial fibrillation and lead to syncope.

Neuroendocrine changes

Plasma renin and aldosterone levels fall with age[35,36] and atrial natriuretic peptide increases five- to nine-fold.[37] The vasopressin response to hypotension may also be reduced.[38] These changes make sodium and water conservation less effective and intravascular volume depletion more frequent, thus increasing the tendency for syncope. In addition, many elderly people have an impaired thirst response to increases in osmolality and do not consume sufficient fluids to prevent hypovolemia.

EFFECT OF AGING ON AUTONOMIC RESPONSE TO STRESS

The most frequent autonomic stress is the cardiovascular adaptation to upright posture and other physiologically induced changes in intravascular volume. Vascular and neurogenic dysfunction, as well as a host of medications, can cause orthostatic hypotension in the elderly. In the Cardiovascular Health study,[39] the prevalence of orthostatic hypotension was 18 percent in subjects age 65 years or older, although only 2 percent of the subjects reported dizziness with standing. There was a modest association with systolic hypertension when supine, carotid stenosis greater than 50 percent, and the use of oral hypoglycemic agents but only a weak association with the use of beta-blockers and no association with other antihypertensive drugs. In other reports, however, as expected, the use of antihypertensive medications was significantly related to postural hypotension in elderly people[40] and discontinuing antihypertensive medications lead to an improvement of orthostatic hypotension.

Orthostatic hypotension

Elderly people have impaired defenses against the fluid shifts that normally accompany upright posture. Their threshold to develop symptomatic orthostatic hypotension is, therefore, lower compared to younger subjects. A variety of symptoms develop with a reduction in blood flow to the brain. Typically, patients will complain of visual disturbances (e.g. blurring, tunneling, or darkening of vision), dizziness, light-headedness, giddiness, feeling faint, as well as a dull neck and shoulder ache (coathanger pain). When orthostatic hypotension is pronounced and cerebral blood flow decreases below a critical level (approximately 25 mL/min per 100 grams), syncope (i.e. loss of consciousness) occurs. A decrease in baroreceptor sensitivity is probably involved in the mild, frequent postural hypotension seen in elderly people. One study, for example, showed a diminished response to tilt (a baroreceptor-mediated response) but not to non-baroreceptor-mediated stimuli such as the cold pressor test or isometric exercise.[41] The reduced baroreceptor response in elderly people (when compared to younger controls) was seen in both hypertensive and normotensive subjects. Insults that would be compensated for in the young may induce symptomatic hypotension in elderly people. For example, drug-induced orthostatic hypotension is the cause of recurrent dizzy spells or syncope in 12–15 percent of elderly patients and should always be suspected.[42] Diuretics, calcium antagonists, angiotensin converting enzyme (ACE) inhibitors, and nitrates are frequently prescribed in elderly patients for the management of hypertension, congestive heart failure and ischemic heart disease. Other pharmacological agents frequently associated with orthostatic hypotension include phenothiazines, antidepressants, sedatives, and narcotics. Similarly, prolonged bed rest is frequent in elderly people and an important cause of cardiovascular deconditioning. Several mechanisms contribute to decreased orthostatic tolerance and syncope after prolonged bed rest.[43] Bed rest reduces extracellular fluid volume, and the skeletal muscle deconditioning impairs the lower limb muscle pump that facilitates venous return in the upright posture. Under normal conditions, important mechanical adjustments to counteract orthostatic pooling of the blood are the muscle and respiratory pumps. Skeletal muscle tone has critical bearing on the volume of blood displaced into the legs when standing. Because intramuscular pressure is decreased after prolonged bed rest, venous pooling augments and venous return to the heart is easily compromised in the standing posture. These conditions need to be ruled out in any patient with symptoms of light-headedness on standing or documented orthostatic hypotension. If the problem persists after adequate measures are taken, a pathological impairment of autonomic function should be considered. The occurrence of orthostatic hypotension in elderly people is predictive of mortality.[44] A study of 3,522 Japanese American men, age 71–93 years, found that orthostatic hypotension, defined as a decrease in systolic blood pressure by 20 mmHg or in diastolic blood pressure by 10 mmHg, was present in 7 percent and increased with age.

Postprandial and heat-induced hypotension

A frequent reason for falls and syncope in elderly people is postprandial and heat-induced hypotension.[45,46] In normal subjects, eating, especially carbohydrates, is accompanied by splanchnic vasodilatation, and hot weather produces cutaneous vasodilatation but there is little change in arterial pressure because of a compensatory increase in sympathetic vasoconstrictor outflow. In elderly people, however, similarly to what occurs in patients with autonomic failure, both eating and hot weather significantly lower blood pressure (even in the supine position) because these subjects cannot compensate for the vasodilatation with an appropriate increase in sympathetic outflow.[47,48] Among elderly residents of nursing homes, for example, 24–36 percent have a 20 mmHg or greater fall in systolic blood pressure within 75 minutes after eating a meal.[49] In patients with autonomic failure, postprandial hypotension occurs within 30 minutes of meal ingestion, lasts about 1.5–2 hours, and can be profound; blood pressure falls of as much as 50–70 mmHg can be observed. This is not only a useful diagnostic test, but it is important to consider the timing of meals when measuring blood pressure in these patients. The initial syncopal episode in patients with chronic autonomic failure is frequently triggered by postprandial hypotension.

DISORDERS OF THE AUTONOMIC NERVOUS SYSTEM IN ELDERLY PEOPLE

Neurally mediated syncopal syndromes

The most frequent cause of hypotension and syncope in otherwise normal subjects is neurally mediated syncope, also referred to as vasovagal, vasodepressor, or reflex syncope. Vasovagal syncope is generally, although not exclusively, observed in patients with no evidence of structural heart disease. Prodromal symptoms include dizziness, blurred vision, nausea, and diaphoresis. This syncope results from acute vasodilatation and bradycardia. According to the apparent trigger mechanism, neurally mediated syncope can be classified in several distinct syndromes: emotional faint, carotid sinus syncope, micturition or gastrointestinal syncope, glossopharyngeal or trigeminal syncope, ventricular or neurocardiogenic syncope, and exercise syncope (commonly seen in aortic stenosis).

Neurally mediated syncope is an acute hemodynamic reaction produced by a sudden change in autonomic nervous system activity.[50] The normal pattern of autonomic outflow that maintains blood pressure in the standing position (increase sympathetic and decreased parasympathetic activity) is acutely reversed. Parasympathetic outflow to the sinus node of the heart increases, producing bradycardia, while sympathetic outflow to blood vessels is reduced resulting in profound vasodilatation.

Classic neurally mediated syncopal syndromes are triggered after compression of carotid baroreceptors in the neck (carotid sinus syncope,[12] following rapid emptying of a distended bladder (micturition syncope)[51] or distension of the gastrointestinal tract.[52] Glossopharyngeal or trigeminal neuralgia can also induce syncope by a similar mechanism.[53,54] It is apparent that in several clinical types of neurally mediated syncope the trigger locus is easily identified but frequently neurally mediated syncope occurs with no obvious trigger. Although in these cases the source of abnormal afferent signals was believed to be sensory receptors in the heart (i.e., neurocardiogenic or "ventricular" syncope,[55,56] neurally mediated syncope has recently been induced in patients with heart transplants, in whom the ventricle is likely to be denervated.[57] Perhaps, sensory receptors in the heart transplant patients are in the arterial tree rather than the ventricle. Similarly, the threshold to trigger neurally mediated syncope can be lowered by a reduction in cardiac preload caused by reduced intravascular volume or excessive venous pooling. Intravascular volume depletion is common in elderly people because sodium and water conservation are less effective, renin and aldosterone levels fall, atrial natriuretic peptide increases, and the vasopressin response to hypotension may be reduced. Moreover, many elderly subjects have an impaired thirst response to increases in osmolality and are prone to hypovolemia, particularly during febrile illnesses. Excessive venous pooling occurs postprandially in the splanchnic circulation, in the skin during exposure to heat, and in the lower limbs due to muscle atrophy when standing after prolonged periods of bed rest, significantly increasing susceptibility to syncope.

Despite the diverse trigger mechanisms of these different types of neurally mediated syncope the efferent reflex response is remarkably similar. There is an increase in parasympathetic efferent activity to the sinus node producing bradycardia or even a few seconds of sinus arrest, and a decrease in sympathetic activity responsible, at least in part, for the fall in blood pressure. Bradycardia is not the only or even the main cause of hypotension because neither atropine nor a ventricular pacemaker, which prevent bradycardia, are able to prevent hypotension and syncope. Blood pressure falls mainly because of vasodilatation. The mechanisms responsible for vasodilatation are incompletely understood. Sympathetic efferent activity decreases as shown by studies using microneurography and measurements of circulating norepinephrine.[58–60] Sympathetic "withdrawal," however, seems an incomplete explanation for profound vasodilatation. Norepinephrine fails to increase but vasopressin, endothelin-1, and angiotensin II vasoconstrictor peptides, important to maintain blood pressure, which should partially compensate for the fall in sympathetic activity, increase normally during neurally mediated syncope.[59] To explain the profound fall in blood pressure, beta-mediated vasodilatation induced by a rise in adrenaline has been postulated.[61] Nitric oxide-mediated vasodilatation due to a rise in cholinergic activity may be involved.[50,62] In summary, current understanding of neurally mediated syncope shows inappropriate reduction in sympathetic nerve activity and norepinephrine release. There is an appropriate increase in epinephrine, angiotensin II, vasopressin, and endothelin release, and preliminary evidence suggests that nitric oxide synthesis is activated.

Baroreflex failure

The most common cause of baroreflex failure is iatrogenic damage during neck surgery or radiation therapy of neural structures that carry afferent input from the baroreceptors. Neurological disorders involving the nucleus tractus solitarii, where these afferents have their first synapse, can also produce baroreflex failure.[4] In a few cases, the underlying cause is not found. Baroreflex function is impaired in essential hypertension, and may be transmitted as a genetic trait.[63] It is not clear if these cases of baroreflex failure of unknown etiology represent the extreme of the spectrum of baroreflex impairment in essential hypertension. Baroreflex failure patients present with severe labile hypertension and hypotension, often accompanied by headache, diaphoresis, and emotional instability. Wide fluctuations of blood pressure are observed, with systolic blood pressure ranging from 50 to 280 mmHg. The hypertensive crises are accompanied by tachycardia, and are due to sympathetic surges, as documented by marked increases in plasma norepinephrine. Treatment with sympatholytics may provide some benefit, attenuating these surges of hypertension and tachycardia, but adequate blood pressure regulation is seldom achieved in the absence of functional baroreflexes. Of interest is that virtually all reported cases are due to bilateral lesions, whereas unilateral lesions are usually clinically silent. This clinical observation underscores the redundancy of the baroreflex system and its importance in cardiovascular regulation.

Chronic autonomic failure

Autonomic failure is divided into primary and secondary forms. Primary autonomic failure is caused by a degenerative process affecting central autonomic pathways (multiple system atrophy, MSA), or peripheral autonomic neurons (pure autonomic failure). Secondary autonomic failure results from destruction of peripheral autonomic neurons in disorders such as diabetes, amyloidosis and other neuropathies, and very rarely by an enzymatic defect in catecholamine synthesis (dopamine beta hydroxylase deficiency). In chronic autonomic failure, orthostatic hypotension and syncope are caused by impaired vasoconstriction and reduced intravascular volume. Vasoconstriction is deficient because of reduced baroreflex-mediated norepinephrine release from postganglionic sympathetic nerve terminals and low circulating levels of angiotensin II caused by impaired secretion of renin.[64] In patients with autonomic failure and central nervous system dysfunction (i.e., MSA), impaired endothelin and vasopressin release also contribute to deficient vasoconstriction in the standing position.[59,65]

Primary autonomic failure

Primary autonomic failure includes several neurodegenerative diseases of unknown cause: pure autonomic failure (PAF), in which autonomic impairment (i.e., orthostatic hypotension, bladder, and sexual dysfunction) occurs alone; MSA (also called Shy–Drager syndrome) in which autonomic failure is combined with an extrapyramidal and/or cerebellar movement disorder; Parkinson's disease (PD) in which autonomic failure is combined with an extrapyramidal movement disorder; and diffuse Lewy body disease (DLB), in which autonomic failure is combined with an extrapyramidal movement disorder, and severe cognitive impairment.

Recent findings suggest that the same neurodegenerative process underlies MSA, PD, DLB, and PAF, as accumulation of alpha synuclein in neuronal cytoplasmic inclusions occurs in all these disorders. A gene encoding for alpha synuclein, a neuronal protein of unknown function, is mutated in autosomal dominant PD.[66] Nonfamilial PD does not have the mutation but alpha synuclein accumulates in Lewy bodies in these patients, suggesting a toxic role for aggregates of this protein.[67] Interestingly, cytoplasmic inclusions in MSA also stain positive for alpha synuclein,[68] and Lewy bodies in PAF[69] are strongly synuclein positive. Thus, abnormalities in the expression or structure of alpha synuclein or associated proteins may cause degeneration of catecholamine-containing neurons. Alpha synuclein, therefore, is an important component of intraneuronal inclusions in PAF, PD, DLB, and MSA neurodegenerative disorders, all of which affect the autonomic nervous system to a variable degree. Thus, these disorders are best classified as alpha synucleinopathies. It is not surprising, therefore, that there is overlap in the clinical presentation of these disorders, and the clinical differences may reflect the type of deposits (forming Lewy bodies or not), and the localization of these deposits within the nervous system. These similarities and differences are discussed below.

Pure autonomic failure (PAF)

Pure autonomic failure, a disorder first described by Bradbury and Eggleston is a sporadic, adult onset, slowly progressive degeneration of the autonomic nervous system characterized by orthostatic hypotension, bladder and sexual dysfunction, and no other neurological deficits. Neuropathological reports of patients with pure autonomic failure showed alpha synuclein-positive intraneuronal cytoplasmic inclusions (Lewy bodies) in brainstem nuclei and peripheral autonomic ganglia.[69,70] These patients are otherwise normal and their prognosis is relatively good. Complications are usually those related to falls and associated disorders.

Multiple system atrophy

Multiple system atrophy (MSA) is a term introduced by Graham and Oppenheimer in 1969 to describe a group of patients with a disorder of unknown cause affecting extrapyramidal, pyramidal, cerebellar, and autonomic pathways. MSA includes the disorders previously called striatonigral degeneration (SND), sporadic olivopontocerebellar atrophy (OPCA), and the Shy–Drager syndrome (SDS). The discovery in 1989 of glial cytoplasmic inclusions in the brain of patients with MSA provided a pathological marker for the disorder (akin to Lewy bodies in Parkinson's disease), and confirmed that SND, OPCA, and SDS are the same disease with different clinical expression.[71] MSA is a progressive neurodegenerative disease of undetermined cause that occurs sporadically and causes parkinsonism, cerebellar, pyramidal autonomic, and urological dysfunction in any combination.[72]

Because parkinsonism is the most frequent motor deficit in MSA, these patients are regularly misdiagnosed as suffering from Parkinson's disease (PD). Data from PD brain banks showed how frequently the diagnosis of PD was incorrect; up to 10 percent of these brains turn out to have MSA.[73] Indeed, even case 1 of James Parkinson's original description (1817), pon which much of his description of paralysis agitans was based, was probably suffering from MSA.

Life expectancy in MSA is shorter than in PD. Ben-Shlomo et al.[74] analyzed 433 published cases of pathologically proven MSA over a 100-year period. Mean age of onset was 54 years (range 31–78) and survival 6 years (range 0.5–24). Survival was unaffected by gender, parkinsonian, or pyramidal features, or whether the patient was classified as SND or OPCA. Survival analysis showed a secular trend from a median duration of 5 years for publications between 1887 and 1970, to 7 years between 1991 and 1994. These figures may be biased toward the worst cases, however.

Parkinson's disease

Autonomic dysfunction in Parkinson's disease is rarely as severe as in patients with MSA. There is a subgroup of patients with PD, however, with severe autonomic failure even early in the course of the disease. In most cases, autonomic failure occurs late in the course of the illness and is associated with levodopa and dopamine agonist therapy. In patients with Parkinson's disease, Lewy bodies are found in central and in peripheral autonomic neurons, and autonomic dysfunction in this disorder may be caused by both pre- and postganglionic neuronal dysfunction.

Diffuse Lewy body disease

The clinical presentation of these patients is that of Parkinson's disease, but dementia often dominates the clinical picture. Autonomic failure is frequently associated with this disorder.

Differential diagnosis among the alpha synucleinopathies

During the early stages of MSA, autonomic deficits may be the sole clinical manifestation, thus resembling PAF, but after a variable period of time, sometimes several years, extrapyramidal or cerebellar deficits or both invariably develop. In PD, extrapyramidal motor problems are the presenting feature, but later in the disease process, patients may suffer severe autonomic failure, making the clinical distinction with MSA difficult. Complicating the distinction further, similar to what occurs in PD, some MSA cases display motor deficits before autonomic failure is apparent. In clinical practice all these possibilities lead to two main diagnostic problems. First, it can't be determined whether a patient who has autonomic failure as the only clinical finding and is believed to have PAF, will develop more widespread nonautonomic neuronal damage and turn out to have MSA. Second, it may be difficult to establish if a patient with autonomic failure and a parkinsonian

movement disorder has PD or MSA. Clinically, the classic parkinsonian resting tremor of unilateral predominance is rarely seen in patients with MSA, in whom bradykinesia and rigidity predominate. Also, with rare exceptions, patients with MSA do not respond as well to antiparkinsonian medications and the progression of disease is faster.

In addition to clinical criteria, several tests have been used to distinguish between PD, PAF, and MSA. For example, vasopressin release in response to hypotension and growth hormone secretion in response to clonidine are blunted in MSA but preserved in PAF and PD, because brainstem–hypothalamic–pituitary pathways are only affected in MSA.[65,75] Plasma norepinephrine concentration while supine is frequently normal in MSA but low in PAF, because postganglionic neurons are normal in MSA.[76] Sphincter EMG shows denervation in MSA, because the Onuf's nucleus in segments S2–S4 of the spinal cord is affected in MSA but is normal in PD.[77]

There are also important differences in cardiovascular control between MSA, PAF, and PD with autonomic failure. Although patients with MSA have substantial CNS degeneration, the brainstem centers where sympathetic tone originates (most likely the rostro ventrolateral medulla) and distal pathways are intact. In support of this postulate, supine plasma norepinephrine is normal or slightly decreased in MSA, but this residual sympathetic activity is not baroreflex-responsive, hence their inability to maintain upright blood pressure. Furthermore, interruption of this residual sympathetic activity with the ganglion blocker trimethaphan leads to profound decrease in supine blood pressure in MSA. In contrast, supine plasma norepinephrine is very low in PAF and treatment with trimethaphan produces small or no changes in blood pressure, indicating that the lesion is distal to brainstem centers.[78]

Similarly, sympathetic cardiac innervation is selectively affected in PD and PAF but is intact in MSA. Several studies using single photon emission computed tomography (SPECT) imaging with ^{123}I metaiodobenzylguanidine (MIBG),[79–81] and positron emission tomography (PET) with 6-[^{18}F] fluorodopamine[82] have shown abnormal cardiac sympathetic innervation in patients with PD, while it was normal in patients with MSA.[83] This may turn out to be a useful diagnostic test to distinguish between PD and MSA because sympathetic innervation of the heart is impaired in PD, and not in MSA. Moreover, in a patient with apparent PAF finding normal sympathetic cardiac innervation should indicate a likely development of MSA.

AUTONOMIC AND NEUROENDOCRINE TESTING Numerous studies have described abnormal cardiovascular reflexes in MSA patients. A characteristic of MSA is that afferent and central autonomic and neuroendocrine reflex pathways are selectively affected, while postganglionic autonomic fibers are spared.[65] Baroreceptor-mediated vasopressin release—a measurement of afferent baroreceptor function, is spared in PAF, and presumably in PD, but is blunted in MSA.[65] Intravenous clonidine, a centrally active alpha 2 adrenoceptor agonist that stimulates growth hormone (GH) secretion, also tests the function of hypothalamic–pituitary pathways. Clonidine raised serum growth hormone in patients with PD and patients with pure autonomic failure but did not in those with MSA. This finding suggests that the growth hormone responses to i.v. clonidine can differentiate MSA from PD and pure autonomic failure and suggest a specific alpha 2 adrenoceptor–hypothalamic deficit in MSA.[75]

BRAIN IMAGING In patients with MSA, magnetic resonance imaging (MRI) of the brain can frequently detect abnormalities of striatum, cerebellum, and brainstem.[84–88] Striatal abnormalities in MSA include putaminal atrophy and putaminal hypointensity (relative to pallidum) on T2 weighted images, as well as slit-like signal change at the posterolateral putaminal margin. The striking slit-like signal change in the lateral putamen corresponds to the area showing the most-pronounced microgliosis and astrogliosis as well as the highest amount of ferric iron at necropsy. This abnormal intensity is frequently asymmetric (Fig. 51-6).

Infratentorial abnormalities in patients with MSA seen on MRI include atrophy and signal change in the pons and middle cerebellar peduncle. The pontine base and the middle cerebellar peduncle may appear as high signal intensity on T2 weighted images and as low intensity on T1, suggesting degeneration and demyelination.

Most if not all these tests are frequently ambiguous and accurate methods to distinguish PD from other diseases with extrapyramidal involvement, particularly MSA, are needed. It is argued that because the diagnosis of MSA during life is based on clinical features, it can only be made with possible or probable certainty, and that definite diagnosis requires pathologic confirmation.

Treatment

There are no known treatments targeted at the underlying degenerative disorder, or therapies that will modify the course of any of these disorders. Treatment of the motor abnormalities in MSA patients remains dismal. As mentioned before, these patients often do not respond to antiparkinsonian medications. Of the autonomic abnormalities, orthostatic hypotension is often treated successfully. An outline of treatment strategies is included later in this chapter.

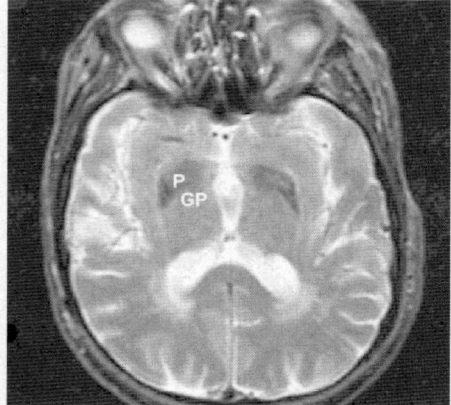

Figure 51-6 Moderate putaminal (P) hypointensity relative to the globus pallidum (GP) in a patient with parkinsonian multiple system atrophy (MSA-P), axial T2 weighting, 1.5 tesla MRI.

Secondary autonomic failure

Cholinergic failure

Botulism and the Lambert–Eaton myasthenic syndrome (LEMS) impair the release of acetylcholine in both somatic and autonomic nerves, producing muscle weakness and cholinergic dysautonomia. Botulism presents as an ascending, predominantly motor polyneuropathy with cranial nerve involvement, beginning 12–36 hours after ingesting food contaminated with the neurotoxins of the anaerobic bacteria *Clostridium botulinum*. The toxin impairs the presynaptic calcium-associated release of acetylcholine leading to symptoms of cholinergic failure: dry eyes, dry mouth, blurred vision, dizziness, paralytic ileus, urinary retention, and anhydrosis. Treatment is supportive; respiratory failure and cardiac arrhythmia can occur. Recovery is often protracted with autonomic dysfunction lasting as long as 6 months after onset.

LEMS is an autoimmune disorder, most commonly paraneoplastic, associated with small-cell lung carcinoma. Autoantibodies to voltage-gated calcium channels, most commonly the P/Q type, have been found in these patients. Electrophysiological and pharmacological studies have reproduced the functional effects of LEMS in passively immunized mice, and confirmed that anti-P/Q-type calcium channel antibodies inhibit transmitter release from autonomic neurons and are likely to be responsible for the autonomic dysfunction in this syndrome.

Dry mouth, erectile dysfunction, proximal muscle weakness, and depressed tendon reflexes are characteristic.[89–91] The risk of developing cancer is estimated to be 62 percent over the next 2 years following diagnosis; this risk decreases over time.[89,92] Autonomic dysfunction is worse in older patients with a carcinoma[90] but improves with treatment of the underlying carcinoma.[91]

Pandysautonomias

Pandysautonomias involve both sympathetic and parasympathetic neurons. Pandysautonomic neuropathies can be divided into preganglionic (most frequently demyelinating) and postganglionic (most frequently axonopathic).[93] These neuropathies are acute or subacute with gradual but often incomplete recovery of autonomic function.[93,94] Patients present with blurred vision, dry eyes and mouth, nausea, vomiting, abdominal pain, diarrhea, constipation, and loss of sweating.

The acute pandysautonomias are uncommon in elderly people and affect almost exclusively healthy young individuals. Those with a protracted course and incomplete recovery are, more frequently, postganglionic axonal.[93,95] The preganglionic demyelinating pandysautonomia with variable involvement of the somatic nervous system is part of a spectrum ranging from pure pandysautonomia—with minimal somatic deficits, to classic Guillain–Barré syndrome[96] and profound muscle weakness and may have a better outcome than the postganglionic axonopathic pandysautonomia.[93] The cause of these pandysautonomias is unknown but a post-infectious or other immune-mediated process is postulated. In some cases they are paraneoplastic[97,98] and many patients have autoantibodies to ganglionic acetylcholine receptors (AChRs). AChRs mediate fast synaptic transmission through autonomic ganglia. It is proposed that ganglionic AChR autoimmunity may cause dysautonomia.[99] Recent reports showed complete recovery in a few patients with apparent postganglionic axonopathic pandysautonomia that were treated early with intravenous immunoglobulin therapy.[100]

Patients with Anti-Hu antibody related paraneoplastic syndrome presenting with progressive dysautonomia have also been described, both with acute onset, and subacute course of neurological symptoms. Autonomic symptoms may improve with treatment of the underlying cancer.

Signs of autonomic hyper- or hypoactivity are present in one- to two-thirds of patients with the acute inflammatory demyelinating polyradiculoneuropathy (AIDP) or Guillain–Barré syndrome (GBS).[101,102] In the majority of cases, there is mild autonomic hypoactivity with resting tachycardia due to decreased parasympathetic activity, and ileus. Urinary retention is less common. With autonomic hyperactivity, sweating is excessive and there can be alternating hyper- or hypotension and alternating brady- or tachycardia. Mortality is increased with significant dysautonomia.[103]

Chronic small fiber (postganglionic) neuropathies can be metabolic (e.g. diabetes or amyloidosis), inherited (e.g. Fabry's disease) or infectious (e.g. HIV). Autonomic dysfunction in both amyloid and diabetes tends to involve all organs. Autonomic failure (orthostatic hypotension and a fixed heart rate) may be the presenting feature. More frequently, patients show a mixed pattern of distal small fiber autonomic and sensory neuropathy or predominantly small fiber sensory neuropathy with only mild autonomic involvement.[97,104] The autonomic symptoms may accompany, precede or follow the somatic neuropathy.[105,106] Alternating diarrhea and constipation, explosive diarrhea, urinary retention, anhydrosis or gustatory hyperhydrosis may be present. Erectile dysfunction is the most common autonomic symptom in diabetes.[107,108] and sudomotor changes may be the earliest sign in diabetic neuropathy.[109–111,112]

Pandysautonomias are commonly associated with the acquired immunodeficiency syndrome (AIDS),[113–115] often combined with a distal sensory polyneuropathy.[116,117] Autonomic symptoms such as bladder and sexual dysfunction are present in up to 60 percent of patients.

Mild, chronic (or subacute) autonomic neuropathies or ganglionopathies, affecting both sympathetic and parasympathetic fibers, are sometimes associated with Sjogren's syndrome.[97,98] Tonic pupils, sudomotor dysfunction, and cases of severe pandysautonomia have been reported.[118]

MANAGEMENT OF ORTHOSTATIC HYPOTENSION

Maintenance of blood pressure in the standing position requires a sustained increase in peripheral vascular resistance (i.e., vasoconstriction) and adequate intravascular volume. In patients with chronic autonomic failure orthostatic hypotension is due to deficient baroreflex-mediated vasoconstriction and also because of reduced intravascular volume. Orthostatic hypotension and syncope occurs in all ages but is most common in elderly people, especially those over 75 years of age. Chronic autonomic failure is associated with central or peripheral nervous system disorders.

> ### Summary of management algorithm
> Stepwise approach to the management of orthostatic hypotension in elderly people
>
> - Remove aggravating factors:
>   - Volume depletion
>   - Drugs (e.g., diuretics, tricyclic antidepressants, venodilators, antihypertensives, insulin in diabetics with autonomic impairment)
>   - Inactivity/prolonged bedrest/deconditioning
>   - Alcohol
> - Nonpharmacological treatment:
>   - Liberalized salt intake
>   - Head-up tilt during the night
>   - Waist-high support stockings
>   - Exercise/physical activity as tolerated
> - Pharmacological treatment:
>   - Sodium chloride 1 g with meals
>   - Fludrocortisone (Florinef) 0.1–0.2 mg/day
>   - Midodrine (Proamitine) 5–10 mg t.i.d.
>   - Yohimbine 5.4 mg t.i.d.

Deficient vasoconstriction

In autonomic failure, vasoconstriction is mainly deficient because of reduced baroreflex-mediated norepinephrine release from postganglionic sympathetic nerve terminals and lack of activation of postsynaptic alpha adrenergic receptors in the vascular wall.[64] Also contributing to blunted orthostatic vasoconstriction in these patients are low circulating levels of angiotensin II resulting from deficient renal sympathetic innervation and reduced secretion of renin.[9,119] In patients with autonomic failure and central nervous system dysfunction (i.e., MSA), impaired endothelin and vasopressin release are also likely to contribute to the deficient vasoconstriction.[59,65]

Reduced intravascular volume

There are several reasons for reduced extracellular fluid volume in patients with autonomic failure. First, impaired sympathetic activation directly decrease sodium reabsorption in the kidney.[120] Second, impaired sympathetic activation inhibits renin secretion so that aldosterone is low and renal sodium reabsorption is decreased.[119] Finally, other hormones involved in fluid homeostasis are also impaired in autonomic failure. For example, hypophyseal vasopressin release in response to hypotension is markedly reduced in patients with autonomic failure caused by CNS lesions (e.g. MSA).[65] Low vasopressin levels prevent water conservation contributing to intravascular volume depletion.

Anemia is a common complication of autonomic failure likely the result of inadequate erythropoietin levels;[121,122] although basal erythropoietin synthesis is not reduced in autonomic failure, the increase in erythropoietin synthesis in response to anemic hypoxia appears to be blunted in these patients. The reason for this abnormality is unknown, but in patients with autonomic failure, the lower the plasma norepinephrine levels in the upright posture, the lower the hemoglobin levels, suggesting some relationship between decreased sympathetic activity and reduced erythropoiesis.[121] Similar to what occurs with the secretion of renin, another renal hormone, decreased renal sympathetic nerve activity may be the cause of impaired erythropoietin response to anemia in patients with autonomic failure. The modest decrease in red blood cell mass is another contributing factor to reduced intravascular volume.

Supine hypertension and diurnal blood pressure variation

In addition to orthostatic hypotension, two distinct features of autonomic failure are hypertension when the patient is supine and marked diurnal variation in blood pressure. The mechanism responsible for supine hypertension is unclear. It is surprising that despite low norepinephrine and low angiotensin levels, systemic vascular resistance is increased in patients with autonomic failure when they are supine. The nocturnal supine hypertension causes pressure-natriuresis. The subsequent reduction in extracellular fluid volume aggravates orthostatic hypotension in the morning. Patients with chronic autonomic failure frequently have elevated supine blood pressure and may be incorrectly diagnosed with arterial hypertension.

Nonpharmacological treatment

A complete medication history should be obtained in order to identify and possibly eliminate agents that can cause orthostatic hypotension such as antihypertensives or diuretics. Levodopa and dopamine agonists exacerbate orthostatic hypotension, especially during the first weeks of treatment. Gradual dosage increases when initiating therapy or dose reductions in established patients can minimize this adverse effect. Dietary sodium and water intake should be maximally increased in these patients. Patients also should be instructed not to lie prone. Lying flat when sleeping at night results in accelerated sodium loss from pressure-natriuresis and reduced renin release leading to loss of intravascular volume. This leads to overnight volume depletion and worsening of orthostatic hypotension in the morning. Elevating the head of the bed is helpful. The beneficial effect of nocturnal head and torso elevation results from lessening supine hypertension, thus reducing "pressure-natriuresis" by the kidney and, in some patients, by increasing renin secretion. Patients should be educated about the hypotensive effects of food, hot weather, and physical exertion. Isotonic exercise produces less hypotension than isometric exercise, and exercise in a pool prevents blood pressure reductions. In patients with autonomic failure, eating can significantly lower blood pressure because the splanchnic vasodilatation induced by food is not appropriately compensated by vasoconstriction in other vascular beds. In some patients, hypotension only occurs postprandially. Thus, patients should eat frequent, small meals with a low carbohydrate content and alcohol intake should be minimized. Caffeine taken with breakfast may be helpful. Hot baths should be avoided, and patients should be especially careful during warm weather. This is because heat-induced vasodilatation still occurs but sympathetic vasoconstriction is impaired. Straining at stool with a closed glottis (i.e., producing a Valsalva maneuver), playing wind instruments, and singing can be particularly

dangerous for patients with hypotension. A high fiber diet is encouraged to prevent constipation. The use of knee-high compressive stockings is not effective, but waist-high stockings (i.e., Jobst stockings) or abdominal binders may be an effective, albeit poorly tolerated, countermeasure for orthostatic hypotension.

Pharmacological treatment

Only patients with symptomatic orthostatic hypotension should be treated pharmacologically. Perhaps because of adaptive cerebral autoregulatory changes, some patients with autonomic failure tolerate very low arterial pressures when standing without experiencing symptoms of cerebral hypoperfusion. Blood pressure levels change throughout the day and from one day to another. Thus, the patient's normal cycle of blood pressure and orthostatic symptoms should be identified before treatment is initiated.

Fludrocortisone

Fludrocortisone, a synthetic mineralocorticoid practically devoid of glucocorticoid effect,[123] is the drug of first choice. Therapy with fludrocortisone (Florinef ™) is initiated with a dose of 0.1 mg per day. At least 4–5 days of treatment are necessary for a therapeutic effect to be evident. Special attention should be given to the development of hypokalemia. Fludrocortisone increases extracellular and intravascular volume by increasing sodium reabsorption by the kidney thus increasing cardiac output and standing blood pressure. The dose of fludrocortisone should be increased slowly. Body weight, blood pressure and the possible development of heart failure due to volume overload should be monitored. Weight gain of 2–5 pounds is expected. A certain degree of pedal edema should not be of concern. Indeed, it may be necessary to support the venous capacitance bed ("water jacket").

Desmopressin

Desmopressin (DDAVP) is a synthetic vasopressin analog which acts specifically on the V2 receptor (renal tubular cell) responsible for the antidiuretic effect of the hormone. At the dose given, DDAVP has no vasoconstrictor effect because it does not activate the V1 receptor which is in vascular smooth muscle.[124] Nocturnal intranasal administration of DDAVP reduces nocturnal polyuria and raises standing blood pressure in the morning without worsening supine hypertension.[125] A problem with the use of DDAVP is the potential development of hyponatremia. Treatment with this drug, therefore, should always be started with caution, and serum sodium should be monitored.

Midodrine

When volume expansion is not sufficient to control symptoms, a pressor agent should be added. The pressor agent of choice is now midodrine, a selective alpha 1 adrenergic agonist which is well absorbed after oral administration and does not cross the blood–brain barrier.[9,126] A 10 mg dose of midodrine is effective in increasing orthostatic blood pressure and ameliorating symptoms in patients with orthostatic hypotension.[127] Because this dose increases pressure for only 4 hours, it can be prescribed two or three times daily, depending upon the physical activity of the patient and can be avoided later in the day as it increases supine blood pressure. An advantage of a pressor agent over fludrocortisone is that its blood pressure raising effect lasts only a few hours. Thus, it can be administered specifically when the patient needs it; typically before breakfast and before lunch and preceding physical activity.[127] Recumbent hypertension is a common side-effect but standing up readily lowers blood pressure. The dose of midodrine should be titrated slowly starting with 2.5 mg. The dose can be quickly increased to 10 mg two or three times a day based on the blood pressure response. Most patients with orthostatic hypotension require chronic treatment with fludrocortisone; it is likely that by adding midodrine to fludrocortisone, the dose of the latter can be reduced. This combination treatment may reduce the long-term complications associated with chronic mineralocorticoid administration. Piloerection and scalp itching are frequent side-effects, and may be used as evidence of a pharmacological effect.

DOPS

DL threo-dihydroxyphenilserine (DL-threo-dops, or DOPS) is an unnatural aminoacid that is converted to norepinephrine through a single decarboxylation step by the enzyme dopa decarboxylase. In patients with autonomic failure due to congenital dopamine beta hydroxylase deficiency (the enzyme that converts dopamine to norepinephrine), DOPS is extremely efficacious in relieving orthostatic hypotension.[128,129] In patients with other forms of autonomic failure, DOPS[130–132] showed a significant pressor effect and significantly ameliorated postprandial hypotension.

Recombinant erythropoietin

Anemia is a common complication of autonomic failure.[121] Because blood pressure in autonomic failure is extremely sensitive to even small changes in intravascular volume, modest decreases in red blood cell mass and blood viscosity may exacerbate orthostatic hypotension. Recent studies in patients with autonomic failure have shown that reversing the anemia using recombinant erythropoietin increases upright blood pressure and ameliorates symptoms of orthostatic hypotension.[121,122,133] Erythropoietin, a polypeptide hormone produced mostly by the kidney, plays a central role in the regulation of red blood cell production. The synthesis of erythropoietin is controlled by a feedback mechanism based on an oxygen sensor.[134] When oxygen delivery to the kidney decreases, as with blood loss or chronic anemia, the synthesis of erythropoietin by renal interstitial cells increases.[135] The hormone is released into the bloodstream and stimulates red cell progenitors in the bone marrow, thereby increasing red cell production. In some patients with autonomic failure, chronic anemia does not produce an adequate increase in serum erythropoietin levels.[121,122,136] This is similar to what occurs in renal disease, malignancy, and other chronic disorders.

A likely mechanism for the increase in blood pressure following erythropoietin treatment is an increase in intravascular volume and blood viscosity due to increased red blood cell mass. In patients with renal failure receiving erythropoietin treatment, however, no correlation was found between increased blood pressure and increased hematocrit;[137] this suggests additional mechanisms for the hypertensive effect of the hormone.

Other agents

Several other agents have been used in the treatment of orthostatic hypotension in autonomic failure. Prostaglandin synthesis inhibitors (indomethacin, ibuprofen),[138,139] and the somatostatin analog octreotide[140,141] are sometimes effective in reducing postprandial hypotension but both agents may induce intolerable gastrointestinal side effects. The dopaminergic blocker metoclopramide increases blood pressure in some patients with autonomic failure,[142,143] but may aggravate or induce extrapyramidal symptoms. Moreover, it was recently reported that metoclopramide infusion acutely lowered blood pressure and worsened orthostatic tolerance in patients with autonomic failure, which should discourage the use of this drug in the treatment of orthostatic hypotension. Beta-blockers with and without intrinsic sympathomimetic activity (propranolol and pindolol) have been used[144] but we have not found them consistently effective. Clonidine, an alpha 2 adrenergic agonist, and yohimbine, an alpha 2 adrenergic antagonist, have been used with occasional success.[145,146] Ergotamine by nasal inhalation has also been reported effective.[147]

Summary

Evaluations of antihypertensive therapy and nonpharmacological interventions are the first steps in treating orthostatic hypotension. Hypotensive therapy should be discontinued if possible. Salt and fluid intake should be increased, and patients should be instructed to elevate the head of the bed and never to lie flat. Education about the effects of eating, hot weather, bathing, exercise, and rising quickly from a prone position will assist in effective behavior modification. If pharmacotherapy is needed, fludrocortisone, midodrine, and erythropoietin (for anemia) may be helpful in normalizing blood pressure regulation.

REFERENCES

1. Ertl AC, Diedrich A, Biaggioni I: Baroreflex dysfunction induced by microgravity: potential relevance to postflight orthostatic intolerance. Clin Auton Res 2000;10:269–277
2. Spyer KM: Neural organisation and control of the baroreceptor reflex. Rev Physiol Biochem Pharmacol 1981;88:24–124
3. Nathan MA, Reis DJ: Chronic labile hypertension produced by lesions of the nucleus tractus solitarii in the cat. Circ Res 1977;40:72–81
4. Biaggioni I, Whetsell WO, Jobe J, Nadeau JH: Baroreflex failure in a patient with central nervous system lesions involving the nucleus tractus solitarii. Hypertension 1994;23:491–495
5. Robertson D, Hollister AS, Biaggioni I et al: The diagnosis and treatment of baroreflex failure. N Engl J Med 1993;329:1449–1455 (see comments)
6. Li YW, Gieroba ZJ, McAllen RM, Blessing WW: Neurons in rabbit caudal ventrolateral medulla inhibit bulbospinal barosensitive neurons in rostral medulla. Am J Physiol 1991;261:R44–51
7. Jeske I, Morrison SF, Cravo SL, Reis DJ: Identification of baroreceptor reflex interneurons in the caudal ventrolateral medulla. Am J Physiol 1993;264:R169–178
8. Ross CA, Ruggiero DA, Park DH et al: Tonic vasomotor control by the rostral ventrolateral medulla: effect of electrical or chemical stimulation of the area containing C1 adrenaline neurons on arterial pressure, heart rate, and plasma catecholamines and vasopressin. J Neurosci 1984; 4:474–494
9. Kaufmann H, Brannan T, Krakoff L, Yahr MD, Mandeli J: Treatment of orthostatic hypotension due to autonomic failure with a peripheral alpha-adrenergic agonist (midodrine). Neurology 1988; 38:951–956

10. Streeten DH, Anderson GH, Jr: Delayed orthostatic intolerance. Arch Intern Med 1992;152:1066–1072

11. Esler M, Jennings G, Lambert G et al: Overflow of catecholamine neurotransmitters to the circulation: source, fate, and functions. Physiol Rev 1990;70:963–985

12. Costa F, Biaggioni I: Microneurographic evidence of sudden sympathetic withdrawal in carotid sinus syncope; treatment with ergotamine. Chest 1994;106:617–620

13. Rudas L, Crossman AA, Morillo CA et al: Human sympathetic and vagal baroreflex responses to sequential nitroprusside and phenylephrine. Am J Physiol 1999;276:H1691–1698

14. Hunt BE, Farquhar WB, Taylor JA: Does reduced vascular stiffening fully explain preserved cardiovagal baroreflex function in older, physically active men? Circulation 2001;103:2424–2427

15. Seals DR, Esler MD: Human ageing and the sympathoadrenal system. J Physiol 2000;528:407–417

16. Morrow LA, Linares OA, Hill TJ et al: Age differences in the plasma clearance mechanisms for epinephrine and norepinephrine in humans. J Clin Endocrinol Metab 1987;65:508–511

17. Supiano MA, Linares OA, Smith MJ, Halter JB: Age-related differences in norepinephrine kinetics: effect of posture and sodium-restricted diet. Am J Physiol 1990;259:E422–431

18. Tanaka H, Davy KP, Seals DR: Cardiopulmonary baroreflex inhibition of sympathetic nerve activity is preserved with age in healthy humans. J Physiol 1999;515:249–254

19. Jones PP, Davy KP, Seals DR: Relations of total and abdominal adiposity to muscle sympathetic nerve activity in healthy older males. Int J Obes Relat Metab Disord 1997;21:1053–1057

20. Monroe MB, Van Pelt RE, Schiller BC, Seals DR, Jones PP: Relation of leptin and insulin to adiposity-associated elevations in sympathetic activity with age in humans. Int J Obes Relat Metab Disord 2000;24:1183–1187

21. Abrass IB, Scarpace PJ: Human lymphocyte beta-adrenergic receptors are unaltered with age. J Gerontol 1981;36:298–301

22. Brodde OE, Zerkowski HR, Schranz D et al: Age-dependent changes in the beta-adrenoceptor-G-protein(s)-adenylyl cyclase system in human right atrium. J Cardiovasc Pharmacol 1995;26:20–26

23. O'Connor SW, Scarpace PJ, Abrass IB: Age-associated decrease of adenylate cyclase activity in rat myocardium. Mech Ageing Dev 1981;16:91–95

24. Taylor JA, Hand GA, Johnson DG, Seals DR: Sympathoadrenal-circulatory regulation of arterial pressure during orthostatic stress in young and older men. Am J Physiol 1992;263:R1147–1155

25. Forman D, Manning W: Perspective on managing atrial fibrillation in the geriatric patient. Cardiovasc Rev Rep 1996;17:49–57

26. Minaker KL, Meneilly GS, Youn GJ et al: Blood pressure, pulse, and neurohumoral responses to nitroprusside-induced hypotension in normotensive aging men. J Gerontol A 1991;46:M151–154

27. Smith JJ, Hughes CV, Ptacin MJ et al: The effect of age on hemodynamic response to graded postural stress in normal men. J Gerontol 1987;42:406–411

28. Lipsitz L. Altered blood pressure homeostasis in advance age: Clinical and research implications. J Gerontol 1989;44:M179–M183

29. Caird FI, Andrews GR, Kennedy RD: Effect of posture on blood pressure in the elderly. Br Heart J 1973;35:527–530

30. Gribbin B, Pickering TG, Sleight P, Peto R: Effect of age and high blood pressure on baroreflex sensitivity in man. Circ Res 1971;29:424–431

31. Lipsitz LA, Mietus J, Moody GB, Goldberger AL: Spectral characteristics of heart rate variability before and during postural tilt. Relations to aging and risk of syncope. Circulation 1990;81:1803–1810

32. Lakatta EG: Cardiovascular regulatory mechanisms in advanced age. Physiol Rev 1993;73:413–467

33. Miyauchi T, Yanagisawa M, Iida K et al: Age- and sex-related variation of plasma endothelin-1 concentration in normal and hypertensive subjects. Am Heart J 1992;123:1092–1093

34. Taddei S, Virdis A, Mattei P et al: Aging and endothelial function in normotensive subjects and patients with essential hypertension. Circulation 1995;91:1981–1987

35. Crane MG, Harris JJ: Effect of aging on renin activity and aldosterone excretion. J Lab Clin Med 1976;87:947–959

36. Weidmann P, De Myttenaere-Bursztein S, Maxwell MH, de Lima J: Effect on aging on plasma renin and aldosterone in normal man. Kidney Int 1975;8:325–333

37. Haller BG, Zust H, Shaw S et al: Effects of posture and ageing on circulating atrial natriuretic peptide levels in man. J Hypertens 1987;5:551–556

38. Rowe JW, Minaker KL, Sparrow D, Robertson GL: Age-related failure of volume-pressure-mediated vasopressin release. J Clin Endocrinol Metab 1982;54:661–664

39. Rutan GH, Hermanson B, Bild DE et al: Orthostatic hypotension in older adults. The Cardiovascular Health Study. CHS Collaborative Research Group. Hypertension 1992;19:508–519

40. Kaplan NM: The promises and perils of treating the elderly hypertensive. Am J Med Sci 1993; 305:183–197

41. Tonkin AL, Wing LM: Effects of age and isolated systolic hypertension on cardiovascular reflexes. J Hypertens 1994;12:1083–1088

42. Lipsitz LA, Pluchino FC, Wei JY, Rowe JW: Syncope in institutionalized elderly: the impact of multiple pathological conditions and situational stress. J Chronic Dis 1986;39:619–630

43. Greenleaf JE: Physiological responses to prolonged bed rest and fluid immersion in humans. J Appl Physiol 1984;57:619–633

44. Masaki KH, Schatz IJ, Burchfiel CM et al: Orthostatic hypotension predicts mortality in elderly men: the Honolulu Heart Program. Circulation 1998;98:2290–2295

45. Lipsitz L: Syncope in the elderly. Ann Intern Med 1983;99:92–105

46. Lipsitz L, Nyqvist R, Wei J, Rowe J: Postprandial reduction in blood pressure in the elderly. N Engl J Med 1983;309:81–83

47. Robertson D, Wade D, Robertson R: Post-prandial alterations in cardiovascular hemodynamics in autonomic dysfunction states. Am J Cardiol 1981;48:1048–1052

48. Mathias C, daCosta D, McIntosh C et al: Differential blood pressure and hormonal effects after glucose and xylose ingestion in chronic autonomic failure. Clin Sci 1989;77:85–92

49. Jansen RW, Lipsitz LA: Postprandial hypotension: epidemiology, patho-physiology, and clinical management. Ann Intern Med 1995;122:286–295

50. Kaufmann H: Neurally mediated syncope: pathogenesis, diagnosis, and treatment. Neurology 1995;45:S12–18

51. Kapoor W, Peterson J, Karpf M: Micturition syncope. A reappraisal. JAMA 1985;253:796–798

52. Palmer E: The abnormal upper gastrointestinal vasovagal reflexes that affect the heart. Am J Gastroenterol 1976;66:513–522

53. Wallin B, Westerberg C, Sundloff G: Syncope induced by glossopharyngeal neuralgia: Sympathetic outflow to muscle. Neurology 1984;34:522–524

54. Ferrante L, Artico M, Nardacci B et al: Glossopharyngeal neuralgia with cardiac syncope. Neurosurgery 1995;36:58–63

55. Mark A: The Bezold-Jarisch reflex revisited: Clinical implications of inhibitory reflexes originating in the heart. J Am Coll Cardiol 1983;1:90–102

56. Abboud FM: Ventricular syncope: is the heart a sensory organ? N Engl J Med 1989;320:390–392

57. Fitzpatrick AP, Banner N, Cheng A, Yacoub M, Sutton R: Vasovagal reactions may occur after orthotopic heart transplantation. J Am Coll Cardiol 1993;21:1132–1137

58. Wallin B, Sundlof G: Sympathetic outflow to muscles during vasovagal syncope. J. Auton Nerv Syst 1982;6:287–291

59. Kaufmann H, Oribe E, Oliver JA: Plasma endothelin during upright tilt: relevance for orthostatic hypotension? Lancet 1991;338:1542–1545

60. Morillo CA, Eckberg DL, Ellenbogen KA et al: Vagal and sympathetic mechanisms in patients with orthostatic vasovagal syncope. Circulation 1997;96:2509–2513

61. Glover W, Greenfield A, Shanks R: The contribution made by adrenaline to the vasodilation in the human forearm during emotional stress. J Physiol (Lond) 1962;161:42P–43P

62. Kaufmann H, Berman J, Oribe E, Oliver J: Possible increase in the synthesis of endothelial derived relaxing factor (EDRF) during vasovagal syncope. Clin Auton Res 1993;3:69 (abstract)

63. Biaggioni I: The autonomic nervous system and heredity. In Appenzeller O (Ed): The autonomic nervous system. Part II: Dysfunctions. Vol 75 (Revised series 31) of Handbook of Clinical Neurology, Vinken PJ, Bruyn GW (Eds). Amsterdam: Elsevier Science, 2000: pp 229–257

64. Ziegler MG, Lake CR, Kopin IJ: The sympathetic-nervous-system defect in primary orthostatic hypotension. N Engl J Med 1977;296:293–297

65. Kaufmann H, Oribe E, Miller M et al: Hypotension-induced vasopressin release distinguishes between pure autonomic failure and multiple system atrophy with autonomic failure. Neurology 1992;42:590–593

66. Polymeropoulos MH, Lavedan C, Leroy E et al: Mutation in the alpha-synuclein gene identified in families with Parkinson's disease. Science 1997;276:2045–2047

67. Spillantini MG, Schmidt ML, Lee VM et al: Alpha-synuclein in pLewy bodies. Nature 1997;388:839–840

68. Gai WP, Power JH, Blumbergs PC, Blessing WW: Multiple-system atrophy: a new alpha-synuclein disease? Lancet 1998;352:547–548 (letter)

69. Kaufmann H, Hague K, Perl D: Accumulation of alpha-synuclein in autonomic nerves in pure autonomic failure. Neurology 2001;56:980–981

70. Hague K, Lento P, Morgello S, Caro S, Kaufmann H: The distribution of Lewy bodies in pure autonomic failure: autopsy findings and review of the literature. Acta Neuropathol (Berl) 1997;94:192–196

71. Papp MI, Kahn JE, Lantos PL: Glial cytoplasmic inclusions in the CNS of patients with multiple system atrophy (striatonigral degeneration, olivopontocerebellar atrophy and Shy–Drager syndrome). J Neurol Sci 1989;94:79–100

72. Gilman S, Low P, Quinn N et al: Consensus statement on the diagnosis of multiple system atrophy. American Autonomic Society and American Academy of Neurology. Clin Auton Res 1998;8:359–362

73. Colosimo C, Albanese A, Hughes AJ, de Bruin VM, Lees AJ: Some specific clinical features differentiate multiple system atrophy (striatonigral variety) from Parkinson's disease. Arch Neurol 1995;52:294–298

74. Ben-Shlomo Y, Wenning GK, Tison F, Quinn NP: Survival of patients with pathologically proven multiple system atrophy: a meta-analysis. Neurology 1997;48:384–393

75. Kimber JR, Watson L, Mathias CJ: Distinction of idiopathic Parkinson's disease from multiple-system atrophy by stimulation of growth-hormone release with clonidine. Lancet 1997;349:1877–1881

76. Goldstein DS, Polinsky RJ, Garty M et al: Patterns of plasma levels of catechols in neurogenic orthostatic hypotension. Ann Neurol 1989;26:558–563

77. Pramstaller PP, Wenning GK, Smith SJ et al: Nerve conduction studies, skeletal muscle EMG, and sphincter EMG in multiple system atrophy. J Neurol Neurosurg Psychiatry 1995;58:618–621

78. Shannon JR, Jordan J, Diedrich A et al: Sympathetically mediated hypertension in autonomic failure. Circulation 2000;101:2710–2715

79. Hirayama M, Hakusui S, Koike Y et al: A scintigraphical qualitative analysis of peripheral vascular sympathetic function with meta-[123I]iodobenzylguanidine in neurological patients with autonomic failure. J Auton Nerv Syst 1995;53:230–234

80. Braune S, Reinhardt M, Schnitzer R, Riedel A, Lucking CH: Cardiac uptake of [123I]MIBG separates Parkinson's disease from multiple system atrophy. Neurology 1999;53:1020–1025

81. Orimo S, Ozawa E, Nakade S, Sugimoto T, Mizusawa H: (123)I-metaiodobenzylguanidine myocardial scintigraphy in Parkinson's disease. J Neurol Neurosurg Psychiatry 1999;67:189–194

82. Goldstein DS, Holmes C, Cannon ROr, Eisenhofer G, Kopin IJ: Sympathetic cardioneuropathy in dysautonomias. N Engl J Med 1997;336:696–702

83. Goldstein DS, Holmes C, Li ST et al: Cardiac sympathetic denervation in Parkinson disease. Ann Intern Med 2000;133:338–347

84. Yagishita T, Kojima S, Hirayama K: [MRI study of degenerative process in multiple system atrophy]. Rinsho Shinkeigaku 1995;35:126–131

85. Schrag A, Good CD, Miszkiel K et al: Differentiation of atypical parkinsonian syndromes with routine MRI. Neurology 2000;54:697–702

86. Konagaya M, Konagaya Y, Honda H, Iida M: A clinico-MRI study of extrapyramidal symptoms in multiple system atrophy—linear hyperintensity in the outer margin of the putamen. No To Shinkei 1993;45:509–513

87. Testa D, Savoiardo M, Fetoni V et al: Multiple system atrophy. Clinical and MR observations on 42 cases. Ital J Neurol Sci 1993;14:211–216

88. Schwarz J, Weis S, Kraft E et al: Signal changes on MRI and increases in reactive microgliosis, astrogliosis, and iron in the putamen of two patients with multiple system atrophy. J Neurol Neurosurg Psychiatry 1996;60:98–101

89. O'Neill JH, Murray NM, Newsom-Davis J: The Lambert-Eaton myasthenic syndrome. A review of 50 cases. Brain 1988;111:577–596

90. O'Suilleabhain P, Low PA, Lennon VA: Autonomic dysfunction in the Lambert-Eaton myasthenic syndrome: serologic and clinical correlates. Neurology 1998;50:88–93

91. Khurana RK, Koski CL, Mayer RF: Autonomic dysfunction in Lambert-Eaton myasthenic syndrome. J Neurol Sci 1988;85:77–86

92. Lennon VA, Kryzer TJ, Griesmann GE et al: Calcium-channel antibodies in the Lambert-Eaton syndrome and other paraneoplastic syndromes. N Engl J Med 1995;332:1467–1474

93. Yokota T, Hayashi M, Hirashima F et al: Dysautonomia with acute sensory motor neuropathy. A new classification of acute autonomic neuropathy. Arch Neurol 1994;51:1022–1031

94. Suarez GA, Fealey RD, Camilleri M, Low PA: Idiopathic autonomic neuropathy: clinical, neurophysiologic, and follow-up studies on 27 patients. Neurology 1994;44:1675–1682

95. Hart RG, Kanter MC: Acute autonomic neuropathy. Two cases and a clinical review. Arch Intern Med 1990;150:2373–2376

96. Low PA, Dyck PJ, Lambert EH et al: Acute panautonomic neuropathy. Ann Neurol 1983;13:412–417

97. McDougall AJ, McLeod JG: Autonomic neuropathy, II: Specific peripheral neuropathies. J Neurol Sci 1996;138:1–13

98. Sodhi N, Camilleri M, Camoriano JK et al: Autonomic function and motility in intestinal pseudoobstruction caused by paraneoplastic syndrome. Dig Dis Sci 1989;34:1937–1942

99. Vernino S, Low PA, Fealey RD et al: Autoantibodies to ganglionic acetylcholine receptors in autoimmune autonomic neuropathies. N Engl J Med 2000;343:847–855

100. Smit AA, Vermeulen M, Koelman JH, Wieling W: Unusual recovery from acute panautonomic neuropathy after immunoglobulin therapy. Mayo Clin Proc 1997;72:333–335

101. Singh NK, Jaiswal AK, Misra S, Srivastava PK: Assessment of autonomic dysfunction in Guillain–Barré syndrome and its prognostic implications. Acta Neurol Scand 1987;75:101–105

102. Tuck RR, McLeod JG: Autonomic dysfunction in Guillain–Barré syndrome. J Neurol Neurosurg Psychiatry 1981;44:983–990

103. Winer JB, Hughes RA: Identification of patients at risk of arrhythmia in the Guillain–Barré syndrome. Q J Med 1988;68:735–739

104. Reyners AK, Hazenberg BP, Haagsma EB et al: The assessment of autonomic function in patients with systemic amyloidosis: methodological considerations. Amyloid 1998;5:193–199

105. Ando Y, Suhr OB: Autonomic dysfunction in familial amyloidotic polyneuropathy (FAP). Amyloid 1998;5:288–300

106. Wang AK, Fealey RD, Gehrking TL, Low PA: Autonomic failure in amyloidosis. Neurology 1999;52:A388

107. Ewing DJ, Clarke BF: Diabetic autonomic neuropathy: present insights and future prospects. Diabetes Care 1986;9:648–665

108. Dyck PJ, Kratz KM, Karnes JL et al: The prevalence by staged severity of various types of diabetic neuropathy, retinopathy, and nephropathy in a population-based cohort: the Rochester Diabetic Neuropathy Study. Neurology 1993;43:817–824 (erratum appears in Neurology 1993;43(11):2345)

109. Fagius J: Microneurographic findings in diabetic polyneuropathy with special reference to sympathetic nerve activity. Diabetologia 1982;23:415–420

110. Maselli RA, Jaspan JB, Soliven BC et al: Comparison of sympathetic skin response with quantitative sudomotor axon reflex test in diabetic neuropathy. Muscle Nerve 1989;12:420–423

111. Hoeldtke RD, Bryner KD, Horvath GG et al: Redistribution of sudomotor responses is an early sign of sympathetic dysfunction in type 1 diabetes. Diabetes 2001;50:436–443

112. Fealey RD, Low PA, Thomas JE: Thermoregulatory sweating abnormalities in diabetes mellitus. Mayo Clin Proc 1989;64:617–628

113. Cohen JA, Laudenslager M: Autonomic nervous system involvement in patients with human immunodeficiency virus infection. Neurology 1989;39:1111–1112

114. Shahmanesh M, Bradbeer CS, Edwards A, Smith SE: Autonomic dysfunction in patients with human immunodeficiency virus infection. Int J STD AIDS 1991;2:419–423

115. Welby SB, Rogerson SJ, Beeching NJ: Autonomic neuropathy is common in human immunodeficiency virus infection. J Infect 1991;23:123–128

116. Freeman R, Roberts MS, Friedman LS, Broadbridge C: Autonomic function and human immunodeficiency virus infection. Neurology 1990;40:575–580

117. Ruttimann S, Hilti P, Spinas GA, Dubach UC: High frequency of human immunodeficiency virus-associated autonomic neuropathy and more severe involvement in advanced stages of human immunodeficiency virus disease. Arch Intern Med 1991;151:2441–2443

118. Wright RA, Grant IA, Low PA: Autonomic neuropathy associated with sicca complex. J Auton Nerv Syst 1999;75:70–76

119. Kaufmann H, Oribe E, Pierotti AR, Roberts JL, Yahr MD: Atrial natriuretic factor in human autonomic failure. Neurology 1990;40:1115–1119

120. Zambrasky E, DiBona G, Kaloyanides G: Specificity of neural effect on renal tubular sodium reabsorption. Proc Soc Exp Biol Med 1976;151:543–546

121. Biaggioni I, Robertson D, Krantz S, Jones M, Haile V: The anemia of primary autonomic failure and its reversal with recombinant erythropoietin. Ann Intern Med 1994;121:181–186

122. Perera R, Isola L, Kaufmann H: Effect of recombinant erythropoietin on anemia and orthostatic hypotension in primary autonomic failure. Clin Auton Res 1995;5:211–213

123. Hickler R: Successful treatment of orthostatic hypotension with 9-alpha fluorohydrocortisone. N Engl J Med 1959;261:788–791

124. Jard S: Vasopressin receptors. In Czernichow P, Robinson A (eds): Diabetes insipidus in man, Vol 13. S. Karger, Basel, 1985:89–104

125. Mathias CJ, Fosbraey P, da Costa DF, Thornley A, Bannister R: The effect of desmopressin on nocturnal polyuria, overnight weight loss, and morning postural hypotension in patients with autonomic failure. Br Med J (Clin Res Ed) 1986;293:353–354

126. Jankovic J, Gilden JL, Hiner BC, et al: Neurogenic orthostatic hypotension: a double-blind, placebo-controlled study with midodrine. Am J Med 1993;95:38–48

127. Wright RA, Kaufmann HC, Perera R et al: A double-blind, dose-response study of midodrine in neurogenic orthostatic hypotension. Neurology 1998;51:120–124

128. Biaggioni I, Robertson D: Endogenous restoration of noradrenaline by precursor therapy in dopamine-beta-hydroxylase deficiency. Lancet 1987;2:1170–1172

129. Man in't Veld AJ, Boomsma F, Moleman P, Schalekamp MA: Congenital dopamine-beta-hydroxylase deficiency. A novel orthostatic syndrome. Lancet 1987;1:183–188

130. Freeman R: Treatment of orthostatic hypotension—midodrine and other pressor drugs. In Robertson D, Low P, Polinsky RJ (eds): Primer on the Autonomic Nervous System. Academic Press, New York, 1996;326–332

131. Kaufmann H, Oribe E, Yahr MD: Differential effect of L-threo-3,4-dihydroxyphenylserine in pure autonomic failure and multiple system atrophy with autonomic failure. J Neural Transm Park Dis Dement Sect 1991;3:143–148

132. Kaufmann H: Could treatment with DOPS do for autonomic failure what DOPA did for Parkinson's disease? Neurology 1996;47:1370–1371

133. Hoeldtke RD, Streeten DH: Treatment of orthostatic hypotension with erythropoietin. N Engl J Med 1993;329:611–615

134. Goldberg M, Dunning S, Bunn H: Regulation of the erythropoietin gene: evidence that the oxygen sensor is a heme protein. Science 1988;242:1412–1415

135. Maxwell A, Lappin T, Bridges J, McGeown M: Erythropoietin production in kidney tubular cells. Br J Haematol 1990;74:535–539

136. Perera R, Isola L, Kaufmann H: Erythropoietin improves orthostatic hypotension in primary autonomic failure. Neurology 1994;44:A363

137. Raine AE, Roger SD: Effects of erythropoietin on blood pressure. Am J Kidney Dis 1991;18:76–83

138. Kochar M, Itskowitz H, Albers J: Treatment of orthostatic hypotension with indomethacin. Am Heart J 1979;98:271–280

139. Crook J, Robertson D, Whorton A: Prostaglandin suppression: Inability to correct severe idiopathic orthostatic hypotension. South Med 1981;73:318–320

140. Hoeldtke RD, Boden G, O'Dorisio TM: Treatment of postprandial hypotension with a somatostatin analogue (SMS 201–995). Am J Med 1986;81:83–87

141. Hoeldtke R, Israel B: Treatment of orthostatic hypotension with octreotide. J Clin Endocrinol Metab 1989;68:1051–1059

142. Kuchel O, Buu N, Gutkowska J, Genest J: Treatment of severe orthostatic hypotension by metoclopramide. Ann Intern Med 1980;93:841–843

143. Lopes de Faria S, Zanella M, Amoriolo A, Ribiero A, Charca A: Peripheral dopaminergic blockade for the treatment of diabetic orthostatic hypotension. Clin Pharmacol Ther 1988;44:670–674

144. Man in't Veld A, Schalekamp M: Pindolol acts as a beta-adrenoceptor agonist in orthostatic hypotension: Therapeutic implications. Br Med J 1981;282:929–931

145. Robertson D, Goldberg M, Hollister A, Wade D, Robertson R: Clonidine raises blood pressure in idiopathic orthostatic hypotension. Am J Med 1983;74:193–199

146. Onrot J, Goldberg MR, Biaggioni I et al: Oral yohimbine in human autonomic failure. Neurology 1987;37:215–220

147. Biaggioni I, Zygmunt D, Haile V, Robertson D: Pressor effect of inhaled ergotamine in orthostatic hypotension. Am J Cardiol 1990;65:89–92

Chapter 52

Parkinsonism and other movement disorders

Jolyon Meara

Material in this chapter contains contributions from the previous edition, and we are grateful to the previous authors for the work done.

The term "movement disorders" is usually restricted to diseases that involve the basal ganglia and its connections such as Parkinson's disease (PD), Huntington's disease, hemiballismus, and torsion dystonia. Movement disorders can be broadly classified into the akinetic–rigid hypokinetic conditions in which voluntary movement is reduced and hyperkinetic conditions in which excess involuntary movements called dyskinesias are present (Table 52-1). Dyskinesias can be further classified into tremor, dystonia, tics, myoclonus, and chorea. This distinction is not absolute as for example, in PD, the commonest akinetic–rigid syndrome, involuntary movements are often present. Akinetic–rigid syndromes are usually associated with poor mobility and difficulty with walking due to the presence of a gait apraxia.

Movement disorders are common in older age and are a significant cause of impairment, disability, and handicap.[1] Once diagnosed, these disorders can often be effectively treated. Older people with movement disorders tend to present late for diagnosis or are detected by chance when the individual presents with another more immediately pressing medical problem. On an average post-take ward round it is not uncommon in older patients to make the diagnoses of hitherto unrecognized essential tremor, parkinsonism, orofacial dyskinesia, or drug-induced movement disorder.

NEUROANATOMY OF THE BASAL GANGLIA

The basal ganglia consist of the paired caudate, putamen, globus pallidus, substantia nigra and subthalamic nuclei.[2–4] The caudate and putamen are sometimes referred to as the *striatum* and with the globus pallidus lie deep in the cerebral hemispheres, closely related to the thalamus and internal

Table 52-1 Classification of movement disorders

- Akinetic–rigid states:
  - Parkinsonism
- Hyperkinetic states:
  - Tremor
  - Chorea
  - Dystonia
  - Myoclonus
  - Complex movement disorders
  - Drug-induced movement disorders (tardive dyskinesia)

capsule. The globus pallidus consists of a lateral (globus pallidus pars externa—GPe) and medial part (globus pallidus pars interna—GPi). The substantia nigra and subthalamic nucleus (STN) lie in close proximity caudal to the other nuclei in the midbrain above the cerebral peduncle and below the thalamus. The substantia nigra consists of a cellular deeply staining melanin containing pars compacta (SNpc) and a less cellular pars reticulata (SNpr). The subthalamic nucleus has a critical role in controlling the normal output from the basal ganglia and in the pathophysiology of the clinical signs of PD and other movement disorders.

CONNECTIONS, NEUROTRANSMITTERS, AND ORGANIZATION OF THE BASAL GANGLIA

Our knowledge of the complex neurochemical, neuroanatomical, and neurophysiological relationships in the basal ganglia in man and animal models has greatly increased in the past decade.[5–11] The basal ganglia receive input from far-reaching areas of the cerebral cortex and project via the thalamus back to specific cortical and brainstem structures. The striatum (caudate and putamen) is the major receiving area of the basal ganglia and in turn projects to the two major output nuclei of the basal ganglia the GPi and SNpr. A further anatomical loop exists in the basal ganglia between the striatum and the GPi/SNpr via the STN and GPe. These two loops provide a direct and indirect pathway between receiving and output nuclei. The output nuclei of the basal ganglia project mainly to the cerebral cortex via specific thalamic nuclei (Fig. 52-1).

Multiple parallel loops pass through the basal ganglia involving voluntary movement (motor loop), eye pursuit movement (oculomotor loop originating from the frontal eye fields), emotional behavior (limbic loop originating from the limbic cortex), and motivational behavior (prefrontal loops). These loops are kept quite distinct in organizational terms within the basal ganglia ("parallel processing").[6] Movement disorders are most clearly associated with the motor loop that links the sensorimotor cortex to the putamen to the GPi/SNPr and back to the supplementary motor area via the ventrolateral thalamus. Within the motor loop, inputs from different anatomical areas appear to be kept separate throughout the basal ganglia. Cortical input to the striatum is glutaminergic and excitatory, whereas the input to GPi/SNpr is inhibitory via a

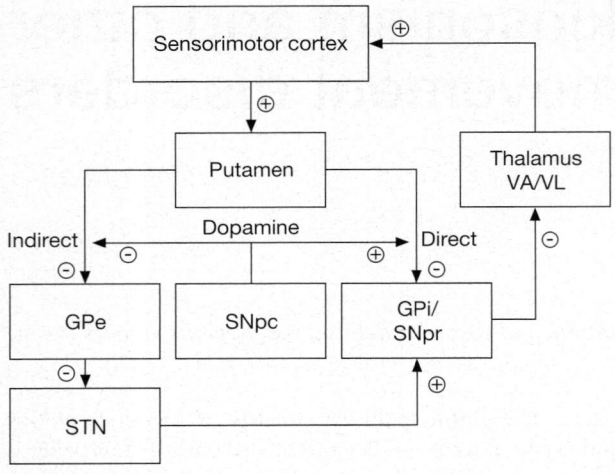

SNpc = Substantia nigra pars compacta
SNpr = Substantia nigra pars reticulata
GPe = Globus pallidus pars externa
GPi = Globus pallidus pars interna
STN = Subthalamic nucleus
VA/VL = Ventro anterior and ventrolateral thalamic nuclei

Figure 52-1 Direct and indirect basal ganglia pathways modulated by dopamine from the nigrostriatal tract. (Reproduced from Meara and Bhowmick,[109] with permission of Cambridge University Press).

GABAergic/substance P direct pathway. The basic output from the thalamus is glutaminergic excitatory to the cortex, though this can be altered by the inputs from the output nuclei of the basal ganglia, which cause tonic inhibition of the thalamus via GABAergic inhibitory input (Fig. 52-2). Normally, tonic thalamic inhibition from the basal ganglia is reduced in preparation for a voluntary movement so that the excitatory thalamic output to the relevant area in the supplementary motor area of the prefrontal cortex can increase. This is achieved by cortical inputs to the putamen that cause inhibition of the output nuclei via the direct pathway. Cortical inputs can also increase the inhibition of the thalamus from the output nuclei by a glutaminergic excitatory input to GPi/SNpr from the STN via the indirect pathway. The balance between the direct and indirect pathways appears to be critically influenced by dopamine released in the striatum from the neurons of the ascending nigrostriatal pathway from the SNpc and from the closely related A8 group of dopaminergic neurons in the midbrain. Dopaminergic input to the striatum is excitatory for the direct and inhibitory for the indirect pathway (Fig. 52-1). In the models of movement disorders that have been proposed the subthalamic nucleus appears to play a critical role in controlling the output from the basal ganglia to the thalamus.[12–14]

Further complexities in the organization of the basal ganglia arise at the cellular level from the finding of two distinct cell populations in the striatum with distinct input/output relationships called the striosome and matrix.[7] Somatosensory input is mainly to the matrix that forms most of the bulk of the putamen, whereas striosomes tend to have input from the limbic system. Both striosomes and matrix receive dopaminergic input from the midbrain but only striosomes send input back to the SNpc. The recognized influence that emotions have on motor behavior can be explained by this interaction at the SNpc which results in limbic inputs controlling activity in the motor loop.

THE AKINETIC–RIGID SYNDROMES

The akinetic–rigid syndromes are a group of disorders characterized by parkinsonism which results from the combination of akinesia, rigidity, and often, but not always, tremor (Table 52-2). Parkinsonism is often associated with impaired balance and a gait apraxia leading to falls and impaired mobility. Primary parkinsonism of no known cause is called idiopathic parkinsonism or PD and accounts for around 70 percent of cases of parkinsonism.[15–17] The remaining secondary causes of parkinsonism are largely due to neuroleptic drug-induced parkinsonism, vascular parkinsonism, and much less frequently, multisystem degenerative conditions, usually referred to as parkinson's-*plus* syndromes. These include conditions such as progressive supranuclear palsy, multiple system atrophy and corticobasal degeneration. With increasing age not only does the risk of parkinsonism increase, but also the likelihood of parkinsonism being due to a cause other than PD.

Table 52-2 **Causes of parkinsonism**

Primary parkinsonism
- Parkinson's disease (idiopathic parkinsonism)

Secondary parkinsonism
- Drug-induced parkinsonism:
  - Neuroleptic drugs
  - Calcium blocker cinnarazine

- Vascular parkinsonism (pseudoparkinsonism)
  - Multi-infarct states
  - Single basal ganglia/thalamic infarct
  - Binswanger's disease

- Multisystem degenerative diseases
  - Progressive supranuclear palsy
  - Multiple system atrophy (striatonigral type)
  - Corticobasal degeneration
  - Alzheimer's disease
  - Wilson's disease (young-onset parkinsonism)
  - Dementia with Lewy bodies
  - Neurofibrillary tangle parkinsonism

- Toxins
  - MPTP
  - Manganese

- Familial parkinsonism

- Post-infectious parkinsonism:
  - Creutzfeldt–Jakob disease
  - AIDS
  - Post-encephalitis (encephalitis lethargica)

- Miscellaneous causes
  - Hydrocephalus
  - Post-traumatic
  - Tumors
  - Metabolic causes (post-anoxic)

PARKINSON'S DISEASE

Although PD can present at any age, and juvenile onset forms are well described, it is a rare disorder outside old age.[18] Cross-sectional prevalence studies of PD and parkinsonism show at least two-thirds of subjects to be over the age of 70 years. PD is usually insidious in onset and may have a long symptomatic phase before eventual diagnosis.

Clinical features

Akinesia is a symptom complex that refers to a lack of spontaneous voluntary movement, slowness of movement (bradykinesia) and faulty execution of movement.[19,20] Voluntary movements tend to be of low amplitude and to show increased fatigability. There is a particular difficulty with sequential and concurrent self-paced movements. Patients when asked to oppose the index finger to the thumb in a tapping motion often start with reasonably fast, large-amplitude movements but the speed and amplitude then rapidly decrease with the movement fading away. Akinesia in the lower limb is best tested by asking the patient to tap the heel of the foot on the floor as rapidly as possible—in this situation akinesia can be heard better than seen. Older patients often find tests for akinesia difficult to execute and may perform poorly because of painful arthritis, restricted joint range or muscle weakness.

Rigidity is an increased resistance of muscle to passive stretch felt by the examiner. Clinically rigidity is best detected at the wrist joint. The subject is asked to relax as fully as possible while the examiner makes flexion and extension movements of the wrist joint with the subject's forearm supported. Passive movements of the head can be used to detect axial rigidity. Parkinsonian rigidity is not velocity dependent and is present to the same degree at all joint positions in flexion and extension ("lead-pipe" rigidity). Activation procedures, akin to the Jendrassik maneuver to enhance tendon jerks, can bring out "activated rigidity" that was not present before. Transient activated rigidity may be a normal finding in anxious individuals. Activated rigidity in the neck muscles may be the first sign of rigidity in PD. The presence of tremor in the upper limb due to any cause will result in a ratchet-like quality of intermittent resistance at the wrist joint called "cog-wheel rigidity" that is not specific for PD.

Tremor is the presenting feature of PD in around 70 percent of cases. Tremor characteristically occurs at rest when the postural muscles are relaxed and has a frequency of around 4–6 Hz. In an anxious patient, postural tremor can easily be misidentified as a resting tremor. Most patients with PD manifest a range of resting, postural, and action tremors. A resting tremor of the hand involving the thumb and index finger described as "pill-rolling" is very suggestive of PD or drug-induced parkinsonism, though can also be seen in multiple system atrophy. Tremor usually begins insidiously in one hand and then may spread to the ipsilateral leg before, often after a delay of a year or more, involving the contralateral hand and chin. Neck and voice tremor is unusual in PD and suggests a diagnosis of essential tremor.

Postural balance can be assessed clinically by asking the patient to stand and then gently pushing the patient forward from behind. Another individual should stand in front of them to prevent a fall. Falls or feelings of imbalance strongly suggest the presence of impaired righting reflexes even if this is not evident at the time of examination.

Neuropathological basis

PD is characterized by cell loss and gliosis in the SNpc and other pigmented brainstem nuclei that is often visible to the naked eye on sectioning the midbrain.[21,22] Aging also results in cell loss in the substantia nigra though the distribution of cell loss is very different to that seen as a result of PD.[23] Tretiakoff, as early as 1919, suggested that degenerative changes in the substantia nigra were linked to PD. Subsequently PD was found to be associated with a deficiency of dopamine in the striatum and the later idenfication of the dopaminergic nigrostriatal tract confirmed Tretiakoff's hypothesis.

Surviving cells in the SNpc contain typical inclusions in the cytoplasm called Lewy bodies.[21,22] Lewy bodies have a dense eosinophilic core surrounded by a pale halo and demonstrate characteristic staining reactions. Lewy bodies are also found in the locus coeruleus, substantia innominata, dorsal vagal motor nucleus, thalamus, hypothalamus, and the peripheral autonomic system and enteric plexus. A different form of Lewy body is also found in the cortex in most patients with PD, particularly in the temporal cortex and insula. Other inclusions have also been described in PD.[24] Lewy bodies can be an incidental finding in up to 10 percent of postmortem examinations in subjects with no apparent history of parkinsonism in life. It is unclear whether such individuals, if they had survived, would have developed PD. Lewy bodies are not completely specific for PD. Lewy body pathology in the substantia nigra does not necessarily lead to the clinical picture of PD and conversely, other pathologies not involving Lewy bodies can give rise to typical PD. However, most experts would agree that the finding of Lewy bodies in the substantia nigra is required for the confirmation of the clinical diagnosis of PD.

The finding of large numbers of cortical Lewy bodies, particularly in association with senile plaques, which are a feature of Alzheimer's disease, suggests the diagnosis of dementia with Lewy bodies.[25] The relationship between PD, dementia with Lewy bodies, and Alzheimer's disease has yet to be established. Plentiful cortical Lewy bodies and vascular changes in the striatum are seen in cases that fulfill pathological criteria for PD but who have atypical clinical features and a poor clinical response to levodopa.[26] PD also involves the ascending serotonergic, noradrenergic, and cholinergic projections to the cortex and basal ganglia.[27] Clinicopathological studies have demonstrated that coexisting neuropathology within the striatum and in other areas of the brain is extremely common in elderly subjects with histologically confirmed PD.[28]

Neurophysiological basis

The loss of dopaminergic modulation in the striatum causes a profound disturbance of voluntary motor control leading to akinesia, tremor, and rigidity. The severity of akinesia and rigidity, but not tremor, appears to be reasonably linked to the degree of striatal dopamine loss in the motor loop. Tremor responds much less well to dopaminergic drug therapy than either akinesia or rigidity, and interestingly, resting tremor is difficult to replicate in animal models of parkinsonism. The loss of dopamine in the striatum increases activity in the indirect pathway, thereby increasing thalamic inhibition and reducing cortical excitability. This provides an explanation, albeit rather simplistic, for akinesia and can account for the failure of the proper execution of automatic learned motor plans that is a central feature of PD.[29] This model is generally supported by neurophysiological evidence, though it fails to explain all the clinical features of PD and the occurrence of levodopa-induced dyskinesia.[30,31] The neurophysiological basis of rigidity[32] and tremor[33] has yet to be fully elucidated. Rigidity appears to result from the enhancement by the basal ganglia of complex tonic stretch reflex circuits at spinal and supraspinal levels. Curiously, the resting tremor of PD can be abolished by lesioning the nucleus ventralis intermedius of the thalamus, which receives no direct input from the basal ganglia. The STN appears to play a critical part in the pathophysiology of PD by providing powerful control over the inhibitory activity of the GPi/SNpr output nuclei. Surgical lesions or supraphysiological stimulation of the STN can improve and sometimes even abolish the akinesia of PD.[34] Interestingly, spontaneous vascular damage to the STN has been known for a long time to cause dyskinesia and hemiballismus.

Clinical diagnosis

The diagnosis of PD is a two-stage process that is still dependent on clinical skills.[35] Firstly, the symptoms of parkinsonism need to be sought in the history and the signs of parkinsonism established by clinical examination. Progressively small handwriting (micrographia) with the written word disappearing into a shaky line is strongly suggestive of parkinsonism, though it is surprising how few people write letters by hand today. Difficulty turning over in bed is also a good clue to the early development of truncal akinesia. A good witness account, usually from a spouse is very useful in confirming the often rather general and nonspecific slowing down seen in older patients with PD. The gradual inability to keep up with a spouse on daily routine walks is again a useful early indication of gait disturbance and akinesia. Secondly, if parkinsonism is detected, consideration has to be given to what type of parkinsonism is present by applying validated clinical diagnostic criteria (Table 52-3).

How good are we at detecting parkinsonism? Epidemiological evidence from community based prevalence studies of parkinsonism suggest that at least 20 percent of apparent cases do not in fact have parkinsonism when examined.[36–39] A recent community based study[17] of 402 subjects in receipt of antiparkinsonian medication found that only 73 percent of this group had clinical evidence of parkinsonism when examined and only 53 percent of the group met diagnostic criteria for clinically probable PD (Table 52-3). The most common cause of misdiagnosis is essential tremor.

In older patients the diagnosis of parkinsonism can be extremely difficult, even in expert hands, particularly when the clinical picture is complicated by other diseases, cognitive impairment, depression, and atypical features. A confident diagnosis of parkinsonism cannot always be made in older people and often a trial of levodopa therapy may be required. However, even the results of a six-week trial of levodopa at adequate dosage (at least 600 mg daily) may be inconclusive. Diagnosis in this difficult area may be improved by use of

DaTSCAN-SPECT imaging of the nigrostriatal tract using a radiolabeled tracer for the dopamine transporter.[40]

How good are experts at distinguishing PD from other types of parkinsonism? Two important clinicopathological brain bank studies have addressed this problem and have demonstrated that diagnostic accuracy for PD at death, which offers the best chance of diagnostic accuracy, was only around 76 percent.[28,41] Neuropathological findings in cases misdiagnosed as PD consisted of multisystem degenerative diseases and more surprisingly a significant number of cases of Alzheimer's disease and Alzheimer-type changes. Diagnostic accuracy in more recent cases referred to a brain bank was shown to have improved to around 84 percent.[42] The use of stringent clinical diagnostic criteria can improve the specificity for the diagnosis of PD to over 90 percent but at the expense of a reduced sensitivity of 70 percent.

Clinical subtypes

Clinical observation suggests that subtypes of PD exist, though surprisingly little scientific study of this phenomenon has been undertaken (Table 52-4).[43–47] Late onset disease (symptoms starting after the age of 70 years) tends to progress more quickly

---

Table 52-3 Guideline diagnostic criteria for Parkinson's disease

A progressive usually nonfamilial disorder with bradykinesia (slowness of initiation of voluntary movement, progressive reduction in speed and amplitude of repetitive movement and difficulty switching smoothly from one motor program to the next) and at least one of the following:
- Muscular rigidity
- Coarse 4–6 Hz resting tremor
- Impaired righting reflexes (not caused by primary visual, vestibular, cerebellar, or proprioceptive dysfunction)

Absolute exclusion criteria are the following:
- Exposure to neuroleptic drugs within the year before the onset of symptoms, or to MPTP
- Presence of cerebellar or corticospinal tract signs
- Past history of encephalitis lethargica or viral encephalitis with oculogyric crises
- Stepwise progression and/or a history of multiple strokes
- Presence of communicating hydrocephalus or a supratentorial tumor
- Presence of severe early autonomic failure
- Supranuclear gaze palsy

Modified with permission from Gibb and Lees.[45]

Table 52-4 Subtypes of Parkinson's disease

Early onset < 50 years old	vs	Late onset > 70 years old
Tremor dominant	vs	Postural imbalance and gait disorder
Benign slow progression	vs	Malignant rapid progression
Unilateral with or without axial disease	vs	Bilateral disease with or without impaired balance

Reproduced from Meara and Bhowmick,[109] with permission of Cambridge University Press.

than early onset disease (symptoms before the age of 40 years) and is more often associated with cognitive impairment.[48] Patients in the longitudinal DATATOP study who were classified as having rapidly progressive disease were older, had more severe bradykinesia and postural imbalance and exhibited less tremor at study entry than the group with slowly progressive disease. Tremor dominant disease was associated with less disability, less cognitive impairment and less depression compared to a group with akinetic rigidity and postural imbalance. The DATATOP analysis suggested that cognitive function and motor deterioration were relatively independent once adjustment for age had taken place.[48] However, patients with late onset disease appear to become demented sooner than patients with early onset disease of similar duration.[49] The risk of levodopa-induced dyskinesias appears to be much lower in patients with late compared with early onset disease. Motor fluctuations are also less evident in late onset disease with the possible exception of end of dose "wearing off" of drug benefit.

The clinical expression and progression of PD with age is likely to reflect the impact of neuropathology in addition to PD as well as possible effects of cell loss due to aging. Vascular and Alzheimer type changes in the striatum and cortex may protect elderly subjects from dyskinesia and motor fluctuations but increase the risk of a poor response to levodopa and cognitive impairment.

Epidemiology

The major causes of neurodegenerative disease, Alzheimer's disease, PD, and motor neuron disease all share a strong age-associated risk and are likely to be an issue of increasing public health concern as a result of the worldwide aging of populations. This is likely to have a particular impact in less industrialized countries that are rapidly developing an elderly population for the first time. Certified deaths from neurodegenerative diseases have been projected to overtake cancer as the second commonest cause of death in the USA by the year 2040.[50]

PD affects all racial groups and, after adjusting crude rates to a standard population and allowing for differences in study methodologies, has a fairly uniform worldwide distribution of around 110 per 100,000.[51] Prevalence is reduced in Africa, China, and Japan. This may reflect both differences in environmental as well as genetic factors. Differences in adjusted prevalence rates may still be explained by differential survival, diagnostic bias, and variable mortality rates. Population-adjusted prevalence rates for PD in European subjects over the age of 65 years have been reported as 2.3 percent for parkinsonism and 1.6 percent for PD.[52] Age-specific prevalence rates for PD increase exponentially with age, though some studies report a falling off in prevalence above the eighth decade, possibly reflecting selection bias by excluding subjects in institutional care.[53] The risk of PD appears to be slightly greater in men.[54] In studies in which all eligible subjects are examined using the total census approach, up to a third or more of subjects ascertained as having PD were medically undiagnosed before the study.[55,56]

The age-adjusted incidence for PD has remained steady over the years 1967–79 based on the longitudinal data from Rochester Minnesota at around 18 new cases per 100,000 subjects per year.[15] A difference in age-specific incidence between older and younger people may have developed over this time without altering the crude incidence rate.[18] In support of this concept, age-specific mortality rates in PD do appear to be increasing in those over 75 years old.[18,50,57] A recent longitudinal study of 4,341 elderly subjects initially free of parkinsonism reported an average annual incidence rate for parkinsonism of 530 per 100,000 and 326 per 100,000 for PD.[54]

Parkinsonism in institutional care has received little research attention. The prevalence of parkinsonism appears to be high in hospitals, nursing homes, and residential/retirement homes.[58] A survey in the United States of 5,000 nursing home residents over the age of 55 years reported a prevalence for medically diagnosed PD of nearly 7 percent.[59] A European study found that 42 percent of cases of PD in elderly subjects living in institutions were medically undiagnosed.[60] Nursing home residents with PD tended to be more disorientated, depressed, and functionally disabled than residents without PD.[61,62] Hallucinations and dementia are the two main factors increasing the risk of admission to nursing homes of elderly people with PD.[61,62]

Etiology

Simple aging is unlikely to be an important factor in the etiology of PD.[63] The finding of inherited familial parkinsonism indicates that parkinsonism can on occasion very rarely arise from a single gene,[64,65] and the 1-methyl-4-phenyl-1,2,2,6-tetrahydropyridine (MPTP) toxin story similarly suggests that on occasion parkinsonism can be caused by exposure to an environmental agent.[66] However, the balance of environmental and genetic factors determining the risk of PD is still unknown.[67–69]

Genetic factors

Familial parkinsonism is now a well-described, albeit rare, condition. The clinical picture and pathological findings in such families indicate little similarity with sporadic PD. In one large kindred with autosomal dominant parkinsonism that is reasonably clinically and pathologically similar to PD, a point mutation in the gene for alpha-synuclein, which is found in Lewy bodies, has been established.[70,71] A similar point mutation in this gene has been described in four further unrelated kindreds. In a form of juvenile parkinsonism, dissimilar clinically to PD, a parkin gene has also been described.[72] The study of the concordance rate of PD in monozygotic and dizygotic twins does not support a major genetic influence on the risk of developing this condition, but likewise cannot exclude a genetic contribution.[73,74] The risk of PD in first-degree relatives of patients does appear to be increased based on case identification and case-control methods.[75,76] Some, but not all, studies have shown an increased risk of PD due to single gene mutations and polymorphisms in genes coding for metabolic enzymes that may be involved in the handling of potential environmental toxins.[77,78] An association between PD and the cytochrome P450 isoenzyme CYP2D6 genotype, whose enzyme product substrates include neuroleptic drugs and MPTP, has been the most widely investigated. The finding of reduced mitochondrial complex 1 activity in the substantia nigra could result directly from a primary mitochondrial genetic deficit.[79]

Environmental factors

Parkinsonism due to environmental toxin exposure, such as that seen in manganese mineworkers, has been recognized for a long time. The worldwide distribution of PD suggests that any potential toxin or protective agent, such as diet, would need to share this widespread distribution. Clinicopathological studies in PD indicate that the rate of cell death in the SNpc is highest in preclinical stages and that cell death begins around 6 years before the onset of clinical disease.[63] However, the search for more widespread environmental agents was accelerated by the description of MPTP parkinsonism in man.[66,80]

The MPTP story also supported the hypothesis that oxidative damage could lead to cell death by inhibition of critical mitochondrial function. MPTP is converted by glial monoamine oxidase-B to a toxic metabolite MPP+. This is then taken up via the dopamine transporter and concentrates in the mitochondria where it inhibits complex 1 activity. In PD there is evidence that the substantia nigra experiences significant oxidative stress.[81,82] Free radicals, normally generated by reactions in the respiratory process, can lead to oxidative cell damage, particularly the peroxidation of membrane lipids, if there is a failure of cell systems to contain them. Free-radical formation would also be enhanced by the accumulation of iron in the SNpc that occurs in PD. Free radicals are also generated by the metabolism and turnover of dopamine. Whether oxidative damage is a primary event or arises secondary to an unknown primary cell insult is unknown. Nigral cell death from any cause will lead to increased dopamine turnover in the surviving neurons that could give rise to evidence of oxidative stress in the substantia nigra such as reduced complex 1 activity that may not in itself be harmful.

Analytical epidemiology has not yet made a major contribution to the understanding of disease etiology.[83,84] Case-control studies investigating risk factors for PD are subject to major sources of bias and confounding. The best designed and conducted studies have suggested a link between the risk of PD and pesticide exposure, prior head injury and having a first-degree relative with the disease. However, such factors may explain only about a third of cases of PD. Most reports have generally pointed to a rather nonspecific risk of rural living. Protective effects, such as a diet rich in antioxidant agents, may reduce the risk of PD in some people.[85] The apparent protective effect of smoking is a fairly robust finding in studies that have addressed this issue by several means.[86,87] The nature of this effect is unclear.[88,89] Smoking may appear to be protective simply because individuals who would have developed PD die from the results of smoking at a premature age, smokers with PD give up smoking or the personality of subjects destined to develop PD makes them less likely to smoke in the first place.[90]

Assessment in PD

Movement disorder clinics can provide a comprehensive assessment of the physical, mental and social functioning of an individual, providing the most important aspect of the long-term management strategy for PD (Fig. 52-2).[91,92] Clinics can access the wide range of health and social care expertise that is usually needed to provide the necessary assessments. Whenever possible, standardized assessment tools should be used. The clinic can provide a means of monitoring the process and outcomes of care and through continual audit the requirements of clinical governance can be met. Assessment in PD should be structured and integrated into the daily working of a multidisciplinary team. In the UK there has been a rapid expansion and development of the role of the PD nurse specialist. Such a post can support the community aspects of care in PD and strengthen expertise in primary care. An effective program of apomorphine therapy also requires the input of specialist nursing. A recently completed randomized controlled trial in the UK of the PD nurse has thus far failed to publish its results other than in abstract form.

The most widely used disease specific assessment scale is the Unified Parkinson's Disease Rating Scale (UPDRS).[93,94]

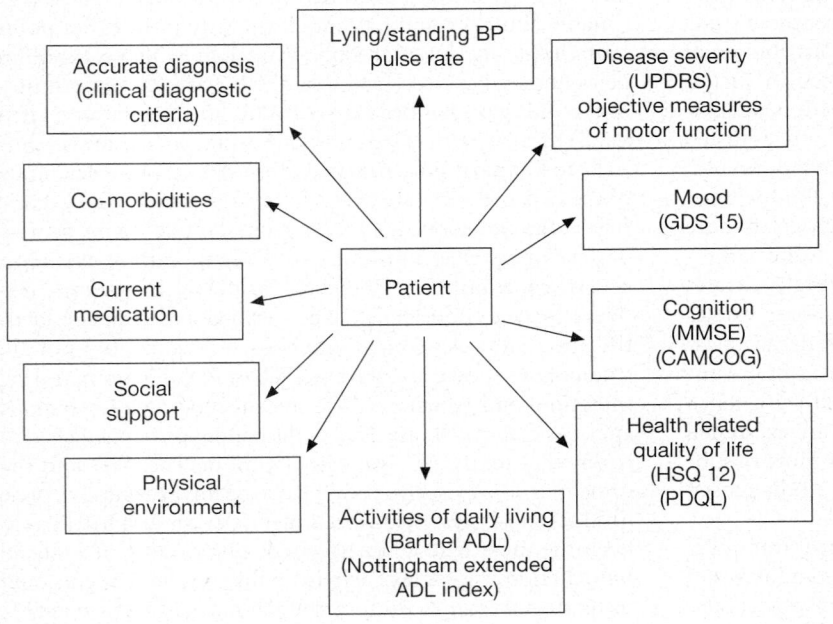

Figure 52-2 Domains in the assessment of Parkinson's disease. (Reproduced from Meara and Bhowmick,[109] with permission of Cambridge University Press.)

The UPDRS covers mood, memory, activities of daily living, motor impairment, and complications of drug therapy, and includes the modified Hoehn and Yahr disease severity scale[95] and the Schwab and England activities of daily living scale.[96] However, the UPDRS remains a subjective tool and fails to clearly distinguish between measures of impairment, disability, and handicap. The higher the score on the UPDRS the greater the impairment, disability, or handicap, but the clinical interpretation and significance of a two- or three-point change in the total score that can range to a total of over 200 points is difficult to glean from published studies using this assessment tool. The UPDRS also takes around 20–25 minutes to administer in routine clinical practice. As an alternative the motor and complications of therapy subsections of the UPDRS could be used as stand-alone measurements with more generic measures used for other domains (Fig. 52-2).[97–103] Lying and standing blood pressure and pulse rate are important measures of autonomic function and risk of postural syncope with anti-parkinsonian medication.

Treatment of the motor symptoms

An increasingly wide and expensive range of drugs is available to treat the motor symptoms of PD (Table 52-5). Detailed discussion of their use can be found in recent reviews of drug therapy[104–106] and in recently published treatment algorithms.[107,108] A summary of management algorithm for the de-novo treatment of older adults with PD is shown. To obtain the best results in older subjects drug treatment should be combined with rehabilitative approaches involving physical therapists, occupational therapists, speech and language therapists, and a range of other allied health and welfare

Table 52-5 Drugs used to treat the motor impairment in Parkinson's disease

Group	Drug	Trade name
Levodopa	Co-careldopa	Sinemet 110
		Sinemet 275
		Sinemet-plus
		Sinemet-S
		Sinemet CR, Half CR
	Co-beneldopa	Madopar 62.5
		Madopar 125
		Madopar 250
		Madopar CR
		Madopar dispersible 62.5/125
COMT inhibitors	Entacapone	Comtess
MAO-B inhibitors	Selegiline	Eldypryl
		Zelapar (sublingual)
Dopamine agonists	Bromocriptine	Parlodel
	Pergolide	Celance
	Ropinirole	Requip
	Cabergoline	Cabasar
	Pramipexole	Mirapexin
	Apomorphine	Britaject
Miscellaneous	Amantadine	Symmetrel
	Anticholinergics	

Table 52-6 Starting levodopa in frail older people

- Baseline measures of disease state and lying/standing blood pressure
- Pretreat for 3 days with domperidone 20 mg three times daily
- Start levodopa 50 mg as co-careldopa/co-beneldopa with food three times daily, 30 minutes after taking the domperidone
- Continue for 4 days before increasing the levodopa by 50 mg increments in divided doses every 4 days until a total daily dose of 300 mg levodopa is reached continuing throughout with the domperidone
- Review patient to assess motor response, side-effects, and postural blood pressure changes
- Continue to slowly build the daily dose of levodopa by 50 mg increments every 4 days in divided doses as before until a total daily dose of 600 mg is reached
- Review to assess motor response and side-effects after 4 weeks of 600 mg levodopa daily
- Adjust levodopa dose to obtain optimal benefit with the smallest dose possible
- In nonresponders increase levodopa slowly as before until limited by side-effects
- Failure to respond to a dose of greater than 1.2 g levodopa daily in the absence of malabsorption makes a diagnosis of Parkinson's disease very unlikely

professionals.[109–114] Drug treatment does not appear from currently available evidence to delay disease progression. It can, however, improve, though rarely abolish, motor impairment. With disease progression, disabling problems develop that do not respond to dopaminergic treatment such as falls, dysarthria, dysphagia, and dementia. These features develop more rapidly in subjects presenting with late onset PD. Today anticholinergic drugs and amantadine have very little role in treating older patients with PD. Both drugs commonly precipitate confusion and worsen pre-existing cognitive impairment. There is conflicting evidence with regard to whether amantadine may improve levodopa-induced dyskinesia.

Drug treatment

Levodopa

The most effective and widely available drug treatment for PD remains levodopa. In order to reduce the side-effects of nausea and vomiting and to increase bioavailability, levodopa is usually combined with an enzyme to prevent peripheral decarboxylation to dopamine (co-careldopa or Sinemet™ and co-beneldopa or Madopar™) and is initially taken with food. Over time most patients become tolerant of this side-effect and the levodopa can then be taken on an empty stomach to improve absorption as levodopa competes with dietary amino acids at duodenal transport sites. The peripheral dopamine receptor antagonist domperidone, used at a dose of 20 mg taken half an hour before the levodopa, can also be effective in controlling levodopa-induced nausea and vomiting. Domperidone also increases levodopa absorption from the gut by improving gastric emptying. Gastric motility and competition by neutral amino acids in the diet influence the absorption of levodopa from the duodenum.[115] There are no hard and fast rules for initiating treatment with levodopa. A suggested regime for initiating levodopa treatment in older frail patients is shown in Table 52-6.

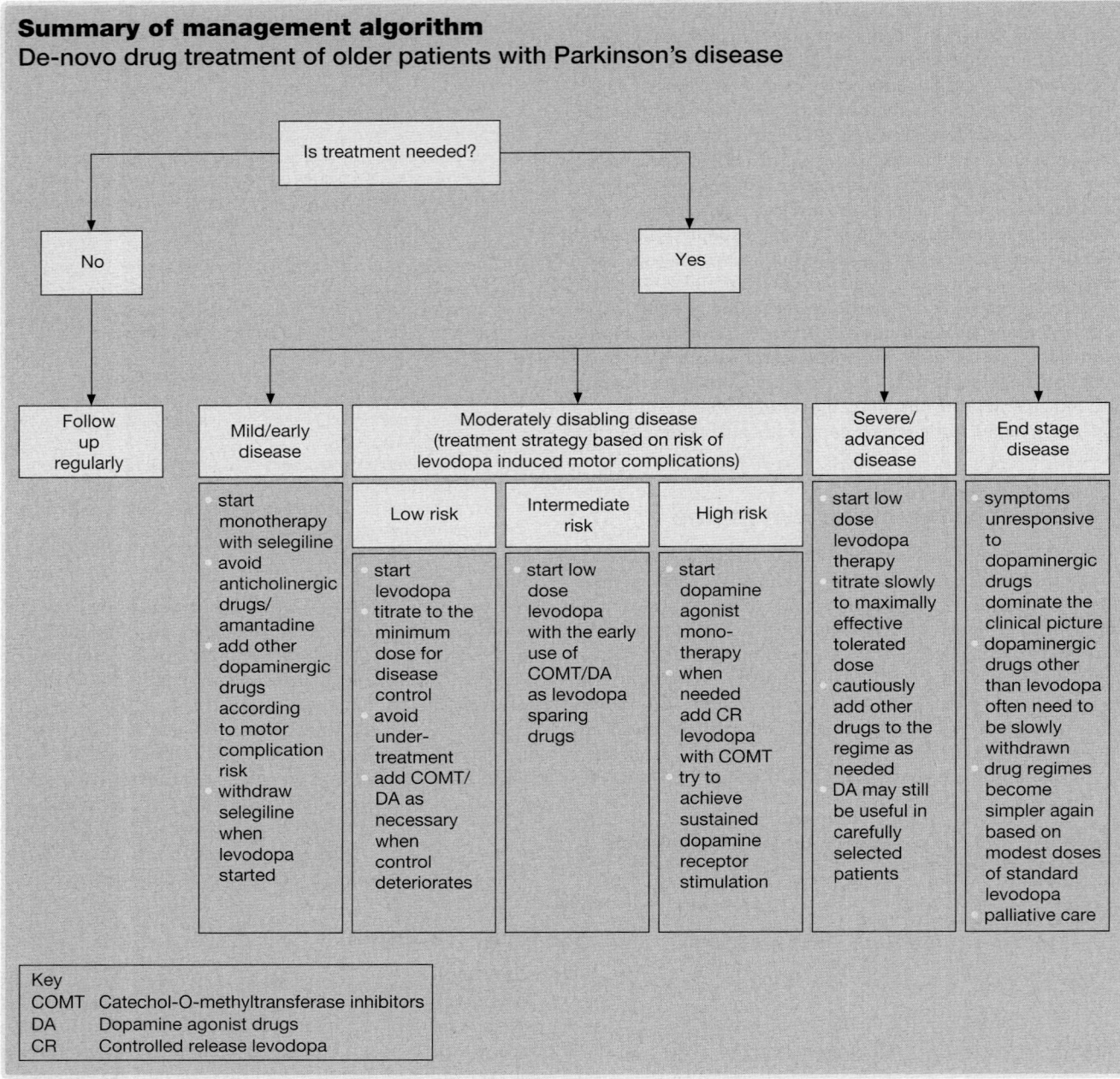

Summary of management algorithm

De-novo drug treatment of older patients with Parkinson's disease

Is treatment needed?

No → Follow up regularly

Yes

Mild/early disease
- start monotherapy with selegiline
- avoid anticholinergic drugs/ amantadine
- add other dopaminergic drugs according to motor complication risk
- withdraw selegiline when levodopa started

Moderately disabling disease (treatment strategy based on risk of levodopa induced motor complications)

Low risk
- start levodopa
- titrate to the minimum dose for disease control
- avoid under-treatment add COMT/ DA as necessary when control deteriorates

Intermediate risk
- start low dose levodopa with the early use of COMT/DA as levodopa sparing drugs

High risk
- start dopamine agonist mono-therapy when needed add CR levodopa with COMT
- try to achieve sustained dopamine receptor stimulation

Severe/ advanced disease
- start low dose levodopa therapy
- titrate slowly to maximally effective tolerated dose
- cautiously add other drugs to the regime as needed
- DA may still be useful in carefully selected patients

End stage disease
- symptoms unresponsive to dopaminergic drugs dominate the clinical picture
- dopaminergic drugs other than levodopa often need to be slowly withdrawn
- drug regimes become simpler again based on modest doses of standard levodopa
- palliative care

Key
COMT   Catechol-O-methyltransferase inhibitors
DA   Dopamine agonist drugs
CR   Controlled release levodopa

Although there is no convincing evidence that levodopa accelerates disease progression, it seems sensible to use the minimum dose of levodopa that leads to an acceptable health-related quality of life for the patient. Many frail patients are unable to tolerate a maximally therapeutic dose of levodopa due to side-effects of nausea and vomiting, postural dizziness, drowsiness, and confusion. Conversely, on presentation to specialists, many elderly patients are undertreated with levodopa, and the first stage in management is often to gently increase levodopa dosage and closely monitor the response. In drug-naive patients it is important to clearly document the response to a 6-week period of adequate levodopa treatment as this can help to clarify the clinical diagnosis and can also give some indication of the likely degree of the future control of the disease.

Delayed release and dispersible preparations

Formulations of delayed or controlled release (CR) levodopa have been developed in conjunction with dopa decarboxylase inhibitors (Sinemet 50/200 CR™, Sinemet 25/100 Half CR™, Madopar CR™). These preparations can lead to a longer duration of action of levodopa and this can be particularly useful in treating "wearing off" motor fluctuations and nocturnal problems that occur over the first few hours of the night.[116] The use of these preparations, although presumably resulting in more sustained and physiological stimulation of striatal dopamine receptors, does not in clinical practice appear to reduce the prevalence of levodopa-associated motor fluctuations and dyskinesias.[117,118] Dispersible forms of levodopa taken in a small volume of water (Madopar Dispersible™) have a more rapid onset of action than conventional levodopa and can be useful in rescuing patients from sudden "off" periods, in treating PD symptoms occurring on waking in the night and in patients with dysphagia.[119]

Levodopa-induced fluctuations and dyskinesia

Chronic levodopa treatment can induce disabling motor fluctuations and dyskinesias.[120–122] Sensory, psychic, cognitive, and autonomic fluctuations can also occur. The mechanisms behind these effects are poorly understood but presumably arise from the abnormal pulsatile stimulation of dopamine receptors resulting from standard drug treatment.[123,124] Pulsatile receptor stimulation could lead to dysregulation of basal ganglia genes and proteins, such as preproencephalin and dynorphin, and the induction of abnormal neuronal discharge in the basal ganglia output nuclei. The half-life of levodopa is only 1–1.5 hours and this may explain why levodopa is so commonly associated with these problems. Longer acting dopaminergic drugs appear to be less likely to cause these problems. Recent clinical studies have shown that motor fluctuations and dyskinesias can be significantly reduced in patients treated with dopamine agonist monotherapy compared with levodopa alone as the initial treatment.[125] Motor complications were also lower in a group of patients in whom levodopa was added to dopamine agonist treatment to improve efficacy compared to levodopa alone.

Clinical impressions suggest that motor fluctuations and dyskinesia are common after five years or so of levodopa exposure. The DATATOP study in 352 de-novo patients reported a prevalence of 50 percent for motor fluctuations and 33 percent for dyskinesia after only a mean of 20 months levodopa exposure.[126] However, a study in 618 patients on levodopa treatment reported motor complications in only 22 percent of the study group overall after nearly 5 years of follow-up.[117] This difference may reflect methodological differences between the two studies in the definitions of motor complications. Factors governing the risk of levodopa-induced complications appear to be the age of the patient at presentation, disease severity, and the dose and duration of levodopa treatment. Young patients presenting before 60 years old appear to be at particular risk of these problems. Older patients appear to be at lower risk of levodopa-induced motor fluctuations and dyskinesia than younger patients, apart from possibly mild "wearing off." The reduced risk in older patients does not appear to result simply from lower exposure to levodopa in terms of dosage and duration of levodopa treatment. Severity of disease is important; monkeys rendered severely parkinsonian by the neurotoxin MPTP rapidly develop severe dyskinesia when exposed to levodopa, and in the rare cases of MPTP parkinsonism in man, similar findings have also been observed. A strong case can be made for delaying the use of levodopa in patients at high risk of developing complications.[127]

COMT inhibition—entacapone

Only the catechol-*O*-methyl transferase (COMT) inhibitor entacapone is currently licensed for use in the UK.[128] Entacapone given at a dose of 200 mg with each daily dose of levodopa prevents the peripheral metabolism of levodopa and increases the uptake of levodopa in the brain. Entacapone increases the area under the concentration–time curve by around 35 percent. A total of 603 patients worldwide have been treated with entacapone in Phase III randomized controlled trials. Entacapone has been shown to increase the duration of the clinical response to both standard and controlled release levodopa.[129–132] These studies have also shown that in patients with motor fluctuations, "on" time was increased and "off" time decreased. Time "off" is generally reduced by around 10–30 percent. Entacapone use allows for a reduction in levodopa dosage of around 12 percent. Entacapone also appears to benefit nonfluctuating patients, though thus far this has been reported only in abstract form. This finding could be highly relevant, if confirmed in other studies, to the use of this drug in older patients, most of whom will be nonfluctuators. Two long-term safety studies confirm that entacapone is well tolerated.[133,134] Entacapone can cause nausea and vomiting, dyskinesias, discoloration of the urine, and diarrhea. The COMT inhibitor tolcapone was recently withdrawn in Europe due to safety issues relating to fatal hepatic toxicity. There is no evidence of any similar risk with entacapone.

MAO-B inhibition—selegiline (deprenyl)

The selective and irreversible monoamine-oxidase B (MAO-B) inhibitor selegiline prevents the breakdown of endogenous dopamine in the brain and has modest direct antiparkinsonian effects. Selegiline at a dose of 5–10 mg daily (possibly 2.5–5 mg in older patients) combined with levodopa is modestly effective in reducing motor fluctuations and improving disability scores, and is levodopa sparing, allowing for a mean reduction in levodopa dose of 20–50 percent.[126,135–137] Despite theoretical neuroprotective activity there is no evidence in man that selegiline delays the progression of clinically evident PD. In the UKPDRG study of 782 patients with early mild disease randomized openly to levodopa, levodopa plus selegiline, or bromocriptine, the combination of levodopa and selegiline was associated with an increased mortality.[138,139] Observational data in general practice in the UK also revealed a small excess mortality in patients on selegiline alone.[140] However, other large long-term studies involving selegiline such as the DATATOP did not observe any excess mortality with selegiline.[141] A possible explanation may lie in the different types of patients recruited to these studies. Older frailer patients appear to have been entered into the UKPDRG study and there was a small excess of sudden deaths, dementia, and falls in the selegiline arm of the study. It seems prudent to avoid the combination of selegiline and levodopa in older patients with cognitive impairment or a history of falls and syncope.[142] A sublingual form of selegiline (Zelaphar™) that results in more stable plasma levels of selegiline with fewer active metabolites is now available. Any advantage over conventional selegiline in older patients remains to be determined.

Dopamine agonists

Six orally active dopamine agonists are now available to treat PD. These include the ergot-derived agonists bromocriptine, lisuride, pergolide, and carbergoline, and the nonergoline agonists ropinirole and pramipexole. In the UK, lisuride and bromocriptine are now rarely used compared with other agonists. Dopamine agonists are being increasingly used either as initial monotherapy or as adjunctive treatment to levodopa.[143–148] In patients with motor fluctuations, studies show that dopamine agonists can reduce "off" time by around 30–50 percent.[149–151]

All dopamine agonists act primarily by stimulating dopaminergic postsynaptic D2 receptors and do not require presynaptic uptake or further metabolism by the surviving nigrostriatal neurons. Some of these drugs also interact with D1 and D3 receptors. Commonly used dopamine agonists have a long duration of action and half-life ranging from ropinirole at 6–8 hours to cabergoline at more than 24 hours. Unfortunately, dopamine agonists are associated with more side-effects than levodopa, particularly in older frailer patients. Agonists can cause nausea and vomiting, drowsiness, headache (sometimes described more as muzziness in the head), postural hypotension, hallucinations, and confusion. Less common side-effects are erythromelalgia, a painful red edema of the lower legs, and reversible pulmonary changes and pleural effusions with the ergot-derived agonists. A baseline chest radiograph is a wise precaution in older patients before starting ergot-derived dopamine agonist drugs. Agonist drugs are usually initiated using special starting packs, as the dose titration over several weeks tends to be quite complex. For many older patients the advised dose titrations are still too rapid and the "start low and go slow" approach is strongly recommended in this patient group.

The role of agonist therapy in older patients is still unclear.[152,153] Physiologically fit and cognitively intact subjects in this age group could reasonably be considered for an initial trial of agonist monotherapy. However, older patients need to be selected with great care before embarking on a trial of agonist therapy as an adjunct to levodopa. Evidence of cognitive impairment or a history of previous levodopa-induced confusion, hallucinations, or sleep disruption indicates that the benefit from the adjunctive use of agonist drugs in this situation is likely to be outweighed by the risk of serious side-effects. A further issue is that although initially tolerated with good benefit in older patients the lifespan of these drugs may be limited at most to six months to a year before side-effects necessitate withdrawal. The clinically useful comparison to help guide therapy in patients with motor fluctuations of agonists vs COMT inhibitors has not yet been reported. Restless legs and nocturnal cramps can be helped by long-acting dopamine agonists such as cabergoline.

Apomorphine

Apomorphine is a particularly valuable and underused, though relatively expensive, dopamine agonist that is currently administered subcutaneously by intermittent injection or continuous infusion. Like levodopa, apomorphine stimulates both D1 and D2 receptors and the magnitude, though not the duration, of the motor response to these two drugs appears to be very similar.[154] Administered by intermittent injection apomorphine has a rapid onset but short duration of action but can be used to rescue patients from distressing motor (immobility, rigidity, tremor) and nonmotor (including sleep disturbance, pain, dyspnea, anxiety, depression, panic, dystonia) symptoms refractory to oral medication. Severe nausea and vomiting is commonly induced by apomorphine and can be controlled by pretreatment for a few days with oral or rectal domperidone 20–30 mg three times daily. The long-term use of apomorphine results in the development of nodules at the injection site in nearly all patients. These nodules can become painful, and rarely break down into ulcers with secondary infection. This is usually only seen in patients on continuous infusions, but can occur with intermittent injection regimes. Rotation of injection sites, massage of the skin before and after injection, reduction of apomorphine dose, and good injection technique can reduce the incidence of complicated nodules.

Continuous administration by pump over the waking hours can decrease "off" time by around 50–70 percent and can also reduce levodopa-induced dyskinesias[155] and neuropsychiatric side-effects. The benefit from apomorphine is maintained over 5 years' follow-up.[156] In addition to open studies,[157,158] the reduction in "off" time has been demonstrated in two recent double-blind placebo-controlled studies. The mean age of patients in all these studies has been around 60 years old.

Elderly frail patients with advanced disease who still appear to get reasonable benefit from their oral drugs for at least some period of the day should be considered for a trial of apomorphine therapy.[159] Hypotension and drowsiness can limit the use of the drug in this situation and predominantly nondopaminergic symptoms such as dysarthria, freezing, and postural imbalance will not be improved by this approach. Apomorphine can be life saving over times such as elective and emergency surgery when oral antiparkinsonian drugs cannot be given. Older patients with disabling disease should probably have a trial of continuous apomorphine infusion before considering neurosurgical intervention.

Other nondopaminergic drug approaches

The progression of PD over time leads to a range of other disabling symptoms that are not usually responsive, and indeed are often exacerbated by dopaminergic drug treatment. Cognitive impairment, depression, anxiety, and symptoms of autonomic dysfunction commonly develop and can usefully be improved in some patients by using a wide range of pharmacological and nondrug interventions. Depression can respond well to selective serotonin reuptake inhibitors such as sertraline[160,161] and citalopram, and low-dose buspirone can help anxiety. Excessive sweating may be controlled by betablockers in some subjects.[162] Postural hypotension that does not improve after simple measures can be managed by the careful use of fludrocortisone.[163] Domperidone can also be useful in this situation. Levodopa-induced neuropsychiatric complications including hallucinations, delusions, and delirium may respond to atypical neuroleptic drugs such as clozapine, olanzapine, and quetiapine started at very low dose and slowly increased.[164–166] Further research evidence is needed to determine whether acetylcholinesterase inhibitors such as rivastigmine and donepezil are useful to treat cognitive impairment in PD.

Drug strategies

Early treatment strategies

The degree to which the disease is interfering with health-related quality of life, not always as easy to determine as it sounds, is probably the yardstick on which early treatment decisions are made by the patient and physician. Although there is no evidence of any drug treatment delaying disease progression, some individuals may elect to start treatment with antioxidants such as vitamins E and C, and possibly the drug selegiline, prior to the development of any handicap.

The most effective drug in relieving motor impairment at all stages of the disease is levodopa. However, as discussed above, after some years of treatment levodopa can cause motor fluctuations and dyskinesias. In subjects felt to be at risk of levodopa-induced complications it seems prudent to start with a long-acting dopamine agonist in order to provide more physiological, continuous dopamine receptor stimulation.[123,124] Due to the reduced efficacy of agonist drugs compared with levodopa and disease progression after a time, nearly all patients will require the addition of levodopa. The agonist studies have demonstrated that only around 30 percent of subjects remain on monotherapy after 3 years of treatment. To pursue the concept of continuous stimulation further it may be sensible to add low-dose levodopa in a controlled release formulation with the additional early use of a COMT inhibitor to improve disease control. To date there is no research-based evidence for this approach.

In patients who have a low risk of levodopa-induced complications the use of levodopa as first-line treatment is usually justified. At first diagnosis, older patients are often already significantly disabled by the disease and may have a reduced life expectancy due to other comorbidities. In this group of patients the dose of levodopa should be titrated to achieve the best possible control of symptoms regardless of levodopa dose. The problems in this group of patients are often poor tolerance of levodopa and a reduced motor response to levodopa.

The best way to initiate treatment in patients presenting with an intermediate risk of long-term levodopa problems is unknown. Treatment could follow the lines for high-risk patients or a decision may be made to commence treatment with low-dose levodopa but to add other agents such as dopamine agonists, selegiline or COMT inhibitors from the outset to act as levodopa-sparing agents. A third approach would be to prescribe higher initial doses of levodopa with the addition of other drugs only as necessary to improve disease control. There are no comparative studies available to show which of these strategies is best at minimizing both the impact of the disease on quality of life and the risk of fluctuations and dyskinesia.

Drug strategies in established disease

As the disease progresses the drug treatment needs to be altered on an individual patient basis to maintain optimal control of symptoms, even in the absence of motor fluctuations. Due to increasing disability, levodopa may need to be commenced in patients in whom the introduction of levodopa has been delayed by the use of dopamine agonists, selegiline or other drugs. In patients already on levodopa the dose of this drug often has to be gently increased in an attempt to maintain benefit. The effectiveness of this approach is unclear. Controlled/delayed release or dispersible formulations of levodopa can be added to or used to replace some of the regime of standard levodopa. The addition of other agents such as COMT/MAO-B inhibitors, or dopamine agonist drugs can also be useful. The combination of the MAO-B inhibitor selegiline with levodopa has raised safety issues as discussed above.

In complex disease, when motor fluctuations and dyskinesias have developed, the dose of levodopa should be reduced to the minimum needed to control the disease and levodopa-sparing agents such as dopamine agonist drugs and COMT inhibitors should be added to the treatment. More frequent doses of levodopa can also be prescribed in this situation but rarely benefit the patient for long and may result in worsening peak dose dyskinesia as well as increasing the burden of frequent tablet taking. The motor fluctuation of "wearing off"/"end-of-dose deterioration" can respond well to the use of controlled/delayed release levodopa, to the addition of COMT/MAO-B inhibitors, or to dopamine agonist drugs. Other types of sudden and less predictable "on/off" motor fluctuations may also respond to this approach. Early morning painful "off" dystonia, usually of the feet, can be improved by long-acting agonists. Fluctuations in nonmotor symptoms (pain, autonomic, sensory, and psychic) and refractory motor "off" periods indicate the need for a trial of apomorphine. Sudden "freezing" episodes do not appear to respond to drug manipulations.

Drug strategies in advanced disease and palliative care

With time, disabling symptoms develop that come to dominate the clinical picture and do not respond to dopaminergic drug treatment. These include dementia, postural imbalance, dysarthria, and dysphagia. Falls become increasingly common, drooling is often a major source of embarrassment and social handicap, and difficulties in communication are common. At this stage in the disease weight loss can be quite marked and appears out of proportion to the difficulties in nutrition caused by dysphagia, and occurs despite apparent adequate intake. Patients at this stage usually become less tolerant of dopaminergic drugs and the insidious onset and development of cognitive impairment results in drug-induced hallucinations, confusion, and psychosis. A common early sign of intolerance of levodopa is drug-induced drowsiness. Drug treatment at this stage is largely limited by the presence and extent of cognitive impairment. All medication needs to be reviewed, and any drugs with anticholinergic activity or known to cause confusion should be slowly withdrawn. Amantadine, selegiline, and dopamine agonist drugs tend to be poorly tolerated at this stage. Finally, if problems persist the dose of levodopa may also have to be reduced and a balance found between mental clarity and mobility.

In advanced stages of the disease, drug regimes often need to be simplified using low doses of standard formulation levodopa to try to maintain mobility as far as possible. Dispersible levodopa can be given by nasogastric tube. Severe rigidity may on occasion respond to intermittent apomorphine used at critical times of the day. Patients approaching the stage of palliative care will often be resident in nursing homes, particularly if cognitive impairment is advanced. The primary care team supported by the PD nurse specialist will need to work closely together to optimize treatment at this time. Pain can be a significant problem in some patients and again may respond to apomorphine. A clear management plan needs to be developed to deal with issues such as the use of antibiotics, the provision of artificial hydration and feeding, cardiopulmonary resuscitation, and the appropriateness of transfer to acute medical facilities.

Nonmotor problems

Depression

The most common neuropsychiatric complication of PD is depression.[167] Studies in hospital-based and community populations using standardized criteria for both depression and PD suggest that the prevalence of depression is around 40 percent,[168–170] though much lower figures have also been reported.[171,172] A complex relationship exists between depression and the disease variables of age at onset, cognitive impairment, and the pattern and severity of motor involvement. It is likely that depression has its origin both in the neurobiology of the disease and in the "reactive" psychological response to a progressive neurological disease. However, motor disability is not strongly linked to depression and the treatment of motor disability with antiparkinsonian drugs is not usually associated with resolution of coexisting depressive symptoms. Depression in PD may be linked to more severe loss of cells in the mesocorticolimbic dopaminergic projection.

There have been only four double-blind studies of the drug treatment of depression in PD, spanning over 30 years, and involving a total of around 100 patients of all ages.[173–176] However, these studies taken together with other studies suggest that drug treatment is effective in the treatment of depression in this disease. The selective serotonin reuptake inhibitors (SSRIs) are better tolerated than tricyclic antidepressant drugs in elderly subjects and are effective in treating depression in PD. Fluoxetine and paroxetine may very rarely cause drug-induced parkinsonism.[177,178] Aggressive treatment of depression in patients with PD may be an important method of reducing carer burden and distress.

Dementia

Dementia is common in patients over the age of 65 years with PD though prevalence figures vary from 10–44 percent depending on the diagnostic criteria used for dementia, PD, and the nature of the study population.[168,179–181] The risk of developing dementia is at least doubled in patients compared to age matched subjects without this disease. The risk of dementia increases exponentially with age such that 65 percent of surviving members of a cohort of patients with this disease over the age of 85 years old are likely to be demented.[182] Depression, cognitive impairment, and age interact in a complex manner and most studies have shown depression to be a risk factor for subsequent dementia.[183] Risk factors for dementia apart from age and depression have been shown to be: late onset disease, postural imbalance and gait disorder subtype, severe motor deficits, rapid progression of PD, and severe facial akinesia/hypomimia.[48,184–187]

Elderly patients with dementia predating parkinsonism by at least 1 year should probably be considered to have a primary dementia, such as Alzheimer's disease (AD), or dementia with Lewy bodies complicated by parkinsonism. Parkinsonism predating dementia by at least 1 year can be considered to be "PD with dementia." In this situation dementia can arise from the same causes as for primary dementia as well as from typical brainstem Lewy-body pathology. The clinicopathological basis of dementia in patients with PD is poorly understood. The striking relationship of age to the risk of dementia in PD indicates the importance of aging changes, Alzheimer-type pathology and cerebrovascular disease.

There remains considerable uncertainty over the nosology of the condition called dementia with Lewy bodies.[188–191] The primary finding at postmortem in this condition is of plentiful Lewy bodies in the limbic areas of the temporal lobe and other cortical areas. Lewy bodies may also be present in subcortical regions. The pathology in older patients with this condition is nearly always complicated by the additional presence of senile plaques and neurofibrillary tangles similar or identical to those found in AD. This condition is variously felt to be an extension of PD,[192,193] to be a type of AD,[194] or to represent a specific type of primary Lewy-body disease.[195]

Psychosis

Acute confusional states, sleep abnormalities, hallucinations, and paranoid delusions are common in PD.[196–198] A classification of psychosis has recently been suggested which emphasizes the distinction between psychosis with and without coexisting delirium and dementia.[199]

Although all antiparkinsonian drugs can provoke these reactions, anticholinergic drugs, dopamine agonists, and selegiline appear to cause problems much more commonly than levodopa itself. Simple hallucinosis that does not distress the patient or carer may be tolerated without reduction in drug treatment.[200] Atypical neuroleptic drugs such as clozapine or olanzapine that act on limbic rather than striatal dopamine receptors may be useful in selected patients to specifically control dopaminometic psychosis and allow a larger dose of levodopa to be prescribed to preserve mobility.[164–166]

Autonomic function

Autonomic function is impaired in older patients with PD. The extent of autonomic failure compatible with a diagnosis of PD has not been established, though the development of severe symptoms of autonomic dysfunction in a patient with parkinsonism within 2 years of the onset of symptoms suggests a true diagnosis of multiple system atrophy.

Postural hypotension was detected in nearly 60 percent of a group of patients attending a specialist clinic[201] and is most commonly drug induced.[142] Postural hypotension should initially be treated by simple measures. Critical review of all prescribed medications can suffice to control symptoms. If this fails, a change in antiparkinsonian drug therapy may be necessary. Occasionally, drugs such as fludrocortisone (0.1 mg to 1 mg per day) and nonsteroidal anti-inflammatory drugs are needed.

Bladder symptoms of urge, urge incontinence, frequency, and distressing nocturia are common. These problems result from bladder detrusor muscle hyperreflexia coupled with abnormalities of the external urethral sphincter. There is still uncertainty about how often urinary dysfunction reflects a specific disease-related urinary dysfunction as opposed to the effects of aging on the bladder and external sphincter.[202] Urological examination of the patient is necessary before embarking on treatment and this should include a rectal examination, a urinary flow rate, and a bladder ultrasound scan to determine residual volume. The anticholinergic drug tolterodine can improve nocturia and urge incontinence though side-effects can be a problem. It is rare for bladder symptoms to be so severe so as to require the use of intermittent self-catheterization or in-dwelling catheters. Immobility, poor diet, drug therapy, poor pelvic floor contractions and autonomic dysfunction with delayed transit time all contribute to the problem of constipation.[203,204] Constipation needs to be managed vigorously to avoid the development of fecal impaction. Loss of the gastrocolic reflex due to constipation may also impair levodopa absorption by delaying gastric emptying. Exercise and a good fluid intake are important aspects of bowel maintenance, though in most patients aperients will also be required.

Balance and falls

Impaired balance with an increasing risk of falls is an ominous development in older patients.[205] The pathogenesis of impaired postural reflexes is unknown but may involve neurotransmitter systems other than dopamine as well as age related changes in the brain and peripheral nervous system. The risk of fracture is additionally increased in PD as the result of reduced bone mineral density.[206,207] More research is needed to explore the apparent poor outcome of surgery following hip fracture.[208] Reducing antiparkinsonian drug treatment may prevent falls due to dyskinesias. The best approach to this problem is to adopt a general preventive strategy[209] coupled with exercise and physiotherapy.[210] Remediable problems with vision, foot care and the environment should be urgently addressed.

Sleep disturbances

Most elderly patients complain of disturbed nights though only around a third complain of poor quality of sleep.[211] In several instances careful questioning can reveal the cause to be due to motor problems (difficulty turning over in bed, painful leg cramps, dystonia, restless legs, leg jerks), more general musculoskeletal problems (back pain), nocturia, vivid dreams, visual hallucinations, and mental restlessness or depression. Difficulty settling down to sleep and restless legs syndrome may respond to dopaminergic treatment last thing at night (controlled release levodopa or a dopamine agonist). Other symptoms such as vivid dreams, dyskinesia and hallucinations may require a reduction in dopaminergic drug treatment later in the day. Hypnotics used every few days, or at most in weekly cycles separated by a fortnight may be justified. There is increasing evidence to suggest that sleep fragmentation is common in PD[212] and that there is a close association between rapid eye movement sleep (REM sleep) abnormalities, vivid dreams and the presence of dopaminergic drug-related hallucinations.[213] The condition of REM sleep behavior disorder is also now well described in PD and may respond well to small doses of clonazepam.[214]

Stereotactic neurosurgery

Stereotactic neurosurgery is becoming increasingly used as a treatment option in PD.[215] The major risks of surgery result from misplacing the lesion, hemorrhage and surgically induced cognitive impairment and depression. It is unclear how many older patients are likely to be suitable for stereotactic neurosurgical interventions as most of these procedures primarily improve drug-induced dyskinesia or improve "off" time in patients with motor fluctuations, neither of which is a common situation in patients with late onset disease. Additionally, cognitive impairment, which is the major contraindication to neurosurgery, is frequently already present in older patients. Many older patients have bilateral disabling disease and predominant axial symptoms for which unilateral lesioning procedures are unlikely to be helpful and bilateral procedures too risky. Furthermore, even in older patients with a good initial response, rapid disease progression may result in any benefit

from neurosurgery being short lived. However, carefully selected physiologically fitter older patients with longstanding disease or with disease starting in earlier old age who have a good objective response to oral medication may benefit from stereotactic neurosurgery and tolerate this procedure remarkably well.

Ablative lesions or deep brain stimulation in the thalamus can control tremor,[216,217] whereas drug-induced dyskinesia responds best to ventrolateral pallidotomy or stimulation.[218–220] However, surgery to the subthalamic nucleus can improve aknesia, rigidity, dystonia, and possibly drug-induced dyskinesia and axial symptoms.[221,222] Subthalamic bilateral deep brain stimulation is increasingly becoming the preferred option to treat this disease in younger patients, with pallidal stimulation being reserved for severe drug-induced dyskinesias. Deep brain stimulation carries a similar immediate risk to unilateral lesioning procedures but has a persistently increased longer term risk and is much more expensive than ablative procedures. The lesion induced by stimulation is reversible as opposed to the permanent nature of ablative procedures. In older patients there would be no risk of side-effects from misplaced ablative lesions, and patients with a good response to stimulation could always later convert to a permanent ablative procedure. Older patients should not be denied access to brain stimulation based on age alone. Exactly when referral in older people should take place is unclear, though a current pilot study of early vs delayed subthalamic stimulation may help answer this question. The long time taken in optimizing drug treatment in older patients over many clinic visits may result in surgical approaches becoming inappropriate due to the progressive cognitive impairment typical of disease in older people. Neurotransplantation with fetal or human transformed cell lines combined with trophic factors remains an experimental but promising prospect for the future.[223] Less encouragingly, results from the first randomized controlled trial of fetal transplantation in 40 patients, using a control arm of sham surgery, suggest that this procedure led to serious side-effects in 15 percent of subjects and only appeared to benefit patients less than 60 years old.[224] The transplantation protocol used by the researchers may have accounted for some of the study's disappointing and worrying results. Gene therapy for PD is a rapidly developing field that may lead in time to new treatment options.[225]

Prognosis in PD

Patients and their families faced with the diagnosis of PD are understandably concerned about what the future holds for them in terms of keeping independent and minimizing disability. As with every chronic progressive disease it is difficult to predict accurately an individual's prognosis. In older people the prognosis may be determined more by concurrent morbidity. The length of time PD symptoms have been present before medical diagnosis is also an important factor. Prognosis needs to be based on a detailed clinical assessment, the physician's clinical experience and judgment and the application of research based evidence. One large prospective clinical study of drug treatment in PD indicated that disability scores based on clinical assessment scales tended to return to pretreatment levels by 4 years of follow-up.[138] This study recruited 782 patients who mostly had mild disease, though it is unclear how long symptoms had been present before study entry. The mean age of patients in this study was around 62 years old.

The UPDRS score of subjects requiring the addition of levodopa in the DATATOP study increased by around 7 points per year over the 3-year follow-up, most of the increase being due to deterioration in the motor subscale.[126] A total of 273 (34 percent) out of the original 800 patients recruited in this study needed to start levodopa treatment after 1 year follow-up. Clinical features associated with more rapid disease progression and a poor prognosis include older age at onset, impaired cognitive function, dominant akinesia–rigidity, and postural imbalance.[48,49] In the absence of poor prognostic features most older patients at diagnosis could reasonably be told to expect a period of 5–6 years of good disease control. Deteriorating cognitive function is likely to determine health-related quality of life more than advancing motor impairment.

Other causes of parkinsonism

Parkinsonism can arise from several causes (Fig. 52-3) though these, with the exception of drug-induced parkinsonism, are much rarer than PD. Even though PD is the commonest cause of parkinsonism, accounting overall for around 70 percent of cases, this proportion falls with increasing age. In young patients presenting with parkinsonism, Wilson's disease must always be excluded by measurement of serum copper and caeruloplasmin levels and, when necessary, urinary copper excretion.[226]

Drug-induced parkinsonism

The most common form of secondary parkinsonism, largely due to the use of neuroleptic (dopamine blocking) drugs in the treatment of serious mental illness, is drug-induced parkinsonism (DIP).[227,228] A total of 32 percent of a series of patients with parkinsonism referred to a neurology clinic were found to have DIP. Older patients, especially women, have increased risk of DIP and may inadvertently be prescribed neuroleptic drugs to treat dizziness (prochloperazine) and gastric upset (metoclopramide). Other non-neuroleptic drugs such as the calcium channel blocker cinnarazine, tetrabenazine, and very rarely lithium, fluoxetine, paroxetine, and amiodarone can cause DIP. Clinically, DIP is indistinguishable from PD. Over 90 percent of cases tend to develop within 3 months of starting the offending drug. After withdrawal of the drug, signs of parkinsonism may take several months to resolve. In some older patients the signs never resolve and careful monitoring reveals the subsequent development of PD. Presumably subclinical PD was "brought on" by the neuroleptic drug. Persisting parkinsonism after neuroleptic withdrawal may also result from the inhibition of mitochondrial complex 1. The treatment of DIP involves whenever possible stopping the causative drug. When this is not possible, anticholinergic medication can help control symptoms, as can amantadine. The value of levodopa is uncertain as it can worsen the mental condition for which the neuroleptic drug may have been originally prescribed and may be ineffective due to the dopamine receptor blockade.

Parkinsonism-plus

Several rare multisystem degenerative conditions, such as progressive supranuclear palsy,[229,230] multiple system atrophy,[231,232] and corticobasal degeneration,[233,234] can present with parkinsonism. Early in the clinical history these conditions can be difficult to distinguish from PD. With time, certain clinical features develop which can help in making the correct diagnosis. However, even at death the diagnostic accuracy for PD in expert hands is at best only around 76 percent.[29] Neuroimaging with CT and MRI can sometimes help in the diagnosis, though this is usually only in advanced disease. Positron emission tomography is helpful in establishing the nature of parkinsonism, though in practice is restricted to being a research tool.[235,236] The response to treatment can also be misleading as both progressive supranuclear palsy and multiple system atrophy can initially respond moderately well to levodopa. Warning signs suggesting the possibility of parkinsonian-*plus* disease are a poor response to levodopa, poor tolerance of levodopa, striking asymmetry of motor signs, early onset of dementia, the presence of pyramidal or cerebellar signs, early onset of falls, rapidly deteriorating mobility, severe autonomic disturbance, and evidence of progressive supranuclear gaze abnormalities. Mild parkinsonism in association with early hallucinations, fluctuant confusion, transient loss of consciousness, and marked sensitivity to neuroleptic drugs would suggest a diagnosis of dementia with Lewy bodies.[237]

Alzheimer's disease

Extrapyramidal signs are a common feature of this disease and parkinsonism is an increasingly well-recognized clinical feature, though the presence of significant cognitive impairment at this time might suggest this diagnosis. Alzheimer-type pathology was the commonest cause of misdiagnosis of PD in one clinicopathological study. Dopaminergic drugs are unlikely to help parkinsonism in association with Alzheimer's disease and are poorly tolerated.

Vascular parkinsonism

Parkinsonism can result from vascular disease of the brain presenting with gait apraxia, truncal ataxia, relative sparing of the upper limb, and absence of tremor.[238–240] A history of hypertension and of other vascular risk factors is often present, and brain imaging usually shows widespread deep white matter ischemic changes. Rarely, infarcts within the basal ganglia can give rise to a condition indistinguishable from PD. The use of DaTSCAN-SPECT may be useful in this situation.

HYPERKINETIC MOVEMENT DISORDERS

Essential tremor

Essential tremor (ET) is the most common involuntary movement disorder and usually presents as a longstanding bilateral persistent postural tremor involving the hands and forearms.[1,241,242] A kinetic tremor is often also present. The head, voice, and legs may also be involved with decreasing frequency. In around a half of cases a family history of similar tremor also exists, as does a temporary improvement of tremor after alcohol. Although usually annoying and embarrassing ET can also result in severe disability and handicap. The prevalence of ET increases with age reaching a crude figure of 39.2/1,000 individuals over the age of 65 years old.[243]

ET is commonly misdiagnosed as PD and is also sometimes confused with dystonic and drug-induced tremor. Dystonic tremor can be easily confused with ET though it tends to be more jerky in nature and is often associated with subtle dystonic posturing of the head.[244] Sometimes a trial of treatment is needed to help distinguish between these two conditions. Head tremor is rare in PD, though jaw tremor is not infrequently found. The distinction between ET and PD in older subjects is made more difficult as a resting tremor can occur in ET and tremor dominant PD can be associated with a postural, rather than resting tremor. A trial of drug therapy may again be needed. In this situation diagnostic difficulty may be resolved by the use of DaTSCAN-SPECT.[40] The prevalence of PD in patients with ET appears to be slightly higher than that expected by chance alone, though this could reflect the diagnostic difficulties in relation to postural tremors.

The treatment of ET is disappointing, though many patients obtain some benefit from beta-adrenergic drugs such as propranolol or the anticonvulsant primidone. Side-effects especially in older subjects limit the usefulness of these drugs. Severe cases of ET may respond to repeated botulinum toxin injections or bilateral thalamic stimulation. Primary orthostatic tremor, a fast palpable but not visible tremor of the thigh and calf, should also be recognized as a rare cause of unsteadiness on standing.[245]

Dystonia

Dystonia is a movement disorder typified by sustained muscle contractions giving rise to twisting and repetitive movements and abnormal postures.[246] Dystonia can present as a specific disorder, such as idiopathic generalized dystonia or the focal dystonia of writer's cramp, or can be a part of the spectrum of abnormal movements found in other diseases such as PD. Dystonia can result from chronic exposure to neuroleptic drugs (tardive dystonia) or as an acute reaction to these drugs. Other drugs, especially levodopa, can also cause dystonia. Most cases of idiopathic generalized dystonia present in childhood or early adult life. In older patients, dystonia most commonly presents as task-specific dystonia such as writer's cramp, blepharospasm, torticollis, dystonic head tremor, laryngeal dystonia, and cranial dystonia. Blepharospasm commonly presents in later life and when severe may respond to botulinum toxin injections. Blepharospasm can also complicate progressive supranuclear palsy and PD. Dystonia can respond to high-dose anticholinergic medication, though older patients tolerate this poorly.

Chorea

The rapid, often jerky, nonrepetitive and dance-like movements that typify chorea are not uncommonly seen in older subjects and require a diagnosis rather than the label of "senile chorea." Drugs are a common cause of this condition, particularly neuroleptics giving rise to tardive chorea. Levodopa also commonly causes choreiform dyskinesias. In older people, chorea can also result from subcortical vascular lesions. Hemiballismus, a high-amplitude form of usually unilateral chorea involving the arm and leg and occasionally the trunk, is seen in older patients as a result of infarction or hemorrhage in the region of the subthalamic nucleus. This movement disorder when severe can be life threatening but is usually self-limiting and responds to neuroleptic drugs and tetrabenazine. Late-onset Huntington's disease must always be excluded.[247] In this situation, chorea is usually associated with cognitive impairment. The diagnosis can be confirmed by genetic testing for evidence of an expanded cytosine–adenosine–guanine (CAG) repeat sequence on the short arm of chromosome four.[248] Other rare causes of chorea include systemic lupus erythematosis, neuroacanthocytosis, polycythaemia rubra vera, hyperthyroidism, and electrolyte disturbances. Orobuccal-lingual choreiform dyskinesia is not uncommon in studies of nursing home residents who have never been exposed to neuroleptic drugs and appears to be related to loss of teeth and failure to wear dentures.[249]

Restless legs syndrome

The condition of unpleasant deep sensory disturbances in the legs associated with irresistible leg movements on trying to get to sleep increases in prevalence with age.[250,251] Subjects with these symptoms usually also have abnormal leg movements in the early stages of pre-REM sleep. Restless legs syndrome occurs in many other neurological diseases as well as in medical conditions such as anemia and renal failure and in response to certain drugs such as lithium and tricyclic antidepressants. This condition can respond to levodopa, dopamine agonist drugs, clonazepam, and codeine.

Drug-induced movement disorders

Drugs commonly cause involuntary movements, usually as a result of the indiscriminate and inappropriate use of neuroleptic drugs in older people.[252,253] A wide range of other

---

> ### KEY POINTS Parkinsonism and other movement disorders
>
> - The prevalence of essential tremor, parkinsonism, and drug-induced movement disorders increases significantly with age.
>
> - Movement disorders in older people often remain undetected and undiagnosed.
>
> - The accurate diagnosis of movement disorders in older people is often difficult and individuals in whom such a diagnosis is considered should be referred for specialist assessment.
>
> - Accurate diagnosis, comprehensive assessment and careful documentation of the response to treatment are key factors in the successful long-term management of these disorders.
>
> - Drugs used to treat movement disorders are usually associated with significant side-effects but polypharmacy and complex treatment regimes are often needed to control symptoms.
>
> - Cognitive impairment, depression, and autonomic dysfunction often leads to considerable handicap and limits the usefulness of drug therapy in Parkinson's disease.

drugs have been linked usually by isolated case reports in the literature to involuntary movements, though it is often difficult to evaluate the clinical significance of such reports. In addition to parkinsonism and acute dystonic reactions, neuroleptics can also cause a wide range of tardive movement disorders including an intense and distressing motor restlessness called akathisia.[254] Neuroleptic malignant syndrome can result from the introduction or increase in dose of a neuroleptic drug or from sudden reduction in dopaminergic drug treatment for PD.[255] This syndrome consists of fever, intense rigidity, confusion, autonomic disturbance and involuntary movements. Rigidity elevates the muscle enzyme creatinine phosphokinase and rhabdomyolysis can develop with associated renal failure. Mortality from this condition can be high. A similar condition, the toxic serotonin syndrome, can result from the combination of a selective serotonin reuptake inhibitor with a monoamine oxidase inhibitor. Many drugs, including lithium, sodium valproate, amiodarone, tetrabenazine, amphetamine, tricyclic antidepressants, and beta agonists can cause tremor. Chorea can result from the use of estrogens, lithium, amphetamine, and myoclonus from tricyclic antidepressants and chlorambucil.

REFERENCES

1. Khatter AS, Kurth MC, Brewer MA et al: Prevalence of tremor and Parkinson's disease. Park Rel Disord 1996;2(4):205–208
2. Carpenter MB: Anatomy of the corpus striatum and brainstem integrating systems. In Brooks VB (ed): Handbook of Physiology, Sect. 1, 2(2). Williams and Wilkins, Baltimore, 1981:947–995
3. Graybeil AM: The basal ganglia. Trends Neurosci 1995;18:60–62
4. Williams PL, Warwick R: Functional Neuro-anatomy of Man. Churchill Livingstone, Edinburgh, 1975
5. Alexander GE, DeLong MR, Strick PL: Parallel organization of functionally segregated circuits linking basal ganglia and cortex. Ann Rev Neurosci 1986;9:357–381
6. Alexander GE, Crutcher MD: Functional architecture of basal ganglia circuits: neural substrates of parallel processing. Trends Neurosci 1990;13:266–271
7. Graybiel AM: Neurotransmitters and neuromodulators in the basal ganglia. Trends Neurosci 1990;13:244–254
8. DeLong MR: Primate models of movement disorders of basal ganglia origin. Trends Neurosci 1990;13:281–285
9. Elble RJ: Motor control and movement disorders. In Jankovic J, Tolosa E (eds): Parkinson's Disease and Movement Disorders. Williams and Wilkins, Baltimore, 1998:15–46
10. McRae A: Neurotransmitters and pharmacology of the basal ganglia. In Jankovic J, Tolosa E. (eds): Parkinson's Disease and Movement Disorders. Williams and Wilkins, Baltimore, 1998:47–66
11. Crossman AR, Sambrook MA: Neural Mechanisms in Disorders of Movement. John Libby, London, 1989
12. Crossman AR: Primate models of dyskinesia: the experimental approach to the study of basal ganglia-related involuntary movement disorders. Neuroscience 1987;21:1–40
13. Albin RL, Young AB, Penney JB: The functional anatomy of basal ganglia disorders. Trends Neurosci 1989;12:366–375
14. Albin RL: The pathophysiology of chorea/ballism and parkinsonism. Park Rel Disord 1995;1:3–11
15. Rajput AH, Offord KP, Beard C et al: Epidemiology of parkinsonism: incidence, classification and mortality. Ann Neurol 1984;16:278–282
16. Morgante L, Rocca WA, Di Rosa AE, et al: Prevalence of Parkinson's disease and other types of parkinsonism: a door-to-door survey in three Sicilian municipalities. Neurology 1992;42:1901–1907
17. Meara RJ, Bhowmick BK, Hobson JP: Accuracy of diagnosis in patients with presumed Parkinson's disease in a community-based disease register. Age Ageing 1999;28:99–102
18. Ben-Shlomo Y: How far are we in understanding the cause of Parkinson's disease? J Neurol Neurosurg Psychiatry 1996;61:4–16
19. Marsden CD: The mysterious motor function of the basal ganglia. Neurology 1982;32:514–539
20. Quinn NP: Parkinson's disease: clinical features. In Quinn NP (ed): Parkinsonism. Ballière's Clinical Neurology; 6: 1. Ballière Tindall, London, 1997:1–14
21. Jellinger K: Overview of morphological changes in Parkinson's disease. Adv Neurol 1986;45:1–18
22. Forno LS: Neuropathology of Parkinson's disease. J Neuropathol Exp Neurol 1996;55:3:259–272
23. Gibb WRG, Lees AJ: Anatomy, pigmentation, ventral and dorsal subpopulations of the substantia nigra, and differential cell death in Parkinson's disease. J Neurol Neurosurg Psychiatry 1991;54:388–396
24. Gibb WRG, Scott T, Lees AJ: Neuronal inclusions of Parkinson's disease. Mov Disord 1991;6:2–11
25. Lennox GG, Lowe JS: Dementia with Lewy bodies. In Quinn NP (ed): Parkinsonism. Ballière's Clinical Neurology; 6: 1. Ballière Tindall, London, 1997:147–166
26. Hughes AJ, Daniel SE, Blankson S et al: A clinicopathological study of 100 cases of Parkinson's disease. Arch Neurol 1993;50:140–148
27. Agid Y, Javoy-Agid F, Ruberg M: Biochemistry of neurotransmitters in Parkinson's disease. In Marsden CD, Fahn S (eds): Movement Disorders 2. Butterworths, London, 1987:166–230
28. Hughes AJ, Daniel SE, Kilford L, Lees AJ: Accuracy of clinical diagnosis of idiopathic Parkinson's disease: a clinicopathological study of 100 cases. J Neurol Neurosurg Psychiatry 1992;55:181–184
29. Delwaide PJ, Gonce M: Pathophysiology of Parkinson's signs. In Jankovic J, Tolosa E (eds): Parkinson's Disease and Movement Disorders. Williams and Wilkins, Baltimore, 1998:159–176
30. DeLong MR, Georgopoulos AP: Motor functions of the basal ganglia. In Brooks VB (ed): Handbook of Physiology, 1, 2, 2. Williams and Wilkins, Baltimore, 1981:1017–1061
31. Bergman H, Wichmann T, Delong MR: Reversal of experimental parkinsonism by lesions of the subthalamic nucleus. Science 1990;249:1436–1438
32. Meara RJ, Cody FWJ: Relationship between electromyographic activity and clinically assessed rigidity studied at the wrist joint in Parkinson's disease. Brain 1992;115:1167–1180
33. Hua S, Reich SG, Zirh AT et al: The role of the thalamus and basal ganglia in parkinsonian tremor. Mov Disord 1998;13(suppl 3):40–42
34. Limousin P, Pollak P, Benazzouz A et al: Effect on parkinsonian signs and symptoms of bilateral subthalamic nucleus stimulation. Lancet 1995;345:91–95
35. Quinn N: Parkinsonism—recognition and differential diagnosis. Br Med J 1995;310:447–452
36. Martila RJ, Rinne UK: Epidemiology of Parkinson's disease in Finland. Acta Neurol Scand 1976;53:81–102
37. Rosati G, Granieri E, Pinna L et al: The risk of Parkinson disease in Mediterranean people. Neurology 1980;30:250–255
38. Graneiri E, Carreras M, Govoni V et al: Parkinson's disease in Ferrara, Italy, 1967 through 1987. Arch Neurol 1991;48:854–857
39. Mayeux R, Marder K, Cote LJ et al: The frequency of idiopathic Parkinson's disease by age, ethnic group, and sex in Northern Manhattan, 1988–1993. Am J Epidemiol 1995;142:820–827
40. Benamer HTS, Patterson J, Grosset DG et al: Accurate differentiation of parkinsonism and essential tremor using visual assessment of [123I]-FP-CIT SPECT imaging. Mov Disord 2000;15:503–510
41. Rajput AH, Rozdilsky B, Rajput A: Accuracy of clinical diagnosis in parkinsonism—a prospective study. Can J Neurol Sci 1991;18:275–278
42. Ansorge O, Lees AJ, Daniel SE: Update on the accuracy of clinical diagnosis of idiopathic Parkinson's disease. Mov Disord 1997;12(suppl 1):S96
43. Zetusky WJ, Jankovic J, Pirozzolo FJ: The heterogeneity of Parkinson's disease: Clinical and prognostic implications. Neurology 1985;35:522–526
44. Goetz CG, Tanner CM, Stebbins GT et al: Risk factors for progression in Parkinson's disease. Neurology 1988;38:1841–1844
45. Gibb WRG, Lees AJ: A comparison of clinical and pathological features of young and old-onset Parkinson's disease. Neurology 1988;38:1402–1406
46. Diamond SG, Markham CH, Hoehn MM et al: Effect of age at onset on progression and mortality in Parkinson's disease. Neurology 1989;39:1187–1190
47. Friedman A: Old-onset Parkinson's disease compared with young-onset disease: clinical differences and similarities. Acta Neurol Scand 1994;89:258–261

48. Jankovic J, McDermott M, Carter J et al: Variable expression of Parkinson's disease: A base-line analysis of the DATATOP cohort. Neurology 1990;40:1529–1534

49. Tanner CM, Kinoria I, Goetz CG et al: Age at onset and clinical outcome in idiopathic Parkinson's disease. J Neurology 1985;232:S25

50. Lilienfeld DE, Chan E, Ehland J et al: Two decades of increasing mortality from Parkinson's disease among the US elderly. Arch Neurol 1990;47:731–734

51. Zhang Z-X, Roman GC: Worldwide occurrence of Parkinson's disease: an updated review. Neuroepidemiology 1993;12:195–208

52. de Rijk MC, Tzourio C, Breteler MMB et al: Prevalence of parkinsonism and Parkinson's disease in Europe: the EUROPARKINSON collaborative study. J Neurol Neurosurg Psychiatry 1997;62:10–15

53. D'Alessandro R, Gamberini G, Graniere F et al: Prevalence of Parkinson's disease in the Republic of San Marino. Neurology 1987;37:1679–1682

54. Baldereschi M, Di Carlo A, Rocca WA et al: Parkinson's disease and parkinsonism in a longitudinal study: two-fold higher incidence in men. Neurology 2000;55:1358–1363

55. Schoenberg BS, Anderson DW, Haerer AF: Prevalence of Parkinson's disease in the biracial population of Copiah County, Mississippi. Neurology 1985;35:841–845

56. Morgante L, Rocca WA, Di Rosa AE et al: Prevalence of Parkinson's disease and other types of parkinsonism: a door-to-door survey in three Sicilian municipalities. Neurology 1992;42:1901–1907

57. Clarke CE: Mortality from Parkinson's disease in England and Wales 1921–1989. J Neurol Neurosurg Psychiatry 1993;48:690–693

58. Moghal S, Rajput AH, Meleth R et al: Prevalence of movement disorders in institutionalised elderly. Neuroepidemiology 1995;14:297–300

59. Mitchell SL, Kiely DK, Kiel DP et al: The epidemiology, clinical characteristics and natural history of older nursing home residents with a diagnosis of Parkinson's disease. J Am Geriat Soc 1996;44:394–399

60. Tison F, Dartigues JF, Dubes L et al: Prevalence of Parkinson's disease in the elderly: a population study in Gironde, France. Acta Neurol Scand 1994;90:111–115

61. Goetz CG, Stebbins GT: Risk factors for nursing home placement in advanced Parkinson's disease. Neurology 1993;43:2227–2229

62. Goetz CG, Stebbins GT: Mortality and hallucinations in nursing home patients with advanced Parkinson's disease. Neurology 1995;45:669–671

63. Fearnley JM, Lees AJ: Ageing and Parkinson's disease: substantia nigra regional selectivity. Brain 1991;114:2283–2301

64. Golbe LI, Do Iorio G, Bonavita V et al: Autosomal dominant Parkinson's disease. Ann Neurol 1990;27:276–282

65. Maraganore DM, Harding AE, Marsden CD: A clinical and genetic study of familial Parkinson's disease. Mov Disord 1991;6:205–211

66. Langston JW, Ballard P, Tetrud JW et al: Chronic parkinsonism in humans due to a product of meperidine analog synthesis. Science 1983;219:979–980

67. Wood N: Genetic aspects of parkinsonism. In Quinn N (ed): Parkinsonism. Ballière's Clinical Neurology; 6: 1. Ballière Tindall, London, 1997:37–53

68. Bandmann O, Marsden CD, Wood NW: Genetic aspects of Parkinson's disease. Mov Disord 1998;13:203–211

69. Ben-Shlomo Y: The epidemiology of Parkinson's disease. In Quinn N (ed): Parkinsonism. Ballière's Clinical Neurology; 6: 1. Ballière Tindall, London, 1997:55–68

70. Polymeropoulos MH, Higgins JJ, Golbe LI et al: Mapping of a gene for Parkinson's disease to chromosome 4q21–q23. Science 1996;274:1197–1199

71. Polymeropoulos MH, Lavedan C, Leroy E et al: Mutation in the alpha-synuclein identified in families with Parkinson's disease. Science 1997;276:2045–2047

72. Saito M, Matsumine H, Tanaka H et al: Clinical characteristics and linkage analysis of autosomal recessive form of juvenile parkinsonism. Nippon-Rinsho 1997;55:83–88

73. Ward CD, Duvoisin RC, Ince SE: Parkinson's disease in 65 pairs of twins and in a set of quadruplets. Neurology 1983;33:815–824

74. Johnson WG, Hodge SE, Duvoisin R: Twin studies and the genetics of Parkinson's disease—a reappraisal. Mov Disord 1990;5:187–194

75. Semchuk KM, Love EJ, Lee RG: Parkinson's disease and exposure to agricultural work and pesticide chemicals. Neurology 1992;42:1328–1335

76. Marder K, Tang MX, Mejia H et al: The risk of developing Parkinson's disease among first-degree relatives: a community based study. Neurology 1996;47:155–160

77. Smith CA, Gough AC, Leigh PN et al: Debrisoquine hydroxylase gene polymorphism and susceptibility to Parkinson's disease. Lancet 1992;339:1375–1377

78. Armstrong M, Daly AK, Chalerton S et al: Mutant debrisoquine hydroxylation genes in Parkinson's disease. Lancet 1992;339:1017–1018

79. Shapira AHV: Evidence for mitochondrial dysfunction in Parkinson's disease—A critical appraisal. Mov Disord 1994;9:125–138

80. Davis GC, Williams AC, Markey SP et al: Chronic parkinsonism secondary to intravenous injection of meperidine analogues. Psych Res 1979;1:249–254

81. Dexter DT, Wells FR, Lees AJ et al: Increased nigral oxygen content and alterations in other metal ions occurring in brain in Parkinson's disease. J Neurochem 1989;52:1830–1836

82. Sian J, Dexter DT, Lees AJ et al: Alterations in glutathione levels in Parkinson's disease and other neurodegenerative disorders affecting the basal ganglia. Ann Neurol 1994;36:348–355

83. Semchuk KM, Love EJ, Lee RG: Parkinson's disease: a test of the multifactorial etiologic hypothesis. Neurology 1993;43:1173–1180

84. Seidler A, Hellenbrand W, Robra BP et al: Possible environmental, occupational and other etiologic factors for Parkinson's disease: a case-control study in Germany. Neurology 1996;46:1275–1284

85. Cerhan JR, Wallace RB, Folsom AR: Antioxidant intake and risk of Parkinson's disease (PD) in older women. Am J Epidemiol 1994;139:S65

86. Doll R, Peto R, Wheatley K et al: Mortality in relation to smoking: 40 years' observations on male British doctors. Br Med J 1994;309:901–911

87. Wang SJ, Fuh JL, Teng EL et al: A door-to-door survey of Parkinson's disease in a Chinese population in Kinmen. Arch Neurol 1996;53:66–71

88. Ben-Shlomo Y: Smoking and neurodegenerative diseases. Lancet 1993;342:1239

89. Riggs JE: Cigarette smoking and Parkinson disease: the illusion of a neuroprotective effect. Clin Neuropharmacol 1992;15:88–99

90. Koller WC: When does Parkinson's disease begin? Neurology 1992;42:27–31

91. Rubenstein LZ, Stuck AE, Siu AL et al: Impacts of geriatric evaluation and management programs on defined outcomes: overview of the evidence. J Am Geriat Soc 1991;39(Suppl):8–16

92. Stuck AE, Siu AL, Wieland GD et al: Comprehensive geriatric assessment: a meta-analysis of controlled trials. Lancet 1993;342:1032–1036

93. Fahn S, Elton RL et al: Unified Parkinson's disease rating scale. In Fahn S, Marsden CD, Calne DB, Goldstein M (eds): Macmillan Health Care Information, New Jersey, 1987:153–164

94. Richards M, Marder K, Cote L et al: Interrater reliability of the Unified Parkinson's Disease Rating Scale motor examination. Mov Disord 1994;9:89–91

95. Hoehn MM, Yahr MD: Parkinsonism: onset, progression and mortality. Neurology 1967;17:427–442

96. Schwab RS, England AC: Projection technique for evaluating surgery in Parkinson's disease. In Gillingham FJ, Donaldson MC (eds): Third Symposium on Parkinson's disease. Livingstone, Edinburgh, 1969:152–157

97. D'Ath P, Katona P, Mullan E et al: Screening, detection and management of depression in elderly primary care attenders. 1: The acceptability and performance of the 15 item Geriatric Depression Scale (GDS-15) and the development of short versions. Fam Pract 1994;11:260–265

98. Folstein MF, Folstein SE, McHugh PR: Mini mental state: a practical guide for grading the mental state of patients for the clinician. J Psych Res 1975;12:189–198

99. Roth M, Tym E, Mountjoy CQ et al: CAMDEX: A standardized instrument for the diagnosis of mental disorder in the elderly with special reference to elderly detection of dementia. Br J Psychiatry 1986;149:698–709

100. Bowling A, Windsor J: Discriminative power of the health status questionnaire 12 in relation to age, sex, and longstanding illness: findings from a survey of households in Great Britain. J Epidemiol Commun Health 1997;51:564–573

101. de Boer AG, Wijker W, Speelman JD et al: Quality of life in patients with Parkinson's disease: development of a questionnaire. J Neurol Neurosurg Psychiatry 1996;61:70–74

102. Collin C, Wade DT, Davis S et al: The Barthel ADL index: a reliability study. Int Disab Stud 1988;10:61–63

103. Nouri FM, Lincoln NB: An extended activities of daily living scale for stroke patients. Clin Rehab 1987;1:301–305

104. Quinn N: Drug treatment of Parkinson's disease. Br Med J 1984;310:575–579

105. Oertel WH, Quinn NP: Parkinsonism. In Brandt T et al (eds): Neurological Disorders—Course and Treatment. Academic Press, San Diego, 1996:715–772

106. Zesiewicz TA, Hauser RA: The drug treatment of Parkinson's disease in elderly people. In Meara J, Koller WC (eds): Parkinson's Disease and Parkinsonism in the Elderly. Cambridge University Press, Cambridge, 2000:134–164

107. Olanow CW, Koller WC: An algorithm for the management of Parkinson's disease: treatment guidelines. Neurology 1998;50(suppl 3)

108. Bhatia K, Brooks DJ, Burn DJ et al: Guidelines for the management of Parkinson's disease. Hosp Med 1998;59:469–480

109. Meara J, Bhowmick BK: Parkinson's disease and parkinsonism in the elderly. In Meara J, Koller WC (eds): Parkinson's Disease and Parkinsonism in the Elderly. Cambridge University Press, Cambridge, 2000:22–63

110. Ward CD: Rehabilitation in Parkinson's disease. Rev Clin Geront 1992;2:254–268

111. Caird FI: Rehabilitation in Parkinson's Disease. Chapman and Hall, London, 1991

112. Ward CD: Rehabilitation in Parkinson's disease and parkinsonism. In Meara J, Koller WC (eds): Parkinson's Disease and Parkinsonism in the Elderly. Cambridge University Press, Cambridge, 2000:165–184

113. Comella CL, Stebbins GT, Brown-Toms N et al: Physical therapy and Parkinson's disease: a controlled clinical trial. Neurology 1994;44:376–378

114. Johnson JA, Pring TR: Speech therapy in Parkinson's disease: a review and further data. Br J Disord Commun 1990;25:183–194

115. Djaldetti R, Baron J, Ziv I et al: Gastric emptying in Parkinson's disease: patients with and without response fluctuations. Neurology 1996;46:1051–1054

116. Wolters EC, Tesselaar HJ: International (NL-UK) double-blind study of Sinemet CR and standard Sinemet (25/100) in 170 patients with fluctuating Parkinson's disease. J Neurol 1996;245:235–240

117. Block G, Liss C, Reines S et al: Comparison of immediate-release and controlled-release Carbidopa/Levodopa in Parkinson's disease. A multicenter 5-year study. Eur J Neurol 1997;37:23–27

118. Dupont E, Andersen A, Boas J et al: Sustained-release Madopar HBS compared with standard Madopar in the long-term treatment of de novo parkinsonian patients. Acta Neurol Scand 1996;93:14–20

119. Steiger MJ, Stocchi F, Bramante L et al: The clinical efficacy of single morning doses of levodopa methylester, dispersible Madopar and Sinemet plus in Parkinson's disease. Clin Neuropharmacol 1992;15:501–504

120. Marsden CD, Parkes JD: 'On-off' effects in patients with Parkinson's disease on chronic levodopa therapy. Lancet 1976;i:292–296

121. Lees AJ, Stern GM: Sustained low dose levodopa therapy in Parkinson's disease. A 3-year follow up. Adv Neurol 1983;37:9–15

122. Quinn NP, Critchley P, Marsden CD: Young onset Parkinson's disease. Mov Disord 1987;1:209–219

123. Nutt JG, Obeso JA, Stocchi F: Continuous dopamine-receptor stimulation in advanced Parkinson's disease. Trends Neurosci 2000;23(suppl):S109–S115

124. Olanow CW, Schapira AHV, Rascol O: Continuous dopamine-receptor stimulation in early Parkinson's disease. Trends Neurosci 2000;23(suppl):S117–S126

125. Rascol O, Brooks DJ, Korczyn AD et al: A five year study of the incidence of dyskinesia in patients with early Parkinson's disease who were treated with ropinirole or levodopa. N Engl J Med 2000;342:1484–1491

126. Parkinson Study Group: Impact of deprenyl and tocopherol treatment on Parkinson's disease in DATATOP subjects not requiring levodopa. Ann Neurol 1996;39:29–36

127. Poewe W: Should treatment of Parkinson's disease be started with a dopamine agonist? Neurology 1998;51(suppl 2):S21–S24

128. Nutt JG: Catechol-O-methyltransferase inhibitors for treatment of Parkinson's disease. Lancet 1998;351:1221–1222

129. Ruottinen HM, Rinne UK: Entacapone prolongs levodopa response in a one month double blind study in parkinsonian patients with levodopa related fluctuations. J Neurol Neurosurg Psychiatry 1996;60:36–40

130. Parkinson Study Group: Entacapone improves motor fluctuations in levodopa-treated Parkinson's disease patients. Ann Neurol 1997;42:747–755

131. Rinne UK, Larsen JP, Siden A et al: Entacapone enhances the response to levodopa in Parkinsonian patients with motor fluctuations. Nomecomt Study Group. Neurology 1998;51:1309–1314

132. Piccini P, Brooks DJ, Korpela K et al: The catechol-O-methyltransferase (COMT) inhibitor entacapone enhances the pharmacokinetic and clinical response to Sinemet CR in Parkinson's disease. J Neurol Neurosurg Psychiatry 2000;68:589–594

133. Myllyla VV and the Filomen Study Group: Long-term safety of entacapone as an adjunct to levodopa in non-fluctuating and fluctuating patients with Parkinson's disease. Mov Disord 1998;13(suppl 2):294

134. Poewe W, Deuschl G, Brandauer E, and the Celomen Study Group: The effect of entacapone in patients with Parkinson's disease (PD): an Austrian-German long-term multicentre study. Eur J Neurol 1999;6(suppl 3):194

135. Presthus J, Hajbe A: Deprenyl (selegiline) combined with levodopa and a decarboxylase inhibitor in the treatment of Parkinson's disease. Acta Neurol Scand 1983;95:127–133

136. Golbe LI, Lieberman AN, Muenter MD et al: Deprenyl in the treatment of symptom fluctuations in advanced Parkinson's disease. Clin Neuropharm 1988;11:45–55

137. Heinonen EH, Rinne UK: Selegiline in the treatment of Parkinson's disease. Acta Neurol Scand 1989;126:103–111

138. Lees AJ on behalf of the Parkinson's Disease Research Group of the United Kingdom: Comparison of therapeutic effects and mortality data of levodopa and levodopa combined with selegiline in patients with early, mild Parkinson's disease. Br Med J 1995;311:1602–1607

139. Ben Shlomo Y, Churchyard A, Head J et al: Investigation by Parkinson's Disease Research Group of the United Kingdom into excess mortality seen with combined levodopa and selegiline treatment in patients with early, mild Parkinson's disease: further results of randomised trial and confidential enquiry. Br Med J 1998;316:1191–1196

140. Thorogood M, Armstrong B, Nichols T et al: Mortality in people taking selegiline: observational study. Br Med J 1998;317:252–254

141. Parkinson Study Group: Mortality in DATATOP: a multicenter trial in early Parkinson's disease. Ann Neurol 1998;43:318–325

142. Churchyard A, Mathias CJ, Boonkongcheun P et al: Autonomic effects of selegiline: possible cardiovascular toxicity in Parkinson's disease. J Neurol Neurosurg Psychiatry 1997;63:228–234

143. Parkinson's Disease Research Group in the United Kingdom: Comparisons of therapeutic effects of levodopa, levodopa and selegiline, and bromocriptine in patients with early, mild Parkinson's disease: three year interim report. Br Med J 1993;307:469–472

144. Montastruc JL, Rascol O, Senard JM et al: A randomised controlled study comparing bromocriptine to which levodopa was later added, with levodopa alone in previously untreated patients with Parkinson's disease: a five year follow up. J Neurol Neurosurg Psychiatry 1994;57:1034–1038

145. Sethi KD, O'Brien CG, Hammerstad JP et al, for the Ropinirole Study Group: Ropinirole for the treatment of early Parkinson's disease. Arch Neurol 1998;55:1211–1216

146. Parkinson Study Group: Safety and efficacy of pramipexole in early Parkinson disease. A randomised dose-ranging study. JAMA 1997;278:125–130

147. Rinne UK, Bracco F, Chouza C et al and the PKDS009 Study Group: Early treatment of Parkinson's disease with cabergoline delays the onset of motor complications. Results of a double-blind levodopa controlled trial. Drugs 1998;55(suppl 1):23–30

148. Hutton JT, Koller WC, Ahlskog JE et al: Multicenter, placebo-controlled trial of cabergoline taken once daily in the treatment of Parkinson's disease. Neurology 1996;46:1062–1065

149. Inzelberg R, Nisipeanu P, Rabey JM et al: Double-blind comparison of cabergoline and bromocriptine in Parkinson's disease patients with motor fluctuations. Neurology 1996;47:785–788

150. Guttman M and the International Pramipexole-Bromocriptine Study Group: Double-blind comparison of pramipexole and bromocriptine treatment with placebo in advanced Parkinson's disease. Neurology 1997;49:1060–1065

151. Rascol O, Lees AJ, Senard JM et al: Ropinirole in the treatment of levodopa-induced motor fluctuations in patients with Parkinson's disease. Clin Neuropharmacol 1996;19:234–245

152. Hindle JV, Meara RJ, Sharma JC et al: Prescribing pergolide in the elderly—an open label study of pergolide in elderly patients with Parkinson's disease. Int J Geriat Psychopharmacol 1998;1:78–81

153. Shulman LM, Minagar A, Rabinstein A et al: The use of dopamine agonists in very elderly patients with Parkinson's disease. Mov Disord 2000;15:664–668

154. Kempster PA, Frankel JP, Stern GM et al: Comparison of motor response to apomorphine and levodopa in Parkinson's disease. J Neurol Neurosurg Psychiatry 1990;53:1004–1007

155. Colzi A, Turner K, Lees AJ: Continuous subcutaneous waking day apomorphine in the long term treatment of levodopa induced interdose dyskinesias in Parkinson's disease. J Neurol Neurosurg Psychiatry 1998;64:573–576

156. Hughes AJ, Bishop S, Kleedorfer B et al: Subcutaneous apomorphine in Parkinson's disease: Response to chronic administration for up to five years. Mov Disord 1993;8:165–170

157. van Laar T, Steur EN, Essink AWG et al: A double-blind study of the efficacy of apomorphine and its assessment in "off" periods in Parkinson's disease. Clin Neurol Neurosurg 1993;95:231–235

158. Ostergaard L, Werdelin L, Odin P: Pen injected apomorphine against off phenomena in late Parkinson's disease: a double-blind, placebo-controlled study. J Neurol Neurosurg Psychiatry 1995;58:681–687

159. Chaudhuri KR, Clough C: Subcutaneous apomorphine in Parkinson's disease. Br Med J 1998;316:641

160. Meara RJ, Bhowmick BK, Hobson JP: An open uncontrolled study of the use of sertraline in the treatment of depression in Parkinson's disease. J Serotonin Res 1996;4:243–249

161. Hauser RA, Zesiewicz TA: Sertraline for the treatment of depression in Parkinson's disease. Mov Disord 1997;12:756–759

162. Tanner CM, Goetz CG, Klawans HL: Paroxysmal drenching sweats in idiopathic parkinsonism: response to propanolol. Neurology 1985;35:918–921

163. Thomas JE, Schirger A, Fealey RD et al: Orthostatic hypotension. Mayo Clin Proc 1981;56:117–125

164. Wolters EC, Hurwitz TA, Make E et al: Clozapine in the treatment of parkinsonian patients with dopaminomimetic psychosis. Neurology 1990;40:832–834

165. Wolters EC, Jansen ENH, Tuynman HG et al: Olanzapine in the treatment of dopaminomimetic psychosis in patients with Parkinson's disease. Neurology 1996;47:1085–1087

166. Meltzer HY, Kennedy J, Dai J et al: Plasma clozapine levels and the treatment of L-dopa-induced psychosis in Parkinson's disease: A high potency effect of clozapine. Neuropsychopharm 1995;12:39–45

167. Cummings JL: Depression and Parkinson's disease: A review. Am J Psychiatry 1992;149:443–454

168. Tison F, Dartigues JF, Auriacombe S et al: Dementia in Parkinson's disease: A population-based study in ambulatory and institutionalized individuals. Neurology 1995;45:705–708

169. Tandberg E, Larsen JP, Aarsland D et al: The occurrence of depression in Parkinson's disease: a community-based study. Arch Neurol 1996;53:175–179

170. Meara RJ, Mitchelmore E, Hobson JP: Use of the GDS-15 geriatric depression scale as a screening instrument for depressive symptomatology in patients with Parkinson's disease and their carers in the community. Age Ageing 1999;28:35–38

171. Madeley P, Biggins CA, Mindham RHS: The psychiatry of Parkinson's disease. In Granville-Grossman K (ed): Recent Advances in Clinical Psychiatry. Churchill Livingstone, London, 1993:63–77

172. Brown RG, MacCarthy B: Psychiatric morbidity in patients with Parkinson's disease. Psychol Med 1990;20:77–87

173. Strang RR: Imipramine in treatment of parkinsonism: a double-blind placebo study. Br Med J 1965;2:33–34

174. Laitinen L: Desipramine in treatment of Parkinson's disease. Acta Neurol Scand 1965;45:109–113

175. Andersen J, Aabro E, Gulmann N et al: Anti depressive treatment in Parkinson's disease. A controlled trial of the effect of nortriptyline in patients with Parkinson's disease treated with L-dopa. Acta Neurol Scand 1980;62:210–219

176. Goetz CG, Tanner CM, Klawans HL: Buproprion in Parkinson's disease. Neurology 1984;34:1092–1094

177. Jiminez-Jiminez FJ, Tejeiro J, Martinez-Junquera G et al: Parkinsonism exacerbated by paroxetine. Neurology 1994;44:2406

178. Steur EN: Increase of parkinson disability after fluoxetine medication. Neurology 1993;43:211–213

179. Cummings JL: Intellectual impairment in Parkinson's disease: Clinical, pathologic, and biochemical correlates. J Geriat Psych Neurology 1988;1:24–36

180. Mayeux R, Denaro J, Hemenegildo N et al: A population-based investigation of Parkinson's disease with and without dementia. Arch Neurol 1992;49:492–497

181. Hobson JP, Meara J: The detection of dementia and cognitive impairment in a community population of elderly Parkinson's disease subjects by use of the CAMCOG neuropsychological test. Age Ageing 1999;28:39–43

182. Mayeux R, Chen J, Mirabello E et al: An estimate of the incidence of dementia in idiopathic Parkinson's disease. Neurology 1990;40:1513–1517

183. Troster AI, Paolo AM, Lyons KE et al: The influence of depression on cognition in Parkinson's disease: A pattern of impairment distinguishable from Alzheimer's disease. Neurology 1995;45:672–676

184. Ebmeier KP, Calder SA, Crawford JR et al: Clinical features predicting dementia in idiopathic Parkinson's disease: A follow-up study. Neurology 1990;40:1222–1224

185. Stern Y, Marder K, Tang MX et al: Antecedent clinical features associated with dementia in Parkinson's disease. Neurology 1993;43:1690–1692

186. Viitanen M, Mortimer JA, Webster DD: Association between presenting motor symptoms and the risk of cognitive impairment in Parkinson's disease. J Neurol Neurosurg Psychiatry 1994;57:1203–1207

187. Marder K, Tang MX, Cote L et al: The frequency and associated risk factors for dementia in patients with Parkinson's disease. Arch Neurol 1995;52:695–701

188. Okazaki H, Lipkin LE, Aronson SM: Diffuse intracytoplasmic ganglionic inclusions (Lewy type) associated with progressive dementia and quadriparesis in flexion. J Neuropathol Exp Neurol 1961;20:237–244

189. Kosaka K: Lewy bodies in cerebral cortex. Report of three cases. Acta Neuropathol 1978;42:127–134

190. Gómez-Tortosa E, Ingraham AO, Irizarry MC et al: Dementia with Lewy bodies. J Am Geriat Soc 1998;46:1449–1458

191. Holmes C, Cairns N, Lantos P et al: Validity of current clinical criteria for Alzheimer's disease, vascular dementia and dementia with Lewy bodies. Br J Psychiatry 1999;174:45–50

192. Gibb WRG, Esiri MM, Lees AJ: Clinical and pathological features of diffuse cortical Lewy-body disease (Lewy-body dementia). Brain 1985;110:1131–1153

193. Lieberman AN: Point of view: Dementia in Parkinson's disease. Park Rel Disord 1997;3:151–158

194. Weiner MF, Risser RC, Cullum CM et al: Alzheimer's disease and its Lewy-body variant: A clinical analysis of postmortem verified cases. Am J Psychiatry 1996;153:1269–1273

195. McKeith IG, Perry RH, Fairbairn AF et al: Operational criteria for senile dementia of Lewy-body type (SDLT). Psychol Med 1992;22:911–922

196. Celesia GG, Wanamaker WM: Psychiatric disturbances in Parkinson's disease. Dis Nerv System 1972;33:577–583

197. Nausieda PA, Glantz R, Weber S et al: Psychiatric complications of levodopa therapy of Parkinson's disease. Adv Neurol 1984;40:271–277

198. Factor SA, Mohlo ES, Podskalny GD et al: Parkinson's disease drug induced psychiatric states. Adv Neurol 1995;65:115–138

199. Peyser CE, Naimark D, Zuniga R et al: Psychoses in Parkinson's disease. Sem Clin Neuropsychiatry 1998;3:41–50

200. Haeske-Dewick HC: Hallucinations in Parkinson's disease: Characteristics and associated clinical features. Int J Geriat Psychiatry 1995;10:487–495

201. Senard JM, Rai S, Lapeyre-Mestre M et al: Prevalence of orthostatic hypotension in Parkinson's disease. J Neurol Neurosurg Psychiatry 1997;63:584–589

202. Gray R, Stern G, Malone-Lee J: Lower urinary tract dysfunction in Parkinson's disease: Changes relate to age and not disease. Age Ageing 1995;24:499–504

203. Edwards LL, Quigley EMM, Harned RK et al: Characterization of swallowing and defecation in Parkinson's disease. Am J Gastroent 1994;89:15–25

204. Byrne KG, Pfeiffer R, Quigley EMM: Gastrointestinal dysfunction in Parkinson's disease. J Clin Gastroent 1994;19:11–16

205. Klawans HL, Topel JL: Parkinsonism as a falling sickness. JAMA 1974;230,11:1555–1557

206. Johnell O, Melton J, Atkinson EJ et al: Fracture risk in patients with parkinsonism: A population-based study in Olmsted County, Minnesota. Age Ageing 1992;21:32–38

207. Taggart H, Crawford V: Reduced bone density of the hip in elderly patients with Parkinson's disease. Age Ageing 1995;24:326–328

208. Gialanella B, Mattioli F, D'Alessandro G et al: Prognosis of femur fractures in parkinsonian patients. In Agnoli A, Fabbrini G, Stocchi F (eds): Parkinson's disease and extrapyramidal disorders. J Libbey, London, 1990:591–594

209. Tinetti ME, Baker DI, McAvay G et al: A multifactorial intervention to reduce the risk of falling among elderly people living in the community. N Engl J Med 1994;331:821–827

210. Campbell AJ, Robertson MC, Gardner MM et al: Randomised controlled trial of a general practice programme of home based exercise to prevent falls in elderly women. Br Med J 1997;315:1065–1069

211. Lees AJ, Blackburn NA, Campbell VL: The nighttime problems of Parkinson's disease. Clin Neuropharm 1988;11:512–519

212. Nausieda PA, Glantz R, Weber S et al: Psychiatric complications of levodopa therapy of Parkinson's disease. Adv Neurol 1984;40:271–277

213. Comella CL, Tanner CM, Ristanovic RK: Polysomnographic sleep measures in Parkinson's disease patients with treatment-induced hallucinations. Ann Neurol 1993;34:710–714

214. Comella CL, Nardine TM, Diederich NJ et al: Sleep-related violence, injury, and REM sleep behaviour disorder in Parkinson's disease. Neurology 1998;51:526–529

215. Obeso JA, Guridi J, DeLong MR: Surgery for Parkinson's disease. J Neurol Neurosurg Psychiatry 1997;62:2–8

216. Tasker RR: Thalamotomy. Neurosurg Clin North Am 1990;1:841–864

217. Koller W, Pahwa R, Busenbark K et al: High-frequency unilateral thalamic stimulation in the treatment of essential and parkinsonian tremor. Ann Neurol 1997;42:292–299

218. Laitinen LV, Bergenhein T, Hariz MI: Leksell's posterventral pallidotomy in the treatment of Parkinson's disease. J Neurosurg 1992;76:53–61

219. Baron MS, Vitek JL, Bakay RAE et al: Treatment of advanced Parkinson's disease by posterior GPi pallidotomy: 1-year results of a pilot study. Ann Neurol 1996;40:335–336

220. Pahwa R, Wilkinson S, Smith D et al: High-frequency stimulation of the globus pallidus for the treatment of Parkinson's disease. Neurology 1997;49:249–253

221. Pollak P, Benabid AL, Limousin P et al: Chronic intracerebral stimulation in Parkinson's disease. Adv Neurol 1997;74:213–220

222. Limousin P, Krack P, Pollak P et al: Electrical stimulation of the subthalamic nucleus in advanced Parkinson's disease. N Engl J Med 1998;339:1105–1111

223. Freeman TB, Olanow CW, Hauser RA et al: Bilateral fetal nigral transplantation into the postcommissural putamen in Parkinson's disease. Ann Neurol 1995;38:379–388

224. Freed CR, Greene PE, Breeze RE et al: Transplantation of embryonic dopamine neurones for severe Parkinson's disease. N Engl J Med 2001;344:710–719

225. Kang UJ: Potential of gene therapy for Parkinson's disease: neurobiologic issues and new developments in gene transfer methodologies. Mov Disord 1988;13(suppl 1):59–72

226. Sternlieb I, Giblin DR, Scheinberg H: Wilson's disease. In Marsden CD, Fahn S (eds): Movement Disorders 2. Butterworths, London, 1987:288–302

227. Montastruc JL, Llau ME, Rascol O et al: Drug-induced parkinsonism: a review. Fund Clin Pharmacol 1994;8:293–306

228. Hubble JP: Drug induced parkinsonism in the elderly. In Meara J, Koller WC (eds): Parkinson's Disease and Parkinsonism in the Elderly. Cambridge University Press, Cambridge, 2000:64–79

229. Litvan I, Agid Y, Jankovic J et al: Accuracy of clinical criteria for the diagnosis of progressive supranuclear palsy (Steele–Richardson–Olszewski syndrome). Neurology 1996;46:922–930

230. Litvan I, Mangone CA, McKee A et al: Natural history of progressive supranuclear palsy (Steele–Richardson–Olszewski syndrome) and clinical predictors of survival: a clinicopathological study. J Neurol Neurosurg Psychiatry 1996;61:615–620

231. Quinn N: Multiple system atrophy—the nature of the beast. J Neurol Neurosurg Psychiatry 1989;52(suppl):S78–S89

232. Wenning GK, Ben-Shlomo Y, Magalhaes M et al: Clinical features and natural history of multiple system atrophy. An analysis of 100 patients. Brain 1994;117:835–845

233. Litvan I, Agid Y, Goetz C et al: Accuracy of the clinical diagnosis of corticobasal degeneration: a clinicopathological study. Neurology 1997;48:119–125

234. Rinne JO, Lee MS, Thompson PD, Marsden CD: Corticobasal degeneration. A clinical study of 36 cases. Brain 1994;117:1183–1196

235. Burn DJ, Sawle GV, Brooks DJ: Differential diagnosis of Parkinson's disease, multiple system atrophy, and Steele–Richardson–Olszewski syndrome: discriminant analysis of striatal ^{18}F-dopa PET data. J Neurol Neurosurg Psychiatry 1994;57:278–284

236. Sawle GV, Brooks DJ, Marsden CD et al: Corticobasal degeneration: A unique pattern of regional cortical oxygen metabolism and striatal flurodopa uptake demonstrated by positron emission tomography. Brain 1991;114:541–556

237. McKeith IG, Galasko D, Kosaka K et al: Clinical and pathological diagnosis of dementia with Lewy bodies (DLB): report of the CDLB international workshop. Neurology 1996;47:1113–1124

238. Thompson PD, Marsden CD: Gait disorder of subcortical arteriosclerotic encephalopathy: Binswanger's disease. Mov Disord 1987;2:1–8

239. Riley DE, Lang AE: Non-Parkinson akinetic-rigid syndromes. Curr Opin Neurol 1996;9:321–326

240. Liston R, Tallis RC: Gait apraxia and multi-infarct states. In Meara J, Koller WC (eds): Parkinson's Disease and Parkinsonism in the Elderly. Cambridge University Press, Cambridge, 2000:98–110

241. Jankovic J, Fahn S: Physiologic and pathologic tremors: Diagnosis, mechanism and management. Ann Intern Med 1980;93:460–465

242. Koller WC: Diagnosis and treatment of tremor. Neurol Clinics 1984;2:499–514

243. Pahwa R, Koller WC: Essential tremor in the elderly. In Meara J, Koller WC (eds): Parkinson's Disease and Parkinsonism in the Elderly. Cambridge University Press, Cambridge, 2000:80–97

244. Jedynak CP, Bonnet AM, Agid Y: Tremor and idiopathic dystonia. Mov Disord 1991;6:230–236

245. Heilman KM: Orthostatic tremor. Arch Neurol 1984;41:880–881

246. Fahn S, Marsden CD, Calne DB: Classification and investigation of dystonia. In Marsden CD, Fahn S (eds): Movement Disorders 2. Butterworths, London, 1987:332–358

247. Myers RH, Sax DS, Schoenfield M et al: Late onset Huntington's disease. J Neurol Neurosurg Psychiatry 1985;48:530–534

248. The Huntington's disease collaborative research group: A novel gene containing a trinucleotide repeat that is expanded and unstable in Huntington's disease chromosomes. Cell 1993;72:971–983

249. Woerner MG, Kane JM, Lieberman JA et al: The prevalence of tardive dyskinesia. J Clin Psychopharmacol 1991;1:34–42

250. Kreuger BR: Restless legs syndrome and periodic movements of sleep. Mayo Clin Proc 1990;65:999–1006

251. Walters AS, Hickey K, Maltzman J et al: A questionnaire study of 138 patients with restless legs syndrome: The "night-walkers" study. Neurology 1996;46:92–95

252. Weiner WJ, Lang AE: Drug Induced Movement Disorders. Futura Publishing, Mount Kisco, NY, 1992

253. Miller LG, Jankovic J: Drug-induced movement disorders: an overview. In Joseph AB, Young RR (eds): Movement Disorders in Neurology and Neuropsychiatry. Blackwell, Oxford, 1992:5–32

254. Jankovic J: Tardive syndromes and other drug induced movement disorders. Clin Neurophamacol 1995;18:197–214

255. Buckley PF, Hutchinson M: Neuroleptic malignant syndrome. J Neurol Neurosurg Psychiatry 1995;58:271–273

Chapter 53

Neuromuscular diseases including myasthenic disorders

Mark E. Roberts

Material in this chapter contains contributions from the previous edition, and we are grateful to the previous author for the work done.

Neuromuscular diseases are, worldwide, an important cause of disability at all ages.[1] This chapter focuses on anterior horn, muscle, and neuromuscular junction disorders that present in older patients. Given the increasing longevity of patients with inherited neuromuscular diseases, these are also briefly discussed. The general clinical approach is outlined, followed by a discussion of individual disorders and their treatment.

APPROACH TO THE PATIENT WITH NEUROMUSCULAR DISEASE

History

Weakness, manifest as an impairment of normal motor function, is the most common presenting symptom of neuromuscular disease. An accurate history documenting the onset, nature and pattern, and progression of weakness is crucial in differentiating diagnostic possibilities, and often requires several consultations with the patient and relatives.

Inquiries into sporting abilities, hobbies, occupational history, and national service often help time the onset of symptoms and aid distinction between common acquired and rare inherited muscle disorders presenting in elderly people. Many patients ascribe their neuromuscular symptoms to normal aging or painful conditions such as arthritis and directive questioning is often required. Questions such as "How far could you walk five years ago?", "When did you first use a stick?", and (in fitter patients) "When could you last run?" are useful since increasing weakness may be present for months and it is only the loss or impairment of some well-established task that brings weakness to the patient's attention.

The nature of weakness is often suggested by the history: difficulties reaching up to a shelf or combing hair suggest upper limb proximal weakness. Proximal lower limb weakness is suggested by difficulty in rising from a low chair, climbing stairs, and stepping up on to a train or bus. Primary neuromuscular disease rarely presents with falls, with the exception of inclusion body myositis (IBM) an inflammatory myopathy often associated with asymmetric quadriceps wasting and weakness which may present with "buckling" around the knees and falls.[2] Catching the foot on stairs or difficulty in depressing car pedals, in turning a key or opening a bottle are suggestive of distal weakness. In myasthenia gravis (MG), power may be reported as being normal at rest with (fatigable) weakness developing with exercise. Symptoms of MG often occur toward the end of the day. Speech and swallowing problems including coughing and choking after ingestion of solids or liquids, and unexplained recurrent pneumonia may suggest weakness of bulbar musculature. Weakness of the cervical muscles will often lead to a complaint of the head falling forward, and many patients will report the necessity of using the hand to support the head. Some patients with cervical muscle weakness present with neck ache reflecting prolonged and ineffectual voluntary attempts to keep the head up. While the causes of dyspnoea are protean, many neuromuscular disorders involve respiratory musculature, and this may be manifest as shortness of breath on exertion and especially on lying flat, due to diaphragmatic involvement. Other symptoms suggestive of neuromuscular hypoventilation include disrupted nocturnal sleep, daytime hypersomnolence and early morning muzziness and headache due to CO_2 retention with associated cerebral vasodilatation.[3]

Myalgia or muscle pain is a relatively nonspecific feature seen in the majority of patients with progressive muscular disease. Patients often find myalgia hard to describe and to differentiate from joint pain. Prominent myalgia is a feature of inflammatory myopathies, polymyalgia rheumatica, and in "metabolic myopathies." Occasionally myalgia is a presenting feature of muscular dystrophies such as fascioscapular humeral dystrophy. Proximal myotonic myopathy (PROMM), a recently recognized myotonic disorder with some similarities to Steinhert's disease, often presents with muscle pain and stiffness.[4] Painful nocturnal muscle cramps often reflect neurogenic diseases including motor neuron disease (MND). Alcohol and drugs, especially those that induce hypokalemia (e.g. diuretics), or those with a structural effect on muscle (e.g. the statins) may induce myalgia. Finally, myalgia may be a prominent symptom in patients with endocrine dysfunction (especially hypothyroidism and hypocalcemia) and those with connective tissue disorders such as systemic sclerosis.[5]

As patients rarely spontaneously report myoglobinuria, specific inquiry is required: the urine may be described as "Coca-Cola" colored. Myoglobinuria may occur in rare acute presentations of inflammatory myopathies, in metabolic muscle diseases such as McArdle's disease, and with drugs including statins and heroin. Myoglobinuria reflects rhabdomyolysis and recognition is important as renal failure can ensue.

Wide-ranging systemic inquiry is essential in patients with suspected neuromuscular disease, as myositis may be a component of many collagen vascular diseases. Myotonic dystrophy, and a related condition PROMM, are multisystem disorders whose manifestations are protean and include diabetes, cataracts as well as muscular weakness and wasting.[6] Cardiac involvement is common in many neuromuscular diseases with symptoms of arrhythmia and or ventricular dysfunction. Early morning headaches may reflect nocturnal hypoventilation. Prominent weight loss is a common feature in MND reflecting both poor nutritional state[7] and loss of muscle bulk.

Many of the neuromuscular diseases are inherited, and it is important therefore to inquire specifically about other family members, and where appropriate about consanguinity. Premature cardiac and respiratory deaths in family members may reflect complications of an inherited neuromuscular disease. It is often useful to examine first-degree relatives in a family suspected of having inherited neuromuscular disorder. The history may not suggest that the elderly relative is affected, whereas this can be confirmed by examination with its clear genetic implications for the wider family. Myotonic dystrophy, because of its marked variability in expression, and the presence of anticipation, may present in older patients with minor manifestations only (e.g. cataracts), compared with major symptoms in siblings.[6,8] The gene defect, which is an expansion of the trinucleotide repeat, is unstable and tends to be magnified from generation to generation particularly via the female line, leading to anticipation with earlier onset and more severe disease in successive generations.

Examination

The aim of examination of the neuromuscular system is to determine the distribution of muscle weakness and to assess its degree. Most acquired and inherited myopathic disorders present with proximal weakness and wasting (a limb girdle distribution). Selective patterns of muscle involvement may suggest facioscapulohumeral dystrophy (FSH), or one of the many subtypes of limb girdle muscular dystrophy, but confirmation relies on DNA and muscle biopsy studies. A scapuloperoneal distribution of weakness may reflect a myopathic disorder, such as FSH, or a neurogenic problem such as spinal muscular atrophy. Myasthenia gravis (MG) presents with a fatigable proximal weakness but without wasting. Lambert–Eaton myasthenic syndrome (LEMS) presents with a fatigable proximal weakness and wasting that can be hard to distinguish clinically from a myopathy. Distal weakness, with involvement of the forearm and hand muscles in the upper limb and the anterior and posterior tibial compartment in the lower limb, is commonly due to a peripheral neuropathy or MND but can be seen in myotonic dystrophy, in IBM, and in very rare distal forms of spinal muscular atrophy and distal myopathies. Weakness of neck flexion occurs in myopathic (e.g. myotonic dystrophy, inflammatory myopathy, FSH), neuromuscular junction (myasthenia gravis), and neurogenic (e.g. MND and Guillain–Barré syndrome) disorders. Paradoxical abdominal movements and indrawing of intercostal muscles on inspiration may indicate respiratory muscle and diaphragm weakness.

Having established the pattern of weakness, the symmetry of involvement is often a guide to the underlying etiology. In myopathic diseases (those involving the muscle fiber per se) symmetry is seen between right and left. In addition, around a joint, all of the muscles will be involved to about the same degree. IBM is a noteworthy exception to this useful general rule as asymmetric quadriceps involvement is common.[2] In neurogenic diseases, such as MND, asymmetry and unequal involvement around a joint are seen.

In primary muscle disorders, tone and reflexes are either normal or, reduced. Increased tone and reflexes should prompt diagnostic re-evaluation, and MND should be considered. Fasciculations are spontaneous involuntary visible worm-like muscle contractions and reflect motor unit instability. Fasciculations are not seen in muscle disease and rather reflect neurogenic disorders such as MND but also peripheral neuropathies where denervation is a feature. As it is seldom possible to differentiate myopathic and neurogenic on symptoms alone a careful search should be made for fasciculations in all patients presenting with neuromuscular weakness. Flicking a muscle may induce fasciculations in normal subjects and is best avoided. Clearly fasciculations may be missed if patients are not undressed fully, and the back, abdomen, and tongue should be inspected as well as the limbs. Difficulty is often encountered in observing fasciculations in the tongue; these are best seen with the tongue lying at rest in the floor of the mouth. Apparent fasciculation may be seen in the normal individual when the tongue is protruded due to anxiety and tongue tremor.

Myotonia (delayed relaxation) is an uncommon complaint in the older patient, and usually signifies myotonic dystrophy. Joint contractures are occasionally due to inherited muscle disease, but foot deformities such as pes cavus reflect very long-standing, usually genetic, peripheral neuropathies.

Investigations

It is rarely possible on the basis of history and examination to make an accurate diagnosis in the majority of cases of neuromuscular disease, not least because of the overlap in clinical signs between neurogenic and myopathic disorders. Confirmation of a neuromuscular diagnosis requires the application of electrophysiological, pathological, biochemical and , increasingly, DNA techniques.[9]

With several caveats, estimation of "muscle enzymes" is useful in patients with neuromuscular disease, and serum creatine kinase (CK) appears to be the most sensitive index of muscle necrosis as occurs in primary muscle necrosis, in polymyositis, but also in secondary myopathic change in longstanding denervation. The magnitude of CK levels give some indication of the nature of the pathology: in denervating conditions such as MND, CK levels are rarely above 1,000 IU/L, whereas they may increase 10, 100, or even 1,000-fold in patients with muscle disease, though clearly overlap occurs. However, CK levels must be interpreted with caution, as "muscle enzymes" are also found in other tissues. For example, CK consists of three separate isoenzymes: MM derived from skeletal muscle, MB derived largely from cardiac muscle, and BB derived mainly from brain. High CK levels may therefore be seen in patients with acute myocardial injury, and occasionally with hepatic disease, as well as in patients with muscle disease. Even so, given that the major isoenzyme of CK is MM, a high CK level is most likely to reflect neuromuscular disease.

Electrophysiology

A detailed description of electrophysiological techniques in the diagnosis of neuromuscular disease is outside the scope of this chapter but will be found in appropriate textbooks.[10] Nerve conduction studies, in which the conduction velocity and amplitudes of motor and sensory (compound) action potentials within peripheral nerves is measured, are used to detect primary pathology in peripheral nerves. The most common method of electrophysiological sampling of muscle is with concentric needle electromyography (CNEMG), which detects characteristic patterns that can be used to distinguish neurogenic and myopathic disorders. Normal muscle is electrically silent at rest. In neurogenic disorders positive sharp waves and fibrillation potentials are seen in CNEMG studies, and on activation a reduced interference pattern is seen reflecting the loss of motor neuron units (denervation). By contrast in myopathies CNEMG reveals small short-duration motor unit potentials. EMG studies may also reveal complex repetitive and myotonic (audible as a "dive bomber" sound) discharges useful in confirming myotonic disorders, and may suggest a previously unsuspected diagnosis such as PROMM where weakness predominates and myotonia is often subclinical.[4]

Repetitive nerve stimulation studies are useful in myasthenic disorders. In both MG and LEMS a decrement in compound muscle action potential response occurs at low frequency stimulation, which mirrors the clinical phenomenon of fatigable weakness. In LEMS a characteristic incremental response occurs with high frequency stimulation, which mirrors the clinical phenomenon of post-tetanic potentiation.[11] Single-fiber EMG (SFEMG) is useful in confirming a neuromuscular junction disorder, particularly in regional forms of MG.[12]

Muscle biopsy

Despite advances in biochemistry, neurophysiology, and genetics, the final diagnosis in patients with muscle disease can often only be made on muscle biopsy. The development of the technique of needle muscle biopsy,[13] which can be undertaken as an outpatient, has made possible one-stop diagnostic neuromuscular clinics with combined clinical, neurophysiological, and muscle sampling. Vastus lateralis, deltoid, and tibialis muscles are commonly biopsied, with care being taken to biopsy a muscle that is clinically affected but not too wasted for fear of seeing only end-stage pathology. Routine histological stains can be employed on both paraffin-embedded and fresh frozen material and permit comment on muscle fiber size, fiber morphology, and the presence or absence of inflammation. Other stains allow differentiation of muscle fiber types and can be used to study the distribution of cellular enzymes and metabolic reserves.[13] Immunohistochemistry on frozen muscle using antibodies directed against sarcolemmal muscle proteins such as dystrophin and the sarcoglycans are crucial in the diagnostic work-up of suspected dystrophinopathies and limb girdle muscular dystrophies and permit a more focused search for genetic abnormalities.[9] Western blotting techniques on muscle are often essential in confirming the suspicion of muscular dystrophies. Direct measurement of enzymic activity in fresh muscle is sometimes useful as in rare metabolic disease such as acid maltase disease, and in mitochondrial myopathies where respiratory chain enzymes can be assayed. Electron microscopy on muscle is useful in confirming suspected mitochondrial abnormalities

seen on light microscopy, and more especially to look for intracellular inclusions as occur in both inherited and acquired muscle disease. Muscle samples are hard to process, and orientate, and degrade rapidly—all of which combines to make the technique unsuitable for routine laboratories. Furthermore, interpretation of muscle biopsies and exclusion of artifactual change is difficult, and it is important therefore that muscle samples are sent to special neuromuscular laboratories or to an experienced pathology center. As percutaneous needle and punch biopsies are far less invasive than open procedures, it is often possible to follow temporal changes in a muscle disease and monitor response to treatment in individual patients using sequential biopsies.

INFLAMMATORY MYOPATHY

Inflammatory myopathy, or myositis, are among the most common muscle disorder presenting in elderly patients and can be subdivided into infective and idiopathic categories. Infective causes, including viral and bacterial pathogens, are the most common causes of myositis worldwide, but tend to be transient. Idiopathic inflammatory myopathies are a significant cause of chronic neuromuscular disease, and constitute a spectrum that includes polymyositis (PM), dermatomyositis (DM) and inclusion body myositis (IBM). PM and DM are related but distinct conditions and are discussed together first.

Etiology of PM and DM

Both PM and DM are autoimmune disorders, though the antigenic targets are ill defined. There is strong circumstantial evidence that PM is an autoimmune (AI) disorder: like most AI disorders, PM is more common in women; PM may arise or fluctuate in pregnancy; PM is often associated with other organ and nonorgan specific AI disorders; a PM phenotype can be triggered by viral illnesses (HIV and HTLV-1) or by certain drugs, especially D-penicillamine; PM responds to immunosuppression and modulation; finally, as further discussed below, muscle biopsies provide evidence of T-cell-mediated cytotoxic process directed against unknown muscle antigens. Similarly, DM is more common in women, may arise or

---

Summary of management algorithm
Inflammatory muscle disease

- *Clinical suspicion*—myalgia, muscle wasting and weakness, skin rash

- *Diagnostic work-up*—CK, EMG, muscle biopsy

- *Treatment*—oral prednisolone (60 mg daily) with second line steroid-sparing immunosupressant either azathioprine (2–2.5 mg/kg body weight daily) or methotrexate, with intravenous immunoglobulin (IVIG) as emergency therapy, taper dose of steroids according to clinical response

- *Reconsider diagnosis*— if failure of response to 3 months of treatment, consider alternative myopathic disorder, e.g., muscular dystrophy or inclusion body myositis

fluctuate in pregnancy, is often associated with other AI disorders, can be triggered by D-penicillamine, responds to immune therapies, and muscle biopsies show damage reflecting a humoral mediated capillary angiopathy.

Clinical features of PM and DM

DM presents in the childhood or elderly years with a female predominance, as with many other AI disorders. PM is rare in children and the majority of patients present in the third and fifth decade.[14] PM and DM present with symptomatic proximal weakness causing functional impairment, diffuse myalgia (especially DM) or a rash. Examination reveals symmetrical proximal weakness and wasting with preserved deep tendon reflexes, and neck and bulbar weakness are common. The pathognomonic rash of DM is a purplish-red butterfly discoloration over the face, often associated with periorbital edema and a heliotrope rash over the eyelids. An additional V-shaped rash may be seen in the sun-exposed areas of the chest. Patients may present with a typical rash of DM without clinically apparent weakness (amyopathic DM), though interestingly these same patients do have subclinical changes evident on muscle biopsy.[15]

Symptomatic myoglobinuria may occur in rare, acute presentations of both PM and DM, and can precipitate acute renal failure.

PM and DM are frequently associated with connective tissue disorders: PM with lupus, Sjögren's syndrome and rheumatoid arthritis; and DM with scleroderma and mixed connective tissue disease.[5] Systemic features including vasculitis of the heart or gut, subcutaneous calcinosis, Gottron's nodules around the knuckles and nail fold capillary changes are seen in DM.[16]

Respiratory muscle weakness occurs rarely in both PM and DM, but fibrosing alveolitis is relatively common in DM, and it is then often associated with antibodies against Jo-1 (t-histidyl transferase synthase).[17] Aspiration pneumonia can occur in patients with severe bulbar weakness, and in DM patients with esophageal involvement.

PM, and more especially DM, can be associated with an underlying malignancy, though estimates of the frequency of this association vary widely from around 5 to 40 percent in published series.[18] This disparity in part reflects differences in case ascertainment: many case reports are anecdotal and there are few prospective and/or retrospective studies. Moreover, diagnostic criteria have also differed between reports, and muscle biopsy has not always been employed to confirm the presence of necrosis. Whatever the true incidence of this association, simple investigations, along with a systemic examination including the breasts, a chest radiograph and an abdominal ultrasound seem appropriate.

Differential diagnosis of PM and DM

Clinical diagnosis of DM is usually straightforward, though lupus associated with a facial rash and motor neuropathy might cause confusion. Differential diagnosis of PM is wider, as it may be confused with inclusion body myositis (see below), chronic neuropathies, motor neuron disease or myasthenia. Of note, however, is that in myasthenia muscle weakness occurs in the absence of muscle wasting, and in motor neuron disease

both upper and lower motor neuron features are apparent. Finally, as inflammatory myopathies presenting in elderly patients can be confused with muscular dystrophies, it is always prudent to take a family history, particularly in those who have not shown the expected response to immunosuppression.

Investigations of PM and DM

Serum creatine kinase (CK) is usually elevated considerably, often 10–50 times the normal value, and this is almost exclusively due to increases in the CK-MM fraction. However, CK values do not correlate well with either myalgia or weakness in PM and DM patients, and occasionally CK values are normal in clinically affected individuals. While the erythrocyte sedimentation rate (ESR) is also usually elevated, this is nonspecific, and it is not a reliable disease marker. An autoantibody screen is worthwhile given the frequent association with collagen vascular disease. Other appropriate baseline investigations include lung function tests, a chest X-ray, and an electrocardiogram.

Neurophysiological investigations are crucial in the evaluation of patients with suspected myositis. Concentric needle EMG studies in PM and DM patients show typical features of a myopathy with short duration myopathic discharges, but with additional indications of muscle irritability: increased insertional activity, and spontaneous activity (including positive sharp waves, and fibrillation potentials) reflecting myogenic denervation secondary to muscle fiber splitting. Nerve conduction and repetitive nerve stimulation studies are useful in excluding motor neuropathy, and neuromuscular junction disorders respectively.

Muscle biopsy is crucial to confirm the diagnosis. As already noted, the biopsy should be performed from a weak but not especially wasted muscle. Almost invariably the muscle biopsies are abnormal in both PM and DM, but if the tissue proves to be surprisingly normal, and a strong clinical suspicion remains, the patient should be rebiopsied as muscle disease can be patchy and sampling errors therefore occur. In PM the pathology consists of a T-cell-mediated cytotoxic necrosis: initially, CD8+ cells and macrophages surround healthy muscle fibers, and subsequently invade them. Muscle fibers show increased HLA Class I expression (normally minimal or absent).[19,20] Endomysial fibrosis is common in PM, and massive fibrosis may underlie some apparently treatment-resistant cases.[20] In DM, circulating antiendothelial antibodies activate complement and C3, triggering further changes in the complement cascade and generating membrane attack complex (MAC) which transverses and destroys endomysial capillaries. With destruction and reduced number of muscle capillaries, ischemia or micro-infarcts occurs in the periphery of the muscle fascicle (watershed area). Finally, as a late event, complement-fixing antibodies, B cells, CD8+ T cells, and macrophages traffic to the muscle.[20] There is often a surprising divergence between clinical and pathological features in DM, and perifascicular atrophy is a useful feature in otherwise bland biopsies.

Treatment of PM and DM

Treatment of PM and DM is largely based on clinical practice and experience. While there have been many studies of immunotherapy in inflammatory myopathies, they often group together adult and childhood DM, PM, and IBM patients. Most studies are retrospective and uncontrolled; and in several studies subjective measures and reduced CK are defined as a response. To date there have only been a few small randomized trials of intravenous immunoglobulin in PM and DM (see discussion in Mastaglia[21]).

Oral prednisolone remains the drug of first choice for patients with both PM and DM. Patients should be started on oral prednisolone 60 mg a day. A clinical response should be evident within 3 months in the majority of patients. Many now advocate coprescription of a second-line immunosuppressive agent such as azathioprine or methotrexate as these have a useful steroid sparing action in the longer term. Intravenous immunoglobulin is useful as a rescue therapy for patients with acute or severe disease, and is occasionally used at intervals for patients with problems related to steroids. A few patients remain resistant to steroids, and if the diagnosis is secure, cyclophosphamide is a useful alternative agent. It is important to remember that the dose of steroids should be tapered according to the clinical response rather than the CK. It can be difficult for doctor and patient alike to detect subtle improvements, and objective physiotherapy assessments including myometry are useful. While it is usually possible to taper off the dose of steroids after about 3 months, many patients do require a maintenance dose of steroids, and timely osteoporosis prophylaxis and regular screening for diabetes and hypertension are therefore advisable.

The prognosis of both DM and PM is generally good, unless associated with an underlying malignancy. Respiratory involvement, and especially fibrosing alveolitis, carries a poor prognosis. If patients fail to respond to steroids at all, IBM may be the diagnosis. Patients should be re-evaluated, and sometimes, rebiopsied.

INCLUSION BODY MYOSITIS

IBM was initially considered to be a rare inflammatory myopathy in elderly people, but it is increasingly emerging as the most important cause of new onset myositis in this age group.[2] The clinical, muscle biopsy, neurophysiological and prognostic features of IBM are different from both PM and DM.

The pathogenesis of IBM is unclear, with features suggesting either an immune-mediated disorder, or a degenerative condition. IBM may be an immune disorder as there is a modest association with other autoimmune disorders such as diabetes, and muscle pathology shows inflammatory features very similar to PM with CD8+ cells, and macrophages, and increased HLA Class I expression. However, IBM may be a degenerative condition as (i) muscle contains increased levels of amyloid, prion protein and other molecules as seen in Alzheimer's disease and (ii) to date there is no evidence of maintained response to immunotherapy in the vast majority of cases.

IBM usually presents as a painless, profound, progressive wasting of quadriceps muscles associated with a characteristic genu recurvatum stance and frequent falls. In a minority of patients weakness and wasting begins in the arms. It is of note that muscle wasting is often asymmetric and may develop over many years.[2] Myalgia and myoglobinuria are rare. Between a quarter and a third of patients have profound distal weakness especially in the forearms associated with a wasting of the volar aspect, and weakness of finger flexes and extensors, and often a floppy, useless thumb. Deep tendon reflexes are often depressed giving rise to confusion with neuropathies. Dysphagia and neck flexion weakness are common in IBM. IBM is not associated with malignancy. There is a male preponderance.

The differential diagnosis of IBM is wide: upper limb presentations of IBM may be confused with cervical radiculopathies, and even MND.[22] The depressed reflexes seen in most IBM patients may cause confusion with neuropathies, but clinical sensory examination is normal. The combination of a wasted quadriceps and a depressed knee reflex may suggest LEMS, but of course in IBM no post-tetanic potentiation of reflexes is seen. The very long history in many patients with IBM may suggest an inherited disorder, but the asymmetry seen in most patients with IBM reflects its acquired nature.

Several investigations are helpful in patients with suspected IBM. Nerve conduction studies are usually normal, but may show features consistent with a mild axonal neuropathy. On EMG studies myopathic, neurogenic or a mixed picture is seen and a high index of clinical suspicion is therefore necessary if the diagnosis is to be considered. CK may be significantly elevated, but more often is normal reflecting the low turnover of muscle cells in this disorder. Muscle biopsies show inflammatory changes, far more marked than one would expect given the often modest elevation of CK, with an infiltration of CD8+ cells, and macrophages. In addition, muscle fibers may contain eosinophilic inclusions and vacuoles with basophilic stippling, hinting at a degenerative process. On electron microscopy, characteristic intracellular filamentous inclusions are seen, as in other degenerative conditions. Immunohistochemistry demonstrates an increased expression of "degenerative" proteins including amyloid precursor protein, prion protein, ubiquitin, and alpha-syneuclinin, prompting comparisons between IBM and Alzheimer's disease.[23] The lack of response to immunotherapy (see below) is surprising, and it may be that the inflammatory changes are secondary to a degenerative process within the muscle, rather than a primary event.

The outcome of treatment of IBM is disappointing and to date all attempts at immunosuppression and immunomodulation have failed to induce a consistent and longlasting benefit. High-dose steroids, methotrexate, azathioprine, cyclophosphamide, and intravenous immunoglobulin (IVIG) have all been tried separately and in various combinations, with inconsistent and largely negative results.[2] Early studies suggested that some patients might benefit from IVIG, but larger randomized studies failed to substantiate this.[24,25] It is not always easy to distinguish IBM from other inflammatory myopathies, particularly as the pathognomic inclusion bodies may be very scanty on biopsy, and my own practice therefore is to give patients a 3-month trial of high-dose oral prednisolone. If there is a suggestion of response, I continue on high-dose steroids adding in a second-line immunosuppressive agent. If no response to steroids is apparent, I reduce these gradually. The lack of response to immunotherapy seen in IBM[26] may reflect the nature of the immune response in the disorder, i.e., a secondary phenomenon related to muscle degeneration. It is important to recognize IBM early, and not to leave patients on high-dose steroids long-term, with all its attendant risks, in the hope of a late response.

DRUG-INDUCED MYALGIA AND MYOPATHY

A large number of drugs induce muscle symptoms but a simple classification is not possible,[27] and an overview with important examples of each is given. Clinical and neurophysiological combinations of a myopathy, neuropathy, and neuromuscular junction abnormalities often suggest a drug-related toxic or endocrine cause.

Several drugs including statins, fibrates, and aminocaproic acid can induce a painful cramping acute or subacute necrotizing myopathy. Statins may cause a painful myopathy a few weeks after starting the drug, and is more common in patients with pre-existent renal and hepatic disease. Unfortunately, clofibrate and other fibrates may also induce a myopathy; a useful etiological clue may be subclinical neurophysiological evidence of associated neuropathy and myotonia. The underlying mechanisms remain unclear, though secondary mitochondrial dysfunction may be important.[27] Statin- and fibrate-induced myopathies might be confused with inflammatory myopathies; drug-induced myopathies evolve quicker and improve, though often slowly, with cessation of the drug.

Antimalarial agents (including chloroquine), amiodarone and perhexilene may all induce a chronic painless proximal myopathy with vacuolar change and lysosmal inclusions on muscle biopsy. Amiodarone-induced neuropathy is more common than a myopathy, though the two may coexist. Similarly, vincristine commonly induces a neuropathy, though some patients also have a myopathy. Diuretics and laxatives may induce muscle pains and or cramps secondary to hypokalemia, and occasionally with very low serum potassium levels can be associated with a painful or painless vacuolar myopathy.

D-Penicillamine may induce an inflammatory myopathy resembling polymyositis, or a myasthenia gravis like illness; both conditions tend to improve on withdrawal of the drug.

Critical illness neuropathy is well recognized and may be associated with a myopathic counterpart. Pathogenesis is unclear and is likely to reflect immobility, steroid treatment, electrolyte imbalance, multiorgan failure, and the toxic effects of antibiotics and paralyzing agents, together with vitamin deficiency.

Excessive alcohol consumption is often associated with neuromuscular disease. Alcohol can induce an acute myopathy, often associated with hypokalemia, and possibly a chronic myopathy, though chronic wasting and weakness is more commonly due to a toxic neuropathy.

ENDOCRINE AND METABOLIC MYOPATHIES
Steroid-induced myopathy

The majority of patients with Cushing disease have clinical and neurophysiological features of a myopathy.[28] Prolonged use of steroids is also often associated with a chronic, painless myopathy and less commonly an acute painful necrotizing (intensive theraphy unit) myopathy. Steroid-induced myopathy is typically associated with obesity, moon facies, and other classical stigmata of glucorticoid excess. Steroid myopathy may be difficult to recognize in patients receiving steroids for inflammatory muscle disease, though steroids are unlikely to be the culprit unless used for more than 4 weeks, when patients will have other stigmata of glucorticoid excess. As CK levels may be normal in both steroid induced and inflammatory myopathies, and EMG findings can be similar, occasionally muscle biopsy is required to distinguish disease activity from iatrogenic myopathy. The pathogenesis of steroid-induced myopathy is complex and involves hypokalemia, and alterations in carbohydrate and protein metabolism. Structural changes on muscle biopsy include type 2 fiber atrophy, though this is nonspecific, lipid deposition, and vacuolation of the muscle. Using second-line immunosupressives such as azathioprine to treat the inflammatory disease in question may facilitate treatment, which consists of slowly withdrawing steroids. Unfortunately, patients recover from steroid-induced myopathy only slowly, and an exercise program may be useful.

Addison's disease and hypoadrenalism

The majority of patients with Addison's disease have significant muscle weakness, which may go unnoticed and be attributed to fatigue. Strength improves gradually with introduction of steroids.

Thyroid dysfunction

Muscle weakness is seen in the vast majority of thyrotoxic patients. Hyperthyroid myopathy may be associated with myalgia and fatigue, and may be readily overlooked in thyrotoxic patients. Weakness may be proximal or generalized, and occasionally involves bulbar and respiratory muscles.[29] Ocular involvement (Graves disease) may occur in patients with hyperthyroidism, and reflects both excessive adrenergic activity and inflammatory changes in extraocular muscle and surrounding orbital tissue.[30] Hyperthyroid myopathy is commonly associated with proximal weakness without wasting, resembling that seen in myasthenia gravis. Patients with autoimmune dysthyroid states may have myasthenia and vice versa. Recognition of such associations is important in targeting treatment. Patients with thyrotoxicosis may also have alterations in deep tendon reflexes and fasciculations which may mimic MND and cause diagnostic confusion. Given these potential diagnostic pitfalls it seems reasonable to recommend initial thyroid function tests in *all* patients presenting with neuromuscular disease.[31] Muscle investigation with serum CK, EMG, and muscle biopsy is usually unhelpful, since there are no specific diagnostic features of the condition, but may be useful in rare cases where dual pathology is suspected, e.g., polymyositis and thyroid myopathy. Occasionally, thyrotoxicosis is associated with a neuropathy, though mixed neuropathic and myopathic features are seen in EMG. The pathogenesis of thyroid myopathy is complex and likely to involve both alterations in muscle metabolism, and electrical properties, principally through increased Na–K–ATP pump activity. Finally, thyrotoxic periodic paralysis[32] is a rare but well-recognized disorder, more common in individuals of oriental descent. (The periodic paralyses are a group of predominately inherited neuromuscular disorders in which paralysis is related to electrolyte imbalances.[33])

Hypothyroidism is also frequently associated with neuromuscular manifestations which may dominate the clinical picture, and rarely may predate the development of overt biochemical abnormalities.[29] A recent prospective study underlies the strength of these associations: in patients with recently diagnosed thyroid dysfunction, 79 percent of hypothyroid patients had neuromuscular complaints including pain and stiffness and 38 percent had clinical weakness.[34] Symptoms did not correlate with serum CK levels and improved slowly with thyroxine therapy. Muscle biopsy shows glycogen accumulation at the periphery of the muscle fiber. The exact relationship between the muscle biopsy and clinical features remains unexplained. Hypothyroid myopathy may cause diagnostic confusion: firstly, patients may have delayed reflex responses and occasionally myotonia (Hoffman's syndrome) simulating features of the genetic myotonic disorders; secondly, occasionally patients have very high CK levels and marked muscle wasting, simulating an inflammatory or inherited muscle disease.[28]

Other metabolic disorders

It is unusual for patients with disorders of glycolytic metabolism to present in old age, but there have been descriptions of patients with acid maltase deficiency presenting with profound respiratory, especially diaphragmatic, muscle weakness in their fifties and sixties, and this possibility needs to be borne in mind when investigating patients with type 2 respiratory failure.

MITOCHONDRIAL DISORDERS

While mitochondrial disorders typically present in childhood and early adult life, these disorders are becoming increasingly recognized in the elderly population as muscle biopsy is becoming more commonplace. Mitochondrial disorders—due to abnormalities in either mitochondrial DNA (mtDNA), or in nuclear DNA (nDNA) encoding mitochondrial proteins—often present with multisystem protean features given the widespread location of mitochondria in many tissues. Patients with mitochondrial disorders may have skeletal or extraocular muscular weakness, deafness, blindness (optic nerve or retinal involvement), diabetes, bone marrow failure, short stature or cardiac arrhythmias—to mention just a few features.[35,36] Because of the familial nature of the mitochondrial disorders with complex patterns of inheritance (mitochondria are inherited through the maternal line), and the variability of clinical expression, there will frequently be the need to investigate some or all members of the family where mitochondrial abnormalities are suspected.[35]

A common phenotype is a chronic progressive external ophthalmoplegia (CPEO) with bilateral ptosis, which may be confused with ocular forms of myasthenia, and the rare oculopharyngeal muscular dystrophy. CPEO is often associated with a slowly progressive skeletal proximal myopathy, and occasionally retinopathy. Muscle biopsies show cytochrome oxidase (COX) negative fibers, reflecting abnormalities in mitochondrial oxidative phosphorylation function, and subsarcolemmal ragged red fibers, which on electron microscopy are seen to be disrupted mitochondria. The majority of CPEO patients have a single large duplication or deletion in their mtDNA; in the remainder, pathogenic mtDNA point mutations are to blame. Mitochondrial disease may also present with exercise intolerance, with or without a clinically apparent proximal myopathy, often associate with a variety of mtDNA point mutations. Kearns–Sayre syndrome rarely presents to geriatricians as this association between a CPEO phenotype with a retinal degeneration and onset before the age of 20 is rapidly progressive, with death occurring before the age of 30, often due to cardiac arrhythmia.

A variety of mitochondrial encephalomyopathies may present to geriatricians: diagnosis requires a strong index of clinical suspicion, particularly as overlap occurs between the various syndromes: mitochondrial encephalomyopathy with lactic acidosis and stroke-like episodes (MELAS), myoclonic epilepsy with ragged red fibers (MERFF), and neuropathy, ataxia, and retinitis pigmentosa (NARP) are just a few of the more common syndromes.[35]

As will be apparent, mitochondrial disease can present in many ways and confirmation is often difficult. Muscle biopsies have a key role both in suggesting the diagnosis with abnormalities of oxidative metabolism, and in providing a rich source of mtDNA (point mutations may not be detected in blood). Respiratory enzyme chain analysis on fresh muscle can be performed in a few centers, and identifies defects in the complex I and other units of the respiratory chain. Direct analysis of respiratory enzyme activity is also useful in the (rare) disorders of fatty acid oxidation pyruvate metabolism. Counseling of patients and families with mitochondrial disease is complex and often best done by a clinical neurogeneticist.

To date there is no effective treatment for mitochondrial disease, and care is largely supportive, taking care to minimize metabolic stress wherever possible. Regular ECG in the majority of patients with mitochondrial disease is recommended.

MYOTONIC DYSTROPHY (MD)

Myotonia or delayed relaxation of muscle after voluntary activation (e.g. gripping or forced eyelid closure) is seen in a number of neuromuscular disorders, and reflects abnormalities of muscle fiber membrane conduction. Myotonia is often temperature dependent, and may rapidly attenuate with repeated muscle activations (so-called "warm-up"). The rare autosomal recessive and dominant congenital myotonic disorders do not affect lifespan, are due to chloride channel mutations, and often respond well to mexiletine.

In contrast, myotonic dystrophy, also known as dystrophia myotonica and Steinhert's disease, is a serious multisystem disorder with significant morbidity.[37] MD is inherited in an autosomal dominant fashion, and is due to an unstable trinucleotide expansion repeat in a protein kinase gene. Like other trinucleotide expansion repeat disorders, MD exhibits anticipation with worsening features presenting at an earlier stage in successive generations.[8] Clinical features of MD are protean and include ptosis, a myopathic faces, neck, bulbar, and distal limb weakness, and areflexia. Patients often walk with a foot-drop gait. Significant systemic associations include cataracts, hypogonadism, hepatic and gastrointestinal disturbances, cardiac arrhythmias, diabetes, hypersomnolence, respiratory failure, premature balding, and cognitive impairment. There is no effective therapy for MD, but regular ECG monitoring is mandatory in view of the risk of cardiac arrhythmias. Recognition of MD in an elderly patient is important as it may prompt clinical and genetic assessment of the family, potentially avoiding the tragedy of a severe, often fatal, congenital form of myotonic dystrophy in subsequent generations.

PROXIMAL MYOTONIC MYOPATHY (PROMM)

This is a related but distinct autosomal dominant multisystem disorder.[4] It is of note that in PROMM myotonia can be precipitated by exercise and paradoxically made worse by high temperature. Muscle wasting is proximal rather than the distal distribution seen in MD. Initial reports suggest PROMM might be more benign than MD, but a spectrum of severity seems likely, and white-matter disease has been described now in this disorder. The genetic cause of PROMM is likely to be identified in the very near future.

MOTOR NEURON DISEASE (MND)

MND is a common, fatal, progressive disorder with degeneration of both upper and lower motor neurons of uncertain cause. Death usually occurs as a consequence of respiratory failure. MND has an incidence of 1–3 per 100,000, and a prevalence of around 4–6 per 100,000.

The etiology of MND is unclear, and a large number of potential mechanisms has been suggested: excessive glutamate, an influx of calcium, and a subsequent excitotoxic cascade triggering cell damage and apoptosis are likely to be important. Abnormalities of superoxide dismutase (SOD 1) gene have been described in a minority of patients with the uncommon familial form of MND, suggesting that free-radical damage and excessive oxidative stress are important.[38]

Clinical features of MND reflect the upper and lower motor neuron involvement. Nocturnal cramps are an early feature, but rarely prompt patients to consult physicians. MND often begins in an asymmetrical fashion in a single body region (arms, legs, trunk, bulbar musculature) but ultimately involves all four regions. Lower motor neuron features include asymmetrical muscle wasting and weakness, fasciculations, and depressed reflexes. Upper motor neuron features include spastic hypertonia, pyramidal weakness, and brisk deep tendon reflexes with extensor plantar responses. A combination of a wasted, weak quadriceps muscle with a pathologically brisk

Summary of management algorithm
Motor neuron disease (MND)

- *Clinical suspicion*—progressive course with cramps, muscle wasting, and weakness; signs are often asymmetrical; need to demonstrate mixed upper and lower motor neuron signs in more than one body region (arms, legs, trunk and bulbar musculature)

- *Diagnostic work-up*—Neurophysiology confirms lower motor neuron involvement and is useful in excluding alternative neuropathic or myopathic causes. Neuroimaging is vital to exclude potential structural explanations for the clinical picture such as spondylosis. Thyroid function tests (TFTs) as dysthyroid states can mimic MND

- *Treatment*—supportive, nutrition (gastrostomy feeding), riluzole (50 mg b.d., need to monitor liver function tests)

- *Reconsider diagnosis*—if clinical course stabilizes, if sensory signs develop, or if unexpected longevity

knee jerk is very suggestive of MND as is the combination of a wasted and fasciculating tongue but with a pathologically brisk jaw jerk. Neck weakness is common in motor neuron disease and may lead to a dropped head posture. Eye movement disorders, sensory signs, and sphincter involvement are all distinctly rare in motor neuron disease and should prompt a review of the diagnosis.

Investigations in MND serve to (i) provide support for the clinical diagnosis, and (ii) exclude structural or other potentially treatable pathologies. Serum CK levels may be modestly increased (<1,000 iu/mL), but are nonspecific. Neurophysiological tests are very useful in excluding a neuropathy or a myopathic process; they also demonstrate neurogenic changes reflecting both denervation and reinnervation. A careful search for nerve conduction block is warranted in patients without upper motor neuron signs, who might have multifocal motor neuropathy, a rare but treatable autoimmune neuropathy frequently associated with antibodies against GM1 ganglioside.[39] Structural imaging, ideally MR scanning, is useful to exclude pathologies such as degenerative disk disease, which may cause both cord and nerve root compression with consequent mixed upper and lower motor neuron signs. Structural imaging is especially important when signs are confined to the limbs, and there are no hard signs "above the neck."

Unfortunately no curative therapies are available, and to date, trials with a variety of nerve growth factors have been disappointing. Riluzole, an antiglutamate agent, produces a moderate prolongation of life and should be considered at an early stage in all patients with possible MND.[40] The lack of curative drug therapy should not be taken to imply that nothing can be done to mitigate the impact of the disease. Rehabilitation utilizing the very different skills of the multidisciplinary team should be available at every stage.[40] Gastrostomy feeding is useful at an early stage both to maintain the patient's nutritional state, and to reduce the chance of aspiration in those with significant bulbar weakness. The role of noninvasive, and formal ventilation in patients with motor neuron disease remains controversial.[41]

MYASTHENIA GRAVIS (MG)

MG is the most common acquired disorder affecting neuromuscular transmission (NMT) and is characterized by fluctuating and fatigable weakness of voluntary muscle. The mechanisms underlying normal NMT are now well understood and the nature of the (motor endplate) defect in MG is well established.[42]

The annual incidence of MG is around 1 per 300,000 with a prevalence of around 1 per 17,000. Overall there is a slight female preponderance, with most young onset patients being female and most elderly onset patients being male.[43]

MG is a chronic autoimmune disorder, with circulating antibodies initiating a blockade, and subsequent complement mediated destruction of nicotinic acetyl choline receptors (nAChR) expressed on the postsynaptic (muscle) aspect of the motor endplate.[44] MG arises because of intolerance to self-antigens generating an aberrant immune response with autoreactive T and B cells.[45,46] The thymus gland is crucial in both the initiation and propagation of MG, and it is notable that primitive cells within the thymus myoid cells express nAChR.[45,46] Serum anti-nAChR antibodies can be detected in most (75–90 percent) patients with generalized MG, and in about 50 percent of patients with purely ocular presentations of MG.[47] Anti-nAChR antibodies are specific for MG.[47] In-vivo and in-vitro work suggests that immune factors are also important in patients with MG but in whom nAChR antibodies cannot be detected (seronegative MG, SNMG).[48] Recent work by the Oxford Group suggests many SNMG patients have a second antibody directed against a second muscle target (muscle specific kinase or MuSK).[49]

Clinical features of MG reflect fatigable muscle weakness and include ocular involvement with ophthalmoplegia, ptosis and diplopia; proximal arm or leg weakness, nasal speech and swallowing difficulties; neck flexion and extension weakness causing a dropped head appearance; and breathlessness. Most patients present with ocular symptoms or signs. In around 20 percent MG remains restricted to the eyes, but in majority of cases it generalizes to other muscle groups, usually within a year of onset of symptoms.[43] Since MG is a fluctuating condition, diagnosis may be difficult and requires a strong clinical suspicion. True binocular diplopia is a very unusual symptom and should always prompt consideration of MG, even if there is no overt paralysis of eye movements. The differential diagnosis of MG is wide and includes nerve (e.g. Guillain–Barré syndrome), other neuromuscular (e.g. botulism) and muscle disorders (e.g. mitochondrial disorders and oculopharyngeal muscular dystrophy). Assessment of isolated bulbar palsy is especially difficult: it is a clinical situation in which treatable MG or progressive MND are the only common diagnoses. Fasciculations are not seen in MG. Diagnosis of MG rests on typical symptoms and signs, and the presence of antibodies.

The Tensilon® test—in which an intravenous bolus of short-acting acetylcholinesterase inhibitor is administered—can help support a clinical diagnosis of MG, especially in patients with ocular MG who are often seronegative. The test is also very useful in the urgent diagnostic evaluation of patients with a flaccid paralysis while the results of antibody and other tests are awaited. Interpretation of the test may not be straightforward, and a blinded observer may be useful. A positive test indicates a neuromuscular component to the patient's symptoms but is not specific to MG, and can be misleading, especially in patients with bulbar palsy. The Tensilon® test is hazardous as acetylcholine levels are elevated throughout the body. Predosing with the muscarinic receptor antagonist atropine reduces the risks of vagally mediated bradyarrhythmias, excessive bronchial secretions, lacrimation, salivation, and gastrointestinal colic. The Tensilon® test should always be conducted with an ECG monitor in place, with access to full resuscitation facilities, and ideally only on the ward.

Neurophysiological tests are also useful in confirming a clinical diagnosis of MG, particularly in those patients who lack antibodies.[12] Repetitive nerve stimulation studies (RNS) at low frequency produce a decremental response mirroring the fatigable weakness seen on examination. RNS studies can be performed on a variety of limb (commonly deltoid), facial (nasalis), and occasionally respiratory (diaphragm) muscles. Single-fiber EMG (SFEMG) studies are technically demanding but very useful in patients with ocular MG where RNS is impractical. An excessive variability in responses between paired muscle fibers ("jitter," or intermittent blocking of neuromuscular transmission) is seen. Abnormalities in RNS and SFEMG are not specific to MG and can be seen in other neuromuscular disorders and occasionally in MND.

Several other tests are recommended in patients with suspected MG. Thoracic imaging with contrast CT or MRI scanning is mandatory given the known association between MG and thymoma. While most thymomas have benign histological appearances, these tumors are locally invasive, and because of their retrosternal location close to crucial structures require timely excision. Given the known association with other autoimmune conditions a full autoantibody screen and thyroid function tests are advisable in MG patients. Finally, CK levels should be considered if concomitant polymyositis is suspected.

Summary of management algorithm
Myasthenia gravis (MG)

- *Clinical suspicion*—fluctuating, fatigable weakness without muscle wasting, affecting eye, bulbar, limb and or respiratory muscles. Deep tendon reflexes are preserved. No sensory signs

- *Diagnostic work-up*—Tensilon test, acetylcholine receptor antibody test, neurophysiology, repetitive nerve stimulation or single fiber EMG. Consider potential mimics, e.g., dysthyroid eye disease (TFTs, thyroid autoantibodies), polymyositis (CK, EMG)

- *Other tests*—CT scan of chest is essential as up to 10 percent of MG patients have a thymoma

- *Treatment*—symptomatic therapy with acetyl cholinesterase inhibitor such as Mestinon 30–60 mg q.d.s., immunological therapy oral prednisolone (initially 60 mg and 0 mg on alternate days) with second line steroid-sparing immunosuppressant, either azathioprine (2–2.5 mg/kg body weight daily) or methotrexate, with intravenous immunoglobulin (IVIG) as emergency therapy, taper dose of steroids according to clinical response. Thymectomy is recommended in patients under the age of 40, and in all patients with thymoma

- *Reconsider diagnosis*—if clinical course progresses, if sensory signs develop, or if no response to immunosuppression

The term myasthenia *gravis* reflects the serious and often fatal prognosis of the condition prior to modern therapies. Nowadays, MG is considered a treatable and largely reversible condition.[50] MG is a chronic disorder and spontaneous remission rare. Most elderly patients require life-long treatment and, because of fluctuations, regular follow-up. Long-acting acetylcholinesterase inhibitors such as Mestinon® (pyridostigmine, typically 30–60 mg q.d.s.) are useful symptomatic therapies, with propantheline cover if required for gastrointestinal side-effects, including colic. Some MG patients with mild symptoms only require Mestinon® but many require more definitive therapy with immunosuppression and or thymectomy. Prednisolone remains the first-line immunosuppressant of choice in MG patients. Ideally, steroids should be started as an inpatient in case there is early, and transient deterioration (the "Drachman" dip). Most patients will show significant improvements within weeks of starting steroids. An alternate day steroid regime and calcium and vitamin D supplements may minimize the risk of osteoporosis; bisphosphonates are also often indicated in elderly patients. Second-line immunosuppressive agents azathioprine or methotrexate have a useful proven, steroid-sparing action but require regular hematological and hepatic monitoring and may take many months to achieve full efficacy.[50] In patients requiring immunosuppression it seems reasonable to use high-dose steroids (60 mg and 0 mg prednisolone on alternate days) and azathioprine from the outset, tapering steroids gradually over the next 6–12 months. Transternal thymectomy has a useful role in younger patients with benign thymic hyperplasia, but its role in the routine management of elderly onset MG patients is controversial. Thymectomy is mandatory in all patients with suspected thymoma. Intravenous immunoglobulin and plasma exchange are both useful as rescue therapy in patients with rapidly deteriorating myasthenia, and occasionally as maintenance therapy in patients intolerant of oral immunosuppression.

KEY POINTS   Neuromuscular diseases including myasthenic disorders

- *History:* close enquiry regarding the temporal evolution of functional impairment may help distinguish acquired from inherited muscle disease.

- *Examination:* the combination of both muscle wasting and weakness may suggest a neurogenic or myopathic disorder.

- *Investigations:* a holistic approach is required in the diagnosis of muscle disease: clinical assessment, serum CK estimates, EMG and muscle biopsy are often all required.

- *Endocrine myopathies:* thyroid function tests are essential in all patients with suspected neuromuscular disease.

- *Mitochondrial disorders:* the manifestations of mitochondrial disease are protean and include muscle wasting and weakness, deafness, visual loss, diabetes, and short stature.

- *Myotonic dystrophy:* recognition of myotonic dystrophy in an elderly patient is crucial, and may prompt an assessment of the wider family that potentially avoids this incurable disorder in successive generations.

LAMBERT–EATON MYASTHENIC SYNDROME (LEMS)

LEMS, like MG, is an acquired, immune-mediated, presynaptic (neuronal) disorder of neuromuscular transmission (NMT) characterized by fatigable weakness of voluntary muscle. In-vivo and in-vitro studies of patients, using a variety of model systems, demonstrate a failure of adequate neurotransmitter release from the presynaptic nerve terminal.[11] LEMS is rare compared to MG, and, in contrast with MG, there is a male preponderance.[51]

LEMS patients have prominent proximal weakness, especially of the legs, which may improve shortly after the onset of voluntary contraction. Ocular and bulbar involvement is comparatively rare. Autonomic features, including a dry mouth, constipation, and pupillary abnormalities, are common. Deep tendon reflexes tend to be absent, but may be elicited after a period of maximal contraction (post-tetanic potentiation), which is in marked contrast with patients with MG who tend to have rather brisk reflexes.

LEMS is frequently associated with an underlying cancer, most commonly with small-cell lung cancer (SCLC). Around 50 percent of LEMS patients have an associated cancer. Given the strength of this association, and as the onset of LEMS can predate tumor detection, it seems prudent to screen patients, especially smokers, regularly for an underlying tumor.[42,51]

As with MG, LEMS is a fluctuating condition and diagnosis may be difficult and requires a strong clinical suspicion, particularly as weakness in patients with known cancer may be wrongly attributed to cachexia. The proximal weakness seen in LEMS may suggest a motor neuropathy, or a lower motor neuron feature of MND. Presynaptic neurotransmission also fails in botulism, but in this condition, unlike LEMS, bulbar features are common.[51]

Diagnosis of LEMS rests on typical symptoms and signs, the Tensilon® test, neurophysiological studies, and the presence of antibodies. The Tensilon® test is positive, consistent with a neuromuscular transmission disorder. Repetitive nerve stimulation (RNS) at low frequency produces a decremental response in recorded compound muscle action potential amplitude (CMAP), similar to that seen in MG, and mirroring the fatigable weakness seen on examination. However, with RNS at high frequency (20–40 Hz) an incremental response is seen with a progressive increase in CMAP amplitudes.[11] Around 85 percent of patients with LEMS have antibodies against P/Q-type neuronal calcium channels,[52] which if detected strongly suggest the disorder. Thoracic imaging with contrast CT or MRI scanning is mandatory given the known association between LEMS and SCLC, but also with thymoma (particularly in those rarer patients with both LEMS and MG).

3,4-Diaminopyridine is a useful symptomatic therapy in LEMS. This drug increases neuronal excitability, through an effect on potassium channels, enhances calcium influx into the nerve and thereby facilitates neurotransmitter release.[53] Acetylcholinesterase inhibitors such as Mestinon® (pyridostigmine, typically 30–60 mg q.d.s.) may provide some symptomatic relief, but are not as effective as in MG.[51] In those patients with an associated tumor removal of this leads to an improvement in the LEMS,[54] suggesting the immune response stimulated by the tumor interferes with neurotransmitter release.

Immunological therapies are often required: Prednisolone remains the first line immunosuppressant of choice in LEMS patients, with a second-line agent such as azathioprine being added if required. Azathioprine should probably be avoided in those patients with a known tumor.[55] Intravenous immunoglobulin and plasma exchange are both useful therapies in LEMS patients.[56]

REFERENCES

1. Hughes RAC: Epidemiology of peripheral neuropathy. Curr Opin Neurol 1995;8:335–338
2. Barohn RJ, Amato AA: Inclusion body myositis. Curr Treat Options Neurol 2000;2:7–12
3. Shneerson JM: Is chronic respiratory failure in neuromuscular diseases worth treating? J Neurol Neurosurg Psychiatry 1996;61:1–3
4. Ricker K, Koch MC, Lehmann-Horn F et al: Proximal myotonic myopathy. Clinical features of a multisystem disorder similar to myotonic dystrophy. Arch Neurol 1995;52:25–31
5. Herrick AL: Neurological involvement in systemic sclerosis. Br J Rheumatol 1995;34:1007–1008
6. Harper P: Myotonic Dystrophy. WB Saunders, London, 2001
7. Turner M: The treatment of motor neurone disease. Practitioner 2001;245:530–532,536-538
8. Harper PS, Harley HG, Reardon W, Shaw DJ: Anticipation in myotonic dystrophy: new light on an old problem. Am J Hum Genet 1992;51:10–16
9. Bushby KM: Making sense of the limb-girdle muscular dystrophies. Brain 1999;122:1403–1420
10. Kimura J: Electrodiagnosis in Diseases of Nerve and Muscle, 5th Ed. FA Davis, Philadelphia,1983
11. Wray D: The Lambert–Eaton myasthenic syndrome. In Vincent A, Wray D (eds): Neuromuscular Transmission: Basic and Applied Aspects. Manchester University Press, Manchester,1990:249–267
12. Stalberg E: Neurophysiological aspects of diagnosis in neuromuscular transmission defects—an update. Electroencephalogr Clin Neurophysiol Suppl 1999;50:377–385
13. Edwards RH, Griffiths RD, Hayward M, Helliwell T: Modern methods of diagnosis of muscle diseases. J R Coll Physicians Lond 1986;20:49–55
14. Rider LG, Miller FW: Idiopathic inflammatory muscle disease: clinical aspects. Baillière's Best Pract Res Clin Rheumatol 2000;14:37–54
15. Callen JP: Dermatomyositis. Lancet 2000;355:53–57
16. Spiera R, Kagen L: Extramuscular manifestations in idiopathic inflammatory myopathies. Curr Opin Rheumatol 1998;10:556–561
17. Brouwer R, Hengstman GJ, Vree Egberts W et al: Autoantibody profiles in the sera of European patients with myositis. Ann Rheum Dis 2001;60:116–123
18. Brown H, Steven M: Myositis and malignancy: is there a true association? Hosp Med 1999;60:51–53
19. Hohlfeld R, Goebels N, Engel AG: Cellular mechanisms in inflammatory myopathies. Baillière's Clin Neurol 1993;2:617–635
20. Hohlfeld R, Engel AG, Goebels N, Behrens L: Cellular immune mechanisms in inflammatory myopathies. Curr Opin Rheumatol 1997;9:520–526
21. Mastaglia FL: Treatment of autoimmune inflammatory myopathies. Curr Opin Neurol 2000;13:507–509
22. Hardiman O: Pitfalls in the diagnosis of motor neurone disease. Hosp Med 2000;61:767–771
23. Lampe JB, Walter MC, Reichmann H: Neurodegeneration-associated proteins and inflammation in sporadic inclusion-body myositis. Adv Exp Med Biol 2001;487:219–228
24. Dalakas MC, Koffman B, Fujii M et al: A controlled study of intravenous immunoglobulin combined with prednisone in the treatment of IBM. Neurology 2001;56:323–327
25. Soueidan SA, Dalakas MC: Treatment of inclusion-body myositis with high-dose intravenous immunoglobulin. Neurology 1993;43:876–879
26. Dalakas MC: Progress in inflammatory myopathies: good but not good enough. J Neurol Neurosurg Psychiatry 2001;70:569–573
27. Argov Z: Drug-induced myopathies. Curr Opin Neurol 2000;13:541–545
28. Anagnos A, Ruff RL, Kaminski HJ: Endocrine neuromyopathies. Neurol Clin 1997;15:673–696
29. Horak HA, Pourmand R: Endocrine myopathies. Neurol Clin 2000;18:203–213
30. Yamada M, Li AW, Wall JR: Thyroid-associated ophthalmopathy: clinical features, pathogenesis, and management. Crit Rev Clin Lab Sci 2000;37:523–549
31. Klein I, Ojamaa K: Thyroid (neuro) myopathy. Lancet 2000;356:614
32. Magsino CH, Jr, Ryan AJ, Jr: Thyrotoxic periodic paralysis. South Med J 2000;93:996–1003
33. Gutmann L: Periodic paralyses. Neurol Clin 2000;18:195–202
34. Duyff RF, Van den Bosch J, Laman DM, van Loon BJ, Linssen WH: Neuromuscular findings in thyroid dysfunction: a prospective clinical and electrodiagnostic study. J Neurol Neurosurg Psychiatry 2000;68:750–755
35. Nardin RA, Johns DR: Mitochondrial dysfunction and neuromuscular disease. Muscle Nerve 2001;24:170–191
36. Pulkes T, Hanna MG: Human mitochondrial DNA diseases. Adv Drug Deliv Rev 2001;49:27–43
37. Harper PS: Trinucleotide repeat disorders. J Inherit Metab Dis 1997;20:122–124
38. Cookson MR, Shaw PJ: Oxidative stress and motor neurone disease. Brain Pathol 1999;9:165–186
39. Pestronk A: Invited review: motor neuropathies, motor neuron disorders, and antyglycolipid antibodies. Muscle Nerve 1991;14:927–936
40. Mitchell JD: Guidelines in motor neurone disease (MND)/amyotrophic lateral sclerosis (ALS)—from diagnosis to patient care. J Neurol 2000;247:7–12
41. Aboussouan LS, Khan SU, Meeker DP, Stelmach K, Mitsumoto H: Effect of noninvasive positive-pressure ventilation on survival in amyotrophic lateral sclerosis [see comments]. Ann Intern Med 1997;127:450–453
42. Newsom-Davis J: Myasthenia gravis and the Lambert–Eaton myasthenic syndrome. Prescrib J 1993;33:205–216
43. Grob D: Natural history of myasthenia gravis. In Engel AG (ed): Myasthenia Gravis and Myasthenic Disorders. Oxford University Press, Oxford,1999:131–141
44. Drachman DB: Myasthenia gravis. N Engl J Med 1994;330:1797–1810
45. Willcox N: Myasthenia gravis. Curr Opin Immunol 1993;5:910–917
46. Willcox N, Baggi F, Batocchi A-P et al: Approaches for studying the pathogenic T cell in autoimmune patients. Ann NY Acad Sci 1993;681:219–237
47. Vincent A: Myasthenia gravis—an autoimmune disorder of neuromuscular transmission. In Vincent A, Wray D (eds): Neuromuscular Transmission: Basic and Applied Aspects. Manchester University Press, Manchester,1990:226–249
48. Yamamoto T, Vincent A, Ciulla TA et al: Seronegative myasthenia gravis: a plasma factor inhibiting agonist-induced acetylcholine receptor function copurifies with IgM. Ann Neurol 1991;30:550–557
49. Hoch W, McConville J, Helms S et al: Auto-antibodies to the receptor tyrosine kinase MuSK in patients with myasthenia gravis without acetylcholine receptor antibodies. Nat Med 2001;7:365–368
50. Seybold M: Treatment of myasthenia gravis. In Engel Ag (ed): Myasthenia Gravis and Myasthenic Disorders. Oxford University Press, Oxford, 1999:167–201
51. Newsom-Davis J, Lang B: The Lambert–Eaton myasthenic syndrome. In Engel AG (ed): Myasthenia Gravis and Myasthenic Disorders. Oxford University Press, Oxford,1999:205–228
52. Motomura M, Johnson I, Lang B, Vincent A, Newsom-Davis J: An improved diagnostic assay for Lambert–Eaton myasthenic syndrome. J Neurol Neurosurg Psychiatry 1994;58:85–87
53. Lundh H, Nilsson O, Rosen I: Treatment of Lambert–Eaton syndrome: 3,4-diaminopyridine and pyridostigmine. Neurology 1984;34:1324–1330
54. Chalk CH, Murray NM, Newsom-Davis J, O'Neill JH, Spiro SG: Response of the Lambert–Eaton myasthenic syndrome to treatment of associated small-cell lung carcinoma. Neurology 1990;40:1552–1556
55. Newsom-Davis J, Vincent A: Antibody-mediated neurological disease. Curr Opin Neurobiol 1991;1:430–435
56. Bain PG, Motomura M, Newsom-Davis J et al: Effects of intravenous immunoglobulin on muscle weakness and calcium-channel autoantibodies in the Lambert–Eaton myasthenic syndrome. Neurology 1996;47:678–683

Chapter 54

Peripheral neuropathies

Brion D. Reichler

The diagnosis of peripheral neuropathy (PN) in elderly people is challenging, inasmuch as the peripheral nervous system (PNS) undergoes clinical and histological changes with normal aging that resemble those of acquired pathology at all ages. The incidental discovery of absent ankle jerks or diminished vibration sensation in the toes, out of the proper clinical context, must be interpreted with caution. However, certain neuropathies occur more frequently in the older population, and others cause increased morbidity in elderly people because of lower "reserve" or complications in other organ systems. In general, the response to all types of nerve injury is impaired with age. Concomitant central nervous system (CNS) disease, which also is more common in elderly people, often complicates the diagnosis and obscures the extent of peripheral contribution to disability. This chapter summarizes the pathophysiological and clinical changes in the PNS with aging, outlines a diagnostic approach to the patient with neuropathy, and provides an overview of neuropathies, which occur with a higher prevalence or are more significant in the geriatric population.

NORMAL CHANGES IN AGING

As it ages, the nervous system undergoes alterations in clinical sensory, reflex, and motor function which resemble those seen in peripheral neuropathy. Possible causes of these changes include defects in neuronal transport mechanisms or protein synthesis, cumulative recurrent trauma, and endoneurial ischemia, as well as a purely biological "axonopathy of aging."[1–3] Advanced glycation endproducts are implicated in oxidative stress and vascular changes which may contribute to the normal aging process.[4] Pathological changes in the peripheral nerves that may be attributable to aging alone include neuronal loss, neuronal and Schwann cell pigment accumulation, demyelination–remyelination, and axon loss in both the peripheral nerves and the dorsal columns.[3,5] The response of nerve to injury is limited in repertoire and becomes impaired with advancing age.[6,7]

Sensory system

Virtually all sensory modalities decline in acuity with age. Potvin et al.[8] reported a 97 percent decrease in quantitative vibration threshold in the lower extremities of normal men between 20 and 80 years of age, but Verillo[9] found diminished sensation only at higher frequencies. Age-adjusted normal values for perception thresholds[10] and perception times[11] have been reported and can be used at the bedside. However, Thomson et al.[12] found that the variability of serially tested quantitative vibratory perception thresholds was unacceptably high in elderly people, limiting their clinical utility.

Thelen et al.[13] found that older women with a mean age of 70 had a 3–4-fold higher threshold for the detection of angular ankle displacement than a group of women with a mean age of 22, and Skinner et al.[14] demonstrated an age effect on joint position sense as far proximally as the knee. However, Pai et al.[15] found that the severity of osteoarthritis had a much greater effect than age on proprioceptive impairment, in patients with bilateral knee disease. Older patients also have impaired integration of propriomuscular input at the spinal cord and higher centers.[16] Nonetheless, this may not translate into clinically testable deficits at the bedside.[17] Age-related decline in temperature,[18–21] pain,[1] and light touch[20,22–24] perception has also been documented, but to a far lesser extent.[25] Therefore, deficits in temperature and pinprick sensation may be better indicators of true pathology.[8,20,25]

Deep tendon reflexes (DTR) depend heavily on an intact sensory arc, involving muscle spindle fibers and large myelinated axons. Reflexes therefore become weaker with advancing age and are eventually lost, beginning at the ankles, and typically involving patellar reflexes last.[26] The reported incidence of ankle areflexia in elderly people varies widely, from 7 to 70 percent, depending on the study.[17,27] In a well-done epidemiological survey in the Republic of San Marino among residents aged 67–87, only 7 percent of subjects had absent ankle reflexes.[17] Yet in another well-executed study combining hospital- and community-based elderly populations and excluding risk factors for PN, the prevalence of ankle areflexia was found to be about 35 percent below age 70, rising steadily to over 50% in patients older than age 85.[25]

Lascelles and Thomas[28] described increased variability of internodal length in the sural nerve in patients over age 65. Asynchronous signal conduction due to the resulting temporal dispersion may explain the early and prominent deficits in reflexes and vibration sensation, which are the two modalities that depend most heavily on a coordinated impulse volley.[28] Other morphological changes in the sensory system involve dorsal root ganglia, nerve, and dorsal columns (predominantly gracile tracts), and are reviewed elsewhere.[1,5,6]

Schmidt et al.[29] determined that loss of mechanoreceptors, rather than nerve dysfunction, accounted for the majority of loss of low-frequency vibration sense with aging. Pacinian corpuscles, which subserve high-frequency vibratory sensation, undergo dropout and morphological changes with age.[9,30] Meissner corpuscles, which mediate light touch and vibration at lower frequencies (< 50 Hz), also degenerate with time.[31] Free nerve endings, which probably mediate temperature and pain sensation, begin to regress as early as the third decade.[1] Changes to muscle spindles include capsular thickening, lamellar fibrosis, and a mild degree of intrafusal fiber loss,[32] and may contribute to the decline in tendon reflexes with age.[27]

Motor system

Quantitatively evaluated muscle strength generally peaks in the third decade, with minimal decline until approximately age 50 and accelerated decline thereafter,[1,33] reaching 20–40 percent of younger levels by age 80.[34] The intrinsic hand and foot muscles are most likely to be clinically weak. However, muscle endurance[35] remains relatively intact. This may be due to selective Type II (fast-twitch) muscle fiber loss, with relative sparing of Type I (slow-twitch) fibers,[35] although this point remains controversial.[34] Mild atrophy, particularly in intrinsic hand, calf, and thigh muscles, is common even in physically active elderly people,[1,33] but asymmetry or the presence of marked fasciculations are pathological. Mild axial or limb rigidity and paratonia may occur with aging[33] and are presumably due to basal ganglia or "extrapyramidal" dysfunction. However, pyramidal signs, such as spastic hypertonia, hyperreflexia, and extensor plantar responses should always be regarded as pathological,[33] as should asymmetrical motor findings.

Histological and physiological changes with aging include decrease in motor neuron,[36] motor unit (MU),[37] and muscle fiber[38] number; increase in motor unit size;[39] selective decrease in Type II fiber diameter; and reduction in motor unit firing rates, particularly at higher force levels.[34] MU number shows a greater than 50 percent decline between ages 20 and 80 years,[40,41] progressing initially at about 1 percent per year and accelerating above age 60.[37] Large myelinated α-motor neurons are preferentially lost, resulting in a disproportionate decrease in the number of large-diameter myelinated motor axons with age.[42] Myelin changes attributable to aging include myelin bubbling, remyelination of axons, and onion bulb formation.[1] There is also a gradual decrease in mean internodal length.[42]

In addition to PNS changes, normal decline of extrapyramidal, cerebellar, and vestibular function may complicate and exacerbate deficits in peripheral motor function. The most conspicuous effect is on gait. These changes include decreased reaction time and balance, slowed rapid alternating movements, and mild dysmetria, and are discussed elsewhere in this volume.

Autonomic system

Manifestations of putative autonomic dysfunction with aging include postural hypotension, insufficiency of thermal regulation, decreased tearing and sluggish pupillary reaction.[43,44] These are similar to the autonomic symptoms that may occur with axonal, demyelinating or pure autonomic neuropathies. However, not all of these age-related abnormalities are necessarily due to primary peripheral nerve dysfunction. The differential diagnosis of autonomic insufficiency includes medications, coincident non-neurological illnesses, and other neurological diseases such as Parkinson's disease and multiple system atrophy. Autonomic dysfunction is discussed at length elsewhere in this book.

Electrophysiology

A detailed discussion of electrodiagnostic principles is beyond the scope of this text. Briefly, the amplitude of the sensory or motor response correlates with the number and size of functioning axons. Conduction velocity (CV) reflects the fastest conducting nerve fibers, and can be diminished by either primary dysfunction of myelin or loss of the larger (faster conducting) axons. Late responses are antidromically stimulated potentials generating a reflex response at the spinal cord, and are therefore more sensitive to pathology along the entire length of the axon. There is a small and progressive decrease in sensory and motor amplitudes and CV from the third to the eighth decade,[45,46] with a fall in CV by about 0.15 m/s per year.[45] In contrast, central (dorsal column) CV declines only after age 60.[45]

PERIPHERAL NEUROPATHY

Epidemiology

The paucity of published data on the prevalence of PN in elderly people betrays the difficulty of clinically distinguishing normal from pathological changes in this age group. Munoz et al.[47] estimated the overall prevalence of PN in a French region with a large geriatric population to be about 1.6 percent. Beghi et al.[48] estimated a much higher prevalence of 3.6 percent for subjects aged 55 and older, and 1.6 percent for those without any known risk factors. The most common causes of PN in elderly people include diabetes (17–27 percent) and neoplasia (12–13 percent), with alcoholism, medications, and idiopathic demyelination accounting for almost one-half of the remaining diagnosed cases.[49,50] The cause of PN could not be determined in approximately one-fourth of patients in these series.[49,50] However, Dyck et al.[51] reported that with intensive evaluation, 76 percent of such "undiagnosed" cases could be properly diagnosed, with the majority having either inherited or idiopathic inflammatory neuropathies.

Table 54-1 enumerates some reasons for the higher prevalence of certain neuropathies in elderly people: (1) PN secondary to medical diseases that are more prevalent in elderly people, (2) PN attributable to progressive pathology or cumulative exposure/trauma, (3) other neuropathies with a higher incidence in old age. Furthermore, peripheral neuropathy

---

Table 54-1 Reasons for increased prevalence of neuropathy in elderly people

Neuropathies secondary to medical conditions more common in elderly people:
- Diabetes, uremia, hypothyroidism
- Neurotoxic medications
- Nutritional deficiencies: thiamine
- Malignancy
- Paraproteinemia
- Vasculitis, collagen vascular disease
- Infection: herpes zoster, hepatitis C virus
- Occlusive vascular disease, peripheral vascular disease

Cumulative effect of progressive disease or exposure over time:
- Progressive disease: inherited neuropathies
- Progressive exposure: alcohol, industrial toxins
- Progressive or repetitive trauma: entrapment neuropathies

Other neuropathies with higher incidence in elderly people:
- GBS
- CIDP

which is subclinical or not age-dependent may have greater functional or neurophysiological salience in elderly people because of: (1) the additive effect of normal aging changes that resemble neuropathy, (2) increased vulnerability of the elderly nervous system and impaired response to injury, (3) the presence of other causes of gait instability (e.g. extrapyramidal, skeletal, and joint changes), and (4) decreased sensory input (e.g. visual, audio, and vestibular).

Functional consequences of neuropathy

One of the main reasons to recognize and treat PN is to limit the associated functional complications. Factors causing falls in the normal elderly include decreased position sense, distal weakness, stooped posture, decreased postural reflexes or reaction time, and impaired balance.[16,52,53] These may be due in part to changes in the visual and vestibular systems, basal ganglia, and cerebellum, but PN is an independent risk factor for falls.[54,55] Other potential complications of PN include foot ulceration and fracture due to loss of pain sensation, deep vein thrombosis and contracture due to immobility from pain or weakness, and life-threatening respiratory compromise

and cardiac arrhythmias. Autonomic dysfunction, including incontinence, impotence and orthostatic hypotension, may be deleterious to both lifestyle and health.

Classification of neuropathies

Table 54-2 presents a schema for the classification of neuropathy based on pathological mechanisms and electrophysiological findings. Length-dependent, or "dying back," neuropathy first involves the distal part of the axon, usually on the basis of toxic, metabolic, or nutritional disorders, with subsequent myelin damage. Wallerian degeneration occurs with focal axonal disruption, leading to concurrent degeneration of the axon and myelin sheath distal to the lesion. Primary sensory neuron damage results in degeneration in both peripheral nerve and dorsal columns.[56] Table 54-3 outlines salient features of the major clinical subtypes, which may exist in combination.

Clinical approach

A detailed history and physical examination are essential. The history should include inquiry into current and prior use of alcohol, intravenous drugs and medications; travel and arthropod exposure; transfusions and occupational exposure; family history of progressive disability; and past vocational and athletic ability. Autonomic symptoms and presence of neck or back pain should be noted. The examination should include inspection of the foot for high arches and palpation of nerves for hypertrophic enlargement at the fibular head or ulnar groove. Vibratory perception time in the toes should be

---

Table 54-2 Classification of neuropathies

Axonal

Distal symmetric ("dying back"):
- Diabetes
- Uremia
- Alcohol
- Toxic/medication
- Nutritional deficiency
- Paraneoplastic
- Paraproteinemic/dysproteinemic
- CMT2

Sensory neuropathy:
- Paraneoplastic
- Sjögren's syndrome
- Cisplatin
- Pyridoxine toxicity

Focal/multifocal (Wallerian degeneration):
- Focal:
  - Entrapment/compression (focal demyelination in early stage)
  - Ischemic: shunt, occlusive vascular disease, PVD
  - Diabetes
  - Herpes zoster
- Multifocal (mononeuritis multiplex):
  - Vasculitic
  - Diabetes
  - Paraproteinemia
  - Infiltrative: leukemia, lymphoma
  - Infectious: Lyme, HIV, HCV

Demyelinating
- Symmetric:
  - GBS
  - CIDP
  - Paraproteinemic (also axonal)
  - CMT1 (Charcot–Marie–Tooth)
- Multifocal:
  - Multifocal motor neuropathy with conduction block
  - Hereditary liability to pressure palsies

Table 54-3 Clinical patterns of neuropathy

Distal sensorimotor (axonal):
- Largest category
- Symmetric distal sensory loss, usually large fiber first
- Distal (ankle) reflex loss first
- Weakness variable

Small-fiber sensory:
- Rarely exists by itself
- Prominent pain: burning, dysesthetic
- Autonomic dysfunction
- Allodynia (painful perception of nonpainful stimuli)

Large-fiber sensory:
- Sensory "gangliononeuronopathies" (see Fig. 54-1)
- Marked vibratory and proprioceptive loss
- Proximal involvement
- Sensory ataxia
- Early reflex loss

Demyelinating:
- Acute, subacute or chronic
- May be distal symmetric, asymmetric or proximal at onset
- Motor signs often predominate (AIDP, CIDP, hereditary neuropathies)
- Early reflex loss

Mononeuritis multiplex:
- Asymmetric, cranial or peripheral nerve involvement (sensory and motor)
- When confluent, may mimic distal polyneuropathy

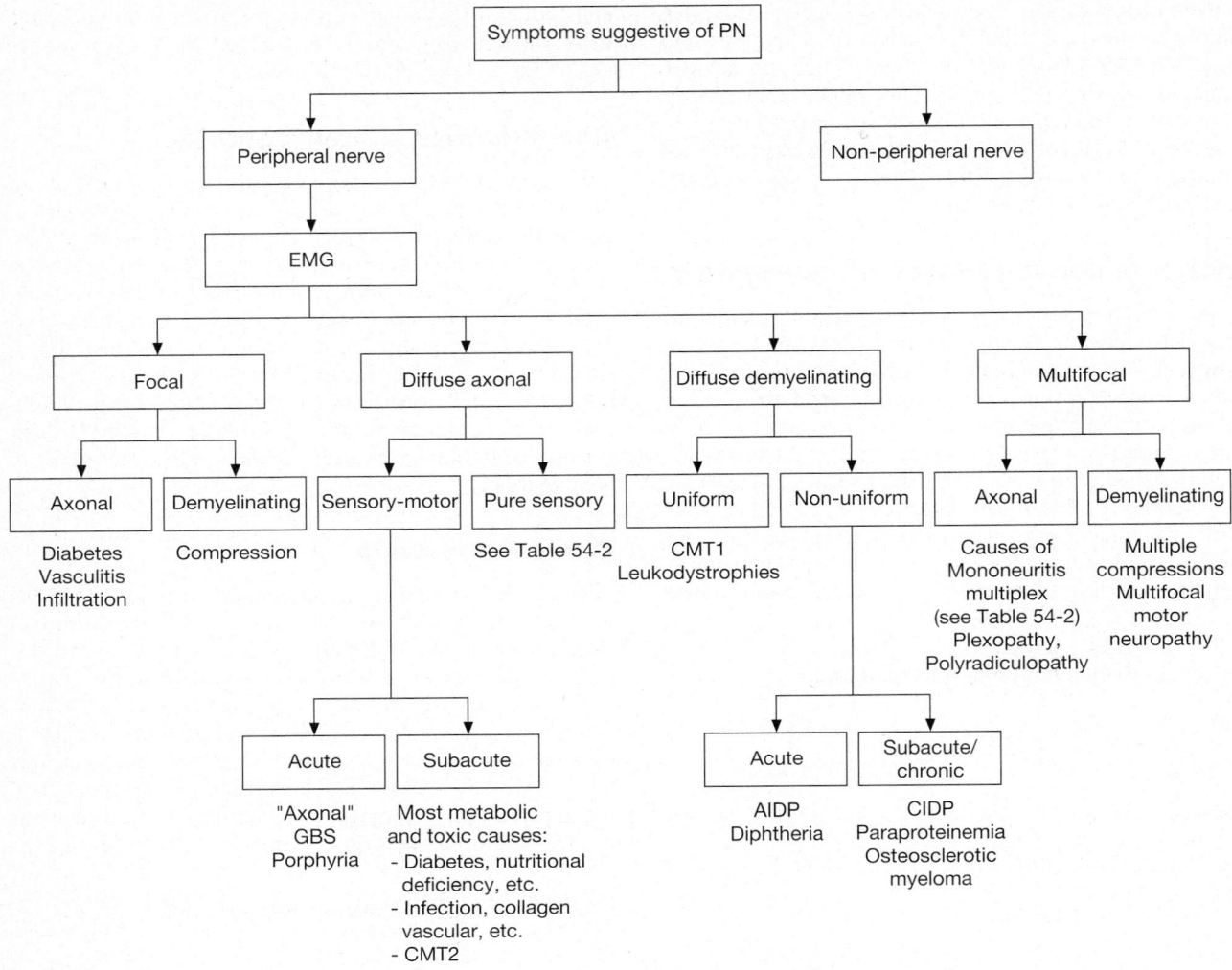

Figure 54-1 Algorithm for the clinical approach to the patient with peripheral neuropathy.

checked, and the pattern of muscle or sensory involvement should be evaluated for symmetry and for conformation to a pattern of multiple nerves or roots.

An algorithm for the diagnostic approach to peripheral neuropathy is presented in Figure 54-1. The first step is to determine whether the problem is in the PNS. Features suggestive of CNS disease include an upper motor neuron pattern of weakness (extensor in arms, flexor in legs), normal or hyperactive tendon reflexes in weak muscles, and extensor plantar responses. Other causes of PNS disease (myopathy, neuromuscular junction disorders, and motor neuron disease) must then be differentiated from PN. Findings suggestive of these disorders include predominantly proximal weakness (including neck flexors), fatiguable weakness on repetitive testing, prominent bulbar (cranial) symptoms, fasciculations, and brisk reflexes. It may be difficult to clinically distinguish confluent multifocal neuropathies from distal symmetric polyneuropathy (DSP), particularly with advanced disease, and certain disorders may present with either pattern.

After an initial clinical evaluation with attention to focality, time course and sensory-motor predominance, electrodiagnostic testing provides valuable diagnostic information, especially in clinically difficult cases. The utility of electromyography (EMG) and nerve conduction testing is several-fold: (1) to confirm neuropathy (vs myopathy, radiculopathy, motor neuron disease, etc.), (2) to distinguish axonal from demyelinating neuropathy and subclassify demyelinating disease, (3) to distinguish symmetric polyneuropathy from mononeuritis multiplex, (4) to establish the approximate duration of nerve pathology, and (5) to grade severity, which is useful in monitoring progression of disease, gauging response to treatment, and determining prognosis. Quantitative sensory threshold testing for thermal and vibratory stimuli, and current perception threshold (CPT) testing, are increasingly available and may provide even greater sensitivity than nerve conduction studies.[57,58] CPT also varies little with age[58] and may therefore be a more specific means of identifying pathology.

Screening blood tests should be ordered even in the presence of a seemingly obvious etiology. For example, because diabetes is common in the elderly population, many cases of concomitant paraproteinemia, cancer, hypothyroidism or hereditary neuropathy could be missed if not specifically searched for. A basic screening battery typically includes hemoglobin A1c, creatinine, thyroid function tests, erythrocyte sedimentation rate, antinuclear antibody, rheumatoid factor, venereal disease research laboratory test, serum B_{12} and folate levels, serum and urine electrophoresis, serum immunofixation, and chest X-ray. Further testing may include anti-Ro and -La antibodies; Lyme, HIV, hepatitis B and hepatitis C titers; cryoglobulins; serum complement levels; antineutrophil cytoplasmic antibodies; paraneoplastic autoantibodies; angiotensin-converting enzyme (ACE) level; heavy metal screen; cerebrospinal fluid (CSF) analysis; and a variety of antiglycolipid antibodies. Of note, specific monoclonal antibody assays may be positive even in the absence of an M-protein detected on immunofixation. However, it is wise to avoid reflexively ordering a battery of expensive antibody tests, including so-called neuropathy "profiles." The subject is reviewed elsewhere.[59]

SPECIFIC NEUROPATHIES BY ETIOLOGY

Diabetes mellitus

Diabetes mellitus (DM) is the most common cause of peripheral nerve dysfunction in developed countries. Two-thirds of all diabetic patients have peripheral neuropathy of some kind, and more than 80 percent of these have evidence of sensorimotor DSP.[60] Patients with insulin-dependent and noninsulin-dependent diabetes mellitus manifest no apparent difference in the incidence or spectrum of disease subtypes.[60,61] Approximately 70 percent of the diabetic population is over 55 years old, and age is an independent risk factor for the occurrence of PN.[62]

Clinical syndromes

It is unclear whether the different forms of diabetic neuropathy represent discrete processes or a continuum,[63] and the tendency for syndromes to overlap renders this question even more difficult.[64] Sensory or sensorimotor DSP is the most common form of PN in DM, and occurs more frequently in the setting of poor glycemic control (see below). Because this neuropathy is length dependent, the distal lower extremities are involved first, followed by the proximal legs, distal arms, and eventually the trunk. The initial complaint is usually of numbness or paresthesias in the feet, which may be accompanied by a burning, stabbing, or dull pain at any point in its progression. There is usually prominent early involvement of large fibers, resulting in sensory ataxia and falling, which may be more pronounced at night or in the shower, when visual feedback is diminished. These features are all common to a variety of sensorimotor neuropathies, and diabetic DSP does not have characteristics that uniquely distinguish it from other causes.

Acute focal mononeuropathies or radiculoneuropathies may involve the limbs, trunk, or cranial nerves, and generally occur without regard to disease duration or severity or degree of glycemic control.[63,65–68] Pain commonly accompanies or precedes the onset of weakness. The prognosis is generally favorable, with spontaneous resolution occurring over months. Mononeuropathies of the third and sixth cranial nerves are common, more often affecting older diabetics with pre-existing

PN.[65] Proximal diabetic neuropathy (also known as diabetic amyotrophy), presents with symmetric or asymmetric lower limb weakness and atrophy, usually preceded by severe proximal leg or pelvic girdle pain.[66] There is typically good spontaneous improvement or response to glycemic control.[63] However, an autoimmune basis has been proposed, in light of a recently discovered inflammatory component,[66,69,70] and there have been anecdotal reports of clinical response to IVIg.[71] Mononeuropathy of an intercostal nerve, or "diabetic truncal radiculoneuropathy," presents as sudden or subacutely progressive unilateral pain and/or dysesthesia around the trunk or in the abdomen and, like proximal diabetic neuropathy, is more common in older men.[66,68,72] There may be abdominal wall weakness suggesting focal swelling, local hypesthesia, or hyperesthesia mimicking abdominal tenderness, which may mislead the physician to search for malignancy. Dermatomal sensory loss is helpful in diagnosis, but often absent. Focal mononeuropathies occurring at common sites of entrapment, especially carpal tunnel syndrome and ulnar neuropathy at the elbow, are far more common, and are responsible for the majority of upper limb symptoms in diabetes.[63,67] Meralgia paresthetica, presenting as pain, dysesthesia, and numbness in the lateral thigh, is also common.[67]

Small myelinated and unmyelinated fibers may be variably involved at all stages of diabetic neuropathy.[63] Veves et al.[73] found that sensory threshold and autonomic testing did not distinguish painful from painless neuropathies. Small-fiber involvement may lead to painless mechanical or thermal injury, including foot ulceration and arthropathy ("Charcot's joint"). Clinical neuropathy is an independent risk factor for ulceration,[74] and is implicated in about 75 percent of all diabetic limb amputations.[75]

Pathogenesis and treatment

The mechanism by which DM causes peripheral nerve dysfunction is the subject of longstanding controversy, principally regarding the relative contributions of ischemic and metabolic factors. Experimental models of diabetic neuropathy suggest prominent roles for oxidative stress,[76] altered ω-6 essential fatty acid metabolism,[77] and accumulation of advanced glycation endproducts,[78] among other mechanisms. However, therapy directed against these mechanisms has largely been limited to the laboratory. Clinical trials of aldose reductase inhibition have had mixed results, but linoleic acid[77] and prostaglandins[79] have enjoyed some success in clinical trials. Glycemic control is the mainstay of preventive treatment, but rarely leads to reversal of disease. Restoration of normoglycemia by pancreatic transplantation stops or even reverses progression of diabetic neuropathy,[80] but is not a practical option for most people. The multicenter Diabetes Control and Complications Trial reported a 64 percent reduction in the incidence of clinically significant neuropathy using "intensive" (continuous infusion or frequent injections) vs conventional therapy in Type I diabetics.[81] Other trials suggest similar results for Type II DM, the most prevalent type in elderly people.[82] However, the risks of insulin-induced hypoglycemia (seizures, coma) may outweigh the benefit of strict control in this population.[82] Treatment with growth factors has shown promise in rat models,[83,84] but the only large-scale Phase III trial of a growth factor (NGF) in humans failed to produce a significant clinical benefit.[85] Focal neuropathies typically demand only supportive treatment, but compression neuropathies may require surgery if severe.[67] Symptomatic treatment of neuropathic pain in DM and other PN may be achieved with tricyclic antidepressants, anticonvulsants (gabapentin, lamotrigine, topiramate), or other agents, including mexiletine, baclofen, and topical lidocaine or capsaicin.[63,86]

Uremia

PN in chronic renal failure occurs in as many as 70 percent of patients requiring treatment,[87] and correlates with disease severity and duration.[88] Although chronic renal failure is more prevalent in the elderly population, age is not an independent risk factor for PN.[89] Clinically, uremic PN resembles that of DM, with insidious symmetric length-dependent sensorimotor dysfunction. Distal dysesthesia is the most common symptom.[90] Muscle cramps are also frequent, but are probably not related to neuropathy.[90] Restless legs syndrome occurs in as many as 40 percent of uremic patients[90] and correlates closely with the presence of neuropathy.[91] PN only develops in patients with glomerular filtration rates below 12 mL/min but the severity of PN does not correlate with serum creatinine or urea concentrations, and no one toxin has been successfully implicated in its pathogenesis.[87] Hemodialysis usually results in stabilization of PN, with frequent complete recovery in mild cases, although response is variable, depending on the severity of disease at onset.[89] In contrast, renal transplantation almost always leads to significant or complete recovery of PN within a year.[87,92]

Toxins

In general, toxic neuropathies are temporally related to exposure and should not progress significantly beyond discontinuation of the implicated substance.[93,94] Industrial chemical and heavy metal exposure is usually evident from the history. Numerous medications may cause PN, including isoniazid, phenytoin, penicillamine, gold, and especially antineoplastic chemotherapeutic agents. Vincristine causes a painful DSP and cisplatin produces an ataxic neuropathy.[95] Amifostine may protect against neurotoxicity from a variety of chemotherapeutic agents.[96]

Nutritional deficiency

Alcohol is one of the most common causes of PN in developed countries.[61] Although there is some epidemiological data to support alcohol as a primary toxin,[97] the weight of evidence points to malnutrition as the principal cause, particularly thiamine deficiency.[98,99] Alcoholic PN presents with distal, symmetric sensory, motor and autonomic findings and often painful dysesthesia. Although abstention from alcohol[100] and initiation of an adequate diet are usually considered critical,[97,98] supplementation with a high bioavailability thiamine alone can improve the PN.[101] Gastrointestinal disease constitutes the other major cause of thiamine deficiency in elderly people.[102] Some studies suggest a high prevalence of symptomatic thiamine deficiency among the elderly population without known risk factors.[103,104] An Irish study found definite or marginal thiamine deficiency in 48 percent of consecutively admitted nonalcoholic geriatric patients, and ankle areflexia was four times more prevalent than in the patients with normal thiamine status.[104] Therefore, although not well studied, patients with idiopathic polyneuropathy might also benefit from empirical thiamine supplementation. PN may also result from deficiencies of pyridoxine (B_6), cobalamin (B_{12}), niacin, folic acid, and vitamin E.[98] Generally, these result in a symmetric, predominantly sensory polyneuropathy, although B_{12} deficiency may present with subacute combined degeneration, involving corticospinal tracts,[105] and vitamin E deficiency often presents with associated spinocerebellar symptoms.[106] Pyridoxine deficiency is responsible for the neurotoxicity of isoniazid, and may also be common among patients on chronic peritoneal dialysis.[107] Notably, excessive ingestion of pyridoxine can result in a pure sensory neuronopathy.[56]

Ischemia and vasculitis

Collagen vascular diseases may present either with DSP, which most likely results from cumulative ischemic lesions summated over the length of the nerve, or more commonly, with mononeuritis multiplex (MNM).[108,109] Vasculitic diseases include polyarteritis nodosa, rheumatoid arthritis, systemic lupus, and Wegener's granulomatosis. Vasculitic neuropathy may respond to corticosteroids with or without cyclophosphamide, although the prognosis is generally poor.[109] PN occurs in 14–22 percent of patients with Sjögren's syndrome and is the presenting manifestation in the majority of cases.[109–111] Garcia-Carrasco et al.[112] reported that 14 percent of their Sjögren's patients had disease onset after age 70 and showed no difference from younger patients in prevalence of PN. However, another study found PNS involvement to be more common in patients older than 50.[111] In addition to trigeminal neuropathy, DSP, and MNM,[109,110] Sjögren's is one of the major causes of "pure sensory" ganglioneuronopathy with prominent ataxia,[56] for which early treatment with intravenous immune globulin (IVIg) may be curative.[113]

Cancer

Neoplasia is an important cause of PN in the elderly, given the increased incidence of cancer with age. Paraneoplastic sensory neuronopathy features prominent proprioceptive loss and sensory ataxia, with minimal if any motor signs.[56] It may precede the diagnosis of cancer by a year or more[61,114] and usually does not respond to successful treatment of the primary tumor.[95,115] It is most commonly associated with primary malignancies of lung, breast, and gastrointestinal tract.[95] DSP may rarely present later in the course of lung cancer.[61] Multiple mononeuropathy may result from leukemic or lymphomatous nerve infiltration, amyloid deposition in multiple myeloma, solid tumor compression of nerve or plexus, and possibly paraneoplastic vasculitis.[95,108]

Infection

Herpes zoster (HZV) infection occurs with greater frequency in elderly and immunocompromised populations.[116] Patients typically present with a painful dermatomal skin eruption associated with or preceded by pain and paresthesia. Dermatomal sensory loss may rarely be present even in the absence of rash. Postherpetic neuralgia and associated motor deficits are more common in elderly people.[116] Hepatitis C virus (HCV) infection constitutes a new worldwide pandemic, which affects about 1.8 percent of the US population.[117] Peripheral nerve involvement is common and ranges in presentation from symmetric or asymmetric painful neuropathies to fulminant MNM, often in association with cryoglobulinemia and vasculitis.[118–120] Although the major risk factors are intravenous drug use and transfusion prior to 1990,[117,121] the prevalence of HCV viremia and antibody response does appear to increase with age.[117] In the population-based Italian Dionysos study, with a population evenly distributed across age groups from 12 to 65, the 56–65 age group accounted for 54 percent of all HCV–RNA positive individuals, with a relative prevalence twice that in the 46–55 age group (26 percent).[122] Accurate data are not available for older age groups, nor are age-related data available for the extrahepatic manifestations. However, we have not observed a higher rate of development of neurological complications in older patients. Antiviral treatment entails use of interferon (interferon α-2b or peginterferon α-2a) with or without ribavirin. The neuropathy has been treated with corticosteroids, cytotoxic agents, plasmapheresis, and IVIg.[123,124] With the above exceptions, most infectious agents are not known to be more prevalent in the elderly, but HIV, Lyme disease, and hepatitis B and C viruses should always be considered in the appropriate clinical setting.

"Inflammatory" neuropathies

Guillain–Barré syndrome

The incidence of Guillain–Barré syndrome (GBS) ranges from 1.2 to 1.7 in 100,000 per year, and constitutes an acute inflammatory demyelinating polyradiculoneuropathy in 85–90 percent of cases in the West.[125–128] Most studies show a linear increase in incidence with age,[127,128] but a bimodal distribution has been described in several series, with the largest peak occurring over age 50.[125,126,128,129] Antecedent conditions include upper respiratory or gastrointestinal (e.g., *Campylobacter jejuni*) infection, vaccination, and surgery.[128] The most common presentation is that of acute sensory loss and prominent weakness, usually in the distal lower extremities, which "ascends" to involve distal arms and eventually the proximal limbs, reaching maximal deficit in under 4 weeks. Weakness may be asymmetric or even proximal at onset, and early involvement of facial muscles is common. At onset, generalized vague pain in the limbs and trunk is common, and sensory complaints, such as paresthesias, often outweigh objective findings. Tendon reflexes are lost early. Other clinical variants, constituting about 17 percent of all cases, include the Miller–Fisher syndrome, ataxia without ophthalmoplegia, and pure bulbar or pure motor syndromes.[125,128] Autonomic instability, marked by cardiac arrhythmias and blood pressure lability, causes serious morbidity. Mechanical ventilation may be necessary in up to 30 percent of patients and is an independent risk factor for poor outcome.[128,130,131] CSF analysis shows high protein with normal cell count, and electrodiagnostic testing suggests segmental demyelination. Depending on presentation, diagnostic testing may include antibodies to *C. jejuni*, GQ1b, GT1a, GM1b, and possibly other gangliosides.[59,128,132] Older patients

tend to have a significantly longer hospital stay and worse prognosis for recovery than younger patients.[128,130,131,133]

Chronic inflammatory demyelinating polyneuropathy (CIDP)

The peak incidence of CIDP is in the fifth and sixth decades.[134] Clinical symptomatology and findings are similar to that of GBS, although facial involvement is uncommon and motor predominance may be less striking.[134] Weakness is usually diffuse, may develop over months or years (by definition longer than 4 weeks), and follows a progressive or relapsing–remitting course, the former being more common in elderly people.[2] Recently, a high incidence of atypical features has been appreciated, including distal predominance, pure sensory involvement, and marked asymmetry.[135] Age at onset is inversely correlated with prognosis.[136]

Treatment

Plasmapheresis is effective in the treatment of both GBS[130,137] and CIDP.[138,139] The efficacy of IVIg in the treatment of CIDP has been demonstrated in double-blind studies,[140,141] and IVIg has been shown to be at least as effective as plasmapheresis in the treatment of GBS,[142,143] although other reports have suggested an unacceptably high relapse rate.[144] Oral corticosteroid therapy is of no benefit over placebo in GBS,[145,146] but has produced improvement in CIDP patients in a controlled trial.[147] Azathioprine is often used for steroid-sparing effect, and in practice it is common to combine two or more modalities (e.g. corticosteroids and plasma exchange). Other agents used in refractory cases include cyclosporine, methotrexate, cyclophosphamide, and recently mycophenolate.[148]

Paraproteinemia

PN associated with monoclonal gammopathy most commonly occurs in the older male population.[149–151] Its clinical manifestations are protean, ranging from mixed DSP to ataxic neuropathy[152] to motor-predominant neuropathy, and are well reviewed elsewhere.[149–151] Associated diseases include multiple myeloma, osteosclerotic myeloma, cryoglobulinemia, Waldenström macroglobulinemia, and amyloidosis.[149,150,153] However, the vast majority of patients have a monoclonal gammopathy of undetermined significance (MGUS), with no other disease association at the time of diagnosis.[149,150,153] MGUS is characterized by a primary demyelinating or mixed neuropathy with predominantly sensory symptoms, and is most commonly associated with an IgM monoclonal protein.[149–151] Patients with IgG and IgA monoclonal proteins often improve with plasmapheresis,[149,153] and may also respond to IVIg or corticosteroids, especially if the phenotype closely resembles CIDP.[153] Patients with IgM monoclonal proteins, with or without anti-myelin-associated glycoprotein, are typically more refractory and may require the addition of other agents, including chlorambucil,[149,153] cyclophosphamide,[149,153] fludarabine,[154] interferon-α, and rituximab.[153] Multiple myeloma may eventually occur in about 17 percent of MGUS patients,[155] but is rarely a direct cause of PN; most such cases are attributable to amyloidosis.[156] Primary (AL) amyloidosis presents at a median age of 65,[156] and may occur alone or in the setting of multiple myeloma. Typical neurological presentations of amyloidosis include a small-fiber type neuropathy and carpal tunnel syndrome,[156] but prominent weakness and atrophy often follow.[157] The presence of PN is considered an adverse prognostic factor for survival.[158]

Hereditary neuropathies

The classic nosology is rapidly becoming obsolete, as our understanding of the molecular basis of the inherited neuropathies has grown exponentially in recent years. The genetics and molecular biology of these disorders are beyond the scope of this chapter, and are reviewed elsewhere.[159,160] Two of the most common clinical forms of hereditary motor and sensory neuropathy receive their designation from the historical eponym "Charcot–Marie–Tooth (CMT) disease." CMT1 is typically a dominantly inherited disorder that causes diffuse and uniformly abnormal myelination. Clinically, it is characterized by distal, symmetric, predominantly motor involvement, with marked wasting in muscles of the feet and calf ("inverted champagne bottle leg," pes cavus) and palpable nerve enlargement. There is early areflexia and stocking-glove sensory loss but usually absence of spontaneous sensory symptoms. Although disease onset is early in life, symptoms are often mild and slowly progressive, and most affected patients do not seek medical consultation.[161] CMT2 is similar to CMT1, but involves primary axon loss. CMT2 is characterized by relative sparing of hand muscles, a lesser degree of hyporeflexia, and later onset, as compared with CMT1. Given the frequency of undiagnosed cases of inherited neuropathy,[51] these entities should always be considered in the differential diagnosis of distal motor weakness in elderly people, and family members should be examined when possible. Genetic testing for a number of the known defects is commercially available.

A common diagnostic problem in elderly people is that of a chronic, slowly progressive, predominantly motor

syndrome with distal muscle wasting and weakness. In addition to CMT2, CIDP, and multiple nerve entrapments, it is important to consider amyotrophic lateral sclerosis and cervical spondylosis, especially when upper motor neuron signs are present.

CONCLUSION

Current trends indicate a progressive increase in mean lifespan in developed countries, which will result in a higher incidence of neurological disease, including PN. Although it is often overshadowed by concurrent systemic or CNS disease, PN may be a major source of disability and discomfort. Appropriate diagnostic measures may establish the specific etiology, and may reveal unsuspected systemic disease. Symptomatic or specific therapies, including neurotrophic factors, may lead to substantial improvement in quality of life.

REFERENCES

1. Schaumburg HH, Spencer PS, Ochoa J: The aging human peripheral nervous system. In Katzman R, Terry RD (eds): The Neurology of Aging. FA Davis, Philadelphia, 1983:111–122
2. Mitchell S: Aging in the peripheral nerves and peripheral neuropathy. In Brocklehurst JC, Tallis RC, Fillit HM (eds): Textbook of Geriatric Medicine and Gerontology, 4th Ed. Churchill Livingstone, Edinburgh, 1992;433–439
3. Thomas PK, Berthold C-H, Ochoa J: Microscopic anatomy of the peripheral nervous system. Nerve trunks and spinal roots. In Dyck PJ, Thomas PK, Griffin JW, Low PA, Poduslo J (eds): Peripheral Neuropathy, 3rd Ed. Saunders, Philadelphia, 1993;28–73
4. Ulrich P, Cerami A: Protein glycation, diabetes, and aging. Recent Prog Horm Res 2001;56:1–21
5. Thomas PK, Scaravilli F, Belai A: Pathologic alterations in cell bodies of peripheral neurons in neuropathy. In Dyck PJ, Thomas PK, Griffin JW, Low PA, Poduslo J (eds): Peripheral Neuropathy, 3rd Ed. Saunders, Philadelphia, 1993:476–513
6. Dyck PJ, Giannini C, Lais A: Pathologic alterations of nerves. In Dyck PJ, Thomas PK, Griffin JW, Low PA, Poduslo J (eds): Peripheral Neuropathy, 3rd Ed. Saunders, Philadelphia, 1993:514–595
7. Spritz N, Singh H, Geyer B: Myelin from human peripheral nerves. Quantitative and qualitative studies in two age groups. J Clin Invest 1973;52:521–523
8. Potvin AR, Syndulko K, Tourtellotte WW, Lemon MS, Potvin JH: Human neurologic function and the aging process. J Am Geriatr Soc 1980;28:1–9
9. Verillo RT: Age related changes in the sensitivity to vibration. J Gerontol 1980;35:185–193
10. Wiles PG, Pearce SM, Rice PJS, Mitchell JMO: Vibration perception threshold: Influence of age, height, sex, and smoking, and calculation of accurate centile values. Diabet Med 1991;8:157–161
11. De Michele G, Filla A, Coppola N et al: Influence of age, gender, height and education on vibration sense: A study by tuning fork in 192 normal subjects. J Neurol Sci 1991;105:155–158
12. Thomson FJ, Masson EA, Boulton AJM: Quantitative vibration perception testing in the elderly—an assessment of variability. Age Ageing 1992;21:171–174
13. Thelen DG, Brockmiller C, Ashton-Miller JA, Schultz AB, Alexander NB: Thresholds for sensing foot dorsi- and plantarflexion during upright stance: effects of age and velocity. J Gerontol A Biol Sci Med Sci 1998;53:M33–38
14. Skinner HB, Barrack RL, Cook SD: Age-related decline in proprioception. Clin Orthop 1984;184:208–211
15. Pai Y-C, Rymer WZ, Chang RW, Sharma L: Effect of age and osteoarthritis on knee proprioception. Arthritis Rheum 1997;40:2260–2265

KEY POINTS Peripheral neuropathies

- Normal aging entails a progressive decline in peripheral sensory and motor function that is steepest after age 50.
- Clinical deficits in pinprick and thermal sensation are more accurate than deficits of vibration and position sense in distinguishing pathological nerve dysfunction from normal aging.
- Peripheral neuropathy is more common in older patients in large part due to an increased prevalence of associated medical conditions, such as diabetes mellitus, cancer, and polypharmacy.
- Peripheral neuropathy is an independent risk factor for falling.
- Screening blood tests for treatable cause of polyneuropathy should be ordered even in the face of an apparently obvious etiology.
- Thiamine deficiency appears to be common and under-recognized in the geriatric population, and patients with idiopathic polyneuropathy may benefit from empirical high bioavailability thiamine supplementation.

16. Hay L, Bard C, Fleury M, Teasdale N: Availability of visual and proprioceptive afferent messages and postural control in elderly adults. Exp Brain Res 1996;108:129–139

17. Benassi G, D'Alessandro R, Gallassi R, Morreale A, Lugaresi E: Neurological examination in subjects over 65 years: an epidemiological survey. Neuroepidemiology 1990;9:27–38

18. Dyck PJ, Curtis DJ, Bushek W, Offord K: Description of "Minnesota Thermal Disks" and normal values of cutaneous thermal discrimination in man. Neurology 1974;24:325–330

19. Jamal GA, Hansen S, Weir AI, Ballantyne JP: An improved automated method for the measurement of thermal threshold. I. Normal subjects. J Neurol Neurosurg Psychiatry 1985;48:354–360

20. Kenshalo DR: Somesthetic sensitivity in young and elderly humans. J Gerontol 1986;41:732–742

21. Heft MW, Cooper BY, O'Brien KK, Hemp E, O'Brien R: Aging effects on the perception of noxious and non-noxious thermal stimuli applied to the face. Aging Clin Exp Res 1996;8:35–41

22. Dyck PJ, Schultz PW, O'Brien PC: Quantitation of touch-pressure sensation. Arch Neurol 1972;26:465–473

23. Thornbury JM, Mistretta CM: Tactile sensitivity as a function of age. J Gerontol 1981;36:34–39

24. Dyck PJ, Karnes J, O'Brien PC, Zimmerman IR: Detection thresholds of cutaneous sensation in humans. In Dyck PJ, Thomas PK, Griffin JW, Low PA, Poduslo J (eds): Peripheral Neuropathy, 3rd Ed. Saunders, Philadelphia, 1993;706–728

25. Thomson FJ, Masson EA, Boulton AJ: The clinical diagnosis of sensory neuropathy in elderly people. Diabet Med 1993;10:843–846

26. Korthals JK: Neuropathies. In Barclay L (ed): Clinical Geriatric Neurology. Lea and Febiger, Philadelphia, 1993;283–293

27. Schmidt JM, Penin F, Cuny G et al: Étude electrophysiologique de l'areflexie achilleenne du sujet agé. Rev Electroencephalogr Neurophysiol Clin 1982;12:357–360

28. Lascelles RG, Thomas PK: Changes due to age in internodal length in the sural nerve in man. J Neurol Neurosurg Psychiatry 1966;29:40–44

29. Schmidt RF, Wahren LK, Hagbarth K-E: Multiunit neural responses to strong finger pulp vibration. I. Relationship to age. Acta Physiol Scand 1990;140:1–10

30. Cauna N, Mannan G: The structure of human digital Pacinian corpuscles (corpuscula lamellosa) and its functional significance. J Anat 1958;92:1–20

31. Bolton CF, Winkelmann RK, Dyck PJ: A quantitative study of Meissner's corpuscles in man. Neurology 1966;16:1–9

32. Swash M, Fox KP: The effect of age on human skeletal muscle: studies of the morphology and innervation of muscle spindles. J Neurol Sci 1972;16:417–432

33. Barclay L, Wolfson L: Normal aging: pathophysiologic and clinical changes. In Barclay L (ed): Clinical Geriatric Neurology. Lea and Febiger, Philadelphia, 1993;13–20

34. Roos MR, Rice CL, Vandervoort AA: Age-related changes in motor unit function. Muscle Nerve 1997;20:679–690

35. Larsson L: Morphological and functional characteristics of the ageing skeletal muscle in man. A cross-sectional study. Acta Physiol Scand Suppl 1978;457:1–36

36. Kawamura Y, O'Brien P, Okazaki H, Dyck PJ: Lumbar motoneurons of man II: the number and diameter distribution of large- and intermediate-diameter cytons in "motoneuron columns" of spinal cord of man. J Neuropathol Exp Neurol 1977;36:861–870

37. Tomlinson BE, Irving D: The numbers of limb motor neurons in the human lumbosacral cord throughout life. J Neurol Sci 1977;34:213–219

38. Lexell J, Taylor CC, Sjostrom M: What is the cause of the ageing atrophy? Total number, size and proportion of different fiber types studied in whole vastus lateralis muscle from 15- to 83-year-old men. J Neurol Sci 1988;84:275–294

39. Stålberg E, Borges O, Ericsson M et al: The quadriceps femoris muscle in 20–70-year-old subjects: relationship between knee extension torque, electrophysiological parameters, and muscle fiber characteristics. Muscle Nerve 1989;12:382–389

40. Brown WF: A method for estimating the number of motor units in thenar muscles and the changes in motor unit count with ageing. J Neurol Neurosurg Psychiatry 1972;35:845–852

41. McComas AJ, Upton ARM, Sica REP: Motoneurone disease and ageing. Lancet 1973;2:1477–1480

42. Stevens JC, Lofgren EP, Dyck PJ: Histometric evaluation of branches of peroneal nerve: technique for combined biopsy of muscle nerve and cutaneous nerve. Brain Res 1973;52:37–59

43. Exton-Smith AN: Disorders of the autonomic nervous system. In Caird FI (ed): Neurological Disorders in the Elderly. Wright, Bristol, 1982:182–201

44. Lye M: Autonomic dysfunction and abnormal vascular reflexes. In Tallis R (ed): The Clinical Neurology of Old Age. John Wiley, Chichester, 1989:191–211

45. Dorfman LJ, Bosley TM: Age-related changes in peripheral and central nerve conduction in man. Neurology 1979;29:38–44

46. Bouche P et al: Clinical and electrophysiological study of the peripheral nervous system in the elderly. J Neurol 1993;240:263–268

47. Munoz M, Boutros-Toni F, Preux PM et al: Prevalence of neurological disorders in Haute-Vienne Department (Limousin Region—France). Neuroepidemiology 1995;14:193–198

48. Beghi E, Monticelli ML: Chronic symmetric symptomatic polyneuropathy in the elderly: a field screening investigation of risk factors for polyneuropathy in two Italian communities. Italian General Practitioner Study Group (IGPST). J Clin Epidemiol 1998;51:697–702

49. George J, Twomey JA: Causes of polyneuropathy in the elderly. Age Ageing 1986;15:247–249

50. Huang CY: Peripheral neuropathy in the elderly: a clinical and electrophysiologic study. J Am Geriatr Soc 1981;29:49–54

51. Dyck PJ, Oviatt KF, Lambert EH: Intensive evaluation of referred unclassified neuropathies yields improved diagnosis. Ann Neurol 1981;10:222–226

52. Bergin PS, Bronstein AM, Murray NMF, Sancovic S, Zeppenfeld K: Body sway and vibration perception thresholds in normal aging and in patients with polyneuropathy. J Neurol Neurosurg Psychiatry 1995;58:335–340

53. Hurley MV, Rees J, Newham DJ: Quadriceps function, proprioceptive acuity and functional performance in healthy young, middle-aged and elderly subjects. Age Ageing 1998;27:55–62

54. Richardson JK, Hurvitz EA: Peripheral neuropathy: a true risk factor for falls. J Gerontol 1995;50A:M211–M215

55. Sabin TD: Peripheral neuropathy: disorders of proprioception. In Masdeu JC, Sudarsky L, Wolfson L (eds): Gait Disorders of Aging: Falls and Therapeutic Strategies. Lippincott, Philadelphia, 1997:273–282

56. Smith BE: Inflammatory sensory polyganglionopathies. Neurol Clin 1992;10:735–759

57. Dyck PJ, O'Brien PC: Quantitative sensation testing in epidemiological and therapeutic studies of peripheral neuropathy. Muscle Nerve 1999;22:659–662

58. Evans ER, Rendell MS, Bartek JP et al: Current perception thresholds in ageing. Age Ageing 1992;21:273–279

59. O'Leary CP, Willison HJ: The role of antiglycolipid antibodies in peripheral neuropathies. Curr Opin Neurol 2000;13:583–588

60. Dyck PJ, Kratz KM, Karnes MS et al: The prevalence by staged severity of various types of diabetic neuropathy, retinopathy, and nephropathy in a population-based cohort: The Rochester Diabetic Neuropathy Study. Neurology 1993;43:817–824

61. Olney RK: Diseases of peripheral nerves. In Tallis R (ed): The Clinical Neurology of Old Age. John Wiley, Chichester, 1989:171–189

62. Naliboff BD, Rosenthal M: Effects of age on complications in adult onset diabetes. J Am Geritar Soc 1989;37:838–842

63. Harati Y: Diabetes and the nervous system. Endocrinol Metab Clin North Am 1996;25:325–359

64. Harati Y: Diabetic peripheral neuropathies. Ann Intern Med 1987;107:546–559

65. Smith BE: Cranial neuropathy in diabetes mellitus. In Dyck PJ, Thomas PK (eds): Diabetic Neuropathy, 2nd Ed. Saunders, Philadelphia, 1999:457–467

66. Said G, Thomas PK: Proximal diabetic neuropathy. In Dyck PJ, Thomas PK (eds): Diabetic Neuropathy, 2nd Ed. Saunders, Philadelphia, 1999:474–480

67. Wilbourn A: Diabetic entrapment and compression neuropathies. In Dyck PJ, Thomas PK (eds): Diabetic Neuropathy, 2nd Ed. Saunders, Philadelphia, 1999:481–508

68. Watkins PJ, Thomas PK: Diabetic truncal radiculoneuropathy. In Dyck PJ, Thomas PK (eds): Diabetic Neuropathy, 2nd Ed. Saunders, Philadelphia, 1999:468–473

69. Said G, Elgrably F, Lacroix C et al: Painful proximal diabetic neuropathy: inflammatory nerve lesions and spontaneous favorable outcome. Ann Neurol 1997;41:762–770

70. Llewelyn JG, Thomas PK, King RMM: Epineurial microvasculitis in proximal diabetic neuropathy. J Neurol 1998;245:159–165

71. Amato AA, Barohn RJ: Diabetic lumbosacral polyradiculoneuropathies. Curr Treat Options Neurol 2001;3:139–146

72. Thomas PK, Tomlinson DR: Diabetic and hypoglycemic neuropathy. In Dyck PJ, Thomas PK, Griffin JW, Low PA, Poduslo J (eds): Peripheral Neuropathy, 3rd Ed. Saunders, Philadelphia, 1993;1219–1250

73. Veves A, Young MJ, Manes C et al: Differences in peripheral and autonomic nerve function measurements in painful and painless neuropathy: a clinical study. Diabetes Care 1994;17:1200–1202

74. McNeely MJ, Boyko EJ, Ahroni JH et al: The independent contributions of diabetic neuropathy and vasculopathy in foot ulceration: How great are the risks? Diabetes Care 1995;18:216–219

75. Boulton AJ: End-stage complications of diabetic neuropathy: foot ulceration. Can J Neurol Sci 1994;21:S18–22

76. Low PA, Nickander KK, Scionti L: Role of hypoxia, oxidative stress, and excitatory neurotoxins in diabetic neuropathy. In Dyck PJ, Thomas PK (eds): Diabetic Neuropathy, 2nd Ed. Saunders, Philadelphia, 1999:317–329

77. Cameron NE, Cotter MA: Role of linoleic acid in diabetic polyneuropathy. In Dyck PJ, Thomas PK (eds): Diabetic Neuropathy, 2nd Ed. Saunders, Philadelphia, 1999:359–367

78. Brownlee M: Advanced glycation end products and diabetic peripheral neuropathy. In Dyck PJ, Thomas PK (eds): Diabetic Neuropathy, 2nd Ed. Saunders, Philadelphia, 1999:353–358

79. Yasuda H, Kikkawa R: Role of antiprostaglandins in diabetic neuropathy. In Dyck PJ, Thomas PK (eds): Diabetic Neuropathy, 2nd Ed. Saunders, Philadelphia, 1999:368–376

80. Navarro X, Sutherland DE, Kennedy WR: Long-term effects of pancreatic transplantation on diabetic neuropathy. Ann Neurol 1998;44:727–736

81. Diabetes Control and Complications Trial Research Group: The effect of intensive treatment of diabetes on the development and progression of long-term complications in insulin-dependent diabetes mellitus. N Engl J Med 1993;329:683–689

82. Skyler JS: Diabetic complications: the importance of glucose control. Endocrinol Metab Clin North Am 1996;25:243–254

83. Brewster WJ, Fernyhough P, Diemel LT et al: Diabetic neuropathy, nerve growth factor and other neurotrophic factors. Trends Neurosci 1994;17:321–325

84. Ishii DN, Lupien SB: Insulin-like growth factors protect against diabetic neuropathy: Effects on sensory nerve regeneration in rats. J Neurosci Res 1995;40:138–144

85. Apfel SC, Schwartz S, Adornato BT et al: Efficacy and safety of recombinant human nerve growth factor in patients with diabetic polyneuropathy: A randomized controlled trial. rhNGF Clinical Investigator Group. JAMA 2000;284:2215–2221

86. Max MB, Culnane M, Schafer SC et al: Amitriptyline relieves diabetic neuropathy pain in patients with normal or depressed mood. Neurology 1987;37:589–596

87. Burn DJ, Bates D: Neurology and the kidney. J Neurol Neurosurg Psychiatry 1998;65:810–821

88. Bolton CF: Peripheral neuropathies associated with chronic renal failure. Can J Neurol Sci 1980;7:89–96

89. Asbury AK: Neuropathies with renal failure, hepatic disorders, chronic respiratory insufficiency, and critical illness. In Dyck PJ, Thomas PK, Griffin JW, Low PA, Poduslo J (eds): Peripheral Neuropathy, 3rd Ed. Saunders, Philadelphia, 1993;1251–1265

90. Nielsen VK: The peripheral nerve function in chronic renal failure. Acta Med Scand 1971;190:105–111

91. Thomas PK: Screening for peripheral neuropathy in patients treated by chronic hemodialysis. Muscle Nerve 1978;1:396–399

92. Bolton CF, Baltzan MA, Baltzan RG: Effects of renal transplantation on uremic neuropathy. N Engl J Med 1971;284:1170–1175

93. Fullerton PM: Toxic chemicals and peripheral neuropathy: clinical and epidemiological features. Proc R Soc Med 1969;62:201–210

94. Schaumburg HH, Berger AR: Human toxic neuropathy due to industrial agents. In Dyck PJ, Thomas PK, Griffin JW, Low PA, Poduslo J (eds): Peripheral Neuropathy, 3rd Ed. Saunders, Philadelphia, 1993:1533–1548

95. Posner JB: Neurologic Complications of Cancer. FA Davis, Philadelphia, 1995

96. Culy CR, Spencer CM: Amifostine: an update on its clinical status as a cytoprotectant in patients with cancer receiving chemotherapy or radiotherapy and its potential therapeutic application in myelodysplastic syndrome. Drugs 2001;61:641–684

97. Behse F, Buchthal F: Alcoholic neuropathy: clinical, electrophysiological, and biopsy findings. Ann Neurol 1977;2:95–110

98. Hillbom M, Wennberg A: Prognosis of alcoholic peripheral neuropathy. J Neurol Neurosurg Psychiatry 1984;47:699–703

99. D'Amour ML, Butterworth RF: Pathogenesis of alcoholic peripheral neuropathy: direct effect of ethanol or nutritional deficit? Metab Brain Dis 1994;9:133–142

100. Windebank AJ: Polyneuropathy due to nutritional deficiency and alcoholism. In Dyck PJ, Thomas PK, Griffin JW, Low PA, Poduslo J (eds): Peripheral Neuropathy, 3rd Ed. Saunders, Philadelphia, 1993:1310–1321

101. Woelk H, Lehrl S, Bitsch R, Köpcke W: Benfotiamine in treatment of alcoholic polyneuropathy: an 8-week randomized controlled study (BAP I Study). Alcohol Alcohol 1998;33:631–638

102. Koike H, Misu K, Hattori N et al: Postgastrectomy polyneuropathy with thiamine deficiency. J Neurol Neurosurg Psychiatry 2001;71:357–362

103. Seligmann H, Halkin H, Rauchfleisch S et al: Thiamine deficiency in patients with congestive heart failure receiving long-term furosemide therapy: A pilot study. Am J Med 1991;91:151–155

104. O'Keeffe ST, Tormey WP, Glasgow R, Lavan JN: Thiamine deficiency in hospitalized elderly patients. Gerontology 1994;40:18–24

105. Victor M, Lear AA: Subacute combined degeneration of the spinal cord. Current concepts of the disease process. Value of serum B_{12} determinations in clarifying some of the common clinical problems. Am J Med 1956;20:896–911

106. Harding AE, Muller DPR, Thomas PK, Willison HJ: Spinocerebellar degeneration secondary to chronic intestinal malabsorption: a vitamin E deficiency syndrome. Ann Neurol 1982;12:419–424

107. Moriwaki K, Kanno Y, Nakamoto H, Okada H, Suzuki H: Vitamin B6 deficiency in elderly patients on chronic peritoneal dialysis. Adv Perit Dial 2000;16:308–312

108. Johnson PC, Rolak LA, Hamilton RH, Laguna JF: Paraneoplastic vasculitis of nerve: a remote effect of cancer. Ann Neurol 1979;5:437–444

109. Rosenbaum R: Neuromuscular complications of connective tissue diseases. Muscle Nerve 2001;24:154–169

110. Gemignani F, Marbini A, Pavesi G et al: Peripheral neuropathy associated with primary Sjögren's syndrome. J Neurol Neurosurg Psychiatry 1994;57:983–996

111. Govoni M, Bajocchi G, Rizzo N et al: Neurological involvement in primary Sjögren's syndrome: clinical and instrumental evaluation in a cohort of Italian patients. Clin Rheumatol 1999;18:299–303

112. Garcia-Carrasco M, Cervera R, Rosas J et al: Primary Sjögren's syndrome in the elderly: clinical and immunological characteristics. Lupus 1999;8:20–23

113. Chen WH, Yeh JH, Chiu HC: Plasmapheresis in the treatment of ataxic sensory neuropathy associated with Sjögren's syndrome. Eur Neurol 2001;45:270–274

114. Horwich MS, Cho L, Porro RS, Posner JB: Subacute sensory neuropathy: a remote effect of carcinoma. Ann Neurol 1977;2:7–19

115. Warenius HM: Paraneoplastic neurological syndromes. In Tallis R (ed): The Clinical Neurology of Old Age. John Wiley, Chichester, 1989:328–334

116. Baringer JR, Townsend JJ: Herpesvirus infection of the peripheral nervous system. In Dyck PJ, Thomas PK, Griffin JW, Low PA, Poduslo J (eds): Peripheral Neuropathy, 3rd Ed. Saunders, Philadelphia, 1993:1333–1342

117. Lauer GM, Walker BD: Hepatitis C virus infection. N Engl J Med 2001;345:41–52

118. Wilson L, Reichler B, Gorevic PD: Cryoglobulinemic and noncryoglobulinemic neuropathy in chronic hepatitis C virus (HCV) infection. Arthritis Rheum 2000;43 (suppl):S192

119. Cacoub P, Maisonobe T, Thibault V et al: Systemic vasculitis in patients with hepatitis C. J Rheumatol 2001;28:109–118

120. Heckmann JG, Kayser C, Heuss D et al: Neurological manifestations of chronic hepatitis C. J Neurol 1999;246:486–491

121. Bellentani S, Miglioli L, Masutti F, Saccoccio G, Tiribelli C: Epidemiology of hepatitis C virus infection in Italy: the slowly unraveling mystery. Microbes Infect 2000;2:1757–1763

122. Bellentani S, Pozzato G, Saccocio G et al: Clinical course and risk factors of hepatitis C virus related liver disease in the general population: report from the Dionysos study. Gut 1999;44:874–880

123. Lin OS, Keeffe EB: Current treatment strategies for chronic hepatitis B and C. Annu Rev Med 2001;52:29–49

124. Zeuzem S, Feinman V, Rasenack J et al: Peginterferon alfa-2a in patients with chronic hepatitis C. N Engl J Med 2000;343:1666–1672

125. Emilia-Romagna Study Group on Clinical and Epidemiological Problems in Neurology. Guillain–Barré syndrome variants in Emilia-Romagna, Italy, 1992–3: incidence, clinical features, and prognosis. J Neurol Neurosurg Psychiatry 1998;65:218–224

126. Cheng Q, Jiang G-X, Fredikson S et al: Incidence of Guillain–Barré syndrome in Sweden 1996. Eur J Neurol 2000;7:11–16

127. Van Koningsveld R, Van Doorn PA, Schmitz PIM et al: Mild forms of Guillain–Barré syndrome in an epidemiologic survey in the Netherlands. Neurology 2000;54:620–625

128. Govoni V, Granieri E: Epidemiology of the Guillain–Barré syndrome. Curr Opin Neurol 2001;14:605–613

129. Alter M: The epidemiology of Guillain–Barré syndrome. Ann Neurol 1990;27(suppl):S7–S12

130. McKhann GM, Griffin JW, Cornblath DR et al: Plasmapheresis and Guillain–Barré syndrome: analysis of prognostic factors and the effect of plasmapheresis. Ann Neurol 1988;23:347–353

131. Fletcher DD, Lawn ND, Wolter TD, Wijdicks EF: Long-term outcome in patients with Guillain–Barré syndrome requiring mechanical ventilation. Neurology 2000;54:2311–2315

132. Yoshino H, Harukawa H, Asano A: IgG antiganglioside antibodies in Guillain–Barré syndrome with bulbar palsy. J Neuroimmunol 2000;105:195–201

133. Sridharan GV, Tallis RC, Gautam PC: Guillain–Barré syndrome in the elderly. Gerontology 1993;39:170–175

134. McCombe PA, Pollard JD, McLeod JG: Chronic inflammatory demyelinating polyradiculoneuropathy. Brain 1987;110:1617–1630

135. Rotta FT, Sussman AT, Bradley WG et al: The spectrum of chronic inflammatory demyelinating polyneuropathy. J Neurol Sci 2000;173:129–139

136. Sghirlanzoni A, Solari A, Ciano C et al: Chronic inflammatory demyelinating polyradiculoneuropathy: long-term course and treatment of 60 patients. Neurol Sci 2000;21:31–37

137. French Cooperative Group of Plasma Exchange in Guillain–Barré Syndrome: Efficiency of plasma exchange in Guillain–Barré syndrome: role of replacement fluids. Ann Neurol 1987;22:753–761

138. Server AC, Lefkowith J, Braine H, McKhann GM: Treatment of chronic relapsing inflammatory polyradiculoneuropathy by plasma exchange. Ann Neurol 1979;6:258–261

139. Dyck PJ, Prineas J, Pollard J: Chronic inflammatory demyelinating polyradiculoneuropathy. In Dyck PJ, Thomas PK, Griffin JW, Low PA, Poduslo J (eds): Peripheral Neuropathy, 3rd Ed. Saunders, Philadelphia, 1993:1498–1517

140. van Doorn PA, Brand A, Strengers PFW, Meulstee J, Vermeulen M: High-dose intravenous immunoglobulin treatment in chronic inflammatory demyelinating polyneuropathy: a double-blind, placebo-controlled, crossover study. Neurology 1990;40:209–212

141. Mendell JR, Barohn RJ, Freimer ML: Randomized controlled trial of IVIg in untreated chronic inflammatory demyelinating polyradiculoneuropathy. Neurology 2001;56:445–449

142. van der Meché FGA, Schmitz PIM, Dutch Guillain–Barré Study Group: A randomized trial comparing intravenous immune globulin and plasma exchange in Guillain–Barré syndrome. N Engl J Med 1992;326:1123–1129

143. Plasma Exchange/Sandoglobulin Trial Group: Randomized trial of plasma exchange, intravenous immunoglobulin, and combined treatment in Guillain–Barré syndrome. Lancet 1997;349:225–230

144. Irani DN, Cornblath DR, Chaudhry V, Borel C, Hanley DF: Relapse in Guillain–Barré syndrome after treatment with human immune globulin. Neurology 1993;43:872–875

145. Hughes RAC, Newsom-Davis JM, Perkin GD, Pierce JM: Controlled trial of prednisone in acute polyneuropathy. Lancet 1978;2:750–753

146. Hughes RAC, Kadlubowski M, Hufschmidt A: Treatment of acute inflammatory polyneuropathy. Ann Neurol 1981;9 (suppl):125–133

147. Dyck PJ, O'Brien PC, Oviatt KF et al: Prednisone improves chronic inflammatory demyelinating polyradiculoneuropathy more than no treatment. Ann Neurol 1982;11:136–141

148. Mowzoon N, Sussman A, Bradley WG: Mycophenolate (CellCept) treatment of myasthenia gravis, chronic inflammatory polyneuropathy and inclusion body myositis. J Neurol Sci 2001;185:119–122

149. Gorson KC: Clinical features, evaluation, and treatment of patients with polyneuropathy associated with monoclonal gammopathy of undetermined significance (MGUS). J Clin Apheresis 1999;14:149–153

150. Ponsford S, Willison H, Veitch J, Morris R, Thomas PK: Long-term clinical and neurophysiological follow-up of patients with peripheral, neuropathy associated with benign monoclonal gammopathy. Muscle Nerve 2000;23:164–174

151. Nobile-Orazio E, Carpo M: Neuropathy and monoclonal gammopathy. Curr Opin Neurol 2001;14:615–620

152. Willison HJ, O'Leary CP, Veitch J et al: The clinical and laboratory features of chronic sensory ataxic neuropathy with anti-disialosyl IgM antibodies. Brain 2001;124:1968–1977

153. Wicklund MP, Kissel JT: Paraproteinemic neuropathy. Curr Treat Options Neurol 2001;3:147–156

154. Wilson HC, Lunn MP, Schey S, Hughes RA: Successful treatment of IgM paraproteinaemic neuropathy with fludarabine. J Neurol Neurosurg Psychiatry 1999;66:575–580

155. Kyle RA: Monoclonal gammopathy of undetermined significance (MGUS). Baillière's Clin Haematol 1995;8:761–781

156. Kyle RA, Dyck PJ: Amyloidosis and neuropathy. In Dyck PJ, Thomas PK, Griffin JW, Low PA, Poduslo J (eds): Peripheral Neuropathy, 3rd Ed. Saunders, Philadelphia, 1993:1294–1309

157. Quattrini A, Nemni R, Sferrazza B et al: Amyloid neuropathy simulating lower motor neuron disease. Neurology 1998;51:600–602

158. Kyle RA, Gertz MA, Greipp PR et al: Long-term survival (10 years or more) in 30 patients with primary amyloidosis. Blood 1999;93:1062–1066

159. Keller MP, Chance PF: Inherited peripheral neuropathy. Semin Neurol 1999;19:353–362

160. Bennett CL, Chance PF: Molecular pathogenesis of hereditary motor, sensory and autonomic neuropathies. Curr Opin Neurol 2001;14:621–627

161. Dyck PJ, Chance P, Lebo R, Carney JA: Hereditary motor and sensory neuropathies. In Dyck PJ, Thomas PK, Griffin JW, Low PA, Poduslo J (eds): Peripheral Neuropathy, 3rd Ed. Saunders, Philadelphia, 1993:1094–1136

Chapter 55

Intracranial tumors

David H. Rosenbaum and Michael L. Gruber

Intracranial tumor ("brain tumor") is perhaps the diagnosis most feared by patients presenting for neurological evaluation. While neoplasms are less common than many of the other conditions that produce neurological symptomatology, their importance in the elderly population becomes proportionately greater because the incidence of brain tumor increases throughout adult life. Furthermore, the incidence and mortality of primary brain tumor have been increasing for at least the last 30 years, and this change has also been most evident in the elderly population.

While the clinical presentation is often suggestive of the diagnosis, the manifestations of brain tumor are protean. The clinical picture may be even more obscure in an elderly person. The introduction of noninvasive brain imaging modalities—computerized X-ray tomography (CT) and magnetic resonance imaging (MRI)—has greatly aided the diagnosis of tumors and intracranial disease in general. While treatment options and prognosis are less favorable in the geriatric age group, recent advances in neurosurgery, radiation treatment, and chemotherapy have to some degree improved this outlook.

CLASSIFICATION

Intracranial tumors are either primary (originating within the calvarium) or metastatic.

Metastatic tumors

Metastatic brain tumors have an incidence in the USA of 150,000 each year. Metastatic lesions are more common in the elderly group.[1,2] Of tumors metastatic to the brain, lung is the most frequent source (50 percent), breast the second. Renal, gastrointestinal tract, and melanomas account for the majority of remaining metastatic brain tumors.

Primary tumors

Primary brain tumors have an incidence of approximately 16,000 each year in the USA.[3] Primary tumors are either parenchymal or extra-axial. Parenchymal tumors are the majority in younger age groups but account for fewer than 50 percent in those aged over 65.[1,4,5] In adults, and particularly the elderly, parenchymal tumors are likely to be malignant, while extra-axial growths are nearly always benign in their pathology. (Note that "malignant" and "benign" are used somewhat idiosyncratically in neuropathology, and the definition of these terms will be discussed later.) The relative incidence of tumor types varies widely from series to series, presumably depending on referral patterns.

Parenchymal primary tumors

Glial-cell-derived growths account for some 90 percent of primary parenchymal tumors. About 85 percent are astrocytomas, and approximately half of these are classified as glioblastoma multiforme, the most malignant of primary brain tumors; 30 percent are in the slightly less malignant category of anaplastic astrocytoma.[1,4,6,7] Glioblastomas and anaplastic astrocytomas together are classified as *malignant gliomas.* The relatively less malignant or "low-grade" tumors account for fewer than 10–15 percent of astrocytomas.[4] Oligodendrogliomas or mixed oligoastrocytomas often calcify and tend to confer a better prognosis; they account for 5–10 percent of adult parenchymal tumors but are less frequent in the geriatric population.[8] Molecular analysis of tissue removed may show deletions of the 1p and/or 19q chromosomes in patients with anaplastic oligodendrogliomas. When present, these findings suggest that the tumor is more likely to respond to chemotherapy, and responders have improved survival.[9,10]

There is a decided shift in incidence towards the more malignant end of the spectrum with advancing age, and some 90 percent of gliomas in those over the age of 65 are glioblastomas.[11,12]

Primary CNS lymphomas account for about 1 percent of parenchymal tumors. They are most often seen in immuncompromised patients (those with AIDS, and the transplant population), are uncommon in the immunologically normal, and occur principally in the sixth and seventh decades of life.[13,14] The incidence is increasing in the elderly population.[15]

Extra-axial tumors

Tumors originating within the skull but outside of brain tissue account for more than half of primary tumors in the older age group. About 80 percent are meningiomas, which become increasingly frequent with age and are as common as glioblastomas.[1,4] Approximately 10 percent are acoustic neuromas and 5–10 percent pituitary adenomas.[1,4,5,7]

EPIDEMIOLOGY

Epidemiological studies indicate that brain tumors of all types are diagnosed with steadily increasing frequency throughout adult life up until the 60s, with a decline in incidence noted after the age of 75.[1,3,16] This apparent decrease may be due to lack of diagnostic aggressiveness in the management of the elderly—if asymptomatic tumors (discovered at autopsy) are included, the incidence is revealed to continue to increase throughout life.

As noted above, the frequency with which certain tumor types are seen also increases with age: malignant lesions—metastatic tumors and malignant gliomas, especially glioblastoma multiforme—become more common,[1,5] as do lymphomas[13] (though the latter remain uncommon). At the benign end of the spectrum, meningiomas (often discovered incidentally) show a striking increase in incidence.[1,5,17] In 5 percent of cases the meningiomas are atypical or malignant.

Epidemiological surveys showed an increase from the 1960s to the 1980s of between two- and eight-fold in deaths from brain malignancy, with the greatest increases in the oldest age groups (over 75 or 80 years).[18–20] While some of the apparent increase is attributable to improved diagnosis consequent to the availability of CT/MRI scanning beginning in the mid-1970s,[18] the trend was already established prior to this time. Changing attitudes towards medical care of the elderly group may account for some portion of the change.[20] A recent study found that the increasing mortality rate from malignant primary brain tumors in the elderly population was directly proportional to the increasing population size of this age group.[21] It proposed a Darwinian differential survival mechanism operating in recent history—in this case, "survival of the less fit"—to account for the observation.

CLINICAL PRESENTATION

A brain tumor is a progressively expanding intracranial mass lesion, and its clinical hallmark is insidious progression of neurological deficits. In up to 10 percent of cases, however, the onset may be abrupt, suggesting a stroke;[22] alternatively, stuttering or paroxysmal symptoms may appear during the course of the illness. These phenomena are occasionally related to intratumoral or peritumoral hemorrhage, secondary vascular compromise, or partial epileptic seizures, but they often remain unexplained. On the other hand, fewer than 1 percent of those presenting with the clinical picture of stroke will be found to have a tumor.[23]

Typically, brain tumors produce progressive dysfunction related to destruction or compression of areas of cortex and subcortical nuclei. With malignant tumors, symptoms develop over weeks to months, while meningiomas may present with insidious progression over months or years.

Primary tumors generally involve the cerebral hemispheres in this age group.[7] Manifestations may include changes in memory, mood, or personality with anterior frontal, deep-seated limbic lesions and temporal tumors; hemiparesis with posterior frontal location; hemisensory loss and hemianopia with parietal lesions; and aphasia with left-sided tumors in the region of the sylvian fissure.

In addition to local effects, since the skull forms a rigid case, the volume increase caused by the tumor and associated edema often raises intracranial pressure. Thalamic tumors may cause obstructive hydrocephalus, leading to the early development of elevated pressure. Intracranial hypertension typically produces both diffuse and remote effects, including headache associated with nausea and vomiting, dizziness, diplopia, gait abnormality and mental changes—most importantly and ominously depressed level of consciousness, suggesting impending brain herniation, which is usually fatal.

While primary tumors of the brainstem and cerebellum are a rarity in the elderly population, about 20 percent of metastatic tumors are located in the posterior fossa, more than 75 percent in the cerebellum.[24] They often present with ataxia or cranial nerve abnormalities.

Acoustic neuromas are very slow-growing Schwann cell tumors of the 8th nerve that produce unilateral hearing loss as the earliest symptom; the adjacent 5th and 7th cranial nerves may be subsequently involved. Only late in their course, with advancing size, do they produce the combination of brainstem and cerebellar signs implicit in their location at the cerebello-pontine angle. Audiometric testing (including brainstem auditory potentials) reveals unilateral retrocochlear hearing loss and indicates the need for an imaging study, ideally contrast-enhanced MRI.[25]

Pituitary adenomas may secrete ACTH, growth hormone, or prolactin, but are more commonly nonfunctioning and produce no symptoms.[26] With progressive enlargement, they may cause headache, change in mental status, or personality, and can produce varying degrees of hypopituitarism. If the tumor grows into the suprasellar cistern, it may compress the optic chiasm and result in bitemporal hemianopia, an almost pathognomonic visual-field defect.

Several factors modify the clinical picture of brain tumor in the elderly person, tending to make the diagnosis less readily evident. The loss of brain parenchymal volume that occurs with age allows tumors to grow for a longer time and become larger without producing an increase in cerebrospinal fluid pressure. Consequently morning headache, with projectile vomiting and papilledema, considered classical signs of brain tumor, are less likely to be prominent in the geriatric patient.[22] Furthermore, elderly individuals are prone to develop mental changes and delirium early in their course and these changes may be phenomenologically indistinguishable from similar states induced by toxic or metabolic disturbances. The clinical picture may at times be difficult to distinguish from degenerative dementia or depression. Such changes in the absence of detectable motor or sensory abnormalities on examination are more likely to occur with meningiomas, which because of their slow growth and extra-axial location allow neural structures to accommodate to their presence. Focal abnormalities on neurological examination in a patient presenting with delirium should, of course, raise the suspicion of tumor, as should progression of a deficit that presents as a "stroke." The most frequent clinical manifestations of brain tumor in the elderly population include motor signs in more than one half, mental changes in a third, and sensory changes, hemianopia or speech abnormalities in one-fifth.[22] The incidence and prevalence of seizures (both partial and secondarily generalized) increase progressively with advancing age, and while vascular lesions account for more than half of the cases of epilepsy beginning after the age of 60, a third are caused by brain tumors.[27]

BENIGN OR MALIGNANT As noted earlier, intracranial neoplasms are classified as benign or malignant and this is conceptually useful for discussion of prognosis and planning of treatment. These terms, however, have a different meaning in neuropathology than they do in general oncology, at least with regard to the primary brain tumors.

Malignancy in primary brain tumors is not defined by the likelihood of metastasis to other organs, which is virtually nil, or even by likely invasion of extraneural structures, but strictly by the ability of the tumor to invade normal neural structures. In this scheme, the vast majority of meningiomas, pituitary adenomas, and acoustic neuromas are potentially benign and surgically curable. However, even these lesions, and meningiomas in particular, may not be surgically approachable because of their location in relation to vital structures (e.g. the carotid artery). "Benign" tumors generally have indolent growth patterns, and even when they are not resectable, often allow for decades of good-quality survival. Low-grade astrocytomas and oligodendrogliomas become a more malignant grade in 5–7 years and should not be considered benign.[9]

INVESTIGATIONS AND DIAGNOSIS

As in the field of neurology in general, a comprehensive history supplemented by a competent neurological examination is likely to bring the clinician close to the correct diagnosis and to suggest the most efficient diagnostic plan. In the elderly person, because of the complexities described above, it is essential that a high index of suspicion be maintained regarding the possibility of brain tumor, particularly since it is generally a treatable and often curable cause of disability.

Brain imaging

Before CT scanning became widely available in the mid-1970s, a definitive evaluation to exclude or diagnose a brain tumor required hospitalization for invasive, uncomfortable, and relatively high-risk procedures—specifically cerebral arteriography and/or pneumoencephalography. Clinicians were reluctant to submit patients, particularly the fragile elderly, to such risks in the absence of clear indications, and patients were often followed clinically without definitive testing as "brain tumor suspects." Today, most experienced neurologists would agree that an individual presenting with a new or progressive neurological deficit or with dementia should, after appropriate clinical evaluation, undergo a definitive brain imaging study. While CT revolutionized the diagnostic evaluation of these patients, contrast-enhanced MRI has proven to be significantly more sensitive in the detection of focal brain lesions and is currently recognized as the optimal screening technique for the detection of most intracranial neoplasms.[25]

Details of the neuroimaging appearances of different types of tumors are beyond the scope of this chapter, but comprehensive reviews are readily available.[25] A few points are worth making here.

By their nature as growing lesions, tumors generally exert a mass effect and displace surrounding structures. Astrocytomas, in addition, infiltrate and replace normal brain parenchyma. A zone of edema typically surrounds a tumor, with characteristic appearance on CT and MRI, though in the case of gliomas some of this "edema" also consists of "fingers" of infiltrating tumor tissue.[28] Because the blood–brain barrier is defective in most tumors, contrast enhancement is an important diagnostic characteristic, though frequently absent in the low-grade gliomas.[25] None of these features, of course, is pathognomonic, and each finding must be interpreted in its clinical context. Contrast enhancement of a parenchymal tumor suggests a

relatively more malignant process, but high-grade pathology can be seen in patients with nonenhancing MRI scans. Multiple lesions, best appreciated with contrast MRI, are typical of metastatic disease but can be seen in 3 percent of astrocytomas. Primary cerebellar tumors are rare in the elderly population and suggest metastasis.

A primary CNS lymphoma is often seen as a densely enhancing lesion in the deep periventricular white matter.[29] In a third of patients the lesions are multiple. In 20 percent of cases there is either evidence of leptomeningeal spread or concomitant vitreal/retinal disease.[30]

Meningiomas are extra-axial in location, and usually have a broad base of attachment to the dura; they show extensive, uniform contrast enhancement and as they enlarge can exert a mass effect.

Functional MRI (perfusion/spectroscopy) is proving very helpful in the initial work-up of a patient with a nonenhancing mass. In a heterogeneous inoperable glioma it can help the surgeon plan the biopsy target. Functional MRI also is used in treated patients to help determine whether findings on conventional MRI are due to tumor progression or radiation necrosis. In some centers it is used to help assess therapeutic response to chemotherapy and other treatments.

CSF examination

Lumbar puncture is *not* indicated for the diagnosis of brain tumor. While elevation of CSF protein is commonly seen, this is a nonspecific finding whose utility has been eclipsed by the advent of noninvasive imaging. Cytological examination may reveal malignant cells and aid in pathological diagnosis, particularly with primary CNS lymphomas, leukemia, or metastases involving the meninges (meningeal lymphomatosis or carcinomatosis).[31] Rarely a glioma will present with a meningeal picture (meningeal gliomatosis) diagnosable by CSF cytology. Since there is a small but real risk that lumbar puncture will cause brain herniation, particularly in the presence of a large tumor and increased intracranial pressure, CT or MR imaging should be performed first to rule out such a situation.

Biopsy

The role of surgery and surgical tumor resection is discussed more fully in the section on treatment. As a rule, a definitive tissue diagnosis should be achieved when practicable. This is both because the particular treatment will depend on the tumor type, and because not all space-occupying lesions seen on brain imaging prove to be neoplastic.[32,33] On the other hand, a recent study of 200 patients undergoing stereotactic biopsy concluded that biopsy may not be needed when a clear presumptive diagnosis can be made on the basis of clinical and neuroimaging evidence.[34] Furthermore, the decision to perform a biopsy must be conditioned by the overall clinical context and the patient's medical and psychosocial status. For example, a patient with known malignancy and uncontrolled systemic metastases who presents with brain lesions typical of metastatic disease does not usually require biopsy; nor does a frail patient with end-stage Alzheimer's disease and a large, radiologically malignant brain tumor. In a patient with a single tumor or multiple brain lesions consistent with metastatic disease, work-up to identify a primary source beyond complete physical examination (with testing for occult blood in stool) and CT scan of chest is often unrevealing and probably not cost-effective.[35] In this situation, biopsy (or resection, if appropriate—see below) would be the logical next step. When biopsy *is* indicated, the procedure of choice is a CT- or MRI-guided stereotactic needle biopsy, which has an overall morbidity of just 2 percent.[36]

TREATMENTS

Surgery

The ideal treatment for brain tumor is total surgical resection resulting in cure. As indicated, this is generally possible only for the "benign" extra-axial lesions: meningioma, acoustic neuroma, and pituitary adenoma. Even here the anatomic location of the tumor or the general health of the patient may preclude aggressive surgery. Age itself is not a contraindication to neurosurgery, and perioperative mortality and morbidity are not necessarily increased after the age of 65.[22] It has also been found that patients over 65 undergoing craniotomy for brain tumor, although sicker and having a higher rate of complications than those under 65, had similar outcomes, including quality-of-life scores.[37] However, since elderly people are more prone to coexisting medical conditions that worsen their prognosis, the approach to treatment is usually balanced toward the less aggressive side, particularly in those who are frail. Since the natural history of "benign" tumors is often measured in decades, an incidentally discovered asymptomatic lesion may not require treatment, and partial removal of a tumor that cannot be completely resected may render the patient asymptomatic for the duration of the lifespan. Stereotactic radiosurgery for unresectable tumors is proving to be an important option (see below). Pituitary adenomas can be treated with a high rate of success and low morbidity by transsphenoidal removal;[38] prolactin-secreting tumors are often effectively treated with bromocriptine[39] or other dopaminergic agents; and tumors that are inoperable or incompletely removed should be treated with radiation (see below). Radiation therapy may also be useful in preventing recurrence of partially resected meningiomas or in treating recurrences.[40]

For malignant tumors and those that cannot be fully removed, and where the clinical situation does not contraindicate an aggressive approach (see discussion above in the section on biopsy), as much of the tumor as is readily accessible should be removed, with care taken not to disturb adjacent brain tissues. Such "debulking" reduces the mass effect, tends to decrease local and diffuse symptoms, often permits a reduction in steroid dose, and may allow the patient to better tolerate the edema that can accompany radiotherapy.[41] Postoperative morbidity is no greater in those undergoing large resections than in those having small resections or biopsies,[42] and large removals, in patients with malignant gliomas, have been shown in some studies to improve survival.[43–45] On the other hand, in the treatment of malignant gliomas many neuro-oncologists feel that resection offers no survival advantage over biopsy, particularly stereotactic serial biopsy.[46] A recent attempt to study this important question from an evidence-based review of the literature found no qualifying studies.[47]

Primary CNS lymphoma patients should be biopsied for accurate diagnosis. If possible the patient should not be on steroids.

In patients with brain metastasis proven by MRI to be solitary and whose primary cancer is controlled, surgical removal followed by radiation has been shown to increase duration of life (40 vs 15 weeks) and to greatly prolong the period of functionally independent survival (38 vs 8 weeks) compared to biopsy plus radiation.[48] Unfortunately, the applicability of this study to geriatrics is unclear, since the median age of the patients was 60 years and none was over 74. As with gliomas, age is a negative prognostic factor for patients with brain metastases. Of note is that, in this study of 54 patients with known systemic cancer and brain lesions diagnosed by CT or MRI to be consistent with brain metastasis, six patients proved to have lesions that were *not* metastatic. Two were abscesses and one was a nonspecific inflammatory reaction[48]— a compelling argument for tissue confirmation of diagnosis prior to treatment.

Low-grade gliomas are uncommon in this population and require treatment only when they become symptomatic. This involves maximal feasible resection followed by local radiotherapy.

Adrenal corticosteroids

Malignant glial tumors, metastatic tumors, and some meningiomas are surrounded by edema, which increases the mass effect, accentuates focal deficits, and produces diffuse signs (headache, and mental and gait abnormalities). This "vasogenic" edema is caused by breakdown of blood–brain barrier secondary to abnormal fenestration of vascular endothelium in the tumor, allowing leakage of water and solutes into and around the tumor.[49] Glucocorticosteroids are effective in reversing this leakiness[50] and have been used as palliative and adjunctive therapy for over 30 years. Significant symptomatic improvement occurs within 24–48 hours in the majority of patients and may be dramatic. Elderly patients respond as well as the young.[51]

Primary CNS lymphoma may disappear when treated with steroids alone, but almost invariably recurs. Best results are obtained with chemotherapy followed by whole-brain radiation.[13,29,52]

Dexamethasone is the standard preparation because of its potency, its relatively minimal mineralocorticoid effect, and because it may cause less psychiatric disturbance than other preparations. It has a prolonged biological half-life that makes it suitable for twice-a-day dosing, and when given with meals, H_2 blockers are needed only for patients with a history of peptic ulcer disease. The usual dose is 16 mg a day, with greater doses given if there is not a satisfactory response. A recent study, however, found that 4 mg a day was as effective as 16 mg (in patients without impending herniation), with significant reduction in toxicity.[53]

The toxicity of glucocorticoids can be quite important, particularly when they are taken for prolonged periods.[54] The most serious relate to immunosuppressive and antipyretic effects, which predispose to infection while masking some of its signs. Weight gain and the development of Cushingoid habitus and facies adversely affect quality of life. Sleep disturbance and emotional lability may occur, the latter to the point of frank psychosis. Hyperglycemia, hypertension, increased gastric acid secretion, and osteoporosis can all lead to major complications. Steroid myopathy, manifesting with proximal muscle weakness, may be quite disabling.[55] The incidence of these toxicities increases with dose and duration of therapy, so that corticosteroids should be used at the lowest effective dose—and tapered, if possible, once definitive therapy has been implemented.

Radiation therapy

External-beam radiotherapy is very important in the treatment of malignant gliomas and metastatic disease; it more than doubles the median survival time in both conditions,[56–58] although the benefit for malignant glioma patients over the age of 70 is significantly diminished.[59] Unfortunately, radiation is toxic to normal brain, and there is evidence that elderly people may be more susceptible.[60] Higher doses are more effective, but also more toxic, with a substantial risk of dementia.[61,62] Particularly in an elderly person, an attempt should be made to restrict treatment to the "involved field" and to treat metastatic disease with smaller fractions over a longer time period (e.g. 4 weeks).

"Involved-field" radiation has replaced whole-brain radiation for malignant gliomas. Primary CNS lymphoma is highly sensitive to radiation, and is generally treated, as noted earlier, with whole-brain radiation,[13] often preceded by chemotherapy.[29,52]

Stereotactic radiosurgery (by linear accelerator or gamma knife) is a widely available technique that concentrates a high-radiation dose into a restricted volume and is less invasive and as effective as brachytherapy.[63] Radiosurgery is an excellent alternative to surgery for metastatic disease provided that the lesions are of appropriate size and volume. As mentioned above, radiosurgery is also useful in the treatment of meningiomas and acoustic neuromas that cannot be completely removed by conventional surgery, although eventual recurrence is likely.[64] In some centers, a combined approach with surgery being the initial procedure, followed by radiosurgery, is the standard of care.

Chemotherapy

The role of chemotherapy in the treatment of brain tumors, particularly in the geriatric population, is limited. It has no place in the therapy of benign extra-axial neoplasms or low-grade astrocytomas, nor has chemotherapy proved to be of much use in the treatment of brain metastases.

BCNU is the most widely used agent in the treatment of malignant gliomas, and a recent meta-analysis has shown it to have a limited effect in prolonging life.[65] Unfortunately even this modest benefit is much diminished in the elderly population.[66,67] New strategies including drugs that may be more effective are currently in clinical trials. Examples are carboplatinum, temozolamide, irinotecan, angiogenesis inhibitors, drugs that target epidermal and platelet-derived growth factor receptors, and tumor vaccines.

Median survival with glioblastoma is less than one year, and only slightly more than two and a half years with anaplastic astrocytoma. The outlook is even more dismal in the elderly population.[68]

In contrast, chemotherapy does seem to prolong survival in those with primary CNS lymphoma (PCNSL),[52,69,70] although again the prognosis is significantly worse in the elderly population.[71] Attempts to treat PCNSL with chemotherapy alone (methotrexate) have shown some initial success.[70] Avoidance of whole-brain irradiation in elderly people is an important goal.[72]

CONCLUSION

While the manifestations of a brain tumor in an elderly person can be subtle and nonspecific, careful attention to the neurological evaluation and appropriate use of brain imaging studies should minimize any delay in diagnosis. It is important to recognize that, ominous as the diagnosis may seem, the majority of primary brain tumors in this population are benign, eminently treatable, and usually curable. Even in the case of malignant tumors, advances in neurosurgical technique, radiation oncology, and chemotherapy have greatly improved the outlook for many elderly patients, in terms of both prolongation of life and enhanced quality of survival. Numerous experimental approaches are currently under investigation, and although a therapeutic breakthrough does not appear imminent, it is to be hoped that in the not-too-distant future more effective treatments for malignant neoplasms of the brain will be found.

Summary of management algorithm
Intracranial tumors

- Enhanced MRI is the diagnostic test of choice.

- Pathological diagnosis is mandatory unless the patient is dying from widespread metastatic disease or has a severe, unrelated neurological or medical condition.

- The geriatric population should not be denied surgery, radiation therapy, or chemotherapy based on age alone.

- All patients who are eligible for clinical trials should be encouraged to participate.

KEY POINTS Intracranial tumors

■ The incidence of all types of brain tumor increases significantly with age.

■ Clinical diagnosis in elderly people may be more difficult and a high index of suspicion is appropriate.

■ Neurological evaluation and MRI scan will nearly always lead to the correct diagnosis.

■ Tissue diagnosis is desirable for treatment planning but, depending on clinical context, is not always necessary.

■ Benign tumors—meningiomas, pituitary adenomas, and acoustic neuromas—are common in the elderly population, usually have a very good prognosis, and are often surgically curable.

■ For malignant growths, surgery may have an important palliative role, but glucocorticoid and radiation therapies are the mainstays. Benefits of chemotherapy have so far been disappointing.

REFERENCES

1. Walker AE, Robins M, Weinfeld FD: Epidemiology of brain tumors: the national survey of intracranial neoplasms. Neurology 1985;35:219–226
2. National Center for Health Statistics, Division of Vital Statistics, Center for Disease Control. Available at: www.edu.gov/nchs.htm (October 2001)
3. Radhakrishnan K, Mokri B, Parisi JE et al: The trends in incidence of primary brain tumors in the population of Rochester, Minnesota. Ann Neurol 1995;37:67–73
4. Jaeckle KA: Central nervous system tumors in the elderly. In Barclay L (ed): Clinical Geriatric Neurology. Lea & Febiger, Philadelphia, 1993
5. Radhakrishnan K, Bohnen NI, Kurland LT: Epidemiology of brain tumors. In Morantz RA, Walsh JW (eds): Brain Tumors. Marcel Dekker, New York, 1993:1–18
6. Walker MD: Malignant Brain Tumors. American Cancer Society, New York, 1975
7. Zulch KJ: Brain Tumors: Their Biology and Pathology. Springer-Verlag, New York, 1986
8. Salcman M: Brain tumors and the geriatric patient. J Am Geriatr Soc 1982;30:501–508
9. Fortin D, Cairncross G, Hammond R: Oligodendroglioma: an appraisal of recent data pertaining to diagnosis and treatment. Neurosurgery 1999;45:1279–1291
10. Glass J, Hochberg FH, Gruber M et al: The treatment of oligodendrogliomas and mixed oligoastrocytomas with PCV chemotherapy. J Neurosurgery 1992;76:741–745
11. Werner MH, Schold CS: Primary intracranial neoplasms in the elderly. Clin Geriatr Med 1987;3:765–779
12. Trouillas P, Menaud G, De The G, Aimard G, Devic M: Etude epidemiologique des tumeurs primitives de neuraxe dans la region Rhone-Alpes. Rev Neurol Paris 1975;131:691–708
13. Murray K, Kun L, Cox J: Primary malignant lymphomas of the central nervous system: results of treatment of 11 cases and review of the literature. J Neurosurg 1986;65:600–607
14. Miller DC, Hochberg FH, Harris NL et al: Pathology with clinical correlations of primary CNS lymphomas: the Massachusetts General Hospital experience. Cancer 1994;74:1383–1397
15. Eby NL, Grufferman S, Flannelly CM et al: Increasing incidence of primary brain lymphoma in the US. Cancer 1988;62:2461–2465
16. Schoenberg BS, Christine BW, Whisnant JP: The descriptive epidemiology of primary intracranial neoplasms: the Connecticut experience. Am J Epidemiol 1976;104:499–510
17. Annegers JF, Schoenberg BS, Okazaki H, Kurland LT: Epidemiologic study of intracranial neoplasms. Arch Neurol 1981;38: 217–219
18. Greig NH, Ries LG, Rancik R, Rapoport SI: Increasing annual incidence of primary malignant brain tumors in the elderly. J Natl Cancer Inst 1990;82:1621–1624
19. Davis DL, Hoel D, Fox J, Lopez A: International trends in cancer mortality in France, West Germany, Italy, Japan, England and Wales, and the USA. Lancet 1990;336:474–481
20. Modan B, Wagener DK, Feldman JJ, Rosenberg HM, Feinleib M: Increased mortality from brain tumors: a combined outcome of diagnostic technology and change of attitude toward the elderly. Am J Epidemiol 1992;135:1349–1357
21. Riggs JE: Rising primary malignant brain tumor mortality in the elderly: a manifestation of differential survival. Arch Neurol 1995;52:571–575
22. Tomita T, Raimondi AJ: Brain tumors in the elderly. JAMA 1981;246:53–55
23. Sandercock P, Molyneux A, Warlow C: Value of computed tomography in patients with stroke. BMJ 1985;290:193–197
24. Posner JB: Management of central nervous system metastases. Semin Oncol 1977;4:81–91
25. Manzione JV, Poe LB, Kieffer SA: Intracranial neoplasms. In Haaga JR, Lanzieri CF, Sartoris DJ, Zerhoumi EA (eds): Computed Tomography and Magnetic Resonance Imaging of the Whole Body, 3rd edn. Mosby, St Louis, 1994
26. Post KD, Jackson JMD, Reichlin S (eds): The Pituitary Adenoma. Plenum Medical, New York, 1980
27. Loiseau J, Loiseau P, Duche B et al: A survey of epileptic disorders in southwest France: seizures in elderly patients. Ann Neurol 1990;27:232–237
28. Halperin EC, Burger PC, Bullard DE: The fallacy of the localized supratentorial malignant glioma. Int J Radiat Oncol Biol Phys 1988;15:505–509
29. DeAngelis LM, Yahalom J, Heinemann MH, Cirrincione C, Thaler HT: Primary CNS lymphoma: combined treatment with chemotherapy and radiotherapy. Neurology 1990;40:80–86
30. Schwaighofer BW, Hesselink JR, Press GA et al: Primary intracranial CNS lymphoma: MR manifestations. AJNR 1989;10:725–729
31. Posner JB, Chernik NL: Intracranial metastases from systemic cancer. In Schoenberg BS (ed): Neurological Epidemiology: Principles and Clinical Applications. Raven Press, New York, 1978
32. Todd NV, McDonagh T, Miller JD: What follows diagnosis by computed tomography of solitary brain tumor? Audit of one year's experience in southeast Scotland. Lancet 1987;i:611–612
33. Patchell RA, Tibbs PA, Walsh JW et al: A randomized trial of surgery in the treatment of single metastasis to the brain. N Engl J Med 1990;322:494–500
34. Vaquero J: Stereotactic biopsy for brain tumors: is it always necessary? Surg Neurol 2000;53:432–437
35. Voorhies RM, Sundresan N, Thaler HT: The single supratentorial lesion: an evaluation of preoperative diagnostic tests. J Neurosurg 1980;53:364–368
36. Bullard DE: Role of streotaxic biopsy in the management of patients with intracranial lesions. Neurol Clin 1985;3:817–830
37. Layon JA, George BE, Hamby B, Gallagher TJ: Do elderly patients overutilize healthcare resources and benefit less from them than younger patients? A study of patients who underwent craniotomy for treatment of neoplasm. Crit Care Med 1995;23:829–834
38. Cohen LC, Bevan JS, Adams CBT: The presentation and management of pituitary tumors in the elderly. Age Ageing 1989;18:247–252
39. Besser GM: Medical management of prolactinomas. In Givens JR (ed): Hormone-Secreting Pituitary Tumors. YearBook Medical, Chicago, 1982
40. Wara WM, Sheline GE, Newman H, Townsend JJ, Boldrey EB: Radiation therapy of meningiomas. Am J Roentgenol Radium Ther Nucl Med 1975;123:453–458
41. Grossman SA, Zeltzman M: Practical considerations in the management of adults with malignant astrocytomas. Neurologist 1996;2:130–138
42. Fadul C, Wood J, Thaler H et al: Mortality and morbidity of craniotomy for excision of supratentorial gliomas. Neurology 1988;38:1374–1379
43. Ammirati M, Vick N, Liao YL, Cirik I, Mikhael M: Effect of the extent of surgical resection on survival and quality of life in patients with supratentorial glioblastomas and anaplastic astrocytomas. Neurosurgery 1987;21:201–206
44. Devaux BC, O'Fallon JR, Kelly PJ: Resection, biopsy and survival in malignant glial neoplasms: a retrospective study of clinical parameters, therapy and outcome. J Neurosurg 1993;78:767–775
45. Simpson JR, Horton J, Scott C et al: Influence of location and extent of surgical resection on survival of patients with glioblastoma multiforme: results of three consecutive Radiation Therapy Oncology Group clinical trials. Int J Radiat Oncol Biol Phys 1993;26:239–244
46. Kelly PJ, Dauma-Duport C, Kispert DB et al: Imaging-based stereotactic serial biopsy in untreated intracranial glial neoplasms. J Neurosurg 1987;66:865–874
47. Metcalfe SE: Biopsy versus resection for malignant glioma. Cochrane Database Syst Rev 2000;(2):CD002034
48. Patchell RA, Tibbs PA, Walsh JW et al: A randomized trial of surgery in the treatment of single metastases to the brain. N Engl J Med 1990;322:494–500
49. Long DM: Capillary ultrastructure and the blood–brain barrier in human malignant tumors. J Neurosurg 1970;32:127–144
50. Delattre JY, Arbit E, Rosenblum MK et al: High-dose versus low-dose dexamethasone in experimental epidural spinal cord compression. Neurosurgery 1988;22:1005–1007
51. Graham K, Caird FI: High-dose steroid therapy of intracranial tumor in the elderly. Age Ageing 1978;7:146–150
52. Glass L, Gruber ML, Hochberg FH: Preirradiation methotrexate chemotherapy of primary CNS lymphoma: long-term outcome. J Neurosurgery 1994;81:188–195
53. Vecht CJ, Hovestadt A, Verbiest HBC, van Vliet JJ, van Putten WLJ: Dose–effect relationship of dexamethasone on Karnofsky performance in metastatic brain tumors: a randomized study of doses of 4, 8, and 16 mg per day. Neurology 1994;44:675–680
54. Weissman DE, Dufer D, Vogel V, Abeloff MD: Corticosteroid toxicity in neuro-oncology patients. J Neurooncol 1987;5:125–128
55. Dropcho EJ, Soong SJ: Steroid-induced muscle weakness in patients with primary brain tumors. Neurology 1991;41:1235–1239
56. Borgelt B, Gelber R, Kramer S et al: The palliation of brain metastases: final results of the first two studies by the Radiation Therapy Oncology Group. Int J Radiat Oncol Biol Phys 1980;6:1–9
57. Walker MD, Green SB, Byar DP et al: Randomized comparisons of radiotherapy and nitrosoureas for the treatment of malignant glioma after surgery. N Engl J Med 1980;303:1323–1329

58. Berk L: An overview of radiotherapy trials for the treatment of brain metastases. Oncology 1995;9:1205–1219

59. Peschel R, Wilson L, Haffty B et al: The effect of advanced age on the efficacy of radiation therapy for early breast cancer, localized prostate cancer and grade III–IV glioma. Int J Radiat Oncol Biol Phys 1993;26:539

60. Stylopoulos LA, George AE, de Leon MJ et al: Longitudinal CT study of parenchymal brain changes in glioma survivors. Am J Neuroradiol 1988;9:517–522

61. Marks JE, Baglan RJ, Prassad SC, Blank WF: Cerebral radionecrosis: incidence and risk in relation to dose, time, fractionation and volume. Int J Radiat Oncol Biol Phys 1981;7:243–252

62. Deangelis LM, Delattre JY, Posner JB: Radiation-induced dementia in patients cured of brain metastases. Neurology 1989;39:789–796

63. Loeffler JS, Alexander E, Shea WM et al: Radiosurgery as part of the initial management of patients with malignant gliomas. J Clin Oncol 1992;10:1379–1385

64. Sawaya R: Neurosurgery issues in oncology. Curr Opin Oncol 1991;3:459–466

65. Fine HA, Dear KBG, Loeffler JS, Black PM, Canellos GD: Meta-analysis of radiation therapy with and without adjuvant chemotherapy for malignant gliomas in adults. Cancer 1993;71:2585–2597

66. Walker MD, Alexander E, Hunt WE et al: Evaluation of BCNU and/or radiotherapy in the treatment of anaplastic gliomas: a cooperative clinical trial. J Neurosurg 1978;49:333–343

67. Green SB, Byar DP, Walker MD et al: Comparisons of carmustine, procarbazine and high-dose methylprednisolone as additions to surgery and radiotherapy for the treatment of malignant glioma. Cancer Treat Rep 1983;67:121–132

68. Salcman M, Kaplan RS, Ducker TB, Abdo H, Montgomery E: The effect of age and reoperation on survival in the combined modality treatment of malignant astrocytoma. Neurosurgery 1982;10:454–463

69. DeAngelis LM, Yahalom J, Thaler HT, Kher U: Combined modality therapy for primary CNS lymphoma. J Clin Oncol 1992;10:635–643

70. Cher LM, Glass J, Hochberg FH et al: Therapy of primary CNS lymphoma with methotrexate-based chemotherapy and deferred whole-brain radiation therapy. Neurology 1994;44(suppl 2):A374–A375

71. Nelson DF, Martz KL, Bonner H et al: Non-Hodgkin's lymphoma of the brain: can high-dose, large-volume radiation therapy improve survival? Report on a prospective trial by the Radiation Tumor Oncology Group: RTOG 8315. Int J Radiat Oncol Biol Phys 1992;23:9–17

Chapter 56

Disorders of the spinal cord and nerve roots

Richard A. Cowie

The majority of the pathological processes affecting the spinal cord in elderly people are related to degenerative diseases of the spinal column, or to insufficiency of the cord's blood supply. However, old age does not exclude many of the disorders that are more commonly seen in other age groups. In most patients, a definite clinical diagnosis can be reached by taking a thorough clinical history and performing a careful examination.

Neurological assessment of an elderly person is sometimes made difficult by failure to obtain a clear history, or by the presence of osteoarthritis of the limb joints and consecutive atrophy of the musculature, which masks weakness and reflex changes. Nonetheless, analysis of the way that a neurological disorder develops and of the pattern of neurological signs should provide a guide to the site of the lesion, both in the transverse plane and in the longitudinal segmental level. A lesion can usually be localized in the cervical, thoracic, lumbar, or sacral segments prior to specialized neuroradiological investigations.

CERVICAL RADICULOPATHY AND MYELOPATHY

General issues

The neuroradiological sequelae of degenerative disease of the cervical spine were established in the 1950s.[1] The degenerative changes of cervical spondylosis begin with desiccation and fragmentation of the intervertebral discs. As the elasticity of the annulus is reduced, the disc height diminishes. Extremes of movement are less well tolerated, and the vertebral endplates are subjected to greater stress. Secondary osteophytic spurs develop circumferentially around the disc, projecting posteriorly into the spinal canal as bony ridges. Parallel degeneration of the hypophyseal joints combines with spurs from the vertebral bodies to reduce the size of the neural foraminae. In most patients there is progressive loss of movement between vertebrae, although in some cases excessive motion between vertebrae and a degree of subluxation may develop. Pathological changes in the ligamentum flavum cause lack of elasticity and a tendency to buckle during extension. The compressive effects of the osteophytic spurs and buckled ligamentum flavum on the spinal cord are greatest when the neck is extended.

These changes bring about restriction of the natural motion of the spinal cord and nerve roots within the spinal canal. Repetitive compression and obstruction of the radicular arteries supplying the cord in the neural foraminae may further compromise cord function. This effect is aggravated if there is occlusive vascular disease of the proximal arteries in the neck. Occasionally, acute rupture of a cervical disc can follow sudden twisting or flexion/extension movements of the neck and cause cord or nerve root compression.[2] The same mechanism can also cause hemorrhage into the spinal cord (hematomyelia).

The older the population, the more these degenerative changes increase in severity and extent. It is clear from epidemiological studies[3] that the prevalence of degenerative changes is increased when heavy laboring work has been undertaken.

Anatomical and radiological studies have shown that the neurological sequelae of cervical spondylosis are more prevalent when the natural size of the spinal canal and neural foraminae is restricted.[4] However, the presence of large osteophytic ridges and subluxation of the vertebrae aggravate the situation. The C5–C6 and C6–C7 levels are most commonly affected at the point of transition from a mobile spine to the fixed section in the upper part of the thorax.[5]

Clinically, there is generally loss of lordosis so that the head is held flexed and downward. However, if the natural kyphosis of the thoracic spine is exaggerated there may be a compensatory extension of the upper cervical spine to maintain forward gaze. Most patients complain of recurrent neck pain and stiffness, together with crepitus on movement. Pain radiates to the occiput, shoulders, and scapula regions.

Radiculopathy

Progressive narrowing of the neural foraminae results from osteophytic ridges alongside the intervertebral discs and hypertrophy of the facet joints, and causes compression and restriction of movement of the nerve root. Pain radiates down the arm in the distribution of the nerve root(s) with a deep, boring quality, aggravated by activities such as lifting and reaching. The pain is generally accompanied by paresthesiae and some sensory loss in the affected dermatomes. In some patients sensory symptoms predominate. Muscular weakness is generally mild, but occasionally wasting can occur. The appropriate reflexes are lost.

Cervical myelopathy

Cervical spondylosis is the most frequent cause of chronic cord compression in the elderly population. The clinical spectrum is wide, depending on many interrelating factors and the pathogenesis of cord damage. Compression leads to atrophy of the anterior horn cells, and the lateral and posterior funiculi of the cord.[6] Most commonly the onset of symptoms and signs is insidious, and a clinical history may extend for many months or years before help is sought. Most frequently there is a mixed picture of lower motor neuron features in the arms, together with long tract signs below.[7]

In the upper limbs, complaints of numb, clumsy hands with weakness and loss of dexterity are common. Muscle wasting follows segmental anterior horn cell damage, affecting proximal muscles when compression is high in the neck, or the intrinsic muscles of the hand when compression is lower. The tendon reflexes in the arms are usually lost at the segmental level of the cord lesion and are exaggerated below. Inversion of the radial reflex occurs when the fifth cervical segment is affected.

In contrast, there is commonly a marked lower limb spasticity when the patient complains of a heavy, leaden weakness and a tendency to drag the limb. Some degree of ataxia may be present with reduction of vibration and joint position sense. Many patients complain of paresthesiae and intermittent numbness in the upper and lower limbs.

Occasionally, symptoms may arise abruptly due to trauma, or sudden extension of the neck. In this situation a central cord syndrome is common, with painless weakness of the upper limbs due to anterior horn cell damage and a mild spastic weakness of the lower limbs as the peripheral regions of the cord are relatively spared. Rarely a Brown–Sequard syndrome can be identified. These neurological disorders can be associated with vertebrobasilar insufficiency, where symptoms are typically related to rotation and extension of the neck. As the clinical presentation of spondylotic myelopathy varies it must be distinguished from other conditions with similar symptoms and signs, including multiple sclerosis, cerebrovascular disease, cord tumor or syrinx, normal pressure hydrocephalus, amyotrophic lateral sclerosis, and peripheral neuropathies.

Investigations

Plain radiographs of the cervical spine reveal narrowing of the intervertebral disc space with sclerosis of adjacent cortical bone. Secondary anterior and posterior osteophytes are demonstrated in Figure 56-1, together with an indication of the size of the spinal canal. Oblique radiographs allow visualization of the neural foraminae. However, several authors[8–10] have shown that degenerative changes increase in frequency with age, and that 70–90 percent of those over 65 years of age have radiological abnormalities. There is poor correlation between symptomatic and asymptomatic groups and the structural changes revealed on plain radiographs.

When the clinical state suggests segmental cord or root compression and surgery is contemplated, then specialized neuroradiological investigation is required. Magnetic resonance imaging (MRI)—which has largely replaced myelography—reveals degeneration of intervertebral discs, the size of osteophytes, and the presence and degree of cord compression (Fig. 56-2). Computerized tomography (CT) reveals the size and shape of the vertebral canals, but cannot give details of vertebral displacements, disc protrusions, and corrugation of the bulging longitudinal ligament, unless intrathecal contrast medium has been injected. Myelography is now performed only when MRI is contraindicated, such as in a patient with an implanted pacemaker or in the presence of cerebral aneurysm clips. Magnetic resonance imaging also allows visualization of intrinsic disorders of the spinal cord (Fig. 56-2).

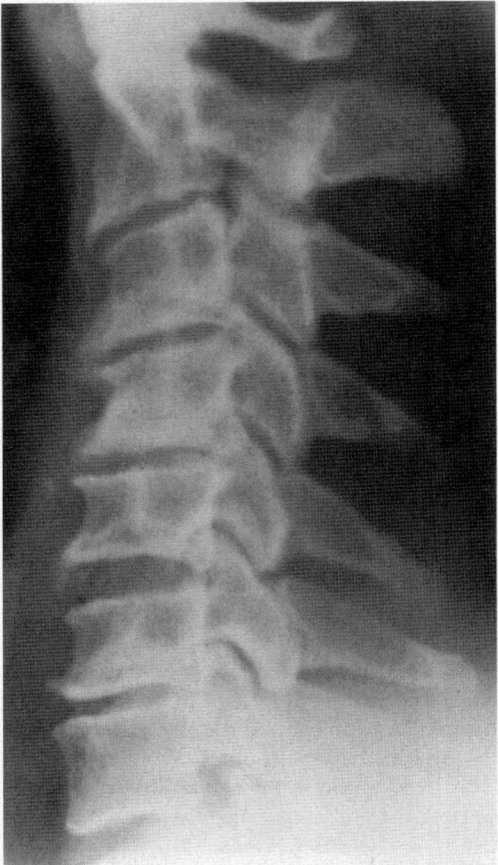

Figure 56-1 Lateral cervical spine radiograph, showing widespread spondylosis. Note the loss of disc height and large anterior osteophytes. This patient has a small spinal canal into which project osteophytes at the posterior margin of the C3–C4 of the 4–5 discs.

Management

Patients with neck pain and radiculopathy generally respond to a treatment regimen that includes a support collar, restriction of upper limb and shoulder movement, and nonsteroidal anti-inflammatory drugs, supplemented by other oral analgesics if necessary. Physical methods of treatment and the application of local heat pads may be soothing. If the symptoms are severe, bedrest and cervical traction may provide some relief. Lees and Turner[12] showed that 22 of 51 patients were symptom-free within a few months and generally remained symptom-free during follow-up. These authors showed that patients with radiculopathy rarely progress to a myelopathic state.

Surgery is not generally required unless progressive motor and sensory deficits lead to loss of function of the upper limbs. Both anterior and posterior approaches can be used to decompress the nerve roots; each carries a good prognosis for neurological recovery,[13–15] although recovery of muscle wasting is rarely satisfactory. The decision to operate is made after taking into account the severity of the disability, its effect on the patient's quality of life, and the patient's ability to withstand surgery.

The natural history of myelopathy complicating cervical spondylosis is variable and unpredictable; many patients run a chronic course characterized by episodes of deterioration

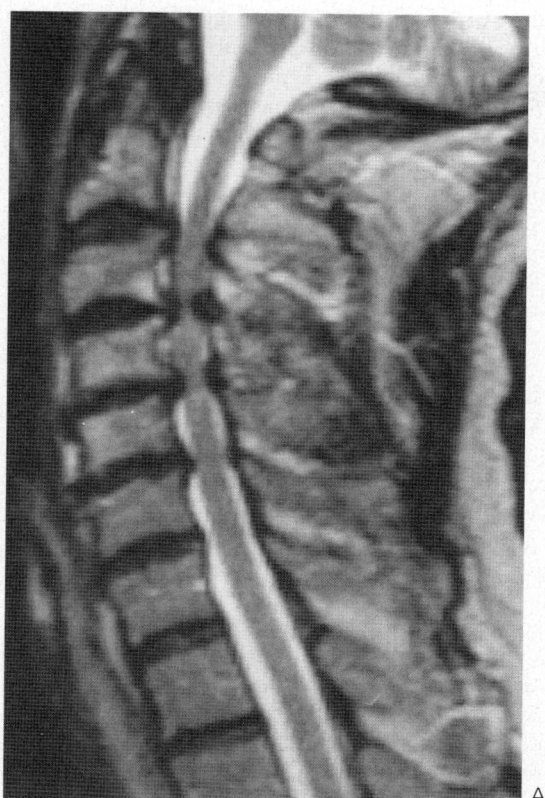

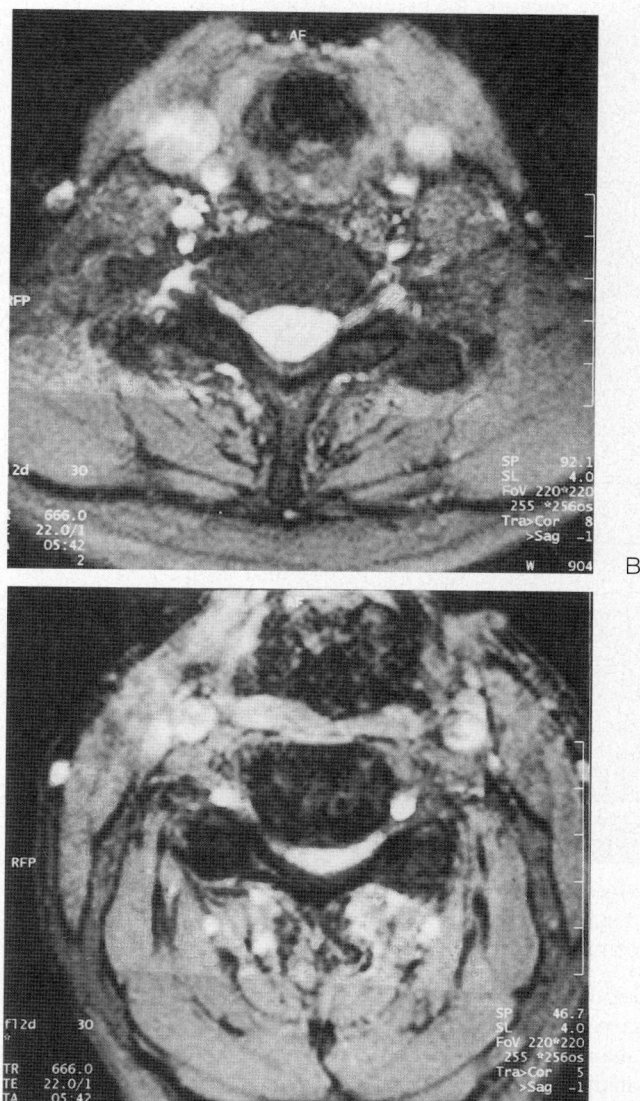

Figure 56-2 (A) Lateral magnetic resonance image of the cervical spine, showing compression of the spinal cord by posterior osteophytes and buckling of the ligamentum flavum. (B) Transverse image of normal cervical spine reveals spinal cord surrounded by cerebrospinal fluid. (C) Transverse image of the patient seen in (A), showing severe narrowing of the spinal canal and compression of the cord.

separated by periods of stability.[7,12] The majority of elderly patients with cervical myelopathy will not need surgical intervention. Surgical treatment is indicated when the myelopathy interferes with daily activities, where there is a short progressive history, or when there is radiological evidence of severe cord compression and/or instability. Anterior decompression of disc and osteophytic spurs is usually carried out when one or two intervertebral levels are affected, whereas laminectomy is indicated for more widespread stenosis and compression of the spinal cord. In general, the prime objective of surgery is to halt the decline in neurological function before irreversible damage to the cord has occurred.

There is poor correlation between the presenting severity, the duration of the symptoms, and the outcome.[4] Hukaka et al.[16] found that posterior decompression gave better results

for more advanced myelopathy and that a short duration of symptoms was associated with better results, although these were not influenced by the age of the patient. Phillips[17] suggested that patients with focal disease who underwent anterior surgery had a better outcome. However, some patients continued to deteriorate, in spite of adequate decompression, possibly because of vascular insufficiency.[7]

CORD COMPRESSION IN RHEUMATOID ARTHRITIS

Neck pain and stiffness are common complaints in patients with progressive rheumatoid arthritis (RA). Radiation of pain to the occipital region and cutaneous numbness at the back of the

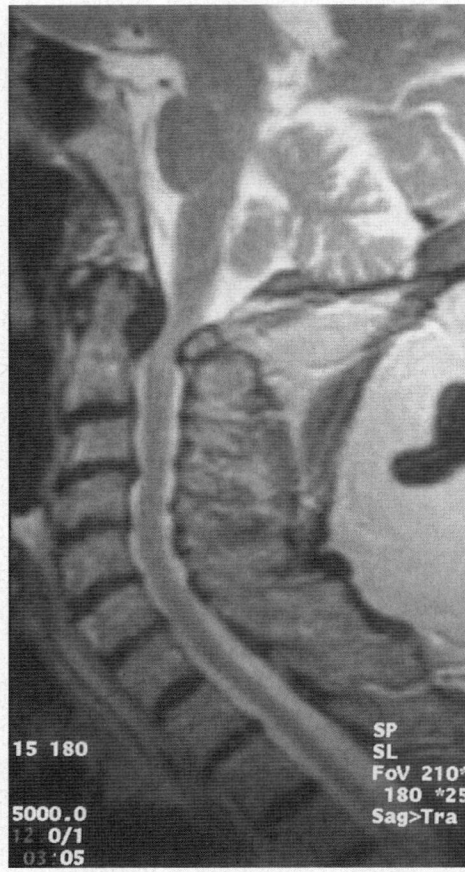

Figure 56-3 MR image of cervical spine, showing rheumatoid pannus at the back of the odontoid peg compressing the spinal cord.

head may occur when the upper cervical nerve roots are compressed. These symptoms may herald the development of atlanto-axial subluxation due to destruction of the transverse atlantal ligament by synovitis. There may be rotatory subluxation, and vertical migration of the odontoid into the foramen magnum of the skull. Atlanto-axial subluxation, which occurs in approximately 33 percent of patients with RA, can be asymptomatic until the slip reaches 8–9 mm when cord compression begins. Once myelopathy develops most patients deteriorate and 50 percent die within 6 months. Approximately 20 percent of patients show subaxial subluxation on cervical radiography, often affecting several segments to produce "staircase" deformity of the vertebrae. Compression of the cord is common.

Most patients present with progressive deterioration of upper limb function, accompanied by tingling, numbness, L'Hermitte's phenomenon, and gait disturbance. It is common for these symptoms to be attributed to severe peripheral joint disease and muscle atrophy. Abnormality of spinothalamic function, hyperreflexia and hypertonia, and extensor plantar responses help differentiate the cause from peripheral nerve lesions. Compression of the trigeminal nucleus and tract at the craniocervical junction may produce facial numbness or paresthesiae.

Radiological assessment requires flexion and extension radiographs of the cervical spine followed by MRI which will reveal compression or distortion of the spinal cord (Fig. 56-3).

Surgical management has to be considered when there is progressive or significant atlanto-axial subluxation, or clinical evidence of increasing neurological morbidity. As most patients have significant medical problems such as pulmonary fibrosis, anemia, atrophic skin, and the effects of prolonged steroid treatment, there is significant risk from surgical intervention. Many patients with subluxation benefit from the use of a collar, though tolerance of use can be limited.

The surgical approach and procedure may consist of an anterior, transoral, or posterior decompression combined with internal fixation.

SPINAL CORD COMPRESSION AND THORACIC DISC PROTRUSION

The central protrusion of a thoracic intervertebral disc is an unusual cause of cord compression, but one that occurs in older age groups as it is associated with degeneration of the disc annulus. Russell[18] noted that 67 percent occurred between the eighth and eleventh interspaces. The majority of patients present with a long history of gradually progressive myelopathy where sensory and motor symptoms are equally common. However, 49 percent of patients complained of radicular symptoms of pain and dysesthesiae. Sometimes the onset is more rapid, leading to a flaccid paraplegia.[19]

The presence of a thoracic disc protrusion is generally recognized when MRI is carried out to investigate the progressive neurological deficit. Cord compression from this source carries a poor prognosis unless surgery is performed. The results of simple decompressive laminectomy are unsatisfactory; either costotransversectomy, transpedicular, or transthoracic approach is recommended.[18,20]

CORD COMPRESSION FROM INTRADURAL TUMORS

Intradural extramedullary tumors cause local compression of the spinal cord and nerve roots. Meningiomas represent approximately 25 percent of primary spinal cord tumors, and 80 percent of them occur in females. They are most commonly seen in the sixth decade, rather later than for neurofibromas; 80 percent occur in the thoracic spine. The majority of patients complain of local or radicular pain, the significance of which often goes unrecognized for a long period until progressive spastic paraparesis, followed by sensory and bladder dysfunction, develops.[21]

Plain radiographs are rarely helpful, and the condition is diagnosed only by myelography or MRI. Results of decompressive surgery are generally good. Levy et al.[22] reported that one-third of paraplegic patients were able to walk after tumor excision. Neurofibromas are slightly more common than meningiomas, but their peak incidence is in younger age groups, so they are less frequently encountered in an elderly patient.[23] Radicular pain is more common, and enlargement of a neural foramen may be seen on plain radiographs if the tumor extends into the paravertebral tissues. Multiple tumors can be encountered in neurofibromatosis. As with meningiomas, surgical excision should be undertaken and carries a good prognosis for neurological recovery.[24]

METASTATIC SPINAL TUMORS

The most common extradural and spinal tumors to cause cord compression are those metastasizing from distant carcinomas or primary hematological tumors. Spread may be hematogenous or via the vertebral venous plexus. Although myeloma and carcinomas of prostate and kidney seem to metastasize preferentially to the spine, in practice the most commonly encountered tumors are those that occur with the greatest frequency in the community. Therefore, primary lung, breast, kidney, and prostate tumors are seen, although in some patients the primary tumor cannot be identified. The thoracic section of the spine is most frequently involved, followed by the lumbosacral and cervical regions.

The majority of patients present with progressive walking difficulty, due to weakness and clumsiness, the significance of which may go unrecognized until the patient is no longer able to bear weight. Many patients have a history of preceding spinal pain, which should always lead to a suspicion of vertebral metastasis in a patient known to have malignant disease. The neurological deficit may develop very rapidly, with collapse of the vertebra, or occlusion of the vascular supply to the cord. An analysis of the level of the sensory deficit helps in assessing the site of the spinal disease and planning the appropriate radiological investigations. However, plain radiographs of all of the spine and chest should be carried out, and may reveal loss of outline of a pedicle, reduction in height of a vertebral body, or a soft tissue mass. MRI of the spine is the investigation of choice. However, CT may reveal evidence of bone destruction and allow percutaneous needle biopsy of the lesion.

There has been considerable debate about the value of decompressive surgery, as a laminectomy alone produces poor results.[25–27] If there has been collapse of the vertebral body, better results may be obtained by an anterior excision of the tumor, insertion of a bone graft, and stabilization of the spine.[28] Alternatively, radiotherapy under steroid cover can be carried out, particularly if the patient presents in the early stages of cord compression and cord compression is incomplete.[29] It has been shown that a long history is associated with a better prognosis after treatment, and that rapid loss of power is associated with a poor outcome.[30] Other features associated with a poor outcome are a paraplegia of greater than 24 hours' duration, collapse of the vertebral body, and metastasis from bronchogenic carcinomas. The prognosis is best in those whose neurological function is preserved prior to surgery, or when there is compression of the cauda equina, rather than the spinal cord.[31]

VASCULAR DISORDERS OF THE SPINAL CORD

The peculiar anatomical arrangement of the arterial blood supply of the spinal cord may protect it from the effects of occlusion of one feeding vessel. The anterior and posterior spinal arteries are fed by radicular arteries, which are branches of vessels arising from either the aorta or the subclavian arteries. There is generally a large feeding artery in the lower thoracic region, most commonly on the left at T10. A watershed lies at the second thoracic segment of the spinal cord, between areas supplied by thoracic vessels and those from the neck.

Interruption of supply can occur in atheroma of the aorta,[32] in dissecting aneurysm,[33] or as a complication of aortic surgery.[34] The extent and severity of the spinal cord neurological deficit varies considerably, probably depending on the anatomical variation of the spinal cord vessels in the individual patient.

The syndrome of the anterior spinal artery arises when this vessel is obstructed by thrombus. The onset is sudden with pain in the back or neck and paresthesiae down the arms. The posterior columns receiving a blood supply from the posterior spinal network are preserved, so that proprioception remains intact, whereas thermal and pain appreciation are impaired. In addition, a lower motor paralysis of the arms is associated with spastic paraparesis, or paraplegia. In some cases, the presence of cervical spondylosis and an osteophytic ridge has been implicated in local occlusion of the anterior spinal artery.[35]

PAGET'S DISEASE

Paget's disease is a generally progressive disorder of bone that causes neurological sequelae of the brain, spinal cord, or peripheral nerves, depending on which bones are involved. It is important to recognize these complications, as many respond to treatment of the underlying disorder. In the spine, pagetic changes may affect one or several vertebrae. The disease is characterized by bony destruction followed by repair, which leads to flattening and expansion of the diameter of the vertebral bodies, and thickening of the pedicles and laminae. Bony projections in the vertebral canal cause spinal cord and nerve root compression. Neurological symptoms may develop suddenly if collapse of a vertebral body occurs.

Spinal cord compression is most common in the thoracic region, and is generally slowly progressive, causing a spastic weakness of the lower limbs combined with sensory symptoms and signs. Pain may be due to local bony changes, malignant degeneration, or nerve root compression. In some patients progressive myelopathy occurs, yet imaging fails to reveal direct compression of the spinal cord. In these patients progressive ischemia may be the cause of neurological deterioration.

When the disease affects the lumbar region, symptoms of single or multiple nerve root compression can develop, producing back pain and sciatica. When the spinal canal is constricted, neurogenic claudication may be the presenting symptom.

Surgical treatment is indicated only when medical treatment fails to control the progression of the neurological sequelae of the condition. However, control of blood loss from the diseased bone during surgery can be very troublesome.[36,37]

NEUROLOGICAL COMPLICATIONS OF DEGENERATIVE DISEASE OF THE LUMBAR SPINE

Spondylosis of the lumbar spine increases in severity and extent with advancing age, often occurring simultaneously with disease in the cervical region.[3] Biochemical and pathological changes are similar at both sites. Loss of disc height and the development of traction spurs and osteophytes are associated

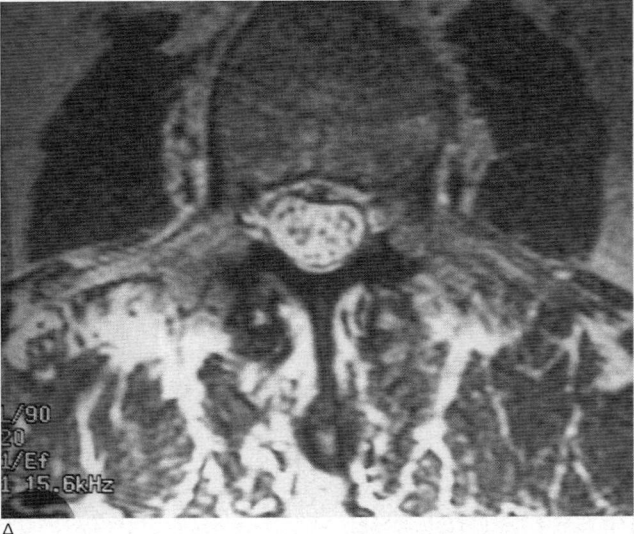

A

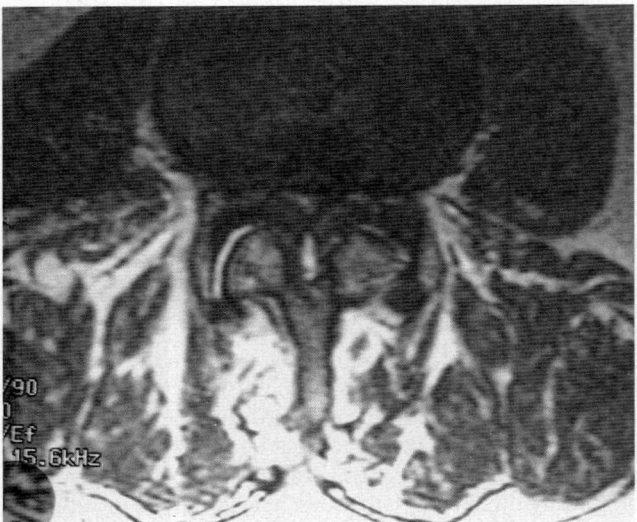

B

Figure 56-4 MR images of (A) normal lumbar spine and (B) severe spinal canal stenosis.

with sclerosis and enlargement of the vertebral bodies. Simultaneous changes in the facet joints occur, with destruction of articular cartilage, laxity of the joint capsule, and osteophytic enlargement of the joint surfaces.[38] This process may be asymmetric, so that rotational subluxation of one vertebra on the other can develop. The lowest intervertebral discs of the lumbar spine are most commonly affected, at the point of transition from the mobile lumbar spine to the fixed sacrum.

A number of discrete neurological conditions may complicate lumbar spondylosis.

Acute nerve root entrapment

True herniation of an intervertebral disc can occur in an elderly person and produce a pattern of symptoms and signs similar to that seen in younger patients.[39] However, compared with the average adult population, elderly people have a higher incidence of motor deficits and are more likely to have a sequestrated disc nucleus.

Chronic nerve root entrapment

Lumbar mono- and polyradiculopathy occur in elderly people, more commonly as a result of nerve root compression in the lateral recess of the spinal canal, and in the neural foramen, than from disc rupture. As degeneration of the intervertebral disc advances, there is loss of disc height and formation of osteophytes that bulge into the neural foramen; hypertrophy of the facet joint further compromises its capacity. At the same time, partial subluxation of the posterior joint with upward and forward movement of the superior articular surface narrows the lateral recess of the spinal canal.[40] At first extension and rotation of the spine aggravate the process, so that dynamic stenosis may produce intermittent compression and symptoms, although, as the condition advances, permanent compression occurs.

Typically, patients complain of pain and stiffness of the back, accompanied by the insidious onset of sciatic pain. These symptoms are generally aggravated by standing or walking and relieved by rest or lying, particularly when the spine is flexed. Patients complain of paresthesiae in the legs, which are also precipitated by the same types of activity. In chronic nerve root entrapment due to stenosis, coughing and straining aggravate the pain, and nerve root stretch tests are generally negative. Some patients show mild weakness of the legs, although objective sensory deficits are rare. The progression of symptoms and signs is generally much slower than for a herniated nucleus pulposus.[41–43]

Nerve root entrapment may complicate degenerative spondylolisthesis. This develops when degeneration of the facet joints and laxity of the disc annulus allow the upper vertebral body to slide forward on the lower. The L4–L5 intervertebral joint is most commonly affected, but other intervertebral levels can be involved[44] and produce sciatic pain and symptoms of nerve root compression.

Neurogenic claudication

Narrowing of the central spinal canal can develop as a result of a combination of degenerative hypertrophy of the facet joints, hypertrophy and corrugation of the ligamentum flavum, and bulging of the disc and osteophytes. As the available space in the spinal canal narrows, there is compression of multiple nerve roots of the cauda equina and its circulation. The symptoms of claudication develop. Bilateral leg pain is precipitated by walking or standing and improved with rest, especially when the spine is flexed or when the patient sits or squats.[43]

Patients frequently develop a stooped posture. As the distance walked increases, a heavy leaden weakness builds up in intensity, accompanied by burning paresthesiae and a fear of the limb giving way.[45] Sometimes neurological signs are present only after an exercise provocation test on a treadmill.

In the elderly population the clinical picture is often confused with the effects of peripheral vascular disease. Sharr et al.[46] reported that urinary symptoms due to a neuropathic bladder often complicate central stenosis of the spinal canal.

Investigations

The extent and severity of degenerative changes of the discs and facet joints is revealed by plain radiographs. Radiculography has been superseded by CT and MRI of the lumbar spine which reveal the cross-sectional anatomy of the spinal and neural canals, and can analyze the degree of degeneration of the disc. However, only MRI can adequately display detail of the neural structures.

Radionuclide scanning is generally not helpful, as increased uptake is common in areas of osteoarthritis, but can exclude spinal infection or neoplasm.

Management

The majority of elderly patients do not require surgical decompression, and their symptoms can be controlled by analgesic and anti-inflammatory medication and modification of their activities of daily living. Rest and physical treatment, combined with restriction of spinal movement, often produce satisfactory results. However, the elderly withstand surgery well, and age alone is rarely a contraindication to operation. Surgery is indicated when sciatic pain and other symptoms significantly reduce a patient's physical capacity, or cannot be controlled by medical treatment. Signs of severe nerve root compression, such as weakness or sensory loss, neurogenic claudication, and cauda equina compression are firm indications for surgical intervention. The aim of surgery is to decompress the spinal canal and neural foraminae, thus freeing the nerve roots. Getty et al.[47,48] obtained satisfactory results in 85 percent of patients after a partial undercutting facetectomy. However, low backache persists after surgery in many patients, owing to the background degenerative changes, and patients must be advised accordingly.[49,50]

KEY POINTS Spinal cord and nerve roots

- Spinal cord compression in the elderly population is most frequently caused by cervical spondylosis or secondary vertebral tumors.

- The clinical presentation of cervical myelopathy is usually either insidious gait disturbance, or numb clumsy hands.

- In patients with advanced rheumatoid arthritis, subluxation at the craniocervical junction may require surgical treatment by internal decompression and fixation.

- Less common causes of cord compression in the elderly population include intraspinal tumor and thoracic disc protrusion.

REFERENCES

1. Brain WR, Northfield D, Wilkinson M: The neurological manifestations of cervical spondylosis. Brain 1952;75:187–225
2. Young S, O'Laoire S: Cervical disc prolapse in the elderly: an easily overlooked, reversible cause of spinal cord compression. Br J Neurosug 1987;1:93–98
3. Lawrence JS: Disc degeneration: its frequency and relationship to symptoms. Ann Rheum Dis 1969;28:121
4. Nurick G: The natural history and the results of surgical treatment of the spinal cord disorder associated with cervical spondylosis. Brain 1972;95:101–108
5. Henderson CM: Posterio-lateral foramenotomy as an exclusive operative technique for cervical radiculopathy: a review of 846 consecutively operated cases. Neurosurgery 1983;13:504–512
6. Ilo T, Oyanagi K, Takahashi H, Takahashi ME: Cervical spondylotic myelopathy clinicopathologic study on the progression pattern and thin myelinated fibres of the lesions of seven patients examined during complete autopsy. Spine 1996;21:827–833
7. Bernhardt M, Hynes RA, Blume HW, White AA: Current concepts review: cervical spondylotic myelopathy. J Bone Joint Surg 1993;75A:119–128
8. Pallis C, Jones AM, Spillaine JD: Cervical spondylosis: incidence and implications. Brain 1954;77:274–289
9. McRae IL: The significance of abnormalities of the cervical spine. Am J Roentgenol 1960;84:3–25
10. Gore DR, Sepic SB, Gardner GM: Roentgenographic findings of the cervical spine in asymptomatic people. Spine 1986;11:521–524
11. Yu YL, du Boulay AH, Stevens JM, Kendall BE: Computed tomography in cervical spondylitic myelopathy and radiculopathy: visualisation of structures, myelographic comparison, cord measurements and clinical ability. Brain 1986;109:421–428
12. Lees F, Turner JW: Natural history and prognosis of cervical spondylosis. BMJ 1963;1:1607–1610
13. Dillin W, Booth R, Cuckler J et al: Cervical radiculopathy: a review. Spine 1985;11:998–991
14. Hunt WE: Cervical spondylosis: natural history and rare indications for surgical decompression. Clin Neurosurg 1980;27:466–480
15. Lundsford DL, Bissonette DJ, Zorub PA, Zorub DS: Anterior surgery for cervical disease. 2: Treatment of cervical spondylotic myelopathy: 32 cases. J Neurosurg 1980;53:12–19
16. Hukaka S, Mochizuki T, Ogata M et al: Operations for cervical spondylotic myelopathy. J Bone Joint Surg 1985;67B:609–615
17. Phillips DG: Surgical treatment of myelopathy with cervical spondylosis. J Neurol Neurosurg Psychiat 1973;36:879
18. Russell T: Thoracic intervertebral disc protrusion: experience of 67 cases and review of the literature. Br J Neurosurg 1989;3:153–160
19. Perot PL: Thoracic disc disease. In Wilkins RH, Rengachary SS (eds): Neurosurgery. McGraw-Hill, New York, 1985
20. Young S, Karr G, O'Laoire S: Spinal cord compression due to thoracic disc heniation: results of microsurgical posterolateral costotransversectomy. Br J Neurosurg 1989;3:31–38
21. Zeidman SM, Ellenbogen RG, Ducker TB: Intradural tumours. Semin Spine Surg 1995;1:323–338
22. Levy WJ, Bay J, Dohn D: Spinal cord meningioma. J Neurosurg 1982;57:804–812
23. Gautier-Smith PC: Clinical aspects of spinal neurofibroma. Brain 1967;90:359–394
24. Nittner KM: In Vinker PJ, Bruyn GW (eds): Handbook of Clinical Neurology, vol 20. North-Holland, Amsterdam, 1976:177–322
25. Findlay GFG: Adverse effects of the management of malignant spinal cord compression. J Neurol Neurosurg Psychiat 1984;47:761–768
26. Findlay GFG: The role of vertebral body collapse in the management of malignant spinal cord compression. J Neurol Neurosurg Psychiat 1987;50:151–154
27. Findlay GFG: Compressive and vascular disorders of the spinal cord. In Miller JD (ed): Northfield's Surgery of the Central Nervous System, 2nd edn. Blackwell, Oxford, 1987
28. Black P: Spinal metastasis: current status and recommended guidelines for management. Neurosurgery 1979;5:726–746
29. Cobb CA, Leavens ME, Eckles N: Indications for non-operative treatment of spinal cord compression due to breast cancer. J Neurosurg 1977;47:653–658
30. Chad HO: In Vinken PJ, Bruyn GW (eds): Handbook of Clinical Neurology, vol 20. North-Holland, Amsterdam, 1976:415–434
31. Seigal T, Seigal T: Neoplastic epidural spinal cord compression: pathophysiology and prognostic factors. Semin Spine Surg 1995;7:269–276
32. Kochar G, Kotler NN, Hartman J et al: Thrombosed aorta resulting in spinal cord ischemia and paraplegia in ischemia cardiomyopathy. Am Heart J 1987;113:1510–1513
33. Braunstein H: Pathogenesis of dissecting aneurysm. Circulation 1963;28:1071–1080
34. Hughes JT: Vascular disorders of the spinal cord. In Tolle JF (ed): Handbook of Clinical Neurology, vol 55. Vascular Diseases, Part III. Elsevier, Amsterdam, 1989
35. Hughes JT, Brownwell B: Cervical spondylosis complicated by anterior spinal artery thrombosis. Neurology 1964;14:1073–1077
36. Douglas DL, Duckworth T, Kanis JA et al: Spinal cord dysfunction in Paget's disease of bone. J Bone Joint Surg 1981;63B:495–503
37. Schmidek HH, Waters A: Neural dysfunction in Paget's disease of bone. In Wilkins RH, Rengachary SS (eds): Neurosurgery. McGraw-Hill, New York, 1985
38. Yong-Hing K, Kirlaldy-Willis WH: The pathophysiology of degenerative disease of the lumbar spine. Orthop Clin North Am 1983;14:491–504
39. Maistrelli GL, Vaughan PA, Evans DC, Barrington TW: Lumbar disc herniation in the elderly. Spine 1987;12:63–66

40. Reynolds AF, Weinstein PR, Wachter RD: Lumbar monoradiculopathy due to unilateral facet hypertrophy. Neurosurgery 1987;10:480–486

41. Ciric I, Mikhael MA, Tarkington JA, Vick NA: The lateral recess syndrome: a variant of spinal stenosis. J Neurosurg 1980;53:433–443

42. Kirkaldy-Willis WH, Wedge JH, Yong-Hing K et al: Lumbar spinal nerve lateral entrapment. Clin Orthop 1992;169:171–178

43. Dillin W, Watkins R: Natural history of lumbar spinal stenosis: clinical features. Semin Spine Surg 1994;6:84–89

44. Cauchoix J, Benoist M, Chassaing V: Degenerative spondylolisthesis. Clin Orthop 1976;115:122–129

45. Paine KWE: Clinical features of lumbar spinal stenosis. Clin Orthop 115:77–82

46. Sharr MM, Garfield JS, Jenkins JD: Lumbar spondylosis and neuropathic bladder: investigation of 73 patients with chronic urinary symptoms. BMJ 1976;1:695–697

47. Getty CJM, Johnson JR, Kirwan EOG, Sullivan MF: Partial undercutting facetectomy for bony entrapment of the lumbar nerve root. J Bone Joint Surg 1981;63B:330–335

48. Getty CJM: Lumbar spinal stenosis: the clinical spectrum and the results of operation. J Bone Joint Surg 1980;62B:481–485

49. Barr JS, Riseborough EJ: Treatment of low back and sciatica pain in patients over 60 years of age. Clin Orthop 1965;26:12–18

50. Simon SD, Silver CM, Litchman HM: Lumbar disc surgery in the elderly (over the age of 60). Clin Orthop 1965;41:157–162

Chapter 57

Head trauma in the geriatric patient

John Bruns, Jr.

Material in this chapter contains contributions from the previous edition, and we are grateful to the previous author for the work done.

The evaluation and management of head injury in the geriatric patient continues to be one of the key high-risk/high-yield key decision-making areas for the clinician. The subtleties and broad spectrum of presentations of occult traumatic brain injury (TBI) results in significant potential for serious errors. For this reason the clinician has to be ever vigilant for the patient with occult central nervous system (CNS) injury as well as the acutely injured and unstable patient.

There is some confusion in the literature regarding head injury and traumatic brain injury. Head injury is best defined as an injury that is externally clinically evident and can occur without TBI. Traumatic brain injury refers to damage to the brain itself and can occur with or without external signs of trauma.

Severe multisystem geriatric trauma is a significant public health problem in the USA with over 800,000 elderly victims of trauma hospitalized and more than 26,000 dying annually. The case fatality proportion for elderly people is significantly higher than in younger trauma victims, with estimates of 50–100 percent higher mortality given similar injury severity scores (ISS).[1,2] The elderly have higher rates of intracranial injuries[3–5] and increased morbidity and mortality from TBI than younger age groups.

Approximately 2 million Americans are victims of head injury annually.[6] In the USA, 1.6 percent of all emergency department (ED) visits are for a head injury, corresponding to 444 new cases of ED-evaluated TBI annually per 100,000 population.[7] TBI is estimated to be the primary cause of death in 40–50 percent of all traumatic deaths. The overall U.S. mortality rate for TBI in 1994 was 19.8 per 100,000;[8] however, it was much higher in elderly people (46.3 per 100,000).[4] For those age 75 and older, the incidence of TBI mortality (per 100,000 population) by mechanism was as follows: falls, 127; firearms, 13; transport related, 38; and assault related, 2. Elderly TBI patients tend to die of multisystem organ failure, while the younger victims usually die from irreversible brain injury.

Geriatric patients with head injuries enter the emergency or geriatric healthcare system in a number of characteristic ways: (1) acute presentation following a fall, other accident, or after being assaulted; (2) subacute presentation in which the patient presents with headache, nausea, or vomiting, with or without a change in mental status several days following an injury; (3) patients presenting with a change in mental status who after work-up are found to have a chronic subdural hematoma.

The high incidence of underlying cardiovascular, pulmonary, and neurological diseases presents an added complexity in determining if the injury was sustained due to a "simple accident" or was caused by a preceding transient loss of consciousness. The patient's traumatic event may have been preceded by a syncopal episode, a transient cardiac rhythm disturbance, a seizure, or a hypoglycemic episode to name but a few common precipitating scenarios.

The evaluation of the geriatric patient with potentially significant head trauma is often difficult because of a pre-existing neurological and cognitive impairment or there may be an acute change in mental status unrelated to the trauma. Neurological evaluations in elderly people may be misleading secondary to: (1) medication effects or side-effects (particularly in the poly-pharmacy patient), (2) dementia, (3) residual focal neurological deficits from prior stroke, or (4) delirium secondary to hypoxemia, metabolic, infectious, and endocrine aberrancies. Obviously, patients with delirium are more likely to sustain injury from falls and on more than one occasion patients will have both a delirium and evidence of a new intracranial injury. There is also epidemiological evidence that previous head trauma is a risk factor for the development of Alzheimer's and Parkinson's diseases.[9–11]

Identification of neurological abnormalities can also be complicated due to sensory impairment. Visual deterioration which is prevalent in elderly people due to: (1) cataracts (70 percent prevalence), (2) glaucoma, and (3) macular degeneration (8 percent prevalence). These occular abnormalities or post-surgical changes may result in abnormal pupillary responses or contribute to patient disorientation. One-third of elderly people are additionally hearing impaired, which can negatively effect orientation and participation in the neurological examination.

Among elderly TBI patients, the greatest comorbidity involves the cardiovascular system. Given the high prevalence of hypertension in this cohort, a blood pressure in the "normal range" for most age groups may be relatively low in this demographic. Anticoagulation and antiplatelet medications increase the risk of hemorrhage. Diuretics decrease intravascular volume and beta-blockers and calcium channel blockers prevent the normal compensatory physiological response to traumatic hemorrhagic hypovolemia.

An obfuscating problem is the relatively high incidence of small intracranial fluid collections in elderly people that are chronic and usually do not have any clinical significance. These include smaller subdural hematomas and subdural hygromas. Lesions should only be thought of as having pathophysiological significance if the patient's presentation and the neurological localization is consistent with the location of the lesion and the neuroimaging study shows localized brain swelling or evidence of mass effect.

These presenting circumstances and comorbidities increase the risk of brain injury after the initial traumatic insult. Reduced systemic physiological reserve, decreased blood oxygen content, reduced cerebral blood flow (CBF) from intracranial and extracranial abnormalities and the confounders of possible antecedent pathology, often questionable and challenging history and physical examination and multiple possible etiologies for neurological or cardiovascular aberrancies all complicate the elder TBI patient's evaluation and management. Therefore, an extremely conservative approach is recommended when caring for elderly TBI patients.

PRIMARY AND SECONDARY BRAIN INJURY

In TBI, all neurological damage does not occur immediately at the moment of impact (primary injury), but evolves over time (secondary injury). This secondary injury results from several extracranial and intracranial perturbations and is largely preventable and is the primary cause of in-hospital mortality. Extracranial insults include systemic hypotension, hypoxemia, hypercarbia, or severe hypocarbia, anemia, and pyrexia. Overall these secondary factors decrease cerebral perfusion and cerebral oxygen delivery or increase cerebral oxygen consumption.

Secondary intracranial insults result from a cascade of pathophysiological biochemical and vascular events that lead to cerebral edema and intracranial hematoma formation, which increases intracranial pressure and reduces cerebral blood flow. In addition, seizures, pyrexia, and, infrequently, intracranial infection can increase cerebral oxygen consumption. Thus, secondary brain injury is ultimately caused by cerebral ischemia and neuronal death.[12]

CLASSIFICATION OF TRAUMATIC BRAIN INJURY

Multiple TBI severity classification schemes exist; however, the Glasgow Coma Scale (GCS) is employed in the majority of studies to define the degree of cerebral impairment.[10] A minor head injury is frequently defined as a patient with a GCS of 13–15 who is alert and back to his or her baseline, but who may have some residual mild cognitive impairment (e.g., retrograde amnesia). This group however, is very heterogeneous and the likelihood of deterioration and need for neurosurgical intervention increases rapidly with divergence from a GCS score of 15.

The Head Injury Interdisciplinary Special Interest Group of the American Congress of Rehabilitation Medicine defines mild TBI to include: (1) any period of loss of consciousness (LOC) of <30 min and GCS score of 13–15 after this period of LOC; (2) any loss of memory of the event immediately before or after the injury, with post-traumatic amnesia (PTA) of <24 hours; (3) any alteration in mental state at the time of the injury (e.g., feeling dazed, disoriented, or confused).

Others use skull fracture or CT evidence of intracranial pathology as exclusionary criteria.

Moderate TBI is often defined as a GCS score of 9–12. There is typically a history of loss of consciousness for more than 5 minutes, and focal neurological deficits may be present. Other authors have used LOC or PTA of 30 minutes–24 hours duration or skull fracture with an otherwise mild TBI as criteria for moderate TBI.

A severe head injured patient has a GCS of 8 or less and will usually be stuporous or comatose. Other classification schemes include the presence of intracranial hematoma, brain contusion, or LOC or PTA of greater than 24 hours duration.

CLASSIFICATION OF HEAD TRAUMA

Traditionally, head trauma has been classified as open (compound) and closed depending on whether there has been a breach of the integrity of the cranial vault. Thus skull fractures associated with an overlying laceration are considered open injuries as are basilar skull fractures. In basilar skull fractures there is the potential for communication between the intracranial contents and a nasal sinus or the nasopharynx with the associated risk of infection. Skull fractures are also defined by whether they are simple (nondisplaced) or whether they are depressed. Thus a patient with a closed head injury may have a compound depressed skull fracture or a linear undisplaced fracture. Penetrating injuries are variants of open head injuries in which a wound has been created by a missile or sharp object that has violated both the cranium and the intracranial structures.

The patient with a skull fracture and/or a scalp laceration has to be considered within the context of the associated signs and symptoms as to whether there is an accompanying intracranial injury. Although these patients require careful investigation for CNS injury, many do not have evidence of an associated intracranial injury or TBI as the energy delivered by the wounding mechanism of injury has been absorbed and dissipated by the scalp and the cranium, which have functioned, as designed, to protect the brain. An exception to this is the situation that obtains with respect to depressed skull fractures. The energy associated with the mechanism of injury directed at the site(s) of injury is proportionately greater than that associated with undisplaced fracture and the likelihood of underlying brain injury is higher, as is the incidence of post-traumatic epilepsy.

OVERVIEW AND MANAGEMENT OF IMPORTANT PATHOLOGICAL AND PATHOPHYSIOLOGICAL ENTITIES
Concussion

Concussion is defined and stratified by three grades and results from a direct blow to the head, or from sudden deceleration or acceleration forces. Grade one or mild concussion occurs when the person does not lose consciousness but may seem slightly disoriented or dazed. A grade two concussion occurs when the patient remains conscious, but has a period of confusion and does not recall the event. A grade three or classic concussion, which is the most severe form, occurs when the person loses consciousness for a brief period of time and is amnesic of the event.

It is now known that post-concussive syndrome may be associated with permanent cognitive and functional impairments. This is an area of current controversy as the differentiation of premorbid deficits, litigation-related factors, and true trauma-related residual deficits is quite difficult to separate. Following the acute concussion, most patients will have subacute to chronic sequelae consisting of persisting headaches, ataxia, vertigo, sleep abnormalities, and mild cognitive impairment. Finally, there are clearly a number of patients with head injuries who have the acute syndrome and the late syndromes who were not unconscious during the period of injury.

Concussed patients who have had serious underlying pathology ruled out by computed tomography (CT) or magnetic resonance imaging (MRI) scans and who continue to have symptoms are a difficult group to manage. By and large they will also improve spontaneously over time, but require support from their physicians, family, friends, and employers. A team approach, managed by the patient's primary physician and including a neurologist, psychologist, neuropsychologist, and other rehabilitation professionals is invaluable.

Diffuse axonal injury

Diffuse axonal injury (DAI) is an entity that merges with and represents a progression from the milder injury of concussion. It too is felt to be caused by the angular or rotational acceleration or deceleration of the brain most often associated with automobile accidents. The neuronal elements of the white matter are stretched and/or torn. This injury is associated with a poor prognosis as it has a proclivity for evolving into a phase where vasogenic cerebral edema is the paramount issue. Patients with severe diffuse axonal injury are usually comatose or at least severely impaired following their injury and deteriorate progressively with the worsening cerebral edema. Management of these patients requires neurosurgical intensive care using intracranial pressure monitoring. Many of these patients will have other brain injuries requiring neurosurgical intervention such as acute subdural hematoma and large intracerebral hematomas, but the lesions of diffuse neural injury themselves are managed nonsurgically.

Subdural hematomas

Subdural hematomas (SDH)[13,14] are classically divided into acute, subacute, and chronic categories. Cerebral atrophy places elderly patients at significant risk for SDH. Stretching of the subdural bridging veins renders them more susceptible to damage after head injury. SDHs result from angular or rotational effects where the shearing forces are vectored at the bridging arterioles and venules in the subdural space. The mechanism of injury for these lesions is similar to that of diffuse axonal injury. Intracerebral hematomas and lacerations often have a polar location at the frontal, temporal, or occipital poles because they often are a part of a coup or contracoup lesion. These patients are usually very severely injured and will require neurosurgical intensive care and evacuation of the hematomas.

Chronic subdural hematomas (CSDH) are often encountered in geriatric patients.[10] The initial traumatic event is usually trivial or unnoticed by the patient and his or her family. Predisposing factors include brain atrophy, atheroscleroses, seizure disorders, and coagulopathy. Falls (74 percent), progressive neurological deterioration (70 percent), head trauma (37 percent), transient neurological deficits (21 percent), seizures (14 percent), and headache (14 percent) were the most common presenting symptom for CSDH in a case series of patients over 75 years old. Forty-two percent of patients had pre-existing confusion and 24 percent were on anticoagulation therapies.[11]

The initial subdural hemorrhage is usually a small collection located over the hemispheres and goes unnoticed perhaps because brain atrophy provides space for hematoma expansion. A capsule forms about the hematoma, becomes chronic and breaks down to a motor oil viscosity. During this phase, the hematoma may resolve spontaneously or continue to grow in volume. The peri-hematoma capsule becomes vascularized. Expansion of the fluid collection when it occurs is either due to microhemorrhages from the fragile capsular vessels, osmotic shifts of fluid into the hematoma, or both mechanisms. As the hematoma enlarges, it eventually reaches a size where the intracranial pressure becomes elevated and results in brain compression and shift causing overt neurological dysfunction.

Late in the course of CSDHs patients become lethargic, somnolent, and develop acute focal neural deficits, which can culminate in herniation syndrome. At this point, immediate evacuation of the hematoma is mandatory in conjunction with temporizing intracranial pressure management techniques. The 6-month mortality for CSDH is about 31 percent with a 37 percent neurosurgical intervention rate.

Epidural hematomas

Epidural hematomas are thought to be caused by a rupture or puncture of a meningeal artery by direct contact with a wounding object, skull fracture fragment or from shearing forces that result in arterial bleeding into the epidural space. About 70 percent of epidural hematomas occur in the temporal area from injury to the middle meningeal artery or vein. Interestingly, epidural hematomas are less frequent in the geriatric population either due to a different mechanism of injury or to the more adherent attachment of the dura to the calvarium in elderly people. Because of the rapid ingress of blood into the epidural space, this process is fast moving following the initial injury and in the concussive period the patient is typically lucid and subsequently deteriorates rapidly. However, some patients with epidural hematomas never have a noticeable lucid interval, enter the hospital in coma, and continue to decline without evacuation of the hematoma.

Missile injuries

The material in this chapter deals with the closed head-injured patient because the survival of all patients who sustain gunshot wounds to the head is quite poor. Kaufman et al.[15] reported that 60 percent of cranial gunshot victims died in the field and only 38 percent of those hospitalized eventually were discharged from the hospital. The mortality rates for hospitalized patients in other studies ranges between 50 and 60 percent. The mortality of geriatric patients with these injuries is substantially higher. The management of these patients requires neurosurgical and intensive care resources, discussions of which are beyond the scope of this chapter.

Associated spinal injuries

A patient with an acute significant head injury has to be considered to have an associated spinal injury until proven otherwise.[16] The exact incidence varies with the series; however, an incidence of about 6 percent is usually given. The vast majority of these are cervical spine injuries. In a series of patients arriving in the emergency department with predominant spinal injuries, 24 percent had associated head injuries. Some of the spinal injuries are potentially unstable but have not as yet affected the spinal cord. Thus the potentially at-risk spinal cord must be protected by full spinal immobilization until the spine has been cleared by physical examination as well as appropriate imaging studies. High-dose methylprednisolone has been found to have a modest effect in lowering the ultimate deficit in spinal-cord-injured patients when administered within 8 hours of injury.

INITIAL EVALUATION AND MANAGEMENT

There is a marked difference between the presentation management options and differential diagnoses of acute and subacute head trauma vs chronic subdural hematomas. While the vast majority of head injury patients have no or mild TBI, the following stresses the evaluation of the more severely injured elderly patient.

Patients with acute and subacute head trauma will present with a history of a recent injury. TBI management includes the rapid recognition and correction of life-threatening conditions, prevention of secondary brain insults, and transportation to the closest appropriate medical facility. Maintaining cerebral perfusion by ensuring adequate blood pressure and oxygenation and serial neurological evaluations are the mainstays of early management. A potential pitfall in the management of the head injury patient is to assume that TBI is entirely responsible for any altered mental status. For all but the most trivial injuries, the patient should receive algorithmic initial management until the resultant CNS injury can be identified and stabilized. A comprehensive approach to the injured patient, particularly the TBI patient, requires consideration of the reversible causes of altered mental status, including hypoglycemia, hypoxemia, hypoperfusion, and drug toxicity, especially in the geriatric population.

In patients with mild TBI, the only historical factors proven to be useful in identifying lesions requiring neurosurgical intervention are LOC and amnesia.[17] A history of alcohol use, anticoagulant therapy, hemophilia, or age over 60 years are additional historical findings that have independently been associated with an increased risk for intracranial pathology. However, pre-existing conditions such as dementia, diabetes, and seizure disorder, or an antecedent event (syncope) or symptom (chest pain, motor deficit) are important historical information in determining the injury etiology and for guiding subsequent diagnostic management decisions.

Several investigations have demonstrated the association of hypoxemia and hypotension with poor outcomes in TBI patients. The Traumatic Coma Data Bank (TCDB) provides the best evidenced definition of hypotension (a single measured SBP <90 mmHg) and hypoxemia (apnea, cyanosis, hemoglobin oxygen saturation <90 percent or arterial pO_2 <60 mmHg).[12] A single episode of hypotension was associated with a doubling of mortality and increased morbidity when compared with nonhypotensive patients. The precise values of hypotension and hypoxemia are unknown, but both must be prevented or immediately corrected to maximize TBI patient outcomes. Serial (preferably continuous) measurements of blood pressure and oxygen saturation should be performed in the prehospital, ED, and intensive care unit settings.

Patient care at the scene of injury begins with a primary survey, including an evaluation of the airway, while maintaining cervical spine control followed by a cardiovascular, brief neurological, abdominal, pelvic, and extremity evaluation. All patients require a minimum assessment of (1) airway and cervical spine, (2) oxygenation, (3) blood pressure, (4) pupils, and (5) the Glasgow Coma Scale (GCS) score. A more detailed examination should be performed during transport and again in the ED.

All head-injured patients have potential cervical spine injury and should be immobilized to a long board and fitted with a cervical collar (e.g. Philadelphia collar) if there is cervical tenderness or pain, neurological deficit, altered mental status, or distracting injuries. As in all injured patients airway protection is the highest priority and a clear airway should be established and maintained. Patient oxygenation is one key to limiting neuronal loss and must be carefully monitored with pulse oximetry. Hypoxemia should be corrected by administering high-concentration supplemental oxygen and endotracheal intubation (ETI) if required.

Indications for intubation in the TBI patient include the inability to protect the airway, failure to ventilate, persistent hypoxemia despite supplemental oxygen administration, and severe TBI (GCS score less than 9). In the later patient group, early endotracheal intubation is associated with a decreased incidence of hypoxemia related secondary brain insults.[18] In most instances, oral ETI will be the employed procedure. Etomidate (0.3 mg/kg) is an induction agent with reduced negative cardiovascular effects in the potentially volume-depleted trauma patient and is employed in the USA with increasing frequency. Multiple studies have demonstrated the safety of using short-acting neuromuscular blockade in the prehospital and ED setting to facilitate definitive airway acquisition.[19,20] In the TBI patient, many rapid-sequence intubation (RSI) protocols recommend that lidocaine (1.5 mg/kg), be administered several minutes prior to direct laryngoscopy. Other central nervous system protectants are also suggested, such as fentanyl (1.5 mg/kg) or thiopental (3–5 mg/kg), as part of the intubation protocol.[21,22] However, these agents may reduce systemic arterial blood pressure, and resultant cerebral

Summary of management algorithm
Geriatric traumatic brain injury

- Obtain a careful history focusing on loss of consciousness, amnesia, use of anticoagulants, pre-existing neurologic impairment, comorbidities, medications, use of intoxicants, and the specific circumstances preceding the injury

- Initially assess the airway, breathing, and circulation of the patient and perform any required interventions before beginning the neurological evaluation

- Consider the cervical spine injured until proven otherwise and appropriately immobilize

- The initial neurological evaluation should include the pupillary examination and GCS score

- Appropriate transport to a medical facility with CT scanning capabilities and in moderate TBI, neurosurgical capabilities and in severe TBI, the additional capabilities of intracranial pressure monitoring and intracranial hypertension management

- Perform a careful physical examination specifically to identify other sites of trauma, signs of pre-existing conditions or comorbidities and the possible antecedent event precipitating the injury

- Perform a complete neurological examination looking for signs of intracranial hypertension, basilar skull fracture, motor abnormalities, and spinal cord syndromes

- Intubate all TBI patients in coma

- Ensure oxygen saturation at >90 percent

- Maintain systolic blood pressure at >90 mmHg

- Obtain an emergent noncontrast head CT on all elderly patients with a history of LOC or PTA or if the history is unclear or suspect

- Normoventilate all intubated patients (target PCO_2 ~35 mmHg) in the absence of signs of cerebral herniation

- Consider the indications for seizure prophylaxis, antibiotics, tetanus prophylaxis, and intracranial pressure monitoring

- Initiate treatment for intracranial hypertension at 20–25 mmHg with mild hyperventilation to a target PCO_2 of ~30 mmHg as a temporizing measure, intermittent bolus mannitol administration, and ventricular CSF drainage

- Prompt evacuation of neurosurgically amenable symptomatic intracranial hematomas

- Corticosteroids are not recommended for TBI in the absence of spinal cord injury

- Provide appropriate written discharge instructions to patients and their families regarding follow-up and the signs or symptoms that should prompt them to seek immediate medical care

- Advise all mild TBI patients of the possibility of post-concussive syndrome

- Above all be proactive in the conservative management of this unique patient population

---

perfusion pressure reductions may contribute to secondary brain injury. Therefore, they should be employed with caution in the hypovolemic or spinal-cord-injured patient.

Routine prophylactic hyperventilation is detrimental and should not be performed.[23] In the absence of intracranial pressure (ICP) monitoring, hyperventilation is only indicated when signs of cerebral herniation, such as extensor posturing or pupillary abnormalities (asymmetric or unreactive), are present after correcting hypotension and hypoxemia. The normal ventilation rate is defined as approximately 10 breaths per minute (bpm) for adults during manual or mechanical ventilation. Determination of arterial partial pressure of CO_2 ($PaCO_2$) should be performed as soon as possible to guide ventilatory parameters. The target $PaCO_2$ in the nonherniating TBI patient should be 30–35 mmHg. In the severe TBI patient with signs of cerebral herniation the temporizing target $PaCO_2$ is 30–35 mmHg. After ensuring the patient's airway, ventilation, and oxygenation, attention is directed to the cardiovascular system.

An initial cardiovascular examination looking for overt or occult hemorrhage, congestive heart failure, rhythm disturbances, and systemic perfusion is the next priority. If the blood pressure is low, suspect hemorrhage, high spinal cord injury, or acute myocardial infarction. Fluid resuscitation in TBI patients should be administered to avoid hypotension or limit hypotension to the shortest duration possible. The most commonly used resuscitation fluid for trauma patients in the acute setting is isotonic crystalloid solution, which should be administered in the volumes required to support blood pressure in the "normal range," although data supporting a specific target blood pressure are lacking. Several studies have demonstrated higher systolic blood pressures and significantly better survival and fewer complications in patients treated with hypertonic saline vs crystalloid resuscitation.[24,25] However, in blunt trauma, current recommendations include the rapid infusion of 2 liters of isotonic fluid, generally Ringer's lactate or normal saline, as the initial fluid bolus in adults.[26] After ensuring adequate airway, breathing, and circulation, attention is focused on the neurological evaluation.

The key signs of neurological function (e.g., pupillary size and reaction, patient's mental state and response to stimulation, as well as the formal GCS). Intracranial hypertension may

Table 57-1 Glasgow coma scale

Eye response		Motor response		Verbal response	
Spontaneous	4	Obeys	6	Oriented	5
To speech	3	Localizes	5	Confused	4
To pain	2	Withdraws	4	Inappropriate	3
None	1	Abnormal flexion	3	Incomprehensible	2
		Extension	2	None	1
		None	1		

result in temporal herniation, compress the third cranial nerve, and cause a unilateral fixed, dilated pupil. Bilaterally dilated and fixed pupils are more indicative of brainstem injury. However, hypoxemia, hypotension, and hypothermia are also associated with dilated and abnormally reactive pupils, requiring that resuscitation and stabilization occur before pupillary assessment commences.[27]

The trauma examination seeks to establish the patient's level of orientation and response to stimulation using the standard GCS[28–30] (Table 57-1) as well as noting the patient's level of neurological functioning and whether there are focal deficits or a sensory or motor level is present. A single GCS score is insufficient to determine the severity of TBI and lacks prognostic value; however, serial GCS scoring is prognostic. A low GCS score that remains low, or a high GCS score that decreases, predicts an increased probability of neurosurgical lesion and a worse outcome than a high GCS score that remains high, or a low GCS score that progressively improves.[29,30] The key to accurately employing the GCS is thorough serial evaluations after the patient has been hemodynamically stabilized, with documentation of all findings.

For the elderly mild TBI patient, the medical facility they are transported to should contain a 911 receiving ED with 24-hour neuroimaging (CT) scanning capabilities. In the moderate or severe TBI patient, the destination medical facility requires 24-hour availability of CT and neurosurgical capabilities. Severe TBI patients should be transported to trauma centers with prompt neurosurgical care and experience in intracranial pressure monitoring and intracranial hypertension management.[31]

HOSPITAL MANAGEMENT

When the patient presents to the receiving medical facility, the primary survey should be repeated and a more thorough secondary survey performed. A basilar fracture should be sought by examining the eyes for a periorbital ecchymosis, the area behind the ear for a hematoma (Battle sign), spinal fluid and otorrhea and hemotypanum, and the nose for spinal fluid rhinorrhea. The back of the head and the entire spine should be palpated for swelling, crepitus, and discongruities (stepoffs). A rapid examination of the cranial nerves and the muscle tone of all four extremities is then carried out. Motor strength and reflexes are recorded, as is rectal tone. Spinal cord injury is suspected when there is loss of rectal tone, loss of reflexes, hypotension, or priapism.

Unless contraindicated, during the secondary evaluation a foley catheter should be inserted to monitor output, and a gastric tube should be placed after endotracheal intubation to decompress the stomach. In patients with penetrating or open head injuries, a short course of broad-spectrum antibiotics is indicated, as is tetanus prophylaxis.

Patients with severe TBIs will usually receive seizure prophylaxis. Specific indications for early seizure prophylaxis (0–7 days post TBI) include a GCS score <10, cortical contusion, depressed skull fracture, epidural hematoma, subdural hematoma, intraparenchymal hematoma, penetrating TBI, or seizure within 24 hours of TBI. Phenytoin or carbamazepine are the typical anticonvulsants of choice for early seizure prophylaxis. The prophylactic use of phenytoin, carbamazepine, phenobarbital, or valproate is not recommended for preventing late (>7 days) post-traumatic seizures.[32]

LABORATORY AND IMAGING STUDIES

In patients with moderate or severe head injury, a baseline complete blood count, SMA7, coagulation profile, type and hold (or cross match), and toxicological and alcohol assays should be considered and are usually obtained. Additional metabolic, endocrine, and cardiac assays are directed by history or clinical suspicion.

To rule out suicidal intent and drug toxicities, toxicological screening is indicated for drugs of abuse and for specific intoxicants if known or suspected. Clues to suicidal behavior include a single-vehicle accident during good weather and lack of skid marks on the road, indicating that the patient did not apply the brakes. The same clues can also be present in patients whose trauma is secondary to loss of consciousness, as in hypoglycemia, epilepsy, or cardiac rhythm disturbances. The cardiopulmonary evaluation includes an electrocardiogram and subsequent electrophysiological and serum assays for cardiac ischemia when indications are present that the injury may have been precipitated by a cardiac dysrrhythmic or a hypoperfusion event.

Imaging studies[33–35] for these patients are carried out once they are initially stabilized and for most patients include a complete cervical spine series: anteroposterior (AP) lateral, and open mouth odontoid views; if these are normal and there is no evidence of a spinal cord injury in the alert patient the immobilization can be removed. An initial lateral film of the cervical spine is taken at the bedside and if all seven cervical vertebrae and the rosteral aspects of the first thoracic vertebrae are seen and appear normal, the AP and open mouth odontoid views are obtained. Often the plain films of the neck are inadequate or show varying degrees of pre-existing subluxation and degenerative changes, abnormalities that will require CT in order to clear the spine.

Elderly patients have been shown to have increased morbidity and mortality from TBI and have been demonstrated to have higher rates of intracranial injuries.[4] In one study, patients older than 60 years with LOC or post traumatic amnesia and a GCS of 15 in the ED had an intracranial lesion in 28 percent of the cases.[36] Therefore, all patients over 60 years of age that have LOC or amnesia regardless of GCS score and patients with moderate or severe head injuries should have an unenhanced head CT. Plain skull films may be useful if a penetrating or depressed skull fracture is suspected, but an unenhanced CT of the head will still be required to evaluate the underlying brain and the skull films are redundant at that point.

DISPOSITION

MILD   Head-injured patients seen in the ED who have a mild head injury, a negative CT, no antecedent event, and are back to baseline can typically be discharged home with a responsible family member and specific written instructions if there is a very stable and supportive home environment and follow-up mechanism. Depending on the particular circumstances however, it may be preferential, to admit these patients for monitoring, neurological checks, and a thorough medical evaluation. Again, when in doubt the conservative approach is recommended in this patient population.

MODERATE   Patients with moderate head trauma are confused or sleepy and are admitted even with a head CT devoid of obvious intracranial pathology. If the CT is abnormal, neurosurgical consultation and observation in a neurosurgical intensive care unit is mandatory in most cases.

SEVERE   Patients with severe head injury will require neurosurgical intensive care. Most of these will be intubated and require a neurosurgical procedure within the first 48 hours. The issue of survivability of the patient with a severe head injury raises the ethical issues of resource utilization and medical futility. These issues are discussed elsewhere in this text as well as in the section on prognosis at the end of this chapter.

CRITICAL CARE ISSUES IN THE MANAGEMENT OF THE HEAD-INJURED PATIENT

Early in their stay in the hospital, the patient's nutritional status and fluid and electrolyte balance have to be considered.[37] We are also concerned about the rapid loss of nitrogen that occurs due to protein breakdown secondary to the stress of trauma and immobilization. To minimize negative nitrogen balance, 10,500 J/day (2,500 calories/day) of carbohydrate and a source of nitrogen are required. Basic fluid replacement consists of about 2,500 cc of fluid per day to cover urine output and insensible losses. Maintenance electrolyte requirements are at least 40 mEq of potassium, 50–100 mEq of sodium per day. Skin care, bowel, and bladder function, as well as mechanical venous thrombosis prophylaxis are even more important in these patients than in other types of acute bedbound patients because of their immobility.

Intracranial pressure (ICP) monitoring should be employed in all patients over 40 years of age with severe TBI regardless of CT findings.[38] TBI patients with ICPs greater than 20–25 mmHg have worse outcomes than those without intracranial hypertension.[37,39] In the emergency management of patients with intracranial hypertension or signs of cerebral herniation several treatment options are available. Temporizing

medical reduction of intracranial pressure consists of hyperventilation to a PCO_2 of 30–35 mm and mannitol (0.5 to 1 g/kg) via intermittent bolus infusion until ventriculostomy with subsequent cerebrospinal fluid drainage or definitive hematoma evacuation (if present) via burr hole or craniotomy can be accomplished.

Patients with head trauma may develop transient or permanent diabetes insipidus manifested by polyuria and severe hypernatremia and prerenal azotemia. This is treated by administering vasopressin (desmopressin) and replacing free water. Other patients will develop the syndrome of inappropriate secretion of antidiuretic hormone and dilutional hyponatremia. This is managed by restricting fluids and infusing furosemide. Adjunctive treatments with demeclocycline, phenytoin, and lithium may be helpful to supplement water restriction.

PROGNOSIS

Aside from the severity of injury, age is probably the single most important variable influencing outcome.[36,40–45] Patients over age 65 have nearly twice the mortality of younger patients with similar injury levels.[38] The issues relating to this worsened prognoses in elderly people is also seen in all categories of major trauma involving other organ systems. In a recent series of geriatric head-injured patients,[43] with an admission GCS of 9 or less and nonsurgical lesions had a mortality of 85 percent. Here, the authors recommend aggressive intensive management and then the limitation of maximal therapy only to those with significant improvement within 24 hours.

In the TCDB study, a marked increase in pre-existing systemic disease was found with increasing age. This pre-existing disease was significantly associated with poor outcomes (death and vegetative) in those patients above 56 years of age (86 vs 50 percent) when compared to the younger age group. In addition, multiple systemic injuries were less likely in the older age group thus emphasizing the importance of the brain injury severity in determining outcome overall.

Advanced age has an important negative influence upon outcome after severe head injury and this is not explained solely by the increased frequency of intracranial complications in older patients.[43] For each level of injury the mortality, morbidity, and failure to return to baseline function are significantly increased in the geriatric population, when comparing similar injury severity. In a study by Vollmer et al.[44] of all patients who had a period of coma following head injury in the 25–35 age group, approximately 30 percent of patients died within 6 months. This mortality rose to 80 percent in patients over age 55. In those who did survive, poor functional outcome was associated with advanced age.[45]

In patients 55 years of age or older sustaining acute head injury complicated by a large extracerebral collection (greater than 15 mL), 89 percent resulted in death or a vegetative state compared to 50 percent in the 16–25 age group.[10] In patients over age 60 with moderate head injury defined as an initial GCS of 9–13, 24 percent made a good recovery, 10 percent had residual moderate disability, 10 percent severe disability, and 55 percent died or were left in a vegetative state.

Other studies[46] suggest that the release of neuroexcitatory transmitters, glutamate and aspartate, may play a role given the diminished neuronal pool and altered receptor availability and sensitivity. Another group of investigators[47] have published a series of experiments on the propensity of the aging brain to respond to direct injury with more gliosis and fibrosis than immature brains. Vascular factors that are thought to be important in prejudicing outcome in elderly people include amyloidangiopathy, atherosclerosis, and fibrosis of vessels, causing them to be less tolerant to shearing forces. Cerebral atrophy, while surrounding the brain with more cerebrospinal fluid, does not adequately protect the brain from the shearing forces if sustained from abrupt accelerating and decelerating forces.

SUMMARY

The challenge of rapidly and accurately diagnosing head-injured geriatric patients is based on creating a medical database that includes early detection of intracranial hematomas and intracranial hypertension and leads to prompt medical and neurosurgical management. It also requires simultaneous, evaluation of non-neurological trauma, which frequently contributes to the systemic etiologies of secondary brain injury.

Of utmost importance is the proactive assessment and rapid management of hypoxemia and hypotension and transport to a medical facility with the equipment and staff to appropriately manage the possible pathologies and complications. What is not unique, but a more frequent confounder in this distinctive cohort are predisposing medical, psychiatric, toxicological, and neurological conditions that may have been antecedent factors in the etiology of the injury. This type of comprehensive assessment and rapid management can improve what is currently a rather poor prognosis for the geriatric patient with a serious head injury. The team approach to the problem should be employed at each stage of the patient's care including the prehospital, ED, intensive care and rehabilitation phases of recovery, maximizing the potential for limiting mortality and lowering the morbidity for these vulnerable patients.

For elderly patients with severe TBI who do not rapidly improve with surgical and intensive medical management over the first few days, there is a dismal prognosis. This situation is no different from other terminal care situations faced by healthcare providers every day and for which there are accepted approaches to limiting futile care. In the head-injured patient, brain death criteria[48,49] (Tables 57-2 and 57-3) are obviously key elements in helping the family and friends in coming to

grips with the loss of their loved one. Patients who are successfully resuscitated from the acute insult to the CNS will require intensive physical and emotional rehabilitation, with a slow response toward baseline, the optimum result that can be expected.

Table 57-3 Confirmatory tests of brain death

Used to shorten period of observation or to help define the patient's status when other factors are involved.
- Four vessel angiography: no cerebral blood flow
- Electroencephalogram: electrocerebral silence
- Cerebral radionuclide angiogram: no isotope in cerebral arteries

---

KEY POINTS Management of geriatric head injury

■ Address airway, breathing, and circulation first.

■ Search for an antecedent etiologic event.

■ Maximize systemic and cerebral perfusion.

■ Obtain an emergent noncontrast head CT on all elderly patients with history or evidence of any traumatic brain injury.

REFERENCES

1. Statistical Abstract of the US, 114th Ed. US Dept of Commerce, Washington, DC, 1994
2. Schiller WR, Knox R, Chleborad W: A five-year experience with severe injuries in elderly patients. Accid Anal Prev 1995;27:167–174
3. van der Sluis CK, Timmer HW, Eisma WH, ten Duis HJ: Outcome in elderly injured patients: injury severity versus host factors. Injury 1997;28:588–592
4. Nagurney JT, Borczuk P, Thomas SH: Elder patients with closed head trauma: a comparison with nonelder patients. Acad Emerg Med 1998;5:678–684
5. Zietlow SP, Capizzi PJ, Bannon MP, Farnell MB: Multisystem geriatric trauma. J Trauma 1994;37:985–988
6. Fife D: Head injury with and without hospital admission: Comparison of incidence and short-term disability. Am J Pub Health 1987; 77:810–812
7. Jager TE, Weiss HB, Coben JH, Pepe PE: Traumatic brain injuries evaluated in U.S. emergency departments, 1992–1994. Acad Emerg Med 2000;7:134–140
8. Thurman DJ, Alverson C, Dunn KA, Guerrero J, Sniezek JE: Traumatic brain injury in the United States: A public health perspective. J Head Trauma Rehabil 1999;14:602–615
9. Chaudra V, Kokman E, Schoenberg BS: Head trauma with loss of consciousness as a risk factor for Alzheimer's disease. Neurology 1989;39:1576–1578
10. Graves AB, White E, Koepsell TD et al: The association between head trauma and Alzheimer's disease. Am J Epidemiol 1990;131:491–501
11. Rassmussen DX, Brandt J, Martin DB: Head injury as a risk factor in Alzheimer's disease. Brain Inj 1995;9:213–219
12. Chesnut RM, Marshall LF, Klauber MR et al: The role of secondary brain injury in determining outcome from severe head injury. J Trauma 1993;34:216–222
13. Stein SC, Ross SE: The value of computed tomographic scans in patients with low-risk head injuries. Neurosurgery 1990;26:638–640
14. Fell DA, Fitzgerald S, Maid RH: Acute subdural hematomas, review of 144. J Neurosurg 1973;42:37–42
15. Kaufman HH, Loyola WP, Makela ME et al: Civilian gunshot wounds: the limits of salvageability. Acta Neurochir 1983;67:115–125

Table 57-2 Diagnosis of brain death in head-injured patient—standard criteria[20,27]

Clinical criteria for cerebral unresponsiveness:
- Patient unresponsive to deep pain
- Patient apneic (there must be a formal test for apnea by preoxygenating the patient and withdrawing the patient from a ventilator for approximately 12 minutes or until the $PaCO_2$ is greater than 60 mm)
- Brainstem reflexes are absent
- Hypothermia and exogenous substances (e.g., alcohol and barbiturates) are absent
- The mechanism and result of the head injury have been documented and are unsurvivable

16. Kraus JF, McArthur DL, Silverman TA: Epidemiology of brain injury. In Nayoyou (ed): Neurotrauma. McGraw-Hill, New York, 1996:14
17. Marshall LF, Gautille T, Klauber MR: The outcome of severe closed head injury. J Neurosurg 1991;75:S28–S36
18. Fearnside M, Cook R, McDougall P: The Westmead Head Injury Project outcome in severe head injury. A comparative analysis of prehospital, clinical and CT variables. Br J Neurosurg 1993;7:267–279
19. Rhee KJ, O'Malley RJ: Neuromuscular blockade-assisted oral intubation versus nasotracheal intubation in the prehospital care of injured patients. Ann Emerg Med 1994;23:37–42
20. Syverud SA, Borron SW, Storer DL: Prehospital use of neuromuscular agents in a helicopter ambulance program. Ann Emerg Med 1998;17:236–242
21. Walls R: Rapid-sequence intubation in head trauma. Ann Emerg Med 1993;22:1008–1013
22. Walls R, Murphy M: Increased intracranial pressure. In Walls R (ed): Emergency Airway Management. Lippincott Williams & Wilkens, Philadelphia, 2000:159–163
23. Muizelaar JP, Marmarou A, Ward JD et al: Adverse effects of prolonged hyperventilation in patients with severe head injury: a randomized clinical trial. J Neurosurg 1991;75:731–739
24. Mattox KL, Maningas PA, Moore EE: Prehospital hypertonic saline/dextran infusion for post-traumatic hypotension. Ann Surg 1991;213:482–491
25. Wade CE, Grady JJ, Kramer GC: Individual patient cohort analysis of the efficacy of hypertonic saline/dextran in patients with traumatic brain injury and hypotension. J Trauma 1997;42:561–565
26. Surgeons ACo: Advanced Trauma Life Support Instructor's Manual. American College of Surgeons, Chicago, 1996
27. Meyer S, Gibb T, Jurkovich G: Evaluation and significance of the pupillary light reflex in trauma patients. Ann Emerg Med 1993;22:1052–1057
28. Teasdale G, Jennett B: Assessment of coma and impaired consciousness. A practical scale. Lancet 1974;2:81–84
29. Oppenheim JS, Camins MB: Predicting outcome in brain-injured patients. Using the Glasgow Coma Scale in primary care practice. Postgrad Med 1992;91:261–264,267–268
30. Jennett B, Teasdale G: Aspects of coma after severe head injury. Lancet 1977;1:878–881
31. Bullock R, Chestnut RM, Clifton G et al: Guidelines for the management of severe head injury. Brain Trauma Foundation. Eur J Emerg Med 1996;3(2):109–127
32. Temkin NR, Dikmen SS, Wilensky AJ et al: A randomized, double-blind study of phenytoin for the prevention of post-traumatic seizures. N Engl J Med 1990;323:497–502
33. Yealy DM, Hogan DE: Imaging after head trauma. Who needs what? Emerg Med Clin North Am 1991;9:707–717
34. Jeret J, Mandell M, Anziska B: Clinical predictors of abnormality disclosed by computed tomography after mild head trauma. Neurosurgery 1993;32:9–15
35. Haydel MJ, Preston CA, Mills TJ et al: Indications for computed tomography in patients with minor head injury. N Engl J Med 2000;343:100–105
36. Luerssen TG, Klauber MR, Marshall LF: Outcome from head injury related to patient's age. A longitudinal prospective study of adult and pediatric head injury. J Neurosurg 1988;68:409–416
37. White RJ, Likavec MJ: The diagnosis and initial management of head injury. N Engl J Med 1992;327:1507–1511
38. Narayan RK, Kishore PR, Becker DP et al: Intracranial pressure: to monitor or not to monitor? A review of our experience with severe head injury. J Neurosurg 1982;56:650–659
39. Kraus JF: Epidemiology of head trauma. In: Cooper, PR (ed): Head Injury. Williams & Wilkins, Baltimore, 1993
40. Conroy C, Kraus JF: Survival after brain injury. Cause of death, length of survival, and prognostic variables in a cohort of brain-injured people. Neuroepidemiology 1988;7:13–22
41. Becker DP, Miller JD, Ward JD et al: The outcome from severe head injury with early diagnosis and intensive management. J Neurosurg 1977;47:491–502
42. Pentland B, Jones PA, Roy CW, Miller JD: Head injury in the elderly. Age Ageing 1986;15:193–202
43. Kotwica Z, Jakubowski JK: Acute head injuries in the elderly. An analysis of 136 consecutive patients. Acta Neurochir 1992;118:98–102
44. Vollmer DG, Torner JC, Eisenberg HM: Age and outcome following traumatic coma: why do older patients fare worse? J Neurosurg Suppl 1991;5:37–49
45. Teasdale G, Skene A, Parker L, Jennett B: Age and outcome of severe head injury. Acta Neurochir Suppl 1979;28:140–143
46. Olneg JW: Excitotoxin medical. Neuronal death in youth and old age. Prog Brain Res 1990;86:37–51
47. Rudge JS, Smith GM, Silver J: An in vitro model of wound healing in the CNS: analysis of cell reaction and interaction at different ages. Exp Neurol 1989;103:1–16
48. Guidelines for the Determination of Death, Report of the Medical Consultants on the Diagnosis of Death to the President's Commission for the Study of Ethical Problems in Medicine and Biomedical and Behavioral Research. JAMA 1981;246:2184–2186
49. Bleak PM: Conception and practical issues in the declaration of death by brain criteria. Neurosurg Clin N Am 1991;2:490–501

Chapter 58

Infections of the central nervous system

Steven L. Berk and James W. Myers

Bacterial meningitis is a disease that presents particular challenges in the elderly patient. The mortality rate from bacterial meningitis is higher in elderly people than in younger adults. Bacterial meningitis has become a more common problem in elderly patients over the past two decades. In 1973, Fraser et al.[1] reported that the mean age of death from meningitis in Olmstead County, Minnesota, had gone from 11.5 years in the period 1935–1946 to 64 years during the period 1959–1970. In the latter period more than one-half of all deaths from meningitis occurred in those over 60 years of age. The incidence of bacterial meningitis rose from 5 cases per 100,000 to 15 cases per 100,000.[1] A Centers for Disease Control survey performed between 1978 and 1981 showed an increasing incidence of meningitis in older patients[2] as did a survey on the incidence of meningitis conducted in Rhode Island.[3] In one review of 445 adults treated for bacterial meningitis at the Massachusetts General Hospital, 56 percent of community-acquired meningitis occurred in patients over 50 years of age.[4] In this study as well as all previous studies the mortality rate was much higher in older patients. The mortality rate in the Massachusetts General Hospital study was 37 in those over 60 years of age compared to 17 in younger adults. In the Rhode Island study, 55 percent of elderly patients died compared with an overall mortality rate of 10.[3]

The increased incidence of meningitis in this age group probably is explained, in part, by the more aggressive care given to elderly patients including more rigorous evaluation of fever, change in mental status, and coma. Nosocomial meningitis particularly related to neurosurgical procedures is also a cause of the increasing incidence of meningitis in this age group. Durand et al.[4] have shown that nosocomial meningitis has increased from 28 percent of all meningitis between 1962 and 1970 to 45 percent of all cases of meningitis from 1980 to 1988. Many of these cases occur in the chronically ill, frequently hospitalized elderly.

Bacteria may reach the subarachnoid space of the elderly patient by several different mechanisms.[5] Elderly patients with focal infections may develop bacteremia and seed the meninges. This occurs, for example, in the elderly patient with pneumococcal pneumonia, or less frequently in the patient with pyelonephritis and Gram-negative meningitis. Meningitis develops by way of direct inoculation of bacteria into the meninges such as occurs in head trauma or after a neurosurgical procedure. Elderly patients are prone to frequent falls and head injuries. *Staphylococcus aureus*, coagulase-negative staphylococci, and Gram-negative bacilli are responsible for most cases of meningitis secondary to head trauma or neurosurgery. Meningitis may occur from contiguous spread of infection to the meninges as in patients with otitis media, sinusitis, or mastoiditis. This mechanism of infection is probably somewhat less common in elderly people, compared with younger adults.

In the bacteremic, elderly patient, symptoms of fever, chills, and rigors will usually be present but afebrile bacteremia in elderly people is well described. Patients with contiguous spread of infection usually complain of localized findings such as ear or facial pain. Bacteria in the subarachnoid space will cause an inflammatory reaction in the pia and arachnoid matter that will manifest itself as neck pain and stiffness with protective reflexes that cause the Kernig and Brudzinski signs. Structures that lie within the subarachnoid space are involved in the inflammatory reaction. Pial arteries and veins may become inflamed and cranial nerve roots damaged.

A diffuse encephalopathy may occur. Abnormal mental status results from cerebral ischemia, edema, or toxic encephalopathy. Confusion, headache, or lethargy is a manifestation of this diffuse, inflammatory process. Papilledema, hydrocephalus, and other focal findings may occur as a result of pus occluding the foramina of Luschka and Magendie resulting in increased intracranial pressure.

The clinical features of meningitis in elderly patients are more subtle than in younger adults. This is a recurring theme in almost all studies that involve older patients with meningitis.[6,7] Most, but not all, studies have found that elderly patients with bacterial meningitis are less likely to have neck stiffness and meningeal signs. At the same time, older patients often have cervical spine disease and poor neck mobility, making interpretation of clinical signs more difficult. Berman et al.[8] found meningismus present in only 58 percent of elderly patients with meningitis. Gorse et al.[9] compared signs and symptoms of patients with meningitis above 50 years of age to those in patients below 50. Older patients had more mental status abnormalities and were more likely to have seizures, neurological deficits, and hydrocephalus. Berk,[6] Roos,[10] Massanari[11] and others have noted that a delay in diagnosis is frequently associated with meningitis in the elderly and this delay may explain the high mortality rate noted in this group of patients.

Elderly patients with bacterial meningitis may not have as pronounced fever or may at times be afebrile. The change in mental status that occurs in elderly people may be attributed to senility, delirium, psychosis, transient ischemia, or stroke. In the elderly patient who has undergone neurosurgery, postoperative lethargy may be mistakenly attributed to an expected postoperative course. A stiff neck in an elderly patient may not arouse the same concern that it would in a young adult.

Physical examination is a critical part of the evaluation of an elderly patient with suspected meningitis. Nuchal rigidity is reported in between 56 and 92 percent of elderly patients depending on the series.[7] When neck stiffness is the result of meningeal irritation, the neck will resist flexion but can be rotated from side to side. A funduscopic and cranial nerve examination are mandatory to alert the clinician to associated increased intracranial pressure or brain abscess. Mental status should be carefully described and followed. Lethargy and coma are poor prognostic signs. Examination of the head should include a search for skull fracture, avulsion, or hematoma. Careful otoscopic examination is also a necessity as otitis media may be missed in the elderly patient, particularly when mental status is abnormal and a history cannot be obtained. The elderly patient may present with pneumonia and concomitant meningitis. Gorse et al.[9] found pneumonia to be much more common in older adults with meningitis. The elderly patient may not complain of respiratory symptoms so examination of the lung may be the first clue to pneumonia. Examination of the heart is necessary to detect underlying valvular heart disease that might predispose the elderly patient to endocarditis with seeding of the meninges. Examination for costovertebral tenderness, decubitus ulcers, and petechial lesions will also provide important information in determining the source and etiologic agent in meningitis.

Performance of a lumbar puncture without delay is the critical element in the diagnosis of bacterial meningitis in both young and old. About 35 percent of elderly patients with meningitis present with focal neurological findings.[9] Because lumbar puncture is contraindicated in patients with brain abscess, computed tomography (CT) or magnetic resonance imaging (MRI) will be necessary in some older patients. However, the high mortality rate from meningitis in the elderly makes time of the essence in the diagnosis and treatment of meningitis in this group. Many infectious disease experts now support the strategy of beginning empirical antibiotic therapy, pending lumbar puncture, particularly when a delay of hours is anticipated due to an imaging study.

There is very little in the literature to suggest that the cerebrospinal fluid (CSF) findings in elderly patients with meningitis differ from young adults with meningitis. Lumbar puncture will show purulent fluid with white blood cell counts between about 500 and 10,000 cu/mm. Polymorphonuclear leukocytes predominate usually making up more than 90 percent of total cell count. Meningitis caused by *Listeria monocytogenes* sometimes has a mononuclear cell predominance. At least one study has shown that elderly patients with meningitis are more likely to have a lack of cellular response in CSF than younger adults.[12] Those elderly patients with meningitis who have few cells in CSF but many bacteria have a poor prognosis.[13] CSF glucose levels are usually low in bacterial meningitis. CSF to serum glucose ratios are usually less than 50 percent. Seventy percent of patients with meningitis will have a ratio less than 31 percent.[14] Spinal fluid protein is elevated above 50 mg/dL. Very high protein levels are associated with poor prognosis. Gram stain of CSF will be positive in 60 to 90 percent of all patients with meningitis.[14] In the study by Berman et al.[8] only 50 percent of elderly patients with meningitis had a positive Gram stain. The Gram stain is most likely to be negative in patients who have received prior antibiotic therapy. In those patients whose Gram stain is negative, a variety of methods to detect bacterial antigen are now in common use. These include latex fixation, coagglutination, and counterimmunoelectrophoresis. The limulus lysate assay has been used to detect Gram-negative meningitis, an important cause of meningitis in elderly people. Other tests such as lactic acid levels and measurement of C-reactive protein have been recommended to help distinguish bacterial from viral meningitis but clinical decisions are rarely based on them.

Blood cultures are recommended in all patients in whom bacterial meningitis is suspected. In the study by Berman et al.[8] almost one-half of all elderly patients with meningitis had concomitant bacteremia. In addition, other cultures such as sputum, urine, and wound may be extremely helpful in determining etiological agent and source of infection.

Streptococcus pneumoniae is the most common organism to cause meningitis in elderly patients.[5] *S. pneumoniae* was responsible for more than one-half of all cases of meningitis in the elderly in several studies.[15–17] The organism caused 43 percent of all cases in the study of Berman et al.[8] and 24 percent of cases in the study of Gorse et al.[9] Gram-negative bacilli cause meningitis in elderly patients both by bacteremic spread of infection such as in urinary tract infection or pneumonia, and as a nosocomial infection after neurosurgery.[18,19] *Escherichia coli* is the most common organism to cause meningitis secondary to bacteremic spread. *E. coli* and *Klebsiella* pneumonia are the more common Gram-negative bacilli to cause meningitis after neurosurgery but more unusual organisms, particularly *Acinetobacter*[20–22] have been more commonly reported. In a review of 581 cases of bacterial meningitis in elderly patients between 1967 and 1980, about 8 percent of cases were caused by Gram-negative bacilli[6] (Fig. 58-1). However, more recent studies have shown Gram-negative bacilli to be responsible for 20–25 percent of cases.[8,9] This increase is not unexpected in light of the reported increase in nosocomial meningitis in all age groups. Gram-negative meningitis occurs at the extremes of life, in the neonate and debilitated elderly people. In a study of 158 patients with Gram-negative meningitis in New York City over one-half of the patients were over 60 years of age. Almost all of these elderly patients died.[23] However, third-generation cephalosporins have replaced chloramphenicol for treatment of Gram-negative meningitis with improvement in overall survival.

L. monocytogenes is also an organism more likely to cause meningitis in elderly people than the younger adult. Because this infection is T-cell mediated, it is possible that immunologic senescence of this system may explain the predisposition of elderly people to this infection. Although *Listeria* accounts for 4–8 percent of all cases of meningitis in elderly people, it is an extremely rare cause of meningitis in young healthy adults. Of 53 cases of *L. monocytogenes* meningitis in New York City, 77 percent of patients were older than 50 and 87 percent of these elderly patients died.[23]

Meningococcal meningitis is the most common cause of meningitis in young adults, but a less common cause of meningitis in elderly people. The incidence of meningococcal meningitis in the elderly patient population varies from one study to another, reflecting the epidemic nature of the disease. Outbreaks have occurred in nursing homes and institutional settings.[24] The infection should be considered in elderly patients who present with meningeal signs and have a petechial or macular rash. No focus of infection will be noted.

Etiologic organism*

Possible source of infection

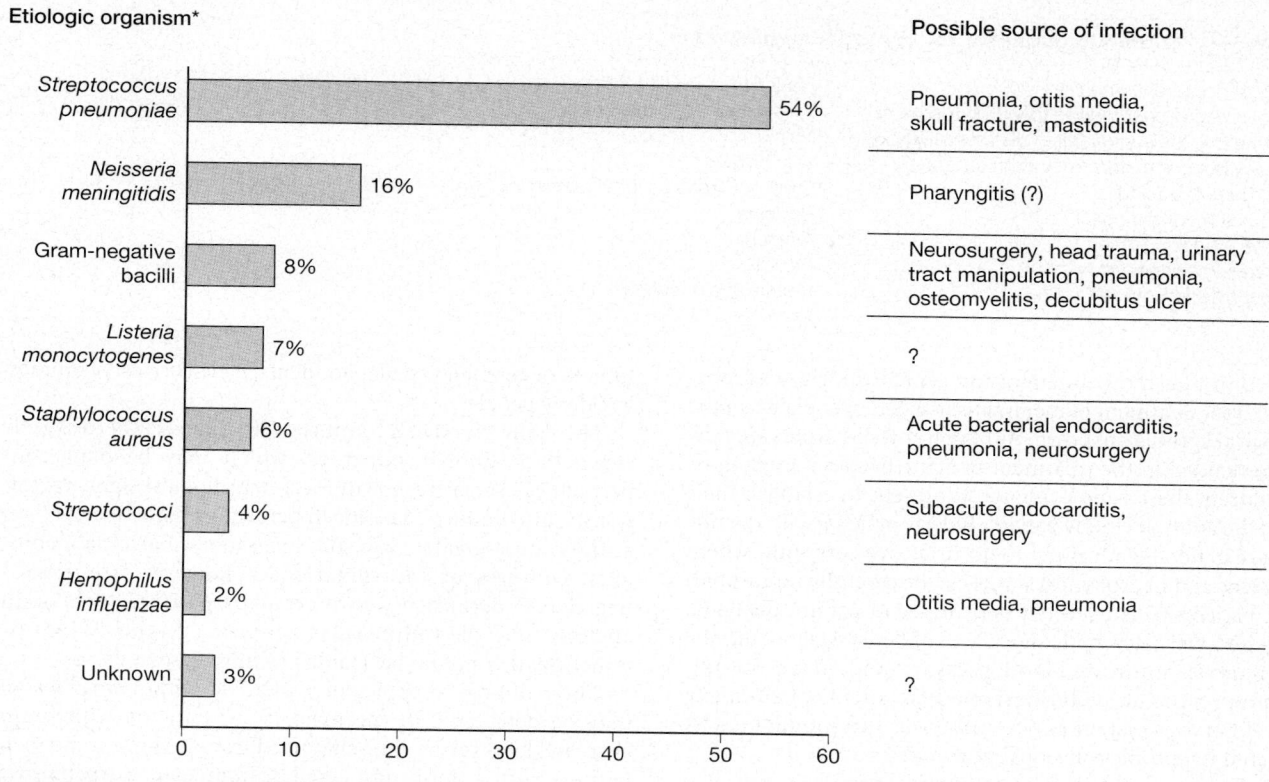

* Based on 581 patients in 7 series

Figure 58-1 Bacterial meningitis in elderly patients. (Modified from Berk and Smith,[5] with permission.)

S. aureus was the most common cause of meningitis in elderly people in a Mayo Clinic study between the years 1948 and 1958.[25] All cases were secondary to neurosurgery. Overall the organism is probably responsible for about 10 percent of cases of meningitis in older patients, either as a neurosurgical infection or part of a complicated staphylococcal sepsis secondary to pneumonia or endocarditis. Coagulase-negative staphylococci have become a more common cause of meningitis in elderly people, being associated with CSF shunts and other neurosurgical procedures.

β-Hemolytic streptococci are a relatively rare cause of meningitis in elderly people. However, this appears to be another organism that causes life-threatening infection and meningitis at the extremes of life.[26] *Hemophilus influenzae*, a cause of meningitis in children, is unusual in adults and elderly people. When *H. influenzae* does occur in older patients, it is usually a nonencapsulated organism.[27] This is in contrast to children, where the type B encapsulated organism is most likely to cause infection.

The treatment of bacterial meningitis requires prompt initiation of antibiotic therapy. The antibiotic chosen must have excellent activity against the etiological agent. Information from the history and physical examination in combination with a careful review of the CSF Gram stain will be the foundation on which the etiological agent will be determined and the optimal antibiotic chosen. An infectious disease specialist, when possible, should be involved in the case as the mortality rate from the disease is high and the margin of error is small. The antibiotic chosen should be bactericidal for the etiological agent and must diffuse across the blood–brain barrier. Table 58-1 lists the etiological agent and the antibiotic generally recommended.

However, the particular epidemiology of the hospital or community of the patient will take on increasing importance in determining the antibiotic of choice. The rapid emergence of penicillin-resistant pneumococci in the United States has created some uncertainty in regard to the initial treatment of pneumococcal meningitis. Given the rising incidence of high-level penicillin-resistant organisms, empirical therapy of pneumococcal meningitis should include vancomycin and a third-generation cephalosporin.[28] Pneumococci with an MIC of ≥2 μg/mL are especially worrisome in that failures have been noted when these patients were treated with cephalosporin alone.[29] The role of dexamethasone, rifampin, and the new fluroquinolones for pneumococcal meningitis is unclear at this time, and infectious disease consultation is advised. In the treatment of Gram-negative meningitis, the antibiotic sensitivity pattern of Gram-negative bacilli at a particular hospital is also critically important. If the infection has occurred after a neurosurgical procedure, the organisms responsible for prior neurosurgical infections should be noted. If *Pseudomonas aeruginosa* is suspected as the etiological agent, ceftazidime is the antibiotic of choice. Cefotaxime or ceftriaxone are generally used for other Gram-negative bacilli including *H. influenzae*. Ampicillin is the drug of choice for *L. monocytogenes*. Oxacillin or nafcillin are drugs of choice for methicillin-sensitive staphylococci; vancomycin is the antibiotic of choice for methicillin-resistant staphylococci and most coagulase-negative staphylococci. As previously noted,

Table 58-1 **Antibiotic of choice for bacterial meningitis**	
Streptococcus pneumoniae	Penicillin
Streptococcus pneumoniae (penicillin resistant)	Vancomycin + ceftriaxone
Staphylococcus aureus (methicillin sensitive)	Nafcillin
Staphylococcus aureus (methicillin resistant)	Vancomycin
Gram-negative bacilli	Third-generation cephalosporin (see text)
β-Hemolytic streptococci	Penicillin
Listeria monocytogenes	Ampicillin
Neisseria meningitides	Penicillin
Hemophilus influenzae	Ceftriaxone or cefotaxime

ampicillin plus a third-generation cephalosporin is recommended for treatment of meningitis in elderly people when the etiological agent is unknown. Although corticosteroids are now recommended in the treatment of acute bacterial meningitis in children, there is no evidence at present to establish their use in the adult or elderly patient. Elderly patients with meningitis are generally admitted to an intensive care unit, where vital signs and neurological status can be carefully monitored. Some patients will be severely dehydrated or volume depleted, and others will be in septic shock. Colloid or crystalloid may be necessary to improve blood pressure and urine output. Inappropriate antidiuretic hormone secretion may accompany central nervous system (CNS) infections but should be self-limited if hypotonic solutions are avoided.

The comatose, elderly patient requires specialized care. The patient may need frequent suctioning, particularly if pneumonia is present. The patient should be turned frequently to avoid decubiti. A condom catheter is preferable to a Foley, unless urinary retention develops. In patients who develop relapsing or prolonged fever, a repeat lumbar puncture is necessary. Drug fever, phlebitis, urinary tract infection, and pulmonary emboli are all possible explanations for prolonged fever.

The currently available pneumococcal vaccine is routinely recommended in all patients over 65 years of age. Although there are no specific data to support the prevention of pneumococcal meningitis in the elderly, it is clear that the vaccine does decrease the incidence of serious pneumococcal respiratory infection. Because most cases of pneumococcal meningitis in older patients are caused by pneumonia as the initial infection, it is likely that a vaccination program in elderly patients would be of benefit in preventing meningitis.

FOCAL LESIONS, ENCEPHALITIS, AND CHRONIC MENINGITIS

Brain abscess

A brain abscess often presents as a mass lesion with focal neurological deficits. Since the advent of the CT scan, mortality has decreased from 30–50 percent to as low as 4–20 percent. The duration of symptoms before hospitalization usually has a mean of 15 days.[30] Risk factors for adverse outcomes include a severe change of mental status on admission, neurological abnormalities on admission, and a short duration between the first symptoms and presentation suggesting a rapid progression. Fever may be absent in 40–50 percent of patients; common symptoms such as headache, change of mental status, and focal neurological deficits may be misdiagnosed as cerebral tumors or cerebral vascular accidents, which are very common in elderly people.

The white blood cell count is ordinarily normal to slightly elevated. A lumbar puncture, which may be dangerous particularly in patients with focal neurological signs, reveals nonspecific findings. Seventeen percent of patients may have a white count greater than 500, suggesting a bacterial meningitis. Cultures of the spinal fluid, however, are usually negative.[30] Because 15–40 percent of patients with brain abscesses may die within 24–48 hours of a diagnostic lumbar puncture, this should be avoided in most cases.

The radiological appearance of a "doughnut ring" lesion may be detectable in the majority of patients with brain abscesses. However, ring-enhanced lesions can also be seen with necrotic tumors and cerebral infarction. Surrounding edema may also be seen on CT scan and might be an indication for corticosteroids.[31,32] In cases of a single abscess, the most common location is generally that of the frontal lobe or parietal lobe rather than the occipital or temporal. Sites of brain abscesses are often independent from presumed origin of infection except for the possibility of ear and sinus infections more often leading to abscesses within the frontal brain.

Generalized seizures can prompt hospitalization of many patients including older adults. Often 50 percent of patients with a brain abscess may have a focal neurological sign such as a hemiparesis or focal seizure. Patients may also present with a diffuse neurological dysfunction such as a coma, generalized seizure, or neuropsychiatric manifestations. Funduscopic examination may also reveal papilledema. In Seydoux and Francioli's study[30] of 39 cases of brain abscesses, predisposing factors were not equally distributed in the different age groups in contrast to previous studies. They were more common in patients less than 50 years of age. Direct spread from a sinus or otological focus appears to be more common with brain abscesses in younger adults, and was infrequently noted in patients older than 60 years of age. A short duration of symptoms before hospitalization also characterized patients between 20 and 60 years of age and was often associated with a poor outcome. The microbiology of brain abscesses does not appear to be significantly different between younger and older patients. Often viridans streptococcus and *Streptococcus milleri* are the most frequently isolated aerobes. *Fusobacterium* and other anaerobes were also common isolates.

Surgery is the only procedure that allows optimal microbiological documentation. Several authors recommend medical therapy, particularly in cases in which abscess is less than 2 cm in diameter and when the lesion is of high density, suggesting a cerebritis. Repeated aspiration and serial CT scans may be required to achieve a satisfactory response.[33-35]

A combination of a β-lactam agent with chloramphenicol or metronidazole generally has been recommended as standard therapy for brain abscesses. Microbiological data obtained from a stereotaxic biopsy will be a further guide to therapy. The optimal duration of brain abscesses has been variable.[36] Usually most authors recommend approximately 4–6 weeks of antibiotics including the combination of parenteral and oral agents. Neurological sequela can be quite high, occurring in as much as 46 percent of cases.[30]

Subdural empyema

Subdural empyema may arise as a complication of a sinusitis or otitis media. Presenting symptoms can often mimic a brain abscess. A contrasted study of the CNS is indicated and neurological drainage is mandatory. Antibiotic therapy is targeted at many of the same organisms that cause brain abscess. Length of therapy is generally several weeks with intravenous antibiotics.

Chronic meningitis

Tuberculosis of elderly people is a serious disorder. Previously this was thought to be a diagnosis of the pediatric age group but recent reports indicate a rising incidence in elderly people.[37] Tuberculosis meningitis is often an insidious disease and may be especially difficult to diagnose in elderly people. Nonspecific symptoms of fatigue, anorexia, nausea, and an altered mental status may suggest dementia in an elderly patient. A miliary picture on chest X-ray may be the only feature that is useful to distinguish tuberculosis meningitis from cryptococcal meningitis. Duration of symptoms may range from 2 days to 6 months. Hospitalization is often precipitated by change in mental status, headache, or fever. Meningeal signs are present in less than one-half of the cases. Ocular palsies, particularly due to involvement of nerve VI, are found in 30–70 percent of cases.

CSF findings often reveal a protein level above 50 and a low glucose below 40. Acid-fast positivity varies among the studies but can range anywhere from 10 to 80 percent depending on how many spinal taps were performed. A chest X-ray and purified protein derivative should be routinely obtained. Several attempts have been made to develop a rapid, common, and specific method for diagnosing tuberculous meningitis.

Adenosine deaminase activity has been detected in the spinal fluid. At levels greater than 9 units/L, the test was found to be sensitive and specific. Levels can also be increased in patients with sarcoid or lymphoma. Levels appear to perhaps correlate with disease activity. Radioimmunoassay has been used for detecting a *Mycobacterium tuberculosis* antigen. The assay becomes negative after therapy.

Tuberculostearic acid, a structural component of *M. tuberculosis*, can be identified by gas–liquid chromatography and may also be useful to diagnoses tuberculosis.[38] Recent methodologies such as polymerase chain reaction (PCR) testing and immunomagnetic enrichment may also prove to be useful for cases of tuberculosis including tuberculosis meningitis.[39-41]

Prognosis is influenced by age, duration of symptoms, and neurological deficits. Mortality is greatest in patients younger than age 5 and older than 50 (60 percent). Clinical staging is often based on neurological status: stage I—rational, no focal neurological signs or hydrocephalus; stage II—confusion, depression, or focal neurological deficits; stage III—stuporous or dense paraplegia or hemiplegia. Isoniozid (INH), pyrazinamide (PZA), and rifampin penetrate the blood–brain barrier to achieve adequate CSF concentrations. Multidrug-resistant tuberculosis may require several drugs.[42] Many authorities recommend the adjunctive use of corticosteroids for stage II and III patients, beginning with the dose of prednisone at 80 mg/d, which may be gradually tapered over 4–6 weeks as guided by the patient's symptoms. If hydrocephalus is present, ventricular shunting procedures may be beneficial.

Cryptococcal meningitis

Cryptococcal meningitis may present in a manner very similar to tuberculosis. Between 20 and 50 percent of patients with *Cryptococcus* may have no underlying disease such as human immunodeficiency virus (HIV). Spinal fluid findings are very similar to tuberculosis in that there is a lymphocyte predominance. The India ink may be positive in 50 percent or more of cases. A cryptococcal antigen is often positive in 90 percent of cases by rapid simple latex fixation test. A CT scan may be helpful to rule out hydrocephalus, which is not uncommon in cryptococcal meningitis.

Poor prognostic signs for cryptococcal meningitis may be related to a high CSF opening pressure, low CSF glucose, fewer than 20 white blood cells in the CSF, and high titers of cryptococcal antigen in a positive India ink, and the presence of HIV disease.

Amphotericin B is the traditional drug of choice for cryptococcal meningitis.[43,44] Flucytosine can serve as a useful adjunct, particularly when trying to lower the dose of amphotericin B to prevent renal insufficiency. However, flucytosine has bone marrow suppressive toxicities. Fluconazole is particularly useful for maintenance therapy but may also be useful as an acute therapy for patients with cryptococcal meningitis as well, particularly for those patients with less poor prognostic parameters.[45] Liposomal amphotericin B is also a new modality that may prove to be useful for treatment for cryptococcal meningitis. Combination therapy with fluconazole and flucytosine has also been investigated in patients with acquired immunodeficiency syndrome.

Coccidiomycosis is another common cause of chronic meningitis syndrome and a careful travel history may be an important clue to disease. Residents of the southwestern United States and Mexico appear to be at increased risk for this disease. Two-thirds of the patients, however, may have no risk factors. Blacks, Filipinos, pregnant women, and patients with HIV disease appear more likely to disseminate. CSF parameters are very similar to cryptococcal and tuberculosis meningitis. Detection of complement fixation antibody in the CSF is specific and sensitive for the diagnosis. Amphotericin B has been the traditional drug of choice. Many experts often recommend the use of an Ommaya reservoir for intraventricular therapy. Newer data suggest that fluconazole may be helpful as an

Summary of management algorithm
Pneumococcal meningitis

- Begin empirical therapy with vancomycin and a third-generation cephalosporin
- Dexamethasone administration is generally not recommended in adults
- Modify therapy based on the organism's MIC to penicillin

Herpes simplex encephalitis

- Begin therapy with high-dose acyclovir pending diagnostic tests
- An abnormal EEG can be suggestive of the diagnosis
- Temporal lobe enhancement on a cranial CT or MRI is high suggestive of the diagnosis
- A positive CSF herpes simplex PCR test can eliminate the need for a brain biopsy

alternative to amphotericin B for long-term treatment of *Coccidioides* meningitis.[46]

Herpes simplex encephalitis

Herpes simplex encephalitis is a serious infection of the CNS most commonly caused by herpes simplex virus type I. Mortality of untreated biopsy proven cases is 60–80 percent, with fewer than 10 percent of the patients being left without any neurological sequelae. This illness occurs in all age groups with an equal number of cases between the sexes. It has no seasonal association. Mortality may be higher in patients over 50 years of age.[47]

Patients may present with an abrupt onset of personality change, altered mental status, fever, and headache. Localizing signs such as speech deficits, olfactory hallucinations, temporal lobe seizures, hemiparesis, and nasal field defects are common and may suggest the diagnosis. The spinal fluid findings are nonspecific with an elevated number of lymphocytes. An elevated number of polymorphonuclear leukocytes may be found early in the disease process. This will later change to a mononuclear site cell predominance as the disease progresses. An elevated red blood cell count can be suggestive of the diagnosis but is not required. The electroencephalogram pattern may consist of slow wave complexes at regular to 2- to 3-second intervals, usually localized to the temporal lobe. CT scanning eventually becomes positive in more than 70 percent of the patients but MRI is more sensitive and results are abnormal earlier in the course of the disease.

The virus cannot usually be isolated from the spinal fluid but newer PCR-based methodology may be helpful in making the diagnosis.[48–51] The definitive diagnosis of herpes simplex encephalitis can be made by brain biopsy and appropriate culture and histology. Effective therapy usually consists of acyclovir at a dose of 10 mg/kg every 8 hours for 10 days, which must be adjusted for renal function in the elderly patients as acyclovir can cause nephrotoxicity, particularly in patients that are dehydrated. Survivals correlate with the patient's level of consciousness at the initiation of treatment. Neurological sequelae are higher if treatment is delayed or the patient is comatose. A high index of suspicion is often required to make the diagnosis and to begin effective therapy for herpes simplex encephalitis. Rarely herpes encephalitis patients may relapse.[52,53]

Spirochetal infections

Neurosyphilis

Several studies have suggested that neurosyphilis remains an important and frequently encountered entity. An estimated two symptomatic cases of neurosyphilis occur per 100,000 patients yearly. Syphilis is often the cause of reversible dementia in an elderly patient. Although neurosyphilis is often felt to be a late manifestation of syphilis, spirochetes invade the nervous system throughout the entire course of syphilis. Syphilitic meningitis may occur at the same time as the rash of the secondary syphilis. Most patients with cerebrovascular syphilis have had a duration of approximately 5–10 years. This can manifest as a stroke in a young person. Elderly patients typically have a presentation of paretic neurosyphilis or tabes dorsalis. The interval between infection and symptoms often ranges from 20 to 30 years for these syndromes. Both races appear easily susceptible. Men, however, have an increased risk as compared to women. The neurological examination may be entirely normal with neurosyphilis, and the diagnosis may only be made by an abnormal CSF examination. As the disease progresses, intellectual function can decline and psychotic changes can occur. Symptoms include irritability, fatigability, personality changes, impaired judgment, depression, confusion, and delusions. Patients may have coarse, movement-induced facial, lingular, and labial tremors. Patients also may have difficulty with distorted handwriting, and abnormal reflexes and focal findings may also occur.[54] Untreated, the disorder is fatal within a few months to 3 or 4 years. Penicillin treatment can effectively reverse the CSF abnormalities and arrest the disease, but the neurological outcome depends on the degree of structural CNS damage that had occurred at the time of therapy.[55] CSF findings in general paresis include an opening pressure between 50 and 300. The cell count is usually less than 100 in 90 percent of the cases. The glucose may be normal or moderately reduced. The protein is greater than 100 in 25 percent of cases. CSF and blood serology are generally positive in greater than 95 percent of cases.[54]

Tabes dorsalis continues to be a common form of CNS syphilis, although the percentage seems to be decreasing. This disease, again, is much more common in men than in women. It has the longest incubation period, being as high as 50 years in some patients. A triad of symptoms including lightning pains, dysuria, and ataxia may be seen in patients. A triad of signs including Argyll Robertson pupils, areflexia, and a loss of proprioception are characteristic of this disorder. Lightning pains last for a few seconds to minutes at a time and usually occur in the lower extremities. These can be separated by interval-free periods of a few months. Pain sensation is often strikingly impaired compared to that of hot and cold sensation.[55] Reduction or loss of ankle or knee jerks can occur in approximately 80–90 percent of patients. Pupillary abnormalities are noted in 79 percent of patients and consist of pupils that accommodate but do not react. In the elderly patient, diabetes can mimic tabes. Other rare causes mimicking tabes include Wernicke's encephalopathy and Charcot–Marie–Tooth disease. As the disease progresses, sensory ataxia becomes a problem. Many patients may have a positive Romberg sign. Less common abnormalities include syphilitic optic atrophy and gastric crises. Characteristic CSF findings of tabes usually include a normal opening pressure in 90 percent of the patients. Only 9–10 percent of patients have a cell count greater than 160. The protein is usually normal to moderately elevated. The majority of patients have an abnormal serum and CSF Verereal Disease Research Laboratory test. In the series by Merritt[54] completely normal findings including an unreactive CSF and blood serology occurred in 2 of the 100 cases reported. In "burned-out" tabes, the fluid may be entirely normal. Penicillin treatment should clear the CSF and arrest progression of the disease; however, findings such as urinary incontinence, lightning pains, and gastric crises may not completely respond to penicillin therapy.

An unreactive peripheral blood FTA-ABS usually excludes the diagnosis of neurosyphilis, and in most cases a CSF examination would not be warranted. Any patient with a positive blood serology for syphilis and neurologic symptoms would warrant a lumbar puncture. An abnormal CSF VDRL test would constitute proof of neurosyphilis. Patients with only an abnormal protein or cell count might also be strongly considered for penicillin therapy. In patients with signs of neurosyphilis but with an unreactive CSF (normal cells and protein), such as in "burned out" neurosyphilis, the neurological deficit is probably due to fixed structural damage and will probably not respond to additional penicillin.[55] A treponemicidal level has been assumed to be 0.3 IU/mL. Comparisons of serum and CSF penicillin levels after benzathine penicillin suggest that benzathine penicillin may not reach adequate treponemicidal levels in the CSF. Adequate levels are achieved by adequate intravenous penicillin doses given for neurosyphilis. The present authors generally tend to treat patients with neurosyphilis with 18–24 million units per day for approximately 10–14 days. Adequate therapy is suggested by a normal spinal fluid cell count and a falling protein count at 6 months following treatment.[56–59] Repeat CSF examination should be performed every 6 months for the next 2 years during which time the protein count should fall and the cell count should remain normal. The VDRL will probably also disappear during this time period or reach a low-level "serofast" state. Any increase in the cell count or major deviation from this response would require retreatment with high-dose penicillin. Neurosyphilis is often an indication to consider desensitization if the patient has a penicillin allergy. Ceftriaxone may be a reasonable alternative in some patients. Penicillin allergy would be an indication for infectious diseases and allergy consultation. Many patients who have a positive serum test and no symptoms could potentially be treated with three injections of benzathine penicillin over a 3-week period. However, this would only be warranted if the physician is sure there is no symptoms of neurosyphilis. A negative CSF would be reassuring to the patient and physician before embarking on this treatment course. Hypothyroidism, cryptococcal and tuberculous meningitis, or other causes of reversible dementia need to be considered in the differential diagnosis of neurosyphilis.

Lyme disease

The CNS effects of Lyme disease are receiving increasing attention in the literature. Lyme disease can cause a meningitis in the second stage weeks to months after the tick exposure. Bell's palsy and peripheral neuropathy syndromes are quite common. A CSF pleocytosis is often found with an elevated protein and a normal to low CSF sugar. Local CSF antibody production occurs. A positive enzyme-linked immunosorbent assay test for Lyme disease is usually recommended to be followed by a Western blot test. Ceftriaxone is generally considered the treatment of choice for the CNS manifestations of syphilis.[60] An exception might possibly be the use of doxycycline for facial nerve palsy.

KEY POINTS Bacterial meningitis: epidemiology and clinical features

- Fifty-six percent of community acquired meningitis occurs in patients over 50 years of age.

- Bacteria reach the subarachnoid space by three mechanisms:

   1. Bacteremia
   2. Head trauma and neurosurgery
   3. Contiguous spread from sinusitis or otitis

- Clinical features may be more subtle in elderly patients.

- CSF findings in elderly patients resemble those of younger adults.

- Streptococcal pneumoniae is the most common organism causing meningitis in elderly patients. Listeria is more likely to cause meningitis in older patients than in young adults.

- Pneumococci may be resistant to β-lactam therapy. The addition of vancomycin to third-generation cephalosporins is recommended initially until culture results are available.

Focal lesions

- Brain abscess often presents as a mass lesion.

- CSF findings are nonspecific.

- Ring-enhancing lesions are detected by CT in the majority of patients.

- Often viride streptococci and *Streptococcus milleri* are isolated.

- A combination of metronidazole and a third-generation cephalosporin is usually recommended.

Subdural empyema

- Arises as a complication of sinusitis and otitis media.

Chronic meningitis

- Tuberculosis

   1. Meningeal signs are often absent.
   2. CSF glucose levels are typically low.
   3. Ocular palsies are common.
   4. Acid fast positively varies.
   5. Prognosis is related to clinical stage.

Cryptococcal meningitis

- India ink is positive about 50 percent of the time.

(continued)

KEY POINTS (continued)

- Poor prognostic signs include a high titer of antigen, and fewer than 20 WBCs/hpf in the CSF.

Herpes simplex encephalitis

- May present as an abrupt personality change, olfactory hallucinations, or temporal lobe epilepsy.

- MRI is more sensitive than CT.

- A CSF PCR test is usually positive.

Spirochetal infections

- Neurosyphilis

  1. Often a cause of reversible dementia.
  2. Elderly patients present with tabes dorsalis or paretic syphilis more often than younger patients.
  3. CSF serology is usually negative.
  4. Patients who have a positive serum FTA-ABS, and an abnormal cell or protein count should be considered for therapy.

Lyme disease

- Bell's palsy is common.

- Ceftriaxone is the therapy of choice for all forms of CNS Lyme disease with the possible exception of facial nerve palsy.

REFERENCES

1. Fraser DW, Henke CE, Feldman RA: Changing patterns of bacterial meningitis in Olmstead County, Minnesota, 1935–1970. J Infect Dis 1973;128:300–307
2. Schlech WF III, Ward JI, Band JD: Bacterial meningitis in the United States, 1978 through 1981: The National Bacterial Meningitis Surveillance study. JAMA 1985;253:1749
3. Aronson SM, DeBuono BA, Buechner JS: Acute bacterial meningitis in Rhode Island: a survey of the years 1976 to 1985. Rhode Island Med J 1991;74:33
4. Durand ML, Calderwood SB, Weber DJ: Acute bacterial meningitis in adults. A review of 493 episodes. N Engl J Med 1993;328:21–28
5. Berk SL, Smith JK: Infectious diseases in the elderly. Med Clin North Am 1983;67:273–293
6. Berk SL: Bacterial meningitis. In Gleckman RA, Gantz NM (eds): Infections in the Elderly. Little Brown, Boston, 1989;235–253
7. Choi C: Bacterial meningitis. Clin Geriatric Med 1992;8:889–902
8. Berman RE, Meyers BR, Mendelson MH: Central nervous system infections in the elderly. Arch Intern Med 1989;149:1596–1599
9. Gorse GO, Trupp LD, Needlewoman KL: Bacterial meningitis in the elderly. Arch Intern Med 1984;144:1603–1607
10. Roos KL: Meningitis as it presents in the elderly: diagnosis and care. Geriatrics 1990;45:63–75
11. Massanari RM: Purulent meningitis in the elderly. Geriatrics 1977;32:55–59
12. Jonson M, Alvin A: A 12 year review of acute bacterial meningitis in Stockholm. Scand J Infect Dis 1971;3:141–150
13. Quaade F: Meningitis in the aged. Geriatrics 1963;18:860–864
14. Marton KI, Gean AD: The spinal tap: a new look at an old test. Ann Intern Med 1986;104:840–848
15. Newton JE, Wilczynski PJG: Meningitis in the elderly. Lancet 1979;1:157–158
16. Swartz MN, Dodge PR: Bacterial meningitis—a review of selected aspects. N Engl J Med 1965;272:725–731
17. Quaade F, Kristensen KP: Purulent meningitis. A review of 658 cases. Acta Med Scand 1962;171:543–550
18. Berk SL, McCabe WR: Meningitis caused by gram-negative bacilli. Ann Intern Med 1980;93:253–260
19. Mangi RJ, Quintiliani R, Andriole VT: Gram-negative bacillary meningitis. Am J Med 1975;59:829–836
20. Berk SL, McCabe WR: Meningitis caused by *Acinetobacter Calcoaceticus var. Antitratus*. A specific hazard in neurosurgical patients. Arch Neurol 1981;38:95–98
21. Nguyen MH, Harris SP, Muder RR, Pasculle AW: Antibiotic-resistant *Acinetobacter* meningitis in neurosurgical patients. Department of Medicine and Pathology, University of Pittsburgh School of Medicine, Pennsylvania. Neurosurgery 1994;35:851–855
22. Siegman IY, Bar-Yosef S, Gorea A, Avram J: Nosocomial *Acinetobacter* meningitis secondary to invasive procedures: report of 25 cases and review. Department of Neurosurgery, Tel Aviv Sourasky Medical Center and Sackler Faculty of Medicine, Tel Aviv University, Israel. Clin Infect Dis 1993;17:843–849
23. Cherubin CE, Marr JS, Sierra MD, Becker S: *Listeria* and gram-negative bacillary meningitis in New York City 1972–1979. Am J Med 1981;71:199–209
24. Young LS, LaForce FM, Head JJ: A simultaneous outbreak of meningococcal and influenza infections. N Engl J Med 1972;287:5–9
25. Eigler JO, Wellman WE, Rooke ED: Bacterial meningitis—a general review. Proc Mayo Clin 1961;26:357–365
26. Dunne DW, Quagliarello V: Group B streptococcal meningitis in adults. Medicine 1993;72:1–10
27. Van Dijk K, Burger A: *Hemophilus influenzae* meningitis in the elderly. J Am Geriatr Soc 1986;34:530–532
28. Paris MM, Ramilo O, McCracken GH: Management of meningitis caused by penicillin-resistant *Streptococcus pneumoniae*. Antimicrob Agents Chemother 1995;39(10):2171–2175
29. Catalan MJ, Fernandez JM, Vasquez A et al: Failure of cefotaxime in the treatment of meningitis due to relatively resistant *Streptococcus pneumoniae*. Clin Infect Dis 1994;18(5):766–769
30. Seydoux CH, Francioli P: Bacterial brain abscesses: factors influencing mortality and sequelae. Clin Infect Dis 1992;15:394–401
31. Scheld WM, Brodeur JP: Effect of methylprednisolone on entry of ampicillin and gentamicin into the cerebrospinal fluid in experimental pneumococcal and *E. coli* meningitis. Antimicrob Agents Chemother 1983;23:108–112
32. Kourtopoulous H, Holm SE, Norrby SR: The influence of steroids on the penetration of antibiotics into brain tissue and brain abscess. An experimental study in rats. J Antimicrob Chemother 1983;11:245–249
33. Rosenblum ML, Hoff JT, Norman D et al: Nonoperative treatment of brain abscesses in selected high-risk patients. J Neurosurg 1980;52:217–225
34. Garvey G: Current concepts of bacterial infections of the central nervous system. J Neurosurg 1983;59:735–744
35. Yamamoto M, Fukushima T, Hirakawa K, Kimura H, Tomonaga M: Treatment of bacterial brain abscess by repeated aspiration—follow up by serial computed tomography. Neurol Med Chir (Tokyo). 2000;40(2):98–104; discussion 104–105
36. Sjölin J, Lilja A, Eriksson N et al: Treatment of brain abscess with cefotaxime and metronidazole: prospective study of 15 consecutive cases. Clin Infect Dis 1993;17:857–863
37. Baran J Jr, Riederer KM, Khatib R: Limits of detection of mycobacterium tuberculosis in spiked cerebrospinal fluid using the polymerase chain reaction in tuberculous meningitis. Eur J Clin Microbiol Infect Dis 2000;19(1):47–50
38. French GL, Teoh R, Chan CY et al: Diagnosis of tuberculosis meningitis by detection of tuberculostearic acid in cerebral spinal fluid. Lancet 1987;2:117–119
39. Lin JJ, Harn HJ, Hsu YD et al: Rapid diagnosis of tuberculous meningitis by polymerase chain reaction assay of cerebrospinal fluid. J Neurol 1995;242(3):147–152
40. Gascoyne-Binzi DM, Hawkey PM: False negative polymerase chain reaction on cerebrospinal fluid samples in tuberculous meningitis. J Neurol Neurosurg Psychiatry 1999;67(2):250
41. Mazurek GH, Reddy V, Murphy D, Ansari T: Detection of mycobacterium tuberculosis in cerebrospinal fluid following immunomagnetic enrichment. J Clin Microbiol 1996;34:450–453
42. Centers for Disease Control and Prevention: Initial therapy for tuberculosis in the era of multidrug resistance: recommendations of the Advisory Council for the elimination of tuberculosis. JAMA 1993;270:694–698
43. Bennett JE, Dismukes WE, Duma RT et al: A comparison of amphotericin B alone and combined with flucytosine in the treatment of cryptococcal meningitis. N Engl J Med 1979;301:126–131
44. Powderly WG: Current approach to the acute management of cryptococcal infections. J Infect 2000;41(1):18–22

45. Larsen RA, Leal MAE, Chan LS: Fluconazole compared with amphotericin B plus flucytosine for cryptococcal meningitis in AIDS: a randomized trial. Ann Intern Med 1990;113:183–187

46. Dewsnup DH, Galgiani JN, Graybill JR et al: Is it ever safe to stop azole therapy for *Coccidioides immitis* meningitis? Ann Intern Med 1996;124:305–310

47. Whitley RJ, Soong SJ, Linneman C Jr et al: Herpes simplex encephalitis: clinical assessment. JAMA 1982;247:317–320

48. Aurelius E, Johansson B, Skoldenberg B et al: Rapid diagnosis of herpes simplex encephalitis by nested polymerase chain reaction of cerebrospinal fluid. Lancet 1991;337:189

49. Domingues RB, Tsanaclis AM, Pannuti CS, Mayo MS, Lakeman FD: Evaluation of the range of clinical presentations of herpes simplex encephalitis by using polymerase chain reaction assay of cerebrospinal fluid samples. Clin Infect Dis 1997;25(1):86–91

50. Domingues RB, Fink MC, Tsanaclis AM et al: Diagnosis of herpes simplex encephalitis by magnetic resonance imaging and polymerase chain reaction assay of cerebrospinal fluid. J Neurol Sci 1998;157(2):148–153

51. Revello MG, Baldanti F, Sarasini A et al: Quantitation of herpes simplex virus DNA in cerebrospinal fluid of patients with herpes simplex encephalitis by the polymerase chain reaction. Clin Diagn Virol 1997;7(3):183–191

52. Skoldenberg B: Herpes simplex encephalitis. Scand J Infect Dis Suppl 1996;100:8–13

53. Barthez-Carpentier MA, Rozenberg F, Dussaix E et al: Relapse of herpes simplex encephalitis. J Child Neurol 1995;10(5):363–368

54. Merritt HH: A Textbook of Neurology, 2nd Ed. Lea & Febiger, Philadelphia, 1950:129–153

55. Simon RP: Neurosyphilis. Arch Neurol 1985;42:606–613

56. Scheck DN, Hook EW: Neurosyphilis. Infect Dis Clin North Am 1994;8(4):769–795

57. Hook EW: Diagnosing neurosyphilis. Clin Infect Dis 1994;18(3):295–297

58. Roos KL: Neurosyphilis. Semin Neurol 1992;12(3):209–212

59. Rolfs RT, Joesoef MR, Hendershot EF et al: A randomized trial of enhanced therapy for early syphilis in patients with and without human immunodeficiency virus infection. The Syphilis and HIV Study Group. N Engl J Med 1997;337(5):307–314

60. Dattwyler RJ, Halperin JJ, Volkmann DJ, Luft BJ: Treatment of late Lyme borreliosis—randomized comparison of ceftriaxone and penicillin. Lancet 1988;1:1191

Chapter 59   Aging and disorders of the eye

Scott E. Brodie

Loss of vision, one of the most feared forms of medical disability, falls disproportionately on elderly people. Unfortunately, the damage to the delicate tissues of the eye from the various metabolic insults that may occur throughout life is generally cumulative. Consequently, most forms of ocular pathology occur ever more frequently, and in more debilitating forms, with increasing age.

Estimates of the prevalence of blindness from all causes vary by perhaps a factor of 13 between industrialized and Third World societies.[1] Nevertheless, regardless of the degree of economic development, the prevalence rate for blindness in any society is typically 100-fold greater among individuals over 65 years of age than among children in the same society.[2] In developed countries, the major causes of blindness are primarily cataract, glaucoma, and retinal disease (mostly macular degeneration and diabetic retinopathy), all of which are strongly related to advancing age. In the Third World, the major causes of blindness are cataract, corneal scarring, glaucoma, and retinal disease.[2,3]

Delivery of adequate eye care to elderly individuals remains an unsolved problem, even in wealthy countries. Recent surveys in the United States have identified significant rates of untreated eye disease among elderly people. The nursing home population appears to be notably underserved.[4,5]

Discussion of age-related ocular problems is conveniently organized by considering the visual apparatus in anatomic order from anterior to posterior.

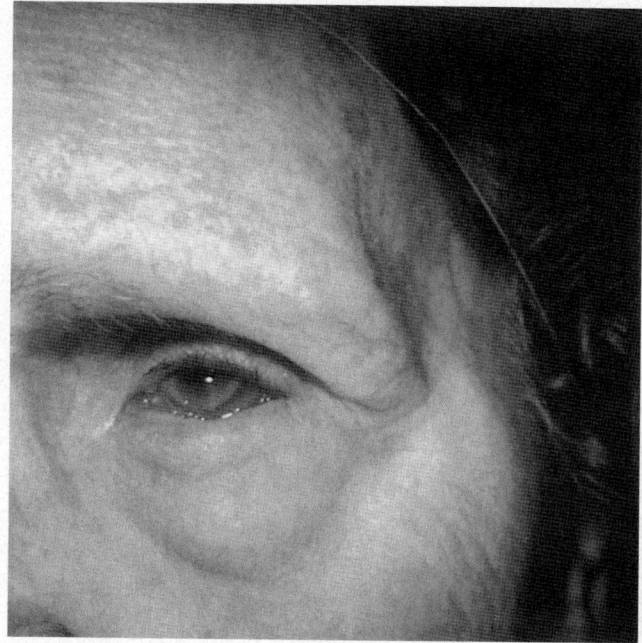

Figure 59-1 Prolapse of orbital fat through atrophic fascial planes in the eyelid produces "bags under the eyes." (Courtesy of Murray Meltzer, MD.)

EYELIDS

The eyelids are vital for the proper circulation of tears and maintenance of the smooth ocular surface necessary for clear image formation by the eye. With increasing age, the skin of the eyelids, as elsewhere, loses elasticity, and the lids become more loosely apposed to the globe. Atrophy of the fascial planes within the eyelids may lead to herniation of the orbital fat into the lid tissue, producing the "bags under the eyes" frequently seen in elderly people (Fig. 59-1). Atrophy or disinsertion of the aponeurosis of the levator palpebrae muscle, which ordinarily supports the upper eyelid, may cause the opened lid to fail to uncover the pupil, as seen in senile ptosis, despite normal levator muscle function (Fig. 59-2; see also Plate 59-1). Senile ptosis must be differentiated from ptosis due to mechanical and neuromuscular causes, such as oculomotor nerve palsies and myasthenia gravis.[6]

Laxity of the lower lid may allow the free lid margin to rotate away from the eyeball, a condition known as ectropion (Fig. 59-3). If severe, the lacrimal punctum may fail to make contact with the pool of tears adjacent to the lower lid. This prevents the normal conduction of tears into the lacrimal sac, which may result in persistent tearing (epiphora) even in the absence of lacrimal duct obstruction. More dangerous is entropion, in which a loosening of the adhesions between tissue planes in the lid allows the muscle tone of the orbicularis oculi to rotate the lid margin inward (Fig. 59-4).[7] Frequently, the lashes come to rub directly against the cornea or conjunctiva, producing irritation or scarring.

The treatment of eyelid malpositions is generally surgical. For senile ptosis, resection of the levator aponeurosis is generally performed.[8] Ectropion and entropion are generally treated by resection of redundant lid tissue.[9]

Of the tumors of the eyelid skin, basal cell carcinomas are the most common. These tumors are frequently a consequence of lifetime exposure to sunlight. If the lesions are detected early, a curative local resection is often possible. In advanced cases, the tumor may cause massive destruction of facial structures by local extension. Metastases are very rare.[10]

LACRIMAL APPARATUS

The lacrimal apparatus consists of the lacrimal glands, which secrete the tears, and the lacrimal sac and ducts, which convey

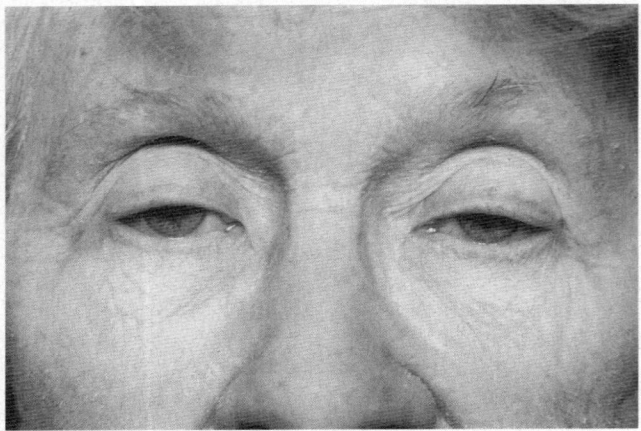

Figure 59-2 Senile ptosis. Note the low lid level and the loss of the normal lid folds. (Courtesy of Murray Meltzer, MD.)

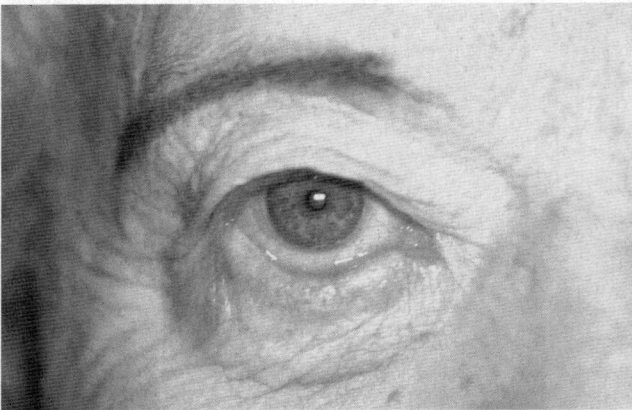

Figure 59-3 Ectropion. Laxity of the lower eyelid allows the lid margin to rotate away from the eyeball. (Courtesy of Murray Meltzer, MD.)

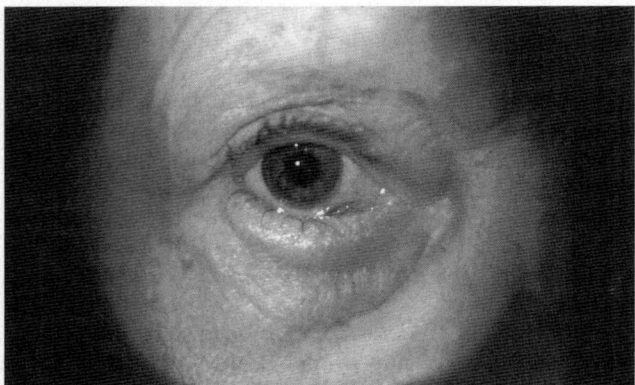

Figure 59-4 Entropion. Breakdown of the adhesion between the tissue planes in the eyelid allows the muscle tone of the orbicularis oculi muscle to rotate the lid margin inward. The eyelashes may chronically irritate the surface of the eyeball. (Courtesy of Murray Meltzer, MD.)

the tears into the nasal cavity. Secretory function of the lacrimal glands declines with age, and many elderly individuals develop "dry eye" syndrome. (This nonspecific reduction in tear production is much more common than the full-fledged Sjögren syndrome, which is an autoimmune disease process affecting both salivary and lacrimal secretion.[11]) Paradoxically, many tear-deficient patients complain of excess tearing, because the chronically irritated eyes may stimulate reflex tear production. Dry eyes are treated with artificial tear eyedrops, as often as needed. In patients whose eyes dry out overnight, lubricant ointment at bedtime may be helpful. In severe cases, small silicone plugs may be placed to obstruct the lacrimal puncta,[12] or surgical occlusion of the lacrimal puncta may be performed, in order to conserve the available tears.

Obstruction of the lacrimal ducts also leads to epiphora. Uncomplicated mechanical stenosis may occasionally be relieved with simple probing, but severe cases (often following bacterial infection of the lacrimal sac) are treated surgically: a dacryocystorhinostomy is performed to anastamose the mucosa of the nasal cavity to the lacrimal sac through an osteotomy made in the lacrimal bone.[13]

CONJUNCTIVA

Subconjunctival hemorrhage, a localized accumulation of blood seen between the conjunctiva and the globe, is frequently encountered in elderly people, either following minor trauma, or occurring spontaneously (Fig. 59-5; see also Plate 59-2). Such hemorrhages are rarely of any consequence, but are often alarming in appearance. They resolve spontaneously without treatment over a period of several days. Occasionally, recurrent hemorrhages may suggest an underlying disease such as hypertension or a coagulation disorder.

Chronic exposure to sunlight, particularly at tropical latitudes, may cause a degeneration of the connective tissue in the exposed sector of the conjunctiva between the eyelids, leading to thickening of the conjunctiva (pingueculum), which may grow over the cornea from the periphery toward the pupil (pterygium). If the growth threatens to cover the visual axis, surgical excision may be indicated. Recurrence after surgery is, unfortunately, not uncommon.[14]

Tumors such as squamous cell carcinoma and melanoma may arise from the conjunctiva. Local excision and cryoablation may be adequate in early cases, but advanced cases may require orbital exenteration.[15]

CORNEA

The eye is unique in its requirement for transparent tissues, including the cornea and crystalline lens. The need for transparency places many constraints on the architecture and metabolism of these ocular structures. In particular, the eye must nourish these tissues with a cell-free fluid, as red blood cells preclude transparency. Similarly, the transparent tissues must rely primarily on anaerobic glycolytic metabolism, as the enzyme systems required for oxidative phosphorylation (aptly named cytochromes) strongly absorb visible light. Even in the absence of these absorbent components, the tissues must be

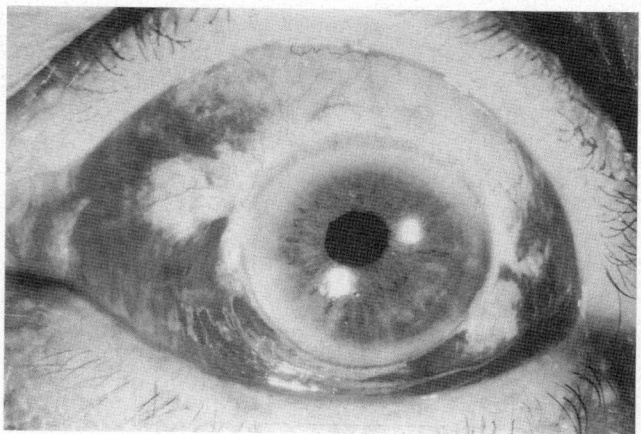

Figure 59-5 Subconjunctival hemorrhage. This small hematoma, seen through the transparent conjunctiva, is benign unless recurrent.

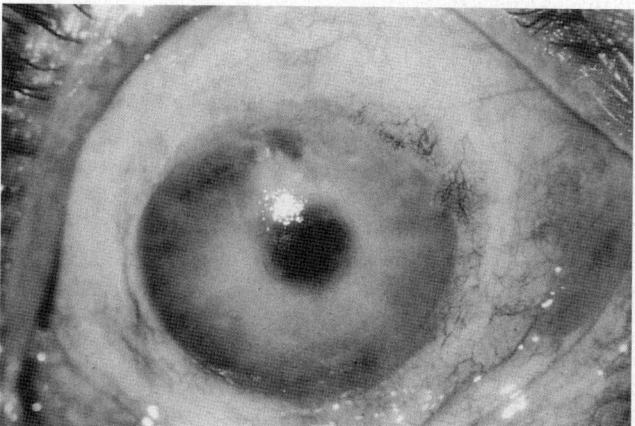

Figure 59-6 Corneal edema. The cornea is thickened and cloudy due to failure of the corneal endothelium to adequately dehydrate the tissue. (Courtesy of Calvin Roberts, MD.)

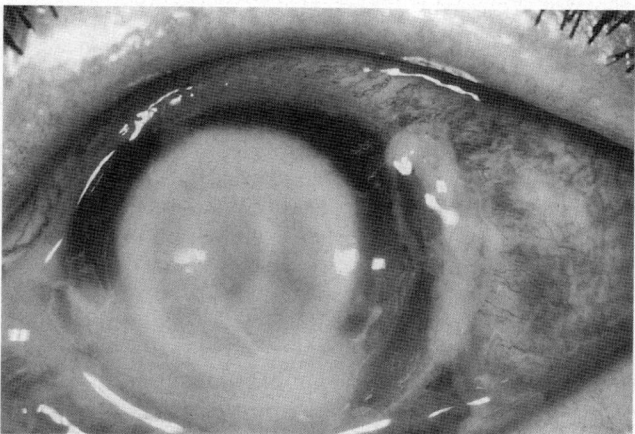

Figure 59-7 Corneal ulcer. A localized infection causes an epithelial defect and attracts an infiltrate of white blood cells. (Courtesy of Michael Newton, MD.)

constructed in a highly compact and regular manner, so that light scattering from tissue organelles does not cause a white, opaque appearance. This requirement is met in the case of the cornea by an active metabolic pump in the corneal endothelial cell layer, which acts to dehydrate the corneal stroma. (Absence of this dehydration mechanism is the main reason that the sclera, which is otherwise histologically very similar to the cornea, is opaque.)[16]

The corneal endothelial cells, on which the dehydration critical for corneal transparency depends, do not divide during adulthood. Indeed, the endothelial cell density declines slowly with age.[17] If the number of endothelial cells falls below a critical level, the cornea imbibes fluid, swells, and becomes cloudy (Fig. 59-6; see also Plate 59-3). Edema fluid percolates to the epithelial surface, and may coalesce into subepithelial bullae. Mild cases may be managed with the use of hypertonic saline eyedrops and ointment to withdraw fluid from the cornea osmotically. If these measures fail, a full-thickness corneal graft, which replaces the deficient endothelium, is necessary to restore vision.[18]

Bacterial ulcers of the cornea (Fig. 59-7; see also Plate 59-4) seem particularly common in elderly people, perhaps reflecting impairments of tear secretion, epithelial integrity, and cellular and humoral immunity, and are associated in elderly people with a poorer prognosis.[19] Intensive antibiotic therapy is generally required.[20]

The ring-shaped deposition of lipid in the far periphery of the cornea, referred to as *arcus senilis*, is completely benign.

UVEAL TRACT

The uveal tract ("uvea") comprises the iris, ciliary body, and choroid, which form a continuous, highly vascular layer inside the sclera. Inflammation of the uvea occurs frequently: as a primary disease process; in response to infections; in many patients with collagen-vascular disease; and as a sequela to accidental or surgical trauma. Clinically, inflammatory cells are seen in the aqueous or vitreous humor. These inflammatory reactions can cause ocular injury by many mechanisms. They may occlude the trabecular meshwork, causing glaucoma. They may accumulate on the inner surface of the cornea as keratic precipitates, where they may injure or destroy the corneal endothelial cells and cause corneal edema. Inflamed tissues often develop pathological adhesions, which may derange normal ocular function. Adhesions between the anterior surface of the peripheral iris and the anterior chamber angle (peripheral anterior synechiae) may occlude the trabecular meshwork, leading to chronic angle-closure glaucoma. Adhesions between the posterior surface of the iris and the anterior surface of the crystalline lens can seal off access of the aqueous humor to the anterior chamber (papillary block), forcing the iris to bow forward (iris bombé). In cases where the peripheral iris becomes apposed to the trabecular meshwork, the egress of aqueous humor from the eye is blocked, resulting in angle-closure glaucoma. In the posterior segment, inflammatory cells in the vitreous humor may obscure vision, and may lead to fibrovascular proliferation that may distort the retina, or even cause a retinal detachment.

Treatment in most cases of uveitis is generally empirical. Dilation of the pupil with cycloplegic eyedrops is generally advisable to prevent posterior synechiae and pupillary block, and to relieve the discomfort (photophobia) caused by light-induced miosis of the inflamed iris. If the inflammation is confined to the anterior segment, topical steroid eyedrops are usually sufficient. In cases involving the posterior segment, retrobulbar steroid injections or systemic administration of steroids are frequently required. In recalcitrant or recurrent cases, a work-up for underlying systemic disease is appropriate. If a treatable systemic condition is discovered, such as syphilis or tuberculosis, specific treatment for the underlying condition may simultaneously cure the uveitis. In refractory cases, some success has been achieved with systemic administration of cytotoxic medications and cyclosporine A.[21]

Intraocular tumors in elderly people occur most frequently within the uveal tract. Melanomas are the most common primary tumor. Treatment is controversial: although prompt enucleation (surgical removal of the eyeball) has been the traditional management, retrospective studies have suggested that there may be an excess mortality which appears to be associated with the enucleation procedure itself, perhaps due to manipulation of the globe during surgery.[22] Many authorities now recommend that, because they have only a very low propensity for metastasis, eyes containing small uveal melanomas be followed closely, rather than enucleated. Enucleation is still often recommended in cases where tumor enlargement is observed.[23] Medium-sized tumors have been successfully treated in many cases with irradiation, either by temporary implantation of a radioactive plaque applied to the overlying sclera,[24] or administered by external beam. A large, prospective, clinical trial recently found no difference in 5-year survival between groups of patients randomized to treatment by radioactive plaque or by enucleation.[25] Primary enucleation is still recommended for large tumors. Metastatic melanoma is usually detected initially in the liver. Regular physical examinations and monitoring of hepatic enzyme activity in the serum are advisable for patients at risk.

Tumors metastatic to the choroid are not uncommon. Lung primaries predominate in men, breast primaries in women.[26] As the eye is seldom the sole site of metastasis, these patients generally require systemic chemotherapy.

GLAUCOMA

Glaucoma is a form of progressive atrophy of the optic nerve, frequently associated with increased intraocular pressure (Figs. 59-8 and 59-9; see also Plates 59-5 and 59-6).

Open-angle glaucoma

In many cases, the primary pathology is presumed to lie in the trabecular meshwork, the ring of porous tissue located in the anterior chamber angle through which aqueous humor drains from the eye. Impaired facility of aqueous outflow through the trabecular meshwork is generally idiopathic (so-called primary open-angle glaucoma). This condition is generally reported to increase in prevalence with increasing age, at least in most Western populations.[27] Loss of outflow facility may also arise

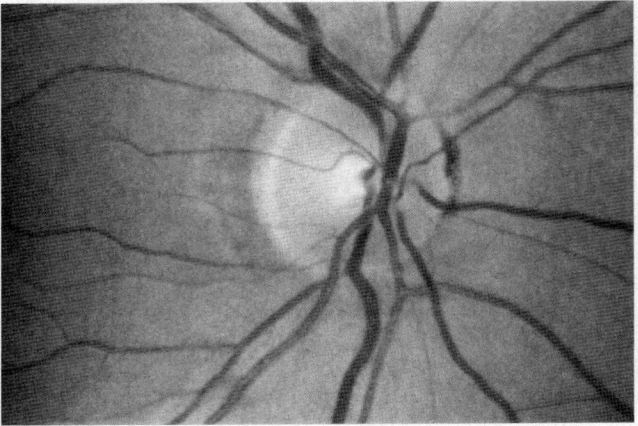

Figure 59-8 Normal optic nerve head. Cup to disk ratio is about 0.3.

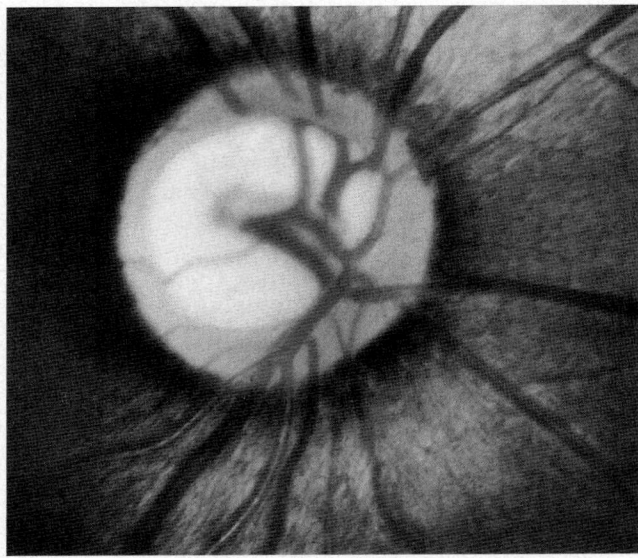

Figure 59-9 Glaucomatous optic nerve head cupping. Loss of neural tissue is seen as narrowing of the neural rim of the optic disk, and enlargement of the central cup. (Compare with Fig. 59-8.)

from various insults to the trabecular meshwork, including trauma, uveitis, hemorrhage, and dispersion of intraocular pigment.

Visual impairment from open-angle glaucoma is generally insidious and chronic, with visual field damage occurring initially in the far periphery, where it is rarely noticeable except by formal testing. Our ability to diagnose this condition in its early stages is quite imperfect. The actual risk of visual field loss in untreated individuals with modestly elevated intraocular pressure is only 1–2 percent per year;[28] conversely, histological studies have shown that as many as 40 percent of the optic nerve fibers must be destroyed before any abnormality of the visual field is detectable by standard techniques.[29]

Initial treatment is usually medical. The goal of therapy is to lower the intraocular pressure with topical or systemic

Treatments for major causes of blindness

- Cataract:
  - Surgical extraction, ideally with intraocular lens implant
- Glaucoma:
  - Initial: lower intraocular pressure with topical, systemic medications
  - Additional options: laser treatment to trabecular meshwork; filtering surgery
- Diabetic retinopathy:
  - Tight control prevents or delays retinopathy in early stages
  - Focal or grid laser treatment for macular edema
  - Pan-retinal laser treatment for proliferative retinopathy
  - Pars-plana vitrectomy for persistent vitreous hemorrhage or traction retinal detachment
- Macular degeneration:
  - Atrophic ("dry"):
    No treatment available
  - Exudative ("wet"):
    (Thermal) laser ablation of neovascular membranes
    Photodynamic therapy
    Macular translocation

medications to a level that is tolerated by the optic nerve, as demonstrated by the arrest of progressive visual field loss. Available medications include parasympathomimetic miotics, anticholinesterase miotics, sympathomimetics, β-adrenergic blockers, carbonic anhydrase inhibitors, and prostaglandin analogs. The potential side-effects of the various topical and systemic pressure-lowering drugs are occasionally serious, particularly in elderly patients (see Systemic Complications of Ophthalmic Medications, below). If medical treatment is unsuccessful, or poorly tolerated, intraocular pressure may be further lowered by laser treatments to the trabecular meshwork, or by "filtering surgery," which creates a fistula between the anterior chamber and the subconjunctival space, allowing easier egress of aqueous humor. Complications of filtering surgery are not infrequent, including hypotony, choroidal effusion, and cataract. Supplementary medical treatment after filtering surgery is often also required. The optimal stage in the disease process for surgical intervention is unclear. Some authors have reported better long-term visual results with earlier surgery.[30] One large study suggests that laser treatment to the trabecular meshwork may also be suitable as initial therapy.[31]

Angle-closure glaucoma

Occasionally, alterations in intraocular anatomy may predispose the iris to cover the trabecular meshwork, suddenly preventing aqueous outflow, and causing an acute elevation of the intraocular pressure. Common scenarios include adhesions between iris and lens (pupillary block), which may cause the iris to bow forward so as to occlude the trabecular meshwork, and dilation of the pupil, such as may occur spontaneously in the dark, or following pharmacological mydriasis. Gradual enlargement of the lens with increasing age or cataract formation is an important factor that predisposes the eye to this process in the elderly. Acute angle-closure glaucoma is generally a dramatic event, with symptoms including severe pain, blurring of

vision, perception of colored haloes around lights, nausea, and vomiting. Diagnosis of acute angle closure is easy once attention is directed to the eye, but may be missed if attention is diverted to the gastrointestinal symptoms. Cases have been reported from the emergency departments of general hospitals where concentration on the nausea and vomiting of a patient with acute angle closure has led to exploratory laparotomy!

The massive elevation of intraocular pressure following acute angle closure (often to triple the normal upper limit of 21 mmHg) may cause permanent optic nerve damage within a matter of weeks. Acute angle closure is generally treated by lowering the intraocular pressure with systemic and topical medications, including miotic eyedrops and systemic osmotic agents. In cases of pupillary block, a small hole (peripheral iridectomy) is made in the iris by laser or invasive surgery to bypass the pupillary block and allow passage of aqueous humor from the posterior segment into the anterior chamber. This prevents subsequent angle-closure attacks. Because the anatomical factors that predispose an eye to acute angle closure are generally found bilaterally, it is usually considered prudent to perform a peripheral iridectomy prophylactically in the fellow eye after an attack of angle closure.

Prolonged episodes of angle-closure may result in permanent damage to the trabecular meshwork, or even adhesions between the iris and sectors of the trabecular meshwork, leading to chronic angle-closure glaucoma. If the angle is sufficiently compromised, filtering surgery may be necessary.

Normal-tension glaucoma

Although elevated intraocular pressure has historically been the hallmark of the diagnosis of glaucoma, it has become clear in recent decades that many patients with otherwise typical glaucomatous optic atrophy and visual field loss seldom if ever are found to have elevated intraocular pressure. Identification and treatment of this so-called low-tension glaucoma (more accurately termed normal-tension glaucoma) remains problematic, although even in this cohort, reduction of intraocular pressure is thought to convey some benefit. This entity is probably more common than previously thought, as population-based surveys have demonstrated a substantial incidence of otherwise typical glaucomatous field loss in patients with normal intraocular pressures.[32]

CRYSTALLINE LENS

The crystalline lens of the eye is a unique ectodermal structure that develops entirely within the primordial lens vesicle. Only the cells on the extreme periphery of the lens divide, adding cells to the outer surface of the growing lens. Thus the center of the adult lens represents the earliest tissue laid down during embryonic development. There is no mechanism by which these cells can turn over, unlike the situation in typical ectodermal structures, such as the skin. The metabolism of the lens is largely confined to anaerobic glycolysis, as neither hemoglobin-mediated oxygen transport nor cytochrome-mediated oxidative phosphorylation is available owing to the need for transparency. The lens is at a further metabolic disadvantage due to the need to maintain a state of great disequilibrium with its surroundings, as the lens must maintain the highest protein concentration, and one of the lowest water concentrations, of any tissue in the body. Thus, relatively modest metabolic insults or osmotic stresses may overwhelm the lens metabolism, resulting in protein denaturation and cataract formation.[33]

The lens of the eye continues to grow and mature throughout life. As the lens ages, it becomes more rigid, and responds less effectively to changes in ciliary muscle tone, decreasing the effectiveness of accommodation, the eye's mechanism for focusing from distant to near objects. This loss of accommodation (presbyopia) is managed with reading glasses or bifocals, or other refractive strategies.

The lens responds to virtually any mechanical or metabolic insult by loss of optical clarity, resulting in the formation of a cataract (Fig. 59-10; see also Plate 59-7). Several patterns of opacities are commonly encountered:

Oxidation ("browning reactions") of lens proteins, particularly in the older, central portions of the lens, is referred to as *nuclear sclerosis*, which may result in alterations in the refractive index of the lens as well as frank opacity. The most common refractive change is in the direction of an increase in myopia or decrease in hyperopia. In some instances, this refractive shift will allow the patient to read without reading glasses (so-called second sight). This improvement in visual performance is usually only temporary, and often heralds the development of a more debilitating lens opacity. Refractive changes in the lens need not be uniform. Patients will occasionally report monocular diplopia due to inhomogeneous refraction by distinct portions of the lens resulting in two distinct images being formed on the retina. (The notion that monocular diplopia is generally indicative of hysteria is incorrect.)

Denaturation of lens proteins in a sector of adjacent cortical lens fibers results in a wedge-shaped or cuneiform cortical opacity. These are often found in the far periphery of the lens, but frequently spare the optical zone near the center.

Aberrant proliferation of lens fibers on the posterior lens capsule produces a posterior subcapsular cataract. These

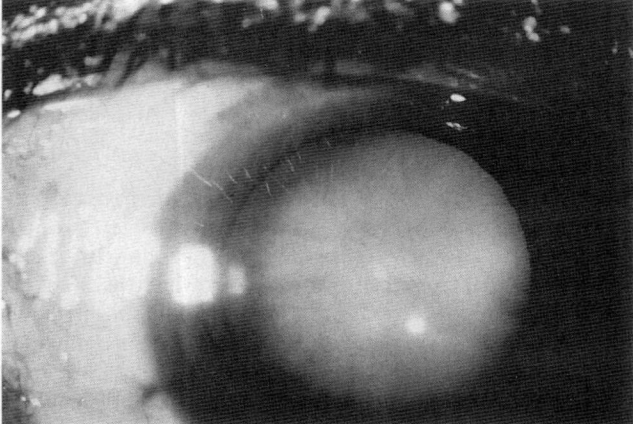

Figure 59-10 Cataract. Loss of transparency of the crystalline lens impairs visual acuity. (Courtesy of Calvin Roberts, MD.)

are often induced by topical or systemic steroid treatment, and are frequently seen in other disease states, such as retinitis pigmentosa.

Treatment of cataract is generally surgical. With rare exceptions, the lens proteins that constitute the opacity are irreversibly denatured, precluding medical treatment.[34] Surgical strategies for removal of the lens material have evolved greatly over recent years. In all cases, an incision must be made in the eyeball. A cataract cannot be removed—even with a laser—without an ocular incision. The simplest operation is to remove the entire lens intact within its lens capsule, a so-called intracapsular procedure. At present, the extracapsular procedure, in which the opaque lens tissue is carefully aspirated from within the lens capsule, has returned to favor, as retention of the capsule to serve as a barrier between the anterior and posterior segments of the eye appears to reduce the rate of complications. Recently, greater emphasis has been placed on the development of minimally invasive surgical methods for cataract extraction. Often, the cataract can be liquefied by the mechanical action of a rapidly vibrating needle (phacoemulsification), and aspirated from the eye through an incision only 3–4 mm in length.[35] Frequently, such wounds can be constructed to be self-sealing, eliminating the need for sutures.[36]

Indications for cataract surgery should be determined in relation to the visual needs of each individual patient. Occasionally, cataract extraction is recommended for technical reasons, such as those rare cases when the lens is itself causing injury to the eye (as in phacolytic glaucoma, when lens proteins leak from a cataractous lens and occlude the trabecular meshwork), or when a cataractous lens prevents adequate visualization or treatment of disease of the posterior segment of the eye, such as diabetic retinopathy. Otherwise, cataract surgery is appropriate whenever the anticipated improvement in visual function would be of benefit to the patient. In general, a visual result of 6/12 (20/40) or better may be anticipated in 90–95 percent of cases without other known concurrent ocular disease; thus, surgery is generally recommended only when the acuity has fallen to the level of 6/15 (20/50) or worse. In some patients, difficulties with glare, contrast sensitivity, diplopia, or specific occupational demands may justify cataract extraction even with less severe loss of visual acuity.

Optical rehabilitation of the aphakic eye requires replacement of the focusing power of the cataractous lens that was removed. Where economic conditions permit, this is usually provided by means of a plastic intraocular lens prosthesis, which is generally implanted at the time of the primary cataract operation. Alternatives include contact lenses (often worn on an extended-wear basis) and thick "aphakic" spectacles, which subject the patient to substantial optical distortions, and (if the aphakia is unilateral) may cause substantial difficulties due to unequal perceived image size in the two eyes. (Indeed, the difficulties with spectacle correction of unilateral aphakes are sufficiently severe that, if spectacle correction is the only modality of optical rehabilitation available, most surgeons recommend deferral of surgery until visual acuity in the *better* eye falls to 6/18 (20/60) or worse.) In some Third World countries, local custom may discourage the use of spectacles after cataract surgery. In these situations, the attitudes of the patient must be taken into account in the decision as to whether or not to perform a cataract extraction.

Some yellowing of the lens proteins is nearly universal with aging. Sufficient opacity to impair visual acuity results in over one million cataract extractions each year in the United States, the vast majority in individuals over 65 years of age. In developing countries, the rate of cataract formation appears to be even higher, so that untreated cataract typically forms the largest single cause of acquired blindness.[3] In India, for example, even at the present rate of millions of cataract procedures each year, present surgical efforts continue to fall behind the rate of new cataract formation in the general population.[37]

Cataract formation may occasionally reflect an underlying metabolic abnormality, such as galactosemia or renal failure. Cataract onset is accelerated in diabetic patients, and may be triggered by various drugs (particularly topical or systemic steroids). In addition to these specific associations, several studies have shown a nonspecific excess mortality among cataract patients, compared with age-matched control patients undergoing other elective surgical procedures.[38] These studies suggest that development of cataracts may reflect a generalized reduction in metabolic competence in these elderly individuals.

RETINA AND VITREOUS
Diabetic retinopathy

Diseases of the retina, particularly diabetic retinopathy and so-called age-related macular degeneration (formerly referred to as "senile macular degeneration") constitute the most frequent cause of acquired blindness, at least in developed countries.

Diabetic retinopathy shows a steady increase in incidence and severity with increasing duration of diabetes mellitus, with significant visual complications rarely occurring before 10 to 15 years after the onset of the disease.[39] Thus, while juvenile-onset (type I) patients may develop severe retinopathy as early as the third decade, the retinal burden of adult-onset (type II) patients is borne largely by the elderly. The disease seems to attack primarily the retinal capillary circulation. Initially, small, innocuous microaneurysms are noted ophthalmoscopically. With time, the retinal capillaries begin to leak fluid into the surrounding tissue, causing retinal edema and precipitation of exudates into the retina, with a concomitant reduction in visual acuity (Fig. 59-11; see also Plate 59-8). At this stage of the disease, loss of visual acuity may be reduced through the use of laser treatments, either directed at leaking microaneurysms or, if the leakage is diffuse, placed in a grid pattern over the leaky sectors of the retinal capillary bed.[40]

In later stages, perfusion of small regions of the retinal capillary bed fails (capillary dropout), leading to localized retinal infarctions, which may be seen ophthalmoscopically as cotton-wool spots. The remaining capillaries are often seen to become dilated, irregular, and leaky. Ultimately, in many patients, the ischemic retina develops a neovascular proliferative response, sprouting new blood vessels that may grow along the retinal surface or along the posterior surface of the vitreous body. These aberrant blood vessels are prone to leaking and hemorrhages. Vision may also be lost through traction exerted on the retina by fibroblastic membranes that accompany the neovascular proliferation (Fig. 59-12; see also Plate 59-9). In severe cases, the neovascular response may extend to the

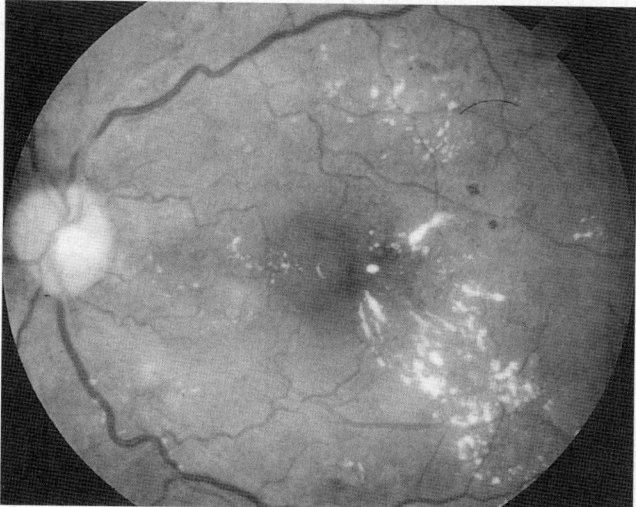

Figure 59-11 Background diabetic retinopathy. Microaneurysms ("dot hemorrhages"), intraretinal hemorrhages ("blot hemorrhages"), and "hard" exudates indicate deterioration of the retinal microcirculation.

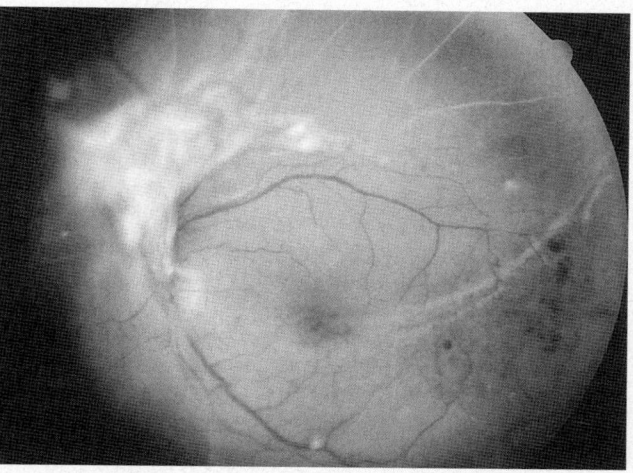

Figure 59-12 Proliferative diabetic retinopathy. A membrane of fibrovascular tissue has sprouted from the optic disk in response to prolonged retinal ischemia.

anterior segment, producing neovascularization on the surface of the iris (rubeosis iridis). If the fibrovascular membrane extends over the anterior chamber angle, it obstructs filtration of aqueous humor through the trabecular meshwork, producing a refractory neovascular glaucoma.

Proliferative retinopathy may often be arrested through the ablation of a large fraction of the peripheral retina with laser photocoagulation.[41] In severe cases, blood in the vitreous cavity and fibrovascular membranes may be removed surgically by introducing mechanized suction-cutter instruments through small scleral incisions over the ciliary body (pars plana vitrectomy).

The benefit of tight control of blood glucose in the management of diabetic retinopathy depends on the stage of the disease. Many attempts to retard the progression of established retinopathy by improving the degree of glucose control have been disappointing.[42] Indeed, in some studies, tight control has been associated with a worsening of retinopathy. Similarly, in one study, successful pancreatic transplantation, with near-perfect normalization of blood glucose levels, failed to improve diabetic retinopathy, compared to the retinal disease in fellow pancreatic transplant patients whose allografts failed, requiring resumption of daily insulin injections, with the usual deficiencies in control of blood glucose.[43] However, it has been demonstrated (albeit in a study enrolling only type I diabetic patients) that better glucose control in recent-onset diabetic patients helps retard the onset of diabetic retinal disease.[44]

Age-related macular degeneration

Age-related macular degeneration is a common cause of impaired vision, although not of total blindness, in the elderly population. In the "atrophic" form, the retinal pigment epithelium and choriocapillaris underlying the macula appear to degenerate, resulting in dysfunction of the overlying photoreceptors (Fig. 59-13; see also Plate 59-10). There is no known treatment. In the "exudative" form, a neovascular net emanates under the macular region of the central retina from the choroidal circulation, proliferating between the retina and the underlying retinal pigment epithelium, or underneath the pigment epithelium.[45] Leakage of plasma components and frank subretinal hemorrhage or scarring cause loss of vision (Fig. 59-14; see also Plate 59-11). In a small portion of cases, laser treatment of neovascular membranes outside of the foveal region may arrest the growth of these membranes before they undermine the central macula, thus helping to preserve central vision.[46]

Some authors have recommended laser treatment of subfoveal membranes, on the theory that it may be possible to thus limit the size and severity of the central scotoma (blind spot) that ultimately results from leakage and scarring. This treatment has gained somewhat limited acceptance, as the immediate effects of the laser treatment frequently include acute loss of central vision, and a net benefit is not apparent until about 2 years after laser treatment.[47]

Photodynamic therapy, an alternative modality of ablation treatment for subretinal neovascularization, has recently been introduced. Patients undergo intravenous infusion of a sensitizing agent which binds selectively to neovascular tissue. The involved retinal sector is then treated with a low-power (nonthermal) ultraviolet laser, which interacts with the sensitizing agent to create highly reactive singlet oxygen species in the target tissue. These molecules exert a cytotoxic effect sufficient in many cases to block perfusion of the subretinal neovascularization.[48] The treatment effect is often only transient, and retreatments are frequently required. Photodynamic therapy has the potential to ablate subretinal neovascular tissue with considerably less destruction of adjacent, healthy retinal tissue than is typically caused by traditional, thermal, laser treatments. In practice, photodynamic therapy appears to be a modest advance over previous ablation techniques, at least in selected patients.[49]

It has also recently become possible to treat selected cases of subretinal neovascularization surgically. One strategy is to make a small incision in the retina, and inject fluid into the

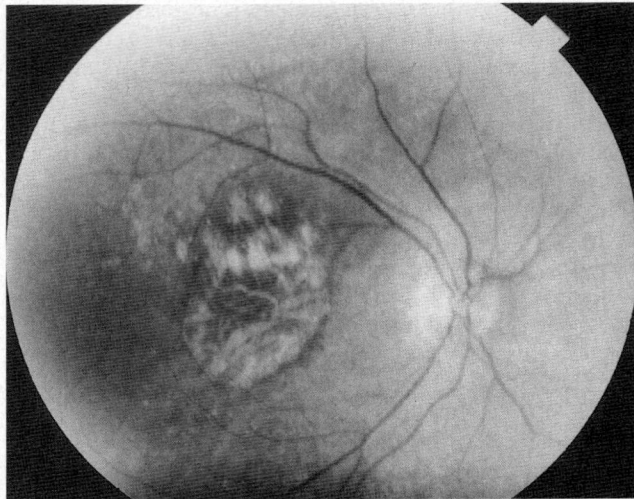

Figure 59-13 Atrophic ("dry") age-related macular degeneration. Geographic atrophy of the retinal pigment epithelium causes loss of central vision.

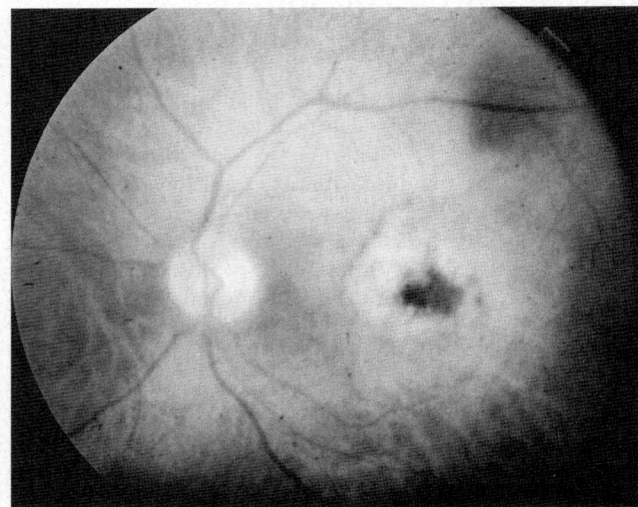

Figure 59-14 Exudative ("wet") age-related macular degeneration. Leakage and scarring from a subretinal neovascular membrane destroys central retinal function.

subretinal space to separate the retina from the underlying tissues. It is often then possible to cause a sufficient distortion of the sclera so that when the retina is reattached, the macula comes to rest over a different, presumably healthier, patch of choroid, better able to support retinal function than the original submacular tissue.[50]

It should be emphasized that these various modalities of treatment for age-related macular degeneration remain on the whole rather unsatisfactory. In most cases, the treatment objective is at best the arrest of the disease process and prevention of further deterioration of vision. Few patients with advanced visual loss are restored to normal or near-normal visual function.

In both atrophic and exudative types of macular degeneration, the pathological process appears to be confined to the posterior pole. These diseases thus spare the peripheral retina in nearly all cases, so that most affected patients indefinitely retain sufficient vision for independent ambulation, and may be reassured that they are not going to go completely blind.

The pale white dots known as *drusen*, frequently seen in the retinas of older patients, are usually benign. They correspond to small deposits of amorphous hyaline material seen histologically between Bruch's membrane and the retinal pigment epithelium. However, these lesions appear to serve as a predisposing factor in the evolution of exudative macular degeneration.[51] Elderly patients with drusen, or who have lost vision in one eye to age-related macular degeneration, may be advised to check their vision every day by examination of an Amsler grid, a 10 cm square of ruled graph paper. Any abnormality or distortion of the central vision should prompt an immediate examination of the retina. This will maximize the chance that a subretinal neovascular net will be discovered before it undermines the fovea, when treatment is most effective.

It may be possible in some cases to slow the progression of macular degeneration by nutritional means. In a major prospective trial, patients aged 55–80 years were randomized to dietary supplementation with either a cocktail of antioxidants (including vitamins C, E, and beta-carotene), zinc, antioxidants and zinc, or placebo, and followed for an average of 6 years. Subjects at high risk for macular degeneration with moderate to severe drusen, or who had already developed substantial visual loss from macular degeneration in one eye, who received antioxidants and/or zinc supplements experienced a reduction in the frequency of development of severe macular degeneration or visual loss of 25–30 percent, compared to the placebo group. The combination of antioxidants and zinc offered greater protection than either supplement alone. Patients with few or no drusen had very little risk of developing frank macular degeneration, and obtained no detectable benefit. None of the supplement regimens offered any protection against the formation or progression of cataract.[52,53]

Retinovascular occlusive disease

Both retinal arteries and retinal veins are subject to sudden occlusive events, particularly in the elderly. Retinal artery occlusions are usually either embolic or arteritic in nature. Embolic occlusions are due to the occlusion of a retinal artery by a small particle derived from the more proximal circulation, most commonly a cholesterol fragment from an ulcerated atherosclerotic plaque. A small refractile cholesterol crystal may often be visualized within a retinal artery (Hollenhorst plaque). Acutely, the affected sector of the retina appears pale and cloudy. Various measures to encourage migration of the occlusive plaque toward the retinal periphery have been recommended, including lowering of intraocular pressure by medical means or by withdrawal of a small amount of fluid from the anterior chamber with a fine needle, and dilation of the retinal arterial tree by breathing an elevated concentration of carbon dioxide. No convincing benefit of these maneuvers has been demonstrated.[54]

Transient obscurations of vision, typically lasting less than 10 minutes (amaurosis fugax) are generally believed to represent embolic arterial occlusions that are quickly dislodged into the far retinal periphery.[55] These attacks indicate an elevated risk of occlusive stroke.[56]

Arteritic disease (e.g., temporal arteritis) may also cause occlusion of the arteries of the retina or optic nerve head. An elevated erythrocyte sedimentation rate is commonly, but not invariably, observed. The diagnosis is usually confirmed by temporal artery biopsy. Prompt treatment with systemic steroids is indicated, and may prevent visual loss in the fellow eye.[57] If the diagnosis of temporal arteritis is suspected, most authorities recommend immediate initiation of systemic steroid treatment; it is unwise to wait until the erythrocyte sedimentation rate and the results of a temporal artery biopsy can be obtained, as the fellow eye may lose vision in the interim. If the tests are negative, the steroid treatment can usually be stopped promptly without a period of tapering doses.

Retinal vein occlusions result in a pattern of vascular tortuosity and intraretinal hemorrhage in the affected sector of the retina. Most retinal vein occlusions seem to be due to compression of a retinal vein by an adjacent retinal artery, frequently exacerbated by hypertension, arteriosclerosis, or glaucoma. Although there is no treatment for the occlusion itself, retinal vein occlusion carries a significant risk of subsequent neovascular complications, particularly glaucoma. In cases where retinal ischemia can be demonstrated (typically by fluorescein angiography or electroretinography), retinal ablation by laser photocoagulation can substantially reduce the risk of subsequent neovascularization.[58]

OPTIC NERVE

Elderly people are particularly susceptible to ischemic injury to the optic nerve. Infarctions of the entire optic nerve head cause sudden obscuration of vision in one eye, and present ophthalmoscopically with optic nerve head swelling and hemorrhages. Many patients present with infarction of only a portion of the optic nerve head, resulting in sudden onset of a monocular visual field defect. As with retinal artery occlusions, it is important to distinguish between arteritic and nonarteritic occlusions,[59] as only the former respond well to systemic steroids.

Ischemic optic neuropathy is also occasionally seen in the period following otherwise uncomplicated cataract extraction. Visual recovery is rare, and the benefit of steroids in this setting is unproved.[60]

The term *papilledema* is reserved in ophthalmic usage for optic disk swelling due to increased intracranial pressure. In these patients, visual acuity is rarely impaired (at least initially); the only visual field abnormality is typically an enlarged blind spot. In chronic papilledema, optic atrophy may ensue, with progressive visual impairment. Treatment is directed at the underlying intracranial cause of the increased pressure. In occasional cases of idiopathic intracranial pressure elevations (pseudotumor cerebri), medical treatment with carbonic anhydrase inhibitors, or surgical decompression of the central nervous system via a shunt or fenestration of the optic nerve sheath, may be of value.[61] Other causes of optic disk swelling that must be distinguished from papilledema include ischemic optic neuropathy, malignant hypertension, and severe uveitis.

NEURO-OPHTHALMOLOGY

The oculomotor nerves and the posterior visual pathways are frequently targets in elderly people for ischemic injury and for compressive injuries due to intracranial mass lesions (typically tumors or aneurysms) and shifts of the intracranial contents. Sudden loss of function of a *single*, isolated cranial nerve is quite common. An isolated trochlear or abducens nerve palsy in a patient otherwise susceptible to atherosclerotic disease is usually a benign event, and spontaneous recovery is frequently seen.[62] Ischemic insults to the oculomotor nerve typically spare the pupillary fibers.[63] Patients with *multiple* cranial nerve deficits, or in whom pupillary dilation has occurred, require a thorough neurological evaluation, preferably including computed tomography or magnetic resonance imaging, if available.

Abnormalities of the visual field should be thoroughly investigated. Scotomas that affect only one eye, or that respect the horizontal meridian, are generally due to injury to the retina, optic disk, optic nerve, or, of course, to glaucoma. Injuries at or posterior to the level of the optic chiasm will impair vision in both eyes. Of particular importance are bitemporal hemianopsias, which suggest compression of the optic chiasm, typically by a pituitary tumor, and highly congruous homonymous field defects, which suggest an injury of the occipital cerebral cortex.

ORBIT

Tumors of the orbit generally present with horizontal, vertical, or anterior displacement of the globe (proptosis). In the elderly, the most frequently diagnosed entities include orbital pseudotumor (idiopathic inflammation of one or more orbital tissues, typically the extraocular muscles, lacrimal gland, or infiltration of the orbital fat), hemangiomas and lymphangiomas, lymphomas, and primary tumors of the lacrimal gland. Management frequently requires orbital exploration for histopathological diagnosis, as well as for anatomical correction.[64]

Thyroid ophthalmopathy (Graves' disease) is a well-known orbital problem. The impairment of ocular motility, lid retraction, and exophthalmos are largely due to the infiltration of the extraocular muscles. The orbital fat is rarely, if ever, involved.[65] Progression of the orbital disease is poorly correlated with the actual thyroid hormone levels, and restoration of the euthyroid state, although desirable for many reasons, is not particularly effective as a tool in the management of the ocular complications. Early cases respond well to systemic steroids. In long-standing cases, patients should be monitored closely for signs of optic nerve compression, and should be promptly offered surgical decompression (generally achieved by fracturing the orbital bones to provide greater room for the swollen orbital contents) if the optic nerve is at risk.[66]

OPHTHALMIC COMPLICATIONS OF SYSTEMIC DISEASES

The vision of elderly patients is at risk, not only from primary ocular diseases, but from the effects of systemic diseases as well.

In addition to the effects of diabetes mellitus and thyroid disease mentioned above, a few of the more prominent disease entities with serious ophthalmic sequelae include hematological disorders (such as leukemia and polycythemia), collagen-vascular diseases (including rheumatoid arthritis, ankylosing spondylitis, and systemic lupus erythematosus), Marfan syndrome, and renal failure. Treatment is usually directed at the primary disease process, but topical or systemic steroids may be needed to control ocular inflammation.

In addition to the local, mechanical effects of metastasis to the eye or orbit, systemic malignancy may also exert a deleterious remote effect on retinal function, greatly impairing vision.[67] Chemotherapy directed at the primary malignancy has occasionally led to visual improvement.

OPHTHALMIC COMPLICATIONS OF SYSTEMIC MEDICATIONS

Many elderly patients receive several concurrent medications, some of which may frequently cause ocular symptoms. A few of the more common problems are described below.[68]

Tricyclic antidepressants have a mild parasympatholytic action, which may cause mydriasis and paralysis of accommodation. Major tranquilizers, such as chlorpromazine, may also cause mydriasis and interfere with accommodation, and may cause a pigmentary retinopathy. Significant visual impairment has generally been reported only with protracted, chronic use. Chloroquine may also cause a "bull's-eye" maculopathy with impairment of central vision, particularly after prolonged use with a total dosage exceeding 100 g of the chloroquine base. Hydroxychloroquine appears to be substantially less retinotoxic than chloroquine.

Systemic steroids may precipitate an open-angle glaucoma (which frequently does not abate until several weeks after cessation of the drug), as well as accelerate the formation of cataracts. Digitalis derivatives may produce various visual disturbances, in addition to the classic "yellow vision" (xanthopsia). Ethambutol is also reported to produce dyschromatopsia, as well as optic atrophy and visual field defects. The anti-impotence drug sildenafil cross-reacts slightly with the retinal isoform of phosphodiesterase, and may cause transient perception of a bluish haze or increased light sensitivity.[69]

Precipitation of an acute angle-closure attack by the mydriatic action of systemic medications is extremely rare.

SYSTEMIC COMPLICATIONS OF OPHTHALMIC MEDICATIONS

Because the dosages of topical eye medications are generally much smaller than the dosages used in systemic treatment, systemic complications from use of eyedrops are very rare. However, these drugs are rapidly absorbed across the conjunctiva and nasal mucous membranes, and occasionally cause systemic complications. Of course, it is also sometimes necessary to treat localized eye disease with systemic medications, which may cause further systemic problems.[68]

The topical anticholinergics used as mydriatic/cycloplegics may occasionally cause the full spectrum of systemic atropinic toxicity. Of the drugs in common use, cyclopentolate appears to cause these problems most frequently. Conversely, the parasympathomimetics, such as pilocarpine, carbachol, and the anticholinesterases, such as echothiophate, may cause such side-effects such as abdominal cramps, diarrhea, and nausea.

Topical adrenergic agents, such as neosynephrine, may cause tachycardia, hypertension, and even frank arrhythmias. Conversely, topical β-blockers, such as timolol maleate, may cause the full spectrum of side effects of β-blockade, including bradycardia, asthma, and hypotension. The use of "cardioselective" β-blockers, such as betaxolol, has not completely eliminated these problems.

Topical use of chloramphenicol has resulted in a few reported cases of aplastic anemia, generally after prolonged treatment. There have also been rare reports of Stevens–Johnson syndrome following topical administration of sulfa antibiotics. Otherwise, there are very few reports of serious systemic toxicity from topical antibiotics, other than hypersensitivity reactions.

Mannitol and glycerine are administered as osmotic agents to lower intraocular pressure in acute glaucoma. The fluid shifts that result may also cause congestive heart failure, renal shutdown, and altered mentation. Patients undergoing repeated treatments should be closely monitored for electrolyte imbalances and signs of renal decompensation.

Systemic carbonic anhydrase inhibitors, such as acetazolamide and methazolamide, are frequently used to treat glaucoma. These are difficult drugs for many patients, frequently causing anorexia, depression, impotence, and paresthesias, in addition to such rare complications as bone marrow depression, gout, and acidosis. Recently, carbonic anhydrase inhibitors have become available in topical formulations, which may reduce or eliminate many of these complications. Patients whose quality of life is intolerable on these medications should be offered medical or surgical alternatives.

LOW-VISION REHABILITATION

The rehabilitation of individuals who have sustained an irremediable loss of vision is an important component of effective medical care, particularly among elderly people. In the United States, over two-thirds of individuals with acuity less than 6/18 are over 65 years of age. Conversely, of individuals over 65 years of age, 7.8 percent are reported to have acuity worse than 6/18, a fraction that increases to 25 percent among individuals over 85 years old. Loss of vision has been ranked as the third most common chronic condition (after arthritis and heart disease) for which individuals over the age of 70 require assistance with the activities of daily living.[70]

Low-vision rehabilitation attempts to allow vision-impaired individuals to make the most effective use of whatever vision they retain, so as to facilitate activities of daily living, prolong independence, and enhance self-confidence. Successful rehabilitation frequently requires the coordinated efforts of a team of care providers, including the ophthalmologist, optometrist, and occupational therapist, as well as the assistance and understanding of the patient's family and friends, or caretakers. Rehabilitation is generally most successful if it is begun as soon as permanent visual disability has been diagnosed. Critical to the functional outcome is the acceptance by the patient of the need to adopt compensatory visual strategies to cope with the loss of vision, rather than to continue vain attempts to reverse the visual loss.

Rehabilitation programs should center on the needs of the patient. A thorough functional history should be obtained. Emphasis should include the patient's perceptions of the impact of the visual disability on accustomed activities, and on goals for the future. Every attempt should be made to identify specific tasks that the patient's visual limitations have curtailed, and whose recovery would be particularly valued. Typical problems include inability to read, mend, or pay bills; loss of independent mobility, and difficulty with distance vision, such as watching television or reading signs.

The severity of the visual deficit should be determined, including measurements of visual acuity, visual fields, and contrast sensitivity. It is often helpful to be more specific in identifying the level of visual acuity than is typical in general ophthalmic practice. Placement of eye charts as close as 1 m may be used to expand the range of acuity testing. It is frequently essential to allow a substantially greater amount of time than usual for visual assessment in low-vision patients, especially elderly people.

Rehabilitation may then proceed.[71] A comprehensive program frequently entails the dispensing and instruction in the use of optical aids (such as spectacles, telescopes, and magnifiers) and nonoptical aids (such as improved lighting, large-print reading materials, high-contrast guides for reading and writing, and closed-circuit television magnifiers). Training in the use of residual vision, such as eccentric viewing for individuals who have lost central macular function, may be attempted, but may require many hours of practice over many months in order to obtain optimal performance. Training in adaptations for activities of daily living, and the introduction of suitable equipment, such as needle threaders or large-print playing cards, can help recapture self-confidence and facilitate independence. Professional counseling, often in a group setting, can play an important role in helping patients deal with the emotional impact of visual disabilities.

KEY POINTS Major causes of blindness in the elderly

- In developed countries:
  - Cataract
  - Glaucoma
  - Diabetic retinopathy
  - Macular degeneration
- In developing countries:
  - Cataract
  - Corneal scarring
  - Glaucoma
  - Diabetic retinopathy
  - Macular degeneration

It is important that the patient adopt reasonable goals for low-vision rehabilitation. In nearly every case, it is impossible to recover the efficiency enjoyed prior to the loss of visual function. Each patient must individually decide whether the results achieved are worth the extra effort that will remain necessary to perform most visual tasks. The best results are achieved when specific tasks are targeted.

REFERENCES

1. World Health Organization: Methods of Assessment of Avoidable Blindness. Geneva, WHO Offset Pub. No. 54, 1980
2. Foster A: Patterns of Blindness. In Tasman W, Jaeger EA (eds): Duane's Clinical Ophthalmology Vol. 5. Lippincott-Raven, Philadelphia, 1984, Ch. 53
3. Lewallen S, Courtright P: Blindness in Africa: present situation and future needs. Br J Ophthalmol 2001;85:897–903
4. Klein R, Klein BEK, Linton KLP et al: The Beaver Dam Eye Study: visual acuity. Ophthalmology 1991;98:1310
5. Tielsch JM, Javitt JC, Coleman A et al: The prevalence of blindness and visual impairment among nursing home residents in Baltimore. N Engl J Med 1995;332:1205–1209
6. Frueh BR: The mechanistic classification of ptosis. Ophthalmology 1980;87:1019–1021
7. Dryden RM, Leibsohn J, Wobig J: Senile entropion: pathogenesis and treatment. Arch Ophthalmol 1978;96:1883–1885
8. Berlin AJ, Vestal KP: Levator aponeurosis surgery. A retrospective review. Ophthalmology 1989;96:1033–1036
9. Smith B: The "lazy-T" correction of ectropion of the lower punctum. Arch Ophthalmol 1976;94:1149–1150
10. Mohs FE: Micrographic surgery for the microscopically controlled excision of eyelid cancers. Arch Ophthalmol 1986;104:901–909
11. van Bijsterveld OP, Mackor AJ: Sjogren's syndrome and tear function parameters. Clin Exp Rheumatol 1989;7:151–154
12. Balaram M, Schaumberg DA, Dana MR: Efficacy and tolerability outcomes after punctal occlusion with silicone plugs in dry eye syndrome. Am J Ophthalmol 2001;131:30–36
13. Rosen N, Sharir M, Moverman DC, Rosner M: Dacryocystorhinostomy with silicone tubes: evaluation of 253 cases. Ophthalmic Surg 1989;20:115–119
14. Vorkas AP: Pterygium. Choice of operation. Trans Ophthal Soc UK 1981;101:192–194
15. Fraunfelder FT, Wingfield D: Management of intraepithelial conjunctival tumors and squamous cell carcinomas. Am J Ophthalmol 1983;95:359–363
16. Edelhauser HF, Van Horn DL, Records RE: Cornea and sclera. In Tasman W, Jaeger EA (eds): Duane's Clinical Ophthalmology Vol. 2. Lippincott-Raven, Philadelphia, 1989, Ch. I
17. Carlson KH, Bourne WM, McLaren JW, Brubaker RF: Variations in human corneal endothelial cell morphology and permeability to fluorescein with age. Exp Eye Res 1988;47:27–41
18. Olson RJ, Waltman SR, Mattingly TP, Kaufman HE: Visual results after penetrating keratoplasty for aphakic bullous keratoplasty and Fuchs' dystrophy. Am J Ophthalmol 1979;88:1000–1004
19. Schaefer F, Bruttin O, Zografos L, Guex-Crosier Y: Bacterial keratitis: a prospective clinical and microbiological study. Br J Ophthalmol 2001;85:842–847
20. Baum J, Barza M: Topical vs. subconjunctival treatment of bacterial corneal ulcers. Ophthalmology 1983;90:162–168
21. Nussenblatt RB, Palestine AG, Chan C-C: Cyclosporine A treatment of intraocular inflammatory disease resistant to systemic corticosteroids and cytotoxic agents. Am J Ophthalmol 1983;96:275–282
22. McLean IW, Foster WD, Zimmerman LE: Uveal melanoma: location, size, cell type, and enucleation as risk factors in metastasis. Hum Pathol 1982;13:123–132
23. Gass JD: Observation of suspected choroidal and ciliary body melanomas for evidence of growth prior to enucleation. Ophthalmology 1980;87:523–528
24. Shields JA, Augsburger JJ, Brady LW, Day JL: Cobalt plaque therapy of posterior uveal melanomas. Ophthalmology 1982;89:1201–1207
25. Diener-West M, Earle JD, Fine SL et al: The Collaborative Ocular Melanoma Study Group. The COMS randomized trial of iodine 125 brachytherapy for choroidal melanoma, III: initial mortality findings. COMS Report No. 18. Arch Ophthalmol 2001;119:969–982
26. Stephens RF, Shields JA: Diagnosis and management of cancer metastatic to the uvea: a study of 70 cases. Ophthalmology 1979;86:1336–1349
27. Shiose Y: Intraocular pressure: new perspectives. Surv Ophthalmol 1990;34:413–435
28. Yablonski ME, Zimmerman TJ, Kass MA, Becker B: Prognostic significance of optic disk cupping in ocular hypertensive patients. Am J Ophthalmol 1980;89:585–592
29. Quigley HA, Addicks EM, Green R: Optic nerve damage in human glaucoma III. Quantitative correlation of nerve fiber loss and visual field defect in glaucoma, ischemic neuropathy, papilledema, and toxic neuropathy. Arch Ophthalmol 1982;100:135–159
30. Jay JL, Murray SB: Early trabeculectomy versus conventional management in primary open angle glaucoma. Br J Ophthalmol 1988;72:881–889
31. The Glaucoma Laser Trial (GLT) and Glaucoma Laser Trial Follow-up Study: 7. Results. Glaucoma Laser Trial Research Group. Am J Ophthalmol 1995;120:718–731
32. Katz J, Tielsch JM, Quigley HA et al: Automated suprathreshold screening for glaucoma: the Baltimore Eye Survey. Invest Ophthalmol Vis Sci 1993;34:3271–3277
33. Olson L: Anatomy and embryology of the lens. In Tasman W, Jaeger EA (eds): Duane's Clinical Ophthalmology. Vol. 1. Lippincott-Raven, Philadelphia, 1978, Ch. 71
34. Cotlier E, Fagadau W, Cicchetti DV: Methods for evaluation of medical therapy of senile and diabetic cataracts. Trans Ophthalmol Soc UK 1982;102,3:416–422
35. Kelman CD: Phaco-emulsification and aspiration of senile cataracts: A comparative study with intra-capsular extraction. Can J Ophthalmol 1973;8:24–32
36. Spaeth GL: No-stitch surgery: good, bad, or both? editorial. Ophthalmic Surg 1991;22:630–631
37. Bachani D, Murthy GV, Gupta KS: Rapid assessment of cataract blindness in India. Indian J Public Health 2000;44:82–89
38. Benson WH, Farber ME, Caplan RJ: Increased mortality rates after cataract surgery. A statistical analysis. Ophthalmology 1988;95:1288–1292
39. Frank RN, Hoffman WH, Podgor MJ et al: Retinopathy in juvenile-onset diabetes of short duration. Ophthalmology 1980;87:1–9
40. Early Treatment Diabetic Retinopathy Study Research Group: Treatment techniques and clinical guidelines for photocoagulation of diabetic macular edema. ETDRS Report No. 2. Ophthalmology 1987;94:761–774
41. Diabetic Retinopathy Study Research Group: Indications for photocoagulation treatment of diabetic retinopathy: DRS report No. 14. Int Ophthalmol Clin 1987;27:239–253
42. Kroc Collaborative Study Group: Blood glucose control and the evolution of diabetic retinopathy and albuminuria. N Engl J Med 1984;311:365–372
43. Ramsey RC, Goetz FC, Sutherland DE et al: Progression of diabetic retinopathy after pancreas transplantation for insulin-dependent diabetes mellitus. N Engl J Med 1988;318:208–214
44. The Diabetes Control and Complications Trial Research Group: The effect of intensive treatment of diabetes on the development and progression of long-term complications in insulin-dependent diabetes mellitus. N Engl J Med 1993;329:977–986
45. Gass JDM: Pathogenesis of disciform detachment of the neuroepithelium, III. Senile disciform macular degeneration. Am J Ophthalmol 1967;63:617–644
46. Macular Photocoagulation Study Group: Argon laser photocoagulation for neovascular maculopathy. Three-year results from randomized clinical trails. Arch Ophthalmol 1986;104:694–701
47. Macular Photocoagulation Study Group: Laser photo-coagulation of subfoveal neovascular lesions in age-related macular degeneration. Results of randomized clinical trial. Arch Ophthalmol 1991;109:1220–1231
48. Schmidt-Erfurth U, Hasan T: Mechanisms of action of photodynamic therapy with verteporfin for the treatment of age-related macular degeneration. Surv Ophthalmol 2000;45:195–214
49. Bressler NM: Photodynamic therapy of subfoveal choroidal neovascularization in age-related macular degeneration with verteporfin: two-year results of 2 randomized clinical trials-tap report 2. Arch Ophthalmol 2001;119:198–207
50. Pieramici DJ, De Juan E Jr, Fujii GY et al: Limited inferior macular translocation for the treatment of subfoveal choroidal neovascularization secondary to age-related macular degeneration. Am J Ophthalmol 2000;130:419–428

51. Gass JDM: Drusen and disciform macular detachment. Trans Am Ophthalmol Soc 1972;70:409–436

52. Age-Related Eye Disease Study Research Group: A randomized, placebo-controlled, clinical trial of high-dose supplementation with vitamins C and E, beta carotene, and zinc for age-related macular degeneration and vision loss. AREDS Report No. 8. Arch Ophthalmol 119:2001;1417–1436

53. Age-Related Eye Disease Study Research Group: A randomized, placebo-controlled, clinical trial of high-dose supplementation with vitamins C and E and beta carotene for age-related cataract and vision loss. AREDS Report No. 9. Arch Ophthalmol 119:2001;1439–1452

54. Augsburger JJ, Magargal LE: Visual prognosis following treatment of acute central retinal artery obstruction. Br J Ophthalmol 1980;64:913–917

55. Bernstein EF (ed): Amaurosis Fugax. Springer-Verlag, New York, 1988

56. Poole CJM, Ross Russel RW: Mortality and stroke after amaurosis fugax. J Neurol Neurosurg Psychiatry 1985;48:902–905

57. Keltner JL: Giant-cell arteritis. Signs and symptoms. Ophthalmology 1982;89:1101–1110

58. Magargal LE, Brown GC, Augsburger JJ, Donoso LA: Efficacy of pan-retinal photocoagulation in preventing neovascular glaucoma following ischemic central retinal vein occlusion. Ophthalmology 1982;89:780–784

59. Glaser JS: Topical diagnosis: pre-chiasmal visual pathways. In Tasman W, Jaeger EA (eds): Duane's Clinical Ophthalmology, Vol. 2. Lippincott-Raven, Philadelphia, 1989, Ch. 5

60. Hayreh SS: Anterior ischemic optic neuropathy, IV. Occurrence after cataract extraction. Arch Ophthalmol 1980;98:1410–1416

61. Sergott RC, Savino PJ, Bosley TM: Modified optic nerve sheath decompression provides long-term visual improvement for pseudotumor cerebri. Arch Ophthalmol 1988;106:1384–1390

62. Rush JA, Younge BR: Paralysis of cranial nerves III, IV, and VI. Cause and prognosis in 1000 cases. Arch Ophthalmol 1981;99:76–79

63. Glaser JS: Infranuclear disorders of eye movement. In Tasman W, Jaeger EA (eds): Duane's ,linical Ophthalmology, Vol. 2. Lippincott-Raven, Philadelphia, 1988, Ch. 12

64. Jones IS, Jakobiec FA, Nolan BT: Patient examination and introduction to orbital disease. In Tasman W, Jaeger EA (eds): Duane's Clinical Ophthalmology, Vol. 2. Lippincott-Raven, Philadelphia, 1976, Ch. 21

65. Trokel SL, Jakobiec FA: Correlation of CT scanning and pathologic features of ophthalmic Graves' disease. Ophthalmology 1981;88:553–564

66. Schorr N, Seiff SR: The four stages of surgical rehabilitation of the patient with dysthyroid ophthalmopathy. Ophthalmology 1986;93:476–483

67. Thirkill CE, Roth AM, Keltner JL: Cancer-associated retinopathy. Arch Ophthalmol 1987;105:372–375

68. Fraunfelder FT: Drug-Induced Ocular Side Effects and Drug Interactions, 3rd Ed. Lea & Febiger, Philadelphia, 1989

69. Marmor MF, Kessler R: Sildenafil (Viagra) and ophthalmology. Surv Ophthalmol 1999;44:153–162

70. Eaglestein A, Rapaport S: Prediction of low vision and usage. J Vis Impair Blindness 1991;85:31–33

71. Rehabilitation: The Management of Adult Patients with Low Vision. American Academy of Ophthalmology, Preferred Practice Pattern, 1995

Color Plates

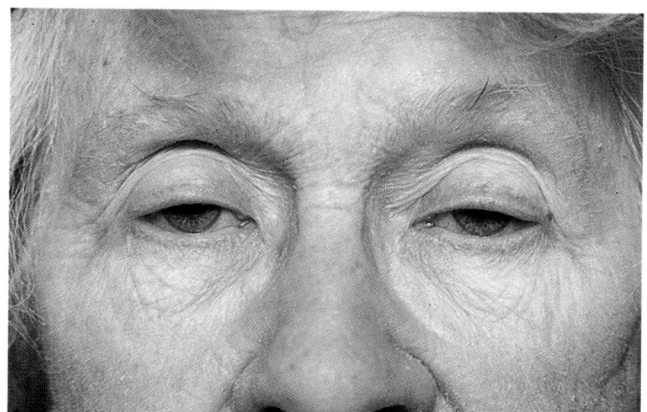

Plate 59-1

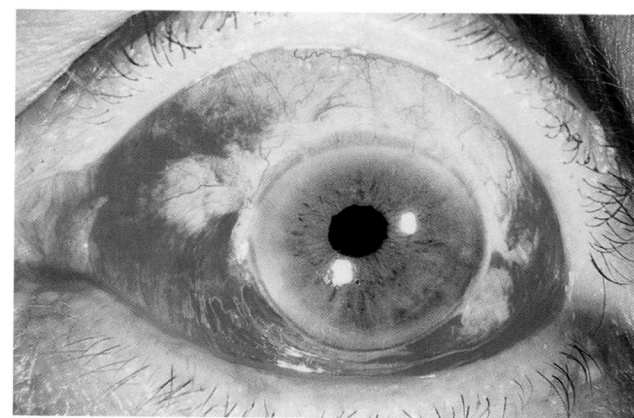

Plate 59-2

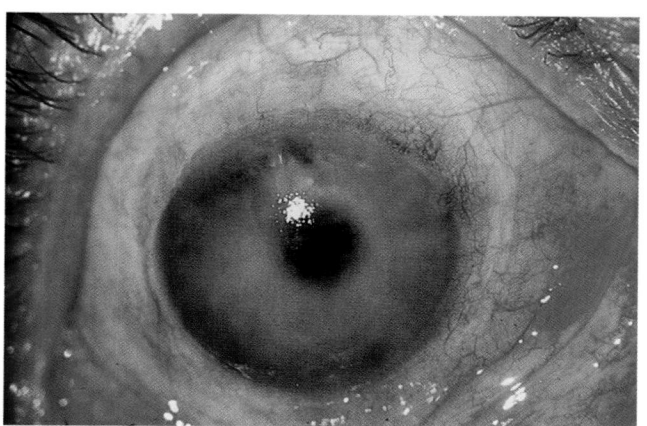

Plate 59-3

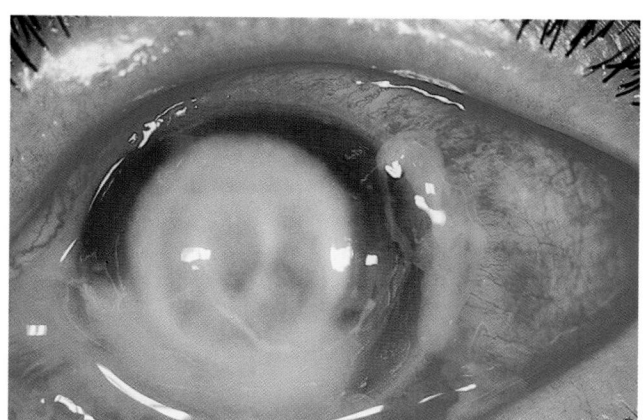

Plate 59-4

Plate 59-1 Senile ptosis. Note the low lid level and the loss of the normal lid folds.
(Courtesy of Murray Melzer, MD.)

Plate 59-2 Subconjunctival hemorrhage. This small hematoma, seen through the transparent conjunctiva, is benign unless recurrent.

Plate 59-3 Corneal edema. The cornea is thickened and cloudy due to failure of the corneal endothelium to adequately dehydrate the tissue.
(Courtesy of Calvin Roberts, MD.)

Plate 59-4 Corneal ulcer. A localized infection causes an epithelial defect and attracts an infiltrate of white blood cells.
(Courtesy of Michael Newton, MD.)

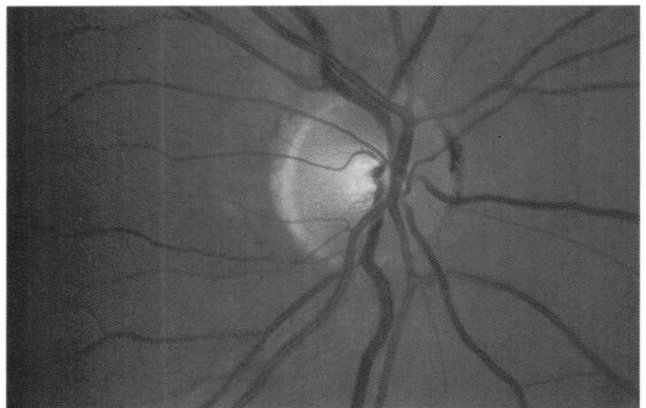

Plate 59-5

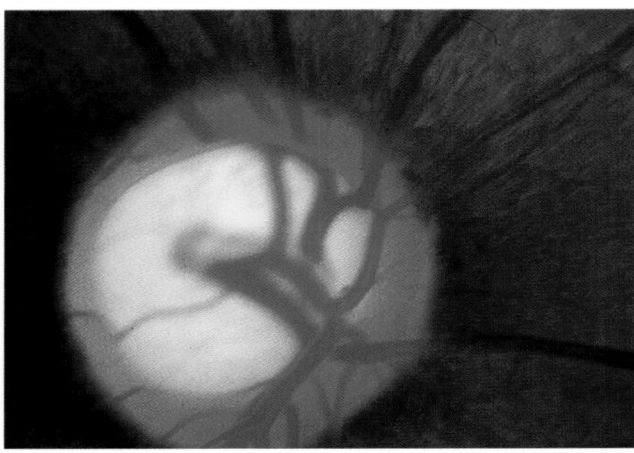

Plate 59-6

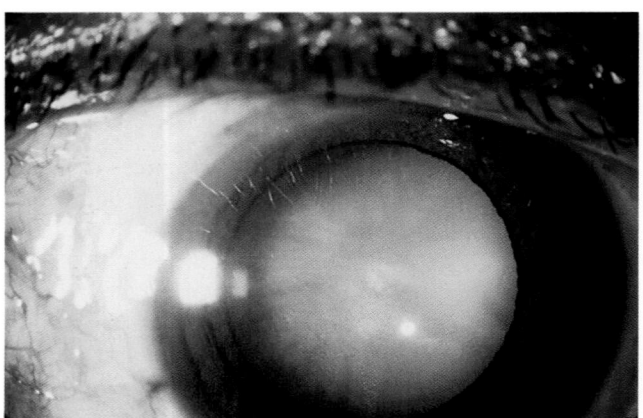

Plate 59-7

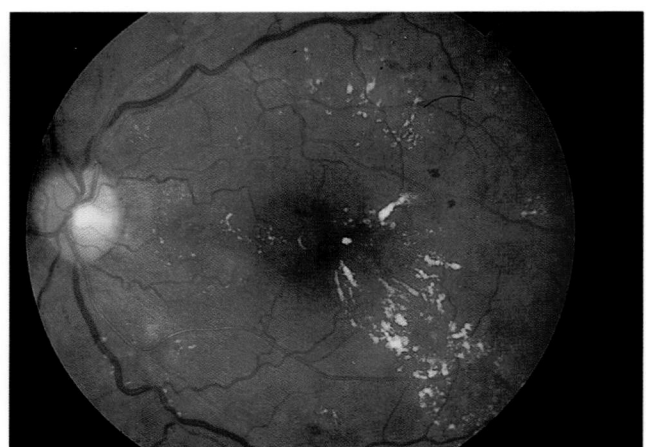

Plate 59-8

Plate 59-5 Normal optic nerve head. Cup to disk ratio is about 0.3.

Plate 59-6 Glaucomatous optic nerve head cupping. Loss of neural tissue is seen as narrowing of the neural rim of the optic disc, and enlargement of the central cup. (Compare with Plate 59-5.)

Plate 59-7 Cataract. Loss of transparency of the crystalline lens impairs visual acuity. (Courtesy of Calvin Roberts, MD.)

Plate 59-8 Background diabetic retinopathy. Microaneurysms ("dot hemorrhages"), intraretinal hemorrhages ("blot hemorrhages"), and "hard" exudates indicate deterioration of the retinal microcirculation.

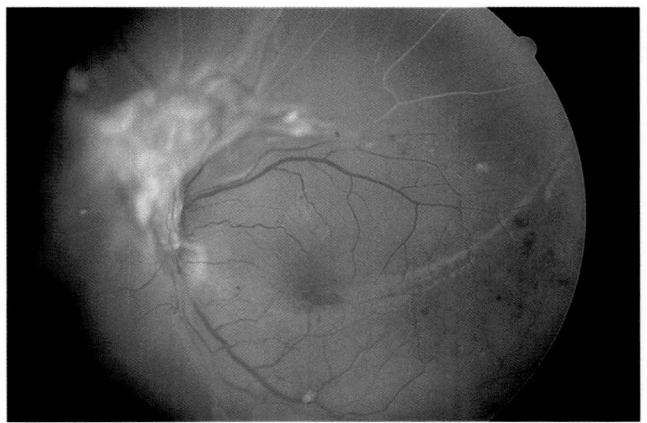

Plate 59-9

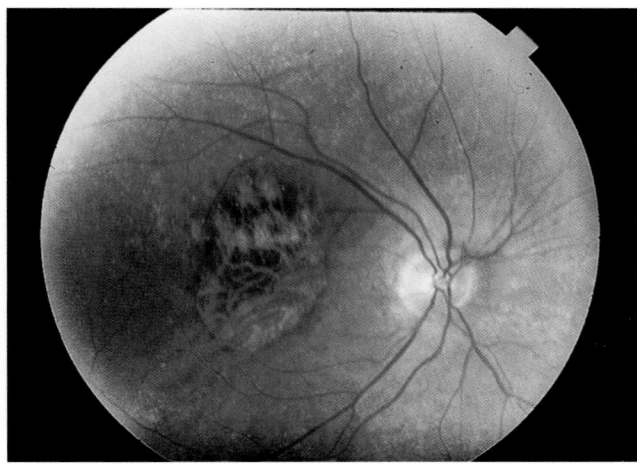

Plate 59-10

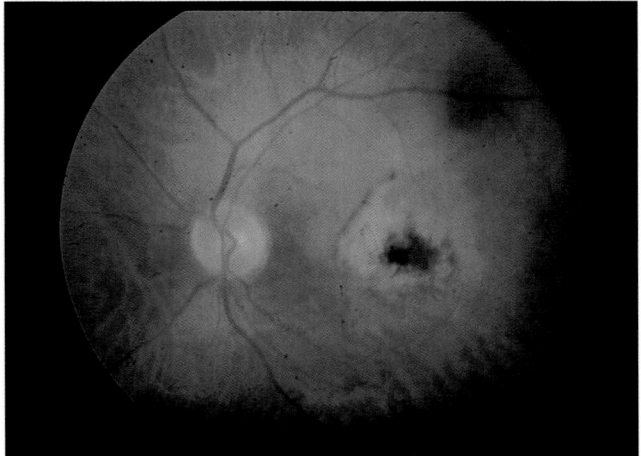

Plate 59-11

Plate 59-9 Proliferative diabetic retinopathy. A membrane of fibrovascular tissue has sprouted from the optic disk in response to prolonged retinal ischemia.

Plate 59-10 Atrophic ("dry") age-related macular degeneration. Geographic atrophy of the retinal pigment epithelium causes loss of central vision.

Plate 59-11 Exudative ("wet") age-related macular degeneration. Leakage and scarring from a subretinal neovascular membrane destroys central retinal function.

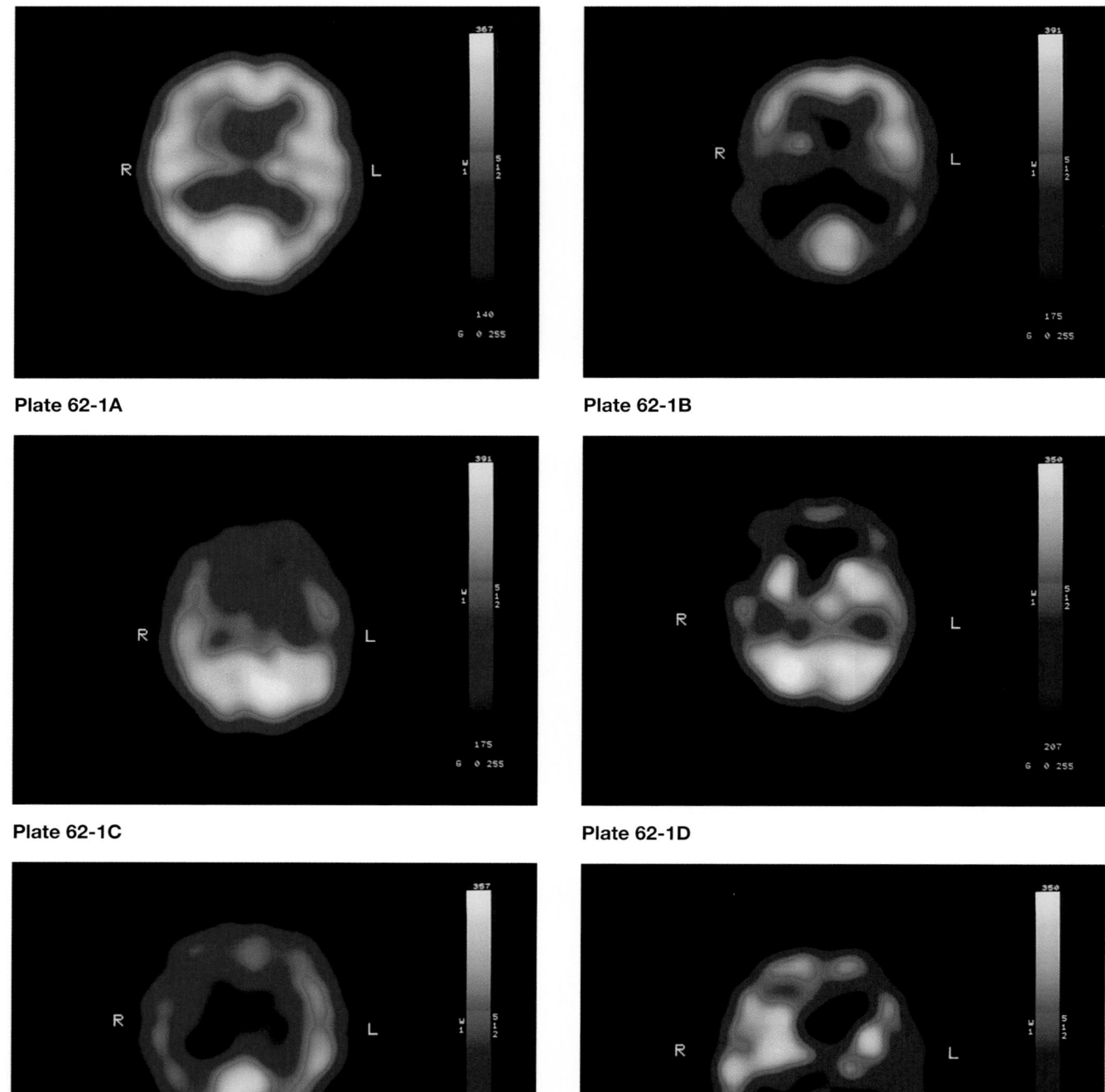

Plate 62-1A

Plate 62-1B

Plate 62-1C

Plate 62-1D

Plate 62-1E

Plate 62-1F

Plate 62-1 Single-photon emission computed tomography (SPECT) scan of (A) normal subject; (B) patient with Alzheimer's disease showing bilateral parietal lobe abnormalities more marked on the right side; (C) patient with frontotemporal dementia, showing bilateral frontal lobe abnormalities; (D) patient with progressive supranuclear palsy, showing bilateral anterior abnormalities; (E) patient with corticobasal degeneration, showing asymmetric right frontoparietal abnormality; (F) patient with Creutzfeldt-Jakob disease, showing multifocal cortical abnormalities.

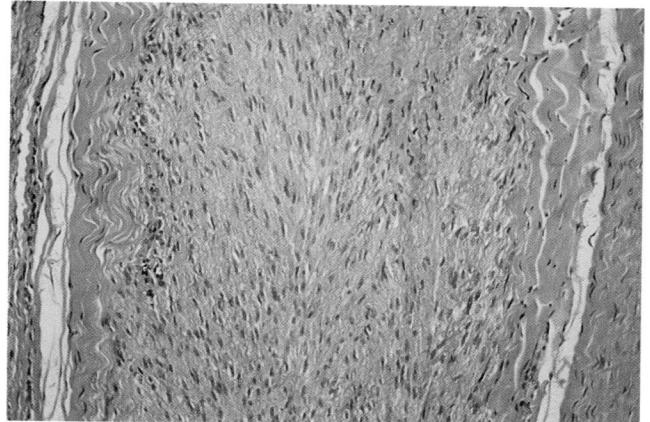

Plate 72-1

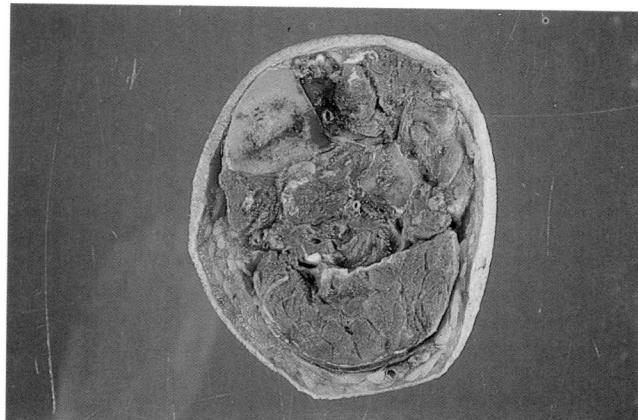

Plate 72-2

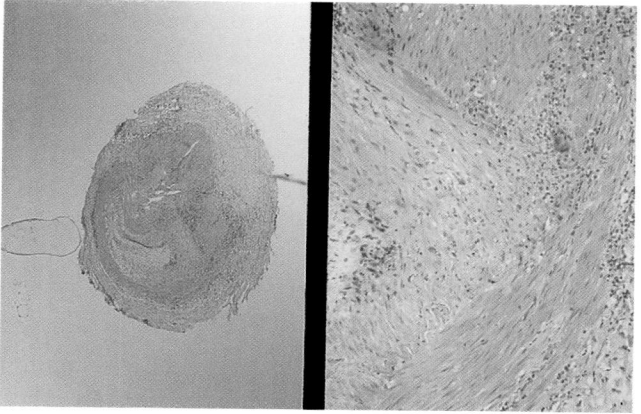

Plate 72-3

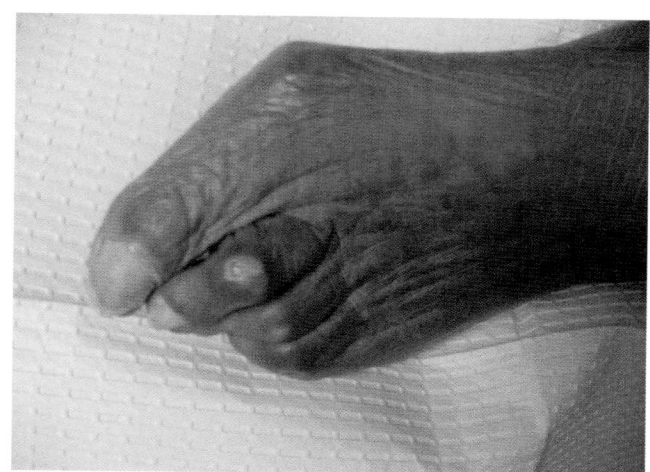

Plate 75-1

Plate 72-1 Cellular proliferation within a Dupuytren's nodule (H&E, x 200).

Plate 72-2 Macroscopic image of a malignant fibrous histocytoma. Diameter approximately 5 cm.

Plate 72-3 Artery from a patient with giant cell arteritis. The left panel shows virtual occlusion of the lumen (H&E. x 10); the right panel shows inflammation including giant cells in the wall (H&E, x 150).

Plate 75-1 A bunion deformity with hammer toe of the second digit. Note pre-ulcerative lesion over proximal phalangeal joint of second toe secondary to shoe pressure.

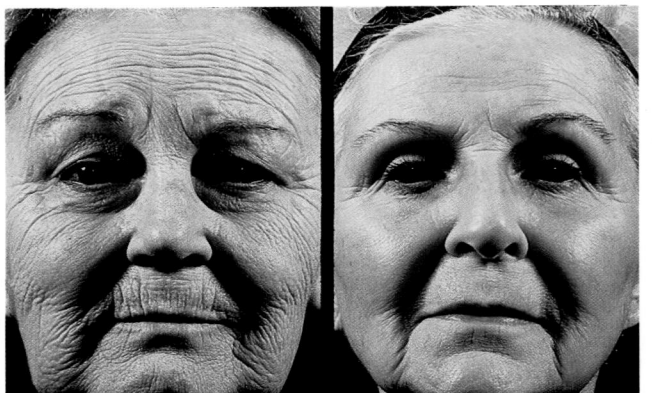

Plate 99-1

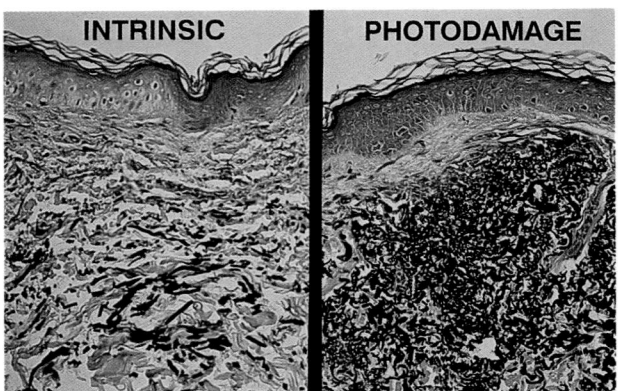

Plate 99-2

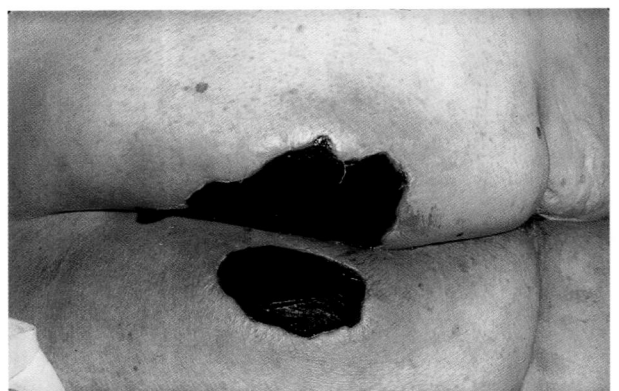

Plate 106-1

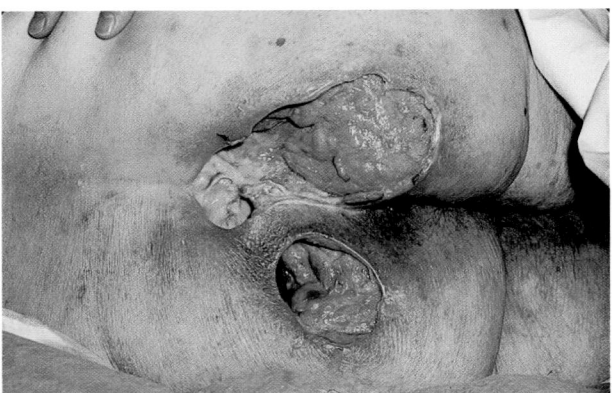

Plate 106-2

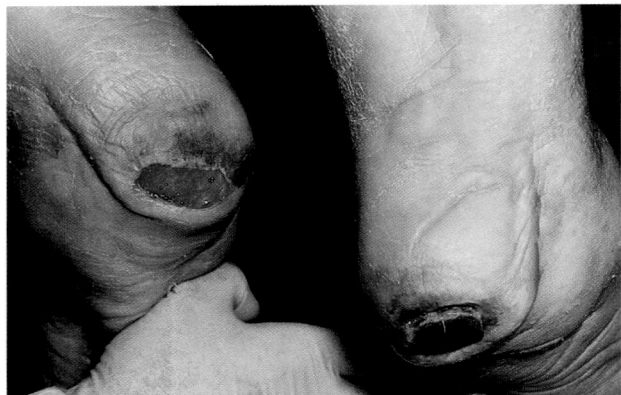

Plate 106-3

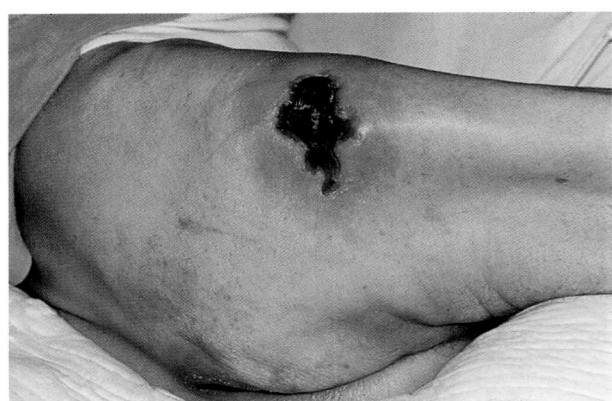

Plate 106-4

Plate 99-1 Faces of two 71-year-old women. The woman on the right has avoided sun exposure for most of her life and the changes are mostly those of intrinsic, chronological aging. The woman on the left has suffered a great deal of sun exposure and the wrinkles and thickened skin are evidence of photoaging. To the untrained observer the woman on the left appears older than her stated age.

Plate 99-2 Photomicrographs of histologic sections of intrinsic and extrinsically aged skin stained with Verhoeff van Giesen stain for elastin. The salient difference is the gross increase in black-staining, elastotic material in the reticular dermis of extrinsic, photoaged skin (x 40).

Plate 106-1 Acute pressure injury over the sacrum and buttocks in an elderly woman.

Plate 106-2 Natural debridement of the pressure injury shown in Plate 106-1 at 2 weeks.

Plate 106-3 Pressure injuries of the heels.

Plate 106-4 Pressure injury over the greater trochanter resulting from lateral turning on a hospital mattress.

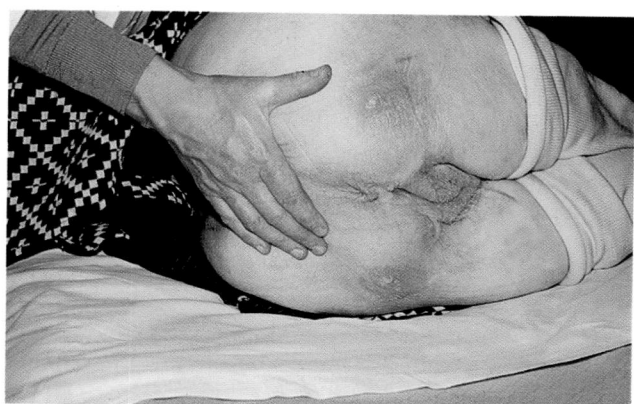

Plate 106-5

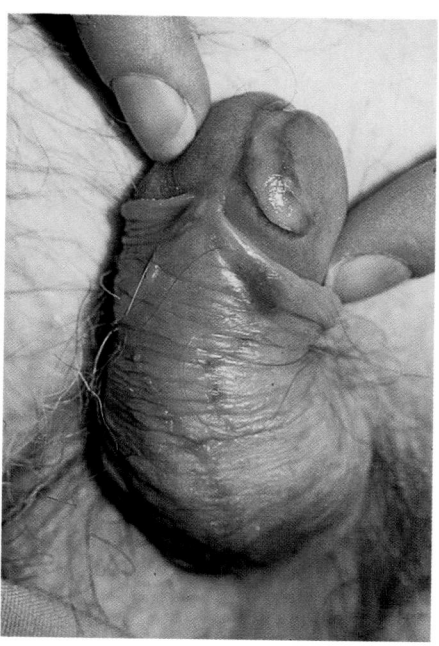

Plate 106-6

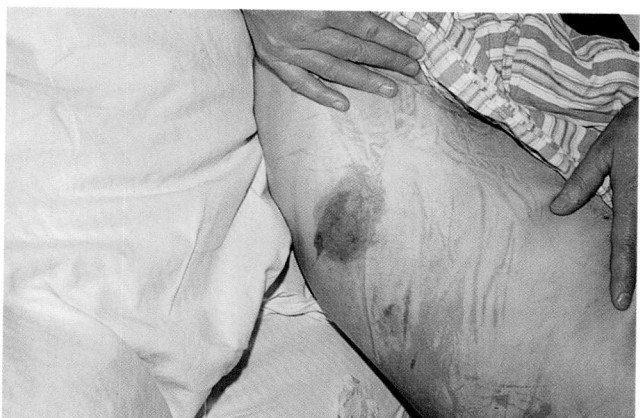

Plate 106-7

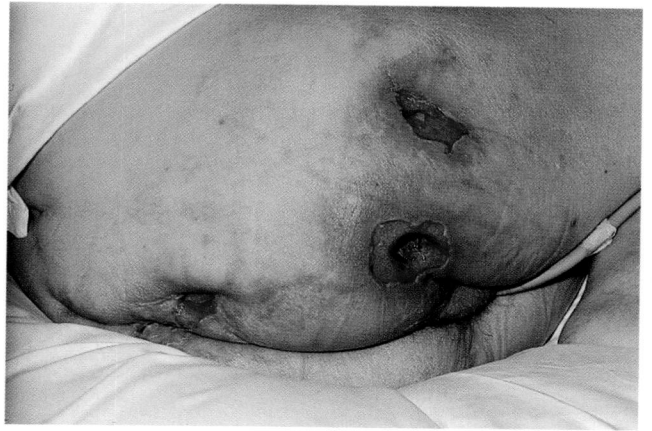

Plate 106-8

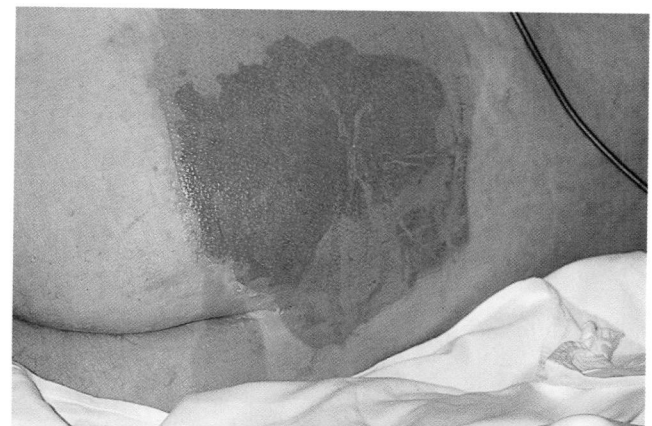

Plate 106-9

Plate 106-5 Pressure injuries over the ischial tuberosities caused by sitting in a chair.

Plate 106-6 Pressure injury on the penis due to a catheter.

Plate 106-7 Early pressure sore over the inferior angle of the scapula.

Plate 106-8 Deep pressure sore with sinuses in a patient with multiple sclerosis.

Plate 106-9 Pressure injury on the back caused by a diathermy plate. (Courtesy of Dr M. Lubbers, Academisch Medisch Centrum, Universiteit van Amsterdam.)

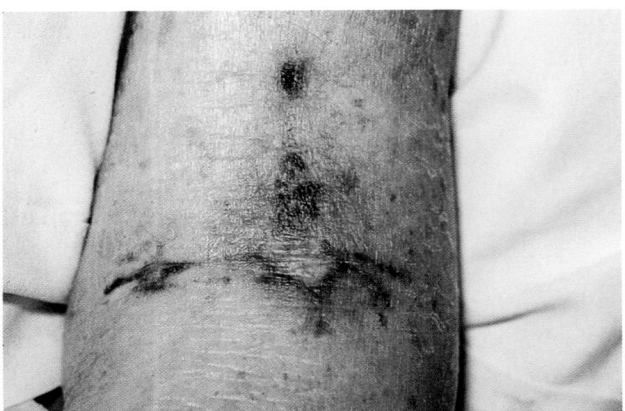

Plate 106-10

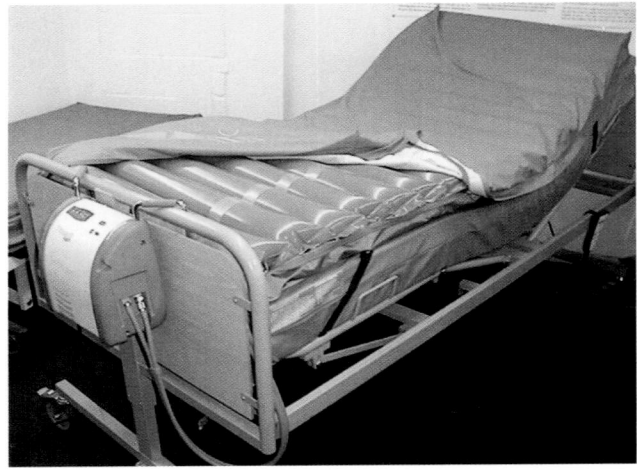

Plate 106-11

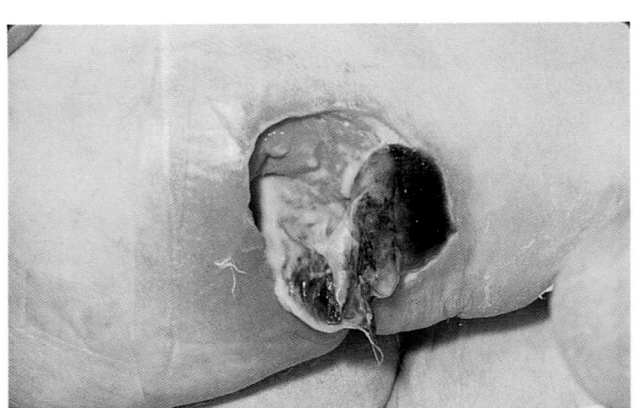

Plate 106-12

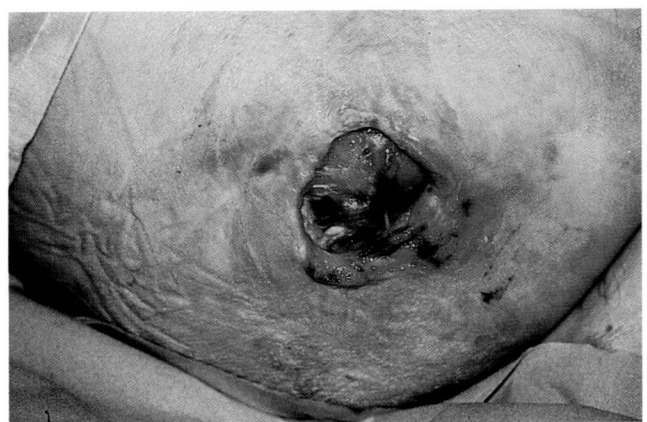

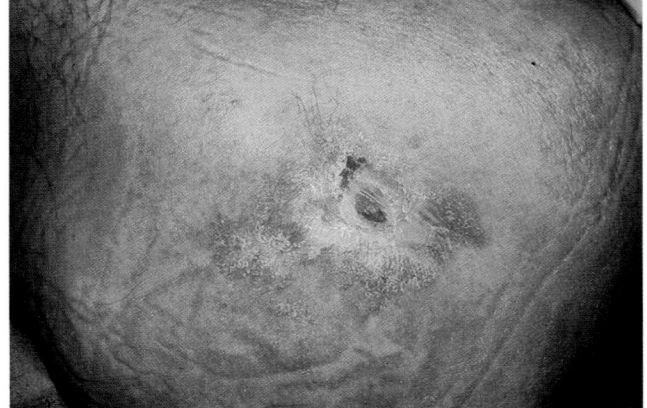

Plate 106-13

Plate 106-10 Pressure injury on the foot due to an antiemboli stocking.

Plate 106-11 An alternating-pressure mattress overlay.

Plate 106-12 Naturally separating slough in a deep pressure sore.

Plate 106-13 Deep pressure injury over the trochanter showing (top) contraction and (bottom) healing.

Chapter 60

Disorders of hearing

Barbara E. Weinstein

DEMOGRAPHICS OF AGING AND HEARING LOSS

Americans are living longer, and are healthier and wealthier than ever before. In 1900, life expectancy at birth was about 49 years. By 1960, life expectancy had increased to 70 years, and in 1997, was 79 years for women and 74 years for men. Life expectancies at ages 65 and 85 have also increased. Under current mortality conditions, people who survive to age 65 can expect to live an average of nearly 18 more years, 5 years longer than persons aged 65 in 1900. The life expectancy of persons who survive to age 85 today is about 7 years for women and 6 years for men. Hence, in the United States half of all people who have ever lived to age 65 are currently alive. The increase in longevity brings with it an increase in the amount of time spent in all major activities including work and retirement. A significant proportion of older adults are gainfully employed well into their 70s, and work part time. Older adults can spend a good deal of life in retirement. In fact, the average man aged 20 today can expect to spend a third of his life in retirement. The ability to communicate effectively with others takes on even greater importance as we move through the twenty-first century because of the lifestyle trends characterizing older adults, increase in average income projected for older adults over the next 40 years, and declining disability rates.

As people age the likelihood of experiencing one or more chronic conditions increases. Hearing impairment, arthritis, and hypertension are among the most prevalent chronic conditions affecting older adults. Overall, the 1995 National Health Interview Survey revealed that 18 percent of noninstitutionalized persons 70 years of age and over were visually impaired (i.e., full or partial blindness or trouble seeing) while one-third of persons 70 years of age and over were hearing impaired.[1] According to the 1995 survey, 25 percent of persons 70–74 years and 50 percent of persons over 85 years of age presented with hearing impairment. In contrast, 13 percent of persons 70–74 years and 31 percent of those over 85 years presented with visual impairment. Hearing loss was more prevalent among whites than blacks, whereas hypertension was more prevalent among blacks than whites. Older white persons were 1.8 times as likely to be hearing impaired as older black persons. Hearing impairment was more prevalent and severe in men, with men having an earlier age of onset than women. The prevalence of visual impairment was comparable for white and black persons over age 70. The high prevalence of hearing impairment among persons over 85 years has implications for nursing home staff as the majority of residents of nursing homes are in their ninth decade of life. That is to say, hearing loss will be the rule rather than the exception among nursing home residents. It is projected that by the year 2030, at least 21 million Americans beyond age 65 will have a hearing impairment.

Given the high prevalence of hearing loss among persons aged 65 years and older, it is no surprise that the majority of persons purchasing hearing instruments are in this age bracket. In fact, 65 percent of hearing instrument consumers are 65 years of age or older whereas only 6 percent are under 18 years of age.[2] Despite the fact that the vast majority of hearing aid users are over 65 years of age, the majority of older adults with handicapping hearing impairment do not use hearing aids.[2a] Specifically three out of five older Americans with hearing loss and six out of seven middle-aged Americans with hearing loss do not use hearing aids. The significant communicative and psychosocial effects of hearing loss, coupled with the fact that a high percentage of older adults suffer from hearing loss that affects ordinary daily life, and the efficacy of hearing aids in reducing the functional consequences of hearing impairment, would indicate that older adults should be encouraged to purchase hearing aids before hearing loss becomes an intolerable burden and less responsive to intervention.[2b] It appears that a number of variables are at play which determine whether an older adult will consider hearing aid use, including the self-perception of severity of hearing impairment, and the perception that one can get along without hearing aids. The high cost of hearing aids, especially digital devices, is a deterrent to older adults on fixed incomes. Unfortunately, third-party reimbursement for hearing aids is quite limited.

AGE-RELATED ANATOMICAL AND PHYSIOLOGICAL CHANGES

The inner ear is composed of several functional components that are vulnerable to the effects of aging. These components comprise the sensory, neural, vascular, supporting, synaptic, and/or mechanical structures within the peripheral and/or central auditory systems.[3] The organ of Corti, which extends spirally from the basal convolution to the cupula or apex of the cochlea, houses the sense organ of hearing. It is the structure most susceptible to age-related histopathological changes. The cochlea rests atop the basilar membrane and is composed of sensory cells (outer and inner hair cells along with their stereocilia), supporting cells, Reisner's membrane, the tectorial membrane, and stria vascularis, among other structures. The fact that various frequencies are registered in different parts of the cochlea is the basis for the tonotopic organization of the auditory system. The organ of Corti is the site of transduction of mechanical to neural energy, and age-related atrophy interferes with the transduction process integral to the reception of sound.

The most critical risk factor for the auditory sense organ is age.[4] The changes the aging ear undergoes have been studied most extensively by Schuknecht.[5–8] In general, hair cell loss is the rule rather than the exception in older adults. Loss of both types of hair cells is most severe in the basal region of the cochlea, with apical and midcochlear involvement of the outer hair cells, as well. Although both outer and inner hair cells tend to degenerate with age, the outer hair cells are more vulnerable than inner hair cells and their degeneration accounts in large part for the "normal" decline in hearing with age.[3]

Recent research[9] clearly demonstrates a relation between age and loss of ganglion cells. As would be expected, neural histopathological studies suggest that age-related loss in ganglion cells is greatest near the base of the cochlea. Similarly, age is associated with a decrease in the average number of fibers in the cochlear nerve with nerve fiber loss greatest within the basal 10 mm of the cochlea.[10] Neural degeneration can occur before and/or independently of sensory cell loss.[10a] That is, loss of nerve fibers in one turn of the cochlea or in all turns has been noted without severe hair cell loss.[3] Stated differently, loss of inner or outer hair cells is not a condition for age-related pathology of ganglion cells.[3] In conclusion, two major age-related structural changes have been observed histologically in the inner ear and auditory nerve. These include extensive atrophy and degeneration of the hair cells, numerous supporting cells, and the stria vascularis, as well as a reduction in the number of functional spiral ganglia and nerve fibers that comprise the auditory portion of the eighth nerve.[10b]

Histological studies of the central auditory nervous system suggest that portions undergo age-related changes as well.[11] These apparent changes, which predominate in the auditory brainstem pathways and the auditory cortex, are not universal across individuals, nor are they universal across the nuclei or tracts within the auditory brainstem. These changes within the central auditory nervous system have profound implications for speech understanding in less than optimal listening conditions and interfere with hearing aid benefit.

In addition to age-related degeneration, a number of other factors can lead to hearing loss in older adults. These include excessive exposure to occupational or recreational noise; genetic factors; acoustic neuroma; trauma; metabolic disease such as kidney problems; vascular disease; infections; and ingestion of ototoxic agents, most notably aminoglycosides, ethacrynic acid, and salicylates. Impacted cerumen, otitis media, glossopharyngeal tumors, and otosclerosis are not uncommon. The latter conditions are associated with conductive hearing loss, yet they can occur in the presence of cochlear involvement. Finally, affective disorders such as depression and cognitive disorders such as senile dementia of the Alzheimer's type are also associated with sensorineural hearing loss. In fact, the prevalence of hearing loss is higher among persons with dementia than among those without it. In addition, inattention or confusion related to depression or dementia may give the impression of significant hearing loss and should be considered in a systematic geriatric assessment. Complete audiometric studies can help identify the existence and etiology of hearing loss in older adults. Hearing loss should be ruled out in individuals being worked up for a cognitive or affective disorder.

BEHAVIORAL IMPLICATIONS OF ANATOMICAL AND PHYSIOLOGICAL CHANGES

The aforementioned age-related changes are associated with decrements in hearing for pure-tone and speech stimuli. In fact, it appears that age and frequency effects emerge in most cross-sectional and longitudinal studies of hearing loss, such that air conduction thresholds became poorer as age or frequency increase.[4,12,13] The majority of recent studies on hearing loss characterizing noninstitutionalized older adults confirm that age-related hearing loss commonly referred to as "presbycusis" has several distinct features. First, pure-tone hearing sensitivity tends to decline with increasing age and the hearing loss tends to be greatest in the frequencies above 1,000 Hz. Further, the hearing loss tends to be bilateral, symmetrical, and sensorineural in origin, associated with damage to the sensory structures within the cochlea. The decline in high-frequency sensitivity appears to be greatest in males, whereas the decline in low-frequency thresholds tends to be greatest in females of comparable age.[4] The average hearing loss in males can be described as mild to moderately severe, bilateral, and sensorineural with a sharply sloping configuration, whereas women tend to present with a mild to moderate gradually sloping bilaterally symmetrical sensorineural hearing loss. Among residents of nursing facilities, the sensorineural hearing loss tends to be more significant, moderately severe sloping to severe, and more prevalent, affecting approximately 70–80 percent of residents. The fact that nursing home residents are older accounts for the high prevalence of more severe hearing loss among residents. Residents of nursing facilities tend to be prone to cerumen impaction which can exacerbate the speech understanding problems in persons with a pre-existing sensorineural hearing loss.

Hallmarks of hearing loss in older adults

- Mild to moderate sensorineural hearing loss
- Difficulty understanding speech in the presence of noise
- Can hear people talking but have difficulty making out the words
- Occasional ringing in the ears (tinnitus)
- Gradual in onset
- Hearing loss is bilateral and symmetrical
- Primarily due to degenerative changes in cochlea, eighth nerve, and auditory brainstem pathways

The pure-tone hearing loss and site of involvement within the cochlea, eighth nerve, auditory brainstem pathways, and auditory cortex determine in large part the nature of the speech understanding problems experienced by older adults. The classic complaint of older adults with presbycusis, namely "I can hear people talking but cannot understand what they are saying, especially in noisy situations," very aptly describes the problems that derive from the reduction in transmission, reception, and perception of the speech signal attributable to sensorineural hearing loss. In fact, these difficulties can easily be predicted from the speech banana and audiograms depicted in Figure 60-1. The speech banana shown in the left panel displays the frequency and intensity levels of typical sounds necessary for speech understanding. Ordinary conversation or the normal speech spectrum is carried out within the range of frequencies from 250 to 6,000 Hz and within the range of decibels from 20 to 60 dBHL. Consonant sounds and diphthongs such as "s," "sh," "th," "k," "t," "p," and "g" are relatively high in frequency or pitch and low in intensity or loudness. Conversely, vowel sounds such as "a," "i," "o," and "u" are concentrated in the lower frequencies and are somewhat higher in intensity.[14] Environmental noise is high in intensity and low in frequency as well. Audibility of the consonant sounds is critical to the understanding of speech. The middle panel depicts a typical hearing loss characterizing older adults suffering from presbycusis.[14]

Those sounds falling below the threshold symbolized by the connected circles are audible (e.g., m, n, e, r, p), whereas those falling above are inaudible (s, t, th). For most older adults with age-related hearing loss, consonants with energy in the high frequencies are frequently inaudible, rendering speech understanding difficult. This difficulty comprehending ordinary conversation is exacerbated in a noisy room, as background noise tends to be audible given good low-frequency hearing, yet consonant sounds important to understanding are inaudible. Further, older adults with good low-frequency hearing can perceive vowels well, even though they may have difficulty with consonant sounds.[14] As a result, older adults claim that they can hear people talking (vowels audible) but they cannot make out the words (consonants inaudible). The goal of hearing aids is to bring consonants into the audible range without amplifying the already audible noise and vowel sounds. This is shown in the right-hand panel in Figure 60-1. Note that the circles in the frequencies above 1,000 Hz, which represent aided air conduction thresholds, are now better than (above) the speech sounds depicted in the banana. The hearing aid has rendered the high-frequency sounds audible.

PSYCHOSOCIAL CONSEQUENCES OF DECREMENTS IN PURE-TONE SENSITIVITY AND SPEECH UNDERSTANDING

The behavioral implications of the speech understanding difficulties characterizing older adults are numerous for the individual, family members, the functioning of nursing facilities, and potentially for society at large. In general, hearing loss in older adults restricts one or more dimensions of quality of life including physical functional status, and cognitive, emotional, and social function.[15–18] Specifically, hearing impairment has been shown to:

* Negatively impact on communicative behavior
* Alter psychosocial behavior
* Strain family relations
* Limit the enjoyment of daily activities
* Jeopardize physical well-being
* Interfere with the ability to live independently and safely
* Interfere with long distance contacts on the telephone, potentially jeopardizing safety and security
* Interfere with medical diagnosis, treatment, and management
* Interfere with compliance with pharmacological regimens, and
* Interfere with therapeutic interventions across all disciplines including social work, speech-language therapy, and physical or occupational therapy

An interesting aspect of the hearing impairment that afflicts older adults is the large variability in response to a given hearing loss. Two individuals with the same level of hearing loss (e.g., mild) will react very differently and will experience different behavioral consequences. Accordingly it is imperative that included in the complete hearing assessment is quantification of the perceived handicapping effects of a given hearing loss on communication and social and emotional function. Items comprising the long or shortened versions of the Hearing

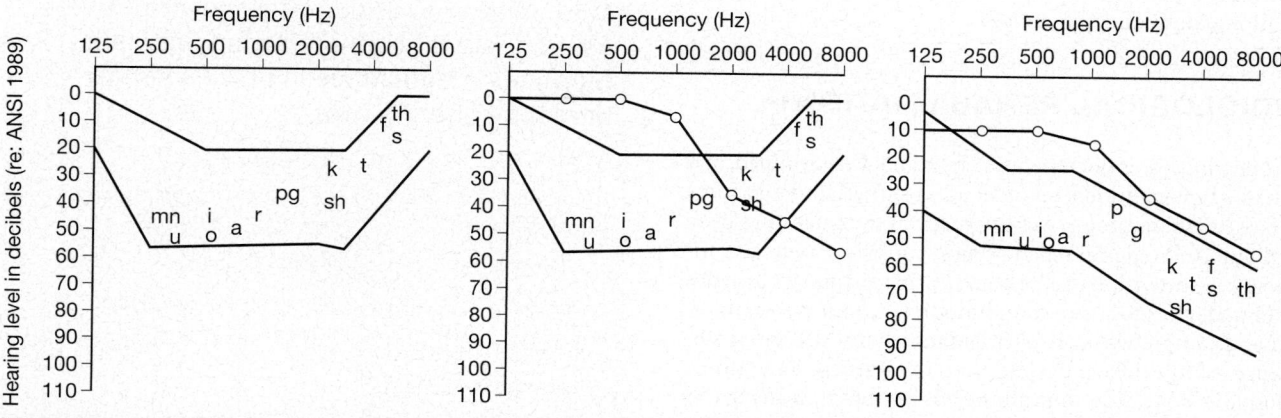

Figure 60-1 Air conduction thresholds of typical presbycusic hearing loss shown relative to typical speech sounds. Also shown are aided air conduction thresholds. (From Bess and Humes[14] with permission.)

Table 60-1 Screening version of the hearing handicap inventory for the elderly (HHIE-S)

Instructions: Answer Yes (4 points), Sometimes (2 points), or No (0 points) for each question. If you are a hearing aid user answer questions according to how you hear with the hearing aid. If the question does not apply merely enter no as your response.

E-1. Does a hearing problem cause you to feel embarrassed when meeting new people?

E-2. Does a hearing problem cause you to feel frustrated when talking to members of your family?

S-1. Do you have difficulty hearing when someone speaks in a whisper?

E-3. Do you feel handicapped by a hearing problem?

S-2. Does a hearing problem cause you difficulty when visiting friends, relatives, or neighbors?

S-3. Does a hearing problem cause you to attend religious services less often than you would like?

E-4. Does a hearing problem cause you to have arguments with family members?

S-4. Does a hearing problem cause you difficulty when listening to TV or radio?

E-5. Do you feel that any difficulty with your hearing limits or hampers your personal or social life?

S-5. Does a hearing problem cause you difficulty when in a restaurant with relatives or friends?

Abbreviations: S, items probe social/situational consequences of hearing loss; E, items probe emotional consequences of hearing loss.

Handicap Inventory for the Elderly (HHIE) are ideal for assessing the perceived handicapping effects of hearing loss. Table 60-1 contains the items comprising the 10-item screening version (HHIE-S).[19] The HHIE/HHIE-S have high test–retest reliability, excellent internal consistency reliability and adequate content, construct, and predictive validity.[19,20] Scores on the questionnaire are highly predictive of hearing aid use such that individuals obtaining a score of 18 or greater on the HHIE-S are considered hearing aid candidates who are likely to purchase and benefit from hearing aid use, irrespective of hearing loss severity. A web site containing the screening version of the Hearing Handicap Inventory for the Elderly can easily be accessed at www.Ph.D.msu.edu/hearing. The web-based version has links to nationwide audiology services.

AUDIOLOGICAL REHABILITATION

Once hearing loss is documented, the etiology determined, and the handicap quantified, an older adult should undergo some form of rehabilitation, assuming medical treatment has been ruled out. Audiological rehabilitation consists of several components: (1) provision of a custom hearing aid and/or assistive listening devices to make sounds audible, comfortable, tolerable, and comprehensible; (2) orientation to the use and maintenance of the hearing aids; and (3) patient and family counseling/education to promote adjustment to hearing loss use of hearing aids and assistive devices.[20a] The greatest barrier to audiological rehabilitation is lack of awareness or acceptance of hearing loss combined with societal agism about the necessity to hear well as we age. Of the components of audiological

rehabilitation, the provision of a hearing aid in the context of a brief counseling session is the most beneficial, improving hearing-related quality of life.[21]

HEARING TECHNOLOGIES
Hearing aids

A host of audiological and nonaudiological variables interact to determine hearing aid candidacy, hearing aid satisfaction, and hearing aid benefit. These include but are not limited to the following: auditory, physical, sociological, psychological, cognitive, and environmental factors. With regard to auditory variables, sensorineural hearing loss of nearly any degree can be remediated via a hearing aid, assuming the client is interested in pursuing amplification. Clinical experience suggests that motivation is one of the most important, yet least well understood, psychological factors that affects rehabilitation potential in general and hearing aid candidacy in particular.[22] It explains why behavior is initiated, why it persists, and why

---

Summary of management algorithm
Technological options

Mild, moderate, moderately severe, severe sensorineural hearing loss, and speech recognition difficulties in quiet and noise

Hearing aids (analog, digitally programmable analog, digital):

- Behind-the-ear
- In-the-ear
- In-the-canal
- Completely in-the-canal

Post-lingual profound sensorineural hearing loss with extreme difficulty understanding speech using hearing aids

Cochlear implant

Mild, moderate, moderately severe, severe sensorineural hearing loss, and speech recognition difficulties in noise—needs unmet by hearing aids

Assistive listening devices:

- Personal listening system (e.g., remote microphone FM system)
- TV listening system (e.g., infrared system)
- Telephone devices (e.g., TDD, telephone amplifiers)
- Interactive pagers
- Fax machines, e-mail
- Alerting devices
- Auditorium-type assistive listening systems

it is attenuated. Motivation to pursue intervention is optimal when an individual (1) knows what he or she wants; (2) expects it can be attained; (3) believes that the rewards are meaningful; and (4) considers that intervention takes place at a reasonable cost.[22] It is incumbent on the audiologist to understand the patient's motivations for pursuing a hearing aid so as to ensure that their needs and expectations are fulfilled. Motivation to purchase amplification can be optimized by emphasizing the positive consequences associated with a hearing aid purchase and instilling realistic expectations regarding the advantages and disadvantages associated with hearing aid use.[22]

Irrespective of the hearing aid style, the philosophy governing all hearing aid fittings is that electroacoustic characteristics should be selected that (1) maximize speech recognition, (2) provide good sound quality, and (3) provide for amplification that is comfortable and compensates for the loss of loudness resulting from the impaired hearing.[23] Simply put, an optimal hearing aid fitting is one that makes speech audible without exceeding the listener's loudness discomfort level and restores the normal loudness relations for speech and other environmental sounds.[24] Prior to selecting the electroacoustic characteristics, hearing aid style and arrangement must be mutually agreed upon.

Hearing aids are basically miniature public address systems with several key components. The components are listed in Table 60-2. The amplifier, along with the microphone, receiver, and battery, make up the central core. In large part, the quality of the signal processing accomplished by the amplifier determines how well a person with handicapping hearing impairment will function with a hearing instrument. An important function of the amplifier, in combination with the receiver and earmold/molded piece, which deliver sound to the ear, is to limit the maximum amount of amplification the user receives. This function is critical as it will minimize the possibility of hearing aid rejection because sound is uncomfortably loud. The size, style, and amplifier type determine which battery powers the hearing aid. All hearing aids take

1.4 volt batteries and at the time the hearing aid is dispensed, the audiologist will advise consumers on the correct battery type for the particular unit. The American Association of Retired Persons is one of the least expensive sources for purchasing batteries.

A variety of hearing aid styles is available to the hearing-impaired older adult once it is mutually decided that hearing aids are the appropriate intervention. The variety of styles available to the consumer is listed in Table 60-3. The simplest way to categorize hearing aids is by the place on the body the hearing aid is worn. The largest and least popular style hearing aid is the body aid. Custom in-the-ear (ITE) hearing aids, which include in-the ear (ITE), in-the-canal (ITC), and completely in-the canal (CIC) represent the largest market share. According to a recent survey of hearing instrument dispensers, 78 percent of all hearing aids sold in 2001 were ITE units and 27 percent were behind-the-ear devices.[2] Approximately, 58 percent of all hearing aids sold in the USA in 2001 were digitally programmable; 30 percent of these were digitally programmable analog units and 19.9 percent were digital signal processing units. Programmable hearing aids have greater flexibility and range over all of the traditional frequencies and intensities typically amplified.[25] In general, programmable instruments employ different circuit options to achieve a variety of sound qualities and performance characteristics. With programmable instruments, hearing aid users have the ability to custom tailor the hearing instrument to their lifestyle, enabling them to benefit from amplification in situations in which previously a hearing aid may have been unusable.[25] Similarly, the dispenser can adjust the low frequencies independent of the high frequencies depending on the hearing configuration and the nature of the input sound, providing for improved speech understanding in favorable and unfavorable listening environments.[25] Table 60-4 contrasts the circuitry available for persons deciding on a hearing aid. As is evident, hearing aids can be classified according to whether they are fully analog, analog with digital control circuits which are fully programmable, or digital. Most hearing aids dispensed today are analog; however, the proportion of dispensers offering and selling digital technology is growing. Anecdotal reports suggest that the hearing impaired favor the digital technology for ease of understanding speech in noise; however, this has not been borne out by systematic investigations. Dual microphone hearing aids which allow the user to switch between an omnidirectional (sensitive to sounds from all directions) or a directional microphone (suppress sounds in the rear) are proving quite effective for individuals having difficulty understanding speech in noise. Currently, directional microphones, whether incorporated into analog or directional hearing aids are the most effective tools for overcoming the detrimental effects of noise.

Custom ITE hearing aids range in size and are identified according to their physical location and their dimensions within the concha of the outer ear or pinna. Custom hearing aids (ITEs, ITCs, and CICs) are completely custom made, taking full advantage of the size and shape of an individual user's ear. For example, a full concha ITE hearing aid, shown in Figure 60-2, completely occupies the external portion of the pinna known as the concha. In contrast, a low-profile unit provides for less protrusion from the concha and a half concha

Table 60-2 Hearing aid components

Components	Function
Microphone	Converts incoming acoustic signals (sound) into an electrical signal
Amplifier	Increases the strength of the electrical signal. It selectively processes the microphone's output signal such that more emphasis tends to be given to high-frequency and weak sounds than to low-frequency intense sounds
Receiver	A miniature loudspeaker which converts the electrical signal back into an acoustic signal (sound)
Earmold/tubing	Delivers the acoustic signal to the hearing aid user's ear(s) or couples the amplified sound into the ear canal
Battery	Provides the power needed by the amplifier

Table 60-3 Hearing aid styles[a]

Style	Characteristics	Candidate	Cost
Behind-the-ear (BTE) units are the largest hearing aids in general use (body aids are rarely recommended). Circuitry is housed in plastic banana-shaped case worn behind the ear and sound is conveyed acoustically by way of a tube which carries a sound to the earmold	Most powerful, least expensive, and most durable of available devices. Larger than in-the-ear units, easy to adjust, easy to change battery	For people with limited dexterity, mild to profound hearing loss Dominant style sold in Europe (65% of European Sales in 2001)	Average cost can range from $796 for an analog nonprogrammable unit to $2,800 for a digital signal processing programmable device with a directional microphone. Analog programmable units can cost between $1,100 to $1,500
In-the-ear (ITE) units are one-piece devices custom fit to the contour of the ear. They are seated in the outer cavity of the ear. All components are built into the shell of a custom mold from an impression of the user's ear(s)	The volume control and battery door are on the faceplate or outer surface of the hearing aids	Can be bulky and the ear can feel uncomfortable in warm weather. Good for persons with mild to moderate hearing loss	Average cost can range from $803 for an analog nonprogrammable device to $2,286 for a digital signal processing programmable unit. Analog programmables cost between $1,150 to $1,550
In-the-canal (ITC) units are about the size of a quarter. They are custom made to fit into the outer one-third or cartilaginous part of the ear canal. All components are housed within the plastic sitting in the canal	Less visible than BTE and ITE and more powerful than CIC hearing aids	Volume control can be difficult to adjust for people with manual dexterity problems or reduced sensation in finger tips. Difficult to insert battery, prone to excessive wax build-up	Average cost can range from $961 for an analog nonprogrammable device to $2,438 for a digital signal processing programmable unit. Analog programmable units cost between $1,300 unit and $1,700
Completely-in-the canal (CIC) units are about the size of a jellybean. All components fit within a plastic shell, molded to fit deep within the ear canal extending into the bony portion	Least visible, a small knob is placed on the end for removal	Difficult to position and remove from the ear. Volume control can be difficult to adjust, although digital circuitry automatically adjusts volume	Average cost can range from $1,300 for an analog nonprogrammable device to $2,700 for a digital signal processing programmable unit. Analog programmable devices cost between $1,600 and $2,000

[a] *Body aids and eyeglass aids are omitted as they represent an extremely small share of the hearing aid market.*

only fills a portion of the concha, namely the concha cavum and the ear canal. Half conchas are smaller and less flexible in that they contain less complicated circuitry and take a smaller size battery (e.g. 312 batteries). Full conchas, on the other hand, are larger, allow for more complex circuit designs, and take a larger battery cell (e.g. #13). ITC hearing aids are smaller than ITE units, having most of their components within the cartilaginous portion of the ear canal. Figure 60-3 shows a canal hearing aid in the user's ear. For the most part, ITCs use small 312 batteries or even smaller size cells (i.e., #10). CIC hearing aids have all of their electronic components deep within the external auditory canal terminating close to the tympanic membrane. Figure 60-4 displays a CIC hearing aid with its tiny components relative to a dime and Figure 60-5 shows a CIC in the user's ear. The only piece visible is the thin piece of plastic extending outward from the faceplate of the hearing aid, which is used to remove the unit. The microphone of CIC hearing aids is located deep in the ear canal providing for a natural high-frequency boost, less wind noise, and

theoretically better speech understanding because of the acoustic advantage provided by the outer ear. CICs use very small batteries, either A10 or A5. Zinc–air batteries, which use zinc and oxygen as their negative and positive electrodes, respectively, are the preferred battery type as they are cheaper and do not have to be changed as often as mercury batteries. Mercury batteries have more adverse environmental consequences than zinc–air batteries when they are discarded. Special devices are now available to assist elderly people to independently insert and remove the small batteries.

Behind-the-ear (BTE) hearing instruments were the hearing aid of choice for hearing impaired consumers in the 1980s and are now enjoying a resurgence. BTEs are ideal for hearing-impaired persons who require high gain (50–70 dBSPL), a strong telecoil for telephone use, larger controls for independent manipulation, or special microphone arrays. Two additional advantages include their flexibility and compatibility with direct audio input microphones. Often, residents of nursing facilities use BTE hearing instruments because of a

Table 60-4 Hearing aid circuitry

Analog	Most basic and least expensive circuitry. Can be adjusted to amplify the range of frequencies most important for speech understanding. Amplifies all sounds, and can mute some background noise. Hearing aid response is changed via screwdriver potentiometers	The electrical voltage is analogous to the acoustic sound pressure. When the sound pressure increases from moment to moment, the electrical signal does, as well.[25] Good for first time hearing aid users
Programmable	Contain a computer chip that stores programs that amplify selected frequencies. Can be reprogrammed as hearing loss severity and configuration change. Parameters of the hearing aids (i.e., frequency emphasis, noise suppression) can be changed electronically through programming. More flexible than analog, fewer mechanical parts so less likely to break down than analog	Remote controls are often used to enable the client or clinician to manipulate the parameters of the hearing aid for different listening needs. They typically employ digital technology to shape and manipulate a signal that has been amplified using analog technology. Contain an analog sound path yet digital control circuits contained within the hearing aid are used to control the characteristics of each of the analog signal processing blocks (e.g., frequency, gain)[25]
Digital signal processing	Greater sound precision, less internal noise. Conversion to a digital form is free of noise and allows for sound to be manipulated in just about any way (i.e., extremely flexible in terms of frequencies amplified, noise suppression, power, etc.). Increasingly, digital aids are gaining a power and size advantage over analog devices	Contain a computer chip which does the work of the amplifier in place of traditional analog circuitry. The digital signal processor performs arithmetic functions to manipulate sound. Difficult to use with cellular phones!

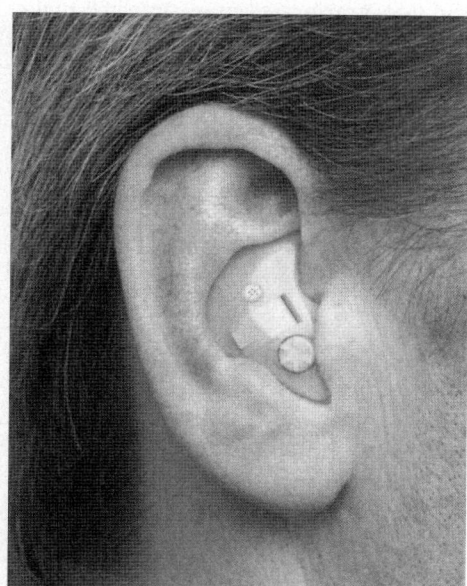

Figure 60-2 In-the-ear hearing aid shown in a user's ear. (Courtesy of Rexton, Inc.)

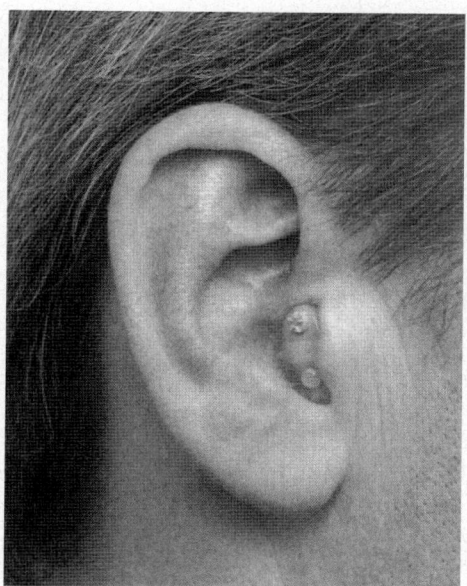

Figure 60-3 Canal hearing aid shown in a user's ear. (Courtesy of Rexton, Inc.)

long history of hearing aid use and because some individuals consider them easier to manipulate and insert comfortably in the ear. It is important to ensure that the earmold is comfortable and rests securely in the ear. New earmolds should be made by the audiologist when the mold routinely becomes unseated or when acoustic feedback is consistently audible. The earmold and hearing aid arrangement should be checked annually to make sure that the hearing-impaired individual is still using the hearing aid and that it is still operating according to

manufacturer specifications. Ideally, the check should be scheduled after 11 months of hearing aid use, as this is within the 1-year warranty period and the consumer is entitled to a free hearing aid overhaul. The latter applies to all hearing aid styles and users.

As is evident from Table 60-3, the average price of a monaural hearing aid in 2000 varied according to the style and the circuitry. It is noteworthy that the cost of hearing aids differs dramatically by dispenser, as well. The average overall price in

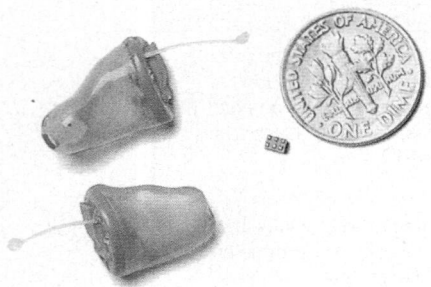

Figure 60-4 Completely in-the-canal hearing aid. (Courtesy of Rexton, Inc.)

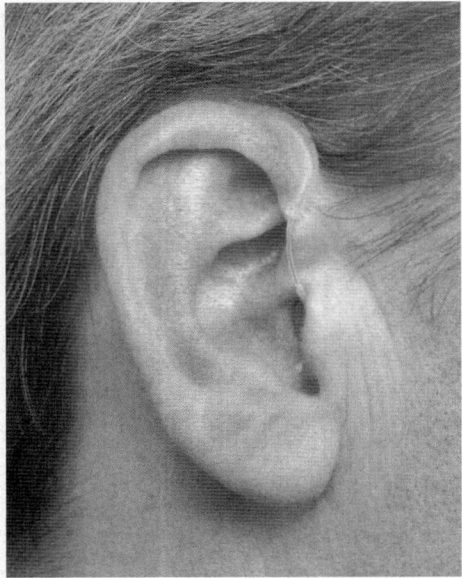

Figure 60–5 Completely in-the-canal hearing aid shown in a user's ear. (Courtesy of Rexton, Inc.)

2000 for an analog nonprogrammable in-the-canal hearing aid was ($1,061) when purchased from a hearing instrument specialist and $938 when purchased from an audiologist. The average price for a digital signal processing programmable BTE hearing aid was $2,396 from a hearing instrument specialist, $2,131 from an audiologist. In part, hearing aids are more costly from hearing instrument specialists because dispensing audiologists tend to charge a separate dispensing fee, whereas hearing instrument specialists tend to bundle professional services into their costs.[26] The considerable financial investment associated with the purchase of hearing aids underlines the importance of referring the consumer to a qualified professional who spends time dispensing the product and orienting the individual and family members to the hearing aid in an effort to optimize the fit.[27] Finally, with the exception of cochlear implant surgery for severely and profoundly impaired individuals, support for hearing care is modest or unavailable in most health plans. However, recently selected managed care plans have introduced some, albeit minimal, coverage toward the purchase of a hearing instrument.

Despite some limitations in their ability to separate out speech from noise, hearing aids have been shown to provide short- and long-term quality-of-life improvements. Hearing aids reduce the social, emotional, and communication dysfunction perceived by older adults with mild to moderately severe sensorineural hearing loss after 6 weeks of hearing aid use and these benefits are sustained after 1 year of use.[15] Compared with the waiting list group, those older adults who received hearing aids demonstrated an 85 percent improvement in social and emotional function, a 68 percent improvement in communication function, and a 26 percent improvement in depressive symptoms as assessed by the Geriatric Depression Scale.[15] Another group of investigators has demonstrated that hearing aids, in conjunction with audiologic rehabilitation, effectively improve psychosocial well-being of persons with handicapping hearing loss.[28] Finally, it has recently been demonstrated that improvements in psychosocial well-being and communication function associated with short-term hearing aid use are comparable for older and younger adults.[29] This finding is an important step toward dispelling the myth that older adults cannot derive significant benefits from hearing aids. Data from a 1999 study completed by the National Council on Aging (NCOA) revealed that hearing aid users are less depressed and more socially engaged than are older adults with comparable hearing loss who do not use hearing aids. Further, the NCOA study revealed that non-hearing-aid users report more negative social effects of hearing loss than users and non-hearing-aid users reported higher levels of anger and frustration than hearing aid users. Finally, it is noteworthy that non-hearing-aid users with significant hearing loss tended to report a loss of interest in activities that at one time gave them pleasure.[29a]

Counseling/hearing aid orientation

When people first put hearing aids in the ear, their own voice and that of others sound very strange.[30] Their own voices tend to have a hollow booming quality as if talking from the bottom of a barrel. The audiologist can make the necessary adjustments to eliminate this sensation. To ensure maximal benefit from hearing aids, older adults must have realistic expectations and patience. Of utmost importance, the new hearing aid user must understand that hearing aids "are not very smart," that they do not always do a good job of discriminating between desirable sounds persons want to hear (i.e., speech) and those undesirable sounds they want to ignore (i.e., background noise).[30] However, this situation is slowly changing with the advent of digital hearing aids and the development of more sophisticated electronics. New hearing aid users should not expect to suddenly hear normally. They should, however, expect to have a reduction in the degree of difficulty they have been having, depending on the acoustics of the listening situation.

Hearing aid users must understand that it takes time to realize the potential benefit from hearing aids, and thus should not become discouraged early. Their ears and their brains must become "re-educated" to hearing selected patterns of sounds that have been made louder by the hearing aid.[30] In a sense, new hearing aid users are suddenly being exposed to or "bombarded with" a world of sounds they have forgotten existed, such as the blare of street noises in the city, and must become reoriented to or acquainted with the location and source of these "new" sounds. To facilitate adaptation to the hearing aid, new hearing users should wear the hearing aids for as many hours during the day that they feel comfortable with the units in their ears. It is advisable that new hearing aid users wear their hearing aids in restricted situations at first, such as while at home with family members, while watching the television, or while eating dinner. Once the individual feels comfortable with amplified sound at home, he or she should venture into new hearing situations, at all times experimenting with the volume control to maintain speech input at a comfortable level and noise at a minimum. Although full-time use should be the goal, there are some exceptions. Persons with mild hearing loss may find their hearing aids useful in business meetings, but may find them burdensome in noisy situations such as restaurants or parties. If patients complain that some intense sounds produce an uncomfortably loud hearing sensation, they should alert the dispensing audiologist at the follow-up visit as a simple adjustment can usually be made to the hearing aid. Many hearing aid users report that although at first they prefer "natural sounding" louder sounds as their ears and mind adjust, they tend to prefer a boost in the high-frequency response of the hearing aid that makes the consonants of speech crisper and easier to understand.[30] It is of utmost importance that new hearing aid users schedule and keep all follow-up appointments (a minimum of 2–4 weeks following receipt of the hearing aid) so that the audiologist can make the necessary adjustments to ensure that sounds are comfortable, audible, tolerable, and understandable. At these visits, the audiologist and new hearing aid user work together to modify the response of the hearing aid for optimal speech understanding. Finally, new hearing aid users should accept their hearing loss and not continue to consider it a disgrace or a stigma. They should not cover their hearing aids as a way of hiding the hearing loss, as hearing aids serve as a signal to others that a hearing loss exists and that they should speak clearly to facilitate speech understanding. According to Ross,[30] an experienced and successful hearing aid

Summary of management algorithm Counseling strategies

Mild, moderate, moderately severe, severe sensorineural hearing loss, and speech recognition difficulties in quiet and noise— new hearing aid user

Counseling:

- Understanding hearing loss
- Accepting handicapping effects of hearing loss
- Overcoming obstacles posed by hearing loss
- Orientation to hearing aids
- Care and maintenance of hearing aids
- Communication skills training—hearing strategies
- Auditory-visual integration training (speech-reading tactics)

Table 60-5 Helpful hints for adjusting to hearing aids

- Allow time to adjust to the hearing aid
- Take advantage of the services of the hearing aid dispenser (e.g., audiologist or hearing instrument specialist)
- Do not get discouraged if the hearing aid does not restore hearing to normal
- Return to the dispenser for reassurance and counseling regarding realistic expectations. Understand that hearing aids will not restore hearing capabilities to normal.
- Allow time to adjust as hearing aids do require time to get used to and to attain maximum performance potential
- At first, wear the hearing aid for as many hours during day as comfortable, part time use may be preferable for some
- Gradually adjust to loud, incoming signals by first using the hearing aid in quiet and small groups. Later moving to larger, less favorable listening situations
- Maintain a diary of listening experiences to share with the audiologist
- Realistic expectations are critical to success
- Family members must adapt their speaking techniques to promote better speech understanding

user and audiologist, the hearing impaired should not worry about people seeing their hearing aids. If the hearing aid users accept their hearing loss and hearing aids, so will persons to whom they are speaking. In short, acceptance of hearing loss, and motivation to overcome its consequences, are conditions for hearing aid satisfaction and success.

The points mentioned above are typically discussed at the individual hearing aid follow-up appointment but are also emphasized in a group hearing aid orientation program made available to consumers upon the purchase of hearing instruments. Although not all professionals provide orientation programs, the consumer organization Self Help For Hard of Hearing People, Inc. (SHHH) recently recommended that all hearing aid dispensers make available and encourage participation in group programs. Group orientation programs should be short term (3–6 weeks), and should provide sufficient time for an instructional component and for the emergence of group exchanges.[31] The instructional component should include (1) discussions about hearing loss and the audiogram; (2) instructions in troubleshooting with hearing aids; (3) discussions about the availability of assistive listening devices to supplement hearing aids; (4) an introduction to speech reading/auditory training; and (5) an overview of coping and conversational repair strategies to facilitate communication. Recently, a few investigators have demonstrated that short-term group programs do in fact promote hearing aid benefit among new hearing aid users above that achieved with just one orientation session. Some helpful hints for adjusting to hearing aids are included in Table 60-5.

Assistive listening devices

Very often hearing aids do not provide for the easy clear listening one desires in all communication environments. The major reason for the lack of a clear acoustic signal in selected situations is that the speech signal (S) is much louder than the background noise (N) yielding an unfavorable S/N ratio.[32] People with normal hearing require the signal to be twice as intense as background noise for speech to be intelligible, whereas people with hearing loss require the primary signal to be 10 times more intense than background sounds to enable them to detect word/sound distinctions, etc. Well-fit hearing aids can provide a favorable S/N ratio if the environment is free of distractions and if the speaker is close to the person with hearing impairment. For the most part, however, the hearing aid microphone at the listener's ear is typically some distance from the sound source, making speech difficult to understand. In essence, the further away from the sound source one is, the softer the sound pressure and the less clear the speech signal.[32] For the most part the listening environments we live in are demanding, and hearing aids alone are insufficient to access auditory events that are not close to the person who is hearing impaired. The use of alternative hearing technologies, known as assistive listening devices, has proven invaluable in overcoming some of the environmental barriers to successful communication. Four categories of devices are available including (1) sound enhancement technology, (2) television enhancement technology, (3) telecommunications technology, and (4) signal alerting technology.[32]

Sound enhancement technologies enable a person with hearing impairment to understand speech clearly when the speaker is at a considerable distance from the listener. This is accomplished by transmitting the signal directly to the ear of the listener, thereby overcoming the barriers posed by distance and environmental noise. Sound enhancement technologies include a remote microphone, placed close to the sound source (within 6 inches), which picks up the signal and via one of several modes of transmission, sends the signal to the listener's ear(s). Signals can be transmitted to the listener via a hard-wired connection between the microphone/amplifier/receiver and the headphones, via wireless radio transmission of signals (i.e., FM unit), via an induction loop system, or via infrared light.

Hard-wired systems that are commercially available and relatively inexpensive (under $50) are ideal in one-to-one situations as in a physician's office, or when being interviewed by a nurse or social worker.[18] Personal FM systems that must be fit by an audiologist are more costly (i.e., greater than $500) yet can facilitate large and small group communication as well as classroom listening. FM systems can be used outdoors and when the speaker and listener are in different rooms. FM systems are widely used by hearing impaired individuals who are members of SHHH. BTE/FM hearing aids have recently been introduced and represent a cosmetically appealing way to enhance speech understanding in a noisy background using an ear-level array (otherwise FM systems require a body-worn receiver that connects in one of several ways to a personal hearing aid). In this arrangement the FM receiver and a conventional hearing aid are both incorporated in a BTE case such that the BTE/FM system can be used as a regular hearing aid, as an FM receiver, or as both together.[33] Older hearing-impaired adults with severe sensorineural hearing loss and/or auditory processing problems should inquire about the availability of BTE/FM systems. They have proven beneficial in restaurants, at lectures, in cars, and at noisy receptions. With this arrangement the FM microphone transmitter is worn close to the source of speech (speaker), and the signal is delivered via FM signals to the listener's ears free of environmental noise. Finally, infrared systems use invisible light, the wavelength of which is outside the range of human visibility, to transmit signals indoors in a single room from the speaker to the listener.[18]

The sound enhancement technology described above can be used with different forms of media including television, stereo systems, and video cassette recorders. Infrared systems provide the best quality sound for radio and television, and are widely used in theaters and concert and lecture halls. Essentially the remote microphone of the system is placed within 6 inches of the media speaker to provide a favorable S/N ratio. Telecaptioning or dialog in the form of captions that run across the bottom of the television screen can also assist in television enjoyment for persons with severe to profound hearing loss. All new televisions manufactured today include telecaptioning capabilities.

Telecommunication technology facilitates communication over the telephone. Options include portable or built-in amplifiers, speakerphones, fax machines, and telecommunication systems for the deaf (TDD). TDDs are invaluable to persons with severe to profound hearing loss for whom it is impossible to discriminate speech over the telephone. TDDs are approximately the size of a typewriter. Individuals communicating over the telephone merely type in their message, or use a relay operator who types in a message, and it is displayed across the listener's TDD. The telephone company provides relay service free of charge for persons wishing to speak with a TDD user. E-mail is also an excellent form of telecommunication technology for persons with hearing impairment unable to communicate comfortably over the telephone. Interactive pagers which offer electronic mail, two-way messaging, fax service and traditional paging have proven to be effective forms of mobile communication for the hearing impaired especially because digital wireless technology is for the most part incompatible with hearing aids and other forms of assistive technology. Finally, signal-alerting technology includes any system that warns, signals, or alerts a person with a hearing loss. They use loud sounds, visual signals, or tactile signals to alert the hearing impaired to sounds in the environment. For example, a vibrator placed under the pillow can awaken the person with hearing loss in the morning, or a strobe light attached to a smoke alarm can alert the hearing impaired person to a fire.[32] Signal-alerting devices are commercially available and are invaluable for hearing-impaired persons who are homebound, for persons with cognitive impairments, and for residents of nursing facilities who cannot hear external events due to hearing loss. Audiologists are well equipped to guide persons and institutions about the system(s) that will best meet their needs and to arrange for the purchase of the necessary assistive listening devices. The hearing impaired often times have to be proactive about assistive techonologies as audiologists sometimes underestimate their value.

SCREENING PROTOCOLS

In light of the psychosocial consequences of acquired hearing loss, and the variety of technologies available to overcome communication difficulties, a variety of major authorities have recently advocated routine screening for hearing impairment among older adults. The American Academy of Family Physicians and US Preventive Services Task Force recommend that persons over 65 years of age undergo periodic hearing evaluations and counseling regarding the availability of hearing aids.[34,35] The Canadian Task Force on the Periodic Health Examination suggests that a hearing screen be considered part of the periodic health examination.[36] Finally, the US Public Health Service recommends that older adults should be questioned about signs of hearing loss.[37] They suggest that a screening questionnaire may be used to screen for communication problems, and social and emotional handicaps stemming from hearing loss. Questionnaires have the advantage of identifying patients who perceive hearing loss to be a problem and who therefore may be particularly motivated to use a hearing aid. They strongly recommend that persons found to have evidence of hearing loss by screening be considered for referral to a specialist, not a hearing aid dealer, for comprehensive audiological evaluation, especially if they feel handicapped by the hearing loss. Because the point of entry into the hearing healthcare system usually involves the primary care physician, he or she has a critical role to play in identifying older persons with handicapping hearing impairments.

A simple, reliable, and valid screening program has been advocated by a number of investigators.[19,38,39] The procedure entails a pure-tone screen and administration of the 10-item screening version of the Hearing Handicap Inventory for the Elderly (HHIE-S). The purpose of the screen should be to identify older persons with handicapping hearing impairment who require audiological testing and intervention.[40] The pure-tone screen involves use of the Audioscope, a hand-held otoscope combined with a screening audiometer that delivers pure tones at 40 dBHL at four frequencies: 500, 1,000, 2,000, and 4,000 Hz. The current cost of the Audioscope is within the range of $500 to $600. A patient fails the screen if he or she does not hear the tones at 1,000 or 2,000 Hz in one or both ears. The patient is instructed to raise his or her finger or hand when the tone is heard. The patient's response should be time-locked to the presentation of the stimulus signaled by a red indicator light on the Audioscope. If otoscopic examination indicates the presence of cerumen impaction, this necessitates a failure and a referral.

Prior to or following the pure-tone screen, the patient should complete the HHIE-S using a face-to-face, paper-and-pencil or computer-assisted presentation. A score of 10 or greater signifies the necessity of a referral. More specifically, scores of 0–8 signify no handicap, scores of 10–22 signify a mild to moderate handicap, and scores of 24–40 suggest significant self-perceived handicap. Scores on the HHIE-S are directly correlated to hearing aid uptake and have been shown to improve after the initiation of hearing aid use.[15] Primary care physicians with first-hand experience with this screening protocol consider it to be simple, cost-effective, quick, and easy to administer.[39]

Fino et al.[41] were among the first investigators to demonstrate that hearing aid candidacy is directly linked to the prefitting score on the HHIE-S.[41] Specifically, they found that the extent of self-perceived hearing handicap on the 10-item (HHIE-S) is predictive of hearing aid candidacy, in that it reliably distinguishes between hearing aid users and nonusers. Irrespective of hearing level (e.g. mild or moderate sensorineural hearing loss), persons who obtain hearing aids tend to be more handicapped as evidenced by higher scores on the HHIE-S, than those who do not. On the average scores on the HHIE-S for new hearing aid users are approximately 18, irrespective of mean hearing level and mean word recognition

ability.[42] Persons with mild and moderately severe hearing levels present with comparable scores on the HHIE-S (i.e., 18). Similarly according to Newman and colleagues, persons with excellent and those with poor scores on a test of word recognition emerged with mean prefitting HHIE-S scores ranging from 16 to 18. Following 3 weeks of hearing aid use, all subjects experienced a dramatic improvement in scores on the HHIE-S such that average postfitting scores were approximately 3.[42] The latter studies demonstrate that self-perceived handicap, identified using a simple and easy screening tool, is linked to hearing aid use and is dramatically reduced following intervention. Weinstein devotes an entire chapter of her textbook to strategies for identifying older adults with hearing loss including multimedia and web based techniques.[43] The NIH website has a link to this chapter as well.

WHEN AND TO WHOM TO REFER

Audiologists and otolaryngologists are hearing healthcare specialists who provide assistance to persons with hearing problems. The otolaryngologist is a medical doctor whose goal is to identify and treat medical diseases of the ear that may be causing a hearing problem. If medical treatment in the form of antibiotic therapy or surgery is not indicated, the person with hearing loss should be seen by an audiologist.[40] The audiologist has a master's or doctoral degree and is trained to evaluate hearing sensitivity/auditory function and to provide services that will improve the ability to communicate. They administer pure-tone tests of middle and inner ear function and measures of speech understanding that help uncover peripheral or central auditory processing problems. Audiologists fit hearing aids in an attempt to help the hearing impaired overcome some of their speech understanding difficulties. Audiologists work in private practice, hospitals, clinics, or rehabilitation centers. Although audiologists can represent the point of entry into the hearing healthcare system, older adults referred to the audiologist by their physician are most likely to purchase audiological services in the form of hearing tests and hearing aids.[44] The latter underlines the role of the physician in assisting older adults in overcoming the effects of hearing loss. A list of three resources physicians may find useful for gaining additional information about hearing loss in older adults appears at the end of the chapter.

CONCLUDING REMARKS

Approximately 30–50 percent of older adults suffer from handicapping hearing impairment that can interfere with the quality of their lives. The advent of technologically sophisticated hearing aids that are more effective than ever before in separating out the speech from noise are a boon to older adults who are living longer and retiring early yet continue to be confronted by difficulty understanding the speech of others, especially in noise. Directional microphones had the key to overcoming the difficulty of understanding speech in noise.[45] Further, the availability of assistive listening devices that compensate for the shortcomings remaining with hearing aids is another avenue for persons with hearing impairment to pursue. The physician has a responsibility and tools in the form of a hand-held Audioscope or reliable and valid questionnaires to identify persons with hearing problems who require and can benefit from the expertise of audiologists. Physicians and audiologists are encouraged to work together to promote the quality of life of the increasing population of older adults suffering from handicapping hearing impairment.

KEY POINTS Disorders of hearing

■ Hearing loss prevalence increases with age such that over 50 percent of person over 80 years of age have a hearing impairment.

■ The majority of residents of nursing facilities have a hearing impairment.

■ The hearing impairment and speech understanding difficulties which are a hallmark of presbycusis are associated with significant functional effects including depression and isolation.

■ Presbycusis arises due to atrophic age related changes in the cochlea, auditory nerve fibers, auditory brainstem pathways and the temporal lobe of the brain.

■ Cerumen impaction is prevalent in older adults and can interfere with the proper functioning of hearing aids.

■ The sensorineural hearing loss affecting a high proportion of older adults is typically not amenable to medical intervention.

■ The most effective treatment for sensorineural hearing loss is hearing aids.

■ Hearing aids are efficacious in ameliorating the functional, social and emotional effects of hearing loss in older adults.

■ The most favorable outcomes with hearing aids take place when a hearing aid is delivered in the context of a counseling oriented rehabilitation program.

REFERENCES

1. National Health Interview Survey, Second Supplement on Aging: In Health, United States, 1999 with Health and Aging Chartbook. U.S. Dept. of Health and Human Services. September, 1999. DHHS Publication number (PHS) 99–1232

2. HJ Report: Hearing J 2001;55:21–34

2a. Popelka M, Cruickshanks K, Wiley T et al: Low prevalence of hearing aid use among older adults with hearing loss: The epidemiology of hearing loss study. J Am Geriatrics Soc 1998;46:1075–1078

2b. Rosenhall U, Jonsson R, Soderlind O: Self-assessed hearing problems in Sweden: A demographic study: Audiology 1999;38:328–334

3. Willott J: Aging and the Auditory System. Singular Publishing, San Diego, 1991

4. Moscicki E, Elkins E, Baum H, McNamara P: Hearing loss in the elderly: an epidemiologic study of the Framingham Heart Study Cohort. Ear Hearing 1985;6:184–190

5. Schuknecht H: Presbycusis. Laryngoscope 1955;65:402–419

6. Schuknecht H: Further observations on the pathology of presbycusis. Arch Otolaryngol 1964;80:369–382

7. Schuknecht H: Pathology of presbycusis. In Goldstein J, Kashima H, Koopman C (eds): Geriatric Otorhinolaryngology. B C Decker, Toronto, 1989

8. Schuknecht H: Pathology of the Ear, 2nd Ed. Lea & Febiger, Philadelphia, 1993

9. Otte J, Schuknecht H, Kerr A: Ganglion cell populations in normal and pathological human cochleae. Implications for cochlear implantation. Laryngoscope 1978;88:1231–1246

10. Crowe S, Guild S, Polvogt L: Observations on the pathology of high-tone deafness. Johns Hopkins Hosp Bull 1934;54:315–380

10a. Walton J, Burkhard R: Neurophysiological manifestations of aging in the peripheral and central auditory nervous system. Anatomical and neurochemical bases of presbycusis. In Hoff, P, Mobbs, C (eds): Functional Neurobiology of Aging. Academic Press, San Diego, CA, 2001:581–596

10b. Frisina R: Anatomical and neurochemical bases of presbycusis. In Hoff P, Mobbs C (eds): Functional Neurobiology of Aging. Academic Press, San Diego, CA, 2001:521–548

11. Hansen C, Reske-Nielsen E: Pathological studies in presbycusis. Arch Otolaryngol 1965;82:115–132

12. Cooper J: Health and Nutrition Examination Survey of 1971–75: Part I. Ear and race effects in hearing. J Am Acad Audiol 1994;5:30–36

13. Gates G, Cooper J, Kannel W, Miller N: Hearing in the elderly: the Framingham Cohort, 1983–1985. Part 1. Basic audiometric test results. Ear Hearing 1991;4:247–256

14. Bess F, Humes L: Audiology, the Fundamentals. 2nd Ed. Williams & Wilkins, Baltimore, 1995

15. Mulrow C, Aguilar C, Endicott J et al: Quality of life changes and hearing impairment: results of a randomized trial. Ann Intern Med 1990;113:188–194

16. Bess F, Lichtenstein M, Logan S: Hearing impairment as a determinant of function in the elderly. J Am Geriatr Soc 1989;37:123–128

17. Uhlmann R, Larson E, Koepsell T: Hearing impairment and cognitive decline in senile dementia of the Alzheimer's type. J Am Geriatr Soc 1986;34:207–210

18. Weinstein B: Auditory testing and rehabilitation of the hearing impaired. In Lubinski R (ed): Dementia and Communication. Singular Publishing, San Diego, 1995

19. Ventry I, Weinstein B: Identification of elderly individuals with hearing problems. ASHA 1983;25:37–42

20. Ventry I, Weinstein B: The hearing handicap inventory for the elderly: a new tool. Ear Hearing 1982;3:128–134

20a. Hanratty B. Lawlor D: Effective management of the elderly hearing impaired—a review. J Pub Health Med 2000;22:512–517 (review)

21. Lavizzo-Mourey R, Siegler F: Hearing impairment in the elderly. J Gen Intern Med 1992;7:191–198

22. Kemp B: The psychosocial context of geriatric rehabilitation. In Kemp K, Brummel-Smith K, Ramsdell J (eds): Geriatric Rehabilitation. Little Brown, Boston, 1990

23. McCandless G: Overview and rationale of threshold based hearing aid selection procedures. In Valente M (ed): Strategies for Selecting and Verifying Hearing Aid Fittings. Thieme-Medical Publishers, New York, 1996

24. Cox R, Alexander G: The abbreviated profile of hearing aid benefit. Ear Hearing 1995;16:176–186

25. Dillon H: Hearing Aids. Thieme Medical Publishers, New York, 2001

26. Kirkwood D: Most dispensers in Journal's survey report greater patient satisfaction with digitals. Hearing J 2001;54:21–32

27. Skafte M: The 1995 hearing instrument market—the dispenser's perspective. Hearing Rev 1996;3:16–34

28. Abrams H, Chisolm T, Guerreiro S, Ritterman S: The effects of intervention strategy on self perception of hearing handicap. Ear Hearing 1992;13:371–377

29. Primeau R: Hearing aid benefit in adults and older adults. In Weinstein B (ed): Seminars in Hearing. Thieme, NY, 1997

29a. Seniors Research Group. The consequences of untreated hearing loss in older persons. The National Council on the Aging. Washington, DC, 1999

30. Ross M: You've done something about it! Helpful hints to the new hearing aid user. SHHH J 1996;17:7–11

31. Self Help for Hard of Hearing People, Inc: Position statement on group hearing aid orientation programs. SHHH J 1996;17:29

32. Flexer C: Access to communication environments through assistive listening devices. Hearsay 1991;6:9–14

33. Ross M: Developments in research and technology. SHHH J 1995;16:32–34

34. American Academy of Family Physicians. Commission on Public Health and Scientific Affairs: Age Charts for Periodic Health Examination. American Academy of Family Physicians, Kansas City, MO, 1993

35. US Preventive Services Task Force: Screening for hearing impairment. In Guide to Clinical Preventive Services. Williams & Wilkins, Baltimore, 1989: Ch 33

36. Canadian Task Force on the Periodic Health Examination: The periodic health examination monograph. Quebec: Ministry: 2. 1984 update. Can Med Assoc J 1984;130:1278–1285

37. U.S. Public Health Service: The Clinician's Handbook of Preventive Services. International Medical Publishing, Virginia, 1994

38. Weinstein B: Validity of a screening protocol for identifying elderly people with hearing problems. ASHA 1986;28:41–45

39. Lichtenstein M, Bess F, Logan S: Validation of screening tools for identifying hearing-impaired elderly in primary care. JAMA 1988;259:2875–2878

40. Jerger J, Chmiel R, Wilson, Luchi R: Hearing impairment in older adults: new concepts. J Am Geriatr Soc 1995;43:928–935

41. Fino M, Bess F, Lichtenstein M, Logan S: Factors differentiating elderly hearing aid wearers and non-wearers. Hearing Instrum 1991;43:6–10

42. Newman C, Jacobson G, Hug G et al: Practical method for quantifying hearing aid benefit in older adults. J Am Acad Audiol 1991;2:70–75

43. Weinstein, B: Health promotion strategies for identifying older adults with handicapping hearing impairment. In: B. Weinstein (ed): Geriatric Audiology. Thieme Medical Publishers, New York, 2000

44. Whelan, C: Key trends are predicted for the next decade in the U.S. hearing aid industry. Hearing J 2001;54:32–35

45. Weinstein, B: Hearing aids in the elderly. Paper presented at N.J. Speech-Language Hearing Association Annual Meeting. Atlantic City, NJ, 2002

Sources of information about hearing loss and hearing aids

American Academy of Audiology: www.audiology.org
American Speech-Language-Hearing Association: www.asha.org
Self Help for Hard of Hearing People: www.shhh.org

Chapter 61

Delirium

Peter Pompei

Material in this chapter contains contributions from the previous edition, and we are grateful to the previous author for the work done.

Delirium is a transient mental syndrome characterized by global disorders of cognition (thinking, perception, memory) and attention (alertness, selectiveness, directiveness).[1,2] The term is derived from Latin where the prefix de- means "out of" and lira refers to "the ridge between two furrows of plowed land" so that together they can be interpreted to mean "off track."[3] The syndrome has been recognized and written about since antiquity. The seriousness of delirium in older persons was described in the aphorisms of Hippocrates, section IV, number 82: "Persons above forty years of age who are affected with frenzy, do not readily recover; the danger is less when the disease is cognate to the constitution and age."[4] Frenzy or phrenitis along with mania, melancholia, and paranoia constituted the major categories in the ancient Greek taxonomy of mental disorders. The presence of fever was an important factor in distinguishing agitated states secondary to physical illness (phrenitis) from those considered psychological in origin (mania).[5] Today, the term delirium often conjures up images of an individual withdrawing from alcohol who is agitated and hallucinating. In fact, this is only one phenotypic variant of a syndrome with diverse clinical manifestations. This variability in clinical presentation, especially among older persons, contributes significantly to the challenges of early recognition, diagnosis, and treatment.

Estimates of the prevalence of delirium vary considerably. In a study of residents of a large city in the eastern United States, 55 years of age and older, the prevalence of delirium was estimated to be about 1 percent.[6] In contrast, among nearly 200 persons 70 years or older seen in the emergency department of an academic medical center in an urban area, 24 percent were judged to have delirium.[7] Arguably, the best estimates of the frequency of delirium are from populations of hospitalized older persons who are being regularly monitored. Even among this group of persons, measurements of the prevalence of delirium range from 14 to 56 percent.[8] If we assume conservatively that 15 percent of older hospitalized persons experience delirium and recognize that, in the United States, 35 percent of older persons spend one or more days in the hospital each year,[9] we would estimate that at least 5 percent of all older Americans experience an episode of delirium each year. Operative therapy especially is associated with an increased risk of delirium. In a systematic review of postoperative delirium in all age groups, the estimated incidence was 36.8 percent (range 0–73.5 percent).[10] The large variance in the estimate of the incidence is due to a number of factors including: differences in definitions of the syndrome, differences in how cognitive changes are measured and differences in the timing of the measurements. Recent studies of postoperative cognitive impairments among older persons have identified a range of clinical syndromes, some of which persist for several months. The term postoperative cognitive dysfunction is being used to describe deficits as diverse as amnesia, concentration impairments, and delirium.[11]

CLINICAL FEATURES OF DELIRIUM

While there is considerable variability in the clinical features of delirium and in the severity of these features, certain manifestations are common. One should expect that patients with delirium will demonstrate perceptual disturbances and changes in level of consciousness. The mental image of the agitated patient suffering from alcohol withdrawal who has visions of wild animals in the room and bugs crawling on the skin helps reinforce the concept of altered perceptions. Older persons may experience more subtle illusions and hallucinations, and they may accommodate to them with less agitation and fear. Alterations in consciousness can range from a hyperalert state to somnolence. Patients who are withdrawn and tend to keep their bedclothes pulled up over their heads are as likely to be delirious as those who are aggressively defending themselves from the intrusion of hospital workers in their rooms. Many patients experience periods of both hypervigilance and somnolence. In a prospective study of delirium among older patients admitted to a general hospital for an acute medical problem, the frequencies of the subtypes were as follows: hyperactive, 15 percent; hypoactive, 19 percent; mixed, 52 percent; and neither 14 percent.[12]

Other characteristic clinical features of delirium are an acute onset, a fluctuating course, and disturbances of the sleep/wake cycle. Unlike the cognitive changes associated with dementia, in delirium the alterations often occur suddenly and may vary considerably over the course of the day. In a study of over 700 persons 75 years of age and older in institutional settings in Sweden, 37 percent of the 315 patients with delirium exhibited symptoms in the afternoon, evening or night, while 47 percent had predominantly morning symptoms.[13] These diurnal variations in mental functioning undoubtedly contribute to the disturbances in the sleep/wake cycle among patients with delirium. Together, these cognitive and behavioral changes can lead to significant alterations in mood. Fear, anxiety, depression, and anger have all been described among patients with delirium. The sudden and sometimes dramatic changes in thinking associated with delirium can be frightening and upsetting for family and friends who witness these changes in their loved-one. When those close to the patient are concerned about changes in thinking and behavior, the clinician should be alerted to the possibility of delirium.

Failure to diagnose delirium is also a characteristic feature of this clinical syndrome. Several studies have found that one-third to one-half of patients with delirium may go unrecognized by health professionals providing their care.[14–17] Certainly, early recognition of the syndrome can be challenging due to the variability of signs and symptoms. Despite these challenges, early recognition and accurate diagnosis of delirium provide important opportunities for us to improve our care of hospitalized older persons. Given the frequency of the syndrome, maintaining a high index of suspicion is an important first step in early detection. An assessment of cognitive function should be a routine part of each visit to the patient's bedside. It is also critical to seek regular input from relatives and friends of the patient and from nurses and other care providers who observe the patient frequently throughout the day.

CRITERIA FOR THE DIAGNOSIS OF DELIRIUM

Scientific societies have contributed significantly to the assessment of delirium by establishing criteria for this syndrome with multiple and sometimes nonspecific clinical features. Both the American Psychiatric Association,[18] and the World Health Organization[19] have published diagnostic criteria. There have been modifications of the criteria by the American Psychiatric Association in its *Diagnostic and Statistical Manual of Mental Disorders* published in 1980, 1987, and 1994.[18,20,21] In the third edition (DSM-III), delirium was distinguished from other so-called organic mental disorders. Many of the characteristic clinical features were reviewed, and inclusion and exclusion criteria were provided. In the revised version of the third edition (DSM-III-R), the term "clouding of consciousness" was eliminated and the focus was shifted to reduced attentiveness and disorganized thinking. The most recent version (DSM-IV) distinguishes between delirium due to a general medical condition, delirium due to substance intoxications or withdrawal, and delirium due to multiple etiologies.[18] In practice, the reason for the delirium often is not known at the time of diagnosis. The criteria for delirium due to a general medical condition are shown in Table 61-1. While having explicit clinical criteria for establishing the diagnosis of delirium is very useful, there are some limitations to this diagnostic approach. The published criteria cannot fully capture the wide array of cognitive impairments and behavioral changes that are commonly seen in patients with this syndrome. In addition, criterion-based diagnoses are dependent on uniform interpretation of clinical features, since there are no objective measures to independently validate the presence of the condition.

These diagnostic criteria are especially helpful in distinguishing delirium from other conditions that should be considered when an older patient experiences confusion or cognitive decline. Dementia is another common condition characterized by global cognitive dysfunction. In contrast to delirium, dementia more commonly has a gradual onset and a course that is progressive over years. The abrupt onset of confusion in the setting of acute illness is most often helpful in distinguishing delirium from dementia. Rarely, a vascular

---

Table 61-1 DSM-IV[18] criteria for the diagnosis of delirium due to a general medical condition

A. Disturbance of consciousness (i.e., reduced clarity of awareness of the environment) with reduced ability to focus, sustain or shift attention

B. A change in cognition (such as memory deficit, disorientation, language disturbance) or the development of a perceptual disturbance that is not better accounted for by a pre-existing, established, or evolving dementia

C. The disturbance develops over a short period of time (usually hours to days) and tends to fluctuate during the course of the day

D. There is evidence from the history, physical examination, or laboratory findings that the disturbance is caused by the direct physiologic consequences of a general medical condition

Reprinted with permission from the Diagnostic and Statistical Manual of Mental Disorders, fourth edition.

Copyright 1994 American Psychiatric Association.

---

dementia can present suddenly in the setting of a new ischemic event, and fluctuating symptoms are sometimes characteristic of Lewy body dementia. The possibility of an acute psychosis should also be considered when a hospitalized patient becomes confused, but this would be rare in an older person without a previous history of significant psychiatric disease. The presence of attention deficits and impaired consciousness should help distinguish delirium from psychosis. Severe depressive disorders can have some of the features of delirium such as cognitive decline and a disturbance of consciousness; acute onset is not characteristic of most cases of depression. Other uncommon syndromes (Charles Bonnet and peduncular hallucinosis) characterized by visual hallucinations can be considered in the differential diagnosis of an acute confusional state, though patients with these syndromes do not meet all the diagnostic criteria for delirium. Rarely, patients being treated with antipsychotic medications develop the neuroleptic malignant syndrome and exhibit features of delirium associated with fever. It is critical for the clinician to be able to distinguish this syndrome from delirium and psychosis. While use of antipsychotic medications to manage the behavioral manifestations of delirium or psychosis can be appropriate, this approach could be fatal for a patient with the neuroleptic malignant syndrome.[22]

STANDARDIZED TOOLS FOR ASSESSING DELIRIUM

A number of different tools have been developed to assist clinicians and researchers identify patients with delirium and quantify the severity of selected features of the syndrome. These instruments most commonly are based on the criteria published in the *Diagnostic and Statistical Manual of Mental Disorders* discussed above. The selection of any assessment tool should be based on how, why, and by whom the tool will be used. Some commonly used instruments with different intended purposes will be reviewed briefly.

The Confusion Assessment Method (CAM) is a standardized instrument that allows nonpsychiatrically trained clinicians to detect delirium.[23] It was developed based on the diagnostic criteria published in the DSM-III-R. Patients are assessed for the presence of each of the following four cardinal features of the syndrome: (1) acute onset and fluctuating course; (2) inattention; (3) disorganized thinking; (4) altered level of consciousness. According to the CAM algorithm, the diagnosis of delirium requires the presence of the first two features plus either one or both of the last two. This tool has been validated when compared to an independent assessment of patients by a psychiatrist and has been mostly studied among older persons. The sensitivity has been reported to range between 94 and 100 percent and the specificity between 46 and 95 percent.[23,24] One advantage of this instrument is the speed with which it can be administered and interpreted.

A number of tools have been developed for use by nurses. The NEECHAM Confusion Scale, published in 1987, includes nursing observations around a number of different patient characteristics: alertness, motor functioning, orientation, hygiene, psychomotor activity, speech, vital signs, oxygen saturation, and continence.[25] Certainly, these last two items have limited specificity for delirium. Total scores are categorized into one of five categories: normal, at risk for confusion, mildly confused, confused, or severely confused. The Clinical Assessment of Confusion also relies on nursing observations of patient behaviors as indicators of delirium.[26] Five dimensions are rated: cognition, general behavior, motor activity, orientation, and psychotic/neurotic behavior. Scores are derived from the ratings, and the patient's degree of confusion is assessed as none, mild, moderate, or severe, based on the score. The Confusion Rating Scale has only four domains for assessment by the nurse: disorientation, inappropriate behavior, inappropriate speech and the presence of illusions or hallucinations.[27] Abnormalities in each domain are rated as absent, mild, or pronounced; the presence of any abnormality is reported as consistent with confusion. It is notable that all of these instruments are easy to use and are designed for nursing staff who generally spend considerably more time with hospitalized patients than either physicians or research assistants. It is important to recognize that these nursing tools are designed to assess the presence and degree of confusion in patients; confusion may or may not be due to delirium.

In contrast, the Delirium Symptom Interview is a standardized script, intended for use by trained interviewers, that includes queries specifically designed to identify delirium.[28] There are questions and required observations that probe the following seven domains: disorientation, sleep disturbance, perceptual disturbance, disturbance of consciousness, incoherent speech, level of psychomotor activity, and fluctuation in behavior. These features were chosen because of their close relationship with the diagnostic criteria for delirium detailed in the DSM-III. Each item in the interview is judged to be either present or absent. The interview takes about 15 minutes to administer. In more severely disturbed individuals who may not be able to answer all the questions, keen observational skills are required, a feature that limits the general usefulness of this instrument. The Delirium Symptom Interview has been modified for use as a telephone assessment tool.[29] In a sample of 41 older patients contacted 1 month after undergoing operative repair of a hip fracture, the test characteristics of the telephone interview version of the instrument were calculated. Six of the 41 patients were considered delirious when evaluated independently using the Confusion Assessment Method diagnostic algorithm. The modified version of the Delirium Symptom Interview for use as a telephone interview had a sensitivity of 100 percent and a specificity of 94 percent in this small sample.

Standardized instruments can be helpful to establish the diagnosis of delirium and to assess the severity of the syndrome. Severity is likely to vary over time, may invoke specific treatments, and may be associated with the outcomes of delirium. The instruments reviewed above have limited value in the assessment of severity since they include items that do not vary over time such as the speed of onset, features that help distinguish delirium from either dementia or psychosis, and aspects of the syndrome that point to an identifiable cause. The Memorial Delirium Assessment Scale (MDAS) was developed specifically to measure severity of delirium among medically ill patients.[30] It is a 10-item scale that includes diagnostic criteria from DSM-IV as well as other clinical features from earlier versions of DSM and from other classification systems of delirium. The clinician rates each item on a scale from 0 (none) to 3 (severe); the total score is the sum of the individual item scores and ranges from 0 to 30. Those who developed the scale found that scores of 13 or more indicate delirium and higher scores indicate greater severity. Others who have used the scale have proposed other cutoff scores; the choice will depend on patient characteristics and the intended use of the tool.[31] There is good correlation between the MDAS, the DRS, the Folstein Mini-Mental State Examination and clinical assessment of delirium severity.[30] A reliable measure of severity may be very useful in predicting outcomes and in measuring the response of patients to preventive and therapeutic interventions. There are many standardized instruments useful for the diagnosis and assessment of patients with delirium.[32] The reason for the assessment should be an important determinant of the choice of the instrument.

NATURAL HISTORY OF DELIRIUM

Some aspects of the natural history of the syndrome are included in its definitions. Delirium is currently defined by the American Psychiatric Association as developing over a short time and fluctuating during the course of the day.[18] Many definitions include the idea that the cognitive changes are transient; there will be improvement in cognitive function among those patients who survive.[1] From the time of Hippocrates (Aphorisms: Section II, number 2), it has been appreciated that patients whose symptoms of confusion resolve quickly are more likely to have a good outcome: "When sleep puts an end to delirium, it is a good symptom."[4] Recent longitudinal studies, however, have called into question the transient nature of delirium. In some patients, evidence of delirium persists even as long as 6 months after discharge.[33] These findings can be interpreted in several ways: delirium may not be as transient as commonly believed, our skill at distinguishing delirium from dementia may be limited, or the coexistence of dementia and delirium confounds our ability to separate the two.[34] The timing of onset and the duration of symptoms have been shown to be highly variable.[35,36] Multiple episodes of delirium during a single hospitalization have been reported more commonly among those patients with several medical problems who are receiving many medications. Another risk factor for multiple episodes of delirium is the severity of the syndrome as measured by the Delirium Rating Scale.[36] As in other medical problems, much of the variability in the timing and intensity of the clinical features is likely related to the underlying pathological derangement, the compensatory mechanisms, comorbid factors, treatments, and environmental stresses. While the heterogeneity of delirium is well recognized, our understanding of the reasons for the variability is incomplete.

RISK FACTORS FOR DELIRIUM

Recognizing clinical factors that are associated with an increased risk of delirium can be helpful in several ways. First, early detection of patients with the syndrome may be possible if those patients at highest risk are more intensively monitored. Second, the risk factors may provide important clues to the underlying pathophysiological mechanisms. Finally, by targeting and reversing risk factors, important preventive and treatment strategies may be discovered to reduce the impact of delirium. Several studies have characterized patient factors that are associated with a baseline vulnerability for developing delirium. While the same risk factors were not evaluated by all investigators, several patient characteristics have been consistently identified in a number of prospective studies of delirium in hospitalized older persons. Dementia has been one of the most consistent risk factors.[37-40] Delirium is not only more common among patients with cognitive impairment, it is also more difficult to recognize, as previously discussed. Illness severity or burden of comorbidity are two other factors that have been associated with an increased risk of developing delirium.[37-40] Other frequently noted risk factors are infections,[15,37,41,42] renal abnormalities,[37,38] metabolic derangements, social stress,[43] and advanced age.[33,41]

Several studies have quantified the predictive value of the presence of these and other risk factors on the likelihood of developing delirium. In a study of 229 patients 70 years of age and older admitted to a teaching hospital in Philadelphia, six risk factors for delirium were identified: abnormal serum sodium, illness severity, dementia, fever or hypothermia, psychoactive drug use, and azotemia.[37] Overall, 22 percent of the patients developed delirium, but among those with three or more of the six risk factors, the rate of delirium was 60 percent. A study at Yale–New Haven Hospital involved patients who were 70 years of age and older and were admitted to the medical wards.[38] There were 107 patients in a development cohort among whom 25 percent developed delirium. Four independent risk factors for delirium were identified: vision impairment, severe illness, cognitive impairment, and a high blood urea nitrogen/creatinine ratio. When a point was assigned for the presence of each risk factor and patients were stratified as low risk (0 points), intermediate risk (1–2 points), and high risk (3–4 points), the rate of delirium in each group was 9, 23, and 83 percent, respectively. In a validation cohort of 174 comparable patients in which the overall rate of delirium was 17 percent, when the patients were stratified into

low-, intermediate-, and high-risk groups the rates of delirium were: 3, 16, and 32 percent. A similar study was conducted at the University of Chicago in a cohort of 432 patients.[39] The four risk factors identified were assigned points based on the strength of their association with delirium: cognitive impairment (2 points), extensive burden of comorbidity (3 points), depression (2 points), and alcoholism (3 points). In a validation cohort, it was shown that by using these criteria, patients in the low-risk category (0–3 points) had an incidence of delirium of 11 compared to 33 percent in a moderate-risk group (4–7 points), and 46 percent in a high-risk group (8–10 points). These studies confirm that admission characteristics can be used to stratify patients according to their risk of developing delirium.

In addition to identifying baseline vulnerability for delirium, patient characteristics present at the time of admission, it is also important to recognize that events that occur during hospitalization can precipitate an episode of delirium. In a study of precipitating events, 196 patients aged 70 years and older, admitted to the medical wards of a university teaching hospital and without baseline delirium, were followed prospectively.[44] Delirium developed in 35 (18 percent) and five independent precipitating factors were identified: use of physical restraints, malnutrition, the addition of more than three new medications, use of a bladder catheter, and any iatrogenic event. Assigning a point for the presence of each precipitating factor, the patients could then be placed into three risk strata: low risk (0 points), intermediate risk (1–2 points), and high risk ($\geq$3 points). The rate of delirium in each group was 3, 20, and 37 percent, respectively. In a validation cohort of 312 comparable patients in which the overall rate of delirium was 15 percent, when the patients were stratified into low-, intermediate- and high-risk groups the rates of delirium were 4, 20, and 35 percent. Again, by taking into account the presence of precipitating factors, one can stratify hospitalized older patients into risk categories for developing delirium.

Delirium among patients undergoing operative therapy is especially prevalent and dangerous. Many studies have been done to characterize the risks of perioperative delirium and recent efforts have been directed at developing clinically useful predictive rules. The task of identifying risk factors for perioperative delirium is especially difficult, since not only are there both predisposing and precipitating patient-specific factors, but there are also different operations and anesthetics to consider. One consistent finding among patients undergoing orthopedic procedures is that the incidence of delirium is greater among patients undergoing urgent operative therapy compared to those who have elective operations.[45,46] The type of anesthetic used, general or epidural, for elective total knee replacement was not found to be associated with the risk of delirium.[47] Among patients undergoing vascular surgery, both the presence of concomitant medical disease and operations involving the aorta are associated with an increased risk of developing delirium.[48,49] In a study of over 800 patients undergoing elective, noncardiac surgery, 9 percent of patients developed delirium postoperatively. Risk factors for delirium were found to be: age 70 years and older, self-reported alcohol abuse, poor cognitive status, poor functional status, markedly abnormal preoperative serum sodium, potassium, or glucose level, noncardiac thoracic surgery, and aortic aneurysm surgery.[49]

Based on the strength of association between these factors and delirium, a prediction rule was developed. Each risk factor was assigned 1 point, except for aortic aneurysm surgery which was assigned 2 points. In a validation study, using an independent sample of 465 comparable patients, the prediction rule successfully stratified patients into groups with low (2 percent), medium (8–13 percent) and high (50 percent) rates of postoperative delirium. The low-risk group had no risk factor points, the medium group had 1 or 2 points, and the high-risk group had 3 or more points. Again, relatively easy to obtain clinical characteristics can be used to stratify hospitalized patients according to their risk of developing delirium.

The syndrome of postoperative cognitive decline is recognized as increasingly important among older patients undergoing surgery. While the relationship of this syndrome to delirium is still debated, there are several common features: acute onset, decline in cognition, and memory impairment. The International Study of Post-Operative Cognitive Dysfunction 1[49a] was a multicenter trial involving over 1,200 patients aged at least 60 years, undergoing major noncardiac surgery, enrolled between 1994 and 1996. The hypothesis of this study was that age, hypoxemia, and arterial hypotension were important risk factors for postoperative cognitive decline. The investigators reported that 25.8 percent of patients exhibited cognitive decline at postoperative day 7 and that factors associated with this decline were: advanced age, duration of anesthesia, little education, a second operation, postoperative infections, and respiratory complications. At 3 months, 9.9 percent of patients showed cognitive impairment that could only be related to advanced age. Neither hypoxemia nor hypotension were identified as risk factors for changes in mental function. A smaller study of 261 patients undergoing coronary artery bypass grafting documented the following rates of cognitive decline: 53 percent at discharge from hospital, 36 percent after 6 weeks, 24 percent after 6 months and 42 percent at 5 years. Later decline was predicted by advanced age, little education, and cognitive decline at the time of discharge.[49b] Is the immediate postoperative cognitive decline observed in these and other studies related to delirium? If so, delirium may be a harbinger of more enduring cognitive decline as is seen in dementia.

CAUSES OF DELIRIUM

According to the DSM-IV criteria for delirium due to a general medical condition, there should be evidence from the history, physical examination, or laboratory findings that the disturbance is caused by the direct physiological consequences of such a condition. Abnormalities in most body systems from many pathological mechanisms have been associated with the syndrome of delirium. Some of the most frequent will be reviewed here. At times, the "medical condition" is an operative therapy and anesthesia as has already been discussed. Other treatments that involve both medications and procedures, such as electroconvulsive therapy[50–53] for depression, have also been associated with delirium.

Exposures to nonmedicinal toxins and adverse effects of medications are among the most common reasons for older hospitalized persons to experience delirium.[54] In Inouye's predictive model of precipitating factors,[44] the addition of three or more medications to the drug regimen of a patient was found to significantly increase the risk of confusion. There are hundreds of reports of delirium associated with medications, though it is often difficult to isolate the effect of the medication from the effect of the condition for which it is being given. Psychotropic medications such as tricyclic antidepressants,[55,56] benzodiazepines,[57–60] and lithium[61] should all be considered as possible causes of delirium. Medications with anticholinergic properties, including topical preparations, commonly have been associated with acute confusional states in older persons.[62,63] Digitalis preparations can cause delirium even when serum concentrations of the drug are in the therapeutic range.[64,65] Other classes of medications associated with delirium are analgesics,[41,60,66] histamine H-2 receptor antagonists,[67,68] nonsteroidal anti-inflammatory medications, and steroids.[69–71]

Delirium in hospitalized older persons is also ascribed to infection, metabolic abnormalities, and serious acute medical problems. Urinary tract infections are frequent in this population of patients and are frequently associated with delirium.[15,72] Many other types of infections have also been linked to acute confusional states.[15,37,41,42,73] Metabolic derangements such as electrolyte abnormalities,[74] renal insufficiency[37,38,75] and dehydration[76] are putative causes of delirium. Thiamine deficiency[77] and hypoalbuminemia[78] have been implicated as causes of confusion, though low albumin levels may be better thought of as a marker of illness severity than a specific metabolic derangement resulting from malnutrition or kidney or liver disease. Hypercalcemia, hypoglycemia, hypoxemia, hyperthyroidism, and hypercortisolism have all been associated with delirium. Patients with any serious illness such as stroke,[79–87] myocardial infarction,[88] cancer,[89] or trauma[90] can experience delirium during the course of their illness. The differential diagnosis of the causes for delirium is very broad. A careful clinical assessment of the patient should focus first on the most common and most serious conditions: adverse drug reactions, infections, metabolic derangements, central nervous system events, and myocardial ischemia.

PATHOPHYSIOLOGICAL MECHANISMS

The path to unraveling the pathophysiological mechanisms of delirium has been a difficult one. For clinicians and investigators alike, delirium is a challenge to recognize and distinguish from other causes of confusion because of its transient and unpredictably fluctuating course, and its diverse and variable clinical manifestations. Even after the patients with the syndrome are identified, they can be very difficult to study because they are typically severely ill with complex interacting medical problems, multiple medications, and, often, underlying brain disease. In the first half of the twentieth century, electroencephalogram (EEG) findings were used to map brain function and particular electrical abnormalities were noted among patients with delirium.[91] The classic abnormalities on EEG have been alpha wave slowing with delta and theta wave intrusions. These abnormal electrical patterns improved with treatment of the presumed medical precipitants of delirium such as by infusioning blood or glucose and by the administration of supplemental oxygen.[92,93] The observation that brain electrical activity normalized when treatments, directed at specific metabolic derangements, were administered gave rise to the theory that delirium was the result of a global failure of brain metabolism. This theory was challenged when delirium was observed among patients with localized strokes or other focal lesions. Recently, functional imaging studies of the brain have been useful in identifying both cortical and subcortical regions affected by delirium. The theory of global cerebral dysfunction is giving way to the notion that delirium is due to focal disruptions of either neural pathways or neurotransmitter systems.[94]

Neurotransmitters have been suspected of playing a key role in the pathophysiology of delirium based on a number of clinical observations. The prevalence of delirium among patients with dementia, a condition in which there is evidence that deficiencies of acetylcholine are causal, and the fact that anticholinergic medications have precipitated acute confusional states[95,96] were important clinical observations to support the cholinergic hypothesis of delirium. Hypoxemia and hypoglycemia, both precipitants of delirium, are known to be associated with a reduction in acetylcholine levels.[97] More recently, it has been possible to document abnormally high levels of serum anticholinergic activity among patients with delirium compared to patients without delirium.[98] Not only are the levels elevated during an episode of delirium, they also return to normal as symptoms resolve.[99] The observation that a drug thought to increase cerebral acetylcholine levels can also cause delirium[100] casts doubt on the notion that the mechanism is as simple as the deficiency in a single neurotransmitter. Indeed, excessive activation of the serotonergic system causes a syndrome of confusion, restlessness, tremor, and diaphoresis that is very similar to delirium.[101,102] In addition, excessive dopamine has also been implicated as a cause of delirium,[103,104] and antipsychotic medications used to treat delirium are dopamine blockers. Rather than the absolute level of any particular neurotransmitter being responsible for delirium, it is possible that altered ratios affecting reciprocal effects of the chemical signals may be most important. The role of altered levels of endogenous opioids and cortisol are also being explored as contributing to the mechanism of delirium.[95]

Mediators of inflammation, such as lymphokines, have been implicated in the pathophysiology of delirium. The prevalence of delirium is increased among patients with infections, cancer, and trauma, all conditions which may raise cytokine levels.[105,106] Whether the release of cytokines contributes to delirium through their effects on neurotransmitters or through direct neurotoxicity is not known.[107,108] The toxic effects of these mediators of inflammation are thought to contribute to dementia syndromes seen in patients in advanced stages of the acquired immunodeficiency syndrome.[109] The observation that acute confusional states sometimes accompany treatment with alpha interferon is supportive evidence for the theory that cytokines play a role in the pathophysiology of delirium.[110]

INTERVENTIONS FOR PREVENTION

Prevention of delirium and other untoward effects of hospitalization should be a goal in caring for older persons. There are reports of interventions that attempt to reduce the occurrence

of delirium through nursing interventions,[111] geriatric consultation,[112] and modifying anesthesia for patients undergoing operative therapy.[113] Most of these interventions have had modest or no success at preventing delirium. One clinical trial has shown convincingly that the rate of delirium can be significantly reduced by addressing selected risk factors.[114] Drawing from previous studies of predisposing and precipitating factors associated with delirium, the investigators selected mutable conditions for which relatively simple interventions were possible. The risk factors and associated interventions are shown in Table 61-2. For patients with baseline cognitive impairment, specific orienting and therapeutic activities were offered three times daily. For patients who had difficulties with sleep, noise reduction and nondrug sleep-enhancing strategies were tried in addition to reducing the use of psychoactive medications. Immobility was addressed with regular activities based on what was safe for the patient and by limiting the use of bladder catheters and physical restraints. Hearing and vision impairments were corrected with adaptive equipment as much as possible. Dehydration was avoided by monitoring volume status and encouraging fluid intake when necessary. By following these relatively simple interventions, the rate of delirium in hospitalized patients was reduced by 40 percent, from 15 percent in the usual-care group to 10 percent in the intervention group. Both number of days of delirium and number of episodes of delirium were reduced. The fact that the incidence of this serious complication among older hospitalized patients can be reduced significantly through relatively simple interventions and modest adjustments in care-plans is very promising. The general application of the intervention and its cost-effectiveness still need to be demonstrated.

EVALUATING THE PATIENT WITH DELIRIUM

An essential first step in the detection of delirium among older hospitalized patients is to maintain a high index of suspicion. Whenever there is a concern about episodes of confusion based on personal observations or on reports from families or care providers, it is important to evaluate the patient thoroughly. Evidence-based guidelines for the evaluation of a patient with delirium do not exist so we must rely on recommendations from reports in the medical literature and expert opinion. Certainly, the evaluation should be individualized according to the specific clinical situation. The presence of delirium as the cause of the confusion should first be documented using either the DSM-IV[18] criteria or a standardized instrument such as the Confusion Assessment Method.[23] Once you are convinced that delirium is the cause of the patient's change in condition, as in most clinical situations, the evaluation begins by obtaining a detailed history. Patients may recognize that there have been periods of confusion and may be able to give useful insights into potential precipitants of their confusion. It is always useful to gather additional input from other informants who know the patient well such as family, friends, or nurses. The focus of the history should be on identifying predisposing and precipitating factors. Starting with a detailed review of medications is often beneficial, since so many episodes of delirium are related to drugs. Otherwise, the history should identify both the extent and severity of

Table 61-2 **Strategies to prevent delirium in hospitalized older persons by targeting risk factors with standardized protocols[114]**

Targeted risk factor and eligible patients	Standardized intervention protocols
Cognitive impairment: All patients, protocol once daily; patients with baseline MMSE score of <20 or orientation score of <8, protocol 3 times daily	Orientation protocol: board with names of care-team members and day's schedule; communication to reorient to surroundings Therapeutic activities protocol: cognitively stimulating activities three times daily (e.g. discussion of current events, structured reminiscence, or word games)
Sleep deprivation: All patients, need for protocol assessed once daily	Nonpharmacological sleep protocol: at bedtime, warm drink (milk or herbal tea), relaxation tapes of music, and back massage Sleep enhancement protocol: unit-wide noise-reduction strategies (e.g. silent pill crushers, vibrating beepers, and quiet hallways) and schedule adjustments to allow sleep (e.g. rescheduling of medications and procedures)
Immobility: All patients, ambulation whenever possible, and range-of-motion exercises when patients chronically nonambulatory, bed or wheelchair bound, immobilized, or when prescribed bed rest	Early-mobilization protocol: ambulation of active range-of-motion exercises three times daily; minimal use of immobilizing equipment (e.g. bladder catheters or physical restraints)
Visual impairment: Patients with <20/70 visual acuity on binocular near-vision testing	Vision protocol: visual aids (e.g. glasses or magnifying lenses) and adaptive equipment (e.g. large illuminated telephone key-pads, large-print books, and fluorescent tape on call bell), with daily reinforcement of their use
Hearing impairment: Patients hearing ≤6 of 12 whispers on whisper test	Hearing protocol: portable amplifying devices, earwax disimpaction, and special communication techniques, with daily reinforcement of these adaptations
Dehydration: Patients with ratio of blood urea nitrogen to creatinine ≥18, screened for protocol by geriatric nurse-specialist	Dehydration protocol: early recognition and volume repletion (i.e., encouragement of oral intake of fluids)

comorbid conditions with special attention directed at common predisposing conditions such as dementia, vascular disease, renal insufficiency, endocrine conditions, alcohol use, and sensory deficits. The current condition of the patient should be fully assessed with focused attention on pain, immobility, the presence of restraints and catheters, and any acute changes that might suggest a cardiopulmonary or neurological event, an infection, or dehydration.

The physical examination should also be focused on uncovering potential causes for the delirium. This can be a challenge if the patient is agitated and resistant. Vital signs and observations of the skin and mucous membranes may be useful in detecting volume depletion. The examination of the lungs and cardiovascular system should be directed at identifying signs of pneumonia, respiratory insufficiency, asthma, dysrhythmias, valvular dysfunction, or congestive heart failure. The abdominal examination can be useful in detecting evidence of obstruction, inflammation, constipation, and urinary retention. Abnormalities on the neurological exam could point to stroke or infections. A simple quantitative assessment of cognitive functioning using the Mini-Mental State Examination[115] will establish a baseline measure of cognition.

The selection of laboratory tests in the evaluation of a patient with delirium should be based on findings from the history and physical examination. Common metabolic abnormalities can be uncovered by measuring electrolytes, glucose, renal and liver function tests, and a thyroid stimulating hormone level. The presence of infection can be assessed initially by obtaining a complete blood count and urinalysis. When congestive heart failure, pulmonary embolism, or respiratory insufficiency are being considered as causes of delirium, it is reasonable to measure either hemoglobin oxygen saturation or the partial pressure of oxygen in arterial blood. Serum drug levels, measures of the hypothalamic–pituitary–adrenal axis, serum ammonia level, and toxin assays should be done only when appropriate based on the clinical setting.

Other diagnostic tests have limited value except among patients in whom specific organ system involvement is suspected.[116] Certainly, when there are cardiac or pulmonary symptoms, an electrocardiogram and a chest radiograph can be helpful. When there is a history of recent head trauma or a focal abnormality on the neurological examination, other than the change in mental status, the yield of brain imaging is highest.[117] Some still recommend an EEG to help confirm the presence of delirium. However, with a false-negative rate of 17 percent and a false-positive rate of 22 percent, this test has a limited diagnostic role.[118] The examination of cerebrospinal fluid in the evaluation of a patient with delirium is not recommended unless there are other symptoms or signs to suspect meningitis or encephalitis.[119] When infection is the suspected cause of delirium, the appropriate cultures should be obtained. It is important to remember that there can be multiple contributing factors to delirium; so once one potential precipitant of delirium, is found, one must remain vigilant to the possibility that other precipitants are also at play. Repeated clinical evaluations may be required to uncover all the important contributing factors to a syndrome as variable, multifactorial, and evanescent as delirium.

OPTIMIZING THE MANAGEMENT

Among patients whose delirium is attributable to an underlying medical condition, a critically important aspect of management is addressing the underlying physical illness. These conditions and patient-specific interventions should be complemented by general measures directed at symptomatic management of this distressing mental state.

Important first steps are to ensure patient safety, preserve functional status as much as possible, and offer an appropriate degree of reassurance to the patient and family.[120] Patients with delirium may exhibit irrational and unsafe behaviors if they become agitated and delusional. Their inability to fully participate in their care, combined with the inclination of health professionals to address the many potential causes of delirium by performing many tests and prescribing symptomatic treatments, increases the risk of iatrogenic injuries. Strategies that have been recommended to maximize patient safety have included regular reorientation of the patient by providing calenders, clocks, familiar objects, a room with a window, and frequent contact by friends, family, and healthcare staff. It is also important to ensure that patients have access to their corrective lenses and hearing aids, if these sensory modalities are impaired, and to avoid unnecessary restraints and catheters. Preserving activity levels as much as possible despite the patient's confusion can be helpful both in reorienting patients to a daily routine and in maintaining their function. Delirium can be a very frightening experience for both patients and family members; explaining the acute and generally reversible nature of the syndrome can be very reassuring. Educating staff about delirium and about how they can support the patients and families has been shown to improve the care of confused patients.[121,122]

Other methods of addressing patient comfort can be very helpful. Pain is often an important contributor to delirium and should be systematically assessed and optimally managed.[123] Sleep is often disturbed in patients with delirium, and non-pharmacological measures to restore the normal sleep–wake cycle should be employed. During the day, patients should be engaged in activities and exposed to an environment with adequate light.[124] At bedtime, excessive noise should be avoided, and calming interventions such as soft music, back rubs, and drinking warm noncaffeinated beverages can be tried. The confusion some patients with delirium experience may be manifest as paranoia; staff should be mindful of their

Summary of management algorithm
Managing patients with delirium

- Prevention
  - Anticipate the problem
  - Avoid unnecessary medications and restraints
  - Optimize sensory input with special attention to vision and hearing
  - Optimize management of chronic medical problems and fluids and electrolytes
- Early diagnosis
  - Maintain a high index of suspicion for delirium
  - Use validated assessment tools for mental status testing
  - Search for the underlying cause and treat promptly
- Supportive care
  - Recognize that delirium can be frightening to patients and families
  - Foster a calm and reassuring environment for the patient
  - Use psychotropic agents sparingly to protect the patient
    - Low-dose antipsychotic medications may be needed for psychotic manifestations such as hallucinations and violent behaviors
    - Benzodiazepines are specifically indicated for alcohol or benzodiazepine withdrawal syndromes

conversations and other actions that may be misinterpreted by patients. As much as possible, the same staff should be assigned to the care of the patient so that a trusting relationship can be developed.

When drug therapy is being considered in the management of patients with delirium, it is important to consider the following. First, delirium is often caused or exacerbated by medications, so it is preferable to eliminate medications rather than add them to the regimen. Second, if drugs are prescribed, the intent should be specifically to manage an unsafe or significantly disruptive behavior that is a manifestation of the syndrome; medications are rarely effective in reversing delirium. Antipsychotic medications are often the first choice for severe agitation and dangerous behaviors.[125] Haloperidol has become a popular choice because it has few anticholinergic side-effects, few active metabolites, and can be administered orally or parenterally. For older persons, dosing usually begins at 0.25–0.5 mg every 4 hours as needed with a slow titration to higher doses for continued agitation. Haloperidol can be administered as a continuous infusion for patients who require frequent dosing. It is rare that older persons require more than about 6 mg of haloperidol per day to alleviate severe behavioral problems associated with delirium, but daily doses of up to 100 mg have been reported to be safe. Other antispychotic medications like droperidol, risperidone, olanzapine, and quetiapine have all been used successfully in the management of patients with delirium. Important side-effects of antipsychotics include excessive sedation, hypotension, extrapyramidal symptoms, neuroleptic malignant syndrome, and a ventricular dysrhythmia, torsades de pointes.[126,127] Whenever the QT c interval on the electrocardiogram is greater than 450 msec or increased by more than 25 percent above baseline, the antipsychotic medication should be discontinued or the dose reduced;

a cardiology consultation may be required for additional management recommendations.

The use of benzodiazepines alone in the management of patients with delirium should be reserved for those cases due to withdrawal from alcohol or sedative hypnotics. There are reports of the combined use of benzodiazepines and antipsychotic medications.[128] The advantage of this combination is that the benzodiazepine may potentiate the effect of the antipsychotic drug, thereby allowing lower doses to be used for patients experiencing undesirable side-effects. As previously mentioned, it is important to have clear therapeutic aims when using drugs in the management of a patient with delirium; benzodiazepines can have anxiolytic, sedating, and hypnotic effects. Lorazepam is the benzodiazepine most commonly recommended because of its rapid onset, short half-life, lack of major active metabolites, and availability in oral and parenteral forms. Dosing often begins at 0.5 mg and is titrated to the patient's condition; though doses in excess of 12 mg per day are uncommon, a total daily dose of 20–30 mg has been used in cases of severe agitation.[125]

Other drug regimens can be used for patients in special circumstances. When anticholinergic medications are felt to be the cause of the delirium, administration of physostigmine may reverse the syndrome.[129] After a dose of 1–2 mg of physostigmine administered parenterally, a rapid improvement in mental status is expected if the cause of delirium is anticholinergic toxicity.[130,131] This intervention has not been fully evaluated in older persons in whom multiple causes of delirium are common and adverse effects of physostigmine such as bronchospasm, vomiting, and bradycardia can be severe. For patients with terminal diseases and in whom pain is an aggravating factor, opioids may provide the best palliation. When vitamin B deficiences are considered a possible cause, replacement of the deficient vitamins is necessary. Some have suggested a role for psychostimulants in patients with hypoactive delirium.[132]

OUTCOMES OF DELIRIUM

When evaluating the outcomes of patients who experience delirium, there are several important timeframes to consider. First are the short-term effects of the syndrome on the patients who experience it. Complications of falls, incontinence, pressure sores, and disruption of various catheters, tubes, and suture lines are common among older hospitalized patients with delirium.[133] Several prospective studies have confirmed that delirium is associated with an increased risk of death during hospitalization.[134–136] Whether the experience of delirium is contributing to the increased mortality or simply a powerful marker of illness severity is still debated.[137] Short of these most serious consequences of this syndrome, as previously mentioned, delirium can be a very upsetting experience for patients.[138] Some may need assistance in coping with an experience in which they felt out of control and may have engaged in uncharacteristic behaviors. In any case, patients who develop delirium should be recognized by physicians and other hospital staff as being at high risk for important untoward events. Not all episodes of confusion resolve by the time of discharge, and patients and families often have to cope with cognitive impairments that last beyond the hospital stay.[33,35]

Since ancient times, there has been speculation that different degrees or manifestations of delirium may be associated with different outcomes. Hippocrates reported in his aphorisms, section IV, number 53: "Delirium attended with laughter is less dangerous than delirium attended with a serious mood."[4] Today, some who study delirium argue that patients with hyperactive behaviors may differ in significant ways from those with a more quiet form of delirium.[12,13,139] If these and other variants of the syndrome can be shown to have different etiologies or outcomes, our treatments may need to be tailored to these behavioral manifestations of the patients.[140]

The untoward outcomes and undesirable effects that delirium has on patients translate into important negative impacts on the healthcare system. Several studies have shown that patients with delirium have significantly longer hospital stays than patients who do not experience delirium.[39,133–135,137] This finding persists even after adjusting for severity of illness or the medical condition for which the patient is hospitalized. There is also a significant association between delirium during hospital stay and discharge to a nursing home.[133,137] One study has noted that readmission rates are increased among patients who experienced delirium.[137] All of these sequelae dramatically increase the cost of caring for patients with delirium.

Finally, many older patients who experience delirium have sobering long-term effects, a finding that suggests the syndrome may be an important marker of poor overall health status. Substantial numbers of patients who experience delirium during a hospital stay are living in an institutional setting 6 months after discharge.[137] The mortality rate after discharge remains very high for patients with delirium.[73,133,136,141] For those who do survive an episode of delirium after an orthopedic procedure, functional status at 6 months can remain significantly impaired.[142,143] Functional decline is seen also in older patients who experience delirium after being admitted to medical and surgical units for a wide array of health problems.[144] While full recovery of cognitive function is the most common outcome of an episode of delirium, many patients have persistent cognitive impairment.[35] This observation has called into question the transient nature of delirium and has blurred the distinction between dementia and delirium.[34] Efforts to identify distinguishing features of the delirium experienced by patients with dementia have not been successful.[145] The increased mortality among patients with dementia who also experience delirium has been confirmed, but this may reflect differences due to the severity of the underlying physical illness.[116,137]

CONCLUSIONS

While major advances have been made in the diagnostic criteria for delirium, in identifying patients at risk based on predisposing and precipitating factors, and in the initial treatment of the behavioral manifestations, there is still much to be learned about this common and important geriatric syndrome. Despite the prevalence and well-recognized adverse outcomes of delirium, the syndrome is still significantly underdiagnosed in most hospitals. In addition to raising the awareness of health professionals to the possibility of delirium among older hospitalized patients, it is important to encourage the regular use of standardized assessment instruments so that there is a uniform and consistent method for establishing the diagnosis. Much is still to be discovered about the pathophysiology of this syndrome with diverse manifestations, multiple precipitants, and varying severity. Uncovering the mechanisms of delirium will continue to be difficult, since the patients who have the condition are often quite frail, ill, and difficult to study. Approaches that combine anatomic and physiological studies with psychological measures may hold the most promise for discovering the pathways that lead to the clinical manifestations of delirium. While many studies have helped us better understand risk factors for delirium, we still do not have a complete understanding of what degree and extent of exposure to a given risk factor might be important in precipitating the syndrome among patients who, themselves, have biological and psychological predispositions to confusion. The description of various subtypes of delirium is intriguing, but we still do not know how or if the manifestations of the syndrome have any relationship to etiology, prognosis, or effect of treatment. There are early reports of effective interventions that can reduce the risk of developing delirium among older hospitalized patients. There will be ongoing advantages from rigorous, systematic studies designed to assess evaluation and treatment strategies that examine both benefits and burdens to patients and healthcare systems.

KEY POINTS Delirium

- Even though delirium affects nearly one out of every six hospitalized older persons and is associated with increased mortality, it is underdiagnosed commonly by most clinicians.

- Easy-to-use, standardized assessment tools exist for both establishing the presence and the severity of delirium.

- Many factors contribute to delirium, and repeated clinical evaluations are needed to uncover all the contributing precipitants and causes.

- Effective preventive strategies focusing on orientation, adequate sleep and hydration, mobility, and sensory input exist to reduce the incidence of delirium in hospitalized older patients.

REFERENCES

1. Lipowski ZJ: Delirium (acute confusional states). JAMA 1987;258:1789–1792
2. Lipowski ZJ: Delirium in the elderly patient. N Engl J Med 1989;320:578–581
3. Hart B: Delirious states. Br Med J 1936; October 17:745–749
4. Adams F: The Genuine Works of Hippocrates. Williams and Wilkins, Baltimore, 1939:292–322
5. Berrios GE: Delirium and confusion in the 19th century: a conceptual history. Br J Psychiatry 1981;139:439–449
6. Folstein MF, Bassett SS, Romanoski AJ et al: The epidemiology of delirium in the community: the Eastern Baltimore Mental Health Survey. Int Psychogeriatr 1991;3:169–176
7. Naughton BJ, Moran MB, Kadah H et al: Delirium and other cognitive impairment in older adults in an emergency department. Ann Emerg Med 1995;25:751–755
8. Inouye SK: Delirium in hospitalized older patients. Clin Geriatr Med 1998;14:745–764
9. Inouye SK, Schlesinger MJ, Lydon TJ: Delirium: a symptom of how hospital care is failing older persons and a window to improve quality of hospital care. Am J Med 1999;106:565–573
10. Dyer CB, Ashton CM, Teasdale TA: Postoperative delirium. A review of 80 primary data-collection studies. Arch Intern Med 1995;155:461–465
11. Ancelin ML, De Roquefeuil G, Ritchie K: Anesthesia and postoperative cognitive dysfunction in the elderly: a review of clinical and epidemiological observations. Rev Epidem Sante Publ 2000;48:459–472
12. Liptzin B, Levkoff SE, Cleary PD et al: An empirical study of diagnostic criteria for delirium. Am J Psychiatry 1991;148:454–457
13. Sandberg O, Gustafson Y, Brannstrom B et al: Clinical profile of delirium in older patients. J Am Geriatr Soc 1999;47:1300–1306
14. Knights EB, Folstein MF: Unsuspected emotional and cognitive disturbance in medical patients. Ann Intern Med 1977;87:723–724
15. Levkoff SE, Safran C, Cleary PD et al: Identification of factors associated with the diagnosis of delirium in elderly hospitalized patients. J Am Geriatr Soc 1988;36:1099–1104
16. Francis J: Delirium in older patients. J Am Geriatr Soc 1992;40:829–838
17. Inouye SK: The dilemma of delirium: Clinical and research controversies regarding diagnosis and evaluation of delirium in hospitalized elderly medical patients. Am J Med 1994;97:278–288
18. American Psychiatric Association. Diagnostic and Statistical Manual of Mental Disorders, 4th Ed. American Psychiatric Association, Washington, DC, 1994
19. World Health Organization. The ICD-10 Classification of Mental and Behavioural Disorders. World Health Organization, Geneva, 1992
20. American Psychiatric Association. Diagnostic and Statistical Manual of Mental Disorders, 3rd Ed. American Psychiatric Association, Washington, DC, 1980
21. American Psychiatric Association. Diagnostic and Statistical Manual of Mental Disorders, 3rd Ed, revised. American Psychiatric Association, Washington, DC, 1987
22. Nicklason FN, Finucane PM, Pathy MJ et al: Neuroleptic malignant syndrome: an unrecognized problem in elderly patients with psychiatric illness? Int J Geriatr Psychiatry 1991;6:171–175
23. Inouye SK, van Dyck CH, Alessi CA et al: Clarifying confusion: the confusion assessment method. A new method for detection of delirium. Ann Intern Med 1990;113:941–948
24. Pompei P, Foreman M, Cassel CK et al: Detecting delirium among hospitalized older patients. Arch Intern Med 1995;155:301–307
25. Champagne MT, Neelon VJ, McConnell ES et al: The NEECHAM Confusion Scale: assessing confusion in the hospitalized and nursing home elderly. Gerontologist 1987;27:4A
26. Vermeersch PE: The clinical assessment of confusion—A. Appl Nurs Res 1990;3:128–133
27. Williams M, Ward S, Campbell E: Confusion: testing vs. observation. J Gerontol Nursing 1988;14:25–30
28. Albert MS, Levkoff SE, Reilly C et al: The delirium symptom interview: an interview for the detection of delirium symptoms in hospitalized patients. J Geriatr Psychiatry Neurol 1992;5:14–21
29. Marcantonio ER, Michaels N, Resnick NM: Diagnosing delirium by telephone. J Gen Intern Med 1998;13:621–623
30. Breitbart W, Rosenfeld B, Roth A et al: The Memorial Delirium Assessment Scale. J Pain Symptom Manage 1997;13:128–137
31. Lawlor PG, Nekolaichuk C, Gagnon B et al: Clinical utility, factor analysis, and further validation of the memorial delirium assessment scale in patients with advanced cancer: Assessing delirium in advanced cancer. Cancer 2000;88:2859–2867
32. Trzepacz PT: A review of delirium assessment instruments. Gen Hosp Psychiatry 1994;16:397–405
33. Levkoff SE, Evans DA, Liptzin B et al: Delirium. The occurrence and persistence of symptoms among elderly hospitalized patients. Arch Intern Med 1992;152:334–340
34. Macdonald AJD, Treloar A: Delirium and dementia: are they distinct? J Am Geriatr Soc 1997;44:1001–1002
35. Rockwood K: The occurrence and duration of symptoms in elderly patients with delirium. J Gerontol A 1993;48:M162–M166
36. Rudberg MA, Pompei P, Foreman MD et al: The natural history of delirium in older hospitalized patients: a syndrome of heterogeneity. Age Ageing 1997;26:169–174
37. Francis J, Martin D, Kapoor WN: A prospective study of delirium in hospitalized elderly. JAMA 1990;263:1097–1101
38. Inouye SK, Viscoli CM, Horwitz RI et al: A predictive model for delirium in hospitalized elderly medical patients based on admission characteristics. Ann Intern Med 1993;119:474–481

39. Pompei P, Foreman M, Rudberg MA et al: Delirium in hospitalized older persons: outcomes and predictors. J Am Geriatr Soc 1994;42:809–815

40. Michel E, Cole MG, Primeau FJ et al: Delirium risk factors in elderly hospitalized patients. J Gen Intern Med 1998;13:204–212

41. Schor JD, Levkoff SE, Lipsitz LA et al: Risk factors for delirium in hospitalized elderly. JAMA 1992;267:827–831

42. Windsor AC: Bacteraemia in a geriatric unit. Gerontology 1983;29:125–130

43. Eriksson S: Social and environmental contributants to delirium in the elderly. Dement Geriatr Cogn Disord 1999;10:350–352

44. Inouye SK, Charpentier PA: Precipitating factors for delirium in hospitalized elderly persons: Predictive model and interrelationship with baseline vulnerability. JAMA 1996;275:852–857

45. Duppils GS, Wikblad K: Acute confusional states in patients undergoing hip surgery: A prospective observational study. Gerontology 2000;46:36–43

46. Andersson EM, Gustafson L, Hallberg IR: Acute confusional state in elderly orthopaedic patients: Factors of importance for detection in nursing care. International J Geriatr Psychiatry 2001;16:7–17

47. Williams-Russo P, Sharrock NE, Mattis S et al: Cognitive effects after epidural vs general anesthesia in older adults. JAMA 1995;274:44–50

48. Bohner H, Schneider F, Stierstorfer A et al: Postoperative delirium following vascular surgery. Anaesthetist 2000;49:427–433

49. Marcantonio ER, Goldman L, Mangione CM et al: A clinical prediction rule for delirium after elective noncardiac surgery. JAMA 1994;271:134–139

49a. Moller JT, Cluitmans P, Rasmussen LS et al: Long-term postoperative cognitive dysfunction in the elderly: ISPOCD1 study. Lancet 1998;351(9106):857–861

49b. Newman MF, Kirshner JL, Phillips-Bute B et al: Longitudinal assessment of neurocognitive function after coronary-artery bypass surgery. N Engl J Med 2001;344(6):395–402

50. Figiel GS, Hassen MA, Zorumski C et al: ECT-induced delirium in depressed patients with Parkinson's disease. J Neuropsychiatry Clin Neurosci 1991;3:405–411

51. Figiel GS, Botteron K, Zorumski CF et al: The treatment of late age onset psychoses with electroconvulsive therapy. Int J Geriatr Psychiatry 1992;7:183–189

52. Martin M, Figiel G, Mattingly G et al: ECT-induced interictal delirium in patients with a history of a CVA. J Geriatr Psychiatry Neurol 1992;5:149–155

53. Kelly KG, Zisselman M: Update of electroconvulsive therapy (ECT) in older adults. J Am Geriatr Soc 2000;48:560–566

54. Francis J: Drug-induced delirium: Diagnosis and treatment. CNS Drugs 1996;5:103–114

55. Kutcher SP, Shulman KI: Desipramine-induced delirium at "subtherapeutic" concentrations: a case report. Can J Psychiatry 1985;30:368–369

56. Meyers BS, Mei-Tal V: Psychiatric reactions during tricyclic treatment of the elderly reconsidered. J Clin Psychopharmacol 1983;3:2–6

57. Zipursky RB, Baker RW, Zimmer B: Alprazolam withdrawal delirium unresponsive to diazepam: case report. J Clin Psychiatry 1985;46:344–345

58. Minichetti J, Milles M: Hallucination and delirium reaction to intravenous diazepam administration: case report. Anesth Prog 1982;29:144–146

59. Rothschild AJ: Disinhibition, amnestic reactions, and other adverse reactions secondary to triazolam: a review of the literature. J Clin Psychiatry 1992;53(suppl):69–79

60. Marcantonio E, Juarez G, Goldman L et al: The relationship of postoperative delirium with psychoactive medications. JAMA 1994;272:1518–1522

61. Brown AS, Rosen J: Lithium-induced delirium with therapeutic serum lithium levels: a case report. J Geriatr Psychiatry Neurol 1992;5:53–55

62. Tune LE, Bylsma FW, Hilt DC: Anticholinergic delirium caused by topical homatropine ophthalmologic solution: confirmation by anticholinergic radioreceptor assay in two cases. J Neuropsychiatry Clin Neurosci 1992;4:195–197

63. Rozzini R, Inzoli M, Trabucchi M: Delirium from transdermal scopolamine in an elderly woman. JAMA 1988;260:478

64. Grubb BP: Digitalis delirium in an elderly woman. Postgrad Med 1987;81:329–330

65. Eisenman DP, McKegney FP: Delirium at therapeutic serum concentrations of digoxin and quinidine. Psychosomatics 1994;35:91–93

66. Steinberg RB, Gilman DE, Johnson F III: Acute toxic delirium in a patient using transdermal fentanyl. Anesth Analg 1992;75:1014–1016

67. Cantu TG, Korek JS: Central nervous system reactions to histamine-2 receptor blockers. Ann Intern Med 1991;114:1027–1034

68. Jenike MA, Levy JC: Physostigmine reversal of cimetidine-induced delirium and agitation. J Clin Psychopharmacol 1983;3:43–44

69. Steele TE, Morton WA: Salicylate-induced delirium. Psychosomatics 1986;27:455–456

70. Allison N, Shantz I: Delirium related to tiaprofenic acid. Can Med Assoc J 1987;137:1022–1023

71. Medical Letter: Drugs that may cause cognitive disorders in the elderly. Medical Lett 2000;42:1–2

72. Manepalli J, Grossberg GT, Mueller C: Prevalence of delirium and urinary tract infection in a psychogeriatric unit. J Geriatr Psychiatry Neurol 1990;3:198–202

73. George J, Bleasdale S, Singleton SJ: Causes and prognosis of delirium in elderly patients admitted to a district general hospital. Age Ageing 1997;26:423–427

74. Koizumi J, Shiraishi H, Ofuku K et al: Duration of delirium shortened by the correction of electrolyte imbalance. Jpn J Psychiatry Neurol 1988;42:81–88

75. Fraser CL, Arieff AI: Nervous system complications in uremia. Ann Intern Med 1988;109:143–153

76. Seymour DG, Henschke PJ, Cape RD et al: Acute confusional states and dementia in the elderly: the role of dehydration/volume depletion, physical illness and age. Age Ageing 1980;9:137–146

77. O'Keeffe ST, Tormey WP, Glasgow R et al: Thiamine deficiency in hospitalized elderly patients. Gerontology 1994;40:18–24

78. Dickson LR: Hypoalbuminemia in delirium. Psychosomatics 1991;32:317–323

79. Benbadis SR, Sila CA, Cristea RL: Mental status changes and stroke. J Gen Intern Med 1994;9:485–487

80. Dunne JW, Leedman PJ, Edis RH: Inobvious stroke: a cause of delirium and dementia. Aust NZJ Med 1986;16:771–778

81. Reding MJ, Gardner C, Hainline B et al: Neuropsychiatric problems interfering with inpatient stroke rehabilitation. J Neurol Rehabil 1993;7:1–7

82. Bogousslavsky J, Regli F: Anterior cerebral artery territory infarction in the Lausanne Stroke Registry. Clinical and etiologic patterns. Arch Neurol 1990;47:144–150

83. Devinsky O, Bear D, Volpe BT: Confusional states following posterior cerebral artery infarction. Arch Neurol 1988;45:160–163

84. Mehler MF: The rostral basilar artery syndrome: diagnosis, etiology, prognosis. Neurology 1989;39:9–16

85. Black DW: Mental changes resulting from subdural haematoma. Br J Psychiatry 1984;145:200–203

86. Velasco J, Head M, Farlin E et al: Unsuspected subdural hematoma as a differential diagnosis in elderly patients. South Med J 1995;88:977–979

87. Balter RA, Fricchione G, Sterman AB: Clinical presentation of multi-infarct delirium. Psychosomatics 1986;27:461–462

88. Bayer AJ, Chadha JS, Farag RR et al: Changing presentation of myocardial infarction with increasing old age. J Am Geriatr Soc 1986;34:263–266

89. Stiefel F, Fainsinger R, Bruera E: Acute confusional states in patients with advanced cancer. J Pain Symptom Manage 1992;7:94–98

90. Zatsick DF, Kang SM, Kim SY et al: Patients with recognized psychiatric disorders in trauma surgery: Incidence, inpatient length of stay, and cost. J Trauma-Injury Infect Crit Care 2000;49:487–495

91. Engel GL, Romano J: Delirium: a syndrome of cerebral insufficiency. J Chronic Dis 1959;9:260–277

92. Romano J, Engel GL: Delirium I. Electroencephalographic data. Arch Neurol Psychiatr 1944;51:356–377

93. Engel GL, Romano J: Delirium II. Reversibility of the electroencephalogram with experimental procedures. Arch Neurol Psychiatr 1944;51:378–392

94. Trzepacz PT: Delirium: Advances in diagnosis, pathophysiology, and treatment. Psychiatr Clin N Am 1996;19:429–448

95. Flacker JM, Lipsitz LA: Neural mechanisms of delirium: Current hypotheses and evolving concepts. J Gerontol A 1999;54:B239–B246

96. Itil T, Fink M: Anticholinergic drug-induced delirium: Experimental medication, quantitative EEG, and behavioral correlations. J Nerv Ment Dis 1966;143:492–507

97. Tune L, Carr S, Cooper T et al: Association of anticholinergic activity of prescribed medications with postoperative delirium. J Neuropsychiatry Clin Neurosci 1993;5:208–210

98. Gibson GE, Blass JP, Huang HM et al: The cellular basis of delirium and its relevance to age-related disorders including Alzheimer's disease. Int Psychogeriatr 1991;3:373–395

99. Mach JR Jr, Dysken MW, Kuskowski M et al: Serum anticholinergic activity in hospitalized older person with delirium: a preliminary study. J Am Geriatr Soc 1995;43:491–495

100. Trzepacz PT, Ho V, Mallavarapu H: Cholinergic delirium and neurotoxicity associated with tacrine for Alzheimer's disease. Psychosomatics 1996;37:299–301

101. Feighner JP, Boyer WF, Tyler DL et al: Adverse consequences of fluoxetine-MAOI combination therapy. J Clin Psychiatr 1990;51:222–225

102. Sternbach H: The serotonin syndrome. Am J Psychiatr 1991;148:705–713

103. Birkmayer W: Toxic delirium after L-dopa medication. J Neural Transm 1978;14(suppl):163–166

104. Cummings J: Behavioral complications of drug treatment of Parkinson's disease. J Am Geriatr Soc 1991;39:708–716

105. Denicoff KD, Rubinow DR, Papa MZ et al: The neuropsychiatric effects of treatment with interleukin-2 and lymphokine-activated killer-cells. Ann Intern Med 1987;107:293–300

106. Hopkins SJ, Rothwell NJ: Cytokines and the nervous system: I. Expression and recognition. Trends Neurosci 1995;18:83–88

107. Rothwell NJ, Hopkins SJ: Cytokines and the nervous system: II. Actions and mechanisms of action. Trends Neurosci 1995;18:130–136

108. Stefano GB, Bilfinger TV, Fricchione GL: The immune-neuro-link and the macrophage: Post-pericardiotomy delirium, HIV-associated dementia and psychiatry. Prog Neurobiol 1994;42:475–488

109. Lipton SA, Gendelman HE: Dementia associated with the acquired immunodeficiency syndrome. N Engl J Med 1995;332:934–940

110. Renault PF, Hoofnagle JH, Park Y et al: Psychiatric complications of long-term interferon alfa therapy. Arch Intern Med 1987;147:1577–1580

111. Williams MA, Campbell EB, Raynor WJ et al: Reducing acute confusional states in elderly patients with hip fractures. Res Nurs Health 1985;8:329–337

112. Cole MG, Primeau FJ, Bailey RF et al: Systematic intervention for elderly inpatients with delirium: a randomized trial. Can Med Assoc J 1994;151:965–970

113. Gustafson Y, Brannstrom B, Berggren D et al: A geriatric-anesthesiologic program to reduce acute confusional states in elderly patients treated for femoral neck fractures. J Am Geriatr Soc 1991;39:655–662

114. Inouye SK, Bogardus ST, Charpentier PA et al: A multicomponent intervention to prevent delirium in hospitalized older patients. N Engl J Med 1999;340:669–676

115. Folstein MF, Folstein SE, McHugh PR: Mini-mental state—a practical method for grading the cognitive state of patients for the clinician. J Psychiatric Res 1975;12:189–198

116. Rummans TA, Evans JM, Krahn LE et al: Delirium in elderly patients: Evaluation and management. Mayo Clin Proc 1995;70:989–998

117. Trzepacz PR: The neuropathogenesis of delirium: a need to focus our research. Psychosomatics 1994;35:374–391

118. Inouye SK: Assessment and management of delirium in hospitalized older patients. Ann Long-Term Care Clin Care Aging 2000;8:53–59

119. Warshaw G, Tanzer F: The effectiveness of lumbar puncture in the evaluation of delirium and fever in the hospitalized elderly. Arch Fam Med 1993;2:293–297

120. Meagher DJ: Delirium: optimising management. Br Med J 2001;322:144–149

121. Simon L, Jewell N, Brokel J: Management of acute delirium in hospitalized elderly: a process improvement project. Geriatr Nurs 1997;18:150–154

122. Foreman MD, Mion LC, Tryostad L et al: Standard of practice protocol: acute confusion/delirium. NICHE Faculty. Geriatr Nurs 1999;20:147–152

123. Lynch EP, Lazor MA, Gellis JE et al: The impact of postoperative pain on the development of postoperative delirium. Anesth Analg 1998;86:781–785

124. Kaneko T, Takahashi S, Naka T et al: Postoperative delirium following gastrointestinal surgery in elderly patients. Japan J Surg 1997;27:107–111

125. American Psychiatric Association: Practice guideline for the treatment of patients with delirium. American Psychiatric Association, Washington, DC, 1999

126. Sharma ND, Rosman HS, Padhi D et al: Torsades de pointes associated with the use of intravenous haloperidol in critically ill patients. Am J Cardiol 1998;81:238–240

127. Jackson T, Ditmanson L, Phibbs B: Torsades de pointes and low-dose oral haloperidol. Arch Intern Med 1997;157:2013–2015

128. Menza MA, Murray GB, Holmes VF et al: Controlled study of extrapyramidal reactions in the management of delirious, medically ill patients: intravenous haloperidol versus intravenous haloperidol plus benzodiazepines. Heart Lung 1988;17:238–241

129. Blitt CD, Petty WC: Reversal of lorazepam delirium by physostigmine. Anesth Analg 1975;54:607–608

130. Granacher RT, Baldessarini RJ, Messner E: Physiostigmine treatment of delirium induced by anticholinergics. Am Fam Physician 1976;13:99–103

131. Goff DC, Garber HJ, Jenke MA: Partial resolution of ranitidine-associated delirium with physostigmine: case report. J Clin Psychiatry 1985;46:400–401

132. Stiefel F, Bruera E: Psychostimulants for hypoactive-hypoalert delirium? J Palliat Care 1991;7:25–26

133. O'Keefe S, Lavan J: The prognostic significance of delirium in older hospital patients. J Am Geriatr Soc 1997;45:174–178

134. Inouye SK, Rushing JT, Foreman MD et al: Does delirium contribute to poor hospital outcomes? A three-site epidemiologic study. J Gen Intern Med 1998;13:234–242

135. Francis J, Kapoor WN: Delirium in hospitalized elderly. J Gen Intern Med 1990;5:65–79

136. van Hemert AM, van der Mast RC, Hengeveld MW et al: Excess mortality in general hospital patients with delirium: a 5-year follow-up of 519 patients seen in psychiatric consultation. J Psychosom Res 1994;38:339–346

137. Cole MG, Primeau FJ: Prognosis of delirium in elderly hospital patients. Can Med Assoc J 1993;149:41–46

138. Mackenzie TB, Popkin MK: Stress response syndrome occurring after delirium. Am J Psychiatry 1980;137:1433–1435

139. Platt MM, Breitbart W, Smith M et al: Efficacy of neuroleptics for hypoactive delirium. J Neuropsychiatry Clin Neurosci 1994;6:66–67

140. Camus V, Gonthier R, Dubos G et al: Etiologic and outcome profiles in hypoactive and hyperactive subtypes of delirium. J Geriatr Psychiatry Neurol 2000;13:38–42

141. Francis J, Kapoor WN: Prognosis after hospital discharge of older medical patients with delirium. J Am Geriatr Soc 1993;40:601–606

142. Dolan MM, Hawkes WG, Zimmerman SI et al: Delirium on hospital admission in aged hip fracture patients: Prediction of mortality and 2-year functional outcomes. J Gerontol A 2000;55:M527–M534

143. Marcantonio ER, Flacker JM, Michaels M et al: Delirium is independently associated with poor functional recovery after hip fracture. J Am Geriatr Soc 2000;48:618–624

144. Murray AM, Levkoff SE, Wetle TT et al: Acute delirium and functional decline in the hospitalized elderly patient. J Gerontol A 1993;48:M181–M186

145. Trzepacz PT, Mulsant BH, Dew MA et al: Is delirium different when it occurs in dementia? A study using the delirium rating scale. J Neuropsychiatry Clin Neurosci 1998;10:199–204

Chapter 62

Classification of the dementias

David Neary and Julie S. Snowden

Dementia is not the name of a disease. It is a generic term that refers to the cognitive and behavioral disorder resulting from chronic brain disease or encephalopathy. Chronic encephalopathies may be nonprogressive, occurring, for example, as a consequence of brain trauma or cerebral hypoxia; or progressive, arising as a result of intrinsic, extrinsic, or metabolic cerebral disorder. The major focus of this chapter are the dementia syndromes that result from progressive intrinsic degenerative and vascular disease. However, extrinsic and metabolic causes of chronic encephalopathy are also considered, because they are important for differential diagnosis.

DEMENTIA SYNDROMES

Traditionally, dementia has been construed as a global deterioration of intellectual function, yet there are good grounds for assuming such a definition to be erroneous. Cerebral diseases do not affect the brain uniformly, but preferentially affect certain brain regions and spare others. Moreover, psychological processes themselves are regionally organized and depend on the functioning of specific brain regions. It follows that different cerebral diseases should be associated with distinctive characteristic neuropsychological syndromes, whose identification can lead to a high degree of accuracy in clinical diagnosis. A useful empirical classification of progressive encephalopathies leading to dementia can be made on the basis of the major distribution of pathology within the brain. This classification is as follows:

* Cortical
* Subcortical
* Corticosubcortical
* Multifocal

Some disorders chiefly affect the cerebral cortex, whereas others predominantly affect subcortical structures. Others affect both cortex and subcortex together. Only a minority have a multifocal distribution, having no respect for functional anatomic systems. These anatomic distinctions are reflected in highly distinct patterns of cognitive and behavioral change, and neurological symptoms and signs. Within the classificatory framework, prototypical syndromes are described in terms of neurological findings, the precise nature of the psychological breakdown, the distribution of cerebral pathology as demonstrated by functional single-photon emission computed tomographic (SPECT) imaging, and the results of the associated electroencephalographic (EEG) recordings. This process of syndrome analysis permits a differential diagnosis of the different forms of dementia.

CORTICAL ENCEPHALOPATHIES
Functional topography of the cortex

Psychological functions are regionally organized in the cerebral cortex (Fig. 62-1). The posterior hemispheres are critical for perceptual and spatial functions, that is, appreciation of the identity of visual percepts (e.g., objects in the environment) and of their spatial relationship with respect to each other and to the individual. Breakdown in visual perception leads to a failure to recognize objects (agnosia) and faces (prosopagnosia), whereas spatial impairment leads to inability to navigate external surroundings (spatial disorientation). Language is dependent on the areas around the sylvian fissure, extending from the frontal into the parietal and temporal lobes in the left hemisphere. Breakdown of language leads to an inability to express and comprehend spoken and written language (aphasia) and to communicate by gesture (gestural apraxia). Parietal lesions of the left hemisphere may be associated with an inability to calculate (acalculia). The superior parietal areas are important for the organization of skilled movements. Failure of executive motor functions leads to difficulties in the purposeful use of the limbs, face, and mouth (apraxia). The medial portion of both hemispheres, designated the limbic system, which includes the hippocampus and amygdala, is essential for the acquisition and retention of information. Damage to limbic structures leads to a failure to learn new information and to recall past experience (amnesia). The anterior, or prefrontal, cortex is essential for the regulation of mental life, including strategic planning and monitoring and evaluation of actions taking place over time. Breakdown in these

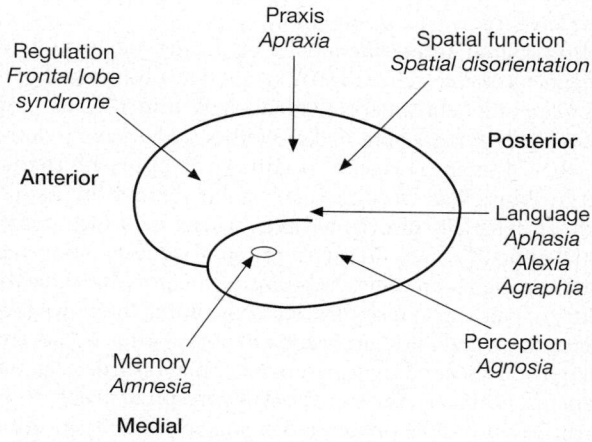

Figure 62-1 Functional topography of the cerebral cortex and the various psychological syndromes arising from breakdown of function of particular cortical areas.

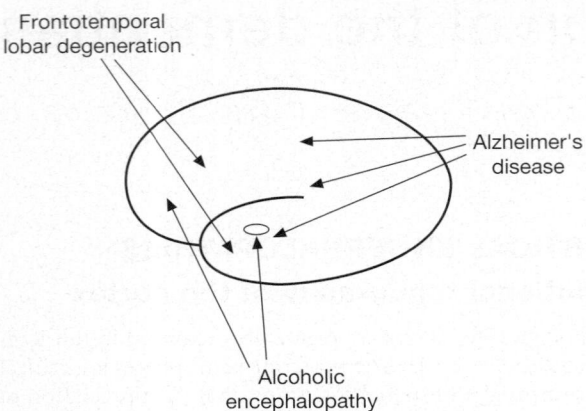

Figure 62-2 Topographic distribution of impaired function in cortical encephalopathies.

regulatory or executive processes leads to aberrant personal and social behavior, change in personality, and an inability to conceive of and successfully achieve behavioral goals.

Cortical encephalopathies give rise to distinct dementia syndromes, reflecting the topographic distribution of pathological change within anterior, medial, and posterior cortices (Fig. 62-2).

Alzheimer's disease

Alzheimer's disease[1] is a cortical dementia, in which the earliest symptom is commonly memory failure, reflecting medial temporal pathology. Patients have difficulty learning new information and are forgetful of day-to-day events. As the disease progresses past memories are also affected, although information from the distant as opposed to the recent past may appear to be relatively well preserved. Amnesia may, in a minority of patients, be the exclusive psychological symptom for many years, reflecting a relatively circumscribed distribution of pathological change within medial temporal lobe structures. Additional cognitive deficits in such patients may emerge only at the late stages.

Visuospatial impairment is a characteristic feature of Alzheimer's disease, reflecting pathological involvement of posterior cerebral hemispheres. Patients have difficulty aligning cutlery when laying a table, folding clothes, and orienting clothing when dressing, because of failure to appreciate spatial relationships. They become lost in their surroundings, and eventually spatially disoriented even within their own home. Spatial difficulties may dominate the clinical presentation and in some patients precede symptoms of memory breakdown. Failure of patients to recognize faces, including their own face in the mirror, and misidentification of objects often occurs late in the disease secondary to visuoperceptual disorder. Spatial problems, however, usually outweigh perceptual problems in the early and middle phase: patients have difficulty locating objects in the environment, which once located are recognized accurately.

When language areas around the perisylvian fissure are involved, language skills are affected. Utterances are halting, reflecting difficulty in finding words and failure to maintain a line of thought. Repetition and comprehension, reading, and writing and calculation are impaired. Alexia, agraphia, and acalculia are compounded by spatial difficulties, because the written word and numerals are poorly organized in space. Breakdown of skilled movements of the arms and legs may be secondary to spatial disorientation, which results in difficulty with copying drawings and designs (constructional apraxia) and with dressing (dressing apraxia). Sometimes there may be severe motor executive difficulties, disproportionate to perceptuospatial impairment, that are sufficient to prevent the manual use of objects and the adoption of postures and appropriate movements on attempted walking.

In contrast to the severe cognitive deficits, social graces are well preserved into the advanced stages of the disease. Indeed, the magnitude of the cognitive disorder is often masked by the patient's normal social facade. Patients rarely complain of symptoms spontaneously, although they may be aware of difficulties when confronted by test failures, and show signs of agitation and distress. The extent of insight is variable and seems to be inversely related to the severity of the patient's amnesia.

Neurological signs in Alzheimer's disease consist of akinesia, rigidity, and myoclonus, which emerge with the gradual involvement of subcortical structures. Physical problems, however, are dwarfed by the momentous psychological disturbance and may be totally absent until the relatively late stages of disease.

The EEG exhibits progressive slowing of waveforms. Computed tomography (CT) reveals nonspecific cerebral atrophy but functional imaging techniques, such as positron emission tomography (PET) and SPECT, reveal characteristic abnormalities of the parietal regions. Abnormalities may be present in the anterior regions, but typically these emerge relatively late in the disease and invariably in the context of posterior hemisphere deficits. Demographic features, the nature and distribution of pathological change, and genetic characteristics are summarized in Table 62-1.

Frontotemporal lobar degeneration

Frontotemporal lobar degeneration refers to a cortical degeneration pathologically distinct from Alzheimer's disease associated with circumscribed atrophy of the frontal and temporal lobes.[2] It encompasses distinct subsyndromes determined by the distribution of pathology within the anterior hemispheres (Fig. 62-3). Bilateral frontal and anterior temporal lobe involvement is characterized by a prominent behavioral disorder (frontotemporal dementia). Asymmetric involvement predominantly of the left dominant anterior hemisphere leads to the syndrome of progressive nonfluent aphasia. Predominant involvement of both temporal lobes leads to a syndrome of fluent aphasia with associative visual agnosia (semantic dementia). These syndromes may be complicated by the development of the amyotrophic form of motor neuron disease. Demographic, pathological, and genetic features are summarized in Table 62-2.

Frontotemporal dementia

Frontotemporal dementia,[1–4] although less common than Alzheimer's disease, accounts for approximately 20 percent of

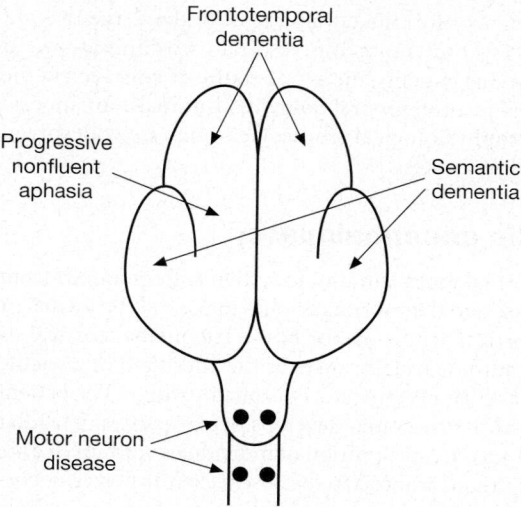

Figure 62-3 The clinical syndromes of frontotemporal lobar degeneration.

Table 62-1 Alzheimer's disease: demographic features, pathology, and genetics

Age of onset	Any age from 30 years onward. Most common after 65 years of age
Sex incidence	Affects females more than males
Duration	Variable, average 8 years, range 2–12 years
Gross pathological features	Generalized cortical atrophy with temporal lobe preference Ventricular dilatation
Histopathology	Numerous deposits of amyloid β/A4 protein in the cerebral cortex, many with dystrophic neurites (neuritic plaques) Amyloid β/A4 protein deposits in cerebellar cortex and basal ganglia Numerous neurofibrillary tangles in cerebral cortex and hippocampus containing tau and ubiquitin Amyloid angiography; β/A4 protein in vessel walls Hirano bodies and granulovacuolar degeneration in hippocampus
Genetics	Point mutations in codons 670/671 and codon 717 of gene for amyloid precursor protein, located on the long arm of chromosome 21 Other genetic loci on chromosome 14, 19 (apolipoprotein E), and 22 segregate with the disease Autosomal dominant inheritance

Table 62-2 Frontotemporal lobar degeneration: demographic features, pathology, and genetics

Age of onset	Usually 45–65 years, range 21–75
Sex incidence	Equal sex incidence
Duration	Variable. Median duration 8 years, range 2–20
Gross features	Atrophy particularly affecting the frontal and/or temporal lobes Bilateral frontal lobe and anterior temporal atrophy (frontotemporal dementia) Asymmetric atrophy of left hemisphere, particularly involving frontal and temporal regions (progressive nonfluent aphasia) Bilateral atrophy of temporal lobes (semantic dementia)
Histopathology	Affected areas of cortex show loss of pyramidal cells, microvacuolation of outer cortical laminae, and mild astrocytosis. No inclusion bodies or swollen neurons *or* Affected cortex shows severe loss of pyramidal cells and severe astrocytosis, sometimes with inclusion (Pick) bodies and swollen (Pick) neurons
Genetics	Up to 50 percent of patients have a positive family history of dementia and autosomal dominant inheritance is demonstrable in the majority. Some familial cases with Parkinsonian features (frontotemporal dementia/Parkinson's disease) show mutations in the *tau* gene on chromosome 17. Cases of frontotemporal dementia with motor neuron disease have shown linkage to chromosome 9

cases of primary cerebral atrophy occurring in the presenium. The striking characteristic is of change in personality and social and personal behavior. Patients rapidly become incapable of managing their own affairs and lose their jobs through irresponsibility and impaired judgment. They may appear apathetic and lacking in motivation, or overactive and disinhibited. Insight is lost and, in contrast to those with Alzheimer's disease, patients show no distress or concern when confronted with task failures. Stereotyped and perseverative behaviors may occur, ranging from simple repetitive actions such as hand rubbing to complex rituals surrounding activities of daily living. Gluttony, food fads, and a preference for sweet foods are common. Speech is economic and concrete, and verbatim copying of what is said by others (echolalia) and repetition of their own responses (perseveration) occur particularly in more apathetic patients. Patients eventually become mute. Severe difficulties in abstraction, mental set shifting, organizational, and strategic skills are elicited on psychological tests sensitive to frontal lobe dysfunction. Despite the severity of their behavioral disorder, patients remain oriented in their environment and show no spatial abnormalities into the terminal stages of the disorder. Neurological signs are minimal and consist of primitive reflexes in the early stages. Akinesia and rigidity occur very late in the disease. The EEG is normal. CT confirms cerebral atrophy, which may be more evident in frontal regions. Preferential involvement of frontal and anterior temporal lobes is typically demonstrable on magnetic resonance imaging (MRI). SPECT confirms selective abnormalities in the frontal and temporal lobes.

Progressive nonfluent aphasia

In this form of lobar degeneration a progressive decline in language occurs in the relative absence of other psychological deficits.[2,5] Speech is nonfluent, effortful, and lacking in prosody, with resemblance to a Broca-type aphasia. Repetition, series speech, and reading aloud are also impaired, with effortful production and sometimes phonemic (literal) paraphasic errors (e.g., "tig" for "big"). Word finding difficulties are prominent. Writing and oral spelling are impaired. Comprehension, at least at the single word level, is relatively preserved. Structural brain imaging using CT and MRI reveals atrophy of the left cerebral hemisphere. Asymmetric left hemisphere abnormalities are also apparent on SPECT imaging. The EEG may be normal or show asymmetric slow waves over the dominant cerebral hemispheres. Behavioral change akin to that of frontotemporal dementia may develop late in the disease, reflecting a spread of pathology to both frontal lobes.

Semantic dementia

Patients with semantic dementia exhibit a multimodal loss of meaning, affecting understanding of words, and face and object identity.[2] Spontaneous speech is fluent, effortless, and grammatically correct, but empty of content and there are semantic (verbal) paraphasias (e.g., "dog" for "pig"), but no sound-based errors. There is a profound anomia and lack of comprehension for spoken and written words. Repetition, reading aloud, and writing to dictation of regularly spelled words are essentially intact, reflecting preservation of phonological and articulatory skills. The pattern of language disturbances closely resembles the transcortical sensory aphasia of focal lesions. Failure to recognize the significance of objects and the identity of faces occurs despite a preserved ability to copy accurately and match objects and faces (associative agnosia). The relative prominence of the semantic disorder for verbal or for visual material reflects the relative involvement of left and right temporal lobes.

In contrast to patients with Alzheimer's disease visuospatial skills are invariably normal. Moreover, day-to-day memorizing is well preserved, contrasting with the striking loss of "semantic" knowledge. Behavioral alterations are common, although they are typically less prominent and socially disruptive than those seen in frontotemporal dementia, and have a more compulsive quality. CT reveals either nonspecific cerebral atrophy or more selective widening of the interhemispheric and sylvian fissures suggesting frontotemporal atrophy, especially involving the temporal lobes. Prominent temporal lobe atrophy is invariably detected by MRI. SPECT shows reduced uptake of tracer in anterior regions. The EEG is normal.

Frontotemporal lobar degeneration and motor neuron disease

Frontotemporal lobar degeneration, in particular the syndrome of frontotemporal dementia, can be complicated by the development of motor neuron disease.[6] This is of the amyotrophic form with bulbar palsy, weakness, wasting, and fasciculations of the limbs, in the absence of significant spasticity of the muscles. Typically the neurological symptoms and signs commence after the development of the dementia and lead to death within 3 years from respiratory complications. In longer-surviving patients, the extrapyramidal signs seen in the late stages of frontotemporal dementia can make an appearance. Electrophysiological studies demonstrate widespread denervation of muscles.

Alcoholic encephalopathy

Both the frontal lobes and limbic system suffer damage from alcohol abuse and therefore alcoholics may exhibit a medial or anterior cortical syndrome, or both. The medial cortical or amnesic syndrome usually arises as the aftermath of an acute neurological crisis (Wernicke's encephalopathy).[7] The patient sinks into stupor or coma, develops ocular palsies, irregular pupils, and ataxia. A proportion of individuals who survive are left with profound amnesia in the absence of the posterior cortical symptoms of aphasia, spatial disorientation, or apraxia (Korsakoff's amnesia or Wernicke–Korsakoff syndrome). They may perform normally on tests sensitive to frontal lobe dysfunction. A proportion of chronic alcohol abusers who neglect their diet present with a progressive dementing syndrome in which there are features both of frontal lobe disturbance and amnesia. Korsakoff's amnesic syndrome is associated with gradual improvement, although this may not be complete in all cases, whereas the more insidious presentation is associated with chronic decline in mental function. CT and MRI evidence of cerebral atrophy is seen in the majority of individuals with both the acute and chronic alcoholic syndromes.

SUBCORTICAL ENCEPHALOPATHIES

Several diseases predominantly affect subcortical structures with relative sparing of the cerebral cortex.[8] These include degenerative disorders such as Parkinson's disease, Huntington's disease, and progressive supranuclear palsy. A similar syndrome also occurs when the subcortical white matter is destroyed by multiple infarcts or is stretched and damaged as a consequence of chronic repeated head trauma and hydrocephalus. Subcortical structures and their projections to the cerebral cortex exert a quantitative and regulatory effect on the pace and organization of psychological functions. Patients with subcortical disorders exhibit slowness and rigidity of thinking (bradyphrenia) with inflexibility and difficulty in switching responses (perseveration). Although forgetful, they do not exhibit a severe amnesia. They have difficulties in planning and sequencing mental events and may fail on tests sensitive to frontal lobe dysfunction, thus showing similarities to patients with anterior cortical disease. They do not, however, show the specific abnormalities of language, visual perception, and spatial functioning seen in cortical disorders. Nor do they typically show the gross behavioral disorder of frontal cortical disease. The exception to this is Huntington's disease, in which personality change and bizarre behavior are not uncommon. Progressive supranuclear palsy represents the prototypical subcortical dementia.

In subcortical disorders the neuropsychological deficits are overshadowed by profound and characteristic neurological symptoms and signs: akinesia, rigidity, and tremor in

Parkinson's disease; involuntary and purposeless jerking movements in Huntington's disease, and paralysis of eye movements in progressive supranuclear palsy. The EEG may be normal or show slight slowing of waveforms but is of no diagnostic significance. CT and MRI may be normal or show nonspecific cerebral atrophy. In progressive supranuclear palsy, PET and SPECT reveal abnormalities in frontal cortex similar to those of frontotemporal dementia.

CORTICOSUBCORTICAL ENCEPHALOPATHY

Two disorders show features of both cortical and subcortical syndromes determined by the spread of pathology to both structures. In Lewy body disease the distribution of pathology is symmetric, whereas in corticobasal degeneration it is highly asymmetric.

Cortical Lewy body disease

Lewy body disease[9] is a disorder of elderly people which is usually sporadic. Mental changes develop before or after parkinsonian symptoms and signs of akinesia, rigidity, and tremor, which are responsive to the administration of L-dopa. Changes in the cerebral cortex may give rise to cortical symptoms of aphasia, agnosia, and apraxia but the dominant feature of the illness is a fluctuating mental state with visual illusions and hallucinations leading to secondary delusions. Such fluctuations, which are presumably due to simultaneous disorder of cortex and subcortex, are highly diagnostic, because they are not characteristic of the cortical or subcortical encephalopathies. When "confusion" does occur in these latter disorders it usually relates to systemic complications, drug toxicity, anesthesia, or the relative sensory deprivation of night-time or unfamiliar surroundings. The EEG in Lewy body disease characteristically reveals severe slowing of waveforms and sometimes periodic wave complexes. CT reveals cerebral atrophy. SPECT reveals reductions of uptake in the cerebral cortex especially in the posterior hemispheres. Demographic features, the nature and distribution of pathological change, and genetic characteristics are summarized in Table 62-3.

Corticobasal degeneration

Corticobasal degeneration[10] is a rare condition in which a cortical neuropsychological syndrome (apraxia) is superimposed on a subcortical dementia and neurological signs of basal ganglia disorder. There is significant left–right asymmetry with respect to the severity of neurological signs and extent of apraxia, reflecting an asymmetric distribution of pathology within cortical and subcortical sites.

Asymmetric akinesia and rigidity affect predominantly the upper limbs, which are also the site of tremor, dystonic movements, and myoclonus. Psychologically there is slowing, inflexibility, and perseveration concordant with a subcortical syndrome. The cortical syndrome is characterized by a profound, asymmetric apraxia, typically most marked in the upper limbs, but gradually involving buccofacial, lower limb, and whole body movements. The limbs progressively lose all

Table 62-3 Lewy body disease: demographic features, pathology, and genetics	
Age of onset	Usually over 40 years. Most common in elderly people
Sex incidence	Affects males at least as often or more than females
Duration	Variable, range 1–12 years. Often more rapid course than Alzheimer's disease
Gross features	Mild generalized cortical atrophy Depigmentation of substantia nigra
Histopathology	Lewy inclusion bodies in cerebral cortical neurons, usually layers V and VI mostly in cingulate and entorhinal cortex Ubiquitin protein Lewy bodies in substantia nigra Numerous cortical deposits of amyloid β/A4 protein in 40 percent of patients A few tangles present, more in the hippocampus and entorhinal cortex, and such patients have an amyloid angiopathy
Genetics	Usually sporadic

executive functions and may develop autonomous movements (alien limb). Additional features of parietal lobe disease, namely visuospatial deficits, may also emerge. CT reveals cerebral atrophy. Functional imaging (PET and SPECT) reveals asymmetric abnormalities of the basal ganglia and associated frontoparietal cortex. EEG changes are of nonspecific asymmetric slow waves.

Vascular encephalopathy

Recurrent completed strokes lead to an accumulated neurological and psychological deficit. The ictal nature of the evolution of the disorder, together with evidence of multiple infarctions or hemorrhages on brain imaging, is not likely to lead to diagnostic confusion.

When vascular lesions predominantly affect the subcortical white matter,[1,8] a characteristic subcortical syndrome (subcortical arteriosclerotic dementia) emerges that is often progressive and lacking ictal events. This syndrome requires differentiation from subcortical neurodegenerative diseases and from communicating hydrocephalus.

In a proportion of patients vascular events occur both in the cortex and the subcortex, but again without evident historical stroke-like events. The clinical picture of multiple (cortical and subcortical) infarct dementia may superficially resemble Alzheimer's disease. CT, MRI, and functional brain imaging reveals asymmetrically distributed focal lesions in the cerebral hemispheres. Demographic features, the nature and distribution of pathological change, and genetic characteristics are summarized in Table 62-4.

MULTIFOCAL ENCEPHALOPATHY

Subacute spongiform encephalopathies (prion disease), such as Creutzfeldt–Jakob disease,[11,12] are rapidly progressive disorders with low familial incidence, which are often terminal within

Table 62-4 **Vascular dementia: demographics, pathology, and genetics**	
Age of onset	Usually after 40 years. Most common in elderly people
Sex incidence	Males affected more often than females
Duration	Variable, up to 12 years
Gross features	Multiple completed infarcts in cerebral cortical and subcortical gray matter and internal capsule *or* White matter demyelination, often with lacunae, usually in frontal and temporal cortex. Incomplete infarction
Histopathology	Completed infarcts, many cases with histopathology of Alzheimer's disease *or* Fibrous and hyaline degeneration of arteries. Stenosis of lumen. Microcystic degeneration around blood vessels sometimes confluent leading to incomplete infarction of white matter. Reactive astrocytosis
Genetics	Spontaneous (associated with atherosclerosis of extracerebral arteries or hypertension and cigarette smoking)

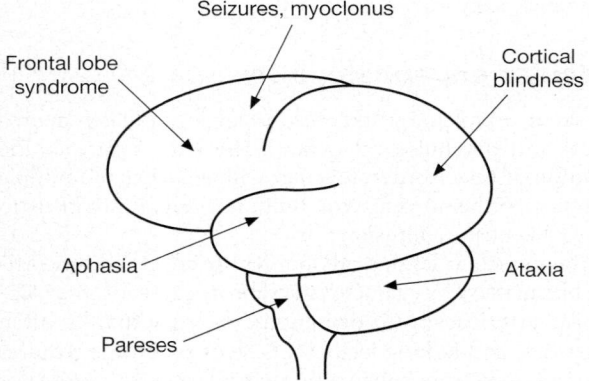

Figure 62-4 Neurological and cognitive disorders associated with multifocal encephalopathy. The figure illustrates the potential widespread cerebral involvement, including cerebellum and brain stem as well as cortical and subcortical areas, resulting in ataxia (unsteadiness) and paresis (paralysis).

approximately 6 months. Longer survival may occur in familial disease forms such as the Gerstmann–Straussler–Scheinker syndrome and in the new variant forms of Creutzfeldt–Jakob disease[13] in young people.

The aggressive disease process seems not to respect anatomic boundaries or functional systems so that a wide variety of psychological and neurological deficits rapidly emerge (Fig. 62-4). Some patients present with neurological symptoms such as a cerebellar syndrome, cortical blindness, sensory motor deficits, myoclonus, and epileptic seizures. Focal psychological syndromes such as aphasia may herald the onset of the disease.

When thalamic structures are preferentially involved the predominant picture may be one of progressive somnolence. In contrast to cortical encephalopathies, in Creutzfeldt–Jakob disease, psychological impairment occurs together with the rapid march of neurological disorder and in an unpredictable manner. However, in the new variant form of Creutzfeldt–Jakob disease, linked to the epidemic of bovine spongiform encephalopathy[13] a "psychiatric" presentation with depression, withdrawal, apathy, or psychosis may precede the onset of ataxia, rigidity, and myoclonus for prolonged periods, prejudicing early diagnosis. In the final stages of Creutzfeldt–Jakob disease episodes of unresponsiveness increase in frequency and duration until akinetic mutism supervenes.

The severe neurological and psychological disorder is reflected in the grossly disturbed EEG in which there is profound slowing of waveforms and characteristic periodic triphasic wave complexes emerge. CT is either normal or reveals nonspecific cerebral atrophy. SPECT imaging reveals a patchy reduction of uptake of tracer in the cerebral cortex.

Diagnostic considerations

Cortical, subcortical, corticosubcortical, and multifocal encephalopathies differ with respect to the relative prominence of associated mental and physical changes in the evolution of disease (Table 62-5), providing a further basis for differential diagnosis of these disorders. Cortical encephalopathies are characterized by profound mental changes in the relative absence of early neurological signs, whereas subcortical encephalopathies are associated with striking physical signs while mental changes may be of relatively lesser significance and tend to emerge later in the disease. In corticosubcortical and multifocal encephalopathies physical symptoms and signs emerge along with the psychological disturbance. Examination of the cerebrospinal fluid is unhelpful, except in sporadic Creutzfeldt–Jakob disease when there may be high levels of 14.3.3 proteinase inhibitor proteins, released from damaged neurons.

The EEG is also of diagnostic significance. In Alzheimer's disease the standard EEG often shows mild slowing of waveforms in the moderately advanced stages of the disease. Frontotemporal dementia is unique in that a normal record is preserved until the latest stages of the disease. Gross slowing of waveforms and periodic complexes are characteristic of the subacute spongiform encephalopathies (with the exception of new variant Creutzfeldt–Jakob disease) and also of cortical Lewy body disease. Whereas CT is useful in delineating structural changes such as the presence of vascular disease or hydrocephalus, it is less useful in differential diagnosis in neurodegenerative disorders because scans may be normal or reveal nonspecific cerebral atrophy. However, high-resolution MRI may be useful in highlighting prominent areas of atrophy, complementing the clinical and SPECT findings. SPECT imaging demonstrates functional change in the brain which is of high diagnostic value in the neurodegenerative disorders, because the abnormalities on imaging closely reflect the topographic distribution of pathology within the cerebrum (Table 62-6). The radioactive tracer crosses the blood–brain barrier and is taken up by cerebral tissue reflecting the cerebral blood flow and perfusion, and hence regional metabolic function. In frontotemporal dementia the characteristic abnormality in the frontotemporal lobes contrasts strikingly

Table 62-5 Nature and relative severity of psychological, neurological, and electroencephalographic (EEG) disorders associated with forms of encephalopathy

Encephalopathy	Cognitive disorder	Neurological disorder	EEG
Cortical	Severe, specific	Mild, specific	Slow (AD); normal (FTLD)
Subcortical	Mild, specific	Severe, specific	Nonspecific
Corticosubcortical	Severe, specific	Severe, specific	Periodic complexes (CLBD)
Multifocal	Severe, nonspecific	Severe, nonspecific	Periodic complexes (CJD)

Abbreviations: AD, Alzheimer's disease; FTLD, frontotemporal lobar degeneration; CLBD, cortical Lewy body disease; CJD, Creutzfeldt–Jakob disease.

Table 62-6 SPECT abnormalities in dementia

Syndrome	Disease	Abnormality
Anterior cortical	Frontotemporal dementia	Anterior deficit
Posterior cortical	Alzheimer's disease	Posterior deficit
Subcortical	Progressive supranuclear palsy	Anterior subcortical deficits
Corticosubcortical	Corticobasal degeneration	Asymmetric fronto-parietal deficits
Multifocal	Subacute spongiform encephalopathy	Diffuse and focal deficits

with the bilateral parietal defects seen in Alzheimer's disease (see Plate 62-1). An asymmetric dominant hemispheric defect characterizes progressive nonfluent aphasia, whereas predominantly bitemporal defects underlie the "semantic" dementia of fluent aphasia and associative agnosia. Subcortical disorders such as progressive supranuclear palsy display an anterior cerebral defect that is less severe than in lobar atrophy. An asymmetric frontoparietal defect is seen in corticobasal degeneration, whereas multifocal lesions are demonstrated in subacute spongiform encephalopathy.

Advances in neurogenetics have permitted the diagnosis from blood samples of specific genetic mutations, accounting for Huntington's disease (huntington gene, chromosome 4) and familial Creutzfeldt–Jakob disease (prion gene, chromosome 20). However, mutations in the presenilin genes in presenile Alzheimer's disease and in the tau gene on chromosome 17 in frontotemporal dementia account for only small numbers of affected families and so cannot be the basis, as yet, of diagnostic tests. Moreover, the detection of risk factors for late onset Alzheimer's disease, such as the apolipoprotein e4 genotype cannot be used diagnostically.

Extrinsic encephalopathy

Extrinsic brain disorders describe the neurosurgical conditions that lead to mechanical compression of the brain and increased space occupation within the cranium, requiring surgical decompressive relief. Two major clinical syndromes are associated with extrinsic compressive disease. The most common results from a space-occupying and expanding lesion within or on the surface of the brain such as a neoplasm, abscess, or hematoma. Here a focal and unilateral neuropsychological syndrome (e.g., aphasia and right hemiparesis) related to the specific site of the lesion in the cerebral cortex or subcortex is compounded by the symptoms and signs of raised intracranial pressure, namely headache and papilledema and progressive confusion and obtundation leading to coma and eventually death due to brain stem failure.

The second extrinsic cortical syndrome is that of hydrocephalus[1] in which, due to obstruction of the flow and absorption of cerebrospinal fluid (CSF), the cerebral ventricles expand under the increased pressure of the CSF. A characteristic syndrome emerges in which bilateral neurological signs reflect the progressive change to the subcortical white matter and nuclei, especially those immediately adjacent to the ventricles. The gait is characteristically slow, shuffling, and wide-based with the feet seemingly rooted to the ground. There is corticospinal (pyramidal) weakness and spasticity of the lower limbs, often with akinesia and rigidity. The upper limbs are less affected, although clumsy and incoordinate, and speech is slow, slurred, and indistinct. Mental function is slowed and inefficient, with response perseverations. Concentration and memory become progressively impaired but "cortical functions" are unaffected, so that aphasia, agnosia, apraxia, and spatial disorientation are absent. This syndrome shares commonalities with the "subcortical dementia" described above. However, in the case of obstructive hydrocephalus usually due to a tumor, progress is rapid, and confusion, obtundation, and coma occur early. In the case of "communicating" hydrocephalus due to impaired CSF absorption the cause is more chronic, consciousness is disrupted later, and therefore the differential diagnosis from neurodegenerative and vascular forms of dementia can be more difficult and requires both structural and functional imaging and physiological studies of the CSF pathways.

Metabolic encephalopathy

Another important group of disorders of general medical significance that must be distinguished from progressive dementia syndromes are those arising when systemic disorders attack a potentially intact nervous system.[14] Cerebral impairment fluctuates in degree as a function of the severity of the general medical disorder, and constitutes a distinct clinical syndrome, referred to as a *confusional state*, intermediate between full arousal and unresponsive coma. The reduced level of arousal leads secondarily to reduced cognitive efficiency. Mental and physical tasks are carried out more slowly, and the ability to sustain attention and attend selectively in the face of distraction are severely compromised. Drowsiness and sleepiness may be evident. Rapid fluctuations of alertness occur.

Before coma supervenes, behavior may be overactive and purposeless (delirium). Language is not frankly dysphasic insofar as grammatical and phonemic paraphasic errors are absent, but patients are unable to maintain a coherent train of thought so that content of speech is irrelevant and often incomprehensible. Written expressions are typically even more incoherent than spoken utterances, and may contain perseverations of words and individual pencil strokes. Naming errors occur, with verbal substitutions and perseverations, although these are inconsistent over repeated trials.

Misperception leads to illusions and hallucinations, often of a fearful aspect. Patients have difficulty carrying out all tasks requiring organizational skills. Constructional tasks such as copying drawings and spatial tasks such as maze-trailing are failed. There is disorientation particularly for time, but often also for place, but never for personal identity. The purposeful regulation of behavior becomes impossible, leading to erratic responses and motiveless wandering. Neurological signs frequently accompanying metabolic encephalopathy are postural tremor, asterixis, and myoclonus. The EEG typically reveals diffuse slow-wave large-amplitude waveforms. Metabolic encephalopathy may be produced by a variety of systemic diseases (Table 62-7). In addition to the characteristic neuropsychological syndrome there is evidence of systemic disease on clinical examination and hematological, biochemical, and endocrine investigation.

Metabolic encephalopathy is likely to account only for a small proportion of the chronic encephalopathies typically encountered by specialists working with the elderly. Nevertheless, recognition of its features is essential so that it can be accurately distinguished from dementia due to progressive intrinsic brain disease. The clinical differentiation is of high therapeutic import because the metabolic encephalopathies are essentially treatable. Diagnosis and treatment of systemic disease, especially in the early stages, can lead to a complete resolution of the metabolic encephalopathy. Moreover, patients with dementia due to intrinsic brain disease, in whom an inexorable decline is inevitable, are themselves not immune, but indeed are more susceptible, to the development of metabolic encephalopathy because they have less cerebral reserve and are more likely to be old and frail.

The development of fluctuations in arousal and especially nocturnal confusion in patients with dementia should instigate a search for systemic complications such as drug intoxication and infection.

CONCLUSION

Dementia is a generic term embracing a number of neuropsychological syndromes characteristic of different brain diseases. Dementia is not a nonspecific end-stage intellectual failure, nor is it a synonym for brain disease. Hierarchical descriptions at the levels of neurological and psychological behavior taken together with the results of brain imaging and electrophysiology permit a rational classification of disorders leading to forms of dementia.

KEY POINTS   Classification of the dementias

- Dementia is not a generalized, nonspecific impairment of intellect; there are unique dementia syndromes associated with specific disease entities.

- The pattern of mental change is determined by the precise distribution of pathology within the brain in different diseases.

- The principal clinical distinctions are between disorders of the neocortex and subcortex and between disorders affecting the posterior and anterior cerebral hemispheres.

- Accurate clinical diagnosis is possible during life and is aided by brain imaging and some recent advances in molecular genetics.

REFERENCES

1. O'Brien J, Ames D, Burns A: Dementia, 2nd Ed. Arnold, London, 2000
2. Neary D, Snowden JS, Gustafson L et al: Frontotemporal lobar degeneration. A consensus on clinical diagnostic criteria. Neurology 1998;51:1546–1554
3. Gustafson L: Frontal lobe degeneration of non-Alzheimer type. II. Clinical picture and differential diagnosis. Arch Gerontol Geriatr 1987;6:209–223
4. Neary D, Snowden JS, Northen B, Goulding PJ: Dementia of frontal lobe type. J Neurol Neurosurg Psychiatry 1988;51:353–361
5. Mesulam M-M: Slowly progressive aphasia without generalized dementia. Ann Neurol 1982;11:592–598
6. Neary D, Snowden JS, Mann DMA, Northern B: Frontal lobe dementia and motor neurone disease. J Neurol Neurosurg Psychiatry 1990;53:23–32
7. Victor M, Adams RD, Collins GH: The Wernicke–Korsakoff Syndrome. Blackwell, Oxford, 1971
8. Cummings JL: Subcortical Dementia. Oxford University Press, London, 1990
9. McKeith IG, Galasko D, Kosaka K et al: Consensus guidelines for the clinical and pathological diagnosis of dementia with Lewy bodies (DLB): report of the Consortium on DLB international workshop. Neurology 1996;47:1113–1124
10. Rinne JO, Lee MS, Thompson PD, Marsden CD: Corticobasal degeneration. A clinical study of 36 cases. Brain 1994;117:1183–1196
11. Matthews WB: Creutzfeldt-Jakob disease. In Frederiks JAM (ed): Handbook of Clinical Neurology. Elsevier, Amsterdam, 1985:289–299
12. Kretzschmar HA, Ironside JW, DeArmond SJ, Tateishi J: Diagnostic criteria for sporadic Creutzfeldt–Jakob disease. Arch Neurol 1996;53:913–920
13. Will RG, Zeidler M, Stewart GE et al: Diagnosis of new variant Creutzfeldt-Jakob disease. Ann Neurol 2000;47:575–582
14. Albert MS, Moss MB: Acute confusional states. In Geriatric Neuropsychology. Guilford Press, New York, 1988:100–114

Table 62-7 Causes of metabolic encephalopathy

Toxic state:
- Systemic infection
- Alcohol, drug overdose

Deficiency state:
- Vitamin B_{12} deficiency

Hepatic encephalopathy

Renal encephalopathy

Cardiorespiratory encephalopathy

Endocrine disorder:
- Diabetic ketoacidosis
- Hypoglycemia
- Hypothyroidism

Electrolyte imbalance:
- Hyper- and hyponatremia
- Hyper- and hypocalcemia

Chapter 63

Presentation and clinical management of dementia

Evelyn M. Russell and Alistair Burns

The purpose of this chapter is to provide an overview of the presentation and clinical management of dementia. The clinical manifestations of dementia can be described in three categories: (1) *neuropsychological*: memory loss (amnesia) is universal and often associated with aphasia (language disorder), apraxia (the inability to carry out motor tasks despite intact motor function), and agnosia (the inability to recognize people and objects despite intact sensory function); (2) *neuropsychiatric*: psychiatric symptoms and behavioral disturbances have become increasingly recognized as important, are distressing to patients and care-givers, and often determine the need for a patient to be institutionalized; (3) *activities of daily living*: loss of the ability to care for oneself can lead to practical difficulties, and loss of independence is probably what people fear most about dementia.

Discussions of the management of dementia usually revolve around drugs to ameliorate the symptoms of cognitive impairment. Although there are agents that have a positive impact on memory loss, there is no curative treatment for most types of dementia. This inevitably encourages a pervasive attitude of therapeutic nihilism. However, there is much that can be done for patients and their families in terms of diagnosis, education, alleviation of excesses of behavior and distressing symptoms, advice, and practical help.

DIAGNOSIS

Definitions of dementia have evolved over the last two decades. They initially encompassed the broad nonspecific concept of an organic brain syndrome characterized by a global deterioration of higher mental functioning which was regarded as progressive in nature and occurred in the absence of delirium.[1]

The most commonly used criteria are those from the *Diagnostic and Statistical Manual* (now in its fourth edition, DSM-IV)[2] which carry definitions of dementia of the Alzheimer type and vascular dementia. The core features of dementia are the development of multiple cognitive deficits manifested by both memory impairment (impaired ability to learn new information or to recall previously learned information) and one (or more) of the following cognitive disturbances: (a) aphasia, (b) apraxia, (c) agnosia, (d) disturbance in executive functioning (i.e., planning, organization, sequencing, abstracting).

The definition includes the fact that the deficits should cause significant impairment in social or occupational functioning and represent a significant decline from a previous level of functioning. The deficits must not occur exclusively during the course of delirium, must not be accounted for by another diagnosis such as depression or schizophrenia, and substance-induced conditions, central nervous system conditions and systemic conditions must all have been excluded. Subtypes are defined both for dementia with Alzheimer's disease and vascular dementia, and those with delirium, with delusions, with depressed mood, and uncomplicated (the absence of these three), and it is allowed to define them further if there is an associated behavioral disturbance. Alzheimer's disease can be further subcategorized into early onset (onset aged 65 years or less) or late onset (65 years or over).

Dementia defines a clinical syndrome affecting brain function in a similar way that jaundice defines a clinical syndrome affecting the liver. As with jaundice, dementia has a number of causes both intra- and extracranial (cf. intrahepatic and extrahepatic). The list of causes is long and includes infection (e.g., Creutzfeld–Jakob disease), metabolic (e.g., thyroid disease), nutritional (e.g., B_{12} deficiency), vascular (e.g., multi-infarct dementia), inflammatory (e.g., systemic lupus erythematosus), malignancy (general effects of carcinoma or the presence of intracranial tumors such as a meningioma), obstructive (e.g., normal pressure hydrocephalus), and degenerative dementias (e.g., Alzheimer's disease and Lewy body dementia).

Differential diagnosis

This includes what are described as the five Ds—*D*epression, *D*elirium, *D*rug, and two other categories, *D*ecline of memory with normal aging and situations where there is *D*iagnostic difficulty (references 3 and 4 present reviews of the differential diagnosis).

The most important differential diagnoses of dementia in older people are delirium (confusional states) and depression. The situation is complicated by the fact that patients may have one or even both of these conditions superimposed on dementia. Delirium can be recognized by the presence of marked fluctuations in the clinical picture of the patient (a change over a day may cause relatives and even staff to suppose a degree of control is being exercised by the patient) and characteristically is associated with impaired concentration, poor attention, over-arousal, changes in behavior, fearful affect, and perceptual abnormalities such as visual hallucinations. Clouding of consciousness was previously the hallmark by which delirium was diagnosed but it is a difficult sign to detect and disorders of attention and concentration tend to be used as proxy measures. It can be difficult to differentiate between delirium and a dementia associated with fluctuating cognitive performance such as vascular dementia or Lewy body dementia.

Depression can mimic dementia and the term *pseudodementia* was coined to describe patients who presented with cognitive impairment in the context of depressive symptoms. Studies using computed tomography (CT) scans have shown that such patients often have evidence of brain atrophy

Summary of management algorithm

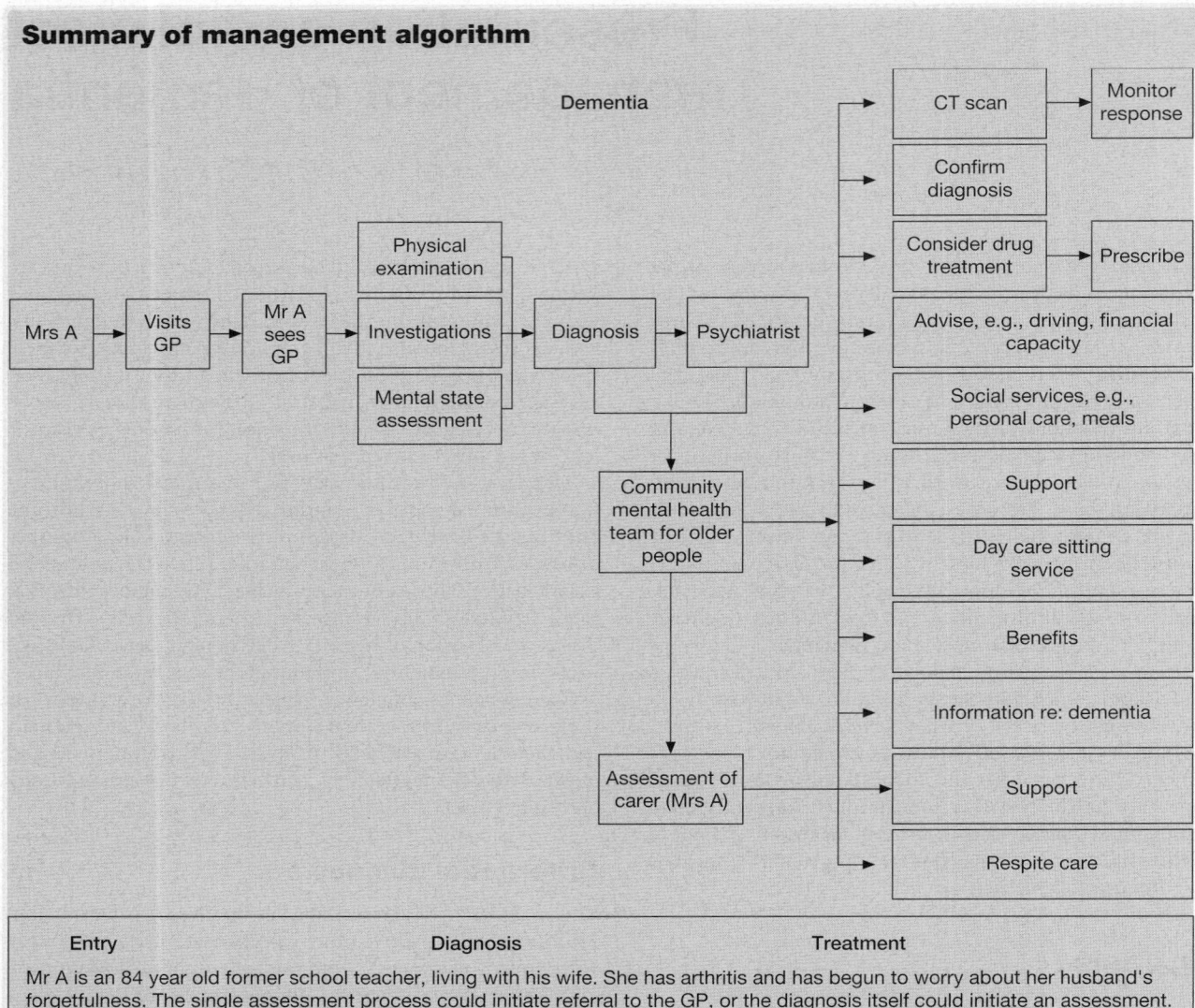

Mr A is an 84 year old former school teacher, living with his wife. She has arthritis and has begun to worry about her husband's forgetfulness. The single assessment process could initiate referral to the GP, or the diagnosis itself could initiate an assessment.

intermediate between normal age-matched controls and patients with dementia. Patients with depression and no associated brain abnormalities may also present with self-neglect and loss of interest and may perform poorly on formal testing of cognitive function, often giving depressive "don't know" answers to questions rather than providing an incorrect answer. The diagnosis of depression can be reached if patients are questioned about their mood, associated neurovegetative symptoms (e.g. diurnal mood variation, poor appetite, early morning wakening, poor concentration, anergia), and negative thoughts about the future and their own self-worth. Older people may not present with feelings of low mood but will admit to experiencing a loss of pleasure (anhedonia) and to giving up their interests over and above what might be normally expected for an older person. Such changes may be explained away by the patient as a natural reaction to growing old or to limitations imposed by physical disability. An informed account of the situation from a relative or care-giver is invaluable in teasing apart the history. The changes in memory which occur with normal aging can be difficult to differentiate from an early dementia. The detailed

neuropsychological differences between the two conditions is outside the scope of this chapter but are discussed elsewhere.[5,5a] The two situations where diagnostic difficulties can arise are when the patient has poor hearing or vision, has been institutionalized for years or has pre-existing cognitive problems (as with a person who has learning difficulties).

Clinical presentation of dementia

Initial presentation

Patients with dementia may present to specialist services when their symptoms are moderately severe and have started to impair independent functioning. By that stage the patient will often be unable to give an accurate history and may deny any difficulties. A collateral history should be obtained from anyone available, preferably a family member. Although dementia may appear to have had a sudden onset, perhaps coinciding with the death of a spouse or a move from a familiar neighborhood, such an impression may have merely brought the condition to the notice of others. Support of the patient by a spouse or other care-giver can minimize problems that become evident to others only after a bereavement. A good history from a son or daughter usually describes the true nature of the sequence of events. Failing cognitive function can be minimized by adherence to rigid routines that are disrupted when the patient moves away from familiar surroundings.

Signs and symptoms of Alzheimer's disease

Common early symptoms of Alzheimer's disease are memory impairment and disorientation in time and place. Oppenheim[6] found that in one-third of patients a psychiatric problem was the presenting complaint. Memory impairment particularly affects short-term memory, and the significance of such a change is sometimes not fully appreciated by families and others (including professionals), being dismissed as a "normal" age-related change. Changes in personality may, retrospectively, be regarded as one of the earliest signs of dementia and are well documented in the later stages. Blessed et al.[7] described 11 types of personality change that are seen: increased rigidity; increased egocentricity; impairment of regard for the feelings of others; coarsening of affect; impairment of emotional control; hilarity in inappropriate situations; diminished emotional responsiveness; sexual misdemeanor; hobbies relinquished; diminished initiative or growing apathy; and purposeless hyperactivity. Impairment of judgment is an important symptom that may put the patient at risk and cause concern to families.

The psychiatric symptoms and behavioral disturbances seen in Alzheimer's disease (and other dementias) comprise a heterogeneous group of phenomena including depression, hallucinations, delusions, agitation, aggression, and wandering. Various shorthand terms have been used to describe them such as noncognitive features (to distinguish them from the cognitive problems of amnesia, aphasia, apraxia, and agnosia), neuropsychiatric features and Behavioural and Psychological Symptoms of Dementia (BPSD).[8]

The overall course of Alzheimer's disease is usually steadily and smoothly progressive with death following usually within 5–7 years when the onset is in later life.[9]

The most cited criteria for the diagnosis of Alzheimer's disease are the NINCDS-ADRD.[10] A number of studies have demonstrated the validity and reliability of these criteria in accurately predicting the presence of Alzheimer's disease at post-mortem in around 90 percent of patients.[11]

Signs and symptoms of vascular dementia

Differentiation between Alzheimer's disease and vascular dementia can be difficult during life and an accurate diagnosis often depends on a reliable informant supplying a collateral history. Classically, the onset of a vascular dementia is sudden and follows a clearly definable cerebrovascular accident. The course is usually described as having a stepwise progression with episodes of clouding of consciousness and subsequently a fluctuating level of cognitive impairment. Commonly they consist of abrupt episodes of hemiparesis, sensory change, dysphasia, or visual disturbances. At first they can be transient and followed by gradual restitution of function but later permanent neurological deficits appear. There is greater mood lability and a greater tendency toward depression and anxiety than is commonly seen in Alzheimer's

disease. Lacunar (small) infarcts can be associated with gradual mental deterioration without focal neurological signs. Other features include somatic symptoms such as headache, dizziness, tinnitus, and syncope, which may be the main complaints for some time prior to diagnosis. The patchy nature of the psychological deficits in contrast to the global impairment of Alzheimer's disease is said to distinguish between the two types of dementia with relative preservation of personality and insight in vascular dementia.

The key features that distinguish between Alzheimer's disease and vascular dementia were described by Hachinski et al.[12] and made into a checklist from which a score (the Hachinski score) is derived. The original score was based on features of vascular dementia in a textbook of psychiatry and studies of the cerebral blood flow in patients with dementia. The initial study group were relatively young and more mildly affected by their illness than are patients seen in most old age psychiatry services. A bimodal distribution of scores was found and suggested that patients with a score below 4 had a dementia of the Alzheimer's type and those having a score of 7 or above a vascular dementia. Patients scoring between 4 and 7 were thought to have a mixed picture. These key features are shown in Table 63-1. More recently the validity of using the Hachinski score to differentiate between vascular dementias and other types of dementias has been questioned. The Hachinski score has been criticized as not being sufficiently sensitive to defect vascular dementia not associated with cerebral infarctions. Also, higher scores on the scale do not mean that a diagnosis of vascular dementia is more likely and the checklist does not take into account results from neuroradiological examinations. Cerebral infarctions are common in older people, including those with Alzheimer's disease, and thus a mixed picture is common.

In DSM-IV[2] the key features of vascular dementia include the presence of focal neurological signs and symptoms (e.g. exaggeration of deep tendon reflexes, extensor plantor response, pseudobalbar palsy, gait abnormalities, weakness of an extremity) or laboratory evidence indicative of cerebrovascular disease (e.g. multiple infarctions involving cortex and underlying white matter) that are etiologically related to the disturbance. Two other sets of diagnostic criteria have been published for the presence of vascular dementia. The ADDTC[13] criteria require evidence of two or more strokes by history, neurological signs and/or neuroimaging or a single stroke with a clear temporal relationship to the onset of dementia and

---

Table 63-1 Hachinski scale

Abrupt onset (2)
Stepwise deterioration (1)
Fluctuating course (2)
Nocturnal confusion (1)
Relative preservation of personality (1)
Depression (1)
Somatic complaints (1)
Emotional incontinence (1)
History of hypertension (1)
History of strokes (1)
Evidence of atherosclerosis (1)
Focal neurological symptoms (2)
Focal neurological signs (2)

evidence of at least one infarct outside the cerebellum on brain imaging. The NINDS-AIREN[14] criteria require evidence of cerebrovascular disease, focal signs on examination, and evidence of cerebrovascular disease by brain imaging, and a relationship between the onset of dementia and cerebrovascular disease as evidenced by dementia occurring within 3 months of a stroke, or abrupt deterioration in cognitive function or fluctuating stepwise course.

Symptoms of Lewy body dementia

Lewy body dementia is characterized by a fluctuating course with distressing psychotic symptoms and marked behavioral disturbance interspersed with periods of lucidity where the degree of cognitive impairment seems relatively minor in relation to the severity of the behavioral disturbance. The diagnosis of Lewy body dementia is made based on the consensus criteria described by McKeith et al.[15,16] consist of the following features. The cardinal feature is the presence of progressive cognitive decline which interferes with normal social or occupational function; deficits on tests of attention and frontal/subcortical skills and visiospatial ability may be prominent, and memory impairment may not necessarily occur in the early stages but may be evident with progression; the core features of dementia with Lewy bodies are fluctuation in cognition with pronounced variations in attention and alertness; spontaneous motor features of parkinsonism; recurrent visual hallucinations which are typically well formed and detailed. Features supportive of the diagnosis are: repeated falls; syncope; transient loss of consciousness; neuroleptic sensitivity; systematized delusions and hallucinations (other than visual).

The psychiatric symptoms may be the presenting feature or may appear in the context of longstanding Parkinson's disease. Sleep disturbance, autonomic lability, and marked sensitivity to neuroleptic drugs are also characteristic of the illness. At times it can be difficult to differentiate between vascular dementia and Lewy body dementia, and as with Alzheimer's disease and vascular dementias a mixed picture is not uncommon.

INVESTIGATIONS

The aim of investigations is to establish a diagnosis and to determine the presence of coexisting disorders. An accurate diagnosis allows discussion of further management and prognosis with the patient and the family. For example, a diagnosis of dementia in a family member may arouse anxieties about genetic implications and it may be that reassurance or referral for genetic counseling is needed, and this depends on the diagnosis. Differentiating between Alzheimer's disease and vascular dementia allows the clinician to give the family information about the course of the illness. Now that drug treatments are available for Alzheimer's disease, a proper diagnosis is an essential prerequisite for treatment.

History

The most helpful investigation is a full history from the patient together with further information from informants. These will include members of the patient's family and close friends, and professionals involved with the patient. The family doctor will be a valuable source of information about the family history, past medical and personal history, premorbid personality, social circumstances, and any dynamics of family relationships.

Discussion with an informant will usually establish the onset and duration of the presenting problem. Difficulties with memory and changes in personality are usual. Problems encountered with hobbies such as following a complicated knitting pattern or playing bridge may be the first change noted. Difficulties may have become apparent after a change in social or personal circumstances when support was removed. The course of the illness is also of importance in distinguishing between vascular dementia and Alzheimer's disease. A detailed account of the difficulties that patients experience in their activities of daily living is important with due attention paid to preserved abilities.

Evidence of memory impairment can be obtained from the patient telling the same story or asking the same questions during the interview as well as from specific questions about whether the patient forgets, unless reminded, family anniversaries or important appointments. Reports of episodes where patients become lost are also important. Language difficulties may be apparent during the interview but are often elicited only on direct questioning. Evidence of dyspraxia can be obtained by judging the patient's ability to use a knife and fork and to dress. Changes in personal habits or interactions with family or friends may indicate a change in personality. Evidence of hallucinations or delusions can also be obtained from family members who may describe the situation when the patient appears to talk to someone when there is no one there, to see things when no one else can, or to have odd ideas, for example, accusing others of stealing from him or her or of not being who they claim.

Other details from the history can be valuable in establishing factors that may be of etiological importance, such as a family history of dementia or vascular risk factors such as hypertension, diabetes, ischemic heart disease, or cerebrovascular disease.

Examination of mental state

Appearance and behavior

Evidence of self-neglect is relevant as is the presence of disinhibited or otherwise inappropriate behavior. Guarded or hostile behavior may indicate paranoid ideas or personality change. Clouding of consciousness is an important clinical sign in differentiating between a delirium and a dementia. It can be difficult to detect and usually a deficit in attention span is taken as indicating clouded consciousness. The patient may look physically ill. Signs that may indicate depression, such as agitation or retardation, may be apparent at interview.

Speech

The patient's speech may reveal evidence of aphasia or dysarthria. Abnormalities of speech such as perseveration (when the patient continues to give the answer to the previous question in response to new questions), pallilalia (when the last word of a question is repeated with increasing frequency), logoclonia (when the last syllable is repeated), or logorrhea (a meaningless outpouring of words) should be noted. The patient may echo the examiner's speech (echolalia) or actions (echopraxia). Often in dementia, speech may be fluent but somewhat banal, giving the impression of lack of content.

Thought content

The content of thought is often impoverished in dementia but careful questioning may reveal the presence of delusions or depressive ideas and the patient may elaborate on psychotic experiences.

Mood

Mood disturbances are often found in association with dementia and can be the presenting feature. Objective evidence of agitation, anxiety, irritability, or low mood should be noted. Subjective symptoms of depression are less likely to be forthcoming but should be sought.

Perceptions

Some patients may be hallucinating at interview but as psychotic symptoms are common in dementia they should be inquired about in all patients by a nondirective question such as "Does your imagination play tricks on you?"

Assessment of cognitive state

Much of the assessment of cognitive function is carried out before formal testing but a quantitative assessment is also important. Two of the most commonly used measures are the Mini-Mental State Examination (MMSE)[17] and the Abbreviated Mental Test Score (AMTS).[18] The AMTS is used widely by geriatricians and the longer MMSE is commonly used by old age psychiatrists. The MMSE, a useful screen for the presence of cognitive impairment, is scored out of 30 points of which 10 are given for orientation in time and place and the remainder for tests of attention, registration, recall, language, manipulating information, and praxis. It has been suggested that a cutoff of 23 or 24 on the MMSE is a satisfactory discriminator between cognitive dysfunction and normality. The MMSE is a useful screening instrument in clinical assessment but is not a substitute for a full history and mental state examination. Normal scores on the MMSE can be found in patients in the early stages of Alzheimer's disease; it can also be normal in patients with quite marked frontal lobe abnormalities as the screen does not include tests of frontal lobe dysfunction. The normal decline is approximately 3 points each year in a patient with Alzheimer's disease. If the history includes symptoms such as loss of interest, poor motivation, or personality change without evidence of a mood disorder then it is worthwhile adding some tests of frontal lobe function. Such tests include asking patients to name four-legged animals or words beginning with F (where 12 or more words in a minute would be considered normal) and asking them to copy sequences of simple hand actions (when patients with frontal lobe problems often have difficulties changing set from one sequence to another).

The clock drawing test is easy to carry out and is regarded as nonthreatening. A number of different ways have been described in which the test can be administered. Usually, the patient is asked to draw a clock face freehand on a plain piece of paper, then put the numbers in and then put the hands to show ten past ten. It is a useful screening test for the presence of cognitive impairment and takes only a minute or two to complete.[19]

Physical examination

Physical examination includes a search for the signs of conditions known to cause dementia. Assessment of vision and hearing is important, not necessarily as causal factors in cognitive impairment but as exacerbating factors. A neurological examination will detect focal neurological signs that are more commonly found in vascular dementias.

There is some controversy as to the extent to which patients with dementia should be investigated. The argument against so doing is the assumed relatively low prevalence of treatable dementias compared to the cost of the investigations. The prevalence of different forms of dementia remains unknown and data from different studies vary greatly because of the way in which cases are selected.[19a] Investigations that are most useful are minimally invasive and relatively inexpensive. A standard screen would include full blood count, erythrocyte sedimentation rate, serum B_{12} and folate, urea and electrolytes, liver function tests, thyroid function tests, and serological tests for syphilis. More detailed investigation by a physician may be indicated in patients with cerebrovascular disease in order to try to prevent further strokes.

NEUROIMAGING

For reviews of the role of neuroimaging in dementia, the reader is referred to Burns and Pearlson,[20] Forstl and Hentschl,[21] and Barber and O'Brien.[22] There are two main types of brain imaging: structural imaging, which reflects the anatomy of the brain, and functional imaging, which assesses cerebral function in relative or absolute terms. This division is useful in attempting to understand the two types of brain imaging, but increasingly there is an integration of the two methods (e.g. by functional magnetic resonance imaging [MRI]). Structural imaging includes computed tomography (CT) and MRI, whereas the two examples of functional imaging are single photon emission computed tomography (SPECT) and positron emission tomography (PET).

Computed tomography

The main use of CT is to exclude intracranial lesions such as tumors (primary or secondary), cerebral infarctions, subdural or extradural hematomata, cerebral abscess, and normal pressure hydrocephalus. Two other features of the CT scan are of particular interest: cerebral atrophy and ventricular enlargement, both as a result of brain shrinkage. Cerebral atrophy (also referred to as sulcal, surface, or cortical atrophy) represents a diminution of the cortex, whereas ventricular enlargement (subcortical or central atrophy) indicates swelling of the ventricular system. The CT scan in dementia can provide useful information on the following: (1) the distribution of cerebral atrophy (frontal atrophy may suggest frontotemporal dementia); (2) the size of the caudate nuclei (gross shrinkage would support a clinical diagnosis of Huntington's disease); and (3) white matter changes (indicative of small vessel vascular disease).

Guidelines for performing CT scans have been discussed by Bradshaw et al.[23] and Larson et al.[24] Alexander et al.[25] performed a study of patients over the age of 65 who had been referred for CT brain scans, reporting the presence of subdural hematoma, hydrocephalus, and intracranial tumor (which was not obviously metastatic). They found that these potentially treatable lesions were rare (145 in 137, 100 person years at risk) and most presented in a way that was clearly distinguishable from typical Alzheimer's disease. Of 59 patients who presented with cognitive impairment, the following clinical features determined the likelihood of finding a lesion with over 90 percent sensitivity: cognitive impairment for 1 month or less, head trauma in the week before mental state change, rapid onset of change over 48 hours, history of cerebrovascular accident, seizures or incontinence, focal neurological signs, papilledema, visual field defects, gait abnormalities, postural instability, or headaches.

Many people mistakenly regard the failure to find a treatable structural lesion as indicating that the scan is superfluous. However, it is important to exclude small vascular lesions such as lacunar infarctions. It is also important to evaluate the distribution of cerebral atrophy and observe the presence of leukoariaosis, which may indicate small vessel disease.

Structural brain imaging reveals the extent of cerebral atrophy. There is considerable overlap between Alzheimer's disease and normal aging. The precision with which brain scans can differentiate, in groups, between normal aging and Alzheimer's disease varies with the method of interpretation. Visual ratings have relatively low discriminatory power, whereas more sophisticated, computer-assisted assessments are superior.[26] Specific analyses of certain cerebral regions have been undertaken in an attempt to improve this discriminatory power (e.g., measurements of the temporal lobe region may be particularly accurate in discriminating patients from normal controls).[27] Volumetric CT scans, and measurements of lateral ventricular and sylvian fissure size achieve satisfactory sensitivity and specificity distinctions between normal aging and mild Alzheimer's disease.[28,29] The entorhinal cortex is known to be affected early in Alzheimer's disease[30] and several studies have concentrated on this area as a site where differences can be found. Jobst et al.[31] found that in 44 patients with Alzheimer's disease, the minimum width of the medial temporal lobe was approximately half that of normal controls.

Magnetic resonance imaging

MRI scanning has several advantages: no radiation is involved, resolution is superior to CT, and there is no bone artifact. There is prolongation of the T1 relaxation in patients with Alzheimer's disease and multi-infarct dementia compared with nondemented age-matched controls.[32] However, the ability of this technique to differentiate Alzheimer's disease from multi-infarct dementia is poor and it is possible that prolongation times represent small infarcts or white matter changes that can occur in both disorders. O'Brien et al.[33] examined MRI scans in 43 patients with Alzheimer's disease and compared them with scans of 32 subjects with major depression. Atrophy ratings (on a four-point scale) were made of temporal lobe structures—hippocampus, amygdala, entorhinal cortex, parahippocampal gyrus, and cerebral cortex—and correct allocation of patients to their respective diagnostic groups was

achieved in nearly 90 percent of cases. Within the dementia group, entorhinal cortex atrophy was significantly correlated with length of history.

White matter changes have been investigated extensively in Alzheimer's disease and normal aging. The exact nature of white matter changes or leukoaraiosis is still uncertain. Subcortical white matter lesions appear to be age related, whereas periventricular lesions are more associated with cognitive decline and are found in Alzheimer's disease.[34,35] The prevalence of leukoaraiosis varies from 20 percent to over 60 percent and specific relationships have been found between the severity of the white matter change and the degree of cognitive impairment, particularly deficits of attention and comprehension.[36]

Single photon emission computed tomography

SPECT involves the administration (usually intravenously) of single photon emitting elements (e.g. technetium-99, xenon-133, iodoamphetamine-123) attached to compounds (e.g., hexamethylpropyleneamineoxime) that are distributed in the brain according to cerebral blood flow. The compound crosses the blood–brain barrier and is trapped within functioning brain cells. The amount of radioactivity present can be measured by a rotating gamma camera (which can be used for any nuclear medicine examination) or by multiple scintillation counters in a machine dedicated to brain imaging. Image reconstruction allows sagittal, coronal, and transverse planes to be viewed, enabling localization of radionucleotide distribution to be made.

The pattern of distribution of tracer in Alzheimer's disease is temporoparietal hypoperfusion and comparative measures of temporoparietal blood flow (often presented as a ratio compared to the cerebellum, traditionally regarded as being unaffected in dementia) have been used to differentiate dementia from normal aging.[37]

Patchy distribution of tracing can often demonstrate marked abnormalities in blood flow that may not be apparent on a CT or even MRI scan. Normal pressure hydrocephalus demonstrates a pattern of blood flow reflecting the underlying structural changes (i.e., a thin area of preservation of blood flow in the cortical rim). Correlations have been found between areas of regional hypoperfusion and cognitive impairment.[38]

Specific relationships have been evaluated and associations have been found between amnesia and temporal hypoperfusion, between apraxia and decreased posterior parietal hypoperfusion, and between aphasia and hypoperfusion throughout the left hemisphere.[39] Other associations have included level of previous education, occupation,[40] and delusions and hallucinations.[41] The technique has also been used to define dementia of the frontal lobe type[42] when anterior deficits in blood flow are prominent, quite different from the posterior hypoperfusion seen in Alzheimer's disease. Diminished uptake in the caudate nuclei has been shown in Huntington's disease. Although SPECT methodology has been used for some time to image the brain and the development of new compounds and imaging systems has greatly advanced the technique, SPECT still remains to be established as a widely used and applicable neuroimaging modality in the diagnosis of dementia. It can be used to assess the response to drug treatment[43] (for a recent review see reference 43a). The combination of functional and structural imaging can increase diagnostic power in relation to the early assessment of Alzheimer's disease.[31]

Positron emission tomography

PET can be used to measure regional cerebral metabolism (as opposed to purely blood flow) in vivo. However, the practicalities of performing a PET scan have thus far precluded use in clinical diagnosis in psychiatry and the value is still primarily as a research tool.[37] The two most common positron emission compounds are ^{15}O and ^{18}F-deoxyglucose.

Frackowiak et al.[44] were the first to use ^{15}O in the investigation of dementia and showed that in Alzheimer's disease there was diminished oxygen consumption in the fronto-temporal and parietal lobes with prominent frontal lobe diminution in severe dementia. Parietal lobe deficits characterized vascular dementia (possibly because of the greater frequency of infarcts in the middle cerebral artery territory). A close link between cerebral blood flow and cerebral oxygen consumption was demonstrated, suggesting that there was no chronic ischemia (which would have led to increased oxygen consumption relative to blood flow) in either vascular or degenerative dementia. Generally, the findings of PET scan studies in dementia have shown the following: there is a decrease in metabolism with increasing age; temporoparietal deficits have been found in Alzheimer's disease; less commonly, frontal lobe defects occur in Alzheimer's disease; focal deficits have been described in vascular disease; specific associations have been demonstrated between clinical features and regional blood flow metabolism (e.g. between apraxia and right-sided hypometabolism, between aphasia and lower left fronto-temporal metabolism, and between personality changes and decreased metabolism in frontal regions).

Asymmetric temporoparietal hypometabolism may indicate the development of cognitive impairment in previously nondemented patients but there is no real evidence that the metabolic changes occur in the absence of detectable cognitive deficits. The two tend to run in parallel, thus reducing the additional value of PET scanning in early diagnosis in Alzheimer's disease (for a recent review see reference 43a).

Electroencephalography

Electroencephalography (EEG) has been used to differentiate dementia from normal aging and more recently quantified EEG studies have been reported. In normal aging the EEG tracing is symmetric and four characteristic waveforms have been described: delta (less than 4 Hz), theta (4–7 Hz), alpha (8–13 Hz), and beta (14–30 Hz). Delta waves predominate in the newborn, theta waves are apparent until age 18 years, and both disappear with increasing age, although some delta activity may occur in the normal adult especially during sleep. Thus, the faster rhythms (predominantly alpha and beta activity) predominate in the young adult. After the age of 60 years the EEG changes. There is slowing of the alpha rhythm from a mean rate of 10 Hz to a rate of about 9 Hz at age 80 years. Theta and delta activity increase after age 75 (theta

activity is mostly focal on the left temporal region and delta activity occurs bilaterally in the anterior regions). Beta activity tends to increase throughout adult life until about age 60 and does not diminish significantly until age 80. There is evidence that increased slow activity may be associated with a number of nonspecific symptoms in elderly people, such as dizziness and headache.

In dementia, the earliest studies of the EEG showed gross abnormalities with a regular slow wave activity. However, many of these patients had advanced disease. When studies of less advanced cases were reported, the abnormalities seen were inconsistent and poorly correlated with the degree of dementia. The EEG then largely fell into disrepute as a diagnostic instrument for dementia. Cummings and Benson[45] describe the situation where a normal EEG in the presence of severe dementia was likely to be indicative of Alzheimer's disease, whereas an abnormal tracing in mild impairment was associated with delirium. The EEG is usually normal in very early stages of Alzheimer's disease but diffuse slowing of the tracing can occur thereafter. As the disease progresses there is progressive slowing of the tracing with alpha and beta activity decreasing symmetrically and delta and theta waves increasing. Soininen et al.[46] found that EEG abnormalities were present in 52 percent of 62 patients with Alzheimer's disease but only 1 of 90 in age-matched controls. The average dominant frequency was 7 Hz in the patient group and 9 Hz in the control group. Another important feature in dementia is the presence of paroxysmal bifrontal delta waves, which are more common in dementia than normal aging. It has been shown in Alzheimer's disease that there was a decrease in the mean frequency of dominant occipital activity[47] of the alpha–theta ratio and an increase of the relative or absolute theta power, whereas delta power increases in the later stages of the illness[48,49] (for a recent review see reference 49a).

TREATMENTS IN DEMENTIA

Treatments can be divided into pharmacological therapies and nonpharmacological interventions. Both can be directed at the cognitive and noncognitive features of the disorder. Management of dementia has recently been reviewed.[49a]

Pharmacological treatments

Treatment of cognitive deficits in Alzheimer's disease

MODIFICATION OF CHOLINERGIC SYSTEMS Among the neurotransmitter abnormalities found in Alzheimer's disease, deficits in the acetylcholine system have been the most consistently found.[50] The synthesis and degradation of acetylcholine is shown in Figure 63-1.

There are three ways in which the concentration of acetylcholine can be increased: (1) loading the substrate; (2) actions on the receptor for acetylcholine; and (3) inhibiting the enzyme responsible for the breakdown of acetylcholine.

1. Substrate loading: Attempts to replace acetylcholine by loading with one of the precursors of acetylcholine, choline,

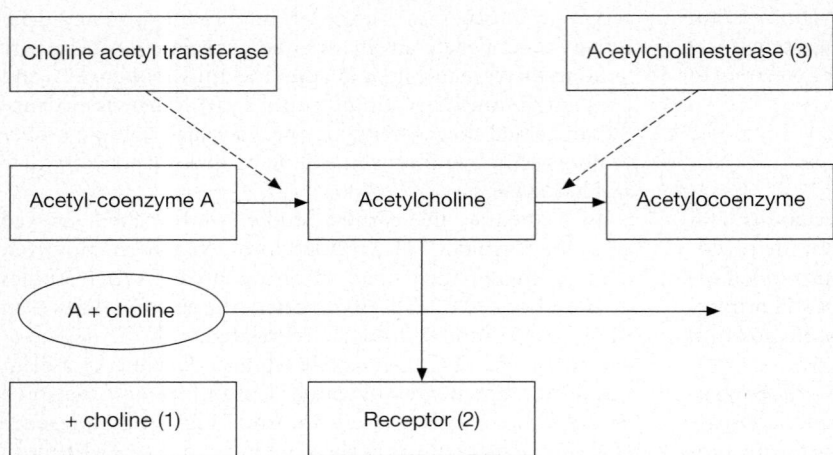

Figure 63-1 Synthesis and degradation of acetylcholine.

produced disappointing results.[51] Increasing the level of the other precursor, acetyl CoA by L-acetylcarnitine has been more successful[52,53] and this also affects the enzyme that catalyzes the formation of acetylcholine and affects the uptake of choline and the release of acetylcholine.

A recent double-blind study[53] suggests that the drug may slow the progression of the disease in younger patients. At present there are inadequate data on the drug for it to be licensed.

2. Acetylcholine receptor agonists: There are two main types of receptors in the cholinergic system: muscarinic receptors, such as those found at the neuromuscular junction, and nicotinic receptors, including those found at synapses within ganglia. In the brain, the system seems even more complicated with at least five different subgroups of muscarinic receptors having been identified. The need to administer some of these drugs parenterally made them unsuitable for clinical use. Overall, studies with muscarinic agonists have produced disappointing results.[54]

Nicotinic receptors are thought to be important in learning and memory and are reduced in the cerebral cortex of patients with Alzheimer's disease. Cigarette smoking increases the number of brain nicotinic receptors in humans and was thought to protect against Alzheimer's disease. However, more recent evidence[55] suggests that the negative effects on blood vessels and action on apolipoprotein E_4 results in smokers having double the risk for dementia and Alzheimer's disease. There is some suggestion that agonists of nicotinic receptors may have some benefit. Studies have used only small samples of patients and have not shown consistent changes, although subcutaneous nicotine may have some effect on cognitive function. Compounds have been developed including the licensed acetylcholinesterase inhibitor, galantamine, which modulate the activity of nicotinic receptors. It is not as yet clear whether the additional activity of this drug will produce benefit in clinical practice.

3. Cholinesterase inhibitors: The most successful strategy for increasing acetylcholine levels in the cortex has been by the inhibition of the enzyme cholinesterase, which is involved in the breakdown of acetylcholine to its component molecules. Cholinesterases are found in two main forms in the brain,

acetylcholinesterase, the most prominent, and butyrylcholinesterase.

Tacrine was the first anticholinesterase drug but the side-effect profile (up to a third of people dropping out of treatment) of cholinergic side-effects (nausea, gastrointestinal disturbance, and dizziness), and elevated liver transaminases makes it unsuitable for prescription. There are currently three anticholinesterase drugs licensed in the UK for the treatment of Alzheimer's disease—donepezil (Aricept), rivastigmine (Exelon), and galantamine (Reminyl).[56] A number of studies have shown that Aricept is effective at improving cognitive function and global rating of dementia over 26 weeks.

Donepezil (Aricept) The development of a drug with a similar efficacy profile to tacrine but free of side-effects was awaited, and donepezil hydrochloride seemed to satisfy this criterion. As a piperidine-based anticholinesterase, it does have the same potential for liver toxicity as the acridine-based compound, tacrine. It was licensed for use in the symptomatic treatment of mild to moderate Alzheimer's disease in the UK in March 1997. A number of studies have demonstrated that donepezil is effective at improving the symptoms of Alzheimer's disease.[56–59]

The magnitude of change (similar in all studies) seen with donepezil is an improvement of around three points on active drug compared to placebo on the Alzheimer's disease assessment scale-Cognitive section (ADAS-Cog), highly statistically significant ($P < 0.0001$). To look at it another way, 42 percent of patients on placebo had worse cognitive function at the end point compared to 20 percent on donepezil. An improvement of 7 points on the ADAS-Cog is regarded as being of clinical significance—on this basis 8 percent on placebo improved, 15 percent on 5 mg and 25 percent on 10 mg. On the Clinician's Interview Based Impression of Change (CIBIC), 11 percent improved in the placebo group compared to 26 percent on 5 mg, 25 percent on 10 mg. The recommended dose is to start with 5 mg per day and titrate after a minimum of 1 month to 10 mg. In the UK, the cost of the drug is £68.32 for 28 × 5 mg tablets and £95.76 for 28 × 10 mg tablets.

Rivastigmine (Exelon R) Rivastigmine was licensed in May 1998 in the European Community for the treatment of mild to moderately severe Alzheimer's disease. Compared to donepezil, there is a larger patient database on which the introduction of the drug was based. A specific program of studies (the ADENA program), consisted of four pivotal trials aimed at overcoming the drawbacks of existing studies, i.e., small numbers of patients, short duration of treatment, and restrictive entry criteria.[60,61] Over 2,000 patients have been examined with a dose range of between 6 and 12 mg (twice daily administration), previous studies having shown that 4 mg was ineffective. The magnitude of the effect is similar to that seen with donepezil. Compared to placebo, 21 percent compared to 12 percent improved on ADAS-Cog, 29 percent compared to 18 percent on the CIBIC plus and 26 percent compared to 17 percent on the PDS. Side-effects of rivastigmine include anorexia, nausea, dizziness, vomiting, appetite, and weight loss. It is not, like donepezil, contraindicated in asthma. The recommended drug dose is to start at 1.5 mg b.d. with the therapeutic dose being between 6 and 12 mg. Rivastigmine is also effective in Lewy body dementia.[62]

Galantamine (Reminyl) This third anticholinesterase was licensed in the UK in autumn 2000. It has a dual action of anticholinesterase function and direct receptor agonist action. Studies show that it is effective in improving cognitive function in Alzheimer's disease as well as activities of daily living and neuropsychiatric features.[63,64,64a] The effective dose seems to be 16 or 24 mg/day.

MANAGED INTRODUCTION—CLINICAL GUIDELINES Guide-lines have been used to manage the introduction of the new drugs for the treatment of Alzheimer's disease.[56] They define diagnostic criteria, suggest clinically relevant inclusion and exclusion criteria based broadly on those used in the clinical trials, and, ideally, should be agreed locally with general practitioners, pharmacists, local purchasers of healthcare, and specialists in the management of Alzheimer's disease.

The UK Government's Standing Medical Advisory Committee (SMAC) has produced guidelines on the treatment of Alzheimer's disease and recommends that treatment should be initiated and supervised by a specialist familiar with the management of the disease and that, generally speaking, the characteristics of patients selected for treatment, should be the same as those in drug trials. Treatment should be assessed after 12 weeks and continued only if there is clear evidence of benefit, a judgment informed by the application of recognized objective tests.

Clinical experience[56] supports the research data showing a modest group effect, but in individual patients marked beneficial effects on functioning and neuropsychiatric features are also seen, and for some patients the striking effects on BPSD may outweigh the effects on cognition. The UK National Institute for Clinical Excellence (NICE) has recently reviewed the available literature[65] on the cholinesterase inhibitors and has advised that all three drugs should be made available in the NHS as one component of the management of patients with Alzheimer's disease and a Mini-Mental State Examination of > 12.

OTHER DRUGS Other drugs have been tested for their efficacy in Alzheimer's disease. Selegiline and vitamin E, alone but not in combination, have been shown to slow the rate of progression in the disorder.[66] Estrogen is a promising treatment in terms of prevention of Alzheimer's disease without any significant benefits in terms of improvement in cognition.[67,68] Hydergine is used by many people in the treatment of dementia.[69] Gingko biloba is used by many patients and can be bought without prescription and there has been a positive study rating efficacy.[70] Piracetam seems to be ineffective in the treatment of dementia.[71] Memantine is beneficial in people with more severe dementia.[72]

Management of noncognitive symptoms of dementia

MOOD DISORDERS Depressive symptoms in a patient with dementia should be treated vigorously. Such symptoms include low mood, anhedonia, pessimism about the future, irritability, sleep disturbance, diurnal variation in mood or behavior, weight loss, and appetite changes. About 60–70 percent of depressed patients derive benefit from treatment regardless of the choice of drug. The side-effect profile and individual preference of the clinician normally govern the choice of drug. The anticholinergic effects of the tricyclics are said to further impair cognitive function but this is rarely a problem in practice. Toxic confusional states can be a result of treatment with tricyclics (as with many drugs in patients with dementia); therefore, starting doses need to be much lower than in younger adults and the patients need careful monitoring for adverse side-effects. Clinical experience shows that a good response to the drug is often found with doses of tricyclics (e.g. amitriptyline 10 mg three times a day), which would be considered well below the therapeutic dose in younger adults. Selective Serotonin Reuptake Inhibitors (SSRIs) seem to be well tolerated in older people and are preferable in patients with cardiac problems or where the anticholinergic effects make tricyclics inadvisable. Some clinicians would choose an SSRI as their first choice of antidepressant and some a tricyclic regardless of the patient's age. The atypical antidepressants such as trazodone, the newer selective reversible monoamine oxidase inhibitors such as moclobemide, and drugs acting on both noradrenergic and serotonin receptors such as venlafaxine, also all have a role in the treatment of depression in patients with dementia. Restlessness and an inner feeling of being driven can also be helped by small doses of a sedating tricyclic antidepressant such as amitriptyline.

In patients with vascular dementia emotional lability can be a problem both for patients and their families and there is some evidence that SSRIs may be helpful in dealing with this symptom.[73]

BEHAVIORAL DISTURBANCES Drugs are commonly prescribed for agitation in dementia. Neuroleptics are widely used for agitation and aggression regardless of the cause of the symptom. These drugs can be useful but do not replace the need for appropriate investigation and treatment of patients and attention to environmental or physical factors such as constipation or a urinary tract infection that may produce a deterioration in behavior. Most studies have shown neuroleptics to be better than placebo in the treatment of symptoms of agitation, overactivity, and restlessness. A meta-analysis of the literature suggests that about 18 percent of agitated patients benefit from treatment with neuroleptics.[74] Thioridazine and haloperidol have been shown to be equally efficacious[75] but thioridazine is no longer licensed for this indication. Side-effects of older neuroleptics include extrapyramidal symptoms of stiffness, tremor and gait disturbance that mimic the symptoms of Parkinson's disease, tardive dyskinesia, postural hypotension, agranulocytosis, liver and cardiac toxicity, sedation, and anticholinergic side-effects. Some side-effects such as the postural hypotension and the anticholinergic effects can be a problem clinically, whereas others such as sedation can be beneficial in some patients.

Anticholinergic drugs such as procyclidine that are used in younger patients to counteract the extrapyramidal side-effects of neuroleptic drugs are best avoided in elderly people with dementia as they can significantly impair cognitive function. Instead the drug dosage should be reduced or the drug stopped completely if side-effects are bothersome. Anticholinergic side-effects are common in older people.[76]

Newer atypical neuroleptics such as risperidone, olanzapine, and quetiapine may also be useful in the treatment of patients with agitation or other behavioral disturbances, particularly in patients who are sensitive to treatment with conventional neuroleptics.[77–79]

Aggression and irritability can also be helped in some patients by SSRIs or trazodone.[80] These effects on aggression and irritability are often seen much earlier than would be expected from an antidepressant effect and it is likely that antidepressant drugs have specific effects in addition to their antidepressant actions. Trazodone also seems to be of benefit in a minority of patients in stopping apparently purposeless shouting.

PSYCHOTIC SYMPTOMS These are common in dementia and if they are distressing or result in disturbances of behavior it is appropriate to treat them. Paranoid ideas are common, often relate to members of the family or other care-givers, and respond well to neuroleptics. Both the older drugs and the newer atypicals are useful. The treatment of the psychotic symptoms and disturbed behavior in patients with Lewy body dementia needs to be considered carefully in view of the increased mortality resulting from neuroleptic treatment.[81] Recommendations from the Committee for Safety of Medicines[82] have emphasized the need for caution. Chlormethiazole can be useful either alone or in conjunction with lorazepam, which is an effective anxiolytic and sedative. Atypical neuroleptics need to be used with caution but can be of benefit.

The cholinesterase inhibitor rivastigmine has been shown to have significant benefit in recent studies, and this class of drugs is being investigated for use in Lewy body dementias.[74]

Pharmacological treatments have recently been reviewed.[83]

Nonpharmacological treatments

Specific treatments for some of the symptoms of dementia have been developed. To maximize the benefit, these treatments should be administered with empathy and understanding of the patient's predicament and a recognition of their past experiences. Patients, even those with quite severe dementia, should be encouraged to participate as fully as they are able with activities of daily living, to make choices, to engage in activities, and to interact socially. Providing such an environment of care requires considerable time and expertise and has financial implications.

Memory training

At present, most patients with dementia are referred to specialist services when their illness is too severe for any benefit to be gained from memory training. However, for people with mild memory impairment the maxim "use it or lose it" is relevant. Techniques to aid memory, for example, by making visual associations, together with the use of prompts have been shown to be helpful. Often, over the early stages of the development of the memory impairment, patients and their families have put such ideas into practice but there are some patients who can benefit from the formal teaching of such techniques either individually or in groups.[84,85]

The use of cholinesterase inhibitors in improving cognitive function may produce a window of opportunity for such psychological treatments to be of benefit.

Behavior modification

The basis of this technique is often described as the ABC of behavior, where A is the antecedent, B the behavior itself, and C the consequences of the behavior. Behavior modification can be useful with a range of undesirable behaviors such as aggression, wandering, screaming, incontinence, lack of cooperation when personal care is being provided, repetitive or stereotyped behavior, and some types of incontinence.

Care-givers are first asked to give a detailed description of the type and circumstances of the undesired behavior. From that information, it may be possible to educate the care-giver as to how they might alter the environment and their actions to reduce the behavior and establish a treatable comorbid condition such as constipation. A valuable part of the therapy is the development of a patient-centered approach to treatment of behaviors and the increased understanding by the care-giver of the patient's needs.

Reality orientation

Disorientation to time and place is an early symptom of dementia and there are two forms of reality orientation, an informal or a 24-hour reorientation when all opportunities are taken to orient the patient to time and place.[86] Orientation boards common in most institutions are examples. A more formal structured reality orientation session consists of a small number of patients undergoing a program of discussion exploring topics of interest. Exponents of formal reality orientation emphasize that these sessions are intended as a supplement to, as opposed to an alternative for, 24 hour reality orientation. It is fundamental in both types of reality orientation that staff or care-givers do not collude with patients in situations where the patient is clearly mistaken.

Although the relationship between patient and therapist is fundamental to all psychotherapeutic interventions including behavioral therapy and reality orientation, such techniques in practice may not encompass important features such as empathy, support, and nonjudgmental listening. Reality orientation may degenerate to sharply worded information about today's date with a lack of sensitivity to the patient's feelings and cognitive impairment. It has been criticized as a "dehumanizing" behavior modification technique solely preoccupied with targeting symptom management. However, evaluations of reality orientation have clearly demonstrated improvements in verbal orientation and have a positive effect on staff and care-givers.[86]

Validation therapy

Validation therapy is a more patient-centered therapy that was designed to validate the patient's past and present experiences and feelings. It was designed for use in elderly patients with dementia and emphasizes the need to interact in "whatever reality they are in, in order to ease distress and restore self-worth."[87] Thus, for example, if a patient became anxious about the need to collect her children from school, the therapist would start by sharing the anxiety associated with these thoughts and then gradually move the patient through that phase of their life to the present day. The precise date is of less importance in this therapy than the patient's stage in the life cycle and a sharing of their past experiences. As with reality orientation these techniques can be used formally in groups or can be incorporated into round-the-clock care for the patient. Although widely used in institutions, especially in the United States, the evidence that they are useful is solely anecdotal.

Reminiscence therapy

A range of other techniques have been used with patients with dementia with the aim of increasing their quality of life. Reminiscence therapy is widely used. It has its roots in psychodynamic theory and ideas about the process of life review in later life where past experiences are reviewed and past conflicts can be looked at again and reintegrated. Most often the technique is applied as a group therapy. Groups of patients normally meet with a therapist and various techniques are used to help patients recall parts of their personal memory. Photographs of past times, music, or other sensory experiences such as smells are used as triggers to memory and then the therapist aims to facilitate discussion. Specifically designed packages of audiovisual material have been produced for use in reminiscence therapy. According to King[88] meeting in groups allows opportunity for socialization and social reintegration, resolution of old conflicts through life review, identification of current concerns and struggles, recognition of self as a survivor, and appreciation of one's own achievements and those of others.

Much of the published work on reminiscence therapy is anecdotal and many of the studies have not included a control group. Reminiscence therapy groups are reported as often being enjoyed by both staff and patients and are important in giving both groups a sense of mastery. The groups are also said to increase staff knowledge of their patients and to increase the quality of interactions between patients and staff. It is not clear to what extent these positive benefits are nonspecific or related to the reminiscence therapy. No lasting effects on memory have been reported in controlled trials.

Expressive therapies

Other techniques are used with patients with dementia, not only to provide interest and occupation, but also to reduce anxiety and aid self-expression, often through nonverbal routes. Art and music are used as are techniques involving physical contact. Hand massage and aromatherapy using specific oils are increasingly used and are likely to have at least some nonspecific benefit. The Snoezelen technique, used for people with learning difficulties,[80] has also been used in severely demented patients with the aim of providing input through a range of senses.

A trial of psychotherapy in early Alzheimer's disease has just been completed in Manchester (Burns, personal communication).

Longer term management of patients with dementia

Dementia affects not only the patient but their family. Many spouses caring for patients with dementia are elderly and frail themselves and many are reluctant to accept help until a crisis point is reached and they can no longer cope. An emergency or unplanned admission to an institution then becomes the only solution. Nonmedical professionals, including community psychiatric nurses, occupational therapists, physiotherapists, psychologists, speech therapists, and social workers all have important roles in the management of dementia. It is important that one professional takes over the role of key worker and is responsible for maintaining good communication between members of the team.

The initial assessment of patients will include their physical, psychological, and social environment. Care will be required for their self-care, shopping, and food preparation. Activity will often be needed and this may be provided within the circle of family and friends; within the wider community, for example, by church or voluntary groups; at a social services day center, or at a day hospital. If the patient is being cared for at home the needs of the family must be considered and it may be important to provide some day care and/or respite care to allow the care-giver to have a break and to encourage the care-giver to join a support group, such as one run by the Alzheimer's Society. Table 63-2 outlines the services that are potentially available to an individual with dementia. The provision of such a package of care requires time and effort to understand the needs of both the patient and his or her family and to tailor the care to those needs. The needs of patients and their care-givers will change over time and the provision of care should be flexible to cope with these changes. New symptoms or behaviors may develop in the course of the illness and these need to be dealt with using the treatments already discussed. Although many patients wish to stay at home and care should be provided for them, institutional care can be beneficial for other patients and should not always be seen as the last resort. Removing the daily burden of care from a relative may enhance the relationship between patient and family and allow both to enjoy the patient's last years or months of life.

MEMORY CLINICS The establishment of memory clinics is likely to be useful in encouraging early referral of patients with cognitive impairment. Many were established in teaching hospitals in which there was an interest in testing treatments for dementia and therefore also served to provide patients with the opportunity to participate in drug trials. However, most clinics regularly referred patients on to district health

Table 63-2 Services available

Primary care team
 General practitioner
 District nurse
 Health visitor
 Practice nurse
 Counseling/psychology

Social services
 Domiciliary care (elderly care team)
  Social work assessment
  Home help
  Meals on wheels
  Sitting services
  Continence service
  Chiropody
  Laundry service
 Other
  Day centers
  Residential care
  Respite care
  Housing

Hospital services
 Geriatric psychiatrist
 Geriatrician
 Psychologist
 Domiciliary assessment
 Hospital admission
 Long-term/respite care
 Community psychiatric nurses
 Day hospitals
 Multidisciplinary team assessment
 Physiotherapy
 Occupational therapy
 Speech therapy

Voluntary agencies
 Alzheimer's Disease Society
 Age Concern
 Housing associations

Others
 Private nursing/residential homes
 DSS—attendance allowance

and social services and 60 percent said that they themselves initiated and monitored nonresearch treatments. Published descriptions show the clinics to be broadly similar in that they are hospital-based multidisciplinary services that provide a detailed first assessment for a small number of patients. Advocates of memory clinics argue that they will play an increasingly important role both in the assessment of patients with possible dementia referred from primary care and in the treatment of dementia.[89]

CONCLUSIONS

The management of dementia is multifaceted, including many techniques ranging from highly technological neuroimaging to hand massage. The first stage in the management is to obtain a definitive diagnosis. Where a reversible etiology is identified this should be treated. For the majority of patients with a progressive and untreatable dementia a long-term management plan needs to be drawn up that employs general therapeutic principles supplemented by specific pharmacological, psychological, and social interventions as necessary to meet the needs of the individual patient and the family. Teamwork is essential for the delivery of such a service. Due recognition must be given to the skills and knowledge both of the various professionals in the team and also of others such as members of the family, friends, community members, care-givers such as home helpers, and voluntary workers, all of whom have important contributions to make to the care of the patient.

KEY POINTS Presentation and clinical management of dementia

- Symptomatic treatments for Alzheimer's disease are effective at alleviating memory loss.

- Early diagnosis of Alzheimer's disease facilitates more effective management.

- Comprehensive community services should be available for people with dementia.

- Psychosocial interventions reduce strain in carers looking after people with dementia.

REFERENCES

1. Lishman WA: Organic Psychiatry: The Psychological Consequences of Cerebral Disorder, 3rd Ed. Blackwell Scientific Publications, Oxford, 1998
2. American Psychiatric Association: Diagnostic and Statistical Manual of Mental Disorders, 4th Ed. American Psychiatric Association, Washington, DC,1994
3. Corey Bloom J, Thal L, Galasko D et al: Diagnosis and evaluation of dementia. Neurology 1995;45:211–218
4. Knopman DS, DeKosky ST, Cummings JL et al: Practice parameter: Early detection of dementia: mild cognitive impairment (an evidence-based review). Neurology 2001;56:1143–1153
5. Petersen RC, Stevens JC, Ganguli M et al: Practice parameter: Early detection of dementia: mild cognitive impairment (an evidence-based review). Neurology 2001;56:1133–1142
5a. Ritchie K, Touchon J: Mild cognitive impairment: conceptual basis of current nosological status. Lancet 2000;355:225–228
6. Oppenheim G: The earliest signs of Alzheimer's disease. J Geriatr Psychiatry Neurol 1994;7:118–122
7. Blessed G, Tomlinson B, Roth M: The association between quantitative measures of dementing and senile change in cerebral grey matter of elderly subjects. Br J Psychiatry 1968;114:797–811
8. Finkel S, Burns A: BPSD: a clinical and research update. Int Psychogeriatr 2000;12(suppl 1):9–18
9. Burns A, Lewis G: Survival in Dementia. In Burns A (ed): Ageing and Dementia: A Methodological Approach. Edward Arnold, London, 1993:125–143
10. McKhann G, Drachman D, Folstein M et al: Clinical diagnosis of Alzheimer's disease. Report of the NINCDS–ADRDA workgroup under the auspices of the Department of Health and Human Services Taskforce on Alzheimer's disease. Neurology 1984;34:939–944
11. Ballard C: Criteria for the Diagnosis of Dementia. In O'Brien J, Ames D, Burns A (eds): Dementia. Arnold, London, 2000
12. Hachinski V, Illiff L, Zilkha E et al: Cerebral blood flow in dementia. Arch Neurol 1975;32:632–637
13. Chui H, Victoroff J, Margolin D et al: Criteria for the diagnosis of ischaemic vascular dementia proposed by the State of California Alzheimer Disease Diagnostic and Treatment Centres. Neurology 1992;42:473–480
14. Roman G, Tatemechi TK, Erkinjuntti T et al: Vascular dementia: diagnostic criteria for research studies. Report of the NINCDS–ADRDA International Workshop. Neurology 1993;43:250–260

15. McKeith I, Galasko D, Kosaka K et al: Consensus Guidelines for the Clinical and Pathologic Diagnosis of Dementia with Lewy Bodies (DLB): Report of the consortium on DLB International Workshop. Neurology 1996;47:1113–1124

16. McKeith I, Perry E, Perry R: Report of the 2nd Dementia with Lewy Body International Workshop. Neurology 1999;53:902–905

17. Folstein MF, Folstein SE, McHugh PR: Mini-Mental State Examination—a practical method for grading the cognitive state of patients for the clinician. J Psychiatr Res 1975;12:189–198

18. Hodkinson M: Mental impairment on the elderly. J R Coll Physician 1973;7:305–317

19. Shulman I: Clock drawing: Is it the ideal cognitive screening test? Int J Geriatr Psychiatry 2000;15:548–561

19a. Philpot M, Burns A: Reversible dementia. In Katona C (ed): Dementia Disorders: Advances and Prospects. Chapman & Hall, London, 1989

20. Burns A, Perlson G: Computed tomography. In O'Brien J, Ames D, Burns A (eds): Dementia. Arnold, London, 2000:101–113

21. Forstl H, Hentschl F: Contributions to the differential diagnosis of dementia 2: neuroimaging. Rev Clin Gerontol 1994;4:317–341

22. Barber R, O'Brien J: Structural and functional magnetic resonance imaging. In O'Brien J, Amers D, Burns A (eds): Dementia. Arnold, London, 2000;115–130

23. Bradshaw J, Thomas J, Campbell M: Computed tomography in the investigation of dementia. Br Med J 1983;286:277–280

24. Larson E, Reifler B, Featherstone J, English D: Dementia in elderly outpatients. A prospective study. Ann Intern Med 198;100:417–423

25. Alexander E, Wagner E, Buchner D et al: Do surgical brain lesions present as isolated dementia? A population based study. J Am Geriatr Soc 1995;43:138–143

26. De Carli C, Kaye J, Horowitc B, Rapoport S: Critical analysis of the use of CT to study human brain in ageing and dementia of the Alzheimer type. Neurology 1990;40:872–873

27. Jobst K, Smith A, Szatmari M et al: Detection in life of confirmed Alzheimer's disease using a simple measurement of medical temporal lobe atrophy by computed tomography. Lancet 1992;340:1179–1183

28. Burns A, Jacoby R, Philpot M, Levy R: CT in Alzheimer's disease—methods of scan analysis comparison with normal controls and clinico-radiological correlations. Br J Psychiatry 1991;159:609–614

29. Forstl H, Zerfass R, Geiger Kabisch C et al: Brain atrophy in normal ageing and Alzheimer's disease. Br J Psychiatry 1995;167:739–746

30. Braak H, Braak E: Neuropathological staging of Alzheimer-related changes. Acta Neuropathol 1991;82:239–259

31. Jobst K, Smith A, Barker C et al: Association of atrophy of the medio-temporal lobe with reduced blood flow in the posterior parieto-temporal cortex in patients with a clinical and pathological diagnosis of Alzheimer's disease. JNNP 1992;55:190–194

32. Besson J, Corrigan F, Foreman E et al: NMR imaging in dementia. Br J Psychiatry 1985;146:31–36

33. O'Brien J, Desmond P, Ames D et al: The differentiation of depression from dementia by temporal lobe magnetic resonance imaging. Psych Med 1994;24:633–640

34. McDonald W, Krishnan K, Doraiswamy P et al: Magnetic resonance findings in patients with early onset Alzheimer's disease. Biol Psychiatry 1991;29:799–810

35. Matsubayashi K, Shimada K, Kawamoto A, Ozawa T: Incidental brain lesions on magnetic resonance imaging and neurobehavioural functions in the apparently healthy elderly. Stroke 1992;23:175–180

36. Kertesz JP, Nalciolglu O, Cotman CW: Cognition and white matter changes on magnetic resonance imaging in dementia. Arch Neurol 1990;47:387–391 (for a review, see Barber and O'Brien[22])

37. Burns A, Tune L, Steele C, Folstein M: Positron emission tomography in dementia—a clinical review. In J Geriatr Psychiatry 1989;4:67–72

38. Gemmil H, Sharpe P, Smith F et al: Cerebral blood flow measured by SPET as a diagnostic tool in the study of dementia. Psychiatric Res 1989;27:327–329

39. Burns A, Philpot MP, Costa DC et al: The investigation of Alzheimer's disease with single photon emission tomography. J Neurol Neurosurg Psychiatry 1989;52:248–253

40. Stern Y, Alexander G, Prohovnik I et al: Relationship between lifetime occupation and parietal flow. Neurology 1995;45:55–60

41. Starkstein et al: 1991

42. Neary D, Snowden J, Northen B, Goulding P: Dementia of frontal lobe type. J Neurol Neurosurg Psychiatry 51:353–361

43. Geaney D, Soper N, Shepstone B, Cowan P: Effect of central cholinergic stimulation on regional cerebral blood flow in Alzheimer's disease. Lancet 1990;335:1484–1487

43a. Jobst K, Wyper B: Single photon emission computed tomography. In O'Brien J, Ames D, Burns A (eds): Dementia, 2nd Ed. Edward Arnold, London, 2000:151–161

44. Frackowiak R, Pozzilli C, Legg N et al: Regional cerebral oxygen supply and utilisation in dementia. Brain 1981;104:753–758

44a. Kennedy A: Positron emission tomography in dementia. In O'Brien J, Ames D, Burns A (eds): Dementia 2nd Ed. Edward Arnold, London, 2000:163–177

45. Cummings J, Benson DF: Laboratory aids in the diagnosis of dementia. In Cummings JL, Benson DF (eds): Dementia—A Clinical Approach. Butterworths, Boston, 1983:285–308

46. Soininen H, Partinen VJ, Helkala EL, Riekken PJ: EEG findings in senile dementia and normal ageing. Acta Neurol Scand 1982;65:59–70

47. Prinz PN, Vitello MV: Dominant occipital (alpha) rhythm frequency in early stage Alzheimer's disease and depression. EEG Clin Neurophysiol 1989;73:427–432

48. Prichep LS, John ER, Ferris SH et al: Quantitative EEG correlates of cognitive deterioration in the elderly. Neurobiol Aging 1994;15:85–90

49. Coben LA, Danziger WL, Berg L: Frequency analysis of the resting awake EEG in mild senile dementia of Alzheimer type. EEG Clin Neurophysiol 1983;55:372–380

49a. Doody RS, Stevens JC, Beck C et al: Practice parameter: management of dementia (an evidence-based review). Report of the Quality Standards Subcommittee of the American Academy of Neurology. Neurology 2001 May 8;56(9):1154–1166

50. Bowen D, Smith C, White P, Davidson A: Neurotransmitter transmitted enzymes as indices of hypoxia in senile dementia and other abiotrophies. Brain 1976;459–496

51. Little A, Levy R, Kidd P et al: A double-blind placebo controlled trial on high dose lecithin in Alzheimer's disease. JNNP 1985;48:736–742

52. Brooks JO, Yesavage JA, Costa A, Brassi D: Acetyl-L-carnitine slows decline in younger patient's with Alzheimer's disease. Psychogeriatrics 1998;10(2):193–203

53. Thal LJ, Calvani MD, Amato A, Carta A: A 1-year controlled trial of acetyl-L-carnitine in early-onset AD. Neurology 2000;55:805–810

54. Spiegel R, Azcona A, Wettstein A: First results with RS86, an orally active muscarinic agonist in health subjects and in patients with dementia. In Wurtman S, Corkin S, Growdon J (eds): Alzheimer's Disease: Advances in Basic Research and Therapy. Center of Basic Sciences and Metabolism Charitable Trust, Cambridge, MA, 1987:391–405

55. Ott A, Breteler MMB, van Harskamap F, Hofman A: Smoking increases the risk of dementia: the Rotterdam study. Neurology 1997;48:A78

56. Burns A, Russell E, Page S: New drugs for Alzheimer's disease. Br J Psychiatry 1999;174:476–479

57. Burns A, Rossor M, Hecker J et al: The effects of donepezil in Alzheimer's disease—results from a multinational trial. Dementia Geriatr Cognit Disord 1999;10:237–244

58. Rogers S, Doody R, Pratt R, Ieni J: Long-term efficacy and safety of donepezil in the treatment of Alzheimer's disease. European Neuropsychopharmacol 2000;20(10):195–203

59. Burks J, Melzer D: Donepezil for mild and moderate Alzheimer's disease (Cochrane Review) The Cochrane Library, Issue 3 Update Software, Oxford, 1999 (www.update-software.com/ccweb/cochrane)

60. Rosler M, Anand R, Cicin-Sain A et al: Efficacy and safety of rivastigmine in patients with Alzheimer's disease: international randomised controlled trial. Br Med J 1999;318:633–640

61. Schneider L, Anand R, Farrow N: Systematic review of the efficacy of rivastigmine on patient with Alzheimer's disease. Int J Geriatr Psychopharmacol 1998;1:S26–S34

62. McKeith I, Del Ser T, Spano P et al: Efficacy of rivastimine in dementia with Lewy bodies. Lancet 2000;356:2031–2036

63. Tariot P, Soloman P, Morris J et al: A five-month randomised placebo-controlled trial of galantamine in Alzheimer's disease. Neurology 2000;54:2269–2276

64. Rasking M, Perskind E, Wessel T et al: Galantamine and AD: a 6-month randomised placebo-controlled trial with a 6-month extension. Neurology 2000;54:2261–2268

64a. Wilcock G, Lilienfeidl S, Gaens E et al: Efficacy and safety of galantamine in patient with mild to moderate Alzheimer's disease: multicentre randomised controlled trial. Galantamine International Study Group

65. NICE Technology Appraisal Guidance No 19. January 2001

66. Sano M, Ernesto MS, Thomas RG et al: A controlled trial of selegiline, alpha-tocopherol or both as treatment for Alzheimer's disease. N Engl J Med 1997;17:1216–1217

67. Mulnard R, Cotman C, Kawas C et al: Oestrogen replacement therapy for treatment of mild to moderate Alzheimer's disease. JAMA 2000;283:1007–1015

68. Henderson V, Paganini Hill A, Miller B et al: Oestrogen for Alzheimer's disease in women. Neurology 2000;54:295–301

69. Schneider L, Olin J: Overview of clinical trials of hydergine in dementia. Arch Neurol 1994;54:787–798

70. Le Bars P, Katz M, Berman N et al: A placebo controlled double blind randomized trial of an extract of gingko biloba for dementia. JAMA 1997;278:1327–1332

71. Flicker L, Evans JG: Piracetam for dementia or cognitive impairment (Cochrane Review). In The Cochrane Library Issue 3. Update Software, Oxford, 1999

72. Winblad B, Portis N: Memantine in severe dementia—results of the M-BEST study (Benefit and Efficacy During Treatment with Memantine). Int J Geriatr Psychiatry 1999;14:135–146

73. Burns A, Russell E, Stratton-Powell H et al: Sertraline in stroke-associated lability of mood. Int J Geriat Psychiatry 1999;14: 681–685

74. Schneider LS, Sobin P: Treatments for psychiatric symptoms and behavioral disturbances in dementa. In Burns A, Levy R (eds): Dementia. Chapman and Hall, London, 1994

75. Steele C, Lucas M, Tune L: Haloperidol vs thioridazine in the treatment of behavioural symptoms in senile dementia of the Alzheimer's type. J Clin Psychiatry 1986;47:310–312

76. Mintzer J, Burns A: Anticholinergic side-effects of drugs in elderly people. J R Soc Med 2000;93:457–462

77. Oberholzer A, Hendriksen C, Monsch A et al: Safety and effectiveness of low dose clozapine in psychogeriatric patients. Int Psychogeriatr 1992;4:187–195

78. De Deyn P, Katz I: Control of aggression and agitation in patients with dementia: efficacy and safety of risperidone. Int J Geriatr Psychiatry 2000;15:S14–S22

79. De Deyn P, Rabheru K, Rasmussen A et al: A randomised trial of risperidone, placebo and haloperidol for behavioural symptoms of dementia. Neurology 1999;53:946–955

80. Wilcock G, Stevens J, Perkins A: Trazodone/tryptophan for aggressive behaviour. Lancet 1987;1:929–930

81. McKeith I, Fairburn A, Perry R et al: Neuroleptic sensitivity in patients with senile dementia of the Lewy body type. Br Med J 1992;305:673–678

82. Committee on Safety of Medicine: Neuroleptic sensitivity in patients with dementia. Curr Prob Pharmacovigil 1994;20(6)

83. Jones R: Drug Treatment in Dementia. Blackwell Science, Oxford, 2000

84. Twining C: Can we train the brain. In Levy R, Howard R, Burns A (eds): Treatment and Care in Old Age Psychiatry. Wrightson Biomedical Publishers, Petersfield, UK, 1993:139–150

85. West R: Compensatory strategies for age associated memory impairment, In Baddely A, Wilson B, Watts F (eds): Handbook of Memory Disorders. John Wiley, Chichester, 1995

86. Bleathman C, Morton I: Psychological treatments. In Burns A, Levy R (eds): Dementia. Chapman & Hall, London, 1994

87. Morton I, Bleathman C: The effectiveness of validation therapy in dementia—a pilot study. In J Geriatr Psychiatry 1991;6:327–330

88. King K: Reminiscing psychotherapy with ageing people. J Psychosoc Nurs Ment Health Serv 1982;20:21–25

89. Lindesay J, Marudkar M, van Diepen E, Wilcock G: The 2nd Leicester survey of memory clinics in the British Isles. Int J Geriatr Psychiatry 2002;117:41–47; BMJ 2000 Dec 9;321(7274):1445–1449

Chapter 64

Alzheimer's disease

Gordon K. Wilcock

Alzheimer first described the disease that now bears his name early last century, publishing his classic account of the neuropathology in 1906.[1] The patient he described was only 51 years of age, and the term "Alzheimer's disease" was subsequently reserved for dementia starting in the presenium, differentiating this from that in older people, where the underlying etiology was assumed to be either a manifestation of aging, or arteriosclerosis, or both. This concept remained largely unchallenged until the late 1960s, when Tomlinson and his colleagues reported their observations on the differences between the brains of nondemented old people and those with dementia.[2,3] This showed conclusively that what we now call Alzheimer's disease was the commonest cause of dementia, irrespective of the sufferer's age.

PREVALENCE OF ALZHEIMER'S DISEASE

The prevalence of dementia, and also of Alzheimer's disease, is probably similar in most, if not all, westernized populations, when studies are adjusted for the relevant variables, e.g. age structure of the cohorts and diagnostic criteria. This has been confirmed in the EURODEM studies.[4] Most of these studies, however, have centered on urban populations in relatively well-developed countries, and it may be that the prevalence is lower in rural and less developed societies.

In a review of 36 prevalence and 15 incidence studies of dementia[5] the overall prevalence of dementia, i.e., not just Alzheimer's disease, is reported to vary between 0.3 and 1.0 per 100 people in individuals aged 60–64 years, increasing to between 42.3 and 68.3 per 100 people in those aged 95 years and older. The incidence varies from 0.8 to 4.0 per 1,000 person years in those aged 60–64 years, rising to 49.8 to 135.7 per 1,000 person years in the population aged 95 years and over. International comparison between the studies revealed that both prevalence and incidence showed little geographical variation, with differences between countries reflecting more methodological than actual differences, a rising incidence and prevalence with increasing age, and the possibility that different dementia types might have different age distributions. In a recent comparison of prevalence figures of dementia across European studies, Lobo et al.[6] quote the prevalence of Alzheimer's disease to be 0.6 percent in the age group 65–69 years, rising to 22.2 percent in those subjects aged 90 years and over. Variation in the prevalence of Alzheimer's disease across the studies was greatest for men. Overall they reported that dementia appeared to be more prevalent in women, and that Alzheimer's disease was the main contributor to the steep increase of prevalence with age.

CLINICAL FEATURES AND DIFFERENTIAL DIAGNOSIS

Clinical features

The history and findings on clinical examination make the largest contribution to diagnosis and also distinguishing probable Alzheimer's disease from other causes of dementia.

Early dementia

The early stages of Alzheimer's disease will be known to all readers, with an onset usually marked by significant impairment of memory and learning, although in a small number of individuals pronounced language impairment and visuoconstructional deficits may be early features. The memory impairment usually affects a number of other cognitive domains, and has an impact on the ability to undertake the activities of daily living. More complex tasks are often affected by central executive impairment with a loss of ability to plan and organize activities, and there is some impairment of judgment. A reduction in verbal fluency and increasing anomia, progressing to quite significant motor language disability, begins to impair communication. As the disease progresses, other, predominantly cortical, neuropsychological deficits become apparent, including constructional apraxia. Spatial disorientation, if it has not already occurred, joins temporal disorientation as a destructive factor in daily life, and will affect driving ability. Noncognitive disturbances, including depression and emotional lability, may occur.

Moderate dementia

The mild stage gives way to the moderate stage, which is characterized by even more marked deterioration in the ability to reason, make sensible judgments, plan, organize, and undertake less complex activities. Communication becomes more difficult as language deteriorates, and reading, and comprehension skills are also affected, as is writing ability in most patients. This leads to a major impact on functional ability for both simple activities of daily living (ADL) skills, as well as the more complicated activities that were affected earlier. Visual agnosia becomes apparent, hallucinations may occur in 10–20 percent of patients, and lack of awareness of their illness sets in, if it has not already occurred. Some sufferers over-react to relatively minor challenges in some circumstances, with what is often described as a "catastrophic reaction," which may imply some limited insight into their predicament. Behavior deteriorates further, with often apparently aimless and restless wandering in some, lack of ability to safely manage gas and electrical appliances in most, and it becomes increasingly clear that an independent existence within the community is no longer possible, unless considerable support can be provided.

Severe dementia

As the disease progresses further, those afflicted enter the final and severest stage, during which it is very difficult to obtain any useful differential diagnostic information. In most cases, however, a person with dementia will have presented considerably earlier in their illness, when the clinical pattern and spectrum of neuropsychological deficits will point in the direction of probable Alzheimer's disease. The severe stage is eventually marked by almost total dependence upon others. There is severe impairment of nearly all cognitive functions, which makes communication difficult, even in relation to the most simple needs. Some patients may develop repetitive and stereotype behavior problems such as calling out, wandering, and aggressive traits. Primitive reflexes may emerge, e.g., snout and grasp reflexes, motor problems may include rigidity and myoclonus, and a small proportion of severely affected individuals experience epileptic seizures (see Chapter 46). Those who become immobile will, of course, be subject to the physical problems that are frequently associated with reduced mobility. It is also important not to forget that difficult behavior may really be an indicator of an underlying problem, e.g., discomfort, that cannot be communicated in any other manner.

Routine clinical investigations

Having established that the clinical picture is compatible with Alzheimer's disease and does not point in the direction of one of the other common causes of dementia, i.e., vascular dementia, dementia associated with Lewy bodies, and importantly, but less commonly in elderly people, a frontotemporal dementia, other contributory factors should be considered. The usual laboratory screen and simple neuroimaging, such as a computed tomography (CT) scan, will exclude potentially reversible conditions such as vitamin deficiencies, hypothyroidism, and, to a large extent, normal pressure hydrocephalus, although the latter will require a magnetic resonance imaging (MRI) scan. A mixed dementia, most usually Alzheimer's disease and vascular dementia coexisting, can easily be missed, and is a frequent cause of incorrect diagnosis in autopsy-validated studies. Often the features of one cause of the dementia will overshadow those of the other, and it is particularly important not to miss a vascular component to the dementia, because attention to risk factors may improve the patient's prognosis. Basic laboratory investigations should include a full blood count, erythrocyte sedimentation rate (ESR) or viscosity, full biochemical screen, thyroid function tests, serology for syphilis, vitamin B_{12} and folic acid levels and any other investigation that seems clinically appropriate. Many physicians would also recommend a baseline ECG, chest X-ray, carotid vessel ultrasonography, and an EEG. However, in the writer's experience, these are worthwhile only where there is a clinical indication. Wherever possible, all patients should have a baseline CT scan, but in many countries this is impractical, and an MRI scan even more so, for the generality of patients. If the diagnosis is in doubt, however, then an MRI and a single-positron emission CT (SPECT) scan will often prove extremely valuable in distinguishing other conditions that may be contributing to the dementia. The value of neuroimaging is further discussed below.

More specific aids to diagnosis

It is important to remember that Alzheimer's disease is not a single homogenous condition, but that there is considerable heterogeneity in its manifestations. This has made it difficult to identify either a clinical or pathological diagnostic approach that has high specificity and sensitivity. Nevertheless the accuracy of a clinical diagnosis of Alzheimer's disease is of the order of 90 percent or so in centers with adequate clinical experience. The two main areas of difficulty are, of course, differentiating it from so-called "normal" intellectual changes of aging on the one hand, and distinguishing it from alternative causes of dementia on the other. The heterogeneity of Alzheimer's disease and the possibility of it coexisting with other conditions exacerbate the latter difficulty.

There is a preclinical phase of Alzheimer's disease in which there is a decrease in cognitive functioning many years before the diagnosis is recognized and this can be difficult to differentiate from "normal aging." A 22-year prospective study of the Framingham cohort, involving 1,076 subjects who were free of dementia at their initial assessment, reported lower scores for measures of new learning, recall, retention, and abstract reasoning during the dementia-free period in those who subsequently developed probable Alzheimer's disease.[7]

A number of different sets of formalized criteria have been proposed to assist with the diagnosis of probable Alzheimer's disease, and two of the most widely used are the DSM-IV criteria for dementia of Alzheimer's type American Psychiatric Association, 1994 and the NINCDS-ADRDA criteria (Table 64-1).[8,9] These include evidence that dementia is present, that the clinical picture is consistent with that expected in someone with Alzheimer's disease, and that alternative causes of dementia have been excluded. The NINCDS-ADRDA criteria have been especially used in clinical trials of new treatments for Alzheimer's disease. The DSM-IV criteria will be well known to many readers on both sides of the Atlantic, and in the UK and elsewhere many will also be familiar with the ICD-10 criteria (Table 64-2), which enshrine similar principles to the others.[10]

There have been many attempts to develop biochemical markers for Alzheimer's disease in blood, cerebrospinal fluid (CSF), and urine, but to date none has proved consistently reliable—similarly for those physiological parameters that have been explored, e.g., olfactory ability and pupillary changes to specific pharmacological challenge. Many of the blood and CSF tests have centered on evaluation of levels of amyloid or tau components. A consensus meeting held in 1997 defined the characteristics of an ideal biomarker, and concluded that at that time none of the available potential tests met the requirements in terms of sensitivity, specificity, and reliability.[11] Although a number of potential tests discriminate reasonably well between a group of people with Alzheimer's disease and an age- and gender-matched control group, their predictive value in an individual patient is limited.

A number of promising approaches, based on the combined levels of amyloid and tau components in the CSF, are still under evaluation, and may prove clinically useful.

The EEG in Alzheimer's disease is usually abnormal, but reveals only relatively nonspecific changes that are of limited diagnostic help. SPECT and positron emission tomography (PET) scanning have been widely evaluated, and although PET

Table 64-1 Criteria for clinical diagnosis of Alzheimer's disease

I. The criteria for the clinical diagnosis of PROBABLE Alzheimer's disease include:
- dementia established by clinical examination and documented by the Mini-Mental Test, Blessed Dementia Scale, or some similar examination, and confirmed by neuropsychological tests;
- deficits in two more areas of cognition;
- progressive worsening of memory and other cognitive functions;
- no disturbance of consciousness;
- onset between ages 40 and 90, most often after age 65; and
- absence of systemic disorders or other brain diseases that in and of themselves could account for the progressive deficits in memory and cognition

II. The diagnosis of PROBABLE Alzheimer's disease is supported by:
- progressive deterioration of specific cognitive functions such as language (aphasia), motor skills (apraxia), and perception (agnosia);
- impaired activities of daily living and altered patterns of behavior;
- family history of similar disorders, particularly if confirmed neuropathologically; and
- laboratory results of:
  - normal lumbar puncture as evaluated by standard techniques,
  - normal pattern or nonspecific changes in EEG, such as increased slow-wave activity, and
  - evidence of cerebral atrophy on CT with progression documented by serial observation

III. Other clinical features consistent with the diagnosis of PROBABLE Alzheimer's disease, after exclusion of causes of dementia other than Alzheimer's disease, include:
- plateaus in the course of progression of the illness;
- associated symptoms of depression, insomnia, incontinence, delusions, illusions, hallucinations, catastrophic verbal, emotional, or physical outbursts, sexual disorders, and weight loss;

- other neurologic abnormalities in some patients, especially with more advanced disease and including motor signs such as increased muscle tone, myoclonus, or gait disorder;
- seizures in advanced disease; and
- CT normal for age

IV. Features that make the diagnosis of PROBABLE Alzheimer's disease uncertain or unlikely include:
- sudden, apoplectic onset;
- focal neurologic findings such as hemiparesis, sensory loss, visual field deficits, and incoordination early in the course of the illness; and
- seizures or gait disturbances at the onset or very early in the course of the illness

V. Clinical diagnosis of POSSIBLE Alzheimer's disease:
- may be made on the basis of the dementia syndrome, in the absence of other neurologic, psychiatric, or systemic disorders sufficient to cause dementia, and in the presence of variations in the onset, in the presentation, or in the clinical course;
- may be made in the presence of a second systemic or brain disorder sufficient to produce dementia, which is not considered to be *the* cause of the dementia; and
- should be used in research studies when a single, gradually progressive severe cognitive deficit is identified in the absence of other identifiable cause

VI. Criteria for diagnosis of DEFINITE Alzheimer's disease are:
- the clinical criteria for probable Alzheimer's disease and
- histopathologic evidence obtained from a biopsy or autopsy

VII. Classification of Alzheimer's disease for research purposes should specify features that may differentiate subtypes of the disorder, such as:
- familial occurrence;
- onset before age of 65;
- presence of trisomy-21; and
- coexistence of other relevant conditions such as Parkinson's disease

Reprinted from McKhann et al.[9]

Table 64-2 ICD-10 definition of dementia

- Dementia is a syndrome due to disease of the brain, usually of a chronic or progressive nature, in which there is disturbance of multiple higher cortical functions, including memory, thinking, orientation, comprehension, calculation, learning capacity, language, and judgment
- Consciousness is not clouded
- The impairments of cognitive function are commonly accompanied, and occasionally preceded, by deterioration in emotional control, social behavior, or motivation
- This syndrome occurs in Alzheimer's disease, in cerebrovascular disease, and in other conditions primarily or secondarily affecting the brain

Source: WHO.[10]

scanning is probably more sensitive than SPECT, it is not available as a clinical tool to the majority of physicians working in this field. SPECT, on the other hand, may show the fairly characteristic picture of temporoparietal hypoperfusion. Although it is not specific to Alzheimer's disease, it does help to discriminate the latter from frontal and/or frontotemporal degenerative conditions and others such as vascular dementia.

The ability of neuroimaging, i.e., CT or MRI scanning in particular, to assist in the diagnosis of Alzheimer's disease, has been extensively explored in the literature. The hippocampus is an early target for the Alzheimer's disease pathology, and many studies have concentrated their attention on hippocampal atrophy, or atrophy of the hippocampus and other medial temporal lobe structures. There is now significant evidence to indicate that medial temporal structures atrophy more rapidly in patients with Alzheimer's disease than in age- and gender-matched control subjects.[12,13] Similarly, serial quantification of brain volume changes differentiates those with Alzheimer's disease from a control group.[14] In general, however, neuroimaging of this nature is probably more useful for quantifying brain atrophy in a clinical trial context, rather than diagnosis in the clinic.

Routine genetic testing

The value of routine genetic screening, in particular determining whether a patient has one or more ApoE4 alleles, has engendered much controversy. In those subjects in whom there is a strong family history, usually younger patients, genetic screening for the known early onset mutations may be helpful for a number of reasons, but should only be undertaken within the context of a properly resourced unit that is able to provide appropriate counseling and support. This is relevant to very few patients, whereas it has been suggested that ApoE4 screening should be undertaken for all people with what appears to be sporadic Alzheimer's disease, and there have been attempts to market kits for this purpose. There is, however, now a general consensus that this is inappropriate. ApoE4 testing is certainly of no value for general population screening, as not all patients with ApoE4 will develop Alzheimer's disease, and 30–40 percent of patients with Alzheimer's disease do not have an ApoE4 allele. This approach will therefore not identify individuals at risk for the subsequent development of Alzheimer's disease at a reasonable level of sensitivity and specificity. In those in whom dementia is already present, however, this approach has greater utility, but it is still inadequate as a useful clinical aid. In a study of well-characterized Alzheimer's disease patients and controls, followed longitudinally and in whom autopsy confirmation of the diagnosis was available, Welsh–Bohmer and coauthors reported that the absence of an ApoE4 allele was of no useful clinical predictive value.[15] In other words, the presence of one or more ApoE4 alleles in a patient with a clinical diagnosis of Alzheimer's disease makes that diagnosis very much more likely, but its absence does not exclude Alzheimer's disease.

Finally, it must be remembered that we are diagnosing probable, rather than definite, Alzheimer's disease, the latter only being possible at autopsy, or in those infrequent situations where biopsy is indicated. This is important, because even if the degree of probability is around 90 percent, there is a 1 in 10 chance that the diagnosis is incorrect and one should be prepared to review the diagnosis from time to time.

THE PATHOLOGY OF ALZHEIMER'S DISEASE

The traditional neuropathological hallmarks of Alzheimer's disease are, of course, the deposition of amyloid protein within the plaques and also lying free within the parenchyma on the one hand, and the intraneuronal neurofibrillary tangles on the other. Both plaques and tangles can be found in small numbers in the brains of apparently normal elderly people, and in some other chronic conditions, but their association with Alzheimer's disease was firmly established by studies showing a significant correlation between the pathology and the severity of both the clinical presentation, and markers of cholinergic activity within the Alzheimer brain.[16–18] The areas most affected by the neuropathology, i.e., the medial temporal structures including the hippocampus and entorhinal cortex, infero-posterior temporal areas, and adjacent areas in the parietal and occipital lobes, among others, relate well to the known early clinical features of the disease. In a very careful study, Braak and Braak[19] charted the topographic distribution of the plaques, tangles, and neuropil threads within the parenchyma, and the way in which the distribution progressed as the severity of the disease increased.

Other important neuropathological changes, which have some overlap with normal aging and other dementias, include abnormalities of neuronal processes and synapses, and changes in glia and white matter. The latter represents the pathological basis of the white matter low attenuation or leukoaraiosis that is visible on neuroimaging and includes partial loss of myelin sheaths, axons, and oligodendrocytes, with mild astrocytosis and small vessel changes but no lacunae. Further links between vascular pathology and Alzheimer's disease are emerging, and readers are referred to a recent review, as space precludes further discussion.[20]

The cholinergic neurochemical pathology of Alzheimer's disease was first established over 20 years ago.[21] Since then our knowledge in this field has increased significantly, including an understanding of the interaction between the cholinergic and other neurotransmitter systems.[22] There are also significant changes in serotonin, noradrenaline, dopamine, and some neuropeptides such as somatostatin, to name but a few other transmitter systems that are affected in Alzheimer's disease. It is always difficult to know whether these are primary or secondary lesions.

An understanding of the neurochemical basis of Alzheimer's disease, particularly the cholinergic deficit, has of course underpinned the development of cholinergic strategies for the symptomatic treatment of Alzheimer's disease, which has led to the availability of donepezil, rivastigmine, and galantamine. Major strides have also been made in understanding the molecular pathology of Alzheimer's disease and its relevance to the clinical features, this relating mainly to β-amyloid production and toxicity, and the role of microtubule-associated proteins in the formation of neurofibrillary tangles. Just as knowledge of the cholinergic deficits led to the development of symptomatic treatment strategies, so our understanding of the molecular pathology of amyloid deposition and neurofibrillary tangle production has led to the development of therapeutic strategies that may be disease modifying. Beta-amyloid is considered by most working in the field to play a central role in the neuronal damage that occurs in Alzheimer's disease, although it is possible that it is a marker for other pathological processes that are more important. This debate will only be completely resolved if it is shown that anti-amyloid strategies have a major impact on the disease process in people with Alzheimer's disease as well as in animal models. The synthesis of β-amyloid from amyloid precursor protein, and the mechanisms of its neurotoxicity and interaction with other factors, including ApoE and other genetic factors, is too complex and intricate to describe here, and the reader is referred elsewhere.[23–27]

The main hallmark of neurofibrillary tangles is the presence of paired helical filaments (PHF), which are found in neurons, neuritic plaques, and dystrophic neurites throughout the neuropil. The major component of the paired helical filaments is a form of tau protein, one of the microtubule-associated proteins that are found within neurons. Hyperphosphorylation of tau protein is thought by many to be an important factor in the assembly of neurofibrillary tangles. There are also links between tau and altered processing of the amyloid precursor protein and the presenilin proteins, which leads to the possibility that strategies to prevent tau aggregation in Alzheimer's disease may be therapeutically important and lead to an arrest, or slowing down, of the neuronal damage and clinical progression of the disease.[28] Tau pathology, and mutations in the tau gene on chromosome 17, appear to play a part in a number of neurodegenerative disorders, but so far there has not been any evidence to support a genetic basis for the abnormal tau processing in Alzheimer's disease.

PHARMACOLOGICAL TREATMENT STRATEGIES

The use of drugs to treat people with Alzheimer's disease is only a small part of the overall management strategy. This section will, however, concentrate on drugs designed to influence the symptoms and basic pathology of Alzheimer's disease, and the reader is referred to Ch. 63 for a wider discussion of the other very important aspects of patient management.

Cholinergic strategies

There have been two main cholinergic approaches to developing treatment in Alzheimer's disease: prolonging the life of the reduced amounts of acetylcholine in the Alzheimer brain on the one hand, and muscarinic receptor agonist strategies on the other. A number of muscarinic agonist compounds have been evaluated, but to date have not stood the test of time. A number of cholinesterase inhibitors, i.e., drugs that block the action of acetylcholinesterase, have now been licensed and are available in many parts of the world for the treatment of mild to moderate dementia caused by Alzheimer's disease. Four have been licensed in the UK and elsewhere, tacrine, donepezil, rivastigmine, and galantamine, and others are under evaluation. The first real evidence that cholinesterase inhibition might be helpful in Alzheimer's disease came from the 1986 report of Summers et al.[29] Although controversial for a number of reasons, it was followed by many studies confirming significant benefit to some sufferers, and the drug in question, tacrine (tetrahydroaminoacridine, THA) eventually received a product license and was used extensively in the USA. Its modest efficacy was confirmed in a recent meta analysis of 12 trials involving nearly 2,000 patients.[30]

A significant number of clinical trials of second-generation cholinesterase inhibitors have all shown similar results, mainly modest but tangible benefits to a proportion (40–50 percent) of those for whom they were prescribed. The adverse event profile is mainly related to gastrointestinal tract symptomatology, and in the majority of individuals is manageable. Most of these trials involve donepezil,[31–33] rivastigmine,[34,35] and galantamine,[36–38] but similar evidence is available for metrifonate,[39,40] although this has not yet been granted a license because of doubts about its adverse event profile. There are claims and counter claims about the superiority of one drug over another. In clinical practice there seems little to choose between them but we are currently awaiting the outcome of comparative studies of one compound against another. Donepezil is the only one that can be given on a once daily dose regime, however.

Evidence is now emerging, mainly from open label studies, that these drugs are also effective and safe for long-term treatment, e.g., up to nearly 3 years in one report,[41] compared to the 3–6 month duration of the pivotal trials. They may have some benefit in controlling noncognitive symptoms of Alzheimer's disease, and their benefit includes help for carers in terms of reduced time needed for assisting and supervising Alzheimer's disease sufferers. Furthermore, a number of European and North American studies have begun to provide some evidence that the prescription of cholinesterase inhibitors is cost-effective.[42–45]

The UK National Institute for Clinical Excellence (NICE), has recently considered the evidence in favor of making donepezil, rivastigmine, and galantamine available with the cost of prescription borne by the UK National Health Service. Although these guidelines were prepared only in relation to prescribing in the UK, the principles involved are sound, and may be helpful to those in other countries. The full guidelines are available in a small publication[46] but the main points are summarized below:

- The diagnosis of probable mild to moderate Alzheimer's disease must be made in a specialist clinic, according to standard diagnostic criteria.
- Pre-prescribing assessment should include tests of cognitive, global, and behavioral functioning, and an assessment of ADL ability. The Mini-mental State Examination (MMSE) score should be above 12 points.
- Compliance should be carefully considered, and in general it would be expected that this would be supervised by a carer or careworker.
- Treatment should be initiated by a specialist, and there should subsequently be a shared-care protocol if general practitioners take over the prescribing.
- A subsequent assessment should be made 2–4 months after maintenance dose of the drug has been reached, and prescription should only be continued where there has been improvement or no deterioration in MMSE score, together with evidence of global improvement on the basis of behavioral and/or functional assessment.
- Those continuing treatment should have 6-month assessments of MMSE score and global functional and behavioral assessment, and in general only remain on treatment while their MMSE score stays above 12 points, and the other assessment parameters indicate that the drug is having a worthwhile effect.
- When the MMSE score falls below 12 points, prescribing should be discontinued unless there are exceptional reasons to indicate otherwise.

Development of antiamyloid and antineurofibrillary tangle-based treatments

Increasing knowledge of the molecular pathology of amyloid deposition and its presumed toxicity has led to the development of a number of different therapeutic strategies. These include the use of protease inhibitors, which block the enzymes that cleave the amyloid precursor protein at the sites which allow the release of the 42 amino acid β-peptide. Reducing the formation of this "building block" should, in turn, reduce the amount of β-amyloid protein formed. Similarly, compounds are being developed that might stop amyloid formation by preventing its aggregation to form the toxic fibrils. Other approaches address the potential mechanisms by which amyloid toxicity may be produced, e.g., the use of antioxidant compounds, antiapoptotic agents, and drugs that block inflammatory processes.

An intriguing and novel approach, which has shown great promise in transgenic mice models of Alzheimer's disease, involves the use of immunization with the β-amyloid peptide. In a relatively small study in transgenic mice, Schenk and colleagues[47] showed that immunization with the β-amyloid peptide significantly reduced amyloid deposits within the brain. Two more recent studies[48,49] supported this and also that immunization was associated with some protection from the "spatial" learning deficits that accompanied plaque formation. Clinical trial in human sufferers of Alzheimer's disease is now in its early stages, and whether the efficacy of this approach in patients matches that in the mouse model will become clear in a few years time. These studies in humans, have, for the time being at least, been discontinued whilst toxicity issues are being explored.

Although the production of amyloid appears central to the brain damage in Alzheimer's disease, there are some who question whether it is the primary cause or a secondary phenomenon. There are a number of reasons for this, including the fact that the deposition of relatively large quantities of amyloid in the brains of the transgenic mouse models seem to produce only very little neuronal damage and loss, and tangles are not formed. This may be the result of species differences in how the potential toxic effects of amyloid are handled by neurons and glia, but this debate will be settled only when antiamyloid strategies are evaluated in human Alzheimer's disease sufferers.

Neurofibrillary tangles are intraneuronal and may represent the final common pathway that leads to neuronal malfunction and eventually death. Their formation probably disrupts the normal intracellular transport mechanisms, and there is some evidence that their presence correlates better with the clinical and neurochemical pathology than does the amyloid load. The intracellular site of the tangle may make it a more difficult target, but potential therapeutic strategies are being developed, although they are further from clinical trial than the antiamyloid approaches.

Other strategies for treating Alzheimer's disease

A number of other strategies have been explored as potential treatments for Alzheimer's disease. Unfortunately space precludes discussion of many of these, but three in particular merit specific comment: estrogen (hormone) replacement therapy (HRT) in post-menopausal women, treatment with anti-inflammatory drugs, and the antioxidant approach.

There is considerable evidence from epidemiological studies that women taking HRT medication are less likely to develop dementia, and possible Alzheimer's disease specifically. In addition, those who develop dementia while taking HRT medication may experience its onset later than those who are untreated, and this protection may be effective in both younger and older onset cases.[50–53] However, this has not been a uniformly consistent finding, e.g., in a population-based case-control study from the UK-based general practice research database.[54] Many of the positive studies have been criticized because they inadequately addressed the biases introduced by education, improved healthcare, and lower exposure to risk factors for cerebrovascular disease in the women who were most likely to take HRT medication, i.e., those who are better educated and belong to higher socio-economic groups.

Two recent studies of the effects of estrogen in women with an existing diagnosis of Alzheimer's disease have failed to show any benefit,[55,56] although they used relatively small numbers of subjects, and were of short duration. Further longer-term studies are required before it will be possible to conclude whether or not the apparent protective effect may indicate that those who have established Alzheimer's disease may also benefit.

Similarly, there is epidemiological evidence suggesting that the use of anti-inflammatory drugs, especially nonsteroidal anti-inflammatory drugs, may be neuroprotective, and this is supported by the demonstration of inflammatory processes that appear to be taking place within the brain in Alzheimer's disease.[57–61] The hypothesis is not that inflammatory processes initiate the disorder, but that once the pathology is under way, amyloid deposition and possibly other factors lead to an inflammatory response which then exacerbates the neuronal damage. This has led to clinical trials of anti-inflammatory regimes in those with established disease but, as in the case of the estrogen trials to date, the response has been disappointing.[62,63] However, again, longer-term studies in larger cohorts of subjects are needed before a definite conclusion can be drawn.

There is considerable evidence linking Alzheimer's disease with oxidative stress, and free radical formation.[64–68] This is clearly an area that needs further exploration, and has implications for lifestyle and long-term preventative strategies, as does the potential value of certain statins, although regarded by some as controversial.[69]

GENETIC ASPECTS OF ALZHEIMER'S DISEASE

This is a field that has literally exploded with new knowledge, since identification of the first mutation in the gene for amyloid precursor protein located on chromosome 21.[70] Since then, a significant number of associated mutations have been described. They are, however, only relevant to a very small proportion of young-onset Alzheimer's disease familial pedigrees. Identification of the presenilin-1 gene mutation in other early-onset families followed[71] and since then more than 40 further mutations have been described in relation to this site on chromosome 14. It is also now known that some of these mutations may occur in those with late-onset Alzheimer's disease, albeit a minority. Like the amyloid precursor protein (APP) mutations, these are autosomal dominant traits, and have nearly complete penetrance in the majority of reports. A second presenilin mutation in the presenilin-2 gene on chromosome 1 was reported in seven families of Volga German ancestry.[72] The presenilins are transmembrane proteins and the mechanism of action of these mutations is not completely understood. However, it seems that they all result in an increased production of the 42 amino-acid amyloid β-peptide essential for the formation of the amyloid protein. This knowledge has been extremely important for our understanding of Alzheimer's disease, and the development of potential therapeutic strategies, but the three mutations together are probably responsible for no more than 1–2 percent of all Alzheimer's disease cases. Recently, another locus has been identified on chromosome 10, which is probably more important in relation to late-onset familial disease than the other mutations.[73–75]

More important for those of us working predominantly with elderly people is, of course, the series of mutations affecting apolipoprotein E on chromosome 19. Since its original description in 1993,[76] many further mutations have been described. Apolipoprotein E is a lipid transporter protein, and genetically there are three common alleles, ε2, ε3, and ε4. The ε4 allele is a risk factor for Alzheimer's disease in elderly individuals, with sporadic Alzheimer's disease, and also in some young-onset cases. Possession of an ε4 allele increases the amyloid load and reduces the age of onset in familial cases, and this appears to be dose related, with two ε4 alleles conferring a worse prognosis than one. The risk is, however, modified by age, sex, and ethnic background. It is very important to remember, as mentioned previously, that the possession of an ε4 allele is neither sufficient, nor necessary, for the presence of Alzheimer's disease. At least one-third of individuals with this condition do not have an ε4 allele, and as many as 50 percent of ε4 homozygotes can live to the age of 80 or over without developing Alzheimer's disease.

There are many other putative genetic risk factors for Alzheimer's disease, the majority being polymorphisms in one of a large number of candidate genes. The literature is full of conflicting reports about the relevance of these, e.g., the low-density lipoprotein receptor-related protein, α_2 macroglobulin on chromosome 12, α_1 antichymotrypsin on chromosome 14, bleomycin hydrolase on chromosome 17, and many others. For further discussion of this complex area, the reader is referred to some excellent recent reviews.[77–80]

RISK FACTORS

Increasing age is the most important risk factor for the development of Alzheimer's disease, but there is some controversy as to whether there is a leveling off in the very old, i.e., age 90 years and over. Similarly, although it is widely quoted that women have a higher prevalence of Alzheimer's disease than men, the literature presents conflicting reports, and even if true, the difference is not very significant. There also appear to be differing degrees of risk in different ethnic groups, and further studies are ongoing to quantify this.

A family history of dementia is, as one would expect, an important risk factor, especially in early-onset disease. There is also a link with Down's syndrome and all those with this condition develop neuropathological features of Alzheimer's disease by the time they reach 40 years of age. However, they do not all develop the clinical syndrome of dementia, and the reason for this is not known.

Other potential factors affecting the risk of developing Alzheimer's disease include the level of education, premorbid intelligence, head trauma, use of certain medications including anti-inflammatory drugs and hormone replacement therapy, pre-existing depression, and levels of stress. Occupational hazards have also been explored, as have environmental factors such as exposure to herpes simplex virus.[81] A recent study has also suggested that the diversity and intensity of activities undertaken in midlife may be a contributory factor, those less active having an increased risk of developing the disease.[82]

It is very difficult to interpret the significance of this type of evidence. It is possible that many of the putative risk factors, and protective mechanisms, may be contributing to the level of brain reserve left in old age, rather than specifically contributing to the development of plaques and tangles. Individuals with more intact neurons as older age approaches may be able to withstand the damaging effects of Alzheimer's disease pathology for longer, with a later onset of the dementia. In some cases death may occur from other causes before significant intellectual deterioration arises. Space precludes detailed discussion of risk factors, but the reader is referred to an excellent review by Jorm.[83]

KEY POINTS Alzheimer's disease

- The diagnosis of probable Alzheimer's disease is still essentially a clinical process.

- It is a "positive" diagnosis rather than one of exclusion, as in the past.

- The diagnosis is likely to have an accuracy of around 90 percent in experienced centers.

- Symptomatic treatment, i.e., anticholinesterase therapy, is now available and effective in a significant proportion of sufferers.

- Previous treatments have suppressed brain activity, e.g., neuroleptics, but the new drugs enhance brain function.

- Knowledge of the underlying molecular pathology has led to the development of disease modifying strategies that are in early evaluation.

- Drug treatment is only a part of the overall management strategy.

- Lifestyle and environmental factors in earlier life may contribute to the risk of developing the disease.

- Early diagnostic tests are yet to be developed.

REFERENCES

1. Alzheimer A: Uber einen eigenartigen schweren Krankheitsprozes der Hirnrinde. Neurologisches Centralblatt 1906;25:113–114
2. Tomlinson BE, Blessed G, Roth M: Observations on the brains of non-demented old people. J Neurol Sci 1968;7:331–356
3. Tomlinson BE, Blessed G, Roth M: Observations on the brains of demented old people. J Neurol Sci 1970;11:205–242
4. Hofman A, Rocca WA, Brayne C et al: The prevalence of dementia in Europe: a collaborative study of 1980–1990 findings. Eurodem Prevalence Research Group. Int J Epidemiol 1991;20:736–748
5. Fratiglioni L, De Ronchi D, Aguero-Torres H: Worldwide prevalence and incidence of dementia. Drugs Aging 1999;155:365–375 (review; 81 refs)
6. Lobo A, Launer LJ, Fratiglioni L et al: Prevalence of dementia and major subtypes in Europe: A collaborative study of population-based cohorts.

Neurologic Diseases in the Elderly Research Group. Neurology 2000;5411(suppl 5):S4–S9

7. Elias MF, Beiser A, Wolf PA et al: The preclinical phase of Alzheimer disease: A 22-year prospective study of the Framingham Cohort. Arch Neurol 2000;576:808–813 (see comments)

8. American Psychiatric Association: Desk Reference to the Diagnostic Criteria from DSM-IV. APA, Washington, DC, 1994

9. McKhann G et al: Clinical diagnosis of Alzheimer's disease: report of the NINCDS-ADRDA work group under the auspices of department of health and human services task force on Alzheimer's disease. Neurology 1984;34:939–944

10. World Health Organization: The ICD-10 Classification of Mental and Behavioural Disorders: Diagnostic Criteria for Research. WHO, Geneva, 1993

11. Growdon JH: Biomarkers of Alzheimer disease. Arch Neurol 1999;5633:281–283 (review; 14 refs)

12. Jack CR, Jr, Petersen RC, Xu YC et al: Medial temporal atrophy on MRI in normal aging and very mild Alzheimer's disease. Neurology 1997;493:786–794

13. Scheltens P: Early diagnosis of dementia: neuroimaging. J Neurol 1999;2461:16–20 (review; 35 refs)

14. Fox NC, Cousens S, Scahill R, Harvey RJ, Rossor MN: Using serial registered brain magnetic resonance imaging to measure disease progression in Alzheimer disease: power calculations and estimates of sample size to detect treatment effects. Arch Neurol 2000;573:339–344 (see comments)

15. Welsh-Bohmer KA, Gearing M, Saunders AM, Roses AD, Mirra S: Apolipoprotein E genotypes in a neuropathological series from the Consortium to Establish a Registry for Alzheimer's Disease. Ann Neurol 1997;423:319–325

16. Blessed G, Tomlinson BE, Roth M: The association between quantitative measures of dementia and of senile change in the cerebral grey matter of elderly subjects. Br J Psychiatry 1968;114:797–811

17. Wilcock GK, Esiri MM, Bowen D, Smith CCT: Alzheimer's disease: Correlation of cortical choline acetyltransferase activity with the severity of dementia and histological abnormalities. J Neurol Sci 1982;57:407–417

18. Wilcock GK, Esiri MM: Plaques, tangles and dementia. A quantitative study. J Neurol Sci 1982;56:343–356

19. Braak H, Braak E: Neuropathological staging of Alzheimer-related changes. Acta Neuropathol Berl 1991;82:239–259

20. Kalaria RN: The role of cerebral ischemia in Alzheimer's disease. Neurobiol Aging 2000;212:321–330 (review; 90 refs)

21. Perry EK, Tomlinson BE, Blessed G et al: Correlation of cholinergic abnormalities with senile plaques and mental test scores in senile dementia. Br Med J 1978;II:1457–1459

22. Francis PT, Palmer AM, Snape M, Wilcock GK: The cholinergic hypothesis of Alzheimer's disease: a review of progress. J Neurol Neurosurg Psychiatry 1999;6622:137–147 (review; 118 refs)

23. Hardy J, Duff K, Gwinn-Hardy K, Perez-Tur J, Hutton M: Genetic dissection of Alzheimer's disease and related dementias: amyloid and its relationship to tau. Nat Neurosci 1998;1:355–358

24. Lansbury PT, Jr: Evolution of amyloid: what normal protein folding may tell us about fibrillogenesis and disease. Proc Natl Acad Sci USA 1999;96:3342–3344

25. Price DL, Sisodia SS, Borchelt DR: Genetic neurodegenerative diseases: the human illness and transgenic models. Science 1998;282:1079–1083

26. Scheper W, Annaert W, Cupers P, Saftig P, De Strooper B: Function and dysfunction of the presenilins. Alzheimer's Rep 1999;2:73–81

27. Sturchler-Pierrat C, Sommer B: Transgenic animals in Alzheimer's disease research. Rev Neurosci 1999;101:15–24 (review; 68 refs)

28. Wischik C, Harrington C: The role of tau protein in the neurodegenerative dementias. In O'Brien J, Ames D, Burns A (eds): Dementia. Arnold, London, 2000:461–492

29. Summers WK, Majovski LV, Marsh GM et al: Oral tetrahydroaminoacridine in long-term treatment of senile dementia, Alzheimer type. N Engl J Med 1986;315:1241–1245

30. Qizilbash N, Whitehead A, Higgins J et al: Cholinesterase inhibition for Alzheimer disease: a meta-analysis of the tacrine trials. Dementia Trialists' Collaboration. JAMA 1998;280:1777–1782

31. Burns A, Rossor M, Hecker J et al: The effects of donepezil in Alzheimer's disease—results from a multinational trial. Dement Geriatr Cognit Disord 1999;10:237–244

32. Rogers SL, Friedhoff LT: Long-term efficacy and safety of donepezil in the treatment of Alzheimer's disease: an interim analysis of the results of a US multicentre open label extension study. Eur Neuropsychopharmacol 1998;81:67–75

33. Rogers SL, Farlow MR, Doody RS, Mohs R, Friedhoff LT: A 24-week, double-blind, placebo-controlled trial of donepezil in patients with Alzheimer's disease. Donepezil Study Group. Neurology 1998;501:136–145

34. Corey-Bloom J, Anand R, Veach J: A randomised trial evaluating the efficacy and safety of ENA 713 rivastigmine tartrate, a new acetylcholinesterase inhibitor, in patients with mild to moderately severe Alzheimer's disease. Int J Geriatr Psychopharmacol 1998;1:55–65

35. Rosler M, Anand R, Cicin-Sain A et al: Efficacy and safety of rivastigmine in patients with Alzheimer's disease: international randomised controlled trial. Br Med J 1999;318:633–638 (see comments)

36. Raskind MA, Peskind ER, Wessel T, Yuan W: Galantamine in AD: A 6-month randomized, placebo-controlled trial with a 6-month extension. The Galantamine USA-1 Study Group. Neurology 2000;5412:2261–2268

37. Tariot PN, Solomon PR, Morris JC et al: A 5-month, randomized, placebo-controlled trial of galantamine in AD. The Galantamine USA-10 Study Group. Neurology 2000;5412:2269–2276

38. Wilcock GK, Lilienfeld S, Gaens E: Efficacy and safety of galantamine in patients with mild to moderate Alzheimer's disease: multicentre randomised controlled trial. Br Med J 2000;321:1445–1449

39. Cummings JL, Cyrus PA, Bieber F et al: Metrifonate treatment of the cognitive deficits of Alzheimer's disease. Metrifonate Study Group. Neurology 1998;505:1214–1221 (see comments)

40. Gelinas I, Gauthier S, Cyrus PA: Metrifonate enhances the ability of Alzheimer's disease patients to initiate, organize, and execute instrumental and basic activities of daily living. J Geriatr Psychiatry Neurol 2000;131:9–16

41. Doody RS, Geldmacher DS, Gordon B, Perdomo CA, Pratt RD: Open-label, multicenter, phase 3 extension study of the safety and efficacy of donepezil in patients with Alzheimer's disease. Arch Neurol 2001;58:427–433

42. Jonsson L, Lindgren P, Wimo A, Jonsson B, Winblad B: The cost-effectiveness of donepezil therapy in Swedish patients with Alzheimer's disease: a Markov model. Clin Ther 1999;217:1230–1240

43. Neumann PJ, Hermann RC, Kuntz KM et al: Cost-effectiveness of donepezil in the treatment of mild or moderate Alzheimer's disease. Neurology 1999;526:1138–1145 (see comments)

44. O'Brien BJ, Goeree R, Hux M et al: Economic evaluation of donepezil for the treatment of Alzheimer's disease in Canada. J Am Geriatr Soc 1999;475:570–578

45. Schumock GT: Economic considerations in the treatment and management of Alzheimer's disease. Am J Health-System Pharmacy 1998;55(suppl 2):S17–S21 (review; 17 refs)

46. National Institute of Clinical Excellence: Guidance on the use of Donepezil, Rivastigmine and Galantamine for the Treatment of Alzheimer's disease. Technology Appraisal Guidance, London, NICE, 2001;19:1–13

47. Schenk D, Barbour R, Dunn W et al: Immunization with amyloid-beta attenuates Alzheimer-disease-like pathology in the PDAPP mouse. Nature 1999;4006740:173–177 (see comments)

48. Janus C, Pearson J, McLaurin J et al: Aβ peptide immunization reduces behavioural impairment and plaques in a model of Alzheimer's disease. Nature 2000;408:979–982

49. Morgan D, Diamond DM, Gottschall PE et al: Aβ peptide vaccination prevents memory loss in an animal model of Alzheimer's disease. Nature 2000;408:982–985

50. Birkhauser MH, Strand J, Kampf C, Bahro M: Oestrogens and Alzheimer's disease. Int J Geriatr Psychiatry 2000;157:600–609 (review; 92 refs)

51. Kawas C, Resnick S, Morrison A et al: A prospective study of estrogen replacement therapy and the risk of developing Alzheimer's disease: the Baltimore Longitudinal Study of Aging Neurology 1997;486:1517–1521 (erratum appears in Neurology 1998;512:654)

52. Slooter AJ, Bronzova J, Witteman JC et al: Estrogen use and early onset Alzheimer's disease: a population-based study. J Neurol Neurosurg Psychiatry 1999;676:779–781

53. Waring SC, Rocca WA, Petersen RC et al: Postmenopausal estrogen replacement therapy and risk of AD: a population-based study. Neurology 1999;525:965–970

54. Seshadri S, Zornberg GL, Derby LE et al: Postmenopausal estrogen replacement therapy and the risk of Alzheimer's disease. Arch Neurol 2001;58:435–440

55. Henderson VW, Paganini-Hill A, Miller BL et al: Estrogen for Alzheimer's disease in women: randomized, double-blind, placebo-controlled trial. Neurology 2000;542:295–301

56. Wang PN, Liao SQ, Liu RS et al: Effects of estrogen on cognition, mood, and cerebral blood flow in AD: a controlled study. Neurology 2000;5411:2061–2066 (see comments)

57. Akiyama H, Barger S, Barnum S et al: Inflammation and Alzheimer's disease. Neurobiol Aging 2000;213:383–421 (review; 635 refs)

58. Beard C, Waring S, O'Brien P, Kurland L, Kokmen E: Nonsteroidal anti-inflammatory drug use and Alzheimer's disease: a case-control study in Rochester, Minnesota, 1980 through 1984. Mayo Clinic Proc 1998;73:951–955

59. In't Veld BA, Launer LJ, Hoes AW et al: NSAIDs and incident Alzheimer's disease. The Rotterdam Study. Neurobiol Aging 1998;196:607–611 (see comments)

60. Lim GP, Yang F, Chu T et al: Ibuprofen suppresses plaque pathology and inflammation in a mouse model for Alzheimer's disease. J Neurosci 2000;2015:5709–5714

61. Eikelenboom P, Rozemuller AJ, Hoozemans JJ, Veerhuis R, van Gool WA: Neuroinflammation and Alzheimer disease: clinical and therapeutic implications. Alzheimer Dis Assoc Disord 2000;14(suppl 1):S54–S61 (review; 83 refs)

62. Aisen PS, Davis KL, Berg JD et al: A randomized controlled trial of prednisone in Alzheimer's disease. Alzheimer's Disease Cooperative Study. Neurology 2000;543:588–593

63. Scharf S, Mander A, Ugoni A, Vajda F, Christophidis N: A double-blind, placebo-controlled trial of diclofenac/misoprostol in Alzheimer's disease. Neurology 1999;531:197–201

64. Butterfield DA, Koppal T, Subramaniam R, Yatin S: Vitamin E as an antioxidant/free radical scavenger against amyloid beta-peptide-induced oxidative stress in neocortical synaptosomal membranes and hippocampal neurons in culture: insights into Alzheimer's disease. Rev Neurosci 1999;102:141–149 (review; 164 refs)

65. Christen Y: Oxidative stress and Alzheimer disease. Am J Clin Nutr 2000;712:621S–629S (review; 117 refs)

66. Repetto MG, Reides CG, Evelson P et al: Peripheral markers of oxidative stress in probable Alzheimer patients. European J Clin Invest 1999;297:643–649

67. Rosler M, Retz W, Thome J, Riederer P: Free radicals in Alzheimer's dementia: currently available therapeutic strategies. J Neural Transmiss Suppl 1998;54:211–219 (review; 52 refs)

68. Sano M, Ernesto C, Thomas RG et al: A controlled trial of selegiline, alpha-tocopherol, or both as treatment for Alzheimer's disease. The Alzheimer's Disease Cooperative Study. N Engl J Med 1997;33617:1216–1222 (see comments)

69. Scott HD, Laake K: Statins for the prevention of Alzheimer's disease. Cochrane Database Rev 2001;(4):CD003160

70. Goate A, Chartier-Harlin MC, Mullan M et al: Segregation of a missense mutation in the amyloid precursor protein gene with familial Alzheimer's disease. Nature 1991;349:704–706 (see comments)

71. Sherrington R, Rogaev EI, Liang Y et al: Cloning of a gene bearing missense mutations in early-onset familial Alzheimer's disease. Nature 1995;375:754–760 (see comments)

72. Levy Lahad E, Wijsman EM, Nemens E et al: A familial Alzheimer's disease locus on chromosome 1. Science 1995;269:970–973 (see comments)

73. Bertram L, Blacker D, Mullin K et al: Evidence for genetic linkage of Alzheimer's disease to chromosome 10q. Science 2000;290:2302–2303

74. Ertekin-Taner N, Graff-Radford N, Younkin LH et al: Linkage of plasma Aβ42 to a quantitative locus on chromosome 10 in the late-onset Alzheimer's disease pedigrees. Science 2000;290:2303–2304

75. Myers A, Holmans P, Marshall H et al: Susceptibility locus for Alzheimer's disease on chromosome 10. Science 2000;290:2304–2305

76. Strittmatter WJ, Saunders AM, Schmechel D et al: Apolipoprotein E: high-avidity binding to beta-amyloid and increased frequency of type 4 allele in late-onset familial Alzheimer disease. Proc Natl Acad Sci USA 1993;90:1977–1981

77. Cruts M, Van Broeckhoven C: Molecular genetics of Alzheimer's disease. Ann Med 1998;3066:560–565 (review; 70 refs)

78. George-Hyslop PH: Molecular genetics of Alzheimer's disease. Biol Psychiatry 2000;473:183–199 (review; 155 refs)

79. Lovestone S: Early diagnosis and the clinical genetics of Alzheimer's disease. J Neurol 1999;2462:69–72 (review; 24 refs)

80. Shastry BS, Giblin FJ: Genes and susceptible loci of Alzheimer's disease. Brain Res Bull 1999;482:121–127 (review; 86 refs)

81. Itzhaki RF, Lin WR, Shang D et al: Herpes simplex virus type 1 in brain and risk of Alzheimer's disease. Lancet 1997;349:241–244 (see comments)

82. Friedland RP, Fritsch T, Smyth KA et al: Patients with Alzheimer's disease have reduced activities in midlife compared with healthy control-group members. Proc Natl Acad Sci USA 2001;98:3440–3445

83. Jorm A: Risk Factors for Alzheimer's Disease. In O'Brien J, Ames D, Burns A (eds): Dementia. Arnold, London, 2000:383–390

Chapter 65

Vascular dementia

Kenneth Rockwood and Timo Erkinjuntti

Our understanding of the concept, diagnosis, and treatment of vascular dementia is undergoing interest and renewal. In its guise as a "multi-infarct dementia," vascular dementia was held to be the second most common cause of acquired, global, chronic progressive cognitive impairment that interfered with daily life.[1] But that view is changing, as a consequence of the re-evaluation of two related facts. The first is that there is more to vascular impairment of cognition than the sum of discrete strokes. Second, while the early criteria for dementia used Alzheimer's disease (AD) as the archetype of clinical expression of that syndrome, profound cognitive impairment which interferes with daily life can occur in the setting of cerebrovascular disease that is not well captured by, or even excluded from, AD-based criteria. This chapter situates present concepts within what has generally been understood to have been the case of vascular dementia, in a way that, it is hoped, will be of some use to clinicians.

HISTORICAL OVERVIEW

Until comparatively recently, it was widely believed that the syndrome of dementia in elderly people came about due to impaired cerebral blood flow resulting from cerebral atherosclerosis ("hardening of the arteries"). The relationship between dementia and age was so well established that the term "senility," which simply means aging, came to be synonymous with impaired cognition. By contrast, AD was held to be a rare cause of dementia, which by definition (as a "presenile" condition) affected only younger patients. Tomlinson et al.[2] drew attention to AD as the most frequent cause of progressive cognitive impairment in elderly people, far exceeding that of arteriosclerotic dementia. Shortly thereafter, Hachinski and colleagues coined the term multi-infarct dementia (MID) to describe the mechanism by which they considered that vascular dementia (VaD) was produced.[3] While now recognized as a subtype of VaD,[4] MID was typically described as the "second most common type" of all dementias, although it was held by some to be overdiagnosed.[5]

The early to mid-1990s, however, saw a reappreciation of the role of VaD, and the more broadly construed vascular cognitive impairment (VCI). The idea of VaD being caused chiefly by many small or large brain infarcts has largely given way to the view of a larger spectrum of vascular causes of cognitive impairment and dementia.[6] Further reconceptualization has focused on the complex interactions between vascular causes, functional and structural changes in the brain, related illnesses and other host factors, and cognition.[7–11] For example, Sultzer and colleagues drew attention to cortical metabolic abnormalities associated with ischemic subcortical structural lesions in VaD.[12] These findings suggest that many lesions previously felt to be "incidental" might be playing (or at the very least, signaling) an important role for ischemia, even in the absence of cortical abnormalities demonstrable by traditional neuroimaging or by clinical examination.

In addition to these considerations, which taken together serve to undermine the importance of frank infarction, in favor of ischemic impairment, Hachinski drew attention to the better opportunities for prevention offered by a more broadly construed conceptualization of how cerebrovascular (and even cardiovascular) illnesses contributes to cognitive impairment.[6] Waiting until a person developed dementia before identifying the cognitive impairment as an illness meant both missing the opportunity to prevent such progression, and excluding those whose clinically important cognitive impairment did not meet criteria for dementia which were modeled on AD.[13–16] In consequence, the term VCI has been proposed, although operational criteria for its scope and use have only recently begun to emerge,[17] and to be formally tested.[18–20]

EPIDEMIOLOGY

The view of how commonly VCI occurs, and what its consequences, is critically dependent on how it is defined.[21–24] It may even be that VCI is the most common cause of chronic progressive cognitive impairment in elderly people, if Alzheimer's disease is understood often to have vascular causes.[25]

Prevalence

The prevalence of VaD (as compared with VCI) is the second most common cause of dementia, accounting for 10–50 percent of dementia cases in various series.[21,24,26] In a recent European collaborative study using population-based studies of persons aged 65 years and older conducted in 1990s the age-standardized prevalence of dementia was 6.4 percent (all causes), 4.4 percent for AD, and 1.6 percent for VaD.[24] In this study, 15.8 percent of the cases had VaD and 53.7 percent AD. A large variation in VaD prevalence was seen across studies. The prevalence ranged from 0.0 to 0.8 percent at age 65–69 years, and from 2 to 8.3 percent at age 90 years and over in different studies. There was a difference in prevalence between men and women; under 85 years of age the prevalence of VaD was higher in men compared to women; and thereafter the prevalence was higher in women. The pooled prevalence for the groups is presented in Figure 65-1, which also shows data from the Canadian Study of Health and Aging (CSHA).

The prevalence of VCI has been estimated at 5 percent of people over age 65 in the CSHA.[18] This included vascular cognitive impairment which did not meet the criteria for dementia. Such patients are a subset of the group said to have

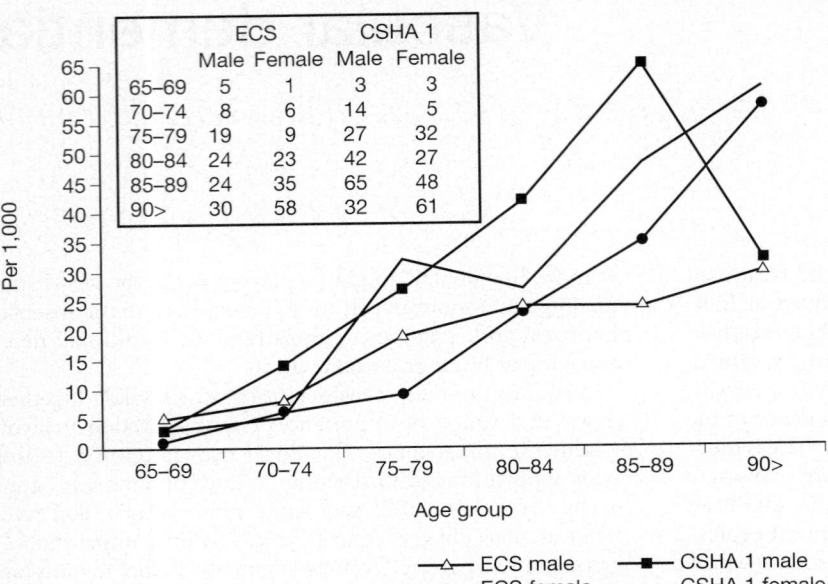

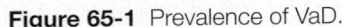

Figure 65-1 Prevalence of VaD.

"Cognitive Impairment, No Dementia" (CIND),[27,28] and herein are called "vascular CIND." The prevalence of vascular CIND was 2.4 percent, the prevalence of mixed AD/VaD was 0.9 percent, and the prevalence of VaD was 1.5 percent. By contrast, in the same study, the prevalence of AD without a vascular component was 5.1 percent, and at all ages up to age 85, was less common than VCI. There was no clear sex differential in VCI or its subtypes.

Incidence

The incidence of VaD has varied between 6 and 12 cases per year in 1,000 persons aged 70 years and older.[26] The incidence of VaD increases with increasing age, without any substantial difference between men and women in a recent European collaborative study.[23] In the European study the pooled incidence rate of VaD per 1,000 person-years for the groups increased with age, as shown in Figure 65-2. In the CSHA, the incidence of VaD was between 0.25 and 0.38 percent (2.5–3.8 per thousand per year).[29]

Prognosis

In the CSHA, the mean duration of survival in VCI was 41 months.[18] Women with VaD experienced the highest 5-year mortality rates (60 percent in those aged 65–74 to 83 percent of those aged 85+ years). Overall, the mortality rate ratio was highest for women with VaD aged 65–74 years, at 10.1 (95 percent c.i. 5.27–19.4).[30] In general, survival from VaD is around 5 years,[26] which is less than that for the general population or for AD.[31,32] Also post-stroke dementia is an independent predictor of mortality.[33] Detailed studies on the natural history of subcortical and cortical VaD are lacking; little is known about their rate and pattern of cognitive decline.[34]

STROKE AND DEMENTIA

Stroke and dementia show numerous points of inter-relatedness. These intersections provide opportunities to advance our

understanding of both syndromes. Stroke increases the risk of dementia. Two studies of the frequency of dementia after stroke yielded comparable estimates: just over one-quarter of patients had dementia, a nine-fold higher proportion than that of stroke-free comparison groups.[35,36] In the Helsinki Stroke Aging Memory Study the frequency of DSM-III dementia 3 months post-stroke was 25 percent and the frequency was in the groups aged 55–64, 65–74, and 75–85 years 19, 24, and 32 percent, respectively.[37]

Dementia occurs more often after stroke than with any other known risk. In the New York study, stroke was the underlying cause of dementia in 56.1 percent of cases of dementia, while 36.4 percent are presumably due to the cumulative effects of stroke and AD.[36] In the Helsinki study the frequency of stroke-related dementia was 67.8 percent.[37] The risk also appears to extend to subcortical strokes. Four years after a first lacunar infarct, 23.1 percent of patients develop dementia, i.e., 4–12 times more than controls.[38] Even after exclusion of patients who are demented 3 months after an ischemic stroke, the relative risk of dementia within 4 years is 5.5.[39] In the community-based Rochester study, the standardized morbidity ratio for new-onset dementia was 8.6 percent for patients in the first year after stroke with the rate of new onset dementia doubling during the follow-up.[40]

Interestingly, dementia also increases the risk of stroke. Cohort studies have shown that prevalent dementia is associated with incident stroke, even after adjustment for other potential cofounders.[40–42] An important interpretation of these data is that they may signal some forms of cognitive impairment as manifestations of cerebrovascular ischemia; alternatively stroke may induce an earlier expression of AD.[25,40]

ETIOLOGY AND PATHOPHYSIOLOGY OF VCI

VCI as a general entity includes many syndromes, which themselves reflect a variety of vascular mechanisms and changes in the brain, with different causes and clinical

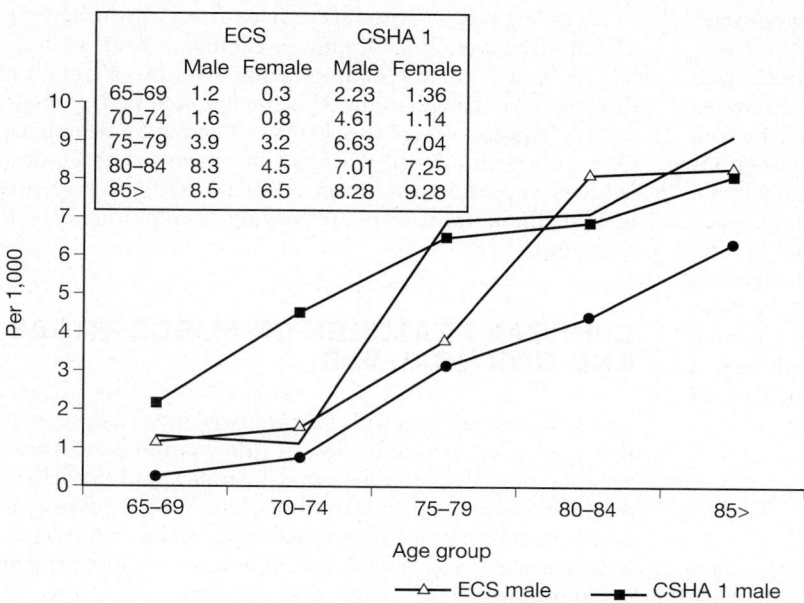

Figure 65-2 Incidence of VaD.

	ECS		CSHA 1	
	Male	Female	Male	Female
65–69	1.2	0.3	2.23	1.36
70–74	1.6	0.8	4.61	1.14
75–79	3.9	3.2	6.63	7.04
80–84	8.3	4.5	7.01	7.25
85>	8.5	6.5	8.28	9.28

—△— ECS male   ─■─ CSHA 1 male
—●— ECS female   ──── CSHA 1 female

manifestations. In addition to multiple strokes, the pathophysiology of VaD incorporates interactions between vascular causes (cardiovascular disease [CVD] and vascular risk factors), brain manifestations of disease expression (white matter lesions [WMLs] atrophy), and host factors (age, education) and cognition.[7–11] Vascular causes of cerebrovascular diseases include large artery disease, cardiac embolic events, and small vessel and hemodynamic mechanisms.[43–47] As noted, there are also risk factors for VCI which of course overlap with risk factors for CVD, stroke, WMLs, as well as with many of those related to AD.[11,29,48] In addition, the CSHA data suggest that eating shellfish is protective for VaD, as is regular exercise for women. In that study, rural residence increased the risk, perhaps as a function of pesticide or fertilizer exposure, which were themselves also found to confer an increased risk of VaD.

The mechanisms by which these risks cause changes in the brain linked to VCI are controversial. While there is good agreement on the role of arterial territorial infarcts, distal field (watershed) infarcts, lacunar infarcts, and ischemic WMLs, there is controversy about incomplete ischemic injury.[7,8,43,47] In its least controversial guise, incomplete injury can arise not as a consequence of focal (around the ischemic lesion) changes, but as a function of remote (disconnection, diaschisis) ischemic injury.[47,49]

While vascular factors predispose to VCI and likely AD, many important questions remain. For example, it is unclear to what extent the type, side, size, site, and tempo of vascular lesions relate to different types of VaD.[7,8,9,47]

HETEROGENEITY OF VCI

As noted, VCI is not a distinct disease, but comprises many heterogeneous syndromes. One method of better understanding this heterogeneity is by the analysis of possible clinical subtypes. Several subtypes are recognized, including vascular CIND, a predominantly cortical VaD (MID), subcortical VaD (also called small vessel dementia), strategic

infarction dementia,[43,44,50–53] and in some classifications, hypoperfusion, or cardiogenic dementia.[43,51,52,54,55] Further subtypes suggested include hemorrhagic dementia, hereditary vascular dementia, and combined or mixed dementia (AD with CVD).[4] These are next reviewed briefly.

Main subtypes

Multi-infarct dementia (MID)
MID is classically diagnosed in the presence of large vessel disease, cardiac embolic events or hypoperfusion. It shows predominantly cortical and cortico-subcortical arterial territorial and distal field (watershed) infarcts. Typical clinical features are lateralized sensorimotor changes and abrupt onset of cognitive impairment and aphasia.[50,56] In addition, various combinations of cortical neuropsychological syndromes have been described.[57,58]

Strategic infarct dementia
Focal, often small, ischemic lesions involving specific sites critical for higher cortical functions have been classified separately. Of the cortical sites, the hippocampal formation, angular gyrus, and gyrus cinguli are examples. The subcortical sites include thalamus, fornix, basal forebrain, caudate, globus pallidus, and the genu or anterior limb of the internal capsule.[8,13,47] Depending on the strategic location in question, the time course and clinical features vary considerably.

Subcortical VaD
"Subcortical" refers to two entities, "the lacunar state" and "Binswanger disease," each of which consists of small vessel disease, lacunar infarcts, focal and diffuse ischemic WMLs, and incomplete ischemic injury.[12,50,57,59] Ischemic lesions affect especially the prefrontal subcortical circuit including prefrontal cortex, caudate, pallidum, thalamus, and the thalamo-cortical circuit (genu or anterior limb of the internal capsule, anterior centrum semiovale, and anterior corona

radiata).[60] Accordingly, the so-called "subcortical syndrome" predominates.[60,61]

Clinically, the subcortical syndrome is characterized cognitively by deficits in executive functioning, bradyphrenia and by a propensity for mood disorders (especially depression, and sometimes emotional lability). Motor manifestations can occur, classically consisting of pure motor hemiparesis, bulbar signs and dysarthria.[57,59,62–64] In some settings, such as memory clinics, these manifestations are less common than the frontal/subcortical cognitive and behavioral disorder.[65] Nevertheless, subcortical VaD/VCI appears to be an important candidate for a more homogeneous subgroup which could be the focus of clinical trials, although a neuroimaging requirement would seem to be particularly important.[61]

MIXED DEMENTIA

The so-called "mixed dementia" syndrome may have been underdiagnosed in our estimation of dementia subtypes.[4,25,58] In addition to simple coexistence, VaD and AD seem to have important interactions, particularly with respect to risk factors,[48,66] disease expression,[67] and such pathogenetic mechanisms as delayed neuronal death and apoptosis.[68]

Given these overlaps, clinical recognition of patients with mixed dementia or AD with CVD is difficult in the absence of a biological marker for AD. Potential markers of some usefulness, given the importance of neuroimaging to a VCI diagnosis include early and significant medial temporal lobe atrophy on magnetic resonance imaging (MRI) or bilateral parietal hypoperfusion on single-photon emission computed tomography (SPECT). In a recent multicenter study of mixed dementia, two diagnostic approaches predominated.[19] In many cases, the presentation is highly suggestive of Alzheimer's disease, but for the presence of one or more features which point to a "vascular" aspect to the diagnosis, as illustrated in Table 65-1. Others appear to use a similar approach.[69]

Table 65-1 Clinical clues to the diagnosis of a vascular contribution to dementia in a patient with an otherwise typical presentation of Alzheimer's disease

Abrupt onset[a]
Step-wise deterioration[a]
Fluctuating course[a]
Prolonged periods of plateau
History of stroke[a]
Focal neurological symptoms[a]
Early onset of a gait disorder
Early onset of a seizure
Early onset of urinary incontinence
Patchy cognitive deficits
Focal neurological signs[a]

[a] Indicates an item from the Hachinski Ischemia Scale Modified from Rockwood K, MacKnight C. Understanding dementia: a primer of diagnosis and management (Halifax: Pottersfield, 2001)[111] and used with permission.

A second pathway was seen in patients with otherwise typical Alzheimer's disease who were found to have ischemic lesions on CT or MR neuroimaging. The most common findings were changes in the white matter, followed by single strokes (equally cortical or subcortical) and multiple lesions. Of note is that almost 4 percent of patients with clinical features suggestive of mixed AD/VaD had no evidence of ischemic lesions on neuroimaging (predominantly CT scanning).

CLINICAL FEATURES OF SUBCORTICAL AND CORTICAL VaD

As noted, subcortical VCI is characterized by (1) a dysexecutive syndrome including slowed information processing, (2) a memory deficit (which may be mild), and (3) behavioral and psychological symptoms. The dysexecutive syndrome in subcortical VCI may be of particular importance. It has been argued that while executive cognitive impairment is common to all dementias, present definitions of dementia, and indeed the most commonly used screening tests of cognition, are biased towards posterior cortical function, as is seen in Alzheimer's disease.[70] By contrast, VCI that spares the temporal and parietal lobes can still have profound consequences for daily life, and for quality of life. Such deficits can result in impairment in goal formulation, initiation, planning, organizing, sequencing, executing, set-shifting and set-maintenance, as well as in abstracting.[52,57,71] The memory deficit in subcortical VaD may be milder than, e.g., in Alzheimer's disease, and is specified by impaired recall, relative intact recognition, less severe forgetting, and better benefit from cues.[71] Behavioral and psychological symptoms include in particular depression, personality change, emotional liability and incontinence, as well as inertia, emotional bluntness, and psychomotor retardation.[51,52,57]

The early cognitive syndrome seen in cortical VCI typically includes memory impairment which is often mild. In addition, heteromodal cortical symptom(s) such as aphasia, apraxia, agnosia, and visuospatial or constructional difficulty are present. Most patients have some degree of the dysexecutive syndrome found in subcortical VCI.

Clinical neurological findings in subcortical VCI include upper motor neuron signs (drift, reflex asymmetry, incordination), gait disorder (apractic–atactic or small stepped), imbalance and falls, urinary frequency and incontinence, dysarthria, dysphagia, as well as extrapyramidal signs (hypokinesia, rigidity).[50,51,59,62,63] These signs can be episodic, and often are subtle,[72,73] which may explain why many patients with mixed AD/VaD appear to have classical AD until neuroimaging reveals otherwise. They also may explain the sensitivity of VaD criteria which require focal signs, as discussed below.

Patients with cortical VCI, as a consequence of multiple cortico-subcortical infarcts, often show more obvious neurological abnormalities, including visual field deficits, facial weakness, lateralized sensimotor changes and gait impairment (classically hemiplegic, apractic–atactic).[50]

Onset and course. In subcortical VCI the onset is variable. For example in the series of Babikian and Ropper[63] 60 percent of patients had a slow, less abrupt onset, and only 30 percent an acute onset of cognitive symptoms. The course was gradual, both without (40 percent) and with (40 percent) acute deficits. Acute stroke alone without progression occurred in 13 percent.[63] Traditionally, cortical VaD (MID) has been characterized by a relatively abrupt onset (days to weeks), a stepwise deterioration (some recovery after worsening), and fluctuating course (e.g., difference between days) of cognitive functions.[51,59,72–75]

DIAGNOSTIC CRITERIA

Despite their widely recognized faults, several sets of diagnostic criteria enjoy widespread use, including the DSM-IV,[76] the ICD-10,[77] the ADDTC criteria,[75] and the NINDS-AIREN criteria.[51] To make this diagnosis, all present criteria include: (1) a definition of the cognitive syndrome of dementia,[22] and (2) a definition of a vascular cause of the dementia.[78–80] All sets of criteria operate in the shadow of Alzheimer's disease, and all are heir to the Hachinski Ischemic Scale.[3]

Variation in how these two critical elements are defined has caused substantial variability in estimating the frequency and characteristics of VCI/VaD, and consequently the nature and extent of brain lesions observed.[22,31,37,65,80,81] Perhaps even more importantly, this heterogeneity may have been a factor for negative results in prior clinical trials on VaD.[61,82]

All the clinical criteria used are consensus criteria, which are neither derived from prospective community based studies on vascular factors affecting the cognition, nor based on detailed natural histories.[51,55,75,79,83] All the cited criteria are mainly based on the ischemic infarct concept and designed to have high specificity, although they have been poorly implemented and validated.[55,83]

The DSM-IV definition for VaD requires focal neurological signs and symptoms or laboratory evidence of focal neurological damage clinically judged to be related to the disturbance.[76] The course is characterized by sudden cognitive and functional losses. The DSM-IV criteria do not specify brain imaging requirements. In short, the DSM-IV definition of VaD is reasonably broad and lacks detailed clinical and radiological guidelines.

The ICD-10 criteria[77] require unequal distribution of cognitive deficits, focal signs as evidence of focal brain damage, and significant cerebrovascular disease judged to be etiologically related to the dementia. These criteria also do not specify brain imaging requirements. The shortcomings of these criteria include lack of detailed guidelines (e.g., unequal cognitive deficits and neuroimaging), lack of etiological cues, and heterogeneity.[78,80]

The ADDTC criteria are exclusively for ischemic vascular dementia (IVD).[75] They require (1) evidence of two or more ischemic strokes by history, neurological signs or neuroimaging studies (CT or T1-weighted MRI), or (2) in case of a single stroke a clearly documented temporal relationship (not specified in detail), and always neuroradiological evidence of at least one infarct outside the cerebellum. Ischemic WMLs on CT or MRI do not qualify as brain-imaging evidence of probable IVD, but may support a diagnosis of possible IVD.

The criteria list features supporting the diagnosis, as well as a list of features casting doubt on a diagnosis of probable IVD.

The NINDS-AIREN research criteria for VaD[51] begin with definitions of the dementia syndrome and cerebrovascular disease and then require a relationship between the two. Cerebrovascular disease is defined by the presence of focal neurological sins and detailed brain imaging evidence of ischemic changes in the brain. A relationship between dementia and cerebrovascular disorder is based on the onset of dementia within 3 months following a recognized stroke, or on abrupt deterioration in cognitive functions or fluctuating, stepwise progression of cognitive deficits. The criteria include a list of features consistent with the diagnosis, as well as a list of features that make the diagnosis uncertain or unlikely. Also different levels of certainty of the clinical diagnosis (probable, possible, definite) are included. The inter-rater reliability of the NINDS-AIREN criteria has been held to be moderate to substantial (kappa 0.46 to 0.72)[84] although more recent estimates for any of the criteria are less persuasive.[85]

Comparison of clinical criteria. The current criteria for VaD are not interchangeable; they identify different numbers and clusters of patients labeled as VaD. The DSM-IV criteria are less restrictive compared to the ICD-10, the ADDTC, and the NINDS-AIREN criteria.[80,86] The ADDTC criteria seem to be more sensitive and the NINDS-AIREN criteria more specific.[87]

As noted, the heterogeneity of the patient populations which are derived by using current criteria has raised a need for more precise systematization. One suggestion has been that, by dividing VaD into subtypes, a more homogeneous group of patients could be identified. A recent development are the new research criteria for subcortical VaD.[88] Alternatively, heterogeneity can be better classified within a more broadly construed VCI syndrome.[4,20,65]

DIFFERENTIAL DIAGNOSIS

The differential diagnosis of VCI includes any of the dementias or other types of mild cognitive impairment. On a population basis, however, the differential diagnosis is chiefly between VaD and AD.

Alzheimer's disease

The clinical approach to dementia has evolved in the last decade. Many physicians traditionally held that Alzheimer's disease was a "diagnosis of exclusion," made only when other conditions had been "ruled out." It is now understood, however, that AD has typical stages both in its neuropathological and clinical expression.[89] Accordingly, AD can be diagnosed with confidence at its various stages. Given that AD is very common, a useful starting point for clinicians working in memory clinics is to determine whether the patient with cognitive impairment conforms to the typical AD profile. In patients who do conform to this profile, the presence of additional focal features or neuroimaging findings would suggest a diagnosis of "mixed AD/VaD."

As noted, at the onset, the traditional concept of dementia has been based on the typical clinical features of AD.[22,90] In consequence, the focus has been on early episodic memory

Table 65-2 Differential diagnosis between vascular dementia and Alzheimer's disease

Vascular dementia	Alzheimer's disease
Early cognitive syndrome	
Dysexecutive syndrome: Impaired planning, sequencing, speed of processing	Impaired episodic memory: Ineffective learning, increased forgetting, impaired recognition, poor response to cues, intrusion errors
Memory impairment (often mild): Preserved recognition, good response cues, perseveration	Ineffective learning, less forgetting
Cortical symptom(s) (variable): Aphasia, apraxia, agnosia, visuospatial and constructive difficulty	Anomia (mild) Visuospatial impairment (mild)
Early clinical features	
Mild UMN signs (motor deficit, decreased coordination, brisk tendon reflexes, Babinski's sign) Gait disorder, imbalance Urine frequency Dysarthria Mood changes, depression	Absence of focal neurological signs Dysthymia, mild depression
Onset	
Variable: relative abrupt, insidious	Insidious
Clinical course	
Variable: fluctuating, stepwise, progressive, stable	Progressive May have plateaus

impairment, followed by a more or less global cognitive syndrome, which typically progresses to impair activities of daily living (ADLs). While these features can also be seen in VaD, they are less common in early cases. Importantly, some patients with isolated cognitive deficits of vascular origin (e.g., aphasia following stroke) can have profound cognitive impairment without ever meeting the AD-based dementia criteria.

The most widely used definition of the cause of the cognitive syndrome includes the NINDS-AIREN for probable VaD[51] and the NINCDS-ADRDA for probable AD.[90] These criteria define a stereotyped set of patient groups: probable VaD characterized by abrupt onset, or fluctuating and stepwise course with clinical signs of CVD and relevant CVD on brain imaging. Conversely, AD is characterized by insidious onset, progressive course, without clinical signs of CVD, and without signs of CVD in brain imaging. Accordingly, in typical cases the differentiation between probable VaD and AD using common clinical tools is direct.[91]

The Hachinski Ischemic Score has been widely used to differentiate patients with VaD and AD.[92] In a large neuropathologically confirmed series by Moroney et al.[93] the independent correlates of VaD were stepwise deterioration (OR 6.1), fluctuating course (OR 7.6), history of hypertension (OR 4.3), history of stroke (OR 4.3), and history of focal neurological symptoms (OR 4.4).

PREVENTION AND TREATMENT OF VASCULAR DEMENTIA

Prevention of VCI conceptually can occur at a number of levels. Most pervasively, *primary prevention* seeks to reduce disease occurrence by eliminating risk factors.[66,94] In VCI, the chief exposures are hypertension, atrial fibrillation, myocardial infarction, coronary heart disease, diabetes, lipid abnormalities and smoking. As noted, some factors may be protective, including estrogen, anti-inflammatory agents and antioxidants,[95] diet and exercise.[29] Nevertheless, the impact of primary prevention of VaD is still scanty.[11,96]

Secondary prevention seeks to prevent established disease from progressing, chiefly through early detection and treatment.[97] For those at risk for VCI, population strategies include (1) early diagnosis and treatment of acute stroke in order to limit the extent of ischemic brain changes and to promote recovery, (2) prevention of stroke recurrence according to the type of stroke, and (3) intensifying treatment of risk factors. The selection of treatment is guided by the supposed etiology of CVD, so that large artery disease (e.g., aspirin, dipyridamole, clopidogrel, carotid endarterectomy), cardiac embolic events (e.g., anticoagulation, aspirin), small-vessel disease (e.g., antiplatelet therapy as in large vessel disease), and hemodynamic mechanisms (e.g., control of hypotension and cardiac arrhythmias)[46,83,98] can all be targeted. Hypoxic ischemic events (cardiac arrhythmias, congestive heart failure, myocardial infarction, seizures, pneumonia) are important risk factors for incident dementia in patients with stroke and should be taken into account in the secondary prevention of VaD.[99]

Detailed knowledge of effects of secondary prevention directed toward the vascular component of VaD is still scanty. In small series of patients with established VaD control of high arterial blood pressure,[100] cessation of smoking,[100] and use of aspirin[101] has improved or stabilized cognition. It has been suggested that lowering of plasma viscosity could also have an effect in VaD.[102] Further, absence of progressive cognitive decline in patients receiving placebo in symptomatic treatment trials of VaD may also reflect an effect of intensified risk factor control.[103] Of some importance has been a recent study suggesting that the treatment of systolic hypertension in elderly people can reduce the incidence of all causes of dementia by half.[104] In addition, studies suggesting a decreased risk of Alzheimer's disease in patients on HMG CoA reductase inhibitors[105,106] may hold out hope for a new strategy in this regard, although considerable caution seems warranted.[107]

Symptomatic treatment (tertiary prevention). A number of drugs have been studied for symptomatic treatment of VaD including cerebro- and vasoactive drugs, nootropics and some calcium antagonists, but these studies have largely shown negative results.[108] The studies have mostly had small numbers, short treatment periods, variations in diagnostic criteria and tools, often included mixed populations, and have had variations in the application of clinical endpoints. Recently both nimodipine,[109] memantine,[110] and propentofylline[103] have raised expectations in the symptomatic treatment of VaD. It is possible that the symptomatic treatment with acetylcholinesterase inhibitors may prove effective also on the cognitive symptoms of VaD. Still, currently there is not a widely accepted standard symptomatic treatment of VaDs.

CONCLUSION

The important problem of VCI is undergoing changes in its conceptualization, measurement, classification, and treatment. Given the large disease burden which likely underlies vascular causes of cognitive illness, the need to think critically about these problems is great. We are at a stage where the criteria must pass from the researchers to active, busy clinicians so that the generalizability and usefulness of these new approaches to VCI can be understood, and so that we can move ever closer to effective treatment and even prevention of this problem.

KEY POINTS Vascular dementia

- There is, as yet, no specific treatment of VCI, but cholinesterase inhibitors appear to hold promise

- Vascular dementia is now understood as part of more broadly construed vascular cognitive impairment

- Vascular cognitive impairment describes three groups: those with vascular dementia, those with mixed Alzheimer's disease/vascular dementia, and those with vascular cognitive impairment that does not meet dementia criteria

- Those with "vascular cognitive impairment, no dementia" (vascular CIND) include patients, akin to people with mild cognitive impairment, who are at an increased risk of dementia, and patients who are cognitively and functionally impaired, but who do not meet dementia criteria (e.g., patients with disability effects of stroke)

- This clinical characterization can be cross-classified by the neuroimaging profile, which includes: multiple/single continual strokes, multiple/single subcortical strokes, and white matter changes

- Vascular risk factors are risks for all causes of late life cognitive impairment, including Alzheimer's disease and not just vascular dementia

REFERENCES

1. Erkinjuntti T, Rockwood K: Vascular cognitive impairment. Psychogeriatrics 2001;1:6–11
2. Tomlinson BE, Blessed G, Roth M: Observations on the brains of demented old people. J Neurol Sci 1970;11:205–242
3. Hachinski VC, Lassen NA, Marshall J: Multi-infarct dementia. A cause of mental deterioration in the elderly. Lancet 1974;ii:207–210
4. Rockwood K, Bowler J, Erkinjuntit T et al: Subtypes of vascular dementia. Alzheimer Dis Assoc Disord 1999;13:S59–S64
5. Brust JC: Vascular dementia is over diagnosed. Arch Neurol 1988;45:799–801
6. Hachinski VC: The decline and resurgence of vascular dementia. Can Med Assoc J 1990;142:107–111
7. Chui HC: Dementia: a review emphasising clinicopathologic correlation and brain-behaviour relationships. Arch Neurol 1989;46:806–814
8. Tatemichi TK: How acute brain failure becomes chronic. A view of the mechanisms and syndromes of dementia related to stroke. Neurology 1990;40:1652–1659
9. Desmond DW: Vascular dementia: a construct in evolution. Cerebrovasc Brain Metab Rev 1996;8:296–325
10. Pasquier F, Leys D: Why are stroke patients prone to develop dementia? J Neurol 1997;244:135–142
11. Skoog I: Status of risk factors for vascular dementia. Neuroepidemiology 1998;17:2–9
12. Sultzer DL, Gray KF, Gunay I: A double-blind comparison of trazodone and haloperidol for treatment of agitation in patients with dementia. Am J Geriatr Psychiatry 1997;5:60–69
13. Erkinjuntti T, Hachinski VC: Rethinking vascular dementia. Cerebrovasc Dis 1993;3:3–23
14. Hachinski V: Preventable senility: a call for action against the vascular dementias. Lancet 1992;340:645–648 (see comments)
15. Rockwood K, Cosway S, Stolee P et al: Increasing the recognition of delirium in elderly patients. J Am Geriatr Soc 1994;42:252–256
16. Bowler JV, Hachinski V: Vascular cognitive impairment: a new approach to vascular dementia. Baillière's Clin Neurol 1995;4:357–376
17. Rockwood K, Ebly E, Hachinski V, Hogan D: Presence and treatment of vascular risk factors in vascular cognitive impairment. Arch Neurol 1997;54:33–39
18. Rockwood K, Wentzel C, Hachinski V et al: Prevalence and outcomes of vascular cognitive impairment. Neurology 2000;54:447–451
19. Rockwood K, MacKnight C, Wentzel C et al: The diagnosis of "mixed" dementia in the Consortium for the Investigation of Vascular Impairment of Cognition (CIVIC). Ann NY Acad Sci 2000;903:522–528
20. Wentzel C, Darvesh S, MacKnight C et al: Inter-rater reliability of the diagnosis of vascular cognitive impairment at a memory clinic. Neuroepidemiology 2000;19:186–193
21. Rocca WA, Hofman A, Brayne C et al: The prevalence of vascular dementia in Europe: facts and fragments from 1980–1990 studies. EURODEM-Prevalence Research Group. Ann Neurol 1991;30:817–824
22. Erkinjuntti T, Ostbye T, Steenhuis R, Hachinski V: The effect of different diagnostic criteria on the prevalence of dementia. N Engl J Med 1997;337:1667–1674
23. Fratiglioni L, Launer LJ, Andersen K et al: Incidence of dementia and major subtypes in Europe: A collaborative study of population-based cohorts. Neurology 2000;54:S10–S15
24. Lobo A, Launer LJ, Fratiglioni L et al: Prevalence of dementia and major subtypes in Europe: A collaborative study of population-based cohorts. Neurology 2000;54:S4–S9
25. Rockwood K: Lessons from mixed dementia. Int Psychogeriatr 1997;9:245–250
26. Hébert R, Brayne C: Epidemiology of vascular dementia. Neuroepidemiology 1995;14:240–257
27. Ebly EM, Hogan DB, Parhad IM: Cognitive impairment in the nondemented elderly. Results from the Canadian Study of Health and Aging. Arch Neurol 1995;52:612–619
28. Graham JE, Rockwood K, Beattie BL et al: Prevalence and severity of cognitive impairment with and without dementia in an elderly population. Lancet 1997;349:1793–1796
29. Hébert R, Lindsay J, Verreault R et al: Vascular Dementia: Incidence and risk factors in the Canadian Study of Health and Aging. Stroke 2000;31:1487–1493
30. Ostbye T, Hill G, Steenhuis R: Mortality in elderly Canadians with and without dementia. Neurology 1999;53:521–526
31. Skoog I, Nilsson L, Palmertz B et al: A population-based study on dementia in 85-year-olds. N Engl J Med 1993;328:153–158
32. Mölsä PK, Marttila RJ, Rinne UK: Long-term survival and predictors of mortality in Alzheimer's disease and multi-infarct dementia. Acta Neurol Scand 1995;91:159–164
33. Tatemichi TK, Paik M, Bagiella E et al: Dementia after stroke is a predictor of long-term survival. Stroke 1994;25:1915–1919
34. Chui HC, Gonthier R: Natural history of vascular dementia. Alzheimer Dis Assoc Disord 1999;13:124–130
35. Suzuki K, Kutsuzawa T, Nakajima K, Hatano S: Epidemiology of vascular dementia and stroke in Akita, Japan. In Hartmann A, Kuchinsky W, Hoyer S (eds): Cerebral Ischemia and Dementia. Springer-Verlag, New York, 1991;16–24
36. Tatemichi TK, Desmond DW, Mayeux R et al: Dementia after stroke: baseline frequency, risks, and clinical features in a hospitalized cohort. Neurology 1992;42:1185–1193
37. Pohjasvaara T, Erkinjuntti T, Vataja R, Kaste M: Dementia three months after stroke. Baseline frequency and effect of different definitions of dementia in the Helsinki Stroke Aging Memory Study (SAM) cohort. Stroke 1997;28:785–792
38. Loch C, Gandolfo C, Croce R, Conti M: Dementia associated with lacunar infarction. Stroke 1992;23:1225–1229
39. Tatemichi TK, Paik M, Bagiella E et al: Risk of dementia after stroke in a hospitalized cohort: results of a longitudinal study. Neurology 1994;44:1885–1891
40. Kokmen E, Whisnant JP, O'Fallon WN et al: Dementia after ischemic stroke: a population-based study in Rochester, Minnesota (1960–1984). Neurology 1996;46:154–159

41. Ferrucci L, Guralnik JM, Salive ME et al: Cognitive impairment and risk of stroke in the older population. J Am Geriatr Soc 1996;44:237–241

42. Zhu L, Fratiglioni L, Guo Z et al: Incidence of stroke in relation to cognitive function and dementia in the Kungsholmen Project. Neurology 2000;54:2103–2107

43. Brun A: Pathology and pathophysiology of cerebrovascular dementia: pure subgroups of obstructive and hypoperfusive etiology. Dementia 1994;5:145–147

44. Wallin A, Blennow K: The clinical diagnosis of vascular dementia. Dementia 1994;5:181–184

45. Pantoni L, Garcia JH: The significance of cerebral white matter abnormalities 100 years after Binswanger's report. A review. Stroke 1995;26:1293–1301

46. Amar K. Wilcock G: Vascular dementia. Br Med J 1996;312:227–231

47. Erkinjuntti T: Clinicopathological study of vascular dementia. In Prohovnik I, Wade J, Knezevic S, Tatemichi TK, Erkinjuntii T (eds): Vascular Dementia. Current concepts. John Wiley, Chichester, 1999;73–112

48. Breteler MM: Vascular risk factors for Alzheimer's disease: an epidemiologic perspective. Neurobiol Aging 2000;21:153–160

49. Mielke R, Herholz K, Grond M et al: Severity of vascular dementia is related to volume of metabolically impaired tissue. Arch Neurol 1992;49:909–913

50. Erkinjuntti T: Types of multi-infarct dementia. Acta Neurol Scand 1987;75:391–399

51. Roman GC, Tatemichi TK, Erkinjuntti T et al: Vascular Dementia: Diagnostic Criteria for Research Studies. Report of the NINDS-AIREN International Work Group. Neurology 1993;43:250–260

52. Cummings JL: Vascular subcortical dementias: clinical aspects. Dementia 1994;5:177–180

53. Loeb C, Meyer JS: Vascular dementia: still a debatable entity? J Neurol Sci 1996;143:31–40

54. Sulkava R, Erkinjuntti T: Vascular dementia due to cardiac arrhythmias and systemic hypotension. Acta Neurol Scand 1987;76:123–128

55. Rockwood K, Parhad I, Hachinski V et al: Diagnosis of vascular dementia: Consortium of Canadian Centres for Clinical Cognitive Research concensus statement. Can J Neurol Sci 1994;21:358–364

56. Erkinjuntti T, Haltia M, Palo J et al: Accuracy of the clinical diagnosis of vascular dementia: a prospective clinical and post-mortem neuropathological study. J Neurol Neurosurg Psychiatry 1988;51:1037–1044

57. Mahler ME. Cummings JL: The behavioural neurology of multi-infarct dementia. Alzheimer Dis Assoc Disord 1991;5:122–130

58. Ballard C, McKeith I, O'Brien J et al: Neuropathological substrates of dementia and depression in vascular dementia, with a particular focus on cases with small infarct volumes. Dement Geriatr Cogn Disord 2000;11:59–65

59. Roman GC: Senile dementia of the Binswanger type. A vascular form of dementia in the elderly. JAMA 1987;258:1782–1788

60. Cummings JL: Fronto-subcortical circuits and human behaviour. Arch Neurol 1993;50:873–880

61. Erkinjuntii T, Inzitari D, Pantoni L et al: Research criteria for subcortical vascular dementia in clinical trials. J Neural Transmiss 2000;59:23–30

62. Ishii N, Nishihara Y, Imamura T: Why do frontal lobe symptoms predominate in vascular dementia with lacunes? Neurology 1986;36:340–345

63. Babikian V, Ropper AH: Binswanger's disease: a review. Stroke 1987;18:2–12

64. Wallin A, Blennow K, Gottfries CG: Subcortical symptoms predominate in vascular dementia. Int J Geriatr Psychiatry 1991;6:137–146

65. Rockwood K, Howard K, MacKnight C, Darvesh S: Spectrum of disease in vascular cognitive impairment. Neuroepidemiology 1999;18:248–254

66. Skoog I, Kalaria RN, Breteler MMB: Vascular factors and Alzheimer's disease. Alzheimer Dis Assoc Disord 1999;13:S106–S114

67. Snowdon DA, Greiner LH, Mortimer JA et al: Brain infarction and the clinical expression of Alzheimer disease. The Nun Study. JAMA 1997;277:813–817 (see comments)

68. Kalaria RN, Ballard C: Overlap between pathology of Alzheimer disease and vascular dementia. Alzheimer Dis Assoc Disord 1999;13:S115–S123

69. Bowler JV, Steenhuis R, Hachinski V: Conceptual background to vascular cognitive impairment. Alzheimer Dis Assoc Disord 1999;13:S30–S37

70. Royall DR: Executive Cognitive Impairment: a novel perspective on dementia. Neuroepidemiology 2000;19:293–299

71. Desmond DW, Erkinjuntti T, Sano M et al: The cognitive syndrome of vascular dementia: implications for clinical trials. Alzheimer Dis Assoc Disord 1999;13:S21–S29

72. Fischer P, Gatterer G, Marterer A et al: Course characteristics in the differentiation of dementia of the Alzheimer type and multi-infarct dementia. Acta Psychiatr Scand 1990;81:551–553

73. Skoog I: Blood pressure and dementia. In Hansson L, Birkenhäger WH (eds): Handbook of Hypertension. Vol 18. Assessment of Hypertensive Organ Damage. Elsevier Science, Amsterdam, 1997; 303–331

74. Erkinjuntti T: Differential diagnosis between Alzheimer's disease and vascular dementia: evaluation of common clinical methods. Acta Neurol Scand 1987;76:433–442

75. Chui HC, Victoroff JI, Margolin D et al: Criteria for the diagnosis of ischemic vascular dementia proposed by the State of California Alzheimer's Disease Diagnostic and Treatment Centers. Neurology 1992;42:473–480

76. American Psychiatric Association: Diagnostic and Statistical Manual of Mental Disorders, 4th Ed. American Psychiatric Association, Washington, DC

77. World Health Organization: ICD-10 Classification of Mental and Behavioural Disorders: Diagnostic Criteria for Research WHO, Geneva, 1993

78. Wetterling T, Kanitz RD, Borgis KJ: The ICD-10 criteria for vascular dementia. Dementia 1994;5:185–188

79. Erkinjuntti T: Clinical criteria for vascular dementia: The NINDS-AIREN criteria. Dementia 1994;5:189–192

80. Wetterling T, Kanitz RD, Borgis KJ: Comparison of different diagnostic criteria for vascular dementia (ADDTC, DSM-IV, ICD-10, NINDS-AIREN). Stroke 1996;27:30–36

81. Erkinjuntti T, Bowler JV, DeCarli C et al: Imaging of static brain lesions in vascular dementia: implications for clinical trials. Alzheimer Dis Assoc Disord 1999;13:S81–S90

82. Inzitari D, Erkinjuntti T, Wallin A et al: Is subcortical vascular dementia a clinical entity for clinical drug trials? Alzheimer Dis Assoc Disord 1999;(3):S66–S68

83. Erkinjuntti T: Vascular dementia: challenge of clinical diagnosis. Int Psychogeriatr 1997;9:51–58

84. Lopez OL, Larumbe MR, Becker JT et al: Reliability of NINDS-AIREN clinical criteria for the diagnosis of vascular dementia. Neurology 1994;44:1240–1245 (see comments)

85. Chui HC, Mack W, Jackson E et al: Clinical criteria for the diagnosis of vascular dementia. A multicenter study of comparability and inter-rater reliability. Arch Neurol 2000;57:191–196

86. Verhey FR, Lodder J, Rozendaal N, Jolles J: Comparison of seven sets of criteria used for the diagnosis of vascular dementia. Neuroepidemiol 1996;15:166–172

87. Gold G, Giannakopoulos P, Montes-Paixao JC et al: Sensitivity and specificity of newly proposed clinical criteria for possible vascular dementia. Neurology 1997;49:690–694

88. Erkinjuntti T, Inzitari D, Pantoni L et al: Research criteria for subcortical vascular dementia in clinical trials. J Neural Transmiss 2000;59:23–30

89. Braak H, Braak E: Neuropathological staging of Alzheimer-related changes. Acta Neuropathol (Berl) 1991;82:239–259

90. McKhann G, Drachman D, Folstein M et al: Clinical diagnosis of Alzheimer's disease: report of the NINCDS-ADRDA Work Group under the auspices of Department of Health and Human Services Task Force on Alzheimer's Disease. Neurology 1984;34:939–944

91. Erkinjuntti T, Haltia M, Palo J et al: Accuracy of the clinical diagnosis of vascular dementia: a prospective clinical and post-mortem neuropathological study. J Neurol Neurosurg Psychiatry 1988;51:1037–1044

92. Hachinski VC, Iliff LD, Zilhka E et al: Cerebral blood flow in dementia. Arch Neurol 1975;32:632–637

93. Moroney JT, Bagiella E, Desmond DW et al: Meta-analysis of the Hachinski Ischemic Score in pathologically verified dementias. Neurology 1997;49:1096–1105

94. Last JM: A Dictionary of Epidemiology, 2nd Ed. Oxford University Press, New York, 1988

95. Mortel KF, Meyer JS: Lack of postmenopausal estrogen replacement therapy and the risk of dementia. J Neuropsych Clin Neurosci 1995;7:334–337

96. Skoog I: The relationship between blood pressure and dementia: a review. Biomed Pharmacother 1997;51:367–375

97. Skoog I: The possibility for secondary prevention of Alzheimer's disease. In Mayeux R (ed): The Epidemiology of Alzheimer's Disease. 1999

98. Konno S, Meyer JS, Terayama Y et al: Classification, diagnosis and treatment of vascular dementia. Drugs Aging 1997;11:361–373

99. Moroney JT, Bagiella E, Desmond DW et al: Risk factors for incident dementia after stroke. Role of hypoxic and ischemic disorders. Stroke 1996;27:1283–1289

100. Meyer JS, Judd BW, Tawaklna T et al: Improved cognition after control of risk factors for multi-infarct dementia. JAMA 1986;256:2203–2209

101. Meyer JS, Rogers RL, McClintic K et al: Randomized clinical trial of daily aspirin therapy in multi-infarct dementia. A pilot study. J Am Geriatr Soc 1989;37:549–555

102. Lechner H: Status of treatment of vascular dementia. Neuroepidemiology 1998;17:10–13

103. Rother M, Erkinjuntti T, Roessner M et al: Propentofylline in the treatment of Alzheimer's disease and vascular dementia: A review of Phase III. Dementia Geriatr Cogn Disord 1998;9:36–43

104. Forette F, Seux ML, Staessen JA: Prevention of dementia in randomised double-blind placebo-controlled Systolic Hypertension in Europe (Syst-Eur) trials. Lancet 1998;352:1347–1351

105. Wolozin B, Kellman W, Ruosseau P et al: Decreased prevalence of Alzheimer disease associated with 3-hydroxy-3-methylglutaryl coenzyme A reductase inhibitors. Arch Neurol 2000;57:1439–1443

106. Jick H, Zornberg GL, Jick SS, Drachman DA: Statins and the risk of dementia. Lancet 2000;356:1627–1631

107. Haley R, Dietschy J: Is there a connection between the concentration of cholesterol circulating in plasma and the rate of neuritic plaque formation in Alzheimer's disease? Arch Neurol 2000;57:1410–1412

108. Knezevic S, Labs KH, Kittner B et al: The treatment of vascular dementia: problems and prospects. In Prohovnik I, Wade J, Knesevich J, Tatemichi TK, Erkinjuntti T (eds): Vascular dementia. Current concepts. John Wiley, Chichester, 1996, 301–312

109. Pantoni L, Carosi M, Amigoni S et al: A preliminary open trial with nimodipine in patients with cognitive impairment and leukoaraiosis. Clin Neuropharmacol 1996;19:497–506

110. Görtelmeyer R, Erbler H: Memantine in treatment of mild to moderate dementia syndrome. Drug Res 1992;42:904–912

111. Rockwood K, MacKnight C: Understanding Dementia: a Primer of Diagnosis and Management. Pottersfield Press, Halifax, Nova Scotia, 2001

Chapter 66

Psychology in the diagnosis and treatment of the dementias

Rajendra Jutagir

The primary role of the psychologist working with older patients is evaluation and treatment of cognitive and emotional disorders. The prevalence of dementia in the community increases with age. One estimate was 3 percent for ages 65–74 years and as high as 47 percent beyond age 85.[1] Apart from dementia there may be cognitive impairment that is not pervasive or does not include memory loss. For example, in vascular disease there is a continuum of cognitive impairment, which may range from subtle, subclinical cognitive loss, up to and including dementia.[2] If one includes more subtle deficits, the rate of cognitive impairment would be very high in older people. Thus the psychologist working with a geriatric population must be knowledgeable about cognitive disorders. This requires a background in neuropsychology, beyond expertise in working with emotional disorders. The first part of this chapter focuses on neuropsychological evaluation of the dementias in geriatric patients. The second part addresses psychological treatment of dementing individuals and their families.

COGNITIVE IMPAIRMENT

Memory loss is one of the most common reasons for referral of geriatric patients for neuropsychological testing, and often leads to a diagnosis of dementia. Dementia is defined as global intellectual impairment, operationalized as memory loss and impairment in at least one other domain of higher cortical functioning (aphasia, apraxia, agnosia, executive functioning), decline in social or occupational functioning, with exclusion of delirium and possible nonorganic causes of cognitive loss.[3] Recently there has been some question as to whether the emphasis on Alzheimer's disease has led to an overstatement of the importance of early memory loss in the dementias, since other dementias may initially show impairment in other abilities (e.g. executive functions) or behaviors (e.g. psychosis, social dysfunction).[4,5] In any event these criteria rely heavily on evaluation of intellectual deficits, which are best documented by neuropsychological testing. The nature and degree of cognitive impairment is uncovered by a test battery that should minimally evaluate the following domains: attention and orientation, learning and memory, language, motor, visuospatial, and executive functions.[6] Additional tests, such as calculations, are helpful in evaluating older people. The neuropsychological profile, consisting of intact and impaired cognitive domains, is used to arrive at a diagnosis. For example, if it shows circumscribed impairment one might suspect a focal event. More widespread deficits in intellectual functioning would suggest a dementia.

The first task in developing the profile is to differentiate impairment from normal aging. Both cross-sectional and longitudinal studies indicate that many cognitive abilities, including memory, undergo normative decline with age.[7–10] Therefore care must be taken to avoid overdiagnosing impairment in older people by attributing normative change to disease, especially in memory disorders where positive findings can be distressing to both patient and family. To avoid this problem, a patient's performance on neuropsychological tasks is compared with normative data derived from others in the same age group. This allows the clinician to judge the likelihood that the patient belongs to a "normal" or "impaired" population. The use of normative data by itself is not always sufficient to make this discrimination. Early in a dementing process, for example, individuals may function below their usual capacity even though they still fall within normal limits for their age group. This is especially likely to occur in individuals of high intellectual capacity.[11] When this occurs, premorbid capacity is estimated from the patient's level of educational or occupational achievement. Premorbid functioning can also be inferred from standardized reading tests or tests of crystallized intelligence such as vocabulary or general information. Even though these show early and progressive decline in dementia,[12–14] they are thought to be less affected by organic deterioration than other tests. Discrepancies between premorbid and current capacity can suggest whether decline has occurred.

Once the neuropsychological profile of intact and impaired cognitive domains is established, it is used to identify the disease process that gave rise to it. There are compelling reasons to differentiate among the dementias. As treatments proliferate, improved diagnosis will ensure appropriate treatment. Iatrogenic illness may be avoided, as in the case of neuroleptic treatment in Lewy body disease.[15] The correct prognosis is valuable in patient management, and improves counseling for families. Finally, accurate diagnosis enhances research, which holds the promise of further improvement in diagnosis and treatment.

Differential diagnosis of the dementias is complicated by the overlap of deficits in different syndromes, which compromises the specificity of the diagnosis. Cortical disorders may have some subcortical involvement, posterior disorders may have some anterior involvement, and different disorders that involve the same regions of the brain (especially degenerative disorders that spread progressively) can show convergence of symptoms. Furthermore, a patient may present with more than one disorder, as in the case of mixed vascular and Alzheimer's dementia,[16] mixed Alzheimer's and Lewy body dementia,[17,18] or mixed Alzheimer's and Parkinson's disease.[19] In addition to clinical ambiguity, there are deficiencies in research efforts to compare the dementias. Some studies have failed to control for the severity of dementia, making it unclear whether the findings represent true differences between disorders, or are merely due to the stage of the disorder. Furthermore, absence of neuropathological confirmation in some studies makes it uncertain whether cases were correctly classified.

The complexity of dementing disorders is matched by the complexity of memory itself. Different theoretical memory systems have been proposed, and attempts made to relate these to underlying brain structures and processes. Memory is broadly divided into primary (short-term) and secondary (long-term) memory. The former refers to temporary storage of material in memory for periods of up to about 30 seconds, whereas secondary memory refers to storage for longer periods. Primary memory has been extensively investigated in the context of "working memory," which is described as a central executive system that integrates and coordinates slave subsystems, two of which are the articulatory loop system and the visuospatial sketchpad.[20]

Secondary memory has been divided into explicit (or declarative) memory, and implicit[21] (or nondeclarative) memory, based on whether stored information is available to conscious awareness, or not. Implicit memory consists of unconscious processing, such as occurs in conditioning, priming, or using information (which may be motoric, perceptual, or cognitive) that enables performance in the world. Explicit memory has been further subdivided into episodic and semantic memory. Tulving[22] proposed that memory consists of three systems that are monohierarchically arranged. Procedural memory is necessary for adaptation to the environment, and stands at the bottom of the hierarchy. Semantic memory has the additional capability of internally representing knowledge of words, concepts, and facts of the world, and constructing mental models. On top of that, episodic memory has the additional capacity of storing autobiographical experiences with specific reference to the time when they occurred. Each system requires the system below it. The distinction between episodic and semantic memory has been criticized, but is regarded as heuristically productive.[23] Secondary memory has also been subdivided into recent and remote memory, the latter referring to the more distant past. These theoretical subdivisions of memory are not universally agreed upon. They have been reviewed elsewhere.[24-26]

The complexity of the brain with regard to its functions and diseases makes the neuropsychological profile a valuable tool in specifying and quantifying the patterns of deficits seen in brain disorders, especially when combined with information derived from detailed inquiry into the nature, onset, duration, and course of symptoms. For this reason it is often included in research diagnostic criteria for the dementias.[16,27-29] Over the last 5 years considerable progress has been made in characterizing the dementias. Standard diagnostic criteria have been adopted, neuropsychological batteries used in research have become more standardized and have been administered to a wider range of patient populations. This has made it possible to compare the neuropsychological profiles of different dementias. Neuropsychological evaluation is perhaps the most sensitive instrument for the detection of early or mild dementia,

when deficits are not grossly apparent, and are too subtle for detection by screening tests. It is essential to the differential diagnosis of the dementias because of its ability to delineate neuropsychological profiles. It may also be of value in identifying progressive dementias in the preclinical stage.[30,31] An interdisciplinary approach to differential diagnosis has also become increasingly necessary, combining neuropsychological testing with medical and neurological evaluation, and neuroradiological procedures.

Dementias have been grouped according to cortical and subcortical symptoms,[32,33] although there is not universal agreement about this distinction. Alzheimer's disease and the focal lobar atrophies[34] would be considered cortical, whereas Parkinson's disease, progressive supranuclear palsy, and Huntington's disease, would be considered subcortical. However, some disorders such as Lewy body disease and vascular dementia may span these categories, producing lesions in both cortical and subcortical areas. Cortical dementias have been grouped along a topographic axis from anterior to posterior regions of the cortex according to presumed location of lesions.[35] Frontotemporal dementias and Pick's disease would be considered anterior, whereas Alzheimer's disease would be posterior. Neuropsychological profiles of the most common dementias found in the elderly are described below. Studies were selected for review with a bias toward the early detection of dementia.

ALZHEIMER'S DISEASE

Alzheimer's disease (AD) is the most common dementia in elderly people.[36] Loss of neuronal cells in the hippocampus is considered responsible for episodic memory deficits, and there is progressive degeneration of cortical tissue in the temporal and parietal lobes. For clinical diagnosis, the *Diagnostic and Statistical Manual* of the American Psychiatric Association (DSM-IV) requires, beyond documentation of a dementia, that there be insidious onset and gradual progression of symptoms.[3] Research criteria for *probable* AD established by the National Institute of Neurologic and Communicative Disorders (NINCDS) and the Alzheimer's Disease and Related Disorders Association (ADRDA) are: dementia established by clinical examination, documented by a screening test for dementia and confirmed by neuropsychological testing; deficits in two or more areas of cognition; progression of memory and other cognitive deficits; no disturbance of consciousness; onset between ages 40 and 90 years; and exclusion of systemic disorders or other brain diseases that could account for progressive cognitive deficits. A diagnosis of *possible* AD is made if there is a concurrent systemic or brain disorder which could produce dementia, or if only one progressive cognitive deficit can be identified.[27] Using these criteria, clinical classification of AD, which included neuropsychological evaluation, was found to be 80–90 percent accurate when compared with the results of postmortem neuropathological testing. Depending on the neuropathological criteria used, sensitivity ranged from 64 to 86 percent and specificity from 89 to 91 percent.[37] A more recent study found 95 percent sensitivity, and 79 percent specificity.[38] As AD remains a diagnosis of exclusion, the requirement that other brain disorders be excluded takes on greater significance with the increased awareness of other dementias such as frontotemporal dementia and diffuse Lewy body disease.

Memory

Episodic memory

Impairment in episodic memory is required for a diagnosis of AD. There is abundant documentation of impairment on a wide variety of episodic memory tasks in AD relative to normal elderly subjects (NE). Numerous studies have shown impairment in immediate and/or delayed recall of wordlists.[30,39–50] This is so even on tasks which provide cognitive support through category cueing.[51–53] Using a grocery list that may have better ecological validity, similar deficits were found.[54] Patients with mild AD retain the capacity to learn new information, although not to the same degree as NE; their learning curve declines as the severity of dementia increases.[55–57] Recognition testing for wordlist items is also impaired in AD.[30,39,40,58] Overall, wordlists that evaluate episodic memory appear to be particularly sensitive in identifying AD.

Impaired performance has also been documented in episodic memory when memoranda consist of stories.[50,59–65] Although patients with mild AD are able to learn to associate pairs of words, performance is deficient relative to NE.[59] This ability is sensitive to severity of dementia, as patients with moderate dementia do not show a learning curve. Only NE and a group of patients who had very mild cognitive deficits showed a learning curve for difficult associates.[66]

Serial-position effects in recall of wordlists are different in AD than in NE. In normal recall, more words are retrieved from the beginning (primacy) and end (recency) than from the middle of a wordlist. In AD, a smaller number of items are recalled from the beginning of lists, indicating that the primacy effect is weaker in AD than in NE.[39,40,46,50,56,67] Closer inspection reveals that in AD there is a primacy effect on shorter lists, which is lost as the list gets longer.[68] This may represent an extension of the finding of impaired immediate recall in AD, because a list that is longer than seven words would exceed the capacity of working memory, necessitating transfer to secondary memory.[69] Similarly, secondary memory has been found to be more impaired in AD than in NE when compared to primary memory if there is a lag of more than six items between presentation and recall.[53,70] The weakening of the primacy effect is related to the severity of dementia.[57,71]

Numerous studies of patients with AD have shown a liberal response bias and retrieval errors on learned wordlists, such that they allow intrusion of items that are not on the list. Patients with AD made more intrusions on cued recall than NE,[30,51] and this effect was also statistically significant in a small subsample of preclinical AD cases.[30] The same effect was found for immediate and delayed free recall in AD.[39,40] Intrusion errors are also more frequent in visual reproduction tasks in patients with AD.[72]

There is disagreement about the mechanism that results in poorer performance in AD on tests of episodic memory. Some investigators believe that storage is impaired, resulting in a more rapid rate of forgetting. Studies that purport to demonstrate this have used a "savings score," which represents the percent of learned material recalled or recognized after delay.[61,62] This is problematic; even if both groups forget the same number of items, it would appear that patients with AD retain a lower proportion, because they initially learn fewer items. A number of studies that have attempted to equate the amount of learning in AD and NE failed to find evidence of an increased rate of forgetting in learned material, suggesting that encoding rather than storage is impaired in AD.[45,73–75] Other data suggest that impairment in wordlist learning is due to a deficit in an active organizational strategy required for cumulative learning, leading to a failure of learning rather than forgetting.[50]

Episodic memory for visual stimuli is also impaired in AD. Deficient reproduction of geometric shapes has been noted in very mild AD, becoming worse with severity of dementia.[76] Nonagenarians with AD performed more poorly than comparably aged NE on an object memory test.[70] Patients with mild but not moderate AD showed a learning curve for visual stimuli.[57] Delayed recall of visual material is worse in patients with AD than in NE,[45,60,64,73–75,77] regardless of severity of dementia.[49] Recognition memory for unfamiliar faces is impaired in AD,[58,70,78] as is learning to associate names with faces.[54]

Semantic memory and semantic knowledge

Semantic memory consists of internal representation of knowledge of words, concepts, facts of the world, and mental models.[22] Performance on a wide variety of tests measuring this construct has been shown to be impaired in AD. Category fluency tests are commonly used, in which subjects are required to name as many exemplars within a given category (animals, fruits, vegetables) as they can within 1 minute. Performance on this task is quite impaired in AD,[47,65,79–90] and has discriminated between mild AD and NE with 100 percent sensitivity and 93 percent specificity.[91] It has even successfully differentiated NE from patients with mild and preclinical AD,[30,49] and people at risk for developing dementia.[92] One prospective study, although limited by a small sample size, found that generating words to category cue was impaired more than 2 years prior to diagnosis of AD.[93] Patients with mild AD generate not only fewer words, but fewer clusters (subcategories) within the category tested,[94] and smaller cluster sizes.[85,95] Patients generate more words early and fewer words later in the recall period than NE.[96] Category fluency declines with the progression of AD.[97] It is more impaired than letter fluency in AD.[91]

In word-finding tasks (confrontation naming), patients look at pictures and are asked to name them. This skill has consistently been found to be impaired in AD,[41,47,63,65,79,84,86,92,98,99] and the deficit increases with severity of dementia.[48,84] Word-finding difficulty occurs even in minimal AD (MMSE = 24–30).[84]

In an early review of semantic memory in AD, Nebes concluded that word finding and certain aspects of concept formation are deficient in patients with AD, and that they benefit less than NE from the effect of semantic context when contextual cues are subtle.[100] Patients with AD may be able to use semantic information to facilitate episodic memory, but perform less well on tests of general world knowledge than do normal individuals. Numerous studies support the idea that semantic memory is impaired in AD, the following being a partial listing. Patients with AD have deficits in making category membership judgments,[101] reading,[13] reading low-frequency words with irregular spelling-to-sound correspondence (e.g., ache),[14] picture vocabulary[102,103] and picture-matching tasks,[49] judging relationships between words,[104] making associations to words,[105] judging the coherence of simple sentences,[106] verifying sentences,[107] and generic knowledge (e.g., number of ounces in a pound).[108] Semantic components of memory for faces were also found to be poorer in AD than NE.[78] Patients with AD gave inaccurate or impoverished definitions of line drawings.[84] The evidence in support of a breakdown in the structure and organization of semantic memory in AD has been reviewed.[109]

Remote memory for public and autobiographical information

There is considerable evidence that remote memory is impaired in AD. Memory for well-known faces[110–113] and names[111,113] is worse in AD than in NE. The same was true for recall and recognition of famous events in a mixed group of AD and vascular dementia.[114] The evidence concerning temporal gradient in AD is mixed, with some finding that memory for famous faces from earlier decades is better preserved in AD,[110,111,113] while others found no significant temporal difference.[112,115,116] Memory of public information is impaired in AD, and shows a temporal gradient.[117,118] The relationship of remote memory for public information to severity of dementia is also mixed, with some showing a decline with increasing severity,[112] and others showing a limited effect.[111]

Autobiographical memory is impaired fairly early on in patients with AD compared to NE.[111,119–122] This has been attributed to defective approach to searching remote memories.[119] Findings concerning temporal gradient are mixed, with some showing the same distribution of recalled events throughout the lifespan,[121] while others have found that earlier life events are more accurately recalled.[112,120,122] Patients with mild AD were better at locating places on a map of the area where they were raised than using a map of the area where they resided, suggesting temporally graded retrograde amnesia.[123] Autobiographical memory is correlated with severity of dementia.[122] With increasing severity not only are autobiographical memories lost, but elicited memories contain fewer details.[124]

Working memory

Deficits due to AD in the components of working memory have been reviewed. The articulatory loop system is essentially intact in AD, and it remains unclear whether the visuospatial sketchpad is impaired. However, there is considerable evidence of dysfunction of the central executive system, which may account for the observed decrement in memory span and vulnerability to distraction in AD.[125] A neural network basis for this dysfunction has been proposed, namely the disruption of fibers that connect the anterior and posterior regions of the brain.[126]

Visuospatial functions and calculations

Copying of a clock[92] and geometric figures[92,127] was found to be impaired relative to NE. Visuoconstructional deficit is correlated with severity of impairment in other cognitive domains, and with overall severity of dementia.[128] Visuospatial performance is worse in patients with AD who are disoriented

or wander.[129,130] Arithmetic calculations are also impaired in early to moderate AD.[59,131] In one sample of mildly demented patients with AD (mean MMSE = 22), the majority fell below the cutoff for normal performance in calculations. Scores did not correlate with episodic memory score for verbal material, which may indicate that working memory is more important than episodic memory in this skill.[132] Working memory was also implicated in executive-attentional skills that were associated with overall arithmetic ability in AD.[131]

Attention and executive functions

Major components of executive functions include volition, planning and attention, self-regulation, and self-monitoring. These have been reviewed in AD.[133] Executive deficits are found early in the disorder, following the onset of episodic memory loss.[134] Some findings are summarized here. Letter fluency, measured by the number of words generated for a given letter in a limited period of time, is impaired in AD.[65,83,87,88,90–92,97,135–137] It is impaired very early in the disease process, as even preclinical cases do less well than NE.[30,92] One study found that letter fluency was not worse in mild AD; however, all but two patients performed below the mean for NE.[82] It declines with the progression of AD.[97]

A lengthy review of the literature on attention concluded that selective and divided attention are adversely affected early in the dementing process, whereas sustained attention is preserved.[138] Digit span is impaired in mild AD.[30,92,136] Studies which have not found reduced spans tend to use small samples,[59,139] suggesting that the effect size in early dementia is small. Ability to shift mental set is impaired in mild AD, both on trailmaking, and card sorting tests.[30,92]

Performance on delayed alternation and subject-ordered pointing tasks which tap skills in planning, anticipation and self-monitoring were also impaired in mild AD.[135,136] Planning and anticipation are impaired in AD as measured by performance on a maze task.[47,65] Response inhibition is impaired in AD.[136,137,140] In patients with AD, two underlying factors accounted for 60 percent of performance in executive functions: inhibition processes, and storage and processing functions.[136] Conceptualization is impaired on a similarities task which requires grouping of stimuli according to abstract criteria even in preclinical cases,[30,59] and in card sorting.[137,140]

Early and preclinical AD

Of particular clinical interest is how early in the dementing process neuropsychological tests are able to make the distinction between AD and NE. The onset of AD is insidious. In theory, cases initially have subtle cognitive changes which progress until they cross a threshold at which time the changes are sufficiently prominent to be diagnosed as AD. Changes below the threshold are considered preclinical or prodromal. Detection of this threshold depends on the sensitivity and specificity of the tests used. This carries with it the implication that as neuropsychological tests improve, the boundary between early (or very mild) AD and preclinical AD will change. Furthermore, tests varying in sensitivity and specificity will yield different findings. The latter problem has blighted some of the literature that attempts to characterize early vs preclinical AD.

Cross-sectional studies using discriminant function analysis are somewhat difficult to compare as the rationale for inclusion of variables is not always clear, and the battery of neuropsychological tests used in different investigations varies. Nonetheless, consistent findings have emerged. Delayed wordlist recall again appears as a sensitive discriminator in mild AD,[43,44,92,141] and beyond this, delayed visual recall adds to discrimination.[92] One study found that a measure of forgetting was the best discriminator between AD and NE; it is likely that this was a proxy for delayed recall.[40] Immediate verbal[12,142] and visual[143] recall were good discriminators in earlier studies, but later studies appear to show that delayed recall is a better measure. Other tests that have shown some discriminative power are trailmaking,[92,142] naming,[12,92] word fluency,[142,143] and visual pattern–location pairings.[65]

A longitudinal strategy for identifying preclinical neuropsychological changes in sporadic AD is to prospectively follow a population, using repeated evaluations at baseline and at specific time intervals afterwards. When incident AD cases are diagnosed, their baseline data can be compared to those of nondementing controls drawn from the same population. Using a variation on this methodology, four tests entered into a logistic regression showed promise in identifying a high proportion of cases that would not develop dementia after 4 years. These were delayed recall on a selective reminding test, category fluency, immediate recall on an object memory test, and digit span.[144] Principal component indices derived from a wordlist incorrectly identified five NE as having AD; all of them went on to develop AD at follow-up. These indices were also successful in differentiating NE with a family history of dementia from those without it.[30] Cases with preclinical AD were more similar to nondemented elderly people in primary memory on a wordlist, whereas secondary memory was worse in preclinical and prevalent AD cases.[53] Reducing the number of tests by statistical methods, different combinations of tests have been found to discriminate best between preclinical AD and nondemented elderly people. These include delayed wordlist recall and trailmaking;[31] immediate recall of an organized wordlist, remote visual memory, and letter fluency;[145] and age, category fluency, delayed verbal and visual recall, general attention, and attention.[146]

In summary, features in the neuropsychological profile that are the most useful in making an early diagnosis of AD are impaired episodic memory in both verbal and visual modalities, in particular poor delayed recall; attenuated primacy effect, such that more words are recalled from the end of a long wordlist or set of memoranda than from the beginning; a liberal response bias and a high rate of intrusions; and poor performance on category fluency tasks, indicating impairment in semantic memory. Given the relentless progression of AD, all neuropsychological skills are devastated by the later stages of the disorder, and the neuropsychological profile may become similar to that of other degenerative diseases. Therefore differential diagnosis is often enhanced if evaluation occurs earlier in the dementing process.

VASCULAR DEMENTIA

Several cerebrovascular diseases cause cognitive impairment in the older person. These include multi-infarct dementia (MID), strategically placed infarcts, multiple subcortical lacunar infarcts, Binswanger's disease, and single or multiple hemorrhagic lesions. These are all subsumed under the diagnosis of vascular dementia (VaD). In addition there are combinations of these disorders, and cases of mixed AD and VaD.[147] DSM-IV clinical criteria for VaD are memory loss and impairment in at least one other domain of higher cortical functioning (aphasia, apraxia, agnosia, executive functioning), decline in social or occupational functioning, focal neurological signs and symptoms or laboratory evidence of cerebrovascular disease, and exclusion of delirium.[3] Research criteria for VaD (from the National Institutes for Neurological Disorders and Stroke and the Association Internationale pour la Recherche et l'Enseignement en Neurosciences) require a decline in memory and intellectual abilities that is associated with impaired functioning in daily living; the existence of cerebrovascular disease as shown by focal signs consistent with stroke, a temporal relationship with symptom onset, and neuropsychological documentation of cognitive decline demonstrated by loss of memory and deficits in at least two other cognitive domains; brain imaging that shows nontrivial infarcts or extensive and diffuse white matter changes, and that correlates with clinical evidence; and supportive clinical features such as abrupt decline within 3 months of a stroke, gait disorder or falls, psychiatric changes, urinary infrequency or incontinence, or other neurological signs and symptoms.[28] These criteria were shown to have sensitivity of 58 percent and specificity of 80 percent.[148]

These diagnostic criteria have been criticized. Failure to differentiate between types of VaD complicates efforts to delineate a neuropsychological profile. In requiring that impairment be sufficiently severe to interfere with daily functioning, the criteria do not recognize that there is a continuum of impairment in cerebrovascular disease that begins with subtle deficits.[2,149–151] This excludes many cases of mild vascular disease, which prevents them from being identified and treated in a timely manner.[152] The criteria are also criticized for being too patterned on AD, a cortical dementia with hippocampal involvement leading to prominent memory loss. As vascular pathology is more varied and memory loss is not as prominent as in AD, the requirement of memory loss excludes cases and has an adverse impact on sensitivity. Indeed, these criteria have been found to diagnose VaD with high specificity but low sensitivity.[148,153] This problem has been addressed by other criteria which do not emphasize memory loss.[154] An alternative term *vascular cognitive impairment* (VCI) has been proposed which would include all levels of cognitive impairment.[2] A recent study of VCI in a memory clinic population included three subsets of patients: vascular cognitive impairment not dementia, VaD, and mixed AD/VaD. About 24 percent of cases did not meet criteria for dementia, illustrating that current criteria for VaD underestimate cognitive deficits in cerebrovascular disease.[155]

The neuropsychological presentation of VaD depends on the extent and region of the brain that is affected. The following review includes several subtypes of VaD, with both cortical and subcortical involvement. As AD is the most common dementia in elderly people, many investigations of VaD have compared its profile to that of AD. Only those which matched patient groups for severity of dementia are included here.

Memory

Episodic, semantic, and remote memory

Compared to NE, wordlist learning is impaired in VaD for both immediate and delayed recall.[47,90,156–161] Patient groups with cortical and subcortical VaD were both impaired on these measures.[162] Patients with very mild VaD show reduced storage and retrieval.[156] Story recall is also impaired relative to NE,[47,151] as is paired associate learning for difficult items.[151]

Studies which have compared VaD to AD, equating for severity of dementia by matching on a screening test, have found that episodic memory is less impaired in VaD. On each of three different wordlists and an object memory task, performance of patients with AD was worse on immediate recall.[90,157,158,160,163] It was also worse in AD on delayed recall.[90,157,158,160,164,165] Storage was found to be better in VaD than in AD, suggesting less early hippocampal involvement.[156] Using stories, patients with Binswanger's disease (BD) had better recall than patients with AD,[166] as did patients with VaD more broadly defined.[47,163] One study found that the primacy effect in wordlist recall was intact in VaD but diminished in AD, whereas the recency effect was spared in both groups.[157] These findings need to be replicated. VaD patients have fewer intrusions than AD patients,[164,167] and fewer false positives on recognition testing.[164] Visual reproduction failed to differentiate VaD from AD.[47,157,160,168] Recognition of unfamiliar faces is impaired, but does not differ between VaD and AD.[70,169] Delayed recall of the Rey–Osterreith Complex Figure (ROCF) is impaired, and worse in AD than in VaD.[159] Delayed recognition for the ROCF was also worse in AD than in VaD.[127]

The findings with regard to semantic memory are less clear-cut. Confrontation naming is impaired in VaD relative to NE.[47,89,151,158,170,171] Some studies report that naming is better in VaD[47,167,171] and BD[172] than in AD, while others have found no statistical difference.[89,158,163–165,168] On an odd-man-out task, VaD was worse than NE but no different than AD.[170] Category fluency is impaired in MID and VaD.[89,90,159] It has been found consistently to be no different in VaD and AD.[47,87–90,159,163,166,167] Word definitions and picture sorting by category were impaired but no different from AD.[89] Store of general information did not differ between VaD and AD.[168]

On a remote memory recognition test of faces of famous people, NE performed better than patients with VaD, who in turn did better than patients with AD. This finding needs replication as the sample with AD was also slightly more demented.[169]

Working memory

The preponderance of evidence is that digit span forward is equivalent in NE, AD, and VaD,[47,90,157,173] and that digit span backward is equally impaired in AD and VaD.[47,90,173] VaD patients do not differ from AD patients on spatial memory spans.[47,168,173] Auditory and visual continuous performance tasks were found to be worse in VaD than in AD.[47] Accuracy on a high load cancellation task was impaired in VaD, but better than in AD.[90] In general, the findings indicate no difference between VaD and AD except for vigilance tasks, where VaD were more impaired.

Visuospatial functions

The findings are mixed with regard to copying. In copying the ROCF, VaD patients were impaired relative to NE.[47,127,159] One study found them to be the same as patients with AD,[47] another found them to be worse,[127] possibly because different scoring systems were used. In one study clock drawing to command and copy were worse in VaD than in AD,[164] but in another they did not differentiate the two patient groups.[167] In yet another study the VaD group was the same as AD in the command condition but worse in the copy condition.[174]

Patients with VaD were worse than patients with AD on timed subtests of the Wechsler Adult Intelligence Scale—Revised (WAIS-R) that require copying symbols and putting together puzzle-like pieces.[168] They were impaired on block design[47] but did not differ from AD.[47,168] They were impaired on visual perception and organization, again about the same amount as patients with AD.[47,169] Copying a star, cube, and house did not differentiate VaD from AD.[90,157]

Speech and language

There are mixed findings with regard to language functions in VaD. One study failed to find any differences between demented patients and NE on a lengthy aphasia battery, nor could VaD patients be discriminated from those with AD.[175] On the other hand, vascular patients with general cerebral dysfunction were found to be impaired on several language measures.[151] Mechanical problems of speech have been reported to be worse in VaD, whereas linguistic changes were more marked in AD.[176] Dysarthria was more common in a sample of patients with subcortical lacunae than in NE.[149] In VaD patients with subcortical lesions only, severity of white matter ischemia was highly correlated with verbal output disturbance consisting of expressive and articulatory deficits.[177]

Executive functions

Frontal-subcortical structures are preferentially affected in VaD,[178] with concomitant decrement in executive functions that is well documented. Card sorting is impaired in VaD, and worse than in AD.[159] Performance on Raven's Matrices is equally impaired in VaD and AD.[47,90] Using a pair of unstructured tasks designed to elicit spontaneity and initiative, VaD patients performed poorly relative to both AD and NE.[158] Initiation and perseveration were impaired and more so than in AD.[179] Ability to shift mental set was impaired in VaD,[149,158] but no difference was found relative to AD.[163,167] Perseveration, difficulty inhibiting responses, and semantic clustering were worse in VaD than in NE.[149] Trailmaking is impaired.[151] Mental control was worse in VaD than in AD.[164] On Similarities, a test of conceptualization, VaD patients made more out-of-set errors than AD, indicating a deficit in executive function which suggests reduced monitoring of responses and reduced ability to sustain mental set.[180] VaD patients make more perseverations than AD patients, and these are associated more with motor and executive functions than with semantic knowledge.[181] VaD patients have also been shown to be impaired on mazes, pattern completion, and auditory and visual continuous performance tests, and they are also worse than AD patients on these tasks. Orientation to time and place was impaired in VaD, but better than in AD.[47] Letter fluency is impaired in VaD relative to NE,[87,88,90,149,164] but may not be in mildly demented cases.[159] Some studies have found that letter fluency in VaD and MID does not differ from AD,[88,90,157,158,167] but others have found that it is worse in VaD.[87,165] Closing-in responses on copying tasks, and global or odd responses to a visual conceptualization task were found to be more frequent in AD than in VaD.[157] Tasks that tap motor or cognitive speed are more impaired in VaD and MID than AD, suggesting subcortical involvement.[90,168] A motor performance index which tapped executive functions, writing, and arrangement of cartoon pictures into stories was found to be more impaired in VaD than AD.[182]

Behavioral disorder

A variety of behavioral disturbances are frequently reported in VaD. Depression is a common finding. A population study found its prevalence to be 21 percent, compared to 3 percent in AD.[183] Another population study found depression present in 32 percent of cases, vs 20 percent in AD.[184] Prevalence of major depression in a hospital dementia registry was 19 percent for VaD and 8 percent for AD.[185] Using a test designed to assess neurobehavioral change, VaD patients were reported to show more motor retardation, and more anxiety and depression than patients with AD who were matched for severity of dementia. VaD patients also had more subjectively experienced symptoms of depression and anxiety, and more neurovegetative signs, as measured by the Hamilton Depression Scale. They were more impaired on a motor inventory that tapped speech, psychomotor speed, posture, gait, and movement.[186] Interestingly, a frontal-subcortical substrate has been implicated in both depression[187] and VaD,[178] raising the possibility that the same pathology underlies both cognitive and behavioral symptoms.

The prevalence of psychosis in clinical samples of VaD patients was estimated at 37 percent.[188] Delusions were present in 8 percent of VaD cases in a free-living population compared to 22 percent of AD cases.[184] In a hospital dementia registry, 46 percent of VaD patients had psychotic symptoms.[185] Agitation/aggression had a prevalence of 32 percent in VaD and was not statistically different from AD.[184] Prevalence of anxiety in VaD in a population study was 17 percent, not significantly different from AD.[184] In a dementia registry it was significantly higher in VaD (71 percent) than in AD (38 percent).[185]

In a population study, prevalence of apathy in VaD was 22 percent, and did not differ significantly from AD.[184] Apathy was observed more frequently in a well-defined sample of patients with subcortical lacunae than in NE.[149] VaD patients had a higher apathy score than AD patients in an outpatient sample.[189] Patients with Binswanger's disease also showed more apathy than severity-matched AD patients.[190]

In summary, immediate recall is impaired in mild VaD, but not as much as in early AD. The same is true of delayed recall. Retrieval deficit may be more prominent than in AD. Some executive functions are more impaired in VaD than in early AD, including planning, shifting set/perseverating, performing unstructured tasks that require initiation of activity, vigilance, orientation to time and place, and motor or cognitive speed. This pattern of better episodic memory but worse executive functions was also found in another review of the neuropsychological profile in VaD.[191] There may be more problems with mechanics of speech in VaD, whereas in mild AD language impairment is likely to be at a deeper, linguistic level.

Behavioral disturbance is common. Depression occurs frequently, and is more likely to occur in VaD than in AD. Agitation and aggression are also common, as is apathy. This pattern of neuropsychological and neurobehavioral deficits reflects a frontal-subcortical distribution of lesions with relative sparing of the hippocampus, which is the reverse of AD.

DEMENTIA WITH LEWY BODIES

The discovery that Lewy bodies are not limited to subcortical areas of the brain, but may be present in neocortex as well, has necessitated reconceptualization of disorders with this neuropathology. It has been proposed that Lewy body disease represents a spectrum of disorders ranging from preclinical states with mild subcortical Lewy body disease, through Parkinson's disease, up to dementia with Lewy bodies in both brainstem and neocortex.[18,192] The terms diffuse Lewy body disease (DLBD)[17] and senile dementia Lewy body type (SDLT)[193] have been applied to the latter condition. However, an international consortium that standardized criteria for this disorder recommended use of the term Dementia with Lewy bodies (DLB),[194] which will be adopted here, except when reviewing research that used different diagnostic criteria for sample selection. Clinically defined DLB cases often show some AD features on neuropathological examination. Cases of pure DLB may be exceptional, one investigation of 245 dementia patients finding only two cases (<1 percent).[195] In addition, clear-cut AD neuropathology often shows some concomitant Lewy body disease, which has been described as a Lewy body variant of AD (LBV).[196] It is likely that most clinical research samples of AD include cases with this variant.

An early review of published cases of DLBD found that dementia, psychosis, and parkinsonism were frequently reported.[197] Neuropsychological testing of 15 SDLT patients who were later identified on neuropathological grounds showed dysphasia, dyscalculia, and visuospatial, constructional, and ideomotor dyspraxia. The primary symptom at presentation was about equally divided between parkinsonism and dementia, but eventually all cases progressed to dementia.[198] Since then the international consortium on DLB recommended the following diagnostic criteria: progressive cognitive decline of sufficient magnitude to affect social or occupational functioning; memory impairment not required early on, but deficits on attentional, frontal-subcortical and visuospatial tests may be prominent; at least two of three core features (fluctuating cognition, visual hallucinations, parkinsonism).[194] Supportive features are falls, syncope, transient loss of consciousness, neuroleptic sensitivity, delusions, and hallucinations. Stroke disease must be excluded, and any other illness that could produce similar symptoms. These criteria include features necessary for a dementia (i.e., global cognitive decline which interferes with social and occupational functioning), with memory loss de-emphasized and executive functions emphasized in the neuropsychological profile. Behavioral and neurological findings assume greater importance than in the diagnosis of AD, and consideration is given to differentiation of DLB from cerebrovascular disease.

Recent findings concerning the neuropsychological profile in DLB have been generally consistent. Cognitive loss is global, with deficits relative to NE in episodic, semantic, and working memory, perceptual and visuospatial skills, executive functions, and attention.[199] Of particular interest are aspects of the profile that distinguish DLB from other dementias. Thus far this research has focused on AD. The studies cited here have controlled for severity of dementia. Episodic memory is not as impaired in DLB as in AD. This has been found using a wide variety of tasks, including immediate and delayed recall of stories,[199] word learning and recall,[200–202] and in screening tests.[203–205] However, one study of neuropathologically confirmed cases showed no statistical difference between AD and LBV cases on episodic memory.[206] Semantic memory is generally equivalent in DLB, AD, and LBV as shown in tasks of naming, category fluency, general information, and vocabulary.[199–202,206,207] Working memory is worse in DLB as measured by digits backwards.[199] A series of investigations of spatial working memory showed that SDLT were more impaired than AD patients on a task that required them to associate patterns with specific locations,[208] on a visual delayed matching-to-sample task,[209] and on a task of self-ordered pointing that required subjects to find hidden tokens.[210] Digit span forward and backward is impaired.[211] Perceptual and visuospatial skills are generally worse in DLB than in AD. This also has been demonstrated in a wide variety of tasks, including block design, copying, object size and form discrimination, overlapping figures, and multiple subtests of the visual object and space perception test.[199–201,203–206,212,213] Some executive functions such as letter fluency, trailmaking, card sorting, motor sequencing, initiation, and perseveration are worse than in AD.[199,201,204,211] Sustained, selective, and divided attention are also worse than in AD.[199] Orientation to date[204] and place[200] are worse in AD than in DLB.

The pattern of deficits in DLB compared to AD is thought to reflect the structural changes known to occur in these two disorders. Preservation of episodic memory in DLB relative to AD is attributed to less involvement of the medial temporal lobe[200] and especially the hippocampus,[201] which are known to be less affected in DLB than in AD. Perceptual and visuospatial deficits have been attributed to occipital cholinergic deficits,[200] and to changes in substantia nigra leading to depletion of dopaminergic input to the striatum in DLB.[201] Attentional deficit may be due to known cholinergic depletion in DLB.[199] Since anterior and inferolateral temporal areas are suspected of involvement in semantic memory, the finding that DLB and AD groups are equivalent on semantic memory tasks has led to the proposal that these regions are equally impaired in both disorders.[199] Compared to VaD, DLB patients did not differ in neuropsychological profile except for recent memory, which was worse in VaD.[203] Additional research is needed to clarify the differences between DLB and VaD. It has been suggested that the neuropsychological deficits in DLB reflect a frontal-subcortical profile, as it does in VaD, which may confound efforts at differential diagnosis.[196,204]

Behavioral and neurological symptoms

Estimates of behavioral disorder in DLB are high. In neuropathologically confirmed cases the prevalence of hallucinations ranges from 56 to 60 percent, delusions from 39 to 60 percent, delusional misidentification was found in 38 percent, anxiety in 84 percent, and anhedonia in 76 percent.[188,214]

Hallucinations, delusions, anxiety, anhedonia, and anergia were significantly more common in DLB than in AD.[214] Masked facies, bradykinesia, and essential tremor were more common in cases of Lewy body variant of AD.[196]

In summary, cases of pure DLB are uncommon. This disorder has been placed on a continuum with Parkinson's disease. Lewy bodies are also found in neuropathologically confirmed AD, which has been referred to as a Lewy body variant of AD. The diagnosis is based on significant decline in cognitive functions, early presentation of visual hallucinations or parkinsonism, and fluctuating course. Patients with DLB may show a frontal-subcortical pattern of neuropsychological deficits, with prominent deficits in attention, working memory, visuospatial skills, and some executive functions, while episodic memory is somewhat impaired though and better than in AD. There may be poor response to neuroleptic medication.

FRONTOTEMPORAL DEMENTIAS

Several degenerative cortical diseases afflict the anterior regions of the brain, leading to a dementia syndrome. Interest in these disorders grew with the description of frontal lobe degeneration of non-Alzheimer type,[215,216] which is neuropathologically distinct from AD, Pick's disease, and dementia with motor neuron disease.[217,218] Functional neuroimaging has demonstrated a reduction in cerebral metabolism in the frontal and anterior temporal lobes.[219,220] Clinical manifestation reflects the topographic distribution of cortical lesions, which may be unilateral on either side, or bilateral. A wide range of behavioral disturbances are reported. Onset is insidious, between age 40 and 70.[35,221,222]

It became clear that the frontal dementia syndrome was a heterogeneous entity, based on the distribution rather than on the nature of underlying pathology, which could be due to different conditions including Pick's disease, AD, motor neuron disease, or nonspecific changes with spongiosis. A consensus group defined three clinical syndromes:[223] frontotemporal dementia (FTD) also known as frontal variant FTD,[224] progressive nonfluent aphasia, and semantic dementia. Behavioral disorder is likely to be the presenting symptom in the first syndrome, whereas speech and language difficulties are more likely to be seen early in the others. The term *frontotemporal dementia* (FTD) is adopted here, as the literature shows it to have the widest currency. The term Pick complex has also been suggested.[225]

Frontal variant FTD

This clinical syndrome is marked by neurobehavioral impairment, with change in personality and social behavior.[223]

Using a scale designed to detect frontal lobe behavioral dysfunction, the most common behavioral changes, found in 70–100 percent of cases of broadly defined FTD, were social and self-neglect, apathy, hyperorality, restlessness, flat affect, irritability, and disinhibition.[228] Many cases initially receive a psychiatric diagnosis.[229]

In more narrowly defined cases, socially undesirable behavior was more common in right-sided than in left-sided FTD in right-handed patients.[231] In one case with frontal variant FTD, the ability to internally represent the thoughts and feelings of others was impaired.[232]

Compared to AD, FTD patients were found to have more major depression, anxiety, agitation, irritability, lability of mood, disinhibition, anergia, and social withdrawal.[233] They had more verbal outbursts and inappropriate activity, and scored higher on a global rating scale of behavioral disturbance.[234] They were more disinhibited, socially awkward, passive/apathetic, and had more executive dysfunction.[235] They showed more stereotypic behavior and eating changes, and loss of social awareness.[236] A study that compared behavioral change in FTD and VaD found that sudden onset, memory disturbance, confusion, and neurological deficits were significantly different in the two groups, all being more prominent in the vascular group.[237]

Neuropsychologically, this disorder can be conceptualized as a dysexecutive syndrome, broadly defined as deficits in skills underlying volition, planning and attention, purposive action and self-regulation, and effective performance or self-monitoring. Pathology is primarily in the frontal lobes, with possible disruption of dorsolateral-prefrontal, orbitofrontal-subcortical, and medial-frontal circuits.[133] The hippocampus is relatively unaffected and posterior areas are preserved. The associated neuropsychological profile is one of severe executive deficit disproportionate to the degree of episodic memory loss, which is mild to moderate, and relative preservation of other cognitive functions.

Documentation of the above profile was provided by early studies of FTD in 89 patients confirmed by pathology or measurement of cerebral metabolism (probably mostly frontal variant FTD). Executive deficits were prominent, found in sorting and shifting mental set, word generation to letter and category cue, divided attention, picture arrangement, and anticipation and planning.[221,222,226,238–240] Episodic memory deficit was in the mild–moderate range, consistent with the idea that the hippocampus is only moderately involved in FTD.[221,240] Drawings and block designs were generally intact or only mildly deficient early on, reflecting minimal parietal or occipital involvement. Speech and language showed expressive rather than receptive deficit.[35,221] Some patients exhibited verbal aspontaneity, and others logorrhea. Stereotypy and impoverishment of speech, progressing to mutism, were reported.[35]

A few studies have helped delineate the neuropsychological profile in narrowly defined frontal variant FTD. Executive functions were found to be impaired relative to NE on letter fluency, card sorting, dual task, map search, counting with distraction, and decision making. Performance on these tasks was worse than in AD. Episodic memory was impaired, but not as badly as in AD. Semantic memory was comparable to NE on several semantic tasks and better than in semantic dementia. Digit span and visuospatial ability were also preserved.[224,227,241]

Semantic dementia and progressive nonfluent aphasia

These disorders were initially grouped under the heterogeneous rubric of primary progressive aphasia (PPA). This was described as a slowly progressing anomic aphasia, and related to left perisylvian deterioration.[243] Longitudinal testing in a sample of these cases revealed that naming, word fluency, and repetition of words and sentences declined over 3–5 years, while episodic memory, visuoperceptual skills, and nonverbal reasoning remained intact.[244] A study of eight cases showed that naming declined more precipitously over serial test administrations, while memory and other cognitive functions declined more slowly.[245] A study that compared PPA, AD, and aphasic patients using an aphasia test battery found that spontaneous speech and object naming were most impaired in PPA.[246] Although the initial cases were reported to progress very slowly, others reported progression to dementia within a few years.[245,246] Symptoms were caused by a variety of diseases, including Pick's disease, AD, Creutzfeldt–Jakob disease and focal spongiform degeneration.[247,248]

Since these initial cases numerous additional cases have been reported, and two patterns have been differentiated, a fluent syndrome (semantic dementia) and a nonfluent syndrome, which have different neuropsychological profiles.[34,249,250]

In *semantic dementia* (SD), the clinical picture is of impairment in naming and comprehension leading to fluent but empty speech. Degeneration is primarily in the left anterior temporal lobe.[223,251] The neuropsychological profile shows impairment in semantic memory, episodic memory preserved for recent events, executive functions intact early on, and preservation of visuoperceptual skills. Impairment in semantic memory is evidenced by poor performance relative to NE on category fluency,[224,252] picture naming,[224,252,253] naming in response to verbal description,[224] awareness of semantic features,[224] picture sorting at different conceptual levels,[224] and associative semantic knowledge.[224,252] Surface dyslexia and surface dysgraphia have also been reported in SD.[254]

In SD, retrograde memory is better for recent or current experience than for remote experience.[255] Episodic verbal memory is impaired relative to NE, but not as badly as in AD.[224,252] SD patients rely more on sensory/perceptual information than on conceptual information to facilitate episodic memory.[253] Performance on executive tests may be intact early on, unlike in frontal variant FTD.[224,252] Digit span[224,252,256] and visuoperceptual ability[252] are intact.

Relative to AD patients at a comparably early stage of dementia, SD patients show more profound impairment in semantic memory. The reverse is true for episodic memory, where greater impairment is found in AD. Recent autobiographical experience is preserved in SD but not in AD. Relative to patients with frontal variant FTD, SD patients are more impaired in semantic memory, but less impaired in executive functions. Behavior in SD is preserved, whereas it is the hallmark of the frontal disorder. Episodic memory is about equally impaired in both of these conditions, and therefore cannot differentiate between them. Digit span and visuoperceptual ability do not appear to discriminate any of the above patient groups.

In *progressive nonfluent aphasia* the clinical picture is of focal impairment in expressive language which progresses over time. Speech is hesitant, articulation may be effortful, phonemic paraphasias or anomia may be present. Mutism may occur late in the process. Agrammatism occurs both in speech and writing. Repetition is impaired, reading and writing are effortful. Comprehension including single word meaning is relatively preserved.[223,250] However, word–picture matching for verbs but not nouns may be impaired.[257] Unlike AD, episodic memory appears to be preserved, although testing requires use of nonverbal tests. Social skills and activities of daily living are preserved. Pathology is primarily in the left peri-sylvian area. Buccofacial and limb apraxia may occur.

In summary, there are three FTD syndromes, associated with the distribution of pathology in frontal and anterior-temporal regions. *Frontal variant FTD* presents with behavioral disorder which may include apathy, social with-drawal, disinhibition, disruption of social conduct, lack of insight, poor planning and judgment, and mood disorder. The neuropsychological profile in these patients consists of prominent executive dysfunction out of proportion to deficit in episodic memory, while semantic memory remains intact. In *semantic dementia* there is a slowly progressing anomia that results in fluent but empty speech. Tests of semantic memory are impaired and decline over time, while episodic memory is less affected and declines more slowly. Executive functions are intact early on. *Progressive nonfluent aphasia* presents with compromised expressive language, including effortful speech and phonemic paraphasias, which can progress to mutism. Episodic memory and social skills appear to be preserved.

DEPRESSION

Depression is known to produce cognitive changes which can be confused with mild dementia. Since depression is treatable, it is important that it be differentiated from dementia. The term "pseudodementia" has been used to describe this condition,[258] but has come under criticism, in part because it implies that the cognitive loss seen in depression is not real.[259–261]

Numerous studies have shown that depressed patients have deficits in episodic memory. Immediate recall of wordlists by severely depressed patients is impaired relative to NE,[46,187,262–266] but is consistently better than in patients with dementia.[46,67,267–269] Delayed recall is impaired,[263,270] and also falls between NE and AD patients.[46,264] On recognition testing, depressed patients are more impaired than NE,[264] but have fewer intrusions and random errors than demented patients.[267,268,271] Similar patterns have been found for visual stimuli.[262,272,273] Immediate recall of stories is also impaired,[263] and worse in dementia than in depression.[77,265,267] Two meta-analyses have summarized the literature on depression and impaired memory performance.[274,275]

Additional neuropsychological findings in depression have been reviewed.[260] Rate of forgetting, which has been shown to be very rapid in AD, is no different in depressed patients relative to NE subjects.[46,265] This suggests that impairment in depression is not due to difficulty with retention, but rather appears to be related to response style and motivational state. Patients with depression make conservative responses that result in more false negatives than AD patients, who have a liberal response bias which produces more false positives.[46,267,272,276] This difference is best elicited by delayed recognition tasks, which allow observation of response style while minimizing effort. Responses of patients with AD favor items at the end of a wordlist over items at the beginning of the list, whereas depressed patients are more like normal subjects in showing both primacy and recency effect,[46,67] the

implication being that secondary memory is basically intact in depression. Semantic memory as measured by confrontation naming was found to be better in patients with depression than in AD, but no different from NE,[277] and better in depressed patients with cognitive loss relative to dementia patients with depression.[278] Category fluency is impaired in depression relative to NE,[77,264,279] but not as deficient as in AD.[265] Recall of events from autobiographical memory showed the same distribution in depressed patients as in AD and NE, but the group with depression recalled more negative memories in recent years.[121]

Several studies suggest that deficits in processing resources mediate episodic memory loss in depression. When processing speed and working memory were entered first as independent variables in a hierarchical regression analysis, they accounted for a significant proportion of variance. Whether subjects were depressed or not failed to account for a significant increment in variance. This was true for each of the three different memory tests that were used: stories, wordlist, and figural memory.[280] A similar result was found with a block design task. P300 latency was longer in depressed patients than in NE, and correlated with tests of executive function.[281] Spatial working memory was also worse in depressed patients.[279] In a population-based sample, processing speed accounted for the largest proportion of variance in a regression analysis using address memory, symbol memory, and picture memory as dependent variables; depression did not account for an appreciable amount of additional variance.[282]

Several studies have examined executive functioning in depression. Significant impairment has been found in dual-task performance,[280] initiation/perseveration,[281] letter fluency,[65,77,264,265,279,281] Stroop test (number correct),[281] card sorting test,[281] attentional set shifting,[65,283] and planning.[65,279,283]

On an aphasia battery, depressed patients showed worse performance than NE on word fluency, reading comprehension, and on a test of syntactic complexity. However they were invariably better than patients with AD.[277]

Performance is sometimes worse on tasks that require effort, leading to the conclusion that depressed patients are less motivated than NE.[284,285] They may do better when challenged, giving rise to the clinical observation that they are sometimes inconsistent, performing better on difficult items than on easy ones.

There is a body of evidence which suggests that a frontal-subcortical substrate mediates the cognitive changes observed in depression.[286] Support for this theory comes from various sources. Patients with depression were successfully classified into two subgroups, one which performed similarly to NE on a verbal learning task, and another which was similar to patients with a subcortical dementia (Huntington's disease).[187] Depression is also common in other dementias with known subcortical lesions, such as vascular dementia and Parkinson's disease.[150,287,288] Finally, investigations using functional brain imaging show a decrease in cerebral metabolism in anterior paralimbic and prefrontal cortex in primary depression.[289] These converging lines of evidence suggest that depression of different etiologies may reflect the same neuroanatomic substrate. However, there is some disagreement.[279,283,290]

In summary, depressed patients have mild cognitive deficits, but their performance on a variety of cognitive tasks is more like that of healthy subjects than patients with mild dementia. Thus the rate of forgetting learned material is similar to that of NE in being less rapid than in AD patients, and the primacy effect is also preserved, unlike in AD. Depressed patients are more likely to show a conservative response bias on delayed recognition testing, with more false negatives, but fewer false positives than AD patients. Episodic memory deficit may be mediated by processing resources including processing speed and working memory. Language functions of depressed patients are also superior to AD patients, and confrontation naming may be slightly worse in early AD than in depression. Additional data that facilitate the differential diagnosis of depression and mild AD come from the patient's history. Sometimes it can be determined that onset of memory loss preceded symptoms of depression. Sometimes true symptoms of depression can be distinguished from apathy or withdrawal secondary to cognitive decline, which are often interpreted by family members as depression.

FORGETFULNESS

Mild cognitive decline with advancing age is of particular interest as many older people complain of some amount of forgetfulness. Proper clinical classification is needed before the causes are understood and interventions can be developed. Since the initial formulation of benign senescent forgetfulness,[291] there have been several attempts to define this condition. The concept of age-associated memory impairment (AAMI) attempts to describe older people with memory loss due to non-disease-related cognitive decline relative to the person's level of functioning at an earlier age. Proposed criteria for AAMI include subjective complaints of memory loss in everyday living, memory test performance at least one standard deviation below the mean established for young adults, adequate intellectual function (verbal IQ estimated to be above the 37th percentile), with exclusion of dementia and psychiatric or other disorders that might impair cognition.[292] Age-associated cognitive decline (AACD) aims to identify similar cases with mild impairment that are not preclinical AD. Diagnosis requires a decline of at least one standard deviation relative to age-matched controls in any cognitive domain.[293] Mild cognitive impairment (MCI) is a more recent concept, developed to describe the transitional state between normal aging and dementia.[294] Diagnostic criteria are memory complaint, abnormal memory for age, normal activities of daily living, normal general cognitive function, and absence of dementia.

The criteria for AAMI have been criticized. Subjective complaint of memory loss, which is required in AAMI, has been linked more to mood than to objective memory loss.[295] In addition there are psychometric shortcomings. Since very early dementia may be below the threshold for sensitive detection (e.g. not global), dementia cases are likely to be included in AAMI samples. Indeed, 42 percent of AAMI cases in one study converted to dementia after 3 years.[296] Consistent with this, another study found that only 59 percent of cases still met AAMI criteria after 3.6 years of follow-up, while 16 percent converted to dementia or showed decline.[297] Additional false positive errors would occur by inclusion of dementing people of high premorbid intellectual capacity who, despite decline, still function within normal limits. Older people of low average intellectual capacity whose memory is unchanged might also be falsely identified as having AAMI by the existing criteria if their performance falls one standard deviation below the average for young adults. This problem could be avoided by the use of appropriate age-referenced norms,[298] and both problems could be addressed by incorporation of educational or occupational achievement as indices of premorbid functioning.[299] In spite of its shortcomings, AAMI does identify some cases of mild memory loss that do not progress.[297] AAMI cases have been found to be impaired relative to NE in other domains than memory, including executive tests,[300] verbal fluency and visuospatial reasoning.[301] There is more extensive cognitive loss in cases identified as AACD than in AAMI.[301] A significant percentage of these progress to dementia.[302]

MCI criteria have been criticized for being too stringent in requiring cognitive deficit in the memory domain alone, which reduces its sensitivity, and for failing to stipulate specific neuropsychological tests for identifying memory loss, as it is known that memory tests vary in sensitivity.[302] Nonetheless, classification of MCI appears to be somewhat successful in identifying people who go on to develop dementia, which is its goal. Up to 12 percent of cases convert to dementia annually.[302,303] Elevated cholesterol level and possibly elevated systolic blood pressure in midlife may increase the risk of developing MCI.[304] White matter lucencies and temporal lobe atrophy may help identify which cases of MCI will progress to dementia.[305]

INTERVENTIONS

A critical moment in the care of the elderly patient with dementia occurs immediately following evaluation, when the provider and patient meet to review the findings. This contact is important because it lays the groundwork that determines the success of later interventions. There is some debate about the wisdom of telling patients their diagnosis in cases of irreversible dementia, AD in particular. In favor of disclosure are the right of patients to self-determination and the need for their full participation in formulating advance directives, financial planning, and other personal affairs while they are still competent to express their wishes. A survey of older people living in a retirement community supported this point of view. It found that 79 percent of respondents said they would want to know if they had AD, and 65 percent would want their spouse to be told if the spouse had the disease.[306] Having the opportunity to do advance and financial planning, to settle family matters, and to get a second opinion were the major reasons cited for wanting to know the diagnosis. Because the subjects were not patients undergoing evaluation for AD, it remains unknown whether they would respond similarly if actually faced with this situation.

Arguing against disclosure has been the uncertainty of the diagnosis, the perceived paucity of therapeutic options, and the fear that the stress of the diagnosis may exacerbate the patient's symptoms. The uncertainty of the diagnosis no longer appears tenable, because antemortem diagnosis of dementia has become increasingly sophisticated. Clinical classification of AD may be 80–90 percent accurate when compared to neuropathological evidence,[37] and there is now a considerable literature contrasting the different dementias. Regarding therapeutic options, treatment is available in the form of psychological and psychosocial interventions, which provide significant reduction of excess disability and enhance the quality of life for both patient and family. In addition, pharmacological agents, although not curative, may be of help to some patients. Unless the diagnosis is discussed, it is difficult to utilize these interventions to maximum effect. The fear that stress caused by knowing the diagnosis may be damaging to the patient deserves consideration. Although the majority of respondents to a survey indicated that they would want to know if they had AD, about 11 percent said they would not want to know, and 2.5 percent would want to know if they had AD so that they could consider suicide.[306] These are complex issues in need of future study. Should not wanting to know the diagnosis be accepted at face value, or treated as denial? What is the rate of suicide upon receiving a poor medical prognosis? Currently many patients are aware of the public debate about assisted suicide, and may reasonably wonder whether this is an alternative they should consider.

The author takes the position that the benefits of frankness in disclosing the diagnosis outweigh the disadvantages. It is generally in the patient's best interest, facilitating adaptation to disability while promoting both self-determination and confidence in the healthcare provider. The diagnosis is best presented by a professional who has established a relationship with the patient, and to whom the patient can turn for follow-up care. Family members should be present for support. If a patient indicates that he or she does not want to know the diagnosis, the reasons should be discussed, with exploration of both pros and cons. In the end the patient's wishes should be respected. Often the patient will allow family involvement, so that interventions to guarantee the patient's health and safety can be implemented anyway.

Clinical judgment regarding the patient's mental status should determine how the diagnosis is presented. If the patient is suicidal or otherwise acutely emotionally disturbed, it would be preferable to withhold the findings until he or she has been stabilized. If the patient is likely to have a less extreme but nonetheless adverse reaction to disclosure, caution should be used. For example, with a few very anxious or depressed patients it may be better to describe a degenerative disorder by using words such as "cognitive impairment," "memory disorder," or even "dementia," which are less alarming than "Alzheimer's disease." They can be told that their symptoms have to be followed in subsequent months to document progression. This allows work to proceed to address the patient's cognitive and emotional difficulties. At a later date, when the patient has become accustomed to the idea of having a disability, a treatment alliance has been formed and social supports are in place, the exact diagnosis can be presented. This strategy should be used sparingly, and deception should be avoided. In all cases the provider should be sensitive to the patient's anxiety about the information that is going to be disclosed, and attentive to his or her response.

Psychotherapy

Psychotherapy can help the dementing patient with the immediate tasks of adjusting to the diagnosis, and becoming engaged in planning for the future. Treatment necessarily includes a psychoeducational component. Thus the professional provides information about the diagnosis and the disease, and makes recommendations, while simultaneously responding to the patient's emotional reactions and mobilization of defenses. When the diagnosis is made early in the dementing process, or suspected preclinically, long-term psychotherapy is also feasible for some patients. Early intervention allows the professional to capitalize on the patient's remaining capacity for insight. Deeper psychodynamic exploration of the personality structure and defenses can help the patient come to terms with unresolved life conflicts. There is a complex interaction between internalized psychic structure and brain deterioration. For example, a chronic weak sense of self could contribute to some AD patients' difficulty in acknowledging the loss of capacity early on, as it might be too fearful to tolerate. It could also account for the agitation seen in some as they lose the capacity to hold themselves together.

Psychotherapy must be adapted to the stage of the disease.[307] With progression there is increased emphasis on loss of function. Having someone to discuss this with is reassuring to the patient and can lead to better coping with deficits. The psychologist may have to be empathic in verbalizing the patient's feelings as self-expression diminishes. Still later, reality testing may become compromised, with evidence of delusions or hallucinations. Knowing that certain experiences are merely the product of a difficulty in interpreting reality can reduce a patient's anxiety. For example, one patient stated that he knew that the bomb next to his bed was probably not real; instead of becoming agitated and trying to flee the bedroom, he turned over and went back to sleep. Psychopharmacological intervention becomes increasingly helpful in this stage of the disorder, although drug holidays are necessary to identify when medication can be discontinued.

Some aspects of family psychoeducational treatment developed for mental illness[308] can be adapted for use with the families of patients with dementia. Examining how family members react to the patient's symptoms can help to manage stresses of caregiving and minimize family burden. The professional also serves an important educational function. What is dementia? What tests were done and what did they show? What are the implications for the future? Will the patient have to go to a nursing home? Will the disease be inherited by family members? These questions are commonly raised by families and can be addressed in this context. Structured recommendations regarding future planning and use of respite or home aides can also be made and clarified. Providing continuity of care is critical so that the family feels supported and knows where to turn for help. Given the multiple needs of the patient with dementia, the establishment of a treatment team is helpful in ensuring that the patient receives comprehensive care. Even when professionals are in private practice, they can establish relationships with healthcare providers in other disciplines who, through consultations and referrals, serve as a team. Connecting family members with a support network (e.g. psychotherapy groups, social agencies) helps to reduce isolation and the sense they often have of enduring difficult times alone.[309]

Dementia bears some similarity to chronic mental illness, and some of the concepts developed in the latter may put the disorder into perspective for the healthcare provider. In one view,[310] families must adapt to chronic mental illness in three primary areas: interpersonal, instrumental, and life course. Interpersonally, many feelings are aroused in family members toward the patient: they may express anger at the patient's behavior, thinking that he or she could perform normally if he or she tried harder. Their anger may be exacerbated by feeling frustrated and let down by a healthcare system that often fails to diagnose dementia adequately, or to provide adequate support. The psychologist can address family anger by clarifying that the patient is functioning as best he or she can, which may require providing concrete evidence of organic dysfunction in the form of test results. Another emotional strain commonly encountered in families when the disease progresses is mourning the loss of the person they knew. Because patients often remain physically healthy while their personality disintegrates under the onslaught of the disease process, families may not readily become aware of their own sense of loss and the emotions that accompany it. The psychologist can bring this feeling into awareness and help the family deal with their grief.

Instrumentally, the family must adapt to behavioral problems. A major source of burden to dementia care-givers is the patient's daily difficulty in functioning (e.g. losing things, inability to get dressed), and problem behaviors (e.g. wandering, combativeness). The psychologist can make practical suggestions about how to deal with these, while at the same time exploring aspects of the care-giver's circumstances or personality that make certain behaviors particularly difficult to cope with. Finally, life-course issues are raised because patients can live for many years with a dementia. A common pattern is for a close family member to become completely consumed by the caregiving task. With support and planning the disease process can become better integrated into family life so that it does not demand the end of a normal existence for this person. Family treatment can explore family resources, build a sense of perspective with regard to the disease, and engender optimism in family members who may have felt that they were unable to continue.

REFERENCES

1. Evans DA, Fukenstein HH, Albert MS et al: Prevalence of Alzheimer's disease in a community population of older persons. JAMA 1989;262(18):2551–2592
2. Hachinski V: Vascular dementia: a radical redefinition. Dementia 1994;5:130–132
3. American Psychiatric Association: Diagnostic and Statistical Manual of Mental Disorders, 4th Ed. American Psychiatric Association, Washington, DC, 1994
4. Knopman DS, DeKosky ST, Cummings JL et al: Practice parameter: Diagnosis of dementia (an evidence-based review). Neurology 2001;56(9):1143–1153
5. Sachdev P: Is it time to retire the term "dementia"? J Neuropsych Clin Neurosci 2000;12(2):276–279
6. White RF: Clinical Syndromes in Adult Neuropsychology: The Practitioner's Handbook. Elsevier Science Publishers, 1992
7. Shock NW, Greulich RC, Costa PT: Normal Human Aging: the Baltimore Longitudinal Study of Aging. NIH publication No. 84-2450, Department of Health and Human Services, Rockville, MD, 1984
8. Schaie KW: The optimization of cognitive functioning in old age: predictions based on cohort-sequential and longitudinal data. In Baltes PB (ed): Successful Aging. Cambridge University Press, Cambridge, 1990:94–117
9. Salthouse T: Age-related changes in basic cognitive processes. In Storandt M, VandenBos G (eds): The adult years: continuity and change. American Psychological Association, Washington, DC, 1989:5–40
10. Schaie KW: Intellectual development in adulthood. In Birren JE, Schaie KW (eds): Handbook of the Psychology of Aging. Academic Press, San Diego, 1996:266–286
11. Naugle R, Cullum CM, Bigler ED: Evaluation of intellectual and memory function among dementia patients who were intellectually superior. Clin Neuropsychol 1990;4(4):355–374
12. Storandt M, Hill RD: Very mild senile dementia of the Alzheimer type: II. Psychometric test performance. Arch Neurol 1989;46:383–386
13. Storandt M, Stone K, LaBarge E: Deficits in reading performance in very mild dementia of the Alzheimer type. Neuropsychology 1995;9:174–176
14. Patterson KE, Graham N, Hodges JR: Reading in dementia of the Alzheimer type: A preserved ability? Neuropsychology 1994;8:395–407
15. McKeith IG, Perry RH, Fairbairn AF, Jabeen S, Perry EK: Operational criteria for senile dementia of Lewy body type (SDLT). Psychol Med 1992;22:911–922
16. Brun A, Englund B, Gustafson L et al: Clinical and neuropathological criteria for frontotemporal dementia. J Neurol Neurosurg Psychiatry 1994;57:416–418

> ## KEY POINTS   Psychology in the diagnosis and treatment of the dementias
>
> - The neuropsychological profile can help in the differential diagnosis of the dementias by characterizing the nature and extent of cognitive impairment in several cognitive domains, including attention and orientation, learning and memory, language, motor, visuospatial, and executive abilities.
> - Dementia is a global cognitive decline (in memory and at least one other cognitive skill) which interferes with social or occupational functioning.
> - Impaired episodic memory is the hallmark of Alzheimer's disease, and occurs early in the dementing process.
> - In vascular dementia, executive dysfunction is prominent and may be out of proportion to memory loss.
> - Dementia with Lewy bodies shows a frontal-subcortical pattern of deficits, with impaired attention, working memory, and visuospatial skills; psychotic features or parkinsonism may appear early, and the course is fluctuating.
> - Frontotemporal dementia (FTD) consists of three syndromes: frontal variant FTD, semantic dementia, and progressive nonfluent aphasia, which are related to the distribution of neuropathology in frontal and anterior temporal lobes.
> - In severe depression there can be global abasement of cognitive functioning, but generally not as much as in Alzheimer's disease.
> - Early detection of dementia is important because treatments are available, including medication, and psychological and psychosocial interventions, that can have a significant impact on the well-being of patients and their families.
> - The benefits of frankness in disclosing the diagnosis to the patient and family outweigh the disadvantages.

17. Kosaka K, Yoshimura M, Ikeda K, Budka H: Diffuse type of Lewy body disease: progressive dementia with abundant cortical Lewy bodies and senile changes of varying degree—a new disease? Clin Neuropathol 1984;3:185–192

18. Olichney JM, Galasko D, Corey-Bloom J, Thal LJ: The spectrum of diseases with diffuse Lewy bodies. Adv Neurol 1995;65:159–170

19. Leverenz J, Sumi S: Parkinson's disease in patients with Alzheimer's disease. Arch Neurol 1986;43:662–664

20. Baddeley A: The concept of working memory: A view of its current state and probable future development. Cognition 1981;10(1–3):17–23

21. Schacter DL: Implicit memory: History and current status. J Exp Psychol Learn Mem Cognit 1987;13(3):501–518

22. Tulving E: How many memory systems are there? Am Psychol 1985;40(4):385–398

23. Tulving E: Precis of elements of episodic memory. Behav Brain Sci 1984;7(2):223–268

24. Butters N, Delis DC, Lucas JA: Clinical assessment of memory disorders in amnesia and dementia. Annu Rev Psychol 1995;46:493–523

25. Morris RG, Kopelman MD: The memory deficits in Alzheimer-type dementia: A review. Special Issue: Human memory. Q J Exp Psychol 1986;38A:575–602

26. Gainotti G, Marra C: Progress and controversies in neuropsychology of memory. Second Congress of the Pan European Society of Neurology (1991, Vienna, Austria). Acta Neurol 1992;14:561–577

27. McKhann G, Drachman D, Folstein M et al: Clinical diagnosis of Alzheimer's disease: report of the NINCDS-ADRDA Work Group under the auspices of Department of Health and Human Services Task Force on Alzheimer's disease. Neurology 1984;34:939–944

28. Roman GC, Tatemichi TK, Erkinjuntti T et al: Vascular dementia: Diagnostic criteria for research studies: Report of the NINDS-AIREN International Workshop. Neurology 1993;43(2):250–260

29. Kumar A, Gottlieb G: Frontotemporal dementias: A new clinical syndrome? Am J Geriatr Psychiatry 1993;1(2):95–107

30. Bondi MW, Monsch AU, Galasko D et al: Preclinical cognitive markers of dementia of the Alzheimer type. Neuropsychology 1994;8:374–384

31. Chen P, Ratcliff G, Belle SH et al: Cognitive tests that best discriminate between presymptomatic AD and those who remain nondemented. Neurology 2000;55(12):1847–1853

32. Albert ML: The 'subcortical dementia' of progressive supranuclear palsy. J Neurol Neurosurg Psychiatry 1974;37:121–130

33. Cummings JL: Vascular subcortical dementias: Clinical aspects. Special Issue: Vascular dementia: Etiological, pathogenetic, clinical and treatment aspects. Dementia 1994;5:177–180

34. Gregory CA, Hodges JR: Dementia of frontal type and the focal lobar atrophies. Int Rev Psychiatry 1993;5(4):397–406

35. Gustafson L: Frontal lobe degeneration of non-Alzheimer type: II. Clinical picture and differential diagnosis. Eric K. Fernstrom Foundation Symposium: Frontal lobe degeneration of non-Alzheimer type (1986, Lund, Sweden). Arch Gerontol Geriatr 1987;6(3):209–223

36. Larson EB, Reifler BV, Sumi SM, Canfield CG, Chinn NM: Diagnostic tests in the evaluation of dementia. A prospective study of 200 elderly outpatients. Arch Intern Med 1986;146:1917–1922

37. Tierney MC, Fisher RH, Lewis AJ et al: The NINCDS:ADRDA Work Group criteria for the clinical diagnosis of probable Alzheimer's disease: A clinicopathologic study of 57 cases. Neurology 1988;38:359–364

38. Lopez OL, Litvan I, Catt KE et al: Accuracy of four clinical diagnostic criteria for the diagnosis of neurodegenerative dementias. Neurology 1999;53(6):1292–1299

39. Tierney MC, Nores A, Snow WG et al: Use of the Rey Auditory Verbal Learning Test in differentiating normal aging from Alzheimer's and Parkinson's dementia. Psychol Assess 1994;6(2):129–134

40. Incalzi RA, Capparella O, Gemma A et al: Effects of aging and of Alzheimer's disease on verbal memory. J Clin Exp Neuropsychol 1995;17:580–589

41. Pillon B, Deweer B, Agid Y, Dubois B: Explicit memory in Alzheimer's, Huntington's, and Parkinson's diseases. Arch Neurol 1993;50:374–379

42. Moss MB, Albert MS, Butters N, Payne M: Differential patterns of memory loss among patients with Alzheimer's disease, Huntington's disease, and alcoholic Korsakoff's syndrome. Arch Neurol 1986;43:239–246

43. Welsh K, Butters N, Hughes J, Mohs R, Heyman A: Detection of abnormal memory decline in mild cases of Alzheimer's disease using CERAD neuropsychological measures. Arch Neurol 1991;48(3):278–281

44. Knopman DS, Ryberg S: A verbal memory test with high predictive accuracy for dementia of the Alzheimer type. Arch Neurol 1989;46:141–145

45. Carlesimo GA, Sabbadini M, Fadda L, Caltagirone C: Forgetting from long-term memory in dementia and pure amnesia: Role of task, delay of assessment and aetiology of cerebral damage. Cortex 1995;31:285–300

46. Gainotti G, Marra C: Some aspects of memory disorders clearly distinguish dementia of the Alzheimer's type from depressive pseudo-dementia. J Clin Exp Neuropsychol 1994;16(1):65–78

47. Villardita C: Alzheimer's disease compared with cerebrovascular dementia. Neuropsychological similarities and differences. Acta Neurol Scand 1993;87:299–308

48. Mitrushina M, Drebing C, Uchiyama C et al: The pattern of deficit in different memory components in normal aging and dementia of Alzheimer's type. J Clin Psychol 1994;50:591–596

49. Hodges JR, Patterson K: Is semantic memory consistently impaired early in the course of Alzheimer's disease? Neuroanatomical and diagnostic implications. Neuropsychologia 1995;33:441–459

50. Greene JDW, Baddeley AD, Hodges JR: Analysis of the episodic memory deficit in early Alzheimer's disease: Evidence from the doors and people test. Neuropsychologia 1996;34(6):537–551

51. LeMoal S, Reymann JM, Thomas V et al: Effect of normal aging and of Alzheimer's disease on episodic memory. Dement Geriatr Cognit Disord 1997;8(5):281–287

52. Brown LB, Storandt M: Sensitivity of category cued recall to very mild dementia of the Alzheimer's type. Arch Clin Neuropsychol 2000;15:529–534

53. Baeckman L, Small BJ: Influences of cognitive support on episodic remembering: Tracing the process of loss from normal aging to Alzheimer's disease. Psychol Aging 1998;13(2):267–276

54. Larrabee GJ, Youngjohn JR, Sudilovsky A, Crook TH: Accelerated forgetting in Alzheimer-type dementia. J Clin Exp Neuropsychol 1993;15(5):701–712

55. Mitrushina M, Satz P, Drebing CE et al: The differential pattern of memory deficit in normal aging and dementias of different etiology. J Clin Psychol 1994;50:246–252

56. Simon E, Leach L, Winocur G et al: Intact primary memory in mild to moderate Alzheimer disease: Indices from the California Verbal Learning Test. J Clin Exp Neuropsychol 1994;16(3):414–422

57. Pollmann S, Haupt M, Romero B, Kurz A: Is impaired recall in dementia of the Alzheimer type a consequence of a contextual retrieval deficit? 36th Annual Meeting of the German Society of Neuropathology and Neuroanatomy (1991, Dusseldorf, Germany). Dementia 1993;4:102–108

58. Diesfeldt HF: Recognition memory for words and faces in primary degenerative dementia of the Alzheimer type and normal old age. J Clin Exp Neuropsychol 1990;12:931–945

59. Pillon B, Dubois B, Lhermitte F, Agid Y: Heterogeneity of cognitive impairment in progressive supranuclear palsy, Parkinson's disease, and Alzheimer's disease. Neurology 1986;36:1179–1185

60. Cullum CM, Butters N, Troster AI, Salmon DP: Normal aging and forgetting rates on the Wechsler Memory Scale—Revised. Arch Clin Neuropsychol 1990;5(1):23–30

61. Butters N, Salmon DP, Cullum CM et al: Differentiation of amnesic and demented patients with the Wechsler Memory Scale—Revised. Special Issue: Initial validity studies of the new Wechsler Memory Scale—Revised. Clin Neuropsychol 1988;2:133–148

62. Troester A, Butters N, Salmon DP et al: The diagnostic utility of savings scores: Differentiating Alzheimer's and Huntington's diseases with logical memory and visual reproduction tests. J Clin Exp Neuropsychol 1993;15(5):773–788

63. van der Hurk PR, Hodges JR: Episodic and semantic memory in Alzheimer's disease and progressive supranuclear palsy: A comparative study. J Clin Exp Neuropsychol 1995;17(3):459–471

64. Becker JT, Boller F, Saxton J, McGonigle Gibson KL: Normal rates of forgetting of verbal and non-verbal material in Alzheimer's disease. Cortex 1987;23(1):59–72

65. Swainson R, Hodges JR, Galton CJ et al: Early detection and differential diagnosis of Alzheimer's disease and depression with neuropsychological tasks. Dement Geriatr Cognit Disord 2001;12(4):265–280

66. Duchek JM, Cheney M, Ferraro FR, Storandt M: Paired associate learning in senile dementia of the Alzheimer type. Arch Neurol 1991;48:1038–1040

67. Baeckman L, Hassing L, Forsell Y, Viitanen M: Episodic remembering in a population-based sample of nonagenarians: Does major depression

exacerbate the memory deficits seen in Alzheimer's disease? Psychol Aging 1996;11(4):649–657

68. Bemelmans KJ, Goekoop JG: The contribution of list length to the absence of the primacy effect in word recall in dementia of the Alzheimer type. Psychol Med 1991;21(4):1047–1050

69. Morris RG, Baddeley AD: Primary and working memory functioning in Alzheimer-type dementia. J Clin Exp Neuropsychol 1988;10:279–296

70. Hassing L, Baeckman L: Episodic memory functioning in population-based samples of very old adults with Alzheimer's disease and vascular dementia. Dement Geriatr Cognit Disord 1997;8(6):376–383

71. Pepin EP, Eslinger PJ: Verbal memory decline in Alzheimer's disease: A multiple-processes deficit. Neurology 1989;39:1477–1482

72. Jacobs D, Salmon DP, Troster AI, Butters N: Intrusion errors in the figural memory of patients with Alzheimer's and Huntington's disease. Arch Clin Neuropsychol 1990;5:49–57

73. Huppert FA, Kopelman MD: Rates of forgetting in normal ageing: A comparison with dementia. Neuropsychologia 1989;27(6):849–860

74. Kopelman MD: Multiple memory deficits in Alzheimer-type dementia: Implications for pharmacotherapy. Psychol Med 1985;15:527–541

75. Freed DM, Corkin S, Growdon JH, Nissen MJ: Selective attention in Alzheimer's disease: Characterizing cognitive subgroups of patients. Neuropsychologia 1989;27(3):325–339

76. Robinson-Whelen S: Benton Visual Retention Test performance among normal and demented older adults. Neuropsychology 1992;6:261–269

77. Hart RP, Kwentus JA, Taylor JR, Harkins SW: Rate of forgetting in dementia and depression. J Consult Clin Psychol 1987;55(1):101–105

78. Lemesle B, Puel M, Demonet JF, Cardebat D: Implicit and explicit memory for faces in dementia of Alzheimer's type. Brain Cognit 1998;37(1):83–85

79. Martin A, Fedio P: Word production and comprehension in Alzheimer's disease: the breakdown of semantic knowledge. Brain Language 1983;19:124–141

80. Bayles KA, Trosset MW, Tomoeda CK, Montgomery EB, Wilson J: Generative naming in Parkinson disease patients. J Clin Exp Neuropsychol 1993;15:547–562

81. Randolph C, Braun AR, Goldberg TE, Chase TN: Semantic fluency in Alzheimer's, Parkinson's, and Huntington's disease: dissociation of storage and retrieval failures. Neuropsychology 1993;7:82–88

82. Mickanin J, Grossman M, Onishi K, Auriacombe S, Clark C: Verbal and nonverbal fluency in patients with probable Alzheimer's disease. Neuropsychology 1994;8:385–394

83. Monsch AU, Bondi MW, Butters N et al: A comparison of category and letter fluency in Alzheimer's disease and Huntington's disease. Neuropsychology 1994;8:25–30

84. Hodges JR, Patterson K, Graham N, Dawson K: Naming and knowing in dementia of Alzheimer's type. Brain Language 1996;54(2):302–325

85. Beatty WW, Testa JA, English S, Winn P: Influences of clustering and switching on the verbal fluency performance of patients with Alzheimer's disease. Aging Neuropsychol Cognit 1997;4(4):273–279

86. Beatty WW, Salmon DP, Testa JA, Hanisch C, Troester AI: Monitoring the changing status of semantic memory in Alzheimer's disease: An evaluation of several process measures. Aging Neuropsychol Cognit 2000;7(2):94–111

87. Carew TG, Lamar M, Cloud BS et al: Impairment in category fluency in ischemic vascular dementia. Neuropsychology 1997;11(3):400–412

88. Crossley M, D'Arcy C, Rawson NSB: Letter and category fluency in community-dwelling Canadian seniors: A comparison of normal participants to those with dementia of the Alzheimer or vascular type. J Clin Exp Neuropsychol 1997;19(1):52–62

89. Bentham PW, Jones S, Hodges JR: A comparison of semantic memory in vascular dementia and dementia of Alzheimer's type. Int J Geriatr Psychiatry 1997;12(5):575–580

90. Gainotti G, Marra C, Villa G: A double dissociation between accuracy and time of execution on attentional tasks in Alzheimer's disease and multi-infarct dementia. Brain 2001;124(4):731–738

91. Monsch AU, Bondi MW, Butters N et al: Comparisons of verbal fluency tasks in the detection of dementia of the Alzheimer type. Neurology 1992;49:1253–1258

92. Cahn DA, Salmon DP, Butters N et al: Detection of dementia of the Alzheimer type in a population-based sample: Neuropsychological test performance. J Int Neuropsychol Soc 1995;1:252–260

93. Weingartner HJ, Kawas C, Rawlings R, Shapiro M: Changes in semantic memory in early stage Alzheimer's disease patients. Gerontologist 1993;33:637–643

94. Binetti G, Magni E, Cappa SF et al: Semantic memory in Alzheimer's disease: an analysis of category fluency. Neuropsychology 1995;17:82–89

95. Troester AI, Fields JA, Testa JA et al: Cortical and subcortical influences on clustering and switching in the performance of verbal fluency tasks. Neuropsychologia 1998;36(4):295–304

96. Rohrer D, Salmon DP, Wixted JT, Paulsen JS: The disparate effects of Alzheimer's disease and Huntington's disease on semantic memory. Neuropsychology 1999;13(3):381–388

97. Salmon DP, Heindel WC, Lange KL: Differential decline in word generation from phonemic and semantic categories during the course of Alzheimer's disease: Implications for the integrity of semantic memory. J Int Neuropsychol Soc 1999;5(7):692–703

98. Lipinska B, Baeckman L: Encoding-retrieval interactions in mild Alzheimer's disease; The role of access to categorical information. Brain Cognit 1997;34(2):274–286

99. Daum I, Riesch G, Sartori G, Birbaumer N: Semantic memory impairment in Alzheimer's disease. J Clin Exp Neuropsychol 1996;18(5):648–665

100. Nebes RD: Semantic memory in Alzheimer's disease. Psychol Bull 1989;106:377–394

101. Grossman M, Robinson K, Biassou N, White-Devine T, D'Esposito M: Semantic memory in Alzheimer's disease: Representativeness, ontologic category, and material. Neuropsychology 1998;12(1):34–42

102. Knotek PC, Bayles KA, Kaszniak AW: Response consistency on a semantic memory task in persons with dementia of the Alzheimer type. Brain Language 1990;38:465–475

103. Crowe SF, Dingjan P, Helme RD: The neurocognitive basis of word-finding difficulty in Alzheimer's disease. Austr Psychol 1997;32(2):114–119

104. Bayles KA, Tomoeda CK, Cruz RF: Performance of Alzheimer's disease patients in judging word relatedness. J Int Neuropsychol Soc 1999;5(7):668–675

105. Abeysinghe SC, Bayles KA, Trosset MW: Semantic memory deterioration in Alzheimer's subjects: Evidence from word association, definition, and associate ranking tasks. J Speech Hear Res 1990;33:574–582

106. Grossman M, Mickanin J, Robinson KM, D'Esposito M: Anomaly judgments of subject-predicate relations in Alzheimer's disease. Brain Language 1996;54(2):216–232

107. Sailor KM, Bramwell A, Griesing TA: Evidence for an impaired ability to determine semantic relations in Alzheimer's disease patients. Neuropsychology 1998;12(4):555–564

108. Norton LE, Bondi MW, Salmon DP, Goodglass H: Deterioration of generic knowledge in patients with Alzheimer's disease: Evidence from the Number Information Test. J Clin Exp Neuropsychol 1997;19(6):857–866

109. Salmon DP, Butters N, Chan AS: The deterioration of semantic memory in Alzheimer's disease. Can J Exp Psychol 1999;53(1):108–116

110. Hodges JR, Salmon D, Butters N: Recognition and naming of famous faces in Alzheimer's disease: a cognitive analysis. Neuropsychologia 1993;31:775–788

111. Greene JDW, Hodges JR: The fractionation of remote memory: Evidence from a longitudinal study of dementia of Alzheimer type. Brain 1996;119(Pt):129–142

112. Dorrego MF, Sabe L, Cuerva AG et al: Remote memory in Alzheimer's disease. J Neuropsych Clin Neurosci 1999;11(4):490–497

113. Fama R, Sullivan EV, Shear PK et al: Extent, pattern, and correlates of remote memory impairment in Alzheimer's disease and Parkinson's disease. Neuropsychology 2000;14(2):265–276

114. Leplow B, Dierks C, Herrmann P et al: Remote memory in Parkinson's disease and senile dementia. Neuropsychologia 1997;35(4):547–557

115. Wilson RS, Kaszniak AW, Fox JH: Remote memory in senile dementia. Cortex 1981;17:41–48

116. Storandt M, Kaskie B, Von Dras DD: Temporal memory for remote events in healthy aging and dementia. Psychol Aging 1998;13(1):4–7

117. Kopelman MD: Remote and autobiographical memory, temporal context memory, and frontal atrophy in Korsakoff and Alzheimer patients. Neuropsychologia 1989;27:437–460

118. Sagar HJ, Cohen NJ, Sullivan EV, Corkin S, Growdon JH: Remote memory function in Alzheimer's disease and Parkinson's disease. Brain 1988;111:185–206

119. Dall'Ora P, Della Sala S, Spinnler H: Autobiographical memory. Its impairment in amnesic syndromes. Cortex 1989;25:197–217

120. Greene JDW, J.R. H, Baddeley A: Autobiographical memory and executive function in early dementia of Alzheimer type. Neuropsychologia 1995;33:1647–1670

121. Fromholt P, Larsen P, Larsen SF: Effects of late-onset depression and recovery on autobiographical memory. J Gerontol 1995;50B:P74–P81

122. Kazui H, Hashimoto M, Hirono N et al: A study of remote memory impairment in Alzheimer's disease by using the Family Line Test. Dement Geriatr Cognit Disord 2000;11(1):53–58

123. Beatty WW, Salmon DP: Remote memory for visuospatial information in patients with Alzheimer's disease. J Geriatr Psychiatry Neurol 1991;4:14–17

124. Fromholt P, Larsen SF: Autobiographical memory in normal aging and primary degenerative dementia (dementia of Alzheimer type). J Gerontol 1991;46:P85–P91

125. Baddeley A, Logie R, Bressi S, Sala SD, Spinnler H: Dementia and working memory. Special Issue: Human memory. Q J Exp Psychol 1986;38A:603–618

126. Morris RG: Working memory in Alzheimer-type dementia. Special Section: Working memory. Neuropsychology 1994;8:544–554

127. Freeman RQ, Giovannetti T, Lamar M et al: Visuoconstructional problems in dementia: Contribution of executive systems functions. Neuropsychology 2000;14(3):415–426

128. Reichman WE, Cummings JL, McDaniel KD, Flynn FG, Gornbein J: Visuoconstructional impairment in dementia syndromes. Behav Neurol 1991;4:153–162

129. Henderson VC, Mack W, Williams BW: Spatial disorientation in Alzheimer's disease. Arch Neurology 1989;46:391–394

130. de Leon MJ, Potegal M, Gurland B: Wandering and parietal signs in senile dementia of Alzheimer's type. Neuropsychobiology 1984;11:155–157

131. Carlomagno S, Iavarone A, Nolfe G, Bourene G, Martin C, Deloche G: Dyscalculia in the early stages of Alzheimer's disease. Acta Neurol Scand 1999;99:166–174

132. Deloche G, Hannequin D, Carlomagno S et al: Calculation and number processing in mild Alzheimer's disease. J Clin Exp Neuropsychol 1995;17:634–639

133. Duke LM, Kaszniak AW: Executive control functions in degenerative dementias: A comparative review. Neuropsychol Rev 2000;10(2):75–99

134. Lafleche G, Albert MS: Executive function deficits in mild Alzheimer's disease. Neuropsychology 1995;9:313–320

135. Bhutani GE, Montaldi D, Brooks DN, McCulloch J: A neuropsychological investigation into frontal lobe involvement in dementia of the Alzheimer type. Neuropsychology 1992;6:211–224

136. Collette F, Van der Linden M, Salmon E: Executive dysfunction in Alzheimer's disease. Cortex 1999;35(1):57–72

137. Dalla Barba G, Nedjam Z, Dubois B: Confabulation, executive functions, and source memory in Alzheimer's disease. Cognit Neuropsychol 1999;16(3–5):385–398

138. Perry RJ, Hodges JR: Attention and executive deficits in Alzheimer's disease: A critical review. Brain 1999;122(3):383–404

139. Lines CR, Dawson C, Preston GC et al: Memory and attention in patients with senile dementia of the Alzheimer type and in normal elderly subjects. J Clin Exp Neuropsychol 1991;13(5):691–702

140. Perry RJ, Watson P, Hodges JR: The nature and staging of attention dysfunction in early (minimal and mild) Alzheimer's disease: Relationship to episodic and semantic memory impairment. Neuropsychologia 2000;38(3):252–271

141. Welsh K, Butters N, Hughes JP, Mohs RC, Heyman A: Detection and staging of dementia in Alzheimer's disease: Use of the neuropsychological measures developed for the Consortium to Establish a Registry for Alzheimer's disease. Arch Neurol 1992;49:448–452

142. Storandt M, Botwinick J, Danzinger WL, Berg L, Hughes C: Psychometric differentiation of mild senile dementia of the Alzheimer type. Arch Neurol 1984;41:497–499

143. Eslinger PJ, Damasio AR, Benton AL, Van Allen M: Neuropsychologic detection of abnormal mental decline in older persons. JAMA 1985;253:670–674

144. Masur DM, Sliwinski M, Lipton RB, Blau AD, Crystal HA: Neuropsychological prediction of dementia and the absence of dementia in healthy elderly persons. Neurology 1994;44:1427–1432

145. Small BJ, Herlitz A, Fratiglioni L, Almkvist O, Bäckman L: Cognitive predictors of incident Alzheimer's disease: A prospective longitudinal study. Neuropsychology 1997;11(3):413–420

146. Nielsen H, Lolk A, Andersen K, Andersen J, Kragh-Sorensen P: Characteristics of elderly who develop Alzheimer's disease during the next two years—A neuropsychological study using CAMCOG: The Odense Study. Int J Geriatr Psychiatry 1999;14(11):957–963

147. Loeb C, Meyer J: Vascular dementia: still a debatable entity? J Neurol Sci 1996;143:31–40

148. Gold G, Giannakopoulos P, Montes-Paixco JC: Sensitivity and specificity of newly proposed clinical criteria for possible vascular dementia. Neurology 1997;49:690–694

149. Wolfe N, Linn R, Babikian VL, Knoefel JE, Albert ML: Frontal systems impairment following multiple lacunar infarcts. Arch Neurol 1990;47:129–132

150. Mahler ME, Cummings JL: Behavioral neurology of multi-infarct dementia. Special Issue: Dementia. Alzheimer Dis Assoc Disord 1991;5:122–130

151. Emery VO, Gillie EX, Ramdev PT: Noninfarct vascular dementia: A new subtype. J Clin Geropsychol 1996;2(3):197–213

152. Bowler JV, Steenhuis R, Hachinski V: Conceptual background to vascular cognitive impairment. Alzheimer Dis Assoc Disord 1999;13(suppl 3):S30–S37

153. Holmes C, Cairns N, Lantos P et al: Validity of current clinical criteria for Alzheimer's disease, vascular dementia and dementia with Lewy bodies. Br J Psychiatry 1999;174:45–50

154. Chui HC, Victoroff JI, Margolin D et al: Criteria for the diagnosis of ischemic vascular dementia proposed by the State of California Alzheimer disease Diagnostic and Treatment Centers. Neurology 1992;42:473–480

155. Rockwood K, Howard K, MacKnight C, Darvesh S: Spectrum of disease in vascular cognitive impairment. Neuroepidemiology 1999;18(5):248–254

156. Batchelder WH, Chosak-Reiter J, Shankle WR, Dick MB: A multinomial modeling analysis of memory deficits in Alzheimer's disease and vascular dementia. J Gerontol B Psychol Sci Social Sci 1997;5:206

157. Gainotti G, Parlato V, Monteleone D, Carlomagno S: Neuropsychological markers of dementia on visual-spatial tasks: a comparison between Alzheimer's type and vascular forms of dementia. J Clin Exp Neuropsychol 1992;14(2):239–252

158. Mendez MF, Ashla Mendez M: Differences between multi-infarct dementia and Alzheimer's disease on unstructured neuropsychological tasks. J Clin Exp Neuropsychol 1991;13(6):923–932

159. Tei H, Miyazaki A, Iwata M et al: Early-stage Alzheimer's disease and multiple subcortical infarction with mild cognitive impairment: Neuropsychological comparison using an easily applicable test battery. Dement Geriatr Cognit Disord 1997;8(6):355–358

160. Zimmer NA, Hayden S, Deidan C, Lowenstein DA: Comparative performance of mildly impaired patients with Alzheimer's disease and multiple cerebral infarctions on tests of memory and functional capacity. Int Psychogeriatr 1994;6(2):143–154

161. Shapiro AM, Benedict RHB, Schretlen D, Brandt J: Construct and concurrent validity of the Hopkins Verbal Learning Test—Revised. Clin Neuropsychol 1999;13(3):348–358

162. Vanderploeg RD, Yuspeh RL, Schinka JA: Differential episodic and semantic memory performance in Alzheimer's disease and vascular dementias. J Int Neuropsychol Soc 2001;7(5):563–573

163. Libon DJ, Swenson RA, Malamut BL et al: Periventricular white matter alterations, dementia, and Binswanger's disease. Dev Neuropsychol 1993;9(2):87–102

164. Libon DJ, Bogdanoff B, Bonavita J et al: Dementia associated with periventricular and deep white matter alterations: A subtype of subcortical dementia. Arch Clin Neuropsychol 1997;12(3):239–250

165. Lafosse JM, Reed BR, Mungas D et al: Fluency and memory differences between ischemic vascular dementia and Alzheimer's disease. Neuropsychology 1997;11(4):514–522

166. Bennett DA, Gilley DW, Lee S, Cochran EJ: White matter changes: neurobehavioral manifestations of Binswanger's disease and clinical correlates in Alzheimer's disease. Dementia 1994;5:148–152

167. Barr A, Benedict R, Tune L, Brandt J: Neuropsychological differentiation of Alzheimer's disease from vascular dementia. Int J Geriatr Psychiatry 1992;7:621–627

168. Almkvist O, Backman L, Basun H, Wahlund LO: Patterns of neuropsychological performance in Alzheimer's disease and vascular dementia. Cortex 1993;29:661–673

169. Ricker JH, Keenan PA, Jacobson MW: Visuoperceptual-spatial ability and visual memory in vascular dementia and dementia of the Alzheimer type. Neuropsychologia 1994;32(10):1287–1296

170. Laine M, Vuorinen E, Rinne JO: Picture naming deficits in vascular dementia and Alzheimer's disease. J Clin Exp Neuropsychol 1997;19(1):126–140

171. Lukatela K, Malloy P, Jenkins M, Cohen R: The naming deficit in early Alzheimer's and vascular dementia. Neuropsychology 1998;12(4):565–572

172. Grosse DA, Gilley DW, Bernard BA, Wilson RS, Bennett DA: Semantic and episodic memory in Binswanger's versus Alzheimer's disease. J Clin Exp Neuropsychol 1991;13:70

173. Carlesimo GA, Fadda L, Lorusso S, Caltagirone C: Verbal and spatial memory spans in Alzheimer's and multi-infarct dementia. Acta Neurol Scand 1994;89:132–138

174. Libon DJ, Malamut BL, Swenson R, Sands LP, Cloud BS: Further analyses of clock drawings among demented and nondemented older subjects. Arch Clin Neuropsychol 1996;11(3):193–205

175. Erkinjuntti T, Laaksonen R, Sulkava R, Syrjalainen R, Palo J: Neuropsychological differentiation between normal aging, Alzheimer's disease and vascular dementia. Acta Neurol Scand 1986;74:393–403

176. Powell AL, Cummings JL, Hill MA, Benson DF: Speech and language alterations in multi-infarct dementia. Neurology 1988;38:717–719

177. Sultzer DL, Mahler ME, Cummings JL et al: Cortical abnormalities associated with subcortical lesions in vascular dementia. Arch Neurol 1995;52:773–780

178. Ishii N, Nishihara Y, Imamura T: Why do frontal lobe symptoms predominate in vascular dementia with lacunes? Neurology 1986;36:340–345

179. Lukatela K, Cohen RA, Kessler H et al: Dementia Rating Scale performance: A comparison of vascular and Alzheimer's dementia. J Clin Exp Neuropsychol 2000;22(4):445–454

180. Giovannetti T, Lamar M, Cloud BS et al: Different underlying mechanisms for deficits in concept formation in dementia. Arch Clin Neuropsychol 2001;16(6):547–560

181. Lamar M, Podell K, Carew TG et al: Perseverative behavior in Alzheimer's disease and subcortical ischemic vascular dementia. Neuropsychology 1997;11(4):523–534

182. Kertesz A, Clydesdale S: Neuropsychological deficits in vascular dementia vs Alzheimer's disease: Frontal lobe deficits prominent in vascular dementia. Arch Neurol 1994;51:1226–1231

183. Newman SC: The prevalence of depression in Alzheimer's disease and vascular dementia in a population sample. J Affect Disord 1999;52(1–3):169–176

184. Lyketsos CG, Steinberg M, Tschanz JT et al: Mental and behavioral disturbances in dementia: Findings from the Cache County Study on Memory in Aging. Am J Psychiatry 2000;157(5):708–714

185. Ballard C, Neill D, O'Brien J et al: Anxiety, depression and psychosis in vascular dementia: Prevalence and associations. J Affect Disord 2000;59(2):97–106

186. Sultzer DL, Levin HS, Mahler ME, High WM, Cummings JL: A comparison of psychiatric symptoms in vascular dementia and Alzheimer's disease. Am J Psychiatry 1993;150:1806–1812

187. Massman PJ, Delis DC, Butters N, Dupont RM, Gillin JC: The subcortical dysfunction hypothesis of memory deficits in depression: Neuropsychological validation in a subgroup of patients. J Clin Exp Neuropsychol 1992;14:687–706

188. Ballard C, Gray A, Ayre G: Psychotic symptoms, aggression and restlessness in dementia. Rev Neurol 1999;155(suppl 4):4S44–4S52

189. Aharon-Peretz J, Kliot D, Tomer R: Behavioral differences between white matter lacunar dementia and Alzheimer's disease: A comparison on the neuropsychiatric inventory. Dement Geriatr Cognit Disord 2000;11(5):294–298

190. Bernard BA, Wilson RS, Gilley DW et al: The dementia of Binswanger's disease and Alzheimer's disease. Neuropsych Neuropsychol Behav Neurol 1994;7:30–35

191. Looi JCL, Sachdev PS: Differentiation of vascular dementia from AD on neuropsychological tests. Neurology 1999;53(4):670–678

192. Filley CM: Neuropsychiatric features of Lewy body disease. Special Issue: Neuropsychological issues in Lewy body disease and related disorders. Brain Cognit 1995;28(3):229–239

193. McKeith IG, Fairbairn AF, Perry RH, Thompson P: The clinical diagnosis and misdiagnosis of senile dementia of Lewy body type (SDLT). Br J Psychiatr 1994;165(3):324–332

194. McKeith IG, Galasko D, Kosaka K et al: Consensus guidelines for the clinical and pathologic diagnosis of dementia with Lewy bodies (DLB): Report of the Consortium on DLB international workshop. Neurology 1996;47(5):1113–1124

195. Lopez OL, Hamilton RL, Becker JT et al: Severity of cognitive impairment and the clinical diagnosis of AD with Lewy bodies. Neurology 2000;54(9):1780–1787

196. Hansen L, Salmon D, Galasko D et al: The Lewy body variant of Alzheimer's disease: a clinical and pathologic entity. Neurology 1990;40:1–8

197. Burkhardt CR, Filley CM, Kleinschmidt-DeMasters BK et al: Diffuse Lewy body disease and progressive dementia. Neurology 1988;38:1520–1528

198. Byrne EJ, Lennox G, Lowe J, Godwin Austen RB: Diffuse Lewy body disease: Clinical features in 15 cases. J Neurol Neurosurg Psychiatry 1989;52(6):709–717

199. Calderon J, Perry RJ, Erzinclioglu SW et al: Perception, attention, and working memory are disproportionately impaired in dementia with Lewy bodies compared with Alzheimer's disease. J Neurol Neurosurg Psychiatry 2001;70(2):157–164

200. Shimomura T, Mori E, Yamashita H et al: Cognitive loss in dementia with Lewy bodies and Alzheimer disease. Arch Neurol 1998;55(12):1547–1552

201. Salmon DP, Galasko D, Hansen LA et al: Neuropsychological deficits associated with diffuse Lewy body disease. Brain Cognit 1996;31(2):148–165

202. Heyman A, Fillenbaum GG, Gearing M et al: Comparison of Lewy body variant of Alzheimer's disease with pure Alzheimer's disease: Consortium to establish a registry for Alzheimer's disease, part XIX. Neurology 1999;52(9):1839–1844

203. Ballard CG, Ayre G, O'Brien J et al: Simple standardised neuropsychological assessments aid in the differential diagnosis of dementia with Lewy bodies from Alzheimer's disease and vascular dementia. Dement Geriatr Cognit Disord 1999;10(2):104–108

204. Connor DJ, Salmon DP, Sandy TJ et al: Cognitive profiles of autopsy-confirmed Lewy body variant vs pure Alzheimer disease. Arch Neurol 1998;55(7):994–1000

205. Walker Z, Allen RL, Shergill S, Katona CLE: Neuropsychological performance in Lewy body dementia and Alzheimer's disease. Br J Psychiatr 1997;170(2):156–158

206. Galasko D, Katzman R, Salmon DP, Hansen L: Clinical and neuropatho-logical findings in Lewy body dementias. Brain Cognit 1996;31(2):166–175

207. Lambon Ralph MA, Powell J, Howard D et al: Semantic memory is impaired in both dementia with Lewy bodies and dementia of Alzheimer's type: A comparative neuropsychological study and literature review. J Neurol Neurosurg Psychiatry 2001;70(2):149–156

208. Galloway PH, Sahgal A, McKeith IG et al: Visual pattern recognition memory and learning deficits in senile dementias of Alzheimer and Lewy body types. Dementia 1992;3:101–107

209. Sahgal A, Galloway PH, McKeith IG et al: Matching-to-sample deficits in patients with senile dementias of the Alzheimer and Lewy body types. Arch Neurol 1992;49:1043–1046

210. Sahgal A, McKeith IG, Galloway PH, Tasker N, Steckler T: Do differences in visuospatial ability between senile dementias of the Alzheimer and Lewy body types reflect differences solely in mnemonic function? J Clin Exp Neuropsychol 1995;17:35–43

211. Gnanalingham K, Byrne E, Thornton A, Sambrook M et al: Motor and cognitive function in Lewy body dementia: Comparison with Alzheimer's and Parkinson's diseases. J Neurol Neurosurg Psychiatry 1997;62:243–252

212. Ala TA, Hughes LF, Kyrouac GA, Ghobrial MW, Elble RJ: Pentagon copying is more impaired in dementia with Lewy bodies than in Alzheimer's disease. J Neurol Neurosurg Psychiatry 2001;70(4):483–488

213. Mori E, Shimomura T, Fujimori M, Hirono N, Imamura T et al: Visuoperceptual impairment in dementia with Lewy bodies. Arch Neurol 2000;57:489–493

214. Rockwell EA, Choure J, Galasko D, Olichney J, Jeste DV: Psychopathology at initial diagnosis in dementia with Lewy bodies versus Alzheimer disease: Comparison of matched groups with autopsy-confirmed diagnoses. Int J Geriatr Psychiatry 2000;15(9):819–823

215. Neary D, Snowden JS, Bowen D et al: Cerebral biopsy in the investigation of presenile dementia due to cerebral atrophy. J Neurol Neurosurg Psychiatry 1986;49:157–162

216. Brun A: Frontal lobe degeneration of non-Alzheimer type. I. Neuropathology. Arch Gerontol Geriat 1987;6:193–208

217. Brun A: Frontal lobe degeneration of non-Alzheimer type revisited. 2nd International Conference: Frontal lobe degeneration of non-Alzheimer type (1992, Lund, Sweden). Dementia 1993;4(3–4):126–131

218. Mitsuyama Y: Presenile dementia with Motor Neuron disease. Dementia 1993;4:137–142

219. Risberg J, Passant U, Warkentin S, Gustafson L: Regional cerebral blood flow in frontal lobe dementia of non-Alzheimer type. 2nd International Conference: Frontal lobe degeneration of non-Alzheimer type (1992, Lund, Sweden). Dementia 1993;4:186–187

220. Neary D, Snowden JS, Shields RA et al: Single photon emission tomography using super(99m)Tc-HM-PAO in the investigation of dementia. J Neurol Neurosurg Psychiatry 1987;50(9):1101–1109

221. Neary D, Snowden JS, Northen B, Goulding P: Dementia of frontal lobe type. J Neurol Neurosurg Psychiatry 1988;51:353–361

222. Miller BL, Chang L, Mena I, Boone K, Lesser IM: Progressive right frontotemporal degeneration: clinical, neuropsychological and SPECT characteristics. Dementia 1993;4:204–213

223. Neary D, Snowden JS, Gustafson L et al: Frontotemporal lobar degeneration: A consensus on clinical diagnostic criteria. Neurology 1998;51(6):1546–1554

224. Hodges JR, Patterson K, Ward R et al: The differentiation of semantic dementia and frontal lobe dementia (temporal and frontal variants of frontotemporal dementia) from early Alzheimer's disease: A comparative neuropsychological study. Neuropsychology 1999;13(1):31–40

225. Kertesz A, Munoz DG: Pick's Disease and Pick Complex. Wiley-Liss, New York, 1998

226. Miller BL, Cummings JL, Villanueva-Meyer J et al: Frontal lobe degeneration: Clinical, neuropsychological, and SPECT characteristics. Neurology 1991;41:1374–1382

227. Perry RJ, Hodges JR: Differentiating frontal and temporal variant frontotemporal dementia from Alzheimer's disease.

228. Pasquier F, Lebert F, Lavenu I, Guillaume B: The clinical picture of frontotemporal dementia: Diagnosis and follow-up. Dement Geriatr Cognit Disord 1999;10(suppl):10–14

229. Gregory CA, Hodges JR: Frontotemporal dementia: Use of consensus criteria and prevalence of psychiatric features. Neuropsych Neuropsychol Behav Neurol 1996;9(3):145–153

230. Perry RJ, Rosen HR, Kramer JH et al: Hemispheric dominance for emotions, empathy and social behaviour: Evidence from right and left handers with frontotemporal dementia. Neurocase 2001;7(2,Pt2):145–160

231. Mychack P, Kramer JH, Boone KB, Miller BL: The influence of right frontotemporal dysfunction on social behavior in frontotemporal dementia. Neurology 2001;56(suppl 4):S11–S15

232. Lough S, Gregory C, Hodges JR: Dissociation of social cognition and executive function in frontal variant frontotemporal dementia. Neurocase 2001;7(2,Pt2):123–130

233. Lopez OL, Gonzalez MP, Becker JT et al: Symptoms of depression and psychosis in Alzheimer's disease and frontotemporal dementia. Neuropsych Neuropsychol Behav Neurol 1996;9(3):154–161

234. Mendez MF, Perryman KM, Miller BL, Cummings JL: Behavioral differences between frontotemporal dementia and Alzheimer's disease: A comparison on the BEHAVE-AD rating scale. Int Psychogeriatr 1998;10(2):155–162

235. Lindau M, Almkvist O, Kushi J et al: First symptoms—frontotemporal dementia versus Alzheimer's disease. Dement Geriatr Cognit Disord 2000;11(5):286–293

236. Bozeat S, Gregory CA, Ralph MAL, Hodges JR: Which neuropsychiatric and behavioural features distinguish frontal and temporal variants of frontotemporal dementia from Alzheimer's disease? J Neurol Neurosurg Psychiatry 2000;69(2):178–186

237. Sjoegren M, Wallin A, Edman A: Symptomatological characteristics distinguish between frontotemporal dementia and vascular dementia with a dominant frontal lobe syndrome. International J Geriatr Psychiatry 1997;12(6):656–661

238. Knopman DS, Mastri AR, Frey WH, Sung JH, Rustan T: Dementia lacking distinctive histologic features: A common non-Alzheimer degenerative dementia. Neurology 1990;40:251–256

239. Frisoni GB, Trabucchi M, Pizzolato G: Frontal lobe dementia. Int J Geriatr Psychiatry 1993;8:357

240. Elfgren C, Passant U, Risberg J: Neuropsychological findings in frontal lobe dementia. 2nd International Conference: Frontal lobe degeneration of non-Alzheimer type (1992, Lund, Sweden). Dementia 1993;4:214–219

241. Rahman S, Sahakian BJ, Hodges JR, Rogers RD, Robbins TW: Specific cognitive deficits in mild frontal variant frontotemporal dementia. Brain 1999;122(8):1469–1493

242. Varma AR, Snowden JS, Lloyd JJ et al: Evaluation of the NINCDS-ADRDA criteria in the differentiation of Alzheimer's disease and frontotemporal dementia. J Neurol Neurosurg Psychiatry 1999;66(2):184–188

243. Mesulam M-M: Slowly progressive aphasia without generalized dementia. Ann Neurol 1982;11:592–598

244. Weintraub S, Rubin NP, Mesulam M-M: Primary progressive aphasia: Longitudinal course, neuropsychological profile, and language features. Arch Neurol 1990;47:1329–1335

245. Green J, Morris JC, Sandson J, McKeel DW, Miller JW: Progressive aphasia: a precursor of global dementia? Neurology 1990;40:423–429

246. Karbe H, Kertesz A, Polk M: Profiles of language impairment in primary progressive aphasia. Arch Neurol 1993;50:193–201

247. Duffy JR, Petersen RC: Primary progressive aphasia. Aphasiology 1992;6:1–15

248. Kirshner HS: Progressive aphasia and other focal presentations of Alzheimer disease, Pick disease, and other degenerative disorders. In Emery VO, Oxman TE (eds): Dementia Presentations, Differential Diagnosis, and Nosology. The Johns Hopkins University Press, Baltimore, 1994:108–122

249. Mesulam M-M, Weintraub S: Primary progressive aphasia: sharpening the focus on a clinical syndrome. In: Boller F (ed): Heterogeneity of Alzheimer's Disease. Springer-Verlag, Heidelberg, 1992:43–66

250. Snowden JS, Neary D, Mann DM, Goulding PJ, Testa HJ: Progressive language disorder due to lobar atrophy. Ann Neurol 1992;31:174–183

251. Hodges JR, Patterson K, Oxbury S, Funnell E: Semantic dementia: progressive fluent aphasia with temporal lobe atrophy. Brain 1992;115:1783–1806

252. Perry RJ, Hodges JR: Differentiating frontal and temporal variant frontotemporal dementia from Alzheimer's disease. Neurology 2000;54(12):2277–2284

253. Graham KS, Simons JS, Pratt KH, Patterson K, Hodges JR: Insights from semantic dementia on the relationship between episodic and semantic memory. Neuropsychologia 2000;38(3):313–324

254. Garrard P, Hodges JR: Semantic dementia: Implications for the neural basis of language and meaning. Aphasiology 1999;13(8):609–623

255. Snowden JS, Griffiths HL, Neary D: Semantic-episodic memory interactions in semantic dementia: Implications for retrograde memory function. Cognit Neuropsychol 1996;13(8):1101–1137

256. Gregory CA, Orrell M, Sahakian B, Hodges JR: Can frontotemporal dementia and Alzheimer's disease be differentiated using a brief battery of tests? Int J Geriatr Psychiatry 1997;12(3):375–383

257. Rhee J, Antiquena P, Grossman M: Verb comprehension in frontotemporal degeneration: The role of grammatical, semantic and executive components. Neurocase 2001;7(2,Pt2):173–184

258. Wells CE: Pseudodementia. Am J Psychiatry 1979;136:895–900

259. Poon LW: Toward an understanding of cognitive functioning in geriatric depression. Special Issue: 1991 IPA Research Awards in Psychogeriatrics: Winning papers and selected outstanding submissions. Int Psychogeriatr 1992;4(suppl 2):241–266

260. Lamberty GJ, Bieliauskas LA: Distinguishing between depression and dementia in the elderly: A review of neuropsychological findings. Arch Clin Neuropsychol 1993;8(2):149–170

261. Folstein MF, Rabins PV: Replacing pseudodementia. Neuropsych Neuropsychol Behav Neurol 1991;4(1):36–40

262. Gibson A: A further analysis of memory loss in dementia and depression in the elderly. Br J Clin Psychol 1981;20:179–185

263. Williams JM, Little M, Scates S, Blockman N: Memory complaints and abilities among depressed older adults. J Consult Clin Psychol 1987;55:595–598

264. King DA, Caine ED, Conwell Y, Cox C: The neuropsychology of depression in the elderly: A comparative study of normal aging and Alzheimer's disease. J Neuropsych Clin Neurosci 1991;3:163–168

265. Hart RP, Kwentus JA, Taylor JR, Hamer RM: Productive naming and memory in depressed and Alzheimer's type dementia. Arch Clin Neuropsychol 1988;3:313–322

266. Crowe SF, Hoogenraad K: Differentiation of dementia of the Alzheimer's type from depression with cognitive impairment on the basis of a cortical versus subcortical pattern of cognitive deficit. Arch Clin Neuropsychol 2000;15:9–19

267. Whitehead A: Verbal learning and memory in elderly depressives. Br J Psychiatry 1973;123:203–208

268. Taylor R, Gilleard CJ: Encoding preferences in memory in dementia. Br J Clin Psychol 1990;29:243–244

269. La Rue A: Patterns of performance on the Fuld Object Memory evaluation in elderly patients with depression or dementia. J Clin Exp Neuropsychol 1989;11:409–422

270. Cipolli C, Neri M, De Vreese LP et al: The influence of depression on memory and metamemory in the elderly. Arch Gerontol Geriatr 1996;23:111–127

271. LaRue A, D'Elia LF, Clark EO, Spar JE, Jarvik LF: Clinical tests of memory in dementia, depression, and healthy aging. J Psychol Aging 1986;1:69–77

272. Miller E, Lewis P: Recognition memory in elderly patients with depression and dementia: a signal detection analysis. J Abnorm Psychol 1977;86:84–86

273. Abas MA, Sahakian BJ, Levy R: Neuropsychological deficits and CT scan changes in elderly depressives. Psychol Med 1990;20:507–520

274. Burt DB, Zembar MJ, Niederehe G: Depression and memory impairment: A meta-analysis of the association, its pattern and specificity. Psychol Bull 1995;117:285–305

275. Kindermann SS, Brown GG: Depression and memory in the elderly: A meta-analysis. J Clin Exp Neuropsychol 1997;19:625–642

276. Niederehe G, Camp CJ: Signal detection analysis of recognition memory in depressed elderly. Exp Aging Res 1985;11:207–213

277. Emery OB, Breslau LD: Language deficits in depression: comparisons with SDAT and normal aging. J Gerontol Med Sci 1989;44:M85–92

278. Hill CD, Stoudemire A, Morris R et al: Dysnomia in the differential diagnosis of major depression, depression-related cognitive dysfunction, and dementia. J Neuropsych Clin Neurosci 1992;4:64–69

279. Elliott R, Sahakian BJ, McKay AP, Herrod JJ: Neuropsychological impairments in unipolar depression: The influence of perceived failure on subsequent performance. Psychol Med 1996;26(5):975–989

280. Nebes RD, Butters MA, Houck PR et al: Dual-task performance in depressed geriatric patients. Psychiatry Res 2001;102(2):139–151

281. Kindermann SS, Kalayam B, Brown GG, Burdick KE, Alexopoulos GS: Executive functions and P300 latency in elderly depressed patients and control subjects. Am J Geriatr Psychiatry 2000;8(1):57–65

282. Luszcz MA, Bryan J, Kent P: Predicting episodic memory performance of very old men and women: Contributions from age, depression, activity, cognitive ability, and speed. Psychol Aging 1997;12(2):340–351

283. Beats BC, Sahakian BJ, Levy R: Cognitive performance in tests sensitive to frontal lobe dysfunction in the elderly depressed. Psychol Med 1996;26:591–603

284. Cohen RM, Weingartner H, Smallberg SA, Pickar D, Murphy DL: Effort and cognition in depression. Arch Gen Psychiatry 1982;39:593–597

285. Weingartner H: Automatic and effort-demanding cognitive processes in depression. In Poon L (ed): Handbook for Clinical Memory Assessment of Older Adults. American Psychological Association, Washington, DC, 1986:218–225

286. Nussbaum PD: Pseudodementia: A slow death. Neuropsychol Rev 1994;4(2):71–90

287. Levin BE, Tomer R, Rey GJ: Cognitive impairments in Parkinson's disease. Neurol Clin 1992;10(2):471–485

288. Raskin SA, Borod JC, Tweedy J: Neuropsychological aspects of Parkinson's disease. Neuropsychol Rev 1990;1(3):185–221

289. Ketter TA, George MS, Kimbrell TA, Benson BE, Post RM: Functional brain imaging, limbic function, and affective disorders. Neuroscientist 1996;2(1):55–65

290. Sahakian BJ: Depressive pseudodementia in the elderly. Special Issue: Affective disorders in old age. Int J Geriatr Psychiatry 1991;6(6):453–458

291. Kral VA: Senescent forgetfulness: Benign and malignant. Can Med Assoc J 1962;86:257–260

292. Crook T, Bartus RT, Ferris SH et al: Age-associated memory impairment: Proposed diagnostic criteria and measures of clinical change: Report of a National Institute of Mental Health work group. Dev Neuropsychol 1986;2(4):261–276

293. Levy R: Aging-associated cognitive decline. Int Psychogeriatr 1994;6:63–68

294. Petersen RC: Normal aging, mild cognitive impairment, and early Alzheimer's disease. Neurologist 1995;1:326–344

295. Kahn R, Zarit S, Hilbert N, Niederehe G: Memory complaint and impairment in the aged: the effect of depression and altered brain function. Arch Gen Psychiatry 1975;32:1569–1573

296. Goldman WP, Morris JC: Evidence that age-associated memory impairment is not a normal variant of aging. Alzheimer Dis Associated Disord 2001;15(2):72–79

297. Haenninen T, Hallikainen M, Koivisto K et al: A follow-up study of age-associated memory impairment: Neuropsychological predictors of dementia. J Am Geriatr Soc 1995;43(9):1007–1015

298. Smith G, Ivnik RJ, Petersen RC et al: Age-associated memory impairment diagnoses: Problems of reliability and concerns for terminology. Psychol Aging 1991;6(4):551–558

299. Larrabee GJ, McEntee W: Age-associated memory impairment: Sorting out the controversies. Neurology 1995;45:611–614

300. Haenninen T, Hallikainen M, Koivisto K et al: Decline of frontal lobe functions in subjects with age-associated memory impairment. Neurology 1997;48(1):148–153

301. Richards M, Touchon J, Ledesert B, Richie K: Cognitive decline in ageing: Are AAMI and AACD distinct entities? Int J Geriatr Psychiatry 1999;14(7):534–540

302. Ritchie K, Artero S, Touchon J: Classification criteria for mild cognitive impairment: A population-based validation study. Neurology 2001;56(1):37–42

303. Petersen RC, Smith GE, Waring SC et al: Mild cognitive impairment: Clinical characterization and outcome. Arch Neurol 1999;56(3): 303–308

304. Kivipelto M, Helkala EL, Haenninen T et al: Midlife vascular risk factors and late-life mild cognitive impairment: A population-based study. Neurol 2001;56(12):1683–1689

305. Wolf H, Ecke GM, Bettin S, Dietrich J, Gertz H-J: Do white matter changes contribute to the subsequent development of dementia in patients with mild cognitive impairment? A longitudinal study. Int J Geriatr Psychiatry 2000;15(9):803–812

306. Holroyd S, Snustad D, Chalifoux Z: Attitudes of older adults on being told the diagnosis of Alzheimer's disease. J Am Geriatr Soc 1996;44:400–403

307. Solomon K, Szwabo P: Psychotherapy for patients with dementia. In Morely J, Coe R, Strong R, Grossberg G (eds): Memory Function and Aging-related Disorders. Springer Publishing, New York, 1992:295–319

308. McFarlane WR: Family psychoeducational treatment. In Gurman AS, Kniskern DP (eds): Handbook of Family Therapy, Vol 2. Brunner/Mazel, New York, 1991:363–395

309. Zarit SH, Zarit JM: Families under stress: interventions for caregivers of senile dementia patients. Psychother Theory Res Pract 1982;19:461–471

310. Smyer MA, Birkel RC: Research focused on intervention with families of the chronically mentally ill elderly. In Light E, Lebowitz B (eds): The Elderly with Chronic Mental Illness. Springer Publishing, New York, 1991:111–130

Chapter 67

Functional psychiatric illness in old age

Cornelius L. E. Katona, Vivienne Watkin, and Gill Livingston

Older people may suffer a wide range of psychiatric difficulties in late life; those with concurrent physical illness are particularly vulnerable. Although these conditions tend to be underdetected and undertreated, their outcome with appropriate management is often excellent. In this chapter the clinical presentation, epidemiology, management, and outcome of depression, the schizophrenia-like psychoses and delusional disorders, mania, the anxiety disorders, alcohol-related problems, and disorders of personality in old age are discussed in some detail, with briefer discussion also of obsessive–compulsive disorder, somatoform disorders, post-traumatic stress disorder, and bereavement.

DEPRESSION

Depression is common and disabling in old age, particularly in people with comorbid physical illness or in institutional care. It is associated with high health and social care costs.[1] Despite this, it is often missed, ignored, or not managed adequately. Patients present needing help but often not complaining of low mood. This is in part a consequence of widely held "agist" assumptions that depression is intrinsic to the aging process, and that treatment is inappropriate, excessively risky, or unlikely to be effective. These assumptions are demonstrably untrue: the majority of older people are not clinically depressed (despite their increased risk of loss and of adversity); those that are respond as well to the range of pharmacological and psychological treatment as do younger depressed patients.

Epidemiology

The prevalence of depression in older people varies widely depending on sample selection, instruments used, and "caseness" criteria. The clinical features of depressive disorder may be complicated by its less than obvious presentation as well as by coexisting medical problems and/or cognitive impairment. It is possible that older individuals with clinically significant depression may not be identified as suffering from major depression as defined by standard diagnostic criteria. Older people in the community appear to have a lower prevalence of *major* depression (as defined within the *Diagnostic and Statistical Manual* [DSM] system) than their younger counterparts.[2] In an early United Kingdom community study, a 10 percent prevalence for depression in community residents was found, but only 1.3 percent met criteria for what would correspond to major depression.[3] In an Australian study,[4] which included individuals living in both community and institutional settings, the rate for depressive episodes as defined by Draft ICD-10 criteria[5] was 3.3 percent. The rate found using DSMIIIR criteria[6] was somewhat higher at 11 percent. Within DSM criteria, rates for dysthymia (chronic mild depression) are far from consistent; whereas in the Epidemiologic Catchment Area Study of United States communities, the prevalence for dysthymia was only 1–1.5 percent in those aged over 65,[7] a Finnish study[8] reported a rate for dysthymia as high as 23 percent.

More consistent results have been achieved using semi-structured interviews and diagnostic algorithms designed to detect depression of a level of severity which would indicate the need for intervention in elderly people. The most extensively validated of these is the Geriatric Mental State (GMS) interview and associated AGECAT computerized diagnostic system.[9] An alternative instrument, the Short-CARE,[10] is also specifically designed for elderly people and is an extensively validated diagnostic interview. It generates very similar findings. The GMS has been used in Hobart, Tasmania, with a reported prevalence of 14.2 percent for moderate to severe depression,[11] as well as in Liverpool,[12] where the prevalence was 11.3 percent, and in a two-center transatlantic study that found rates of 16.2 percent in New York City and 19.5 percent in London.[13] In these studies, the overall depression prevalence rates for women were about 50 percent greater than for men. The rates for severe depression were, however, similar in male and female subjects. An inner London community-based study using the Short-CARE[14] reported a prevalence of pervasive depression of 15.9 percent; this study also involved a follow-up that revealed an annual new incidence rate of 3.8 percent.

The comprehensive review by Beekman et al.[15] reported a point prevalence for depression ranging between 0.4 and 35 percent with an average prevalence of 13.5 percent. They also reported consistent evidence for higher prevalence rates for women and among older people living under adverse socio-economic circumstances. Similarly, the review by Copeland et al.[16] compared nine European studies using a standardized psychiatric interview in the community and found an overall prevalence of 12.3 percent (women 14.2 percent; men 8.6 percent).

The prevalence of depressive illness appears higher among those older people who attend their general practitioner (GP). Rates as high as 31 and 34 percent have been reported.[17,18] There is an established inter-relationship between depression, physical disability, and contact with services.[19] Livingston et al.[14] noted a statistically significant association in community subjects between depression and frequency of GP attendance, suggesting that frequent attendance may be a "marker" of increased likelihood of depression. Not all studies, however, report higher prevalence of depression in primary care attenders.[20]

In the hospitalized elderly, the prevalence of depression rises further, with a reported range between 12 and 45 percent.[21] Similarly, the prevalence of depressive disorders among elderly people in long-term institutional care is in excess of 20 percent.[22]

Depression in old age may be complicated by underlying cerebral pathologies. The range of reported depression in people with Alzheimer's disease varies between 19 and 87 percent.[23] Studies that screen out individuals with cognitive impairment may miss clinically significant depression, although such depressive symptoms may be relatively likely to remit spontaneously.[24]

Etiology

Demographic, social, and biological factors have all been implicated in the etiology of depression in old age.

Gender and age

Most community studies find significantly higher rates for depression in women than in men—this is particularly clear in the meta-analysis by Copeland et al.[16] The relationship between depression and age itself within the elderly population is not clear-cut; some studies find depression to be more common in the very old,[11] whereas others find the reverse to be true.[25]

Genetic susceptibility

Genetic factors are generally reported to be less important in elderly patients with depression than in their younger counterparts.[26] However, some studies have found a positive family history for depression in about one-third of patients whose depression had its first onset after the age of 60 years.[27,28]

Neurobiological risk factors

Brain electrical activity has shown some discriminatory power in elderly patients with depression. A study using sleep electroencephalogram recordings found depression in older subjects to be associated with reduced rapid eye movement (REM) latency and increased proportion of REM sleep.[29] A study of auditory evoked potentials[30] demonstrated increased P300 variability in older subjects with depression.

Neuroendocrine responses, such as the dexamethasone suppression test (DST), are more likely to be abnormal in older than in younger patients with depression.[31] The DST is, however, unhelpful in distinguishing depression from dementia because it may be abnormal in both conditions.[32]

In both depression and aging, there may be decreased non-adrenergic responsiveness with compensatory increases in postsynaptic receptor number. A positive correlation has been noted between age and platelet alpha-2 adrenergic binding capacity in controls but not in subjects with depression.[33] Aging may enhance depression-associated changes in serotonergic responsiveness as evidenced by reduced platelet ^{3}H-imipramine binding[34] and blunted prolactin responses to the 5HT precursor L-tryptophan.[35] It has been hypothesized that cholesterol might be an important factor in the relationship between serotonergic dysfunction and depression, through alterations in synaptosomal membrane properties. However, a meta-analysis of the outcome of elderly patients participating in clinical trials of cholesterol-lowering agents revealed no significant associations between low cholesterol concentration and severity of depressive symptoms.[36]

Imaging techniques have been widely used in the study of depression in old age. A recent review of structural imaging studies in depression in old age concluded that ventricular enlargement, and arteriosclerotic and ischemic changes are more frequently found in patients whose first onset of depression was after age 60.[37] An important study using single-photon emission computed tomography (SPECT) demonstrated that, at rest, elderly patients with depression had lower regional cerebral blood flow (rCBF) than controls, particularly in the left hemisphere.[38] However, rCBF failed to correlate with severity of depressed mood but there was a positive correlation between rCBF and severity of psychotic symptoms and negative correlations with somatic symptoms and anxiety. Reduced anterior frontal and temporal blood flow but an increase in occipital flow have also been shown in elderly depressed patients.[39] Studies using positron emission tomography (PET) reveal that depression in elderly people is associated with a reduction in whole brain glucose metabolic rate.[40]

Physical health

Depression is more common in physically ill than in healthy older people. As physical illness and depression both often present with physical features (such as sleep disturbance, loss of appetite and pain) then the use of screening tests which use biological symptoms can lead to false positives. The prevalence range varies from 6 to 25 percent when diagnostic interviews validated among elderly people are used.[41] The main risk factors for depression appear to be the severity of physical illness, the degree of disability, coexisting cognitive impairment, and a positive past psychiatric history. Physical disability seems to be particularly strongly associated with depression in institutional settings.[22]

Although illness in general is a risk factor, stroke and Parkinson's disease have been associated with a particularly high likelihood of developing depression. This is illustrated by a study which found much higher rates of significant depressive symptoms (45 vs 10 percent) in stroke patients compared with orthopedic patients with similar levels of disability.[42] Reported relationship with lesion size and site of stroke have been inconsistent.[43] As many as 70 percent of people with Parkinson's disease have been reported to be affected, with risk being higher in those with predominantly left-sided disease or with a prominent tremor.[44] Depression in elderly medical patients frequently becomes chronic, and in turn appears to have an adverse effect on the physical prognosis, especially in terms of likelihood of successful rehabilitation.[45] In addition, older medical patients with depression consume more healthcare resources, have longer admissions, a higher mortality, and are more likely to be transferred to residential care.[46] However, depression in elderly medical patients is frequently overlooked by medical staff, despite high rates of depressive symptomatology.[47] Its detection may be facilitated by simple screening tests (see below).[48] The management of depression in physically ill elderly patients is essentially the same as for depression in general; the possibility of adverse consequences or interactions between antidepressants and other drug treatments must be considered carefully. There is some clinical trial evidence to suggest that newer antidepressants may be of value. Citalopram has been found superior to placebo both in post-stroke depression and post-stroke pathological crying;[49,50] fluoxetine has been trialed against placebo in older depressed medical patients unselected by medical diagnosis but was found to be significantly superior only in post-hoc analyses of those with more severe physical illness and those able to complete 5 weeks of treatment.[51] Patients with depression should be discouraged from making decisions about life-sustaining therapy until after their depression is treated.[52]

Personality

Those individuals with late-onset depressive illness have more robust personalities than those with recurrent depression arising earlier.[53] Dependent, anxious, and avoidant personality traits have, however, been reported to be associated with late life depression.[54]

Social factors

The most striking social vulnerability factors identified in community surveys are poverty, bereavement, and social isolation. Life events often precipitate depression in old age.[55] Several community studies have emphasized the importance of the concept of loss in understanding the depressions of old age. Illness, chronic disability, social isolation, bereavement, and poverty are correlates of depressive symptoms.[56] The importance of physical illness has already been discussed. Social losses have been implicated in the etiology of depressive illness; a confidant may act as a buffer against such loss-related depression, particularly in women.[55] This research area is particularly problematic because of the lack of cause/effect clarity: Does poor support render persons liable to depression, or does depression lead to the loss of support? Personality variables are likely to be important mediators. Those individuals who are separated, divorced, or widowed exhibit more depressive illness than single or married subjects.[57] Depression is associated with recent deaths and accidents in near relatives.[58] Several studies have found that being a care-giver for someone with dementia or depression is associated with an increased risk of depression in the care-giver; this is particularly marked in women, in spouse care-givers, where the premorbid relationship was poor, and where there are prominent behavioral problems such as aggression.[59,60]

Clinical features

Depression often presents in a less typical fashion in old age with the core complaint of low mood being less prominent or even absent. This clearly has implications for the under- or misdiagnosis of depression in elderly people. Older patients tend to have an increase in somatic complaints, sleep disturbance (initial insomnia), and agitation.[61] Depressive symptomatology is often found in older subjects without frank depressive illness; the psychological symptoms frequently elicited include dysphoria, sleep disturbance, thoughts of death, anergy, impaired concentration, agitation, and retardation.[62] Prince et al.[63] demonstrated two main symptom clusters: "affective suffering" which included low mood, tearfulness, and the wish to die, and a "motivational" cluster comprising loss of interest, poor concentration, and lack of enjoyment.

Symptom patterns have been found to differ by gender. Depressed mood, guilt, anxiety, and diurnal mood variation were found to be more common in women than in men with depression.[64] Age-related differences in symptom patterns have been reported within elderly people. Items relating to low self-esteem showed an inverse relationship with age, whereas the presence of hypochondriasis was positively correlated with age.[65] Subjects whose first episode of depression occurred in late life are less likely to display psychotic features, and are also more likely to display cognitive impairment.[66] However, the latter finding may be a reflection of the greater age of the late first-onset group.

Depression and dementia

Cognitive impairment is frequently found in association with depression in older subjects. Its presence may be important not only in terms of hindering diagnosis, but more positively, as an etiologic and prognostic pointer and an element in a possible specific approach to the subtyping of depression in old age. Prominent cognitive dysfunction that initially reverses with successful antidepressant treatment is the essential clinical feature in the minority of elderly depressed patients with "depressive" pseudodementia.[67] Subtle cognitive impairment may, however, be present in a broad spectrum of depressed elderly people and may in any case not be as consistently reversible as had been thought.[68] Conventional teaching suggests that "don't know" responses are helpful in distinguishing such depressive pseudodementia from true dementia but a recent study suggests that this may not be so.[69]

The evolution of cognitive and depressive symptoms in people in whom these coexist is not always straightforward. Depressive symptoms may present as early or even prodromal symptoms of dementia, particularly vascular dementia. In a study of people aged over 75 years with declining cognitive function, mood disturbance first increased, then decreased.[70] Lack of motivation increased sharply with decreasing cognitive function, and increasing disability was associated with deterioration in both mood and motivation symptoms. Cognitive impairment in elderly inpatients with depression tended to be associated with late-onset depression. This suggests that people with the combination of cognitive impairment and late first onset of depression may represent a distinct subgroup whose depression reflects cortical pathology. This is further supported by the finding that subjects becoming depressed for the first time in late life have a distinct pattern of symptoms and are less likely to have first-degree relatives with depression.[61] In addition, late first-onset depression has been reported to be associated with more frequent cognitive impairment, suboptimal treatment response, and a higher rate of brain imaging abnormalities.[40] There is increasing evidence that a past history of depression may increase vulnerability to dementia,[71,72] though this has been disputed.[73] A recent twin pair study[74] found that prior depressive episodes (particularly when these occurred shortly before the onset of cognitive impairment) were associated with increased risk of subsequently developing Alzheimer's disease.

Depression may also be an important cause of disability in people with primary dementia. It frequently presents as part of the prodrome of Alzheimer's disease as well as complicating both early and late stages of dementia.[23] Depression within dementia appears to be clinically relevant and amenable to treatment.[75] Three trials of newer antidepressants in patients with coexistent depression and dementia attest to the efficacy of moclobemide[76] and of citalopram[77] against placebo. Paroxetine and imipramine were both found effective in another recent trial without a placebo arm,[78] with paroxetine being somewhat better tolerated than imipramine. There is also emerging evidence that cholinesterase inhibitors may ameliorate mood as well as cognition in Alzheimer's disease.[79]

The detection of depression in subjects with dementia is difficult. The subject finds it difficult as dementia progresses to articulate emotional distress. There are, however, rating scales specifically designed to detect depression in subjects with dementia; the best of these is probably the Cornell Scale.[80]

Screening for depression in older people

The distinctive clinical features of depression in old age, particularly the frequent absence of overt depressed mood and the coexistence of apparent or real cognitive impairment render its detection particularly difficult. One option for increasing recognition rates (both on medical wards as discussed above and in primary care) is the use of screening questionnaires. Depression in older people is undoubtedly a legitimate screening target given that it is common, disabling, frequently persistent, and eminently amenable to treatment. Several depression screening instruments have been developed specifically for use in older people.

Sensitivities for the GDS30 and GDS15 in medical patients range between 70 and 100 percent, with specificities of 64–90 percent.[81] The best results are for a five-item version of the GDS developed specifically for use in medically ill people. This has a sensitivity of 97 percent and specificity of 85 percent.[82] An alternative which may be particularly useful where privacy or hearing impairments hinder interviewing is the BASDEC which is the Brief Assessment Schedule as a Deck of Cards.[83] It has a sensitivity of 71 percent and a specificity of 88 percent. In its shorter 15-item form[84] it is highly acceptable: D'Ath et al.[85] reported that 98 percent of older primary care attenders completed it successfully by interview, with only 12 percent finding the process difficult or stressful. The Geriatric Depression Scale is sensitive and specific in both the hospital[52] and primary care[85] settings, is quick to administer and highly acceptable to patients,[85] and has been extensively validated. Arthur et al.[86] examined the practicality of using the GDS15 as part of a nurse administered health check to all patients aged 75 and over and found that only 25 percent of screening positive subjects had any record of depressive symptoms in their general practice case notes. Other scales validated to some degree in identifying depression in older primary care patients include scales originally designed for use in younger adults such as the 12-item General Health Questionnaire,[87] the 20-item Center for Epidemiologic Studies Depression Scale,[88] and the 12-item SelfCARE(D).[89]

The management of depression in old age

Community and primary care studies suggest that only a small minority of older patients with depression receive treatment.

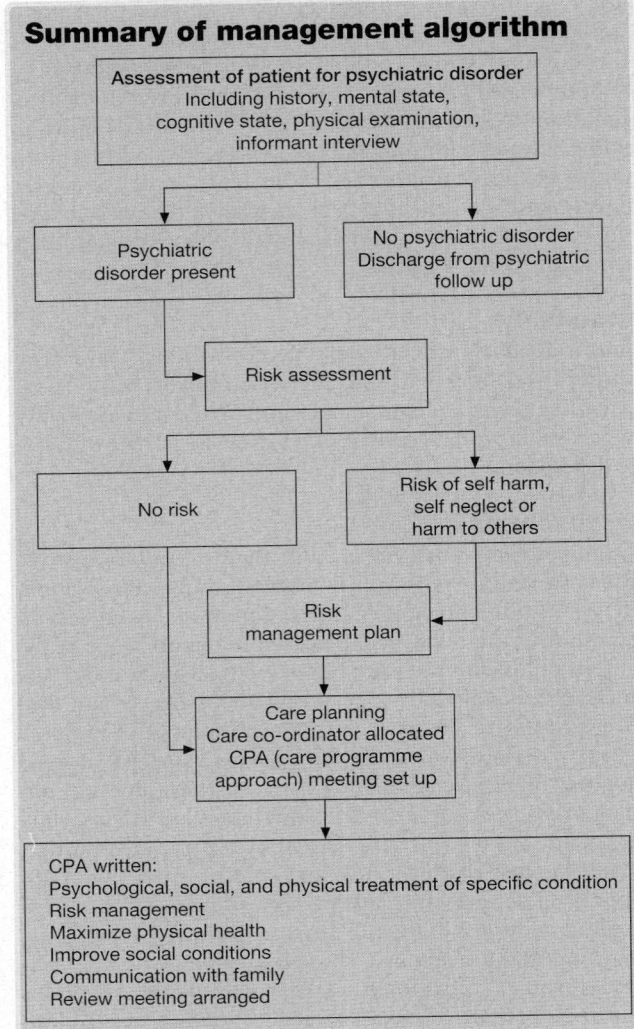

Summary of management algorithm

Assessment of patient for psychiatric disorder
Including history, mental state, cognitive state, physical examination, informant interview

Psychiatric disorder present

No psychiatric disorder
Discharge from psychiatric follow up

Risk assessment

No risk

Risk of self harm, self neglect or harm to others

Risk management plan

Care planning
Care co-ordinator allocated
CPA (care programme approach) meeting set up

CPA written:
Psychological, social, and physical treatment of specific condition
Risk management
Maximize physical health
Improve social conditions
Communication with family
Review meeting arranged

A community study found that only 13 percent of subjects with depression were being treated with antidepressants; at follow-up the figure remained virtually the same at 14 percent.[14] Similarly, only 10 percent of patients with depression identified from consecutive primary care attenders were receiving treatment for depression.[17] However, their general practitioners were aware of depression in 95 percent of cases. This suggests that GPs may conceptualize depression in old age as a legitimate and unavoidable consequence of aging and associated adversity, which is recognizable but not seen as treatable, or may believe drug treatment is highly toxic or ineffective.

This failure to treat depression in old age is unfortunate because treatment is clearly efficacious. Reviews of the many controlled trials of tricyclic and newer antidepressants against each other and against placebo[90] have consistently demonstrated superior efficacy for active drug (response rate about 50 percent) over placebo (about 25 percent).

Antidepressants are undeniably more hazardous in old age, because of age-related pharmacokinetic changes and the high frequency in older people of coexistent medical problems and coadministered drugs which may adversely interact with antidepressants. Some of the adverse effects of antidepressants, particularly falls, are potentially much more serious in old age. Vulnerability to falls relates mainly to the potency of older tricyclic antidepressants as alpha-1 adrenergic receptor blockers aggravate postural hypotension. Selective serotonin reuptake inhibitors (SSRIs) also have important side-effects, such as headache, nausea, hyponatremia and sexual dysfunction. Not all antidepressants within a class have identical side-effects. Nortriptyline, for example, causes relatively little postural hypotension and is widely used in old age psychiatry practice in the USA, and lofepramine is relatively free of anticholinergic side-effects, causes little cognitive impairment, and is very safe in overdose.

A recent meta-analysis of controlled trials of the main classes of antidepressant drugs (tricyclics, SSRIs, reversible monoamine oxidase inhibitors and atypical antidepressants) found all to be superior to placebo but no significant differences between classes.[91] This may in part reflect the reduced statistical power of such meta-analyses as well as the blurring of differences between drugs within a class. Looking at individual antidepressant–antidepressant and antidepressant–placebo comparisons in terms of "number needed to treat" does in fact suggest important differences between individual drugs. Paroxetine shows significant superiority over fluoxetine, and there is a trend in favor of SSRIs and venlafaxine over tricyclics. Fluoxetine and moclobemide perform relatively badly (in contrast to other antidepressants) compared with placebo.[92]

In "real-life" practice, newer antidepressants may, because of their better side-effect and safety profile have greater advantage than is apparent in the "super-fit, super-depressed" subjects eligible for clinical trials. There is some evidence that antidepressants may take as long as 10–12 weeks to show clinical improvement in older subjects.[92]

Electroconvulsive therapy (ECT) remains an important treatment option in very severe or treatment resistant depression in old age. A meta-analysis of published studies revealed a 62 percent recovery and 21 percent substantial improvement.[93] It is indicated particularly where depressive delusions are present, where retardation is marked, in patients whose fluid intake (secondary to loss of appetite and self-neglect) is poor enough to threaten renal function, and where suicide risk is considered high. Good anesthetic support is essential; ECT may have to be delayed in very frail patients until their physical condition improves. ECT may be lifesaving, particularly in the context of dehydration or suicidality. Its safety profile in older patients with depression is surprisingly good.[94] A wide spectrum of clinical response, including anxiety symptoms, has been demonstrated. Unilateral electrode placement appears as effective as bilateral in older patients, but there is clearer evidence that unilateral electrode placement is associated with fewer memory-related side-effects in this age group.[95]

Psychological treatments are also underused in old age. This is partly because their availability is often limited. There is also a misconception that older people lack the psychological flexibility to benefit from psychotherapeutic interventions.[96] Elderly people appear to respond particularly well to cognitive therapy for depression;[97] this is effective both in an individual setting and (more economically) in groups. The focus is often on real or threatened losses (bereavement, physical health, financial security) and on fears of impending death. Interpersonal psychotherapy (IPT), which is widely used in the

United States and increasingly so in Europe has been shown to be effective in acute, continuation, and maintenance treatment of depression in older people.[98,99]

Depression in old age frequently fails to respond to initial treatment. Patients with apparent treatment resistance should be fully re-evaluated, with consideration of whether the original diagnosis was correct, previous treatment was adequate (dosage and duration), and adherence was satisfactory. Possible physical (e.g., hypothyroidism, poorly controlled pain) or psychosocial (isolation, poor marital relationship) maintenance factors should also be considered. A variety of pharmacological approaches to refractory depression in older people have been evaluated.[100] Within these, lithium augmentation has the strongest evidence base[101] despite lithium's high risk of neurotoxicity in old age, particularly in the context of comorbid dementia and/or Parkinson's disease.

There have been relatively few studies of longer term treatment following good initial response. In general, antidepressants should where possible be continued (without any dose reduction) for at least 6 months after clinical recovery. Following this, antidepressant treatment may be tapered slowly. In view of the high risk of depressive recurrence (see below), opportunistic monitoring of depressive symptoms should form part of any subsequent clinical contact. In people with other previous episodes of depression, continued antidepressant treatment has been shown to be effective in preventing relapse for at least 2–3 years. The Old Age Depression Interest Group[102] reported a relapse rate 2.5 times higher at 2 years in patients maintained on placebo than in those on dothiepin. Reynolds et al.[99] found nortriptyline to be similarly effective over 3 years, as has citalopram. Though most published trials have lacked placebo control, there is consistent open trial evidence that both TCA and SSRI antidepressants have similar prophylactic effect. Psychological therapies, such as cognitive-behavioral therapy (CBT)[103] and supportive psychotherapy[104] may also reduce relapse rate, with the most powerful prophylactic effect resulting from combined antidepressant and psychotherapy.[99]

Suicide and depression in old age

Suicide in old age is far from rare. Suicide rates in most countries are highest in elderly people.[105] In the United Kingdom the rate in those over 65 years is approximately three times that in the 15–24-year age group, and in men continues to rise into the ninth decade. In the United Kingdom, suicide attempts in old age are usually by overdose. Violent means (hanging, firearms, etc.) are more frequently used by men to commit suicide.[106] Suicide is much more closely associated with depression in older than in younger subjects. Cattell and Jolley[107] found evidence for recent depression in 60 percent in a series of 100 consecutive suicides aged 65 and over. Forty-three percent had seen their GP in the previous month but only 25 percent were prescribed antidepressants and as few as 14 percent were in contact with psychiatric services. Other factors associated with suicide in old age include bereavement, increasing social isolation, deteriorating physical health, and pain.

Attempted suicide closely resembles completed suicide in elderly people.[108,109] Psychiatric illness is prominent in most cases. The predominant psychiatric diagnosis is depression.

Comorbid diagnoses include delirium and mild dementia. Minor depression and personality dysfunction are associated with suicide attempts of relatively low intent and higher levels of psychosocial stresses. There is an interaction with physical illness, psychosocial stress, age, and gender. Hopelessness persisting after remission of other depressive symptoms is associated with suicide attempts and completed suicide.[110]

Suicidal ideation is surprisingly common in depressed older people. Schulberg et al.[111] found that 21 percent of a primary care sample of older patients with significant depressive symptoms expressed some degree of suicidal ideation; this was the case in as many as 42 percent of those with major depression. The close association between depression, deliberate self-harm, and completed suicide in old age carries a clear message that all such behavior in older patients should be taken seriously with particular attention to the exclusion or treatment of underlying depressive illness.

The prognosis of depression in old age

Cole and Bellavance[112] reviewed all available and methodologically sound studies of prognosis in older depressed subjects. Hospital-based studies generated a total of 1,487 subjects, with a further 249 subjects identified and followed up in the community. Overall, 60 percent of the hospital subjects had recovered (though many had subsequently relapsed) and 14–22 percent had been depressed throughout the follow-up period. In the community cohorts, 19–34 percent were well at follow-up, 27 percent had remained ill through the follow-up period, and most of the remainder had died. The mortality rate is considerably higher in elderly patients with depression than in age- and sex-matched controls.[113] O'Brien and Ames[114] consider that the important "direct" effects of depression on mortality in old age are depression-related impairments of the hypothalamo-pituitary-adrenal axis and immune function, the consequences of depression-related psychomotor retardation and the greater risk of poor compliance with physical treatment in depressed elders. Unsurprisingly, mortality is particularly high in the context of comorbid physical illness. Cole and Bellavance[115] reviewed studies of physically ill older depressed patients and found that at 3-month follow-up only 1/5 were psychiatrically well. At follow-up of a year or more, over 50 percent had died and only 19 percent had recovered from their depression. Persistent depression was associated with long admission, poor physical rehabilitation, and transfer to residential or nursing care.

Cole and Bellavance[112] concluded that the main factors predictive of persistence of depression were physical illness, cognitive impairment, and initial severity of the depression. Bruce et al.[116] and Callahan et al.[117] both emphasize the importance of deterioration in physical health as a marker for persistence of depression. Livingston et al.[118] confirmed the association between initial severity of depression and its persistence. They also found depression to be more persistent in older women than in men, and that comorbid anxiety was associated with decreased likelihood of recovery from depression.

Although depression in old age does not necessarily have a worse prognosis than earlier in life, there is considerable room for improvement. This improvement could result from optimizing treatment. Continuing treatment appears to have a protective effect against relapse. This has been shown most clearly for maintenance antidepressant drugs,[102] but the efficacy of supportive group psychotherapy has also been shown.[104] The combination of antidepressants and psychotherapy appears more effective than either alone.[99]

LATE LIFE PSYCHOSIS

The onset of schizophrenia-like psychotic illness later in life not due to an organic or affective disorder has been referred to as *paraphrenia, late paraphrenia,* and *late-onset schizophrenia*. More circumscribed delusional disorders also occur in late life; these are referred to below as *persistant delusional disorders*. In addition, the challenges posed by patients with longstanding psychotic illness (usually schizophrenia) who "graduate" to old age are also considered within this section. Finally, it should be borne in mind that psychosis in older people is often due to an organic illness, particularly dementia, which is discussed in detail elsewhere in this book. Other neuropsychiatric syndromes associated with psychosis include Parkinson's disease and its treatment (see Chapter 52).

Paraphrenia

The original concept of paraphrenia referred to the first onset of persecutory delusions and associated hallucinations after the age of 60 years in the absence of an affective or organic psychosis.[119] It may thus be viewed as schizophrenia or a schizophrenia-like illness in old age and is referred to as late-life schizophrenia in ICD X.

Epidemiology

In an early study[119] paraphrenia was estimated to account for 10 percent of psychogeriatric admissions; this is probably an overestimate. Data from admissions to psychiatric units reveal an age-related increase in first admission rates for schizophrenia and paranoid states from 8.7 per 100,000 in subjects aged 65–74 years to 14.5 per 100,000 in the 75-plus age group.[120] Studies in community samples of older people have found prevalences of paranoid delusions ranging from 2.0 to 13 percent.[121–128] Christenson and Blazer[121] report that their study only detected pervasive delusional systems and therefore their prevalence figures were likely to be an underestimate. Community studies, however, often find either no cases at all of late-life schizophrenia or prevalence rates of less than 2 percent, possibly because people with paranoid symptoms are more likely to refuse interview.[124] Recent community studies found 2–4 percent of the population had delusions or hallucinations over the past month.[124,125]

Hospital admission data also probably underestimate prevalence because patients with paraphrenia tend only to be admitted compulsorily and in the context of particularly severe behavioral disturbance. There is relatively good consensus that late-onset schizophrenia is more common in women than in men.[124]

Etiology

About 10 percent of the relatives of patients developing schizophrenia in middle age also have the disease; this is similar to the proportion for patients with early-onset schizophrenia.[124] In family studies of paraphrenia, however, the rate of schizophrenia in first-degree relatives is much lower, generally less than 5 percent.[125] Standardized instruments were not used in the paraphrenia studies, however, so the data are not directly comparable to those from fully operationalized family studies of younger subjects.

The influence of personality, social, and environmental factors, in association with genetic predisposition is clearly complex.[128] Patients with paraphrenia are often socially isolated and live alone.[129] They are more likely to have paranoid and/or schizoid premorbid personalities that are characterized by suspicion, sensitivity to setback and disappointment, and preoccupation with what others may think about them.[130] Their isolation is often chronic and may well be secondary to personality traits. They are predominantly unmarried women without close family or personal attachments. Those who do marry often end up divorced or separated. Fertility seems markedly reduced. This social isolation creates an environment allowing the individual to become preoccupied in her own world.

The social isolation can be further accentuated by sensory impairment. There is a confirmed association between deafness and late paraphrenia in particular. Many patients suffer conductive hearing loss contracted in early life to such a degree as to impair social interaction resulting in "social deafness."[131] Visual impairment may be present but there is dispute as to whether it is more common than in normal elderly people.[120,125,128] Patients with paraphrenia have been found to come from the lower social classes and/or socio-economic groups;[129] this may result from social deterioration secondary to the disease, as also occurs in younger people with schizophrenia. Other reported risk factors are disability and black ethnicity.[121,122]

Presentation and clinical features

Patients often come to the attention of services because they complain to the police and neighbors with bizarre accusations over a period of time or because of neighborly concern triggered by extreme self-neglect. On mental state assessment there are no qualitative differences between the symptoms of early and late-onset schizophrenia. The clinical presentation of late-life schizophrenia is quite varied. Patients are in clear consciousness. Usually their affective state is normal although occasionally a secondary depressive mood is found. The history may be difficult to elicit from patients who tend to be distrustful and hostile.

Delusions are central. Organized delusional systems are common,[132] with the frequency of paranoid and systematized delusions increasing in line with age.[133] Sexual themes are common in women. The patient usually accuses a man or men of entering her bed at night and molesting her sexually. Delusions of influence and passivity phenomena are frequently reported.[134] Patients may describe their bodies as being controlled, or complain that some power affects them and they are made to do things against their will. Thought insertion, withdrawal, and broadcasting are, however, fairly rare, and formal thought disorder is almost nonexistent.

Hallucinations are frequently experienced.[130] These are often in several modalities. Auditory hallucinations are the most common and usually have an accusatory and/or insulting content. The voices speak in the second or the third person with "running commentary" occasionally encountered. Hallucinations of bodily sensation are also found. Patients complain of being vibrated, raped, or forced to have sexual intercourse. Olfactory hallucinations often relating to poisonous gas are encountered. Visual hallucinations are rarer and if present should raise a suspicion of an underlying organic state.

Patients are much less likely to have negative symptoms (such as apathy, withdrawal, decreased speech, and flattening of affect) than those who developed early-onset schizophrenia.[132]

At the time of initial presentation, the cognitive function of patients with late-life schizophrenia is often mildly impaired on formal testing. Although such impairment is to a much lesser degree than found in dementia, it is nevertheless significantly greater than in psychiatrically healthy age-matched controls.[134] Decline may not occur, with only a small group of patients entering the dementia range at 3-year follow-up.

Brain imaging studies

A representative CT study has reported increased mean ventricle to brain ratio with cortical sulcal appearances remaining within normal limits.[134] Magnetic resonance imaging (MRI) has demonstrated an excess of deep white matter changes,[135] although these findings have failed to be consistently replicated[136,137] and may have reflected the over-representation of individuals with cerebrovascular disease risk factors.

A number of studies using PET have shown increased basal ganglia dopamine D2 receptors in late-onset schizophrenia.[138] However, these findings have not been consistently replicated, particularly in drug-naive subjects, suggesting that some of the differences initially reported may have reflected treatment, rather than disease-induced receptor alteration.

Neuropsychological testing

Patients with late-life schizophrenia have been shown to perform less well on the Mental Test Score and Digit Copying Test than age-matched controls. Deficiencies have also been shown on full-scale IQ tests, tests of frontal lobe function, and verbal memory tasks.[130] The presence of brain abnormalities was not associated with particularly low neuropsychological test scores.

Assessment, treatment, and course

The initial management of late late-life schizophrenia involves evaluation and engagement.[129] Patients should be assessed at home (rather than in a clinic) both because they are unlikely to comply with outpatient appointments and because their psychopathology may be strongly triggered by cues within their normal environment and less obvious away from it. It is also not surprising on this basis that hospital admission commonly results in an apparent complete remission followed by relapse on return home. Health workers may initially find it difficult to gain access to the home of the patient. Once initial access is gained, patients are often glad to gain a new audience for the expression of their delusional beliefs.

It used to be said that late-life schizophrenia tends to run a chronic course.[139] One review article, however, found that studies report a short-term complete remission of between 27 and 48 percent and no relapses in 65 percent of survivors during a mean 3.7 year follow-up and thus the response is as good or better than for younger onset schizophrenia.[140] Attempts at treatment should begin in the community wherever possible, with hospital admission reserved for patients with particularly severe or dangerous behavioral disturbance or poor self-care. Medication, psychosocial intervention, and ECT have all been reported to produce temporary remission. Adequate neuroleptic treatment produces improvement in psychotic symptoms but not much improvement to the patient's pretreatment level of social functioning. Dosages of neuroleptics are much lower than those used in younger patients with schizophrenia; older people are often very sensitive to extrapyramidal side-effects.[139] Atypical antipsychotics may produce less side-effects and be more tolerable. Compliance is a major problem in these patients who usually live alone and do not have any insight into treatment necessity. Even when compliance is assured, many patients remain psychotic, although they may be less distressed by their symptoms and less disturbed in their behavior.[123] Community psychiatric nurses administering depot preparations are most likely to ensure a favorable response but side-effects are common.

An attempt should be made to correct remediable physical or environmental contributory factors, particularly through alleviating sensory and/or social isolation. A flexible approach is required, and patients' characteristic insistence on remaining isolated (as they have often been for much of their lives) must be respected. Patients' importuning requests for rehousing should, if secondary to delusional beliefs, be resisted; although symptoms may improve or even abate in a new home setting this is usually a temporary respite. Old "tormentors" re-emerge or have "phoned ahead" and new ones may be acquired. Antipsychotic medication is a vital component of the total therapeutic package but is far from the whole answer; improvisation and ingenuity in engaging these patients and then retaining them in long-term follow-up is crucial to maintain both compliance and an optimal level of social functioning and to reduce risk of symptomatic relapse. The benefits of long-term neuroleptics in reducing relapse rate must be weighed against the increased risk of tardive dyskinesia in old age.

Late-life delusional (paranoid) disorder

Persecutory ideas are common in older people. It has been estimated that 4 percent of a community-living elderly population experience some persecutory beliefs of delusional intensity.[123] Such beliefs are commonly associated with a neuropsychiatric disorder. A primary delusional disorder is present when there is evidence of persistent, nonbizarre delusions that are not attributable to another psychiatric disorder or any organic cause.[141] Persistent delusional disorder refers to persistent delusions without evidence of schizophrenia, schizophreniform, or mood disorders. There is no evidence of organic dysfunction. The distinction between such disorders and late-life schizophrenia reflects the relative absence of schizophrenia-like features other than delusions in the late-life delusional group. Persistent delusional disorder occurs in middle as well as late life. It is not different from late-life schizophrenia in terms of demographic factors or treatment responsiveness and there is continuing discussion regarding the classification.[142]

Pathogenesis and etiology

An increased evidence of schizophrenia has been observed in families of patients with persistent delusional disorder.[143] Individuals with avoidant, paranoid, or schizoid personality disorders may be more susceptible to developing a delusional disorder. There is an association between hearing loss and delusional disorder in the elderly.[144] Immigration or low socio-economic status may also predispose individuals to delusional disorder.[145] There is an increased frequency of women, immigrants, or children of immigrants with somatic delusions diagnosed as part of a delusional disorder. There may be a possible association of early-life trauma and the failure to reproduce progeny with the development of delusions in later life.[148]

Management and outcome

The optimal approach encompasses drug treatment, psychotherapy, and environmental change.[147] Neuroleptics may be effective in decreasing the intensity of the delusions, but noncompliance is a common problem. Intramuscular depot neuroleptics may be preferable. Antidepressant drugs and ECT have been used with variable success in delusional patients, particularly those with coexistent depressive symptoms. The provision of alternative explanations for patients' delusional beliefs may be a useful psychotherapeutic approach. There are few outcome data available, but the overall outcome is often poor.[148]

GRADUATES

The term *graduates* is used to refer to patients with long-standing mental illness who have "graduated" to elderly status.[149] Many graduates entered a mental hospital when relatively young and remained in institutional care. Many such patients have now returned to the community as the large psychiatric hospitals close. This group of patients are now becoming rarer as very few people remain in long-term care in a mental hospital. There is no separate term for people with psychiatric illness enduring from adulthood into old age who have received or will receive care in the community. Although the latter group is likely to be less institutionalized, there is likely to be considerable overlap in terms of both current clinical presentation and care needs, and these people may also usefully be considered as graduates.

The largest subgroup of graduates have schizophrenia. Most of the remainder have primary diagnoses of affective psychoses, learning disability, or personality disorder. Disability in the graduate population is varied. Some patients may require total nursing care, whereas others remain physically fit and relatively competent in daily living skills. Many have some degree of cognitive impairment. There are associations between negative symptoms (social withdrawal, slowness, underactivity, poverty of speech, lack of interest, and poor self-care), cognitive deficit, and structural brain abnormality. This highlights the issue of the long-term cognitive effects of schizophrenic illness. Some of the deficits of chronic schizophrenia are probably integral to the illness process and may manifest at a relatively early stage in the evolution of the illness over time. Social disability may be due not only to the effects of the illness itself but secondary to the deleterious effects of institutional care on the capacity to return to independent living. It has been suggested that in some patients a phenomenon of "burn-out" in schizophrenia (an amelioration of positive symptoms after the age of 55) may occur, but this is still disputed.[150] The lowered prevalence of positive symptoms in this group may be due to reduced exposure to the stresses and strains of everyday life rather than either the effects of medication or the natural history of schizophrenia.

There is a high prevalence of physical disability and handicap among long-stay patients. This increases with age but is not confined to elderly patients or those with the longest duration of stay. The presence of neurological abnormalities referred to as "soft" neurological signs, including disorders of posture and tone, motor performance, inappropriate activity, abnormal movements, automatic movements, and speech production, seem to be intrinsic to the schizophrenic process and cannot be attributed to hospitalization, physical treatment, or undiagnosed neurological illness.[151] Incontinence of urine and, less often, of faeces is a problem in long-stay patients. Likely contributory factors include physical disability, inefficient bladder emptying, and colonic fecal stasis.[152] These problems, particularly constipation, are difficult to manage and require individual assessment and particularly tailored programs. Graduates may also suffer from the range of physical problems to which older people are vulnerable. Cardiovascular and respiratory disease is found relatively frequently reflecting the heavy smoking in this patient group. The mortality rates of long-stay patients are disputed. Patients with schizophrenia are considered either to have a life expectancy similar to the general population or a higher mortality attributable to suicide or to the effects of rapid and inadequately planned transfers from their familiar hospital surrounding into the community.[153]

The care of graduate patients encompasses elements of good practice within old age psychiatry, psychiatric rehabilitation, and medicine.[149] It is vital for the multidisciplinary teams caring for such patients in the hospital setting, and now, increasingly, in the community, to overcome the negative attitudes traditionally held about elderly long-stay patients. The needs of graduates are very different from those of patients with severe dementia and they should not be cared for in the same settings. Patients' skills should be identified and cultivated as part of a rehabilitative process, in the context of working toward an improved quality of life by improving the physical and social environment. Residential options in the community are varied and should be determined by the individual's present and likely future physical and mental health needs. Medication regimens often need review, and many patients benefit from cautious reduction or withdrawal of antipsychotic drugs that have often been prescribed in substantial amounts over the years or by changing to an atypical antipsychotic which has fewer extrapyramidal side-effects.

MANIA
Epidemiology

The reported prevalence and new incidence of mania in old age varies widely; studies to date are reviewed by Shulman.[154]

Several studies have suggested that mania only rarely occurs de novo in old age, with approximately 90 percent of patients with a manic episode in old age having been identified as bipolar by 50 years of age. National statistics from the United States for first admission to psychiatric hospitals, however, suggest that the number of first admissions with mania does not reduce with age but rather increases in older men. The initial Epidemiological Catchment Area (ECA) data revealed no manic cases in the community[155] and a more recent ECA study reported a prevalence of only 0.1 percent compared with 1.4 percent in young adults.[156] This does not reflect clinical experience, however, because manic and hypomanic illnesses are quite commonly encountered on old age psychiatry units, representing 12 percent of all admissions with affective disorders.[156] The discrepancies between these results may reflect that mania in old age has different clinical features than those found in younger people; this is reviewed below.

Older patients with mania typically had their first manic episode in their mid- to late fifties.[157] Most older people with episodes of mania live alone, are unmarried and impoverished, and are maintained in the community.[158] People with mania of earlier onset are under-represented in these hospitalized samples; possible explanations for this include effective treatment with lithium, "burn-out" after many years, and higher mortality rates among younger patients with bipolar disorder. In about one-half of elderly patients with mania, the first episode of mental illness is depression,[159] with many years latency before mania becomes manifest.

Clinical features

Many of the clinical features of mania are similar to those found in younger patients but dramatic physical overactivity, violence, criminal behavior, infectious euphoria, and grandiosity are less common.[160] Clinical experience suggests that mixed mood states are more commonly found in older subjects, but this has not been substantiated in a controlled study.[161] Adverse life events, particularly episodes of illness, more commonly appeared to precipitate mania in older subjects. Subjective confusion or perplexity is relatively prominent in elderly people. First-episode mania in very late life with no previous psychiatric history was frequently associated with comorbid neurological disorder.

Secondary mania

This concept refers to an episode of mania causally associated with medical illness, exogenous substances, and organic cerebral dysfunction.[161] First-onset mania in old age should be considered to have an underlying organic cause until proven otherwise. The frequent presence of some degree of nonprogressive cognitive impairment in secondary mania reflects its heterogeneous etiology. Even if no acute cause is discovered, there is still a greater prevalence of coexisting neurological illness. Stroke is the most characteristic precipitant of secondary mania, and long-standing cerebrovascular disease is also over-represented, with white matter hyperintensities often found on MRI scanning. Family history and prior psychiatric disturbance are uncommon in secondary mania.

The treatment of mania in old age

The drug treatment of elderly people with mania is similar to that in younger patients.[162] However, drug doses will generally be smaller. Neuroleptics are the mainstay of acute treatment. In secondary mania treatment is also directed at the underlying medical cause. Prophylactic treatment is with lithium, although the risks of neurotoxicity are higher, even at relatively low serum lithium levels.[163] The acute antimanic effect may also be useful in older people. The anticonvulsants carbamazepine and sodium valproate are increasingly widely used for their mood stabilizing effects, but few data have been reported in older people with mania. One retrospective naturalistic study comparing valproate with lithium found that the number of patients who improved was significantly greater in the lithium group.[164] When the response rates for those whose drug levels were in the therapeutic ranges were compared the rates were similar, with 82 percent of those taking lithium responding and 75 percent taking valproate. The therapeutic range reported for valproate was 65–90 μm. It is unclear from the study report whether valproate was used in those who had not tolerated or not responded to lithium or whether it was a first-line drug. The long-term use of neuroleptics should be avoided due to the increased risks of tardive dyskinesia.

The acute outcome is similar to that in younger patients. Studies are contradictory as to whether mania with first onset in old age has a poorer or better long-term prognosis than mania recurring in old age. The picture is confounded by the greater likelihood of comorbid physical disease and/or cognitive impairment.[156, 158]

ANXIETY DISORDERS
Epidemiology

Several studies have examined the prevalence of anxiety disorders in community-based populations.[165–169] The prevalence rates for phobias range between less than 1 and 11.7 percent; for generalized anxiety the range is between 1.4 and 7.3 percent. The variability in these findings probably reflects the use in some studies of specific case-finding instruments designed for elderly subjects. There is good consensus that panic disorder is extremely rare in old age. Jorm[170] concludes in a review of epidemiological studies across the lifespan that there is some evidence that susceptibility to anxiety (and depression) reduces with age and that this decrease is not accounted for by selective institutionalization of people with the symptoms. Longitudinal studies are needed to distinguish the effects of aging from cohort effects.

Phobic disorders

Phobic disorders consist of persistent or recurrent irrational fear of an object, activity, or situation that results in the compelling desire to avoid the phobic stimulus.[171] This reduces the fear and is thus rewarding and therefore avoidance increases. In old age they are associated with higher rates of medical and of other psychiatric morbidity, but are frequently found in the absence of other psychiatric disorder.[165] Most specific phobias are early onset and then continue into adult life.[119,171] Most late-onset phobias are agoraphobic and are precipitated by traumatic experiences or acute physical ill-health.[119,171]

At six-month follow-up in a community sample, most of whom have not been treated, more than two-thirds still have phobic anxiety. Persistence of the disorder is predicted by female gender and stand-alone phobic anxiety (without comorbid depression).[119,171] Individuals with one phobia may develop another. Fear of crime is particularly common in old age, leading to fear of going out and to night-time fearfulness. Social phobias in old age have usually developed earlier in life and persisted; they tend to be chronic and unremitting.[173] Comorbidity with agoraphobia, specific phobia, depression, and alcohol abuse is common.[174] Older people rarely seek treatment, and phobias do not in general seem to reduce life satisfaction.[119] Cognitive-behavioral treatment is favored over pharmacological interventions, although antidepressants may be useful. Drug treatment alone is not acceptable to older people with phobic disorders.[172] Anxiolytics provide only symptomatic relief and are best avoided because of their dependency potential.[171]

Generalized anxiety disorder

Generalized anxiety disorder consists of generalized, persistent anxiety, with motor tension, restlessness, tachycardia, tachypnea, other autonomic symptoms, apprehensiveness, and hypervigilance.[174] It usually runs a chronic course.[175] It is hard to diagnose in older people because of its high degree of comorbidity with depression. Coexistent medical conditions can complicate the situation. Patients are high service users although they may not present complaining of anxiety.[1,176] Benzodiazepines have been the mainstay of treatment, but dependence and adverse effects should limit their use to very short-term management only. Antidepressants and cognitive-behavioral strategies may be useful.[177]

Panic disorder

Panic disorder is characterized by recurrent attacks of panic, with intense fear often of death accompanied by severe somatic anxiety symptoms. The patient often feels that s/he must escape from the situation. It usually runs a chronic course[178] but may remit spontaneously or become less disabling secondary to reduced rates of social interaction in old age. It may, albeit rarely, occur de novo in older people.[179] Panic disorder with onset earlier in life is associated with depression,[179] alcohol abuse,[180] increased suicide risk,[181] and higher cardiovascular morbidity.[182] Rarely it is due to an underlying endocrine abnormality. Part of the explanation for the low prevalence in the elderly may be that sufferers may not survive into old age. Antidepressants are the pharmacological antipanic agents of choice with SSRIs increasingly used in preference to tricyclics. Benzodiazepines are efficacious for symptom control, but can be used only very short term because of undesirable side-effects and dependence. Cognitive-behavioral therapy can be effective. Long-term outcome is improved by a combination of drug and cognitive-behavioral approach.

Post-traumatic stress disorder and bereavement

Post-traumatic stress disorder (PTSD) occurring earlier in life can be associated with disabilities persisting into old age; traumatic events in old age can trigger similar PTSD reactions to those occurring in younger victims.[183] The symptom profile is the same as: younger people in re-experiencing the trauma; hyperarousal and avoidance. Symptoms may be persistent or intermittent.[184] The intensity of the physiological response to the original trauma may be the most significant predictor of a poor outcome. Further stressful life events can slow recovery, which may also be hindered by drug and alcohol abuse, which may themselves be triggered by PTSD.[185] PTSD can impair people's ability to deal with subsequent life stresses, and symptoms may therefore resurface among older veterans in healthcare settings.[186] PTSD probably responds best to a combination of a supportive therapeutic relationship, antidepressants, and cognitive-behavioral therapy. There are no controlled trials in this age group.

Bereavement is, sadly, an all-too-common experience for older people. Although depressive symptomatology is very common in the weeks immediately after bereavement, most subjects experience a gradual diminution of these symptoms without developing a full-blown depressive illness. Persistent, severe depression following bereavement is most strongly associated with a past history of depression. Surprisingly, only weak statistical associations are found with quality of the relationship with the lost partner or with level of post-bereavement social support.[187]

Obsessive–compulsive disorder

Obsessive–compulsive disorder (OCD) has a prevalence rate of 0.5–1.5 percent in older people.[168,188] The onset is usually earlier in life, with persistence into old age but those patients seen in old age usually have had a relatively late age of onset.[174,188] There is no difference in the severity of symptoms but older patients have less concern about symmetry and counting, while handwashing and fear of sinning are more common.[188] OCD is often resistant to treatment, but the use of clomipramine, SSRIs, and cognitive-behavioral techniques has improved the outlook.[189] In elderly people, it is important to bear in mind both that obsessive–compulsive phenomena frequently occur within a primary depressive illness, and that the development of obsessional orderliness may indicate the onset of dementia.[191]

Somatoform disorders

Older people often develop exaggerated bodily complaints in the context of real physical illness. Physically ill patients may also present with generalized anxiety or panic symptoms. The common medical disorders producing anxiety symptoms are endocrine, cardiovascular, pulmonary, and neurological conditions. A thorough history must be taken in an attempt to establish the temporal relationship of psychiatric symptomatology and the onset of medical illness.

Somatoform disorders are those in which physical symptoms occur in the absence of any or sufficient organic pathology to account for them. Psychological contributory factors can usually be identified. Although the onset of somatoform disorder is usually in early life and runs a chronic course, somatizing patients avoid psychiatrists in youth and adulthood and so not uncommonly present for the first time in old age.[190] Older people presenting with somatoform disorders in

general practice also frequently have a comorbid major depression.[88] Such patients usually have clear symptoms of depression and/or anxiety; their bodily complaints tend to be restricted to one or two body organs or systems. They are preoccupied with the possibility of serious physical illness. They demand investigation rather than treatment. In contrast, hypochondriacal preoccupation presenting for the first time in old age is likely to be secondary to anxiety and depression. Elderly patients only rarely present with hysterical amnesia or conversion reactions in response to stressful experience.

ALCOHOL ABUSE
(See also Chapter 80)

The average alcohol intake of older people is less than that of younger adults. Fewer drink regularly[191] and abstinence is more common.[192] Social and psychological factors may contribute to a decrease in alcohol intake with age; these include reduced social opportunities and financial constraints. Older people are, however, more vulnerable to the effects of alcohol because of physiological changes and the increased presence of pathological processes. Despite this general downward trend, drinking (and past drinking) is an important contributor to mental and physical ill health in some old people.[193,194]

Epidemiology and etiology

American studies suggest that the prevalence of abusive or dependent drinking is about 5 percent in the population aged 65 years and over, with a male preponderance of about 4:1.[195] A British community study reported a 1 percent prevalence of problem drinking.[196] In the hospital setting, elderly patients who abuse alcohol are concentrated in general medical settings and in psychiatric settings; one study[197] identified 14 percent of elderly emergency admissions as having current alcohol abuse. Similarly, one-third of patients aged 60 and over discharged from a psychiatric hospital in the USA had comorbid substance abuse.[198] Cultural, ethnic, and socioeconomic factors, differences between countries, and regional variation may influence drinking behavior and related problems, resulting in variable prevalence.

The rates of alcohol abuse in the elderly are related to the levels of consumption by the community as a whole.[199] Psychiatric disorder and personality attributes predispose to alcohol abuse. In particular, those older people with a late onset of alcohol abuse tend to have a past history of harmless drinking patterns, with consumption increased in the context of depression, bereavement, lack of social support, and/or deteriorating physical health.[193,200] Elderly people with insomnia and/or chronic pain, those previously dependent on alcohol, and those with current depression or dementia seem particularly vulnerable to alcohol-related problems in old age.[201] Persisting social problems perpetuate the cycle of loneliness and further drinking.[199]

Clinical features

The diagnosis of alcohol abuse may be difficult because the presentation may be masked, unsuspected, or atypical.[202]

In a general medical setting the prevalence is higher and the index of suspicion should be raised.[203] In particular, alcohol abuse must be suspected in the assessment of otherwise unexplained falls. Alcohol abuse may present with a wide range of neuropsychiatric complications.[189] Patients can present with cognitive impairment, problems due to mixed intoxication with drugs, or unrecognized withdrawal states. Alcohol abuse is also associated with functional psychiatric disorder.[204] Up to one-third of elderly persons who break the law abuse alcohol or are dependent on it.[205] They are often under the influence of alcohol when the crime is committed.

There is little information regarding the clinical course and prognosis. Light to moderate use of alcohol is associated with a decreased mortality in elderly people. The benign course of "normal" drinking seems very different, however, from that of the problem drinkers in old age, who often present when brain damage or social breakdown supervenes. A past history of alcohol-related problems is associated with both depression and dementia in later life. Depression and anxiety are major comorbid diagnoses.

Management

As already noted, alcohol abuse in older people is probably often undetected, particularly in patients presenting with medical conditions. Screening at-risk groups[206] may identify individuals at risk of alcohol abuse. Screening instruments used for younger people are probably limited in their value in elderly people; a recent review by Beresford[195] presents one such screening test designed for older people, the Michigan Alcoholism Screening Test (MAST)—Geriatric Version, although this has yet to be extensively validated. A recent study in the UK suggested that the CAGE (stands for *C*ut down, *A*nnoy, *G*uilty *E*ye opener)and the MAST screening too have low sensitivity in older UK medical inpatients.[207]

When an individual is recognized as having an alcohol-related problem, several services may need to be involved. Home visits are often invaluable in the initial assessment.[208] Hospital admission may be needed to break the drinking routine, reduce risks associated with acute alcohol withdrawal,[209] and allow for full physical and psychiatric assessment. Alcohol withdrawal symptoms become more severe with age, and detoxification is more likely to be complicated by intercurrent illness. Withdrawal seizures may occur within 24 hours. Tremor, tachycardia, hypertension, anxiety, nausea, and insomnia are prominent features of the alcohol withdrawal syndrome in old age. The patient should be nursed in a calm, well-lit environment. Shorter acting benzodiazepines and chlormethiazole are preferred for sedation. The dosage for older patients undergoing detoxification should begin at about one-third of that used for a fit younger person and should then be titrated against the clinical response.

A long-term management plan needs to be formulated with either abstinence or controlled drinking as a goal. Elderly people respond better to social intervention than intensive confrontation. Amelioration of social stresses, group socialization, family work, medical treatment, and management of depression are all part of the approach needed. Disulfiram is not recommended in older people because of the increasing medical risks involved with ingesting alcohol while taking the drug.[210]

PERSONALITY DISORDERS IN OLD AGE

Personality disorders are generally recognizable by adolescence or earlier and continue throughout most of adult life, although they become less obvious in middle or old age.[211] Some patients with life-long subclinical personality traits may present clinically in old age as a result of experiencing increasing stress and adversity. Global well-being, life satisfaction, and the capacity to cope with illness and loss in old age are also critically influenced by personality and its adaptation to old age.[212] Personality traits may be critical in adapting to the adverse life events all too often encountered by older people.

Epidemiology

An individual's personality is essentially stable over time[213] (see also Chapter 63). Introversion has, however, been shown to increase with age,[214] whereas extraversion, neuroticism, and openness to experience decrease.[215] Older people tend to have higher scores on scales for orderliness, social conformity, and emotional stability and lower scores for activity and energy.[216] A decline in sociopathy and criminality has been documented.[217] Few large-scale studies of personality disorder in old age have been performed. An early epidemiological survey[3] reported a prevalence of 3.6–10.6 percent for personality disorders in subjects aged 65 years and over. More recent surveys of older community-living individuals using standardized diagnostic schedules have found lifetime prevalence rates for personality disorder ranging between 2.1 and 18 percent.[218]

Senile self-neglect (Diogenes syndrome)

Patients with senile self-neglect may present to units for medicine of elderly people. This syndrome has also been called senile squalor syndrome, senile breakdown, and litter-hoarding syndrome. The syndrome can be understood as an expression of abnormal personality traits, in reaction to stress and loneliness or as the end stage of longstanding reclusiveness.[219] It is also sometimes secondary to psychosis, dementia, frontal lobe syndrome, or obsessional compulsive disorder.[220] The clinical picture is of very gross self-neglect not accompanied by any psychiatric or physical disorder sufficient to account for the squalor in which the individual lives. Some early organic cerebral impairment or mild depressive symptoms may be present. The prognosis of such cases is not good. Compulsory hospitalization is difficult to accomplish and mortality is high; apparently successful rehabilitation is usually followed by relapse.[220,221] Day care might maintain an individual but some form of institutional care usually becomes necessary.

Outcome of personality disorder in old age

Clinical experience suggests that patients with personality disorders do not cause as much trouble for themselves, their families, and healthcare professionals when they reach old age.[222] Formal long-term follow-up studies are, however, sparse. Immature personality disorders including antisocial, impulsive, histrionic, dependent, and narcissistic improve with time. Mature personality disorders, including anancastic, paranoid, schizoid, and schizotypal, tend to persist into later life. Deterioration may become evident in the obsessive–compulsive patient becoming increasingly rigid, the paranoid patient more suspicious and isolated and the schizotypal/schizoid patient old age more withdrawn and anxious. This view, however, has not been adequately substantiated by follow-up studies.

The high suicide rate of patients with borderline personality precludes their frequent graduation to the care of psychiatrists. In those who do survive into old age, the criteria for borderline personality disorder are still rare because self-mutilation is so uncommon. Good global outcome in such patients is associated with high intelligence, attractiveness, artistic talent, and coexisting obsessive–compulsive traits.[223] The highly subjective "likeability" seems also to confer good prognosis. Poor outcome is associated with a history of parental brutality, impulsivity, poor premorbid functioning, and coexistent schizotypal/antisocial personality disorder.[224]

In patients with antisocial personality disorder, there is a tendency toward spontaneous remission so that these individuals are rarely encountered over the age of 60.[211] Patients with schizotypal and schizoid personality disorder rarely seek treatment, so little is reported on their long-term outcome but the outlook is probably poor.[225] There is also little information on the outcome of histrionic, narcissistic, obsessive–compulsive, and depressive personality disorders.[211]

Management of personality disorder in old age

There has been little formal study of treatment approaches to personality disorders in old age.[211] The psychotherapeutic treatment of elderly patients is unpromising for individuals with longstanding personality disorders who cannot realistically be expected to resolve a lifetime of failed relationships and missed opportunities. However, the general principles of psychiatric treatment of older people apply to patients with primary personality psychopathology. Concurrent disorders should be optimally treated with medication or other means. The use of medication per se in personality disorders in old age has not been formally studied.

KEY POINTS Functional psychiatric illness in old age

- There is a wide range of functional psychiatric disorders
- These disorders are common especially in the presence of physical illness
- They are frequently undetected and/or untreated
- Most patients with functional psychiatric disorders improve with appropriate management
- The conditions if untreated lead to significant distress, increased care costs, and increased physical morbidity and mortality

REFERENCES

1. Livingston G, Manela M, Katona C: Cost of community care for elderly people. Br J Psychiatry 1997;171:56–59
2. Myers JK, Weissman MM, Tischler GL et al: Six-month prevalence of psychiatric disorders in three communities. Arch Gen Psychiatry 1984;41:959–967
3. Kay DWK, Beamish P, Roth M: Old age mental disorders in Newcastle upon Tyne. Part I: a study of prevalence. Br J Psychiatry 1964;110:146–158
4. Henderson AS, Jorm AF, Mackinnon A et al: The prevalence of depressive disorders and the distribution of depressive symptoms in later life: a survey using draft ICD-10 and DSM-III R. Psychol Med 1993;23:719–729
5. World Health Organization: International Classification of Mental Disorders, 10th Ed. World Health Organization, Geneva, 1992
6. American Psychiatric Association: Diagnostic and Statistical Manual of Mental Disorders, 3rd Ed, revised. American Psychiatric Association, Washington, DC, 1987
7. Weissman MM, Leaf PJ, Bruce ML, Florio L: The epidemiology of dysthymia in five communities—rates, risks, co-morbidity and treatment. Am J Psychiatry 1988;145:815–819
8. Kivela S-L, Pahkala K, Laippala P: Prevalence of depression in an elderly population in Finland. Acta Psychiatr Scand 1988;78:401–413
9. Copeland JRM, Dewey ME, Griffiths-Jones HM: A computerized psychiatric diagnostic system and case nomenclature for elderly subjects: GMS and AGECAT. Psychol Med 1986;16:89–99
10. Gurland BJ, Golden RR, Teresi JA, Challop J: The Short-CARE: an efficient instrument for the assessment of depression, dementia and disability. J Gerontol 1984;39:166–169
11. Kay DWK, Henderson AS, Scott R et al: Dementia and depression among the elderly living in the Hobart community: the effect of a diagnostic criteria on the prevalence rates. Psychol Med 1985;15:771–778
12. Copeland JRM, Dewey ME, Wood N et al: Range of mental illness among the elderly in the community: prevalence in Liverpool using the GMS-AGECAT package. Br J Psychiatry 1987;150:815–823
13. Copeland JRM, Gurland BJ, Dewey ME et al: Is there more dementia, depression and neurosis in New York? A comparative community study of the elderly in New York and London using the community diagnosis AGECAT. Br J Psychiatry 1987;151:466–473
14. Livingston G, Hawkins A, Graham N et al: The Gospel Oak Study: prevalence rates of dementia, depression and activity limitation among elderly residents in inner London. Psychol Med 1990;20:137–146
15. Beekman AT, Copeland JR, Prince MJ: Review of community prevalence of depression in later life. Br J Psychiatry 1999;174:307–311
16. Copeland JR, Beekman AT, Dewey M et al: Depression in Europe. Geographical distribution among older people. Br J Psychiatry 1999;174:312–321
17. Macdonald AJD: Do general practitioners "miss" depression in elderly patients? Br Med J 1986;292:1365–1367
18. Evans S, Katona CLE: The epidemiology of depressive symptoms in elderly primary care attenders. Dementia 1993;4:327–333
19. Iliffe S, Tai SS, Haines A et al: Assessment of elderly people in general practice. 4. Depression, functional ability and contact with services. Br J Gen Pract 1993;431:371–374
20. Callahan MC, Hui SL, Niebauer NA et al: Longitudinal study of depression and health service use among elderly primary care patients. J Am Geriatr Soc 1994;42:833–838
21. Koenig HG, Meador KG, Cohen HJ, Blazer D: Depression in elderly hospitalised patients with medical illness. Arch Intern Med 1988;148:1929–1936
22. Ames D: Depression among elderly residents of local-authority residents homes: its nature and the efficacy of intervention. Br J Psychiatry 1990;156:667–676
23. Wragg RE, Jeste DV: Overview of depression and psychosis in Alzheimer's disease. Am J Psychiatry 1989;146:577–586
24. Ballard CG, Patel A, Solis M et al: A one-year follow-up study of depression in dementia sufferers. Br J Psychiatry 1996;168:287–291
25. Heeren TJ, van Hemert AM, Lagaay AM, Rooymans HGM: The general population prevalence of non-organic psychiatric disorders in subjects aged 85 years and over. Psychol Med 1992;22:733–738
26. Mendlewicz J: The age factor in depressive illness: some genetic considerations. J Gerontol 1976;31:300–303

27. Baldwin R: Age of onset of depression in the elderly. Br J Psychiatry 1990;156:445–446

28. Beekman AT, Copeland JR, Prince MJ: Review of community prevalence of depression in later life. Br J Psychiatry 1999;174:307–311

29. Reynolds CF, Kupfer DJ, Houck PR et al: Reliable discrimination of elderly depressed and demented patients by electroencephalographic sleep data. Arch Gen Psychiatry 1988;45:258–264

30. Patterson JV, Michalewski HJ, Storr A: Latency variability of the components of auditory event-related potentials to infrequent stimuli in aging, Alzheimer-type dementia and depression. Electroencephalogr Clin Neurophysiol 1988;71:450–460

31. Schneider LS: Biologic features of geriatric affective disorder. Clin Geriatr Med 1992;8:253–265

32. Katona CLE, Aldridge CR: The dexamethasone suppression test and depressive signs in dementia. J Affect Disord 1985;8:83–89

33. Stahl SM, Lemoine PM, Ciaranello RD, Berger PA: Plateletadrenergic receptor sensitivity in major depressive disorders. Psychiatry Res 1983;10:157–164

34. Mellerup ET, Plenge P: Imipramine binding in depression and psychiatric conditions. Acta Psychiatr Scand 1988;78(suppl 345):61–68

35. Heninger GR, Charney DS, Sternberg GE: Serotonergic function in depression: prolactin response to intravenous tryptophan in depressed patients and healthy subjects. Arch Gen Psychiatry 1984;41:398–402

36. Guraluik JM, Kohout FJ: Low cholesterol concentrations and severe depressive symptoms in elderly people. Br Med J 1994;308:1328–1332

37. Philpot MP, Banerjee S, Needham-Bennett H et al: tc-HMPAO single photon emission tomography in late-life-depression: a pilot study of regional cerebral blood flow at rest and during a verbal fluency task. J Affect Disord 1993;28:233–240

38. Beats B, Levy R: Imaging and affective disorder in the elderly. Clin Geriatr Med 1992;8:267–274

39. Kumar A: Functional brain imaging in late-life depression. J Clin Psychiatry 1993;54(suppl):21–25

40. Baldwin RC: Late life depression and structural brain changes: a review of recent magnetic resonance imaging research. Int J Geriatr Psychiatry 1993;8:115–123

41. Kok RM, Heeren TJ, Hooijer C et al: The prevalence of depression in elderly medical inpatients. J Affect Disord 1995;33:77–82

42. Folstein MF, Mailberger R, McHugh P: Mood disorder as a specific complication of stroke. J Neurol Neurosurg Psychiatry 1977;40:1018–1020

43. Katona C, Livingston G: Comorbid Depression and Physical Illness in Older People. Martin Dunitz, London, 1997:1–81

44. Ring HA, Trimble MR: Affective disturbance in Parkinson's disease. Int J Geriatr Psychiatry 1991;6:385–393

45. Koenig HG, Shelp F, Goli V et al: Survival and health care utilization in elderly medical inpatients with major depression. J Am Geriatr Soc 1989;37:599–606

46. Cooper B: Psychiatric disorders among elderly patients admitted to hospital medical wards. J R Soc Med 1987;80:13–16

47. Koeing HG, Meador KG, Cohen HJ et al: Self-rated depression scales and screening for major depression in the older hospitalized patient with medical illness. J Am Geriatr Soc 1988;36:699–706

48. Yesavage JA, Brink TL, Rose TL, Lum O: Development and validation of a geriatric depression screening scale: a preliminary report. J Psychiatric Res 1983;17:37–49

49. Anderson G, Vestgaard K, Riis J: Citalopram for poststroke pathological crying. Lancet 1993; 342:837–839

50. Anderson G, Vestgaard K, lauritzen L: Effective treatment of post stroke depression with the selective serotonin uptake reinhibitor citalopram. Stroke 1994;25:1099–1104

51. Evans M, Hammond M, Wilson K et al: Placebo-controlled trial of depression in elderly physically ill patients. Int J Geriatr Psychiatry 1997;12:817–824

52. Ganzini L, Lee MA, Heintz RT et al: The effect of depression treatment on elderly patients' preferences for life-sustaining medical therapy. Am J Psychiatry 1994;151:1631–1636

53. Roth M: The natural history of mental disorder in old age. J Ment Sci 1955;101:281–301

54. Abrams RC, Alexopoulos GS, Young RC: Geriatric depression and DSMIII R personality disorder criteria. J Am Geriatr Soc 1987;35:383–386

55. Murphy E: Social origins of depression in old age. Br J Psychiatry 1982;141:135–142

56. Kennedy GJ, Kelman HR, Thomas C et al: Hierarchy of characteristics associated with depressive symptoms in an urban elderly sample. Am J Psychiatry 1989;146:220–227

57. Murrell SA, Himmelfarb SA, Wright K: Prevalence of depression and its correlates in older adults. Am J Epidemiology 1983;117:173–185

58. Linn MW, Hunter K, Harris R: Symptoms of depression and recent life events in the community elderly. J Clin Psychology 1980; 36:675–682

59. Livingston G, Manela M, Katona C: Depression and other Psychiatric Morbidity in the carers of elderly people. Br Med J 1996;312:153–156

60. Murray J: The Prevention of Anxiety and Depression in Vulnerable Groups. Gaskell, London, 1995

61. Brown RP, Sweeney J, Loutsch E et al: Involutional melancholia revisited. Am J Psychiatry 1984;137:439–444

62. Fredman L, Schoenbach VJ, Kaplan BH et al: The association between depressive symptoms and mortality among older participants in the Epidemiologic Catchment area—Piedmont Health Survey. J Gerontol 1989;44:S149–S156

63. Prince MJ, Reisches F, Beekman ATF et al: Development of the Euro-D scale—a European initiative to compare symptoms of depression in fourteen European centres. Br J Psychiatry 1999;174:330–338

64. Kivela SL, Pahkala K: Symptoms of depression in old people in Finland. Z Gerontol 1988;21:257–263

65. Wallace J, Pfohl B: Age-related differences in the symptomatic expression of major depression. J Nerv Ment Dis 1995;183:99–102

66. Burvill PW, Hall WD, Stampfer HG, Emmerson JP: A comparison of early-onset and late-onset depressive illness in the community. Br J Psychiatry 1989;155:673–679

67. Alexopoulos GS: Late-life depression and neurological brain disease. Int J Geriatr Psychiatry 1989;4:187–190

68. Abas MA, Sahakian BJ, Levy R: Neuropsychological deficits and CT scan changes in elderly depressives. Psychol Med 1990;20:507–520

69. O'Boyle M, Amadeo M: "Don't know" responses in elderly demented and depressed patients. J Geriatr Psychiatr Neurol 1989;2:83–86

70. Forsell Y, Jorm AF, Winblad B: Association of age, sex, cognitive dysfunction and disability with major depressive symptoms in an elderly sample. Am J Psychiatry 1994;151:1600–1604

71. Jorm AF, van Duijn CM, Chandra V et al: Psychiatric history and related exposures as risk factors for Alzheimer's disease. International J Epidemiol 1991;20(suppl 2):43–47

72. Devanand DP, Sano M, Tang MX et al: Depressed mood and the incidence of Alzheimer's disease in the elderly living in the community. Arch Gen Psychiatry 1996;53:175–182

73. Henderson AS, Korten AE, Jacomb PA et al: The course of depression in the elderly: a longitudinal community-based sample in Australia. Psychol Med 1997;27:119–129

74. Wetherell JL, Gatz M, Johansson B, Pedersen NL: History of depression and other psychiatric illness as risk factor for Alzheimer's disease in a twin sample. Alzheimer's Dis Assoc Disord 1999;13:47–52

75. Allen NHP, Burns A: The non-cognitive features of dementia. Rev Clin Gerontol 1995;5:57–75

76. Roth M, Mountjoy CI, Amrein R et al: Moclobemide in elderly patients with cognitive decline and depression: an international double-blind, placebo controlled trial. Br J Psychiatry 1996;8:270–275

77. Nyth AL, Gottfries CG, Lyby K et al: A controlled multicenter clinical study of citalopram and placebo in elderly depressed patients with and without concomitant dementia. Acta Psychiatr Scand 1992;86:138–145

78. Katona CLE, Hunter BN, Bray J: A double-blind comparison of the efficacy and safety of paroxetine and imipramine in the treatment of depression with dementia. International J Geriatr Psychiatry 1998;13:100–108

79. Kaufer DI, Cummings JL, Christine D: Effect of tacrine on behavioral symptoms in Alzheimer's disease: an open-label study. J Geriatr Psychiatry Neurol 1996;9:1–6

80. Alexopoulos GS, Abrams RC, Young RC, Shamoian CA: Cornell Scale for Depression in Dementia. Biol Psychiatry 1988;23:271–284

81. Katona C, Livingston G: Impact of screening older people with physical illness for depression. Lancet 2000;366(8):91

82. Hoyl MT, Alessi CA, Harker JO et al: Development and testing of a 5 item version of the geriatric depression scale. J Am Geriatr Soc 1999;47:873–878

83. Adshead F, Cody DD, Pitt B: BASDEC—a novel screening instrument for depression in elderly medical patients. Br Med J 1992;305:397

84. Sheikh JA, Yesavage JA: Geriatric depression scale (GDS): Recent findings and development of a shorter version. In Brink TL (ed): Clinical gerontology: a guide to assessment and intervention. Howarth Press, New York, 1986

85. D'Ath P, Mullan M, Katona P et al: Screening, detection and management of depression in elderly primary care attenders. 1: The acceptability and performance of the 15 item Geriatric Depression Scale (GDS15) and the development of short versions. Fam Pract 1994;11:260–266

86. Arthur A, Jagger C, Lindesay J, Graham C, Clarke M: Using an annual over-75 health check to screen for depression: validation of the short Geriatric Depression Scale (GDS15) within general practice. Int J Geriatr Psychiatry 1999;14:431–439

87. Turrina C, Caruso R, Este R et al: Affective disorders among elderly general practice patients: a two-phase survey in Brescia, Italy. Br J Psychiatry 1994;165:533–537

88. Lyness JM, Noel TK, Cox C, King DA: Screening for depression in elderly primary care patients: a comparison of the Center for Epidemiologic Studies-Depression Scale and the Geriatric depression Scale. Arch Intern Med 1997;157:449–454

89. Banerjee S, Shamash K, Macdonald AJD, Mann AH: The use of the SelfCARE(D) as a screening tool in the clients of local authority home care services—a preliminary study. International J Geriatr Psychiatry 1998;13:695–699

90. Rockwell E, Lam RW, Zisook S: Antidepressant drug studies in the elderly. Psychiatr Clin N Am 1988;11:215–233

91. Mittmann N, Herrmann N, Einarson TR et al: The efficacy, tolerability of antidepressants in late life depression: a meta-analysis. J Affect Disord 1997;46:191–217

92. Georgotas A, McCue RE, Cooper TB et al: Factors affecting the delay of anti-depressant effect in responders to nortriptyline and phenelzine. Psychiatr Res 1989;28:1–9

93. Mulsant BH, Rosen J, Thornton JE, Zubenko GS: A prospective naturalistic study of electroconvulsive therapy in late-life depression. J Geriatr Psychiatry Neurol 1991;4:3–13

94. Benbow SM: The role of electroconvulsive therapy in the treatment of depressive illness in old age. Br J Psychiatry 1989;155:147–152

95. Fraser RM, Glass IB: Unilateral and bilateral ECT in elderly patients: a comparative study. Acta Psychiatr Scand 1980;62:13–31

96. Morris RG, Morris LW: Cognitive and behavioural approaches with the depressed elderly. Int J Geriatr Psychiatry 1991;6:407–413

97. Koder D-A, Brodaty H, Anstey KJ: Cognitive therapy for depression in the elderly. Int J Geriatr Psychiatry 1996;11:97–107

98. Reynolds CF, Frank E, Perel JM et al: Combined pharmacotherapy and psychotherapy in the acute and continuation treatment of elderly patients with recurrent major depression. Am J Psychiatry 1992;149:1687–1692

99. Reynolds CF, Frank E, Perel JM et al: Nortriptyline and interpersonal psychotherapy as maintenance therapies for recurrent major depression: a randomised controlled trial in patients older than 59 years. J Am Med Assoc 1999;281:39–45

100. Flint A, Rifat S: Augmentation strategies in refractory depression. Int J Geriatr Psychiatry 1995;10:137–146

101. van Marwijk HWJ, Bekker FM, Nolen WA et al: Lithium augmentation in geriatric depression. J Affect Disord 1990;20:217–223

102. Old Age Depression Interest Group: How long should the elderly take antidepressants? A double-blind placebo-controlled study of continuation/prophylaxis therapy with dothiepin. Br J Psychiatry 1993;162:175–182

103. Morris RG, Morris LW: Cognitive and behavioural approaches with the depressed elderly. Int J Geriatr Psychiatry 1991;6:407–413

104. Ong YK, Martineau F, Lloyd C, Robbins I: A support group for the depressed elderly. Int J Geriatr Psychiatry 1987;2:119–123

105. Lindesay J: Suicide in the elderly. Int J Geriatr Psychiatry 1991;6:355–361

106. Pierce D: Deliberate self-harm in the elderly. Int J Geriatr Psychiatry 1987;2:105–110

107. Cattell H, Jolley DJ: One hundred cases of suicide in older people. Br J Psychiatry 1995;166:451–457

108. Barraclough BM, Bunch J, Nelson B et al: One hundred cases of suicide—clinical aspects. Br J Psychiatry 1974;125:355–373

109. Draper B: Suicidal behaviour in the elderly. Int J Geriatr Psychiatry 1994;9:655–661

110. Rifai AH, George CJ, Stack JA et al: Hopelessness in suicide attempters after acute treatment of major depression in late life. Am J Psychiatry 1994;151:1687–1690

111. Schulberg HC, Mulsant B, Schulz R et al: Characteristics and course of major depression in older primary care patients. Int J Psychiatry Med 1998;28:421–436

112. Cole M, Bellavance F: The prognosis of depression in old age. Am J Geriatr Psychiatry 1997;5:4–14

113. Millard P: Depression in old age. Br Med J 1983;267:375–376

114. O'Brien JT, Ames D: Why do the depressed elderly die? Int J Geriatr Psychiatry 1994;9:689–693

115. Cole M, Bellavance F: Depression in elderly medical inpatients: a meta-analysis of outcomes. Can Med Assoc J 1997;157:1055–1060

116. Bruce ML, Seeman TE, Merrill S et al: The impact of depressive symptoms on physical disability. Am J Pub Health 1994;84:1796–1799

117. Callahan CM, Wolinsky FD, Stump TE et al: Mortality, symptoms and functional impairment in late-life depression. J Gen Intern Med 1998;13:746–752

118. Livingston G, Watkin V, Milne B, Manela MV, Katona C: The natural history of depression and the anxiety disorders in older people: the Islington community study. J Affect Disord 1997;46:255–262

119. Kay DWK, Roth M: Environmental and hereditary factors in the schizophrenias of old age ("late paraphrenia") and their bearing on the general problems of causation in schizophrenia. J Ment Sci 1961;107:649–686

120. DHSS (Department of Health and Social Security): Mental Health Statistics. HMSO, London, 1985

121. Christenson R, Blazer D: Epidemiology of persecutory ideation in an elderly population in the community. Am J Psychiatry 1984;141:9:1088–1091

122. Blazer D, Hays J, Salive M: Factors associated with paranoid symptoms in a community sample of older adults. Gerontologist 1996;36:1:70–75

123. Forsell Y, Scott Henderson A: Epidemiology of paranoid symptoms in an elderly population. Br J Psychiatry 1998;172:429–432

124. Howard R: Late paraphrenia. Int Rev Psychiatry 1993;5:455–460

125. Lyketsos CG, Steinberg M, Tschanz JT et al: Mental and behavioral disturbances in dementia: findings from the Cache County Study on memory and aging. Am J Psychiatry 2000;157:708–714

126. Livingston G, Kitchen G, Manela M, Katona C, Copeland J: Persecutory symptoms and perceptual disturbance in a community sample of older people: the Islington study. Int J Geriatr Psychiatry 2001;16:462–468

127. Blazer D, Hays J, Salive M: Factors associated with paranoid symptoms in a community sample of older adults. Gerontologist 1996;36(1):70–75

128. Castle D, Howard R: What do we know about the aetiology of late-onset schizophrenia? Eur Psychiatry 1992;7:99–108

129. Herbert ME, Jacobson S: Late paraphrenia. Br J Psychiatry 1967;113:461–469

130. Howard R, Levy R: Personality structure in the paranoid psychoses of later life. Eur Psychiatry 1993;8:59–66

131. Naguib M, Levy R: Paranoid states in the elderly and late paraphrenia. In Jacoby R, Oppenheimer C (eds): Psychiatry in the Elderly. Oxford University Press, Oxford, 1991:758–778

132. Castle DJ, Wessely S, Howard R, Murray RM: Schizophrenia with onset at the extremes of adult life. Int J Geriatr Psychiatry 1997;12:712–717

133. Hafner H, Hambrecht M, Loffler W et al: Is schizophrenia a disorder of all ages? A comparison of first episodes and early course across the life cycle. Psychol Med 1998;28:351–356

134. Naguib M, Levy R: Late paraphrenia—neuropsychological impairment and structural brain abnormalities on computed tomography. Int J Geriatr Psychiatry 1987;2:83–90

135. Levy R, Naguib M: Late paraphrenia. Br J Psychiatry 1985;146:451

136. Howard RJ, Almeida O, Levy R: Phenomenology, demography and diagnosis in late-paraphrenia. Psychol Med 1994;24:397–410

137. Roth M, Kay DWK: Late paraphrenia: A variant of schizophrenia manifest in late life or an organic clinical syndrome? A review of recent evidence. Int J Geriatr Psychiatry 1998;13:775–784

138. Miller BL, Lesser IM, Boone K et al: Brain white matter lesions and psychosis. Br J Psychiatry 1991;158:76–82

139. Krull AJ, Press G, Dupont R et al: Brain imaging in late onset schizophrenia and related psychoses. Int J Geriatr Psychiatry 1991;6:651–658

140. Lesser IM, Miller BL, Schwartz TR et al: Brain imaging in late-life schizophrenia and related psychoses. Schizophr Bull 1993;19:773–782

141. Post F: Persistent Persecutory States of the Elderly. Pergamon Press, Oxford, 1966

142. Jeste DV, Harris MJ, Pearlson GD et al: Late onset schizophrenia. Studying clinical validity. Psychiatr Clin N Am 1988;11:1–13

143. Lacro JP, Harris MJ, Jeste DV: Late-life psychosis. In Murphy E, England, Alexopoulou G (eds): Geriatric Psychiatry, Vol. 18. John Wiley, Chichester, UK, 1995:231–244

144. Kendler S, David KL: The genetics and biochemistry of paranoid schizophrenia and other paranoid psychoses. Schizophr Bull 1981;7:689–709

145. Cooper AF, Curry AR: The pathology of deafness in the paranoid and affective psychoses of later life. J Psychosom Res 1976;20:97–105

146. Rockwell E, Krull AJ, Dimsdale J, Jeste DV: Late-onset psychosis with somatic delusions. Psychosomatics 1992;35:66–72

147. Gurian BS, Wexler D, Baker EH: Late-life paranoia: possible association with early trauma and infertility. Int J Geriatr Psychiatry 1992;7:277–284

148. Greene JA, Taylor SE: Paranoid states in the elderly. Clin Rep Aging 1989;3:8–11

149. Campbell P: Graduates. In Jacoby R, Oppenheimer C (eds): Psychiatry in the Elderly. Oxford University Press, Oxford, 1991:779–818

150. Bridge TP, Cannon HE, Wyatt RJ: Burned-out schizophrenia: evidence for age effects on schizophrenia symptomatology. J Gerontol 1978;33:835–839

151. Rogers D: The motor disorders of severe psychiatric illness: a conflict of paradigms. Br J Psychiatry 1985;147:221–232

152. Carrick J, Ramchurn L, Malone-Lee D: Urinary incontinence in a large psychiatric hospital. Health Trends 1988;20:118–119

153. Ciompi L: Aging and schizophrenic psychosis. Acta Psychiatr Scand 1985;136:413–420

154. Shulman KI: Mania in the elderly. Int Rev Psychiatry 1993;5:445–453

155. Kramer M, German PS, Anthony JC et al: Patterns of mental disorders among the elderly residents of Eastern Baltimore. J Am Geriatr Soc 1985;33:236–245

156. Weissman MM, Leaf PJ, Tichler GL et al: Affective disorders in five United States communities. Psychol Med 1988;18:141–153

157. Winokur G: The Iowa 500: heterogeneity and course in manic depressive illness (bipolar). Compr Psychiatry 1975;16:125–131

158. Meeks S: Bipolar disorder in the latter half of life: symptom presentation, global functioning and age of onset. J Affect-Disord 1999;J52(1–3):161–167

159. Shulman K, Tohen M, Satlin A et al: Mania compared to unipolar depression in old age. Am J Psychiatry 1992;149:341–345

160. Collins CC: Affective disorders in old age. In Joyce PR, Romans SE, Ellis PM, Silverstone TS (eds): Affective Disorders. University of Otago, Christchurch, New Zealand, 1995:257–280

161. Young RC, Kleinman GL: Mania in late life: focus on age at onset. Psychiatry 1992;149:867–876

162. Manela M, Katona C, Livingston G: How common are the anxiety disorders in old age? Int J Geriatr Psychiatry 1996;11:65–70

163. Finch EJL, Ktona C: Lithium augmentation of refractory depression in old age. Int J Geriatr Psychiatry 1989;4:41–46

164. Chen ST, Altshuler LL, Melnyk KA et al: Efficacy of lithium vs. valproate in the treatment of mania in the elderly: a retrospective study. J Clin Psychiatry 1999;60(3):181–186

165. Myers JK, Weissman M, Tischler GL: Six month prevalence of psychiatric disorders in three communities—1980–1982. Arch Gen Psychiatry 1984;41:959–967

166. Lindesay J, Briggs C, Murphy E: The Guy's/Age Concern Survey. Prevalence rates of cognitive impairment, depression and anxiety in an urban elderly community. Br J Psychiatry 1989;155:317–329

167. Lindesay J: Phobic disorders in the elderly. Br J Psychiatry 1991;159:531–541

168. Beekman AT, Bremmer MA, Deeg DJ et al: Anxiety disorders in later life: a report from the Longitudinal Aging Study Amsterdam. Int J Geriatr Psychiatry 1998;13(10):717–726

169. Schaub RT, Linden M: Anxiety and anxiety disorders in the old and very old—results from the Berlin Aging Study (BASE). Compr Psychiatry 2000;41(2 suppl 1):48–54

170. Jorm AF: Does old age reduce the risk of anxiety and depression? A review of epidemiological studies across the adult life span. Psychol Med 2000;30(1):11–22

171. Lindesay J: Phobic disorders in the elderly. Br J Psychiatry 1991;159:531–541

172. Stevens T, Katona C, Manela M, Watkin V, Livingston G: Drug treatment of older people with affective disorders in the community: lessons from an attempted clinical trial. Int J Geriatr Psychiatry 1999;14(6):467–472

173. Blazer D, George LK, Hughes D: The epidemiology of anxiety disorders: an age comparison. In Salzman C, Lebavitz BD (eds): Anxiety in the Elderly. Springer, New York, 1991:17–30

174. Sheikh JI, Salzman C: Anxiety in the elderly. Psychiatr Clin N Am 1995;18:871–883

175. Lindesay J: Anxiety disorders in the elderly. In Jacoby R, Oppenheimer C (eds): Psychiatry in the Elderly, Vol. 22. Oxford University Press, Oxford, 1991:735–757

176. de Beurs E, Beekman AT, van Balkom AJ et al: Consequences of anxiety in older persons: its effect on disability, well-being and use of health services. Psychol Med 1999;29(3):583–593

177. Stanley MA, Novy DM: Cognitive-behavior therapy for generalized anxiety in late life: an evaluative overview. J Anxiety Disord 2000;14(2):191–207

178. Sheikh JI, King RJ, Taylor CB: Comparative phenomenology of early-onset versus late-onset panic attacks: a pilot survey. Am J Psychiatry 1991;148:1231–1233

179. Sheikh JI, Taylor CB, King RJ et al: Panic attacks and avoidance behaviour in the elderly. In Proceedings of the 141st Annual Scientific Meeting of the American Psychiatric Association, Montreal, 1988

180. Katon W, Vitiliane P, Anderson K et al: Panic disorder: residual symptoms after the acute attacks abate. Compr Psychiatry 1987;28:151–158

181. Kushner MG, Sher KJ, Beitman BD: The relation between alcohol problems and the anxiety disorders. Am J Psychiatry 1990;147:685–695

182. Weissman MM, Kleinman GL, Markovitz JS et al: Suicidal ideation and suicide attempts in panic disorder and attacks. N Engl J Med 1989;321:1209–1214

183. Coryell W: Mortality of anxiety disorders. In Noyes R Jr, Roth M, Burrows GP (eds): Handbook of Anxiety. Vol. 2. Classification, Etiological Factors and Associated Disturbances. Elsevier Science, Amsterdam, 1988:311–320

184. Weintraub D, Ruskin PE: Posttraumatic stress disorder in the elderly: a review. Harv Rev Psychiatry 1999;7(3):144–152

185. Van der Kolk B: Psychopharmacological issues in post-traumatic stress disorder. Hosp Commun Psychiatry 1983;34:683–691

186. Snell FI, Padin-Rivera E: Post-traumatic stress disorder and the elderly combat veteran. J Gerontol Nurs 1997;23(10):13–19

187. Katona CLE: The aetiology of depression in old age. In Katona CLE (ed): Depression in Old Age. John Wiley, Chichester, UK, 1994:43–62

188. Kohn R, Westlake RJ: Clinical features of obsessive compulsive disorder in elderly patients. Am J Geriatr Psychiatry 1997;5(3):211–215

189. Rasmussen SA, Eisen JL, Pato MT: Current issues in the pharmacological management of obsessive compulsive disorder. J Clin Psychiatry 1993;54(suppl 6):4–9

190. Lindesay J: Neurotic disorders in the elderly. Int Rev Psychiatry 1993;5:461–467

191. Wattis JP: Alcohol and old people. Br J Psychiatry 1983;143:306–307

192. Busby WJ, Campbell AJ, Borrie MJ, Spears GFS: Alcohol use in a community-based sample of subjects aged 70 years and older. J Am Geriatr Soc 1988;36:301–305

193. Brody JA: Aging and alcohol abuse. J Am Geriatr Soc 1982;30:123–126

194. Friedmann PD, Jin L, Karrison T et al: The effect of alcohol abuse on the health status of older adults seen in the emergency department. Am J Drug Alcohol Abuse 1999;25(3):529–542

195. Beresford TP: Alcoholism in the elderly. Int Rev Psychiatry 1993;5:477–483

196. Saunders PA, Copeland JRM, Dewey ME et al: Alcohol use and abuse in the elderly: findings from the Liverpool Longitudinal Study of continuing health in the community. Int J Geriatr Psychiatry 1989;4:103–108

197. Adams WL, Magruder-Habib K, Trued S, Broome HL: Alcohol abuse in elderly emergency department patients. J Am Geriatr Soc 1992;40:1236–1240

198. Blixen CE, McDougall GJ, Suen LJ: Dual diagnosis in elders discharged from a psychiatric hospital. Int J Geriatr Psychiatry 1997;12(3):307–313

199. Ticehurst S: Alcohol and drug abuse. In Lindesay J (ed): Neurotic Disorders in the Elderly, Vol. 10. Oxford University Press, Oxford, 1995:172–192

200. Rosin AJ, Glass MM: Alcohol excess in the elderly. Q J Studies Alcohol 1971;32:53–55

201. King MB: Alcohol abuse and dementia. Int J Geriatr Psychiatry 1983;1:31–36

202. Zimburg S: Diagnosis and management of the elderly alcoholic. In Atkinson RM (ed): Alcohol and Drug Abuse in Old Age. American Psychiatric Press, Washington, DC, 1984:23

203. Wattis JP: Alcohol problems in the elderly. J Am Geriatr Soc 1981;24:131–134

204. Schuckit MA, Pastor PA: The elderly as a unique population: alcoholism. Alcoholism Clin Exp Res 1978;2:31–38
205. Taylor J, Parrott JM: Elderly offenders. Br J Psychiatry 1988;152:340–346
206. Zimberg S: Diagnosis and treatment of the elderly alcoholic. Alcoholism Clin Exp Res 1978;2:27–29
207. Luttrell S, Watkin V, Livingston G et al: Screening for alcohol misuse in older people. Int J Geriatr Psychiatry 1997;12(12):1151–1154
208. Jolley D, Hodgson S: Alcoholism in the elderly: a tale of women and our times. In Isaacs B (ed): Recent Advances in Geriatric Medicine, 3rd Ed. Churchill Livingstone, Edinburgh 1986:3–12
209. Liskow BI, Rinck C, Campbell J, De Souza C: Alcohol withdrawal in the elderly. J Studies Alcohol 1989;50:414–421
210. Dunne FJ, Schipperheijn JAM: Alcohol and the elderly. Br Med J 1989;298:1660–1661
211. Howard R, Bergmann K: Personality disorders in old age. Int Rev Psychiatry 1993;5:469–475
212. Abrams RC: Personality disorders. In Lindesay J (ed): Neurotic Disorders in the Elderly, Vol. 9. Oxford University Press, Oxford, 1995:154–171
213. Costa PT, McCrae RR: Still able after all these years: personality as a key to some issues in adulthood and old age. In Baltes PB, Brinn OG (eds): Lifespan Development and Behavior. Academic Press, New York, 1980
214. Gutman GM: A note on the MMPI: age and sex differences in extroversion and neuroticisms in a Canadian sample. Br J Social Clin Psychol 1996;5:128–129
215. Costa PT, McCrae RR, Zonderman AB et al: Cross-sectional studies of personality in a national sample: 2. Stability in neuroticism, extroversion and openness. Psychol Aging 1986;1:149
216. Stoner SB, Panek PE: Age and sex differences with the Courey Personality Scales. J Psychol 1985;119:137–142
217. Vaillant GE, Vaillant CO: Natural history of male psychosocial health XII. A 45 year study of predictors of successful aging at age 65. Am J Psychiatry 1990;147:31–37
218. Casey P: The epidemiology of personality disorder. In Tyrer P (ed): Personality Disorders: Diagnosis, Management and Care. Wright, London, 1988
219. Post F: Functional disorders. Description, incidence and recognition. In Levy R, Post F (eds): The Psychiatry of Later Life. Blackwell, Oxford, 1982
220. Rosenthal M, Stelian J, Wagner J, Berkman P: Diogenes syndrome and hoarding in the elderly: case reports. Israeli J Psychiatry Relat Sci 1999;36(1):29–34
221. Sidkar S: Diogenes syndrome: a case report. Hosp Med 1999; 60(9):679
222. Bergmann K: Psychiatric aspects of personality in older patients. In Jacoby R, Oppenheimer C (eds): Psychiatry in the Elderly, Vol. 24. Oxford University Press, Oxford, 1991:852–871
223. Woolcott P: Prognostic indicators in the psychotherapy of borderline patients. Am J Psychother 1985;39:17–29
224. Links P, Mittan JE, Steiner M: Predicting outcome for borderline personality disorder. Compr Psychiatry 1990;31:490–498
225. Stone MH: Long-term outcome in personality disorders. Br J Psychiatry 1993;162:299–313

Chapter 68   Exercise for successful aging

William J. Evans

Advancing age is associated with a remarkable number of changes in body composition. Reductions in lean body mass have been well characterized. This decreased lean body mass occurs primarily as a result of losses in skeletal muscle mass.[1,2] This age-related loss in muscle mass has been termed *sarcopenia*.[3] Loss in muscle mass accounts for the age-associated decreases in basal metabolic rate, muscle strength, and activity levels, which, in turn is the cause of the decreased energy requirements of elderly people. In sedentary individuals, the main determinant of energy expenditure is fat-free mass, which declines by about 15 percent between the third and eighth decade of life. It also appears that declining caloric needs are not matched by an appropriate decline in caloric intake, with the ultimate result an increased body fat content with advancing age. Increased body fatness along with increased abdominal obesity are thought to be directly linked to the greatly increased incidence of Type II diabetes among elderly people. This review discusses the extent to which regularly performed exercise can affect nutritional needs (with particular emphasis on protein needs) and functional capacity in elderly people.

MUSCLE STRENGTH AND MASS

Sarcopenia, the age-associated loss of muscle mass,[3] is a direct cause of the age-related decrease in muscle strength. Our laboratory[1] examined muscle strength and mass in 200 healthy 45–78-year-old men and women, and concluded that muscle mass (not function) is the major determinant of the age and sex-related differences in strength. This relationship is independent of muscle location (upper vs lower extremities) and function (extension vs flexion). Reduced muscle strength in elderly people is a major cause of their increased prevalence of disability. With advancing age and very low activity levels seen in very old people, muscle strength and power are critical components of walking ability.[4] The high prevalence of falls among institutionalized elderly people may be a consequence of their lower muscle strength.

The question that we have been attempting to address is: To what extent are these changes inevitable consequences of aging? Data examining young and middle-aged endurance-trained men demonstrate that body fat stores and maximal aerobic capacity were not related to age, but rather the total number of hours these men were exercising per week.[5] Even among sedentary individuals, energy spent in daily activities explains more than 75 percent of the variability in body fatness among young and older men.[6] These data and the results of other investigators indicate that levels of physical activity are important in determining energy expenditure and ultimately body fat accumulation. However, cross-sectional data of Klitgaard et al.[7,8] indicated that older endurance athletes (runners and swimmers) display fat-free mass and muscle strength similar to that seen in sedentary aged-matched controls, an indication that endurance exercise alone may not prevent sarcopenia.

AEROBIC EXERCISE

Maximal aerobic capacity ($\dot{V}O_{2max}$) declines with advancing age.[9] This age-associated decrease in $\dot{V}O_{2max}$ has been shown to be approximately 1 percent per year between the ages of 20 and 70 years old. This decline is likely due to a number of factors, including decreased levels of physical activity, changing cardiac function (including decreased maximal cardiac output), and reduced muscle mass. Flegg and Lakatta[10] determined that skeletal muscle mass accounted for most of the variability in $\dot{V}O_{2max}$ in men and women above the age of 60 years old. Recently, Rosen et al.[11] examined predictors of this age-associated decline in $\dot{V}O_{2max}$. They found that $\dot{V}O_{2max}$ declines at the same rate in athletic and sedentary men and that 35 percent of this decline is due to sarcopenia.

Aerobic exercise has long been an important recommendation for the prevention and treatment of many of the chronic diseases typically associated with old age. These include non-insulin-dependent diabetes mellitus, or NIDDM (and those with impaired glucose tolerance), hypertension, heart disease, and osteoporosis. Regularly performed aerobic exercise increases insulin action. The responses of initially sedentary young (age 20–30) and older (age 60–70) men and women to 3 months of aerobic conditioning (70 percent of maximal heart rate, 45 minutes/day, 3 days per week) were examined by Meredith et al.[12] They found that the absolute gains in aerobic capacity were similar between the two age groups. However, the mechanism for adaptation to regular submaximal exercise appears to be different between old and young people. Muscle biopsies taken before and after training showed a more than two-fold increase in oxidative capacity of the muscles of the older subjects, while that of the young subjects showed smaller improvements. In addition, skeletal muscle glycogen stores in the older subjects, significantly lower than those of the young men and women initially, increased significantly. The degree to which elderly people demonstrate increases in maximal cardiac output in response to endurance training is still largely unanswered. Seals and coworkers[13] found no increase after 1 year of endurance training while, more recently, Spina et al.[14] observed that older men increased maximal cardiac output, while healthy older women demonstrated no change in response to endurance exercise. If these gender-related differences in cardiovascular response are real, it may explain the lack of response in maximal cardiac output when older men and women are included in the same study population.

EXERCISE AND CARBOHYDRATE METABOLISM

The 2-hour plasma glucose level during an oral glucose tolerance test (OGTT) increases by an average of 5.3 mg/dl per decade, and fasting plasma glucose increases by an average of 1 mg/dl per decade.[15] The NHANES II study demonstrated a progressive increase of about 0.4 mM/decade of life in mean plasma glucose value 2 hours after a 75 g OGTT ($n = 1,678$ men and 1,892 women).[16] Shimokata and coworkers[17] examined glucose tolerance in community-dwelling men and women ranging in age between 17 and 92. By assessing level of obesity, pattern of body fat distribution, and activity and fitness levels, they attempted to examine the independent effect of age on glucose tolerance. They found no significant differences between the young and middle-aged groups; however, the old groups had significantly higher glucose and insulin values (following a glucose challenge) than young or middle-aged groups. They concluded that "The major finding of this study is that the decline in glucose tolerance from the early-adult to the middle-age years is entirely explained by secondary influences (fatness and fitness), whereas the decline from mid-life to old age still is also influenced by chronological age. This finding is unique. It is also unexplained." However, it must be pointed out that anthropometric determination of body fatness becomes increasingly less accurate with advancing age and does not reflect the intra-abdominal and intramuscular accumulation of fat that occurs with aging.[18] The results of this study may be due more to an underestimate of true body fat levels than age, per se. These age-associated changes in glucose tolerance can result in NIDDM and the broad array of associated abnormalities. It has been estimated that 13 percent of men and women between the ages of 60 and 74 had impaired glucose tolerance and an additional 17 percent had NIDDM. In a large population of older men and women (over 55 years), serum glucose and fructosamine levels were seen to be higher in subjects with retinopathy compared with those without, and within the groups with retinopathy, serum glucose was significantly associated with the number of hemorrhages.[19] These relationships were independent of body composition, abdominal obesity, or the presence of NIDDM.

The effects of exercise intensity on insulin action and risk of diabetes are not clear. Epidemiological evidence has shown that increased physical activity can prevent type 2 diabetes in those at greatest risk of the disease.[20] However, most clinical studies use high-intensity exercise in the belief that this intensity is necessary to produce the largest effect. Kirwan and coworkers[21] found that 9 months of endurance training at 80 percent of the maximal heart rate (4 days/week) resulted in reduced glucose-stimulated insulin levels; however, no comparison was made with a lower-intensity exercise group. Hughes and coworkers[22] demonstrated that regularly performed aerobic exercise without weight loss resulted in improved glucose tolerance, rate of insulin-stimulated glucose disposal and increased skeletal muscle GLUT-4 levels in older glucose intolerance subjects. In this investigation, a moderate intensity aerobic exercise program was compared with a higher-intensity program (50 vs 75% of maximal heart rate reserve, 55 min/day, 4 days/week, for 12 weeks). No differences were seen between the moderate and higher-intensity aerobic

exercise on glucose tolerance, insulin sensitivity, or muscle GLUT-4 (the glucose transporter protein in skeletal muscle) levels, indicating, perhaps that a prescription of moderate aerobic exercise should be recommended for older men or women with NIDDM or a high risk for NIDDM to help to ensure compliance to the program.

Endurance training and dietary modifications are generally recommended as the primary treatment in the non-insulin-dependent diabetic. Cross-sectional analysis of dietary intake supports the hypothesis that a low carbohydrate/high-fat diet is associated with the onset of NIDDM.[23] This evidence, however, is not supported by prospective studies where dietary habits have not been related to the development of NIDDM.[24,25] The effects of a high-carbohydrate diet on glucose tolerance have been equivocal.[26,27] Hughes et al.[28] compared the effects of a high-carbohydrate (60 percent CHO and 20 percent fat)/high-fiber (25 g dietary fiber/1,000 kcal) diet with and without 3 months of high-intensity (75 percent max. heart rate reserve, 50 min/day, 4 days/week) endurance exercise in older, glucose-intolerant men and women. Subjects were fed all of their food on a metabolic ward during the 3 month study and were not allowed to lose weight. These investigators observed no improvement in glucose tolerance or insulin-stimulated glucose uptake in either the diet or the diet-plus-exercise group. The group on exercise plus high-carbohydrate diet demonstrated a significant and substantial increase in skeletal muscle glycogen content and at the end of the training, the muscle glycogen stores would be considered to be saturated. Since the primary site of glucose disposal is skeletal muscle glycogen stores, the extremely high muscle glycogen content associated with exercise and a high-carbohydrate diet likely limited the rate of glucose disposal. Thus, when combined with exercise and a weight maintenance diet, a high-carbohydrate diet had a counter-regulatory effect. It is likely that the value of a high-carbohydrate/high-fiber diet in the treatment of excess body fat may be an important cause of the impaired glucose tolerance. Schaefer and coworkers[29] demonstrated that older subjects consuming an ad libitum high-carbohydrate diet lost weight.

There appears to be no attenuation of the responses of elderly men and women to regularly performed aerobic exercise when compared with those seen in young subjects. Increased fitness levels are associated with reduced mortality and increased life expectancy. It has also been shown[20] to prevent the occurrence of NIDDM in those who are at the greatest risk for developing this disease. Thus regularly performed aerobic exercise is an important way for older people to improve their glucose tolerance.

Aerobic exercise is generally prescribed as an important adjunct to a weight loss program. Aerobic exercise combined with weight loss has been demonstrated to increase insulin action to a greater extent than weight loss through diet restriction alone. In the study by Bogardus et al.,[30] diet therapy alone improved glucose tolerance, mainly by reducing basal endogenous glucose production and improving hepatic sensitivity to insulin. Aerobic exercise training, on the other hand, increased carbohydrate storage rates, and therefore, "diet therapy plus physical training produced a more significant approach toward normal." However, aerobic exercise (as opposed to resistance training) combined with a hypocaloric diet has been demonstrated to result in a greater reduction in resting metabolic rate (RMR) than diet alone.[31] Heymsfield and coworkers[32] found aerobic exercise combined with caloric restriction did not preserve fat-free mass (FFM) and did not further accelerate weight loss when compared with diet alone. This lack of an effect of aerobic exercise may have been due to a greater decrease in RMR in the exercising group. In, perhaps, the most comprehensive study of its kind, Goran and Poehlman[33] examined components of energy metabolism in older men and women engaged in regular endurance training. They found that endurance training did not increase total daily energy expenditure due to a compensatory decline in physical activity during the remainder of the day. In other words, when elderly subjects participated in a regular walking program, they rested more, so that activities outside of walking decreased and thus 24 hour calorie expenditure was unchanged. However, older individuals who have been participating in endurance exercise for most of their lives have been shown to have a greater RMR and total daily energy expenditure than age-matched sedentary controls.[34] Ballor et al.[35] compared the effects of resistance training with those of diet restriction alone in obese women. They found that resistance exercise training results in increased strength and gains in muscle size as well as a preservation of FFM during weight loss. These data are similar to the results of Pavlou et al.[36] who used both aerobic and resistance training as an adjunct to a weight loss program in obese men.

STRENGTH TRAINING

While endurance exercise has been the more traditional means of increasing cardiovascular fitness, strength or resistance training is currently recommended by the American College of Sports Medicine as an important component of an overall fitness program. This is particularly important in elderly people where loss of muscle mass and weakness are prominent deficits.

Strength conditioning or progressive resistance training is generally defined as training in which the resistance against which a muscle generates force is progressively increased over time. Progressive resistance training involves few contractions against a heavy load. The metabolic and morphological adaptations resulting from resistance and endurance exercise are quite different. Muscle strength has been shown to increase in response to training between 60 and 100 percent of the one repetition maximum (1RM). This is the maximum amount of weight that can be lifted with one contraction. Strength conditioning will result in an increase in muscle size and this increase in size is largely the result of increased contractile proteins. The mechanisms by which the mechanical events stimulate an increase in RNA synthesis and subsequent protein synthesis are not well understood. Lifting weight requires that a muscle shorten as it produces force. This is called a concentric contraction. Lowering the weight, on the other hand, forces the muscle to lengthen as it produces force. This is an eccentric muscle contraction. These lengthening muscle contractions have been shown to produce ultrastructural damage that may stimulate increased muscle protein turnover.[37]

Our laboratory examined the effects of high-intensity resistance training of the knee extensors and flexors (80 percent 1RM, 3 days/week) in older men (age 60–72 years). The average increases in knee flexor and extensor strength were 227 percent and 107 percent respectively. Computed tomography (CT) scans and muscle biopsies were used to determine muscle size. Total muscle area by CT analysis increased by 11.4 percent, while the muscle biopsies showed an increase of 33.5 percent in Type I fiber area and 27.5 percent increase in Type II fiber area. In addition, lower body $\dot{V}_{O_2max}$ increased significantly, while upper body $\dot{V}_{O_2max}$ did not, indicating that increased muscle mass can increase maximal aerobic power. It appears that the age-related loss in muscle mass may be an important determinant in the reduced maximal aerobic capacity seen in elderly men and women.[10] Improving muscle strength can enhance the capacity of many older men and women to perform many activities such as climbing stairs, carrying packages, and even walking.

We have applied this same training program to a group of frail, institutionalized elderly men and women (mean age 90 ± 3 years, range 87–96).[38] After 8 weeks of training, the 10 subjects in this study increased muscle strength by almost 180 percent and muscle size by 11 percent. More recently,[39] a similar intervention on frail nursing home residents demonstrated not only increased muscle strength and size, but increased gait speed, stair climbing power, and balance. In addition, spontaneous activity levels increased significantly, while the activity of a nonexercised control group was unchanged. In this study the effects of a protein/calorie supplement (240 mL liquid supplying 360 kcal in the form of carbohydrate (60 percent), fat (23 percent), and soy-based protein (17 percent) was designed to augment caloric intake by about 20 percent and provide one-third of the RDA of vitamins and minerals) combined with exercise was also examined. While no interaction was seen with muscle strength, functional capacity, or muscle size (no differences in improvements between the supplemented group and a nonsupplemented control group), the men and women that consumed the supplement and exercised gained weight compared to the three other groups examined (exercise control, nonexercise supplemented, and nonexercise control). The nonexercising subjects who received the supplement reduced their habitual dietary energy intake so that total energy intake was unchanged. It should be pointed out that this was a very old, very frail population with diagnoses of multiple chronic diseases. The increase in overall levels of physical activity have been a common observation in our studies.[39–41] Since muscle weakness is a primary deficit in many older individuals, increased strength may stimulate more aerobic activities like walking and cycling. In this study population, Singh[42] found that resistance exercise significantly reduced symptoms of depression and concluded, "Progressive resistance training is an effective antidepressant in depressed elders, while also improving strength, morale, and quality of life."

Strength training may increase balance through the improvement in strength of muscle involved in walking. Indeed ankle weakness has been demonstrated to be associated with increased risk of falling in nursing home patients.[43] However, balance training, which may demonstrate very little improvement in muscle strength, size, or cardiovascular changes has also been demonstrated to decrease the risk of falls in older people.[44] Tai chi, a form of dynamic balance training that requires no new technology or equipment, has been demonstrated to reduce the risk of falling in older people by almost 50 percent.[45] As a component of the National Institute on Aging FICSIT trials (Frailty and Injuries: Cooperative Studies of Intervention Techniques), individuals aged 70+ were randomized to tai chi (TC), individualized balance training (BT), and exercise control education (ED) groups for 15 weeks.[46] In a follow-up assessment 4 months post-intervention, 130 subjects responded to exit interview questions asking about perceived benefits of participation. Both TC and BT subjects reported increased confidence in balance and movement, but only TC subjects reported that their daily activities and their overall life had been affected; many of these subjects had changed their normal physical activity to incorporate ongoing TC practice. The data suggest that when mental as well as physical control is perceived to be enhanced, with a generalized sense of improvement in overall well-being, older persons' motivation to continue exercising also increases. Province et al.[47] examined the overall effect of many different exercise interventions in the FICSIT trials on reducing falls. While each intervention was insufficient to make conclusions about its effects, they did conclude that "all training domains, taken together under the heading of 'general exercise' showed an effect on falls, this probably demonstrates the 'rising tide raises all boats' principle, in which training that targets one domain may improve performance somewhat in other domains as a consequence. If this is so, then the differences seen on fall risk due to the exact nature of the training may not be as critical compared with the differences in not training at all." Recently, the use of a community-based exercise program for frail older people was examined.[48] Participants were predominantly sedentary women over age 70 with multiple chronic conditions. The program was conducted with peer leaders to facilitate its continuation after the research demonstration phase. In addition to positive health outcomes related to functional mobility, blood pressure maintenance, and overall well-being, this intervention was successful in sustaining active participation in regular physical activity through the use of peer leaders selected by the program participants.

In addition to its effect on increasing muscle mass and function, resistance training can also have an important effect on energy balance of elderly men and women.[49] Men and women participating in a resistance training program of the upper and lower body muscles required approximately 15 percent more calories to maintain body weight after 12 weeks of training when compared to their pretraining energy requirements. This increase in energy needs came about as a result of an increased resting metabolic rate, the small energy cost of the exercise, and what was presumed to be an increase in activity levels. While endurance training has been demonstrated to be an important adjunct to weight loss programs in young men and women by increasing their daily energy expenditure, its utility in treating obesity in elderly people may not be great. This is because many sedentary older men and women do not spend many calories when they perform endurance exercise, due to their low fitness levels. Thirty to forty minutes of exercise may increase energy expenditure by only 100–200 kcal with very little residual effect on calorie expenditure. Aerobic exercise training will not preserve lean body mass to any great extent during weight loss. Because resistance training can preserve or even increase muscle mass during weight loss, this type of exercise for those older men and women who must lose weight may be of genuine benefit.

BONE HEALTH

The increased calorie need resulting from strength training may be a way for elderly people to improve their overall nutritional intake when the calories are chosen as nutrient dense foods. In particular, calcium is an important nutrient to increase, since calcium intake was found to be one of the only limiting nutrients in the diet of free-living elderly men and women in the Boston nutritional status survey which assessed free-living and institutionalized elderly men and women.[50] Careful nutritional planning is needed to reach the recommended calcium levels of 1,500 mg/day for post-menopausal women with osteoporosis or using hormone replacement therapy, and 1,000 mg/day for post-menopausal women taking estrogen. An increased calorie intake from calcium-containing food is one method to help achieve this goal.

In one of the very few studies to examine the interaction of dietary calcium and exercise, we studied 41 post-menopausal women consuming either high calcium (1,462 mg/day) or moderate calcium (761 mg) diets. Half of these women participated in a year-long walking program (45 min/day, 4 days/week, 75 percent of heart rate reserve). Independent effects of the exercise and dietary calcium were seen. Compared with the moderate calcium group, the women consuming a high-calcium diet displayed reduced bone loss from the femoral neck, independent of whether the women exercised. The walking prevented a loss of trabecular bone mineral density seen in the nonexercising women after 1 year. Thus, it appears that calcium intake and aerobic exercise are both independently beneficial to bone mineral density at different sites. The effects of 52 weeks of high intensity resistance exercise training was examined in a group of 39 post-menopausal women.[40] Twenty were randomly assigned to the strength training group (2 days/week, 80 percent 1RM for upper and lower body muscle groups). At the end of the year significant differences were seen in lumbar spine and femoral bone density between the strength-trained and sedentary women. However, unlike other pharmacological and nutritional strategies for preventing bone loss and osteoporosis, resistance exercise affects more than just bone density. The women who strength trained improved their muscle mass, strength, balance, and overall levels of physical activity. Thus, resistance training can be an important way to decrease the risk for an osteoporotic bone fracture in post-menopausal women.

PROTEIN NEEDS AND AGING

Previous estimates of dietary protein needs of elderly people using nitrogen balance have ranged from 0.59 to 0.8 g·kg^{-1}·d^{-1}.[51–53] However, the low value was reported by Zanni et al. who preceded their 10-day dietary protein feeding with a 17-day protein-free diet, which was likely to improve nitrogen retention during the 10-day balance period. Recently, we[54] reassessed the nitrogen balance studies mentioned above using the currently accepted, 1985 WHO[55] nitrogen-balance formula. These newly recalculated data were combined with nitrogen balance data collected on 12 healthy older men and women (age range 56–80 years, 8 men and 4 women) consuming the current RDA for protein or double this amount (0.8 g·kg^{-1}·d^{-1} and 1.6 g·kg^{-1}·d^{-1}, respectively) in our laboratory. Our subjects consumed the diet for 11 consecutive days and nitrogen balance (mg N·kg^{-1}·d^{-1}) was measured during days 6 to 11. The estimated mean protein requirements from the three retrospectively assessed studies and the current study can be combined by weighted averaging to produce an overall protein requirement estimate of 0.91 ± 0.043 g·kg^{-1}·d^{-1}. The combined estimate excluding the data from our 12 subjects is 0.894 ± 0.048 g protein·kg^{-1}·d^{-1}.

The current Recommended Dietary Allowance (RDA) in the United States of 0.8 g·kg^{-1}·d^{-1} is based on data collected, for the most part, on young subjects. The RDA includes an upward adjustment based on the coefficient of variability of the average requirement established in these studies (0.6 g·kg^{-1}·d^{-1}). Based on the CV previously established for N balance studies, an adequate dietary protein level for 97.5 percent of the elderly population would be provided by an intake of 25 percent (twice the SD) above the mean protein requirement. Our data suggest that the safe protein intake for elderly adults is 1.25 g·kg^{-1}·d^{-1}. On the basis of the current and recalculated short-term N-balance results, a safe recommended (high-quality) protein intake for older men and women should be set at 1.0–1.25 g·kg^{-1}·d^{-1}. It has been reported[50] that approximately 50 percent of 946 healthy free-living men and women above the age of 60 living in the Boston, Massachusetts area consume less than this amount of protein and 25 percent of the elderly men and women in this survey consume < 0.86 and < 0.81 g·kg^{-1}·d^{-1}, respectively. A large percentage of homebound elderly people consuming their habitual dietary (mixed) protein intake (0.67 g·kg^{-1}·d^{-1}) have been shown[56] to be in negative N-balance.

We examined the effects of marginial dietary protein intake in 12 sedentary healthy women, aged 66–79. They were admitted into a 9-week metabolic study and consumed a meat-free diet with a protein content of 0.45 or 0.93 g·kg^{-1}·d^{-1}. The nonprotein energy in the diet was provided by carbohydrates (65 percent) and fat (35 percent). Six-day nitrogen balance periods were measured during study days 16–21 (week 3), and 56–61 (week 9). In addition to N-balance, body composition (total body potassium, body density (underwater weighing), and dual-energy X-ray absorptiometry), whole-body leucine kinetics ([1-^{13}C]leucine infusion), muscle fiber area, immune function (delayed hypersensitivity), urinary creatinine and 3-methylhistidine, muscle strength, and plasma IGF-1 was measured while the women consumed protein at 1.2 g·kg^{-1}·day^{-1} at baseline and after adaptation to the two different dietary protein levels (week 9). This study demonstrated that long-term adaptation to protein consumption of 0.45 g·kg^{-1}·d^{-1} resulted in an accommodation resulting in reductions in ^{40}K (active cell mass), skeletal muscle mass, muscle strength, and immune function. Leucine oxidation rate was a more sensitive index of the adequacy of protein intake than synthesis, flux, or metabolic rate. N-balance was negative in the low-protein group. The greatest losses in body nitrogen occurred during the first balance period; however, the women on the low-protein intake remained in negative N-balance throughout the

trial. The change in IGF-1 levels was significantly associated with the change in nitrogen balance, body cell mass, muscle fiber size, and skeletal muscle and immune function. Inadequate dietary protein intake may be an important cause of sarcopenia. These data demonstrate that the compensatory response to long-term decreases in dietary protein intake is a loss in lean body mass.

We recently examined adequacy of the current RDA for protein for healthy elderly men and women by examining the effects of long-term (15 weeks) consumption of a eucaloric diet providing protein at 0.8 g·kg^{-1}·d^{-1}. CT scans of the thigh muscle shows that the subjects who consumed the RDA for protein and did not exercise lost a significant amount of skeletal muscle, confirming our hypothesis that the RDA for protein is inadequate for older individuals. Muscle biopsies taken from the m. vastus lateralis confirm the CT scan data by demonstrating a significant reduction in muscle fiber area of Type IIa muscle cells in the sedentary group of subjects.

High-intensity resistance training appears to have profound anabolic effects in elderly people. Data from our laboratory demonstrate a 10–15 percent decrease in N-excretion at the initiation of training that persists for 12 weeks. That is, progressive resistance training improved N-balance, thus older subjects performing resistance training have a lower mean protein requirement than do sedentary subjects. These results are somewhat at variance to our previous research[57] demonstrating that regularly performed aerobic exercise causes an increase in the mean protein requirement of middle-aged and young endurance athletes. This difference likely results from increased oxidation of amino-acids during aerobic exercise that may not be present during resistance training.

We recently examined the effects of resistance training on nitrogen balance in subjects with mild to moderate chronic renal failure (CRF): 5 women (62 ± 10 years old, body mass index (BMI) = 30.3 ± 4 kg/m^2, creatinine clearance = 56 ± 22 mL/min) were studied before and after a 4-week resistance training protocol (2 upper body and 3 lower body exercises, 3 sets of 8 repetitions, at 80 percent 1RM, 3 days per week). All of the women consumed a diet providing 0.6 g·kg^{-1}·d^{-1} protein for 3 weeks before and during the training period. Body weight was maintained at ± 0.5 kg of baseline weight. At week 3 of baseline and week 4 of resistance training, 24-hour urine collections and food homogenates were collected during 4 consecutive days, and analyzed for total nitrogen by the Kjeldahl method. With resistance training, strength increased 11 ± 6 percent for upper body ($P < 0.05$) and 17 ± 6 percent ($P < 0.01$) for the lower body. Glomerular filtration rate estimated by inulin clearance (57 ± 26 mL/min), renal plasma flow estimated by p-aminohyppurate clearance (277 ± 146 mL/min), and percent body fat (42.3 ± 6.2 percent) and fat-free mass estimated by underwater weighing (44.8 ± 4.2 kg) did not change during the intervention. Urinary nitrogen excretion decreased 10.7 ± 7.9 percent (0.56 ± 0.4 g N/day, $P < 0.05$) and estimated nitrogen balance increased from −0.34 ± 0.58 to 0.08 ± 0.41 g N/day, $P < 0.05$. These results demonstrate that resistance training in CRF patients is safe, increases nitrogen retention, and reduces renal handling of nitrogen. Strength training may, therefore, be an important clinical tool in the treatment of CRF, especially to prevent muscle wasting.

MUSCLE STRENGTH TRAINING IN ELDERLY PEOPLE

Muscle strength training can be accomplished by virtually anyone. Many healthcare professionals have directed their patients away from strength training in the mistaken belief that it can cause undesirable elevations in blood pressure. With proper technique, the systolic pressure elevation during aerobic exercise is far greater than that seen during resistance training. Muscle strengthening exercises are rapidly becoming a critical component to cardiac rehabilitation programs as clinicians realize the need for strength as well as endurance for many activities of daily living.

In conclusion, there is no other group in our society that can benefit more from regularly performed exercise than elderly people. While both aerobic and strength conditioning are highly recommended, only strength training can stop or reverse sarcopenia. Increased muscle strength and mass in the elderly people can be the first step toward a lifetime of increased physical activity and a realistic strategy for maintaining functional status and independence.

KEY POINTS Exercise for successful aging

- Increasing age is associated with decreased fat-free mass, the principal component of which is skeletal muscle.

- This loss of skeletal muscle with advancing age has been termed "sarcopenia."

- Sarcopenia is associated with decreased bone density, resting metabolic rate, decreased energy requirements, and reduced functional capacity.

- Regularly performed aerobic exercise will increase insulin sensitivity, decrease the risk for cardiovascular disease, and increase life-expectancy. However, it will not prevent sarcopenia.

- Progressive resistance exercise improves muscle strength and size, total daily energy needs, bone density, and balance. It has also been demonstrated to decrease symptoms of depression in very old nursing home residents.

- Exercise is both safe and effective for people of all ages.

REFERENCES

1. Frontera WR, Hughes VA, Evans WJ: A cross-sectional study of upper and lower extremity muscle strength in 45–78 year old men and women. J Appl Physiol 1991;71:644–650
2. Tzankoff SP, Norris AH: Longitudinal changes in basal metabolic rate in man. J Appl Physiol 1978;33:536–539
3. Evans W: What is sarcopenia? J Gerontol 1995;50A (special issue):5–8
4. Bassey EJ, Fiatarone MA, O'Neill EF et al: Leg extensor power and functional performance in very old men and women. Clin Sci 1992;82:321–327
5. Meredith CN, Zackin MJ, Frontera WR, Evans WJ: Body composition and aerobic capacity in young and middle-aged endurance-trained men. Med Sci Sports Exerc 1987;19:557–563
6. Roberts SB, Young VR, Fuss P et al: What are the dietary energy needs of elderly adults? Int J Obesity Related Metab Disord 1992;16:969–976
7. Klitgaard H, Mantoni M, Schiaffino S et al: Function, morphology and protein expression of ageing skeletal muscle: a cross-sectional study of elderly men with different training backgrounds. Acta Physiol Scand 1990;140:41–54
8. Klitgaard H, Zhou M, Schiaffino S et al: Ageing alters the myosin heavy chain composition of single fibres from human skeletal muscle. Acta Physiol Scand 1990;140:55–62
9. Buskirk ER, Hodgson JL: Age and aerobic power: the rate of change in men and women. Fed Proc 1987;46:1824–1829
10. Flegg JL, Lakatta EG: Role of muscle loss in the age-associated reduction in VO2max. J Appl Physiol 1988;65:1147–1151
11. Rosen MJ, Sorkin JD, Goldberg AP, Hagberg JM, Katzel LI: Predictors of age-associated decline in maximal aerobic capacity: A comparison of four statistical models. J Appl Physiol 1998;84:2163–2170
12. Meredith CN, Frontera WR, Fisher EC et al: Peripheral effects of endurance training in young and old subjects. J Appl Physiol 1989;66:2844–2849
13. Seals DR, Hagberg JM, Hurley BF, Ehsani AA, Holloszy JO: Endurance training in older men and women: cardiovascular responses to exercise. J Appl Physiol Respir Environ Exerc Physiol 1984;57:1024–1029
14. Spina RJ, Ogawa T, Kohrt WM et al: Differences in cardiovascular adaptation to endurance exercise training between older men and women. J Appl Physiol 1993;75:849–855
15. Davidson MB: The effect of aging on carbohydrate metabolism. A review of the English literature and a practical approach to the diagnosis of diabetes mellitus in the elderly. Metabolism 1979;28:688–705
16. Hadden WC, Harris MI: Prevalence of diagnosed diabetes, undiagnosed diabetes, and impaired glucose tolerance in adults 20–74 years of age: United States, 1976–1980. DHHS PHS publ. no. 87–1687. US Govt. Printing Office, Washington, DC, 1987
17. Shimokata H, Muller DC, Fleg JL et al: Age as independent determinant of glucose tolerance. Diabetes 1991;40:44–51
18. Borkan GA, Hultz DE, Gerzoff AF: Age changes in body composition revealed by computed tomography. J Gerontol 1983;38:673–677
19. Stolk RP, Vingerling JR, de Jong PTVM et al: Retinopathy, glucose and insulin in an elderly population: The Rotterdam study. Diabetes 1995;44:11–15
20. Helmrich SP, Ragland DR, Leung RW, Paffenbarger Jr. RS: Physical activity and reduced occurrence of non-insulin-dependent diabetes mellitus. N Engl J Med 1991;325:147–152
21. Kirwan JP, Kohrt WM, Wojta DM, Bourey RE, Holloszy JO: Endurance exercise training reduces glucose-stimulated insulin levels in 60- to 70-year-old men and women. J Gerontol A 1993;48:M84–M90
22. Hughes VA, Fiatarone MA, Fielding RA et al: Exercise increases muscle GLUT 4 levels and insulin action in subjects with impaired glucose tolerance. Am J Physiol 1993;264:E855–E862
23. Marshall JA, Hamman RF, Baxter J: High-fat, low-carbohydrate diet and the etiology of non-insulin-dependent diabetes mellitus: the San Luis Valley Diabetes Study. Am J Epidemiol 1991;134:590–603
24. Feskens EJM, Kromhout D: Cardiovascular risk factors and the 25-year incidence of diabetes mellitus in middle-aged men. Am J Epidemiol 1989;130:1101–1108
25. Lundgren J, Benstsson C, Blohme G et al: Dietary habits and incidence of noninsulin-dependent diabetes mellitus in a population study of women in Gothenburg, Sweden. Am J Clin Nutr 1989;52:708–712
26. Garg A, Grundy SM, Unger RH: Comparison of effects of high and low carbohydrate diets on plasma lipoprotein and insulin sensitivity in patients with mild NIDDM. Diabetes 1992;41:1278–1285
27. Borkman M, Campbell LV, Chisholm DJ, Storlien LH: Comparison of the effects on insulin sensitivity of high carbohydrate and high fat diets in normal subjects. J Clin Endocrinol Metab 1991;72:432–437
28. Hughes VA, Fiatarone MA, Fielding RA et al: Long term effects of a high carbohydrate diet and exercise on insulin action in older subjects with impaired glucose tolerance. Am J Clin Nutr 1995;62:426–433
29. Schaefer EJ, Lichtenstein AH, Lamon-Fava S et al: Body weight and low-density lipoprotein cholesterol changes after consumption of a low-fat ad libitum diet. JAMA 1995;274:1450–1455
30. Bogardus C, Ravussin E, Robbins DC et al: Effects of physical training and diet therapy on carbohydrate metabolism in patients with glucose intolerance and non-insulin-dependent diabetes mellitus. Diabetes 1984;33:311–318
31. Phinney SD, LaGrange BM, O'Connell M, Danforth Jr E: Effects of aerobic exercise on energy expenditure and nitrogen balance during very low calorie dieting. Metabolism 1988;37:758–765
32. Heymsfield SB, Casper K, Hearn J, Guy D: Rate of weight loss during underfeeding: relation to level of physical activity. Metabolism 1989;38:215–223

33. Goran MI, Poehlman ET: Endurance training does not enhance total energy expenditure in healthy elderly persons. Am J Physiol 1992;263:E950–E957

34. Withers RT, Smith DA, Tucker RC, Brinkman M, Clark DG: Energy metabolism in sedentary and active 49- to 70-year-old women. J Appl Physiol 1998;84:1333–1340

35. Ballor DL, Katch VL, Becque MD, Marks CR: Resistance weight training during caloric restriction enhances lean body weight maintenance. Am J Clin Nutr 1988;47:19–25

36. Pavlou KN, Steffee WP, Lerman RH, Burrows BA: Effects of dieting and exercise on lean body mass, oxygen uptake, and strength. Med Sci Sports Exerc 1985;17:466–471

37. Evans WJ, Cannon JG: The metabolic effects of exercise-induced muscle damage. In Holloszy JO (ed): Exercise and Sport Sciences Reviews. Williams & Wilkins, Baltimore, 1991:99–126

38. Fiatarone MA, Marks EC, Ryan ND et al: High-intensity strength training in nonagenarians. Effects on skeletal muscle. JAMA 1990;263:3029–3034

39. Fiatarone MA, O'Neill EF, Ryan ND et al: Exercise training and nutritional supplementation for physical frailty in very elderly people. N Engl J Med 1994;330:1769–1775

40. Nelson ME, Fiatarone MA, Morganti CM, Trice I, Greenberg RA, Evans WJ: Effects of high-intensity strength training on multiple risk factors for osteoporotic fractures. JAMA 1994;272:1909–1914

41. Frontera WR, Meredith CN, O'Reilly KP, Evans WJ: Strength training and determinants of VO2 max in older men. J Appl Physiol 1990;68:329–333

42. Singh NA: A randomized controlled trial of progressive resistance training in depressed elders. J Gerontol A 1997;52:M27–M35

43. Whipple RH, Wolfson LI, Amerman PM: The relationship of knee and ankle weakness to falls in nursing home residents. J Am Geriatr Soc 1987;35:13–20

44. Wolfson L, Whipple R, Judge J, Amerman P, Derby C, King M: Training balance and strength in the elderly to improve function. J Am Geriatr Soc 1993;41:341–343

45. Wolf SL, Barnhart HX, Kutner NG, McNeely E, Coogler C, Xu T: Reducing frailty and falls in older persons: an investigation of Tai Chi and computerized balance training. Atlanta FICSIT Group. Frailty and Injuries: Cooperative Studies of Intervention Techniques. J Am Geriatr Soc 1996;44:489–497 (see comments).

46. Kutner NG, Barnhart H, Wolf SL, McNeely E, Xu T: Self-report benefits of Tai Chi practice by older adults. J Gerontol B 1997;52:P242–P246

47. Province MA, Hadley EC, Hornbrook MC et al: The effects of exercise on falls in elderly patients: A preplanned meta-analysis of the FICSIT trials. JAMA 1995;273:1341–1347

48. Hickey T, Sharpe PA, Wolf FM et al: Exercise participation in a frail elderly population. J Health Care Poor Underserved 1996;7:219–231

49. Campbell WW, Crim MC, Young VR, Evans WJ: Increased energy requirements and body composition changes with resistance training in older adults. Am J Clin Nutr 1994;60:167–175

50. Sahyoun N: Nutrient intake by the NSS elderly population. In Hartz SC, Russell RM, Rosenberg IH (eds): Nutrition in the Elderly: The Boston Nutritional, Status Survey. Smith-Gordon and Company, London, 1992:31–44

51. Gersovitz M, Munro H, Scrimshaw N, Young V: Human protein requirements: assessment of the adequacy of the current recommended dietary allowance for dietary protein in elderly men and women. Am J Clin Nutr 1982;35:6–14

52. Uauy R, Scrimshaw N, Young V: Human protein requirements: nitrogen balance response to graded levels of egg protein in elderly men and women. Am J Clin Nutr 1978;31:779–785

53. Zanni E, Calloway D, Zezulka A: Protein requirements of elderly men. J Nutr 1979;109:513–524

54. Campbell WW, Crim MC, Dallal GE, Young VR, Evans WJ: Increased protein requirements in the elderly: new data and retrospective reassessments. Am J Clin Nutr 1994;60:167–175

55. WHO/FAO/UNU. Energy and protein requirements. WHO Tech. Rep Ser 1985:724

56. Bunker V, Lawson M, Stansfield M, Clayton B: Nitrogen balance studies in apparently healthy elderly people and those who are housebound. Br J Nutr 1987;57:211–221

57. Meredith CN, Zackin MJ, Frontera WR, Evans WJ: Dietary protein requirements and body protein metabolism in endurance-trained men. J Appl Physiol 1989;66:2850–2856

Chapter 69

Bone and joint aging

Jonathan H. Tobias and Mo Sharif

The musculoskeletal system serves three primary functions: (1) it enables an efficient means of limb movement; (2) it acts as an endoskeleton, thereby providing overall mechanical support and the protection of soft tissues; and (3) it serves as a reservoir of mineral for calcium homeostasis. In the elderly population the first two of these functions frequently become compromised, as illustrated by the fact that musculoskeletal problems are the major cause of pain and physical disability in people over the age of 65 years,[1] and by observations that fracture incidence rises steeply with age (Fig. 69-1).

Several factors contribute to the age-related decline in musculoskeletal function, including the following (see also the accompanying box):

1. There are aging effects on components of the musculoskeletal system (i.e. articular cartilage, the skeleton, and soft tissues). These effects are responsible for the increasing incidence of osteoporosis and osteoarthritis with age, for the reduced range of joint movement, and for the stiffness and difficulty in initiating movement.
2. There is the age-related rise in the prevalence of common musculoskeletal disorders that begin in young adulthood or in middle age, and cause increasing pain and disability without shortening lifespan.
3. There is a high incidence of certain musculoskeletal disorders in the elderly, such as polymyalgia rheumatica and Paget's disease of bone.

A number of interrelated hypotheses have been advanced to explain the high prevalence of bone, muscle, and joint problems in older human:[2-5]

1. The long lifespan of humans results in increasing accumulation of mechanical damage to the musculoskeletal system.
2. There is a lack of genetic investment in the repair of age-related tissue damage that develops in the post-reproductive phase of life.
3. The musculoskeletal system in humans has not adapted fully to the upright posture and prehensile grip because of lack of evolutionary pressure to do so, with the result that many of our bones and joints are inappropriately shaped and "underdesigned" to be able to cope with the stresses applied.

Some factors contributing to the high prevalence of musculoskeletal problems in the elderly population

Aging effects on components of the musculoskeletal system, leading to osteoarthritis and osteoporosis:
- The skeleton
- Articular cartilage
- Soft tissues (i.e. muscle, ligaments, tendons, meniscus, joint capsule)
- Neurological function (e.g. joint proprioception)

Common disorders with peak incidence in younger adults, but which cause increasing pain and disability with age, without shortening lifespan:
- Rheumatoid arthritis
- Seronegative spondarthritides
- Musculoskeletal trauma

Other disorders of the musculoskeletal system with a high incidence:
- Paget's disease of bone
- Crystal-related arthropathies
- Polymyalgia rheumatica

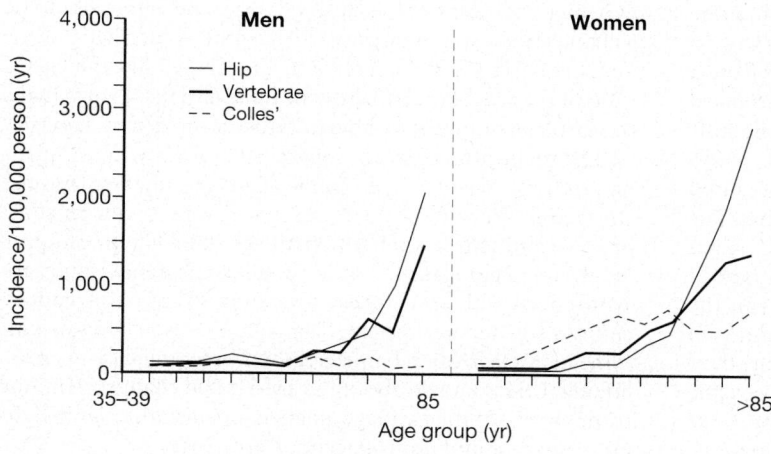

Figure 69-1 Age-specific incidence rates for hip, vertebral, and distal forearm (Colles') fracture in Rochester, Minnesota, men and women. Adapted from Cooper and Melton,[32] with permission.

4. By virtue of their sedentary lifestyle, modern humans tend to be exposed to less mechanical stress than their ancestors. Because musculoskeletal strength is governed by the mechanical inputs to which that individual is exposed, this may result in modern humans having a weaker musculoskeletal system, which is not well adapted for episodes of sudden major stress.

Several different mechanisms are apparently involved in musculoskeletal tissue aging,[6] including:

- reduced synthetic capacity of differentiated cells such as osteoblasts and chondrocytes, with a consequent loss of ability to maintain matrix integrity;
- a decline in the mesenchymal stem cell populations;
- post-translational modification of structural proteins such as collagen;
- the accumulation of degraded molecules, such as proteoglycan fragments, in musculoskeletal tissue matrices;
- decreased circulating and local levels of trophic hormones, growth factors, and cytokines, such as insulin-like growth factor-1 (IGF-1), involved in maintaining tissue integrity;
- a decreased capacity for wound healing and tissue repair, which may be the result of some or all of the mechanisms described above.

The major tissues that have received the most attention, and which are pivotal to the integrity of the system, are articular cartilage, the skeleton, and soft tissues. Age-related changes in these structures are now described in more detail.

ARTICULAR CARTILAGE

The structure of a mammalian synovial joint is summarized in Figure 69-2. Much of its function derives from the properties of articular cartilage, which cushions the subchondral bone and provides a low-friction surface necessary for free movement. Articular cartilage contains very few cells, is aneural and avascular, and yet its integrity is maintained throughout a lifetime of biomechanical stress. With increasing age the cartilage surface often starts to break down, leading to osteoarthritis (OA). This is associated with changes in other tissues of the joint (Fig. 69-3). Whether the latter directly cause OA, or are a necessary predisposition to OA, or are unrelated to the disorder remains controversial, but current opinion favors some relationship between the two processes.

With age, articular cartilage thins and changes color from a glistening white to a dull yellow. In addition, the mechanical features of the tissue change. There is a decrease in tensile stiffness, fatigue resistance, and strength, but no significant change in the compressive properties. These changes are partly caused by the decrease in water content that accompanies aging. The morphology and function of the cells (chondrocyte) and nature of the two main matrix components, aggrecan and type II collagen, also change with age. The density of cells in the tissue changes little, but their morphology alters with an increase in intracytoplasmic filaments, and they change their secretion of matrix components, producing more variable proteoglycans. Aging is also associated with alterations in the response of the chondrocytes to anabolic and catabolic

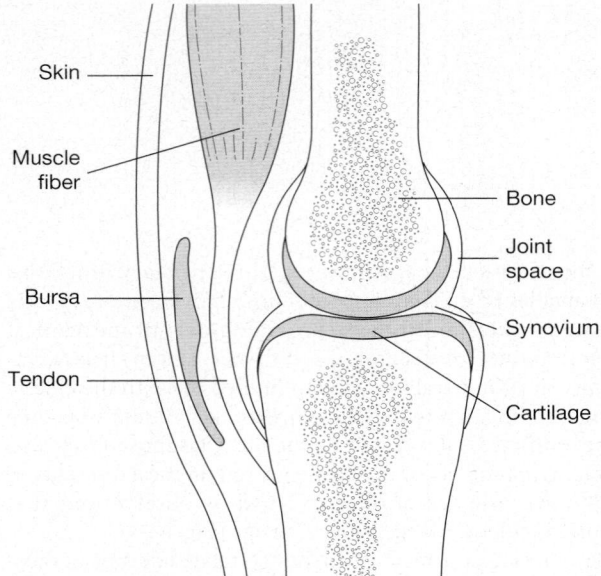

Figure 69-2 The synovial joint. The histological appearances of the main tissues are highlighted. Courtesy Drs J. H. Klippel and P. A. Dieppe.

stimuli such as IGF-1 and interleukin-1 action. For example, immature cartilage degrade more readily when stimulated with interleukin-1.

Depletion of cartilage proteoglycan is one of the earliest signs of articular cartilage loss in OA. Proteoglycans consist of a protein core and two major glycosaminoglycan (GAG) side-chains, chondroitin sulfate (CS) and keratan sulfate. The CS is the predominant GAG chain in human articular cartilage. It is made up of oligosaccharide (sugar) chains containing a basic disaccharide repeat of two sugar molecules (N-acetylgalactosamine and glucuronic acid). These sugar molecules carry a sulfate group on either the sixth (C6) or fourth (C4) carbon atom of the sugar ring. Such sulfation patterns are often called C6 and C4 sulfation and show marked changes with aging and in OA.[7,8] More than 90 percent of the CS in adult human articular cartilage is the C6, which is thought to interact with collagen and other extracellular matrix macromolecules and help maintain the integrity of the cartilage.[7] C4 accounts for less than 10 percent of the adult cartilage and is thought to be a characteristic of immature cartilage. In OA cartilage there is an increase in C4 and decrease in C6. Changes in the C6:C4 ratio of the articular cartilage with aging and in OA may make the cartilage more susceptible to cytokine-mediated damage.[8]

The main proteoglycan—aggrecan—binds with hyaluronan to form massive, hydrophilic aggregates that expand the collagen framework of the tissue, to provide it with its compressive and tensile strength. With age there is reduced proteoglycan aggregation, and smaller proteoglycans are synthesized with an increase in keratan sulfate and reduced chondroitin sulfate content. The collagen also changes, with some increase in fiber diameter, as well as an increase in cross-linking. Less is known about the age-related changes in minor components of the cartilage, such as small-molecular-weight proteoglycans and noncollagenous proteins.

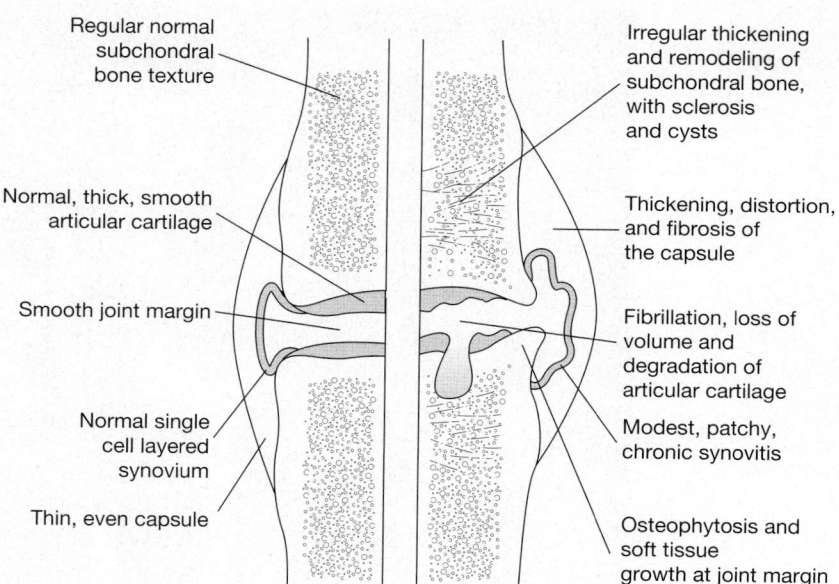

Regular normal
subchondral
bone texture

Normal, thick, smooth
articular cartilage

Smooth joint margin

Normal single
cell layered
synovium

Thin, even capsule

Irregular thickening
and remodeling of
subchondral bone,
with sclerosis
and cysts

Thickening, distortion,
and fibrosis of
the capsule

Fibrillation, loss of
volume and
degradation of
articular cartilage

Modest, patchy,
chronic synovitis

Osteophytosis and
soft tissue
growth at joint margin

Figure 69-3 Normal versus osteoarthritic synovial joint. Courtesy Drs J. H. Klippel and P. A. Dieppe.

Cell death in cartilage

An age-related decrease in articular cartilage cellularity has been associated with cartilage fibrillation, thinning, and an increased prevalence of OA in elderly people.[9,10] Recent studies investigating the mechanisms of cell death in articular cartilage suggest that the chondrocytes may be dying by apoptosis.[10,11] Apoptosis is a normal physiological process involved in the removal of potential carcinogenic and damaged cells. The process is also involved in development; for example, during endochondral ossification of the hyaline cartilage, cells (chondrocytes) die by apoptosis.[12] Chondrocyte death may contribute to the pathogenesis of OA and currently there is a great deal of research interest in this area. Possible mechanisms by which apoptosis may play a significant role in the pathogenesis of OA involves cartilage matrix degradation by apoptotic bodies. These bodies are the result of cell death by apoptosis and normally cleared from tissues by phagocytic cells. However, in articular cartilage there are no phagocytic cells and therefore the apoptotic bodies are likely to accumulate in the cartilage matrix and promote matrix damage. Age-related decreases in cellularity in human cartilage may reduce the ability of the hypocellular tissue to maintain and repair itself and thus contribute to age-related degeneration and development of OA.

THE SKELETON

Weight-bearing bones consist of an outer shell of cortical bone, an arrangement that is designed for maximum strength. In addition, certain sites, such as vertebrae and metaphyses, contain an inner meshwork of trabecular bone to act as an internal scaffold (Fig. 69-4). Microscopically, the skeleton is made up of interconnecting fibrils of type I collagen, which provide tensile strength. Hydroxyapatite crystals, which are made up of calcium and phosphate, are deposited in holes within the collagen fibrils, giving bone its rigidity.

Adult bone continuously undergoes self-renewal. This process, which is known as bone remodeling, occurs at discrete

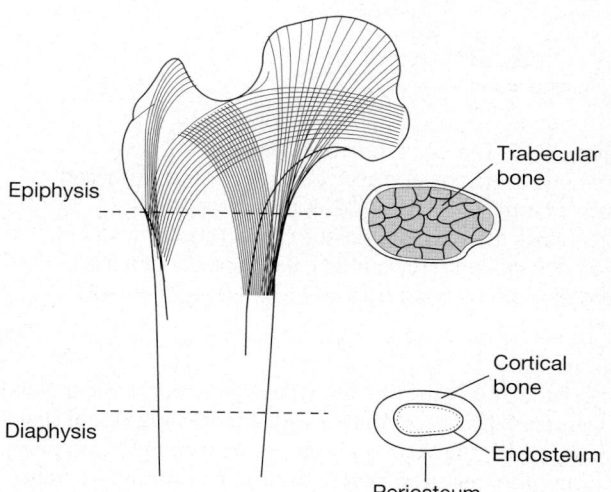

Epiphysis

Diaphysis

Trabecular
bone

Cortical
bone

Endosteum

Periosteum

Figure 69-4 The macroscopic organization of bone. Courtesy Drs J. H. Klippel and P. A. Dieppe.

sites throughout the skeleton called bone remodeling units. Bone remodeling involves the coordinated activity of those cells responsible for bone formation and resorption (i.e. osteoblasts and osteoclasts, respectively) (Fig. 69-5). Although the signals which direct bone remodeling to specific sites remain unclear, local fatigue damage and mechanical strain are thought to represent important influences. Osteoclasts differentiate from hematopoietic precursors shared with macrophages under the influence of RANK ligand and related cytokines.[13] Osteoblasts arise from mesenchymal precursors which also give rise to fibroblasts, stromal cells, and adipocytes. The transcription factor Cbfa1 has recently been identified as playing a critical role in this process of osteoblast differentiation.[14]

Structural changes in the skeleton

Once middle age is reached, the total amount of calcium in the skeleton (i.e. bone mass) starts to decline—a process that is

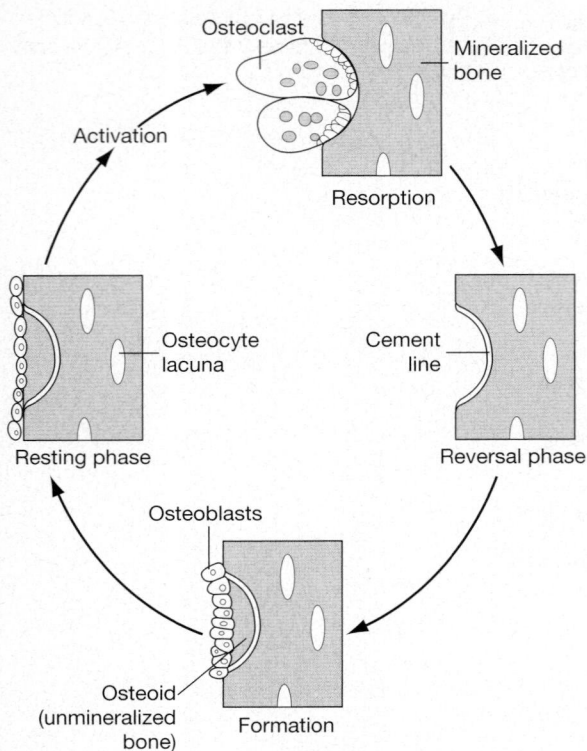

Figure 69-5 The bone remodeling sequence. This commences with osteoclastic bone resorption, following which a cement line is laid down (reversal phase). Osteoblasts then fill up the resorption cavity with osteoid, which subsequently mineralizes, the bone surface finally being covered by lining cells and a thin layer of osteoid.

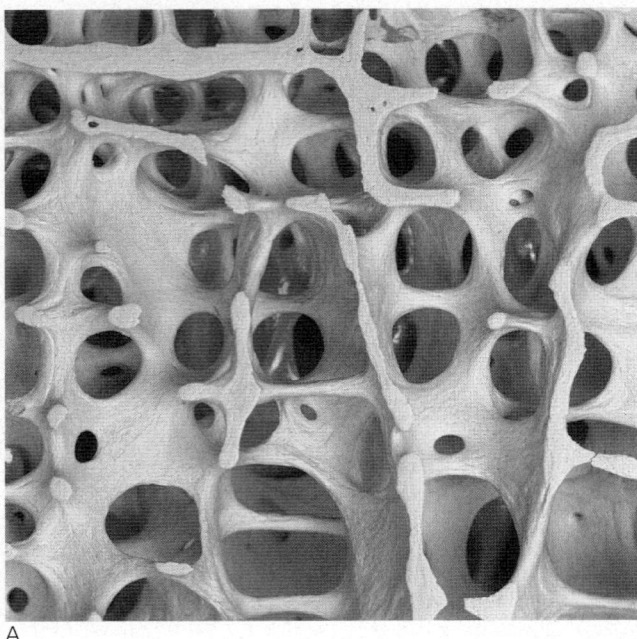

A

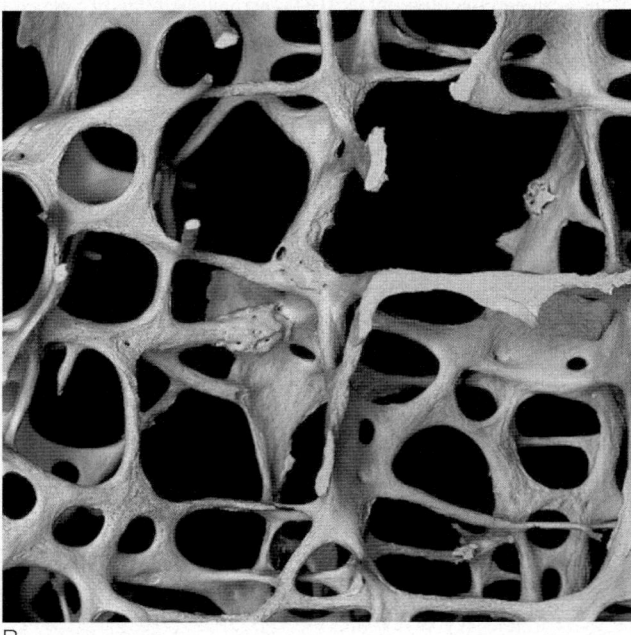

B

Figure 69-6 Changes in trabecular structure associated with osteoporosis. Scanning electron micrographs of lumbar vertebrae (magnification × 20) obtained from: (A) 31-year-old male. (B) An 89-year-old female. Note the loss of bone tissue, associated with thinning and removal of trabecular plates. Kindly supplied by Professor A. Boyde, Department of Anatomy and Developmental Biology, University College London.

accelerated during the first few years following the menopause in women.[15] This is associated with changes in skeletal structure, by which the skeleton becomes weaker and more prone to sustaining fractures. Where these alterations affect trabecular bone, individual trabeculae undergo thinning followed by perforation and ultimately removal, leading to disruption of the trabecular network (Fig. 69-6).

The bony cortex also becomes considerably weaker during aging, through a combination of thinning as a result of expansion of the inner medullary cavity, and an increase in size and number of Haversian canals. The latter represent the end-result of bone remodeling within cortical bone (Fig. 69-7). Recent evidence suggests that clustering of Haversian canals causes increased skeletal fragility at the femoral neck in elderly women who sustain hip fractures.[16] As well as deterioration in skeletal architecture, the material strength of bone may also decline significantly with age. For example, microfractures are thought to accumulate within bone tissue with increasing age, representing the accumulation of fatigue damage.[17] In addition, adverse biochemical changes may occur, such as a decline in efficiency of the cross-linking process required for stabilizing collagen fibrils.[18]

Changes in skeletal metabolism
Bone loss in the elderly population is largely a result of excess osteoclast activity,[19] which causes both an expansion in the total number of remodeling sites and an increase in the amount of bone resorbed per individual site—resulting in a bone remodeling imbalance. The rise in osteoclast activity in older women partly reflects the decline in ovarian hormone

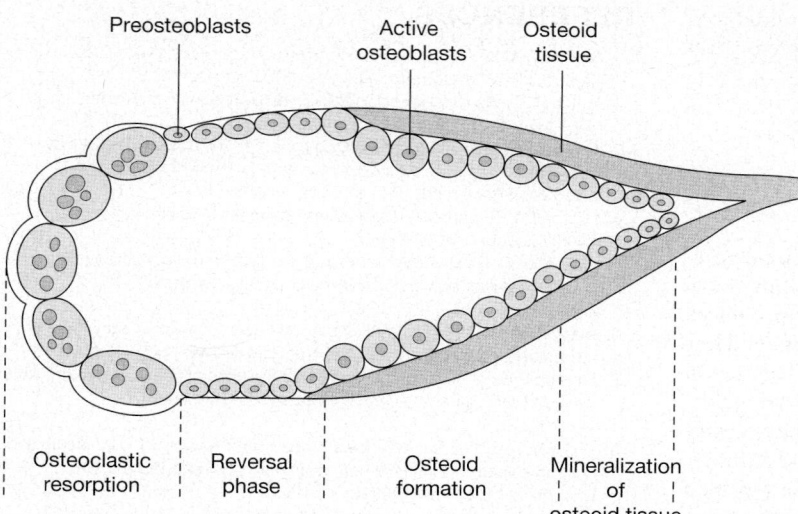

Figure 69-7 A cortical bone remodeling unit, illustrating how a cortical osteon is formed by a cutting cone resulting from osteoclastic bone resorption. Courtesy Drs J. H. Klippel and P. A. Dieppe.

production following the menopause, because estrogens exert an important restraining influence on bone resorption.[20] Endogenous estrogen levels in elderly women are also thought to influence bone metabolism, based on evidence that post-menopausal women with undetectable serum estradiol concentrations and high sex hormone-binding globulin have increased risk of hip and vertebral fracture.[21] Observations that the lifetime risk of fractures in women is approximately three times that of men[22] may reflect the fact that androgens exert an important protective effect on the skeleton in men. On the other hand, in elderly men, serum estradiol levels appear to exert a greater influence on bone mass than does testosterone.[23]

In addition, osteoclast activity may be elevated in the elderly population as a consequence of dietary vitamin D insufficiency combined with reduced sunlight exposure, which leads to mild secondary hyperparathyroidism.[24] Despite subclinical evidence of osteomalacia, many of these patients present in the same way as osteoporosis, for example, with fractures of the femoral neck. As well as reduced vitamin D intake, the tendency to develop vitamin D insufficiency in the elderly population is also thought to reflect an age-related decline in efficiency of renal 1α hydroxylation of vitamin D. These effects of vitamin D insufficiency on bone metabolism are aggravated by a tendency for dietary intake of calcium to be reduced, and by an age-related decline in efficiency of gastrointestinal calcium absorption.

Bone loss is also thought to involve an age-related decline in the recruitment and synthetic capacity of osteoblasts. This may partly reflect the reduction in physical activity associated with aging, thereby reducing the quality and quantity of mechanical inputs into the skeleton that are important in maintaining osteoblast activity. Additionally, age-related changes in the bioavailability of important regulatory factors such as IGF-1 have been suggested to contribute to impaired osteoblast function.[25] Animal models of osteoporosis also suggest that in the aging skeleton, there is an increased tendency to produce adipocytes rather than osteoblasts, leading to the accumulation of bone marrow fat at the expense of trabecular bone.[26] Finally, it is likely that important interactions exist between changes in skeletal metabolism associated with aging and genetic determinants of osteoporosis, such as polymorphisms in the collagen type Iα1 gene.[27]

SOFT TISSUES

Age-related changes occur in other bone and joint tissues, largely as a result of reduced synthesis and post-translational modification of collagen. For example, the tensile strength of tendons and ligament–bone complexes declines with age, and integrity of joint capsules may be lost. This may result in disorders such as loss of the rotator cuff of the shoulder, which may be associated with communications between the shoulder joint and subachromial bursa. In addition, there is a gradual loss of connective tissue resistance to calcium crystal formation in the elderly population, leading to an increase in the incidence of crystal-related arthropathies. Functional impairment in soft tissues may also adversely affect biomechanics of the joint, which may be an important initiating factor in the development of osteoarthritis. For example, age-related changes have been described in the metabolism and composition of the extracellular matrix in the meniscus,[28] which may contribute to the development of knee osteoarthritis.

Back and neck pain and stiffness are common complaints in the elderly population, which are likely to reflect age-related changes in intervertebral discs. The latter consist of an outer fibrous ring called anulus fibrosus and an internal gelatinous (semi-fluid) structure called nucleus pulposus. As people get older the diameter of the nucleus pulposus and the hydrostatic pressure within this region decreases, resulting in increased compressive stress within the anulus.[29] Thus with age the intervertebral disc becomes more compressed, causing a decrease in the intervertebral space and therefore an overall decrease in height of the individuals. The extracellular matrix of the disc contains a network of collagen fibers (both type I and II) which are responsible for the tensile strength, and aggregating proteoglycans that help the disc to resist compressive forces. Age-related changes in the distribution and concentrations of these macromolecules can also significantly alter the mechanical properties of the disc. In many ways extracellular matrix metabolism in the disc is rather similar to articular cartilage; for example, with age there is increased degradation and reduced synthesis of type II collagen, and the glycosaminoglycan and collagen contents of the disc are decreased.[30]

CONSEQUENCES OF BONE AND JOINT AGING

Musculoskeletal problems cause a huge burden of pain and physical disability in older people. The most important functional impairments include the marked loss of muscle strength, reduced range of movements of the spine and peripheral joints, and loss of joint proprioception contributing to problems of balance. In addition, spinal osteoporosis causes progressive kyphotic deformity and height loss which in some individuals may be relatively asymptomatic. The key symptoms include pain and stiffness. Although pain thresholds may increase, there is also a very high prevalence of musculoskeletal pain. For example, some 25 percent of those individuals over the age of 55 years complain of current knee pain. Stiffness and difficulty in initiating movement are almost universal in those over the age of 70 years.

Changes in the bone and soft tissues make the whole system more susceptible to trauma. Periarticular pain syndromes and spinal disorders related to minor trauma are common, but by far the most important result is the high incidence of fractures. These partly reflect the age-related increase in skeletal fragility that characterizes osteoporosis, and partly the age-related increase in falls, which is thought to be multifactorial (see Chapter 105). Osteoporosis predisposes to an increased risk of fracture at all skeletal sites other than flat bones such as the skull, although fractures of the vertebrae, distal radius, and hip are by far the most common (Fig. 69–1). The relative increase in hip fractures in the very elderly may be related to changes in the pattern of falling, since older subjects may be more likely to fall sideways rather than forwards onto an outstretched arm.

The extent of the disability related to musculoskeletal changes is well described in community surveys. Problems with reaching and with locomotion are particularly frequent, the latter contributing extensively to the isolation of elderly people. In addition, it is well recognized that in those who sustain a hip fracture the majority fail to regain their previous level of functioning, and there is also an appreciable excess mortality.[31]

KEY POINTS Bone and joint aging

- Musculoskeletal problems cause a huge burden in elderly people, through a combination of pain and functional impairment.

- These problems result partly from the increased incidence of common musculoskeletal disorders in the elderly, such as rheumatoid arthritis and polymyalgia rheumatica.

- The high burden of musculoskeletal disease in elderly people also reflects the impact of the aging process on tissues which make up the musculoskeletal system, such as articular cartilage and bone.

- There have been considerable advances in recent years in understanding of the cellular and molecular mechanisms which underlie these age-related changes.

REFERENCES

1. Martin J, White A: The prevalence of disability among adults. OPCS survey of disability in Great Britain, report 1. HMSO, London, 1988
2. Hutton CW: Generalised osteoarthritis: an evolutionary problem? Lancet 1987;1:1463–1465
3. Lim KKT, Rogers J, Shepstone L, Dieppe PA: The evolutionary origins of osteoarthritis: a comparative skeletal study of hand disease in two primates. J Rheumatol 1995;22:2132–2134
4. Dieppe PA: Therapeutic targets in osteoarthritis. J Rheumatol 1995;22(suppl 43):136–139
5. Alexander C: Relationship between the utilisation profile of individual joints and their susceptibility to primary osteoarthritis. Skeletal Radiol 1989;18:199–205
6. Buckwalter JA, Woo S L-Y, Goldberg VM et al: Soft tissue aging and musculoskeletal function. J Bone Joint Surg Am 1993;75A:1533–1548
7. Mourao PAS: Distribution of chondroitin 4-sulfate and chondroitin 6-sulfate in human articular and growth cartilage. Arthritis Rheum 1988;31:1028–1033
8. Sharif M, Osborne DJ, Meadows K et al: The relevance of chondroitin and keratan sulphate markers in normal and arthritic synovial fluid. Br J Rheumatol 1996;35:951–957
9. Mankin HJ, Dorfman H, Lipiello L, Zarins A: Biochemical and metabolic abnormalities in articular cartilage from osteoarthritic hips. J Bone Joint Surg 1971;53:523–537
10. Hashimoto S, Ochs RL, Komiya S, Lotz M: Linkage of chondrocyte apoptosis and cartilage degradation in human osteoarthritis. Arthritis Rheum 1998;41:1632–1638
11. Clements KM, Bee ZC, Crossingham GV et al: How severe must repetitive loading be to kill chondrocytes in articular cartilage? Osteoarthritis Cartilage 2001;9:499–507
12. Gibson GJ, Kohler WJ, Schaffler MB: Chondrocyte apoptosis in endochondral ossification of chick sterna. Dev Dyn 1995;203:468–476
13. Lacey DL, Timms E, Tan H-L et al: Osteoprotegerin ligand is a cytokine that regulates osteoclast differentiation and activation. Cell 1998;93:165–176
14. Ducy P, Zheng R, Geoffroy et al: Osf2/Cbfa1: a transcriptional activator of osteoblast differentiation. Cell 1998;89:747–754
15. Pouilles JM, Tremollieres F, Ribot C: Effect of menopause on femoral and vertebral bone loss. J Bone Miner Res 1995;10:1531–1536
16. Jordan GR, Loveridge N, Bell KL: Spatial clustering of remodeling osteons in the femoral neck cortex: a cause of weakness in hip fracture? Bone 2000;26:305–313
17. Todd RC, Freeman MAR, Price CJ: Isolated trabecular fatigue fractures in the femoral neck. J Bone Joint Surg Br 1972;54B:723–728
18. Oxlund H, Mosekilde L, Ortoft G: Reduced concentration of collagen reducible cross-links in human trabecular bone with respect to age and osteoporosis. Bone 1996;19:479–484
19. Garnero P, Sornay-Rendu E, Chapuy MC, Delmas PD: Increased bone turnover in late postmenopausal women is a major determinant of osteoporosis. J Bone Miner Res 1996;11:337–349
20. Stepan JJ, Presl J, Broulik P, Pacovsky V: Serum osteocalcin levels and bone alkaline phosphatase isoenzyme after oophorectomy and primary hyperparathyroidism. J Clin Endocrinol Metab 1987;64:1079–1084
21. Cummings SR, Browner SW, Bauer D et al: Endogenous hormones and the risk of hip and vertebral fractures among older women. N Engl J Med 1998;339:733–738
22. Melton LJ, Chrischilles EA, Cooper C et al: How many women have osteoporosis? J Bone Miner Res 1992;7:1005–1010
23. Amin S, Zhang Y, Sawin CT et al: Association of hypogonadism and estradiol levels with bone mineral density in elderly men from the Framingham study. Ann Int Med 2000;133:951–963
24. Chapuy MC, Arlot ME, Duboeuf F et al: Vitamin D3 and calcium to prevent hip fractures in elderly women. N Engl J Med 1992;327:1637–1642
25. Rosen C, Donahue LR, Hunter S et al: The 24/25-kDa serum insulin-like growth factor-binding protein is increased in elderly women with hip and spine fractures. J Clin Endocrinol Metab 1992;74:24–27
26. Nuttall ME, Gimble JM: Is there a therapeutic opportunity to either prevent or treat osteopenic disorders by inhibiting marrow adipogenesis? Bone 2000;27:177–184
27. Uitterlinden AG, Burger H, Huang Q et al: Relation of alleles of the collagen type Iα1 gene to bone density and the risk of osteoporotic fractures in postmenopausal women. N Engl J Med 1998;338:1016–1021

28. McAlinden A, Dudhia J, Bolton MC et al: Age-related changes in the synthesis and mRNA expression of decorin and aggrecan in human meniscus and articular cartilage. Osteoarthritis Cartilage 2001; 9:33–41

29. Adams MA, McNally DS, Dolan P: "Stress" distributions inside intervertebral discs. J Bone Joint Surg Br 1996;78B:965–972

30. Antoniou J, Steffen T, Nelson F et al: The human lumbar intervertebral disc: evidence for changes in the biosynthesis and denaturation of the extracellular matrix with growth, maturation, aging, and degeneration. J Clin Invest 1996;98:996–1003

31. Keene GS, Parker MJ, Pryor GA: Mortality and morbidity after hip fractures. BMJ 1993;307:1248–1250

32. Cooper C, Melton LJ: Epidemiology of osteoporosis. Trends Endocrinol Metab 1992;3:224–229

Chapter 70

Metabolic bone disease

Roger M. Francis

Although the popular image of the skeleton is of an inert structure supporting the rest of the body, bone is a dynamic tissue which undergoes constant remodeling throughout life. This remodeling is necessary to allow the skeleton to increase in size during growth, respond to the physical stresses placed on it, and repair damage due to structural fatigue or fracture. In addition to its mechanical properties, bone plays an important role in calcium homeostasis, acting as a mineral reservoir which can be drawn upon to maintain normocalcemia. The skeleton comprises two types of bone: cortical or compact, and trabecular or cancellous bone. Cortical bone is predominantly found in the shafts of the long bones, whilst trabecular bone is mainly located in the vertebrae, pelvis, and the ends of long bones, where it forms a lattice-like structure within bone. Trabecular bone has a larger surface area, undergoes greater remodeling, and is therefore more responsive to changes in mineral metabolism than is cortical bone. The respective proportion of cortical and trabecular bone varies with the anatomical site, though overall the skeleton is composed of 80 percent cortical and 20 percent trabecular bone.

The three major cell types involved in bone remodeling are osteoclasts, osteoblasts, and osteocytes. Osteoclasts are multinucleate cells derived from macrophage–monocyte precursors which resorb bone, releasing mineral and removing degraded organic material. Osteoblasts are derived from fibroblast precursors and synthesize bone matrix or osteoid, which is subsequently mineralized around foci of crystal formation known as matrix vesicles. The matrix vesicles are extruded from osteoblasts by exocytosis and contain promoters of crystal formation such as alkaline phosphatase and pyrophosphatase. Osteocytes are mature osteoblasts which become trapped within calcified bone. These are interconnected by long dendritic processes, possibly providing a communication network to transmit information about mechanical forces and direct bone resorption and formation.

Bone remodeling is initiated by a period of bone resorption lasting about 2 weeks, when osteoclasts erode an area of bone. Osteoblasts are then attracted to the resorption cavity, where over the subsequent 3 months new bone matrix is deposited and mineralized. The processes of bone resorption and bone formation are usually closely coupled, probably through local humoral factors, though bone formation exceeds resorption during skeletal growth and resorption outstrips bone formation after involutional bone loss starts. Bone remodeling may be influenced by mechanical forces applied to the skeleton, by local humoral factors, and by circulating hormones such as estrogen, testosterone, calcitonin, parathyroid hormone (PTH) and 1,25-dihydroxyvitamin D ($1,25(OH)_2D$).

Bone mass changes throughout life in three major phases: growth, consolidation, and involution. Up to 90 percent of the ultimate bone mass is deposited during skeletal growth, which lasts until the closure of the epiphyses. There is then a phase of skeletal consolidation lasting for up to 15 years, when bone mass increases further until the peak bone mass is achieved in the mid-thirties. Involutional bone loss then starts between the ages of 35 and 40 in both sexes, but in women there is an acceleration of bone loss in the decade after the menopause. Overall, women lose 35–50 percent of trabecular and 25–30 percent of cortical bone mass with advancing age, whilst men lose 15–45 percent of trabecular and 5–15 percent of cortical bone.

OSTEOPOROSIS

Osteoporosis is characterized by a reduction in bone density, associated with skeletal fragility and an increased risk of fractures. The World Health Organization (WHO) has quantitatively defined osteoporosis as a bone mineral density (BMD) 2.5 standard deviations or more below the mean value for young adults, whereas the terms *severe* or *established* osteoporosis indicates that there has also been one or more fragility fracture.[1]

The three major osteoporotic fractures are those of the forearm, vertebral body, and femoral neck, but fractures of the humerus, tibia, pelvis, and ribs are also common in patients with osteoporosis. These fractures are a major cause of mortality, morbidity, and health and social service expenditure in elderly people, but this is particularly the case with hip fractures. The annual cost of osteoporotic fractures in the UK has been estimated at £942 million, of which 87 percent is attributable to hip fractures.[2]

There is a strong inverse relationship between bone density and fracture risk, with a 2–3 fold increase in fracture incidence for each standard deviation reduction in BMD.[3] The risk of fracture is also determined by other skeletal risk factors, such as bone turnover, trabecular architecture, skeletal geometry, and previous fragility fracture.[4–6] Nonskeletal risk factors for fracture include postural instability, physical and mental frailty, and conditions associated with falling.[7–9]

Prevalence of osteoporosis

Using the WHO definition, the prevalence of osteoporosis in the hip increases in white women in the USA from 8 percent in the seventh decade to 47.5 percent in the ninth decade, whilst the prevalence of osteoporosis in the forearm, spine, or hip rises from 21.6 to 70 percent.[1,10] An alternative approach is to determine the prevalence of osteoporotic fractures. It has been estimated that the lifetime risk of fracture for a 50-year-old white woman in the USA is 16.0 percent for the forearm, 15.6 percent for the vertebra, and 17.5 percent for the proximal femur, whilst the corresponding figures for a 50-year-old man are 2.5, 5.0, and 6.0 percent.[10]

Pathogenesis of osteoporosis

Bone mass at any age, and therefore the risk of fracture, is determined by the peak bone mass, the age at which bone loss starts, and the rate at which it progresses.

PEAK BONE MASS Genetic factors account for as much as 80 percent of the variance in peak bone mass.[11] Recent work suggests that polymorphism of the vitamin D receptor, estrogen receptor, and collagen genes may have an important effect on bone density and fracture risk. Other potential determinants of peak bone mass include exercise, dietary calcium, smoking, alcohol consumption, and hormonal factors.[12,13]

INVOLUTIONAL BONE LOSS Bone loss starts between the ages of 35 and 40 in both sexes, possibly related to impaired new bone formation, owing to declining osteoblast function. The onset of bone loss is likely to be genetically predetermined, and the subsequent rate of bone loss may also be influenced by genetic factors. Bone loss increases in the decade following the menopause in women, owing to the marked reduction in the circulating estradiol concentrations. Other causes of age-related bone loss include low body weight, smoking, excess alcohol consumption, physical inactivity, declining vitamin D concentrations, and secondary hyperparathyroidism.[12,13]

Body weight is an important determinant of bone density and fracture risk, as bone loss is more rapid in post-menopausal women with low body weight and individuals with osteoporotic fractures are lighter than expected.[9,14] The protective effects of high body weight on bone density and fracture risk may be due to the stimulation of bone formation by greater mechanical loading, increased conversion of adrenal androgens to estrogens in fat, and the shock-absorbing properties of subcutaneous fat.

Smoking may increase bone loss by reducing the age at menopause by several years, decreasing plasma estrogen levels by increasing their metabolism, and possibly depressing osteoblast function. The deleterious effect of smoking on the skeleton may also be due in part to the association with low body weight. Although alcoholism is a recognized cause of osteoporosis, the effect of modest alcohol consumption on bone density remains unclear.

The decline in physical activity with advancing age is also likely to cause further bone loss. Physical activity is important to the skeleton since the associated weight-bearing and muscular activity stimulates bone formation and increases bone mass, whilst immobilization leads to rapid bone loss. The importance of physical activity is underlined by a number of studies which show that physical inactivity is associated with an increased risk of hip fracture.[9,15,16]

The role of dietary calcium intake in the pathogenesis of bone loss remains controversial. Although there is a relationship between dietary calcium and bone mass in adolescence, studies show little correlation between calcium intake and bone density or bone loss in post-menopausal women. Other nutrients which have been suggested as potential determinants of the rate of bone loss include fluoride, protein, and sodium, but their importance is still uncertain.

There is a reduction in circulating 25-hydroxyvitamin D (25OHD) and $1,25(OH)_2D$ concentrations with advancing age, owing to decreased cutaneous production and impaired metabolism of vitamin D. This is likely to contribute to the observed increase in circulating parathyroid hormone (PTH) with age.[17] There is a weak relationship between serum 25OHD and bone density in middle-aged women, with an inverse correlation between bone density and serum PTH, suggesting that vitamin D status may influence bone loss.[18] Other studies show that vitamin D insufficiency and secondary hyperparathyroidism are common in older patients with osteoporosis and fractures.[19,20]

Secondary osteoporosis

In addition to the factors influencing the attainment of peak bone mass and subsequent involutional bone loss, there are a number of conditions which may accelerate the development of osteoporosis. Secondary causes of osteoporosis may be found in up to 35 percent of women and 55 percent of men with symptomatic vertebral crush fractures.[21,22] The most frequently encountered are oral steroid therapy, male hypogonadism, hyperthyroidism, myeloma, skeletal metastases, and anticonvulsant therapy.

Clinical features of osteoporosis

Osteoporosis is generally considered to be asymptomatic until fractures occur. Fractures of the forearm and hip are usually easy to diagnose, but vertebral crush fractures are more difficult to detect clinically. Only 30 percent of patients come to medical attention after a vertebral fracture, and there are many other causes of acute back pain. Classically, however, a vertebral fracture is associated with an acute episode of back pain lasting for 6–8 weeks before settling to a more chronic backache. The pain may radiate anteriorly but rarely radiates to the hips or legs. Individuals with vertebral fractures may also be aware of loss of height of several inches and notice the development of a kyphosis. Physical signs include a kyphosis, local tenderness over the spine, and horizontal skin creases and abdominal protrusion owing to the loss of trunk height.

Diagnosis of osteoporosis

Prior to the development of techniques which accurately measure bone density, osteoporosis was usually detected only after a fracture had occurred. The term "osteoporosis" was therefore reserved for the fracture syndrome resulting from reduced bone density. With the advent of bone densitometry and the development of effective treatments which decrease fracture risk, the term "osteoporosis" is now increasingly used to describe reduced BMD before fractures have occurred.

Although accurate measurements of lumbar spine and femoral BMD can be made using dual-energy X-ray absorptiometry (DXA), population-based bone-density screening cannot be advocated for the prevention of osteoporotic fractures. A number of indications for BMD measurements are recognized, but their relevance in older people remains uncertain.[23,24] It is also important to appreciate that spine BMD may be spuriously elevated in elderly people, because of degenerative changes and aortic calcification.

The most important indication for BMD measurement in an older person is fracture after minimal trauma in a previously fit individual. This may confirm the diagnosis of osteoporosis, provide an assessment of the risk of future fractures, and allow the most appropriate use of expensive treatments such as bisphosphonates.[24] Other indications include early menopause in women up to the age of 70 years, underlying causes of secondary osteoporosis, particularly if the results are likely to alter management, and radiological evidence of osteopenia.[24]

BMD measurements are of limited value in the assessment of frail elderly patients with hip and other fractures, as the vast majority will have osteoporosis and the results are unlikely to influence management. Early menopause is not necessarily an indication for bone-density measurement in women over the age of 70 years, as the impact of this risk factor diminishes with advancing age. Bone densitometry may also be unnecessary in patients on prolonged oral steroid therapy, as a Consensus Group from the UK has recently recommended that all people over the age of 65 years on 7.5 mg prednisolone daily should be offered treatment for osteoporosis.[25]

BMD measurements may be expressed as standard deviation units above or below the mean value for normal young adults or relative to the mean value for control subjects of the same age, to give T and Z scores, respectively. Although the WHO definition of osteoporosis ($T < -2.5$) may be useful in epidemiological studies, it does not necessarily represent a threshold for treatment. This is important as 70 percent of women above the age of 80 years have a T score under -2.5, but only a proportion of these will sustain an osteoporotic fracture.[1] It may therefore be more appropriate to use Z scores in interpreting BMD measurements in older people, to identify individuals whose bone density is lower than expected for their age and who are at particularly high risk of osteoporotic fractures.

Investigation of osteoporosis

In patients with probable long-bone fractures, X-rays are generally performed to confirm that a fracture has occurred and to determine its position prior to subsequent fixation. As vertebral fractures are more difficult to diagnose, spine X-rays should be considered in patients with acute back pain, loss of height, or kyphosis, to look for evidence of vertebral deformation, degenerative arthritis, or other pathology. Such X-rays may also show lytic or sclerotic lesions, which suggest the possibility of neoplastic disease. Whilst spine X-rays are useful in the diagnosis of vertebral fracture, they are unreliable in the assessment of bone density.

In patients with vertebral fractures, causes of secondary osteoporosis should be identified by careful history, physical examination, and appropriate investigation (Table 70-1), as specific treatment of underlying conditions such as

---

Table 70-1 Investigations for secondary osteoporosis in older people with fractures after minimal trauma or low BMD (Z score < −2.0)

- Full blood count
- ESR or CRP
- Biochemical profile
- Thyroid function tests
- Serum testosterone, sex hormone binding globulin, LH, FSH (men)
- Serum and urine electrophoresis (vertebral fractures)
- ? 25OHD and PTH

---

hyperthyroidism, hypogonadism, or hyperparathyroidism increases bone density by up to 15 percent. Underlying causes of secondary osteoporosis should also be sought in elderly men and women presenting with hip and other nonvertebral fractures after minimal trauma. Routine biochemical profile is probably worthwhile, as hypocalcemia and hypophosphatemia may indicate possible osteomalacia, although these measurements lack diagnostic specificity or sensitivity. Serum 25OHD and intact PTH measurements may be useful in the diagnosis of vitamin D deficiency in patients with limited sunlight exposure, previous gastric resection, malabsorption, or anticonvulsant treatment. These measurements are probably unnecessary if calcium and vitamin D supplementation is planned. Investigations for secondary osteoporosis should also be performed in patients found to have a BMD below the normal range for their age (Z score under −2.0), to identify underlying causes of bone loss which may be modified.

Management of osteoporosis

All patients with osteoporotic fractures should be given general advice on lifestyle measures to decrease further bone loss, including eating a balanced diet rich in calcium, moderating tobacco and alcohol consumption and, if possible, maintaining regular physical activity and exposure to sunlight. As bone loss continues into old age in both men and women, specific treatment for osteoporosis should be considered in all patients with osteoporotic fractures. Furthermore, treatment of osteoporosis is likely to be more cost-effective in older people, because of their higher fracture rate.

Treatments for osteoporosis may be classified into antiresorptive agents, such as hormone replacement therapy (HRT), tibolone, raloxifene, bisphosphonates, calcitonin, calcium and vitamin D, and calcitriol, and anabolic agents like anabolic steroids, fluoride salts, and PTH. Although antiresorptive agents decrease bone resorption, the transient uncoupling of resorption and formation leads to a modest increase in bone density of 5–10 percent, predominantly in the first year of treatment. Many of these antiresorptive agents have also been shown to decrease the incidence of fractures. In contrast, anabolic agents increase bone density by up to 50 percent, but this has not been associated with a consistent reduction in fracture risk.

In the UK, the Royal College of Physicians (RCP) and Bone and Tooth Society have recently published guidelines on the management of osteoporosis.[23] Their recommendations are graded on the levels of evidence for each therapeutic intervention. Grade A recommendations are based on randomized controlled trials, whereas grade B recommendations result from controlled studies without randomization, studies with a quasi-experimental design, and epidemiological studies. Grade C recommendations are based on expert committee reports or the clinical experience of recognized authorities.

Hormone replacement therapy, tibolone, raloxifene, bisphosphonates, calcitonin, calcium and vitamin D, and calcitriol all have grade A recommendations for a beneficial effect on BMD.[23] The Royal College of Physicians recommendations on the efficacy of these treatments in the reduction of vertebral, nonvertebral, and hip fractures is shown in Table 70-2.[23] Although the grading of the strength of the recommendations based on study design is clearly useful,

Table 70-2 Effect of interventions on the incidence of vertebral, nonvertebral, and hip fractures. Grading of recommendations is adapted from the UK Royal College of Physicians' Clinical Guidelines for Prevention and Treatment of Osteoporosis[23]

	Vertebral fractures	Nonvertebral fractures	Hip fractures
Estrogen	A	A	B
Raloxifene	A	ND	ND
Etidronate	A	B	B
Alendronate	A	A	A
Risedronate	A	A	A
Calcitonin	A	B	B
Calcium and vitamin D	ND	A	A
Calcitriol	A	A	ND
Hip protectors	–	–	A

ND indicates that a beneficial effect on fracture incidence has not been demonstrated.

this takes no account of study size, the magnitude of the treatment effect, and the patient groups studied. It is therefore important to consider these issues at this stage.

HORMONE REPLACEMENT (HRT) A number of small controlled trials each involving less than 150 women show that HRT prevents the rapid bone loss that occurs at the menopause.[23] Epidemiological studies suggest that HRT also decreases the risk of fractures.[26,27] A recent 5-year randomized controlled trial in 464 post-menopausal women shows that HRT reduces the risk of nonvertebral fractures by 71 percent.[28] Unfortunately, the benefit of previous long-term HRT on bone density decreases progressively once treatment is stopped and may be lost completely by the age of 75 years.[29]

HRT may be more useful in older women or those with established osteoporosis, where the reduction in fracture risk may be apparent earlier. Two small studies of older women with established osteoporosis (subject numbers 40 and 78, with mean age 65 and 68 years, respectively) showed that HRT increases spine BMD by about 5 percent.[30,31] One of these studies also showed a reduction in vertebral fracture incidence of 60 percent.[31]

TIBOLONE Tibolone has weak estrogenic, progestogenic, and androgenic actions. One study of 91 normal women who had been post-menopausal for over 10 years, and another of 107 osteoporotic women with a mean age of 63 years, showed that tibolone increases BMD, but there is no information on its effect on fracture incidence.[32,33]

RALOXIFENE Raloxifene is a selective estrogen receptor modulator (SERM), which has estrogen agonist actions on the skeleton and lipid profile, but acts as an estrogen antagonist on the breast and endometrium. In a study of 601 normal women aged between 45 and 60 years, it has been shown to prevent post-menopausal bone loss and improve the lipid profile, without stimulating the endometrium.[34] In a study in 7,705 post-menopausal women aged 31–80 years with osteoporosis,

raloxifene increased lumbar spine and femoral neck BMD by 2–3 percent, reduced the risk of vertebral fractures by 30–50 percent, and decreased the incidence of breast cancer by 76 percent.[35,36] There is no evidence that raloxifene decreases the incidence of nonvertebral fractures.

BISPHOSPHONATES These are analogs of naturally occurring pyrophosphate which, although poorly absorbed from the bowel, localize preferentially in bone where they bind to hydroxyapatite crystals. Bisphosphonates decrease bone resorption by reducing osteoclast recruitment and function. As bisphosphonates persist in the skeleton for many months, their duration of action is prolonged beyond the period of administration.

Two studies of women aged up to 75 years with established osteoporosis (involving 66 and 423 women, respectively) showed that intermittent cyclical etidronate increases spine BMD by 5 percent and reduces the incidence of further vertebral fractures by about 60 percent.[37–39] Cyclical etidronate also increased femoral neck BMD by 2 percent compared with the control group,[38] but there are no interventional studies investigating the effect of treatment on hip fracture incidence.

In a randomized controlled trial of 994 women with osteoporosis aged between 45 and 80 years, alendronate has been reported to increase BMD by up to 8.8 percent at the lumbar spine and by 5.9 percent at the femoral neck.[40] This study also showed a 48 percent reduction in the proportion of women with new vertebral fracture. Results from the Fracture Intervention Trial, in 2,027 women (aged 55–81 years) with low hip-bone density and at least one vertebral fracture, show that alendronate significantly increases BMD at the forearm, spine, and femoral neck and decreases the incidence of fractures at these sites by 48, 55, and 51 percent, respectively.[41] In a further 4,432 women with low hip BMD but no prevalent vertebral fracture, taking part in the clinical fracture arm of the Fracture Intervention Trial, alendronate decreased the incidence of vertebral deformation by 44 percent.[42] This second part of the Fracture Intervention Trial showed no overall reduction in clinical fractures with alendronate, but there was a significant reduction in women with baseline femoral-neck bone density more than 2.5 standard deviations below the young adult mean.[42]

In a further study in 359 women with osteoporosis, aged between 60 and 85 years, alendronate was as well tolerated and effective in increasing bone density in women above the age of 70 years as in younger women.[43] This suggests that there is no attenuation of the effect of alendronate with advancing age. A recent comparative study shows similar increases in lumbar-spine and proximal-femur BMD in women with osteoporosis treated with alendronate 70 mg once weekly and those receiving alendronate 10 mg daily.[44] The use of weekly alendronate may be more appropriate and improve compliance in certain patients, particularly those who dislike the fasting involved in the daily administration of an oral bisphosphonate.

Risedronate has been shown, in two randomized controlled trials involving 2,458 and 1,226 post-menopausal women with osteoporosis, to increase lumbar-spine and femoral-neck BMD and decrease the incidence of vertebral and nonvertebral fractures by 41–49 percent and 33–39 percent, respectively.[45,46] The Hip Intervention Programme was a randomized controlled trial, comparing the effect of risedronate with placebo on hip fracture incidence in 9,331 women.[47] This study recruited 5,445 women aged between 70 and 79 years with a low femoral-neck BMD (group 1) and 3,886 women aged 80 years and above with either a nonskeletal risk factor for hip fracture or low femoral-neck BMD (group 2). Overall, there was a 30 percent reduction in hip fracture incidence with risedronate, but no significant decrease in fracture risk was seen in group 2. There was a 40 percent reduction in hip fractures in group 1, which increased to 60 percent if vertebral fractures were present at baseline.[47]

The results of the risedronate Hip Intervention Programme and the alendronate Fracture Intervention Trial suggest that bisphosphonates are particularly useful in patients with low BMD and/or a prevalent vertebral fracture, as they have a high fracture incidence and show the largest reduction on treatment.

CALCITONIN Calcitonin is a potent antiresorptive agent, with a rapid but short-lived effect on osteoclast function. A dose–response study of intranasal calcitonin (100–400 iu daily) in the treatment of 208 women (mean age 70 years) with reduced forearm BMD showed significant increases in spine BMD of 1–3 percent over 2 years, associated with a reduction in the number of vertebral fractures of 64–68 percent.[48] Another study of 60 post-menopausal women with vertebral fractures (mean age 68 years) demonstrated that cyclical intramuscular calcitonin (100 iu daily) and oral calcium supplements (500 mg elemental calcium daily) for 10 days every 4 weeks decreased the incidence of vertebral fractures by 60 percent over 2 years, compared with an increase in 35 percent in a group receiving calcium alone.[49] The Prevent Recurrence Of Osteoporotic Fractures (PROOF) study of 1255 women with established osteoporosis showed only marginal improvements in BMD with intranasal calcitonin.[50] Although there was a 36 percent reduction in new vertebral fractures with doses of 200 iu calcitonin daily, no significant decrease in fractures was seen with 100 or 400 iu/day.[50]

CALCIUM Calcium supplements were previously used alone in the treatment of osteoporosis, but this is probably no longer appropriate as more effective treatments are available. Two studies showed that calcium supplementation decreases bone loss in normal post-menopausal women (subject numbers 120 and 122, with mean age 56 and 58 years, respectively), but is less effective than hormone replacement therapy.[51,52] Calcium supplements have been reported to prevent bone loss from the femoral shaft and decrease vertebral fractures in a study of 159 elderly women (mean age 75 years) who were vitamin D replete.[53] One study also showed a reduction in vertebral fracture incidence in 94 elderly women with a mean age of 75 years with prevalent fractures and a dietary calcium intake of less than 1 g daily.[54]

CALCIUM AND VITAMIN D Calcium and vitamin D supplementation may be the most appropriate treatment for frail elderly patients with osteoporosis, as vitamin D deficiency and secondary hyperparathyroidism are common in this situation. A French study in 3270 women (mean age 84 years) living in nursing homes and apartment blocks for the elderly showed that 800 iu vitamin D_3 and 1.2 g elemental calcium daily decreases parathyroid hormone, increases femoral neck BMD, and reduces the risk of hip fracture by 27 percent.[55,56] A smaller American study of 389 elderly men and women (mean age 70 years) living at home demonstrated that 700 iu vitamin D_3 and 500 mg elemental calcium daily had a modest beneficial effect on BMD and decreased the incidence of nonvertebral fractures by 54 percent.[57] It is unclear if the benefits of treatment seen in these studies were due to vitamin D, calcium, or the combination of both. A Finnish study showed that an annual intramuscular injection of 150,000–300,000 iu vitamin D decreased the risk of fractures in 1186 elderly people by 25 percent.[58] In contrast, a Dutch study showed a small increase in hip BMD with 400 iu vitamin D_3 daily, but no effect on the incidence of hip fractures in 2,578 elderly people.[59]

VITAMIN D METABOLITES Patients with established osteoporosis have lower calcium absorption than age-matched control subjects, which may be due to reduced serum $1,25(OH)_2D$ concentrations or to relative resistance to the action of vitamin D metabolites on the bowel.[60] Malabsorption of calcium in osteoporosis can be overcome by pharmacological doses of parent vitamin D or by low doses of the vitamin D metabolites, calcitriol and alfacalcidol. Studies of the effect of treatment with vitamin D metabolites on BMD and fracture incidence in established osteoporosis have produced conflicting results.[60] A study comparing calcitriol with calcium supplementation in 622 women with vertebral fractures (mean age 64 years) showed a significantly lower incidence of new vertebral fractures with calcitriol, but this was due to an increase in fracture rate with calcium rather than a reduction with calcitriol.[61] The potential risk of hypercalcemia and the need for regular monitoring of serum calcium and renal function limit the use of calcitriol in the management of osteoporosis.

FLUORIDE SALTS Initial studies showed that sodium fluoride increased spine bone density by up to 35 percent over 4 years in women with vertebral osteoporosis, but this appeared to be at the expense of cortical bone loss.[62,63] There was no reduction in vertebral fracture incidence, but the number of nonvertebral fractures increased with fluoride.[62,63] These studies also showed that sodium fluoride is potentially toxic, causing nausea, vomiting, indigestion, and lower-extremity bone pain.[62,63] A more recent study using lower-dose, slow-release sodium fluoride in 110 women with vertebral fractures (mean age 68 years) shows smaller increases in spine and hip bone density, without adverse effects on forearm bone mass.[64] This study also showed a significant reduction in vertebral fracture incidence, without the side-effect profile described with the higher dose treatment. Nevertheless, the therapeutic window for fluoride appears narrow and this agent cannot yet be advocated for the management of osteoporosis.

ANABOLIC STEROIDS Anabolic steroids such as stanozolol and nandrolone increase bone mass in osteoporosis by 5–10 percent.[65,66] This has previously been attributed to increased bone formation, but may be due to decreased bone resorption. Anabolic steroids may be associated with androgenic side-effects and fluid retention, whilst prolonged administration may lead to abnormal liver function tests and even hepatocellular tumors. Their use in the management of osteoporosis cannot be advocated, particularly as there is no evidence of a reduction in fracture incidence.

PARATHYROID HORMONE Initial studies with PTH showed large increases in trabecular bone density, but these were accompanied by cortical bone loss.[67] Recent work suggests that the combination of PTH with calcitonin or HRT increases spine bone density without adverse effects on cortical bone mass.[68,69] A randomized controlled trial in 34 post-menopausal women with osteoporosis on HRT (mean age 62 years) demonstrated that 3 years' treatment with PTH (400 iu daily by subcutaneous injection) increased BMD by 13 percent at the spine and by 2.7 percent in the hip.[69] Although this study lacked the statistical power to accurately assess the effect of treatment on fracture incidence, there was a significant reduction in new vertebral deformities. Pending the results of larger studies examining the effect of PTH on fracture incidence, this treatment should be regarded as promising but experimental.

FALLS ASSESSMENT All patients with a past history of fractures and recurrent falls should undergo a falls assessment. Risk factors for falling are divided into intrinsic factors (including poor vision, neurological disease, and medication) and extrinsic or environmental factors (such as trailing wires, loose carpets, and ill-fitting footwear). Intrinsic causes of falls should be sought by history, examination, and review of medication; extrinsic or environmental causes may be identified from the history and home visit. In elderly patients with unexplained falls or syncope, tilt testing may also be useful.

A number of randomized controlled trials have assessed the effect of modifying risk factors for falling, although the results have not all been consistent. In an American study of 301 elderly patients with an apparent risk factor for falling, the intervention group underwent geriatric assessment, with modification of risk factors for falling, whereas the control group had the usual healthcare and social visits.[70] Over the 12 months' follow-up period, 35 percent of the intervention group had falls compared to 47 percent in the control group. A more recent British study examined the effectiveness of a detailed medical and occupational therapy assessment in 397 older patients presenting to an accident and emergency department with a fall.[71] There was a significant 61 percent reduction in the risk of falls in the intervention group over 12 months, compared with the control group. Although both studies showed a significant decrease in falls, neither had the statistical power to detect a meaningful reduction in fracture incidence.[70,71]

EXTERNAL HIP PROTECTORS An alternative approach to fracture prevention is to decrease the impact of falls using external hip protectors, which are incorporated into specially designed underwear. A Danish study block randomized 665 elderly residents of nursing homes to receive external hip protectors or to serve as controls.[72] Over the 12-month study there was a reduction in hip fracture risk of over 50 percent in those using the hip protectors. In the group randomized to receive

hip protectors, the only patients who fractured were not using hip protectors at the time. A systematic review of five randomized controlled trials of hip protectors has recently been published, involving 1,681 participants living in a nursing or residential home.[73] This showed an overall prevalence of hip fractures of 2.1 percent in the hip protector group, compared with 6.2 percent in the control group. Owing to the large number of participants allocated to intervention by cluster randomization, it was not possible to demonstrate conclusively that this difference between groups was statistically significant.

Although external hip protectors are potentially one of the most promising interventions for the prevention of hip fractures, they are bulky and uncomfortable, so may be unacceptable to many elderly people at risk of hip fracture.[74]

Choice of treatment

In considering the choice of treatment in the individual patient, a number of factors are important. These include the underlying pathogenesis of bone loss, the evidence of efficacy in any particular situation, the cost-effectiveness of treatment, tolerability, and patient preference. Hormone replacement and other hormonal treatments are likely to be more effective in younger post-menopausal women with osteoporosis, where bone loss is largely due to estrogen deficiency. In contrast, calcium and vitamin D supplementation may be more appropriate in frail elderly people, who are likely to have vitamin D insufficiency and secondary hyperparathyroidism. Bisphosphonates are effective across a wide age range, but may be inappropriate in individuals with cognitive impairment, because of difficulties in coping with the complex instructions on administration. The use of alendronate in particular may be precluded in older patients with hiatus hernia, esophageal disease, or peptic ulcers, because of concern about the risk of esophagitis.

A number of factors may influence compliance and tolerability. Conventional HRT causes regular vaginal bleeding in 90 percent of women. Although this may be tolerated in women close to the menopause, it is less well accepted in older women. Although continuous-combined estrogen/progestogen preparations offer the prospect of the benefits of HRT without the need for regular bleeds, these cause some spotting in the early months of treatment, which is unacceptable to some women. HRT is also likely to cause breast tenderness in older women,

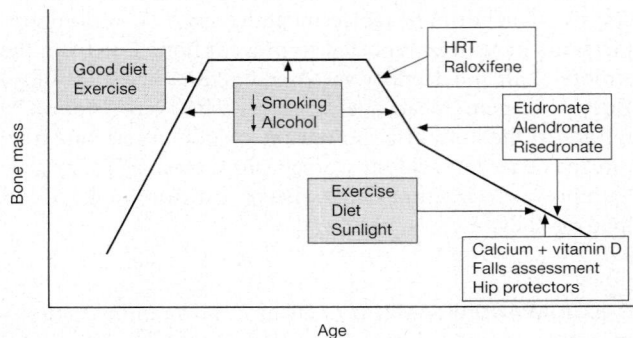

Figure 70-1 Schematic of the major therapeutic options in patients with osteoporosis of different ages, together with lifestyle measures in the shaded boxes.

who may also be concerned about the risk of breast cancer with prolonged HRT. Raloxifene is likely to aggravate hot flushes, particularly in women close to the menopause, so may be more appropriate in older post-menopausal women. Bisphosphonates have complex instructions for administration, which can preclude their use in unsupervised patients with cognitive impairment. Calcium and vitamin D supplements may be poorly tolerated in some individuals because of bowel symptoms.

A schematic representation of the management of osteoporosis is provided in Figure 70-1. All individuals should be given lifestyle advice on diet, exercise, tobacco and alcohol consumption, and exposure to sunlight. In younger post-menopausal women with osteoporosis, the treatment of choice may be HRT or raloxifene, because of the skeletal and nonskeletal benefits. In women who are unable or unwilling to take HRT, or in older patients, bisphosphonates are probably most appropriate. In the frail elderly, calcium and vitamin D supplementation would appear to be the treatment of choice. In patients with a past history of recurrent falls, measures should be taken to reduce the incidence of falls. Consideration should also be given to the use of external hip protectors.

OSTEOMALACIA

Osteomalacia is a generalized bone disorder characterized by an impairment of mineralization leading to accumulation of unmineralized matrix or osteoid in the skeleton.[75,76] There are a number of causes of osteomalacia but the majority of cases are due to vitamin D deficiency, abnormal vitamin D metabolism, or hypophosphatemia (Table 70-3).

Adequate amounts of calcium and phosphate are essential for mineralization of osteoid to proceed normally, and whilst vitamin D is important in the homeostasis of calcium and phosphate, the precise role of the vitamin D metabolites in mineralization remains uncertain. The major source of vitamin D is from cutaneous production, following the exposure of the precursor 7-dehydrocholesterol to ultraviolet irradiation.[77,78] The diet provides much smaller amounts of vitamin D, but this becomes essential when cutaneous production is limited. Vitamin D itself has little biological activity, and is metabolized in the liver to 25OHD, the major circulating form of vitamin D. This undergoes further hydroxylation in the kidneys to form $1,25(OH)_2D$, the hormonally active metabolite of vitamin D, which regulates calcium absorption from the bowel, influences bone remodeling, and affects muscle function.[79,80]

Vitamin D deficiency osteomalacia predominantly occurs because of reduced cutaneous production of vitamin D due to lack of exposure to sunlight or increased skin pigmentation. It is therefore particularly seen in the housebound elderly or Asian immigrants, particularly when the dietary intake of vitamin D is poor.[75,76] Vitamin D deficiency osteomalacia is also seen with malabsorption or after gastric surgery, and is related to reduced sunlight exposure, decreased absorption of vitamin D, and malabsorption of calcium or phosphate.[75,76] Anticonvulsant therapy and hepatic disease are also associated with low plasma 25OHD levels and the development of vitamin D-deficiency osteomalacia.[75,76]

Anticonvulsants induce liver enzymes which metabolize vitamin D to biologically inactive polar metabolites, whereas liver disease may be associated with impaired 25 hydroxylation of vitamin D. In addition, patients with epilepsy or liver disease may be less exposed to sunlight and therefore have reduced cutaneous production of vitamin D.

Renal impairment leads to the development of osteomalacia because of reduced production of $1,25(OH)_2D$, malabsorption of calcium, and low plasma calcium, though plasma 25OHD concentration may also be low because of reduced sunlight exposure. Hypophosphatemic osteomalacia may result from decreased renal tubular reabsorption of phosphate as in familial, tumor-associated, and sporadic cases, or from phosphate depletion associated with the use of phosphate binders.[75,76]

Osteomalacia in the elderly population

Vitamin D deficiency is the commonest cause of osteomalacia in the elderly population. Renal failure is a smaller but significant cause in this age group. There is a reduction in plasma 25OHD with advancing age,[81] which is mainly due to reduced sunlight exposure, though decreased capacity for cutaneous production, low dietary intake, poor absorption, and impaired hepatic hydroxylation of vitamin D may also contribute to this.[77,78,82,83] Plasma 25OHD concentrations are lower in individuals living in residential care than in people living in the community, and lowest in residents of long-term geriatric wards.[84,85] The reduction in renal function with age is associated with decreased plasma $1,25(OH)_2D$ concentrations which may contribute to the development of osteomalacia in the elderly group.[86]

Osteomalacia is essentially a histological diagnosis, so there is little information on its overall prevalence in the elderly population. Nevertheless, as mentioned above, low 25OHD concentrations are common in the elderly, particularly in subjects who are housebound or institutionalized. As about 10 percent of elderly people are housebound, a significant proportion are at risk of developing osteomalacia because of absent cutaneous production of vitamin D, and several investigators have shown that osteomalacia occurs in about 4 percent of elderly people admitted to hospital.[87,88] A histological study from Leeds, UK, suggested that up to 40 percent of patients with hip fracture had evidence of osteomalacia, though the criteria used for this diagnosis were either excess osteoid or decreased calcification fronts.[89] Using the stricter diagnostic criteria of the combination of

Table 70-3	**Classification of the major causes of osteomalacia**	
Deficiency	**Cause**	**Clinical form**
Vitamin D	↓ Sunlight exposure ↓ Dietary vitamin D Malabsorption	Housebound elderly Asian immigrants Small bowel disease
25OHD	Abnormal vitamin D metabolism	Anticonvulsants Liver disease
1,25 (OH$_2$)D	↓ 1α-hydroxylase activity	Renal failure
Phosphate	↓ Tubular reabsorption	Familial Tumoral Sporadic
	Phosphate depletion	Use of phosphate binders

increased osteoid seam width and reduction in calcification fronts, a subsequent study from Cardiff, Wales, showed osteomalacia in only 2 percent of patients with hip fracture.[90]

Clinical features of osteomalacia

The presentation of osteomalacia may be variable, and the diagnosis may be easily missed in the early stages of the disease, because of the vague nature of the symptoms. The patient may complain of aches and pains, aggravated by muscular contraction, but tending to persist after rest. Although there is a propensity for fracture in osteomalacia, the soft elastic bone also deforms easily, leading to kyphosis, scoliosis, and deformity of the rib cage, pelvis, and long bones. The patient may also develop a proximal myopathy, causing a waddling gait and difficulties rising from a chair or climbing stairs. Occasionally, the hypocalcemia associated with osteomalacia leads to latent tetany, with paresthesiae of the hands and around the mouth, cramps, a main d'accoucheur appearance of the hands, and positive Chvostek's and Trousseau's signs.

Investigations in osteomalacia

RADIOLOGY   The classical radiological appearances of osteomalacia are relatively rare and may not be found in the early stages of the disease. Osteomalacic bone is softer than normal and so becomes easily deformed. The intervertebral discs balloon out and deform the adjacent vertebrae to give them a uniformly biconcave codfish appearance. Similar deformity may occur in osteoporosis, but the biconcavity is more regular in osteomalacia than with osteoporosis, where the extent of vertebral deformity is variable. There may be radiological evidence of deformity of the rib cage, pelvis, and long bones (Figs 70-2 and 70-3). A characteristic finding in osteomalacia is the Looser's zone or pseudofracture, which consist of a large area of osteoid. These appear as bands of decalcification surrounded by more dense bone, which occur perpendicular to the bone surface, often where nutrient arteries enter bone (Fig. 70-4). Looser's zones are seen particularly in the proximal femur, humeral neck, pubic rami, ribs, metatarsals, and the outer border of the scapula. There may also be radiological evidence of secondary hyperparathyroidism, with subperiosteal erosions in the metacarpals or phalanges.

BIOCHEMICAL FINDINGS   The biochemical findings in the major types of osteomalacia are shown in Table 70-4. In vitamin D-deficiency osteomalacia, the plasma calcium tends to be low because of reduced calcium absorption resulting from low plasma 25OHD and 1,25(OH)$_2$D concentrations. The hypocalcemia leads to secondary hyperparathyroidism, which in turn stimulates the renal tubular reabsorption of calcium and reduces tubular reabsorption of phosphate. Plasma phosphate is therefore often low in osteomalacia because of reduced absorption from the bowel and decreased renal tubular reabsorption. The secondary hyperparathyroidism also increases bone remodeling, which is reflected in elevation of the plasma alkaline phosphatase and urine hydroxyproline excretion. Not all patients with vitamin D-deficiency osteomalacia will have hypocalcemia, hypophosphatemia, and raised alkaline phosphatase; these abnormalities may occur individually in an elderly person with intercurrent illness—so they lack specificity in the diagnosis of osteomalacia in the elderly population.[91]

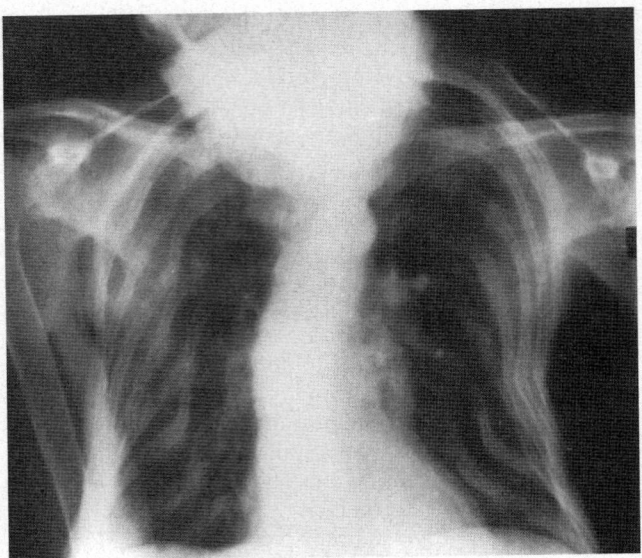

Figure 70-2   Chest X-ray of a woman with osteomalacia, showing deformity of the rib cage due to bone softening.

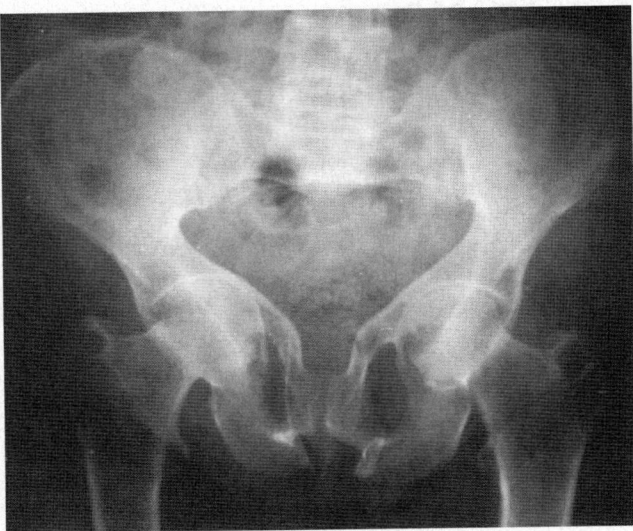

Figure 70-3   X-ray of the pelvis of a woman with osteomalacia, showing deformity of the pelvic bones due to bone softening.

In osteomalacia associated with renal failure, hypocalcemia is seen in the majority of cases, though the plasma phosphate is normal or high because of reduced urinary excretion of phosphate. The plasma 1,25(OH)$_2$D is low because of impaired production by the kidneys, though the plasma 25OHD may also be reduced because of inadequate exposure to sunlight. Plasma alkaline phosphatase is raised in the vast majority of cases, and the serum PTH is invariably elevated.[75]

In hypophosphatemic osteomalacia, the major biochemical abnormality is a low plasma phosphate, though this may vary in severity. A few cases may also show hypocalcemia, low plasma 1,25(OH)$_2$D, and elevation of serum PTH (Table 70-4).

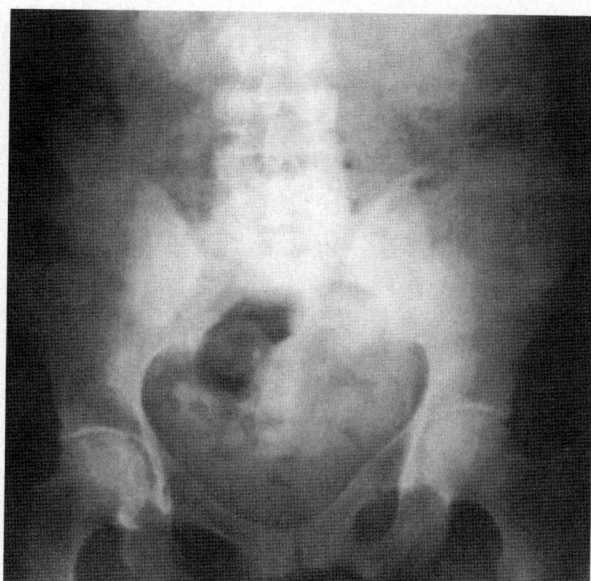

Figure 70-4 X-ray of the pelvis of a woman with osteomalacia, showing Looser's zones in the pubic rami.

Table 70-4 Biochemical abnormalities in major types of osteomalacia. Data are derived from Peacock[76]

	Vitamin D deficiency (%)	Renal failure (%)	Hypophosphatemic (%)
Hypocalcemia	59	63	9
Hypophosphatemia	68	0	73
↑ Alkaline phosphatase	88	88	27
↓ 25OHD	80	58	0
↓ 1,25(OH)$_2$D	75	81	36
↑ PTH	90	100	11

Diagnosis of osteomalacia in the elderly population

The only definite way of diagnosing osteomalacia is by histological examination of undecalcified bone and demonstrating excess osteoid and reduced calcification fronts or mineralization rate. Histological confirmation of the diagnosis is required in the minority of cases, however. In patients with a typical history of bone pain and muscle weakness, with radiological evidence of Looser's zones or typical biochemical changes, there is little indication for bone biopsy. When the diagnosis is less clear-cut, measurement of plasma 25OHD and serum PTH may be useful, as the combination of low plasma 25OHD and elevated PTH is a strong indicator of the presence of osteomalacia. An alternative approach is to use a therapeutic trial of vitamin D in subjects likely to have osteomalacia, and to monitor any subsequent clinical and biochemical improvement.

Treatment of osteomalacia

In cases of vitamin D-deficiency osteomalacia, the condition will heal with ultraviolet irradiation or vitamin D treatment.

Treatment with vitamin D is more practical and can either be given orally in a regular daily dose of 25 µg (1,000 units) or as a single intramuscular injection of 7.5 mg (300,000 units) vitamin D, which should be repeated every 6–12 months to prevent recurrence. Although a single intramuscular injection may be convenient, there is considerable variation in bioavailability with this method of administration. Furthermore, oral vitamin D is often given in combination with a calcium supplement, to increase the dietary calcium intake by about 1,000 mg/day.

In patients with osteomalacia associated with malabsorption, the metabolites of vitamin D should be given, in a dose of 1–4 µg daily of either alfacalcidol or calcitriol. Calcium supplements may also be required, but the serum calcium should be monitored to avoid the development of hypercalcemia. Magnesium supplements may also be necessary if hypomagnesemia is present. If malabsorption is due to bacterial overgrowth, pancreatic insufficiency, or celiac disease, appropriate treatment of the underlying disorder with antibiotic therapy, pancreatic enzyme supplements, or gluten-free diet should be instituted.

In patients with osteomalacia and renal impairment, either alfacalcidol or calcitriol should be used in a dose of 1 µg daily, together with calcium supplements as required. Serum calcium and renal function should be monitored regularly on this treatment.

Treatment of osteomalacia leads to a resolution of the proximal myopathy and any symptoms of hypocalcemia within a few weeks, though the bone pain may take longer to improve. The biochemical abnormalities also persist for up to 6 months after treatment is started, and the bone remains histologically and structurally abnormal during this time. Care should therefore be taken to avoid falls during rehabilitation, as these may easily lead to fractures of the abnormal bone. The plasma calcium and phosphate returns to normal within a few weeks, whilst the plasma alkaline phosphatase rises further on treatment and may take many months to return to normal. Serum PTH also remains elevated for up to 6 months. Ultimately, radiological abnormalities such as Looser's zones and changes of secondary hyperparathyroidism will resolve on treatment, though deformity will persist despite the remodeling of bone.

PAGET'S DISEASE

Prevalence of Paget's disease

Paget's disease of bone (osteitis deformans) is a common but poorly understood condition which causes significant morbidity in elderly patients.[92] Studies of its prevalence are limited by the fact that many cases are asymptomatic, but radiographic surveys in hospital patients over age 55 suggest an overall prevalence of up to 4 percent in England and the USA, compared with less than 0.1 percent in Asia and Africa.[93] By the age of 85, up to 20 percent of men and 10 percent of women in the UK have evidence of the condition.[94]

Etiology and pathophysiology

The etiology of Paget's disease remains unclear. There is a significant genetic component to the condition, as there is some evidence of HLA linkage and about 25 percent of patients have a family history of the condition. The clustering of cases of

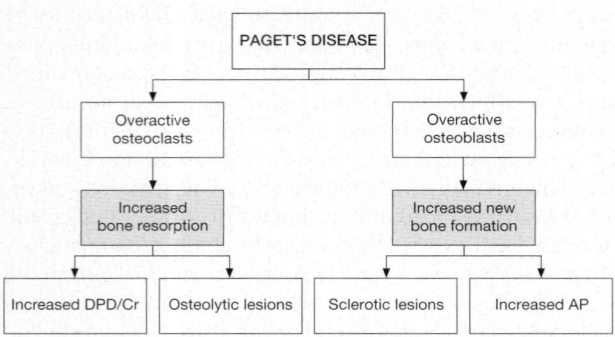

Figure 70-5 Pathophysiology of Paget's disease of bone.

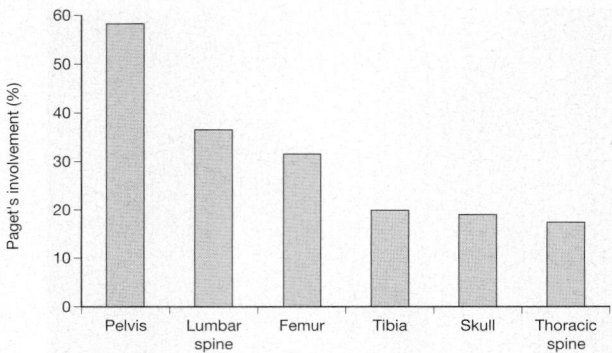

Figure 70-6 Skeletal involvement in 889 patients with Paget's disease. Data are derived from Davie et al.[99]

Paget's disease within families includes spouses, so may reflect not only genetic factors but also shared environment. It has been suggested that Paget's disease may result from a slow virus infection, which either causes the disease or triggers it in a susceptible individual.[95,96] Inclusion bodies resembling paramyxoviruses have been seen in affected osteoclasts, but their role in the pathogenesis of Paget's disease remains uncertain.

Paget's disease is characterized by increased bone resorption mediated by enlarged, hyperactive osteoclasts.[97] This leads secondarily to increased osteoblastic activity and new bone formation (Fig. 70-5). The rapid bone turnover leads to the deposition of woven bone, which is structurally weak, more vascular, and prone to fracture.

Clinical features of Paget's disease

Paget's disease may present at any age over 30, but is most often diagnosed in the sixth decade of life. The condition is more common in men than women. The majority of people with radiological evidence of Paget's disease are asymptomatic and do not come to medical attention. The condition is therefore often an incidental finding in patients having X-rays for an unrelated reason.

It is characteristic of the condition that only a few bones are affected in any one individual. The bones most commonly involved are the pelvis, spine, femur, tibia, and skull (Fig. 70-6), although the distribution of the disease is usually asymmetrical.[97,98] The extent of skeletal involvement is generally constant, with previously unaffected bones rarely becoming involved long after diagnosis. The commonest presentation is with pain, which may be due to the Pagetic changes in the bone itself or to the effects of skeletal deformity on surrounding structures. The cause of bone pain in Paget's disease may be difficult to determine. It may be due to periosteal stretching, microfractures, or to direct nerve stimulation by substances released by osteoclasts during bone resorption.

Paget's disease may also cause skeletal deformity, as the affected bones thicken, enlarge, and become more elastic. Classically this causes frontal bossing of the skull, bowing of the long bones, and deformity of the pelvis (protrusio acetabuli). Pagetic bone is more likely to fracture and fissure fractures may also occur on the outer aspect of bowed long bones.

Thickening of the skull may cause compression of the cranial nerves, particularly the auditory nerves, resulting in deafness. Other cranial nerves are only rarely involved in Paget's disease. The increased vascularity of Pagetic bone may also result in neurological deficit because of a "vascular steal" syndrome. Softening of the base of the skull may rarely lead to basilar invagination, causing brain stem compression. Vertebral involvement may result in crush fractures or more rarely spinal cord compression.

A major management problem is the development of secondary degenerative arthritis in joints adjacent to involved bone. This is frequently more disabling than the Paget's disease itself, and will not respond to treatment of the underlying bone disease. Other complications of Paget's disease include high output cardiac failure, due to the increased vascularity of the affected bone, which although often described is rarely seen. Sarcomatous change also occurs only rarely, but has a poor prognosis.[98,99]

Diagnosis and investigation of Paget's disease

The diagnosis of Paget's disease is reached through a combination of clinical assessment and selected investigations. Although the history rarely leads directly to a diagnosis of Paget's disease, it is very important to seek clues to other conditions which may coexist with or masquerade as it. Examination may reveal skeletal deformity, especially of the skull or long bones, which may feel warm to the touch. There may also be signs of associated degenerative arthritis. A full neurological assessment is advisable in symptomatic patients, though abnormalities other than deafness are not often found.

The diagnosis of Paget's disease is usually confirmed radiologically. X-rays may show an increase in size of affected bones, alteration of bone texture with areas of sclerosis and lucency (Fig. 70-5), skeletal deformity, and evidence of degenerative arthritis in adjacent joints. The radiological appearances are often said to be pathognomonic, but skeletal metastases from occult carcinoma of the prostate or breast should be considered in the differential diagnosis. Prostate-specific antigen should therefore be measured in all men with probable Paget's disease. Rarely, bone biopsy may be required if the diagnosis remains uncertain.

The extent of the bone disease can be assessed by isotope bone scan, although X-rays of areas with increase uptake may be advisable, if there is any doubt about the diagnosis. Serum alkaline phosphatase (AP) and urine deoxypyridinoline/creatinine (DPD/Cr) are often markedly raised in Paget's disease, reflecting increased osteoblast and osteoclast activity respectively (Fig. 70-5), so may be used to assess the activity of the condition and its response to treatment.

Treatment of Paget's disease

Treatment of Paget's disease is directed at suppressing the over-activity of osteoclasts, thereby decreasing bone turnover. Although calcitonin has been used for several decades in management of the disease, bisphosphonates have now become the treatment of choice.[92] These agents are generally used in patients with symptomatic Paget's disease, but their role in asymptomatic individuals is unclear.

CALCITONIN Calcitonin has a direct, receptor-mediated action on osteoclast function. In-vivo studies show that within 30 minutes of calcitonin administration, osteoclasts cease synthetic activity and begin to detach from bone. Recruitment of osteoclasts and fusion of precursor cells is also halted, resulting in a rapid reduction in bone resorption. Calcitonin has a short half-life, so osteoclast activation recommences as soon as local concentrations return to basal levels. Nevertheless, calcitonin has proved to be useful in the management of Paget's disease, where it decreases bone pain and reduces the biochemical markers of bone turnover.[100] Salmon and porcine preparations of calcitonin are weakly antigenic, and neutralizing antibodies are formed during treatment by some patients, which may limit the treatment's long-term efficacy. Calcitonin may be given by subcutaneous injection or by intranasal administration, although the latter is not available throughout the world.

BISPHOSPHONATES Oral antiresorptive therapy for Paget's disease became practical for the first time with the introduction of etidronate in the late 1970s. Disodium etidronate 400 mg daily decreases the biochemical markers of bone turnover by 40–60 percent.[92] Unfortunately, prolonged therapy with etidronate leads to impaired mineralization, so courses of treatment should not exceed 6 months. There is also evidence that previous treatment with etidronate decreases the efficacy of subsequent courses of treatment.[101,102]

Intravenous infusions of pamidronate decrease the biochemical markers of bone turnover by 60–70 percent, resulting in prolonged remission in many patients.[92,103] Pamidronate may be given by weekly infusion of 30 mg for 6 weeks, or by three fortnightly infusions of 60 mg. The intravenous route of administration avoids the potential problems of oral bisphosphonates, such as poor absorption from the bowel, the need to take medication in a fasting condition, and gastrointestinal side-effects. These advantages are offset by the need for intravenous infusion and influenza-like symptoms which may follow treatment.

Oral tiludronate 400 mg daily for 3 months decreases the biochemical markers of bone turnover by at least a half in 70 percent of patients.[104] This may avoid the need for further treatment for at least 18 months. A comparative study in 234 patients with Paget's disease showed that significantly more responded to 3 or 6 months' treatment with tiludronate 400 mg daily (60.3 and 70.1 percent, respectively), than to 6 months' etidronate 400 mg daily (25.3 percent).[102] This study also showed an attenuated response to etidronate, in patients who had previously received this bisphosphonate.

A North American study randomized 123 men and women with documented Paget's disease with risedronate 30 mg daily for 2 months or etidronate 400 mg daily for 6 months.[101] At 12 months, alkaline phosphatase decreased into the normal range in 73 percent of patients who had taken risedronate, compared to 18 percent with etidronate. Previous treatment with etidronate had no significant effect on the subsequent response to risedronate, but resulted in a blunted response to further etidronate. There was a significant reduction in pain with risedronate, whereas etidronate was associated with insignificant improvement.

Although bisphosphonates decrease bone pain and reduce the activity of Paget's disease, there is currently no evidence that any treatment will prevent skeletal deformity, fractures, or other complications of the condition. The choice of bisphosphonate for the management of Paget's disease also depends on the potential advantages and disadvantages in the individual patient. Despite its low cost, etidronate should no longer be used, because it is much less effective than other bisphosphonates. The main choice lies between intravenous pamidronate and oral risedronate, as tiludronate is more expensive but has no greater efficacy.

FRACTURES IN THE ELDERLY POPULATION

The mechanical properties of an individual bone are determined by the amount of bone present, skeletal architecture, and bone quality. Aging is associated with a reduction in bone mass, disruption of trabecular architecture, and an increased prevalence of disorders such as osteomalacia and Paget's disease which adversely affect the quality of bone. Nevertheless, the risk of fracture is determined not only by skeletal factors, but also by nonskeletal risk factors including postural instability, physical and mental frailty, and conditions associated with falling.[7–9] It is therefore not surprising that the incidence of fractures increases with advancing age. Whilst fractures in young adults usually occur after extensive trauma, fractures in the elderly population may result from minimal trauma, such as falling from standing height. The major fractures occurring in elderly people are those of the forearm, vertebral body, humerus, pelvis, and hip.[105,106] The incidence of these fractures increases with advancing age and is higher in women than men, because of their lower peak bone mass, more rapid bone loss, and greater risk of falls.

There is considerable geographical variation in fracture incidence around the world,[105] which may reflect differences in bone mass due to race, smoking, alcohol consumption, and physical activity. The absolute number of fractures in the elderly population is rising rapidly, due in part to the increasing numbers of elderly people and a rising age-specific incidence of fractures.[106–109] If present demographic trends continue in the UK, the number of young elderly will remain reasonably constant over the next few decades, whilst the number of people over the age of 85 will increase considerably.[110] Many of these elderly people will be frail, and therefore particularly at risk of fractures. There is also evidence of a rising age-specific incidence of fractures of the forearm, vertebral body, humerus, and hip, which has been attributed to the increased survival of frail individuals and secular changes in smoking, alcohol consumption, diet, and physical activity.[107,108]

Forearm fractures

These are the commonest fractures before the age of 75.[105] The incidence rises steeply at the menopause in women and then plateaus above the age of 65, whilst the incidence changes little with age in men.[111] It has been suggested that the rise in incidence at the menopause is due to an increase in postural instability and therefore falls in women at this age.[111,112] The absence of a further increase in incidence of forearm fractures after the age of 65 may be due to the fact that the arm is less likely to be used to break a fall. About 50 percent of postmenopausal women with Colles' fracture have evidence of osteoporosis at the forearm, spine, or hip.[113] Forearm fractures are also associated with an increased risk of vertebral and hip fractures in both men and women.[114–116]

Vertebral fractures

The incidence and prevalence of vertebral fractures is difficult to quantify, as many patients with this fracture do not seek medical attention.[117] The European Vertebral Osteoporosis Study (EVOS) shows that the overall prevalence of vertebral deformity increases in women from 5 percent at the age of 50 years to 25 percent at 75 years, whereas the corresponding figures for men are 10 and 18 percent.[118] The higher prevalence of vertebral deformity in young men compared with women may be due to greater exposure to trauma.[119] There is also a large variation in the prevalence of vertebral fractures across Europe, which may reflect differences in physical activity and other lifestyle factors.[118]

In addition to back pain, loss of height, and kyphosis, vertebral fractures may also result in loss of energy, emotional problems, sleep disturbance, social isolation, and reduced mobility.[120] There is also an increased mortality associated with vertebral crush fractures of about 18 percent at 5 years, but this may be due to coexisting conditions associated with osteoporosis, rather than the fracture itself.[117]

It has been estimated that the acute cost of vertebral fractures in the UK is £12 million per year,[2] but the real cost may be substantially higher than this, because of the associated long-term morbidity. Patients with symptomatic vertebral fracture consult their GPs 14 times more than control subjects in the year following fracture,[2] so are likely to continue to use health and social service resources at an increased rate.

Hip fractures

This is the most important fracture in the elderly population since it causes greater mortality, higher morbidity, and more expenditure than all other fractures combined.[105] The incidence of this fracture rises steeply with age in both sexes, though it is considerably higher in women than men.[107] Using current age-specific incidence rates for England and Wales, it has been estimated that 12 percent of women and 5 percent of men will have sustained a hip fracture by the age of 85.[109]

The risk of hip fractures is determined not only by bone mineral density, but also by nonskeletal risk factors. Studies show an increased risk of hip fracture with causes of secondary osteoporosis, such as oral corticosteroid therapy, thyroid disease and hypogonadism, and with conditions associated with falling, such as previous stroke, Parkinson's disease, and dementia.[9,121–125] Hip fractures are associated with a considerable mortality, particularly in older, more dependent individuals.[117] This excess mortality following femoral neck fractures has been reported to be about 17 percent over 5 years, though most deaths occur within 6 months of fracture.[117] In addition to the excess mortality, femoral fractures are associated with considerable morbidity, with many patients becoming more immobile and more dependent. Between 25 and 50 percent of individuals are more dependent after fracture, with deterioration occurring more often in women over the age of 75, those with a poor clinical result, and those who were already dependent before fracture.[126–128] It is estimated that the average cost of hip fracture in the UK is £12,000, of which £4,800 is due to acute costs.[2]

KEY POINTS Metabolic bone disease

- Fractures are a major cause of excess mortality, morbidity, and health and social service expenditure in elderly people.

- The risk of fracture is determined by both skeletal and nonskeletal risk factors.

- The incidences of osteoporosis, osteomalacia, and Paget's disease increase with advancing age.

- Osteoporosis, osteomalacia, and Paget's disease can be diagnosed and treated in elderly people.

REFERENCES

1. World Health Organization Study Group: Assessment of Fracture Risk and its Application to Screening for Postmenopausal Osteoporosis. WHO, Geneva, 1994
2. Dolan P, Torgerson DJ: The cost of treating osteoporotic fractures in the United Kingdom female population. Osteopor Int 1998;8:611–617
3. Marshall D, Johnell O, Wedel H: Meta-analysis of how well measures of bone mineral density predict occurrence of osteoporotic fractures. BMJ 1996;312:1254–1259
4. Garnero P, Hausherr E, Chapuy MC et al: Markers of bone resorption predict hip fracture in elderly women: the EPIDOS prospective study. J Bone Miner Res 1996;11:1531–1538
5. Faulkner KG, Cummings SR, Black D et al: Simple measurement of femoral geometry predicts hip fracture: the study of osteoporotic fractures. J Bone Miner Res 1993;8:1211–1217
6. Ross PD, Davis JW, Epstein RS et al: Pre-existing fractures and bone mass predict vertebral fracture incidence in women. Ann Intern Med 1991;114:919–923
7. Nguyen T, Sambrook P, Kelly P et al: Prediction of osteoporotic fractures by postural instability and bone density. BMJ 1993;307:1111–1115
8. Dargent-Molina P, Favier F, Grandjean H et al: Fall-related factors and risk of hip fracture: the EPIDOS prospective study. Lancet 1996;348:145–149
9. Cummings SR, Nevitt MC, Browner WS et al, for the Study of Osteoporotic Fractures research group: Risk factors for hip fracture in white women. N Engl J Med 1995;332:767–773
10. Melton LJ, Chrischilles EA, Cooper C et al: How many women have osteoporosis? J Bone Miner Res 1992;7:1005–1010
11. Slemenda CW, Christian JC, Williams CJ et al: Genetic determinants of bone mass in adult women: a reevaluation of the twin model and the potential importance of gene interaction on heritability estimates. J Bone Miner Res 1991;6:561–567

12. Compston JE: Risk factors for osteoporosis. Clin Endocrinol 1992;36:223–224
13. Scane AC, Francis RM: Risk factors for osteoporosis in men. Clin Endocrinol 1993;38:15–16
14. Christiansen C, Riis BJ, Rodbro P: Predictions of rapid bone loss in postmenopausal women. Lancet 1987;i:1105–1108
15. Cooper C, Barker DJP, Wickham C: Physical activity, muscle strength, and calcium intake in fracture of the proximal femur in Britain. BMJ 1988;297:1443–1446
16. Boyce WJ, Vessey MP: Habitual physical inertia and other factors in relation to risk of fracture of the proximal femur. Age Ageing 1988;17:319–327
17. Endres DB, Morgan CH, Garry PJ et al: Age-related changes in serum immunoreactive parathyroid hormone and its biological action in healthy men and women. J Clin Endocrinol Metab 1987;65:724–731
18. Khaw KT, Sneyd MJ, Compston J: Bone density parathyroid hormone and 25-hydroxyvitamin D concentrations in middle aged women. BMJ 1992;305:273–277
19. Baker MR, McDonnell H, Peacock M et al: Plasma 25-hydroxy vitamin D concentrations in patients with fractures of the femoral neck. BMJ 1979;i:589
20. Sahota O, Masud T, San P et al: Vitamin D insufficiency increases bone turnover markers and enhances bone loss at the hip in patients with established vertebral osteoporosis. Clin Endocrinol (Oxf) 1999;51:217–221
21. Caplan GA, Scane AC, Francis RM: Pathogenesis of vertebral crush fractures in women. J Royal Soc Med 1994;87:200–202
22. Baillie SP, Davison CE, Johnson FJ et al: Pathogenesis of vertebral crush fractures in men. Age Ageing 1992;21:139–141
23. UK Royal College of Physicians and Bone and Tooth Society of Great Britain: Osteoporosis clinical guidelines for prevention and treatment. Update on pharmacological interventions and an algorithm for management. Royal College of Physicians, London, 2000
24. Francis RM: Management of established osteoporosis. In Hosking DJ, Ringe JD (eds): Treatment of Metabolic Bone Disease. Martin Dunitz, London, 2000:143–162
25. Eastell R, Reid DM, Compston J et al: A UK Consensus Group on the management of glucocorticoid-induced osteoporosis: an update. J Int Med 1998;244:271–292
26. Torgerson DJ, Bell-Syer SE: Hormone replacement therapy and prevention of nonvertebral fractures: a meta-analysis of randomized trials. JAMA 2001;285:2891–2897
27. Hoidrup S, Gronbaek M, Pedersen AT et al: Hormone replacement therapy and hip fracture risk: effect modification by tobacco smoking, alcohol intake, physical activity, and body mass index. Am J Epidemiol 1999;150:1085–1093
28. Komulainen MH, Kroger H, Tuppurainen MT et al: HRT and Vit D in prevention of non-vertebral fractures in postmenopausal women: a 5 year randomized trial. Maturitas 1998;31:45–54
29. Felson DT, Zhang Y, Hannan MT et al: The effect of postmenopausal estrogen therapy on bone density in elderly women. N Engl J Med 1993;329:1141–1146
30. Lindsay R, Tohme J: Estrogen treatment of patients with established postmenopausal osteoporosis. Obstet Gynecol 1990;76:1–6
31. Lufkin EG, Wahner HW, O'Fallon WM et al: Treatment of postmenopausal osteoporosis with transdermal estrogen. Ann Intern Med 1992;117:1–9
32. Bjarnason NH, Bjarnason K, Haarbo J et al: Tibolone: prevention of bone loss in late postmenopausal women. J Clin Endocrinol Metab 1996;81:2419–2422
33. Pavlov PW, Ginsburg J, Kicovic PM et al: Double-blind, placebo-controlled study of the effects of tibolone on bone mineral density in postmenopausal women with and without previous fractures. Gynecol Endocrinol 1999;13:230–237
34. Delmas PD, Bjarnason NH, Mitlak BH et al: Effects of raloxifene on bone mineral density, serum cholesterol concentrations, and uterine endometrium in postmenopausal women. N Engl J Med 1997;337:1641–1647
35. Ettinger B, Black DM, Mitlak BH et al, for the Multiple Outcomes of Raloxifene Evaluation (MORE) investigators: Reduction of vertebral fracture risk in postmenopausal women with osteoporosis treated with raloxifene: results from a 3-year randomized clinical trial. JAMA 1999;282:637–645
36. Cummings SR, Eckert S, Krueger KA et al: The effect of raloxifene on risk of breast cancer in postmenopausal women: results from the MORE randomized trial. JAMA 1999;281:2189–2197
37. Storm T, Thamsborg G, Steinich T et al: Effect of intermittent cyclical etidronate therapy on bone mass and fracture rate in women with postmenopausal osteoporosis. N Engl J Med 1990; 322:1265–1271
38. Watts NB, Harris ST, Genant HK et al: Intermittent cyclical etidronate treatment of postmenopausal osteoporosis. N Engl J Med 1990;323:73–79
39. Harris ST, Watts NB, Jackson RD et al: Four-year study of intermittent cyclic etidronate treatment of postmenopausal osteoporosis: three years of blinded therapy followed by one year of open therapy. Am J Med 1993;95:557–567
40. Liberman UA, Weiss SR, Broll J et al: Effect of oral alendronate on bone mineral density and the incidence of fractures in postmenopausal osteoporosis. N Engl J Med 1995;333:1437–1443
41. Black DM, Cummings SR, Karpf DB et al: Randomised trial of effect of alendronate on risk of fracture in women with existing vertebral fractures. Lancet 1996;348:1535–1541
42. Cummings SR, Black DM, Thompson DE et al: Effect of alendronate on risk of fracture in women with low bone density but without vertebral fractures: results from the Fracture Intervention trial. JAMA 1998;280:2077–2082
43. Bone HG, Downs RW, Tucci JR et al: Dose-response relationships for alendronate treatment in osteoporotic elderly women. J Clin Endocrinol Metab 1997;82:265–274
44. Schnitzer T, Bone HG, Crepaldi G et al: Therapeutic equivalence of alendronate 70 mg once-weekly and alendronate 10 mg daily in the treatment of osteoporosis. Aging Clin Exp Res 2000;12:1–12
45. Harris ST, Watts NB, Genant HK et al, for the Vertebral Efficacy with Risedronate Therapy (VERT) study group: Effects of risedronate treatment on vertebral and nonvertebral fractures in women with postmenopausal osteoporosis: a randomized controlled trial. JAMA 1999;282:1344–1352
46. Reginster J, Minne HW, Sorensen OH et al, for the Vertebral Efficacy with Risedronate Therapy (VERT) study group: Randomized trial of the effects of risedronate on vertebral fractures in women with established postmenopausal osteoporosis. Osteoporosis Int 2000;11:83–91
47. McClung MR, Geusens P, Miller PD et al, for the Hip Intervention Program study group: Effect of risedronate on the risk of hip fracture in elderly women. N Engl J Med 2001;344:333–340
48. Overgaard K, Hansen MA, Jensen SB et al: Effect of salcatonin given intranasally on bone mass and fracture rates in established osteoporosis: a dose–response study. BMJ 1992;305:556–561
49. Rico H, Henandez ER, Revilla M et al: Salmon calcitonin reduces vertebral fracture rate in postmenopausal crush fracture syndrome. Bone Miner 1992;16:131–138
50. Chesnut CH, Silverman S, Andriano K et al, for the Prevent Recurrence Of Osteoporotic Fractures (PROOF) study: A randomized trial of nasal spray salmon calcitonin in postmenopausal women with established osteoporosis. Am J Med 2000;109:267–276
51. Prince RL, Smith M, Dick IM et al: Prevention of postmenopausal osteoporosis. A comparative study of exercise, calcium supplementation and hormone-replacement therapy. N Engl J Med 1991;325:1189–1195
52. Reid IR, Ames RW, Evans MC et al: Effect of calcium supplementation on bone loss in postmenopausal women. N Engl J Med 1993;328:460–464
53. Chevalley T, Rizzoli R, Nydegger V et al: Effects of calcium supplements on femoral neck bone mineral density and vertebral fracture rate in vitamin D replete elderly patients. Osteoporosis Int 1994;4:245–252
54. Recker RR, Hinders S, Davies KM et al: Correcting calcium nutritional deficiency prevents spine fractures in elderly women. J Bone Miner Res 1996;11:1961–1966
55. Chapuy MC, Arlot ME, Duboeuf F et al: Vitamin D₃ and calcium to prevent hip fractures in elderly women. N Engl J Med 1992;327:1637–1642
56. Chapuy MC, Arlot ME, Delmas PD et al: Effect of calcium and cholecalciferol treatment for three years on hip fractures in elderly women. BMJ 1994;308:1081–1082
57. Dawson-Hughes B, Harris SS, Krall EA et al: Effect of calcium and vitamin D supplementation on bone density in men and women 65 years of age and older. N Engl J Med 1997;337:670–676
58. Heikinheimo RJ, Inkovaara JA, Harju EJ et al: Annual injection of vitamin D and fractures of aged bones. Calcif Tissue Int 1992;51:105–110
59. Lips P, Graafmans WC, Ooms ME et al: Vitamin D supplementation and fracture incidence in elderly persons: a randomized, placebo-controlled clinical trial. Ann Int Med 1996;124:400–406

60. Francis RM, Boyle IT, Moniz C et al: A comparison of the effects of alfacalcidol treatment and vitamin D$_2$ supplementation on calcium absorption in elderly women with vertebral fractures. Osteoporosis Int 1996;6:284–290

61. Tilyard MW, Spears GFS, Thompson J et al: Treatment of postmenopausal osteoporosis with calcitriol or calcium. N Engl J Med 1992;326:357–362

62. Riggs BL, Hodgson SF, O'Fallon WM et al: Effect of fluoride treatment on the fracture rate in postmenopausal women with osteoporosis. N Engl J Med 1990;322:802–809

63. Kleerekoper M, Peterson EL, Nelson DA et al: A randomized trial of sodium fluoride as a treatment for postmenopausal osteoporosis. Osteoporosis Int 1991;1:155–161

64. Pak CYC, Sakhaee K, Adams-Huet B et al: Treatment of postmenopausal osteoporosis with slow release sodium fluoride. Ann Int Med 1995;123:401–408

65. Chesnut CH, Ivey JL, Gruber HE et al: Stanozolol in postmenopausal osteoporosis: therapeutic efficacy and possible mechanisms of action. Metabolism 1983;32:571–580

66. Need AG, Chatterton BE, Walker CJ et al: Comparison of calcium, calcitriol, ovarian hormones and nandrolone in the treatment of osteoporosis. Maturitas 1986;8:275–280

67. Reeve J, Meunier PJ, Parsons JA et al: Anabolic effect of human parathyroid hormone fragment on trabecular bone in involutional osteoporosis: a multicentre trial. BMJ 1980;280:1340–1344

68. Hodsman AB, Fraher LJ, Watson PH et al: A randomized controlled trial to compare the efficacy of cyclical parathyroid hormone versus cyclical parathyroid hormone and sequential calcitonin to improve bone mass in postmenopausal women with osteoporosis. J Clin Endocrinol Metab 1997;82:620–628

69. Lindsay R, Nieves J, Formica C et al: Randomised controlled study of effect of parathyroid hormone on vertebral-bone mass and fracture incidence among postmenopausal women on oestrogen with osteoporosis. Lancet 1997;350:550–555

70. Tinetti ME, Baker DI, McAvay G et al: A multifactorial intervention to reduce the risk of falling among elderly people living in the community. N Engl J Med 1994;331:821–827

71. Close J, Ellis M, Hooper R et al: Prevention of falls in the elderly trial (PROFET): a randomised controlled trial. Lancet 1999;353:93–97

72. Lauritzen JB, Petersen MM, Lund B: Effect of external hip protectors on hip fractures. Lancet 1993;341:11–13

73. Parker MJ, Gillespie LD, Gillespie WJ: Hip protectors for preventing hip fractures in the elderly. Cochrane Library, issue 3, 2000

74. Villar MTA, Hill P, Inskip H et al: Will elderly rest home residents wear hip protectors? Age Ageing 1998;27:195–198

75. Francis RM, Selby PL: Osteomalacia. In Reid IR (ed): Baillière's Clinical Endocrinology and Metabolism: Metabolic Bone Disease. Baillière Tindall, London, 1997;11(1):145–163

76. Peacock M: Osteomalacia. In Nordin BEC (ed): Metabolic Bone and Stone Disease, 2nd edn. Churchill Livingstone, Edinburgh, 1984:72–111

77. Poskitt EME, Cole TJ, Lawson DEM: Diet, sunlight and 25 hydroxyvitamin D in healthy children and adults. BMJ 1979;i:221–223

78. Lawson DEM, Paul AA, Black AE et al: Relative contributions of diet and sunlight to vitamin D state in the elderly. BMJ 1979;ii:303–305

79. Fraser DR, Kodicek E: Unique biosynthesis by kidney of biologically active vitamin D metabolite. Nature 1970;228:764–766

80. Kodicek E, Lawson DEM, Wilson PW: Biological activity of polar metabolite of vitamin D$_3$. Nature 1970;228:763–764

81. Baker MR, Peacock M, Nordin BEC: The decline in vitamin D status with age. Age Ageing 1980;9:249–252

82. Barragry JM, France MW, Corless D et al: Intestinal cholecalciferol absorption in the elderly and in younger adults. Clin Sci 1989;55:213–220

83. Skinner RK: 25 hydroxylation of vitamin D in the elderly. In Norman AW, Schaefer K, Herrath DV et al (eds): Vitamin D: Basic Research and Its Clinical Application. Walter de Gruyter, Berlin, 1979:1011–1013

84. Dunnigan MG, McIntosh WB, Ford JA et al: Acquired disorders of vitamin D metabolism. In Heath DA, Marx SJ (eds): Clinical Endocrinology. 2: Calcium Disorders. Butterworths, London, 1982:125–150

85. Corless D, Beer M, Boucher BJ et al: Vitamin D status in long stay geriatric patients. Lancet 1975;ii:1404–1406

86. Francis RM, Peacock M, Barkworth SA: Renal impairment and its effects on calcium metabolism in elderly women. Age Ageing 1984;13:14–20

87. Anderson I, Campbell AER, Dunn A et al: Osteomalacia in elderly women. Scott Med J 1966;2:429–436

88. Campbell GA, Kemm JR, Hosking DJ et al: How common is osteomalacia in the elderly? Lancet 1984;ii:386–388

89. Aaron JE, Gallagher JC, Anderson J et al: Frequency of osteomalacia and osteoporosis in fractures of the proximal femur. Lancet 1974;i:229–232

90. Compston JE, Vedi S, Croucher PI: Low prevalence of osteomalacia in elderly patients with hip fracture. Age Ageing 1991;20:132–134

91. Campbell GA, Hosking DJ, Kemm JR et al: Timing of screening for osteomalacia in the acutely ill elderly. Age Ageing 1986;15:156–164

92. Hosking D, Meunier PJ, Ringe JD et al: Paget's disease of bone: diagnosis and management. BMJ 1996;312:491–494

93. Siris ES: Paget's disease of bone. In Favus MJ (ed): Primer on the Metabolic Bone Diseases and Disorders of Mineral Metabolism. American Society for Bone and Mineral Research, Kelseyville, CA, 1990:253–259

94. Barker DJP, Clough PW, Guyer PB et al: Paget's disease of bone in 14 British towns. BMJ 1977;i:1181–1183

95. O'Driscoll JB, Anderson DC: Past pets and Paget's disease. Lancet 1985;ii:919–921

96. Gordon MT, Anderson DC, Sharpe PT: Canine distemper virus localised in bone cells of patients with Paget's disease. Bone 1991;12:195–201

97. Kanis JA: Pathophysiology and treatment of Paget's disease of bone. Martin Dunitz, London, 1991

98. Frassica FJ, Tiegs RD, Unni KK et al: Paget's sarcoma of bone: clinicopathologic features and treatment in 51 cases. In First International Symposium on Paget's Disease of Bone. Paget's Disease Foundation, 1992:25

99. Davie M, Davies M, Francis R et al: Paget's disease of bone: a review of 889 patients. Bone 1999;24(Suppl):11S–12S

100. Cantrill JA, Anderson DC: Treatment of Paget's disease of bone. Clin Endocrinol 1990;32:507–518

101. Miller PD, Brown JP, Siris ES et al: A randomized, double-blind comparison of risedronate and etidronate in the treatment of Paget's disease of bone. Am J Med 1999;106:513–520

102. Roux C, Gennari C, Farrerons J et al: Comparative prospective, double-blind, multicenter study of the efficacy of tiludronate and etidronate in the treatment of Paget's disease of bone. Arthritis Rheum 1995;38:851–858

103. Anderson DC, Richardson PC, Kingsley Brown J et al: Intravenous pamidronate: evolution of an effective treatment strategy. Semin Arthritis Rheum 1994;23:273–275

104. Fraser WD, Stamp TC, Creek RA et al: A double-blind, multicentre, comparative study of tiludronate and placebo in Paget's disease of bone. Postgrad Med J 1997;73:496–502

105. Cummings SR, Kelsey JL, Nevitt MC et al: Epidemiology of osteoporosis and osteoporotic fractures. Epidemiol Rev 1985;7:178–208

106. Francis RM, Sutcliffe A: Implications of osteoporotic fractures in the elderly. In Drife JO, Studd JWW (eds): Hormone Replacement Therapy and Osteoporosis: Proceedings of the 22nd Study Group of the Royal College of Obstetricians and Gynaecologists. Springer-Verlag, Berlin, 1990:87–93

107. Boyce WJ, Vessey MP: Rising incidence of fracture of the proximal femur. Lancet 1985;i:150–151

108. Obrant KJ, Bengner U, Johnell O et al: Increasing age-adjusted risks of fragility fractures: a sign of increasing osteoporosis in successive generations? Calcif Tissue Int 1989;44:157–167

109. UK Royal College of Physicians: Fractured neck of femur. RCP, London, 1989

110. UK Office of Population Census and Surveys: 1991 Census Report for Great Britain. HMSO, London, 1993

111. Winner SJ, Morgan CA, Evans JG: Perimenopausal risk of falling and incidence of distal forearm fracture. BMJ 1989;298:1486–1488

112. Crilly RG, Richardson LD, Roth JH et al: Postural stability and Colles' fractures. Age Ageing 1987;16:133–138

113. Earnshaw SA, Cawte SA, Worley A et al: Colles' fracture of the wrist as an indicator of underlying osteoporosis in postmenopausal women: a prospective study of bone mineral density and bone turnover rate. Osteoporos Int 1998;8:53–60

114. Cuddihy MT, Gabriel SE, Crowson CS et al: Forearm fractures as predictors of subsequent osteoporotic fractures. Osteoporosis Int 1999;9:469–475

115. Mallmin H, Ljunghall S, Persson I et al: Fracture of the distal forearm as a forecaster of subsequent hip fracture: a population-based cohort study with 24 years of follow-up. Calcif Tissue Int 1993;52:269–272

116. Lauritzen JB, Schwarz P, McNair P et al: Radial and humeral fractures as predictors of subsequent hip, radial or humeral fractures in women, and their seasonal variation. Osteoporosis Int 1993;3: 133–137

117. Cooper C: Epidemiology and public health impact of osteoporosis. In Reid DM (ed): Baillière's Clinical Rheumatology: Osteoporosis. Baillière Tindall, London, 1993;7:459–477

118. O'Neill TW, Felsenberg D, Varlow J et al: The prevalence of vertebral deformity in European men and women: the European Vertebral Osteoporosis study. J Bone Miner Res 1996;11:1010–1018

119. Silman AJ, O'Neill TW, Cooper C et al: Influence of physical activity on vertebral deformity in men and women: results from the European Vertebral Osteoporosis study. J Bone Miner Res 1997;12:813–819

120. Scane AC, Francis RM, Sutcliffe AM et al: Case–control study of the pathogenesis and sequelae of symptomatic vertebral fractures in men. Osteoporosis Int 1999;9:91–97

121. Nguyen T, Sambrook P, Kelly et al: Prediction of osteoporotic fractures by postural instability and bone density. BMJ 1993;307:1111–1115

122. Cooper C, Mitchell M, Wickham C: Rheumatoid arthritis, corticosteroid therapy and the risk of hip fracture. Ann Rheum Dis 1995;54:49–52

123. Poor G, Atkinson EJ, O'Fallon WM et al: Predictors of hip fractures in elderly men. J Bone Miner Res 1995;10:1900–1907

124. Jackson JA, Spiekerman AM: Testosterone deficiency is common in men with hip fracture after simple falls. Clin Res 1989;37:131–136

125. Grisso JA, Kelsey JL, Strom BL et al: Risk factors for falls as a cause of hip fracture in women. N Engl J Med 1991;324:1326–1331

126. Jensen JS, Bagger J: Long-term social prognosis after hip fractures. Acta Orthop Scand 1982;53:97–101

127. Thomas TG, Stevens RS: Social effects of fractures of the neck of femur. BMJ 1974;3:456–458

128. Beals RK: Survival following hip fracture: long follow up of 607 patients. J Chron Dis 1972;25:235–244

Chapter 71

Arthritis in the elderly

David L. Scott

Rheumatic diseases are common in elderly people and are often undiagnosed or undertreated. Elderly patients have the same types of musculoskeletal disorders as younger age groups. However, there are differences in the pattern, severity, and effect of these diseases and variations in their optimal treatment. A few disorders such as polymyalgia rheumatica are far more common in elderly people.

Problems in elderly patients with arthritis include the insidious nature of musculoskeletal symptoms, associated comorbidity and muscle weakness, slow response to treatment, poorer outcome, and greater propensity to adverse drug reactions. The main rheumatic diseases of the elderly, summarized in Table 71-1, include inflammatory arthritis, degenerative arthritis, connective tissue diseases, soft tissue rheumatism, and back pain.

Arthritis is the most common cause of disability in people aged over 75 years.[1] The most common cause of terminal dependency due to loss of mobility, confinement in bed or in the house, is also arthritis and rheumatism. One hospital-based survey in London showed that 76 percent of patients admitted to an acute elderly unit had peripheral arthritis, 48 percent had arthritis directly contributing to their functional disability, and 19 percent did not volunteer information about their joint disease.[2] The prevalence rate of disabling joint diseases increases as people age, osteoarthritis being the most common type of joint disease in the elderly population.[3]

DISEASE MECHANISMS

The pathological changes of arthritis

Arthritis involves cell adhesion and migration, T- and B-cell activation, cytokine release, and joint destruction. Synovial lining cells, derived from macrophages and fibroblasts, show variable increases in rheumatoid synovia resulting from proliferation and recruitment of macrophage-like cells. The underlying subintimal layer contains many blood vessels, reticular connective tissue components, tissue macrophages, and occasional giant cells, and a variable lymphocytic and plasma cell infiltrate. At the margins of the synovium is the pannus, which overlies articular cartilage. Most cells of the pannus are large and mononuclear and some have fibroblastic appearances. The main features of rheumatoid synovitis are summarized in Table 71-2. The features of synovial inflammation are similar in different arthropathies.

The cells involved

T-lymphocytes have a central pathological role in synovitis.[4] The concept of a pathologic T-cell response in rheumatoid arthritis (RA) is supported by the demonstration that removing T-cells by thoracic duct drainage, lymphapheresis, or total lymphoid irradiation ameliorates arthritis. Germline T-cell receptor complex polymorphisms may contribute to genetic susceptibility to arthritis.[5]

Synovial lining cell hyperplasia and mononuclear cell infiltration are conspicuous in the earliest stages of synovitis.[6] Macrophage-like synoviocytes originate in the bone marrow, as do other mononuclear phagocytes, and are constantly replaced via the circulation.[7] In the rheumatoid synovium, about 80 percent of the lining cells are macrophage-like cells functioning as antigen-processing and antigen-presenting cells to T-lymphocytes.

Signaling between cells: cytokines and growth factors

Cytokines, cytokine inhibitors, and growth factors are important mediators of inflammation and joint destruction in

Table 71-1 The main musculoskeletal disorders of the elderly

Type of disorder	Examples
Inflammatory synovitis	Rheumatoid arthritis Gout Pseudogout Septic arthritis
Degenerative arthritis	Osteoarthritis
Vasculitis and connective tissue diseases	Polymyalgia rheumatica Temporal arteritis Systemic lupus erythematosus
Soft tissue rheumatism	Rotator cuff shoulder lesions Frozen shoulder
Back pain	Mechanical back pain Lumbar spondylosis and spondylolisthesis Spinal stenosis Osteoporotic vertebral fracture Spinal malignancy

Table 71-2 The main pathologic features of rheumatoid arthritis

Synovial lining cell hyperplasia
Superficial fibrin deposition
Vascular proliferation
Lymphocytic infiltration and variable lymphocytic aggregation
Macrophages and plasma cells in subintimal synovium
Variable synovial fibrosis
Marginal pannus over articular cartilage
Destruction of adjacent articular cartilage and bone

Table 71-3 Cytokines and growth factors involved in arthritis

Cytokines influencing synovial cells	Cytokines influencing neutrophils	Growth factor influencing synovial cells
Interleukin-1 Interleukin-6 Tumor necrosis factor-α	Interleukin-8	Platelet-derived growth factor Insulin-like growth factor Fibroblast growth factor Transforming growth factor β

arthritis.[8] Several classes of peptides are involved, including interleukins, tumor necrosis factors, interferons, and a variety of peptide regulatory factors. These are summarized in Table 71-3.

Interleukin-1 (IL-1) is a small protein produced by monocytes and macrophages.[9] Its systemic effects include fever and anorexia. In arthritis, local effects may be important such as augmentation of T- and B-lymphocyte function and chemotaxis of neutrophils and other cells. IL-1 may contribute to joint scarring and fibrosis by stimulating fibroblast proliferation either directly or indirectly through the induction of platelet-derived growth factor and other peptide regulatory factors. A variety of natural IL-1 inhibitors have been identified in cell supernatants and in human urine.[10]

Tumor necrosis factor-α (TNF-α) is another small peptide produced by monocytes and macrophages. It is secreted together with IL-1, although its production is regulated independently. As monocytes mature into macrophages their ability to produce IL-1 decreases while TNF-α production is relatively unaffected. TNF-α binds to separate receptors on target cells, although it has similar biological functions to IL-1. TNF-α is present in synovial fluid and is synthesized by synovial tissue.[11] Similar to IL-1, the local effects of TNF-α may be counteracted by regulatory or inhibitory proteins.

Interleukin-6 (IL-6) is a further small polypeptide from monocytes, T-lymphocytes and fibroblasts.[12] IL-1 and TNF-α induce its synthesis and secretion. IL-6 has similar actions to IL-1, but it is a more potent inducer of hepatic synthesis of acute-phase proteins and of immunoglobulin production by B-lymphocytes. High levels of IL-6 are present in arthritic synovial fluids. IL-6 may both amplify some of the effects of IL-1 and TNF-α and also induce the synthesis of acute-phase proteins and rheumatoid factors.

Interleukin-8 (IL-8) is a different cytokine that activates neutrophils. It is also known as neutrophil-activating peptide-1.[13] It induces a range of responses in neutrophils, including the expression of surface adhesion molecules and the production of reactive oxygen metabolites. IL-8 is a product of mononuclear phagocytes and also fibroblasts and other cells. In arthritis, IL-8 could bring about the accumulation of neutrophils that are considered a major source of cartilage-degrading enzymes. IL-8 levels are high in synovial fluids from patients with RA.[14]

How are the large number of different cytokines in the inflamed synovium regulated? Studies on synovial biopsies show persistent expression of mRNA to IL-1, TNF-α, IL-6 and other cytokines. This stability and persistence of cytokine production suggests it plays an important role in the pathogenesis of the chronicity of synovitis in rheumatoid disease. There is evidence that TNF-α is the dominant signal regulating IL-1 production,[15] although other noncytokine signals such as immune complexes may also be significant.

Many other growth factors are implicated in synovitis. Fibroblast growth factors, which have some homology with IL-1, effect angiogenesis and are intracrine growth factors.[16] Synovial cells may stimulate their own proliferation in an autocrine manner through modulators like basic fibroblast growth factor (FGF). Transforming growth factor β, which is present in lymphocytes and macrophages, has potent immunomodulatory effects.[17] Platelet-derived growth factor, which is released from the α granules of platelets during blood clotting,[18] is mitogenic for fibroblasts and chondrocytes.

Adhesion molecules

Adhesion molecules are involved in cell–cell adhesion, antigen recognition, lymphocyte activation, and cell trafficking.[19] There are three main groups of adhesion molecules each binding to different ligands: molecules of the immunoglobulin supergene family, the integrins, and the selectins (Table 71-4). The integrins are the key adhesion molecules, which are widely distributed and interact with extracellular matrix components. They are important in wound healing and cell migration in tissue remodeling and repair. Several extracellular and intracellular factors modify adhesion molecule expression.[20] These include exposure to cytokines,[21] adhesion to extracellular matrix proteins,[22] and lymphocyte activation. Adhesion molecules are widely distributed in the inflamed synovium and are involved in lymphocyte localization.

The extracellular matrix

The cells of the synovium interact closely with their surrounding extracellular matrix, which acts as a scaffolding and also controls activities like migration, division, and differentiation.[23] The main components of the extracellular matrix are summarized in Table 71-5.

Collagen is a ubiquitous protein and in connective tissues the main forms are collagens I, II, and III, which are fiber-forming collagens with a triple helical structure. Collagens I and III are found in the synovium and collagen II is the main collagen of cartilage. Collagen and its breakdown products are chemotactic for monocytes and fibroblasts, attracting them to

Table 71-4 Classification of adhesion molecules

Families	Subfamilies	Examples
Immunoglobulin Supergene	T-cell receptor/CD3 CD2 receptor/LFA3	
Integrins	β₁ integrins β₂ integrins β₃ integrins	VLA 1–6 LFA 1 Mac-1 p150,95 Vitronectin receptor Platelet glycoprotein IIb/IIIa
Selectins	ELAM-1 LAM-1 PADG-EM	

Table 71-5 Main components of the extracellular matrix

Type of component	Examples	Distribution
Collagen	Collagens I and III	Interstitial connective tissues
	Collagen II	Cartilage
	Collagen IV	Basement membranes
	Collagen V	Pericellular extracellular matrix
Noncollagenous structural glycoproteins	Fibronectin	Widely distributed in connective tissue
	Laminin	Basement membrane component
	Vitronectin	More limited pericellular distribution
Proteoglycans and glycosaminoglycans	Hyaluronic acid	Widely distributed
	Heparan sulfate	Basement membranes proteoglycan
	Keratan sulfate	Cartilage

sites of tissue damage in the early phases of inflammation. Immunohistochemical studies have localized the various collagens in normal and inflamed synovia from RA and other arthropathies.[24,25] Collagen type II is present in synovial phagocytes from patients with rheumatoid synovial fluids,[26] and it is a potential marker of cartilage erosion in RA phagocytic cells in joint damage.

Glycosaminoglycans include hyaluronic acid, chondroitin sulfate, dermatan sulfate, keratan sulfate, and associated molecules. Hyaluronate is responsible for many of the viscous properties of synovial fluid, but it is also involved in many reactions in the tissues and is involved with a specific cell adhesion molecule.[27] The interaction between hyaluronate, its cell surface receptor, and the cell cytoskeleton may have important pathogenic roles in determining the chronic inflammatory response.[28] There is a marked increase in hyaluronate with free binding sites for its associated link protein in the rheumatoid synovium.[29] Hyaluronic acid is also present in the serum and its levels are high in rheumatoid disease.

Proteolytic enzymes

Proteolytic enzymes, activators and inhibitors, are the key factors in the resorption of connective tissues during joint destruction. Collagenase is the most specific metalloproteinase (Table 71-6). Fibroblast collagenase is synthesized in a latent form that is activated by removal of part of the polypeptide chain.[30] Other enzymes involved include stromelysin and gelatinase.

Connective tissue metalloproteinases are inhibited by a tissue inhibitor of metalloproteinase (TIMP), a low-molecular-weight protein.[31] Metalloproteinases are also inhibited by α_2-macroglobulin. In the inflammatory response of RA, α_2-macroglobulin concentrations rise in plasma and there is greater capillary permeability, allowing it to reach sites such as synovial tissues. The metalloproteinases are controlled by the synthesis of the latent enzyme, by the need for an activation mechanism, and by the presence of inhibitory TIMPs. Expression of metalloproteinase and TIMP by cultured connective tissue cells is regulated by cytokines, growth factors, and hormones.

Symptoms and signs of arthritis

Local symptoms comprise pain, tenderness, swelling and stiffness in the joints, periarticular tissues, ligaments and

Table 71-6 Metalloproteinase enzymes of human connective tissue

Enzyme	Size (latent), kD	Size (active), kD	Substrates
Collagenase	55	43	Collagens I, II, and III
Stromelysin	57	48	Proteoglycan core protein Collagen IV Fibronectin Laminin Elastin Denatured collagens
Gelatinase	72	66	Denatured collagens Collagens IV, V, VII

tendons, and muscles. Pain is the predominant symptom. Usually persistent and moderately severe, it is often worse on movement and it invariably limits patients' lifestyles.

Stiffness is the most characteristic arthritic symptom. It comprises both early morning stiffness and post-exercise stiffness. Morning stiffness points towards inflammatory arthritis or polymyalgia rheumatica. It usually lasts over 60 minutes and can be very prolonged. Post-exercise stiffness points more towards osteoarthritis. Tenderness and swelling of the joints or tendons usually go together and indicate an inflammatory synovitis or tendonitis. They vary from very subtle to gross symptoms. Some elderly patients minimize the extent of their joint swelling, even though it is extensive on examination. Bony swelling of the joints usually indicates osteoarthritis.

Systemic symptoms vary. In rheumatoid arthritis or polymyalgia rheumatica they can be quite marked and include malaise, anorexia, weight loss, and depression. Low-grade fevers can occur, especially in connective tissue disorders.

The goal of the examination is to identify the presence and extent of joint swelling and tenderness, the numbers of joints or soft tissue structures involved, the distribution of joint inflammation, its severity, and the presence of effusions and deformities. Extra-articular features such as subcutaneous nodules should be sought. Regional problems such as back pain or shoulder problems require specific attention to those sites. Comorbidity is common in elderly patients with arthritis, so a general physical examination is essential.

Investigations

Investigations range from full blood counts and routine biochemistry to immunological measures of rheumatoid factor and analysis of synovial fluid for crystals. The main tests are summarized in Table 71-7.

RHEUMATOID FACTOR   Rheumatoid factors are antibodies against the Fc fragment of IgG. Rheumatoid factors react against different species of IgG, including human and rabbit. Rheumatoid factors can involve different immunoglobulin classes, giving IgM, IgG, and IgA rheumatoid factors. Different subclasses of antibody can also be involved, such as IgA_1 and IgA_2 rheumatoid factors. Most tests detect IgM rheumatoid factor. There is some evidence that IgA rheumatoid factor is more related to joint destruction. Rheumatoid factor positivity goes with worse disease and poorer outcome in rheumatoid arthritis and is associated with subcutaneous nodules, vasculitis, and other extra-articular features. Osteoarthritis, gout, and psoriatic arthritis should all be negative on tests for rheumatoid factor.

OTHER IMMUNOLOGICAL TESTS   Antinuclear antibodies are more important in connective tissue diseases, although rheumatoid arthritis is a common cause of low-titer positive antinuclear antibodies. There are many types of antinuclear antibodies and the less specific IgM subclass are more often seen in RA. Osteoarthritis, gout, and psoriatic arthritis should be negative for antinuclear antibodies.

The other main area of testing is for acute-phase changes. An elevated C-reactive protein level, together with a high erythrocyte sedimentation rate (ESR) and changes in several serum proteins characterizes active RA. It is termed the *acute-phase response*. It is mediated by the cytokine network, especially IL-1 and IL-6. The levels of these cytokines can be measured directly but they are labile and secreted in pulses and thus are poor measures of disease activity in many cases. The range of immunological tests and methods are summarized in Tables 71-8 and 71-9.

CHANGES IN DEGENERATIVE ARTHRITIS   Osteoarthritis and inflammatory arthritis are characterized by cartilage damage and collagen turnover. Unfortunately the markers of this process are not ideal and at present no tests have a major role, but investigations based on connective tissue biochemistry will be available in the future. They comprise measures of derivatives of collagen metabolism, cartilage breakdown products, and mediators of connective tissue turnover. Excluding crystal deposition disease by synovial fluid microscopy also helps in the differential diagnosis.

Collagen degradation leads to pyridinoline and deoxypyridinoline cross-link fragments in blood and urine, which can be measured in chromatographic or immunochemical assays. They are the most widely used markers in osteoarthritis,[32] although they have not extended beyond clinical trials (Table 71-10). Other potential markers include measuring the products of cartilage damage such as keratan sulfate, which is a glycosaminoglycan in cartilage, and collagen propeptide fragments.

IMAGING IN ARTHRITIS   Imaging arthritic joints has a variety of aims that depend on the specific circumstances.

Table 71-7   Laboratory investigations

Class of test	Category	Example of abnormality
Hematology	Hemoglobin	Anemia in rheumatoid arthritis
	White cell count	Leucocytosis in septic arthritis
	Platelet count	Thrombocytopenia in systemic lupus erythematosus
	ESR	Elevated in polymyalgia rheumatica
Biochemistry	Creatinine	High with involvement in systemic vasculitis
	Uric acid	Elevated in gout
	CPK	Elevated in polymyositis
Immunology	Rheumatoid factor	Positive in rheumatoid arthritis
	Antinuclear antibody	Positive in systemic lupus erythematosus
	C-reactive protein	Elevated in rheumatoid arthritis
	Immunoglobulins	Elevated in Sjögren's syndrome
	Complements C_3 and C_4	Low in active systemic lupus erythematosus
Synovial fluid microscopy	Crystals	Present in gout and pyrophosphate crystal deposition disease
Culture	Bacteria in septic arthritis	

Table 71-9   Immunological methods

Method	Example of use
Agglutination	IgM rheumatoid factor
Nephelometry	IgM rheumatoid factor
ELISA	IgA and IgG rheumatoid factors
Radial immunodiffusion	C-reactive protein
Immunodiffusion	ENA (e.g. Sm and RNP)
Immunofluorescence	ANA, crythidea
Radio-immunoassay	DNA binding

Table 71-8   Immunological investigations

Acute-phase changes	Immunoglobulins	Complement	Cytokines
ESR	IgG	C_3	TNF-α
C-reactive protein	IgA	C_4	IL-1
Serum amyloid A protein	IgM		IL-6

Table 71-10 Laboratory investigations in osteoarthritis

Type of test	Example
Synovial fluid analyses	Cell counts Crystals (in chondrocalcinosis) Cartilage damage markers (e.g. keratan sulfate)
Blood	Cartilage damage markers (e.g. keratan sulfate) Collagen turnover markers (e.g. collagen propeptides)
Urine	Collagen damage markers (e.g. pyridinium cross-links)

Table 71-11 Imaging methods

Modality	Example
Plain radiology	X-rays of hands in rheumatoid arthritis
Magnetic resonance imaging	Imaging of knee joint to show internal derangement
Computed tomography	Imaging of sacroiliac joint if infection suspected
Bone scan	Showing active joints in inflammatory synovitis
DEXA	Identifying osteoporosis with inflammatory synovitis

Table 71-12 Nonsteroidal anti-inflammatory drugs

Oldest	Modern	Newest
Cheap	Modest price	Premium price
Very effective	Effective	Effective
Relatively toxic	Safe	Very safe
Examples:	*Examples:*	*Examples:*
Ibuprofen	Nabumetone	Rofecoxib
Indomethacin	Etodolac	Celecoxib
Diclofenac	Meloxicam	

leukocytes, allows the assessment of joint inflammation.[38] Labeled immunoglobulin may also be useful. The resolution of detectors allows better images of large joints such as the knee.

Densitometry has many advantages for assessing bone changes.[39] It can be either whole-body densitometry or localized views of specific joints or regions. Until now it has mainly focused on assessing the effects of drugs on bone mineral density and the relation to fracture risk. The introduction of new systems may be more advantageous for looking at specific joints.

Drug therapy in arthritis

Conventionally, antirheumatic drugs have been divided into nonsteroidal anti-inflammatory drugs (NSAIDs), slow-acting drugs, and steroids. Slow-acting drugs are often thought capable of modifying the course of RA and are sometimes termed "disease modifying" drugs. The belief that such drugs affect the course of RA is based on their effects on the radiological progression of joint damage. There is evidence that some slow-acting drugs may reduce the rate of progression but the situation is not straightforward. Concerns have led to the suggestion that the classification of antirheumatic drugs should be changed and the concept of "disease control" introduced.[40]

Disease control implies a beneficial effect on inflammatory synovitis, leading to reduced anatomical damage, improved and maintained function, and an amelioration of systemic rheumatoid disease over a long period. Disease control must relate as much to an overall management strategy or drug combination as to a single drug.[41] Most antirheumatic drugs are symptomatically effective and this should be one determinant of their classification. If a drug or a therapeutic strategy then meets the criteria for disease control it can be reclassified accordingly. At least 12 months of disease-controlling activity is needed to predict improved long-term outcome.

Anti-inflammatory drugs

Ibuprofen, the first non-aspirin NSAID, was identified in the early 1950s, and by the 1970s it was being widely prescribed for the treatment of arthritis. Subsequently a large number of NSAIDs were identified. NSAIDs such as diclofenac, ibuprofen, and naproxen are well established and have been available for many years. New drug development has concentrated on reducing side-effects while maintaining efficacy. The main NSAIDs are summarized in Table 71-12.

These drugs are now among the most widely prescribed of all therapeutic agents, but they also have a history of toxicity

These include diagnosis, assessing progression and the effects of drugs, looking at early rapid changes in the extent of synovitis, and looking at joints at risk of progression and damage.

The modalities of imaging are summarized in Table 71-11. Currently plain joint radiographs remain the most widely used method for determining the extent and nature of structural changes in arthritis. The main radiological changes include periarticular osteoporosis and sclerosis, loss of joint space (reflecting cartilage damage), juxta-articular erosions, marginal osteophytes, joint destruction, and ankylosis.[33] Although joint radiographs are one of the most objective methods of assessing joint destruction, many investigators have failed to demonstrate a significant correlation between the severity of radiographic findings on hand radiographs and functional status.[34]

Magnetic resonance imaging (MRI) gives the opportunity for far greater information to be gained from imaging joints. It will probably be the gold standard for evaluating the nature and extent of pathological changes within the joints in future years. However, experience is still at an early stage. Essential information needs to be obtained before the place of MRI in the assessment of arthritis can be fully defined.[35,36]

Physiological measurements and diagnostic assessments can both be achieved using nuclear medicine techniques and densitometry. The role of these alternative imaging procedures must not be overlooked. Most experience has been gained from using bone scans.[37] These examine a combination of bone blood flow and osteoblastic activity. Their resolution is poor and this is a limiting factor. The three-phase bone scan looks at initial uptake, the blood pool interval, and subsequent localization within the bones. The use of labeled white cells, such as indium-labeled

and adverse effects. Nevertheless, NSAIDs remain the central focus of antirheumatic therapy. They reduce the signs and symptoms of acute synovitis and relieve pain and are widely used in RA, osteoarthritis, gout, back pain, and soft tissue rheumatism.

The NSAIDs exert their anti-inflammatory effect by inhibition of the enzyme cyclo-oxygenase (COX); this mechanism is the basis for their therapeutic effect as well as their toxicity. Gastrointestinal irritation, ulceration, and hemorrhage; fluid retention and exacerbation of hypertension; and exacerbation of bronchospasm and anaphylaxis are their most serious adverse effects, although many others have been recorded. In recent years it has become clear that COX exists in two isoforms, constitutive COX-1 and inducible COX-2. Drugs that selectively inhibit the COX-2 isoform are much less likely to cause the adverse effects of COX-1 inhibition. These agents offer the promise of efficacy with less toxicity.[42]

The main adverse effect of NSAIDs is their gastrointestinal toxicity, and their propensity to cause ulcers accounts for the peptic ulcers, bleeding, and perforations associated with their use. There is a significant morbidity and mortality. There are several strategies to reduce these adverse effects. The most widely used is coprescribing with misoprostol, a synthetic prostaglandin that reduces the gastrointestinal side-effects of NSAIDs and both prevents and heals NSAID-associated ulcers.[43] It can be given by itself or in a combined fixed-dose combination with diclofenac. Reducing gastric acid by H_2-antagonists such as ranitidine also heals NSAID-associated ulcers and has a role in their prevention. There is debate about whether all NSAIDs cause the same frequency of ulcers, and the evidence suggests that some NSAIDs such as azapropazone may be more likely to result in gastrointestinal adverse effects. Newer NSAIDs have intrinsically fewer gastrointestinal adverse reactions. An example is a prodrug like nabumetone, which does not itself cause gastric damage.

NSAIDs cause many different adverse effects and these are summarized in Table 71-13. In addition to gastrointestinal problems, renal and central nervous system reactions can be a special problem. The mild reactions of dizziness and confusion can be a particular difficulty in elderly patients already taking many different medications and can lead to considerable disorientation.

The value of NSAIDs for symptomatic treatment in osteoarthritis is an area of controversy. Although most clinicians use them, the supporting evidence is not strong. Dieppe et al.[44] highlighted the lack of randomized placebo-controlled trials of NSAIDs; the majority of trials in osteoarthritis compare one NSAID with another. One large study by Bradley et al.[45] compared ibuprofen against paracetamol in patients with osteoarthritis of the knee and suggested that there was no convincing evidence in favor of the NSAID. Brandt[46] has outlined in detail the deficiencies in the case for using NSAIDs in osteoarthritis. But the absence of good evidence for their use does not mean NSAIDs are ineffective; it merely indicates the inadequacy of randomized clinical trials in the area.

Disease-controlling drugs and immunosuppression

Disease-controlling drugs and immunosuppression are mainly used to treat RA. The assessment of their effect includes

Table 71-13 Adverse effects of NSAIDs

Type of adverse reaction	Example
Gastrointestinal	Indigestion Erosions Peptic ulcer Hemorrhage and perforation Small bowel enteropathy
Hepatic	Hepatocellular damage Cholestasis
Renal	Acute renal failure Interstitial nephritis
Hematologic	Thrombocytopenia Neutropenia Hemolytic anemia
Skin	Photosensitivity Urticaria Erythema multiforme
Chest	Bronchospasm Pneumonitis
Central nervous system	Headache Dizziness Confusion

clinical, laboratory, functional, and radiological approaches. A central theme of therapy—disease control—is based on overcoming the inflammatory synovitis and thus reducing the progression of joint damage. The effects of generalized inflammation indicated by the acute-phase response on the progression of RA are well known, as is the association between radiological progression and acute-phase proteins such as C-reactive protein. Otterness[47] has shown that drugs that reduce C-reactive protein give the best outcomes. However, normalizing an elevated acute-phase response may be insufficient, and only patients who consistently maintain low ESR and C-reactive protein levels have less radiological progression. Further work is needed to define whether it is most important to control local or systemic inflammation in RA. Despite such uncertainties, there is a clear need both to control symptoms of inflammatory synovitis and reduce the elevated acute-phase response. Therapy with slow-acting drugs has this as a combined aim.

Aggressive RA or the early onset of erosions are indications for early treatment with a slow-acting drug. Most rheumatologists use sequential monotherapy, with one slow-acting drug following another in an attempt to control the disease without excessive side-effects. The concurrent use of several second-line drugs is controversial. Wilke et al.[48] argued that as the long-term outcome of sequential monotherapy has been disappointing, specific goals of treatment should be established and aggressive treatment given in a logical manner in early disease. As RA rarely remits, refractory disease is common and in this situation the therapeutic options include cyclosporine A, high-dose methotrexate, combination second-line agents, and tailored use of corticosteroids.

Gold, penicillamine, and sulfasalazine perform similarly, with about 60 percent of patients continuing to receive each drug for at least 1 year.[49] Patients with a longer disease duration showed a greater tendency to stop treatment. The median percentage improvement was 33 percent in pain score and 50 percent in ESR. Methotrexate has proved a major advance from the 1980s in the treatment of RA. Used initially in patients with psoriatic arthritis because of their skin disease, it induced improvement in synovitis. A subsequent placebo-controlled trial in RA confirmed its efficacy. Alarcon et al.[50] reviewed the clinical and radiological effects of methotrexate and questioned its effects on X-ray progression. They performed a meta-analysis of 353 methotrexate-treated subjects and 205 controls and computed a monthly rate of disease progression. The rates of disease progression were similar for methotrexate-treated cases and controls. A new agent for use in nonresponding RA is ciclosporin A, which controls the symptoms of early and late RA.[51] Ciclosporin A slows radiological progression in advanced disease.[52]

The use of several antirheumatic drugs concurrently is routine clinical practice. NSAIDs, slow-acting drugs, and steroids are often used together, and therapy may also include hormone replacement. But the concept of combination therapy with two slow-acting drugs is more controversial. Tugwell et al.[53] have shown that the combination of ciclosporin A and methotrexate appear to be effective and this is an important focus of future therapy.

Steroids
In RA, the efficacy of corticosteroids was demonstrated in early clinical trials. But their long-term side-effects, particularly osteoporosis, have remained a substantial obstacle limiting their routine use. Short courses of oral prednisolone or a depot intramuscular injection are often used in active disease when commencing therapy with a slow-acting drug, to control symptoms before the slow-acting drug has an appreciable effect.[54] Pulse therapy with intravenous steroids such as 0.5–1.0 g methylprednisolone has a rapid onset of action, but its advantage is often not maintained and its use remains in some doubt.[55] The more prolonged use of oral steroids has been shown to be advantageous in early disease. Kirwan[56] reported that, in early RA patients, low-dose prednisolone (7.5 mg/day) when used in conjunction with disease-modifying antirheumatic drugs reduced the progression of erosive disease. More studies are needed to establish the risks and benefits of steroids in this situation.

Hormone replacement therapy
The widespread use of hormone replacement therapy (HRT) has been an important advance in the management of osteoporosis, and there is evidence that HRT should also be used as part of the integrated management of rheumatoid arthritis. Hall et al.[57] assessed the effect of HRT on bone mass in 200 post-menopausal female patients with RA treated with and without steroid therapy. Hormone replacement therapy increased spinal bone mineral density and maintained femoral bone mineral density. HRT is also effective in preserving bone mass in patients taking low-dose corticosteroids.

Supportive nondrug therapy
Physiotherapy, occupational therapy, supplying aids and appliances such as walking sticks, modifying footwear such as fitting insoles and providing surgical shoes, and chiropody all have important roles. Of equal importance is providing patient education and general advice about arthritis, together where possible with simple exercise programs.

RHEUMATOID ARTHRITIS

Rheumatoid arthritis is a chronic inflammatory synovitis of peripheral joints. It is usually polyarticular and symmetrical in distribution. Many patients have radiological evidence of juxta-articular erosions and are seropositive for rheumatoid factor. Extra-articular features such as subcutaneous nodules are common.

Epidemiology of RA
Rheumatoid arthritis is a common disorder. We know the incidence of new cases of RA from prospective studies such as the Norfolk Arthritis Register; there will be in the region of 50 new cases of inflammatory synovitis each year per 100,000 population in the UK.[58] Most of these will be due to RA. There is also a considerable amount of information about the prevalence of established RA. In Europe this varies from 0.5 to 2 percent or more depending on the exact population studied.[59] Some populations in North America have higher prevalence rates (Table 71-14).

The prevalence of RA increases with age and it is especially frequent in elderly women. A study in North America in the early 1960s showed that it was rare in men before the age of 45 years and in women before the age of 35 years. In the over-65 age group its prevalence increased to 1.8 percent in males and 4.9 percent in females.[60]

Disease onset and course of RA
The most common presentation is an insidious onset.[61,62] Up to three-quarters of cases start in this way. The characteristic features of an inflammatory synovitis are present, including joint swelling, joint tenderness, and morning stiffness. These usually involve multiple sites in a symmetrical distribution. There are often systemic features such as malaise and fatigue. A small number of cases, about 5–10 percent, have an acute onset with an "explosive" beginning and a rapid onset of symptoms over a few days or even less. Between these two extremes there is an intermediate onset of the symptoms over days and weeks; this is seen in nearly 20 percent of cases.

Table 71-14 **Prevalence of rheumatoid arthritis in different populations**	
Population	**Prevalence (%)**
Europe	
United Kingdom	1.1
Netherlands	0.9
Finland	2.0
Denmark	0.8
North America	
US National Health Survey	1.0
Inuit Indians (Canada)	0.6
Pima Indians (United States)	5.3

Table 71-15 The course of rheumatoid arthritis

Disease type	Frequency (%)	Description
Progressive course	70	Chronic disease with invariable progression and some fluctuations in severity
Intermittent course	25	Intermittent attacks of arthritis, often less than 1 year, and intermissions for variable periods of time
Brief remissions		Lasting less than 1 year in 10% of cases
Long remissions		Lasting over 1 year in 10% of cases
"Malignant" disease	Less than 5	Uncommon form of RA with severe extra-articular disease, especially vasculitis; often fatal

Table 71-16 Extra-articular features of rheumatoid arthritis

Extra-articular feature	Specific example
Subcutaneous nodules	Pressure area at elbow In wall of olecranon bursa At sacrum
Pulmonary	Pleural effusion Interstitial fibrosis
Cardiac	Pericarditis Valvular disease
Ocular	Keratoconjunctivitis sicca Episcleritis Scleritis
Neurological	Carpal tunnel syndrome Mononeuritis multiplex Peripheral neuropathy Cervical myelopathy
Renal	Amyloidosis Drug toxicity
Vasculitis	Nail-fold infarctions Leg ulcers Systemic vasculitis
Hematological	Anemia Felty syndrome

Early RA usually involves the proximal interphalangeal joints of the hands together with the wrists. The metatarsophalangeal joints of the feet are also commonly involved. A small number of patients have an atypical onset. These include intermittent episodes of arthritis termed *palindromic rheumatism*, polymyalgic and monoarticular onsets. Patients with a polymyalgic onset have predominant shoulder girdle symptoms with muscle pain and prolonged morning stiffness. Palindromic arthritis, which can develop into RA, is more a symptom complex than a disease entity.[63] Its features are transient synovial inflammation, involvement of different joints, and asymptomatic periods without synovitis. When there is a monoarticular onset the knee is usually involved.

Rheumatoid arthritis is usually divided into progressive disease, an intermittent course, and cases with long clinical remissions, which form a variant of intermittent disease. A few patients with severe extra-articular disease can be described as having "malignant" RA. These different patterns are summarized in Table 71-15.

Clinical features of RA

Persistent joint inflammation is the central diagnostic feature of RA. The joints are swollen, tender, and stiff. Morning stiffness is prolonged and may last over an hour. The joint involvement is symmetrical and usually involves the hands (proximal interphalangeal and metacarpophalangeal joints), wrists, and feet (proximal interphalangeal and metatarsophalangeal joints). The elbows, knees, and ankles are often involved as well.

The synovitis is accompanied by systemic features of ill-health with malaise, weight loss, occasional intermittent fever, and constitutional upset in many cases. As the arthritis progresses there are characteristic destructive changes—for example, ulnar deviation and the Swan neck and Boutonierre deformities of the fingers.

Subcutaneous nodules are a classic extra-articular feature. They are found on extensor surfaces such as the elbows or sites of pressure such as the lower back or in some parts of the hands. They occur in about 20 percent of cases. Other extra-articular features are summarized in Table 71-16.

The main clinical problems result from rheumatoid vasculitis. This is due to an inflammatory infiltration of small and medium-sized vessels. It usually occurs after 10 years or more of the disease in patients with high levels of rheumatoid factor and destructive disease.[64]

Assessment of RA

CLINICAL ASSESSMENT The core dataset, which has been agreed internationally,[65] is summarized in the accompanying box. The measures give a good overall picture of RA and permit assessment of progression and response to treatment.

Disease activity can be assessed by counting the number of active joints. The best joint count has been an area of recent investigation. Prevoo et al.[66] contrasted several available

Core dataset in rheumatoid arthritis

- Number of swollen joints
- Number of tender joints
- Pain assessed by the patient
- Patient's global assessments of disease activity
- Physician's global assessments of disease activity
- Laboratory evaluation of an acute-phase reactant (ESR, C-reactive protein, or equivalent)
- Self-administered functional assessment (such as the Health Assessment Questionnaire)

methods. The various indices had similar reliability and validity and no joint index was superior for measuring disease activity. The implication is that the simplest index, the 28-joint count, is best. Other studies have also concluded that the 28-joint count gives all the necessary information.

Patients can assess their disease activity in RA. A self-report measure of disease activity was developed by Stewart et al.[67] based on an articular index. The measure was sensitive to therapeutic change when completed by patients both before and after intra-articular corticosteroid injection. Although a self-report articular index has the potential to provide an inexpensive method for monitoring disease activity or treatment response in RA, it may be affected by confounding variables such as the patient's mood. Further work by Stucki et al.[68] has confirmed the value of patients' self-assessments.

Because RA is multidimensional its activity should be assessed in several areas or domains. There are apparent advantages in using a single index that pools several outcome measures to provide one overall measure. Examples include the disease activity index derived by van der Heijde et al.,[69] the Stoke index,[70] and the Mallya and Mace index.[71] Pooled indices may be difficult to calculate and interpreting their results may present problems.

IMAGING   Joint imaging includes plain radiology, MRI, bone scans and isotope labeling methods, and DEXA scans for periarticular osteoporosis. Conventional X-rays remain the gold standard for diagnosis and determining drug efficacy. MRI will be the future method of choice for defining cartilage and synovial changes in single joints. Isotope methods give the best indication of synovial inflammation.

Radiographs of the hands and feet can be scored by simple standardized methods. The most widely used methods are those of Sharp et al.[72] and Larsen et al.[73] Both methods are reproducible[74] and are composite indices combining joint space loss, erosions, and other changes. Their disadvantage is that they combine diverse changes in a single score and assign numerical values to qualitative changes. Radiographic changes in hands and wrists reflect changes in major joints. In early RA, 70 percent of patients have radiographic damage at 3 years.[75] By 10 years, X-ray progression is invariable in severe disease.[76]

FUNCTIONAL ASSESSMENT   The most familiar instruments used in RA are the Health Assessment Questionnaire (HAQ)[77] and the Arthritis Impact Measurement Scale (AIMS).[78] Both were developed specifically for RA. There are also several questionnaires designed to be relevant to a wide range of health problems, the so-called generic measures. A number of these generic instruments have been used to assess health status in RA,[79] including the Sickness Impact Profile, the Nottingham Health Profile (NHP), the Quality of Well-Being Scale, and the SF-36. The NHP and the Medical Outcome Study Short Form-36 (SF-36) have been widely used in RA.[80,81]

LABORATORY ASSESSMENT   Rheumatoid factor levels assist in both diagnosis and assessment of severity. There are many different measures available, including particle assays (e.g. latex test and RA particle agglutination), radio-immunoassays, and enzyme-linked immuno-sorbent assays (ELISAs). They use a variety of immunoglobulin sources, including rabbit and human IgG, and different classes of rheumatoid factors are measured. Traditional assays such as the latex test measure mainly IgM rheumatoid factor. ELISAs measure both IgG and IgA rheumatoid factor as well as IgM.

Rheumatoid factor status is an important prognostic indicator in all cases. Isomaki[82] reviewed follow-up results of unselected adult arthritis cases and found outcome was worst in seropositive rheumatoid patients and best in seronegative oligoarthritis of unknown etiology. Increased rheumatoid factor levels in early RA, especially a high level of IgA rheumatoid factor within 3 years of the onset of symptoms, was prognostic for a more severe disease outcome 6 years after the onset of symptoms. The importance of rheumatoid factor status has been confirmed in many other studies.[83]

Single measures showing a high ESR or C-reactive protein level indicate a poor prognosis. A combination of measures or multiple values are better. Hassell et al.[84] evaluated disease activity annually over 7 years in 127 patients and found significant correlations between "areas under the curve" for the ESR and other disease activity measures and destructive RA.

General demographic features, predictive of a poor response in most disease, include age, gender, and disease duration. Kaarela[85] evaluated predictors of outcome in 442 patients with recent arthritis and compared 22 variables recorded at the onset of arthritis. Destructive RA was predicted by symmetrical polyarthritis, female sex, and old age.

Rheumatoid arthritis is related to HLA DR4, but there is debate about its value in predicting response. Some studies have shown little effect. Silman et al.[86] found no evidence that HLA DR4 was a useful indicator of subsequent outcome, but van der Heijde et al.[87] considered HLA typing to be useful in predicting the outcome in early RA. Emery[88] suggests that the combination of polyarthritis, high C-reactive protein levels, and genetic markers, especially DR4 status, will all help define the course of early disease.

Van Zeben et al.[89] looked at prognostic factors in early RA. A combination of three commonly available variables—number of swollen joints, IgM rheumatoid factor, and the erosion score—predicted outcome well. Corbett et al.[90] reported predictors of death, survival, and function after 15 years; outcome could be correctly predicted in 73 percent of cases from a combination of early erosive change, seropositivity, poor grip strength, and cervical subluxation.

Clinical outcomes in RA

Studies of antirheumatic therapy tend to show that it is successful in the short term whereas there are poor results in the longer term. This was first highlighted by Pincus.[91] Prospective long-term clinical studies show that most patients first seen as inpatients are moderately or severely impaired by 20 years, and the average outpatient has a 30 percent chance of severe disability.[92]

Not all studies show that RA has a poor outcome. A review of 64 survivors from a prospective study of early RA found that, after 15 years, 60 percent of survivors had relatively normal function. In another study, 128 RA patients who developed the disease in 1985 were studied after 6–7 years: 32 percent had no articular swelling; 23 percent had normal X-rays and 31 percent had no erosions: and 31 percent had normal function. Rheumatoid factors and nodules were related to more severe outcomes.[93]

Rheumatoid arthritis leads to premature mortality. In hospitalized patients with RA, nearly 20 percent of deaths are directly caused by RA. Wolfe et al.[94] reported results from a large study examining 922 deaths in 3501 patients with RA. The standardized mortality ratio was 2.3. The causes of mortality in RA do not differ much from those in the normal population, although there is an increase in infection and lymphatic malignancies as a cause of death. The average shortening of life is in the region of 4–5 years. Patients with severe RA are most likely to die early.

Specific problems in the elderly population

Rheumatoid arthritis is increasingly becoming a disease of later life. The most common time for developing the disease is the sixth decade, and as it lasts 10 to 20 years many patients with RA are over 65 years old. When its onset is in old age it is often overlooked or ignored by patients and physicians. It is difficult to manage complex RA in an elderly person, especially if he or she has other problems with mobility. RA is frequently associated with other diseases and such comorbidity can be a serious clinical problem. Finally, elderly people have increased risks of adverse effects with antirheumatic drugs such as nonsteroidal anti-inflammatory agents, and this makes management more complex.

OSTEOARTHRITIS

Osteoarthritis (OA) is a heterogeneous condition with a variety of causes and patterns of expression. It is analogous to kidney or heart failure in which similar clinical and pathological features develop irrespective of the underlying causes, and could be considered as "joint failure." Older age is the most significant factor in its development in a general population.[95] The joint most commonly affected is the knee, and osteoarthritis of the knee is one of the most common causes of pain and disability in the community. There is a rise in the annual consultation rate for osteoarthritis,[96] and this may reflect not only an increased incidence of disease but also decreased tolerance of joint problems.

Osteoarthritis can be considered as a synovial joint syndrome rather than a single disease. Pathologically it is characterized by a loss of, and change in, the composition of cartilage proteoglycans leading to failure of normal responses to stress. The results include cartilage fibrillation and loss, bone exposure, and a clinical syndrome of pain and disability. Rare forms of heritable chondrodysplasia lead to premature osteoarthritis but, in most instances, its cause is either excess, inappropriate, or insufficient mechanical demand, or traumatic, infective, inflammatory, endocrine, or metabolic disease. There remain idiopathic ("primary") cases in which no cause is demonstrable.[97]

Epidemiology of osteoarthritis

The prevalence of osteoarthritis rises steeply with age. Its frequency has been evaluated in both clinical and radiography studies. X-ray evidence of osteoarthritis exceeds its clinical frequency. In Europe and North America there is a similar prevalence, rising from less than 1 percent of those aged under 35 years to over 30 percent of those aged over 75 years.[98,99] Both hand and knee osteoarthritis are more common in women than men. Hip osteoarthritis is less common and its prevalence rates in men and women appear to be more similar. The incidence of symptomatic osteoarthritis has been studied less often. One study from North America showed the incidence of knee and hip osteoarthritis was 200 per 100,000 person-years.[100] Felson et al.[101] evaluated 869 patients from the Framingham osteoarthritis study and found rates of incident disease were 1.7 times higher in women than in men, progressive disease occurred slightly more often in women, but rates did not vary by age. Among women, approximately 2 percent per year developed incident radiographic disease, 1 percent per year developed symptomatic knee osteoarthritis, and about 4 percent per year experienced progressive knee osteoarthritis.

Clinical features of osteoarthritis

Osteoarthritis is characterized by articular pain, bony joint swelling, morning and inactivity stiffness, and associated functional disability and radiography changes (see the accompanying box). Pain is the predominant symptom in osteoarthritis. It varies in severity and its exact nature both between patients and in individual cases over a period of time. Although pain is more marked in patients with severe joint destruction on X-rays, there is often no close relationship between pain and radiography abnormalities. Causes of pain in osteoarthritis include raised intraosseous pressure, inflammatory synovitis, periarticular problems, periosteal elevation, muscular changes, fibromyalgic amplification, and central neurogenic changes. There is often relatively little relationship between the severity and clinical importance of pain, stiffness, and physical function.[102]

Stiffness is experienced by most patients with osteoarthritis. "Stiffness" may refer to difficulty initiating movement, problems in completing a full range of movement, or the ache or pain of a joint on movement. It is often present first thing in the morning, but lasts only 10–25 minutes in many cases. More characteristically it comes on after inactivity, when it is frequently termed "gelling" of a joint.

Many patients have loss of movement or instability of one or more joints. Sometimes patients note that a joint will suddenly "give way." In some joints there is a sensation of inflammation due to an associated synovitis and the joint is swollen, tender, and warm.

On examination there is firm or bony swelling around the joint and crepitus on movement. The most characteristic bony swellings are the Heberden's and Bouchard's nodes of hand osteoarthritis. Coarse "crepitations" are usually felt on movement of the involved joint. In severe disease they can be

Clinical features of osteoarthritis

- Pain
- Stiffness
- Bony swelling and crepitus
- Loss of movement
- Instability
- Loss of function

audible. Effusions occur in some cases, especially in knee osteoarthritis. It is possible to use an articular index to standardize the clinical assessment of osteoarthritis and such an index was developed by Doyle et al.,[103] but assessment remains difficult to reproduce.

There are problems in diagnosing osteoarthritis. Although a set of clinical criteria has been developed,[104] these have been criticized for using rheumatoid patients who had not been age- and sex-matched as controls, using osteophytes as a feature of osteoarthritis, for circularity, and for inadequate validation.[105] Loss of cartilage on X-rays has been reported as the one feature present in all attempted definitions, but these are based on pathological changes that are not often available to the clinician making the diagnosis.[106] Furthermore the relationship between the incidence of symptoms and the degree of radiological change is not clear. Almost the entire population over the age of 65 years have at least one joint with evidence of radiographic osteoarthritis but the proportion with symptoms varies with joint, age, and sex.

Clinical subgroups with OA

Osteoarthritis includes several different subgroups that may all have different natural histories, patterns of joints affected, and different rates of disease progression. These include knee/hand osteoarthritis (often known as "generalized osteoarthritis"), inflammatory/erosive osteoarthritis, rapidly progressive osteoarthritis, secondary osteoarthritis, hypertrophic and atrophic osteoarthritis, and destructive osteoarthritis of the elderly. Set against the classification of osteoarthritis into such distinct subgroups are the findings of Cushnaghan and Dieppe,[107] who found a strong relationship between age and the number of involved sites. This was thought to be due to the slow addition of new joint sites with age. However, there was no evidence of well-defined clinical subsets of patients.

Inflammatory osteoarthritis and destructive disease in the elderly deserve special consideration. Destructive osteoarthritis with radiographic findings of rapid severe joint destruction can be a diagnostic problem. The X-ray changes mimic septic arthritis, rheumatoid, and seronegative arthritis. Rapid progression of pain and disability are consistent clinical features. The condition mainly effects the shoulder, knee, and hip.[108] Progression to complete joint destruction takes only 1–2 years. Most patients are elderly women.

Laboratory markers of OA

Several biochemical markers such as keratan sulfate and pyridinoline have been investigated but there have been difficulties with all of these systems.[109] One of the major problems is that

---

Radiological features of osteoarthritis

- Loss of joint space
- Marginal osteophytes
- Subchondral sclerosis
- Tibial spiking
- Loss of alignment

---

most of the body cartilage is in the intervertebral discs and costochondral junctions, and the joints that are affected by osteoarthritis form a small proportion of this total, and may develop only subtle biochemical changes in early disease. In addition, the concentration of cartilage degradation products depends on many factors, including rate of release of the compounds, diurnal variation, the route via which they reach the blood, and their distribution in the different body pools.

Imaging in osteoarthritis

X-rays are the main investigation (see the accompanying box). Several changes are observed. The most important are loss of joint space, marginal osteophytes, subchondral sclerosis, cysts, tibial spiking (in the knees), and loss of alignment.

Several scoring systems quantify the radiographic changes in osteoarthritis. The first one, developed by Kellgren and Lawrence in 1957,[110] grades the disease on a scale of 0 to 4 in comparison to a set of standard films. Later methods of grading have paid less attention to osteophytosis, which may be related to normal aging. In 1987 the American Rheumatism Association reviewed the radiographic criteria commonly used in the assessment of progression in the hand, hip, and knee.[111] It showed that in knee osteoarthritis early joint space narrowing and changes in subchondral bone were more significant indicators of progression than a lone osteophyte.[112] Joint space narrowing appears to be the most reproducible feature of knee osteoarthritis.[113]

POLYMYALGIA RHEUMATICA AND GIANT CELL ARTERITIS

Polymyalgia rheumatica and giant cell arteritis, which is also known as temporal arteritis, are related diseases that form two ends of a single spectrum. They are both diseases of the elderly population and their mean age of onset is 70 years, with a range from 50 to 90 years. Their onset is characteristically dramatic and many patients can give the exact date and hour of their first symptoms. Occasionally the onset is insidious and the symptoms may have been present for months or longer prior to the diagnosis.

Paulley and Hughes,[114] in 1962, were the first to link these two conditions, suggesting polymyalgia has many of the manifestations of temporal arteritis. Since then most authorities recognize the relationship between the two conditions.

Epidemiology

These diseases are relatively uncommon. One study from North America suggested the annual incidence of biopsy-proven giant cell arteritis between 1950 and 1985 in North America was 17 in 100,000 people aged over 50 years.[115] It was approximately three times more frequent in women. Studies from Europe suggest an incidence of 16.8 per 100,000.[116] In the UK the prevalence of polymyalgic symptoms in people over 65 years of age is approximately 330 per 100,000.[117]

Clinical features

Both polymyalgia rheumatica and giant cell arteritis are associated with fever, fatigue, anorexia, weight loss, and depression. Occasionally patients present with a fever.

Polymyalgia rheumatica The onset usually involves pain and stiffness in the muscles of the shoulder and neck. There is eventual involvement of the pelvic girdles in some patients. The symptoms are bilateral and symmetric. Stiffness is a predominant feature especially after rest or in the morning, and usually lasts for longer than an hour. Muscle pain is diffuse, movement accentuates the pain, and it can be worse at night. Muscle strength is usually unimpaired although the pain makes testing difficult. There is often an associated synovitis especially of the knees, wrists, and small joints of the hands. It is usually transient and mild and erosive changes are unusual. The arthritis may overlap with rheumatoid disease in an elderly person.

Giant cell arteritis Headache is a predominant symptom and is present in a majority of cases (see Chapter 47). It often begins early in the course of the disease and may be a presenting symptom. Pain is severe and localized to the temple; there may be associated scalp tenderness. Visual disturbance is described in about 25 percent of cases; visual loss is less common and can involve 5–10 percent, but blindness remains a significant risk owing to involvement of the ophthalmic artery, which is an end artery. Rare features of giant cell arteritis include hemiparesis, peripheral neuropathy, and deafness. Involvement of the coronary artery occasionally leads to myocardial infarction.

Investigations

The ESR is usually but not always elevated, so it is unusual to make the diagnosis of polymyalgia rheumatica or giant cell arteritis in the presence of a normal ESR. There is often an associated rise in the C-reactive protein levels and a mild anemia. Rheumatoid factor is usually negative. Biopsies of the temporal arteries should be undertaken in cases of giant cell arteritis and if there is diagnostic doubt. These will show the distinctive giant cell arteritis. However, skip lesions mean that a normal biopsy can occur despite the presence of the disease.

Treatments

Corticosteroids are the mainstay of therapy. A high dose of corticosteroids should be used in giant cell arteritis, 60 mg daily being a reasonable initial dose. A lower dose (10–15 mg daily) is used in patients with polymyalgia rheumatica. In both diseases the steroids should be gradually withdrawn over a period of 12–18 months. Not all patients respond to steroids alone. Sometimes symptomatic treatment with an NSAID is needed and in some cases an additional disease-modifying drug such as azathioprine or methotrexate can be used. There is some evidence that intramuscular depomedrone may control symptoms with less risk of adverse reactions in polymyalgia rheumatica than conventional steroids, and this is an area of ongoing research.

GOUT

Gout is a syndrome caused by an inflammatory response to the formation of urate crystals. These crystals develop secondary to hyperuricemia. Gout can occur in both acute and chronic forms.

The hyperuricemia may be due to environmental or genetic factors. Although it most frequently affects middle-aged males, there is an increasing frequency in elderly females taking diuretic tablets. The acute form is usually relapsing and self-limiting. The chronic form is associated with tophus formation and bone and joint destruction.

Epidemiology of gout

Hyperuricemia has been investigated in many populations. In males the prevalence of hyperuricemia rises steeply after puberty and in females after the menopause, although levels in women are usually lower than in men.[118] It is difficult to determine the precise incidence and prevalence of gout as it is a remitting and relapsing disease and patients frequently are misdiagnosed. It is rare in children and pre-menopausal women. It is uncommon in men under the age of 30, and the peak onset in men is between 40 and 50 years. In women it occurs later.

The epidemiology of gout is changing, with an increasing number of females having the disease. This is probably due to changes in lifestyle, drug therapy, and increased longevity. Gout remains the most common inflammatory arthritis in males over 40 years of age.[119] The prevalence of gout is between 5 and 28 per thousand males and between 1 and 6 per thousand females. The annual incidence is between 1 and 3 per thousand males and 0.2 per thousand females. The plasma urate concentration is the most important determinant of the risk of developing gout.[120] An important identifiable cause is concomitant thiazide diuretic therapy.

Clinical features of gout

Asymptomatic hyperuricemia is far more frequent than gout. The risk of gout increases with a rising level of serum uric acid. However, many years of hyperuricemia may precede the onset of acute gout and many individuals with hyperuricemia do not develop the disease. When there is a severe acute overproduction of urate, as for example occurs with cytotoxic chemotherapy, there is a high risk of acute gout.

Acute gout is characterized by the rapid onset of pain, its exquisite nature, and the swelling and associated redness around the affected joint. The classic presentation is in the first metatarsophalangeal joint and in time this is affected in over 80 percent of patients with gout. Many joints may be involved. The lower limbs are involved more frequently than the upper limbs. Redness over the affected joints is a feature that sets gout apart from most other noninfective causes of arthritis. The swelling can be very marked over the entire region. The natural history of acute gout varies: mild attacks may resolve within 1 or 2 days. More severe attacks may last 1 or 2 weeks. Approximately 90 percent of initial attacks of gout are monoarticular. Concurrent features are mild or absent.[121]

Sometimes gout presents early in its course with polyarticular involvement and it can then be easily confused with other forms of arthritis. In the elderly population, gout is often more indolent and is frequently mistaken for osteoarthritis, which results in a delay in diagnosis.[122] In elderly people, polyarticular gout can be the presenting feature of an attack, especially in elderly women. Acute gout can be precipitated by a variety of factors, including acute illness, trauma, surgery, and alcohol and drugs, which increase the uric acid concentration.

Incomplete resolution of acute gout normally indicates a concurrent arthropathy, especially osteoarthritis. However, a substantial proportion of patients with acute gout go on to develop a chronic phase of the disease. This is characterized by the formation of tophi. These are firm nodular or fusiform swellings that can occur at most sites of the body but are especially common on the hands and feet and around the ear. The inflammatory process in chronic gout is often mild although there can be supra-added acute episodes. Most of the disability is due to the presence of tophi that can become ulcerated and infected. Long-term problems with chronic gout are usually due to the deposition of tophi in the kidney or other sites; allopurinol therapy (see below) has a role in preventing such renal involvement.

Associated disorders Gout is associated with obesity, hypertension with diuretic therapy, excess alcohol intake, hyperlipidemia, and other vascular disorders. There may also be an association with diabetes mellitus.

Investigations in gout

The diagnosis of gout is based on identification of urate crystals in synovial fluid on polarizing light microscopy. This is usually undertaken on fresh synovial fluid. Occasionally material from a gouty tophus can be examined in a similar way.

Serum uric acid concentrations are usually elevated. It is very uncommon for acute gout to occur unless the uric acid level is high. On the other hand, an elevated uric acid level does not necessarily mean the patient has gout.

There are often characteristic features on radiography. During an acute attack there may be soft tissue swelling or effusions. Most characteristic features are large erosions that are classically called "punched out" and are some distance from the joint surface. In late disease, extensive erosive change may be difficult to differentiate from rheumatoid arthritis.

Treatment of gout

Therapy is directed towards controlling the symptoms in acute episodes, and preventing further attacks and complications in chronic gout.[123]

Acute episodes of gout normally respond to short-term treatment with relatively large doses of NSAIDs. An example is to give indomethacin 50 mg four times a day. Occasionally colchicine is used, but that is less satisfactory as it has a therapeutic dose relatively close to the toxic one: normally 1 mg of colchicine is given initially followed by 0.5 mg every 2–3 hours until the attack tends to settle or diarrhea and vomiting occur. An alternative approach is to give intra-articular steroids, which can be very effective in the early stages of gout.

Preventing further episodes of gout is normally achieved by allopurinol, which inhibits the enzyme xanthine oxidase. The dosage varies from 100 to 600 mg daily: it is usual to start with a low dose and build up. The initiation of allopurinol may lead to an acute episode of gout and it is conventional to start allopurinol at the same time as giving NSAID therapy. Allopurinol may make an acute attack of gout worse so it is used subsequent to control of the joint inflammation with NSAIDs. Rarely patients develop hypersensitivity to allopurinol. In these circumstances a uricosuric drug can be used, such as sulfapyrazone. Treatment in this situation is less satisfactory.

CALCIUM PYROPHOSPHATE CRYSTAL DEPOSITION (CPCD)

This disease is associated with calcium pyrophosphate dihydrate crystal deposition. Although it is usually sporadic, there are familial forms and it can be associated with other metabolic disturbances. It is predominantly a disease of the elderly population, presenting with an acute self-limiting arthritis that is termed "pseudogout." There is a strong association and overlap with osteoarthritis. It mainly involves the large joints such as the knees and wrists. There is a spectrum of pathology. In some cases there is only chondrocalcinosis, which is the deposition of calcium in articular cartilage, and is usually asymptomatic. In other patients there is more widespread deposition of pyrophosphate dihydrate and an associated synovitis develops. Thus, although many patients with pseudogout have chondrocalcinosis, the latter can occur by itself and be asymptomatic or it may be seen against the background of osteoarthritis.

Epidemiology

Chondrocalcinosis has a female preponderance and is associated with aging. It is rare under the age of 50 years. In those aged between 65 to 75 years it affects 10–15 percent of the population, and over the age of 85 years it affects up to 60 percent of the population.[124] The large population-based radiographic survey from Framingham,[125] which looked at a population ranging in age between 63 and 93 years, found an overall prevalence of 8 percent. No epidemiological data exist for pyrophosphate arthropathy, although it is generally thought to occur in the elderly with a female preponderance. Most studies show that the mean age of presentation is between 65 and 75 years. It is rare in younger cases although occasionally seen. There are many associated conditions, including diabetes, anemia, Paget's disease, and hypothyroidism. The strongest association is with hemochromatosis.[126]

Clinical features of CPCD disease

Pyrophosphate crystal deposition disease can present as an acute synovitis, as chronic arthritis, or as an incidental finding. The classic presentation is the acute synovitis of pseudogout, which is the most common cause of an acute monoarthritis in the elderly population. The typical attack develops with severe pain, stiffness, and swelling maximal between 6 and 24 hours after the onset. The patient often describes the pain as very severe. There may be overlying erythema. Examination shows a tender joint with signs of marked synovitis such as warmth, a large intense effusion, joint line tenderness, and restriction of movement. Fever is common and this can be marked. Elderly patients often appear unwell and mildly confused. The acute attacks are self-limiting and usually resolve within 1–3 weeks.

Chronic pyrophosphate arthropathy is also predominantly found in elderly and female patients. It mainly involves the knees, wrists, and shoulder joints. Presentation is with chronic pain, early morning and inactivity stiffness, reduced movement, and functional impairment. Acute attacks may be superimposed upon this chronic history. Symptoms are often restricted to just a few joints, but occasionally multiple joint involvement is seen. Affected joints usually reveal signs of osteoarthritis, such as bony swelling, crepitus, and varying degrees of synovitis. Knee joints may be warm with some tenderness, effusion, and soft tissue thickening.

Examination may show more widespread evidence of osteoarthritis. There may also be occasionally more severe inflammatory features and the presentation may develop into pseudo-RA, although the infrequency of tenosynovitis and the absence of extra-articular disease normally allows distinction.

Most patients present a benign course and a majority show stabilization of symptoms.[127] Occasionally, progressive severe destructive arthritis may occur, especially involving the knees, shoulders, or hips. This is almost entirely confined to elderly women, usually accompanied by severe night and rest pain and associated with a poor outcome.[128]

Atypical presentations include marked shoulder pain and stiffness that might suggest polymyalgia rheumatica; or severe spinal stiffness that may present with similarities to ankylosing spondylitis, tendonitis and tenosynovitis, bursitis, and even tophaceous or tumoral calcium pyrophosphate deposition.

Investigations

Aspiration of synovial fluid and identification of calcium pyrophosphate crystals on microscopy are the key to the diagnosis. The crystals can be difficult to see in some cases and it is usually best to examine fresh synovial fluid.

Standard radiographs show both the osteoarthritic pattern of joint destruction and calcification associated with crystal deposition disease. The latter occurs most commonly in fibrocartilage such as the knee menisci or triangular ligament of the wrist. It can also be seen in hyaline cartilage, particularly the knee and hip joints. Severe pseudogout can trigger a moderate acute-phase response with elevation of the ESR and acute-phase reactant such as C-reactive protein. The white cell count may also be elevated.

Management

The aspiration of synovial fluid in acute synovitis associated with calcium pyrophosphate crystal deposition disease can markedly improve the initially severe symptoms. Analgesics and NSAIDs are usually given and these also rapidly improve symptoms. Colchicine is effective but rarely warranted. For severe polyarticular attacks unresponsive to aspiration and injection, oral steroids may be considered although their efficacy is unproven. Once the synovitis is settling, active mobilization with attention to muscle training is worthwhile.

Unlike with gout, there is no specific therapy for chronic pyrophosphate arthropathy. Treatment of the underlying metabolic disease has little effect on outcome. The main objective is to reduce symptoms, and maintain and improve function. Exercise programs, a reduction in obesity, and building up muscle strength are all immensely valuable. If osteoarthritic joint damage is a particular problem, surgical replacement must be considered.

APATITE DEPOSITION DISEASE

Periarticular deposits of calcific material that are predominantly carbonated apatites or intra-articular deposits of a variety of basic calcium phosphates, also predominantly apatites, are seen in a variety of disease settings. Calcific periarthritis and the acute synovitis associated with apatite deposition have different etiologies and clinical courses but are united by the presence of calcium deposits in bone.

The presence of calcific periarthritis has been recognized for many years. However, the relationship between apatite deposition and joint diseases is more recent and was not described in detail until 1976.[129]

Epidemiology of apatite deposition disease

Calcific periarthritis is relatively common. In one large study of office workers, published in the 1940s, there was a prevalence of 2.7 percent of shoulder calcification.[130] Subsequent studies have found relatively similar high levels of shoulder calcification. There have been few studies of the epidemiology of articular apatite deposition mainly because the relationship between pathological and radiological findings and symptoms of arthritis or the presence of an arthopathy or acute synovitis is uncertain. However, that apatite particles were found in 30–60 percent of osteoarthritic synovial fluids may be of some pathological relevance.[131]

Clinical features of apatite deposition disease

Calcific deposits around the shoulder and elsewhere are often asymptomatic. They may be associated with a number of clinical syndromes. The most striking presentation is acute calcific periarthritis.[132] Over 70 percent of attacks occur around the shoulder, although other sites may be involved. The episode may be preceded by mild trauma or illness but is often spontaneous. Patients present with a sudden onset of severe pain described as "acute hyperalgia." Within hours there is often associated swelling that might be hot and red. There is extreme local tenderness. Movement around the shoulder is very limited. The condition appears to be initiated by a rupture of the calcific deposit leading to crystals being shed into the adjacent periarticular tissues. Sites other than the shoulder that may be involved include the greater trochanter, the epicondyle, the wrist, and around the knee.[133]

Our understanding of the relationship between intra-articular apatite crystals and clinical symptoms is poor. It is possible that the deposition of apatite in aging articular cartilage is relatively common and usually benign. In some patients there may be an acute synovitis associated with the presence of apatite crystals and this may be a causal relationship. Chronic monoarthritis is also sometimes seen. More commonly apatite crystals are associated with osteoarthritis.[134]

The most important potential relationship is with large-joint destructive arthropathies. In 1981, McCarty et al.[135] described this entity in some detail and used the term "Milwaukee shoulder." They suggested that the apatite crystals were implicated in much of the damage. Others subsequently confirmed this finding and suggested that "apatite-associated destructive arthritis" may be more descriptive. The clinical picture is characteristic.[136] Patients may or may not have a preceding history of chronic joint disease, they are usually over 70 years of age, and 90 percent are female. They present with a relatively short history over a few weeks and months of increasing pain, swelling, and loss of function of the affected joint which is usually a shoulder. Aspiration of the effusion reveals a large quantity of synovial fluid. It may be blood-stained and apatite crystals are found on evaluation.

Investigations

Plain joint radiology will show the presence of calcific periarthritis or associated changes within the joint. Aspiration and microscopy of the synovial fluid confirms the presence of apatite crystals. Other investigations add little, although alternative imaging modalities including MRI may be advantageous in due course.

Management

If calcific periarthritis or periarticular calcium deposits are found, asymptomatic individuals need no treatment. In an acute attack of calcific periarthritis, high doses of NSAIDs or even colchicine can be used initially. Local steroid injections also have a role, although their exact place is controversial as they may increase calcification and make recurrent attacks more likely. Patients with chronic arthritis and osteoarthritis who have apatite deposition must be managed in the same way as for the underlying condition.

The destructive arthritis associated with "Milwaukee shoulder" is a difficult management problem. Anti-inflammatory drugs, analgesics, and local steroids have all been used but they are often ineffective. However, as symptoms do appear to be reduced in a majority of patients over a few months, conservative and simple symptomatic measures may eventually allow a resolution of the symptoms to occur as part of the natural history of the disease.

DIFFUSE IDIOPATHIC SKELETAL HYPEROSTOSIS

Diffuse idiopathic skeletal hyperostosis (DISH), also known as Forestier's disease, is a ubiquitous condition that predominantly affects the spine. It is a chronic age-related condition characterized by new bone growth. There may be a stiffening peripheral arthropathy. Growth factors, particularly insulin, are implicated in its pathogenesis. It is mainly identified on X-rays, which reveal hyperostosis and an increase in bone mass generally. It is associated with diabetes, gout, hypertension, obesity, and anemia.

Epidemiology of DISH

DISH is rare before the age of 45 years. In Scandinavia the incidence is estimated at 700 per 100,000 person-years with approximately half the risk in women.[137] Prevalence rates suggest it involves approximately 10 percent of males and 8 percent of females over the age of 65 years.

Clinical features of DISH

DISH is diagnosed principally on radiological findings. It is characterized by new bone formation with an increased amount of normal bone, heterotopic bone formation, and the presence of new bone growth into the entheses, where tendons,

ligaments, joint capsules, and annulus fibrosus fibers insert into bone.[138] This is seen most commonly in the spine, especially the thoracolumbar spine. Other areas of the skeleton are involved, including phalangeal tufting and increase in size of the sesamoid bones.[139]

The deposition of new bone in DISH is often asymptomatic apart from increased stiffness in the neck, back, and peripheral joints. Pain may be present when there is a peripheral enthesopathy such as a calcaneal spur. The relationship between the radiological changes and the symptoms of pain is uncertain. DISH is often associated with degenerative hip disease and may modify the skeletal response to inflammatory and traumatic conditions.[140]

Investigations

DISH is diagnosed radiologically. Occasionally associated diseases may be diagnosed, such as maturity-onset diabetes or hyperlipidemia.

Management

In many cases of DISH no specific treatment is needed other than reassuring the patient. In patients where there is obesity or other problems, weight reduction may help. Local tender points can be treated by corticosteroid injections. This is especially true of patients with enthesopathies. Analgesics or anti-inflammatory drugs are of limited value.

SPONDYLOARTHROPATHIES

This group of diseases includes ankylosing spondylitis, reactive arthritis, the arthritis associated with Crohn's disease and ulcerative colitis, Reiter's syndrome, and psoriatic arthritis. These diseases principally involve young men and are rare in the elderly population. They are characterized by sacroiliitis and inflammatory back disease and the presence of oligoarthritis involving large joints and occasionally with an enthesopathy.

There are extra-articular features, such as uveitis or upper lobe pulmonary fibrosis in ankylosing spondylitis, and conjunctivitis and urethritis in Reiter's syndrome. Some elderly patients may have the end results of pre-existing ankylosing

---

KEY POINTS Arthritis in the elderly

- Arthritis is common in the elderly.
- The prevalence of osteoarthritis exceeds 30 percent of women aged over 75 years.
- The prevalence of rheumatoid arthritis exceeds 5 percent of women aged over 75 years.
- Arthritis causes substantial pain and disability and is a major factor in limiting quality of life.
- The treatment of arthritis is similar in elderly and younger people, although drug therapy requires greater caution in the elderly population.
- Aggressive treatment of inflammatory arthritis is effective in elderly people and there is no reason not to prescribe disease-modifying drugs for these patients.

spondylitis but it is very unusual for the disease to present in old age.

Psoriatic arthritis is more frequently seen in the elderly population but it still has a peak incidence under the age of 50 years. It is an inflammatory arthritis associated with psoriasis, has a variety of forms including a peripheral polyarthritis, which is a symmetric or inflammatory involvement of the distal phalangeal joints, and uncommonly a characteristic mutilating arthritis associated with telescoping of the fingers.

The treatment of seronegative spondyloarthropathies involves education and advice, analgesia, and anti-inflammatory medication, sulfasalazine and local steroid injections in some patients, and exercise programs in the majority of cases.

REFERENCES

1. Abrahams M: Three Score Years and Ten. Age Concern, London, 1977
2. Jenkinson ML, Bliss MR, Brain AT, Scott DL: Peripheral arthritis in the elderly: a hospital study. Ann Rheum Dis 1989;48:227–231
3. Zeidler H: Epidemiology of musculoskeletal conditions in the geriatric population. Eur J Rheumatol Inflamm 1994;14:3–6
4. Salmon M, Gaston JS: The role of T-lymphocytes in rheumatoid arthritis. Br Med Bull 1995;51:332–345
5. Bowness P, Bell J: T-cell receptors and rheumatic disease: approaches to repertoire analysis. Br J Rheumatol 1992;31:3–8
6. Zvaifler NJ, Boyle D, Firestein GS: Early synovitis: synoviocytes and mononuclear cells. Sem Arthritis Rheum 1994;23(suppl 2):11–16
7. Cutolo M, Sulli A, Barone A et al: Macrophages, synovial tissue and rheumatoid arthritis. Clin Exp Rheumatol 1993;11:331–339
8. Arend WP, Dayer J-M: Cytokines and cytokine inhibitors or antagonists in rheumatoid arthritis. Arthritis Rheum 1990;33:305–315
9. Dinarello CA: Interleukin-1 and its biologically related cytokines. Adv Immunol 1989;44:153–205
10. Larrick JW: Native interleukin1 inhibitors. Immunol Today 1989;10:61–66
11. Yocum DE, Esparza L, Dubry S et al: Characteristics of tumour necrosis factor production in rheumatoid arthritis. Cell Immunol 1989;122:131–145
12. Wong GG, Clark SC: Multiple actions of interleukin 6 within a cytokine network. Immunol Today 1988;9:137–139
13. Baggiolini M, Walx A, Kunkel SL: Neutrophil-activating peptide-1/interleukin 8, a novel cytokine which activates neutrophils. J Clin Invest 1989;84:1045–1049
14. Seitz M, Dewald B, Gerber N, Baggiolini M: Preferential production of interleukin-8 in rheumatoid arthritis. Clin Rheumatol 1990;9:569
15. Brennan FM, Field M, Chu CQ et al: Cytokine expression in rheumatoid arthritis. Br J Rheumatol 1991;30(suppl 1):76–80
16. Logan A: Intracrine regulation at the nucleus: a further mechanism of growth factor activity? J Endocrinol 1990;125:339–343
17. Wahl SM, McCartney-Francis N, Mergenhagen SE: Inflammatory and immunomodulatory roles of TGF-beta. Immunol Today 1989;10:258–261
18. Deuel TF, Tong BD, Huang JS: Platelet-derived growth factor: structure, function and roles in normal and transformed cells. Curr Top Cell Regul 1985;26:51–64
19. Springer TA: Adhesion molecules of the immune system. Nature 1990;346:425–434
20. Arnout MA: Leucocyte adhesion molecule deficiency: its structural basis, pathophysiology and implications for modulating the inflammatory response. Immunol Rev 1990;114:145–180
21. Rothlein R, Czajkowski M, O'Neill MM et al: Induction of intercellular adhesion molecule-1 on primary and continuous cell lines by pro-inflammatory cytokines. J Immunol 1988;141:1665–1669
22. Dougherty GJ, Murdoch S, Hogg N: The function of human intercellular adhesion molecule-1 (ICAM-1) in the generation of an immune response. Eur J Immunol 1988;18:35–40
23. Shimizu Y, Van Seventer GA, Horgan KJ, Shaw S: Role of adhesion molecules in T cell recognition: fundamental similarities between four integrins on resting human T cells (LFA-1, VLA-4, VLA-5, VLA-6) in expression, binding and costimulation. Immunol Rev 1990;114:109–143
24. Linck G, Stocker S, Grimaud J-A et al: Distribution of immunoreactive fibronectin and collagen (type I, II, IV) in mouse joints. Histochemistry 1983;77:323
25. Okada Y, Naka K, Minamoto T et al: Localization of type VI collagen in the lining cell layer of normal and rheumatoid synovium. Lab Invest 1990;63:647–656
26. Moreland LW, Stewart T, Gay RE et al: Immunohistologic demonstration of type II collagen in synovial fluid phagocytes of osteoarthritis and rheumatoid arthritis patients. Arthritis Rheum 1989;32:1458–1464
27. Miyake K, Underhill CB, Lesley J, Kincade PW: Hyaluronate can function as a cell adhesion molecule and CD44 participates in hyaluronate recognition. J Exp Med 1990;172:69–75
28. Lacy BE, Underhill CB: The hyaluronate receptor is associated with actin filaments. J Cell Biol 1987;105:1395
29. Worrall JG, Bayliss MT, Edwards JCW: Distribution of hyaluronan in rheumatoid synovium. Br J Rheumatol 1989;28(suppl 2):62
30. Doherty AJP, Murphy G: The metalloproteinase family and the inhibitor TIMP: a study using cDNAs and recombinant proteins. Ann Rheum Dis 1990;49:469–479
31. Cawston TE: Protein inhibitors of metalloproteinases. In Barrett AJ, Salveson G (eds): Protein Inhibitors. Elsevier, Amsterdam, 1986:589–610
32. MacDonald AG, McHenry P, Robins SP, Rid DM: Relationship of urinary pyridinium crosslinks to disease extent and activity in osteoarthritis. Br J Rheumatol 1994;33:16–19
33. Scott DL, Adebajo AO, El-Badaway S et al: Disease controlling anti-rheumatic therapy: preventing or significantly decreasing the rate of progression of structural joint damage. J Rheumatol 1994;41:36–40
34. Regan-Smith MG, O'Connor GT, Kwoh CK et al: Lack of correlation between the Steinbroker staging of hand radiographs and the functional health status of individuals with rheumatoid arthritis. Arthritis Rheum 1989;32:128–133
35. Yanagawa A, Takano K, Nishioka K et al: Clinical staging and gadolinium-DTPA enhanced images of the wrist in rheumatoid arthritis. J Rheumatol 1993;20:781–784
36. Jevtic V, Watt I, Rozman B et al: Precontrast and postcontrast (Gd-DTPA) magnetic resonance imaging of hand joints in patients with rheumatoid arthritis. Clin Radiol 1993;48:176–181
37. al-Janabi MA: The role of bone scintigraphy and other imaging modalities in knee pain. Nucl Med Commun 1994;15:991–996
38. Rydgren L, Wollmer P, Hultquist R, Gustafson T: 111-Indium-labelled leukocytes for measurement of inflammatory activity in arthritis. Scand J Rheumatol 1991;20:319–325
39. Deodhar AA, Brabyn J, Jones PW et al: Measurement of hand bone mineral content by dual energy x-ray absorptiometry: development of the method, and its application in normal volunteers and in patients with rheumatoid arthritis. Ann Rheum Dis 1994;53:685–690
40. Edmonds JP, Scott DL, Furst DE et al: Anti-rheumatic drugs: a proposed new classification. Arthritis Rheum 1993;36:336–339
41. Edmonds JP, Scott DL, Furst DE, Paulus HE: New classification of anti-rheumatic drugs: the evolution of a concept. J Rheumatol 1993;20:585–587
42. Mitchell JA, Akarascreenont P, Theimermann C et al: Selectivity of nonsteroidal antiinflammatory drugs as inhibitors of constitutive and inducible cyclooxygenase. Proc Natl Acad Sci USA 1993;90:11693–11697
43. Ballinger A, Kumar P, Scott DL: Misoprostol and the prevention of gastroduodenal damage due to non-steroidal anti-inflammatory drugs. Ann Rheum Dis 1992;51:1089–1093
44. Dieppe PA, Frankel SJ, Toth B: Is research into the treatment of osteoarthritis with non-steroidal anti-inflammatory drugs misdirected? Lancet 1993;341:353–354
45. Bradley JD, Brandt KD, Katz BP et al: Comparison of an anti-inflammatory dose of ibuprofen, an analgesic dose of ibuprofen, and acetaminophen in the treatment of patients with osteoarthritis of the knee. N Engl J Med 1991;325:87–91
46. Brandt KD: Should nonsteroidal anti-inflammatory drugs be used to treat osteoarthritis? Rheum Dis Clin North Am 1993;19:29–44
47. Otterness I: The value of C-reactive protein measurement in rheumatoid arthritis. Sem Arthritis Rheum 1994;24:91–103
48. Wilke WS, Sweeney TJ, Calabrese LH: Early, aggressive therapy for rheumatoid arthritis: concerns, descriptions, and estimate of outcome. Sem Arthritis Rheum 1993;23(suppl):26–41

49. Capell HA, Porter DR, Madhok R, Hunter JA: Second line (disease modifying) treatment in rheumatoid arthritis: which drug for which patient? Ann Rheum Dis 1993;52:423–428

50. Alarcon GS, Lopez-Mendez A, Walter J et al: Radiographic evidence of disease progression in methotrexate treated and nonmethotrexate disease modifying antirheumatic drug treated rheumatoid arthritis patients: a meta-analysis. J Rheumatol 1992;19:1868–1873

51. Dougados M: Cyclosporin in rheumatoid arthritis. Clin Exp Rheumatol 1994;12(suppl 11):S75–78

52. Forre O, the Norwegian Arthritis Study Group: Radiologic evidence of disease modification in rheumatoid arthritis patients treated with cyclosporin: results of a 48-week multicentre study comparing low dose cyclosporin with placebo. Arthritis Rheum 1994;37:1506–1512

53. Tugwell P, Pincus T, Yocum D et al: Combination therapy with cyclosporin and methotrexate in severe rheumatoid arthritis. N Engl J Med 1995;333:137–141

54. Corkill MM, Kirkham BW, Chikanza IC et al: Intra-muscular depot methylprednisolone induction of chrysotherapy in rheumatoid arthritis: a 24 week randomised controlled trial. Br J Rheumatol 1990;29:274–279

55. Hansen TM, Kryger P, Elling H et al: Double blind placebo controlled trial of pulse treatment with methylprednisolone combined with disease modifying drugs in rheumatoid arthritis. BMJ 1990;301:268–270

56. Kirwan J: The effect of glucocorticoids on joint destruction in rheumatoid arthritis. N Engl J Med 1995;333:142–146

57. Hall GM, Daniels M, Doyle DV, Spector TD: Effect of hormone replacement therapy on bone mass in rheumatoid arthritis patients treated with and without steroids. Arthritis & Rheum 1994;37:1499–1505

58. Symmons DPM, Barrett EM, Bankhead CR et al: The incidence of rheumatoid arthritis in the United Kingdom: results from the Norfolk Arthritis Register. Br J Rheumatol 1994;33:735–739

59. Silman AJ, Hochberg MC: Epidemiology of the Rheumatic Diseases. Oxford University Press, Oxford, 1994

60. Engel A, Roberts J, Burch TA: Rheumatoid arthritis in adults: United States, 1960–1962. Vital and Health Statistics, National Centre for Health Statistics, DHEW, series 11, no 17, 1966

61. Fleming A, Crown JM, Corbett M: Early rheumatoid disease. I: Onset. Ann Rheum Dis 1976;35:357–360

62. Fleming A, Crown JM, Corbett M: Incidence of joint involvement in early rheumatoid arthritis. Rheumatol Rehab 1976;15:92–96

63. Schumacher HR: Palindromic onset of rheumatoid arthritis. Arthritis Rheum 1982;25:361–369

64. Scott DGI, Bacon PA, Tribe CR: Systemic rheumatoid vasculitis: a clinical and laboratory study of 50 cases. Medicine 1981;60:288–296

65. Felson DT, Andersen JJ, Boers M et al: The American College of Rheumatology preliminary core set of disease activity measures for rheumatoid arthritis clinical trials. Arthritis Rheum 1993;36:729–740

66. Prevoo ML, van Riel PL, van't Hof MA et al: Validity and reliability of joint indices: a longitudinal study in patients with recent onset rheumatoid arthritis. Br J Rheumatol 1993;32:589–594

67. Stewart MW, Palmer DG, Knight RG: A self-report articular index measure of arthritic activity: investigations of reliability, validity and sensitivity. J Rheumatol 1990;17:1011–1015

68. Stucki G, Stucki S, Bruhlmann P et al: Comparison of the validity of self-reported articular indices. Br J Rheumatol 1995;34:760–766

69. van der Heijde DMFM, van't HofMA, van Riel PLCM et al: Judging disease activity in clinical practice in rheumatoid arthritis: first step in the development of a disease activity score. Ann Rheum Dis 1990;49:916–920

70. Davis MJ, Dawes PT, Fowler PD et al: Comparison and evaluation of a disease activity index for use in patients with rheumatoid arthritis. Br J Rheumatol 1990;29:111–115

71. Mallya RAK, Mace BEW: The assessment of disease activity in rheumatoid patients using a multivariate analysis. Rheumatol Rehabil 1982;20:14–17

72. Sharp JT, Lidsky MD, Collins LC et al: Methods of scoring the progression of radiological changes in rheumatoid arthritis. Arthritis Rheum 1971;14:706–720

73. Larsen A, Dale K, Eek M: Radiographic evaluation of rheumatoid arthritis and related conditions by standard reference films. Acta Radiol (Diagn) 1977;18:481–491

74. Grindulis KA, Scott DL, Struthers GR: The assessment of radiological changes in the hands and wrists in rheumatoid arthritis. Rheumatol Int 1983;3:39–42

75. van der Heijde DM, van Leeuwen MA, van Riel PL et al: Biannual radiographic assessments of hands and feet in a three year follow up of patients with early rheumatoid arthritis. Arthritis Rheum 1992;35:26–34

76. Scott DL, Coulton BL, Popert AJ: Long term progression of joint damage in rheumatoid arthritis. Ann Rheum Dis 1986;45:373–378

77. Fries J, Spitz P, Young D: The dimensions of health outcomes: the Health Assessment Questionnaire disability and pain scales. J Rheumatol 1982;9:789–793

78. Meenan R, Gertman P, Mason J: Measuring health status in arthritis: the Arthritis Impact Measurement Scales. Arthritis Rheum 1980;23:146–152

79. Fitzpatrick R, Fletcher A, Gore S et al: Quality of life measures in health care. 1: Applications and issues in assessment. BMJ 1992;305:1074–1077

80. Fitzpatrick R, Ziebland S, Jenkinson C et al: A comparison of the sensitivity to change of several health status instruments in rheumatoid arthritis. J Rheumatol 1993;20:429–436

81. Fitzpatrick R, Ziebland S, Jenkinson C et al: Transition questions to assess outcomes in rheumatoid arthritis. Br J Rheumatol 1993;32:807–811

82. Isomaki HA: An epidemiologically based follow-up study of recent arthritis: incidence, outcome and classification. Clin Rheumatol 1987;6(suppl 2):53–59

83. van-Schaardenburg D, Hazes JM, de Boer A: Outcome of rheumatoid arthritis in relation to age and rheumatoid factor at diagnosis. J Rheumatol 1993;20:45–52

84. Hassell AB, Davis MJ, Fowler PD: The relationship between serial measures of disease activity and outcome in rheumatoid arthritis. QJM 1993;86:601–607

85. Kaarela K: Prognostic factors and diagnostic criteria in early rheumatoid arthritis. Scand J Rheumatol Suppl 1985;57:1–54

86. Silman AJ, Reeback J, Jaraquemada D: HLA-DR4 as a predictor of outcome three years after onset of rheumatoid arthritis. Rheumatol Int 1986;6:233–235

87. van der Heijde DM, van't HofMA, van Riel PL et al: Validity of single variables and composite indices for measuring disease activity in rheumatoid arthritis. Ann Rheum Dis 1992;51:177–181

88. Emery P: Assessment of rheumatoid arthritis: a clinician's viewpoint. J Rheumatol 1994;42(suppl):20–24

89. van Zeben D, Hazes JM, Zwinderman AH et al: Factors predicting outcome of rheumatoid arthritis: results of a follow-up study. J Rheumatol 1993;20:1288–1296

90. Corbett M, Dalton S, Young A et al: Factors predicting death, survival and functional outcome in a prospective study of early rheumatoid disease over fifteen years. Br J Rheumatol 1993;32:717–723

91. Pincus T: The paradox of effective therapies but poor long-term outcomes in rheumatoid arthritis. Sem Arthritis Rheum 1992;21(suppl 3):2–15

92. Scott DL, Symmons DPM, Coulton BL, Popert AJ: The long-term outcome of treating rheumatoid arthritis: results after 20 years. Lancet 1987;1:1108–1111

93. Suarez-Almazor ME, Soskolne CL, Saunders LD, Russell AS: Outcome in rheumatoid arthritis: a 1985 inception cohort study. J Rheumatol 1994;21:1438–1446

94. Wolfe F, Mitchell DM, Sibleg J et al: The mortality of 3501 persons with rheumatoid arthritis in the ARAMIS data banks. Arthritis Rheum 1991;34(suppl):D109

95. Acheson RM, Collart AB: New Haven survey of joint diseases. XVII: Relationship between some systemic characteristics and osteoarthrosis in a general population. Ann Rheum Dis 1975;34:379–387

96. Croft P: Osteoarthritis: review of UK data on the rheumatic diseases. Br J Rheumatol 1990;29:391–395

97. Gardner DL: Problems and paradigms in joint pathology, review. J Anat 1994;184(3):465–476

98. Van Saase JLCM, van Romunde LKJ, Cats A et al: Epidemiology of osteoarthritis: Zoetmeer survey. Comparison of radiological osteoarthritis in a Dutch population with that in 10 other populations. Ann Rheum Dis 1989;48:271–280

99. Felson DT: The epidemiology of osteoarthritis: results from the Framingham osteoarthritis study. Semin Arthritis Rheum 1990;20(suppl 1):42–50

100. Wilson MG, Michet CJ, Ilstrup DM, Melton LJ: Idiopathic symptomatic osteoarthritis of the hip and knee: a population-based incidence study. Mayo Clin Proc 1990;65:1214–1221

101. Felson DT, Zhang Y, Hannan MT et al: The incidence and natural history of knee osteoarthritis in the elderly: the Framingham osteoarthritis study. Arthritis Rheum 1995;38:1500–1505

102. Bellamy N, Wells G, Campbell J: Relationship between severity and clinical importance of symptoms in osteoarthritis. Clin Rheumatol 1991;10:138–143

103. Doyle DV, Dieppe PA, Scott J, Huskisson EC: An articular index for the assessment of osteoarthritis. Ann Rheum Dis 1981;40: 75–78

104. Altman RD, Bloch DA, Bole GG et al: Development of clinical criteria for osteoarthritis. J Rheumatol 1987;suppl 14:3–6

105. McAlindon T, Dieppe P: Osteoarthritis: definitions and criteria. Ann Rheum Dis 1989;48:531–532

106. McAlindon T, Dieppe P: The medical management of osteoarthritis of the knee: an inflammatory issue? Br J Rheumatol 1990;29: 471–473

107. Cushnaghan J, Dieppe PA: Study of 500 patients with limb joint osteoarthritis. I: Analysis by age, sex and distribution of symptomatic joint sites. Ann Rheum Dis 1991;50:8–13

108. Rosenberg ZS, Shankman S, Steiner GC et al: Rapid destructive osteoarthritis: clinical, radiographic, and pathologic features. Radiology 1992;182:213–216

109. Brandt KD: A pessimistic view of serologic markers for diagnosis and management of osteoarthritis: biochemical immunologics and clinicopathologic barriers. J Rheumatol 1989;18:39–42

110. Kellgren JH, Lawrence JS: Radiological assessment of osteoarthrosis. Ann Rheum Dis 1957;16:494–502

111. Altman R, Asch E, Bloch D et al: Development of criteria for the classification and reporting of osteoarthritis: classification of osteoarthritis of the knee. Arthritis Rheum 1986;29:1039–1049

112. Altman RD, Fries JF, Bloch DA et al: Radiographic assessment of progression in osteoarthritis. Arthritis Rheum 1987;30:1214–1225

113. Cooper C, Cushnaghan J, Kirwan J et al: Radiographic assessment of the knee joint in osteoarthritis. Br J Rheumatol 1990;29:37

114. Paulley JW, Hughes JP: Giant cell arteritis or arthritis of the aged. BMJ 1962;15:62–67

115. Machedo EBV, Michet CJ, Ballard DJ et al: Trends and incidence in clinical presentation of temporal arteritis. Olmsted Country, Minnesota 1950–85. Arthritis Rheum 1988;31:745–749

116. Nordberg E, Bengtsson BA: Epidemiology of biopsy proven giant cell arteritis. J Intern Med 1990;227:233–236

117. Kyle V, Silverman B, Silman A et al: Polymyalgia rheumatica, giant cell arteritis and general practice. BMJ 1985;13:385–388

118. Mikkelsen WM, Dodge HJ, Valkenburgh Hiems S: The distribution of serum uric acid value in a population unselected as to gout or hyperuricaemia. Ann J Med 1965;39:242–251

119. Rubenoff R: Gout and hyperuricaemia. Rheum Dis Clin North Am 1990;16:539–550

120. Campion VW, Glynn RG, DeLabre LO: Asymptomatic hyperuricemia. Am J Med 1987;82:421–426

121. Lawry GV, Fan BT, Blueston ER: Polyarticular versus monoarticular gout; the prospective comparative analysis of clinical features. Medicine (Baltimore) 1988;67:335–343

122. Tear Borg EJ, Rasker JJ: Gout in the elderly: a separate entity? Ann Rheum Dis 1987;46:72–76

123. Wallace SL, Singer JZ: Therapy in gout. Rheum Dis Clin North Am 1988;14:441–447

124. Doherty M, Dieppe PA: Clinical aspects of calcium pyrophosphate dihydrate deposition. Rheum Dis Clin North Am 1988;14:395–414

125. Felson DT, Anderson JJ, Naimarka Cannel W, Meenan RF: The prevalence of chondrocalcinosis in the elderly and its associations with knee osteoarthritis: the Framingham study. J Rheumatol 1989;16:1241–1245

126. Hamilton EBD: Diseases associated with CPPD deposition disease. Arthritis Rheum 1976;19:353–357

127. Mayer RA, Bush DC, Harrington TM: Acute calcific tendonitis of the hand and wrists. J Rheumatol 1989;16:198–202

128. Pinals RS, Short CL: Calcific periarthritis involving multiple sites. Arthritis Rheum 1966;9:566–574

129. Dieppe PA, Huskisson EC, Crocker P, Willoughby DA: Apatite deposition disease: a new arthropathy. Lancet 1976;1:266–269

130. Boswood BM: Calcium deposits in the shoulder and sub acromial bursitis: a survey of 12,222 shoulders. JAMA 1941;116:2477–2482

131. Halverson P, McCarty DJ: Identification of hydroxy apatite crystals in synovial fluid arthritis. Arthritis Rheum 1979;22:389–395

132. Swannel AJ, Underwood FA, Dixon AStJ: Periarticular calcific deposits mimicking acute arthritis. Ann Rheum Dis 1970;29:380–385

133. Mayer RA, Bush DC, Harrington TM: Acute calcific tendonitis of the hands and wrists. J Rheumatol 1989;16:198–202

134. Deippe PA, Watt I: Crystal deposition in osteoarthritis: an opportunistic event. Clin Rheum Dis 1985;11:367–391

135. McCarty DJ, Halverson PB, Carrera GF et al: Milwaukee shoulder association of microsteroids containing hydroxyapartite crystals, active collaginase and neutral protease with rotator cuff defects. Arthritis Rheum 1981;24:464–491

136. Campion GV, McCrae F, Alwan W et al: Idiopathic destructive arthritis of the shoulder. Semin Arthritis Rheum 1988;70:232–245

137. Julkunen H, Heinoneno P, Knekt P, Maatela J: The epidemiology of hyperostosis of the spine together with its symptoms in related mortality in a general population. Scand J Rheumatol 1973;45:81–91

138. Littlejohn GO: More emphasis on the enthesis. J Rheumatol 1989;16:1020–1022

139. Littlejohn GO, Urowitz MB, Smythe HA, Keystone EC: Radiographic features of the hands in diffuse idiopathic skeletal hyperostosis (DISH): a comparative study with normals and acromegalics. Radiology 1981;140:623–629

140. Arlet J, Jacqueline F, Depeyre M et al: Le hanche dans l'hyperostose vertebrale. Rev Rheumal Osteoartic 1978;45:17–26

Chapter 72

Connective tissue disease

Anthony J. Freemont

The term *connective tissues* encompasses a wide variety of different body materials derived from mesoderm; they support mammalian organs and tissues physically and chemically.[1] The majority of connective tissues consist of a matrix of insoluble complexed proteins,[2] the most abundant of which is collagen, in which are embedded cells. The main connective tissues are bone, cartilage, fibrous tissue, smooth and skeletal muscle, and fat. By and large the proportional volume of cells to matrix is less than 50 percent. The one major exception to these generalizations is adipose tissue in which the apparent matrix, fat, is intracellular.

The age-related changes in connective tissues are described in Chapter 10 in this volume. These changes clearly contribute to the pathology of the tissue, although there must always be debate as to the relative contributions of "age-related"[3,4] and "non-age-related" phenomena to any perceived pathology; and indeed, whether an appearance should be assessed as being "pathological" relative to the "young normal" or "age-related normal."[5]

Diseases of three of the connective tissues—bone, articular cartilage, and skeletal muscle—together with some of the consequences of alterations in the connective tissue components of elements of the cardiovascular system, are described in detail in Chapters 30 and 68–71; blood and skin (of which connective tissue is an important part) are discussed in Chapters 98 and 100. This chapter concentrates on the common disorders of the connective tissues not already covered, and their associations with aging.

There is a very marked relationship between certain types of connective tissue disease and age. Most of the disorders of connective tissues have their highest incidence in the young and middle-aged. If they are not the cause of significant mortality, these disorders can continue into the older age groups; however, these are not the diseases specific to old age. The number of connective tissue disorders, or their variants, that characteristically have an onset in the elderly age group rather than any other age group is surprisingly small.

The reasons why certain connective tissue diseases arise in the elderly population are not known. There are as many anomalies. Why, for instance, should one form of fibroblastic proliferation, Dupuytren's disease, be common in the elderly age group, when another, keloid, is not? Why does the incidence and range of malignant epithelial neoplasms increase in this age group whereas the diversity of malignant connective tissue neoplasms is so low?

In this chapter only those disorders characterized by a peak age of onset in the elderly population are discussed. Coverage cannot be exhaustive or comprehensive, but important issues and diseases affecting elderly people are highlighted.

NONMETABOLIC DISEASES OF BONE

The major nonmetabolic diseases of bone are fracture, osteomyelitis, Paget's disease, avascular bone necrosis, and bone neoplasms.

Fracture (see also Chapter 73)

There is a higher incidence of metastasizing neoplasms in the elderly population. Such metastases often produce factors that stimulate osteoclasts leading to local osteopenia. This, together with the effects of osteoporosis, both in men and women, leads to a high incidence of pathological fracture in this age group.[6] These disorders are dealt with in more detail elsewhere.

Osteomyelitis

With age, the decrease in native immunity increases the risk of developing infection. Osteomyelitis is an infection in bone marrow that usually reaches the bone by hematogenous spread from a primary site elsewhere.[7] In the elderly population, as in other age groups, the most common organism causing pyogenic osteomyelitis is *Staphylococcus aureus*. Mycobacterial infections, particularly of the spine, are increasingly common.

The inflammatory process is destructive, giving rise to loss of bone and increased risk of fracture. Inflammatory cells produce digestive enzymes that destroy bone directly and stimulate osteoclasts. If the inflammation breaks out of bone, non-osteoclast-mediated tissue degradation may result in damage to adjacent structures, such as the intervertebral discs in the spine, and articular structures in the synovial joints.

Paget's disease

Paget's disease (see also Chapter 70) is a disorder of unknown etiology that causes an increase in the size of one or, rarely, more than one bone. Although sometimes classified with the metabolic bone disease, which are generalized skeletal disorders, it is this one characteristic of the disease that shows it as a separate entity. It is believed to develop slowly, manifesting itself predominantly in the elderly population.[8] Initially, perhaps in every case, there is a decrease in bone mass, which is only later followed by an increase. Only in the late stages do clinical features usually manifest themselves. Even then probably as few as 10 percent of affected individuals present clinically.

ETIOLOGY AND PATHOLOGY The incidence varies widely in Britain, being greatest in north-west England where at post-mortem as many as 10 percent of individuals over 70 years of age show histological changes of the disease. Histologically there is a generalized increase in bone cell activity that, in severe cases, leads to disruption of the normal lamellar structure of the collagen fiber arrays and uncoupling of osteoblastic and osteoclastic activity.[9] Together these two factors lead to the laying down of excessive quantities of weak bone. The bone marrow is very vascular and the normal hemopoietic marrow is replaced by fibrous tissue. By electron microscopy the osteoblasts are seen to contain viral particles, and modern research techniques, including immunohistochemistry and in-situ hybridization, have shown that all bone cells are infected by a virus (Fig. 72-1). There is considerable controversy over the nature of this virus, which has been identified variously as measles, respiratory syncytial virus, and canine distemper virus.[10] Recent studies have shown that the viral infection causes profound changes in the function of osteoclasts and particularly their responsiveness to interleukin (IL)-6.[11] The implication of these findings indicates that the disease process is driven by inadequately controlled osteoclasts that are driving themselves through a viral-mediated novel autocrine loop.

CLINICAL FEATURES, DIAGNOSIS, AND MANAGEMENT

The abnormal bone matrix leads to weakness that manifests as bone pain and fracture.[12] The increased bone cell turnover, particularly of the osteoblast lineage, causes an increased risk of developing bone malignancies, most commonly osteosarcoma. The high vascularity within the affected bone or bones can, particularly in an elderly individual and others with poor cardiac function, lead to high output cardiac failure.[13]

The excessive bone cell activity causes an increase in the serum alkaline phosphatase and urinary collagen breakdown products. The bone itself is thicker, both clinically and radiologically, and the skin over the bone is warm to touch. As the disease is driven by the osteoclast, symptomatic relief can be obtained by the use of drugs that suppress osteoclast function, notably bisphosphonates and calcitonin.[14]

Avascular bone necrosis

With the exception of the form of avascular bone necrosis that follows fracture of the femoral neck or the carpal scaphoid, there is no form of avascular bone necrosis that particularly affects the elderly population.[15]

CARTILAGE DISORDERS

Most cartilage is present within joints, either the articular surfaces of the synovial joints, or cartilaginous joints (e.g. the costosternal joints). The disease of these structures is covered in Chapter 71. Cartilage is present outside the joints mainly within the upper respiratory tract and the pinnae. There are few disorders of these cartilages, and the most common, chondrosarcoma and relapsing polychondritis, are not disorders specifically of the elderly population.

The cartilage does, however, change its physical properties with age. As the water content increases so the compliance decreases.[16] In addition there is progressive dystrophic calcification and even ossification that can affect the function and load response characteristics of these tissues.[17] Finally, crystals other than hydroxyapatite, such as monosodium urate and calcium pyrophosphate, can be deposited within this cartilage (see below).

DISORDERS OF FIBROUS TISSUE, LIGAMENTS, AND TENDONS

Disorders of fibrous tissue, particularly the organized fibrous tissues of ligaments and tendons, are very common. They include proliferations such as keloid and the fibromatoses; trauma, either to the structure itself or to its insertion into bone (the enthesis); myxoid degeneration (ganglion formation); and metaplasia.

Keloid

Because of the changes that occur in fibroblast function with age, keloid[18] is rare in the elderly population, even in those ethnic groups in which it is most frequently encountered.

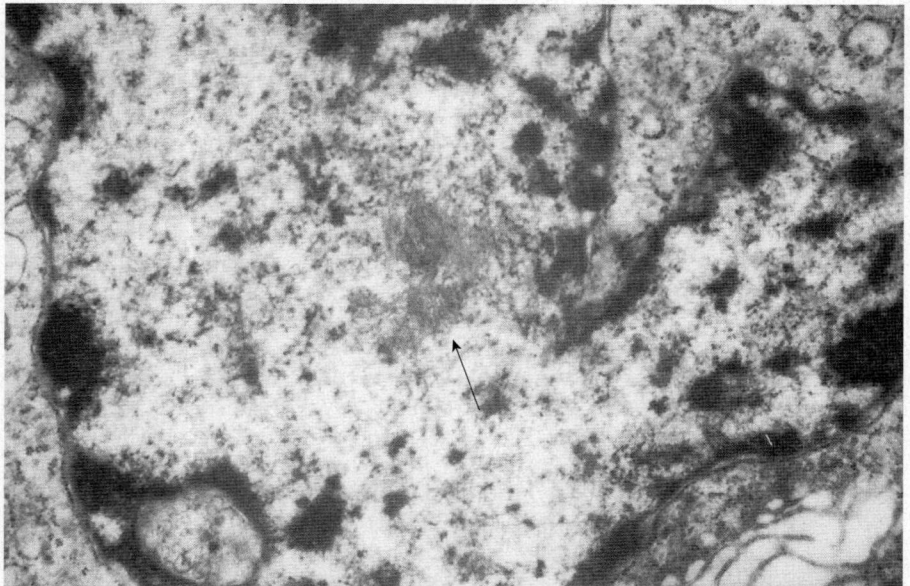

Figure 72-1 Osteoclast nucleus containing viral inclusions (arrowed) in Pagetic bone (×27,000).

The same applies to other fibrotic disorders such as Morton's metatarsalgia.

Dupuytren's disease

Dupuytren's disease[19] is a disorder in which there is a nodular proliferation of fibroblasts within the palmar fascia and its digital extensions, leading to dense collagen deposition, thickening and contracture within the fascia, and permanent deformity of the adjacent finger.[20]

ETIOLOGY AND PATHOLOGY   Many theories have been put forward to explain Dupuytren's disease. They include changes induced by mast cell and epidermal chemical mediators, alterations in the vasculature, and paraneoplastic changes in DNA. None has been unequivocally accepted.

Within the palmar fascia the fibroblastic proliferation is focal, leading to small nodules of very active fibroblasts (Fig. 72-2; Plate 72-1). The nodular proliferation flits from area to area of the fascia, resulting in a generalized increase in collagen deposition. As the collagen "matures," internal fiber cross-linking leads to an overall reduction in fiber length and consequent contracture.[21]

CLINICAL FEATURES, DIAGNOSIS, AND MANAGEMENT
The patient complains of a slowly progressive, painless nodule in the fascia that, as it worsens, shortens the affected ligament, causing further thickening and fascial contracture. Each fascial slip is attached to a finger and the contracture leads to a permanent flexion deformity of the digit.

The clinical presentation is diagnostic, as are the biopsy appearances. Surgical excision is the treatment of choice, but the potential progression of the disease is not affected. The pathogenesis is unknown, indeed puzzling, as the fibroblast proliferation is difficult to reconcile with the behavior of skin fibroblasts from older people, which divide more slowly than those from younger individuals in vitro. There are other forms of non-neoplastic proliferation of fibroblasts within fascia, such as nodular fasciitis, proliferative fasciitis, and plantar fibromatosis (Lederhose's disease), but they all typically affect younger people.

Trauma

One consequence of alterations in fibroblast function with age is abnormal deposition and polymerization of collagen.[22] In addition, with increasing age, there is fatty infiltration of ligaments. Together these factors predispose elderly people to an increased risk of complete and partial ligamentous tears. The general decrease in excessive physical activity counters this risk to some extent, as does the very high degree of cross-linking (and therefore increased strength) of the older collagen fibers.

Enthesopathies

Enthesopathy is the name given to a disparate group of disorders that occur at the entheses. The most striking of these are the inflammatory enthesopathies, seen in ankylosing spondylitis (AS)[23] and rheumatoid arthritis (RA).[24] Active enthesopathic AS is not a disease of elderly people, and RA is discussed in Chapter 71.

There are two other major causes of enthesopathy, hyperparathyroidism and trauma. Although the incidence of primary hyperparathyroidism peaks in elderly women, it is a mild form of the disease and the abnormal activity of the parathyroid glands is brought under control by an early resetting of the homeostatic mechanisms while the serum calcium is still within the normal range. There is therefore little of the bone erosion that is seen in the classically described histological feature of the disease. In more severe disease, hyperosteoclasis at the enthesis can weaken the insertion, leading to pain and ligament failure.

The changes in the collagen structure of the ligament/tendon and in the cartilage and bone at the enthesis make the incidence of partial or complete physical failure during exercise much higher in the increasingly fit elderly population.

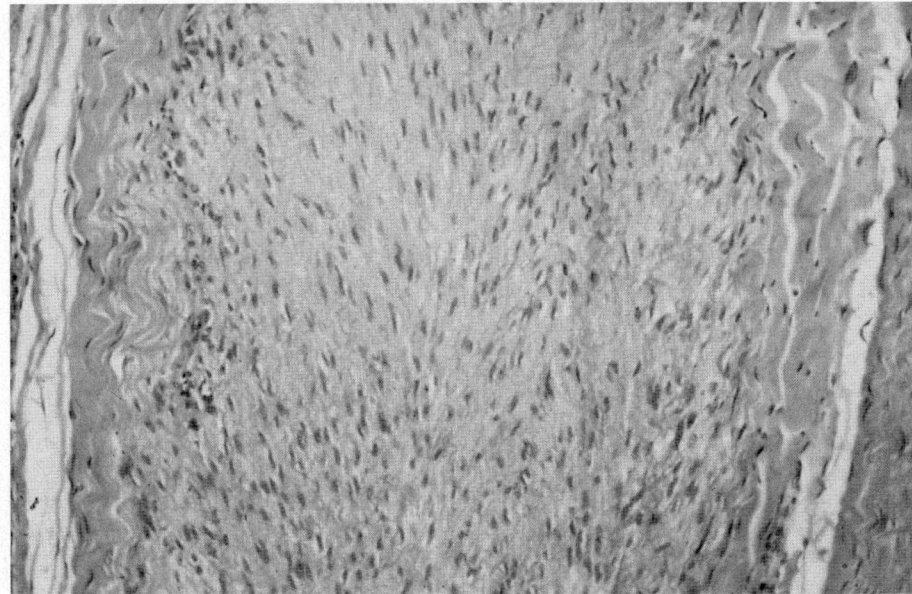

Figure 72-2 Cellular proliferation within a Dupuytren's nodule (H&E ×200).

Traumatic damage and even avulsion leads to a repair process, with development of bone outgrowths called "traction spurs" particularly at sites of maximum load—the insertion of the plantar fascia into the calcaneum, the insertion of the Achilles tendon, and the insertions of the long ligaments of the spine into vertebral bodies.

Elastosis

An increase in elastic fibers is a common feature of the skin of elderly persons.[25] It happens in other connective tissues, notably cartilage. Its significance in disease terms is not known.

Adipose tissue (see also Chapter 85)

The major disorders of fat, other than changes in its amount and distribution and the effects of trauma, are the inflammatory disorders, of fat itself and its septae known as panniculitis and neoplasms.[26] These are not disorders specifically of the elderly population.

NEOPLASMS OF CONNECTIVE TISSUE

The most common neoplasms, generally, of the connective tis-sues are secondary malignant tumors.[27,28] As the incidence of primary malignancies increases with age, so too does the number of secondary neoplasms within connective tissues. The bone, or more accurately the bone marrow, is a common site of secondary epithelial malignancies, most commonly from primaries in the breast, bronchus, prostate, bowel, thyroid, and kidney.

Hemic neoplasms, leukemias, lymphomas, and myeloma also metastasize to, or arise within, bone marrow and other connective tissues, where they may mimic secondary carcinomas. In bone tumor, cell production of cytokines stimulates bone cells (most commonly osteoclasts, but more rarely osteoblasts[29]), leading to local changes in bone mass. Increased osteoclasis leads to local bone loss and increased risk of fracture.

Although many benign and malignant connective tissue neoplasms are seen in the elderly population, only very rare primary benign and malignant connective tissue neoplasms have their peak incidence in this age group. Some, such as lipoma, persist if not treated, and therefore appear to increase in incidence with age, but there are others that are truly neoplasms of the elderly.[30] "Benign" neoplasms include atypical fibroxanthoma; malignant neoplasms include malignant fibrous histiocytoma, cutaneous angiosarcoma, and osteosarcoma arising in Paget's disease.

Atypical fibroxanthoma

Atypical fibroxanthoma is a neoplasm that occurs principally on the actinic-damaged skin of the head and neck of elderly persons. It is not really correct to place it with benign neoplasms as its local behavior and histological appearances are indistinguishable from malignant fibrous histiocytoma (see below). It responds exceptionally well to local excision.

Malignant fibrous histiocytoma

Malignant fibrous histiocytoma is the most common sarcoma of late adult life and is found predominantly in the skeletal muscle of the extremities or in the retroperitoneum.

ETIOLOGY AND PATHOLOGY Malignant fibrous histiocytoma can be caused by radiation, but most cases are idiopathic. The tumor varies in size depending on site and growth rate. It is typically solitary and multilobulated but may spread long distances along fascial planes (Fig. 72-3; Plate 72-2). It may be firm or myxoid and contains areas of hemorrhage and necrosis. Histologically it consists of spindle-shaped cells arranged in a cartwheel or storiform pattern with scattered multinucleate cells. The spindle cells have an indeterminate phenotype whereas the multinucleate cells react with macrophage markers. The cell of origin of this neoplasm has yet to be determined. Malignant fibrous histiocytoma metastasizes predominantly to the lungs (82 percent). The 2-year survival is 60 percent, but of the survivors one-third will be expected to have a recurrence or metastasis.

CLINICAL FEATURES, DIAGNOSIS, AND MANAGEMENT The patient usually presents with a painless swelling of a few months' duration. The diagnosis is suggested by magnetic resonance imaging and made by biopsy. Wide local excision is the treatment of choice.

Cutaneous angiosarcoma

Unlike other forms of angiosarcoma, cutaneous angiosarcoma primarily affects the elderly population.

ETIOLOGY AND PATHOLOGY The neoplasm arises on the head and neck, raising the possibility of sun exposure as a causative agent. The tumor consists of irregularly shaped

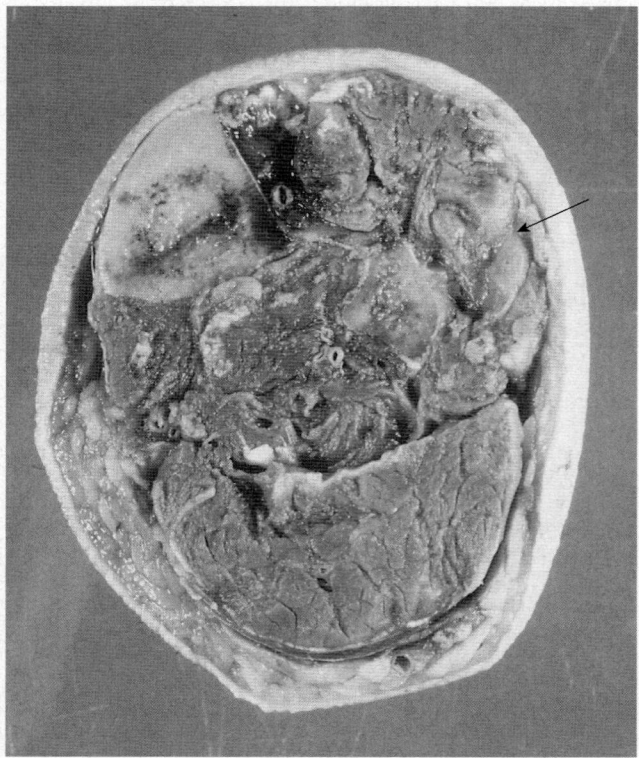

Figure 72-3 Macroscopic image of a malignant fibrous histiocytoma (arrowed) in the lower leg. Diameter approximately 5 cm. See also Plate 72-2.

vascular channels lined by atypical endothelial cells. About 40 percent of patients die of their disease. Metastasis is to the lung and liver.

CLINICAL FEATURES, DIAGNOSIS, AND MANAGEMENT

The neoplasm present as small nodules resembling blood blisters or blue–red macules. The lesions are often multiple and painless but may later ulcerate and bleed. The tumors respond only poorly to radiotherapy; but wide local excision, the treatment of choice, is often very difficult on the face, head, and neck.

Paget's sarcoma

Malignant change within a stem line occurs as a consequence of mutation within replicating DNA. The change of mutation is a function of the rate of replication of the stem cell line. In Paget's disease, excessive production of cytokines induces rapid stem cell recruitment, particularly in the cells of the osteoblast lineage. As a consequence the opportunity for malignant transformation of osteoprogenitor stem cells is high. Approximately 1 in 40 of all patients with Paget's disease will develop a sarcoma within the affected bone, and the overwhelming majority will be osteosarcomas.

IMMUNE-MEDIATED CONNECTIVE TISSUE DISORDERS

This group of clinicopathological entities is characterized by an immune response against "self-antigens," leading to damage to "connective tissues" and blood vessels in multiple organs, notably joints, skin, glomeruli, and large and small blood vessels. Pathogenetically all these disorders exhibit immune complex deposition, and/or formation, within affected organs (usually on basement membranes) and consequent tissue damage. The intriguing thing about these disorders is that the balance of the organs affected by the disease process varies from condition to condition, so that in rheumatoid disease the joints are most commonly and severely affected, whereas in polyarteritis nodosa it is the blood vessels and in systemic lupus erythematosus, the skin and kidney.

Clinically all the "connective tissue diseases" are associated with nonspecific constitutional disturbances coupled with patterns of organ involvement and circulating antigens that determine the clinical designation. The major members of this group are rheumatoid disease, systemic lupus erythematosus, the vasculitides (including polyarteritis nodosa and giant cell arteritis), systemic sclerosis, and polymyositis.

Like all autoimmune diseases they most commonly present in young adult women. Some, such as rheumatoid disease (discussed in Chapter 71), can present at any age and in the elderly population may have a different presentation and course from that in the young. Others, notably giant cell arteritis and polymyalgia rheumatica, present in the elderly population and are truly disorders of this age group.

Systemic lupus erythematosus

Although the majority of cases of systemic lupus erythematosus occur in young adults,[31,32] approximately 15 percent of cases present in those over the age of 60 years. The disease is characterized by the development of autoantibodies to nuclear antigens, especially double-stranded DNA and Sm. The antigens/antibody complexes form, or are deposited, on the basement membranes of the epidermis, joints, renal glomeruli, arteries, and the microvasculature in a variety of organs. Vascular injury and stimulation of the clotting mechanism lead to thrombosis and functional disturbances in the affected organ.

Disease starting in elderly patients is often insidious in onset and associated with a relatively high incidence of interstitial lung disease and a lower incidence of renal disease.

Vasculitides

The vasculitides are a group of disorders in which inflammation in the blood vessel wall leads to its damage, extravasation of vascular contents, and thrombosis. These disorders may be restricted to blood vessels or may be part of a broader spectrum of disease.[33] The vascular element may be classified in a number of ways, but the simplest is on the basis (1) of the type of vessel involved (artery, microvasculature, etc.), and (2) by the nature of the inflammatory cell infiltrate (lymphocytic, granulocytic, etc.).

The inflammation is believed to be caused by immune complex deposition in the wall of the blood vessel, but this is only infrequently possible to prove. Of the many types of vasculitis only one occurs specifically in the elderly population: giant cell or temporal arteritis.

Giant cell arteritis and polymyalgia rheumatica

Giant cell arteritis (see also Chapter 71) is a relatively uncommon disorder (approximately 1:1,000 over 60 years) manifesting as an arterial vasculitis with a predilection for the arteries of the head,[34] particularly the external carotid and the retinal branch of the internal carotid arteries, in elderly women (F:M = 3:1).

ETIOLOGY AND PATHOLOGY   The American College of Rheumatology has proposed diagnostic criteria.[35] Early in the disorder there is a leukocytoclastic vasculitis, so called because the vessel wall contains viable polymorphs and polymorph debris, evidence of complement activation, and generation of toxic polymorph products. Not only do polymorphs perish in this environment but so too do the smooth muscle cells of the arterial wall, leading to segmented mural necrosis. Later the distinctive but rarely seen picture of chronic inflammation with giant cells within the wall of the vessel appears. The giant cells are of two types including (1) immune-competent cells, primed to an unknown antigen, and (2) foreign-body type cells that are phagocytosing the internal elastic lamina. Thrombosis is commonly seen. The disease has a focal distribution within the vessel and, in any one location, a short time course. After the inflammation has spontaneously settled the vessel wall undergoes fibrosis; if extensive this can indicate earlier destructive inflammation. The presence of fibrosis and loss of the internal elastic lamina cannot always be taken as evidence of previous inflammation, however, because fibrosis of arterial walls is a "normal" finding in the elderly population.

The etiology of the vasculitis is not known. There is familial aggregation[36] and association with HLA DR4.[37] In the serum there are raised levels of IgG, total complement, C3, and C4.

Circulating immune complexes have been demonstrated in up to 90 percent of patients.[38] They have also been seen attached to the internal elastic lamina, perhaps by absorbence.

CLINICAL FEATURES, DIAGNOSIS, AND MANAGEMENT

Classically, but not universally, the patient complains of a severe headache, often in the temple. The external carotid artery is characteristically firm, tortuous, and pulseless (Fig. 72-4; Plate 72-3). The erythrocyte sedimentation rate (ESR) is elevated, arteriograms may be abnormal, and arterial biopsy sometimes shows the typical histological appearances. Biopsy is less commonly performed nowadays because the focal nature of the disease and sometimes nonspecific features make the diagnostic yield low,[39] and even if an abnormality is found there is poor correlation between the biopsy findings and disease activity.[40] Instead, response to therapy is used as a diagnostic test. Steroids are the treatment of choice and the symptoms settle rapidly on adequately large doses. Early management is seen as essential if the most feared complication, retinal artery thrombosis and blindness, is to be prevented.

Polymyalgia rheumatica

The local disorder, giant cell arteritis, is associated with a generalized condition known as polymyalgia rheumatica.[41] It is characterized by low-grade fever, weight loss, ill-defined pain and stiffness in the shoulder girdle, upper arms, and neck, malaise, and fatigue. Movement accentuates the pain, which is worst at night. Affected joints, particularly the knees and sternoclavicular joints, are actively inflamed. There is an increase in the number of cells within the synovial fluid and a normochromic, normocytic anemia. The ESR is very high but there is no leukocytosis. Tests for autoantibodies are negative. It also responds to steroids.

METABOLIC AND ENDOCRINE DISORDERS

Prominent among the metabolic disorders are the crystal deposition diseases due to the accumulation within connective tissues of monosodium urate and calcium pyrophosphate. Other metabolic products can accumulate in the connective tissues, notably abnormal proteins such as glycosylated proteins in diabetes, and proteins with a β-pleated sheet molecular structure, the hallmark of amyloid. Although there are many metabolic disorders, the following are the most common in the elderly population.

Gout

Uric acid is a breakdown product of purine metabolism.[42] Most is excreted by the kidney.[43] Alteration in uric acid excretion, either idiopathic or secondary to diuretic therapy, leads to an increase in monosodium urate in the blood and extracellular fluid and its precipitation in the tissues. Cartilage, particularly articular fibrocartilage and nonarticular hyaline cartilage, and subcutaneous connective tissue are the most common sites of its accumulation. Here aggregates of the crystals induce a macrophage response. These "tophi" may ulcerate. In elderly people, tophaceous or nontophaceous gout occurs either due to an idiopathic decrease in urate secretion, generalized deterioration in renal function, or the use of certain diuretics.

Calcium pyrophosphate deposition disease

Unlike monosodium urate deposition disease, calcium pyrophosphate crystals precipitate out most commonly within joints, notably fibrocartilage.[44] Their anomalous activation of either macrophages and neutrophils, and the disease so caused,[45] are discussed in Chapter 71.

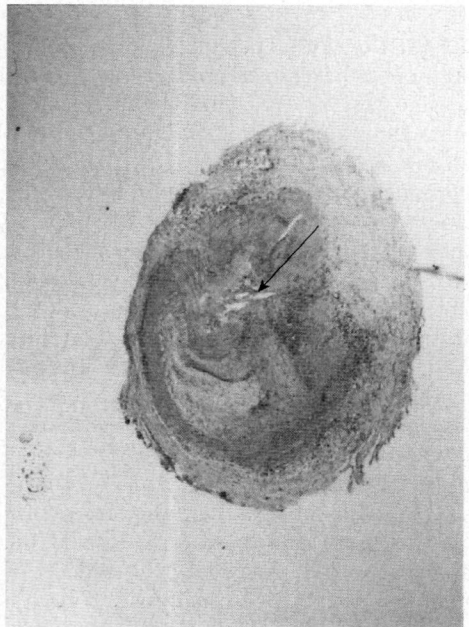 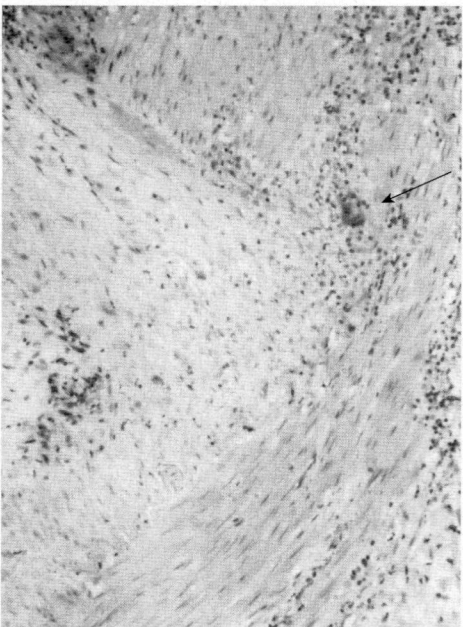

Figure 72-4 Artery from a patient with giant cell arteritis. The left panel shows (arrowed) virtual occlusion of the lumen (H&E, ×10). The right panel shows inflammation including giant cells (arrowed) in the wall (H&E, ×150).

Diabetes

The effects of diabetes on connective tissues are much the same as those elsewhere. Both by nonenzymic glycosylation and alteration of intracellular metabolism, diabetes results directly in the production and deposition of abnormal proteins. This is most prominent in bone in which structural and physicochemical changes in the matrix lead to deposition of an autofluorescent matrix. In addition, effects on the vasculature and nerves cause traumatic, infective, and infarctive events in connective tissues.

Amyloid

Proteins normally have a tertiary molecular structure in the form of an α-helix. In certain circumstances (including old age) the tertiary structure of a particular protein changes to a β-pleated sheet configuration.[46] In this form the protein is less readily degraded and therefore accumulates within the tissue. Certain proteins are more prone to undergoing β-pleated sheet configuration. Prominent among them are immunoglobulin light chains, the acute-phase protein (protein A), certain hormones (e.g. insulin and calcitonin), and—particularly in old age—a family of proteins similar to prealbumin and designated amyloid S. These accumulate most commonly in the myocardium, synovium, cartilage, ligaments, menisci, and brain. These proteins accumulate preferentially within the walls of blood vessels, leading to poor perfusion, and in connective tissues such as fat, and articular cartilage. Their unique protein structure means they take up certain histological dyes (such as Congo red) particularly well, and the parallel arrangement of these dye molecules attached to the β-pleated sheet makes the stained product birefringent.

The most common site for amyloid S to assimilate in the elderly is in cartilage and synovium and there is a strong association between amyloid deposition and osteoarthritis.

SUMMARY

The connective tissues are the most abundant in the whole body. Diseases of connective tissue can occur at any time of life and most present first during middle age. There are some that are specific to the elderly population, including Paget's disease of bone, Dupuytren's disease, malignant fibrous histocytoma, cutaneous angiosarcoma, giant cell arteritis and polymyalgia rheumatica, and senile amyloid, discussed here; and osteoporosis and osteoarthritis, two of the most common noninfective diseases in the Western world, which are discussed in other chapters. Many are significant causes of morbidity and even mortality.

KEY POINTS Connective tissue disease

- Connective tissues are found in every organ as are their diseases.
- Few diseases of connective tissues are restricted to the elderly population.
- The increased incidence of connective tissue diseases with increasing age is usually a reflection of the general changes in immune surveillance, environmental exposure, and senescence that underlie many diseases of old age.

REFERENCES

1. Wainwright SA, Biggs WD, Currey JD, Gosline JM: Mechanical Design in Organisms. Edward Arnold, London, 1976
2. Hukins DSL, Weston SA, Humphries M, Freemont AJ: Extracellular matrix. In Bitter EE, Bitter N (eds): Principles of Medical Biology. JAI Press, Greenwich, CT, 1995:181–230
3. Rehman MTA, Hoyland JA, Denton J, Freemont AJ: Age related histomorphometric changes in bone in normal British men and women. J Clin Pathol 1994;47:529–534
4. Hoyland JA, Jayson MIV: Age related changes in the structures within and bordering the intervertebral foramen: associations with low back pain. In Hukins DW, Nelson MA (eds): The Ageing Spine. Manchester University Press, Manchester, 1987:94–110
5. Freemont AJ: Bone histomorphometry. In Tovey FI, Stamp T (eds): The Measurement of Metabolic Bone Disease. Parthenon Publishing Group, New York, 1995:77–90
6. Hall BK: Fracture repair and regeneration. In Hall BK (ed): Bone, vol. 5. CRC Press, Boca Raton, FL, 1992:55–62
7. Freemont AJ: Inflammation. In Byers P, Salisbury J, Woods C (eds): Diseases of Bones and Joints. Chapman & Hall, London, 1994:126–162
8. Paget J: On a form of chronic inflammation of bones (osteitis deformans). Trans Med Chir Soc Lond 1877;60:37–63
9. Freemont AJ: The pathology of Paget's disease of bone. In Sharpe P (ed): The Molecular Biology of Paget's Disease. RC Landes, 1996
10. Mee AP, Dixon JA, Hoyland JA et al: Detection of canine distemper virus in 100% of Paget's disease samples by in situ–reverse transcriptase–polymerase chain reaction. Bone 1998;23(2):171–175
11. Hoyland JA, Freemont AJ, Sharpe P: Interleukin 6 (IL-6), IL-6 receptor and IL-6 nuclear factor gene expression in Paget's disease. J Bone Min Res 1994;9:75–80
12. Drake WM, Kendler DL, Brown JP: Consensus statement on the modern therapy of Paget's disease of bone from a Western Osteoporosis Alliance symposium. Clin Ther 2001;23:620–626
13. Rothschild BM: Paget's disease of the elderly. Compr Ther 2000;26:251–254
14. Theriault RL, Hortobagyi GN: The evolving role of bisphosphonates. Semin Oncol 2001;28:284–290
15. Pavelka K: Osteonecrosis. Best Pract Res Clin Rheumatol 2000;14:399–414
16. Hamerman D: Biology of the aging joint. Clin Geriatr Med 1998;14:417–433
17. Huber M, Trattnig S, Lintner F: Anatomy, biochemistry, and physiology of articular cartilage. Invest Radiol 2000;35:573–580
18. Haverstock BD: Hypertrophic scars and keloids. Clin Podiatr Med Surg 2001;18:147–159
19. Dupuytren G, le Baron: De la rétraction des doigts par suite d'une affection de l'aponeurose palmaire, opération chirurgicale qui convient dans ce cas. J Universal et Hebdomadaire de Médecine et de Chirurgie Pratiques 1831;5(2 ser):352–365
20. Mackenzie DH: The Differential Diagnosis of Fibroblastic Disorders. Blackwell Scientific, Oxford, 1970:44–49
21. Kloen P: New insights in the development of Dupuytren's contracture: a review. Br J Plast Surg 1999;52:629–635
22. Gardner DL: Pathological Basis of the Connective Tissue Diseases. Edward Arnold, London, 1992
23. Gran JT, Husby G: Clinical, epidemiologic, and therapeutic aspects of ankylosing spondylitis. Curr Opin Rheumatol 1998;10:292–298
24. Freemont AJ: The Pathology of Rheumatoid Arthritis. In Henderson B, Pettifer R, Edwards J (eds): Mechanisms and Models in Rheumatoid Arthritis. Academic Press, New York, 1995:83–114
25. Robert L, Jacob MP, Frances C et al: Interaction between elastin and elastases and its role in the aging of the arterial wall, skin and other connective tissues: a review. Mech Aging Dev 1984;28:155–166
26. Scharffetter-Kochanek K, Brenneisen P, Wenk J et al: Photoaging of the skin from phenotype to mechanisms. Exp Gerontol 2000;35:307–316
27. Huvos AG: Bone Tumors, Diagnosis, Treatment and Prognosis, 2nd edn. WB Saunders, Philadelphia, 1991
28. Enzinger FM, Weiss SW: Soft Tissue Tumors, 4th edn. CV Mosby, St Louis, 2001
29. McCullum P, Freemont AJ, Geary C, Liu Yin JA: A case of IgD myeloma presenting as diffuse osteosclerosis. J Clin Pathol 1988;41:486–489
30. Hartley AL, Blair V, Harris M et al: Sarcomas in North West England. II: Incidence. Br J Cancer 1991;64:1145–1150

31. Kammer GM, Mishra N: Systemic lupus erythematosus in the elderly. Rheum Dis Clin North Am 2000;26:475–492

32. Kono DH, Theofilopoulos AN: Genetic studies in systemic autoimmunity and aging. Immunol Res 2000;21:111–122

33. Cid MC, Vilardell C: Tissue targeting and disease patterns in systemic vasculitis. Best Pract Res Clin Rheumatol 2001;15:259–279

34. Horton BT, Magath BT, Brown GE: An undescribed form of arteritis of the temporal vessels. Arch Intern Med 1934;53:400–409

35. Hunder GG, Bloch DA, Michel BA et al: The American College of Rheumatology 1990 criteria for the classification of giant cell arteritis. Arthritis Rheum 1990;33:1122–1128

36. Liang GC, Simkin PA, Hunder GG et al: Familial aggregation of polymyalgia rheumatica and giant cell arteritis. Arthritis Rheum 1975;17:19–24

37. Gonzalez-Gay MA: Genetic epidemiology: giant cell arteritis and polymyalgia rheumatica. Arthritis Res 2001;3:154–157

38. Huang D, Zhou Y, Hoffman GS: Pathogenesis: immunogenetic factors. Best Pract Res Clin Rheumatol 2001;15:239–258

39. Nordborg C, Nordborg E, Petursdottir V: The pathogenesis of giant cell arteritis: morphological aspects. Clin Exp Rheumatol 2000;18:S18–S21

40. Nordborg E: Epidemiology of biopsy-positive giant cell arteritis: an overview. Clin Exp Rheumatol 2000;18(4 suppl 20):S15–S17

41. Hunder GG, Allen GL: The relationship between polymyalgia rheumatica and temporal arteritis. Geriatrics 1973;28:134–142

42. Agudelo CA, Wise CM: Gout: diagnosis, pathogenesis, and clinical manifestations. Curr Opin Rheumatol 2001;13:234–239

43. Agudelo CA, Wise CM: Crystal-associated arthritis in the elderly. Rheum Dis Clin North Am 2000;26:527–546

44. Rosenthal AK: Pathogenesis of calcium pyrophosphate crystal deposition disease. Curr Rheumatol Rep 2001;3:17–23

45. Fam AG: What is new about crystals other than monosodium urate? Curr Opin Rheumatol 2000;12:228–234

46. Bridger J, Wright NA: Amyloidosis. In McGee JO'D, Isaacson PG, Wright NA (eds): Oxford Textbook of Pathology. Oxford University Press, Oxford, 1992:406–412

Chapter 73

Orthopedic geriatrics

Jesse Eisler, Jessica Gallina, Erik Johnson,

Asit Shah, Karen Wu, and Elton Strauss

EVALUATION AND TREATMENT OF HAND, WRIST, AND ELBOW PROBLEMS IN THE GERIATRIC POPULATION

History

The evaluation of the patient with hand, wrist, or elbow pain begins with a careful history. The location, nature, and duration of pain should be evaluated, as well as any alleviating or exacerbating symptoms. The exact location of pain can be clarified by having the patient point with a single finger to the point of maximum tenderness. Radiation of pain can also be shown in this manner. Often the patient's use of anatomic terms is quite different from yours; misunderstanding is best prevented by having the patient simply point. The nature of the pain should also be described. Tingling, radiating, or burning pain is often due to nerve irritation, whereas a dull aching pain is more typical of tendinitis or osteoarthritis. Throbbing pain that wakens the patient at night accompanied by erythema and swelling is typical of infection, whereas night pain in the absence of obvious infection can be due to a neoplastic process. The duration of the symptoms must also be carefully assessed, particularly in relation to any trauma or new activities. Although a recent fall is easily recognized as a cause for symptoms, less obvious are new exercise regimens, hobbies, or changes in lifestyle. Activities that specifically worsen and alleviate the pain should be described or demonstrated. Inquiries should be made concerning the presence of similar symptoms in the past; patients will often surprisingly forget to mention that they had the exact problem 10 years ago, or more recently on the other side. Finally, ask about neck pain, as problems in the hand or elbow may be due to a cervical etiology.

Physical examination

The physical examination of the upper extremity is similar to a general physical examination in that a specific order should be followed. Establishing a routine promotes efficiency and also prevents inadvertent omissions of portions of the exam. One should create a screening exam to which more detailed and pertinent examination techniques may be added depending on positive findings and the patient's specific complaint.

Begin with inspection of the involved area. Note changes in the color and texture of the skin, as well as swelling, erythema, ecchymosis, and muscle atrophy. It is useful to compare the affected side to the normal limb. Inspection leads to the evaluation of circulation. Begin by examining the fingertips and assessing color and capillary refill. Capillary refill should be approximately 1 second; faster or slower times can indicate

venous and arterial insufficiency, respectively. The radial and ulnar arteries should also be palpated. A normal ulnar pulse may not be palpable. The Allen's test can assess ulnar artery contribution to hand circulation. With the patient's fist clenched to exsanguinate the hand, occlude the radial and ulnar arteries by applying pressure with your fingers. When the patient opens his or her hand, it should be blanched. Release of the ulnar artery should lead to quick reperfusion of the hand (noticeable by color change) if ulnar artery supply is intact. Checking the circulation is often forgotten; doing it early helps to prevent this oversight.

Testing of sensation should also begin in the fingertips. It can be tested quickly in a gross fashion by gently stroking the patient's fingers and asking if it feels "normal" or "funny." Alternatively, ask the patient if it feels the "same" or "different" from testing of the unaffected side. It is often difficult for the patient to verbalize numbness or parasthesias more specifically. Abnormalities should be quantified by testing two-point discrimination on both the radial and ulnar aspects of the finger pulp. Normally, a patient should be able to differentiate between two points on the fingertip that are 1 cm apart. Unbend a paper clip so that its two ends are 1 cm apart. Touch the patient's fingertip with either one or two and ask the patient if he or she feels one or two points. You should also determine if sensory complaints are consistent with specific nerve dermatomes. In general, the sensory distribution of the radial nerve includes the dorsum of the radial side of the hand, thumb, index, middle, and radial half of the ring fingers. The median nerve supplies the palmar surfaces of these structures. The ulnar nerve supplies the ulnar side of the hand, 5th finger, and the ulnar half of the ring finger.

The motor examination should measure individual muscle strength as well as the deep tendon reflexes. Active and passive range of motion should also be performed. Finger flexion can be quickly recorded by measuring the distance from the fingertip to the distal palmar crease. When measuring the range of motion of the wrist and elbow, one should remember to include supination and pronation in addition to flexion and extension. A passive range of motion greater than the active range of motion can indicate tendon rupture, whereas decrease in both active and passive range of motion is suggestive of contracture.

Next proceed to palpation of bony and soft tissue structures. Here again the single finger method is useful. It forces the physician to be both accurate and gentle. Masses should be looked for, and if found carefully described as to location, size, and firmness. Mobility in relation to underlying structures is also important, including assessment if a mass appears to move with tendon excursion.

Further work-up

After the history and physical examination, the diagnosis will be apparent in the majority of cases. Further studies may be necessary if the diagnosis remains unknown, or to assist in the planning of treatment. Radiographs are usually the first step in imaging. In cases of trauma with suspected fracture, radiographs are obviously indicated. Further studies such as bone scans, computed tomography (CT), magnetic resonance imaging (MRI), or electromyogram (EMG) are more appropriately ordered by the specialist. These studies for the large part should be used to confirm or rule out specific diagnoses from a short differential list, which has already been formulated. Or they can provide additional information, for example visualizing details, which help with operative planning. Some of the more common uses of these studies are as follows:

- Bone scan: diagnosis of nondisplaced scaphoid fracture, avascular necrosis of the lunate, suspicion of metastatic disease (whole body scan).
- CT: occasionally for complex intra-articular distal radius fracture. Also for bony tumors.
- MRI: used for ligamentous and triangular fibrocartilage injuries of the wrist. Also for soft tissue tumors.
- EMG: commonly ordered to confirm carpal tunnel syndrome or help determine the location of a neurological lesion.

Treatment

Although the treatment of hand, wrist, and elbow disorders is beyond the scope of this text, a description of the more commonly encountered problems will help illustrate some of the options and dilemmas faced by the hand surgeon.

Fracture

Distal radius fractures are the most common upper extremity fracture in elderly people, with approximately 250,000 annually in the US. These represent a pathological fracture due to osteoporosis, which increases the difficulty of treating these injuries. Historically, treatment of distal radius fractures in elderly patients consisted of closed reduction and casting, based on the belief that good clinical outcomes were obtained even with malunion. However, it is now recognized that the final outcome regarding pain, range of motion, and function are directly related to the adequacy of not initial, but final reduction. This point is critical, as almost all fractures can be temporarily reduced and placed in plaster. However, due to the compressive and comminuted nature of these fractures in osteoporotic bone, collapse in the cast is practically inevitable. Techniques to combat this now include percutaneous pinning, external fixation, open reduction and internal fixation, and bone grafting. These modalities can be used in almost any combination depending on the individual patient. Although the current trend is toward more aggressive fixation, how much is too much is yet to be answered. Finally, one should not forget that treatment of these fractures includes medical treatment of the osteoporosis.

Carpal tunnel syndrome

Carpal tunnel syndrome is due to compression of the median nerve in the carpal tunnel. Increased public awareness of carpal tunnel syndrome has given rise to a large number of patients who present with a "chief complaint" of carpal tunnel syndrome. One must confirm that the patient's signs and symptoms are consistent with median nerve deficits at the level of the carpal tunnel. Other neurological findings indicate a more proximal problem. Initial complaints of carpal tunnel syndrome include numbness and tingling in the thumb, index, and middle fingers. Eventually, thenar muscle atrophy can result. Patients will often note dropping tea or coffee cups due to the sensory and motor changes. Patients also typically have worsening of symptoms at night. This is due to the usual flexed or extended position of the wrist while sleeping, both of which greatly increase carpal tunnel pressure. Phalen's test and Tinel's sign are helpful physical exam tests. To perform Phalen's test, hold the wrist in maximal flexion. The development of paresthesias in the median nerve distribution of the hand is suggestive of carpal tunnel syndrome. A positive Tinel's sign is the production of median nerve parasthesias with lightly tapping over the median nerve in the carpal tunnel at the base of the palm. EMG is usually not indicated, but may be helpful with atypical presentations. Initial treatment consists of nonsteroid anti-inflammatory drugs (NSAIDs) to reduce presumed tenosynovitis, activity modification, and wrist splinting in the neutral position. Steroid injections have obtained mixed long-term results; however, most agree that a good short-term response to injection is an excellent prognostic indicator of surgical release. Surgical carpal tunnel release is indicated after conservative measures have failed. Additionally, if there are signs of thenar atrophy at initial presentation, surgical release should not be delayed, as return of motor function is poor.

Tenosynovitis: trigger finger

Patients often present with a combination of carpal tunnel syndrome and trigger finger, as both are usually due to tenosynovitis. In the trigger finger, a portion of the flexor tendon becomes enlarged so that it barely fits through the A1 pulley located at the metacarpophalangeal (MCP) joint. This enlargement can be palpated and is often tender. The strong finger flexors are able to pull the enlarged portion of the tendon through the tight tunnel, but the weak extensor tendons cannot pull it back through, resulting in a finger stuck in flexion. The patient will report either the need to strenuously extend the finger or to open the finger with the other hand, usually with a painful popping sensation. Patients will sometimes only complain of pain in the region of the proximal interphalangeal (PIP) joint; specific questions can lead to the diagnosis. Permanent relief can be obtained with steroid injection; however, surgical release is sometimes necessary.

Tenosynovitis: De Quervain's

De Quervain's tenosynovitis affects the first extensor tendon compartment, through which run the abductor pollicis longus and extensor pollicis brevis tendons. Patients present with pain over the distal lateral aspect of the radius, worsened by active wrist extension and radial deviation. Finkelstein's test (placing the thumb in fist and the wrist in ulnar deviation) also reproduces pain in this area. Initial treatment consists of thumb and wrist bracing, occupational therapy, and steroid injection. Surgical release of the tendon compartment is indicated for recalcitrant cases.

Dupuytren's disease

Dupuytren's disease is a fibromatosis of the palmar fascia leading to finger contracture. It typically presents with painless progressive flexion contracture of the ring or small finger, although it can involve all fingers. Palpable nodules and cords are present. Family history may be positive. The disease is found more commonly in men, smokers, diabetics, and those with liver disease. Steroid injection can be used, but the standard treatment is surgical excision of the diseased fascia. Surgical intervention is indicated when metacarpophalangeal joint contracture reaches 30 degrees or there is any proximal interphalangeal joint contracture present.

Osteoarthritis

The chief complaint in osteoarthritis is pain with activity. The two most common sites of osteoarthritis in the upper extremity are the thumb carpometacarpal (CMC) or basal joint, and the distal interphalangeal (DIP) joints. Radiographs are diagnostic, with the presence of subchondral sclerosis, subchondral cysts, joint interval narrowing, and osteophytes. Initial treatment is symptomatic, with acetaminophen or NSAIDs and activity adjustment. Splints can be effective in basal joint arthritis. Treatment for failure of conservative therapy of the DIP joints usually consists of fusion. For the basal joint, partial or complete resection of the trapezium with ligament reconstruction and/or tendon interposition can be performed. Silicone implants have fallen out of favor in osteoarthritis, although they still play a role in rheumatoid arthritis.

Osteoarthritis can also affect the elbow. The usual presenting symptoms are pain and flexion contracture. Medical treatment as described above also applies here. Additionally, there is a growing role for arthroscopy in the treatment of osteoarthritis of the elbow. Debridement, removal of loose bodies and osteophytes, olecranon fossa fenestration, and capsular release can all be achieved via arthroscopy. Studies have shown successful improvement in pain as well as an average of 20–30 degrees increase in range of motion with these arthroscopic techniques;[1] however, elbow arthroscopy is a technically demanding procedure. Although safe and effective, arthroscopy requires training and experience, it is gaining in popularity in treating osteoarthritis of the elbow.[2,3] Interest is fueled by recent reports of positive outcomes and the need for more treatment modalities due to the limitations of total elbow arthroplasty. Because of the high complication rate of elbow arthroplasty, it is more commonly indicated for treatment of rheumatoid arthritis and is discussed in the section below.

Rheumatoid arthritis

Rheumatoid arthritis, like osteoarthritis, presents with pain. Characteristic complaints are of morning pain and stiffness caused by synovitis. With disease progression, the rheumatoid synovium invades and destroys surrounding tendons, ligaments, cartilage, and bone. Deformity results. Radiographic findings also differ from osteoarthritis. There is generalized osteopenia, periarticular bone erosion and subluxation or even dislocation of joints.

Treatment is based on pharmacological control of the disease, bracing, and physical therapy. Surgical treatment is aimed at both preventing deformity and correcting deformity already present. Routinely, initial procedures involve the removal of synovium surrounding joints and tendons. The goal is to alleviate pain, prevent further destruction, and restore function.

In contrast to osteoarthritis, the PIP and MCP joints are most commonly involved in the rheumatoid hand. Ulnar deviation of the digits at the MCP joints is the most common deformity. Patients also frequently develop swan neck or boutonniere deformities of the fingers. Treatment of the deformities in the fingers and thumb is by a combination of fusion, occasional silicone arthroplasty, and ligament and tendon rebalancing.

In the wrist, synovitis commonly is found around the extensor tendons. Often a transverse indentation in the swelling can be seen on the dorsum of the wrist. This is due to the restraining effect of the dorsal retinaculum. Extensor tendon damage may be caused by direct invasion of the synovium and by fraying over the dorsally displaced ulna. (This migration of the ulna occurs as synovium also destroys ligaments of the distal radioulnar joint.) As a result, the most common pattern of extensor tendon involvement is the small finger first, followed by the ring, middle, and index fingers. A single extensor tendon rupture may present with only a mild extension lag due to the juncturae tendinea; however, subsequent ruptures will result in a more marked loss of range of motion and function. Function can be restored by performing tendon transfers, but this becomes increasingly difficult with increasing number of tendon ruptures. It is preferable to perform tenosynovectomy prior to tendon rupture. Thus, failure to control the synovitis with medical therapy over a period of 6 months is an indication for synovectomy.[4] If dorsal migration of the ulna is present, this must also be addressed in order to prevent future tendon damage.

Synovitis surrounding the flexor tendons presents with pain, symptoms of median nerve compression, and loss of motion. The swelling usually is not as prominent as on the dorsum of the wrist, and only a slight loss of the skin creases may be seen. Flexor tendon ruptures occur less commonly than extensor tendon ruptures. Most often the thumb and index finger are involved due to fraying over bony spur on the scaphoid. Treatment consists of synovectomy, tendon repair or transfer, and removal of any offending bony spurs.[5]

Synovectomy of the wrist joints themselves remains somewhat more controversial. Although tenosynovectomy prevents tendon rupture, synovectomy of the wrist joints has not been firmly shown to prevent the progressive destruction of the joint, and has also been found by some to result in a loss of range of motion.[5,6] However, it is generally agreed that for synovitis not responsive to medical treatment, in the presence of minimal cartilage and bone destruction, synovectomy will provide significant pain relief.[6–8]

Once significant cartilage and bone destruction have occurred, surgical options include arthrodesis and arthroplasty. Each of these options has several variations with specific advantages and disadvantages. Although wrist fusion gives a stable and pain-free wrist, bilateral wrist fusions in the rheumatoid patient can cause significant difficulty with activities of daily living. Partial fusions are another option. Because the pattern of joint destruction frequently shows severe radiocarpal disease with maintenance of the midcarpal joint, a fusion of just the radiocarpal joint leaving the midcarpal joint intact will relieve pain, yet retain 25–50 percent of wrist motion.

Numerous other partial fusions may also be performed, the concept being to limit fusion to the diseased joints while preserving motion in the healthier joints.

Joint replacements have taken the form of either silicone or metal and plastic implants. While retaining motion, significant problems have been encountered. These include silicone synovitis, dislocation and breakage of the implants, progression of bone destruction, and infection. In addition, candidates must have adequate bone stock for the implant and functioning wrist extensors. High-demand patients also do more poorly after joint replacement. This must be kept in mind in a population that may require ambulatory aids. Silicone wrist implants have shown disappointing long-term results. Many surgeons now recommend their use only in very low-demand patients who specifically require wrist motion, for example patients who have bilateral wrist disease or significant loss of motion in their elbows and shoulders such that further loss of motion with wrist fusion would compromise function. In the patient with failed wrist arthroplasty, wrist fusion remains as a salvage procedure.

The elbow is affected in 20–50 percent of patients with rheumatoid arthritis. Initial presentation is with synovitis causing pain, swelling, and loss of range of motion. Synovitis may cause so much swelling as to cause compression of surrounding structures, including the posterior interosseus and ulnar nerves.[9] Synovectomy prior to evidence of bone and ligament involvement has shown good relief of pain for 5 years in 70–80 percent of patients.[10–12] Some patients will also show some improvement in the range of motion. There is some controversy regarding the use of synovectomy in patients with joint destruction; although increases in the range of motion cannot be expected, many have reported significant pain relief in this group of patients.[11,12] Radial head excision at the time of synovectomy is also a point of controversy.[13] It is advocated by some to both improve exposure and to prevent future painful supination and pronation due to radiohumeral joint destruction.[14] Others have proposed that removal of the radial head will destabilize the elbow, and with newer arthroscopic techniques, is unnecessary to facilitate adequate synovectomy.[15] Patients with more severe joint destruction and instability or stiffness are candidates for one of the forms of arthroplasty.

Arthroplasty in the elbow can be performed using interposition of biological material, nonconstrained metal components, or semiconstrained metal and plastic prostheses. A requirement for interpositional arthroplasty is adequate bone stock; this is often not present in the rheumatoid. Prosthetic replacement results in pain relief in more than 90 percent of patients. Functional range of motion is also a predictable outcome. However, total elbow arthroplasty has considerable limitations. Complications include loosening, infection, neuropraxia, and instability. Although results have improved with new prosthetic designs, loosening rates are still reported in 9–30 percent of patients. Infection rates of 3–36 percent are reported, due partly to the subcutaneous nature of the joint. Neuropraxias of the ulnar nerve are seen in 7–26 percent of patients. Instability is found in about 5 percent of patients.[16–19] Complication rate is much higher and lifespan much more limited than that of total hip and knee arthroplasty. For the properly selected patient, total elbow arthroplasty can be confidently predicted to provide relief of pain and a functional range of motion.

EVALUATION AND TREATMENT OF GERIATRIC DISORDERS OF THE SHOULDER

This section discusses the relatively common conditions of osteoarthritis, rheumatoid arthritis, rotator cuff disease, and the stiff shoulder in the geriatric population. It should be noted that these conditions may coexist and be related to each other. Understanding the relationship between these disease processes is key to formulating an effective treatment plan.

History and physical examination

Pain is the most common chief complaint, and is almost always associated with a functional deficit. Ask the patient to point to the exact location of pain as well as describe or demonstrate activities that cause pain. Pain secondary to shoulder pathology may radiate down the upper arm and forearm, or upward to the neck and trapezial area. Specifically inquire about any history of trauma, weakness, and limits in range of motion. Pathology in the neck may refer pain to the shoulder, usually to the superior or posterior aspects of the shoulder. Examination of the neck and a careful neurological examination should help identify a cervical etiology.

Some key features of the physical examination of the shoulder are presented here. Begin with inspection for swelling, asymmetry, and periscapular muscle atrophy. Palpation should be performed along the glenohumeral joint line, acromioclavicular (AC) joint line, bicipital groove, periscapular muscles, as well as over specific areas of pain. Active and passive range of motion should be assessed for abduction, adduction, flexion, extension, and internal and external rotation. Strength testing should be sure to include initial and midrange abduction, internal rotation, and external rotation. Neurological testing should include sensory exam of the axillary nerve distribution (lateral shoulder).

Osteoarthritis and rheumatoid arthritis

Pain due to glenohumeral arthritis is exacerbated by use of the extremity and relieved with rest. Pain at night is common with sleeping on the affected side and as the patient becomes aware of daytime activity joint irritation. Patients often must sleep with multiple pillows for comfort. Inspection of the arthritic shoulder may reveal varying degrees of periscapular atrophy. Pain upon palpation of the joint line is common. Tenderness of the AC joint is a reliable indicator of AC joint arthritis. Range of motion is painful and limited, and may be associated with palpable crepitus. Crepitus anteriorly and superiorly may indicate the presence of a massive rotator cuff tear with glenohumeral and humeroacromial arthritis (cuff tear arthropathy). Strength of the shoulder musculature may be preserved unless compromised by rotator cuff tear or pain.

Radiographic evaluation of the arthritic shoulder consists of true anteroposterior (AP) views in both internal and external rotation and an axillary view. The AP views are helpful in assessing the degree of joint interval narrowing and the presence of osteophytes. The axillary view is used to assess posterior glenoid wear, which may alter the surgical technique. The radiographic pathoanatomy of osteoarthritis of the shoulder is similar to that of any disarthroid joint; narrowing of the joint interval, subchondral sclerosis, peripheral osteophytes, and subchondral cyst formation. The largest osteophytes are usually located inferiorly. Osteophytes can enlarge the head of the humerus significantly and lead to a mechanical block to motion. Advanced cases are often associated with posterior glenoid wear from concomitant posterior shoulder instability.

Shoulder involvement in rheumatoid arthritis is common, affecting 50–60 percent of patients with the disease. However, the course and severity of the disease varies greatly from individual to individual. All of the tissues about the shoulder are usually affected in rheumatoid arthritis. The subdeltoid–subacromial bursa can develop a painful bursitis that coexists with rotator cuff pathology. Attrition of the glenohumeral joint capsule and ligaments can lead to instability. The radiographic appearance of the proximal humerus and glenoid may vary from normal appearance to the demonstration of extensive erosions that parallel the degree of synovitis.

Conservative measures should be undertaken for initial treatment of mild to moderately severe shoulder arthritis. In addition, patients with severe disease who are poor surgical candidates because of medical comorbidities must also be managed nonoperatively. Physical therapy protocols designed to stretch and strengthen the rotator cuff and periscapular musculature are useful for increasing the range of motion and strength of the arthritic shoulder. Local modalities (e.g. heat, ice, ultrasound) and nonsteroidal anti-inflammatory medication may help control swelling and pain. Because night-time pain and the resultant sleep deprivation are common problems the prescription of sleep medication may provide invaluable relief. Additionally, medical management of rheumatoid arthritis should be maximized.

Surgical treatment of the arthritic shoulder ranges from minimally invasive arthroscopic synovectomy to total shoulder replacement. Arthroscopic synovectomy can provide pain relief for patients with rheumatoid arthritis, especially if attempted early in the course of their disease. Prosthetic arthroplasty of the shoulder, if properly performed, provides predictable relief of pain with good or excellent functional results in more than 90 percent of patients. The treatment of glenohumeral arthritis associated with rotator cuff tears must take into consideration the biomechanical alteration of joint kinematics. Insertion of a glenoid component has been associated with a high rate of loosening and failure. Therefore, hemiarthroplasty with a large-headed humeral component has become the accepted treatment for these patients. Other surgical options with less predictable outcomes include capsular release, osteotomy, resection arthroplasty, and shoulder arthrodesis.

Rotator cuff tear

The rotator cuff consists of the tendinous insertions of the supraspinatus, infraspinatus, teres minor, and subscapularis muscles on the humeral head. It functions to both rotate the humeral head about its axis as well as to compress the humeral head into the concavity of the glenoid fossa, thus providing a fulcrum against which the powerful deltoid muscle can abduct, extend, and forward flex the humerus. As noted earlier, the rotator cuff is frequently involved in arthritis of the shoulder,

but tears frequently present in the geriatric population without concomitant glenohumeral arthritis. The tendons of the rotator cuff are highly resistant to tearing in young patients, and full-thickness rotator cuff tears rarely occur in patients younger than 40 years of age. With increasing age and disuse, failure of the cuff tendons is more likely.

The patient will typically present with the insidious onset of pain and weakness of shoulder abduction and external rotation. Complaints of inability to sleep on the affected side, place the hand behind the head (e.g. when combing hair), and place objects on high shelves are common. Physical examination may reveal atrophy of the affected muscles in chronic cases. Occasionally, the cuff defect may be palpated by rotating the humeral head underneath the examiner's fingers. Strength in abduction and external rotation is decreased, and the patient may exhibit a positive "drop-arm" test (inability to maintain active shoulder abduction against manual downward pressure).

The radiographic analysis of patients with isolated rotator cuff tears is not as revealing as those associated with glenohumeral arthritis. Chronic tears may be associated with subacromial or greater tuberosity sclerosis or cyst formation. The coracoacromial ligament and/or cuff tendon insertion may be partially calcified. Ultrasound and magnetic resonance imaging are useful modalities to confirm the presence and evaluate the extent of cuff pathology.

The treatment of a full-thickness rotator cuff tear must be tailored to the functional demands of the patient, the patient's symptoms, and the ability to achieve a durable and functional repair. Low-demand patients with minimal symptoms may be treated nonoperatively with nonsteroidal anti-inflammatory medications and physical therapy. However, arthroscopic surgery can play a role in providing pain relief via joint debridement and decompression. Healthy patients with greater functional demands benefit significantly from surgical repair of the torn tendon edges to their anatomic insertion sites on the proximal humerus. As in any chronic condition, surgical repair is not an emergency and may be reserved for those patients who fail to respond favorably to nonoperative treatment.

Stiff shoulder

The stiff shoulder is a common complaint in the geriatric population. Reeves subdivided the stiff shoulder, which is not a result of arthritic disease, into the idiopathic frozen shoulder and the post-traumatic stiff shoulder.[20] The frozen shoulder is the result of an idiopathic and global contracture of the joint capsule. As the name implies, the post-traumatic stiff shoulder results from injury or trauma. After the shoulder sustains an insult, potential constraints to joint mobility are adhesions within the joint, capsular fibrosis, and contracture of the surrounding musculotendinous structures.[20]

Patients with frozen shoulder present with a several month history of pain with progressive stiffness. By definition, there is no history of trauma to the joint and the loss of range of motion exists in all planes. Although idiopathic, frozen shoulder is associated with several medical conditions, including diabetes mellitus, thyroid disease, and pulmonary disease. In contrast, the post-traumatic stiff shoulder is preceded by trauma to the joint (e.g. rotator cuff tear, fracture, contusion, surgery) which is often followed by prolonged immobilization.

Limitation in range of motion is usually global, but may be limited to certain planes.

Treatment protocols are similar for both idiopathic and post-traumatic stiff shoulder. Prevention is key; avoidance of extended immobilization should be avoided when possible. Treatment begins with physical therapy combined with a home exercise program to work on range of motion. Nonsteroidal anti-inflammatory drugs are used to treat pain and allow the patient to move the shoulder. A steroid injection may also be used as an adjunct to treat inflammation. Nonoperative management is successful in the majority of patients, especially those with idiopathic frozen shoulder. Post-traumatic stiff shoulder more often requires surgical release of the contracture. Operative management is indicated after 3–6 months of failed nonoperative measures. Surgical modalities include manipulation under anesthesia and arthroscopic and open release.

CONDITIONS OF THE HIP AND KNEE
Total hip arthroplasty

Hip pain is a common complaint in the geriatric population. Many times the history is vague and the orthopedist must rely on the clinical presentation, physical, and radiographic studies to narrow the differential diagnosis. The physical examination should include not only the affected hip, but also evaluation of the back, pelvis, and knees.

Contusion about the pelvis and hip region may be very painful and disabling. Because of the subcutaneous location of the iliac crests and greater trochanters, these regions are at risk of injury during falls. A contusion over the greater trochanter may cause persistent bursitis, tenderness directly over the greater trochanter, and increased pain with abduction of the leg. Females are more prone to trochanteric bursitis because of their broader pelvis. A hip pointer is a very painful contusion over the iliac crest that occurs after direct trauma following a fall. It must be differentiated from an avulsion fracture of the iliac crest or a tear of the muscle aponeurosis. Profuse bleeding may occur leaving a painful persistent hematoma. For contusions over the greater trochanter and hip pointers, treatment consists of application of ice and decreased activities. Padding may be helpful to prevent recurrent injuries. The prognosis is good.

The majority of hip pain in the geriatric population is usually due to trauma or arthritis. Fractures of the hip constitute a medical, social, and economic challenge for the healthcare industry. Approximately 250,000 hip fractures occur in the US each year, resulting in healthcare costs exceeding eight billion dollars per annum.[21] As the average life expectancy of the population increases, the number of hip fractures is predicted to double by the year 2050.[22] Treatment consists of stable internal fixation or joint replacement.

Total hip arthroplasty (THA) has been one of the major successes of 20th century medicine. First popularized by Sir John Charnley, joint arthroplasty has revolutionized the treatment of degenerative arthritis. Today, more than 120,000 primary THAs are performed in the USA each year at an estimated cost of over 2.5 billion dollars. Because most hip replacements are done in patients older than 65 years of age, the number of procedures is expected to increase as the population ages.

The primary reason for elective THA in the geriatric population is arthritis. The many forms of arthritis produce similar consequence in the involved joints including pain, loss of motion, and deformity. Reconstructive surgery may be indicated to treat any of these sequelae with the goal being pain relief and restoration of joint function. Secondary indications for THA in the geriatric population include fractures of the hip or pelvis, osteonecrosis of the femoral head, and polytrauma patients requiring early mobilization. In these instances, implantation of orthopedic prostheses can stabilize the situation, but introduce a new set of challenges in ensuring that interactions between the bone and implant are stable.

Joint replacement components can be fixed to the host skeleton with the use of acrylic polymers (i.e., polymethyl methacrylate), termed "cement fixation," or through bone regeneration and subsequent osseointegration. In the latter process, the design of the implant takes advantage of the bone's natural ability to repair itself. This type of fixation is called "cementless" and has the theoretic advantage of providing a living, self-repairing environment. The stated reasoning for a trend toward noncemented fixation in THA is the reported higher rates of loosening in young active patients treated with cemented components.[23] In the geriatric population, the majority of THAs is cemented with low failure rates reported in long-term studies.[24–26]

A common problem associated with the introduction of prosthetic devices in orthopedic surgery is the eventual loosening of these implants as a result of lack of ingrowth, cement failure, or the presence of biomaterial wear debris.[22,27] In either case, failure of the implant results in bone resorption at the metal–bone interface. This causes the need for replacement of the endoprosthesis in order to restore functional capability of the joint.[28]

Complications in total hip arthroplasty

The major complications associated with THA include infection, thromboembolism, heterotopic ossification, and dislocation. Infection remains the most devastating complication following total hip arthroplasty. The incidence of infection following THA was 3.2 percent a decade ago, but with advances in surgical technique, the use of body-exhaust suits during surgery, and perioperative antibiotics, the accepted infection rate approaches 1 percent for primary THA and 3–4 percent for revision THA.[29] Increased risks of infection have been shown to occur in patients with rheumatoid arthritis (1.2 percent), psoriatic arthritis (5.5 percent), and diabetes mellitus (5.6 percent). The average cost to the medical community exceeds 250 million dollars per year for treating infected total hips.[21]

Infection following THA may lack the classic symptoms of fever and chills, and physical examination may not show signs of warmth, redness, or wound drainage. The erythrocyte sedimentation rate (ESR) and C-reactive protein (CRP) are both acute phase reactants that when elevated are not specific for the infectious process but are helpful. Other procedures or tests available to help confirm an infected prosthesis include joint aspiration, polymerase chain reaction (PCR), nuclear scans including technetium Tc 99m and gallium 67 citrate scan, and surgical exploration of the joint with frozen section analysis. The most common organisms are Gram-positive isolates including *Staphylococcus aureus* and *Staphylococcus epidermidis*. Recently, there has been a growing incidence of methicillin-resistant *Staph. aureus* (MRSA) infected THA.

Treatment of infection is predicted on identification of the organism and sensitivity patterns, host defenses, and fixation of implant. The primary treatment of an infected THA involves an immediate exchange arthroplasty or a delayed two-staged reimplantation with the use of an interval antibiotic impregnated cement spacer.[30] Success rates for staged exchange approach 97 percent. Principles of reimplantation are based on the condition and physiological age of the patient, the sensitivity of the organism to antibiotics, and the absence of active infection. An early postoperative superficial infection must be drained completely. Failure to adequately control an infection will eventually lead to an amputation for unsalvageable cases or resection arthroplasty, which provides a pain-free alternative and allows ambulation using external support.

Despite the use of routine anticoagulation measures postoperatively (warfarin, heparin, low-molecular-weight heparin, aspirin), thromboembolism remains the most common complication following THA and is the leading cause of postoperative morbidity.[31] The incidence of DVT ranges from 8 to 70 percent, with a fatal pulmonary embolus to occur in 1–2 percent of patients left untreated.[32] The highest incidence of DVT is reported to be on postoperative day 4. The classic presentation of pulmonary embolus consists of shortness of breath, pleuritic chest pain, and mental status changes.[33] Secondary signs include the presence of calf tenderness (Homan's sign), low-grade fever, fatigue, tachycardia, and diaphoresis. The "gold standard" for detecting a pulmonary embolus is still the pulmonary angiogram. Standard treatment for a pulmonary embolus includes immediate anticoagulation. The use of the Greenfield filter is an alternative approach in selected patients in whom anticoagulation is contraindicated.[34] Aggressive anticoagulation may lead to wound hematoma and subsequent infection.

The incidence of hetertopic ossification (HO) following THA has been reported to be between 0.6 and 61.7 percent. HO after THA most commonly affects males. Predisposing factors include hypertrophic osteoarthritis, ankylosing spondylitis, diffuse idiopathic skeletal hyperostosis, post-traumatic arthritis, and history of head trauma. HO is more commonly seen with the direct lateral approach to the hip. HO limits hip motion when pronounced, but it generally does not cause pain or muscle weakness. Reoperation to remove HO is not recommended unless there is severe restriction of hip range or pain from impingement is severe. Recurrence is likely unless prophylactic measures are taken. Once HO is seen radiographically, there is no treatment to prevent further progression. Instead, treatment for HO is directed toward identifying those patients at high risk for developing HO and treating this subgroup prophylactically. Prophylactic treatment is limited to low-dose radiation and NSAIDs.[35]

The overall incidence of dislocation following THA is reported to be 3 percent.[36] There is a slight predisposition to dislocation in patients that have had a posterior approach for a THA.[37] Treatment of the dislocated total hip depends on the reason for dislocation. Many factors have been implicated as increasing the risk of postoperative dislocation. Patients with a previous history of dislocation, neuromuscular problems, and poor compliance are at increased risk of dislocating. Approximately two-thirds of patients with a dislocated total hip can be treated successfully with a closed reduction and a period of hip immobilization. Adherence to the postoperative regimen of restricted motion is mandatory, to allow time for formation of a pseudocapsule. An acute traumatic dislocation responds well to reduction. Recurrent painful dislocations, however, often require revision to be ultimately corrected.

Revision total hip replacement

Revision hip surgery is difficult and complex. It is estimated that of the more than 120,000 THAs performed each year in the USA, 18 percent of these are revision cases. The results of revision arthroplasty are less satisfactory than in primary hip replacement. Postoperative complications of infection, dislocation, nerve palsy, fracture, thromboembolism, and heterotopic bone formation are higher than in primary THA.[38] The surgical goals in revision hip replacement are (1) removal of loose components without significant destruction to host bone and tissue, (2) reconstruction of bone defects with bone graft and/or metal augmentation, (3) stable revision implants, and (4) restoration of normal hip center of rotation. A variety of cemented and noncemented implants are currently available for revision arthroplasty. Neither type is appropriate in all situations, but instead should be selected depending on the patient's age, activity level, remaining bone stock, and reason for revision.

Revision THR is indicated for a number of reasons. Mechanisms of failure of a primary THA include material failure, loss of fixation, mechanical failure, wear debris, infection, recurrent dislocation, instability of components, and periprosthetic fractures. The materials used to construct THR implants must be able to sustain loads of 2–3 times body weight with routine activity and peak loads approaching 6–8 times body weight. The materials must be biologically inert and have acceptable wear rates to minimize the generation of wear debris. Current alloys superior to the original designs of stainless steel include forged cobalt chrome and titanium with variable surface textures. Despite advances in THR design, osteolysis induced by polyethylene debris remains the major cause of implant loosening and revision.

Loss of fixation with cemented THR can result from fracture of the cement mantle surrounding the stem. When cement is subjected to high stress over time, it may undergo fatigue failure, resulting in fracture, fragmentation, and ultimately osteolysis and/or implant loosening. Cementless THR was introduced to eliminate the potential of bone cement failure and hopefully achieve longer-lasting fixation. However, even with primary THR, cementless replacements are prone to failure if intraoperative implant stability is not achieved leading to micromotion along the implant stem.

Finally, recurrent dislocation is a major cause of early revision. Inappropriate sizing of components, poor surgical technique, poor component alignment, and postoperative patient compliance have all been associated with increased dislocation. Prior to revision, the reason for the dislocation must be addressed so that appropriate corrections can be made the second time around.

Following revision surgery, patients should be mobile as quickly as possible. Patients with cemented components can bear weight as tolerated, while press-fit components require a period of toe-touch weight bearing for 6 weeks. An abduction brace should be used if there are concerns regarding hip stability and is used for 6–12 weeks after surgery until there has been enough healing of the pericapsular tissues to prevent dislocation.

Osteoarthritis of the knee

Osteoarthritis of the knee is one of the most prevalent conditions in the geriatric population that threatens their independence. Currently, there are more than 13 million Americans with symptomatic osteoarthritis of the knee that requires medical attention.[39] As the American geriatric population grows, so does the number of patients with osteoarthritis of the knee.

Arthritis may be primary with an unknown etiology, or secondary to rheumatoid arthritis, post-traumatic arthritis, or an infectious process. Primary osteoarthritis is a progressive degenerative process that increases in prevalence nonlinearly with age after 50 years. It is estimated that 85 percent of persons over the age of 65 years have radiographically detectable osteoarthritis.[40] Currently, there is no cure for this disease. Treatment options include conservative measures such as activity modification, or surgical salvage procedures such as total knee arthroplasty.

A comprehensive history focusing on patient's employment, activity level, other comorbidities, and symptoms are important in determining appropriate treatment options. Patients with osteoarthritis of the knee commonly present with diffuse pain in the knee region. The pain is exacerbated with activity and alleviated with rest. Pain may be limited to one compartment in the knee when the patient presents early in the disease process, or the pain may be diffuse in more advanced disease. The physical exam should be organized and systematic. The patient's body habitus and gait pattern are initially evaluated. Ipsilateral joints are inspected to assess involvement of ankle and/or hip joints. Referred pain from the ipsilateral hip is a common occurrence, so the hip examination may detect hip pathology. Visualization of the knee may reveal gross varus/valgus deformity suggesting severe disease. Range of motion of the knee is evaluated on both extremities to ascertain flexion or extension contractures. Greater restriction in motion is usually associated with advanced disease. All three knee joint compartments are palpated (medial, lateral, patellofemoral). This helps determine unicompartmental disease from panarthritis of the knee.

Radiographic examination of the affected and unaffected knees is the key diagnostic tool in evaluating patients with osteoarthritis. Common radiographs include standard anteroposterior and lateral standing views with the patient fully erect. However, a 45-degree flexion weight-bearing posteroanterior view may help diagnose early signs of osteoarthritis. The radiographic findings in osteoarthritis include loss of articular cartilage between the femoral condyle and tibial plateau, subchondral sclerosis, peripheral osteophyte formation, and subchondral cysts.

Conservative treatment options

Osteoarthritis usually progresses slowly, which allows for a stepwise treatment protocol. With more of the US population living longer and healthier lives, treatments needs to be tailored to the patient's physiological age rather than chronological age. Prosthetic joint replacement is not an emergency procedure, thus conservative treatment may be maximized prior to surgical treatment. Nonsurgical treatment options include medical management, lifestyle modifications, physical therapy, bracing, and orthotics.

One of the primary goals in lifestyle modification is patient education. Patients will benefit from taking frequent breaks during periods of prolonged standing and avoiding high-impact activities. Low-impact activities such as swimming and bicycling should be encouraged along with proper dieting to reduce body weight. Obesity has been linked to osteoarthritis and patient education regarding weight loss will decrease the stress on the knees.

Physical therapy is appropriate for strengthening the periarticular muscles to help stabilize the knee joint. Range of motion exercises help reduce the occurrence of contractures around the knee. Special modalities such as ultrasound and heat massage work through reflex-mediated pathways reducing the pain experienced by the patient.

Knee sleeves may provide a sense of stability to osteoarthritic knees, possibly through enhanced proprioceptive feedback. In patients with unicompartmental osteoarthritis, "unloader" braces may reduce joint reactive forces in the involved compartment. Limitations in bracing include the relative expense and inability of patients to tolerate wearing these cumbersome braces continuously.

Medical management includes administration of acetaminophen, NSAIDs, and the newer Cox-2 inhibitors. The NSAIDs help reduce the inflammatory response by inhibiting the production of prostaglandins and leukotrienes. Some of the common side-effects of NSAIDs include dyspepsia, gastrointestinal ulceration, renal toxicity, hepatotoxicity, and cardiac failure. Especially with the geriatric population where many patients have associated comorbidities, these patients must be closely monitored for side-effects. The Cox-2 inhibitors help reduce the risks of gastric ulcers, thus allowing a greater margin of safety among high-risk patients.

Chondroprotective oral supplements have recently been shown to be beneficial to patients with osteoarthritis of the knee.[41] Glucosamine and chondroitin sulfate act synergistically when taken together to help reduce pain and inflammation within synovial joints. These medications are believed to work by their effect on stimulating chondrocyte and synovial metabolism and inhibiting degradative enzymes within the joint. Randomized clinical trials are underway to better understand their role in treatment of osteoarthritis. One of the major drawbacks is the relative high expense for the medications.

Intra-articular injection of corticosteroid may be indicated for patients who fail medical therapy or who have contraindications to NSAIDs. Medical management should be tried for 6–8 weeks prior to administration of these medications. Steroids should be limited to three injections per year, as the risk of complications increases with each additional injection. The corticosteroids work by inhibiting the inflammatory pathway, thus temporarily reducing the amount of pain the patient perceives.

Viscosupplementation has recently gained acceptance in the treatment of osteoarthritis of the knee. There are two brands of viscosupplementation that are currently available in the USA, Hyalgan and Synvisc. Many clinical studies have shown intra-articular injection of hyaluronate therapy to be safe and nontoxic.[42,43] Studies have shown that patients treated with viscosupplementation have improved long-term pain relief, reduced disability, and improved quality of life.[44] Patients receive weekly injections for a series of 3–5 weeks. Patients may receive up to 6 months of pain relief depending on the severity of osteoarthritis. The appropriate indication for viscosupplementation is for a patient with mild osteoarthritis with short duration of symptoms, and minimal deformity of the extremity.

Surgical treatment

The role of arthroscopic debridement and lavage of osteoarthritic knees has been evolving over the past decade. Under the appropriate conditions, the literature supports arthroscopic lavage.[45,46] The beneficial effects consist of diluting and washing away proinflammatory cytokines. The patients that will benefit the most are those who have a history of mechanical symptoms such as locking or catching, short duration of symptoms (<6 months), normal knee alignment, and only minimal radiographic evidence of osteoarthritis.[45–47] As in viscosupplementation, the effects are often short lived, lasting from a few weeks to months. Thus patients should be educated regarding arthroscopic lavage of osteoarthritic knees and its temporary pain relief.

Osteotomy around the knee joint has a limited role in the geriatric patient. The primary goal of osteotomies is to unload the affected compartment. In patients with medial compartment arthritis, a high tibial valgus osteotomy is performed under the appropriate indications. Contraindications include panarthritis involving all three knee compartments, restricted range of motion, and inflammatory arthritis. For lateral compartment arthritis, either a high tibial lateral closing wedge osteotomy or distal femoral osteotomy may be used. Similar contraindications exist as for valgus osteotomies.

In patients with osteoarthritis limited to one compartment, unicompartmental knee replacements have favorable results. This procedure is a reasonable option for patients who have relatively normal range of motion and normal alignment. Excellent results have been reported in 5–10-year follow-up, with 70 percent satisfactory results.[48–50]

The definitive surgical procedure for osteoarthritis of the knee is total knee arthroplasty. Knee arthroplasty is indicated in patients who have failed a course of medical treatment or in patients who are unwilling to change their lifestyle. Pain is the most common indication to perform a joint replacement in the geriatric population. Cemented total knee arthroplasty remains the gold standard among the total knee prostheses.[51,52] The routine use of patellar resurfacing devices remains a topic of debate because of the potential complications, including patellar fracture, patellar instability, and implant loosening. The suggested indications for patellar resurfacing include grade IV patellofemoral arthritis, especially associated with patellar subluxation or dislocation. Knee replacement has been shown to offer predictable long-term pain relief with improved function in elderly patients with osteoarthritis.[53,54] With better designs and modern technology, the knee prostheses have a longer survivorship. Patients report a decrease in pain and increased mobility following knee replacements. However, some patients may encounter complications associated with the procedure including infection, blood loss with subsequent transfusions, wound complications, and deep vein thrombosis. The procedure is not without complications, so the patients must be educated regarding the risks and benefits of total knee replacement prior to embarking on surgical intervention.

Osteoarthritis of the knee is a debilitating disease that compromises a patient's independence. Carefully prescribed conservative measures such as activity modification, medications, and injections may be successful. However, these treatments are often palliative. Osteoarthritis is usually progressive, with more definitive procedures such as total knee arthroplasty being more predictable and successful in reducing a patient's pain.

CONDITIONS OF THE FOOT AND ANKLE

Foot and ankle pain are a common complaint in the geriatric patient. There are many potential sources for this pain. This section will review the more common foot and ankle pathology seen in the geriatric population.

One etiology of foot and ankle pain in the geriatric patient is arthritis. There are many types of arthritis, including osteoarthritis, inflammatory arthritis, neuropathic arthropathy, post-traumatic arthritis, and infectious arthritis. Radiography is helpful in differentiating the types of arthritis. The X-ray of a patient with osteoarthritis will show osteophyte formation, joint space narrowing, subchondral bone cysts, and subchondral sclerosis. Inflammatory arthritis is categorized by symmetric joint space narrowing, osteopenia, and juxta-articular erosions. Post-traumatic arthritis is seen after an intra-articular fracture. Neuropathic arthrosis (Charcot neuropathy) develops in the weight-bearing joints, including the midfoot and ankle.[55] The X-ray reveals numerous fractures, in various stages of healing, and loss of the normal bony anatomy.[56]

The initial treatment of each type of arthritis is the same. The patient is prescribed a nonsteroidal anti-inflammatory and an orthotic or specialized shoe to offload the affected joint. Physical therapy can be prescribed for gait training, strengthening, and to maintain range of movement. An injection of half lidocaine and half corticosteroid can be both diagnostic and therapeutic.

If conservative treatment fails, surgery may be considered. Operative treatment for ankle arthritis includes ankle arthroscopy, ankle arthrodesis, and total ankle arthroplasty.

Ankle arthroscopy has become a useful technique for treating a wide range of ankle pathology. Improvements in instrumentation and technique are expanding the diagnostic and therapeutic indications for ankle arthroscopy.[57] Diagnostic indications include unexplained pain, swelling, stiffness, instability, hemarthrosis, and locking or popping. Therapeutic indications include injuries of the articular cartilage and soft tissue, bone impingement, debridement of soft tissue lesions, synovectomy and loose body removal, arthrofibrosis, ankle fractures, and osteochondral defects. It has been used to perform ankle stabilization procedures, arthrodesis, and irrigation and debridement of septic arthritis.[56] The decreased morbidity and faster recovery times make ankle arthroscopy an appealing alternative to open arthrotomy.

Patients with painful ankle arthritis and a deformity who do not respond to nonoperative treatment modalities may be candidates for ankle arthrodesis.[58]

Ankle arthrodesis is considered by many to be the standard operative treatment for end-stage ankle arthritis.[59] However, there are numerous complications that may result from arthrodesis including subtalar arthrosis, delayed union, malunion, nonunion, and infection. For these patients, total ankle arthroplasty may be a good option.

Total ankle arthroplasty was developed in the 1970s after the success of total knee and total hip arthroplasty. Initially, total ankle arthroplasty had not been as successful as replacement of other joints. Long-term follow-up from initial studies showed that most ultimately failed.[60] As a result, total ankle arthroplasty was abandoned during the 1980s because of the poor long-term results and high complication rate. Newer second-generation design techniques have had excellent results in experienced hands.[61]

The painful heel

Heel pain is a common problem. There are multiple etiologies, and successful treatment requires proper diagnosis of the cause of the pain. Heel pain can be divided into two main categories: subcalcaneal pain syndrome and posterior heel pain syndromes.

Patients with subcalcaneal pain syndrome generally complain of an insidious onset of pain along the plantar medial aspect of the heel without distal radiation or paresthesias. The pain is typically most severe upon arising out of bed in the morning. The pain may also increase with increasing activity throughout the day. Complaints of numbness, paresthesias, or proximal or distal radiation are suggestive of nerve entrapment. The physical exam will usually reveal tenderness at the origin of the plantar fascia. Tenderness just distal to the origin of the abductor hallucis muscle is suggestive of compression of the lateral plantar nerve. The range of motion of the hindfoot should also be assessed. Standing AP, lateral, and oblique radiographs of the foot should be obtained. Radiographs may reveal a heel spur. The relationship between a heel spur and heel pain has not been clearly established. The majority of patients with subcalcaneal heel pain will respond to conservative management. Cushioning materials, like heel cups and well-padded shoes, should be used. The patient should be instructed to avoid impact loading activities, and taught exercises to increase the flexibility of the heel cord and plantar fascia. It is important to tell the patient that it may take between 6 months and 1 year for their symptoms to resolve. The patient should be re-evaluated after approximately 6 weeks. If there is no response to the stretching program, a dorsiflexion night splint can be prescribed. If this is unsuccessful, a steroid injection can be considered. It should be given with extreme caution because there is a risk of atrophy of the plantar fat pad and iatrogenic rupture of the plantar fascia. Conservative therapy should be used for at least 1 year before considering surgical intervention, because the natural history has been shown to be self-limiting. Surgical success in between 50 and 100 percent of patients has been reported. Both open and endoscopic release of the plantar fascia have been used.

Pain in the posterior portion of the calcaneus should be distinguished from subcalcaneal heel pain. The etiology of posterior heel pain includes retrocalcaneal bursitis, Achilles insertional tendinitis, adventitial bursitis, or complications of Haglund's deformity. The history associated with these entities is often similar. Patients complain of pain on the posterior aspect of the heel with shoe wear, morning pain upon awakening, and increased pain with activity. The proper diagnosis can be ascertained through the physical exam. Pain along the Achilles tendon down to its insertion is indicative of insertional tendinosis. Pain over the anterior border of the Achilles tendon is consistent with retrocalcaneal bursitis. Adventitial bursitis is pain between the skin and the achilles tendon, rather than deep to the tendon. A Haglund's deformity can be palpated through the skin. It is an enlargement of the posterior aspect of the calcaneus, with associated irritation over the bony prominence. There is often an overlying callus. The treatment of these entities is usually conservative. This includes the use of a nonsteroidal anti-inflammatory medication, use of a small heel lift, and a stretching program. Injection of steroid in this area is generally not advisable, since it could result in rupture of the tendon.

The Achilles tendon

Patients with Achilles tendinitis complain of pain over the Achilles tendon. Treatment should include heel cord stretching, a heel lift, and a nonsteroidal anti-inflammatory.

Complete rupture of a healthy Achilles tendon is seen in association with forceful dorsiflexion of a plantarflexed ankle. Many patients have pre-existing tendinitis. Steroid therapy, gout, and fluoroquinolone antibiotics are associated with Achilles tendon ruptures. Patients often report hearing a pop or a snap. A defect in the Achilles tendon may be palpable. The Thompson test is performed by squeezing the calf with the patient prone and the ankle free. If the Achilles tendon is intact, the foot will plantar flex. Ultrasound and MRI can be used if the diagnosis is questionable. Surgical treatment of a complete Achilles tendon rupture is recommended unless the patient has compromised wound healing because of peripheral vascular disease, diabetes, or chronic steroid use. Surgical treatment results in better motion and strength. There is also a lower risk of rerupture. Surgical complications include infection, skin slough, and sural nerve laceration.

Posterior tibial tendon

Posterior tibial tendon dysfunction includes a spectrum of pathological change which include paratendinitis, pure tendinosis, and tendon rupture. Patients usually report the gradual onset of a flatfoot deformity. The patient is tender with palpation over the medial aspect of the ankle, along the tendon sheath, or at the attachment of the tendon on the under surface of the navicular. With weight bearing, there may appear to be a flatfoot deformity because of the valgus alignment of the hindfoot and increased abduction of the forefoot. The patient may be unable to perform a single heel rise.

The treatment of posterior tibial tendon dysfunction depends on the patient's age, weight, systemic factors, length of time of disease course, and the extent of foot collapse. Initial treatment consists of rest, a nonsteroidal anti-inflammatory, and immobilization for 6–8 weeks. Most patients can then progress to a stiff-sole shoe or an ankle–foot orthosis. If the patient's symptoms persist, surgical intervention may be necessary. The patient with an acute injury can often be treated successfully with a soft tissue procedure. A delay in presentation usually necessitates an osseous procedure to correct the deformity and align the foot. A talonavicular arthrodesis is indicated for the flexible flatfoot deformity without degenerative changes in the subtalar joint.[56]

Hallux valgus

Hallux valgus is valgus angulation of the great toe on the first metatarsal.[56] While taking the history from a patient with hallux valgus, it is important to determine why the patient is seeking medical attention. The patient may complain of pain over the medial eminence with certain types of shoewear. The patient should be examined standing. The severity of the great toe deformity and any lesser toe deformities should be noted. Standing AP and lateral X-rays will show the severity of the deformity. Initial treatment can usually be conservative, including wider shoewear and placing pads or mole skin over painful areas. Patients who want to wear a pointed shoe should wear a larger size, made from soft material that can expand. Athletic shoes should not have a seam over the medial eminence. If the lesser toes are involved, a toe sling may be used.[62] Surgical correction of a hallux valgus deformity should be considered when the patient is no longer able to function comfortably.

DISORDERS OF THE SPINE IN THE GERIATRIC POPULATION

This section reviews the most common and important causes and symptoms of neck and back pain in the older patient and summarizes the diagnostic approaches used in assessment. It also examines the clinical attributes of and distinctions between the acute and chronic pain conditions, in addition to briefly addressing the consequences of radiculopathy and myelopathy. Pharmacological and other treatment approaches are discussed.

Cervical spondylosis

Narrowing of the cervical canal or neural foramina due to degeneration of the intervertebral disk and the annulus and to formation of bony osteophytes.

The major clinical manifestations of degenerative disease of the cervical spine include axial neck pain, and radiculopathy. Narrowing may ultimately lead to spinal cord compression, which typically causes a progressive myelopathy, characterized by a spastic gait. If a painful cervical root syndrome predominates, radicular signs often indicate the most involved dermatome, usually one between C-5 and C-6 or between C-6 and C-7. Neural foraminal root compression causes arm weakness and atrophy with segmental reflex loss; spinal cord compression causes hyper-reflexia, increased tone, vibratory impairment, and plantar extensor responses in the legs. Facet joint disease may lead to neck pain, crepitus and decreased range of motion.[63]

Spinal X-rays, including oblique views of the neural foramina, reveal degeneration with osteophytes and disk-space narrowing. If the sagittal diameter of the cervical canal is <10 mm, spinal cord compression is likely. CT defines the diameter of the canal, and myelography, or MRI determines the level and extent of the epidural compression.[64]

Often, signs improve spontaneously. Conservative therapy includes a soft collar, cervical traction, anti-inflammatory drugs, and mild analgesics. Cervical facet injections may be both diagnostic and therapeutic. Decompressive laminoplasty or laminectomy in the presence of cervical lordosis is used to halt disease progression or to stabilize myelopathy in severe and progressive cases.[46,65]

Although data regarding the benefits of physical therapy and traction are conflicting, these methods may provide relief for some patients. For patients suffering from acute neck pain, a regimen that seems too demanding or painful can undermine potential rehabilitation. In these cases, reducing the duration of sessions and lowering the recommended poundage for weights lifted can be beneficial.

Most cases of neck pain stem from benign muscular strain and will resolve without intervention in 2–3 weeks. Determining the existence of radiculopathy or myelopathy is a key assessment objective. Effective initial management of pain symptoms can be achieved through conservative use of NSAIDs, whereas radiculopathy and myelopathy may require use of mild narcotics and short-term corticosteroid therapy.[66–68] Intra-articular steroid injections are less reliable in chronic pain conditions.[69] For radicular arm pain that persists, initiate a short-term regimen of corticosteroid therapy (methylprednisolone [Medrol], 5- to 7-day regimen with a dose taper). Antacids should be taken with the corticosteroid.[70]

Imaging studies produce important diagnostic information, but because most cases of neck pain resolve within several weeks, such studies should be used conservatively.[71] If neck pain persists for more than a few months or if radicular arm pain progresses for several weeks, then MRI and plain films are appropriate.[72] Patients with myelopathy should be imaged as soon as the diagnosis is entertained.[73]

Some patients can benefit from physical therapy, massage, and other nonpharmacological approaches to pain management. When MRI studies show compression of nerves or spinal cord or evidence of other structural problems such as tumor, fracture, or syrinx, a neurosurgeon can help guide subsequent patient management.

Spinal stenosis

A narrowing of the spinal canal, causing pressure on the nerve roots and occasionally on the cord.

Aging of the spine, as with other joints of the body, can bring on bony and ligamentous changes. The pressure on the spinal cord may result from bony or soft tissue encroachment on the spinal cord or lumbosacral nerve roots. This may be congenital or acquired, as in traumatic or degenerative stenosis. Degenerative narrowing of the disk spaces and hypertrophy of the ligamentum flavum and facet joints are accompanied by narrowing of the spinal canal. Absolute (anteroposterior canal diameter <10 mm) or relative (10–13 mm diameter) stenosis in the cervical spine predisposes the patient to the development of radiculopathy, myelopathy, or both from relatively minor soft- or hard-disk pathology or trauma.[39] Minor trauma such as hyperextension may lead to a central cord syndrome, even without obvious skeletal injury. Neurogenic claudication (i.e., aching pain with or without paresthesia or numbness in the buttocks, thighs, or calves) is characteristic of lumbar stenosis. Discomfort is caused by prolonged lumbar extension (e.g. while walking) and relieved by lumbar flexion (e.g. while sitting or leaning forward). Mild to moderate low-back pain and symptoms of radicular nerve root compression may be present. Physical findings are often nonspecific. A thorough history will often be sufficient to differentiate between neurogenic and vascular claudication. Neurogenic pain commonly goes from proximal to distal, while vascular claudication is distal to proximal, and occurs quite suddenly. The presence of brisk peripheral pulses on examination also helps exclude peripheral vascular disease as a diagnosis.[74]

Diagnosis can be confirmed by CT or MRI. However, many asymptomatic elderly persons have the pathological changes of spinal stenosis on imaging studies. Thus, careful clinical judgment must be used to determine whether spinal stenosis found on X-ray is the cause of the patient's symptoms.

Treatment

Treatment for most patients includes an initial course of analgesics and exercise. Moist heat, use of a cervical collar, and cervical traction have been found to be helpful.[75] If a patient does not respond to this approach or if function is severely compromised, with signs of myelopathy with motor/gait impairment or radiculopathy with persistent disabling pain and weakness, then surgical decompression is indicated.[76]

Rheumatoid spondylitis

The cervical spine contains many synovial articulations, making it a common site of manifestations in rheumatoid arthritis (RA). It is common with longstanding disease and multiple joint involvement. Neck pain, decreased range of motion, crepitation, and occipital headaches are the most common complaints. Neurological impairment in patients with RA usually occurs gradually (weakness, decreased sensation, hyperreflexia) and is often attributed to other joint disease.[64,77]

Treatment

Indications for surgical stabilization include instability, pain, neurological deficit due to neural compression, impending neurological deficit, or some combination of these.[78] Patients with RA should have flexion/extension radiographs before elective surgery.

Diffuse idiopathic skeletal hyperostosis

Widespread calcification and ossification of the anterolateral ligaments of the spine, which may give rise to ankylosis.

Widespread calcification and ossification of the anterolateral ligaments of the spine are characteristic and may result in bony ankylosis. Peripheral joints may also be involved, with evidence of osteophyte or spur formation and ligamentous calcification (enthesopathy). The incidence is about 0.5 percent/year in elderly patients. The male/female distribution is 2:1.

The pathogenesis is unknown. Some studies have found a possible link to increases in the plasma concentrations of insulin and growth hormone. Others have postulated a relationship to increases in the concentration of vitamin A and retinoic acid derivatives; this finding is interesting because the X-ray abnormalities of diffuse idiopathic skeletal hyperostosis (DISH) resemble those of chronic hypervitaminosis A.[74]

Typically, patients report stiffness and pain (usually mild) localized mainly to the thoracic spine. Pain may be noted years before X-ray manifestations appear. In about 15 percent of patients, cervical spine involvement leads to dysphagia. More than one-third of patients exhibit peripheral joint manifestations; the most commonly involved sites are the heels (characterized by spur formation), elbows, knees, and shoulders. Spinal stenosis and neurological manifestations are uncommon.

Physical examination shows few abnormalities. Thoracolumbar and cervical spine mobility may be mildly or moderately decreased, and tenderness may be present over the thoracic spine. Occasionally, anterior cervical osteophytes can be palpated at the posterior aspect of the pharynx. Laboratory findings are usually normal; about 40 percent of patients have asymptomatic hyperglycemia or overt diabetes mellitus.

Early in the disease, X-rays of the peripheral joints may suggest DISH, but X-rays of the spine may show normal findings. Later in the disease, rheumatic abnormalities are extensive, but pain is often minimal and spinal motion is only moderately limited. X-rays of the peripheral joints show new bone formation (whiskering) and large bone spurs, particularly on the calcaneus and olecranon process. Advanced ligamentous calcification can be seen in the iliolumbar and patellar ligaments. Periarticular osteophytes are usually conspicuous. X-rays of the spine typically show flowing ossification along the anterolateral aspect of at least four contiguous vertebral bodies, preservation of disk height, and the absence of marginal sclerosis and apophysial joint ankylosis.

Treatment

Treatment is symptomatic; physical therapy, massage, and nonopioid analgesics may be sufficient. Painful spurs may be managed by orthotics or local corticosteroid injections. Patients should be reassured that DISH does not cause permanent disability.

Kyphosis

Kyphosis in the geriatric population may be idiopathic, posttraumatic, secondary to ankylosing spondylitis, or a result of metabolic bone disease. Progressive kyphosis secondary to multiple osteoporotic compression fractures is usually treated with exercises, bracing, and medical management of the underlying bone disease. Evaluation with MRI is sensitive for determining the presence of tumor. Recently, interest in a percutaneous procedure to augment and possibly correct painful kyphosis with bone cement has gained popularity. Vertebroplasty, or kyphoplasty accomplish lengthening and kyphosis correction in the case of kyphoplasty as well as pain relief in well chosen patients with painful osteoporotic compression fractures. This is a new procedure that was first used in France in 1984 and is now gaining favor.[79,80]

MUSCULOSKELETAL ONCOLOGY IN THE GERIATRIC POPULATION

General considerations

The overwhelming majority of destructive bone lesions in the geriatric population will be caused by metastatic bone disease. The differential diagnosis will also include multiple myeloma, lymphoma, and primary mesenchymal tumors. The primary mesenchymal tumors include chondrosarcoma, which is the most common, malignant fibrous histiocytoma, and osteosarcoma. Other considerations in the diagnosis of destructive bone lesions in a geriatric patient include Paget's disease, sarcoma in Paget's disease, post-irradiation sarcoma, and hyperparathyroidism.

Metastatic bone disease

Metastatic bone disease should be the leading diagnosis as the cause of a destructive lesion in the adult. It may have insidious and nonspecific onset. Patients may describe rest pain, and pain at night. Pain may also be experienced with weight bearing, especially when a lesion exists in the hip. When bone pain exists in a patient with a history of cancer, the clinician must always consider possible metastases as the cause. There are about 1.3 million new cases of cancer per year in the USA. About one-half are either breast, prostate, lung, or renal in origin. When autopsy studies are performed on cancer patients with no known clinical metastasis, a high incidence of metastasis is found in breast and prostate disease. Metastasis is found in 84 percent of prostate patients, 73 percent of breast patients, 50 percent of thyroid patients, and 32 percent of lung cancer patients.[81] Common carcinomas which metastasize to bone are breast, prostate, renal, and lung disease. Cancers with uncommon metastases to bone are from skin, the oral cavity, esophagus, cervix, stomach, and colon.

Radiographic evaluation

The radiographic appearance of bony metastases is variable. Lesions may be purely lytic, as is the case for lung, renal, and some breast cancers. Lesions may be purely sclerotic as in prostate, and breast metastasis. Or they may be a mix of lytic and sclerotic which is the most common presentation.[82] Technetium bone scans are positive in 95 percent of cases when metastasis is present. However, multiple myelomas, and some highly aggressive lesions, such as melanoma, and lung or renal carcinomas, may yield false negatives.[83]

Effect on the skeletal system

Metastatic disease commonly causes destructive lesions that predispose the bone to fracture under normal physiological loading. This creates a situation known as an impending fracture. Impending fractures may be due to stress risers or open sections. A stress riser is created by a cortical defect which weakens the bone in both bending and torsion. Eccentric

lesions weaken the bone with twice the effect of central lesions. An open section occurs when the length of a defect in bone exceeds 3/4 of the diameter of the bone. This leads to a 90 percent reduction in torsional strength. Several authors have developed specific criteria for determining the risk of fracture in a metastatic lesion.[84–86] The following criteria are generally well accepted. Those lesions with more than 50 percent cortical bone destruction are at high risk. Certain anatomic areas bear high stress, making them high-risk sites, such as the femoral subtrochanteric region, the femoral diaphysis, the humeral diaphysis, and the humeral anatomic neck. Purely lytic lesions are high risk. Weight-bearing pain, and pain following irradiation are also important signs of impending fracture.

Effect on the hematopoietic system

A normocytic/normochromic anemia often results from metastatic disease derived from breast, prostate, lung, and thyroid cancer. The peripheral blood smear will demonstrate teardrop and fragmented cells. Immature cells will be present as well as a white blood cell shift. The patient may need a transfusion for a platelet count of less than 50,000/mm³. Surgery should be avoided during neutropenia (absolute WBC less than 500/mm³). Patients with metastatic bone disease should have a hematocrit of 30 percent prior to surgery.

Effect on mineral metabolism

Hypercalcemia is common with certain tumors, especially myeloma, lymphoma, lung, and breast carcinoma. On early presentation, patients may appear flu-like and have symptoms of polyuria/polydipsia, anorexia, easy fatiguability, and weakness. Late symptoms might include apathy, irritability, depression, profound muscle weakness, nausea, vomiting, abdominal pain, visual disturbances, and even coma.[87] The treatment is hydration and bisphosphonates. Intravenous pamidronate is the drug of choice and will correct the condition within 48 hours.[88]

Surgical treatment

Internal rigid fixation is the treatment of choice for metastatic bone disease. Before any surgical decisions are made it is important to visualize the entire bone so that implant devices do not end at the level of a lesion. Prosthetic devices requiring resection of bone and lesion are indicated when rigid fixation cannot be achieved with internal fixation, when the articular surfaces have been destroyed, after failure of internal fixation and with progressive disease despite irradiation of the lesion. Surgeons will commonly use intramedullary rods, plates, or prosthetic devices.[89]

Preoperative and postoperative care

As mentioned, a radiograph of the entire bone in question is important so as not to miss another lesion. The cervical spine must be examined with either plain radiographs or a technetium bone scan for intubation purposes. A preoperative calcium level is required to evaluate hypercalcemia.

Prophylactic antibiotics are used pre- and postoperatively as there is a 3–5 percent infection rate. Proper pain management should be ensured. Likewise, an effective bowel protocol, incorporating a laxative and stool softener twice daily, must be instituted.

Evaluation of an unknown primary lesion

A standard history and physical examination asking for a previous history of cancer and checking the breast, prostate, abdomen, and thyroid are critical. The radiographic studies include a chest radiograph, a bone scan to look for primary lesions, and a CT chest and abdomen looking for lung and renal carcinoma, and lymphoma. A bone scan will show a solitary bone lesion in 2/3 of patients with metastatic carcinoma with unknown primary.[90] Laboratory studies include a CBC, and ESR are helpful as myeloma patients frequently have hemoglobin levels below 10, and an elevated ESR. A serum protein electrophoresis is performed for myeloma, and a chemistry, including calcium and phosphorous will identify hyperparathyroidism.

Post-irradiation sarcoma

Sarcomas may occur in any area of previous irradiation. Destructive lesions occur in the irradiated field. This is common with breast cancer, lymphoma, urogenital cancers, and Ewing's sarcoma. Postradiation sarcomas may appear between 2 and 20 years after the initial treatment.[91,92]

Bone pain in the cancer patient

Whenever a cancer patient complains of bone pain, several entities should come to mind. The symptoms may be caused by metastatic bone disease, post-irradiation sarcoma, or from radiation injury to bone. Radiation injury may demonstrate bone atrophy, or multiple lucencies with an intact cortex, and stress fractures may also occur.

Differential diagnosis

The differential diagnosis of a solitary destructive lesion in an adult (over 40 years old) consists of the benign lesions, Paget's disease and hyperparathyroidism, and the malignant lesions, metastatic bone disease, myeloma, lymphoma, primary mesenchymal tumors, chondrosarcoma, malignant fibrous histiocytoma, Paget's disease sarcoma, and post-irradiation sarcoma.

If there is any question that a bone lesion is not a metastasis, consultation with an orthopedic oncologist is in order for management, including diagnosis of a primary bone tumor. A general orthopedist is qualified in managing metastatic bone disease.

Soft tissue tumors

Soft tissue sarcomas are as likely to be found in a patient over 55 years as in a patient under 55.[93] It is difficult to distinguish between benign and malignant soft tissue sarcomas. The presentation can be insidious and nonspecific. The cells of origin are nonepithelial extraskeletal tissue from muscle, fat, blood vessels, nerves, or fibrous tissues. Soft tissue sarcomas are classified according to their differentiation patterns. They can be fibrous, fibrohistiocytic, fat, smooth muscle, skeletal muscle, synovial, or neural. Benign lesions can be neoplasms or reactive conditions. Lipoma and schwannoma are examples of benign lesions, while nodular fascitis and myositis ossificans are reactive conditions. It is important to use proper caution when a soft tissue mass presents, and appropriate referral is warranted.

REFERENCES

1. Kim SJ, Shin SJ: Arthroscopic treatment for limitation of motion of the elbow. Clin Orthop 2000;375:140–148
2. Ogilvie-Harris DJ, Gordon R, MacKay M: Arthroscopic treatment for posterior impingement in degenerative arthritis of the elbow. Arthroscopy 1995;11(4):437–443
3. Osborn AG: Diagnostic Neuroradiology. Mosby, St. Louis, 1994
4. Ryu J, Saito S, Honda T, Yamamoto K: Risk factors and prophylactic tenosynovectomy for extensor tendon rupture of the rheumatoid hand. J Hand Surg [Br] 1998;23(5):658–661
5. Thirupathi RG, Ferlic DC, Clayton ML: Dorsal wrist synovectomy in rheumatoid arthritis—a long-term study. J Hand Surg [Am] 1983;8(6):848–856
6. Chantelot C, Fontaine C, Flipo RM et al: Synovectomy combined with the Sauve–Kapandji procure for the wrist. J Hand Surg [Br] 1999;24(4):405–409
7. Tulp NJ, Winia WP: Synovectomy of the elbow in rheumatoid arthritis. Long-term results. J Bone Joint Surg Br 1989;71(4):664–666
8. Adolfsson L, Frisen M: Arthroscopic synovectomy of the rheumatoid wrist. A 3.8 year follow-up. J Hand Surg [Br] 1997;22(6):711–713
9. O'Driscoll SW: Operative treatment of elbow arthritis. Curr Opin Rheumatol 1995;7(2):103–106
10. Ferlic DC, Patchett CE, Clayton ML, Freeman AC: Elbow synovectomy in rheumatoid arthritis. Long-term results. Clin Orthop 1987;220:119–125
11. Brumfield RH Jr, Resnick CT: Synovectomy of the elbow in rheumatoid arthritis. J Bone Joint Surg Am 1985;67(1):16–20
12. Turk DC, Flor H: Etiological theories and treatments for chronic back pain. II. Psychological models and interventions. Pain 1984;19(3):209–233
13. Summers GD, Webley M, Taylor AR: A reappraisal of synovectomy and radial-head excision in rheumatoid arthritis. Br J Rheumatol 1987;26(1):59–61
14. Tabor OB Jr, Tabor OB: Unicompartmental arthroplasty: A long-term follow-up study. J Arthroplasty 1998;13:373–379
15. Rymaszewski LA, Mackay I, Amis AA, Miller JH: Long-term effects of excision of the radial head in rheumatoid arthrits. J Bone Joint Surg Br 1984;66(1):109–113
16. Hildebrand KA, Paterson SD, Regan WD, MacDermid JC, King GJ: Functional outcome of semiconstrained total elbow arthroplasty. J Bone Joint Surg Am 2000;82-A(10):1379–1386
17. Mansat P, Morrey BF: J Bone Joint Surg Am 2000;82(9):1260–1268
18. Schneeberger AG, Hertel R, Gerber C: Total elbow replacement with the GSB III prosthesis. J Shoulder Elbow Surg 2000;9(2):135–139
19. Rozing P: Souter–Strathclyde total elbow arthroplasty. J Bone Joint Surg Br 2000;82(8):1129–1134
20. Goldberg VM, Figgie HE III, Heiple KG et al: Use of a total condylar knee prosthesis for treatment of osteoarthritis and rheumatoid arthritis. Long-term results. J Bone Joint Surg [Am] 1988;70:802–811
21. Sculco TP: Cost reduction in total joint arthroplasty. Orthopedics 1998;21(9):1053–1054
22. Barrack RI, Folgueras A, Munn B, Tvetden D, Sharkey P: Pelvis lysis and polyethylene wear at 5–8 years in an uncemented total hip. Clin Orthop 1997;335:211–217
23. Zicat B, Engh CA, Gokcen E: Patterns of osteolysis around total hip components inserted with and without cement. J Bone Joint Surg 1995;77A:432–439
24. Berger RA, Kull LR, Rosenberg AG, Galante JO: Hybri total hip arthroplasty 7- to 10-year results. Clin Orthop 1996;333:134–146
25. Capello WN, D'Antonio JA, Feinberg JR, Manley MT: Hydroxyapatite-coated total hip femoral components in patients less than fifty years old:

Clinical and radiographic results after five to eight years of follow-up. J Bone Joint Surg 1997;79A:1023–1029

26. Dowdy PA, Rorabeck CH, Bourne RB: Uncemented total hip arthroplasty in patients 50 years of age or younger. J Arthroplasty 1997;12:853–862

27. Schmalzried TP, Callaghan JJ: Wear in total hip and knee replacements. J Bone Joint Surg 1999;81A:115–136

28. Wouters E, Bassett FH III, Hardaker WT Jr et al: An algorithm for arthroscopy in the over-50 age group. Am J Sports Med 1992;20:141–145

29. Garvin KL, Hanssen AD: Infection after total hip arthroplasty: Past, present, and future. J Bone Joint Surg 1995;78A:1576–1588

30. Masteron EL, Masri BA, Duncan CP: Treatment of infection at the site of total hip replacement. J Bone Joint Surg 1997;79A:1740–1749

31. Pellegrini VD Jr, Clement D, Lush-Ehmann C, Keller GS, Kevarts CM: Natural history of thromboembolic disease after total hip arthroplasty. Clin Orthop 1996;333:27–40

32. Sikorski JM, Hampson WG, Staddon GE: The natural history and etiology of deep vein thrombosis after total hip replacement. J Bone Joint Surg 1981;63B:171–177

33. White AA, Panjabi MM: Biomechanical considerations in the surgical management of cervical spondylotic myelopathy. Spine 1988;13:856–860

34. Johnson R, Green JR, Charnley J: Pulmonary embolism and its prophylaxis following total hip replacement: Clin Orthop 1977;127:123–132

35. Knelles D, Barthel T, Karrer A et al: Prevention of heterotopic ossification after total hip replacement. J Bone Joint Surg 1997;79B:596–602

36. Helundh U, Hybbinette CH, Fredin H: Influence of surgical approach on dislocations after Charnley hip arthroplasty. J Arthroplasty 1995;10:609–614

37. Morrey BF: Difficult complications after hip replacement: Dislocation. Clin Orthop 1997;344:179–187

38. Pellici PM, Wilson PD Jr, Sledge CB: Long-term results of revision total hip replacement. A follow-up report. J Bone Joint Surg 1985;67A:513–516.

39. Arthritis Foundation: Osteoarthritis Fact Sheet. August 6, 1997

40. Chang RW, Falconer J, Stulberg SD et al: A randomized, controlled trial of arthroscopic surgery versus closed-needle joint lavage for patients with osteoarthritis of the knee. Arthritis Rheum 1993;36:289–296

41. Muller-Fabbender H, Bach GL, Haase W et al: Glucosamine sulfate compared to ibuprofen in osteoarthritis of the knee. Osteoarthritis Cartilage 1994;2:61–69

42. Adams ME, Atkinson MH, Lussier A et al: The role of viscosupplementation with hylan G-F 20 (Synvisc) in the treatment of osteoarthritis of the knee: a Canadian multicenter trial comparing hylan G-F 20 alone, hylan G-F 20 with nonsteroidal anti-inflammatory drugs (NSAIDs) and NSAIDs alone. Osteoarthritis Cartilage 1995;3:213–226

43. Jones AC, Pattrick M, Doherty S et al: Intra-articular hyaluronic acid compared to intra-articular triamcinolone hexacetonide in inflammatory knee osteoarthritis. Osteoarthritis Cartilage 1995;3:269–273

44. Raynauld JP: A prospective, randomized, effectiveness and cost-effectiveness evaluation of appropriate care with Synvisc compared to appropriate care without Synvisc in the treatment of patients with osteoarthritis of the knee. Safety and effectiveness data. In: Program and Abstracts of OARSI 1999 4th World Congress, September 17, 1999; Vienna, Austria. (abstract)

45. Merchan ECR, Galindo E: Arthroscope-guided surgery versus nonoperative treatment for limited degenerative osteoarthritis of the femorotibial joint in patients over 50 years of age: A prospective comparative study. Arthroscopy 1993;9:663–667

46. Yonenobu K, Hosono N, Iwasaki M, Asano M, Ono K: Laminoplasty versus subtotal corpectomy: A comparative study of results in multisegmental cervical spondylotic myelopathy. Spine 1992;17:1281–1284

47. Yang SS, Nisonson B: Arthroscopic surgery of the knee in the geriatric patient. Clin Orthop 1995;316:50–58

48. Tan JC, Nordin M: Role of physical therapy in the treatment of cervical disk disease. Orthop Clin North Am 1992;23(3):435–449

49. Newman JH, Ackroyd CE, Shah NA: Unicompartmental or total knee replacement? Five-year results of a prospective, randomized trial of 102 osteoarthritic knees with unicompartmental arthritis. J Bone Joint Surg [Br] 1998;80:862–865

50. Marmor L: Unicompartmental knee arthroplasty: Ten- to 13-year follow-up study. Clin Orthop 1988;226:14–20

51. Rand JA: Cement or cementless fixation in total knee arthroplasty? Clin Orthop 1991;273:52–62

52. Ranawat CS, Flynn WF Jr, Deshmukh RG: Impact of modern technique on long-term results of total condylar knee arthroplasty. Clin Orthop 1994;309:131–135

53. Colizza WA, Insall JN, Scuderi GR: The posterior stabilized total knee prosthesis. Assessment of polyethylene damage and osteolysis after 10-year-minimal follow-up. J Bone Joint Surg [Am] 1995;77:1713–1720

54. Goldberg BA, Scarlat MM, Harryman DT II: Management of the stiff shoulder. J Orthop Sci 1999;4:462–471

55. Frykberg RG, Armstrong DG, Giurini J et al: Diabetic foot disorders. A clinical practice guideline for the American College of Foot and Ankle Surgeons and the American College of Foot and Ankle Orthopedics and Medicine. J Foot Ankle Surg 2000;Suppl:1–60

56. Myerson MS: Foot and Ankle Disorders. WB Saunders 2000:212

57. Stetsib WB, Ferkel RD: Ankle arthroscopy I. Technique and complications. J Am Acad Orthop Surg 1996;4(1):17–23

58. Abidi NA, Gruen GS, Conti SF: Ankle arthrodesis: indications and techniques. J Am Acad Orthop Surg 2000;8(3):200–209

59. Coester LM, Saltzman CL, Leupold J, Pontarelli W: Long term results following ankle arthrodesis for post-traumatic arthritis. J Bone Joint Surg Am 2001;83(2):219–228

60. Hansen S: Functional Reconstruction of the Foot and Ankle. Lippincott Williams & Wilkins, 2000.

61. Neufeld SK, Lee TH: Total ankle arthroplasty: indications, results, and biomechanical rationale. Am J Orthop 2000;29(8):593–602

62. Mothershed RA, Strapp MD, Smith TF: Talonavicular arthrodesis for correction of posterior tibial tendon dysfunction. Clin Podiatr Med Surg 1999;16(3):501–526

63. Depalma AF, Subin DK: Study of the cervical syndrome. Clin Orthop 1985; 38:135–142

64. Bridwell KH, Dewald RL. Keith H: The Textbook of Spinal Surgery. 2nd Ed. Vols I, II. Lippincott-Raven, Philadelphia, 1997.

65. Benzel EC: Spine Surgery: Techniques, Complication Avoidance, and Management, 1st Ed. Vols 1,2. Churchill Livingstone, New York, 1999.

66. Dillin W, Uppal GS: Analysis of medications used in the treatment of cervical disk degeneration. Orthop Clin North Am 1992;23(3):421–433

67. Goodman LS, Gilman A, Gilman AG: Goodman and Gilman's The Pharmacological Basis of Therapeutics (7th Ed). New York, Macmillan, 1985

68. Pilowsky I, Chapman CR, Bonica JJ: Pain, depression, and illness behavior in a pain clinic population. Pain 1977;4(2):183–192

69. Barnsley L, Lord SM, Wallis BJ, Bogduk N: Lack of effect of intraarticular corticosteroids for chronic pain in the cervical zygopophyseal joints. N Engl J Med 1994;330(15):1047–1050

70. DiPalma JR, DiGregorio GJ: Management of low back pain and neck pain by analgesics and adjuvant drugs: An update. Mt Sinai J Med 1994; 61(3):193–196

71. Kriss TC, Kriss VM: Neck pain: Primary care work-up of acute and chronic symptoms. Geriatrics 2000;55(Jan):47–57

72. Pasternak G: Psychotropic drugs and chronic pain. In Hendler NH, Long DM, Wise TN (eds): Diagnosis and Treatment of Chronic Pain, Wright Publishing, Littletown, MA, 1982:35–50

73. Shapiro S: Approach to the patient with neck pain, with and without associated arm pain. In Biller J (ed): Practical Neurology. Lippincott-Raven, Philadelphia, 1997:229–237

74. Menezes, AH, Sonntag VKH: Principles of spinal surgery, Vols 1, 2. McGraw-Hill, Health Professions Division, New York, 1996.

75. Rath WW: Cervical traction: A clinical perspective. Orthop Rev 1984;8:430–449

76. Wilkins RH, Rengachary SS: Neurosurgery, 2nd Ed. McGraw-Hill, Health Professions Division, New York, 1996

77. Labbe EE, Goldberg M, Fishbain D et al: Behavioral Health Inventory norms for chronic pain patients. J Clin Psychol 1989;45(3):383–390

78. Benzel EC: Biomechanics of Spine Stabilization: Principles and Clinical Practice. New York, McGraw-Hill, 1995

79. Mathis JM, Barr JD, Belkoff SM et al: Percutaneous vertebroplasty: a developing standard of care for vertebral compression fractures. AM J Neuroradiol 2001;22(2):373–381

80. Cyteval C, Sarrabere MP, Roux JO et al: Acute osteoporotic vertebral collapse: open study on percutaneous injection of acrylic surgical cement in 20 patients. Am J Roentgenol 1999;173:1685–1690

81. Landis SH, Murray T, Bolden S, Wingo PA: Cancer Statistics, 1999. CA Cancer J Clin 1999;49(1):8–31

82. Kamholtz R, Sze G: Current imaging in spinal metastatic disease. Semin Oncol 1991;18(2):158–169

83. British Association of Surgical Oncology Guidelines: The management of metastatic bone disease in the United Kingdom: the Breast Specialty Group of the British Association of Surgical Oncology. Eur J Surg Oncol 1999;25:3–23

84. Hipp JA, Springfield DS, Hayes WC: Predicting pathologic fracture risk in the management of metastatic bone defects. Clin Orthop 1995;312:120–135

85. Beals RK, Lawton GD, Snell WE: Prophylactic internal fixation of the femur in metastatic breast cancer. Cancer 1971;28:1350–1354

86. Mirels H: Metastatic disease in long bones: A proposed scoring system for diagnosing impending pathologic fractures. Clin Orthop 1989;249:256–264

87. Walls J, Bundred N, Howell A: Hypercalcemia and bone resorption in malignancy. Clin Orthop 1995;312:51–63

88. Warwck D, Williams MH, Bannister GC: Death and thromboembolic disease after total hip replacement. J Bone Joint Surg 1995;77B:6–10

89. Sim FH, Frassica FJ, Chao EY: Orthopaedic management using new devices and prostheses. Clin Orthop 1995;312:10–172. Spivak JM: Degenerative lumbar spinal stenosis. J Bone Joint Surg Am 1998;80:1053–1066

90. Galasko CS: Diagnosis of skeletal metastases and assessment of response to treatment. Clin Orthop 1995;312:6475.

91. Frassica DA, Gunderson LL: Principles of radiation therapy in the treatment of bone metastases. Orthopedics 1992;15:579–581

92. Harrison LB, Franzese F, Gaynor JJ, Brennan MF: Long-term results of a prospective randomized trial of adjuvant brachytherapy in the management of completely resected soft tissue sarcomas of the extremity and superficial trunk. Int J Radiat Oncol Biol Phys 1993;27:259–265

93. Fleming JB, Berman RS, Cheng SC et al: Long-term outcome of patients with American Joint Committee on Cancer stage IIB extremity soft tissue sarcomas. J Clin Oncol 1999;7:2772–2780

Chapter 74

Injury in elderly people

Michael A. Horan

To consider trauma as a condition confined to the young is wrong. Although injuries are certainly more common in younger people than in the older population, older people are much more likely to die as a result of their injuries, virtually regardless of injury severity.[1–8] People aged over 65 years account for about 28 percent of all fatal injuries, despite constituting only about 12 percent of the total population.[9] Falls are the cause of the majority of injuries in older people[10] but falls are common in all age groups. In one study, older people accounted for only about 14 percent of fall-related injuries but for about 50 percent of fall-related deaths.[11] Road traffic accidents account for the majority of multiple injuries.[10,12] American figures for 1986 report that 38 percent of hospital bed-days for all patients in whom injury was the primary reason for hospital admission were accounted for by those over the age of 65 years.[5] Using 1986 average daily costs in the hospital ($500) and in intensive care units ($1,200 to $2,000), their hospital expenses were estimated to exceed $4.4 billion. Despite these huge resource implications, most research has focused on younger victims of trauma and older victims of trauma have almost certainly received suboptimal treatment.

DEFINING AND MEASURING INJURY

The transfer of energy at rates and in amounts above the tolerance of tissues is the necessary and specific cause of injury. The amount of energy concentration outside the limits of tissue tolerance determines the severity of injury. Thus, injury generally refers to the damage to cells, tissues, and organs but may also include the nature and magnitude of the various physiological responses in the recipient of the injury.

The measurement of injury is as important for planning management and studying outcomes, as is measurement in any other disease where a variety of grading and staging systems may be used. The systems used for injury utilize either the anatomical extent of the injury, the (patho)physiological responses of the recipient of the injury, or some hybrid of these two.

Anatomical indexes (e.g. Abbreviated Injury Scale, Injury Severity Score, Anatomical Profile), which require complete and accurate diagnosis, are of only limited use in the immediate management of an injured patient because full information is rarely available until much later. However, they are very useful in evaluating trauma systems and outcome assessment. Scoring systems based on the response of the injured individual (e.g. Glasgow Coma Scale, Revised Trauma Score, Simplified Acute Physiology Score, APACHE) are particularly useful for triage and/or patient management. The most commonly used hybrids are the TRISS (Revised Trauma Score + Injury Severity Score) and ASCOT (A Severity Characterization

of Trauma), the latter having been developed in response to the limitations of the anatomical component of TRISS and which appears to be a much better predictor of survival. None of the available systems is entirely satisfactory for all purposes, particularly for the prediction of outcomes other than death.[5,13] The shortcomings of the TRISS methodology are particularly apparent for falls from a low height: adverse outcomes are very poorly predicted.[14]

The data used to derive most of these scoring systems come mainly from injured younger people, and the systems may not perform well for old people.[6,15,16] Possible reasons for this are discussed by Horan et al.[17] Because old bones are weaker than young ones, less energy will be needed to exceed breaking tolerance and the associated soft tissue damage is likely to be less extensive, and thus anatomical scoring systems tend to overestimate the anatomical severity of injury. However, any age-related attenuation of the physiological responses of the recipient of the injury would tend to underestimate the severity of the injury. This seems to be of only theoretical importance because old people tend to present greater physiological perturbations (SAPS) for all but the most extreme anatomical injury severity scores (ISS).[18] Once age groups are stratified for SAPS score, age ceases to be an important outcome predictor, provided equivalent treatments are employed. A similar conclusion was reached in a study designed to validate the APACHE III scoring system, which showed that age alone accounted for very little of the variation of outcome; physiological derangements and comorbid factors were much more important.[19]

Although well recognized, the deficiencies of the generally used scoring systems when applied to elderly people have not been adequately addressed. DeMaria et al.[16] devised a Geriatric Trauma Survival Score that was 92 percent accurate in predicting survival. This system is based on the ISS plus cardiac and infective complications as well as ventilator dependence. Other studies to address the utility of this scoring system seem not to have been done and it is not widely used.

INJURIES AT SPECIFIC SITES
Head injuries

As the brain ages, its dura becomes tightly adherent to the skull, which makes epidural hematomas uncommon. A progressive loss of brain volume leads to an increase in the space around the brain that is thought to protect it against contusions, but makes subdural hematomas more likely. Intraparenchymal hemorrhage is also more common in elderly people. The epidemiology of head injuries has been reviewed.[20] Two aspects are particularly worthy of note: First, there is a modest increase in incidence rates after the age of about 60 years and, second, head injuries are more common in men than in women, even in extreme old age. Thus, crude figures, unadjusted for sex, may underestimate the importance of head injuries among older people owing to the preponderance of women in older age groups.

Head injuries in older people can be devastating. Severe injuries (Glasgow Coma Scale less than 8) have a fatality rate of about 90 percent.[21] Those who survive the initial injury have long hospital stays and more severe residual neurological deficits. In a study comparing 33 younger patients with acute subdural hematomas with 34 older patients with similar lesions, none of the older patients with a GCS less than 13 made a functional recovery. It is widely believed that elderly people also have poorer outcomes after minor head injuries (GCS 13 or greater on presentation) but there is little published evidence to support this conclusion.

It is not clear why older people have such poor outcomes after head injuries. It is likely that comorbid factors, suboptimal management, and a predisposition to systemic complications play important roles, although a recent study suggests that there is a reduced capacity of the aging brain to recover from injuries.[22]

Thoracic trauma

Older people with isolated chest injuries have a two to three times greater risk of death than similarly injured younger people[2,23,24] and low rib fractures may be associated with liver or spleen injuries. Rib fractures often complicate even mild blunt trauma to the chest in older people. Similarly, insignificant falls or blows to the chest may cause occult pneumothorax or hemothorax, and pulmonary contusions often accompany even mild thoracic injuries. Prompt mechanical ventilation is warranted in older patients showing signs of respiratory distress in any of these circumstances. A history of rapid deceleration should alert one to the possibility of traumatic rupture of the aorta in all older patients. Mediastinal widening or an ill-defined aortic knuckle are characteristic radiographic appearances. Although more than 80 percent of those with this complication die at the accident scene, the remainder may be hemodynamically stable on presentation.

Abdominal trauma

The death rate in older patients with visceral injuries is about 80 percent.[6] The principles of management of abdominal injuries change little with age. However, it should be borne in mind that the old are intolerant of both shock and unnecessary laparotomy and their management demands a sense of urgency and a high degree of clinical acumen. Those with a history of previous significant abdominal surgery, young or old, should have either a computed tomography scan or ultrasound scan rather than diagnostic peritoneal lavage.

Fall-related fractures

The nature of the fall dictates the nature of the fracture. Fractures of the wrist and proximal humerus are believed to be associated with falls on an outstretched arm, implying that the person was moving reasonably fast at the time of the fall.

Falls from a stationary position or during slow locomotion are generally considered most likely to result in proximal femoral fractures, and it is these that account for most of the old-age peak in trauma deaths.[25] Falls also account for the majority of cervical spine fractures in older people.[26] Frail older people may sustain long bone fractures without a clear history of injury or falls.[27] These have been termed *minimal trauma fractures* and the only precipitating factor clearly identified is severely impaired mobility.

Falls have four distinct phases: (1) loss of balance, (2) a phase of descent, (3) an impact phase, and (4) a postimpact phase during which the faller eventually comes to rest.[28] Most work on falls and fall prevention has concentrated on the first of these (why people fall) and the results emphasize the importance of gait disorders, dementia, visual impairment, neurological and musculoskeletal disorders, orthostatic hypotension, drugs, and environmental hazards. By contrast, little is known about the other three phases (how people fall) and how this relates to the risk of fracture. Cummings and Nevitt[29] consider that for a hip fracture to occur, there must be (1) impact near the hip, (2) failure of active protective mechanisms, and (3) insufficient passive energy absorption by local soft tissues. Under these conditions they suggest that sufficient force can be transmitted to the proximal femur to exceed its fracture load. Others have reported that in a typical fall, more than enough energy will be available to fracture an elderly hip.[30,31]

Experimental systems have been developed to get more precise measurements of the forces involved in falls under different experimental conditions. It was shown that fall in a state of muscle contraction (mainly trunk and back muscles) considerably increases impact force.[32] However, more physiological studies on experimental falls suggest that eccentric contractions of these muscle groups can dissipate up to two-thirds of the available potential energy with further contributions from stiffness and damping in the hip and knee.[33] Thus, although falls among elderly subjects are associated with available potential energies between 400 J and 700 J, the actual energy available at impact could be only about one-third of these values. The strength of the proximal femur has been measured in cadaveric specimens tested in a loading configuration that simulated a fall with impact on the greater trochanter. It was found that fracture load is linearly related to bone mineral density.[34]

Nevitt and Cummings[35] compared fallers sustaining fractures with those who did not. Those who sustained fractures were more likely to have fallen sideways or straight down (odds ratio 3.3) and to have landed on or near the hip (odds ratio 32.5). For those who fell on their hip, the risk of fracture approximately doubled for every standard deviation decrease in bone mineral density at the hip. Similarly, Greenspan et al.[36] found that falling to the side increased fracture risk six-fold; increasing the potential energy of the fall by one standard deviation increased the risk three-fold; and a reduction of body mass index by one standard deviation increased fracture risk two-fold. A decrease in bone mineral density by one standard deviation increased fracture risk three-fold.

The combined data from the above studies show an average impact force of about 5,600 N[33] and an average fracture load of about 4,170 N. Thus, those who do not sustain fractures under these conditions *must* employ energy absorbing/dissipating mechanisms to reduce the force delivered to the femur: eccentric contraction of large muscles, use of the outstretched hand, and energy absorption by soft tissues. These studies also suggest that pharmacological interventions to increase proximal femur bone mineral density would have to show substantial effects in order to increase fracture load above the likely impact forces and interventions to prevent falls would probably have a much greater impact on fracture incidence.

Multiple injuries

Visceral injuries in the absence of fractures are very rare in older trauma victims.[1] The bony injuries that present the most immediate threats to life are skull fractures (with underlying brain injury) and fractures of the pelvis. The main problem with pelvic fractures is massive bleeding from lacerations to the pelvic venous plexus, but this can generally be controlled by external fixators. About 15 percent of older people with closed pelvic fractures die, whereas for open fractures the death rate is approximately 80 percent.[37] Long-bone fractures, especially of the tibia, are common and must be stabilized early to control blood loss, reduce the risk of fat embolism, and enable early mobilization. Older people do not tolerate delays before surgical stabilization well,[38] even after isolated hip fractures.[39,40]

Injuries associated with restraints

Physical restraints have been used, usually in cognitively impaired patients, with the intention of preventing wandering or falls. However, most study findings indicate that the use of restraints does not reduce either the risk or incidence of falls, other accidents, or disruption of medical care when appropriate alternative interventions are provided. In fact, research suggests that the use of restraints causes more problems than it prevents, including exacerbation of agitation and wandering, falls from a greater height than would have otherwise occurred, and even death (for example by asphyxiation when trapped between bed rails).

RESPONSES TO INJURY
The ebb and flow phases

The general response to physical injury is complex and is conventionally divided into two phases: the ebb phase and the flow phase.[41] In general, the ebb phase is one of increased fuel production and reduced metabolic rate, whereas the flow phase is characterized by increased metabolic rate, catabolism, and fuel utilization. Because responses to injury in older people have not been systematically studied, it is impossible to give a complete account and so I will concentrate on those aspects that are best understood and those that seem of particular clinical importance.

The hypothalamic–pituitary–adrenal axis

One of the most rapid effects of injury is to provoke well-known neuroendocrine responses. The activity of the sympathoadrenal system and the hypothalamic–pituitary–adrenal (HPA) axis, and the secretion of a number of other hormones (growth hormone, prolactin, vasopressin, aldosterone, and glucagon), are increased. In some systems, such as the sympathoadrenal, the magnitude of the initial response increases with injury severity and may not be detectable at all with minor injuries. For other systems, such as the HPA axis, it is the duration of the response that increases with injury severity. Aging does not appear to impair these early neuroendocrine responses.

It has been repeatedly shown that the plasma cortisol concentration remains elevated at 2 weeks after proximal femur fracture, by which time it has returned to normal in younger patients with injuries of similar, and even greater, severity[42] and the difference from healthy or bed-ridden elderly control subjects can persist for at least 8 weeks.[43] Compared with healthy elderly women, patients 2 weeks after hip fracture have increased rates of cortisol production and urinary free cortisol excretion.[44]

The reason for the continued cortisol production is unclear. The early HPA response to injury may be provoked by a number of signals (volume depletion, hypotension, nociception, hypoxia, circulating cytokines), the relative importance of which will depend on the nature and severity of the injury. In patients with simple fractures, such stimuli should soon cease as appropriate treatments are instituted, and this is consistent with the short-lived cortisol response in younger patients. We believe that older people have an impaired ability to down-regulate the response after resolution of the stimulus rather than a more persistent stimulus. Such a defect is observed in old rats and results from loss of corticosteroid receptors in the hippocampus, which play a role in feedback inhibition.[45] Evidence for the same process in humans comes from patients with Alzheimer's dementia, who have extensive hippocampal neuron loss and show impaired feedback inhibition of the HPA axis as measured by the dexamethasone suppression test. Resistance to dexamethasone suppression in depression is more common among elderly than among young patients and is associated with cognitive impairment.[45] We have found marked resistance to dexamethasone suppression in elderly patients with hip fracture,[43,46] suggesting that their hypercortisolemia may also be due to degenerative changes in the hippocampus. Whether or not some older people are particularly predisposed to a prolonged cortisol response to stress is not known. Genetic factors have not been sought but early life events might dictate responses in later life. Recently, Barker[47] has drawn attention to the importance of perinatal events and the development of disease in later life. Levitt et al.[48] have shown that administration of glucocorticoids to rats in the last week of pregnancy leads to reduced numbers of hippocampal glucocorticoid receptors and the development of hypertension when the offspring reach adulthood. Likewise, their administration in the first week of life leads to similarly reduced numbers of hippocampal glucocorticoid receptors in adulthood.

It is still not known whether the persistent hypercortisolemia is maladaptive or a necessary adaptive response, but if the cause(s) is/are essentially pathological, the former possibility is the more likely. The acute adrenocortical response helps protect against the effects of hypovolemia by increasing blood glucose and promoting compensatory fluid movement.[49] However, once fluid loss has been corrected, there is little evidence that a sustained elevation in cortisol concentration (as opposed to basal levels, which are known to protect against circulatory collapse) is required to maintain cardiovascular integrity.

If the response is a beneficial adaptation it might be expected that there would be evidence of acquired resistance to glucocorticoid effects, which has already been described in Alzheimer's disease[50] and as a transient phenomenon in depression, septic shock, and acquired immunodeficiency syndrome as well as in corticosteroid-resistant asthma, colitis, and rheumatoid disease.[51] Our own unpublished work has shown no evidence of resistance to glucocorticoid effects in circulating lymphocytes or polymorphonuclear leukocytes.

If it is a maladaptive response, we would expect to see evidence of its effects in the form of insulin resistance, muscle proteolysis, immune suppression, impaired wound healing, etc. Such effects are well known in patients with Cushing's disease and are found also in patients with major depression.[52] Animal experiments with glucocorticoid antagonists have shown that endogenous glucocorticoids have protein-catabolic and immunosuppressive effects soon after injury, when their concentrations are elevated.[53,54]

Metabolic changes

Like the early neuroendocrine responses, the early metabolic changes after injury are not attenuated with aging. Plasma glucose concentrations rise with injury severity but plasma insulin fails to rise commensurately owing to suppression of insulin secretion by circulating catecholamines. Concentrations of lipid metabolites and lactate are also similar in young and old people after injury, although there is evidence that older people have higher rates of lipolysis and re-esterification of free fatty acids within adipose tissue for reasons that are not clear.

The flow phase is associated with elevations in metabolic rate and urinary nitrogen excretion caused by muscle protein catabolism. Older hip fracture patients show the expected rise in metabolic rate and nitrogen excretion.[55–57] The patients in these studies accumulated an energy and nitrogen deficit over about a week that was estimated to be preventable in most patients by dietary supplementation of about 300 kcal/day energy and 20 g/day protein. Those patients with a more marked protein deficiency had a reduced probability of survival.[56]

The flow phase also affects carbohydrate and fat metabolism. There is a shift from carbohydrate to fat as the preferred fuel and patients are resistant to the effects of insulin. The magnitude of insulin resistance in injured elderly people is reported to be significantly greater than in the young.[58] The cause of this exaggerated insulin resistance is unknown but it seems highly likely that the high cortisol concentrations are at least partly responsible.

RECOVERY FOLLOWING INJURY

Recovery following injury has at least three components: (1) resolution of the catabolic flow phase and restoration of the energy and protein deficits, (2) return of function of injured body parts, and (3) the psychosocial adjustment of the injured patient.

The phase of anabolism

It is not known whether the catabolic flow phase gives way to the phase of anabolism and recovery occurs simply by the passive termination of the signals that maintain the flow phase or whether it is actively driven by positive signals. Moore,[59] studying recovery from major surgery in younger patients, considered that the anabolic phase could not occur without the resumption of feeding but that this is not the signal that initiates it. He also thought that protein synthesis proceeds at its maximum rate and could not be increased further by endocrine manipulations or forced feeding. Only after the nitrogen debt is repaid and lean body mass is restored is fat deposited. Failure to increase dietary intake results in a failure to gain weight and recovery becomes stalled. Interestingly, even healthy older women fed an energy-replete but marginally protein-deficient diet over 9 weeks developed significant losses of lean body mass, muscle strength, and immune functions.[60]

The studies of Moore have not been confirmed. Indeed, it is surprising how little work has been done in this important area in patients of any age. Humberstone and Shaw[61] studied glucose and protein kinetics in eight patients aged 56–79 years following major surgery and showed that these patients were unable completely to oxidize glucose to carbon dioxide and there was increased glucose recycling to lactate. Glucose oxidation was reduced by about 40 percent. Glucose production was increased and this was not suppressed normally by the infusion of glucose. Basal insulin concentrations were elevated with a reduced response to glucose infusion.

The only other aspect of the whole body response to injury studied beyond the flow phase is fatigue.[62] Although there are modest reductions in isokinetic endurance and isometric strength of skeletal muscles during convalescence from moderate surgery, a sensation of fatigue is a very prominent symptom that persists for a month or more, at least in younger patients. Its cause is not known and the phenomenon has not been studied specifically in older trauma patients or patients undergoing elective surgery.

The importance of proper nutrition for older people, the high prevalence of undernutrition in older people in the hospital, and the severe morbidity and mortality associated with undernutrition are all well known, and yet undernutrition continues to be overlooked.[63] Many older people admitted with hip fractures already have evidence of undernutrition at the time of presentation[64,65] and it has been suggested that thinness[48] and weight loss after age 50 years[66] increase fracture risk through poorly understood mechanisms that presumably include a reduced ability to dissipate energy on impact.[29,36] Surprisingly, it has been reported that one-third of orthopedic surgeons in the north of England did not feel that malnutrition was an important problem in their patients with hip fractures.[67]

People presenting with hip fractures who are already undernourished fare worse than their well-nourished counterparts[65] and nutritional support seems to improve their condition.[68,69] Bastow et al.[68] used overnight nasogastric feeding and Delmi et al.[69] claim impressive results with oral supplements, although oral supplements in large quantities are not well tolerated by older patients with hip fracture.[70] Although the concept of nutritional support for patients with hip fractures is well established, we do not know how best to tailor it to the needs of individual patients. The shortcomings of these, and other, studies have been highlighted in a Cochrane review,[71] which concluded that the strongest evidence of the effectiveness of nutritional supplementation exists for oral multinutrient feeds, but the evidence is very weak. The benefits of nasogastric feeding are even less certain, and it should probably be reserved for the very malnourished, with extremely poor intakes not responsive to oral supplementation.

Return of function

Recent studies have shown that only about 40 percent of patients with hip fractures who were ambulant without a walking aid before the injury returned to that state.[72,73] Interestingly, the degree of impairment in lower extremity fractures accounts for only about half the variance in functional outcome.[74] Lamb et al.[75] studied previously healthy patients with hip fractures and showed that extensor muscle power in the fractured leg was the most important determinant of walking speed and stair-climbing time and that the most important determinant of leg extensor power was pain. Other factors are also important. Comorbid conditions including depression and dementia, malnutrition, social supports, and prefracture functional abilities and fitness predict eventual functional recovery.[65,76–84]

Although many of the factors mentioned above are ameliorable, the only intervention that has actually been shown to modify recovery is nutrition. We, and others, are interested in the use of anabolic agents and other pharmacological interventions, but none has been properly studied in the injured elderly population. Nevertheless, it would seem prudent to optimize management of comorbid conditions and take steps to prevent complications, for example by heparin prophylaxis for venous thromboembolism, perioperative antibiotics, and competent fluid resuscitation. Early mobilization is also to be encouraged as immobilization results in further deconditioning,[85] muscle wasting, body fluid shifts, and in an increased risk of venous thrombosis and decubitus ulcers. Some orthopedic surgeons delay weight-bearing after insertion of a rigid fixation device. Such devices maintain good reduction of the fracture but reduce the callus response and slow fracture healing with the attendant risk of fixation failure. However, at least for hip fractures, this may not be a very important consideration. A recent study has shown that early, complete weight-bearing is not associated with a high risk of failure of fixation, nonunion, osteonecrosis, or prosthetic dislocation.[79] The optimal rehabilitation approach to get people safely back on their feet and walking again has not been established. People may be asked to rest in bed, restrict weight-bearing, or restrict particular activities and different physiotherapy and exercise programs may be used. A recent Cochrane review found there was not enough evidence from randomized trials to show the effects of these different strategies for helping people walk after hip fracture surgery.[86]

Psychosocial adjustment

The importance of psychological factors on recovery from illness and surgery has recently been stressed[87] but little is known about this in older people in any clinical setting. Only depression has been addressed in any detail.[78,88,89] It is common, often undiagnosed, and contributes to the syndrome of "failure to thrive."[90] Adequate screening instruments and effective treatments for depression are readily available but it has not yet been shown whether either preventive strategies or early detection and treatment will improve the quality, or accelerate the rate, of recovery.

CONCLUSION

Injuries are common in older people and are poorly tolerated. There is evidence that, because of the greater physiological disturbances induced by the injuries and because older patients (age greater than 50 years) are particularly predisposed to develop multiple organ failure,[91] a lower threshold for invasive monitoring will enhance survival. Indeed, aggressive treatment with early invasive monitoring has already been reported to be beneficial for outcome.[18,91,92] A recent study in the USA, where there are well-organized trauma teams, has suggested that an age of 70 years or more in an injured patient should be sufficient to trigger trauma team activation.[93] There is also evidence that some aspects of the endocrine-metabolic response may be maladaptive and may be amenable to therapeutic interventions (e.g. by controlled inhibition of glucocorticoid synthesis). Other factors that predispose to suboptimal outcomes are also known and are more readily amenable to modification (e.g. nutritional support, antidepressants, prevention of complications, treatment of comorbid conditions), although the ultimate benefits that might result have only been demonstrated for nutritional interventions. Early mobilization should also be done because the theoretical objections have been shown to be of little importance. However, we do not yet know what constitutes an optimal rehabilitation strategy after hip fracture, let alone after other injuries in the elderly population. Even if we did know what should be done, could we deliver?[94]

REFERENCES

1. Oreskovich MR, Howard JD, Copass MK, Carrico CJ: Geriatric trauma: injury patterns and outcome. J Trauma 1984;24:565–572
2. Allen JE, Schwab CW: Blunt chest trauma in the elderly. Am Surg 1985;51:697–700
3. Evans JG: Falls and fractures. Age Ageing 1988;17:361–364
4. Osler T, Hales K, Baack B et al: Trauma in the elderly. Am J Surg 1988;156:537–543
5. Champion H, Copes W, Buyer D et al: Major trauma in geriatric patients. Am J Public Health 1989;79:1278–1282
6. Finelli FC, Jonsson J, Champion H et al: A case control study for major trauma in geriatric patients. J Trauma 1989;29:541–548
7. McCoy GF, Johnstone RA: Injury to the elderly in road traffic accidents. J Trauma 1989;29:494–497
8. Sklar DP, Demarest GB, McFeeley P: Increased pedestrian mortality among the elderly. Am J Emerg Med 1989;7:387–390
9. Lonner JH, Koval KJ: Polytrauma in the elderly. Clin Orthop Rel Res 1995;318:136–143
10. Zietlow SD, Capizzi PJ, Bannon MP, Farnell MB: Multisystem geriatric trauma. J Trauma 1994;37:985–988
11. Mosenthal AC, Livingston DH, Elcavage J et al: Falls: epidemiology and strategies for prevention. J Trauma 1995;38:753–756
12. van der Sluis CK, Klasen HJ, Eisma WH, ten Duis HJ: Major trauma in young and old: what is the difference? J Trauma 1996;40:78–82
13. Champion HR, Sacco WJ, Copes WS: Injury severity scoring again. J Trauma 1995;40:78–82

14. Kennedy RL, Grant PT, Blackwell D: Low-impact falls: demands on a system of trauma management, prediction of outcome, and influence of comorbidity. J Trauma 2001;51:717–724

15. Horst HM, Obeid FN, Sorensen UJ, Bivins BA: Factors influencing survival of elderly trauma patients. Crit Care Med 1986;14:681–684

16. DeMaria EJ, Kenney P, Merrian MA et al: Survival after trauma in geriatric patients. Ann Surg 1987;206:738–743

17. Horan MA, Barton RN, Little RA: Ageing and the response to injury. In Evans JG, Caird FI (eds): Advanced Geriatric Medicine 7. Wright, Bristol, 1988:101–135

18. Shabot MM, Johnson CL: Outcome from critical care in the "oldest old" trauma patients. J Trauma 1995;39:254–259

19. Knaus WA, Wagner DP, Draper EA et al: The APACHE III prognostic system: risk prediction of hospital mortality for critically ill hospitalized adults. Chest 1991;100:1619–1636

20. Jennett B: Epidemiology of head injury. J Neurol Neurosurg Psychiatr 1996;60:362–369

21. Amacher AL, Bybee DE: Tolerance of head injury by the elderly. Neurosurgery 1987;20:954–958

22. Vollmer DG, Torner JC, Jane JA et al: Age and outcome following traumatic coma: why older patients fare worse. J Neurosurg 1991;75:S37–S49

23. Kulshrestha P, Iyer KS: Chest injuries: a clinical and autopsy profile. J Trauma 1988;28:844–847

24. Shorr RM, Rodriguez A, Indeck MC et al: Blunt chest trauma in the elderly. J Trauma 1989;29:234–237

25. Tubbs N: A comparison of deaths from injury: 1947–56 compared with 1962–71. Injury 1976;7:233–241

26. Lieberman IH, Webb JK: Cervical spine injuries in the elderly. J Bone Joint Surg 1994;76B:877–881

27. Kane RS, Burns EA, Goodwin JS: Minimal trauma fractures in older nursing home residents: the interaction of functional status, trauma, and site of fracture. J Am Geriatr Soc 1995;43:891–894

28. Hayes WC, Myers ER, Morris JN et al: Impact near the hip dominates fracture risk in elderly nursing home residents who fall. Calcif Tissue Int 1993;52:192–198

29. Cummings SR, Nevitt MC: A hypothesis: the causes of hip fracture. J Gerontol A 1989;44:M107–M111

30. Frankel VH, Burstein AH: Orthopaedic Biomechanics. Lea & Febiger, Philadelphia, 1970

31. Muckle DS, Bentley G, Deane G, Kemp FH: Basic science of the hip. In Muckle DS (ed): Femoral Neck Fractures and Hip Joint Injuries. Wiley, New York, 1978:53–58

32. Robinovitch SN, Hayes WC, McMahon TA: Prediction of femoral impact forces in falls on the hip. J Biomech Eng 1991;113:366–374

33. Hayes WC, Myers ER: Biomechanics of fractures. In Riggs BL, Melton L (eds): Osteoporosis—Etiology, Diagnosis and Management. Lippincott-Raven, Philadelphia, 1995:93–114

34. Courtney AC, Wachtel EF, Myers ER, Hayes WC: Effects of loading rate on strength of the proximal femur. Calcif Tissue Int 1994;55:53–58

35. Nevitt MC, Cummings SR: Type of fall and risk of hip and wrist fractures: the study of osteoporotic fractures. J Am Geriatr Soc 1993;41:1226–1234

36. Greenspan SL, Myers ER, Maitland LA et al: Fall severity and bone mineral density as risk factors for hip fracture in ambulatory elderly. JAMA 1994;324:1326–1331

37. Martin RE, Teberian G: Multiple trauma and the elderly patient. Emerg Med Clin North Am 1990;8:411–420

38. Riska EB, Myllynen P: Fat embolism in patients with multiple injuries. J Trauma 1982;22:891–894

39. Rogers FB, Shackford SR, Keller MS: Early fixation reduces morbidity and mortality in elderly patients with hip fractures from low-impact falls. J Trauma 1995;39:261–265

40. Zuckerman JD, Skovron ML, Koval KJ et al: Postoperative complications and mortality associated with operative delay in older patients who have a fracture of the hip. J Bone Joint Surg 1995;77A:1551–1556

41. Cuthbertson DP: Observations on disturbance of metabolism produced by injury to the limbs. Q J Med 1932;25:233–246

42. Frayn KN, Stoner HB, Barton RN, Heath DF: Persistence of high plasma glucose, insulin and cortisol concentrations in elderly patients with proximal femoral fractures. Age Ageing 1983;12:70–76

43. Roberts NA, Barton RN, Horan MA, White A: Adrenal function after upper femoral fracture in elderly people: persistence of stimulation and the roles of adrenocorticotrophic hormone and immobility. Age Ageing 1990;12:70–76

44. Barton RN, Weijers JWM, Horan MA: Increased rates of cortisol production and urinary free cortisol excretion in elderly women 2 weeks after proximal femur fracture. Eur J Clin Invest 1993;23:171–176

45. Seeman TE, Robbins RJ: Aging and hypothalamic-pituitary-adrenal response to challenge in humans. Endocr Rev 1994;15:233–259

46. Doncaster HD, Barton RN, Horan MA, Roberts NA: Factors influencing cortisol–adrenocorticotrophin relationships in elderly women with upper femur fractures. J Trauma 1993;34:49–55

47. Barker DJP: Mothers, Babies and Disease in Later Life. BMJ Publishing Group, London, 1994

48. Levitt NS, Lindsey RS, Holmes MC, Seckl JR: Dexamethasone in the last week of pregnancy attenuates hippocampal glucocorticoid receptor gene expression and elevates blood pressure in the adult offspring in the rat. Neuroendocrinology 1996;64:412–418

49. Drucker WR, Chadwick CD, Gann DS: Transcapillary refill in haemorrhage and shock. Arch Surg 1981;116:1344–1353

50. Linder J, Nolgaård P, Näsman B et al: Decreased peripheral glucocorticoid sensitivity in Alzheimer's disease. Gerontology 1993;39:200–206

51. Brönegaård M, Stierna P, Marcus C: Glucocorticoid resistant syndromes— molecular basis and clinical presentations. J Neuroendocrinol 1996;8:405–415

52. Sternberg EM, Chroussos GP, Wilder RL, Gold PW: The stress response and the regulation of inflammatory disease. Ann Intern Med 1992;117:854–866

53. Hall-Angeraås M, Angeraås U, Zamir O et al: Effect of the glucocorticoid receptor antagonist RU38486 on muscle protein breakdown in sepsis. Surgery 1991;109:468–473

54. Cech AC, Shore J, Gallagher H, Daly JM: Glucocorticoid receptor blockade reverses post-injury macrophage suppression. Arch Surg 1994;129:1227–1232

55. Jallut D, Tappy L, Kohut M et al: Energy balance in elderly patients after surgery for a femoral neck fracture. JPEN 1990;14:563–568

56. Patterson BM, Cornell CN, Carbone B et al: Protein depletion and metabolic stress in elderly patients who have a fracture of the hip. J Bone Joint Surg 1992;74A:251–260

57. Nelson KM, Richards EW, Long CL et al: Protein and energy balance following femoral neck fracture in geriatric patients. Metabolism 1995;44:59–66

58. Watters JM, Moulton SB, Clancey SM et al: Aging exaggerates glucose intolerance following injury. J Trauma 1994;37:786–791

59. Moore FD: Bodily changes in surgical convalescence 1. The normal sequence: observations and interpretations. Ann Surg 1953;137:289–315

60. Castaneda C, Charnley JM, Evans WJ, Crim ML: Elderly women accommodate to a low-protein diet with losses of body cell mass, muscle function, and immune response. Am J Clin Nutr 1995;62:30–39

61. Humberstone DA, Shaw JH: Isotopic studies during surgical convalescence. Br J Surg 1989;76:154–158

62. Christiansen T, Kehlet H: Postoperative fatigue. World J Surg 1993;17:220–225

63. Cedersholm T, Jägrén C, Hellström K: Outcome of protein-energy malnutrition in elderly medical patients. Am J Med 1995;98:67–74

64. Older MWJ, Delyth E, Dickenson JWT: A nutrient survey in elderly women with femoral neck fracture. Br J Surg 1980;67:884–886

65. Bastow MD, Rawlings J, Allison SP: Undernutrition, hypothermia and injury in elderly women with fractured femur: an injury response to altered metabolism? Lancet 1983;1:143–145

66. Langlois JA, Harris T, Looker AC, Madans J: Weight change between age 50 years and old age is associated with risk of hip fracture in white women aged 67 years and older. Arch Intern Med 1996;156:989–994

67. Hussein A, Barer D: Nutritional assessment in patients admitted with proximal femoral fractures. Gerontology 1994;40:289

68. Bastow MD, Rawlings J, Allison SP: Benefits of supplementary tube feeding after fractured neck of femur: a randomised controlled trial. Br Med J 1983;287:1589–1592

69. Delmi M, Rapin C-H, Bengoa J-M et al: Dietary supplementation in elderly patients with fractured neck of the femur. Lancet 1990;335:1013–1016

70. Stableforth PG: Supplementary feeds and nitrogen and calorie balance following femoral neck fracture. Br J Surg 1986;73:651–655

71. Avenell A, Handoll HHG: Nutritional supplementation for hip fracture aftercare in the elderly. Cochrane Musculoskeletal Injuries Group. Cochrane Database of Systematic Reviews, Issue 3, 2001 (systematic review)

72. Keene GS, Parker MJ, Pryor GA: Mortality and morbidity after hip fractures. Br Med J 1993;307:1248–1251

73. Marottoli RA, Berkman LF, Cooney LM: Decline in physical function following hip fracture. J Am Geriatr Soc 1992;40:861–866

74. Mock C, Mackenzie E, Jurkovich G et al: Determinants of disability after lower extremity fracture. J Trauma 2000;49:1002–1011

75. Lamb SE, Morse RE, Evans JG: Mobility after proximal femoral fracture: the relevance of leg extensor power, postural sway and other factors. Age Ageing 1995;24:308–314

76. Ions GK, Stevens J: Prediction of survival in patients with femoral neck fractures. J Bone Joint Surg 1987;69B:384–387

77. Jette AM, Harris A, Cleary PD, Campion EW: Functional recovery after hip fracture. Arch Phys Med Rehabil 1987;68:735–740

78. Mossey JM, Mutran E, Knott K, Craik R: Determinants of recovery 12 months after hip fracture: the importance of psychosocial factors. Am J Public Health 1989;79:279–286

79. Koval KJ, Skovron ML, Polatsch D et al: Dependency after hip fracture in geriatric patients: a study of predictive factors. J Orthop Trauma 1996;8:531–535

80. Mossey JM, Knott K, Craik R: The effects of persistent depressive symptoms on hip fracture recovery. J Gerontol A 1990;45:M163–M168

81. Bernardini B, Meinecke C, Pagani M et al: Comorbidity and adverse clinical events in the rehabilitation of older adults after hip fracture. J Am Geriatr Soc 1995;41:894–898

82. Svensson O, Strömberg L, Öhlén G, Lindgren U: Prediction of the outcome after hip fracture in elderly patients. J Bone Joint Surg 1996;78B:115–118

83. Myers AH, Palmer MH, Engel BT et al: Mobility in older patients with hip fractures: examining prefracture status, complications, and outcomes from the acute-care hospital. J Orthop Trauma 1996;10:99–107

84. Ponzer S, Bergman B, Brismar B, Johansson LM: A study of patient-related characteristics and outcome after moderate injury. Injury 1996;27:549–555

85. Shahar A, Powers KA, Black JS: The risk of postoperative deconditioning in older adults. J Am Geriatr Soc 1996;44:471

86. Parker MJ, Handoll HHG, Dynan Y: Mobilisation strategies after hip fracture surgery in adults. Cochrane Musculoskeletal Injuries Group. Cochrane Database of Systematic Reviews, Issue 3, 2001 (systematic review)

87. Johnston M: Psychological factors in recovery from illness and from surgery. Proc R Coll Physicians Edinb 1996;26:451–460

88. Billig N, Ahmed SW, Kenmore P et al: Assessment of depression and cognitive impairment after hip fracture. J Am Geriatr Soc 1986;34:499–503

89. Fox KM, Hawkes WG, Magaziner J et al: Markers of failure to thrive among older hip fracture patients. J Am Geriatr Soc 1996; 44:371–376

90. Sarkisian CA, Lachs MS: "Failure to thrive" in older adults. Ann Intern Med 1996;124:1072–1078

91. DeMaria EJ, Kenney PR, Merrian MA et al: Aggressive trauma care benefits the elderly. J Trauma 1987;27:1200–1205

92. Scalea TM, Simm HM, Duncan AO: Geriatric blunt trauma: improved survival with early invasive monitoring. J Trauma 1990;30:29–34

93. Demetriades D, Sava J, Alo K et al: Old age as a criterion for trauma team activation. J Trauma 2001;51:754–756

94. Hanspal R, Wright M, Proctor D et al: Failure to deliver the formal therapy prescribed in an NHS rehabilitation unit. Clin Rehab 1994;8:161–165

Chapter 75

Podiatry

Katherine Ward, Mark A. Kosinski, and Bryan Markinson

As the new millennium brings a population explosion of older people, particular attention must be paid to the multiple and complex disorders that impair functional independence and compromise quality of life. One of the most important and sometimes overlooked topics is that of proper foot health and function. It has been estimated that 70 percent of the population over 65 years of age suffers from a foot problem.[1] Foot pain can easily jeopardize an individual's ability to perform many of the important instrumental activities of daily living including cooking, shopping, housekeeping, doing laundry, and using transportation.

Foot pain in elderly people may be caused by changes in gait, hereditary problems, or previous foot conditions that were not treated or treated inadequately. Changes in mental status, nutritional deficiencies, systemic and local disease, hospitalization and confinement to bed, polypharmacy, and other common elderly life situations may complicate the picture.

The myriad of changes associated with aging results in a diminished homeostatic reserve, commonly manifested with loss of ambulation. The ability of an individual to remain ambulatory may be the only dividing line between institutionalization and remaining an active and viable member of society.[2]

Proper foot care must be provided for elderly patients in an attempt to promote pain-free ambulation. The consequences of immobility in this age group (bladder infections, pulmonary problems, and venous thrombosis) certainly underscores this point. Podiatric problems are often preventable or readily treatable. Podiatric care is just part of the comprehensive and interdisciplinary nature of geriatric medicine.

In this chapter, the diagnosis, treatment, and prevention of common pedal problems are discussed.

ORTHOPEDIC/BIOMECHANICAL DISORDERS

Lower extremity joint impairment and painful foot disorders also represent major causes of treatable gait disturbances. Heel pain is a common complaint of older individuals, especially as the older population exercises more. Recent weight gain, increased walking or standing activities, hard floors or surfaces, and biomechanical abnormalities are the factors that predispose to the development of plantar calcaneal pain. Plantar calcaneal spurs (diagnosed by a lateral radiograph of the foot) are often aggravated by an atrophied fat pad. Conservative treatment includes rest, stretching exercises, nonsteroidal anti-inflammatory drugs (NSAIDs), and biomechanically sound footwear, such as a sneaker or running shoe, with a thick shock-absorbing insole. Viscoelastic heel cushions or heel cups (available commercially) can be inserted into existing shoes to provide cushioning. Prescription custom-made orthoses may be indicated to support the arch and to reduce traction of the plantar fascia from its origin on the calcaneus. Accordingly, shoe modification and orthoses are prescribed for the long term. Stretching of the Achilles tendon and plantar fascia may help diminish symptoms more rapidly. Recalcitrant cases may require a series of local injections (local anesthetic combined with a corticosteroid) into the area of maximum tenderness (usually the anteromedial tubercle of the calcaneus). Acute plantar heel pain can become a chronic condition, especially in patients who are overweight or have bilateral symptoms.[3]

When appropriate therapy fails to achieve expected results (especially within 3–6 months), one should consider systemic disease as a possible etiology of heel pain. Diseases such as rheumatoid arthritis, ankylosing spondylitis, psoriatic arthritis, and Reiter's syndrome can also cause heel pain.

Another common musculoskeletal problem in elderly people, which is often misdiagnosed, is posterior tibial tendon dysfunction. Suspect this in a presentation of sudden asymmetry in arch height. There may be swelling and tenderness on palpation of the tendon insertion around the medial and plantar aspect of the navicular, and these findings often extend along the course of the tendon proximally behind the medial malleolus. If not already present, an actual tear or even rupture of the tendon may result. Orthotics can control minor cases, but depending on the level of activity of the patient and the degree of discomfort, custom-made braces or surgical correction may be the best option.

The joints of the feet are also prone to osteoarthritis. Diagnosed by limited and painful range of motion with or without crepitation, this condition usually responds well to conservative measures. Joint space narrowing on radiographs is often a late finding. Shoe modifications such as balanced inlay orthoses and a forefoot rocker sole angled to follow the progression of gait provide good local treatment. Topical preparations such as capsaicin (Zostrix) cream have been shown to relieve pain caused by degenerative joint disease, and may augment NSAID therapy which is the mainstay of treatment.

Joint pains from hallux valgus, hammer toes, and mallet toes are also common lower extremity problems in elderly people (see Fig. 75-1; see also Plate 75-1). The myth that these are caused by ill-fitting shoegear is disproven by the studies of populations in the world who typically live their lives unshod. The same incidence of these deformities occur, pointing to a more biomechanical/genetic etiology. Indeed, shoes aggravate these conditions and make them painful, with the development of corns and adventitious bursae. A hammer toe is one in which there is a flexion contracture at the proximal interphalangeal joint. An extensor contracture at the metatarsophalangeal joint may coexist. A mallet toe is contracted at the distal interphalangeal joint, and a claw toe is contracted at

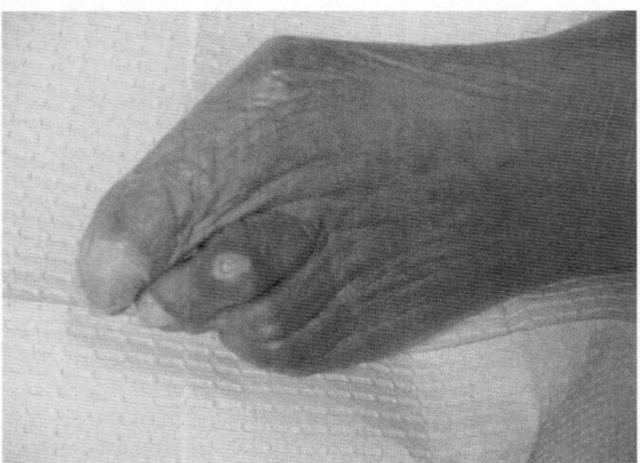

Figure 75-1 A bunion deformity with hammer toe of the second digit. Note pre-ulcerative lesion over proximal phalangeal joint of second toe secondary to shoe pressure.

both. The most common problem associated with these deformities is the formation of corns dorsally over areas of prominence as well as medial and lateral, and interdigitally. If the above-mentioned conservative measures fail to alleviate the pain, surgical correction may be considered. Foot surgery can provide improvement of function and quality of life, even in the presence of chronic illnesses. Of course, a prudent comprehensive surgical work-up in conjunction with the primary care physician, as well as an anesthesiologist, would be obligatory. Fortunately, many forefoot procedures require only local anesthesia and are done on an ambulatory basis.

Your examination should always include watching the patient walk. Gait disturbances are a common sequela of age-related changes in the central and peripheral nervous systems. Senile ataxia is a gait pattern characterized by a flexed posture with wide-based gait in men, and a waddling, narrow-based gait in women.[4] This is seen in neurologically healthy individuals and has no known etiology.

Features of pathologically induced gait disturbances are frequently nonspecific and overlap with those of senile ataxia, giving little clue as to the primary pathology. In Parkinson's disease and cerebellar atrophy, gait characteristics are specifically helpful in establishing the diagnosis. Shuffling and abducted gaits also produce increased stress and pressure on the soft tissues leading to dermal lesions (see dermatology section below).

It is important to search for an underlying etiology in the physical assessment, as approximately 25 percent of geriatric gait disturbances do have a treatable cause.[5] Serum studies may reveal vitamin B_{12} deficiency, hypothyroidism, osteomalacia, or drug toxicity. Radiographic studies assist in excluding bone disease. Remember that stress fractures may not be evident at the time of injury. If signs and symptoms are consistent with fracture, treat as such and repeat the radiograph in 10–14 days. Computed tomography, magnetic resonance imaging, myelography, and electrophysiological studies may offer a definitive diagnosis in cases of primary central nervous system pathology. Common etiologies of gait disorders include neurological (cerebrovascular accident, dementia, Parkinson's

disease, etc.), musculoskeletal (arthritis, osteoporosis, myopathy, etc.), vascular, endocrine (hypothyroidism, diabetes), psychological (depression, fear of falling), as well as medications. Demonstration of poor gait, difficulty with chair transfer, and a loss of balance when standing on tiptoe suggests an underlying neurological or musculoskeletal disorder.[6]

DERMATOLOGICAL DISORDERS

Hyperkeratotic lesions (corns and calluses) are the most common podiatric complaints of elderly people. They frequently arise in areas of increased pressure or friction and over bony prominences. Although these conditions are common among all age groups, degenerative joint disease, atrophy of the plantar fat pad, and decreased pain threshold predispose elderly people to increased frequency of complaints. Depending on their depth and severity, there may be an associated adventitious bursa formation. Treatment consists of aseptic debridement and weight or pressure dispersion. Lesions on the plantar aspect of the foot should also be treated with a shock-absorbing insert to disperse the weight-bearing forces and augment an atrophic or displaced plantar fat pad.

It is especially important to debride chronic hyperkeratotic lesions in patients with vascular or neurological impairment, as untreated lesions may give rise to soft tissue breakdown, ulcerations, and bone infection. As noted earlier in this chapter, sneakers or running shoes are ideal footgear for biomechanical as well as dermatological problems. A wide and high toe box is important for preventing pressure on the digits, and abundant cushioning on the sole of the foot is required to mitigate the excessive plantar pressures that cause the hyperkeratotic lesions.

Well-cushioned shoegear is also required to mitigate the consequences of atrophied subcalcaneal or submetatarsal fat pads. When the natural fat found on the plantar aspect of the feet atrophies, the underlying bony structures become more prominent and cause pain. When such pain occurs under the plantar aspect of the metatarsal head, it is called metatarsalgia. The complaint is frequently a callus or inflammation of the area (bursitis). Diagnosis can be made by clinical examination, and radiographs may reveal underlying bone pathology. Treatment consists of debridement of hyperkeratotic lesions with padding to disperse the weight. Long-term treatment includes the use of soft tissue supplements such as plastizote, which can be added to foot orthotics or inserted directly into the shoe.

Expensive custom-molded shoes are often unnecessary for all but the most severe foot deformities. If they are indeed indicated, they should include a high, wide toe box, a bunion last, and an extra depth feature to accommodate weight-dispersive orthoses. Surgical correction should always be considered as the last resort, after all conservative measures have failed.

Maceration and fissuring of the interspaces is another common dermatological finding in the elderly population. Vision and dexterity loss make it difficult to examine and care for the feet, and digital deformities precipitate moisture accumulation between the toes. The dark and moist environment between the toes predisposes the area to fungal and bacterial infection, which range from a mild annoyance to a severe debilitating infection. A Wood's light can be used to detect coral red fluorescence suggestive of *Corynebacterium minutissimum*, which is usually treated with topical erythromycin. Macerated toe web spaces may also be due to a fungal or yeast infection that can be treated with ciclopirox (Loprox) or clotrimazole solution (Lotrimin, Mycelex) applied interdigitally twice daily for 2–4 weeks. Of course, meticulous cleaning and drying of the area while bathing is also necessary. If lamb's wool or gauze is used to separate the toes, never encircle a digit; such dressings may become constrictive and severely compromise the circulation.

Interdigital tinea pedis (described above), inflammatory tinea pedis, and chronic dry scaly tinea pedis are the three main categories of pedal dermatophyte infections. Inflammatory tinea pedis, which is an acute vesicular eruption that has a particular predilection for the long arch, is caused by the dermatophyte *Trichophyton mentagrophytes*. It is usually severely pruritic, it may weep, and the severest of cases may require bed rest in addition to topical and/or oral antifungal therapy. The chronic form of tinea pedis, usually caused by *Trichophyton rubrum*, has a predilection for the arch as well, but is mainly confined to the lateral surfaces of the sole. Sometimes the entire plantar aspect is involved in what is classically described as a moccasin distribution. In contrast to the inflammatory type, these lesions are scaly and erythematous, and commonly display an arcuate shape.

There is also a decrease in skin hydration as aging progresses. Combined with diminished sebaceous and eccrine activity, dry, scaly, and hyperkeratotic skin often results. Peripheral heel hyperkeratosis is very common, but when fissures occur, severe pain and infection may ensue. This is a serious problem in the face of arterial insufficiency. Management includes debridement of the tissue, hydration of the skin, and avoidance of backless footwear. Chemical cautery with silver nitrate is often necessary to close a bleeding fissure. It is momentarily painful but works very effectively. Heel fissuring is more prevalent in the obese, and tends to be a chronic problem. In patients who have had total joint replacement, the presence of heel fissures should not be trivialized (see Fig. 75-2).

Ulcerations of the leg, feet, and toes are also seen frequently in the geriatric population. The differential diagnosis of pedal ulcers includes arteriosclerosis obliterans, neurotrophic, chronic pernio, gout, mycobacterium tuberculosis, Raynaud's disease/phenomenon, scleroderma, and neoplasms, in addition to those caused by biomechanic, iatrogenic, or patient-induced diseases.[7]

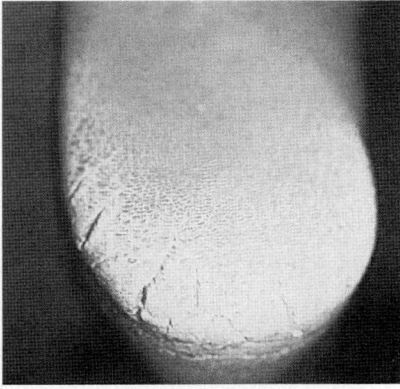

Figure 75-2 Severe xerosis causing fissuring of the heels.

Ischemic ulcers typically occur on the distal aspect of digits and over bony prominences. Symptoms include severe pain, often worse at night and relieved by dependency. They are characterized by poor granulation tissue, poor color of tissue (cyanotic, gray, or black), and poor bleeding upon debridement.

Neurotrophic ulcers commonly occur beneath pressure points or hyperkeratotic lesions. There is usually no pain, as the patient is typically neuropathic. The ulcers are characterized by punched-out lesions with a red granular base and white fibrotic rim. Due to the high incidence of diabetic ulcers and their coexisting morbidity, this topic will be discussed thoroughly in a separate section within this chapter.

Venous stasis ulcerations often follow chronic stasis dermatitis, which is secondary to incompetent venous circulation in the leg, as further described in Chapter 40. Poor arterial circulation is an added risk factor that will impair healing and increase the chance of infection.

Treatment of these ulcers must address their etiology, and therefore requires a multidisciplinary approach. An ischemic ulcer requires a vascular consult as soon as possible, with possible revascularization. Neurotrophic ulcers require weight dispersion, debridement of devitalized tissue, and use of antibiotics when appropriate. Edema can be reduced with elevation of the foot (above heart level), as well as with compressive boots and stockings. Individuals with a history of venous stasis ulcers should wear elastic supports daily. Wound care must be performed regularly to ensure a clean, moist granular bed of the ulcer. Aerobic and anerobic cultures must be performed if infection is suspected, followed by the appropriate antibiotic coverage.

It is important to keep in mind that a chronic ulceration, especially if it is not responding to appropriate therapy, has the potential for malignant degeneration. This is especially true for the common venous stasis ulcer. Any suspicious ulcer should be biopsied to include the most ominous border, along with normal skin for comparison.

NAIL DISORDERS

Identification of a fungal nail infection is easily performed with a KOH prep and fungal culture. The PAS (Periodic Acid Schiff Stain) test is also used to detect the presence of viable or degenerating fungus organisms, and its sensitivity may be higher than that of the KOH test. Mycotic nail infections tend to respond poorly to topical therapy. The advent of safer oral agents such as Sporanox (itraconazole, Janssen Pharmaceutica) and Lamisil (terbinafine hydrochloride, Novartis) may help to achieve a cure in some patients, although the success of systemic agents is directly related to the vascular supply to the nail bed. A new topical antifungal, Penlac solution, 8 percent (ciclopirox, Dermik Laboratories), was approved by the FDA in 2000, and is indicated for mild to moderate onychomycosis due to *Trichophyton rubrum*. Older patients usually do well with serial nail debridement, which not only maintains comfort but decreases the chance of soft tissue infection, infected ingrown toenails, and subungual corns or ulceration.

It is important to differentiate mycotic nail infections from nail dystrophies secondary to systemic disease, vascular insufficiency, and trauma. For example, poor nutritional status can lead to toenails that are atrophic, thin, brittle, and lackluster, with possible longitudinal ridges. Other systemic diseases associated with common nail dystrophies include diabetes mellitus, syphilis, psoriasis, Reiter's syndrome, ischemia, gout, rheumatoid arthritis, and systemic lupus erythematosus.

Although patients invariably attribute periungual pain as being secondary to an ingrown or incurvated nail, it is important to rule out ischemia as the etiology of the nail pain. Ischemic changes of the digit can often mimic nail pain and mislead both patient and physician.

Nail fold infections often exhibit adjacent chronic granulation tissue. In chronic infections, it may be prudent to biopsy such lesions. We are aware of patients in whom Kaposi's sarcoma, amelanotic melanoma, and squamous cell carcinoma of the nail groove have given the appearance of a pyogenic granuloma.

Subungual hematomas are not uncommon in older individuals, and usually result from microtrauma secondary to improperly fitting shoegear. However, it is prudent to consider any subungual hyperpigmented lesion a melanoma until proven otherwise. In such cases, debride the nail plate as proximal as possible: many times part of the nail can be removed to reveal subungual debris consistent with previous hemorrhage or fungal infection. If a melanotic process is suspected, a biopsy must be performed.

FOOT PROBLEMS IN PATIENTS WITH DIABETES

Neuropathy, peripheral vascular disease, and immunopathy all play a role in the development of foot pathology in patients with diabetes. These three factors, combined with the reduced vision and mobility that impair the ability of older patients to inspect and care for their feet, can have disastrous consequences. When left unrecognized and therefore untreated, many minor foot problems (such as corns and calluses) progress to ulcerations and infections, producing the well-known morbidity associated with diabetes. Risk factors for diabetic foot ulcers include sensorimotor and autonomic neuropathy, peripheral vascular disease, limited joint mobility, high plantar pressures, bony deformities, history of previous ulceration, and visual or functional impairment.

Chronic sensory neuropathy is one of the most common long-term complications of diabetes mellitus. Symptoms frequently include numbness, dysesthesia, lancinating pain, burning, and hypersensitivity. Sensory loss is typically in a stocking-glove distribution and is often of insidious onset. In its early stages, patients may be unaware that a decrease in sensorium even exists. In those patients without diabetes, pedal neuropathy may be secondary to alcoholism, a herniated nucleus pulposus, heavy metals, vitamin deficiencies, and collagen diseases, among other systemic conditions.

Sensory neuropathy is often accompanied by a motor component. In the foot of a patient with diabetes, loss of motor fibers may lead to intrinsic muscle atrophy and imbalance between flexor and extensor muscles. Clawing of the toes, prominent metatarsal heads, and anterior displacement of an already atrophied plantar fat pad may increase the patient's risk for pressure-induced lesions.[8,9] Glycation of collagen leads

to thickening and increased cross-linking of collagen bundles, resulting in thin, tight, and waxy skin and further restriction of joint movement.[10] Dry and atrophic skin is also caused by the autonomic neuropathy, which leads to denervation of the sweat glands. Cracks and fissures violate the skin defenses, leaving the patient vulnerable to bacterial infection.

Ulcerations may be caused by an acute event or repetitive minor trauma. It has been shown that constant pressure of 5–7 pounds per square inch over a bony prominence can cause ischemic necrosis in less than 7 hours.[11] If an ulcer is indeed caused by pressure or a biomechanical problem, it will never resolve if weight is not dispersed from the affected area, regardless of how much debridement of local wound care is given.

Peripheral vascular disease is 20 times more common in patients with diabetes than in nondiabetic individuals.[12] Micro- and macrovascular disease puts the patient at risk for gangrene and ulceration by reducing the perfusion pressure where tissue ischemia occurs. Diabetic occlusive disease has a predilection for the tibial and peroneal arteries, and tends to be bilateral and multisegmental. Ankle/brachial index and pulse volume recordings may be of questionable value in assessing peripheral circulation in patients with diabetes, but they are useful if they are low.[10] In general, be suspicious if the ankle/brachial index

---

Summary of management algorithm
Diabetic foot ulcers

1. Evaluation
   a. Clinical appearance
   b. Depth of penetration
   c. X-rays to detect
      1) foreign body
      2) osteomyelitis
      3) subcutaneous gas
   d. Location
   e. Biopsy
   f. Blood supply (noninvasive vascular studies)

2. Debridement, radical

3. Bacterial cultures (aerobic and anerobic)

4. Metabolic control

5. Antibiotics
   a. Oral
   b. Parenteral

6. Do not soak feet

7. Decrease edema

8. Non-weight-bearing
   a. bed rest
   b. crutches
   c. wheelchair
   d. special sandals
   e. contact casting

9. Improve circulation (vascular surgery)

Source: Levin ME: The diabetic foot: Pathophysiology, evaluation, and treatment. In Levin ME, O'Neal LW, Bowker J (eds): The Diabetic Foot, 5th Ed. Mosby Year Book, St. Louis, MO, 1993:17–60. Reproduced with permission

is greater than 1.0. A reading of less than 0.5 indicates serious arterial compromise and poor healing potential.

The best treatment for the foot of a patient with diabetes is patient education and thorough, frequent foot examinations. The foot examination should be a regular part of each office visit. Both shoes and socks should be removed and the feet should be checked for trophic and pretrophic skin changes, thickened or incurvated nails, and hyperkeratosis. Hemorrhage within a callus may be suggestive of ulcer formation. The interspaces should be carefully inspected for maceration or fissuring. Legs and feet should be evaluated for diabetic skin markers such as bullous diabeticorum, diabetic dermopathy, and necrobiosis lipoidica, some of which may herald vasculopathy and retinopathy.

The neurological examination should include evaluation of deep tendon reflexes, sharp/dull discrimination, light touch, proprioception, vibratory sensation using a 128 Hz tuning fork, and protective threshold using the Semmes–Weinstein monofilament. In fact, patients can do monofilament tests themselves. Vibratory sensation and proprioception, both carried by the posterior columns, are the first to be affected by diabetic neuropathy. Keep in mind that decreased vibratory sensation may also occur as part of normal aging. Diminished or absent knee and ankle jerk reflexes are also common with aging, and in the absence of other pathology do not require further evaluation. Autonomic neuropathy can be recognized clinically by the absence of sweating, a relatively fixed heart rate, and postural hypotension.

A palpable popliteal pulse may be an unreliable indicator of circulation in the lower extremity, as 40 percent of patients with diabetes presenting with distal gangrene have a popliteal pulse.[13] Similarly, a palpable dorsalis pedis or posterior tibial pulse is an unreliable indication of circulation in the toes. Twenty percent of patients with diabetes with palpable pedal pulses have significant small-vessel disease. Temperature gradient, capillary filling time, rubor on dependency, and pallor on elevation are useful adjunctive tests for assessing distal lower extremity circulation.

The pain of diabetic neuropathy is another common complaint of patients with diabetes. It is difficult to control, especially in patients with poor glucose control. Topical capsaicin (Zostrix) applied 2 or 3 times a day may provide some relief. Tricyclic antidepressants and nonsteroidal anti-inflammatories may also prove advantageous, as are new drugs on the horizon.

Patients play an important role in preventing their foot problems. The following recommendations should be made at each office visit: stop smoking, inspect feet daily for cuts and blisters, inspect the inside and outside of shoes for foreign objects, do not walk barefooted, cut toenails straight across, avoid temperature extremes on the feet, and notify a physician of any problems immediately.

SUMMARY

Successful patient management must extend beyond diagnosis and disease treatment and include promotion of function and prevention of decline.[14] The podiatrist can be a valuable team member in the multidisciplinary approach of geriatric assessment; he or she can deliver proactive and preventive care

that maintains or improves quality of life for older patients. The simple ability to ambulate comfortably is critical for our patient's feelings of overall well-being, self-esteem, and ability to interact in society. In addition, elderly people have become increasingly engaged in athletic activities, making them more prone to overuse, repetitive motion, and traumatic injuries. It is therefore necessary to prevent and treat the pedal manifestations of vascular, neurological, musculoskeletal, and metabolic disorders in order to improve quality of life and ambulatory ability, while reducing pain and foot morbidity.

KEY POINTS Podiatry

- Orthopedic/biomechanical disorders:
  heel pain
  posterior tibial tendon dysfunction
  osteoarthritis
  digital deformities
  pathological gait

- Dermatological disorders:
  hyperkeratotic lesions
  bacterial infections
  tinea pedis
  xerosis/fissuring
  ulcerations

- Nail disorders:
  fungal nail infections
  nail dystrophies

- Foot problems in patients with diabetes:
  neuropathy
  ulcerations
  peripheral vascular disease

REFERENCES

1. DellaCorte MP, Tsouris J, Buffone WF: Geriatrics. In Birrer RB, DellaCorte MP, Grisafi PJ (eds): Common Foot Problems in Primary Care. Hanley & Belfus, Philadelphia, 1992:73
2. Helfand A: Care of the foot. In Steinberg FU (ed): Care of the Geriatric Patient. CV Mosby Company, St. Louis, 1983:406
3. Wolgin M, Cook C, Graham C, Mauldin D: Conservative treatment of plantar heel pain: long-term follow up. Foot Ankle 1995;15:97–102
4. Rubine FA: Gait disorders in the elderly. Postgrad Med 1993;94:185–190
5. Sudarsky L, Ronthal M: Gait disorders among elderly patients: a survey of 50 patients. Arch Neurol 1983;40:740–743
6. Tideiksaar R: Geriatric falls: assessing the cause, preventing recurrence. Geriatrics 1989;44:57–64
7. Kosinski M, Ramcharitar S: In-office management of common geriatric foot problems. Geriatrics 1994;49:43–47
8. Cavanaugh PR, Derr JA, Ulbrecht JS et al: Correlates of structure and function in the diabetic foot. Diabetologia 1991;34(suppl 2):A39
9. Boulton AM: The diabetic foot. Med Clin North Am 1988;72:1513–1530
10. Goodfield MJB, Millard LG: The skin in diabetes mellitus. Diabetologia 1988;31:567–575
11. Sage R: Diabetic ulcers: evaluation and management. Clin Podiatr Med Surg 1987;4:383–393
12. Gibbons GW, Freeman D: Vascular evaluation and treatment of the diabetic. Clin Podiatr Med Surg 1987;4:377–381
13. Bulat T, Kosinski M: Diabetic foot: strategies to prevent and treat common problems. Geriatrics 1995;50:46–55
14. Cassel CK: Successful aging; how increased life expectancy and medical advances are changing geriatric care. Geriatrics 2001;56:35–39

Chapter 76

Geriatric gastroenterology: overview

Robert E. Tepper and Seymour Katz

Over 20 percent of our population is expected to exceed 65 years of age by 2030,[1] with the most rapidly growing segment over 85 years of age.[2] Of necessity, gastroenterologists will be increasingly confronted with digestive diseases in elderly patients. Gastrointestinal disease is the second most common indication for hospital admission of elderly patients,[3] who account for four times as many hospitalizations as do younger patients.[1] In the outpatient setting, patients 75 and older visit internists six times more frequently than do younger adults.[3]

NORMAL PHYSIOLOGY OF AGING

With a few notable exceptions, the digestive system maintains normal functioning in elderly people. In order to distinguish between the expected age-related alterations of the gut and symptoms attributable to pathological conditions, the clinician must have an understanding of the normal physiology of aging. One must also appreciate the interactions between the gastrointestinal (GI) tract and longstanding exposures to environmental agents (e.g. medications, tobacco, and alcohol) and chronic non-GI disease states (e.g. congestive heart failure, diabetes mellitus, chronic obstructive pulmonary disease, dementia, depression).[4] With this knowledge, it will become apparent that most new GI complaints in otherwise healthy older people are due to disease rather than to aging alone and therefore merit appropriate investigation and treatment.

Aging is not associated with a difference in either the desire to eat or the hunger response prior to meal intake, but postprandial hunger and desire to eat are reduced.[5,6] One explanation may be that fasting and intraduodenal lipid-stimulated plasma concentrations of cholecystokinin (CCK), a physiological satiety factor, have been found to be higher in older than in younger men.[7] However, anorexia in older individuals should not be attributed to advanced age alone. This symptom warrants evaluation to exclude a medical or psychological cause or a medication-induced adverse effect.[5]

Up to 40 percent of healthy elderly people subjectively complain of a dry mouth. Although baseline salivary flow probably decreases with aging, stimulated salivation is unchanged in both healthy and edentulous geriatric patients.[8–11] Chewing power is diminished, probably because of decreased bulk of the muscles of mastication,[12,13] though perhaps attributable in part to preclinical manifestations of neurological disease rather than to the normal aging process.[11] While many older patients are edentulous to some degree, better dental care has enabled more of them to have intact teeth now than in the past.[5,14,15]

Gustatory and olfactory sensation tend to decrease with aging. The ability to detect and discriminate between sweet, sour, salty, and bitter tastes deteriorates as one gets older.[5,16] Thresholds for salt and bitter taste show age-related elevations, while that for sweet taste appears stable.[5,17] By the ninth decade, the olfactory threshold increases by about 50 percent, contributing to poor smell recognition.[5,18]

Despite early data to the contrary, the physiological function of the esophagus in otherwise healthy individuals is well-preserved with increasing age, with the exception of very old patients.[19,20] Studies from the early 1960s introduced the concept of the "presbyesophagus" based on cineradiographic and manometric data,[21,22] but the term has been abandoned.[23] A more recent study that excluded patients with diabetes or neuropathy found no increase in dysmotility in elderly men.[24] Investigators have also found that minor alterations may occur in some octogenarians, including decreased pressure and delayed relaxation of the upper esophageal sphincter and reduction in the amplitude of esophageal contractions.[25,26] In addition, in a study comparing esophageal manometry and scintigraphic examinations of gastroesophageal reflux in groups of healthy volunteers ranging from 20 to 80 years of age, it was determined that while the number of reflux episodes per volunteer was similar in the various age groups, the duration of reflux episodes was longer in the older volunteers. The older participants had impaired clearance of refluxed materials due to a high incidence of defective esophageal peristalsis.[27]

Most studies on gastric histology have found evidence of an increased prevalence of atrophic gastritis in people over 60.[28] Consequently, it has been suggested that aging results in an overall decline in gastric acid output.[19,29,30] However, more recent data have demonstrated that gastric atrophy and hypochlorhydria are not normal processes of aging. Rather, *Helicobacter pylori* infestation, which is common in the elderly, not advancing age itself, appears to be the more likely cause of these histological and acid secretory changes.[31–34] The literature remains conflicted over the issue of whether aging alone, rather than factors such as increased *H. pylori* infestation and decreased smoking, leads to altered pepsin secretion.[6,33,35] Intrinsic factor secretion is usually maintained into advanced age and is retained longer in the setting of gastric atrophy than is acid or pepsin secretion.[36] Gastric prostaglandin synthesis, bicarbonate, and nonparietal fluid secretion may diminish, making the elderly more prone to nonsteroidal inflammatory drug (NSAID)-induced mucosal damage.[5,6] Finally, most (but not all) studies have shown that gastric emptying of solids remains intact in the elderly, although liquid emptying is prolonged.[37–40]

Small bowel histology[41,42] and transit time[43–45] do not appear to change with age in humans, although increased epithelial proliferation in response to cellular injury has been found in a rodent model.[46] Splanchnic blood flow is reduced in the elderly population.[6] Small bowel absorptive capacity for most nutrients remains intact, but there are some exceptions. No change with aging was found in duodenal brush border membrane enzyme activity of glucose transport.[47] D-xylose absorption testing remains normal after correction for renal impairment, except perhaps in octogenarians.[48,49] Jejunal lactase activity decreases with age, while that of other disaccharidases remains relatively stable, declining only during the seventh decade.[50] Protein digestion and assimilation[19] and fat absorption remain normal with aging, although the latter has a more limited adaptive reserve capacity.[51–54] Absorption of the fat-soluble vitamin A is increased in the elderly population,[55] while vitamin D absorption may be impaired[56,57] and a reduction in vitamin D receptor concentration and responsiveness occurs.[5,18] Absorption of the water-soluble vitamins B_1 (thiamine),[58] B_{12} (cyanocobalamin),[51,53,59] and C (ascorbic acid)[60] remains normal, while disparate data exist on folate absorption with aging.[61,62] Iron absorption is maintained in the healthy elderly people who are not hypochlorhydric,[63] but absorption of zinc[64] and calcium[65–67] declines with age.

Several histological changes have been demonstrated in the colon, including increased collagen deposition,[6] atrophy of the muscularis propria with an increase in the amount of fibrosis and elastin,[19,68] and an increase in proliferating cells especially at the superficial portions of the crypts.[46,69] Some studies have found that colonic transit time increases with aging to varying degrees,[70] while others have not shown any change.[71,72] Current thinking holds that colonic motility and the colon's response to feeding are largely unaffected by healthy aging. Prolonged transit time in older people with constipation is due to factors associated with aging (e.g. comorbidity, immobilization, drugs) rather than aging per se.[73]

Anorectal physiological changes have been well-documented. Aging is associated with decreased resting anal sphincter pressure in both sexes and decreased maximal sphincter pressure in women.[74] This may be due in part to age-related changes in muscle mass and contractility and in part to pudendal nerve damage associated with perineal descent in elderly women.[75] The closing pressure—that is, the difference between the maximum resting anal pressure and the rectal pressure—also falls in elderly women.[76] Maximum squeeze pressure declines with age, particularly in postmenopausal women,[8] as does rectal wall elasticity.[77] An age-dependent increase in rectal pressure threshold producing an initial sensation of rectal filling has also been demonstrated.[78] Defecation dynamic studies in older women show a significant failure of rectal evacuation because of insufficient opening of the rectoanal angle and an increased degree of perineal descent compared with younger women.[73] Histological[79] and endosonographic[80] studies on anorectal structure revealed that the internal anal sphincter develops fibro-fatty degeneration and increased thickness, respectively, with aging.

The pancreas undergoes minor histological changes with aging.[19] There also appears to be a steady increase in the caliber of the main pancreatic duct, with other branches showing areas of focal dilatation or stenosis without any apparent disease.[81] In fact, 69 percent of patients older than 70 years of age without pancreatic pathology have a "dilated" duct when criteria developed for younger patients are applied.[82]

High echogenicity of the pancreas is a normal finding on ultrasonography.[83] Aging reduces exocrine pancreatic flow rate and secretion of bicarbonate and enzymes, and the rate falls significantly with repeated stimulation.[8,84]

Anatomical studies on the liver reveal an age-related decrease in weight, both absolute and relative to body weight, as well as in the number and size of hepatocytes.[85–86] Lipofuscin accumulation, bile duct proliferation, fibrosis, and nonspecific reactive hepatitis are histological changes more common in the elderly population.[86] The major functional changes in older patients are reduction in hepatic blood flow, altered clearance of certain drugs, and delayed hepatic regeneration after injury.[87] The altered drug clearance is due to age-related reductions in phase I reactions (e.g. oxidation, hydrolysis, reduction), first-pass hepatic metabolism, and serum albumin binding capacity. Phase II reactions (e.g. glucuronidation, sulfation), however, remain unaffected by aging.[85–88] There are no age-specific alterations in conventional liver blood tests.[89]

While an early cholecystographic study found that gallbladder emptying remained stable with increasing age,[90] more recent data showed that gallbladder contraction in an elderly person may be less responsive to CCK.[91] Increases in the proportions of the phospholipid and cholesterol components of bile raise the lithogenicity index,[92,93] leading to increased occurrence of gallstones in the aged.[19] Choledocholithiasis is particularly common; in elderly patients who have undergone an emergency cholecystectomy, the incidence of bile duct stones approaches 50 percent.[94] Even in the absence of bile duct stones or other pathology, older patients generally have larger common bile duct diameters than do younger patients.[95]

ALTERED MANIFESTATIONS OF ADULT GASTROINTESTINAL DISEASE

While there are certain disorders that occur almost exclusively in the elderly population, the majority of diseases afflicting older people are those that affect younger adults as well. However, these illnesses may have atypical features which must be recognized by clinicians and represent a formidable challenge. In elderly people with an "acute abdomen," the initial diagnostic impression has been found to be incorrect in up to two-thirds of patients,[96] and the mortality in octogenarians is 70 times that in young adults.[97]

Acute abdominal pain appears to mute with age.[36] Theories explaining this phenomenon include increased endogenous opiate secretion, a decline in nerve conduction, and mental depression.[98] Pain localization is often atypical in elderly patients. For example, in a study on acute appendicitis, 21 percent of patients over 60 years of age presented with atypical pain distribution, while this occurred in only 3 percent of patients under 50 years of age.[99] The causes of acute abdominal pain differ as well. Acute cholecystitis, rather than nonspecific abdominal pain or acute appendicitis, was found to be the most common cause in one large survey.[97] In this series, 10 percent of patients over 70 years of age were found to have a vascular etiology for their pain, such as mesenteric ischemia, embolus, or infarction, an abdominal aortic aneurysm, or a myocardial infarction. A multicenter review found that 25 percent of emergency patients over the age of 70 had cancer (usually colorectal in Europe and North America, and hepatocellular in tropical regions)[97] as the etiology of pain, whereas patients below age 50 had malignancy as the explanation in fewer than 1 percent of cases.[100]

Acute appendicitis may have few overt abdominal signs[99,101] and may therefore progress more frequently to gangrene and perforation.[102] Other intra-abdominal inflammatory conditions, such as diverticulitis, may have rather nonspecific symptoms including anorexia, altered mental status, low-grade or absence of fever, relatively little tenderness, and late-stage complications (e.g. hepatic abscess). Even perforation of a viscus may lack the typical dramatic manifestations.[98,103] Possible explanations for the paucity of tenderness in some cases include altered sensory perception, use of psychotropic drugs, and absence of chemical peritonitis if the patient is hypochlorhydric.[36] The site of perforation also differs with age. Colonic perforation is more common than perforated peptic ulcer disease or appendicitis, the two most common causes for generalized peritonitis in younger patients.[97]

Studies vary regarding whether or not there is a higher prevalence of *gastroesophageal reflux disease* (GERD) in the elderly population,[104–106] but several studies suggest that the frequency of GERD complications is significantly higher in older people.[104] Severe esophagitis is much more common in patients beyond the age of 65 than in young people. Esophageal sensitivity seems to decrease with age,[107] so very severe esophagitis may be associated with a relative paucity of symptoms. Therefore, manifestations of GERD are more likely to be late-stage complications such as bleeding from hemorrhagic esophagitis,[108] dysphagia from a peptic stricture, or adenocarcinoma in the setting of Barrett's esophagus. GERD-induced chest pain may mimic or occur concomitantly with cardiac disease; thus reflux must be excluded in any elderly patient with all but very typical angina.[20] Aspiration from occult GERD should be considered in elderly patients with recurrent pneumonia or exacerbations of underlying chronic obstructive pulmonary disease.[20] Early endoscopy is indicated in all elderly patients with GERD, regardless of symptom severity. The medical and surgical treatment of GERD in the elderly follows the same principles as for young patients,[104] although the elderly may require a greater degree of acid suppression than young patients to heal their esophagitis.[106]

Gastroduodenal ulcer disease has a several-fold greater incidence, hospitalization rate, and mortality in the elderly,[109,110] with up to 90 percent of ulcer-related mortality in the USA occurring in patients over 65.[111] This is due to an increase in injurious agents (e.g. *H. pylori* and NSAIDS, two factors which do not seem to act synergistically)[112] and to impaired defense mechanisms (e.g. lower levels of mucosal prostaglandins).[113] There may be a paucity or distortion of classic burning epigastric pain, temporal features related to food intake, and typical patterns of radiation.[36] Pain was absent in one-third of elderly hospitalized patients with peptic ulcer disease.[114] As a result, elderly patients more frequently develop complications like bleeding or perforation. Giant benign ulcers of the elderly can mimic malignancy by presenting with weight loss, anorexia, hypoalbuminemia, and anemia. Despite the increased morbidity and mortality of upper GI bleeding in the elderly, endoscopic and clinical criteria have been reported which would allow for successful outpatient management.[115,116]

The manifestations of *celiac sprue* differ considerably in the elderly since features are generally more subtle than in young patients.[36] Only one-quarter of newly diagnosed elderly patients with celiac disease present primarily with diarrhea and weight loss.[117] Vague symptoms including dyspepsia or an isolated folate or iron deficiency may be the patient's sole manifestation. Severe osteopenia and osteomalacia and a bleeding diathesis due to hypoprothrombinemia are more common in the elderly than in the young.[36] Small bowel lymphoma may be particularly common when celiac disease occurs in the elderly person.[118] Therefore, elderly patients with persistent symptoms including weight loss, pain, and bleeding, despite strict adherence to a gluten-free diet, require careful evaluation to exclude GI malignancy.[119]

Constipation is perceived by elderly patients to be straining during defecation rather than decreased bowel frequency,[120] and it may be manifested in unusual ways. Excessive defecatory straining in patients with underlying cerebrovascular disease or impaired baroreceptor reflexes can present as syncope or a transient ischemic attack. When unrelieved constipation progresses to fecal impaction, an overflow "paradoxical" diarrhea may occur, even in patients with relatively normal anal sphincter pressures. If the clinician does not recognize this and prescribes standard antidiarrheal therapy, the underlying impaction will only worsen and potentially lead to other serious complications, such as stercoral ulcers and bleeding.

Crohn's disease of new onset in elderly people has been commonly reported to be limited to the colon more often than it is in young patients.[121] The colitis is more often left-sided in the elderly, whereas proximal colonic involvement is more common in the young.[122] Older patients are less likely to have close relatives affected by Crohn's disease and to have abdominal pain as a presenting symptom.[123] Crohn's disease in the elderly group develops more rapidly and is characterized by a shorter time interval between onset of symptoms and first resection.[123] Elderly patients with Crohn's disease may suffer fewer relapses,[36] and their postoperative recurrence rate is lower than, or equal to, that of young people.[121] However, in older patients who do have postoperative recurrence, it occurs more rapidly than in younger patients.[123] Whereas those few young Crohn's disease patients who die do so of their disease, death in older patients is usually due to unrelated causes.[121] Older patients are more prone to steroid-induced osteoporosis:[119] bisphosphonates prevent and effectively treat bone loss in these patients[124] and their use must be strongly considered in this setting.

The manifestations of *ulcerative colitis* are generally the same in the young and the old. In the elderly person, *proctosigmoiditis* is more common, while *pancolitis* and the need for surgery are less common.

The most common manifestations of *gallstone disease* in the elderly population are acute cholecystitis and cholangitis.[36] Cholecystitis in the elderly person may have nonspecific symptoms, including vague mental and physical disability.[125,126] Pain may be muted or absent even in the presence of gallbladder empyema, leading to a delay in hospitalization.[127] Typical features of cholangitis may be absent. Therefore, blood cultures are critical to exclude bacteremia as the sole evidence of an infected biliary tract which can result in greater mortality in the elderly.[128,129] Elderly patients who require emergency cholecystectomy have a higher mortality rate than younger patients, but can do well with elective operations aside from longer operative times and postoperative hospital stays.[130] Thus, surgery should not be denied to the healthy elderly patient with recurrent biliary colic based on age alone.[94] Minimally invasive procedures such as endoscopic retrograde cholangiopancreatography and laparoscopic cholecystectomy should be used whenever possible.[94]

The clinical course of *liver disease* in the elderly is usually similar to that in the young, though complications are tolerated less well.[36,131] Chronic hepatitis C, along with alcoholic liver disease, is emerging as the most common cause of chronic parenchymal liver disease in the elderly population.[89] Viral hepatitis more commonly has a prolonged and cholestatic picture in the elderly, although data are equivocal on whether older people are more or less likely to suffer severe or fulminant hepatitis.[86] While the risk of death from fulminant liver failure from acute hepatitis A infection appears to increase with age, acute hepatitis B in elderly patients is usually a mild, subclinical disease and the risk of fulminant disease is not increased.[132] Advanced age at the onset of infection with hepatitis C is associated with an increased mortality rate.[132] When fulminant hepatic failure develops from any cause, advanced age is an adverse prognostic variable.[89] Certain conditions, including alcoholic liver disease, hemochromatosis, primary biliary cirrhosis, and hepatocellular carcinoma, are often seen in more advanced stages when they first present in older patients.[86]

GASTROINTESTINAL PROBLEMS UNIQUE TO THE ELDERLY POPULATION

Certain gastrointestinal symptoms and diseases occur primarily, or even exclusively, in the elderly population.

In the esophagus, a posterior hypopharyngeal (Zenker's) diverticulum may form as a result of reduced muscle compliance of the upper esophageal sphincter.[133] Neurological disorders, particularly cerebrovascular insult and Parkinson's disease, account for 80 percent of cases of oropharyngeal dysphagia in elderly people.[134] Dysphagia aortica is a syndrome in which symptoms are caused by extrinsic compression of the esophagus by a large thoracic aneurysm or a rigid atherosclerotic aorta.[26] While cervical osteophytes are common in the elderly population, they are thought to be a very rare cause of dysphagia.[26]

Stomach disorders generally confined to elderly people include atrophic gastritis, with or without pernicious anemia. As mentioned previously, prolonged *H. pylori* infection rather than aging alone may be responsible for this condition. A Dieulafoy's lesion, resulting from a nontapering ectatic submucosal artery, may be an obscure etiology of upper GI bleeding in patients of all ages but is particularly frequent in the elderly population.[135]

The prevalence of small bowel diverticulosis increases greatly in older people. The condition may be limited to a single large duodenal diverticulum or may be characterized by numerous diverticula throughout the jejunum. While most cases are completely asymptomatic, some lead to perforation, hemorrhage, or bacterial overgrowth-induced malabsorption.[36]

Chronic mesenteric ischemia, manifested by intestinal angina, is a very rare form of mesenteric vascular disease seen in elderly patients with atherosclerosis. Aortoenteric fistula, an uncommon cause of life-threatening GI hemorrhage, occurs in elderly patients with prior graft placement for an abdominal aortic aneurysm (AAA) or, rarely, with an untreated AAA. NSAID-induced enteropathy, characterized by ulceration leading to acute or occult bleeding, ileal stenosis, strictures, protein loss, or iron deficiency, has been increasingly recognized.[119]

Age is a strong risk factor for colon polyps and cancer. Guidelines which advise colorectal screening examinations beginning at age 50 in average-risk patients and at age 40 for certain high-risk patients do not provide upper age constraints for colorectal screening. Some experts have suggested an age cutoff at 80 years for screening[136] and 85 years for surveillance for patients who have had only small tubular adenomas.[137] Since these ages are somewhat arbitrary, colorectal screening and surveillance in the elderly group must be individualized based on comorbidity and life expectancy. Colonoscopic polypectomy, rather than surgery, has been advocated for the treatment of large polyps in healthy elderly patients up to 90 years old in whom the life expectancy is at least 5 years.[136]

Several other colonic disorders are seen far more commonly in older patients than in younger patients. These include colonic diverticulosis, a condition found on postmortem examination in more than 50 percent of people over the age of 70;[138] segmental colitis associated with sigmoid diverticulosis;[139,140] sigmoid volvulus; vascular ectasia of the cecum,[141] stercoral ulcer in the setting of fecal impaction; fecal incontinence,[120,142] a common reason for institutionalization among the elderly;[75] and *Clostridium difficile* infection, the most frequent cause of diarrhea in older people.[140,143]

The majority of elderly patients with jaundice have biliary tract obstruction as the cause, rather than hepatocellular disease. Malignancy is more common than choledocholithiasis as a cause of obstruction. Since an elderly person with malignant obstructive jaundice rarely survives more than 4 months, endoscopic rather than surgical biliary decompression is appropriate.[94] In this setting, endoscopic biliary stenting for palliation of the jaundice has been advocated to restore a sense of well-being, to avoid early liver failure and encephalopathy, and to improve the patient's nutritional and immunological status.[94] When acute hepatitis occurs, it is more commonly drug-induced and not viral as in young people.[86] Pyogenic liver abscesses primarily affect elderly patients, and should be considered in the differential diagnosis of fever or bacteremia of unclear etiology.[132]

SUMMARY

The gastrointestinal tract generally maintains normal physiological functioning in the elderly population. Most new GI symptoms in otherwise healthy older patients are due to pathology rather than to the aging process alone. These patients merit attentive and expeditious evaluation and management since their ability to tolerate illness is lower than that of younger patients.

KEY POINTS Evaluation and treatment of GI disorders

■ Normal physiological changes in the aged gastrointestinal tract are few, so clinicians must seek out and actively treat GI disorders (e.g. oropharyngeal dysphagia, malabsorption, abnormal liver enzymes) and not ascribe these signs and symptoms to the aging process.

■ Elderly patients have diminished reserve capacity to accommodate illness and should be thoughtfully evaluated and treated early in the course of disease to prevent irreversible deterioration.

■ Goals of treatment must be realistic and individualized, with an emphasis on returning the patient to a functional lifestyle.

■ Comorbid conditions and concomitant medications have a dramatic effect on the presentation and prognosis of GI disease in elderly people.

■ In order to improve compliance, clinicians must avoid prescribing medications that are expensive and/or are taken frequently throughout the day if alternatives are available, because elderly patients may be on a fixed income, subject to "polypharmacy," or have memory impairment.

■ Clinicians should avoid prescribing drugs more likely to cause adverse effects (e.g. isoniazid, corticosteroids, opiates, mineral oil, NSAIDs, anticholinergics) if reasonable alternatives are available, and avoid overprescribing tranquilizers and antidepressants for symptoms thought to be due to somatization.

■ While irritable bowel syndrome of new onset may occur in the elderly, 90 percent of cases first appear before the age of 50. Therefore, this diagnosis should be rendered only after thorough evaluation to exclude other disease, including malignancy or ischemia.

■ Endoscopy and abdominal surgery can be performed safely in the elderly. Morbidity and mortality are related to the degree of concomitant disease and the emergent or elective nature of the procedure. An unnecessary delay in surgery is often lethal.

■ Chronological age need not be an absolute contraindication to aggressive therapeutic measures, such as chemotherapy or organ transplantation, as the tolerance of these interventions correlates more with the overall physiological condition.

REFERENCES

1. Katz S: Gastrointestinal diseases of the elderly: introduction to the series. Pract Gastroenterol 1993;17:9
2. Lubitz JD, Egger PW, Gornick ME et al: Demography of aging. In Cobbs EL, Duthie EH, Murphy JB (eds): Geriatric Review Syllabus. Kendall/Hunt, Iowa, 1999:1–5
3. Almy TP: The gastroenterologist and the graying of America. Am J Gastroenterol 1989;84:464–468
4. Farthing M, James O: Aging and the alimentary tract. Gut 1997;41:421 (editorial)
5. Dharmarajan TS, Pitchumoni CS, Kokkat AJ: The aging gut. Pract Gastroenterol 2001;25:15–27
6. Blechman MB, Gelb AM: Aging and gastrointestinal physiology. Clin Geriatr Med 1999;15:429–438
7. MacIntosh CG, Andrews JM, Jones KL et al: Effects of age on concentration of plasma cholecystokinin, glucagon-like peptide 1 and peptide YY and their relation to appetite and pyloric motility. Am J Clin Nutr 1999;69:989–1006
8. Lovat LB: Age related changes in gut physiology and nutritional status. Gut 1996;38:306–309
9. Shern RJ, Fox PC, Li SH: Influence of age on the secretory rates of the human minor salivary glands and whole saliva. Arch Oral Biol 1993;38:755–761
10. Gilbert GH, Heft MW, Duncan RP: Mouth dryness as reported by older Floridians. Community Dent Oral Epidemiol 1993;21:390–397
11. Baum BJ, Bodner L: Aging and oral motor function: evidence for altered performance among older persons. J Dent Res 1983;62:2–6
12. Karlsson S, Persson M, Carlsson GE: Mandibular movement and velocity in relation to. state. of dentition and age. J Oral Rehabil 1991;18:1–8
13. Newton JP, Yemm R, Abel RW et al: Changes in human jaw muscles with age and dental state. Gerodontology 1993;10:16–22
14. Dharmarajan TS, Ugalino JT, Kathpalia R: Anorexia in older adults: consequence of aging or disease? Pract Gastroenterol 1999;23:82–92
15. Bergdahl M: Salivary flow and oral complaints in adult dental patients. Community Dent Oral Epidemiol 2000;28:59–66
16. Kaneda H, Maeshima K, Goto N: Decline in taste and odor discrimination abilities with age, and relationship between gustation and olfaction. Chem Senses 2000;25:331–337
17. Duffy VB: Smell, taste, and somatosensation in the elderly. In Chernoff R (ed): Geriatric Nutrition, 2nd edn. Aspen Publishers, Maryland, 1999:170–211
18. Dharmarajan TS, Ugalino JT: The aging process. In Dreger D, Krumm B (eds): Hospital Physician Geriatric Board Review Manual. Turner White, Pennsylvania, 2000:(1)1–12
19. Baime MJ, Nelson JB, Castell DO: Aging of the gastrointestinal system. In Hazzard WR, Bierman EL, Blass JP et al (eds): Principles of Geriatric Medicine and Gerontology, 3rd edn. McGraw-Hill, New York, 1994:665–681
20. Brandt LJ: In Capell MS, Upper gastrointestinal diseases and the elderly: an interview. Intern Med World Rep 1995;10(suppl):1–2
21. Soergel KH, Zboralske FF, Amberg JR: Presbyesophagus: esophageal motility in nonagenarians. J Clin Invest 1964;43:1972–1979
22. Zboralske FF, Amberg JR, Soergel KH: Presbyesophagus: cineradiographic manifestations. Radiology 1964;82:463–464
23. Tack J, Vantrappen G: The aging oesophagus. Gut 1997;41:422–424
24. Hollis JB, Castell DO: Esophageal function in elderly men: a new look at "presbyesophagus." Ann Intern Med 1974;80:371–374
25. Fulp SR, Dalton CB, Castell JA et al: Aging related alterations in human upper esophageal sphincter functions. Am J Gastroenterol 1990;85:1569–1572
26. Schroeder PL, Richter JE: Swallowing disorders in the elderly. Pract Gastroenterol 1994;18:19–41
27. Ferriolli E, Oliveira RB, Matsuda NM et al: Aging, esophageal motility, and gastroesophageal reflux. J Am Geriatr Soc 1998;46:1534–1537
28. Bird T, Hall MR, Schade RO: Gastric histology and its relation to anaemia in the elderly. Gerontology 1977;23:309–321
29. Baron JH: Studies of basal and peak acid output with an augmented histamine meal. Gut 1963;4:136–144
30. Grossman MI, Kirsner JB, Gillespie IE et al: Basal and histolog-stimulated gastric secretion in control subjects and in patients with peptic ulcer or gastric ulcer. Gastroenterology 1963;45:14–26
31. Dooley CP, Cohen H, Fitzgibbons PL et al: Prevalence of *Helicobacter pylori* infection and histologic gastritis in asymptomatic persons. N Engl J Med 1989;321:1562–1566
32. Goldschmiedt M, Barnett CC, Schwarz BE et al: Effect of age on gastric acid secretion and serum gastrin concentrations in healthy men and women. Gastroenterology 1991;101:977–990
33. Feldman M, Cryer B, McArthur KE et al: Effects of aging and gastritis on gastric acid and pepsin secretion in humans: a prospective study. Gastroenterology 1996;110:1043–1052
34. Kawaguchi H, Haruma K, Komoto K et al: *Helicobacter pylori* infection is the major risk factor for atrophic gastritis. Am J Gastroenterol 1996;91:959–962
35. McCloy RF, Arnold R, Bardhan KD et al: Pathophysiological effects of long-term acid suppression in man. Dig Dis Sci 1995;40(suppl):96S–120S
36. Holt P: Approach to gastrointestinal problems in the elderly. In Yamada T (ed): Textbook of Gastroenterology. Lippincott-Raven, Philadelphia, 1991:882–899
37. Moore JG, Tweedy C, Christian PE et al: Effect of age on gastric emptying of liquid–solid meals in man. Dig Dis Sci 1983;28:340–344

38. Riezzo G, Pezzolla F, Giorgio I: Effects of age and obesity on fasting gastric electrical activity in man: a cutaneous electrogastrographic study. Digestion 1991;50:176–181

39. Kao CH, Lai TL, Wang SJ et al: Influence of age on gastric emptying in healthy Chinese. Clin Nucl Med 1994;19:401–404

40. Tougas G, Eaker EY, Abell TL et al: Assessment of gastric emptying using a low fat meal: establishment of international control values. Am J Gastroenterol 2000;95:1456–1462

41. Warren PM, Pepperman MA, Montgomery RD: Age changes in small-intestinal mucosa. Lancet 1978;ii:849–850

42. Corazza GR, Frazzoni M, Gatto MR et al: Ageing and small-bowel mucosa: a morphometric study. Gerontology 1986;32:60–65

43. Kim SK: Small intestine transit time in the normal small bowel study. Am J Roentgenol 1968;104:522–524

44. Kupfer RM, Heppell M, Haggith JW et al: Gastric emptying and small bowel transit rate in the elderly. J Am Geriatr Soc 1985;33:340–343

45. Nobles LB, Marcuard SP, Farrior ES et al: No effect of fiber and age on oral cecum transit time of liquid formula diets in women. J Am Diet Assoc 1991;91:600–602

46. Atillasoy E, Holt P: Gastrointestinal proliferation and aging. J Gerontol A 1993;48:B43–B49

47. Wallis JL, Lipski PS, Mathers JC et al: Duodenal brush-border mucosal glucose transport and enzyme activities in aging man and effect of bacterial contamination of the small intestine. Dig Dis Sci 1993;38:403–409

48. Kendall MJ: The influence of age on the xylose absorption test. Gut 1970;11:498–501

49. Montgomery RD, Haeney MR, Ross IN et al: The ageing gut: a study of intestinal absorption in relation to nutrition in the elderly. QJM 1978;47:197–224

50. Welsh JD, Poley JR, Bhatia M et al: Intestinal disaccharidase activities in relation to age, race, and mucosal damage. Gastroenterology 1978;75:847–855

51. Webster SG, Wilkinson EM, Gowland E: A comparison of fat absorption in young and old subjects. Age Ageing 1977;6:113–117

52. McEvoy A: In Evans JG, Laird FI (eds): Advanced Geriatric Medicine. Pitman, London, 1982;100

53. Arora S, Kassarjian Z, Krasinski SD et al: Effect of age on tests of intestinal and hepatic function in healthy humans. Gastroenterology 1989;96:1560–1565

54. Holt PR, Balint JA: Effects of aging on intestinal lipid absorption. Am J Physiol 1993;264:G1–G6

55. Krazinski SD, Russell RM, Dallal GE et al: Aging changes vitamin A absorption characteristics. Gastroenterology 1985;88:1715(abstract)

56. Barragry JM, France MW, Corless D et al: Intestinal cholecalciferol absorption in the elderly and in younger adults. Clin Sci Mol Med 1978;55:213–220

57. Gallagher JC, Riggs BL, Eisman J et al: Intestinal calcium absorption and serum vitamin D metabolites in normal subjects and osteoporotic patients: effect of age and dietary calcium. J Clin Invest 1979;64:729–736

58. Thomson AD: Thiamine absorption in old age. Gerontol Clin 1966;8:354

59. McEvoy AW, Fenwick JD, Boddy K et al: Vitamin B_{12} absorption from the gut does not decline with age in normal elderly humans. Age Ageing 1982;11:180–183

60. Booth JB, Todd GB: Subclinical scurvy: hypovitaminosis C. Geriatrics 1972;27:130

61. Elsborg L: Reversible malabsorption of folic acid in the elderly with nutritional folate deficiency. Acta Haematol 1976;55:140–147

62. Baker H, Jaslow SP, Frank O: Severe impairment of dietary folate utilization in the elderly. J Am Geriatr Soc 1978;26:218–221

63. Marx JJ: Normal iron absorption and decreased red cell uptake in the aged. Blood 1979;53:204–211

64. Turnlund JR, Durkin N, Costa F et al: Stable isotope studies of zinc absorption and retention in young and elderly men. J Nutr 1986;116:1239–1247

65. Bullamore JR, Wilkinson R, Gallagher JC et al: Effect of age on calcium absorption. Lancet 1970;ii:535–537

66. Ireland P, Fordtran JS: Effect of dietary calcium and age on jejunal calcium absorption in humans studied by intestinal perfusion. J Clin Invest 1973;52:2672–2681

67. Ambrecht HJ, Zenser TV, Bruns ME et al: Effect of age on intestinal calcium absorption and adaption to dietary calcium. Am J Physiol 1979;236:E769

68. Yamajata A: Histopathological studies of the colon due to age. Jpn J Gastroenterol 1965;62:224

69. Roncucci L, Ponz de Leon M, Scalmati A et al: The influence of age on colonic epithelial cell proliferation. Cancer 1988;62:2373–2377

70. Madsen JL: Effects of gender, age, and body mass index on gastrointestinal transit times. Dig Dis Sci 1992;37:1548–1553

71. Melkerssen M, Andersson H, Bosaeus I et al: Intestinal transit time in constipated geriatric patients. Scand J Gastroenterol 1983;18:593–597

72. Merkel IS, Locher J, Burgio K et al: Physiologic and psychologic characteristics of an elderly population with chronic constipation. Am J Gastroenterol 1993;88:1854–1859

73. Camilleri M, Seong Lee J, Viramontes B et al: Insights into the pathophysiology and mechanisms of constipation, irritable bowel syndrome, and diverticulosis in older people. J Am Geriatr Soc 2000;48:1142–1150

74. McHugh SM, Diamant NE: Effect of age, gender, and parity on anal canal pressures. Dig Dis Sci 1987;32:726–736

75. Wald A: Managing constipation and fecal incontinence in the elderly. Pract Gastroenterol 1994;18:28H–37H

76. Haadem K, Dahlstrom JA, Ling L: Anal sphincter competence in healthy women: clinical implications of age and other factors. Obstet Gynecol 1991;78:823–827

77. Ibre T: Studies on anal function in continent and incontinent patients. Scand J Gastroenterol 1974;25:1–64

78. Akervall S, Nordgren S, Fasth S et al: The effects of age, gender, and parity on rectoanal functions in adults. Scand J Gastroenterol 1990;25:1247–1256

79. Klosterhalfen B, Offner F, Torf N: Sclerosis of the internal anal sphincter: a process of ageing. Dis Colon Rectum 1990;33:606–609

80. Papachrysostomou M, Pye SD, Wild SR et al: Significance of the thickness of the anal sphincters with age and its relevance in faecal incontinence. Scand J Gastroenterol 1994;29:710–714

81. Sahel J, Cros RC, Lombard C et al: Morphometrique de la pancreatographie endoscopique normal du sujet age. Gastroenterol Hepatol 1979;15:574–577

82. Hastier P, Buckley MJM, Dumas R et al: A study of the effect of age on pancreatic duct morphology. Gastrointest Endosc 1998;48:53–57

83. Glaser J, Steinecker K: Pancreas and aging: a study using ultrasonography. Gerontology 2000;46:93–96

84. Gullo L, Ventrucci M, Naldoni P et al: Aging and exocrine pancreatic function. J Am Geriatr Soc 1986;34:790–792

85. Mooney H, Roberts R, Cooksley WG et al: Alterations in the liver with aging. Clin Gastroenterol 1985;14:757–771

86. Keefe EB: Abnormal liver tests and liver disease in the elderly. Pract Gastroenterol 1993;17:16A–17A

87. Popper H: Aging and the liver. In Popper H, Schaffner F (eds): Progress in Liver Disease, vol 8. Grune & Stratton, Orlando, 1986:659–683

88. Kenichi K: Aging and the liver. In Popper H, Schaffner F (eds): Progress in Liver Disease, vol 9. WB Saunders, Philadelphia, 1990:603–623

89. James OFW: Parenchymal liver disease in the elderly. Gut 1997;41:430–432

90. Boyden EA, Grantham SA: Evacuation of the gallbladder in old age. Surg Gynecol Obstet 1936;62:34

91. Khalil T, Walder JP, Wiener I et al: Effect of aging on gallbladder contraction and release of cholecystokinin-33 in humans. Surgery 1985;98:423–429

92. Trash DB, Ross PE, Murison J et al: Proceedings: the influence of age on cholesterol saturation of bile. Gut 1976;17:394

93. Valdivieso V, Palma R, Wunkhaus R et al: Effect of aging on biliary lipid composition and bile acid metabolism in normal Chilean women. Gastroenterology 1978;74:871–874

94. Siegel JH, Kasmin FE: Biliary tract diseases in the elderly: management and outcomes. Gut 1997;41:433–435

95. Affronti J: Biliary disease in the elderly patient. Clin Geriatr Med 1999;15:571–578

96. Oliver N: Abdominal pain in the elderly. Aust Fam Physician 1984;13:402–404

97. deDombal FT: Acute abdominal pain in the elderly. J Clin Gastroenterol 1994;19:331–335

98. Phillips SL, Burns GP: Acute abdominal disease in the aged. Med Clin North Am 1988;72:1213–1224

99. Arnbjornsson E: Recognizing appendicitis in the elderly. Geriatr Med Today 1984;3:72

100. Telfer S, Fenyo G, Holt PR et al: Acute abdominal pain in patients over 50 years of age. Scand J Gastroenterol 1988;23:47–50

101. Hangos G, Thurzo R: Appendicitis in the aged. Gerontol Clin 1961;3:55–67

102. Arnbjornsson E, Adren-Sandberg A, Bengmark S: Appendicectomy in the elderly: incidence and operative findings. Ann Chir Gynaecol 1983;72:223–228

103. Narayanan M, Steinheber FU: The changing face of peptic ulcer in the elderly. Med Clin North Am 1976;60:1159–1172

104. Richter JE: Gastroesophageal reflux disease in the older patient: presentation, treatment, and complications. Am J Gastroenterol 2000;95:368–373

105. Locke GR, Talley NJ, Fett SL et al: Prevalence and clinical spectrum of gastroesophageal reflux: a population-based study in Olmsted County, Minnesota. Gastroenterology 1997;112:1448–1456

106. Collen MJ, Abdulian JD, Chen YK: Gastroesophageal reflux disease in the elderly: more severe disease that requires aggressive therapy. Am J Gastroenterol 1995;90:1053–1057

107. Lasch H, Castell DO, Castell JA: Evidence for diminished visceral pain with aging: studies using graded intraesophageal balloon distention. Am J Physiol 1997;272:G1–G3

108. Zimmerman J, Shohat V, Tsvang E et al: Esophagitis is a major cause of upper gastrointestinal hemorrhage in the elderly. Scand J Gastroenterol 1997;32:906–909

109. Schoon IM, Mellstrom D, Oden A et al: Incidence of peptic ulcer disease in Gothenburg, 1985. BMJ 1989;299:1131–1134

110. Holt PR: Are gastrointestinal disorders in the elderly important? J Clin Gastroenterol 1993;16:186–188

111. Holt PR: Perspectives on upper gastrointestinal disease in the elderly: symposium on perspectives on upper GI diseases in the elderly: strategies for treatment. Pract Gastroenterol 1988;12:5–12

112. Cullen DJE, Hawkey GM, Greenwood DC et al: Peptic ulcer bleeding in the elderly: relative roles of *Helicobacter pylori* and non-steroidal anti-inflammatory doses. Gut 1997;41:459–462

113. Lee M, Feldman M: The aging stomach: implications for NSAID gastropathy. Gut 1997;41:425–426

114. Clinch D, Banerjee AK, Ostick G: Absence of abdominal pain in elderly patients with peptic ulcer. Age Ageing 1984;13:120–123

115. Cebollero-Santamaria F, Smith J, Gioe S et al: Selective outpatient management of upper gastrointestinal bleeding in the elderly. Am J Gastroenterol 1999;94:1242–1247

116. Laine L, Cohen H, Brodhead J et al: Prospective evaluation of immediate versus delayed refeeding and prognostic value of endoscopy in patients with upper gastrointestinal hemorrhage. Gastroenterology 1992;102:314–316

117. Swinson CM, Levi AJ: Is coeliac disease underdiagnosed? BMJ 1980;281:1258–1260

118. Swinson CM, Clavin G, Coles EC et al: Coeliac disease and malignancy. Lancet 1983;i:111–115

119. Nagar A, Roberts IM: Small bowel diseases in the elderly. Clin Geriatr Med 1999;15:473–486

120. DeLillo AR, Rose S: Functional bowel disorders in the geriatric patient: constipation, fecal impaction, and fecal incontinence. Am J Gastroenterol 2000;95:901–905

121. Kadish SL, Reinus J: Inflammatory bowel disease in the elderly. Pract Gastroenterol 1994;18:23–30

122. Carr N, Schofield PF: Inflammatory bowel disease in the older patient. Br J Surg 1982;69:223–225

123. Wagtmans MJ, Verspaget HW, Lamers CBHW et al: Crohn's disease in the elderly: a comparison with young adults. J Clin Gastroenterol 1998;27:129–133

124. Saag KG, Emkey R, Schnitzer TJ et al: Alendronate for the prevention and treatment of glucocorticoid-induced osteoporosis. N Engl J Med 1998;339:292–299

125. Croker JR: Biliary tract disease in the elderly. Clin Gastroenterol 1985;14:773–809

126. Cobden I, Lendrum R, Venables CW et al: Gallstones presenting as mental and physical disability in the elderly. Lancet 1984;i:1062–1064

127. Thornton JR, Heaton KW, Espiner HJ et al: Empyema of the gallbladder: reappraisal of a neglected disease. Gut 1983;24:1183–1185

128. Madden JW, Croker JR, Beynon GP: Septicaemia in the elderly. Postgrad Med J 1981;57:502–506

129. Esposito AL, Gleckman RA, Cram S et al: Community acquired bacteremia in the elderly: analysis of 100 consecutive episodes. J Am Geriatr Soc 1980;28:315–319

130. Ido K, Suzuki T, Kimora K et al: Laparoscopic cholecystectomy in the elderly: analysis of preoperative risk factors and postoperative complications. J Gastroenterol Hepatol 1995;10:517–522

131. Gibinski K, Fojit E, Suchan S: Hepatitis in the aged. Digestion 1973;8:254–260

132. Varanasi RV, Varanasi SC, Howell CD: Liver diseases. Clin Geriatr Med 1999;15:559–570

133. Cook IJ, Gabb M, Penagopoulos V et al: Pharyngeal (Zenker's) diverticulum is a disorder of upper esophageal sphincter opening. Gastroenterology 1992;103:1229–1235

134. Pulliam JT, Richter JE: Dysphagia and esophageal obstruction. In Renkel RE (ed): Conn's Current Therapy. WB Saunders, Philadelphia, 1990:428–436

135. Wootton FT, Johnson DA: Gastrointestinal bleeding in the elderly. Pract Gastroenterol 1994;18:11–19

136. Miller KM, Waye JD: Approach to colon polyps in the elderly. Am J Gastroenterol 2000;95:1147–1151

137. Ransohoff DF: Sigmoidoscopic screening in the 1990s. JAMA 1993;269:1278–1281

138. Almy TP, Howell D: Diverticular disease of the colon. N Engl J Med 1980;302:324–331

139. Van Rosendaal GMA, Andersen MA: Segmental colitis complicating diverticular disease. Can J Gastroenterol 1996;10:361

140. Lindner AE: Inflammatory bowel disease in the elderly. Clin Geriatr Med 1999;15:487–497

141. Boley SJ, DiBiase A, Brandt LJ et al: Lower intestinal bleeding in the elderly. Am J Surg 1979;137:57–64

142. Romero Y, Evans JM, Fleming KC et al: Constipation and fecal incontinence in the elderly population. Mayo Clin Proc 1996;71:81–92

143. James EM, MacGowan AP: Back to basics in management of *Clostridium difficile* infection. Lancet 1998;352:505

Chapter 77

Aging and the orofacial tissues

Hugh Devlin and Mark W. J. Ferguson

Some of the world's greatest artists have depicted the face of old age. Leonardo Da Vinci's sketchbooks and Rembrandt's self-portraits over a lifetime illustrate the gnarled features, the wrinkles, the compressed lips, the sunken jaws and prominent chin, the changes in pigmentation, and the moles that mark the aging face. Indeed, it would be surprising if the tissues in and around the mouth did not suffer the abuses of wear and tear. A lifetime of eating and drinking, of talking and breathing, of smiling and frowning, and of exposure to heat, cold, wind, and rain—as well as a lifetime's vigilance in warding off threats to the body at its main portal of entry—is bound to leave a mark, even on tissues that are uniquely equipped for self-preservation and defense of the body. Oral tissues have high rates of turnover and repair, rich sensory and motor networks for testing the environment and reacting appropriately, and elaborate general and specific immune defenses, while the teeth themselves contain highly specialized and unique tissues such as enamel, dentine, pulp, cementum, and the periodontal ligament, all of which have their own specific diseases and aging changes. Moreover, the oral cavity can serve as a window to the rest of the body. Many age changes and disorders that occur elsewhere in the body affect the oral tissues, often first, making them useful diagnostic indicators. The accessibility and variety of the oral tissues makes them useful model systems for investigating a number of issues related to aging from the clinical to the molecular and from the physiological to the pathological.

Despite a rapidly emerging body of literature, the ease of examination of the oral cavity, and recent significant improvements in dental health, even in the elderly population, there remain large reservoirs of ignorance and neglect of the oral tissues among both the public and healthcare providers. Many believe that tooth loss in old age, either through caries or periodontal diseases, is inevitable. Many believe that alterations of tooth color, dry mouth, burning sensations, and changes in oral function such as speech, mastication, and swallowing are inevitable consequences of aging. Nothing could be further from the truth. Even many tooth and gum disorders are preventable, but stop individuals from enjoying a normal active life. All too often, elderly patients with head or neck cancer undergo life-saving surgery or radiation only to suffer unnecessary pain, rampant tooth decay, acute infection, and osteoradionecrosis. Those elderly individuals who would regard themselves as reasonably healthy may have oral symptoms resulting from their medication. Those forced to take daily medication to control blood pressure, heart problems, depression, or other systemic conditions may suffer adverse oral effects. The side-effects of dry mouth (xerostomia) associated with approximately 500 over-the-counter and prescription drugs may go completely unmentioned by the patient or be dismissed by the examining physician, an oversight that indicates how little is appreciated about the role of saliva in protecting, preserving, and lubricating the oral tissues. Most people recognize the beneficial effects of fluoride treatment—in the water supply, by self-medication (e.g. mouthwashes, toothpaste, tablets), or by professional administration—in controlling and preventing dental diseases in children. What is not generally appreciated is that these beneficial effects extend into old age and that similar preventative programs are required to care for the aging dentition in elderly patients who have lost some of their natural defenses. The diet of many elderly people is often soft, mushy, and carbohydrate-rich, which renders their teeth more susceptible to periodontal disease and caries—often of a unique kind (e.g. root caries) not seen commonly in younger patients.

This chapter summarizes the effects of normal aging on the principal cells and tissues of the oral cavity and suggests how the effect of these changes on the functional capacity of the tissues can be minimized. It also summarizes epidemiological data outlining the extent of oral problems in the elderly population, concentrating on American data, which are the most up to date and comprehensive in the world. Common conditions affecting the oral cavity in elderly people, including those induced iatrogenically, are described, as are the oral effects of systemic aging. Whenever possible, recent developments and future changes in the clinical management of dentistry are mentioned: geriatric dentistry is a rapidly emerging speciality as evidenced by the recent establishment of university chairs, consultancies, and departments of gerontology, and the publication of journals and textbooks (e.g. *Colour Atlas and Text of Dental Care of the Elderly*[1]).

TISSUES OF THE ORAL CAVITY

The mucous membrane (epithelium and underlying connective tissue) of the gingivae covers the roots of the teeth and their surrounding alveolar bone. The outside of the crown of each tooth is covered by hard, dense, white enamel (the most highly mineralized tissue—97 percent—in the body). The cells that form the enamel are present on its outermost surface before eruption but are lost on eruption; consequently, once erupted in the oral cavity, enamel contains no living cells. The inorganic enamel matrix does, however, participate in mineral exchange with the saliva and oral contents and is capable of limited chemical repair (remineralization) after acid attack (e.g. in dental caries). This property is the biological basis for topical fluoride therapy and the evolution of caries-minimizing dietary regimes.

Beneath the enamel lies the yellow dentine. It contains no cell inclusions (only nerve fibers and odontoblast processes) but is resilient in nature and forms the basic shape outline of the crown and root. Dentine is permeated by millions ($30,000/mm^2$) of tiny tubules which contain the cytoplasmic processes of the cells that form the dentine (odontoblasts, whose cell bodies lie in the pulp) together with tissue fluid and nerves. Movement of fluid within the dentinal tubule stimulates the nerve endings, which accounts for dentine's extreme sensitivity (to hot, cold, osmotic, or pressure stimuli) which is usually perceived as pain. As dentine contains the living cellular processes of the odontoblasts, it undergoes a number of age changes and reparative responses to injury. Covering the external surface of the dentine on the root lies a thin layer of cementum which resembles bone in composition. The collagen fibers of the periodontal ligament attach the tooth to the bone inserted into the cementum on one side and to bone on the other side. Cementum contains living cells and is continually deposited throughout life. The periodontal ligament consists mostly of collagen fibers, blood vessels, nerves, and lymphatics. Most of the collagen fibers run obliquely from the bone toward the apex of the root of the tooth. The periodontal ligament is thin (0.2 mm) and has the highest rate of collagen turnover anywhere in the body. It also contains numerous proprioceptive nerve endings essential for precise regulation of oral function in eating, speaking, swallowing, and so on. At the apex of the root of the tooth, vessels and nerves pass into the central pulp via the apical foramen. The pulp of the tooth contains a rich supply of blood vessels, sensory nerves, lymphatics, fibroblasts, undifferentiated mesenchyme cells, extracellular matrix, and cell bodies of the odontoblasts adjacent to the dentine.

The alveolar bone completely surrounds the roots of the teeth and is contiguous with the underlying basal bone of the mandible. Alveolar bone develops from part of the embryonic dental follicle and is critically dependent on the presence of teeth for its persistence in the adult—when teeth are extracted the alveolar bone disappears. Clinical experience would indicate that surgery involving the jaws is more difficult in elderly people as a result of age changes. The mandibular bone becomes denser with age, which can be surprising in a shrunken edentulous mandible.

The soft tissues of the gum and the hard tooth tissues meet at the gingival margin. This junction is highly specialized and critical for maintenance of the dentition. Close apposition of the gum to the tooth depends on many factors but chiefly on an intact network of supporting collagen fibers from the tooth root and bone to the overlying gingival cuff. The epithelium adjacent to the tooth is highly specialized and very permeable—numerous immunoglobulins and leukocytes pass out in the continual flow of gingival (crevicular) fluid from the gum margin. This junction between living, rapid-turnover gingiva and dead, highly mineralized enamel must be tight at the micrometer level to prevent ingress of micro-organisms or food debris.

Elsewhere the tissues of the oral cavity are covered by mucous membrane, the structure of which varies according to the region of the oral cavity. The epithelium covering the hard palate is nonpermeable, keratinized, stratified squamous with a thick lamina propria densely bound down to the alveolar bone, whereas that lining the floor of the mouth (beneath the tongue) is thin, permeable, and nonkeratinized, with a loose elastic submucosa. These marked regional variations in oral epithelial differentiation are regulated by the underlying fibroblasts and stroma via epithelial mesenchymal interactions.

Injury to the oral mucosa usually results in a regenerative scar-free mode of wound healing typical of the embryo.[2] There is usually little inflammation, and healing occurs rapidly. Fibroblasts from the papillary region of the gingiva resemble embryonic mesenchymal cells[3] in the way they migrate into the three-dimensional matrices of collagen gels and produce migration stimulating factor (MSF). This protein has sequence homology with the gelatin-binding domain of fibronectin.[4] MSF-producing fibroblasts in the gingival papillae may contribute to the advantageous healing pattern in the mouth. Healthy adult skin fibroblasts and larger fibroblasts from the deeper, reticular region of the gingiva do not exhibit a fetal-like migratory phenotype or produce MSF. The matrix of the gingival papillary layer also differs from that of the reticular layer in having a greater predominance of collagen type III fibers (which are also more abundant in fetal than in adult skin).

Saliva is secreted from the parotid, submandibular, and sublingual salivary glands and from a multitude of minor salivary glands in the cheeks and palate. It is a complex secretion with the unique feature that 70 percent of the secreted protein comprises salivary-specific, proline-rich proteins.[5] Saliva is rich in mucin; lubricating proteins; immunoglobulins; blood group antigens; antibacterial, antifungal, and antiviral agents (e.g. lactoferrin, lysozyme, histatins); amylase enzymes; and proteins which protect against dietary factors (e.g. tannins,[6] epidermal growth factor, and nerve growth factor). Of special importance are remineralization proteins which allow calcium and phosphate salts to exist in a supersaturated solution, thereby preventing teeth from dissolving in saliva by the laws of mass action. Saliva has neutral or alkaline pH, with buffers to neutralize proton production by cariogenic bacteria, and is an aqueous solvent of appropriate viscosity for such functions as dissolving tastants, hydrating the oral mucosa, and contributing to food bolus formation.

AGE CHANGES IN THE OROFACIAL TISSUES

Teeth

Many of the changes encountered in teeth are not due to age changes alone but are the result of incremental effects of wear, habit, and disease (Fig. 77-1). The most conspicuous feature is loss of tooth substance due to wear. Tooth surface wear is extremely variable and is related to diet, occlusion, habits, occupation, and the composition of the enamel itself. Occlusal wear may be due to attrition (tooth–tooth contact), abrasion (tooth–food contact or contact with other exogenous particles, such as abrasive toothpaste) or erosion (acid). Occlusal attrition gradually increases the occlusal areas of the teeth that are in direct contact; it is claimed that this relates to more efficient food processing in the older dentition. The length of the tooth is maintained by deposition of cementum, which is thickest on the apical surface of the root. The thickness of apical cementum on single-rooted teeth is approximately tripled between ages 10 and 70 years.[7] Attrition also occurs at contact points between teeth because of their movement during mastication. Interproximal attrition may result in the loss of as much as 1 cm from the overall arch circumference by the age of 40, the teeth

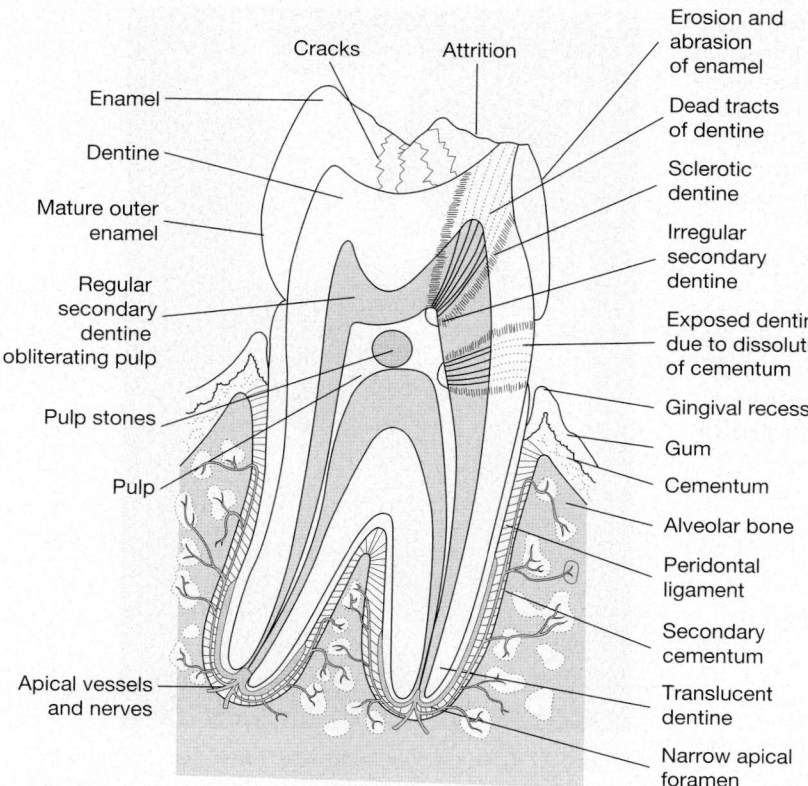

Cracks — Attrition

Enamel —

Dentine —

Mature outer enamel —

Regular secondary dentine obliterating pulp —

Pulp stones —

Pulp —

Apical vessels and nerves —

Erosion and abrasion of enamel

Dead tracts of dentine

Sclerotic dentine

Irregular secondary dentine

Exposed dentine due to dissolution of cementum

Gingival recession

Gum

Cementum

Alveolar bone

Peridontal ligament

Secondary cementum

Translucent dentine

Narrow apical foramen

Figure 77-1 Age changes in teeth and surrounding bone and gums. Adapted from Ferguson,[14] with permission.

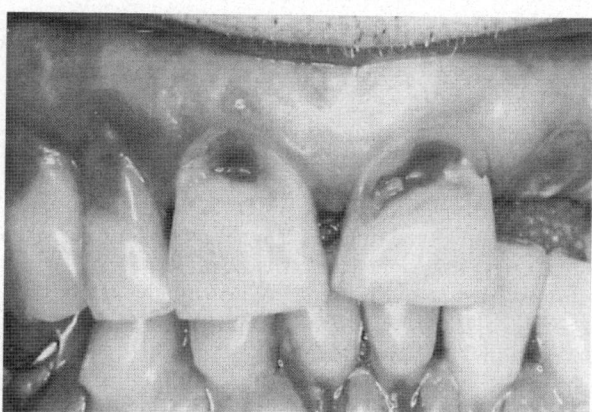

Figure 77-2 Severe abrasion of the tooth crown and root, probably caused by incorrect toothbrushing technique and abrasive toothpaste. The dark stained areas represent the onset of root caries.

maintaining their contacts through mesial drift. Abrasion of the buccal and lingual surfaces of the enamel tends to thin the enamel, allowing the underlying yellowish dentine to show through (Fig. 77-2). This, together with extrinsic staining of the enamel means that teeth tend to darken with age.

Loss of tooth substance by erosion is caused by acids in the diet or in medicines, or as a result of regurgitation. Regurgitation erosion may occur in older patients as a result of esophageal reflux or hiatus hernia. Hydrochloric acid replacement therapy, vitamin C, aspirin, or pure fruit juices used habitually can all cause tooth erosion.

Vertical hairline cracks running from the occlusal surface of the enamel are prevalent in older teeth. These are probably the result of age changes in the dentine which result in it becoming less aqueous, shrinking, and also becoming less resilient, consequently becoming unsupportive of the overlying enamel. Importantly, the fluoride content of surface enamel increases with age.[8] This has important implications for resistance to dental caries and for restorative dental procedures.

Two age changes take place in dentine: continued growth, called "regular secondary dentine formation," which progressively reduces the volume of the pulp chamber; and gradual obliteration of the dentinal tubules by deposition of intratubular dentine, called "dentine sclerosis."[7] What remains of the diminishing dental pulp tends to become less cellular, more fibrous, less vascular, and less innervated with increasing age.[9,10] Dystrophic calcification, often in the form of pulp stones, frequently occurs in the pulps of older teeth. Collectively, these changes result in the teeth being less sensitive (elderly patients may require no anesthesia for restorative dental procedures) and more brittle with increasing age.[9]

With increasing age, the gingival margin tends to migrate apically, leading to exposure of the entire anatomic crown of the tooth and eventually of part of the cementum-covered root (Fig. 77–2). This often causes loss of the more soluble cementum and exposure of the underlying dentine which, if rapid, results in marked sensitivity to hot and cold substances. It also results in a dental disease—root caries—almost unique to old people (Fig. 77–2). Severson et al.[11] investigated histologically the age changes in 80 periodontal ligaments from 24 human cadavers aged 20 to 90 years and found that the older specimens had a decreased fiber and fibroblast content and an increase in the size of interstitial compartments but no change in collagen orientation. Diffuse calcification is also frequent.[12] The rate of collagen synthesis decreases, and the collagen fibers become thicker and more stable, exhibiting increased insolubility, thermal stability, and mechanical strength.[12,13] Investigations of changes in the width of the periodontal ligament with age yield equivocal data,[12] probably because of differences in the functional loading of the teeth studied.

Teeth are exceptionally useful in determining the age of mutilated or otherwise unrecognizable bodies and also in archeological studies. Up to the age of 20, the developing and erupting teeth provide a useful estimate of an individual's age.[14] Beyond that age or when only individual teeth are available, an estimate can be made by considering a number of parameters from longitudinal ground sections of the teeth, particularly the following:

- degree of attrition;
- degree of secondary dentine formation;
- presence or absence of translucent dentine and its extent;
- position of the epithelial attachment;
- thickness of cementum on the root of the tooth;
- condition of the apical foramen;
- size and shape of the pulp cavity.

Various tables exist for translating these data into age approximations. Perhaps the best known method is that of Gustafsen (summarized by Ferguson[14]).

Jaw bone and temporomandibular joint

With age, attrition of the molar cusps enables the lower jaw to move forward relative to the upper jaw, thereby tending to establish an edge-to-edge occlusion for the incisors, which accelerates attrition of the latter. In general, bone turnover is lower in old age than in young individuals and, like many other bones in the skeleton, the jaw bones in females may be subject to post-menopausal osteoporosis.[15,16] However, by far the greatest age change in the jaw bones is that accompanying tooth extractions, particularly when several teeth are removed: atrophy of the alveolar bone occurs (Figs 77-3 and 77-4), resulting in a decrease in the face height and characteristic changes in the facial profile. If all the teeth are extracted, the upper and lower gums at first cannot come into contact but, with time, this becomes possible due to stretching of the ligaments and capsules of temporomandibular joints. Loss of the posterior teeth also results in overclosure of the oral cavity and a "Punch-and-Judy" appearance.

Patients seeking treatment of symptoms attributable to their temporomandibular joint are normally young. The prevalence of disc displacement and osteoarthritis of this joint increases with age but is not usually accompanied by an increase in patient symptoms.[17] However, some surveys of selected elderly populations have found a high prevalence of joint symptoms.[18] Perhaps elderly people assume that painful temporomandibular joints, deviation of the jaw to one side on opening, or joint noises are all part of growing old and therefore do not seek treatment.[19] Osteoarthritis of the temporomandibular joint is characterized by erosion and flattening of the condylar surface and is a common finding in radiographic surveys of elderly cadaver specimens.[20]

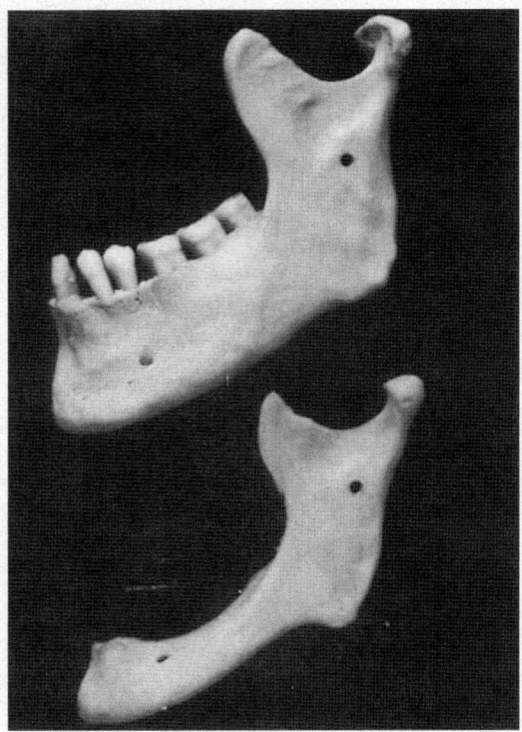

Figure 77-3 Comparison between dried mandibles from elderly dentate (top) and edentulous (bottom) individuals. In the edentulous specimen, note the loss of alveolar bone with the mental foramen approaching the crest of the jaw bone, thinning of the coronoid process, narrowing of the ramus, and the characteristic notching at the inferior border.

Continued resorption of the jaw bones following tooth extraction is especially severe in the mandible, often resulting in a pencil-thin mandible. Loss of mandibular teeth usually results in atrophy of the muscles of mastication and the muscular processes of the bones concerned; for example, the coronoid process becomes narrow and pointed and the mandibular angle widens (Fig. 77–3). There is a measurable reduction in masseter and medial pterygoid muscle bulk with age.[21] Old people are also less precise in their contraction of masticatory muscles,[22] suggesting that, overall, masticatory muscles become less efficient with age.

These changes in bone and muscle, together with associated age changes in the dermis and epidermis, give rise to the typical appearance of the drooping, aged face and lips: numerous plastic surgical procedures have been devised to "lift" the appearance of the aging face to resemble that of its young predecessor.[23,24]

The soft tissues

Clinically, the oral mucosa and skin differ between young and old subjects. With age, the oral mucosa becomes increasingly thin, smooth, and dry,[25] has a satin-like, edematous appearance with loss of elasticity and stippling,[26] and is more susceptible to injury.[27] Often, the tongue appears smooth, with the loss of filiform papillae, apparent disturbance of taste, and occurrence of occasional burning sensations. Perceived

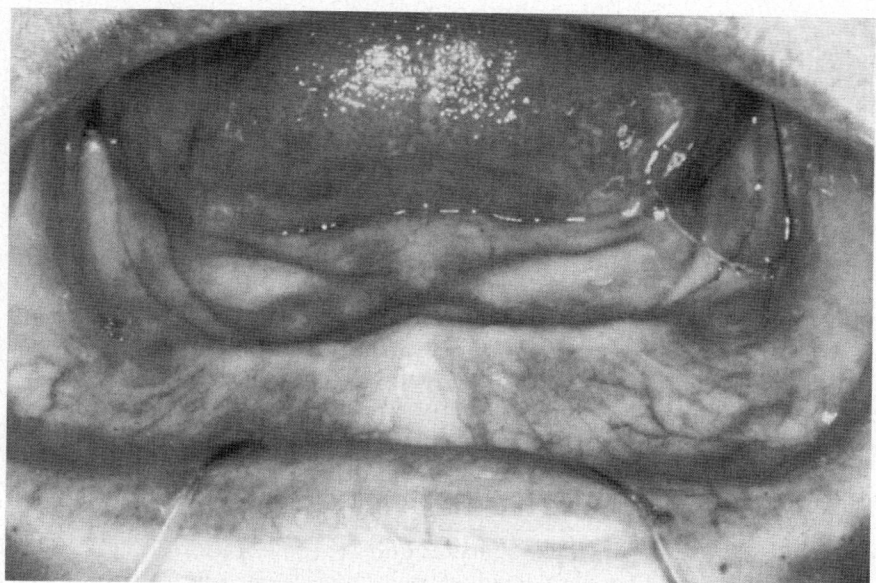

Figure 77-4 Intraoral view of the edentulous lower jaw of an elderly patient. There is almost no dental ridge on which to construct a denture. This massive loss of alveolar bone contributes to the difficulties of denture wearing and can be further compounded by tranquilizers and other drugs that reduce the amount of lubricating saliva.

alterations in taste may relate not only to structural changes and atrophy in the taste buds but also to alterations in diet and masticatory efficiency. Sodium chloride detection levels increase with age,[28] but early reports exaggerated the loss of salt taste acuity. Elderly people rarely complain that they are unable to detect tastes (probably because of the small changes in perceived threshold) but report alterations in the intensity of the stimulation. Perceived taste intensity rises more steeply with stimulus concentration in young adults than in the elderly.[29] Age reduces the perceived intensity of taste sensations, but the changes are small. Age-related changes in taste perception are not uniform for all taste qualities, for all taste performances, or for all populations of elderly individuals.[30] Apparently, the mechanisms underlying the four basic taste qualities age independently, but deficits reflect age-related sensory loss.[30] Further, aging alters not only chemosensory sensitivity but also chemosensory preference,[31] which may be significant in the context of nutrition. Dietary deficiencies, such as lack of iron or B vitamins, can also lead to atrophic changes of the oral mucosa. In post-menopausal women, mucosal atrophy and the associated clinical symptoms (e.g. a burning mouth) may be reversed by estrogen therapy,[32] suggesting systemic influences rather than intrinsic age changes. Changes in the blood vessels with age, particularly the development of varicosities in the cheeks, lips, and especially sublingually are part of the normal aging process and are not associated with cardiovascular disease.[33]

Elderly patients often complain of a burning sensation in the tongue, palate, and denture bearing area, but the tissues appear normal. This condition is termed "burning mouth syndrome" (BMS). In one form of this condition, the patient is rarely wakened by pain during the night, but pain severity increases during the day (type-1 BMS). In type-2 BMS, the burning sensation is present on waking and throughout the day. Patients with type-3 BMS have symptom-free periods.[34]

Allergy to food preservatives or flavoring agents, as well as emotional instability, are important in the etiology of type-3 BMS. The symptoms can also be caused by local denture trauma, nutritional inadequacies, diabetes, or anemia. The patient may consult a medical practitioner, suspecting oral cancer. It is important that the medical practitioner liaise with dental colleagues to investigate and treat BMS.

Structural changes in human oral epithelia with aging include thinning of the epithelial cell layers (e.g. thinning of the lingual epithelium[35]), diminished keratinization, and simplification of epithelial structure.[36] In addition there are alterations in the morphology of the connective tissue–epithelial interface, with a more papillary (rather than ridge) architecture[37] of shortened rete pegs.[13] Age changes in the rate of cell renewal in human oral epithelia are controversial, with both increases and decreases reported.[12] The age of the patient per se does not affect the results of surgical periodontal therapy,[38] suggesting that the healing capacity of healthy oral mucosa is not functionally impaired with increasing age (as reviewed elsewhere[39]).

Many clinically apparent changes in the oral mucosa with age are probably the result of changes in the dermis rather than the epithelia, particularly as the connective tissue lamina propria is considered responsible for signaling and maintaining the regional specific epithelial differentiation patterns of the oral mucosa.[35,40] A thickening of the collagen and elastin fibers[41] probably reduces flexibility and resilience with age, while changes in staining characteristics suggest alterations in the proteoglycan composition.[12] The fibroblasts appear reduced in size, and the matrix collagen denser and more heavily cross-linked. Gingival fibroblasts derived from donors of different ages show a decrease in proliferative activity, proteoglycan synthesis,[42] and protein and collagen synthesis.[43] The concept of heterogeneity in a population of fibroblasts is now receiving much attention, with the description of differentiation of human skin fibroblasts along a seven-stage lineage, each with distinctive phenotypes.[44] Fibroblast populations aged in vitro or obtained from old donors have higher proportions of stage 7 large, epithelioid-like cells. Such changes in fibroblast heterogeneity with aging are particularly relevant to the oral mucosa which already shows marked differences in fibroblast morphology, growth requirements, metabolism of steroid hormones, and biosynthetic activity according to site of origin in the oral cavity.[45,46] Alterations in fibroblast clonal heterogeneity are probably important in the development, aging, and pathogenesis of various diseases.[47] Much more is known about age changes in the skin than in the oral mucosa.[12]

Saliva

The stereotype that growing old is associated with decreased salivary flow, dry mouth, and its associated pathologies has its basis in several clinical studies conducted some time ago. These investigations did not distinguish among healthy, diseased, or drug-consuming individuals and had numerous methodological and analytical errors.[48] The decreased salivary gland function reported in nearly all studies before 1980 probably reflects pathological or pharmacologically induced gland dysfunction and not normal aging.[48]

Histological studies of aging salivary glands show a gradual loss of acinar elements, a relative increase in the proportion of ductal elements, an increase in inflammatory infiltrates, and an increase in fibrofatty tissue.[49–51] These changes are present not only in the submandibular gland (where up to half of the acini may be lost between youth and old age), the sublingual gland, and the parotid gland, but also in the numerous minor salivary glands.[52–55] Despite these structural changes, the effects of aging on salivary flow rate are still controversial. Since 1981, several reports[48,53] have indicated no reduction in parotid salivary flow rates with age; others have reported marked decreases[56] or little reduction[57,58] in submandibular salivary output in healthy subjects. Generally, it appears that in the major salivary glands, extensive secretory tissue is lost with age but without significant decreases in salivary flow, presumably because of the large secretory reserve in the major glands. However, the function of the numerous minor salivary glands is reduced,[52,57] which may be of considerable functional significance in view of their unique biochemical constituents.[56] Studies on the composition of either major or minor gland saliva with aging are scanty,[58–62] but they do indicate a diminution in sodium concentration and no alteration in potassium concentration, total protein concentration, or anionic proline-rich protein content. The perception of xerostomia probably results from reduced minor gland function, nutritional disturbances, side-effects of medication, or oral or systemic diseases.[63] For patients with real xerostomia induced by any of these factors, commercially available artificial saliva may be useful.

SYSTEMIC DISORDERS AND THE ORAL CAVITY

Many systemic diseases have oral manifestations which often appear before the full-blown systemic condition; as such the oral cavity provides a unique diagnostic window. Jones and Mason[64] provide an excellent analysis of the oral manifestations of systemic diseases; what follows is a brief summary of the more important age-related diseases and disorders.

Osteoporosis

The mandible is largely composed of thick cortical plates and a thin sandwich of trabecular bone. Age-related bone loss in both the edentulous mandible[65] and long bones[66] consists of a thinning of the cortex rather than an increase in cortical porosity.

Generalized skeletal osteoporosis results in an increased incidence of hip, vertebral, and wrist fractures as the study population ages. Age-related loss of bone is a normal feature of advancing years, but this atrophy does not affect the skeleton uniformly at all sites.

Several groups of clinical investigators have suggested a relationship between severe mandibular atrophy of edentulous subjects and metabolic bone disease.[67,68] Cadaver studies have demonstrated relationships between the specific gravity of femoral bone and edentulous alveolar bone[69] and between the specific gravity of slices of edentulous mandible and the radius.[45] Clinical studies have used quantitative computed tomography and have shown significant relationships between the bone mineral density of the buccal (outer) mandibular cortex and that of the femur and lumbar spine.

Many radiographs are taken by dentists investigating patients' complaints unrelated to osteoporosis. It would be beneficial if radiographic investigations undertaken by a dental surgeon could provide a useful screening function, allowing referral of those suspected of osteoporosis to specialist centers for definitive investigation. Measurement of bone loss from the jaws is handicapped by the methodological problems of obtaining accurate reproducible data. Routine radiographic diagnosis of bone loss is too insensitive since a reduction of less than 20 percent of bone calcium cannot be detected radiographically. The condition of the cortical part of the mandible is more predictive of the general bone status than that of the trabecular portion,[70] but measurement of mandibular cortical width has low sensitivity and specificity and cannot accurately predict osteoporosis risk.[71]

Diabetes mellitus

In cross-sectional randomized surveys, the proportion of diabetics in the population increases with age. Surprisingly high numbers of patients with symptoms of altered taste, burning, dryness, or gingival tenderness have glucose intolerance. Unfortunately, the correlation of blood glucose levels with those of glucose in the saliva is poor. Some diabetics with xerostomia may have a measurable reduction in salivary flow, and others have no change in salivary flow rate. Despite one-third of patients, in one study, complaining of a dry mouth, none had alterations in salivary flow rate.[72] Changes in salivary flow rate may be due to increased urination, dehydration, or atherosclerosis of the salivary blood vessels; enlargement of the parotid gland (sialosis) is sometimes present. Diabetics have an increased incidence and severity of periodontal diseases, possibly because of gingival microangiopathy, altered polymorphonuclear leukocyte function, or an increased rate of collagen breakdown.

Iron-deficiency anemia

Hypochromic anemia is a significant problem in elderly people. The oral mucosa has a yellowish pallor and may be associated with atrophy and aphthous ulceration, angular cheilitis, dysphagia, or candidiasis. In the tongue, atrophy of the filiform papillae occurs, followed by atrophy of the fungiform papillae. This produces the characteristic raw, red, painful tongue.

If the patient has an unsatisfactory dentition or dentures, he or she may choose easily masticated, poorly nutritious food, which can only exacerbate anemia (see later).

Benign mucous membrane pemphigoid
Benign mucous membrane pemphigoid is a disease that principally affects those over 40 years of age. Subepidermal vesiculobullous blisters may appear on the oral cavity, conjunctiva, or skin and on the mucous membranes of the vagina, penis, anus, or pharynx. The oral blisters eventually rupture, leaving a raw, ulcerated surface.

Lichen planus
Lichen planus has both oral and skin manifestations, with most patients in the 30 to 60 year age group. About three-quarters of patients with oral lichen planus are over the age of 50 years. Many different types of lesions have been described, but the most common (the reticular type) is characterized by a white lacework pattern on the buccal mucosa (Fig. 77-5).

Other variations in presentation are seen with the predominance of either papular, plaque, atrophic, or ulcerative lesions. The painful erosions of lichen planus are treated by local steroid application.

Sjögren's syndrome
Primary Sjögren's syndrome (or sicca syndrome) is associated with dry mouth and dry eyes. When a connective tissue disease is also present (most commonly rheumatoid arthritis) then a secondary Sjögren's syndrome is diagnosed. Other connective tissue diseases may be associated and include primary biliary cirrhosis, systemic sclerosis, and mixed connective tissue disease. Oral ulceration is common, and because of the absence of lubrication, swallowing food may be particularly difficult.

Diagnosis is made from a comprehensive clinical history, combined with special tests for diminished lacrimation (Schirmer test), biopsy of the lower lip salivary glands, and sialectasis with sialography.

The oral dryness can be treated with a lubricant mouthwash, such as 2% methylcellulose, or by encouraging the patient to take regular sips of water.

Orofacial pain in the elderly patient
See also Chapter 59.

PSYCHIATRIC DISEASE   Atypical facial pain has a significant psychogenic background. Patients complain of chronic, continuous pain of the maxillary region, but no organic disease is present. The pain is often poorly localized and persistent over many years. The symptoms often become easier with eating, which is in contrast to pain from ulcers which is made worse by eating. A psychiatric assessment may be beneficial, with many patients responding to antidepressant drug therapy.

TRIGEMINAL NEURALGIA   Elderly persons are most often affected by this excrutiatingly painful condition. The pain is usually unilateral, very severe and spasmodic, and lasts for a few seconds or minutes. There are pain-free intervals between the attacks. It is initiated by touching a trigger zone within the distribution of the trigeminal nerve. The pain can also be initiated by toothbrushing or even smiling. Carbamazepine, an anticonvulsant, is effective if given continuously, but not if taken as an analgesic. The patient requires a neurological assessment to eliminate other conditions with similar pain symptoms.

GLOSSOPHARYNGEAL NEURALGIA   This neuralgia primarily affects middle-aged and elderly people, but is rare. Severe, unilateral pain is triggered by swallowing or chewing. It affects the base of the tongue, tonsil, and nasopharynx. The condition may respond to carbamazepine.

POSTHERPETIC NEURALGIA   This neuralgia affects mainly the elderly population. It occurs after herpes zoster infection

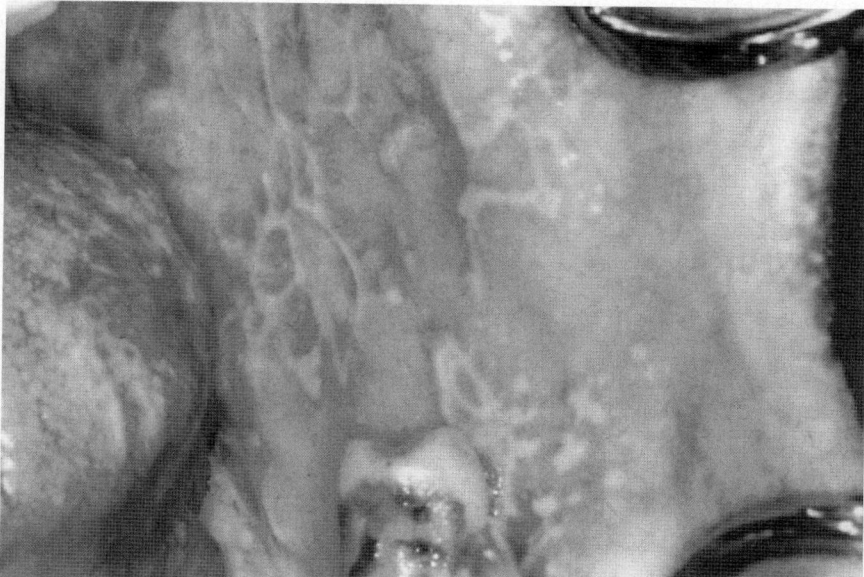

Figure 77-5 Typical reticulated pattern of nonerosive lichen planus on the inside of the cheek of an elderly patient.

affecting the trigeminal nerve. The pain is severe, continuous, and of a burning nature. Analgesia is required, but tricyclic antidepressants or carbamazepine may be necessary. Systemic aciclovir, if started at the onset of the infection, can markedly reduce the prevalence of postherpetic neuralgia.

DRUG-INDUCED PROBLEMS

The tongue undergoes changes in color or texture in a number of age-related disorders and also as a result of pharmacological therapy. For example, antibiotic administration may result in elongation of the filiform papillae which become darkly stained—the so-called black hairy tongue.

A number of drugs (e.g. salicylates, corticosteroids, pancreatic enzymes, emepromium, tetracycline, clindamycin) can cause ulcerations of the oral mucosa, particularly if they are not swallowed immediately.[73] Oral herpes often occurs during immunosuppressive treatment; similarly, oral candidal infections occur during therapy with corticosteroids and antibiotics, as well as in a variety of compromising systemic conditions.

The dental complications of drug-induced decreased salivary secretion and consequent dry mouth include rampant dental caries (Fig. 77-6), loss of fillings, poorly fitting dentures,[74] oral ulcers, glossitis, stomatitis, acute parotitis, candida, and other mucosal infections. Dry mouth occurs during therapy with drugs with an anticholinergic effect, for example antihistamines, cyclic antidepressants (particularly amitriptyline, imipramine, and doxepin), high doses of neuroleptics, some opiates, and disopyramide.[75] Lithium also induces dry mouth and thirst, owing to its diuretic effect. Management of tricyclic-induced dry mouth may include dose reduction or substitution of a nonanticholinergic drug (e.g. fluoxetine), as well as artificial saliva substitutes.[76]

Systemic diseases and therapies in elderly people may markedly affect the nature and type of dental treatment.[73–78]

AGE-RELATED DISEASES OF THE ORAL CAVITY

Surveys of elderly people have shown that a large percentage have some pathological lesion present in their mouth, ranging in severity from localized inflammation, ulceration, and leukoplakia to carcinoma. Hoad-Reddick[79] examined 233 elderly subjects living in Cheshire, England, and found 41 percent of the sample had an oral pathological lesion. The highest incidence of oral pathology was present in those living in the community with no assistance (over 60 percent). Medical practitioners and carers must therefore be aware of the oral problems of older people and educate them to the value of regular oral examination.

Oral cancer

The oral cavity is easily examined, and oral cancer can therefore be diagnosed early (Fig. 77-7). The prognosis for patients with oral cancer improves dramatically when the lesion is small and there is an absence of metastases to the lymph nodes in the neck. Unfortunately though, about half of patients with oral cancer will die from it. Oral cancer is often painless, has a variable clinical appearance, and can mimic denture trauma. Chronic lesions with associated induration or fixation to underlying tissue should be investigated urgently.

Squamous cell carcinoma is the most common oral malignant tumor; its incidence increases sharply with age, most cases occurring in the over-60 age group.[80] The lower lip is the most commonly affected site, the tumor manifesting in a variety of ways—a large exophytic growth, a deep ulcer, swelling of the vermilion border, or a crusty inconspicuous lesion.[80] An important feature of oral mucosal cancers is the induration palpable at the periphery of the tumor.

The tongue is the next most common site of cancer, with a variety of clinical manifestations—leukoplakia, exophytic growth, ulcer, or asymptomatic. Three-quarters arise on the lateral borders and inferior surface of the anterior two-thirds

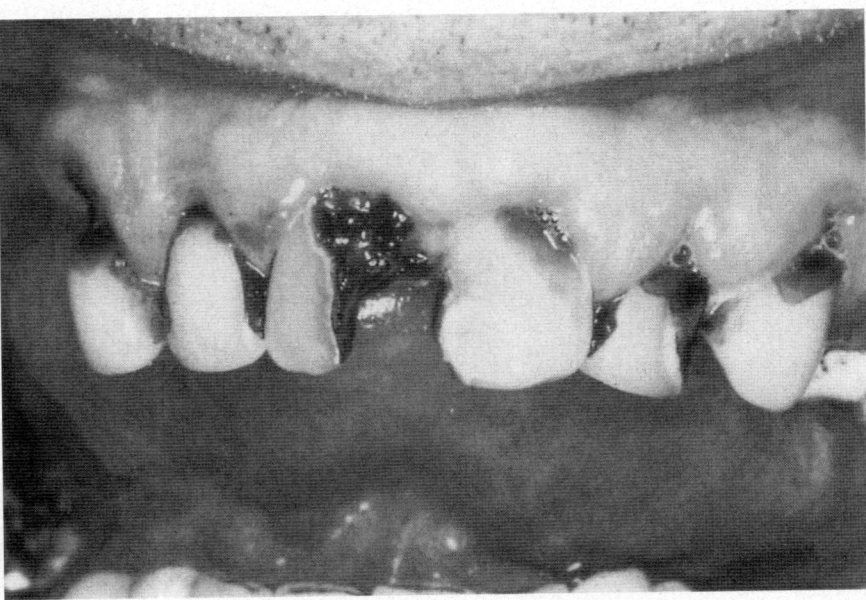

Figure 77-6 Advanced, rapidly destructive dental caries in an elderly person. This was almost certainly induced by the damaging effects of reduced salivary gland secretion as a result of oral tranquilizer use.

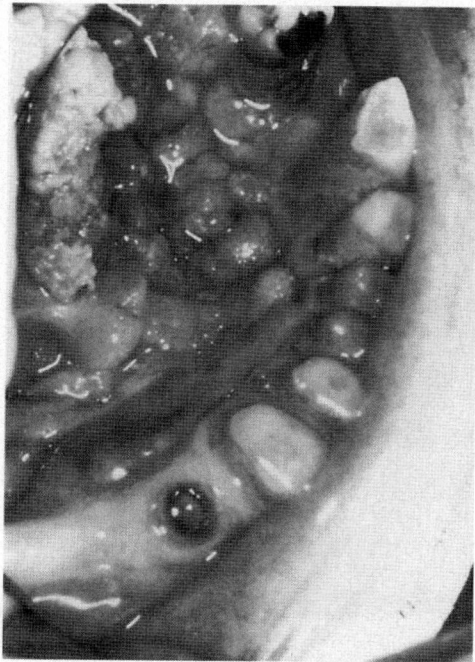

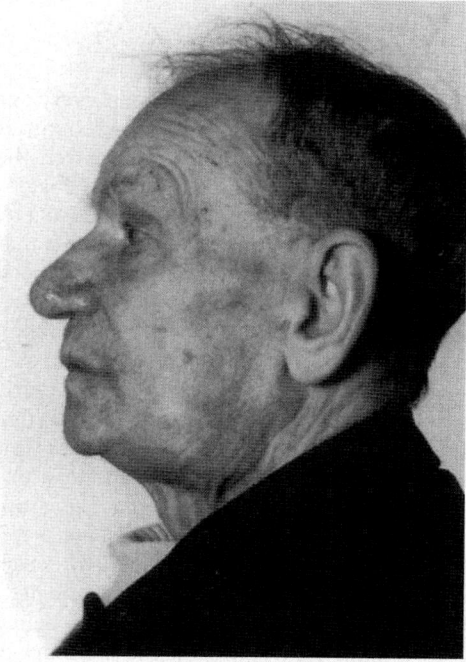

Figure 77-7 Intraoral and extraoral views of an advanced squamous cell carcinoma of the anterior floor of the mouth. Note the fungating appearance of the carcinoma, and the hard, fixed lump on the lower border of the mandible, visible in the external view.

of the tongue. The highest incidence is in the sixth to eighth decades. Cancer of the buccal mucosa and floor of the mouth is common in the seventh decade, usually as an ulcerated lesion with raised and indurated margins near the frenum.

All oral cancers are more frequent in men than in women, but the pattern is changing. In Manchester, England, the male/female ratio decreased from 13:1 in 1932–39 to 4:1 in 1960–69, probably because of an increased consumption of cigarettes and alcohol by women.[81] Both smoking and alcohol consumption (and sunlight for lip cancer) are important risk factors, with a synergistic effect occurring between the two. Using betel quid and habitually placing snuff in the buccal sulcus (snuff dipping) are also associated with oral cancer.

Regular oral examination, every year or two, provides an efficient screening service for intraoral lesions and vastly improves the patient's prognosis. Both the incidence and mortality from oral cancer vary widely: for example, the 1985 male mortality per 100,000 population for oral cancer was 19.6 in France and 3.0 in the Netherlands.[82] Importantly, white (leukoplakia) or red (erythroplakia) patches in the mouth are important early signs and must be regarded as premalignant lesions until proven otherwise. Biopsy of oral red and white patches is mandatory.

Treatment of oral cancer usually involves surgery and/or radiotherapy. Surgical reconstruction techniques have been revolutionized by the use of titanium implants, which have done much to minimize aesthetic and functional defects.

Oral premalignancy

Some premalignant conditions, such as Plummer–Vinson syndrome, predispose to oral cancer. This syndrome consists of iron deficiency, spoon-shaped nails, and dysphagia.

Premalignant lesions are those in which carcinoma may develop. Large, longstanding white lesions with areas of redness, speckling, or ulceration indicate a high risk. A detailed history, examination of the clinical features and biopsy of the lesion are necessary to assess the malignancy potential. High-risk sites include the floor of the mouth, the retromolar area, the posterolateral surface of the tongue, and the anterior pillar of the fauces. Treatment of the high-risk lesions is usually by surgical excision.

Denture-associated pathology

Denture stomatitis is an inflammatory lesion of varying severity beneath upper dentures and may occur in up to 60 percent of elderly denture-wearing patients.[80] Causes include ill-fitting, dirty dentures, often with superimposed yeast infection, such as the opportunistic pathogen *Candida albicans*. Treatment involves adjustment or replacement of the denture, instructing the patient to remove the denture at night and clean it, and fungistatic Miconazole oral gel applied to the denture four times daily. Miconazole gel should be avoided if the patient is currently taking oral anticoagulants (acenocoumarol [nicoumalone] or warfarin) as serious interactions may occur. Hematological investigations are essential to exclude predisposing factors such as iron, vitamin B_{12}, and folate deficiencies and undiagnosed diabetes mellitus.

Elderly denture wearers often develop painful lateral lip fissures (prevalence about 16 percent), which are frequently infected by *Candida albicans* and *Staphylococcus aureus* (Fig. 77-8). Predisposing factors include iron, vitamin B_{12}, and folate deficiencies, diabetes mellitus, sagging cheeks with deepened labial angles constantly moistened by saliva, and poor dentures.

Denture-irritation hyperplasia manifests itself as folds and excesses of oral mucosa at the periphery of the dentures, which

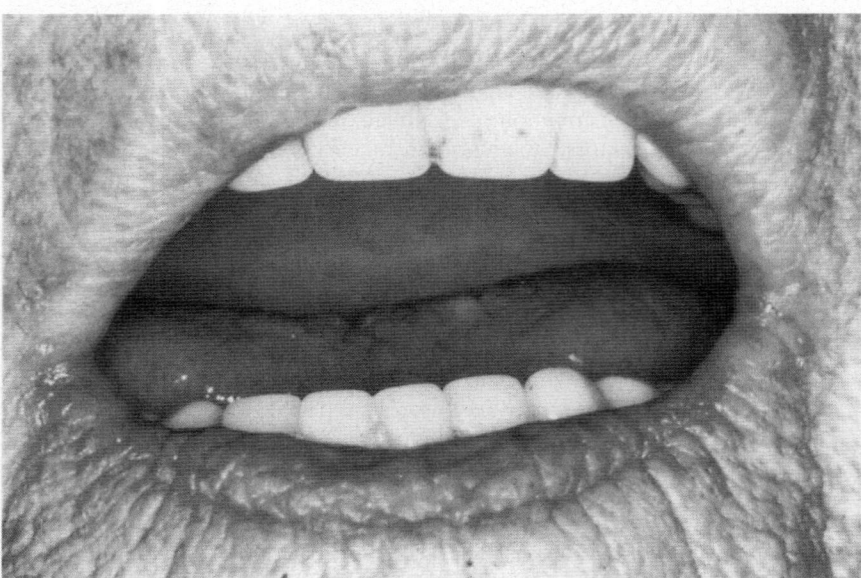

Figure 77-8 Angular cheilitis in an elderly patient. This condition is often associated with denture stomatitis, candida infection, and poorly fitting dentures.

have usually been ill-fitting over a long period. Its incidence varies from 3 to 26 percent.[80,82]

In extensive surveys of elderly patients, generally less than one-third of dentures examined have been considered acceptable by the examining clinicians.[72,83] Most have been worn for a considerable time without replacement—60 percent were at least 10 years old and a further 30 percent in excess of 20 years old.[84,85] It is generally accepted among dentists that dentures need regular checking and replacement every 5–10 years. Health professionals must communicate this message more clearly to patients.

Candidiasis

Old age, ill-health, and malignancy predispose an individual to oral candidiasis because the person is unable to mount an effective immune response. Severely reduced immunocompetence may lead to systemic candidiasis, which is a life-threatening condition. Such patients should receive a prophylactic antifungal agent.

DENTAL HEALTH IN THE ELDERLY POPULATION

Professionals from all branches of medicine, politicians, and the elderly people themselves all have a role to play in dental health promotion. Numerous surveys have demonstrated that the main problems associated with aging are loss of teeth, periodontal disease, oral mucosal lesions,[86] and root surface caries.[87,88] Good oral hygiene, avoidance of a confectionery or a starchy diet, and regular visits to the dentist will improve dental health. Chlorhexidine rinses are recommended for confused and physically handicapped elderly people.[89] Rinsing with fluoride solutions may encourage remineralization of early carious lesions.[90] Fluoridation of the public water supply is inexpensive, does not require active cooperation from those who benefit, and at optimal levels has no harmful effects. Deaths from oral cancer could be reduced with regular oral

examination of elderly people because diagnosis could be made while the lesions are small.

Dental caries and fluoride

The prevalence of tooth decay and edentulism at every age interval has dropped significantly in most developed countries over the last 20 years, and will continue to decrease over the next 20 years (Fig. 77-9). This is primarily due to the widespread use of toothpastes containing fluoride. Advertising by the oral care industry has established amongst patients that twice-daily toothbrushing is a socially desirable, beneficial activity. Research has shown that there is an additional 6 percent reduction in dental caries for every 500 parts per million (ppm) increase in the fluoride concentration of toothpaste over the range 1000–2500 ppm.[91] Elderly people are particularly prone to gum recession which exposes tooth root surfaces that are susceptible to caries. In the USA, fluoride dentifrices containing 5000 ppm are available on prescription, and this concentration may be particularly effective in remineralizing root caries in elderly subjects.

Elderly people living in "fluoridated areas" experience much less root surface decay than those living in "nonfluoridated" communities.[92] Water fluoridation can benefit the dental health of the elderly population by reducing the incidence of dental decay and preventing the onset of caries throughout life.[93] It is estimated that 145 million people in the USA alone benefit from a fluoridated water supply,[94] which is therefore an important public health measure.

There is also strong evidence that water fluoridation reduces the incidence of hip fractures. A recent meta-analysis of 29 studies showed that water fluoridation over 10 years in duration was associated with fewer bone fractures.[95] Phipps et al.[96] examined over 7000 white women aged over 65 years and obtained information on their exposure to fluoridated water from 1950 to 1994. Women with continuous fluoride exposure had a 31 percent reduction in risk of hip fracture and a 27 percent reduction in risk of vertebral fracture compared to subjects

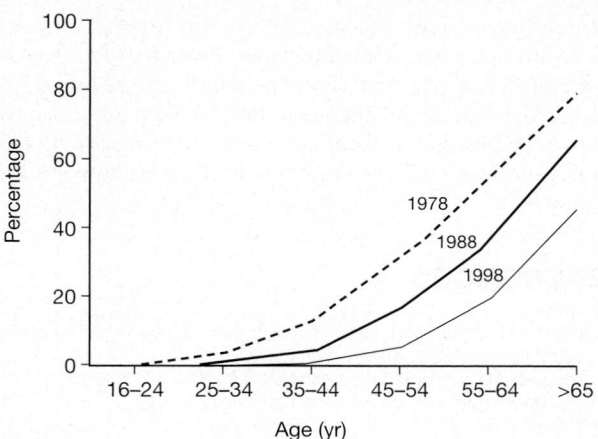

Figure 77-9 Percentage of edentulous adult individuals among the UK population. Three study periods are indicated: 1978, 1988, and 1998. Note the general improvement in this 20-year period. Reproduced by permission from the "Adult Dental Health Survey" National Statistics, © Crown Copyright 2001.

with no exposure to fluoride. In addition, subjects with continuous exposure to fluoridated water had a hip-bone mineral density which was significantly greater than in those with no fluoride exposure ($P < 0.001$). Many previous studies did not control for estrogen use, smoking, and body weight and, not surprisingly, tended to show that fluoridated water had no benefit in reducing the incidence of hip fractures.

The beneficial effect of adding a small amount of fluoride to the water supply is in marked contrast to the detrimental effect of high doses of fluoride used in the treatment of established osteoporosis. In a recent systematic review,[97] high therapeutic doses of fluoride, usually given concurrently with calcium, were associated with an increased risk of nonvertebral fractures and gastrointestinal side-effects.

The need for dental care

The presence of 20 or 21 teeth has been used as an oral health goal by the World Health Organization.[98] In the UK, the percentage of elderly people with no natural teeth varies from 57 percent in the north of England to 33 percent in the south.[99] Even within a particular region, variations in the level of dental health correlate with income, social class, pattern of visits to the dentist, and degree of social independence of the elderly group.[100] Several subgroups, such as the mentally ill or extremely old, may have a yet higher dental treatment need.

In one survey in 1986, fewer than 20 percent of the elderly subjects visited a dentist regularly, and over 30 percent had not visited a dentist for more than 20 years.[86] Moreover, although some surveys indicate a huge need for dental treatment in the elderly population, other surveys recording self-assessment reveal a markedly low level of demand for dental care. For example, 60–90 percent were satisfied with dentures that clinically were ranked unacceptable. One conclusion could be that old people accept the degeneration of oral tissues as part of the normal aging process and do not seek dental treatment, perhaps because of apathy or financial and logistical considerations, and

because dental treatment is perceived as irrelevant by a person of limited life expectancy. Denture usage decreases as patients' dependence on others increases, with those living at home leading more active lives and caring more about their appearance and eating ability than those in institutions. The large differences between dentist-assessed and patient-perceived needs for dental care are of the utmost importance in planning geriatric dental health education and preventative or curative procedures.

Medical practitioners should be aware that dentures require regular assessment of their function and appearance. They should be inspected by a dental surgeon at least every 2 years. Successive surveys have shown that chronic trauma and poor denture hygiene account for an astonishing amount of oral pathology in the elderly population. Nursing staff and dental hygienists can be invaluable in instructing and assisting with oral hygiene. For example, surprisingly few elderly patients realize that dentures should be removed, cleaned, and left in water overnight. In nursing homes, elderly patients' dentures can be mislaid or jumbled with others, but proprietary denture-marking kits are available to mark the patient's name on their surface. Other easy temporary methods are available for marking dentures for identification where no proprietary kit is available. For example, the person's name can be written in pencil on the roughened denture surface and protected with clear nail varnish.

Radical new approaches to the organization and delivery of dental care to elderly people (both in the community and in institutions) are being pioneered worldwide.[101] The implementation of such schemes is being expedited by financial and demographic changes, including a reduction in the birthrate and marked improvements in the dental health of children (thereby allowing diversion of labor and resources from children to old people), the increasing number of old people, and the emergence of the new elderly—better educated, healthier, and more demanding of dental services. These individuals will reach old age with more teeth at risk of dental decay, further straining government-funded dental services. From this emerging group of old people, large increases in demand for an increasingly wide range of complex dental restorative treatments (e.g. implants for tooth replacement, aesthetic procedures) are predicted.

ORAL DISEASE AND QUALITY OF LIFE

The aim of dental care is a healthy, functional dentition providing good esthetics and speech. The established approach has been to restore as many teeth as possible and provide dentures routinely where extractions have been necessary. However, this treatment approach for elderly people has undergone re-examination recently because of the costs involved to patients and to healthcare systems.[102] Anterior and premolar teeth are essential for speech and good esthetics,[103] and restorative care should be concentrated on preserving these strategic parts of the dentition.[104] Elderly people can function satisfactorily with a reduced dentition consisting of 10 or fewer occluding teeth.[105]

There are important correlations between oral health and the psychological and social functioning of an elderly individual. Smith and Sheiham[106] reported that 40 percent of elderly individuals with inadequate dentition claimed that the length of time they took to eat a meal was a source of embarrassment to them, 32 percent reported oral discomfort, and 30 percent had difficulty chewing. In many cases, individuals were so concerned about their dental state that they avoided eating in company, which in turn led to social isolation and depression. These difficulties often cause dentally handicapped patients to avoid particular foods, many of which contain high levels of protein and vitamins.[107] Recent studies indicate that, following dental treatment, 75 percent of elderly patients felt that they had benefited, with greatest improvements in self-image and social interaction.[107,108] Recent surveys of the new elderly indicate a change of attitude, with a high percentage perceiving the loss of teeth and the provision of dentures as requiring high levels of psychosocial readjustment.[109] Unfortunately, though, it is not always possible to restore the dentition to satisfactory levels of function. For example, gross bone resorption of the jaws, poor neuromuscular control, and a lack of displaceable tissue can limit an individual's ability to wear dentures.

When planning geriatric healthcare programs, the quality of life of elderly people could be improved with more attention to the present high levels of oral disease in this group.[110] Carers provide an essential role in preventing oral disease in the dependent elderly population, but many studies have shown that they have little knowledge about good oral healthcare practice. Oral healthcare instruction in nurse training establishments is also often neglected.[111] In some residential nursing homes, well-meaning but poorly educated and trained carers provide the day-to-day care. Even where oral healthcare training of carers is provided, combined with continued support from dental personnel, little positive improvement in oral health may be observed. Simons et al.[112] involved management of the residential nursing homes in their comprehensive oral health training program for carers, together with practical instruction to carers, but found little improvement in the oral health of the residents. Intensive efforts by all managerial, medical, nursing, and dental personnel are required for any effective behavioral change in oral hygiene provision by carers to be possible. A team approach involving dental and medical specialists will therefore provide the best outcome for patients.

REFERENCES

1. Drummond J, Newton J, Yemm R: Colour Atlas and Text of Dental Care of the Elderly. Mosby–Wolfe, London, 1995
2. Longaker MT, Whitby DJ, Ferguson MW et al: Adult skin wounds in the fetal environment heal with scar formation. Ann Surg 1994;219:65–72
3. Irwin CR, Picardo M, Ellis I et al: Inter- and intra-site heterogeneity in the expression of fetal-like phenotypic characteristics by gingival fibroblasts: potential significance for wound healing. J Cell Sci 1994;107:1333–1346
4. Schor SL, Grey AM, Ellis I et al: Migration stimulating factor: its structural homology to the gelatin-binding domain of fibronectin, mode of action and possible function in health and disease. Symp Soc Exp Biol 1993;47:235–251
5. Bennick A: Structural and genetic aspects of proline rich proteins. J Dent Res 1987;66:457–461
6. Mehansho H, Butler LG, Carlsson DM: Dietary tannins and salivary proline-rich proteins: interaction, induction and defence mechanisms. Ann Rev Nutr 1987;7:423–440
7. Mjor IA: Age changes in the teeth. In Holm-Pedersen P, Loe H (eds): Geriatric Dentistry. Munksgaard, Copenhagen, 1986:94–101
8. Arends J: Enamel. In Reaction Patterns in Human Teeth. CRC Press, Boca Raton, FL, 1983:47–62
9. Fried K: Changes in innervation of dentine and pulp with age. In Ferguson DB (ed): The Aging Mouth. Karger, Basel, 1987:63–84
10. Nielsen CJ: Collagen changes in dental pulp. In Ferguson DB (ed): The Aging Mouth. Karger, Basel, 1987:111–125
11. Seversen JA, Moffett BC, Kokich V et al: A histological study of age changes in the adult human periodontal joint (ligament). J Periodontol 1987;49:189–200
12. MacKenzie IC, Holm Pedersen P, Karring T: Age changes in the oral mucous membranes and periodontium. In Holm-Pedersen P, Loe H (eds): Geriatric Dentistry. Munksgaard, Copenhagen, 1986:102–113
13. Shklar G: The effects of ageing upon oral mucosa. J Invest Dermatol 1986;47:115–120
14. Ferguson MWJ: The dentition through life. In Elderton RJ (ed): The Dentition and Dental Care. Heinemann, Oxford, 1990:1–48
15. Henrikson PA, Wallenius K: The mandible and osteoporosis. J Oral Rehabil 1974;1:67–74
16. Wowern NV, Stoltze J: Pattern of age-related bone loss in mandible. Scand J Dent Res 1978;88:134–146
17. Ow RKK, Loh T, Neo J, Khoo J: Symptoms of craniomandibular disorder among elderly people. J Oral Rehabil 1995;22:413–419
18. Galan D, Odlum O, Grymoupre R, Brecx M: Medical and dental status of a culture in transition: the case of the Inuit elderly of Canada. Gerodontology 1993;10:44–50
19. Penreira FJ Jr, Lundh H, Westesson PL: Morphologic changes in the temporomandibular joint in different age groups: an autopsy investigation. Oral Surg Oral Med Oral Pathol 1994;78:279–287
20. Ebner KA, Otis LL, Zakhary R, Danforth RA: Axial temporomandibular joint morphology: a correlative study of radiographic and gross anatomic findings. Oral Surg Oral Med Oral Pathol 1990;69:247–252
21. Newton JP, Abel KW, Robertson EM et al: Changes in human masseter and medial pterygoid muscle with age: a study using computed tomography. Gerodontics 1987;3:151–154
22. Yemm R, Newton JP, Lewis GR: Age changes in human muscle performance. In Lisney SJW, Matthews B (eds): Current Topics in Oral Biology. University of Bristol Press, Bristol, 1985:17–25
23. Fanous N: Ageing lips: aesthetic analysis and correction. Facial Plast Surg 1987;4:179–183
24. Gonzalez-Ulloa M: The Ageing Face. Williams & Wilkins, Baltimore, MD, 1987
25. Kydd WL, Daly CH: The biological and mechanical effects of stress on oral mucosa. J Prosthet Dent 1982;47:317–329

KEY POINTS Aging and the orofacial tissues

- Drugs with an anticholinergic action (such as antihypertensive or antidepressant drugs) often have the unpleasant side-effect of a dry mouth. This, in turn, may result in rampant dental caries, poorly fitting dentures, and oral ulceration.

- The prognosis for patients with oral cancer improves where the lesion is detected early. Premalignant lesions are those in which carcinoma may develop. Large, longstanding white lesions with areas of redness, speckling, or ulceration are at high risk and require immediate referral to a specialist.

- [Fluoridation]

  Fluoridation of the public water supply dramatically reduces the incidence of tooth decay and bone fractures.

- [Dentition]

  In the future, more elderly people will retain their dentition longer, but despite this the frail, homebound group are vulnerable and effective oro-dental health care programs are necessary.

26. Pickett HG, Appleby RG, Osborn MO: Changes in denture supported tissues associated with ageing. J Prosthet Dent 1972;27:35–42

27. Corbet EF, Holmgren CJ, Phillipsen HP: Oral mucosal lesions in 65–74 year old Hong Kong Chinese. Community Dent Oral Epidemiol 1994;22:392–395

28. Grzegorczyk PB, Jones SW, Mistretta CM: Age related differences in salt taste acuity. J Gerontol 1979;34:834–840

29. Bartoshuk LM, Rifkin B, Marks LE et al: Taste and ageing. J Gerontol 1986;41:51–57

30. Weiffenbach JM: Taste perception mechanisms. In Ferguson DB (ed): The Ageing Mouth. Karger, Basel, 1987:151–167

31. Murphy C: Ageing and chemosensory perception. In Ferguson DB (ed): The Ageing Mouth. Karger, Basel, 1987:135–150

32. Belding JH, Tate WH: Evaluation of epithelial maturity in hormonally related stomatitis. J Oral Med 1978;33:17–19

33. Ettinger RL, Manderson RD: A clinical study of sublingual varices. Oral Surg 1974;40:540–545

34. Lamey PJ, Lewis MAO: Oral medicine in practice: burning mouth syndrome. Br Dent J 1989;167:197–200

35. MacKenzie IC: Epithelial connective tissue relationships and development and maintenance of structure. In Meyer J, Squier CA, Gerson SJ (eds): The Structure and Function of the Oral Mucosa. Pergamon Press, New York, 1984:119–139

36. Scott J, Valentine JA, Hill CA et al: A quantitative analysis of the effect of age and sex on human lingual epithelium. J Biol Bucal 1983;11:303–315

37. Loe H, Karring T: The three dimensional morphology of the epithelium-connective tissue interface of the gingiva as related to age and sex. Scand J Dent Res 1971;79:315–326

38. Lindhe J, Socransky S, Nyman S et al: Effect of age on healing following periodontal therapy. J Clin Periodontol 1985;12:774–787

39. Ashcroft GS, Horan MA, Ferguson MW: The effects of ageing on cutaneous wound healing in mammals. J Anat 1995;187:1–26

40. Mackenzie IC, Binnie WH: Recent advances in oral mucosal research. J Oral Pathol 1983;12:389–416

41. Rossa B: Quantitative changes in the elastic fibres of the human oral mucosa of the hard palate and cheek of various ages. Zahn Mund Kieferhalbid 1984;72:217–222

42. Bartold PM, Boyd RR, Page RC: Proteoglycans synthesized by gingival fibroblasts derived from human donors of different ages. J Cell Physiol 1986;126:37–46

43. Johnson BD, Page RC, Narayanen AS et al: Effects of donor age on protein and collagen synthesis in vitro by human diploid fibroblasts. Lab Invest 1986;55:490–496

44. Bayreuther K, Roredmann HP, Hommel R et al: Human skin fibroblasts in vitro differentiate along a terminal cell lineage. Proc Natl Acad Sci USA 1988;85:5112–5116

45. Otsuka K, Pitarn S, Overall CM et al: Biochemical comparison of fibroblast populations from different periodontal tissues: characterisation of matrix protein and collagenolytic enzyme synthesis. Biochem Cell Biol 1988;66:167–176

46. Somerman MJ, Archer SY, Imm GR et al: A comparative study of human periodontal ligament cells and gingival fibroblasts in vitro. J Dent Res 1988;67:66–70

47. Schor SL, Schor AM: Clonal heterogeneity in fibroblast phenotype: implications for the control of epithelial–mesenchymal interactions. Bioassays 1988;7:200–204

48. Baum BJ: Saliva secretion and composition. In Ferguson DB (ed): The Ageing Mouth. Karger, Basel, 1987:126–134

49. Scott J: Structure and function in ageing human salivary glands. Gerodontology 1986;5:149–158

50. Scott J: Structural age changes in salivary glands. In Ferguson DB (ed): The Ageing Mouth. Karger, Basel, 1987:40–62

51. Drummond JR: Morphological changes in human salivary glands. In Ferguson DB (ed): The Ageing Mouth. Karger, Basel, 1987:31–39

52. Drummond JR, Chisholm DM: A qualitative and quantitative study of ageing human labial salivary glands. Arch Oral Biol 1984;29:151–155

53. Baum BJ: Salivary gland function during ageing. J Am Geriatr Soc 1989;37:453–458

54. Pederson W, Izutsu K, Schubert M: Age dependent decreases in human submandibular gland flow rates as measured under resting and post stimulation conditions. J Dent Res 1985;64:822–825

55. Tylenda CA, Ship JA, Baum BJ: Evaluation of submandibular flow rate in different age groups. J Dent Res 1988;67:1225–1228

56. Slomiany BL, Zolebska E, Murty VLN et al: Lipid composition of human labial salivary gland secretions. Arch Oral Biol 1981;28:711–714

57. Gandara BK, Izutsu KT, Truelore EL et al: Age related salivary flow rate changes in controls and patients with oral lichen planus. J Dent Res 1985;64:1149–1151

58. Baum BJ, Kousrelari EE, Oppenheim FG: Exocrine protein secretion from human parotid glands during ageing; stable release of the acidic proline rich proteins. J Gerontol 1982;37:392–395

59. Dagogo JS: Epidermal growth factor EGF in human saliva: effect of age, sex, race, pregnancy and sialogogue. Scand J Gastroenterol Suppl 1986;124:47–54

60. Fox PC, Heft MW, Herrerd M et al: Secretion of antimicrobial proteins from the parotid glands of different aged healthy persons. J Gerontol 1987;42:466–469

61. Kim SX: Protein synthesis in salivary glands as related to ageing. In Ferguson DB (ed): The Ageing Mouth. Karger, Basel, 1987:90–110

62. Smith DJ, Taubman MA, Ebersile JL: Ontogeny and senescence of salivary immunity. J Dent Res 1987;66:451–456

63. Wavazesh M: Xerostomia in the aged. Dent Clin North Am 1989;33:75–80

64. Jones JH, Mason DK: Oral manifestations of systemic disease, 2nd edn. Baillière Tindall, London, 1990

65. Bras J, van Ooij CP, Abraham-Inpijn L et al: Radiographic interpretation of the mandibular angular cortex: a diagnostic tool in metabolic bone loss. I: Normal state and postmenopausal osteoporosis. Oral Surg Oral Med Oral Pathol 1982;53:541–545

66. Thompson DD: Age changes in bone mineralization, cortical thickness, and Haversian canal area. Calcif Tissue Int 1980;31:5–11

67. Bays RA, Weinstein RS: Systemic bone disease in patients with mandibular atrophy. J Oral Surg 1982;40:270–272

68. Bras J, Ooij CPV, Duns JV et al: Mandibular atrophy and metabolic bone disease: a radiographic analysis of 126 edentulous patients. Int J Oral Surg 1983;12:309–313

69. Dyer MRY, Ball J: Alveolar crest recession in the edentulous. Br Dent J 1980;149:290–292

70. Klementti E, Kolomakov S, Heiskanen P et al: Panoramic mandibular index and bone mineral densities in postmenopausal women. Oral Surg Oral Med Oral Pathol 1993;75:774–779

71. Klementti E, Kolmakov S, Kroger H: Pantomography in assessment of the osteoporosis risk group. Scand J Dent Res 1994;102:68–72

72. Stuck AE, Chappuis C, Flury H et al: Dental treatment needs in an elderly population referred to a geriatric hospital in Switzerland. Community Dent Oral Epidemiol 1989;17:267–272

73. Molhulm-Hansem P, Kampmann D: Pharmacology and ageing. In Holm-Pedersen P, Loe H (eds): Geriatric Dentistry. Munksgaard, Copenhagen, 1986:195–204

74. Kreher JM, Graser GN, Handelman SL: The relationship of drug use to denture function and saliva flow rate in a geriatric population. J Prosthet Dent 1987;57:631–638

75. Baker KA, Ettinger RL: Intra-oral effects of drugs in elderly persons. Gerodontics 1985;1:111–116

76. Borson S, Finkel SI: Essentials of geropsychiatry for the dental profession. In Holm-Pedersen P, Loe H (eds): Geriatric Dentistry. Munksgaard, Copenhagen, 1986:205–217

77. Irvine PW: Diseases in the elderly with implications for oral stratum and dental therapy. In Holm-Pedersen P, Loe H (eds): Geriatric Dentistry. Munksgaard, Copenhagen, 1986:179–186

78. Gottfries CG: Psychiatric disorders in old age. In Holm-Pedersen P, Loe H (eds): Geriatric Dentistry. Munksgaard, Copenhagen, 1986:187–194

79. Hoad-Reddick GA: Oral pathology and prostheses—are they related? Investigation in an elderly population. J Oral Rehabil 1989;16:75–87

80. Pindborg JJ: Pathology and treatment of diseases in oral mucous membranes and salivary glands. In Holm-Pedersen P, Loe H (eds): Geriatric Dentistry. Munksgaard, Copenhagen, 1986:290–306

81. Easson EC, Palmer MK: Prognostic factors in oral cancer. Clin Oncol 1976;2:191–202

82. Hamilton FA, Sarl DW, Grant AA et al: Dental care for elderly people by general dental practitioners. Br Dent J 1990;168:108–112

83. Wilson GN, Salway DJ, McLaughlin EA: The dental needs and demands of an elderly population living in care in South Cumbria. Community Dent Health 1987;4:395–405

84. Farmer PE, Drummond JR, Yemm R: Dental state, dental needs and demands of an elderly population of residential homes in Tayside: a pilot study. J Dent Res 1986;65:1151–1156

85. Hoad-Reddick GA, Grant AA, Griffiths C: Knowledge of dental service provided: investigations in an elderly population. Community Dent Oral Epidemiol 1987;15:137–140

86. Kandelman D, Bordear JM, Simard P et al: Dental needs of the elderly a comparison between some European and North American surveys. Community Dent Health 1986;3:19–39

87. Banting DW: Epidemiology of root caries. Gerodontology 1986;5:5–11

88. Wallace MC, Retief DH, Bradley EL: Prevalence of root caries in a population of older adults. Gerodontics 1988;4:84–89

89. de Baat C, Kalk W, Schuil GR: The effectiveness of oral hygiene for elderly people: a review. Gerodontology 1993;10:109–113

90. Youngs G: Risk factors for and the prevention of root caries in older adults. Spec Care Dentist 1994;14:68–70

91. O'Mullane DM, Kavangh D, Ellwood RP et al: A three-year clinical trial of a combination of trimetaphosphate and sodium fluoride in silica toothpastes. J Dent Res 1997;76:1776–1778

92. O'Mullane D, Whelton H: Oral Health of Irish Adults 1989–1990. The Stationery Office, Dublin, 1992

93. Murray JJ: Adult dental health in fluoride and non-fluoride areas. Br Dent J 1971;131:391–395

94. Hausen HW: Fluoridation, fractures and teeth: fluoride does not cause fractures but its benefits may vary. BMJ 2000;321:844–845

95. McDonagh MS, Whiting PF, Wilson PM et al: Systematic review of water fluoridation. BMJ 2000;321:855–858

96. Phipps KR, Orwoll ES, Mason JD, Cauley JA: Community water fluoridation, bone mineral density, and fractures: prospective study of effects in older women. BMJ 2000;321:860–864

97. Haguenauer D, Welch V, Shea B, Tugwell P, Wells G: Fluoride for treating osteoporosis. The Cochrane Library, issue 4, 2000

98. World Health Organization: A Review of Current Recommendations for the Organisation and Administration of Community Oral Health Services in Northern and Western Europe. WHO, Copenhagen, 1982

99. Steele JG, Walls AWG, Ayatollahi SMT, Murray JJ: Major clinical findings from a dental survey of elderly people in three different English communities. Br Dent J 1996;180:17–23

100. Hoad-Reddick GA, Grant AA, Griffiths C: Knowledge of dental service provided: investigations in an elderly population. Community Dent Oral Epidemiol 1987;15:137–140

101. Holm-Pedersen P, Loe H (eds): Geriatric Dentistry. Munksgaard, Copenhagen, 1986

102. Kayser AF, Meeuwissen R, Meeuwissen JH: An occlusal concept for dentate geriatric patients. Community Dent Oral Epidemiol 1990;18:319

103. Kayser AF: The shortened dental arch: a therapeutic concept in reduced dentitions and certain high-risk groups. Int J Periodontics Restorative Dent 1989;9:427–438

104. Kayser AF, Witter DJ: Oral functional needs and its consequences for dentulous older people. Community Dent Health 1985;2:285–291

105. Kayser AF: How much reduction of the dental arch is functionally acceptable for the ageing patient? Int Dent J 1990;40:183–188

106. Smith JM, Sheiham A: How dental conditions handicap the elderly. Community Dent Oral Epidemiol 1979;7:305–310

107. Ettinger RL: Oral disease and its effect on the quality of life. Gerodontics 1987;3:103–106

108. Friske J, Gillier S, Watson RM: The benefit of dental care to an elderly population assessed using a sociodental measure of oral handicap. Br Dent J 1990;168:153–156

109. Bergendal B: The relative importance of tooth loss and denture wearing in Swedish adults. Community Dent Health 1989;6:103–111

110. Beck JD, Hunt RJ: Oral Health status in the United States: problems of special patients. J Dent Educ 1985;49:407–426

111. Longhurst RH: A cross-sectional study of the oral health care instruction given to nurses during their basic training. Br Dent J 1998;184:453–457

112. Simons D, Baker P, Jones B, Kidd EAM, Beighton D: An evaluation of an oral health training programme for carers of the elderly in residential homes. Br Dent J 2000;188:206–210

Chapter 78

The upper gastrointestinal tract

David A. Greenwald and Lawrence J. Brandt

Symptoms of gastrointestinal disorders are frequently mentioned by older Americans during visits to the doctor, and the digestive diseases producing these symptoms are among the most common hospital discharge diagnoses for elderly patients in the United States.[1,2] As the elderly population expands and the demand by older individuals for medical care grows, it becomes increasingly important for physicians to be acquainted with the manifestation of diseases of the upper gastrointestinal tract in members of this age group.

THE ORAL CAVITY

The most proximal of the digestive organs traditionally is considered to be the esophagus; patients with complaints thought to originate within the oral cavity or pharynx are referred to a dentist or a specialist in disorders of the ear, nose, and throat. The oral cavity, however, is examined easily by the general practitioner and may reveal the cause of unexplained or apparently unrelated abnormalities; thus evaluation of the upper gastrointestinal tract should begin with the mouth.

The mouth and nutrition

Changes in the oral cavity occasionally limit the ability of elderly people to eat and enjoy a normal diet. Problems with eating sometimes are severe enough to cause malnutrition and prompt a search for a wasting illness.[3] The number of general oral health problems has been shown to be a strong predictor of involuntary weight loss in elderly people.[4]

A variety of abnormalities of oral structure and function may contribute to malnutrition. The muscles of mastication may become impaired during aging as the result of a decrease in (lean) body mass.[5] Eating occasionally becomes difficult because of tooth loss due to periodontal disease, poor dentition, or loosening of dentures caused by resorption of mandibular bone.[6]

A reduction in food intake by elderly individuals is sometimes related to a change in taste perception. The number of taste buds decreases after age 45, resulting in a decrease in taste sensation, especially the ability to appreciate salty and sweet foods.[7–9] Diminished perception of sour and bitter tastes is associated with palatal defects and typically occurs in patients who wear dentures. Taste sensation may also be altered directly by medications or indirectly affected by a drug's unpleasant flavor. Agents associated with abnormal taste perception (dysgeusia) include tricyclic antidepressants, sulfasalazine, clofibrate, L-dopa, gold salts, lithium, and metronidazole. Medications with anticholinergic properties interfere with taste by reducing salivary gland secretions and producing xerostomia. Age alone, however, is not associated with a reduction in stimulated saliva flow in nonmedicated subjects.[10]

While abnormal perception may lead to deficient nutrition, some primary nutritional disorders may be responsible for dysgeusia and glossitis. For example, vitamin B_{12} and niacin deficiency are associated with a "bald" or magenta-colored tongue, respectively. Taste sensation and eating habits also are disturbed by processes that interfere with the sense of smell, which typically is diminished substantially by age 70.[11]

Vascular lesions

Diminutive vascular lesions of the upper gastrointestinal tract are poorly understood and rarely reported. The nomenclature for these lesions is confusing, and the terms *arteriovenous malformation, vascular ectasia, angiodysplasia*, and *telangiectasia* are usually used interchangeably with little regard as to their true meanings.

The lips are a frequent site of senescent vascular lesions resembling those of hereditary hemorrhagic telangiectasia (Osler–Weber–Rendu disease), and involvement often includes the upper gastrointestinal tract. In addition to this form of small vascular abnormality, patients often have sublingual varices, or "caviar lesions" (Fig. 78-1). The walls of these dilated

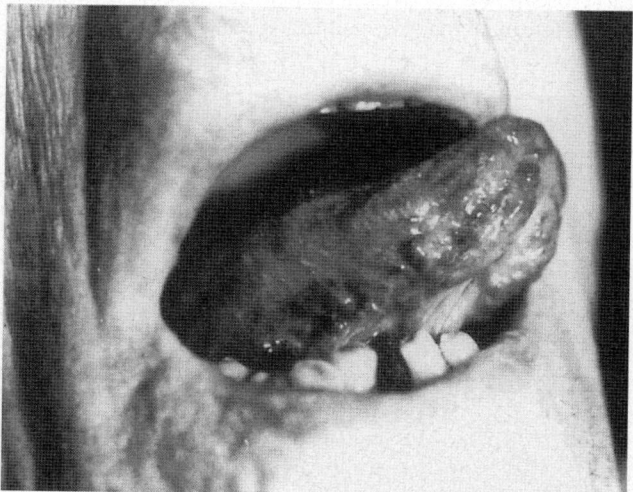

Figure 78-1 Caviar lesion (sublingual varices) in a patient with occult upper gastrointestinal bleeding. (Reproduced from Brandt.[154])

vessels are thick, but the endothelial lining is hypoplastic.[12] In males, sublingual varices may be associated with the occurrence of capillary phlebectasias, or Fordyce lesions, of the scrotal skin (Fig. 78-2).

Because vascular abnormalities are often responsible for cryptogenic gastrointestinal bleeding, their presence in the mouth should suggest that similar lesions elsewhere in the gastrointestinal tract may be responsible for blood loss in such cases.[13] Not every individual, however, with bleeding vascular lesions of the gastrointestinal tract has involvement of oral structures, and the presence of oral lesions does not preclude existence of an unrelated distal bleeding lesion.

The oral mucosa

A number of abnormalities of the oral mucosa are encountered in elderly patients. These changes may be the result of medical therapy, signify the presence of a systemic disease, or represent premalignant changes.

Candidiasis

Candidiasis is usually caused by the fungus *Candida albicans*. This organism is part of the normal gastrointestinal flora, and its presence is not sufficient by itself to produce disease. Mucosal candidiasis occurs only after a change in other constituents of the normal flora or in the presence of an immunological abnormality. In elderly patients, the widespread use of antibiotics and immunosuppressive chemotherapy for malignancies is most often responsible for the development of mucosal candidiasis.

The typical oral lesions of candidiasis are soft, white plaques which resemble cottage cheese. Characteristically, these plaques can be peeled from the mucosa, leaving the underlying surface raw and bleeding. This observation is important because most other white, plaquelike lesions, for example, leukoplakia, cannot be stripped off the mucosa.

A diagnosis of candidiasis is made by smearing scrapings of the lesion on a glass slide, macerating them with 20 percent potassium hydroxide, and examining this preparation under a microscope for the presence of typical hyphae. A definitive diagnosis can be made by culture on selected media.

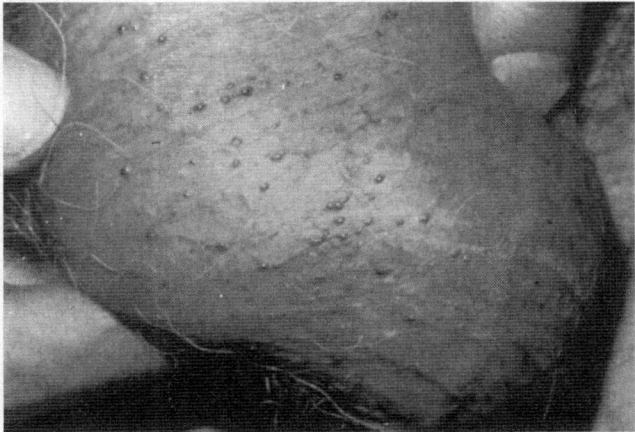

Figure 78-2 Phlebectasias in the scrotum of the same patient as in Figure 78-1. (Reproduced from Brandt.[154])

Therapy usually consists of re-establishing the normal microbiological flora by discontinuing antibiotics. In the immunocompromised host and the individual with significant morbidity, topical therapy with nystatin suspensions or troches is usually successful, although treatment with absorbable oral agents such as fluconazole may be required. Antifungal agents may be supplemented by the use of topical anesthetics to provide symptomatic relief (see below).

Stomatitis

Cancer patients treated with radiation or chemotherapy frequently develop painful inflammation and erosions of the oropharyngeal mucosa. Stomatitis complicating cancer therapy is the direct consequence of drug and radiation toxicity to susceptible, rapidly dividing cell populations of the upper gastrointestinal tract and the indirect consequence of neutropenia, which impairs regeneration of injured tissues. Radiation to the head and neck also causes xerostomia secondary to fibrosis of the salivary glands. An absence of lubrication by saliva further aggravates mucosal damage, and a lack of salivary IgA permits overgrowth of bacteria and fungi. Oral lesions may become infected, contributing to persistent injury, discomfort, and poor nutrition and posing a risk of more widespread infection in immunocompromised individuals.

The initial therapy for stomatitis is promotion of good oral hygiene. Brushing and flossing are contraindicated in neutropenic patients because of the risk of disseminated infection. Instead, mouthwashes containing dilute hydrogen peroxide or a salt and soda solution are used to reduce mucosal bacterial and fungal colonization.

A number of therapeutic mouthwash "cocktails" have been recommended to relieve symptoms, promote healing, and treat superficial mucosal infection in patients with stomatitis.[14] Some of these cocktails have been tested in controlled trials, but the use of most is empirical, based on the known analgesic, antibiotic, and protective effects of widely available liquid medicines. Viscous lidocaine (2 percent) is frequently used as a topical anesthetic, as is diphenhydramine, which is often mixed with oral antacis or kaolin–pectin. Many recipes include sucralfate suspension because it coats damaged epithelium and promotes the production of mucus and protective prostaglandins. Antibiotics used alone or in combination in mouthwash cocktails to treat superficial infection include chlorhexidine gluconate, nystatin, tetracycline, neomycin, vancomycin, and clindamycin. Hydrocortisone and other glucocorticoids also have been added to reduce inflammation, but rapid absorption across the denuded oral mucosa into the systemic circulation may compromise the patient's immune defenses. Artificial saliva replacements (Salivart, Moi-Stir, Xero-Lube) are also available for patients with xerostomia.

"Hairy tongue"

"Hairy tongue" is characterized by hypertrophy of the filiform papillae of the tongue and a lack of normal desquamation. In this condition, the color of the tongue varies from yellow to brown or black, depending on staining by exogenous substances such as tobacco or food and on the presence of various chromogenic microorganisms.[15,16] Hairy tongue is frequently seen in patients who have had extensive radiotherapy to the head and neck. While these individuals are usually asymptomatic, some complain of nausea, dysgeusia, and halitosis. On occasion, the lingual papillae reach such considerable length that they brush against the soft palate, gagging the patient.

Many organisms have been cultured from papillary scrapings from this entity; there is, however, no proof of a cause-and-effect relationship with any microorganism, and invasion of the lingual epithelium has not been demonstrated. Species of microorganisms that have been isolated are, in all probability, simply colonizing an already abnormal, excessively papillated tongue.

Therapy for this disorder consists of vigorous brushing of the tongue to promote desquamation and to remove accumulated debris. In extreme cases, topical treatment with podophyllin, an alcoholic extract of the mayapple, may result in a dramatic response.

Leukoplakia

The term *leukoplakia* was introduced by Schwimmer in 1877 to describe any white plaque. Today, some authors use this term to refer to histological zones of hyperkeratosis, acanthosis, and chronic inflammation, while others reserve it to describe malignant dyskeratosis and epithelial atypia. Although leukoplakia is considered by many clinicians to be a premalignant condition, its natural history is uncertain because of a lack of uniform definition in case selection. The term should be abandoned because of its lack of specificity. Any persistent white lesion of the oral mucosa should be biopsied in an attempt to make a specific histological diagnosis.

Leukoplakia is more common in men than in women, and most often occurs during the sixth and seventh decades.[17] It can be found anywhere in the oral cavity, although it is most common on the buccal mucosa, tongue, and floor of the mouth. Leukoplakia varies in appearance, partly depending on the age of the lesion. Some investigators consider verrucous patches to be of higher malignant potential than smooth plaques, whereas others believe that granular pinkish-gray to red islands, also called erythroplakia, are most likely to be associated with carcinoma in situ or even invasive malignancy. Such controversy stresses the importance of biopsy in the management of all such lesions. Approximately 10 percent of patients with leukoplakia have or will develop invasive carcinoma in the lesion.[17–19]

Once the diagnosis of leukoplakia has been substantiated by microscopic examination of a biopsy specimen, therapy is initiated. When dysplasia is present, or when the lesion fails to resolve after a source of physicochemical trauma has been eliminated, treatment consists of ablation.

Epidermoid carcinoma

Approximately 5 percent of human cancers arise in the mouth; 95 percent of oral malignancies are epidermoid carcinomas.[18,19] The lower lip is the most common site of malignancy in the area of the oral cavity. Epidermoid carcinoma of the lip occurs almost exclusively in elderly men; etiologic factors include actinic radiation, syphilis, and tobacco use, especially pipe smoking.

Carcinoma of the lip varies in clinical appearance and may be bulky or ulcerated. It metastasizes slowly, usually to the ipsilateral submental or submaxillary lymph nodes. Surgical resection or radiation therapy produces equally good results, with cures in approximately 80 percent of affected individuals. Successful treatment depends on the duration of symptoms, size of lesion, and presence of metastases.

Within the oral cavity, one-half of epidermoid carcinomas originate in the tongue, and the rest arise with equal frequency in the palate, buccal mucosa, floor of the mouth, and gingiva. The disease is seen mainly in older individuals and occurs most often in males. Factors suspected of contributing to the development of oral cancer include tobacco, alcohol, nutritional deficiencies, syphilis, and miscellaneous forms of physicochemical trauma, such as irritation from pipe stems and dentures. Almost 90 percent of patients have a combination of predisposing factors.

Intraoral epidermoid carcinomas display a considerable amount of histological variation, although lesions tend to be moderately well differentiated. Early carcinomas arising in the tongue typically are painless, even though they may ulcerate. Pain develops later, as the lesions grow, especially if they become secondarily infected. Tumors are usually located on the lateral or ventral surface of the tongue. The site of the primary lesion is of prognostic importance because cancers of the posterior aspect of the tongue tend to be more aggressive. Nodal metastases are located on either or both sides of the neck. Tumors also spread by direct invasion. Early detection is mandatory if patients are to survive more than a year after diagnosis.

Keratoacanthoma is a spontaneously resolving benign lesion often mistaken for epidermoid carcinoma.[20] It occurs most frequently in adults 50–70 years of age, involves the upper and lower lips equally, and usually presents as a painful umbilicated lesion seldom more than 1–1.5 cm in diameter. It initially appears as a small nodule which reaches full size within 4–8 weeks. It persists as a static lesion for another 4–8 weeks, after which the keratin core is expelled and the mass resorbed over a period of 6–8 weeks. Recurrence is rare.

THE OROPHARYNX

The oropharyngeal phase of swallowing is exceedingly complex, requiring the participation of multiple distinct structures in the mouth, pharynx, and esophagus coordinated by six cranial nerves and orchestrated by the swallowing center of the central nervous system. After food has been masticated and moistened with saliva, the tongue initiates swallowing by thrusting the food bolus into the oropharynx. The soft palate prepares for the arrival of the bolus by elevating, so that material from the mouth cannot enter the nasal passages. The glottis also shuts, and the epiglottis tilts downward to prevent the bolus from entering the trachea. Relaxation of the upper esophageal sphincter in association with contraction of the pharyngeal muscles allows propulsion of food into the esophagus[21] (Table 78-1).

Striated muscle involved in the oropharyngeal phase of swallowing, like the muscles of mastication, may be impaired during aging by a decrease in lean body mass. A radiographic study of 100 individuals beyond the age of 65 suggested that 22 had pharyngeal muscle weakness as well as abnormal cricopharyngeal relaxation with pooling of barium in the valleculae and

Table 78-1 Causes of oropharyngeal dysphagia in elderly people

Malignancy—pharyngeal carcinoma

Central nervous system disease—tumor, Parkinson's disease, stroke

Peripheral nervous system disease—diabetes mellitus

Muscle disease—hypothyroidism

Mechanical—strictures, osteophytes, thyromegaly

Postoperative—laryngectomy

Medications

Motility disorders of the upper esophageal sphincter

pyriform sinuses.[22] Several individuals also were noted to have tracheal aspiration of barium. All the subjects, however, were asymptomatic. Thus, although functional changes in the oropharyngeal phase of swallowing may occur with aging, these changes have not been identified as a cause of morbidity in elderly people.

Oropharyngeal dysphagia

Patients with oropharyngeal (cervical or "transfer") dysphagia complain of difficulty shifting food from the front of the mouth into the back of the throat, or of trouble initiating a swallow once the food bolus has been positioned in the oropharynx. Symptoms may be most severe when the patient attempts to swallow liquids. Signs of transfer dysphagia include nasal regurgitation or aspiration of oral contents during swallowing as a result of a failure to seal the nasopharynx or the trachea by appropriate muscle contraction. Inasmuch as oropharyngeal dysphagia may be due to a neuromuscular disorder, the patient may display other signs of neuromuscular dysfunction including dysarthria, nasal speech, cranial nerve dysfunction, weakness, or sensory abnormalities.[23]

A variety of conditions interfere with the transfer of food from the mouth to the esophagus.[24] Mechanical lesions, including tumors, abscesses, and strictures, may block passage of the food bolus or disrupt structures that directly mediate the oropharyngeal phase of swallowing. A neoplasm, infection, or cerebrovascular accident may damage the central nervous system, producing brain stem or pseudobulbar palsy and associated transfer dysphagia. The initiation of swallowing also may be impaired by degenerative diseases of the central or peripheral nervous system, the motor end plate, or the muscle itself. Finally, oropharyngeal dysphagia is often caused by a failure of upper esophageal sphincter function. Many of these problems are encountered in older individuals.

Cricopharyngeal achalasia

The term *cricopharyngeal achalasia*, partly derived from the Greek word meaning "absence of slackening," is a misnomer, as the cricopharyngeus muscle of patients with this disorder is capable of relaxing. The problem in cricopharyngeal achalasia is failure of the muscle to function in synchrony with other elements of the swallowing mechanism. As a result, the pharyngeal muscles propel all or part of the food bolus against a closed sphincter, producing symptoms of cervical dysphagia.

Cricopharyngeal achalasia is usually encountered in elderly individuals. Many disorders may cause this problem, but central nervous system diseases predominate. The clinical features are those of oropharyngeal dysphagia in general. Depending on the cause, the onset of symptoms may be sudden, as with a cerebrovascular accident, or intermittent, as with more insidious disorders such as diabetic neuropathy. The natural history of cricopharyngeal achalasia is also variable, again probably reflecting its many causes: dysphagia may diminish, remain unremitting, or follow a relapsing, remitting course. Most individuals with this disorder have more difficulty swallowing liquids than solids. Many patients have a pulmonary presentation with laryngitis, bronchitis, recurrent pneumonia, bronchiectosis, and pulmonary abscesses as the sequelae of otherwise quiet cricopharyngeal dysfunction.[25] In some patients, symptoms result in such a fear of eating that weight loss, malnutrition, and psychological problems overshadow the motility disorder.

Postintubation dysphagia

Special mention must be made of cervical dysphagia occurring as a sequela of endotracheal intubation. Unilateral vocal cord weakness is a common complication of endotracheal intubation and, because the vocal cords are important to the formation of a tight laryngeal seal during the oropharyngeal phase of glutition, patients with vocal cord weakness may experience coughing and aspiration with swallowing. Individuals who have undergone a tracheostomy also may develop symptoms of oropharyngeal dysphagia. Scar formation from a tracheostomy occasionally prevents normal elevation and anterior rotation of the larynx, causing decreased pharyngeal contraction and incomplete upper esophageal sphincter relaxation during swallowing.

Management of oropharyngeal dysphagia depends only in part on its etiology. Any underlying disorder, such as parkinsonism, should be treated. If dysphagia persists despite such therapy, or if significant complications result from impairment of the swallowing mechanism, treatment can be directed at the esophagus itself.

Bougienage of the upper esophageal sphincter with mercury-weighted rubber dilators is beneficial to some patients but often gives only temporary relief. This technique is contraindicated by the presence of a pharyngoesophageal diverticulum because of the high risk of perforation (see below).

Many individuals with cricopharyngeal achalasia benefit from surgical interruption of the upper esophageal sphincter.[26] Failure to respond is observed most often in patients with central nervous system disease or peripheral neuropathy, although even these individuals are occasionally relieved of symptoms by this procedure. Serious complications following cervical myotomy are rare. Botulinum toxin injection and balloon dilation also have been employed. Gastroesophageal reflux or severe distal esophagitis indicating reflux is an absolute contraindication to cricopharyngeal myotomy unless the lower esophageal defect is corrected first.

Pharyngeal diverticula

Zenker's diverticulum

Zenker's diverticulum (Fig. 78-3) is a posterior herniation of the hypopharynx through the triangular area just above the upper esophageal sphincter where the oblique and transverse fibers of the cricopharyngeus muscle join. It is seen once in every 1,000 routine upper gastrointestinal series and is more frequent in males. Approximately 85 percent of cases occur in individuals over the age of 50.[27]

Symptoms of Zenker's diverticulum usually develop insidiously. An annoying irritation in the back of the throat is an early complaint which may be followed later by the more classic symptoms of oropharyngeal dysphagia. Occasionally, an affected individual complains of a noise like the "roar of the ocean" or a "washing machine" during swallowing. Postcibal and nocturnal regurgitation of undigested food are common complaints. Obstructive symptoms may be caused by associated cricopharyngeal achalasia or, rarely, by compression of the esophagus by a large diverticulum.

Incoordination and incomplete relaxation of the upper esophageal sphincter during swallowing have been described in association with Zenker's diverticulum, lending support to the theory that cricopharyngeal dysfunction leads to high pharyngeal pressures which result in the formation of hypopharyngeal diverticula. Many patients with a Zenker's diverticulum, however, have normal function of the upper esophageal sphincter or even reduced upper esophageal sphincter pressure, suggesting that high pharyngeal pressures may be due to stiffening of the pharyngeal muscles with loss of compliance.[28]

Zenker's diverticula most often are seen during X-ray examination but when small may be missed in the posteroanterior view because of superimposition over the main column of barium in the esophagus; this problem can be avoided by rotating the patient during the study (Fig. 78-3). Endoscopic examination of the upper gastrointestinal tract in the presence of a hypopharyngeal diverticulum may be associated with an increased risk of perforation; however, this danger is minimized by passage of the instrument under direct vision.

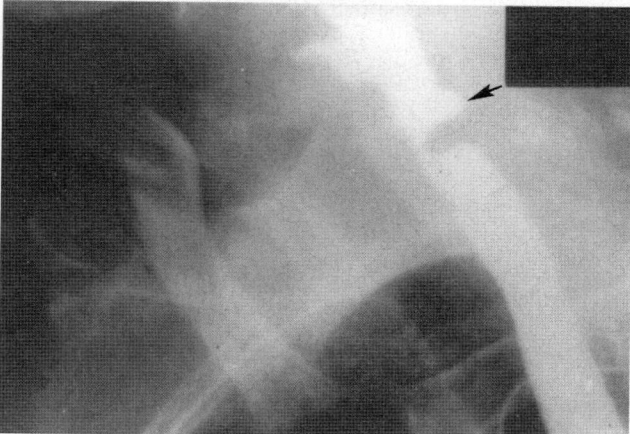

Figure 78-3 Oblique view of a barium-filled esophagus showing a small Zenker's diverticulum (arrow) proximal to a hypertrophied cricopharyngeus. (Reproduced from Brandt.[154])

Complications include compression and obstruction of the distal esophagus by a large diverticulum, respiratory difficulties caused by aspiration of diverticular contents, and diverticulitis with perforation. Rarely, carcinoma may develop in a Zenker's diverticulum.[29] Worsening of dysphagia, weight loss, and the appearance of blood in regurgitated material suggest the development of a malignant neoplasm.

The therapy for a symptomatic Zenker's diverticulum includes surgical excision alone or cricopharyngeal myotomy with or without removal of the diverticulum.[30] Endoscopic techniques for the treatment of Zencker's diverticulum also have been described.[31]

Lateral pharyngeal diverticula

Lateral pharyngeal diverticula, or pharyngoceles, occur with increased frequency in elderly people and are especially common in men.[32] They develop in the gap between the superior and middle pharyngeal constrictors. Symptoms are the same as those of a Zenker's diverticulum. In addition, patients may complain of a neck mass that enlarges with a Valsalva maneuver. Increased intrapharyngeal pressure may be an important etiologic factor, as exemplified by the frequency of this entity in muezzins and wind instrument players. Surgical repair is safe and effective.

THE ESOPHAGUS

The muscularis propria of the esophagus is composed of striated muscle fibers proximally and smooth muscle fibers distally. The central nervous system governs the activity of the striated muscle by means of sequential activation of extrinsic nerves. In humans, the dominant mechanism for control of the smooth muscle of the esophagus is unknown; both central and intramural neural pathways have been demonstrated. Orderly peristaltic contractions of esophageal muscle are necessary for normal esophageal function.

Although no information is available about the effects of aging on the regulation of esophageal muscle activity, alterations in esophageal muscle function have been identified manometrically in elderly individuals. These changes were described first in 1964 by Soergel and colleagues,[33] who referred to motility disturbances in the elderly as "presbyesophagus." Soergel and his coworkers studied 15 subjects beyond the age of 90 and found a variety of abnormalities; 13 of their patients, however, had diseases known to affect esophageal motility. Subsequent studies have confirmed that, in the absence of other disorders, esophageal motility may be abnormal in elderly individuals, but the only manometric change identified in all the published work is a reduction in the amplitude of muscle contraction after a swallow.[34–36]

Elderly people also may be noted to have disordered motility, or "tertiary contractions," during a barium esophagram, but this finding is rarely associated with symptoms.[37] Because motility changes that develop with aging do not appear to have clinical importance, the diagnosis of presbyesophagus should be abandoned. Elderly patients with dysphagia should be evaluated for the presence of disease processes involving the esophagus, and complaints should not be ascribed to motility changes occurring as a result of age alone.

Dysphagia and heartburn

Dysphagia and heartburn (pyrosis) are the principal symptoms of esophageal diseases; patients with esophageal disorders, especially elderly people, also may complain of respiratory difficulties, painful swallowing (odynophagia), chest pain resembling the pain of myocardial ischemia, regurgitation, and vomiting.[38–40]

Dysphagia is caused by impaired passage of food through the esophagus and is experienced immediately after the act of deglutition. Patients often complain that food "sticks on the way down." Since sensation in the esophagus is referred proximally, lesions at the gastroesophageal junction often appear as symptoms experienced at the level of the sternal notch. When a patient has symptoms apparently originating in the area of the proximal esophagus, evaluation of the entire esophagus, often with both esophagoscopy and barium radiography, is required.

The pattern of dysphagia frequently suggests the nature of the underlying disease.[41] Schatzki observed that a correct diagnosis can be made after taking a careful history in up to 85 percent of patients with this complaint.[42] Thus, intermittent dysphagia connotes a motility disorder or a pliant mechanical obstruction such as an esophageal web. Progressive dysphagia often represents a neoplasm. Individuals who experience difficulty in swallowing liquids as well as solid foods usually have a primary neuromuscular abnormality and disordered esophageal motility, while dysphagia produced only by solid foods is associated with mechanical obstruction of the esophagus.

Heartburn is a manifestation of the reflux of gastric contents into the esophagus and, as its name suggests, is described as being a hot sensation behind the sternum or in the left parasternal area. Pyrosis is relieved by antacids and intensified by bending at the waist or lying supine, especially when the stomach is full. Pyrosis also may be aggravated by some medications, smoking, and ingestion of alcohol, fruit juices, caffeine, chocolate, or peppermint. Discomfort is often accompanied by regurgitation of gastric contents, belching, vomiting, or secretion of saliva (water brash). The nature or extent of esophageal abnormalities associated with gastroesophageal reflux and heartburn cannot be predicted on the basis of the intensity of symptoms, especially in elderly people; severe reflux disease as evidenced by esophageal ulcers may be present in the absence of substantial symptoms.[43]

Esophageal motility disorders

After individuals with structural lesions have been excluded, over 50 percent of adults of all ages with a complaint of dysphagia are found to have esophageal motility disorders.[44,45] These abnormalities may be primary or secondary and are classified according to their manometric signatures. Most often, adults with dysphagia have disordered motility with nonspecific and inconsistent manometric features.

Nonspecific secondary motility disorders

In elderly people, nonspecific disorders of esophageal motility frequently are secondary to a systemic disease. Examples of generalized disorders sometimes responsible for esophageal dysmotility are myxedema, amyloidosis, connective tissue diseases, and diabetes mellitus.

Approximately 50 percent of patients with diabetic neuropathy have abnormal esophageal motility. Findings in these individuals include a decrease in the amplitude of muscle contraction, delayed esophageal emptying, esophageal dilation, and reduced lower esophageal emptying sphincter pressure. In patients with diabetes, the severity of motility changes correlates with the severity of other neuropathic complications; however, affected individuals usually do not have significant dysphagia. For this reason, esophageal symptoms in a diabetic must be fully evaluated and not simply attributed to diabetes.

Primary and secondary achalasia

Primary achalasia is the second most common motility disorder diagnosed in patients with nonstructural dysphagia, but it is rare in elderly people.[46] In persons beyond the age of 50, achalasia is most often secondary to gastric adenocarcinoma (Fig. 78-4); pancreatic adenocarcinoma, oat cell carcinoma, reticulum cell sarcoma, and anaplastic lymphoma are responsible for isolated cases.[47,48] Manometric findings in secondary achalasia are identical to those in the primary disorder: absence of esophageal peristalsis, usually in association with elevation of resting lower esophageal sphincter pressure and failure of the lower esophageal sphincter to relax following an appropriate stimulus. The elevation of resting lower esophageal sphincter pressure typical of achalasia is less pronounced in elderly people, who also experience less chest pain in association with this disorder than do younger patients.[49]

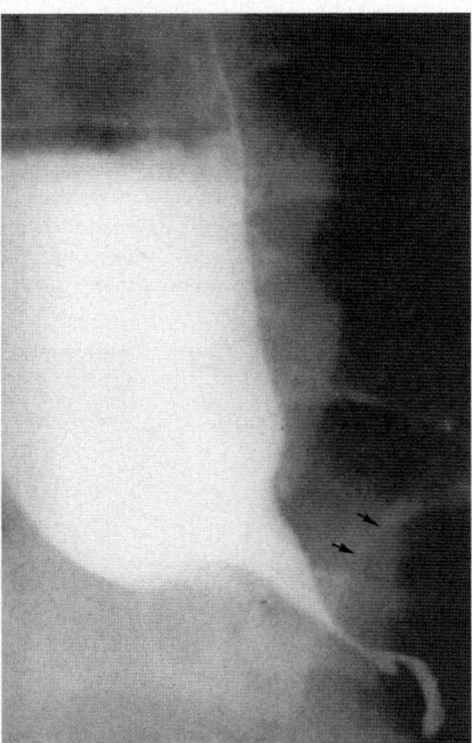

Figure 78-4 Barium esophagram showing tapering of the distal esophagus simulating achalasia. The subtle presence of a mass in the gastric fundus (arrows) suggested a diagnosis of carcinoma. (Reproduced from Brandt.[154])

Patients with both primary and secondary achalasia may experience progressive difficulty in swallowing. Food collects in the esophagus, which may become distended and tortuous even when the patient has an underlying carcinoma. In the absence of proximal dilation of the esophagus, a diagnosis of malignancy is favored. When the patient reclines, pooled food flows out of the esophagus back into the pharynx, resulting in coughing and aspiration. Affected individuals, therefore, may present with aspiration pneumonia. In addition to an infiltrate, a chest X-ray may reveal an air–fluid level in the esophagus and absence of the gastric air bubble. Because the presentations of primary and secondary achalasia may be identical, malignancy must be excluded in an elderly patient with this syndrome. Computed tomographic X-rays of the chest and upper abdomen, as well as endoscopy with biopsy of the distal esophagus, are recommended.[50] Endoscopic ultrasound may be helpful in differentiating primary from secondary achalasia.

The pathogenesis of secondary achalasia is unknown. Submucosal infiltration of the distal esophagus by tumor has been noted in some cases and normal histology in others.[51] It is possible that, in the absence of tumor infiltration, the motility disorder reflects a paraneoplastic neuropathy; manometric and roentgenographic abnormalities may disappear after resection of a gastric carcinoma or therapy for a lymphoma.[52,53]

Diffuse esophageal spasm

Although primary esophageal motility disorders usually occur in middle-aged individuals, manometric recordings in elderly persons with intermittent dysphagia occasionally display the pattern of diffuse esophageal spasm.[38] In this motility disturbance, the patient has simultaneous, repetitive muscle contractions of prolonged duration occurring spontaneously or after a swallow. Normal peristalsis is present most of the time, explaining the intermittent nature of symptoms, which may be triggered by hot or cold foods, pills, or carbonated beverages. The pathogenesis of diffuse esophageal spasm is obscure; on the basis of case reports, some have speculated that in some cases this disorder represents a stage in the development of achalasia.

"Nutcracker" esophagus and noncardiac chest pain

It is usually assumed that in persons free of significant coronary artery disease with chest pain resembling the pain of myocardial ischemia, symptoms are due to an esophageal motility disorder. Such patients, however rarely have chest pain during esophageal manometry, and provocative testing may be used to precipitate symptoms. Provocative testing with intravenous edrophonium chloride and infusion of acid into the esophagus causes chest pain in about 30 percent of subjects with a history of noncardiac chest pain.[54] A similar number of patients with noncardiac chest pain have been found to have an esophageal motility disorder, but only 25 percent of these individuals have symptoms during provocative testing.[44] It is often difficult, therefore, to prove that the esophagus is the source of the patient's complaints.

The most common motility disorder found in patients with noncardiac chest pain is "nutcracker" esophagus.[44] This abnormality is characterized by peristaltic muscle contractions of extremely high amplitude and long duration in the distal portion of the esophagus. A defect in esophageal transit can be demonstrated in many affected patients using a radionuclide marker. In one large series of individuals with noncardiac chest pain, 50 percent of patients with a motility disorder had nutcracker esophagus; other symptomatic individuals were found to have diffuse esophageal spasm.[44] A causal role for these motility defects in the production of chest pain has not been proved. In recent studies, many patients with noncardiac chest pain were found to have musculoskeletal disorders.

A number of medications have been used to treat primary esophageal motility disorders, especially diffuse esophageal spasm and nutcracker esophagus. Nitrates, anticholinergics, calcium channel blockers, or sedatives are occasionally effective in relieving symptoms of dysphagia and chest pain; their benefit in this setting, however, has never been evaluated in an appropriately designed trial. Some patients also obtain relief from dysphagia after bougienage. Pneumatic dilation is the treatment of choice for primary achalasia.

Hiatus hernia

The incidence of hiatus hernia (Fig. 78-5) increases with each decade of life from less that 10 percent of those under age 40 to approximately 40 percent in the sixth and seventh decades and 70 percent in patients beyond the age of 70. Symptoms such as pyrosis and regurgitation formerly attributed to the hernia are now known to be due to lower esophageal sphincter dysfunction. Sphincter dysfunction and gastrointestinal reflux are independent of the presence of a hiatus hernia, and the common "sliding" hiatus hernia is not considered by itself to be pathogenic.

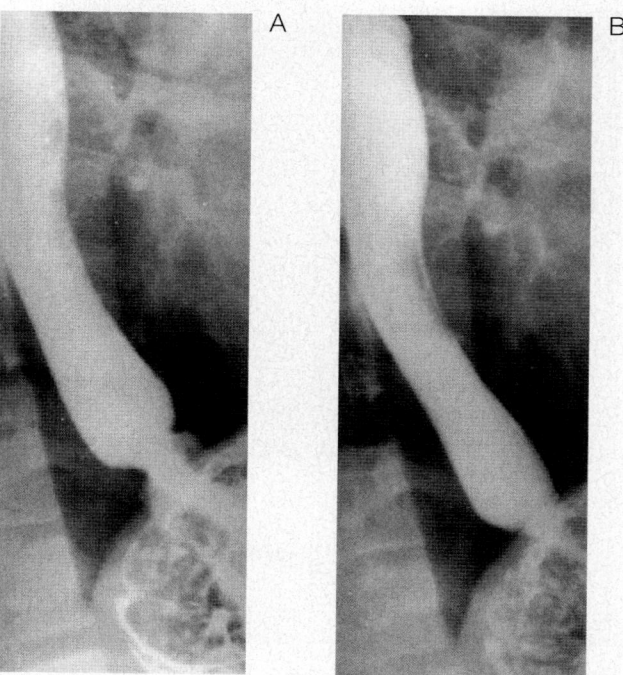

Figure 78-5 A small hiatus hernia (A) sliding in and (B) out of the thorax. The esophagogastric junction is seen above the diaphragm. (Reproduced from Brandt.[154])

One type of hiatus hernia that deserves special mention is the paraesophageal hernia (Fig. 78-6), an uncommon hernia that occurs most often in persons between the ages of 60 and 70. Paraesophageal hernias often result in significant complications and therefore are of major importance. These hernias are frequently asymptomatic or cause only nagging discomfort until mechanical entrapment occurs. Such a catastrophe is associated with progressive distension of the incarcerated segment, vascular embarrassment, hemorrhage, gangrene, and perforation. In the absence of contraindications, a paraesophageal hernia demands surgical repair.

Reflux esophagitis

The only notable change in the lower esophageal sphincter seen with aging is a reduction in the amplitude of postdeglutative contraction or relaxation. Nevertheless, because the secretion of gastrin, which potentiates contraction of the lower esophageal sphincter, increases with age, and because gastric acid secretion declines with age in many individuals, it is unusual for reflux esophagitis to appear for the first time in elderly people.[55] The nature or extent of esophageal injury associated with gastroesophageal reflux cannot be predicted on the basis of the intensity of symptoms in older patients.[43] Complications of chronic, asymptomatic reflux such as stricture formation may be the initial clinical presentation of

esophagitis in about 20 percent of affected elderly patients. When an aged individual complains of the recent onset of pyrosis, other causes of esophageal symptoms, such as candidiasis, must be considered. The therapy of reflux in elderly patients is the same as in younger patients, however, attention must be paid to the potential development of adverse effects of medications (see below).[56]

Barrett's metaplasia

In patients with Barrett's metaplasia, the lower esophagus is lined for a variable distance by columnar, rather than the usual stratified squamous, epithelium.[57] The metaplastic columnar epithelium may be continuous with the columnar epithelium of the stomach and extend in tongues into the distal esophagus, or it may be present in islands surrounded by normal sequamous epithelium. The importance of Barrett's metaplasia lies in its association with reflux esophagitis, (deep) esophageal ulcers, (high) esophageal strictures (Fig. 78-7), and adenocarcinoma. The metaplastic columnar lining is believed to develop as a consequence of gastroesophageal reflux. Esophageal squamous epithelium damaged by exposure to gastric contents is replaced by a specialized columnar epithelium (intestinal metaplasia), a junctional-type epithelium, or a gastric fundic-type epithelium. Each of these three cell types may be seen alone or in combination with the others.

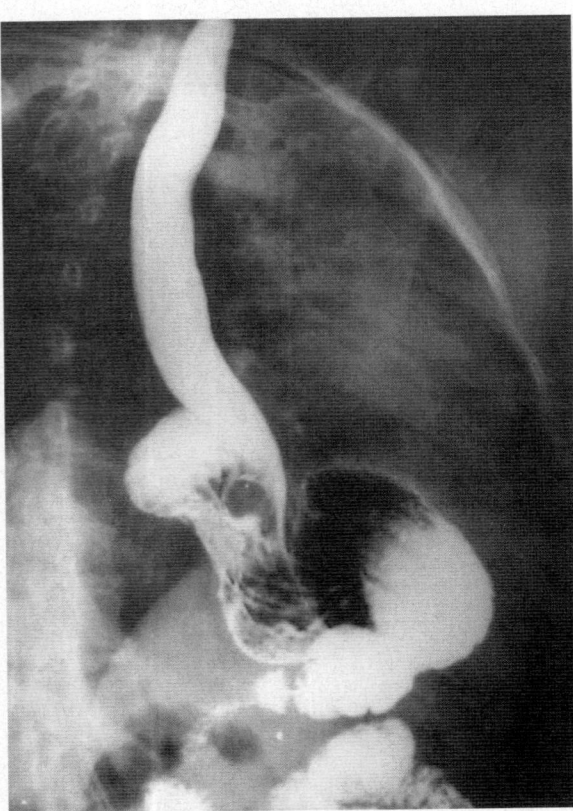

Figure 78-6 Barium esophagram demonstrating a paraesophageal hernia with the gastric fundus above the diaphragm. The esophagogastric junction is at the level of the diaphragm. (Reproduced from Brandt.[154])

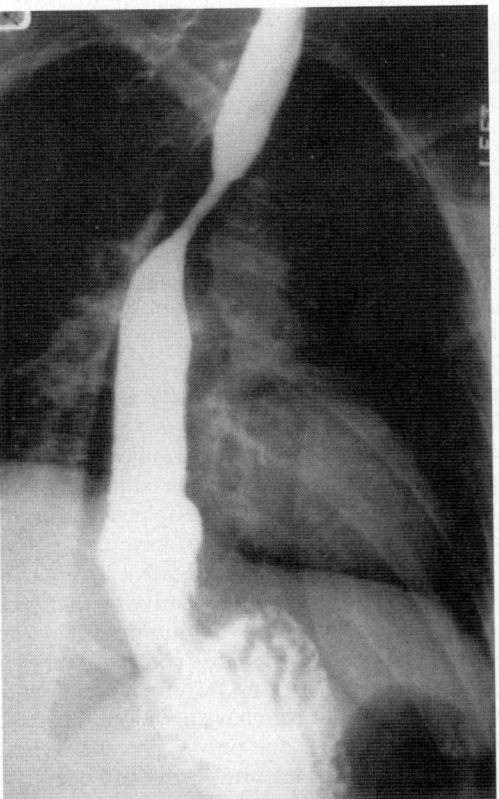

Figure 78-7 Barium esophagram revealing a stricture of the esophagus at the level of the aortic arch in a patient with Barrett's esophagus. A hiatus hernia is also present. (Reproduced from Brandt.[154])

Most cases of Barrett's esophagus probably occur between the ages of 50 and 70; the exact incidence is unknown. The most common symptoms are those related to the reflux of stomach contents, and the entity is diagnosed best by esophagoscopy with multiple biopsies. The presence of specialized columnar epithelium establishes the diagnosis of Barrett's esophagus.[57] If the columnar epithelium in the biopsy specimen is one of the other two types, the biopsy must have been made at least 3 cm above the gastroesophageal junction to make the diagnosis. Intestinal metaplasia can be recognized in situ by staining with Alcian blue.

Stricture and neoplasia are long-term complications of Barrett's esophagus. There is increasing evidence that cancer arises only in the specialized columnar epithelium. By careful screening using esophagoscopy with directed biopsy every 1–2 years, premalignant dysplastic changes can usually be detected.[58,59] The development of severe dysplasia or carcinoma in situ requires resection of the involved esophagus. Thermal ablation of Barrett's epithelium with multipolar electrocoagulation, laser coagulation, or argon plasma coagulation has been investigated. Destruction of the Barrett's epithelium by these techniques is successful initially, but recurrence of the Barrett's tissue may occur. Therapy of reflux usually results in symptomatic improvement, but regression of the columnar epithelium does not occur without surgery.

Lower esophageal ring

A lower esophageal or Schatzki ring (Fig. 78-8) is a thin, annular ridge of mucosa projecting perpendicularly into the esophageal lumen at or near the squamocolumnar junction.[60–62] A Schatzki ring may be asymptomatic, found incidentally during evaluation of the upper gastrointestinal tract for unrelated reasons, or it may cause intermittent episodes of dysphagia and an uncomfortable sticking or pressing sensation due to food lodging above the ring. Episodes commonly occur during hurried meals, meals requiring a great deal of mastication, or meals consumed with alcohol, hence the appellation "steakhouse syndrome." As the lumen of the ring diminishes to less than 12 mm (0.047 in.) in diameter, attacks become more frequent. Attacks usually last several minutes or more until the patient regurgitates the food bolus or flushes it into the stomach with a beverage.

Total obstruction of the esophagus secondary to food impaction frequently brings patients to the emergency department. Relaxation of the esophagus by administration of a small dose of intravenous benzodiazepine or 1 mg of glucagon is occasionally effective in relieving the impaction. Papain solution (meat tenderizer) should not be used to try to digest the meat, as its use has been associated with esophageal perforation. If the impacted bolus does not pass, it must be removed by esophagoscopy. Alternatively, it may be gently nudged into the stomach if a patent lumen can be seen distally, the esophageal mucosa is intact, and there is no bone or other sharp object present. Multiple biopsies to disrupt the ring or dilation with bougies are techniques used to treat symptomatic rings.

Dysphagia aortica

Degenerative changes in the aorta may produce compression of the esophagus and dysphagia. Obstruction of the upper

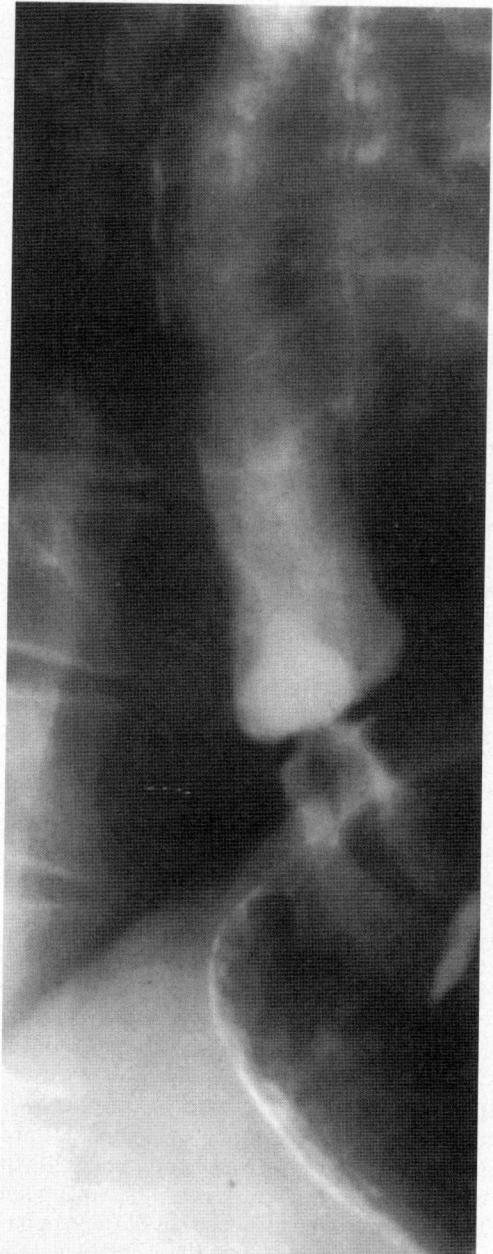

Figure 78-8 A Schatzki ring prevents passage of a barium pill in a patient with intermittent dysphagia. (Reproduced from Brandt.[154])

esophagus is occasionally caused by a thoracic aneurysm, while the distal esophagus may be squeezed between an atherosclerotic aorta posteriorly and the heart or esophageal hiatus anteriorly. Most patients are women beyond the age of 70.[63–65] Symptoms are usually prevented by having the patient thoroughly masticate solid foods, but occasionally the obstruction is severe enough to warrant surgical mobilization of the esophagus at the hiatus.[66]

Medication-induced esophageal injury

Esophageal injury can occur as a result of the local caustic effects of medications.[67,68] The most frequent offenders are antibiotics, especially tetracyclines, potassium chloride, ferrous sulfate, nonsteroidal anti-inflammatory drugs, alendronate, and quinidine.

Most patients with medication-induced esophageal injury have no underlying esophageal disorder. Some individuals, however, have nonspecific, asymptomatic disorders of esophageal motility, peptic strictures, esophageal compression from left atrial enlargement, a prominent aortic knob, or mediastinal adhesions following thoracic surgery. Pills commonly lodge in the esophagus at the level of the aortic knob or the lower esophageal sphincter without the patient's knowledge. Many cases of pill-induced esophageal injury probably remain unrecognized with full recovery. The most frequent symptoms of medication-induced esophageal injury are odynophagia and retrosternal pain. Symptoms usually resolve within 6 weeks of stopping the medication or changing it to a liquid formulation; damage, however, may result in esophageal stricture formation or, occasionally, hemorrhage or perforation. Pills should always be taken with a generous amount of water, and elderly patients should not take pills immediately before bedtime, as a decrease in salivation and esophageal motor activity accompanies sleeping.[69]

Esophageal diverticula

Diverticula of the esophagus are much less common than diverticula of other parts of the gastrointestinal tract. In a review of 20,000 barium studies on the upper gastrointestinal tract, Wheeler noted only six midesophageal (traction-type) and three epiphrenic (pulsion-type) diverticula, as compared with 1,020 duodenal diverticula.[70] The terms *traction* and *pulsion* refer to commonly accepted theories regarding the pathogenesis of esophageal diverticula. Traction diverticula are thought to be caused by the effects of fibrotic disease in structures contiguous with the esophagus, while pulsion diverticula are hypothesized to result from increased intraluminal pressure. Pseudodiverticulosis of the esophagus also has been described.

Midesophageal diverticula (traction diverticula)
Traction diverticula occur most commonly in the middle third of the esophagus, where a large group of lymph nodes lies in direct contact with the esophageal wall. Nodal inflammation of this area may lead to periesophagitis, fixation of the esophagus to the lymph nodes, and distortion of the esophageal wall. In the past, tuberculosis was the most common etiology for this process; any infection with lymph node involvement, however, may lead to the formation of a traction diverticulum.

Traction diverticula usually occur in patients of middle age or older and are slightly more common in men. They rarely cause symptoms, perhaps because they are small, have a broad neck, and can contract and empty because they contain all the layers of the esophageal wall including muscle.

Epiphrenic diverticula (pulsion diverticula)
Pulsion diverticula are found in the lower 10 cm of the esophagus, usually on the right wall. Like traction diverticula, they contain all the layers of the esophageal wall; the muscular layer, however, may be quite attenuated.

Epiphrenic diverticula usually develop in males during middle age. Patients may complain of dysphagia or chest pain,

but symptoms are probably due to an associated esophageal motor abnormality such as achalasia or diffuse esophageal spasm.[71] The occurrence of an epiphrenic diverticulum without an underlying motility disorder or a hiatus hernia appears to be rare.

Many epiphrenic diverticula are asymptomatic, and in these instances no therapy is required.[72] Treatment of esophageal reflux or an underlying, motility disorder may afford the patient symptomatic relief.[73,74] In cases of larger diverticula, surgical resection may be necessary.[75]

Intramural pseudodiverticulosis
In esophageal pseudodiverticulosis, dilation of the excretory ducts of submucosal glands causes multiple small (1 to 3 mm) invaginations of the esophageal wall.[76,77] These defects involve all, or segments of, the esophagus in a circumferential fashion. Pseudodiverticula are best detected by barium contrast studies; their roentgenographic appearance is quite characteristic (Fig. 78-9). Pseudodiverticulosis is usually diagnosed during the seventh decade of life in patients with dysphagia. In at least 20 percent of cases, gastroesophageal reflux, a motility disorder, or a malignancy is found, and in approximately one-half of patients, smears or cultures of the esophageal mucosa reveal *Candida albicans*. Stenoses, or areas of reduced distensibility, are found in up to 90 percent of cases of pseudodiverticulosis and preferentially seem to involve the upper esophagus. Surprisingly, there is no fixed relationship between the narrowed area and the segment involved with pseudodiverticula.

The etiology of pseudodiverticulosis is unknown. The term *adenosis* has been used to refer to this entity because the number of deep esophageal mucous glands is markedly increased. Therapy consists of treatment of associated abnormalities. Coexisting strictures should be evaluated to ensure that they are benign.

Esophageal candidiasis

Infection of the esophagus is rare in patients without acquired immunodeficiency syndrome, with the exception of infection with *C. albicans*. *Candida albicans* is a normal inhabitant of the alimentary tract; the yeast form is found in almost 50 percent of oral washings and 80 percent of stool samples.[78] The population of *C. albicans* is suppressed in healthy adults by other intestinal flora. Comparison of fecal specimens from subjects aged 70–100 with those of individuals aged 20–69 have revealed fungi to be more common in the elderly group. This finding may be explained by a diminution in esophageal peristalsis, a reduction in gastric acid secretion, and age-related alterations in cellular and humoral immunity.

In the absence of antibiotic therapy or an underlying immune disorder, esophageal candidiasis is a disease of elderly people. Most cases in this age group, however, occur in association with predisposing conditions, including malignancy, therapy with immunosuppressive or cytotoxic drugs, diabetes mellitus, malnutrition, and treatment with broad-spectrum antibiotics.[79,80]

In the proper clinical setting, dysphagia, odynophagia, substernal burning, or an awareness of food passing down the esophagus should suggest the possibility of candida infection, although even in the presence of infection with *C. albicans*,

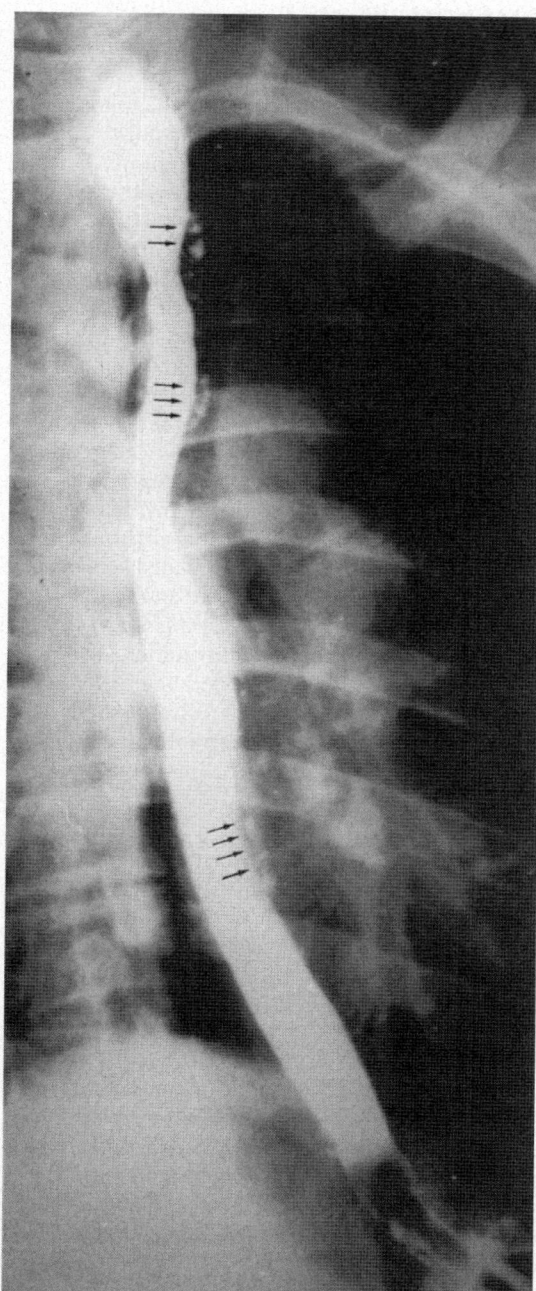

Figure 78-9 Intramural pseudodiverticulosis with multiple outpouchings (arrows) on a barium esophagram. (Reproduced from Brandt.[154])

confused with that of exudative esophagitis, and therefore the diagnosis must be confirmed by brushings and biopsies. Typical hyphae are revealed under the microscope in scrapings placed on a glass slide and macerated with 20 percent potassium hydroxide.

In the appropriate setting, a trial of therapy may be initiated without attempting an invasive diagnosis. As in oral and vaginal candidiasis, therapy usually consists of promoting the re-establishment of normal microbiological flora by discontinuing antibiotics. In an immunocompromised host or in an individual with significant morbidity, fluconazole is considered the drug of choice. Odynophagia can be treated with viscous lidocaine or with a "swish-and-swallow" preparation of the type used to treat stomatitis (see above). Failure to respond to simple treatment necessitates endoscopic confirmation of the diagnosis and, often, systemic therapy with additional antifungal agents.

Esophageal neoplasms

Esophageal cancer (Fig. 78-10) occurs most frequently after age 55 and is three times more common in males than in females in the USA, and two times more common in males than in females in the UK.[1] In the USA, it accounts for approximately 2 percent of all reported cancers. Factors associated with the development of esophageal cancer include alcohol and tobacco use, thermal irritation, poor oral hygiene, and esophageal stasis.[1,81,82] Furthermore, an association has been noted with certain esophageal diseases, notably achalasia, Barrett's esophagus, lye stricture, Plummer–Vinson syndrome, and also with previous gastric surgery.[83–85]

Surveillance, epidemiology, and end results (SEER) data show an increase in adenocarcinoma from 8 to 18 percent of all esophageal cancers during the years 1973–1984; it now represents the most rapidly increasing malignancy in the US.[86] Esophageal adenocarcinoma is either cancer of the gastric fundus or a malignancy that has developed in a segment of Barrett's esophagus. Squamous cell carcinoma most commonly involves the middle third of the esophagus. Local spread occurs early, and, because the esophagus dilates so readily, dysphagia, the most common complaint at the time of diagnosis, is a late symptom.

In elderly people an important manifestation of esophageal cancer is an achalasia-like syndrome. Primary achalasia is uncommon in patients beyond the age of 50. Elderly individuals who present with symptoms of achalasia of less than 1 year's duration associated with marked weight loss should be suspected of having a malignancy, most often gastric adenocarcinoma. The pathogenesis of secondary achalasia is unknown; in some cases the lower esophagus is infiltrated with tumor cells, but in other cases achalasia may reflect a paraneoplastic process.

The prognosis for esophageal cancer is dismal. Management is directed at relieving progressive obstruction.[87–89] Surgical resection and radiation are the accepted modes of treatment. Surgical resection offers the only chance for long-term survival, but fewer than half of all patients presenting with esophageal cancer have a respectable lesion. If there is evidence of nodal or distant metastases, a thoracotomy should be

up to one-half of patients may be asymptomatic. Esophageal candidiasis often results from the extension of oral lesions, and a careful examination of the oral cavity is important in any debilitated patient complaining of esophageal symptoms.

A diagnosis of candida esophagitis may be suggested by an abnormal barium esophagram, although a normal study does not exclude the presence of this organism. Esophagoscopy is the best method for detecting candida infection; raised white plaques, hyperemia, ulceration, and friability are characteristic. The gross appearance of candida esophagitis may be

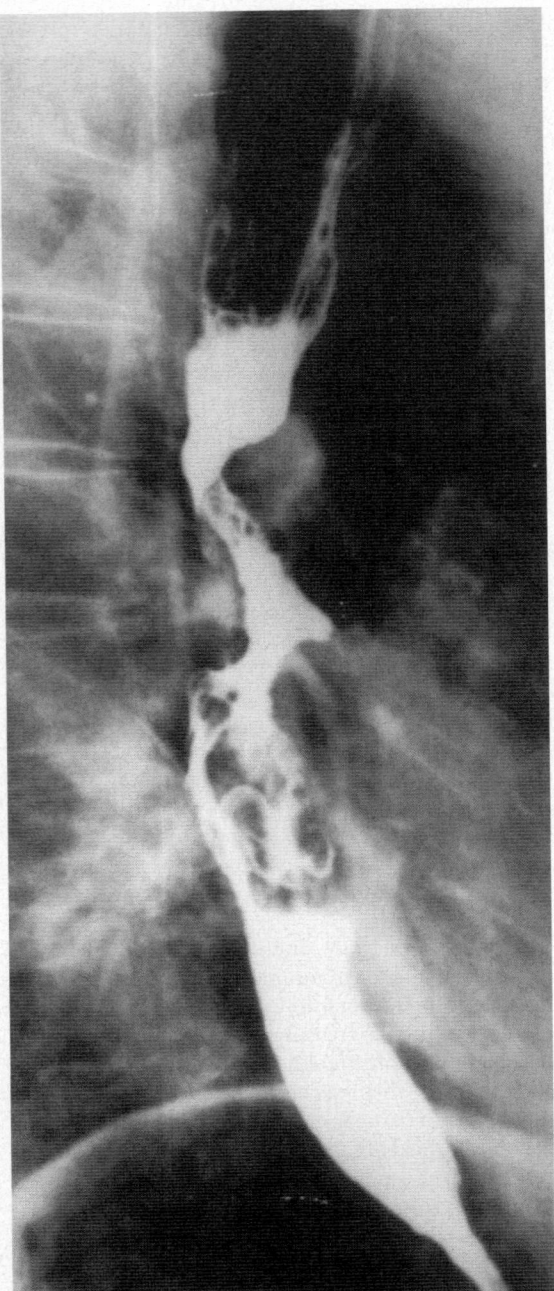

Figure 78-10 Barium esophagram demonstrating an ulcerating esophageal carcinoma. (Reproduced from Brandt.[154])

avoided. Thoracic radiation, while useful, may be followed by the development of esophagitis, usually within 3 weeks of initiating therapy and continuing for several weeks after its completion. Chemotherapy may result in symptomatic improvement but does not substantially prolong survival. New chemotherapeutic agents should be administered under an investigational protocol. Combined modality therapy may offer advantages over more traditional approaches. Palliative therapy with endoscopically placed stents, lasers, or photodynamic therapy is often very useful and has improved the quality of life for many patients, albeit without prolonging survival.

THE STOMACH

Aging is associated with alterations in both the motor and secretory functions of the stomach but, as in other parts of the gastrointestinal tract, changes in gastric physiology attributable to age alone rarely are responsible for symptoms.

The motor activity of the stomach allows it to behave as two individual, albeit coordinated, organs: one that processes liquids and another that processes solids. The fundus and proximal body of the stomach serve as a reservoir for liquids. In contrast, the distal gastric body and the antrum grind solids into small particles and pump them into the duodenum. The activities of both the proximal and distal stomach are controlled by complex neural and hormonal mechanisms. Studies employing food labeled with radioactive isotopes suggest that gastric emptying of liquids is prolonged in elderly persons, while emptying of solids is unaffected by age.[90,91]

Changes in gastric secretion also occur in individuals as they grow older. In the past, almost every study on gastric acid production showed a decline in basal and stimulated acid output with advancing age.[92] Work by Goldschmiedt and colleagues,[93] however, suggests that, in the absence of *Helicobacter pylori* infection, aging is actually associated with an increase in gastric acid secretion. Previous confusion about the effect of aging on gastric acid secretion is probably related to the high incidence of *H. pylori* infection and chronic atrophic gastritis with secondary achlorhydria in older individuals (see below).[94]

Gastric and duodenal mucosal injury

Advances in our understanding of the pathobiology of gastric and duodenal mucosal injury, and improvements in our ability to examine the upper gastrointestinal tract and detect diseases responsible for mucosal injury, make it important for physicians to use descriptive and diagnostic terminology carefully in clinical practice.[95,96] Unless diagnostic findings are reported with a precision that accurately reflects current understanding of mucosal injury, the benefits of medical advances made during the past few decades may be lost to patients.

In usual cases of gastric or duodenal mucosal injury, endoscopic inspection often reveals the presence of gross epithelial defects. Small epithelial defects, or erosions, do not penetrate the muscularis mucosae. Ulcers are defined as being larger than 3 mm in diameter and extend a variable distance through the muscularis mucosae, in some instances freely perforating into the peritoneal cavity or penetrating into an adjacent organ. A typical ulcer is composed of four layers or zones: a superficial layer of fibrinopurulent debris overlying a zone of inflammation, a layer of granulation tissue, and, at its base, a collagenous scar. Both erosions and ulcers may be sources of bleeding.

Diffuse mucosal erythema, a common finding at endoscopy, in most instances represents microvascular congestion and, although it is interpreted by many endoscopists as indicating the presence of "gastritis," this conclusion is unjustified. Mucosal erythema due to microvascular congestion is caused by a variety of factors and is without any specific etiologic significance or clinical association.[96] Conversely, patients often have histological gastritis without the presence of mucosal erythema.

The term *gastritis* implies the presence of inflammation and should not be used unless examination of a biopsy specimen has revealed typical mucosal inflammatory changes, including infiltration of the lamina propria with polymorphonuclear leukocytes and mononuclear cells. Neutrophils are seen early in the course of inflammation (acute gastritis). With the passage of time, mononuclear cells, mainly plasma cells, and eosinophils appear in increasing numbers (chronic gastritis). Most patients with gastritis have a predominance of mononuclear cells in the lamina propria with a lesser number of neutrophils (chronic active gastritis).[97] The inflammatory changes of gastritis are accompanied by signs of cell injury and regeneration. Cell damage and death cause submucosal hemorrhage and edema and lead to development of epithelial defects. Hemorrhage and edema may be visible grossly at endoscopy as well as evident on microscopic examination of biopsy specimens, as are erosions and ulcers. In response to injury, the epithelium regenerates by proliferation and differentiation of mucous neck cells, a process that leads to elongation and tortuosity of the gastric pits (foveolar hyperplasia). The vast majority of cases of gastritis are caused by infection with *H. pylori* (type B gastritis). Gastritis also may be due to other less common bacterial infections, granulomatous disease, autoimmune disease (type A gastritis), and hypersensitivity reactions.

Other agents of gastric injury damage the mucosa without exciting an inflammatory response. This gastropathy is sometimes referred to as type C gastritis, an unfortunate misnomer given the noninflammatory nature of the process.[98] Microscopic examination of biopsy specimens from patients with gastropathy typically reveals vascular congestion and edema of the lamina propria, hypertrophy of the muscularis mucosae, and mucosal regenerative changes with foveolar hyperplasia.[99] As in gastritis, cell damage and death are accompanied by submucosal hemorrhage and edema and lead to the development of epithelial defects. The latter changes are all often grossly visible on endoscopy. The most common causes of gastropathy are ingestion of nonsteroidal anti-inflammatory drugs (NSAIDs) and ethanol.

Helicobacter pylori, gastritis, and peptic ulcer disease

Infection with *H. pylori*, a spiral Gram-negative microaerophilic rod, is the most common chronic bacterial disease in humans. This organism attaches to receptors on the surface of gastric mucous neck cells and is also found on metaplastic gastric epithelium in the duodenum but not on the duodenal mucosa itself or on metaplastic duodenal mucosa in the stomach (Fig. 78-11).[100] *Helicobacter pylori* causes alterations in cell structure and function, inflammation, metaplasia, and cell death.[101] A number of virulence factors, including urease, make it possible for the organism to colonize the stomach and produce disease.[102]

Helicobacter pylori infection is the most common cause of chronic gastritis (type B antral gastritis) and is one of the two principal causes of peptic ulcer disease, the other being ingestion of NSAIDs. More than 90 percent of patients with duodenal ulcer and more than 75 percent of patients with gastric ulcer also have *H. pylori* infection and chronic active gastritis.[1] The relationship between ulcer disease and gastritis was recognized long before the etiological role of *H. pylori* in the pathogenesis of peptic ulcer disease was understood.

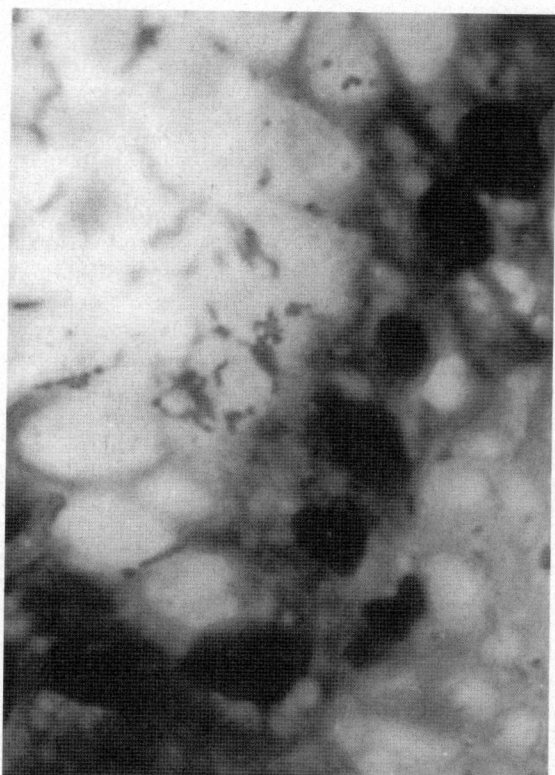

Figure 78-11 Gastric biopsy showing *H. pylori* in the surface mucous layer (Giemsa stain, 1,000×). (Courtesy of Sumi Mitsudo.)

Helicobacter pylori infection also has been linked to the development of gastric cancer, another gastritis-associated disease.[103]

Infection with *H. pylori* is usually acquired during childhood and occurs most often in persons living under conditions of poverty, crowding, and inadequate sanitation.[104] The prevalence of *H. pylori* infection in the United States and in the nations of western Europe increases with advancing age, a result of the poorer living conditions in these countries during the early years of the twentieth century.[105] Thus, regardless of present socioeconomic status, infection is most prevalent in older individuals. The incidence of peptic ulcer disease also increases progressively with advancing age, reflecting the age-related increase in *H. pylori* infection.

Under experimental conditions, acute infection with *H. pylori* causes transient dyspeptic symptoms accompanied by the development of active antral gastritis.[106] Mucosal inflammation apparently may resolve spontaneously in the minority of patients or become chronic, gradually spreading proximally into the body and fundus of the stomach. As the disease progresses, inflammation extends into the deeper, glandular part of the epithelium containing the gastric secretory cells; these include parietal cells which make hydrochloric acid an intrinsic factor, chief cells which make pepsin, pylorocardiac gland cells which make mucus, and endocrine G cells which make gastrin. Normal glands are gradually destroyed and replaced by metaplastic glands (intestinal metaplasia) or by atrophic gastric mucosa (atrophic gastritis), a process that takes many years. Atrophic gastritis often is associated with low serum gastrin levels and antibodies to gastrin-secreting cells. Patients with chronic active gastritis frequently also have submucosal hemorrhage, edema, epithelial erosions (erosive gastritis), and peptic ulcers.

Individuals with active gastritis and gastric mucosal atrophy are usually asymptomatic but may complain of intermittent dyspepsia, abdominal pain, distension, nausea and vomiting (nonulcer dyspepsia). The relationship, if any, between symptoms of nonulcer dyspepsia and gastritis is unclear (see below); many persons with dyspepsia do not have gastritis, and many persons with gastritis do not have dyspepsia.[107] Dyspeptic symptoms may be due to the development of a gastric or duodenal ulcer, although, at least 50 percent of patients with acute ulcers are asymptomatic.

Helicobacter pylori infection may be diagnosed by a transendoscopic pinch biopsy of the stomach. Microscopic examination of biopsy specimens from infected individuals reveals chronic active gastritis and typical spiral Gram-negative rods in the mucus coating the surface epithelium (Fig. 78-11). The absence of gastritis strongly argues against *H. pylori* infection, while its presence suggests that a failure to identify *H. pylori* is due to sampling error. Tissue also may be implanted in commercially available agar plates containing urea and a pH indicator. If *H. pylori* is present in the tissue specimen, bacterial urease will split the urea into bicarbonate and ammonia, raising the pH and producing a color change. Because infection may be patchy, testing several specimens obtained from different parts of the stomach improves the sensitivity of the assay.

Noninvasive diagnosis of *H. pylori* infection can be made by detecting serum antibody to bacterial antigens. This method of diagnosis is satisfactory—presuming there is no indication for endoscopy—if the patient has not previously been treated with antibiotics to which *H. pylori* is sensitive. Antibody titers decrease gradually after eradication of infection, but qualitative serology remains positive for a number of years, leaving what has been referred to as an "immunological scar." The presence of an immunological scar makes it impossible to use antibody testing to assess the effectiveness of therapy or the occurrence of reinfection. This problem is avoided by using the urea breath test, which is positive only in a setting of active infection. In the urea breath test, the patient is given an oral dose of urea labeled with either a stable (^{13}C) or unstable (^{14}C) isotope of carbon. If the patient is infected with *H. pylori*, the urea will be metabolized by bacterial urease to ammonia and bicarbonate, and bicarbonate containing the isotopic tracer will be converted to CO_2 and expired. The presence of labeled CO_2 in samples of expired gas indicates active *H. pylori* infection. A stool assay for detection of *H. pylori* also is available commercially.

Simultaneous treatment with a combination of two antibiotics and a proton pump inhibitor is the most consistently effective means of curing *H. pylori* infection.[108] *Helicobacter pylori* is sensitive to a variety of antimicrobial agents, including metronidazole, tetracyclines, macrolides, some quinolones, β-lactams, and bismuth preparations, as well as to proton pump inhibitors. The most commonly used regimen is a combination of a amoxicillin, clarithromycin, and a proton pump inhibitor. Regimens containing metronidazole are limited by the frequent occurrence of bacterial resistance to this agent. Because of the morbidity caused by *H. pylori* infection, the

National Institutes of Health Consensus Development Panel has published guidelines mandating treatment of all *H. pylori*-infected ulcer patients, including those currently without an active ulcer crater or dyspeptic symptoms.[109] The significant treatment failure rate makes it desirable to document cure by conducting a urea breath test 4 weeks after the completion of therapy. In addition to antibiotic therapy for *H. pylori* infection, patients with acute ulcers should be treated with an antisecretory agent to promote ulcer healing.

Nonsteroidal anti-inflammatory drugs, gastropathy, and peptic ulcer disease

Nonsteroidal anti-inflammatory drugs (NSAIDs) are among the most frequently prescribed medicines in the world. Approximately 3 million people in the USA, or 1.2 percent of the population, take at least one NSAID daily. Uncounted others regularly use over-the-counter NSAID preparations, including aspirin. As a result, NSAID-related morbidity is exceedingly common; each year 2 to 4 percent of chronic NSAID users have a serious drug-induced complication involving the gastrointestinal tract.[110] The use of NSAIDs and complications of NSAID use are most prevalent in elderly people.[111–113] In the UK, NSAID prescription rates for the entire population increased steadily from 1967 to 1985 and did so in direct proportion to the age of the recipient, with progressively more prescriptions being written for progressively older patients.[114] Thus, in 1985, an astonishing 1,400 NSAID prescriptions were written for every 1,000 women in the UK aged 65 years or older. These chronic NSAID users are estimated to have a two- to three-fold greater mortality than nonusers because of drug-related gastrointestinal complications.

Each and every nonselective NSAID is capable of injuring the gastrointestinal mucosa and does so in a dose-dependent fashion roughly proportional to its anti-inflammatory effect. Virtually 100 percent of patients who take a NSAID preparation, including aspirin, develop acute gastropathy during the first 1–2 weeks of therapy.[115] This gastropathy has the typical histological features described above and characteristically is associated with submucosal hemorrhage and some degree of edema, both of which are often grossly visible at endoscopy. Many NSAIDs, like aspirin, are weak acids which remain nonionized as the tablets break up and are dispersed in low-pH gastric secretions. Because they are nonionized, NSAIDs move easily across the membranes of epithelial cells and then ionize at the neutral pH of the cytoplasm. In the ionic form, they interact with cell constituents and cause cell damage and death.[116] Dead epithelial cells leave shallow mucosal defects (erosions) which may bleed. Patients often have dyspeptic symptoms during this acute phase of injury.

In a significant minority of chronic NSAID users, mucosal defects enlarge and form true ulcers; approximately 12–30 percent of patients develop a gastric ulcer, and 2–19 percent of patients develop a duodenal ulcer.[117] Elderly people seem to be particularly vulnerable to the harmful effects of NSAIDs. In a study of peptic ulcer disease in persons aged 65 and older, Griffin and colleagues[118] found that almost 30 percent of ulcers diagnosed in these individuals may have been caused by NSAIDs. The principal mechanism by which NSAID use leads to the development of peptic ulcers is dose-dependent systemic inhibition of prostaglandin synthesis. Prostaglandins protect the upper gastrointestinal mucosa by stimulating the secretion of bicarbonate and mucus, increasing mucosal blood flow, and promoting a number of cellular processes crucial to mucosal defense and repair. A decrease in prostaglandin synthesis tips the balance between defensive and aggressive factors in the upper gastrointestinal tract in favor of those that injure the mucosa, leading to the formation of ulcers and the possible development of complications including hemorrhage, obstruction, perforation, and penetration into an adjacent organ.

The cycloxygenase-2 (COX-2) specific agents have been shown to be equally efficacious as nonselective NSAIDs in the treatment of both osteoarthritis and rheumatoid arthritis, but with significantly fewer gastrointestinal side-effects. These agents have a greater affinity for COX-2 as compared to COX-1; COX-2 is induced in response to inflammation, whereas COX-1 is a constitutive enzyme that functions in a variety of maintenance and housekeeping roles. Many studies have demonstrated a decreased incidence of both gastric and duodenal ulcers in patients taking COX-2 selective agents as compared to those using nonselective NSAIDs. The use of COX-2 selective agents is associated with ulceration rates in the gastrointestinal tract that are no different than placebo.[119]

A variety of treatment strategies for preventing the development of gastric and duodenal ulcers in patients on chronic NSAID therapy have been tested.[120] Many commonly used medicines are without any demonstrable prophylactic benefit in this setting. Ranitidine and omeprazole have been shown to prevent duodenal but not gastric ulcers in arthritis patients taking NSAIDs.[120–122] Similar results were obtained by Taha and coworkers[123] in arthritis patients treated with prophylactic famotidine; however, in the same study high-dose famotidine reduced the incidence of both duodenal and gastric ulcers.[123] An alternative approach to ulcer prevention in patients who require chronic NSAID therapy is prostaglandin replacement with an oral synthetic prostaglandin E analog. The prostaglandin E_1 analog, misoprostol, like famotidine, has been shown to prevent development of both duodenal and gastric ulcers.[124] This agent also reduces the incidence of bleeding, perforation, and gastric outlet obstruction in patients on chronic NSAID therapy.[112] The use of misoprostol has been limited by its tendency to cause loose stools, abdominal cramps, and flatulence in a significant minority of individuals during initiation of treatment.

The large number of eligible patients makes it impossible to prescribe prophylactic famotidine or misoprostol for every NSAID user, or to use COX-2 selective agents in all. Instead, an effort should be made to identify and treat those who both require chronic NSAID therapy and are at greatest risk for developing a significant NSAID-related complication. Included in this high-risk group are elderly people, as well as persons with a history of peptic ulcer disease or previous upper gastrointestinal bleeding, individuals also taking steroids, and patients with cardiovascular disease.[112,113] Once an ulcer develops, a serious complication is often the first sign of its presence in as many as approximately 50 percent of persons with ulcers have no dyspeptic symptoms. Patients taking NSAIDs who have dyspeptic symptoms require evaluation for

ulcer disease as well as possible *H. pylori* infection, and those with ulcers should be treated with an antisecretory agent and also antibiotics, if indicated.

Peptic ulcer disease in elderly people

Ulcer disease, whether due to *H. pylori* infection, NSAID use, or some other less common cause, frequently exhibits a virulent course in elderly people with more complications and mortality than in the young.[125–127] Duodenal ulcer occurs two to three times more frequently than gastric ulcer, but the latter is responsible for two of every three deaths from peptic ulcer disease in older individuals, and the death rate increases with advancing age.

The presentation of ulcer disease in elderly people tends to be acute, often with bleeding or perforation, but symptoms may be subtle; this is particularly true of gastric ulcers. Gastric ulcers produce chronic blood loss more commonly than duodenal ulcers, and resultant anemia may lead to cardiac or neurological symptoms. Weight loss and fatigue suggesting malignancy may be the only complaints, a presentation characteristic of giant ulcers. So-called geriatric ulcers (Fig. 78-12) high in the cardia may cause misleading symptoms such as dysphagia mimicking esophageal neoplasm or chest pain suggesting angina. A history of NSAID use is commonly obtained from elderly patients with peptic ulcer disease.

The complication rate of peptic ulcer disease rises progressively from 31 percent in patients 60–64 years of age to 76 percent in those 75–79 years of age. Surgery should not be withheld

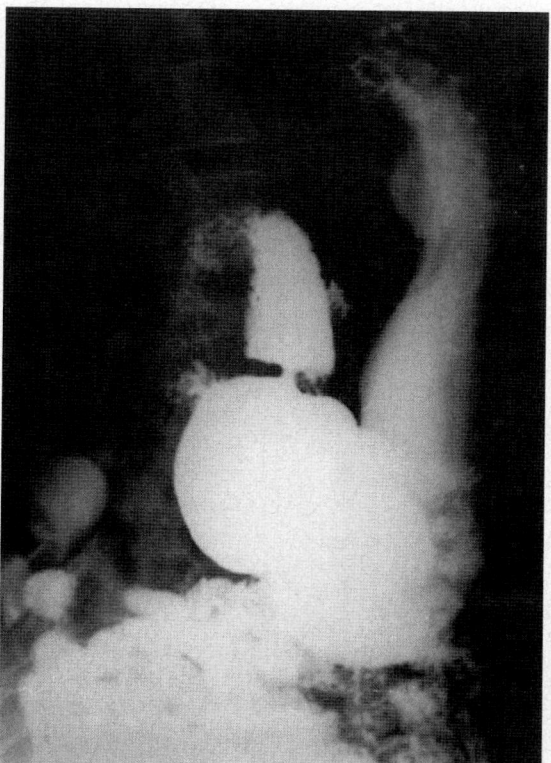

Figure 78-12 Upper gastrointestinal series revealing a large benign "geriatric ulcer" high on the lesser curvature. (Reproduced from Brandt.[154])

or delayed solely because of advanced age because it is often life-saving in older patients. Bleeding, the most common complication, accounts for one-half to two-thirds of all fatalities (see below). Perforation is the second most common complication of peptic ulcers in elderly people. The presentation of a perforated ulcer is subtle in this age group, delaying the correct diagnosis and contributing to the high mortality. Gastric outlet obstruction complicates ulcer disease in 10–15 percent of patients beyond 60 years of age, generally occurring in those with a long history of disease; an obstructing malignant lesion must be excluded in such patients.

Duodenal ulcers greater than 2 cm in diameter were once considered a distinct entity because of their poor prognosis, but it is probable that most of these "giant" duodenal ulcers are caused by either *H. pylori* infection or NSAID use, just like smaller lesions. Giant duodenal ulcers occur most often in men over 70 years of age who have no prior history of peptic ulcer disease. The most frequent complaint is of abdominal pain radiating to the back or right upper quadrant, suggesting pancreatic or biliary disease. Pain may be relieved by antacids, but aggravated by eating, and is often accompanied by significant weight loss. The ulcer crater is so large that it sometimes is mistaken for the duodenal bulb on an upper gastrointestinal series (Fig. 78-13). While giant duodenal ulcers were often fatal 30 years ago, today they usually respond to therapy with histamine antagonists or proton pump inhibitors and with antibiotics when indicated by the presence of *H. pylori* infection.

Giant gastric ulcers have a diameter of over 3 cm.[128,129] They also are most likely caused by either *H. pylori* infection or NSAID use. Giant gastric ulcers are slightly more common in males and are usually seen in patients over 65 years of age. Pain is not a prominent complaint, but only about 10 percent of patients are completely free of pain. Pain may radiate to the chest, periumbilical region, or lower abdomen. Morbidity and mortality rates are high, with hemorrhage being the most common complication. These ulcers are usually benign and can be treated with histamine antagonists or proton pump inhibitors

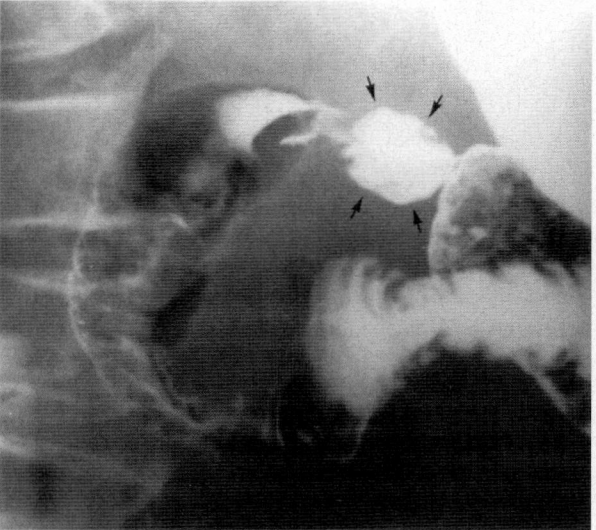

Figure 78-13 Upper gastrointestinal series demonstrates a giant duodenal ulcer resembling the duodenal bulb (arrows). (Reproduced from Brandt.[154])

as well as with antibiotics when there is documented *H. pylori* infection. Patients should be followed carefully with endoscopy to demonstrate healing. Candidiasis of the ulcer crater may delay healing and requires adjunctive antifungal therapy.

A number of potential problems must be considered in prescribing acid-suppressive therapy for elderly patients with peptic ulcer disease. Many antacid preparations contain large amounts of mineral salts which may produce undesirable effects, such as fluid retention, diarrhea, or constipation. Aluminum hydroxide forms insoluble chelates with a number of drugs, including digoxin, quinidine, and tetracycline, interfering with their absorption. Histamine antagonists variably inhibit the oxidative metabolism of many drugs, prolonging their duration of action. Cimetidine impairs the elimination of lidocaine, nifedipine, phenytoin, propranolol, quinidine, theophylline, and warfarin, to mention a few. Ranitidine is a less potent inhibitor of mixed-function oxidases than cimetidine, and alterations in drug metabolism caused by ranitidine are usually not associated with pharmacological effects. Famotidine has no effect on the oxidative metabolism of drugs. Intravenous administration of cimetidine in elderly patients with impaired renal function may produce mental confusion in a dose-related fashion. Cimetidine may also cause a mild elevation of serum creatinine levels unassociated with impairment of renal function. Ranitidine is a rare cause of hepatitis, and ranitidine and famotidine may cause headache. Sucralfate frequently causes constipation in elderly individuals. The National Institutes of Health Consensus Development Panel has published guidelines mandating antibiotic treatment of all ulcer patients infected with *H. pylori*, including those without an active ulcer crater or dyspeptic symptoms.[109]

Nonulcer dyspepsia

Patients with nonulcer dyspepsia suffer from chronic, recurrent upper abdominal pain and nausea which may or may not be related to meals and which occurs in the absence of an ulcer crater.[130] Nonulcer dyspepsia is at least twice as common as true peptic ulcer disease. Most patients with this problem have no recognizable pathological abnormality, although many have histological gastritis.[107] Nonulcer dyspepsia is further defined by the absence of reflux esophagitis, disease of the biliary tract or pancreas, or most symptoms of irritable bowel syndrome. The criteria used to select patients for inclusion in clinical studies of nonulcer dyspepsia are very inconsistent, perpetuating confusion about this diagnosis among physicians and patients.[131]

The etiology of nonulcer dyspepsia is unknown; numerous explanations have been proposed for this syndrome, including psychosocial factors, altered sensation, abnormal gastrointestinal motility and compliance, and *H. pylori* infection.[130,131] Gas washout studies show that individuals with nonulcer dyspepsia do not have increased gas in their digestive tracts, and therefore complaints of bloating are probably explained by sensitivity to normal volumes of gas; in some, the transit of infused gas is abnormal, suggesting a motility disorder. Gastric antral hypomotility and impaired gastric emptying of solids have been observed in 40–50 percent of patients with nonulcer dyspepsia, and treatment with drugs that affect upper gastrointestinal motility relieves symptoms in many patients.[132–134] Thirty to 50 percent of patients with symptoms of nonulcer dyspepsia have chronic active gastritis, even when the gastric mucosa appears grossly normal at endoscopy. It has been suggested that nonulcer dyspepsia is part of the spectrum of disease caused by *H. pylori*, which includes chronic active gastritis, duodenitis, and peptic ulcer disease. The successive development of nonulcer dyspepsia, duodenitis, and duodenal ulcer disease has been termed Moynihan's disease.[135] *Helicobacter pylori* infection, however, has not been shown to be the etiology of nonulcer dyspepsia, nor has a definite relationship between nonulcer dyspepsia and peptic ulcer disease been proved.[136]

In practice, therapy for nonulcer dyspepsia is the same as for peptic ulcer disease, despite the fact that in double-blind, placebo-controlled trials, histamine antagonists, and proton pump inhibitors are only a little better than a placebo in treating this disorder, and the role of gastric acid hypersecretion in nonulcer dyspepsia is unproved by formal measurements of basal and peak acid outputs.[137,138] Peptic ulcer disease, NSAID use, *H. pylori* infection, and gastric cancer must be excluded in elderly patients who present with dyspeptic complaints.

Upper gastrointestinal bleeding

Thirty-five to 45 percent of all cases of acute upper gastrointestinal hemorrhage occur in patients beyond age 60, and of these, half are caused by peptic ulcer disease.[139–141] Other important causes of gross upper gastrointestinal bleeding in elderly people are gastric erosions and esophagitis; these two entities in combination with peptic ulcer disease account for 70–80 percent of hospital admissions for upper gastrointestinal bleeding in older patients.

It is unclear whether elderly patients with upper gastrointestinal hemorrhage frequently have a long history of underlying acid-peptic disease, for example, chronic peptic ulcer disease, or whether they usually bleed from newly developed lesions. In one series, 36 percent of older individuals admitted to the hospital with acute upper gastrointestinal bleeding gave no history of preceding symptoms.[139] Alternatively, some patients complain of prior epigastric pain, pain in other parts of the abdomen, anorexia, dyspepsia, pyrosis or, simply, weight loss. Elderly patients with acute upper gastrointestinal bleeding usually present with hematemesis, although 30 percent of patients have only melena.[139] Hemorrhage is often seen in persons with chronic medical illnesses, the most common being degenerative joint disease. Therapy with NSAIDs for rheumatological and other problems has been found to be an important cause of upper gastrointestinal bleeding in elderly patients.[141,142] Other causes include disease found in younger patients, as well as entities seen almost exclusively in older individuals. Geriatric ulcers and giant duodenal ulcers are not associated with an unusually high incidence of hemorrhage, while giant gastric ulcers frequently do bleed.[129]

Aortoenteric fistula is an uncommon cause of gastrointestinal hemorrhage seen most often in men during the seventh and eighth decades of life. The most common etiology is rupture of an arteriosclerotic abdominal aortic aneurysm. Other causes of aortoenteric fistulas include graft-enteric fistula, aortitis, mycotic aneurysm, carcinoma, trauma, foreign body, and peptic ulceration.[143,144] The overwhelming majority of fistulas between the aorta and the alimentary tract occur in the duodenum and, as a result, usually produce upper gastrointestinal bleeding. Other reported sites of communication include the esophagus, stomach, distal small bowel, and colon. Most patients experience an initial self-limited or "sentinel" bleed, followed hours to days later by massive hemorrhage. Mortality is very high but may be reduced by early endoscopic detection of the fistula during investigation of the cause of bleeding. An elderly patient with an aortic graft who has upper gastrointestinal bleeding, no matter how trivial, must undergo immediate endoscopy because of the possible presence of a graft-enteric fistula.

Another rare cause of massive upper gastrointestinal hemorrhage in elderly people is a dilated gastric artery with an overlying mucosal defect, typically located within 2 cm of the cardioesophageal junction. This lesion, called exulceratio simplex, or the ulcer of Dieulafoy, often requires surgical therapy, although it has been treated effectively with electrocautery, laser, argon plasma coagulation, and banding.[145,146]

Occasionally, vascular abnormalities of the type found in Osler–Weber–Rendu syndrome (hereditary hemorrhagic telangiectasia) may also be responsible for upper gastrointestinal bleeding in elderly people. There may be no history of childhood epistaxis and no family history of similar occurrences, although typical telangiectactic lesions are often found in the oral cavity, lips, nailbeds, and skin.

The hospital course of elderly patients with upper gastrointestinal bleeding is similar to that of younger patients with respect to duration, amount of blood transfused, and frequency of surgery.[147,148] Older patients, however, suffer significantly more morbidity than do younger patients; complications include cardiac, neurological, and renal disease, sepsis, and reactions to medications and transfusions. Elderly patients are more likely than young patients to die during a hospital admission for gastrointestinal bleeding, especially if peptic ulcer is the cause.

The evaluation and treatment of upper gastrointestinal bleeding in elderly people is the same as in younger individuals. Age per se is not a contraindication for surgery; the decision to operate on an individual patient must be made in the context of the clinical setting. Early surgery should be contemplated for elderly patients who have bled from ulcers, who have signs of major hemorrhage (e.g. hypotension), and when endoscopic findings imply a significant risk of recurrent bleeding.

Volvulus of the stomach

Volvulus of the stomach is a relatively rare condition occurring most often after age 50 and requires relaxation of the gastric ligaments for its development.[149,150] Gastric volvulus may be responsible for chronic abdominal symptoms or may be manifested acutely with strangulation and gangrene.

Gastric volvulus is classified according to the axis around which the stomach rotates: torsion about a longitudinal axis formed by a line connecting the cardia and pylorus is known as organoaxial volvulus; rotation about a vertical axis passing through the middle of the lesser and greater curvatures is referred to as mesenteroaxial volvulus. Approximately 60 percent of affected patients have the organoaxial type, 30 percent have the mesenteroaxial type, and 10 percent have a combination form. Rotation may be partial or complete; complete twists often severely impair gastric blood flow and may cause gangrene, while partial twists may be asymptomatic or responsible for chronic symptoms.

Organoaxial volvulus usually has an acute presentation and often is associated with the presence of a large paraesophageal hiatus hernia or eventration of the diaphragm. Patients complain of the abrupt onset of upper abdominal or lower thoracic pain. Vomiting gives way to retching, and it is difficult to pass a nasogastric tube beyond the gastroesophageal junction. This group of symptoms and signs has been referred to as Borchardt's triad. Roentgenograms may reveal a gas-filled viscus in the chest or an "upside-down stomach" in the upper abdomen (Fig. 78-14). Gangrene ensues in approximately 5 percent of cases, mostly in individuals with a traumatic diaphragmatic hernia. Organoaxial volvulus usually requires surgical correction.

Mesenteroaxial volvulus is often intermittent and incomplete. Affected persons complain of chronic postprandial pain, belching, bloating, vomiting, and early satiety; strangulation is rare. Diagnosis is made by barium roentgenogram. Decompression with a nasogastric tube may return the stomach to its normal position. Surgery is indicated for persistent symptoms. Some patients have been successfully treated by fixation of the stomach with two percutaneous endoscopic gastrostomy tubes; these are removed after adhesions fix the stomach to the anterior abdominal wall.

Benign gastric tumors

The incidence of benign gastric tumors increases with age. A hyperplastic polyp accounts for 75–90 percent of such growths and typically is a small, solitary lesion at the junction of the gastric body and antrum.[151] Hyperplastic polyps are not considered true neoplasms and are not premalignant. They rarely produce symptoms and thus are found incidentally in an evaluation of the upper gastrointestinal tract. In contrast, adenomatous polyps are true neoplasms and account

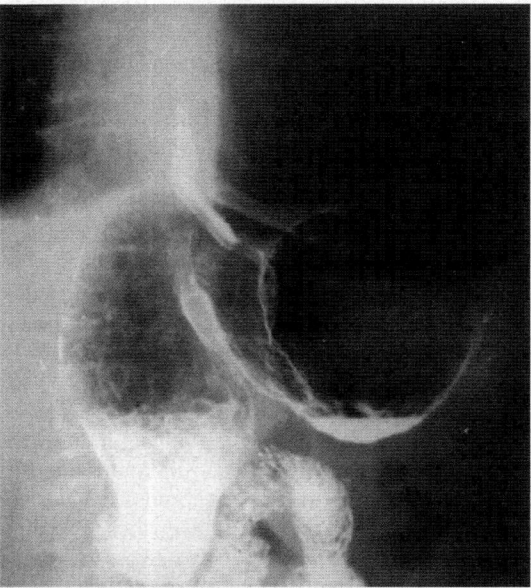

Figure 78-14 An organoaxial volvulus of the stomach identified on upper gastrointestinal series. (Reproduced from Brandt.[154])

for 10–25 percent of gastric polyps. The mean incidence of malignant change in gastric adenomas is reported to be anywhere from 6 to 75 percent, probably reflecting their heterogeneity in size, age, and histology (tubular, villous, or mixed).

Gastric polyps may occur in some gastrointestinal polyposis syndromes, but the only one appearing in older individuals is the Cronkhite–Canada syndrome. This disorder is acquired, not inherited, and is characterized by diffuse gastrointestinal polyposis, protein-losing enteropathy, and ectodermal abnormalities, including hyperpigmentation, alopecia, and dystrophic nail changes. Polyps in this syndrome are hamartomas composed of tubules and mucus-filled cysts.

Mesenchymal tumors, including leiomyomas, fibromas, and tumors of neural origin, account for a significant percentage of benign gastric tumors. Symptoms of these tumors are usually related to their size and not their type. Pain and bleeding are the most common manifestations.

Malignant gastric tumors

Gastric adenocarcinoma

Inexplicably, the incidence of gastric cancer is decreasing in elderly people, while relatively more cases are being diagnosed in younger patients.[152] Nevertheless, the vast majority of gastric cancers occur in patients beyond 60 years of age.[1] Carcinoma of the stomach is usually incurable by the time symptoms appear because symptoms often do not develop until the tumor is large. Initial symptoms are often mild and nonspecific. The tendency to treat dyspepsia in older patients without a diagnostic evaluation prompted Sir Heneage Ogilvie to say in the early 1900s, "in carcinoma of the stomach, alkalis are the undertaker's best friend."

Vague epigastric discomfort, anorexia, early satiety, and weight loss are the most frequent symptoms of gastric cancer. Physical examination may reveal enlarged left axillary and supraclavicular lymph nodes, an umbilical nodule, or a hard palpable left hepatic lobe. Rarely, the patient develops acanthosis nigricans, dermatomyositis, or an explosive outbreak of skin tags or keratotic lesions (sign of Leser–Trélat), raising the suspicion of a visceral neoplasm. Laboratory abnormalities are nonspecific.

Surgical excision is the only potentially curative treatment. Seventy to 90 percent of patients with gastric cancer are considered suitable for laparotomy, but only half are found to be eligible for potentially curative resections and death occurs in most of these individuals within 1 year. Five-year survival rates are 5–15 percent. Combined chemotherapy and irradiation may be of some benefit, but irradiation alone is ineffective except for palliation of bone pain from metastases.

Gastric lymphoma

The stomach is the most frequent site of primary, extranodal lymphoma and accounts for one-half to three-fourths of patients with lymphoma of the gastrointestinal tract. Gastric lymphoma produces nonspecific symptoms, but epigastric pain with weight loss and a palpable mass in a patient who is otherwise well is typical. Radiographically, lymphoma resembles carcinoma in up to two-thirds of cases (Fig. 78-15). Large, ulcerated masses, hyperrugosity, polypoid lesions, or antral narrowing suggests lymphoma. A definitive diagnosis cannot be made from gastroscopic brush cytology and biopsy, and laparotomy

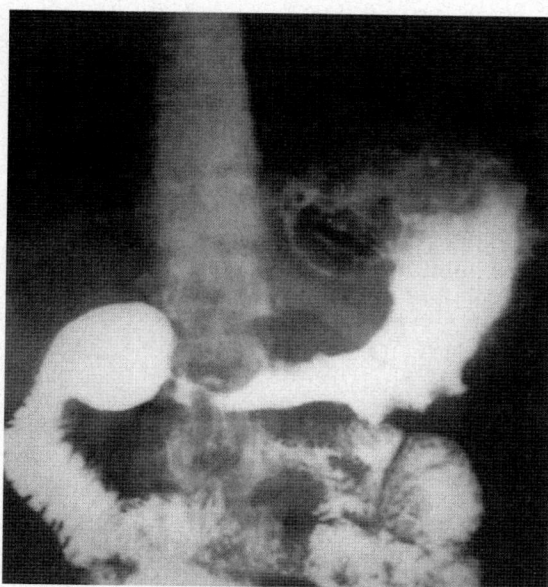

Figure 78-15 Upper gastrointestinal series showing a gastric lymphoma with antral narrowing mimicking an adenocarcinoma. (Reproduced from Brandt.[154])

may be necessary. Therapy is wide excision followed by radiation and leads to a 5-year survival of about 40–50 percent.

SYSTEMIC DISEASES
Diabetes mellitus

Patients with long-standing diabetes mellitus often have profound abnormalities of gastrointestinal motility, including delayed gastric emptying of solids.[153] Such abnormalities are frequently without clinical manifestations, although difficulty controlling plasma glucose, due to an inconstant and unpredictable rate of gastric emptying, may be a subtle indication of gastroparesis. Gastric atony may be manifested by a gradual onset of upper abdominal fullness, satiety, and vomiting. Gastroparesis and accompanying hypochlorhydria probably underlie the development of gastric bezoars and bacterial and fungal overgrowth in this population.

Diabetic gastroparesis is caused by an abnormality of the autonomic nervous system almost always associated with peripheral or autonomic neuropathy. Metoclopramide has been used to improve gastric motility and relieve symptoms but causes intolerable central nervous system effects in many patients.

Amyloidosis

The gastrointestinal tract is involved in 50–75 percent of patients with amyloidosis, and in approximately one-half of these cases the stomach is affected. It is unusual for signs and symptoms of gastrointestinal involvement to be directly attributable to the amyloidosis per se. Outlet obstruction may be caused by an obstructing mass of amyloid in the distal stomach. Amyloid may also diffusely infiltrate the gastric wall, making surgery difficult, and may be associated with giant gastric ulcers resistant to medical therapy. Prognosis is related to that of the primary disease.

REFERENCES

1. Everhart JE (ed): Digestive Diseases in the United States: Epidemiology and Impact. US Department of Health and Human Services, Public Health Service, National Institutes of Health, National Institute of Diabetes and Digestive and Kidney Diseases. NIH Publication 94–1447. US Government Printing Office, Washington, DC, 1994
2. Cohen RA, Van Nostrand JF: Trends in the Health of Older Americans: United States, 1994. National Center for Health Statistics 1995; Vital Health Stat 3(30)
3. Shay K, Ship JA: The importance of oral health in the older patient. J Am Geriatr Soc 1995;43:1414–1422
4. Sullivan DH, Martin W, Flaxman N et al: Oral health problems and involuntary weight loss in a population of frail elderly. J Am Geriatr Soc 1993;41:725–731
5. Finch CE, Hayflick L: Muscle: Handbook of the Biology of Aging. Van Nostrand Reinhold, New York, 1977:709
6. Jensen GL, McGee M, Binkley J: Nutrition in the elderly. Gastroenterol Clin North Am 2001;30:313–334
7. Morley JE: Anorexia of aging: physiologic and pathologic. Am J Clin Nutr 1997;66:760–773
8. Henkin RI, Graziadei PP, Bradley DF: The molecular basis of taste and its disorders. Ann Intern Med 1969;71:791–821
9. Rolls BJ: Aging and appetite. Nutr Rev 1992;50:422–426
10. Baum BJ: Evaluation of stimulated patroid saliva flow rate in different age groups. J Dent Res 1950;29:686
11. Doty RL, Shaman P, Applebaum SL et al: Smell identification ability: changes with age. Science 1984;226:1441–1443
12. Bean WB: The changing incidence of certain vascular lesions of the skin with aging. Geriatrics 1956;11:97–102
13. Kjeldsen AD, Kjeldsen J: Gastrointestinal bleeding in patients with hereditary hemorrhagic telangiectasia. Am J Gastroenterol 2000;95:415–418
14. Carnel SB, Blakeslee DB, Oswald SG et al: Treatment of radiation- and chemotherapy-induced stomatitis. Otolaryngol Head Neck Surg 1990;102:326–330
15. Mirbod SM, Ahing SI: Tobacco-associated lesions of the oral cavity: Part I. Nonmalignant lesions. J Can Dent Assoc 2000;66:252–256
16. Levine N: Dark discoloration of the tongue. Geriatrics 1996;51:20
17. Reichart PA, Langford A, Gelderblom HR et al: Oral hairy leukoplakia: Observations in 95 cases and review of the literature. J Oral Pathol Med 1989;18:410–415
18. Fantasia JE: Diagnosis and treatment of common oral lesions found in the elderly. Dent Clin North Am 1997;41:877–890
19. Salisbury PL: Diagnosis and patient management of oral cancer. Dent Clin North Am 1997;41:891–914
20. deSantana EJ, Rodrigues CB, Consolaro A: Keratoacanthoma versus squamous cell carcinoma of the lip. Ann Dent 1990;49:9–13
21. Buchholz DW, Boxma JF, Donner MW: Adaptation, compensation, and decompensation of the pharyngeal swallow. Gastrointest Radiol 1985;10:235–239
22. Piaget F, Fouillet J: Le pharynx et l'oseuphage séniles: stude clinique radiogique et radiocinematographique. J Med Lyon 1959;40:951
23. Tack J, Vantrappen G: The aging oesophagus. Gut 1997;41:422–424
24. Robbins J, Hamilton JW, Lof GL et al: Oropharyngeal swallowing in normal adults of different ages. Gastroenterology 1992;103:823–829
25. Cook IJ: Diagnosis and management of cricopharyngeal achalasia and other upper esophageal sphincter opening disorders. Curr Gastroenterol Rep 2000;2:191–195
26. Lindgren S, Ekberg O: Cricopharyngeal myotomy in the treatment of dysphagia. Clin Otolaryngol 1990;15:221–227
27. Achkar E: Zenker's diverticulum. Dig Dis 1998;16:144–151
28. Knuff TE, Benjamin SB, Castell DO: Pharyngoesophageal (Zenker's) diverticulum: a reappraisal. Gastroenterology 1982;82:734–736
29. Huang B, Unni KK, Payne WS: Long-term survival following diverticulectomy for cancer in pharyngoesophageal (Zenker's) diverticulum. Ann Thorac Surg 1984;38:207
30. Sideris L, Chen LQ, Ferraro P: The treatment of Zenker's diverticulum: A review. Semin Thorac Cardiovasc Surg 1999;11:337–351
31. Bremnar CG, DeMeester TR: Endoscopic treatment of Zenker's diverticulum. Gastrointest Endosc 1999;49:126–128
32. Norris CW: Pharyngoceles of the esophagus. Laryngoscope 1979;89:1788–1807

33. Soergel KH, Zboralske FF, Amberg JR: Presbyesophagus: Esophageal motility in nonagenarians. J Clin Invest 1964;43:1472

34. Hollis JB, Castell DO: Esophageal function in elderly men: a new look at "presbyesophagus." Ann Intern Med 1974;80:371

35. Khan TA, Shragge BW, Crispin JS et al: Esophageal motility in the elderly. Am J Dig Dis 1977;22:1049–1054

36. Richter JE, Wu WC, Johns DN et al: Esophageal manometry in 95 healthy adult volunteers: variability of pressures with age and frequency of "abnormal" contraction. Dig Dis Sci 1987;32:583–592

37. Grishaw EK, Ott DJ, Frederick MG et al: Functional abnormalities of the esophagus: A prospective analysis of radiographic findings relative to age and symptoms. Am J Roentgenol 1996;16:719–723

38. Castell DO: Dysphagia. Gastroenterology 1979;76:1015–1024

39. Shaker R, Staff D: Esophageal disorders in the elderly. Gastroenterol Clin North Am 2001;30:335–361

40. Triadafilopoulos G, Sharma R: Features of symptomatic gastroesophageal reflux disease in elderly patients. Am J Gastroenterol 1997;92:2007–2011

41. Edwards DA: Discriminative information in the diagnosis of dysphagia. J R Coll Physicians Lond 1975;9:257

42. Schatzki R: Panel discussion on diseases of the esophagus. Am J Gastroenterol 1959;31:117–119

43. Collen MJ, Abdulian JD, Chen YK: Gastroesophageal reflux disease in the elderly: More severe disease that requires aggressive therapy. Am J Gastroenterol 1995;90:1053–1057

44. Katz PO, Dalton CB, Richter JE et al: Esophageal testing of patients with noncardiac chest pain or dysphagia: Results of three year's experience with 1161 patients. Ann Intern Med 1987;106:593–597

45. Adler DG, Romero Y: Primary esophageal motility disorders. Mayo Clin Proc 2001;76:195–200

46. Mayberry JF, Atkinson M: Studies on the incidence and prevalence of achalasia in the Nottingham area. Q J Med 1985;56:451–456

47. Kahrilas PJ, Kishik SM, Helm JF et al: Comparison of pseudoachalasia and achalasia. Am J Med 1987;82:439

48. Tracey JP, Traube M: Difficulties in the diagnosis of pseudoachalasia. Am J Gastroenterol 1994;89:2014–2018

49. Clouse RE, Abramson BK, Todorczuk JR: Achalasia in the elderly: Effects of aging on clinical presentation and outcome. Dig Dis Sci 1991;36:225–228

50. Carter M, Deckmann RC, Smith RC et al: Differentiation of achalasia from pseudoachalasia by computed tomography. Am J Gastroenterol 1997;92:624–628

51. Kolodny M, Schrader ZR, Rubin W: Esophageal achalasia probably due to gastric carcinoma. Ann Intern Med 1968;69:569–572

52. Menin R, Fisher RS: Return of esophageal peristalsis in achalasia secondary to gastric cancer. Dig Dis Sci 1981;26:1038–1044

53. Davis JA, Kantrowitz PA, Chandler HL et al: Reversible achalasia due to reticulum cell sarcoma. New Engl J Med 1975;293:130–132

54. Richter JE, Hackshaw BT, Wu WC et al: Edrophonium: A useful provocative test for esophageal chest pain. Ann Intern Med 1985;103:14–21

55. Richter JE: Gastroesophageal reflux disease in the older patient: Presentation, treatment, and complications. Am J Gastroenterol 2000;95:368–373

56. Katz PO: Gastroesophageal reflux disease. J Am Geriatr Soc 1998;46:1558–1565

57. Spechler SJ, Goyal RK: The columnar-lined esophagus, intestinal metaplasia, and Norman Barrett. Gastroenterology 1996;110:614–621

58. Spechler SJ: Endoscopic surveillance for patients with Barrett esophagus: Does the cancer risk justify the practice? Ann Intern Med 1987;106:902–904

59. Cameron AJ: Epidemiology of columnar-lined esophagus and adenocarcinoma. Gastroenterol Clin North Am 1997;26:487–494

60. Schatzki R, Gary JE: Dysphagia due to a diaphragm-like localized narrowing in the lower esophagus ("lower esophageal ring"). Am J Radiol 1953;70:911

61. Goyal RK, Bauer JL, Spiro HM: The nature and location of lower esophageal ring. New Engl J Med 1971;284:1775

62. Hendrix TR: Schatzki ring, epithelial junction, and hiatal hernia—an unresolved controversy. Gastroenterology 1980;79:584

63. Birnholz JC, Ferrucci TT, Wyman SM: Roentgen features of dysphagia aortica. Radiology 1974;111:93–96

64. Mucklow EH, Smith OE: Dysphagia and unusual radiographic appearances associated with the variable relationships of the aorta and lower oesophagus. J Fac Radiol 1954;6:88–95

65. Pearson RH, Bessell EM, Bowely NB: Compression of oesophagus by tortuous dilated aorta. Br Med J 1981;282:1032–1033

66. McMillin IK, Hyde I: Compression of the oesophagus by the aorta. Thorax 1969;24:32–38

67. Kikendall JW, Friedman AC, Oyewole M et al: Pill-induced esophageal injury: Case reports and review of the medical literature. Dig Dis Sci 1983;28:174–182

68. Bott S, Prakash C, McCallum RW: Medication-induced esophageal injury: Survey of the literature. Am J Gastroenterol 1987;82:758

69. Channer KS, Virjee JP: The effect of size and shape of tablets on their esophageal transit. J Clin Pharmacol 1986;26:141

70. Wheeler D: Diverticula of foregut. Radiology 1947;49:476–481

71. Debas HT, Payne WS, Cameron AJ et al: Physiopathology of lower esophageal diverticulum and its implications for treatment. Surg Gynecol Obstet 1980;151:593–600

72. Habein H, Moersch H, Kirklin J: Diverticula of the lower part of the esophagus. Arch Intern Med 1956;97:768–777

73. Bender MK, Haddad JK: Disappearance of multiple esophageal diverticula following treatment of esophagitis. Gastrointest Endosc 1973;20:19–22

74. Schima W, Schober E, Stacher G et al: Association of midoesophageal diverticula with oesophageal motor disorders: Videofluoroscopy and manometry. Acta Radiol 1997;38:108–114

75. Benacci JC, Deschamps C, Trastek VF et al: Epiphrenic diverticulum: results of surgical treatment. Ann Thorac Surg 1993;55:1109–1113

76. Flora KD, Gordon MD, Lieberman D et al: Esophageal intramural pseudodiverticulosis. Dig Dis 1997;15:113–119

77. van der Putten AB, Loffeld RJ: Esophageal intramural pseudodiverticulosis. Dis Esophagus 1997;10:61–63.

78. Gorback SL, Nahas L, Lerner PI et al: Studies of intestinal microflora: Effects of diet, age and periodic sampling on numbers of fecal microorganisms in man. Gastroenterology 1967;53:845–855

79. Kodsi BE, Wickremesinghe PC, Kozinn PJ et al: Candida esophagitis: A prospective study of 27 cases. Gastroenterology 1976;71:715–719

80. Scott BB, Jenkins D: Gastro-oesophageal candidiasis. Gut 1982;23:137–139

81. Wienbeck M, Berges W: Oesophageal lesions in the alcoholic. Clin Gastroenterol 1981;10:375

82. La Vecchia CL, Liati P, Decarli A et al: Tar yields of cigarettes and the risk of oesophageal cancer. Int J Cancer 1986;38:381

83. Carter R, Brewer LA: Achalasia and esophageal carcinoma: Studies in early diagnosis for improved surgical management. Am J Surg 1975;130:114

84. Appelqvist P, Salmo M: Lye corrosin carcinoma of the esophagus. Cancer 1980;45:2655

85. Hameeteman W, Tytgat GN, Houthoff HJ et al: Barrett's esophagus: Development of dysplasia and adenocarcinoma. Gastroenterology 1989;96:1249–1256

86. Sondik EJ, Dessler LG, Ries LA: Cancer Statistics Review 1973–1986, Including a Report on the Status of Cancer Control. National Cancer Institute, Division of Cancer Prevention and Control, Surveillance Program. NIH Publication. 89-2789. U.S. Government Printing Office, Washington, DC, 1989

87. Lerut T, Coosemans W, De Leyn P et al: Treatment of esophageal carcinoma. Chest 1999;116:463S–465S

88. Thomas P, Doddoli C, Neville P et al: Esophageal cancer resection in the elderly. Eur J Cardiothorac Surg 1996;10:941–946

89. Reed CE: Endoscopic palliation of esophageal carcinoma. Chest Surg Clin N Am 1994;4:155–172

90. Evans MA: Gastric emptying rate in the elderly: Implications for drug therapy. J Am Geriatr Soc 1981;29:201

91. Moore JG, Tweedy C, Christian PE et al: Effect of age on gastric emptying of liquid-solid meals in man. Dig Dis Sci 1983;28:340

92. Blackman AH, Lambert DL, Thayer WR et al: Computed normal values for peak acid output based on age, sex and body weight. Am J Dig Dis 1970;15:783–789

93. Goldschmiedt M, Barnett CC, Schwarz BE et al: Effect of age on gastric acid secretion and serum gastrin concentrations in healthy men and women. Gastroenterology 1991;101:977–990

94. Hurwitz A, Brady DA, Schaal SE et al: Gastric acidity in older adults. JAMA 1997;278:659–662

95. Misiewixz JJ, Price AB, Tytgat GN: Working party report to the World Congresses of Gastroenterology, Sydney, 1990. J Gastroenterol Hepatol 1991;6:207–234

96. Carpenter HA, Talley NJ: Gastroscopy is incomplete without biopsy: Clinical relevance of distinguishing gastropathy from gastritis. Gastroenterology 1995;108:917–924

97. Yoshida N, Granger DN, Evans DJ Jr et al: Mechanisms involved in *Helicobacter pylori*-induced inflammation. Gastroenterology 1993;105:1431–1440

98. Hawkey CJ, Hudson N: Mucosal injury caused by drugs, chemicals, and stress: In Haubrich WS, Schaffner F (eds): Bockus, Gastroenterology, 5th Ed. WB Saunders, Philadelphia, 1995:656–699

99. Wyatt JL, Dixon MF: Chronic gastritis: A pathogenetic approach. J Pathol 1988;154:113–124

100. Smoot DT: How does Helicobacter pylori cause mucosal damage? Direct mechanisms. Gastroenterology 1997;113:S31–S34

101. Blaser MJ: *Helicobacter pylori* and the pathogenesis of gastroduodenal inflammation. J Infect Dis 1990;161:626–633

102. Peterson WL: Helicobacter pylori and peptic ulcer disease. N Engl J Med 1991;11;324:1043–1048

103. Asghar RJ, Parsonnet J: Helicobacter pylori and risk for gastric adenocarcinoma. Semin Gastrointest Dis 2001;12:203–208

104. Dooley CP, Cohen H, Fitzgibbons PL et al: Prevalence of *Helicobacter pylori* infection and histologic gastritis in asymptomatic persons. N Engl J Med 1989;321:1562–1566

105. Banatvala N, Mayo K, Megraud F et al: The cohort effect and *Helicobacter pylori*. J Infect Dis 1993;168:219–221

106. Warren JR: Gastric pathology associated with *Helicobacter pylori*. Gastroenterol Clin North Am 2000;29:705–751

107. Talley NJ, Axon A, Bytzer P et al: Management of uninvestigated and functional dyspepsia: A Working Party report for the World Congresses of Gastroenterology 1998. Aliment Pharmacol Ther 1999;13:1135–1148

108. Cohen H: Peptic ulcer and Helicobacter pylori. Gastroenterol Clin North Am 2000;29:775–789

109. NIH Consensus Development Panel on *Helicobacter pylori* in Peptic Ulcer Disease: *Helicobacter pylori* in peptic ulcer disease. JAMA 1994;272:66–69

110. Wolfe MM, Lichtenstein DR, Singh G: Gastrointestinal toxicity of nonsteroidal antiinflammatory drugs. N Engl J Med 1999;340:1888–1899

111. Griffin MR: Epidemiology of nonsteroidal anti-inflammatory drug-associated gastrointestinal injury. Am J Med 1998;104:23S–29S; discussion 41S–42S

112. Silverstein FE, Graham DY, Senior JR et al: Misoprostol reduces serious gastrointestinal complications in patients with rheumatoid arthritis receiving nonsteroidal anti-inflammatory drugs. Ann Intern Med 1995;123:241–249

113. Laine L: Approaches to nonsteroidal anti-inflammatory drug use in the high-risk patient. Gastroenterology 2001;120:594–606

114. Walt R, Katschinski B, Logan R et al: Rising frequency of ulcer perforation in elderly people in United Kingdom. Lancet 1986;2:489–492

115. Graham DY, Smith JL, Spjut HJ et al: Gastric adaptation: Studies in humans during continuous aspirin administration. Gastroenterology 1988;95:327–333

116. Graham DY, Smith JL: Aspirin and the stomach. Ann Intern Med 1986;104:390–398

117. Fries JF, Miller SR, Spitz PW et al: Toward an epidemiology of gastropathy associated with nonsteroidal anti-inflammatory drug use. Gastroenterology 1989;96:647–655

118. Griffin MR, Piper JM, Daughterty JR et al: Nonsteroidal anti-inflammatory drug use and increased risk for peptic ulcer disease in elderly persons. Ann Intern Med 1991;114:257–263

119. Langman MJ, Jensen DM, Watson DJ et al: Adverse upper gastrointestinal effects of rofecoxib compared with NSAIDs. JAMA 1999;282:1929–1933

120. Dajani EZ, Agrawal NM: Prevention and treatment of ulcers induced by nonsteroidal anti-inflammatory drugs: An update. J Physiol Pharmacol 1995;46:3–16

121. Ehsanullah RS, Page MC, Tildesley G et al: Prevention of gastroduodenal damage induced by non-steroidal anti-inflammatory drugs: Controlled trial of ranitidine. Br Med J 1988;297:1017–1021

122. Robinson MG, Griffin JW, Bowers J et al: Effect of ranitidine gastroduodenal (sic) mucosal damage induced by nonsteroidal antiinflammatory drugs. Dig Dis Sci 1989;34:424–428

123. Taha AS, Hudson N, Hawkey CJ et al: Famotidine for the prevention of gastric and duodenal ulcers caused by nonsteroidal anti-inflammatory drugs. N Engl J Med 1996;334:1435–1439

124. Graham DY, White RH, Moreland LW et al: Duodenal and gastric ulcer prevention with misoprostol in arthritis patients taking NSAIDs. Ann Intern Med 1993;119:257–262

125. Linder JD, Wilcox CM: Acid peptic disease in the elderly. Gastroenterol Clin North Am 2001;30:363–376

126. Borum ML: Peptic ulcer disease in the elderly. Clin Geriatr Med 1999;15:457–471

127. Pilotto A: Helicobacter pylori-associated peptic ulcer disease in older patients: Current management strategies. Drugs Aging 2001;18:487–494

128. Raju GS, Bardhan KD, Royston C et al: Giant gastric ulcer: its natural history and outcome in the H_2RA era. Am J Gastroenterol 1999;94:3478–3486

129. Strange SL: Giant innocent gastric ulcer in the elderly. Geront Clin 1963;5:171–189.

130. Talley NJ, Phillips SF: Non-ulcer dyspepsia: Potential causes and pathophysiology. Ann Intern Med 1988;108:865–879

131. Mc Namara DA, Buckley M, O'Morain CA: Nonulcer dyspepsia. Current concepts and management. Gastroenterol Clin North Am 2000;29:807–818

132. Camilleri M, Malagelada JR, Kao PC et al: Gastric and autonomic responses to stress in functional dyspepsia. Dig Dis Sci 1986;31:1169–1177

133. Greydanus MP, Vassallo M, Camilleri M et al: Neurohormonal factors in functional dyspepsia: Insights on pathophysiological mechanisms. Gastroenterology 1991;100:1311–1318

134. Talley NJ: Therapeutic options in nonulcer dyspepsia. J Clin Gastroenterol 2001;32:286–293

135. Spiro HM: Moynihan's disease? The diagnosis of duodenal ulcer. N Engl J Med 1974;291:567–569

136. Talley NJ: A critique of therapeutic trials in *Helicobacter pylori*-positive functional dyspepsia. Gastroenterology 1994;106:1174–1183

137. Dobrilla G, Comberlato M, Steele A et al: Drug treatment of functional dyspepsia: A meta-analysis of randomized controlled clinical trials. J Clin Gastroenterol 1989;11:169–177

138. Collen MJ, Loebenberg MJ: Basal gastric acid secretion in nonulcer dyspepsia with or without duodentitis. Dig Dis Sci 1989;34:246–250

139. Farrell JJ, Friedman LS: Gastrointestinal bleeding in the elderly. Gastroenterol Clin North Am 2001;30:377–407.

140. Gostout CJ: Gastrointestinal bleeding in the elderly patient. Am J Gastroenterol 2000;95:590–595

141. Rosen AM: Gastrointestinal bleeding in the elderly. Clin Geriatr Med 1999;15:511–525

142. Laszlo A, Kelly JP, Kaufman DE et al: Clinical aspects of upper gastrointestinal bleeding associated with the use of nonsteroidal antiinflammatory drugs. Am J Gastroenterol 1998;93:721–725

143. Antinori CH, Andrew CT, Santaspirt JS et al: The many faces of aortoenteric fistulas. Am Surg 1996;62:344–349

144. Dossa CD, Pipinos II, Shepard AD et al: Primary aortoenteric fistula: Part I. Ann Vasc Surg 1994;8:113–120

145. Fockens P, Tytgat GN: Dieulafoy's disease. Gastrointest Endosc Clin N Am 1996;6:739–752

146. Schmulewitz N, Baillie J: Dieulafoy lesions: A review of 6 years of experience at a tertiary referral center. Am J Gastroenterol 2001;96:1688–1694

147. Guttmacher AE, Marchuk DA, White RI Jr: Hereditary hemorrhagic telangiectasia. N Engl J Med 1995;333:918–924

148. Segal WN, Cello JP: Hemorrhage in the upper gastrointestinal tract in the older patient. Am J Gastroenterol 1997;92:42–46

149. Godshall D, Mossallam U, Rosenbaum R: Gastric volvulus: Case report and review of the literature. J Emerg Med 1999;17:837–840

150. Schaefer DC, Nikoomenesh P, Moore C: Gastric volvulus: An old disease process with some new twists. Gastroenterologist 1997;5:41–45

151. Lau CF, Hui PK, Mak KL et al: Gastric polypoid lesions—illustrative cases and literature review. Am J Gastroenterol 1998;93:2559–2564

152. Sial SH, Catalano MF: Gastrointestinal tract cancer in the elderly. Gastroenterol Clin North Am 2001;30:565–590

153. Kong MF, Horowitz M: Gastric emptying in diabetes mellitus: Relationship to blood-glucose control. Clin Geriatr Med 1999;15:321–328

154. Brandt LJ: Gastrointestinal Disorders of the Elderly, 1st Ed. Lippincott-Raven, New York, 1986

Chapter 79

The pancreas

Vishal Kaushik and Alistair Makin

Material in this chapter contains contributions from the previous edition, and we are grateful to the previous authors for the work done.

ACUTE PANCREATITIS

The incidence of acute pancreatitis is approximately 100 cases per 100,000 population[1] and this incidence is increasing.[2,3] This rise may reflect increasing alcohol intake or the upward trend of gallstone disease. Three percent of all admissions with abdominal pain in the UK will be due to acute pancreatitis and some cases are diagnosed only at post mortem. Age in itself is not a risk factor for the development of this condition, but elderly people experience a more severe disease. Eighty percent of cases of acute pancreatitis will run a mild course with a self-limiting disease, whereas the remaining 20 percent will suffer a severe illness with multiorgan involvement.

Pathogenesis and pathophysiology

"Acute pancreatitis" is a pathological diagnosis that describes an acute inflammatory process of the pancreas. The term encompasses a range of organ dysfunction and is not limited to the pancreas alone but extends to peripancreatic tissues and distant organs. Systemic inflammatory response syndrome (SIRS), acute respiratory distress syndrome (ARDS), multiorgan dysfunction syndrome (MODS), and disseminated intravascular coagulation (DIC) are grave complications of acute severe pancreatitis.

The pancreas requires a trigger (usually extrapancreatic, e.g. alcohol or a passage of stone in biliopancreatic duct) but the exact mechanism of induction of pancreatitis by these agents is not known. One of the earliest events in acute pancreatitis is blockade of secretion of pancreatic enzymes while synthesis continues. Acute pancreatitis results from the intra-acinar activation of these proteolytic enzymes, which progresses to an autodigestive injury to the gland. This sets up a cycle of active enzymes damaging cells, which then release more active enzymes and the destruction spreads along the gland and into the peripancreatic tissue.[4]

Etiology

The etiological factors for acute pancreatitis are outlined in Table 79-1. Alcohol and gallstones are responsible for up to 80 percent of attacks. In elderly people gallstone disease is the commonest cause. The amount of alcohol, type of beverage, duration of intake (from 5 to 20 years), and drinking pattern (binge or steady) has no consistent correlation to the precipitation of pancreatitis, which usually occurs after several hours of an alcohol binge. Biliary sludge has been noted in up to 32 and 75 percent of patients with nonalcoholic and idiopathic pancreatitis, respectively.[5,6] Biliary pancreatitis typically follows a meal. In elderly people, other risk factors—including

Table 79-1 Etiology of acute pancreatitis

Alcohol
Gallstone disease
Postoperative: major abdominal or cardiac surgery
Metabolic:
- Hypertriglyceridemia (often at levels > 50 mg/L)
- Hypercalcemia

Medications:[a]
- Immunosuppressives, e.g. azathioprine, 6-mercaptopurine
- Corticosteroids
- Oral 5-aminosalicylate, sulfasalazine
- Antibacterials, e.g. tetracycline, metronidazole, nitrofurantoin, sulfonamide, erythromycin
- Diuretics, e.g. thiazides, frusemide
- Angiotensin converting enzyme inhibitors
- Methyldopa
- Estrogens
- Valproic acid
- Pentamidine
- Antiretroviral agents, e.g. didanosine

ERCP
End stage renal failure
Ischemia
Pancreatic or ampullary tumors
Pancreas divisum (found in 5–7 percent of population)
Periampullary diverticulum
Penetrating posterior peptic ulcer
Infections, e.g. TB, aspergillosis, candidiasis, mumps, HIV
Trauma
Hypothermia
Smoke inhalation
Hereditary
Biliary cholesterol crystals
Sphincter of Oddi dysfunction
Idiopathic

[a] Reference 7 of Folsch et al.[20]

pancreatic ischemia, particularly following vascular surgery, e.g. aortic or renal grafts, coronary artery bypass grafts, vasculitis, medication, atypical infections and endoscopic retrograde cholangiopancreatography (ERCP)—are associated with acute pancreatitis. Hereditary pancreatitis is a disease of the young and is characterized by recurrent attacks that commence any time from infancy to the 50s. Inheritance is autosomal dominant and the gene responsible is the human cationic trypsinogen gene.[7] Cystic fibrosis is another inherited cause. Identification of the underlying cause of an attack is important to prevent further episodes. Despite extensive investigation in up to 10 percent of cases referred to specialist centers, no obvious cause will be found, and this group is labeled as having idiopathic acute pancreatitis.

There are no significant differences in the outcome of acute pancreatitis caused by various etiological factors. Morbidity may differ, as pancreatic pseudocyst formation and chronic pancreatitis are much more common in alcoholic as opposed to biliary pancreatitis.

Clinical presentation

Abdominal pain is the most common feature in the presentation of acute pancreatitis. The pain is characteristically in the upper abdomen and is steady and boring, with radiation through to the back. It builds up in intensity to a peak in a few minutes and lasts for several hours or days. The patient acquires a typical posture of comfort, leaning forward with the knees flexed. In elderly people, pain may be absent, particularly in the postoperative period when receiving strong analgesia. An acute confusional state or even coma may be the first indication of an attack. Nausea and vomiting are present in 75–90 percent of patients. Mild jaundice is common and does not always indicate biliary pancreatitis. Examination findings vary in an acute attack, from minimal tenderness to rebound or guarding, abdominal distension and/or discoloration. Central ecchymosis (around umbilicus) is known as Grey Turner's sign, whereas lateral ecchymosis (in flanks) is Cullen's sign. Abdominal wall discoloration that appears after 48–72 hours is associated with mortality.[8] Ileus is common and is potentiated by opiate use. Shifting dullness is a sign of hemorrhagic necrosis, but in the later stages of the disease it may represent hypoalbuminemia or a pancreatic fistula. The patient may be severely dehydrated due to reduced intake and vomiting or fluid losses into the retroperitoneal space. Pleural effusions can be uni- or bilateral. Widespread crackles in the lung fields may indicate ARDS or congestive cardiac failure. A palpable epigastric mass suggests the development of an inflammatory mass or fluid collection. Acute pancreatitis should be considered in any case of unexplained shock or metabolic acidosis.

Diagnosis

The most important diagnostic test is the serum amylase. Hyperamylasemia occurs shortly after the onset and peaks within 24 hours. The levels return to normal in 1–4 days due to rapid excretion from the kidneys. The degree of serum amylase elevation does not correlate with the disease severity. Total serum amylase has a low specificity of <70 percent as it is elevated in other conditions (Table 79-2) and it may be interpreted as low in patients with lipemic serum. Serum amylase more than three times the upper limit of normal has more than 90 percent specificity of making an accurate diagnosis. Serum lipase activity of twice the normal is more specific and sensitive (>95 percent) than serum amylase but is less widely available and takes longer to be processed. Lipase levels remain elevated until 6–7 days after onset. Serum levels of pancreatic isoamylase, trypsin or elastase are of no additional value in the diagnosis. More recently, urinary trypsinogen-2 has been shown to be a useful screening test.

Hematocrit may be high due to dehydration and there is often leukocytosis. Abnormal liver function tests indicate the likelihood of biliary pancreatitis. An alanine transaminase (ALT) rise of three-fold or greater is more sensitive than

Table 79-2 Differential diagnosis

Abdominal causes:
- Acute hepatitis[a]
- Acute cholecystitis[a]
- Acute cholangitis[a]
- Biliary[a] and renal colic
- Bowel obstruction, strangulation, or perforation[a]
- Perforated peptic ulcer[a]
- Dissecting or ruptured aortic aneurysm[a]
- Acute mesenteric ischemia[a]
- Acute appendicitis
- Diverticulitis
- Splenic rupture
- Ruptured ectopic pregnancy or ovarian cyst[a]

Extra-abdominal causes:
- Myocardial infarction
- Pulmonary embolism
- Basal pneumonia
- Esophageal rupture
- Porphyria
- Herpes zoster
- Familial mediterranean fever
- Lead poisoning

[a]A recognized nonpancreatic cause of elevated amylase.

elevated bilirubin in predicting common bile duct stones as the cause (positive predictive value of 95 percent).[9] Hyperglycemia and hypoalbuminemia are common and there may be evidence of renal impairment. Blood gases show metabolic acidosis and hypoxemia. A plain abdominal X-ray may show ileus, sentinel loop (air-filled loop of jejunum next to the pancreas), or calcification in the pancreas suggesting chronic pancreatitis. An abdominal ultrasound scan (USS) should be obtained as early as possible as it may reveal gallstones, biliary tree dilatation, or an enlarged pancreas, and it is good at detecting fluid collections. A nonionic contrast-enhanced computed tomography (CT) scan of the abdomen gives ideal views of the pancreas and is more sensitive than USS (almost 100 percent at day 3–5) in identifying necrosis[10]—defined as a hypoperfused, nonenhancing area of > 30 percent or >3 cm in diameter on a CT scan[11] (see Fig. 79-1). A CT scan is not necessary in mild cases. CT scanning is mandatory in severe disease to assess the extent of necrosis and to investigate clinical deterioration in both mild and severe disease.[12] An MR scan of the pancreas and the biliary tree avoids use of a potentially harmful contrast, particularly in renal impairment, and also identifies biliary tree dilatation. Endoscopic ultrasound (EUS) is better than USS in detecting biliary sludge (95 vs 55 percent), but is rarely used during an acute attack. Laparotomy is now rarely required for diagnosis of acute pancreatitis. Once the diagnosis has been established by biochemical and radiological investigations, the severity and the cause of the attack should be documented.

Severity markers

These prognostic aids help in the management and appropriate use of healthcare resources. There are three main systems available—Acute Physiological and Chronic Health Evaluation (APACHE II), Ranson's criteria, and Glasgow score. APACHE score (75 percent sensitivity and 92 percent specificity) is

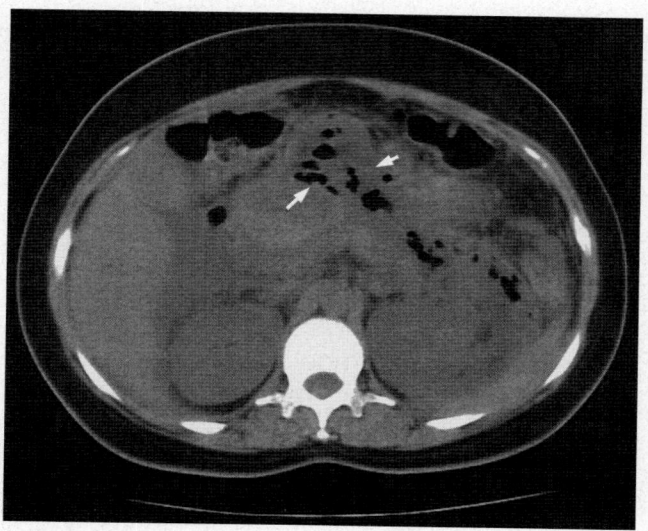

Figure 79-1 Infected pancreatic necrosis. CT scan showing nonenhancing pancreas with gas in retroperitoneum (white arrows).

available on admission, unlike Ranson's (72 percent sensitivity and 76 percent specificity) and Glasgow score, which are most suitably applied at 48 hours. Glasgow score, along with CRP (C-reactive protein), has a sensitivity of 80 percent and specificity of 87 percent and is relatively easy to use. A CT grading system can also be used: Grade A is normal pancreas and indicates minimal oedematous pancreatitis; Grade B reveals focal or diffuse enlargement of the gland; Grade C shows peripancreatic inflammation and <30 percent nonenhancement of the gland; Grade D has single fluid collection and 30–50 percent necrosis; and in Grade E there are multiple fluid collections and >50 percent necrosis of the gland.

Newer tests for assessment of severity include elevated serum polymorphonuclear cell elastase, serum phospholipase A2 urinary trypsin activation peptide and carboxypeptidase activation peptide. These await routine clinical use.

Treatment

Acute pancreatitis continues to have a significant mortality. An impact on this outcome will depend on early identification of the condition, an accurate assessment of its severity, and a multidisciplinary approach to the severe cases. Severe cases should be managed in a specialist setting (Fig. 79-2).

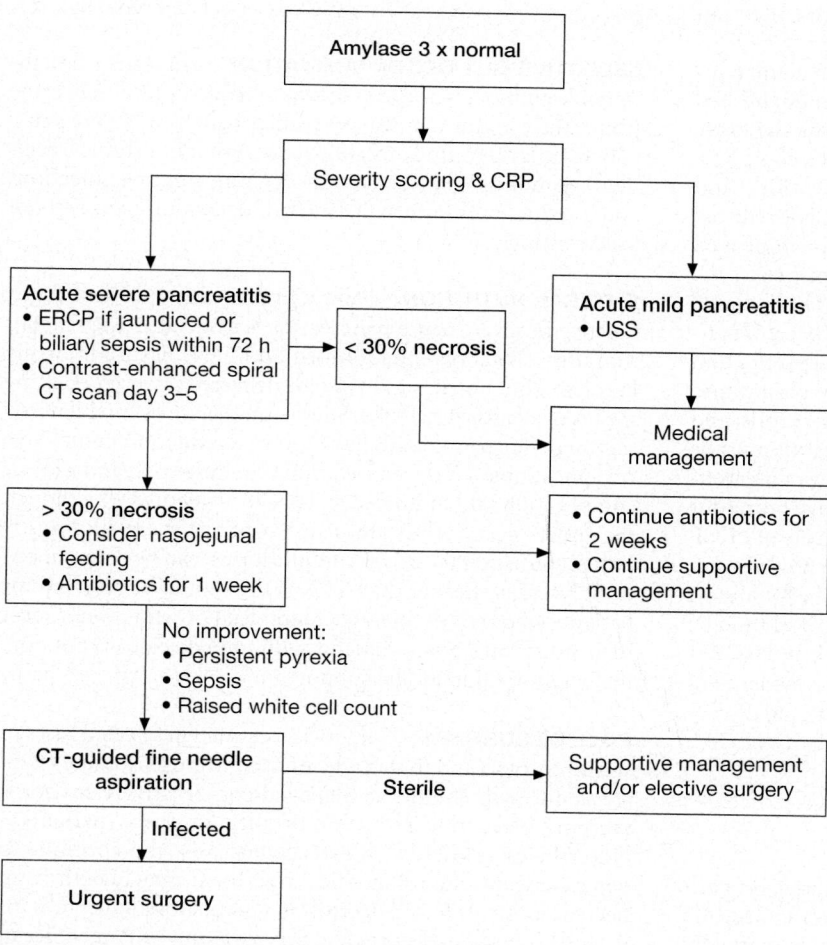

Figure 79-2 Management of acute pancreatitis.

Mild acute pancreatitis

A mild attack of pancreatitis can be managed on a general ward. Supportive measures include nil by mouth, intravenous fluids, and pain relief with opiates. We use patient-controlled analgesia (PCA) and prefer diamorphine for its superior analgesic properties. Daily review of the patient along with blood tests to ensure clinical and biochemical recovery is important. Rarely, a mild attack of pancreatitis will progress to a severe attack. Patients usually require 3–7 days of inpatient care.

Severe acute pancreatitis

The same simple supportive measures as mentioned above apply to patients with severe disease. Fluid resuscitation is particularly important because these patients suffer a significant intravascular volume loss. Inadequate hydration can lead to hypotension and acute tubular necrosis. Renal failure requiring hemofiltration or dialysis may persist beyond the acute stage. Fluid replacement needs to be carefully monitored to prevent peripheral and pulmonary edema, and inotropic support is often required. Hypoxia and lung injury are a common sequelae of severe pancreatitis. There is a significant intrapulmonary shunt, which, combined with ARDS, results in prolonged ventilation. Patients with severe disease are best managed on an intensive care unit in a specialist center, as a prolonged illness is not uncommon. The input of an expert multidisciplinary team is one of the few factors that can improve the outcome of these patients.

A variety of other therapies have been tried in acute pancreatitis. Antiprotease treatment has not yet been established in clinical practice. Aprotinin showed no benefit. Gabexate mesilate does not affect mortality but may reduce complications.[13] Meta-analysis of somatostatin, octreotide, and gabexate mesilate also suggested that gabexate mesilate reduced complications and octreotide and somatostatin improved outcome,[14] but the benefit of octreotide has not been confirmed in a subsequent study.[15] PAF antagonist (Lexipafant) and anti-inflammatory cytokine agents have not been of benefit in the clinical situation. Enhanced free-radical production and increased concentration of lipid peroxides in plasma and tissue have been found in patients with acute pancreatitis, and antioxidant trials are under way. Gallstone pancreatitis must be actively sought, as appropriately timed therapeutic intervention may alter the course of the disease. There have been four randomized controlled studies investigating the role of ERCP in biliary pancreatitis.[16–19] Three of these studies showed a significant reduction in complications, duration of hospital stay, and mortality.[16–18] These results suggest that ERCP should be performed within 72 hours of disease onset. Early ERCP is indicated only in severe pancreatitis where there is evidence of biliary sepsis or progressive jaundice. Those with mild disease and nonbiliary pancreatitis do not benefit from early ERCP.

Treatment of complications

Necrosis

This is characterized by focal or diffuse areas of nonviable pancreatic parenchyma. Mortality is very low when the necrotic area is not infected (sterile necrosis) but increases markedly once infection becomes established (infected necrosis) which occurs in approximately 30 percent of cases.[20] Infected necrosis should be suspected if there is a persistent fever, raised white cell count, high platelet count or deterioration of the clinical picture into the second week or thereafter. CT may suggest the diagnosis but confirmation by fine needle aspiration (FNA) and culture of an organism from the necrotic collection is needed. A single organism is responsible in 75 percent of cases and the majority of the organisms involved are gut derived. A quarter of patients develop infected necrosis in the first week but this figure increases to 70 percent by week 3.[21] Different approaches have been taken to reduce the rate of infected necrosis and are gaining wider acceptance.

PROPHYLACTIC ANTIBIOTICS Initial studies were disappointing as they invariably used antibiotics that exhibit poor penetration into the pancreas. Third-generation cephalosporins, fluoroquinolones, metronidazole, piperacillin, or imipenem are the antibiotics of choice.[22] More recent studies using combinations of these antibiotics have shown a significant reduction in infectious complications and a reduction in mortality.[23–25] A meta-analysis of eight controlled trials concluded that prophylactic antibiotics reduced mortality only in patients with severe acute pancreatitis who were treated with appropriate antibiotics.[26] Antibiotics should be commenced on admission in severe acute pancreatitis. Fungal infections occur in < 10 percent of patients. Antifungals are often used early in severe pancreatitis if there is associated renal failure.

SELECTIVE GUT DECONTAMINATION The use of nonabsorbable antibiotics has been shown to reduce infection in acute liver failure and it may have a similar benefit in severe acute pancreatitis. One study of gut decontamination (topical regimen) demonstrated a reduction in Gram negative infections and a reduction in mortality but gut decontamination is not used routinely.[27]

ENTERAL NUTRITION Failure to provide positive nitrogen balance in severe acute pancreatitis is associated with higher mortality. Total parenteral nutrition (TPN) has traditionally been used but nutrition can also be delivered safely enterally by means of a nasojejunal tube. Studies on the use of enteral nutrition in severe pancreatitis have shown a reduction in infective complications, a reduced inflammatory response, and a lower complication rate compared to TPN-fed patients,[28,29] although the most recent study does not confirm these findings.[30] Enteral nutrition has fewer complications, can be commenced earlier, and is cheaper than TPN. TPN should be reserved for patients who do not tolerate enteral feed or who do not meet their nutritional goals. Patients with mild disease do not normally require nutritional support.

ROLE OF SURGERY Surgery is indicated in selected cases of sterile necrosis and to debride infected necrosis. Patients with sterile necrosis should be managed conservatively as necrosectomy does not reduce mortality in these patients.[21] Nevertheless, patients with sterile necrosis who continue to deteriorate despite full medical treatment may benefit from necrosectomy. Infected necrosis is a mandatory indication for surgery and requires complete necrosectomy with a choice of lavage, drainage, secondary closure, and reoperation, all of which have similar outcome.

Cholecystectomy should be performed during the same admission or within 4 weeks in mild biliary pancreatitis to avoid recurrent attacks. In severe biliary pancreatitis, this should be delayed until complications settle, or performed during surgery if this is required to deal with other complications.

Pseudocyst

Acute fluid collections arising in or next to the pancreas that persist beyond 4 weeks become encased by a well defined wall of fibrous and granulation tissue, termed acute pseudocyst. Acute fluid collections occur in 30–50 percent of cases of which more than 50 percent will resolve spontaneously. Prolonged hyperamylasemia suggests development of a pseudocyst, but may also indicate continuing necrosis or abscess. Up to 60 percent of the asymptomatic pseudocysts will resolve spontaneously within 1 year. Those producing symptoms in the form of pain, fever, and biliary or duodenal obstruction require intervention in one of three ways: radiological percutaneous drainage, surgical drainage (internal or external), or endoscopic drainage. Percutaneous drainage has a high rate of recurrence of 63 percent and overall failure rate of 54 percent.[31] It is now rarely performed. Surgical external drainage is associated with a recurrence rate of 22 percent and mortality of 6 percent.[32] Internal drainage is by cystogastrostomy, cystoduodenostomy or Roux-en-Y cystojejunostomy with a recurrence rate of 0–17 percent, complication rate of 25 percent and mortality of 6 percent.[31,32] The trend in last few years has been toward using endoscopic techniques to deal with the pseudocysts, as the morbidity and mortality are lower.[33] Transpapillary cyst drainage is useful when the pseudocyst communicates with the pancreatic duct, which occurs in only 20 percent of cases. In this procedure, pancreatic sphincterotomy is performed with subsequent placement of a stent into the cyst that is left in situ for about 3 months. Transenteric drainage, either cystgastrostomy or cystduodenostomy, requires that the distance between pseudocyst and gastric or duodenal wall should be <1 cm and there should be a clear bulge into the lumen of the gut. A needle knife is used to puncture the cyst and stents are inserted to allow free drainage into the gut. The stents can be left in or removed with resolution of the cyst. Endoscopic techniques achieve resolution in over 80 percent of cases with recurrence rates of 6–18 percent and no mortality. The success of this technique is related to the expertise of the endoscopist. Pseudocysts, if left untreated may bleed, leak, rupture, or become infected. Infected pseudocyst or pancreatic abscess requires prolonged drainage but traditionally is treated by surgical intervention.

PANCREATIC DUCT LEAK Pancreatic fistulas arise from an area of duct disruption or from a leaking pseudocyst and may cause ascites, pleural effusion or mediastinal pseudocyst. External fistulae result from surgery or radiological intervention, whereas internal fistulae occur spontaneously. Treatment is by medical measures in the form of nil by mouth, TPN, nasojejunal feeding, octreotide, endoscopic stents, and surgery that entails a distal pancreatectomy or cystjejunostomy.

Prognosis

The overall mortality of acute pancreatitis has remained unchanged at 10–20 percent for the past two decades.[1] Mild acute pancreatitis has a low complication and death rate. The majority of the deaths (95 percent) occur in the severe form of the disease. Sterile necrosis has a mortality of 0–11 percent, whereas infected necrosis has mortality of at least 40 percent.[20] One-third of deaths related to severe acute pancreatitis occur within the first week of onset of the disease from multiorgan failure. The majority of deaths thereafter, are due to infections, particularly from infected pancreatic necrosis, which accounts for up to 80 percent of deaths in the group with necrotizing pancreatitis. Even before severity scoring, patients with significant comorbidity,[34] elderly patients,[35] obese patients with body mass index (BMI) >30, and cases due to certain causes, such as postoperative acute pancreatitis have the highest mortality.[36]

CHRONIC PANCREATITIS

Chronic pancreatitis (CP) is a progressive chronic inflammatory condition that leads to an irreversible destruction of pancreatic tissue, which can result in a loss of both exocrine and endocrine function. It was believed that CP was an inexorable process leading to pancreatic destruction. Current evidence suggests that the characteristic histological and functional features of CP are usually irreversible but the disease itself does not inevitably progress to pancreatic failure.

Pathology and pathogenesis

CP is characterized morphologically by varying degrees of edema, acute inflammation, and necrosis. These acute changes are superimposed on a background of chronic changes that include fibrosis, inflammation, and loss of exocrine tissue.[37] The ducts may be dilated and can contain protein plugs. These plugs are an early feature of CP produced by the precipitation of protein within the ducts and intraductal stones develop when calcium carbonate is deposited into the plugs.

A number of studies have tried to locate a single abnormal function that initiates the process of CP and ties in all the pathological features. Recent evidence suggests that there may be more than one defect needed to produce CP.[38] A reduction in ductal bicarbonate secretion is one of the earliest defects in CP, and in alcoholics there is a hypersecretion of protein.[39] It is postulated that this process is mediated by either an autoimmune process—CP is associated with other autoimmune diseases such as Sjögren's syndrome, primary biliary cirrhosis, and primary sclerosing cholangitis—or by a defect in the protein encoded by the cystic fibrosis gene (the cystic fibrosis transmembrane conductance regulator [CFTR]). CFTR functions as a cyclic adenosine monophosphate (c-AMP)-regulated chloride channel that enhances bicarbonate, sodium, and water movement across ductular epithelium. A defect in the CFTR function prevents adequate alkalinization and dilution of the pancreatic juice.[40] The protein-rich acinar secretions become increasingly viscous and inspissated causing plugs that obstruct the ducts. Protein plugs are an early finding in CP, and their endoscopic removal can improve a patient's pain.[41] CFTR mutations have been identified in 10–20 percent of patients with idiopathic chronic pancreatitis (normal prevalence 2.5–5 percent), which suggests a role in the disease.

The protein GP2, released from the apical cell, aggregates at pH < 7 contributing to plug formation in the nonalkalinized juice of early chronic pancreatitis. Pancreatic juice, which is supersaturated with calcium, contains inhibitors of calcium precipitation, which include lithostathine. Lithostathine production by apical cells is reduced in alcoholics with calcific chronic pancreatitis and may be a factor in the formation of pancreatic stones, although other factors including pH and citrate concentration may be involved.[38]

Sphincter of Oddi dysfunction, ischemia, and deficiency of antioxidants have also all been implicated in the pathophysiology of chronic pancreatitis but as yet no definite evidence of their respective roles have been demonstrated. Recurrent attacks of acute pancreatitis may result in chronic pancreatitis. The evidence for this assertion is anecdotal, as chronic pancreatitis is found in both alcohol-induced and hypertriglyceridemia-related acute pancreatitis. The transition of acute pancreatitis to CP has been more clearly defined in hereditary pancreatitis. In this disorder a mutation of the cationic trypsinogen gene facilitates premature activation of trypsin in the pancreas which results in autodigestion and attacks of acute pancreatitis. Chronic pancreatitis develops in the subset most seriously affected by acute pancreatitis, suggesting that recurrent inflammation may lead to fibrosis.[42]

Etiology

The prevalence of chronic pancreatitis is increasing, particularly in women, and the age of onset is decreasing. The frequency of the disease is lower in developed countries than in the Third World. In developed countries alcohol accounts for 60–70 percent of all cases and occurs most frequently in men aged 35–40 years. There is usually a long history (>6 years) of heavy alcohol consumption although the type of alcoholic beverage and the pattern of consumption—binge or continuous—varies. Tropical pancreatitis develops in young patients within 30° of the equator and is characterized by marked calcification, pancreatic insufficiency, and diabetes. It is believed to be due to either protein deficiency or ingestion of pancreatotoxins—cyanogens from cassava root.

Obstruction of the main pancreatic duct by tumor, posttraumatic scarring, pseudocysts or congenital abnormalities, such as pancreas divisum, can also produce chronic pancreatitis. This form of the disease is characterized by pancreatic duct dilatation, an absence of calcification, and exocrine dysfunction. These changes may improve when the obstruction is relieved.

Defects in the CFTR gene are commoner in patients with non-alcohol-induced chronic pancreatitis and the proposed role has been discussed previously. Hereditary pancreatitis—a defect in the cationic trypsinogen gene—is a familial disease that has a young age of onset where chronic pancreatitis develops following multiple attacks of acute pancreatitis.[7] Rarer causes of chronic pancreatitis include hyperlipidemia, hyperparathyroidism, and sclerosing pancreatopathy associated in up to 30 percent of cases of primary sclerosing cholangitis.

Where no obvious cause can be found, up to a third of cases, the disease is labeled as "idiopathic" chronic pancreatitis which has a peak incidence among 15–30-year-olds and a second peak in 50–70-year-olds.[37]

Clinical presentation

Persistent epigastric pain radiating through to the back is the main symptom of chronic pancreatitis. The pain is often associated with nausea and vomiting and is exacerbated by eating. Initially there may be discrete episodes of acute pain that gradually increase in frequency and may become continuous.[43] Colicky pain is unusual. The pain is multifactorial and due to a combination of increased intraductal pressure, increased pancreatic tissue pressure, pancreatitis-associated neuritis, pancreatic ischemia and ongoing pancreatic inflammation.[43] Pain disappears spontaneously in 30 percent of patients and does appear to be associated with an increase in exocrine insufficiency.[44]

Exocrine insufficiency occurs only when pancreatic lipase secretion is reduced to less than 10 percent of normal.[45] Patients with advanced exocrine insufficiency cannot digest or absorb the breakdown products of complex foods. Steatorrhea, due to maldigestion of fat, presents with the passage of loose, greasy, offensive stools that are difficult to flush away. Bloating, excessive flatus, and colicky abdominal pain are often present. In advanced chronic pancreatitis, lack of proteolytic enzyme production results in protein malnutrition and significant weight loss.

Glucose intolerance is not uncommon in chronic pancreatitis and diabetes develops late in the course of the disease. Diet and oral hypoglycemic agents usually suffice initially but 40 percent of all cases will progress to become insulin dependent. As the α-cells that produce glucagon are also affected, diabetic control is often brittle, and patients are at increased risk of treatment-related hypoglycemia.[46]

Investigation

Chronic pancreatitis is not a clinical diagnosis. There has to be some evidence of morphological or functional abnormality to substantiate the diagnosis (see Fig. 79-3).

Serum concentrations of pancreatic enzymes—amylase and lipase—are often raised in chronic pancreatitis but can be normal in more advanced disease. C-reactive protein is a good indicator of ongoing inflammation but is not specific. Abnormal liver function tests suggest a biliary stricture which occurs in 5–10 percent of cases or merely indicates coexistent liver disease. Fat malabsorption is demonstrated by measurement of a daily fecal fat excretion of >20 g/day (normal ≤ 7 g/day) while the patient eats a diet containing 100 g of fat per day.

Pancreatic calcification seen on plain abdominal X-ray confirms the diagnosis but is only found in 30 percent of cases (Fig. 79-4). USS has a reported sensitivity and specificity of 60 and 80 percent, respectively in detecting diagnostic features of chronic pancreatitis. CT is the imaging method of choice as it has a greater sensitivity and specificity (80 and 90 percent) and is superior for the detection of complications. Magnetic resonance cholangiopancreatography (MRCP), originally described in 1991, may become the standard diagnostic test for pancreatic duct morphology.[47] It is a useful tool for detecting main pancreatic duct abnormalities. MRCP is relatively insensitive for picking up early structural changes which are confined to the side branches and the normal main pancreatic duct may not be visualized in 20 percent of cases.[47] The main use for MRCP is where ERCP has failed, where there is an obstructed main pancreatic duct, or where the pancreatic

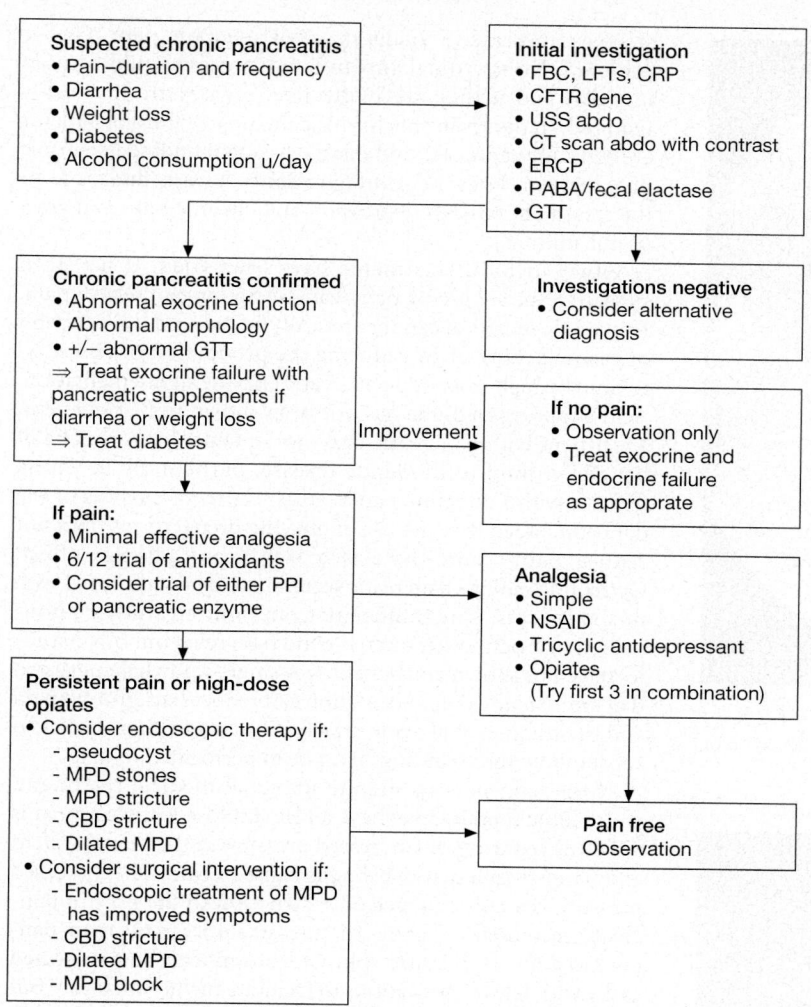

Figure 79-3 Management of chronic pancreatitis. FBC: full blood count LFT: liver function test; GTT; glucose tolerance test; MPD: main pancreatic duct; CBD: common bile duct; PPI: proton pump inhibitor.

duct is inaccessible endoscopically, i.e., post surgery. In most centers ERCP is still the "gold standard" imaging procedure for diagnosing chronic pancreatitis as it can demonstrate abnormalities of both the side branches and the main pancreatic duct (Fig. 79-5). Under the age of 60 a dilated main pancreatic duct and cyst-like abnormalities of the second-order ducts support the diagnosis of chronic pancreatitis. These findings may be normal in elderly people, so evidence of more gross ductal abnormalities is needed in this age group to establish the diagnosis.[48] Fat malabsorption can be demonstrated by measurement of a daily fecal fat excretion of >20 g/day (normal ≤ 7 g/day) while the patient eats a diet containing 100 g of fat per day. Endoscopic ultrasound (EUS) is a useful adjunct to other imaging techniques in the diagnosis of chronic pancreatitis.[49] In expert hands not only can EUS prove to be the best diagnostic tool but it also allows tissue diagnosis and therapy to be undertaken.

Pancreatic exocrine insufficiency was traditionally investigated by analysis of pancreatic secretions collected following duodenal intubation and stimulation with either hormones or a Lundh test meal. These "direct" pancreatic function tests have been superseded by less invasive and cumbersome "indirect"

tests. The two most commonly used tubeless tests—pancreolauryl and PABA (*N*-benzoyl-L-tyrosyl-*p*-aminobenzoic acid)—rely on pancreatic enzymes to cleave the compounds and release their respective markers which are recovered in the urine and measured. They both provide a good index of moderate to severe pancreatic insufficiency but are not valid in the presence of liver disease, renal failure, or intestinal malabsorption. Recently, measurement of the pancreatic enzyme elastase in stool samples has provided a simple and reliable method of assessing pancreatic exocrine function. It is also important to assess pancreatic endocrine function using a standard glucose tolerance test. Tests of pancreatic morphology and exocrine and endocrine function should be seen as complementary in establishing the diagnosis and monitoring the progression of chronic pancreatitis.

Treatment

Pain is present in up to 85 percent of cases and is the main symptom that requires treatment. The pain is multifactorial and often difficult to treat medically in 40 percent of cases.[50]

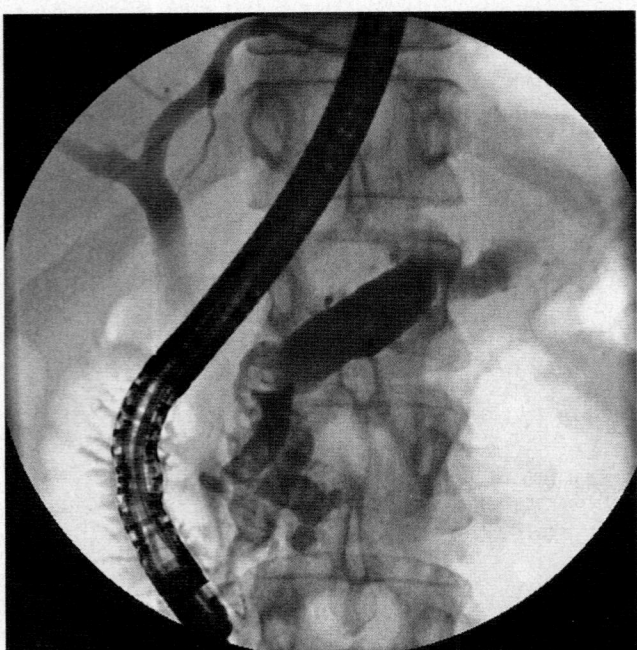

Figure 79-4 Chronic pancreatitis. ERCP demonstrating a grossly dilated main pancreatic duct, containing large stones, and ectatic side branches.

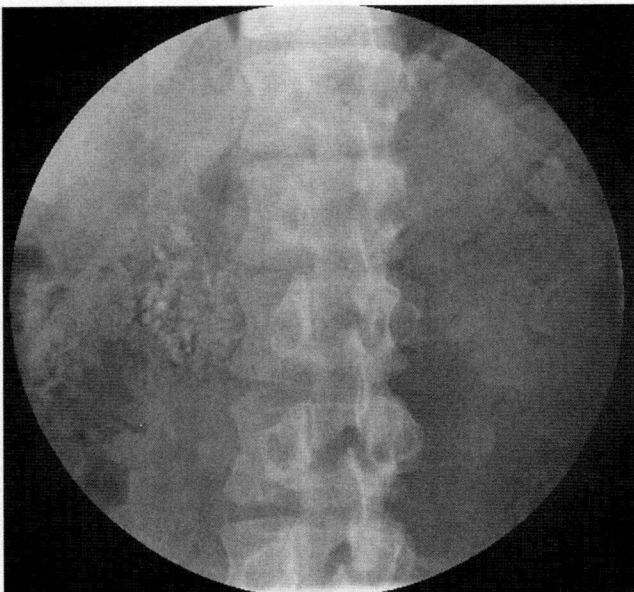

Figure 79-5 Pancreatic calcification on plain abdominal X-ray.

Once other causes of the pain have been ruled out the initial step in alcohol-induced disease is to stop smoking and alcohol consumption. This reduces the frequency and severity of painful attacks resulting in a better prognosis.[44,50] Acute exacerbations accompanied by vomiting often require hospital admission. In the acute setting, patient-controlled analgesia enables rapid pain relief and is a good indication of the progress of the attack. The treatment of chronic pain requires a stepwise increase in analgesia until adequate pain relief is achieved. Nonsteroidal anti-inflammatories should be used initially, and if they are ineffective, opiates are invariably required. In the setting of chronic pain, up to a third of patients are clinically depressed, and this is a frequent finding in chronic pancreatitis. Tricyclic antidepressants have a dual role in the treatment of both depression and chronic pain and are a useful adjunct.

Other medical treatments have been tried. It has been suggested that reducing pancreatic secretion can relieve pain. Pancreatic secretion can theoretically be reduced by reduction of gastric acidity or by reducing the production of cholecystokinin by high-dose oral pancreatic enzyme supplementation. Acid suppression alone has not been shown to be of benefit. Treatment with pancreatic enzymes in tablet form may be of benefit in mild to moderate disease, particularly in young females with idiopathic pancreatitis.[51] A meta-analysis of the data concluded that the use of enzyme preparations does not reduce pain[52] and there is a significant placebo effect. Octreotide inhibits pancreatic secretion and has been tried with mixed success. One multicenter randomized study demonstrated that octreotide offered good pain relief but other studies have not shown any benefit.[43] A single study has suggested that antioxidant supplementation can reduce background pain and the frequency of acute attacks[53] but no further studies to substantiate these findings have been performed to date.

If the pain persists despite maximal medical treatment, endoscopic therapy may have a role. Endoscopic treatment is aimed at reducing the increased pressure in the ductal system and parenchyma that may be the cause of pain. The increased pressure is a consequence of obstruction to the flow of pancreatic secretions either by strictures or stones in the main pancreatic duct. Pancreatic sphincterotomy can be performed easily with few complications to facilitate further therapy[54] but pain relief can be predicted if main pancreatic duct reduces in size immediately post sphincterotomy.[43] Strictures can be dilated but as stricture relapse is common pancreatic stent insertion is invariably required.[55] There are almost 400 pancreatic stent placements reported in the literature with a 10 percent complication rate.[54,55] Clinical improvement was observed in 50–93 percent of cases. When duct morphology was taken into account, obstruction with dilation was the most likely to predict a response to stenting, which may in turn predict a good response to surgical drainage.[55] Stenting the main pancreatic duct has never been subjected to a randomized controlled trial and is not without complication as the stents block at 4–6 months or produce further strictures that can alter the course of the disease.[54] For these reasons pancreatic duct stenting should only be performed in expert endoscopy centers in selected patients as a prelude to definitive surgery.

Pancreatic stones can obstruct the main pancreatic duct and their removal may improve symptoms. Patients with intermittent acute attacks and proximal mobile stones without evidence of pancreatic duct strictures are the most likely to benefit.[56] When endoscopic extraction alone fails it can be combined with extracorporeal shock-wave lithotripsy. Using these two techniques, stones can be removed in at least 50 percent of cases and pain relief achieved in up to 75 percent,[44,56] and in 50 percent of cases this may be long-term.

Surgery should be considered in chronic pancreatitis when severe pain persists despite full medical and endoscopic therapy. When there is a dilated duct a longitudinal pancreaticojejunostomy produces pain relief in about 65–80 percent of cases and may delay the progress of the disease.[57] A mass in the head of the pancreas, disease predominantly in the head or small duct disease are indications for pancreatic resection. Whipple procedure or duodenum-preserving resection of the head of the pancreas are both used in this setting and can produce pain relief in up to 90 percent of cases, with a mortality rate of <5 percent.[57] When longitudinal pancreaticojejunostomy is combined with a local resection of the head of the pancreas, similar results are achieved in terms of pain relief but there is a lower post-surgical rate of endocrine and exocrine insufficiency.[57]

Complications

Pseudocysts

A pseudocyst is a walled-off collection of pancreatic secretion that occur in up to 25 percent of patients with chronic pancreatitis (Fig. 79-6). Most pseudocysts are asymptomatic but only 9 percent resolve spontaneously and complications occur in up to 50 percent of cases—infection, rupture, obstruction, and hemorrhage—which cause 5–10 percent of all deaths in chronic pancreatitis.[33,58] Indications for drainage are presence of symptoms, enlargement of cyst, complications, or suspicion of malignancy.[33] There are three methods of pseudocyst drainage—percutaneous, surgical, and endoscopic. Percutaneous drainage under ultrasound or CT guidance is a simple and safe method of drainage. Aspiration alone has a high rate of recurrence and failure (>50 percent), and ideally continuous drainage via a catheter should be achieved, which has a success rate of >80 percent and a recurrence rate of <10 percent.[33]

Percutaneous drainage may result in a permanent external fistula, which is more likely if there is a stricture of the main pancreatic duct. Surgical treatment, usually cystgastrostomy or cystjejunostomy, is widely used. It has a high success rate and a low recurrence rate, but does have a small mortality rate. Percutaneous and surgical drainage have been compared and there appears to be no difference in the failure rates, rate of recurrence, or the need for subsequent surgery, but mortality rates were higher in the surgical group.[33] Endoscopic therapy is gaining increasing acceptance as it has a high success rate, low morbidity and mortality, and recurrence rates of <10 percent, but these figures are dependent on the expertise of the endoscopist. Endoscopic ultrasound-guided drainage can further advance this technique.[59] It is suggested that endoscopic drainage is the method of choice unless the pseudocyst contains debris or is recurrent. Percutaneous catheter drainage is the first choice for immature or infected pseudocysts and for poor-risk patients. Surgery is indicated for recurrent or multiple pseudocysts, if there is a suspicion of malignancy or when other methods have failed.

Pancreatic ascites

Pancreatic juice can leak into the peritoneal cavity either from a ruptured duct or pseudocyst. The high amylase content of the fluid is diagnostic. Nonmedical treatment, including aspiration, octreotide, nil by mouth, and parenteral nutrition is successful in half the cases but results in prolonged morbidity.[37] Surgery is inevitable when medical treatment fails but is often technically difficult and has limited success. Endoscopic decompression of the pancreatic duct by means of a transpapillary stent is safe and effective—90 percent resolution at 6 weeks—and should be considered as the initial management.[60]

Pseudoaneurysm

Pseudoaneurysms are the result of enzymatic or infective disruption of arterial walls. The arteries most frequently involved are splenic, gastroduodenal, pancreatoduodenal and hepatic. They occur in up to 5 percent of cases of chronic pancreatitis and carry a significant (90 percent) mortality if untreated.[45] All pseudoaneurysms require treatment either by radiological embolization or surgery.

Common bile duct and duodenal obstruction

Common bile duct obstruction as a result of fibrosis in the head of the pancreas occurs in up to 10 percent of cases. It presents with increased pain, fever, jaundice, or abnormal liver function tests, and initially requires endoscopic biliary stenting. If the stricture does not resolve then surgical biliary drainage is required.

Clinically significant duodenal stenosis causing pain and vomiting occurs in up to 5 percent of cases. Medical management is of little use and either endoscopic balloon dilatation or definitive surgery is required.

Cancer

Cancer complicates alcoholic and tropical chronic pancreatitis and hereditary pancreatitis carries a 40 percent risk of cancer by the age of 70. As yet there is no effective screening method and the development of a mass in the head of the pancreas associated with chronic pancreatitis remains a diagnostic dilemma.

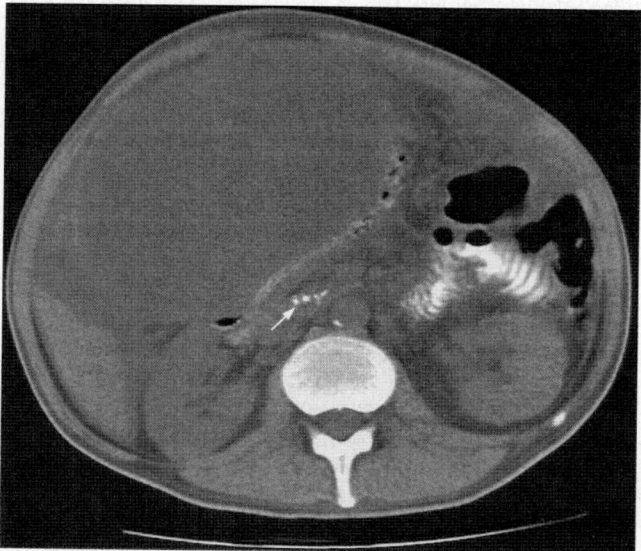

Figure 79-6 Pancreatic pseudocyst. Huge pseudocyst occurring in chronic pancreatitis. Pancreatic calcification clearly seen (white arrow).

Conclusions

Chronic pancreatitis is becoming more common. The diagnosis is often made on clinical grounds and not substantiated by full investigation. The chance of symptom relief is perceived as poor and treatment limited. A multidisciplinary approach involving thorough investigation and a logical progression of treatment in specialist centers can offer relief and hope to the majority of cases, and as more is understood about the pathogenesis the outlook is more optimistic.

CARCINOMA OF PANCREAS

Pancreatic adenocarcinoma is the tenth most common cancer and the fifth leading cause of death from all adult cancers in the Western world. In the last decade, the incidence in England and the USA has averaged an age-standardized incidence of 9 per 100,000 with slight preponderance in men.[61,62] The majority of the patients (about 60–70 percent) newly diagnosed with this disease are over 65 years of age. In the USA in 1996, there were 27,800 pancreatic cancer-related deaths, which correlated closely with the figures for newly diagnosed cases (26,300) in the following year.

Prognosis

Pancreatic carcinoma has a poor prognosis, as 85 percent of patients at the time of diagnosis will have an unresectable tumor. The overall 5-year survival remains 2–5 percent and has not changed significantly despite improved diagnosis and availability of newer adjuvant therapy.[63] Patients undergoing curative resection of histological proven disease have a 5-year survival of 10 percent (up to 20 percent in specialist centers).[62] Outcome is related to the size of the tumor, with tumors of ≤ 2 cm carrying the best prognosis.[64] Patients with locally invasive disease have a median survival of well under a year, and less than 6 months for metastatic disease.

Etiology and risk factors

As with most cancers, the etiology of pancreatic carcinoma is multifactorial. There are several known etiological and risk factors in the development of this cancer (Table 79-3). Early diagnosis provides the best chance of successful therapy. The development of a screening program aimed at detecting resectable tumors needs adequate identification of these risk factors.

Pathology

Pancreatic cancer arises from ductal cells of the exocrine portion in over 85 percent of cases. The commonest site is the head of the gland (about 70–80 percent). This often results in obstruction to the flow of the pancreatic juices and occasionally distal pancreatitis. The associated areas of papillary hyperplasia suggest multicentric origin of these cancers but this has not been confirmed. K-*ras* mutation is implicated in pathogenesis of up to 90 percent of pancreatic cancers. Other mutations, in p53 and CDKN2 genes, are found in 50–60 percent

Table 79-3 Risk factors for carcinoma of the pancreas

Age
Male
Black
Cigarette smoking (constitutes probably a quarter of all cases; the relative risk is double compared to nonsmokers)
Diet (increased risk with high fat, high in meat and fish, and low in fruit and vegetable)
Heavy coffee consumption (inconclusive evidence)
Occupational exposure to industrial toxins (nitrosamines, solvents, petroleum compounds)
Longstanding diabetes mellitus (DM) (likely to be a result rather than cause, due to hormonal alterations induced by the tumor)
Alcoholism
Chronic pancreatitis
Tropical pancreatitis
Inherited predisposition
- Hereditary pancreatitis (compared to the general population, 53-fold higher incidence, with cumulative risk of ≈ 40 percent by age 70)
- Lynch syndrome II
- Familial adenomatous polyposis (FAP)
- Peutz Jeghers syndrome
- Von Hippel Lindau disease
- Ataxia telangiectasia
- Gardner's syndrome
- Familial atypical multiple-mole melanosis syndrome (FAMMM)
- Familial pancreatic cancer (BRCA2 gene germline mutation)
Intraductal papillary mucinous tumor
Cystic fibrosis
Alzheimer's disease (inconclusive evidence)

of cancers.[65] The remaining 15 percent of the exocrine and nonexocrine tumors of the pancreas may arise in the acinar or the islet cells (endocrine tumors). Acinar carcinomas are rare and have mixed cellular differentiation.

It is important to differentiate between the rare cystadenocarcinomas that are ductal in origin and have a better prognosis (5-year survival is 50 percent), than adenocarcinomas.[66] Lymphomas (nonepithelial tumors) represent 5 percent of all pancreatic tumors and appear as large masses (>6 cm) with extrapancretic extension and prominent retroperitoneal lymph nodes. Surgery should be avoided and diagnosis made by fine needle aspiration, as these respond well to chemotherapy.

Clinical presentation

Patients with pancreatic carcinoma may be discovered incidentally or may present with myriad of symptoms. The classical presentation is with a triad of weight loss, painless obstructive jaundice and a palpable gall bladder (Courvoisier's sign). However, only a few cases present in this manner. The intractable pain in the upper abdomen passes through to the back, often follows a meal and is worse in reclining position; a feature found in only 30 percent of advanced cases. Ascites, if present, is almost invariably due to peritoneal carcinomatosis, but portal vein occlusion or hypoalbuminemia may also contribute. In elderly people, a new onset of diabetes can be the initial sign of pancreatic cancer. In about 10–15 percent, glucose intolerance develops 6–12 months before the diagnosis.

Differential diagnosis

The nonspecific presentation often results in a delayed diagnosis. Ampullary carcinoma can present similarly but is often accompanied by blood loss in addition to jaundice. Jaundice could be due to cholangiocarcinoma or due to benign disease such as common bile duct stones or intrahepatic cholestasis. In 5–10 percent of resected specimens for pancreatic cancer, chronic pancreatitis will be the only finding (and vice versa).[66] Pancreatic pseudocysts should be needled with caution to avoid a misdiagnosis of cystic adenocarcinomas. The history and CT findings should help, but if in doubt surgical biopsy of the wall should be obtained.

Investigations

Work-up of pancreatic cancer includes making a diagnosis followed by staging to assess respectability. Transabdominal ultrasound scan is often the first-line test, particularly in a jaundiced patient, as it effectively demonstrates the presence of biliary tree dilatation. Doppler probe will determine the portal venous flow. However, in about 10 percent of cases, views of the pancreas may be limited by overlying bowel gas.[67] USS is also unable to detect small liver metastases and provides little information on the anatomical layout and resectability. Dual-phase contrast-enhanced helical (spiral) CT scan is universally accepted as the best mode of investigation for diagnosis and assessment of resectability of pancreatic cancer (Fig. 79-7). It has a sensitivity of 98 percent for diagnosis (of tumors >2 cm) and specificity of 70 percent. In one study, 75 percent of patients were resectable when judged to be so on helical CT.[67] It gives reasonably accurate findings about tumor invasion, liver metastases bigger than 1 cm, vascular involvement, and the presence of ascites. However, lymph node involvement and peritoneal seedling smaller than 2 mm may be missed on the spiral CT. Magnetic resonance imaging (MRI) with gadolinium contrast offers little advantage over dual-phase spiral CT other than an increased sensitivity in identifying smaller peritoneal metastases (1–2 mm).[66] Of the several tumor markers that are available, CA 19–9 is the most widely used. It has varying degrees of sensitivity (40–92 percent) and specificity (60–99 percent), and is also elevated in pancreatitis and other tumors like biliary, gastric, colon.[68] The higher the level of CA19-9, the more sensitive and specific the test appears to be. At a level of 250 u/mL, the specificity is of the order of 95 percent.[68] This test is more valuable during follow-up of treatment, rather than as a diagnostic or screening tool.

The value of ERCP lies in its diagnostic and therapeutic abilities. Diagnostic ERCP is useful in those with equivocal or negative CT and has a sensitivity of 90–97 percent and specificity of 81–90 percent.[69] ERCP can help differentiate chronic pancreatitis from pancreatic cancer as it allows for bushings, fluid aspirates or biopsies to be taken with a yield of 92–100 percent specificity, but only 30–79 percent sensitivity.[70] Findings supportive of pancreatic cancer are "double duct sign" where there is an abrupt cutoff of both pancreatic and biliary duct (Fig. 79-8), or irregular stenosis of the main pancreatic duct. Therapeutic ERCP, with placement of biliary stents in a patient with jaundice should be restricted to palliative care and episodes of cholangitis or delay in surgery, and should be avoided in patients imminently proceeding to surgical resection (anecdotal risks of introducing infection).

EUS has taken the work-up of pancreatic cancer a step further with its sensitivity greater than 90 percent and staging accuracy of 80–97 percent.[71] It offers superior visualization of local tumor invasion and lymph node involvement compared to spiral CT. Laparoscopy and laparoscopic ultrasound may allow better assessment of resectability and of peritoneal involvement but their cost-effectiveness remains unconfirmed

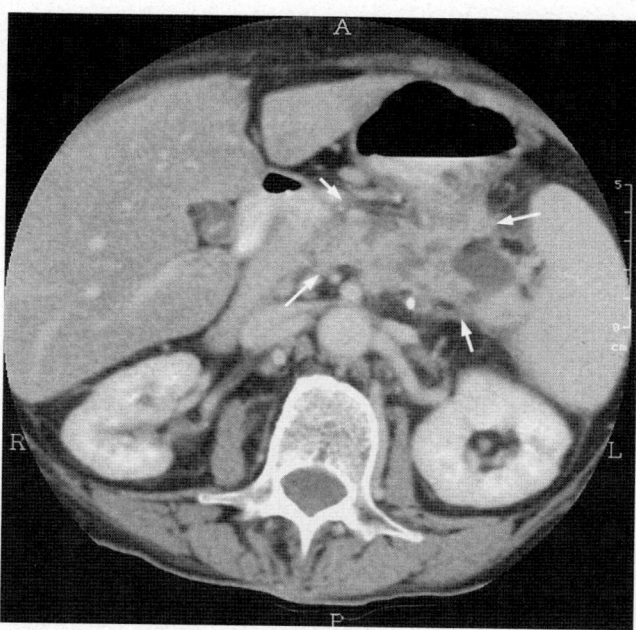

Figure 79-7 Carcinoma of the pancreas. Large heterogenous mass in body of pancreas (white arrows).

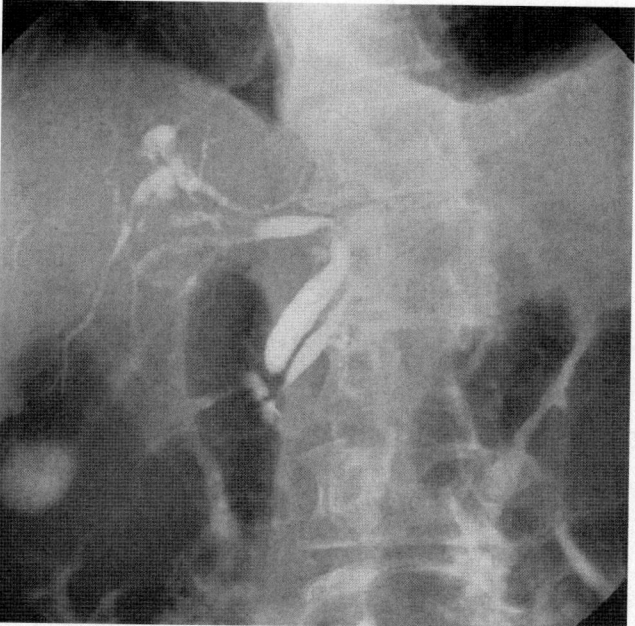

Figure 79-8 "Double duct" sign in carcinoma of the pancreas. Stricture of both common bile duct and main pancreatic duct.

and they are invasive and require skill. Angiography used to be performed to assess vascular anomalies and invasion, but with the advent of spiral CT it is now only performed in selected cases. CT or US guided fine-needle biopsy of suspected pancreatic cancer is best avoided in resectable cases because of concerns, albeit less evidence-based, of tumor cell seeding of the needle tract or peritoneal spread. In inoperable cases or when there is possibility of another cause for a mass in the pancreas, e.g., lymphoma, a tissue biopsy for histological diagnosis is advisable. EUS guided needle biopsy shares similar sensitivity (about 90 percent) to CT guided biopsy and may obviate the risk of tumor seeding of the needle tract.[72]

Treatment (Fig. 79-9)

Resectable disease

Curative surgical resection of pancreatic cancer is the only treatment that achieves long-term survival. Only 10–15 percent of newly diagnosed cancers will be found resectable on spiral CT. The CT criteria for resectability are: absence of extrapancreatic tumor spread; patent superior mesenteric and portal vein confluence; and no direct tumor invasion of coeliac axis or superior mesenteric artery. Pancreaticoduodenectomy (Whipple procedure) is the surgical procedure of choice for cancer in the head of the gland. The perioperative morbidity and mortality of this procedure has been found to be higher in elderly people over 70 years of age compared to younger patients, 39.1 vs 21.5 percent and 4.3 vs 1.9 percent, respectively. Distal pancreatectomy is performed for tumors in the body and tail of pancreas. The outcome of surgery will depend on the preoperative condition of the patient. Associated comorbid diseases and the nutritional state, which are frequent concerns in elderly people, influence this. Local recurrence occurs in up to 85 percent of patients undergoing surgery. Further clinical responses can be achieved with the use of postoperative adjuvant or neoadjuvant chemotherapy or chemoradiotherapy (combined modalities). Postoperative adjuvant therapy was developed with intentions of eradicating residual disease. Initial enthusiasm for the use of single agents such as fluorouracil (5-FU), chlorambucil, and mitomycin gave way to disappointment with the advent of CT assessment of tumor response. Subsequently, external-beam radiation therapy

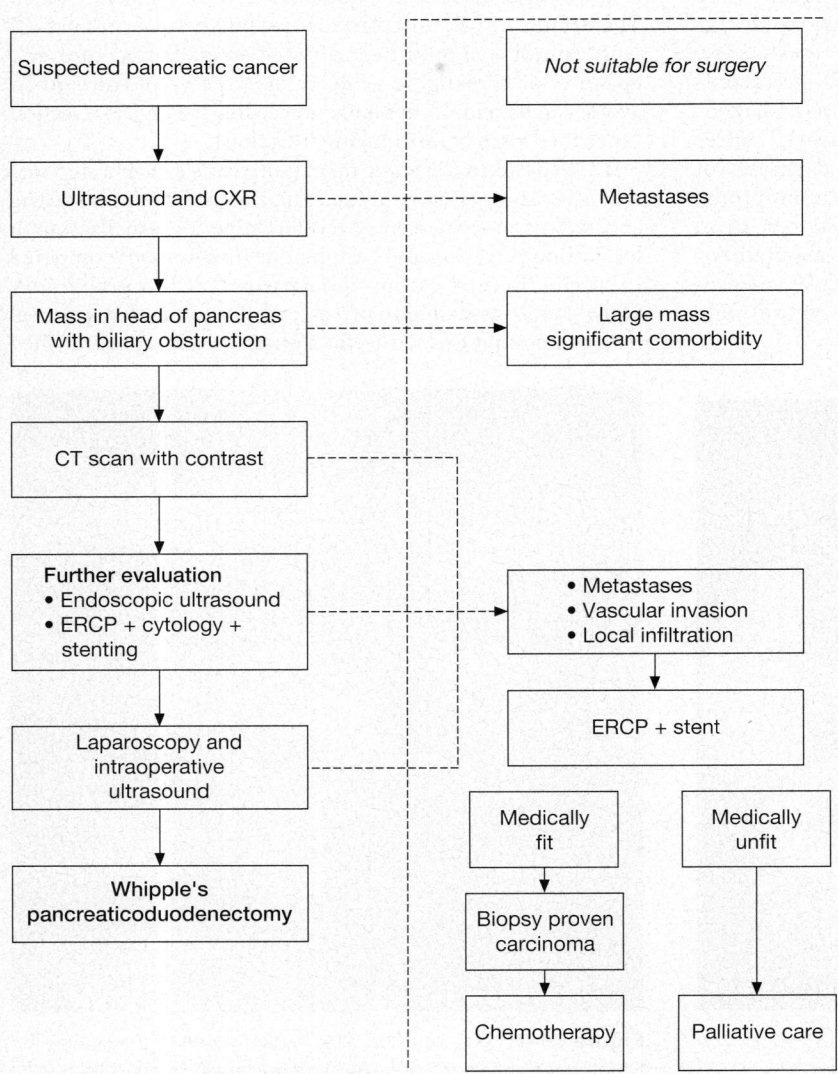

Figure 79-9 Diagnosis and management of carcinoma of the pancreas.

combined with 5-FU (postoperative neoadjuvant chemoradiation) showed prolongation of survival by 4–6 months compared to surgery alone, but without significant impact on the 5-year survival.[73] Further data are awaited from a European trial comparing surgery alone, chemoradiation with 5-FU, 5-FU based chemoradiation followed by systemic 5-FU and leucovorin, and 5-FU with leucovorin alone.[74] Neoadjuvant (preoperative) chemoradiotherapy is currently only available in protocol setting. The rationale of this treatment is several-fold: to detect undetectable metastasis (repeat CT after treatment revealed liver metastasis in 25 percent); to turn unresectable into resectable disease; to improve survival of resectable tumors with the advantage of avoidance of delay in commencing therapy in prolonged postoperative recovery.

Nonresectable disease

Locally invasive and metastatic pancreatic cancer markedly reduces survival and quality of life of the patients. Palliative treatment is indicated, aimed at prolonging survival and improving the symptoms. Not every patient is suitable for what may be an invasive or relatively toxic treatment, and they should be carefully selected with paramount importance to their best interests. The available modes of palliative therapy are: chemotherapy, radiotherapy, endoscopy, and surgery.

Much has been achieved in control of pain associated with terminal cancers. Nonsteroidals and opiates, coeliac plexus block or thoracic splanchnisectomy, and radiotherapy (which will help pain in 60 percent)[75] are various means of providing pain relief. Chemotherapy using 5-FU or gemcitabine alone, or in combination with radiotherapy (chemoradiotherapy) can prolong survival by few months. Gemcitabine has been found to produce a clinical benefit in 24 percent, with a survival of 5.7 months compared to 4.4 months with 5-FU monotherapy in the treatment of advanced disease.[76] Chemoradiation (using 5-FU) has been shown to prolong survival for 10 months vs 5.5 months with radiotherapy alone in locally advanced disease.[77] However, 2-year survival remained unchanged in both groups.

Endoscopy is a useful method of inserting stents for symptomatic biliary obstruction. This may also be performed as a prophylactic measure in asymptomatic individual commencing chemotherapy. Metal stents, although more expensive than plastic stents, last longer (half-life of 6 months vs 3 months). The percutaneous transhepatic approach may be necessary when endoscopic access has failed. Subsequent stenting can either be performed percutaneously or combined with endoscopy. Palliative gastrojejunostomy is a surgical procedure undertaken for palliative treatment of gastric outlet obstruction but endoscopic placement of a duodenal metal stent achieves the same result with less morbidity and mortality.

Adequate analgesia, invariably with opiates, is a vital aspect of terminal care that needs careful and sympathetic management. Other measures that are necessary include treatment of diabetes (requires insulin), of steatorrhea (pancreatic enzyme supplements), and of pruritus (with bile salt binders—cholestyramine or ursodeoxycholic acid, anti-histamines and opiates if severe) and enteral supplements for nutrition. Hospice care is required to support the patient and family when all other measures fail.

REFERENCES

1. Beckingham IJ, Bornman PC: ABC of diseases of liver, pancreas and biliary system: acute pancreatitis. Br Med J 2001;322:595–598
2. Wilson C, Imrie CW: Changing patterns of incidence and mortality from acute pancreatitis in Scotland, 1961–1985. Br J Surg 1990;77(7):731–734
3. Corfield AP, Cooper MJ, Williamson RC: Acute pancreatitis: a lethal disease of increasing incidence. Gut 1985;26(7):724–729
4. Steer ML: Pathogenesis of acute pancreatitis. Digestion 1997;58(suppl 1):46–49
5. Ros E, Navarro S, Bru C, Garcia-Puges A, Valderrama R: Occult microlithiasis in "idiopathic" acute pancreatitis: prevention of relapses by cholecystectomy or ursodeoxycholic acid therapy. Gastroenterology 2001;101(6):1701–1709
6. Lee SP, Nicholls JF, Park HZ: Biliary sludge as a cause of acute pancreatitis. N Engl J Med 1992;326:589–593
7. Whitcomb DC: The spectrum of complications of hereditary pancreatitis. Pancreas update. Gastroenterol Clin North Am 1999;28(3):525–541
8. Dickson AP, Imrie CW: The incidence and prognosis of body wall ecchymosis in acute pancreatitis. Surg Gynecol Obstet 1984;159(4):343–347
9. Tenner S, Dubner H, Steinberg W: Predicting gallstone pancreatitis with laboratory parameters: a meta-analysis. Am J Gastroenterol 1994;89(10):1863–1866
10. Larvin M, Chalmers AG, McMahon MJ: Dynamic contrast enhanced computed tomography: a precise technique for identifying and localising pancreatic necrosis. Br Med J 1990;300:1425–1428
11. Bradley EL: A clinically based classification system for acute pancreatitis. Summary of the International Symposium on Acute Pancreatitis, Atlanta, Ga, September 11–13, 1992. Arch Surg 1993;128(5):586–590
12. Balthazar EJ, Robinson DL, Megibow AJ, Ranson JH: Acute pancreatitis: value of CT in establishing prognosis. Radiology 1990;174:331–336
13. Messori A, Rampazzo R, Scroccaro G: Effectiveness of gabexate mesilate in acute pancreatitis. A meta-analysis. Dig Dis Sci 1995;40:734–738
14. Andriulli A, Leandro G, Clemente R: Meta-analysis of somatostatin, octreotide and gabexate mesilate in the therapy of acute pancreatitis. Aliment Pharmacol Ther 1998;12:237–245
15. Uhl W, Buchler M, Malfertheiner P et al: A randomised, double blind, multicentre trial of octreotide in moderate to severe acute pancreatitis. Gut 1999;45:97
16. Widdison AL, Karanjia ND: Pancreatic infection complicating acute pancreatitis. Br J Surg 1993;80:148–154
17. Fan ST, Mok FP, Lo CM, Zheng SS, Wong J: Early treatment of acute biliary pancreatitis by endoscopic papillotomy. N Engl J Med 1993;328(4):228–232
18. Neoptolemos JP, Carr-Locke DL, London NJ et al: Controlled trial of urgent endoscopic retrograde cholangiopancreatography and endoscopic sphincterotomy versus conservative treatment for acute pancreatitis due to gallstones. Lancet 1988;2:979–983
19. Nowak A, Nowakowsca-Dulawa E, Marek TA, Rybicka J: Final results of the prospective, randomised, controlled study on endoscopic sphincterotomy versus conventional management in acute biliary pancreatitis. Gastroenterology 1995;108:A380 (abstract)
20. Folsch UR, Nitsche R, Ludtke R, Hilgers RA, Creutzfeldt W: Early ERCP and papillotomy compared with conservative treatment for acute biliary pancreatitis. The German Study Group on Acute Biliary Pancreatitis. N Engl J Med 1997;336(4):237–242

21. Bradley EL, Allen K: A prospective longitudinal study of observation versus surgical intervention in the management of necrotizing pancreatitis. Am J Surg 1991;161(1):19–24

22. Buchler M, Malfertheiner P, Freiss H: Human pancreatic tissue concentration of bactericidal antibiotics. Gastroenterology 1987;103:1902–1908

23. Pederzoli P, Bassi C, Vesentini S, Campedelli A: A randomized multicenter clinical trial of antibiotic prophylaxis of septic complications in acute necrotizing pancreatitis with imipenem. Surg Gynecol Obstet 1993;176(5):480–483

24. Sainio V, Kemppainen E, Puolakkainen P et al: Early antibiotic treatment in acute necrotising pancreatitis. Lancet 1995;346:663–667

25. Delcenserie R, Yzet T, Ducroix JP: Prophylactic antibiotics in treatment of severe acute alcoholic pancreatitis. Pancreas 1996;13(2):198–201

26. Golub R, Siddiqi F, Pohl D: Role of antibiotics in acute pancreatitis: A meta analysis. J Gastrointest Surg 1998;2:496–503

27. Luiten EJ, Hop WC, Lange JF, Bruining HA: Controlled clinical trial of selective decontamination for the treatment of severe acute pancreatitis. Ann Surg 1995;222:57–65

28. Kalfarentzos F, Kehagias J, Mead N, Kokkinis K, Gogos CA: Enteral nutrition is superior to parenteral nutrition in severe acute pancreatitis: results of a randomized prospective trial. Br J Surg 1997;84(12):1665–1669

29. Windsor AC, Kanwar S, Li AG, Barnes E et al: Compared with parenteral nutrition, enteral feeding attenuates the acute phase response and improves disease severity in acute pancreatitis. Gut 1998;42(3):431–435

30. Powell JJ, Murchison JT, Fearon KC, Ross JA, Siriwardena AK: Randomized controlled trial of the effect of early enteral nutrition on markers of the inflammatory response in predicted severe acute pancreatitis. Br J Surg 2000;87(10):1375–1381

31. Gumaste UV, Dave PB: Pancreatic pseudocyst drainage—the needle or the scalpel? J Clin Gastroenterol 1991;13(5):500–505

32. Bradley EL, Gonzalez AC, Clements JL Jr: Acute pancreatic pseudocysts: incidence and implications. Ann Surg 1976;184(6):734–737

33. Pitchumoni CS, Agarwal N: Pancreatic pseudocysts: when and how should drainage be performed? Gastroenterol Clin North Am 1999;28(3):615–639

34. De Bolla AR, Obeid ML: Mortality in acute pancreatitis. Ann R Coll Surg Engl 1984;66(3):184–186

35. Fan ST, Choi TK, Lai CS, Wong J: Influence of age on the mortality from acute pancreatitis. Br J Surg 1988;75(5):463–466

36. Thompson JS, Bragg LE, Hodgson PE, Rikkers LF: Postoperative pancreatitis. Surg Gynecol Obstet 1988;167(5):377–380

37. Steer ML, Waxman I, Freedman SD: Chronic pancreatitis. New Engl J Med 1995;332:1482–1490

38. Freedman SD: New concepts in understanding the pathophysiology of chronic pancreatitis. Int J Pancreatol 1998;24(1):1–8

39. Sahel J, Sarles H: Modifications of pure human pancreatic juice induced by chronic alcohol consumption. Dig Dis Sci 1979;24:897–905

40. Cohn JA, Bornstein JD, Jowell PS: Cystic fibrosis mutations and genetic predisposition to idiopathic chronic pancreatitis. Med Clin North Am 2000;84(3):621–631

41. Harada H, Miyake H, Miki H, Kibayashi T, Sasaki T: Role of endoscopic elimination of protein plugs in the treatment of chronic pancreatitis. Gastroenterol Jap 1982;17:463–468

42. Whitcomb DC: The spectrum of complications of Hereditary Pancreatitis. Pancreas Update. Gastroenterol Clin North Am 1999;28(3):525–541

43. Pitchumoni CS: Chronic pancreatitis: Pathogenesis and management of pain. J Clin Gastroenterol 1998;27:101–107

44. Naruse S, Kitagawa M, Ishiguro H et al: Chronic pancreatitis: Overview of medical aspects. Pancreas 1997;16:323–328

45. Banks PA, Feldman M, Scharschmidt BF, Sleisenger MH: (eds): Acute and chronic pancreatitis. Sleisenger & Fordtran's Gastrointestinal and Liver Disease, 6th Ed. WB Saunders Company, Philadelphia, 1998:809–862

46. Mergener K, Baillie J: Chronic pancreatitis. Lancet 1997;350:1379–1385

47. Barish MA, Yucel EK, Ferrucci JT: Magnetic resonance cholangiopancreatography. New Engl J Med 1999;341(4):258–264

48. Jones SN, McNeil NI, Lees WR: The interpretation of retrograde pancreatography in the elderly. Clin Radiol 1984;40:393–396

49. Zuccaro G, Sterling MJ, Van Dam I, Sivak MV (eds): Endosonography in pancreatic disease. Gastrointestinal Endosonography, 1st Ed. WB Saunders Company, Philadelphia, 1999:235–243

50. Gullo L: Medical treatment of chronic pancreatitis. Ann Ital Chir 2000;LXXI:33–37

51. Apte MV, Keogh GW, Wilson JS: Chronic pancreatitis: complications and management. J Clin Gastroenterol 1999;29(3):225–240

52. Brown A, Hughes M, Tenner S, Banks PA: Does pancreatic enzyme supplementation reduce pain in patients with chronic pancreatitis: a meta-analysis. Am J Gastroenterol 1997;92:2032–2035

53. Uden S, Bilton D, Nathan L et al: Antioxidant therapy for recurrent pancreatitis: placebo-controlled trial. Aliment Pharmacol Ther 1990;4:357–371

54. Jakobs R, Riemann JF: The role of endoscopy in pancreatitis and pancreatic cancer. Gastroenterol Clin North Am 1999;28(3):783–800

55. Geenen JE: Benign pancreatic duct strictures: medical and endoscopic therapy. Can J Gastroenterol 2000;14(2):127–129

56. Howell DA: Pancreatic stones: treat or ignore? Can J Gastroenterol 1999;13(6):461–465

57. Izbicki JR, Bloechle C, Knoefel WT, Rogiers X, Kuechler T: Surgical treatment of chronic pancreatitis and quality of life after operation. Surg Clin North Am 1999;79(4):913–944

58. Levy P, Milan C, Pignon JP, Baetz A, Bernades P: Mortality factors associated with chronic pancreatitis. Gastroenterology 1989;96:1165–1172

59. Pitchumoni CS, Agarwal N: Pancreatic pseudocysts: when and how should drainage be performed? Gastroenterol Clin North Am 1999;28(3):615–639

60. Chak A: Endosonographic-guided therapy of pancreatic pseudocysts. Gastrointest Endosc 2000;52(6(suppl)):S23–S27

61. Bracher GA, Manocha AP, De Banto JR et al: Endoscopic pancreatic duct stenting to treat pancreatic ascites. Gastrointest Endosc 1999;46(6):710–715

62. Bramhall SR, Allum WH, Jones AG et al: Treatment and survival in 13,560 patients with pancreatic cancer, and incidence of the disease, in the West Midlands: an epidemiological study. Br J Surg 1995;82(1):111–115

63. Niederhuber JE, Brennan MF, Menck HR: The National Cancer Data Base report on pancreatic cancer. Cancer 1995;76(9):1671–1677

64. Conlon KC, Klimstra DS, Brennan MF: Long-term survival after curative resection for pancreatic ductal adenocarcinoma. Clinicopathologic analysis of 5-year survivors. Ann Surg 1996;223(3):273–279

65. Nitecki SS, Sarr MG, Colby TV, van Heerden JA: Long-term survival after resection for ductal adenocarcinoma of the pancreas. Is it really improving? Ann Surg 1995;221(1):59–66

66. Howe JR, Conlon KC: The molecular genetics of pancreatic cancer. Surg Oncol 1997;6(1):1–18

67. Evans JD, Morton DG, Neoptolemos JP: Chronic pancreatitis and pancreatic carcinoma. Postgrad Med J 1997;73:543–548

68. Gloor B, Todd KE, Reber HA: Diagnostic workup of patients with suspected pancreatic carcinoma: the University of California-Los Angeles approach. Cancer 1997;79(9):1780–1786

69. Niederau C, Grendell JH: Diagnosis of pancreatic carcinoma. Imaging techniques and tumor markers. Pancreas 1992;7(1):66–86

70. Shemesh E, Czerniak A, Nass S, Klein E: Role of endoscopic retrograde cholangiopancreatography in differentiating pancreatic cancer coexisting with chronic pancreatitis. Cancer 1990;65(4):893–896

71. McGuire DE, Venu RP, Brown RD et al: Brush cytology for pancreatic carcinoma: an analysis of factors influencing results. Gastrointest Endosc 1996;44(3):300–304

72. Chang KJ, Nguyen P, Erickson RA, Durbin TE, Katz KD: The clinical utility of endoscopic ultrasound-guided fine-needle aspiration in the diagnosis and staging of pancreatic carcinoma. Gastrointest Endosc 1997;45(5):387–393

73. Brugge WR: The role of endoscopic ultrasound in pancreatic disorders. Int J Pancreatol 1996;20(1):1–10

74. Yeo CJ, Abrams RA, Grochow LB et al: Pancreaticoduodenectomy for pancreatic adenocarcinoma: postoperative adjuvant chemoradiation improves survival. A prospective, single-institution experience. Ann Surg 1997;225(5):621–633

75. Neoptolemos JP, Baker P, Beger H et al: Progress report. A randomized multicenter European study comparing adjuvant radiotherapy, 6-mo chemotherapy, and combination therapy vs no-adjuvant treatment in resectable pancreatic cancer (ESPAC-1). Int J Pancreatol 1997;21(2):97–104

76. Watanapa P, Williamson RC: Surgical palliation for pancreatic cancer: developments during the past two decades. Br J Surg 1992;79(1):8–20

77. Burris HA 3rd, Moore MJ, Andersen J et al: Improvements in survival and clinical benefit with gemcitabine as first-line therapy for patients with advanced pancreas cancer: a randomized trial. J Clin Oncol 1997;15(6):2403–2413

78. Moertel CG, Frytak S, Hahn RG et al: Therapy of locally unresectable pancreatic carcinoma: a randomized comparison of high dose (6000 rads) radiation alone, moderate dose radiation (4000 rads + 5-fluorouracil), and high dose radiation + 5-fluorouracil: The Gastrointestinal Tumor Study Group Cancer. Cancer 1981;48(8):1705–1710

Chapter 80

The liver

Oliver F. W. James

STRUCTURE, FUNCTION, AND AGE

Structure

The liver reaches maximum size in early adult life, and thereafter there is a decrease in liver volume, both in absolute terms and in relation to body weight, which is more marked from about the age of 60 onward. This reduction has been estimated to be about 37 percent between ages 24 and 90.[1] Liver blood flow also declines by about 35 percent from early adult life to the age of 90.[2] Furthermore, liver perfusion (liver blood flow per unit volume liver) also falls over this age range by about 10 percent. The liver becomes a darker brown color with advanced age as a result of the accumulation of fluorescent brown pigmented lipofuscin granules in lysosomes within hepatocytes. The deposition of this protein is due to decreased intracellular proteolysis with age. Lipofuscin is also deposited elsewhere in advanced age—notably in the brain.[3,4]

Although liver size declines with age, human hepatocytes increase in size, unlike the situation in liver atrophy accompanying starvation. Liver cell nuclei show polyploidy and increased nuclear size; as in other organelles, mitochondria are also enlarged.[5–7] It is unclear whether the increased intracellular protein is functionally active or whether it represents the accumulation of "junk" within liver cells. A number of studies have reported that the hepatocellular concentration of smooth endoplasmic reticulum declines during senescence; this corresponds to lower yields of hepatic microsomes and, at least in rats, this in turn correlates with reduced drug metabolizing capacity.[8] In the absence of disease, hepatocytes divide only two or three times during the human life span. The space of Disse between liver cells is enlarged in aging, and there is a corresponding increase in the amount of collagen. However, the nature of the collagen appears unaltered.[9]

Liver function

As with the morphological changes described above, it is useless to extrapolate alteration in hepatic function found in aging from experimental animals to humans. Conventional liver blood tests do not change with age. There has been little examination of the changes in hepatic synthetic function with age, but there is a significant negative correlation between peak urea synthesis and age;[10] and hepatic conversion of α-amino-nitrogen to urea nitrogen—functional hepatic nitrogen clearance—declines by about 50 percent in advanced age. This appears to be greater than the concomitant decline in liver volume.[11] Hepatic synthesis of cholesterol is reduced in old age, and there is a reduction in total bile acid pool and possibly synthesis of bile acid from cholesterol.[12] With normal aging, galactose elimination, a cytosolic function, is reduced at the same rate as liver size.[2]

It is conceivable that the capacity of the liver for regeneration is impaired in advanced age, and this may reduce its ability to "repair" itself. Interestingly, in serial transplantation experiments, cells from young and old mice appear to be equally efficient in their ability to repopulate damaged livers derived from selective genetic knockout animals.[13] Fausto has speculated that apparently "senescent" diploid and tetraploid hepatocytes located throughout the liver lobule retain a remarkable capacity to proliferate even in old animals. Furthermore, the number of replications in these serial transplantation experiments exceeds that expected for mammalian cells. It is unclear why these cells apparently do not obey the normal rules of senescence. As Fausto has written, "This topic is ready for scientific experimentation given the recent advances on telomerases and the mechanisms of ageing."[13]

In man there is an age-related decline in mitogen-activated protein kinase activity in hepatocytes stimulated by epidermal growth factor; furthermore, an age-associated two-fold increase in DNA bases damaged by oxidative modification has also been observed in rat liver.[14,15]

While the significance of the above animal experiments in relation to aging and man remains obscure, clinical experience suggests that there is a decline in the ability of the human liver to regenerate and repair itself.

What is urgently needed now are studies to bring together our increasing knowledge of mechanisms of aging with modern understanding of liver injury, regeneration, and cell death.

Drug metabolism

This is the most widely studied aspect of aging and the human liver. The clearance of drugs whose metabolism is dependent on the cytochrome P450 group of liver enzymes declines variably between 0 and 50 percent according to age.[16] It seems probable that when such lifetime environmental variables as diet, smoking, and nutrition are taken into account, there is a broad decline in hepatic drug metabolism of between 5 and 30 percent from adulthood to old age.[17,18] It is probable that the decline of metabolism of such model drugs as antipyrene, aminopyrene, and caffeine can largely be accounted for by the decline in liver blood flow already described.[19]

INVESTIGATIONS OF HEPATOBILIARY DISEASE

A good history, particularly a history of medications including nonprescribed and herbal remedies, together with clinical examination are of paramount importance in the diagnosis of possible liver disease in elderly people. While there are no major differences in this respect between old and young patients, selection of appropriate investigations, particularly those that are invasive, may differ according to age. Specific points relating to history and examination will arise in relation to the diseases discussed later. It is the purpose of this section to propose a rational system for the investigation of elderly patients with possible hepatic disease. For further more detailed accounts of individual modes of investigation, readers are referred to major texts on liver disease.[20–22]

Laboratory investigations

Serum biochemistry
Routine serum biochemical tests—liver function tests (LFTs)—include determinations of serum bilirubin, serum alkaline phosphatase (ALP), and serum aspartate aminotransferase (AST) or alanine aminotransferase (ALT). In general, elevated ALP indicates cholestasis, whereas elevated transaminase indicates liver cell damage. In addition, serum γ-glutamyl transpeptidase (γ-GT) can be used to indicate cholestasis. Since ALP originates not only in the biliary tree but also in bone and intestine—relevant sources in some elderly patients—measurement of γ-GT may confirm or refute suspected cholestasis in a patient with isolated elevated ALP. γ-GT activity may be increased by a wide range of enzyme inducers, including many medications, hence care must be taken in interpreting elevated γ-GT. Since alcohol is itself a hepatic enzyme inducer, elevated γ-GT has been used as a possible marker for alcoholism. Unfortunately, this test has limited specificity and sensitivity.

Serum transaminases are elevated in most liver diseases. A recent district hospital study of marked elevation of AST (< 400 U/L) found that 47 percent of patients were older than age 70. The commonest cause for very elevated AST was hepatic ischemia, associated with sepsis, heart failure, hypoxia, or hypotension. This was much commoner in elderly patients. Pancreaticobiliary disease may also lead to very elevated transaminase particularly when associated with infection.[23]

Elevation of serum bilirubin leads to the most obvious sign of clinical liver disease—jaundice. This is normally clinically detectable when serum bilirubin is elevated above about 50 mmol/L or 3 mg percent (three times the normal range). Bilirubin may be elevated in cholestatic or hepatocellular disease; unfortunately, as with other biochemical LFTs, its degree of elevation does not correspond closely with the severity of liver disease. Furthermore, hemolysis—leading to increased red cell breakdown and formation of bilirubin—which may accompany some liver diseases, may also contribute to elevation of serum bilirubin.

Serum albumin is often reduced in chronic liver disease. Although albumin is synthesized by the liver, serum albumin level reflects not only synthesis but also dietary protein intake and absorption. Nonetheless, since serum albumin reflects hepatic synthetic function, it should be regarded as an important LFT.

Serum globulin levels do not reflect liver function. Persistent elevation of total globulin and particularly γ-globulin is associated with autoimmune liver disease, elevated IgA with alcoholic liver disease (ALD), and elevated IgM with primary biliary cirrhosis (PBC). None of these is more than indicative.

Probably the best routine test of hepatic synthetic function is prothrombin time (or ratio), since the liver synthesizes clotting factors I (fibrinogen), II (prothrombin), V, VII, IX, and X. Because these factors are normally present in excess in human serum, impairment of coagulation, dependent on one or more of them, may indicate quite profound liver cell dysfunction. In cholestasis or in circumstances in which fat malabsorption occurs, coagulation may be deficient not because of impairment of clotting factors themselves but because of lack of procoagulant function. In these circumstances, parenteral vitamin K (usually one or two 10 mg injections) should restore normal clotting function. Indeed, in patients with moderate impairment of prothrombin, time correction by parenteral K is itself highly suggestive of a cholestatic, usually obstructive, cause of the liver disease under investigation.

How to use LFTs in elderly patients
All elderly patients with suspected liver disease should have the blood tests indicated in the liver screen. In the presence of elevated serum ALP, γ-GT is more reliable than ALP electrophoresis in confirming cholestasis (i.e., intra- or extrahepatic obstruction). In the evaluation of abnormal liver enzyme results in asymptomatic patients, and with otherwise negative liver screen blood tests, alcoholic liver disease, nonalcoholic steatohepatitis (NASH), and an hepatic adverse drug reaction are the commonest primarily liver diseases to be considered.[24] At the same time careful exclusion of heart failure and occult infection should be made. It is important to remember that mild abnormalities in one or more of the liver enzymes are present in diabetes, a variety of generalized inflammatory disorders (e.g. rheumatoid arthritis and polymyalgia rheumatica), in several malignancies not directly affecting the liver, and in thyroid disease.[25]

Faced with an apparently isolated abnormality of the LFTs (notably alkaline phosphatase or transaminase) in the absence of any other positive information from the liver screen or from the considerations above, the clinician may decide to reassure their elderly patient after a period of observation, particularly if ultrasound examination of the liver and biliary tree shows no abnormality. It is poor practice, however, merely to ignore abnormal LFTs in an elderly patient who is otherwise well. Such patients should certainly receive some follow-up.

Hematology
Blood count and blood film are mandatory in the investigation of suspected liver disease. In chronic liver disease with hypersplenism associated with portal hypertension, there is depressed erythropoiesis and shortened red cell life. Splenic enlargement may lead to reduced platelet levels and in severe instances to reduced white blood cell count and anemia. The toxic effects of ALD result from a combination of the direct effect of alcohol on the bone marrow, the liver disease and portal hypertension, together with the frequent concomitant undernutrition. Macrocytosis, frequently with normal serum folate and red blood cell folate, is seen in all forms of chronic liver disease, not just in patients with ALD, but persistently elevated mean corpuscular volume (MCV) > 105 with normal B_{12} and folate measurements is certainly suggestive of alcohol in the setting of chronic liver disease. Blood loss from esophageal varices or portal gastropathy can occur in all forms of chronic liver disease, while bleeding from esophagitis, gastritis, and duodenitis occurs particularly in ALD or in severe acute or

chronic liver damage associated with impaired clotting. The hematology of liver disease is complex, and readers are referred to an excellent monograph by Berk.[26]

Hepatobiliary radiology and scanning

Ultrasound

In patients with signs, symptoms, or LFTs suggesting biliary obstruction, ultrasound examination should be the first imaging procedure employed. It is fast, safe, and noninvasive. Its use in detection of biliary obstruction and extrahepatic biliary disease is discussed elsewhere (Chapter 81). In relation to investigation of intrinsic liver disease, ultrasound may be carried out for three reasons: (1) to detect space occupying lesions within the liver; (2) to assess the texture, size, and shape of the liver in evaluation of chronic liver disease (this should include assessment of the spleen and other upper abdominal organs); (3) to assess the patency and anatomy of the hepatic vascular tree.[27,28] Modern color ultrasound with Doppler and now other modalities such as three-dimensional imaging and vascular enhancement are increasingly enabling more sophisticated noninvasive evaluation of the liver and its circulation.[29] It is best to be cautious about overconfident interpretation of the appearances of lesions within the liver. For example, the distinction between a small tumor and a regeneration nodule in a patient with cirrhosis may be extremely difficult, as may the interpretation of ultrasound findings in patients with fatty liver.[28] In routine clinical practice ultrasound is seldom helpful in making a histological diagnosis beyond reporting the existence of a shrunken irregular liver highly suggestive of cirrhosis, particularly in conjunction with an enlarged spleen, distended portal vessels, or ascites.[27,28]

Computed tomography

Computed tomography (CT), now spiral CT, is, with few exceptions, the best noninvasive imaging technique for the liver parenchyma. CT with vascular enhancement is particularly useful in detecting tumors within the liver. In the evaluation of primary hepatocellular cancer (HCC), CT may be carried out 2 weeks following lipiodol angiography (see below).[30,31] CT should be regarded as a complementary investigation to ultrasound.

Magnetic resonance imaging

Magnetic resonance imaging (MRI) can now produce images of almost comparable definition to the best CT scans. There are three specific indications in which MRI is particularly suited. Gadolinium enhancement provides reliable non-operator-dependent information about vascular flow. MR cholangiography has reduced the need for endoscopic retrograde cholangiography (ERC) and is noninvasive. MRI also provides information about the texture of the liver, for example in the detection of hemochromatosis in which excessive iron deposition is easily observed.[32,33]

Guided liver biopsy

Liver biopsy is now very frequently carried out under guidance of one of the above imaging techniques, usually ultrasound. With the advent of portable ultrasound machines, it is now perceived as good practice for many liver biopsies, not just those carried out to sample specific focal lesions within the liver, to be carried out under ultrasound guidance.[34]

Angiography

In clinical practice in older patients, angiography involving the liver has two purposes—diagnostic and therapeutic. Therapeutic angiography will be considered below with respect to its clinical indications. Angiography is an invasive and uncomfortable procedure which carries morbidity and (extremely rarely) mortality risks. It should not, therefore, be undertaken except after the use of other imaging techniques or in circumstances where specific information available only from angiography is required. It is particularly useful in the assessment of patients who may have liver tumors.[35] Most tumors whether benign or malignant, primary or secondary, exhibit an abnormal vascular pattern within the liver. The diagnostic value of hepatic angiography has been enhanced by the use of injection into the angiographic catheter of the radiodense contrast medium Lipiodol. Lipiodol is selectively retained in or around tumor tissue in the liver and can best be detected 1–2 weeks after angiography by obtaining a subsequent CT scan.[31] This technique is reasonably sensitive and specific and is particularly important where resection of small primary liver cancers is being considered since it may reveal previously unsuspected multiple tumors or greater extent of single tumors. Angiography is mandatory before major hepatic surgery.

Venography of the vessels associated with the liver is now less commonly used. Occasionally, in the assessment of suspected hepatic vein occlusion (Budd–Chiari syndrome) inferior venacavography or hepatic venography is used, although color Doppler is now superseding this indication.[29] Hepatic vein catheter pressures may demonstrate the level of portal hypertension in cirrhotic patients but the technique is, at present, of little diagnostic or therapeutic value in older patients except in relation to transjugular intrahepatic portal system shunt (see below).

Transjugular intrahepatic portal systemic shunt (TIPS)

This radiological technique in which a stent is placed angiographically between the hepatic vein and a major branch of the portal vein within the liver, thus creating the equivalent of a surgical portosystemic shunt, has received a great deal of attention and evaluation in the past few years. The treatment should be carried out only at highly experienced centers. It is currently recommended for treatment of intractable repeated bleeding from esophageal or esophogastric varices where injection and/or banding has been unsuccessful or of repeated bleeding from portal gastropathy where these techniques are inapplicable. In patients with resistant ascites occasionally with associated large recurrent plural effusion this procedure may also represent an alternative to repeated abdominal paracentesis. For both indications advanced age is an independent risk factor for mortality. In patients with Child's grade C status, mortality following TIPS is in excess of 70 percent at 6 months. In patients with any degree of chronic hepatic encephalopathy, TIPS is almost always followed by deterioration. The place of TIPS in the management of elderly patients with complications of portal hypertension is thus unproven. Nonetheless, in patients with a previous good quality of life and with good hepatic function (normal serum albumin, good clotting) who develop intractable bleeding from portal hypertension, the treatment may be highly effective even in elderly patients.[36,37]

ERCP

This mode of investigation is discussed in Chapter 81.

Percutaneous transhepatic cholangiography

This mode of investigation is considered in Chapter 81.

Laparoscopy

Laparoscopy, like other invasive investigational techniques already described, is increasingly being used in elderly patients because it offers opportunities for immediate therapeutic intervention where appropriate.[38] It should be carried out only at a center where the technique is in routine use. Its particular virtues are (1) direct visualization of lesions within or adjacent to the liver, (2) enhancing or speeding up diagnosis of some disseminated intra-abdominal conditions (e.g. metastases or infections), (3) undertaking biopsies with direct vision, and (4) using laparoscopic ultrasound to further delineate "difficult" lesions, particularly within the hilum of the liver.[39]

Liver biopsy

The histological assessment of liver disease is fundamental to understanding its pathogenesis and thus its treatment. Physicians caring for elderly patients with liver disease must not hesitate to carry out needle biopsies of the liver with appropriate safeguards concerning clotting, and where appropriate, under ultrasound-guided control or via laparoscopy, the procedure is extremely safe. Complications include hemorrhage, perforation of the gallbladder with biliary peritonitis, pneumothorax and septicemia.

In a recent survey of 1,500 liver biopsies from district hospitals throughout England and Wales, the median decade for biopsy was 60–69 years, 6 percent of the patients were over the age of 80, and mortality was 0.13 percent.[40] Accurate pathological assessment of liver histology is critical in the following circumstances.

1. Documentation of neoplastic disease: This is critical both in confirming the nature of a disease and in planning treatment. In the recent England and Wales study, 50 percent of liver biopsies in persons over 65 were carried out because of suspected malignant disease.[40] While tissue diagnosis of tumor within the liver is often justifiable and necessary, it is emphasized that if surgical excision of the focal lesion within the liver is contemplated then biopsy with its risk of tumor spread is best avoided. Characterization of the lesion should be carried out with the scanning and angiographic procedures described above. Serum α-fetoprotein (see below) is elevated in 70+ percent of primary HCCs and can be regarded as diagnostic in a patient with a focal intrahepatic lesion at a level of above 500 IU/L or where successive values over a 1-month period show a significant rise. Biopsy of intrahepatic neoplastic disease should also be avoided in cases where widespread disseminated malignancy is already established or where the likely nature of the hepatic lesion is already known because of the previous histological diagnosis of a distant primary neoplasm.

2. Classification of chronic liver disease: In chronic viral or autoimmune liver disease, while serological markers are extremely important, the gold standard is liver biopsy. Increasingly, staging (degree of fibrosis) and grading (degree of inflammation, necrosis, and other features) are observed and recorded on the initial liver biopsy. This is true not only for hepatitis C[41] but autoimmune hepatitis[42] and NASH.[43]

It is often invaluable in estimating prognosis and formulating strategy to know the histological stage of a specific progressive liver disease. For example, the likelihood of progression toward cirrhosis may be calculated in patients with hepatitis C taking into account age, alcohol consumption, and male sex.[44] ALD and PBC are other cases in point.

3. Evaluation of treatment programs: Again the gold standard for evaluation of the success of treatment is a baseline biopsy (for the reasons above) with follow-up biopsy or biopsies after a defined period of treatment. Even in relatively elderly patients this practice may be desirable and justifiable, particularly in evaluating new therapies or in monitoring possible drug hepatotoxicity.

4. Evaluation of abnormal LFTs: In elderly patients with consistently abnormal LFTs or in whom there is diagnostic doubt concerning the nature of their liver disease, liver biopsy is important. A recent study to investigate histological findings in individuals who had persistently abnormal LFTs in the absence of diagnostic serology found that 26 percent of 354 patients had some degree of fibrosis and 6 percent were cirrhotic.[45] The commonest findings were NASH in 34 percent and simple fat (32 percent) but drug hepatotoxicity including Chinese herbal remedies and nonprescription nonsteroidal anti-inflammatory drugs, autoimmune liver disease, and unexpected alcohol-related liver disease were all found in significant numbers, as was cryptogenic cirrhosis.

Other serological tests (Table 80-1)

Viral markers

HEPATITIS A HAV IgM is a reliable marker for recent or current infection with hepatitis A virus (HAV).

HEPATITIS B HBsAg indicates the presence of the surface protein of hepatitis B virus (HBV) in the serum. In patients with acute type B hepatitis this protein is often associated with the presence of the whole virus in the blood and thus infectivity.

Table 80-1 **Blood tests for suspected liver disease (the liver screen)**
Blood count and film (note ↑ MCV)
LFTs (ALP, ALT, bilirubin)
Proteins (albumin, total globulin)
Prothrombin time (or ratio)
HBsAg anti-HBc, anti-HCV
Autoimmune profile (AMA, SMA, ANA)
Ferritin (if ↑ check HFE genotype)
Random blood ethanol
Urea, creatinine, electrolytes

In patients with chronic liver disease, after incorporation of the viral genome into hepatic nuclear material, production of the HBsAg protein and its presence in the serum give no indication of infectivity or of stage of illness. Anti-HBs is usually present in low titer following initial infection with HBV. It may or may not persist for months or years following an initial infection. Anti-HBc—an antibody to the core of the virus—is the most reliable indicator of past infection. It gives no indication of current infectivity or when initial infection took place. HBeAg, the e antigen, is distinct from HBsAg and anti-HBc but is closely associated with the virion core. Presence of the e antigen in the serum is indicative of the presence of whole virus and thus of infectivity. In patients found to be HBsAg positive these other markers must then be sought to indicate likelihood of infectivity. Having said this, a few patients are now being identified in whom e antigen is not detected but in whom HBV DNA may be found (by molecular diagnostic assays). Serum HBV DNA is thus now the gold standard to assess infectivity.[46]

HEPATITIS C Anti-HCV merely indicates past or present infection with the hepatitis C virus (HCV), giving no indication of either prognosis or infectivity. Anti-HCV does not become detectable in the serum until a number of weeks after initial exposure. Third-generation enzyme-linked immunosorbent assays (ELISA) and recombinant immunoblot assays (RIBA) have excellent sensitivity and specificity. The detection of HCV RNA in the serum by reverse transcriptase PCR is nowadays considered the gold standard for the diagnosis of HCV infection and for assessing the antiviral response to therapy.[47] This may also be used for the early diagnosis of acute HCV infection and to detect the minority of anti-HCV positive patients with past resolved HCV infection who are no longer infectious.[48]

Autoimmune markers
These are summarized in Table 80-2.

ANTIMITOCHONDRIAL ANTIBODIES These are nontissue and nonspecies specific but highly disease specific for PBC. The group of antigens against which AMAs are directed have recently been isolated. Both indirect immunofluorescent tests and more specific ELISA tests are being carried out; for the radioimmunoassay a titer of 1 in 40 or greater on more than one occasion, particularly in the absence of other autoantibodies is considered highly suggestive of PBC.[49]

Table 80-2	**Second-line tests for suspected liver disease**
In hepatitis	HAV IgM; plus if HBsAg positive, then e antigen or e antibody; anti-HCV
In hyperbilirubinemia To confirm cholestasis	Conjugated vs unconjugated γ-Glutamyl transpeptidase
For HCC For immune disease	α-Fetoprotein Immunoglobulins; anti-M$_2$AMA, LKM, ANA, SMA
α$_1$-Antitrypsin deficiency	α$_1$-Antitrypsin phenotype

SMOOTH MUSCLE ANTIBODY (SMA) AND LIVER KIDNEY MICROSOMAL ANTIBODY (LKM) SMA and LKM together with the newer soluble liver antigen (SLA) are usually indicators of autoimmune chronic hepatitis. LKM is extremely rare in patients over age 65.[50]

ANTINUCLEAR ANTIBODIES (ANAs) These are a group of antibodies detected by various indirect immunofluorescent techniques. They are seen in the full spectrum of autoimmune liver diseases, particularly in so-called autoimmune cholangiopathy—AMA negative PBC. In a recent study of autoimmune hepatitis in elderly patients, 14 of 18 were ANA positive.[50] ANAs may also be seen in primary sclerosing cholangitis.

SERUM α-FETOPROTEIN This marker is elevated in about 70 percent of patients with primary HCC. Normally, values are < 10 mmol/L in adults; in patients with chronic liver disease and cirrhosis this level may rise to 50 mmol/L. Values above 500 mmol/L in the context of an elderly patient with cirrhosis and a possible liver tumor are virtually diagnostic of primary liver cancer. A rising value above about 50 mmol/L over a period of months in a patient with cirrhosis is also highly suggestive of development of primary HCC. Unfortunately, about one-third of primary hepatic tumors do not synthesize this fetal protein, hence a normal serum value by no means excludes such a tumor.

SERUM FERRITIN, IRON BINDING CAPACITY, HFE GENE Combinations of these measures are used in the diagnosis of hereditary hemochromatosis. In a patient with elevated serum ferritin and increased iron saturation, as indicated by iron binding capacity, genotyping for the HFE genes, homozygosity for the common HFE mutation C282Y or compound heterozygosity C282Y/H63D should be sought. Both evidence of phenotypic iron overload (raised ferritin and iron saturation) and the genotypes above should be confirmed to make the diagnosis of hemochromatosis.[51] Serum ferritin is an acute phase reactant protein and hence can be elevated in other hepatic inflammation, infection, or malignancy. The normal value for men and women is up to 300 ng/mL.

SPECIFIC DISEASES OF THE LIVER
Toxic damage: alcoholic liver disease (ALD) in elderly people

Although ALD is perceived as being uncommon in older people, a British series showed that 28 percent of patients with this disease presented for the first time over the age of 60 and 7 percent over the age of 70.[52] In France a large retrospective study found that 20 percent of patients were over the age of 70.[53] In the United States one study among white males showed that the peak decade for presentation with cirrhosis was the seventh.[54] In our experience older patients present with a higher proportion of signs and symptoms suggestive of the complications of severe liver disease—jaundice, hypoproteinemia, ascites, or bleeding for esophagogastric varices. Almost all patients over the age of 70 who are referred to hospital for the first time with alcoholic liver disease already have cirrhosis, whereas this proportion is less than 50 percent among those presenting under age 50. Prognosis of ALD is related to age. Mortality among under 60-year-olds at presentation in unselected series is around 5 percent at 1 year and 24 percent at 3 years, whereas of those patients of ours presenting over age 70, 75 percent were dead at 1 year, 90 percent at 3 years.[52] It is unclear why older patients present with more severe clinical features and have a worse prognosis. It may be that family doctors are more reluctant to refer elderly individuals with minor signs or symptoms of possible ALD to hospitals; this may be understandable—even correct—in the social context in which patients find themselves. Older patients presumably present further down the clinical path than younger ones; for one reason or another they have not received medical attention until the disease has become decompensated.

It has also been suggested that with advanced age there is increased susceptibility of the liver to the toxic effect of alcohol. Recent careful pharmacokinetic studies have shown that blood ethanol area under the curve (AUC) in both men and women is significantly greater in older subjects following ingestion of ethanol in the fasting state. But, interestingly, not when ethanol is given following a meal.[55] This observation may imply a decline in one or more mechanisms responsible for rapid ethanol metabolism within the first hour after ingestion, but the reason for this is unclear, particularly as there are no age-related changes in the specific activity of total hepatic alcohol dehydrogenase.

Investigation

Elderly patients with ALD usually have deranged LFTs but there is no characteristic diagnostic pattern; as with other parenchymal liver diseases the LFTs may be rather more cholestatic than in younger individuals. Routine investigation of an old person with suspected ALD should also include serum albumin, blood film (note raised mean corpuscular volume [MCV]), and clotting screen. The ratio of AST to ALT is usually > 1. Random blood or urine ethanol is also useful. Liver biopsy provides diagnostic and prognostic information and should be carried out except where there is marked ascites or where clotting is impaired or platelets markedly reduced (prothrombin time prolonged by 4 seconds or more, platelet count below 70,000). In these circumstances, particularly if there is doubt about the diagnosis, patients may have a transjugular liver biopsy carried out in an experienced center. In the presence of ascites a diagnostic tap should be carried out since spontaneous bacterial peritonitis (SBP) is a common complication of advanced cirrhosis in these patients and carries a high mortality. A polymorphonuclear white cell count of > 250/cm³ acitic fluid is considered diagnostic of SBP. Fluid should be submitted for aerobic and anaerobic culture. Liver imaging with ultrasound or CT is particularly important in elderly patients with suspected alcoholic cirrhosis, since a significant proportion may have complicating HCC. Liver pathology can be regarded in terms of three stages but two or all three may coexist.

1. Fatty liver Some patients may show fatty change alone perhaps with minor steatonecrosis or fibrosis in zone 3. This is usually reversible but where significant fibrosis or alcoholic hepatitis coexists the prognosis is worse. In the few individuals who, despite drinking to great excess for many years, have only mildly abnormal LFTs with liver histology showing only fatty change the prognosis is good, and for an old person advice concerning future alcohol consumption need not be too prescriptive.

2. Alcoholic hepatitis This may have a mild to an extremely aggressive histological appearance and concomitantly may occur in individuals who have few clinical symptoms or signs as well as those with deep jaundice who are very seriously ill. In general, alcoholic hepatitis usually accompanies cirrhosis in elderly patients. The histological appearance is of a polymorph infiltrate of the liver parenchyma often with fibrosis. Continuing ethanol consumption, particularly in women, leads to a poor prognosis; the vast majority of patients progress to cirrhosis.

3. Alcoholic cirrhosis This is an irreversible condition. Recent population surveys have suggested that even among elderly people up to 40 percent of individuals with alcoholic cirrhosis may have few signs or symptoms. Once decompensation occurs, however, the prognosis is poor.

The clinical findings in elderly patients with ALD are shown in Table 80-3. They are the same as for other patients with other chronic liver disease.

Treatment

By far the most important treatment for ALD is abstinence or, in the case of mild disease, a return to sensible drinking levels (ethanol < 28 units per week for men, 21 units for women, preferably taken with meal and on several days in the week rather than as a "binge"). By far the single most important prognostic factor in ALD is drinking behavior.

Acute alcohol withdrawal should be treated with chlordiazepoxide, up to 20 mg q.d.s., although elderly patients may need less. The β-blocker atenolol is beneficial in preventing peripheral manifestations of alcohol withdrawal—tremor and hypertension in particular, and 50 mg daily is the recommended dose for the first week in hospital. Benzodiazepines should be withdrawn before or shortly after hospital discharge.[56] The only study that examined alcohol withdrawal specifically in elderly subjects suggested that it was more severe and that higher doses of chlordiazepoxide were required to control symptoms.[55]

Table 80-3 **Clinical findings in alcoholic liver disease**	
Compensated	**Decompensated**
Telangiectasia	Encephalopathy
Parotid enlargement	Alcohol withdrawal symptoms
Spider naevi	Jaundice
Loss of body hair	Fetor hepaticus
Gynecomastia	Ascites
Hepatomegaly ±	Dilated abdominal veins
Splenomegaly ±	Asterixis
Vertebral (plus rib) fractures	Peripheral edema
Liver palms	
Clubbing plus leukonychia	
Muscle wasting	
Testicular atrophy	

If liver disease is assessed to be very severe on clinical and biochemical grounds, particularly if bilirubin is markedly elevated and there is significant impairment of clotting, consideration should be given to treatment with corticosteroids—40 mg prednisolone daily for 4 weeks. This is based upon several studies showing benefit in survival for up to 1 year in patients with severe alcoholic hepatitis defined by a discriminant function of > 32 (a formula based on elevation of bilirubin and prolongation of clotting). Intercurrent infection or coincident variceal bleeding are absolute contraindications to initiation of steroid treatment.[57] Nutritional support, initially with intravenous vitamins (particularly thiamine) together with maintenance of blood glucose is vital. Longer-term restoration of normal nutrition with high-protein diet containing sufficient calories is also important, although studies of enteral or parenteral nutrition as treatment for acute severe ALD have failed to show definite benefit.[58]

No studies of long-term treatment of ALD specifically in elderly patients have been conducted. It is recommended that elderly patients with established ALD receive regular follow-up for the following reasons:

1. To encourage abstinence
2. To check on possible complications of therapy (diuretics, lactulose, etc.)
3. To maintain biochemical and nutritional supervision
4. To monitor for possible development of HCC in cirrhotic patients.

It has been recently estimated that the annual risk of development of HCC in older patients with alcoholic cirrhosis is 4 percent per year.[59]

Drug-induced liver disease

Although adverse drug reactions (ADRs) are said to be commoner in elderly people it is possible that much of this impression is created by increased prescribing for individuals and the increased number of drugs they receive.[60] Alterations in pharmacodynamics and pharmacokinetics with advancing age may alter the response to drugs.[61] Furthermore, older patients have more intercurrent illness with impaired cardiac or renal function which may directly or indirectly potentiate the adverse effects of some drugs on the liver. For whatever reason, drug-induced liver disease is encountered with increased frequency in parallel with advancing age. For example, in Denmark the overall incidence of drug-induced hepatitis is 20 per 1 million person years but the incidence increases to a maximum of 50 per 1 million person years in individuals aged 70–79 years.[62]

Increased likelihood of age-related susceptibility to drug-induced liver damage has been shown for a few drugs—for example isoniazid, halothane, and the nonsteroidal anti-inflammatory drug benoxoprofen (now withdrawn).[63] The exact mechanism for the increased severity of drug-induced liver damage in elderly people has not been elucidated. But, because most severe hepatic ADRs are idiosyncratic, age-related decline in drug clearance is probably irrelevant.

Viral hepatitis

Hepatitis A

Probably because of a cohort effect due to improved sanitation the proportion of the older adult population in Western countries who have not acquired immunity to hepatitis A is rising. While hepatitis A virus (HAV) infection is usually a mild disease with acute liver failure occurring in less than 0.35 percent of adults and while acute HAV is encountered relatively rarely in patients older than age 65, outbreaks of HAV among older adult populations are now being described and older people have been shown to be more susceptible to clinically severe disease with serious complications, acute hepatic failure, and higher mortality compared to younger patients.[64–66] In the UK, the ratio of death from HAV to notification rose from 7 per 10,000 persons age 15–24 to more than 400 per 10,000 in persons over age 65. In 1984, 5 of 11 deaths from HAV in the UK were in patients older than age 70.[66] The basis for the worse outcome of fulminant viral hepatitis with advancing age, as with all fulminant liver failure, is unclear but higher prevalence of comorbidity and age-related impaired resistance to stress are likely to play a part.

For all these reasons HAV vaccination is strongly recommended for elderly patients traveling to areas endemic for HAV although the cost effectiveness of vaccination has not been evaluated.[67]

Hepatitis B virus (HBV)

Routine testing for HBsAg in donor blood and blood products for over 30 years together with the fact that the major risk groups for acute hepatitis B in Europe and the United States (homosexuals, intravenous drug abusers) are not highly represented in the geriatric population means that acute hepatitis B among elderly people has become much less common, although sporadic cases and rare outbreaks may still occur. Although only a small proportion of immunocompetent adults with acute HBV infection overall progress to chronic infection, in one outbreak of acute HBV in a nursing home in Japan 59 percent of patients mean age 77 years ultimately became HBV carriers.[68]

Recently, incorporation of highly immunogenic pre-S antigens into HBV vaccine has improved the immunogenicity of vaccine and may lead to increased seroconversion rates in older patients.[69] Elderly travelers to the Far East and Africa should now be vaccinated with these safe effective newer vaccines.[70]

Chronic hepatitis B

Older patients may present with signs and symptoms of chronic liver disease in which chronic HBV infection is the underlying cause. Among those over 65, such patients are usually HBsAg positive, e antigen negative, sometimes e antibody positive, thus indicating lack of infectivity. However, among elderly patients receiving cancer chemotherapy, reactivation of hepatitis B virus replication readily occurs.[71] Among elderly patients with HBV-associated cirrhosis, development of HCC may be 5 percent per year.

In considering treatment of elderly patients with chronic HBV the objectives and the nature of the treatment, as well as the likelihood of success, should be borne in mind. In pre-cirrhotic patients in general the two goals of treatment are to prevent progression to cirrhosis and to reduce or abolish infectivity. Furthermore, successful treatment in such patients has now been shown to reduce risk of subsequent hepatic decompensation or the development of HCC. Patients who are HBsAg positive with evidence of viral replication (HBe antigen positive, serum HBV DNA positive) with normal ALT levels (indicating immune tolerance of the virus) should not be treated. More recently, the availability of lamivudine which is generally well tolerated has broadened the indications for treatment of patients with chronic HBV to encompass patients with clinical cirrhosis. Although the rate of post-treatment relapse is high, the clinical and histological benefits of 6 months lamivudine treatment warrant its consideration for use in patients with HBe antigen negative cirrhosis.

In general, the still developing field of treatment of chronic hepatitis B with interferon and emerging antiviral treatment is best left to specialist centers.[72]

Hepatitis C

The worldwide total of people infected with hepatitis C virus is probably about 170 million; in Western Europe and the United States where nearly 4 million people are thought to be infected, it is much the commonest hepatitis virus.[73] Acute hepatitis C in older people seems usually to have a benign course but there are few recent studies. The seroprevalence of anti-HCV among patients over 65 varies between different countries in Europe and North America. In the United States, seroprevalence of anti-HCV has been estimated at 1 percent in persons over 70 vs 3 percent in persons age 30–40.[74] As the cohort of the middle-aged population who acquired hepatitis C through blood transfusion or IV drug abuse moves into older age we can anticipate that in many countries the numbers of elderly people affected by hepatitis C will increase over the next 20 years or so before falling away, hopefully as treatments improve further.[75,76]

Following acute acquisition of HCV over 80 percent patients become chronic carriers but the long-term prognosis for the disease is still controversial. Advanced age is one of the main independent risk factors associated with more rapid progression of chronic HCV infection as are male gender, regular alcohol consumption and (probably) obesity. Studies by Poynard et al.[77] and by Roudot-Thoraval et al. have both shown that both rates of progression of fibrosis toward cirrhosis and the risk of cirrhosis are related independently to increased age at the time of exposure to the HCV virus. The prevalence of cirrhosis was 46.8 percent in patients who acquired HCV over age 60 in the Roudot-Thoraval study.[78]

The availability of reliable serological tests for anti-HCV means that all older patients with abnormal LFTs should be screened at the time of first presentation. Despite advances in interferon therapy treatment of HCV infection in elderly patients is still controversial. Furthermore, variations between the six main genotypes of HCV (type 1–6) further complicate questions of treatment in older patients. Only three studies have specifically addressed the use of interferon treatment in elderly patients, all were before the advent of the use of the antiviral agent ribavirin and more recently pegylated interferons (summarized in ref 63). Regimes of treatment are changing rapidly but the combination of pegylated (PEG) interferon alpha (IFN-α) with ribavirin for between 24 and 48 weeks in noncirrhotic patients has been shown to produce sustained virological response in over 50 percent patients with concomitant improvement of liver histology.[79] Unfortunately, ribavirin is relatively contraindicated in patients with a history of heart disease, which may exclude a number of elderly patients with hepatitis C. The questions of efficacy, tolerability, and cost effectiveness of newer combination chemotherapies have not been addressed in older patients. Since a high proportion of patients aged over 70 have cirrhosis or near cirrhosis at diagnosis the question of treatment of patients with hepatitis-C-related cirrhosis with IFN is controversial. Referral for consideration of treatment to a major center in such patients should be considered.

Pyogenic liver abscess

Almost 50 percent of European and North American patients presenting with pyogenic liver abscess are aged 70 or older.[80–82] Such patients frequently have very nonspecific symptoms—epigastric pain, weight loss, shortness of breath and rigors—although the last-mentioned symptoms have been reported as being less common in very elderly people. General malaise, nausea and vomiting, diarrhea, and pleuritic pain may also be encountered in an elderly patient with pyogenic liver abscess. The conditions most commonly associated with liver abscess are now biliary tract obstruction and cholangitis. But distant abdominal sepsis, often associated with paracolic abscess, is still seen in many elderly patients with "cryptogenic" liver abscess. There appears to be an increased incidence in individuals with diabetes mellitus and metastatic cancer.

Diagnosis

The diagnosis of pyogenic liver abscess is often delayed or missed. Many patients have anemia and over 75 percent have an elevated leukocyte count. Serum ALP is elevated in almost all patients, but other LFTs are more inconsistent; serum albumin is often low and globulin elevated. On examination the liver or lower ribs over the liver are often tender. Diagnosis should be made by high-quality ultrasound, often followed by CT scan. The abscess is often loculated or multiple and ill formed. Sometimes debris is shown in the middle of the abscess and these features can make distinction from multicentric tumor more difficult. In most series of elderly patients *Escherichia coli* is the organism most commonly isolated.

Treatment

Several recent series have shown that, excluding individuals with associated malignancy, and those where the abscess was found only at post mortem, prognosis for older patients is no different from that for younger ones. The strong consensus of many series describing the management of liver abscess is that percutaneous needle aspiration, usually, in patients with well-delineated abscess, with subsequent continuous catheter drainage is now the treatment of choice rather than open surgical drainage.[83] Antibiotic treatment, which should initially be intravenous, may be carried out with intravenous cephalosporin or ciprofloxacin, and metronidazole. This treatment should be continued intravenously for about 2 weeks and then followed by 2–3 months of oral treatment. The catheter should be removed when drainage becomes negligible, usually after a few days, and the treatment progress monitored with repeat ultrasound examinations. Subsequent investigation, first of the hepatobiliary tree and then (if indicated) of the colon, should be carried out to detect the source of primary infection. Rapid treatment of pyogenic liver abscess by drainage and antibiotics is vital, since in untreated cases mortality is extremely high. It is emphasized that in sick elderly patients with nonspecific symptoms, such as those referred to above, and with abnormal LFTs (particularly elevated serum ALP), together with a raised white cell count, the index of suspicion should be high and early ultrasound of the liver is mandatory.

Liver abnormalities in systemic infections

Abnormal LFTs may be associated with systemic infections of almost all types. In addition, distant localized infections in which there is no overt evidence of bacteremia may be associated with LFT abnormalities. Sites of infection include appendicitis, diverticulitis, renal disease, endocarditis, or soft tissue abscesses.[84,85] In lobar pneumonia in elderly people, raised serum ALP and sometimes even jaundice are not infrequent. However, the reasons for this are quite unclear. In Gram-negative bacterial infection endotoxinemia may be contributory. While in younger patients systemic or distance infection may be a rare cause of abnormal LFTs in otherwise largely asymptomatic patients (where the commonest cause by far is fatty liver or nonalcoholic steatohepatitis)[24,25] the picture is quite different in very elderly patients in whom systemic or distant infection is one of the most frequent causes of unexplained abnormal LFTs.[86] In an elderly patient with a known infection, for example pneumonia, nonspecific abnormalities of LFTs need not be investigated unless they persist following the treatment and resolution of the infective illness. In one unselected series of mainly elderly general hospital patients with abnormal LFTs the abnormality was ascribed to nonhepatic bacterial infection in almost 15 percent of cases.[86]

AUTOIMMUNE LIVER DISEASE
Primary biliary cirrhosis

PBC must now be recognized as an important disease in middle aged and elderly women. The mean age of presentation in the largest published series of 1,023 patients was 61 years with 397 (40 percent) patients presenting at or over the age of 65.[87] Increasing age has been shown to be an independent prognostic indicator for PBC, whether deaths from liver disease or overall deaths are considered.[88] Not surprisingly, overall mortality is higher among patients presenting over age 65 (in the largest published series 59 vs 33 percent of those presenting under age 65) but the annual risk of dying from liver disease was also found to be 2.4 times higher in those presenting over 65, with an annual liver mortality of over 3 percent compared to 1.3 percent among those presenting under 65.[87]

Asymptomatic disease

Physicians now make a diagnosis of PBC in asymptomatic patients either based upon the finding of a positive AMA on an autoimmune profile for some other suspected disease—often because of joint pains or suspected thyroid disease—or based upon the unexpected finding of persistently elevated serum ALP on biochemical screening, often in an elderly woman. In women over the age of 50 with positive AMA and persistently elevated serum ALP the diagnosis of PBC is highly likely.[87] Recently, it has been shown that strongly positive AMA alone, even in the absence of raised serum ALP or signs or symptoms of liver disease, is a strong indication that an individual will ultimately develop biochemically and clinically apparent PBC.[89] The prognosis for patients with asymptomatic PBC is now thought to be little different from those presenting with symptoms of liver disease with an excess of deaths from nonhepatic causes in the asymptomatic cases balancing the increased likelihood of dying from liver disease among initially symptomatic individuals.[90]

Symptomatic disease

Most patients present with symptoms of malaise, lethargy, upper abdominal pain, or more specially, pruritus or jaundice. There are no differences in the proportion of patients presenting with these symptoms among older or younger patients, nor in the proportion presenting with complications (around 15 percent). In a patient, particularly a woman, over age 50 with one or more of these symptoms, a positive AMA, and deranged LFTs, the diagnosis of PBC is very likely indeed. Except in very elderly or frail patients the diagnosis should still, however, be confirmed by liver biopsy after any conceivable extrahepatic biliary obstruction has been excluded by ultrasound examination.

In addition to age, other factors with prognostic importance in symptomatic patients are: serum bilirubin, presence or absence of cirrhosis on liver biopsy, presence or absence of complications of portal hypertension, and serum albumin. About 50 percent of PBC patients presenting with or developing symptoms of liver disease will die within 5 years without therapeutic intervention. Death usually arises from complications of portal hypertension or sepsis; very rarely, primary HCC supervenes.[91]

Complications

Apart from the complications of portal hypertension (bleeding varices and ascites—see below) and of hepatocellular failure (encephalopathy, undernutrition, and susceptibility to infections) the prolonged cholestasis of PBC and possibly additional malabsorption due to associated pancreatic hyposecretion occasionally lead to weight loss. In the elderly age group, osteoporosis is probably slightly more common in PBC patients, particularly those with prolonged profound cholestasis, than in the normal elderly female population, but this difference is not very great.[92] A wide variety of autoimmune diseases have been associated with PBC, the most important of which are Sjögren's syndrome, rheumatoid arthritis, thyroid disease (hypo or hyper), mixed connective tissue disease or scleroderma, and fibrosing alveolitis.[92]

Treatment

The treatment for late-stage PBC in cirrhotic patients with complications is liver transplantation. Indeed, PBC is one of the major indications for transplantation in a person over the age of 60. Several studies have now shown that in very carefully selected patients, over the age of 60, overall 1-year graft and patient survival rate equal those achieved in younger patients.[93,94] Only a very few patients over age 70 with PBC have now received successful transplants, however, and such patients must undergo an exhaustive assessment to ensure that they have no other medical contraindications to this very major surgery. As technology and technique advance, debate as to the ethical and economic consequences of more widespread availability of liver transplantation for patients over 70 years old must take place.

The only medical therapy presently licensed in most countries for treatment of PBC is the bile acid ursodeoxycholic acid (URSO). This treatment at doses of 12–15 mg/kg body weight has been suggested to improve survival.[95] However, a recent meta-analysis has cast doubt upon the efficacy of URSO.[96] Nonetheless, since this treatment appears almost free of adverse effects beyond dose-related looseness of bowels, it should be considered in patients with symptomatic disease. Pruritus is usually effectively treated with cholestyramine 4–12 g daily. Prophylaxis against the development of osteoporosis should be considered using bisphosphonates. Hormone replacement therapy, where indicated, appears to have no cholestatic adverse effect.

Autoimmune hepatitis

Autoimmune hepatitis (AIH) is defined as chronic inflammation of the liver with a mainly lymphocytic and plasma cell infiltrate, expanding outward from the portal tracts into the liver lobules with accompanying piecemeal necrosis of liver cells. In severe disease fibrotic scarring and bridging between the portal tracts and central veins, leading to cirrhosis, is seen. In addition to these histological features chronic AIH is accompanied by the presence of one or more autoantibodies in the serum, in older patients usually SMA or ANA, occasionally SLA.[97]

AIH has been thought to be uncommon in elderly people, but recently, groups of patients presenting with the disease over the age of 65 have been described.[97–99] Perhaps because of the perception that this disease usually occurs in younger individuals, time to diagnosis may be longer in older patients. Presentation may be with jaundice. Insidious development of fatigue and fluid retention are typical. Initial histology may be more severe than in younger patients.

Diagnosis of AIH is made using criteria laid down by the International Autoimmune Hepatitis Group.[100] These include the presence of autoantibodies, elevation of transaminase and gamma globulin and some histological criteria. The importance of making a diagnosis which fulfils all or most of these parameters is that this may help predict response to treatment. AIH is also a diagnosis of exclusion, by absence of markers for hepatitis B and C for example. Physical signs of AIH are similar to those for other chronic liver diseases.

Prognosis and treatment

In all the recently published series, prognosis for older AIH patients was similar to that for younger ones, or even better from the point of view of liver morbidity and mortality. Treatment of AIH is normally with prednisolone, beginning with 20 mg daily and tapering to maintenance dose around 10 mg daily. In younger patients azothiaprine is also used, but there appears to be more intolerance of this drug in older patients.[97]

There is some overlap between AIH and PBC, occasionally primary sclerosing cholangitis (PSC), but this is extraordinarily rare in older patients.

Primary sclerosing cholangitis (PSC)

PSC is often associated with ulcerative cholitis and may be an indolent disease, especially if it only affects the small intrahepatic bile ducts rather than (as is normally the case) the larger intra- and extrahepatic biliary tree.[101,102] Occasionally, an elderly patient, usually a man, presents with persistent LFT abnormalities, usually cholestatic and with positive ANA, together with symptoms and signs of chronic liver disease often accompanying ulcerative cholitis. The diagnosis rests on:

1. Diagnostic appearance of the biliary tree on ERCP
2. Compatible liver histology
3. The persistent cholestatic LFT abnormality with exclusion of other possible causes of liver disease.

PSC may be complicated by development of cholangiocarcinoma and since signs and cholangiographic appearances may be similar the diagnosis of cholangiocarcinoma is often not made until late.

At present, despite numerous clinical trials, no treatment has been shown to be of definite benefit. If a "critical stricture" of the extrahepatic biliary tree is demonstrated it can be stented. Recurrent attacks of cholangitis should be energetically treated with antibiotics.

NONALCOHOLIC STEATOHEPATITIS

In the past 5 years it has become clear that nonalcoholic steatohepatitis (NASH) is an important cause of progressive liver disease. The term NASH was coined by Ludwig et al. in 1980 to describe patients who had all the histological features of alcoholic steatohepatitis but who did not drink alcohol.[103] We now recognize that the spectrum of non-alcoholic fatty liver disease includes simple fatty liver alone as well as features of steatonecrosis and hepatitis as well as fibrosis leading to cirrhosis.[104] It is still unclear what the prevalence of nonalcoholic fatty liver disease (NAFLD) is but estimates suggest that in Western countries abnormalities of liver blood tests or ultrasound scans showing fatty liver attributable to NAFLD may occur in 2–15 percent of the adult population.[105] Nonalcoholic fatty liver disease appears to be very strongly associated with obesity and type 2 diabetes; indeed almost all patients with this disorder have insulin resistance, thus making it a component of the group of diseases associated with Western overnutrition including type 2 diabetes, obesity, and hypertension.[106]

The pathogenesis of NASH may occur in two stages. It seems that the presence of fat in the liver, often associated with central obesity, is necessary together with insulin resistance. The development of steatonecrosis and fibrosis leading ultimately to cirrhosis may result from oxidative stress/lipid peroxidation and/or the effects of the inflammatory cytokine cascade initiated by (possibly gut-derived) endotoxin and TNFα release.[107] These mechanisms, in many ways parallel to the development of alcoholic liver disease may, like alcoholic liver disease, be modulated by genes associated with liver metabolism and susceptibility to oxidative stress or inflammation.

Natural history

Our understanding of the natural history of NAAFLD is still emerging and remains slightly speculative. It seems likely that while an increasingly high proportion of the young adult population in Western countries may have fat in the liver only an unknown proportion of these will go on to develop steatohepatitis, necrosis and fibrosis. Increasing age over 40, marked obesity, and presence of overt type 2 diabetes appear to be predictors of those who will go on to develop more serious liver disease.[108–110]

Of great interest is the emergence of the connection between NASH in middle age and cryptogenic cirrhosis arising in over 60-year-olds.[111,112] Recent studies on patients with cryptogenic cirrhosis, the vast majority over age 60, many over age 70, suggest that obesity and/or type 2 diabetes were associated with cryptogenic cirrhosis in over 70 percent of cases (vs perhaps 20–30 percent in other forms of cirrhosis). Cryptogenic cirrhosis in which viral, autoimmune, and other identifiable causes have been excluded is probably increasingly common in older patients and, if predictions for the rapid rise in prevalence of NASH prove correct, we may expect to see an enormous increase in "cryptogenic" cirrhosis—actually associated with burnt-out NASH—among elderly patients in future years. Very recently the development of HCC in these cryptogenic cirrhosis patients has been described. This appears to occur with comparable frequency in these cryptogenic cirrhosis patients to many other forms of cirrhosis but at an older age (median age probably around 70).[113]

Diagnosis

The diagnosis of NASH or NASH-related cryptogenic cirrhosis is effectively a diagnosis of exclusion. The presence of associated features—obesity, particularly central obesity (measured by waist/hip ratio), and/or type 2 diabetes and hyperlipidemia—is important. Exclusion of significant ethanol consumption (over 2 units per day), and of other liver diseases by the usual serological tests is mandatory. Patients usually have moderate elevation of serum transaminase (in mild cases ALT/AST ratio is >1, whereas in ALD this ratio is <1). Gamma GT may also be elevated. Patients with milder disease usually have few signs or symptoms but persistent tiredness and/or right upper abdominal pain in the absence of gallstones may be seen in up to one-third. In patients over 50 with suspected NASH or cryptogenic cirrhosis liver biopsy is mandatory, since ultrasound or other liver imaging, while demonstrating fat, cannot demonstrate the presence of inflammation or fibrosis. In late-stage disease in which cryptogenic cirrhosis has supervened the clinical and laboratory findings are similar to those of any other advanced liver disease.

Treatment

At present no treatment has been shown in randomized control trials to prevent progress of NASH to cirrhosis. In view of the association between NASH and obesity/insulin resistance, sensible weight reduction and exercise (which improves insulin resistance) seem logical and are currently being evaluated in control trials. Metformin may also be used to improve insulin resistance (again this is the subject of current control trials); however, in elderly patients with significant liver disease the use of metformin may be hazardous in view of the possibility of development of hypoglycemia. In patients presenting with cryptogenic cirrhosis, treatment and monitoring are as for other forms of cirrhosis.

HEMOCHROMATOSIS

The only inherited disease of the liver that is of importance in elderly people is hereditary hemochromatosis (HHC). Wilson's disease is not known to occur in individuals over the age of 50 and other important inborn errors of metabolism causing liver injury usually lead to death well before the age of 60, or, as in the case of α1 antitrypsin deficiency are of doubtful relevance in patients over 60.

HHC results from increased inappropriate absorption of iron with increase hepatic uptake of iron from transferrin. It is characterized by progressive iron loading of parenchymal cells of the liver, pancreas, heart, and other organs, ultimately leading to cirrhosis and deterioration of function of these other organs.[51] The hemochromatosis gene (HFE gene) is located on chromosome 6. HHC is associated with homozygosity of a mutation at position C282Y on the HFE gene or of compound heterozygosity in positions 282Y/H63D (this latter compound mutation being rare). HHC occurs in about one person in 400 in populations with largely white and particularly Celtic origin. The principal genetic mutation (C282Y) has variable phenotypic expression. This is still poorly understood. It is the most common autosomal recessive gene of importance.[114] The mean age of presentation with first symptoms attributable to hemochromatosis is probably around 50 years but in individuals with no previous known family history, detection may be made up to 75 years. Similarly, screening of families in which newly detected cases have been observed can reveal asymptomatic subjects over the age of 65 or 70. Diagnosis of hemochromatosis is now made using the triad of genotyping, iron studies (raised ferritin and iron saturation), and liver biopsy (appearance of excess stainable iron). Liver biopsy is important for assessment of severity of liver injury. While in very young individuals found on screening to have HHC liver biopsy is not necessary, in patients over 60, liver biopsy should be carried out. In Mediterranean countries some patients with hereditary hemochromatosis do not have the classical mutations (presumably others are involved); some patients who have received excessive blood transfusions or treatment with iron over many years may develop secondary hepatic hemosiderosis very comparable to HHC.

Typically symptoms are weakness, abdominal pain, and lethargy. Arthralgia, loss of libido or impotence, cardiac failure, and symptoms of diabetes represent nonhepatic manifestations of the illness. Clinical diabetes is present in over 50 percent of older patients. Occasionally, older patients present for the first time with the complications or portal hypertension or liver failure superimposed upon evidence of cirrhosis; this is often associated with the development of HCC. In general, elderly patients presenting with cirrhosis rapidly develop severe complications of portal hypertension and liver cell failure. Suspicion should be extremely high that these individuals already have or will shortly develop HCC.[115] For this reason family screening, even for elderly family members, is mandatory after detection of an individual with hemochromatosis and may be carried out now by routine genotyping where the genotype of the proband is known.[51]

Treatment is with venesection. About 500 mL blood should be removed at 2-weekly intervals until serum ferritin falls within the normal range. Despite frequent venesection, anemia very seldom occurs. Once serum ferritin has been returned to normal, follow-up may be two or three times per year with repeat serum ferritin; if ferritin rises above the normal range venesection may be carried out again. In pre-cirrhotic patients venesection prevents progression to cirrhosis. In cirrhotic patients it reduces the likelihood of hepatocellular failure; unfortunately it does not prevent development of HCC. Up to 30 percent of patients with hemochromatosis and cirrhosis die of HCC.[115] Venesection also prevents the onset of nonhepatic complications of hemochromatosis if they have not already occurred.

LIVER CYSTS

It is unclear whether many liver cysts within the liver are congenital or arise during life. It is convenient to consider them under this section on inherited disorders. Liver cysts are defined for this purpose as a liver enclosed space or spaces which may contain air, liquid, or a small amount of solid.[116]

Solitary cysts

These cysts are now being detected much more frequently because of increased use of abdominal ultrasound. They are almost always under low pressure, seldom grow with any speed, and are rarely associated with symptoms. Occasionally, an elderly patient with abdominal pain of unknown origin may be shown to have one or several such cysts. It may be worth aspirating such a cyst by percutaneous needle aspiration under local anesthetic on one occasion, particularly if symptoms are localized and repeat ultrasound shows some change in size. If the treatment produces relief of symptoms consideration can be given to marsupialization since, following aspiration, cysts almost always reform. Unfortunately, the connection between right-sided upper abdominal pain and liver cysts, even of moderate size is still quite unclear. These cysts are always benign and despite considerable size almost never rupture without abdominal trauma.

Adult fibropolycystic disease

Multiple cysts from three or four up to several hundred within the liver are frequently associated with polycystic kidneys.[116] There is an overlap among the conditions of congenital hepatic fibrosis, intrahepatic biliary cystic disease (Caroli's disease), and simple polycystic disease. Occasionally, such cystic diseases of the liver appear in elderly adults, and there may be a question of distinguishing between such cysts and malignant lesions. Polycystic disease of the liver is compatible with long life and no specific treatment is indicated. Occasionally in young adults the number and size of these symptoms lead to the development of portal hypertension and its complications. In extraordinarily rare circumstances there may be malignant transformation of such cysts.

THE LIVER IN SYSTEMIC CONDITIONS

It has already been mentioned that in conditions such as severe cardiac failure and systemic (essentially nonhepatic) bacterial infections the liver may become involved showing abnormal blood tests, impaired function, and abnormal histology.[24,25,45] In addition there are several systemic diseases in which, while the liver is not the origin of the illness, nor indeed the prime target organ, clinically important or vital hepatic abnormalities may occur, occasionally being life threatening in their own right. These conditions will be briefly reviewed specifically in relation to liver disease of old age.

Liver in heart failure

Hepatomegaly is present in over 90 percent of patients with chronic right heart failure and since splenomegaly, peripheral edema, plural effusions, and ascites may also be present in chronic right heart failure as well as in cirrhosis, there are occasionally difficulties in making the differential diagnosis in an elderly patient with these signs. With improved treatments for severe heart failure now available the development of fibrosis (so-called nutmeg liver) and ultimately cirrhosis in chronic heart failure now very rarely occurs.[117] In patients with acute left heart failure accompanied by hypotension, hepatic hypoperfusion may occur giving rise to a sudden very sharp elevation in liver enzymes, particularly transaminases. It is now recognized that this may be the commonest cause of very elevated transaminase in elderly people,[23] and may occur not only in the setting of acute myocardial infarction but following major abdominal surgery.

Connective tissue diseases

While certain specific liver diseases (like PBC) are found in association with a variety of connective tissue diseases (for example rheumatoid arthritis and primary Sjögren's syndrome), in many instances nonspecific abnormalities in LFTs and histology are noted. In particular elevations of serum, ALP may be observed in up to 50 percent of patients with rheumatoid arthritis. In some of these individuals the ALP may be of bony origin, in some it may be related to medications, and in some it may be attributable to asymptomatic PBC. Nonetheless, variable elevation of serum ALP over time is seen in elderly patients with rheumatoid arthritis for whom none of the above explanations is applicable.[118] Liver histology in such patients shows mild nonspecific and nonprogressive changes. Similar abnormalities in LFTs and liver histology are frequently found in elderly patients with polymyalgia rheumatica. Unless an additional separate liver disease is expected, therefore, it is unnecessary to investigate mild abnormalities of LFTs in older patients with rheumatic or collagen vascular disorders beyond the conventional screen of liver blood tests.

Hodgkin's lymphoma and non-Hodgkin's lymphomas

The liver is significantly involved in perhaps 5 percent of patients with Hodgkin's lymphoma and in a higher proportion (about 25 percent) with non-Hodgkin's lymphomas. Such liver involvement can vary from mild abnormalities in serum ALP seen in up to 40 percent of Hodgkin's disease patients, but with no clinical significance, to gross hepatic enlargement due to massive infiltration of the liver or obstructive jaundice due to hilar lymph node enlargement.[119] Occasionally in the investigation of pyrexia of unknown origin liver biopsy reveals the presence of the Reed–Sternberg cells of Hodgkin's disease or the highly abnormal lymphocytes of non-Hodgkin's lymphoma. The treatment of such patients is the same as for other elderly patients with lymphoma (see Chapter 98). For further consideration of liver involvement in systemic diseases see relevant chapters in refs 20–22.

HEPATOCELLULAR CANCER

It is becoming increasingly clear that primary HCC is largely a disease of aging in Western countries, like the United States and even in England.[120,121] In elderly people it is almost always associated with cirrhosis, regardless of the underlying cause, and it is probable that the length of time for which an individual has had cirrhosis is an important determining factor. In Britain, about half of HCC patients with cirrhosis present over the age of 65, although in only a minority of those presenting over 65 was the underlying cirrhosis known prior to first presentation of HCC. Worldwide the main underlying causes of cirrhosis are HBV and HCV.[122] In the United Kingdom, an area with low prevalence of HBV infection, about 20 percent of HCC patients over 65 years old show markers of previous HBV infection and about 40 percent have evidence of previous presumed HCV infection.[123] In Japan, where HCV is common, Ikeda et al. showed that the incidence of HCC increases with age in Japanese patients with cirrhosis.[124] However, in individuals over age 80, incidence of HCC appears to decline again for reasons that are unclear.[125] In European populations the combination of alcohol consumption with markers for previous HBV or HCV infection appears to be particularly potent in leading to the development of HCC in elderly cirrhotics. Now, the development of HCC in cryptogenic cirrhosis, hemochromatosis, and even primary biliary cirrhosis is recognized. Among men, risk of development of HCC in cirrhosis varies from 1 to 5 percent per year depending upon the underlying cause of cirrhosis. Among women, development of HCC is less common.

Diagnosis and presentation

AFP is the most important tumor marker for the diagnosis of HCC, being present in 70 percent of most series. Other tumor markers have been proposed but none is used routinely.[122] Great advances have been made in imaging of HCCs. Differential diagnosis has improved by using combination of several modalities with contrast material. Ultrasound angiography has most recently been shown to detect even small HCCs (<3 cm in diameter) in over 90 percent of cases; elsewhere conventional angiography or lipiodol CT are most widely used.[126,127] If curative surgery is contemplated, biopsy of suspected HCC lesions should not be carried out.

Elderly patients with HCC frequently present with the complications of cirrhosis—bleeding varices, ascites, and encephalopathy—and it is only during subsequent observation of the underlying cause of their disease and the reason for its sudden decompensation that HCC becomes apparent. There should be a high suspicion of underlying HCC in all individuals over 70 years presenting for the first time with complications of what is clearly cirrhosis.

Management

Patients with known cirrhosis, particularly men, should now be followed to try to detect the development of very early HCC. Routine screening with serum αFP at 6-monthly intervals is a minimal requirement. This should be accompanied by annual liver ultrasound screening, although the results of such screening are still debatable.[122] In patients with hepatitis-C-related cirrhosis, initial observations have suggested that treatment with interferon, whether successful in eliminating the HCV or not, appears to halve the risk of carcinogenesis.[128] Since the prognosis for elderly patients with HCC is dreadful—in a recent UK review, mean survival following diagnosis was 10.5 weeks in those over 65[123]—heroic treatments may be considered, but such treatment should be balanced against likelihood of improvement and overall likely efficacy of treatment in frail elderly patients. Older patients presenting with worse prognostic features (raised bilirubin ascites, extrahepatic spread, multiple and large tumors) should, at present therefore probably only receive palliative treatment. In patients with small (<3 cm) lesions, even if there are two or three of these, percutaneous ethanol injection or, more recently thermocoagulation, may yield more palliative results with survival of up to several years.[129,130] In larger tumors, consideration may be given to infusion into the hepatic artery branches of chemotherapy (adriamycin or cisplatin) using lipiodol as a vehicle to deliver the chemotherapy to the lesion; this may be accompanied by arterial embolization, particularly in Child's Grade A patients.[131] Very occasionally in extremely fit elderly patients, particularly those rare individuals without cirrhosis, local resection of small HCCs may be considered.[131] Liver transplantation is also used in carefully selected patients with HCCs <5 cm and very rigorous exclusion of extrahepatic spread, but this is extraordinarily rarely undertaken in patients over 65.

METASTATIC CANCER

Hepatic metastases from distant primary sources, often in the gut, are far more common in elderly individuals than primary tumors. In a recent audit of patients admitted to Newcastle hospitals with all liver diseases 10 percent of admissions were for metastatic cancer; mean age was 65 (personal observation). Such metastases are usually detected in one of three ways:

1. As part of routine screening following detection of a primary tumor elsewhere—before colonic surgery for carcinoma of the colon for example
2. In the investigation of an elderly patient with abnormal LFTs
3. In the investigation of a patient presenting with an abdominal mass revealed to be an enlarged liver.

In any event, histological confirmation of a lesion detected by one imaging technique or another must be obtained unless the source of a presumed distant primary tumor is already established or unless surgical resection of the hepatic lesion is contemplated. The reason for biopsy is that whereas multiple metastases from pancreatic or gastric primary adenocarcinomas carry an extremely poor prognosis, this is not the case for some ovarian tumors, carcinoid tumors, or lymphoma. The management of these conditions is considered elsewhere.

COMPLICATIONS OF CIRRHOSIS

It should be remembered that while cirrhosis and its complications are the major factor influencing prognosis in elderly patients with chronic liver disease, the impact of concurrent diseases unrelated to the liver on mortality in elderly patients is of great importance. Thus, in a Japanese study of 135 patients aged 80 or older, only 37 percent of deaths were liver related even though 28 patients had HCC at the time of death.[125]

Portal hypertension

The pathogenesis and anatomy of portal hypertension are well described in standard major texts on liver disease. This section will deal with acute and long-term management of the two major complications of portal hypertension—bleeding varices, and ascites. Portal hypertension may result from cirrhosis of any cause and may also occur following occlusion of the hepatic vein (Budd–Chiari syndrome) or, more commonly in elderly patients, occlusion of the portal vein (portal vein thrombosis). Budd–Chiari syndrome is extremely rare in elderly patients but may occasionally occur in association with a hypercoagulable state associated with a myeloproliferative disorder. Far more common is the development of portal hypertension in elderly patients without parenchymal liver disease as a result of portal vein thrombosis. This may occur following abdominal sepsis (for example a diverticular abscess) or following abdominal surgery with associated hypotension. Portal vein thrombosis is manifested by ascites. LFTs are often normal or near normal and liver biopsy reveals no serious hepatic abnormality. Diagnosis can now be made by Doppler ultrasound and confirmed by MRI.[132]

Bleeding esophageal and gastric varices

The definitive cause of bleeding in a patient who may have had esophageal varices for several years is still unclear. What can be said is that large varices are more likely to bleed than smaller ones, as are varices in patients with more severe liver disease (as reflected by Child's classification). Bleeding from varices almost never occurs until the hepatic vein pressure gradient (HVPG) exceeds 12 mmHg. This is defined as "clinical significant portal hypertension."[133] The appearance of red wale markings on the varices suggests increased likelihood of hemorrhage. Varices may also form in the stomach, often after endoscopic obliteration of esophageal varices. Effectively these varices merge into so-called portal hypertensive gastropathy in which there is increased gastric mucosal blood flow associated with increased portal pressure, often following obliteration of other varices. In severe gastropathy chronic blood loss may occur as well as the sudden blood loss associated with true varices.[134]

Patients bleeding from varices may present with sudden hematemasis or melena and occasionally only with the signs and symptoms of severe anemia. About 5 percent of first-time upper gastrointestinal bleeders admitted to general hospitals are bleeding from varices. If it is assumed that on admission to the hospital, bleeding has been recent and overt, the twin tracks of diagnosis and treatment run side by side. Acute treatment of bleeding from varices is as for other upper gastrointestinal hemorrhage, with emergency resuscitation initially with plasma expanders until blood has been cross-matched and is available. In severe circumstances this may need to be via a central venous line which in patients with chronic liver disease and potential clotting abnormalities should be placed by a highly experienced person. Once blood pressure has been restored in a patient with suspected varices still actively bleeding, upper gastrointestinal endoscopy should take place. If bleeding is confirmed, start intravenous infusion of the somatostatin analog octreotide (50 mg/hr for up to 48 hours intravenously).[135] If bleeding does not stop with this treatment, balloon tamponade with a Sengstaken–Blakemore triple lumen tube should be used. There is a high rate of complications with this or a similar device (the Minnesota tube), and placement should preferably take place in an experienced center following at least partial control of bleeding with octreotide infusion. If possible, at the time of first endoscopy, direct injection of varices should be made with sclerosant or banding of each varix should be carried out but this is difficult and hazardous in actively bleeding patients.[134]

Longer-term treatment

The incidence of bleeding in cirrhotic patients who have not previously bled is probably about 5 percent per year; if patients have already bled there is a 70 percent chance of rebleeding within 1 year without prophylactic treatment. For these reasons long-term treatment for the varices either to prevent a first bleed or to prevent rebleeding is strongly recommended in elderly patients. There are four main treatment options; each has its advocates. It is vital that whichever is used it is carried out in an experienced center. Briefly, treatment options are as follows.

1. **Pharmacological:** Nonselective beta-blockers significantly reduce the risk of first hemorrhage and significantly improve survival rates when compared to placebo and are currently the treatment of choice to prevent first bleeding. The risk is reduced by 40–50 percent. Propranolol therapy may also reduce mortality; certainly it reduces bleeding-related deaths.[136]

2. **Sclerotherapy:** A course of injection sclerotherapy into the varices at roughly weekly intervals until the veins are eradicated has until relatively recently been the most popular treatment. The problems with sclerotherapy are more frequent hospital inpatient stays, the development of portal gastropathy, and the development of sclerotherapy ulceration itself leading to recurrent bleeding. In acute bleeding, sclerotherapy may help to prevent early rebleeding, thus allowing time for consideration of other treatments.[134] In long-term prophylaxis the place of sclerotherapy has now been largely taken by endoscopic banding. In the past few years, ligation of varices using endoscopic banding apparatus has advanced considerably and

is now the endoscopic treatment of choice, although the relative efficacy of banding against pharmacological treatment is still not clear.[134]

3. TIPS: Transjugular intrahepatic portal systemic shunting (TIPS) is a technical masterpiece but despite early enthusiasm for its use, particularly in patients with refractory bleeding, its place in the treatment of elderly patients is very limited. For reasons that are not clear, prognosis in patients aged over 65 following TIPS is extremely bad, with 80+ percent 6-month mortality. It should, therefore, only be considered in the last resort as a rescue procedure in patients failing medical treatment.

In summary, for both primary and secondary prevention of bleeding in an elderly patient, if there are no other contraindications, long-term nonselective beta-blockade with propranolol is probably the treatment of choice. If beta-blockers are contraindicated then banding, if necessary after control of initial bleeding, is now recommended. Although the prognosis for upper gastrointestinal bleeding is generally worse in elderly patients, at centers with experience in treating bleeding varices immediate mortality and the proportion of elderly patients leaving hospital following an admission with bleeding varices is little different than for younger ones.[137,138]

Cirrhotic ascites

Ascites may be classified conveniently in terms of its causation as transudate or exudate. Transudative causes include severe right-sided heart failure, tricuspid incompetence and constrictive pericarditis, uncomplicated cirrhosis, and portal venous obstruction. Ascites is clearly a transudate if ascitic fluid protein is less than about 15 g/L. Exudative causes include intraperitoneal carcinomatosis, intraperitoneal infectious chylous ascites, and pancreatic ascites; these are unequivocal above 25 g/L. Unfortunately, there is considerable overlap among many of the above conditions but the distinction is still of value.

INVESTIGATION   Investigation of ascites starts with a diagnostic tap which can be carried out with a venepuncture needle. Fluid should be submitted for protein content, microscopy, cytology, and culture. In the investigation of ascites of unknown origin the overwhelming majority of cases are caused by (1) cirrhosis, (2) right-sided heart failure, (3) hepatic venous or portal venous obstruction, and (4) disseminated intra-abdominal carcinomatosis.

Bacterial infection of ascitic fluid without an overt primary source of infection—spontaneous bacterial peritonitis (SBP)—is a common complication in patients with a cirrhosis and carries a serious prognostic implication. Up to 20 percent of patients admitted to a hospital with alcoholic cirrhosis and ascites have occult SBP, now thought to be due to translocation of bacteria from the gut lumen. Specific signs and symptoms of infection are rather lacking, although abdominal pain, fever, and tenderness in a patient with ascites are highly suggestive. If there is a polymorphonuclear white blood cell count over $250/cm^3$, or total white cell count over $50/cm^3$, irrespective of culture positivity, the diagnosis is highly likely and urgent antibiotic treatment should be started immediately.

Treatment with ciprofloxacin, cefotaxime, or norfloxacin is advised. Up to 76 percent of patients developing SBP die within 1 year of its first occurrence.[139]

TREATMENT   Ascites treatment should not necessarily be aimed at completely abolishing all ascitic fluid. Such an objective often leads to overtreatment with consequent risks of electrolyte imbalance and renal impairment. This is particularly true in older patients. Cirrhotic ascites is often accompanied by sodium retention; hence the first step in its treatment is moderate restriction of sodium intake. In ill elderly patients with cirrhosis, malnutrition and ascites often go hand in hand and a high protein intake is desirable. Hence a balancing act must be carried out between providing enough salt to make protein palatable and not giving an excess thus worsening a tendency toward ascites. Since impaired water excretion frequently accompanies cirrhotic ascites paradoxical hyponatremia may also develop—particularly in patients treated with diuretics.[140] Patients in whom serum sodium falls below 125 mmol (125 m equivalent/L) should have water intake restricted to 1 L per day. Intravascular volume can be replaced in these patients with modest infusions of salt poor albumin (2 units every 2 days until serum sodium rises and water restriction can be lifted).

The two mainstays of therapy for ascites are diuretic treatment and abdominal paracentesis. Because hyperaldosteronism is a concomitant of cirrhotic ascites, the use of spironolactone which opposes the action of aldosterone and blocks tubular reabsorption of sodium is the recommended first-line treatment of ascites. Dosage should be cautiously increased from 50 mg/day up to a maximum of 600 mg/day (normally 200–400 mg/day is sufficient). In patients with peripheral edema as well as ascites, a loop diuretic such as frusemide may be added. Thiazide diuretics, which cause natriuresis as well as excretion of potassium and metabolic alkalosis, are not recommended for cirrhotic patients. The progress of diuretic therapy should be monitored by daily weighing at first. A patient with abdominal ascites and without peripheral edema should not lose more than about half a kilogram per day or the risk of renal impairment (hepatorenal syndrome, see below) or development of encephalopathy (see below) will be greatly increased. Bed rest adds to the likely efficacy of this treatment.[140]

Large volume abdominal paracentesis with simultaneous intravenous infusion of albumin is now the most commonly used treatment for severe ascites. This procedure has been shown to be followed by no greater incidence of side-effects than conventional diuretic treatment.[141] Its advantage is that it relieves the patient of discomfort more quickly and may shorten their hospital stay. In elderly patients with end stage liver disease, repeated 24-hour hospital stays with abdominal paracentesis followed by moderate diuretic treatment at home seems sensible and pragmatic. During abdominal paracentesis, 4–6 L of fluid are removed over 1–2 hours and replaced with plasma volume expansion (8 g albumin per liter drained) given intravenously. A peritoneal dialysis catheter is used but must be removed immediately following the paracentesis since leaving it in place greatly increases the risk of subsequent infection. A further treatment is now available for the management of intractable ascites. This is TIPS, already mentioned in connection with treatment of bleeding varices.

The procedure is also highly effective in treatment of ascites, but in patients with very severe liver disease as reflected by Child's Grade C status or, over age 70, complications of infection encephalopathy, other manifestations of hepatocellular failure or renal failure frequently supervene in the months following the TIPS procedure. It is stressed that this procedure is extremely technically demanding and should be carried out only in a very experienced center.[142]

Hepatorenal syndrome

Hepatorenal syndrome (HRS) represents the extreme expression of a systemic circulatory dysfunction in cirrhosis. These patients have arterial hypotension, very low systemic vascular resistance, very high plasma renin and vasoconstriction of the kidneys. This is often exacerbated by diuretic treatment and has, until relatively recently, been thought to carry an extremely adverse prognosis. Now it has been shown that the administration of a vasoconstrictor—one of the vasopressin analog like terlipressin—together with plasma volume expansion (which should be monitored using central venous pressure measurement) may remarkably reverse hepatorenal syndrome.[142] This exciting treatment development should be carried out in an experienced center.

Hepatic encephalopathy

Hepatic encephalopathy is the reversible decrease of consciousness seen in patients with severe liver disease; at the worse end of the spectrum it results in coma. Encephalopathy may be acute, chronic, or episodic. In patients with cirrhosis it is usually precipitated by an adverse event—infection, gastrointestinal bleeding, constipation, electrolyte disturbance, or incorrect medication. In hepatic encephalopathy lethargy, confusion, and stupor are characteristic. At an early stage the characteristic asterixis (flapping tremor) may be seen although it is not specific to hepatic encephalopathy—occasionally being seen in other metabolic encephalopathies. It is sometimes important to distinguish hepatic encephalopathy from the confusion of alcohol withdrawal. In the latter, agitation with anxiety and sweating, tachycardia, hypertension, and tremulousness are important features, whereas somnolence distinguishes encephalopathy. The clinical course of encephalopathy depends on the rapidity with which steps are taken to reverse it, the nature of the precipitative cause and the severity of the underlying liver disease. The greater the depression of conscious level the greater the corresponding risk. The pathogenesis of hepatic encephalopathy is still controversial but although increased levels of such toxins as ammonia and mercaptans may well be contributory or sensitizing factors it is becoming clear that the major mechanism involved in induction of encephalopathy concerns the inhibitory neurotransmitter gamma-aminobutyric acid (GABA) and its receptor. The GABA receptor whose molecular structure has recently been described also appears to be the receptor for benzodiazepine and benzodiazepine-like substances.[143] It now seems that benzodiazepine receptors themselves are increased in brains of individuals with hepatic encephalopathy.[144] Regardless of the exact pathogenesis of hepatic encephalopathy standard treatment is aimed at lowering ammonia. This is carried out by oral administration of lactulose or lactitol. Some attempts have been made at improving the neurological status of patients with encephalopathy using benzodiazepine receptor antagonists and dopamine agonists but these have had controversial results and are not recommended in routine management.[145,146]

REFERENCES

1. Wynne HA, Cope E, Mutch E et al: The effect of age upon liver volume and apparent liver blood flow in healthy man. Hepatology 1989;9:297–301
2. Marchesini G, Bua V, Brunori A et al: Galactose elimination capacity and liver volume in ageing man. Hepatology 1988;8:1079–1083
3. Kitani K: Ageing and the liver. In Popper H, Schaffner F (eds): Progress in liver diseases, Vol 9. WB Saunders, Philadelphia 1990:606–623
4. Ivy GO, Schottler F, Baudrey M et al: Inhibition of lisomosal enzymes: accumulation of lipofuscin like dense bodies in the brain. Science 1984;226:985–987
5. David H, Reinke P: Liver morphology with ageing. In Bianchi L, Holt P, James OFW, Butler RN (eds): Ageing in Liver and Gastrointestinal Tract. MTP Lancaster, UK, 1988:143–159
6. Watanabe T, Tanaka Y: Age related alteration in the size of human hepatocytes: study of mononuclear and binuclear cells. Virchows Archiv 1982;39:9–20
7. Sato T, Tauchi H: The formation of enlarged and giant mitochondria in the ageing process of human hepatic cells. Acta Pathol Jpn 1975;25:403–412
8. Schmucker DL: Hepatocyte fine structure during maturation and senescence. J Electron Microsc Techniques 1990;14:106–110
9. Popper H: Ageing and the liver. In Popper H, Schaffner F (eds): Progress in Liver Diseases, Vol VIII. Grune and Stratton, New York 1986:659–683
10. Marchesini G, Bianchi GP, Fabbri A et al: Synthesis of urea after a protein rich meal in normal man in relation to ageing. Age Ageing 1990;19:4–10
11. Fabbri A, Marchesini A, Bianchi G et al: Functional hepatic urea clearance in advanced age. Liver 1994;14:288–292
12. Einarsson K, Nilsell K, Leijd B et al: Influence of age on secretion of cholesterol and synthesis of bile acids by the liver. N Engl J Med 1985;313:277–282
13. Fausto N: Liver regeneration. J Hepatol 2000;32(suppl 1):19–31
14. Liu Y, Guyton KZ, Gorospe M et al: Age related decline in mitogen activated protein kinase activity in epidermal growth factor stimulated rat hepatocytes. J Biochem 1996;271:3603–3607
15. Wang E: Senescent human fibroblasts resist programmed cell death and failure to suppress bc 12 is involved. Cancer Res 1995;55:2284–2292
16. Greenblatt DJ, Sellers EM, Schader RI: Drug disposition in old age. N Engl J Med 1982;306:1081–1088
17. Woodhouse KW, James OFW: Hepatic drug metabolism and ageing. Br Med Bull 1990;46:22–35
18. Vestal RA: Ageing and determinates of hepatic drug clearance. Hepatology 1989;9:331–334
19. Schnegg MI, Lauterberg BH: Quantitative liver function in the liver assessed by galactose elimination capacity, amino pyrene demethylation and caffeine clearance. J Hepatol 1986;3:164–171
20. Zakim D, Boyer TD (eds): Hepatology: A Textbook of Liver Disease, 4th Ed. WB Saunders, Philadelphia 2002
21. Sherlock S, Dooley JS: Diseases of the Liver and Biliary System, 11th Ed. Blackwell, Oxford, 2002
22. McIntyre N, Benhamou JP, Bircher J et al: Oxford Textbook of Clinical Hepatology, 2nd Ed. Oxford Medical Publications, Oxford, 1997
23. Whitehead MW, Hawkes ND, Hainsworth I et al: A prospective study of the causes of notably raised aspartate aminotransferase of liver origin. Gut 1999;45:129–133
24. Pratt DS, Kaplan MM: Evaluation of abnormal liver enzyme results in asymptomatic patients. New Engl J Med 2000;342:1266–1271
25. Daniel S, Ben-Menachem C, Vasudevan G et al: Prospective evaluation of unexplained chronic liver transaminase abnormality in asymptomatic or symptomatic patients. Am J Gastroenterol 1999;94:3010–3014
26. Berk PD. Hematologic issues in contemporary hepatology. Semin Liver Dis 1987;7:169–277
27. Taylor KJW, Holland S: Doppler ultrasound 1, basic principles instrumentation and pitfalls. Radiology 1990;174:297–308

28. Scoutt IM: Doppler ultrasound 2, clinical applications. Radiology 1990;174;309–330
29. Ralls PW, Johnson MB, Radins DR et al: Budd–Chiari syndrome: detection with colour Doppler sonography. Am J Radiol 1992;159:112–117
30. Jacobs JE, Birnbaum BA, Shapiro MA et al: Contrast enhanced helical CT of liver. Am J Radiol 1998;171:659–664
31. Raby N, Karani R, Mitchell M et al: Lipiodol enhanced CT scanning in assessment of hepatocellular carcinoma. Clin Radiol 1989;40:4480–4485
32. Siegelam ES, Outwater EK: MR imaging of the liver. Radiol Clin Am 1998;36:263–286
33. Siegelman ES, Rosen MA: Imaging of hepatic steatosis. Semin Liver Dis 2001;21:71–80
34. Grant A, Neuberger J: Guidelines on the use of liver biopsy in clinical practice. British Society of Gastroenterology Gut 1999;45(suppl 4)
35. Ueda K, Matsui O, Kawamori Y et al: Hypervascular hepatocellular carcinoma: evaluation of haemodynamics with dynamic CT during hepatic arteriography. Radiology 1998;206:161–166
36. Pomier-Layrargues G: TIPS and hepatic encephalopathy. Semin Liver Dis 1996;16:315–320
37. Rossle MR, Haag K, Ochs A et al: The transjugular intrahepatic shunt procedure for refractory ascites. N Engl J Med 1995;332:1192–1197
38. Lightdale CJ: Laparoscopy. In Zakim D, Boyer TD (eds): Hepatology: A Textbook of Liver Disease. WB Saunders, Philadelphia, 1996;833–844
39. Lightdale CJ: Laparoscopy. In Zakim D, Boyer TD (eds): Hepatology: A Textbook of Liver Disease 4th Ed. WB Saunders, Philadelphia, 2002
40. Gilmore IT, Burroughs A, Murray Lion IM et al: Indications, methods and outcomes of percutaneous liver biopsy in England and Wales. Gut 1995;30:437–441
41. Bedossa P, Poynard T, Metvia R: Coop study group. An algorithm for the grading of activity in chronic hepatitis C. Hepatology 1996;24:289–293
42. Obermayer-Straub P, Strassburg CP, Manns MP: Autoimmune hepatitis. J Hepatol 2000;32(suppl 1):181–197
43. Brunt EM: Non-alcoholic steatohepatitis: Definition and pathology. Semin Liver Dis 2001;21:3–16
44. Poynard T, Bedossa P, Opolon P: Natural history of liver fibrosis progression in patients with chronic hepatitis C. Lancet 1997;349:825–832
45. Skelly MM, James PD, Ryder SD: Findings on liver biopsy to investigate abnormal liver function tests in the absence of diagnostic serology. J Hepatol 2001;35:195–199
46. Lok ASF: Hepatitis B infection: pathogenesis and management. J Heptol 2000;32(suppl 1):89–97
47. Pawlotsky JM, Longjon I, Hezode C, Raynard B et al: What strategy should be used for diagnosis of hepatitis C virus infection in clinical laboratories? Hepatology 1998;27:1700–1702
48. Boyer N, Marcellin P: Pathogenesis diagnosis and management of hepatitis C. J Hepatol 2000;32(suppl 1):98–112
49. James OFW: Natural History and Demography of PBC. In Lindor KD, Heathcote EJ, Poupo R (eds): Primary Biliary Cirrhosis. Kluwer, Dordrecht, 1998:3–10
50. Schramm C, Kanzler S, Meyer zum Buschenfelde KM, Galle PR, Lohse AW: Autoimmune hepatitis in the elderly. Am J Gastrol 2001;96:1587–1590
51. Powell LW, Subramainian VN, Yapp TR: Hemochromatosis in the new millennium. J Hepatol 1999;32(suppl 1):48–62
52. Potter JR, James OFW: Clinical features and prognosis of alcoholic liver disease in respect of advancing age. Gerontology 1987;33:380–387
53. Aron E, Dupin M, Jobard P: Les cirrhoses du troisieme age. Ann Gastroenterol Hepatol 1979;15:558–563
54. Garagliano CF, Lilienfeld AM, Mendelhof AI: Incidence rates of liver cirrhosis and related diseases in Baltimore and selected areas of the United States. J Chron Dis 1979;32:543–554
55. Beresford TP, Lucey MR: Ethanol metabolism and intoxication in the elderly. In Beresford TP, Gomberg E (eds): Alcohol and Ageing. Oxford University Press, New York, 1995:117–127
56. Kraus ML, Gottlieb LD, Horwitz RI et al: Randomised clinical trial of atenolol in patients with alcohol withdrawal. N Engl J Med 1985;313:905–909
57. Mathurin P, Duchatelle V, Ramond MJ et al: Survival and prognosis factors in patients with severe alcoholic hepatitis treated with steroids. Gastroenterology 1996;110:1847–1853
58. Cabre E, Rodriguez-Iglesias P, Caballeria J et al: Short and long term outcome of severe alcohol-induced hepatitis is treated with steroids or enteral nutrition. Hepatology 2000;32:36–42
59. Nair S, Eason JD, Loss GER, Mason AL: Relative risk of hepatocellular carcinoma in cirrhosis. Hepatology 2001;34:462A
60. Woodhouse KW, Mortimer O, Wiholm BE: Hepatic adverse drug reactions—the effect of age. In Kitani K (ed): Liver and Ageing. Elsevier, Amsterdam, 1986:75–80
61. Nolan L, O'Malley K: Prescribing for the elderly. Part I. Sensitivity of the elderly to adverse drug reactions. J Am Geriat Soc 1998;36:142–150
62. Almdal TP, Sorensen TIA: Incidence of parenchymal liver disease in Denmark 1981–1885. Analysis of hospitalisation registry data. Hepatology 1990;13:650–654
63. Regev A, Schiff ER: Liver disease in the elderly. Gastroenterol Clin N America 2001;30:547–563
64. Willner IR, Howard SC, Williams EQ et al: Serious hepatitis A: an analysis of patients hospitalised during an urban epidemic in the United States. Ann Intern Med 1998;128:111–114
65. Lee WM, Schiodt FV: Fulminant hepatic failure. In Schiff ER, Sorrel MF, Maddrey WC (eds): Schiff's Diseases of the Liver, 8th Ed. Philadelphia, Lippincott-Raven, 1999:879
66. Forbes A, Williams R: Increasing age—an important adverse prognostic factor in hepatitis A virus infection. JR Coll Physicians Lond 1988;22:237–239
67. James OFW: Parenchymal liver disease in the elderly. Gut 1997;41:430–432
68. Condo Y, Tsukada K, Takeuchi T et al: High carrier rate after hepatitis B virus infection in the elderly. Hepatology 1993;18:768
69. Waters JA, Bailey C, Love C et al: A study of the antigenicity and immunogenicity of a new hepatitis B vaccine using a panel of monoclonal antibodies. J Med Virol 1998;54:1–6
70. Lemon SM, Thomas DL: Vaccines to prevent viral hepatitis. N Engl J Med 1997;336:196–204
71. Saif MW, Little RF, Hamilton JM, Allegra CJ, Wilson WH: Reactivation of chronic hepatitis B infection following intensive chemotherapy. A case report and review of the literature. Ann Oncol 2001;12:123–129
72. Lynn SM, Sheen IS, Schien RN, Chu CM, Liaw YF: Long term beneficial effect of interferon therapy in patients with chronic hepatitis virus infection. Hepatology 1999;29:971–975
73. WHO: Hepatitis C: Global prevalence. Weekly Epidemiol Rec 1997;72:341
74. Markus EL, Kaspa RT: Viral hepatitis in older adults. JAGS 1997;45:755–763
75. Hoshida Y, Ikeda K, Kobayashi M et al: Chronic liver disease in the extremely elderly of 80 years or more: clinical characteristics, prognosis and patient survival analysis. J Hepatol 1999;31:860–866
76. Alter MJ, Kruszon-Moran D, Nainan OV et al: The prevalence of hepatitis C virus infection in the United States 1988 through 1994. N Engl J Med 1999;341:556–560
77. Poynard T, Bedossa P, Opolon P: Natural history of liver fibrosis progression in patients with chronic hepatitis C. Lancet 1997;349:825–832
78. Roudot-Thoraval F, Bastie A, Pawlotsky JM et al: Epidemiological factors affecting the severity of hepatitis C virus related liver disease. Hepatology 1997;26:485–490
79. Reddy KR, Wright TL, Pockros PJ et al: Efficacy and safety of pegylated interferon α-2a compared with interferon α-2a in non-cirrhotic patients with hepatitis C. Heptology 2001;33:433–438
80. Sridharan GV, Wilkinson SP, Promrose WR: Pyogenic liver abscess in the elderly. Age Ageing 1990;19:199–203
81. Smoger SH, Mitchell CK, McClave SA: Pyogenic liver abscesses: a comparison of older and younger patients. Age Ageing 1998;27:443–448
82. Greenstein AJ, Lowenthal D, Hammer JS et al: Continuing changing patterns of disease in pyogenic liver abscess. A study in 38 patients. Am J Gastroenterol 1984;79:217–222
83. Bertel CR, Van Heerden JA, Sheedy PF: Treatment of pyogenic hepatic abscess, surgical vs percutaneous drainage. Arch Surg 1986;121:554–562
84. Zimmerman HJ, Fang M, Utili R et al: Jaundice due to bacterial infection. Gastroenterology 1979;77:362–369
85. Miller DJ, Keeton GR, Webber JL et al: Jaundice in severe bacterial infection. Gastroenterology 1976;71:94–98
86. Parker SG, James OFW, Young ET: Causes of raised serum alkaline phosphatase in elderly patients. Mod Trends Ageing Res 1986;147:153–157
87. Newton JL, Jones DE, Metcalf JV et al: Presentation and mortality of PBC in older patients. Age Ageing 2000;29:305–309
88. Grambsch PM, Dickson ER, Kaplan MM et al: Extramural cross validation of the Mayo PBC model. Hepatology 1989;10:846–850
89. Metcalf JV, Mitchison HC, Palmer JM et al: Natural history of early primary biliary cirrhosis. Lancet 1996;348:1399–1402

90. Prince MI, Chetwynd A, Craig WL et al: Clinical features, prognosis and symptom progression in a large population based cohort of patients with PBC. Lancet 2002 (in press)

91. Kaplan MM: Primary biliary cirrhosis. N Engl J Med 1996;335:1570–1580

92. Newton J, Francis R, Prince M et al: Osteoporosis in primary biliary cirrhosis revisited. Gut 2001;49:282–287

93. Ruddich S, Busuttil R: Similar outcomes morbidity and mortality for orthotopic liver transplantation between the very elderly and the young. Transplant Proc 1999;31:523–528

94. Zetterman RK, Belle SH, Hoofnagle JH et al: Age and liver transplantation: a report of the liver transplantation database. Transplantation 1998;66:500–504

95. Poupon RE, Lindor KD, Cauch Duduk K et al: Combined analysis of randomed control trials of UDCA in primary biliary cirrhosis. Gastroenterology 1997;113:884–890

96. Goulis J, Leandro G, Burroughs AK: Randomised control trials of ursodeoxycholic acid therapy for primary biliary cirrhosis: a meta-analysis. Lancet 1999;354:1053–1060

97. Schramm C, Kanzler S, Meyer zum Buschenfelde K-H, Galle PR, Lohse AW: Spectrum of autoimmune hepatitis in older individuals. Am J Gastrol 2001;1587–1591

98. Newton JL, Burt AD, Park JB et al: Autoimmune hepatitis in older patients. Age Ageing 1997;26:441–444

99. Parker DR, Kingham JGC: Type 1 autoimmune hepatitis is primarily a disease of later life. QJ Med 1997;90:289–296

100. Alvarez F, Berg PA, Bianchi FB et al: International autoimmune hepatitis group report: review of criteria for diagnosis of autoimmune hepatitis. J Hepatol 1999;31:929–938

101. Ben-Ari Z, Czaja AJ: Autoimmune hepatitis and its variant syndromes. Gut 2001;49:589–594

102. Broome U, Olsson R, Loof L et al: Natural history and prognostic factors in 305 Swedish patients with PSC. Gut 1996;38:610–615

103. Ludwig J, Viggiano TR, McGill DB, Ott BJ: Nonalcoholic steatohepatitis. Mayo Clinic Proc 1980;55:4334–4338

104. Falck-Ytter Y, Younossi ZM, Marchesini G, McCullough AJ: Clinical features and natural history of non-alcoholic steatosis syndromes. Semin Liver Dis 2001;21:17–26

105. Reid AE: Nonalcoholic steatohepatitis. Gastroenterology 2001;121:710–723

106. Day CP, James OFW: Steatohepatitis: a tale of two "hits"? Gastroenterology 1998;114:842–845

107. Chitturi S, Farrel GC: Etiopathogenesis of non-alcoholic steatohepatitis. Semin Liver Dis 2001;21:27–41

108. Matteoni CA, Younossi ZM, Gramlich T et al: Non-alcoholic fatty liver disease: a spectrum of clinical and pathological severity. Gastroenterology 1999;116:1413–1419

109. Angulo P, Keach JC, Battz KP, Lindor KD: Independent predictors of liver fibrosis in patients with non-alcoholic steatohepatitis. Hepatology 1999;30:1356–1362

110. Raziu V, Girai P, Charlotte F et al: Liver fibrosis in overweight patients. Gastroenterology 2000;118:1117–1123

111. Caldwell S, Oelsner D, Lezzoni J et al: Cryptogenic cirrhosis: clinical characterization and risk factors for underlying disease. Hepatology 1999;29:664–669

112. Poonawalon A, Nair SP, Thuluvath PJ: Prevalence of obesity and diabetes in patients with cryptogenic cirrhosis: A case-control study. Hepatology 2000;32:689–692

113. Ratziu VD, Bonyhay L, Cavallaro L et al: Hepatocellular carcinoma, liver failure, and liver mortality in obesity related cryptogenic cirrhosis. Hepatology 2001;34:458A

114. Bacon BR, Powell LW, Adams PC, Kresina TF, Hoofnagle JH: Molecular medicine and haemochromatosis: at the crossroads. Gastroeneterology 1999;116:193–207

115. Niederau C, Fisher R, Sonnenberg A et al: Survival and causes of death in cirrhotic and non-cirrhotic patients with primary haemochromatosis. N Engl J Med 1985;313:1256–1262

116. Somerfield JA, Nagafuchi Y, Sherlock S et al: Hepatobiliary fibropolycistic disease: a clinical and histological review of 51 patients. J Hepatol 1986;2:141–149

117. Clain DJ: Liver disease in the elderly. In Gelb AM (ed): Clinical Gastroeneterology in the Elderly. Dekker, New York, 1996:167–183

118. Thompson PW, Houghton BJ, Clifford C et al: The source and significance of raised serum enzymes in rheumatoid arthritis. Q J Med 1970;28:869–881

119. Jaffe ES: Malignant lymphomas: pathology of hepatic involvement. Semin Liver Dis 1987;7:257–268

120. El Serag HB, Mason AC: Rising incidence of hepatocellular carcinoma in the United States. N Engl J Med 1999;340:745–750

121. Taylor-Robinson SD, Foster GR, Arrora S, Hargreaves S, Thomas HC: Increase in primary liver cancer in the UK 1979–1994. Lancet 1997;350:1142–1143

122. Okuda K: Hepatocellular carcinoma. J Hepatol 2000;32(suppl 1):225–237

123. Collier JD, Curless R, Bassendine MF, James OFW: Clinical features and prognosis of hepatocellular carcinoma in Britain in relation to age. Age Ageing 1994;23:22–28

124. Ikeda K, Saitoh S, Suzuki Y et al: Disease progression and hepatocellular carcinogenesis in patients with chronic viral hepatitis: a prospective observation of 2215 patients. J Hepatol 1998;28:930–932

125. Hoshida Y, Ikeda K, Kobayashi M et al: Chronic liver disease in the extremely elderly of 80 years or more, clinical characteristics, prognosis and patient survival analysis. J Hepatol 1999;31:860–864

126. Kudo M: Imaging diagnosis of hepatocellular carcinoma and pre-malignant borderline lesions. Semin Liver Dis 1999;19:235–241

127. Yumota Y, Ginno K, Tokuyama K et al: Hepatocellular carcinoma detected by iodised oil. Radiology 1985;154:19–24

128. Ikeda K, Saitoh S, Arase Y et al: Effective interferon therapy on hepatocellular carcinogenesis in patients with chronic hepatitis type C. A long term observation study of 1643 patients using statistical bias correction with proportional hazards analysis. Hepatology 1999;29:1124–1130

129. Livraghi T, Giorgio A, Marin G et al: Hepatocellular carcinoma and cirrhosis in 746 patients. Long-term results of percutaneous ethanol injection. Radiology 1995;197:101–108

130. Goldberg SN, Gazelle GS, Solbiati L: Ablation of liver tumours using percutaneous RF therapy. Am J Roentgenol 1998;170:1023–1028

131. Bismuth H: Hepatocellular carcinoma in the elderly. Results of surgical and non-surgical management. Am J Gastoenterol 1999;94:2336–2340

132. Merckel C, Sacerdoti D, Bolognesi M, Bombonato G, Gatta A: Doppler sonography and hepatic vein catheterisation in portal hypertension: Assessment of agreement in evaluating severity and response to treatment. J Hepatol 1998;28:622–630

133. de Franchis R: Updating consensus in portal hypertension: Report of the Baveno III Consensus Workshop on Definitions, Methodology and Therapeutic Strategies in Portal Hypertension. J Hepatol 2000;33:846–852

134. Bosch J, Garcia-Pagan JC: Complications of cirrhosis I portal hypertension. J Hepatol 2000;32(suppl 1):141–156

135. Garcia-Pagan JC, Escorsell A, Moitinho E, Bosch J: Influence of pharmacological agents of portal haemodynamics. Semin Liver Dis 1999;19:427–438

136. Poynard T, Cales P, Pasta L et al: Beta-adrenergic anatagonist drugs in the prevention of gastrointestinal bleeding in patients with cirrhosis and oesophageal varices. N Engl J Med 1991;324:1532–1538

137. Bullimore DW, Miloszewski KJ, Losowsky MS: The prognosis of elderly subjects with oesophageal varices. Age Ageing 1989;18:35–39

138. del Olmo, JA, Pena A, Serra MA et al: Prediction of morbidity and mortality after the first episode of upper gastrointestinal bleeding in liver cirrhosis. J Hepatol 2000;32:19–26

139. Navasa M, Rimola A, Rodes J: Bacterial infections in liver disease. Semin Liver Dis 1997;17:323–333

140. Arroyo V, Jimenez W: Complications of cirrhosis II. J Hepatol 2000;32(suppl 1):157–170

141. Arroyo V, Gines P, Gerbes AL et al: Definition and diagnostic criteria of refractory ascites and hepatorenal syndrome in cirrhosis. Hepatology 1996;23:164–176

142. Arroyo V, Cardenas A: TIPS in the treatment of refractory ascite. In Arroyo V, Bosch J, Bruguera M, Rodes J, Sanchez Tapias JM (eds): Treatment of Liver Diseases. Masson, Barcelona, 1999:43–51

143. Guevara M, Gines P, Fernandez-Esparrach G et al: Reversibility of hepatorenal syndrome by prolonged administration of ornipressin and plasma volume expansion. Hepatology 1998;1:35–41

144. Basile AE, Gammal SH, Mullen KD et al: Hepatic encephalopathy: Evidence for the involvement of an endogenous benzodiazepine receptor ligand. Hepatology 1987;7:1103–1110

145. Butterworth RF: Complications of cirrhosis III hepatic encephalopathy. J Hepatol 2000;32(suppl 1):171–180

146. Ferenci P, Herneth A, Steindl P: Newer approaches to therapy of hepatic encephalopathy. Semin Liver Dis 1996;16:329–338

Chapter 81

Biliary tract diseases

Maria Luisa Raimondo and Andrew Burroughs

Jaundice, or icterus, is the yellow discoloration of sclerae, mucous membranes, and skin caused by accumulation of bilirubin: clinically, it is not obvious until the bilirubin concentration in the blood exceeds 51 µmol/L (3 mg/dL).

The appearance of jaundice is also related to the circulatory status and any accompanying edema. Particularly in elderly people, paralytic and edematose limbs tend not to have the typical pigmentation and it is possible to observe a one-sided icterus in patients with hemiplegia.

Jaundice can be classified in different ways, depending on:

- prevalent form of bilirubin detectable in serum: unconjugated, mixed, or conjugated hyperbilirubinemia
- site of impairment in bilirubin production and/or excretion pathway: it is classically divided into prehepatic, hepatocellular, and obstructive.

From a practical point of view, it is useful clinically to consider conditions that lead to icterus under the following categories:

- isolated disorders of bilirubin metabolism
- liver disease
- obstruction of the bile ducts.

ISOLATED DISORDERS OF BILIRUBIN METABOLISM

In these conditions there is an increase in bilirubin production (hemolysis, ineffective erythropoiesis, blood transfusion, resorption of hematomas) or decreased hepatocellular uptake or conjugation (congenital hyperbilirubinemias); liver function is otherwise normal and hyperbilirubinemia is often characterized by a predominant elevation in unconjugated bilirubin.

Jaundice resulting from hemolysis is usually mild with a serum bilirubin of 68–102 µmol/L (or 4–6 mg/dL) as normal liver function can easily handle the increased bilirubin derived from excessive breakdown of red cells. Unconjugated bilirubin is not water-soluble and therefore will not pass into the urine; hence the term "acholuric jaundice." Urinary urobilinogen is increased. Causes of hemolytic jaundice are those of hemolytic anemia. Investigations show raised unconjugated bilirubin but normal serum alkaline phosphatase, transferase, and albumin, and serum haptoglobins are low.

Most of the congenital and inherited defects are diagnosed in young people; the only condition that could incidentally be found in older patients is Gilbert's syndrome, the most common familial hyperbilirubinemia. It is asymptomatic and is usually detected as an incidental finding of a slightly raised bilirubin 17–102 µmol/L (or 1–6 mg/dL) on a routine check. No signs of liver disease are present. There is a family history of jaundice in 5–15 percent of patients.

Hepatic glucuronidation is approximately 30 percent of normal, resulting in an increased proportion of bilirubin monoglucuronide in bile. Most patients have reduced levels of UDP-glucuronosyl transferase activity, the enzyme that conjugates bilirubin with glucuronic acid. Recent evidence[1–3] has shown mutations in the gene encoding this enzyme with an expanded nucleotide repeat consisting of two extra bases in upstream 5' promoter element. The abnormality appears to be necessary, but is not in itself sufficient for the phenotypic expression of the syndrome.[4]

The major importance of establishing this diagnosis is to inform the patient that it is not a serious disease and to prevent unnecessary investigations. Tests show only a raised unconjugated bilirubin, which is further raised on fasting, during mild illnesses, infections, after surgery or consumption of large amounts of alcohol; the reticulocyte count is normal. No treatment is necessary.

LIVER DISEASE

Primary sclerosing cholangitis (PSC) is a chronic cholestatic disease characterized by progressive obliterating fibrosis of the biliary tree. It affects primarily young men. Etiology is still unclear: both immune (genetic) and nonimmune (infections, toxins, ischemic damage) mechanisms have been postulated. There is a strong association between PSC and inflammatory bowel diseases (IBD): 60–80 percent of PSC patients have coexisting ulcerative colitis (UC) and in 2–6 percent of UC patients, PSC is also present. However, there is no correlation between severity of PSC and IBD, nor a temporal relation between the onset of the diseases.

Usually PSC presents as an acute cholangitis, with right upper quadrant pain, fever, rigors, and jaundice, with recurrent attacks; in advanced disease, jaundice is constantly present.

Serum alkaline phosphatase levels are raised in the majority of patients; perinuclear antineutrophil cytoplasmic antibodies (pANCA) may be detected in 26–85 percent of PSC cases, but since they are present in other autoimmune liver diseases or IBD without concomitant PSC they lack specificity for diagnosis.

Despite emerging evidence supporting a role for magnetic resonance imaging in diagnosing PSC,[5,6] endoscopic retrograde cholangiopancreatography (ERCP) is still the gold standard, although it is invasive: typical findings are multifocal strictures of the biliary tree alternating with normal segments and ectatic ducts; liver biopsy shows fibro-obliterative ductal lesions in one-third of cases. There is no correlation between histological severity and radiological findings.

An estimated median survival of 12 years has been reported for PSC: for symptomatic patients there is a significant reduction in life expectancy (112 months).[7] There is a well established risk of developing cholangiocarcinoma, especially in patients with coexisting UC; these patients are also considered to carry a higher risk of developing colorectal cancer, but evidence is less clear.

Different drugs (antifibrotic such as methotrexate or colchicin, penicillamine, UDCA) have been used, but none of them has proven to be effective in improving liver function tests, symptoms or survival.

Currently liver transplantation is the only life-extending treatment available, with 5-year survival rates of 75–85 percent.

OBSTRUCTION OF BILE DUCTS

Obstruction can be mechanical or anatomical and is commonly due to stones, intrinsic disorders of the biliary tree (e.g. cholangiocarcinoma) or extrinsic compression, usually by pancreatic carcinoma.

Clinically, there is a considerable rise of serum conjugated bilirubin, alkaline phosphatase (ALP), and cholesterol. In contrast to what happens in cirrhosis, serum bilirubin levels rarely exceed 600 μmol/L, with a trend to a plateau, as, when conjugated bilirubin concentration increases, glomerular filtration and excretion also increase. In complex cases with prolonged partial obstruction, hepatocytes function is also affected, thus producing a mixed biochemical picture, with elevation of circulating unconjugated bilirubin. Patients do not usually have signs of chronic liver disease but may have signs indicating malignancy, and pruritus is usual.

On examination, in the presence of obstructive jaundice a palpable gallbladder may be found: this is due to malignant obstruction of the biliary tree, usually pancreatic head carcinoma (Courvoisier's sign) or to a stone impacted in Hartman's pouch, leading to a mucocele or an empyema (Mirizzi's syndrome).

Signs of infection such as fever, abdominal pain, and chills are common. Steatorrhea is responsible for weight loss and malabsorption of fat-soluble vitamins A, D, E, and K and calcium.

Gallstones

Diseases affecting the gallbladder and bile ducts occur commonly in elderly people. By the age of 70, cholelithiasis and choledocolithiasis are found in 13–50 percent of the population and the figures rise to 38–53 percent above the age of 80. There is geographical variation: gallstones are rare in the Far East and Africa and very common in native North Americans, in Chile and Sweden. They occur twice as frequently in women as in men but this difference decreases with increasing age.

Gallstones can be divided into those composed of cholesterol and those composed of bile pigment. Cholesterol stones, which account for 80 percent of all gallstones in the West, contain more than 70 percent cholesterol, often with some bile pigment and calcium (mixed stones). Pure cholesterol stones are often solitary. They develop only in bile that has an excess of cholesterol relative to bile salts and phospholipids (supersaturated bile). This may either occur because of excess of cholesterol or because of a decrease in bile salts.

There is a reduced bile salt pool in some patients with cholesterol gallstones and the pool circulates more frequently: this may account for the reduction in the rate-limiting cholesterol-7a-hydroxylase found in some patients (feedback inhibition). Diminished bile salt synthesis is not the only cause of supersaturated bile; there appears to be an increase in HMG-CoA reductase with an increase in cholesterol secretion into bile in some patients. In supersaturated bile the bile acids solubilize phospholipids from the unilamellar vehicles more than cholesterol. This results in unstable vehicles which are more prone to aggregate, fuse, and form multilamellar vesicles, from which cholesterol crystals can nucleate. Factors other than cholesterol saturation are required to form gallstones, as supersaturated bile is found in normal subjects during an overnight fast. The rate of cholesterol crystallization and gallbladder motor dysfunction also plays a role. Glycoproteins in bile promote nucleation of cholesterol crystals, leading to stone formation, but why this occurs only in bile from patients with gallstones is unclear. The role of infection is unknown.

Patients with spontaneous gallstone disease also have prolonged large bowel transit time, more colonic Gram-positive anaerobes, increased bile acid metabolizing enzymes and higher intracolonic pH values than stone-free controls. Together, these changes lead to increased deoxycholic acid formation, solubilization, and absorption.

Black pigment stones contain calcium salts of bilirubin, phosphate, and carbonate in addition to bilirubin polymers and mucin glycoproteins. The biliary lipids are normal. These stones form in the gallbladder and are seen in patients with chronic hemolysis (e.g. hereditary spherocytosis and sickle cell disease) where there is an increase in bilirubin, and also in cirrhosis.

Brown pigment stones have layers of cholesterol, calcium salts of fatty acids (mainly palmitate) and calcium bilirubinate. They form in the common bile duct as a result of stasis and infection, usually in the presence of *E. coli* and *Klebsiella* spp., which produce β glucuronidase that converts soluble conjugated bilirubin back to the insoluble unconjugated state prone to precipitation with calcium. They are also found with strictures, sclerosing cholangitis and Caroli's syndrome.

The commonest presentation of gallstone disease is biliary pain. This occurs in the epigastrium and right hypocondrium and does not fluctuate, but persists from 15 minutes up to 24 hours, subsiding spontaneously or with opioid analgesics; it may radiate round to the back in the interscapular region.

Acute cholecystitis, common duct stones, and cholangitis

Acute cholecystitis occurs when a gallstone impacts in the neck of the gallbladder or in the cystic duct, leading to distension and inflammation. The inflammation is usually sterile, but within 24 hours gut organisms can be cultured from the gallbladder. Occasionally inflammation may be mild and quickly subside, sometimes leaving a gallbladder distended by mucus (mucocele). More commonly, the inflammation is severe, involving the whole wall and giving rise to localized peritonitis and acute pain. The gallbladder can become distended by pus (empyema) and rarely, an acute gangrenous cholecystitis occurs with perforation and a more generalized peritonitis.

The patient is usually ill with fever and shallow respirations. Right hypochondrial tenderness is present, being worse on inspiration (Murphy's sign). There is guarding and rebound tenderness.

The presentation of biliary colic in the elderly patient with diabetes and diabetic neuropathy is obfuscated and atypical. In such patients, a condition as serious as gangrenous cholecystitis can present with minimal temperature increases, without significant leukocytosis and few, if any, abdominal complaints. Consequently, clinically significant cholecystitis can be interpreted as an episode of mild biliary colic.

At ultrasound (US) examination, the detection of gallstones alone is insufficient for a diagnosis of acute cholecystitis. Additional criteria are:

- sonographic Murphy's sign (focal tenderness directly over the visualized gallbladder)
- distension of gallbladder
- presence of biliary sludge
- pericholecystic fluid
- gallbladder wall thickening (but not specific for acute disease)

Common bile duct stones are frequently found in elderly patients who present with concomitant cholecystitis. In the general population, 5 percent of patients presenting with cholecystitis have coexisting bile duct stones, but this figure raises to 10–20 percent in elderly people. Presentation can be with one or all of the triad of abdominal pain, jaundice, and fever. The pain is usually severe and situated in the epigastrium and right hypochondrium and may be accompanied by vomiting; it usually lasts for a few hours and then clears up, only to return days, weeks or even months later. Between attacks the patient is well.

The jaundice is variable in degree, depending on the amount of obstruction. Urine is dark and the stools are pale. High fever and rigors indicate cholangitis. The liver is enlarged if the obstruction lasts for more than a few hours. Prolonged biliary obstruction or repeated attacks lead to secondary biliary cirrhosis, but this is now rare.

US examination reveals a dilated common bile duct, but stones are detected in only about 75 percent of cases. Endoscopic ultrasound, when available, is a more accurate method of detecting a stone.

Acute cholangitis is due to bacterial infection of the bile ducts and is always secondary to bile duct abnormalities. The most frequent causes are common duct stones, biliary strictures, neoplasms or following ERCP in the presence of large duct obstruction.

Symptoms are fever, often with a rigor, upper abdominal pain, and jaundice. Older patients can present with collapse and Gram-negative septicemia.

Initial therapy of acute cholecystitis and cholangitis is directed toward general support of the patient, including fluid and electrolyte replacement, correction of metabolic imbalances and antibacterial therapy. In all but mild cases, pain relief with an opiate is required. In the absence of vomiting, the patient can soon tolerate oral fluids and nasogastric aspiration is not often required.

Antimicrobial therapy is usually empirical. Initial therapy should cover the Enterobacteriaceae, in particular *E. coli*, and anaerobes, especially in elderly people and in patients with previous bile-duct–bowel anastomosis. In patients with moderate clinical severity, monotherapy with a ureidopenicillin—mezlocillin or piperacillin—is at least as effective as the combination of ampicillin plus aminoglycoside. In severely ill patients with septicemia, an antibacterial combination is preferable. Therapy with aminoglicosides, mostly for *Pseudomonas aeruginosa*-related infections, should not exceed a few days because the risk of nephrotoxicity is increased during cholestasis.

Relief of biliary obstruction is mandatory,[8] even if there is clinical improvement with conservative therapy, because cholangitis is most likely to recur with continued obstruction. Cholecystectomy[9,10] is the treatment of choice for virtually all patients with gallbladder stones and symptoms. Laparoscopic cholecystectomy is thought by many to be the operation of choice.[11] The mortality is less than 0.1 percent and the patients can leave hospital in 24–48 hours. Complications are low and include wound sepsis, bile duct injury (0.5 percent) and retained gallstones in the common bile duct. Some surgeons prefer the "mini laparotomy" approach, with a small surgical incision, so that the length of stay in hospital and return to full activity is similar to that of laparoscopic surgery.

Endoscopic techniques provide an effective alternative for removing bile duct stones by sphincterotomy and stone extraction, and may be safer than surgery in elderly people,[12] as the associated morbidity and mortality are unchanged regardless of age. Stent insertion with bypass of common bile stones may be needed if stones cannot be removed or sphincterotomy is unsafe. Endoscopic nasobiliary drainage may be required as a first step to relieve obstruction in the presence of sepsis, with a second therapeutic endoscopy to remove stones.

Malignant obstruction

Obstructive jaundice can result from neoplasms of the gastrointestinal tract, arising from the biliary tree or most frequently from the pancreas. The usual presentation of this syndrome in the elderly consists of the insidious development of cholestasis and jaundice.

Pancreatic carcinoma

Pancreatic carcinoma is the most common cause of malignant biliary obstruction in the USA, where it accounts for nearly 27,000 cases each year and it has become the fifth leading cause of death from cancer, but its incidence has increased worldwide. Usual presentation is in the sixth and subsequent decades of life.

Primary adenocarcinoma of the gallbladder

Primary adenocarcinoma of the gallbladder represents less than 1 percent of all cancers; it occurs chiefly in patients over 70 years of age, more commonly in women and has striking genetic, racial, and geographic characteristics, with an extremely high prevalence in Native Americans and Chileans. Gallstones are usually present but a definite relationship is uncertain. Polyps that are >1 cm, single, sessile, and echopenic are associated with a higher risk of malignancy. Anomalous junction of pancreaticobiliary ducts and porcelain gallbladder are additional factors that predispose to cancer. Lesser associations include chronic bacterial infections, certain occupational and environmental carcinogens, and hormonal changes. Occasionally a mass can be palpable in the right hypochondrium.

The majority of cases are discovered during exploration for presumed gallstone disease and cholecystectomy is performed if possible. Few patients survive 1 year.

Cholangiocarcinoma

Cholangiocarcinoma is the most common primary tumor of the biliary tree; it is quite uncommon compared to hepatocellular carcinoma, representing less than 3 percent of gastrointestinal cancers in the year 2000,[13] but is increasing in incidence in several countries.[14] There is no association with cirrhosis or viral hepatitis, while in the Far East it may be associated with infestation with *Clonorchis sinensis* or *Opisthorchis viverrini*. Long-standing inflammation and chronic injury of the biliary epithelium seem to be important as risk factors: 10–20 percent of patients with primary sclerosing cholangitis will go on to develop a cholangiocarcinoma.[15]

It usually develops at the hepatic hilum, from the junction between right and left hepatic duct; more rarely the tumor arises from the common bile duct or intrahepatic ducts. Despite the central site of obstruction, the two hepatic lobes can present different degrees of dilatation of the biliary ductal system, with the left lobe usually more involved. Local invasion and proximity of vital structures within the porta hepatis contribute to the difficulty in achieving complete resectability, so that curative surgical resection is rarely possible: only one-third of cases are suitable after staging; patients usually die within 6 months.[16–18]

Liver transplantation is not a current option, with 5-year survival of 23 and 84 percent recurrence of tumor after 2 years.[19]

Ampullary tumors

Malignant tumors of the ampulla present with a cholestatic jaundice, which may occasionally be intermittent. They may ulcerate and produce gastrointestinal hemorrhage or chronic anemia. The diagnosis is usually made at ERCP. Carcinoma of the ampulla can sometimes be resected, with a 5-year survival rate of 40 percent.

The main goal in treating patients with malignant biliary diseases, presumed to be unresectable, is to provide palliation of jaundice, to avoid early liver failure due to chronic obstruction and improve the patient's nutritional and immunological status. Surgical therapy consists of either attempting a curative resection of the tumor or performing a palliative operation. Unfortunately, the surgical cure rate of these tumors is less than 5 percent.

Staging techniques should be used in elderly people in order to select carefully those patients who are likely to have resectable disease. Endoscopic ultrasound (EUS) is probably the most sensitive diagnostic modality currently available for predicting resectability.[20]

Palliative surgery is directed toward relieving jaundice by creating a biliary-enteric anastomosis. However, given the morbidity and 30-day mortality (up to 20 percent) for bypass procedure, nonoperative techniques of palliation are preferred in aged populations, unless there is a concomitant or impending duodenal obstruction.

Endoscopic relief of jaundice has been used successfully for over 20 years, and endoscopic techniques have a high rate of success (up to 90–95 percent of attempts). Greater success is achieved when treating distal bile ducts obstruction as complications occur less frequently. With tumors affecting the bifurcation of the hepatic ducts (Klatskin tumors), stents can be placed into both the right and left intrahepatic ducts to provide decompression.

Plastic stents placed endoscopically have a propensity to clog or occlude within 6 months of placement, thus requiring exchange. Expandable metal stents seem to delay stent occlusion, but they are not removable and are more expensive than plastic stents. However, with a limited lifespan in many patients, metallic stents offer a one-step procedure with excellent palliation.

INVESTIGATIONS OF THE BILIARY TRACT

Liver ultrasound

This is the imaging technique of choice in the evaluation of jaundice. In acute jaundice, if clinical history and laboratory test suggest obstructive etiology, liver ultrasound should be the first imaging modality and can be considered as the "stethoscope" of the hepatologist. It can demonstrate changes in size and shape of the liver. Fatty changes and fibrosis produce a diffuse increased echogenicity. In established cirrhosis there may be marginal nodularity of the liver surface and distortion of the arterial vascular architecture. The patency and diameter of the portal and patency of hepatic veins can be evaluated. The sensitivity of abdominal ultrasonography for the detection of biliary obstruction in jaundiced patients ranges from 55 to 91 percent and the specificity from 82 to 95 percent. US can demonstrate cholelithiasis and space occupying lesions in the parenchyma greater than 1 cm in diameter, as well as enlargement of pancreatic head suggestive of carcinoma.

Ampullary carcinomas are usually too small to be directly visualized, but they can be suspected when a simultaneous dilatation of pancreatic and biliary duct is found without any other abnormality ("double duct sign"). Dilatation of the common biliary duct, which usually indicates biliary tract obstruction, is also common in patients who have undergone previous cholecystectomy. The major advantages of ultrasound are that is noninvasive, portable, and relatively inexpensive. The major disadvantages are that it is operator dependent, and the images may be difficult to interpret in obese patients or patients with overlying bowel gas.

Computed tomography of the abdomen (CT)

This is useful in all hepatobiliary problems and is complementary to US. Pancreatic disease, enlargement of regional lymph nodes and lesions in the porta hepatis can be visualized. Abdominal CT permits accurate measurements of the caliber of the biliary tree, with a sensitivity of 63–96 percent and specificity of 93–100 percent for detecting biliary obstruction. Spiral (helical) CT improves the diagnostic accuracy of this method in relation to space occupying lesions of the liver: it involves rapid acquisition of a volume of data during or immediately after i.v. contrast injection. Data can thus be acquired in both arterial and portal phases of enhancement, enabling more precise characterization of a lesion and its vascular supply.

It remains the main imaging technique for the study of the liver, including screening for focal lesions, as it can detect nodules as small as 5 mm, differentiating benign masses from malignant and helping in staging HCC in patients undergoing hepatic resection.

CT is not as operator dependent as US and provides technically superior images in obese patients in whom the biliary tree is obscured by bowel gas. CT is not as accurate as US in detecting cholelithiasis, because only calcified stones can be seen clearly. Other considerations in the use of abdominal CT in patients with jaundice are its lack of portability, requirement for intravenous contrast, and expense.

Magnetic resonance imaging (MRI)

This is an increasingly useful investigation of hepatobiliary disease, especially in diagnosing and staging malignant disease. Alteration in weighting of the image leads to prominence of the ductal system in the biliary tree and pancreas, known as magnetic resonance cholangiopancreatography (MRCP). The basic principle of MRCP is to utilize T2-weighted images in which stationary or slowly moving fluid, including bile, is high in signal intensity and all surrounding tissues including retroperitoneal fat and solid visceral organs are lower in signal. MRCP provides detail of the liver parenchyma and biliary tree; it can be employed when there are contraindications to PTC or ERCP, if therapeutic intervention is unlikely to be required, or as a first imaging test when there is a previous biliary-enteric or Billroth II anastomosis. MRCP has 95 percent sensitivity for detecting obstruction though it is inaccurate in assessing the grade of obstruction. Similarly strictures cannot be well characterized due to a signal dropout. Its accuracy is equal to ERCP in determining the level of obstruction and whether it is due to a neoplastic process. Unlike PTC or ERCP, MRCP enables the biliary tract to be visualized above and below a complete obstruction. MRCP has an advantage over ERCP in being noninterventional and non-operator dependent, and does not require contrast injection, although unlike ERCP it is purely diagnostic. MRCP has already replaced direct cholangiography in many clinical circumstances, but PTC and ERCP remain the tests of choice when a therapeutic intervention is necessary. MRCP has proven to be a useful tool for diagnosis of primary sclerosing cholangitis (PSC), with reported sensitivity of 83 percent and specificity of 98 percent;[6] it can also provide information about the periductal tissue, allowing for a single modality to provide both diagnosis of PSC and screening for cholangiocarcinoma. Due to its lack of complications compared to ERCP, MRCP could find application particularly in older patients, who are often in worse clinical conditions.

Endoscopic retrograde cholangiopancreatography (ERCP)

This permits direct visualization of the biliary tree as well as the pancreatic ducts. The technique involves the passage of an endoscope into the second part of the duodenum and cannulation of the ampulla; contrast is then injected into both systems and the patient is screened radiologically. In comparison with abdominal US and CT, ERCP is more invasive and requires conscious sedation.

It is highly accurate in the diagnosis of biliary obstruction, with a sensitivity of 89–98 percent and specificity of 89–100 percent. In addition to providing radiographic images, other diagnostic and therapeutic procedures can be carried out in the same session:

- Common bile duct stones can be removed after balloon dilatation (if small) or diathermy cut to the sphincter has been performed to facilitate their withdrawal. Sphincterotomy has a complication rate of 8–12 percent: acute pancreatitis in 5 percent of cases, severe hemorrhage in 2 percent, with an overall mortality of 0.5–1 percent.[21] Endoscopic balloon dilatation preserves biliary sphincter function and is safer.
- The biliary system can be drained by passing a tube (stent) through an obstruction, or placement of a nasobiliary drain.
- Biopsy specimens and brushing for cytology study can be obtained.

Periampullary lesions are often diagnosed only at ERCP. The rates of morbidity and mortality with ERCP from untoward events such as respiratory depression, aspiration, bleeding, perforation, cholangitis and pancreatitis are 3 percent and 0.2 percent, respectively.[22]

Percutaneous cholangiography (PTC)

This is a procedure that complements ERCP. Contraindications are as for liver biopsy. Under a local anesthetic a fine flexible needle is passed into the liver. Contrast is injected slowly until a biliary radicle is identified and then further contrast is injected to outline the whole of the biliary tree. In the presence of obstruction, bile can be aspirated and a guidewire can be passed to allow stenting.

Its sensitivity (98–100 percent) and specificity (89–100 percent) are comparable with those of ERCP. In difficult cases the two techniques are sometimes combined, PTC showing the biliary anatomy above the obstruction, with ERCP showing the more distal anatomy. It is the procedure of choice when

---

KEY POINTS Biliary tract diseases

- Jaundice is clinically evident when the bilirubin concentration exceeds 50 µmol/L.

- A careful history, physical examination, and review of the standard laboratory tests should allow a physician to make an accurate diagnosis in 85 percent of cases.

- In acute jaundice, liver ultrasound should be the first imaging modality, particularly in elderly people.

- If there is any evidence of biliary obstruction and a therapeutic intervention is planned, ERCP or PTC are the investigations of choice.

- MRCP should follow ultrasound if this has been technically difficult or obstruction has not been ruled out or therapeutic intervention is not needed.

- Liver biopsy is needed to confirm presence, cause, and severity of chronic liver disease.

interventional procedures are needed, such as balloon dilatation and stent placement to relieve focal obstructions of the biliary tree. PTC is potentially advantageous under conditions in which the level of biliary obstruction is proximal to the common hepatic duct or in which altered anatomy precludes ERCP. PTC may be technically limited in the absence of dilatation of the intrahepatic bile ducts. The rates of morbidity (3 percent) and mortality (0.2 percent) are similar to ERCP and are due to major complications: biliary leakage, sepsis, perforation, and bleeding.

REFERENCES

1. Koiwai O, Nishizawa M, Hasada K et al: Gilbert's syndrome is caused by a heterozygous missense mutation in the gene for bilirubin UDP-glucuronosyltransferase. Hum Mol Genet 1995;4(7):1183–1186
2. Borlak J, Thum T, Landt O, Erb K, Hermann R: Molecular diagnosis of a familial nonhemolytic hyperbilirubinemia (Gilbert's syndrome) in healthy subjects. Hepatology 2000;32(4 Pt 1):792–795
3. Ishihara T, Gabazza EC, Adachi Y, Sato H, Maruo Y: Genetic basis of fasting hyperbilirubinemia. Gastroenterology 1999;116(5):1272
4. Persico M, Persico E, Bakker CT et al: Hepatic uptake of organic anions affects the plasma bilirubin level in subjects with Gilbert's syndrome mutations in UGT1A1. Hepatology 2001;33(3):627–632
5. Fulcher AS, Turner MA, Franklin KJ et al: Primary sclerosing cholangitis: evaluation with MR cholangiography—a case-control study. Radiology 2000;215(1):71–80
6. Angulo P, Pearce DH, Johnson CD et al: Magnetic resonance cholangiography in patients with biliary disease: its role in primary sclerosing cholangitis. J Hepatol 2000;33(4):520–527
7. Broome U, Olsson R, Loof L et al: Natural history and prognostic factors in 305 Swedish patients with primary sclerosing cholangitis. Gut 1996;38(4):610–615
8. Tseng LJ, Tsai CC, Mo LR et al: Palliative percutaneous transhepatic gallbladder drainage of gallbladder empyema before laparoscopic cholecystectomy. Hepatogastroenterology 2000;47(34):932–936
9. Maxwell JG, Tyler BA, Rutledge R et al: Cholecystectomy in patients aged 80 and older. Am J Surg 1998;176(6):627–631
10. Borzellino G, de Manzoni G, Ricci F et al: Emergency cholecystostomy and subsequent cholecystectomy for acute gallstone cholecystitis in the elderly. Br J Surg 1999;86(12):1521–1525
11. Montori A, Boscaini M, Gasparrini M et al: Gallstones in elderly patients: impact of laparoscopic cholecystectomy. Can J Gastroenterol 2000;14(11):929–932
12. Sugiyama M, Atomi Y: Endoscopic sphincterotomy for bile duct stones in patients 90 years of age and older. Gastrointest Endosc 2000;52(2):187–191
13. Greenlee RT, Murray T, Bolden S, Wingo PA: Cancer statistics, 2000. CA Cancer J Clin 2000;50(1):7–33
14. Taylor-Robinson SD, Toledano MB, Arora S et al: Increase in mortality rates from intrahepatic cholangiocarcinoma in England and Wales 1968–1998. Gut 2001;48(6):816–820
15. Chapman RW: Risk factors for biliary tract carcinogenesis. Ann Oncol 1999;10(suppl 4):308–311
16. Blom D, Schwartz SI: Surgical treatment and outcomes in carcinoma of the extrahepatic bile ducts: the University of Rochester experience. Arch Surg 2001;136(2):209–215
17. Launois B, Reding R, Lebeau G, Buard JL: Surgery for hilar cholangiocarcinoma: French experience in a collective survey of 552 extrahepatic bile duct cancers. J Hepatobiliary Pancreat Surg 2000;7(2):128–134
18. Reed DN, Vitale GC, Martin R et al: Bile duct carcinoma: trends in treatment in the nineties. Am Surg 2000;66(8):711–714
19. Meyer CG, Penn I, James L: Liver transplantation for cholangiocarcinoma: results in 207 patients. Transplantation 2000;69(8):1633–1637
20. Erickson RA, Garza AA: Impact of endoscopic ultrasound on the management and outcome of pancreatic carcinoma. Am J Gastroenterol 2000;95(9):2248–2254
21. Freeman ML, Nelson DB, Sherman S et al: Complications of endoscopic biliary sphincterotomy. N Engl J Med 1996;335(13):909–918
22. Cotton PB: Critical appraisal of therapeutic endoscopy in biliary tract diseases. Annu Rev Med 1990;41:211–222

Chapter 82

The small bowel

Christopher A. Rodrigues

Diseases of the small bowel can be divided into two categories for clinical purposes. Diffuse processes such as celiac disease result in the malabsorption syndrome, whereas discrete diseases like small bowel tumors produce focal manifestations. Some diseases like Crohn's disease and radiation enteritis can cause a combination of malabsorption and focal features. The true prevalence of malabsorption in elderly people is not known, but it occurred in 7 percent of elderly residents of a home[1] and in 30 and 5 percent of elderly patients in two hospital series.[2,3] Fat absorption was impaired in 29 elderly patients with congestive heart failure and weight loss.[4] Three conditions account for most cases of malabsorption in the elderly: bacterial overgrowth syndrome, chronic pancreatitis, and celiac disease. The causes of malabsorption in three series are listed in Table 82-1.

Steatorrhea, the typical symptom of fat malabsorption, is much less likely to occur in elderly patients[7] who may even be constipated despite an increased stool volume. This is probably due to low dietary fat intake and slower transit of intestinal contents with aging. Carbohydrate malabsorption causes watery diarrhea, abdominal distention, borborygmi, and flatulence. These symptoms are due to the action of bacteria on carbohydrate residues in the colon. Lactose malabsorption is common in healthy elderly individuals[8] and also complicates many diffuse small bowel diseases.

Since frank steatorrhea is rare in elderly people, the clinical presentation of malabsorption is nonspecific. It consists of a variable combination of the following: fatigue, poor mobility, anorexia, nausea, diarrhea, anemia, weight loss, depression, and confusion.[1,3,9] Peripheral edema may develop due to hypoproteinemia. Vague generalized body ache and muscle weakness can be early clinical indicators of osteomalacia. Vitamin K deficiency may cause bruising, petechiae, and bleeding manifestations. Abdominal discomfort and distention are common but abdominal pain is relatively rare. Recurrent abdominal pain occurs with chronic pancreatitis, inflammation as in Crohn's disease, subacute obstruction due to strictures, or chronic mesenteric ischemia.

The diagnosis of malabsorption should therefore be considered in elderly patients with clinical and anthropometric evidence of undernutrition even in the absence of gastrointestinal symptoms. A dietary assessment is important in determining whether the malnutrition can reasonably be attributed to inadequate nutrient intake. The details of previous surgical procedures should be ascertained: gastric surgery or intestinal bypass procedures can result in the bacterial overgrowth syndrome, and extensive small bowel resection can cause malabsorption due to a critical reduction in the mucosal absorptive surface area.

INVESTIGATION OF SMALL BOWEL DISORDERS

Screening tests

Routine blood tests are often helpful in the diagnosis of small bowel disease. The full blood count and blood film may show anemia with macrocytosis, an iron deficient picture, or a dimorphic film. Macrocytosis, leukopenia, and thrombocytopenia are suggestive of megaloblastic anemia. Ferritin, vitamin B_{12}, and red cell folate levels should be measured in patients with suspected malabsorption even with a normal blood film, as typical changes may not be present in early deficiency. A low B_{12} level and normal or increased red cell folate raise the possibility of small bowel bacterial overgrowth. Howell–Jolley bodies in the blood film are an indicator of splenic atrophy which occurs in association with celiac disease. Osteomalacia results in a raised alkaline phosphatase with low calcium and phosphate levels and is confirmed by a low serum 25-hydroxycholecaliferol. Vitamin K deficiency prolongs the international normalized ratio (INR). Hypoalbuminemia is a common though nonspecific finding, as it also occurs with poor dietary intake, injury, sepsis, and malignancy. Malabsorption is unlikely if these screening tests are completely normal.

Tests of absorption

These tests confirm impaired absorption of nutrients, but do not provide any information about the underlying disease

Table 82-1 **Causes of malabsorption in three series of patients more than 65 years old**[a]

Cause	Montgomery[5] (1986)	McEvoy[3] (1983)	Price[6] (1977)
Pancreatic insufficiency	14 (20%)	2 (8%)	7 (44%)
Celiac disease	8 (11%)	2 (8%)	4 (25%)
Bacterial overgrowth	48 (69%)	17 (71%)	3 (19%)
Small bowel diverticula	12	9	1
Postgastric surgery	11	4	2
Normal small bowel	15	4	
Crohn's disease	3		
Scleroderma	2		
Miscellaneous	5		
Short-bowel syndrome		1 (4%)	
Tropical sprue			2 (13%)
Unknown (refused further investigation)		2 (8%)	
Totals	70	24	16

[a] *Percentages do not add up to 100 because of rounding.*

process. They are cumbersome to perform or are relatively insensitive, often giving equivocal results. Protein absorption studies are particularly difficult to carry out and are not routinely used in clinical practice.

FAT ABSORPTION Detection of excess fecal fat in stool samples by Sudan staining is simple and inexpensive but is reliable only in patients with moderate or severe steatorrhea. The steatocrit is the relative quantity of fat in a stool sample expressed as a percentage of total stool solids. It has been validated in adults as a test of malabsorption—when fat excretion exceeds 10 g/day[10]—and may therefore be a useful screening test in elderly patients.

Measurement of fecal fat over a 72-hour period with the patient taking a 100-g fat diet is the standard method of quantifying fat malabsorption. Values of less than 7 g (20 mmol) of stool fat per day are normal. The test is unpopular with patients and staff, and older patients are often unable to tolerate a high-fat diet. The [14C]triolein breath test is easier to carry out as it does not involve either a special diet or stool collection.[11] This radiolabeled triglyceride releases $^{14}CO_2$ after undergoing digestion, absorption, and metabolism. After an overnight fast, 5 μCi of [14C]triolein are administered with a test meal, and $^{14}CO_2$ is measured in breath samples collected hourly for 6–8 hours. The test cannot be used when there are coexistent disorders (such as diabetes mellitus) that alter the conversion of fatty acids to CO_2, and in chronic lung diseases which lower breath CO_2 excretion. The results are affected by age, probably because of delayed rather than decreased absorption with aging, but normal reference ranges have been defined for the elderly population.[12] Fecal fat estimation and the triolein breath test do not distinguish between fat malabsorption due to small bowel disease and maldigestion resulting from pancreatic insufficiency.

CARBOHYDRATE ABSORPTION Xylose is a pentose sugar which is absorbed unchanged in the proximal jejunum. The amount absorbed is proportional to the surface area of normal mucosa and this is the basis of the xylose tests. After an overnight fast, 25 g of D-xylose is administered orally, urine is collected for 5 hours, and a 1-hour venous blood sample taken. Abnormal function is indicated by a 5-hour urinary excretion of less than 4 g or a serum level of less than 25 mg/dL.[13] Urinary xylose excretion declines with age because of declining renal function.[14–16] This can be corrected for by performing oral and intravenous xylose tolerance tests on separate days since renal function affects both tests to the same degree,[14–16] but this is impractical for clinical use. The alternative is to use the 1-hour serum level, either after 25 g of xylose[13] or after a 5-g dose with a correction for body surface area.[17] Earlier studies found decreased xylose absorption in hospital inpatients over 70 years of age even after correcting for altered renal function,[16,18] but more recent work in healthy elderly people showed no change in absorption up to the ninth decade.[19,20] The xylose breath hydrogen test is another method of measuring xylose absorption and is independent of renal function.[21] After an oral dose of 25 g, end-expiratory breath samples are collected every 30 minutes for 5 hours. Malabsorption of xylose results in fermentation of the sugar by colonic flora, producing a rise in breath hydrogen at about 3 hours. A rise in breath hydrogen

also occurs in patients with small bowel bacterial overgrowth, though usually much earlier than in patients with jejunal mucosal disease. Between 3 and 25 percent of individuals are not colonized by hydrogen-producing colonic flora and hence have a false negative test.

Lactose intolerance can be confirmed by a wide variety of tests.[22] In the lactose tolerance test, blood glucose levels are measured at half-hourly intervals for 2 hours after the ingestion of 50 g of lactose. A rise of less than 1.1 mmol/L indicates lactose intolerance. Alternatively, a breath test can be used as described above for xylose.

VITAMIN B$_{12}$ ABSORPTION The Schilling test distinguishes vitamin B$_{12}$ (cobalamin) malabsorption due to terminal ileal disease from that due to lack of intrinsic factor. A modification of the procedure requires only a single 24-hour urine collection, as two separate radioisotopes of cobalt are used—one to label vitamin B$_{12}$ and the other to label the vitamin B$_{12}$-intrinsic factor complex.[23] Pernicious anemia causes B$_{12}$ deficiency only in a small minority of elderly people.[24,25] Food-cobalamin malabsorption, due to impaired release of the vitamin from food because of atrophic gastritis or the use of acid suppressing drugs, is much more common. It can be detected with a Schilling test using radiolabeled cobalamin bound to food protein.[26]

Tests for bacterial overgrowth

The gold standard for the diagnosis of small bowel bacterial overgrowth is quantitative aerobic and anaerobic culture of fasting small bowel fluid: normal jejunal bacterial counts are less than 10^5/mL, and ileal counts less than 10^8/mL.[27,28] Collection of jejunal fluid can be carried out either by intubation under radiological control[29] or, more conveniently, during esophagogastroduodenoscopy (EGD).[3,30,31] The invasive procedure and cumbersome culture techniques involved have led to the development of noninvasive tests. In the [14C]glycocholate breath test, 5–10 μCi of glycocholic acid, a conjugated bile acid, radiolabeled with 14C is administered with a test meal.[32,33] Bacterial deconjugation results in separation of [14C]glycine from cholic acid, and $^{14}CO_2$ produced from the former is measured in breath samples collected over the next 4–8 hours. Terminal ileal disease or resection also results in a positive test since the bile acid is not reabsorbed and is then metabolized by colonic flora. The two conditions can be distinguished by measuring fecal 14C radioactivity,[32] but this complicates an otherwise simple, convenient test. The alternative is to use the 75Se-homotaurocholate (SeHCAT) test, an isotopic method for diagnosing bile acid malabsorption.[34] False negative results with the glycocholate breath test have been reported in as many as 30–40 percent of patients with culture-proven overgrowth.

Breath hydrogen measurement after ingestion of 50–80 g of glucose or 10–12 g of lactulose can also be used in the diagnosis of small bowel bacterial overgrowth.[27,35] Metabolism of either carbohydrate by the abnormal bacterial population produces hydrogen which can be detected by breath testing. The timing of the hydrogen rise is crucial for the lactulose test since this sugar is not absorbed in the small bowel and produces a second "colonic" hydrogen peak. A recent small study in healthy volunteers has shown that a 10 g dose accelerates small bowel transit,[36] and so the glucose–hydrogen breath test is probably more reliable. Breath hydrogen tests have low sensitivity and specificity rates,[27,29] and false negative results occur in individuals not colonized by hydrogen-producing flora. The [14C]xylose breath test[37] was developed to avoid these problems and is more accurate than the hydrogen breath test.[38] Elevated CO_2 levels appear in breath samples within 60 minutes of taking 10 μCi of [14C]xylose with 1 g of unlabeled xylose by mouth. Xylose is a better substrate than glycocholic acid or lactulose since it is absorbed in the jejunum and is less likely to reach the colon. Colonic "dumping" of xylose does occur, but the false positive result due to colonic fermentation can be detected using technitium-99m, a transit marker which does not alter small bowel motility.[39] However, studies in patients with bacterial overgrowth have produced conflicting results,[34,38,40] and in more recent work the test failed to detect overgrowth reliably.[41–45] Thus the search for the ideal breath test continues.

A conjugate of ursodeoxycholic acid and p-aminobenzoic acid (UDCA–PABA) has been used as an alternative method for detecting small bowel bacterial overgrowth.[46] The bile acid UDCA is split from PABA by small bowel bacteria and the latter is then absorbed and excreted in the urine.

Radiology and endoscopy

Double-contrast barium follow-through examination and enteroclysis (small bowel enema) are the two radiological contrast techniques used to investigate the small bowel. Enteroclysis is probably more accurate but is more invasive. The role of abdominal computed tomography (CT) scanning and mesenteric angiography is described in the relevant sections.

EGD is the usual method for collecting fluid for culture and for obtaining biopsies from the distal duodenum. The detection of villous atrophy at endoscopy can be improved by viewing the duodenal mucosal surface at high magnification after spraying with indigo carmine.[47] Small bowel enteroscopy is now used more widely for the investigation of gastrointestinal (GI) bleeding, in patients with malabsorption or unexplained diarrhea, as well as to confirm and biopsy abnormalities detected by contrast studies.[48–50] Three methods are available:

- The sonde enteroscope reaches the ileum in 75 percent, and the ileocecal valve in 10 percent of examinations but has no biopsy channel and takes 4–8 hours to complete.
- The push enteroscope can be inserted 60–120 cm beyond the ligament of Treitz and has an instrument channel for therapeutic procedures.
- Intraoperative enteroscopy, in which the small bowel is "pleated" over an endoscope at laparotomy, is the most accurate technique but has a significant complication rate.

Enteroscopy is helpful in the investigation of patients with obscure GI bleeding, in whom endoscopy of the upper and lower GI tracts and small bowel radiology have failed to locate the source. Small bowel arteriovenous malformations and tumors are the most common abnormalities encountered. However, most studies have shown that a significant proportion of lesions, mostly vascular ectasias, are actually situated in the stomach or proximal duodenum and were missed on the original EGD.

Wireless endoscopy has just been introduced[51] and is currently being tested for clinical use.[52] It consists of a capsule endoscopy system which is swallowed and propelled by peristalsis, transmitting color video images as it passes through the gastrointestinal tract. This safe, ambulatory procedure has the potential to revolutionize investigation of small bowel diseases.

SMALL BOWEL DISEASES

The five common clinical conditions affecting elderly patients are discussed below.

Celiac disease

In celiac disease, sensitivity to dietary gluten in cereals like wheat, barley, and rye leads to a characteristic small bowel mucosal lesion, hyperplastic villous atrophy. The disease affects the proximal small bowel, decreases in severity distally, and may spare the distal jejunum and ileum. The wider use of serological screening tests has altered our understanding of the epidemiology of the disease.[53] It appears to be much more common than previously appreciated with current prevalence rates of 1 in 200–300. Only 30–40 percent of patients are symptomatic, the rest have clinically silent disease. This variable clinical picture is probably related to the extent of affected bowel. Although classically a disease of early childhood, presentation in adult life is common with a second peak in women in the fourth decade and men in the sixth and seventh decades.[54] The female to male ratio in adults is 2:1. The proportion of people with celiac disease who are elderly has increased from 2–7 percent in series reported about 30 years ago[55] to 19–34 percent more recently.[54,56,57] Celiac disease is present in 8–25 percent of patients over the age of 65 years who have malabsorption (Table 82-1).[3,5,6]

Many elderly patients, like adults with celiac disease, are either asymptomatic or have trivial or nonspecific symptoms. In a recent series, only 45 percent of patients had diarrhea, the rest presenting with abdominal distention and flatulence, fatigue, anemia, or dermatitis hepetiformis.[56] The diagnosis should be considered in patients with unexplained anemia, macrocytosis, or evidence of splenic atrophy on the blood film.[55] Folate deficiency is the most common cause of anemia, but malabsorption of iron or vitamin B_{12} can occur. Osteoporosis and osteomalacia are common, the former occurring in about 50 percent of patients.[58]

Celiac disease is associated with a large number of conditions, the most important being insulin-dependent diabetes mellitus, autoimmune thyroid disease, Sjögren's syndrome, inflammatory bowel disease, and primary biliary cirrhosis.[53,59] Dermatitis herpetiformis can be regarded as an extraintestinal manifestation of celiac disease as virtually all patients have an enteropathy, mostly villous atrophy. Neurological disorders such as epilepsy, cerebellar syndrome, dementia, peripheral neuropathy, myopathy, and hyporeflexia have been reported in celiac disease.[57] More than 90 percent of celiac patients have the HLA class 2 molecule DQ2, and at least 1 in 10 first-degree relatives are affected.

DIAGNOSIS The diagnosis is confirmed by proximal small bowel biopsy. The mucosal surface is flattened as a result of subtotal or total villous atrophy, with stunting of (or an absence of) the brush border and hyperplastic crypts. The intraepithelial lymphocyte count is increased, and the lamina propria is infiltrated mainly with plasma cells and lymphocytes. These changes, accompanied by a clinical response to a gluten-free diet, are adequate to establish the diagnosis. A repeat biopsy to confirm histological remission is required only in asymptomatic patients or in those with an equivocal clinical response. Rebiopsy after a gluten challenge is rarely carried out now but may be necessary in cases where there is diagnostic difficulty, such as when the original biopsy was done on a gluten-free diet. Tests of nutrient absorption are unhelpful, but serological markers are useful for screening patients for biopsy. Currently, endomysial antibody is the best test[60] and is probably as reliable in the elderly population.[61] Antibody titers decrease or disappear with treatment, thus adding support to the diagnosis as well as being useful in monitoring dietary compliance. Tissue transglutaminase (tTG) has recently been identified as the antigen for endomysial antibody,[62] and anti-tTG antibody is being introduced as an alternative, simpler screening test.

MANAGEMENT   Most elderly patients respond to a well-balanced gluten-free diet and cope well with the change in lifelong eating habits.[56] It is now generally accepted that patients can take a moderate amount of oats, up to 50 g daily. Lactose intolerance can cause apparently resistant disease in some patients. However, milk and milk products are an important source of calcium and should be restricted only if they exacerbate symptoms—ideally after confirming the diagnosis with an objective test. Patients should receive supplements to correct nutrient deficiencies, as complete recovery of mucosal function can take months. Elderly patients with celiac disease should be given multivitamins and a calcium supplement initially. Bone mineral densitometry should be carried out at diagnosis in all patients with celiac disease. Bone mass improves, but does not normalize, in adult and elderly patients on a gluten-free diet and other therapeutic measures are often required.[58] A few individuals, some of whom develop small intestinal ulcers and strictures (ulcerative enteritis), fail to respond to gluten withdrawal or relapse after an initial remission.[63,64] Most patients with refractory disease have a cryptic T-cell lymphoma of the intraepithelial lymphocytes.[65] Some respond to corticosteroids or immunosuppressive agents, but in general the prognosis is poor. Patients with ulcerative enteritis often require surgery for complications such as perforation or obstruction.

NEOPLASMS   Overall mortality in celiac disease is approximately twice that of the general population and is largely due to the development of malignant complications. T-cell lymphoma of the small intestine is the commonest tumor, but there is an increased risk of developing squamous cell carcinomas of the esophagus, mouth, and pharynx, and adenocarcinoma of the small bowel.[66,67] The incidence of lymphoma rises with age, and patients in their sixth, seventh, and eighth decades have a 1 in 10 chance of developing the tumor.[68] Lymphoma may be the first manifestation of celiac disease, but the diagnosis should also be considered in patients known to have celiac disease whose condition is either resistant to, or relapses on, a strict gluten-free diet. Weight loss is the commonest symptom, and patients also experience profound lethargy and muscle weakness, abdominal pain, and diarrhea. A gluten-free diet, adhered to for at least 5 years, has a protective effect against the development of malignancy in celiac disease.[59,66]

Bacterial overgrowth syndrome

Bacterial counts normally increase aborally and bacterial populations vary in different sections of the gastrointestinal tract: the jejunum is colonized by Gram-positive aerobes and facultative anaerobes, ileal flora contain some strict anaerobes as well, and the colon is heavily populated by predominantly anaerobic bacteria.[27,28] Malabsorption can occur when the small bowel population increases and becomes more anaerobic. This is partly due to direct injury to the intestinal mucosa, but uptake or binding of major nutrients and vitamin B_{12} by the proliferating bacteria also play a part. In addition, fat absorption is affected by deconjugation of bile salts by anaerobic bacteria, resulting in impaired micelle formation. Folic acid and vitamin K are synthesized by bacteria, and folate levels are often normal or raised when bacterial overgrowth is present. Two factors are largely responsible for regulating bacterial growth: gastric acid and intestinal motility.[27,28,69] Gastric acid secretion destroys micro-organisms ingested with food and saliva. The interdigestive migrating motor complex, a cyclic fasting motility pattern, regularly propels luminal contents towards the colon, thus preventing stagnation and bacterial overgrowth.[70] Gut immune defenses[69] and interactions between microbial populations[28] also play a part in limiting bacterial growth.

PATHOGENESIS   The classic disorders associated with bacterial overgrowth are those in which grossly disordered intestinal motility permits abnormal proliferation of bacteria; examples are diabetic autonomic neuropathy, late radiation enteropathy, collagen diseases such as scleroderma, and the numerous causes of chronic intestinal pseudo-obstruction. Partial small bowel obstruction due to strictures, radiation damage, or adhesions has a similar effect. Bacterial overgrowth occurs in abnormal reservoirs that permit stagnation of luminal contents—for example, small bowel diverticula and the afferent limb of a Billroth II gastrectomy. Abnormal communications between the proximal and distal intestine result in contamination of the former by denser, more anaerobic bacterial populations. Examples of this group include gastrocolic and jejunocolic fistulas, resection of the ileocecal valve, and surgical bypass of obstructed or diseased intestinal segments.

Overgrowth of bacteria in the small bowel also occurs under conditions that impair gastric acid secretion, such as atrophic gastritis, treatment with acid-reducing drugs, or after surgery for peptic ulcer disease. The prevalence of atrophic gastritis rises with age, largely as a result of *Helicobacter pylori* infection,[71] and probably affects 20–30 percent of otherwise healthy elderly people.[72,73] Nutrient malabsorption occurs only in a minority,[41,42] probably in those with an additional risk factor that results in the proliferation of anaerobic or Gram-negative flora. Simple colonization[72] without malabsorption is common in elderly people, occurring in 15–59 percent of healthy individuals,[20] hospital patients,[74–76] and people in residential care.[77] In one series, 21 of 39 malnourished patients had high duodenal bacterial counts, but only seven had clinically significant bacterial overgrowth.[78] However, subclinical malabsorption may occur: eight asymptomatic subjects in residential care with overgrowth gained weight after antibiotic treatment.[77] Simple colonization is also common in adults and elderly patients on proton pump inhibitors, affecting 43–53 percent even after short-term treatment.[76,79,80] Most patients are asymptomatic, but acid suppression can promote proliferation of fecal-type anaerobic flora,[81] and a recent study in 40 subjects demonstrated deconjugation of bile acids and fat malabsorption after 5 weeks use of omeprazole.[82]

Since 1977, bacterial overgrowth and malabsorption have been reported in small numbers of elderly patients with an anatomically normal small bowel (Table 82-1).[3,5,30,78,83] These individuals have normal gastric acid secretion and a prolonged mouth-to-cecum transit time.[30] Asymptomatic small bowel stasis is common in healthy elderly people[84] and appears to be more important than atrophic gastritis in the pathogenesis of this unique syndrome, though the two conditions must coexist in some cases.

CLINICAL PICTURE   As already noted, bacterial overgrowth is the commonest cause of malabsorption in elderly patients. Apart from overgrowth associated with a normal small bowel, some of the predisposing conditions, such as small bowel diverticula, become more common with increasing age.[85] Most patients who have undergone surgical procedures for peptic ulcer disease are now elderly.[86] The clinical picture of bacterial overgrowth syndrome may be changing. In a retrospective review of 100 patients, 90 percent had gastroparesis, irritable bowel syndrome, or chronic pancreatitis—rather than the conditions hitherto associated with the syndrome.[87] Patients with confirmed overgrowth should have a small bowel X-ray series to look for abnormal communications or reservoirs. It is essential to confirm the presence of malabsorption, preferably by evaluating fat absorption. The nonspecific clinical picture in patients who have a high prevalence of simple colonization may otherwise lead to unnecessary, and possibly harmful, treatment with antibiotics.

MANAGEMENT   The conditions underlying bacterial overgrowth are rarely amenable to surgical correction, and the mainstay of treatment is antibiotics.

Tetracycline was traditionally used to reduce bacterial flora, but about two-thirds of patients do not benefit from this drug. Chloromycetin and clindamycin are rarely used now because of their toxicity. Co-amoxyclav and norfloxacin are effective in standard doses given for 7–10 days, as is metronidazole in combination with one of the cephalosporins.[88,89] In some patients, a single course produces a satisfactory response lasting for months, but many patients need cyclic courses given at monthly intervals for 4–6 months.[30] Octreotide, a long-acting analog of somatostatin, has been tested in small numbers of patients with connective tissues diseases and chronic intestinal pseudo-obstruction. It improves motility and appears to be highly effective on its own[90,91] or in combination with erythromycin.[92]

Prokinetic agents may play a role in the management of bacterial overgrowth, particularly in elderly patients with prolonged small bowel transit.[69] Clinicians should avoid using acid-suppressing agents in elderly people without a clear indication: apart from their possible role in promoting clinically significant bacterial overgrowth, these drugs can also cause food-cobalamin malabsorption.

Crohn's disease

Crohn's disease is a chronic relapsing disorder characterized by transmural inflammation and ulceration occurring in a segmental distribution. Intestinal ulceration ranges from superficial aphthoid ulcers to deep fissures, and the course is often complicated by the formation of strictures, abscesses, and fistulas. The disease predominantly affects teenagers and young adults, but most surveys describe a second smaller peak from the sixth to the eighth decades.[93–97] The proportion of patients with Crohn's disease aged 60 years or more at the time of diagnosis ranges from 7 to 26 percent, and these figures are likely to increase.[98] Small bowel involvement is less common in this age group, occurring in 40–67 percent of elderly patients[99–102] compared to the overall frequency of 75–80 percent. However, in a recent large epidemiological study of 1936 patients over a 35-year period, approximately three-quarters of both elderly (60 years or more) and young subjects had small bowel disease. Elderly patients were more likely to have isolated small bowel involvement without colonic disease.[97]

CLINICAL PICTURE   The clinical features of Crohn's disease,[100–103] including the extraintestinal manifestations,[101] are no different in elderly patients. Extensive small bowel disease is rare,[99] but the terminal ileum is affected in most individuals. Right iliac fossa pain, diarrhea, weight loss, fever, and an abdominal mass are typical features. Abdominal pain may be less common in elderly patients. Stricture formation can lead to subacute or acute obstruction, and fistulas to a wide variety of manifestations. In some series,[99,101,102] elderly patients have presented more frequently with acute complications, such as obstruction and perforation, needing early or emergency surgery. This may be due to delays in diagnosis,[102,104] which is made only when a stricture, severe inflammation, or perforation results in acute illness. Terminal ileal Crohn's disease can mimic acute appendicitis or an appendiceal abscess; the differential diagnosis in older patients includes cecal diverticulitis, colonic carcinoma, and small bowel ischemia. Intercurrent infections, smoking, and nonsteroidal anti-inflammatory drugs can all precipitate relapse.[105]

The radiological features of Crohn's disease in the elderly do not differ from those in younger patients.[100] The distribution, extent, and severity of disease are usually well visualized on double-contrast barium follow-through or enteroclysis.[106,107] Abdominal CT scanning demonstrates bowel wall thickening and is more accurate than contrast studies in detecting fistulas other than entero-enteric communications. CT and ultrasound scans are both used to outline phlegmons (inflammatory masses) and abscess cavities. Surgical drainage of intra-abdominal abscesses can be avoided in more than 50 percent of cases by carrying out percutaneous CT or ultrasound-guided drainage.[106,107] Labeled leukocyte scanning is a noninvasive method of assessing disease activity and complements other imaging techniques. It is more accurate in the investigation of colonic disease but can be used to differentiate luminal narrowing due to inflammatory changes from fibrous strictures. Magnetic resonance (MR) imaging may be helpful in the evaluation of small bowel involvement but is currently largely used for complex perianal disease.

MANAGEMENT The management of Crohn's disease consists of both the induction and maintenance of remission. Elderly patients with small bowel disease respond as well to medical treatment as do younger patients.[100,101] Aminosalicylates are used in mild or moderate disease, but sulfasalazine is not consistently effective in small bowel Crohn's disease without colonic involvement. This is probably because the active component, mesalazine or 5-aminosalicylate, is released from its "carrier" sulfapyridine by the action of colonic bacteria. Mesalazine preparations coated with a pH-sensitive resin or in ethylcellulose-coated granules start releasing the drug in the small bowel and are effective in achieving remission at doses of 3.2–4 g daily.[105,108,109] Clinical trials and meta-analyses of the value of aminosalicylates in maintaining remission have not produced consistent results. They appear to be more effective after surgical resection than in patients in whom remission has been induced with steroid treatment.[105,108] Corticosteroids like prednisolone are largely used for moderate-to-severe disease in daily doses of 40–60 mg. They cause many side-effects[110,111] and approximately 50 percent of treated patients become steroid-dependent or resistant. Budesonide, a topically active steroid with extensive first-pass metabolism in the liver, is probably less effective than prednisolone but has a better side-effect profile. Steroids have no role in maintaining remission in Crohn's disease.

Immunosuppressive agents such as azathioprine and 6-mercaptopurine are used as steroid-sparing agents which enable the dose of corticosteroids to be reduced or tapered off. They are effective in maintaining remission after steroid therapy for up to 4 years.[105,108,112] They should be used cautiously in the elderly given their potential for serious toxicity, although in clinical trials 6-mercaptopurine has been tolerated by patients in the seventh decade as well as their younger counterparts.[112] Methotrexate, ciclosporin, mycophenolate mofetil, and tacrolimus are immunosuppressive agents which are being increasingly used in patients with refractory disease who are intolerant to other drugs. Metronidazole is not effective in Crohn's disease limited to the small bowel, but can be used for patients with ileocolic disease. Ciprofloxacin is as effective as mesalazine when used alone, and is as effective as methylprednisolone when used with metronidazole for active disease.[105,108,113] Infliximab, a chimeric monoclonal antibody against tumor necrosis factor alpha (TNF-α), has recently been introduced for the treatment of moderate-to-severe Crohn's disease and for fistulas, usually in patients who are refractory or intolerant to conventional treatment. A single infusion of 5 mg/kg can have beneficial effects lasting up to 12 weeks, and multiple infusions can be used to maintain remission.[114] Patients with Crohn's disease are prone to osteopenia and osteoporosis.[103] Bone loss occurs due to malabsorption of calcium and vitamin D, as a direct result of the inflammatory process and with corticosteroid use.[110,111] Comprehensive guidelines for the detection and management of osteoporosis in inflammatory bowel disease have been published.[58]

Malnutrition is common in small bowel Crohn's disease and is due to a variable combination of reduced nutrient intake, malabsorption, and increased energy requirements resulting from inflammation, sepsis, or surgery. In most patients nutrient intake can be increased by using small, frequent, low-fiber meals and supplementary polymeric sip feeds. Some patients benefit from tube feeding, and a few need parenteral nutrition. Enteral nutrition, with either elemental or polymeric diets, can also be used as a primary treatment for Crohn's disease and induces remission in approximately 60 percent of patients. It is less effective than corticosteroids and is also less acceptable to patients.[115]

Surgery is required for obstruction due to strictures, for suppurative complications, and for disease that is refractory to medical treatment. Elderly patients usually tolerate surgery well,[99,100,116,117] except those presenting more acutely with severe disease, among whom postoperative mortality is high.[102] Thus early surgery, usually a limited right hemicolectomy and terminal ileal resection, is advisable in elderly patients not responding to medical treatment. Postoperative recurrence rates are lower than those in younger patients.[99,100,116] Adenocarcinoma of the small bowel can complicate small bowel Crohn's disease and is more likely to arise in the distal jejunum and ileum, affected by longstanding chronic active disease.[118]

Mortality rates in elderly people with Crohn's disease are similar to those in age-matched controls.[119]

Small bowel ischemia

Small bowel ischemia, which can be acute or chronic, is predominantly a disease of the elderly population. The diagnosis and management of these conditions is currently largely based on clinical experience as randomized controlled trials have not been carried out.[120–122]

Acute mesenteric ischemia

Acute arterial mesenteric ischemia is due to embolism, thrombus formation, or nonocclusive ischemia of the superior mesenteric artery (SMA) or its territory. Complete occlusion of the SMA, which supplies the entire small bowel and the right half of the colon, has catastrophic effects. Patients who survive frequently require long-term nutritional support and may need parenteral nutrition depending on the length of residual jejunum. Embolism accounts for 40–50 percent of cases and usually occurs in elderly people with predisposing causes such as atrial fibrillation, left-sided cardiac chamber enlargement, or myocardial infarction. Nonocclusive mesenteric ischemia occurs in 20–30 percent of cases and is due to vasoconstriction of the mesenteric circulation following a low-output state or circulatory collapse, for example, severe congestive cardiac failure (CCF), hypotension, cardiac arrhythmias or following cardiac arrest. This form of ischemia may be on the increase: 47 percent of patients were affected in a recent series.[123] Thrombosis (20–30 percent) occurs in the setting of widespread vascular disease, and 20–50 percent of patients have a history of abdominal angina in the proceeding weeks to months.

The mortality rate of 71 percent (range 59–93 percent) has not altered over the last 70 years. The outlook is much better when the diagnosis is made before irreversible infarction occurs.

DIAGNOSIS Patients present with severe abdominal pain but examination is initially either normal or reveals only tenderness. This disparity between symptoms and physical signs in an elderly patient with vascular disease or a hypercoagulable state is highly suggestive of mesenteric ischemia. Up to 25 percent of patients have abdominal distention or gastrointestinal bleeding without pain. Signs of peritonitis, hypotension, vomiting, fever, gastrointestinal bleeding, increasing distention, leukocytosis and metabolic acidosis are features of intestinal infarction. About a third of elderly patients may present with an acute confusional state.[124] Raised serum levels of amylase, alkaline phosphatase, and phosphate have been reported but are not reliable markers. Fluid levels and dilated loops of bowel on plain abdominal films occur in up to a third of patients, but more specific radiological features such as gas in the intestinal wall or portal vessels are rare. Patients with abnormal films have a poor prognosis as even nonspecific changes usually signify intestinal necrosis. Mesenteric angiography is the gold standard for establishing the diagnosis and should ideally be performed before signs of infarction appear. It can, however, be difficult to differentiate between acute and longstanding vascular changes on an angiogram.

The difficulties of performing angiography in sick elderly patients with few objective clinical signs has led to the use of noninvasive tests. Duplex ultrasonography has a specificity of 92–100 percent but a sensitivity of only 70–89 percent in identifying severe stenosis or occlusion of the SMA. Contrast-enhanced CT scanning is accurate only in the diagnosis of mesenteric vein thrombosis. Magnetic resonance imaging is promising, but clinical experience is limited to date.

MANAGEMENT Management warrants aggressive measures in the appropriate patients, and initial resuscitation includes monitoring of central pressures, correction of hypovolemia, and inotropic support. Splanchnic vasoconstrictors, mainly norepinephrine (noradrenaline) and digitalis preparations, should be avoided. Broad-spectrum antibiotics are given empirically to treat the septicemia resulting from bacterial translocation across infarcted bowel. Patients with established signs of infarction need emergency surgery with resection of infarcted bowel and embolectomy, thrombectomy, or arterial reconstruction. A second-look operation is often indicated 12–24 hours later to differentiate between viable and nonviable intestine. When the diagnosis is suspected before clinical signs of infarction have developed, emergency angiography should be performed first. Intra-arterial infusions of the vasodilator papaverine relieve the associated mesenteric arterial spasm and improve perfusion perioperatively. Full anticoagulation with heparin is started after surgery. Thrombolytic therapy can be successful in patients with a more distal SMA embolus, if carried out within 12 hours of the onset of symptoms.

Thrombosis of the superior mesenteric vein (SMV) is present in 5–10 percent of patients with acute mesenteric ischemia.[125–127] Hypercoagulable states and previous abdominal surgery are the most common predisposing conditions, but no cause is identified in 20–35 percent of patients. The clinical picture is less acute and more variable than that of arterial insufficiency, and thus the diagnosis even more difficult to establish. The thrombus is visualized on contrast-enhanced CT in the majority[127] and fewer than 10 percent of patients require angiography.

Patients without peritoneal signs can be treated with anticoagulation alone. Those with peritonism require laparotomy and resection of nonviable bowel as described above. Mesenteric venous thrombectomy has been reported but should be carried out only if there is fresh thrombus in the proximal superior mesenteric vein. There are a few case reports of successful thrombolytic therapy. All patients require anticoagulation for at least 6 months. Mesenteric vein thrombosis generally has a better prognosis than the other ischemic syndromes, but published mortality rates show wide variation from 20 to 80 percent. Focal segmental ischemia causes localized infarction, often at multiple sites, and can be due to vasculitis, cholesterol, or atheromatous emboli and various nonvascular diseases.

Comprehensive algorithms for the diagnosis and management of intestinal ischemia have been published.[122]

Chronic mesenteric ischemia

The syndrome of abdominal or intestinal angina is a rare condition that develops as a result of atherosclerosis of the splanchnic circulation.[120–122] Mesenteric blood flow fails to meet the increased metabolic demand that occurs after meals, resulting in pain with or without malabsorption and disordered motility. The pain begins within 30 minutes of a meal and increases gradually to a plateau which lasts for up to 3 hours. It is located in the upper abdomen, can radiate to the back and is gnawing or cramping in character. It is sometimes relieved by lying prone or squatting. Constipation, diarrhea, steatorrhea, abdominal bloating and flatulence may also occur. Patients may miss or restrict meals in order to avoid provoking symptoms, and hence lose weight.

DIAGNOSIS Clinical assessment often reveals evidence of widespread vascular disease. An abdominal systolic bruit may be present but is not a specific finding. Individuals with advanced atherosclerotic disease can have severe stenosis or occlusion of two or even all three main mesenteric arterial trunks and remain asymptomatic.[128] Diagnosis therefore depends on history as well as angiographic findings of proximal stenosis in at least two of the main mesenteric trunks, with a collateral circulation indicating chronic ischemia. Occlusion of two vessels was found in 91 percent, and three-vessel involvement in 55 percent of patients with chronic mesenteric ischemia.[129] It is important to exclude atypical angina pectoris and other causes of recurrent abdominal pain such as gallstone colic, and peptic ulcer disease. Noninvasive indirect measurements of splanchnic blood flow—such as duplex ultrasonography, MR angiography, MR oximetry, and intestinal oxygen consumption—are used to screen patients for angiography.

MANAGEMENT Surgical revascularization relieves symptoms in most patients who fulfill the above criteria and prevents acute thrombotic occlusion.[120,121,130] Percutaneous transluminal mesenteric angioplasty is being used for high-risk patients, but experience with this technique is limited and recurrence rates are higher than after surgery.

Chronic mesenteric vein thrombosis is asymptomatic, and requires no treatment, when an adequate collateral system prevents the development of portal hypertension. Management of patients with portal hypertension largely consists of the prevention of variceal hemorrhage.

Small bowel tumors

Small bowel tumors are relatively rare, accounting for only 1–2.4 percent of all gastrointestinal neoplasms.[131],[132] Adenomas, leiomyomas, and lipomas are the most common benign tumors. Adenomas usually arise in the duodenum and proximal jejunum, lipomas are more frequent in the ileum.[131] Leiomyomas are distributed more evenly in the small bowel but have a slight jejunal preponderance.[133] More than 50 percent of benign tumors are asymptomatic, the rest present with obstruction, intussuception, or occult bleeding. Adenomas situated within reach of an enteroscope should be snared and removed since, as with colonic adenomas, they have malignant potential.[134] The treatment of distal adenomas and leiomyomas is surgical resection. Asymptomatic lipomas discovered incidentally can be left in situ as malignant transformation is unknown.

The most common forms of malignancy involving the small bowel are metastases from distant sites, together with direct spread from adjacent organs such as pancreas and colon.[134] Primary malignant small bowel tumors are more common in men and increase in frequency with age, with a peak incidence in the sixth and seventh decades.[131],[135],[136] Adenocarcinomas (24–42 percent of tumors), carcinoid tumors (27–41 percent), leiomyosarcomas (10–11 percent), and lymphomas (20–22 percent) are the four major histological types encountered.[135–137] Adenocarcinomas usually arise in the duodenum and proximal jejunum,[137] whereas carcinoid tumors are predominantly ileal.[138],[139] Leiomyosarcomas are slightly more common in the jejunum compared to the ileum and less than one-fifth involve the duodenum.[133] Most B-cell lymphomas occur in the ileum whereas the majority of T-cell lymphomas are jejunal.[140],[141] One-quarter of B-cell and 50 percent of T-cell tumors are multifocal with up to 10 lesions.[140]

PRESENTATION AND DIAGNOSIS Abdominal pain, bleeding, intestinal obstruction, and weight loss are the major manifestations, a palpable abdominal mass being less frequent.[142] Perforation occurs in about 10 percent of cases, periampullary tumors can present with obstructive jaundice, and diarrhea is more common in patients with lymphoma.[131] With small bowel carcinoids, the carcinoid syndrome comprising flushing, telangiectasiae, diarrhea, bronchospasm and, less commonly, right heart failure, occurs only when hepatic metastases are present.[138],[139]

The diagnosis of small bowel malignancy is often delayed because of the nonspecific history and the absence of clinical signs. Enteroclysis is far more sensitive than barium follow-through in detecting tumors.[142] Abdominal CT scanning visualizes larger lesions, particularly sarcomas, and is important for staging the disease. Push enteroscopy is being increasingly used to confirm radiological abnormalities and to investigate patients with iron-deficiency anemia and obscure gastrointestinal bleeding as described above. Mesenteric angiography will also detect some small bowel tumors in the latter group. However, the diagnosis is often established only at laparotomy despite these investigative techniques.

MANAGEMENT Adenocarcinomas and leiomyosarcomas are both treated by surgical resection in the appropriate patients without disseminated disease. Duodenal tumors usually require pancreatoduodenectomy, whereas jejunal and ileal lesions are amenable to segmental resection. Radiotherapy and chemotherapy are not effective, even as adjuvant therapy.[133],[137] These tumors have a poor prognosis. Overall disease-specific 5-year survival in 4995 patients with adenocarcinoma was 30.5 percent, but was even less in patients over aged 75 years and in those with duodenal disease.[137] Five-year survival was 27.8 percent in 708 patients with leiomyosarcoma reported from 22 series.[133]

Carcinoid tumors grow slowly and are compatible with prolonged survival even with incurable disease. The 5-year survival rate after surgical resection is 80 percent, and even patients with hepatic metastases have a median survival of 3 years with 30–38 percent alive at 5 years.[138],[143] Overall 5-year survival rates for small bowel carcinoids range from 50 to 60 percent.[139],[144] Octreotide is an effective, albeit temporary, palliative treatment for the carcinoid syndrome. Cyproheptadine, an antihistamine with antiserotonergic activity, and the serotonin antagonists ondansetron and tropisetron, are also used for symptomatic control. In patients in whom curative resection is not possible, multimodal therapy including debulking procedures, hepatic artery embolization for metastases, chemotherapy, and interferon-α can produce good long-term results.[143]

Two-thirds of primary small bowel lymphomas are of the B-cell type, the remainder being T-cell in origin.[140] Approximately 50 percent of T-cell lymphomas are associated with enteropathy, mainly celiac disease. Twenty percent of B-cell lymphomas are low-grade tumors of mucosa-associated lymphoid tissue (MALT lymphomas). Treatment is primarily by surgical resection, but the optimal treatment strategy with adjuvant chemoradiotherapy has not yet been established.[141],[145] T-cell tumors have a worse prognosis, with 5-year survival rates of 25 percent compared to 50 percent for high-grade and 75 percent for low-grade B-cell lymphomas, respectively.[140]

The overall 5-year survival in a population-based study of 328 primary small bowel tumors over a 25-year period was 54 percent.[135]

KEY POINTS Small bowel disease

- Celiac disease, small bowel bacterial overgrowth, and chronic pancreatitis are the main causes of malabsorption in older patients.

- Celiac disease can affect all age groups and more than 50 percent of patients are asymptomatic.

- Small bowel bacterial overgrowth must be distinguished from simple colonization without malabsorption, as the latter is common in elderly people and in those taking acid-reducing drugs.

- Crohn's disease has a bimodal distribution with a second peak in the elderly population.

- The mortality rate of about 71 percent in acute mesenteric ischemia has remained unaltered for many years.

- Small bowel tumors are rare and account for only 1–2.4 percent of all gastrointestinal neoplasms.

REFERENCES

1. Pelz KS, Gottfried SP, Soos E: Intestinal absorption studies in the aged. Geriatrics 1968;23:149–153
2. Montgomery RD, Haeney MR, Ross IN et al: The ageing gut: a study of intestinal absorption in relation to nutrition in the elderly. QJM 1978;47:197–211
3. McEvoy A, Dutton J, James OFW: Bacterial contamination of the small intestine is an important cause of malabsorption in the elderly. BMJ 1983;287:789–793
4. King D, Smith ML, Chapman TJ, Stockdale HR, Lye M: Fat malabsorption in elderly patients with cardiac cachexia. Age Ageing 1996;25:144–149
5. Montgomery RD, Haboubi NY, Mike NH et al: Causes of malabsorption in the elderly. Age Ageing 1986;15:235–240
6. Price HL, Gazzard BG, Dawson AM: Steatorrhoea in the elderly. BMJ 1977;1:1582–1584
7. Ryder JB: Steatorrhoea in the elderly. Gerontol Clin 1963;5:30–37
8. Goulding A, Taylor RW, Keil D et al: Lactose malabsorption and rate of bone loss in older women. Age Ageing 1999;28:175–180
9. Riordan SM, McIver CJ, Wakefield D et al: Small intestinal bacterial overgrowth in the symptomatic elderly. Am J Gastroenterol 1997;92:47–51
10. Sugai E, Srur G, Vazquez H et al: Steatocrit: a reliable semiquantitative method for the detection of steatorrhea. J Clin Gastroenterol 1994;19:206–209
11. Newcomer AD, Hofmann AF, DiMagno EP et al: L-Triolein breath test: a sensitive and specific test for fat malabsorption. Gastroenterology 1979;76:6–13
12. Mylvaganam K, Hudson PR, Herring A, Williams CP: ^{14}C triolein breath test: an assessment in the elderly. Gut 1989;30:1082–1086
13. Craig RM, Atkinson AJ: D-Xylose testing: a review. Gastroenterology 1988;95:223–231
14. Kendall MJ: The influence of age on the xylose absorption test. Gut 1970;11:498–501
15. Kendall MJ, Nutter S: The influence of sex, body weight, and renal function on the xylose test. Gut 1970;11:1020–1023
16. Webster SGP, Leeming JT: Assessment of small bowel function in the elderly using a modified xylose tolerance test. Gut 1975;16:109–113
17. Haeney MR, Culank LS, Montgomery RD, Sammons HG: Evaluation of xylose absorption as measured in blood and urine: a one-hour blood xylose screening test in malabsorption. Gastroenterology 1978;75:393–400
18. Mayersohn M: The "xylose test" to assess gastrointestinal absorption in the elderly: a pharmacokinetic evaluation of the literature. J Gerontol 1982;37:300–305
19. Johnson SL, Mayersohn M, Conrad K: Gastrointestinal absorption as a function of age: xylose absorption in healthy adults. Clin Pharmacol Ther 1985;38:331–335
20. Arora S, Kassarjian Z, Krasinski SD et al: Effect of age on tests of intestinal and hepatic function in healthy humans. Gastroenterology 1989;96:1560–1565
21. Casellas F, Chicharro L, Malagelada JR: Potential usefulness of hydrogen breath test with D-xylose in clinical management of intestinal malabsorption. Dig Dis Sci 1993;38:321–327
22. Arola H: Diagnosis of hypolactasia and lactose malabsorption. Scand J Gastroenterol Suppl 1994;29:26–35
23. Bell TK, Bridges JM, Nelson MG: Simultaneous free and bound radioactive vitamin B_{12} urinary excretion test. J Clin Pathol 1965;18:611–613
24. Holt PR: Diarrhea and malabsorption in the elderly. Gastroenterol Clin North Am 2001;30:427–444
25. Carmel R: Cobalamin, the stomach, and aging. Am J Clin Nutr 1997;66:750–759
26. Aimone-Gastin I, Pierson H, Jeandel C et al: Prospective evaluation of protein bound vitamin B_{12} (cobalamin) malabsorption in the elderly using trout flesh labelled in vivo with ^{57}Co-cobalalmin. Gut 1997;41:475–479
27. King CE, Toskes PP: Small intestine bacterial overgrowth. Gastroenterology 1979;76:1035–1055
28. Simon GL, Gorbach SL: Intestinal flora in health and disease. Gastroenterology 1984;86:174–193
29. Corazza GR, Menozzi MG, Strocchi L et al: The diagnosis of small bowel bacterial overgrowth. Gastroenterology 1990;98:302–309
30. Haboubi NY, Montgomery RD: Small-bowel bacterial overgrowth in elderly people: clinical significance and response to treatment. Age Ageing 1992;21:13–19
31. Bardhan PK, Gyr K, Beglinger C et al: Diagnosis of bacterial overgrowth after culturing proximal small-bowel aspirate obtained during routine upper gastrointestinal endoscopy. Scand J Gastroenterol 1992;27:253–256
32. Fromm H, Hofmann AF: Breath test for altered bile-acid metabolism. Lancet 1971;ii:621–625
33. James OFW, Agnew JE, Bouchier IAD: Assessment of the ^{14}C-glycocholic acid breath test. BMJ 1973;3:191–195
34. Suhr O, Danielsson A, Horstedt P, Stenling R: Bacterial contamination of the small bowel evaluated by breath tests, ^{75}Se-labelled homocholic-tauro acid, and scanning electron microscopy. Scand J Gastroenterol 1990;25:841–852
35. Rhodes JM, Middleton P, Jewell DP: The lactulose hydrogen breath test as a diagnostic test for small-bowel bacterial overgrowth. Scand J Gastroenterol 1979;14:333–336
36. Miller MA, Parkman HP, Urbain JL et al: Comparison of scintigraphy and lactulose breath hydrogen test for assessment of orocecal transit: lactulose accelerates small bowel transit. Dig Dis Sci 1997;42:10–18
37. King CE, Toskes PP, Spivey JC et al: Detection of small intestinal bacterial overgrowth by means of a ^{14}C-D-xylose breath test. Gastroenterology 1979;77:75–82
38. King CE, Toskes PP: Comparison of the 1-gram [^{14}C]xylose, 10-gram lactulose-H_2, and 80-gram glucose-H_2 breath tests in patients with small intestine bacterial overgrowth. Gastroenterology 1986;91:1447–1451
39. Lewis SJ, Young G, Mann M, Franco S, O'Keefe SJ: Improvement in specificity of [^{14}C]D-xylose breath test for bacterial overgrowth. Dig Dis Sci 1997;42:1587–1592
40. Rumessen JJ, Gudmand-Hoyer E, Bachmann E, Justesen T: Diagnosis of bacterial overgrowth of the small intestine. Scand J Gastroenterol 1985;20:1267–1275
41. Husebye E, Skar V, Hoverstad T, Melby K: Fasting hypochlorhydria with Gram positive organisms is highly prevalent in healthy old people. Gut 1992;33:1331–1337
42. Saltzman JR, Kowdley KV, Pedrosa MC et al: Bacterial overgrowth without clinical malabsorption in elderly hypochlorhydric subjects. Gastroenterology 1994;106:615–623
43. Husebye E, Skar V, Hoverstad T et al: Abnormal intestinal motor patterns explain enteric colonization with Gram-negative bacilli in late radiation enteropathy. Gastroenterology 1995;109:1078–1089
44. Valdovinos MA, Camilleri M, Thomforde GM, Frie C: Reduced accuracy of ^{14}C-D-xylose breath test for detection of bacterial overgrowth in gastrointestinal motility disorders. Scand J Gastroenterol 1993;28:963–968
45. Riordan SM, McIver CJ, Duncombe VM, Bolin TD, Thomas MC: Factors influencing the 1-g ^{14}C-D-xylose breath test for bacterial overgrowth. Am J Gastroenterol 1995;90:1455–1460
46. Zsuzsanna FK, Wölfling J, Csati S et al: The ursodeoxycholic acid-p-aminobenzoic acid deconjugation test: a new tool for the diagnosis of bacterial overgrowth syndrome. Eur J Gastroenterol Hepatol 1997;9:679–682
47. Siegel LM, Stevens PD, Lightdale CJ et al: Combined magnification endoscopy with chromoendoscopy in the evaluation of patients with suspected malabsorption. Gastrointest Endosc 1997;46:226–230
48. Lewis B: Radiology versus endoscopy of the small bowel. Endoscopy 1998;30:412–415
49. Waye JD: Small-bowel endoscopy. Endoscopy 1999;31:56–59
50. Oates BC, Morris AI: Enteroscopy. Curr Opin Gastroenterol 2000;16:121–125
51. Appleyard M, Fireman Z, Glukhovsky A et al: A randomised trial comparing wireless capsule endoscopy with push enteroscopy for the detection of small-bowel lesions. Gastroenterology 2000;119:1431–1438
52. Appleyard M, Glukhovsky A, Gan S, Swain P: The wireless endoscope: first clinical trials in patients with GI bleeding. Gut 2001;(suppl 1)48:A13
53. Parnell NDJ, Ciclitira PJ: Coeliac disease and its management. Aliment Pharmacol Ther 1999;13:1–13 (review)
54. Swinson CM, Levi AJ: Is coeliac disease underdiagnosed? BMJ 1980;281:1258–1260
55. Anonymous: Coeliac disease in the elderly. Lancet 1984;i:775–776
56. Hankey GL, Holmes GKT: Coeliac disease in the elderly. Gut 1994;35:65–67
57. Beaumont DM, Mian MS: Coeliac disease in old age: "a catch in the rye". Age Ageing 1998;27:535–538

58. Scott EM, Gaywood I, Scott BB: Guidelines for osteoporosis in coeliac disease and inflammatory bowel disease. Gut 2000;46(suppl 1):i1–i8

59. Collin P, Reunala T, Pukkala E et al: Coeliac disease: associated disorders and survival. Gut 1994;35:1215–1218

60. Ferreira M, Lloyd Davies S, Butler M et al: Endomysial antibody: is it the best screening test for coeliac disease? Gut 1992;33:1633–1637

61. Attia L, Holt PR: Serological testing for celiac disease in the elderly. Gastroenterology 1995;109:2053

62. Dieterich W, Ehnis T, Bauer M et al: Identification of tissue transglutaminase as the autoantigen of celiac disease. Nat Med 1997;3:797–801

63. O'Mahoney S, Howdle PD, Losowsky MS: Management of patients with nonresponsive coeliac disease. Aliment Pharmacol Ther 1996;10:671–680 (review)

64. Ryan BM, Kelleher D: Refractory celiac disease. Gastroenterology 2000;119:243–251

65. Isaacson PG: Relation between cryptic intestinal lymphoma and refractory sprue. Lancet 2000;356:178–179

66. Holmes GKT, Prior P, Lane MR et al: Malignancy in coeliac disease: effect of a gluten free diet. Gut 1989;30:333–338

67. Swinson CM, Slavin G, Coles EC, Booth CC: Coeliac disease and malignancy. Lancet 1983;ii:111–115

68. Cooper BT, Holmes GKT, Cooke WT: Lymphoma risk in coeliac disease of later life. Digestion 1982;23:89–92

69. Holt PR: Clinical significance of bacterial overgrowth in elderly people. Age Ageing 1992;21:1–4

70. Vantrappen G, Janssens J, Hellemans J, Ghoos Y: The interdigestive motor complex of normal subjects and patients with bacterial overgrowth of the small intestine. J Clin Invest 1977;59:1158–1166

71. Lovat LB: Age related changes in gut physiology and nutritional status. Gut 1996;38:306–309

72. Holt PR, Rosenberg IH, Russell RM: Causes and consequences of hypochlorhydria in the elderly. Dig Dis Sci 1989;34:933–937

73. Saltzman J: Epidemiology and natural history of atrophic gastritis. In Holt PR, Russell R (eds): Chronic Gastritis and Hypochlorhydria in the Elderly. CRC, Boca Raton, 1993:31–47

74. Lipski PS, Kelly PJ, James OFW: Bacterial contamination of the small bowel in elderly people: is it necessarily pathological? Age Ageing 1992;21:5–12

75. Hellemans J, Joosten E, Ghoos Y et al: Positive $^{14}CO_2$ bile acid breath test in elderly people. Age Ageing 1984;13:138–143

76. Hutchinson S, Logan R: The effect of long-term omeprazole on the glucose-hydrogen breath test in elderly patients. Age Ageing 1997;26:87–89

77. Lewis SJ, Potts LF, Malhotra R, Mountford R: Small bowel bacterial overgrowth in subjects living in residential care homes. Age Ageing 1999;28:181–185

78. Donald IP, Kitchingmam G, Donal F, Kupfer RM: The diagnosis of small bowel bacterial overgrowth in elderly patients. J Am Geriatr Soc 1992;40:692–696

79. Thorens J, Froehlich F, Schwizer W et al: Bacterial overgrowth during treatment with omeprazole compared with cimetidine: a prospective randomised double blind study. Gut 1996;39:54–59

80. Pereira SP, Gainsborough N, Dowling RH: Drug-induced hypochlorhydria causes high duodenal bacterial counts in the elderly. Aliment Pharmacol Ther 1998;12:99–104

81. Fried M, Siegrist H, Frei R et al: Duodenal bacterial overgrowth during treatment in outpatients with omeprazole. Gut 1994;35:23–26

82. Shindo K, Machida M, Fukumura M, Koide K, Yamazaki R: Omeprazole induces altered bile acid metabolism. Gut 1998;42:266–271

83. Roberts SH, James O, Jarvis EH: Bacterial overgrowth syndrome without "blind loop": a cause for malnutrition in the elderly. Lancet 1977;ii:1193–1195

84. Haboubi NY, Hudson P, Rahman Q et al: Small-intestine transit time in the elderly. Lancet 1988;i:933

85. Akhrass R, Yaffe MB, Fischer C, Ponsky J, Shuck JM: Small bowel diverticulosis: perceptions and reality. J Am Coll Surg 1997;184:383–388

86. Mellstrom D, Rundgren A: Long-term effects after partial gastrectomy in elderly men. Scand J Gastroenterol 1982;17:433–439

87. Kumar A, Forsmark CE, Toskes PP: Small bowel bacterial overgrowth: the changing face of an old disease. Gastroenterology 1996;110:A340

88. Bouhnik Y, Alain S, Attar A et al: Bacterial populations contaminating the upper gut in patients with small intestinal bacterial overgrowth syndrome. Am J Gastroenterol 1999;94:1327–1331

89. Attar A, Flourie B, Rambaud JC et al: Antibiotic efficacy in small intestinal bacterial overgrowth-related chronic diarrhea: a crossover randomised trial. Gastroenterology 1999;117:794–797

90. Soudah HC, Hasler WL, Owyang C: Effect of octreotide on intestinal motility and bacterial overgrowth in scleroderma. N Engl J Med 1991;325:1508–1509

91. Perlemuter G, Cacoub P, Chaussade S, Wechsler B, Couturier D, Piette J-C: Octreotide treatment of chronic intestinal pseudo-obstruction secondary to connective tissue diseases. Arthritis Rheum 1999;42:1545–1549

92. Verne GN, Eaker EY, Hardy E, Sninsky CA: Effect of octreotide and erythromycin on idiopathic and scleroderma-associated intestinal pseudoobstruction. Dig Dis Sci 1995;40:1892–1901

93. Rose JDR, Roberts GM, Williams G et al: Cardiff Crohn's disease jubilee: the incidence over 50 years. Gut 1988;29:346–351

94. Stowe SP, Redmond SR, Stormont JM et al: An epidemiologic study of inflammatory bowel disease in Rochester, New York. Gastroenterology 1990;98:104–110

95. Ekbom A, Helmick C, Zack M, Adami H: The epidemiology of inflammatory bowel disease: a large, population-based study in Sweden. Gastroenterology 1991;100:350–358

96. Kyle J: Crohn's disease in the northeastern and northern isles of Scotland: an epidemiological review. Gastroenterology 1992;103:392–399

97. Lapidus A, Bernell O, Hellers G, Persson P-G, Löfberg R: Incidence of Crohn's disease in Stockholm County, 1955–1989. Gut 1997;41:480–486

98. Grimm IS, Friedman LS: Inflammatory bowel disease in the elderly. Gastroenterol Clin North Am 1990;19:361–389

99. Fabricius PJ, Gyde SN, Shouler P et al: Crohn's disease in the elderly. Gut 1985;26:461–465

100. Shapiro PA, Peppercorn MA, Antonioli DA et al: Crohn's disease in the elderly. Am J Gastroenterol 1981;76:132–137

101. Softley A, Myren J, Clamp SE et al: Inflammatory bowel disease in the elderly patient. Scand J Gastroenterol Suppl 1988;23:27–30

102. Lee FI, Giaffer M: Crohn's disease of late onset in Blackpool. Postgrad Med J 1987;63:471–473

103. Robertson DJ, Grimm IS: Inflammatory bowel disease in the elderly. Gastroenterol Clin North Am 2001;30:409–426

104. Foxworthy DM, Wilson JAP: Crohn's disease in the elderly: prolonged delay in diagnosis. J Am Geriatr Soc 1985;33:492–495

105. Hanauer SB, Sandborn W: Management of Crohn's disease in adults. Am J Gastroenterol 2001;96:635–643

106. Wills JS, Lobis IF, Denstman FJ: Crohn disease: state of the art. Radiology 1997;202:597–610

107. Carroll K: Crohn's disease: new imaging techniques. Ballière's Clin Gastroenterol 1998;12:35–72

108. Regueiro MD: Update in medical treatment of Crohn's disease. J Clin Gastroenterol 2000;31:282–291

109. Feagen BG: Aminosalicylates for active disease and in the maintenance of remission in Crohn's disease. Eur J Surg 1998;164:903–909

110. Akerkar GA, Peppercorn MA, Hamel MB, Parker RA: Corticosteroid-associated complications in elderly Crohn's disease patients. Am J Gastroenterol 1997;92:461–464

111. Thomas TPL: The complications of systemic corticosteroid treatment in the elderly. Gerontology 1984;30:60–65

112. Rutgeerts P, Baert F: Immunosuppressive drugs in the treatment of Crohn's disease. Eur J Surg 1998;164:911–915

113. Gionchetti P, Rizzello F, Campieri M: Probiotics and antibiotics in inflammatory bowel disease. Curr Opin Gastroenterol 2001;17:331–335

114. Bell SJ, Kamm MA: The clinical role of anti-TNFα antibody treatment in Crohn's disease. Aliment Pharmacol Therap 2000;14:501–514 (review)

115. Cabré E, Gassull MA: Nutrition in inflammatory bowel disease: impact on disease and therapy. Curr Opin Gastroenterol 2001;17:342–349

116. Tchirkow G, Lavery IC, Fazio VW: Crohn's disease in the elderly. Dis Colon Rectum 1983;26:177–181

117. Norris B, Solomon MJ, Eyres AA et al: Abdominal surgery in the older Crohn's population. Aust NZ J Surg 1999;69:199–204

118. Bernstein D, Rogers A: Malignancy in Crohn's disease. Am J Gastroenterol 1996;91:434–440

119. Munkholm P, Langholz E, Davidsen M, Binder V: Intestinal cancer risk and mortality in patients with Crohn's disease. Gastroenterology 1993;105:1716–1723

120. Greenwald DA, Brandt LJ, Reinus JF: Ischemic bowel disease in the elderly. Gastroenterol Clin North Am 2001;30:445–473

121. Brandt LJ, Boley SJ: AGA technical review on intestinal ischemia. Gastroenterology 2000;118:954–968

122. Anonymous: American Gastroenterological Association medical position statement: guidelines on intestinal ischemia. Gastroenterology 2000;118:951–952

123. Newman TS, Magnuson TH, Ahrendt SA, Smith-Meek MA, Bender, JS: The changing face of mesenteric infarction. Am Surg 1998;64:611–616

124. Finucaine PM, Arunachalam T, O'Dowd J, Pathy MSJ: Acute mesenteric infarction in elderly patients. J Am Geriatr Soc 1989;37:355–358

125. Grendell JH, Ockner RK: Mesenteric venous thrombosis. Gastroenterology 1982;82:358–372

126. Hassan HA, Raufman J: Mesenteric vein thrombosis. Southern Med J 1999;92:558–562

127. Rhee RY, Gloviczki P, Mendonca CT et al: Mesenteric venous thrombosis: still a lethal disease in the 1990s. J Vasc Surg 1994;20:688–697

128. Croft RJ, Menon GP, Marston A: Does "intestinal angina" exist? A critical study of obstructed visceral arteries. Br J Surg 1981;68:316–318

129. Moawad J, Gewertz BL: Chronic mesenteric ischemia: clinical presentation and diagnosis. Surg Clin North Am 1997;132:357–370

130. Marston A, Clarke JMF, Garcia Garcia J, Miller AL: Intestinal function and intestinal blood supply: a 20-year surgical study. Gut 1985;26:656–666

131. O'Riordan BG, Vilor M, Herrera L: Small bowel tumours: an overview. Dig Dis 1996;14:245–257

132. Martin RG: Malignant tumours of the small intestine. Surg Clin North Am 1986;66:779–785

133. Blanchard DK, Budde JM, Hatch GF et al: Tumours of the small intestine. World J Surg 2000;24:421–429

134. Buckley JA, Jones B, Fishman EK: Small bowel cancer: imaging features and staging. Radiol Clin North Am 1997;35:381–402

135. DiSario JA, Burt RW, Vargas H, McWhorter WP: Small bowel cancer: epidemiological and clinical characteristics from a population-based registry. Am J Gastroenterol 1994;89:699–701

136. Gabos S, Berkel J, Robson D, Whittaker H: Small bowel cancer in western Canada. Int J Epidemiol 1993;22:198–206

137. Howe JR, Karnell LH, Menck HR, Scott-Conner C: Adenocarcinoma of the small bowel: review of the National Cancer Data Base 1985–1995. Cancer 1999;86:2693–2706

138. Moertel CG: An odyssey in the land of small bowel tumours. J Clin Oncol 1987;5:1503–1522

139. Modlin IM, Sandor A: An analysis of 8305 cases of carcinoid tumours. Cancer 1997;79:813–829

140. Domizio P, Owen RA, Shepherd NA et al: Primary lymphoma of the small intestine: a clinicopathological study of 119 cases. Am J Surg Pathol 1993;17:429–442

141. Crump M, Gospodarowicz M, Shepherd FA: Lymphoma of the gastrointestinal tract. Semin Oncol 1999;26:324–337

142. Maglinte DDT, Reyes BL: Small bowel cancer: radiologic diagnosis. Radiol Clin North Am 1997;35:361–380

143. Neary PC, Redmond PH, Houghton T, Watson GRK, Bouchier-Hayes D: Carcinoid disease: review of the literature. Dis Colon Rectum 1997;40:349–362

144. Stinner B, Kisker O, Zielke A, Rothmund M: Surgical management for carcinoid tumours of small bowel, appendix, colon and rectum. World J Surg 1996;20:183–188

145. Ha CS, Cho M, Allen PK et al: Primary non-Hodgkin lymphoma of the small bowel. Radiology 1999;211:183–187

Chapter 83

The large bowel

Arnold Wald

ANATOMY

The colon is a large, hollow organ that is derived embryologically from the primitive mid- and hindguts.[1] The appendix and transverse and sigmoid colons have mesenteries, whereas the ascending and descending colons do not. Like the stomach and small intestine, the colon has both circular and longitudinal smooth muscle layers, but uniquely, the longitudinal muscle of the colon is separated into three bundles known as taenia. The configuration of the taenia causes the colon to be divided into haustral folds which presumably help to slow the passage of fecal material and thus facilitate absorption.

The superior mesenteric artery supplies the right colon to the midtransverse colon, whereas the inferior mesenteric artery supplies the left colon.[2] The anorectum derives its blood supply from branches of the internal iliac arteries.[3] In the distal transverse to middescending colon, the superior and inferior mesenteric arteries are linked by a series of anastomoses known as the marginal artery of Drummond. This anatomical arrangement increases the vulnerability of this area to ischemic damage.

Innervation of the colon is via the autonomic nervous system and the enteric neurons.[4] Parasympathetic innervation is by the vagus nerve in the right colon and by sacral parasympathetics from the second, third, and fourth sacral nerves. Sympathetic innervation is derived from the lowest cervical to the third lumbar nerves via the splanchnic nerves. However, colon function may persist even after vagal or splanchnic interruption because of the presence of a well-developed enteric nervous system which can function in the absence of extrinsic innervation.

FUNCTIONS AND SYMPTOMS

The principal functions of the colon and rectum are to store fecal wastes for prolonged periods of time and to expel them in a socially appropriate manner. Storage is facilitated by adaptive compliance of the bowel and by muscular contractions of colonic smooth muscle, which retard the forward movement of stool, thereby promoting electrolyte and water absorption and reducing stool volume. Forward movement occurs principally by relatively infrequent peristaltic contractions which move intraluminal contents over long distances. Continence is maintained by recognition of rectal filling and coordinated function of the anal sphincters and pelvic floor muscles to defer defecation until socially appropriate. Colonic motility and transit in healthy elderly people are similar to that in younger individuals,[5] whereas aging is associated with diminished anal sphincter tone and strength as well as a less compliant rectum.[6,7] The latter changes may lead to greater susceptibility to fecal incontinence in elderly people (see Ch. 103).

The major symptoms of colonic and rectal disorders are constipation, diarrhea, pain, and rectal bleeding. The conditions that produce these symptoms are not unique to the elderly population; those occurring with increased frequency in elderly people include diverticulosis, neoplasms, ischemic colitis, vascular ectasias, fecal incontinence, constipation, and antibiotic-associated diarrhea and colitis. Inflammatory bowel diseases occur in all age groups, but onset of these diseases is less likely in the elderly population.

DIAGNOSTIC TESTING
Radiology

Contrast studies

Contrast examination of the large intestine is done by using barium sulfate in either a single- or a double-contrast technique in which a thickened barium suspension is used to coat the mucosa followed by insufflation to expand the viscus. Alternatively, water-soluble contrast agents can be used if perforation is suspected.

The single-contrast technique is preferred when studying patients with suspected obstruction, diverticulitis, or fistula, whereas the double-contrast technique is preferred for demonstrating fine mucosal lesions and neoplasms. There continues to be controversy concerning the choice of barium contrast or colonoscopy when investigating colonic diseases, although most clinicians favor colonoscopy for its greater sensitivity and opportunity for biopsy and therapy. Contrast studies may be indicated in cases where severe stricturing disease or adhesions make colonoscopy hazardous, where conditions such as diverticulitis are suspected, if the location and nature of a colonic obstruction requires assessment, and if functional as well as structural information is required. A barium enema should not be attempted when increases in colon pressure may worsen the patient's condition, for example, in patients with suspected toxic megacolon or those with peritoneal signs that suggest ischemic colitis.

When patients complain of constipation or a recent change in bowel habit, barium radiographs complement sigmoidoscopy in detecting organic causes and are also useful in diagnosing functional megacolon and megarectum. Complete filling of the colon with barium is neither necessary nor desirable in patients with megacolon. However, conventional barium studies provide limited information about colonic motor function in most patients with chronic constipation.[8] Moreover, they are frequently inadequate in frail or hospitalized elderly patients.[9,10]

Imaging techniques

ABDOMINAL COMPUTED TOMOGRAPHY This procedure allows visualization of the thickness of the bowel wall, the solid viscera within the abdomen, the mesenteries, and soft tissues adjacent to the bowel. It offers a modest advance in the diagnosis of diverticulitis by demonstrating inflammation of pericolic fat, abscesses that may contain collections of fluid and gas, and intramural sinus tracts. Fistulas to other organs can be identified when gas is found within the bladder or vagina. It also can identify extension of disease at a distance from the colon, including unsuspected intra-abdominal abscesses.

Computed tomography is also valuable when evaluating and managing complications of Crohn's disease, including abscesses, fistulas, and involvement of psoas muscles and ureters, and occasionally for percutaneous drainage of collections. Other complications, including sacral osteomyelitis, cholelithiasis, nephrolithiasis, and vascular necrosis of the femoral head associated with corticosteroid therapy, can also be diagnosed.

In appendicitis (and cecal diverticulitis, which is usually misdiagnosed as appendicitis), computed tomography may augment the clinical diagnosis by showing the periappendicular inflammatory process and differentiating phlegmon from abscess.[11] Occasionally, appendicoliths are identified, which are considered pathognomonic of appendicitis when associated with periappendicular inflammatory signs.

ANAL AND RECTAL ENDOSONOGRAPHY This new technique accurately delineates the layers of the rectal wall, the internal and external anal sphincters, and the levator muscles.[12] Several studies suggest that endosonography is potentially useful in evaluating pelvic floor structures in many patients with fecal incontinence to detect occult sphincter injuries arising from childbirth or other conditions associated with potential injury to continence mechanisms.[13,14]

Endoscopic ultrasonography has been used to image rectal polyps, focal malignancy within polyps, tumor masses penetrating into the bowel wall, and extramural lesions such as prostatic tumors and ovarian lesions. Perirectal fistulas and abscesses can also be evaluated (including determining whether there is destruction of pelvic muscles).

Colonoscopy and flexible sigmoidoscopy

These procedures are usually performed in the prepared colon except when evaluating diarrheal illnesses. Colonoscopic examinations provide unparalleled evaluation of the mucosal surfaces and opportunities for biopsy and therapy. These include diagnosis and determining extent of inflammatory bowel disease, evaluation of patients with overt or occult gastrointestinal bleeding, evaluation of chronic watery diarrhea, endoscopic sampling and removal of polyps, decompression of sigmoid volvulus or functional megacolon, and ablation of vascular lesions. Colonoscopy is generally done under conscious sedation, whereas flexible sigmoidoscopy usually is not.[15] In many elderly patients, the physician must be aware of their increased sensitivity to sedatives and analgesic medications. As elderly people are susceptible to hypotension and respiratory depression, careful monitoring of the patient during the procedure is especially important. Even in elderly patients, such procedures are generally safe in experienced hands and when done in units that monitor blood gases and cardiorespiratory functions. Major complications include bleeding and perforation, which should not occur more than 2 or 3 times in 1,000 routine procedures.

Histopathology

Mucosal biopsies are often indicated when evaluating undiagnosed diarrhea, in longstanding ulcerative colitis during surveillance for precancerous dysplasia, in obtaining tissue for viral culture, and in evaluating polypoid or ulcerated lesions. In inflammatory disorders of the colon and rectum, biopsies serve to establish the presence, extent, and distribution of colitis and to differentiate ulcerative from Crohn's colitis and these disorders from other inflammatory conditions such as infectious colitis. Biopsies should be obtained from endoscopically normal as well as abnormal areas, as characteristic changes may be patchy and therefore missed if too few biopsies are obtained. This is especially true in pseudomembranous, collagenous, and lymphocytic colitis in which the distal colon may be spared. As hypertonic phosphate enemas and purgative laxatives may induce mucosal changes that can be mistaken for mild colitis, they should be avoided when evaluating suspected inflammation of the colon.

Fecal occult blood testing

Fecal occult blood tests (FOBTs) identify hemoglobin or altered hemoglobin compounds in the stool. Foods containing peroxidases, such as melon and uncooked broccoli, horseradish, cauliflower, and turnips, may produce false positive results, whereas reducing agents such as ascorbic acid may decrease sensitivity.[16] Tests that extract the protoporphyrin from hemoglobin, such as Hemo Quant, are more specific and are quantitative but are also more time-consuming and expensive. Rehydration of Hemoccult slides increases sensitivity but decreases specificity and is not recommended. A weakly positive slide may become negative after 2–4 days of storage. Oral iron supplements do not interfere with any of these tests.

COLONIC DIVERTICULOSIS

Colonic diverticula are herniations of colonic mucosa through the smooth muscle layers. Diverticula occur in areas of anatomic weakness of the circular smooth muscle created by penetration of blood vessels to the submucosa. They are most commonly found in the sigmoid and descending colons and rarely, if ever, in the rectum.[17]

This disorder has been recognized with increasing frequency in modern Western countries.[18] Colonic diverticula are present in about one-third of persons by age 50 and about two-thirds by age 80. Dietary fiber insufficiency and the increased longevity of modern Western populations have been hypothesized to explain the increased prevalence of diverticulosis. Dietary factors may promote increased colonic motor activity and intraluminal pressures, whereas aging may lead to structural weakness of the colonic muscle.[17] As diverticula are asymptomatic in most individuals, caution must be taken before attributing nonspecific gastrointestinal symptoms to them.[19]

Painful diverticular disease

Painful diverticular disease is characterized by crampy discomfort in the left lower abdomen. Symptoms are often associated with constipation or diarrhea as well as with tenderness over the affected areas. These symptoms are similar to those of irritable bowel syndrome as well as partial bowel obstruction due to tumors or ischemia. In contrast to diverticulitis, there is no fever, leukocytosis, or rebound tenderness.

Diverticulitis

Diverticulitis develops in approximately 10–25 percent of individuals with diverticulosis who are followed for 10 years or more; however, less than 20 percent of these patients require hospitalization. Inflammation begins at the apex of the diverticulum when the opening of a diverticulum becomes obstructed (e.g. with stool), leading to micro- or macroperforation of a diverticulum.[20] The presence of a palpable mass, fever, leukocytosis, and/or rebound tenderness indicates an inflammatory process which often remains localized in the adjacent pericolic tissues but may progress to a peridiverticular abscess.[21] Other complications include fibrosis and bowel obstruction, fistula formation to the bladder, vagina, or adjacent small intestine, and free perforation with peritonitis. The frequency of complications rises to about 60 percent with recurrent attacks of diverticulitis.

Making a clinical distinction between painful diverticular disease and diverticulitis carries a sizable rate of error.[20] In an elderly or debilitated patient, the absence of fever, leukocytosis or rebound tenderness does not exclude diverticulitis.[21]

Other disorders such as carcinoma, inflammatory bowel disease, and ischemia may mimic symptomatic diverticular disease. Diagnostic studies include barium enema, computerized tomography, ultrasonography, and colonoscopy. In most cases of suspected diverticulitis, barium enema should be delayed for about a week to allow some resolution of the inflammatory process. A single-contrast study should be performed cautiously to minimize the risk of perforation. Radiographic findings suggesting diverticulitis include longitudinal fistulas connecting diverticula over segments of colon, fistula into adjacent organs, a fixed eccentric defect in the colon wall, contrast outside the lumen of the colon or diverticulum, and intraluminal defects representing abscesses.[17] Computed tomography and ultrasonic imaging of the abdomen provide superior definition of colonic wall thickness and extraluminal structures and are preferred at the time of initial evaluation. Colonoscopy is a less attractive option during an acute episode and is best employed to exclude tumors or other conditions if other diagnostic tests are inconclusive.

The treatment of painful diverticular disease is designed to reduce symptoms based on smooth muscle spasm, in contrast to the treatment of diverticulitis which is designed to treat bacterial infection (Table 83-1). Patients with severe pain, nausea and vomiting or complications should be hospitalized and given intravenous antibiotics until clinical improvement occurs.

Surgery is recommended for patients with diverticulitis who fail to respond to medical therapy within 72 hours, often for those who have had two or more attacks of diverticulitis, for immunocompromised patients,[23] and those who have fistula to the bladder with pneumaturia and urinary infection or fistula to the vagina with discharge of stool into the vagina. A one-stage operation, in which the diseased segment of bowel is resected and continuity restored by a primary anastomosis, is preferred.[24] In cases of generalized peritonitis or emergent surgery for perforation with abscess or high-grade obstruction, a two-stage procedure requiring a diverting colostomy should be used.[25] Large abscesses can often be drained percutaneously by an interventional radiologist using computerized tomography or ultrasonography as a guide.[26,27] Elective surgery can then be performed after 2–3 weeks of antibiotic therapy.

Emergent surgery is required for generalized peritonitis or persistent high-grade bowel obstruction. Most patients with complicated diverticular disease require surgery, even if clinical recovery occurs, since there is a high risk of recurrent attacks.

Bleeding

Bleeding associated with diverticula is typically brisk and painless and usually arises in the right colon. Bleeding is thought

Table 83-1 Medical treatment of diverticular disease

Measure	Painful diverticulosis	Diverticulitis
Diet	Increase fiber	Reduce fiber (or NPO)
Bulk laxatives	Sometimes effective	Not indicated
Analgesics	Avoid narcotics	Avoid morphine; meperidine is best
Antispasmodics	Propantheline bromide (15 mg tid); dicyclomine hydrochloride (20 mg tid); hyoscyamine sulfate (0.125–0.250 mg q4h)	Not indicated
Antibiotics	Not indicated	Oral: amoxicillin/clavulanate K⁺ (750 mg tid) Parenteral (1) gentamycin or tobramycin (5 mg/kg/d) plus clindamycin (1.2–2.4 g/d) or (2) (2) cefoxitin (4–6 g/d) (3) ampicillin/sulbactam sodium (6–12 g/d)

Modified from Wald.[17] with permission

to occur when a fecalith erodes into a vessel in the neck of the diverticulum or there is rupture of the penetrating arteriole in its course around the diverticular sac.[17]

An important indication for emergent colonoscopy is to identify the source of bleeding in patients with diverticula, as other lesions not seen by contrast studies may be the actual source.[22] If bleeding is brisk, a bleeding scan or selective mesenteric angiography can locate the site of bleeding, and the latter can be used to infuse vasoactive substances to control bleeding (see Lower Gastrointestinal Bleeding).

APPENDICITIS

Elderly patients with appendicitis are at increased risk (about 60 percent) for perforation. They have a higher mortality and often do not exhibit a fever or elevated white blood cell count.[28]

The onset of abdominal pain is abrupt, begins in the mid-abdomen, relocates to the right lower quadrant, and is often associated with nausea, vomiting, and fever. Physical examination characteristically reveals signs of local peritonitis in the right lower quadrant, and the white blood cell count is frequently elevated. The differential diagnosis includes pyelonephritis, Crohn's disease, gastroenteritis, pelvic inflammatory disease, ovarian cyst, and cecal diverticulitis. In elderly patients, appendicitis may occur in association with colon cancer in which low-grade obstruction results in distention of the appendix and mimics true appendicitis.

If the diagnosis is uncertain, ultrasonography has been shown to have positive and negative predictive values of about 90 percent for appendicitis and is also useful in identifying another cause of symptoms in patients with right lower quadrant pain.[29] One sonographic criterion for acute appendicitis is visualization of a noncompressible appendix with a diameter of greater than 6 mm.

INFECTIOUS DISEASES
Clostridium difficile

The vast majority of cases are associated with two protein exotoxins (A and B) produced by *Clostridium difficile*. Toxin A is an enterotoxin which triggers diarrhea, epithelial necrosis, and a characteristic inflammatory process in animals, whereas toxin B is a cytoxin in tissue culture but does not by itself cause toxicity in animals.[30] The disease spectrum ranges from mild diarrhea, with little or no inflammation, to severe colitis, often associated with pseudomembranes which are adherent to necrotic colonic epithelium. Acquisition of *C. difficile* occurs most frequently in elderly persons in hospitals or nursing homes, potentially because of environmental contamination with *C. difficile* and spores carried on the hands of hospital or institutional personnel.[31] Acquisition is often asymptomatic but may have clinical consequences if elderly patients receive certain antibiotics or chemotherapeutic agents. Other possible risk factors include surgery, intensive care, nasogastric intubation, and length of hospital stay. A smaller number of patients have antibiotic-associated diarrhea but no evidence of *C. difficile* infection.

Although virtually all antibiotics have been implicated, the most common are cephalosporins, ampicillin or amoxicillin, and clindamycin.[32] Less commonly mentioned antibiotics include other penicillins, erythromycin, and fluoroquinolones.

The typical clinical picture of *C. difficile*-associated colitis includes nonbloody diarrhea, lower abdominal cramps, fever, and leukocytosis. Fever is usually low grade although, on occasion, it can be quite high. In severe cases, dehydration, hypotension, hypoproteinemia, toxic megacolon, or even colonic perforation may occur.

In severely ill patients, the diagnostic test of choice is flexible sigmoidoscopy or colonoscopy. As the distal colon is involved in the majority of cases, flexible sigmoidoscopy is usually satisfactory; however, changes may be confined to the right colon in up to one-third of cases, making colonoscopy necessary if less extensive procedures do not confirm a suspected diagnosis. The yellowish-gray pseudomembranes are densely adherent to the underlying colonic mucosa, interspersed with mucosa that appears normal. Mucosal biopsies may exhibit characteristic findings of epithelial necrosis and micropseudomembranes ("volcano lesions") even when pseudomembranes are not grossly visible. Endoscopy should be performed in severely ill patients who present atypically and therefore require a rapid diagnosis.[33]

Several tests identify *C. difficile* or its toxin. The enzyme immunoassay (EIA) for toxin A and/or B is the preferred test to detect toxin. On average, EIA tests range in sensitivity from 70 to 95 percent in confirmed cases of *C. difficile* diarrhea. Thus, it should be emphasized that a negative EIA test does not exclude a diagnosis of *C. difficile* colitis.

The offending drug should be discontinued if possible. If symptoms persist or are severe, patients should receive oral metronidazole 250 mg qid for 7–10 days or oral vancomycin 125 mg PO qid for 7–10 days. If oral intake is not possible, metronidazole 500 mg IV q6h is given until oral administration can be accomplished. Metronidazole and vancomycin appear to be therapeutically comparable, but metronidazole costs less and there are current concerns about vancomycin resistant enterococcus.[34] In general, fever resolves within 24 hours and diarrhea decreases within 4–5 days.

Relapses average about 20–25 percent following successful treatment with either agent,[35] often involving sporulation which leads to relapse within 4 weeks after completion of successful treatment. These episodes invariably respond to another course of antibiotic therapy. About 5–10 percent of patients have multiple relapses. In such individuals, metronidazole or vancomycin in conventional doses should be followed by a 3-week course of cholestyramine 4 g tid and/or Lactinex 500 mg PO qid, or vancomycin 125 mg PO every other day. Others advocate a 6-week schedule consisting of a 2-week course of vancomycin or metronidazole given daily in the standard dose, a 2-week course in the same dose given every other day, followed by a 2-week course at the same dose given every third day. Currently, trials are being conducted to explore the efficacy of a nonpathogenic yeast, *Saccharomyces boulardii*, and preliminary results appear to be promising.[36] It has been shown that this yeast inhibits the binding of toxin A to rat ileum, with consequent prevention of enterotoxicity.

Table 83-2 Practice guidelines for prevention of _Clostridium difficile_ diarrhea

1. Limit the use of antimicrobial drugs.
2. Wash hands between contact with all patients.
3. Use enteric (stool) isolation precautions for patients with _C. difficile_ diarrhea.
4. Wear gloves when contacting patients with _C. difficile_ diarrhea/colitis or their environment.
5. Disinfect objects contaminated with _C. difficile_ with sodium hypochlorite, alkaline glutaraldehyde or ethylene oxide.
6. Educate the medical, nursing and other appropriate staff members about the disease and its epidemiology.

From Fekety,[33] with permission.

Guidelines for prevention of _C. difficile_ diarrhea and colitis are based upon a few simple practices and attitudes and are shown in Table 83-2.[33]

Shigella

These organisms consist of four groups: A (_Shigella dysenteriae_), B (_S. flexneri_), C (_S. boydii_), and D (_S. sonnei_), the last of which accounts for most clinical infections in Western countries. In contrast to other enteric pathogens, very few organisms are needed to produce infection, which is spread by fecal–oral transmission between humans and which continues to occur despite high standards of water purification and sewage disposal. The precise virulence factor(s) of this organism is (are) unknown. Disease is caused by invasion of colonic epithelial cells, perhaps in part mediated by cytotoxins produced by _S. dysenteriae_ and _S. flexneri_, but enterotoxins may also contribute to early symptoms of nondysenteric diarrhea.[37] Enterotoxins have also been hypothesized to mediate the hemolytic–uremic syndrome associated with severe colitis caused by _S. dysenteriae_ type I.

Symptoms

Colitis is heralded by the passage of bloody mucoid stools associated with urgency, tenesmus, abdominal cramping, fever, and malaise. The frequency of stools is highest during the first 24 hours of illness and gradually diminishes thereafter.

Diagnosis

Stool examination reveals numerous polymorphonuclear cells, and leukocytosis is common. Stool culture grown on selective media is the definitive diagnostic study. Sigmoidoscopy is usually not necessary, but if done, will demonstrate a friable hyperemic mucosa. Barium contrast studies are not indicated.

Treatment

If the illness is mild and self-limited, antibiotics can be withheld. As resistance to sulfonamides, ampicillin, tetracycline, and even trimethoprim-sulfamethoxazole is now common, treatment with a fluoroquinolone (e.g. ciprofloxacin 500 mg twice daily for 5 days) is indicated in elderly or debilitated patients with acute disease to shorten the illness and the period of fecal excretion of the organism.[38] Antidiarrheal agents prolong the clinical illness and carrying of the organism and should not be administered.[39] The development of a chronic carrier state is rare and difficult to treat.

Toxigenic _Escherichia coli_

This organism commonly causes disease in developed countries and is a major cause of diarrhea in tourists visiting underdeveloped countries. As older individuals increasingly engage in overseas travel, this organism can become a major impediment to a successful trip.

Low-grade fever, anorexia, and watery diarrhea are characteristic and are caused by plasmid-controlled enterotoxins which are both heat-stable and heat-labile. Strictly speaking, this organism does not affect the colon directly. The presence of dysentery or other manifestations of colitis should suggest another cause of diarrhea. Preventive measures include eating cooked food only while it is still hot and avoiding local water, including fruits and vegetables washed with local water. In elderly tourists, the disease can be shortened by prompt use of trimethoprim-sulfamethoxazole or a fluoroquinolone.[40]

Escherichia coli 0157:H7

This organism has been identified as a major pathogen in the United States and Canada.[41] In addition to sporadic infections, epidemics have been traced to consumption of undercooked and raw ground beef, and infections have also been associated with exposure to patients with bloody diarrhea, contaminated water supplies, and nonpreserved apple cider. Clinical manifestations include nonbloody diarrhea, hemorrhagic colitis, and hemolytic–uremic syndrome (HUS).[42] Unlike most bacterial enteric diseases, _E. coli_ 0157:H7 is often characterized by low-grade fever or the absence of a fever.[43] The pathogenesis of colitis has been linked to Shiga-like toxins (verocytotoxins 1 and 2) which bind to a glycolipid on the surface of colonocytes, but adherence factors may also play a role. Older age is both a risk factor for this infection and increases the risk of HUS and death. It is generally believed that antibiotics are not indicated for active infections and appear to predispose to hemolytic–uremic syndrome.[42]

Campylobacter species

Campylobacter jejuni and _C. coli_ are among the most common bacterial causes of diarrhea and can be manifested by gastroenteritis, pseudoappendicitis, or colitis. These organisms are usually transmitted from animals to humans through contaminated food and water and sometimes by direct contact with pets. Constitutional symptoms usually precede diarrhea and abdominal cramps by up to 24 hours, and colitis may be characterized by fever and dysentery lasting for a week or more. Diagnosis is made by stool culture. Convalescent carriage up to a mean of 5 weeks is common after the onset of illness and is significantly reduced by antimicrobial treatment.

Although the infection is usually self-limited, antibiotics may be given if the illness is severe or in patients who are immunosuppressed.[44] Treatment consists of erythromycin or fluoroquinolones; newer macrolides such as azithromycin and clarithromycin show excellent in vitro activity. Resistance to fluoroquinolones has been reported in Europe.

Entamoeba histolyticia

This organism remains a primary cause of dysentery which may be complicated by fulminant colitis, toxic megacolon, bleeding, stricture, and perforation. Severe disease is more common in elderly people and in patients who are immunosuppressed or debilitated.[45] The disease is typically acquired by ingesting cysts from contaminated water or fresh vegetables but can also be transmitted venereally through sexual practices that promote fecal–oral transmission. Studies on germ-free animals suggest that intestinal disease does not develop unless bacteria are present. This may partly account for the effectiveness of metronidazole, which is also active against anaerobic bacteria.

Three separate stool specimens should be examined if the diagnosis is suspected. A wet preparation should be performed within 30 minutes of passage to look for motile trophozoites which may contain ingested red blood cells. A Formalin–ethyl acetate concentration preparation should be examined for cysts. Barium, bismuth, kaolin compounds, magnesium hydroxide, castor oil, and hypertonic enemas all interfere with the ability to detect the parasite in stools.[45]

Colonoscopy may reveal erythema, edema, friability of the mucosa, and scattered ulcers 5–15 mm in diameter, covered with a yellow exudate. These ulcers may occur anywhere in the colon but are most common in the cecum and ascending colon. Biopsies from the edge of these ulcers may reveal typical "hourglass" ulcers containing trophozoites. Cathartics and enemas should not be used because they interfere with identification of the parasite.

As these techniques may miss identifying the parasite, serological tests for antiamebic antibody should also be obtained in suspected cases. The indirect hemagglutination assay (IHA) is positive in almost 90 percent of patients with amebic dysentery and in virtually all patients with amebic liver abscesses. The IHA remains positive for years after treatment of invasive amebiasis.[46]

Treatment of acute amebic dysentery consists of metronidazole 750 mg three times daily for 10 days or, if not tolerated orally, by the intravenous route. This should be followed by luminal acting oral drugs such as paromomysin 500 mg three times daily for 7 days or iodoquinol 650 mg three times daily for 20 days to eliminate all cysts and prevent possible relapse.[47]

Cytomegalovirus

Cytomegalovirus (CMV) is a member of the herpes virus family which enters a lifelong latent phase after primary infection in immunocompetent persons. In patients who are immunocompromised with diminished T-cell function, reactivation may occur and may become persistent, with reappearance of IgM anti-CMV antibodies in the serum. Among the gastrointestinal syndromes associated with CMV are focal and diffuse colitis.

CMV colitis is associated with severe small-volume diarrhea, abdominal pain, and fever. Colonoscopy may reveal variable degrees of focal erythema, petechial hemorrhage, erosions, and in advanced cases, scattered ulcers. Mucosal biopsy may reveal characteristic intranuclear inclusions ("owl-eye" lesions) or cytoplasmic inclusions in vascular endothelial cells. In cases in which biopsy is not diagnostic, immuno-histological or in-situ hybridization techniques may be helpful, together with serum IgM anti-CMV antibodies.

The treatment of choice is ganciclovir (5 mg/kg IV q12h for 21 days) to achieve remission.[48] For patients who relapse after discontinuation of the drug, chronic maintenance therapy (6 mg/kg five times per week) may be instituted. As the drug has hematological side-effects such as neutropenia, regular blood counts should be obtained. Human immunodeficiency virus (HIV)-infected patients with CMV colitis should be placed on maintenance therapy indefinitely. Foscarnet is used in patients who do not respond to ganciclovir or who cannot tolerate its toxicity.

INFLAMMATORY BOWEL DISEASE

Both ulcerative colitis and Crohn's disease are more common in early adulthood but are found with increased frequency in the elderly population. In part, this is because increasing numbers of patients with inflammatory bowel disease (IBD) now live into old age. In addition, both ulcerative colitis and Crohn's disease exhibit a bimodal age of onset,[49,50] the peak incidence occurring in the third decade and the second between the ages of 50 and 80 years; over 10 percent of cases have their onset after the age of 60. This pattern persists even when other diseases that mimic inflammatory bowel disease, such as ischemic colitis and infectious causes, have been excluded. The reasons for this bimodal pattern are unknown.

Ulcerative colitis

Ulcerative colitis is a chronic inflammatory process of unknown etiology which affects the mucosa and submucosa of the colon in a continuous distribution.

Histopathology

Histologically, there are diffuse ulcerations and epithelial necrosis, depletion of mucin from goblet cells, and a polymorphonuclear and lymphocytic infiltration involving the superficial layers of the colon to the muscularis mucosa.[51] The finding of crypt microabscesses is characteristic but not pathognomonic. The inflammatory process invariably involves the rectum and extends proximally for variable distances but does not involve the gastrointestinal tract proximal to the colon.

Symptoms and signs

Symptoms in elderly patients are similar to those seen in younger persons.[52] The severity of ulcerative colitis may be classified as mild, moderate, and severe and is generally proportional to the extent of colonic inflammation (Table 83-3). Most patients exhibit diarrhea, with or without blood in the stools, although older patients with proctitis only occasionally present with constipation or hematochezia. Systemic manifestations occur during more severe attacks and carry a poorer prognosis. Indeed, despite the occurrence of less extensive disease in older patients, elderly persons more often present with a severe initial attack and have higher mortality and morbidity than do younger patients.[53]

Toxic megacolon is a feared complication of ulcerative colitis which occurs more frequently in elderly patients. Abdominal radiographs show colonic dilatation, often to impressive proportions, and patients may exhibit mental confusion, high fever, abdominal distension, and overall deterioration.[54]

Extraintestinal manifestations may occur in ulcerative colitis, including arthralgias, erythema nodosum, pyoderma gangrenosum, uveitis, and migratory polyarthritis. These disorders occur less frequently than in Crohn's disease and are generally associated with increased disease activity.

Diagnosis

The diagnosis is made by sigmoidoscopy and rectal mucosal biopsies since the disorder invariably involves the rectum. The extent of the disease is determined by colonoscopy or barium radiography, both of which should be avoided in patients who are severely ill because of the danger of inducing perforation or toxic megacolon. The characteristic findings are diffuse erythema, granularity, and friability of the mucosa without intervening areas of normal mucosa. Inflammatory pseudopolyps indicate more severe erosion of the mucosa and must be distinguished from true polyps.

Particularly in elderly people, it is important to exclude other diseases that may mimic ulcerative colitis, including Crohn's colitis (see below), ischemic colitis, radiation proctocolitis, and diverticulitis. In acute presentations, infectious agents should be excluded with appropriate stool cultures, including *Salmonella, Campylobacter, Shigella*, amebiasis, *Yersinia*, and *E. coli* 0157:H7. Finally, *C. difficile*-associated diarrhea and pseudomembranous colitis should be considered in elderly persons, particularly those who have recently been treated with antibiotics, reside in institutions, or have recently been hospitalized.

Treatment

The treatment of ulcerative colitis is based on the extent and the severity of the disease (Table 83-4). Medical therapy consists of a number of effective drugs which are administered

---

Table 83-3 Proposed criteria for assessment of disease activity in ulcerative colitis

Factor	Severe[a]	Mild
Bowel frequency	≥6 daily	≤4 daily
Blood in stool	++	±
Temperature	>37.5°C on 2 of 4 days	Normal
Pulse rate (beats/min)	>90	Normal
Hemoglobin (allow for transfusion)	≤75%	Normal or near normal
Erythrocyte sedimentation rate (mm in 1 h)	>30	≤30

[a]Moderate disease is intermediate between severe and mild classifications.
(Data from Truelove and Witts, British Medical Journal 1955;2:4941–4948, with permission.)

Table 83-4 Medical treatment of ulcerative colitis

Indication	Drug	Dosage
Mild to moderate distal disease	Hydrocortisone enemas	hs
	5-ASA enemas	hs
	Sulfasalazine	2–4 g/d PO
Mild to moderate disease extensive disease	Sulfasalazine	2–4 g/d PO
	Mesalamine[a]	2.4–4.8 g/d PO
	Balsalazide[a]	6.75 g/d PO
	Prednisone	40–60 mg/d PO
Severe disease (recently receiving steroids)	Prednisolone	60–80 mg/d IV
	Hydrocortisone	300 mg/d IV
Severe disease (not recently receiving steroids)	Corticotropin (ACTH)	120 units/d IV
Maintenance of remission		
Distal disease	5-ASA (mesalamine) enemas	o.n. or q 3rd night
Pancolonic	Sulfasalazine	2 g/d PO
	Mesalamine[a]	1.2–2.4/d PO
	Balsalazide[a]	3 gm/d PO
	Azathioprine	2–2.5 mg/kgBW/d PO
	6-Mercaptopurine	1–2 mg/kgBW/d PO

Abbreviations: ASA, aminosalicylate; ACTH, adrenocorticotrophic hormone.
[a]If patient is intolerant of sulfasalazine.

intravenously, orally, or rectally. The major classes of drugs are corticosteroids, 5-aminosalicylate (5-ASA) products, and immunomodulators.[55] In elderly people, some drugs must be used more carefully than in younger patients. For example, corticosteroids have a higher risk of complications, whereas sulfasalazine, 5-ASA products, and immunomodulators are generally tolerated well.[53]

SEVERE DISEASE Patients with severe or fulminant disease, including toxic megacolon, should be hospitalized for intravenous therapy. This treatment consists of hydrocortisone or adrenocorticotrophic hormone (ACTH) infused in fluids containing sufficient amounts of potassium to avoid hypokalemia. One study suggests that ACTH is superior for treating patients who have not previously received corticosteroids, whereas hydrocortisone tends to be more effective in those who have.[56] If ACTH or hydrocortisone does not produce significant improvement within 2–3 days, IV cyclosporin may be attempted with close monitoring of renal function, an especially important consideration in an elderly patient. Once improvement is noted, the patient should be converted to oral therapy (see below). However, in most cases, surgery is preferred unless the patient is an extremely poor operative risk.

MODERATELY SEVERE DISEASE Oral corticosteroids are used to achieve remission or to sustain remission after intravenous therapy. Initial therapy should be 40–60 mg/d in divided doses, followed by conversion to a single morning dose. Corticosteroids should be viewed as acute phase drugs and should not be used as long-term maintenance therapy because of significant side-effects related to both the dose and duration of therapy. Diabetes, congestive heart failure, osteoporosis, cataracts, and hypertension are common in elderly people and may be exacerbated by corticosteroids.[53] Corticosteroid reduction should be accomplished in stepwise fashion while monitoring clinical activity and appropriate laboratory studies.

5-ASAs may be started together with oral corticosteroids. Sulfasalazine is quite effective and inexpensive but is somewhat limited by side-effects which are often dose-dependent and occur in as many as 30 percent of patients. Side-effects include nausea, anorexia, headache, and, less commonly, a generalized rash; in most cases, these conditions are due to the inactive sulfapyridine carrier rather than the 5-ASA moiety. If side-effects occur, patients should be switched to the more expensive 5-ASA products such as mesalamine. Diarrhea is a potential side-effect of all 5-ASA drugs.

If patients fail to respond to 5-ASA drugs and cannot be weaned from oral corticosteroids, a trial of azathioprine or 6-mercaptopurine should be considered an alternative to surgery.[57] These drugs act slowly and have a response time ranging from 3 to 6 months. Complete blood counts should be monitored frequently when these agents are used.

MILD DISEASE Patients with mild disease can be treated effectively with 5-ASA drugs which can be administered orally, by enema in cases of left-sided disease, or by suppositories in patients with proctitis. Corticosteroid enemas are also effective in left-sided disease but in general are not more effective than 5-ASA products. As up to 60 percent of the rectal corticosteroid may be absorbed, they also are less suitable

for maintenance therapy. Budesonide is a nonsystemic steroid with a significant first-pass hepatic metabolism which does not affect the adrenal–pituitary–hypothalamic axis. It is available outside the USA in both enema and oral controlled ileal release formulations.[55]

MAINTENANCE THERAPY For patients in remission, long-term maintenance with a 5-ASA product reduces the frequency of relapses.[58] The usual maintenance dose of sulfasalazine is 1 g bid with little or no long-term adverse effects. For patients who are intolerant to sulfasalazine, mesalamine 1.2 mg/day is also effective. For those with ulcerative proctitis or left-sided colitis, 5-ASA suppositories and enemas, respectively, are very effective when given every night to every third night. Nonsteroidal anti-inflammatory drugs have been reported to activate quiescent inflammatory bowel disease and should be avoided if possible.[59]

Surgery

Indications for surgery include failure of medical therapy for acute fulminant disease, inability to wean patients from long-term corticosteroid therapy, development of precancerous colonic lesions identified during surveillance studies, and suboptimal response to medical therapy in chronic ulcerative colitis.

The surgical procedure most commonly performed for acute fulminant colitis in all age groups is subtotal colectomy and ileostomy. In the elderly patient, proctocolectomy and ileostomy also remains the most popular choice for chronic failure of medical treatment or because of the development of premalignant changes. Although procedures that avoid ileostomy, such as the ileoanal reservoir, are a viable choice for many younger patients, the increased morbidity of the treatment minimizes its use in elderly patients who also are at greater risk for fecal incontinence because of age-associated changes in anal sphincter function.

Risk of colon cancer

The risk of developing colorectal cancer in elderly patients with ulcerative colitis is approximately nine times that of the general population of that age group.[60] The risk in all age groups increases substantially about 8 years after the onset of the disease and is greatest in those with universal colitis. Carcinoma almost always develops many years after quiescent disease has been present and occurs at an earlier age than in the general population. For this reason, yearly colonoscopy has been recommended to detect mucosal dysplasia, which is considered a premalignant lesion in ulcerative colitis. Biopsies are obtained randomly throughout the colon and in areas that appear suspicious. Despite some shortcomings in the interpretation of biopsies and in the outcome of surveillance programs, all patients with longstanding ulcerative colitis should receive periodic colonoscopy and biopsy to look for evidence of mucosal dysplasia. The presence of low-grade dysplasia in the absence of active inflammation is an indication for proctocolectomy.[60]

Crohn's disease

Crohn's disease is a chronic inflammatory process of unknown etiology which most often affects the terminal ileum and/or colon and is characterized by transmural inflammation of the bowel wall, often with linear ulcerations and granulomas.

Histopathology

Histologically there is transmural inflammation affecting all layers of the bowel and often associated with submucosal fibrosis. Other features that serve to distinguish this disease from ulcerative colitis are linear ulcerations, fissures, fistulas, discrete mucosal ulcers, granulomas, skip areas, and frequent rectal sparing.[51] The disease can involve all areas of the gastrointestinal tract, from the mouth to the anus, but most frequently involves the ileum and colon. According to most published series, Crohn's disease confined to the colon (Crohn's colitis) occurs more frequently in elderly than in younger persons, and left-sided colitis appears to be prevalent in elderly women.[53]

Symptoms and signs

As with ulcerative colitis, the clinical picture in elderly patients is similar to that in younger individuals and includes rectal bleeding, diarrhea, fever, abdominal pain, and weight loss. In patients with colorectal involvement, perianal disease, including fistulas, may be an early manifestation. The prevalence of extraintestinal manifestations such as migratory arthritis, pyoderma gangrenosum, iritis, and erythema nodosum is similar to that in younger patients. Common laboratory abnormalities such as anemia, leukocytosis, hypoalbuminemia, and elevated sedimentation rate vary with the severity of the illness. Rarely, the disease may be manifested by peritonitis due to bowel perforation, but this occurs more commonly with ileal disease. In elderly patients, peritonitis may occur atypically with mild abdominal pain, often minimal abdominal findings, and mental confusion. Uncommonly, Crohn's colitis is characterized by massive lower gastrointestinal bleeding or bowel obstruction.

Diagnosis

Prolonged delays in diagnosis probably occur more frequently in elderly patients. It has been speculated that there is a tendency for Crohn's colitis to appear in a more indolent fashion than does ileal or ileocolonic involvement.[53]

As the disease may often not involve the rectum and the distribution in the colon is often not confluent, colonoscopy and barium radiography are the diagnostic tests of choice. Both procedures can identify the characteristic ulcerations, skip lesions, and areas of colonic narrowing. Barium studies are superior for identifying fistulas from the intestine to adjacent visceral organs, whereas colonoscopy provides superior examination of the mucosa and allows mucosal biopsies to be obtained. Biopsies should also be obtained from grossly normal-appearing mucosa to help distinguish Crohn's colitis from other diseases that may mimic it. This is particularly important because of the increased frequency with which diverticula occur in elderly people and because of the tendency for ischemic colitis to occur in a discontinuous distribution.

Computed tomography provides superior definition of the wall of the colon and can identify extraintestinal abdominal pathology, such as abscesses in patients with fever or palpable masses. Computed tomography and ultrasonography can also identify renal lithiasis or ureteral obstruction, which often occur silently.

Perianal involvement is a well-recognized manifestation of Crohn's disease and may be characterized by rectal or anal strictures, fissures, fistulas, abscesses, prominent skin tags, and ulcers. Venereal disease (uncommon in elderly people) and carcinoma should be excluded, particularly as the latter may complicate long-standing Crohn's proctitis. Infectious agents should be excluded by appropriate studies.

Treatment

As with ulcerative colitis, treatment of Crohn's disease is based on its extent and severity as well as its distribution. Medical therapy encompasses all the drugs used in treating ulcerative colitis;[55] in addition, selected antibiotics are helpful in some patients (Table 83-5).

Table 83-5 Medical treatment of Crohn's colitis

Indications	Drug	Dosage
Ileocolitis or colitis	Sulfasalazine	2–4 g/d PO
	Mesalamine[a]	2.4–4.8 g/d PO
	Metronidazole	10–20 mg/kg/d PO
	Prednisone	40–60 mg/d PO
Perineal disease	6-Mercaptopurine or	50 mg/d up to 1.5 mg/kg/d
	Azathioprine or	50 mg/d up to 2.5 mg/kg/d PO
	Metronidazole or	1–2 g/d PO
	Ciprofloxacin	500 mg bid PO
	Inflixmab	5 mg/kg/IV
Refractory disease	6-Mercaptopurine or	50 mg/d to 1.5 mg/kg/d PO
	Azathioprine or	50 mg/d up to 2.5 mg/kg/d PO
	Infliximab or	5 mg/kg/IV
	Methotrexate	25 mg IV/week
Maintenance of remission	Sulfasalazine or	2 g/d PO
	Mesalamine[a]	800–1,200 mg/d PO
	6-Mercaptopurine or azathioprine	50 mg/d up to 1.5 or 2.5 mg/kg/d, respectively
	Methotrexate	15 mg IV/week

[a]If patient is intolerant of sulfasalazine.

ILEOCOLITIS AND COLITIS Patients with mild to moderate disease often respond to sulfasalazine, or if they are intolerant to the drug, to one of the newer 5-ASA products in doses similar to those used for ulcerative colitis. If the disease remains mild or only moderate in severity but responds inadequately to 5-ASA drugs, metronidazole 125–250 mg three times daily or ciprofloxacin 500 mg once or twice daily can be tried before using immunomodulator agents.[61]

If the disease worsens despite conservative therapy or if the patient has moderate to severe symptoms, corticosteroids are begun in doses similar to those used in ulcerative colitis. After remission is induced, prednisone is tapered at rate of 5 to 10 mg/wk until a dose of 20 mg/d is achieved. Subsequently, prednisone should be reduced by 5 mg/d every 3 weeks while monitoring clinical activity and laboratory studies.

Approximately 60 percent of patients who cannot be weaned from oral corticosteroids respond to azathioprine (up to 2.5 mg/kg per day) or 6-mercaptopurine (up to 1.5 mg/kg per day). Response may not occur for 6–9 months.[62] These drugs can be continued indefinitely, but at least one attempt should be made to discontinue them after 1 year of therapy to see if quiescence can be maintained. Methotrexate 25 mg IM weekly appears to be effective in many patients who are resistant or intolerant to azathioprine or 6-mecaptopurine and has been used successfully to maintain remission.[63]

PERIANAL DISEASE Perianal fistulas and abscesses can be terribly debilitating and frustrating to treat. Although perianal disease often improves with standard therapy for bowel inflammation and control of diarrhea, some patients continue to have persistent symptoms. Short-term success has been reported with metronidazole in doses of 1.5 to 2 g/d, but side-effects at these doses are not uncommon and relapses occur when the drug is discontinued or tapered.[64] Ciprofloxacin 500 mg twice daily is a more expensive alternative, albeit one with fewer side-effects, but again there is a high relapse rate when the drug is discontinued. If an abscess develops, incision and drainage should be performed.

If perianal disease remains unresponsive to therapy, surgical diversion of the colon may be performed in an attempt to allow healing, but this too may be unsuccessful. Azathroprine or 6-mercaptopurine may be helpful in some patients with refractory disease.[65] Infliximab, a monoclonal antibody directed at human tumor necrosis factor-α has been reported to be effective in severe Crohn's disease and those with resistant fistula.[55]

SURGERY Unlike ulcerative colitis, Crohn's disease cannot be cured by surgery. Therefore, surgical procedures should be reserved for patients who do not respond to medical therapy.

Protocolectomy with ileostomy is the best surgical option for patients with extensive Crohn's colitis. In elderly patients who are debilitated or malnourished, an initial subtotal colectomy with ileostomy is less debilitating and permits weight gain and improved physical well-being. If proctectomy is subsequently required, it can be done with a low complication rate but may not be necessary if rectal disease is mild or absent. More limited colonic resections may be appropriate if severe disease is localized or obstructive symptoms are caused by relatively circumscribed bowel involvement.

Lymphocytic and collagenous colitis

Lymphocytic and collagenous colitis are uncommon disorders characterized by chronic watery diarrhea and histological evidence of chronic mucosal inflammation in the absence of endoscopic or radiological abnormalities of the large bowel. They comprise two histologically distinct disorders which have been grouped under the term "microscopic colitis" and which differ principally by the presence or absence of a thickened collagen band located in the colonic subepithelium.[66,67] Both lymphocytic and collagenous colitis occur most commonly between ages 50 and 70 years, with a strong female predominance and a frequent association with arthritis, celiac disease, and autoimmune disorders.

In both lymphocytic and collagenous colitis, there is a modest increase in mononuclear cells within the lamina propria and between crypt epithelial cells, primarily consisting of CD8+T lymphocytes, plasma cells, and macrophages.[68] In collagenous colitis, there is a thickened subepithelial collagen layer which may be continuous or patchy. Although inflammatory changes occur diffusely throughout the colon, the characteristic collagen band thickening is highly variable, occurring in the cecum and transverse colon in over 80 percent of cases and less than 30 percent of the time in the rectum. Although involvement of the left colon appears to be less intense, multiple biopsies of the left colon above the rectosigmoid during flexible sigmoidoscopy is sufficient to make the diagnosis in about 90 percent of cases.

Patients with collagenous and lymphocytic colitis usually present with chronic watery diarrhea, with an average of eight stools each day, often with nocturnal stools, ranging from 300 to 1,700 g/24 hours, occasional fecal incontinence, abdominal cramps, and decreased symptoms when fasting.[69] Nausea, weight loss, and fecal urgency have also been reported but are variable. Diarrhea is generally longstanding, ranging from months to years, with a fluctuating course of remissions and exacerbations. In one series of 172 patients, the median time from onset of symptoms to diagnosis was 11 months, whereas in another of 31 patients, it was 5.4 years. Physical examinations are usually unremarkable and blood in the stool is absent. Routine laboratory studies are also normal.

Examination of fresh stools showed fecal leukocytes in 55 percent of 116 patients with collagenous colitis. Mild steatorrhea, mild anemia, low serum vitamin B_{12} levels, hypoalbuminemia, and mild steatorrhea have been reported in variable numbers of patients but are not characteristic. Autoimmune markers which have been identified in patients with collagenous colitis include antinuclear antibodies (up to 50 percent), pANCA in 14 percent, rheumatoid factor, and increased C_3 and C_4 complement components.

Colonoscopic examinations are usually normal. Infectious agents should be excluded by testing for stool ova and parasites, standard stool cultures, and *Clostridium difficile* toxin assays. Many patients have been diagnosed to have irritable bowel syndrome, a disorder which can be excluded by the abnormal colonic biopsies and the finding of increased stool volume, both of which are not characteristic of irritable bowel syndrome.

There have been very few controlled trials for either collagenous or lymphocytic colitis and therapy is largely empiric.[70] Most reports of treatments suggest that no single agent works for all cases. About one-third of patients respond to antidiarrheal agents such as loperamide or diphenoxylate with atropine as well as bulk agents such as psyllium or methylcellulose; however, they do not exhibit improvement in inflammation or collagen thickness. In a recent open-label trial of bismuth subsalicylate in 12 patients,[71] eight chewable tablets per day for 8 weeks resulted in resolution of diarrhea and reduction of stool weight within 2 weeks, and in nine patients, colitis resolved, including disappearance of collagen band thickening. Although the basis for its efficacy is unknown, bismuth subsalicylate possesses antidiarrheal, antibacterial, and anti-inflammatory properties.

The majority of other treatment trials for collagenous colitis and lymphocytic colitis have studied 5-ASA compounds, corticosteroids, and bile acid resins. Alone or in combination, these agents appear to improve diarrhea and inflammation in some but certainly not all treated patients.[70] Although corticosteroids given in either the oral or enema route provide symptomatic improvement and decreased inflammation in over 80 percent of cases, relapse usually occurs quickly after stopping the drug.[69] Moreover, long-term corticosteroids have undesirable effects, especially in older patients.

COLONIC ISCHEMIA

The blood supply to the colon is derived mainly from branches of the superior and inferior mesenteric arteries and is characterized by a rich collateral circulation, except for the potentially susceptible marginal artery of Drummond and the arc of Riolan located at the peripheral junction of the two mesenteric arteries.[72] Occlusion of a major artery results in immediate opening of collateral vessels to maintain an adequate blood supply to the bowel. Intestinal ischemia may occur as a result of generalized reduction of blood flow (nonocclusive ischemia), redistribution of blood flow (e.g. vessel obstruction with poor collateral circulation), or a combination of the two. Colonic ischemia is the most common vascular disorder of the intestines in the elderly population and one that is often misdiagnosed unless there is a high index of suspicion and an aggressive diagnostic approach is used in patients suspected of having this disorder.[73]

The clinical spectrum of colonic ischemia includes a vast array of presentations and may be associated with a number of potentiating factors. Ischemia may be classified as reversible and irreversible; the former may present with submucosal or intramural hemorrhage or transient ischemic colitis which completely resolves within weeks to months, depending on the severity of the process. Irreversible ischemia may be characterized by chronic ulcerations, strictures of varying lengths, colonic gangrene, or fulminant transmural colitis.[74]

In most cases, the etiology of colonic ischemia cannot be established with certainty and no vascular occlusions can be identified. A significant minority of patients are found to have a potentially obstructing process in the colon such as a benign stricture, diverticulitis, or carcinoma. Other contributing factors include hypotension, dehydration, congestive heart failure, use of digitalis, polycythemia, volvulus, and cardiac arrhythmias.

Symptoms and signs

The most common manifestation is the sudden onset of mild to moderately severe left lower abdominal cramping pain; this is often accompanied by bloody diarrhea or hematochezia which may not appear until 24 hours later. Frank hemorrhage is not characteristic of ischemia. Physical examination reveals tenderness at the site of the involved bowel; these sites encompass the distal transverse, splenic flexure, and/or descending colons in about two-thirds of patients. Peritoneal signs may last for several hours, but persistence beyond that time suggests a transmural process. Fever, leukocytosis, absence of bowel sounds, and abdominal distension also suggest the possibility of bowel infarction.

Diagnosis

If the diagnosis is suspected on clinical grounds, colonoscopy with minimal insufflation with air has replaced barium enema as the most common diagnostic procedure and should be performed within 48 hours. Barium studies may reveal "thumbprinting" in the affected areas of the colon, which represents submucosal or mucosal hemorrhages and edema during the early phase of the process. This corresponds to the hemorrhagic nodules noted on colonoscopic examination. Later radiographic findings include segmental ischemia which may or may not return to normal within weeks or months; such findings correspond to segmental necrosis, inflammation, ulcerations, or mucosal sloughing on endoscopic studies. There is no meaningful role for mesenteric angiography in patients with colon ischemia, unless there is involvement of the right colon with suspected mesenteric ischemia of the small intestine.

Treatment

Patients should be managed with bowel rest, intravenous fluids, or plasma expanders, and in severe cases, systemic antibiotics such as gentamycin and clindamycin.[75,76] Corticosteroids are of no benefit and should not be administered. In mild disease, symptoms resolve within several days, and radiological healing occurs within several weeks, although some patients may not heal for up to 6 months.

If the patient continues to have diarrhea, bleeding, or significant obstructive symptoms for more than several weeks, surgical resection is usually indicated. If colonic infarction is suspected, emergency laparotomy with resection of nonviable bowel is needed.[75]

Prognosis

Recurrent episodes of colonic ischemia occur in less than 10 percent of patients. Attempts should be made to correct or remove underlying conditions that predispose to this disorder.

COLONIC PSEUDO-OBSTRUCTION

Acute colonic pseudo-obstruction, sometimes termed Ogilvie's syndrome, is characterized by nonobstructive, nontoxic dilatation of the colon.[77] This condition may develop after surgical procedures, especially orthopedic ones, and also occurs in a setting of serious coexisting illness, including sepsis, pneumonia, acute pancreatitis, spinal cord injury, or administration of anticholinergic, narcotic, or psychotropic drugs. This disorder can compromise respiratory status and cause cecal perforation. The risk of cecal perforation is said to rise when the diameter of the cecum increases beyond 10 cm. A variant of this disorder is "megasigmoid syndrome," often described in psychotic patients but not exclusively seen within this group.

After obstruction has been excluded, treatment includes correction of electrolyte imbalances, discontinuation of offending drugs, treatment of underlying infection or inflammation, nasogastric suction, a rectal or colonic decompression tube with positioning of the patient on the right and left sides at intervals of several hours, or medical treatment with intravenous neostigmine.[78] Decompression with colonoscopy may be attempted if there is severe dilatation and no response to medical therapy.[79] Surgical decompression under local anesthesia using a stab-wound cecostomy can be performed if other measures fail. Post-decompression X-ray films should be obtained for several days to document continued resolution.

Chronic colonic pseudo-obstruction, with or without colonic dilatation (megacolon), may be associated with amyloidosis, muscular dystrophy, myxedema, dementia, multiple sclerosis, Parkinson's disease, quadriplegia, and schizophrenia, as well as idiopathic visceral neuropathy and myopathy. There may be esophageal, gastric, small intestinal, and genitourinary dysfunction. Although most patients have constipation, diarrhea occurs if there is small bowel bacterial overgrowth or overflow around a fecal impaction.

Subtotal colectomy may be necessary in some patients with refractory symptoms and if anorectal function is normal. If anorectal dysfunction is present, proctocolectomy with ileostomy is indicated. Sigmoid resection may be all that is necessary in patients with megasigmoid syndrome. Most patients can be treated conservatively.

VOLVULUS

Factors thought to contribute to colonic volvulus include increasing age, chronic constipation, fecal retention, poor peritoneal fixation during embryological rotation of the hindgut, and, in some areas of the world, diets very high in fiber.[1] The clinical setting typical of a sigmoid volvulus is an elderly institutionalized individual with a history of chronic constipation or laxative abuse.[80]

The sigmoid colon, with its copious mesentery, is most commonly involved, but cecal volvulus can occur when fixation to the posterior parietal wall is incomplete. Volvulus of the transverse colon is by far the least common. Patients have a sudden onset of severe abdominal pain, followed by rapid and marked abdominal distension. Compromise of blood flow occurs as a result of twisting of the mesentery and marked distension of the loop.

Abdominal X-rays reveal massive distension of a single loop of bowel; the obstructed loop frequently is shaped like a coffee bean, with the concavity marking the point of torsion. The concavity points to the left lower quadrant in patients with sigmoid volvulus, and to the right lower quadrant when cecal volvulus is present. Administering contrast through the rectum confirms the diagnosis by the appearance of the pointed twist of the contrast column.

Closely related to a cecal volvulus is a cecal bascule in which malfixation allows the cecum to fold anteriorly and in a cephalad direction, which can result in a flap-valve obstruction with cecal distension. Abdominal X-rays reveal distension of the cecum, but no "bird beak" is seen on a barium enema, as in volvulus. However, treatment is identical to that for conventional cecal volvulus.

Attempts to untwist a sigmoid volvulus may be made by gently inserting an endoscope as far as the twisted segment.[81] Successful detorsion must be followed by careful observation should the bowel continue to be ischemic. Nonoperative decompression is more successful with a sigmoid than with a cecal volvulus; indeed, attempts to treat a cecal volvulus by nonoperative means can be dangerous. Opinion is divided as to whether the first episode of sigmoid volvulus should be treated with resection. Fixation without resection is not considered a useful option. Certainly, patients with more than one episode of sigmoid volvulus should have resection.

In patients with cecal volvulus, early surgical intervention to untwist the volvulus followed by cecal fixation (cecopexy) is frequently all that is necessary unless bowel necrosis is present. If the latter is present, resection with ileostomy is indicated.

NEOPLASTIC LESIONS

Colonic polyps may be classified into: (1) neoplastic polyps which include adenomatous polyps and carcinomas; (2) nonneoplastic polyps which include hyperplastic, inflammatory, and hamartomatous types; and (3) submucosal tumors such as lipomas, leiomyomas, hemangiomas, fibromas, lymphoid polyps, and carcinoids.[82]

Most (80–90 percent) colonic polyps are either adenomatous or hyperplastic, and of these about 75 percent are adenomas. However, when only polyps less than 5 mm are considered, half are hyperplastic and most are found in the rectosigmoid colon. Current evidence suggests that hyperplastic polyps are not of clinical importance.[83] In contrast, it is widely accepted that most carcinomas arise from adenomas.

Adenomatous polyps

These polyps arise from mucosal glandular epithelium and can be described based on the following characteristics.

1. **Size:** Approximately 25 percent of adenomas are larger than 1 cm, and over 80 percent of large adenomas occur in the left colon and rectum.

2. **Architecture:** Over 80 percent of adenomas are tubular, 3–6 percent are villous, and the rest are tubulovillous. Those with a higher proportion of villous elements tend to be larger and carry a higher risk of malignant transformation.

3. **Dysplasia:** All adenomas are dysplastic, but high-grade dysplasia is strongly associated with malignancy.

In the United States, prevalence rates in men and women are similar. Except in familial syndromes, colonic adenomas are rare before the age of 40, increase steadily, and reach a peak after the age of 60. Population studies suggest that the environment strongly contributes to adenoma prevalence and probably to the frequency of colon cancer as well.[84]

It is logical to identify and remove all benign adenomas at an early stage to prevent progression to carcinoma. In one study, screening and polyp removal by rigid sigmoidoscopy during the previous 10 years resulted in a 70 percent reduction in the risk of fatal cancer of the rectum and distal colon compared to the outcome in nonscreened subjects.[85] In the National Polyp Study, colonoscopic polypectomy reduced the incidence of colorectal cancer by 76–90 percent during a follow-up of almost 6 years.[86] These findings form the basis for current screening recommendations.

There is epidemiological evidence that aspirin and other, nonsteroidal anti-inflammatory drugs (NSAIDs) may reduce the risk of colorectal cancer.[87] Several large studies, although not all, have found a significant reduction in death rates from colon cancer among both men and women who use NSAIDs on a regular basis. Such observations are supported by laboratory studies demonstrating that aspirin and other cycloxygenase inhibitors demonstrate chemopreventive effects in animal models of colon carcinogenesis. There currently are insufficient data supporting the use of NSAIDs as colorectal cancer chemopreventive agents outside appropriately designed trials.

Management of polyps

Criteria for the adequacy of colonoscopic polypectomy are well established for pedunculated malignant polyps.[88,89] In patients having favorable criteria, the risk of residual tumor is 0.3 percent for pedunculated lesions and 1.5 percent for sessile lesions, whereas the risk is 8.5 percent for those having unfavorable criteria. Surgery is therefore strongly considered in the latter situation, although recommendations should be individualized based on patient age and comorbid conditions.

The following recommendations for treatment after polypectomy are based on recent information.[90]

1. Patients should undergo complete colonoscopy at the time of polypectomy and removal of all synchronous polyps.
2. In 3 years the first follow-up colonoscopy should be performed to check for missed synchronous and or metachronous adenomas. It has been suggested that if the results are negative, subsequent surveillance intervals may be increased to 5 years.
3. Selected patients with multiple adenomas or those with large sessile polyps (> 3 cm) or those with suboptimal initial clearing examinations may require colonoscopy at 1 year or sooner and again 3 years later if the colon is clear.

Screening strategies

A clear consensus does not exist concerning recommendations for screening of asymptomatic subjects at *average risk* for colorectal cancer. Although a yearly FOBT for all patients 50 years and older has been suggested, controversy exists regarding the cost and benefits of such a policy. The sensitivity of Hemoccult II tests for detecting asymptomatic colorectal cancer ranges from 45 to 80 percent in mass-screened populations and is less than 25 percent for detecting polyps 1 cm or larger in diameter.[91,92] Thus, a FOBT is a relatively effective way to screen for asymptomatic cancers but is ineffective in detecting even sizable premalignant polyps.[93] Moreover, at least 50 percent of screened individuals over the age of 40 are false positive or have an upper gastrointestinal source of bleeding. However, the specificity of an unrehydrated FOBT is about 98–99 percent.

More recent data suggest that an annual FOBT with rehydration and colonoscopy in patients who screen positive for FOBT has a 90 percent sensitivity in detecting colorectal cancer and is associated with a decrease of 33 percent in 13 years' cumulative mortality from colorectal cancer.[94] This benefit was largely lost by increasing the screening interval to 2 years. However, rehydration resulted in a decrease of specificity to 90 percent with a positive predictive value (true positive/true positive plus false positive) of only 2.2 percent. As almost 10 percent of the screened population had a positive FOBT when rehydrated, cost-effectiveness was significantly and adversely affected.

Since January, 1998, colorectal cancer screening services have been provided by law for all Medicare patients in the USA. The American Cancer Society currently recommends an annual FOBT and flexible sigmoidoscopy every 5 years. Some studies suggest that colonoscopy should be performed only when flexible sigmoidoscopy detects high-risk adenomas, tentatively defined as adenomas larger than 1 cm and all tubulovillous or villous adenomas, as well as subjects with multiple adenomas. There is indirect evidence that colonoscopy every 10 years may be a viable option.[89]

Colorectal cancer

Colorectal cancer is the second most common cause of cancer death in the USA (140,000 new cases and 56,000 deaths in 1999). Epidemiological evidence strongly suggests that colon cancer is an acquired genetic disease produced by chronic exposure to environmental carcinogens. Thus, deaths from colon cancer increase slowly by middle age and rise steeply thereafter. Moreover, immigrants from areas of low incidence acquire, within a single generation, the increased risks of the indigenous population in areas of higher incidence.[95] Except for the increased risk for colorectal cancer among individuals with ulcerative colitis and those with a family history of colorectal cancer, no high-risk exposures have consistently been identified in the USA. However, epidemiological evidence implicates both decreased dietary fiber and increased consumption of animal protein and fat. That colorectal cancer is caused by cumulative alterations in the cellular genome, and not by a single genetic alteration, may explain the long latency period between initial exposure to carcinogen(s) and the appearance of cancer.[96]

In about 80 percent of cases, somatic mutations in the APC gene on chromosome 5 are the earliest recognized genetic alterations in sporadic colonic carcinogenesis and are found in the smallest adenomas. These mutations permit unregulated proliferation at the base of the colonic crypt. A multistep genetic model for sporadic colorectal tumorigenesis involves sequential mutations in cellular oncogenes (e.g. *K-ras* gene) and tumor suppressor genes.[96,97] Two cellular proteins associated with the APC gene have recently been identified and appear to be involved in cell adhesion, which may provide an important clue to the mechanism of tumor initiation.

In about 20 percent of cases, a colon cancer "susceptibility gene" on the short arm of chromosome 2 has been identified in patients with families with hereditary nonpolyposis colon cancer (HNPCC) and in sporadic colon cancers as well. Widespread mutations in short, repeated DNA sequences due to defective or mutant DNA mismatch repair enzymes have been identified on chromosome 2p. At least four such repair genes have now been identified in the pathogenesis of colon cancer.[98] These tumors appear to have a genetic pathogenesis different from that of the hereditary polyposis syndromes that probably result in different clinical features and less aggressive behavior.

Colonic cancers can be classified by gross appearance, histology (well to poorly differentiated, mucinous, signet-ring type) or by DNA content.[95] In general, poorly differentiated carcinomas have a somewhat worse prognosis than well-differentiated tumors. More helpful is staging, for example, by the Astler and Coller modified Dukes (Dukes–Turnbull) classifications: A, tumor extends no further than muscularis mucosa; B1, tumor penetrates muscularis propria or, B2, extends through serosa into pericolic fat; C1, four or fewer regional lymph node metastases or, C2, greater than four nodes involved; and D, distant metastases. Actuarial 5-year survival rates diminish from 85–95 percent for Dukes A lesions to less than 5 percent for Dukes D lesions. As expected, prognosis is much poorer when there is vascular or neural invasion.

The primary treatment for colorectal cancer is surgical resection. Preoperative studies include a complete evaluation of the colon, preferably by colonoscopy and a chest X-ray. Routine measurement of carcinoembryonic antigen (CEA) probably is not as cost-effective as a primary screening test. Although serial measurements of CEA have been advocated to detect early recurrences after surgery, cancer cures attributable to CEA monitoring appear to be infrequent[99] and it must be questioned whether such a practice is justified in view of the substantial cost or the emotional stress that CEA testing may cause patients. Abdominal imaging studies are most useful for detecting advanced disease (i.e., hepatic metastases) but are less useful in finding localized extracolonic spread. However, such information can be obtained directly at the time of surgery, and the presence of metastases does not influence the need for surgery or the type of surgery that is performed. In contrast, rectal endosonography appears to be superior to computed tomography and magnetic resonance imaging in staging rectal cancers.[100]

There is no benefit from adjunctive radiation therapy for colon cancer outside the rectum. However, adjuvant chemotherapy with fluorouracil and levamisole[101] or fluorouracil and leucovorin has been associated with a significant reduction in tumor recurrence and enhanced survival in patients with Dukes C colon cancer[102] as well as many patients with Dukes B colon cancer. These data support the use of postoperative adjuvant chemotherapy in both Dukes B and C colon cancers. In contrast, adjuvant combined radiotherapy and chemotherapy improve postsurgical survival in patients with rectal carcinoma, albeit with increased and often severe toxicity.[103] Some patients with unresectable rectal cancer may become surgical candidates following radiation therapy.

LOWER GASTROINTESTINAL BLEEDING

The two most frequent causes of acute lower gastrointestinal bleeding in elderly patients, defined as originating below the ligament of Trietz, are diverticulosis and vascular ectasias (angiodysplasia).[104] These two entities account for two-thirds of hemodynamically significant lower gastrointestinal bleeding (Table 83-6). The most common causes of chronic lower gastrointestinal bleeding are hemorrhoids, angiodysplasia, and colonic neoplasms. Known causes of acute lower gastrointestinal bleeding other than angiodysplasia and diverticulosis make up perhaps 25 percent of all bleeding episodes. These include neoplasm; radiation enterocolitis; ischemic, ulcerative, and Crohn's colitis; solitary rectal ulcer syndrome; and internal hemorrhoids. Less frequently reported causes of bleeding include small intestinal and Meckel's diverticula, vasculitis, and Dieulafoy lesions of the small intestine and colon.

Angiodysplasia

Angiodysplasia are small clusters of dilated and tortuous veins which appear in the mucosa of the colon as well as in the small intestine.[105] They are thought to result from age-associated degeneration of colonic submucosal veins, are often multiple, and are an important cause of lower gastrointestinal bleeding in the elderly population; two-thirds of patients with angiodysplasia are over 70 years of age. The principal theory concerning their development is that repeated episodes of low-grade partial obstruction of submucosal veins occur during muscular contraction or from increased intraluminal pressure,

---

Table 83-6 Clinical presentation of common causes of lower gastrointestinal bleeding

Symptom	Young adult	Middle age	Elderly
Abdominal pain	IBD	IBD	Ischemia, IBD
Painless	Meckel's diverticula, Polyp	Diverticulosis, polyp, cancer	Angiodysplasia, diverticulosis, polyp, cancer
Diarrhea	IBD, infection	IBD, infection	Ischemia, infection, IBD
Constipation	Hemorrhoids, fissure, rectal ulcer	Hemorrhoids, fissure	Cancer, hemorrhoids, fissure

Abbreviation: IBD, inflammatory bowel disease.

resulting in dilatation and tortuosity of the vein.[106] This process may extend to the mucosal veins which are drained by the submucosal vein. Finally, the precapillary sphincter becomes incompetent, and a small arteriovenous communication with an ectatic tuft of vessels develops. The tendency of vascular ectasias to occur in the right colon is best explained by the greater tension on the bowel wall, as expressed by Laplace's law relating tension to the diameter of the bowel lumen. A review of the literature casts doubt on a causal association between vascular ectasias and aortic stenosis.[107] Nevertheless, it has been reported that recurrent bleeding from these lesions decreases after replacement of a stenotic aortic valve.[108]

Vascular ectasias remain asymptomatic in most individuals. The usual manifestation is that of painless subacute or recurrent bleeding which stops spontaneously in most cases. Bleeding may consist of bright red blood, maroon stools or (rarely) melena, or may be occult.[104] About 10–15 percent of patients have episodes of brisk blood loss, and up to half exhibit iron deficiency anemia.

Diagnosis may be made by colonoscopy or angiography; of the two, colonoscopy is preferred, since it can exclude other causes of bleeding and can be used for therapeutic interventions.[109,110] As lesions are small, often multiple, and difficult to see, thorough cleansing of the colon is necessary to provide adequate visualization of the mucosa. Colonoscopy is usually performed after bleeding has stopped and within 48 hours to permit identification of other bleeding sources.

Mesenteric angiography is the diagnostic procedure of choice when acute bleeding is brisk. The finding of tortuous, densely opacified clusters of small veins that empty slowly represents the advanced ectatic process. Early filling of the vein, indicative of the presence of an arteriovenous communication, is found in most patients who are studied for bleeding. Extravasation of contrast into the bowel lumen is seen when there is active bleeding at a rate of at least 0.5 mL/min; as bleeding is often intermittent, a bleeding site is identified by angiography in only a minority of patients.

Bleeding can be controlled acutely by intra-arterial administration of vasopressin in doses ranging from 0.2 to 0.6 units/min. This often permits stabilization of the patient and appears to be more effective when bleeding is from the right colon. When bleeding cannot be controlled, surgery is required. Colonoscopic therapeutic modalities generally involve thermal ablation techniques, but rebleeding remains a significant problem.[111] A right hemicolectomy is performed if bleeding from the right colon has been identified by angiography or colonoscopy and if other sources of bleeding have not been identified. The extent of resection should not be influenced by the presence of left colonic diverticulosis. Recurrent bleeding, probably due to undetected ectasias, occurs in up to 20 percent of patients who may require either more extensive colonic resection or exploratory laparotomy.

Treatment should be conservative whenever possible and consists of blood or iron replacement as appropriate. For recurrent bleeding, transcolonoscopic electrocoagulation or laser coagulation may be attempted; difficulties include identifying the ectatic lesion(s) and excluding other causes of blood loss if bleeding has stopped. Perforation of the right colon with coagulation therapy is a hazard.[112]

The development of small bowel enteroscopy may eventually reduce the need for diagnostic laparotomy in patients with recurrent bleeding from obscure sites.

Vasculitis

Inflammation and necrosis of blood vessels may lead to ischemia and ulceration, resulting in pain and/or bleeding. Polyarteritis nodosa, Churg–Strauss syndrome, Henoch–Schonlein purpura, systemic lupus erythematosus, rheumatoid vasculitis, Behcet's disease, and essential mixed cryoglobulinemia have all been reported to produce gastrointestinal bleeding and are best diagnosed with endoscopic procedures in the appropriate clinical setting.

Dieulafoy lesions

Recently, these lesions have been reported to cause bleeding, in several cases massive, in the small intestine and colon.[113] They are characterized by a small mucosal defect with minimal inflammation and a congenitally large, tortuous, thick-walled arteriole at the base which ruptures into the bowel lumen. The histology of these vessels is normal, and their abnormality is their size relative to their superficial location. Bleeding can be localized with angiography, although occasionally colonoscopy can identify the lesion if bleeding has stopped and the colon is well prepared. Surgical resection or embolization therapy is the treatment of choice.

Evaluation and management of lower gastrointestinal bleeding

The first goal of management is to rapidly assess the severity of bleeding and cardiovascular status of the patient and to resuscitate those with major blood loss (Fig. 83-1). Vital signs reflecting orthostatic changes and other signs of hypovolemia should be checked immediately and at frequent intervals thereafter. If signs of shock or hypovolemia are present, one or two large-bore intravenous catheters should be placed to facilitate fluid resuscitation. Initial blood work, including hemogram, platelet count, coagulation profiles, routine blood chemistries, and type and cross-match should be obtained immediately. Only after these critical tasks are completed should a more detailed history and physical examination be performed to help determine the site of bleeding and potential etiologies. Another important step is to distinguish acute bleeding from active bleeding superimposed on chronic blood loss—this is best done with the hematocrit and mean corpuscular volume; if the latter is low, chronic bleeding should be suspected.

The third step is to consider the location of the gastrointestinal bleed based on characteristics of the bleeding and a BUN/creatinine ratio.[114] Although hematochezia, defined as the passage of red blood through the rectum, suggests a lower gastrointestinal source, up to 20 percent of patients with upper gastrointestinal bleeding may present with hematochezia because of the rapid passage of large amounts of blood through the small and large intestines.[115] Such patients always show evidence of severe hemodynamic compromise, and most have a BUN/creatinine ratio greater than 25 on initial evaluation.[114] On the other hand, melena is often characteristic of upper gastrointestinal bleeding but can also be seen in patients with bleeding from the small intestine or right colon when colonic transit is slow. Fresh unclotted blood dripping into the toilet after defecation suggests a very distal anorectal source, whereas blood streaking the stool suggests origin in the left colon.

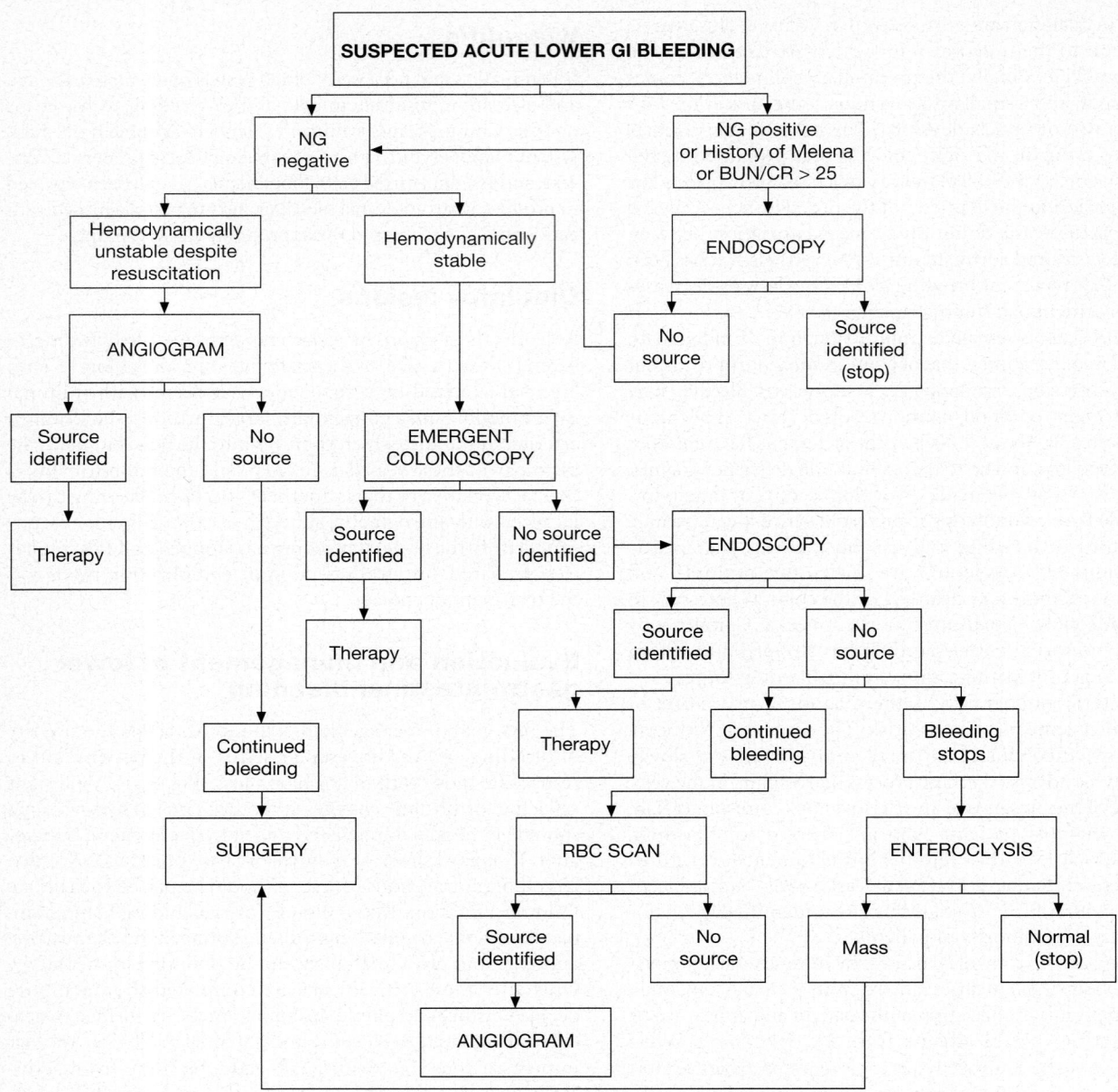

Figure 83-1 Suspected acute lower gastrointestinal bleeding.

Exclusion of an upper gastrointestinal site begins with passage of a nasogastric tube and examination of gastric contents for red blood, coffee ground material, and bile. The presence of bile and an absence of blood or coffee ground materials significantly diminishes but does not exclude bleeding proximal to the duodenojejunal junction; thus, an upper endoscopy should be performed in a setting compatible with an upper gastrointestinal source. There is no role for occult blood testing of a nasogastric aspirate in the absence of coffee grounds or bloody material. Finally, hemorrhoidal and low rectal bleeding should be excluded by sigmoidoscopy in patients thought to have lower gastrointestinal hemorrhage.

When evaluating stable patients with acute lower gastrointestinal hemorrhage, colonoscopy preceded by oral bowel preparation is preferred in identifying and potentially treating a colonic bleeding source.[22] If an emergency colonoscopy is to

be considered, the nasogastric tube should be left in place to permit rapid administration of a polyethylene glycol electrolyte solution to cleanse the colon.

If bleeding is active and bowel preparation cannot be done, scintigraphy with ^{99m}Tc-labeled red blood cells can be used to locate a bleeding site. This technique detects active bleeding at rates of approximately 0.1 mL/min, and the patient can be serially scanned for up to 36 hours if bleeding is intermittent. Site localization may be impaired if delayed films are taken too infrequently and, of course, the patient must be actively bleeding at the time of the study. Although there were initial enthusiastic reports of an approximately 90 percent rate of detection of active bleeding, subsequent studies have yielded conflicting results.[116,117] These latter reports have raised serious concerns regarding a rigid policy of routinely performing nuclear scintigraphy prior to mesenteric angiography, particularly in high-risk patients for whom rapid diagnosis is preferred. It may be more accurate if upper gastrointestinal bleeding has been excluded.[117] If bleeding is active and severe and/or scintigraphy is not diagnostic, selective mesenteric angiography can be used to detect extravasated contrast into the bowel when bleeding rates are 0.5 to 1.0 mL/min, or to demonstrate vascular lesions, neovascularity, or tumors in the absence of extravasation.[118] Sensitivity declines when bleeding is recurrent or chronic. Attempts have been made to increase diagnostic sensitivity and accuracy by using systemic heparinization, intra-arterial vasodilators, or thrombolytic agents during angiography if the initial study is negative.[119] More extensive experience is needed to determine whether the increased yield justifies the increased risk of bleeding complications.

Angiography also offers the potential for local therapy, provided selective catheterization can be achieved. These modalities include infusion of vasopressin to control acute arterial bleeding in colonic diverticular disease or angiodysplasia,[120] as well as selective embolization of an identified bleeding site with a gelatin sponge, vascular coils, or polyvinyl alcohol particles.[121] Complications include electrolyte disturbances, cardiovascular complications, and bowel ischemia with vasopressin infusion and bowel infarction following embolization. The latter should be attempted only at centers that have the expertise to perform superselective catheterization. Some investigators report that urgent colonoscopy is superior to selective mesenteric angiography in identifying the source of severe lower gastrointestinal bleeding. If bleeding is massive, emergent surgery with or without intraoperative endoscopy may be the best option. There is little or no place in modern surgical practice for blind colonic resection.

If no source of bleeding is detected by colonoscopy and no further bleeding occurs, a small bowel enteroscopy and/or enteroclysis should be performed. Enteroscopes can often be passed to 60–100 cm past the ligament of Treitz if the procedure is done by experienced personnel.[122] The diagnostic yield has varied from 30 to 60 percent, with arteriovascular malformations accounting for most of the causes of bleeding.

Barium enema has no role in the evaluation of patients with acute lower gastrointestinal bleeding. It is unable to demonstrate active bleeding and interferes with attempts to perform colonoscopy or mesenteric angiography. Even if a lesion is detected, there is no proof that it is the source of the acute bleed.

KEY POINTS   The large bowel

- Principal functions of the colon are to store fecal wastes and to expel them in an appropriate manner. Colonic dysfunction may result in constipation, diarrhea, or fecal incontinence.

- Making a clinical distinction between painful diverticular disease and diverticulitis carries a sizable rate of error in elderly people. Computerized tomography and ultrasonography often help in this process which is important as treatment approaches are very different.

- Both ulcerative colitis and Crohn's disease are found with increased frequency in elderly people. There are more and better drugs to treat these patients, both acutely and to maintain remissions.

- Colonic ischemia is often underdiagnosed in elderly people, is characterized by the sudden onset of abdominal pain and bleeding and often is benign and reversible. Colonoscopy is the diagnostic procedure of choice.

- Colon cancers are a frequent but often preventable cause of death in both men and women. The aggressive use of colonoscopy to detect premalignant polyps is the gold standard for prevention and should begin at age 50 in persons of normal risk.

- Lower gastrointestinal bleeding in elderly people is most often associated with angiodysplasias and diverticulosis. Colonoscopy is the preferred diagnostic test, whereas scintigraphy and angiography are helpful if no source of bleeding is seen or if bleeding is so brisk as to exclude colonoscopy.

REFERENCES

1. Cohn SM, Birnbaum EH: Colon: Anatomy and structural anomalies. In Yamada T (ed): Textbook of Gastroenterology, 3rd Ed. JB Lippincott, Philadelphia, 1999:1761–1774
2. Sonneland J, Anson B, Beaton L: Surgical anatomy of the arterial supply to the colon from the superior mesenteric artery based upon a study of 600 specimens. Surg Gynecol Obstet 1958;106:385
3. Boxall TA, Smart P, Griffiths JD: The blood supply of the distal segment of the rectum in anterior resection. Br J Surg 1963;50:399
4. Hasler WL: Motility of the small intestine and colon. In Yamada T (ed): Textbook of Gastroenterology, 3rd Ed. JB Lippincott, Philadelphia, 1999:215–245
5. Merkel IS, Locher J, Burgio K et al: Physiologic and psychologic characteristics of an elderly population with chronic constipation. Am J Gastroenterol 1993;88:1854–1859
6. McHugh SM, Diamant NE: Effect of age, gender and parity on anal canal pressure: contribution of impaired anal sphincter function to fecal incontinence. Dig Dis Sci 1987;32:726–736
7. Bannister JJ, Abouzekry I, Read NW: Effect of aging on anorectal function. Gut 1987;28:353–357
8. Patriquin H, Martelli H, Devroede G: Barium enema in chronic constipation: is it meaningful? Gastroenterology 1978;75:619–622
9. Tinetti ME, Stone L, Cooney L, Kapp MC: Inadequate barium enemas in hospitalized elderly patients. Arch Intern Med 1989;149:2014–2016
10. Gurwitz JH, Noonan JP, Sanchez M, Prather W: Barium enemas in the frail elderly. Am J Med 1992;92:41–44
11. Mulholland MW: Approach to the patient with acute abdomen. In Yamada T (ed): Textbook of Gastroenterology, 3rd Ed. JB Lippincott, Philadelphia, 1999:826–841
12. Law PL, Bartram CI: Anal endosonography: technique and normal anatomy. Gastrointest Radiol 1989;14:349–353
13. Cuesta MA, Meijer S, Derksen EJ et al: Anal sphincter imaging in fecal incontinence using endosonography. Dis Colon Rectum 1992;35:59–63
14. Sultan AH, Kamm MA, Hudson CN et al: Anal sphincter disruption during vaginal delivery. N Engl J Med 1993;329:1905–1911
15. Foutch PG: Flexible fiberoptic sigmoidoscopy. Pract Gastroenterol 1988;12:25–31
16. Ransohoff DF, Lang CA: Improving the fecal occult-blood test. N Engl J Med 1996;334:189–190
17. Wald A: Colonic diverticulosis. In Winawer SJ (ed): Management of Gastrointestinal Diseases. Gower Medical Publishing, Edinburgh, 1992:34.1–34.18
18. Painter NS, Burkitt DP: Diverticular disease of the colon: a 20th-century problem. Clin Gastroenterol 1975;4:3–25
19. Thompson WG: Do colonic diverticula cause symptoms? Am J Gastroenterol 1986;81:613–614
20. Morson BC: Pathology of diverticular disease. Clin Gastroenterol 1974;4:37–52
21. Wahlby L, Knutsen OH: Leukocyte counts, ESR and fever in the diagnosis of diverticulitis. Acta Chir Scand 1982;148:623–624

22. Richter JM, Christensen MR, Kaplan LM et al: Effectiveness of current technology in the diagnosis and management of lower gastrointestinal hemorrhage. Gastrointest Endosc 1995;41:93–98

23. Perkins JD, Shield CF, Chang FC, Farha GJ: Acute diverticulitis: comparison of treatment in immunocompromised and nonimmunocompromised patients. Am J Surg 1984;745–748

24. Rodkey GV, Welch CE: Changing patterns in the surgical treatment of diverticular disease. Ann Surg 1984;200:466–478

25. Ferzoco LB, Raptopoulos V, Silen W: Acute diverticulitis. N Engl J Med 1998;338:1521–1526

26. vanSonnenberg E, Mueller PR, Ferrucci JT Jr: Percutaneous drainage of 250 abdominal abscesses and fluid collections. I. Results, failures and complications. Radiology 1984;151:337–341

27. Stabile BE, Puccio E, vanSonnenberg E, Neff CC: Preoperative percutaneous drainage of diverticular abscesses. Am J Surg 1990;159:99–104

28. Lewis FR, Holcroft JW, Boey J, Dunphy JE: Appendicitis: a critical review of diagnosis and treatment in 1000 cases. Arch Surg 1975;110:677

29. Puylaert JBCM, Rutgers PH, Lalisang RI et al: A prospective study of ultrasonography in the diagnosis of appendicitis. N Engl J Med 1987;317:666–669

30. Kelly CP, Pothoulakis C, LaMont JT: Clostridium difficile colitis. N Engl J Med 1994;330:257–262

31. McFarland LV, Mulligan ME, Kwok RYY, Stamm WE: Nosocomial acquisition of Clostridium infection. N Engl J Med 1989;320:204–210

32. Settle CD, Wilcox MH: Review article: antibiotic-induced Clostridium difficile infection. Aliment Pharmacol Ther 1996;10:835–841

33. Fekety R: Guidelines for the diagnosis and treatment of Clostridium difficile associated diarrhea and colitis. Am J Gastroenterol 1997;92:739–750

34. Teasley DG, Gerding DN, Olson MM et al: Prospective randomized trial of metronidazole versus vancomycin for Clostridium difficile-associated diarrhea and colitis. Lancet 1983;2:1043–1046

35. Walters BAJ, Roberts R, Stafford R, Seneviratne E: Recurrence of antibiotic associated colitis: endogenous persistence of C. difficile during vancomycin therapy. Gut 1983;24:206–212

36. McFarland LV, Surawicz CM, Greenberg RN et al: A randomized placebo-controlled trial of Saccharomyces boulardii in combination with standard antibiotics for Clostridium difficile disease. JAMA 1994;271:1913–1918

37. LaMont JT: Bacterial infections of the colon. In Yamada T (ed): Textbook of Gastroenterology, 2nd Ed. JB Lippincott, Philadelphia, 1995:1891–1911

38. Bennish ML, Salam MA, Khan AM: Treatment of shigellosis. III. Comparison of one- or two-dose ciprofloxacin with standard 5-day therapy: a randomized blinded trial. Ann Intern Med 1992;117:727

39. DuPont HL, Hornick RB: Adverse effect of Lomotil therapy in shigellosis. JAMA 1973;226:1525

40. Ericsson CD, Johnson PC, DuPont HL et al: Ciprofloxacin or trimethoprim-sulfamethoxazole as initial therapy for traveler's diarrhea. Ann Intern Med 1987;106:216

41. MacDonald KL, O'Leary MJ, Cohen ML et al: Escherichia coli 0157:H7, an emerging gastrointestinal pathogen: results of a one year, prospective, population based study. JAMA 1988;259:3567–3570

42. Wong CS, Jelacic S, Habeeb RL et al: The risk of the hemolytic-uremic syndrome after antibiotic treatment of Escherichia coli 0157:H7 infections. N Engl J Med 2000;342:1930–36

43. Griffin PM, Ostroff SM, Tauxe RV et al: Illnesses associated with Escherichia coli 0157:H7 infections: a broad clinical spectrum. Ann Intern Med 1988;109:705–712

44. Cornick NA, Gorbach SL: Campylobacter. Infect Dis Clin North Am 1988;2:643

45. Hill DR, Petri WA, Guerrant RL: Parasitic diseases: protozoa. In Yamada T (ed): Textbook of Gastroenterology, 2nd Ed. JB Lippincott, Philadelphia, 1995:2343–2348

46. Kagan IG: Serologic diagnosis of parasitic diseases. N Engl J Med 1970;282:685–686

47. Kozarsky PE, Jernigan JA: Amebiasis. In RE Rakel (ed): Conn's Current Therapy. WB Saunders, Philadelphia, 1996:66–69

48. Meyers JD: Prevention and treatment of cytomegalovirus infections. Ann Rev Med 1991;42:179

49. Garland CF, Lilienfeld AM, Mendeloff AM et al: Incidence of rates of ulcerative colitis and Crohn's disease in fifteen areas of the United States. Gastroenterology 1981;81:1115

50. Kyle, J: An epidemiological study of Crohn's disease in Northeast Scotland. Gastroenterology 1971;61:826

51. Kirsner JB, Shorter RG: Inflammatory Bowel Disease, 3rd Ed. Lea and Febiger, Philadelphia, 1988

52. Softley A, Myren J, Clamp SE et al: Inflammatory bowel disease in the elderly patient. Scand J Gastroenterol 1988;23(suppl 144):27

53. Holt PR: Approach to gastrointestinal problems in the elderly. In Yamada T (ed): Textbook of Gastroenterology, 2nd Ed. JB Lippincott, Philadelphia, 1995:968–988

54. Danovitch SH: Fulminant colitis and toxic megacolon. Gastroenterol Clin N Am 1989;18:73

55. Stein RB, Hanauer SB: Medical therapy for inflammatory bowel disease. Gastroenterol Clin N Am 1999;28:297–321

56. Meyers S, Sachar DB, Goldberg JD, Janowitz HD: Corticotropin versus hydrocortisone in the intravenous treatment of ulcerative colitis. Gastroenterology 1983;85:351–357

57. Adler DJ, Korelitz BI: The therapeutic efficacy of 6-mercaptopurine in refractory ulcerative colitis. Am J Gastroenterol 1990;85:717–722

58. Azad Khan AK, Howes DT, Piris J, Truelove SC: Optimum dose of sulphasalazine for maintenance treatment in ulcerative colitis. Gut 1980;21:232–240

59. Kaufman HJ, Taubin HL: Nonsteroidal anti-inflammatory drugs activate quiescent inflammatory bowel disease. Ann Intern Med 1987;107:513–516

60. Lewis JD, Deren JJ, Lichtenstein GR: Cancer risk in patients with inflammatory bowel disease. Gastro Clin N Am 1999;28:459–477

61. Sutherland L, Singleton J, Sessions J et al: Double-blind placebo controlled trial of metronidazole in Crohn's disease. Gut 1991;32:1071–1075

62. Present DH, Korelitz BI, Wisch N et al: Treatment of Crohn's disease with 6-mercaptopurine. N Engl J Med 1980;302:981–987

63. Feagan BG, Fedorak RN, Irvine EJ et al: A comparison of methotrexate with placebo for the maintenance of remission in Crohn's disease. N Engl J Med 2000;342:1627–1632

64. Brandt LJ, Bernstein LH, Boley SJ, Frank MS: Metronidazole therapy for perineal Crohn's disease: a follow-up study. Gastroenterology 1982;83:383–387

65. Korelitz BI, Present DH: Favorable effect of 6-mercaptopurine on fistulae of Crohn's disease. Dig Dis Sci 1985;30:58–64

66. Sylwestrowicz T, Kelly JK, Hwang WA et al: Collagenous colitis and microscopic colitis: the watery diarrhea-colitis syndrome. Am J Gastroenterol 1989;84:763–768

67. Tremaine WJ: Collagenous colitis and lymphocytic colitis. J Clin Gastroenterol 2000;80:245–249

68. Lazenby AJ, Yardley JH, Giardiello FM et al: Lymphocytic ("microscopic") colitis: a comparative histopathologic study with particular reference to collagenous colitis. Hum Pathol 1989;20:18–28

69. Bohr J, Tysk C, Eriksson S, Abrahamsson H, Jarnerot G: Collagenous colitis: a retrospective study of clinical presentations and treatment in 163 patients. Gut 1996;39:846–851

70. Zins BJ, Sandborn WJ, Tremaine WJ: Collagenous and lymphocytic colitis: Subject review and therapeutic alternatives. Am J Gastroenterol 1995;90:1394–1400

71. Fine KD, Lee EL: Efficacy of open label bismuth subsalicylate for the treatment of microscopic colitis. Gastroenterology 1998;114:29–36

72. Binns JC, Isaacson P: Age related changes in the colonic blood supply: their relevance to ischemic colitis. Gut 1978;19:384–390

73. Robert JH, Mentha G, Rohner A: Ischemic colitis: two distinct patterns of severity. Gut 1993;34:4–6

74. Brandt LJ, Boley SJ: Colonic ischemia. Surg Clin N Am 1992;72:203–229

75. Kaleva RN, Boley SJ: Colonic ischemia. In Fazio VW (ed): Current Therapy in Colon and Rectal Surgery. BC Decker, Toronto, 1990:324–329

76. Bower TC: Ischemic colitis. Surg Clin N Am 1993;73:1037–1053

77. Rex DK: Acute colonic pseudo-obstruction (Ogilvie's syndrome). Gastroenterologist 1994;2:233–238

78. Ponec RJ, Saunders MD, Kinney MB: Neostigime for the treatment of acute colonic pseudo-obstruction. N Engl J Med 1999;341:137–141

79. Jetmore AB, Timmcke AE, Gathright JB et al: Ogilvie's syndrome: colonic decompression and analysis of predisposing factors. Dis Colon Rectum 1992;35:1135–1142

80. Ballantyne GH, Brandner MD, Beart RW et al: Volvulus of the colon: incidence and mortality. Ann Surg 1985;202:83–92

81. Morrissey KP: Sigmoid volvulus: is it a difficult twist to manage? In Barkin JS, Rogers A (ed): Difficult Decisions in Digestive Diseases. Yearbook Medical Publishers, Chicago, 1989:543–550

82. O'Brien M, Winawer SJ, Waye JD: Colorectal polyps. In Winawer, SJ (ed): Management of Gastrointestinal Diseases. Gower Medical Publishing, New York, 1992:26.1–26.45

83. Provenzale D, Garrett JW, Condon SE, Sandler RS: Risk for colon adenomas in patients with rectosigmoid hyperplastic polyps. Ann Intern Med 1990;113:760–763

84. Correa P: Epidemiology of polyps and cancer. In Morson BC (ed): The Pathogenesis of Colorectal Cancer. WB Saunders, Philadelphia, 1978:126–152

85. Selby JV, Friedman GD, Quesenberry CP, Weiss NS: A case-control study of screening sigmoidoscopy and mortality from colorectal cancer. N Engl J Med 1992;326:653–657

86. Winawer SJ, Zauber AG, Ho MN et al: Prevention of colorectal cancer by colonoscopic polypectomy. N Engl J Med 1993;329:1977–1981

87. Janne PA, Mayer RJ: Chemoprevention of colorectal cancer. N Engl J Med 2000;342:1960–1968

88. Cranley JP, Petras RE, Carey WD et al: When is endoscopic polypectomy adequate therapy for colonic polyps containing invasive carcinoma? Gastroenterology 1986;91:419–427

89. Cooper HS, Deppish LM, Gourley WK et al: Endoscopically removed malignant colorectal polyps: clinicopathologic correlations. Gastroenterology 1995;108:1657–1665

90. Winawer SJ, Stewart ET, Zauber AG et al: A comparison of colonoscopy and double-contrast barium enema for surveillance after polypectomy. N Engl J Med 2000;342:1766–1772

91. Allison JE, Tekawa IS, Ransom LJ, Adrain AL: A comparison of fecal occult-blood tests for colorectal cancer screening. N Engl J Med 1996;334:155–159

92. St John DJB, Young GP, Alexeyeff MA et al: Evaluation of new occult blood tests for detecting colorectal neoplasia. Gastroenterology 1993;104:1661–1668

93. Selby JV, Friedman GD, Quesenberry CP, Weiss NS: Effect of fecal occult blood testing on mortality from colorectal cancer. Ann Intern Med 1993;118:1–6

94. Mandel JS, Church TR, Ederer F et al: Colorectal cancer mortality: The effectiveness of biennial screening for fecal occult blood. J Natl Cancer Inst 1999;91:434

95. Bond JH: Colorectal cancer update: Prevention, screening, treatment and surveillance for high risk groups. Med Clin N Am 2000;84:1163–1182

96. Fearon ER: Molecular genetic studies of the adenoma-carcinoma sequence. Adv Intern Med 1994;39:123–147

97. Scott N, Quirke P: Molecular biology of colorectal neoplasia. Gut 1995;34:289–292

98. Rustgi AK: Hereditary gastrointestinal polyposis and nonpolyposis syndromes. N Engl J Med 1994;331:1694–1702

99. Moertel CG, Fleming TR, MacDonald JS et al: An evaluation of the carcinoembryonic antigen (CEA) test for monitoring patients with resected colon cancer. JAMA 1993;270:943–947

100. Milsom JW, Graffner H: Intrarectal ultrasonography in rectal cancer staging and in the evaluation of pelvic disease: clinical uses of rectal ultrasound. Ann Surg 1990;212:602–606

101. Moertel CG, Fleming TRD, MacDonald JS et al: Fluorouracil plus levamisole as effective adjuvant therapy after resection of stage III colon cancer. Ann Intern Med 1995;122:321–326

102. MacDonald JS: Adjuvant therapy of colon cancer. CA Cancer J Clin 1999;49:202–219

103. O'Connell MJ, Martenson JA, Wieand HS et al: Improving adjuvant therapy for rectal cancer by combining protracted-infusion fluorouracil with radiation therapy after curative surgery. N Engl J Med 1994;331:502–507

104. Sharma R, Gorbien MJ: Angiodysplasia and lower gastrointestinal bleeding in elderly patients. Arch Intern Med 1995;155:807–812

105. Duray PH, Marcel JM Jr, Livolsi VA et al: Small intestinal angiodysplasia in the elderly. J Clin Gastroenterol 1984;6:311–319

106. Parkes BM, Oberd FN, Sorensen VJ et al: The management of massive lower gastrointestinal bleeding. Ann Surg 1993;59:676–678

107. Imperiale TF, Ransohoff DF: Aortic stenosis, idiopathic gastrointestinal bleeding and angiodysplasia: is there an association? Gastroenterology 1988;95:1670–1676

108. Cappell MS, Lebwohl O: Cessation of recurrent bleeding from gastrointestinal angiodysplasias after aortic valve replacement. Ann Intern Med 1986;105:54–57

109. Richter JM, Hedbert SE, Athanasoulis CA et al: Angiodysplasia: clinical presentation and colonoscopic diagnosis. Dig Dis Sci 1984;29:481–485

110. Fallah MA, Prakash C, Edmundowicz S: Acute gastrointestinal bleeding. Med Clin North Am 2000;84:1183–1208

111. Richter JM, Christensen MR, Colditz GA, Nishioka NS: Angio-dysplasia: natural history and efficacy of therapeutic interventions. Dig Dis Sci 1989;34:1542–1546

112. Foutch PG: Colonic angiodysplasia. Gastroenterologist 1997;5:148–156

113. Abdulian JD, Santor MJ, Chen YK et al: Dieulafoy-like lesions of the rectum presenting with exsanguinating hemorrhage: successful endoscopic sclerotherapy. Am J Gastroenterol 1993;88:1939–1941

114. Snook JA, Holdstock GE, Bamforta J: Value of a simple biochemical ratio in distinguishing upper and lower sites of gastrointestinal hemorrhage. Lancet 1986;1:1064–1065

115. Zuckerman GR, Prakash C, Stodkilde H: Acute lower intestinal bleeding: Part 1. Clinical presentation and diagnosis. Gastrointest Endosc 1998;48:606–616

116. Hunter JM, Pezim ME: Limited value of technetium^{99m} labelled red cell scintigraphy in localization of lower gastrointestinal bleeding. Am J Surg 1990;159:504–506

117. Dusold R, Burke K, Carpentier W, Dyck WP: The accuracy of technetium^{99m} labeled red cell scintigraphy in localizing gastrointestinal bleeding. Am J Gastroenterol 1994;89:345–348

118. Schapiro MJ: The role of the radiologist in the management of gastrointestinal bleeding. Gastroenterol Clin N Am 1994;23:123–181

119. Koval F, Brenner KG, Rosch J et al: Aggressive angiographic diagnosis in acute lower gastrointestinal hemorrhage. Dig Dis Sci 1987;32:248–253

120. Gomes AS, Lois JF, McCoy RD: Angiographic treatment of gastrointestinal hemorrhage: comparison of vasopressin infusion and embolization. Am J Gastroenterol 1986;146:1031–1037

121. Rosen RJ, Sanchez G: Angiographic diagnosis and management of gastrointestinal hemorrhage. Current concepts. Radiol Clin North Am 1994;32:951–967

122. Morris AJ: Small bowel investigation in occult gastrointestinal bleeding. Semi Gastrointest Dis 1999;2:65–70

Chapter 84

Nutrition

Anita J. Thomas

Elderly people are at risk of malnutrition because reduction in food intake may be accompanied by changes in gut function, inefficient metabolism, failing homeostasis, and defective nutrient utilization. The coincidence of acute or chronic illness, trauma, hypercatabolic state, infection, and drug therapy change nutrient requirements. Such factors may cause a critical deterioration in nutritional status which impairs tissue repair and immune function, and from which recovery is difficult if not impossible.

Nutrition has been a neglected subject in clinical practice, and in many medical undergraduate and postgraduate educational programs,[1,2] though this may be changing.[3] Institutional malnutrition is a particular concern.[4–6] Estimates of the incidence of malnutrition in hospital inpatients vary from 15 to 40 percent.[7] Diagnosis of inadequate nutritional status depends on the availability of appropriate and validated assessment tools, and comparisons between studies are complicated by the use of different outcome measures.[8,9] Identification of inadequate nutritional status is not always followed by appropriate action.[7]

The true incidence of malnutrition in the institutionalized elderly population is poorly defined, yet good nutritional status is fundamental to clinical management, rehabilitation, and recovery. The provision of appropriate hydration and nutrition is an ethical and legal duty of basic clinical care, but tube feeding and artificial hydration are regarded as medical treatments and careful consideration must be given to such intervention (see also Chapter 24).[10] Nutritional supplementation may improve nutritional indices, but the evidence base for effective intervention is incomplete[11] and extrapolation of findings from studies of younger individuals to older people is not valid. Current research initiatives in nutrition and aging in health and disease are likely to affect clinical practice significantly. New discoveries, such as the basis of nutrient–gene interaction and the influence of genetic polymorphism, herald many exciting research opportunities.[12,13]

DEMOGRAPHY AND THE SOCIAL CONTEXT

Taking the UK as an example, the number of people aged 60 years and over is predicted to increase from 12 million (20 percent of the population) in 2001 to 18.6 million (30 percent) in 2031, with concomitant two- to three-fold increase in those suffering a chronic disease or disability, and those unable to carry out four activities of daily living.[14] People aged 65 years and over are the largest low-income group in the UK, with the poorest spending less than £25 per week on food, and about 20 percent having no central heating.[15] There are large differences in morbidity between the young old, the middle old, and the old old.[16] In 1996, 50 percent of women

and 25 percent of men aged 85 years and over were unable to cook a main meal without help, yet only 10 percent received a home-delivered hot meal (Meals on Wheels). Twenty percent reported difficulty seeing even with eyeglasses, 10 percent were unable to walk down the road or manage stairs, and 17 percent were unable to manage household shopping.[17]

Still in the UK, there will be a great increase in numbers of elderly people suffering from dementia (from 1 million in 1996 to 2 million in 2036) and from fractured neck of femur (doubling between 1996 and 2021 from approximately 40,000 annually to 80,000 and almost doubling again by 2051).[14] These are major challenges for health and social care provision and will prompt development of new preventive and therapeutic interventions. Dementia and disability are risk factors for malnutrition, and admission to hospital with acute or acute-on-chronic illness, such as fractured neck of femur, often results in a further nutritional insult compromising recovery and increasing mortality (see below). Homebound individuals are particularly vulnerable.[18,19] In 1998, 20 percent of people aged 75 years or over reported an inpatient stay in the preceding 12 months.[20]

In 1979, the UK Committee on Medical Aspects of Food (COMA) Panel on Nutrition of the Elderly drew attention to the fall in dietary intake with age and links between poor socioeconomic status, disease, and overt malnutrition in hospitals.[21] The survey showed a 7 percent incidence of malnutrition diagnosed on clinical and biochemical grounds in otherwise healthy subjects living in their own homes. The incidence doubled in those aged at least 80 years. The multicenter survey in England and Scotland in 1967/68, using dietary recall and diaries, provided data on 764 people over 65 years old. In 1972/73, the 365 traceable survivors from the earlier study were re-examined. These studies, which excluded people in institutional care, showed that well older people in general ate a diet that was similar to that of younger people, and identified several risk factors for the development of malnutrition.

The recent National Diet and Nutrition Survey (NDNS) of people aged 65 years or over in the UK[22] confirms these trends and includes information on institutionalized people. Important findings include biochemical vitamin D deficiency in 8 percent of free-living and in 37 percent of institutionalized older people, with further evidence of deficiency in significant proportions of the study population for folate (15–40 percent), iron (30–40 percent), and vitamin C (40 percent). The oral health section of the NDNS reported 50 percent of free-living and 80 percent of institutionalized people to be edentulous; 8 percent had nonmatching dentures, and the average age of dentures was 17 years (one set was 68 years old!).

In the NDNS, geographical and social inequalities were linked to poorer vitamin C status, lower consumption of vitamins present in fruit and vegetables, and higher sodium and lower potassium intakes. Important research challenges were identified.[23] A European project—the Survey in Europe on Nutrition in the Elderly: a Concerted Action (SENECA)—has collected anthropometric, laboratory, dietary, health and lifestyle data on almost 2,000 subjects longitudinally, with similar findings.[24]

MALNUTRITION IN CLINICAL PRACTICE

Early influences

Nutritional status in fetal and infant life has been linked to some of the major diseases of middle and late life. In the UK, Barker and colleagues have provided evidence suggesting that heart disease, stroke, diabetes, hypertension, and obstructive pulmonary disease may be determined by programming in early life. The death rate from ischemic heart disease in men from one area whose body weight at 1 year of age was 8.2 kg or less was three times that of men from the same area who had attained 12.2 kg or more.[25,26] Swedish work supports the association of impaired fetal growth with adult hypertension, particularly in those who become obese, and it is suggested that this may be mediated by metabolic disturbances such as insulin resistance.[27]

Malnutrition is frequently associated with the major diseases of older people. There is evidence of malnutrition in about one-third of patients with COPD (particularly emphysema), one-half of patients with fractured femur, and one-third to one-half of patients with stroke.

The "thrifty phenotype hypothesis" predicts an increasing incidence of heart disease and glucose intolerance in populations where low birthweight and high body mass index in later life coexist; just such a pattern is emerging in India.[28]

Stroke and coronary heart disease

Lifestyle and dietary habits may reduce the incidence of important diseases in later life, such as coronary heart disease and stroke.[29,30] Gariballa[31] has reviewed recent evidence regarding nutritional factors in stroke prevention and treatment. Interventions for dysphagia in acute stroke await the results of further studies (such as the FOOD and PEGASUS trials), but present work suggests that percutaneous endoscopic gastrostomy (PEG) feeding may improve outcome and nutrition compared with nasogastric tube (NGT) feeding.[32]

Bone health

In the area of calcium metabolism and bone health, the interactions of genotype, lifestyle,[33] dietary intake,[34,35] hormone status, body composition,[36] and interindividual variation[37] are well illustrated. Between 60 and 70 percent of variability in bone mass can be accounted for by genetic variability and 30–40 percent by environmental factors.[38] The high incidence of biochemical vitamin D deficiency in the institutionalized elderly population in the UK should prompt implementation of the widely ignored guidelines for vitamin D supplementation in this group given by the COMA subgroup some years previously.[21] Large randomized trials currently under way will clarify the effectiveness of vitamin D supplementation in fracture prevention.[39]

Elderly people are often malnourished at the time of hip fracture, and nutritional status worsens after admisson with low energy and protein intakes in many patients.[40] Studies of nutritional supplementation after hip fracture are hampered by small sample sizes, methodology, and outcome assessment, but they do suggest a reduction in overall unfavorable outcomes (death or complications) though not demonstrating a clear effect on mortality.[40]

Dementia

Patients with dementia often have poor access to food and reduced intake, sometimes with increased levels of physical activity; these factors are thought to contribute to weight loss rather than to a hypermetabolic state, as suspected in the past.[41] Deficiencies of B vitamins and folic acid are associated with Alzheimer's disease, but it is unclear whether the deficiencies contribute to neurocognitive decline or are a consequence of poor intake or inefficient metabolism.[42] An education program for carers is currently being evaluated as a way of preventing weight loss.[43]

Chronic obstructive pulmonary disease

Weight loss in COPD is associated with higher resting energy expenditure, poor pulmonary function, lower diaphragmatic mass, lower exercise capacity, and higher mortality.[44] Approximately one-third of patients with COPD are malnourished to some degree, and there may be a relationship between metabolic change and inflammatory mediators—though no significant effects of nutritional supplementation have been shown to date in randomized controlled trials.[45]

Age-related macular degeneration

It has been suggested that a diet high in antioxidant vitamins and minerals is associated with a lower incidence of age-related mascular degeneration. However, supplementation seems to have no effect on incidence or progression of the disease, so further trials are awaited.[46]

Immunity

The immune response may not simply be diminished with aging. Cell-mediated immunity is affected more than humoral, there are changes in the relative ratios of T-cell subsets, and other factors also contribute to the effectiveness of the immune response.[47] The immune response is blunted in protein energy malnutrition, the effect being proportional to the degree of malnutrition. Vitamin and mineral supplementation improve immunity in both healthy and institutionalized elderly people.[47]

ASSESSMENT OF NUTRITIONAL STATUS

The nutritional status of individuals and of populations can be assessed by the following:

- dietary assessment;
- laboratory tests of biochemical status or of function;
- measurements of body size and composition (including anthropometry);
- clinical assessment.

A simple model of a nutrient deficiency suggests the evolution of an initial predisposition, then subclinical deficiency, and finally clinical disease. Dietary inadequacy at the predisposition stage may be revealed by dietary assessment, followed by a decrease in tissue reserves, body fluids, or nutrient-dependent enzymes, or in function revealed by biochemical or anthropometric methods. Clinical symptoms and signs are the last manifestation of nutrient deficiency.

Estimates of nutrient requirements—and thus guidelines for adequate intake—are derived from various sources, including metabolic balance studies, prevention or cure of deficiency states, and biochemical or enzymatic indexes of adequacy.[48]

In clinical practice, there are often deficiencies of more than one nutrient, sometimes at different stages of development. Biochemical tests of status or function are not widely available for all nutrients. Gibson[49] provides an authoritative account of nutritional assessment, but a basic summary is provided below to allow interpretation of the often sparse information available for the senior age group.

Dietary assessment

Food consumption can be assessed at the national, group, or individual level. Information is collected on the food available per capita nationally and at the household level in the UK National Food Survey. Food consumption of individuals can be measured over a defined time period either qualitatively (a dietary history or food frequency questionnaire) or quantitatively (recall, written, or weighed record). Such methods require the subject to have a good memory, to be numerate and literate, and to have a stable diet during the study period. Interpretation necessitates reference to food tables[50] that have been compiled over many years with changing methods of food preparation, preservation, and analysis and which are probably reliable for macronutrients though not accurate for some micronutrients. Chemical analysis of duplicate meals is the most accurate method of assessing actual intake of nutrients and forms part of the metabolic balance study in which all output is also chemically analyzed (including urine, feces and sometimes sweat, menstrual loss, and semen). Such information has been used to estimate human requirements for individual nutrients, such as nitrogen, iron, and calcium. Bioavailability should be taken into account in the application of guidelines for dietary intake.[51]

COMA's most recent guidelines for dietary intake of food energy and nutrients for all ages includes a comprehensive literature review[48] in which dietary reference values (DRVs) replace the earlier recommended dietary allowances (RDAs). Figure 84-1 shows the derivation of DRVs: assuming a normal distribution, the notional mean requirement is designated the estimated average requirement (EAR). The mean plus two standard deviations is the reference nutrient intake (RNI), and intakes above this amount "will almost certainly be adequate." The lower reference nutrient intake (LRNI) represents intakes that are at or below the mean minus two standard deviations and that are "almost certainly inadequate for most individuals." The data available for formulating these recommendations vary in

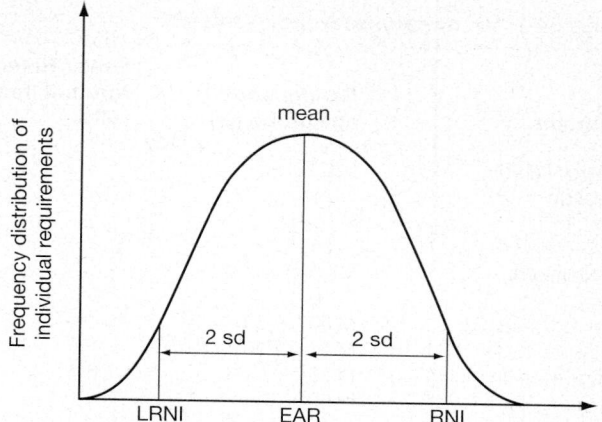

Figure 84-1 Dietary reference values. SD, standard deviation; EAR, estimated average requirement; LRNI, lower reference nutrient intake; RNI, reference nutrient intake.

amount and quality and are sparse for the older population. Historically many recommendations depended on extrapolation from data for younger age groups. Table 84-1 summarizes the dietary recommendations for energy, protein, and most minerals, and DRVs for older people for vitamins can be found in Table 84-2. In 1992, COMA published a more specialized and detailed review entitled "The Nutrition of Elderly People," which endorsed the DRVs for the population aged 50 or older years and made specific recommendations.[52]

The 1994/95 National Diet and Nutrition Survey assessed dietary, anthropometric, and biochemical variables for all age groups, including a sample of people aged 65 years or over living at home and in institutions.[22] A summary of results is presented in Figures 84-2 and 84-3. Later, Tables 84-3 to 84-5 give more detail.

Laboratory tests of biochemical status and physiological function

Biochemical tests of nutrient status measure the concentration of a nutrient in biological tissue or fluid, the most common being blood or a blood component (such as plasma, erythrocytes, or leucocytes). Plasma and serum levels tend to reflect acute changes in nutritional status and are affected by factors as varied as recent dietary intake, diurnal variation, concomitant medication, infection, inflammation, and stress. Erythrocyte nutrient levels are difficult to analyze and seldom useful. Leucocyte levels may be helpful, but laboratory analysis is time-consuming and requires relatively large blood samples. Invasive biopsy of tissue storage sites such as bone for calcium, adipose tissue for vitamin E or liver, and bone marrow for iron may be useful in some clinical settings.

Trace element analysis is particularly challenging, and the use of hair or nails is not generally acceptable. Urinary excretion of the nutrient or a metabolite may reflect acute nutritional status and can be useful in estimating vitamin C and water-soluble B vitamin status as well as for some minerals and nitrogen.

Table 84-1 UK dietary reference values[48]

Nutrient	Gender and age group (yr)	Lower Reference Nutrient Intake, LRNI	Estimated Average Requirement, EAR	Reference Nutrient Intake, RNI
Energy (MJ/d)	M 65–74		9.71 (2330)	
(kcal/d)	75+		8.77 (2100)	
	F 65–74		7.96 (1900)	
	75+		7.61 (1810)	
Protein (g/d)	M 50+			53.3
	F 50+			46.5
Calcium (mmol/d)	M 50+, F 50+	10	13.1	17.5
Phosphorus (mmol/d)	M 50+, F 50+			17.5
Magnesium (mmol/d)	M 50+	7.8	10.3	12.3
	F 50+	6.2	8.2	10.9
Sodium (mmol/d)	M 50+, F 50+	25		70
Potassium (mmol/d)	M 50+, F 50+	50		90
Chloride (mmol/d)	M 50+, F 50+			70
Iron (μmol/d)	M 50+, F 50+	80	120	160
Zinc (μmol/d)	M 50+	85	110	145
	F 50+	60	85	110

Abbreviations: M, male; F, female.

Table 84-2 Vitamins

Vitamin	Reference Nutrient Intake[a]	Metabolic role	Laboratory test	Clinical features of deficiency
A: retinol	M, 700 μg/d; F, 600 μg/d	Formation of rhodopsin	Dark adaptation, colorimetric or fluorimetric assay, serum retinol	Night blindness, follicular hyperkeratosis, xeropthalmia
B: thiamin	M, 0.9 mg/d; F, 0.8 mg/d	Thiamin pyrophosphate (TPP) is coenzyme for oxidative decarboxylation of pyruric acid	Erythrocyte transketolase activity before/after TPP	Polyneuropathy (dry beri beri), cardiomyopathy (wet beri beri), encephalopathy (Wernicke–Korsakoff syndrome)
Niacin: nicotinic acid equivalent	M, 16 mg/d; F, 12 mg/d	Component of respiratory enzymes (NAD, NADP)	HPLC urinary excretion of N-methylnicotinamide	Pellagra—symmetric, pruritic erythema on light-exposed skin, chronic dry scaly dermatitis, delirium, dementia, neuropathy
B_2: riboflavin	M, 1.3 mg/d; F, 1.1 mg/d	Component of flavin adenine dinucleotide (FAD), oxidation reduction reactions	Erythrocyte glutathione reductase activity before/after FAD	Angular stomatitis, glossitis, cheilosis, nasolabial seborrhea
B_6: pyridoxine	M, 1.4 mg/d; F, 1.2 mg/d	Coenzyme for amino acid decarboxylation and transamination reactions	Plasma pyridoxal 5-phosphate	Peripheral neuropathy (e.g. isoniazid)
B_{12}: cyanocobalamin	M, 1.5 μg/d; F, 1.5 μg/d	Synthesis of thymine (DNA base) from deoxyuridine, proprionate metabolism	Serum vitamin B_{12} (radioassay)	Macrocytic anemia, subacute combined degeneration of cord
Folate	M, 200 μg/d; F, 200 μg/d	Thymin synthesis	Serum, erythrocyte folate (microbiologic or radioassay)	Macrocytic anemia
C: ascorbic acid	M, 40 mg/d; F, 40 mg/d	Antioxidant	Colorimetric or fluorimetric assay, plasma or (better) leucocyte ascorbic acid	Scurvy—gingvitis (if not edentulous), perifollicular petechiae, corkscrew hairs, bruises, sheet hemorrhages in skin, ocular hemorrhage, femoral neuropathy, sudden death

(continued)

Table 84-2 **Vitamins** (continued)				
Vitamin	Reference Nutrient Intake[a]	Metabolic role	Laboratory test	Clinical features of deficiency
D: cholecalciferol	M and F 65+ years, 10 µg/d	Promotes calcium and phosphate absorption, calcium release from bone (PTH-dependent)	Competitive binding assay of 25OHD	Bone tenderness, spontaneous fractures, proximal myopathy

Abbreviations: M, male; F, female; HPLC, high-pressure liquid chromatography; PTH, parathormone.

[a]*Aged 50+ years unless otherwise stated. RNI assumes protein = 14.7 percent EAR for energy.*

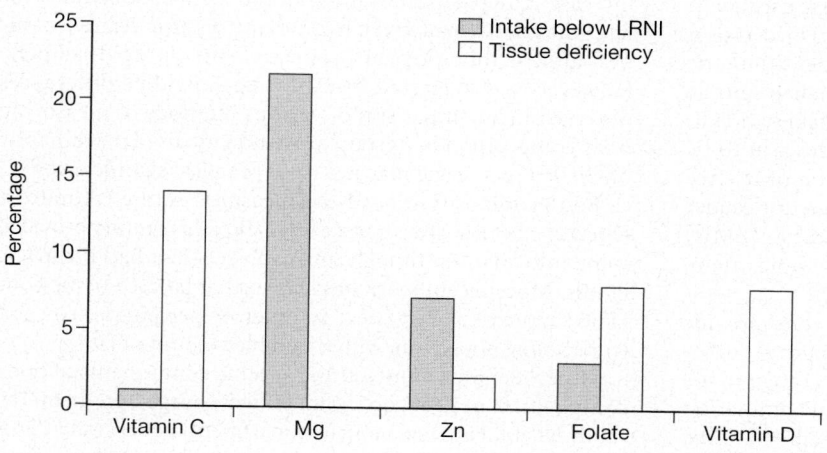

Figure 84-2 Micronutrient intake and status in free-living elderly people (aged 65+).

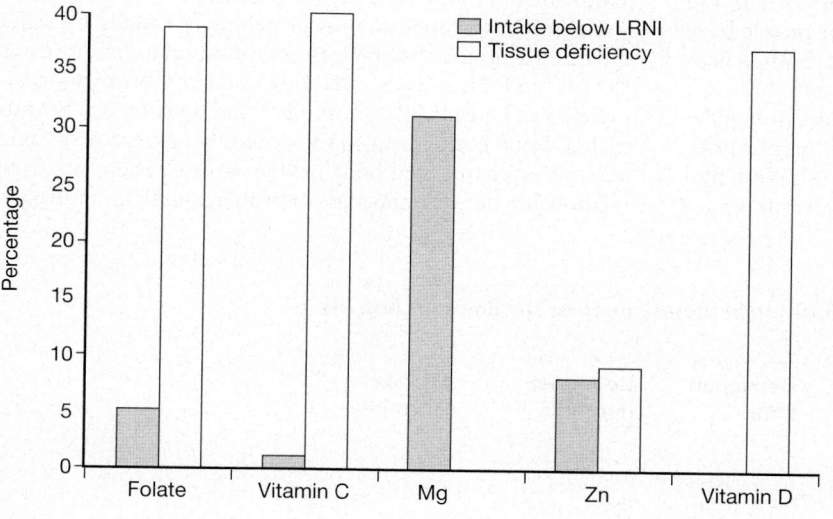

Figure 84-3 Micronutrient intake and status in institutionalized older people (aged 65+).

Biochemical tests of physiological function include in-vivo responses (such as dark adaptation for vitamin A), in-vitro and in-vivo induced responses, and loading tests, and the more familiar measurements of enzymatic activity or concentration of another blood component dependent on the nutrient (such as erythrocyte transketolase activity for thiamin or hemoglobin concentration for iron).

Measurements of body size and composition

Body weight is one of the simplest and most neglected clinical parameters. Baseline measurements and regular monitoring can identify significant weight loss or gain at an early stage. Visual impressions of significant weight change are unreliable.

The translation of body weight measurement into a useful measure of body fatness, taking account of height and body shape, produced a series of anthropometric indexes. The first of these was the indice ponderale (weight$^{1/3}$/height) derived using physical scaling principles (as the size of a spherical body increases, the weight varies according to the cube of the diameter).[53] Hydrodensitometry (underwater weighing) allowed calculation of body fat content. Assuming a lean body mass (LBM) with a constant density of 1.10, weighing individuals in air and then under water with a correction for residual lung volume allows body volume and percentage of body fat to be calculated.[54] It is not surprising to find that few elderly people were included in these studies.

Skinfold thickness measurements from different sites (triceps, biceps, subscapular, suprailiac) were first used as an estimate of subcutaneous fat by Jelliffe[55] in the Third World and have shown a close correlation with hydrodensitometric measurements in youth and middle life. Mean arm muscle circumference (MAMC) with triceps skinfold thickness (TSF) allows calculation of muscle area (assuming the arm to be circular in cross-section) and thence a derivation of fat-free mass (FFM). Corrections for "bone-free" FFM and for gender are available.[56,57] Comparisons of body mass indexes (BMIs) are valid within groups of the same gender and ethnic origin, though there may be inter-regional differences.[58]

Population studies on adults in the Western world provide reference data; for example, the Dietary and Nutritional Survey of British Adults in the United Kingdom (age range 16–64 years), the US National Health and Nutrition Examination Surveys (25–74 years), and the Nutrition Canada National Survey (20–69 years).[53]

The use of anthropometry in ill older people has presented problems,[59] though some information is available for TSF and conventional BMI values.[60] Low BMIs in older people have been associated with an increased mortality risk, both in general[61–63] and specifically after fracture of the femur.[64]

Modifications of anthropometric indexes for use in an older population may improve interpretation. Height may be difficult to measure or unreliable because of kyphosis, vertebral collapse, or unsteadiness, and other surrogate measures have been suggested.[65] Demispan shows a close correlation with height and is measured from the finger web to the sternal notch with the arm outstretched.[66] Indexes have been developed for use in older men and women using demispan as a measure of stature in the UK[67] and Canada.[68] Demiquet (weight[kg]/demispan^2) is used for men, and Mindex (weight[kg]/demispan) for women. The Nottingham Ageing and Activity Survey[67] provides information on a randomly selected sample of 890 free-living people aged 65–74 years and 75–94 years and is summarized in Table 84-3.

Anthropometric variables such as TSF and MAMC should be interpreted with caution in elderly populations. There are age-related changes in body composition which may affect interpretation. These include a fall in FFM,[69,70] a relative increase in deposition of internal rather than subcutaneous fat,[71] the relative paucity of hydrodensitometric reference values, and methodological problems with skinfold calipers. However, it is suggested that the interindividual differences observed in a comparison of various methods of measuring body composition in a group of 60 individuals predominantly under 75 years of age may not be of practical significance.[72]

Body composition has been measured in the laboratory. Direct chemical analysis of cadavers earlier this century provided some information, though most subjects had had a chronic illness. More recent work has shown that fat-free tissue contained approximately 72 percent water, 20 percent protein, and 69 mmol/kg potassium, with a variable amount of fat.[73]

Other methods of measuring specific components of body composition depend on either a two-compartment model (body fat and FFM) or a four-compartment model (water, protein, minerals, and fat). Estimation of total body potassium measures the γ-radiation emitted by naturally occurring ^{40}K as a measure of FFM. One study has used multi-isotope dilution and elimination kinetics in older people.[74] Total body water can be measured with a stable isotope dilution technique using ^{18}O, ^3H, and ^2H, and since all body water comprises approximately 73.2 percent FFM, both FFM and body fat can be estimated. Total body nitrogen measured by neutron activation analysis estimates total body protein because there is a fixed relationship between the mass of protein and that of nitrogen

Table 84-3 Weight, demispan, and derived ratios in elderly people: Nottingham Activity and Ageing Survey

Age range (yr)	Number	Weight (kg)[a]	Demispan (cm)[a]	Demiquet (kg/m²)[a]	Mindex (kg/m)[a]
Men					
65–74	205	72.5 ± 12.6 (39–114)	81.6 ± 4.05 (71.5–92.7)	108.8 ± 17.2 (68.6–162.6)	
75–91	153	68.6 ± 11.4 (43–94)	80.4 ± 4.1 (71.5–91.3)	106.0 ± 15.1 (72.0–153.6)	
Women					
65–74	257	64.5 ± 13.3 (35–124)	73.8 ± 3.6 (63.3–84.0)		87.3 ± 17.4 (49.9–168)
75–94	275	59.7 ± 11.6 (35–102)	72.7 ± 3.5 (64.2–84.8)		82.1 ± 15.2 (49.3–86.8)

[a]Mean values ± 1 standard deviation are shown in parentheses.

Data from Department of Health[52] and Lehmann et al.[67]

(1 g of N to 6.25 g of protein). Plethysmography estimates body volume without underwater weighing, the disadvantages of which were mentioned above. Differences in the electrical conductivity of fat and FFM allow the development of total body electric conductivity and bioelectric impedance as measures. Imaging techniques such as ultrasound, computed tomography (CT), and magnetic resonance imaging (MRI) are currently under review.[75–78] These more recently developed methods are still research tools and have not yet been validated in clinical practice.

Little information from older subjects is available, and many of the inherent assumptions regarding the use of anthropometry in older people have been challenged. The development of simple, noninvasive methods for measuring body composition in this age group would be an important advance.[72,79]

Clinical assessment

Clinically evident malnutrition represents the culmination of months or years of nutrient deficiency. Multiple pathology and nonspecific presentation of disease complicate the diagnosis of specific nutrient deficiencies which rarely exhibit pathognomonic features even in a younger population. A proper clinical (including social) history and examination will reveal the presence of risk factors for malnutrition.[21] Factors influencing nutritional status in older people are summarized as follows.

- *Acquisition of food*: poverty, immobility, social isolation, and choice may be limited by dietary traditions, by impaired appetite, taste, smell, vision, and hearing, and by inadequate cooking facilities.
- *Ingestion of food*: affected by dentition and oral health[80] as well as conditions such as dysphagia.
- *Digestion and absorption*: influenced by previous surgery (e.g. partial gastrectomy and malabsorption syndromes).
- *Utilization of nutrients and tissue requirements*: may vary with age, physical activity, drugs, and disease.

Physical examination should therefore note conditions that may affect individual ability to acquire, ingest, digest, absorb, and efficiently utilize nutrients, as well as physical signs arising as a consequence of poor nutrition. The factors predisposing to malnutrition and some clinical consequences are represented in Figure 84-4. Single indexes used in nutritional assessment, such as serum transferrin or delayed cutaneous hypersensitivity, have low sensitivity, specificity, and predictive value. Indexes based on a composite of several parameters such as prognostic nutritional index (PNI) and hospital prognostic index (HPI) have been used in some clinical settings. Subjective global assessment based on history and physical examination may be as effective.[49]

SPECIFIC NUTRIENTS

Tables 84-4 to 84-6 provide data from the National Diet and Nutrition Survey (NDNS, 1994/95) for macro- and micronutrient intake and status indicators for people aged 65 years or over.

Energy

Energy requirements, and thus the dietary intake needed to meet them, are determined by the level of energy expenditure. Total energy expenditure (TEE) is determined by basal metabolic rate (BMR) and physical activity (with a small contribution from thermogenesis). A decrease in the mass of metabolically active tissue and a reduction in physical activity result in a fall in TEE with increasing age.[81] Energy requirements may decrease by about a third between the ages of 30 and 80 years, mainly because of reduced physical activity, the moderate decline in BMR being a consequence of a decrease in total FFM.[82] There is no fall in BMR per kilogram FFM, and the interindividual variation in energy intake and expenditure seen earlier in life persists into old age.[83,84] Neuromuscular inefficiency with age[85] or disability[86] may increase the energy cost of apparently light physical activity, though adaptation may occur.[87] Declining energy expenditure may compromise adequate intake of nutrients, and maintaining an active lifestyle has other potential benefits for older individuals.[88]

Resting metabolic rate in the very old may not be lower than in younger old people, and differences in total energy expenditure are likely to be due to much reduced physical activity.[89] Malnutrition and a negative energy balance are common in hospitalized older people[90–92] in comparison with healthy older people.[19] The coexistence of low intake and increased BMR, such as may occur with surgery, acute infection, and disability producing mechanical inefficiency in activities of daily living, contribute to the vulnerability of the hospital patient.

Protein

Total body protein in LBM declines with age, and the rates of protein synthesis, turnover, and degradation decrease.[93–95] Utilization of protein and homeostatic mechanisms such as increased albumin synthesis with adequate dietary protein intake may also be inefficient.[96,97] The equilibrium between protein synthesis and degradation may be affected by illness, sepsis, trauma, and immobility.[95,98,99] Protein malnutrition impairs cellular and humoral immunity.[100]

The decline in functional capacity and muscle strength in old age may be largely attributable to age-related changes in body composition but is not irreversible, and physical training may produce profound improvement in strength as well as increased protein requirement.[101] Skeletal muscle protein (somatic protein) and visceral protein (blood cells, serum proteins, and solid organs such as heart and liver) comprise the metabolically available protein. Noncellular structural proteins (e.g. cartilage) in skeletal tissue are not metabolically available. Total body nitrogen and potassium are measures of whole-body protein; anthropometric indexes (see above) and creatinine and 3-methylhistidine excretion can indicate changes in somatic (skeletal muscle) protein. Visceral protein status is estimated from serum levels of albumin, transferrin, thyroxine binding prealbumin (TBPA), and retinol binding protein (RBP) which are all of hepatic origin. Serum TBPA and RBP levels are most reliable for monitoring short-term changes in visceral protein status during recovery from acute illness since they have a relatively smaller body pool, have a shorter half-life, and are less confounded by the often coexistent problems of sepsis, stress, and dehydration than are albumin and

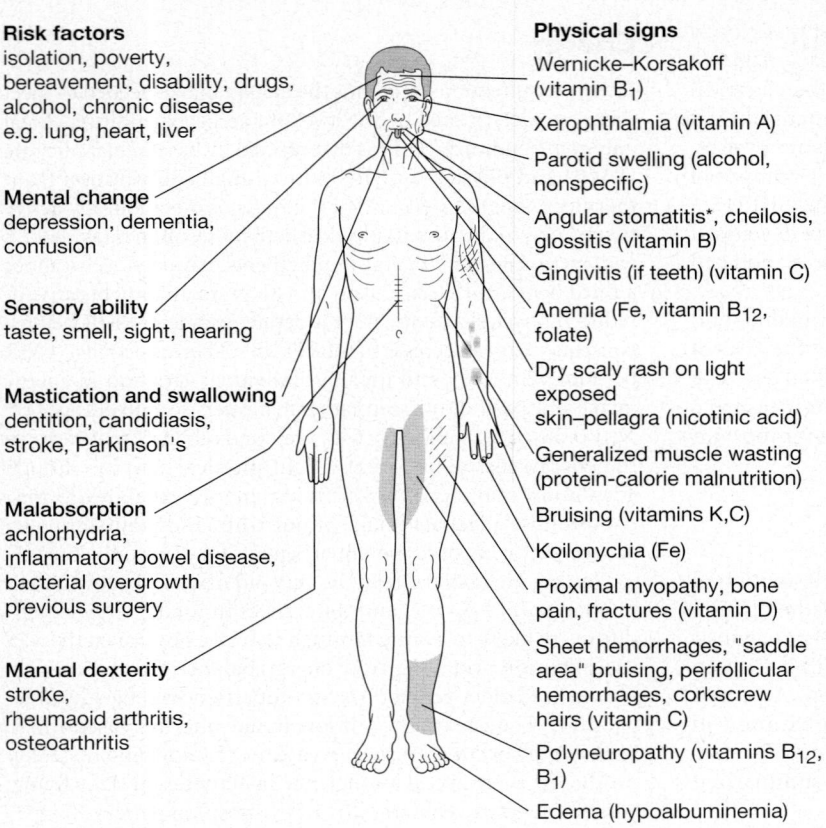

Risk factors
isolation, poverty, bereavement, disability, drugs, alcohol, chronic disease e.g. lung, heart, liver

Mental change
depression, dementia, confusion

Sensory ability
taste, smell, sight, hearing

Mastication and swallowing
dentition, candidiasis, stroke, Parkinson's

Malabsorption
achlorhydria, inflammatory bowel disease, bacterial overgrowth previous surgery

Manual dexterity
stroke, rheumaoid arthritis, osteoarthritis

Physical signs
Wernicke–Korsakoff (vitamin B_1)

Xerophthalmia (vitamin A)

Parotid swelling (alcohol, nonspecific)

Angular stomatitis*, cheilosis, glossitis (vitamin B)

Gingivitis (if teeth) (vitamin C)

Anemia (Fe, vitamin B_{12}, folate)

Dry scaly rash on light exposed skin–pellagra (nicotinic acid)

Generalized muscle wasting (protein-calorie malnutrition)

Bruising (vitamins K,C)

Koilonychia (Fe)

Proximal myopathy, bone pain, fractures (vitamin D)

Sheet hemorrhages, "saddle area" bruising, perifollicular hemorrhages, corkscrew hairs (vitamin C)

Polyneuropathy (vitamins B_{12}, B_1)

Edema (hypoalbuminemia)

Figure 84-4 Clinical assessment of nutritional status. Parentheses indicate associated nutrient deficiency. Ill-fitting dentures are the most common cause of angular stomatitis(*).

Table 84-4 National Diet and Nutrition Survey, UK: Average daily macronutrient intake in adults aged 65+ years

	Free-living		Institutionalized	
	M	**F**	**M**	**F**
Energy (MJ)	8.02	5.98	8.14	6.94
Protein (g)	71.5	56	66.5	56.7
Total CHO (g)	232	175	256	222
Total sugar	103	79	131	118
Starch	129	96	125	104
NSP	13.5	11	11	9.5
Total fat	74.7	58	76.9	65.5
Saturated fat (%)	14.6	15.3	15.2	15.4

Abbreviations: M, male; F, female; CHO, carbohydrate; NSP, nonstarch polysaccharides.

Source: OPCS (1998),[22] with permission.

Table 84-5 National Diet and Nutrition Survey, UK: Average daily vitamin intake in adults aged 65+ years

	Free-living		Institutionalized	
	M	**F**	**M**	**F**
Vitamin A (μg)	1173	969	1054	962
Thiamin (mg)	1.49	1.19	1.34	1.14
Riboflavin (mg)	1.74	1.43	1.8	1.62
Niacin (eq. u)	32	24.8	27.3	23.3
Vitamin B_6 (mg)	2.1	1.6	1.9	1.6
Vitamin B12 (μg)	6.1	4.5	4.9	4.6
Folate	270	207	235	197
Vitamin C (mg)	66.9	60.7	49.6	47.6
Vitamin D (μg)	4.07	2.92	3.79	3.31
Vitamin E (mg)	9	6.8	7.8	6.6

Abbreviations: M, male; F, female.

Source: OPCS (1998),[22] with permission.

transferrin.[49] Nitrogen balance is an example of one metabolic index of body protein, and muscle strength has been used as a functional measure—though handgrip dynamometry used to measure muscle strength has obvious problems in an older population with a high prevalence of joint disease. Immunological tests such as delayed cutaneous hypersensitivity and T-lymphocyte count are affected by protein malnutrition but, as already noted, are of low sensitivity and specificity as functional indexes.

Nitrogen balance studies have been the traditional method of estimating protein requirements, and metabolic equilibrium for protein in elderly people has been observed with daily intakes of between 0.59 and 0.80 g/kg body weight,[102,103] though 0.80 g daily was found inadequate by others.[97] Healthy elderly people living at home in the UK and eating a self-selected diet were in equilibrium with daily intakes equivalent to 0.97 g/kg body weight.[19] Hospitalized elderly patients studied by the

Table 84-6 National Diet and Nutrition Survey, UK: Average daily mineral intake in adults aged 65+ years

	Free-living		Institutionalized	
	M	F	M	F
Iron (mg)	11	8.6	9.6	8.2
Calcium (mg)	836	690	953	861
Phosphorus (mg)	1237	989	1199	1055
Magnesium (mg)	254	197	215	188
Sodium (mg)	2695	2053	2714	2207
Potassium (mg)	2715	2207	2426	2141
Zinc (mg)	8.8	6.9	8.4	7.1
Copper (mg)	1.12	0.87	0.94	0.84

Abbreviations: M, male; F, female.

Source: OPCS (1998),[22] with permission.

same methods had inadequate energy and protein intakes.[90] Current DRVs are shown in Table 84-1 and agree with the WHO/FAO/UNU recommendation of not less than 0.75 g of good-quality protein per kilogram body weight per day. However, these recommendations have been challenged with more recent work suggesting that a safe daily protein intake for older people is 1.0–1.25 g/kg body weight.[104,105] Mean daily protein intakes in the NDNS appeared satisfactory (Table 84-4).

In recent years the model for protein metabolism has undergone a conceptual re-evaluation, and it is proposed that dietary amino acids not only function as a substrate for protein synthesis but also have a regulatory role, exerting an anabolic drive.[106] Isotopic studies on amino acid oxidation are prompting reassessment of current recommendations for protein adequacy as well as enabling organ-specific measures of protein turnover.[107,108] Understanding demand, adaptation, and nutrient–nutrient interactions in amino acid metabolism will define protein requirement in growth, aging, health, and disease.[109]

Fats

The essential fatty acids are linoleic and α-linoleic acid, which are components of phospholipids and thus important in maintaining the structure and function of cell membranes. Adult Western diets provide 8–15 g per day, and adipose tissue provides a reserve of 500–1,000 g. Clinical deficiency is rare but has been reported in adults with small bowel failure due to surgery or disease receiving inadequate nutritional therapy. Current recommendations are that intake of linoleic acid be at least 1 percent of total food energy, and of α-linoleic acid at least 0.2 percent.[48]

LIPID PEROXIDATION, FREE RADICALS, AND ANTI-OXIDANTS Highly reactive oxygen-derived species such as hydrogen peroxide and the free radicals (superoxide and hydroxyl are examples) produced in the course of normal metabolism may cause oxidation, and iron is one catalyst of the damage. Naturally occurring antioxidants either prevent

free radical formation (such as iron chelators) or scavenge free radicals (such as superoxide dismutase and vitamins A and C). The selenium-dependent enzyme glutathione peroxidase converts lipid peroxides to fatty acids. There is a balance between free radical and antioxidant activity in healthy tissue. Free-radical damage has been implicated in normal aging[110] and in the pathology of chronic degenerative disease and is thought to be a primary cause of tissue ischemia or reoxygenation injury. Lipid peroxidation may sometimes be a sequel to tissue damage mediated by another pathology.[111]

It is not yet clear how dietary intake of antioxidants affects antioxidant status. Supplementation studies have not suggested a consistent effect on mortality from cardiovascular disease or cancer and re-emphasize the importance of complementing observational and epidemiological studies with clinical trials and empirical research.[112]

Insofar as dietary fat is considered, COMA recommend that saturated fat should provide an average of 10 percent of the population's total dietary intake. Despite recent concerns, there is no clear evidence that a higher intake of polyunsaturated fatty acid (PUFA) contributes to human disease, but the current COMA recommendation is that PUFA should constitute not more than 10 percent total food intake.[48] The biological effects of isomeric fatty acids are unclear, and the current recommendation is that daily intake should not exceed 5 g, or 2 percent of dietary energy.[48]

The major environmental risk factors for coronary heart disease (CHD) are smoking, hypertension, and serum cholesterol. International differences in mortality from CHD relate to dietary fat intake and correlate most strongly with saturated fat intake which in turn correlates with serum cholesterol. Contrary to earlier beliefs, serum cholesterol level remains predictive of mortality from CHD in elderly people, justifying the recommendation that "older people adopt a diet that moderates their serum cholesterol."[52] Since long-chain fatty acids may reduce thrombogenicity and there are some clinical and epidemiological data suggesting a possible cardioprotective effect of a higher intake of n-3 fatty acid, it has also been suggested that older people should eat more oily fish.[52]

Intakes of saturated fat in the NDNS study were well in excess of the COMA recommendation (Table 84-4).

Carbohydrates (sugars and complex carbohydrates)

Sugars

Glucose, fructose, and galactose (monosaccharides) and sucrose, lactose, and maltose (disaccharides) are soluble carbohydrates (sugars) and a valuable source of energy. Classified according to their metabolic availability, intrinsic sugars are those naturally integrated into the cellular structure of food, and extrinsic sugars are those that are free in food or added to it. Extrinsic sugars comprise milk sugars found in milk and milk products (e.g. lactose) and nonmilk sugars (e.g. honey, fruit juices, added sugar). The COMA panel on dietary sugars[113] recommended a reduction in the intake of nonmilk extrinsic sugars, noting the association with dental caries and (at intakes above 30 percent of total food energy) adverse metabolic responses. Average daily intake of extrinsic sugars by institutionalized older people in the NDNS study (mainly from table sugar and sweet spreads and preserves) was approximately 18 percent of daily food energy intake, and correlated with root decay.[22]

Older people probably consume more nonmilk extrinsic sugar than younger ones, and though edentulousness increases with age, remaining teeth are important and abnormal metabolic responses to a sucrose load more common.[52] As the quantity of food eaten falls with age, the quality is all the more important, and consumption of large amounts of sugar may threaten the adequacy of the diet overall. Nutrient density expresses the nutrient content of food as a ratio of the energy content and is a helpful index of dietary quality.

Complex carbohydrates

Dietary polysaccharides comprise starches (long-chain or branched α-glucan polysaccharides) and nonstarch polysaccharides (nondigestible and nonabsorbable plant cell-wall carbohydrates). The latter represent the majority of what was previously described as "dietary fiber," a term now considered obsolete because of imprecision in definition and analysis.[48]

STARCHES Cereals and cereal products contributed approximately 70 percent of total starch intake, with vegetables, including potatoes accounting for approximately 20 percent in the recent NDNS. Current recommendations for adults, which are probably equally beneficial for older individuals, suggest that starches and intrinsic and milk sugars should contribute 37 percent of the total dietary energy for the population.[113]

NONSTARCH POLYSACCHARIDES Increasing daily dietary intake of nonstarch polysaccharides from 12 g to 18 g benefits older people in the prevention of constipation, diverticular disease, and colonic cancer, though other potential benefits are not yet proven.[52] The NDNS revealed lower levels of intake in both free-living and institutionalized older people (Table 84-4). The consumption of large amounts of raw bran can reduce bioavailability of essential minerals such as iron, calcium, zinc, and copper because phytate binds to divalent mineral cations.

Vitamins

Table 84-2 summarizes the metabolic role, features of clinical deficiency states, and reference nutrient intakes for vitamins A, B_1 (thiamin), B_2 (riboflavin), niacin, B_6 (pyridoxine), B_{12}, folic acid, C (ascorbic acid), D, and E. Detailed discussions of measures of status,[49] deficiency states,[114] and illustrations of clinical signs[115] can be found in other texts. Clinical deficiencies of vitamins D and C, folic acid, and vitamins B_{12} and B_1 are seen in older people, particularly in institutions,[116] but are rare or undefined for the other vitamins. Metabolic evidence of vitamin deficiencies may be seen with normal serum levels.[117] Comparison of the UK and US literature should be made with the knowledge that the use of vitamin supplements is more common in the USA, though the NDNS showed that approximately a third of people aged 65 years or over take nonprescribed dietary supplements.

VITAMIN A AND VITAMIN E Average intakes of vitamins A and E were above the RNI and minimum safe level, respectively, though about one in twenty free-living older people had intakes below the LRNI for vitamin A. The mean dietary ratio of α-tocopherol to PUFA was above the minimum safe level recommended for American diets.[22] Statutory fortification of yellow fats other than butter is endorsed since it provides an additional source of intake from a group of foods favored by elderly people.[52] Since deficiencies of vitamins A and E are rare in the Western world, and there is no substantial literature relating to older people, no further discussion is presented here except to observe that, with increasing interest in the antioxidant role of these two vitamins, toxicity may occur at doses which are 10 times the recommended intake for vitamin A.

VITAMIN B_1 (THIAMIN) The mean thiamin intake for elderly men and women in the recent NDNS appeared adequate, though intakes have been lower than for the adult population aged 16–64 years.[21,22] Fortified cereals are an important source,[118] and thiamin intakes have increased since the 1972/73 study possibly because of increased fortification of breakfast cereals.[22] Thiamin intake is closely related to dietary energy intake, and assessment of biochemical adequacy is limited. Thiamin intake may become inadequate if energy intake falls in ill institutionalized older people,[119–121] and it was suggested that confusional states in older orthopedic patients might be partly attributable to poor thiamin status.[122] Between 10 and 15 percent of the NDNS sample had poor biochemical thiamin status.[22] Thiamin deficiency does not appear common in elderly patients with cardiac failure.[123] Interactions occur between thiamin and other B vitamins, as well as with drugs. Alcohol abuse is associated with thiamin deficiency and the clinical syndromes of Korsakoff's psychosis (short-term memory loss, confabulation) and Wernicke's encephalopathy (acute confusion, ophthalmoplegia, and ataxia).

VITAMIN B_2 (RIBOFLAVIN) Dietary intake levels of riboflavin in the NDNS were in keeping with current recommendations.[48] Although some indication of biochemical insufficiency was found in previous studies,[21,119] and in 40 percent of the NDNS sample, the relationship between vitamin intake and biochemical status is complex,[124] and inadequate riboflavin status is probably not a common problem for elderly people.[93]

NIACIN Pellagra is the clinical syndrome of niacin deficiency and is rare in the Western world. Adequate protein intake usually ensures adequate niacin intake, and flour is fortified with niacin. Intakes appeared adequate in the NDNS.[22] No functional measure of niacin status exists.

VITAMIN B_6 Plasma levels of pyridoxal phosphate (PLP) fall with age, but the activity of erythrocyte aspartate aminotransferase (for which PLP is a coenzyme) does not. While there may be a higher absolute requirement in elderly subjects,[126] COMA found that there was no evidence supporting a higher recommended intake[48] and intakes appeared adequate in the NDNS.

VITAMIN B_{12} Dietary inadequacy is relatively rare, and deficiency is more commonly caused by absorption dysfunction, whether due to pernicious anemia and absence of the specific binding protein gastric intrinsic factor or to small intestinal malabsorption secondary to disease, surgery, or bacterial overgrowth. Vitamin B_{12} absorption does not decline with age,[127] and healthy older populations in general do not seem to have lower serum vitamin B_{12} levels than younger groups.[128] However, 6 percent of free-living and 9 percent of institutionalized older people in the NDNS had vitamin B_{12} serum levels below 118 pmol/L (i.e. subnormal) and 4 percent of the institutionalized had levels below 90 pmol/L.[22] Vitamin B_{12} deficiency may appear as macrocytic anemia or subacute combined degeneration of the cord, but current diagnostic methods are insensitive indexes of status and atypical presentation in older people may lead to important delays in diagnosis and treatment.[129] Microbiological methods and radioassay are the most commonly used techniques.

FOLIC ACID Folic acid is destroyed by prolonged cooking, and the dietary lifestyle of some disabled or ill older people may not allow a sufficient intake of folate-rich foods. Malabsorption can occur, as in the case of vitamin B_{12}. Serum folate levels reflect recent dietary intake, and erythrocyte levels reflect tissue status. Metabolism of vitamin B_{12} and of folate are interrelated,[130] and since vitamin B_{12} deficiency can result in low erythrocyte folate levels, it is important to measure both serum and erythrocyte folate levels. Metabolic consequences of folate deficiency in advance of macrocytic anemia are indicated by abnormal deoxyuridine suppression tests on bone marrow and peripheral blood lymphocytes.[49] Borderline erythrocyte folate levels were seen in a fifth of the healthy older people studied in the 1972/73 study, and 1 in 20 had subnormal levels. In the NDNS, 16 percent of the institutionalized group had levels of red cell folate below 230 nmol/L. Dietary folate deficiency is not considered a major factor in anemia in healthy elderly people, but it may be important in people who abuse alcohol, in the prescription of certain drugs (e.g. phenytoin), or in hospitalization.[131]

VITAMIN C Vitamin C is a water-soluble antioxidant which is rapidly oxidized with prolonged heating. Over 20 years ago it was reported that hot food provided in the UK by Meals on Wheels lost over 90 percent of its vitamin C content before delivery,[132] and foods high in vitamin C content often require preparation and chewing, thus making them relatively less accessible for some older people. In the 1972/73 UK study, mean daily intake of vitamin C was at the level of the RNI, with 2 percent of men and 6 percent of women eating less than the LRNI of 10 mg, and there were three cases of frank scurvy in this community-based study. In the USA intakes were higher, reflecting the more widespread use of supplements,[133] and vitamin C intake in the older population in the UK has increased substantially.[22] Patients in continuing-care settings are vulnerable,[134] with 40 percent of the institutionalized study population in the NDNS having biochemical vitamin C deficiency. Chronic marginal vitamin C status may have quite different pathophysiological effects on acute severe deficiency.[135] Vitamin C intake has been related to cognitive impairment, atherogenesis,[136] and death from stroke;[137] and serum ascorbate levels have been shown to have a strong inverse correlation with plasma fibrinogen and factor VIIC, providing support for the suggestion that a high intake of vitamin C may be cardioprotective.[138]

VITAMIN D Vitamin D_3 (cholecalciferol) is synthesized in the skin by the action of sunlight (ultraviolet radiation of wavelength 290–310 nm) on 7-dehydrocholesterol and converted in the liver to 25-hydroxyvitamin D (25OHD). This compound is then further hydroxylated in the kidney to 1,25-dihydroxyvitamin D (1,25[OH]$_2$D), the active form of the vitamin which promotes intestinal calcium and phosphate absorption and ensures adequate bone mineralization via its effects on bone resorption and renal reabsorption of calcium and phosphate. Dietary sources of vitamin D include eggs and margarine and oily fish. Vitamin D_3 from the skin is the major source of the vitamin in UK adults, with diet contributing an approximate average of 3 µg daily (DRV). Solar radiation varies with season, latitude, and time of day. Limited skin exposure makes dietary contribution relatively more important, and older people, particularly those who are institutionalized and housebound, are vulnerable to subclinical and clinical vitamin D deficiency. Malabsorption, gastric surgery, anticonvulsant therapy, and hepatic disease can compromise vitamin D status. Levels of 25OHD$_3$ reflect vitamin D status[13] and decline with age,[139] probably reflecting less exposure to the sun. Levels of 25OHD below 10 nmol/L (4.1 ng/mL) (with an associated rise in parathormone levels) are seen in osteomalacia. Plasma 25OHD levels are maintained above the level associated with osteomalacia when daily dietary intake is 5–10 µg in the absence of skin synthesis of the vitamin.[140] Seasonal post-menopausal bone loss can be favorably influenced by vitamin D supplementation.[141] The COMA recommendation that elderly people seek some exposure to sunlight from May to September is complemented by advice to provide supplements ensuring a total daily intake of 10 µg of vitamin D for homebound or institutionalized individuals.[48,52] European work supported this concept, indicating that older people were at substantial risk of vitamin D deficiency,[142] and the NDNS found biochemical vitamin D deficiency in over one-third of the institutionalized older people studied.[22]

Minerals

Calcium

Ninety-nine percent of body calcium is found as a vital structural component of bone, and the remaining 1 percent is found in tissues and serum involved with enzyme activity, blood clotting, and the expression of hormonal effects via cyclic adenosine monophosphate. Milk is an important source of dietary calcium, particularly in older people, and the recognition that milk consumption in this age group is falling has led to the recommendation that doorstep deliveries of milk should continue.[52] Intestinal absorption of calcium declines with age,[143,144] probably partly as a consequence of vitamin D status[145–147] since this is the major factor controlling calcium absorption. Phytate, oxalates, and fiber also reduce calcium absorption, and bioavailability must be taken into account when assessing adequacy of calcium in the diet, though intakes in the older population seem to meet current recommendations.[22] Aging is accompanied by reduced ability to adapt to low calcium intake.[148]

The current RNI for daily calcium intake is 17.5 mmol (700 mg) for all adults over 50 years of age, assuming a mean intestinal absorption of 30 percent, but it is recognized that the data on which this recommendation is based are particularly sparse for people over 60 years of age.[48,149] Elderly subjects in the community were found to be in metabolic equilibrium with an intake of 25 mmol (1000 mg) daily,[19] and calcium requirements determined by metabolic balance may rise to as much as 37 mmol (1480 mg) daily perimenopausally.[150] There is no convenient biochemical test for estimating calcium status; serum calcium concentrations are homeostatically tightly controlled, and serum ionized calcium levels are not widely available. Measurement of bone mineral mass by absorptiometry or imaging techniques indicates body calcium stores.

Hypocalcemia may result in cardiac arrhythmias and neuromuscular dysfunction. Adequate dietary calcium intake is important in the achievement of peak adult bone mass,[151] but the relevance of calcium in the diet to the development of osteoporosis in later life and the place of dietary calcium supplements in the management of osteoporosis remain unclear.[152–156]

Magnesium

Mean national daily intake magnesium in free-living men in the NDNS accords with the level at which balance was seen in a healthy elderly group, though the average intake in women in this group was below 200 mg/day—somewhat lower than in a previous study.[19,22,157] Dietary magnesium deficiency is rare, and malabsorption due to surgery or gut dysfunction or increased losses, such as occur with diuretic therapy,[158,159] are a more common cause of a clinical deficiency. Magnesium deficiency may occur in alcoholism and congestive cardiac failure, and physical signs of deficiency include muscle weakness, cardiac arrhythmias, and neurological signs such as muscle fasciculation, spasm, and fits. Serum magnesium levels are of low specificity and sensitivity but may be a guide to magnesium status in clinical practice, though leucocyte and muscle magnesium levels are probably a better reflection of total body status.[49] Older people may be vulnerable to deficiencies because of the coincidence of poor diet, disease, and drug treatment. Between 20 and 25 percent of free-living older people and nearly 40 percent of those living in institutions were taking diuretics.[22]

Sodium

The UK RNI for sodium is 70 mmol (4 g), and average daily intakes for adults in the UK are 9 g, well above current WHO guidelines for population intakes. Debate continues regarding the dietary guideline for sodium intake.[160,161] Hypertension is related to dietary salt intake,[128] and convenience foods have a high salt content. It is recommended that elderly people should follow the same guidelines as other adults in reducing their level of salt consumption.[52] Eighty-five percent of free-living older people taking part in the NDNS study added salt to food in cooking, and approximately half of the men and a quarter of the women also added salt at the table.[22]

Iron

Heme iron in the diet is better absorbed than nonheme iron, and vitamin C enhances absorption. Cereals and meat are important dietary sources in the UK. Achlorhydria and previous gastric surgery may reduce dietary iron absorption, and bioavailability may be lower with diets containing complex carbohydrates, phytate, or even tannins in tea.[48] Gut mucosal absorption of iron is responsive to body iron status, and different mechanisms may operate in the iron-sufficient and iron-deficient states.[163,164] Advancing age is associated with reduced iron absorption[165] and inefficient tissue utilization of iron, perhaps as a result of ineffective erythropoiesis or increased hepatic retention of iron.[166] The DRV of iron for men and women over 50 years of age (daily EAR and RNI = 120 μmol and 160 μmol) is the same as for younger men; older women may have depleted iron stores from their pre-menopausal years, and recent work suggests that this age group may be iron-replete.[167] Hospitalized and homebound older people, particularly women, may have low intakes compared to free-living healthy subjects even with comparable dietary iron densities.[133] The NDNS reported biochemical iron deficiency in 30–40 percent of institutionalized older subjects.

The hypochromic microcytic anemia of iron deficiency is the best recognized of any micronutrient deficiency, but iron deficiency can result in other less well-defined effects such as muscle dysfunction, tiredness, impaired cellular immunity, and abnormalities in catecholamine metabolism.[134] Progressive changes in the indexes of iron status in the development of deficiency begin with depletion of storage iron manifested by low serum ferritin levels, but with normal hemoglobin and transport iron levels indicated by normal transferrin saturation. Later, iron-deficient erythropoiesis is seen, accompanied by a decrease in transferrin saturation. Last, frank iron deficiency anemia occurs.[135] Serum ferritin is the most sensitive index of early iron deficiency but may be raised in chronic inflammation. Simultaneous measurement of iron binding capacity reveals a low level of transferrin saturation, and thus it may be important in some circumstances to use two or more indexes of iron status. Iron deficiency without anemia may be a common but unrecognized problem in homebound older women and hospitalized older people.[133] Gastrointestinal blood loss is a major cause of iron deficiency in hospitalized elderly people[136] and is often due to a remediable pathology,[137] justifying a careful evaluation before attributing anemia to dietary deficiency. In the NDNS study about half of the institutionalized men and a third of the women had hemoglobin levels below 13 g/dL and 12 g/dL, respectively; one tenth had low ferritin levels.[22]

Zinc

Zinc is essential for the function of major metabolic pathways because it is involved in many enzymatic reactions, in maintaining the integrity of biomembranes, and in DNA and RNA synthesis. Zinc deficiency in the adult can cause hypoguesia (reduced or abnormal taste), neuropsychiatric symptoms, dermatitis, and impaired cellular immunity. Deficiency may be seen in clinical practice as a complication of other conditions such as alcoholic liver disease and inflammatory bowel disease. The daily RNI for zinc (145 μmol for men and 110 μmol for women aged 50+ years) is similar to that of iron (160 μmol) but clinical deficiency is rarely recognized, perhaps partly because of difficulties with biochemical assessment (serum levels are of low specificity and sensitivity) and poorly defined symptoms and signs.[49] Institutionalized older people are at risk of zinc deficiency;[90,173] plasma zinc levels below 10 μmol/L were seen in 15 percent of institutionalized men and in 7 percent of the women in the NDNS study.[22] Supplementation in a proven state of zinc deficiency improves wound healing, but indiscriminate use of zinc supplements may produce adverse effects such as gastritis.[52]

KEY POINTS Nutrition

- Elderly people are at risk of malnutrition for many reasons.

- Ill-health, disability, and institutionalization compound the problems.

- Differences in assessment methods and outcome measures make comparisons between studies difficult.

- Malnutrition is seen in 15–40 percent of hospitalized patients in the UK.

- Nutritional supplementation may improve indices, but the effect on clinical outcome is unclear.

REFERENCES

1. UK Department of Health: The Health of the Nation. Nutrition: Core Curriculum for Nutrition in the Education of Health Professionals. HMSO, London, 1994

2. Garrow J: Starvation in hospital. BMJ 1994;308:934

3. Lo C: Integrating nutrition as a theme throughout the medical school curriculum. Am J Clin Nutr 2000;72(suppl):882S–889S

4. McWhirter JP, Pennington CR: Incidence and recognition of malnutrition in hospital. BMJ 1994;308:945–948

5. Bender AE: Institutional malnutrition. BMJ 1984;288:92–93

6. Kelly IE, Tessier S, Cahill A et al: Still hungry in hospital: identifying malnutrition in acute hospital admissions. QJM 2000;93:91–98

7. Elia M, Stratton RJ: How much undernutrition is there in hospitals? Br J Nutr 2000;84:257–259

8. Corish CA, Kennedy NP: Protein-energy undernutrition in hospital inpatients. Br J Nutr 2000;83:575–591

9. Corish CA, Flood P, Mulligan S, Kennedy NP: Apparent low frequency of undernutrition in Dublin hospital inpatients: should we review the anthropometric thresholds for clinical practice? Br J Nutr 2000;84:325–335

10. Lennard-Jones JE: Giving or withholding fluid and nutrients: ethical and legal aspects. J R Coll Physicians 1999;33:39–45

11. Potter J, Langhorne P, Roberts M: Routine protein energy supplementation in adults: systematic review. BMJ 1998;317:495–501

12. Young VR, Adjami AM: Metabolism 2000: the emperor needs new clothes. Proc Nutr Soc 2001;60:27–44

13. Dauncey MJ, White P, Burton KA et al: Nutrition–hormone receptor–gene interactions: implications for development and disease. Proc Nutr Soc 2001;60:63–72

14. Khaw K-T: How many, how old, how soon? BMJ 1999;319:1350–1352

15. UK Office of Population Censuses and Surveys: Family Expenditure Survey 1999–2000. HMSO, London, 2000

16. The Medical Research Council Cognitive Function and Ageing Study (MRC CFAS): Health and ill-health in the older population in England and Wales. Age Ageing 2001;30:53–62

17. UK Office of Population Censuses and Surveys: Living in Britain: Results from the 1994 General Household Survey. HMSO, London, 1996

18. Exton-Smith AN, Stanton BK, Windsor ACM: Nutrition of Housebound Old People. King Edward's Hospital Fund, London, 1972

19. Bunker VW, Clayton BE: Research review: studies in the nutrition of elderly people with particular relevance to essential trace elements. Age Ageing 1989;18:422–429

20. UK Office of Population Census and Surveys: Living in Britain: Results from the 1998 General Household Survey. HMSO, London, 1999

21. UK Department of Health and Social Services: Nutrition and Health in Old Age: Report on Health and Social Subjects. HMSO, London, 1979

22. UK Office of Population Census and Surveys: The National Diet and Nutrition Survey: People Aged 65 Years and Over. HMSO, London, 1998

23. Bates, CJ, Prentice A, Cole TJ et al: Micronutrients: highlights and research challenge from the 1994–5 National Diet and Nutrition Survey of people aged 65 years and over. Br J Nutr 1999;82:7–15

24. SENECA: Nutrition and the elderly in Europe. Eur J Clin Nutr 1991;45(suppl 3):1–196

25. Barker DJP: Fetal origins of coronary heart disease. BMJ 1995;312:171–174

26. Barker DPJ, Osmond C, Winter PD et al: Weight in infancy and death from ischaemic heart disease. Lancet 1989;ii:577–580

27. Leon DA, Koupilova I, Lithell HO et al: Failure to realise growth potential in utero and adult obesity in relation to blood pressure in 50 yr old Swedish men. BMJ 1996;312:401–441

28. Robinson R: The fetal origins of adult disease. BMJ 2001;322:375–376

29. Gubitz G, Sandercock P: Prevention of ischaemic stroke. BMJ 2000;321:1455–1459

30. Stampfer MJ, Hu FB, Manson JA et al: Primary prevention of coronary heart disease in women through diet and lifestyle. N Engl J Med 2000;343:16–22

31. Gariballa SE: Nutritional factors in stroke. Br J Nutr 2000;84:5–17

32. Bath PMW, Bath FJ, Smithard DG: Interventions for dysphagia in acute stroke. The Cochrane Library, issue 1, 2001

33. Anderson JJB: The important role of physical activity in skeletal development: how exercise may counter low calcium intake. Am J Clin Nutr 2000;71:1384–1386

34. Rapuri PB, Gallagher JC, Balhorn KE et al: Alcohol intake and bone metabolism in elderly women. Am J Clin Nutr 2000;72:1206–1213

35. Olson RE: Osteoporosis and vitamin K intake. Am J Clin Nutr 2000;71:1031–1032

36. Wortsman J, Matsuoka LY, Chen TC et al: Decreased bioavailability of vitamin D in obesity. Am J Clin Nutr 2000;72:690–693

37. Nordin BEC: Calcium requirement is a sliding scale. Am J Clin Nutr 2000;71:1381–1383

38. Prentice A: The relative contribution of diet and genotype to bone development. Proc Nutr Soc 2001;60:45–52

39. Gillespie WJ, Avenell A, Henry DA et al: Vitamin D and vitamin D analogues for preventing fractures associated with involutional and post-menopausal osteoporosis. The Cochrane Library, issue 1, 2001

40. Avendoll A, Handoll HHG: Nutritional supplementation for hip fracture aftercare in the elderly. The Cochrane Library, issue 1, 2001

41. Poehlmann ET, Dvorak RV: Energy expenditure, energy intake and weight loss in Alzheimer disease. Am J Clin Nutr 2000;71(suppl):650S–655S

42. Selhub J, Bagley LC, Miller J et al: B vitamins, homocysteine, and neurocognitive function in the elderly. Am J Clin Nutr 2000;71(suppl):614S–620S

43. Gillette-Guyonnet S, Nourhashemi F, Andrieu S et al: Weight loss in Alzheimer disease. Am J Clin Nutr 2000;71(suppl):637S–642S

44. Ezzell L, Jensen GL: Malnutrition in chronic obstructive pulmonary disease. Am J Clin Nutr 2000;72:1415–1416

45. Ferreira IM, Brooks D, Lacasse Y et al: Nutritional supplementation for stable chronic obstructive pulmonary disease. The Cochrane Library, issue 1, 2001

46. Evans JR, Henshaw K: Antioxidant vitamin and mineral supplementation for preventing age-related macular degeneration. The Cochrane Library, issue 1, 2001

47. Lesourd B, Mazari L: Nutrition and immunity in the elderly. Proc Nutr Soc 1999;58:685–695

48. UK Department of Health: Dietary Reference Values for Food Energy and Nutrients for the United Kingdom. Report on Health and Social Subjects 41. HMSO, London, 1991

49. Gibson RS: Principles of Nutritional Assessment. Oxford University Press, New York, 1990

50. Paul NA, Southgate DAT: McCance and Widdowson's The Composition of Foods, 4th edn. HMSO, London, 1985

51. Traber MG: The bioavailability bugaboo. Am J Clin Nutr 2000;71:1029–1030

52. UK Department of Health: The Nutrition of Elderly People: Report on Health and Social Subjects. HMSO, London, 1992

53. Micozzi MS, Albanes D, Jones Y, Chumlea WC: Correlations of body mass indices with weight, stature, and body composition in men and women in NHANES I and II. Am J Clin Nutr 1986;44:725–731

54. Durnin JVGA, Rahaman MM: The assessment of the amount of fat in the human body from measurements of skinfold thickness. Br J Nutr 1967;21:681–689

55. Jelliffe DB: The assessment of the nutritional status of the community (WHO monograph 53). World Health Organization, Geneva, 1966

56. Frisancho AR: Triceps skinfold and upper arm muscle size norms for assessment of nutritional status. Am J Clin Nutr 1974;27:1052–1058

57. Heymsfield SB, McManus C, Smith J et al: Anthropometric measurement of muscle mass: revised equations for calculating bone free arm muscle area. Am J Clin Nutr 1982;36:680–690

58. Delarue J, Constans T, Malvy D et al: Anthropometric values in an elderly French population. Br J Nutr 1994;71:295–302

59. Kemm JR, Allcock J: The distribution of supposed indicators of nutritional status in elderly patients. Age Ageing 1984;13:21–28

60. Burr ML, Phillips KM: Anthropometric norms in the elderly. Br J Nutr 1984;51:165–169

61. Freidman PJ, Campbell AJ, Caradoc-Davies TH: Prospective trial of a new diagnostic criterion for severe wasting malnutrition in the elderly. Age Ageing 1985;14:149–154

62. Mattila K, Haavisto M, Rajala S: Body mass index and mortality in the elderly. BMJ 1986;292:867–868

63. Campbell AJ, Spears GFS, Brown JS et al: Anthropometric measurements as predictors of mortality in a community population aged 70 years and over. Age Ageing 1990;19:131–135

64. Delmi M, Rapin CH, Bengoa JM et al: Dietary supplementation in elderly patients with fractured neck of the femur. Lancet 1990;335:1013–1016

65. Han TS, Lean MEJ: Lower leg length as an index of stature in adults. Int J Obesity 1996;20:21–27

66. Bassey EJ: Demispan as a measure of skeletal size. Ann Hum Biol 1986;13:499–502

67. Lehmann AB, Bassey EJ, Morgan K, Dalluso HM: Normal values for weight, skeletal size and body mass indices in 890 men and women aged over 65 years. Clin Nutr 1991;10:18–22

68. Smith WDF, Cunningham DA, Paterson DH, Koral JJ: Body mass indices and skeletal size in 394 Canadians aged 55–86 years. Ann Hum Biol 1995;22:305–314

69. Snead DB, Birge ST, Kohrt WM: Age related differences in body composition by hydrodensitometry and dual x-ray absorptiometry. J Appl Physiol 1993;74:770–775

70. Paolisso G, Gambardella A, Balbi V et al: Body composition, body fat distribution and resting metabolic rate in healthy centenarians. Am J Clin Nutr 1995;62:746–750

71. Durnin JVGA, Womersley J: Body fat assessment from total body density and its estimation from skinfold thickness measurement in 481 men and women aged 16–72 years. Br J Nutr 1974;32:77–92

72. Reilly JJ, Murray LA, Wilson J, Durnin JVGA: Measuring the body composition of elderly subjects. Br J Nutr 1994;72:33–44

73. Garrow JS: Indices of adiposity. Nutr Abstr Rev 1983;53:697–708

74. Fulop T, Worum I, Csongor J et al: Body composition in elderly people. Gerontology 1985;31:6–14

75. Lukaski HC: Methods for the assessment of human body composition: traditional and new. Am J Clin Nutr 1987;46:537–556

76. Fuller MF, Fowler PA, McNeill G, Foster MA: Body composition: the precision and accuracy of new methods and their suitability for longitudinal studies. Proc Nutr Soc 1990;49:423–436

77. Campbell IT, Watt T, Withers D et al: Muscle thickness, measured with ultrasound may be an indicator of lean tissue wasting in multiple organ failure in the presence of oedema. Am J Clin Nutr 1995;62:533–539

78. Houtkooper LB, Going SB, Sproul J et al: Comparison of methods for assessing body composition changes over 1 y in postmenopausal women. Am J Clin Nutr 2000;72:401–406

79. Bergsma-Kadijk JA, Baumeister B, Deurenberg P: Measurement of body fat in young and elderly women: comparison between a four compartment model and widely used reference methods. Br J Nutr 1996;75:649–657

80. Moynihan PJ: The relationship between diet, nutrition and dental health: an overview and update for the 90's. Nutr Res Rev 1995;8:193–224

81. Shock NW: Energy metabolism, caloric intake and physical activity in the aging. Symposia of the Swedish Nutrition Foundation. X: Nutrition in Old Age Swedish Nutrition Foundation. Uppsala, Sweden, 1972;12–23

82. McGandy KB, Barrows CH, Spanias A et al: Nutrient intake and energy expenditure in men of different ages. J Gerontol 1966;22:581–587

83. Durnin JVGA: Body composition and energy expenditure in elderly people. Bibl Nutr Dieta 1983;33:16–30

84. Prentice AM: Energy expenditure in the elderly. Eur J Clin Nutr 1992;46(suppl 3):521–528

85. Bassey EJ, Terry AM: The oxygen cost of walking in the elderly. J Physiol 1986;373:42P

86. Isakov E, Suzak Z, Becker E: Energy expenditure and cardiac responses in above knee amputees while using prostheses with open and locked knee mechanisms. Scand J Rehabil Med Suppl 1985;12:108–111

87. Didier JP, Mourey F, Brondel L et al: The energetic cost of some daily activities: a comparison in a young and old population. Age Ageing 1993;22:90–96

88. Fiatarone MA, O'Niell EF, Ryan ND et al: Exercise training and nutritional supplementation for physical frailty in very elderly people. N Engl J Med 1994;330:1769–1775

89. Rothenberg EM, Bosaeus IG, Westerturp KR et al: Resting energy expenditure, activity energy expenditure and total energy expenditure at age 91–96 years. Br J Nutr 2000;84:319–324

90. Thomas AJ, Bunker VW, Hinks LJ et al: Energy, protein, zinc and copper status of twenty-one elderly inpatients: analysed dietary intake and biochemical indices. Br J Nutr 1988;59:181–191

91. Roberts M, Reilly JJ, Klipstein K, Potter J: The nutritional status and clinical course of acute admissions to a geriatric unit. Age Ageing 1995;24:131–136

92. Klipstein-Grobusch, Reilly JJ, Potter J, Edwards CA, Roberts MA: Energy intake and expenditure in elderly patients admitted to hospital with acute illness. Br J Nutr 1995;73:323–334

93. Uauy R, Winterer JC, Bilmazes C et al: The changing pattern of whole body protein metabolism in aging humans. J Gerontol 1978;33:663–671

94. Golden MHN, Waterlow JC: Total protein synthesis in elderly people: a comparison of results with ^{15}N glycine and ^{14}C leucine. Clin Sci Mol Med 1977;53:277–288

95. Lehmann AB, NM Johnston C, James OFW: The effects of old age and immobility on protein turnover in human subjects with some observations on the possible role of hormones. Age Ageing 1989;18:148–157

96. World Health Organisation: Energy and Protein Requirements: Report of a Joint FAO/WHO/UNU Expert Consultation (WHO technical report series 724). WHO, Geneva, 1985

97. Gersovitz M, Motil K, Munro HN et al: Human protein requirements: assessment of the adequacy of the current recommended allowance for dietary protein in elderly men and women. Am J Clin Nutr 1982;35:6–14

98. Reeds PJ, James WPT: Protein turnover. Lancet 1983;i:571–574

99. Rennie M, Harrison R: Effect of injury, disease and malnutrition on protein metabolism in man: unanswered questions. Lancet 1984;i:323–325

100. Chandra RK: The relation between immunology, nutrition and disease in elderly people. Age Ageing 1990;19:S25–S31

101. Fielding RA: Effects of exercise training in the elderly: impact of progressive resistance training on skeletal muscle and whole-body protein metabolism. Proc Nutr Soc 1995;54:665–675

102. Uauy R, Scrimshaw NS, Young VR: Human protein requirements: nitrogen balance response to graded levels of egg protein in elderly men and women. Am J Clin Nutr 1978;31:779–785

103. Zanni E, Calloway DH, Zezulka AY: Protein requirements of elderly men. J Nutr 1979;109:513–524

104. Young VR: Amino acids and proteins in relation to the nutrition of elderly people. Age Ageing 1990;19:S10–S24

105. Campbell WW, Crim MC, Dallal GE et al: Increased protein requirement in elderly people: new data and retrospective reassessments. Am J Clin Nutr 1994;60:501–509

106. Millward DJ, Price GM, Pacy PJH, Halliday D: Maintenance protein requirement: the need for conceptual re-evaluation. Proc Nutr Soc 1990;49:473–487

107. Millward DJ, Price GM, Pacy PJH, Halliday D: Whole body protein and amino acid turnover in man: what can we measure with confidence? Proc Nutr Soc 1991;50:197–216

108. Garlick PJ, Wernerman J, McNurlan MA, Heys SD: Organ specific measurements of protein turnover in man. Proc Nutr Soc 1991;50:217–225

109. Jackson AA: Human protein requirement: policy issues. Proc Nutr Soc 2001;60:7–11

110. Meydani SN, Wu D, Santos MS, Heyck MG: Antioxidants and immune response in aged persons, an overview of present evidence. Am J Clin Nutr 1995;62:1462S–1476S

111. Halliwell B, Gutteridge JMC: Free Radicals in Biology and Medicine, 2nd edn. Clarendon Press, Oxford, 1989

112. Greenberg ER, Sporn MB: Antioxidant vitamins, cancer and cardiovascular disease. N Engl J Med 1996;334:1189–1190

113. UK Department of Health: Dietary Sugars and Human Disease: Report on Health and Social Subjects. HMSO, London, 1989

114. Thurnham DI: The interpretation of biochemical measurements of vitamin status in the elderly. In Kemm J, Ancill R (eds): Vitamin Deficiency in the Elderly. Blackwell, London, 1985;46–67

115. McLaren DS: A Colour Atlas of Nutritional Disorders. Wolfe Medical, London, 1981

116. Baker H, Frank O, Thind IS et al: Vitamin profiles in elderly persons living at home or in nursing homes versus profile in healthy young subjects. J Am Geriatr Soc 1979;XXVII:444–449

117. Naurath HJ, Joosten E, Reizler R et al: Effects of vitamin B_{12}, folate and vitamin B_6 supplements in elderly people with normal serum vitamin concentrations. Lancet 1995;346:85–89

118. Anderson SH, Vickery CA, Nicol AD: Adult thiamine requirements and the continuing need to fortify processed cereals. Lancet 1986;ii:85–89

119. Vir SC, Love AHG: Nutritional status of institutionalised aged in Belfast, Northern Ireland. Am J Clin Nutr 1979;32:1934–1947

120. Thomas AJ, Finglas P, Bunker VW: The B vitamin content of hospital meals and potential low intake by elderly inpatients. J Hum Nutr Diet 1988;1:309–320

121. O'Rourke NP, Bunker VW, Thomas AJ et al: Thiamine status of healthy and institutionalised elderly subjects: analysis of dietary intake and biochemical indices. Age Ageing 1990;19:325–329

122. Older MJW, Dickerson JWT: Thiamine and the elderly orthopaedic patient. Age Ageing 1982;11:101–197

123. Kwok T, Falconer Smith JF et al: Thiamine status of elderly patients with cardiac failure. Age Ageing 1992;21:67–71

124. Rutishauser IHE, Bates CJ, Paul AA et al: Longterm vitamin status and dietary intake of healthy elderly subjects. Br J Nutr 1979;42:33–42

125. Garry PJ, Goodwin JS, Hunt WC: Nutritional status in a healthy elderly population: riboflavin. Am J Clin Nutr 1982;36:902–909

126. Vir SC, Love AHG: Vitamin B_6 status of hospitalised aged. Am J Clin Nutr 1978;31:1383–1391

127. McEvoy AW, Fenwick JD, Boddy K, James OFW: Vitamin B_{12} absorption from the gut does not decline with age in normal elderly humans. Age Ageing 1982;11:180–183

128. Garry PJ, Goodwin JS, Hunt WC: Folate and B_{12} status in a healthy elderly population. J Am Geriatr Soc 1984;32:719–726

129. van Goor LP, Woiski MD, Lagaay AM et al: Cobalamin deficiency and mental impairment in elderly people. Age Ageing 1995;24:S36–S42 (review)

130. Shane B, Stokstad ELR: Vitamin B_{12} folate interrelationships. Ann Rev Nutr 1985;5:115–141

131. Rosenberg IH, Bowman BB, Cooper BA et al: Folate nutrition in the elderly. Am J Clin Nutr 1982;36:1060–1066

132. Stanton BR: Meals for the Elderly. King Edward's Hospital Fund for London. London, 1971

133. Garry PJ, Goodwin JS, Hunt WC, Gilbert BA: Nutritional status in a healthy elderly population. Am J Clin Nutr 1982;36:332–339

134. Andrews J: Vitamin C status of elderly long stay hospital patients. Gerontol Clin 1973;15:221–226

135. Ginter E: Chronic marginal vitamin C deficiency: biochemistry and pathophysiology. World Rev Nutr Diet 1979;33:104–141

136. Gale CR, Martyn CN, Cooper C: Cognitive impairment and mortality in a cohort of elderly people. BMJ 1996;312:608–611

137. Gale CR, Martyn CN, Winter PD, Cooper C: Vitamin C and risk of death from stroke and coronary heart disease in a cohort of elderly people. BMJ 1995;310:1563–1565

138. Khaw KT, Woodhouse P: Interrelation of vitamin C, infection, haemostatic factors and cardiovascular disease. BMJ 1995;310:1559–1563

139. Dattani JT, Exton Smith AN, Stephen JM: Vitamin D status of the elderly in relation to age and exposure to sunlight. Hum Nutr Clin Nutr 1984;38C:131–137

140. Krall EA, Sahyoun N, Tannenbaum S et al: Effect of vitamin D intake on seasonal variations in parathyroid hormone secretion in post-menopausal women. N Engl J Med 1989;321:1777–1783

141. Dawson-Hughes B, Dallas GE, Krall EA et al: Effect of vitamin D supplementation in winter-time and overall bone loss in healthy post-menopausal women. Ann Intern Med 1991;115:505–512

142. Van der Wielen RPJ, Lowik MRH, Van der Berg H et al: Serum vitamin D concentrations among healthy elderly people in Europe. Lancet 1995;346:207–210

143. Avioli LV, McDonald JE, Lee SW: The influence of age on the intestinal absorption of ^{47}Ca in women and its relation to ^{47}Ca absorption in postmenopausal osteoporosis. J Clin Invest 1965;44:1960–1967

144. Bullamore JR, Wilkinson R, Gallagher JC et al: Effect of age on calcium absorption. Lancet 1970;ii:535–537

145. Francis RM, Peacock M, Storer JH et al: Calcium malabsorption in the elderly: the effect of treatment with oral 25-hydroxyvitamin D. Eur J Clin Invest 1983;13:391–396

146. Francis RM, Peacock M, Barkworth SA: Renal impairment and its effects on calcium metabolism in elderly women. Age Ageing 1984;13:14–20

147. Nordin BEC, Baker MR, Horsman A, Peacock M: A prospective trial of the effect of vitamin D supplementation on metacarpal bone loss in elderly women. Am J Clin Nutr 1985;42:470–474

148. Ireland P, Fortran JS: Effect of dietary calcium and age on jejunal calcium absorption in humans studied by intestinal perfusion. J Clin Invest 1973;52:2672–2682

149. Wood RJ, Suter PM, Russell RM: Mineral requirements of elderly people. Am J Clin Nutr 1995;62:493–505

150. Heaney RP, Recker RR, Saville PD: Menopausal changes in calcium balance. J Lab Clin Med 1978;92:953–963

151. Matkovic V, Kostial K, Simonovic I et al: Bone status and fracture rates in two regions of Yugoslavia. Am J Clin Nutr 1979;32:540–549

152. Hegsted DM: Calcium and osteoporosis. J Nutr 1986;116: 2316–2319

153. Stevenson JC, Whitehead MI, Padwick M et al: Dietary intake of calcium and postmenopausal bone loss. BMJ 1988;297:15–17

154. Kanis JA, Passmore R: Calcium supplementation of the diet I. BMJ 1989;298:137–140

155. Kanis JA, Passmore R: Calcium supplementation of the diet II. BMJ 1989;298:205–208

156. Nordin BEC, Heaney RP: Calcium supplementation of the diet: justified by present evidence. BMJ 1990;300:1056–1060

157. Lewis J, Buss DH: Trace nutrients. 5. Minerals and vitamins in the British household food supply. Br J Nutr 1988;60:413–424

158. Lim P, Jacob E: Magnesium deficiency in patients on longterm diuretic therapy for heart failure. BMJ 1972;3:620–622

159. Dykner T, Wester PO: The relation between intra and extracellular electrolytes in patients with hypokalaemia and/or diuretic treatment. Acta Med Scand 1978;204:269–282

160. Kaplan NM: The dietary guideline for sodium: should we shake it up? No. Am J Clin Nutr 2000;71:1020–1026

161. McCarron DA: The dietary guideline for sodium: should we shake it up? Yes! Am J Clin Nutr 2000;71:1013–1019

162. Elliott P, Stamler J, Nichols R et al: Intersalt revisited: further analysis of 24 hour sodium excretion and blood pressure within and across populations. BMJ 1996;312:1249–1253

163. Bjorn Rasmussen E: Iron absorption: present knowledge and controversies. Lancet 1983;i:914–916

164. Valberg LS, Flanagan PR: Intestinal absorption of iron and related metals. In Sarkar B (ed): Biological Aspects of Metals and Metal-Related Diseases. Raven Press, New York. 1983;41–66

165. Jacobs AM, Owen GM: The effect of age on iron absorption. J Gerontol 1969;24:95–96

166. Marx JJM, Dinant HJ: Ferrokinetics and red cell iron uptake in old age: evidence for increased liver iron retention. Haematologica 1982;67:161–168

167. Fleming DJ, Jacques PF, Tucker KL et al: Iron status of the free living elderly Framingham Heart study cohort: an iron replete population with a high prevalence of elevated iron stores. Am J Clin Nutr 2001;73:638–646

168. Thomas AJ, Bunker VW, Stansfied MF et al: Iron status of hospitalised and housebound elderly people: dietary intake, metabolic balance, haematological and biochemical indices. QJM 1989;262:175–184

169. Dallman PR: Manifestation of iron deficiency. Semin Hematol 1982;19:19–29

170. Cook JD, Finch CA: Assessing iron status of a population. Am J Clin Nutr 1979;32:2115–2119

171. Croker JR, Beynon G: Gastrointestinal bleeding: a major cause of iron deficiency in the elderly. Age Ageing 1981;10:40–43

172. Calvey HD, Castleden CM: Gastrointestinal investigations for anaemia in the elderly: a prospective study. Age Ageing 1987;16:399–404

173. Senapati A, Jenner G, Thompson RPH: Zinc in the elderly. QJM 1989;70:81–87

Chapter 85

Obesity

Cyril Weinkove

Since this chapter appeared in the fifth edition there have been some interesting and important developments:

1. The prevalence of obesity in the developed world has reached epidemic proportions making a significant contribution to the increase in malignant disease.[1]
2. We have a better understanding of the biochemical mechanisms, by which obesity increases mortality and morbidity. Fat can no longer be regarded as merely a storage form of energy. It must now be seen "as a complex metabolically active endocrine tissue secreting bioactive peptides and cytokines, which may contribute to the onset and severity of age-associated diseases."[2]
3. More evidence has accumulated that intra-abdominal fat is mainly responsible for the pathologies associated with obesity and that this is reflected by waist circumference. In future we should use waist circumference rather than weight or weight height ratios as an index of adiposity.
4. Caloric restriction, certainly in rodents and possibly in nonhuman primates, has been shown to increase longevity. Some of the disorders commonly associated with advancing years may now be ascribed to the concomitant increase in intra-abdominal fat.
5. The genetic basis of some of the rarer causes of obesity have been elucidated, but is currently not deemed relevant to the obese elderly population.

The effects and causes of obesity in elderly people are little different from those in younger adults, and the subject has been well reviewed[3] in other texts. This chapter should be read in conjunction with Ch. 84, nutrition, which defines the body compartments, the nutritional requirements of elderly people, and methods of measuring body adiposity.

This chapter stresses the clinical importance of obesity in elderly people, describes the difficulties in helping patients lose weight, corrects some of the obesity mythology, and explains the pivotal role of the medical profession in the management of overweight and obese elderly patients.

DEFINITION

By convention, the weights of males and females of different heights as shown by the 1983 Metropolitan Life Insurance Company tables have been accepted as normal. These tables, however, offer no correction for the age of the subjects.

In the United Kingdom, people weighing in excess of 110 percent of the accepted normal weight for their height are referred to as overweight, those weighing in excess of 120 percent of the accepted normal weight are referred to as obese, and those weighing more than 130 percent of the accepted limit are described as suffering from morbid obesity.

It is now generally agreed that it is not only the degree of obesity that determines the pathological outcome but also the distribution of the excess fat (see later). Central obesity with fat concentrated around the abdominal viscera (an "apple shape") is accepted as being more hazardous than excess fat concentrated around the buttocks, hips, and thighs (a "pear shape").

MEASUREMENT

Instead of referring to standard tables of heights and weights, most clinicians quote a patient's body mass index (BMI) or Quetelet's index. This figure is calculated by dividing the patient's weight in kilograms by the square of their height in meters (kg/m^2). In Europe patients with a BMI between 25 and 30 kg/m^2 are considered overweight. In this text, as in many publications, the BMI units (kg/m^2) will be omitted. Individuals with a BMI greater than 30 are obese, and those with a BMI greater than 40 are regarded as suffering from morbid obesity. In the United States the cutoff point for overweight is 27.8 in men and 27.3 for women, with severe overweight occurring in men with a BMI greater than 31.1 and in women with a BMI greater than 32.3. In the United States morbid obesity has been defined as a BMI of 39 or greater.[4] In this text I will use the European cutoff points of 25 and 30 to separate the overweight from the obese.

BODY FAT DISTRIBUTION

Both obesity and central body fat distribution are related to multiple adverse changes in cardiovascular risk factors. By dividing the waist circumference, at the level of the umbilicus, by the hip circumference at the level of the iliac crest, the waist/hip ratio[5] (WHR) can be calculated. This ratio correlates positively with the amount of visceral fat mass, which has metabolic characteristics that are unique in comparison with other adipose tissues.[6]

Visceral adipose tissue is associated with hyperinsulinism, insulin resistance, and high amounts of free fatty acids.[7] This leads to an impairment of glucose tolerance,[8] high total triglyceride and low high-density lipoprotein (HDL) cholesterol concentrations,[9] and hypertension.[10]

Thus central body fat distribution is associated with an increased risk for non-insulin-dependent diabetes mellitus (NIDDM) in middle-aged subjects even after accounting for overall obesity.[11,12] In the same population central body fat distribution has been consistently shown to be associated with an increased risk of coronary heart disease, again independently of obesity.[13,14]

Although the effect of obesity and fat distribution on glucose tolerance and cardiovascular risk factor levels has been thoroughly investigated in middle-aged subjects, little is known about this effect in elderly people.

The relationship between body fat distribution and aging

Lean body tissue steadily declines after the age of 20, whereas the level of body fat increases and peaks at around 60, after which both lean body tissue and fat mass decline.[15] This will influence the mathematical relationship between height and weight used to calculate BMI and its use as an indicator of adiposity. One can envisage an older person with a "normal" BMI but increased intra-abdominal fat.

Mykkänen and coworkers[16] have re-examined the relationship between obesity and waist/hip ratio in elderly people. They concluded that obesity per se rather than its distribution was a more significant determinant of glucose and insulin as well as total triglyceride and HDL cholesterol levels in elderly subjects. This observation could be explained by the fact that, with advancing age, fat tends to be distributed around the abdomen in both males and females.

In a large complicated statistical study using more than 7,000 subjects in the UK and the Netherlands (stratified into four groups from 20 to 59) Han and coworkers[17] analyzed the interdependence of age, weight, height, and waist circumference. They concluded that waist measurement alone may be used to indicate adiposity or to reflect metabolic risk factors in their subjects. In contrast, the influence of height on body weight was found to be less important. Their subjects were less than 60 years old and it could be argued that the relationship does not extend beyond the age of 60.

PREVALENCE OF OBESITY

One of the Health of the Nation policy targets was "to reduce the percentages of men and women aged 16–64 who are obese by at least 25% for men and at least 33% for women by 2005 (from 8% for men and 12% for women in 1986/87 to no more than 6% and 8% respectively)."[18] It is interesting to note that elderly people were excluded from these goals.

In a thorough review of obesity and aging, Kotz, Billington, and Levine[19] remind us that obesity prevalence is increasing in the world. The United States data, stratified by age and sex from 1960 through 1994, show that the increase applies to all age groups in both sexes. However, the prevalence of obesity peaks in the 50–59 year group and falls in those between 60–69 and 70–79. The cause of the relative fall in the prevalence of obesity after the age of 60 is unclear. It may be due to obesity-related deaths in the younger group or the physiological anorexia of aging.

CAUSES OF OBESITY

Overweight and obesity arise when the total energy intake exceeds the energy output. There is *no* other cause. Many patients attending obesity clinics feel that they are unique in that they eat little and yet continue to gain weight, ascribing this to an abnormally low metabolic rate. In a comprehensive summary of the causes of and associations with obesity, Kopelman[20] points out that less than 10 percent of patients have a primary endocrine condition or a secondary endocrine disorder associated with obesity.

In general only two endocrine causes of obesity need be considered: hypothyroidism and Cushing's syndrome. The latter should be clinically apparent from the history and physical signs. Weight gain after steroid treatment is more common. Hypothyroidism is also more common than Cushing's syndrome but impossible to exclude on clinical grounds. Thyroid function tests should be done on *all* overweight individuals prior to medical treatment. We have identified two new covert hypothyroid patients attending our weight management clinic. Like other known obese hypothyroid patients, they require a restricted caloric intake as well as thyroxine, to help them lose weight.

To understand the mechanism of excessive weight gain one must review the two components of the metabolic equation, energy expenditure and energy intake.

ENERGY EXPENDITURE

Three components of energy expenditure can be easily identified by measuring the metabolic rate under varying conditions.

Resting metabolic rate

The lowest or the basal metabolic rate (BMR)[21] occurs transiently during the early morning hours of deep sleep. In clinical practice this transient basal rate has little influence on total energy requirements and is often impractical to measure. Another state of metabolism is the resting metabolic rate (RMR) which occurs while a person is resting and fasting. The RMR is the best predictor of the person's overall requirements and usually approximates 65–70 percent of the daily energy requirements of most ambulatory humans; it also reflects almost all the energy requirements of bedridden hospitalized patients.[22] In healthy elderly people body weight alone predicted RMR when compared with other indexes of body composition. The influence of age on RMR was trivial, and regional distribution of fat had no influence. There were wide 95 percent confidence limits of RMR in both lean and obese subjects. Thus metabolic efficiency was not necessarily or exclusively related to obesity.

Dietary-induced thermogenesis

Dietary-induced thermogenesis (DIT) is the increase in energy associated with eating and digesting a meal and accounts for 10 percent of total daily energy expenditure.

Thermic effect of physical activity

The thermic effect of physical activity is the most variable component of daily energy expenditure and includes less conscious muscular activity, such as shivering and fidgeting, as well as purposeful exercise.

Poehlman[23] has shown that all these components of daily expenditure decline with age. Energy intake also declines with age, but intake and expenditure do not decline proportionally, leading to an energy imbalance characterized by obesity or leanness. This is at variance with the findings of Owen[22] mentioned above.

ENERGY INTAKE

Until recently it has been impossible to obtain a true measure of a patient's dietary intake. In the past we were dependent on the patient providing an accurate dietary history or else observing the individual under unnatural conditions, such as in a metabolic unit. Now, using a doubly labeled water ($^2H_2^{18}O$) technique, it is possible to measure total daily energy expenditure in free-living subjects. Prentice[24] and others using this method have convincingly demonstrated that, despite claims to the contrary, the obese grossly misreport their caloric intake. Dietary histories can no longer be accepted as accurate, since the obese underestimate their dietary intake by as much as 40 percent.[25]

CONSEQUENCES OF OBESITY

Obesity causes, or is associated with, many complications (Table 85-1), all generally recognized to increase mortality and morbidity. In the absence of complicating factors the clinician has to decide whether treating obesity is warranted, particularly in light of some evidence that longevity is increased in the overweight. For example, a 5-year longitudinal study performed by Matilla et al.[26] (1986) in 526 people over the age of 85 showed that overweight elderly people (BMI greater than 30, 53 percent mortality) survived longer than those with the lowest weight (BMI less than 20, 87 percent mortality).

Similarly, in another study on the hypertensive elderly, total mortality and cardiovascular and noncardiovascular terminating events were highest in patients in the leanest BMI quintile. Thus these workers report that the association between BMI and cardiovascular end points was U-shaped.[27]

Kinney and Caldwell[28] have pointed out that not all mortality studies on elderly people have controlled for cigarette smoking, hypertension, glucose intolerance, or subclinical disease. When early deaths were excluded (presumably due to subclinical disease) in subjects over 75 years old, the only variable significantly related to survival was age. Interestingly they concluded that there was no ideal weight per se for aged men. The lowest BMI was associated with decreased survival, but none of the aged men had a BMI greater than 36.5. They suggest that men with a high BMI might die before reaching 75 years of age.

Most clinicians agree that obesity in diabetic and hypertensive patients requires treatment, but they may hesitate before treating the "healthy" obese. Hubert[29] has reviewed publications concerned with the relationship between obesity and cardiovascular disease. It is well established that obesity is associated with elevated blood pressure and high levels of blood lipids, lipoproteins, and blood glucose and that changes in body weight are accompanied by changes in these risk factors for cardiovascular disease. Both clinical and epidemiological evidence suggests that even mild obesity may "lie at the beginning of the chain of events leading to disease causation" and that preventive strategies that include weight control need to be encouraged.

Some studies suggest that the increased risk observed in heavier individuals is due primarily to the influence of the associated risk factors and not to the degree of obesity per se. This has been interpreted as suggesting that obesity is benign when it exists without other major risk factors for disease.

The Framingham Study[30] and other long-term prospective studies[31,32] concerned with the independent role of obesity in cardiovascular risk challenge this notion. Some may argue that the physician treating the elderly patient is not primarily concerned with disease prevention and that managing obesity is the work of others. I do not believe that obesity is a benign condition for reasons outlined below. Intra-abdominal obesity in elderly persons should be taken seriously and treated should they wish it.

MECHANISMS BY WHICH OBESITY INCREASES MORTALITY AND MORBIDITY

Barzilai[2,33] has summarized the biological functions of fat, which can no longer be regarded as a silent energy depot. Fat tissue is a very active endocrine gland which secretes a variety of peptides (such as leptin and plasminogen activator inhibitor-1 [PAI-1]), cytokines (such as tumor necrosis factor alpha [TNF-α]) and complement factors (such as D, C3, and B). Fat-derived TNF-α is directly involved in insulin resistance. PAI-1 released from fat cells also will lead to thrombotic episodes in obese patients with a reduction in weight reversing this effect.[34]

Leptin acting on the hypothalamus should reduce caloric intake and help to maintain weight. This action is overriden in humans who regularly have meals regardless of their plasma leptin levels and the degree of their appetite.

The cytokines have important neuroendocrine effects and influence the immune response, as well as body composition and energy balance. It is the visceral (intra-abdominal) fat which is mostly responsible for producing these deleterious peptides leading to diabetes, strokes, malignant disease, and heart attacks, seen more commonly in elderly people.

Table 85-1 **Risks associated with obesity**	
Disorders directly caused by obesity	**Disorders aggravated by obesity**
Diabetes mellitus (NIDDM)[51]	All cardiorespiratory disorders
Hypertension	Esophagitis
Ischemic heart disease	Anesthetic risk
Hernias and uterine prolapse	Postoperative complications
Sleep apnea (Pickwickian syndrome)	Arthritis
Malignant disease	Hyperlipidemia

NIDDM: non-insulin-dependent diabetes mellitus.

It is reasonable to ask how much of the mortality and morbidity of advanced years can be explained by an increase in abdominal obesity which accompany the aging process. In a recent review[35] caloric restriction has been found to be the most useful and reproducible method of increasing longevity in short lived animals. A 40 percent decrease in caloric intake of rodents increased their mean and maximum longevity by about 50 percent with a decrease in the cardiovascular changes observed with advancing age. In these calorie-restricted animals bone loss was diminished, and the incidence of age-associated illnesses such as chronic renal disease, cardiomyopathies, gastric ulcers, hypertension, neoplastic diseases, autoimmune disorders, and cataracts were reduced.

It is interesting to note that surgical removal of abdominal fat in rodents[2] (not possible with liposuction in humans) decreased insulin resistance when compared to sham-operated controls. This is strong supportive evidence for the role of intra-abdominal fat in the pathological consequences of obesity and aging.

THE VALUE OF TREATING OBESITY IN ELDERLY PATIENTS

Clinicians and patients demand evidence of the benefits of medical intervention. However, it is impossible to conduct "placebo-controlled" double-blind trials demonstrating the long-term benefits of weight loss, and whether the healthy obese should be treated is an unresolved issue.

According to Garrow,[36] "obesity is associated with serious morbidity and mortality, and the more overweight and the younger the patient the more severe the health implications. Since many of the diseases related to obesity are crippling rather than killing diseases, so the mortality figures tend to underestimate the importance of obesity as a public health problem." Some of the obese middle-aged may live long enough to present with problems in old age.

My experience running an obesity clinic for 15 years leads me to believe that healthy obese patients are the exception rather than the rule. Obesity, like hypothyroidism, has a gradual onset, and most obese patients remain unaware of their increasing incapacity. Even in the absence of overt cardiovascular or respiratory disease, these patients all comment on improved breathing, exercise tolerance, and well-being following a small (5 percent) reduction in weight (unpublished data). Others have measured pulmonary function before and following weight loss and demonstrated improvement in asthmatic[37] and nonasthmatic[38] obese patients. Lazarus and coworkers[39] reported differential effects of obesity and fat distribution on ventilatory function. There are a variety of mechanisms by which excess body fat might directly influence ventilatory function. These include impeding descent of the diaphragm and interfering with chest wall movement. I suspect that the increased metabolic rate associated with weight gain puts greater demands on pulmonary function.

Results in elderly patients are no different from those in younger patients. We found that elderly patients responded just as well as younger patients to a very low-calorie treatment regimen (Table 85-2) provided they gained some clinical advan-

Table 85-2 The effect of age on the response to a very low-calorie diet[a]

Age (years)	Total no.	Patients with weight loss of			
		< 0	0–10%	10–20%	> 20%
< 65	559	33 (6%)	280 (50%)	152 (27%)	94 (17%)
> 65	47	1 (2%)	23 (49%)	17 (36%)	6 (13%)

[a]All subjects were managed on a very low-calorie diet (Lipotrim, Howard Research Foundation, Cambridge, UK) at the Hope Hospital Weight Management Clinic.

tage to offset the inconvenience of weekly visits to the clinic. The prospect of hip or knee replacement is a strong motivating factor. In our experience, minimal weight loss leads to an improvement in patients' breathing, angina, diabetes, and hypertension, with a corresponding reduction in drug dosage. Olefsky and coworkers[40] found a 33 percent decrease in insulin resistance and a 40 percent decrease in very low-density triglyceride production in obese subjects after weight reduction. They observed no difference in this objective biochemical response between the five most and the five least obese men in their experimental group after an average weight loss of 11 kg. They concluded that modest decreases in weight can initiate profound metabolic changes. Thus patients do not have to achieve their ideal body weight to benefit clinically and biochemically from weight loss.

PRACTICAL MANAGEMENT OF OBESE ELDERLY PEOPLE

In getting patients to lose weight, one must examine both parts of the energy equation, energy intake and energy output.

Increasing energy output appears to be a reasonable way to get elderly people to lose weight. However, to dissipate 420 kJ (100 kcal) the patient would have to walk or run 1 mile, which is not an easy option in a less mobile elderly patient.

A study by Reed et al.[41] measured physical exercise by questionnaire, body adiposity by anthropometry and bioelectric impedance, and muscle strength using a hand-held dynamometer in 213 healthy ambulatory patients over the age of 60 (mean age 70). Muscle strength increased with the increase in physical exercise. However, the level of reported physical exercise over the range of 0 to 6,418 kJ/d (0 to 1,520 kcal/d) did not predict body adiposity in the healthy elderly population. Those exercising were probably eating more, and the authors conclude that "to decrease body fat without modifying caloric consumption in elderly individuals would require a more intensive exercise regimen."

Decreasing energy intake is not an easy option. In 1958, Stunkard[42] summarized the results of the previous 30 years of experience of treating obesity as follows: "Most obese persons will not stay in treatment for obesity. Of those who stay in treatment, most will not lose weight, and of those who do lose weight, most will regain it."

Summary of management algorithm

- Dietary restriction is the only safe way for elderly people to lose weight

- As little as a 10 percent reduction in body weight will improve the well-being of the clinically obese

- Vitamin and mineral supplements are recommended during caloric restriction

- Doctors and health workers treating obese patients should be positive, supportive, and prepared to see them regularly

- A program of weight maintenance must be established after weight loss

This depressing finding continues to be the experience of clinicians referring their obese patients to dietitians for treatment on conventional diets. It is not surprising that few doctors are interested in directly managing their obese patients despite the fact that, as with other lifestyle changes (e.g. smoking cessation and blood pressure control), even minimal physician involvement may enhance outcome.[43]

However, there is some good news. Reviewing the results of clinical research trials, Wadden[44] revealed that patients treated in randomized trials using a conventional 5,040 kJ/d (1,200 kcal/d) reducing diet, combined with behavior modification, lost approximately 8.5 kg in 20 weeks, maintaining approximately two-thirds of this weight loss 1 year later. Patients treated under medical supervision using a very low-calorie diet (1,680 to 3,360 kJ/d [400 to 800 kcal/d]) lost approximately 20 kg in 12–16 weeks and maintained one-half to two-thirds of this loss in the following year. These results are certainly better than the earlier experience of Stunkard.

Two other issues need to be addressed: why patients fail to lose weight and whether repeated dieting can lead to weight gain by decreasing the lean body mass (LBM), thereby reducing the patient's caloric requirement.

Why patients fail to lose weight

Most doctors do not understand why many of their obese patients fail to lose weight on conventional low-calorie diets. They and their patients are too ready to accept the idea that the obese suffer from some abnormality in metabolic rate. This problem has been thoroughly dealt with by Kreitzman,[45] who makes the following points.

- The rapid initial weight loss on any reduced-calorie diet consists predominantly of water, with every pound of glycogen (7,560 kJ [1,800 kcal]) catabolized releasing 4 lb of water. To lose an equivalent weight (5 lb) of fat would require a 73,500-kJ (17,500-kcal [5 × 3,500]) deficit.
- Any restriction of caloric intake is countered by up to a 15 percent reduction in RMR.
- The RMR is linearly related to the patient's weight. Hence with increasing weight loss the RMR decreases, and even further reductions in caloric intake are necessary to maintain weight loss.
- Dietitians, let alone patients, cannot accurately calculate the caloric content of a conventional food diet. In one study[46] 4,200-kJ (1,000-kcal) diet sheets prepared by hospital dietitians were found, after careful examination by nutrition experts, to provide 4,305–6,917 kJ (1,025–1,647 kcal).

It is easy to see why many dieting patients lose heart rather than weight. The initial encouraging weight loss (predominantly fluid) is followed by a much slower weight loss which diminishes even further with time. Excessive fluid loss in the early phases of dieting may lead to a diminished circulating blood volume and a fall in blood pressure. The patient may feel "faint" and "weak," erroneously attributing this to a need for food rather than a requirement for fluid. It is therefore important that the dieting patient understand the pathophysiology of weight loss and that fluid intake be carefully monitored, especially if very low-calorie diets are used.

The calorie content of a "natural" diet varies enormously with the type of food eaten. Any unintentional miscalculation of dietary caloric content may cause patients to gain weight, which makes them depressed and unhappy. They begin to overeat in earnest and then blame dieting for damaging their metabolic rate permanently and being the *cause* of their obesity. It is for this reason that I favor the use of commercially prepared, prepackaged, very low-calorie diets in elderly patients who fail to lose weight on normal diets. No calculation of calories is required, the macro- and micronutrient content of the diet is known, and portions do not have to be carefully weighed. Thus the dieting process is considerably simplified.

Effects of weight cycling on body composition

Many patients seeking help for weight loss give a history of weight regain being substantially greater after periods of successful weight loss. It has been argued that it is the repeated cycles of weight loss and regain that make people fat,[47] the mechanism allegedly being an inappropriate and irreversible loss of LBM. Prentice and colleagues[48] present good animal and human, clinical, and experimental evidence against this commonly accepted myth. They have shown that natural weight cycling in a rural Gambian population does not lead to a more rapid age-related loss of lean mass than occurs in better nourished, noncycling populations. Furthermore, the substantial published animal studies, which they review, are remarkable in agreeing that body composition is unaffected by weight cycling. Their own study of experimental yo-yo dieting in humans revealed no evidence of excessive lean tissue loss and in fact provided some indication of the reverse.

Why then do patients tend to regain more weight after bouts of restricted intake? The majority of overweight people look forward to returning to their "normal" diet once they have lost weight. They fail to appreciate that having lost weight they can never go back to their previous eating habits. Doctors and dietitians do not stress the simple physiological fact that lighter people need fewer calories to maintain their weight than do heavier subjects. The previously obese patient who returns to their normal eating habits rapidly regains weight, becomes depressed, eats even more and, as already noted, attributes their failure to loss of LBM and a damaged metabolism.

TREATMENT OF OBESITY IN ELDERLY PEOPLE

The use of drug therapy for treating obesity in elderly people has been well reviewed by Dvorak and coworkers.[49] They discuss the mechanisms of action of the various compounds but conclude that few drugs have produced and sustained a significant body weight loss. Most patients are on a host of other medications for concomitant illnesses and it is debatable whether obesity in elderly people should be treated with drug intervention. There are similar objections to surgical procedures. This leaves dietary restriction as the only really effective way to lose a significant amount of weight.

The danger of undernutrition and osteoporosis is used as a reason for not treating obese elderly patients with caloric restriction. This can be countered by providing adequate vitamin and mineral supplements regardless of the type of diet which is prescribed.

There are some who reason that elderly people should not be treated for obesity because of the difficulties outlined above. This is rational if neither the patient nor the clinician sees any long- or short-term advantage to offset the discomfort imposed by dietary restriction. On the other hand, the benefits conferred by a relatively small amount of weight loss makes this discomfort worthwhile. Even those who claimed that they felt well before dieting, report an improvement in their breathing and mobility after losing 5 percent of their body weight. The clinician will note a rapid improvement in glycemic control, hypertension, respiration, and exercise tolerance in their patients.

Commercial prepackaged vitamin- and mineral-supplemented meal replacements are the only way to ensure that elderly patients receive adequate replacement of micronutrients. The author has successfully used very low-calorie diets (less than 3,360 kJ/d [800 kcal/d]) in such patients. It is important to maintain careful medical monitoring at weekly intervals of the patients' weight, blood pressure, fluid intake, and drug therapy, which will need alteration with weight loss. These diets may or may not be supplemented by small (prepackaged) standard meals of known macronutrient content.

There is no need to aim for a BMI of 25 kg/m², since the lower the final weight, the more difficulty the patient will have maintaining this weight. Caloric intake can be increased once the patient feels better and the desired effect on blood pressure, angina, or breathing has been obtained. The patient will then need to be re-educated regarding their eating habits and seen regularly at a weight maintenance clinic. Increased exercise can help to maintain the weight loss.

Many large patients are self-conscious when their abdominal girth is measured, but if embarassment can be avoided, waist circumference is a better index of the complications of obesity than the patient's BMI.[17,50] While the clinicians aim is to reduce the risks of obesity there is no doubt that vanity is the best motivator for weight maintenance. All our patients notice the change in their dress (or trouser) size. We try and encourage this self-awareness and pride.

SUMMARY

Obesity is not as common in elderly people as in younger adults, perhaps because obesity is associated with a higher mortality in the young. Excessive weight is more incapacitating in elderly people than in the young because of the general decrease in muscle mass and the additional pathology associated with aging. Sadly there has been no dramatic improvement in our methods of treating obesity. Our new understanding of the mechanisms of tissue damage induced by obesity may lead to novel therapeutic agents to combat the effects, if not the cause of obesity.

Clinicians are unwilling to subject elderly patients to rigorous dietary regimens because they feel that the risks outweigh the advantages and because most overweight patients (regardless of age) do badly on diets. The negative attitude of the physician (and dietitian) is readily apparent to the patient, and failure is guaranteed.

If physicians took a more active, positive role in the management of obesity in elderly patients, patients' hospital stays and medication could be reduced and the quality of their life improved. Those caring for elderly people must accept that obesity is a chronic recurrent problem requiring lifelong management and that even minimal but sustained weight loss has clinical benefits, fully justifying their efforts.

KEY POINTS Obesity

- Obesity is increasing in all age groups (including elderly people) in the developed world.

- Obesity is a major contributor to many diseases including diabetes, hypertension, ischemic heart disease, arthritis, and arterial and venous thrombosis, found in elderly people.

- Fat is not just a passive calorie storage organ but releases potent peptides and cytokines which contribute to the ill-effects listed above and to the aging process itself.

- Intra-abdominal fat is the villain and can be simply monitored by measuring waist circumference.

- Weight loss, even in elderly people, can reverse many of the adverse effects of abdominal obesity.

- Obesity is a chronic relapsing condition requiring a lifetime of support.

REFERENCES

1. Josefson D: BMJ News: Obesity and inactivity fuel global cancer epidemic. Br Med J 2001;1322:945
2. Barzilai N: Obesity: age-associated weight gain and the development of disease. Geriatrics 1999;54:61–64
3. Morley JE, Glick Z: Obesity. In Morley JE, Glick Z, Rubinstein LZ (eds): Geriatric Nutrition. Raven Press, New York, 1995:245–255
4. Kuczmarski RJ: Prevalence of overweight and weight gain in the United States. Am J Clin Nutr 1992;55:495S–502S
5. Kalkoff RK, Hartz AH, Rupley D et al: Relationship of body fat distribution to blood pressure, carbohydrate tolerance and plasma lipids in healthy obese women. J Lab Clin Med 1983;102:621–627
6. Seidell JC, Björntorp P, Sjöström L et al: Regional distribution of muscle and fat mass in men—new insight into the risk of abdominal obesity using computed tomography. Int J Obes 1989;13:289–303

7. Reaven GM: Role of insulin resistance in human disease. Diabetes 1988;37:1595–1607
8. Fujioka S, Matsuzawa Y, Tokunaga K, Tarui S: Contribution of intra-abdominal fat accumulation to the impairment of glucose and lipid metabolism in human obesity. Metabolism 1987;36:54–59
9. Despres JP, Moorjani S, Lupien PJ et al: Regional distribution of body fat, plasma lipoproteins and cardiovascular disease. Arteriosclerosis 1990;10:497–511
10. Peiris AN, Sothmann MS, Hoffmann RG et al: Adiposity, fat distribution, and cardiovascular risk. Ann Intern Med 1989;110:867–872
11. Ohlson LO, Larsson B, Svärdsudd K et al: The influence of body fat distribution on the incidence of diabetes mellitus: 13.5 years of follow-up of participants in the study of men born in 1913. Diabetes 1985;34:1055–1058
12. Lundgren H, Bengtsson C, Blohme G et al: Adiposity and adipose tissue distribution in relation to incidence of diabetes in women: results from a prospective population study in Gothenburg, Sweden. Int J Obes 1989;13:413–423
13. Larsson B, Svärdsudd K, Welin L et al: Abdominal adipose tissue distribution, obesity and risk of cardiovascular disease and death: 13 year follow-up of participants in the study of men born in 1913. Br Med J 1984;288:1401–1404
14. Lapidus L, Bengtsson C, Larsson B et al: Distribution of adipose tissue and risk of cardiovascular disease and death: a 12 year follow-up of participants in the population study of women in Gothenburg, Sweden. Br Med J 1984;289:1257–1261
15. Muller DC, Elahi D, Tobin JD et al: The effect of age on insulin resistance and secretion: A review. Semin Nephrol 1996;16:289–298
16. Mykkänen L, Laakso M, Pyörälä K: Association of obesity and distribution of obesity with glucose tolerance and cardiovascular risk factors in the elderly. Int J Obes 1992;16:695–704
17. Han TS, Seidell JC, Currall JE et al: The influences of height and age on waist circumference as an index of adiposity in adults. Int J Obes Relat Metab Disord 1997;21:83–89
18. The Health of the Nation: A Strategy for Health in England. HMSO, London, 1992
19. Kotz CM, Billington CJ, Levine AS: Obesity and aging. Clin Geriatr Med 1999;15:391–412
20. Kopelman PG: Investigation of obesity. J Clin Endocrinol 1994;41:703–708
21. Ravussin E, Burnand B, Schutz Y, Jequier E: Twenty-four-hour energy expenditure and resting metabolic rate in obese, moderately obese and control subjects. Am J Clin Nutr 1982;35:566–573
22. Owen OE: Resting metabolic requirement of men and women. Mayo Clin Proc 1988;53:503–510
23. Poehlman ET: Energy expenditure and requirements in aging humans. J Nutr 1992;122:2057–2065
24. Prentice AM: Assessing food intake in obese people. Micrographia 1994;16:29–32
25. Bandini LG, Schoeller DA, Cyr HN, Dietz WH: Validity of reported energy intake in obese and nonobese adolescents. Am J Clin Nutr 1990;52:421–425
26. Matilla K, Haavisto M, Rajala S: Body mass index and mortality in the elderly. Br Med J 1986;292:867–868
27. Tuomilehto J: Body mass index and prognosis in elderly hypertensive patients: a report from the European Working Party on High Blood Pressure in the Elderly. Am J Med 1991;90(suppl 3A):34S–41S
28. Kinney EL, Caldwell JW: Relationship between body weight and mortality in men aged 75 years and older. Southern Med J 1990;83:1256–1258
29. Hubert HB: The nature of the relationship between obesity and cardiovascular disease. Int J Cardiol 1984;6:268–274
30. Hubert HB, Feinleib M, McNamara PM et al: Obesity as an independent risk factor for cardiovascular diseases: a 26 year follow up of participants in the Framingham Heart Study. Circulation 1983;67:968–977
31. Manson JE, Colditz GA, Stampfer MJ et al: A prospective study of obesity and risk of coronary heart disease in women. N Engl J Med 1990;332:882–889
32. Rabkin SW, Mathewson FAL, Hsu PH: Relation of body weight to development of ischaemic heart disease in a cohort of young North American men after a 26 year observation period: the Manitoba Study. Am J Cardiol 1977;39:452–458
33. Barzilai N, Gupta G: Revisiting the role of fat mass in the life extension induced by caloric restriction. J Gerontol A 1999;54:B89–B96
34. Calles-Escandon J, Ballor D, Harvey-Berino J et al: Amelioration of the inhibition of fibrinolysis in elderly, obese subjects by moderate energy intake restriction. Am J Clin Nutr 1996;64:7–11
35. Nicolas AS, Lanzmann-Petithory D, Vellas B: Caloric restriction and aging. J Nutr Health Aging 1999;3:77–83
36. Garrow JS: Obesity and Related Diseases. Churchill Livingstone, Edinburgh, 1988
37. Stenius-Aarniala B, Poussa T, Kvarnstrom J et al: Immediate and long term effects of weight reduction in obese people with asthma: randomised controlled study. Br Med J 2000;320:827–832
38. Womack CJ, Harris DL, Katzel LI et al: Weight loss, not aerobic exercise, improves pulmonary function in older obese men. J Gerontol A 2000;55:M453–M457
39. Lazarus R, Sparrow D, Weiss ST: Effects of obesity and fat distribution on ventilatory function: the normative aging study. Chest 1997;111:891–898
40. Olefsky J, Reaven GM, Farquhar JW: Effects of weight reduction on obesity: studies of lipid and carbohydrate metabolism in normal and hyperlipoproteinaemic subjects. J Clin Invest 1974;53:64–76
41. Reed RL, Yochum K, Pearlmutter L et al: The interrelationship between physical exercise, muscle strength and body adiposity in a healthy elderly population. J Am Geriatr Soc 1991;39:1189–1193
42. Stunkard AJ: The management of obesity. NY State J Med 1958;58:79–87
43. Blackburn GL: Comparison of medically supervised and unsupervised approaches to weight loss and control. Ann Intern Med 1993;119:714–718
44. Wadden TA: Treatment of obesity by moderate and severe caloric restriction: results of clinical research trials. Ann Intern Med 1993;119:688–693
45. Kreitzman SN: Why patients fail to lose weight. In Brown JS, Gray DJP, Home RA, McBride M (eds): The Royal College of General Practitioners Members' Reference Book 1993. Sabrecrown Publishing, London, 1993:430–433
46. Stordy BJ: Data presented at Physician Conference on Obesity Management. Swiss Cottage, London, 1991
47. Cannon G, Einzig H: Dieting Makes You Fat. Century Publishing, London, 1983
48. Prentice AM, Jebb SA, Goldberg GR et al: Effects of weight cycling on body composition. Am J Clin Nutr 1992;56:209S–216S
49. Dvorak R, Starling RD, Calles-Escandon J, Sims EA, Poehlman ET: Drug therapy for obesity in the elderly. Drugs Aging 1997;1:338–351
50. Ashwell M, Cole TJ, Dixon AK: Ratio of waist circumference to height is strong predictor of intra-abdominal fat. Br Med J 1996;313:559–560
51. West KM: Epidemiology of Diabetes and Its Vascular Complications. Elsevier, New York, 1978

Chapter 86

Aging of the urinary tract

Sarbjit Vanita Jassal and Dimitrios G. Oreopoulos

The study of the aging process in the kidney is beset by difficulties. One major problem, as in all gerontological research, is to distinguish between changes influenced by "normal" aging, and those influenced by disease.

With the possible exception of respiratory function, the changes in kidney function with normal aging are the most dramatic of any human organ or organ system. In a normal young adult, renal capacity far exceeds the ordinary demands for solute and water conservation and excretion. In old age, renal function, although substantially diminished, still provides adequate regulation of the volume and composition of extracellular fluid under ordinary circumstances. However, the reduced function of the kidney has important clinical implications for diagnosis and treatment of many disorders, and clearly reduces the individual's capacity to respond to a variety of physiological and pathological stresses.

There is still a lack of basic information about epidemiology and symptomatology of renal disease in elderly people, diagnostic difficulties, and response to treatment. In general, renal disease in the aged is caused by several concomitant pathoanatomical changes. Atherosclerosis, infection, and age-induced changes might occur simultaneously. The diagnostic entities are not so clear cut as in younger individuals.

ANATOMIC CHANGES
Changes in the nephron

Age-induced renal changes are manifested microscopically by a reduction in weight of the kidney and a loss of parenchymal mass. According to Oliver,[1] the average combined weight of the kidneys in different age groups is as follows: 60 years, 250 g; 70 years, 230 g; 80 years, 190 g. The decrease in weight of the kidneys corresponds to a general decrease in the size and weight of all organs.[2] Microscopically, the most impressive changes are a reduction in the number and size of nephrons in the cortex of the kidney, with a relative sparing of the medullary zones. Loss of parenchymal mass leads to widening of the interstitial spaces between the tubules and an increase in the interstitial connective tissue. The increase in connective tissue material is caused by deposition of laminin β_1, thrombospondin (an extracellular glycoprotein associated with a variety of cellular processes including growth and embryogenesis) and fibronectin.[3] Deposition of collagen I and III, but not II or IV, has been noted in focal areas, suggesting that the fibrotic stimulus in aging differs from that seen in response to inflammation.

The total number of identifiable glomeruli falls with age, roughly in accord with the changes in renal weight.[4] The number of sclerotic glomeruli identified on light microscopy increases from 1 to 2 percent during the third to fifth decade and to 12 percent after age 70.[5,6] Aging is associated with glomerular sclerosis and loss of lobulation of the glomerular tuft, thus decreasing effective filtering surface. Although the total number of nuclei per glomerulus is unchanged with age, the filtering surface is diminished after 40 years by a progressive increase in the number of mesangial cells, and a reciprocal decrease in the number of epithelial cells. In response to the decrease in the filtering surface, the remaining nonsclerosed glomeruli enlarge in size and begin to hyperfilter in accordance with the hyperfiltration theory (see below). The mesangium, which accounts for roughly 8 percent of total glomerular volume at age 45 years, increases by age 70 years to nearly 12 percent.[7] Thrombospondin deposition in the glomerular basement membrane (GBM) occurs during aging, causing a thickening of the membrane.[8] The functional significance of the thickened GBM is unclear as studies of glomerular filtration characteristics show no differences in permeability with aging.[9] Biochemical changes such as sulphation of basement membrane glycosaminoglycans and nonenzymatic glycolation of proteins have also been documented.[10]

Darmady et al. have observed an interesting change in the distal convoluted tubule:[8] an increase with age of the number of diverticulae in the distal tubules. They reasoned that these diverticulae might play a part in the pathophysiology of pyelonephritis, by harboring organisms and contributing to the recurrence of renal infection often seen in elderly people. It has been suggested that these diverticulae represent the origin of the simple retention cysts commonly seen in elderly people.[4]

Vascular changes

Changes in the intrarenal vasculature, independent of hypertension or other renal diseases, are likely responsible for a majority of clinically relevant changes in renal function in elderly people. Normal aging is associated with variable sclerotic changes in the walls of the larger renal vessels. These sclerotic changes are augmented in the presence of hypertension.[5] Smaller vessels appear to be spared, with fewer than 20 percent of senescent kidneys from nonhypertensive individuals displaying arteriolar changes.[11]

Combined microangiographic and histological studies have identified very distinctive patterns of change in arteriolar–glomerular units with senescence.[12,13] In the cortex, hyalinization and collapse of the glomerular tuft is associated with obliteration of the lumen of the preglomerular arteriole, and a resultant loss in blood flow. Changes in the juxtamedullary area are characterized by the development of anatomic continuity between the afferent and efferent arterioles during glomerular sclerosis. The result is loss of the glomerulus and shunting of blood flow from afferent to the efferent arteriole. Blood flow is maintained to the arteriolar recta vera, the primary vascular supply of the medulla, which do not decrease in number with age (Fig. 86-1).

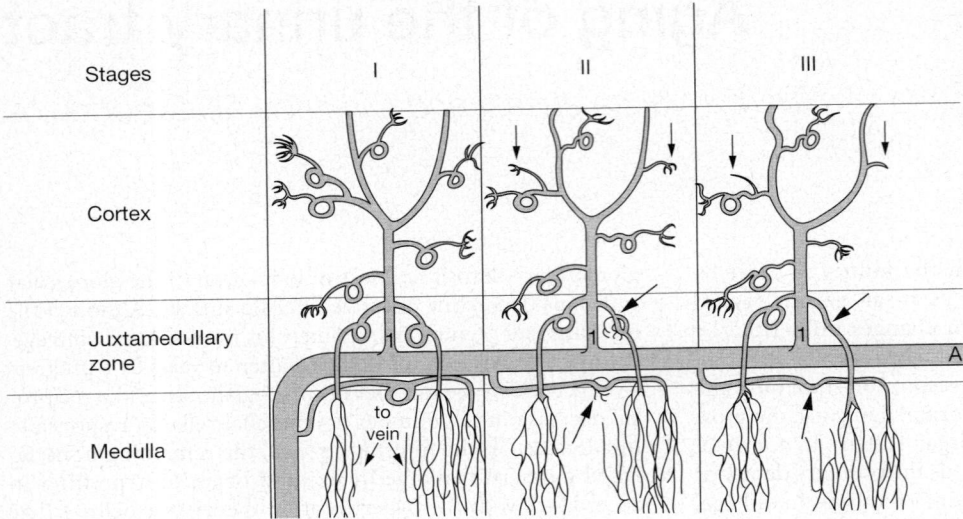

Figure 86-1 Changes in the intrarenal arterial pattern with age. (A, arcuate artery. 1, interlobular artery.) Stage I—basic adult pattern showing glomerular arterioles; stage II—partial degeneration of some glomeruli. Two cortical afferent arterioles ramify into remnants of glomerular tufts (small arrows). Two juxtamedullary arterioles pass through partially degenerated glomeruli (large arrows). There is slight spiraling of interlobular arteries and afferent arterioles. Stage III—two cortical afferent arterioles now end blindly (small arrows), and two juxtamedullary arterioles are agromerular (large arrows). The corresponding glomerular tufts have degenerated completely. The spiraling of interlobular arteries and afferent arterioles is now more pronounced. (From Ljungqvist and Lagergren,[13] with permission of Cambridge University Press.)

In humans, it is difficult to differentiate between age-induced changes and changes caused by past renal insult. Changes due to arteriosclerosis associated with hypertension, diabetes, and pyelonephritis are very common. The histological appearance of kidney structure in elderly people without any evidence of pathology is rare. According to Brocklehurst,[14] an analysis of 100 consecutive autopsies on geriatric patients at Farnborough Hospital, England, showed normal histology in only 3 percent of the cases.

FUNCTIONAL CHANGES

Renal blood flow

A progressive reduction in renal plasma flow of approximately 10 percent per decade from 600 mL/min in young adulthood to 300 mL/min by 80 years of age is well established.[15,16] Detailed studies indicate selective loss of cortical vasculature with preservation of medullary flow. These cortical vascular changes likely account for the patchy cortical defects commonly seen on renal scans in healthy older adults. Filtration occurs mainly in the juxtamedullary nephrons, with only a small contribution from the cortical nephrons. As a result of the differential decrease in renal perfusion to the cortex, there is little change in the filtration fraction (the fraction of renal plasma flow that is filtered at the glomerulus), despite a decrease in the total renal blood flow with age.

Local changes in the vascular tone of both afferent and efferent renal arterioles control renal blood flow and glomerular filtration rate (GFR). Thus alterations in renal vascular reactivity to circulating and local mediators cause hemodynamic alterations in aged kidneys. Baseline renin levels are approximately 50 percent lower in elderly people, as are angiotensinogen II levels and aldosterone levels. Stimulation of renin, using a variety of different experimental techniques that normally promote renin release, cause a lesser response in older individuals compared with that seen in younger persons. However, in animal studies, the use of an ACE inhibitor or an angiotensin II inhibitor causes a more marked effect, suggesting that the angiotensin-related vasoconstrictive tone is greater with age.[17–20] These vascular responses, however, are further complicated by changes in G-protein signaling in the vascular smooth muscle cell, as well as newly identified vasoconstrictors and vasodilators, e.g., platelet activating factor, thromboxane A_2 and prostaglandin I_2 and by the role of nitric oxide levels.[21] Although the literature is incomplete, and in some cases contradictory, an overall picture of increased vasoconstriction and decreased vasodilator reserve of the renal vascular bed is seen with age.

Glomerular filtration rate

Contrary to general belief, the glomerular filtration rate (GFR) does not always decline with age. The Baltimore longitudinal study showed an overall linear decrease of about 8.0 mL/min per 1.73 m²/decade from the middle of the fourth decade of life (Fig. 86-2). However, approximately one-third of these patients did not have a decline in GFR over time. Fliser et al. similarly found that in many cases the creatinine clearance may underestimate GFR as measured by inulin clearance in healthy elderly subjects.[22]

The decrease in GFR with age is not matched by an elevation in serum creatinine.[23] Since muscle mass, from which creatinine is derived, falls with age at roughly the same rate as

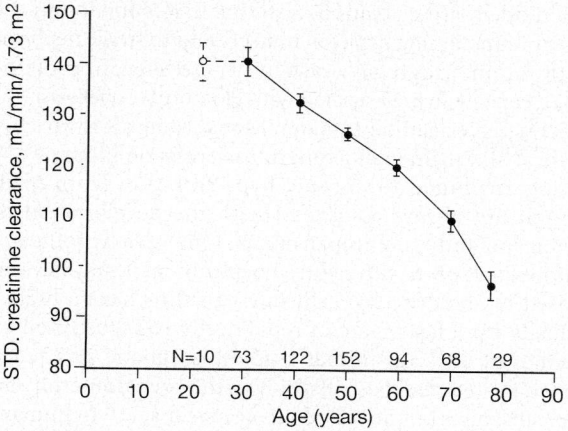

Figure 86-2 Cross-sectional differences in standard creatinine clearance with age. The number of subjects in each age group is indicated above the abscissa. Values plotted indicate mean ± SEM. The data represent creatinine clearance determinations based on measure of true creatinine. Creatinine autoanalyzer determinations in common clinical use will yield creatinine clearance values approximately 20–25 percent lower than results shown here. Values in women are approximately 20 percent lower than men. (From Rowe et al.[23] Copyright © The Gerontological Society of America. Reproduced by permission of the publisher.)

GFR, the rather drastic age-related loss of renal function is not reflected by an elevation of serum creatinine. Thus serum creatinine often overestimates GFR in elderly people.

Although methods for estimating creatinine clearance based on normative data employing various formulae have been developed,[24,25] the reliability of these formulae has been questioned.[17,26,27] Up to one-third of elderly patients may have no decline in GFR with aging, and some individuals actually demonstrate an increase in GFR with aging.[28] As the individual rate of decline cannot be predicted, creatinine clearance should not be estimated using only the serum creatinine. Even the most commonly used formula, published by Cockcroft and Gault,[24] leads to a mean underestimation of measured creatinine clearance of 12.1 mL/min in a healthy group of patients.[27] In a comparison of 15 equations, used to estimate creatinine clearance in healthy elderly patients, none correlated closely to measured clearance. The average bias ranged from −33.1 mL/min to +19.6 mL/min. Newer methods have similar limitations. For example, cystatin C had been advocated as a good marker of inulin clearance in elderly patients. However, the testing range of serum creatinine and of GFR was limited, restricting the use of the test to those with near-normal renal function.[29] Equations were variable in their erroneous placement of individuals into renal function categories.[27] Elderly patients with apparently normal serum creatinine and blood urea nitrogen levels were seen to have clearance of 60 mL/min or less, even in the ambulatory and healthy elderly. Additionally, individual variation may be very high. In severely ill elderly patients on medications, the reliability of such estimations may be low, and since the frail elderly are the most susceptible to the dangers of overestimation of creatinine clearance when prescribing medications, the formulae should be

used with caution. Timed urine collections, of short duration, for creatinine clearance are therefore recommended.[27,30] Depressions of GFR, so severe as to result in elevation of serum creatinine above 132 mmol/L (1.5 mg/dL), are rarely due solely to normal aging, and generally indicate the presence of an additional disease state.

Renal reserve function, a measure of the ability of the kidney to increase GFR in response to an increased protein or amino acid load, appears to be well preserved in elderly people.[31,32] In a study of 10 patients with a median age of 70 years, the basal inulin clearance, C_{in} (a measure of GFR) and para-aminohippurate clearance, C_{pah} (a measure of effective renal blood flow) was lower than that of individuals aged 23–32 years. However, after an infusion of amino acid to stimulate the renal reserve function, the increase in GFR was similar in both young and old adults, demonstrating an increase from 102 to 118 mL/min per 1.73 m² and 122 to 146 mL/min per 1.73 m² in the older and younger subjects respectively.[33]

Tubular function

Both excretory and reabsorptive capacities of the renal tubules decrease as age increases.[34–36] The decrease in tubular secretion of diodrast and para-aminohippuric acid in elderly people reveals a decrease in tubular function. The kidney of an old individual is, however, generally capable of maintaining a normal electrolyte and acid–base balance unless stressed.

Salt and water handling is impaired in stress states in the elderly individual. The ability to both conserve and excrete sodium is impaired. Animal and human studies show abnormal resorption of salt in the ascending loop of Henle,[37] reduced serum aldosterone secretion,[38,39] and a relative resistance to both aldosterone and angiotensin II.[40] In the laboratory setting, older adults took 31 hours to decrease their sodium excretion in response to a salt restricted diet, in comparison to 17 hours for younger adults. Similarly, after a sodium load (given as intravenous saline), older adults took longer to excrete the excess sodium absorbed.[21] The resultant effect is that older persons can generally maintain sodium balance in steady state but, when under stress such as salt depletion or dehydration, they are unable to defend their intravascular and intracellular volume and osmolality.

As with salt regulation, regulation of water balance takes longer. Older individuals are not able to either concentrate or dilute urine maximally. Antidiuretic hormone levels tend to rise with increasing age, yet the maximal osmolality of urine falls by 5 percent every 10 years. Animal models show conflicting results, often depending on the strain studied, making it difficult to establish whether the defect is in the production, storage or release of the hormone or because of down-regulation of receptor sensitivity. Emerging evidence also suggests that the defect in concentrating ability is related to the aquaporins. In one model, aging was accompanied by a decrease in the abundance of aquaporin-2 and aquaporin-3 proteins in the distal tubule and collecting duct.[41] If representative of the human kidney, this may explain why the diluting capacity decreases with age.

The elderly individual has difficulty maintaining potassium and phosphate balance in stress states. This is of clinical relevance in the setting of hospitalized patients. An overall reduction in total body potassium by around 20 percent[42] predisposes the individual to hypokalemia, especially when given diuretics.

An acid load in the elderly patient causes a prolonged decrease in the pH and pCO_2, compared with younger individuals. Basal ammonium excretion appears unchanged although a slower adaptive response is seen.[43–45]

Mechanisms of age-related reductions in renal function

The hyperfiltration theory,[46–48] has been proposed as a mechanism for the progressive glomerulosclerosis seen with aging.[49] However, recent data suggest it may not be the sole contributory factor. Within the glomerulus, capillary blood flow rate and intracapillary hydraulic pressure are finely regulated, by changes in vascular tone, to maintain a stable filtration pressure gradient. The term "single nephron glomerular filtration rate" (SNGFR) has been coined to describe the filtration rate across the basement membrane of each individual nephron. A reduction in nephron number causes increased blood flow to each nephron and therefore increased SNGFR. The hyperfiltration hypothesis[47] proposes that, in a kidney with a reduced number of glomeruli, there is increased capillary blood flow through each glomerular capillary bed, and thus a correspondingly high intracapillary pressure. This high pressure (often referred to as shear stress) results in local endothelial cell damage and resultant glomerular injury. Contrary to initial reports, there is no alteration in systemic hemodynamics.[47] As small increases in blood flow, seen with increased SNGFR, lead to disproportionate increases in pressure, endothelial cell damage occurs, causing platelet aggregation and thrombin production. Activation of platelets leads to release of growth factors including platelet-derived growth factor (PDGF), epidermal growth factor (EGF), fibroblast growth factor (FGF) and tumor necrosis factor beta (TNF_β), which are associated with increased fibroblast collagen production and mesangial cell sclerosis.[50–52] At the same time, shear stresses cause a disruption in the ion exchange, changes in cell membrane voltage and altered protein transcription within the endothelial cells.[53] Alterations in the endothelin-derived relaxing factor (EDRF)/endothelin axis upset vascular hemodynamics and increase angiotensin II secretion. As glomeruli become sclerosed, the amount of blood flow directed to each of the remaining nephrons increases, further potentiating the damage.

In support of this theory, a reduction in glomerular capillary pressure associated with restricted protein intake decreases glomerular injury and can prolong the time to doubling of serum creatinine in patients with impaired creatinine clearances.[53,54] Similarly, antihypertensives which reduce single nephron GFR (e.g. ACE inhibitors and angiotensin II blockers) reduce glomerular injury more than antihypertensives, which solely control systemic blood pressure at comparable levels.[55] Experimentally, both reduced protein intake and ACE inhibitors cause local hemodynamic changes and decrease angiotensin II. However, animal studies have not consistently shown an increased intraglomerular pressure with senescence, suggesting that it may not be the sole contributor.

A reduced nephron mass at the time of birth is believed to contribute to the natural progression of renal disease. In animal models, renal ablation, resulting in a reduction in the number of functioning nephron units, results in single nephron hyperfiltration, progressive systemic hypertension, proteinuria, and renal failure associated with glomerular sclerosis.[46,54] Patients with congenital unilateral renal agenesis invariably show focal and segmental glomerulosclerosis on biopsy,[56–60] a finding attributed to chronic hyperfiltration from birth (although not always associated with the development of hypertension and renal impairment). One may hypothesize that individuals born with reduced nephron mass may have an increased tendency to hyperfiltrate and thus have a higher propensity for a faster rate of renal decline as illustrated by Lindeman et al.[28] In animal studies, pregnant rats fed a restricted protein diet had offspring with fewer glomeruli and tubular structures but increased connective tissue.[61] In humans this has not been shown, although epidemiological data demonstrate a correlation between low birth weight and hypertension.[62]

Other theories are also attractive. The genetic theory proposes that each individual has a predetermined rate of cellular apoptosis.[21] A number of genes have been shown to be related to age-related pathological appearances, though not specifically in the kidney. Alternatively, some authors have shown that as a cell replicates, the whole length of the chromosome is not replicated, leading to an eventual shortening of the telomere, and loss of DNA. Thus after a predetermined number of replications, DNA loss may lead to an inability to further replicate. Alternatively, if cellular replication was associated with a risk of injury to the genetic code, the older an individual became, the more at risk they are of significant injury and cellular malfunction.

The "toxin-mediated" theory proposes that the by-products of normal metabolism may progressively damage the kidney.[21] The theory seems attractive because it can explain both the structural and functional changes seen with age. Toxins, for example reactive oxygen species (ROS), advanced glycosolation end-products (AGE) and advanced lipoxidation end-products (ALE), can cause similar pathological changes in renal tissue. In high concentrations ROS cause necrosis, while in lower concentrations they can induce mesangial cell proliferation and autocoid release. Recent data show an increase in the in-vitro ROS synthesis in glomerular and mesangial cells derived from old rats. Furthermore, inactivation of nitric oxide

---

KEY POINTS Aging of the urinary tract

- Age-related renal changes include a decrease in the size and weight of the kidney with a proportionally greater loss of cortical tissue than medullary tissue.

- Glomerular filtration tends to decrease in the majority of older individuals but remains constant over time in a small proportion.

- Renal tubular handling of a sodium, potassium, or water load is impaired.

- Estimates of GFR using mathematical calculations based on serum markers may lead to an error of −33.1 mL/min to +19.6 mL/min.

has been suggested as an effect of certain ROS, an observation that would explain some of the abnormal vasoconstrictor tone seen in renal vessels of older animals. It is plausible that all three theories of renal aging are simultaneously active and that the rate of renal decline, if present, is dependent on a complex interaction of all these processes. Until the etiology of age related renal decline is better understood, the only interventions of value for the elderly individual with known renal impairment are ACE inhibitor drugs and possibly a reduction in the amount of dietary protein or the use of angiotensin II blocking drugs.

REFERENCES

1. Oliver J: Urinary system. In Cowdry EV (ed): Problems of Aging. Williams & Wilkins, Baltimore, 1952

2. Roessle R, Roulet F: (eds): Mass und Zahl in der Pathologie. Springer, Berlin, 1932

3. Abrass CK, Adcox MJ, Raugi GJ: Aging-associated changes in renal extracellular matrix. Am J Pathol 1995;146(3):742–752

4. McLachlan MS: The ageing kidney. Lancet 1978;2(8081):143–145

5. McLachlan MSF, Guthric JC, Anderson CK: Vascular and glomerular changes in the aging kidney. J Pathol 1977;121:65

6. Kaplan C, Pasternack B, Shah H, Gallo G: Age-related incidence of sclerotic glomeruli in human kidneys. Am J Pathol 1975;80(2):227–234

7. Sorenson F: Quantitative studies of the renal corpuscles. Acta Med Scand 1977;85:356

8. Darmady EM, Offer J, Woodhouse MA: The parameters of the ageing kidney. J Pathol 1973;195–209

9. Artursen G, Groth T, Grotte G: Human glomerular membrane porosity and filtration pressure: dextran clearance data analyzed by theoretical models. Clin Sci 1971;40:137–158

10. Cohen MR, Kin L: Age-related changes in sulfation of basement membrane glycosaminoglycans. Exp Gerontol 1983;18:461–469

11. Mortiz AR, Oldt MR: Arteriolar sclerosis in hypertensive and non-hypertensive individuals. Am J Pathol 1973;13:679

12. Takazakura E, Sawabu N, Handa A et al: Intrarenal vascular changes with age and disease. Kidney Int 1972;2:224–230

13. Ljungqvist A, Lagerggen C: Normal intrarenal arterial pattern in adult and aging human kidney. J Anat 1962;96:285

14. Brocklehurst JC: Clinical geriatrics. In Rossman L (ed): Lippincott-Raven, Philadelphia, 1971:227

15. Holtenberg NK, Adams DF, Solomon HS, et al: Senescence and the renal vasculature in normal man. Circ Res 1974;34:309–316

16. Hollenberg NK, Moore TJ: Age and the renal blood supply: renal vascular responses to angiotension converting enzyme inhibition in healthy humans. J Am Geriatr Soc 1994;42:805–808

17. Epstein M: Aging and the kidney. J Am Soc Nephrol 1996;7:1106–1102

18. Sharma K, Ziyadeh FN: The emerging role of transforming growth factor-B in kidney diseases. Am J Physiol 1994;266:F829–F842

19. Mulkerrin E, Brain A, Hampton D et al: Reduced renal haemodynamic response to atrial natriuretic peptide in elderly volunteers. Am J Kidney Dis 1993;22:538–544

20. Rockelhoff JF, Manning RD: Role of endothelium-derived nitric oxide in control of renal microvasculature in aging male rats. Am J Physiol 1993;265:R1126–R1131

21. Rodriguez-Puyol D: The aging kidney. Kidney Int 1998;54:2247–2265

22. Fliser D, Bischoff I, Hanses A et al: Renal handling of drugs in the healthy elderly. Creatinine clearance underestimates renal function and pharmacokinetics remain virtually unchanged. Eur J Clin Pharmacol 1999;55(3):205–211

23. Rowe JW, Andres A, Tobin JD, Norris AH, Shock NW: The effect of age on creatinine clearance in men: a cross-sectional and longitudinal study. J Gerontol 1976;32(2):155–163

24. Cockcroft DW, Gault MH: Prediction of creatinine clearance from serum creatinine. Nephron 1976;16(1):31–41

25. Lott RD, Hayton WL: Estimation of creatinine clearance from serum creatinine concentration: a review. Drug Intell Clin Pharm 1978;12:140

26. Friedman JR, Norman DC, Yoshikawa TT: Correlation of estimated renal function parameters versus 24 hour creatinine clearance in ambulatory elderly. J Am Geriatr Soc 1989;37:145–149

27. Malmrose LC, Gray SL, Pieper CF et al: Measured versus estimated creatinine clearance in a highly functioning elderly sample: MacArthur Foundation study of successful aging. J Am Geriatr Soc 1993;41:715–721

28. Lindeman RD, Tobin JD, Shock NW: Longitudinal studies on the rate of decline in renal function with age. J Am Geriatr Soc 1985;33:278–285

29. Fliser D, Eberhard R: Serum cystatin C concentration as a marker of renal dysfunction in the elderly. Am J Kidney Dis 2001;37(1):79–83

30. Goldberg TH, Finkelstein MS: Difficulties in estimating glomerular filtration rate in the elderly. Arch Intern Med 1987;147:1430

31. Desanto NG, Anastasio P, Coppola S et al: Age related changes in renal reserve and tubular changes in healthy humans. Nephrol Urol 1991;11:33–40

32. Bohler J, Gloer D, Reetze-Bonorden P, Keller E, Schollmeyer PJ: Renal functional reserve in elderly patients. Clin Nephrol 1993;39:145–150

33. Fliser D, Zeler M, Nowack R, Ritz E: Renal functional reserve in healthy elderly subjects. J Am Soc Nephrol 1993;3:1371–1377

34. Kunin CM, White LV, Hua TH: A reassessment of the importance of "low-count" bacteriuria in young women with acute urinary symptoms. Ann Intern Med 1993;119:454–460

35. Frocht A, Fillit H: Renal disease in the geriatric patient. J Am Geriatr Soc 1984;32:28–43

36. Meyer BR: Renal function in aging. J Am Geriatr Soc 1989;37:791–800

37. Macias Nunez JF, Garcia Iglesias C, Bondia Roman A et al: Renal handling of sodium in old people: a functional study. Age Ageing 1978;7:178–181

38. Sambhi MP, Crane MG, Genest J: Essential hypertension: new concepts about mechanisms. Ann Intern Med 1973;79:411–424

39. Tsunoda K, Abe K, Goto T et al: Effect of age on the renin angiotensin-aldosterone system in normal subjects: simultaneous measurement of active and inactive renin, renin substrate, and aldosterone in plasma. J Clin Endocrino Metabol 1986;62:384–389

40. Duggan J, Nussberger J, Kilfeather S, O'Malley K: Aging and human hormonal and pressor responsiveness to angiotensin II infusion with simultaneous measurement of exogenous and endogenous angiotensin II. Am J Hypertens 1993;6:641–647

41. Nielsen S, Kwon TH, Christensen BM et al: Physiology and pathophysiology of renal aquaporins. J Am Soc Nephrol 1999;10(3):647–663

42. Cox JR, Shalaby WA: Potassium changes with age. Gerontology 1981;27:340–344

43. Adler S, Lindeman RD, Yiengst MJ, Beard E, Shock NW: Effect of acute acid loading on urinary acid excretion by the aging human kidney. J Lab Clin Med 1968;72(2):278–289

44. Agarwal BN, Cabebe FG: Renal acidification in elderly subjects. Nephron 1980;26:291–295

45. Shuck O, Nadvornikova H: Short acidification test and its interpretation with respect to age. Nephron 1987;46:215–216

46. Hostetter TH, Olson J, Rennke HG et al: Hyperfiltration in remnant nephrons: a potentially adverse response to renal ablation. Am J Physiol 1981;241:F85–F93

47. Brenner BM: Nephron adaptation to renal injury or ablation. Am J Physiol 1985;249:F324–F337

48. Neuringer JR, Brenner BM: Haemodynamic theory of progressive renal disease: a 10 year update in brief review. Am J Kidney Dis 1993;22:98–104

49. Brenner BM, Chertow GM: Congenital oligonephropathy and etiology of adult hypertension and progressive renal injury. Am J Kidney Dis 1994;23:171–175

50. Klahr S: Chronic renal failure management. Lancet 1991;338:423–427

51. Wardle EN: Cytokine growth factors and glomerulonephritis. Nephron 1991;57:257–261

52. Wardle EN: Cellular biology of glomerulosclerosis. Nephron 1992;61:125–128

53. LaBarbera M: How fluid dynamics channel natural selection. Sci NY Acad Sci 1991;31:30–37

54. Brenner BM, Meyer TW, Hostetter TH: Dietary protein intake and the progressive nature of kidney disease: the role of haemodynamically mediated glomerular injury in the pathogenesis of progressive glomerular sclerosis in aging, renal ablation and intrinsic renal disease. N Engl J Med 1982;307:652–659

55. Zucchelli P, Zuccala A, Borghi M et al: Long-term comparison between captopril and nifedipine in the progression of renal insufficiency. Kidney Int 1992;42(2):452–458

56. Thorner PS, Arbus G, Celermajer DS, Baumal R: Focal segmental glomerulosclerosis and progressive renal failure associated with unilateral kidney. Pediatrics 1984;73:806–810

57. Bhathena DB, Julian BA, McMorrow RG, Baehler RW: Focal sclerosis of hypertrophied glomeruli in solitary functioning kidneys of humans. Am J Kidney Dis 1985;5:226–232

58. Weinstein T, Zevin D, Gafter U, Ben-Bassat M, Levi J: Proteinuria and chronic renal failure associated with unilateral renal agenesis. Isr J Med Sci 1985;21:919–921

59. Rugiu C, Oldrizzi L, Lupo A et al: Clinical features of patients with solitary kidneys. Nephron 1986;43:10–15

60. Gutierrez-Millet V, Nieto J, Praga M et al: Focal glomerulosclerosis and proteinuria in patients with solitary kidneys. Arch Intern Med 1986;46:705–709

61. Zeman FJ: Effects of maternal protein restriction on the kidney of the newborn young of rats. J Nutr 1968;94:111–116

62. Simpson MA, Mortimer JG, Silva PA et al: Correlates of blood pressure in a cohort of Dunedin seven-year old children. Onesti G, Kim KE (eds): Hypertension in the Young and Old. Grune & Stratton, New York, 1981:191–205

Chapter 87

Diseases of the aging kidney

Sarbjit Vanita Jassal, Howard M. Fillit, and

Dimitrios G. Oreopoulos

DIAGNOSTIC PROBLEMS OF RENAL DISEASE IN ELDERLY PEOPLE

The diagnosis of renal disease in elderly people poses a unique challenge to the clinician and indeed calls for sensitivity and attention to detail. Unlike younger patients, older patients often present with nonspecific symptoms which may lead to diagnostic and therapeutic delays. Additionally, the concomitant occurrence of diseases other than renal, such as diabetes, cardiac failure, and arteriosclerotic vascular disease, confuse both the clinical picture and the symptomatology, and as a result the clinician often overlooks renal disease. The interpretation of clinical findings, urinary findings, and clearance estimations, are often difficult without specialist knowledge of the aging process.

These diagnostic difficulties indicate the need for a high index of suspicion for renal disease in elderly people. A prevalence of renal disease has been well documented in this age group.[1,2] The basic examinations which must be performed as a matter of routine on all elderly patients should include: hemoglobin (or hematocrit), blood urea nitrogen and/or serum creatinine, urinalysis for albumin, sugar, and pH, and microscopic examination of the urinary sediment, with additional screening for bacteria.

Collection of urine samples

Although it may seem trivial, obtaining a clean urine sample for examination is of special importance, since there is frequent contamination of the sample, particularly in elderly women. The bedridden female patient of advanced age is the most difficult subject, and the nursing staff therefore needs special training in collecting urine samples. According to Roberts et al.,[3] the best method is to clean the periurethral area with water without adding any disinfecting agent. The specimen is best obtained in the morning when the urine has been in the bladder for some time. A large diuresis might reduce the concentration of bacteria and therefore impede interpretation of the bacteria count. It is of the utmost importance that the laboratory data be obtained under controlled conditions.

The incontinent elderly patient can, with careful nursing care, provide a clean catch specimen of urine.[4,5] Occasionally, single or intermittent catheterization is necessary. The use of sterile technique provides no superior benefit over the standard clean method of catheterization.[6] Catheterization must only be performed when necessary, as it can itself infect the urinary tract in up to 5.6 percent of cases.[7] As a last resort, bladder puncture and suprapubic aspiration may be used. Suprapubic aspiration is both safe and accurate, but it is technically difficult in elderly patients and has a consistent success rate of only 65 percent, making it impractical as a routine procedure.[8] According to Moore-Smith, the mid-stream urine (MSU) has an incidence of doubtful results between 17.5 and 28 percent, while frankly contaminated results may be as high as 31 percent.[8]

Interpretation of urinary sediment

As with younger patients, the interpretation of urinary sediment helps identify glomerular disease and vasculitis. Casts, dysmorphic red cells, high levels of proteinuria and hematuria all call for further investigation by a nephrologist. The addition of salicylic acid to urine causes precipitation of protein, not normally identified with albumin dipsticks, if light chain protein excretion in myeloma is significant. In elderly patients, microscopic examination of sediment most commonly reveals an increased number of leukocytes and epithelial cells. If the bacteriological findings reveal a mixed infection, then contamination must be suspected, although mixed infection may occur especially in patients with indwelling catheters. In these cases, the urinary tests should be repeated. An increase in the number of leukocytes—more than 10 per milliliter—is regarded as pathological in younger patients, but is not always a sign of an infection of the urinary tract in elderly patients. Conversely, the occurrence of a normal number of leukocytes does not exclude the possibility of infection. It should be recognized that there are several sources of error in the examination of the urinary sediment.[9] These include the volume of urine being sampled and the presence of bacteria in the urinary sediment with a negative culture suggesting the presence of lactobacilli and corynebacteria. Additionally, variations in the number of white blood cells seen under the microscope depend upon (a) how the specimen was obtained (i.e. the degree of vaginal or urethral contamination), (b) the urine flow rate at the time of collection, (c) the intensity of the tissue reaction of the uroepithelial surfaces to the disease process, (d) the volume, time, and speed of centrifugation, and (e) the volume in which the observer suspends the sediment.

Screening for bacteria

Screening for bacteria in the urine is traditionally done using the colony count method described by Kass.[10] In this series, screening of young healthy women revealed that a bacterial count of more than 10^5 organisms/mL was associated with a ~80 percent probability of representing true bacteriuria rather than contamination. Strictly speaking, the definition applies only to *Escherichia coli* and *Proteus* spp., which do not grow in clumps or chains. However, the definition has traditionally become synonymous with the presence of a urinary tract infection. As urine samples are more difficult to obtain in elderly persons, a high false positive rate is seen when this definition is used,[11] and the use of urine culture as a screening test for urinary tract infection has been brought into question.[12] Lower counts of bacteriuria may also be significant, and bacterial invasion of the bladder wall has been recorded with fewer than 10^5 colonies of bacteria/mL.[13]

A number of chemical and microscopic methods for rapid screening of urine for infection are in use. These include dipstick testing for urinary nitrites, leukocyte esterase, and ward-based urine microscopy for urinary leukocytes. No one screening test has adequate sensitivity and specificity; however, the use of two or more tests together increase the sensitivity to over 90 percent when one or more tests is positive, and over 95 percent specificity when all are negative. These tests should not be used after urinary catheterization or any urological procedure as they have unacceptably low sensitivity and specificity rates.[14]

DISEASES OF THE KIDNEY IN ELDERLY PEOPLE

Elderly people are prone to the same diseases of the kidney as younger patients. The difference lies in the presentation, which may be less overt or confounded by the presence of multisystem disease. Common presentations of renal disease in elderly people include:

- an acute deterioration in renal function (often related to hospitalization or other illness);
- gradual deterioration in renal function (often an incidental finding);
- proteinuria, sometimes in the form of nephrotic syndrome;
- hypertension and renal vascular disease;
- systemic disease with renal involvement;
- infection of the urinary tract.

There is poor correlation between clinical presentation and the etiology of disease in many cases. The following sections, however, do attempt to cover both clinical presentation and etiology collectively.

Acute renal failure

Acute renal failure (ARF) is seen more frequently in older patients probably because of common inciting events. In a prospective observational study of all patients aged 60 years or more admitted to a single institution with stable renal function, 1.4 percent developed a rise in serum creatinine to greater than 177 μmol/L or a rise of greater than 138 μmol/L during their hospital stay.[15] Patients with impaired renal function who remained stable or those admitted because of a rising serum creatinine were excluded. Of note, nephrotoxic drugs contributed towards the acute renal injury in 66 percent of cases, with sepsis and hypoperfusion contributing to another 46 percent of cases. Radiocontrast nephrotoxicity and postoperative renal failure were seen in 17 and 25 percent of cases respectively. As can be seen from these data, disease is often due to multifactorial causes. In addition, age-related changes in renal function, including tubular changes resulting in alterations in water and electrolyte balance, predispose elderly people to acute renal failure.

The incidence of acute renal insufficiency is estimated to be around 6–10 percent of all elderly admissions to an acute medical service. In a prospective study, of patients over 65 years of age, 6.8 percent of all hospital admissions had a serum urea $\geq$17 mmol/L and/or creatinine $\geq$160 μmol/L at presentation.[16] Fifty-five percent of patients had a prerenal etiology and had an excellent rate of renal recovery. The majority of patients had mild renal impairment with only 24 percent presenting with serum urea $\geq$31 mmol/L and/or creatinine $\geq$400 μmol/L. Patients with intrinsic renal failure had a higher mortality rate (48 percent) than expected, possibly because of a delay in recognition of the disease. In contrast to other studies, however, a higher mortality was seen in patients with obstructive renal disease. This appears to be because of a disproportionately high number of patients with pelvic neoplasia and may reflect some sampling bias.

In another study of patients requiring admission to an intensive care unit, ARF was due to cardiogenic or septic shock in 17 percent of cases, post-surgical causes in 13 percent and ischemia and hypovolemic shock in 22 percent.[17] Overall, mortality rates correlate with the severity of the clinical disease state and range between 40 and 60 percent, with the highest mortality seen with hepatic failure, shock, renal parenchymal, and renovascular disease. The prognosis for patients with acute renal failure resulting from aortic aneurysm repair is poor, with a 100 percent mortality in some series.[17–21] Good recovery is expected when ARF is caused by hypercalcemia or medication. Mortality appears to correlate closely to the serum creatinine and urea levels. When dialysis is started the prescription should be tailored to ensure serum blood urea nitrogen (BUN) levels are maintained lower than 15 mmol/L.[19,22] Age itself does not have a significant impact on the prognosis of the patient with acute renal failure. Hypophosphatemia and hypokalemia are associated with an unexpectedly high death rate, and it remains unclear if this reflects the severity of the underlying disease or malnutrition.[23–25] Of those patients who survive to discharge, 58 percent have complete recovery of renal function and 39 percent have some degree of renal impairment but do not require dialysis.[17]

The management of acute renal failure in elderly people is complex and demanding. The aged kidney retains the capacity to recover from acute ischemic or toxic insults over the course of several weeks. As the recovering kidney is vulnerable to additional insults which can prolong recovery, care should be taken to avoid nephrotoxins such as aminoglycoside antibiotics and radiocontrast agents, as well as volume depletion. Renal function, as reflected in serum BUN and creatinine levels, is impaired for several days after a brief hypotensive episode associated with surgery, sepsis, overmedication or volume depletion, or after the administration of nephrotoxic radiographic contrast agents. After a brief period of azotemia, renal function gradually can return to its previous level. Oliguria is not a prominent component of the clinical picture in this age group, although if present, it is associated with a poorer outcome. Since the clinical hallmark of renal failure is generally thought to be a dramatic reduction in urine output, cases of nonoliguric acute renal failure may go unrecognized. This may result in the inadvertent overdose of patients with renally excreted medications, including digitalis preparations and aminoglycoside antibiotics such as gentamicin.

Standard intermittent hemodialysis, peritoneal dialysis or slow continuous methods of hemodialysis are all reported to be successful in older patients, though no data exist as to the most preferable method. Aside from the initiation of dialysis, careful attention to the balance of several factors is necessary. Water and salt balance must be monitored carefully. Due to catabolism, the usual patient with acute renal failure will lose about 0.5 kg of body mass per day. Attempts to keep body weight constant will result in the gradual expansion of the extracellular fluid and consequent increase in blood pressure and risk of precipitation of cardiac failure. Similarly, overzealous fluid restriction will impair the patients' general condition and central nervous system function and may delay the recovery of renal function. Nutritional support should be implemented at an early stage.

Glomerular diseases

Although glomerular disease was previously believed to be rare in older patients, this may have reflected a lack of routine urine testing and a reluctance to refer older individuals to a nephrologist. More recent data indicate a similar or slightly higher incidence of primary glomerular disease in elderly people (8.5 patients per 10^5 population per year in those over 75 years old compared with 8.4 per 10^5 population per year in younger adults).[26] The disease spectrum seen in the older individual is as diverse as in the younger population. As in the younger population, the main presenting features of glomerular disease are proteinuria and hematuria, with or without hypertension and renal dysfunction. The clinical syndromes often used to describe the common patterns include the terms nephritic, nephrotic, and secondary diseases. These, though useful in some settings, often do not correlate with etiology or histological features, resulting in complex classifications. To simplify the schema we use the following terminology: nephrotic syndrome (describing a predominantly proteinuric presentation), proliferative syndromes including cresentic nephritis (which describe a clinical picture of hematuria and proteinuria, often with cellular casts) and systemic disorders causing glomerular disease.

The diagnosis of glomerular disease is often based on the clinical features and serology. The gold standard for diagnosis, however, is renal biopsy. Renal biopsy appears to be safe in those over 60 years old. Most attempts at biopsy in elderly patients are successful, and reported complication rates vary from 2.2 to 9.8 percent.[27,28] Interpretation of the tissue is more difficult, as arteriolar sclerosis and global sclerosis associated with chronic ischemia and aging may be difficult to differentiate from previously healed proliferative glomerulonephritis (GN) or focal sclerosing GN. A recent large prospective biopsy series showed that most patients undergoing a biopsy present with nephrotic syndrome or acute renal failure. Of those with biopsies, 30 percent had a diagnosis of pauci-immune glomerulonephritis, 22 percent of acute interstitial nephritis and 13.5 percent of vascular disease.[29] Details of the clinical presenting features are given in Table 87-1.[30] Administrative data show differing results. In 7,086 cases collected over a 13-year period,

825 biopsies were from patients aged over 65 years old.[31] Renal biopsy was 3.5 times less likely to be done in older patients in the earlier years than in the latter years, and, when compared to younger patients, older patients were more likely to have impaired renal function and heavier proteinuria at the time of biopsy. In this series, idiopathic GN was the most common underlying diagnosis for all ages, with secondary GN and unclassified being the next most common diagnoses seen in the older cohort. Few elderly patients were biopsied to help establish a diagnosis of diabetic nephropathy. Disorders associated with a proliferative picture on histology, including pauci-immune GN, were rarer, suggesting either that pauci-immune was less often considered a diagnosis or that there is a change over time in the disease spectrum seen in aged individuals.

Nephrotic syndrome

Nephrotic syndrome is the most common reason given for performing a renal biopsy in those over 75 years old. The commonest cause of nephrotic syndrome is membranous nephropathy, with minimal change disease (MCD) and nephrotic syndrome secondary to amyloidosis and myeloma being the next most common diagnoses. Based on data from a 15-year prospective study,[32] the annual incidence of membranous nephropathy in patients aged 60 years or more was 2.5 patients per 10^5 population per year, a figure almost three times as high as the overall incidence of membranous nephropathy. Bias arising from a reluctance to biopsy older patients may have been present, but this would tend to skew the data toward an even higher incidence in elderly patients. Focal segmental glomerulosclerosis and IgA nephropathy are less common than in younger patients.

Membranous nephropathy

Seventy-five to 80 percent of cases of membranous nephropathy are idiopathic, with the remaining 20–25 percent being secondary to solid organ tumors and drugs. The clinical presentation is fairly typical with proteinuria, often greater than 3 g/24 hours. In contrast to younger patients, 40 percent of older patients have associated hypertension, 30–90 percent haematuria and 15 percent renal impairment at the time they are first seen. Although an association with solid organ malignancy is recognized, the current recommendations call only for a full clinical examination, chest X-ray, and stool for occult bloods. In heavy smokers, a CT scan of the chest may be appropriate.[33] Further work-up is not indicated unless symptoms or signs suggestive of a neoplastic lesion are present. The natural history of membranous nephropathy appears similar to that in younger individuals, although the presence of subclinical glomerulosclerosis may make the prognosis in older patients appear worse than that of younger patients. In a small retrospective study, older patients with membranous nephropathy responded favorably to treatment with prednisone and chlorambucil.[34] The time to remission was often longer and the incidence and severity of side-effects higher than in younger patients, but in contrast, remission rates were lower. Response rates for patients treated conservatively or with corticosteroids alone were poor. On this basis, the recommended treatment for the older patient is low dose chlorambucil (0.1 mg/kg/per day) for a 3–6 month period with or without low-dose corticosteroid therapy.

Table 87-1 Clinical data in cases of acute renal insufficiency by diagnosis and age group

Renal biopsy diagnosis	Age (y)	Sex (M/F)	Serum creatinine (mg/dL)	Proteinuria (g/24 h)	Nephrotic-Range proteinuria (%)	Hematuria (%)	Hypertension (%)
Pauci-immune crescentic GN	71.9 ± 6.6 (79) (60–90)	38/41	6.3 ± 3.7 (79) (1.8–20.9)	2.8 ± 2.4 (54) (0.1–11.0)	14/54 (25.9)	74/75 (98.7)	53/74 (71.6)
Acute interstitial nephritis	70.9 ± 9.4 (47) (60–98)	23/24	6.7 ± 3.3 (45) (2.5–18.6)	2.8 ± 3.0 (30) (0.1–9.0)	10/30 (30.0)	25/36 (69.4)	31/45 (68.9)
ATN with nephrotic syndrome	72.1 ± 6.2 (19) (62–84)	15/4	4.7 ± 2.7 (18) (1.9–11.9)	14.1 ± 10.0 (19)* (5.2–42.0)	19/19 (100)	7/15 (46.7)	17/19 (89.5)
Atheroemboli	71.5 ± 7.4 (18) (60–88)	13/5	6.6 ± 3.7 (18) (3.5–20.0)	2.0 ± 2.2 (15) (0.2–6.6)	3/15 (20.0)	11/14 (78.6)	17/18 (94.4)
ATN	72.9 ± 7.6 (17) (61–85)	9/8	7.3 ± 5.6 (17) (2.0–25.8)	0.9 ± 0.7 (19) (0.1–2.0)	0/10 (0)	7/12 (58.3)	11/14 (78.6)
Light chain cast nephropathy	75.6 ± 7.2 (15) (63–86)	8/7	9.8 ± 3.6 (14)* (4.5–16.3)	2.1 ± 1.8 (8) (0.9–5.0)	3/8 (37.5)	4/10 (40.0)	9/14 (64.3)
Postinfectious GN	69.7 ± 6.7 (14) (60–82)	10/4	7.8 ± 4.2 (12) (2.7–16.0)	5.2 ± 5.7 (8) (1.5–15.0)	5/8 (62.5)	12/12 (100)	12/14 (85.7)
Anti-GBM nephritis	72.0 ± 7.1 (10) (61–82)	4/6	10.4 ± 5.4 (10)* (2.8–18.0)	1.9 ± 1.4 (7) (0.3–4.0)	1/7 (14.3)	9/9 (100)	5/9 (55/6)
IgA Henoch–Schönlein nephropathy	72.7 ± 8.1 (9) (60–84)	6/3	5.5 ± 2.5 (2.7–11.1)	3.8 ± 3.6 (8) (0.7–13.0)	4/8 (50.0)	9/9 (100)	7/8 (87.5)
Age group (y)							
60–69	64.7 ± 2.0 (107) (60–69)	51/56	7.3 ± 4.4 (103) (1.9–20.9)	3.5 ± 5.1 (72) (0.1–36.0)	23/72 (31.9)	78/95 (82.1)	70/99 (70.7)
70–79	73.7 ± 2.9 (113) (70–79)	65/48	6.6 ± 3.8 (109) (1.8–25.8)	4.5 ± 6.4 (74) (0.1–42.0)	25/74 (33.8)	69/86 (80.2)	82/102 (80.4)
≥80	83.7 ± 3.6 (39) (80–98)	22/17	6.6 ± 3.3 (38) (2.0–18.0)	3.1 ± 3.0 (24) (0.1–10.0)	10/24 (41.7)	23/27 (85.2)	31/39 (79.5)
All cases	71.8 ± 7.4 (259) (60–98)	138/121	6.9 ± 4.0 (250) (1.8–25.8)	3.9 ± 9.5 (170) (0.1–42.0)	58/170 (34.1)	170/208 (81.7)	183/240 (76.3)

*Significantly different (P ≤ 0.002) from mean value for all cases by t-test.

Age, serum creatinine level, and 24-hour urine protein level are expressed as the mean ± SD for the number of cases listed directly afterward in parentheses. Hematuria includes gross and/or microscopic hematuria. Values listed in parentheses for each diagnosis and age group after the number of cases represent the range of values (for age, serum creatinine level, and proteinuria) or the percentage of patients with the specified finding (for nephrotic-range proteinuria, hematuria, and hypertension).

Reproduced with permission from Haas et al: Am J Kid Dis 2000;35:433–447.

Minimal change nephropathy

Minimal change nephropathy, as with younger patients, typically presents with the features of the nephrotic syndrome. The incidence of microscopic hematuria, hypertension, and renal impairment at the time of presentation is much higher than in younger patients. Oliguria usually heralds a poor prognosis, often with progression to death or renal replacement therapy. Further complications resulting from hypoalbuminemia, hyperlipidemia, and hypercoagulability include thrombotic events, infection, and progressive cardiovascular disease. As with membranous nephropathy, standard therapeutic regimes can be used. Treatment with oral corticosteroid therapy frequently needs to be prolonged for up to 16 weeks. Corticosteroid resistant cases may benefit from the introduction to chlorambucil, cyclophosphamide, or cyclosporine A, although the risk of bone marrow depression is high.

A history of nonsteroidal anti-inflammatory drug usage should be actively sought, as minimal change nephropathy secondary to drugs may partially remit without aggressive immunosuppressive therapy.

Focal and segmental glomerulosclerosis

Focal and segmental glomerulosclerosis (FSGS) is much less commonly seen in elderly people. It can be difficult to distinguish from ischemic changes without electron microscopy. Patients present with heavy proteinuria and often have some degree of renal insufficiency. A trial of corticosteroids or immunosuppressive medication may be offered on the basis of the results of a small study of FSGS in the older patient.[35] Therapy should be given for a 3-month trial period, and if successful tapered gradually over the next month. Those with no response should be treated for a further 3-month period.[33] Angiotensin-converting enzyme inhibitors and nonsteroidal anti-inflammatory agents are both effective antiproteinuric drugs but can lead to significant elevations in serum creatinine and must be used with caution.

Proliferative syndromes

Proliferative GN includes glomerular diseases caused by immune complex deposition, the antineutrophil cytoplasmic antibody (ANCA) associated syndromes and antiglomerular basement membrane (anti-GBM) antibody-mediated disease. The clinical characteristics and rate of deterioration are similar to those seen in younger patients, though the diagnosis is best confirmed with renal biopsy. The older patient tends to present with much higher serum creatinine levels and at a later stage of the disease. Immunosuppression is not well studied in this population, and no randomized controlled studies of therapy in those over 65 years old exist. Most therapeutic studies are small but appear to show a good short-term prognosis with standard regimes of therapy. Observational data suggest that older patients are at higher risk of septic and gastrointestinal complications with immunosuppression.[36] Some also report a higher incidence of refractory renal impairment and hypertension compared to younger patients.

Cresentic GN is a pathological lesion which occurs in a range of renal and systemic disorders. In some series it is more common in older individuals than the younger patient.[28,35,36] Cresentic GN is a histological diagnosis, which can be subdivided into those with immune deposits, as seen in severe IgA nephropathy or lupus nephritis, or pauci-immune disease where no immune deposits are seen. The differential diagnoses of a pauci-immune picture includes Wegener's granulomatosis, anti-GBM disease and polyarteritis nodosa, while those with immune deposits characteristically include systemic lupus erythematosus and mesangiocapillary glomerulonephritis. Henoch–Schönlein disease and IgA nephropathy, though recognized in older patients, are less commonly seen (approx 3.8 percent of all biopsied lesions). Cryoglobulinemia should always be suspected in patients presenting with a palpable purpuric rash and features of a mesangiocapillary GN. The clinical presentation is variable with nonspecific complaints of nausea, anorexia, and malaise, edema, arthalgia and myalgia. Symptoms of pyrexia, rash, and hemoptysis are more typical of systemic vasculitis. The renal manifestations include microscopic (and macroscopic) hematuria, hypertension, and oliguria. The majority of patients present with significant renal failure and become dialysis-dependent in the early course of their disease. The data presented by Haas et al. suggest that serum ANCA levels are a good marker for pauci-immune glomerulonephritis.[29] In their series, 92 percent of all patients who had biopsy-proven pauci-immune GN had an elevated ANCA (either perinuclear or cytoplasmic), with 71 percent having elevated perinuclear ANCA level. In this series, only eight patients (from a total of 228) had a positive serum ANCA level in the absence of pathological disease, although it is unclear what proportion of patients were tested. Serum ANCA levels, anti-GBM levels, antinuclear factor, complement, immunoglobulin levels, and renal biopsy help distinguish the different syndromes (Table 87-1). Treatment with pulsed steroids and cyclophosphamide is indicated in most cases.

Systemic disorders causing glomerular disease

Many systemic diseases can be associated with glomerular disease, in particular diabetes, myeloma, and systemic lupus erythematosus. The presentation and course of these diseases are similar in both old and young patients.

Although the classical description of temporal arteritis does not include renal disease, glomerular involvement has been described in the literature from as early as 1958.[37–39] Azotemia in giant-cell arteritis is recognized, although renal disease may also be secondary to involvement of the aorta, with dissection of the renal artery or renal artery thrombosis. Azotemia and renal involvement in giant-cell arteritis is responsive to immunosuppressive therapy.

Chronic or acute systemic bacterial infection may cause immune complex formation and thus active glomerular proliferative disease. Acute poststreptococcal glomerulonephritis (APSGN) has also been reported in elderly people.[40–43] However, APSGN in elderly people tends to originate more often from pyodermal streptococcal infections rather than streptococcal throat infections. Since the antistreptolysin O titer may fail to rise after a pyodermal infection, antideoxyribonuclease B titers may be of more value in assessing precedent streptococcal infections in elderly patients with APSGN. In addition, oliguria may be more common in elderly patients with APSGN, perhaps because of underlying age-related changes. However, the outcome of APSGN in elderly patients is similar to younger age groups, with most patients recovering renal function. Thus, dialysis is generally of value, when required, in elderly patients with APSGN and acute renal failure.

RENOVASCULAR DISEASE

Ischemic nephropathy

Ischemic nephropathy is a generic term used to describe renal disease associated with poor renal perfusion. It can manifest either as macrovascular disease (renal artery stenosis) where the vascular disease predominantly affects one or both renal arteries, or microvascular disease, where diffuse disease affects the intrarenal arteries. The latter is poorly studied and the exact prevalence of ischemic nephropathy causing end-stage renal disease in older patients remains unknown. It has, however, been implicated in a large number of cases of "end-stage renal disease of unknown etiology."

Renal artery stenosis (RAS) is a common and often undetected disorder seen particularly in patients older than 55 years. If left untreated, progression of the stenotic lesion is seen in up to 30–40 percent of cases over a 4 year period with a corresponding decrease in the renal size. The prevalence is difficult to estimate. In an autopsy series, 5 percent of those examined had incidental severe renal artery stenosis. However, angiography studies of both hypertensive and nonhypertensive populations give estimates between 11 and 25 percent. Differences in the prevalence rate reported may be influenced by the population studied and the characteristics of the population. Age, hypertension, diabetes, and vascular disease (particularly coronary artery disease and peripheral vascular disease) increase the risk of clinically significant renal artery stenosis.

Screening for RAS is indicated in patients who present with flash pulmonary edema, severe unresponsive hypertension and in those with generalized vascular disease and renal impairment of unknown etiology. In addition, patients who develop acute renal failure after a mild hypotensive or hypovolemic episode or in response to angiotensin-converting enzyme inhibitor (ACEi) drugs should also be considered for investigation. Patients commonly have other manifestations of vascular disease at the time of presentation. In the latter cases, the acute renal failure often resolves with appropriate fluid resuscitation or withdrawal of the ACEi. Methods of screening are listed in Table 87-2. Initial screening with captopril renography or color Doppler sonography is appropriate unless accessory renal arteries are suspected.[44] Recent work showing that a "resistance index" may help identify patients who would benefit from intervention seems promising.[45]

The two main treatments available for RAS are surgery and angioplasty. The latter is occasionally supplemented by stent insertion to improve long-term vessel patency. Recent studies show similar radiological success rates with either treatment, though surgery is favored particularly for technically difficult lesions. Traditional surgical methods include aortorenal bypass surgery and transaortic renal endarterectomy. However, other methods currently being used include hepatorenal or gastroduodenal renal bypass for right-sided stenoses, splenorenal bypasses for left-sided lesions, extra-anatomic revascularization or ex-vivo reconstruction, and autotransplantation.[46]

Renal function improves after surgical revascularization in approximately 50 percent, although values varying between 22–65 percent are reported.[47] With angioplasty, initial patency rates are high (90–95 percent) at and around the time of the procedure, but restenosis rates are as high as 9–25 percent by 6–12 months. In addition, the clinical benefits are not so clear. Most reports estimate that renal function improves in approximately 25 percent, with a further 50 percent having stable renal function. Stents, inserted into the renal artery at the point of maximal stenosis have improved the long-term results, with up to 70 percent of patients having a short-term stabilization in creatinine clearance after stenting.[48] Despite these impressive results, treatment for RAS is not always recommended because of the progressive decline in renal function seen even with successful revascularization.[49]

Atheroembolic disease

Atheroembolism is an important, though uncommon, cause of both acute and chronic renal failure in elderly people.[50] Renal arterial emboli occur in any setting associated with peripheral embolization, such as acute myocardial infarction, chronic atrial fibrillation, subacute bacterial endocarditis, and aortic surgery or aortography. Renal embolization in elderly people varies from a clinically silent event to a full-blown syndrome of severe flank pain and tenderness, hematuria, hypertension, pyrexia, marked reduction in renal function, and elevations of serum lactate dehydrogenase. Small emboli are very difficult to detect, since renal scans may show focal perfusion defects in many apparently normal elderly patients. Major emboli are suggested by findings of differential contrast excretion on pyelography and confirmed by renal scan and aortography. Thrombolytic therapy, given intra-arterially, is now the treatment of choice, and few cases warrant surgical intervention.[51] The degree and duration of occlusion does not affect outcome and the final level of renal function often correlates with the degree of collateral renal blood flow.[51] In patients where renal function is discernibly impaired, improvement may occur over several weeks to months. When atheroembolism causes acute renal failure, dialysis can maintain the patient through the critical period of recovery.

Renal dysfunction secondary to cholesterol embolism is seen in older individuals with diffuse atheromatous disease. The classical presentation is that of a sudden increase in serum creatinine, typically after arterial catheterization or systemic heparinization. As urine microscopy is often bland and clinical examination unremarkable, the diagnosis can be easily overlooked. On occasion, an active urinary sediment, signs of peripheral embolism in the limbs, fluctuating confusional state, gut ischemia and peripheral eosinophilia can be seen. The diagnosis is confirmed if intravascular cholesterol crystals are seen on renal biopsy, skin biopsy, or muscle biopsy.

Systemic diseases involving the kidney

Diabetic nephropathy

Nephropathy is a common complication of diabetes at all ages. In elderly people, type 2 diabetes is more commonly seen, and the incidence of nephropathy at the time of diagnosis is high. It is usual for the nephropathy to present with microalbuminuria, or more commonly, proteinuria. The National Kidney

Table 87-2 Screening and diagnostic tests for renal artery stenosis

	Sensitivity (%)	Specificity (%)	Comments
Rapid sequence intravenous pyelogram	74.5	86.2	
Nuclear imaging:			
With captopril	83	93	Improved sensitivity and specificity with captopril challenge. High negative predictive value for unilateral renal disease, but high false positive rate. Less value if impaired renal function
Without captopril	75	85	
Renal artery color doppler sonography	66–98	86–98	Sensitivity varies on cutoff for stenosis. Requires technical expertise. Low detection of accessory renal artery if present. Diagnostic value has been improved by using ACEi before and after the examination, though technique limited to certain centers
Selective renal vein renin sampling	77–80	62–75	Not useful for bilateral disease but may help predict hypertensive response to revascularization. Invasive
Peripheral plasma renin sampling with or without captopril	52–100	85–95	High false negative and false positive results but good for detection of bilateral disease, especially in transplant renal artery stenosis
	44–62	17–93	
Angiography:			
Standard angiography	Gold Standard		
Carbon dioxide angiography	87–100	91–97	No need for contrast use. Technically complex
Magnetic resonance angiography	94–100	92–100	No need for contrast use. Expensive
Spiral computed angiography	92–99	83–98	Detects aberrant vessels in addition to normal vessels

Foundation recommends that all individuals, aged 70 years or less, with non-insulin-dependent diabetes mellitus (NIDDM) have their urine tested for microalbuminuria at yearly intervals.[52] Microalbuminuria, which indicates early diabetic nephropathy, is defined as an albumin excretion of 30–300 mg/24 hours in at least two urine samples evaluated within a 6–12 week period. Strict glycemic control, the introduction of ACE inhibitor (ACEi) therapy, and reduction of blood pressure to less than 130/80 mmHg are advised if microalbuminuria or proteinuria is present.[53] Diabetic dyslipidemia has been proposed as a further independent risk factor in the progression of renal disease, but a reduced rate of disease progression has not been demonstrated with the introduction of lipid-lowering agents. Although the disease course can be modified by the early introduction of ACEi,[54] the elderly diabetic patient is at a high risk of subclinical renal artery stenosis, and close monitoring of serum creatinine and serum potassium levels is therefore mandatory.

The antihypertensive protocol recommended by the National Kidney Foundation Hypertension and Diabetes Working Group suggests that a combination of ACEi and diuretics is the best initial therapy. The combination of ACEi and β-blockers has not shown benefit unless the patient manifests a resting pulse rate greater than 84/min or coexistent cardiac disease warrants it, in which case calcium channel blockers are recommended as third-line agents. A self-limited decline in renal function (as measured by serum creatinine) of up to 30 percent within the first 4 months of starting an ACEi is acceptable in individuals with a baseline creatinine of 250 μmol/L or less. Long-term follow-up studies suggest a continued benefit even after 3 years in this group.[53]

Multiple myeloma

Multiple myeloma (MM) is seen predominantly in the older population and is the primary renal disease in 1 percent of patients on chronic renal replacement therapy.[55] Estimates put the incidence of MM at 3.8–11.3 per 100,000 hospitalized patients overall, with an increase to 5 percent in those older than 80 years of age. Renal failure is estimated to occur in 20–60 percent of patients with myeloma.[56–58] There are a variety of reasons for renal disease in patients with MM. These include myeloma glomerulopathy, tubular toxic effects of light chains, light chain cast formation with intratubular obstruction (myeloma kidney), hypercalcemia, hyperuricemia, cryoglobulinemia and the additive effect of dehydration and nephrotoxic drugs. In a significant proportion of patients, the renal failure is reversible, and careful attention should be therefore paid to the prevention of further renal insult. Hyperuricemia secondary to chemotherapy, hypercalcemia, and radiocontrast nephrotoxicity should be avoided by adequate hydration and the use of allopurinol if needed. Patients who present with myeloma and renal disease are often not biopsied as the management usually involves chemotherapy directed at the myeloma with renal support, regardless of etiology of renal disease. Although biopsy may not alter therapy, a recent report has suggested that it may help predict prognosis.[59] In a series of 118 patients, the authors found that biopsy showed myeloma kidney in 41 percent of cases, AL-amyloidosis in 35 percent and light chain deposit disease in 19 percent. Survival correlated with the biopsy diagnosis (light chain deposit disease hav-

ing the best prognosis), the stage of the myeloma, and the type of chemotherapy used. Estimated survival in this series was better than in most, with a 1-year survival with myeloma kidney, 2 years with AL-amyloid, and up to 4 years when diagnosed with light chain deposit disease. Although successful case reports of both hemodialysis and peritoneal dialysis are published, some authors recommend peritoneal dialysis (PD) as the treatment of choice.[60] PD has the advantage of clearing a small fraction of the immunoglobulin load, particularly if rapid exchanges are used. This may confer a theoretical benefit with a reduction in tubular toxic effect of the light chains, the incidence of hyperviscosity syndrome and amyloidosis.[61,62] The long-term survival of patients with myeloma commenced onto renal replacement therapy has improved as a result of better chemotherapeutic regimes. Recent studies have shown that the presence and degree of azotemia does not correlate with outcome and that there is a good survival of patients with myeloma on chronic dialysis.[63–67]

Obstructive nephropathy

The most common cause of urinary obstruction in old age is prostatic hypertrophy.[50,68] Olbrich et al.[69] reported a 30–50 percent decrease of glomerular filtration rate and renal plasma flow in aged males with prostatic hypertrophy. After prostatectomy, renal plasma flow increased slightly, but glomerular filtration rate did not change. The increased intrapelvic pressure caused by urinary obstruction has been considered to be transmitted back through the tubular lumina and induce pressure atrophy of the renal parenchyma. Renal failure caused by obstruction is restored after removal of obstruction if the renal trauma is not irreversible. Age does not have a major effect on the likelihood or clinical presentation of nephrolithiasis, renal tumors or renal tuberculosis. Obstructive renal disease occasionally presents in old age with hematuria, recurrent urinary infections, or azotemia. The progress is usually slow. Treatment of urinary tract infection and hypertension is indicated in patients with this disorder.[70]

Urinary tract infections and pyelonephritis

The significance of bacteriuria in elderly people

There are four clinical categories which describe the relationship between bacteriuria and urinary tract infection. These include symptomatic infection, asymptomatic infection (asymptomatic bacteriuria), relapsing or persisting infection, and reinfection.[71] The relationship between bacteriuria, lower urinary tract infection, and upper urinary tract infection (or pyelonephritis) in these categories of patients is not clear, and methods for making the distinction between upper and lower urinary tract infection are not completely reliable. Significant bacteriuria occurs in up to 20 percent of the population aged 65 and over.[72,73] In the institutionalized patient, the incidence of bacteriuria increases to 43 percent in noncatheterized patients,[74] and 50.6 percent in patients catheterized intermittently[75] The risk of bacteriuria increases with age, non-self-catheterization (in males) and infrequently practiced catheterization routines.[75] The commonest organisms seen on urine culture in uncomplicated urinary tract infections are

E. coli, *Klebsiella* spp., *Staphylococcal saphrophyticus*, *Enterococcus* spp., and *Proteus* spp. Catheter-associated infections with *Pseudomonas* and *Candida* species are not uncommon. Bacterial virulence factors that promote survival of the organism, and thus increase the incidence of symptomatic urinary tract infection, include pili or fimbria which increase the attachment of the organism to cells, toxins secreted by the organism (α-hemolysis, cytotoxic necrotizing factor-1, and enterobactin) and proteins which allow the organism to alter complement activation. These virulence factors are modulated by genes, triggered by such signals as temperature, pH and the oxygen level of the tissues.[76] No long-term sequelae of bacteriuria are seen in the elderly.[12,77–80] The older, sicker, and less mobile patients are more prone to urinary infections, leading to an initial impression of a causal relationship between increased mortality and bacteriuria.[81] This has since been proven to be purely a reflection of the general condition of the patient rather than a causal relationship. Antimicrobial therapy does not improve mortality and neither screening for, nor treatment of, asymptomatic urinary tract infections is warranted in elderly patients.[73]

Asymptomatic bacteriuria

Asymptomatic bacteriuria is defined as $\geq$ 100,000 colony-forming units/mL urine on two or more consecutive occasions in the absence of any clinical symptoms. It assumes that samples are collected using aseptic techniques and that the chance of contamination is minimized using standard protocols. The test specificity is estimated at 90 percent. Regardless of whether the patient is catheterized or not, a leukocyte count of >10 white blood cells/mm^3 in the urine does not correlate strongly with infection and should not be used as diagnostic criteria.[82–84]

The prevalence of asymptomatic bacteriuria increases with age and functional debility and is estimated at 9.3 percent in women aged 65 years or more, increasing to 20–50 percent in those aged over 80 years. In men the incidence, although lower, is still significant, with a prevalence of 6–20 percent in those aged $\geq$ 80 years.[85] In diabetics the incidence, although higher, does not appear to correlate with diabetic control or renal function.

Screening for asymptomatic bacteriuria should not be routine because of the high asymptomatic prevalence. In patients with nonspecific fever, without an indwelling catheter, urine culture is appropriate only if there are some clinical indicators of urinary tract infection (incontinence, frequency, etc.). The therapeutic approach recommended in these circumstances is of nontreatment and close clinical follow-up. Treatment is only indicated in the following circumstances: in patients with frequent episodes of symptomatic urinary tract infection who are noted to have asymptomatic infection; in those with a structural defect or a history of renal transplantation; and prior to urological interventions. Treatment should be given for 2 weeks and urine bacteriology checked at 4 weeks. In post-menopausal women with recurrent urinary tract infection, an intravaginal application of vaginal estrogen cream may be beneficial.

Pyelonephritis

The prevalence of pyelonephritis in the aged has been extensively studied in autopsy series. Raaschou[86] studied an autopsy series of 3,107 patients aged 10 years and over. He reported pyelonephritis in 28 percent of the patients. Baumanis and Russell,[87] who studied a series of 900 autopsies obtained from a hospital for chronic disease, reported chronic pyelonephritis in 185 instances, or 20 percent of the patients. Ascending infection is most common, with only 12 percent being acquired by hematogenous spread. The ages of the subjects varied from 50 to 101 years. Bruckel and Wincker[88] reported that pyelonephritis occurred in 28 percent of an autopsy series obtained from a hospital for chronic diseases. Numerous other authors reported a similar prevalence of acute and chronic pyelonephritis.[89–93] Discrepancies in the reports may be due to the different populations studied and the various interpretations placed on the findings. Low bacterial counts may result from early urinary infection with progression or subsequent infection over a period of a few days,[94–96] because of invasion and inflammation of the bladder wall in cases when shedding of bacterial material into the urine is minimal, or because of infection with fastidious organisms. In a cohort of 51 women with a history of recurrent urinary symptoms and negative culture, Maskell et al.[97] showed an increased presence of fastidious organisms, principally lactobacilli, associated with symptoms. Infection with these organisms persisted for some time after symptoms disappeared, suggesting a slower return to normal commensal flora than with the more common aerobic organisms. Other fastidious organisms seen include *Ureaplasma urealyticum*,[98] *Gardnerella vaginalis*,[99] *Staphylococcus saphrophyticus*,[100] *Corynebacteria* spp.[101,102] and certain strains of *streptococcus* spp.[103,104]

An important feature of chronic pyelonephritis in the old is the asymptomatic course of the disease. Kass[105] claimed that pyelonephritis is clinically diagnosed in one-fifth of those patients detected at autopsy. Many cases of chronic pyelonephritis in elderly patients are detected when the patients have been admitted into hospital for other reasons and the disease has often attained an advanced level with uremia. In a few cases, viruses may have caused the infections, although such cases presumably are rare. Endotoxins and immunological mechanisms, producing free oxygen radical species, cytokines, and other mediators of inflammation, such as leukotrienes, thromboxanes, prostacyclins, and prostaglandins, can induce prolonged damage in the renal interstitium after the disappearance of detectable bacteria in the tissue.[106]

Predisposing factors for urinary tract infections

Escherichia coli causing urinary tract infection mostly originate in the intestine. Because of special affinity for the urogenital mucosa or abundance in the stool flora,[107–109] bacteria proceed to colonize the outer genital[110] and periurethral areas[111] and ascend the urinary tract. Bacteria ascend and remain in the urinary tract despite the urine flow. Predisposing factors include structural and functional abnormalities of the urinary tract, invasive manipulation, underlying diseases causing relative immunosuppression, and bacterial virulence. The most common cause of a functional abnormality is obstruction because of prostatic hypertrophy or carcinoma in older men.[72] Digital examination of the prostate is not satisfactory—even an apparently normal finding does not exclude enlargement of the prostate and bladder neck obstruction. Obstruction can also be promoted by changes in the bladder neck, malformations, nephro- and ureterolithiasis, and neoplasms. In women, prolapse conditions and even slight descensus of the vagina increase the possibility of urinary tract infection.[112] The vast majority of infected female patients show no evident obstruction. Some of these patients have coexistent prolapse conditions.[112] The occurrence of recurrent and therapy-resistant infections correlated with the presence of laxity of the vaginal wall and definite vaginal or uterine prolapse. Patients with recurrent urinary tract infection are, apparently, influenced by anatomical changes of the bladder, and frequently show cystocele caused by vaginal descensus of uterine prolapse. Bladder capacity is often decreased in such patients, as is shown by cystometry. Patients who are resistant to therapy are less influenced by these changes and are represented in equal proportions in all groups. In both sexes, neurological disorders and diabetes are important factors in the development of urinary tract infection, since an atonic bladder is at risk of infection. This is of particular importance in patients with stroke, Parkinson's disease, motor neuron disease, and spinal injury.

Another important factor promoting urinary tract infection is the use of indwelling catheters in elderly people.[113,114] Removal of all indwelling catheters is recommended at the earliest time, as the longer a catheter is left in situ, the more likely a patient is to develop bacteriuria, polymicrobial bacteriuria, or chronic pyelonephritis. In a prospective single center series, the prevalence of chronic pyelonephritis at death was 10 percent if catheterized more than 90 days during their last year of life but zero when catheterized less than or equal to 90 days.[114] Other predisposing factors for infection include female gender, failure to maintain a closed drainage system and failure to administer antibiotics prior to catheter removal. Although antibiotics given at the time of or before catheter removal can reduce the incidence of subsequent urine infection, they also increase antimicrobial resistance rates and are currently not recommended.[50,115] In patients catheterized for less than 2 weeks, both silver-impregnated and antibiotic-impregnated urinary catheters have been shown to reduce the infection rate, by approximately 20–50 percent.[116] Cost savings of the silver-impregnated catheter were estimated to be around $4 US per patient.[117] As these studies focused on short-term catheterization, the benefit in patients with long-term indwelling catheters and those resident in nursing homes are less clear.

The increased incidence and severity of urinary tract infections in geriatric patients may be influenced by any comorbid illness causing immunosuppression. Thus, diabetic patients and those with neoplasia or on immunosuppressive drugs are at higher risk of urine infections. The immune response is impaired with senescence[118] and mucosal immunity may be altered.[119] Seneca and Grant[120] have shown that older patients are more susceptible to the consequences of instrumentation and surgical operations involving the genitourinary tract. Bacterial virulence factors affect the ability of an organism to attach to human uroepithelial cells in vitro and are related to the severity of infection produced in vivo.[121] Pathogenicity factors help promote survival in the urinary space for example by secreting toxins which inactivate the complement mediated response to infection and by decreasing the colonization of the urinary tract. Such promoters include both fimbria and nonfimbrial adhesions factors (e.g. type 1, P and S fimbrae, the Dr hemagluttins, AFA-I and AFA-III adhesion fimbrae).

Treatment of urinary tract infections

In both complicated and uncomplicated urinary tract infections, the main therapeutic objectives should be to eradicate microorganisms invading the renal parenchyma and blood, and to prevent chronic infection and scarring. In uncomplicated infections, cotrimoxazole (a combination of sulfamethoxazole 800 mg and trimethoprim 160 mg) or amoxycillin is recommended.[122] Catheter-associated infections require both penicillin and aminoglycoside therapy, or treatment with a quinolone, because of the increased chance of pseudomonas infection. Acute pyelonephritis is traditionally treated with intravenous antibiotics given for a 2-week period. Recently, patients without sepsis have been successfully treated with oral therapy only.[123] Antibiotic therapy with ampicillin and an aminoglycoside, a third-generation cephalosporin or a quinolone is recommended. As in younger patients, an evaluation for reversible causes of urinary tract infection and pyelonephritis should be sought, including obstruction, nephrolithiasis, cysts, and neoplasia.

Although patients who have various distressing symptoms should, as is the case with younger age groups, be given adequate therapy with antimicrobial drugs,[11,124] elderly patients without subjective complaints of urinary infections should not be treated. Therapy for significant bacteriuria is unnecessary in protecting against renal damage, but is helpful in mitigating distressing symptoms. There are, however, some patients with significant bacteriuria and nonspecific symptoms, like fatigue, dizziness, cognitive deterioration, who perhaps can benefit from treatment of the urinary infection. A short-term course of antibiotic therapy for elderly patients manifesting significant bacteriuria for the first time seems indicated regardless of the symptoms. Foul smell and social handicap can be important problems for elderly people, and successful treatment of urinary tract infection is of great importance for these patients.

Long-term treatment of urinary tract infections is appropriate only in patients with distressing symptoms and a high recurrence rate. The benefits have been reported in a randomized controlled trial comparing cotrimoxazole (sulfamethoxazole 800 mg and trimethoprim 160 mg daily), divided into two doses, with placebo. With a long-acting sulfonamide, Sourander et al.[125] found that 65 percent of patients were free of bacteriuria after a 6-month course of treatment. The urine of the patients in the first group was sterile for an average of 195 days, compared to an average of 113 days in the placebo-treatment group. There is obviously a great need for a critical attitude and a restrictive treatment policy for the use of antibiotics in hospitals. Gruenberg and Bendall[109] reported a hospital outbreak of plasmid-borne trimethoprim resistance in pathogenic coliform bacteria, which was associated with heavy use of cotrimoxazole, sulfonamides, and ampicillin, but was controlled by isolation of the patients and restriction of antibiotic use. These observations have not been confirmed in old age, but it seems highly probable that the frequent occurrence of multiple-resistant E. coli strains, causing urinary tract infections and pyelonephritis in the aged, is not simply a result of treatment of urinary infections with antibiotics and chemotherapeutic agents: it is also related to the treatment of other infections, with a change in the fecal bacterial resistance-pattern and subsequent reinfection of the urinary tract. This might explain the high degree of recurrent urinary tract infection with multiple resistant bacterial strains in geriatric hospitals, as well as the failure of the long-term administration of sulfonamides to prevent reinfection. Failure of therapy is mostly because of reinfection with a new pathogen, bacterial resistance or the use of appropriate antibiotics for an insufficient period of time. Reinfection with a new pathogen can be responsible for up to 20 percent of the failures observed.[106] Resistance, identified after culture of the organism, should prompt the clinician to change to a more suitable antibiotic. The organisms more often associated with resistance are *Pseudomonas, Enterobacter, Citrobacter, Serratia, Proteus* and *Klebsiella* spp. Treatment with aminoglycosides, the newer third-generation cephalosporins, carbapenems (including imipenem), quinolones, and monobactams has reduced this problem significantly.[126] Tissue penetration of the various antibiotics used in the management of pyelonephritis cannot be predicted from blood or urine samples.[106,127] Intracellular concentrations should be above the minimum inhibitory concentrations for effective therapy. Bergeron[128] has shown that the accumulation of tissue aminoglycoside or quinolone concentration is increased during pyelonephritis or endotoxemia. In contrast, betalactams have lower tissue levels and high tubular secretion. Pharmacological synergism may have an important role in the therapy of pyelonephritis. When ampicillin was administered after a short course of intravenous aminoglycoside therapy, in a randomized controlled study, the results were equivalent to those seen with intravenous and oral quinolones suggesting synergism. Over 80 percent of patients had clinical and bacteriological cure with both regimes. The ideal duration of therapy is not well determined but most reports suggest a course of treatment lasting between 5 and 14 days.[129–131]

Miscellaneous causes of renal disease

Allergic interstitial nephritis

Medication use is a common and important cause of renal disease in elderly people, particularly frail elderly patients who are subject to polypharmacy. A wide variety of medications may cause interstitial nephropathies, in addition to various forms of glomerular disease. Presenting features include renal impairment, often with urinary white blood cells in the absence of infection. Classically patients also show features of allergy—eosinophilia, rash and pruritus, temporally associated with the introduction of a new drug. The most common medications causing interstitial nephropathy are antibiotics, particularly the penicillin and sulfonamide derivatives, analgesics, and anti-inflammatory medications, although other offending agents include anticoagulants, diuretics, anticonvulsants, allopurinol, various metals (particularly lithium), and azathioprine and other immunosuppressives.[132] Nonsteroidal anti-inflammatory (NSAID) agents have been demonstrated to induce renal dysfunction via several mechanisms, including interference with renal prostaglandin release, particularly in patients, with underlying renal impairment. In addition, NSAIDs may cause an acute or chronic allergic interstitial reaction often without the classical features of allergy or eosinophilia. Interstitial nephritis should be considered as a differential diagnosis in patients with heavy proteinuria and taking anti-inflammatory medication on a regular basis. Withdrawal of the offending

drug is usually sufficient, though a trial of steroid therapy may be warranted in some situations.

COX-2 inhibitors and the kidney

The newer COX-2 inhibitors have been advocated as having a better drug side-effect profile compared to NSAIDs. However, from a renal perspective, they must still be used with care in the older population. Older patients are prone to increased salt retention and decreased glomerular filtration rate when dehydrated, or suffering from congestive cardiac failure, liver disease with ascites, or nephrotic syndrome. Both NSAIDs and COX-2 inhibitors inhibit renin release and promote sodium retention equally and therefore the renal consequences are no different. As with NSAIDs, COX-2 inhibitors can decrease proteinuria and may have an immunomodulatory effect in inflammatory kidney disease.[133]

Radiocontrast nephrotoxicity

Radiocontrast materials cause vacuolization of the cells in the proximal tubule and hence interstitial disease, possibly by inducing intense local vasoconstriction. The healthy kidney does not appear to be at risk of damage. Age itself is not a risk factor for the nephrotoxic effects of radiocontrast materials.[134] However, as age increases the incidence of subclinical renal disease, a higher incidence of radiocontrast nephrotoxicity is higher in the older patient. Predisposing factors include diabetes,[135–137] particularly if associated with reduced renal function,[138,139] severe congestive cardiac failure,[140] dehydration, the volume of contrast used[136,141] (higher volumes causing increased risk) and the use of high-osmolality nonionic contrast media.[142,143] The literature describing an increased risk of contrast-mediated nephrotoxicity with the administration of contrast media to patients with multiple myeloma is weak. Often the renal impairment can be attributed to the myeloma or the complications of the disease and its treatment.[132] The overall incidence of contrast-associated nephropathy varies according to the population studied and the definition used, but most data report 1–7 percent incidence of radiocontrast-mediated nephrotoxicity.[144]

Nephrotoxicity may be prevented with prior hydration with saline or hypotonic saline for a minimum of 12 hours.[145–148] The addition of an oral dose of *N*-acetylcysteine to a regime of hydration has been shown to decrease the chances of an acute rise in the serum creatinine level at 48 hours in patients with chronic renal impairment and stable creatinine.[149] Other methods used to limit the nephrotoxicity associated with interventional radiology include the use of low volume, low ionic contrast media, the use of carbon dioxide as a contrast, and more recently the use of fenoldopam (a specific dopamine agonist) at the time of the procedure.[150] The use of agents to increase intra-tubular urine flow rates, for example mannitol or frusemide, or the use of renal vasodilatory agents, including theophylline or calcium channel blockers does not improve outcome, and in some studies is associated with a poorer prognosis.[145]

Renal papillary necrosis

Renal papillary necrosis is not an uncommon complication of urinary infection in elderly people. The disease can be defined as a severe form of chronic pyelonephritis with ischemic necrosis of the papillae and the medullary pyramid. Necrotic papillae migrate through the urinary passages and are often detected macroscopically in the urine. The patients suffer from hematuria, urinary colic, and very often from fever, which may be high. The disease often has a quite rapid course resulting in uremia and death. Vascular diseases, including unilateral renal artery stenosis, are important etiological factors.[151] Diabetes is no longer believed to be a predisposing factor to the development of papillary necrosis. Consumption of analgesics—especially phenacetin—may play an important role. Clinical experience favors the opinion that continuous prolonged use of analgesics is connected with the development of papillary necrosis in elderly people. In the majority of cases, relief of the obstruction caused by the necrotic papilla leads to improved renal function. On rare occasions patients present with end-stage renal disease and may require renal replacement therapy.

CHRONIC RENAL FAILURE AND END-STAGE RENAL DISEASE (ESRD)

The most common primary diagnoses in newly treated elderly ESRD patients are nephrosclerosis, diabetes, and renal disease of unknown etiology. The incidence of ESRD secondary to tubulointerstitial disease, glomerulonephritis and polycystic kidney disease is lower in the over 65-year-old patient group than in the age group 15–65 years.[55,152,153]

Predialysis management

As the number of older patients with advanced renal failure increases, the importance of continued follow-up at a predialysis clinic grows. Early referral to a nephrologist is recognized to improve long-term survival,[154,155] and family physicians and general internists are encouraged to refer all patients, regardless of age, for specialist follow-up at an early stage.[156] Although the literature suggests an age-related bias still persists in referral patterns, the tendency to deny older patients specialist access is less with increasing awareness of the benefits of dialysis in elderly people. In the ideal situation patients are reviewed in predialysis clinics where the four main aims are:

- to decrease the rate of renal deterioration
- to control predialysis uremic complications including hyperkalemia, fluid balance, anemia, hypertension, and renal osteodystrophy early in the disease course
- to educate and prepare both the patient and family for dialysis
- to identify a suitable time to start dialysis and prevent an acute event precipating urgent dialysis.

The rate of deterioration of renal function is stable with time. Shorter kidney survival is seen in patients with glomerulonephritis, diabetes mellitus, and nephrosclerosis, while those with tubulointerstitial disease have a slower renal decline. Like their younger counterparts, strict control of blood pressure, prevention of hyperglycemia, and moderate protein restriction in elderly patients, is essential in the preservation of residual renal reserve. Recent studies addressing the question of protein restriction have only been able to demonstrate a small benefit from moderate protein restriction in patients with mildly impaired renal function (defined as a glomerular filtration rate, GFR, of 25–55 mL/min).[155,157] As the older patient is more prone to malnutrition, dietary restriction to less than 0.86 g/kg body weight is controversial.[158] Blood pressure control is of greater benefit than dietary restriction, especially when ACE inhibitors are used.

The assessment and control of symptoms in the older patient with advanced renal disease is confounded by the poor correlation between serum creatinine and glomerular filtration rate. More frequent monitoring of creatinine clearance is necessary, therefore clinicians are advised to place increased emphasis on symptom control. Furthermore, as elderly patients are increasingly prone to minor changes in sodium and fluid balance precipitating either dehydration or symptoms of pulmonary edema, close attention to fluid balance is required. When used with clinical examination of the jugular venous pressure and fluid balance charts regular weight records can be an easy approximation of fluid changes over a day, particularly in the inpatient setting. Fluid overload can usually be controlled by the use of high-dose loop diuretics (e.g. 80–120 mg frusemide), although in some patients, addition of metolazone is necessary to augment the diuretic effect of either frusemide or ethacrynic acid. Severe, and often refractory, constipation can exacerbate the hyperkalemia of chronic renal failure as a larger percentage of potassium is lost via the gastrointestinal system. In such situations simple therapies directed toward correction of the constipation are often sufficient. If ion-exchange resins are required they must be given with sufficient doses of sorbitol (for example a dose of 30 mL of 70 percent sorbitol with each 15 g of calcium resonium).

Since the introduction of human recombinant erythropoietin (rh-Epo), anemia is less frequently encountered in the dialysis patient. Few studies have been directed specifically at the over 65-year-old population, nevertheless, the older patient appears to have similar dose responses to those seen in younger patients. Erythropoetin administration has been shown to improve the patient quality of life, appetite, exercise capacity, and sleep quality in addition to prevention of LV hypertrophy, decreased angina and a decrease in episodes of congestive cardiac function. More recent studies show that rh-Epo also has an effect on cognitive function and restless legs and sleep apnea. Current guidelines suggest commencing rh-Epo at a dose of 80–120 u/kg per week (approximately 6,000 u per week in divided doses) in predialysis patients, if symptoms attributable to anemia (fatigue, decreased exercise tolerance, angina, congestive heart failure, diminished work performance, and symptomatic peripheral vascular disease) are present in patients with a GFR greater than 15 mL/min.[159] Anemia associated with chronic renal failure often requires more aggressive management in elderly patients because of coexisting cardiac disease. Red cell indices are not a reliable estimate of iron deficiency in uremia. Iron deficiency should be excluded by evaluation of transferrin saturation (target > 20 percent) and ferritin (target > 100 and < 800 ng/mL). Oral or parenteral iron supplements should be administered if indicated. In rare cases, patients can be rh-Epo unresponsive and require blood transfusion. Particularly in elderly people, transfusion can lead to acute pulmonary edema. Packed red cells are better tolerated than whole blood. Ideally hemoglobin should be maintained around 11–12 g/dL to achieve the optimal cost–benefit ratio.[159]

The predialysis patient is at risk for renal osteodystrophy and malnutrition. As serum phosphate rises, phosphate-binding antacids (e.g. calcium carbonate) should be given, with meals, in order to suppress hyperphosphatemia, hypocalcemia, and the resultant adverse effects on bone. As serum phosphate falls in response to treatment, serum calcium will generally rise toward the normal range. If hypocalcemia persists after normalization of phosphate this should be treated with preparations of vitamin D or its active metabolites. As aluminum toxicity is well recognized, aluminum hydroxide should no longer be used as a phosphate binder.

Dietary management of elderly people with chronic renal failure is often overdone, leading to malnutrition. Protein and salt restriction is often needed in young individuals to suppress the volume expansion and BUN elevations. Many elderly patients ingest only 60–70 g of protein daily and 4–5 g of salt under normal conditions, and strict limitation of these dietary constituents is often unnecessary. Similarly, hyperkalemia should be avoided and dietary potassium controlled, but the reductions required in elderly patients are often moderate.

Pruritus is a major problem in elderly uremic patients, especially in the presence of coexisting xerosis. In addition to skin moisteners, ultraviolet light treatments have been found effective and safe. Administration of so-called "antipruritic" agents such as antihistamines is rarely helpful, since they act primarily by causing sedation and may have adverse nervous system effects in elderly people.

Chronic dialysis therapy

As renal replacement therapy becomes increasingly common in elderly patients, there is a growing awareness that this population poses a unique set of problems. Many types of dialysis are available—in-center hemodialysis (IHD), home hemodialysis, continuous ambulatory peritoneal dialysis (CAPD), intermittent peritoneal dialysis (IPD), and continuous cycling peritoneal dialysis (CCPD). All forms of peritoneal dialysis (PD) and home hemodialysis are grossly underused in this age group, especially within the USA.[160–162] The provision of transplantation as a means of treatment for the elderly patient with end stage renal disease remains limited, despite its demonstrated success.

The acceptance criteria used for older patients worldwide have been liberalized over the years. This is reflected by an increased number of older patients accepted onto renal replacement therapy programs. The percentage of patients aged 65 years or more who start dialysis therapy ranges from 27 percent in the UK to 43 percent in Italy, with a mean worldwide acceptance rate of 34 patients aged over 65 years per million population per year.[161] In fact, the 65–74-year-old age group show the fastest rate of growth of all age groups.[160,163,164] Acceptance rates across the world differ for many reasons. Some differences result from resource restrictions (for example, in the UK where dialysis is funded by the government) but some differences are due to selection bias (for example, Japan and New Zealand where there is a high overall acceptance rate but a relatively lower population of aged dialysis patients). There is a growing concern, that, without adequate provision of specialized services targeted at elderly people, a medical and ethical crisis is imminent.[162,165]

One-year survival rates are around 70 percent in maintenance hemodialysis patients aged 65 years or more.[55] Five-year survival rates range from 20 to 25 percent. Patients on peritoneal dialysis have an average survival rate of 75 and 22 percent at 1 and 5 years respectively.[55,166–172] As most national databases define chronic dialysis patients as patients who are dialysis dependent for "more than 90 days," early deaths are not accounted for. Hence the true mortality rate in older patients is much higher than reported. Eleven percent of patients aged 65–69 years die within the first 90 days of treatment.[173,174] As expected, the early mortality rate increases linearly with age (14, 18, 19, and 26 percent for age groups 70–74 years, 75–79 years, 80–84 years and 85+ years respectively).[162] In the United States, a 40 percent higher mortality risk is seen in older patients compared with Japanese patients of equal age. A similar, but less marked survival advantage is seen in European patients even after adjustment for age and diabetes. The reason for this survival advantage is not known but may relate to differences in comorbidity and severity of coexisting disease or other factors. Comorbidity increases with increasing age.[55,175] This does not appear to impact on the initial choice of dialysis modality among elderly patients, but does influence the long-term outcome of the individual, regardless of age. Mortality increases with increasing comorbid conditions. The strongest predictors of survival are high predialysis functional state, good nutritional status and low comorbidity. Diabetes, cardiac disease, and underdialysis are predictors of poor outcome. The choice of dialysis modality (usually IHD vs CAPD) is based on patient preferences, clinical history, functional capabilities, and social circumstances. Most studies show similar survival in both hemodialysis and peritoneal dialysis patients, despite differences in comorbidity; however, recent data have led to some doubt about the effectiveness of CAPD in the long term. A USRDS study showed a marginal survival advantage in elderly patients managed on hemodialysis.[176] In contrast, however, a 0.76 risk advantage (confidence interval 0.69–0.83) was seen in Canadian patients aged 65+ on PD, even after correction for age and the number of comorbid illnesses.[55] Older female diabetic patients appear to have better outcome if treated with hemodialysis.[177,178] Unlike younger patients, technique failure is no higher with peritoneal dialysis.[168,177] Peritoneal dialysis is ideal for patients with good family support, where a family member is prepared to assist with dialysis exchanges. The introduction of CCPD (Continuous cyclic peritoneal dialysis), where a preprogrammed machine performs the exchanges during the night, provides more flexibility for family members who may work during the day. Peritoneal dialysis has been performed successfully in the nursing home.[179]

Medical advantages of peritoneal dialysis include better cardiovascular stability, reduced dialysis-induced arrhythmias, easier control of hypertension, and preservation of residual renal function. The physician may favor peritoneal dialysis if vascular access difficulties arise repeatedly. Other disadvantages of PD in elderly patients include poor tissue turgor and wound healing, which cause abdominal wall herniae and catheter leaks. Protein losses in dialysate exacerbate malnutrition and may increase abnormal bone mineralization and reduce immune function.

Hospitalization rates are higher in the elderly dialysis patient. The median number of days spent in hospital for the

65+-year-old dialysis patient was 15 days per year compared with 9.75 days for younger patients. The frequency of hospitalization is also higher (1.89 and 1.43 admissions per year for 65+-year-old patients and 45–64-year-old patients respectively).[164] Most admissions are precipitated by fluid overload or access-related problems although cardiac disease accounts for over 25 percent of admissions.[153] In peritoneal dialysis, the rate of peritonitis is similar to that of the center where the patient is based;[169,170,180] however, patients over 80 years of age tend to have a prolonged hospital stay with peritonitis.[181] There is no difference in admission rates between HD and PD patients.

The experience with vascular access creation in the older patient is variable and may reflect partly the skill and enthusiasm of the surgeon and the patient selection criteria. There are conflicting data about the success rate for arteriovenous (AV) fistulae creation, with over 80 percent of patients having a functional access creation in some series[182,183] and 25–30 percent in others.[153,183] Fistula survival rates are poor, with a less than 10 percent success rate at one year.[182,183] In contrast prosthetic graft survival averages around 60–80 percent at 1 year and 50–70 percent at 2 years.[182–185] One problem, more common in elderly patients, is poor wound healing after fistula or graft creation. Elective vascular access surgery should be considered as early as possible in the elderly patient to allow adequate healing and maturation of the fistula or graft. Although the guidelines suggest access creation when the creatinine clearance reaches a GFR less than 25 mL/min, a plasma creatinine concentration greater than 354 μmol/L, or a rapid rate of progression should lead to prompt evaluation for vascular access creation.[159] Despite the apparently poor patency rate of fistulae in the elderly patient, some suggest an initial attempt at access creation should be with a native vessel fistula rather than prosthetic graft. As with younger dialysis patients temporary hemodialysis access can be gained using double lumen catheters placed in the internal jugular vein, femoral vein, or (less commonly) subclavian vein.

Specific problems resulting from the vascular access are rare but include high-output cardiac failure and steal syndrome. The incidence of high-output cardiac failure as a result of fistula or graft creation is low. Temporary occlusion of the fistula leading to a reduction in heart rate or increase in ejection fraction, as measured by 2D echocardiogram, may help to identify those few patients who would benefit from banding or ligation of the fistula. Steal syndrome is seen in patients with severe peripheral vascular disease where small arterial vessels have compromised perfusion. In these cases the creation of a fistula or graft further exacerbates the problem by diverting blood away from the extremity. This may result in gangrenous changes which, often only partially, respond to ligation of the access.

Intradialytic problems in elderly patients are similar to those seen in younger patients. However, two complications (hypotension and hypoxemia) occurring during hemodialysis and one (protein loss) during peritoneal dialysis merit mention here. Both hypotension and hypoxemia, though temporary, may reduce functional independence in an older compromised patient and may affect the rate of rehabilitation. Hypotension may be reduced or minimized by frequent assessment of dry weight, maintaining hemoglobin greater than

or equal to 100 g/L (or hematocrit greater than 30 percent), and the avoidance of rapid ultrafiltration and of antihypertensive medications prior to dialysis. The consumption of food during and immediately before dialysis may exacerbate hypotension. Dialysis prescriptions with sequential ultrafiltration and sodium ramping may be used. In addition both hyperparathyroidism and uremia can cause a functional cardiomyopathy and consequently hypotension. Hypoxemia can be prevented by the use of biocompatible membranes and bicarbonate-buffered dialysate and is less frequently seen nowadays. Hemodialysis-related arrhythmias are more common in the older patient.[186]

High protein loss in peritoneal dialysate is recognized in certain groups of patients and may contribute to hypoalbuminemia, malnutrition and hyperlipidemia of renal failure. Malnutrition has been reported in up to 20 percent of older hemodialysis patients[187] and 30–35 percent of peritoneal dialysis patients.[188,189] Predisposing factors include low income, social isolation, ill-fitting dentures, depression, uremic anorexia and impaired taste acuity, constipation, frequent and prolonged hospitalization, recurrent peritonitis, and prolonged underdialysis. It may remain unrecognized for some time and be very profound at the time of diagnosis. Consequently, active assessments should be performed at 6-monthly intervals. The recommended nutritional intake is > 35 Kcal/kg per day for energy expenditure and 1.0–1.2 g/kg per day protein. Fluid restriction, traditionally, is imposed to prevent more than 5 percent interdialytic weight gain. This is being brought into question as current data show improved nutritional indices in patients with higher intradialytic weight gain. Vitamin supplementation should be introduced early as dialysis causes a loss of water-soluble vitamins. Weight loss remains the simplest and most accurate indicator of malnutrition, although measurement scales, for example, the subjective global assessment scale, are highly recommended as formal measures of nutritional status. Other indices include bodyweight < 80 percent of ideal bodyweight, serum albumin < 35 g/L, serum cholesterol concentration less than 2.6 mmol/L and a low serum creatinine or serum urea in patients without residual renal function. Low predialysis serum potassium and phosphorus, and a protein catabolic rate less than 0.8 g/kg per day are also useful nonspecific biochemical markers of malnutrition. Recent studies reveal an early alteration in growth hormone and insulin-like growth factor-1 (IGF-1) function,[190] with clinical evidence of growth hormone resistance despite normal or increased serum levels. Newer techniques to improve nutrition include amino-acid-based peritoneal dialysate,[191,192] parenteral nutrition (containing amino acid, lipid, and dextrose solutions) given during hemodialysis,[193] the use of anabolic steroids,[194] and subcutaneous injection of human recombinant growth hormone or recombinant human IGF-1.[190] Some of these methods are in clinical use and seem promising, although further randomized controlled studies are needed to establish an improvement in long-term outcome.

Other complications in dialysis patients include gastric bleeding, hyperparathyroidism, rapidly progressive cardiac disease, left ventricular hypertrophy, and falls. Falls, particularly those occurring post dialysis, may cause subdural bleeding because of the heparin used during hemodialysis. Accelerated athlerosclerosis is seen in all patients with advanced renal disease, and recent research data implicate advanced glycosylation end-products (AGE) in the pathogenesis of the rapidly progressive disease course.[195] These glycosylation products nonenzymatically bind to amine groups and can increase oxidative damage, cause cellular growth and matrix formation via cytokine activation, or cause protein crosslinks and increased connective tissue rigidity.[188,189,196,197] In animal studies the administration of AGE-peptides cause increased vascular permeability and impaired vasodilatation responses. Normally AGEs are detected and cleared by scavenger cells including endothelial cells, macrophages, monocytes, T-cells and renal mesangial cells among others. However, in diabetes, the hyperglycemic milieu allows an increased generation of AGEs, while in renal failure the clearance of the AGEs is impaired.[198,199] Advanced age is associated with increased levels of AGE. Although promising, further research into AGEs and aminoguanide (which inhibits the final stages of the glycosylation pathway) is required before its role in advanced atherosclerosis can be fully understood.[200,201]

Functional independence is one of the strongest predictors of outcome in the elderly patient starting renal replacement therapy. It has repeatedly been shown to correlate with both mortality and morbidity.[77] Although commonly measured using the Karnofsky scale, this scale is not sensitive to change over time and more appropriate and sensitive tests suggested include the Functional Independence Measure (FIM), six-minute-walk test, or the timed-up-and-go test.[202–205]

The prevalence of disability is high in ESRD patients. In an inner-city practice a group of HD patients, mean age 56 years (range 21–92 years), 36 percent were unable to perform routine living chores without assistance.[206] The presence of either diabetes or increased age increases this proportion to over 70 percent.[207] In the past relatively fewer older patients were accepted into nursing homes for long-term care because of various issues and the complexity of their medical history.[208] However, newer policies, specialized training and novel approaches to care has resulted in a growth in the long-term care facilities now offering dialysis care. The cost effectiveness of such programs is reported.[209]

Exercise programs have been widely reported to improve functional status in younger patients, increase dialysis clearance and decrease the morbidity associated with dialysis. Programs specific to elderly people are not described; however, exercise has been used in these age groups. Both muscle function and maximal oxygen consumption (peak $\dot{V}_{O_2}$) dialysis patients, increase with exercise suggesting some reversibility. Interestingly, little correlation has been found between the activity level, recorded using an accelerometer, and K_t/V suggesting no direct correlation between uremia and disability.[210]

The quality of life of elderly patients on dialysis depends on the comparison group used. When compared with younger dialysis patients, older patients have more disability but show a more positive psychological outlook and higher satisfaction with life.[211–214] Westlie et al. report that 40 percent of respondents felt they were in better health than other 70-year-old people.[215] In contrast, in studies using objective measures of quality of life in an age-matched control population, older dialysis patients, had significantly lower life satisfaction[216] and it is now recognized that age is one of the main determinants of quality of life.[216]

Transplantation

Transplantation is becoming an increasingly favored option for renal replacement therapy in the younger age group. The ethical dilemma revolving around the paucity of cadaver kidneys continues and some nephrologists still advocate the restriction of transplantation to younger individuals. The recent literature, however, is in favor of the use of cadaver kidneys harvested from older donors as well as transplantation as a therapy for ESRD in elderly patients.

The use of kidneys from older donors for cadaveric transplantation is well established.[217–228] Although the best results are seen with donor kidneys from patients aged 16–45 years of age, the outcome from kidneys from donors over the age of 55 years is good. As the incidence of concomitant disease is higher with increasing age, the number of patients aged over 60 years at the time of death who are suitable for organ donation is lower than in a comparable, but younger population. Nevertheless the criteria used for acceptance of a kidney is the same as that applied to younger donors. In particular, there should be no past history of renal disease, normal serum creatinine, and an inactive urinary sediment. In cases of doubt, a renal biopsy, done at the time of harvesting, is helpful. Kidneys with less than 20 percent glomerulosclerosis are acceptable.[227] Biopsies showing more than 20 percent sclerosis are predictive of an increased incidence of delayed graft function, a lower baseline renal function, and need for early transplant nephrectomy. Graft survival ranges from 62–94 percent at 1 year[217,228–230] and patient survival 80–91 percent at 1 year.[217,228,231,232] Variations reflect the different age groups studied and the differing criteria for patient acceptance. No difference is seen in graft survival or function when the outcome of transplantation with kidneys from donors aged 55–64 are compared with donors aged 65 years or more.[224]

The use of older kidneys is associated with a similar incidence of primary nonfunction, delayed graft function, acute rejection, and acute tubular necrosis to that seen in kidneys from younger donors.[218–222,224,228] The baseline serum creatinine tends to be higher in patients receiving older cadaveric transplant kidneys, suggesting reduced functional renal reserve.[233] If transplanted into highly sensitized patients, older kidneys appear to have a higher risk of rejection and their sensitivity to prolonged ischemia is greater.[226] As older individuals are less immunologically efficient, they tend to have a lower incidence of high sensitization, and some authors advocate the use of older kidneys for older patients.[226] The reverse philosophy has also been proposed—the avoidance of older, higher-risk, kidneys in older (also higher-risk) patients. Neither practice has been validated and the restriction of certain kidneys to particular age groups of donors is not recommended. Age matching of the donor kidney to within 5 years of the age of the recipient does not change outcome.[234] Results from living related donors aged 65 years or more are similar to those from younger living related donors.

Kidney transplantation is increasingly offered to elderly patients.[228,235] In the pre-cyclosporin era, the patient and graft outcomes were significantly poorer than those of younger patients[236] and transplantation was not recommended in patients over 55 years old. More recent data show comparable censored graft survival rates (calculated as graft loss not including loss due to patient death with a functioning graft) in both those under 65 and over 65 years old.[55,164,228] In comparison, patient survival is lower in older patients. Both transplant recipients aged 40–55 and those aged 55 years or more have a higher risk of death compared with patients aged 18–40 years (relative risk of death of 1.94 and 4.86 respectively).[231] The incidence of acute rejection is lower, possibly because of compromised immunocompetence with increasing age.[217] Live donor transplants still have the best outcome, though as with cadaveric donors, the baseline serum creatinine is higher in older recipients.[217]

The increased rate of patient death is mostly attributable to higher rates of infection and cardiac disease. Additionally, older patients treated for acute rejection have almost twice the mortality rate of those without rejection.[231] Sepsis is not only more common, but also associated with increased mortality. Altered immune function results in increased sensitivity to immunosuppressive therapy with age and centers with higher reported patient survival often use lower doses of immunotherapy.[237] The most appropriate regime for immunosuppression has not been studied but the general opinion is that older patients should be treated with lower doses of immunosuppression, particularly low-dose steroids. Cyclosporin A has been recommended and is shown to reduce the number of episodes of acute rejection.

The acceptance criteria for transplantation in patients over 65 years old remain poorly defined and although the frequency of transplantation in elderly patients is increasing, services remain restricted. The published literature illustrates a definite sociodemographic selection bias with fewer diabetic patients, fewer patients over 70 years old, and fewer patients with one or more concomitant illnesses being transplanted. Increased comorbidity alone does not account for the reduced numbers of elderly patients reaching transplantation.[217] Most reports compare the survival rates of older patients with younger patients and are therefore of limited use in the clinical setting. In contrast, Schaubel et al.[235] compared the survival of older patients treated with transplantation with similarly aged patients remaining on dialysis. The study shows a lower mortality rate in transplanted patients, although the comparison groups (dialysis and transplant patients) were dissimilar. Subgroup analysis of a better-matched group of patients without comorbid illness showed that the survival advantage was still present. No information regarding psychosocial data or dialysis adequacy was included and a selection bias cannot be excluded.

Physical fitness and strength does not appear to improve with transplantation, possibly because of corticosteroid-related myopathy.[238] Increased quality of life[239] and freedom for the patient is, however, well recognized, and transplantation should be a considered option in the older dialysis patient.

ETHICAL ISSUES ASSOCIATED WITH THE PROVISION OF RENAL REPLACEMENT THERAPY IN ELDERLY PATIENTS

The ethical issues surrounding the question of renal replacement therapy in elderly patients are complex and are influenced by society as well as by personal experiences. No answers exist and, to date, no guidelines outlining the most suitable patients for either dialysis or transplantation have been published.

Political arguments revolve around limited healthcare resources and increasing costs, with elderly patients often being the first group to be considered expendable. Recent surveys show that financial limitations have a powerful impact on patient selection for dialysis: for example, in a survey of dialysis directors, 10 percent would reject patients on the basis of age alone, while 85 percent indicated that they would do so under significant scarcity.[240,241] Is this a valid argument? Should we, as physicians, be involved in the allocation of finances as well as having primary responsibility for the care of the individual?

Elderly people are a heterogeneous group in whom chronological age does not match physiological age. No two patients are alike and each should be assessed individually. Few would argue that renal replacement therapy has little role in a patient in whom treatment is futile or where the quality of life is felt, by the patient, to be unacceptable. The problem lies in identifying these patients. There are no criteria for futility, and the assessment of quality of life is so individualized that we, as healthcare workers, are unable to accurately assess life satisfaction on behalf of our patients. It is interesting to note that in one ethicist's eyes, dialysis in elderly patients was "at the price of a doubtful or poor quality of life."[242] This assumption is false, and in fact, most elderly dialysis patients see their lives as better than, or at least as good as, those not on dialysis.[212–214]

So what is the best management of the elderly patient with ESRD? Should we offer dialysis or transplantation to our older patients? One dogma is that "individualism should give way to a community-based and affirmed notion of the value of the aged in the society…."[242] Is our role to serve society or is our responsibility to the patient? This question remains unanswered. Our recommendation is that a treatment trial should be offered to all patients, and that appropriate outcome objectives be established from the outset.[243] If, after such a trial, treatment is not beneficial, the physician can discontinue dialysis and direct his/her energy to reducing uremic symptoms and easing the patient to a more dignified end. Careful attention to symptom relief, psychological support of the patient, and support for the patient's family and the nursing staff is essential.

The question of stopping therapy also arises in those patients well established on chronic dialysis. Respect for the patient's autonomy dictates that dialysis be withdrawn at his or her own request. Indeed dialysis withdrawal is becoming one of the leading causes of death in the ESRD patient.[244] However, the case is less clear when the patient suffers some catastrophic medical event (e.g. a severe disabling stroke) and has not previously expressed his/her wishes. The discussion and introduction of an "advance directive" or "living will" at an early stage of treatment helps both the physician and the patient plan therapy in such an event. Strict guidelines in the preparation and execution and frequent review of the directive can prevent abuse by either the physician or the family.

Physicians, as their patients' advocates, have an obligation to advocate for the needs of their elderly patients and each must strive to avoid discrimination or "agism."

> ## KEY POINTS Diseases of the aging kidney
>
> ■ Older patients often present with nonspecific symptoms, thus causing diagnostic delay and a delay in starting treatment.
>
> ■ Glomerular and vasculitic causes of acute renal insufficiency are increasingly recognized in elderly people.
>
> ■ Acute interstitial nephritis, caused by drugs, is common in elderly people.
>
> ■ Survival with dialysis and transplantation is improving with acceptable mortality statistics.

REFERENCES

1. Canadian Institute for Health Information: Annual Report 2000, Dialysis and Transplantation, Canadian Organ Replacement Register, Vol 1. Ottawa, Ontario, 2000

2. National Institute of Diabetes and Digestive and Kidney Diseases: US Renal data systems, Annual Data Report (on CD). Researchers Guide, reference tables and ADR slides. United States Renal Data System Coordinating Center, Ann Arbor, MI, 2001

3. Roberts AP, Robinson RE, Beard RW: Some factors affecting bacterial colony counts in urinary tract infection. Br Med J 1967;1:400–403

4. Ouslander JG, Schapira M, Fingold S, Schnelle J: Accuracy of rapid urine screening tests among incontinent nursing home residents with asymptomatic bacteriuria. J Am Geriatr Soc 1995;43:772–775

5. Ouslander JG, Schapira M, Schnelle JF et al: Does eradicating bacteriuria affect the severity of chronic urinary incontinence in nursing home residents? Ann Intern Med 1995;122:749–754

6. Duffy LM, Clearly J, Ahern S et al: Clean intermittent catheterisation: safe, cost-effective bladder management for male residents of VA nursing homes. J Am Geriatr Soc 1995;43:865–870

7. Bakke A, Vollset SE, Hoistaeter PA, Irgens LM: Physical complications in patients treated with clean intermittent catheterisation. Scand J Urol Nephrol 1993;27:55–61

8. Moore-Smith B: The treatment of urinary tract infections in elderly women. Mod Geriatr 1974;4:408–414

9. Stamey TA: Diagnosis, localization and classification of urinary infections. In Stamey TA (ed): Pathogenesis and Treatment of Urinary Tract Infections. Williams & Wilkins, Baltimore 1980:1–51

10. Macdonald RA, Levitin H, Mallory GK, Kass EH: Relation between pyelonephritis and bacterial counts in the urine: an autopsy study. N Engl J Med 1957;256:915–922

11. Brocklehurst JC, Bee P, Jones D, Palmer M: Bacteriuria in geriatric hospital patients: its correlates and management. Age Ageing 1977;6:240–245

12. Clauge JE, Horan MA: Urine culture in the elderly: scientifically doubtful and practically useless? Lancet 1994;344:1035–1036

13. Dontas AS, Parasaki I, Petrikkos G, Giamarelou H: Diuresis bacteriuria in physically dependent women. Age Ageing 1977;6:240–245

14. Mills SJ, Ford M, Gould FK, Burton S, Neal DE: Screening for bacteriuria in urological patients using reagent strips. Br J Urol 1992;70:314–317

15. Kohli HS, Bhaskaran MC, Muthukumar T et al: Treatment-related acute renal failure in the elderly: A hospital-based prospective study. Nephrol Dial Transplant 2000;15:212–217

16. McInnes EG, Levy DW, Chaudhuri MD, Bhan GL: Renal failure in the elderly. Q J Med 1987;64:583–588

17. Druml W, Lax F, Grimm G et al: Acute renal failure in the elderly 1975–1990. Clin Nephrol 1994;41:342–349

18. Gornick CC, Kjellstrand CM: Acute renal failure complicating aortic aneurysm surgery. Nephron 1983;35:145–157

19. Bellomo R, Farmer M, Boyce N: The outcome of critically ill elderly patients with severe renal failure treated by continuous hemodiafiltration. Int J Artif Org 1994;17:466–472

20. Lamiere N, Dekeyterk N, Pauwels W: Acute renal failure in the elderly. In Oreopoulos DG (ed): Geriatric Nephrology. Martinus Nijhoff Publishers, Dordrecht, 1986;103–116

21. Lamiere N, Matthys E, Vanholder R et al: Causes and prognosis of acute renal failure in elderly patients. Nephrol Dial Transplant 1987;2:316–322

22. Hakim RW, Lazarus JM: Haemodialysis in acute renal failure. In Brenner BM, Lazarus JM (eds): Acute Renal Failure. Churchill Livingstone, New York 1988:767–807

23. Rosenfeld JB, Shobat J, Grosskopf I, Borner G: Acute renal failure: A disease of the elderly. Adv Nephrol 1987;16:159–168

24. Pascual J, Orofino L, Liano F: Incidence and prognosis of acute renal failure in older patients. J Am Geriatr Soc 1990;38:25–30

25. Gentric A, Cleded J: Immediate and long term prognosis in acute renal failure in the elderly. Nephrol Dial Transplant 1991;6:86–90

26. Simon P, Charasse C, Autuly V: Epidemiology of primary glomerular disease in the elderly: A prospective study during a 15 year period. In Sessa A, Meroni M, Battini G (eds): Contributions in Nephrology. S. Karger, Basel 1993:161–166

27. Stiles KP, Yuan CM, Chung EM et al: Renal biopsy in high-risk patients with medical diseases of the kidney. Am J Kidney Dis 2000;36(2):419–433

28. Levison SP: Renal disease in the elderly: the role of the renal biopsy. Am J Kidney Dis 1990;16:300–306

29. Haas M, Spargo BH, Wit E-JC, Meehan SM: Etiologies and outcome of acute renal insufficiency in older adults: A renal biopsy study of 259 cases. Am J Kidney Dis 2000;35(3):433–447

30. Johnson PA, Coulshed SJ, Davison AM: Renal biopsy findings in patients older than 65 years of age presenting with the nephrotic syndrome. A report from the MRC Glomerulonephritis Registry. In Sessa A, Meroni M, Battini G (eds): Glomerulonephritis in the Elderly. S. Karger, Basel, 1993:127–132

31. Labeeuw M, Cailette A, Colon S et al: Renal biopsy in elderly adults over 75 years of age. Ger Nephrol Urol 1995;4:177–181

32. Bolton KW: Nephrotic syndrome in the aged. In Cameron JS, Glassock RJ (ed): The Nephrotic Syndrome. Marcel Dekker, New York: 1988 523–554

33. Kunis CL, Teng SN: Treatment of glomerulonephritis in the elderly. Semin Nephrol 2000;20(3):256–264

34. Passerini P, Como G, Vigano E: Idiopathic membranous nephropathy in the elderly. Nephrol Dial Transplant 1993;8:1324–1325

35. Nagai R, Cattran DC, Pei Y: Steroid therapy and prognosis of focal segmental glomerulosclerosis. Clin Nephrol 1994;42:18–21

36. Jeffrey RF, Gardiner DS, More IA et al: Cresentic glomerulonephritis: experience of a single unit over a five year period. Scot Med J 1992;37:175–178

37. Wagner HP, Hollenhorst RW: The ocular lesions of temporal arteritis. Am J Ophthalmol 1958;45:617–630

38. Truong L, Kopelman RG, Williams GS, Pirani CL: Temporal arteritis and renal disease. Case report and review of the literature. Am J Med 1985;78:171–175

39. Pascual J, Quereda C, Liano F et al: End-stage renal disease after necrotising glomerulonephritis in an elderly patient with temporal arteritis. Nephron 1994;66:236–237

40. Samily AG, Field RA, Merrill JP: Acute glomerulonephritis in elderly patients: report of seven cases over sixty years of age. Ann Intern Med 1961;54:603–609

41. Moorthy AV, Zimmerman SW: Renal disease in the elderly: clinicopathologic analysis of renal diseases in 115 elderly patients. Clin Nephrol 1980;14:223–229

42. Montoliu J, Darnell A, Torras A, Revert L: Primary acute glomerular disorders in the elderly. Arch Intern Med 1980;140:755–756

43. Melby PC, Musick WD, Luger AM, Khanna R: Poststreptococcal glomerulonephritis in the elderly; report of a case and review of the literature. Am J Nephrol 1987;7:235–240

44. Pedersen EB: New tools in diagnosing renal artery stenosis. Kidney Int 2000;57:2657–2677

45. Radermacher J, Chavan A, Bleck J et al: Use of Doppler ultrasonography to predict the outcome of therapy for renal-artery stenosis. New Engl J Med 2001;344(6):410–417

46. Sicard GA, Reilly JM, Picus DD, Allen BT: Alternatives in renal vascularisation. Curr Probl Surg 1995;32:571–652

47. Griffiths GJ, Robinson KB, Cartwright GO, McLachlan MS: Loss of renal tissue in the elderly. Br J Radiol 1976;49(578):111–117

48. Tuttle KR, Chouinard RF, Webber JT et al: Treatment of atherosclerotic ostial renal artery stenosis with the intravascular stent. Am J Kidney Dis 1998;32(4):611–622

49. Scoble JE: Atherosclerotic nephropathy. Kidney Int (suppl) 1999;71:S106–S109

50. Sotto A, De Boever CM, Fabbro-Peray P et al: Risk factors for antibiotic-resistant *Escherichia coli* isolated from hospitalized patients with urinary tract infections: A prospective study. J Clin Microbiol 2001;39(2):438–444

51. Gasparini M, Hofman R, Stoller M: Renal artery embolism: clinical features and therapeutic options. J Urol 1992;147:567–572

52. Bennett PH, Haffner S, Kasiske BL et al: Screening and management of microalbuminuria in patients with diabetes mellitus: Recommendations to the scientific advisory board of the National Kidney Foundation from an ad hoc committee of the council on diabetes mellitus of the National Kidney Foundation. Am J Kidney Dis 1995;25:107–112

53. Bakris GL, Williams M, Dworkin L et al: Preserving renal function in adults with hypertension and diabetes: A consensus approach. Am J Kidney Dis 2000;36(3):646–661

54. Lewis EJ, Hunsicker LG, Bain RP, Rhode RD: The effect of angiotensin converting enzyme inhibition on diabetic nephropathy. N Engl J Med 1993;329:1456–1462

55. Canadian Institute for Health Information: Annual Report 1999, Dialysis and Transplantation, Canadian Organ Replacement Register, Vol. 1. Ottawa, Ontario, 1999

56. Blade J, Fernandez-Llama P, Bosch F et al: Renal failure in multiple myeloma: presenting features and predictors of outcome in 94 patients from a single institution. Arch Intern Med 1998;158(17):1889–1893

57. Sakhuja V, Jha V, Varma S et al: Renal involvement in multiple myeloma: a 10-year study. Renal Failure 2000;22(4):465–477

58. Knudsen LM, Hjorth M, Hippe E: Renal failure in multiple myeloma: reversibility and impact on the prognosis. Nordic Myeloma Study Group. Eur J Haematol 2000;65(3):175–181

59. Montseny J-J, Kleinknecht D, Meyrier A et al: Long-term outcome according to renal histological lesions in 118 patients with monoclonal gammopathies. Nephrol Dial Transplant 1998;13:1438–1445

60. Shetty A, Oreopoulos DG: CAPD in the treatment of end stage renal disease in myeloma patients. Nephrol Urol 1995;5:3–8

61. Rosansky SJ, Richards FW: Use of peritoneal dialysis in the treatment of patients with renal failure and paraproteinemia. Am J Nephrol 1985;5:361–365

62. Solling K: Clearances of Bence Jones proteins during dialysis or plasmapheresis in myelomatosis associated with renal failure. Contrib Nephrol 1988;68:259–262

63. Misiani R, Tiraboschi G, Mingardi G, Mecca G: Management of myeloma kidney: an anti-light chain approach. Am J Kidney Dis 1987;10:28–33

64. Nissenson AR, Port FK: Outcome of ESRD in patients with rare causes of renal failure. I. Inherited and metabolic disorders. Q J Med 1989;73:1055–1061

65. Port FK, Nissenson AR: Outcome of ESRD in patients with rare causes of renal failure. II. Renal systemic neoplasms. Q J Med 1989;73:1162–1166

66. Alexanian R, Baslogie B, Dixon D: Renal failure in multiple myeloma. Arch Intern Med 1990;150:1693–1695

67. Iggo N, Parsons V: Renal disease in multiple myeloma: Current prospectives. Nephron 1990;56:229–233

68. Mukamel E, Nissenkorn I, Boner G: Occult progressive renal damage in the elderly male due to benign prostatic hypertrophy. J Am Geriatr Soc 1979;27:403–406

69. Olbrich O, Woodford-Williams E, Irvine RE, Webster D: Renal function in prostatism. Lancet 1957;i:1322

70. Ralston AJ: Renal disease. Mod Geriatr 1975;5:10–14

71. Choudhury SL, Brocklehurst JC: Urinary tract infection in old age. In Macias Nunez JF, Cameron JS (eds): Renal Function and Disease in the Elderly. Butterworths, London, 1987:254–281

72. Sourander L: Urinary tract infection in the aged. An epidemiological study. Ann Med Intern Fed 1966;55(45): 1–55

73. Brocklehurst JC, Dillane JB, Griffith L, Fry J: The prevalence and symptomatology of urinary infection in an aged population. Gerontol Clin 1968;10:242–253

74. Eberlye CM, Winsemius SE: Risk factors and consequences of bacteriuria in non-catheterized nursing home residents. J Gerontol A 1993;48:M266–M271

75. Bakke A, Vollset SE: Risk factors for bacteriuria and clinical urinary tract infection in patients treated with intermittent catheterisation. J Urol 1993;149:527–531

76. Stein G, Funfstuck R: Asymptomatic bacteriuria—What to do. Nephrol Dial Transplant 1999;14:1618–1621

77. Nicolle LE, Mayhew WJ, Bryan L: Prospective randomized comparison of therapy and no therapy of asymptomatic bacteriuria in institutionalized elderly women. Am J Med 1987;83:27–33.

78. Kirkland JL, Robinson J: Bacteriuria and survival in old age. N Engl J Med 1981;305:586–587

79. Nordenstam GR, Ake Brandenberg O, Oden AS et al: Bacteriuria and mortality in an elderly population. N Engl J Med 1986;314:1152–1156

80. Abrutyn E, Mossey J, Berlin JA et al: Does asymptomatic bacteriuria predict mortality and does antimicrobial treatment reduce mortality in elderly ambulant women? Ann Intern Med 1994;120:827–833

81. Dontas AS, Kasavaki-Charvati P, Papanayiotou PC: Bacteriuria and survival in old age. N Engl J Med 1981;304:939–943

82. Tambyah PA, Maki DG: The relationship between pyuria and infection in patients with indwelling urinary catheters: A prospective study of 761 patients. Arch Intern Med 2000;160(5):673–677

83. Orr PH, Nicolle LE, Duckworth WC et al: Febrile urinary infection in the institutionalized elderly. Am J Med 1996;100:71–77

84. Nicolle LE: Urinary tract infections in the elderly: Symptomatic or asymptomatic? Int J Antimicrob Agents 1999;11:265–268

85. Mellito KF: Asymptomatic bacteriuria in older adults: when is it necessary to screen and treat? Nurse Pract 1995;20:50–66

86. Raaschou F: Studies of Chronic Pyelonephritis with Special Reference to Kidney Function. Munksgaard, Copenhagen, 1948

87. Baumanis J, Russell HK: Pyelonephritis in a chronic disease hospital. Geriatrics 1959;14:25–37

88. Bruckel RW, Wincker HJ: Clinical aspects of urinary tract infections in geriatrics. 6th International Congress of Gerontology (Excerpta Medica Congress Series 57). Copenhagen, 1963

89. Lieberthal F: Pyelonephritic contracture of the kidney. Surg Gynecol Obstet 1939;69:159–171

90. Bell ET: Exudative interstitial nephritis (pyelonephritis). Surgery 1942;2:261–280

91. Jackson GG, Dallenbach F, Kipnis GP: Symposium on clinical advances in medicine; pyelonephritis: correlation of clinical and pathologic observations in antibiotic era. Med Clin North Am 1955;39:297

92. Sanjuro LA: The problem of chronic pyelonephritis. Med Clin North Am 1959;43:1601–1610

93. Kleeman SE, Freedman LR: The finding of chronic pyelonephritis in males and females at autopsy. N Engl J Med 1960;263:988–992

94. Fihn SD, Johnson C, Stamm WE: *Escherichia coli* urethritis in women with symptoms of acute urinary infection. J Infect Dis 1988;157:196–199

95. Kunin CM, White LV, Hua TH: A reassessment of the importance of "low-count" bacteriuria in young women with acute urinary symptoms. Ann Intern Med 1993;119:454–460

96. Arav-Boger R, Leibovici L, Danon YL: Urinary tract infections with low and high colony counts in young women. Arch Intern Med 1994;154:300–304

97. Maskell R, Pead L, Sanderson RA: Fastidious bacteria and the urethral syndrome: a 2-year clinical and bacteriological study of 51 women. Lancet 1983;2:1277–1280

98. Fairly KF, Birch D: Detection of bladder bacteriuria in patients with acute urinary symptoms. J Infect Dis 1989;159:131–226

99. Wilkins E, Payne SR, Pead PJ et al: Interstitial cystitis and urethral syndrome: a possible answer. Br J Urol 1989;64:39–44

100. Pead L, Maskell R, Morris J: *Staphyloccus saphrophyticus* as a urinary pathogen: a six year prospective survey. Br Med J 1985;291:1157–1159

101. Maskell R, Pead L: Corynebacteria as urinary pathogens. J Infect Dis 1990;162:782–783

102. Soriano F, Fernandez-Roblas R: Infections caused by antibiotic-resistant *Corynebacterium* Group D2. Eur J Clin Microbiol Infect Dis 1988;7:337–341

103. Brumfitt W, Gargan RA, Hamilton-Miller J: Diagnosis and cure of recurrent urinary infection with microaerophilic and anaerobic bacteria. Br Med J 1980;281:909–910

104. Collins LE, Clarke RW, Maskell R: Streptococci as urinary pathogens. Lancet 1986;2(479):481

105. Kass EH: Chemotherapeutic and antibiotic drugs in management if infection of urinary tract. Am J Med 1955;18:764–781

106. Bergeron MG: Treatment of pyelonephritis in adults. Med Clin North Am 1995;79:619–649

107. Truck M, Petersdorf RG, Fournier MR: The epidemiology of non-enteric *Escherichia coli* infections: prevalence of serological groups. J Clin Invest 1962;41:1760–1765

108. Lidin Janson G, Hanson LA, Kaijser B: Comparison of *Escherichia coli* from bacteriuric patients with those from feces of healthy school children. J Infect Dis 1977;136:346–353

109. Gruenberg RN, Bendall MJ: Hospital outbreak of trimethoprim resistance in pathogenic coliform bacteria. Br Med J 1979;2:7–9

110. Stamey TA, Timothy M, Miller M, Mihara G: Recurrent urinary infections in adult women. The role of introital enterobacteria. California Med 1971;115:1–19

111. Bollgren I, Winberg J: The periurethral aerobic flora in girls highly susceptible to urinary infection. Acta Paediatr Scand 1976;65:81–87

112. Sourander L, Ruikka I, Gronroos M: Correlation between urinary tract infection, prolapse conditions and function of the bladder in the aged female hospital patient. Gerontol Clin 1965;7:179–184

113. Carty M: Bacteriuria and its correlates in old age. Gerontology 1981;27:72–75

114. Warren JW, Muncie H, Jr, Hebel JR, Hall-Craggs M: Long-term urethral catheterization increases risk of chronic pyelonephritis and renal inflammation. J Am Geriatr Soc 1994;42:1286–1290

115. Nicolle LE: Prevention and treatment of urinary catheter-related infections in older patients. Drugs Aging 1994;4(5):379–391

116. Karchmer TB, Giannetta ET, Muto CA, Strain BA, Farr BM: A randomized crossover study of silver-coated urinary catheters in hospitalized patients. Arch Intern Med 2000;160:3294–3298

117. Saint S, Veenstra DL, Sullivan SD, Chenoweth C, Fendrick AM: The potential clinical and economic benefits of silver alloy urinary catheters in preventing urinary tract infection. Arch Intern Med 2000;160(17):2670–2675

118. Saltzman R, Perterson PK: Immunodeficiency of the elderly. Rev Infect Dis 1987;9:1127–1139

119. Wade AW, Szewczuk MR: Changes in the mucosal-associated B cell response with age. In Goidl EA (ed): Aging and the Immune Response. Marcel Dekker, New York, 1987:95–127

120. Seneca H, Grant J, Jr: Urologic sepsis/shock. J Am Geriatr Soc 1976;24:292–300

121. Svanborg EC: Attachment of *Escherichia coli* to human uroepithelial cells. An in vitro test system applied in the study of urinary tract infection. Scand J Infect Dis 1978;15(suppl):1–74

122. Isada CM, Kasten BL, Goldman MP et al: Infectious Diseases Handbook. LexiComp, Hudson, Cleveland, 1995

123. Pinson AG, Philbrick JT, Lindbeck GH, Schorling JB: Oral antibiotic therapy for acute pyelonephritis: a methodologic review of the literature. J Gen Intern Med 1992;7:544–553

124. Brocklehurst JC, Dillane JB, Griffiths L, Fry J: A therapeutic trial in urinary infection of old age. Gerontol Clin 1968;10:345–347

125. Sourander L, Kasanen A: En dos langtids' sulfonamid i veckan (4-sulfanilamido-5-6-dimetoxypyrimidin) vid behandling av urinvagsinfektionen hos aldringar. Nord Med 1965;74:1229–1230

126. Chamberland S, L'Ecuyer J, Lessard C et al: Antibiotic susceptibility profiles of 941 gram negative bacteria isolated from septicaemic patients throughout Canada. Clin Infect Dis 1992;15:615–628

127. Bergeron MG: Therapeutic potential of high renal levels of aminoglycosides in pyelonephritis. J Antimicrob Chemother 1985;15:4–8

128. Bergeron MG, Marois Y: Benefit from high levels of gentamycin in the treatment of E. coli pyelonephritis. Kidney Int 1986;30:481–487

129. Mouton Y, Ajana F, Chidiac C et al: A multicenter study of lomefloxacin and trimethoprim/sulfamethoxazole in the treatment of uncomplicated acute pyelonephritis. Am J Med 1992;92:87S–90S

130. Cox CE, Gentry LO, Rodriguez-Gomez G: Multicenter open-label study of parenteral ofloxacin in treatment of pyelonephritis in adults. Urology 1992;39:453–456

131. Bailey RR, Lynn KL, Robson RA et al: Comparison of ciprofloxacin with netilmicin for the treatment of acute pyelonephritis. NZ Med J 1992;105:102–103

132. McCarthy CS, Becker JA: Multiple myeloma and contrast media. Radiology 1992;183:519–521

133. Kramer BK: Cyclo-oxygenase-2 and renal function. Nephrol Dial Transplant 2001;16:180–183

134. Moore RD, Steinberg EP, Powe NR et al: Frequency and determinants of adverse reactions induced by high-osmolality contrast media. Radiology 1989;170:727–732

135. Weisberg LS, Kurnik PB, Kurnik BR: Risk of radiocontrast nephropathy in patients with and without diabetes mellitus. Kidney Int 1994;45:259–265

136. Manske CL, Sprafka JM, Strong JT, Wang Y: Contrast nephropathy in diabetic patients undergoing coronary arteriography. Am J Med 1990;89:615–620

137. Weinrauch LA, Healy RW, Leland OS et al: Coronary angiography and acute renal failure in diabetic azotemic nephropathy. Arch Intern Med 1977;86:56

138. Berkseth RO, Kjellstrand CM: Radiolic contrast-induced nephropathy. Med Clin North Am 1984;68:351–370

139. Cochran ST, Wong WS, Roe DJ: Predicting antiographic induced acute renal impairment: Clinical risk model. Am J Radiol 1983;141:1027–1033

140. Taliercio CP, Vliestra R, Fisher LD, Burnett JC: Risks of renal dysfunction with cardiac angiography. Ann Intern Med 1986;104:501–504

141. Porter GA: Contrast associated nephropathy. Am J Cardiol 1989;64:22E–26E

142. Barrett BJ, Carlisle E: A meta-analysis of the relative nephrotoxicity of high and low-osmolality contrast media. J Am Soc Nephrol 1992;3:719

143. Moore RD, Steinberg EP, Powe NR et al: Nephrotoxicity of high-osmolality versus low-osmolality contrast media: randomised clinical trial. Radiology 1992;182:649–655

144. Porter GA: Contrast-associated nephropathy: presentation, pathophysiology and management. Min Electrolyte Metab 1994;20:232–243

145. Soloman R, Werner C, Mann D et al: Effects of saline, mannitol, and furosemide to prevent acute decreases in renal function induced by radiocontrast agents. N Engl J Med 1994;331:1416–1420

146. Weinstein JM, Heyman S, Brezis M: Potential deleterious effect of furosemide in radiocontrast nephropathy. Nephron 1992;62:413–415

147. Weisberg LS, Kurnik PB, Kurnik BR: Dopamine and renal blood flow in radiocontrast-induced nephropathy in humans. Ren Fail 1993;15:61–68

148. Erley CM, Duda SH, Schlepckow S et al: Adenosine antagonist theophylline prevents the reduction of glomerular filtration rate after contrast media application. Kidney Int 1994;45:1425–1431

149. Tepel M, van der GM, Schwarzfeld C et al: Prevention of radiographic-contrast-agent-induced reductions in renal function by acetylcysteine N Engl J Med 2000;343(3):180–184

150. Bakris GL, Lass NA, Glock D: Renal hemodynamics in radiocontrast medium-induced renal dysfunction: A role for dopamine-1 receptors. Kidney Int 2001;56(1):206–210

151. Eknoyan G: Renal papillary necrosis. In Massry SG, Glassock RJ (eds): Textbook in Nephrology. Wilkins & Wilkins, Baltimore, 1989:1910–1916

152. Blagg CR: Chronic renal failure in the elderly. In Oreopoulus DG (ed): Geriatric Nephrology. Martinus Nijhoff, Boston, 1986;117–126

153. Challah S, Wing AJ, Bauer R et al: Negative selection of patients for dialysis and transplantation in the United Kingdom. Br Med J 1984;288:1119–1122

154. Dalzeil M, Garrett C: Intraregional variation in the treatment of end stage renal failure. Br Med J 1987; 294:1382–1383

155. Khlar S, Levey AS, Beck G et al: The effects of dietary protein restriction and blood pressure control on the progression of chronic renal disease. N Engl J Med 1994;330:877–884

156. Mendelssohn DC, Barrett BJ, Brownscombe LM et al: Elevated levels of serum creatinine: recommendations for management and referral. Can Med Assoc J 1999;161(4):413–417

157. Petersen JC, Alder S, Burkart JM et al: Blood pressure control, proteinuria and the progression of renal disease. The modification of diet in renal disease study. Ann Intern Med 1995;123:754–762

158. National Kidney Foundation: Dialysis Outcomes Quality Initiative Guidelines. National Kidney Foundation, Washington, 1997

159. Weinstein MC, Stason WB: Cost-effectiveness of interventions to prevent or treat coronary heart disease. Ann Rev Public Health 1985;6:41–63

160. Nissenson AR: Chronic peritoneal dialysis in the elderly. Ger Nephrol Urol 1991;1:3–12

161. D'Amico G, Striker GE: Proceedings from the symposium on renal replacement therapy throughout the world: the registries. Comparability of the different registries on renal replacement therapy. Am J Kidney Dis 1995;25:113–118

162. Ismail N, Hakim RM, Oreopoulos DG, Patrikarea A: Renal replacement therapies in the elderly: Part 1. Hemodialysis and chronic peritoneal dialysis. Am J Kidney Dis 1993;22(6):759–782

163. US Renal Data System: USRDS 1989 Annual Report. Bethesda, Maryland, The National Institutes of Health, National Institute of Diabetes and Digestive and Kidney Diseases. Am J Kidney Dis 1989;17–20

164. National Institute of Diabetes and Digestive and Kidney Diseases. US Renal data systems, Annual Data Report. Researchers Guide, reference tables and ADR slides. United States Renal Data System Coordinating Center, Ann Arbor, MI, 1999

165. Agodoa LY, Eggers PW: Renal replacement therapy in the United States: data from the United States Renal Data System. Am J Kidney Dis 1995;25(1):119–133

166. Benevent D, Benzakour M, Peyronnet P et al: Comparison of continuous ambulatory peritoneal dialysis and haemodialysis in the elderly. Adv Perit Dial 1990;6(suppl):68–71

167. Walls J: Dialysis in the elderly: Some UK experience. Adv Perit Dial 1990;6(suppl):68–71

168. Piccoli G, Quarello F, Salomone M et al: Dialysis in the elderly: comparison of different dialytic modalities. Adv Perit Dial 1990;6(suppl):72–81

169. Nissenson AR, Gentile DE, Soderblom R: CAPD in the elderly: Southern California/South Nevada experience. Adv Perit Dial 1990;6(suppl):51–55

170. Gokal R: CAPD in the elderly: European and UK experience. Adv Perit Dial 1990;6(suppl):38–40

171. Williams AJ, Nicholl JF, El-Nahas AM et al: Continuous ambulatory peritoneal dialysis and haemodialysis in the elderly. Q J Med 1990;274:215–223

172. Segoloni GP, Salamone M, Piccoli GB: CAPD in the elderly. Italian multicenter study experience. Adv Perit Dial 1990;6(suppl):41–46

173. Khan IH, Catto GRD, Edward N, MacLeod AM: Death during the first 90 days of dialysis: a case control study. Am J Kidney Dis 1995;25:276–280

174. Metcalfe W, Khan IH, MacLeod AM, Simpson K: Can we improve early mortality in patients receiving renal replacement therapy? Kidney Int 2000;57(6):2539–2545

175. Jassal SV, Douglas JF, Stout RW: Prognostic markers for one year survival in elderly dialysis patients. Nephrol Dial Transplant 1996;11:1052–1057

176. Held PJ, Port FK, Turenne MN et al: Continuous ambulatory peritoneal dialysis and haemodialysis: comparisons of patient mortality with adjustment for comorbid conditions. Kidney Int 1994;45:1163–1169

177. Winston DJ, Imagawa DK, Holt CD et al: Long-term gancyclovir prophylaxis eliminates serious cytomegalovirus disease in liver transplant recipients receiving OKT3 therapy for rejection. Transplantation 1995;60(11):1357–1360

178. Conti DJ, Singh TP, Gruber SA et al: Gancyclovir prophylaxis of cytomegalovirus disease. ASTP Abstract Book 1996 (abstract)

179. Michel C, Bindi P, Viron B: CAPD with private home nurses: an alternative treatment for elderly and disabled patients. Adv Perit Dial 1990;6(suppl):92–94

180. Nolph KD, Lindblad AS, Noval JW, Steinberg SM: Experiences with the elderly in the national CAPD registry. Adv Perit Dial 1990;6(suppl):33–37

181. Jagose JT, Afthentopoulos IE, Shetty A, Oreopoulos DG: Successful use of CAPD in octagenarians. Adv Perit Dial 1996;12:126–131

182. Wing AJ, Brunner FP, Brynger H: Combined report on regular dialysis and transplantation in Europe, IX 1978. Proc Eur Dial Trans Assoc 1979;13:2–52

183. Hinsdale JG, Lipcouritz GS, Hoover EL: Vascular access in the elderly: Results and perspectives in a geriatric population. Dial Trans 1985;14:560–562

184. Pourchez T, Moriniere P, St Priest A: Outcome of vascular access for haemodialysis in the elderly (<75 years). Proc Eur Dial Trans Assoc 1990;27:160

185. Munda R, First MR, Alexander JW et al: Polytetrafluorethylene graft survival in hemodialysis. JAMA 1983;249:219–222

186. Gruppo Emodialisi e Pathologie Cardiovascolari: Multicentre cross-sectional study of ventricular arrhythmias in chronically haemodialysed patients. Lancet 1988;6:305–308

187. Sherman RA, Cody RP, Rodgers ME, Solanchick JC: Inter dialytic weight gain and nutritional parameters in chronic haemodialysis patients. Am J Kidney Dis 1995;25:579–583

188. Schnider SI, Kohn RR, Cerami A: Effects of age and diabetes mellitus on the solubility of collagen from human skin, tracheal cartilage and dura mater. Exp Gerontol 1982;17:185–194

189. Monnier VM, Vishwantath V, Frank KE et al: Relation between complications of type I diabetes mellitus and collagen-linked fluorescence. N Engl J Med 1986;314:403–408

190. Blake PG: Growth hormone and malnutrition in dialysis patients. Perit Dial Int 1995;15:210–216

191. Jones MR, Martis L, Algrim CE et al: Amino acid solutions for CAPD: rationale and clinical experience. Min Electrolyte Metab 1992;18:309–315

192. Kopple KD, Bernard D, Messana J et al: Amino acid solutions for CAPD patients with an amino acid based dialysate. Kidney Int 1995;47:1148–1157

193. Chertow GM, Ling J, Lew NL et al: The association of intradialytic parenteral nutrition administration with survival in haemodialysis patients. Am J Kidney Dis 1994;24:912–920

194. Dombros NV, Digenis GE, Soliman G, Oreopoulos DG: Anabolic steroids in the treatment of malnourished patients: a retrospective study. Perit Dial Int 1994;14:344–347

195. Bucala R, Vlassara H: Advanced glycosylation end products in diabetic renal and vascular disease. Am J Kidney Dis 1995;26:875–888

196. Skolnik EY, Yang Z, Makita Z et al: Human and rat mesangial cell receptors for glucose-modified proteins: potential role in kidney tissue remodelling and diabetic nephropathy. J Exp Med 1991;174:931–938

197. Doi T, Vlassara H, Kirstein M et al: Receptor-specific increase in extracellular matrix production in mouse mesangial cells by advanced glycosylation end products is mediated via platelet-derived growth factor. Proc Natl Acad USA 1992;89:2873–2877

198. Sell DR, Moonier VM: End stage renal disease and diabetes catalyse the formation of a pentose-derived crosslink from aging human collagen. J Clin Invest 1990;685:380–384

199. Makita Z, Raddoff S, Rafield EJ et al: Advanced glycosylation end products in patients with diabetic nephropathy. N Engl J Med 1991;325:836–842

200. Vlassara H, Fuh H, Makita Z et al: Endogenous advanced glycosylation end products induce complex vascular dysfunction in normal animals; a model for diabetic and aging complications. Proc Natl Acad USA 1992;89:12043–12047

201. Fuh H, Yang D, Striker G, Vlassara H: In vivo AGE-peptide injection induces kidney enlargement and glomerular hypertrophy in rabbits; prevention by aminoguanidine. Diabetes 1992;41:9A(abstract)

202. Willenheimer R, Erhardt LR: Value of 6-min walk test for assessment of severity and prognosis of heart failure. Lancet 2000;355:515–516

203. Fitts SS, Guthrie MR: Six-minute walk by people with chronic renal failure: Assessment of effort by perceived exertion. Am J Phys Med Rehab 1995;74(1):54–58

204. Podsiadlo D, Richardson S: The timed "up & go": A test of basic functional mobility for frail elderly persons. J Am Geriatr Soc 2001;39(2):142–148

205. Weiner DK, Duncan PW, Chandler J, Studenski SA: Functional reach: A marker of physical frailty. J Am Geriatr Soc 1992;40(3):203–207

206. Burd RS, Gillingham KJ, Farber MS et al: Diagnosis and treatment of cytomegalovirus disease in pediatric renal transplant recipients. J Pediatr Surg 1994;29(8):1049–1054

207. Nakazato PZ, Burns W, Moore P et al: Viral prophylaxis in hepatic transplantation: preliminary report of a randomized trial of acyclovir and gancyclovir. Transplant Proc 1993;25(2):1935–1937

208. Anderson JE, Kraus J, Sturgeon D: Incidence, prevalence, and outcomes of end-stage renal disease patients placed in nursing homes. Am J Kidney Dis 1993;21(6):619–627

209. Roscoe JM: Haemodialysis in the nursing home. Presented at the 4th International Conference on Geriatric Nephrology. Toronto, 1996;19:2

210. Johansen KL, Chertow GM, Ng AV et al: Physical activity levels in patients on hemodialysis and healthy sedentary controls. Kidney Int 2000;57(6):2564–2570

211. Evan RW, Manninen DL, Garrison LP et al: The quality of life of patients with end stage renal disease. N Engl J Med 1985;312:553–559

212. Stout JP, Gokal R, Hillier VF et al: Quality of life of high risk and elderly dialysis patients in the UK. Dial Trans 1987;16:674–677

213. Moody H, Moody C, Szabo E et al: Are old dialysis patients happy and can they fend for themselves or not? XII Int Congr Nephrol, Jerusalem, 1993 (abstract)

214. Horina JH, Holzer H, Reisinger EC et al: Elderly patients and chronic haemodialysis. Lancet 1992;339:183

215. Westlie L, Umen A, Nestrud S, Kjellstrand CM: Mortality, morbidity and life satisfaction in the very old dialysis patient. ASAIO J 1984;30:21–30

216. Neves PL: Chronic haemodialysis in elderly patients. Nephrol Dial Transplant 1995;10(suppl):69–71

217. Jassal SV, Opelz G, Cole E: Transplantation in the elderly: A review. Ger Nephrol Urol 1997;7:157–165

218. Wyner LM, McElroy JB, Hodge EE, Peidmonte M, Novick AC: Use of kidneys from older cadaver donors for renal transplantation. Urology 1993;41:107–110

219. Kumar MS, Stephan R, Chui J et al: Donor age and graft outcome in cadaver renal transplantation. Trans Proc 1993;25:3097–3098

220. Cacciarelli TV, Sumrani N, Scriven R et al: Influence of donor and recipient age on renal allograft survival time. Transpl Proc 1993;25:3140–3142

221. Lloveras J, Arais M, Puig JM et al: Long-term follow-up of recipients of cadaver kidney allografts from elderly donors. Transpl Proc 1993;25:3175–3176

222. Phillips AO, Bewick M, Snowdon SA, Hillis AN, Hendry BM: The influence of recipient and donor age on the outcome of renal transplantation. Clin Nephrol 1993;40(6):352–354

223. Shmueli D, Nakache R, Lustig S et al: Renal transplant from live donors over 65 years old. Trans Proc 1994;26:2139–2140

224. Alexander JW, Bennett LE, Breen TJ: Effect of donor age on outcome of kidney transplantation. A two-year analysis of transplants reported to the United Network for Organ Sharing Registry. Transplantation 1994;57:871–876

225. Hayashi T, Koga S, Higashi Y et al: Living related renal transplantation from elderly donors (older than 66 years of age). Transpl Proc 1995;27:984–985

226. Cecka JM, Terasaki PI: Optimal use for older kidneys: older recipients. Transpl Proc 1995;27:801–802

227. Gaber LW, Moore LW, Alloway PR et al: Glomerulosclerosis as a determinant of posttransplant function of older donor renal allografts. Transplantation 1995;60(4):334–339

228. Albrechtson D, Leivestad T, Sodal G et al: Kidney transplantation in patients older than 70 years of age. Transpl Proc 1995;27(1):86–88

229. Tesi RJ, Elkhammas EA, Davies EA, Henry ML, Ferguson RM: Renal transplantation in older people. Lancet 1994;343:461–464

230. Ismail N, Hakim R, Helderman JH: Renal replacement therapies in the elderly: Part II, renal transplantation. Am J Kidney Dis 1994;23(1):1–15

231. Cole EH, Farewell VT, Aprile M et al: Renal transplantation in older patients: the University of Toronto experience. Ger Nephrol Urol 1995;5:85–92

232. Pirsch JD, Stratta RJ, Armbrust MJ et al: Cadaveric renal transplantation with cyclosporine in patients more than 60 years of age. Transplantation 1989;47:259–261

233. Andreu J, de la Torre M, Oppenheimer F et al: Renal transplantation in elderly recipients. Transpl Proc 1992;24:120–121

234. Cardella CJ, Harding ME, de Veber GA: A controlled trial comparing sequential anti-lymphocyte serum and cyclosporine therapy in renal transplant patients. Transpl Proc 1987;19:1996–1998

235. Schaubel D, Desmeules M, Mao Y, Jeffery J, Fenton SS: Survival experience among elderly end-stage renal disease patients. Transplantation 1995;60(12):1389–1394

236. Ost L, Groth C-G, Lindholm B et al: Cadaveric renal transplantation in patients of 60 years of age and above. Transplantation 1980;30:339–340

237. Vivas CA, Hickey DP, Jordan ML et al: Renal transplantation in patients 65 years old or older. J Urol 1992;147:990–993

238. Nyberg G, Norden G, Hadimeri H, Wrammer L: Physical performance does not improve in elderly patients following successful kidney transplantation. Nephrol Dial Transplant 1995;10:86–90

239. Laupacis A, Keown P, Pus N et al: A study of the quality of life and cost-utility of renal transplantation. Kidney Int 1996;50:235–242

240. McKenzie JM: Survey of Canadian Directors. Canadian Society of Nephrology, 1993

241. Kilner JF: Selecting patients when resources are limited: a study of US medical directors of kidney dialysis and transplantation facilities. Am J Pub Health 1988;78:144–147

242. Callaghan D: Setting Limits: Medical Goals in an Aging Society. Simon and Schuster, New York, 1987

243. Oreopoulos DG: Should the elderly be denied dialysis. Ger Nephrol Urol 1994;4:67–70

244. Churchill DN, Taylor DW, Cook RJ et al: Canadian haemodialysis morbidity study. Am J Kidney Dis 1992;19:214–234

Chapter 88

Disorders of water and electrolyte metabolism

Catherine L. Kelleher

Material in this chapter contains contributions from the previous edition, and we are grateful to the previous author for the work done.

Anatomical and physiological changes in the aging kidney have been detailed in earlier chapters and are only briefly reviewed below. The impact of these age-associated changes on the day-to-day ability of the kidney to maintain fluid and electrolyte homeostasis is usually not clinically significant. However, under environmental and disease-related stresses such as volume changes, severe infection, or illness, the aging kidney is more sensitive, less flexible, and slower to respond to maintain normal homeostasis. It is under these conditions that electrolyte abnormalities develop. The development of electrolyte abnormalities may be further compounded by the comorbidity associated with the aging process, including vascular disease, diabetes, and cardiac disease which place older adults at increased risk for a renal insult. At the same time, older adults may be on multiple medications that can increase the risk of a renal insult even further.

The ultimate goal in geriatric medicine is to help older adults maintain a level of function and independence they find satisfying. In the case of water and electrolyte abnormalities, the goal is to try to prevent the occurrence of these abnormalities altogether by understanding the impact of disease on renal function, the contribution of comorbid conditions, and the slowed response of the kidney in maintaining homeostasis. Understanding the age-associated changes in renal function as well as changes in body composition with aging is critical in understanding age-associated alterations in water and electrolyte metabolism, and in preventing clinically significant alterations in electrolyte abnormalities.

AGE-ASSOCIATED CHANGES IN THE KIDNEY

Briefly, age-associated changes include a decrease in kidney size and mass primarily through glomerular atrophy in the renal cortex with sparing of the medulla.[1–4] The glomeruli show mesangial matrix expansion, and an increase in basement membrane thickness with the deposition of hyaline and ultimately collapse of the glomerular tuft. In the cortex, there is sclerosis of the afferent and efferent arterioles. However, in the juxtamedullary area the arterioles appear to form direct connections which may explain the normal or relative increase in medullary blood flow seen in older kidneys (although renal blood flow overall appears to decrease).[1–3] There is also a decrease in tubular number with atrophy of tubular epithelium and tubular dilation, interstitial fibrosis, and arteriolar vascular changes.[1–3] Diverticula have been observed to increase in number in the distal convoluted tubules where they communicate directly with the tubular lumen.[4]

It is important to remember that, although there is loss of glomerular mass with aging, the loss of tubular mass is proportional and so the glomerular–tubular balance is usually maintained.[1,2] Equally important, it is not at all clear that renal function declines with "normal aging." The most frequently utilized and most useful measure of renal function is an estimate of the glomerular filtration rate (GFR), as decreases in all other functions (tubular functions, concentrating ability, acid excretion, etc.) tend to parallel decreases in GFR.[1,2] Interestingly, data from the Baltimore Longitudinal Study of Aging[5] showed that while two-thirds of aging individuals followed for up to 24 years showed a decline in renal function as measured by the glomerular filtration rate, one-third had no decline in GFR. This suggest that a decline in renal function is not "normal aging" but more likely the result of the accumulation of the described renal anatomical and physiological age-associated changes in the setting of comorbidity (including unrecognized clinical disease) and medication. In addition, age-associated changes in the hormones that regulate intravascular volume may contribute. The influence of diet and metabolism may also be substantial. Genetic background is also likely to play a role.

AGE-ASSOCIATED CHANGES IN BODY COMPOSITION

There are characteristic changes in body composition that are important to consider when evaluating renal functioning. Bodyweight is composed of primarily two components: fat and fat-free mass. Lean body mass is that component of the fat-free mass less the weight of bone and nonadipose fat.[6] While precise definitions of lean body mass vary slightly depending on measurement methods, for the purposes of this review, fat-free and lean body mass will be taken as equivalent; age changes in lean body mass and bones are essentially parallel so that no significant systematic errors will be introduced.[7] Numerous cross-sectional studies using different techniques have consistently demonstrated a significant increase in body fat in older adults,[8,9] a change that has not been observed in primitive populations.[10] At the same time, in all populations, a decline in lean body mass has been noted (Fig. 88-1).

This decrease in lean body mass is important to consider when evaluating an older individual's renal functioning. In an effort to estimate renal function the glomerular filtration rate (GFR) is calculated. The creatinine clearance is the most reproducible measure of GFR available for clinical decision-making. Creatinine production decreases with age in relation

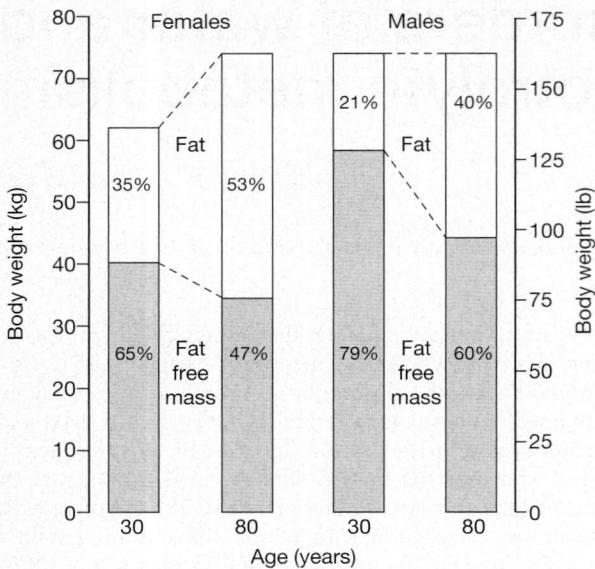

Figure 88-1 Effects of age on body composition in healthy adults.

to the decrease in lean body mass. Therefore, there may be no change in the serum creatinine despite a decline in renal function. The relationship between serum creatinine and GFR has prompted a number of investigators to suggest one could properly correct for the confounding variables, so they have developed formulas to estimate creatinine clearance as a measure of GFR. The most widely utilized formula is that of Cockcroft and Gault:[11]

$$Ccr \, (mL/min) = \frac{(140 - age \, in \, years) \times (weight \, in \, kg)}{72 \times (serum \, creatinine \, in \, mg/dL)}$$

This Ccr is multiplied by 0.85 for women.

This formula was developed and validated on very selected samples of older adults that did not include many very old people. Only moderate correlations have subsequently been found between calculated and actual creatinine clearances, especially in older populations.[12–14] Currently, no available method of estimating GFR from easily obtainable variables such as age, sex, weight, and serum creatinine is very accurate, and no method will be available until we have an easy method for estimating muscle mass. It should also be remembered that some creatinine is secreted by the renal tubule, so the creatinine clearance overestimates the GFR. Nevertheless, in clinical practice, use of an estimated GFR from the Cockcroft–Gault formula will provide a prompt and reasonable guide for clinical decision-making in most situations.

Understanding how well the kidneys are functioning helps identify individuals at risk for an electrolyte abnormality in any given clinical situation, including acute illness, change in volume status, or medication. Whenever possible, it is best to measure serum drug levels to assist with accurate dosing. It is also important to recognize that certain commonly prescribed drugs (trimethoprim–sulfamethoxazole, cimetedine, and cefoxitin) compete with creatinine for tubular secretion, thereby increasing the serum creatinine concentration without changing the GFR.

BODY COMPARTMENTS

Total body water (TBW) accounts for approximately 60 percent of bodyweight in young individuals. It is divided between the intracellular space (30–40 percent) and the extracellular space (20 percent).

Changes in the intracellular fluid volume result primarily from changes in plasma osmolality or the serum sodium concentration. The serum sodium concentration reflects the hydration status of individual cells.

The extracellular space is divided into the plasma, the interstitial space, and the transcellular space (spaces divided by a layer of epithelium such as the intraocular or the pleural space). The intravascular space or plasma determines the effective circulating volume. In general, the plasma reflects the extracellular fluid (ECF) volume (although not in some patients with edema). Alterations in the ECF volume reflect changes in the absolute amount of sodium or salt present in the body.

Total body water decreases with age in proportion to total bodyweight, so the loss or gain of one liter of water represents proportionately a larger change in older adults than in young adults. For example, in a young man, the TBW makes up approximately 59 percent of the total bodyweight, compared with approximately 55 percent in an older man. For young women, TBW constitutes 53 percent of total bodyweight compared with 45 percent in an older woman.

The etiology, clinical presentation, and treatments of predominantly intracellular versus extracellular fluid problems are different. Usually, abnormalities with sodium content and water balance coexist. However, as they represent different physiological processes, they should be evaluated as separate problems to assure proper treatment.

ACID–BASE BALANCE

In normal healthy indivduals, the hydrogen ion content of the arterial blood, usually measured as pH, is kept constant in spite of changes in acid load produced by many metabolic processes and exercise. The acid–base balance is regulated acutely by the excretion of CO_2 with respiration, and over several days by renal excretion of fixed acids. Some clinical data suggest that older adults develop a mild metabolic acidosis characterized by a slight fall in serum bicarbonate.[15] However, this abnormality is largely reported in older adults with a decline in renal function,[15] and it probably reflects the latter as suggested by the associated elevation in serum chloride (no change in unmeasured anions).

It is not clear what the biological effects, if any, of this mild metabolic acidosis might be with regard to bone, protein catabolism, and muscle wasting. What is important to remember is that, as a general rule, the older kidney is able to maintain acid–base homeostasis. However, in response to an increased acid load, as from exercise or infection, the aging kidney is slower to excrete the acid, probably secondary to decreased ammonia production in the tubular cells. As the older kidney is less able to defend against an acid load, this must be taken into account when caring for the very ill older individual. When it is clinically necessary to correct an acid–base disturbance, as for example in the case of dangerously low pH, it is important to treat cautiously and measure the result of interventions. Whenever possible, it is best to correct the underlying cause of the disturbance as this usually also corrects the acid–base abnormality.

CHANGES IN ELECTROLYTES WITH AGING

Serum measurements of sodium, potassium, chloride, and bicarbonate do not significantly change with increasing age.[15,16] However, clinically significant alterations in the serum sodium and potassium concentration are common in older individuals and contribute to increased morbidity and mortality.

Sodium

Sodium homeostasis

As noted above, serum sodium concentration does not change with increasing age. It is important that the serum sodium concentration should remain within defined limits (generally 137–143 mEq/L) because sodium is the primary cation in the extracellular fluid and the major determinant of plasma osmolality. An elevated serum sodium concentration or elevated plasma osmolality means that the patient has a free-water deficit relative to the amount of sodium present, and the individual cells are dehydrated. A low serum sodium concentration or low plasma osmolality means that free water is present in excess of sodium and individual cells are overhydrated.

In interpreting an abnormal serum sodium, it is important to know whether the reported sodium is an accurate reflection of serum osmolality. Plasma osmolality may be calculated using a standard formula:

$$\text{Plasma osmolality} = 2 \times \text{serum sodium} + \frac{\text{glucose}}{18} + \frac{\text{blood urea nitrogen}}{2.8}$$

or it may be measured.[17] As blood urea nitrogen moves freely through most plasma membranes it is, in general, not an effective osmol and does not contribute to cell hydration. The effective plasma osmolality may thus be estimated by:

$$\text{Effective plasma osmolality} = 2 \times \text{serum sodium (mEq/L)} + \frac{\text{glucose}}{18}$$

Pseudohyponatremia may be seen with hyperglycemia, hyperproteinemia, and hyperlipidemia. When insulin is given to a hyperglycemic patient, glucose moves intracellularly and water follows down its osmotic gradient, returning the serum sodium concentration to normal. One formula that may be used to calculate the effect of hyperglycemia on the serum sodium concentration is to add 1.6 mEq/L for every

100 mg/dL rise in blood glucose.[17] With hyperlipidemia and hyperproteinemia, the measured plasma osmolality is normal. Hyponatremia secondary to hyperlipidemia and hyperproteinuria is rare but may be associated with multiple myeloma.[18] If pseudohyponatremia is a concern, a measured serum osmolality should be compared with a calculated serum osmolality.

The concentration of serum sodium (as opposed to total body sodium content) is primarily controlled by the excretion or absorption of water in the kidney in response to arginine vasopressin (ADH) and to the sensation of thirst. When the serum sodium concentration rises, the increase in plasma osmolality is sensed by hypothalamic osmoreceptors. In response, ADH is produced by the supraoptic and paraventricular nuclei in the hypothalamus. In aging rats, no known degenerative changes in these nuclei have been appreciated,[19] nor does there appear to be a decrease in neurosecretory material with age.[20] In fact, there are data to suggest that the activity of these nuclei increase with age.[21–23] There are some mouse data suggesting a reduction in the neuroaxonal transport of ADH.[24] These changes in the nucleus might explain the clinical observation that in response to an osmotic stimulus, many older adults produce almost twice the ADH as do younger individuals.[25] However, in response to a volume stimulus with orthostasis, many older individuals show a decrease in ADH secretion, possibly owing to alterations in the afferent limb of the baroreceptor reflex arc.[26]

ADH then binds to the V2 receptors in the principal cells of the collecting duct in the kidney, and through stimulation of G-alpha-s heterotrimeric proteins activates adenylyl cyclase. This leads to increased cAMP levels, activation of protein kinase A, and ultimately fusion of aquaporin 2 channels with the luminal membrane, increasing water absorption with a return of plasma osmolality to normal. In animals, an age-associated decrease in cAMP production has been observed.[27] The clinical impact of these changes in uncertain. What is known, based on clinical studies, is that the ability of the aging kidney to concentrate urine in response to water deprivation is decreased.[28,29] In individuals studied after 12–24 hours of water deprivation, the maximal urine osmolality in younger individuals (aged 20–39) was 1109 mOsm/kg, compared with 882 mOsm/kg in older individuals.[29] Why this happens is not clear. One contributing factor might be the decline in renal function observed in two-thirds of aging individuals.[5] It is also possible that the renal responsiveness to ADH is decreased, an hypothesis suggested by data from aging rats.[30] It is also possible that with the age-associated increase in medullary blood flow compared to juxtaglomerular flow, the medullary countercurrent concentrating gradient is washed out. In addition, morphological data from rats suggest that tubular compromise with aging occurs first in the long looped medullary tubules which help maintain the medullary osmolality necessary for the countercurrent system.[31]

Another point of interest is clinical data suggesting that the normal circadian rhythm of ADH release (with increased production during the night) is attenuated with aging.[32] The circadian pacemaker in humans is the suprachiasmatic nucleus, and it appears that with aging there is a significant decline in cell volume and number of these nuclei.[32] This might help to explain the nocturnal diuresis experienced by many older individuals.

The urinary diluting ability of the kidney is also thought to decline with age but is less well studied. Again, on a day-to-day basis these changes do not generally cause problems unless the renal system is challenged or under stress. The sensation of thirst is also very important in maintaining the serum sodium concentration and, as discussed below, decreases with age.

The second clinically important problem seen with alterations in sodium homeostasis involves changes in the absolute amount of sodium (total body sodium) and water in the ECF (as opposed to their relative concentrations). Renal excretion of sodium is determined by the interplay among several neural hormonal systems, including atrial natriuretic peptide (ANP), the renin–angiotensin–aldosterone system, the sympathetic nervous system, and other factors. ANP is released from atrial myocytes in response to atrial stretch. This results in an increase in renal sodium excretion. ANP also suppresses aldosterone. Serum ANP levels increase with aging.[33,34] Renin is synthesized in the juxtaglomerular cells in the afferent arterial in response to changes in transmural pressure. In the circulation, renin combines with angiotensinogen to make angiotension I which is converted to angiotension II in the liver. Angiotension II stimulates aldosterone excretion from the adrenal gland, which then acts at the distal renal tubule and collecting duct to increase sodium absorption and increase potassium excretion.

Clinical studies suggest that the aging kidney is slower to conserve sodium when sodium-deprived than is a younger kidney. When older adults and young individuals are placed on low-sodium diets, the kidneys of the older persons take significantly longer to decrease sodium excretion.[35] Data from clinical studies suggest that with age there is decreased sodium reabsorption at the distal tubule.[36] This may be related to the clinical observation that active renin and renin activity as well as aldosterone levels (likely secondary to decrease in renin) also decrease with aging.[37,38] Data from rat studies suggest that both renin synthesis and release are decreased in the aging kidney.[39] Although this decrease on the basis of age alone may not reach clinical significance, it is easy to imagine how introducing a drug or disease that further inhibits renin, such as a non-steroidal anti-inflammatory medication (NSAID), might reduce the renin to a clinical significant level and be associated with a hyporenin–hypoaldosterone state. Furthermore, given these age-associated changes, it is also understandable why older adults become hypovolemic when orders for "nothing by mouth" are written for an extended period in preparation for a diagnostic study. This problem is easily avoided with maintenance fluids during that period.

Just as the aging kidney is slow in decreasing sodium excretion when faced with a need to conserve, so the aging kidney is slower in excreting a sodium load than its younger counterpart.[40]

Hypernatremia

Hypertonic dehydration (serum sodium >148 mmol/L) is common in older adults, especially among acutely hospitalized patients. Clinical data collected on hospitalized persons aged over 59 years showed that 1.1 percent had an elevated serum sodium concentration (Na greater than 1148 mEq/L).[41] Of these patients, 56 percent developed hypernatremia in the hospital, and the remaining were hypernatremic at the time of admission.[41] Of note, the mortality rate among the hypernatremic patients was seven times that of age-matched controls and was not related to the severity of the hypernatremia.[41] In another clinical analysis, the incidence of hypernatremia in febrile nursing home patients was 25 percent and was associated with hypernatremia and impaired oral intake.[42] Another group found that after a 24-hour period of water deprivation, the older individuals had significant increase in serum sodium, plasma osmolality, and vasopression when compared to younger individuals.[43]

The important point is that hypernatremia is often avoidable. Understanding how age-associated changes contribute to hypernatremia helps the clinician identify individuals at risk and institute preventive measures. As previously noted, these factors include the age-associated decrease in body water as a proportion of total bodyweight because of the relative increase in fat content of normal older adults. However, probably most important is the decrease in thirst experienced by older individuals.[43,44] Thirst is an important component in regulating plasma osmolality. It is regulated centrally but sensed peripherally. The "cue" to drink is the sensation of thirst. In older adults, the blunted thirst response may be due to a defect in the opioid-associated drinking drive.[45] This thirst response is even more impaired in patients with cerebral disease.

Along with decreased thirst, the ability of many older adults to obtain free water is further limited because of decreased mobility, poor visual acuity, cognitive impairment, swallowing disorders, or alterations in thirst from medications. Older persons with urinary incontinence may limit their consumption of water to avoid the embarrassment and inconvenience associated with daytime urinary incontinence. In particularly warm weather, especially in the absence of air conditioning, it is important to make sure older adults know to increase their consumption of fluids—particularly given the age-associated decrease in thirst. Often, it is helpful to give older adults a specific amount to drink each day. In the institutionized older adult, particularly one with decreased mobility (decreased access to water) or a decline in cognitive function, placing a specific amount of fluid within easy reach, and assuring it is gone by the end of the day, is helpful. In addition, on the very hot days, it is often wise to hold or decrease the dose of diuretics in selected individuals.

Other clinical situations that are associated with hypernatremia in older adults include poorly controlled diabetes mellitus, not severe enough to develop a ketoacidosis, where the urinary loss of glucose results in an osmotically obligated water loss which causes hypernatremia. In a patient with diabetes insipidus, as seen with lithium therapy, in the setting of acute illness the individual may not be able to keep up with free water needs, resulting in hypernatremia. In addition, an increase in protein consumption with tube feedings may increase free water excretion, as for every gram of nitrogenous waste excreted, the kidney must also excrete 40–60 mL of water.

Symptoms of hypernatremia (obtundation, lethargy, coma) are predominantly neurological, presumably due to shrinkage of the brain cells. Because intravascular volume is preserved at the expense of cell water, changes in blood pressure, pulse rate, and skin turgor may not be prominent early in the process. To prevent recurrent hypernatremia, a fluid prescription (defined quantity of fluid to be ingested daily) may be an important component of treatment.

Hyponatremia

Surveys of older adults in both acute and chronic care facilities show a high prevalence of hyponatremia (serum sodium < 132 mmol/L). Among older adult patients in the acute hospital setting, 11 percent have hyponatremia.[46] In the chronic care setting, prevalence studies show 22 percent of patients have chronic hyponatremia.[47]

The initial evaluation of hyponatremia should always include a careful history and physical examination to help determine whether the patient is hypervolumeic, hypovolumeic, or euvolumeic. By definition, these individuals all have an excess of water relative to solute. In older adults, hypervolumia hyponatremia may be suggested by a change in clothing size, tight belts or clothing, or symptoms suggestive of congestive heart failure, ascites, or nephrosis. In older adults, volume depletion may be suggested by evidence of loose clothing or new dizziness on standing suggesting orthostatic blood pressure changes. Thirst, when present, is helpful, but as noted it is often depressed in older adults. The history will often suggest a source of fluid loss. This includes gastrointestinal losses from vomiting, nasogastric suction, diarrhea, laxative abuse, and enemas. Volume depletion from renal losses in older adults is usually associated with diuretic use. However, one must keep in mind that glycosuria, diabetes insipidus (as noted above, important to consider in older adults with a history of lithium use), radiographic contrast agents, or suppression of vasopression with drugs such as phenytoin, may also contribute. There are some situations in older adults where a history of loss of a sodium-containing fluid may not be obvious. For example, older patients on a sodium-restricted diet may become severely sodium-depleted with diuretic therapy, especially a thiazide diuretic.

On physical examination, the evaluation of volume status in older adults is similar to that in younger individuals, with a few exceptions. First, orthostatic hypotension is common in older adults and may be related to medication or prolonged bedrest and does not always represent true volume depletion. As above, the history is helpful to ascertain whether the patient has developed new symptoms to suggest this diagnosis Skin turgor, commonly used to assess volume status in young individuals, is less reliable in older people, secondary to age-associated changes observed in the skin.

In differentiating hypovolemia from euvolemia, the urine sodium concentration and fractional excretion of sodium may be useful. In response to hypovolumia, the kidney normally increases sodium absorption and the fraction of excreted sodium is less than 1 percent. The fraction of excreted sodium is usually greater than 1 percent in the setting of euvolumia. These measurements are generally not helpful in evaluating volume status in patients taking diuretics.

The syndrome of inappropriate ADH (SIADH) is probably the most common cause of hyponatremia in older adults. In this condition, free water excretion by the kidney is depressed secondary to increased ADH levels. ADH levels may be elevated in many clinical settings, including neuropsychiatric disorders, with pulmonary disease including pneumonia, with severe pain, vomiting, in postoperative patients, and with many medications. Medications such as tricyclic antidepressants,[48] amitriptyline, bromocriptine, haldoperidol, carbamazepine, or thioridazine may also lead to increased production of ADH.[17] Other medications that may potentiate the effects of ADH include chloropropamide, carbamazepine, tolbutamide, and intravenous cyclophosphamide.[17] Some cancers, in particular small-cell carcinoma of the lung, secrete ectopic ADH. Some clinical data suggest the possibility that in adults aged over 80 years there is a subset of individuals with SIADH secondary to unknown age-associated change in physiology.[49] SIADH should be suspected when an older adult has euvolumeic hyponatremia and hypo-osmolality together with an inappropriately high urine osmolality. Recall that when the serum sodium concentration is low, ADH should be suppressed to allow the kidney to excrete a maximally dilute urine until the serum osmolality normalizes. Laboratory findings in SIADH include: (1) a urine osmolality greater than 100 mOsm/kg, (2) urine sodium greater than 40 mEq/L, (3) normal adrenal, thyroid, and renal function, and (4) normal acid–base and potassium balances. As older adults may not maximally dilute their urine, the urine osmolality it is often greater than 100 mOsm/kg making this a less reliable factor. Cerebral salt wasting may be confused with SIADH but is suggested by the findings of mild volume depletion, whereas with SIADH individuals are euvolumic.

Another important diagnosis to consider in older adults with euvolemic hyponatremia is hypothyroidism. In younger persons, hyponatremia rarely occurs in the absence of clinical evidence of hypothyroidism. However, in older individuals, the symptoms and physical findings of hypothyroidism may be occult and hyponatremia may, in fact, be the presenting sign. Therefore, unless an otherwise obvious cause is identified, a thyroid-stimulating hormone (TSH) level should be obtained in screening older adults with hyponatremia. The signs and symptoms of adrenal insufficiency are similar in old and young individuals.

Another important problem to consider in older adults with hyponatremia is the decreased ability of the aging kidney to excrete a free water load, resulting in a rapid decrease in the serum sodium concentration.[50] This observation, supported by clinical studies, has been observed without significant differences in minimum urine osmolality or ADH levels between old and young individuals after the administration of hydrochlorothiazide.[51] A free water load may occur when hypertonic solutions such as mannitol, glycine, or sorbitol are administered. The absorption of these fluids is variable but after metabolism they leave behind a free water load. Glycine is sometimes used to flush the bladder after a transurethral resection of the bladder or prostate.[52] There is also a risk of ammonia toxicity with glycine metabolism.[52,53] Other clinical situations where hyponatremia may develop secondary to a free water load include the rapid administration of intravenous medication in a hypotonic fluid. Tapwater enemas are used by many older adults and may result in a free water load and hyponatremia. The relatively rapid development of hyponatremia may also be seen when older postsurgical patients are given hypotonic intravenous fluids to replace insensible losses and avoid sodium-containing fluids.[54]

Medications commonly used in older adults may compound the problem of free water excretion. Thiazides have been shown in clinical studies to exacerbate the ability of the aging kidney to excrete water.[50] Nonsteroidal anti-inflammatory drugs inhibit renal prostaglandins and limit the ability of the kidney to excrete a dilute urine.[55] In addition, laxatives may deplete the extracellular volume—which, when replaced with water alone, decreases the serum sodium concentration.

When evaluating hyponatremia one must consider the possibility of water intoxication as well as the entity of reset osmostat. Water intoxication is caused by compulsive drinking of water or other hypotonic fluids where a large amount of water is consumed so rapidly it overwhelms the kidney. This problem is generally seen in psychiatric patients regardless of age. Medications used to treat psychiatric illness cause a dry mouth which may compound the problem. Complicating the issue, these same medications may directly stimulate ADH. The diagnosis of water intoxication is supported by a very low urine specific gravity (less than 1.003) or a urine osmolality below 100 mOsm/kg. These values are indicative of both a maximally dilute urine and complete suppression of ADH. If the patient is water-restricted the urine osmolality will remain low until the serum sodium concentration normalizes.

A reset osmostat refers to a condition where the patient responds normally to changes in osmolality but releases ADH at a lower threshold. It is associated with a number of conditions including hypovolemia, psychosis, malnutrition, and the syndrome of inappropriate ADH secretion.[17] In this setting, water restriction will stimulate secretion of ADH and cause a slight rise in the serum sodium concentration. The urine osmolality will show some increase in response to ADH.

Clinically, the rate at which the serum sodium concentration falls tends to correlate with the severity of symptoms. The osmotic gradient produced by the decrease in the extracellular serum sodium concentration causes fluid to move intracellularly into brain cells. The resulting edema in the brain cells gives rise to the observed symptoms. More severe symptoms are associated with a more rapid decline in serum osmolality. When the serum sodium concentration is between 125 and 130 mEq/L, patients may be asymptomatic, although decreased appetite, confusion, muscle cramps, headache, nausea, and vomiting are often reported. Once a diagnosis of hyponatremia is made, it is important to immediately restrict the intake of free water to prevent a further decline in serum osmolality. Restricting free water will generally raise the serum sodium concentration whatever the etiology. Intravenous medications are often given in free water, and this needs to be included in the free water restriction. Treatment should be directed at correcting the underlying etiology as soon as it is known. Any potentially offending medications should be stopped if possible. As the serum sodium concentration falls below 120 mEq/L, symptoms are more severe with confusion, coma, seizures, and even death. In older adults, especially with significant chronic hyponatremia, a general vague uncomfortable feeling is sometimes reported. For example, some older adults report a feeling that they are wearing tight pants and are unable to find a comfortable position. Patients with chronic severe hyponatremia are, over time, able to compensate for these changes in osmolality. Rapid correction of the serum sodium concentration places a patient at risk for myelinolysis, which is now thought to include both central and extrapontine myelinolysis.[56,57] This devastating syndrome usually presents several days after rapid correction of the serum sodium concentration and is characterized by upper motor neuron symptoms, quadriparesis, paraparesis, dysarthria, and coma.[17,56,57]

It is more likely to occur with rapid correction of chronic hyponatremia as opposed to acute hyponatremia.

The treatment of severe hyponatremia is the subject of some controversy. The rate at which the hyponatremia developed, the severity of the condition, and the patient's symptoms are all used to guide therapy. As patients with longstanding hyponatremia may have partially adapted to the changes in osmolality, in general, the serum sodium should be increased slowly. For example, it is reasonable to increase the serum sodium concentration by 0.5 mEq/L hourly. With acute symptomatic hyponatremia, the goal is to increase the serum sodium concentration by approximately 1.0 mEq/L hourly. However, with severely symptomatic patients, many would advocate a more rapid increase until the serum sodium is 120 mEq/L, and then slowing the rate of rise to no more than 0.5 mEq/L each hour. In addition to water restriction, therapeutic options for hyponatremia include the administration of sodium. With severe symptomatic hyponatremia, sodium is usually cautiously administered. It requires careful monitoring of the patient's volume status to prevent volume overload. It is important to check the serum sodium concentration often to assure that the rate of correction is not more rapid than expected. Sodium may be administered as normal saline, hypertonic saline, or sodium chloride tablets. It should be remembered that giving normal saline to an individual with SIADH may actually lower the serum sodium concentration as the kidney will excrete the solute and hold on to the water. Once the serum sodium is greater than 120 mEq/L, the administration of sodium is generally stopped or slowed and free water restriction continued. The exception to this is the patient with a true decrease in the amount of total body sodium with decreased perfusion of vital organs; obviously, in this case, rapid administration of fluid with sodium is imperative.

Potassium

Potassium homeostasis

Whereas sodium is the primary cation in the extracellular fluid, potassium is the primary cation in the intracellular fluid where 98 percent of the total body potassium is found. It therefore contributes to the osmolality of the intracellular fluid and cell volume. It is very important in maintaining the resting membrane potential which is in part mediated by the ATPase sodium–potassium exchange pump. Potassium is also involved in cell metabolism.

Potassium homeostasis within the body compartments is primarily under the control of epinephrine, insulin, and the acid–base environment. It is these systems that operate to maintain a normal extracellular potassium concentration in the setting of a potassium load either from dietary intake or secondary to cell damage. However, it is the kidney that is responsible for the excretion of potassium and ultimately for potassium balance. This is augmented by the actions of aldosterone in the distal tubule. Serum aldosterone levels decrease with aging (as noted above, likely to be secondary to decreased renin). Aldosterone is released from the adrenal gland in response to angiotensin II (as described above) and also by hyperkalemia directly (independently from the renin–angiotensin pathway). However, angiotensin II appears to potentiate the effect of hyperkalemia on the adrenal gland.

Interestingly, clinical data show that older adults when given a potassium infusion had depressed aldosterone response compared with younger persons.[58] Although this is in part secondary to the depressed renin levels observed in older adults, the elevated ANP levels observed in older adults are also likely to contribute.

There is conflict in the literature regarding the effect of age on serum potassium level. As the serum potassium level is tightly maintained in the normal range (3.5–5.5 mEq/L) with aging, any changes that do occur are unlikely to be clinically significant. However, it appears that total body potassium content decreases with age.[59] The reason for this is not clear and is the subject of speculation. Although most of the potassium is in muscle, it was thought that the decrease in muscle mass with aging was responsible for the decline in total body potassium. However, when the potassium content is adjusted for the decrease in muscle mass, the difference in content between young and old increases. While there are no described changes in potassium homeostasis, it is clear that the older adult is at increased risk for both hypokalemia and hyperkalemia. Again, this reflects the lack of flexibility and slow response of the aging kidney to disease states and medications. The extent to which a decrease in potassium content contributes is unclear.

Hypokalemia

There is a long list, often multifactorial, of etiologies for hypokalemia in older adults. Again, a careful medical history and physical examination are critical in guiding the diagnostic work-up and identifying underlying and contributory mechanisms of hypokalemia.

Usually hypokalemia represents total body potassium depletion resulting from gastrointestinal or renal losses. A history of diarrhea, nasogastric suction, excessive laxative abuse, or fistula drainage would suggest gastrointestinal potassium losses. Villous adenomas of the colon or rectum may also present with profuse diarrhea and hypokalemia. Stool electrolytes are useful in making this diagnosis. Although there is some potassium loss with vomiting, the role of increased aldosterone in response to volume loss plays a larger role in producing hypokalemia. Vomiting also produces a metabolic alkalosis which shifts potassium into cells.

In older adults, excessive renal potassium losses are usually secondary to diuretic therapy. Hypokalemia secondary to diuretic use generally appears within 1–2 weeks of initiating therapy. After this period the patient reaches a steady state. Therefore, in older adults who develop hypokalemia after taking diuretics beyond this period, another source of potassium loss should be sought. For example, it would not be unusual for an older adult on diuretics to begin taking laxatives or using enemas and develop diarrhea. Urine potassium may be helpful. In the setting of hypokalemia the kidney should be conserving potassium and the urine potassium should be low (<10 mEq/L). If a patient is actively taking diuretics then the urine potassium is generally high (>30 mEq/L). Other causes of hypokalemia, such as Cushing's disease, Bartter's syndrome, and renal tubular acidosis, are not common in older adults. Hypomagnesemia-induced hypokalemia with ongoing renal potassium wasting is also seen with diuretic usage. Other medications associated with hypokalemia include both parental and inhaled bronchodilators (β2-adrenergic stimulation),[60]

sodium carbenicillin which creates a gradient for potassium excretion, and aminoglycosides. Excessive licorice ingestion may cause a hypokalemic, metabolic alkalosis with a high urinary chloride. Primary and secondary aldosteronism (the latter from renal artery stenosis or volume contraction resulting from diuretic usage in patients with cardiac, hepatic, or renal disease) are further common contributing factors. Other less common states associated with hypokalemia include low thyrotropin levels as well as overt thyrotoxicosis. Nonendocrine tumors such as an oat-cell carcinoma of the bronchus may produce ectopic ACTH and present with severe hypokalemic alkalosis.[61] The local administration of acetozolamide used to treat chronic glaucoma may produce persistent hypokalemia by increasing bicarbonate delivery to the distal tubule and creating a gradient favorable to potassium excretion.

As noted above, it is the ratio of the potassium concentrations between the intracellular and extracellular fluids that determines the transmembrane potential. The rate at which this transmembrane potential is altered determines the severity of the symptoms, with the rapid development of hypokalemia associated with marked changes in this potential and more acute symptoms. Potassium deficiency most importantly affects the cardiovascular system, neurological system, muscles, and kidneys. Persistent minor hypokalemia may present with apathy, nonspecific weakness, or confusion. As the serum potassium decreases, more widespread and severe manifestations are apparent with paresis and ileus or constipation leading to fecal impaction, and clinically significant arrhythmyias. Renal effects include polyuria and development of a metabolic alkalosis with paradoxical aciduria. Chronic hypokalemia may cause significant impairment of renal tubular function, which is initially reversible, but if prolonged may become permanent.

Since an alkalosis (chloride depletion) usually accompanies hypokalemia and is responsible for a shift of potassium intracellularly, replacement therapy should be with potassium chloride. The exception is the patient with renal tubular acidosis where the alkaline salts of potassium should be given.

Hyperkalemia

Hyperkalemia is defined as a serum potassium greater than 5.5 mEq/L. In evaluating hyperkalemia, it is important to make sure the blood specimen was not hemolyzed, as this would falsely elevate the serum potassium level. At the same time significant thrombocytosis and leukocytosis may also cause spurious hyperkalemia.[62] Clearly, treating hyperkalemia under these circumstances would be dangerous. However, any individual with an elevation in serum potassium should have an immediate ECG whether they are symptomatic or not, and be treated accordingly.

Most episodes of hyperkalemia are seen in patients with impaired renal function. However, patients with chronic renal failure and good urine flow rates generally do not develop significant hyperkalemia until the renal failure is significant (GFR 10–20 mL/min) or another factor contributes such as an increased endogenous or ingested potassium load, severe acidosis, administration of a diuretic to block sodium–potassium exchange (triamterene, spironolactone), a deficiency of endogenous aldosterone or mineralocorticoid, or (importantly) administration of drugs. Many medications may cause hyperkalemia. It is important not only to be aware of this risk but also to know how to identify individuals at risk for complications. Heparin is directly toxic to the adrenal zona glomerulosa; the exact mechanism is not clear, but it attenuates aldosterone.[63] This affect has been observed with low-dose heparin[64] and even with low-molecular-weight heparin.[65] Salt substitutes are associated with hyperkalemia especially if used in conjunction with potassium-sparing medication.[66] Trimethoprim is now a recognized cause of hyperkalemia as it blocks the amiloride-sensitive sodium channel in the distal nephron, thus inhibiting potassium excretion.[67] There are numerous medications known to cause hyperkalemia and a careful review of medications in individuals with hyperkalemia is critical.

One entity that is probably overlooked in older adults is failure of the renin–aldosterone system or hyporenin–hypoaldosteronism. This syndrome is characterized by an elevated serum potassium, mild metabolic acidosis with a normal anion gap; it is also referred to as type IV renal tubular acidosis.[68] It is not uncommon and is associated with renal insufficiency, diabetes, chronic interstitial nephritis, and medications such as NSAIDs.

ABNORMALITIES ASSOCIATED WITH NSAID USE

As nonsteroidal anti-inflammatory drugs (NSAIDs) are widely used by older adults, it is worth a brief review of their potential effects on the kidneys. They are used frequently both because of their effectiveness in relieving pain in a variety of common, chronic musculoskeletal disorders and because they may be purchased without a doctor's prescription. Older individuals are more predisposed to the adverse renal effects of NSAIDs because of (1) the age-associated decline in renal function observed in many individuals, (2) the increased prevalence of such comorbid conditions as heart failure, hypertension, diabetes, and renal insufficiency, and (3) the high utilization of concomitant drugs that affect kidney function (e.g. diuretics, antihypertensives). It should be possible to use these drugs safely in older adults and maintain a low risk-to-benefit ratio as individuals at risk for NSAID-induced renal disease may be identified and monitored.

NSAIDs inhibit prostaglandins. Prostaglandins increase renin release and influence renal blood flow through their affects on autoregulation. They also antagonize the antidiuretic hormone and inhibit active chloride transport by the medullary thick ascending limb. Therefore, inhibiting prostaglandins leads to maximal urine concentration and decreased excretion of free water. Adding an NSAID to thiazide therapy appears to enhance this affect and may lead to significant hyponatremia. Sodium retention and hypertension are also associated with NSAID usage. NSAIDs have also been associated with hyperkalemia when they are used in the setting of mild renal insufficiency. They may also induce a variety of acute and chronic renal lesions including acute interstitial nephritis (AIN) and the nephrotic syndrome. Patients taking NSAIDs for months or years may develop papillary necrosis, chronic interstitial nephritis, and even end-stage renal disease. Impaired medullary circulation and direct toxicity due to a drug metabolite appear

to play a critical role in inducing interstitial fibrosis, which can be facilitated by a sustained production of some growth factors and cytokines.

COMORBIDITY

In preventing the development of electrolyte abnormalities in older adults, the impact of comorbid conditions must always be considered. The treatment of hypertension, cardiac disease, diabetes, and the use of medications may all alter renal function and therefore increase the risk of electrolyte abnormalities.

Therefore, before beginning any medication in older adults it is important to know all the other medications they are taking to review for potential drug interactions. It is useful to have patients bring all their medications from home on the first visit—including over-the-counter medications. It is surprising how many old prescriptions are saved. Many of these old medications may be outdated, easily confused with current medications, and potentially interact with the new medication being prescribed. It is important to strongly encourage the elimination of all old and outdated medications. For the purpose of assessing compliance, and to assure that what is prescribed is being taken, it is helpful to have the patient also bring in their medications on each subsequent visit.

KEY POINTS Water and electrolyte metabolism

- Although two-thirds of the individuals in the Baltimore Longitudinal Study of Aging developed a decline in renal function when studied over a 20-year period, the other third showed no such decline.

- On a day-to-day basis, the aging kidney is able to maintain fluid and electrolyte homeostasis.

- The aging kidney is more sensitive, less flexible, and slower to respond to maintain normal homeostasis in the setting of a physiological challenge—as seen with illness, infection, and with many medications.

- Electrolyte abnormalities, including hyponatremia, hypernatremia, hypokalemia, and hyperkalemia, occur commonly in older adults. Understanding the potential impact of disease and medications in this age group helps to identify individuals at risk for an electrolyte abnormality and to prevent their occurrence altogether.

REFERENCES

1. Meyer BR: Renal function in aging. J Am Geriatr Soc 1989;37:791–800
2. Lindeman LD: Renal physiology and pathophysiology of aging. Am J Kidney Dis 1990;4:275–282
3. Rodriguez-Puyol D: The aging kidney. Kidney Int 1998;53:2247–2265
4. Darmady EM, Offer J, Woodhouse MA: The parameters of the ageing kidney. J Pathol 1973;109:195–207
5. Lindeman RD, Tobin JD, Shock NW: Longitudinal studies on the rate of decline in renal function with age. J Am Geriatr Soc 1985;33:278–285
6. Bevier WC, Wiswell RA, Pyka G: Relationship of body composition, muscle strength, and aerobic capacity to bone mineral density in older men and women. J Bone Min Res 1989;4:421–432

7. Munro HN: Nutrition and ageing. Br Med Bull 1981;37:83–88
8. Shimokata H, Tobin JD, Muller DC: Studies in the distribution of body fat. I: Effects of age, sex and obesity. J Gerontol 1989;44:M66–M73
9. Silver AJ, Guillen CP, Kahl MJ, Morley JE: Effect of aging on body fat. J Am Geriatr Soc 1993;41:211–213
10. Glanville EV, Geerdink RA: Skinfold thickness, body measurements and age changes in Trio and Wajana Indians of Surinam. Am J Phys Anthropol 1970;32:454–460
11. Crockcroft DW, Gault HM: Prediction of creatinine clearance from serum creatinine. Nephron 1976;16:31–41
12. Malmrose LC, Gray SL, Peiper CF et al: Measured verses estimated creatinine clearance in a high functioning elderly sample: MacArthur Foundation study of successful aging. J Am Geriatr Soc 1993;41:715–721
13. Drusano GL, Muncie AL, Hoopes JM et al: Commonly used methods of estimating creatinine clearance are inadequate for debilitated nursing home patients. J Am Geriatr Soc 1988;36:437–441
14. Goldberg TH, Finkelstein MS: Difficulties in estimating glomerular function rate in the elderly. Arch Int Med 1987;147:1430–1433
15. Frassetto LA, Morris RC, Sebastian A: Effect of age on blood acid–base composition in adult humans: role of age-related renal functional decline. Am J Physiol 1996;F1112–F1121.
16. Leask RGS, Andrews GR, Caird FI: Normal values for sixteen blood constituents in the elderly. Age Ageing 1973;2:14–23
17. Osterlind PO, Alafuzoff I, Lofgren A-C et al: Blood components in an elderly population. Gerontology 1984;30:247–251
18. Rose BD: Hypoosmolar states: hyponatremia. In: Rose BD, Post TW (eds): Clinical Physiology of Acid–Base and Electrolyte Disorders, 4th edn. McGraw-Hill, New York, 1994:650–694
19. Hsu HK, Peng MT: Hypothalamic neuron number of older female rats. Gerontology 1978;24:434
20. Froklis VV, Golovchenko SF, Medved VI et al: Vasopression and the cardiovascular system in aging. Gerontology 1982;28:290
21. Flier E, Swaab DF: Activation of vasopressinergic and oxytocinergic neurons during aging in the Wistar rat. Peptides 1983;4:165
22. Flier E, Swaab DF, Pool Chw et al: The vasopression and oxytocin neurons in the human supraoptic and paraventricular nucleus: changes with aging and in senile dementia. Brain Res 1985;342:45
23. Hoogendijk JE, Flier E, Swaab DF et al: Activation of vasopressin neurons in the human supraotic and paraventricular nucleus in senescence and senile dementia. J Neurol Sci 1985;69:291
24. Fotheringham AP, Davidson YS, Davies I et al: Age-associated changes in neuroaxonal transport in the hypothalamo-neurohypophyseal system of the mouse. Mech Ageing Dev 1991;59:113
25. Helderman JH, Vestal RE, Rowe JW et al: The response of arginine vasopressin to intravenous ethanol and hypertonic saline in man: the impact of aging. J Gerontol 1989;33:39
26. Rowe JW, Minaker KL, Sparrow D, Robertson GL: Age-related failure of volume–pressure mediated vasopressin release in man. J Clin Endocrinol Metab 1982;54:661–663
27. Beck N, Yu BP: Effect of aging on urinary concentrating mechanism and vasopressin dependant cAMP in rats. Am J Physiol 1982;243:F121
28. Lindeman RD, Van Buran C, Raisz LG: Osmolar renal concentrating ability in healthy young men and hospitalized patients without renal disease. N Engl J Med 1959;261:1306
29. Rowe JW, Shock NW, Defronzo RA: The influence of age on the renal response to water deprivation in man. Nephron 1976;17:270–278
30. Bengele HH, Mathias RS, Perkins JH et al: Urinary concentrating defect in the aged rat. Am Physiol Soc 1981;F147–F150
31. Greenfield Z, Stillman IE, Brezis M et al: Medullary injury in the ageing rat kidney: functional–morphometric correlations. Eur J Clin Invest 1997;27:346–351
32. Swaab DF, Hofman MA, Honnebier MBOM: Development of vasopressin neurons in the human suprachiasmatic nucleus in relation to birth. Dev Brain Res 1990;51:289
33. Ohashi M, Fujio N, Nawata H et al: High plasma concentration of atrial natriuretic polypeptide levels in aged men. J Clin Endocrinol Metab 1987;64:81–85
34. Clark BA, Elahi D, Epstein FH: The influence of gender, age, and menstrual cycle on atrial natriuretic peptide levels in man. J Clin Endocrinol Metab 1990;70:349–352
35. Epstein M, Hollenberg NK: Age as a determinant of renal sodium conservation in man. J Lab Clin Med 1976;87:411–417
36. Nunez JFM, Iglesias CG, Roman AB et al: Renal handling of sodium in old people: a functional study. Age Ageing 1978;7:178–181
37. Tsunoda K, Abe K, Goto T et al: Effect of age on renin–angiotensin–aldosterone system in normal subjects: simultanous measurements of active and inactive renin, renin substrate, and aldosterone in plasma. J Clin Endrocrin Metab 1986;61:384–389
38. Hegstad R, Brown R, Jiang N et al: Aging and aldosterone. Am J Med 1983;74:442–417
39. Jung FF, Kenneflick TM, Ingelfinger JR et al: Down-regulation of the intrarenal renin–angiotensin system in the aging rat. J Am Soc Nephrol 1995;5:1573–1580
40. Luft FC, Weinberger MH, Fineberg NS et al: Effects of age on renal sodium homeostasis and its relevance to sodium sensitivity. Am J Med 1987;82:9–15
41. Synder NA, Feigal DW, Afieff AI: Hypernatremia in elderly patients. Ann Intern Med 1987;107:309–318
42. Weinberg AD, Pals JK, Leveque PG et al: Dehydration and death during febrile episodes in the nursing home. J Am Geriatr Soc 1994;42:968–971
43. Phillips PA, Rolls BJ, Ledingham JJG et al: Reduced thirst after water deprivation in elderly healthy men. N Engl J Med 1984;311:752–758
44. Miller PD, Krebs RA, Neal BJ et al: Hypodipsia in geriatric patients. Am J Med 1982;73:354–356
45. Silver AJ, Morely JE: Role of the opioid in hypodipsia with aging. J Am Geriatr Soc 1992;40:546–550
46. Nunez JFM, Roman AB, Commes JLR: Physiology and disorders of water balance and electrolytes in the elderly. In: Nunez JFM, Cameron JS (eds): Renal Function and Disease in the Elderly. Butterworth, London, 1987:67–93
47. Kleinfeld M, Casimar M, Borra S: Hyponatremia as observed in a chronic disease facility. J Am Geriatr Soc 1979;27(4):155–160
48. Mitsch RA, Lee AK: Syndrome of inappropriate antidiuretic hormone with imipramine. Drug Intell Clin Pharm 1986; 20:787–789
49. Anpalahan M: Chronic idiopathic hyponatremia in older people due to syndrome of inappropriate antidiuretic hormone secretion possibly related to aging. Am Geriatr Soc 2001;49:788–792
50. Crowe MJ, Forsling ML, Rolls BJ: Altered water excretion in healthy elderly men. Age Ageing 1987;16:285–293
51. Clark BA, Shannon RP, Rosa RM, Epstein FH: Increased susceptibility to thiazide-induced hyponatremia in the elderly. J Am Soc Nephrol 1994;5:1106–1111
52. Ayus JC, Arieff AI: Glycine-induced hypo-osmolar hyponatremia. Arch Intern Med 1997;157:223–226
53. Roesch RP, Stoelting RK, Lingeman FE et al: Ammonia toxicity resulting from glucine absorption during a transurethal resection of the prostrate. Anesthesiology 1983;57:567–569
54. Tolias CM: Severe hyponatremia in elderly patients: cause for concern. Ann R Coll Surg Engl 1995;77:346–348
55. Clive DM, Stoff JS: Renal syndromes associated with nonsteroidal antiinflammatory drugs. N Engl J Med 1987;310:553–572
56. Laureno R, Karp BI: Myelinolysis after correction of hyponatremia. Ann Intern Med 1997;126:56–61
57. Sterns RH, Riggs JE, Schochet SS: Osmotic demyelination syndrome following correction of hyponatremia. N Engl J Med 1986;314:1525–1542
58. Mulkerrin E, Epstein F, Clark BA: Aldosterone response to hyperkalemia in healthy elderly humans. J Am Soc Nephrol 1995;6:1459–1462
59. Novak LP: Aging, total body potassium, fat free mass, and cell mass in males and females between ages 18 and 85 years. J Gerontol 1972;27:438–443
60. Gelmont DM, Balmes JR, Yee A: Hypokalemia induced by inhaled bronchodilators. Chest 1988;94:763–766
61. Rees LH: The biosynthesis of hormones by non-endocrine tumors: a review. J Endocrinol 1975;67:143–175
62. Spurious hyperkalemia associated with severe thrombocytosis and leukocytosis. Can J Anesth 1991;38:603–605
63. Gonzalez-Martin G, Diaz-Molinas MS, Martinez AM, Ortiz M: Heparin-induced hyperkalemia: a prospective study. Int J Clin Pharmacol Ther Toxicol 1991;29:446–449
64. Sherman RA, Ruddy MC: Suppression of aldosteron production by low-dose heparin. Am J Nephrol 1986;6:165
65. Canova CR, Fischler MP, Reinhart WH: Effect of low-molecular-weight heparin on serum potassium. Lancet 1997;348:1447
66. Ray K, Dorman S, Watson R: Severe hyperkalemia due to the concomitant use of salt substitutes and ACE inhibitors in hypertension: a potentially life threatening interaction. J Hum Hypertens 1999;13:717–720
67. Perlmutter EP, Sweeney D, Herskovits G, Kleiner M: Case report: severe hyperkalemia in a geriatric patient receiving standard doses of trimethoprim–sulfamethoxazole. Am J Med Sci 1996;311:84–85
68. Tan SY, Burotn M: Hyporeninemic hypoaldosteronism: an overlooked cause of hyperkalemia. Arch Intern Med 1981;141:30–33

Chapter 89

The prostate gland

Nicholas J. R. George

The prostate gland lies between the bladder base and pelvic floor and is intimately associated with each structure. Secretions of the seminal vesicle and vas deferens are conducted through its substance to the ejaculatory duct, which terminates in the urethra at the verumontanum. Exocrine secretion products, largely under androgenic control, are discharged into prostatic acini and include zinc, citric acid, and numerous enzymes—acid phosphatase, coagulases, fibrinolysins, and proteolytic enzymes—that form a significant part of the seminal plasma acting to support the physiological changes required for transport of spermatozoa.

DEVELOPMENT

The embryonic prostate differentiates in response to androgen secretion by the fetal testis commencing at about the eighth week of intrauterine life.[1] Androgenic activity at the time of puberty results in rapid growth to a weight of approximately 20 g by the age of 20 years. Thereafter, weight remains reasonably constant until 40–50 years of age when growth of benign adenomatus (prostatic) hyperplasia (BPH) becomes increasingly common with advancing years. Autopsy studies reveal BPH in more than 40 percent of men in their 50s and almost 90 percent of men in their 80s;[2] figures are confirmed by community-based studies involving transrectal ultrasound estimation of prostatic volume.[3]

Castration prior to puberty prevents prostatic development as well as the later emergence of both BPH and prostate cancer. Removal of testes in the adult leads to involution of the gland,[4] but replacement reactivates growth though only to and not beyond the normal adult size.

The action of androgen on the prostate cell is highly complex and only partially understood. Within the prostate testosterone is converted to its active metabolite, 5α-dihydrotestosterone (DHT) by the 5α-reductase enzyme located on the nuclear membrane. Most evidence suggests that prostatic epithelial cells per se are unresponsive to DHT, which acts via signaling between stromal and epithelial components of the tissue; epidermal growth factor (Fig. 89-1) and transforming growth factor-α (TGF-α) providing the most potent mitogenic stimulus.[5] The importance of DHT to prostatic growth has been illustrated by the studies of Imperato-McGinley and colleagues[6] into males from the Dominican Republic with an autosomal recessive form of male pseudohermaphroditism caused by deficiency of the 5α-reductase enzyme. These children develop phenotypically into men at puberty with normal serum testosterone, but with prostates that remain impalpable.[6] These observations form the basis of the development of the 5α-reductase inhibitors presently widely prescribed for men with early symptomatic BPH.

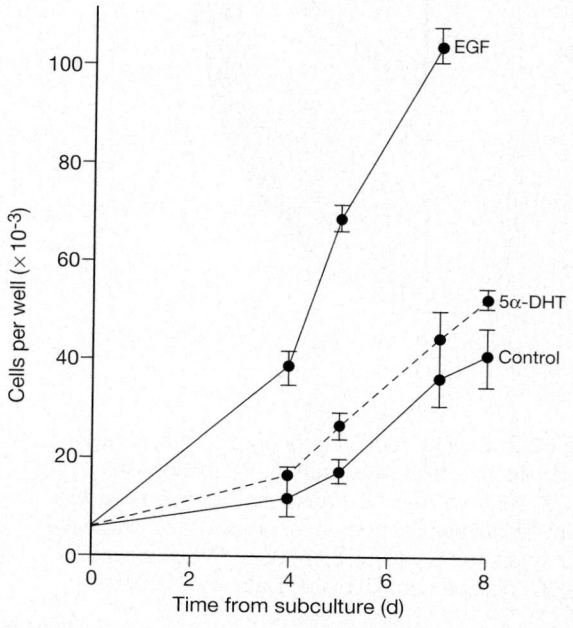

Figure 89-1 Prostate epithelial cells (CAPE-1) in culture. 5-α-DHT stimulation is no greater than control while EGF stimulation leads to significantly enhanced stimulation.

MORPHOLOGY

Early work by Lowsley[7] concerning the anatomy of the prostate has been superseded in recent years by the extensive studies of McNeal and associates.[8] They described peripheral and central zones of the gland (Fig. 89-2) as distinct from earlier lobe terminology: the central zone, approximately one-third of the gland mass, completely surrounds the ejaculatory ducts, while the peripheral zone extends to the apex and wraps around the central zone like an egg-cup. The benign prostatic hypertrophy mass arises from the periurethral zone (within the transitional zone) and this extends from the bladder neck to the region of the verumontanum, but never caudal to that structure. By contrast, prostate cancer usually arises from the peripheral zone, explaining the difficulties in identifying early disease endoscopically via the urethra (see below).

Much confusion has been created by this conflicting prostatic terminology over the years. Surgeons refer to "lateral" and "middle" lobes at operation, but clearly these are all contained within the periurethral transitional zones. The true exocrine prostate is not removed in operations for BPH, although patients frequently assume—not unnaturally—that "prostatectomy" means removal of the entire gland. The operation of radical prostatectomy for cancer does, however,

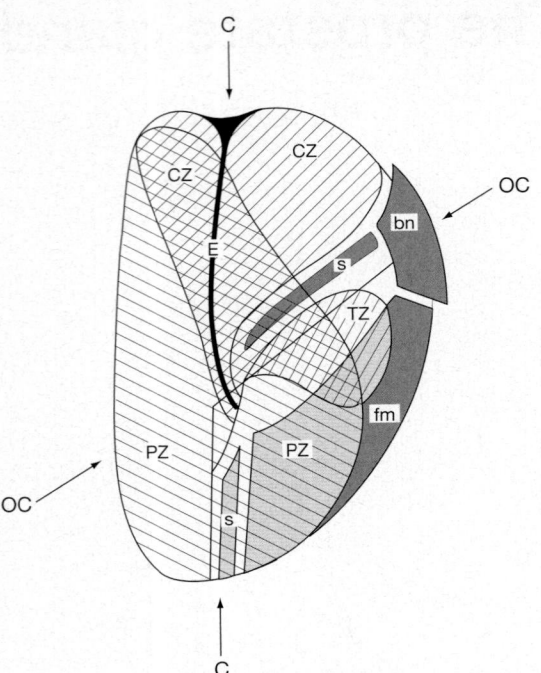

Figure 89-2 Sagittal section through prostate, showing zonal architecture relative to urethra. PZ, peripheral zone; CZ, central zone; TZ, transitional zone; bn, bladder neck; fm, fibromuscular stroma; s, preprostatic, and distal striated sphincter; E, ejaculatory ducts; C, true coronal plane; OC, oblique coronal plane. Data from McNeal.[9]

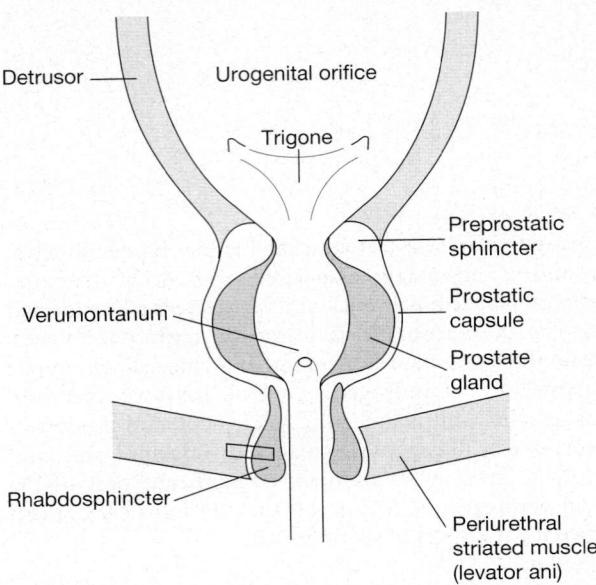

Figure 89-3 Distal sphincter and bladder neck mechanism in the male. P, periurethral striated muscle (levator ani); R, rhabdosphincter; V, verumontanum; PG, prostate gland; PC, prostatic capsule; PPS, preprostatic sphincter; T, trigone; UO, ureteric orifice; D, detrusor. Adapted from George et al.,[71] with permission.

involve extirpation of all prostatic tissue—each zone and contained BPH tissue en bloc.

The substance of the prostate consists of glandular tissue, stroma, and smooth muscle. The preprostatic sphincter lies at the bladder neck (Fig. 89-3) and is responsible for preventing retrograde ejaculation during intercourse. This α-adrenergic muscle is inevitably removed during the operation of transurethral resection (TUR) for BPH, but lack of leakage following the procedure shows, however, that this sphincter is not normally responsible for urinary continence. α-Adrenergic fibers are present throughout the gland and may be implicated in the etiology of chronic inflammatory conditions of the gland (see below); pharmacological manipulation by α-adrenergic blocking agents provides a useful therapeutic approach to patients with mild prostatic obstruction.

The continence mechanism lies intimately related to the apex of the prostate at the level of the pelvic floor. Studies by Gosling[10] and coworkers clearly show that the true external urethral sphincter lies within a sleeve of connective tissue, which separates it from the periurethral striated (levator ani) pelvic floor muscle (Fig. 89-3). This latter muscle is innervated via the pudendal nerve and is responsible for emergency extra voluntary effort required for continence, such as occurs during laughing, coughing, or sneezing. The nerve supply to the (slow twitch) specialized external urethral sphincter remains debatable; horseradish peroxidase techniques have suggested it travels via the pelvic nerve to terminate in the ventral horn of S2–S3 on Onuf's nucleus X.[11] Damage to

this sphincter, which by anatomical definition must be distal to the verumontanum, during TUR by inexperienced surgeons will inevitably lead to postoperative genuine stress incontinence.

ASSESSMENT OF THE PROSTATE

The prostate is relatively accessible to a number of techniques that may confirm normal or abnormal morphological features. In a broader sense, prostatic investigations may also encompass assessment of vesicourethral dysfunction, the gland being intimately involved in the storage and voiding disorders of the lower urinary tract.

Rectal examination

Digital rectal examination (DRE) can by definition only assess the posterior aspect of the peripheral zone of the prostate. The periphery of the gland and the midline sulcus, as well as the texture of the gland, may be recorded, but inevitably the experience of the examiner is crucial for accuracy of diagnosis. Rectal examination gives a poor indication of prostatic size; glands may protrude variably into the rectal lumen, and other factors, such as a full bladder in acute or chronic retention of urine, may displace the bladder base and prostate downward leading to an erroneous assessment of volume. Additionally, prostatic size is not related to the presence or absence of outflow tract obstruction,[12] but nevertheless the examination remains an essential technique of assessment, particularly with regard to the detection of neoplastic change.

Plain X-ray of abdomen

A single film showing kidneys, ureter, and bladder (KUB) may frequently be performed prior to prostatic surgery, chiefly to exclude bladder stone. Although the size of the gland cannot be assessed on these films, abnormalities such as calcification may be seen within the gland substance, perhaps indicating past inflammatory disease within the prostatic ducts.

Intravenous urogram

For many years urography was routinely performed prior to prostatectomy,[13] and although it is now accepted that this is unnecessary in the majority of cases,[14] radiologists continue to report on the size of the prostate as judged by shadows on bladder films (Fig. 89-4). Clinical experience suggests that such assessment can be very misleading, not only because of other causes of intravesical impressions (i.e. bladder tumor), but because of technical factors such as the variable angle of incidence of the X-rays through the pelvis.

Transrectal ultrasound

Transrectal ultrasound (TRUS) imaging of a prostate is now accepted as the principal method by which accurate anatomical detail of the gland may be obtained. Modern machines linked to sophisticated software packages may give high resolution in both multiple transverse and sagittal planes. Additionally, computer-assisted guided needle biopsies may retrieve tissue from exactly specified areas of the gland to distinguish between benign and malignant disease.

In practice, TRUS technology is rarely applied unless it is necessary to exclude or confirm the presence of carcinoma. Patients with straightforward symptom complexes thought on the basis of tests including prostate-specific antigen (PSA) to be due to BPH are likely to be offered therapy without the need further to image the gland and its appendices.

By contrast, TRUS is an essential preoperative investigation in patients with a suspicious prostate on rectal examination and in those (often younger) patients in whom PSA tests indicate the possibility of cancer. Most cancers are seen as hypoechoic lesions, although approximately one-fourth may be isoechoic.

Additionally, the images may identify capsular bulge (Fig. 89-5) or extension, indicating tumorous spread that will restrict treatment options.[15,16] Spread of cancer to the seminal vesicles can also be imaged with relative ease. TRUS-guided biopsies have been shown to be more accurate than digitally guided biopsies for both palpable and impalpable tumors. Recent reports[17] reveal the standard sextant biopsy technique to be inadequate and suggest extended field biopsies to enhance cancer detection.

Computed tomography

Computed tomography (CT) scanning is not commonly employed in the diagnosis of prostatic disorders. Although relatively good resolution may be obtained with modern machines, the technique does not offer major advantages over other radiological investigations, and precise interpretation of capsular spread and seminal vesicle invasion has been difficult.[18]

Magnetic resonance imaging

In recent years, developing magnetic resonance imaging (MRI) technology has been used extensively in an attempt to make an early and reliable diagnosis of prostate cancer. Magnetic resonance images give a reasonably clear capsular outline (Fig. 89-6), although the accuracy of local staging is presently no better than with TRUS.[19] T2-weighted images show internal architecture of the gland, but disappointingly it has not proved possible with accuracy to distinguish carcinoma from other disorders such as inflammatory foci of prostatitis. Nevertheless, within the UK, MRI is commonly used as part of the objective database assembled for patients undergoing therapeutic trials in early prostate cancer.

SERUM MARKERS OF PROSTATIC DISEASE

Acid phosphatase

Since the report of Gutman and Gutman[20] noting high acid phosphatase levels in men with metastatic prostate disease, acid phosphatase estimations have been widely used in the staging

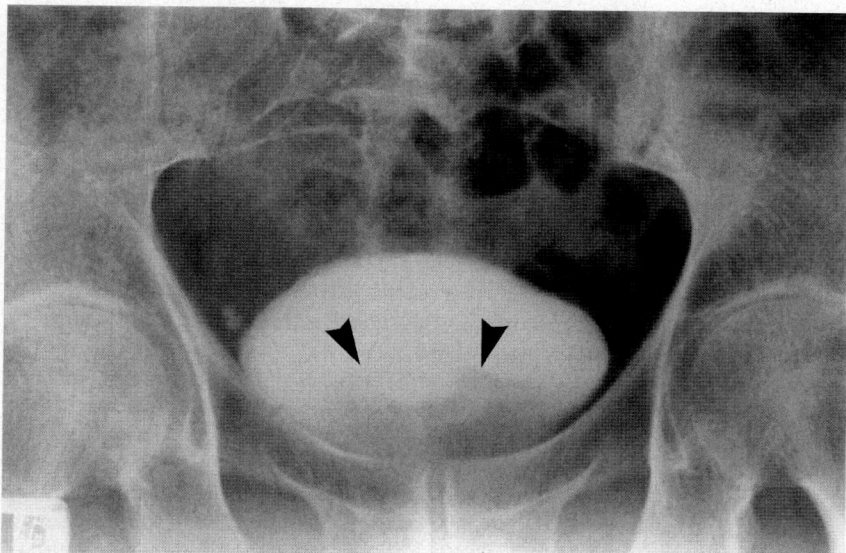

Figure 89-4 Bladder film from intravenous urogram series. Shadows at base of bladder (arrows) are a poor indicator of prostatic size and may represent bladder tumor or other intravesical pathology.

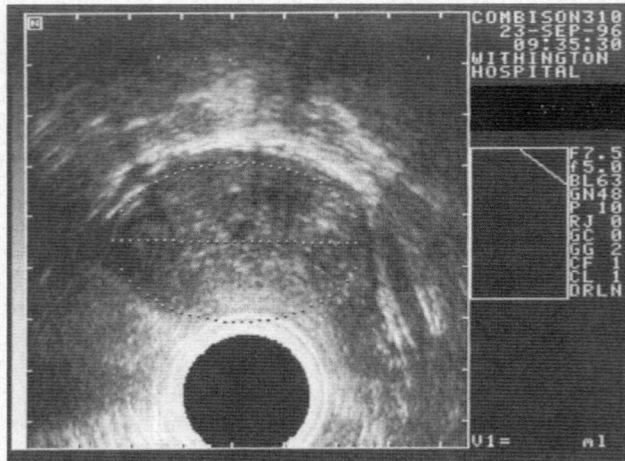

Figure 89-5 Transrectal ultrasound scan of prostate, showing relatively homogeneous pattern within, but with loss of capsular definition on the left. Biopsy from this area showed well-differentiated prostatic cancer.

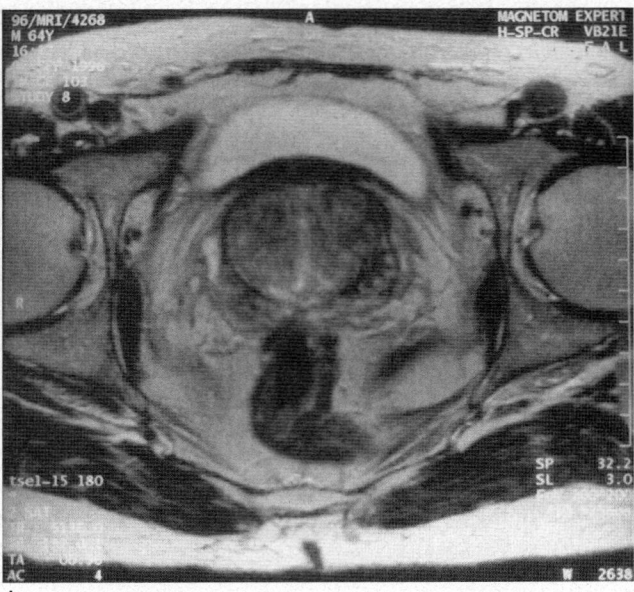

A

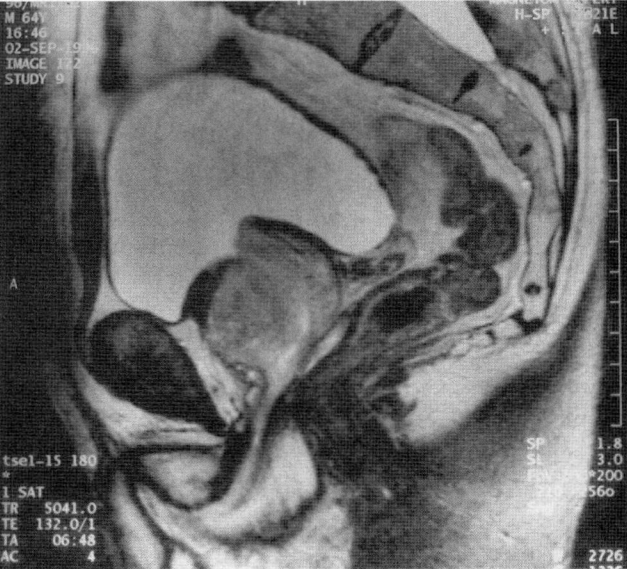

B

Figure 89-6 MRI scans. (A) Transverse (axial) section through prostate. In the peripheral zone on the left, a 1.5 cm lesion is identified adjacent to, but probably not penetrating, the capsule. (B) Sagittal section through same case as in (A). The architecture and relations of bladder, prostate, and urethra are clearly shown.

of prostate cancer. Unfortunately, lack of sensitivity with regard to localized disease precluded its use for cancer detection and the test has now effectively been replaced by prostate-specific antigen, although it is still employed by some authorities to monitor results of therapy in patients with proven bony metastatic disease.

Prostate-specific antigen

This serum protease was isolated from prostatic tissue in 1979 by Wang and associates[21] and has rapidly emerged as the most important marker of prostatic epithelial activity. Contrary to widespread public opinion, this marker is not cancer-specific (Fig. 89-7), but may be elevated in other pathologies such as inflammation or benign hyperplasia. Prostate-specific antigen varies with the proportion of ductal epithelial cells, so it is not surprising that higher values are found in patients with larger glands and that age-adjusted ranges have been proposed.[22] Damage to epithelial cells either by inflammation or other means such as elective prostate biopsy may elevate levels markedly, often for some weeks, making interpretation difficult in an already cancer-anxious patient.

In general, PSA levels correlate with advancing stage of prostate cancer. Levels under 4 ng/mL (but allow for age-adjusted range in an elderly patient—see above) are usually associated with benign disease. Approximately 33 percent of patients with values between 4 ng and 10 ng per milliliter are later found on biopsy to have cancer whilst, overall, two-thirds of cases with levels over 10 ng/mL have neoplastic change. Most patients presenting with a PSA above 50 ng/mL will have skeletal metastases (Fig. 89-7).

The level of PSA at presentation carries therapeutic implications for those later found to have biopsy-confirmed prostate cancer. High surgical margin positivity following radical prostatectomy determines that this treatment option is usually offered only to patients with a PSA under 10 ng/mL; rarely (see below) is surgery performed for patients with a PSA above 20 ng/mL. Not surprisingly, surgery is usually reserved for patients with cancer discovered at an early age (<70 years), but extended life-expectancy has led many surgeons, particularly in the USA, to offer this modality to otherwise fit men between 70 and 80 years of age.

FREE AND BOUND PROSTATE-SPECIFIC ANTIGEN Recent studies have extended the utility of PSA by showing that it may exist in the serum in two modes—free and bound or complexed forms.[23] Determination of these fractions has added new impetus to the search for a test that can distinguish between BPH and cancer; tumor cells may stimulate

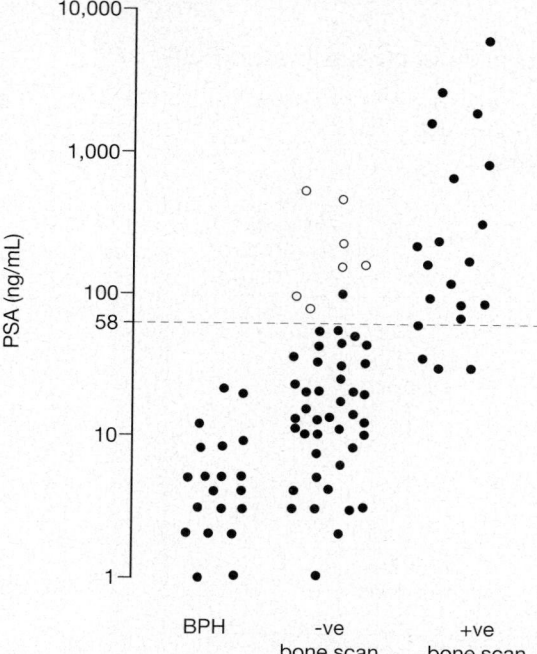

Figure 89-7 Prostate-specific antigen levels in patients with benign prostatic hyperplasia, localized prostate cancer (bone scan negative), and metastatic prostate cancer. Open circles represent seven patients with raised acid phosphatase suggesting metastatic disease despite apparently negative scans. The degree of overlap between the values can be clearly seen, illustrating that PSA is a marker of prostate epithelium and not a specific indicator of prostate cancer. Dotted line: discriminant analysis identifies 58 ng/mL as optimum cutoff distinguishing between skeletal and nonskeletal disease. See text for details. Data from Pantilides et al.,[72] with permission.

production of α-chymotrypsin (ACT) with which binding may occur, leading to higher levels of complexed PSA–ACT than is detected in patients with simple BPH.[24] The determination of the free or complex forms in practical terms is usually limited to the most difficult diagnostic group of patients—those with a presenting PSA between 4 and 10 ng/mL. Above this level the chances of cancer are so high (see above) that sophisticated biochemical analysis is rarely required to make a histological diagnosis.

CLINICAL ASPECTS OF PROSTATIC DISEASE

Prostatitis

Inflammation of the prostatic ducts and acini may occur at any age, although it is more common in its typical form in the third, fourth, and fifth decades. The infection, commonly by coliform organisms, may lead to severe systemic illness with high fever, rigors, and acute perineal discomfort. More chronic forms of the disorder may be difficult to eradicate and it is suggested that spasm of α-adrenergic smooth muscle as well as general pelvic floor tension may contribute to poor duct drainage, and

hence, persisting symptoms. Combination therapy using both antibiotics and smooth/striated muscle relaxants has been advocated in such cases.[25]

In older men, prostatic infection is usually related to the presence of residual urine and outflow tract obstruction. Infection commonly spreads distally down the vas deferens leading to epididymo-orchitis; in earlier times bilateral vasectomy was commonly performed at the time of (open) prostatic surgery to prevent this almost inevitable consequence of the infected residual. In general, the presence of lower urinary tract infection associated with poor bladder emptying will demand surgical intervention after a period of suitable antibiotic treatment so as to reduce the residual volume. In some patients in whom surgery is inappropriate or contraindicated, direct installation of antibiotics into the bladder by a self-catheterization has been described[26] and tried in the elderly group, with some success.

Benign prostatic hyperplasia

Symptom complexes and terminology

It has already been noted that BPH arises chiefly in the periurethral zone and affects a high proportion of men as part of the aging process. It is essential to appreciate, however, that the presence of hyperplasia per se does not imply either significant obstruction to the lower urinary tract or association with particular clinical symptom complexes that may be related to vesicourethral dysfunction rather than the enlarged prostate gland.

These three components—hyperplasia, symptoms, and obstruction—have been brought together in a classic diagram by Hald[27] (Fig. 89-8) demonstrating that, while all three may be found in a minority of cases, each may exist alone or with one another in a random association.

Urologists have argued for many years against the usage of the common phrase "prostatism" employed to describe a wide range of symptoms relating to the male lower urinary tract. Not only does this imply, often wrongly, that the symptoms may be due to the hyperplasia, but it also suggests that therapeutic attention to the gland will cure the patient.

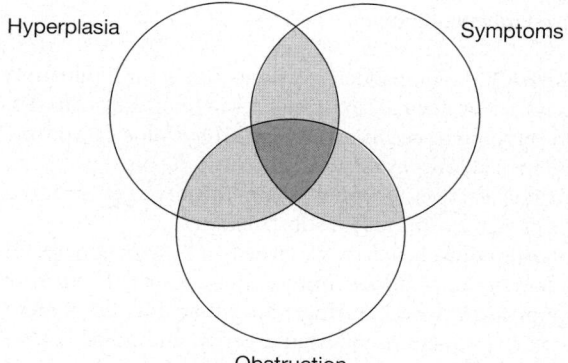

Figure 89-8 Interlocking diagram demonstrating the interdependence of lower urinary tract symptoms, outflow tract obstruction, and hyperplastic tissue when considering symptoms of patients with "prostatism." Significant volumes of hyperplasia may not necessarily be associated either with obstruction or symptoms, while all three may be present in some cases. Adapted from Hald,[27] with permission.

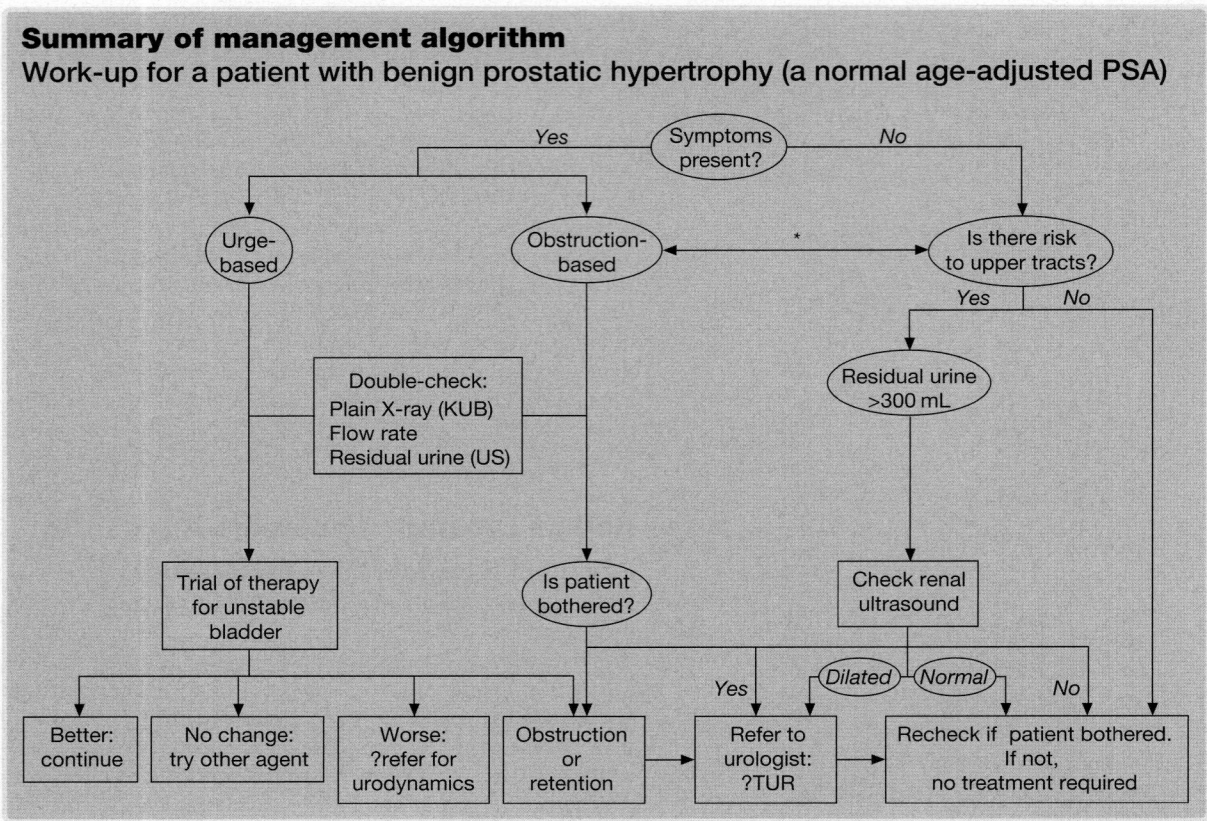

Summary of management algorithm
Work-up for a patient with benign prostatic hypertrophy (a normal age-adjusted PSA)

"Obstruction" should be reserved for those patients proven to be obstructed by urodynamic tests—lower urinary tract symptoms (LUTS) more exactly describe the symptom complex that may or may not be associated with the gland.[28]

Associated detrusor dysfunction

The reaction of the bladder to the presence of emergent BPH is responsible for the symptom complexes which are associated with the condition. These changes are best understood if the filling and voiding segments of the micturition cycle are considered independently.

FILLING PHASE The bladder, receiving urine at 1 mL/min from the kidneys under normal circumstances in temperate climates, normally responds by accommodating the physiological volume (400/500 mL) at low (<5 cmH2O) intrinsic detrusor pressure. This normal reaction to filling may be observed even in the presence of significant outflow obstruction.

More commonly, however, the growth of the emerging gland may give rise to *bladder instability*—abnormal intrinsic detrusor pressure waves during filling that lead the patient to experience frequency, nocturia, urgency, and possibly urge incontinence. Unfortunately, not all bladder instability is related to prostatic obstruction, there being a significant association with old age and neurological disorder (when instability is correctly called "detrusor hyper-reflexia"). Careful studies have shown that approximately two-thirds of older men being investigated for "prostatic" symptoms have bladder instability, and of these only two-thirds will lose their instability following prostatectomy.[29] Unfortunately, there is no test at present that can detect

preoperatively which patients will not lose their bladder instability postoperatively. Persistence of the disorder following surgery leaves a very unhappy patient with significantly worse urge symptoms that may take many months to settle (Fig. 89-9).

VOIDING PHASE As with the filling phase, significant prostatic hyperplasia may not necessarily affect vesicourethral function. This observation presumably explains in part the large number of elderly men who have apparently enlarged glands on rectal examination, but who deny any impairment to micturition performance. More typically, however, two types of bladder dysfunction are found in association with BPH—typical *high-pressure* obstructed voiding or relatively *low-pressure* underactive detrusor function.

High-pressure/low-flow voiding is the classic reaction to mechanical blockage of the urethra by BPH leading to typical symptoms of hesitancy, poor stream, and gradually increasing frequency by day and night. Additionally (see above) symptoms of bladder instability may superimpose problems related to urgency and urge incontinence.

Low-pressure/low-flow underactive bladders have been recognized only since the 1980s, but may account for 20–25 percent of patients with outflow tract symptomatology. The reason for the abnormal detrusor function remains unknown, although the condition has been likened to a nonobstructive myopathy.[30] Men with low-flow voiding also complain of frequency and poor stream (often prolonged and interrupted), which is impossible to separate from high-pressure/low-flow voiding except by invasive urodynamic tests. It has been recognized increasingly that inclusion of such

Patient A

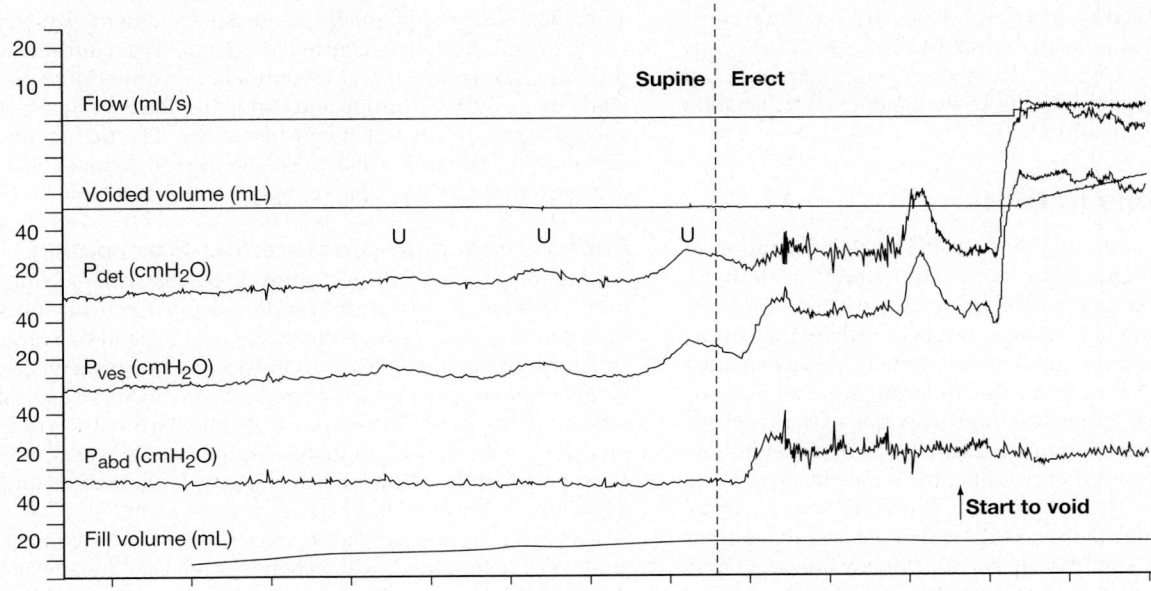

Patient B

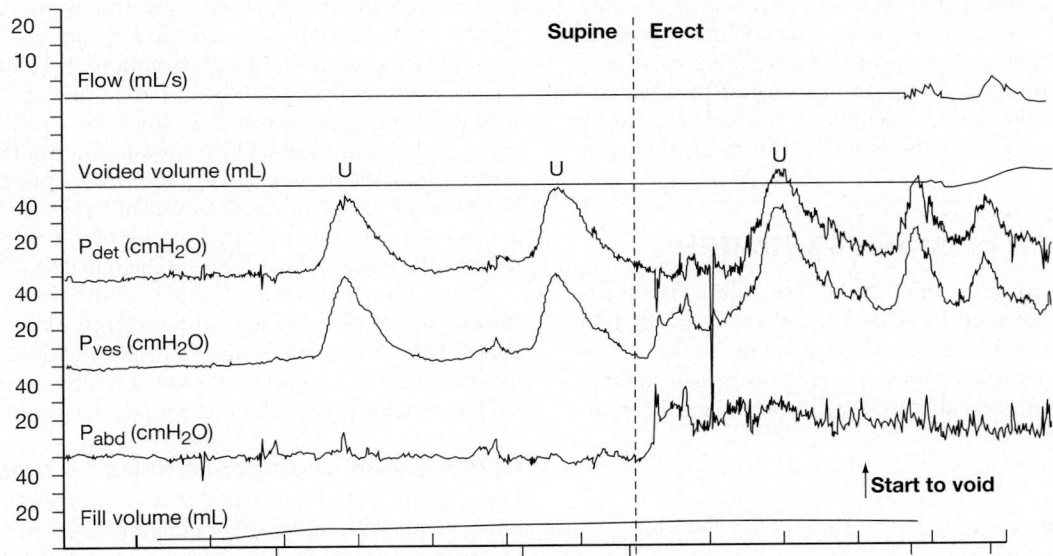

Figure 89-9 Urodynamic (cystometry) traces from patients with (A) bladder instability probably associated with obstruction, and (B) bladder instability probably not associated with obstruction. In both cases the patient presented with urgency, frequency, and a poor flow. It remains extremely difficult to determine which patient might benefit from outflow tract surgery without urodynamic investigation. In the cases illustrated, patient A would probably benefit significantly from surgery whilst patient B would probably become signficantly worse. P_{det}, intrinsic detrusor pressure; P_{ves}, pressure within bladder; P_{abd}, pressure within abdomen (rectal line). U: patient experienced urgency sufficient to mention to the investigator. Vertical dotted line: commencement of move from supine to erect investigation position.

low-pressure/low-flow patients in prostatectomy series leads to the impression of poor outcomes from the procedure.[31,32]

Retention and bladder dysfunction

Sudden increase in prostate size, such as may occur during hemorrhage or infarction, may cause acute (painful) retention of urine, but these conditions are unusual. It is a common observation that patients on urological waiting lists for outflow tract obstruction rarely present in acute retention; by contrast men admitted with this condition have usually not seen their general practitioner previously and the precipitating factor seems often to relate to acute fluid loading and subsequent overstretching of the unrelieved bladder—as happens for example during a long coach trip.

Chronic (painless) retention of urine is broadly divided into two forms: the low-pressure "floppy" bladder, which may become complicated by infection, but which has normal upper tracts; and the high-pressure "tense" bladder, which frequently is seen in patients with few if any lower tract symptoms, but which is usually associated with bilateral upper tract dilatation and obstructive uropathy.[33]

Investigations in BPH

In recent years, audit studies have led to rationalization of investigations required to assess the patient with BPH. Frequency/volume charts filled in by the patient at home are helpful in revealing nonprostatic causes of urinary tract disorders such as fluid excretion patterns related to cardiovascular disease or excessive tea drinking. Following urine microscopy and culture, rectal examination, and palpation of the abdomen for chronic retention of urine, plain X-ray of the abdomen (KUB) will detect potential operative problems such as bladder calculus. An independent flow-rate test, correctly performed (greater than 150 mL voided, no valsalva pushes permitted) is mandatory (Fig. 89-10). Intravenous urography is no longer advised unless the patient complains of, or is found on urine testing to suffer from, significant hematuria. Five percent of patients with high-pressure obstruction develop upper tract dilatation and may be uremic;[34,35] for this reason, if a residual urine of greater than 300 mL is detected abdominally, upper tract ultrasound is advised to assess renal anatomy. In summary, audit studies suggest that patients without blood in their urine or significant residual urine do not require any form of upper tract studies prior to consideration for surgery.

Management of patients with BPH

Many patients come to their doctor because a friend has recently been admitted in acute painful retention or they have seen a television program about prostate cancer. A negative work-up followed by reassurance permits these patients to return to their normal lifestyle without the need for any intervention.

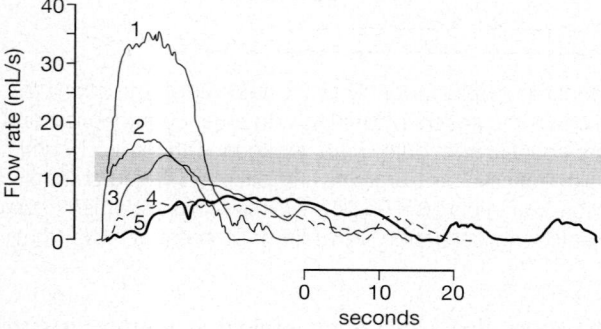

Figure 89-10 Independent flow rate traces. 1: normal flow rate, younger male. 2,3: normal flow rates, older male (>70 years). 4,5: poor flow rate. It is not possible to determine whether the reduced rate is related to outflow tract obstruction or underactive detrusor function—see text for details. Stippled line: lower limit of normality.

Patients with incontinence

Stress incontinence is very rare in neurologically normal males and when observed is usually the result of prostatic surgery where the sphincter mechanism has been damaged during the procedure. By contrast, urge incontinence is common, particularly in the older age group and is chiefly related, in the presence of sterile urine, to bladder instability. The therapeutic approach to instability has been mentioned below and is discussed more fully in Chapter 104.

Patients with high-pressure/low-flow voiding

Advice for patients with uncomplicated obstructive symptoms—hesitancy, poor stream, and moderate frequency/nocturia (no urge or urge incontinence)—will depend to a large extent on the patient's own circumstances and preferences. Frequency may not trouble a retired man as much as a clerical officer at his desk. Reassurance, particularly concerning prostate cancer, may be all that is required and it is tempting to propose that the reduction in α-adrenegic periprostatic tone might be responsible for the noted improvement.

More usually, however, active intervention will be required, and typically the choice will be between medical therapy and operation (transurethral resection of the prostate). Two forms of medical therapy are presently in common use, but both suffer from a relatively slow onset of action with resultant modest increment in urine flow rate. Nevertheless, for patients with smaller prostates who have equivocal symptoms or for those who wish to avoid the risks of operation, these drugs can be effective. A number of α-blockers are available (Table 89-1) with varying degrees of uroselectivity.[35] Most of the α-blockers exert their full effect within 1 month, whereas the α-reductase inhibitors[36] may take up to 3 months for clinical effect to be noticeable. Recently, a controversial report has considered α-blockade to be significantly superior to α-reductase inhibition, which was equal in efficacy only to placebo.[37]

For patients with severe "simple" obstruction, TUR offers the unquestioned "gold standard" in terms of measured outcomes. Despite the significant comorbidity of the elderly treatment population, a rapid resolution of symptoms ensures that the great majority are delighted with the results of treatment.

Patients with underactive detrusor function

It has already been emphasized that it is not possible to separate patients with underactive function from those with true obstruction unless full preoperative urodynamic tests are performed;[31] and hence, overall, it is not surprising that in the

Table 89-1 **Alpha-blockers**
Nonselective α-blocker Phenoxybenzamine
Selective α-blockers Prazosin Alfusozin Indoramin
Selective long-acting α-blockers Terazosin Doxazosin Tamsulosin

absence of such tests some patients are not satisfied with their postoperative micturition performance.[32] Nevertheless, some improvement is seen and the disappointment is a relative measure of the difference in postoperative flow rates between obstructive and underactive groups. The reversibility of medical therapy makes it ideal for a trial of treatment in this group, and transurethral resection may be reserved for those who are dissatisfied or who cannot tolerate blockade therapy.

Patients with irritative symptoms

As previously noted, bladder instability is very common in men with either obstructed or unobstructed bladders. Although a complete diagnostic picture may be obtained by urodynamic tests on each patient, few units can afford the academic luxury of this purist approach. Hence, trials of therapy are commonly practiced in elderly patients with the frequency urge syndrome.

Physiological bladder contraction is mediated by a stimulation of postganglionic parasympathetic cholinergic receptors on detrusor smooth muscle, and the M_3 subtype is thought to be the most important form of muscurinic receptor for bladder contraction.[38] Hence, atropine and atropine-like agents will induce a lessening of the contraction wave with corresponding decrease in detected urgency by the patient. Trials of such agents[39] or musculotropic relaxation agents such as oxybutynin chloride[40] show reasonable efficacy, and recently a modified-release formulation of this drug given once daily has been shown to be as effective as conventional dosage and may be better tolerated.[41] Other muscurinic receptor antagonists include tolterodine which may demonstrate an improved side-effect profile (dry mouth, dry eyes, blurred vision, headache) although maximum efficacy may require up to 10 weeks treatment[42] in older patients. Most recently trospium chloride, a quaternary ammonium nonselective muscurinic blocker, has been promoted with a further improvement in side-effect profile.[43,44] Nevertheless, many will be familiar with the statement about any treatment for instability: "one is always surprised when it works."

New modalities for treatment

While it is accepted that transurethral resection remains the gold standard for treatment of patients with obstructive BPH,[45] a number of new modalities have been introduced, including prostate incision, laser therapy, stent therapy, and varieties of thermotherapy. All these techniques have their vociferous supporters; but for the patient with a significant volume of hyperplastic tissue obstructing the bladder outlet, endoscopic transurethral resection remains the treatment of choice. The need for critical evaluation of the new technology in terms of outcome measures continues to be debated in urological circles.

Prostatic surgery in the elderly population

Recent advances in anesthetic techniques have allowed a complete reappraisal of treatment options in the elderly group, and it is now rare for a patient to be refused prostatectomy on anesthetic grounds alone. While many patients over 100 years of age have been treated satisfactorily—an unnecessary urethral catheter is undesirable at any age—the chief contraindication to operation is presently the inability of the patient mentally to appreciate what is being offered to alleviate his symptoms.

Hence, apart from a very few seriously compromised patients, modern anesthesia permits straightforward decisions to be made about the elderly patient and "lesser" operative techniques such as urethral stent insertion[46] hold little advantage over simple transurethral resection.

PROSTATE CANCER

Prostate cancer has developed into a significant and increasing health problem.[47,48] Presently second only to lung cancer as a cause of cancer mortality, greater public awareness and the development of cancer detection programs utilizing prostate-specific antigen (PSA) have ensured that the problem will not diminish in the foreseeable future.

However, the very slow growth of some tumors means that, unlike many other neoplasms, not every prostate cancer is a life-threatening event for the patient. Many older men die *with* rather than *of* their prostate cancer, but the prediction as to whether the disease as identified in any one individual patient carries a good prognosis remains extremely difficult. This problem is not helped by the very wide difference between the *incidence* and *mortality* of the disease in many Western countries. In the USA in 1995, the incidence/mortality ratio was 1:7.8, and in Holland it was 1:2.1 (Holtgrewe and Schröder, personal communication, 1996), demonstrating that the diagnostic tests were detecting many more individuals with cancers than were later dying of the disease. The essential question relates to whether or not all detected cancers are capable of progressing and leading eventually to the death of the patient.

SITE OF DISEASE   Anatomically, most cancers (70–75 percent) are found in the peripheral zone of the gland (Fig. 89-2). Approximately 20 percent of lesions are thought to originate in the transitional zone, while the remainder are located in the central zone. Thus, most nodules or palpable lesions should be detected by the educated finger on rectal examination, while in a minority the transurethral resection of the transitional zone (i.e. for an obstructive lesion thought to be "BPH") may occasionally eradicate unsuspected tumor in that area.

EPIDEMIOLOGICAL STUDIES   Prostatic disease is rare in the Far East, Japan, and China. Migratory studies have clearly shown, however, that the incidence of the disease increases as males move to a more Western lifestyle. Significant racial differences also exist; within the San Francisco Bay area, Japanese Americans are eight times less likely to suffer from the disease than African Americans.[49]

PROSTATE CANCER AND THE ELDERLY   It has already been mentioned that the disease is presently being diagnosed at an earlier stage in younger men. At the present time, the question of whether to screen for prostate cancer and which treatment to offer for the cases so detected remains at the forefront of medical debate. Views are strongly expressed because a tumor discovered at age 53, however indolent its growth pattern, is likely to lead to death within the patient's natural lifespan. For the older person, however, the decision criteria are different and it is in this context that the following variants of disease presentation are discussed.

Summary of management algorithm
Assessment and treatment of a patient with prostate cancer suspected on the grounds of a digital rectal exam and PSA

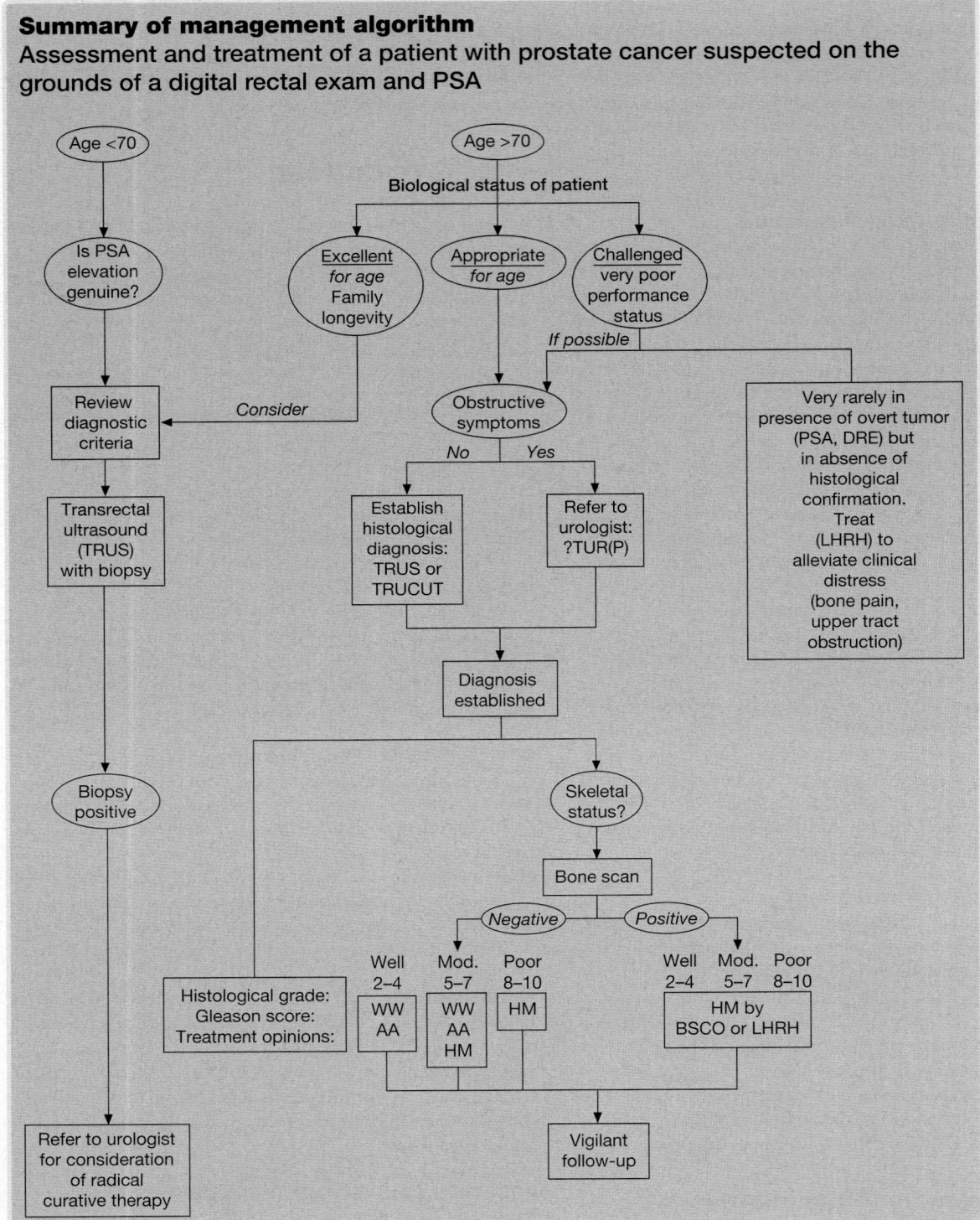

Localized prostate cancer

Localized prostate cancer may be detected incidentally or it may be discovered as part of the investigation of a man with developing lower urinary tract symptoms. PSA-led ultrasound biopsy may reveal carcinoma (stage Tlc; see Table 89-2) in a patient who presented merely with anxiety, no symptoms, and a normal rectal examination (i.e. BPH in texture). However,

in the elderly man, lower urinary tract symptoms (irritation or obstruction) are more often the reason for a first visit to his doctor. At this time, digital rectal examination may or may not reveal obvious neoplastic change, and it is likely that histological confirmation will need to await specialist referral and subsequent TRUS biopsy or transurethral resection. The absence of bony metastatic disease may be confirmed by isotope bone scan,

Table 89-2 TNM staging of prostate cancer—1997 revision

Primary tumor, clinical (T)	Primary tumor, pathologic (pT)	Regional lymph nodes (N)	Distant metastasis (M)
TX Primary tumor cannot be assessed	pT2 Organ confined	NX Regional lymph nodes cannot be assessed	MX Distant metastasis cannot be assessed
T0 No evidence of primary tumor	pT2a Unilateral	N0 No regional lymph node metastasis	M0 No distant metastasis
T1 Clinically inapparent tumor not palpable or visible by imaging	pT2b Bilateral	N1 Metastasis in regional lymph node or nodes	M1 Distant metastasis
T1a Tumor incidental histological finding in 5% or less of tissue resected	pT3 Extraprostatic extension		M1a Nonregional lymph nodes
T1b Tumor incidental histological finding in more than 5% of tissue resected	pT3a Extraprostatic extension		M1b Bone(s)
T1c Tumor indentified by needle biopsy (e.g. because of elevated PSA)	pT3b Seminal vesicle invasion		M1c Other site(s)
T2 Palpable tumor confined within prostate	pT4 Invasion of bladder, rectum		
T2a Tumor involves one lobe			
T2b Tumor involves both lobes			
T3 Tumor extends through the prostatic capsule			
T3a Extracapsular extension (unilateral or bilateral)			
T3b Tumor invades seminal vesicles			
T4 Tumor is fixed or invades adjacent structures other than seminal vesicles: bladder neck, external sphincter, rectum, levator muscles, and/or pelvic wall			

but it has been recently suggested that PSA is a superior predictor of a negative scan if levels are less than 20 ng/mL, and so the time-consuming and expensive scan may be avoided.[50]

Treatment of local disease

Four options are available for older men with apparently localized disease: watchful waiting, conventional radiotherapy, brachytherapy, or radical prostatectomy. The therapeutic choice will depend *inter alia* on the histological grade of the tumor, the PSA level at diagnosis, and the biological age of the patient.

WATCHFUL WAITING Studies from Scandinavia[51] and England[52] have shown that long symptom-free intervals may be obtained by observation policies if the histological grade is favorable. Originally, the concept of "latent" cancer was introduced for cancers that apparently failed to progress; but observational studies have clearly demonstrated that local advance, albeit slow, does occur in nearly all prostate cancers.[52] These findings have been confirmed by PSA data that are requested at 6-month intervals during routine follow-up. Histological grade is acknowledged as the most important prognostic indicator for progression; Figure 89-11 shows survival and time to metastasis data for patients from north-west England on a

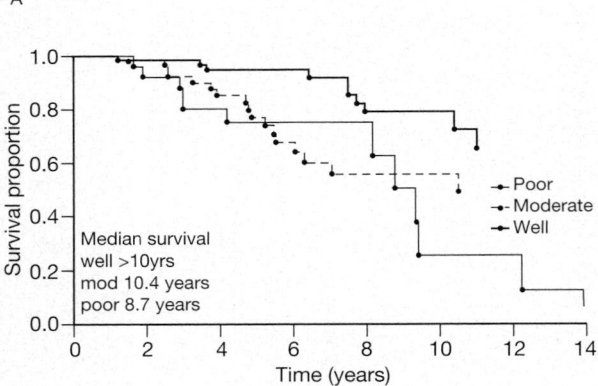

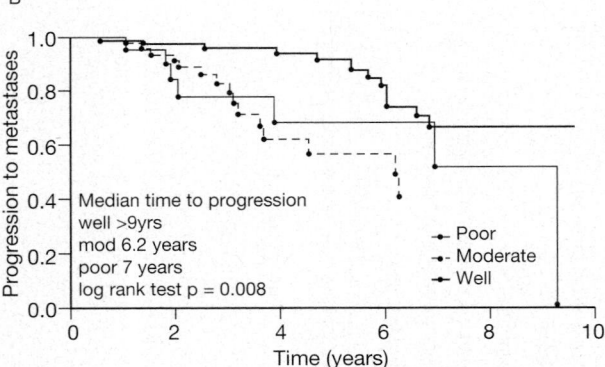

Figure 89-11 Disease-specific Kaplan–Maier analysis of localized prostate cancer in the Manchester series, 1980–95.[52] The importance of histological grade can be seen, as (A) the median times to survival and (B) progression to bony metastases (the most significant cause of morbidity) has not yet been reached for patients with well-differentiated tumors.

watchful waiting protocol. In this series,[52] the mean age at presentation was 74.5 years and it can be seen that patients with well-differentiated tumors had not yet reached the median point at 10 years. The survival data also emphasize that many moderate and all high-grade tumors are not suited to a watch-and-wait policy.

CONVENTIONAL RADIOTHERAPY In the UK, radiotherapy has traditionally been the mode of treatment for those patients with localized disease in whom markers—grade or stage (as judged by rectal examination)—pointed to the need for local primary control. Recently, the efficacy of this treatment modality has been questioned, particularly in the context of younger patients. Additionally, results of comparative trials with surgery have not been favorable, but it is generally agreed that patients entered to the radiotherapy arm of such trials are poorly staged when compared to those submitted to radical surgery. Of late, however, centers in the USA have reported more favorable outcomes with intensity-modulated conformal radiotherapy,[53] an approach which is acknowledged to provide the most efficacious treatment to the gland itself with the minimal toxicity to the surrounding structures. Hence, for the older man in whom watchful waiting or radical surgery are contraindicted, radiotherapy remains an acceptable method of treatment usually without serious short- or long-term complications.

BRACHYTHERAPY The implantation of an interstitial radiation source within the prostate has gained rapid popularity in both younger and older men with localized prostate cancer. Relative simplicity, short (if any) inpatient stay, and rapid return to normal activity constitute the unarguable attractions of the technique. Within the USA it is estimated that brachytherapy, chosen by only 4 percent of men with localized prostate cancer in 1996, will soon be the choice of 50 percent.[54]

Selection criteria for men suitable for brachytherapy are strict. A large prostate (>60 mL), prominent median lobes, previous transurethral resection of the prostate (risk of incontinence), and significant comorbidity (previous pelvic irradiation, diabetes) are contraindications.

Whether brachytherapy will be shown in the long term to be superior to standard treatment remains a matter of active debate.[55] The technique requires specialist equipment and expertise to obtain optimum results.[56,57]

RADICAL SURGERY Radical prostatectomy has always been the first choice in the USA for the treatment of localized prostate cancer, particularly in younger men. Recently, enthusiasm has been taken to extremes with a rapid increase in the numbers of procedures performed even in men aged over 75 years.[58] Many would regard this as overtreatment, as the complications of surgery—incontinence and impotence—are not insignificant in the elderly population, particularly when the procedure is performed by an inexperienced surgeon. Nevertheless, the treatment preference of biologically fit elderly men with 10-year life expectancy should be respected.

SUMMARY Observational studies incorporating histological grade have shown that the biological age of the patient is the most important factor in making a decision between the treatment options. Whereas there is little doubt that the man of 55 years should be offered radical therapy on the basis of the 10- to 15-year predicted survival data, for men over 70 the choice widens to include more conservative approaches such as watchful waiting. Patient preference remains a very important part of the therapeutic decision process.

Extensive local disease

Many patients with large (T3+) local tumors also have metastatic spread to bone. However, since the advent of PSA testing (case finding by primary care physicians) an increasingly large proportion of elderly patients are presenting with advanced (i.e. not curable by radical treatment) local disease but a negative bone scan, and this group probably represents now the majority of new patients presenting for treatment within the UK. Prostate-specific antigen data may show these lesions to be slow-growing, but it is most likely that treatment should be offered—usually in addition to transurethral resection to cure outflow tract symptoms. Typically, hormone manipulation by medical (LHRH) or surgical (bilateral subcapsular orchidectomy) means is usually found to be very satisfactory in these cases. Resection or estrogen therapy (intravenous Honvan) may be required occasionally when local tumor advance leads to blockage of the lower ends of the ureters with resultant abnormalities of renal function.

Two important radomized prospective studies have addressed the treatment of bone-scan-negative patients with locally advanced disease. In these trials, neo-adjuvant[59] and adjuvant[60] LHRH therapy was found significantly to improve local control in patients treated with external-beam radiotherapy. Although it might be expected that patients randomized to early hormone therapy might show a treatment advantage, further studies are under way specifically to test the efficacy of radiotherapy in advanced localized disease. It seems likely that these trials will produce highly relevant data for treatment of this important group of patients within a reasonable time.

Bicalutamide is a nonsteroidal antiandrogen that has been tried in patients with locally advanced and metastatic prostate cancer.[61] The treatment was not effective for the latter group but subsequently has been shown to be as efficacious (150 mg dose) as castration (medical and surgical) for patients with localized disease.[62] Recently the large early prostate cancer (EPC) trials were halted by AstraZeneca after the first protocol analysis showed a significant (42 percent) reduction in objective progression in the bicalutamide (Casodex) arm.[63] Naturally the same caveat observed above for the Bolla study apply to the EPC trial outcomes, and this important trial will probably not now be able to detect whether such antiandrogen therapy results in a survival advantage for the treatment group. Nevertheless antiandrogen monotherapy is clearly developing as an important treatment modality for patients with locally advanced nonmetastatic disease.

Metastatic disease

It is an unfortunate fact that until very recently the majority of patients with prostate cancer presented with bone metastases, so treatment could be regarded only as palliative rather than curative. Worldwide it is accepted that even with immediate treatment the survival for such patients is approximately 50 percent at 2 years and 10–14 percent at 5 years.[52,64]

Treatment of metastatic disease

HORMONAL MANIPULATION Androgen deprivation has (since 1940 when Huggins discovered the hormone-dependent nature of the tumor) been the mainstay of treatment for metastatic prostate cancer. Remission occurs for a variable period—usually 9–12 months—before prostate markers, which usually fall following treatment, start to rise again. Approximately 10–15 percent of patients fail to respond significantly to the hormonal manipulation, which may be achieved by either medical or surgical means.

Bilateral subcapsular orchidectomy has been the traditional approach to androgen deprivation, and the serum testosterone rapidly falls into the "castrate" range. Medical therapy by LHRH analogue[65] has, however, become widely established,[66] although the injections are expensive and the serum testosterone does not fall for 8–10 days, which may be of clinical importance. It has to be emphasized to the patients that the side-effect profile of these two treatments—impotence and hot flushes—is identical, a point not always well made by the manufacturers. Diethylstilboestriol (DES) at a dose of 5 mg was for many years used to achieve the required hormonal manipulation. Well-publicized cardiac toxicity, however, has led many to avoid this medication even at the lower 1 mg dose, although some continue to advocate the approach in combination with daily aspirin (75 mg).

NONSTEROIDAL ANTIANDROGENS These have the attraction of blocking the action of testosterone peripherally without the major side-effect problems associated with traditional hormonal manipulation. Each compound, however, has particular drawbacks. Flutamide leads to significant gastrointestinal upset and diarrhea, while bicalutamide, which has the attraction of once-daily dosage,[67] also causes some breast tenderness and leads to elevation of serum testosterone owing to a central agonist action effecting a rise in luteinizing hormone. Bicalutamide is also licenced for the treatment of metastatic disease in conjunction with LHRH analogues.

Timing of treatment

Some debate has surrounded the ideal timing for treatment of metastatic prostate cancer. Surprisingly, some patients with positive bone scans remain entirely asymptomatic, and it was argued that, as the patients were feeling well, it was not possible to improve their situation and treatment should await the onset of symptoms.

In the UK, the Medical Research Council Early/Delayed Treatment Trial has addressed this issue.[68] The trial showed clearly that delayed therapy in patients with metastatic disease was associated with significantly worse morbidity, so there seems little doubt that therapy should be commenced without delay in such patients with disease in bone even if no symptoms are present. Conclusions relating to patients with nonmetastatic disease were more controversial, and a recent follow-up analysis (reported at Société International d'Urologie, Singapore, 2000) has suggested that no significant advantage could be attributed to early treatment in this patient group.[68]

Bone pain

Bone pain remains the most troublesome aspect of the disease for the patient, and it is often difficult to manage. Radiotherapy remains the basis of local control, although promising results[69] have been noted with strontium-89 and disphosphonate (antiosteoclast) infusions,[70] among other approaches.

CONCLUSION

In the elderly population, prostate cancer may manifest as an almost benign slow-growing local tumor or as an aggressive spreading disease that almost invariably leads to a painful and distressing death. Surgical relief of obstruction plays a major part in each of these variants, but for the latter group an approach involving hospital specialists, the palliative care team, and the general practitioner is most likely to result in meaningful support for both the patient and his family.

KEY POINTS The prostate

- Anatomical knowledge of the sphincter apparatus assists understanding of continence mechanisms.

- Physicians offering prostate-specific antigen (PSA) tests to patients should fully understand the implications of an abnormal result.

- "Prostatic" symptoms may not be related to disease of the prostate gland.

- Elderly patients with localized prostate cancer have a wide range of therapeutic options.

- Elderly patients with metastatic prostate cancer should be treated, even if no symptoms are present.

REFERENCES

1. Cunha GR, Donjacour AA, Cooke PS et al: The endocrinology and developmental biology of the prostate. Endocr Rev 1987;8:338–362
2. Berry SJ, Coffey DS, Walsh PC et al: The development of human benign prostatic hypertrophy with age. J Urol 1984;132:474–477
3. Garraway WM, Collins GN, Lee RJ: High prevalence of benign prostatic hypertrophy in the community. Lancet 1991;338:469–471
4. Lee C: Physiology of contraction induced regression in rat prostate. In Murphy GP, Sandberg AA, Carr JP (eds): Prostate Cell: Structure and Function. Alan R Liss, New York, 1981:145–159
5. Hiramatsu M, Kashimata M, Minami N: Androgenic regulation of epidermal growth factor in the mouse ventral prostate. Biochem Int 1988;17:311–314
6. Imperato-McGinley J, Guerrero L, Gautier T, Peterson RE: Steroid 5α reductase deficiency in men: an inherited form of male pseudohermaphroditism. Science 1974;186:1213–1215
7. Lowsley OS: The development of the human prostate gland with reference to the development of other structures at the neck of the urinary bladder. Am J Anat 1912;13:299–304
8. McNeal JE: Normal histology of the prostate. Am J Surg Pathol 1988;12:619–626
9. McNeal JE: Origin and evolution of benign prostatic hypertrophy. Invest Urol 1978;15:340
10. Gosling J: Structure of the bladder and urethra in relation to function. Urol Clin North Am 1979;6:31–38
11. Schroder HD: Onuf's Nucleus X: a morphological study of a human spinal nucleus. Anat Embryol 1981;162:443–453
12. Simonsen O, Moller-Madsen B, Dorflinger T et al: Significance of age on symptoms and urodynamic findings in benign prostatic hypertrophy. Urol Res 1987;15:355–361
13. Butler MR, Donnelly B, Komaranchat A: Intravenous urography in evaluation of acute retention. Urology 1978;12:464
14. Pinck BD, Corrigan MJ, Jasper P: Preprostatectomy excretory urography: does it merit the expense? J Urol 1980;123:390–394
15. Scardino PT, Shinohara K, Wheeler TM et al: Staging of prostate cancer: value of ultrasonography. Urol Clin North Am 1989;16:713–734
16. Ohori M, Egawa S, Shinohara K et al: Detection of microscopic extracapsular extension prior to radical prostatectomy for clinically localised prostate cancer. Br J Urol 1994;74:72–79
17. Babaian RJ: Extended field prostate biopsy enhances cancer detection. Urology 2000;55:453–456
18. Platt IF, Bree RL, Schwab RE: Accuracy of CT in staging of carcinoma of prostate. Am J Radiol 1987;149:315–318
19. Rifkin MD, Zerlouri EA, Gatsonis CA et al: Comparison of MRI and ultrasonography in staging early prostate cancer. N Engl J Med 1990;323:611–625
20. Gutman AB, Gutman EB: An "acid" phosphatase occurring in the serum of patients with metastatic carcinoma of the prostate gland. J Clin Invest 1938;17:473–477
21. Wang MC, Valenzuela LA, Murphy GP et al: Purification of a human prostate specific antigen. Invest Urol 1979;17:159
22. Oesterling JE, Jacobsen SJ, Chute CG et al: Serum prostate specific antigen in a community based population of healthy men: establishment of age specific reference ranges. JAMA 1993;270:840–864
23. Lilja H, Christensson A, Dahlen U et al: Prostate specific antigen in serum occurs predominantly in complex with an alpha 1 chymotrypsin. Clin Chem 1991;37:9–14
24. Christensson A, Bjork T, Nilsson O et al: Serum PSA complexed to alpha 1 chymotrypsin as an indicator of prostatic cancer. J Urol 1993;150:100–105
25. George NJR, Reading C: Sympathetic nervous system and dysfunction of the lower urinary tract. Clin Sci 1986;70:69–76
26. McGuire EJ, Savastano JA: Treatment of intractable bacterial cystitis with intermittent catheterization and antimicrobial installation. J Urol 1987;137:495–496
27. Hald T: Urodynamics in benign prostatic hypertrophy: a survey. The Prostate 1989;(suppl 2):69–77
28. Abrams PH: New words for old: lower urinary tract symptoms for "prostatism". BMJ 1994;308:929
29. Abrams PH, Farrar DJ, Turner-Warwick RT et al: The results of prostatectomy: a symptomatic and urodynamic analysis of 152 patients. J Urol 1979;121:640–642
30. Holm-Bentzen M, Larsen S, Hainan B, Howells T: Non obstructive detrusor myopathy. Scand J Urol Nephrol 1985;19:21–26
31. Jensen K-ME, Jorgensen JP, Mogensen P: Urodynamics in prostatism II: prognostic value of pressure flow study. Scand J Urol Nephrol 1988;114:72–77
32. Neal DE, Ramsden PD, Sharples L: Outcome of elective prostatectomy. BMJ 1989;299:762–767
33. George NJR, O'Reilly PH, Barnard RJ, Blacklock NJ: High pressure chronic retention. BMJ 1983;286:1780–1783
34. Abrams PH, Roylance J, Fenerley RCL: Excretion urography in the investigation of "prostatism". Br J Urol 1976;48:681–684
35. Kirby RS, Coppinger SWC, Corcoran MO et al: Prazosin in the treatment of prostatic obstruction. Br J Urol 1987;60:136–142
36. Stoner E, Finasteride Study Group: Three year safety and efficacy data on the use of finasteride in the treatment of BPH. Urology 1994;43:284–292
37. Lepor H, Willford W, Barry MJ et al: Efficacy of terazosin, finasteride or both in BPH. N Engl J Med 1996;335:533–539
38. Nilvebrant L, Hallén B, Larsson G: Tolterodine—a new bladder selective muscurinic receptor antagonist: pre-clinical pharmacological and clinical data. Life Sci 1997;60:1129–1136
39. Benson GS, Sarshik SA, Baezer DM: Comparison of the effects and mechanisms of action of atropine, propantheline, flavoxate and imipramine. Urology 1977;9:31–37
40. Moisey C, Stephenson TR, Brendler C: The urodynamic and subjective result of treatment of detrusor instability with oxybutimin chloride. Br J Urol 1980;52:472–475
41. Binns J, Lukkari E, Malone-Lee JG et al: A randomised controlled trial comparing the efficacy of controlled-release oxybutynin tablets (10 mg once daily) with conventional oxybutynin tablets (5 mg twice daily) in patients whose symptoms were stabilized on 5 mg twice daily. BJU Int 2000;85:793–798

42. Malone-Lee JG, Shaffu B, Anand C, Powell C: Tolterodine: superior tolerability than and comparable efficacy to oxybutynin in individuals 50 years old or older with overactive bladder: a randomised controlled trial. J Urol 2001;165:1452–1456

43. Madersbacher H, Stöhrer M, Richter R et al: Trospium chloride versus oxybutynin: a randomised, double blind, multi-centre trial in the treatment of detrusor hyper-reflexia. Br J Urol 1995;75:452–456

44. Cardozol, Chapple CR, Toozs-Hobson P et al: Efficacy of trospium chloride in patients with detrusor instability: a placebo control, randomised, double blind, multi-centre clinical trial. BJU Int 2000;85:659–664

45. Holtgrewe HL: Transurethral prostatectomy. Urol Clin North Am 1995;22:357–368

46. Milroy E, Chapple CR: The UroLume stent in the management of BPH. J Urol 1993;150:1630–1635

47. Carter HB, Coffey DS: The prostate: an increasing medical problem. The Prostate 1990;16:39–48

48. CRC Fact Sheet 20, London, 1994

49. Waterhouse JA, Murir CS, Shanmugaratuam K et al: IARC Scientific Publication 15, Lyon, 1982

50. Chybowski FM, Larson-Keller JJ, Bergstrath EJ et al: Predicting bone scan findings in patients with newly diagnosed untreated prostate cancer: PSA is superior to all other parameters. J Urol 1991;145: 313–318

51. Johansson J, Adami H, Andersson S et al: High ten-year survival rate in patients with early untreated prostate cancer. JAMA 1992;267:2191–2196

52. George NJR: Natural history of localised prostate cancer treated by conservative therapy alone. Lancet 1988;1:494–497

53. Zelefsky M, Fuks Z, Hunt M et al: High dose radiation delivered by intensity modulated conformal radiotherapy improves the outcome of localised prostate cancer. J Urol 2001;166:876–881

54. Nag S: Brachytherapy for prostate cancer: summary of American Brachytherapy Society recommendations. Semin Urol Oncol 2000;18:133–136

55. Turner CD, Brendla CB: Ultrasound-guided brachytherapy: is it really better? Urology 1999;53:869–872

56. Blasko JC, Wallner K, Grimm PD et al: PSA-based disease control following ultrasound guided ^{125}iodine implantation for stage T1/T2 prostate carcinoma. J Urol 1995;154:1096–1099

57. Gelblum DY, Potters L: Rectal complications associated with transperineal interstitial brachytherapy for prostate cancer. Int J Radiat Oncol Biol Phys 2000;48:119–121

58. Lu-Yao GL, McClerran D, Wasson J et al: An assessment of radical prostatectomy. JAMA 1993;269:2633–2636

59. Pilepich MD, Sause WT, Shipley WU et al: Androgen deprivation with radiation therapy compared with radiation therapy alone for locally advanced prostatic carcinoma: a randomised comparative trial of the radiation therapy oncology group. Urology 1995;45:616–623

60. Bolla M, Gonzalez D, Ward EP et al: Improved survival in patients with locally advanced prostate cancer treated with radiotherapy and goserelin. N Engl J Med 1997;337:295–300

61. Tyrrell CJ, Kaisary AV, Iversen P et al: A randomised comparison of "Casodex" (bicalutamide) 150 mg monotherapy versus castration in the treatment of metastatic and locally advanced prostate cancer. Eur Urol 1998;33:447–456

62. Iversen P, Tyrell CJ, Kaisary AV et al: Bicalutamide monotherapy compared with castration in patients with non-metastatic locally advanced prostate cancer: 6.3 years of follow-up. J Urol 2000;164:1579–1582

63. Data reported at EPC Investigator Meeting (Bicalutamide 150 mg), Montreux, Switzerland, 2001

64. Sandhu DPS, Mayor PE, Sambrook P, George NJR: Increased survival of patients with massive lymphadenopathy and prostate cancer: evidence of heterogenous tumour behaviour. Br J Urol 1990;66:415–419

65. Peeling WB: Phase III studies to compare goserelin (Zoladex) with orchidectomy and DES in the treatment of prostatic carcinoma. Urology 1989;33:45–52

66. Cassileth BR: Patients choice of treatment in stage D prostatic cancer. Urology 1989;33:57–59

67. Furr BA, Valcaccia B, Curry B: ICI 176334: a novel non-steroidal peripherally selective antiandrogen. J Endocrinol 1987;113:R7–R9

68. MRC Prostate Cancer Working Party Investigator's Group: Immediate versus deferred treatment for advanced prostatic cancer: initial results of the Medical Research Council Trial. Br J Urol 1997;79:235–246

69. Crawford ED, Balmar C, Kozlowski JM et al: Strontium^{89} for palliation of pain for bone metatases associated with hormone refractory prostate cancer. Urology 1994;44:481–485

70. Clarke NW, Halbrook J, McClure J et al: Effects of osteoclast inhibition by pamidronate in metastatic bone disease from prostate cancer. Br J Cancer 1991;63:420–423

71. George NJR: Bladder and urethra: function and dysfunction. In Weiss RM, George NJR, O'Reilly PH (eds): Comprehensive Urology. Mosby, London, 2001:67–79

72. Pantilides ML, Bowman SP, George NJR: Levels of PSA that predicts skeletal spread in prostate cancer. Br J Urol 1992;17:299–303

Chapter 90

Gynecological disorders

Alan D. G. Brown and Tara K. Cooper

CHANGES IN THE GENITAL TRACT WITH AGING

The female physiological aging process accelerates after the menopause, particularly in the genital tract.

Hormonal changes

In peri-menopausal women the ovary becomes less responsive to gonadotrophins. This results in a gradual increase in the circulating level of follicular stimulating hormone (FSH) and, later, luteinizing hormone (LH), and a subsequent decrease in estradiol concentration. The FSH level can fluctuate markedly several years before menses cease, so is a poor diagnostic test; but eventually follicular development fails completely, estradiol production is no longer sufficient to stimulate the endometrium, amenorrhea ensues, and FSH and LH levels are persistently elevated, reaching peaks 3–5 years after the menopause. Thereafter there is a gradual decline to pre-menopausal levels 20 years later.[1] In the reproductive years the ovary has three components for steroid biosynthesis: the maturing follicle, functioning corpus luteum, and the stroma. After the menopause the stroma is the only source of estrogen.

Estrone is the major post-menopausal estrogen and it is derived from the conversion of androgens, mainly androstenedione, produced by the ovaries and adrenal glands. The efficiency of this process increases with age and estrone levels rise to four times that found in young women. This conversion also correlates with weight as fat has the ability to aromatize androstenedione to estrone.[2]

The other post-menopausal estrogens include estriol, which is weak and does not seem to have a significant role, and estradiol. Although estradiol secretion is minimal, with blood levels being reduced by 90 percent, it has ten times greater biological activity than estrone so has an important role to play in maintaining hormone-dependent tissues.[3]

Progesterone is derived mainly from the adrenal glands and levels fall steadily. Production of testosterone remains relatively unchanged, so surgical oophorectomy will result in a decrease of serum testosterone levels of up to 50 percent.[4]

Anatomical changes

The major anatomical change is atrophy, which results in smaller and smoother structures, flattened epithelial surfaces, and fibrous stroma with much reduced vascularization and fat content.

OVARY The post-menopausal ovary is small and sclerotic with absence of follicular activity. The cortex involutes and germinal inclusion cysts are found. Lipid droplets may be seen in the stroma as evidence of continuing steroidogenesis.

UTERUS There is a marked reduction in uterine size so that the uterine body to cervix ratio reverts from 4:1 of reproductive life to the 2:1 of childhood. In the myometrium there is interstitial fibrosis and thickened blood vessels due to obliterative, subintimal sclerosis. The endometrium is a single layer of cuboidal cells with a few inactive glands, which may be dilated due to blocked ducts.

CERVIX AND VAGINA The cervix becomes more flush with the vaginal vault. The squamocolumnar junction recedes into the endocervical canal; this can cause stenosis of the external os.

VULVA Post-menopausal changes are characterized by skin shrinkage, loss of prominent landmarks, and sparse, graying hair. The epidermis is thinner although there is increased keratinization. These features may coincide with a vulval epithelial disorder (see below).

PELVIC FLOOR Aging produces pelvic floor weakness. Damage to the nerve supply starts with parturition[5] and progressive denervation is found with prolapse.[6] An important element of pelvic floor support is collagen, which diminishes after the climacteric.

THE MENOPAUSE

The cessation of ovarian function at the menopause has many short- and long-term consequences. Early menopausal symptoms (e.g. mood swings, hot flushes, and night sweats) affect most women to varying degrees and those who have problems can be treated effectively by hormone replacement therapy (HRT).

More serious is the prolonged effect of estrogen deficiency post-menopausally. The average age of the menopause has remained around 51 years for centuries. With female life expectancy now reaching over 80 years there has been a massive increase in the number of post-menopausal women, and the morbidity/mortality from ovarian failure becomes increasingly important. At present there is poor correlation between early symptoms and late consequences, so it is not possible to select women for prophylactic HRT to obtain the most beneficial outcome. The protective influence of HRT against cardiovascular disease and derangement of connective tissue in bone and skin is well documented. Widespread HRT use has been advocated to improve the quality of life and slow down the female aging process,[7] but it is not without its drawbacks and is not accepted universally.

Osteoporosis

In post-menopausal women there is accelerated bone loss, so that by the age of 70 years 50 percent of bone mass is lost, whereas men lose only 25 percent by 80 years.[8] The loss is due to increased bone absorption by osteoclasts. Altered calcium metabolism may be a contributory factor, but the primary defect is generalized connective tissue loss with reduced bone mineral content following breakdown of the organic collagen matrix.[9] The resultant osteoporosis increases the elderly female fracture rate dramatically: 50 percent of women aged 75 years will have sustained one or more fractures at the most common sites of wrists, vertebral bodies (resulting in the classical "Dowager's hump"), and neck of femur. The latter is the most significant consequence of osteoporosis because of its high morbidity and mortality: there is a 20 percent death rate within the first year and half of the survivors will fail to regain their independence.[10]

Hormone replacement therapy for 2 years results in a 66 percent reduction in hip fracture in the subsequent 2 years,[11] and taken for 10 years produces a 60 percent reduction in the overall mortality rate related to osteoporotic fractures.[12] HRT can also protect dentition.

Cardiovascular disease

Heart disease is five times more common in men than in pre-menopausal women, but by age 70 years the sex difference is lost. In younger women estrogen exerts cardioprotective effects through a vasodilatory effect and an alteration in lipid metabolism. Ovarian failure causes increased levels of cholesterol, triglyceride, and low-density lipoprotein (LDL), and a reduction in high-density lipoprotein (HDL). These changes contribute to an increased predisposition to ischemic heart disease.[13] Estrogen therapy can reverse these effects, and observational studies have shown a 30–50 percent reduction in mortality from ischemic heart disease and stroke.[14] The recent HERS study[15] showed less clear-cut benefits in secondary protection, and reported a slight increase in cardiovascular events in the first year of treatment.

Skin changes

Skin changes have been attributed to the aging process, but estrogen deficiency and light exposure also are significant factors. Skin thickness declines after the menopause by 30 percent in the first 10 years, which is comparable to bone loss over the same time.[16] When HRT is started early there is maintenance of skin collagen and thickness.

Postmenopausal bleeding

Postmenopausal bleeding (PMB) is defined as bleeding from the genital tract after 1 year's amenorrhea. The causes are set out in Table 90-1. It must be considered to be due to malignancy until proved otherwise. One percent of isolated episodes and 10 percent of recurrent episodes have a malignant etiology, which is predominantly endometrial carcinoma.[17] More usually, however, the cause is benign, including atrophic vaginitis (greater than 40 percent), endometrial and cervical polyps, decubitus ulceration secondary to prolapse, and vaginal infection. Rarer problems are vulval or vaginal carcinoma and hormone-secreting ovarian tumors that produce endometrial hyperplasia and hence bleeding (see below). Many women in this age group are on tamoxifen therapy for breast cancer, and the drug can have estrogen-like effects on endometrial receptors resulting in hyperplasia, polyp formation, and carcinoma.[18] Selective estrogen receptor modulators (SERMs) such as

Table 90-1 Etiology of post-menopausal bleeding	
Atrophic vaginitis	Neoplastic lesions:
Vaginal infection	Vulval
Benign cervical lesions	Vaginal
Polyp	Cervical
Ectropion/erosion	Uterine
Iatrogenic	Ovarian
HRT	
Tamoxifen	
Extragenital:	
Hematuria	
Rectal bleeding	

raloxifene may prevent this problem. The medical history should include details of any HRT or tamoxifen use.

Examination may be difficult in an elderly patient, and further complicated by obesity and arthritic changes. Investigations include a cervical smear if appropriate and outpatient endometrial sampling, although this can be difficult in the older woman due to cervical stenosis. Vaginal ultrasound measurement of endometrial thickness can be helpful in directing the need for biopsy, with a measurement of less than 5 mm being reassuring.[17]

Hysteroscopy is now the "gold standard" investigation of post-menopausal bleeding. The procedure can be carried out under general anesthesia or as an outpatient, although again cervical stenosis may cause failures. It should be mandatory in cases of recurrent bleeding, and cystoscopy and sigmoidoscopy may also be necessary if there is any doubt about the bleeding source. Laparoscopy and even hysterectomy may be the only way to exclude a small ovarian tumor.

Treatment depends on the cause and is outlined in the appropriate section below. Bleeding after hysterectomy is usually due to atrophic vaginitis or vaginal vault granulation tissue. This can be treated with silver nitrate applications.

HORMONE REPLACEMENT THERAPY

Estrogen therapy is the appropriate treatment for the consequences of ovarian failure, either for symptom relief or prevention of long-term effects. It may be given orally or parenterally (i.e. transvaginally, transdermally, or subcutaneously). There is an additional need for progesterone in women with an intact uterus because unopposed estrogen therapy causes endometrial hyperplasia, which may lead to adenocarcinoma; progesterone for 12–14 days each month reduces these risks[19] and may be administered orally or transdermally. When HRT is given in this cyclical sequential regime there is a withdrawal bleed at the end of each course. In post-menopausal women, progesterone can be given continuously; it prevents endometrial proliferation, so there is no bleeding. The levonorgestrel intrauterine system can fulfill this role.

Oral estrogen

Oral administration is the most widely used route and is convenient, relatively inexpensive, and generally well tolerated. Many combinations are available commercially, both cyclical and continuous. In peri-menopausal women who do not wish frequent withdrawal bleeds, a 3-monthly bleed preparation can

Summary of management algorithm
Work-up in a patient with post-menopausal bleeding

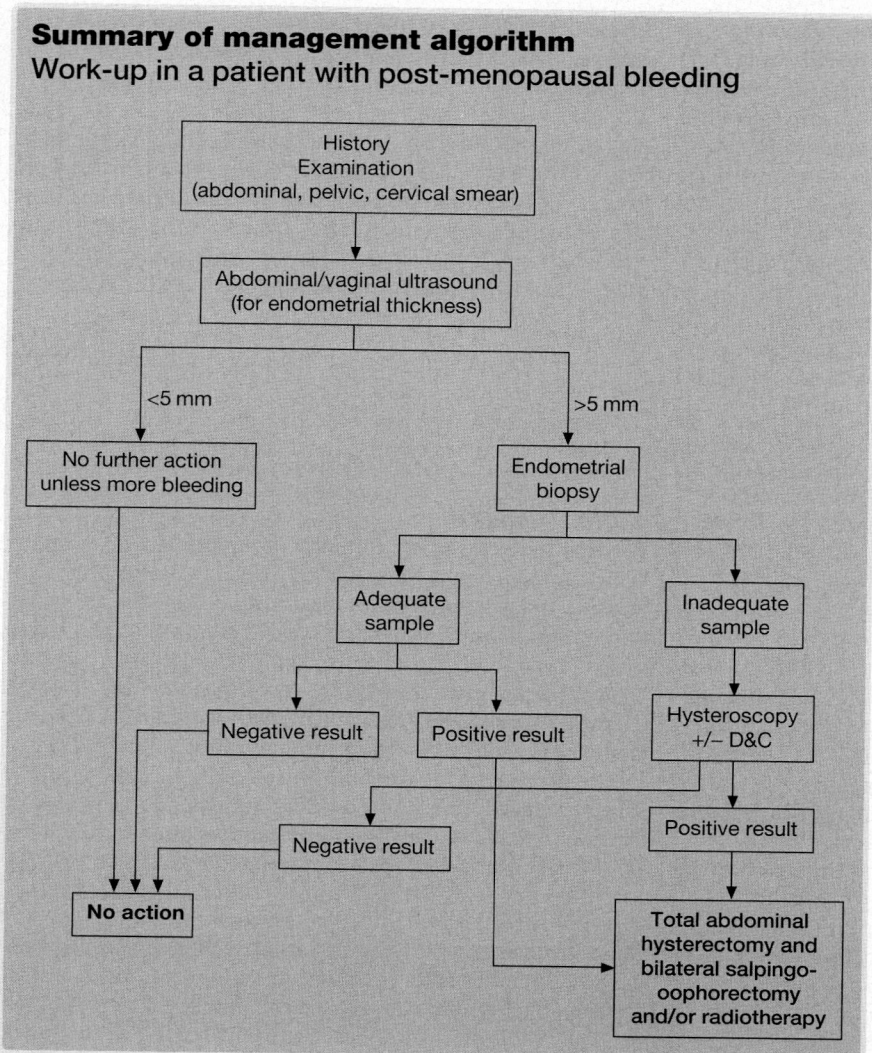

be tried. Tibolone is a synthetic steroid with estrogenic, progestogenic, and androgenic properties and acts as a continuous combined product. It also improves libido and may have fewer effects on breast tissue.[20]

The main disadvantage of the oral route is that estrogen passes directly to the liver, where it is inactivated and partially metabolized to the less effective estrone. This is called the "first-pass" effect and means that higher doses are required than with parenteral therapy. It may also result in altered hepatic metabolism with changes in clotting factors, and increased renin substrate which predisposes to hypertension.

Transdermal estrogen
Transdermal patches may be matrix or reservoir in type and require changing once or twice weekly. Combination patches with progesterone are also available. Estradiol is delivered at a controlled rate depending on surface area. The first-pass effect is avoided and hepatic metabolism not affected, thus reducing the risk of thrombosis. The main problems are with adhesion, and transient skin reactions can occur in up to 30 percent of women; the frequency is less with matrix patches. A transdermal gel may be used instead.

Topical estrogen
Vaginal creams and pessaries are used primarily for treating atrophic vaginitis. Systemic absorption is minimal, but if use is prolonged, progesterone therapy should be considered. In general a short course is adequate: a 14-day course should be followed by two nights' application each week for up to 6 weeks. A problem with this route in the elderly population is reduced acceptability and impaired manual dexterity for self-administration. A district nurse may help, or a slow-release soft vaginal ring provides 3 months' therapy. Other alternatives include a low-dose hydrophilic vaginal tablet which has a fine, prelubricated and preloaded applicator.

Subcutaneous implants
Estradiol implants are inserted in the lower abdominal wall under local anesthesia, and serum levels are sustained for several months depending on the dose. Levels tend to be higher and symptoms tend to return more quickly despite therapeutic serum levels, requiring more frequent implants (tachyphylaxis). This method has become less popular with the introduction of patches but can increase bone mass because of the higher estradiol level.[21]

Contraindications to HRT

There are few contraindications to HRT, which provides estrogen replacement at below the normal pre-menopausal plasma concentrations and the high-dose synthetic steroids used in the combined oral contraceptive pill. The main contraindications are estrogen-dependent breast or endometrial cancers, although women with treated breast cancer and debilitating menopausal symptoms may be given HRT under specialist supervision, and there is no evidence of increased recurrence rates.[22]

Recent reports have suggested a small increase in the risk of venous thromboembolism with HRT, which was not thought previously to exist.[23] Patients with other risk factors should therefore be treated with caution and preferably with transdermal HRT. It is not necessary to stop HRT prior to surgery as most patients will fall into a moderate-risk category (in view of their age) and receive antithrombosis prophylaxis.

HRT may be given where there are pre-existing gynecological conditions (e.g. endometriosis and fibroids), but fibroids may fail to shrink and cause heavier withdrawal bleeds.

Duration of treatment

There is no limit to the duration of HRT. It may be given to women in their sixties and beyond for the first time if they have significant osteoporosis. The principle is to start with the lowest dose available and titrate against symptoms. Long-term therapy requires regular screening of blood pressure and of the breasts with mammography. There is no indication to continue cervical screening longer than normal.

The benefits of HRT are considerable and the question is not so much whether it should be given but when it should be stopped. The chief concern with long-term therapy is that studies have shown a modest increase in breast cancer risk related to use for greater than 10 years.[24] Also, although initially protective against endometrial cancer, use over more than 10 years again causes a modest increase in this cancer too.[25] It therefore seems reasonable to advocate HRT use for 5–10 years to obtain the many benefits, and only continue thereafter in patients willing to accept the risks. Changing to continuous combined HRT as soon as appropriate reduces the endometrial risk.[26] The cardioprotective benefits and reduction in mortality from osteoporosis outweigh the cancer risk, but the latter is more emotive and provokes more fear.

Despite extensive educational products and improved therapies such as "no-bleed" continuous HRT, compliance is poor and 50 percent of patients do not remain on HRT 12 months after starting treatment, even when at risk of osteoporosis.[27]

VULVAL DISORDERS

The vulva is affected by many conditions specific to the area or as part of a more widespread problem, such as psoriasis. Vulval skin is more sensitive than other epithelium because it is subjected to increased heat, friction, and occlusion.[28] Aging is also a factor and some chronic vulval disorders represent an advanced stage of atrophic change.

It is necessary to diagnose vulval pathology accurately, in particular malignancy and infection because, even in the elderly, genital warts, herpes, and *Chlamydia* may be detected.

Therefore, local/general examination and investigation of urine and vaginal discharge, and biopsies of abnormal areas may be required. Vulval epithelial disorders are important because of the severity and chronicity of symptoms (most commonly itching, soreness, and irritation), and the association with carcinoma. There have been conflicting views about pathogenesis, diagnosis, and terminology, but a classification[28] has been agreed by the two international societies for the study of vulval disease and of gynecological pathologists for non-neoplastic epithelial disorders of vulval skin and mucosa. This is:

- lichen sclerosis;
- squamous-cell hyperplasia—when hyperplasia is not attributable to another cause;
- other dermatoses—a noninfective, non-neoplastic skin condition which is recognized as a dermatological entity.

Lichen sclerosis

Lichen sclerosis (LS) is a common problem affecting the aging vulva. The etiology is uncertain but there is an association with genetic and hormonal factors and autoimmune disease.[29] In a study of 350 women with LS, Meyrick Thomas et al. found that lesions were noted at the vulva and elsewhere (97.5 percent), vulva and perianal skin only (44 percent), and vulva alone (38 percent). The vulval appearance varies but the characteristic lesions are a figure-of-eight configuration around the vulva of white plaques of keratin with purple areas where keratin is much reduced; the condition does not extend to the vagina. Fusion of tissue occurs: for example the prepuce to the clitoris and the labia minora, which may lead to introital stenosis. The picture is complicated by chronic scratching, so the skin may be thickened (i.e. lichenified). Although the clinical appearance varies there are characteristic histological features, including an atrophic epidermis with hyalinization and areas of thickening (hyperkeratosis), and inflammation.

The histological pattern varies throughout the vulva. Punch biopsies under local anesthetic should be taken of any suspicious areas to exclude atypical change. Squamous carcinoma is more likely when there is ulceration, raised lesions, or lymph node involvement. The most effective treatment is the range of anti-inflammatory topical steroids, such as betamethasone valerate 0.1% or, if necessary, clobetasol propionate 0.05%, which arrests epithelial reaction. Although the condition is associated with atrophy, topical estrogen is ineffective and should be considered only for vaginal use. Simple vulvectomy has been used for intractable problems, but it is contraindicated because the epithelial changes and symptoms invariably recur.

The risk of LS undergoing change to squamous carcinoma is 5–10 percent.[29] These patients, therefore, should report alteration in symptoms and be checked 6-monthly to yearly.

Vulval discomfort (vulvodynia)

This chronic and complex problem is well known in elderly women and is characterized by pain, burning and rawness of the vulva, or extreme tenderness to touch in that area. The etiology is uncertain but it is now recognized that there are both psychological and physical factors.[30] Specific causative agents have been suggested such as genetic, infective, traumatic, allergic, neurological, and other factors.[31] Depression is a possible factor as these people often live alone. Assessment includes neurological and local examinations with urethral, vaginal, and endocervical swabs to exclude infections. Pathology is rarely found.

Initial treatment consists of local applications used empirically but under strict control and in the short term, such as estrogen, topical steroid, and anesthetic cream. The use of pelvic floor exercises to improve muscle tone and blood supply, and antidepressants, should be considered. It is now widely accepted that a multidisciplinary approach is essential particularly for intractable cases.[32,33] This may involve referral to specialists in psychiatry, pain relief, and gynecological dermatology.

UTEROVAGINAL PROLAPSE

Prolapse of the anterior and posterior vaginal walls occurs independently or together, resulting in any combination of urethrocele, cystocele, rectocele, and enterocele, which are displacements of the underlying urethra, bladder, rectum, and pouch of Douglas (and any contents) respectively. Uterine descent may predominate but usually it is associated with some degree of vaginal laxity. Prolapse is most commonly related to childbirth and post-menopausal hormone deficiency when lack of estrogen causes collagen loss and ligament atrophy.[34] Congenital weakness of sustaining structures and the natural aging process are other factors.

The main supports of the uterus and upper vagina are the transverse cervical, or cardinal, ligaments, which arise from the supravaginal cervix and upper vagina and are inserted into the pelvic side-walls. These ligaments extend anteriorly to form the pubocervical fascia, which supports the bladder base, urethra, and anterior vaginal wall as it travels to insertion in the symphysis pubis; their posterior extensions—the uterosacral ligaments—contribute minimally to uterine support. The lower vagina is buttressed by fibers of the levator ani which are inserted into its side-walls, the urogenital diaphragm, and perineal muscles. In the erect posture the anterior vagina rests on the posterior wall which is strengthened by the rectovaginal fascia and perineal body.

PRESENTATION Major degrees of prolapse are less common now because of lower parity and improved obstetric management. The patient presents with a dragging, or bearing down, sensation of gradual onset which is worse with activity and settles with rest, and a lump may be seen or felt. Urinary symptoms such as frequency, urgency, incontinence and incomplete/slow emptying result from distortion of the prolapsed bladder and urethra, but they may also be due to atrophy, infection, or detrusor overactivity[35]—previously called "detrusor instability." Digital replacement of the anterior or posterior vaginal wall is sometimes necessary before micturition or defecation, respectively, may proceed.

For extensive prolapse problems, dynamic fluoroscopic techniques have been developed which involve different contrast mediums being used to delineate the elements of the prolapse. In one study,[36] 11 of 30 patients had their surgery modified as a result of the radiographic findings.

With prolonged uterine descent, edema occurs owing to interference with venous and lymphatic drainage, leading to epithelial hyperkeratinization and decubital ulceration. Bleeding may result, but carcinoma rarely develops.

MANAGEMENT The management of prolapse depends on the severity of the symptoms, the degree of incapacity, and the patient's operative fitness. Surgery is most effective and includes, as appropriate, anterior colporrhaphy, amputation of the elongated cervix or vaginal hysterectomy, and posterior colpoperineorrhaphy. It is now standard practice to give subcutaneous heparin pre- and postoperatively to reduce venous thromboembolism risk. Most patients tolerate surgery well because of improved anesthetics and minimal postoperative morbidity, and the procedures lead to greater mobility and return to an independent life.

When surgery is contraindicated or declined, conservative measures may be used. A polyvinyl ring pessary is inserted, and inspection and cleaning/renewing every 4–6 months are necessary because mucosal ulceration occurs; in this event the ring should be removed for a few weeks and local estrogen used daily to allow epithelial healing (see the HRT section).

URINARY INCONTINENCE

Urinary incontinence is particularly disabling and distressing, but with modern investigations and treatment symptoms may be alleviated in the elderly population. (See also Chapter 104.) Uninhibited detrusor muscle contractions are usually the cause in geriatric patients owing to age-related changes in the central nervous system. Brading and Turner[37] have shed light on this troublesome condition. Leakage may be due also to weakness, or dysfunction, of the urethral closure mechanism (i.e. genuine stress incontinence) which is a common cause in reproductive or early post-menopausal years.

ASSESSMENT This has reached a high degree of sophistication. Examples are combined video cystourethrography with pressure and flow studies to diagnose detrusor overactivity with/without outlet obstruction.[38] However, static cystometry, where the tests are performed in a combination of lying, standing, or sitting positions, is known to have poor sensitivity and specificity compared with ambulatory monitoring.[39] In this investigation, telemetry is performed over 2–3 hours during which such maneuvers as walking, climbing stairs, hand-washing etc. are performed. The significance of the increased incidence of bladder overactivity with this technique is unclear as asymptomatic control patients have been shown to exhibit overactivity. In an elderly person, however, such simple and noninvasive tests as daily urinary frequency/volume and incontinence charts are important, because the patient or attendants can provide accurate and objective information about bladder habit and function.[40]

MANAGEMENT The treatment of genuine stress incontinence should be nonoperative initially, and the best results for mild/moderate leakage are with pelvic floor exercises.[41] The urethra has two striated muscles within and immediately adjacent to it, and regular, active contraction has been shown to improve leakage and reduce frequent urination. There is limited value in estrogen therapy for either type of leakage,[42] but it has a place when urinary symptoms are associated with significant estrogen deficiency.

GYNECOLOGICAL CANCER

An association has been noted between aging and gynecological cancer development, and there is a tendency for cancers to be at a more advanced stage at presentation.[43] Also, aggressive disease may be more common in older women.[44] Female genital cancer affects four main sites: the vulva, vagina, uterus, and ovary.

The management of gynecological cancer patients is now mostly centralized in units staffed by experienced gynecological oncologists where the care and outcome are improved.

Vulval cancer

Vulval cancer is seen most frequently in the 60–70 year age group and accounts for about 5 percent of genital neoplasia. Early symptoms are pruritis or an asymptomatic lump, but late presentation is more common because of embarrassment and is usually in the form of bleeding and/or an offensive discharge.

Ninety-five percent of tumors are squamous in type, but occasionally malignant melanoma can occur. The lesion commonly arises in the labium majus and spreads directly to the regional lymph glands—the superficial inguinal and prefemoral nodes. Lateral tumors tend to spread to the ipsilateral nodes but centrally placed tumors may involve the contralateral nodes.

Radical vulvectomy with bilateral groin node dissections is the treatment of choice, and it is generally well tolerated even in the elderly patient as there are few postoperative complications. It is curative in 80–90 percent of patients with early-stage disease. The primary tumor is resected and separate groin node dissections are performed rather than the previous conventional butterfly incision, which had increased problems with infection and wound healing.

Wide excision of advanced or recurrent lesions may be used as palliation in patients unfit for radical surgery. If a large vulval defect results, repair may be possible using a myocutaneous flap with rectus abdominus or gracilis muscle. Pelvic radiotherapy is available for extensive nodal involvement, but dosage determination is difficult because of the anatomical site. Chemotherapy is not commonly used in this condition, but topical regimens have been developed, for example 5-fluorouracil.

Nursing management may be difficult owing to increasing problems with catheterization and foul-smelling discharge.

Vaginal cancer

Primary vaginal squamous cancer is rare and virtually confined to the elderly population. Usually vaginal malignancy is metastatic adenocarcinoma with blood or lymphatic spread from the uterus and, rarely, kidney, breast, or colon. Direct invasion may occur from bladder, cervical, or vulval lesions. Presenting symptoms are post-menopausal bleeding, offensive discharge, and eventually fistula formation. Diagnosis is by biopsy and the treatment is usually radiotherapy, although vaginectomy can be considered for primary lesions. Other surgical measures include urinary diversion for a fistula or palliative vaginal closure (colpocleisis). Endometrial metastases show some response to high-dose progesterone.

Cancer of the uterus
CERVIX Worldwide, cervical cancer is the most common gynecological malignancy. In developed countries the incidence is falling significantly as a result of screening programs, although premalignant disease of the cervix is increasing.[45] Screening programs stop at 60 years, but if an abnormal smear is found in a woman over this age it is 16 times more likely to lead to a diagnosis of invasive cancer compared with women aged under 30 years.[46] Etiological factors are early age of coitus, many sexual partners, and a history of sexually transmitted disease. The human papilloma virus (HPV) types 16 and 18 have been incriminated in the pathogenesis of invasive squamous carcinoma and are detectable in over 90 percent of cases. New methods of screening to include detection of HPV are being developed.

Elderly patients will present with such symptoms as offensive vaginal discharge and post-menopausal or post-coital bleeding. Pain is experienced late and related usually to diffuse pelvic infiltration or bony metastases. The first sign of this cancer may be obstructive renal failure from hydronephrosis due to advanced disease.

Diagnosis is by biopsy of suspicious areas, preferably under general anesthesia so that clinical staging and evaluation of histological tumor grade is achieved. Squamous-cell cancer accounts for more than 80 percent of cases. Lymphatic metastases occur quickly, so up to 50 percent of early lesions have pelvic spread at presentation.

Tumors confined to the cervix may be treated by radical hysterectomy and pelvic node dissection, or radiotherapy. Both treatments carry similar 5-year survival rates in early stages, but in elderly patients radiotherapy has been more commonly used because of the fear of radical surgery complications. However, a fit elderly patient will tolerate the procedure well and should not be denied it on the basis of age alone. In advanced disease the tumor may infiltrate locally, causing fistula formation to the bladder or rectum. As in other squamous carcinomas, the success of chemotherapy is limited.

CORPUS UTERI Endometrial adenocarcinoma is the most common gynecological malignancy in the elderly population. The mean age at presentation is 62 years.[47] Post-menopausal bleeding is the most frequent symptom and occurs early, so the prognosis tends to be good. There are significant associations with celibacy, nulliparity and late menopause, and with obesity, hypertension, and diabetes mellitus (Saint's Triad). The etiological role of estrogen is established with endometrial proliferation occurring which may result in carcinoma. This may be from such endogenous sources as polycystic ovary syndrome, hormone-producing ovarian tumors, or exogenous unopposed estrogen.[48] This latter process is opposed by adding cyclical or continuous progesterone to hormone replacement therapy regimens.[49] Although this confers protection, new data suggest that long-term use of cyclical hormones will cause a duration-dependent increase in endometrial cancer, so patients should be changed to continuous combined regimens as soon as is appropriate.[25]

More rarely sarcomatous and mixed mesodermal tumors occur and they have a poorer prognosis.

Diagnosis and clinical staging are achieved using examination under anesthesia, usually with hysteroscopy and curettage. The majority of cancers are in the early stage and are treated by total abdominal hysterectomy and bilateral salpingo-oophorectomy. Postoperative radiotherapy is given when the myometrium is invaded beyond the inner third or if there is poor differentiation; usually it is a combination of vaginal radiotherapy to reduce vault recurrence, which occurs in up to 12 percent,[50] and external radiotherapy. Tumors extending to the cervix may require preoperative irradiation or Wertheim hysterectomy, but this increases the morbidity with no improvement in results.

Advanced cancers are treated with radiotherapy and then surgery if the response is good. Progestational agents cause regression of endometrial hyperplasia and carcinoma-in-situ, and are used as adjunctive therapy. This may control vaginal bleeding associated with advanced disease and reduce pain from bony metastases.

Ovarian cancer

Ovarian cancer remains the most lethal gynecological malignancy and is currently the fifth leading cause of female cancer deaths. It affects those aged 65 years and older more frequently than younger women, with almost 50 percent of ovarian tumors occurring in this age group. More of the older women are likely to present with advanced disease and are less likely to be offered radical surgery and chemotherapy. The onset and progress is often insidious, so a high index of suspicion is necessary in post-menopausal women with nonspecific symptoms such as abdominal discomfort and swelling, malaise, and weight loss. In a post-menopausal woman with ascites, ovarian cancer should be the diagnosis until proved otherwise. Currently there is no satisfactory screening method for ovarian neoplasia, but women with a family history of breast or ovarian cancer should be offered regular ultrasonic assessment. The tumor marker CA125 is an indicator of ovarian malignancy and is elevated in about 90 percent of carcinomas. It is used for confirmation of diagnosis or suspicion of recurrence, but is being studied in conjunction with ultrasound as a screening tool.

Ninety percent of ovarian malignancies in older women are epithelial adenocarcinomas, but other ovarian components may become malignant and give rise to such histological types as sex-cord and germ-cell tumors; also metastases may be seen from elsewhere, particularly colon and breast.

Granulosa cell tumor is the most common sex-cord malignancy and up to 60 percent occur after the menopause. Hormone production can cause vaginal bleeding due to endometrial hyperplasia. This association is also often seen with a benign thecoma arising from cortical stroma.

ASSESSMENT Investigations include hematological and biochemical profiles, chest X-ray, and ultrasound screening of the pelvis and renal tract which can be diagnostic as ascites and solid areas within an ovarian cyst are strongly suggestive of malignancy. Laparotomy establishes the diagnosis, and examination of abdominal contents provides accurate staging which will influence treatment and prognosis.

MANAGEMENT Patients with suspected ovarian cancer should have their primary surgery carried out by a gynecological oncologist. Debulking of the tumor with bilateral salpingo-oophorectomy, total hysterectomy, and omentectomy is the mainstay of treatment. Complete tumor removal may be difficult, but the greater the reduction of tumor bulk the more effective is adjuvant therapy, and ascites is better controlled.

Postoperative chemotherapy is used in all but stage 1 disease, and indeed many patients will have residual disease after surgery. Cisplatin and carboplatin remain the agents of choice; they are toxic and side-effects include myelosuppression and nephro- and neurotoxicity, and severe emetogenesis. They are given by intermittent intravenous therapy with sufficient antiemetics and fluids to minimize problems. Between 40 and 50 percent of patients with extensive disease will have complete remission with platinum, but the majority relapse within 2 years.[51] A less aggressive option is the oral alkylating agent, chlorambucil, which is sometimes used in the elderly patient.

Failure of first-line treatment is ominous as recurrent disease is often resistant to further therapy, but taxanes are tried in these patients with some success. Recurrent ascites is a major problem and requires repeated paracentesis; spironolactone may reduce the fluid and limit recurrence. Radiotherapy is limited to unresectable tumors and patients with symptomatic recurrence and is used only for palliation.

SEXUALITY AND AGING

There is a view that sexuality in elderly people is irrelevant and sexual activity unnecessary. The facts are, however, that sexual drive is not exhausted with aging, and as life expectancy increases it is necessary to recognize that continued sexual activity is an important requirement of old age to promote satisfactory relationships, personal well-being, and quality of life. There will be an increasing demand from this age group for advice and expert help on sexual matters.[52] Many older people have problems because they grew up in sexually restricted times so that ignorance is widespread.[53] Society now has an obsession with youth and its sexuality while largely stereotyping elderly people and ignoring their difficulties in this area. In addition, as is generally the case with disabled people, the organization of institutions for elderly people does not recognize their sexuality, so their needs (e.g. opportunities for privacy) are ignored.[54]

A longitudinal study[55] has shown that sexual activity remains relatively constant within a stable relationship and declines only following a negative event particularly for the male partner, for example the death of the spouse. Many factors contribute to changing sexuality such as age, physical appearance, self-image, culture, education, and social attitudes.

Sexual behavior and age in men

A steady reduction in male sexuality from early and middle years has been observed.[56] A common phenomenon in older men is erectile dysfunction due to penile arterial insufficiency and/or the effect of such drugs as antihypertensives, and illnesses like diabetes.[57] Brecher[58] noted that 75 percent of 70-year-old men continued to have some sexual activity. A Danish study showed that in men aged 51–95 years the related phenomena of sexual interest and morning erections diminished with age;[59] coital activity declined dramatically whereas masturbation did to a lesser extent, indicating that the latter is the most common outlet in the very old.

Waning sexuality with age is also related to previous experience.[60] Those who have high levels of activity in early life experience less change with age, whereas low interest in young men is associated with increased problems later.

Sexual behavior and age in women

An early study observed little change in women's capacity for sexual activity until later life.[61] However, questionnaires[62,63] from both sexes between ages 45 and 71 were analyzed. A greater reduction was noted in sexual interest and activity in women, the most significant change being between 50 and 60 years. At 66 to 71 years, 50 and 10 percent of women and men, respectively, had no sexual interest. Perrson[64] noted that only 16 percent of 70-year-old women were having intercourse compared with 46 percent of men at the same age. As with men, low activity levels in youth are associated with decreased activity in later life.[65]

Sexual interest also depends on the availability of a partner. Women who tend to marry older men who die before them are often left alone and may experience difficulty finding a new partner.[53] Thus masturbation may become a more regular activity. It has been found that female sexual activity was highest in those currently married and it progressively reduced in the divorced, widowed, and never-married.[66] Resumption of interest a year after widowhood is more likely when death was expected, there had been extramarital experience, and in younger women; activity diminished when the marriage had been sexually satisfying and there was still a strong attachment to the lost partner.[67]

The role of the menopause has been studied in 800 Swedish women aged 38–54 years.[68] With advancing years there was reduced sexual interest, orgasmic capacity, and coital frequency. It was shown that decline in interest was the result rather than the cause of infrequent coitus, and diminished activity was due to the menopause and not to aging.

A common problem following post-menopausal lack of estrogen is vaginal atrophy and dryness causing dyspareunia,[58] which leads to a loss of interest and activity. It has been observed[69] that the more sexually active woman (with coitus and masturbation) has less vaginal atrophy, suggesting that activity protects the vagina by stretching and possibly stimulating hormone production. The use of HRT has been studied.[70] Estrogen, androgen, and a combination of both and placebo were compared in oopherectomized women. The results indicated a beneficial effect of androgen alone or with estrogen on sexual motivation and coital frequency. Thus the evidence suggests that female sexuality is affected by aging but initially less so than by the menopause, and the hormones involved are estrogen and androgen. Testosterone treatment has been recommended in women where other therapeutic and counseling techniques have not helped.[71] Tibolone is an oral HRT preparation which contains androgen and has been shown to improve sexual problems, including reduced libido.[72] Alternatively, a 6-week trial of testosterone undecanoate, 40 mg daily, may be used and if there is no beneficial effect the drug should be stopped. A subcutaneous implant of 50 mg testosterone is also effective. With either treatment there is little risk of masculinizing effects such as hirsutism or deepening of the voice; however, if these symptoms occur treatment should be discontinued.

Sexual response and aging

It has been noted[71] that with age vasocongestive changes following sexual stimulation develop more slowly in both sexes; these alterations are gradual so that the couple adjusts to activity that is less intense but may be as enjoyable. In older men, morning erections are less frequent, they develop slowly, and pyschic stimulation is less effective, so direct tactile stimulation is often required although sensitivity to touch is reduced.[53] Maintenance of the erection is not as good and if lost is more difficult to regain. Also ejaculation is less forceful, with a small volume and fewer contractions; scrotal and testicular changes are reduced, the postorgasmic resolution phase is rapid, and the refractory period prolonged.

In women, vaginal lubrication diminishes and takes longer, and there is less vaginal elasticity so that there is shrinkage in the absence of coitus. There are changes elsewhere; for example, nipple erection and breast engorgement are less marked and orgasm is associated with fewer contractions, but orgasmic capacity may not be reduced.[58] Another study suggested a decrease in orgasmic capacity post-menopausally;[73] also the sense of touch in the genital area may be reduced or experienced as unpleasant or painful, which can further inhibit orgasm.

Management of couples with sexual problems

The management of sexual problems should be guided by the same principles irrespective of age and condition of the patient, though the emphasis may vary. Both partners should take part in therapy because although one usually presents a problem the other invariably contributes to it, and the treatment is obviously facilitated by cooperation. After an initial discussion the couple should be seen separately so that confidential interviews are obtained, including information not to be disclosed to the partner. A preliminary medical and social history may suggest contributing factor(s) and helps rapport to be established before turning to more sensitive questions.

The sexual history concerns the couple's problems, their duration, and current activity. Their past life together is relevant, particularly the emotional relationship which has a profound effect on sexual function. Information is required about early experience, including masturbation, difficulties with previous partners, and any episode of sexual assault is most important. Negative parental and religious sexual attitudes have profound effects on development and are often major factors causing future disorder. Examination and investigation will depend on whether a physical basis is suggested, particularly in men where sexuality is most commonly affected by such problems. For example, in a study[74] where 262 patients with erectile dysfunction were investigated, 52 percent had organic disease, the most common being arterial and urological disorders.

Behavioral techniques include stressing the couple's mutual responsibility for their shared problem, and changing negative attitudes resulting from parental or religious influences or past experiences. Ignorance about sexuality is common so there is a need for basic education and permission to experiment, for example, with different methods of stimulation and coital positions. Couples, particularly older ones, frequently have difficulty talking to each other about sexual anxieties or needs, and discussion with the therapist increases their mutual understanding and ability to communicate.

A series of touching exercises called "sensate focus"[53,71] have been devised to improve lovemaking and analyze the couple's emotional response. An initial ban on intercourse and fondling the breasts and genitals is advised to reduce performance anxiety because many problems relate to difficulties with erection, intercourse, and orgasm. The initial exercises, therefore, are not goal-oriented, and they allow each partner to experiment with touching the other in a pleasurable and nondemanding way and to communicate through touch. The sensations and any problems encountered are discussed together and later with the therapist, and when difficulties are overcome progress is allowed slowly with genital contact and then coitus. Thus sensate focus is a gradual relearning of sexual or courting behavior, which initially involves touching and kissing, leading to intercourse. It forms the basis for treatment of most disorders and the results are generally good.[75]

Treatment of erectile dysfuntion

For men with psychogenic, organic, or mixed erectile dysfunction (ED) a variety of treatments have become available in recent years. A concise account of these is available.[76] After a full assessment to screen for conditions associated with ED, the following main options have been successful.

SYSTEMIC THERAPY Sildenafil (prostaglandin E1) is a type-5 phosphodiesterase inhibitor which prevents the breakdown of cyclic GMP and prolongs corporeal smooth muscle relaxation. The standard dose of 50–100 mg improves erectile quality compared with placebo.[77] The common mild side-effects are headache, flushing, and dyspepsia with, rarely, a temporary loss of blue color discrimination. Sildenafil should not be used with organic nitrates or nitric oxide donors (e.g. amyl nitrite) because of the risk of profound hypotension; also a lower dose of 25 mg should be used with such drugs as cimetidine and erythromycin which significantly increase sildenafil concentrations, and the protease inhibitors (e.g. ritonavir) because of pharmacokinetic interaction. Other systemic therapy now available includes apomorphine hydrochloride which stimulates dopamine receptors in the hypothalmus and mid-brain, and enhances erection.

LOCAL THERAPY Until the introduction of sildenafil, intracavernosal alprostadil was the only ED treatment licenced in the UK. It is available in doses of 2.5–40 µg and is titrated from an initial level of 2.5–5 µg to find the most effective dose. Men can be taught to self-inject the drug, but instructions are required in the event of prolonged erection (4–6 hours) with such measures as exercise and ice-pack application. If these are unsuccessful the patient should attend the nearest Emergency department for aspiration of the corpora. The intracavernosal technique is still used when sildenafil is ineffective.

A further local treatment is the intraurethral insertion of alprostadil using the "MUSE" (Medicated Urethral System for Erection) technique. The pellets are available in 250–1,000 µg of the drug and good results have been achieved,[78] but generally this technique has not been widely accepted.

In the UK, there are currently limitations to the prescribing of ED drugs in the National Health Service; they are allowed only in men who have had, for example, prostate surgery, renal failure, spinal cord injury, diabetes mellitus, multiple sclerosis, and some other specific medical conditions. Those suffering severe emotional stress due to ED are entitled to a prescription, but many health authorities have not provided funding so the men have to rely on a private script from their hospital clinic or general practitioner.

Mechanical devices have been tried for ED such as vacuum cylinders and penile prostheses. The latter technique involves referral to a specialist urologist for detailed counseling and management.

KEY POINTS Gynecological disorders

- The female aging process accelerates after the menopause, particularly in the genital tract as a result of cessation of ovarian estrogen production.

- An elderly patient with gynecological cancer should be offered the same surgical treatment recommended to younger women.

- In most cases of itchy or painful vulva, the diagnosis will be made following a detailed history/examination and biopsy when indicated. Appropriate treatment is likely to be successful.

- There is no age limit to the expression of sexuality. The range of counseling and other treatments for sexual problems is appropriate in the elderly population.

REFERENCES

1. Speroff L, Glass RH, Kase NG: Clinical Gynaecology Endocrinology, and Infertility, 5th edn. Williams & Wilkins, Baltimore, 1994:101–111
2. Upton GV: The menopause: physiologic correlates and clinical management. J Reprod Med 1982;27:1–27
3. Morse AR, Hutton JD, Jacob HS et al: Relation between karyopyknotic index and plasma oestrogen concentrations after the menopause. Br J Obstet Gynaecol 1979;86:981–983
4. Judd HL, Judd GE, Lucas WE et al: Endocrine function of the post-menopausal ovary: concentrations of androgens and oestrogens in ovarian and peripheral blood. J Clin Endocrinol Metab 1994;39:102–104
5. Smith ARB, Hosker GL, Warrell DW: Partial denervation of the pelvic floor in aetiology of genital tract prolapse. J Obstet Gynaecol 1989;96:25–29
6. Allan RE, Hosker GL, Smith ARB, Warrell DW: The role of pregnancy and childbirth in partial denervation of the pelvic floor. Neurol Urodyn 1988;7:237–239
7. Whitehead MI, Studd JWW: Selection of patients for treatment: which therapy and for how long? Menopause 1988;116–129
8. Grimley Evans J: The significance of osteoporosis. In Smith R (ed): Osteoporosis. Royal College of Physicians, London, 1990:1–8
9. Savvas M, Brincat M, Studd JWW: Postmenopausal osteoporosis. Br J Hosp Med 1987;38:16–18,22,24
10. Cummings SR, Kelsey JL, Nevitt MC et al: Epidemiology of osteoporosis and osteoporotic fractures. Epidemiol Rev 1985;7:178–208
11. Keil DP, Felson DP, Anderson JJ et al: Hip fracture and the use of estrogens in postmenopausal women: the Framingham Study. N Engl J Med 1987;317:1169–1174
12. Ross RK, Pike PC, Henderson BE et al: Stroke prevention and oestrogen replacement therapy. Lancet 1989;1:505
13. Whitehead MI: The climacteric. In Studd JWW (ed): Progress in Obstetrics and Gynaecology, vol 3. Churchill Livingstone, London, 1985:338–339
14. Wolff PH et al: Reduction of cardiovascular disease-related mortality among postmenopausal women who use hormones: evidence from a national cohort. Am J Obstet Gynecol 1991;164:489–494
15. Hulley S, Gray GD, Bush T et al: Randomized trial of estrogen plus progestin for secondary prevention of coronary heart disease in postmenopausal women: Heart and Estrogen/progestin Replacement Study (HERS) Research Group. JAMA 1998;280:605–613
16. Brincat M, Moniz CJ, Studd JWW et al: Long term effects of menopause and sex hormones on skin thickness. Br J Obstet Gynaecol 1985;92:256–259

17. McKay Hart D: Postmenopausal bleeding. In: Medical Dialogue 362, 1992
18. Love CDB, Muir BB, Scrimgeour JB et al: Investigation of endometrial abnormalities in asymptomatic women treated with tamoxifen and an evaluation of the role of endometrial screening. J Clin Oncol 1999;17:2050–2054
19. Studd JWW, Magos A: Oestrogen therapy and endometrial pathology. Menopause 1988;18:197–212
20. Gompel A, Kandouz M, Siromachkova M et al: The effect of tibolone on proliferation, differentiation and apoptosis in normal breast cells. Gynecol Endocrinol 1997;1:77–79
21. Savvas M, Studd JWW, Fogelman I et al: Skeletal effect of oral oestrogen compared with subcutaneous oestrogen and testosterone in postmenopausal women. BMJ 1988;297:331–333
22. Vassilopoulou-Sellin R, Theriault RL: Randomised prospective trial of oestrogen replacement therapy in women with a history of breast cancer. J Natl Cancer Inst Mongr 1994;16:153–159
23. Daly E, Vessey MP, Hawkins MM et al: Risk of venous thromboembolism in users of hormone replacement therapy. Lancet 1996;348:977–980
24. Sillero-Arenas M, Delgado-Rodriguez M, Rodriguez-Conteras R et al: Menopausal hormone replacement therapy and breast cancer: a meta-analysis. Obstet Gynecol 1992;79:286–294
25. Beresford SAA, Weiss NS, Voight LF et al: Risk of endometrial cancer in relation to use of oestrogen combined with cyclic progestogen therapy in postmenopausal women. Lancet 1997;349:458–461
26. Sturdee DW, Ulrich LG, Barlow DH et al: The endometrial response to sequential and continuous oestrogen–progestogen replacement therapy. Br J Obstet Gynaecol 200;107:1392–1400
27. Hope S, Wager E, Rees M: Survey of British Women's views on the menopause and HRT. J Br Menopause Soc 1998;4(1):33–36
28. Ridley CM: Dermatological conditions of the vulva. In Stanton SL (ed): Clinical Obstetrics and Gynaecology. Baillière Tindall, London, 1988:317–339
29. Meyrick Thomas RH, Ridley CM, McGibbon DH et al: Lichen sclerosis et atrophicus and autoimmunity: a study of 350 women. Br J Dermatol 1988;118:41–46
30. Nunns D: Vulvodynia: the basic facts. CME Bull Gynaecol 1999;1(2):36–37
31. Wylie KR, Hallam-Jones R, Coan A et al: A review of psychophenomenological aspects of vulval pain. Sex Marital Ther 1999;14(2):151–164
32. Bradley JJ, Ridley CM: Historical and psychological considerations: subjective and traumatic conditions of the vulva. In Ridley CM (ed): The Vulva. Churchill Livingstone, London, 1988
33. Graziottin A: Organic and psychological factors in vulval pain; implications for management. Sex Marital Ther 1998;13:329–338
34. Brincat M, Moniz CF, Studd JWW et al: Sex hormones and skin collagen content in postmenopausal women. BMJ 1983;287:1337–1338
35. Wyndaele JJ: The overactive bladder. BJU Int 2001;88:135–140
36. Nager C, Kumar D, Stanton S: Female pelvic floor investigations: a review. The Diplomate 1998;5:167–173
37. Brading AF, Turner WH: The unstable bladder: towards a common mechanism. Br J Urol 1994;73:3–8
38. Bates CP, Whiteside CG, Turner-Warwick RT: Synchronous cine-pressure flow cystourethography with special reference to stress and urge incontinence. Br J Urol 1970;42:714–723
39. Bristow SE, Neal DE: Ambulatory urodynamics. Br J Urol 1996;77:333–338
40. Brown ADG: The GP's role in the management of female urinary incontinence. Practitioner 1988;232:768–769
41. Wilson PD, Al Samarrai T, Deakin M et al: An objective assessment of physiotherapy for female genuine stress incontinence. Br J Obstet Gynaecol 1987;94:575–582
42. Wilson PD, Farragher B, Butler B et al: Treatment with oral piperazine oestrone sulphate for genuine stress incontinence in postmenopausal women. Br J Obstet Gynaecol 1987;94:568–574
43. Lawton FG, Hacker NF: Surgery for invasive gynecologic cancer in the elderly female population. Obstet Gynecol 1990;76:287–289
44. Merino MJ, Jaffe G: Age contrast in ovarian pathology. Cancer 1993;71:634–637
45. Hackama M: Trends in the incidence of cervical cancer in the Nordic countries. In Magnus K (ed): Trends in Cancer Incidence. Hemisphere Publishing, Washington, DC, 1982:279–292
46. Shingleton HM, Partridge EE, Austin JM: The significance of age in the colposcopic evaluation of women with atypical Papanicolaou smears. Obstet Gynecol 1977;49:61–64

47. Studd JWW, Tom M: Oestrogens and endometrial cancer. In Studd JWW (ed): Progress in Obstetrics and Gynaecology. Churchill Livingstone, London, 1981:182–188
48. Whitehead MI, Lane G, Dyer G et al: Estradiols: the predominant intranuclear estrogen in the endometrium of estrogen-treated postmenopausal women. Br J Obstet Gynaecol 1981;88:914–918
49. Studd JWW, Magos A: Oestrogen therapy and endometrial pathology. Menopause 1988;18:197–212
50. Kilstad P: Advances in the treatment of carcinoma of the cervix and corpus uteri. In Bonner J (ed): Recent Advances in Obstetrics and Gynaecology, vol 14. Churchill Livingstone, Edinburgh, 1982:325–340
51. Wiltshaw E, Kroner T: Phase II study of cis-diaminodichloroplatinum (III) 9NSC 119875 in advanced adenocarcinoma of the ovary. Cancer Treat Rep 1960:50–60
52. Webster L: Sex and ageing. Br J Sex Med 1992;19:124–126
53. Bancroft J: Human Sexuality and Its Problems, 2nd edn. Churchill Livingstone, Edinburgh, 1989
54. White CB: Sexual interest, attitudes, knowledge and sexual history in relation to sexual behaviour in the institutionalised aged. Arch Sex Behav 1982;11:11–22
55. George L, Weiler SJ: Sexuality in middle and late life. Arch Gen Psych 1981;38:919–923
56. Kinsey AC, Pomoroy WB, Martin CE: Sexual Behaviour in the Human Male. WB Saunders, Philadelphia, 1948
57. Pentimone F, Del Corso L: Male impotence in old age. Minerva Medica 1994;85:261–264
58. Brecher EM: Love, Sex and Aging: A Consumer's Union Report. Little Brown, Boston, 1984
59. Hegelar S, Mortensen M: Sexuality and Ageing. Br J Sex Med 1978;5:16–19
60. Martin CE: Factors affecting sexual functioning in 60–79 year old married males. Arch Sex Behav 1981;10L399–420
61. Kinsey AC, Pomoroy WB, Martin CE et al: Sexual Behaviour in the Human Female. WB Saunders, Philadelphia, 1953
62. Pheiffer E, Davis GC: Determinants of sexual behaviour in middle and old age. J Am Geriatr Soc 1972;20:151–158
63. Pheiffer E, Verwoerdt A, Davis GC: Sexual behavior in middle life. Am J Psych 1972;128:1262–1267
64. Persson G: Sexuality in the 70-year old urban population. J Psychosom Res 1990;24:335–342
65. Christenson CV, Gagnon JH: Sexual behaviour in a group of older women. J Gerontol 1965;20:351–356
66. Corby N, Solnick RL: Psychosocial and physiological influences in sexuality in the older adult. In Birren JE, Sloane RE (eds): Handbook of Mental Health and Aging. Prentice-Hall, Englewood Cliffs, NJ, 1980
67. Kansky J: Sexuality of widows: a study of sexual practices of widows during the first 14 months of bereavement. J Sex Marital Ther 1986;12:307–321
68. Halstrom T: Mental Disorders and Sexuality in the Climacteric. Scandinavian University Books, Goteborg, 1973
69. Lieblum S, Bachman G, Kemmann E et al: Vaginal atrophy in the postmenopausal woman: the importance of sexual activity and hormones. JAMA 1983;249:2195–2198
70. Sherwin BB, Gelfand MM: The role of androgen in the maintenance of sexual functioning in oopherectomised women. Psychosomat Med 1987;49:397–409
71. Griffin M: The sexual health of women after the menopause. Sex Marital Ther 1995;10:277–291
72. Rhymer JM, Chapman M, Fogelman I et al: A study of the effect of tibolone on the vagina in postmenopausal women. Maturitas 1994;18:127–133
73. McCoy NL, Davidson JM: A longitudinal study of the effects of the menopause on sexuality. Maturitas 1985;7:203–210
74. Masters WH, Johnson VE: Human Sexual Response. Churchill Livingstone, London, 1966
75. Warner P, Bancroft J and Members of the Edinburgh Human Sexuality Group: A regional clinical service for sexual problems: a 3-year survey. Sex Marital Ther 1987;2:115–126
76. Williams G: Male erectile dysfunction. Prescriber's J 2000;40:49–58
77. Goldstein I, Lue TF, Padma-Nathan H et al: Oral sildenafil in the treatment of erectile dysfunction: Sildenafil Study Group. N Engl J Med 1998;338:1397–1404
78. Williams G, Abbou C-C, Amar AT et al: Efficacy and safety of transurethral alprostadil therapy in men with erectile dysfunction: MUSE Study Group. Br J Urol 1998;81:889–894

Chapter 91

Carcinoma of the breast

Robert E. Mansel

Management of elderly patients with cancer of the breast is often directed toward preservation of quality of life, with less emphasis on "cure" than is usual with younger patients. Achieving a balance between minimizing intervention, which may reduce quality of life temporarily, and securing lasting relief from local and systemic effects of the cancer can present the clinician with several difficulties.

PRESENTATION, DIAGNOSIS, AND STAGING

Carcinoma of the breast can present in various ways, as follows.

PAINLESS LUMP Any discrete mass within the breast of a patient over 65 years old is likely to be malignant whether it displays overt signs of malignancy or not. Cysts are uncommon as the normal age range for these is 35–60 years. A "cyst" in a patient over the age of 65 is more likely to be a cancer with a necrotic center. Ancient fibroadenomas may present as the surrounding breast tissue undergoes involution but these are normally heavily calcified and easily visible on mammography. The incidence of inflammatory masses related to duct ectasia decreases from the seventh decade onward.[1] Fat necrosis can simulate a malignant mass, but is usually preceded by a history of trauma and extensive bruising.

DISCHARGE FROM THE NIPPLE A persistent serous or blood-stained discharge from a single duct is usually associated with a benign ductal papilloma, but the proportion of patients with such a discharge who have a carcinoma rises to about 30 percent in the seventh decade.[2]

PERSISTENT LOCALIZED PAIN Five to 15 percent of carcinomas present with pain or tenderness.[1,3] Most will also have a palpable mass.

PAGET'S DISEASE Any eczema-like eruption on the nipple should be viewed with suspicion. Although there may be no palpable mass, all cases are associated with ductal carcinomas. If neglected the rash spreads outward onto the skin of the breast.

FUNGATION A majority of patients presenting with neglected, locally advanced tumors are elderly. The appearance may vary from a shrunken ulcerated plaque (automastectomy) to a cavitating mass with bleeding, purulent exudate, slough, and offensive odor.

EFFECTS OF METASTASIS Rarely patients may present with symptoms due to metastases (e.g. bone pain or shortness of breath).

Diagnosis

With fine-needle aspiration cytology, needle biopsy, and mammography it is usually possible to confirm malignancy without the need for open biopsy. Modern triple assessment using ultrasound imaging has increased the accuracy of preoperative diagnosis. The stage of the tumor can be assessed clinically (Table 91-1) and is a guide to the prognosis (Fig. 91-1). More recently core needle biopsy using a 14 gauge needle with ultrasound guidance has become the preferred diagnostic method. The rate of preoperative diagnosis has risen steadily throughout the 1990s and was recorded as 92 percent in the latest NHS Breast Screening Programme Review in 1999.

Screening by mammography

The initial design of the National Health Screening Programme imposed an upper limit of 64 years on women invited for screening and there have been recent calls for extension of the program to older women. Women who reach 64 years while in the program can elect to continue to be screened. Recent studies indicate that older women do respond to screening invitations as readily as younger women. Extending screening to older women has major financial implications in view of the growing proportion of elderly women in the population. The detection rate for elderly women is higher than that for women under 65 years (13.1 cancers per 1,000 mammograms vs 5.9; NHS Screening Programme Review, 1999).

TREATMENT
Early (Stage I and II) cancer

The standard surgical treatment in the past for "early" cancer of the breast was some form of mastectomy. More recently

---

Table 91-1 Clinical staging of cancer of the breast

Stage I: Only breast parenchymal tissue is involved
  Palpable tumor in breast, not involving skin or fixed to deep structures; no palpable nodes
Stage II: Breast parenchymal + ipsilateral axillary node involvement
  Primary tumor as stage I, with palpable, mobile, discrete, ipsilateral axillary nodes[a]
Stage III: Local extension beyond breast or axillary nodes
  Deep fixation or involvement of skin of breast (infiltration, ulceration, edema, or satellite nodules) and/or axillary nodes fixed to chest wall or to skin of axilla or matted to each other
Stage IV: Distant spread
  Any more distant disease

[a] *Histological confirmation of nodal involvement gives better prognostic discrimination.*

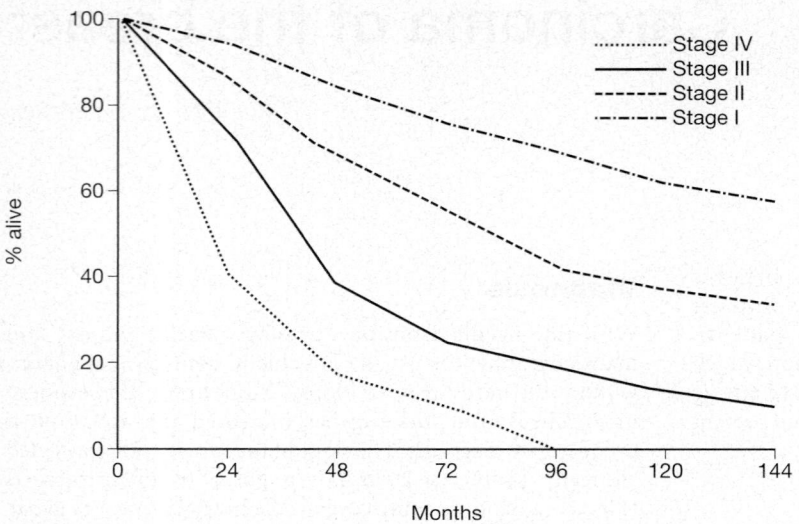

Figure 91-1 Survival of patients with breast cancer stratified by clinical stage (South Manchester data, 1976–1990).

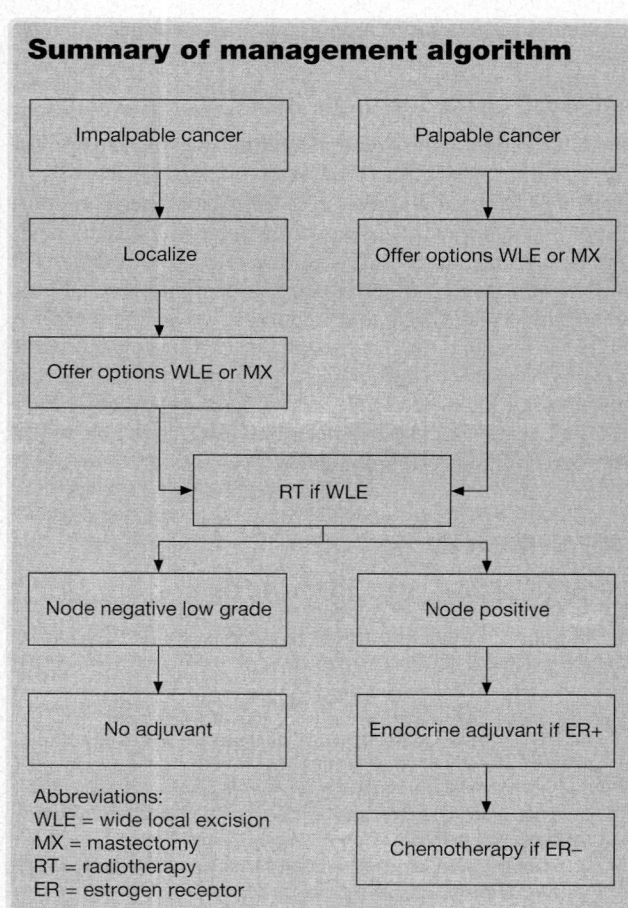

Summary of management algorithm

Impalpable cancer

Palpable cancer

Localize

Offer options WLE or MX

Offer options WLE or MX

RT if WLE

Node negative low grade

Node positive

No adjuvant

Endocrine adjuvant if ER+

Chemotherapy if ER–

Abbreviations:
WLE = wide local excision
MX = mastectomy
RT = radiotherapy
ER = estrogen receptor

there has been a trend for reducing the extent of surgery because studies have shown that wide excision of the cancer with postoperative radiotherapy gives similar results in terms of local recurrence and mortality as does mastectomy.[4] This approach is also relevant in the older woman provided that she is fit for a general anesthetic.

Simple (total) mastectomy

Simple mastectomy comprises removal of all breast tissue without dissection of axillary nodes. It is unsuitable as sole treatment for patients with suspiciously enlarged axillary nodes. With retention of axillary nodes, locoregional recurrence occurs in 30–40 percent of patients within 10 years of primary treatment.[5] For patients aged 80 years or over this is less than the risk of death in the same period,[6,7] and it could be argued that simple mastectomy would be the only treatment needed. However, there is an increasing trend of treating elderly patients who are fit for anesthetic in the same way as younger patients. For younger patients this balance of risk is reversed. Simple mastectomy carries no significant morbidity or mortality in patients who are otherwise fit for surgery.

Modified radical (Patey) mastectomy

In this operation axillary nodes are cleared in continuity with a total mastectomy but without the extensive removal of skin and muscle of the classic Halsted radical mastectomy. This results in a low incidence of local recurrence, which is usually confined to the skin flaps. The disadvantage is related to the extensive axillary dissection that results in longer admissions than simpler procedures, and a risk of reduced mobility at the shoulder joint with sensory disturbances in the upper arm. With attention to postoperative exercises the risk of long-term disability is low. Although published evidence suggests that elderly patients tolerate extensive surgery well, radical surgery is used selectively in patients over 75 years of age. Since only around 25 percent of patients with screen detected cancer will have positive axillary nodes the alternative strategy of targeted node biopsy (sentinel node biopsy) using a radiopharmaceutical such as technetium labeled colloid, and blue dye is being explored. The technique removes only 1–2 nodes and early studies suggest that a sentinel node can be found in around 90 percent of patients with a prediction of the true axillary status in 95 percent. The efficacy, morbidity, and economics of this technique are being examined in several randomized trials currently.[8]

Local excision

Although local excision alone is superficially attractive as a treatment for operable cancer in elderly patients, experience has shown that local relapse occurs in 29–40 percent of patients within 5 years of presentation.[9–12] For this reason local excision is usually offered in combination with either radiotherapy or endocrine treatment to enhance control. Rare exceptions include localized in-situ carcinoma, and small tubular pattern lesions, which have an excellent prognosis.

Local excision and radiotherapy

The high local recurrence rate after excision alone can be reduced by postoperative radiotherapy, providing adequate surgical clearance has been obtained and the disease is not multifocal.[13] When surgical clearance of axillary nodes is carried out, radiotherapy can be confined to the residual ipsilateral breast. Axillary node clearance virtually abolishes the risk of uncontrolled axillary recurrence seen from time to time with other treatments but carries the same problems of rehabilitation discussed earlier. This program of therapy may need to be abandoned in favor of mastectomy when the histological margins are positive after local excision. In addition, some radiotherapists enforce an upper age limit for treatment because radiotherapy is not tolerated well by elderly patients.

Local excision and tamoxifen

Tamoxifen is effective as a treatment for advanced disease, and as an adjuvant agent.[14,15] There are few data on the value of tamoxifen after local excision but it is reasonable to assume that patients with endocrine-responsive tumors will benefit.

Tamoxifen as sole agent in operable breast cancer

The efficacy of tamoxifen in advanced disease has led to its use as sole agent initially in patients unfit for surgery and lately in fit elderly patients. Early studies have reported regression rates of 61–81 percent in this context,[16–19] while surgical salvage remains possible for patients who show no sign of response within 3–6 months. Formal trials comparing tamoxifen alone with surgery have produced differing conclusions. In one study there was no difference in rates of local relapse although surgical management was inadequate relying on local excision alone.[20] In another, subtotal "anterior" mastectomy was superior to tamoxifen although the ultimate prevalence of relapse was higher than would be expected after total mastectomy.[9]

With median durations of response of 18–25 months,[16,18] even responders are likely to suffer further progression of disease and present for surgery eventually. A randomized trial comparing surgery against primary tamoxifen showed higher rates of local failure in the tamoxifen-treated arm, although there was no demonstrable effect on survival.[21] However, longer follow-up in this trial has now shown a worse mortality in the tamoxifen alone arm. This suggests that tamoxifen alone should be reserved for patients with a very limited expectation of life for other reasons.

Adjuvant treatment

Adjuvant treatment is given after potentially curative treatment to reduce the rate of relapse. Cytotoxic treatment is tolerated poorly in elderly post-menopausal patients.[15,22] and

offers little benefit over hormone therapy in the adjuvant setting. Recent updating of the overview of breast cancer treatments confirms the benefit of tamoxifen in mortality at 15 years (Oxford overview 2000 presented in Oxford 2001). Although post-menopausal patients were offered tamoxifen empirically in the past, it is now recommended that all tumors are assayed for estrogen receptor levels and tamoxifen offered to patients who have positive receptor levels.

The preliminary analysis of the largest trial of adjuvant hormone therapy ever performed (ATAC—Arimidex against Tamoxifen And the Combination), involving over 9,000 post-menopausal patients was recently reported (San Antonio breast cancer conference 2001). This showed that the aromatase inhibitor Arimidex was significantly superior in terms of ipsilateral breast recurrences and new contralateral breast tumors to both tamoxifen alone or the combination of tamoxifen and Arimidex. The follow-up is not yet mature enough to know if these early promising results will translate into mortality advantage.

Locally advanced (Stage III) disease

There are two aims of treatment of patients with locally advanced disease: control of primary disease and systemic control.

Surgical clearance may be possible when the disease is not fixed firmly onto the chest wall or involving skin widely. Radiotherapy is also valuable, particularly for localized unresectable tumors. Irrespective of primary treatment, dissemination and local relapse occur frequently. Endocrine therapy reduces the rate both of relapse and mortality. In hormone-sensitive tumors tamoxifen may produce a dramatic response in advanced tumors.

Metastatic (Stage IV) cancer

Palliation is the principal aim. The best management should be decided by consultation between surgeon, oncologist, and primary care palliation team. There are three treatment modalities that can be used, as follows.

Radiotherapy

Radiotherapy is particularly useful for painful bone deposits. A single treatment to a painful area usually relieves pain within 10–14 days. Spinal deposits that threaten paraparesis can also be treated, although preliminary decompression is necessary when symptoms are severe or progress rapidly. Bony disease is improved by bisphosphonates, which are also the agents of choice in hypercalcemia secondary to bony metastases.

Endocrine therapy

About half of patients who have endocrine therapy will benefit. These results are even better in elderly patients who tend to have estrogen receptor positive tumors. Tamoxifen is the first choice. Second-line endocrine therapy is achieved by suppression of peripheral synthesis of estrogens by aromatase enzyme inhibition. Aminoglutethamide was the first-line aromatase inhibitor but side-effects including adrenocortical suppression were common and the agent is no longer used. Newer agents such as formestane 250 mg by injection every 2 weeks or anastrozole 1 mg daily or letrozole 2.5 mg daily, or exemestane 25 mg daily given orally are highly effective suppressants of aromatase but without the side-effects of adrenal suppression. These second-line agents can produce useful complete responses, especially where there was a previous documented first-line response to tamoxifen or another hormonal agent. Recent studies in advanced disease comparing the orally active aromatase inhibitors have shown that these agents are superior to tamoxifen and are thus likely to become the first-line agents in due course.[23,24] About one-half of patients who have responded once (regression or stability) respond again. Megestrol acetate (160 mg od) can be used as third-line therapy, but causes fluid retention.

Cytotoxic chemotherapy

Cytotoxic chemotherapy is tolerated poorly by elderly patients. Although developments of less morbid forms of treatment, for example, oral combination of cyclophosphamide, methotrexate, and fluorouracil, are tolerated better than intravenous therapy,[21] such treatment is generally reserved for younger patients with visceral metastases, and for symptomatic patients who fail to respond to endocrine therapy.

KEY POINTS Carcinoma of the breast

■ Breast cancer in elderly women behaves the same as younger women.

■ Surgery should still be used for operable cancer if the patient is fit.

■ Endocrine treatments are the best adjuvant treatments in older women as they tend to have ER positive tumors.

REFERENCES

1. Haagensen CD: Disease of the Breast, 3rd Ed. WB Saunders, Philadelphia, 1986:357
2. Seltzer MH, Perloff LJ, Kelly RI et al: The significance of age in patients with nipple discharge. Surg Gynecol Obstet 1970;131:519–522
3. Yorkshire Breast Cancer Group: Symptoms and signs of operable breast cancer 1976–1981. Br J Surg 1983;70:350–351
4. Fisher B, Redmond C, Poisson R et al: Eight year results of a randomised clinical trial comparing total mastectomy and lumpectomy with or without radiation in the treatment of breast cancer. N Engl J Med 1989;320:822–828
5. Murray JG, Mitchell JR, Gresham GA: Management of early cancer of the breast: report on an international multicentre trial supported by the Cancer Research Campaign. Br Med J 1976;1:1035–1037
6. Office of Population Census and Surveys (OPCS): Mortality Statistics for 1985. HMSO, London
7. Herbsman H, Feldman J, Seldera J et al: Survival following breast cancer in the elderly. Cancer 1981;47:2358–2363
8. Guiliano AE, Kirgan DM, Guenther GM, Morton DL: Lymphatic mapping and sentinel lymphadenectomy for breast cancer. Ann Surg 1994;220:391–401
9. Reed MWB, Morrison JM: Wide local excision as the sole primary treatment in elderly patients with carcinoma of the breast. Br J Surg 1989;76:898–900
10. Robertson JFR, Todd JH, Ellis IO et al: Comparison of mastectomy with tamoxifen for treating elderly patients with operable breast cancer. Br Med J 1988;297:511–514
11. Fisher B, Bauer M, Margolese R et al: Five year results of a randomised clinical trial comparing total mastectomy and segmental mastectomy with or without radiation in the treatment of breast cancer. New Engl J Med 1985;312:665–673
12. Tagart R, Bratherton D, Hartley L, Sikora K: Partial mastectomy alone in early breast cancer. Br Med J 1985;290:434
13. Schnitt SG, Connolly JL, Harries JR et al: Pathological predictors of early local recurrence in stage I and stage II breast cancer treated by primary radiation therapy. Cancer 1984;53:1049–1057
14. Nolvadex Adjuvant Trial Office (NATO): Controlled trial of tamoxifen as single adjuvant agent in the management of early breast cancer. Lancet 1985;1:836–839
15. Early Breast Cancer Trialists Group: Systemic treatment of early breast cancer by hormonal, cytotoxic or immune therapy. Lancet 1992;339:1–15,71–85
16. Bradbeer JW, Kyngdon J: Primary treatment of breast cancer in elderly women with tamoxifen. Clin Oncol 1983;9:31–34
17. Preece PE, Wood RAB, Mackie CR, Cuschieri A: Tamoxifen as initial sole treatment of localised breast cancer in elderly women: a pilot study. Br Med J 1982;284:869–870
18. Allan SG, Rodger A, Smyth JF et al: Tamoxifen as primary treatment of breast cancer in elderly or frail patients: a practical management. Br Med J 1985;290:358
19. Helleberg A, Lundren B, Norin T, Sanders S: Treatment of early localised breast cancer in elderly patients by tamoxifen. Br J Radiol 1982;55:511–515
20. Gazet J-C, Markopoulos C, Ford HT et al: Prospective randomised trial of tamoxifen versus surgery in elderly patients with breast cancer. Lancet 1988;1:679–681
21. Bates T, Riley D, Houghton J et al: Breast cancer in elderly women; a Cancer Research Campaign trial comparing treatment with tamoxifen and optimal surgery with tamoxifen alone. Br J Surg 1991;78:591–594
22. Howell A, Bush H, George WD et al: Controlled trial of adjuvant chemotherapy with cyclophosphamide, methotrexate and fluorouracil for breast cancer. Lancet 1984;2:307–311
23. Bonneterre J, Buzdar A, Nabholtz J-M et al: Anastrozole is superior to tamoxifen as first line therapy in hormone receptor positive advanced breast cancer. Cancer 2001;92:2247–2258
24. Buzdar A: Exemestane in advanced breast cancer. Anti-Cancer Drugs 2000;11:609–616 (review)

Chapter 92

Aging and the endocrine system

Ioan Davies

The endocrine system detects and integrates humoral and sensory information to regulate physiological function—the process of homeostasis. Age-associated declines in physiological performance are well known, and it is accepted that the basis of this decline is a *failure of homeostasis* at either a molecular or system level.

The conventional view is that "normal" aging changes predispose to age-related disease, and contribute to the poor recovery of elderly people after illness, or after severe stresses such as surgery. The results of early studies of age changes in endocrine function were frequently contradictory because investigators often failed to take sufficient account of confounding factors. This subject has been dealt with at length elsewhere.[1,2] Measuring hypothalamic or pituitary function by assessing suppression, or stimulation, of secretion is a matter of routine, but in aging research the importance of the confounding effect of serious illness must be appreciated.[3] Many changes in the pituitary gland are related to illness, and laboratory reference ranges for pituitary function obtained from young ambulatory subjects are not appropriate for hospital inpatients over 75 years of age.[4] Interfering factors are well recognized, and researchers attempting to define underlying age-related changes in human subjects are using increasingly sophisticated selection procedures to identify individuals free from disease, particularly when attempting to define normative measures. Lighthart and his coworkers established the *Senieur* protocol[5,6] for the selection of subjects to study the function of the aged immune system, and the criteria have been used to define "normal" subjects for research in other areas of bodily function. Subject selection and screening is rightly a high priority for quality research, but as usual the application of the screen must be related to the scientific question being asked. This matter has been debated recently and anyone involved in the study of age-related changes in humans should make themselves familiar with the arguments for the use of rigorous criteria in this endeavor.[7–10]

The role of the endocrine system in aging is complex. Reproductive senescence, particularly in the female, has focused attention on the potential role of the endocrine system in the aging process. Whether changes in the endocrine system are the cause of senescence is a more difficult question to answer. What is clear is that many elderly people have significant endocrine-mediated modifications in mineral, glucose, water, and electrolyte metabolism. Perhaps surprisingly, the equilibrium concentrations of the principal hormones are not necessarily altered with age,[11] but what may differ as we get older are the regulatory processes involved in maintaining equilibrium hormone concentrations, and the ways that hormones act on target tissues. Thus, with advancing age,

significant alterations in hormone production, metabolism, and action are found.[12] The scale of the age-related changes is highly variable and sex-dependent. Whereas only subtle changes occur in pituitary dynamics, adrenal gland physiology, and thyroid function, the changes in glucose homeostasis, reproductive function, and calcium metabolism are more apparent.[11]

This chapter is very selective and is about changes in the way that certain components of the endocrine system are regulated in old age, and how this may affect other functions in the body. Since changes in body composition and metabolism are important in elderly people, the focus is on control factors in the hypothalamus and pituitary (the neuroendocrine system), and the regulation of growth hormone (GH) secretion.

THE HYPOTHALAMUS AND PITUITARY

Hypothalamic structure

Early studies in laboratory rodents and humans of the numbers of neurons in the hypothalamus have found no consistent, age-related loss of cells in this region of the brain. Most of the principal neuroendocrine nuclei in the hypothalamus are structurally intact in old age, although there is some loss of morphological integrity of the suprachiasmatic nucleus (SCN) (see below).[13] Morphological variables (e.g. the size of neuron cell bodies, neuronal nuclear diameter, and neuronal number) that have been associated with increased functional activity have been measured in the supraoptic nucleus (SON), lateral tuberal nucleus (LTN), and lateral mammillary nucleus (LMN), and in the SCN. Some age-related alterations were observed in all of these nuclei, most obviously the LTN, but the size of neuron cell bodies and the number of neurons did not decline significantly with age.[14]

Neurons in the paraventricular nucleus (PVN) of elderly people seem activated based on morphological criteria.[15] The cells that produce antidiuretic hormone, arginine vasopressin (ADH, or AVP), increase in size, and the number of neurons that express both ADH and corticotrophin-releasing hormone (CRH) increase with age.[15] These data have important implications for vasopressinergic innervation of the brain, the modulation of neuronal function in the CNS, and possibly the endocrine control of water metabolism. However, the supraoptic nucleus in healthy older people shows increased sensitivity by releasing significantly more ADH in response to an osmotic challenge in health-status-defined elderly people.[16,17] Neuronal hypertrophy in a subpopulation of neurons in the infundibular nucleus also correlates with changes in the sex hormone secretion of post-menopausal women.[18] Studies in rodents have shown a reduced sensitivity of the hypothalamic–pituitary system to ovarian sex steroid feedback with increasing age, and recent research suggests that in post-menopausal women a similar process is taking place.[19,20] It has been argued that the hypothalamus of post-menopausal women shows impaired negative-feedback sensitivity to ovarian sex steroids, which interferes with the central neurotransmitter activity governing gonadotrophin-releasing hormone (GnRH) secretion.[20] However, despite the development of intrinsic age-related defects, at all levels of the hypothalamic–pituitary–testicular axis reproductive capacity is maintained in most healthy elderly men,[21] but the frequency of sexual activity declines dramatically with age.

Measurement of function

The hypothalamus has a central homeodynamic role, but direct examination of its function in the living human subject is difficult. Advances in molecular biological techniques are changing this situation and we now have excellent probes for the measurement of hypothalamic hormones. It has been proposed that sophisticated testing of pituitary function may be better achieved using a cocktail of hypothalamic releasing hormones.[22] For clinical studies it was proposed that the following releasing hormones should be used: growth-hormone-releasing hormone (GHRH), CRH, GnRH, and thyrotrophin-releasing hormone (TRH).[22] An investigation using this protocol showed that elderly men had lower baseline plasma concentrations of testosterone, free tri-iodothyronine, and insulin-like growth factor I (IGF-I) than young men, while 17β-estradiol and inhibin were not significantly different, although all the values were within normal laboratory limits. However, after challenge with intravenous GHRH, CRH, GnRH, and TRH, the elderly men differed from young men only for GH and prolactin release at a single time point.[22]

Regulation of circadian rhythms

The morphological alterations observed in the SCN correlate with reduced control of circadian rhythms. One autopsy study showed alterations in the diurnal oscillations of AVP immunoreactive neurons in the SCN of elderly people.[13] Others have investigated circadian rhythms of plasma melatonin. ACTH, cortisol, and oral temperature in healthy young and old women.[23] The elderly women showed a reduction in their mean oral temperature, and of the amplitude of its circadian rhythm. The mean plasma concentrations of ACTH and cortisol were increased, and nocturnal melatonin secretion was selectively impaired. The elderly subjects also showed a reduced sensitivity to the dexamethasone suppression test. These changes may be due to age-related modifications in the CNS, or alterations in the metabolic clearance of hormones.[23]

Many studies of the anterior pituitary show unchanged output of stimulating hormones, although the plasma concentrations of hormones produced by target tissues have decreased. The evidence suggests that age-related changes in endocrine regulation are not simply to do with concentrations of hormones in the hypothalamus, anterior pituitary, or peripheral circulation, but also with rhythms in their secretion. Twenty-four-hour profiles of cortisol, thyroid-stimulating hormone (TSH), melatonin, prolactin (PRL), and GH were compared in healthy young and old men.[24] Mean plasma concentrations of cortisol in the older men were normal, but the amplitude of the circadian rhythm was reduced. Circulating plasma concentrations of day- and night-time TSH and GH were greatly diminished in the older age group. In contrast, PRL and melatonin concentrations were decreased during the night only. The circadian rises of cortisol, TSH, and melatonin occurred 1–1.5 hours earlier in elderly subjects, and the distribution of rapid eye movement (REM) stages during sleep was similarly advanced, suggesting that circadian timekeeping is modified in normal senescent subjects. Despite perturbations of sleep, sleep-related release of GH and PRL occurred in all elderly men. Age-related decreases in the plasma concentrations of these hormones were associated with a decrease in the amplitude, but not the frequency, of secretory pulses. These findings imply that the aging process influences central mechanisms controlling the timing of hormone release.[24]

Hypothalamic regulation: receptors and neurotransmitters

The hypothalamus is robust in both morphology and physiological function. For example, the distribution and properties of α_2-adrenoreceptors are not affected by age.[25] However, there are many gaps in our knowledge regarding age changes in neurotransmitter functioning. Most of the data have been derived from the study of laboratory rodents, but uncertainties far outnumber demonstrated causative relationships between changes in neurotransmitter release and age-associated changes in hormone secretion.[26] A decline in function of the tubero-infundibular dopamine system is responsible, in part, for the age-related elevation in prolactin secretion, and may be involved in the decline in luteinizing hormone (LH) secretion. An age-associated reduction in hypothalamic noradrenaline turnover plays a role in the reduced LH and GH secretion, and may be involved in altered TSH secretion with age. The postulated decline in the circadian activity of SCN serotoninergic neurons may account for the age-associated blunting of circadian rhythms of several anterior pituitary hormones.[26] A recent study of healthy human brains at autopsy showed reduced catecholamine neurotransmitter concentrations in the hypothalamus.[27] Other areas of hypothalamic regulation will become more accessible with improvements in brain functional imaging and the arrival of new molecular probes.

Clearly, a qualitative preservation of hypothalamic and pituitary secretion has emerged from these investigations, but the critical feature of hypothalamic–pituitary regulation is the timing and size of the secretory bursts. The temporal organization of the hormone secretions is critical, and this is what may be affected in both rodents and humans. For example, optimum reproductive physiology in males and females depends on carefully timed surges of hormone secretion; so is it this aspect of endocrine regulation that is most affected with age? Recent studies are drawing attention to alterations in feedback sensitivity in the hormonal pathways involved in male reproductive senescence,[28] and are summarized more broadly as a breakdown in the "orderliness" in the regulatory pathways of several important systems.[29] The remainder of this chapter is confined to a discussion of the regulation of the growth-hormone/insulin-like growth factor (GH/IGF) system, where there have been major developments over the past few years.

GROWTH HORMONE AND AGING

The somatotrophic effects of growth hormone (GH) are mediated directly and through the actions of insulin-like peptides. The insulin-like growth factors I and II (IGF-I, IGF-II) account for most of the circulating somatotrophic activity in humans, and in addition they can exert their actions by autocrine or paracrine effects. Growth hormone increases the plasma concentration of IGF-I, but IGF-II is less sensitive to alterations in GH. In humans, circulating IGF-I is low at birth, rises progressively during childhood, and peaks during mid-adolescence. The normal increase in stature during adolescence is probably the result of the increase in circulating IGF-I. Following adolescence, plasma concentrations of IGF-I fall progressively with age, and is associated with a decreased secretion of GH. Changes in IGF-II are small as a function of increasing age.[30]

Regulation of circulating growth hormone concentrations

Figure 92-1 illustrates the major control points in the regulation of the secretion of GH with the major age-associated changes

that take place. GHRH is produced in the hypothalamus and stimulates the somatotrophs in the anterior pituitary to release GH. GH then stimulates IGF-I production by the liver. IGF-I stimulates the release of somatostatin in the hypothalamus, which causes the somatotrophs to reduce release of GH. In addition, IGF-I reduces the output of GH from the somatotrophs directly. Clearly, there are several critical points that could be susceptible to an age-related decline in function. The age-associated decrease in GH may be due to either increased hypothalamic somatostatin release, or to decreased secretion of GHRH. An alternative explanation could be that the somatotrophs are less responsive to GHRH because of a lack of receptors, or a decline in signal transduction mechanisms. The following discussion examines the basic facts about the age-associated decline in GH release and then investigates some of the current research on the cause of the deficit.

Circulating GH concentrations in man fluctuate widely due to pulsatile GH secretion by the pituitary. Time-series analysis of plasma GH concentrations shows dynamic fluctuations of more than three orders of magnitude.[31] GH pulses occur with an average frequency of about 13 per day in both sexes, with a dominant, but not strictly periodic, 2-hourly rhythm.

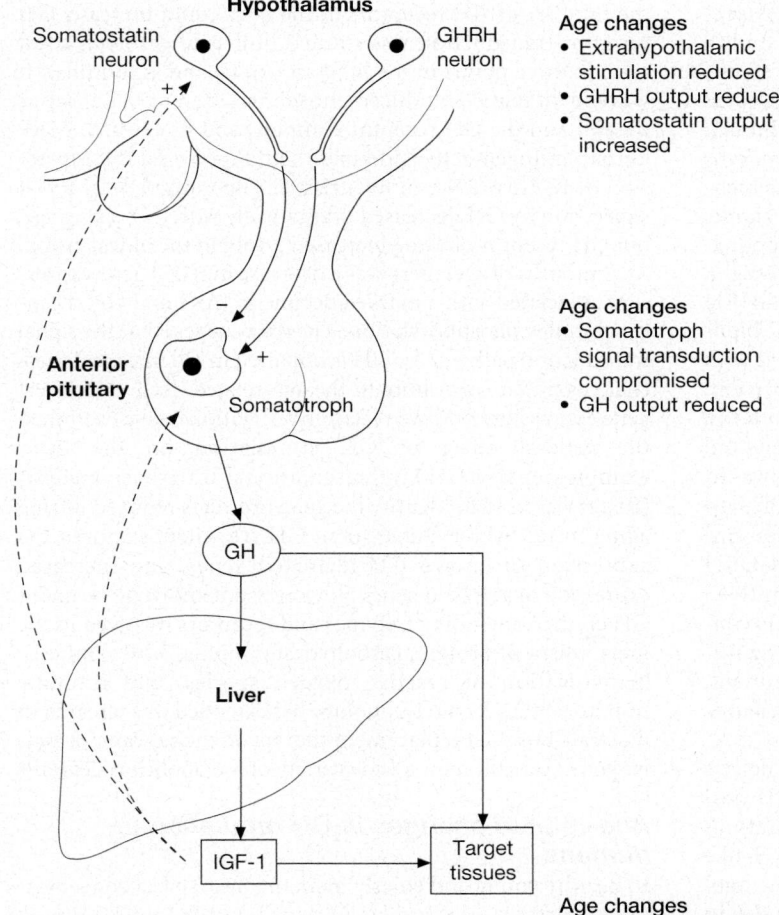

Figure 92-1 Regulation of the GH/IGF-I pathway.

Age changes
- Extrahypothalamic stimulation reduced
- GHRH output reduced
- Somatostatin output increased

Age changes
- Somatotroph signal transduction compromised
- GH output reduced

Age changes
- Changes in IGFBPs
- Changes in IGF receptors
- Changes in GH receptors

Thus, the pulsatile secretion of GH in man is oscillatory rather than episodic.[31] IGF-I concentrations decrease substantially with age in healthy men, which may be partially responsible for the age-associated catabolic effects on muscle and bone.[32,33] It was proposed that the declining activity of the GH/IGF-I axis with advancing age may contribute to the age-associated decrease in lean body mass, and the increase in adipose tissue mass.[32] Reduced plasma concentrations of GH are also a feature of old age in other primates,[34] and in rats, although the decrease is seen at an earlier age in females.[35,36]

Age-related changes in GH regulation in laboratory animals

In rats there is a marked decline in the pituitary response to GHRH that contributes to the decline in amplitude of GH pulses with age.[37] At the receptor-signal transduction level in the somatotrophs of the anterior pituitary, a diminished cAMP response to GHRH has been recorded,[38] and GHRH-stimulated adenylate cyclase activity is reduced by 50 percent in senescent rats.[39] The data suggested an age-associated, selective loss of functional GHRH receptors, but much of the postreceptor signal transduction mechanism was intact.[39] The GH response to an intravenous bolus of GHRH, morphine, and clonidine is dramatically reduced, or absent in old male and female rats,[36] and age-associated changes in GHRH-binding sites may precede, or even initiate, the GH impairment.[40] A recent study[41] investigated the sensitivity of somatotrophs to GHRH stimulation in 2- and 18-month old rats. The animals were injected subcutaneously for 14 days with an active fragment of human GHRH (0.5 or 1.0 mg/kg bodyweight), or saline. At 2 months of age, the lower dose of GHRH increased the number of high-affinity somatotroph binding sites 2-fold and hypothalamic somatostatin content by 45 percent. It did not affect hypothalamic GHRH content, serum total IGF-I, or gain in bodyweight. Treatment of the young rats with the higher dose of GHRH decreased the number of high-affinity pituitary GHRH-R-binding sites by 2.4-fold compared with that in rats treated with 0.5 mg/kg, decreased circulating levels of IGF-I by 13 percent, and slowed the growth rate by 17 percent. In the 18-month-old rats, treatment with the lower dose of GHRH for 14 days did not increase somatotroph GHRH binding variables. However, treatment with 1.0 mg/kg GHRH restored the affinities of high-and low-affinity classes of GHRH-binding sites to values similar to those found in 2-month-old rats. The high-dose GHRH treatment increased GHRH receptor messenger RNA (mRNA) transcripts that were typically reduced in the 18-month-old control animals. Serum IGF-I levels were also increased significantly in old rats after the high-dose GHRH treatment, although no effect was observed on bodyweight, hypothalamic somatostatin, or GHRH content.[41]

Senescent male rats are thought to have a number of defects in their hypothalamic neurosecretory neurons. GHRH synthesis is impaired in the hypothalamus of aged male rats, as shown by reductions in GHRH mRNA and GHRH-like immunoreactivity. This alteration may be due to the age-related changes in neurotransmitters and neuropeptides in hypothalamic and extrahypothalamic structures, especially the catecholaminergic and acetylcholinergic neurons.[42] Although somatostatin gene expression seems to decrease with age in the rat hypothalamus, secretion and activity of this hormone is increased, resulting in an altered relationship between GHRH and somatostatin gene expression and secretion. Age-associated variations in the mRNAs of GH and somatostatin have been measured in rats of both sexes by quantitative in-situ hybridization with cDNA probes.[43,44] There is a gradual decline in somatostatin mRNA in adult and senescent rats of both sexes, suggesting that aging in the GH/IGF axis is probably not a consequence of increased somatostatin activity.[44] Furthermore, GHRH-induced GH secretion is differentially affected by the inhibiting action of somatostatin, suggesting a loss of pituitary sensitivity to somatostatin in the presence of a high concentration of GHRH. Old rats stimulated with both GHRH and a synthetic GHRH-6 show a robust and immediate GH secretion when compared with animals challenged only with GHRH. These data suggest that the cellular processes involved in GH secretion are intact in old rats, and that age-related decrements in GH secretion may result from inadequate stimulation, rather than simply defective GH synthesis and release.[45] Increases in our knowledge of the regulation and synthesis of GH, such as the role of transcriptional activator protein (PIT-1), will enable more detailed research of the regulatory components of this pathway with advancing age.[46]

The release of IGF-I by the liver has now been studied in some depth in the mouse.[47] While it is known that there is a decline in GH secretion with age,[37] it has been suggested that the number of GH receptors in the liver could increase. GH receptor transduction was studied in liver slices from adult mice at three points in the lifespan (10, 17, and 31 months). It was shown that GH induced phosphorylation of JAK2 (Janus kinase) and the GH receptor complex, and it activated MAP kinase (mitogen-activated kinase), and increased the expression of IGF-I mRNA in liver tissue. The induction of IGF-I expression by GH decreased dramatically with increasing age, but GH receptor binding increased 2-fold in the oldest group. At 31 months of age, there was a decrease in IGF-I gene expression associated with a marked decline in JAK2 and GH receptor complex phosphorylation. The data suggest that the signal transduction pathway for GH is impaired in old mice and these changes might contribute to the age-related decline in IGF-I gene expression.[47] More recent investigations have examined the general effect of GH stimulation on the liver. Complementary DNA representational difference analysis (RDA) was used to identify the gene products reduced during aging in rat liver.[48] Subsequent GH treatment restored the expression of known GH-regulated genes, and increased expression of at least 11 genes previously not known to be under GH control, including enzymes and receptors involved in the metabolism of protein, carbohydrates, lipids, ATP synthesis, detoxification of reactive oxygen species, and immune response.[48] DNA chip technology has extended this research to illustrate how GH replacement therapy in the rat can normalize gene expression for a wide variety of metabolic processes.[49]

Age-related changes in GH regulation in humans

In healthy young and elderly men, the mean basal concentration of plasma GH is similar. Over 24 hours the total GH peak area, and the amplitude of the peaks, is significantly lower in elderly men, although the frequency of secretory pulses is unchanged. However, plasma IGF-I concentrations are significantly lower in elderly men[24,50,51] and women.[51] This suggests that a threshold concentration of plasma GH, which is required to stimulate IGF-I release, is not reached in older people. In addition, despite obvious sleep perturbations the sleep-related release of GH occurred in all elderly men.[24] These, and other data related to age-associated diurnal variations in neuro-endocrine control, suggest that circadian timekeeping is modified with age in humans. Similarly, aged nonhuman primates (rhesus monkeys) experience a reduction in plasma GH and fewer nocturnal GH pulses.[52]

RESPONSE OF SOMATOTROPHS TO GHRH A critical question is whether the anterior pituitary in healthy elderly people can respond to stimulation by GHRH. There seems to be a consensus that GH secretion in this age group increases after injection of GHRH.[53,54] In addition, GH secretion also increases in response to direct stimulation of the GH receptor on somatotrophs by synthetic ligands[55,56] in healthy elderly people. Priming GH secretion with a β-blocker (propranolol) caused a significant rise in both basal and peak GHRH-stimulated increases in GH despite old age.[57] This latter treatment is likely to affect the basal GH secretory tone and not simply GHRH-stimulated GH secretion. A priming dose of human pituitary GHRH (hpGHRH) also increased the GH response to GHRH. This implies an age-associated decline in the sensitivity of somatotrophs to GHRH stimulation, and that repetitive administration of GHRH could restore the attenuated response.[58] Low doses of either intravenous or oral arginine also can enhance the output of GH to GHRH stimulation in elderly subjects.[59] The GH response is dose-dependent and it was subsequently shown that a dosing regime involving intravenous injection of arginine combined with GHRH maintained the high GH response for up to 15 days.[60]

EFFECT OF MANIPULATING HYPOTHALAMIC SECRETION OF SOMATOSTATIN AND GHRH Somatostatin secretion is inhibited by the cholinergic system, and several investigators have tried to increase "central cholinergic tone."[61,62] GH secretion, after treatment with physostigmine, a cholinergic agonist, is increased with age.[63] Alpha-glyceryl-phosphorylcholine (a putative acetylcholine precursor) has a potentiating effect on GH secretion that is more pronounced in elderly people.[64] Others have examined the effect of intravenous injection of GHRH, either alone, or in combination with pyridostigmine (a cholinesterase inhibitor), or arginine, on GH release.[65] GHRH induced an increase in GH in young and old groups but the response was lower in the older age group.[65] Injection of pyridostigmine significantly increased the GH response to GHRH in both groups, but the response was lower in the older subjects. Simultaneous administration of arginine potentiated the GHRH-induced release of GH, in both young and old groups. The increase was greater than that found after pyridostigmine and GHRH in the elderly group, but not in young subjects. Of the elderly subjects, 61.3 percent had a GH peak below the limit observed for normal young adults after combined pyridostigmine and GHRH administration, while arginine with GHRH elicited a normal GH peak in all but one older person.[65] Finally, it has been shown that pyridostigmine treatment followed by an intravenous injection of TRH can stimulate the release of GH in euthyroid, old subjects.[66] In healthy elderly men (65–88 years), the GH response to G-DAMME (a guanyl derivative of an opioid analogue) was reduced or absent, while prompt GH release was found in all young men.[67]

REGULATION OF IGF-I The end of the GH/IGF pathway, the synthesis of IGF-I by the liver, has also been investigated in some detail. Investigations have covered the relationship between IGF-I and the following: age; total and regional adiposity, as assessed by body mass index and waist-to-hip ratio; lean body mass; bone mineral density; and circulating levels of parathyroid hormone, 1,25-$(OH)_2$ D_3, 25-OHD, and osteocalcin. Serum IGF-I levels declined significantly with age in both healthy men and women, although the manner of the decline differed between the sexes. In men, there was a linear decline in IGF-I concentrations. In women, IGF-I decreased more rapidly in those under 45-years of age than in either older women or men.[51] However, after adjustment for age, IGF-I was not significantly related to the various indices of body composition in either men or women, leading to the conclusion that advancing age, rather than declining serum levels of IGF-I, appears to be a major determinant of lifetime changes in body composition and bone mineral density (BMD) in either sex.[51]

Numerous studies have aimed to elevate plasma concentrations of IGF-I in elderly people. An early paper showed increased circulating IGF-I concentrations in response to GHRH-induced GH production in different age groups, with no age-dependent alterations in the magnitudes of these responses. These data suggest that increasing age in adult men has little effect on the response of pituitary somatotrophs to GHRH.[53] Other studies have been less conclusive. Serum IGF-I concentration was significantly lower in older subjects, and the GHRH-induced GH increase was lower in elderly people.[65] Oral administration for 4 days of the so-called GH-secretagogue, GH receptor peptide 6 (GHRP-6), in normal elderly subjects showed only a trend towards an increase in IGF-I concentrations after treatment.[59] It is now known that a certain fragment of GHRH (1–29), and GHRP-6 and related compounds, can produce a sustained stimulation of the GH axis; and in contrast to GH itself, they preserve feedback regulation at the pituitary level and stimulate a near-physiological pulsatile pattern of GH release. Short-term treatment with GHRH and the GHRPs can enhance GH secretion and elevate IGF-I and IGFBP-3 levels, and the agents are generally well tolerated. A major practical issue is that the GHRPs, and their nonpeptide analogues, are also active when given orally.[68]

The effects of IGF-I on tissues throughout the body is mediated by two specific receptors.[69] The availability of IGF-I to the tissue receptors is mediated by six serum IGF-binding proteins (IGFBPs); these are present in high concentrations so that there is little or no free IGF-I in the blood. The intrinsic bioactivities of the IGFBPs are still being determined; in general, all six of these proteins inhibit IGF action but stimulatory effects have been established for IGFBP-1, -3 and -5, although the precise mechanism for this action is unknown.[70] Age-related changes have been investigated in all of these binding proteins. Of the three IGFBPs with potential dual roles (inhibition and stimulation), IGFBP-1 increases[71] and IGFBP-3 and IGFBP-5 both decrease with increasing age.[72] Of the two inhibitory proteins, IGFBP-2 tends to decline with increasing age, and IGFBP-4 increases significantly.[73] The role of these binding proteins in the overall regulation of the GH axis in advanced age remains unclear, although interactions between the IGFBPs, and the concentrations of ovarian steroid hormones, have been implicated in osteoporosis.[72]

Replacement therapy with growth hormone

From the data described above, it is clear that there are a number of age-associated alterations in the regulation of the GH axis at every level. The reduction of muscle mass and strength observed in normal aging is well described and has stimulated clinical interventions in the GH axis in an attempt to reverse the situation (see the box). It is well known from experimental studies in aged rodents, and human diploid fibroblasts, that protein turnover (synthesis and degradation) is also reduced with increasing age.[74] Myofibrillar protein synthesis in skeletal muscle is reduced in healthy elderly men under resting[75] and exercise[76] conditions. Early studies suggested that the reduced muscle mass of old age could be increased by treatment with GH.[77] Treatment of men, with GH concentrations below 350 U/L, by subcutaneous injections of biosynthetic human GH for 6 months led to significant increases in plasma IGF-I, lean body mass, and lumbar vertebral bone density, and a decrease in adipose tissue mass. Skin thickness tended to increase. However, no significant change in bone density of the radius or proximal femur was detected. In controls, lean body mass, the mass of adipose tissue, skin thickness, and bone density during treatment remained unchanged.[77] Malnourished elderly people (weight 20 percent below average bodyweight, and serum albumin less than 3.8 g/dL) benefited from daily intramuscular injections of recombinant human GH for 21 days.[78] During this period mid-arm muscle circumference increased an average of 0.6 cm in the treated group, compared with a fall in saline injected controls. Weight increased by an average of 2.2 kg in the group treated with GH, but decreased by an average of 2.2 kg in the controls. Urinary nitrogen retention occurred only in the GH-treated subjects. IGF-I rose significantly in those treated with GH, but was unchanged in the controls. Furthermore, there was a significant association between weight change and IGF-I concentration. Neither clinical edema nor hyperglycemia was noted. These findings suggested that GH might be an effective way of maintaining and enhancing weight in malnourished older people.[78]

Direct studies of the effect of GH on muscle mass and strength in men aged over 60 years show that improvements take place on both these variables; it is not due to a change in the rate of myofibrillar protein synthesis.[79] In addition, there is no evidence for an increase in IGF-I mRNA abundance in skeletal muscle after injection of GH in people over 60 years of age.[80] There has been great interest in the possibility that elevating the levels of GH in elderly people may provide anabolic stimulation to achieve increased bone mass, but the practical benefits of treatment with GH alone seem to be questionable.[81] Clearly, some aspects of the age-associated changes in body composition can be reversed by GH therapy. However, even though there might be benefits of treating old people with GH deficiency, the criteria for deciding which patients to treat are not clear,[82] and the standard insulin stress test (IST) is unpleasant and potentially dangerous. At present, combination therapies involving GH and IGF-I would appear to be the most rational way forward,[80,83] but the complexity of the GH axis offers considerable scope for developing other strategies for its stimulation—for example, the incorporation of strength training regimens.[84]

Treatment of the human "somatopause"

- Recombinant human GH (by injection) in healthy elderly men with low IGF-I
  - Increase in lean body mass
  - Increase in vertebral body mineral density
  - Increase in muscle strength—uncertain
  - *Side-effects include carpal tunnel syndrome*

- GH secretagogues
  - GHRH (by injection) elevates GH and IGF-I
  - GH-releasing peptides and analogues
    - Orally active
    - Elevate GH and IGF-I
    - Effect on lean body mass unknown

KEY POINTS   Aging and the endocrine system

- Age changes in endocrine function are affected by numerous confounding factors, especially disease.

- Evidence suggests that neurotransmitters and neuroendocrine factors regulating hypothalamic function, and thus, anterior pituitary hormone secretion, are intimately involved in the aging process.

- Equilibrium concentrations of principal hormones are not necessarily altered with age, but there are changes in endocrine regulatory processes and signal transduction processes in target tissues.

- Over 24 hours the peak area of plasma GH decreases substantially with age. Plasma IGF-I concentrations also decrease substantially with age.

- There is a marked decline in the pituitary somatotroph response to GHRH that contributes to the decline in amplitude of GH pulses with age.

- GHRH and somatostatin regulation is impaired with age.

- In rodents the signal transduction pathway for GH is impaired with age contributing to the age-related decline in IGF-I gene expression.

- Circulating IGF-I concentrations do not seem to be significantly related to various indices of body composition in either men or women. Advancing age, rather than declining serum levels of IGF-I, seems to be a major determinant of late-life changes in body composition and bone mineral density in both sexes.

- Serum IGF-binding proteins mediate the availability of IGF-I to tissue receptors but the role of these binding proteins in the overall regulation of the GH-axis in advanced age remains unclear.

- In rodents GH replacement therapy can normalize gene expression for various metabolic processes.

- Early studies suggested that the reduced muscle mass of old age was increased by treatment with GH.

- Elevating the levels of GH in older people may provide anabolic stimulation to achieve increased bone mass but the practical benefits of treatment with GH alone seem to be questionable, although some aspects of the age-associated changes in body composition can be reversed by GH therapy.

CONCLUSION

The evidence discussed above gives support to the idea that manipulation of the endocrine milieu can influence some aspects of age-associated change. It is also evident, at least circumstantially, that neurotransmitters and neuroendocrine factors regulating hypothalamic function—and thus, anterior pituitary hormone secretion—must be intimately involved in aging. The age-related decrease in turnover of hypothalamic noradrenaline (norepinephrine) is involved in the decline of LH and GH secretion. The age-associated decline in circadian activity of 5-HT neurons in the suprachiasmatic nucleus may account for altered circadian rhythms in the secretions of several anterior pituitary hormones. Drugs that increase hypothalamic noradrenaline and dopamine activity can delay or reverse these events.[26] The hyposomatotropism of aging has been linked to a progressive defect in hypothalamic neurons producing GHRH, although alterations of somatostatin-producing neurons have also been implicated.[85,86]

The neuroendocrine system seems to be a major factor in the age-associated failure in homeostasis. The maintenance of life relies on correct gene expression, and in order to function appropriately the organism has to integrate gene expression in a large number of systems simultaneously. Although neuroendocrine and endocrine effects may not be the primary cause of the age-associated decline in function, they are capable of modifying certain of the associated phenomena, and can restore certain functions. The introduction of therapeutic measures designed to re-establish homeostatic control might ameliorate the rate of deterioration in aging organisms, leading to modification of the effects of advancing age and improving quality of life. However, studies of the biology of aging in the nematode *Caenorhabditis elegans* are implicating hormonal regulation of lifespan, particularly of an insulin/IGF-I like pathway.[87] Although *C. elegans* is a long way from the complexity of a mammal, research in this area may crucially improve our understanding of the genetic and cellular regulatory processes involved. Readers are referred to Chapters 6 and 7 for further information on the biology of aging and genetic mechanisms.

REFERENCES

1. Rowe JW: Clinical research on aging: strategies and directions. N Engl J Med 1977;297:1332–1336
2. Minaker KL, Meneilly GS, Rowe JW: Endocrine systems. In Finch CE, Schneider EL (eds): Handbook of the Biology of Aging. Van Nostrand Reinhold, New York, 1985:433–456
3. Van den Berghe G, de Zegher F, Lauwers P et al: Luteinizing hormone secretion and hypoandrogenaemia in critically ill men: effect of dopamine. Clin Endocrinol 1994;41:563–569
4. Impallomeni M, Yeo T, Rudd A et al: Investigation of anterior pituitary function in elderly in-patients over the age of 75. QJM 1987;63:505–515
5. Ligthart GJ, Corberand JX, Fournier C et al: Admission criteria for immunogerontological studies in man: the Senieur protocol. Mech Age Devel 1984;28:47–55
6. Ligthart GJ, Corberand JX, Geertzen HGM et al: Necessity of the assessment of health status in human immunogerontological studies: evaluation of the Senieur protocol. Mech Age Devel 1990; 55:89–105
7. Castle SC, Uyemura K, Makinodan T: The Senieur protocol after 16 years: a need for a paradigm shift? Mech Age Devel 2001;122:127–130
8. Ershler WB: The value of the Senieur protocol: distinction between "ideal aging" and clinical reality. Mech Age Devel 2001;122:134–136
9. Ligthart GH: The Senieur protocol after 16 years: the next step is to study the interaction of ageing and disease. Mech Age Devel 2001;122:136–140
10. Pawelec G, Ferguson FG, Wikby A: The Senieur protocol after 16 years. Mech Age Devel 2001;122:132–134
11. Mooradian AD, Morley JE, Korenman SG: Endocrinology in aging. Dis Mon 1988;34:393–461
12. Mobbs CV, Hof PR: Functional Endocrinology of Aging. S. Karger AG, Basel, 1998
13. Hofman MA, Swaab DF: Alterations in circadian rhythmicity of the vasopressin-producing neurons of the human suprachiasmatic nucleus with aging. Brain Res 1994;651:134–142
14. Morys J, Dziewiatkowski J, Switka A et al: Morphometric parameters of some hypothalamic nuclei: age-related changes. Folia Morphol (Warsz) 1994;53:221–229
15. Raadsheer FC, Hoogendijk WJ, Stam FC et al: Increased numbers of corticotropin-releasing hormone expressing neurons in the hypothalamic paraventricular nucleus of depressed patients. Neuroendocrinology 1994;60:436–444
16. Davies I, O'Neill PA: Aging in the hypothalamo-neurohypophysial-renal system. Geriatr Nephrol Urol 1993;3:93–106
17. Davies I, O'Neill PA, McLean KA et al: Age-associated alterations in thirst and arginine vasopressin in response to a water or sodium load. Age Ageing 1995;24:151–159
18. Rance NE: Hormonal influences on morphology and neuropeptide gene expression in the infundibular nucleus of postmenopausal women. Prog Brain Res 1992;93:221–235
19. Rossmanith WG, Reichelt C, Scherbaum WA: Neuroendocrinology of aging in humans: attenuated sensitivity to sex steroid feedback in elderly postmenopausal women. Neuroendocrinology 1994;59:355–362
20. Rossmanith WG: Gonadotropin secretion during aging in women: review article. Exp Gerontol 1995; 30:369–381
21. Tsitouras PD, Bulat T: The aging male reproductive system. Endocr Metab Clin North Am 1995; 24:297–315
22. Pontiroli AE, Ruga S, Maffi P et al: Pituitary reserve after repeated administrations of releasing hormones in young and elderly men: reproducibility on different days. J Endocrinol Invest 1992;15:559–566
23. Ferrari E, Magri F, Dori D et al: Neuroendocrine correlates of the aging brain in humans. Neuroendocrinology 1995;61:464–470
24. van Coevorden A, Mockel J, Laurent E et al: Neuroendocrine rhythms and sleep in aging men. Am J Physiol 1991;260:E651–E661
25. Meana JJ, Barturen F, Garcia-Sevilla JA: Characterization and regional distribution of alpha 2-adrenoceptors in postmortem human brain using the full agonist [3H]UK 14304. J Neurochem 1989; 52:1210–1217
26. Meites J: Neuroendocrine biomarkers of aging in the rat. Exp Gerontol 1988;23:349–358
27. Arranz B, Blennow K, Ekman R et al: Brain monoaminergic and neuropeptidergic variations in human aging. J Neural Trans 1996;103:101–115
28. Hermann M, Untergasser G, Rumpold H et al: Aging of the male reproductive system. Exp Gerontol 2000;35:1267–1279
29. Veldhuis JD: Nature of altered pulsatile hormone release and neuroendocrine network signalling in human ageing: clinical studies of the somatotropic, gonadotropic, corticotropic and insulin axes. Novartis Found Symp 2000;227:163–185; discussion 185–189
30. Hammerman MR: Insulin-like growth factors and aging. Endocrinol Metab Clin North Am 1987;16:995–1011
31. Winer LM, Shaw MA, Baumann G: Basal plasma growth hormone levels in man: new evidence for rhythmicity of growth hormone secretion. J Clin Endocrinol Metab 1990;70:1678–1686
32. Rudman D: Growth hormone, body composition and aging. J Am Geriatr Soc 1985;33:800–807
33. Florini JR, Prinz PN, Vitiello MV et al: Somatomedin-C levels in healthy young and old men: relationship to peak and 24-hour integrated levels of growth hormone. J Gerontol 1987;40:2–7
34. Wheeler MD, Schutzengel RE, Barry S et al: Changes in basal and stimulated growth hormone secretion in the aging rhesus monkey: a comparison of chair restraint and tether and vest sampling. J Clin Endocrinol Metab 1990;71:1501–1507
35. Takahashi S, Gottschall PE, Quigley KL et al: Growth hormone secretory patterns in young, middle-aged and old female rats. Neuroendocrinology, 1987;46:137–142
36. Millard WJ, Romano TM, Simpkins JW: Growth hormone and thyrotropin secretory profiles and provocative testing in aged rats. Neurobiol Aging 1990;11:229–235
37. Sonntag WE, Gough MA: Growth hormone releasing hormone induced release of growth hormone in aging male rats: dependence on pharmacological manipulation and endogenous somatostatin release. Neuroendocrinology 1988;47:482–488

38. Ceda GP, Valenti G, Butturini U et al: Diminished pituitary responsiveness to growth hormone-releasing factor in aging male rats. Endocrinology 1986;118:2109–2114

39. Robberecht P, Gillard M, Waelbroeck M et al: Decreased stimulation of adenylate cyclase by growth hormone-releasing factor in the anterior pituitary of old rats. Neuroendocrinology 1986;44:429–432

40. Abribat T, Deslauriers N, Brazeau P et al: Alterations of pituitary growth hormone-releasing factor binding sites in aging rats. Endocrinology 1991;128:633–635

41. Girard N, Boulanger L, Denis S et al: Differential in-vivo regulation of the pituitary growth hormone-releasing hormone (GHRH) receptor by GHRH in young and aged rats. Endocrinology 1999;140:2836–2842

42. Müller EE, Cella SG, De Gennaro Colonna V et al: Aspects of the neuroendocrine control of growth hormone secretion in ageing mammals. J Reprod Fertil 1993;46:99–114

43. Crew MD, Spindler SR, Walford RL et al: Age-related decrease of growth hormone and prolactin gene expression in the mouse pituitary. Endocrinology 1987;121:1251–1255

44. Martinoli MG, Ouellet J, Rheaume E et al: Growth hormone and somatostatin gene expression in adult and aging rats as measured by quantitative in-situ hybridization. Neuroendocrinology 1991;54:607–615

45. Walker RF, Yang SW, Bercu BB: Robust growth hormone (GH) secretion in aged female rats co-administered GH-releasing hexapeptide (GHRP-6) and GH-releasing hormone (GHRH). Life Sci 1991;49:1499–1504

46. Tuggle CK, Trenkle A: Control of growth hormone synthesis. Domest Anim Endocrinol 1996;13:1–33

47. Xu X, Bennett SA, Ingram RL et al: Decreases in growth hormone receptor signal transduction contribute to the decline in insulin-like growth factor I gene expression with age. Endocrinology 1995;136:4551–4557

48. Tollet-Egnell P, Flores-Morales A, Odeberg J et al: Differential cloning of growth hormone-regulated hepatic transcripts in the aged rat. Endocrinology 2000;141:910–921

49. Tollet-Egnell P, Flores-Morales A, Stahlberg N et al: Gene expression profile of the aging process in rat liver: normalizing effects of growth hormone replacement. Mol Endocrinol 2001;15:308–318

50. Vermeulen A: Nyctohemeral growth hormone profiles in young and aged men: correlation with somatomedin-C levels. J Clin Endocrinol Metab 1987;64:884–888

51. O'Connor KG, Tobin JD, Harman SM et al: Serum levels of insulin-like growth factor-I are related to age and not to body composition in healthy women and men. J Gerontol A 1998;53:M176–M182

52. Kaler LW, Gliessman P, Craven J et al: Loss of enhanced nocturnal growth hormone secretion in aging rhesus males. Endocrinology 1986;119:1281–1284

53. Pavlov EP, Harman SM, Merriam GR et al: Responses of growth hormone (GH) and somatomedin-C to GH-releasing hormone in healthy aging men. J Clin Endocrinol Metab 1986;62:595–600

54. Giusti M, Lomeo A, Marini G et al: Role of aging on growth hormone and prolactin release after growth hormone-releasing hormone and domperidone in man. Horm Res 1987;27:134–140

55. Chapman IM, Hartman ML, Pezzoli SS et al: Enhancement of pulsatile growth hormone secretion by continuous infusion of a growth hormone-releasing peptide mimetic, L-692,429, in older adults: a clinical research center study. J Clin Endocrinol Metab 1996;81:2874–2880

56. Chapman IM, Bach MA, Van-Cauter E et al: Stimulation of the growth hormone (GH)-insulin-like growth factor I axis by daily oral administration of a GH secretogogue (MK-677) in healthy elderly subjects. J Clin Endocrinol Metab 1996;81:4249–4257

57. Lang I, Kurz R, Geyr G et al: The influence of age on human pancreatic growth hormone releasing hormone stimulated growth hormone secretion. Horm Metab Res 1988;20:574–578

58. Iovino M, Monteleone P, Steardo L: Repetitive growth hormone-releasing hormone administration restores the attenuated growth hormone (GH) response to GH-releasing hormone testing in normal aging. J Clin Endocrinol Metab 1989;69:910–913

59. Ghigo E, Ceda GP, Valcavi R et al: Low doses of either intravenously or orally administered arginine are able to enhance growth hormone response to growth hormone releasing hormone in elderly subjects. J Endocrinol Invest 1994;17:113–117

60. Ghigo E, Ceda GP, Valcavi R et al: Effect of 15-day treatment with growth-hormone-releasing hormone alone or combined with different doses of arginine on the reduced somatotrope responsiveness to the neurohormone in normal aging. Eur J Endocrinol 1995;132:32–36

61. Giusti M, Marini G, Sessarego P et al: Effect of cholinergic tone on growth hormone-releasing hormone-induced secretion of growth hormone in normal aging. Aging (Milano) 1992;4:231–237

62. Giusti M, Marini G, Sessarego P et al: Growth hormone secretion in aging: effect of pyridostigmine on growth hormone responsiveness to growth hormone-releasing hormone. Recent Prog Med 1991;82:665–668

63. Raskind MA, Peskind ER, Veith RC et al: Differential effects of aging on neuroendocrine responses to physostigmine in normal men. J Clin Endocrinol Metab 1990;70:1420–1425

64. Ceda GP, Ceresini G, Denti L et al: Alpha-glycerylphosphorylcholine administration increases the GH responses to GHRH of young and elderly subjects. Horm Metab Res 1992;24:119–121

65. Ghigo E, Goffi S, Arvat E et al: A neuroendocrinological approach to evidence an impairment of central cholinergic function in aging. J Endocrinol Invest 1992;15:665–670

66. Giusti M, Giovale M, Sessarego P et al: Cholinergic modulation of growth hormone, prolactin and thyroid stimulating hormone responses to thyrotropin-releasing hormone in normal aging. Recent Prog Med 1995;86:341–344

67. Giusti M, Delitala G, Marini G et al: The effect of a met-enkephalin analogue on growth hormone, prolactin, gonadotropins, cortisol and thyroid stimulating hormone in healthy elderly men. Acta Endocrinol (Copen) 1992;127:205–209

68. Merriam GR, Buchner DM, Prinz PN et al: Potential applications of GH secretagogs in the evaluation and treatment of the age-related decline in growth hormone secretion. Endocrine 1997;7:49–52

69. Rother KI, Accili D: Role of insulin receptors and IGF receptors in growth and development. Pediatr Nephrol 2000;14:558–561

70. Baxter RC: Insulin-like growth factor (IGF)-binding proteins: interactions with IGFs and intrinsic bioactivities. Am J Physiol 2000;278:E967–E976

71. Donahue LR, Hunte SJ, Sherblom AP et al: Age-related changes in serum insulin-like growth factor-binding proteins in women. J Clin Endocrinol Metab 1990;71:575–579

72. Rosen CJ, Glowacki J, Craig W: Sex steroids, the insulin-like growth factor regulatory system, and aging: implications for the management of older postmenopausal women. J Nutr Health Aging 1998;2:39–44

73. Honda Y, Landale EC, Strong DD et al: Recombinant synthesis of insulin-like growth factor-binding protein-4 (IGFBP-4): development, validation, and application of a radioimmunoassay for IGFBP-4 in human serum and other biological fluids. J Clin Endocrinol Metab 1996;81:1389–1396

74. Levine RL, Stadtman ER: Protein modifications with aging. In Schneider EL, Rowe JW (eds): Handbook of the Biology of Aging. Academic Press, San Diego, 1996:184–197

75. Welle S, Thornton C, Jozefowicz R et al: Myofibrillar protein synthesis in young and old men. Am J Physiol 1993;264:E693–E698

76. Welle S, Thornton C, Statt M: Myofibrillar protein synthesis in young and old human subjects after three months of resistance training. Am J Physiol 1995;268:E422–E427

77. Rudman D, Feller AG, Nagraj HS et al: Effects of human growth hormone in men over 60 years old. N Engl J Med 1990;323:1–6

78. Kaiser FE, Silver AJ, Morley JE: The effect of recombinant human growth hormone on malnourished older individuals. J Am Geriatr Soc 1991;39:235–240

79. Welle S, Thornton C, Statt M et al: Growth hormone increases muscle mass and strength but does not rejuvenate myofibrillar protein synthesis in healthy subjects over 60 years old. J Clin Endocrinol Metab 1996;81:3239–3243

80. Welle S, Thornton C: Insulin-like growth factor-I, actin, and myosin heavy chain messenger RNAs in skeletal muscle after an injection of growth hormone in subjects over 60 years old. J Endocrinol 1997;155:93–97

81. Marcus R: Skeletal effects of growth hormone and IGF-I in adults. Endocrine 1997;7:53–55

82. Bates AS, Evans AJ, Jones P et al: Assessment of GH status in adults with GH deficiency using serum growth hormone, serum insulin-like growth factor-I and urinary growth hormone excretion. Clin Endocrinol 1995;42:425–430

83. Borst SE, Lowenthal DT: Role of IGF-I in muscular atrophy of aging. Endocrine 1997;7:61–63

84. Bermon S, Ferrari P, Bernard P et al: Responses of total and free insulin-like growth factor-I and insulin-like growth factor binding protein-3 after resistance exercise and training in elderly subjects. Acta Physiol Scand 1999;165:51–56

85. Simpkins JW, Millard WJ: Influence of age on neurotransmitter function. Endocrinol Metab Clin North Am 1987;16:893–917

86. Cocchi D: Age-related alterations in gonadotropin, adrenocorticotropin and growth hormone secretion. Aging Clin Exp Res 1992;4:103–113

87. Guarente L, Kenyon C: Genetic pathways that regulate ageing in model organisms. Nature 2000;408:255–262

Chapter 93

Adrenal and pituitary disorders

Paul Belchetz and Peter Hammond

DISORDERS OF THE ADRENAL CORTEX

The need for normal adrenal functioning continues into old age. After decades of speculation, there is now firm evidence that the patterns of basal and stimulated levels of cortisol secretion are substantially unchanged in the healthy aging population. Subtle age-related changes have been described related to the metabolism of adrenal hormones, and morphological features such as nodules appear quite commonly in the aging adrenal glands. Their importance arises from much readier and often serendipitous recognition as advanced imaging techniques are more widely used. It is, therefore, relevant to open this chapter with a resumé of the physiological and biochemical actions of adrenal steroids, mechanisms controlling their secretion, and techniques available for assessing the function and anatomy of the adrenal glands.

Physiological responses to adrenocortical steroids

Of the multitude of steroids found in the adrenal cortex, only the secretion of cortisol and aldosterone have undisputed and vital endocrine roles. The distinction between glucocorticoid and mineralocorticoid hormone actions is based on physiological observations, backed by differential effects on critical enzyme systems in target tissues.

Glucocorticoids

Cortisol (hydrocortisone) is the natural glucocorticoid of humans and most other mammals (but not the rat, which is unable to synthesize cortisol and uses corticosterone instead). It has long been recognized that cortisol, especially in high doses, has mineralocorticoid properties and this has led to the widespread use of dexamethasone, a synthetic glucocorticoid, effectively without mineralocorticoid properties as the "benchmark" glucocorticoid.[1]

This practice has passed from laboratory experiments to clinical investigation, as will be discussed below. There are growing reasons to question the validity of such assumptions, although the pragmatic clinical tests have proven value. There has previously been a tendency to subdivide the actions of glucocorticoids into those seen at low doses and termed physiological, and those seen with high doses, classically causing cushingoid side-effects, as pharmacological. There is no sound scientific basis for this differentiation as new effects are not seen with high doses, although the clinical sequelae are, of course, striking.

The term *glucocorticoid* derives from the effects on carbohydrate metabolism: antagonism of insulin action, promotion of hepatic glycogen synthesis, and participation in the defenses against hypoglycemia. It may affect resource utilization by virtue of tissue differences in response of the key glycolytic enzyme, phosphoenol pyruvate carboxykinase.[2] Glucocorticoids have many other actions, often permissive in nature. These include vascular and renal responses affecting control of blood pressure and extracellular water content. Other critical roles include actions on protein and lipid synthesis and complex interactions with the immune system. In addition there is the well-recognized but poorly characterized function that enhanced glucocorticoid secretion plays in combating stress. The stimuli recognized as stressful and capable of evincing enhanced cortisol secretion are numerous, including: fever, trauma, hemorrhage, and plasma-volume depletion, hypoglycemia, and even psychological disturbance. A unifying hypothesis is thus hard to achieve; but with regard to inflammatory processes, it is now widely believed that the role of glucocorticoids is to curtail the effects of the rapidly responding cytokine and acute-phase protein production, which if protracted could be potentially damaging.[3]

Mineralocorticoids

The action of aldosterone is ostensibly simpler, operating primarily via renal mechanisms to control extracellular sodium and potassium levels with secondary consequences on fluid balance and blood pressure. The effects of mineralocorticoids on other tissues such as the colon, brain, and pituitary are documented, but their significance is much less certain. The secretion of aldosterone and its circadian rhythm are maintained in the elderly despite a decrease in tonic levels of renin, its principal regulator.[4]

Adrenal androgens

The adrenal cortex also synthesizes androgens. These include androstenedione and dehydroepiandrosterone; much of the latter is conjugated and secreted as the sulfate. The function of adrenal androgens remains obscure, although much has been made of the phenomenon in childhood of the so-called "adrenarche," when enhanced amounts are made from about the age of 7 years. By contrast with cortisol production, there is a well-documented fall in adrenal androgen production in old age, to as little as 5 percent of young adult levels, with decreased ACTH responsiveness, which has been termed the "adrenopause."[5]

Apart from effects on body hair, it is not at all clear what function the secretion of adrenal androgens serves in normal adults. It has been postulated that the decline in dehydroepiandrosterone levels is, in part, responsible for the increased atherogenesis and, hence, cardiovascular disease in old age, but recent evidence does not support this hypothesis.[6] It appears more likely that dehydroepiandrosterone has an immunomodulatory, and possibly antioncogenic, action. Dehydroepiandrosterone replacement in an elderly person increases natural killer (NK) cell cytotoxicity and is claimed to dramatically improve the sense of physical and psychological well-being.[7]

Biochemical actions of steroid hormones

The effects of hormones on tissues depend on the distribution of specific receptors. Recent advances in knowledge have simultaneously clarified aspects of steroid hormone action and raised paradoxes that await definitive resolution. Steroids are lipophilic and readily enter cells: steroid receptors are intracellular. The classic model of steroid action is that steroid hormones bind to cytoplasmic receptors, forming activated complexes that are translocated to the nucleus where specific genes are activated, leading eventually to protein products as the end-point of hormone influence.[8] A similar pattern was proposed for the structurally dissimilar thyroid hormones. Molecular cloning techniques have not only revealed that all steroid hormone receptors show strong homologies to each other and the proto-oncogene c-erb-A, but that the latter actually appears to be a thyroid-hormone receptor. All these receptors share homologies, both in the hormone and the DNA-binding domains, and can be regarded as constituting a superfamily of genes, whose products are transcriptional regulatory proteins evolved from a common ancestor gene.[9] The steroid-hormone receptor is bound to a protein complex containing the heat-shock proteins hsp 90, hsp 70, and hsp 65. Exposure to steroid hormone leads to dissociation of the receptor from the complex so that the receptor is able to bind the hormone.[10]

The new complex of hormone plus receptor adopts a different molecular conformation, exposing the DNA-binding domain of the receptor. Thus far, the generalized scheme for steroid hormones applies to glucocorticoids. When it comes to identifying the molecular basis for mineralocorticoid and glucocorticoid actions, difficulties arise. The type-1 receptor—originally considered to bind mineralocorticoids with higher affinity than glucocorticoids—shows no such distinction with more modern techniques. Indeed, there is a marked kinship shown at the molecular level as well.[11,12] A possible explanation for the failure of the great molar excess of cortisol to swamp the type-1 receptor with regard to aldosterone binding has been suggested for tissues such as kidney, gut, and salivary glands. These tissues possess a potent 11-hydroxysteroid dehydrogenase enzyme system, which rapidly converts cortisol to cortisone, and cortisone does not bind measurably to the receptor.[13]

Acting through the genome, glucocorticoids enhance several key metabolic enzymes such as hepatic tyrosine aminotransferase[14] and tryptophan oxygenase.[15] In addition to this classic mode of action, it has also been suggested that many of the actions of glucocorticoids on the immune system are mediated by a specific protein product termed *lipocortin*, which acts as a second messenger.[16] The major site of action of lipocortin is thought to be on phospholipase A_2 and blocking the arachidonic acid pathways to prostaglandins and other inflammatory mediators.

Regulation of adrenal function

Regulation of glucocorticoid production

Cortisol secretion is under the immediate control of pituitary ACTH secretion acting to promote the conversion of cholesterol to pregnenolone by the removal of the six-carbon fragment from the cholesterol side-chain. These steps occur within the mitochondrion. A complex cascade of cytochrome-P450 variants has been implicated as steroidogenesis proceeds, shuttling from mitochondrion to endoplasmic reticulum and back. The chronic effects of ACTH affect many more steps in steroidogenesis than just cholesterol side-chain cleavage.[17]

Physiological control of ACTH secretion involves three major areas: circadian rhythms, stress, and negative-feedback inhibition by cortisol. ACTH is synthesized as part of a large 31-kDa precursor polypeptide pro-opiomelanocortin.[18] This is cleaved and the major fragments, including ACTH and β-endorphin, are usually cosecreted in equimolar proportions. The stimulus to ACTH release is from the hypothalamus by way of the hypothalamopituitary portal vessels conveying corticotrophin-releasing factors.[19]

These are a complex of polypeptides, the major constituent of which is a 41-residue moiety, corticotrophin-releasing hormone (CRH). However, this alone has less potent ACTH-releasing properties than crude hypothalamic extracts. It has been shown that vasopressin (AVP) and probably other, as yet unidentified, compounds act synergistically with CRH.[20] The secretion of these corticotrophin-releasing factors appears to be pulsatile-driving pulses—driving pulses of ACTH and cortisol in turn. The circadian rhythm is composed of pulses of varying amplitudes and frequency, with a nadir reached at midnight, but the onset of activity at about 0300 to 0400 hours reaching a peak at 0800 to 0900 hours. The pulses of ACTH and cortisol decline in size and frequency thereafter, although there is often a secondary rise at about lunchtime which seems to be related to food ingestion.[21]

As mentioned earlier, there is a formidable array of apparently unrelated stressors that can stimulate the release of ACTH and cortisol. There is preliminary evidence that the relative importance of CRH, AVP, and oxytocin varies according to the stimulus.[22] Where inflammation is involved, there is growing evidence for interleukin-1, interleukin-6, and tumor necrosis factor (TNF) having the capacity to stimulate the hypothalamic–pituitary–adrenal axis, thus providing a loop to suppress their own production.[23]

Reports suggesting extrahypothalamic production of ACTH secretagogues lack confirmation of authenticity or physiological significance.

Negative feedback of cortisol on ACTH production constitutes a sensitive homeostatic regulatory mechanism. The sites of negative feedback include not only the ACTH-producing cells of the anterior pituitary itself, but also higher centers including the hypothalamus and CA3 field of the hippocampus.[24]

Regulation of aldosterone production

Aldosterone is produced by the distinct outer part of the adrenal cortex, the zone glomerulosa. In humans this is found in cell clusters rather than in a distinct zone. The main regulation of aldosterone is by the renin–angiotensin system. The stimuli to renin release from the juxtaglomerular cells of the kidney are low-renal perfusion pressure, sodium depletion, and hypokalemia, although hyperkalemia acting directly on the zona glomerulosa is a more potent stimulus to aldosterone release than hypokalemia. Renin acts on renin substrate or angiotensinogen, released into the circulation from the liver, to form angiotensin-I. This decapeptide is converted to the octapeptide angiotensin-II by angiotensin-converting enzyme (ACE), which is of widespread distribution, but most importantly found in the pulmonary bed.[25]

Angiotensin-II, apart from being a powerful arteriolar vasoconstrictor, stimulates aldosterone secretion from the adrenal cortex. Aldosterone, as mentioned earlier, acts powerfully to retain salt (and obligatorily water), but promotes kalliuresis, hence closing the homeostatic feedback loop. There are other minor influences recognized as acting on aldosterone secretion, including ACTH, dopamine, and serotonin.

Adrenocortical function in normal aging

Numerous studies indicate that basal, circadian, and stimulated cortisol secretion remains intact well into old age.[26–32] This is particularly important with regard to the ability to withstand stress, and the cortisol response to exogenous ACTH has been shown to be normal in elderly patients following myocardial infarction.[33] There are well-documented changes in the metabolism of corticosteroids with age-related decrease in the catabolism of cortisol.[34,35] Because of the intact negative feedback mechanisms there is a commensurate reduction in cortisol production rate. Aldosterone secretion is also normally well preserved in the healthy geriatric population.[36] The recognized decline in adrenal androgen production[29,37–40] has been referred to earlier.

Tests of adrenal function

Tests of adrenal function in elderly people are for the foregoing reasons largely those established for the younger adult population. The diminishing reliance on urinary collections is beneficial for practical reasons, and also means that some of the physiologically irrelevant changes alluded to earlier will not prove distracting. The key to successful and safe investigation is careful selection.

Adrenal insufficiency

To investigate possible adrenal insufficiency, the basal measurement of greatest value is the plasma cortisol, measured at the circadian peak of 0800 to 0900 hours. Measurement of midnight cortisol is uninformative. If the 0900 cortisol is less than 150 nmol/L, the diagnosis of adrenal insufficiency is made, and if greater than 450 nmol/L the patient is normal. For values in between, adrenal reserve should be assessed by measuring plasma cortisol before the intramuscular administration of 250 μg tetracosactrin (synthetic $ACTH_{1-24}$) and then 30 minutes after. If secondary adrenal insufficiency is suspected, central mechanisms need assessing. While the insulin-induced hypoglycemia test is still the "gold standard" for younger patients, and indeed, has been used successfully in the elderly,[41] there are serious hazards attending its use. If the 0900-hour plasma cortisol is not greater than 180 nmol/L, if there is a history of epilepsy, or if there is a

significant risk of ischemic heart disease (surely present in all elderly patients), the test is contraindicated.

Alternative tests have been suggested, including several varieties of the metyrapone (metopirone) test. This drug blocks the 11-hydroxylase enzyme, which is a crucial step in cortisol biosynthesis. If negative-feedback mechanisms are intact, metyrapone provokes enhanced ACTH secretion, which drives adrenal synthesis of 11-desoxycortisol. In the classic version, the adrenal response is measured by urinary 17-oxogenic steroid excretion,[42,43] but altered production of urinary metabolites in old age plus the nonstandardized assays used for the measurements diminish the value of this approach. Other investigators have proposed measurement of the plasma 11-desoxycortisol response, but this, too, has not been fully validated, especially in the elderly age group.[44–46] Finally, it has been proposed that the ACTH level should be directly monitored, and this has been evaluated in a geriatric population.[47] The difficulties of ACTH measurements are many, standardization nonexistent, and the assay is costly and not widely available; thus, as a practical test this version does not bear further consideration. Most importantly, it does not assess what one needs to know: the capacity to secrete cortisol adequately in the face of stress. It is popular in North America, but for reasons of tradition rather than sound science.

A test by which contrast has much to recommend is the glucagon stimulation test. In the most widely used version, 1 mg of glucagon is injected subcutaneously and blood samples then taken basally at 90 minutes and thereafter at 30-minute intervals up to 240 minutes. As with the insulin test, the patient fasts overnight. There is no correlation between the cortisol response (or growth hormone response, because it is a reliable test of reserve of this hormone) and blood glucose changes. The diagnostic power of the test closely approaches the insulin stress test.[48] Glucagon is, however, safe to use even in the presence of heart disease and in epilepsy. The length of sampling period is dictated by the variable time taken to reach peak cortisol secretion—this adds inconvenience and expense. The use of intramuscular glucagon has been a simpler, more reliable version requiring samples only at 0, 150, and 180 minutes.[49] It is a more reliable test than the short Synacthen test when compared to the insulin tolerance test as the reference.[50] As with the insulin tolerance test, a peak plasma cortisol of 550 nmol/L or higher is regarded as a satisfactory response to glucagon.

Another useful aid in distinguishing primary and secondary hypoadrenalism is the long ACTH-stimulation test using depot tetracosactrin 1 mg intramuscularly and sampling at 0, 30, and 60 minutes as with the short test, but taking further samples at 4, 8, 16, and 24 hours.[51] The atrophied adrenals following ACTH deficiency can usually be stimulated, albeit subnormally, over this time span—in contrast to the flat response in Addison's disease.

Glucocorticoid excess

Adrenal hyperfunction usually means cortisol excess or Cushing's syndrome. Conventional methods of investigation are employed first to establish the presence of the syndrome. The 24-hour urine-free cortisol is a simple and reliable test.[52,53] Its value derives from the fact that at normal levels of plasma cortisol is much bound to a high-affinity cortisol-binding globulin (CBG). The free cortisol level (though thought to be the biologically active fraction) is generally small, and is readily excreted in the urine. Because the capacity of CBG is limited, and saturated with even minor degrees of cortisol hypersecretion, there tends to be a nonlinear and marked rise in urinary-free cortisol. The overnight dexamethasone suppression test is much used, but also much criticized for unacceptable error rates.[54] If a patient is genuinely thought to have Cushing's syndrome, inpatient investigation is usually required. The low-dose dexamethasone test (0.5 mg orally taken strictly every 6 hours for 48 hours) and high-dose dexamethasone test (2 mg every 6 hours for 48 hours) were originally described in terms of suppression of urinary cortisol metabolites and proved useful in the differential diagnosis of pituitary-dependent Cushing's syndrome from other causes of the syndrome, namely adrenal tumors (benign and carcinoma) and ectopic ACTH secretion from a wide variety of neoplasms.[55] More commonly, the plasma cortisol response is relied upon these days.[56] The basis of this test is that in Cushing's syndrome the pituitary lesion, most commonly a microadenoma only a few millimeters in diameter, is not truly autonomous, but shows blunted suppression of ACTH secretion, especially with high-dose dexamethasone. The plasma cortisol is an accurate index of ACTH secretion because its measurement is not affected by the concomitant presence of dexamethasone. (This useful property of dexamethasone can be used to assess adrenal reserve in seriously ill patients with suspected Addison's disease in whom glucocorticoid therapy may need to be given empirically, and the cortisol response to tetracosactrin assessed at the same time to establish diagnosis.) There is increasing use of synthetic CRH, either of ovine or human composition.[57,58] Though many investigators find this a helpful and safe test, as with all tests used in Cushing's syndrome it is not infallible.[59] Nevertheless, it is useful to know that there is a preservation of response in the healthy elderly population.[32]

In cases of adrenal carcinoma it is not unusual to have mixed patterns of steroid excess. Virilization in women is not uncommon, and plasma testosterone is raised. A striking rise in dehydroepiandrosterone sulfate is characteristic of adrenal carcinoma,[60] and this large production of a weak androgen may greatly raise the urinary 17-oxosteroid excretion.[61]

Mineralocorticoids

The mineralocorticoid status can be monitored by measurement of plasma aldosterone and also plasma renin activity both lying and standing (if clinically possible). The latter measurement of renin requires prior consultation with the laboratory so that rapid handling can be arranged to prevent artefactual results. Primary hyperaldosteronism is very uncommon in the elderly population and is diagnosed by raised aldosterone and suppressed plasma renin activity in hypertensive patients who usually exhibit hypokalemic alkalosis. The much more frequent occurrence of secondary hyperaldosteronism is indicative of disease outside the adrenals, such as renal artery stenosis, cardiac failure, or hepatic cirrhosis leading to raised renin, driving the normal zona glomerulosa to secrete high levels of aldosterone.

Hyporeninemic hypoaldosteronism occurs predominantly in the elderly population and is characterized by hyperkalemia, a hyperchloremic metabolic acidosis, and moderate hyponatremia. It is more common in men, and is often associated with diabetes mellitus, particularly in the presence of autonomic failure or renal impairment. It is aggravated by potassium-sparing diuretics, β-blockers, and nonsteroidal anti-inflammatory drugs.[62]

Imaging techniques in adrenal disease

The adrenal glands are readily visualized using CT scanning, especially if the patient is at all obese. Ultrasound can be useful, but is much less valuable than CT.[63] There is growing experience with magnetic resonance imaging (MRI), which may provide an indication of the likely functional status of any lesion. However, potential pitfalls arise with the exquisite sensitivity but nonspecificity of this and advanced CT scanning techniques.[64]

There remains a small role for isotopic scintigraphy in the diagnosis of adrenal hyperfunction, perhaps more for extra-adrenal or bilateral pheochromocytomas using metaiodobenzylguanidine than the use of selenocholesterol or its variants in Cushing's and Conn's syndromes.[65] Angiography is invasive, but much less so with the advent of digital venous imaging (DVI), which can be useful in adrenal disease. The pituitary may require imaging in Cushing's disease—often the tiny size of the tumor defies even the latest generation CT scanners,[66] but it does seem that MRI with gadolinium enhancement offers a slight edge.[67] In cases of hypopituitarism, CT scanning may be valuable.

As a final resort, venous sampling under radiographic control may be useful in the diagnosis of adrenal, pituitary, or ectopic sites of hormone production.[68] This approach in the elderly patient should be undertaken only if, after the most careful consideration, a balance of cost–benefit factors points inescapably in this direction. In practice this will rarely be the case.

CLINICAL PATTERNS OF ADRENAL DISORDERS

The patterns of adrenal disease do not differ greatly in the elderly population from those in younger adults. Because these are well-described in standard textbooks of clinical medicine and endocrinology, full descriptions will not be given here in all cases. Instead, emphasis will be placed on points particularly relevant to an elderly person.

Adrenal insufficiency

Primary adrenal failure (Addison's disease) characteristically begins insidiously with nonspecific symptoms, although gastrointestinal features, including weight loss, are often prominent, and in the elderly person functional status may be diminished.[69] Though the characteristic ACTH-mediated pigmentation is a useful feature if present, it is occasionally absent.[70] A large survey suggested that in elderly patients Addison's disease was not only more likely to be tuberculous than in younger patients, but likely to prove fatal and the diagnosis be made at post mortem.[71] Other rarer causes of adrenal failure, such as hemorrhage and amyloid, should be borne in mind.[72]

Though metastases are commonly found in the adrenal glands, they only exceptionally compromise cortisol secretion.[73] The therapeutic dividend from diagnosing Addison's disease is so great that the cortisol response to tetracosactrin should be assessed at the slightest suspicion. It is emphatically not necessary for the electrolytes to be disturbed or random cortisol to be "subnormal" for the significant adrenal insufficiency to be present. Secondary adrenal insufficiency is considered later.

Cushing's syndrome and adrenal carcinomas

Cushing's syndrome is rare in elderly people. It is most frequently due to ectopic ACTH production, usually by small-cell carcinoma of the lung, but these patients typically present with cachexia and profound hypokalemia, rather than the characteristic cushingoid appearance. If due to pituitary-dependent disease, trans-sphenoidal surgery may be considered because it causes little constitutional disturbance. Nevertheless, in mild cases medical treatment with metyrapone alone may suffice and be more appropriate. This mode of treatment is certainly appropriate with other forms of Cushing's syndrome, such as ectopic ACTH secretion. The mixed picture of Cushing's syndrome and virilization in adrenal carcinoma may be difficult to recognize: the hirsuties and thinning of capital hair may be much more prominent than the features of cortisol excess (Fig. 93-1). Indeed, the main features of Cushing's syndrome may be skin atrophy and fragility with spontaneous bruising. Obesity and plethora may be conspicuously absent. In the elderly person certain features are more marked, particularly impaired cognitive function, myopathy,

osteoporosis, and diabetes. Hypokalemia is common in all forms of Cushing's syndrome other than pituitary-dependent, although a patient with the nodular hyperplasia variety of Cushing's disease was diagnosed following an admission precipitated by an acute diarrheal illness in which the plasma potassium fell to 1.2 mmol/L.

Adrenal carcinomas may occasionally secrete estrogen. This was retrospectively recognized in a youthful looking elderly woman with Cushing's syndrome (Fig. 93-2) following removal of her large adrenal tumor (Fig. 93-3) when she had a brisk vaginal blood loss. Rescue of preoperative urine specimens revealed high estrogen levels. Treatment is primarily surgical unless there are widespread metastases. The use of opDDD is probably helpful, but may be associated with severe side-effects, in which case it should not be persevered with.[74]

Iatrogenic glucocorticoid excess

The most common cause of Cushing's syndrome in an elderly person is the exogenous administration of steroids for a variety of medical disorders. The side-effects of steroid therapy, often aggravating pre-existing problems, are usually more marked in the elderly group. Particular problems include decreased cognitive function, emotional lability, and dysphoria; osteoporotic fractures; myopathy and muscle wasting with limitation of mobility; skin fragility; and impaired glucose tolerance. Furthermore, patients on maintenance steroids (>10 mg prednisolone daily or equivalent for more than 2 weeks) are at risk of adrenal insufficiency in the event of intercurrent illness, and the daily steroid dose should be doubled for at least 3 days in these circumstances.

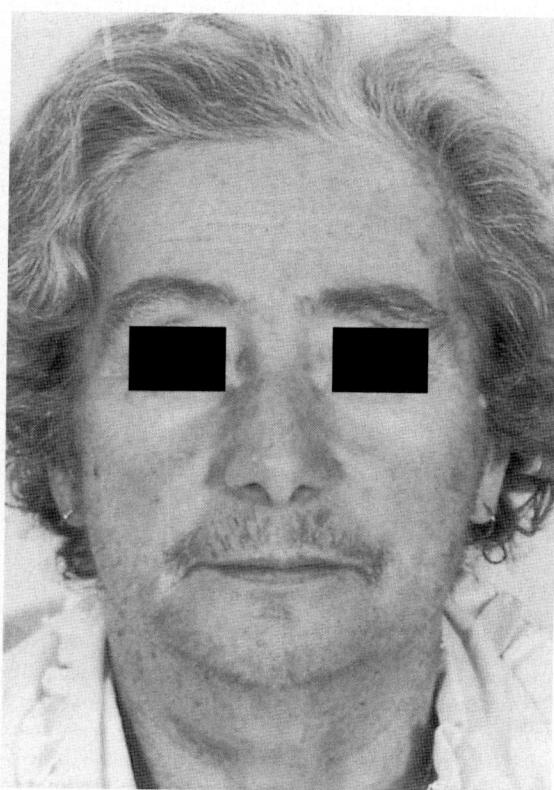

Figure 93-1 Patient with a metastasizing adrenal carcinoma causing virilization and Cushing's syndrome. Note hirsuties, slight scalp recession, but absence of cushingoid facies.

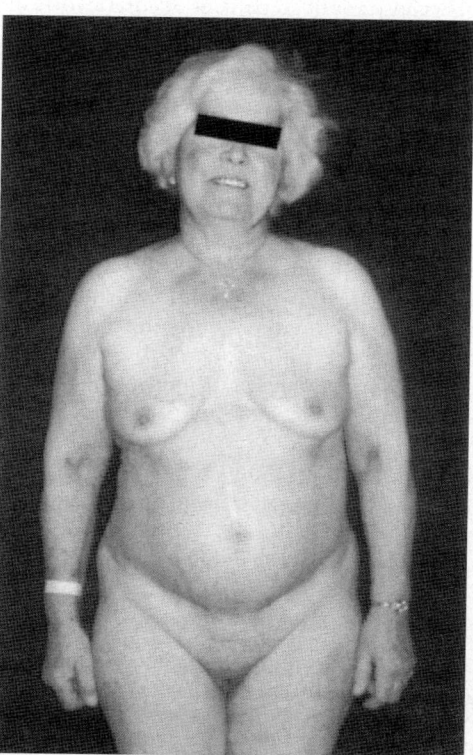

Figure 93-2 Patient with adrenal carcinoma causing Cushing's syndrome and feminization.

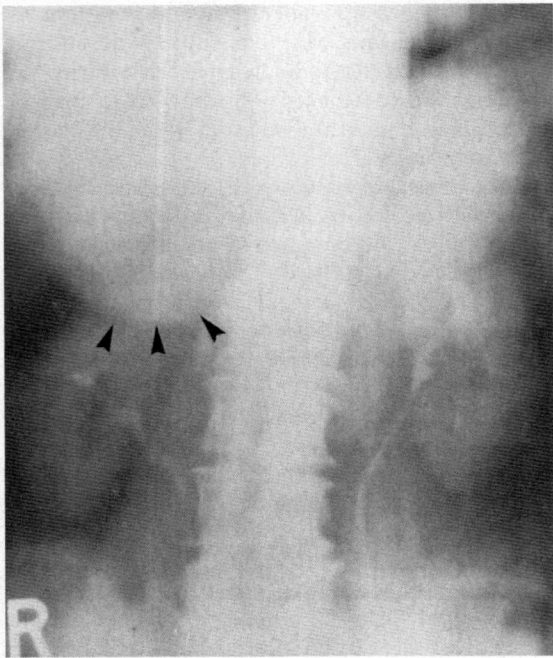

Figure 93-3 Intravenous pyelogram, showing large right-sided adrenal mass depressing the right kidney.

Incidentalomas

Last, but very far from least, is the vexed problem of what to do with a patient who for usually quite unrelated reasons has an abdominal ultrasound or CT scan that reveals an unsuspected adrenal mass.[75,76] Because about 20 percent of adrenocortical carcinomas are nonfunctioning in the absence of any clinical endocrine syndrome, it is probably prudent to repeat the scans at intervals, particularly for lesions greater than 3 cm diameter, since lesions progressing to greater than 6 cm diameter are almost always malignant. However, the problem must be kept in proportion. Adrenal cancer is rare, with an annual incidence approximately 2 per million.[77] Autopsy studies show that benign nodules are extremely common, especially with advancing age, and particularly in hypertensives.[78] Most are microscopic, but lesions of greater than 1 cm are found in approximately 1 percent of patients undergoing abdominal CT.[64] Clearly, there is a need for biochemical screening to exclude pheochromocytoma, Conn's, and also Cushing's syndrome. Hypertension and hypokalemia are particularly good indicators of functioning lesions. It has been estimated that the frequency of these conditions in 100,000 patients with an adrenal incidentaloma would be 6,500 pheochromocytomas, 7,000 Conn's syndrome, and only 35 Cushing's syndrome. However, subclinical cortisol hypersecretion has been reported in up to 25 percent of patients with adrenal tumors incidentally discovered on CT in a number of studies.[79,80]

PITUITARY DISORDERS
Pituitary tumors

Pituitary tumors are increasingly uncommon in the elderly population, with the exception of nonfunctioning (null-cell)

adenomas, which increase in incidence over the age of 50. These tumors present with local complications—usually due to compression of the optic chiasm causing bitemporal hemianopia, or more rarely due to invasion into surrounding structures, such as the cavernous sinus—or with features of hypopituitarism (see below). Functioning pituitary tumors are associated with the characteristic syndromes of hormone excess, notably, acromegaly and Cushing's disease, and behave in a similar fashion to tumors in younger patients, although it has been suggested that the somatotroph adenomas causing acromegaly are more benign in the elderly person, and thus medical therapy could be considered as a first-line option.[81] However, advances in neurosurgical techniques mean that almost all tumors can be at least debulked by the trans-sphenoidal approach; the relative simplicity and low morbidity and mortality of this procedure make it the treatment of choice for even the very elderly patient, especially one presenting with visual field defects.[82]

Other sellar lesions are very rare, although two occur more commonly in the elderly. Pituitary metastases may present like nonfunctioning tumors. Pituitary incidentalomas—adenomas, usually less than 1 cm diameter, without clinical sequelae—may be identified on CT or MRI scan performed for other indications, in the same way as adrenal incidentalomas, and have a prevalence of up to 10 percent in the over-80 age group, but intervention is not required in such cases.

Hypopituitarism

Hypopituitarism may be caused by pituitary adenoma as in younger age groups. A valuable clue in post-menopausal women is finding inappropriately low gonadotrophin levels, although it has been reported that these can be depressed in nonspecific illness in the extremely elderly.[47] More important, because subtler and more difficult to diagnose, is idiopathic hypopituitarism, in which the pituitary fossa is normal in size. Key features may be orthostatic hypotension, hyponatremia (reflecting adrenal and thyroid insufficiency causing water overload, possibly from inappropriate ADH secretion), or hypothyroidism with inappropriately low TSH.[83] Computed tomograph scanning may indicate a number of abnormalities ranging from a thickened pituitary stalk to empty sella.[84] Replacement therapy with hydrocortisone and thyroxine is gratifyingly effective. As with patients on steroid therapy, those patients needing replacement hydrocortisone should be advised to double the dose of hydrocortisone for 3 days with intercurrent illnesses, and they need parenteral steroids if they cannot tolerate oral medication while unwell.

Growth hormone deficiency

Growth hormone secretion declines by about 15 percent per decade from a peak at about 30 years of age,[85] and stimulated growth hormone secretion, using both pharmacological agents and physiological stimuli, such as exercise, is diminished in elderly people. This fall in growth hormone secretion is due to a decline in the frequency[85] and amplitude[86] of growth hormone pulses, probably the result of an increase in somatostatinergic tone. Furthermore, there is a decrease in circulating levels of insulin-like growth factor-I (IGF-I), the peripheral mediator of the somatic effects of growth hormone—although, in contrast to young adults, the IGF-I levels do not show as strong a correlation with 24-hour growth hormone secretion.[87]

Some of the features of aging are similar to the characteristics of adult growth hormone deficiency, such as the decrease in lean body mass and bone mineral density, the increase in fat mass,[88] and possibly, neuropsychological sequelae and increased cardiovascular mortality.[89] The availability of recombinant growth hormone has made the treatment of adult growth hormone deficiency possible, and recently there has been interest in its effects on the healthy elderly individual. In those with low IGF-I levels, administration of growth hormone increases lean body mass, skin thickness, lumbar spine bone density, and nitrogen retention, and decreases adipose tissue. No effect was seen on bone density at other sites or on serum cholesterol, and nonsignificant increases in blood pressure and fasting glucose have been reported. Side-effects of fluid retention, in some cases causing bloating or carpal tunnel syndrome, arthralgia, headaches, lethargy, and gynecomastia may occur.[88,90]

At present, the only group for whom growth hormone therapy can be recommended are those with pituitary disease, requiring at least one form of pituitary hormone replacement therapy, in whom growth hormone deficiency has been demonstrated using a pharmacological stimulation test and who have symptoms of growth hormone deficiency. Elderly patients with hypothalamic–pituitary disease and growth deficiency are distinguishable from elderly controls with respect to lipid profiles, body composition, and quality of life.[91] They respond as positively to growth hormone replacement as do younger patients.[92]

Isolated ACTH deficiency

Less frequent is the development of isolated ACTH deficiency. This has been seen in an octogenarian who developed frequent hypoglycemic comas associated with raised insulin levels. The clue that this was not due to an insulinoma came from the equimolar secretion of insulin and C-peptide. Replacement therapy with hydrocortisone completely abolished the hypoglycemic episodes.[93]

REFERENCES

1. Funder JW: On mineralocorticoid and glucocorticoid receptors. In Anderson DC, Winter JSD (eds): Adrenal Cortex. Butterworth, London, 1985:86–95
2. Feldman D, Funder JW, Loose D: Is the glucocorticoid receptor identical in various target organs? J Steroid Biochem 1978;9:141–145
3. Munck A, Guyre, Holbrook NJ: Physiological functions of glucocorticoids in stress and their relation to pharmacological actions. Endocrinol Rev 1984;5:25–44
4. Cugini P, Lucia P, Di Palma L et al: Effect of aging on circadian rhythm of atrial natriuretic peptide, plasma renin activity, and plasma aldosterone. J Gerontol 1992;47:214–219
5. Dewis P, Anderson DC: The adrenarche and adrenal hirsutism. In Anderson DC, Winter JSD (eds): Adrenal Cortex. Butterworth, London, 1985:96–119
6. Casson PR, Andersen RN, Herrod HG et al: Oral dehydroepiandrosterone in physiologic doses modulates immune function in postmenopausal women. Am J Obstet Gynecol 1993;169:1536–1539
7. Morales AJ, Nolan JJ, Nelson JC, Yen SS: Effects of replacement dose of dehydroepiandrosterone in men and women of advancing age. J Clin Endocrinol Metab 1994;78:1360–1367
8. Gorski J, Gannon F: Current models of steroid hormone action: a critical review. Ann Rev Physiol 1976;38:425–450
9. Green S, Chambon P: A superfamily of potentially oncogenic hormone receptors. Nature 1986;324:615–617
10. Joab I, Radanyi C, Renoir M et al: Common non-hormone binding component in non-transformed chick oviduct receptors of four steroid hormones. Nature 1984;308:850–853
11. Gustafsson J-A, Carlstedt-Duke J, Poellinger L et al: Biochemistry, molecular biology, and physiology of the glucocorticoid receptor. Endocrinol Rev 1987;8:185–234
12. Arriza JL, Weinberger C, Cerelli G et al: Cloning of human mincralocorticoid receptor complementary DNA: structural and functional kinship with the glucocorticoid receptor. Science 1987;237:268–275
13. Edwards CRW, Burt D, Stewart PM: The specificity of the human mineralocorticoid receptor: clinical clues to a biological conundrum. J Steroid Biochem 1989;32:213–216
14. Ernest MJ, Feigelson P: Multihormonal control of tyrosine transferase in isolated liver cells. In Baxter JD, Rousseau GG (eds): Glucocorticoid Hormone Action. Springer-Verlag, Heidelberg, 1979:219–241
15. Schultz G, Beato M, Feigelson P: Messenger RNA for hepatic tryptophan oxygenase: its partial purification, its translation in a heterologous cell-free system, and its control by glucocorticoid hormones. Proc Natl Acad Sci USA 1973;70:1218–1221
16. Flower RJ: Background and discovery of lipocortins. Agents Actions 1986;17:255–262
17. Waterman MR, Simpson ER: Cellular mechanisms involved in the acute and chronic actions of ACTH. In Anderson DC, Winter JSD (eds): Adrenal Cortex. Butterworth, London, 1985:57–85
18. Eipper BA, Mains RE: Structure and biosynthesis of proadrenocorticotropin/endorphin and related peptides. Endocrinol Rev 1980;1:1–27
19. Harris GW: Neural control of the pituitary gland. Physiol Rev 1948;28:139–173
20. Gillies GE, Linton EA, Lowry PJ: Corticotropin releasing activity of the new CRF is potentiated several times by vasopressin. Nature 1982;299:355–357
21. Weitzman ED, Fukushima D, Nogeire C et al: Twenty-four hour pattern of the episodic secretion of cortisol in normal subjects. J Clin Endocrinol Metab 1971;33:14–22
22. Antoni FA: Hypothalamic control of adrenocorticotropin secretion: advances since the discovery of 41-residue corticotropin-releasing factor. Endocrinol Rev 1986;7:351–378
23. Tsagarikis S, Gillies G, Rees LH et al: Interleukin-1 directly stimulates the release of corticotropin-releasing factor from rat hypothalamus. Neuroendocrinology 1989;49:98–101
24. Sopolsky RM, Krey IC, McEwen BS: The neuroendocrinology of stress and aging: the glucocorticoid cascade hypothesis. Endocrinol Rev 1986;7:284–301
25. James VHT: Adrenal cortex physiology. In Besser GM, Cudworth AG (eds): Clinical Endocrinology: An Illustrated text. Gower, London, 1987:6.2–6.10
26. West C, Brown H, Simons E et al: Adrenocortical function and cortisol metabolism in old age. J Clin Endocrinol Metab 1961;21:1197–1207
27. Touitou YK, Sulon J, Bogdan A et al: The adrenocortical hormones, aging and mental condition: seasonal and circadian rhythm of plasma 18-OH-11-DOC total and free cortisol and urinary corticosteroids. J Endocrinol 1983;96:53–64
28. Grad B, Rosenberg G, Liberman H et al: Diurnal variation of serum cortisol level of geriatric subjects. J Gerontol 1971;26:351–357
29. Serio M, Piolanti P, Cappelli G et al: The miscible pool and turnover rate of cortisol with aging and variations in relation to time of day. Exp Gerontol 1969;4:95–101
30. Tourigny-Rivard M, Raskind M, Rivard D: The dexamethasone suppression test in an elderly population. Biol Psych 1981;16:1173
31. Ohashi M, Kato K, Nawata H, Ibayashi H: Adrenocortical responsiveness to graded ACTH infusions in normal young and elderly human subjects. Gerontology 1986;32:43–51
32. Ohashi M, Fujio N, Kato K et al: Aging is without effect on the pituitary adrenal axis in men. Gerontology 1986;32:335–339
33. Jensen BA, Sanders S, Frlund B, Hjortrup A: Adrenocortical function in old age as reflected by plasma cortisol and ACTH test during the course of acute myocardial infarction. Arch Gerontol Geriat 1988;7:289–296
34. Romanoff LP, Morris CW, Welch P et al: The metabolism of cortisol-4-14C in young and elderly men. I: Secretion rate of cortisol and daily excretion of tetrahydrocortisol, allotetrahydrocortisol, tetrahydrocortisone and cortolone (20α and 20β). J Clin Endocrinol Metab 1961;21:1413–1425

35. Abbo FE: The 17-ketosteroid/17-hydroxycorticosteroid ratio as a useful measure of the physiological age of the human adrenal cortex. J Gerontol 1966;21:112–114

36. Lebel M, Grose JH: Angiotensin II effect on plasma steroids in selective hypoaldosteronism. Horm Metab Res 1982;14:432–436

37. Hamburger C: Normal urinary excretion of neutral 17-ketosteroids with special reference to age and sex variations. Acta Endocrinol (Copen) 1948;1:19–37

38. Migeon C, Keller A, Lawrence B, Shepard T: DHA and androsterone levels in human plasma. Effect of age and sex: day-to-day and diurnal variations. J Clin Endocrinol Metab 1957;17:1051–1061

39. Parker LN, Odell WD: Decline of adrenal androgen production as measured by radioimmunoassay of urinary unconjugated dehydroepiandrosterone. J Clin Endocrinol Metab 1978;47:600–602

40. Vermeulen A, Deslypere JP, Schelflhout W et al: Adrenocortical function in old age: response to acute adrenocorticotropin stimulation. J Clin Endocrinol Metab 1982;54:187–191

41. Muggeo M, Fedele D, Tiengo A et al: Human growth hormone and cortisol response to insulin stimulation in aging. J Gerontol 1975;30:546–551

42. Liddle GW, Estep HL, Kendall JW et al: Clinical application of a new test of pituitary reserve. J Clin Endocrinol Metab 1959;19:875–894

43. Gold EM, DeRaimondo VC, Forsham PH: Quantitation of pituitary corticotropin reserve in man by use of adrenocortical 11 β-hydroxylase inhibitor (SU-4885). Metabolism 1960;9:3–20

44. Jubiz W, Matsukara S, Meikle AW: Plasma metyrapone, adrenocorticotropic hormone, cortisol, and deoxycortisol levels: sequential changes during oral and intravenous metyrapone administration. Arch Intern Med 1970;125:468–471

45. Nattrass M, Smith J, Wood PJ, Marks V: Plasma corticosteroid determinations for assessment of pituitary response to metyrapone. Lancet 1972;ii:903–904

46. Blicher-Toft M, Hummer L: Serum immunoreactive corticotropin and response to metyrapone in old age in man. Gerontology 1977;23:236–243

47. Impallomeni M, Yeo T, Rudd A et al: Investigation of anterior pituitary function in elderly inpatients over the age of 75. QJM 1987;63:493–503

48. Spathis GS, Bloom SR, Jeffcoate WJ et al: Subcutaneous glucagon as a test of the ability of the pituitary to secrete GH and ACTH. Clin Endocrinol 1974;3:175–186

49. Rao RH, Spathis GS: Intramuscular glucagon as a provocative stimulus for the assessment of pituitary function: growth hormone and cortisol responses. Metabolism 1987;36:658–663

50. Orme SM, Peacey SR, Barth JH, Belchetz PE: Comparison of tests of stress-released cortisol secretion in pituitary disease. Clin Endocrinol 1996;45:135–140

51. Galvao-Teles A, Burke CW, Fraser RT: Adrenal function tested with tetracosactrin depot. Lancet 1971;i:557–560

52. Burke CW, Beardwell CG: Cushing's syndrome: an evaluation of the clinical usefulness of urinary free cortisol and other urinary steroid measurements in diagnosis. QJM 1973;42:175–204

53. Crapo L: Cushing's syndrome: a review of diagnostic tests. Metabolism 1979;28:955–977

54. Cronin C, Igoe D, Duffy MJ et al: The overnight dexamethasone test is a worthwhile screening procedure. Clin Endocrinol 1990;33:27–33

55. Liddle GW: Tests of pituitary–adrenal suppressibility in the diagnosis of Cushing's syndrome. J Clin Endocrinol Metab 1960;20:1539–1560

56. Ashcraft MW, van Herle AJ, Vener SL, Geffner DL: Serum cortisol levels in Cushing's syndrome after low- and high-dose dexamethasone suppression. Ann Intern Med 1982;96:21–26

57. Chrousos GP, Schulte HM, Oldfield EH et al: The corticotropin releasing factor stimulation test: an aid in the evaluation of patients with Cushing's syndrome. N Engl J Med 1984;310:622–626

58. Hermus AR, Picters GF, Pesman GJ et al: The corticotropin-releasing hormone test versus the high-dose dexamethasone test in the differential diagnosis of Cushing's syndrome. Lancet 1986;ii:540–544

59. Orth DN: The old and the new in Cushing's syndrome. N Engl J Med 1984;310:649–651

60. Freeman DA: Steroid hormone-producing tumors in man. Endocr Rev 1986;7:204–220

61. Hutter AM, Kayhoe DL: Adrenal cortical carcinoma: clinical features of 138 patients. Am J Med 1966;41:572–580

62. Holland OB: Hypoaldosteronism: disease or normal response? N Engl J Med 1991;324:488

63. Abrams HL, Siegelman SS, Adams DF et al: Computed tomography versus ultrasound of the adrenal: a prospective study. Radiology 1982;143:121–128

64. Glazer GM, Francis IR, Quint LE: Imaging of the adrenal glands. Invest Radiol 1989;23:3–11

65. Hawkins LA, Britton KE, Shapiro B: Selenium 75 selenomethyl cholesterol: a new agent for quantitative functional scintigraphy of the adrenals: physical aspects. Br J Radiol 1980;53:883–889

66. Semple CG, Thomson JA, Teasdale GM: Transsphenoidal microsurgery for Cushing's disease. Clin Endocrinol 1984;21:621–629

67. Kulkarni MV, Lee KF, McArdle CB et al: 1.5-T MR imaging of pituitary microadenomas: technical considerations and CT correlation. AJNR 1988;9:5–11

68. Findling JW, Aron DC, Tyrrell JB et al: Selective venous sampling for ACTH in Cushing's syndrome: differentiation between Cushing's disease and the ectopic ACTH syndrome. Ann Intern Med 1981;94:647–652

69. Tobin MV, Aldridge SA, Morris AI et al: Gastrointestinal manifestations of Addison's disease. Am J Gastroenterol 1989;84:1302–1305

70. Nerup J: Addison's disease: clinical studies: a report of 108 cases. Acta Endocrinol (Copen) 1974;76:127–141

71. Mason AS, Meade TW, Lee JAH, Morris JN: Epidemiological and clinical picture of Addison's disease. Lancet 1968;ii:744–747

72. Edwards OM: Adrenal apoplexy: the silent killer. J R Soc Med 1993;86:1–2

73. Cedermark BJ, Sjoberg HE: The clinical significance of metastases to the adrenal glands. Surg Gynaecol Obstet 1981;152:607–610

74. Luton J-P, Cerdas S, Billaud L et al: Clinical features of adrenocortical carcinoma, prognostic factors, and the effects of mitotane therapy. N Engl J Med 1990;322:1195–1201

75. Geellhoed GW, Druy EM: Management of the adrenal 'incidentaloma'. Surgery 1982;92:866–874

76. Prinz RA, Brookes MH, Churchill R et al: Incidental asymptomatic adrenal masses detected by computed tomographic scanning: is operation required? JAMA 1982;248:701–704

77. Dobbie JW: Adrenocortical nodular hyperplasia: the aging adrenal. J Pathol 1969;99:1–18

78. Virkkala A, Valimaki M, Pelkonen R et al: Endocrine abnormalities in patients with adrenal tumours incidentally discovered on computed tomography. Acta Endocrinol (Copen) 1989;121:67–72

79. Osella G, Terzolo M, Borretta G et al: Endocrine evaluation of incidentally discovered adrenal masses (incidentalomas). J Clin Endocrinol Metab 1994;79:1532–1539

80. Reincke M, Nieke J, Krestin GP et al: Preclinical Cushing's syndrome in adrenal 'incidentalomas': comparison with adrenal Cushing's syndrome. J Clin Endocrinol Metab 1992;75:826–832

81. Lamberts SWJ: Medical treatment of acromegaly. In Wass JA (ed): Treating Acromegaly. Society for Endocrinology, Bristol, 1992

82. Benbow SJ, Foy P, Jones B, Shaw D, MacFarlane IA: Pituitary tumours presenting in the elderly: management and outcome. Clin Endocrinol 1997;46:657–660

83. Belchetz PE: Idiopathic hypopituitarism in the elderly. BMJ 1985;291:247–248

84. Belchetz PE: Clinical recognition of idiopathic hypopituitarism in the geriatric patient. Geriatr Med Today 1987;6:27–42

85. Iranmanesh A, Lizarraide G, Veldhuis JD: Age and relative adiposity are specific negative determinants of the frequency and amplitude of growth hormone (GH) secretory bursts and the half-life of endogenous GH in healthy men. J Clin Endocrinol Metab 1991;73:1081–1088

86. van Coevorden A, Mookel J, Laurent E et al: Neuroendocrine rhythms and sleep in aging men. Am J Physiol 1991;260:E651–E656

87. Rudman D, Vintner MH, Rogers CM et al: Impaired growth hormone secretion in the adult population: relation to age and adiposity. J Clin Invest 1981;67:1361–1369

88. Rudman D, Feller AG, Nagray HS et al: Effects of human growth hormone in men over 60 years old. N Engl J Med 1990;323:1–6

89. Rosen T, Bengtsson B-A: Premature mortality due to cardiovascular disease in hypopituitarism. Lancet 1990;336:285–288

90. Thompson JL, Butterfield GE, Marcus R et al: The effects of recombinant human insulin-like growth factor-1 and growth hormone on body composition in elderly women. J Clin Endocrinol Metab 1995;80:1845–1852

91. Li Voon Chong JSW, Benbow SJ, Foy P et al: Elderly people with hypothalamic–pituitary disease and growth hormone deficiency: lipid profiles, body composition and quality of life compared with control subjects. Clin Endocrinol 2000;53:551–559

92. Monson JP, Abs R, Bengtsson B-A et al: Growth hormone deficiency and replacement in elderly hypopituitary adults. Clin Endocrinol 2000;53:281–289

93. Orme SM, Belchetz PE: Isolated ACTH deficiency. Clin Endocrinol 1991;35:213–217

Chapter 94

Disorders of the thyroid

Myron Miller

Although thyroid disorders occur over the entire age range, many appear to be increasingly common with advancing age. It is important to recognize that the clinical features of thyroid disease may be significantly altered in the aged individual so that symptoms and physical findings typical in young persons may be modified, different, or absent in the elderly population.

The diagnosis of a thyroid disorder may be further influenced by the age of the patient as a consequence of normal aging-associated changes in thyroid physiology. Of even greater importance is the impact of nonthyroidal illnesses that frequently occur in the elderly person on many of the tests used to assess thyroid function.[1]

NORMAL AGING

Morphology

The normal aging process is accompanied by changes in the gross and microscopic appearance of the thyroid gland. Early studies based on autopsy data indicated that overall mass declines from the normal range of 15–25 g so that with increasing age a progressively larger proportion of individuals will have glands weighing less than 20 g.[2] In recent years, data obtained by ultrasound in healthy subjects reveal that aging results in little change in size of the thyroid.[3]

With advancing age, there is progressive fibrosis, the appearance of lymphocytes, a decrease in follicle size, and a reduction in the amount of colloid.[4] Although these changes are common in the elderly population, they are by no means characteristic of all aged persons. More importantly, there does not appear to be a decline in thyroid function concomitant to the morphological changes, and neither weight nor histological appearance correlate with common measures of thyroid function.[5]

Hypothalamic–pituitary–thyroid regulation

The production of thyroid hormones is regulated by the hypothalamic–pituitary–thyroid axis. Thyrotropin-releasing hormone (TRH) is synthesized in the hypothalamus and functions to stimulate release of thyroid-stimulating hormone (TSH) from the anterior pituitary by binding to receptors on the cell membrane of TSH-producing thyrotropes. Thyroid-stimulating hormone is regulated by the negative feedback of the thyroid hormones thyroxine (T4) and tri-iodothyronine (T3) acting on the pituitary gland.

The neuroendocrine mechanisms controlling TSH release may be altered during the normal aging process. Thus, serum TSH concentration, which undergoes circadian variation, exhibits smaller fluctuations in elderly than in young men.[6] The ability of TRH to stimulate TSH release may be affected by both the age and gender of the individual. Several studies have documented that elderly men have an impaired TSH response to TRH stimulation with peak serum TSH values in men over the age of 60 showing approximately a 40 percent reduction compared with young men.[7–12] In women, however, there does not appear to be an effect of age on TSH responsiveness.[13]

The ability of the pituitary gland to synthesize TSH does not appear to be diminished by the aging process, as reflected by the observation that pituitary TSH content undergoes no significant change over the lifespan.[14] The 24-hour TSH secretion has been reported to be decreased in healthy elderly men,[10] but the secretion rate of TSH has also been reported to be higher in elderly subjects than in young individuals.[15] However, circulating levels of TSH remain constant with advancing age, and the elevations that are commonly seen in elderly persons must be considered as evidence for failing thyroid function.[16]

Thyroid-stimulating hormone exerts its effects by binding to the membrane of thyroid follicular cells. The response of these cells to TSH stimulation is not impaired by aging, as reflected by T4 and T3 release into the circulation following either TRH or TSH administration.[17]

Within the thyroid gland, T4 and T3 synthesis results from the trapping of iodide by follicular cells, subsequent oxidation of iodide leading to iodination of tyrosine, and coupling of two iodinated tyrosines. In the normal adult, approximately 80 μg of T4 and 30 μg of T3 are produced daily.[18] In elderly individuals, T4 and T3 production decline to approximately 60 and 20 μg per day, respectively. These changes may be related to the decrease in thyroidal iodide accumulation, which has been observed with aging.[19]

Thyroid hormone secretion and metabolism

In response to TSH stimulation, T4 and T3 stored in thyroid follicles are hydrolyzed from thyroglobulin and released into the circulation where they are bound to albumin, thyroid-binding prealbumin (TBPA), and thyroid-binding globulin (TBG) with less than 0.1 percent of the hormones circulating in the free form. Thyroid-binding globulin is the primary thyroid hormone transport protein, carrying about 70 percent of bound hormone, and its levels do not appear to differ between healthy young and old individuals.[9] A greater T4-binding capacity of TBG has been observed in the elderly population but appears to be without clinical significance.[20,21]

The small proportion of T4 and T3 in the free state (FT4 and FT3) are the biologically active forms of the hormones and are responsible for peripheral thyroid hormone action and metabolism. Circulating levels of both FT4 and FT3 remain constant over the age span and a decrease in concentration, especially FT3, should be considered a consequence of illness rather than due to normal aging.[9,16,17,20,22] Approximately 20–30 percent of circulating T3 is directly secreted by the thyroid gland, with the remaining 70–80 percent resulting from 5′-monodeiodination of the outer ring of T4 in peripheral tissues.[18] T4 degradation is decreased with advancing age so that, by age 90, the degradation rate is approximately 50 percent that of young subjects.[17,23,24] This change appears to be due to an age-related reduction in the activity of mono-deiodinase enzymes in peripheral tissue.[25] T3 degradation is less affected by aging.[17,25] A consequence of these changes is a decline in T4 metabolic clearance rate and an increase in the half-life of circulating T4 from approximately 6 days in young persons to over 9 days in individuals who have reached their ninth decade.[23,24,26] Since serum T4 concentration is not affected by aging, the prolongation of T4 half-life implies that there is an aging-related decline in T4 production by the thyroid gland.

Part of T4 degradation involves 5-monodeiodination of the inner ring of the molecule and results in the generation of the biologically inactive reverse T3 (rT3).[18,27] The outer-ring 5′-monodeiodinase is sensitive to a variety of influences including starvation, febrile illness, elevation of glucocorticoid concentration, and drugs such as propranolol, amiodarone, and iodinated contrast materials.[18,28] As a result of inhibition of the enzyme activity, there is impaired T4 conversion to T3, with a decline in serum T3 concentration and a parallel rise in rT3 concentration. Serum rT3 is not affected by normal aging, and an increase must be considered to be a consequence of illness or drug-induced alteration in T4 degradation.[22,25,29] Figure 94-1 shows the structures of T4, T3, and rT3.

Thyroid hormone action

The primary thyroid hormone acting on peripheral tissue and responsible for the broad range of thyroid actions is FT3. FT3, and to a lesser amount FT4, act on peripheral tissue cells by binding to specific nuclear receptors and subsequently affect DNA transcription, RNA formation, and new protein synthesis.[30–32] There are two T3 receptor genes, located on chromosomes 17 and 3, whose products are a group of T3 receptors.[32] Protein products coded for by the c-*erb*-A gene family, the cellular counterpart of the viral oncogene v-*erb*-A, have been demonstrated to be nuclear receptors for thyroid hormone.[33,34] At the level of the pituitary, thyroid hormone action results in inhibition of synthesis and release of TSH.[35,36]

Thyroid hormone action appears to be diminished as part of the aging process. Oxygen consumption is decreased and is reflected clinically by a decline in basal metabolic rate.[37] In aging animals, there is decreased ability to stimulate hepatic enzyme synthesis following exposure to thyroid hormone.[38] Clinical support for diminished thyroid hormone action is provided by the observation that typical features of hyperthyroidism are often absent in the elderly population of patients.

Thyroid function in advanced aging

Studies in healthy centenarians ranging in age from 100 to 110 years provide further information regarding the extent to which aging alone contributes to change in measures of thyroid function. There was no difference in serum FT4 of the centenarians as compared to both healthy elderly (aged 65–80 years) and healthy younger adults (aged 20–64 years), but serum FT3 was reduced in the centenarians. Serum TSH was also lower in the centenarians, and for the older groups as a whole there was an inverse relationship between serum TSH and age. Serum rT3 was increased in the centenarians, suggesting that there was reduced outer-ring deiodination of T4. Thus, in healthy aging persons, thyroid function was preserved into the eighth decade, while advanced old age was associated with reduced thyroid activity that was likely to be due to a decrease in TSH secretion and impairment of peripheral 5′-deiodination.[1,39]

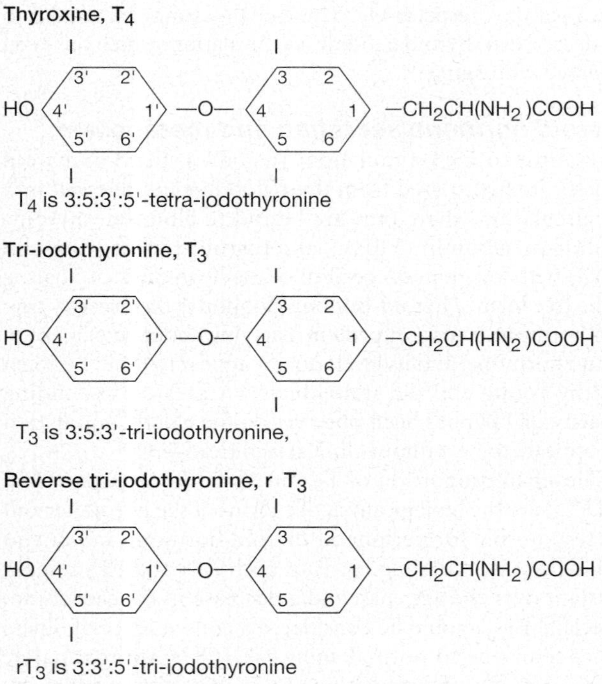

ASSESSMENT OF THYROID FUNCTION

Circulating thyroid hormones

Screening of the secretory status of the thyroid gland can be accomplished by measurement in the blood of TSH, total circulating T4 and T3 concentrations, and FT4 and FT3 concentrations through use of radioimmunoassay or immunometric assays.[12] The development of "super sensitive" immunoassays for TSH have allowed differentiation of normal from suppressed levels of the hormone so that this single measurement can provide evidence supporting a diagnosis of primary hypothyroidism, secondary hypothyroidism, or hyperthyroidism.[40–42] It now appears that this assay may be the best initial test of thyroid function in evaluating patients for suspected under- or overactivity of the thyroid gland.[40] Although it has been suggested that the generally accepted value of 5 mIU/L as the upper limit of normal for the adult population may actually be as high as 10 mIU/L in individuals who have reached their eighth decade, it is more likely that TSH values between 5 and 10 mIU/L are indicative of mild thyroid dysfunction.[42]

Total and free concentrations of T4 and T3 are commonly used to document the status of thyroid secretory activity. It appears to be well supported that the normal range for these

Thyroxine, T4

T4 is 3:5:3′:5′-tetra-iodothyronine

Tri-iodothyronine, T3

T3 is 3:5:3′-tri-iodothyronine,

Reverse tri-iodothyronine, r T3

rT3 is 3:3′:5′-tri-iodothyronine

Figure 94-1 Structures of thyroxine (T4), triiodothyronine (T3), and reverse triiodothyronine (rT3).

hormones is unaffected by aging and that deviations from normal must be considered as evidence for thyroid disease or for other illness or states that may affect hormone measurement.[16,17,20,22,25,43]

Serum-free T4 is best measured by equilibrium dialysis,[44,45] or more easily by the use of T4-specific antibodies.[46,47] Less reliable estimates of FT4 concentration can be obtained from the FT4 index, which involves measurement of both total T4 and a measure of thyroid hormone-binding protein capacity such as the T3 resin uptake.

Low T₄ states

In addition to the expected reduction in total T4 seen in primary or secondary hypothyroidism, total T4 may be low due to a variety of other causes. Levels of TBPA may be acutely lowered in the presence of infectious disease, protein wasting states, surgery, and malnutrition with accompanying decline in total T4. More importantly, TBG levels can be depressed as a result of X-linked congenital deficiency, severe catabolic illness, chronic hepatic disease, glucocorticoids, and androgen administration.[48] Binding of T4 to TBG can be inhibited by drugs such as furosemide and high-dose salicylates.[49] The anticonvulsants carbamazepine and phenytoin can reduce serum T4 by stimulating an increase in hepatic enzyme metabolizing activity.[49] In from 20 to 74 percent of patients with nonthyroidal illness, an inhibitor of T4 binding to TBG has been detected, which may contribute to the measurement of a low T4 in these patients.[48,50]

The finding of a low T4 concentration in the presence of nonthyroidal illness has been termed the "euthyroid sick syndrome."[51] In mild to moderate forms, measurement of FT4 will be normal even though total T4 concentration is reduced.[45,48] However, severe illness can result in marked reduction of both total and free T4 concentrations. When this circumstance occurs, the prognosis of the patient is poor with a mortality rate of approximately 80 percent having been reported.[52] The ability to differentiate these patients from those with hypothyroidism can be difficult.[53] Although serum TSH is usually in the normal range, occasionally mild to moderately elevated concentrations are found. This is especially true in the recovery phase of the illness when values can rise to as high as 20 mIU/L. Within 4–20 weeks after clinical recovery, all measures of thyroid function usually will have returned to normal.[54]

Low T₃ states

The serum concentration of total T3 is easily affected by many nonthyroidal illnesses, and low values are often seen in elderly ill patients, giving rise to the "low T3 syndrome." This consequence of systemic illness is the earliest and most common of the alterations in thyroid hormone levels.[16,17,28,43,48,53,55,56] In response to many acute illnesses, there is decreased peripheral 5′-monodeiodination of T4 to T3 with consequent reduction in serum T3 concentration and increase in serum rT3. Lowering of TBPA and TBG in the presence of acute and chronic illness further contributes to the marked fall in serum T3 characteristic of the sick elderly person. Often, the possibility of a diagnosis of hypothyroidism is raised and can usually be excluded by the absence of an increase in TSH and by the demonstration of normal or increased serum levels of rT3.

Cytokines such as interleukin-1, interleukin-6, and tumor necrosis factor (TNF) could be involved as intermediaries in the development of low T4 and T3 states. Many patients with nonthyroidal illnesses and low T4 and/or T3 also have elevated serum concentrations of cytokines.[57,58] Experimental increase of TNF-α has been observed to induce low serum concentrations of T4, T3, and TSH.[59]

High T₄ states

Although less common than low thyroid hormone states, nonthyroidal factors can result in elevation of serum T4 concentration.[53,60] A euthyroid increase in total T4 can occur as a result of overproduction of TBG, a disorder that may be familial.[61] More commonly, TBG is increased due to therapy with estrogen or tamoxifen or as a transient acute-phase reactant during acute hepatocellular injury. In these circumstances, serum-free T4 will be normal. On occasion, mild to moderate levels of illness can increase FT4 in the patient with euthyroid sick syndrome as a result of impaired T4 monodeiodination by peripheral tissues.[48,51]

Thyrotropin-releasing hormone test

The response of serum TSH to exogenously administered TRH is a useful method of assessing the dynamics of the pituitary–thyroid axis. In the normal individual, the bolus intravenous administration of 500 µg TRH results in a prompt rise in serum TSH, with peak values achieved in 30 minutes.[7,8] The minimal normal response should be an increase of greater than 2 mIU/L over the basal value, with many normal subjects reaching peak concentrations up to 30 mIU/L.[12] As previously stated, many elderly males respond less well to TRH stimulation than younger subjects or women at all ages.[7–13] Failure to respond to TRH is supportive of a diagnosis of hyperthyroidism, while a normal response will exclude the diagnosis. Subnormal responses may be seen in patients with severe illness, depression, or hypercortisolism as well as in euthyroid patients with thyroid adenomas or multinodular goiter. An exaggerated response of serum TSH is characteristic of primary hypothyroidism.[42]

Measures of iodine uptake

The ability of the thyroid gland to trap iodide and other ions such as technetium (Tc) has been the basis for assessment of both thyroid gland function and morphology. The oral administration of ^{131}I to normal individuals results in accumulation of 5–25 percent of the dose in the gland by 24 hours.[62,63] Because of considerable overlap between normal and hypothyroid subjects, low values for 24-hour ^{131}I uptake are of lesser diagnostic usefulness in establishing a diagnosis of hypothyroidism. Further, exposure to increased amounts of iodide in the diet or to iodine-containing drugs or radiographic contrast media will result in marked reduction of ^{131}I uptake. Elevated values are useful in supporting a diagnosis of hyperthyroidism, although some elderly patients with toxic nodules may have 24-hour ^{131}I uptake values within the normal range. The 24-hour ^{131}I uptake is usually obtained in a patient with an established diagnosis of hyperthyroidism in order to calculate the dose of ^{131}I to be given for ablation therapy.

Thyroid scanning with [99mTc] is useful in the evaluation of the patient with a palpable single thyroid nodule where demonstration of activity within the nodule markedly reduces the likelihood of the nodule representing an area of malignancy. In the elderly hyperthyroid patient, scanning can be used to differentiate a diffusely overactive thyroid from the gland with single or multiple toxic nodules.[64]

Other thyroid imaging procedures

High-quality anatomical detailing of thyroid structure can be achieved by currently available imaging techniques, including real-time ultrasonography, CT, and MRI. These procedures can be useful in evaluating patients with single and multiple nodules by identifying cysts, areas of hemorrhage, and tissue calcification. Ultrasonography may be of value in determining which regions of the thyroid are most appropriate for fine-needle aspiration. Both CT and MRI are expensive and have few clinical indications at present, but may be of occasional value in assessing the extent of tracheal compression by a thyroid mass, in determining the extent of substernal goiters, and in determining the extent of local invasion or metastasis by thyroid cancers.[65]

Antithyroid antibodies

Many thyroid disorders, including hyperthyroidism of the Graves' disease type[66] and hypothyroidism of the Hashimoto type, are believed to be the result of autoimmune disease.[12,67] As a consequence, high levels of serum antibodies to both thyroglobin and to microsomes are commonly found in patients with thyroid disease. Low levels of antithyroglobulin antibody (titer less than 1:100) may be present in patients without clinical signs of a thyroid disorder. Moderate to high titers (1:1,600 to 1:25,600) can be found in patients with nonthyroid autoimmune disorders.[12]

Thyroid antibodies in the serum increase in incidence progressively with increasing age, reaching a peak incidence of 20–25 percent in women above the age of 50 years and 5–10 percent in similarly aged men.[68,69] However, in a highly selected population of healthy elderly individuals ranging from 65 to 110 years, the prevalence of antithyroid antibodies was low and did not differ from the prevalence in healthy young persons.[1] This finding suggests that the high incidence of antithyroid antibodies in aging populations is a reflection of disease, and is not a consequence of normal aging. In many patients, the findings of high-serum antithyroglobulin and/or antimicrosomal antibody titers is accompanied by elevation of basal serum TSH concentration and reduced levels of serum T4, suggesting the presence of an autoimmune thyroiditis and a failing thyroid gland.[70]

From a diagnostic standpoint, high titers of antithyroid antibodies are commonly found in patients with documented hypothyroidism and suggest a diagnosis of chronic lymphocytic or Hashimoto's thyroiditis. In patients with hyperthyroidism, elevated antithyroglobulin and antimicrosomal antibody titers are more characteristic of patients with Graves' disease than of those with toxic nodules.

Thyroid-stimulating thyrotropin receptor antibodies

Thyroid-stimulating activity similar to that of TSH can be found in the IgG portion of serum obtained from many patients with hyperthyroidism due to Graves' disease. These immunoglobulins have been demonstrated to be antibodies directed against the TSH receptor.[66] Thyroid-stimulating thyrotropin receptor antibodies can be detected by both radioreceptor assays utilizing radiolabeled TSH and by bioassay based on stimulation of cyclic AMP release from isolated thyroid cell cultures.[71–75] Both methods reveal positive tests for TSH receptor antibodies in over 85 percent of patients with untreated Graves' disease and in essentially 100 percent of patients with severe Graves' ophthalmopathy. Positive tests are infrequent in Hashimoto's disease and rare in nodular thyroid disease, including toxic nodular goiter. Monitoring of antibody levels may be useful in predicting the likelihood of sustained remission in patients with Graves' disease who are treated with antithyroid drugs.[76]

Serum thyroglobulin

Thyroglobulin involved in intrathyroidal synthesis of T4 and T3 can gain entry to the circulation where it can be detected in normal individuals at low levels by means of immunometric assays.[77] Many elderly people have circulating antithyroglobulin antibodies which can interfere with accurate estimation of thyroglobulin concentration. Normal individuals have been found to have serum concentrations of thyroglobulin of less than 5 μg/L and levels appear to be unaffected by age. Concentrations can be increased in patients with hyperthyroidism, benign nodules, and inflammatory disorders, such as subacute thyroiditis. High levels are found in the majority of patients with thyroid cancer.

In patients with thyroid cancer previously treated by surgical or radioiodine ablation, measurement of serum thyroglobulin appears to be a sensitive indicator of tumor recurrence, either locally or by metastases. However, caution must be observed in interpreting blood levels because elevations above normal can be found in patients whose ablation has not been complete and have been left with small remnants of nonmalignant thyroid tissue.[77]

SCREENING FOR THYROID DYSFUNCTION

Disorders of thyroid function become increasingly common with advancing age and include both overt and subclinical hyperthyroidism and hypothyroidism (see below). As a consequence, a number of organizations have recommended that screening for thyroid dysfunction be initiated in the general population as a means of early detection of altered thyroid function. The American College of Physicians has recommended that women over the age of 50 should have serum TSH testing followed by measurement of free thyroxine if the TSH level is undetectable or greater than 10 mU/L.[78,79] The American Academy of Family Physicians recommends that thyroid function be measured periodically in all older women. Most recently, the American Thyroid Association has published guidelines for the detection of thyroid dysfunction which recommend that all adults, both men and women, be screened with measurement of serum TSH starting at age 35 and then repeated every 5 years thereafter, with more frequent screening for individuals who may be at higher risk of developing thyroid dysfunction.[80]

HYPERTHYROIDISM

Overproduction of thyroid hormone leads to the clinical condition of hyperthyroidism. This disorder, also referred to as thyrotoxicosis, is accompanied by a broad array of symptoms and signs that can differ markedly between young and old patients.

Demography

In the past, hyperthyroidism has been regarded as a disorder with preferential expression in young to middle-aged individuals, especially women. It is now clear that this disorder is also common in the elderly population.[78] The proportion of patients with hyperthyroidism who are over 60 years of age is estimated to be 15–20 percent.[81,82–85] Many studies confirm that hyperthyroidism is far more common in women than men, with estimates of female preponderance ranging from 4:1 to as high as 10:1.[81,84,86]

Etiology

In young persons, Graves' disease remains the most common cause of hyperthyroidism and is the consequence of thyroid receptor antibodies, which have stimulatory effects on the thyroid gland.[66,72,74,75] With increasing age, there is a change in etiology so that more cases are due to multinodular toxic goiter and fewer to Graves' disease.[81,87] It is estimated that more than 50 percent of hyperthyroid patients over the age of 60 years have thyroxicosis due to multinodular toxic goiters. Multinodular goiters are common in the elderly population and may not be clinically apparent.[5] Many clinical observations support the concept that longstanding euthyroid multinodular goiters may undergo change to become overproductive of thyroid hormones[81] (Table 94-1).

Another less common cause of hyperthyroidism in the elderly population is toxic adenoma (Plummer's disease), usually identifiable on thyroid scanning by the demonstration of a solitary hyperfunctioning nodule with suppression of activity in the remainder of the thyroid gland.[88,89] Hyperthyroidism can occur in a previously euthyroid person following ingestion of iodide or iodine-containing substances (Jod Basedow phenomenon). This is usually a self-limiting disorder lasting several weeks to several months.[90] Most commonly, this occurs following exposure to iodinated radiocontrast agents and to amiodarone.[91] Up to 40 percent of persons taking amiodarone will have serum T4 levels above the normal range but only

about 5 percent will develop clinical hyperthyroidism.[92] Amiodarone is fat-soluble and has a long half-life so that drug-induced hyperthyroidism can be prolonged and difficult to treat.[93,94]

The possibility of hyperthyroidism must always be considered in the elderly person who is receiving thyroid hormone, especially if the dose is greater than 0.15 mg of L-thyroxine daily. Patients who have received such doses for many years without evidence for hyperthyroidism may insidiously develop features of hyperthyroidism as they age past 60 years due to age-associated slowing in thyroid hormone metabolism.[95]

Rare causes of hyperthyroidism in the elderly population include TSH-producing pituitary tumors[96,97] and ectopic TSH production by nonpituitary tumors. These can be recognized by the finding of unsuppressed levels of serum TSH in the presence of increased amounts of circulating thyroid hormone. An additional uncommon cause of hyperthyroidism is overproduction of thyroid hormone by metastatic follicular carcinoma.

Transient hyperthyroidism may occur in patients with subacute thyroiditis as a result of increased discharge of thyroid hormone into the circulation during the inflammatory phase of the illness.[98] In a similar fashion, radiation injury to the thyroid can be accompanied by transient increase in circulating thyroid hormone levels with associated symptoms.

T3 TOXICOSIS   In a small proportion of cases of hyperthyroidism, measurement of serum thyroid hormone concentrations will result in the expected increase in serum T3, but with the finding that serum T4 is within the normal range, although often at the upper end. This circumstance has been designated as "T3 toxicosis" and can occur with any type of hyperthyroidism, but more commonly in patients with toxic multinodular goiter or solitary toxic adenoma.[89] The diagnosis will not be missed if T3 is measured in patients with clinically suspected hyperthyroidism who do not demonstrate elevated levels of serum T4.

Clinical presentation of hyperthyroidism

As with other disorders occurring in the elderly person, the clinical presentation of hyperthyroidism often differs from the classic description of the disease in younger individuals[81,82,99–101] (Table 94-2). Presenting features may be progressive functional decline, including weakness, fatigue, changes in mental status, loss of appetite, weight loss, cardiac arrhythmia, and congestive heart failure. A symptom complex peculiar to the geriatric hyperthyroid patient is "apathetic hyperthyroidism," in which the patient lacks the hyperactivity, irritability, and restlessness common to the young patient with thyrotoxicosis and presents instead with weakness, lethargy, listlessness, depression, and the appearance of a chronic, wasting illness. Often, the initial impression in such patients is that of depression, malignancy, or cardiovascular disease.[102,103]

The elderly patient with Graves' disease often differs from younger patients in nature and severity of expected classic symptoms and in physical findings. Clinically detectable thyroid enlargement, present in almost all younger patients, is absent in as many as 37 percent of elderly patients.[81] Infiltrative ophthalmopathy with severe proptosis and exophthalmos occur infrequently in the elderly group. Thus, none of the

Table 94-1   Etiology of hyperthyroidism and hypothyroidism in the elderly population

Hyperthyroidism	Hypothyroidism
Toxic multinodular goiter	Autoimmune disease
Graves' disease	Radioiodine or surgical thyroid ablation
Toxic adenoma	
Iodine-induced	Hypothalamic/pituitary disease
Exogenous thyroid hormone	Iodine-induced
Subacute thyroiditis (early)	Iodine deficiency
	Subacute thyroiditis (late)
	Inborn disorder of thyroid hormone synthesis

Table 94-2 Frequency of symptoms and signs of hyperthyroidism

| Symptom/sign | Kawabe et al[99] (%) | | Davis and Davis[81] (%) |
	Young (n = 48)	Elderly (n = 45)	Elderly (n = 85)
Palpitation	100	60	63
Goiter	98	58	64
Tremor	96	71	55
Excessive perspiration	92	66	38
Weight loss	73	85	69
Eye signs	71	28	57
Arrhythmias (atrial fibrillation and VPC)	4.6	16.4	62

From Griffin and Solomon,[100] with permission of Blackwell Science, Inc.

elements of the classic triad of Graves' disease (clinical hyperthyroidism, diffuse goiter, and infiltrative ophthalmopathy) may be recognizable in the elderly patient in whom the diagnosis may be suspected only on the basis of laboratory studies.[81,99,100]

Several reports have attempted to compare symptoms and objective physical findings in young and elderly patients with hyperthyroidism. Symptoms less commonly present in the elderly group include nervousness, increased sweating, tremor, increased appetite, and increased frequency of bowel movements. Symptoms more common include marked weight loss, present in over 80 percent of patients, poor appetite, worsening angina, edema, agitation, and confusion. Similarly, physical findings differ in elderly patients. In addition to absence of palpable goiter and eye signs of exophthalmos, pulse rate is slower, and reflexes are often not hyper-reflexic. Cardiac arhythmias, especially atrial fibrillation and ventricular premature beats, are more common. Lid lag and lid retraction are frequently seen.[81,99–104]

The spectrum of symptoms and findings due to thyroid hormone excess is broad and can involve almost all body systems. Thyroid hormones act on the myocardium to sensitize the heart to β-adrenergic stimulation with resultant increase in heart rate, stroke volume, cardiac output, and shortened left ventricular ejection time.[104–106] These changes underlie the clinical consequences of increased risk of atrial fibrillation, often with a slow ventricular response, exacerbation of angina in patients with pre-existing coronary artery disease, and precipitation of congestive heart failure, which responds less readily to digoxin treatment owing to increased renal clearance of the drug.

Gastrointestinal consequences of hyperthyroidism in an elderly person include weight loss, poor appetite, and occasionally abdominal pain, nausea, and vomiting.[81,82] Diarrhea and increased frequency of bowel movements resulting from thyroid hormone action on intestinal motility can occur, but are often absent in the elderly in whom constipation is likely to be present. Hepatic actions of thyroid hormone can lead to alterations in liver enzymes, including elevation of alkaline phosphatase and γ-glutamyl transpeptidase levels, which return to normal following restoration of thyroid function to normal.

Weakness, especially of the proximal muscles, is a major feature of hyperthyroidism in elderly patients and is often accompanied by muscle wasting.[81,103] As a consequence, disorders of gait, postural instability, and falls can be significant symptoms. Tremor occurs in over 70 percent of elderly thyrotoxic patients, but this sign must be distinguished from other causes of tremor common in the elderly which are usually more coarse or primarily present at rest.[99,100] A rapid relaxation phase of the deep tendon reflexes is common in young patients, but is often difficult to assess in the older patient. Central nervous system manifestations may be a prominent component of the symptom complex of the elderly patient and include confusion, depression, forgetfulness, irritability, and a shortened concentration span.[87,107] These cognitive impairments may point to a diagnosis of dementia and failure to consider the presence of hyperthyroidism.

Other clinical manifestations of hyperthyroidism in the elderly population may include glucose intolerance and, occasionally, the unmasking of latent diabetes mellitus. Mild elevations of serum calcium can occur and hyperthyroidism can cause the development of osteoporosis.

Diagnosis of hyperthyroidism

Because of the altered clinical presentation of hyperthyroidism in an elderly person, suspicion must always be high and the laboratory should be used for any patient with possible symptoms. It is not uneconomical to employ screening tests for thyroid status in all geriatric patients undergoing initial clinical evaluation.[78,104]

Serum T4 or free T4 and measurement of serum TSH by modern ultrasensitive methods are the preferable screening procedures for thyroid dysfunction.[42,109] The findings of a normal serum T4 with suppressed serum TSH raises the possibility of T3 toxicosis and calls for measurement of serum T3.[47,48,87] Determination of FT4 concentration by one of the direct measurement techniques may be useful when there is reason to suspect an alteration in thyroid-binding proteins.[44,47] Demonstration of anti-TSH receptor antibodies can be helpful in making a diagnosis of Graves' disease.[66,72,75]

The TRH stimulation test can be useful in evaluating the patient with borderline laboratory tests.[8,12] A significant rise in serum TSH will exclude the likelihood of hyperthyroidism, but an inadequate rise of TSH can only be considered as supportive of the diagnosis.

Thyroid scanning with ^{99m}Tc and measurement of ^{131}I uptake can be useful in distinguishing Graves' disease from toxic multinodular goiter.[62,63] Scanning may demonstrate the presence of a small diffusely active goiter that could not be detected on physical examination. Very low ^{131}I uptake in a patient with elevated circulating thyroid hormone levels suggests exogenous thyroid hormone ingestion (factitious hyperthyroidism), the hyperthyroid phase of subacute thyroiditis, or iodine-induced hyperthyroidism.

Management of hyperthyroidism

The first step in management of the patient with hyperthyroidism is to determine the underlying etiology and to exclude the possibility of one of the transient forms that may require supportive therapy directed toward the primary process (hormone ingestion, iodine exposure, subacute thyroiditis). While the vast majority of patients with either Graves' disease or toxic multinodular goiter can be treated using antithyroid drugs, radioactive iodine, or surgery, radioactive iodine ablation is the preferred treatment in the elderly patient.[110,111]

In the patient with suspected hyperthyroidism who is still undergoing investigation, a useful initial step in treatment is the administration of β-adrenergic blocking agents such as propranolol, metoprolol, or atenolol. These agents are especially indicated in patients who have palpitations, tachycardia, angina, or agitation as symptoms since use of the β-blockers can lead to quick symptom control. These drugs act by interfering with some peripheral actions of thyroid hormone, but do not correct the hypermetabolic state. The drugs, however, do not interfere with laboratory assessment of thyroid function and can allow control of symptoms until definitive treatment can be undertaken.

Once a diagnosis of Graves' disease or a toxic nodular goiter is established, treatment should be started with one of the antithyroid drugs, propylthiouracil or methimazole.[112] These agents impair biosynthesis of thyroid hormone and will lead to depletion of intrathyroidal hormone stores and consequently to decreased hormone secretion. A decline in serum-T4 concentration is usually seen by 2–4 weeks after initiation of antithyroid drug therapy, and the dose can be tapered once thyroid hormone levels reach the normal range in order to avoid development of hypothyroidism. In 1–5 percent of patients, the antithyroid drugs may cause fever, rash, and arthralgia. Drug-induced agranulocytosis occurs more commonly in the elderly population and is most likely to occur within the first 3 months of treatment, especially in patients who receive more than 30 mg/day of methimazole.[113] Periodic monitoring of the white blood cell count should be done and the drugs discontinued if there is evidence of neutropenia. Long-term antithyroid drug administration can be used as a primary therapy in patients over the age of 60 with Graves' disease, who appear to respond more rapidly and have a greater likelihood of long-lasting remission than younger persons.[114,115] Long-term antithyroid drugs are rarely successful in inducing sustained remission in elderly patients with toxic multinodular goiter.

The recommended definitive treatment in the elderly group is thyroid ablation through use of [131]I.[110,111] Once the patient has been rendered euthyroid by antithyroid drugs, these agents should be stopped for 3–5 days, following which ^{131}I is given orally. Therapy with β-blockers can be maintained and antithyroid agents can be restarted 5 days after radiotherapy and continued for 4–10 weeks until the effect of radioiodine is achieved.

Many therapists will attempt to calculate a dose that will render the patient euthyroid without subsequent development of hypothyroidism. These calculations are based on clinical estimate of thyroid gland size, 24-hour ^{131}I uptake, and whether the gland is diffusely overactive or contains toxic nodules. In spite of this approach, many patients will still develop permanent hypothyroidism following ^{131}I therapy.[116] It is not unreasonable to treat all elderly patients with a large dose of ^{131}I to assure ablation of thyroid tissue and avoid the possibility of recurrence of hyperthyroidism. Using this approach, patients are monitored following treatment until their serum thyroid hormone levels reach the hypothyroid range and are then put on permanent replacement therapy with exogenous thyroid hormone. Hypothyroidism may be evident as early as 4 weeks after treatment and can occur at any time after treatment. With all dosing regimens, by 12 months posttherapy 40–50 percent of patients are hypothyroid and hypothyroidism continues to occur thereafter at the rate of 2–3 percent per year.[117]

Periodic monitoring of thyroid status is a necessity for any patient treated with ^{131}I who has not yet become hypothyroid.

Surgery is not recommended as a primary choice for treatment of hyperthyroidism in the elderly patient. The frequent accompaniment of hyperthyroidism by many coexisting disorders, including cardiac, pulmonary, and CNS disease, puts the patient at increased operative risk. In addition, postoperative complications of hypoparathyroidism and recurrent laryngeal nerve damage represent significant problems, especially when surgery is performed by surgeons not highly experienced in thyroidectomy.[118] Surgery may be of value for the rare patient with tracheal compression secondary to a large goiter.

ATRIAL FIBRILLATION This condition occurs in 10–15 percent of hyperthyroid patients, most of whom are elderly.[106] In a retrospective study of 163 hyperthyroid patients with atrial fibrillation, approximately 60 percent had spontaneous reversion to sinus rhythm after becoming euthyroid. Most of these reversions occurred with 3 weeks of becoming euthyroid, while no patient reverted if atrial fibrillation was still present after 4 months of euthyroidism or if atrial fibrillation had been present for more than 13 months before becoming euthyroid.[119] Thus, the patient who remains in atrial fibrillation beyond 16 weeks of return to the euthyroid state is a candidate for cardioversion.

While in the hyperthyroid state, the patient with atrial fibrillation is more sensitive to the anticoagulant effect of warfarin, resulting in a greater lowering of activity of coagulation factors II and VII and greater increase in prothrombin ratio and partial thromboplastin time.[120] Many older persons with hyperthyroidism and atrial fibrillation are at increased risk for thromboembolic events, especially those with a prior history of thromboembolism, hypertension, or congestive heart failure or who have evidence of left atrial enlargement or left ventricular dysfunction.[106] In the absence of contraindications, anticoagulant therapy should be given with warfarin in a dose which will increase the international normalization ratio (INR) to 2.0–3.0. Warfarin should be continued until euthyroidism has been achieved and there has been return to a normal sinus rhythm.[105]

ACUTE HYPERTHYROIDISM

Acute hyperthyroidism or "thyroid storm" can occur in the patient with either known or undiagnosed hyperthyroidism who is subjected to acute stress such as an operative procedure, trauma, or infection or who is exposed to iodine-containing drugs. It can also occur in the elderly patient treated with ^{131}I who did not receive adequate antithyroid medication prior to therapy.[121] In these patients, features of severe hyperthyroidism may develop over several hours and include fever, tachycardia, vomiting, diarrhea, dehydration, severe restlessness, and disorientation. Patients with cardiac disease are at especially high risk for acute heart failure or acute myocardial ischemia.

Thyroid storm is a life-threatening condition and must be treated vigorously and promptly.[122,123] Immediate treatment involves administration of antithyroid drugs and iodide to interfere with thyroid hormone production. Propylthiouracil is given in an initial dose of 900–1,200 mg followed in several hours with sodium iodide or oral Lugol's solution. High-dose β-blockers such as propranolol and high-dose corticosteroids are also given to blunt peripheral action of thyroid hormones and to inhibit T4 to T3 conversion in peripheral tissues. Supportive measures include sedation, fluids, antipyretics, and cooling blankets, plus antibiotics if infection is present.[122]

SUBCLINICAL HYPERTHYROIDISM

The finding of suppressed or nondetectable serum TSH along with normal serum T4 and/or T3, often in the upper end of the normal range, is defined as subclinical hyperthyroidism. Etiology ranges from excessive thyroid hormone replacement therapy to thyroid disease, with the most common cause in the elderly person being longstanding multinodular goiter.

Individuals with thyroid function values indicating the presence of subclinical hyperthyroidism generally have no or only mild clinical features suggestive of hyperthyroidism.[124] The finding of subnormal TSH concentrations in the elderly is not infrequent. In a study of 1,210 persons in England, low TSH was found in 6.3 percent of women and 5.5 percent of men.[125] However, repeat measurements of serum TSH 1 year later showed a return of TSH to the normal range in the majority of cases. Several studies suggest that the conversion rate to overt hyperthyroidism ranges from 1.5 to 13 percent within one year.[125–127] Thus, the natural history of subclinical hyperthyroidism is variable, sometimes disappearing over time. However, persons with subclinical hyperthyroidism are at increased risk of developing atrial fibrillation as reflected by a cumulative incidence of 28 percent over a 10-year period in individuals over the age of 60 years, representing a 3-fold increase in risk.[127] There may be other cardiac consequences of persistent subclinical hyperthyroidism including increased prevalence of atrial premature beats, increased heart rate, increased left ventricular mass, enhanced systolic function, and impaired diastolic function.[128]

Many studies suggest that apparently asymptomatic individuals with subclinical hyperthyroidism have accelerated loss of bone mineral which is benefited by treatment.[129–131] Post-menopausal women with subclinical hyperthyroidism and nodular goiter who were treated with ^{131}I with subsequent normalization of serum TSH had an increase in bone mineral density at the spine and hip after 2 years of follow-up while a similar group of women who were not treated showed progressive bone loss.[132] Therefore, the finding of suppressed TSH and normal T4 in an asymptomatic elderly person calls for periodic retesting of thyroid function, including measurement of FT4. In the presence of significant osteopenia or if there is subsequent development of clinical features of hyperthyroidism, atrial fibrillation or increased thyroid hormone production, restoration of thyroid function to normal should be undertaken. Normalization of thyroid function tests has been suggested as an appropriate intervention in all persons with persistent subclinical hyperthyroidism in order to prevent later development of osteoporosis or cardiac dysfunction.[128,133]

HYPOTHYROIDISM

Hypothyroidism is the clinical state that results from inadequate peripheral tissue response to thyroid hormone action. Most commonly, this occurs as a consequence of decreased thyroid hormone production from the thyroid gland,[134,135] but in rare instances can result from tissue unresponsiveness to the presence of adequate amounts of thyroid hormone in the circulation.[136,137] Deficient thyroid hormone release most commonly is the result of disease or dysfunction of the thyroid gland itself and is referred to as "primary hypothyroidism." In some patients, pituitary TSH release is inadequate, leading to failure of the thyroid gland and "secondary hypothyroidism." Rare cases of "tertiary hypothyroidism" have been identified in which the underlying mechanism is failure of synthesis or release of hypothalamic TRH.

Demography

Hypothyroidism is relatively common in the general population and shows a clear sex and age relationship.[78,83] The Whickham, England, study identified hypothyroidism, based on measurement of serum TSH, in 19 per 1,000 women with a mean age at diagnosis of 57 years and a prevalence 10-fold more common in women than in men. The incidence rate of elevated serum TSH showed a direct relationship to age in women, increasing from 4.0 to 5.7 percent of women under age 45 to 17.4 percent of women over the age of 75 years. In men, elevated serum TSH was present in 1.6–3.5 percent of those under age 65 and increased to 3.5–6.9 percent in persons over the age of 65 years.[84] Similarly, study of the Framingham population in the USA revealed clear elevation of serum TSH in 5.9 percent of women between the ages of 60 and 89 years and borderline elevation in an additional 7.7 percent. Men of the same age had elevated serum TSH in 2.4 percent of subjects, with another 3.3 percent showing borderline levels.[138]

Many population studies carried out in Great Britain, Sweden, Switzerland, West Germany, Japan, and the USA confirm the high frequency of hypothyroidism in the population, its predominance in women, and its progressive increase with advancing age.[78,85,108,139–145] Based on the clear influence of age on the risk of development of hypothyroidism, it is reasonable to screen all elderly individuals for the possible presence of the disorder through measurement of serum TSH.[78]

Etiology

Hypothyroidism can arise as a consequence of inborn or acquired disorders/diseases of the thyroid gland, from exposure to agents affecting thyroid-hormone synthesis, and from disease or disturbance of hypothalamic–pituitary production of TRH and TSH (Table 94-1). In the elderly population, the most common cause of thyroid failure is Hashimoto's disease.[135] This autoimmune disorder is characterized histologically by continuous replacement of normal thyroid tissue with lymphocytic and fibrous tissue, ultimately leading to a reduced mass of functional thyroid elements and decline in hormone production.[4] Many patients can be identified by demonstrating the presence of antithyroglobulin and antimicrosmal antibodies in their serum.[67,68,71] Much evidence has accumulated for the presence of another family of immunoglobulins that are capable of blocking the action of TSH on thyroid cells either by interfering with TSH binding to its receptor or by blocking both pre- and postreceptor processes.[67,146]

There is a question over whether or not the presence of antithyroid antibodies in the serum can predict the subsequent development of hypothyroidism.[147] In a study of subjects with demonstrated thyroid antibodies, hypothyroidism developed at a rate of 5 percent per year. Other reports do not support the predictive value of antithyroid antibodies, although they document the strong association of the antibodies with the presence of increased serum TSH and clinical hypothyroidism.[148]

Some patients with previously diagnosed Graves' disease may go on to develop an autoimmune hypothyroidism.[149] This consequence may be related to the presence of TSH-blocking antibodies. Other forms of thyroiditis, such as subacute and silent thyroiditis, may progress from a transient hyperthyroid state to euthyroidism, and finally, to permanent hypothyroidism.

A major cause of hypothyroidism is the prior treatment of hyperthyroidism, especially Graves' disease, by either radioiodine[116,117] or subtotal thyroidectomy.[150] Both treatments have been demonstrated to be followed by a continuous, life-long risk of development of hypothyroidism, with a rate 1 year after initial treatment of 20–40 percent and an annual incidence of 2–4 percent each year thereafter. Any patient with a prior history of surgical or radioiodine treatment of hyperthyroidism should have yearly monitoring of thyroid status with serum TSH and/or T4.

Iodide and iodine-containing drugs can result in inhibition of thyroid-hormone synthesis (Wolff–Chaikoff effect) with ensuing hypothyroidism, which is usually reversible when the source of exogenous iodine or iodide is removed.[151] Common sources of iodine ingestion are expectorants (potassium iodide), topical antifungal or antiseptic agents (betadine), iodine-containing radiographic contrast agents, and the antiarrhythmic agent, amiodarone.[152] Long-term lithium therapy can also lead to impaired thyroid hormone synthesis and to inhibition of thyroid hormone release. As many as 20 percent of patients taking lithium may develop hypothyroidism.[49]

Impairment of production or release of TSH from the anterior pituitary or of TRH from the hypothalamus leads to secondary and tertiary hypothyroidism, respectively. These alterations can be the consequence of pituitary or hypothalamic tumors, surgical or traumatic injury, radiotherapy, or infiltrative diseases such as histiocytosis, sarcoidosis, tuberculosis, or amyloidosis. These patients may have isolated abnormalities of the TRH–TSH–thyroid axis or, more commonly, other associated disorders of hypothalamic, anterior, and posterior pituitary function.

Iodine deficiency in the past accounted for many cases of hypothyroidism, usually with an accompanying goiter. With the routine use of iodized salt and common exposure to many iodine-containing agents in the diet, this is now a rare cause of hypothyroidism in the USA. However, in many underdeveloped parts of the world, iodine deficiency remains as a common cause of failure of thyroid hormone production.

Clinical presentation of hypothyroidism

Hypothyroidism, particularly in the elderly population, is a disorder with insidious onset characterized by the emergence of symptoms and signs over many years, so that neither the patient nor close associates may be aware of the process.[153,154] Consequently, the manifestations of hypothyroidism are often attributed to "old age" or to other disorders common in the elderly person. Depending on recognition of the "classic" clinical features of hypothyroidism will invariably result in failure to make the diagnosis in many symptomatic patients.[155] In one study, only 10 percent of patients with a laboratory-confirmed diagnosis were recognized as being hypothyroid on clinical examination.[156] Similar results have been found in other investigations.[138,139,141,157]

Central nervous system manifestations are a significant consequence of hypothyroidism in the elderly population. Mental slowing is common, along with complaints of fatigue and excessive sleepiness. The possibility of psychiatric disorder is raised by patients who present with depression, delerium, or paranoid ideation.[139,158,159] So-called "myxedema madness" with psychotic behavior is infrequent. Alterations in level of consciousness can occur with confusion and coma. An acute decline in mental status may be precipitated by the stress of infection or trauma, exposure to the cold, or to drugs such as sedatives and narcotics.[160] Seizures can occasionally be due to severe hypothyroidism. The possibility that hypothyroidism may be a cause of reversible dementia has led to much study of patients undergoing dementia evaluation. Most reports confirm that while hypothyroidism is common in patients with dementia, only rarely is the dementia truly reversible with thyroid hormone therapy, although there may be overall improvement in the patients' functional state.[139]

Classic cold intolerance and diminished sweating are often present in the elderly hypothyroid patient, but these symptoms are also common in euthyroid elderly. Hypothermia may be found. Dry skin, puffiness of the face, periorbital edema, coarsened and thinned hair, thinning of the outer parts of the eyebrows, brittle nails, and yellowing of the skin are common features of the patient, but also occur with great frequency in patients of advanced age whose thyroid function appears normal.

Coarsening of the voice with slow and sometimes slurred speech should increase the awareness of possible hypothyroidism. Hearing impairment may be due to thyroid insufficiency or, more commonly, hypothyroidism may aggravate a hearing disorder of other cause.

An important feature of thyroid deficiency in the elderly group is physical slowing with accompanying symptoms of fatigue, weakness, and occasionally muscle stiffness. Arthralgia can also lead to physical slowing. Entrapment neuropathy with paresthesias can occur, especially involving the carpal tunnel.[161] Other aspects of neurological involvement in hypothyroidism include impairment of reflex function leading to the classic delayed or "hung-up" relaxation phase of the reflex. Not infrequently, there may be hyporeflexia or complete loss of reflexes, especially of the achilles tendon.

In the elderly patient, assessment of changes in weight may give little insight into a possible diagnosis of hypothyroidism. Weight gain may occur, but decrease in appetite may be sufficient to result in weight loss. Bowel motility may be slowed with resultant constipation but, here again, this is a common complaint of the nonhypothyroid elderly.

The myocardium is affected by thyroid-hormone deficiency, with the most common changes being bradycardia and narrowed pulse pressure. Reduced cardiac output is the consequence of slowed heart rate, decreased ventricular filling, and decrease in ventricular contractility.[106,162] The myocardium may undergo myxedematous infiltration with resultant cardiac enlargement, symptoms of ischemic heart disease, and development of pericardial effusion.[163] Electrocardiographic abnormalities may be seen including slow heart rate, low voltage of the QRS complex, flattening or inversion of T waves, and ventricular arrhythmias.[106] Alterations in peripheral vascular resistance can lead to hypertension. Reduced cardiac output results in decrease of glomerular filtration rate, and consequent renal retention of sodium and water, so that peripheral edema may develop even in the absence of overt congestive heart failure.

Hematological, metabolic, and other systemic impacts of hypothyroidism are more likely to be detected by laboratory evaluation than by clinical examination.[164] Anemia of the normocytic or macrocytic type can be found in about one-third of patients,[139] appears to be mediated by insufficient production of erythropoietin, and is directly attributable to the lack of thyroid hormone. Serum iron may be low in some patients, but serum levels of folic acid and B_{12} are usually normal. Pernicious anemia occurs frequently in association with autoimmune forms of hypothyroidism and should be looked for in hypothyroid patients with persistent anemia after hormonal treatment or in patients with macrocytosis and low serum B_{12}.

Hyponatremia occurs frequently in elderly individuals and may be found in patients with hypothyroidism. The clinical picture is that of the syndrome of inappropriate antidiuretic-hormone secretion—that is, dilutional hyponatremia, concentrated urine, normal or expanded intravascular volume, and sodium excretion in the urine. The mechanism appears to be due to increased release of antidiuretic hormone as well as to altered renal blood flow with increased tubular reabsorption of sodium and water.

Evidence suggestive of myopathy is provided by elevated levels of serum-creatine phosphokinase (CPK), which may be very high. The increased levels are largely contributed to by decreased renal clearance of the enzyme.

MYXEDEMA COMA This condition is an extreme, life-threatening form of hypothyroidism that occurs almost exclusively in the elderly population. Presentation is that of an elderly person with rapid development of stupor, seizures, or coma, often in association with infection, stress, exposure to the cold, or following administration of sedatives, tranquilizers, or narcotics.[160] History or symptoms of hypothyroidism may have been present for a long time. Hypothermia of profound degree is often present along with more common signs of hypothyroidism. Respiratory depression with hypoxia and carbon dioxide retention is commonly present and may necessitate intubation and ventilatory assistance. Blood pressure may be low, along with bradycardia and features of shock. Laboratory data will reveal, in addition to marked hypothyroxinemia, hyponatremia, hypoglycemia, elevation of serum CPK, and evidence of respiratory acidosis with increase in P_{CO_2}. Recognition of the syndrome and prompt initiation of therapy is essential, the mortality rate probably being in excess of 50 percent.

Laboratory diagnosis of hypothyroidism

The findings of low serum T4 concentration along with elevation of serum TSH clearly establish a diagnosis of primary hypothyroidism and these two findings require no further investigation.[42] Measurement of serum T3 in an elderly patient is of little diagnostic value because many disorders or drugs common in this age group lead to reduced concentrations of T3.[28] Conversely, in some patients with hypothyroidism, serum T3 levels may remain in the normal range.

The failure to find elevation of serum TSH in a patient with reduced serum T4 and/or T3 concentrations and clinical features suspicious for hypothyroidism requires that more extensive laboratory evaluation be carried out. The differentiation between secondary or tertiary hypothyroidism and the various "sick euthyroid" syndromes may be difficult. Normal values of FT4 point against hypothyroidism, but low FT4 may be seen in both conditions. Measurement of rT3 may be useful because its concentration will be low in true hypothyroidism and is generally normal or increased in nonthyroidal illness.[28]

The TRH test may occasionally be of value because patients with secondary hypothyroidism will show blunted or absent rise in TSH, while the sick euthyroid individual usually will respond to TRH with a rise. The measurement of antithyroid antibodies may provide indirect support for a diagnosis of hypothyroidism if the titers are high, but the levels themselves cannot indicate the functional state of the thyroid gland.

Therapy for hypothyroidism

The establishment of a diagnosis of hypothyroidism generally calls for initiation of thyroid hormone replacement. In the vast majority of patients, the preferred form of treatment is with synthetic L-thyroxine. There is little role for treatment with T3 because peripheral conversion of T4 to T3 is capable of providing adequate amounts of T3.

It is now well-established that the usual replacement dose of T4 is lower in the elderly than in the young patient, largely as a result of an age-related reduction in the rate of T4 clearance.[165–169] The mean daily dose of T4 for patients over the age of 65 years has been estimated to be 0.110 mg (1.6 μg/kg), but it varies in individual patients from 0.05 to 0.2 mg. Determination of the optimum T4 dose is based on monitoring of serum TSH and is defined as the dose of T4 that will reduce serum TSH into the normal range.[170] There is a suggestion that the magnitude of initial serum TSH elevation correlates with the final T4 replacement dose.[169]

Excessive thyroid hormone replacement should be avoided. Elderly patients treated with L-thyroxine in standard doses and with serum T4 in the normal range have often been found to have suppressed serum TSH. Even though clinically evident features of hyperthyroidism are not detectable, metabolic effects of increased thyroid hormone can occur, and include increased nocturnal heart rate, shortened systolic time interval, increased urinary sodium excretion, and increased hepatic and muscle enzyme activity.[171,172] Of even greater consequence is the observation that patients on thyroid hormone replacement who have suppressed serum TSH also have evidence for increased bone resorption with consequent risk of accelerated rate of osteoporosis and, possibly, increased risk of fracture.[172–174]

In the elderly patient, initiation of hormone replacement should be with small doses, which are then slowly increased until full replacement has been achieved.[165,166] For most older patients, a dose of 0.025 mg daily of L-thyroxine is an appropriate starting amount. Subsequent increases can be in increments of 0.025 mg daily at 4–8 week intervals until normalization of serum TSH has been accomplished. It is not usual for the decline in TSH to lag behind the attainment of normal values for serum T4. This approach to treatment will minimize the risk of possible adverse effects of thyroid therapy, which include provocation of anginal pain, myocardial infarction, congestive heart failure, and arrhythmias.

Special attention must be given to the patient who, in addition to hypothyroidism, has an established diagnosis of ischemic heart disease. In this circumstance, it may be different to achieve full hormone replacement without provoking cardiac symptoms. Attempt should be made to maximize the antianginal regimen, including administration of β-blockers, vasodilator agents, and calcium-channel blockers.[175,176] Should this approach fail, the patient should undergo evaluation for the possibility of angioplasty or coronary artery bypass surgery.[177]

In the patient who is thought to have secondary or tertiary hypothyroidism, consideration must be given to the possibility that there may be coexistent ACTH deficiency with resultant hypoadrenalism. Because the increased metabolic state resulting from thyroid replacement can precipitate the clinical picture of adrenal insufficiency, glucocorticoid replacement should be started concomitantly with thyroid hormone if there is any likelihood that ACTH deficiency is present. Some patients with longstanding, severe primary hypothyroidism may also develop signs of adrenal insufficiency following initiation of thyroid hormone, owing to metabolic impairment of adrenal hormone production from the hypothyroidism itself. Should any features of hypoadrenalism be suspected, prompt treatment with physiological doses of glucocorticoids should be started. After a euthyroid state has been achieved, the steroid dose may be tapered and discontinued. In some patients, it may be prudent to start treatment with both thyroid and glucocortocoid hormones and discontinue the latter as the patient approaches euthyroidism.

The treatment of *myxedema coma* warrants special consideration. The patient should be cared for in an intensive-care setting.[122,178,179] If the diagnosis is suspected, therapy must be started at once, even though laboratory confirmation has not yet been obtained.[122,178,179] Treatment with thyroxine is necessary to correct the hypothyroid state with an initial dose of 300–500 µg given intravenously, because both intestinal and intramuscular absorption are likely to be unreliable.[178,179] In a review of 87 patients with myxedema coma, initial thyroxine doses greater than 500 µg were associated with a mortality rate of 53 percent, whereas the mortality rate in patients treated with an initial dose less than 500 µg was 9 percent. Mortality was highest in those patients over the age of 65 years.[180] Once there is evidence of a clinical response such as rise in body temperature and heart rate, the daily dose of thyroxine should be reduced to 50–100 µg, given orally as soon as possible and adjusted further as necessary by monitoring of serum TSH.[179] T3 or combinations of T4 and T3 are not recommended in an elderly patient since the acute metabolic impact of T3 can lead to cardiac arrhythmia or myocardial infarction.

Adrenal insufficiency can be present in patients with myxedema coma. In life-threatening situations, blood for measurement of cortisol should be drawn and intravenous stress doses of glucocorticoids should be given and continued until there is laboratory confirmation of status of adrenal function. A decision can then be made to either continue treatment for adrenal insufficiency or to taper and discontinue the glucocorticoid.

Supportive therapy must be promptly initiated and may include ventilatory support for respiratory failure, antibiotics for infection, external rewarming for hypothermia, and correction of hypotension by fluid replacement or dopamine. Hyponatremia, if severe, should be treated.

SUBCLINICAL HYPOTHYROIDISM

As a result of a number of large laboratory survey studies, a significant population of individuals has been identified who have serum levels of TSH above the accepted upper limits of normal, but in whom serum concentrations of T4 and T3 are normal, and symptoms of hypothyroidism are usually mild or lacking.[78,83,157] This syndrome has been termed "subclinical hypothyroidism" and is most commonly found in women above the age of 60 years.[181–184] It is thought that the failing thyroid gland responds with an increase in TSH secretion which, in turn, is capable of further driving the thyroid to maintain normal levels of T4 and T3 until true thyroid failure ensues. In the Framingham study, 5.9 percent of subjects over the age of 60 years had clearly elevated serum-TSH concentrations (>10 mIU/L) with normal serum T4 levels, and an additional 14.4 percent had slightly elevated serum TSH (5–10 mIU/L) with normal serum T4.[138]

Of primary clinical importance is the question of what the likelihood is that the person with laboratory criteria for subclinical hypothyroidism will go on to develop clinical hypothyroidism. In a long-term follow-up study, women who initially had antithyroglobulin and antimicrosomal antibodies along with a serum TSH of greater than 6 mIU/L developed overt hypothyroidism at the rate of 5 percent per year. No cases developed in women with borderline elevation of TSH only (6–10 mIU/L), and only one case developed in the 67 women who had antithyroid antibodies with normal TSH levels.[182]

Other studies support progression to overt hypothyroidism at the rate of 7 percent per year in women with elevated serum TSH and high titers of antithyroid antibodies with ranges from 1 percent to 20 percent per year.[76,185,186] It is clear that the presence of antithyroid antibodies constitutes a significant risk factor for the development of clinically apparent hypothyroidism in women who are found to have isolated elevated values of serum TSH.[84,146]

Women with hypercholesterolemia have an increased likelihood of having coexisting subclinical hypothyroidism.[187] Patients with subclinical hypothyroidism have been noted to have a relative increase in low-density lipoprotein and decrease in high-density lipoprotein with a higher prevalence of ischemic heart disease.[188] In a large group of elderly women with evidence of aortic atherosclerosis, 13.9 percent were found to have subclinical hypothyroidism; and in those women with a history of myocardial infarction, 21.5 percent had subclinical hypothyroidism.[184] Similarly, the presence of subclinical hypothyroidism was accompanied by a high prevalence of both aortic atherosclerosis and myocardial infarction, with an even higher prevalence in those who also had detectable antimicrosomal antibodies.

Thus, attention must be given to the question of whether or not the detection of subclinical hypothyroidism warrants treatment. Treatment with L-thyroxine has resulted in improved systolic and diastolic functioning, improvement in left ventricular ejection fraction with exercise, and decrease in systemic vascular resistance.[189,190] Several studies have reported that treatment with L-thyroxine results in decrease in total and LDL cholesterol, increase in serum high-density lipoproteins, and decrease in low-density lipoproteins and apolipoprotein B, and some sense of improved well-being and performance on psychometric testing.[191–198] There are no substantive data as yet to indicate that early treatment of subclinical hypothyroidism with thyroid hormone replacement is effective in reducing the risk for subsequent development of atherosclerosis or coronary artery disease. At present, a conservative approach is to monitor patients identified with the syndrome with serum TSH and T4 at 6–12 month intervals. Replacement therapy with thyroxine should be given to those patients with serum TSH greater than 10 mIU/L and to those with TSH between 5 and 10 mIU/L who have either high levels of antimicrosomal antibodies or symptoms consistent with mild hypothyroidism.

NODULAR THYROID DISEASE AND NEOPLASIA

The development of thyroid nodules is an age-related process that occurs more commonly in women than in men.[84,199–201] Autopsy studies have demonstrated that thyroid nodules are frequently found in the elderly population, even when clinical examination of the neck has failed to reveal abnormality.[199,201] Autopsy data reveal that an increase in frequency of nodules is evident in women and men over age 30 with a rapid increase to a frequency of 90 percent in women and 50 percent in men aged over 70 years.

Clinical presentations

Thyroid nodules most commonly are asymptomatic and may be discovered accidentally by the patient or are found by the physician during the course of a physical examination. Of greatest concern is the finding of a single palpable nodule, which raises the possibility of thyroid malignancy. In many such patients, further evaluation will reveal the presence of multiple nodules. Although a single nodule is more likely to harbor a malignancy than a multinodular thyroid, only approximately 10 percent of clinical single nodules will, in fact, be malignant.

Patients with thyroid nodules should be questioned for the history of external radiation exposure of the head, neck, and upper thorax. It is well-established that radiation of the thyroid results in a marked increase in risk of developing thyroid malignancy. In the USA, it was common practice for many years up to the 1950s to treat facial acne, tonsillar enlargement, cervical adenitis, and thymic enlargement with external radiation. It is estimated that several million people were irradiated, many of whom are entering or are now in the over-60 age group. Although a history of irradiation in a patient with nodular thyroid increases the likelihood of malignancy, it is important to note that irradiation also increases the development of benign nodules. Of individuals who as children received low-dose head and neck irradiation, 87 percent have ultrasound-detectable nodules, from 16 to 29 percent will develop palpable thyroid nodules and, of these, approximately one-third will be malignant.[202,203] Nodules are apparent after a latency of 10–20 years and the incidence of malignant nodules reaches a peak 20–30 years after exposure.[200,202]

Occasionally, a thyroid nodule will be associated with acute onset of neck pain and tenderness. This circumstance may be the result of acute or subacute thyroiditis or hemorrhage into a pre-existing nodule.

The finding of multinodular thyroid is increased in areas of iodine deficiency. Often there is a history of goiter dating back to childhood or young adult years. Very large multinodular goiter, particularly those with a sizable substernal component, may compress the trachea and lead to complaints of dyspnea. Disturbances of swallowing may also occur. This presentation is most common in older women. A large substernal goiter sometimes is first recognized when the patient has had a chest radiogram and is noted to have compression or deviation of the trachea or a superior mediastinal mass.[204]

Differential diagnosis

The entities that present as thyroid nodules are many. The vast majority are the result of benign thyroid lesions and include follicular and colloid adenomas, acute and subacute thyroiditis, Hashimoto's thyroiditis, and thyroid cysts. Malignant thyroid neoplasms include papillary, follicular, medullary, and anaplastic carcinomas, as well as thyroid lymphoma and metastases to the thyroid. Nonthyroid lesions may also present as apparent thyroid nodules and include lymph nodes, aneurysms, parathyroid adenomas and cysts, and thyroglossal duct cysts.[205]

The likelihood that a single nodule is malignant is increased if there is a history of radiation exposure, if it occurs in a man, has been observed to undergo increase in size, is accompanied by hoarseness of the voice suggestive of impingement on the recurrent laryngeal nerve, and is stony hard on palpation.

Age appears to be a risk factor for the development of thyroid cancer. The National Cancer Data Base of 53,856 patients with thyroid cancer indicates that approximately 25 percent of all thyroid cancers are first diagnosed in individuals who are older than 60 years.[206,207] The overall histological distribution of thyroid cancer is 79 percent papillary, 13 percent follicular, 3 percent Hurthle cell, 3.5 percent medullary, and 1.7 percent anaplastic.[206] Age is a factor in predicting histological type of malignancy.[206,208] (Table 94-3). In patients over the age of 60 years, papillary carcinoma accounts for approximately 67 percent of thyroid cancers. Follicular carcinoma, the next most common histological type, has a peak frequency in both the fourth and sixth decades of life with a mean age at diagnosis of 44 years. It, along with Hurthle-cell carcinoma, makes up approximately 23 percent of the thyroid malignancies in the over-60 age group. Medullary carcinoma has a peak incidence in the fifth and sixth decades and accounts for 5 percent of thyroid cancers in the elderly population.[206,209]

Anaplastic carcinoma of the thyroid is almost exclusively a disease of older persons and accounts for approximately 6 percent of thyroid cancers in this age group. It is invariably fatal in a short period of time from its first diagnosis, especially when greater than 5 cm in diameter.[210] Clinically, it often arises in an area of previous thyroid disease and is recognized by its rapid growth, rock-like consistency, and local invasiveness with recurrent laryngeal nerve involvement and tracheal compression.

Lymphoma and metastatic cancers make up the remaining thyroid malignancies in elderly people. Lymphoma is characterized by a rapidly enlarging painless neck mass which may cause compressive symptoms and initially may be difficult to differentiate from anaplastic carcinoma on clinical appearance alone. Hashimato's thyroiditis is commonly present in patients with lymphoma.[211]

The rapid onset of a painful, tender thyroid mass with accompanying fever and leukocytosis is highly suggestive of acute suppurative thyroiditis. Similarly, the development of a painful, tender, firm thyroid mass without fever and leukocytosis points towards a diagnosis of subacute or granulomatous thyroiditis. History of an antecedent upper-respiratory tract infection with sore throat is further supportive of the diagnosis. This disorder may be accompanied in its acute phase by transient hyperthyroidism as a result of leakage of thyroid hormones from damaged follicular cells. Another consideration in the patient with acute onset of a painful, tender neck mass is hemorrhage into a previously asymptomatic thyroid cyst or adenoma.

Evaluation of a thyroid nodule

The major objective of evaluation in the patient who is found to have a thyroid nodule, especially an apparently single nodule, is to determine if the nodule is benign or malignant. A number of diagnostic modalities are available.

Blood tests of thyroid function will usually give normal results, with the exception of the patient with a hyperfunctioning adenoma or toxic multinodular goiter. In some patients with nodular disease secondly to Hashimato's thyroiditis, serum TSH may be increased. Measurement of serum thyroglobulin is often elevated in patients with thyroid cancer, but cannot reliably differentiate malignancy from benign adenoma or thyroiditis.[77] Its major usefulness is in the early recognition of recurrence or metastasis in patients with papillary or follicular carcinoma who had previously undergone total thyroidectomy. Elevation of serum calcitonin concentration is highly supportive of a diagnosis of medullary carcinoma.[212]

Determination of functional status of a nodule by isotope imagining is useful. Malignant tissue rarely is able to take up iodine, so that identification of a nodule as "warm" or "hot" by ^{123}I or technetium scanning makes the likelihood of malignancy in the nodule remote. In addition, scanning may reveal that an apparent single nodule is, in fact, part of a multinodular thyroid, again decreasing the risk of malignancy. The finding of a nonfunctioning or "cold" nodule does not establish a diagnosis of malignancy since 95 percent of thyroid nodules are cold and, of these, the incidence of malignancy is 5 percent.[213] For this reason, isotopic scanning is no longer considered as an initial diagnostic test.

High-resolution ultrasonography can detect lesions as small as 2 mm and can permit classification of a nodule as solid, cystic, or mixed solid–cystic.[214] The technique will often demonstrate multinodularity in a gland with a single palpable nodule. The value of ultrasonography in establishing a diagnosis of malignancy is limited because there is considerable overlap in the ultrasound characteristics of benign and malignant nodules. The procedure may be useful in detecting recurrent or residual thyroid cancer and in screening individuals who have had a history of irradiation exposure. It may also be of value in the patient suspected of having thyroid lymphoma since this malignancy often produces a characteristic asymmetrical pseudocystic pattern.[215]

Computed tomography and MRI can provide detailed information on thyroid anatomy. These procedures are expensive and appear to add little to initial clinical assessment

Table 94-3 Occurrence of thyroid malignancy in the older patient, and 10-year survival

| Cancer type | Percentage of cancer patients | | Percentage 10-year survival[a] |
	> Age 40	> Age 64	
Papillary/mixed	79	60–67	<65
Follicular	13	20–25	<57
Medullary	3	5	<63
Anaplastic	2	6	0
Lymphoma	3	5	≤100

[a]Age at diagnosis > 60 years.

for malignancy.[65] However, they may be useful in determining the extent of disease in patients with anaplastic carcinoma or lymphoma of the thyroid. Additionally, CT and MTI can provide information about size and substernal extent of large goiters and compression of neck structures.

In patients with nontoxic nodular goiter, thyroid hormone has been used to suppress TSH on the assumption that benign lesions were more likely to be TSH-dependent and, therefore, likely to decrease in size. The procedure involves giving L-thyroxine in a dose sufficient to suppress serum TSH and monitoring of size of the thyroid nodule for a period of 3–6 months. Because of the subjective nature of assessment of thyroid nodular size, and the demonstration that suppressive therapy had little significant effect on goiter or nodule size during several well-controlled trials of L-thyroxine, there does not appear to be justification for future use of this procedure.[216,217] In addition, the administration of suppressive doses of L-thyroxine to elderly patients carries substantial risk for precipitation or aggravation of ischemic heart disease and for acceleration of bone loss.

Fine-needle aspiration (FNA) of the thyroid to obtain tissue for cytological or histological examination appears to be the most reliable and accurate method of separating benign from malignant disease.[218–220] FNA is indicated in any patient with a solitary nodule and when there is suspicion of thyroid malignancy from clinical, ultrasound, or scanning findings. In skilled hands, the procedure is safe, inexpensive, and capable of determining the presence or absence of malignancy with 95 percent accuracy. The reliability of FNA can be further increased if done in conjunction with real-time sonographic guidance. The cytopathological findings from FNA are assigned to four categories: positive for malignancy, suspicious for malignancy, negative for malignancy, and nondiagnostic. In the case of a nondiagnostic aspirate, repeat FNA is recommended. Surgery is recommended for all patients with a malignant cytological diagnosis. For patients with a suspicious interpretation of the FNA, thyroid scanning is recommended with surgical excision to follow if the lesion is hypofunctioning. The patient with benign cytology can be managed subsequently by observation. The patient with clinical or FNA features suggestive of lymphoma should have a large-needle or surgical biopsy done to confirm the diagnosis.[215]

Management of thyroid nodules

The management of thyroid nodules is largely dependent on the results of the diagnostic evaluation, especially the determination as to whether the nodule has a high risk of being malignant.[221] Nodules identified as being "warm" and with associated normal thyroid hormone production and no compressive symptoms warrant only observation with examination at intervals of 6–12 months. "Hot" nodules are managed similarly as long as thyroid function is normal. If evidence for hyperthyroidism is found, then appropriate treatment for this condition should be initiated.

Subtotal thyroidectomy has been the traditional therapy for compressive goiter.[222] However, large compressive goiters can respond to ablation doses of [131]I (25–125 mCi) with significant shrinkage of the thyroid and accompanying relief of compressive symptoms such as stridor, dyspnea, and dysphagia.[204,217,223,224] In these patients, replacement doses of

L-thyroxine sufficient to keep serum TSH within the normal range should be given following either surgery or radioiodine treatment to maintain suppression of thyroid tissue and to avoid the late development of hypothyroidism.

If acute, suppurative thyroiditis is suspected, treatment with antibiotics is called for. The micro-organisms most commonly responsible are *Staphylococcus aureus*, *Streptococcus hemolyticus*, *Escherichia coli*, *Pneumococcus*, and *Salmonella*. Rarely, surgical drainage of a fluctuant mass will be necessary. Nodules found in association with subacute thyroiditis require no special care and may diminish in size as the disease resolves.

Management of the "cold" nodule is more complex.[225] When possible, FNA biopsy should be performed.[218–220] Demonstration of benign cytology in either a solid or cystic nodule indicates that the patient can be managed subsequently by observation. The combination of suspicious cytology by FNA and cold appearance on scanning should lead to recommendation of surgical excision. If FNA reveals malignant cells, operation is recommended with little need for further study.

Surgery for thyroid carcinoma should be performed only by a surgeon experienced in the procedure. If a diagnosis of malignancy has not been firmly established preoperatively, the nodule should be removed with a wide margin of uninvolved tissue and examined by frozen section. If a diagnosis of papillary or follicular carcinoma is confirmed or has been made prior to surgery, near-total thyroidectomy should be carried out because of the high frequency of multicentricity of malignancy and the need to remove functional thyroid tissue in order to monitor the patient with whole-body radioiodine scanning in the future.[207,221,226–228] Regional lymph nodes should be explored and removed if there is evidence of metastatic involvement. Postoperatively, attention must be paid to the possible complications of recurrent laryngeal nerve injury and hypoparathyroidism, which may be transient or permanent. Almost certainly, patients will become hypothyroid following surgery and will require hormone replacement, which should be in a dose sufficient to suppress serum TSH to levels below normal, if clinically tolerated.

Postoperatively, and at 6–12 month intervals thereafter, it will be necessary to discontinue thyroid replacement for a period of up to 6 weeks to allow endogenous serum TSH levels to rise sufficiently high to promote tissue uptake of [131]I. Alternatively, replacement thyroid hormone can be continued and recombinant human TSH (rhTSH) can be given intramuscularly at 24-hour intervals for two doses.[229] Twenty-four hours after the second dose of rhTSH or after the period of thyroid hormone withdrawal, blood is obtained for measurement of thyroglobulin and then large scanning doses of ^{131}I are administered and neck and total-body scans are performed at 24, 48, and 72 hours. If serum thyroglobulin is elevated, or if areas of uptake are found, large ablative doses of ^{131}I are then administered and replacement therapy reinstituted 48 hours later. This approach reduces the recurrence rate of both papillary and follicular carcinoma and prolongs survival.[207,227,228,230] The 10-year survival rate when initial diagnosis is made over the age of 60 years is estimated to be less than 65 percent for patients with papillary carcinoma, while 10-year survival falls to less than 57 percent in older patients with follicular carcinoma and is lower yet for patients with medullary carcinoma.[208,231] In patients with follicular carcinoma, increased size (greater than 3 cm) was associated with increased recurrence, and distant metastases at time of diagnosis predicted a high risk of subsequent death.[209]

For medullary carcinoma, the operative procedure of choice is total thyroidectomy because the disease is often multicentric. Routine dissection of the lymph modes is also recommended. The majority of medullary carcinomas do not respond to ^{131}I therapy so that patients with inoperable residual or recurrent disease are treated palliatively with external irradiation. The survival declines with increase in age at time of initial diagnosis, being substantially lower in patients over age 60 years. In patients in their seventh decade, approximately two-thirds will have persistent disease after surgery.[232] The efficacy of surgery can be monitored postoperatively by measurement of blood calcitonin concentration, both in the basal state and after stimulation.[212] Survival rates for thyroid malignancy initially diagnosed in patients over the age of 60 years are given in Table 94-3.

The management of anaplastic carcinoma of the thyroid remains unsatisfactory.[230] Relief of symptoms of compression can sometimes be achieved by surgery followed by high-dose (45–60 Gy) external irradiation.[233] Chemotherapy with doxorubicin may be beneficial in combination with surgery and external irradiation.[210,234]

Patients with thyroid lymphoma should have clinical staging carried out by means of CT or MRI. The survival rate can approach 100 percent in response to aggressive external irradiation in combination with CHOP (cytoxan, adriamycin, vincristine, prednisone) chemotherapy.[215]

Summary of management algorithm
Hyperthyroidism

- Use β-blockers for rate control of tachyarrhythmias.

- [131]I ablation is preferred treatment.

- If atrial fibrillation is present:
Use anticoagulants.
Use cardioversion if normal sinus rhythm has not occurred by 16 weeks after normalization of thyroid function.

- Use high dose antithyroid drugs plus iodide for thyroid storm.

Subclinical hyperthyroidism

- Normalize thyroid function if:
Atrial fibrillation occurs.
There is evidence for osteoporosis.

Hypothyroidism

- Treat with L-thyroxine:
Start with low-dose 12.5–25 µg daily.
Increase by 12.5–25 µg at 2–4 week intervals.

- Monitor treatment response with serum TSH.

- If coronary artery disease and angina are present, start β-blocker along with L-thyroxine.

- For myxedema coma:
Provide supportive care in intensive-care setting.
Treat immediately with IV L-thyroxine 300–500 µg.
Give IV glucocorticoids until adrenal status is determined.

Subclinical hypothyroidism

- Initiate treatment with L-thyroxine if:
TSH is >10 mIU/L.
Antithyroid antibody titers are >1:1600.
Dyslipidemia is present.
Coronary artery disease is present.
Symptoms suggestive of mild hypothyroidism are present.

Thyroid nodules/malignancy

- If suspicious nodule is present, do FNA biopsy.

- If positive diagnosis is made of differentiated thyroid cancer:
Treat with near-total thyroidectomy.
Follow with ^{131}I ablation of any thyroid remnant.
Subsequent yearly follow-up with ^{131}I scans and serum thyroglobulin.

KEY POINTS   Disorders of the thyroid

- Both disease states and drugs commonly used in the elderly can affect measures of thyroid function.

- Disorders of thyroid function increase in prevalence with increasing age.

- Since aging can alter the clinical presentation of both hyperthyroidism and hypothyroidism, screening for thyroid dysfunction is warranted for all persons over the age of 50 years.

- Treatment of both subclinical hyperthyroidism and subclinical hypothyroidism may prevent the later occurrence of significant adverse clinical events.

- Treatment of both hyperthyroidism and hypothyroidism in elderly people differs from the approach to treatment in younger persons.

- Thyroid malignancy increases in prevalence with increasing age, and initial diagnosis in the older person carries higher risk of subsequent recurrence and/or decreased survival.

REFERENCES

1. Mariotti S, Franceschi C, Cossarizza A, Pinchera A: The aging thyroid. Endocrinol Rev 1995;16:686–715
2. Mochizuki Y, Mowafy R, Pasternak B: Weights of human thyroids in New York City. Health Phys 1963;9:1299–1301
3. Hegedus L, Perrild H, Poulsen LR et al: The determination of thyroid volume by ultrasound and its relationship to body weight, age and sex in normal subjects. J Clin Endocrinol Metab 1983;56:260–263
4. Blumenthal HT, Perlstein IB: The aging thyroid. I: A description of lesions and an analysis of their age and sex distribution. J Am Geriatr Soc 1987;35:843–854
5. Denham MJ, Wills EJ: A clinco-pathological survey of thyroid glands in old age. Gerontology 1980;26:160–166
6. Barreca T, Franceschini R, Messina U et al: 24-hour thyroid-stimulating hormone secretory pattern in elderly men. Gerontology 1985;31:119–123
7. Snyder PJ, Utiger RD: Response to thyrotropin releasing hormone (TRH) in normal man. J Clin Endocrinol Metab 1972;34:380–385
8. Utiger RD: Thyrotropin-releasing hormone and thyrotropin secretion. J Lab Clin Med 1987;109:327–335
9. Harman SM, Whemann RE, Blackman MR: Pituitary-thyroid hormone economy in healthy aging men: basal indices of thyroid function and

thyrotropin responses to constant infusion of thyrotropin releasing hormone. J Clin Endocrinol Metab 1984;58:320–326

10. Van Coevorden A, Laurent E, Decoster C et al: Decreased basal and stimulated thyrotropin secretion in healthy elderly men. J Clin Endocrinol Metab 1989;69:177–185

11. Targum SD, Marshall LE, Magac-Harris K, Martin D: TRH tests in a healthy elderly population: demonstration of gender differences. J Am Geriatr Soc 1989;37:533–536

12. Hay ID, Klee GG: Thyroid dysfunction. Endocrinol Metab Clin North Am 1988;17:473–509

13. Snyder PJ, Utiger RD: Thyrotropin response to thyrotropin releasing hormone in normal females over forty. J Clin Endocrinol Metab 1972;34:1096–1098

14. Ryan M, Kovaks K, Ezrin C: Thyrotrophs in old age: an immunologic study of human pituitary glands. Endokrinologie 1979;73:191–198

15. Cuttelod S, Lemarchand-Beraud T, Magnenat P et al: Effect of age and role of kidneys and liver on thyrotropin turnover in man. Metabolism 1974;23:101–113

16. Olsen T, Laurberg P, Weeke J: Low serum triiodothyronine and high serum reverse triiodothyronine in old age: an effect of disease not age. J Clin Endocrinol Metab 1978;47:1111–1115

17. Hermann J, Heinen E, Kroll HJ et al: Thyroid function and thyroid hormone metabolism in elderly people. Low T3-syndrome in old age? Klin Wochenschr 1981;59:315–323

18. Chopra IJ, Solomon DH, Chopra U et al: Pathways of metabolism of thyroid hormones. Rec Prog Horm Res 1978;34:521–567

19. Hansen JM, Skovsted L, Siersboek-Nielsen K: Age dependent changes in iodine metabolism and thyroid function. Acta Endocrinol (Copenhagen) 1975;79:60–65

20. Braverman LE, Dawber NA, Ingbar SH: Observations concerning the binding of thyroid hormones in serum of normal subjects of varying age. J Clin Invest 1966;45:1273–1279

21. Hesch RD, Gatz J, Juppner H, Stubbe P: TBG dependency of age-related variations of thyroxine and triiodothyronine. Horm Metab Res 1977;9:141–146

22. Kabadi UM, Rosman PM: Thyroid hormone indices in adult healthy subjects: no influence of aging. J Am Geriatr Soc 1988;36:312–316

23. Gregerman RI, Gaffney GW, Shock NW: Thyroxine turnover in euthyroid man with special reference to changes with age. J Clin Invest 1962;41:2065–2074

24. Ingbar SH: Effect of aging on thyroid economy in man. J Am Geriatr Soc 1976;24:49–53

25. Nishikawa M, Inada M, Naito K et al: Age-related changes of serum 3, 3′-diiodothyronine, 3′-5′-diiodothyronine, and 3,5-diiodothyronine concentrations in man. J Clin Endocrinol Metab 1981;52:517–552

26. Gambert SR, Tsitouras PD: Effect of age on thyroid hormone physiology and function. J Am Geriatr Soc 1985;33:360–365

27. Engler D, Burger AG: The deiodination of the iodothyronines and of their derivatives in man. Endocrinol Rev 1984;5:151–184

28. Chopra IJ, Hershman JM, Pardridge MD et al: Thyroid function in nonthyroidal illnesses. Ann Intern Med 1983;98:946–957

29. Chopra IJ: Euthyroid sick syndrome: is it a misnomer? J Clin Endocrinol Metab 1997; 82: 329–334

30. Dillman WH: Mechanism of action of thyroid hormones. Med Clin North Am 1985;69:849–861

31. Oppenheimer JH: Thyroid hormone action at the nuclear level. Ann Intern Med 1985;102:374–384

32. Brent GA: The molecular basis of thyroid hormone action. N Engl J Med 1994;331:847–853

33. Sap J, Munoz A, Damm K et al: The c-erb-A protein is a high affinity receptor for thyroid hormone. Nature 1986;324:635–640

34. Weinberger C, Thompson CC, Ong ES et al: The c-erb-A gene encodes a thyroid hormone receptor. Nature 1986;324:641–646

35. Leonard JL, Kohrle J: Intracellular pathways of iodothyronine metabolism. In Braverman LE, Utiger RD (eds): Werner & Ingbar's The Thyroid, 8th edn. Lippincott Williams & Wilkins, Philadelphia, 2000:136–173

36. Larsen PR, Silva JE, Kaplan MM: Relationships between circulating and intracellular thyroid hormone: physiological and clinical implications. Endocrinol Rev 1981;2:87–102

37. Denckla WD: Role of the pituitary and thyroid glands on the decline of minimal oxygen consumption with age. J Clin Invest 1974;53:572–581

38. Gambert SR, Ingbar SH, Hagen TC: Interaction of age and thyroid hormone status on Na+–K+ATPase in rat renal cortex and liver. Endocrinology 1980;108:27–30

39. Mariotti S, Barbesino G, Caturegli P et al: Complex alteration of thyroid function in healthy centenarians. J Clin Endocrinol Metab 1993;77:1130–1134

40. Spencer CA: Clinical utility and cost effectiveness of sensitive thyrotropin assay in ambulatory and hospitalized patients. Mayo Clin Proc 1988;63:1214–1222

41. Franklyn JA, Black EG, Betteridge J, Sheppard MC: Comparison of second and third generation methods for measurement of serum thyrotropin in patients with overt hyperthyroidism, patients receiving thyroxine therapy, and those with nonthyroidal illness. J Clin Endocrinol Metab 1994;78:1368–1371

42. Klee GG, Hay ID: Assessment of sensitive thyrotropin assays for an expanded role in thyroid function testing: proposed criteria for analytic performance and clinical utility. J Clin Endocrinol Metab 1987;64:461–471

43. Burrow AW, Shakespear RA, Hesch RD et al: Thyroid hormones in the elderly sick: "T4 euthyroidism." BMJ 1975;4:437–439

44. Kaptein EM, MacIntyre SS, Weiner JM et al: Free thyroxine estimates in nonthyroidal illness: comparison of eight methods. J Clin Endocrinol Metab 1981;52:1073–1077

45. Surks MI, Hupart KH, Pan C, Shapiro LE: Normal free thyroxine in critical nonthyroidal illnesses measured by ultrafiltration of undiluted serum and equilibrium dialysis. J Clin Endocrinol Metab 1988;67:1031–1039

46. Csako G, Zweig MH, Benson C, Ruddel M: On the albumin dependence of measurements of free thyroxine. I: Technical performance of seven methods. Clin Chem 1986;32:108–115

47. Spencer CA: Clinical evaluation of free T4 techniques. J Endocrinol Invest 1986;9(suppl 4):57–66

48. Wiersinga WM: Nonthyroidal illness. In Braverman LE, Utiger RD (eds): Werner & Ingbar's The Thyroid, 8th edn. Lippincott Williams & Wilkins, Philadelphia, 2000:281–295

49. Surks MI, Sievert R: Drugs and thyroid function. N Engl J Med 1995;333:1688–1694

50. Chopra IJ, Huang T-S, Beredo A et al: Serum thyroid hormone binding inhibitor in nonthyroidal illnesses. Metabolism 1986;35:152–159

51. Wartofsky L, Burman KD: Alterations in thyroid function in patients with systemic illnesses: the "euthyroid sick syndrome." Endocrinol Rev 1982;3:164–217

52. Slag MF, Morley JE, Elson MK et al: Hypothyroxinemia in critically ill patients as a predictor of high mortality. JAMA 1981;245:43–45

53. Gavin LA: The diagnostic dilemmas of hyperthyroxinemia and hypothyroxinemia. Adv Int Med 1988;33:185–203

54. Hamblin PS, Dyer SA, Mohr VS et al: Relationship between thyrotropin and thyroxine changes during recovery from severe hypothyroxinemia of critical illness. J Clin Endocrinol Metab 1986;62:717–722

55. Tibaldi JM, Surks MI: Effects of nonthyroidal illness on thyroid function. Med Clin North Am 1985;69:899–911

56. Simmons RJ, Simon JM, Demers LM, Santen RJ: Thyroid dysfunction in elderly hospitalized patients. Effect of age and severity of illness. Arch Intern Med 1990;150:1249–1253

57. Bartalena L, Brogioni S, Grasso L et al: Relationship of the increased serum interleukin-6 concentration to changes of thyroid function in nonthyroidal illness. J Clin Invest 1994;17:269–274

58. Rogy MA, Coyle SM, Oldenburg HSA et al: Persistently elevated soluble tumor necrosis factor receptor and interleukin-1 receptor antagonist levels in critically ill patients. J Am Coll Surg 1994;178:132–138

59. Pang XP, Hershman JH, Mirell CJ, Pekary AE: Impairment of hypothalamic–pituitary–thyroid function in rats treated with human recombinant tumor necrosis factor-α (cachectin). Endocrinology 1989;125:76–84

60. Borst CG, Eil C, Burman KD: Euthyroid hyperthyroxinemia. Ann Intern Med 1983;98:366–378

61. Ruiz M, Rejatanavin R, Young RA et al: Familial dysalbuminemic hyperthyroxinemia: a syndrome that can be confused with thyrotoxicosis. N Engl J Med 1982;306:635–639

62. Robertson JS, Nolan NG, Wahner HW, McConahey WM: Thyroid radioiodine uptakes and scan in euthyroid patients. Mayo Clinic Proc 1975;50:79–84

63. Khafagi FA, MacFarlane DJ, Shapiro B, Gross MD: Nuclear medicine. In Moore WT, Eastman RC (eds): Diagnostic Endocrinology, 2nd edn. Mosby-YearBook, St Louis, 1996:451–492

64. McDougall IR, Cavalieri RR: In-vivo radionuclide tests and imaging. In Braverman LE, Utiger RD (eds): Werner & Ingbar's The Thyroid, 8th edn. Lippincott Williams & Wilkins, Philadelphia, 2000:355–375

65. Hegedus L: Nonisotopic techniques of thyroid imaging. In Braverman LE, Utiger RD (eds): Werner & Ingbar's The Thyroid, 8th edn. Lippincott Williams & Wilkins, Philadelphia, 2000:432–440

66. Zakarija M, McKenzie JM: The spectrum and significance of autoantibodies reacting with the thyrotropin receptor. Endocrinol Metab Clin North Am 1987;16:343–363

67. Dussault JH, Rousseau F: Immunologically mediated hypothyroidism. Endocrinol Metab Clin North Am 1987;16:417–429

68. Robuschi G, Safran M, Braverman LE et al: Hypothyroidism in the elderly. Endocrinol Rev 1987;8:142–153

69. Blumenthal HT, Perlstein IB: The aging thyroid. II: An immunocytochemical analysis of the age-associated lesions. J Am Geriatr Soc 1987;35:855–863

70. Spaulding SW: Age and the thyroid. Endocrinol Metab Clin North Am 1987;16:1013–1025

71. Delespesse G, Hubert C, Gausset P, Govaerts A: Radioimmunoassay for human antithyroglobulin antibodies of different immunoglobulin classes. Horm Metab Res 1976;8:50–54

72. Massart C, Hody B, Mouchel L et al: Assay for thyrotropin-receptor binding and thyroid-stimulating antibodies in sera from patients with Graves' disease. Clin Chem 1986;32:1332–1335

73. Kasagi K, Konishi J, Iida Y et al: A sensitive and practical assay for thyroid-stimulating antibodies using FRTL-5 thyroid cells. Acta Endocrinol (Copen) 1987;115:30–36

74. Rees Smith B, McLachlan SM, Furmaniak J: Autoantibodies to the thyrotropin receptor. Endocrinol Rev 1988;9:106–121

75. Weetman AP: Graves' disease. N Engl J Med 2000;343:1236–1248

76. Wilson R, McKillop JH, Henderson N et al: The ability of the serum thyrotropin receptor antibody (TRAB) index and HLA status to predict long term remission of thyrotoxicosis following medical therapy for Graves' disease. Clin Endocrinol (Oxf) 1986;25:151–156

77. Spencer CA, Takeuchi M, Kazarosyan M: Current status and performance goals for thyroglobulin assays. Clin Chem 1996;42:164–173

78. Helfand M, Redfern CC: Screening for thyroid disease: an update. Ann Intern Med 1998;129:144–148

79. American College of Physicians: Screening for thyroid disease. Ann Intern Med 1998;129:141–143

80. Ladenson PW, Singer PA, Ain KB et al: American Thyroid Association guidelines for detection of thyroid dysfunction. Arch Intern Med 2000;160:1573–1575

81. Davis PJ, Davis FB: Hyperthyroidism in patients over the age of 60 years: clinical features in 85 patients. Medicine 1974;53:161–182

82. Ronnov-Jessen V, Kirkegaard C: Hyperthyroidism: a disease of old age? BMJ 1973;1:41–43

83. Canaris GJ, Manowitz NR, Mayor G, Ridgway EC: The Colorado thyroid disease prevalence study. Arch Intern Med 2000;160:525–534

84. Tunbridge WMG, Evered DC, Hall R et al: The spectrum of thyroid disease in a community: the Whickham survey. Clin Endocrinol (Oxf) 1977;7:481–493

85. Bagchi N, Brown TR, Parish JD: Thyroid dysfunction in adults over age 55 years: a study in an urban US community. Arch Intern Med 1990;150:785–787

86. Furszyfer J, Kurland LT, McConahey WM et al: Epidemiologic aspects of Hashimoto's thyroiditis and Graves' disease in Rochester, Minnesota (1935–1967), with special reference to temporal trends. Metabolism 1972;21:197–204

87. Martin FIR, Deam DR: Hyperthyroidism in elderly hospitalized patients: clinical features and treatment outcomes. Med J Aus 1996;164:200–203

88. Ferriman D, Hennebry TM, Tassopoulos CN: True thyroid adenoma. QJM 1972;41:127–139

89. Marsden P, Facer P, Acosta M, McKerron CG: Serum triiodothyronine in solitary autonomous nodules of the thyroid. Clin Endocrinol (Oxf) 1975;4:327–330

90. Fradkin JE, Wolff J: Iodine induced thyrotoxicosis. Medicine 1983;62:1–20

91. Daniels GH: Amiodarone-induced thyrotoxicosis. J Clin Endocrinol Metab 2001;86:3–8

92. Harjai KJ, Licata AA: Effects of amiodarone on thyroid function. Ann Intern Med 1997;126:63–73

93. Bartolana L, Brogioni S, Grasso L et al: Treatment of amiodarone-induced thyrotoxicosis, a difficult challenge: results of a prospective study. J Clin Endocrinol Metab 1996;81:2930–2933

94. Dickstein G, Shechner C, Adawi F et al: Lithium treatment in amiodarone-induced thyrotoxicosis. Am J Med 1997;102:454–458

95. Banovac K, Papic M, Bilsker MS et al: Evidence of hyperthyroidism in apparently euthyroid patients treated with levothyroxine. Arch Intern Med 1989;149:809–812

96. Smallridge RC: Thyrotropin-secreting pituitary tumors. Endocrinol Metab Clin North Am 1987;16:765–792

97. Beck-Peccoz P, Mariotti S, Guillausseau PJ et al: Treatment of hyperthyroidism due to inappropriate secretion of thyrotropin with the somatostatin analog SMS 201–995. J Clin Endocrinol Metab 1989;68:208–214

98. Hay ID: Thyroiditis: a clinical update. Mayo Clin Proc 1985;60:836–843

99. Kawabe T, Komiya I, Endo T et al: Hyperthyroidism in the elderly. J Am Geriatr Soc 1979;27:152–155

100. Griffin MA, Solomon DH: Hyperthyroidism in the elderly. J Am Geriatr Soc 1986;34:887–892

101. Trivalle C, Doucet J, Chasogne P et al: Differences in the signs and symptoms of hyperthyroidism in older and younger patients. J Am Geriatr Soc 1996;44:50–53

102. Thomas FB, Mazzaferri EL, Skillman TG: Apathetic thyrotoxicosis: a distinctive clinical and laboratory entity. Ann Intern Med 1970;72:679–685

103. Tibaldi JM, Barzel US, Alben J et al: Thyrotoxicosis in the very old. Am J Med 1986;81:619–622

104. Ladenson PW: Recognition and management of cardiovascular disease related to thyroid dysfunction. Am J Med 1990;88:638–641

105. Aronow WS: The heart and thyroid disease. Clin Geriatr Med 1995;11:219–229

106. Klein I, Ojamaa K: Thyroid hormone and the cardiovascular system. N Engl J Med 2001; 344:501–509

107. Salzman C, Shader RI: Depression in the elderly. I: Relationship between depression, psychologic defense mechanisms and physical illness. J Am Geriatr Soc 1978;26:253–260

108. Livingston EH, Hershman JM, Sawin CT, Yoshikawa TT: Prevalence of thyroid disease and abnormal thyroid tests in older hospitalized and ambulatory persons. J Am Geriatr Soc 1987;35:109–114

109. Bayer MF, Macoviak JA, McDougall IR: Diagnostic performance of sensitive measurements of serum thyrotropin during severe nonthyroidal illness: their role in the diagnosis of hyperthyroidism. Clin Chem 1987;33:2178–2184

110. Orgiazzi J: Management of Graves' hyperthyroidism. Endocrinol Metab Clin North Am 1987;16:365–389

111. Solomon B, Glinoer D, Lagasse R, Wartofsky L: Current trends in the management of Graves' disease. J Clin Endocrinol Metab 1990;70:1518–1524

112. Cooper DS: Antithyroid drugs. N Engl J Med 1984;311:1353–1362

113. Cooper DS, Goldminz D, Levin AA et al: Agranulocytosis associated with antithyroid drugs: effects of patient age and drug dose. Ann Intern Med 1983;98:26–29

114. Yamada T, Aizawa T, Koizumi Y et al: Age-related therapeutic response to antithyroid drug in patients with hyperthyroid Graves' disease. J Am Geriatr Soc 1994;42:513–516

115. Allahabadia A, Daykin J, Holder RL et al: Age and gender predict the outcome of treatment for Graves' hyperthyroidism. J Clin Endocrinol Metab 2000;85:1038–1042

116. Sridama V, McCormick M, Kaplan EL et al: Long-term follow-up study of compensated low-dose 131I therapy for Graves' disease. N Engl J Med 1984;311:426–432

117. Holm LE: Changing annual incidence of hypothyrodism after iodine-131 therapy for hyperthyroidism, 1951–1975. J Nucl Med 1982;23:108–112

118. Palestini N, Valori MR, Carlin R et al: Mortality, morbidity and long-term results in surgically treated hyperthyroid patients: review of 597 cases. Acta Chir Scand 1985;151:509–513

119. Nakazawa HK, Sakurai K, Hamada N et al: Management of atrial fibrillation in the post-thyrotoxic state. Am J Med 1982;72:903–906

120. Kellet HA, Sawers JS, Boulton FE et al: Problems of anticoagulation with warfarin in hyperthyroidism. QJM 1986;58:43–51

121. McDermott MT, Kidd GS, Dodson LE et al: Radio-iodine induced thyroid storm. Am J Med 1983;75:353–359

122. Gavin LA: Thyroid crises. Med Clin North Am 1991;75:179–193

123. Burch HB, Wartofsky L: Life threatening thyrotoxicosis: thyroid storm. Endocrinol Metab Clin North Am 1993;22:263–277

124. Stott DJ, McLellan AR, Finlayson J et al: Elderly persons with suppressed serum TSH but normal free thyroid hormone levels usually have mild thyroid overactivity and are at increased risk of developing overt hyperthyroidism. QJM 1991;78:77–84

125. Parle JV, Franklyn JA, Cross KW et al: Prevalence and follow-up of abnormal thyrotropin (TSH) concentrations in the elderly in the United Kingdom. Clin Endocrinol (Oxf) 1991;34:77–83

126. Sawin CT, Geller A, Kaplan MM et al: Low serum thyrotropin (thyroid-stimulating hormone) in older persons without hyperthyroidism. Arch Intern Med 1991;151:165–168

127. Sawin CT, Geller A, Wolf PA et al: Low serum thyrotropin concentrations as a risk factor for atrial fibrillation in older persons. N Engl J Med 1994;331:1249–1252

128. Biondi B, Palmieri EA, Fazio S et al: Endogenous subclinical hyperthyroidism affects quality of life and cardiac morphology and function in young and middle-aged patients. J Clin Endocrinol Metab 2000;85:4701–4705

129. Mudde AH, Reijnders FJL, Nieuwenhuijzen Kruseman AC: Peripheral bone density in women with untreated multinodular goitre. Clin Endocrinol 1992;37:35–37

130. Kumeda Y, Inaba M, Tahara H et al: Persistent increase in bone turnover in Graves' patients with subclinical hyperthyroidism. J Clin Endocrinol Metab 2000;85:4157–4161

131. Bauer DC, Ettinger B, Nevitt MC, Stone KL: Risk for fracture in women with low serum levels of thyroid-stimulating hormone. Ann Intern Med 2001;134:561–568

132. Faber J, Jensen IW, Petersen L et al: Normalization of serum thyrotrophin by means of radioiodine treatment in subclinical hyperthyroidism: effect on bone loss in postmenopausal women. Clin Endocrinol 1998;48:285–290

133. Cooper DS: Subclinical thyroid disease: a clinicians' perspective. Ann Intern Med 1998; 129:135–138

134. Havard CWH: The thyroid and aging. Endocrinol Metab Clin North Am 1981;10:163–178

135. Hurley JR: Thyroid disease in the elderly. Med Clin North Am 1983;67:497–516

136. Refetoff S, DeGroot LJ, Barsano CP: Defective thyroid hormone feedback regulation in the syndrome of peripheral resistance to thyroid hormone. J Clin Endocrinol Metab 1980;51:41–45

137. Cooper DS, Ladenson PW, Nisula BC et al: Familial thyroid hormone resistance. Metabolism 1982;31:504–509

138. Sawin CT, Castelli WP, Hershman JM et al: The aging thyroid: thyroid deficiency in the Framingham study. Arch Intern Med 1985;145:1386–1388

139. Bahemuka M, Hodkinson HM: Screening for hypothyroidism in elderly inpatients. BMJ 1975;1:601–603

140. Falkenberg M, Kogedal B, Norr A: Screening of an elderly female population for hypo and hyperthyroidism by use of a thyroid hormone panel. Acta Med Scand 1983;214:361–365

141. Riniker M, Tiechl M, Lupi GA et al: Prevalence of various degrees of hypothyroidism among patients of a general medical department. Clin Endocrinol (Oxf) 1981;14:69–74

142. Herrmann J: Prevalence of hypothroidism in the elderly in Germany: a pilot study. J Endocrinol Invest 1981;4:327–330

143. Inada M, Nisikawa M, Kawai I: Hypothyroidism associated with positive results of the perchlorate discharge test in elderly patients. Am J Med 1983;74:1010–1015

144. Okamura K, Ueda K, Sone H et al: A sensitive thyroid stimulating hormone assay for screening of thyroid functional disorder in elderly Japanese. J Am Geriatr Soc 1989;37:317–322

145. Campbell AJ, Reinken J, Allan BC: Thyroid disease in the elderly in the community. Age Ageing 1981;10:47–52

146. Konishi J, Iida Y, Kasagi K et al: Primary myxedema with thyrotrophin-binding inhibitor immunoglobulins: clinical and laboratory findings in 15 patients. Ann Intern Med 1985;103:26–31

147. Tunbridge WMG, Brewis M, French J: Natural history of autoimmune thyroiditis. BMJ 1981;282:258–262

148. Sawin CT, Bigos ST, Land S, Bacharach P: The aging thyroid: relationship between elevated serum thyrotropin level and thyroid antibodies in elderly patients. Am J Med 1985;79:591–595

149. Hirota Y, Tamai H, Hayashi Y et al: Thyroid function and history in forty-five patients with hyperthyroid Graves' disease in clinical remission more than 10 years after thionamide drug treatment. J Clin Endocrinol Metab 1986;62:165–169

150. Max MH, Scherm M, Bland KI: Early and late complication after thyroid operations. South Med J 1983;76:977–980

151. Roti E, Vagenakis AG: Effect of excess iodide: clinical aspects. In Braverman LE, Utiger RD (eds): Werner & Ingbar's The Thyroid, 8th edn. Lippincott Williams & Wilkins, Philadelphia, 2000:316–329

152. Martino E, Safran M, Aghini-Lombardi F et al: Environmental iodine intake and thyroid dysfunction during chronic amiodarone therapy. Ann Intern Med 1984;101:28–34

153. Tachman ML, Guthrie GP: Hypothyroidism: diversity of presentation. Endocrinol Rev 1984;5:456–465

154. Bastenie PA, Bonnyns M, Vanhaelst L: Natural history of primary myxedema. Am J Med 1985;79:91–100

155. Doucet J, Menard JF, Bercoff E: Does age play a role in clinical presentation of hypothyroidism. J Am Geriatr Soc 1994;42:984–986

156. Lloyd WA, Goldberg IJL: Incidence of hypothyroidism in the elderly. BMJ 1961;2:1256–1259

157. Rai GS, Gluck T, Luttrell S: Clinical presentation of hypothyroidism in older persons. J Am Geriatr Soc 1995;43:592–593

158. Hall RCW: Psychiatric effects of thyroid hormone disturbance. Psychosomatics 1983;24:7–18

159. Logotheis J: Psychiatric behavior as the initial indicator of adult myxedema. J Nerv Ment Dis 1963;136:561–568

160. Zellman HE: Unusual aspects of myxoedema. Geriatrics 1968;23:140–148

161. Rao SN, Katiyar BC, Nair KRP, Misra S: Neuromuscular status in hypothyroidism. Acta Neurol Scand 1980;61:167–177

162. Buccino RA, Spann JF, Pool PE et al: Influence of the thyroid state on the intrinsic contractile properties and the energy stores of the myocardium. J Clin Invest 1967;46:1669–1682

163. Vanhaelst L, Neve P, Chailly P, Bastenie P: Coronary artery disease in hypothyroidism. Lancet 1967;ii:800–802

164. Horton L, Coburn RJ, England JM, Himsworth RL: The haematology of hypothyroidism. QJM 1976;45:101–124

165. Rosenbaum RL, Barzel US: Levothyroxine replacement dose for primary hypothyroidism decreases with age. Ann Intern Med 1982;96:53–55

166. Sawin CT, Herman T, Molitch ME et al: Aging and the thyroid: decreased requirement for thyroid hormone in older hypothyroid patients. Am J Med 1983;75:206–209

167. Davis FB, LaMantia RS, Spaulding SW et al: Estimation of a physiologic replacement dose of levothyroxine in elderly patients with hypothyroidism. Arch Intern Med 1984;144:1752–1754

168. Cunningham JJ, Barzel US: Lean body mass is a predictor of the daily requirement for thyroid hormone in older men and women. J Am Geriatr Soc 1984;32:204–207

169. Kabadi UM: Optimal daily levothyroxine dose in primary hypothyroidism: its relation to pretreatment thyroid hormone indexes. Arch Intern Med 1989;149:2209–2212

170. Mandel S, Brent GA, Larsen PR: Levothyroxine therapy in patients with thyroid disease. Ann Intern Med 1993;119:492–502

171. Toft AD: Thyroxine therapy. N Engl J Med 1994;331:174–180

172. Oppenheimer JH, Braverman LE, Toft A et al: Thyroid hormone treatment: when and what? J Clin Endocrinol Metab 1995;80:2873–2883

173. Stall GM, Harris S, Sokoll LJ, Dawson-Hughes B: Accelerated bone loss in hypothyroid patients overtreated with L-thyroxine. Ann Intern Med 1990;113:265–269

174. Solomon BL, Wartofsky L, Burman KD: Prevalence of fractures in postmenopausal women with thyroid disease. Thyroid 1993;3:17–23

175. Steinberg AD, Schrader ZR: Myxoedema with angina pectoris treated with propranolol and triiodothyronine. Lancet 1971;ii:213

176. Levine HD: Compromise therapy in the patient with angina pectoris and hypothyroidism. Am J Med 1980;69:411–418

177. Becker C: Hypothyroid and atherosclerotic heart disease: pathogenesis, medical management and the role of coronary artery bypass surgery. Endocrinol Rev 1985;6:432–440

178. Ridgway EC, McCammon JA, Benotti J, Maloof F: Acute metabolic responses in myxedema to large doses of intravenous L-thyroxine. Ann Intern Med 1972;77:549–555

179. Jordan RM: Myxedema coma. Pathophysiology, therapy, and factors affecting prognosis. Med Clin North Am 1995;79:185–194

180. Yamamoto T, Fukuyama J, Fujiyoshi A: Factors associated with mortality of myxedema coma: report of eight cases and literature survey. Thyroid 1999;9:1167–1174

181. Evered DC, Ormston BJ, Smith PA et al: Grades of hypothyroidism. BMJ 1973;1:657–662

182. Tunbridge WMG, Brewis M, French J et al: Natural history of autoimmune thyroiditis. BMJ 1981;282:258–262

183. Jayme JJ, Ladenson PW: Subclinical thyroid dysfunction in the elderly. Trends Endocrinol Metab 1994;5:79–86

184. Hak AE, Pols HAP, Visser TJ et al: Subclinical hypothyroidism is an independent risk factor for atherosclerosis and myocardial infarction in elderly women: the Rotterdam study. Ann Intern Med 2000;132:270–278

185. Lazarus JH, Burr ML, McGregor AM et al: The prevalence and progression of autoimmune thyroid disease in the elderly. Acta Endocrinol 1984;106:199–202

186. Rosenthal MJ, Hunt WC, Garry PJ, Goodwin JS: Thyroid failure in the elderly: microsomal antibodies as discriminant for therapy. JAMA 1987;258:209–213

187. Bindels AJ, Westendorp RG, Frolich M et al: The prevalence of subclinical hypothyroidism at different total plasma cholesterol levels in middle aged men and women: a need for case finding? Clin Endocrinol (Oxf) 1999;50:217–220

188. Biondi B, Fazio S, Palmiere EA et al: Left ventricular diastolic dysfunction in patients with subclinical hypothyroidism. J Clin Endocrinol Metab 1999;84:2064–2067

189. Monzani F, Di Bello V, Caraccio N et al: Effect of levothyroxine on cardiac function and structure in subclinical hypothyroidism: a double blind, placebo-controlled study. J Clin Endocrinol Metab 2001;86:1110–1115

190. Althous BU, Staub JJ, Ryff-de-Leche A et al: LDL/HDL changes in subclinical hypothyroidism: possible risk factors for coronary heart disease. Clin Endocrinol (Oxf) 1988;28:157–163

191. Bell GM, Todd WTA, Forfar JC et al: End-organ responses to thyroxine therapy in subclinical hypothyroidism. Clin Endocrinol (Oxf) 1985;22:83–89

192. Cooper DS, Halpern R, Wood LC et al: L-thyroxine therapy in subclinical hypothyroidism. A double blind placebo-controlled trial. Ann Intern Med 1984;101:18–24

193. Nystrom E, Caldahl K, Fager G et al: A double-blind cross-over 12 month study of L-thyroxine treatment of women with "subclinical" hypothyroidism. Clin Endocrinol (Oxf) 1988;29:63–75

194. Arem R, Patsch W: Lipoprotein and apolipoprotein levels in subclinical hypothyroidism: effect of levothyroxine therapy. Arch Intern Med 1990;150:2097–2100

195. Caron P, Calazel C, Parra HJ et al: Decreased HDL cholesterol in subclinical hypothyroidism: the effect of L-thyroxine therapy. Clin Endocrinol (Oxf) 1990;33:519–523

196. Jaeschke R, Guyatt G, Herstein H et al: Does treatment with L-thyroxine influence health status in middle-aged and older adults with subclinical hypothyroidism. J Gen Intern Med 1996;11:744–749

197. Lindeman RD, Schade DS, La Rue A: Subclinical hypothyroidism in a biethnic, urban community. J Am Geriatr Soc 1999;47:703–709

198. Danese MD, Ladenson PW, Meinert CL, Powe NR: Effect of thyroxine therapy on serum lipoproteins in patients with mild thyroid failure: a quantitative review of the literature. J Clin Endocrinol Metab 2000;85:2993–3001

199. Mortensen JD, Woolner LB, Bennett WA: Gross and microscopic findings in clinically normal thyroid glands. J Clin Endocrinol Metab 1955;15:1270–1280

200. Vander JB, Gaston EA, Dawber TR: The significance of nontoxic thyroid nodules: final report of a 15-year study of the incidence of thyroid malignancy. Ann Intern Med 1968;69:537–540

201. Ezzat S, Sarti DA, Cain DR, Braunstein GD: Thyroid incidentalomas: prevalence by palpation and ultrasonography. Arch Intern Med 1994;154:1838–1840

202. Schneider AB, Bekerman C, Leland J et al: Thyroid nodules in the follow-up of irradiated individuals: comparison of ultrasound with scanning and palpation. J Clin Endocrinol Metab 1997;82:4020–4027

203. DeGroot LJ: Clinical review. II: diagnostic approach and management of patients exposed to irradiation to the thyroid. J Clin Endocrinol Metab 1989;69:925–928

204. Huysmans DAKC, Hermus ARMM, Corstens FHM et al: Large, compressive goiters treated with radioiodine. Ann Intern Med 1994;121:757–762

205. Mazzaferri EL: Management of a solitary thyroid nodule. N Engl J Med 328;1993:553–559

206. Hundah SA, Fleming ID, Fremgen AM, Menck HR: A National Cancer Data Base report on 53,856 cases of thyroid carcinoma treated in the US, 1985–1995. Cancer 1998;83:2638–2648

207. Mazzaferri EL, Kloos RT: Current approaches to primary therapy for papillary and follicular thyroid cancer. J Clin Endocrinol Metab 2001;86:1447–1463

208. Molitch ME, Beck JR, Dreisman M et al: The cold thyroid nodule: an analysis of diagnostic and therapeutic options. Endocrinol Rev 1984;5:185–199

209. DeGroot LJ, Kaplan EL, Shukla MS et al: Morbidity and mortality in follicular thyroid cancer. J Clin Endocrinol Metab 1995;80:2946–2953

210. Kobayashi T, Asakawa H, Umeshita K et al: Treatment of 37 patients with anaplastic carcinoma of the thyroid. Head Neck 1996;18:36–41

211. Holm L-E, Blomgren H, Lowhagen T: Cancer risks in patients with chronic lymphocytic thyroiditis. N Engl J Med 1985;312:601–604

212. Rude RK, Singer R: Comparison of serum calcitonin levels after a 1-minute calcium injection and after pentogastrin injection in the diagnosis of medullary thyroid carcinoma. J Clin Endocrinol Metab 1977;44:980–985

213. Burch HB: Evaluation and management of the solid thyroid nodule. Endocrinol Metab Clin North Am 1995;24:663–710

214. James EM, Charboneau JW: High frequency (10 MHz) thyroid ultrasonography. Sem Ultrasound CT MR 1985;6:294–309

215. Matsuzuka F, Miyauchi A, Katayama S et al: Clinical aspects of primary thyroid lymphoma: diagnosis and treatment based on our experience of 119 cases. Thyroid 1993;3:93–99

216. Gharib H, Mazzaferri EL: Thyroid suppressive therapy in patients with nodular thyroid disease. Ann Intern Med 1998;128:386–394

217. Wesche MFT, Tiel-v Buul MMC, Lips P et al: A randomized trial comparing levothyroxine with radioactive iodine in the treatment of sporadic nontoxic goiter. J Clin Endocrinol Metab 2001;86:998–1005

218. Gharib H, Goellner JR: Evaluation of nodular thyroid disease. Endocrinol Metab Clin North Am 1988;17:511–526

219. Gharib H, Goellner JR: Fine-needle aspiration biopsy of the thyroid: an appraisal. Ann Intern Med 1993;118:282–289

220. Leenhardt L, Hejblum G, Franc B et al: Indications and limits of ultrasound-guided cytology in the management of nonpalpable thyroid nodules. J Clin Endocrinol Metab 1999;84:24–28

221. Mazzaferri EL: An overview of the management of papillary and follicular thyroid carcinoma. Thyroid 1999;9:421–427

222. Gardiner KR, Russell CFJ: Thyroidectomy for large multinodular colloid goiter. J R Coll Surg Edinb 1995;40:367–370

223. Bonnema SJ, Bertelsen H, Mortensen J et al: The feasibility of high dose iodine-131 treatment as an alternative to surgery in patients with a very large goiter: effect on thyroid function and size and pulmonary function. J Clin Endocrinol Metab 1999;84:3636–3641

224. Hermus HR, Huysmans DA: Treatment of benign nodular thyroid disease. N Engl J Med 1998;338:1438–1447

225. Singer PA, Cooper DS, Daniels GH et al: Treatment guidelines for patients with thyroid nodules and well-differentiated thyroid cancer. Arch Intern Med 1996;156:2165–2172

226. Hay ID, Grant CS, Taylor WF, McConahey WM: Ipsilateral lobectomy versus bilateral lobar resection in papillary thyroid carcinoma: a retrospective analysis of surgical outcome using a novel prognostic scoring system. Surgery 1987;102:1088–1095

227. Beierwaltes WH: The treatment of thyroid carcinoma with radioactive iodine. Sem Nucl Med 1978;8:79–94

228. Robbins J, Merino MJ, Boice JD et al: Thyroid cancer: a lethal endocrine neoplasm. Ann Intern Med 1991;115:133–147

229. Haugen BR, Pacini F, Reiners C, Schlumberger M et al: A comparison of recombinant human thyrotropin and thyroid hormone withdrawal for the detection of thyroid remnant or cancer. J Clin Endocrinol Metab 1999;84:3877–3885

230. Thoresen SO, Akslen LA, Glattre E et al: Survival and prognostic factors in differentiated thyroid carcinoma: a multivariate analysis of 1055 cases. Br J Cancer 1989;59:231–240

231. Schlumberger MJ: Papillary and follicular thyroid carcinoma. N Engl J Med 1998;338:297–306

232. Ball DW, Baylin SB, De Bustros AC: Medullary thyroid carcinoma. In Braverman LE, Utiger RD (eds): Werner & Ingbar's The Thyroid, 8th edn. Lippincott Williams & Wilkins, Philadelphia, 2000:930–943

233. Simpson WJ: Anaplastic thyroid carcinoma: a new approach. Can J Surg 1980;23:25–27

234. Kim JH, Leeper RD: Treatment of locally advanced thyroid carcinoma with combination doxorubicin and radiation therapy. Cancer 1987;60:2372–2375

Chapter 95

Disorders of the parathyroids

Peter Hammond and Paul Belchetz

There are usually four parathyroid glands, but a larger number may sometimes be found which poses potential problems for the surgeon. The usual positions are behind the upper and lower poles of the thyroid in each side of the neck, but they may be enwrapped by thyroid tissue. The normal parathyroid gland weighs about 35 mg and thus may be quite inconspicuous. In embryonic life the glands originate from the third and fourth branchial pouches, but the initial upper glands migrate to a final lower position and indeed may be taken into the mediastinum with the associated descent of the thymus.

PARATHYROID HORMONE (PTH)

Regulation of PTH synthesis and secretion

The circulating level of ionized calcium acting directly on parathyroid tissue largely regulates the normal parathyroid. Advances in molecular biology have led to a deeper understanding of normal functioning parathyroid tissue and pathophysiology of adenomas. It is now known in some detail that the parathyroid gene consists of three exons and these transcribe to form a large messenger RNA (mRNA) species with a polyadenylate tail. Following a series of specific splicings this is translated outside the nucleus on ribosomes to form the large precursor pre-proPTH. This undergoes a series of cleavages before and after reaching the Golgi apparatus where the 84-residue parathyroid hormone is packaged into granules for storage prior to secretion.[1] Raised levels of ionized calcium suppress the messenger RNA for PTH in normal bovine parathyroid glands and adenomatous tissue, but PTH secretion is unsuppressed from adenomas in vitro.[2] It has recently been demonstrated that calcium ions act to suppress PTH synthesis and secretion via specific cell-membrane G-protein coupled receptors. Inactivating mutations of this receptor elevate the set point for PTH secretion, causing familial hypocalciuric hypercalcemia, a benign condition associated with mild hypercalcemia.[3]

The normal parathyroid mRNA production is also regulated by 1,25-dihydroxy-vitamin D levels, but adenomatous cells fail to give this response.[4] It is possible that at normal levels of ionized calcium the rate of gene transcription is maximal, so the response to hypocalcemia may be regulated by liberating a normally inaccessible pool of mRNA bound to riboprotein, hence increasing the rate of translation without changes in steady-state levels in mRNA.

PTH secretion and age-related bone loss

Serum PTH concentrations are increased in the elderly population by about 30 percent. This increase correlates with a decline in vitamin D level, and treatment with

1,25-dihydroxy-vitamin D results in a decrease in the circulating PTH level.[5] The increase in serum PTH with age is thought to account for age-related bone loss, and this is supported by the observation that the hypoparathyroid state protects against such loss.[6] This provides the rationale for using vitamin D, with or without calcium supplements, in elderly people with type II osteoporosis. Such treatment has proved effective in reducing the risk of hip fractures in the elderly population.[7]

Actions of parathyroid hormone

PTH raises the ionized calcium levels in the blood through actions on the kidney, gut, and bones. The major renal action is to increase tubular reabsorption of calcium via activation of adenylate cyclase mechanisms.[8] This mediation can be uniquely observed because of the liberation of cyclic AMP (cAMP) into the tubular luminal fluid, allowing its ready measurement in the excreted urine. PTH also exerts a phosphaturic effect, enhancing tubular secretion of phosphate. PTH has a complex action on bone which is partly dose-dependent. High levels are catabolic with increased bone resorption, but lower levels may exert an overall anabolic effect. This is discussed in greater detail below.

PTH enhances the gastrointestinal absorption of calcium. Some of this effect is mediated by the promotion of 25-hydroxy-vitamin D 1-hydroxylation to form the active metabolite 1,25-dihydroxy-vitamin D,[9] which has actions on gut absorption, on bone, and indeed on many tissues. PTH has complex relationships with magnesium. PTH enhances magnesium absorption, but hypomagnesemia can significantly suppress PTH secretion.[10] A low magnesium level can also inhibit renal production of 1,25-dihydroxy-vitamin D, so blocking this important action of PTH.[11] Finally it appears that PTH may have independent and important effects on vascular tone.

HYPERPARATHYROIDISM

It is commonly believed that hyperparathyroidism is rare and that the nature of the disease is changing. The disease, which Fuller Albright described over half a century ago, was a fulminating disorder with devastating effects on bone which led to its ready recognition. This form of the disease is exceedingly rare today. With time came diagnostic refinement and the recognition of the frequent causative role of hyperparathyroidism in renal calculus formation associated with hypercalciuria. The most dramatic change came with the widespread availability of accurate plasma calcium measurements.[12]

Currently the great majority of cases of hyperparathyroidism are detected incidentally or in screening. This trend may be reversed if economic pressures restrict chemical tests performed to the few specifically requested by the clinician.

The definitive audit has yet to be performed as to whether this would matter. It is indisputable that most of these cases have only modest degrees of hypercalcemia, especially in the elderly female population where the incidence of hyperparathyroidism soars to about 2 per thousand.[13]

Etiology of hyperparathyroidism

Hyperparathyroidism is most commonly caused by a single benign adenoma. Involvement of two glands is not uncommon, and when it occurs the histological appearance in the two glands may be strikingly different. There is some dispute whether involvement of more than one gland in fact represents parathyroid hyperplasia: histological distinction of adenoma from hyperplasia based on the presence of a rim of normal, if sometimes compressed gland, is not totally reliable.[14] True hyperplasia is an important diagnosis since surgery must be radical if early relapse is to be avoided. The presence of hyperplasia is a pointer to possible multiple endocrine neoplasia type 1 (MEN-1) which is inherited as an autosomal dominant trait with high penetrance.[15] In this syndrome, hyperparathyroidism is very much the rule, affecting 97–100 percent of subjects at risk in affected families.[16]

The other affected glands are the neuroendocrine tissues of the duodenum and pancreas, with insulinoma and gastrinoma as the most frequently represented tumor types, and the anterior pituitary gland where functionless tumors and prolactinomas occur most often, but acromegaly is not uncommon.[17] The gene which is mutated in MEN-1, found on the long arm of chromosome 11 in the region q11.13, has recently been characterized; it is a transcription factor and has been termed *menin*.[18]

Molecular biology is proving informative in both the sporadic adenomatous and hyperplastic forms of hyperparathyroidism. In the case of tumors appearing in the context of MEN-1, it is proposed that loss of one *menin* allele from the germline leads to hyperplasia.[19,20] A further somatic loss of the allele from the second chromosome 11 may occur later, and is associated with larger, clonal tumor development. In the case of the more common sporadic parathyroid adenomas, there appear to be somatic mutations involving both chromosomes 11. The gene for parathyroid hormone itself is localized to the short arm of chromosome 11, and in at least some cases of sporadic parathyroid adenoma there is a rearrangement of genetic material on chromosome 11 between regions containing the MEN-1 gene and the locus for the parathyroid hormone.[21] In other cases of sporadic hyperparathyroidism, no obvious changes in chromosome 11 have been observed.

Clinical features of hyperparathyroidism

Symptoms attributable to hyperparathyroidism range widely and nonspecifically. Overall, 50 percent of patients have minimal or no symptoms, although elderly patients more often have neuropsychiatric or neuromuscular symptoms or suffer osteoporotic fractures. Common features caused by the ensuing hypercalcemia include polyuria and the consequent polydipsia. The increased urine volume partly results from the overall increased urinary calcium excretion exerting an osmotic diuresis: hypersecretion of PTH increases tubular reabsorption but this does not compensate for the greatly raised glomerular filtration of calcium caused by the hypercalcemia. Hypercalcemia also can induce varying degrees of tubular

resistance to vasopressin, leading to nephrogenic diabetes insipidus. Sustained hypercalcemia may lead to nephrocalcinosis with impaired renal function, or promote the formation of renal calculi. Calculi may be passed, or they may impact, for example at the vesico ureteric junction, causing pain and hematuria. Stones may be associated with pyelonephritis which is difficult to eradicate, especially if staghorn calculi form. Stones may require removal surgically or by lithotripsy.

Symptoms of fatigue, lethargy, loss of vitality, and varying degrees of mental impairment are also common in hyperparathyroidism. These symptoms are nonspecific and common in the aging community in general, so it is often hard to predict in which cases surgical cure of the hyperparathyroidism will improve such problems.

This is a vexed question, as a causal relationship has been claimed even in cases with biochemically mild disease; yet it is clearly true that resection of a parathyroid adenoma with restoration of normocalcemia is not invariably successful. This problem is further discussed below. Rare patients show a marked and reversible neuromuscular syndrome, characterized histologically by type II muscle fiber atrophy.[22]

More florid manifestations of hyperparathyroidism are less common. They include gastrointestinal features of anorexia and nausea. This rarely can proceed to vomiting, with a danger of a hypercalcemic crisis when loss of extracellular fluid exacerbates the hypercalcemia and vomiting, causing a vicious spiral, termed "disequilibrium hypercalcemia," which can prove fatal. Hypercalcemia per se may increase gastrin secretion and gastric acid production, with dyspepsia and peptic ulceration. This occurs separately from the independent association with gastrin-producing tumors (Zollinger–Ellison syndrome). There is a well-recorded, although rare, association with acute pancreatitis.

Hyperparathyroidism is also associated with cardiovascular disease, especially hypertension. It is far from certain what the nature of this link is, although endothelial vasodilatory dysfunction has been shown.[23] There is also controversy over whether the cure of hyperparathyroidism has any beneficial effect on blood pressure control. It has been suggested that there are delayed benefits on mortality from cardiovascular disease following surgery for hyperparathyroidism, although these are probably greatest in younger people.[24]

Hyperinsulinism reflecting insulin resistance is being increasingly recognized as a cardiovascular risk factor, and this has been linked with hyperparathyroidism.[25] It is not certain whether this is a function of hypercalcemia or an independent effect of hypophosphatemia, whether or not part of primary hyperparathyroidism.[26]

ASYMPTOMATIC DISEASE The management of asymptomatic disease, diagnosed following request for a biochemical profile, continues to cause heated discussion. The frequently cited need for controlled prospective randomized trials combined with quite varied criteria for determining a conservative approach versus surgery are the main reasons for this continuing uncertainty.[27] At one extreme lie the advocates for surgery in virtually all cases of hyperparathyroidism, including prevention or arrest of bone disease in the arguments.[28] This is highly dubious as discussed below. Several reviews conclude that mild disease is stable and does not lead to progressive renal failure or bone disease.[29,30] Judging mild hyperparathyroidism truly asymptomatic may be difficult as the features may be slight and nonspecific even in severe cases, and those labeled asymptomatic may feel better following parathyroidectomy.

Case report A 70-year-old woman developed profuse diarrhea for a week while away from home on holiday. She had a long history of angina and, on having an attack, collapsed following use of her nitro lingual spray. On admission to hospital she was dehydrated and found to be in hyperosmolar nonketotic precoma with a blood glucose of 33 mmol/L. Subsequent routine biochemical screening revealed a plasma calcium of 4.32 mmol/L, which fell to 3.73 mmol/L only after vigorous rehydration; intravenous pamidronate lowered the level further to 2.5 mmol/L. She then developed a massive anterior myocardial infarction and pump failure, dying despite prompt thrombolysis and resuscitative measures. Prior to this, systematic enquiry did not reveal any specific features of hypercalcemia. Autopsy revealed a not-unexpected severe triple coronary artery disease. It also disclosed a massive parathyroid adenoma weighing 52 g in the right side of her neck (Fig. 95-1). Her bones showed osteitis fibrosa (Fig. 95-2) and there was widespread nephrocalcinosis (Fig. 95-3).

This patient had severe hyperparathyroidism which would certainly have been treated surgically had she survived. There was nevertheless a striking lack of symptoms which could be directly attributed to her hyperparathyroidism. It is noteworthy that her hypercalcemia responded rapidly to a bisphosphonate, pamidronate.

The consensus opinion is that in an elderly patient with asymptomatic hyperparathyroidism, a serum calcium of less than 3 mmol/L, normal renal function, no stones, and no obvious bone disease, then a conservative approach has much to commend it, with serum calcium and renal functioning being monitored at 6-monthly intervals.

BONE DISEASE The possibility of developing bony complications has been cited as a reason for surgical intervention. It is generally believed that hyperparathyroidism particularly affects the cortical bone of the appendicular skeleton, with bone loss particularly evident in the forearm. Careful studies indicate a lack of continued accelerated bone loss in hyperparathyroidism or excess of vertebral fractures.[31] Indeed there is demonstrable preservation of cancellous bone structure,[32] consonant with the demonstration of increased bone mass in osteoporotic patients treated with parathyroid hormone (rhPTH 1-34).[33] The apparent diminishing frequency of severe bone complications such as giant-cell or brown tumors is incompletely explained, but it has been linked with improving nutrition especially leading to less concomitant vitamin D deficiency.

MENTAL SYMPTOMS The spectrum of mental symptoms which have been attributed to hypercalcemia is wide and include fatiguability, failing memory, poor concentration, sleep disturbance, aggression, and depression. It is generally agreed that elderly people are especially susceptible to such changes even with modest degrees of hyperparathyroidism. This may be particularly true when there is multiple pathology.

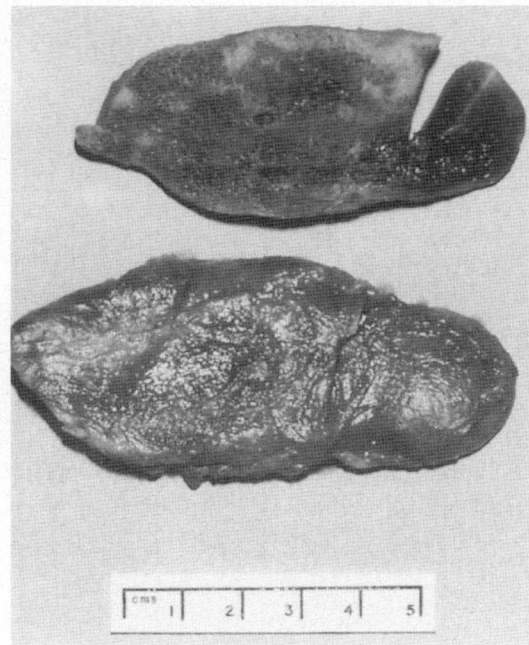

A

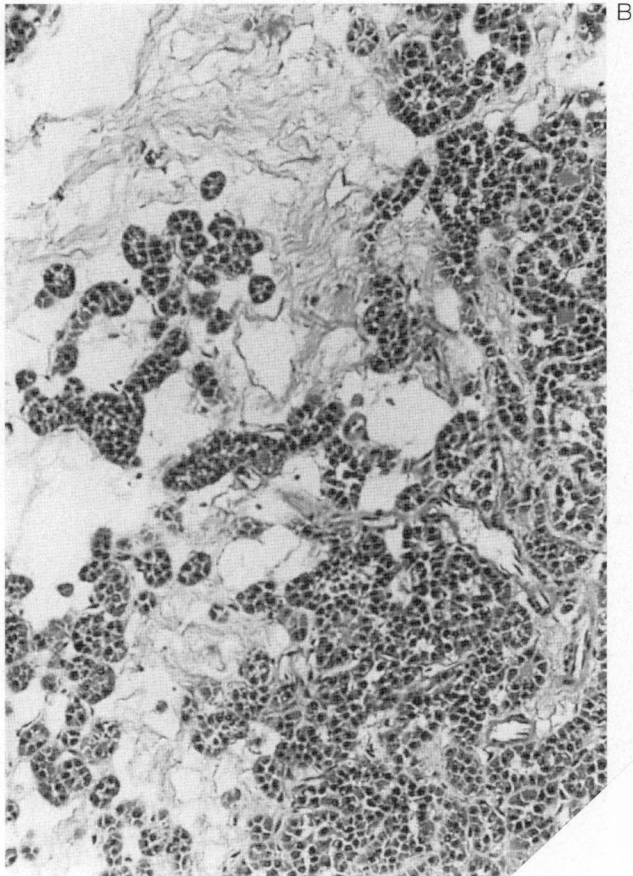

B

Figure 95-1 (A) Macroscopic view of a mass adenoma. At the top is a cut surface, abov surface. (B) Parathyroid (H&E, × 78). Loc oxyphilic "chief cells" extend into an edem.

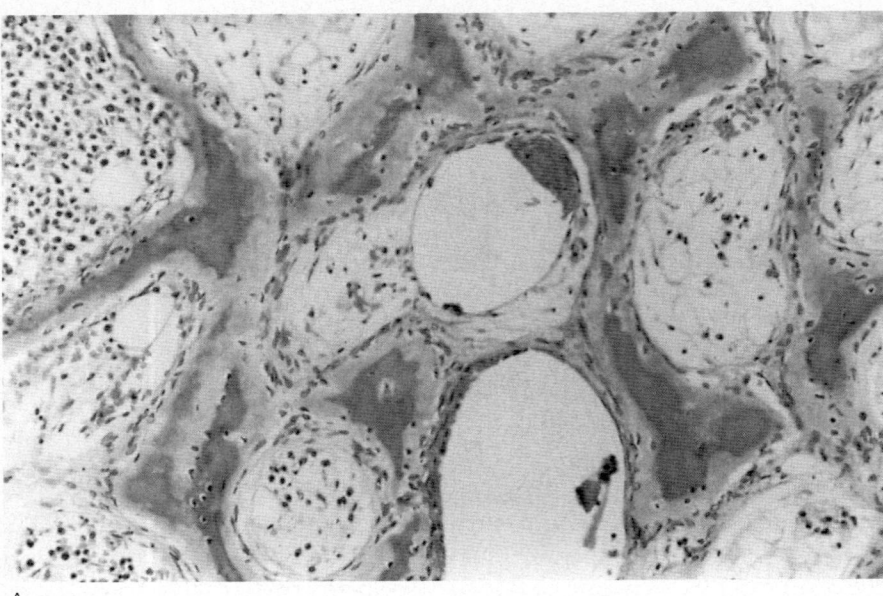

A

Figure 95-2 (A) Lumbar vertebrae (H&E, ×78). There is a prominent resorption with osteitis fibrosa. (B) Lumbar vertebrae (H&E, ×250). There is a lacunar reabsorption of the bony trabeculum with small osteoclasts.

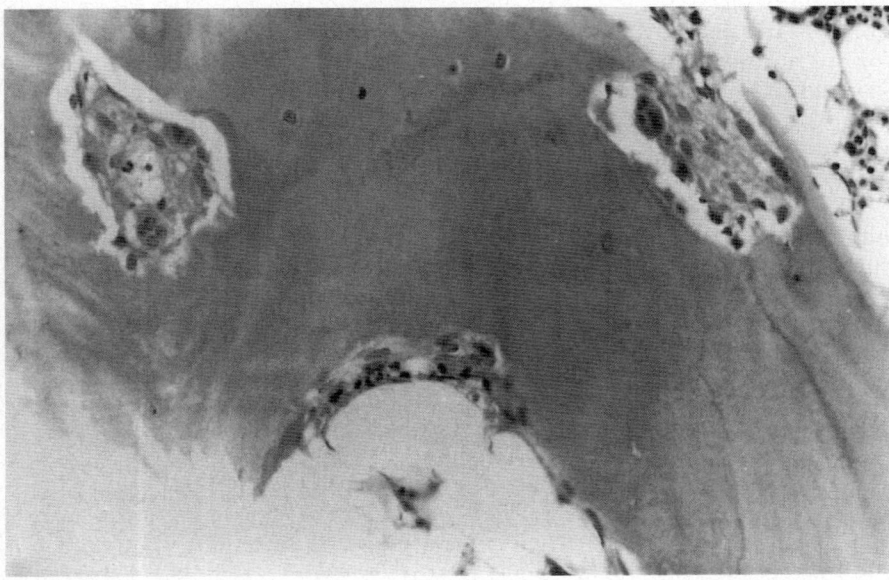

B

Case reports A 70-year-old man developed acute confusion. Hydrocephalus was diagnosed and a ventriculo-peritoneal shunt relieved symptoms. Mild hyperparathyroidism was detected during follow-up. He then suddenly became euphoric and disorientated in time and space. Neurosurgical causes were excluded. Surgical correction of his hypercalcemia normalized his mental state. Formal psychometric assessment reported: "Intellectually he is functioning within the high average range of intelligence. Compared to his preoperative state, the mild confusion, poor remote memory, slight disorientation, and confabulation have all improved. In addition there is now no evidence of the short-term memory impairment previously reported."

A 46-year-old woman developed noncirrhotic portal hypertension and underwent portacaval anastomosis. Thirteen years later she developed confusion and anemia. Mild

hyperparathyroidism was also diagnosed, but a conservative approach was adopted. After 5 years, serum calcium rose to 2.94 mmol/L. She was widowed, living alone, and had frequent falls. She was also encephalopathic with hyperammonemia. A year later she fractured her left humerus. After a further 2 months, right upper parathyroid adenomectomy rendered her normocalcemic and greatly improved her mental state.

Diagnosis of hyperparathyroidism

Hyperparathyroidism is now a relatively straightforward diagnosis to make with the advent of sensitive immunoradiometric assays for PTH.[34] These have largely overcome the problems posed by circulating PTH fragments without biological activity, but which were sometimes read in the older radioimmunoassays. A normal PTH level is inappropriate in

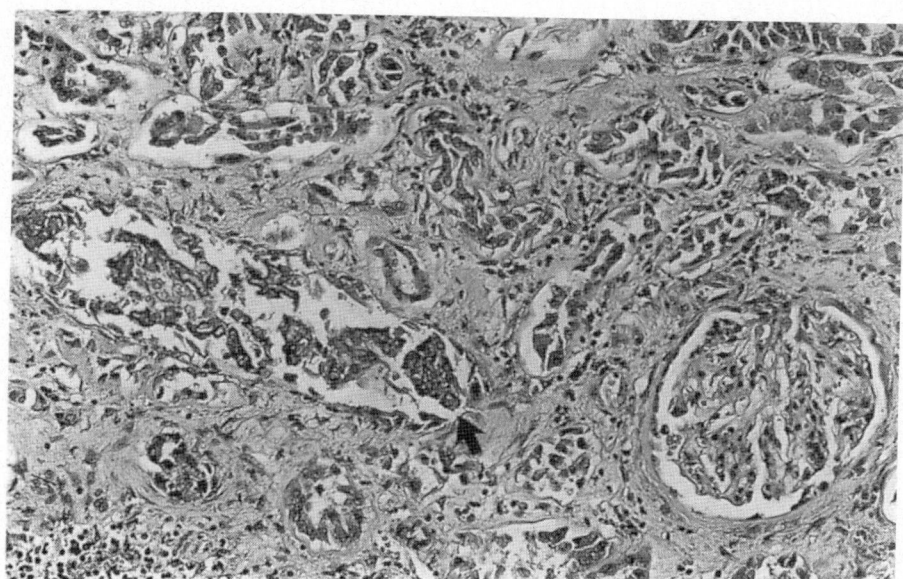

Figure 95-3 Kidney (H&E, ×160). There is advanced interstitial fibrosis and ischemic contracture of the glomerular tuft with periglomerular fibrosis. A dilated tubule contains a granular deposit of calcium phosphate (arrow).

the face of hypercalcemia and confirms hyperparathyroidism; although, using intact PTH assays, serum PTH levels are usually unequivocally raised as parathyroid adenoma cells secrete a higher proportion of intact molecule than do normal cells, which secrete more PTH fragments. The combination of inappropriately elevated PTH measurements using these techniques in the presence of bona fide hypercalcemia is highly reliable evidence. It may be prudent to check urinary calcium excretion to exclude hypocalciuric hypercalcemia.[35,36] The other major cause of hypercalcemia is malignancy, with or without bony metastases. The clinical diagnosis is usually not difficult, and common causes include carcinoma of the lung (usually squamous), breast, or kidney, and hematological malignancies including multiple myeloma. It must be remembered that malignancy and hyperparathyroidism may occasionally coincide.[37]

Treatment of hyperparathyroidism

There is little controversy about the need for surgical intervention in those with complications of hyperparathyroidism (Table 95-1), but it is more difficult to be certain about the potential benefits in those with mild or asymptomatic disease. Older patients gain as much benefit from surgery as do younger patients. A study from California[38] showed little difference between the populations preoperatively, except for an excess of hypertension in the elderly group (age >60). Postoperatively, fewer than 2 percent of elderly patients remained hypercalcemic, whilst 82 percent had significant relief of preoperative symptoms—including, in the older population, fatigue (50 percent), muscle weakness (49 percent), and joint pain (41 percent). There was minimal perioperative morbidity and no deaths.

It is often helpful to localize the parathyroid tumor preoperatively. Favored methods include magnetic resonance imaging (MRI), ultrasound, and isotopic scanning.[39] None is universally accurate, but isotopic scanning with ^{99m}Tc-sestamibi, which has replaced thallium–technetium subtraction scanning, is probably the most sensitive and specific.[40]

Table 95-1 **Indications for surgery in primary hyperparathyroidism**
Definite
Serum calcium >3.0 mmol/L
Renal impairment
Nephrocalcinosis/nephrolithiasis
Significant hypercalciuria
Parathyroid bone disease
Osteoporosis: *Z* score < −2.0
Age <50
Possible
Neuropsychiatric or neuromuscular symptoms
Age <70
Reproduced from reference 45.

Selective venous sampling for high PTH levels is now usually restricted to cases where the first neck exploration has failed to identify the tumor. The experienced surgeon can usually identify the normal parathyroid gland. Scanning techniques are often unhelpful with the smaller tumors weighing less than 400 mg, which is just when their assistance is most needed. The surgery for a single adenoma is straightforward. In hyperplasia the intraoperative frozen section reports may not always easily provide conclusive information. In this situation it is common practice to remove $3\frac{1}{2}$ out of 4 identified glands, or all four glands, transplanting one to the forearm.

Medical treatment is increasingly sought in cases of relatively mild hyperparathyroidism in the elderly patient. Estrogen can be used in women, both reducing PTH secretion and inhibiting bone resorption. Bisphosphonates, such as intermittent pamidronate or clodronate, can control hypercalcemia acutely, but a rebound increase in PTH secretion occurs so repeated doses are necessary.[41] Oral clodronate can be used as chronic treatment, but is poorly tolerated because of gastrointestinal side-effects. Calcium-receptor agonists have been developed, which suppress PTH

Table 95-2 **Monitoring required for patients with primary hyperparathyroidism managed conservatively**

Six-monthly
Assessment of symptoms
Blood pressure
Serum calcium, creatinine

Twelve-monthly
Abdominal radiograph/ultrasound
ECG ± echocardiogram/exercise test
24-hour urine calcium
Bone densitometry (interval may be more prolonged)

Reproduced from reference 45.

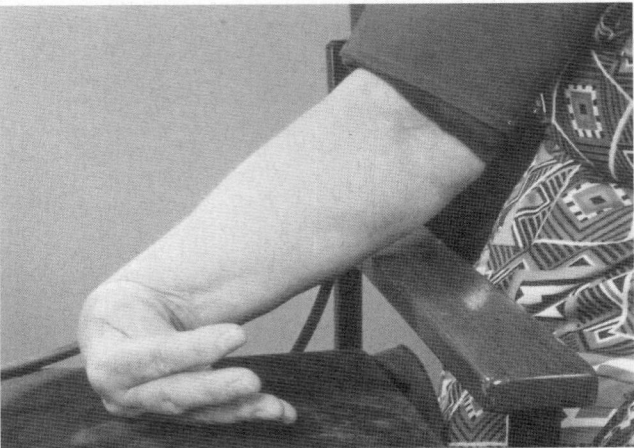

Figure 95-4 Hand held in the "main d'accoucheur" position, a positive Trousseau sign.

secretion from normal parathyroid cells, but it remains to be determined whether they will control secretion from adenomatous cells. Interventional radiology, with ultrasound-guided ethanol injection of parathyroid adenomas, also has its advocates.

If a conservative approach to managing the condition is adopted, patients should be monitored regularly for evidence of complications which would indicate the need for surgical intervention (Table 95-2).

HYPOPARATHYROIDISM

Hypoparathyroidism leads to hypocalcemia and hyperphosphatemia. The clinical hallmark of low ionized calcium is tetany. This neuromuscular hyperexcitability can cause carpopedal spasm and rarely, but dangerously, laryngeal spasm causing stridor and even respiratory arrest. Mild forms present with paresthesiae which are characteristically perioral. Latent tetany may be elicited by Trousseau's sign: inflating a sphygmomanometer cuff above systolic pressure for up to three minutes. Discomfort is to be expected, but the involuntary flexion of the fingers and thumb or "main d'accoucheur" which constitutes a positive response (Fig. 95-4) is intensively painful and the cuff must be immediately deflated when this sign is elicited. Chvostek's sign is elicited by tapping the facial nerve just as it emerges into the cheek in front of the parotid gland. The positive response of ipsilateral twitching of the corner of the mouth is too commonly seen in normal people for this sign to have much value. It must be recalled that tetany may also result from hypomagnesemia, hypokalemia, and hyperventilation. Hypocalcemia may cause central problems with mental depression, fits,[42] and even reversible dementia[43] in the elderly population.

The most common cause of hypoparathyroidism is iatrogenic following neck surgery, but an idiopathic variety is increasingly recognized in elderly people. Two forms of pseudo-hypoparathyroidism exist where there is end-organ resistance to the action of PTH: in the first form the generation of cyclic AMP is impaired, and in the second form that is normal and the defect lies distal to this within the target cells.

Treatment of hypoparathyroidism

When hypoparathyroidism occurs after neck surgery, it is often transient and the postoperative administration of short-term calcium supplementation may be all that is needed. If it persists then vitamin D administration is required. This is commonly given as one of the 1-alpha hydroxylated preparations which act rapidly and directly. There is no justification for the continued use of pharmacological doses of cholecalciferol. This is because the ever-present danger in vitamin D therapy is unpredictable hypercalcemia. Cholecalciferol is a fat-soluble prohormone and it is difficult to remove from stores if calcium levels rise excessively.[44] Reversibility is normally easy and quick following withdrawal of the more polar 1-hydroxylated compounds. It must be emphasized that dangerous hypercalcemia can develop quite asymptomatically with potentially disastrous effects on renal function. It is therefore mandatory to measure serum calcium levels regularly: approximately 2-monthly is a reasonable routine interval, lifelong for patients treated in this way for hypoparathyroidism.

Summary of management algorithm
Primary hyperparathyroidism

- Surgery ± preoperative localization.
- Medical management, usually with bisphosphonates, if unfit for surgery.
- Conservative management for mild/asymptomatic disease.
- ? Percutaneous, ultrasound-guided ethanol injection into parathyroid adenoma.

KEY POINTS Primary hyperparathyroidism

- The disease is more common in elderly women, with an annual incidence of 2 per 1000 (age >60).
- It is usually present with mild hypercalcemia—calcium <3.0 mmol/L
- Severe bone or renal disease now are very rare.

(Continued)

KEY POINTS (Continued)

- Neuropsychiatric and neuromuscular symptoms are common but may be difficult to discriminate from signs of normal aging.

- Elderly patients benefit from surgery as much as do younger patients.

REFERENCES

1. Farrow SM, O'Riordan JLH: Regulation of parathyroid hormone gene expression. Bone (Clin Biochem News Rev) 1990;7:51–53

2. Farrow SM, Karmali R, Gleed JH et al: Regulation of preproparathyroid hormone messenger RNA and hormone synthesis in human parathyroid adenomata. J Endocrinol 1988;117:133–138

3. Brown EM, Pollak M, Seidman CE et al: Calcium-ion-sensing cell-surface receptors. N Engl J Med 1995;333:234–239

4. Karmali R, Farrow S, Hewison M et al: Effects of 1,25-dihydroxy-vitamin D, and cortisol on bovine and human parathyroid cells. J Endocrinol 1989;123:137–142

5. Quesada JM, Coopmans W, Ruiz B et al: Influence of vitamin D on parathyroid function in the elderly. J Clin Endocrinol Metab 1992;75:494–501

6. Fujiyama K, Kiriyama T, Ito M et al: Attenuation of postmenopausal high bone loss in patients with hypoparathyroidism. J Clin Endocrinol Metab 1995;80:2135–2138

7. Chapuy MC, Arlot ME, Duboeuf F et al: Vitamin D_3 and calcium to prevent hip fractures in elderly women. N Engl J Med 1992;333:1437–1443

8. Agus ZS, Wasserstein A, Goldfarb S: PTH, calcitonin, cyclic nucleotides, and the kidney. Ann Rev Physiol 1981;41:583–595

9. Garabedian M, Holick MF, De Luca HF, Boyle IT: Control of 25-hydroxycholecalciferol metabolism by the parathyroid glands. Proc Natl Acad Sci USA 1972;69:1673–1676

10. Anast CS, Mohs JM, Kaplan SL, Burns PW: Evidence for parathyroid failure in magnesium deficiency. Science 1972;177:606–608

11. Fraser DR, Kodicek E: Unique biosynthesis by kidney of a biologically active vitamin D metabolite. Nature 1979;228:764–766

12. Mundy GR, Cove DH, Fisken RA: Primary hyperparathyroidism: changes in the pattern of clinical presentation. Lancet 1980;i:1317–1320

13. Heath H, Hodgson SF, Kennedy MA: Primary hyperparathyroidism: incidence, morbidity and potential economic input in a community. N Engl J Med 1980;302:189–193

14. Black WC III, Utley JR: The differential diagnosis of parathyroid adenoma and chief cell hyperplasia. Am J Clin Pathol 1968;49:761–775

15. Trump D, Farren B, Wooding C et al: Clinical studies of multiple endocrine neoplasia type I (MEN I). QJM 1996;89:653–669

16. Jung RT, Grant AM, Davie M et al: Multiple endocrine adenomatosis (type I) and familial hyperparathyroidism. Postgrad Med J 1978;54:92–94

17. Leshin M: Multiple endocrine neoplasia. In Wilson JD, Foster DW (eds): Williams Textbook of Endocrinology, 7th edn. WB Saunders, Philadelphia, 1985:1274–1289

18. Chandrasekharappa SC et al: Positional cloning of the gene for multiple endocrine neoplasia type 1. Science 1997;276:404–407

19. Friedman E, Sakaguchi K, Bale AE et al: Clonality of parathyroid tumors in familial multiple endocrine neoplasia type I. N Engl J Med 1989;321:213–218

20. Thakker RV, Bouloux P, Wooding C et al: Association of parathyroid tumors in multiple endocrine neoplasia type I with loss of alleles on chromosome 11. N Engl J Med 1989;321:218–224

21. Arnold A, Staunton CE, Kim HG: Monoclonality and abnormal parathyroid hormone genes in parathyroid adenomas. N Engl J Med 1988;318:658–662

22. Patten BM, Bilezikian JP, Mallette LE et al: The neuromuscular disease of hyperparathyroidism. Ann Intern Med 1974;80:182–194

23. Nilsson I-L, Aberg J, Rastad J, Lind L: Endothelial vasodilator dysfunction in primary hyperparathyroidism is reversed after parathyroidectomy. Surgery 1999;126:1049–1055

24. Palmer M, Adami H-O, Bergstrom R et al: Mortality after surgery for primary hyperparathyroidism: a follow-up of 441 patients operated on from 1956 to 1979. Surgery 1987;102:1–7

25. Kim H, Kalkhoff RK, Costrini NV et al: Plasma insulin disturbances in primary hyperparathyroidism. J Clin Invest 1971;50:2596–2605

26. DeFronzo RA, Lang R: Hypophosphatemia and glucose intolerance: evidence for tissue insensitivity to insulin. N Engl J Med 1980;303:1259–1263

27. Potts JR: Management of asymptomatic hyperparathyroidism. J Clin Endocrinol Metab 1990;70:1489–1493

28. Stevenson JC, Lynn JA: Time to end a conservative treatment for mild hyperparathyroidism. BMJ 1988;296:1016–1017

29. Paterson CR, Burns J, Mowat E: Long-term follow-up of untreated primary hyperparathyroidism. BMJ 1984;289:1261–1263

30. Sampson MJ, van't Hoff W, Bicknell EJ: The conservative management of primary hyperparathyroidism. QJM 1987;65:1009–1014

31. Rao DS, Wilson RJ, Kleerekoper M, Parfitt AM: Lack of biochemical progression or continuation of accelerated bone loss in mild asymptomatic primary hyperparathyroidism: evidence for biphasic disease course. J Clin Endocrinol Metab 1988;67:1294–1298

32. Parisien M, Silverberg SJ, Shane E et al: The histomorphometry of bone in primary hyperparathyroidism: preservation of cancellous bone structure. J Clin Endocrinol Metab 1990;70:930–938

33. Neer RM et al: Effect of parathyroid hormone (1–34) on fractures and bone mineral density in postmenopausal women with osteoporosis. N Engl J Med 2001;344:1434–1441

34. Nussbaum SR, Zahradnik RJ, Lavigne JR et al: Highly sensitive two-site immunoradiometric assay of parathyrin, and its clinical utility in evaluating patients with hypercalcemia. Clin Chem 1987;8:1364–1367

35. Paterson CR, Gunn A: Familial benign hypercalcaemia. Lancet 1981;ii:61–63

36. Marx SJ, Spiegel AM, Levine MA et al: Familial hypocalciuric hypercalcemia: the relation to primary parathyroid hyperplasia. N Engl J Med 1982;307:416–426

37. Drezner MK, Lebovitz HE: Primary hyperparathyroidism in para-neoplastic hypercalcaemia. Lancet 1978;i:1004–1006

38. Uden P et al: Primary hyperparathyroidism in younger and older patients: symptoms and outcome of surgery. World J Surg 1992;16:791–797 (review)

39. Heath DA: Localization of parathyroid tumours. Clin Endocrinol 1995;43:523–524

40. Arici C et al: Can localization studies be used to direct focused parathyroid operations? Surgery 2001;129:720–729

41. Hamdy NAT, Gray RES, McCloskey E et al: Clodronate in the medical management of hyperparathyroidism. Bone 1987;8(Suppl 1):569–577

42. Graham K, Williams BO, Rowe MJ: Idiopathic hypoparathyroidism: a cause of fits in the elderly. BMJ 1979;i:1460–1461

43. Eraut D: Idiopathic hypoparathyroidism presenting as dementia. BMJ 1974;i:429–430

44. Hossain M: Vitamin-D intoxication during treatment of hypoparathyroidism. Lancet 1970;i:1149–1151

45. National Institutes of Health conference: Diagnosis and management of asymptomatic primary hyperparathyroidism: consensus development conference statement. Ann Intern Med 1991;28:95–100

Chapter 96

Diabetes mellitus

Alan J. Sinclair and Simon C. M. Croxson

There is ample proof of the economic, social, and health burden of diabetes in the elderly population.[1–4] Despite this recognition, there has been relative neglect in the medical literature, with few detailed studies of older diabetic patients.[1,5] For example, articles on diabetes research specifically involving older patients accounted for fewer than 5 percent of those published between 1978 and 1988.[5] Thus our care of the elderly diabetic subject, whose health status may range from fitness to total dependency, is often evidence-*biased* rather than evidence-based. For many possible reasons, the present state of diabetic care for older adults is essentially unstructured, poorly coordinated, often inappropriate, and therefore in great need of reorganization.[6]

Recent initiatives justify optimism that care is improving.[7] In particular, there is more recognition that older patients with diabetes may be different from younger counterparts;[8] for example, they have a high degree of comorbidity, an age-related impairment of functional ability, and an increased vulnerability to hypoglycemia and its consequences. They may also require a different approach to management, which involves spouses and other carers to a greater extent.[9] Along with these developments has come an appreciation of new aims of care for the older patient[6] which are far more comprehensive than previous aims that focused only on avoiding hypoglycemia and keeping the patient symptom-free. This chapter provides an account of the scientific and clinical basis of managing older people with diabetes, so enabling the reader to implement practical steps to improve care. However, this is a very large topic, and indeed there are whole books on the subject.[10] This chapter can provide only a basic text within the space provided. The essential point is that basic care—glycemic control, and prevention of vascular disease, especially blood pressure control and care of the eyes, feet, and kidneys—should be within the reach of all practitioners (Table 96-1).

DIABETES DEFINITION, CLASSIFICATION, AND DIAGNOSIS

Diabetes is defined by hyperglycemia and the tendency to develop specific complications, particularly retinopathy; indeed, the "gold standard" test for diabetes would be to leave the subject untreated for several years after which the presence of retinopathy is diagnostic.[11–13] The diagnostic criteria were developed to diagnose type 2 diabetes mellitus (previously known as non-insulin-dependent diabetes mellitus), since type 1 diabetes (previously known as insulin-dependent diabetes mellitus) is generally obvious clinically. A venous plasma glucose level equal to or exceeding 11.1 mmol/L (200 mg/dL)[14,15] following glucose challenge identifies those subjects who have a dramatically increased risk of retinopathy.[11–13,16] This cutoff value is derived from Whitehall civil servants,[16] residents of Bedford,[13] and Pima Indians of all ages.[11,12] If one examines populations with a very high incidence of type 2 diabetes, such as the Pima Indians or Nauru Islanders, who have not previously been diagnosed as diabetic, then mass glucose tolerance testing reveals a bimodal distribution of 2-hour glucose values at all ages, including elderly people, which is not seen in populations with small numbers of undiagnosed diabetic subjects.[17,18] The cutoff value of 11.1 mmol/L does actually separate normoglycemic and diabetic populations (each with a Gaussian distribution of 2-hour values) in different age groups, suggesting that the World Health Organization criteria (see below) apply in elderly people as well as the young. However, the 11.1 mmol/L cutoff has never been tested by long-term follow-up in the elderly population to confirm its validity.

Use of modern diagnostic criteria

Measure venous plasma glucose:

Fasting ≥7.0 mmol/L
or
Random ≥11.1 mmol/L
or
2-hour post 75 g glucose load ≥11.1 mmol/L

suggests diabetes, which should be confirmed by:

Classical osmotic symptoms of polyuria/polydispia
or
Specific complication (which means retinopathy)
or
Another elevated plasma glucose level on a different day.

One can use other blood specimens, but venous plasma glucose is the standard. Stress hyperglycemia can complicate any acute illness and a diagnosis made at this time should be reviewed 6 weeks after the illness.

The majority of elderly diabetic people have type 2 diabetes, but type 1 does occur[19] and the age-specific incidence of type 1 is the same from 30 to 80 years of age.[20] Type 1 diabetes in the elderly population may have a very insidious onset, when it is termed "latent autoimmune diabetes of the aged" (LADA). LADA has been shown to be quite common in some series (e.g. 10–15 percent of diabetic adults and 50 percent of the

Table 96-1 Aims in managing the elderly diabetic person

- Maintain well-being and quality of life
- Avoid symptoms of hyperglycemia including hyperglycemic malaise
- Assess and ameliorate comorbid conditions, particularly vascular disease
- Avoid adverse drug events, particularly hypoglycemia
- Maintain acceptable bodyweight
- Prevent, screen for, and treat complications
- Recognize disability and limit handicap

nonobese type 2 diabetic subjects[21]); the autoantibody screen is not used in routine clinical practice in elderly people because it is not particularly predictive. One should be very suspicious of an elderly diabetic person who is not obese and who does not seem to respond to oral hypoglycemic agents. Diabetes may also be secondary to or exacerbated by other conditions such as pancreatic disease, endocrine disease such as Cushing's syndrome, acromegaly, or thyrotoxicosis, and (most commonly) drug therapy with high-dose thiazide diuretics, oral glucocorticosteroids, and oral β-blockers. A comprehensive list of diabetogenic drugs is given in the National Diabetes Data Group criteria.[14] The majority of subjects with secondary diabetes are elderly.[22] A simple classification of diabetes mellitus in the elderly population is given in Table 96-2.

Impaired glucose tolerance (IGT) is a state between normal and diabetic glucose tolerance. In itself it does not lead to diabetic-specific complications; but it is a significant risk factor for large-vessel disease, and over 10 years, 10 percent will progress to diabetes in British residents.[23] Far more will progress in populations with a high prevalence of diabetes, such as the Pima Indians,[24] in whom 6 percent convert per year. It is, however, possible to regress from IGT to normal

glucose tolerance. Although the cutoff between diabetic and nondiabetic glucose tolerance is based on the risk of specific complications, the cutoff between IGT and normal glucose tolerance is more arbitrary and was reached by consensus of experts.[26] One should note that diabetic complications are divided into specific complications (e.g. retinopathy) which are related to degree and duration of hyperglycemia, and nonspecific complications (e.g. large-vessel disease) which occur in normal glucose-tolerant subjects, but are more common with any degree of abnormal glucose tolerance, including IGT.[23,25]

Recently, the diagnostic criteria were revised by both the American Diabetes Association (ADA)[27] and the WHO[28]—see Table 96-3 and www.diabetes.org.uk/info/carerec/newdiagnotic.htm. These revisions have attempted to make screening for diabetes easier, but the ADA criteria have created pitfalls for the unwary. Both sets of criteria lower the threshold for an abnormal fasting plasma glucose (FPG) from 7.8 to 7.0 mmol/L, which addresses the low sensitivity of the fasting plasma glucose to detect an elevated 2-hour post-challenge glucose. Many studies have shown that this decrease in FPG increases the sensitivity of the FPG (e.g. from 65 to 81 percent in Bristol, UK), but the test still misses diabetic subjects with elevated 2-hour plasma glucose levels.[29] Isolated post-challenge hyperglycemia is not a benign mild condition: it carries increased risk of death.[30] The ADA criteria embrace the FPG fully, but the WHO do point out their reservations. Usefully, both sets of criteria emphasize that one needs confirmatory evidence (classical osmotic symptoms, or specific complications or a further diagnostic plasma glucose level on a different day) to make the diagnosis. Finally, the ADA reintroduced the concept of impaired fasting glucose (IFG) for subjects with a fasting glucose of 6.0–6.9 mmol/L. It is true that the risk of macrovascular disease increases once the FPG exceeds 6.0 mmol/L, but these IFG subjects have 2-hour post-challenge glucose levels putting them clearly into normal, IGT, or diabetic categories which require different management. In the

---

Table 96-2 Classification of diabetes in elderly people

Primary
Type 1
Type 2
  Obese
  Nonobese
  Maturity-onset diabetes of the young

Secondary
Pancreatic disease
Drugs (e.g. steroids)
Other endocrine conditions (e.g. Cushing's syndrome, acromegaly, thyrotoxicosis)

Table 96-3 WHO values for diagnosis of diabetes mellitus and other categories of hyperglycemia[28]

| | Glucose concentration (mmol/L) | | |
| | Whole blood | | |
	Venous	**Capillary**	**Plasma (venous)**[a]
Diabetes mellitus:			
Fasting *or*	≥6.1	≥6.1	≥7.0
2 hours after glucose load	≥10.0	≥11.1	≥11.1
Impaired Glucose Tolerance (IGT):			
Fasting (if measured) *and*	<6.1 *and*	<6.1 *and*	<7.0 *and*
2 hours after glucose load	6.7–9.9	7.8–11.0	7.8–11.0
Impaired fasting glycemia (IFG):			
Fasting *and* (if measured)	5.6 *and* <6.1	5.6 *and* <6.1	6.1 *and* <7.0
2 hours after glucose load	<6.7	<7.8	<7.8

[a] *Corresponding values for capillary plasma are:*
    For diabetes mellitus: fasting, 7.0; 2-h, 12.2.
    For impaired glucose tolerance: fasting, <7.0; and 2-h, 8.9 and <12.2.
    For impaired fasting glycemia: 6.1 and <7.0, and if measured, 2-h, <8.9.
For clinical purposes, the diagnosis of diabetes should always be confirmed by repeating the test on another day unless there is unequivocal hyperglycemia with acute metabolic decompensation or obvious symptoms.

predominantly European population of Bristol,[29] one-third of IFG subjects have each category of glucose tolerance, whereas in the high-risk Gujerati population of Leicester, UK, all IFG subjects have either diabetes or IGT on the 2-hour PG.[31] These facts are important if the FPG is used for diagnosing diabetes.

IMPAIRMENT OF GLUCOSE TOLERANCE WITH AGING

The prevalence of diabetes mellitus increases with advancing age and is predominantly type 2. As early as 1921, Spence[32] reported observations relating to an impairment of glucose tolerance in the elderly population. This age-related impairment has been confirmed by more recent studies indicating that glucose intolerance begins in the third decade and continues throughout adulthood.[33–36] The magnitude of the rise has been estimated to be 0.33–0.72 mmol/L (5.9–13.0 mg/dL) per decade in 1- and 2-hour post-glucose ingestion samples. The rise is more pronounced in women (about 0.55 mmol/L [9.9 mg/dL] higher than in men).[36] The National Health and Nutrition Examination Survey (NHANES III) of US residents found a rise in prevalence of impaired glucose tolerance (IGT) of 11.9 percent in those aged 40–49 years to 20.7 percent in those aged 60–74 years;[37] this survey also demonstrated increasing prevalence rates of diabetes with age from 3.4 to 24.4 percent (Fig. 96-1).

Several possible mechanisms may contribute to glucose intolerance during aging and these are listed in Table 96-4. The impairment is clearly multifactorial, being characterized by delays in glucose-mediated insulin secretion, insulin-induced suppression of hepatic glucose output, and a rise in insulin-mediated glucose uptake. From the results of glucose clamp techniques,[38,39] the major disturbance appears to be impaired insulin-mediated glucose uptake, with skeletal muscle being the principal site of this defect.[36] Because insulin receptor numbers or binding are not generally affected by age, the impairment is due primarily to a postreceptor defect. Of the factors indicated in the accompanying list that may modify muscle uptake of glucose, none appears to exert a major influence. The postreceptor defect may comprise abnormalities of glucose transport within the cell, or defective insulin internalization and intracellular metabolism. Age-associated glucose intolerance has been considered to be specific for the aging process and

> **Table 96-4 Mechanisms of decreased glucose tolerance in old age**
>
> - Delayed/decreased glucose induced insulin secretion
> - Impaired insulin-mediated glucose uptake in skeletal muscle and adipose tissue due to predominantly postreceptor defect
> - Other factors:
>   - Increased body fat
>   - Decreased physical activity
>   - Reduced dietary carbohydrate
>   - Impaired renal function
>   - Hypokalemia
>   - Increased sympathetic nervous system activity
>   - Diabetogenic drugs

distinct from those defects that are seen in obesity and type 2 diabetes mellitus, but others disagree.[40] A detailed description of the mechanisms mentioned above is available.[41]

EPIDEMIOLOGY OF DIABETES MELLITUS IN THE ELDERLY POPULATION

Estimates of the incidence and prevalence of diabetes in the elderly population are subject to error because approximately 50 percent may be undiagnosed.[42] However, even studies of subjects with previously diagnosed diabetes can provide useful information. For instance, the surveys of Poole, Oxford, and Southall (UK) of European subjects with diagnosed diabetes[43] reveals that 60 percent of known diabetic subjects are aged 60 years or more. However, when considering the overall prevalence of diabetes, one should include only studies using adequate survey methods, which basically means using the glucose tolerance test. Different investigators have studied different age groups. Some have not analyzed the result by the different ethnic groups in their sample and presentation of results is quite variable. In the past, studies used different diagnostic criteria, prior to the major changes in 1979/1980,[14,26] and some studies pre-screened with a simple test (e.g. urinalysis) to select subjects for further study.

The prevalence of diabetes rises from youth to old age (Fig. 96-1). However, the Melton (UK) screening survey,[44] the

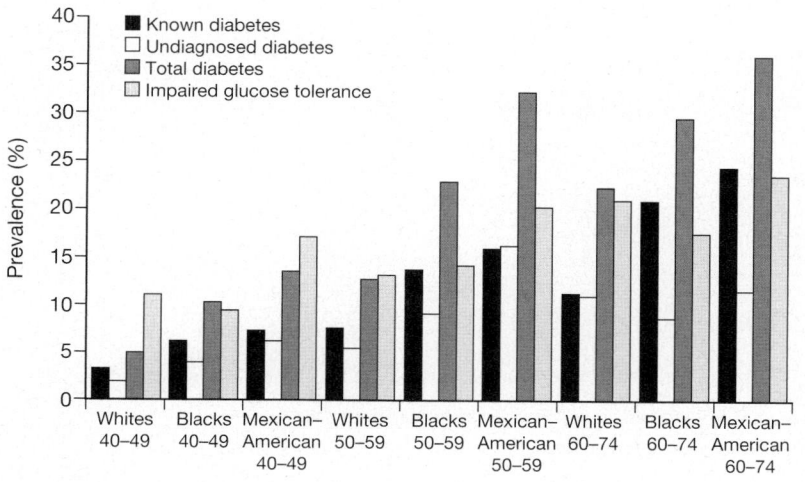

Figure 96-1 Data from NHANES III: rising abnormalities of glucose tolerance with age. From Harris et al.[37]

East & West Finland screening survey,[45] and a survey of Pima Indians[46] found static prevalences from age 65 to 85, suggesting that the age-related increase in diabetes prevalence levels off after age 65. Most developed countries have a prevalence of approximately 17 percent in their elderly white population and around 25 percent in nonwhite populations.[15,37,45–57] The prevalence in white British elderly people is only around 9 percent,[44,58] although the prevalence in nonwhite British elderly people is still approximately 25 percent,[59] and the prevalence in care-home residents is 25 percent.[60]

The prevalence of previously diagnosed diabetes in the UK elderly population has increased over the last few decades and one could argue that this is due to a higher rate of ascertainment, rather than a true increase.[61] However, data from Poole show an increase in diagnosed diabetes from 1983 to 1996, approximately doubling in subjects aged 60 to 69 years;[62] some of this increase may indeed be due to a higher rate of diagnosis, but evidence from screening in Glostrup shows an increased true prevalence in the Danes due to increased obesity and decreased exercise,[63] and NHANES III has shown a true increase in prevalence[37] from NHANES II[42] (Table 96-5).

The risk of developing type 2 diabetes is increased by parental history,[42,57,64] obesity,[42,55,57,63,64] hypertension,[55,64] lack of exercise,[55,64] and nonwhite race.[37,42] In subjects with these risk factors, exercise seems to protect against the development of diabetes.[64] This is important when advising the offspring of patients who are told to stay slim, avoid refined carbohydrates, exercise more (climb 15 flights of stairs per day), and be aware of their risk of diabetes and hypertension.[64] Targeted screening of at-risk individuals is now also advised (e.g. fasting venous plasma glucose every 3 years for offspring of diabetic patients, after the age of 40 years),[27] remembering to advise the subjects to buy life insurance before the test rather than after.

In summary, not only are many elderly people diabetic, many subjects with known diabetes are elderly.

IMPACT OF DIABETES MELLITUS IN THE ELDERLY POPULATION

Overview

Older patients with diabetes appear to have 2–3 times more need for hospital care than the general population[65] for various conditions such as heart failure, stroke, and coronary heart disease. This increase occurs from middle age onwards.[66] Older people with diabetes also use primary care services 2–3 times more than nondiabetic controls.[66,67] Damsgaard's primary care study from Denmark[67] indicated that insulin-treated patients accounted for more than half of the service provision, mainly

Table 96-5 Prevalence of diabetes in different screened elderly populations

Study	Year	Ref.	Age	Sex	Ethnic origin	Diabetes rate (%)	IGT rate (%)
Melton, UK	1991	44	65–85	MF	White	9.1	7.1
Coventry, UK	1988	59	60–79	MF	White	7.0	–
Coventry, UK	1988	59	60–79	MF	South Asian	27.8	–
NHANES II, US	1976–1980	42	65–74	MF	White	17.9	23.0
NHANES II, US	1976–1980	42	65–74	MF	Nonwhite	26.4	14.5
NHANES III, US	1988–1994	37	60–74	MF	White	22.3	20.9
NHANES III, US	1988–1994	37	60–74	MF	Black	29.5	17.6
NHANES III, US	1988–1994	37	60–74	MF	Hispanic	36	23.5
California, US	1972–1974	47	60–89	MF	White	16.1	–
Tampere, Finland (F)	1977	48	85	MF	White	17.0	–
Fredericia, Denmark (F)	1981–1982	53	60–74	M	White	7.2	–
Glostrup, Denmark (U)	1967	54	70	MF	White	10.0	25
Glostrup, Denmark (U)	1977	54	80	MF	White	12.0	36
Glostrup, Denmark	1996–1997	63	60	M	White	12.3	15.9
Glostrup, Denmark	1996–1997	63	60	F	White	6.8	13.1
East/west Finland (pm gtts)	1984	45	65–84	M	White	29.8	31.8
Gothenburg, Sweden	1980	55	67	M	White	10.8	14.2
Amsterdam, Holland (D)	1985	56	65	MF	White	23.6	–
Kuopio, Finland	1986–1988	57	65–74	MF	White	17.8	20.8

Abbreviations: F, FBG-based survey; D, recruitment details scanty; pm gtts, testing performed in afternoon, which may increase diabetes prevalence; U, previously undiagnosed diabetic subjects only recorded.

due to chronic vascular disease, with a correspondingly high number of hospital clinic visits. The average number of bed-days occupied per person per year was 6.8 for males and 8.2 for females, whereas the figures for insulin-treated type 2 diabetic patients was 23.9, which was considerably higher than for insulin-treated patients with type 1 diabetes (15.2).[65] Similar bed-occupancy rates for patients with known diabetes have been reported by others.[68]

Several studies have defined the prevalence of elderly patients in hospital diabetic populations. In a study from Edinburgh Royal Infirmary, elderly patients aged 65 years and over with diabetes accounted for 60 percent of the overall bed-occupancy due to diabetes, giving a mean hospital prevalence of 4.6 percent.[2] A Cardiff-based study of three district general hospitals found a hospital prevalence (pooled data) of 8.4 percent with a mean age of 65 years.[69]

Diabetes in older subjects is associated with considerable morbidity, mainly due to the long-term complications.[70–73] A population-based study from Oxford[70] measured the incidence of complications over a median period of 6 years in 188 patients aged 60 years and over by using a structured questionnaire and clinical examination. Incidence rates of ischemic heart disease, stroke, and peripheral vascular disease were 56, 22, and 146 per 1,000 person-years, which are slightly higher than found in the Framingham study,[74] since the Oxford study involved an older age group. Retinopathy occurred at a rate of 60 and cataract at 29 per 1,000 person-years, while proteinuria (albumin concentration greater than 300 mg/L) was 19 per 1,000 person-years. Incidence rates appeared to be unrelated to sex or duration of diabetes, but stroke and peripheral vascular disease rose significantly with age.

In Poole, a coastal town in southern England, the prevalence of diabetic neuropathy, an important cause of foot ulceration and amputation, was determined in 1,077 diabetic subjects,[71] who comprised 94 percent of the known diabetic population. Neuropathy was diagnosed by the presence of neuropathic symptoms plus one or more physical findings such as loss of light touch or impairment of pain sensation. The overall prevalence of neuropathy was 16.3 percent (compared with 2.9 percent in nondiabetic controls) with similar values in both type 1 and type 2 diabetes patients. Three-quarters of patients reported symptoms. Duration of diabetes and metabolic control were significant predictors of neuropathy. The prevalence of neuropathy increased with age in all groups, with one in four type 2 diabetes patients aged 80 years and over being affected.

A community survey from Nottingham, UK,[72] of 98 elderly diabetic patients (mean age 73 years) registered with two inner-city general practices, studied the impact of diabetes in terms of complications and frequency of hospital and general practice contacts. Figure 96-2 shows that diabetic subjects had significantly higher prevalences of stroke, cognitive impairment, diminished leg pulses, visual impairment, and absent vibration senses (vibration perception threshold greater than 50 V at one or more sites, as a marker of neuropathy) compared with nondiabetic controls. Disability was present in four out of five patients. Cataract was the most common cause of disability associated with visual impairment.

The prevalence of some diabetic complications has been reported to increase with advancing age.[11,75–77] In a cross-sectional study of type 2 diabetes patients aged 53 to 80 years,[77] the prevalence of retinopathy, peripheral neuropathy, and hypertension were evaluated at different ages. Logistic regression demonstrated a significant increase in the prevalence of retinopathy with aging, independent of the effects of metabolic control, duration of disease, and other risk variables. Age was also related to the prevalence of peripheral neuropathy, hypertension, and impotence. The independent contribution of age, per se, to retinopathy was not seen in a study by Ballard et al.[76] in 1988 in Minnesota, who found a positive relationship with persistent proteinuria only, nor in a study in 1986 by Knuiman et al.,[75] who studied both type 1 and type 2 diabetes patients and found independent associations of age with renal impairment, macrovascular complications, and sensory neuropathy only.

Visual loss

Diabetic retinopathy was the third main cause of blindness and partial sight registration in one epidemiological study in Avon, UK.[78] However, the diabetic person also has a greater risk of cataract, glaucoma, retinal artery thrombosis, and retinal vein

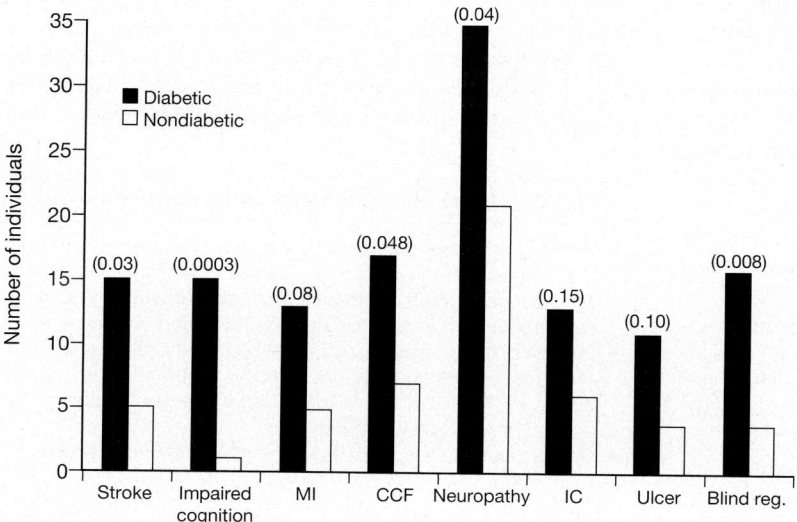

Figure 96-2 Comparison of morbidity between diabetic and nondiabetic individuals. *P* values are shown in parentheses. From Dornan et al.[72]

thrombosis. Thus, it is no surprise that blind registrations for diabetic subjects in Nottingham, UK, are eight times higher than the subjects not known to have diabetes,[71] with 16 percent of elderly diabetic subjects having blind or partial-sight registrations. The diabetic blind registration is predominantly due to maculopathy, which is treatable, unlike most forms of age-related macular degeneration, the main cause of blind registration in the elderly population.

The underlying problem in diabetic retinopathy is capillary occlusion,[79] which may cause a hypoxic area of retina with new vessel formation. However, other capillaries become dilated; this causes microaneurysms if focal, or leakage from the capillaries if generalized. It is this capillary leakage that causes exudative and edematous maculopathies that are the main forms of sight-threatening retinopathy in the older subject with type 2 diabetes.

Many cross-sectional studies show that good glycemic control is associated with less chance of developing retinopathy.[80,81] The UK Prospective Diabetes Study has now shown, in a prospective randomized controlled trial of aggressive versus conventional (when the trial was started) treatments, that both blood glucose lowering and blood pressure lowering decrease the risk of retinopathy.[82–85] Duration of disease is also associated with increased risk of retinopathy. Because the elderly diabetic subject has often had type 2 diabetes for at least 5–7 years before diagnosis,[86] it is not surprising that diabetic retinopathy is already present at diagnosis in 10.5 percent of elderly subjects in whom only one pupil was dilated;[87] 23.8 percent of subjects of all ages in the UK Prospective Diabetes Study had retinopathy at presentation.[88]

Laser photocoagulation can preserve vision in edematous and exudative maculopathies if visual acuity is 6/9 or better,[89,90] and it has been calculated that screening and treating diabetic retinopathy would prevent 56 percent of blind registrations that are due to the retinopathy.[91] Interestingly, the EURODIAB controlled trial of lisinopril in insulin-dependent diabetes (EUCLID) showed a 50 percent reduction in progression of retinopathy in type 1 diabetic subjects randomized to ACE inhibitor.[92]

Cataract has been shown to be more common in diabetic subjects[93,94] even at the time of diagnosis,[95] and its presence predicts increased mortality.[96] However, The UK Prospective Diabetes Study showed that aggressive blood glucose reduction decreased the rate of cataract extraction.[82]

Although some studies show an association of diabetes with open-angle glaucoma,[97] other studies do not.[98–100] There is some evidence that glaucoma is associated with worse retinopathy[101] and neovascularization is associated with glaucoma,[102] particularly if there is rubreosis iridis. It is well accepted that retinal venous thrombosis is a complication of diabetes,[103] and there is some evidence that retinal artery thrombosis is associated with diabetes.[95,104]

Age-related macular degeneration seems very common in diabetic patients; the theoretical reasons for this are discussed in the paper by Klein et al.[105] However, most studies show no such association,[106–108] and only one study has shown such an association in men aged 75 or more.[105]

The "gold standard" ophthalmological assessment is slit-lamp examination by an experienced user,[109] but this is often not practicable. Mydriatic retinal photography has a sensitivity of detection of eye disease of 89 percent, which is significantly better than the sensitivity of direct ophthalmoscopy of 65 percent.[109] If photography is not available, subjects need measurements of visual acuity and dilated fundoscopy by experienced observers each year; this is probably worth doing opportunistically anyway because even photography misses 11 percent of retinopathy. Although exudative maculopathy is easy to spot in the dilated eye (exudates around or within one disk's diameter of the macula), macular edema is practically impossible to distinguish from a normal eye by ophthalmoscopy; hence, the importance of measuring the corrected visual acuity. Reasons for referral to an ophthalmologist are set out in Table 96-6.

Foot disease

Limb amputation remains an important health problem in the diabetic population with the rate of lower limb amputation being 15 times higher than for nondiabetic patients.[110] It is three times higher in diabetic men than in women.[111] Elderly people are particularly affected.[112]

Management of diabetic limb disease is expensive. Even in 1986 the total annual cost of major leg amputations in diabetic patients in the UK was estimated to be in excess of £13 million;[113] in the USA, the direct medical care costs for all amputations in the diabetic populations, not including rehabilitation, exceeded $500 million.[114] A recent study from the Netherlands[115] estimated the direct costs associated with diabetes-related lower limb amputations and found it to be over £10,000 per hospitalization, with a mean inpatient stay of 42 days. This study identified increasing age and a higher level of amputation as important factors leading to increases in both the period of hospitalization and the associated costs (Table 96-7).

The mortality rate for amputees is high, with a 1952 study suggesting that 40–70 percent of diabetic patients die within 5 years of surgery.[116] Thirty percent require amputation of the remaining lower limb within 3 years, with one in two patients not surviving the subsequent 5 years. More recent evidence indicates that the 3-year survival following lower extremity amputation is about 50 percent,[117] with a median life expectancy after amputation of less than 2 years.[111] Only 5 percent of elderly amputees become fully independent postoperatively.[118]

In about 70 percent of cases, amputation is precipitated by foot ulceration[119,120] whose principal antecedents include peripheral vascular disease and peripheral neuropathy, both

---

Table 96-6 Reasons for referral to an ophthalmologist

- Cataract either obscuring examiner's view of fundus or impairing patient's vision
- Diabetic maculopathy as evidenced by exudates within 1 disk diameter of macula or any unexplained loss of visual acuity
- Preproliferative changes, such as intraretinal microvascular abnormalities, venous changes (beading, loops, dilatation), six cotton wool spots in one quadrant, large blot hemorrhages, arteries replaced by white lines
- Proliferative changes, such as new vessels visible or vitreous hemorrhage
- To complete blind registration

Table 96-7 Duration of hospitalization for lower-extremity amputations, and mean costs of hospitalization (including hospital stay and surgery) by age group in the diabetic population

Age group	Duration of hospitalization[a]	Mean costs of hospitalization (£)	Number of cases
<45	25.5 ± 20.5	6,516	53
45–64	38.7 ± 36.0	9,734	346
65–74	43.5 ± 37.2	10,996	521
75	43.3 ± 42.9	10,928	655
Total	41.8 ± 39.1	10,531	1,575

[a] *Results expressed as mean ± SD in days.*

of which increase with age. Other "at-risk" groups include those with limited joint mobility, bony abnormalities, diabetic nephropathy, excess alcohol intake, visual impairment, and patients living alone.[112]

Various risk factors that increase the likelihood of foot ulceration have been identified (Table 96-8). Peripheral sensorimotor neuropathy is the primary cause or contributory factor in 90 percent of cases.[121,122] Both small (often unmyelinated) and large (usually myelinated) nerve fibers are affected, which leads to the common symptoms of numbness, lancinating and burning pain, "pins and needles," and hyperesthesia, which is typically worse at night.[112] Physical examination reveals a glove and stocking loss of pain, fine touch and thermal sensation (small fibers), with coexisting vibration and proprioceptive loss (large fibers). Small muscle atrophy in the foot can also occur due to motor fiber loss, which can cause flexor/extensor muscle imbalance resulting in clawed toes, prominent metatarsal heads, and forward displacement of the metatarsal foot pads.[123] This can lead to abnormally high foot pressures developing, which can increase the risk of foot ulceration and lead to gait disturbances. In elderly patients with peripheral neuropathy, this may give rise to further foot injuries and falls. The presence of visual loss may exacerbate the situation.[124] A trivial foot injury in a patient with severe neuropathy can eventually lead to the development of a Charcot joint, which is a chronic neuroarthropathy whose prevalence varies from 0.15–7 percent depending on the study population.[112] The majority of cases have had diabetes for at least 10 years, and most are elderly people.

Peripheral blood flow in patients with diabetes is disturbed, with loss of blood flow autoregulation, increased arteriovenous shunting, and changes in capillary blood flow. Some of these abnormalities may be reversible or ameliorated by improved glycemic control.[125] Chronic change in peripheral blood vessels is usually manifested by atherosclerosis, with the pattern of vascular disease tending to involve vessels below the knee more often in diabetic than in nondiabetic individuals.[126] Risk factors for peripheral vascular disease include smoking, hypertension, and hypercholesterolemia, with prevalence increasing with both advancing age and duration of diabetes. Symptoms include intermittent claudication and/or rest pain with lower limb ulceration or gangrene being important clinical outcomes. Radiological investigation may show medial arterial calcification, which has been reported to be associated with both diabetic peripheral somatosensory and autonomic neuropathy.[127] Objective assessment of limb blood flow by Doppler ultrasound can be affected by extensive medial calcification, giving rise to a misleadingly high ankle-pressure index.[128]

Table 96-8 Risk factors for foot ulceration in the elderly population

- Peripheral sensorimotor neuropathy
- Autonomic neuropathy
- Peripheral vascular disease
- Limited joint mobility
- Foot pressure abnormalities
- Previous foot ulcer
- Smoking and alcohol

It seems logical that interventions designed to prevent diabetic foot disease and amputations in patients with diabetes should be directed to the prevention of peripheral neuropathy and peripheral vascular disease and the prevention, early detection, and treatment of foot lesions. Several studies using staff and patient education and a multidisciplinary approach to foot care have demonstrated a reduction in diabetes-related amputations.[129,130] However, elderly people require more assistance than the young because they have difficulty perceiving foot problems and touching their feet.[131] By incorporating an intensive multidisciplinary approach in a diabetes foot clinic,[129] a London-based study demonstrated a 44 percent decline in amputation rate after 2 years. By use of suitable-fitting shoes, the recurrence rate of foot ulcers was reduced from 83 to 26 percent. At the University Hospital of Geneva, an 85 percent reduction in the rate of below-knee amputations was seen over a 4-year observation period by a combination of education and training in foot care in patients with diabetes.[130] A 12-year retrospective study from Sweden[120] evaluated the changes in diabetes-related lower extremity amputations following the introduction of a multidisciplinary program for preventing and treating diabetic foot ulcers. The number of major amputations decreased by 75 percent, the number of minor amputations rose from 28 to 53 percent, and the reamputation rate decreased from 36 to 22 percent. The incidence of major amputations fell from 16.1 to 3.6 per 100,000 inhabitants per year. Many factors were identified as possible contributing influences on the observed changes. These included increased availability of preventative foot care and protective footwear, new healing strategies, use of noninvasive vascular tests, use of strict amputation criteria, and a consistent follow-up service. Along with these, other factors such as changing prevalence of diabetes, smoking habits, and changes in surgical and vascular techniques will also have influenced the results.

With many elderly patients having great difficulty in performing the most routine foot care,[131] often as a result of poor vision and reduced mobility, it becomes very important to design strategies that enable partners and other carers to have a role in prevention and treatment of foot lesions. Educational material needs to be concise and repeated regularly,[112] and video presentations may also be helpful. The accompanying box provides general principles of foot care reflecting a positive approach that can be adapted to many patients in clinical settings.

General principles of foot care education

- Target the level of information to the needs of the patient. Those not at risk may require only general advice about foot hygiene and shoes.
- Assess the ability of the patient to understand and perform the necessary components of foot care. If this is limited, then the spouse or carer should be involved at the beginning of the process.
- Suggest a positive approach to foot care with "do's" rather than "don't"—the principle of active rather than passive food care is more likely to be successful and acceptable to the patient.
  - Do inspect the feet daily.
  - Do report any problems immediately.
  - Do have your feet measured every time new shoes are bought.
  - Do buy shoes with a square toe box and laces.
  - Do inspect the inside of shoes for foreign objects every day before putting them on.
  - Do attend a fully trained chiropodist regularly.
  - Do cut your nails straight across and not rounded.
  - Do keep your feet away from heat (fires, radiators, and hot water bottles) and check the bath water before stepping into it.
  - Do wear something on your feet to protect them at all times and never walk barefoot.
- Repeat the advice at regular intervals and check that it is being followed.
- Disseminate advice to other family members and other healthcare professionals involved in the care of a patient.

Mortality

It is a widely held belief that diabetes mellitus confers little or no excess mortality risk in older patients, with life expectancy being similar to nondiabetic risk after age 70–75 years.[132–134] This apparent finding was explained by a shorter life in elderly subjects with other competing causes of death minimizing the effect of diabetes.[135] In line with this, most early reports indicated that the ratio of death rates in diabetics to rates in the general population falls progressively with age especially in those aged 65 years and over, though it remains above unity up to the age 80 years.[135] More recently, one study actually found a significantly lower mortality in patients aged 75 years and over (mortality ratio 0.88) compared with the general population,[136] and these contradictory findings have created uncertainty about the true impact of this metabolic disorder on the older diabetic population.

Few of the studies on diabetic mortality in the population employed universal screening using an oral glucose tolerance test (or other methods of confirming the presence of diabetes). It is possible that actual mortality in any given population may be underestimated because known diabetic subjects are compared to the general population which contains subjects with undiagnosed diabetes or impaired glucose tolerance; undiagnosed diabetes and IGT were associated with increased mortality compared to normal glucose tolerance subjects in Melton Mowbray, UK,[137] which would inappropriately raise the mortality rate in the subjects not known to be diabetic. Other methodological variations have prevented consistent comparisons across different diabetic populations. It is important to determine whether premature death due to diabetes is observable in elderly patients because this evidence would provide guidance to those responsible for providing health services on how best to focus their resources. An unequivocal finding of increased mortality would argue for a more sustained commitment to diabetic healthcare provision and research. Alternatively, the absence of excess mortality could redirect care strategies toward reducing morbidity and disability only.

A recent literature review by the present authors has confirmed that diabetes in later life imposes an excess mortality risk[138] associated with a reduction in life expectancy in both sexes, even in patients aged 75 years and over. The pattern of excess mortality is relatively consistent, even though the duration of follow-up varied between studies. In the Melton study by Croxson et al.[137] a substantial increase in excess mortality was seen in diabetic subjects aged 65 years and over (Fig. 96-3), and impaired glucose tolerance was found to be associated with a relative risk of death of 1.7 (95 percent confidence interval 0.8–3.5). Most studies report a higher mortality in female diabetics and in both sexes; excess mortality is predominantly due to macrovascular disease.

Dementia

Studies have shown that elderly diabetic subjects have impaired cognitive function,[139–143] but these studies were generally not population-based, excluded subjects with dementia,[140–143] and generally used a large battery of tests to show the deficit.[139,141–143] Worse cognitive function in these tests was associated with worse glycemic control.[139–143]

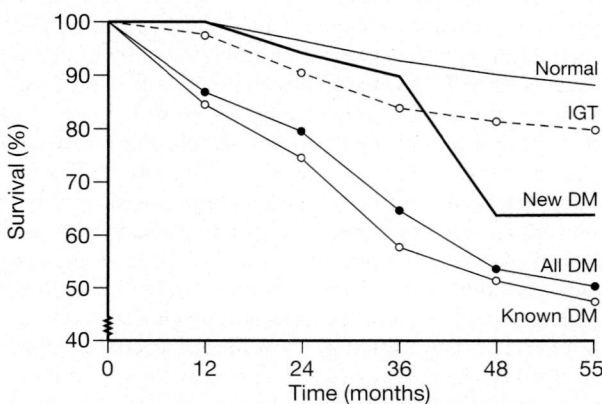

Figure 96-3 Mortality of elderly subjects in Melton Mowbray, according to glucose tolerance status. From Croxson et al.[137]

Community-based studies in both Melton Mowbray,[144] Nottingham,[72] Wales,[145] Rotterdam,[146] and Minnesota,[147] and nursing-home studies from Wales[148] and New York,[149] have shown worse cognitive function in elderly diabetic subjects using simple tests such as the Folstein MMSE and Hodkinson AMT with diagnosed diabetes carrying a 2–3 fold increased chance of dementia. However, other workers have found no decreased cognitive function in elderly diabetic subjects.[150,151]

There are several possible explanations for the lower cognitive function in the known diabetic subjects, apart from abnormal plasma glucose levels. First, depression has been found to be associated with known diabetes.[152,153] Second, hypertension is associated with diabetes and insulin resistance[154] and is itself associated with decreased cognitive function;[155] there is even evidence to suggest that among hypertensive subjects, hyperinsulinemia is associated with worse cognitive function.[156] Third, cerebrovascular disease is 2–3 times more common in people with known diabetes,[72,157] which again might be associated with cognitive impairment. Fourth, there is evidence that cortical atrophy is associated with diabetes. A small population-based study found temporal atrophy to be greater in diabetic subjects, which was most marked for drug-treated rather than diet-treated diabetic subjects;[158] a second study of routine CT scans of hospital patients found that diffuse cerebral and cortical atrophy was associated with diabetes even allowing for the effect of age, hypertension, and cerebrovascular disease.[159] Some studies suggest that the excess dementia is due to vascular disease,[149] whereas others suggest an excess of Alzheimer-type dementia.[146] It is likely that the current diagnosis and classification of dementia in diabetic subjects is inaccurate owing to the multiple risk factors present.[160] However, it is vitally important to exclude iatrogenic hypoglycemia (e.g. from longacting sulfonylureas) as a cause of confusion because it is eminently treatable, although the authors have seen patients rendered permanently confused by a single episode of profound hypoglycemia.

Does hyperglycemia contribute directly to cognitive impairment? Two studies have shown that tightening control in poorly controlled subjects does improve cognitive function, but the level of baseline hyperglycemia was quite high. Many studies show an association between cognitive function and indices of long-term glycemic control. Some studies have shown that cognitive impairment is worsened by increasing duration of diabetes, and cognitive impairment may be associated with peripheral neuropathy, which is a specific complication associated with duration of disease and poor glycemic control.[140,161,162] Thus, cognition may be impaired as a diabetic-specific complication. Although cognitive impairment in younger subjects with insulin-dependent diabetes is associated with hypoglycemia,[161,162] the high levels of glycemia found in community studies of the elderly diabetic person[72] suggest that this is not a major contributory factor in the elderly, but there is little research on this area.

Whatever the reason, known diabetic subjects appear to have poorer cognitive function than subjects not known to have diabetes. It is interesting to note the two studies that suggest that improving glycemic control improves cognitive function.[163–165] Impaired cognitive function should be borne in mind when treating elderly diabetic subjects because it has implications for their safe treatment. It may cause difficulty with glycemic control as a result of erratic taking of diet and medication. This may present with hypoglycemia where patients forget that they have taken medication and repeat the dose. One should enlist the help of family and services to optimize glycemic control to see if this makes any difference; if it does not, accept that one has to change glycemic targets to less strict, but safer control.[166] It is important to consider screening for other treatable causes of cognitive impairment.

RESIDENTIAL CARE AND THE HOUSEBOUND

Several studies have shown that diabetes is an independent risk factor for admission to a care home.[167,168] Again, the number of diabetic residents identified is just the tip of the iceberg. These were prevalences of 12 percent diagnosed and 15 percent undiagnosed diabetes in a study of Birmingham residential care homes,[60] and in Canada a routine screening program led to 30 percent of residents being diagnosed as diabetic.[169] Residence of nursing home is a risk factor for hyperosmolar nonketotic coma and carries increased mortality.[170] Compared to the nondiabetic residents, the diabetic residents have increased rates of stroke, peripheral vascular disease, amputation, urinary catheter, foot ulcer, renal impairment, and dementia.[60,171] They suffer poor nutrition, with 20 percent of residents being at least 20 percent underweight[172] in the USA; in the UK, a survey using 3-day dietary record showed that the residents obtain only 50 percent of their energy requirement (Sue Benbow, personal communication). Diabetes is a risk factor for pressure sores,[173] although this is less of a problem in rural American nursing homes,[174] so it may be preventable.

Interestingly, glycemic control is better in American nursing home residents than in free-range diabetic elders, with less hypoglycemia;[172] cynically, one might suggest that this is because the subjects have uniform energy expenditure (very little) and uniform dietary intake (very little); however, it has been noted that institutionalizing a brittle elderly diabetic does resolve the brittle diabetes.

It is very clear that the residents of care homes receive inadequate diabetes care compared with their noninstitutionalized peers;[171,175,176] see Table 96-9. Housebound elderly people were marginalized in their own homes, and were significantly ($P < 0.001$) less likely to have HbA1c, feet, eyes, urine, smoking habits, or blood pressure checked[177] compared with the mobile elders. Various common problems make diabetes management more complex in these patients.[178] The following are some of the problems.

Table 96-9 Care received by diabetic subjects in care home or free living[176]

	Care home (%)	Free range (%)
Annual review	44[a]	84
Chiropody	60[a]	96
Optician	36[a]	76
Dietician	48	60[b]

[a] $P < 0.05$ care home resident versus free range elder.
[b] Not significant.

- There may be irregular oral intake owing to: (a) confusion and/or a poor appetite due to concurrent illness; or (b) dysphagia due to stroke or other neurological or gastroenterological disorders. Lack of regular calorific intake can be particularly troublesome for insulin-treated patients.
- Recurrent urinary, chest, and other infections can render the diabetic person liable to hyperglycemia, and possibly ketosis with poor metabolic control.
- Leg ulcers and pressure sores may deteriorate rapidly.
- Dysphasia, dysarthria, deafness, or blindness can all make it difficult to communicate. Needs are thus unrecognized and unmet.
- There can be an increased vulnerability to hypoglycemia (especially in those taking sulfonylureas or insulin) owing to poor appetite and difficulties in ensuring sufficient and regular calorific intake, lack of glucose monitoring (urine or blood), lack of knowledge of symptoms and signs of hypoglycemia that may be attenuated in older people with diabetes, polypharmacy, and recurrent acute illness.
- Concurrent pathology (especially cardiac and renal failure) increases the likelihood of adverse drug reactions to prescribed medications. This may be exacerbated by infrequent review of existing medications.
- There may be inadequate facilities to cater for the dietary needs of residents with diabetes, and inadequate knowledge on the part of catering staff—including the need for snacks outside main meals.
- Adequate arrangements for regular diabetes review may be lacking, particularly for those discharged from hospital clinics and who are unable to visit their primary care physician.
- There may be lack of experience and training of institutional staff in diabetes care, which does not allow glucose monitoring to be undertaken correctly and which prevents useful assistance with insulin administration. This is often worsened by the high turnover of staff.
- There may be insufficient provision of health professional input, particularly of specialist nurses, dieticians, dental surgeons, opticians, and state-registered chiropodists and doctors, including hospital specialists.
- In the UK there is an artificial split between nursing home care and residential care, so that people in residential homes tend to get even less nursing care.

The British Geriatrics Society (Special Interest Group in Diabetes)[179] and the British Diabetic Association[180] have both published guidelines. In particular the BDA monograph is an excellent reference work on the subject and an incentive to improve care.

The accompanying box makes suggestions for improving care within residential and nursing home settings.

GLUCOSE CONTROL IN DIABETES MELLITUS
Overview

This is a vast subject, so this chapter can address only the most salient points. It is possible to discuss different aspects of care (e.g. metabolic, vascular, rehabilitative),[181] underlining how elderly diabetic people vary immensely in terms of physical and mental abilities and healthcare needs. Guidelines must be applied in the context of the individual elderly person following a comprehensive assessment.

A major trial to guide us is the UK Prospective Diabetes Study. The initial outcomes of intensive blood glucose control[83] were disappointing, with sulfonylurea or insulin use reducing microvascular end-points from 11.4 to 8.6 percent (i.e. by approximately one-quarter) at 10 years. However, it is important to realize that this was a comparison of two intensities of treatment, rather than two different treatments; and because of the limitations of treatments in use at the time, only a 0.9 percent difference in HbA1c separated the two groups. When one looks at the benefit from a 1 percent decrease in HbA1c,[82] one finds significant reductions in any diabetes end-point (21 percent decrease), diabetes-related death (21 percent decrease), all-cause mortality (14 percent decrease), any MI (14 percent decrease), any stroke (12 percent decrease), microvascular end-points (37 percent decrease), cataract extraction (19 percent decrease), amputation or peripheral vascular disease death (43 percent decrease), and heart failure (16 percent decrease). The UK study looked at intensive control from time of diagnosis; however, the recent Kumamoto intervention study in middle-aged Japanese subjects with type 2 diabetes for 6–10 years found that intensive insulin treatment with good control delayed the onset and progression of specific diabetic complications;[182] that study suggests that the thresholds for developing specific complications are: HbA1c 7 percent, fasting plasma glucose 6.7 mmol/L, and postprandial plasma glucose 10 mmol/L.

Importantly for the elderly person, several studies have now shown that improved glycemic control leads to improved cognitive function[163,165,166,183] and quality of life,[184,185] although one study[186] contradicted the improvement in quality of life.

The main concern is that striving for normoglycemia using insulin or sulfonylurea drugs might result in hypoglycemia. Compared with younger subjects, aging individuals perceive

Improving care within residential and nursing home settings

- Each resident should have an individual diabetes care plan agreed between patient (or relative), doctor (who is responsible for diabetic care) and home care staff.
- There should be increased community support from experienced health professionals such as diabetes specialist nurses and dieticians.
- Diabetic patients living in residential and nursing homes should have ready access to other specialist health professionals.
- Each resident with diabetes should be reviewed by either the family doctor or a hospital consultant physician/geriatrician at least once a year.
- Patients in residential and nursing homes should be included in any local audit of diabetic care.

fewer symptoms of hypoglycemia, need a lower plasma glucose level to elicit symptoms, exhibit a reduced counter-regulatory response to hypoglycemia, and recover more slowly from the hypoglycemic insult.[187–190] Thus the elderly person may have few symptoms of hypoglycemia until developing neuroglycopenia,[191] when nothing can be done about it. Hypoglycemia may be missed entirely or misdiagnosed, especially as one-third of hypoglycemic events in the elderly have nonspecific symptoms.[192] Although age is an independent risk factor for drug-induced hypoglycemia,[193] elderly people are taught very little about it.[194] In the Diabetes Control and Complications Trial and Kumamoto studies,[182,195] the risk of hypoglycemia increased dramatically, as the HbA1c decreased below the upper normal limit. However, the usual control of the elderly diabetic person's glycemia is poor.[72]

Sensible and appropriate diabetic care requires a considered judgment of the risks and benefits of treatment. A framework for this management is assisted by the aims of care, which are:

- achieve metabolic targets at lowest daily doses of therapeutic agents;
- avoid hypoglycemia;
- reduce and limit other associated adverse drug reactions;
- limit weight gain on sulfonylureas and insulin therapy;
- ameliorate microvascular complications;
- attend to macrovascular risk factors and disease.

Unless there are other reasons to treat the elderly diabetic individual differently from the younger diabetic person, aim for an HbA1c level between upper limit normal to upper limit normal plus 1, fasting plasma glucose 6.0–7.0 mmol/L, and random plasma glucose less than 11.1 mmol/L. See the accompanying box.

Initial care plan for the older adult with diabetes

- Set realistic glycemic goals.
- Agree upon the frequency of diabetic follow-up by primary or secondary healthcare team.
- Organize monitoring of glycemic control by the patient and/or carer; for example, by home urine or blood glucose monitoring or, if the patient cannot manage this, by regular review.
- Advise on stopping smoking, on exercise (ideally a minimum of three weekly brisk walks of 30–45 min duration), and on alcohol intake.
- Refer to social or community services as appropriate.

Pathological basis for the treatment of type 2 diabetes

Type 2 diabetes mellitus accounts for more than 90 percent of cases of diabetes in old age,[196] with the remainder being predominantly type 1. Type 2 diabetes has been characterized by a combination of insulin resistance (at both hepatic and peripheral tissue levels) due to a potentially decreased number of insulin receptors and a postreceptor defect, and β-cell dysfunction characterized by defective insulin secretion.[197] It is important to note that hyperglycemia worsens

β-cell function and insulin resistance, so that a period of good glycemic control may lead to unexpected hypoglycemia. Other disturbances are often associated with hyperglycemia, including hypertension, dyslipidemia, and obesity; this is referred to as Syndrome X, Reaven's syndrome, or the Deadly Quartet.[198] Syndrome X is associated with increased risk of large vessel disease, and further abnormalities associated with this syndrome and increased vascular risk are being described (e.g. microalbuminuria, abnormal plasminogen activator inhibitor-1 levels etc.). Thus, the main objectives of treatment include not only reducing hyperglycemia, but also treatment of these associated defects where appropriate. It is also very apparent that the β-cell function continues to deteriorate with time, needing more hypoglycemic treatment.[199,200] Although type 2 diabetes is characterized by the combination of insulin resistance and β-cell dysfunction, in the slim type 2 diabetic person, β-cell dysfunction is the major factor.[201]

Treatments for glucose control

Specific treatments aim to reverse or ameliorate the above defects of glucose control in one or more of the following ways: improvement of β-cell dysfunction; decrease of insulin resistance; limitation of dietary intake of monosaccharides (see the box).

Treatments to improve glucose control

Improve β-cell dysfunction by:
- stimulating pancreatic β-cells to secrete more insulin, for example by the use of sulfonylureas or other insulin secretogogues;
- lowering circulating levels of glucose, for example by dietary modification;
- introducing exogenous insulin to replace the function of the failing β-cell.

Decrease insulin resistance by:
- using drugs which decrease insulin resistance (e.g. metformin, peroxisome proliferator activated receptor γ agonists, and probably a minor effect of some sulfonylureas);
- directly reducing hyperglycemia, for example by dietary modification.

Limit the dietary intake of monosaccharides, for example by:
- diet;
- drugs that delay the absorption of monosaccharides by inhibiting breakdown of polysaccharides (e.g. α-glucosidase inhibitors such as acarbose).

Dietary treatment

The foundation of any treatment in diabetes is diet.[202] Complex carbohydrates should comprise 50–55 percent of the energy intake, and come from foods high in fiber (bread, pasta, rice, and potatoes). Up to 25–50 gm of added sucrose is allowed, but one would generally not advertise this since refined carbohydrate is very prevalent in the British diet. The diet should contain as much fiber as possible, but realistically one is looking at a maximum of 30 g per day. Fat intake should be limited to 30–35 percent of energy intake. Reduction in energy intake is the most important aim in the overweight subject. It is vital to ensure that the elderly individual is actually receiving an adequate diet—it is not unknown for patients having meals delivered to their homes (mobile meals or meals on wheels) to have none on Sundays, leading to profound hypoglycemia.

Although diet is vitally important, it is unlikely to achieve glycemic targets when used alone. In the UK Prospective Diabetes Study, only 6 percent of subjects were controlled on diet at the end of the second year.[203] It may well be compliance with diet which is the problem, rather than the diet itself. In a study looking at 66 elderly subjects with type 2 diabetes failing on diet plus oral agents, control improved enough to avoid insulin treatment in 44 by admitting them to hospital for 6 days of re-education.[204]

In most cases, diet alone will fail, and most patients will need oral hypoglycemic drugs. Although there are many hypoglycemic drugs available, the mainstays are metformin and sulfonylureas as these are relatively cheap.

Sulfonylureas

Sulfonylureas bind to a specific sulfonylurea receptor on the pancreatic β-islet cell which blocks ATP-sensitive potassium channels and hence stimulates insulin release.[205] This action requires that there be residual β-cell activity to achieve a hypoglycemic effect. Some sulfonylureas may also reduce insulin resistance, but just increasing insulin levels and decreasing plasma glucose will decrease insulin resistance.

Sulfonylureas are often felt to be the oral agent of choice for the elderly diabetic subject failing on diet alone,[206] because they are generally well tolerated (apart from the risk of hypoglycemia) without the risk of gastrointestinal upset associated with other oral agents. In-depth reviews of these drugs are available.[207,208] Hypoglycemia is the main side-effect of note, and risk factors for hypoglycemia are given in Table 96-10.

Glibenclamide appears particularly likely to cause hypoglycemia and death, more so than other sulfonylureas[209–212] including chlorpropamide[83,212] and metformin.[213] The deaths of elderly patients from hypoglycemia in a Swedish study,[214] and the finding that some elderly subjects experience a prolonged hypoglycemic effect from it,[215] has placed a question mark over glipizide. Gliclazide has a low (but not zero) risk of hypoglycemia;[216–221] it may be less likely to cause weight gain, the other common problem with sulfonylureas,[216,218–221] and achieves glycemic targets with low rates of secondary failure.[219,221] Gliclazide is undoubtedly safer than glibenclamide,[222] as are all other sulfonylureas. If hypoglycemia is a major worry, then tolbutamide has the lowest risk[210,211] and can be used if

the patient's creatinine is over 200 μmol/L.[207] If compliance is a problem, then glimepiride is useful since the tablet range means that the dose for all patients is one tablet before breakfast. However, there are currently no good comparisons between this and gliclazide.[223]

Metformin

Metformin, the biguanide in common use, reduces insulin resistance particularly in the liver, and so decreases hepatic glucose output by decreasing gluconeogenesis.[224] Any discussion of biguanides revolves around concerns over lactic acidosis. Metformin decreases gluconeogenesis from lactate, but plasma lactate levels stay stable since metformin increases oxidation of lactate.[224] However, older biguanides decreased oxidation of lactate—hence the unpredictable high risk of lactic acidosis. Lactic acidosis is a condition of the elderly group.[225] Metformin is predictable and safe if used correctly.[213] The contraindications[207,208] are given in Table 96-11 and they must be observed.

Particular advantages of metformin are that it does not cause hypoglycemia on its own, it does not cause weight gain, and it is inexpensive. It probably decreases HbA1c by about 1–1.5, and fasting plasma glucose by 4–5 mmol/L,[226–229] which is similar to sulfonylureas. In the UK Prospective Diabetes Study, metformin was used in obese subjects; all-cause mortality, and any diabetes-related end-point were significantly lower on intensive treatment with metformin than with insulin or a sulfonylurea.[228]

Metformin has been shown to be an effective treatment in the elderly population, with results similar to tolbutamide.[229] The usual dose required is approximately 1.7 g,[227] and it is as effective in the lean as in the plump.[227]

Apart from lactic acidosis, other side-effects include gastrointestinal disturbance which may be minimized by gradual introduction of the agent. Metformin may also cause vitamin B_{12} malabsorption, so it is wise to check B_{12} level every 5 years, and particularly if the subject has neuropathy.

Acarbose

This is an α-glucosidase inhibitor which inhibits the breakdown of polysaccharides in the small bowel, which are then digested or fermented more distally. This leads to lower but more susptained postprandial glucose levels and flatulence, which is the main limiting factor in the use of acarbose. Its advantages are low risk of hypoglycemia on its own (though if the patient is rendpered hypoglycemic by coprescription of a sulfonylurea, polysaccharides will be slower to correct this), and little weight gain.

Since only 1–2 percent of oral acarbose is absorbed, it is relatively free of systemic side-effects. Its main contraindications are inflammatory bowel disease and subacute obstruction.

Table 96-10 **Risk factors for hypoglycemia**[209,210]
• Choice of sulfonylurea/insulin
• Tight glycemic control
• Increasing age
• Male gender
• Recent discharge from hospital
• Polypharmacy
• Change of or new hypoglycemic treatment
• Impaired renal function
• Excess alcohol
• Hepatic impairment
• Cardiac failure

Table 96-11 **Contraindications to metformin**
• Renal impairment (creatinine > 120 μmol/L)
• Hepatic impairment (including alcohol abuse) as indicated by abnormal liver function tests
• Cardiac failure, even if treated
• Critical limb ischemia
• Any acute illness
• Use of intravenous radiological contrast media

Diagnosis is based on demonstrating acidosis (arterial pH less than 7.2), and a raised lactate level (either plasma lactate greater than 5 mmol/L or anion gap greater than 18 mmol/L). The anion gap, $(Na^+ + K^+) - (Cl^- + HCO_3^-)$, may also be increased by ketones, salicylates, urea, methanol, and ethylene glycol.

The standard treatment is to infuse 1.4% sodium bicarbonate until the pH reaches 7.2; however, the evidence that this improves mortality (60–70 percent unless shocked, when mortality approaches 100 percent) is lacking.[279] Mortality correlates more with plasma lactate levels than with the degree of acidosis.[279]

BLOOD PRESSURE CONTROL IN DIABETES MELLITUS
See also Chapter 35

Hypertension is very common in elderly people with type 2 diabetes (up to 50 percent prevalence in some studies, and becoming more prevalent as the target blood pressure decreases). The UK Prospective Diabetes Study[84] showed that a 10 mmHg systolic BP reduction led to significant reductions in any diabetes end-point (12 percent reduction), diabetes related death (17 percent), all-cause mortality (12 percent), myocardial infarction (12 percent), stroke (19 percent), microvascular end-points (13 percent), amputation or death from peripheral vascular disease (16 percent), and heart failure (12 percent). The UK study used either ACE-inhibitor-based or β-blocker-based regimens to similar effect, although the ACE inhibitor was better tolerated.

The Systolic Hypertension in Europe trial (Syst-Eur)[280] showed that a regimen based on a calcium-channel blocker achieved greater benefit in diabetic than nondiabetic patients. In the diabetic group, active treatment significantly reduced total and cardiovascular death, all cardiovascular events, and strokes. Furthermore, this treatment reduced adverse outcomes in the treated diabetic subjects to the level of that in the treated nondiabetic subjects, and showed a reduction in development of dementia.[281]

In the Systolic Hypertension in Elderly People (SHEP) trial[282,283] and the Hypertension Optimal Treatment (HOT) trial,[284] the relative benefit in avoiding adverse cardiovascular events was similar in diabetic and nondiabetic subjects, but the absolute benefit was far greater in the diabetic subjects. For instance, in SHEP there was a relative risk reduction of 34 percent in each group, but the diabetic absolute risk reduction was 101 per 1,000 patients, compared with 51 per 1,000 in nondiabetic patients. In HOT the rate of cardiovascular events and deaths in diabetic subjects in the <90 and <85 mmHg diastolic BP groups were higher than in the diastolic BP <80 mmHg group. Hypotensive treatment is therefore beneficial, but there is still some uncertainty about the target blood pressure.

The UK Prospective Diabetes Study suggested that there was no J-shaped curve for systolic blood pressure.[84,85] The active-treatment arm of SHEP did better than the placebo arm with mean BPs of 143/72 mmHg versus 155/72 mmHg. The HOT target group (<80 mmHg systolic) did better than those with higher BPs, on a mean BP of 140/81 mmHg. In the UK study, the intensive BP control group did better than the less-intensive control group on a BP of 143–144/81–83 mmHg

compared to 154/87 mmHg. These figures are reflected in the British Hypertension Society guidelines[285] of 140/80 for type 2 diabetic subjects with no nephropathy (120/70 if nephropathy present). One further point from the UK study protocol[85] is that, once the diagnosis of hypertension was made, treatment was increased if blood pressure was greater than 150 mmHg systolic; in other words, control was tight.

Which agent should be used? Given the HOPE, UK, Syst-Eur, and SHEP studies, one could make a case for ACE inhibitor, long-acting dihydropyridine calcium-channel blocker or thiazide diuretic as first-line agent of choice. If the systolic pressure is more than 10 mmHg from target, then 98 percent of patients will need at least two agents to control their blood pressure, so the question is academic: patients will be taking as many as they can tolerate. One worry is the diabetogenic effect of thiazide diuretics; in SHEP the whole thiazide group's mean glucose rose 1 mmol/L, but we do not know how many needed an escalation of their hypoglycemic medication. If glycemic control is borderline, we generally use indapamide instead of a thiazide since indapamide is said to be metabolically inactive. The main worry about ACE inhibitors (and sartans) is atheromatous renal artery stenosis which is common in diabetic people with peripheral vascular disease.[286] In practice we look at the peripheral circulation and creatinine and, if worried, request Doppler ultrasound of renal arteries.[287] We are undecided about β-blockers as a hypotensive agent, although they are useful for angina and postmyocardial infarction prophylaxis. One analysis shows that they reduce blood pressure but not adverse vascular events[288] in the elderly, whilst a meta-analysis of β-blocker use in diabetic subjects for hypertension concluded that they were as good as other agents.[289] Thus we tend to use β-blockers as an adjunct to hypertension treatment, but not first line in the elderly diabetic person.

LIPID CONTROL IN DIABETES MELLITUS
See also Chapter 32

The Established Populations for Epidemiologic Studies of the Elderly study group showed that a high total to HDL cholesterol ratio was associated with increased mortality, predominantly from vascular disease, in people (diabetic and nondiabetic analysed jointly) aged 70–79 years;[290] although other studies show conflicting results, probably due to methodology and subject selection. In New Zealander subjects aged over 70 with type 2 diabetes, hyperlipidemia was associated with an increased mortality.[291]

Diabetic dyslipidemia is characterized by high triglycerides, low HDL-cholesterol, and an LDL-cholesterol which is rich in highly atherogenic, small, dense LDL particles which contribute to cardiovascular risk.[292] Can we alter this? The Scandinavian Simvastatin Survival Study (4S)[293] included 2,282 subjects with angina or previous myocardial infarction aged 60–70 years with hypercholesterolemia (total cholesterol >5.5 mmol/L) randomized to placebo or simvastatin to achieve total cholesterol below 5.2 mmol/L; this resulted in a 27 percent lowering of risk of death and a 29 percent lowering of risk of a coronary endpoint (nonfatal MI or CHD death). Subgroup analysis examined the diabetic subjects of all ages, and showed a much greater absolute risk reduction in diabetic than in nondiabetic people,[294] with very similar relative risk reductions—emphasizing the much greater benefit of addressing vascular risk in the diabetic than the nondiabetic subject.

The Cholesterol And Recurrent Events (CARE) study[295] took subjects with an acute myocardial infarction in the preceding 3–20 months with total cholesterol below 6.2 mmol/L (mean 5.4 mmol/L) who were randomized to placebo or pravastatin 40 mg per day. In 2,129 subjects aged 60–75 years, pravastatin resulted in a 27 percent relative risk reduction of major coronary events over the 5 year follow-up. The elderly subgroup benefited more than average from the pravastatin.

Thus it appears that lipid reduction benefits the elderly diabetic person. In secondary prevention, a total cholesterol level more than 5.0 mmol/L indicates the need for treatment. In primary prevention, risk assessment is based on age, gender, blood pressure, and microalbuminuria using the color charts.[296]

All the CARE and 4S studies excluded subjects with short life expectancy or moderate failure of any system.[293,296] Treatment needs to be targeted appropriately. We would not measure lipids in subjects aged more than 80 years, because there is at present no evidence that dyslipidemia has an adverse effect at that age. One should attend to other cardiovascular risk factors and consider whether the dyslipidemia is secondary to thyroid, hepatic, or renal disease. The diet for lipid reduction is the same as the diabetic diet, and thus diet intervention is generally ineffective.[297] It is believed that improved glycemic control improves the lipids; in the UK Prospective Diabetes Study this did significantly improve triglycerides, but total cholesterol fell by only 0.28 mmol/L in men and 0.09 mmol/L in women.[298] Thus a statin is frequently used and the choice is generally governed by cost.

VASCULAR PROPHYLAXIS

Data from Nottingham[72] shows increased risk of stroke in the elderly diabetic person. Aggressively treated diabetics in the HOT study[284] had worse major cardiovascular event outcomes than the conventionally treated nondiabetic subjects. Data from Melton[299] and Hoorn[300] show increased vascular death rate and coronary heart disease death rate in the diabetic groups, respectively. Overall, diabetic patients have a 2–3 fold increase in the rate of cerebrovascular accidents or myocardial infarctions, and have a worse outcome than nondiabetic people from either myocardial infarction or stroke.[301] Since the diabetic person does so badly, any intervention with a similar relative risk reduction to that in a nondiabetic person will have a greater absolute benefit for the diabetic person.[302] Similarly, the older person has more to gain than the young.[303] Reducing the risk of vascular disease by glucose, blood pressure, and lipid control has been discussed, but there are several more possible interventions.

Aspirin should be used as secondary prophylaxis in all diabetic people with evidence of macrovascular disease, and it should be strongly considered as primary prevention in diabetic subjects with other risk factors for macrovascular disease such as hypertension, cigarette smoking, dyslipidemia, obesity, and albuminuria (macro or micro).[304] Because of the platelet defects associated with diabetes, it is recommended that the dose of aspirin should be 300 mg per day,[304–306] although the American Diabetes Association's position statement (http://www.diabetes.org/DiabetesCare/supplement198/s45.htm) advocates a dose of 81–325 mg enteric-coated aspirin per day. The HOT study showed similar benefit in diabetic and nondiabetic subjects with just 75 mg of aspirin per day.[284] It may be that larger doses of aspirin do not carry increased risk of gastrointestinal hemorrhage.[307] It is important to control blood pressure first before commencing aspirin.[308] If the patient cannot tolerate aspirin, then clopidogrel[309] can be used. A subgroup analysis in abstract form suggests that clopidogrel may confer greater benefit in diabetic than in nondiabetic subjects.

The elderly diabetic person is at increased risk of atrial fibrillation (odds ratio: 1.4 for men and 1.6 for women)[310] and at 2-fold increased risk of thromboembolism from atrial fibrillation.[311,312] We can find no subgroup analysis of the major atrial fibrillation trials to examine the benefits of warfarin specifically in older diabetic subjects. It appears that the adverse event rate in diabetic people drops from 8.6 events per 100 patients per year to 2.8 events with warfarin use.[312] It is important to check for retinal new vessels when diabetic subjects are placed on warfarin, although the Early Treatment Diabetic Retinopathy Study[313] showed no excess vitreous or preretinal hemorrhages in subjects given aspirin for vascular prophylaxis.

The MicroHOPE substudy of HOPE[314] randomized 3,577 diabetic patients aged 55 or over with one other cardiovascular risk factor (hypertension, smoking, microalbuminuria, dyslipidemia, or previous cardiovascular disease) to ramipril 10 mg daily or placebo for 4.5 years. The primary end-point of stroke or myocardial infarction, fatal or nonfatal, was reduced from 20 to 15 percent, with significant reductions in total mortality (from 14 to 11 percent), revascularization, and diabetic nephropathy. The direct benefit of ACE inhibition versus blood pressure reduction is complicated by the minor BP reduction with the ACE inhibitor. Although it has recently been pointed out that the placebo group on MicroHOPE had higher baseline vascular risk, HOPE was set up because a meta-analysis of heart failure trials had shown a 25 percent reduction in myocardial infarction with ACE inhibitor, and ACE inhibitors in other situations (e.g. after myocardial infarction and in nephropathy) have shown similar reductions in rate of myocardial infarction.

Several trials have examined the role of sartans in limiting diabetic nephropathy. It has to be noted that the outcome in type 2 diabetic subjects with microalbuminuria (the hallmark of early nephropathy) is frequently a macrovascular event, fatal or nonfatal.[315] The recently reported Reduction of Endpoints in NIDDM with the Angiotensin II Antagonist Losartan (RENAAL) trial randomized subjects with type 2 diabetes and overt nephropathy to losartan or calcium-channel blocker regimens to achieve target BP. Unfortunately the trial was halted early on ethical grounds, because the HOPE study indicated that these subjects should be on an ACE inhibitor. There was, however, a suggestion of fewer myocardial infarctions ($P = 0.08$), cardiac failure ($P = 0.005$), and cardiovascular events ($P = 0.25$). Similarly, the Irbesartan Microalbuminuria trial (IRMA) using 300 mg irbesartan versus placebo showed fewer cardiovascular events in the treatment group. Unfortunately these trials were examining the reduction of nephropathy (which occurred significantly) rather than reduction in large-vessel disease, for which they did not have the power.

Given that ACE inhibitors and sartan have an additive effect in blood pressure and microalbuminuria reduction,[316] we now need a comparative trial of these agents on their own and in combination to prevent vascular events. A placebo control group would now be unethical.

Despite our efforts, patients are still likely to suffer myocardial infarction. The Diabetes Mellitus, Insulin Glucose infusion in Acute Myocardial Infarction (DIGAMI) study[317,318] reported on treating subjects with acute myocardial infarction and either diabetes or raised random plasma glucose (i.e. not necessarily diabetic) with either an intensive insulin infusion and then a four-times daily insulin regimen or conventional treatment. Over a mean follow-up of 3.4 years, there was a 33 percent death rate in the treatment group compared to a 44 percent death rate in the control group, an absolute reduction in mortality of 11 percent. The effect was greatest among the subgroup without previous insulin treatment and at a low cardiovascular risk. Evidence is continuing to accumulate that the diabetic person should have a glucose/insulin infusion after a myocardial infarction.

Diabetic people have as least as much to gain as nondiabetic patients with acute myocardial infarction from thrombolysis,[319] post-MI ACE inhibitor,[320] and β-blockade.[321] There are no subgroup analyses of elderly diabetic subjects available from these studies.

CARE ISSUES AND FUTURE INITIATIVES

Diabetes mellitus in old age is increasingly recognized to be a specialist area. It demands skills and commitment often not available to hard-pressed general physicians attempting to cope with the dramatic increase in scientific knowledge and the escalation of clinical involvement required by most employers, whether in hospital or primary care settings. This final section explores several topical themes within the emerging discipline of "geriatric diabetology" which focuses on service delivery.[322]

Models of care

Four models of care are usually defined in relation to managing older adults with diabetes.[323] In the first, where there is effectively a breakdown in patient and doctor education and communication, the patient is essentially self-caring. In one survey, about 7 percent of elderly patients were managed in this way. This model should be avoided. A primary-care-based approach is a common and often an acceptable model as long as there is an enthusiastic and informed commitment to diabetes care. It has several advantages, including increased convenience for both patients and relatives, familiarity with practice staff, and continuity of care. Disadvantages such as lack of on-site specialist input and unstructured follow-up practices may lead to suboptimal care. In one group of patients discharged to primary care,[324] 14 percent were not followed-up at all and 20 percent apparently thought they were cured! In another study of patients similarly discharged,[325] only 5 percent achieved acceptable glycemic control, and mortality was three times higher than in those followed in a hospital specialist clinic.

Hospital-service-based is a third model and has the advantage of regular specialist input, but has two main disadvantages. These are the lack of clinic time to deal with the vast numbers of patients needed to be seen, and the fact that junior medical staff are often expected to provide this "expert" opinion. The extra inconvenience for patients traveling large distances and the excessive waiting times discourage many patients from being involved in this practice. Primary care physicians should always be involved.

The fourth model is the present authors' favored one and consists of a "shared care" approach between the hospital (diabetologist or geriatrician) and primary care. Joint management policies are essential for this to be a worthwhile and effective partnership, with an emphasis on early referral to secondary care when problems develop. Good communication is important and a common diabetes record card is mandatory. Clear boundaries of responsibility need to be established, and educational strategies should form the basis of a common approach to management.

Diabetes specialist nurses for elderly people

Diabetes specialist nurses are an invaluable addition to a diabetes service and can act as a link between primary and secondary care sectors.[326] They have many other roles (see the accompanying box) and we feel strongly that some of these specialist nurses should be appointed specifically to manage older diabetic patients. In conjunction with the primary care physician, community dietician, social worker, chiropodist, geriatric liaison sister, and geriatrician (or diabetologist), they should constitute a "Community Diabetes Team" that will provide multiprofessional diabetes healthcare.

> ### Roles of the diabetic specialist nurse for elderly people
>
> - To teach, advise, and counsel patients and carers both in the clinic and in the patient's home.
> - Where possible, to educate patients to achieve self-care.
> - To teach self-monitoring of blood glucose (or urinalysis, if appropriate) and instruct in the use of special monitoring techniques for patients with physical problems, partial-sightedness, or blindness.
> - Teaching and advising on insulin administration.
> - To liaise with and refer to other health professionals, chiropodists, community nurses, general practitioners, etc.
> - To commence insulin treatment in the patient's home.
> - To advise and guide residential and nursing home staff to manage patients with diabetes.
> - To provide continuing support and advice to patients and healthcare providers when specific problems arise relating to diabetes.

The role of geriatricians in elderly diabetic care

The specialist geriatric service can also provide important care provision for elderly diabetic patients.[178] Geriatricians with experience in diabetic care can contribute in a number of ways (see the accompanying box). They are often in an ideal position to liaise with specialist nurses to coordinate the care a patient receives both inside and outside of the hospital. Both authors participate in older adult diabetic clinics that see

Roles of the geriatrician in elderly diabetic care

- To assess coexisting disease that impacts on diabetes management.
- To manage increasing dependency and disability.
- To recognize and manage cognitive impairment.
- To assess and treat urinary incontinence.
- To liaise between hospital and community support services.
- To provide respite programs for spouses and carers.
- To be a member of a hospital diabetic clinic team.

patients on the basis of need and dependency levels rather than age alone. In these clinics, functional status is measured as routinely as a blood glucose level and these clinics are delivered by senior doctors.

Diabetes mellitus remains an exciting challenge for all health professionals involved in clinical geriatrics, and progress is being made in improving all aspects of the care of this common and serious condition.

KEY POINTS Diabetes mellitus

■ Diabetes is very common in elderly people, and is frequently undiagnosed.

■ Type 2 predominates, but type 1 and secondary diabetes also occur.

■ Diabetes has considerable associated morbidity (predominantly macrovascular disease and conditions with mixed etiology such as dementia and foot ulcers) and increased mortality.

■ Glycemic targets are a compromise between improved cognition and quality of life with a lower plasma glucose level, and risks of drug side-effects with still lower target levels.

■ Control of vascular risk factors using hypotensive and lipid-lowering drugs and antiplatelet and anticoagulant drugs is vitally important.

■ There must be secondary amelioration of complications such as eye and foot disease.

REFERENCES

1. Tattersall RB: Diabetes in the elderly: a neglected area? Diabetologia 1984;27:167–173
2. Harrower ADB: Prevalence of elderly patients in a hospital diabetic population. Br J Clin Pract 1980;34:131–133
3. Neil HAW, Thompson AV, Thorogood M et al: Diabetes in the elderly: the Oxford community diabetes study. Diab Med 1989;6:608–613
4. Damsgaard EMS: Known diabetes and fasting hyperglycaemia in the elderly: prevalence and economic impact upon health services. Dan Med Bull 1990;37:530–546
5. Sinclair AJ: Initial management of non-insulin-dependent diabetes mellitus in the elderly. In Finucane P, Sinclair AJ (eds): Diabetes in Old Age. John Wiley, Chichester, 1995
6. Sinclair AJ, Barnett AH: Special needs of elderly diabetic patients. BMJ 1993;306:1142–1143
7. Sinclair AJ: Diabetes care in the aged: time for reappraisal. Pract Diab 1994;11:60–63
8. Hendra TJ, Sinclair AJ: Improving the care of the elderly diabetic patients: the final report of the St Vincent Joint Task Force for Diabetes. Age Ageing 1997;26:3–6
9. Sinclair AJ, Woodhouse KW: Meeting the challenge of diabetes in the aged. (Editorial: Diabetes in the aged.) J R Soc Med 1994;87:607–608
10. Sinclair AJ, Finucane P (eds): Diabetes in old age, 2nd edn. John Wiley, Chichester, 2000
11. Dorf A, Ballintine EJ, Bennett PH, Miller M: Retinopathy in Pima Indians: relationships to glucose level, duration of diabetes, age at diagnosis of diabetes, and age at examination in a population with a high prevalence of diabetes mellitus. Diabetes 1976;25:554–560
12. Pettitt DJ, Knowler WC, Lisse JR, Bennett PH: Development of retinopathy and proteinuria in relation to plasma glucose concentrations in Pima Indians. Lancet 1980;2:1050–1052
13. Jarrett RJ, Keen H: Hyperglycaemia and diabetes mellitus. Lancet 1976;1009–1012
14. National Diabetes Data Group: Classification and diagnosis of diabetes mellitus and other categories of glucose intolerance. Diabetes 1979;28:1039–1057
15. WHO Study Group: Diabetes Mellitus (Technical Report Series 727). WHO, Geneva, 1985
16. Sayegh HA, Jarrett RJ: Oral glucose-tolerance tests and the diagnosis of diabetes. Lancet 1979;2:431–433
17. Zimmet P, Whitehouse S: The effect of age on glucose tolerance: studies in a Micronesian population with a high prevalence of diabetes. Diabetes 1979;28:617–623
18. Rushforth NB, Bennett P, Steinberg A et al: Diabetes in the Pima Indians. Diabetes 1971;20:756–765
19. Sturrock ND, Page SR, Clarke P, Tattersall RB: Insulin dependent diabetes in nonagenarians. BMJ 1995;310:1117–1118
20. Molbak AG, Christau B, Marner B, Borch-Johnsen K, Nerup J: Incidence of insulin-dependent diabetes mellitus in age groups over 30 years in Denmark. Diab Med 1994;11:650–655; erratum 1995;12:288
21. Zimmet P, Turner R, McCarty D, Rowley M, Mackay I: Crucial points at diagnosis: type 2 diabetes or slow type 1 diabetes. Diab Care 22(suppl 2):B59–B64
22. Melton LJ, Palumbo PJ, Chu CP: Incidence of diabetes mellitus by clinical type. Diab Care 1983;6:75–86
23. Jarrett RJ, Keen H, McCartney P: The Whitehall study: ten year follow-up report on men with impaired glucose tolerance with reference to worsening to diabetes and predictors of death. Diab Med 1984;1:279–283
24. Saad MF, Knowler WC, Pettitt DJ et al: The natural history of diabetes mellitus in the Pima Indians. N Engl J Med 1988;319:1500–1506
25. Jarrett RJ, McCartney P, Keen H: The Bedford Survey: ten year mortality rates in newly diagnosed diabetics, borderline diabetics and normoglycaemic controls and risk indices for coronary heart disease in borderline diabetics. Diabetologia 1982;22:79–84
26. WHO Study Group: Diabetes Mellitus (Technical Report Series 646). WHO, Geneva, 1980
27. Expert Committee on the Diagnosis and Classification of Diabetes Mellitus: Report. Diab Care 1997;20:1183–1197
28. WHO committee: Definition, Diagnosis and Classification of Diabetes Mellitus and its Complications. WHO, Geneva, 1999
29. Croxson SCM, Thomas P: Glucose tolerance tests reappraised using recent ADA criteria. Pract Diab Int 1998;15(6):178–180
30. Barrett-Connor E, Ferrara A: Isolated postchallenge hyperglycemia and the risk of fatal cardiovascular disease in older women and men: the Rancho Bernardo Study. Diab Care 1998;21:1236–1239
31. Davies MJ, Muehlbayer S, Garrick P, McNally PG: Potential impact of a change in the diagnostic criteria for diabetes mellitus on the prevalence of abnormal glucose tolerance in a local community at risk of diabetes: impact of new diagnostic criteria for diabetes mellitus. Diab Med 1999;16:343–346
32. Spence JW: Some observations on sugar tolerance with special reference to variations found at different ages. QJM 1921;14:314–326
33. Davidson MB: The effect of ageing on carbohydrate metabolism: a review of the English literature and a practical approach to the diagnosis of diabetes mellitus in the elderly. Metabolism 1979;28:688–705
34. Andres R: Aging and diabetes. Med Clin North Am 1971;55:835–845
35. Jackson RA, Blix PM, Matthews JA et al: Influence of ageing on glucose homeostasis. J Clin Endocrinol Metab 1982;55:840–848
36. Jackson RA: Mechanisms of age-related glucose intolerance. Diabetes Care 1990;13(suppl 2):9–19
37. Harris MI, Flegal KM, Cowie CC et al: Prevalence of diabetes, impaired fasting glucose, and impaired glucose tolerance in US adults: the Third National Health and Nutrition Examination Survey, 1988–1994. Diab Care 1998;21:518–524

38. De Fronzo RA: Glucose intolerance and aging: evidence for tissue insensitivity to insulin. Diabetes 1979;28:1095–1101
39. Fink RI, Kolterman OG, Griffin J, Olefsky JM: Mechanisms of insulin resistance in aging. J Clin Invest 1983;71:1523–1535
40. Villareal DT, Morley JE: Prevention of diabetes in elderly people. In Finucane P, Sinclair AJ (eds): Diabetes in Old Age. John Wiley, Chichester, 1995;45–67
41. Stout RW: Ageing and glucose tolerance. In Finucane P, Sinclair AJ (eds): Diabetes in Old Age. John Wiley, Chichester, 1995;21–44
42. Harris MI, Hadden WC, Knowler WC, Bennett PH: Prevalence of diabetes and impaired glucose tolerance and plasma glucose levels in US population aged 20–74 years. Diabetes 1987;36:523–534
43. Neil HAW, Gatling W, Mather HM et al: The Oxford Community Diabetes Study: evidence for an increase in the prevalence of known diabetes in Great Britain. Diab Med 1987;4:539–543
44. Croxson SCM, Burden AC, Bodlington M, Botha JL: The prevalence of diabetes in elderly people. Diab Med 1991;8:28–31
45. Tuomilehto J, Nissinen A, Kiveiä S-L et al: Prevalence of diabetes mellitus in elderly men aged 65 to 84 years in eastern and western Finland. Diabetologia 1986;29:611–615
46. Knowler WC, Bennett PH, Hamman RF, Miller M: Diabetes incidence and prevalence in Pima Indians: a 19-fold greater incidence than in Rochester, Minnesota. Am J Epidemiol 1978;108:497–505
47. Wingard DL, Sinsheimer P, Barrett-Connor EL, McPhillips JB: Community based study of prevalence of NIDDM in older adults. Diab Care 1990;13(suppl 2):3–8
48. Haavisto MV, Mattila KJ, Rajala SA: Blood glucose and diabetes mellitus in subjects aged 85 years or more. Acta Med Scand 1983;214:239–244
49. Falconer DC, Duncan LJP, Smith C: A statistical and genetical study of diabetes. 1: Prevalence and mortality. Ann Hum Genet 1971;34:347–369
50. Walker JB, Kerridge D: Diabetes in an English Community. Leicester University Press, Leicester, 1961
51. College of General Practitioners: A diabetes survey. BMJ 1962;1:1497–1503
52. College of General Practitioners: Glucose tolerance and glycosuria in the general population. BMJ 1963;2:655–659
53. Damsgaard EM, Faber OK, Froland A et al: Prevalence of fasting hyperglycaemia and known non-insulin-dependent diabetes mellitus classified by plasma C-peptide. Diab Care 1987;10:26–32
54. Agner E, Thorsteinsson B, Eriksen M: Impaired glucose tolerance and diabetes mellitus in elderly subjects. Diab Care 1982;5:600–605
55. Ohlson LO, Larsson B, Eriksson H et al: Diabetes mellitus in Swedish middle aged men. Diabetologia 1987;30:386–393
56. Cromme PVM, van der Veen EA, Bezemer PD, Kuik DJ: Serum fructosamine assessment as a screening test for diabetes mellitus. Neth J Med 1987;30:202–203
57. Mykkänen L, Laakso M, Uusitua M, Pyörälä K: Prevalence of diabetes and impaired glucose tolerance in elderly subjects and their association with obesity and family history of diabetes. Diab Care 1990;13:1099–1105
58. Forrest RD, Jackson CA, Yudkin JS: Glucose intolerance and hypertension in North London: the Islington Diabetes Study. Diab Med 1986;338–342
59. Simmons D, Williams DRR, Powell MJ: Prevalence of diabetes in a predominantly Asian community: preliminary findings of the Coventry diabetes study. BMJ 1989;298:18–21
60. Sinclair AJ, Croxson SCM, Gadsby R, Bayer AJ, Penfold S: Prevalence of diabetes in care home residents. Diab Care 2001;24:1066–1068
61. Gatling W, Budd S, Walters D et al: Evidence of an increasing prevalence of diagnosed diabetes mellitus in the Poole area from 1983 to 1996. Diab Med 1998;15:1015–1021
62. Sinclair AJ, Croxson SCM: Diabetes mellitus in the older adult. In Tallis R, Fillit H, Brocklehurst JC (eds): Brocklehurst's Textbook of Geriatric Medicine and Gerontology, 5th edn. Churchill Livingstone, Edinburgh, 1998;1051–1072
63. Drivsholm T, Ibsen H, Schroll M, Davidsen M, Borch-Johnsen K: Increasing prevalence of diabetes mellitus and impaired glucose tolerance among 60-year-old Danes. Diab Med 2001;18:126–132
64. Helmrich SP, Ragland DR, Leung RW, Paffenbarger RS: Physical activity and reduced occurrence of non-insulin-dependent diabetes mellitus. N Engl J Med 1991;325:147–152
65. Damsgaard EM, Froland A, Green A: Use of hospital services by elderly diabetics and fasting hyperglycaemic patients aged 60–74 years. Diab Med 1987;4:317–322
66. Currie CJ, Williams DRR, Peters JR: Patterns of in and out-patient activity for diabetes: a district survey. Diab Med 1996;13:273–280
67. Damsgaard EM, Froland A, Holm A: Ambulatory medical care for elderly diabetics: the Fredericia survey of diabetic and fasting hyperglycaemic subjects aged 60–74 years. Diab Med 1987;4:534–538
68. Williams DRR: Hospital admissions of diabetic patients: information from hospital activity analysis. Diab Med 1985;2:27–32
69. Hudson CN, Lazarus J, Peters J et al: An audit of diabetes care in three district general hospitals in Cardiff. Pract Diab Intern 1996;13:29–32
70. Cohen DL, Neil HAW, Thorogood M, Mann JL: A population based study of the incidence of complications associated with type 2 diabetes in the elderly. Diab Med 1991;8:928–933
71. Walters DP, Gatling W, Mullee MA, Hill RD: The prevalence of diabetic distal sensory neuropathy in an English Community. Diab Med 1992;9:349–353
72. Dornan TL, Peck GM, Dow JDC, Tattersall RB: A community survey of diabetes in the elderly. Diab Med 1992;9:860–865
73. Watkins PJ: Chronic complications of diabetes. In Finucane P, Sinclair AJ (eds): Diabetes in Old Age. John Wiley, Chichester, 1995;119–127
74. Kannel WB, McGee DL: Diabetes and cardiovascular disease: the Framingham Study. JAMA 1979;241:2035–2038
75. Knuiman MW, Welborn TA, McCann VJ et al: Prevalence of diabetic complications in relation to risk factors. Diabetes 1986;35:1332
76. Ballard DJ, Humphrey LL, Melton LJ et al: Epidemiology of persistent proteinuria in type II diabetes mellitus: population based study in Rochester, Minnesota. Diabetes 1988;37:405–412
77. Naliboff BD, Rosenthal M: Effects of age on complications in adult onset diabetes. J Am Geriatr Soc 1989;37:838–842
78. Grey RHB, Burns-Cox CJ, Hughes A: Blind and partial sight registration in Avon. Br J Ophthalmol 1989;73:88–94
79. Kohner EM: Diabetic retinopathy. BMJ 1993;307:1195–1199
80. Howard-Williams J, Hillson RM, Bron A et al: Retinopathy is associated with higher glycaemia in maturity onset type diabetes. Diabetologia 1984;27:198–202
81. Nathan DM, Singer DE, Godine JE et al: Retinopathy in older type 2 diabetics. Diabetes 1986;35:797–801
82. Stratton IM, Adler AI, Neil HAW et al, for the UKPDS group: Association of glycaemia with macrovascular and microvascular complications of type 2 diabetes (UKPDS 35): prospective observational study. BMJ 2000;321:405–412
83. Anonymous, for the UKPDS group: Intensive blood-glucose control with sulphonylureas or insulin compared with conventional treatment and risk of complications in patients with type 2 diabetes (UKPDS 33). Lancet 1998;352:837–853
84. Adler AI, Stratton IM, Neil HAW et al, for the UKPDS group: Association of systolic blood pressure with macrovascular and microvascular complications of type 2 diabetes (UKPDS 36): prospective observational study. BMJ 2000;321:412–420
85. Anonymous, for the UK PDS group: Tight blood pressure control and risk of macrovascular and microvascular complications in type 2 diabetes: UKPDS 38. BMJ 1998;317:703–713
86. Harris MI, Klein R, Welborn TA, Knuiman MW: Onset of NIDDM occurs at least 4–7 yrs before clinical diagnosis. Diab Care 1992;15:815–821
87. Soler NG, Fitzgerald MG, Malins JM, Summers ROC: Retinopathy at diagnosis of diabetes with special reference to patients under 40 years of age. BMJ 1969;3:567–569
88. Aldington SJ, Kohner EM, Nugent Z: Retinopathy at entry in the United Kingdom Prospective Diabetes Study of maturity onset diabetes. Diab Med 1987;4:355 (abstract)
89. British Multicentre Study Group: Photocoagulation for diabetic maculopathy. Diabetes 1983;32:1010–1016
90. Kohner EM, Barry PJ: Prevention of blindness in diabetic retinopathy. Diabetologia 1984;26:173–179
91. Rohan TE, Frost CD, Wald NJ: Prevention of blindness by screening for diabetic retinopathy: a quantitative assessment. BMJ 1989;299:1198–1201
92. Chaturvedi N, Sjolie AK, Stephenson JM et al: Effect of lisinopril on progression of retinopathy in normotensive people with type 1 diabetes: the EUCLID study group. Lancet 1998;351:28–31
93. Hiller R, Sperduto RD, Ederer F: Epidemiologic associations with cataract in the 1971–1972 National Health and Nutrition Survey. Am J Epidemiol 1983;118:239–249
94. Caird FI, Hutchinson M, Pirie A: Cataract and diabetes. BMJ 1964;2:665–668

95. Croxson SCM: Complications in screened diabetic subjects. Age Ageing 1995;24(suppl 1):30 (abstract)

96. Cohen DL, Neil HAW, Sparrow J et al: Lens opacity and mortality in diabetes. Diab Med 1990;7:615–617

97. Klein BE, Klein R, Jensen SC: Open-angle glaucoma and older-onset diabetes: the Beaver Dam Eye Study. Ophthalmology 1994;101:1173–1177

98. Wormald RP, Basauri E, Wright LA, Evans JR: The African Caribbean Eye Survey: risk factors for glaucoma in a sample of African Caribbean people living in London. Eye 1994;8:315–320

99. Leske MC, Connell AM, Wu SY et al: Risk factors for open-angle glaucoma: the Barbados Eye Study. Arch Ophthalmol 1995;113:918–924

100. Tielsch JM, Katz J, Quigley HA, Javitt JC, Sommer A: Diabetes, intraocular pressure, and primary open-angle glaucoma in the Baltimore Eye Survey. Ophthalmology 1995;102:48–53

101. Schranz AG, Zarabinska L: Retinopathy in Maltese type 2 diabetic patients. Diab Med 1995;12:441–444

102. Sanders RJ, Wilson MR: Diabetes-related eye disorders. J Natl Med Assoc 1993;85:104–108 (review)

103. Newell FW: Ophthalmology: Principles and Concepts. CV Mosby, St Louis, 1986

104. Duker JS, Sivalingam A, Brown GC, Reber R: A prospective study of acute central retinal artery obstruction. Arch Ophthalmol 1991;109:339–342

105. Klein R, Klein BE, Moss SE: Diabetes, hyperglycemia, and age-related maculopathy: the Beaver Dam Eye Study. Ophthalmology 1992;99:1527–1534

106. Gibson JM, Shaw DE, Rosenthal AR: Senile cataract and senile macular degeneration: an investigation into possible risk factors. Trans Ophthalmol Soc UK 1986;105:463–468

107. Hyman LG, Lilienfeld AM, Ferris FL, Fine SL: Senile macular degeneration: a case control study. Am J Epidemiol 1983;118:213–227

108. Ferris FL: Senile macular degeneration: review of epidemiologic features. Am J Epidemiol 1983;118:132–151

109. Harding SP, Broadbent DM, Neoh C et al: Sensitivity and specificity of photography and direct ophthalmoscopy in screening for sight threatening eye disease: the Liverpool Diabetic Eye Study. BMJ 1995;311:1131–1135

110. Most RS, Sinnock P: The epidemiology of lower extremity amputations in diabetic individuals. Diab Care 1983;6:87–91

111. Deerochanawong C, Home PD, Alberti KGMM: A survey of lower limb amputation in diabetic patients. Diab Med 1992;9:942–946

112. Young MJ, Boulton AJM: The diabetic foot. In Finucane P, Sinclair AJ (eds): Diabetes in Old Age. John Wiley, Chichester, 1995:139–179

113. Connor H: The economic impact of diabetic foot disease. In Connor H, Boulton AJM, Ward JD (eds): The Foot in Diabetes. John Wiley, Chichester, 1986:150–159

114. Bild DE, Selby JV, Sinnock P et al: Lower-extremity amputation in people with diabetes: epidemiology and prevention. Diab Care 1989;12:24–31

115. Van Houtum WH, Lavery LA, Harkless LB: The costs of diabetes-related lower extremity amputations in the Netherlands. Diab Med 1995;777–781

116. Silbert S: Amputation of the lower extremity in diabetes mellitus. Diabetes 1952;1:297–299

117. Palumbo PJ, Melton LJ: Peripheral vascular disease and diabetes. In Diabetes in America: Diabetes Data Compiled 1984. US Government Printing Office, Washington, DC, 1985:1–21

118. Houghton AD, Taylor PR, Thurlow S, Rootes E, McColl I: Success rates for rehabilitation of vascular amputees. Br J Surg 1992;79:753–755

119. Pecoraro RE, Reiber GE, Burgess EM: Pathways to diabetic limb amputation. Basis for prevention. Diab Care 1990;13:513–521

120. Larsson J, Apelqvist J, Agardh DD, Stenstrom A: Decreasing incidence of major amputation in diabetic patients: a consequence of a multidisciplinary footcare team approach? Diab Med 1995;12:770–776

121. Assal JP, Gfeller R, Ekoe JM: Patient education in diabetes. In: Recent Trends in Diabetic Research. Almquist & Wiksell, Stockholm, 1982:276–289

122. Thomson FJ, Veves A, Ashe H et al: A team approach to diabetic foot care: the Manchester experience. Foot 1991;1:75–82

123. Cavanagh PR, Young MJ, Adams JE et al: Correlates of structure and function in the diabetic foot. Diabetologia 1991;34(suppl 2):A39

124. Cavanagh PR, Simoneau GG, Ulbrecht JS: Ulceration, unsteadiness and uncertainty: the biomechanical consequences of diabetes mellitus. J Biomech 1993;26(suppl 1):23–40

125. Flynn MD, Boolell M, Tooke J, Watkins PJ: The effect of insulin infusion on capillary blood flow in the diabetic neuropathic foot. Diab Med 1992;9:630–634

126. Logerfo FW, Coffman JD: Vascular and microvascular disease of the foot in diabetes: implications for foot care. N Engl J Med 1984;25:1615–1619

127. Euerhart JE, Pettitt DJ, Knowler WC et al: Medial arterial calcification and its association with mortality and complications of diabetes. Diabetologia 1988;31:16–23

128. Dormandy J (ed): European Consensus Document on Critical Limb Ischaemia. Springer-Verlag, Berlin, 1989

129. Edmonds ME, Blundell MP, Morris HE et al: The diabetic foot: impact of a foot clinic. QJM 1986;232:763–771

130. Assal JP, Muhlhauser I, Pernet A et al: Patient education as a basis for diabetes care in clinical practice. Diabetologia 1985;28:602–613

131. Thomson FJ, Masson EA: Can elderly diabetic patients co-operate with routine foot care? Age Ageing 1992;21:333–337

132. Panzram G: Mortality and survival in type 2 (non-insulin-dependent) diabetes mellitus. Diabetologia 1987;30:123–131

133. Fitzgerald MG, Kilvert A: Diabetes mellitus. In Brocklehurst JC (ed): Textbook of Geriatric Medicine and Gerontology, 3rd edn. Churchill Livingstone, Edinburgh, 1985:715–730

134. Krolewski AS, Warram JH, Christlieb AR: Onset, course, complications, and prognosis of diabetes mellitus. In Marble A, Krall LP, Bradley RF et al (eds): Joslin's Diabetes Mellitus, 12th edn. Lea & Febiger, Philadelphia, 1985:251–277

135. Keen H, Fuller JH: The epidemiology of diabetes. In Exton-Smith AN, Caird FI (eds): Metabolic and Nutritional Disorders in the Elderly. John Wright, Bristol, 1980:146–160

136. Wong JSK, Pearson DWM, Murchison LE et al: Mortality in diabetes mellitus: experience of a geographically defined population. Diab Med 1991;8:135–139

137. Croxson SCM, Price D, Burden M et al: Mortality of elderly people with diabetes. Diab Med 1994;11:250–252

138. Sinclair AJ, Robert IE, Croxson SCM: Mortality in older people with diabetes mellitus. Diab Med 1997;14:639–647

139. Reaven GM, Thompson LW, Nahum D, Haskins E: Relationship between hyperglycaemia and cognitive function in older NIDDM patients. Diab Care 1990;13:16–21

140. Perlmuter LC, Hakami MK, Hodgson-Harrington C et al: Decreased cognitive function in aging non-insulin-dependent diabetic patients. Am J Med 1984;77:1043–1048

141. U'Ren RC, Riddle MC, Lezak MD, Bennington-Davis M: The mental efficiency of the elderly person with type 2 diabetes mellitus. J Am Geriatr Soc 1990;38:505–510

142. Mooradian AD, Perryman K, Fitten J et al: Cortical function in elderly non-insulin dependent diabetic patients: behavioural and electrophysiological studies. Arch Intern Med 1988;148:2369–2372

143. Jagust W, Cramon DY, Renner R, Hepp KD: Cognitive function and metabolic state in elderly diabetic patients. Diab Nutr Metab 1992;5:265–274

144. Croxson S, Jagger C: Diabetes and cognitive impairment: a community based study of elderly subjects. Age Ageing 1995;24:421–424

145. Sinclair AJ, Girling AJ, Bayer AJ: Cognitive dysfunction in older subjects with diabetes mellitus: impact on diabetes self-management and use of care services. All Wales Research into Elderly (AWARE) study. Diab Res Clin Pract 2000;50:203–212

146. Ott A, Stolk RP, Hofman A et al: Association of diabetes mellitus and dementia: the Rotterdam study. Diabetologia 1996;39:1392–1397

147. Leibson CL, Rocca WA, Hanson VA et al: Risk of dementia among persons with diabetes mellitus: a population-based cohort study. Am J Epidemiol 1997;145:301–308

148. Sinclair AJ, Allard I, Bayer A: Observations of diabetes care in long-term institutional settings with measures of cognitive function and dependency. Diab Care 1997;20:778–784

149. Tariot PN, Ogden MA, Cox C, Williams TF: Diabetes and dementia in long-term care. J Am Geriatr Soc 1999;47:423–429

150. Richardson-Tchabo EA: A longitudinal study of cognitive performance in non-insulin dependent (type 2) diabetic men. Exp Gerontol 1986;21:459–467

151. Atiea JA, Moses JL, Sinclair AJ: Neuropsychological function in older subjects with non-insulin-dependent diabetes mellitus. Diab Med 1995;12:679–685

152. Tun PA, Perlmuter LC, Russo P, Nathan DM: Memory self-assessment and performance in aged diabetics and non-diabetics. Exp Aging Res 1987;13:151–157

153. Palinkas LA, Barrett-Connor E, Wingard DL: Type 2 diabetes and depressive symptoms in older adults: a population based study. Diab Med 1991;8:532–539

154. Reaven GM: Role of insulin resistance in human disease. Diabetes 1988;37:1595–1607

155. Kalra L, Jackson SHD, Swift CG: Neuropsychological test performance as an indicator of silent cerebrovascular disease in elderly hypertensives. Age Ageing 1994;23:517–523 (review)

156. Kuusisto J, Koivisto K, Mykkanen L et al: Essential hypertension and cognitive function: the role of hyperinsulinemia. Hypertension 1993;22:771–779

157. Palumbo PJ, Elveback LR, Whisnant JP: Neurologic complications of diabetes mellitus: transient ischemic attack, stroke and peripheral neuropathy. Adv Neurol 1978;19:593–601

158. Soininen H, Puranen M, Helkala E-L et al: Diabetes mellitus and brain atrophy: a computed tomography study in an elderly population. Neurobiol Ageing 1992;13:717–721

159. Pirtilla T, Jarvenpaa R, Laippala P, Frey H: Brain atrophy on computerized axial tomography scans: interactions of age, diabetes and general morbidity. Gerontology 1992;38:285–291

160. Stewart R, Liolitsa D: Type 2 diabetes mellitus, cognitive impairment and dementia. Diab Med 1999;16:93–112 (review)

161. Amiel S: Diabetes and dementia: a causal association? Diab Med 1994;11:430–431

162. Ryan CM, Williams TM, Finegold DN, Orchard TJ: Cognitive dysfunction in adults with type 1 (insulin dependent) diabetes mellitus of long duration: effects of recurrent hypoglycaemia and other chronic complications. Diabetologia 1993;36:329–334

163. Jagust W, Cramon DY, Renner R, Hepp KD: Tight metabolic control improves cerebral function in older type 2 diabetic patients. Diabetologia 1987;30:535A (abstract)

164. Gradman TJ, Laws A, Thompson LW, Reaven GM: Verbal learning and/or memory improves with glycaemic control in older subjects with non-insulin dependent diabetes mellitus. J Am Geriatr Soc 1993;41:1305–1312

165. Meneilly GS, Cheung E, Tessier D, Yakura C, Tuokko H: The effect of improved glycemic control on cognitive functions in the elderly patient with diabetes. J Gerontol A 1993;48:M117–M121

166. Bayer AJ, Johnston J, Sinclair AJ: Impact of dementia on diabetic care in the aged. J R Soc Med 1994;87:619–621

167. Tsuji I, Whalen S, Finucane TE: Predictors of nursing home placement in community-based long-term care. J Am Geriatr Soc 1995;43:761–766

168. Rockwood K, Stolee P, McDowell I: Factors associated with institutionalization of older people in Canada: testing a multifactorial definition of frailty. J Am Geriatr Soc 1996;44:578–582

169. Gobin W: Diabetes in the aged: under-diagnosis and overtreatment. Can Med Assoc J 1970;103:915–923

170. Wachtel TJ: The diabetic hyper-osmolar state. Clin Geriatr Med 1990;6:797–806

171. Benbow SJ, Walsh A, Gill GV: Diabetes in institutionalised elderly people: A forgotten population? BMJ 1997;314:1868–1869

172. Mooradian AD, Osterweil D, Petrasek D, Morley JE: Diabetes mellitus in elderly nursing home patients: a survey of clinical characteristics and management. J Am Geriatr Soc 1988;36:391–396

173. Brandeis GH, Wee Lock Ooi, Hossain M, Morris JN, Lipsitz LA: A longitudinal study of risk factors associated with the formation of pressure ulcers in nursing homes. J Am Geriatr Soc 1994;42:388–393

174. Spector WD, Fortinsky RH: Pressure ulcer prevalence in Ohio nursing homes: clinical and facility correlates. J Aging Health 1998;10:62–80

175. Tong P, Baillie SP, Roberts SH: Diabetes care in the frail elderly. Pract Diab 1994;11(4):163–165

176. Taylor C, Hendra T: The prevalence of diabetes mellitus and quality of diabetic care in residential and nursing homes: a postal survey. Age Ageing 2000;29:447–450

177. Farooqi A, Sorrie R: Monitoring of elderly housebound and mobile diabetic patients in 31 Leicestershire practices: a comparative study. Pract Diab Int 1999;16(4):114–116

178. Turnbull CJ, Sinclair AJ: Modern perspectives and recent advances. In Finucane P, Sinclair AJ (eds): Diabetes in Old Age. John Wiley, Chichester, 1995

179. Sinclair AJ, Croxson SCM, Turnbull CJ: Document of diabetes care for residents in residential and nursing homes. Postgrad Med J 1997;73:611–612

180. Working Party of the BDA (chairman AJ Sinclair): Guidelines of Practice for Residents with Diabetes in Care Homes. British Diabetes Association, London, 1999

181. Sinclair AJ: Diabetes in old age: changing concepts in the secondary care arena. J R Coll Physicians Lond 2000;34:240–244

182. Ohkubo Y, Kishikawa H, Araki E et al: Intensive insulin therapy prevents the progression of diabetic microvascular complications in Japanese patients with non-insulin-dependent diabetes mellitus: a randomized prospective 6-year study. Diab Res Clin Pract 1995;28:103–117

183. Testa MA, Simonson DC: Health economic benefits and quality of life during improved glycemic control in patients with type 2 diabetes mellitus: a randomized, controlled, double-blind trial. JAMA 1998;280:1490–1496

184. Reza M, Taylor C, Towse K, Ward JD, Hendra TJ: Insulin treatment in elderly subjects with non-insulin-dependent diabetes mellitus: quality of life and impact on carers. Diab Med 1998;15(suppl 1):S17 (abstract)

185. Taylor R, Foster B, Kyne-Grzebalski D, Vanderpump M: Insulin regimes for the non-insulin dependent: impact on diurnal metabolic state and quality of life. Diab Med 1994;11:551–557

186. Tovi J, Engfeldt P: Well being and symptoms in elderly type 2 diabetes patients with poor metabolic control: effect of insulin treatment. Pract Diab Int 1998;15:73–77

187. Meneilly GS, Cheung E, Tuokko H: Altered responses to hypoglycemia of healthy elderly people. J Clin Endocrinol Metab 1994;78:1341–1348

188. Meneilly GS, Cheung E, Tuokko H: Counterregulatory hormone responses to hypoglycemia in the elderly patient with diabetes. Diabetes 1994;43:403–410

189. Brierley EJ, Broughton DL, James OF, Alberti KG: Reduced awareness of hypoglycaemia in the elderly despite an intact counter-regulatory response. QJM 1995;88:439–445

190. Marker JC, Cryer PE, Clutter WE: Attenuated glucose recovery from hypoglycaemia in the elderly. Diabetes 1992;41:671–678

191. Matyka K, Evans M, Lomas J et al: Altered hierarchy of protective responses against severe hypoglycemia in normal aging in healthy men. Diab Care 1997;20:135–141

192. Jaap AJ, Jones GC, McCrimmon RJ, Deary IJ, Frier BM: Perceived symptoms of hypoglycaemia in elderly type 2 diabetic patients treated with insulin. Diab Med 1998;15:398–401

193. Shorr RI, Ray WA, Daugherty JR, Griffin MR: Incidence and risk factors for serious hypoglycemia in older persons using insulin or sulfonylureas. Arch Intern Med 1997;157:1681–1686

194. Thomson FJ, Masson EA, Leeming JT, Boulton AJ: Lack of knowledge of symptoms of hypoglycaemia by elderly diabetic patients. Age Ageing 1991;20:404–406

195. Diabetes Control and Complications Trial Research Group: The effect of intensive treatment of diabetes on the development and progression of long-term complications in insulin-dependent diabetes mellitus. N Engl J Med 1993;329:977–986

196. Laakso M, Pyorala K: Age of onset and type of diabetes. Diab Care 1985;8:114–117

197. De Fronzo RA: Pathogenesis of type 2 (non-insulin-dependent) diabetes mellitus: a balanced overview. Diabetologia 1992;35:389–397

198. Reaven GM: Resistance to insulin-stimulated glucose uptake and hyperinsulinanaemia: role of non-insulin-dependent diabetes, high blood pressure, dyslipidaemia and coronary heart disease. Diab Metab 1991;17:78–86

199. Levy J, Atkinson AB, Bell PM, McCance DR, Hadden DR: Beta-cell deterioration determines the onset and rate of progression of secondary dietary failure in type 2 diabetes mellitus: the 10-year follow-up of the Belfast Diet Study. Diab Med 1998;15:290–296

200. Turner RC, Cull CA, Frighi V, Holman RR: UKPDS 49. Glycaemic control with diet, sulphonylurea, metformin and insulin therapy in patients with type 2 diabetes: progressive requirement for multiple therapies. JAMA 1999;281:2005–2012

201. Meneilly GS, Elliott T, Tessier D, Hards L, Tildesley H: NIDDM in the elderly. Diab Care 1996;19:1320–1325

202. Nutrition Subcommittee of the British Diabetic Association's Professional Advisory Committee: Dietary recommendations for people with diabetes: an update for the 1990s. Diab Med 1992;9:189–202

203. United Kingdom Prospective Diabetes Study group: UKPDS 13: relative efficacy of randomly allocated diet, sulphonylurea, insulin, or metformin in patients with newly diagnosed non-insulin dependent diabetes followed for three years. BMJ 1995;310:83–88

204. Tindall H, Bodansky HJ, Stickland M, Wales JK: A strategy for selection of elderly type 2 diabetic patients for insulin therapy and a comparison of two insulin preparations. Diab Med 1988;5:533–536

205. Cook DL: The beta-cell response to oral hypoglycemic agents. Diab Res Clin Pract 1995;28(suppl):S81–S9

206. Barnett AH: Tablet and insulin therapy in type 2 diabetes in the elderly. J R Soc Med 1994;87:612–614

207. Krentz AJ, Ferner RE, Bailey CJ: Comparative tolerability profiles of oral antidiabetic agents. Drug Safety 1994;11:223–241

208. Croxson S: Diabetes mellitus and common endocrine conditions in the elderly. In Crome P, Ford G (eds): Drugs and the Older Population. Imperial College Press, London, 2000:453–531

209. Asplund K, Wilholm B-E, Lithner F: Glibenclamide-associated hypoglycaemia: a report on 57 cases. Diabetologia 1983;24:412–417

210. Shorr RI, Ray WA, Daugherty JR, Griffin MR: Individual sulfonylureas and serious hypoglycemia in older people. J Am Geriatr Soc 1996;44:751–755

211. Jennings AM, Wilson RM, Ward JD: Symptomatic hypoglycaemia in NIDDM patients treated with oral hypoglycaemic agents. Diab Care 1989;12:203–208

212. Clarke BF, Campbell IW: Long term comparative trial of glibenclamide and chlorpropamide in diet failed maturity onset diabetics. Lancet 1975;1:246–247

213. Campbell IW: Metformin and glibenclamide: comparative risks. BMJ 1984;289:289

214. Asplund K, Wiholm BE, Lundman B: Severe hypoglycaemia during treatment with glipizide. Diab Med 1991;8:726–731

215. Kobayashi KA, Bauer LA, Horn JR et al: Glipizide pharmacokinetics in young and elderly volunteers. Clin Pharm 1988;7:224–228

216. Shaw KM, Wheeley M St G, Campbell DB, Ward JD: Home blood glucose monitoring in non-insulin dependent diabetics: the effect of gliclazide on blood glucose and weight control, a multicentre trial. Diab Med 1985;2:484–490

217. Martin B, Kesson CM: Dietary control of elderly diabetics patients: a case for review. Pract Diab 1986;3:146–148

218. Palmer KJ, Brogden RN: Gliclazide: an update of its pharmacological properties and therapeutic efficacy in non-insulin dependent diabetes mellitus. Drug Eval 1993;46:92–115

219. Harrower A, Wong C: Comparison of secondary failure rate between three second generation sulphonylureas. Diab Res 1990;13:19–21

220. Harrower ADB: Comparison of efficacy, secondary failure rate, and complications of sulphonylureas. J Diab Comp 1994;8:201–203

221. Harrower ADB: Comparison of diabetic control in type 2 (non-insulin dependent) diabetic patients treated with different sulphonylureas. Curr Med Res Opin 1985;9:676–680

222. Tessier D, Dawson K, Tetrault JP, Bravo G, Meneilly GS: Glibenclamide vs gliclazide in type 2 diabetes of the elderly. Diab Med 1994;11:974–980

223. Schneider J, Chaikin P: Glimepiride safety. Postgrad Med J 1997;33–44 (special report)

224. Stumvoll M, Nurjhan N, Perriello G, Dailey G, Gerich JE: Metabolic effects of metformin in non-insulin-dependent diabetes mellitus. N Engl J Med 1995;333:550–554

225. Luft D, Schmülling RM, Eggstein M: Lactic acidosis in biguanide-treated diabetics. Diabetologia 1978;14:75–87

226. De Fronzo RA, Goodman AM, and the Multicenter Metformin Study Group: Efficacy of metformin in patients with non-insulin-dependent diabetes mellitus. N Engl J Med 1995;333:541–549

227. Dornan TL, Heller SR, Peck GM, Tattersall RB: Double-blind evaluation of efficacy and tolerability of metformin in NIDDM. Diab Care 1991;14:342–344

228. UK Prospective Diabetes Study (UKPDS) group: Effect of intensive blood-glucose control with metformin on complications in overweight patients with type 2 diabetes (UKPDS 34). Lancet 1998;352:854–865

229. Josephkutty S, Potter JM: Comparison of tolbutamide and metformin in elderly diabetic patients. Diab Med 1990;7:510–514

230. Coniff RF, Shapiro JA, Robbins D et al: Reduction of glycosylated hemoglobin and postprandial hyperglycemia by acarbose in patients with NIDDM: a placebo-controlled dose-comparison study. Diab Care 1995;18:817–824

231. Jenney A, Proietto J, O'Dea K et al: Low-dose acarbose improves glycemic control in NIDDM patients without changes in insulin sensitivity. Diab Care 1993;16:499–502

232. Rosak C, Nitzsche G, Konig P, Hofmann U: The effect of the timing and the administration of acarbose on postprandial hyperglycaemia. Diab Med 1995;12:979–984

233. Chiasson JL, Josse RG, Hunt JA et al: The efficacy of acarbose in the treatment of patients with non-insulin-dependent diabetes mellitus: a multicenter controlled clinical trial. Ann Intern Med 1994;121:928–935

234. Bayraktar M, Van Thiel DH, Adalar N: A comparison of acarbose versus metformin as an adjuvant therapy in sulfonylurea-treated NIDDM patients. Diab Care 1996;19:252–254

235. Calle-Pascual AL, Garcia-Honduvilla J, Martin-Alvarez PJ et al: Comparison between acarbose, metformin, and insulin treatment in type 2 diabetic patients with secondary failure to sulfonylurea treatment. Diabete Metab 1995;21:256–260

236. Coniff RF, Shapiro JA, Seaton TB, Bray GA: Multicenter, placebo-controlled trial comparing acarbose (BAY g 5421) with placebo, tolbutamide, and tolbutamide-plus-acarbose in non-insulin-dependent diabetes mellitus. Am J Med 1995;98:443–451

237. Hoffmann J, Spengler M: Efficacy of 24-week monotherapy with acarbose, glibenclamide, or placebo in NIDDM patients: the Essen Study. Diab Care 1994;17:561–566

238. Petrie J, Small M, Connell J: "Glitazones," a prospect for non-insulin-dependent diabetes. Lancet 1997;349:70–71

239. Lebovitz HE, Dole JF, Patwardhan R et al, for the Rosiglitazone Clinical Trials study group: Rosiglitazone monotherapy is effective in patients with type 2 diabetes. J Clin Endocrinol Metab 2001;86:280–288

240. Einhorn D, Rendell M, Rosenzweig J et al: Pioglitazone hydrochloride in combination with metformin in the treatment of type 2 diabetes mellitus: a randomized, placebo-controlled study. The Pioglitazone 027 Study Group. Clin Therapeut 2000;22:1395–1409

241. Fonseca V, Rosenstock J, Patwardhan R, Salzman A: Effect of metformin and rosiglitazone combination therapy in patients with type 2 diabetes mellitus: a randomized controlled trial. JAMA 2000;283:1695–1702

242. Wolffenbuttel BH, Gomis R, Squatrito S, Jones NP, Patwardhan RN: Addition of low-dose rosiglitazone to sulphonylurea therapy improves glycaemic control in type 2 diabetic patients. Diab Med 2000;17:40–47

243. King AB: A comparison in a clinical setting of the efficacy and side effects of three thiazolidinediones. Diab Care 2000;23:557

244. Owens DR: Repaglinide—prandial glucose regulator: a new class of oral antidiabetic drugs. Diab Med 1998;15(suppl 4):S28–S36

245. Tronier B, Marbury TC, Damsbo B, Windfield K: A new oral hypoglycaemic agent, repaglinide, minimises risk of hypoglycaemia in well controlled NIDDM patients. Diabetologia 1995;38:A752

246. Damsbo P, Marbury TC, Hatorp V, Clauson P, Muller PG: Flexible prandial glucose regulation with repaglinide in patients with type 2 diabetes. Diab Res Clin Pract 1999;45:31–39

247. Moses R, Slobodniuk R, Donnelly T et al: Additional treatment with repaglinide provides significant improvement in glycaemic control in NIDDM patients poorly controlled on metformin. Diab Care 1997;46(suppl 1):93A

248. Raskin P, Jovanovic L, Berger S et al: Repaglinide/troglitazone combination therapy: improved glycemic control in type 2 diabetes. Diab Care 2000;23:979–983

249. Keilson L, Mather S, Walter YH, Subramanian S, McLeod JF: Synergistic effects of nateglinide and meal administration on insulin secretion in patients with type 2 diabetes mellitus. J Clin Endocrinol Metab 2000;85:1081–1086

250. Choudhury S, Hirschberg Y, Filipek R, Lasseter K, McLeod JF: Single-dose pharmacokinetics of nateglinide in subjects with hepatic cirrhosis. J Clin Pharmacol 2000;40:634–640

251. Horton ES, Clinkingbeard C, Gatlin M et al: Nateglinide alone and in combination with metformin improves glycemic control by reducing mealtime glucose levels in type 2 diabetes. Diab Care 2000;23:1660–1665

252. Hanefeld M, Bouter KP, Dickinson S, Guitard C: Rapid and short-acting mealtime insulin secretion with nateglinide controls both prandial and mean glycemia. Diab Care 2000;23:202–207

253. Tattersall RB, Gale EAM (eds): Diabetes: Clinical Management. Churchill Livingstone, Edinburgh, 1990

254. Garg SK, Carmain JA, Braddy KC et al: Pre-meal insulin analogue insulin Lispro vs Humulin R insulin treatment in young subjects with type 1 diabetes. Diab Med 1996;13:47–52

255. Schernthaner G, Equiluz-Bruck S, Wein W et al: Postprandial Insulin Lispro. Diab Care 1998;21:570–573

256. Taylor R: Insulin for the non-insulin dependent. BMJ 1988;296:1015–1016

257. Roland JM, Lewin IG, O'Brien AD et al: A comparative study of once daily insulin injection regimes in the treatment of elderly diabetics. Diab Res 1987;4:131–134

258. Taylor R, Davies R, Fox C et al: Optimal insulin treatment for type 2 diabetes: a multicentre randomised crossover trial. Diab Med 1999;16(suppl 1):9 (abstract)

259. Tattersall RB, Scott AR: When to use insulin in the maturity onset diabetic. Postgrad Med J 1987;63:859–864
260. Riddle MC: Evening insulin strategy. Diab Care 1990;13:676–686
261. Yki-Jarvinen H, Kauppila M, Kujansuu E et al: Comparison of insulin regimens in patients with non-insulin-dependent diabetes mellitus. N Engl J Med 1992;327:1426–1433
262. Little J, Battison S, Walker JD: Nocturnal isophane insulin in patients with NIDDM: clinic based as opposed to research results. Diab Med 1997;14(suppl 4):S5 (abstract)
263. Yki-Jarvinen H, Dressler A, Ziemen M for the HOE 901/300s study group: Less nocturnal hypoglycemia and better post-dinner glucose control with bedtime insulin glargine compared with bedtime NPH insulin during insulin combination therapy in type 2 diabetes. HOE 901/3002 study group. Diab Care 2000;23:1130–1136
264. Pugh JA, Wagner ML, Sawyer J et al: Is combination sulfonylurea and insulin therapy useful in NIDDM patients? A meta-analysis. Diab Care 1992;15:953–959
265. Johnson JL, Wolf SL, Kabadi UM: Efficacy of insulin and sulfonylurea combination therapy in type II diabetes: a meta-analysis of the randomized placebo-controlled trials. Arch Intern Med 1996;156:259–264
266. McNulty SJ, Mangnall M, Benbow SJ, Hardy KJ: Metformin vs gliclazide in combination with daily NPH insulin in poorly controlled type 2 diabetic patients: 1–2 year follow-up data. Diab Med 1998;15(suppl 1):S9 (abstract)
267. Relimpio F, Pumar A, Losada F et al: Adding metformin versus insulin dose increase in insulin treated but poorly controlled type 2 diabetes mellitus: an open-label randomised trial. Diab Med 1998;15:997–1002
268. Meneilly GS, Milberg WP, Tuokko H: Differential effects of human and animal insulin on the responses to hypoglycemia in elderly patients with NIDDM. Diabetes 1995;44:272–277
269. Croxson S, France J, Oxley J: Clinico-pathological conference: hypoglycaemia in an elderly lady. Pract Diab Int 2002;19(3):87–89
270. Croxson SCM: Metabolic decompensation. In Sinclair AJ, Finucane P (eds): Diabetes in Old Age, 2nd edn. John Wiley, Chichester, 2000:49–62
271. Alberti KGGM: Diabetic emergencies. Br Med Bull 1989;45:242–263
272. Basu A, Close CF, Jenkins D et al: Persisting mortality in diabetic ketoacidosis. Diab Med 1993;10:282–284
273. Leutscher PDC, Svendsen KN: Svaer ketoacidose hos en ikke-insulinkraevende diabetes mellitus patient. Ugeskr Laeger 1991;253:2634–2635
274. Gerich JE, Martin MM, Recant L: Clinical and metabolic characteristics of hyper-osmolar nonketotic coma. Diabetes 1971;20:228–238
275. Berger W, Keller U: Treatment of diabetic ketoacidosis and non-ketotic hyperosmolar diabetic coma. Baillière's Clin Endocrinol Metab 1992;6:1–22
276. Fonseca V, Phaer DN: Hyperosmolar non-ketotic diabetic syndrome precipitated by treatment with diuretics. BMJ 1982;284:36–37
277. Hamblin PS, Topliss DJ, Chosich N et al: Deaths associated with diabetic ketoacidosis and hyperosmolar coma. Med J Aust 1989;151:439–444
278. Barnett DM, Wilcox DS, Marble A: Diabetic coma in persons over 60. Geriatrics 1962;17:327–336
279. Stacpoole PW: Lactic acidosis: the case against bicarbonate therapy. Ann Intern Med 1986;105:276–279
280. Tuomilehto J, Rastenyte D, Birkenhager WH, Thijs L et al: Effects of calcium channel blockade in older patients with diabetes and systolic hypertension. N Engl J Med 1999;340:677–684
281. Forette F, Seux ML, Staessen JA, Thijs L et al: Prevention of dementia in randomised double-blind placebo-controlled Systolic Hypertension in Europe (Syst-Eur) trial. Lancet 1998;352:1347–1351
282. SHEP cooperative research group: Prevention of stroke by antihypertensive drug treatment in older persons with isolated systolic hypertension: final results of the Systolic Hypertension in the Elderly Program (SHEP). JAMA 1991;265:3255–3264
283. Curb JD, Pressel SL, Cutler JA et al, for the Systolic Hypertension in the Elderly Program cooperative research group: Effect of diuretic-based antihypertensive treatment on cardiovascular disease risk in older diabetic patients with isolated systolic hypertension. JAMA 1996;276:1886–1892
284. Hansson L, Zanchetti A, Carruthers SG et al, for the HOT study group: Effects of intensive blood-pressure lowering and low-dose aspirin in patients with hypertension: principal results of the Hypertension Optimal Treatment (HOT) randomised trial. Lancet 1998;351:1755–1762
285. Ramsay LE, Williams B, Johnston GD et al: Guidelines for management of hypertension: report of the third working party of the British Hypertension Society. J Human Hypertens 1999;13:569–592
286. Missouris CG, Buckenham T, Cappuccio FP, MacGregor GA: Renal artery stenosis: a common and important problem in patients with peripheral vascular disease. Am J Med 1994;96:10–14
287. Carr S: ACE inhibition and renovascular disease. Diab Med 2001;18 (suppl 1):4–6
288. Messerli FH, Grossman E, Goldbourt U: Are beta-blockers efficacious as first-line therapy for hypertension in the elderly? A systematic review. JAMA 1998;279:1903–1907
289. Grossman E, Messerli FH, Goldbourt U: High blood pressure and diabetes mellitus: are all antihypertensive drugs created equal? Arch Intern Med 2000;160:2447–2452
290. Corti MC, Guralnik JM, Salive ME et al: HDL cholesterol predicts coronary heart disease mortality in older persons. JAMA 1995;274:539–544
291. Florkowski CM, Scott RS, Moir CL, Graham PJ: Lipid but not glycaemic parameters predict total mortality from type 2 diabetes mellitus in Canterbury, New Zealand. Diab Med 1998;15:386–392
292. Dean JD, Durrington PN: Treatment of dyslipoproteinaemia in diabetes mellitus. Diab Med 1996;13:297–312
293. Scandinavian Simvastatin Survival Study Group: Randomised trial of cholesterol lowering in 4444 patients with coronary heart disease: the Scandinavian Simvastatin Survival Study (4S). Lancet 1994;344:1383–1389
294. Pyörälä K, Pedersen TR, Kjekshus J et al, for the Scandinavian Simvastatin Survival Study Group: Cholesterol lowering with simvastatin improves prognosis of diabetic patients with coronary heart disease. Diab Care 1997;20:614–620
295. Sacks FM, Pfeffer MA, Moye LA et al: The effect of pravastatin on coronary events after myocardial infarction in patients with average cholesterol levels. N Engl J Med 1996;335:1001–1009
296. Yudkin JS, Chaturvedi N: Developing risk stratification charts for diabetic and nondiabetic subjects. Diab Med 1999;16:219–227; erratum 16:972–973
297. Neil HA, Roe L, Godlee RJ et al: Randomised trial of lipid lowering dietary advice in general practice: the effects on serum lipids, lipoproteins, and antioxidants. BMJ 1995;310:569–573
298. Manley SE, Stratton IM, Cull CA et al, for the United Kingdom Prospective Diabetes study group: Effects of three months' diet after diagnosis of type 2 diabetes on plasma lipids and lipoproteins (UKPDS 45). Diab Med 2000;17:518–523
299. Croxson S: Diabetes in the Elderly (MD thesis). University of Leicester, Leicester, 1995
300. de Vegt F, Dekker JM, Ruhe HG et al: Hyperglycaemia is associated with all-cause and cardiovascular mortality in the Hoorn population: the Hoorn Study. Diabetologia 1999;42:926–931
301. Yudkin JS, Hendra TJ: Vascular events and diabetes: acute myocardial infarction and stroke. In Alberti KGGM, DeFronzo RA, Keen H, Zimmet P (eds): International Textbook of Diabetes Mellitus. John Wiley, Chichester, 1992:1185–1210
302. Yudkin JS: How can we best prolong life? Benefits of coronary risk factor reduction in non-diabetic and diabetic subjects. BMJ 1993;306:1313–1318
303. European Arterial Risk Policy Group on behalf of the International Diabetes Federation European Region: A strategy for arterial risk assessment and management in type 2 (non-insulin-dependent) diabetes mellitus. Diab Med 1997;14:611–621
304. American Diabetes Association: Position Statement: Aspirin therapy in diabetes mellitus. Diabetes Care 1997;20:1772–1775
305. Antiplatelet Trialists' Collaboration: Collaborative overview of randomised trials of antiplatelet therapy. I: Prevention of death, myocardial infarction, and stroke by prolonged antiplatelet therapy in various categories of patients. BMJ 1994;308:81–106
306. Yudkin JS: Assessing the evidence on aspirin in diabetes mellitus. Gemini or Libra; lumping or splitting; surrogate or hard; low or high; interventionist or nihilist. Diabetologia 1996;39:1407–1408
307. Derry S, Loke YK: Risk of gastrointestinal haemorrhage with long term use of aspirin: meta-analysis. BMJ 2000;321:1183–1187
308. Meade TW, Brennan PJ: Determination of who may derive most benefit from aspirin in primary prevention: subgroup results from a randomised controlled trial. BMJ 2000;321:13–17
309. Anonymous: A randomised, blinded trial of clopidogrel versus aspirin in patients at risk of ischaemic events (CAPRIE). CAPRIE Steering Committee. Lancet 1996;348:1329–1339

310. Benjamin EJ, Levy D, Vaziri SM et al: Independent risk factors for atrial fibrillation in a population-based cohort: The Framingham Heart Study. JAMA 1994;271:840–844

311. Morley J, Marinchak R, Rials SJ, Kowey P: Atrial fibrillation, anticoagulation, and stroke. Am J Cardiol 1996;77:38A–44A

312. The atrial fibrillation investigators: Risk factors for stroke and efficacy of antithrombotic therapy in atrial fibrillation. Arch Intern Med 1994;154:1449–1457

313. Chew EY, Klein ML, Murphy RP, Remaley NA, Ferris FL: Effects of aspirin on vitreous/preretinal hemorrhage in patients with diabetes mellitus: Early Treatment Diabetic Retinopathy Study report 20. Arch Ophthalmol 1995;113:52–55

314. Anonymous: Effects of ramipril on cardiovascular and microvascular outcomes in people with diabetes mellitus: results of the HOPE study and MICRO-HOPE substudy. Heart Outcomes Prevention Evaluation Study Investigators. Lancet 2000;355:253–259

315. Miettinen H, Haffner SM, Lehto S et al: Proteinuria predicts stroke and other atherosclerotic vascular disease events in nondiabetic and non-insulin-dependent diabetic subjects. Stroke 1996;27:2033–2039

316. Mogensen CE, Neldam S, Tikkanen T et al, for the CALM study group. Randomised controlled trial of dual blockade of renin–angiotensin system in patients with hypertension, microalbuminuria, and non-insulin dependent diabetes: the candesartan and lisinopril microalbuminuria (CALM) study. BMJ 2000;321:1440–1444

317. Malmberg K and the DIGAMI (Diabetes Mellitus, Insulin Glucose Infusion in Acute Myocardial Infarction) study group: Prospective randomised study of intensive insulin treatment on long term survival after acute myocardial infarction in patients with diabetes mellitus. BMJ 1997;314:1512–1515

318. Malmberg K, Ryden L, Efendic S et al: Randomized trial of insulin–glucose infusion followed by subcutaneous insulin treatment in diabetic patients with acute myocardial infarction (DIGAMI study): effects on mortality at 1 year. J Am Coll Cardiol 1995;26:57–65

319. Lynch M, Gammage MD, Lamb P, Nattrass M, Pentecost BL: Acute myocardial infarction in diabetic patients in the thrombolytic era. Diabetic Medicine 1994;11:162–165

320. Zuanetti G, Latini R, Maggioni AP et al: Effect of the ACE inhibitor lisinopril on mortality in diabetic patients with acute myocardial infarction: data from the GISSI-3 study. Circulation 1997;96: 4239–4245

321. Gundersen T, Kjekshus J: Timolol treatment after myocardial infarction in diabetic patients. Diab Care 1983;6:285–290

322. Sinclair AJ: Geriatric diabetes: concerns and celebrations. State of the Art Lecture, Autumn Meeting, Medical and Scientific Section, British Diabetic Association, Harrogate, England, 5 October 1995

323. Hill RD: Models of care for the elderly diabetic. J R Soc Med 1994;87:617–619

324. Wilkes E, Laughton EE: The diabetic, the hospital and primary care. J R Coll Gen Pract 1980;30:199–206

325. Hayes T, Harries J: Randomised control trial of routine hospital clinic care versus routine general practice care for type 2 diabetics. BMJ 1984;289:728–730

326. Sinclair AJ, Turnbull CJ, Croxson SCM: Document of care for older people with diabetes. Postgrad Med J 1996;72:334–338

Chapter 97

Aging and the blood

Maria H. Gilleece

CELLULAR COMPONENTS OF BLOOD AND SITES OF BLOOD PRODUCTION

The cellular content of the blood comprises a diverse population with a wide range of functions that contribute significantly to normal homeostasis. The erythrocytes transport hemoglobin, the major oxygen binding protein, and play a key role in respiratory gas exchange. Age, sex, and hypoxia influence their numbers. Granulocytes, namely neutrophils, eosinophils, and basophils, are important components of the response to bacterial, protozoan, and fungal infections. Monocytes and their derivatives, macrophages, are also a crucial part of the inflammatory response to infection, and both granulocytes and monocytes have the capacity to migrate from blood to the tissues. Lymphocytes orchestrate many of these responses and form an important part of the adaptive immune response, for example, by the production of microorganism-specific antibodies by B-lymphocytes and the targeted killing of cells bearing foreign antigen by cytotoxic T-lymphocytes. Dendritic cells form a minor compartment of peripheral blood but are of key importance in facilitating the presentation of antigen to the effector cells of the immune system. Platelets contribute to the constant process of repair and remodeling as, following activation, they interact with endothelial cells lining blood vessels and soluble coagulation profactors found in plasma to repair breaches in the endothelial wall.

The constituent cells of blood have their origin in the bone marrow, but other organs make major contributions at varying stages of development. During the first 6–8 weeks of embryonic life, hemopoiesis occurs in the yolk sac but following this stage the liver becomes the prime site with some contribution from the spleen. During late gestation the bone marrow is the major site of hemopoietic development and in normal physiological states it is the exclusive site after birth. The liver and spleen retain some capacity to support hemopoiesis as may be seen in pathological states such as the thalassemias or chronic myeloid leukemia when extramedullary hemopoiesis may prevail. In the case of T-lymphocytes, pre-T-cells emanate from the bone marrow and pass through the thymus where they undergo further development before reaching maturity and then, like B-lymphocytes, disseminate throughout the blood and lymphoid tissue.

Bone marrow

The stromal microenvironment of the bone marrow includes fibroblasts, adipose cells, macrophages, reticular cells, and endothelial cells, and is essential for maintenance of hemopoiesis.[1] Bone marrow trephine histology,[2] reveals the orderly arrangement of the developing cells in which early granulocytic cells can be found along the trabecular margins, while erythroid islands, megakaryocytes, and occasional lymphoid nodules are positioned in the intertrabecular spaces. These features suggest that within the stroma there are "niches" where particular developmental events are favored by the local arrangement of stromal cells, growth factors, and hemopoietic progenitor cells.

At birth all marrow is red hemopoietically active tissue, but then there is an orderly retreat of this tissue and replacement by yellow, hemopoietically inactive adipose marrow, beginning in the diaphysis and continuing in the distal metaphysis of each long bone and then in the proximal metaphysis.[3,4] These reversible changes can be triggered by decreased temperature and perfusion.[5,6] By early adulthood red marrow predominates only in the flat bones and vertebral bodies, with remnants in the proximal humeral and femoral bones. Gradual involution of red marrow continues but is especially marked after the age of 70 years when iliac crest marrow cellularity is reduced to about 30 percent of that found in young adults.[7,8] Nuclear magnetic resonance[5] is more sensitive to changes in cellularity than conventional microscopy and suggests that mechanical stress at the cervical and lumbar spine vertebral body endplates and medial portion of the femoral neck accelerates this conversion. At the same time, there is an increase in marrow necrosis and fibrosis, loss of bone substance, which allows further expansion of adipose tissue with age, an increase in bone marrow iron stores,[9] a fall in the number of normoblasts,[10] and an accumulation of benign lymphoid aggregates.[7]

LYMPHOID DEVELOPMENT

Normal lymphoid development occurs in two distinct stages. The first is antigen independent and occurs in bone marrow or thymus, the primary lymphoid organs, while the second is antigen dependent and occurs within secondary lymphoid organs such as the spleen, lymph nodes, Peyer's patches or Waldeyer's ring. Lymphocytes that have undergone antigen independent development are immunocompetent but naïve. They are, however, programmed to interact with specific antigen, a process that occurs in the secondary lymphoid organs, when they will undergo terminal proliferation and differentiation to become effector cells with helper or cytotoxic functions. Naïve lymphocytes develop within the periphery of the bone marrow parenchyma and migrate centrally to the vascular sinuses where they are discharged. Subsequently they are released into the peripheral circulation from which they will penetrate the secondary lymphoid organs. However, T-cell development requires a further intrathymic phase before the cells are equipped to respond to antigen stimulation.

The thymus contains a cortex and medulla. The cortex is densely populated by lymphocytes, constituting 85 percent of the cellularity, in association with epithelial cells that include the dendritic cells whose function it is to present antigen.

The medulla contains a diverse population of epithelioid cells, macrophages that direct thymocyte maturation (phagocytosis, antigen presentation, cytokine production), interdigitating dendritic cells (of bone marrow origin, typical of interdigitating dendritic cells found in T-cell-dependent areas of peripheral lymphoid organs), myoid cells (fetal thymus), and lymphocytes (comprising 15 percent of the thymic medullary population). Prothymocytes leave their origin in bone marrow and migrate to the subcapsular region of the thymus and from there to the deep cortex and then to the medulla from which they are launched into the peripheral circulation once more. When the prothymocytes enter the thymus they express CD34 and CD7 at the cell surface, but maturation within the thymus is associated with loss and down-regulation, respectively of these markers. Maturation within the cortex of the thymus produces distinct $\alpha\beta$ and $\gamma\delta$ lineages due to rearrangement of T-cell receptor genes, a process that also confers antigen specificity. The $\alpha\beta$ lineage becomes the dominant lineage in the peripheral blood and the cells progress through a CD4– CD8– double negative stage to a double positive CD4+ CD8+ within the cortex. These double positive cells then become subject to a positive or negative selection process that results in survival of single positive CD4+ or CD8+ T-lymphocytes that also express the CD45RA "naïve" cell marker. Following antigenic exposure, naïve T-cells proliferate to produce effector cells and also memory cells, the latter expressing CD45RO rather than CD45RA. However, there is some RO–RA reversion in this phenotype so that CD45RA expression cannot always guarantee the naïve status.

Secondary lymphoid organs are structured to provide distinct microenvironments that direct naïve lymphocytes to interact with specialized antigen presenting cells, segregate T- and B-lymphocytes and allow recirculation of antigen activated or memory cells. Lymph node architecture is defined as a cortical area, comprising a superficial and a deep paracortical zone and a medullary area. The cellular components are supported by the reticulum made up of endothelial and fibroblast elements. The cortex contains lymphocyte follicles constituted of uniform small lymphocytes in primary follicles; secondary follicles have an additional blastic population and a germinal center that is indicative of antigen stimulation. The base of the germinal center, the dark zone, contains the centroblasts derived from naïve B-lymphocytes. They proliferate and differentiate to centrocytes occupying the upper, apical, germinal center. Surrounding the germinal center is the mantle zone, an area that contains a mixture of naïve B-lymphocytes, B-lymphocytes that are post-T-cell-independent antigen stimulation, memory B-cells, and CD5+ B-cells. Beyond this, and abutting the medulla is the paracortex. Similar to the diffuse cortical area existing between lymphoid follicles, this area is T-cell rich, particularly CD4+ cells. The cells of the medullary region, lymphocytes, macrophages, and plasma cells, are arranged as cordlike structures adjacent to vascular sinuses. Antigen presentation is effected by macrophages within sinus walls that are able to phagocytose and present antigen, follicular dendritic cells within follicles that present antigen to B-cells and interdigitating dendritic cells within the paracortex that present antigen to T-cells.

The spleen has multiple functions in addition to its role as a secondary lymphoid organ: it provides a microenvironment for terminal differentiation of reticulocytes, platelets, and monocytes; it removes aged or deformed erythrocytes and it acts as a reservoir for erythrocytes and granulocytes. There are two dominant areas—the white pulp, densely populated with lymphocytes, and the red pulp, rich in vascular sinuses and cellular cords. The white pulp may be further subdivided into a periarteriolar lymphatic sheath (PALS) and a marginal zone. The PALS contains a central area rich in T-cells and interdigitating dendritic cells and a peripheral area containing B-cells, T-cells, and secondary follicles bounded by a mantle zone. The marginal zone separates the white pulp from the red pulp and, containing the marginal sinus lined by macrophages, constitutes a major site of antigen localization and lymphocyte trafficking.

Naïve lymphocytes may migrate in and out of secondary lymphoid organs via the high endothelial venules without site preference. However, activated lymphocytes and memory cells migrate specifically to the site where antigen was first encountered. Thus T memory cells will tend to migrate to the extranodal or tertiary lymphoid tissues within the gut, respiratory tree or to sites of inflammation within skin or synovium. Homing of lymphocytes is influenced by the expression of adhesion molecules, chemokines, and their ligands.

The thymus undergoes rapid involution during puberty with pronounced loss of cortical thymocytes and atrophy of epithelial cells. There is at least partial replacement by fat tissue contributed by mesenchymal cells found in connective tissue supporting the capsule and vasculature. By the age of 45, more than 50 percent of the thymus is replaced by adipose tissue. However, thymic function may be more persistent than has been previously accepted: Naïve T-cells undergo random rearrangement and partial excision of T-cell receptor (TCR) DNA prior to clonal expansion. This ensures the specificity and the sensitivity of the T-cell response to antigenic stimulation. The excised DNA, known as a TCR rearrangement excision circle (TREC), is not duplicated during mitosis or expelled from the nucleus. Instead, it is retained by one daughter cell in each generation as the clone expands. Since expansion is exponential, the TREC positive cells are rapidly diluted. Douek et al.[11] exploited this feature of T-cell development to distinguish clones that were recent thymic emigrants (RTE) from memory T-cells. They studied the relationship between age and TREC dominance and reported a cohort of newborn to 73-year-old subjects in which there was a 1–1.5 $\log_{10}$ drop in the number of TRECS in contrast to a four-fold drop in cells deemed naïve by virtue of cell surface phenotype. TREC numbers were also reduced in athymic subjects compared to euthymic controls. The fall in TREC numbers is more likely to reflect reduced thymic function rather than peripheral expansion of naïve cells. Using a broadly similar approach, Poulin et al.[12] confirmed the presence of excised TCR DNA remnants within the CD4+CD45RA+CD62L+ naïve cell compartment up until the age of 76 years. Similarly to Douek's observations, RTE numbers fell with age at a faster rate than the cells identified as naïve by phenotypic markers. Although these data do confirm a decline in thymic function with age they suggest, surprisingly, that more function is preserved than had hitherto been suspected and also that the naïve cell compartment, as defined phenotypically, is heterogenous.

STEM CELL BIOLOGY

Mature cells representing individual lineages circulate in the body for a finite period ranging from a few hours for neutrophils to many years for memory lymphocytes. Maintenance of homeostasis imposes a massive proliferative demand on the hemopoietic system, which must produce more than 10^{11} new cells each day. Additionally, the numbers of differentiating cells within each lineage require regulation simultaneous with retention of the capacity to increase production of specific subpopulations in response to external stresses. Metcalf[13] has divided the hemopoietic system into three hierarchical populations. One contains mature cells, readily identifiable as belonging to a particular lineage, and these have a limited capacity to proliferate. Their precursors are progenitor cells characterized by a substantial proliferative potential but a stringent limitation to differentiation into specific lineages. More primitive still are the totipotential hemopoietic stem cells that have the capacity both for self-replicative division to prevent exhaustion of the totipotential stem cell compartment and for proliferation and differentiation via the process of lineage commitment to produce lineage-restricted progenitor cells. This model predicts that, despite the diversity of function and phenotype, blood cells have a common stem cell of origin whose self-replicative capacity ensures the maintenance of the mature compartment. Thus, a single multipotential stem cell can, in an appropriate environment, give rise to a variety of more developmentally restricted and lineage-restricted progenitor cells capable of producing cells of different mature hemopoietic cell types.[14] Crucially, the self-replicative capacity of the totipotent stem cells guarantees the sustained production of mature blood cells throughout life. Hemopoiesis is polyclonal in healthy young adults,[15–17] indicating that more than one stem cell clone contributes to the production of mature cells from the marrow at any one time. While maturation of some cells such as T-lymphocytes and monocytes may occur outside the bone marrow, the process of stem cell renewal and lineage commitment appears almost entirely confined to the bone marrow.

The hierarchical conformation of hemopoietic cell populations is central to hemopoietic hemostasis but the interaction of the totipotent hemopoietic stem cells and their progeny with their stromal microenvironment and growth factor molecules is also significant. The proliferation and differentiation of hemopoietic progenitors and mature cells is regulated by cell-to-cell interactions within the local microenvironment and by the binding of secreted peptide growth factors to high-affinity receptors expressed at the cell surface during sequential stages of development.

Early evidence for the existence of hemopoietic cells with multipotential differentiating ability came from the work of Till and McCulloch.[18] They showed that in mice whose hemopoietic capacity was ablated by radiotherapy, donor hemopoietic cells could seed recipient hemopoietic tissue. They studied the spleen and found that single donor cells generated colonies of mixed hemopoietic lineages. Such splenic colony-forming

units (CFU-S) were multipotent rather than totipotent and were thus not able to maintain hemopoiesis indefinitely. Recognition of this short-term repopulating capacity led to mixing experiments in which short-term repopulating cells were infused together with purified populations of hemopoietic progenitor cells. The presence of progenitors with short-term repopulating capacity permitted maintenance of hemopoiesis during the lag phase that occurred before very primitive long-term repopulating cells, stem cells, could contribute progenitors committed to individual lineages. The frequency of such stem cells in murine bone marrow has been estimated at 1 in 10,000–100,000 mononuclear cells.[19,20] Evidence for a human equivalent may be deduced from the results of hemopoietic allogeneic stem cell transplantation in which there is successful reconstitution of the cellular elements of blood by purified donor cells following myeloablative therapy of the host.[21]

Demonstration of the existence of the totipotential hemopoietic stem cell then led to investigation of the relative contributions of individual stem cells to hemopoiesis. This was investigated by using the murine transplant model again. Donor cells, however, were "marked" prior to transplant:[22] retroviral infection was used to introduce proviral DNA into the genome of the donor cells. The integration sites were random and inherited by daughter cells, and restriction enzymes could be used to generate DNA fragments whose size was influenced by the site of proviral integration. Since the progeny of a single cell would share a common proviral integration site it became feasible to look at the contribution made by individual clones to hemopoiesis following transplantation. This technique revealed the dominance exerted by some clones in contributing to long-term hemopoiesis in all lineages. Other clones were strongly represented in the early post-transplant phase and then disappeared while some made no initial contribution but appeared later. This study was important in its demonstration of sequential recruitment rather than conscription of the entire stem cell pool to the function of hemopoietic reconstitution.

Although theoretical models have been proposed[23,24] to explain the hierarchy of mechanisms by which stem cells re-enter the cell cycle to self-renew or to differentiate and undergo eventual clonal extinction, how the stem cell environment regulates self-renewal and differentiation of stem cells remains an enigma. Recent data[25] tend to favor a so-called "stochastic"[26] over a "deterministic" process.[27] While definitive data to settle the debate are lacking it is now widely believed that the stochastic processes predominate in early stem cell commitment to self-renewal, differentiation, or death, and that deterministic processes become more relevant in cells that are already lineage restricted.[28,29] However, the contribution made by individual stem cells throughout an entire lifespan and the self-renewal capacity of the stem cell pool at a given point during that lifespan remain the focus of considerable debate. Some data suggest that stem cells have a finite proliferative capacity that falls progressively with age and can be accelerated by damage—a model that would explain the permanent reduction in marrow reserve caused by busulfan[30] and the limited capacity for repopulation in serial bone marrow transplantation.[31] Other data, however, support the idea that for all practical purposes stem cells have an indefinite capacity for self-renewal.[32–36] There is little evidence one way or the other to indicate that there is a physiologically meaningful decline in the self-renewal or differentiating capacity of hemopoietic stem cells with age in humans. In mice, however, careful studies have shown that there is no decline in stem cells or their ability to regenerate hemopoiesis with age within a single lifespan.[33,37]

THE ROLE OF LINEAGE-RESTRICTED PROGENITOR CELLS

Stem cells are relatively few in number (perhaps 1 in 50,000 bone marrow cells)[13] and adequate production of mature cells is met by amplification and development of the more developmentally restricted progeny of the stem cells. Much more is known about the regulation of growth and development of the myeloid progenitor cells (colony forming unit-granulocyte erythroid monocyte macrophage [CFU-GEMM], granulocyte macrophage-colony forming cell [GM-CFC], macrophage-colony forming cell [M-CFC], granulocyte-colony forming cell [G-CFC], burst forming unit-erythroid [BFU-E], and colony forming unit-erythroid [CFU-E] than of the stem cells. Some of these progenitors retain the ability to produce multiple cell lineages (CFU-GEMM and GM-CFC), while others are committed to differentiation along only one cell lineage. Human lymphoid progenitors are relatively difficult to grow in vitro.

All these myeloid progenitor cells can be cultured in vitro using liquid medium containing essential growth factors.[13] Under these conditions they undergo clonal extinction associated with further proliferation and differentiation to produce mature blood cells. The requirement of these cells for growth factors is absolute, and in the absence of appropriate growth factors these progenitors die by apoptosis (programmed cell death).[38] It has been reported that in-vitro colony formation from bone marrow derived from an aged population was inversely proportional to marrow cellularity.[39] Marley et al.[40] have observed a correlation of increasing bone marrow GM-CFC with increasing age. Interestingly, these GM-CFC show a decline in proliferative capacity that is also linked to advancing age and these changes have their onset at birth. These data suggest the possibility that as mitotic capacity of the hemopoietic stem cell population diminishes with age, equilibrium between renewal and differentiation shifts away from self-renewal in order to preserve peripheral blood function. This tends to predict the emergence of monoclonal hemopoiesis in elderly people, and this has in fact been described recently using analysis of X-chromosome inactivation patterns.[41] However, similar techniques applied to the study of monozygotic and dizygotic twins has revealed that acquisition of skewed X-chromosome inactivation with age may also be, in part, genetically determined.[42]

More primitive myeloid progenitors can be grown in long-term bone marrow cultures (LTBMC)[43] when cultured in association with stromal cells. These stromal cells support the survival and development of the hemopoietic progenitor cells forming the characteristic "cobblestone" areas of hemopoietic foci within the stroma. The primitive cells that initiate hemopoiesis in LTBMC, the long-term culture initiating cells (LTCIC), are multipotent and have at least a limited self-renewal capacity allowing them to generate CFU-GEMM, GM-CFC, G-CFC, M-CFC, BFU-E, and CFU-E for periods extending to several months. In other words, the LTCIC have many characteristics in common with stem cells, and because of this the LTBMC system has been used to assess the function of the stromal layer and its interaction with primitive hemopoietic cells and their progeny and to measure the responses of hemopoietic cells to growth factors. In appropriate circumstances, however, the stromal cells can support the proliferation of "non-self" hemopoietic cells, and these secondary cultures have proved to be useful models for detecting possible age-related changes in model systems.[33,37,44–47]

GROWTH FACTORS IN HEMOPOIESIS

Growth inhibitory and stimulatory molecules are produced or sequestered by the stromal cells and hemopoietic cells within the bone marrow, and such factors clearly play an important role in hemopoietic cell development.[13] Receptors with a high affinity for these growth factors are expressed by hemopoietic cells and transduce signals which can influence the cell cycle status and/or induce or facilitate differentiation and activation of mature cells. The type of growth factor, its concentration, the presence or absence of the appropriate receptor, the differentiation status of the cell, and the presence of other costimulatory or inhibitory growth factors are all important in determining the response of the target cells, that is, whether or not to enter the cell cycle, to self-renew, or to differentiate.[13] Furthermore, it is also now known that a major role of growth factors is to suppress apoptosis; indeed this may be one of the primary mechanisms that regulate normal levels of cell proliferation in the bone marrow and that is responsible for greater or fewer cells being released into the circulation.

In studies designed to investigate whether or not the response of hemopoietic cells to growth factors undergoes age-related changes[48] it was found that in elderly patients (who had a hematological malignancy or chronic disease or had received myelotoxic drugs), the hemopoietic response in vivo to recombinant hemopoietic growth factors was well conserved compared to that in young patients. However, an in-vitro study of bone marrow from healthy elderly (70–80 years old) and healthy young (20–30 years old) volunteers revealed a decline in the proliferative response to G-CSF in the elderly group.[49] Another in-vitro study has shown that stromal cells from healthy elderly subjects are less responsive to interleukin-1-induced expression of GM-CSF or G-CSF genes than younger subjects.[49a] Apart from impaired responses due to aging, however, there may be changes in the relative importance of growth factors during a normal lifespan—it is known, for example, that interleukin-9[50] and interleukin-11[51] are of more importance in fetal than in adult hemopoiesis.

PERIPHERAL BLOOD

Early studies on red cell indexes in aging populations suggested that a fall in hemoglobin and a decrease in red cell mass were age related,[52–55] and it was hypothesized that they might be secondary to the reduced oxygen demand associated with a sedentary lifestyle.[56] The confounding effects of intercurrent illness on red cell parameters were not fully appreciated until 1984 when agreement was reached regarding a definition of the healthy elderly population provided by the Senieur guidelines.[57] Even these suggested the use of a hemoglobin range lower than that applied to the rest of the adult population, based on an earlier study by Landahl et al.[58] Recent studies using the clinical recommendations of the Senieur protocol indicate that red cell indexes are well preserved even in centenarians.[59,60]

However, aging is associated with impairment of cellular and humoral immunity, so-called immunosenescence, and this is reflected in an increase in the incidence of infections that accompanies aging. This has been attributed to a decline in T-cell function, since T-cells from aged compared to young subjects are less responsive to mitogens, less responsive to antigen stimulation, and less able to promote B-cell activation and differentiation. There is a fall in total numbers and shifts in the contributions made to the total count by T-cell subpopulations. Further, there is evidence of age-dependent variation in intracellular signal transduction events.[61]

CD4 T-helper cells, responsible for major histocompatibility complex class II restricted recognition of foreign antigen and subsequent activation of CD8 T-suppressor, B-lymphocyte, and granulocyte effector cells of the immune response, show an overall decline with age,[62,63] accompanied by a reduction in capacity to produce naïve CD4CD45RA+ T-cells[63,64] but an expansion in CD45RO+ memory T-cells. The latter changes may be a consequence of stem cell exhaustion (considered unlikely in view of the apparently normal myelopoiesis occurring in these patients) or a defect in the ability of the stem cells to undergo differentiation to produce pre-T-cells or the absence of a thymus or thymus-like microenvironment. There is also a statistically significant increase in the CD4+ CD8+ subset during aging in humans.[65] Coincident with this is a clonal expansion of the CD8+ CD28− subset, particularly after the age of 50. The absence of the CD28 costimulatory antigen may contribute to the lack of responsiveness of T cells to antigen in the aged. It is also speculated that they represent the CD8+ CD28+ subset in its senescent state or that they are a wholly independent suppressor T-cell lineage. Nociari et al.[66] cite experimental evidence to support their hypothesis that CD8+ CD28− population is antigen experienced, despite their frequent coexpression of CD45RA, and is associated with the age-related decline in immune function, since it secretes suppressor cytokines such as IL-10, capable of inhibiting immune responses. Consequently, this raises the possibility that these age-related changes are genetically programmed rather than the net result of a response to accumulation of damaged DNA. (See, however, Chapter 4.)

Another likely cause for immune unresponsiveness to antigen is the age-related reduction in human leukocyte antigen (HLA) expression on T lymphocytes, B lymphocytes, and monocytes.[67] Class I HLA expression is reduced in all three populations; class II HLA-DR expression is increased overall within the T-cell population but decreased in individual cells, while it is reduced overall in the B-cell population, although positive cells express normal numbers. These phenotypic changes would be predicted to result in impaired antigen presentation via Class II HLA and a reduction in the effector T-cell response mediated by Class I HLA restriction. Since HLA-mediated presentation of foreign antigen is a crucial component of host defense to infection these observations help to explain the susceptibility of elderly people to infection. Adhesion molecules contribute to T-cell activation in a non-antigen-specific manner and expression of CD50 (ICAM-3) and CD62L (L selectin homing receptor) is up-regulated in naïve and memory T cells in aged populations: De Martinis et al.[68] speculate that this may be a compensatory mechanism that redresses decreased responsiveness and a greater requirement for activation signals.

Sansoni et al.[60] made a careful study of lymphocyte subsets and natural killer (NK) activity in the healthy elderly and showed that while the number of CD4 and CD8 T-cells fell with age, there was a rise in the number of activated T cells of CD3+HLA-DR+ phenotype and a rise in the number of functional NK CD16+CD57− and CD16−CD57+ cells in healthy centenarians. Curiously, a control group of middle-aged subjects (range 50–68 years) had relatively low NK activity compared to that of the centenarians and young subjects (range 19–30 years), and this has prompted speculation that maintenance of NK activity may be related to a "longevity phenotype." B-lymphocyte numbers in peripheral blood decline with age,[60] but this may represent a redistribution of cells into lymphoid follicles[7] since immunoglobulins and IgG subclasses rise with age in the absence of malignancy.[69–71]

In terms of functional relevance to the aged individual, a Swedish longitudinal study of a cohort of very old subjects aged 86–92 years at baseline has linked certain of the immunological parameters with a reduction in survival. Their initial study[72] defined the differences in immune function in their study cohort as compared to a control group of healthy middle-aged subjects. The most prominent changes were a reduction in proliferative responses to the T-cell mitogen conconavalin A and total CD3+ numbers. When the cohort was reviewed after a 2-year interval,[73] it became apparent that a cluster of immune characteristics defined the nonsurvivors, namely, poor T-cell proliferative responses, high CD8+ T-cell percentages, and low CD4+ T-cell CD4+:CD8+ ratio and CD19+ B-cell percentages. This constellation was more significant than any single parameter taken in isolation. Additionally, subjects who developed this profile in subsequent years of the study[74] acquired the risk for higher mortality. An underlying cellular mechanism to explain the phenotypic and functional features of immune senescence is not yet identified with any certainty. Extrapolation of murine data predicts that failure of interleukin-2 production and dysregulated apoptotic pathways lead to expansion of hyporesponsive and senescent cells within the aging immune system.[75,76]

TELOMERES, CELLULAR SENESCENCE, AND HUMAN AGING

The acceptance of the existence of the totipotential stem cell that is capable of maintaining peripheral blood components throughout life raises further questions about the capacity of that stem cell in terms of the total number of self-renewing cell divisions it can make and whether these are sufficient for the human life span. Normal somatic cells appear to have a finite number of cell divisions available to them: in, 1961, Leonard Hayflick and Paul Moorhead described experiments that generated the concept of the Hayflick limit[77]—that each cell has a predetermined number of cell divisions that it can undergo before entering a resting phase called senescence. These post-mitotic cells do not die upon entering senescence but instead may survive for several years with normal function. During this phase, they may accumulate fibronectin, apolipoprotein J and p21, all of which have been associated[42] with the senescent state.[78] Thus, primary cultures of fibroblasts derived from fetal human lung tissue undergo 40–60 population doublings before reaching senescence. That this was intrinsic to the cells rather than the culture conditions was demonstrated by co-culture of cells derived from the forty-ninth passage of a male cell strain with those from the thirteenth passage of a female strain: after a further 17 subcultures male cells were no longer detectable within the limits of the techniques available.[77]

Elucidation of the cellular biochemistry that underlies the Hayflick limit may eventually be gained from the greater understanding that has been achieved in the last decade of the role of the telomere in cell division. (See also Chapter 8.) Telomeres are the G-rich hexanucleotide repeat sequences that are found at the termini of eukaryotic chromosomes. Their length varies according to cell lineage but in general telomeres derived from germ cells or fetal cells are longer than those of adult somatic cells.[79–81] In normal somatic cells, cell division is associated with a shortening of telomere length.[79,80,82] The likely explanation of this phenomenon is the "lagging strand end replication problem" hypothesis advanced by James D. Watson.[83] It proposes that the inability of DNA polymerases to replicate the 3′ end of linear DNA molecules due to their requirement for a primer sequence imposes attrition of the terminal region with successive rounds of cell division. In vertebrates, the repetitive sequence is TTAGGG and it is believed that the function of the telomeres is to protect the chromosomal terminal from potentially destabilizing events such as illegitimate recombination. Telomeres may also be responsible for the silencing of subtelomeric genes, thereby regulating and stabilizing chromosomal expression.[84] Telomeres appear to be closely involved in the regulation of the replicative capacity of the cell and, in some species of yeast, loss of telomeres causes cell cycle arrest.[85,86] In human cells telomere erosion may ultimately trigger an array of DNA damage responses. The resultant activation of p53 and Rb dependent cell cycle checkpoints causes exit from cell cycle and cellular senescence.[79,80] Some cells, notably germ line cells, maintain telomere length via the action of several telomere related proteins such as the reverse transcriptase complex telomerase,[87] and the DNA-sequence specific duplex binding proteins RAP1[88–90] and TRF.[91] Telomerase, comprising telomerase RNA (TR) and a telomerase reverse transcriptase protein (TERT), facilitates RNA-dependent synthesis of telomeric repeats, thereby overcoming the end replication problem[87] in the cells in which it is expressed. Forced overexpression of the catalytic subunit of telomerase, TERT, in cultured human fibroblasts permits the state of cell senescence to be bypassed and confers a state of apparent immortality.[92,93] Extrapolation of these data suggests that telomere attrition may precipitate the state of senescence in human cells (reviewed by Sherr and DePinho[94]).

The hemopoietic system is notable for its rapid turnover and capacity for proliferative responses and this has stimulated several studies of telomere attrition and telomerase activity in hemopoietic cells. The central question is the extent to which the totipotential hemopoietic cell is affected by telomere erosion during its cycles of self-renewal and whether this has biological relevance to the individual. Murine models are of limited significance in this setting, since telomeres in mice are, at 60 kilobases, approximately five times longer than their human counterparts. However, in genetically engineered telomerase-deficient mice that are studied over successive breeding generations, telomeres show progressive shortening.[95] In later generations it is noteworthy that aberrant hemopoietic stem cell function develops together with splenic cell atrophy, impaired B- and T-lymphocyte proliferation in response to mitogens, and impairment of germinal center formation following immunization.

Hastie et al.[80] reported age-related reduction in telomere length in peripheral blood DNA obtained from 47 healthy subjects aged 20–79 and estimated an annual loss of 33 base pairs. This was in keeping with the assumption that telomere loss was an inevitable feature of somatic cell division but an unexpected revelation was the detection of telomerase in normal somatic cells.[96–98] A larger study of 80 subjects aged 4–95[99] confirmed the age-related erosion of telomere length in peripheral blood mononuclear cells but identified two distinct phases of loss. Their data indicated an average attrition rate of 84 base pairs per year between the ages of 4 and 39 years but a deceleration after the age of 40 years to a rate of 41 base pairs per year. Telomerase activity was also studied and found to decline steadily between the ages of 4 and 39 years but in older individuals one of two patterns was observed: 65 percent of those over 41 years had stable but low levels of telomerase and the remainder had none detectable. It seems probable that the reduction in peripheral blood cell telomere length with age may reflect the net effect of the replicative history of the cell and a decay in telomerase activity. Frenck[100] went on to show that the rate of telomerase shortening in human peripheral blood mononuclear cells is greatest in children up to the age of 4 years (>1 kilobase per year), slows between the ages of 4 and 20, and then declines gradually during the rest of life. Rufer et al.[101] confirmed and extended these observations by studying the telomere lengths of distinct lineages within peripheral blood mononuclear cells taken from more than 500 subjects ranging from infants to 90-year-olds. They found that telomere length decreased as a function of age for granulocytes as well as T-lymphocytes. The maximum rate of telomerase loss in granulocytes, and naïve and memory CD4 and CD8 T-cells was seen in early childhood and was in the region of 1–3,000 base pairs per year. After this period, the rate of loss fell to 30–60 base pairs per year and was relatively constant throughout life. The increased rate of telomere loss seen in early life may reflect increased telomere loss per cell division or an increased rate of cell division: Frenck et al.[100] postulate that telomere loss is differentially regulated in leukocytes of young children and adults.

In trying to map the relationship of precursor cells to distant progeny in terms of numbers of cell divisions that separate the two populations it may be necessary to consider the possibility of intermittent resurgence of telomerase activity. The naïve B-lymphocyte will, upon appropriate stimulation of its Ig receptor, undergo proliferation and differentiation to generate germinal center centroblasts and centrocytes and, eventually, plasma cells or memory cells. The telomere length of successive generations does not fall in the linear pattern predicted by the early model in which successive cell division was linked to successive cell division.[79,80] Instead, the germinal center B-cells have telomeres that are longer than the precursor naïve B-cells or their later descendants, memory cells. Significantly, telomerase activity is detectable in the germinal center but barely present or absent in the naïve or memory B-cells.[14] T-lymphocytes cultured in vitro display high telomerase activity alongside the presence of maintained telomere lengths and this is characteristic of early stages of culture and T-cell activation.[98,102] The opposite is true of the late stages of culture in which telomerase activity is lost and telomeres are lost rapidly.

Consequently, the decline in telomerase activity in peripheral blood cells with age may have been due to the reduced contribution made by activated lymphocytes or primitive hemopoietic stem cells to peripheral blood in older subjects. While stem cells constitute less than 0.01 percent of bone marrow mononuclear cells advances in cell biology permit recognition of hemopoietic stem cell phenotypes. Subsets of primitive hemopoietic progenitor cells may be purified by virtue of the pattern of intensity of expression of the cell surface glycoproteins or proteins such as CD34 or CD38 as well as the absence of markers that denote commitment to differentiation to distinct hemopoietic lineages (Lin$^-$). Vaziri et al.[103] studied DNA derived from CD34$^+$CD38$^{lo/-}$Lin$^-$ primitive hemopoietic progenitors purified from human bone marrow and compared it to similar extracts from umbilical cord blood and fetal liver, tissues that are greatly enriched in primitive hemopoietic cells. Telomere sequence analysis indicated that mean telomere length was shorter in DNA derived from adult than fetal or perinatal tissue. When these cells were cultured in vitro in the presence of cytokine combinations designed to promote proliferation it was confirmed that each population doubling was associated with a mean loss of telomere length. These data are suggestive of telomere loss within the stem cell compartment associated with aging of the organism. However, a confounding possibility is that, even within these highly selected cells thought to be representative of primitive hemopoietic stem cells, there is considerable heterogeneity and that many cells are already committed to differentiation at the expense of self-renewal.

The nature of telomerase expression and associated telomere length in human hemopoietic stem cells was also addressed by Engelhardt et al.[104] who extracted highly purified populations of CD34+ CD38– and CD34+CD38+cells from fetal liver, cord blood, adult bone marrow, and peripheral blood (the latter obtained from patients with newly diagnosed neoplasms and enriched in primitive hemopoietic progenitors as part of high-dose chemotherapy protocols). Cells were analyzed at baseline and after culture in cytokine combinations chosen to maximize stem cell self-renewal in vitro. Mean telomere lengths were analyzed in cord, marrow, and peripheral blood CD34+cells and found to be longest in cord cells at 10.4 kilobase pairs (kbp) compared to 7.4 and 7.6 kbp in marrow and blood CD34+cells. Telomere shortening was observed in all populations after culture in vitro for 4 weeks. However, telomere loss was significantly lower in the first 2 weeks of culture than the last 2 weeks and this was associated with the up-regulation of telomerase activity that was observed in the early life of the culture. While baseline telomerase activity was higher in bone marrow and peripheral blood CD34+ cells than cord or fetal liver CD34+ cells and very low in CD34– cells, all cultures showed up-regulation of telomerase activity within 48–72 hours of exposure to optimal cytokine combinations. Activity peaked at 1 week and then decayed rapidly to baseline levels and was associated with G_1-S phase progression of the cell cycle and induction of expression of the proteins pRb and G_1/S cyclins A and D1. Comparison of CD34+ CD38– with the less primitive CD34+ CD38+ cell population revealed that telomerase activity was absent in the former but detectable in the latter and that the cultured CD34+ CD38+ generated more cells and mature colony forming cells after exposure to cytokines. While telomerase activity was inducible in the CD34+ CD38– stem cell fraction, this population was relatively quiescent in comparison to the CD34+CD38+ early progenitor fraction. A fall in telomerase activity and rapid telomere shortening might be a consequence of progressive differentiation. However, extraction of CD34+ cells from established cultures allowed the analysis of secondary CD34+ cell characteristics, which had a reduced capacity for up-regulation of telomerase activity, and this served to support the hypothesis that inducible telomerase activity in the most primitive hemopoietic cells reduces but does not prevent telomere shortening on proliferation. In fact, telomerase activity seemed to be repressed in G_0 stem cells and terminally differentiated cells but inducible in conditions that promoted CD34+ cell expansion and also proliferation. The inexorable loss of telomere length in successive generations of hemopoietic stem cells may indicate that hemopoietic stem cells are not truly self-renewing, yet it remains possible that subpopulations not detectable in bulk culture fulfill this role.

Interpretation of in-vitro studies of cell growth characteristics is handicapped by the unquantifiable effects of the culture conditions themselves. However, in the case of the human hemopoietic system, in-vitro studies of the relationship of senescence, aging, and telomeres have been supplemented by information gained from the routine clinical application of allogeneic hemopoietic stem cell transplantation (ASCT) following myeloablation in the treatment of neoplastic or hemopoietic stem cell disease. In this scenario, a finite, and relatively small, number of hemopoietic stem cells must repopulate the entire hemopoietic system and thereby overcome a direct challenge to the self-renewing capacity of the hemopoietic system. Thus, Notaro et al.[105] studied 11 fully engrafted transplant recipients in tandem with their donors. Specifically, they analyzed telomere length by single chromosome analysis in peripheral blood granulocytes, thereby selecting a leukocyte subpopulation that has a rapid turnover in contrast to long-lived and heterogeneous lymphocytes. They found that telomeres in engrafted granulocytes extracted from the transplant recipient were significantly shorter than those found in the donor's own peripheral circulation. The age of the donor and the time that had elapsed since transplant bore no relation to the extent of telomere shortening but the number of nucleated cells, and hence the number of stem cells, infused demonstrated a significant correlation with the extent of telomere shortening. The fewer the number of stem cells infused, the greater the number of replications that must be achieved in order to repopulate the hemopoietic organs. These extra replications may occur within the stem cell compartment or more distally but are inevitably accompanied by telomere shortening. Notaro's study comprised almost entirely adult donors, but an analysis of telomere shortening in children post-ASCT[106] revealed that patients who received ASCT from donors older than 18 years had significantly shorter telomeres than those transplanted from donors younger than 18 years. Long-term follow-up studies are required to assess the eventual impact of this upon hemopoiesis. These observations of the in-vivo situation tend to support the in-vitro data and imply that hemopoietic stem cell proliferation is associated with telomere loss. However, late graft failure is an unusual complication following successful hemopoietic stem cell transplant and this suggests that there is ample hemopoietic stem cell capacity for an individual lifespan.

The link between replicative senescence occurring at the cellular level and organismal aging is not fully clear. Replicative senescence does not necessarily explain post-mitotic tissue aging or even stem cell aging. However, advances in investigative techniques as described above are proving useful tools in the study of human aging. This will allow a better understanding of the mechanisms of aging, and to what extent they can be remedied, as well as advances in therapeutic strategies in many fields, particularly infectious diseases, cancer, and transplantation.

REFERENCES

1. Dexter TM, Moore MAS: In vitro duplication and "cure" of haemopoietic defects in genetically anaemic mice. Nature 1977;269:412–414
2. Bain B, Clark D, Lampert IA: Bone Marrow Pathology. Blackwell Scientific Publications, Oxford, 1992
3. Kricun ME: Red-yellow marrow conversion: its effect on the location of some solitary bone lesions. Skeletal Radiol 1985;14(1):10–19
4. Moore SG, Dawson KL: Red and yellow marrow in the femur: age-related changes in appearance at MR imaging. Radiology 1990;175(1):219–223
5. Ricci C, Cova M, Kang YS et al: Normal age-related patterns of cellular and fatty bone marrow distribution in the axial skeleton: MR imaging study. Radiology 1990;177(1):83–88
6. Kita K, Kawai K, Hirohata K: Changes in bone marrow blood flow with ageing. J Orthop Res 1987;5:569–575
7. Liu PI, Takanari H, Yatani R, Nelson G: Comparative studies of bone marrow from the United States and Japan. Ann Clin Lab Sci 1989;19(5):345–351
8. Hartsock RJ, Smith EB, Petty CS: Normal variations with ageing of the amount of hematopoietic tissue in bone marrow from the anterior iliac crest: a study made from 177 cases of sudden death examined by necropsy. Am J Clin Pathol 1965;43:326–331
9. Yip R, Johnson C, Dallman PR: Age-related changes in laboratory values used in the diagnosis of anemia and iron deficiency. Am J Clin Nutr 1984;39(3):427–436
10. Lipschitz DA, Udupa KB, Milton KY, Thumpson CO: Effect of age on hematopoiesis in man. Blood 1984;63(3):502–509
11. Douek DC, McFarland RD, Keiser PH et al: Changes in thymic function with age and during the treatment of HIV infection. Nature 1998;396(6712):690–695
12. Poulin JF, Viswanathan MN, Komanduri KV et al: Direct evidence for thymic function in adult humans. J Exp Med 1999;190(4):479–486
13. Metcalf D: The Colony Stimulating Factors. Elsevier, Amsterdam, 1984
14. Dexter TM: Growth and differentiation in the haemopoietic system. Biochem Soc Trans 1991;19(2):303–306
15. Fialkow PJ: Primordial cell pool size and lineage relationships of five human cell types. Ann Hum Genet 1973;37(1):39–48
16. Vogelstein B, Fearon ER, Hamilton SR et al: Clonal analysis using recombinant DNA probes from the X-chromosome. Cancer Res 1987;47(18):4806–4813
17. Gale RE, Wheadon H, Linch DC: X-chromosome inactivation patterns using HPRT and PGK polymorphisms in haematologically normal and post-chemotherapy females. Br J Haematol 1991;79(2):193–197
18. Till JE, McCulloch EA: A direct measurement of normal mouse bone marrow cells. Radiat Res 1961;14:213–222
19. Harrison DE, Zhong RK: The same exhaustible multilineage precursor produces both myeloid and lymphoid cells as early as 3–4 weeks after marrow transplantation. Proc Natl Acad Sci USA, 1992;89(21):10134–10138
20. Szilvassy SJ, Humphries RK, Lansdorp PM et al: Quantitative assay for totipotent reconstituting hematopoietic stem cells by a competitive repopulation strategy. Proc Natl Acad Sci USA 1990;87(22):8736–8740
21. Aversa F, Tabilio A, Velardi A et al: Treatment of high-risk acute leukemia with T-cell-depleted stem cells from related donors with one fully mismatched HLA haplotype. N Engl J Med 1998;339(17):1186–1193
22. Lemischka IR, Raulet DH, Mulligan RC: Developmental potential and dynamic behavior of hematopoietic stem cells. Cell 1986;45(6):917–927
23. Brown G, Jones NA, Bunce CM et al: Haemopoiesis: a lottery or genomic determinism? Br J Haematol 1991;79(3):527–529
24. Dexter TM, Spooncer E: Growth and differentiation in the hemopoietic system. Annu Rev Cell Biol 1987;3:423–441
25. Fairbairn LJ, Cowling GJ, Reipert BM, Dexter TM: Suppression of apoptosis allows differentiation and development of a multipotent hemopoietic cell line in the absence of added growth factors. Cell 1993;74(5):823–832
26. Blackett N, Gordon M: "Stochastic"—40 years of use and abuse. Blood 1999;93(9):3148–3149
27. Curry JL, Trentin JJ: Haemopoietic spleen colony stimulating factors. Science 1967;236:1229–1237
28. Metcalf D: Lineage commitment and maturation in hematopoietic cells: the case for extrinsic regulation. Blood 1998;92(2):345–347 (discussion 352)
29. Enver T, Heyworth CM, Dexter TM: Do stem cells play dice? Blood 1998;92(2):348–351 (discussion 352)
30. Hellman S, Botnick LE: Stem cell depletion: an explanation of the late effects of cytotoxins. Int J Radiat Oncol Biol Phys 1977;2(1–2):181–184
31. Ogden DA, Micklem HS: The fate of serially transplanted bone marrow cell populations from young and old donors. Transplantation 1976;22:287–290
32. Lajtha LG, Schofield R: Regulation of stem cell renewal and differentiation: possible significance in ageing. In Strehler BL (ed): Advances in Gerontological Research. New York, Academic Press, 1971
33. Schofield R, Dexter TM, Lord BI, Testa NG: Comparison of haemopoiesis in young and old mice. Mech Ageing Dev 1986;34(1):1–12
34. Schofield R, Lord BI, Kyffin S et al: Self-maintenance capacity of CFU-S. J Cell Physiol 1980;103(2):355–362
35. Harrison DE, Astle CM: Loss of stem cell repopulating ability upon transplantation. Effects of donor age, cell number, and transplantation procedure. J Exp Med 1982;156(6):1767–1779
36. Jordan CT, Lemischka IR: Clonal and systemic analysis of long-term hematopoiesis in the mouse. Genes Dev 1990;4(2):220–232
37. Tejero C, Testa NG, Hendry JH: Decline in cycling of granulocyte-macrophage colony-forming cells with increasing age in mice. Exp Hematol 1989;17(1):66–67
38. Williams GT, Smith GT, Spooncer E et al: Haemopoietic colony stimulating factors promote cell survival by suppressing apoptosis. Nature 1990;343(6253):76–79
39. Resnitzky P, Segal M, Barak, Dassa C et al: Granulopoiesis in aged people: inverse correlation between bone marrow cellularity and myeloid progenitor cell numbers. Gerontology 1987;33(2):109–114
40. Marley SB, Lewis JH, Pairdson RJ et al: Evidence for a continuous decline in haemopoietic cell function from birth: application to evaluating bone marrow failure in children. Br J Haematol 1999;106(1):162–166
41. Gale RE, Fielding AK, Harrison CN et al: Acquired skewing of X-chromosome inactivation patterns in myeloid cells of the elderly suggests stochastic clonal loss with age. Br J Haematol 1997;98(3):512–519
42. Vickers MA, McLeod E, Spector TD et al: Assessment of mechanism of acquired skewed X inactivation by analysis of twins. Blood 2001;97(5):1274–1281
43. Dexter TM, Allen TD, Lajtha LG: Conditions controlling the proliferation of haemopoietic stem cells in vitro. J Cell Physiol 1977;91(3):335–344
44. Boggs DR, Patrene KD: Hematopoiesis and ageing III: Anemia and a blunted erythropoietic response to hemorrhage in aged mice. Am J Hematol 1985;19(4):327–338

45. Inoue T, Cronkite EP: The influence of in vivo incubation of aged murine spleen colony-forming units on their proliferative capacity. Mech Ageing Dev 1983;23(2):177–190

46. Lipschitz DA, Udupa KB: Age and the hematopoietic system. J Am Geriatr Soc 1986;34(6):448–454

47. Mauch P, Botnick LE, Hannon EC et al: Decline in bone marrow proliferative capacity as a function of age. Blood 1982;60(1):245–252

48. Shank WA, Jr, Balducci L: Recombinant hemopoietic growth factors: comparative hemopoietic response in younger and older subjects. J Am Geriatr Soc 1992;40(2):151–154

49. Chatta GS, Andrew RG, Rodger E et al: Hematopoietic progenitors and ageing: alterations in granulocytic precursors and responsiveness to recombinant human G-CSF, GM-CSF, and IL-3. J Gerontol A 1993;48(5):M207–M212

49a. Lee MA, Segal GM, Bagby GC: The hematopoietic microenvironment in the elderly: defects in IL-1-induced CSF expression in vitro. Exp Hematol 1989;17:952–956

50. Holbrook ST, Ohls RK, Schibler KR et al: Effect of interleukin-9 on clonogenic maturation and cell-cycle status of fetal and adult hematopoietic progenitors. Blood 1991;77(10):2129–2134

51. Schibler KR, Yang YC, Christensen RD: Effect of interleukin-II on cycling status and clonogenic maturation of fetal and adult hematopoietic progenitors. Blood 1992;80(4):900–903

52. McLennan WJ, Andrew GR, Macleod C et al: Anaemia in the elderly. Q J Med 1973;42(165):1–13

53. Hill RD: The prevalence of anaemia in a rural practice. Practitioner 1967;217:961–963

54. Piomelli S, Nathan DG, Cummins JF et al: The relationship of total red cell volume to total body water in octogenarian males. Blood 1962;19:89–92

55. Myers MA, Saunders CRG, Chalmers DG: The haemoglobin of fit elderly people. Lancet 1968;2:261–263

56. Besa EC: Approach to mild anemia in the elderly. Clin Geriatr Med 1988;4(1):43–55

57. Ligthart GJ, Corberand JX, Fournier C et al: Admission criteria for immunogerontological studies in man: the SENIEUR protocol. Mech Ageing Dev 1984;28(1):47–55

58. Landahl S, Jagenburg R, Svanborg A: Blood components in a 70-year-old population. Clin Chim Acta 1981;112(3):301–314

59. Baldwin JJ: True anaemia: incidence and significance in the elderly. Geriatrics 1989;44:33–36

60. Sansoni P, Cossarizza A, Brianti V et al: Lymphocyte subsets and natural killer cell activity in healthy old people and centenarians. Blood 1993;82(9):2767–2773

61. Di Pietro R, Miscia S, Cataldi A et al: Age-dependent variations in the expression of PLC isoforms upon mitogenic stimulation of peripheral blood T cells from healthy donors. Br J Haematol 2000;111(4):1209–1214

62. Roberts-Thomson IC, Whittingham S, Youngchaiyud U et al: Ageing, immune response, and mortality. Lancet 1974;2(7877):368–370

63. Weinberg K, Parkman R: Age, the thymus, and T lymphocytes. N Engl J Med 1995;332(3):182–183

64. Mackall CL, Fleisher TA, Brown MR et al: Age, thymopoiesis, and CD4+ T-lymphocyte regeneration after intensive chemotherapy. N Engl J Med 1995;332(3):143–149

65. Laux I, Khoshran A, Tindell C et al: Response differences between human CD4(+) and CD8(+) T-cells during CD28 costimulation: implications for immune cell-based therapies and studies related to the expansion of double-positive T-cells during ageing. Clin Immunol 2000;96(3):187–197

66. Nociari MM, Telford W, Russo C: Postthymic development of CD28–CD28+ T cell subset: age-associated expansion and shift from memory to naive phenotype. J Immunol 1999;162(6):3327–3335

67. Le Morvan C, Cogne M, Troutand D et al: Modification of HLA expression on peripheral lymphocytes and monocytes during ageing. Mech Ageing Dev 1998;105(3):209–220

68. De Martinis M, Modesti M, Profeta VF et al: CD50 and CD62L adhesion receptor expression on naive (CD45RA+) and memory (CD45RO+) T lymphocytes in the elderly. Pathobiology 2000;68(6):245–250

69. Radl J, Sepers JM, Skvaril F et al: Immunoglobulin patterns in humans over 95 years of age. Clin Exp Immunol 1975;22(1):84–90

70. Radl J: Effects of ageing on Immunoglobulins. In Ritzmann S, (ed): Pathology of Immunoglobulins. Alan R Liss, New York, 1982:52–69

71. Paganelli R, Quinti I, Fagiolo U et al: Changes in circulating B cells and immunoglobulin classes and subclasses in a healthy aged population. Clin Exp Immunol 1992;90(2):351–354

72. Wikby A, Johansson B, Ferguson F et al: Age-related changes in immune parameters in a very old population of Swedish people: a longitudinal study. Exp Gerontol 1994;29(5):531–541

73. Ferguson FG, Wikby A, Maxson P et al: Immune parameters in a longitudinal study of a very old population of Swedish people: a comparison between survivors and nonsurvivors. J Gerontol A 1995;50(6):B378–B382

74. Wikby A, Maxson P, Olsson J et al: Changes in CD8 and CD4 lymphocyte subsets, T cell proliferation responses and non-survival in the very old: the Swedish longitudinal OCTO-immune study. Mech Ageing Dev 1998;102:187–198

75. Linton PJ, Haynes L, Tsui L et al: From naive to effector—alterations with ageing. Immunol Rev 1997;160:9–18

76. Mountz JD, Wu J, Zhou T et al: Cell death and longevity: implications of Fas-mediated apoptosis in T-cell senescence. Immunol Rev 1997;160:19–30

77. Hayflick L, Moorhead P: The serial cultivation of human diploid cell strains. Exp Cell Res 1961;25:585–621

78. Mondello C, Petropoulou C, Monti D et al: Telomere length in fibroblasts and blood cells from healthy centenarians. Exp Cell Res 1999;248(1):234–242

79. Harley CB, Futcher AB, Greider CW: Telomeres shorten during ageing of human fibroblasts. Nature 1990;345(6274):458–460

80. Hastie ND, Dempster M, Dunlop MG et al: Telomere reduction in human colorectal carcinoma and with ageing. Nature 1990;346(6287):866–868

81. Lindsey J, McGill NI, Lindsey LA et al: In vivo loss of telomeric repeats with age in humans. Mutat Res 1991;256(1):45–48

82. Allsopp RC, Vaziri H, Patterson C et al: Telomere length predicts replicative capacity of human fibroblasts. Proc Natl Acad Sci USA 1992;89(21):10114–10118

83. Watson JD: Origin of concatemeric T7 DNA. Nat New Biol 1972;239(94):197–201

84. Hande MP, Samper E, Lansdorp P et al: Telomere length dynamics and chromosomal instability in cells derived from telomerase null mice. J Cell Biol 1999;144(4):589–601

85. Lundblad V, Szostak JW: A mutant with a defect in telomere elongation leads to senescence in yeast. Cell 1989;57(4):633–643

86. Sandell LL, Zakian VA: Loss of a yeast telomere: arrest, recovery, and chromosome loss. Cell 1993;75(4):729–739

87. Greider CW, Blackburn EH: Identification of a specific telomere terminal transferase activity in Tetrahymena extracts. Cell 1985;43 (2 Pt 1):405–413

88. Kyrion G, Boakye KA, Lustig AJ: C-terminal truncation of RAP1 results in the deregulation of telomere size, stability, and function in *Saccharomyces cerevisiae.* Mol Cell Biol 1992;12(11): 5159–5173

89. Krauskopf A, Blackburn EH: Control of telomere growth by interactions of RAP1 with the most distal telomeric repeats. Nature 1996;383(6598):354–357

90. McEachern MJ, Blackburn EH: Runaway telomere elongation caused by telomerase RNA gene mutations. Nature 1995;376 (6539):403–409

91. Chong L, van Steensel B, Broccoli D et al: A human telomeric protein. Science 1995;270(5242):1663–1667

92. Jiang XR, Jimenez G, Chang E et al: Telomerase expression in human somatic cells does not induce changes associated with a transformed phenotype. Nat Genet 1999;21(1):111–114

93. Bodnar AG, Oule He M, Frolkis M et al: Extension of life-span by introduction of telomerase into normal human cells. Science 1998;279(5349):349–352

94. Sherr CJ, DePinho RA: Cellular senescence: mitotic clock or culture shock? Cell 2000;102(4):407–410

95. Blasco MA, Lee HW, Handz MP et al: Telomere shortening and tumor formation by mouse cells lacking telomerase RNA. Cell 1997;91 (1):25–34

96. Broccoli D, Young JW, de Lange T: Telomerase activity in normal and malignant hematopoietic cells. Proc Natl Acad Sci USA 1995;92(20):9082–9086

97. Hiyama K, Hirai Y, Kyoizumi S et al: Activation of telomerase in human lymphocytes and hematopoietic progenitor cells. J Immunol 1995;155(8):3711–3715

98. Buchkovich KJ, Greider CW: Telomerase regulation during entryinto the cell cycle in normal human T cells. Mol Biol Cell 1996;7(9):1443–1454

99. Iwama H, Ohyashiki K, Ohyashiki JH et al: Telomeric length and telomerase activity vary with age in peripheral blood cells obtained from normal individuals. Hum Genet 1998;102(4):397–402

100. Frenck RW, Jr, Blackburn EH, Shannon KM: The rate of telomere sequence loss in human leukocytes varies with age. Proc Natl Acad Sci USA 1998;95(10):5607–5610

101. Rufer N, Brumonendorf TH, Kolvraa S et al: Telomere fluorescence measurements in granulocytes and T lymphocyte subsets point to a high turnover of hematopoietic stem cells and memory T cells in early childhood. J Exp Med 1999;190(2):157–167

102. Brousset P, al Saati T, Chaouche et al: Telomerase activity in reactive and neoplastic lymphoid tissues: infrequent detection of activity in Hodgkin's disease. Blood 1997;89(1):26–31

103. Vaziri H, Dragowska W, Allsopp RC et al: Evidence for a mitotic clock in human hematopoietic stem cells: loss of telomeric DNA with age. Proc Natl Acad Sci USA 1994;91(21):9857–9860

104. Engelhardt M, Kumar R, Albanell J et al: Telomerase regulation, cell cycle, and telomere stability in primitive hematopoietic cells. Blood 1997;90(1):182–193

105. Notaro R, Cimmino A, Tabarini D et al: In vivo telomere dynamics of human hematopoietic stem cells. Proc Natl Acad Sci USA 1997;94(25):13782–13785

106. Akiyama M, Hoshi Y, Sakurai S et al: Changes of telomere length in children after hematopoietic stem cell transplantation. Bone Marrow Transplant 1998;21(2):167–171

Chapter 98

Blood disorders and their management in old age

Mary Lynn R. Nierodzik, David Sutin, and

Michael L. Freedman

DISEASES OF THE RED BLOOD CELLS
Anemia

Anemia can be defined as a reduction in the number of circulating red cells below the normal range. A US national health and nutrition study defined the normal range of hemoglobin to be 13.3–17.7 g/dL for men and 11.7–15.7 g/dL for women[1,2] in the United States. The World Health Organization criteria for diagnosing anemia are a hemoglobin level of less than 14 g/dL in men and 12 g/dL in women.[3] A subsequent report[4] recommended that for males the critical hemoglobin level be reduced to 13 g/dL. In recent years, there has been considerable controversy regarding whether an "anemia of senescence"[2–15] exists. In order to examine this controversy, the physiological variables affecting blood count in humans must be considered.

The normal red cell number, hematocrit, and hemoglobin levels can be raised by smoking, obesity, altitude, exertion, and stress.[16–20] Most normal men living at or near sea level whose red cell counts are above $6.0 \times 10^6/\mu L$ are smokers. This rise in red cells may be largely attributed to elevated carboxyhemoglobin[20] and chronic pulmonary disease.

The use of hematocrit and hemoglobin concentration to define anemia may be very misleading. When the peripheral blood is examined, it is assumed that the plasma volume remains constant; however, the plasma volume is the most variable portion of the whole blood (Table 98-1).[21–23]

Changes in plasma volume occur throughout the day and are dependent on daily activities. Exercise and activity tend to lower plasma volume and raise hematocrit and hemoglobin levels. The lack of exercise in elderly people tends to raise the plasma volume and therefore lower hemoglobin levels. Bed rest has a dual effect on hemoglobin levels. At first, there is a fall in plasma volume (an increase in hemoglobin due to an initial diuresis resulting from a decrease in antidiuretic hormone [ADH] secretion).[24] This is caused by an increase in thoracic blood volume which is followed by a decrease in extravascular (lymphatic) return of proteins and a further reduction in plasma volume and a rise in hemoglobin. Prolonged bed rest eventually, however, leads to a decrease in erythropoiesis and a lower red cell mass, as there is a decrease in oxygen demand.[25] Thus, after prolonged bed rest a person eventually develops an anemia.

When a young person stands up after being recumbent overnight, the plasma volume falls by about 300 mL.[26] This response is blunted in normal elderly people, presumably because of a defect in the afferent arm of the baroreceptor reflex arc distal to the vasomotor center.[27]

Elderly people also do not respond in the same way as the young when exposed to high-altitude hypoxia. When a young person is exposed to high-altitude hypoxia, in the first 24–48 hours there is an increase in hemoglobin concentration due to a decrease in plasma volume,[28] an increase in 2,3-diphosphoglycreate (2,3-DPG),[29] and an elevation of serum erythropoietin.[30] These changes result in a rapid increase in the oxygen delivery capabilities of the blood which is followed by an erythropoietin-stimulated increase in bone marrow, and eventually in a polycythemic state.[31]

The decrease in plasma volume probably reflects a shift in intravascular fluid from blood to intracellular or extravascular spaces caused by vasoconstriction resulting from increased venomotor tone.[32] The increased venomotor tone in young people can be relieved by breathing 100 percent oxygen.[33] This hemoconcentration in young people is delayed in older people at high altitudes.[34,35]

When measuring the red cell parameters in older people, all the variables must be taken into account. Very few studies have controlled for bed rest, exercise, altitude, time of day, fluid intake, salt intake, or plasma proteins. In addition, many drugs, particularly diuretics and antihypertensives can theoretically alter plasma volume and erythropoiesis.[32] Any antihypertensive medication that blocks the autonomic nervous system can decrease venomotor tone and therefore raise plasma volume (lower hemoglobin levels). Diuretics lower plasma volume but in renal failure may have the opposite effect. The chronic effect of any drug on erythropoiesis has not been carefully studied.

Table 98-1 Factors affecting plasma volume and red cell parameters

Increased physiological factor	Plasma volume	Red cell parameter
Capillary permeability	Decrease	Increase
Hormones:		
Antidiuretic hormone	Increase	Decrease
Aldosterone	Increase	Decrease
Osmotic pressure (plasma protein)	Increase	Decrease
Venomotor tone:		
Exercise	Decrease	Increase
Bed rest (prolonged)	Increase	Decrease

Red cell parameter = RBC, hemoglobin, or hemocrit.

Thus, any measurement of red cell parameters with age must control for medications, which has not been done.

Aging does have an effect on blood production. There is evidence from both animal and human studies for the following age-related changes in bone marrow function.

1. The ratio of bone marrow cells to marrow fat decreases in elderly people,[36] although marrow from older people can be maintained by serial transplantation in tissue culture just as long as marrow from younger people; the number of normoblasts and committed erythroid stem cells (CFU-E) is lower, however. The number of earlier stem cells (BFU-E) was normal in elderly people.[37–39]

2. Iron incorporation into bone marrow cells from older people in vitro is the same as that from younger people. When stimulated with erythropoietin, an older person's marrow increases its iron incorporation to a lesser degree.[40]

3. Older animals do not respond to bleeding or hypoxia with increased erythropoiesis as well as younger animals.[41–42] It is not clear if the defect is in the hematopoietic elements themselves or is due to age-related changes in the marrow environment.

4. In humans, even though iron absorption from the gut is normal, an increase in ineffective erythropoiesis results in impaired incorporation of iron into heme in red cell precursors.[43]

There does seem to be a slightly lower red cell mass in very elderly people.[44] Red cell mass correlates best with lean body mass. It seems that the main determinant of red cell mass in the young is tissue oxygen requirements. Therefore, the decline in lean body mass and tissue oxygen requirements may explain at least part of the fall in red blood cell mass. However, the correlation between lean body mass and red cell mass also decreases with age.[44]

Elderly people respond to testosterone in pharmacological doses, indicating that marrow function is preserved;[45] responsiveness to the hormone is not decreased. Red cell 2,3-DPG has been shown to decrease in aging men, indicating a decrease in the oxygen demand of the tissues.[29] It has been postulated that the "thermostat" for red cell production is set at a lower level, thus lowering the level at which red cell production is turned on. Red blood cell survival remains normal with advancing age.[46]

Normal, healthy young men have a hematocrit[13–15] of about 46 percent and a hemoglobin level of about 15.6 g/dL. By age 60, the normal hemoglobin has slipped approximately 1 g/dL and in subsequent years may fall as much as 1 g per decade. The decline for black men is even steeper than that for white men. The opposite is seen in women. Between age 30 and 60 women show an increase in hemoglobin level of 0.6 g/dL per decade.[47–49] After age 60, their red cell parameters decline in parallel to those of men. Black women at any age have red cell levels about 2 percent lower than those of white women. The difference between whites and blacks may represent nutritional differences or indicate thalassemia minor.[50]

In spite of these changes, most older people still have normal red cell counts, hemoglobin levels, and hematocrits.[13–15] Certainly, if older patients with hemoglobin levels less than 12 g/dL or hematocrits less than 36 percent are investigated, an underlying cause of the anemia is usually discovered.[10] The diagnostic work-up for a mild anemia includes checking for blood loss, hemolysis, nutritional deficiencies, malignancy, infection, renal disease, any chronic disease, and any cause of an increase in plasma volume. Since all these factors are considered as part of a comprehensive geriatric assessment, the physician must always think in terms of what is causing the anemia. Even though there may be some very elderly people who have an anemia due to aging alone, most anemic elderly people have an underlying illness.

Classification of anemia in elderly people

Anemia can be classified either by morphology (Table 98-2) or by etiology (Table 98-3). However, in geriatric clinical practice, these two groups must be allowed to overlap to be of practical value. As discussed below, early in certain anemias, the morphology may be normocytic. For example, the microcytosis of iron deficiency is a late finding, as in the macrocytosis of vitamin B_{12} or folate deficiency. It is possible to diagnose these anemias long before morphological changes appear in the blood smear or the RBC indices become abnormal.

Clinical features

The symptoms and signs of anemia are the same in elderly people as in younger people, but the emphasis differs. Cardiovascular and cerebral features predominate, although many anemic patients have no complaints. Breathlessness and ankle edema are common manifestations and may be due to frank congestive cardiac failure. Left ventricle failure may occur, but angina is rare. Dizziness is common, and mental

---

Table 98-2 Morphological classification of anemia

Microcytic:
1. Iron deficiency
2. Anemia of chronic disease (often normocytic)
3. Sideroblastic anemia (often normocytic or macrocytic)
4. Thalassemia

Macrocytic:
1. Megaloblastic
   (a) B_{12} deficiency
   (b) folic acid deficiency
   (c) myelodysplasia
2. Normoblastic
   (a) chronic liver disease
   (b) alcoholism
   (c) hypothyroidism
   (d) leukemia and myelodysplasia
   (e) aplastic anemia
   (f) increased reticulocytes

Normocytic:
1. Blood loss
2. Hemolysis
3. Early stage iron deficiency or megablastic anemia
4. Anemia of chronic disease
5. Anemia of renal disease
6. Anemia of liver disease
7. Anemia of endocrine disorders
8. Scurvy
9. Collagen-vascular disease
10. Bone marrow infiltration

Table 98-3 **Etiological classification of anemia**

Blood loss—acute or chronic
Excessive red cell destruction (hemolytic anemia)
Impaired red cell formation:

1. Deficiency of substances essential for erythropoiesis
   (a) iron deficiency
   (b) vitamin B_{12} deficiency
   (c) folic acid deficiency
   (d) vitamin C deficiency
   (e) protein malnutrition
   (f) heme deficiency

2. Disturbance of marrow function
   (a) aplastic anemia
   (b) myelophthisis
   (c) myelodysplasia

changes are important but are nonspecific. Apart from confusion there may be apathy and depression, leading to self-neglect or agitation, even with delusions and hallucinations.

The tongue is often smooth and pale, and the patient may complain of a burning sensation on the tongue; but a sore tongue may be due to associated nutritional deficiencies rather than to the anemia itself. In such cases, there may be angular stomatitis or cheilosis. However, wearing an upper denture may produce lesions indistinguishable from angular stomatitis, which may be misleading.

Pallor, especially if recent, is important but is rarely offered as a symptom. The skin of elderly people may be very difficult to assess, and attention should be paid to the color of the buccal and lingual mucosae and the nailbeds. Changes in the nails are rarely of help.

A spleen tip may be felt in severe longstanding anemia, but other causes must be excluded. Associated features should be sought, for example, bone tenderness, abdominal mass, lymphadenopathy, signs of neuropathy, or spinal cord lesions.

The essential feature of the chronic anemias—which are those most commonly seen in old age—is the insidious onset of symptoms and signs. Physiological changes can compensate to some extent for the reduction in hemoglobin (e.g. an altered oxygen dissociation curve of hemoglobin to the right), allowing increased availability of oxygen to the tissues.[51–54] This allows the anemia to become marked before symptoms become troublesome. Furthermore, many old people are adverse to seeking medical (or other) help and may endure various symptoms without complaining. Thus, by the time an anemia is actually diagnosed in elderly people, the patient may in fact be very ill. In milder cases, untoward symptoms or failing general health may be accepted philosophically as part of "the burden of old age."

Investigation of anemia

A full blood count is a valuable routine investigation in all elderly patients. If anemia is found, it must be investigated before any attempt at treatment is made. Indiscriminate use of hematinics before investigation can cause further morbidity and make accurate diagnosis extremely difficult or delayed.

It is necessary to determine the type and cause of the anemia. Examination of the peripheral blood film may suggest the likely cause and indicate the type of anemia present. The cause is finally determined by careful history and exami-

nation, blood findings, and further investigations as required. Every initial geriatric assessment should include a complete blood count (CBC), and some authors advocate yearly testing. A healthy hemoglobin provides a basis for reassurance in a health-conscious population, whereas a hemoglobin in the anemic range (less than 12 g/dL in women and 13.5 g/dL in men is often used) alerts the physician to the potential presence of a disease process requiring early intervention.[55]

Once an anemia has been identified, the next step is to further characterize it utilizing the information already available from the CBC. An anemia accompanied by abnormalities in white blood cell and platelet counts suggests a primary marrow production problem, including aplastic anemia, marrow filled with tumor or infection, drug- or toxin-suppressed marrow, or nutrient-deprived marrow. The mean corpuscular volume (MCV) provides a clue to the red blood cell size, an important feature in classifying anemias. An MCV above 100 fL is considered macrocytic, an MCV less than 80 fL microcytic, and one 80–100 fL normocytic. However, one should never rely entirely on the MCV for defining cell size. Examination of the peripheral blood smear is necessary to confirm automated counter measurements; what the counter identifies as macrocytic may actually be an abundance of reticulocytes with a typical polychromatophilic appearance on visual inspection. Likewise, a mixed population of macrocytes and microcytes might yield a MCV calculated in the normocytic range by the counter.[55] Red cell diameter width (RDW), a measure of anisocytosis, is often unreliable in elderly people.[56–57]

Examination of the peripheral blood smear is essential in establishing red cell morphology. With the aid of an atlas, even a nonhematologist can identify pathological shapes such as teardrops, schistocytes, ovalocytes, poikilocytes, and burr cells—crucial clues to the pathogenesis of the anemia. Cell color (hypo- or normochromic) reflects the hemoglobin concentration and thereby also distinguishes the type of anemia.[55]

After review of the CBC and inspection of the peripheral smear, one additional useful test involves special staining of the peripheral blood cells for a reticulocyte count. Reticulocytes, or young erythrocytes, should be abundantly produced and released in situations of blood loss, such as bleeding or hemolysis, but are scarce in situations in which anemia is due to inadequate marrow production. A low reticulocyte count may be misleading in situations where blood loss has outstripped the supply of nutrients in the marrow, resulting in secondary marrow failure. Reticulocyte count norms are relative to the degree of anemia: the more anemic, the greater the reticulocyte count. The absolute reticulocyte count, corrected reticulocyte count, and reticulocyte production index (RPI) help one to assess the adequacy of the bone marrow response in the face of anemia. The RPI can be calculated in anemic patients in the following way:

$$RPI = \frac{\text{corrected reticulocyte count}}{2}$$

$$\text{Corrected reticulocyte count} = \text{reticulocytes (\%)} \times \frac{\text{patient hematocrit}}{\text{normal hematocrit}}$$

The usual normal hematocrit used is 0.45 L/L. The factor 2 in the denominator is used in anemic patients to take account of shift reticulocytes, prematurely released reticulocytes that take longer to lose their reticulin than normal reticulocytes. An adequate bone marrow response is usually indicated by an RPI greater than 3, and an inadequate one by an RPI less than 2.[58]

With the data accrued from one tube of blood (CBC, MCV, smear, and reticulocyte count), the anemia can usually be characterized.[55]

A bone marrow examination is rarely necessary in the initial evaluation of anemia in older patients. The vast majority of uncomplicated anemias can be diagnosed without a bone marrow examination. However, this procedure should be performed when the anemia is accompanied by abnormalities in white blood cells or platelets or when marrow infiltration is suspected. The examination is no more dangerous or painful in older people than in younger people.

Treatment of anemia—general principles

The first step is to identify and treat the underlying cause of the anemia. For example, in iron deficiency, the source of blood loss must be found and the bleeding stopped. After the cause of the anemia is found, a specific hematinic may be prescribed. If a rapid correction of the anemia is required, a red cell transfusion must be given after diagnostic blood tests have been performed.

Specific hematinics are iron, vitamin B_{12}, folic acid, and perhaps ascorbic acid and pyridoxine. Nonspecific hematinics include hormones such as androgens and growth factors such as erythropoietin and colony stimulating factors.

Following an accurate diagnosis the specific hematinic required should be used alone whenever possible, and the response to full doses assessed. This helps in confirming the diagnosis and simplifies the treatment. Combination preparations or hematinic "cocktails" are to be avoided, as they obscure the diagnosis.

The main indications for blood transfusion are when hematinic therapy will be ineffectual or inappropriate, when the gravity of the patient's condition precludes undue delay, or prior to surgery. Usually when the hematocrit is less than 25 percent or the hemoglobin concentration is below 8 g/dL, transfusion is necessary in patients over the age of 65. When transfusion becomes necessary in elderly people, every attempt must be made to avoid overloading the circulation. This is accomplished by using packed red cells in small volumes at a slow rate (e.g. 0.5 L in 6–8 hours), often adding a diuretic, and by careful clinical observation to avoid pulmonary congestion and a rise in venous pressure.

Microcytic anemias

Iron deficiency anemia

A microcytic (MCV less than 80 fL) hypochromic anemia in an elderly individual means iron deficiency due to blood loss until proven otherwise. The current recommended daily allowance for iron in elderly patients in the United States is 10 mg.[59] The most common anemia in elderly people is rarely due to dietary deficiency in industrialized nations because of the prevalence of iron fortification in wheat as well as a diet heavy in meat containing heme iron.[60] According to the Second National Health and Nutrition Examination Survey, 1976–1980, carried out by the US National Center for Health Statistics, mean iron intake was 13 mg/d for men and 10 mg/d for women over 70 years of age.[61] In fact, since the body salvages and recycles heme iron and stores absorbed dietary iron, elderly people usually have accumulated ample stockpiles of iron over their lifetime. In addition, about one-third of the absorbed iron in the elderly is not utilized for erythropoiesis but is deposited in nonerythroid tissues, predisposing them to iron overload. Therefore, the only rationale for the use of iron supplements in the aged individual is for replacement therapy after a diagnosis of iron deficiency has been appropriately made or for dietary supplementation in an individual with low iron stores who malabsorbs dietary iron (e.g. status postgastrectomy).

STAGES OF IRON DEFICIENCY There are four well-described stages of iron deficiency (Table 98-4), only the last two of which are reflected in the red blood cell indexes.[60,62] Before the overt hematological effects of iron deficiency manifest themselves, only bone marrow stains for iron or serum ferritin can be used to detect the two earlier stages reliably. In the first stage, known as iron depletion, serum ferritin is the most useful indicator because it is not practical to use bone marrow aspiration as a screening test. As iron deficiency progresses, bone marrow iron remains reduced or absent and serum ferritin remains low, while other biochemical and hematological changes occur later. In the second stage, iron deficiency without anemia, there is a fall in serum iron with a corresponding rise in transferrin. In early iron deficiency anemia, the third stage, bone marrow iron is absent but red blood cells are usually still normocytic and normochromic. Additionally,

Table 98-4 **Four stages of iron deficiency**					
	Bone marrow iron	Serum ferritin	Serum Fe/TIBC	Erythrocyte protoporphyrin	RBC morphology
Iron depletion	Low	Low	Normal	Normal	Normal
Iron deficiency without anemia	Low/absent	Low	Normal or low	Normal	Normal
Early iron deficiency anemia	Absent	Low	Low	High	Normal or slightly microcytic
Late iron deficiency anemia	Absent	Low	Low	High	Microcytic hypochromic

the supply of transport iron for heme synthesis becomes limited and erythrocyte protoporphyrin is elevated. In the fourth and final stage of iron deficiency, the classic hematological findings of microcytic, hypochromic anemia are seen.[60,62]

DIAGNOSIS OF IRON DEFICIENCY Tests used to detect iron deficiency have various levels of diagnostic accuracy (Table 98-5),[62] and the limitations of each measurement must be kept in mind. Using anemia as a screening test for iron deficiency is limited because it is a late finding and does not distinguish it from other causes of anemia. Decreased MCV is also a relatively late finding. Additionally, other anemias that may be microcytic and difficult to distinguish from iron deficiency based on MCV alone are thalassemia minor, anemia of chronic disease (ACD), and sideroblastic anemia.

Other tests useful in detecting iron deficiency before overt anemia develops can present several problems from the standpoint of diagnostic accuracy. Whereas a low serum ferritin level always indicates iron deficiency, a normal level does not ensure adequate iron stores, as serum ferritin is often elevated into the normal range in the presence of chronic inflammation and liver disease. In a study by Guyatt et al.[63] on anemic patients over 65 years of age, a ferritin level less than or equal to 18 µg/L had a likelihood ratio of 41 for iron deficiency, and a level of 19 to 45 µg/L had a likelihood ratio of 3. Low transferrin saturation is unreliable because iron and serum transferrin levels are often decreased in elderly people as well as in those with chronic disease. Serum iron may be inaccurate because it can fluctuate depending on the time of day. Free erythrocyte protoporphyrin level increases at about the same time that microcytosis develops and is therefore a relatively late finding. Additionally, high levels of erythrocyte protoporphyrin may not distinguish iron deficiency from lead poisoning.

Thompson et al.[56] have evaluated the accuracy of RDW, MCV, and transferrin saturation in the diagnosis of iron deficiency in hospitalized patients. RDW measures the variability in red cell size (anisocytosis). In contrast to previous reports, the authors found that none of these tests was sensitive or specific enough to be considered an accurate screening test for the diagnosis of iron deficiency anemia in hospitalized patients and elderly people.

In cases where the diagnosis is in doubt, a bone marrow biopsy showing depletion of iron stores is diagnostic, and in the occasional patient who refuses a bone marrow biopsy, a trial of iron therapy for 1 month can be used.

METABOLIC ROLE OF IRON Iron is essential by itself and as a portion of the heme molecule in many metabolic processes. Iron is present at the subcellular level, both by itself and in heme, where it functions as a component of various enzymes. The presence of iron is essential in mitochondria for generation of energy in the form of adenosine triphosphate (ATP) by oxidative phosphorylation. Several enzyme components of the respiratory electron transport chain contain iron, including cytochrome oxidase (containing two heme groups), succinate dehydrogenase (an iron flavoprotein), and other non-heme-containing compounds.[64] By itself, iron exerts a controlling effect on protein synthesis in the mitochondrion and may help maintain the integrity of the organelle.[65–82] The cytoplasmic concentration of heme exerts crucial control of protein synthesis initiation and polyribosome formation in immature red cells,[68] and probably in all cells.[69–72]

DRUG METABOLISM AND IRON Cytochrome P450 is another heme protein and is an important component of the hepatic drug metabolizing enzyme system which usually stays normal with aging. Heme production is regulated in hepatocytes by the balance between heme synthesis, controlled by ALA-S, and heme degradation, controlled by microsomal heme oxygenase. In aged rats, there is decreased hepatic heme synthesis caused by a decrease in ALA-S.[83] In addition, there is an increase in heme oxygenase and heme degradation.[84] In spite of this, heme levels and cytochrome P450 levels stay normal,[84,85] suggesting that an alternative pool of heme exists (such as tryptophan, pyrrolase, or hemopexin) which is increasingly used with age.[84,85] The net result is that with aging, cytochrome P450 is maintained by utilizing dietary heme. However, with iron deficiency, clearly cytochrome P450 is ultimately decreased.[85]

Iron overload also induces heme oxygenase and degrades heme,[86] leading to a decrease of cytochrome P450.[87] Since there is a degree of iron overload with aging, this may explain why

Table 98-5 **Limitations of tests used to diagnose iron deficiency**	
Test	**Limitation**
Hemoglobin/hematocrit	Anemia is a late finding Not specific
Microcytosis (MCV)	Late finding Not specific
Serum ferritin	Normal level not accurate with concurrent chronic disease or liver disease
Transferrin saturation	Low transferrin also found in elderly people and those with chronic disease
Serum iron	Levels may fluctuate during the day
Free erythrocyte protoporphyrin	Late finding, not specific
Red cell distribution width (RDW)	Not sensitive or specific enough for screening

in some elderly individuals there are problems in handling medications metabolized by cytochrome P450.[85]

TISSUE IRON DEFICIENCY In iron deficiency, it also has been shown that there is decreased activity of cytochrome c, cytochrome oxidase, succinic dehydrogenase, aconitase, xanthine oxidase, myoglobin, and other enzymes, including ribonucleotide reductase necessary for DNA synthesis.[60,80–94] Iron deficiency, therefore, is not manifested just as an anemia. In addition to its contributions to red blood cell production, iron is an important regulator of many cellular functions, including protein synthesis and energy production in all cells. Because of iron's ubiquitous involvement in many aspects of cell metabolism, its deficiency results in alterations in many tissues, as summarized in Table 98-6.

A lack of tissue iron seems to have a profound effect on various mucosal surfaces, resulting in several clinical entities. The mouth has been found to be affected by iron deficiency in a number of ways, including glossitis and angular stomatitis.[95] Additionally, several reports have described altered histology in the buccal mucosa of iron-deficient patients.[96–97]

The effects of iron deficiency on the esophagus have received much attention, beginning with the reports of Paterson,[98] Kelly,[99] and Vinson.[100] Sideropenic dysphagia, also known as Paterson–Kelly–Vinson syndrome, is characteristically associated with a mucosal web found in the postcricoid region of the hypopharynx. Although in most cases the web is found to consist of normal epithelium, carcinoma in situ is occasionally demonstrated.[101] Several investigators consider the postcricoid obstruction of Paterson–Kelly–Vinson syndrome to be a premalignant lesion.[97,102–103] This syndrome has also been found to be associated with a variety of autoimmune disorders, including Sjögren's syndrome, Hashimoto's thyroiditis, and pernicious anemia, all of which are common in elderly people.[104–106] Patients may develop pagophagia,[107–108] or ice and starch eating, presumably as a mechanism for soothing irritated mucosal surfaces.[107–108]

The integrity of the gastric mucosa is affected adversely by a lack of iron. Iron deficiency is associated with a high frequency of atrophic gastritis. The loss of normal acid production in iron-deficient subjects may be secondary to the development of autoantibodies to gastric parietal cells.[104,109] Atrophic gastritis and achlorhydria seem to be reversible when iron is replaced before the age of 30, but the changes appear to be permanent when treatment occurs after that age.[110,111] Iron deficiency may also affect the mucosa of the small intestine; mucosal changes similar to those seen in sprue have been observed in children with iron deficiency anemia; however, the mucosa can revert to normal following iron replacement.[112]

There is evidence that adequate tissue levels of iron are necessary for normal growth and skeletal development. Iron-deficient children have been shown to be significantly underweight, and when iron was replaced, weight gain occurred.[113]

As previously mentioned, iron appears to be necessary to maintain the normal integrity of mitochondria, and when iron is deficient, gross abnormalities of mitochondrial structure are seen.[114,115] Mitochondria are found to be enlarged and to have cristae that are sparse, broken, deformed, and swollen. Inadequate tissue iron levels seem to be responsible for structural abnormalities of lymphocytes and may explain susceptibility to infection.[112]

FUNCTIONAL EFFECTS OF IRON DEFICIENCY Iron deficiency results in a decrease in work capacity out of proportion to the degree of anemia. The anemia compromises cardiovascular function by impairing the capacity to perform brief, intense forms of exercise as reflected by the $\dot{V}_{O_2\,max}$. Loss of iron at the cellular level results in a reduction in levels of muscle oxidative enzymes, resulting in impairment in the performance of endurance-type exercises.[116–124] Studies have shown that iron-deficient rats have impaired work performance even when the anemia is corrected by exchange transfusion. During exercise, possibly as a result of depletion in iron-containing mitochondrial enzymes (e.g. α-glycerophosphate oxidase), they accumulate excessive lactate which seems to impair physical activity.[125]

Iron deficiency predisposes individuals to certain infections. Decreases in both cellular immunity[126–130] and neutrophil function have been reported.[130–132]

In contrast to the evidence linking iron deficiency with a predisposition to infection, there are data suggesting that rapid correction of iron deficiency may promote certain bacterial and parasitic infections, particularly if iron-dextran[62,130,133–140] is used. In the tropics, where iron deficiency is widespread and life-threatening, it has been suggested that severely anemic patients be protected against malaria while they are being treated with iron. In addition, such patients must be watched carefully for bacterial infections and treated aggressively if they occur. In otherwise healthy populations, there does not seem to be any reason to withhold iron therapy. However, in very sick elderly patients, it is advisable to closely monitor for infection during treatment for iron deficiency. In those with active infections, it seems prudent to treat the infection first and to limit the use of parenteral iron-dextran.

There is considerable evidence linking iron deficiency to central nervous system (CNS) dysfunction in animals and humans.[60,62,141–162] Studies have been performed on younger people and animals, but to date there have been no studies

Table 98-6 Consequences of tissue iron deficiency

Tissue	Defect
Mouth	Glossitis, angular stomatitis altered histology
Esophagus	Premalignant webs
Stomach	Atrophic gastritis
Small intestine	Malabsorption
Fingernails	Koilonychia
Lymphocytes	Poor function, leading to immunodeficiency
Heart	Hypertrophy
Muscle	Impaired endurance and ability to exercise
Brain	Decreased mentation
Catecholamine metabolism	Hypothermia

on elderly people. Certainly iron deficiency should be treated in elderly people and should be tested for as part of the evaluation of a dementia or altered mental status.

Abnormalities in catecholamine metabolism and thermogenesis have been found in iron-deficient humans.[60,62,163–168] Elevated catecholamine levels have been reported in iron-deficient humans even in the absence of anemia. Additionally, impaired temperature maintenance has been demonstrated in iron-deficient individuals exposed to mild hypothermia.

ABSORPTION OF IRON   Normally, iron is absorbed by specific mucosal receptors located in the duodenum and upper jejunum. To be absorbed, iron must be in the form of heme, soluble ferrous salts, or ferric chelates.[60]

Heme is released by hydrolysis from food hemoglobin or myoglobin by HCl and intramural proteases. The heme is then auto-oxidized to hemin (ferri heme). Hemin enters upper mucosal cells intact, after which heme oxygenase releases the iron for entry into the bloodstream where it is bound to transferrin. Small amounts of heme may be carried by hemopexin directly to the bone marrow[169] (the alternative pool). With age the absorption of heme becomes increasingly important, emphasizing the need for heme-containing foods such as meat in the diet.[170–175]

Most food iron is in the form of ferric iron. For it to remain soluble and absorbable, HCl, reducing agents and low molecular weight weak chelates (such as sugars and amino acids) must be present.[176–178] In the absence of these factors, ferric hydroxide or insoluble complexes with phosphates and phytates form. Ferrous iron is actively transported into mucosal brush border cells by receptor-mediated endocytosis. Divalent metal transporter 1 is a protein that transfers iron across the apical membrane and into cells through a proton-coupled process.[179] Virtually no food iron is in the ferrous form, although medicinal iron is. Thus in achlorhydric older patients, there may be difficulty in absorbing food iron but not medicinal iron. Ascorbic acid has been shown to increase inorganic iron absorption in persons with iron deficiency,[180] and tea, coffee, phytates, and possibly calcium to reduce it. In healthy elderly people, iron absorption seems normal.[43,60]

Body iron is regulated within very narrow limits through iron absorption. It is hypothesized that an exchange equilibrium between transferrin iron and the iron content of mucosal cells regulates total body iron content.[80] Total body iron appears to rise modestly with increasing age. The average diet has 10–15 mg of iron, of which approximately 8 percent is absorbed.[61] A dietary deficiency of iron is extremely rare in elderly people, and takes 3–7 years to develop.[60,181]

CAUSES OF IRON DEFICIENCY IN ELDERLY PEOPLE   The diagnosis of iron deficiency in the absence of any history of hemorrhage should be taken as evidence of occult gastrointestinal bleeding, and gastrointestinal tract evaluations should be performed. Any hemorrhagic lesion of the gastrointestinal tract may be responsible. In a recent study by Rockey and Cello,[182] on 100 patients with iron deficiency anemia who underwent gastrointestinal examinations, an upper gastrointestinal tract bleeding source was found in 37 patients, 19 of which were peptic ulcers; colonic lesions were found in 26, 11 of which were cancers.[182] There is some evidence that low

serum ferritin, even in the absence of anemia, may be a useful aid in detecting patients harboring occult gastrointestinal tract lesions[183,184] and therefore might have some utility as a screening test for these lesions. In selected patients other sites of bleeding or malabsorption should be considered.[179]

TREATMENT OF IRON DEFICIENCY ANEMIA   The first step is to find and to stop the source of bleeding. The iron deficiency is usually treated with oral ferrous iron.[55] Salts and enteric-coated or sustained-release preparations should be avoided, as they are not well absorbed. The simplest oral preparation is ferrous sulfate, 300 mg, which contains 60 mg of iron per tablet. One tablet taken three times a day, 1 hour before meals, supplies 180 mg of iron. As this preparation may cause constipation and gastric irritation, it is sometimes wise to begin with one tablet per day and increase the dose gradually over 1–2 weeks. Patients who are unable to tolerate ferrous sulfate because of gastrointestinal side-effects may tolerate the iron polysaccharide complex (e.g. Niferex). Liquid preparations are available for those who are unable to swallow pills. It is important to appreciate that iron therapy may reduce the absorption of a wide variety of other drugs the patient may be taking, including L-dopa, ciprofloxacin, and thyroxine.[185,186] Response to treatment is monitored by hemoglobin, hematocrit, and ferritin levels, and it usually requires 6 months or more to replenish iron stores if bleeding has stopped (to restore the ferritin to normal). Hemoglobin and hematocrit levels can be raised to their normal levels in 2 months. In the patient who has severe malabsorption, who cannot tolerate oral iron, whose iron stores need rapid replenishing, or who has active bleeding, parenteral iron may be best.[55] Parenteral iron is available as iron-dextran and can be given intravenously or by deep intramuscular injection. This therapy has been associated with anaphylactic shock, and a test dose of 0.5 mL should be given before treatment begins. The maximum recommended dose is 2.0 mL per day (intravenously), which delivers 100 mg of iron (using InFed, as available in the USA). Intravenous infusion should proceed no faster than at a rate of 1 mL/min. Side-effects of iron-dextran include pain at the injection site, fever, and arthralgias. Intramuscular injections have been found under experimental conditions to produce sarcomas in various animals. The most expensive and potentially hazardous way to replenish iron, of course, is by transfusion. Each milliliter of transfused red blood cells delivers 1 mg of iron.

Other causes of microcytic anemia

Anemias caused by abnormal hemoglobins (e.g. sickle cell anemia) are usually not first diagnosed in old age but obviously may be. Thalassemia minor, since it is asymptomatic, may first be found in old age. Thalassemia minor occurs in individuals who are heterozygous for genes that produce none or very little of the α- or β-hemoglobin chain. These conditions result in either microcytosis without anemia or a mild microcytic anemia with hypochromia, target cells, anisocytosis, poikilocytosis, polychromatophilia, and basophilic stippling of red blood cells on the peripheral blood smear. There is no reticulocytosis, and serum iron, total iron binding capacity (TIBC) and ferritin are all normal. Hemoglobin electrophoresis may reveal an increase in the minor hemoglobins, A_2 and F, in β-thalassemia, but in α-thalassemia no increase in these hemoglobins is seen. No treatment is usually required for these conditions. Iron therapy is contraindicated as it may produce iron overload.[58]

The anemia of chronic disease may be microcytic, but it is more commonly normocytic and will be discussed along with the normocytic anemias. Sideroblastic anemia may be microcytic, normocytic, or even macrocytic and will be discussed in the section on myelodysplastic syndromes.

Normocytic anemias

Anemia of chronic disease

The most common normocytic (MCV 80–100 fL) anemia in elderly people is the anemia secondary to other chronic diseases. The anemia is mild to moderate, with variable hypochromia and hypoferremia despite abundant stores of iron in the body.[187] Approximately one-half of these anemias are caused by chronic inflammatory disorders such as infection, and the other half are caused by neoplasms. ACD is about 40 percent as common as iron deficiency anemia in people of European extraction of all ages.[188] It is probably more common in older people, as they have more chronic diseases.

Within 1–2 months of onset of a chronic inflammation or neoplasm, a modest anemia develops which tends to correlate in severity with the underlying disease but never progresses to severe anemia. Typically, hematocrit levels decline to about 30–40 percent (average about 34 percent).[189] The anemia is usually normocytic and in more than 50 percent of cases is hypochromic. Occasionally, microcytosis is seen. The most characteristic pathogenic change is impairment of iron flow from the macrophage to the plasma.

In ACD, apoferritin synthesis by mononuclear phagocytes is increased by a cytokine (probably interleukin-1 [IL-1]).[190–192] This excess apoferritin directs newly mobilized iron to the storage pool, thereby blocking its release from the macrophage. The red cell precursors are then prevented from obtaining the iron necessary to form heme and hemoglobin. In addition, lactoferrin is released into the plasma from neutrophils during inflammation. Plasma lactoferrin binds to specific receptors on macrophages and competes with transferrin for iron,[193] which certainly contributes to the movement of iron away from the bone marrow and into storage in macrophages of the reticuloendothelial system.[194] This shifting of iron into storage is thought to represent a primitive immune mechanism for starving pathogens of necessary iron.[190–195]

Another factor that plays a role in the pathogenesis of ACD includes a modest reduction of erythrocyte survival without an adequate compensatory increase in the rate of red cell production. The reduced red blood cell survival is probably related to an increase in phagocytic activity by activated macrophages. IL-1 (which is increased in many chronic conditions) is also believed to act on T-lymphocytes to produce γ-interferon which is believed to directly inhibit erythroid colony-forming units.[196] Tumor necrosis factor is likewise felt to inhibit erythroid colony forming units in some cases,[197] possibly partly through interferon-beta. Erythropoietin secretion often appears to be less than optimal, and administration of this hormone results in an increasing hematocrit in certain individuals.[196] The mechanism for the blunted erythropoietin response to anemia with systemic disorders is thought to be through inhibition of erythropoietin gene transcription by inflammatory cytokines such as interleukin 1 and tumor necrosis factor.[197]

DIAGNOSIS OF ACD In addition to the mild anemia and hypochromia, the reticulocyte count is also low. Serum iron is low, and in contrast to the situation in iron deficiency, so is iron binding capacity (transferrin levels). Serum ferritin is elevated, and bone marrow shows abundant iron.

TREATMENT OF ACD Since the anemia is usually mild to moderate, no treatment is necessary in most instances. Occasionally blood transfusion may hasten the healing of wounds and stubborn infections. As a rule, however, the hazards of transfusion outweigh any potential benefits. Certain groups of patients, for example, HIV-infected patients with severe anemia on zidovudine and with erythropoietin levels less than 500 mUnits/mL, may respond to erythropoietin.[196] Unless the underlying disease is accompanied by iron deficiency, the administration of oral iron or parenteral iron is contraindicated. Hypoferremia does not appear to be dangerous and may represent a beneficial response on the body's part to protect against infection.[60,62,190,195] The only therapy usually necessary is treating the underlying inflammation or neoplasm.

Anemia of renal disease

In renal insufficiency a normochromic anemia develops which is very similar to ACD. In this condition there is a deficiency of erythropoietin production,[198] and there is evidence that the administration of erythropoietin, when the anemia is severe, can partially improve the condition. Improvement is usually not complete, as nonspecific substances accumulate in renal insufficiency that suppress hematopoiesis.[199] In addition, specific inhibitors may accumulate in uremia.[200,201] However, in patients on hemodialysis, erythropoietin is very effective in correcting the anemia, as these inhibitors are removed. It is important to correct any concomitant nutritional deficiencies such as those involving iron or folic acid, which are common in renal disease. In rare cases, blood transfusions may be necessary to protect the patient's cardiovascular status.

Anemia of liver disease

In liver diseases a normocytic or macrocytic anemia develops. There are many causes of anemia in liver disease, including bleeding, iron deficiency, folate deficiency, hypersplenism, and sideroblastic anemia. Even when these are excluded, anemia is often present that is similar to ACD. In liver disease, however, serum iron is increased and there is an increase in transferrin saturation. Serum ferritin is also increased and often reflects total body iron overload.[202]

Anemia of endocrine disorders

Endocrine disorders that commonly produce anemia are hypothyroidism, hypopituitarism, and adrenal insufficiency. In all three cases the anemia is normocytic and normochromic but may be macrocytic. Hypothyroidism is commonly complicated by iron deficiency,[203] resulting in microcytosis and hypochromia, or by associated megaloblastic anemia,[204] in which the cells are macrocytic and normochromic. Unless a specific deficiency of iron, vitamin B$_{12}$, or folate is identified, the therapy for the anemia is again that for the underlying disorder.

Anemia of collagen vascular diseases

ACD appears in collagen vascular diseases such as rheumatoid arthritis, polyarteritis, dermatomyositis, systemic lupus erythematosus, and temporal arteritis (including polymyalgia rheumatica). The latter is essentially a disease of geriatric patients. The anemia responds to steroid treatment as well as the entire symptom complex does.

"Unexplained anemia" of elderly people

A mild, normochromic, normocytic anemia with a hemoglobin concentration usually between 11 and 12 g/dL has been reported in people over the age of 70. This anemia cannot be accounted for by any underlying disease or deficiency, and the bone marrow does not contain ringed sideroblasts. This unexplained anemia is said to account for over 30 percent of the anemias in this age group.[126] It is associated with low neutrophil, lymphocyte, and platelet counts, and there is an increased red blood cell 2,3-DPG level, implying that this condition is not merely a normal age-related variant. The significance of this type of anemia is presently unknown, but it is probably a myelodysplastic syndrome.

Hemolytic anemias

Frank hemolytic anemias are not common in elderly people, even though a shortened red cell survival is found in various types of anemia. The hereditary forms of hemolytic anemias are usually diagnosed in childhood or in early adolescence and are discussed in any standard textbook of hematology.

Acquired hemolytic anemia (i.e., hemolysis not due to congenital abnormalities of the red blood cell) is a normochromic, normocytic anemia which can occur at any age. The incidence of this disorder increases with advancing age. Peripheral destruction of red cells results in increased production of young red cells by the bone marrow, resulting in an increased reticulocyte count and polychromatophilia on the peripheral blood smear. As reticulocytes are larger than mature red cells, if the reticulocytosis is brisk enough, the indexes may become macrocytic. Red cell destruction results in increased serum unconjugated bilirubin, serum glutamic oxaloacetic transaminase (SGOT), and lactate dehydrogenase (LDH), decreased serum haptoglobin, and increased urine urobilinogen. If the hemolysis is intravascular, urine hemosiderin is increased as well. The direct antiglobulin test (Coombs' test) is used to detect antibody and/or complement on the red blood cell, and it can also identify the antigen to which the antibody is reacting.[205]

Causes of acquired hemolytic anemia

Idiopathic autoimmune hemolysis may be a result of warm-reaction antibodies of the IgG class or cold agglutinins which are usually of the IgM class. Idiopathic cold agglutinin disease is primarily a disease of old age. At times the cold agglutinin may be of the IgG class, or a nonagglutinin may be found.

Immune hemolysis may also be secondary to a variety of other illnesses. Approximately 30 percent of secondary immune hemolytic anemias are caused by lymphoproliferative diseases, including chronic lymphocytic leukemia, non-Hodgkin's lymphoma, Hodgkin's disease, and multiple myeloma. Agnogenic myeloid metaplasia, systemic lupus erythematosus, viral infections, mycoplasma pneumoniae infection, syphilis, and various nonhematologic malignancies are also associated with immune hemolytic anemia. This condition is more common in women, and the incidence of the secondary varieties rises with age.[206]

Another major cause of hemolytic anemia is a drug reaction. Elderly people are more prone to develop this problem simply because they generally take more medications than younger individuals. Several types of drug-induced hemolysis have been described.[207–210]

Treatment of autoimmune hemolytic anemia

Idiopathic autoimmune hemolysis secondary to warm-reaction antibodies of the IgG class responds to steroid therapy approximately 75 percent of the time.[211] Prednisone in a dose of 60 mg/d is the initial treatment, although occasionally 100 mg is needed. A rise in the hemoglobin and hematocrit and a drop in the reticulocyte count usually occur in the first 3–14 days, but the response may be delayed by as much as 8 weeks. Once remission occurs, steroids may be tapered by 5 mg/wk, but relapse requires increasing the dose by 15–20 mg followed by a more gradual taper in dose. Some patients continue to require a small daily dose or alternate-day therapy for long periods of time. If there is no response to 60 mg of prednisone per day after 4–8 weeks, higher doses may be tried or the blocked androgen, danazol, may be added.[212–214] If therapy still fails, the next step is usually splenectomy, which results in long-term remission in 50–75 percent of cases.[214] For patients who either do not respond to the above measures or are poor surgical candidates, immunosuppressive agents cyclophosphamide or azathioprine may be useful.[215] Most patients with warm antibody immune hemolysis do not require transfusion, but for those who are extremely symptomatic because of their anemia, transfusion can be considered. Cross-matching blood is problematic, and the autoantibodies of course reduce the survival of the transfused red blood cells. Plasmapheresis is usually not successful, as IgG has a very large distribution in the body, but has been reported to work sometimes.

Idiopathic cold agglutinin disease due to IgM requires avoidance of exposure to the cold. Steroids and splenectomy are usually not useful, although they have been used with some success in small numbers of patients with disease due to either low-titer IgM or to IgG.[205,214] Plasmapheresis may provide temporary improvement, as the IgM is confined to the intravascular space.[216,217] Disease caused by cold-activated IgG hemolysin is also treated by avoiding exposure to the cold. In both diseases, transfusion should be done if necessary with washed red blood cells that have been warmed. Immune hemolytic anemia secondary to other diseases usually improves only with treatment of the underlying disease. If this strategy is not possible, therapy may be tried as described above, but success is less likely than in idiopathic disease.

As stated previously, treatment of drug-induced hemolytic anemia usually consists of simply discontinuing the responsible medication. In rare instances, methyldopa autoimmune hemolysis continues long enough to require a course of steroids as described above.

Occasionally, intravascular hemolysis may be due to trauma, such as in patients with prosthetic heart valves or prolonged marching, and treatment in these patients should focus on the etiology.

Macrocytic anemias

Macrocytic anemia is described as an anemia in which the MCV is greater than 100 fL. MCV increases slightly with increasing age but usually not enough to produce significant macrocytosis.[10] Relatively few disorders routinely result in macrocytic anemia (Table 98-2). The two common disorders that produce macrocytosis are megaloblastic anemias due to either vitamin B_{12} or folate deficiency.

Vitamin B_{12} deficiency

Vitamin B_{12} (also known as cobalamin) deficiency, has been reported to account for up to 9 percent of anemias in elderly populations. Vitamin B_{12} is found in most animal tissues but not in plants. A normal diet contains up to 5–30 µg/d. Vitamin B_{12} is stable in normal cooking and most of it is available for absorption, but only 2 µg can be absorbed from a single meal, as this is the limit for the ileal receptors.[218] B_{12} loss from the body is very small, being only about 0.1–0.2 percent of the total B_{12} pool daily regardless of the size of the pool.[219] Once absorbed, B_{12} is stored in the liver, which normally contains over 1 mg of the vitamin. Other organs also store this vitamin, so that total body B_{12} is 2–5 mg.[220,221] As a person becomes B_{12}-deficient, less B_{12} is lost than in normal people and less is required to maintain the steady state. This may explain why in latent B_{12} deficiency (B_{12} depletion) with mild malabsorption of B_{12}, an overt megaloblastic anemia may not occur (see below).

Vitamin B_{12} is usually absorbed by active transport with intrinsic factor (IF). Vitamin B_{12} in nature is always bound to R proteins (cobalophilin), which are present in virtually all body secretions as well as in food. R proteins are so named because they have rapid electrophoretic mobility, in contrast to IF, which has slow (S) mobility.

The cobalamin R complex is degraded partially in the stomach by acid peptic digestion and partially in the upper small intestine by pancreatic enzymes,[222] thus allowing formation of the cobalamin–IF complex. IF, a glycoprotein of 50,000 molecular weight, is secreted by the gastric parietal cells and binds cobalamin after it has been released from its R binder by digestive action. Once IF binds cobalamin, the IF–cobalamin complex travels to the terminal ileum where there are specific receptor binding sites for IF.[223,224] As the cobalamin-IF complex crosses the intestinal mucosa, IF is lost and cobalamin is transferred to the cellular R proteins.[224]

The second mechanism available for the absorption of cobalamin involves simple diffusion of the vitamin within the lumen of the gut. This process accounts for only 1–3 percent of the absorption of cobalamin under normal circumstances but may increase in significance when larger amounts, such as 1 mg of free vitamin are ingested. This situation might occur when pharmacological, not physiological, doses of vitamin B_{12} are being ingested. However, with usual dietary intake, if IF is absent, a deficiency of B_{12} eventually occurs.

Even though only 2–5 µg of cobalamin is absorbed daily, because of an extremely efficient enterohepatic circulation which recycles vitamin B_{12} from bile and other intestinal secretions,[225,226] the daily loss is only about 1–2 µg/d (half-life of cobalamin in the body is about 1,360 days). In fact, in cases of pure IF deficiency, such as after total gastrectomy, it may take up to 3–5 years to become overtly B_{12}-deficient.

TCII is the dominant carrier of vitamin B_{12} immediately after its absorption and separation from IF.[227–229] The complex is rapidly cleared from the plasma and taken up by the tissues. TCI and TCIII are thought to be the storage proteins. The physiological transporter TCII is responsible for about 25 percent of the cobalamin circulating in plasma, and the rest is on other transcobalamins.[230,231] Once inside the cell, B_{12} is converted to methylcobalamin and adenosylcobalamin.[223] Adenosylcobalamin is the coenzyme of L-methylmalonyl-CoA mutase, an enzyme catalyzing the first step in the pathway of propionic acid metabolism, in which methylmalonyl-CoA is converted to succinyl-CoA. Thus, B_{12} deficiency leads to an increase in methylmalonic acid. Methylcobalamin is the coenzyme for methionine synthase needed to convert homocysteine to methionine. In the absence of B_{12}, homocysteine levels also increase. It is unclear whether deficient activity in one or both of these enzyme systems results in the neurological abnormalities seen in B_{12} deficiency. The conversion of 5-methyltetrahydrofolate (which is how folate is stored in the body) to tetrahydrofolate is coupled to B_{12}, requiring conversion of homocysteine to methionine. Tetrahydrofolate is then converted to 5,10-methylene tetrahydrofolate, which is necessary for thymidylate and DNA synthesis. Thus, a deficiency of either B_{12} or folate leads to deficient DNA synthesis and to subsequent hematological manifestation of megaloblastosis.[232]

Vitamin B_{12} is stored in the liver in large quantities, so that after a lesion occurs that prevents B_{12} absorption, it takes many years to develop a B_{12} deficiency. For this reason, patients who are B_{12}-deficient may present with profound anemias which are well tolerated, with no volume depletion or orthostatic hypotension. In fact, these patients will be at risk for the development of congestive heart failure if they are transfused.

ETIOLOGY OF VITAMIN B_{12} DEFICIENCY Pernicious anemia (autoimmune disease) is the classically described cause of cobalamin deficiency. There is an overall prevalence of 1 percent occurring equally in men and women. It is more common in Scandinavians but can be found in any ethnic or racial group; it is usually diagnosed in people aged 60 or over.

Pernicious anemia appears to be an autoimmune disease with production of antibodies directed against gastric parietal cells and IF. It occurs more frequently in people who have another autoimmune disease, such as hypothyroidism, Graves' disease, Addison's disease, vitiligo, or hypoparathyroidism. Symptoms of pernicious anemia may be no more specific than fatigue due to profound anemia. Characteristically, however, patients develop glossitis with a smooth red tongue, mild jaundice, and neurological changes, the typical lemon yellow color of the skin is due to a combination of mild jaundice and pallor. The neurological findings include paresthesias, abnormal position and vibration sensation, gait ataxia due to degeneration of the posterolateral columns of the spinal cord, and various psychiatric disorders including dementia and personality changes. These neurological changes are not always corrected when the deficiency is treated.[50]

Laboratory abnormalities accompanying pernicious anemia include macrocytosis and hypersegmented polymorphonuclear leukocytes on the peripheral blood smear and increased serum bilirubin and LDH due to ineffective erythropoiesis. The platelet count and white blood cell count may be reduced, and the serum vitamin B_{12} level is low. Approximately 30 percent of patients with B_{12} deficiency have elevated serum folate levels. The bone marrow, if examined, will show characteristic megaloblastic changes.[232]

In pernicious anemia, there is a deficiency of IF produced in the stomach, resulting in malabsorption of cobalamin. The Schilling test,[50] which measures the oral absorption of radiolabeled vitamin B_{12} with and without the addition of oral IF, differentiates between pernicious anemia and other causes of B_{12} deficiency such as malabsorption and bacterial intestinal overgrowth. In pernicious anemia, the absorption of oral B_{12} alone is abnormal but can be corrected with IF. If absorption is not corrected with IF, the patient is treated for a few weeks with a broad-spectrum antibiotic and the test is then repeated. If absorption becomes normal, the problem is bacterial overgrowth. If the patient really has pernicious anemia and has been B_{12}-deficient for some time, however, they may malabsorb B_{12} because of malfunction of the small intestine as a result of B_{12} deficiency. To test this possibility, the patient should have the Schilling test repeated after a few months of B_{12} supplementation. If it is still abnormal, the patient has intestinal malabsorption.[50] Treatment of B_{12} deficiency usually requires lifetime parenteral B_{12} administration. There are a variety of regimes that consist of initial replenishment followed by maintenance therapy, a convenient one is to give 1,000 μg daily for the first week, then weekly for 4 weeks or until the hemocrit is normal, and then monthly for life. There is some evidence that daily doses of vitamin B_{12} (1,000–2,000 μg) per day orally may be sufficient therapy, with enough B_{12} being absorbed even in the absence of IF.[233,234] The response to treatment is usually evidenced by a brisk reticulocytosis within 1 week. While the anemia should be corrected within 1 month, peripheral blood smear abnormalities, particularly hypersegmented neutrophils, may persist for 1 year. Hypokalemia and hypophosphatemia may occur early in therapy, and serum phosphate and potassium should be monitored and supplementation given if necessary. Transfusion may produce volume overload, and if necessary, should be given slowly with careful monitoring of the patient. It should also be noted that misdiagnosis of B_{12} deficiency as folate deficiency and consequent treatment with folate alone may improve the hematological disorder but does not treat the neurological changes of B_{12} deficiency. It is, therefore, to be avoided at all costs.

Patients with pernicious anemia have been shown to be at increased risk of cancer of the stomach (2.9 standardized incidence ratio in a recent Swedish study), gastric carcinoids, and possibly other cancers as well.[235] Surveillance upper endoscopy can help locate tumors while they are still curable: two small gastric adenocarcinomas as well as two gastric carcinoids were found in 56 patients undergoing gastroscopy in a Finnish study.[236] The role, frequency, and cost of routine endoscopy is still being debated; however, all patients should clearly receive stool occult blood testing and endoscopy for any gastrointestinal symptoms.

Another frequent cause of vitamin B_{12} deficiency in elderly people is an inability to free B_{12} from its binding to dietary proteins. HCl and pepsin contribute to the release of cobalamin from dietary proteins so that B_{12} can bind to IF and thus be available for absorption. If there is a lack of either HCl or pepsin, B_{12} is not liberated from the protein and therefore not bound to IF. These patients have a normal Schilling test, as the B_{12} in the test is free and not bound to protein. It has been shown that omeprazole, a potent inhibitor of gastric acid secretion, decreases B_{12} absorption.[237] It has also been demonstrated that about 30 percent of patients with a history of gastric surgery will become B_{12}-deficient.[238] Patients with B_{12} deficiency due to a lack of HCl can be treated with oral vitamin B_{12} on an empty stomach, as the B_{12} is free and not bound and therefore will be available to bind with IF.

Other causes of B_{12} deficiency such as bacterial overgrowth and ileal diseases may occur as well and have been alluded to above. There is also some recent evidence that metformin, an oral hypoglycemic, may reduce B_{12} absorption because of calcium-dependent ileal membrane antagonism.[239]

LOW SERUM B_{12} LEVELS IN ELDERLY PEOPLE—RELATIONSHIP TO DEMENTIA The dementia of vitamin B_{12} deficiency can be identical to that of Alzheimer's disease. The most important unanswered questions in vitamin B_{12} research concern the frequency of dementia induced by cobalamin deficiency and how often neuropsychiatric changes occur in the absence of any hematologic abnormalities. These questions are still incompletely answered, but recent work has shown that 30 percent or more of patients with B_{12} deficiency and neuropsychiatric abnormalities that respond to B_{12} therapy have normal hemoglobin levels and MCVs.[240,241] It has also been suggested that patients whose duration of symptoms is less than 1 year have better responses to therapy than those whose cognitive deficits have lasted more than 1 year, suggesting a possible time-limited window of opportunity for maximum effect of therapy.[240]

It is generally agreed that patients with organic brain syndrome, unexplained psychosis, unexplained peripheral neuropathy, prior gastrectomy, hypersegmentation of the neutrophils on the peripheral blood smear, or unexplained macrocytosis should be tested for vitamin B_{12} deficiency. It has been demonstrated that sole reliance on these criteria may result in cases of B_{12} deficiency being missed. The absence of an elevated MCV, which was previously felt to be a hallmark of B_{12} deficiency, has now been described by a number of authors.[240–245] RDW has been proposed as a useful screening test for B_{12} deficiency;[246,247] however, this deficiency does occur in patients with normal RDWs.[248] Hypersegmentation on the blood smear is more useful than either MCV or RDW as a screen for B_{12} deficiency.[243,248]

About 8 percent of patients hospitalized on an inpatient medical service had low serum vitamin B_{12} levels.[242,249,250] This included people who were elderly, but also younger people, particularly those with acquired immunodeficiency syndrome (AIDS).[241]

In an ambulatory elderly population, low serum vitamin B_{12} is found in 3–21 percent of those tested. In two studies, a 3 percent incidence was reported.[251,252] Other studies found the incidence to be about 7 percent.[253–255] Even higher incidences have been reported,[256–260] including 21.3 percent in people with early signs and symptoms of dementia.[261] The observation that holotranscobalamin II levels decline with age and that the percentage of vitamin B_{12} binding to transcobalamin II is less suggests that low serum B_{12} truly represents a body deficiency of cobalamin.[253] Demonstrations that B_{12} levels, holotranscobalamin II, and binding of B_{12} to transcobalamin II are lower in some people with dementia,[261,262] and that in these patients an abnormal deoxyuridine suppression test[250] or elevated methylmalonic acid and homocysteine levels[243] are found, and most importantly that some patients with cobalamin deficiency, neuropsychiatric abnormalities, normal hemoglobin, and mean red cell volumes improved with cobalamin replacement[240,241] are strong evidence that in some people the symptoms of B_{12} deficiency are neuropsychiatric rather than hematological.[261]

EVALUATION OF A LOW SERUM VITAMIN B_{12} LEVEL Low serum vitamin B_{12} levels are frequently not investigated.[242,263] As the consequences of B_{12} deficiency can be devastating, all low serum cobalamin levels should be further evaluated. Gallium scans, red cell mass tests, thyroid scans, ^{32}P treatment, and bone scans can falsely elevate the radioactivity count and produce a falsely low B_{12} value. Other causes of falsely low B_{12} levels include pregnancy, folate deficiency, ingestion of high doses of absorbic acid, and multiple myeloma.[264,265] Numerous tests have been proposed to investigate low B_{12} levels, including Schilling and food Schilling tests, serum methylmalonic acid and homocysteine levels, deoxyuridine suppression testing of bone marrow, tests for anti-IF antibody assays, and holotranscobalamin II and transcobalamin II saturation with B_{12}.

Schilling tests are frequently used to evaluate low serum vitamin B_{12} levels. The two-stage Schilling test is superior to the one-stage test.[266] Carmel et al.[267] have recently shown that the food Schilling test is frequently abnormal in patients with a low B_{12} level and a normal fasting Schilling test. It appears that many elderly patients are unable to split off B_{12} from the R proteins in food because of either hypochlorhydria or pancreatic insufficiency. One of the biggest problems with Schilling tests is accurate collection of 24-hour urine specimens. This is especially problematic in geriatric patients who may experience urinary incontinence or have cognitive difficulties.

Both methylmalonic acid and homocysteine serum levels increase with vitamin B_{12} deficiency.[243] In a study by Savage et al.[268] only 1 patient out of over 400 patients with cobalamin deficiency had normal levels of both metabolites, 98 percent had elevation of methylmalonic acid levels, and 96 percent had elevated homocysteine levels. In a study by Stabler et al.[241] only 5 patients out of 86 who responded to cobalamin therapy did not have an elevated level of one of these metabolites, and these patients had an improvement in only one out of four parameters assessed.[240] Testing for these metabolite levels has therefore become very valuable in assessing patients' cobalamin status. Methylmalonic acid levels may also be elevated in renal insufficiency. Homocysteine levels may be increased in folate deficiency, pyridoxine deficiency, or renal insufficiency[269] or because of a variety of genetic defects including cystathionine synthase.

The deoxyuridine suppression test of bone marrow DNA synthesis is felt to be a reliable measure of vitamin B_{12} status.[270,271] Carmel et al.[267] described 18 patients with abnormal deoxyuridine suppression levels, all of whom had normal levels of methylmalonic acid and homocysteine in their urine and only one of whom had a hypersegmented blood smear. Some patients had abnormal Schilling tests, and abnormal food Schilling tests were even more common. Two patients with normal test results had abnormal results 1 year later. Thus, deoxyuridine suppression tests appear to be useful in diagnosing metabolic abnormalities early in the course of B_{12} deficiency. The main disadvantage of the test is that it requires a bone marrow examination and is still restricted to special laboratories. If developed commercially, it is likely to be more expensive than serum measurement of methylmalonic acid or homocysteine. The specificity of the test seems to be excellent,[272] although there is some suggestion that malnutrition and certain drugs may cause false positive results.[273,274]

Antibodies to gastric parietal cells and to IF are common in classic autoimmune pernicious anemia. Parietal cell antibodies lack sufficient specificity to be useful; antibodies to IF are quite specific for pernicious anemia but have a sensitivity of only about 50 percent.[275] A positive test is very helpful, but a negative test should prompt further investigation. It is not known how many patients with low vitamin B_{12} levels have early autoimmune pernicious anemia. Many of these elderly people may not be able to absorb food B_{12} secondary to hypochlorhydria or a decrease in pancreatic enzymes and may never show anti-IF antibodies.

THE STAGES OF VITAMIN B_{12} DEFICIENCY One of the most intriguing developments in the study of vitamin B_{12} deficiency has been the model presented by Herbert.[276] It is proposed that there are four stages in the development of B_{12} deficiency: negative B_{12} balance,[277,278] B_{12} depletion, B_{12}-deficient erythropoiesis, and B_{12} deficiency anemia (Table 98-7). The first two stages are characterized by reduced holotranscobalamin II and decreased transcobalamin II saturation. The deoxyuridine suppression test is said to be normal, there is no hypersegmentation, and the methylmalonic acid level is normal. In the stage of B_{12}-deficient erythropoiesis, hypersegmentation of neutrophils occurs and the deoxyuridine suppression test becomes abnormal. Holotranscobalamin II and transcobalamin II saturation fall further. The patient's hemoglobin and MCV are still normal, and methylmalonic acid may be increased. Only in the final stage does the patient become anemic and develop an elevated MCV. The model makes intuitive sense and has received some preliminary support, but as the authors acknowledge, it remains to be tested in a sufficiently large patient group.[276–278]

One of the most important questions related to this model concerns the stage at which myelin and brain damage occur. If it can occur prior to the development of hypersegmentation and methylmalonic acid elevation, this strongly argues for screening all elderly people for B_{12} levels and ordering holotranscobalamin II levels and transcobalamin II saturations for all those with low or borderline results. Another important question is whether all patients who are in negative B_{12} balance or in the stage of B_{12} depletion will proceed to B_{12}-deficient erythropoiesis, neurological damage, and dementia if untreated. This is an especially important question in regard to elderly people, as transcobalamin II saturation is low in many patients, even those with normal B_{12} levels.[253]

Elevated homocysteine levels have been associated with both arterial[279–281] and venous[280,282] occlusive disease. Naurath

Table 98-7 Proposed four stages of vitamin B$_{12}$ deficiency

Stage	Vitamin B$_{12}$ level	Holo-transcobalamin II levels	Transcobalamin II-B$_{12}$ binding	Methyl-malonic acid and homo-cysteine levels	Hyper-segmented neutrophils	Thymidine uptake in DUST[a]	Mean cell volume	Hemoglobin
1. Negative vitamin B$_{12}$ balance	Low or Normal	Low	Low	Normal	None	Normal	Normal	Normal
2. Vitamin B$_{12}$ depletion	Low or Normal	Low	Low	Normal or High	None	Normal	Normal	Normal
3. Vitamin B$_{12}$ deficient hematopoiesis	Low	Low	Low	High	Few	High	Normal	Normal
4. Vitamin B$_{12}$ deficiency anemia	Low	Low	Low	High	Many	High	High	Low

[a]DUST: deoxyuridine suppression test.

et al.[283] have shown that treating patients with elevated homocysteine levels with a mixture of vitamin B$_{12}$, folate, and pyridoxine, even in the absence of lowered pretreatment values of these vitamins, often lowers the homocysteine level. The question of routine screening of elderly people for elevated homocysteine levels must therefore be raised.

Current recommendations

1. We recommend screening all older adults for vitamin B$_{12}$ deficiency. Many patients with this deficiency have normal hemoglobin and MCVs, and the cognitive dysfunction associated with B$_{12}$ deficiency may have only a short, time-limited window of opportunity for optimal response to therapy.[240] Elevated homocysteine levels, often found in B$_{12}$ deficiency, have been associated with both arterial[279–281] and venous[280,282] occlusive disease. Patients with low B$_{12}$ levels have been shown to have impaired antibody response to pneumococcal vaccine.[284] The above data suggest that all older patients may benefit from screening.

2. Serum vitamin B$_{12}$ levels should be used in routine screening of elderly patients. A B$_{12}$ of less than 350 pg/mL should be taken as evidence that further screening is required.[269] A study by Pennypacker et al.[285] in an outpatient geriatric clinic found elevated methylmalonic acid or homocysteine levels in 56 percent of patients with B$_{12}$ levels from 201 to 300 pg/mL, compared to 62 percent of patients with lower serum cobalamin levels (less than or equal to 200 pg/mL),[285] suggesting that the higher level should be used as the cutoff value for patients requiring further screening.

3. Patients with B$_{12}$ levels less than 350 pg/mL should then have their serum methylmalonic acid and homocysteine levels measured. An elevation to greater than three standard deviations above the mean in normal subjects is highly suspicious for vitamin B$_{12}$ deficiency.[268]

4. Some patients have elevated metabolite levels due to other causes. Methylmalonic acid levels may be elevated in renal insufficiency, and homocysteine levels may be increased in folate deficiency, pyridoxine deficiency, renal insufficiency,[269] and a variety of genetic defects; therefore in the appropriate context these causes should be sought. A reduction to normal or to less than 50 percent of the pretreatment value of the metabolites is usually found in cobalamin-responsive patients.[241]

5. The use of further testing such as a Schilling test or determining anti-IF antibodies should be determined on an individual basis.

Issues that require further information include the following:

1. Some patients with vitamin B$_{12}$ levels greater than 300 pg/mL have elevated methylmalonic acid and homocysteine levels. In the study by Pennypacker et al.[285] seven subjects who met these criteria and were treated with B$_{12}$ had decreases in their metabolite levels.[285] Whether patients should be screened with these metabolites and their responses to therapy routinely monitored is an important issue.

2. Many patients with vitamin B$_{12}$ levels less than 200 pg/mL have normal levels of homocysteine and methylmalonic acid, for example, 38 percent in the study by Pennypacker et al.[285] Rare patients with low B$_{12}$ levels and normal serum metabolites seem to respond to B$_{12}$ therapy (see section on evaluation above). It is not known whether the response of these rare patients was just due to random variations in test results and was not a true response, as might be suggested by the fact that the five cobalamin-responsive patients who had normal metabolite levels studied by Stabler et al.[241] had a response in only one out of four parameters assessed. However, it seems appropriate to give these patients B$_{12}$ therapy. Patients with B$_{12}$ depletion and no deficiency can usually be treated with oral B$_{12}$ initially and their responses closely monitored.

3. The cost-effectiveness of different screening strategies, as compared to routine oral vitamin B$_{12}$ supplementation needs to be assessed.

4. The role of gastroscopic surveillance in detecting early neoplasms needs to be clarified.

Folate deficiency

Folic acid deficiency produces changes on the peripheral blood smear and in the bone marrow that are indistinguishable from those due to vitamin B_{12} deficiency. There is controversy concerning the incidence of folate deficiency in elderly people, partly because different groups define the lower limits of normal differently and because there are several different ways to determine folate levels.[286–295] Serum folate levels fluctuate rapidly and do not necessarily reflect body stores. Red blood cell folate levels are more reliable, but both radioimmunoassay and microbiological methods are available for measuring both red blood cells and serum folate and there is frequently a discrepancy between the results from these methods.[295] Normal body stores of folate can be depleted in less than 6 months, and several conditions can cause folate deficiency to occur rapidly. These include malabsorption, poor nutrition, alcoholism, and states of increased folate utilization such as hemolytic anemia and neoplasia. Furthermore, drugs can cause folate deficiency, including anticonvulsants, antineoplastic drugs, trimethoprim, and nitrofuration. Many older people with psychiatric illnesses become folate-deficient because they do not eat a varied diet. If the above-mentioned conditions are excluded, the vast majority of community-dwelling elderly are folate-replete.[295] Age does not predispose one to folate deficiency; disease states and medications are the reasons people become deficient. Certainly, if people do not eat, they become folate-deficient rapidly. However, even poor elderly people in the USA seem to have diets with sufficient amounts of this vitamin.[295]

Folate deficiency may result in neurological changes which are virtually indistinguishable from those produced by vitamin B_{12} deficiency.[295] Included among the neuropsychiatric problems of folate-deficient individuals are intellectual impairment, confusion, psychosis, depression, stupor, coma, cerebral ischemia, and paraplegia.[295–317] Diagnosis of anemia due to folate deficiency rests on a peripheral blood smear with macrocytic red blood cells and hypersegmented neutrophils, a normal serum B_{12} level, and low serum folate and/or red blood cell folate. Serum homocysteine levels are elevated in 90 percent of patients with folate deficiency, but methylmalonic acid levels are normal.[268] If methylmalonic acid levels are high, coexisting B_{12} deficiency must be considered. Bone marrow, if examined, will be indistinguishable from that seen in B_{12} deficiency. Treatment of folate deficiency consists of 1 mg of folic acid orally, and a parenteral form is available for patients with severe malabsorption. Again, it should be noted that treatment of a patient with megaloblastic anemia secondary to B_{12} deficiency with folate alone may correct the anemia but does not reverse, and may worsen the neurological damage.

Macrocytosis can also be found in a number of other conditions, such as artifactual macrocytosis due to cold agglutinins; reticulocytosis may cause macrocytosis because these cells are larger than older red cells. A variety of medications such as hydroxyurea and zidovudine, myelodysplastic syndromes, alcoholism, liver disease, and hypothyroidism are all associated with macrocytosis as well.[318]

DISEASES OF WHITE BLOOD CELLS AND THE RETICULOENDOTHELIAL SYSTEM

Leukopenia and agranulocytosis

The causes of a decrease in white cells are similar in any age group: infection, medications, viral illness, or an autoimmune or a primary hematological disorder.

Acute leukemia

Acute leukemia is an accumulation of immature lymphoid or myeloid cells in the bone marrow and peripheral blood, tissue invasion by these cells, and associated bone marrow failure. Untreated, median survival is 3 months.

Acute leukemias are classified grossly as either acute lymphocytic leukemia (ALL) or acute nonlymphocytic leukemia (ANLL) based on the morphology, histochemical staining, immunological markers, and cytogenetics. The French–American–British Cooperative Group (FAB) classification of acute leukemias is the system most widely used.[319] This classification is shown in Table 98-8.

Incidence

Acute leukemia is primarily a disease of elderly people.[320] Leukemia has an incidence of about 15 per 100,000 in all age groups. The incidence begins to rise at age 40 and by age 80 is approximately 160 per 100,000. Eighty percent of adults with acute leukemia have acute nonlymphocytic leukemia (i.e., acute myeloid leukemia [AML]), whereas 80 percent of all children with acute leukemia have ALL. In spite of this, the incidence of ALL is four times higher in elderly people than in children.

Table 98-8 French–American–British classification of acute leukemias and myelodysplasia

A. Acute nonlymphocytic leukemia
  1. M1: myeloblastic without maturation
  2. M2: myeloblastic with maturation
  3. M3: promyelocytic
  4. M4: myelomonocytic
  5. M5: monocytic
       M5a: poorly differentiated (monoblastic)
       M5b: monocytic
  6. M6: erythroleukemia
  7. Other (megakaryoblastic, basophilic, eosinophilic)

B. Acute lymphoblastic leukemia
  1. L1: small cells predominate
  2. L2: large heterogeneous cells
  3. L3: large homogeneous cells (Burkitt's type)

C. Myelodysplasia syndrome
  1. Refractory anemia
  2. Refractory anemia with ringed sideroblasts (>15% ringed forms in the marrow)
  3. RAEB[a] (5–20% blasts in the marrow, <5% circulating blasts)
  4. Chronic myelomonocytic leukemia (monocytosis $\geq 1,000/mm^2$ in association with RAEB)
  5. RAEB in transformation (20–30% blasts in marrow, $\geq 5\%$ circulating blasts)

[a]RAEB: refractory anemia with excess blasts.

Etiology

The etiology is unclear in most cases of acute leukemia. Radiation exposure has been implicated in some cases. Atomic bomb survivors from Hiroshima and Nagasaki had a 10–20 percent increased incidence of AML. Diagnostic radiologists and patients who received radiation therapy for ankylosing spondylitis in the earlier part of this century had a 2.5- and 14-fold increased risk, respectively, of AML. High-level benzene exposure in the workplace has also been strongly implicated.[321] Long-term, low-dose therapy with alkylating agents can cause acute leukemia, mostly AML.[322] The combination of chemotherapeutic drugs and radiation increases the risk of developing leukemia. Chronic bone marrow disorders such as myelodysplastic syndromes, polycythemia vera, paroxysmal nocturnal hemoglobinuria, and aplastic anemia sometimes culminate in a rapidly progressive leukemic phase.[320] Viruses have been suspected to be the cause of some acute leukemias.[323] Recent molecular genetic studies have demonstrated that oncogenes, the cellular homologs of retroviral transforming genes, appear to have a role in the induction and maintenance of the malignant state. Cytogenetic and molecular biological techniques have shown that specific oncogenes are involved in nonrandom chromosome translocations or are found on deleted or reduplicated chromosomes.[324–326]

Pathophysiology and signs and symptoms

Primitive white blood cells accumulate rapidly in the bone marrow and may result in severe anemia, thrombocytopenia and a paucity of normal leukocytes. Blasts may invade tissues including the liver, lungs, spleen, lymph nodes, skin, and central nervous system (CNS). Therefore patients may present with acute fever, bleeding, anemia, lymphadenopathy, organomegaly, dyspnea, or mental status changes.

In elderly people, the disease can develop insidiously, with progressive weakness, pallor, a change in the sense of well-being, and delirium.[327]

Laboratory data and diagnosis

The total white blood count may be low, normal, or elevated, usually with blasts in the peripheral blood smear. A bone marrow aspiration confirms the diagnosis with an excess of blast cells (>30 percent) and with decreased or absent normal erythroid, granulocytic, and megakaryocytic cells. Histochemical stains, surface antigen markers, and cytogenetics are also useful to identify the type of leukemia. These also help prognosticate remission rates and choose appropriate chemotherapy.

Prognosis

Untreated, the average patient will die within 4–6 months from clinical presentation. Some patients die within days of the onset of the illness. Infection, bleeding, advanced age, high blast counts, and chromosomal abnormalities have all been proposed as poor prognostic indicators, while the presence of Auer rods (in AML) and the development of hepatitis have been reported to be advantageous. Recent work has tried to define morphological, cytogenetic and in-vitro growth characteristics as prognosticators.[320,327]

Advanced age (>50 years) is a poor prognostic sign. Elderly people also have more complex karyotype abnormalities than younger patients,[320,328] and more of them have underlying primary marrow disorders such as myelodysplasia.[320] The presence of a prior hematological marrow disorder (e.g. myelodysplasia or polycythemia vera) or a leukemia that is secondary to prior alkylating agent therapy seems to be a poor prognostic sign.[329,330] Much of the problem in treating elderly people seems to be their inability to tolerate the prolonged pancytopenia that accompanies aggressive induction chemotherapy regimens.

Treatment

Older patients with ALL have a poor long-term survival compared to children, who have an excellent prognosis. The older patient with ALL usually is defined as high risk and often has a white blood cell count of more than 20,000/mm^3, a mediastinal mass, L2/L3 morphology, T-cell or B-cell leukemia, and meningitis. Therapy usually consists of a combination of drugs including vincristine, prednisone, and additional drugs that may include, among others, doxorubicin, cyclophosphamide, and L-asparaginase.[331] Most older people relapse within the first year of treatment. At the present time, therefore, there is no standard combination therapy.[320,327]

In AML, complete remission must first be obtained. The induction phase is the most crucial time because the patient is often infected and bleeding, and has a large tumor burden with little normal hematopoiesis. Complete remission is defined as the reduction of leukemic blasts to an undetectable level in the bone marrow (<5 percent blasts). Many induction regimens are currently being studied; the standard combination is cytarabine at 100–200 mg/m^2 per day as a continuous intravenous infusion for 7 days and daunorubicin 45 mg/m^2 intravenously for the first 3 days.[331] By supporting the patient with cytokines, platelets, red blood cells, and antibiotics, the current complete remission rate in people over age 60 is reported to be 40–76 percent.[320] The median survival is 1–2 years. New protocols are studying the value of different maintenance and consolidation chemotherapeutic regimens. Idarubicin 12 mg/m^2 in combination with cytarabine has demonstrated superior first remission rates, and remission duration in patients <60 years old.[329,330,332]

Infections are the major cause of mortality and morbidity in acute leukemias because of the severe leukopenia and the destruction of normal cutaneous and mucosal barriers. Approximately 500–1,000 polymorphonuclear leukocytes per cubic millimeter are necessary for protection against infection. In many patients the endogenous bowel flora is the source of the infection. The pharynx, lungs, perirectal areas, and skin are also common sites of infection. The genitourinary tract and meninges are less common sites. Since the source of the infection is endogenous organisms, reverse isolation is of limited value. Viruses, protozoa, and anaerobic bacteria are uncommon pathogens early in therapy. Fungal infections usually occur after 7–14 days of antibiotic therapy in neutropenic patients.[333] The choice of antibiotic depends on the predominant organisms causing infection in a given hospital. Usually an aminoglycoside and a semisynthetic penicillin or cephalosporin are the drugs of choice, as the most common organisms in most hospitals are *Pseudomonas* and *Escherichia coli*. Recently, trimethoprim-sulfamethoxazole as prophylaxis has been suggested, particularly in patients who have had frequent admissions with fever and neutropenia.[334]

Metabolic problems are common during induction therapy. Hyperuricemia from the release of uric acid from the dead blasts is treated prophylactically with allopurinol 300 mg/d. Hypokalemia can occur as a result of natriuresis and/or proximal renal tubular dysfunction. A renal tubular acidosis-like syndrome with hypokalemia, amino aciduria, and hyperphosphaturia occurs but is probably not related to lysozyme. Metabolic alkalosis, metabolic acidosis, hypocalcemia, and hyperphosphatemia are all common complications. Patients should be treated routinely with vigorous hydration, alkalinization of the urine, and allopurinol.[335,336]

Aggregates of blasts and thrombi may occlude small blood vessels throughout the body, particularly in the brain and lungs. Therapy revolves around hydration and rapid reduction of the blast count, usually with prompt treatment with a chemotherapeutic agent such as hydroxyurea, which rapidly lowers the white cell count.[337] Leukopheresis and cranial irradiation may be temporizing measures.[338,339]

The CNS is the most common site of extramedullary relapse in acute leukemia. The need for prophylactic meningeal therapy with cranial irradiation and intrathecal methotrexate or cystosine arabinoside has not yet been formally addressed in elderly people. Therefore, these methods must be used with extreme caution at the present time. Spinal cord compression, when it occurs, is usually responsive to local radiation. T-cell acute lymphocytic leukemias are most likely to cause either CNS or gonadal invasion. However, the role of prophylactic testicular radiation is currently unclear in elderly people.[320,326]

Disseminated intravascular coagulation is an uncommon complication and is mainly seen in M3 (promyelocytic leukemia). In general, it is self-limited and is most problematic during the rapid cell lysis of induction chemotherapy. The use of prophylactic heparin continues to be controversial.

Bone marrow transplant is rarely used in older individuals. The presence of poor prognostic karyotypes and the high frequency of blast cells with multidrug-resistant glycoprotein MDR1 may be the reason for the poor prognosis in elderly people. Intensive induction therapy and cytarabine combined with growth factor support and eventually MDR1 modulators may offer the best treatment in elderly people.[332]

Chronic leukemias

Chronic leukemia is a neoplastic accumulation of mature lymphoid (chronic lymphocytic leukemia +[CLL]) or myeloid elements (chronic myeloid leukemia + [CML]) of the blood which usually progresses more slowly than an acute leukemia. CML will be discussed in the section on myeloproliferative disorders.

Chronic lymphocytic leukemia

CLL is primarily a disease of elderly people, while CML usually occurs in the third or fourth decade, as well as in old age. In more than 95 percent of all cases CLL involves neoplastic proliferation of B-cells.[340]

Incidence

CLL is the most common leukemia in Western society, accounting for 25–40 percent of all leukemias. Ninety percent of all patients are over the age of 50, with the vast majority being over age 60. Men are affected twice as often as women.[340]

Etiology

Ionizing radiation plays no part in the etiology of CLL. There seems to be a genetic component, as the illness is more common in certain families, and in some of these families, there are immunological abnormalities. Chronic viral infections (retroviruses) have been suggested as possible candidates.[341]

Pathophysiology and signs and symptoms

There is an accumulation of monoclonal lymphocytes in peripheral blood, bone marrow, lymphoid tissue, and sometimes other organs. The cells appear morphologically mature, but the presence of receptors for mouse erythrocytes, HLA-DR antigens, and a small amount of surface immunoglobin suggests some degree of immaturity. Trisomy 12 has been described as a chromosomal abnormality in some cases (25 percent), and abnormalities of other chromosomes including 6, 11, and 13 have been described as well.[342] Infiltration of the bone marrow may eventually result in pancytopenia. Normal B-cells are not present in adequate numbers, which often leads to bacterial infection. Transformation into diffuse large-cell lymphoma (Richter's syndrome) or prolymphocytic leukemia may occur as a terminal event.[327,340]

The presentation is highly variable. Over 25 percent of patients have asymptomatic disease that is discovered on routine physical examination or blood analysis. The most common initial symptoms are fatigue, malaise, and decreased exercise tolerance. In many older people, exacerbation of coronary artery or cerebrovascular disease may be the initial manifestation.

Some patients report enlarged lymph nodes most commonly found in the cervical, axillary, and supraclavicular areas, while inguinal adenopathy is rare. Splenomegaly is found in 50 percent of patients at presentation, and hepatomegaly may develop as the disease progresses. Some patients complain of abdominal pain or early satiety due to splenomegaly. Lymphocyte infiltration can occur in any organ. Jaundice usually suggests hemolysis even though periportal lymph node enlargement with biliary tract obstruction can occur. In late-stage disease ecchymoses and petechiae from thrombocytopenia may be seen. Fever is usually secondary to infection, but late in the disease the possibility of transformation into acute prolymphocytic leukemia or aggressive lymphoma should be considered. Clinical hyperviscosity is rare and occurs only when the white blood cell count is 800,000/mm³ or greater.[327,340]

Laboratory data and diagnosis

The diagnosis of CLL requires the demonstration of sustained lymphocytosis and bone marrow lymphocyte infiltration in the absence of other causes. The absolute lymphocyte count is generally above 15,000/mm³, although newer classification systems accept a level of 5,000/mm³.[343] Cells are mature in appearance, and there is a tendency for these lymphocytes to smudge on preparation of the blood smear. In B-cell CLL, the T- and B-cells are both increased in absolute number. However, B-cells are preferentially increased and make up 40–90 percent of all lymphocytes. The B-cells form rosettes with mouse erythrocytes; they are of monoclonal origin and express surface immunoglobins of one light-chain class. The surface immunoglobin is usually IgM but less commonly is IgD.

Immunophenotypically, they also express the cell markers CD5+, CD19+, CD20+, CD23+, FMC7–/+, and CD22–/+.[342] In B-cell CLL, the ratio of helper to suppressor T-cells is reversed because of an increase in the number of suppressor cells. This is thought to account for development of the pure red cell aplasia described in a few patients.[344]

Approximately 1 percent of patients have lymphocytes that form rosettes with sheep red blood cells, and their disease is classified as T-cell CLL. Both helper (T4+) and suppressor (T8+) forms are seen. The lymphocytes often demonstrate cytoplasmic azurophilic granules. Massive splenomegaly, marked neutropenia, skin infiltration, modest bone marrow infiltration, and a rapid clinical course leading to death are seen in less than one-half of these patients.[345] There is a high concurrence with rheumatoid arthritis.[345] Most cases, however, have indolent courses.

Red blood cell morphology is usually normal. Anemia is found in 10–20 percent of all patients and is most often normochromic and normocytic. The anemia may be due to marrow replacement, hypersplenism, or suppressor mechanisms. The Coombs test reveals IgG coating of red blood cells in about 20 percent of cases; however, immune hemolytic anemia is seen only 8 percent of the time. Thrombocytopenia is found in 10–20 percent of cases and may be due to marrow replacement, hypersplenism, or antiplatelet antibodies. Autoimmune thrombocytopenia occurs in about 5 percent of patients. Bone marrow morphology shows interstitial or nodular infiltration in early disease and diffuse infiltration in advanced stages.[346,347]

In about 5 percent of cases, immunoglobin found on the cell surface is the same as that found in the serum as a monoclonal protein. About 50–75 percent of patients are hypo- or agammaglobulinemic.

Prognosis

On the basis of physical examination and a CBC, the patient can be staged clinically (Table 98-9).[343] Group A patients have fewer than three areas of lymphoid enlargement, including cervical, axillary, supraclavicular, or inguinal lymph nodes or liver or spleen. Generally, disease progression follows a stepwise pattern from mild to more severe illness. Patients in group C with anemia (less than 10 g/dL) or thrombocytopenia (less than 100,000/mm³) usually survive less than 2 years.

Other poor prognostic signs include diffuse replacement of bone marrow, IgM surface immunoglobin rather than IgD, and a lymphocyte doubling time of under 12 months.[348] Chromosomal aberrations also affect survival with 17p deletions having the worst prognosis, followed by 11q deletions, 12q trisomy, and normal karyotypes, whereas patients with 13q deletions as the only karyotypic abnormality had the longest survival.[349]

Although survival in CLL is often prolonged, the overall 5-year survival is only about 50 percent.

Treatment

Patients in group A usually do not require any treatment until their disease progresses. This approach is usually extended to individuals in group B, as the complications of chemotherapy such as infection or development of acute nonlymphocytic leukemia may be more deleterious than the CLL.[350]

In stage C,[340] chlorambucil is the agent most often used. It can be given daily (often at doses of 6–8 mg orally) or every 2 weeks (0.4–0.8 mg/kg body weight): response rates range from 40 to 70 percent, but complete responses are rare.[342] Patients who fail to respond can be given other chemotherapy (e.g. fludarabine).[342] Fludarabine when used as initial therapy in CLL yields higher response rates and longer remission duration and progression-free survival than chlorambucil but overall survival is not enhanced.[351] Maintenance therapy is not usually employed. Steroids are often used for the treatment of patients with autoimmune hemolytic anemia or thrombocytopenia, and radiation therapy is used to reduce local bulky disease, vital organ compromise, or painful bone lesions. Newer agents include CAMPATH-1H (alemtuzumab), a human immunoglobulin IgG1 anti-CD52 monoclonal antibody that binds to nearly all B- and T-cell leukemias and has shown significant activity in patients with advanced and chemotherapy-resistant CLL.[352] Rituximab, IDEC C$_2$-B$_5$, a monoclonal antibody against CD20 and used in the treatment of follicular lymphoma, is under study for the treatment of CLL.

The most common complications of CLL are bacterial infections, with pneumonia and urinary tract infections occurring most frequently. Gram-positive cocci, Gram-negative rods, *Listeria*, fungi, and *Pneumocystis carinii* infection all occur. In addition to the appropriate antibiotics, some patients with hypogammaglobulinemia may benefit from regular infusions of immune globulin; however, the cost of this therapy is very high.[353] Patients with CLL have at least a four-fold risk of developing a carcinoma.

When transformation into either a prolymphocytic leukemia or into an aggressive lymphoma occurs, there is generally a poor response to chemotherapy or radiation.

Multiple myeloma

Multiple myeloma is a neoplastic disorder resulting from the proliferation and accumulation of immature plasma cells in the bone marrow. Its major manifestations, which ultimately lead to death, result from both the direct effect of these cells

---

Table 98-9 International workshop on staging of chronic lymphocytic leukemia

Stage	Definition
A	No anemia or thrombocytopenia and fewer than three areas of lymphoid enlargement, median survival >7 years
B	No anemia or thrombocytopenia with three or more involved areas, median survival <5 years
C	Anemia (hemoglobin <10 g/dL) and or thrombocytopenia (<100,000/μL) regardless of the number of areas of lymphoid enlargement, median survival <2 years

and the characteristic proteins produced by them, as well as their secondary effects on other organ systems.[354–356]

The neoplastic plasma cells almost always synthesize abnormal amounts of monoclonal immunoglobulin (IgG, IgA, IgD, or IgE) κ or λ light chains. They are, therefore, usually classified by their immunoglobulin class. Rarely, there are cases in which there is no detectable secretion of immunoglobulin.[356]

Incidence

The annual incidence of multiple myeloma is approximately 3 per 100,000. However, at age 80, the incidence rises to 37 per 100,000. The disease is more common in blacks than in whites, and the incidence is slightly greater in men. Multiple myeloma usually occurs in people over the age of 50 and the incidence increases progressively with age.[354–356]

Etiology

There is an increased incidence of myeloma in first-degree relatives. This, together with the higher frequency of the 4C complex of HLA antigens in myeloma patients and the increased incidence in blacks, suggests that genetic factors play a role.[357–360]

There seems to be an enhanced risk of developing myeloma after high radiation exposure, as shown in Hiroshima and Nagasaki atomic bomb survivors.[361] Other etiological possibilities suggested have included chronic antigenic stimulation such as cholecystitis, osteomyelitis, repeated allergen injections, rheumatoid arthritis, hereditary spherocytosis, and Gaucher's disease.[362–375] Asbestos and viral illnesses such as Aleutian mink disease have also been implicated.[376–381]

Since myeloma is also age related, one possible influence might be the decrease in the T-lymphoid arm of the immune system. As T-cells decrease, B-cell clones may proliferate excessively. Because of such monoclonal expansions, there may then be a higher probability of either spontaneous or externally induced genetic alteration of one such clone, allowing it to proliferate and secrete its immunoglobulin. This activity would still remain under control of the immune system and thus would be considered "benign monoclonal gammopathy." Finally, a second external oncogenic event could result in uncontrolled proliferation of these cells, and multiple myeloma would ensue.

Much interest has recently been focused on a number of cytokines that may play a role in multiple myeloma. IL-6 has been suggested to be a myeloma cell growth factor, and high levels of IL-6 have been associated with a poor outcome in some studies on multiple myeloma.[363,382] There has been some recent discussion of the role of herpesvirus 8 found in some of the nonmalignant stromal cells (IL-6-producing cells) in myeloma patients. The virus was found to encode an IL-6 homolog that can stimulate human myeloma cells but causality remains to be proved.[383]

Pathophysiology and signs and symptoms

The consequences of abnormal plasma cell growth cell tumors include osteolysis, hematopoietic suppression, hypogammaglobulinemia, paraproteinemia, paraproteinuria, and renal disease.[354–356]

Plasma cell tumors usually develop in areas of hematopoietically active bone marrow. They can be seen in virtually any bone and rarely in extraskeletal sites. In most instances, even plasmacytomas that seem solitary eventually become generalized.

Osteolytic lesions are very common and are thought to result from the release of osteoclast activating factor (possibly IL-6) from the neoplastic plasma cell,[384] which stimulates osteoclasts to resorb bone.

Marrow function is impaired in proportion to the number of plasma cells in the bone marrow. Anemia is most common, but neutropenia and thrombocytopenia also occur.

In multiple myeloma, the single species of abnormal plasma cells produces a single type of immunoglobulin or portion of the immunoglobulin molecule in excess. There is concomitant suppression of the other classes of normal immunoglobulin, resulting in actual or functional hypogammaglobulinemia. In over 50 percent of patients, the monoclonal protein is an IgG, in 20 percent IgA, and 12 percent IgM (macroglobulinemia). IgD is found in about 2 percent of cases, and IgE is very rare. About 10 percent of patients produce only light chains, and less than 1 percent produce only heavy chains. In rarer cases patients produce two or more monoclonal proteins, and about 1 percent of patient do not have any monoclonal protein in their serum or urine.[354–356]

About one-half of patients with multiple myeloma have renal disease. Urinary tract infections, glomerular deposits of amyloid, stones from hypercalcemia and hyperuricemia, and plasma cell infiltration of the kidney all may occur. However, the major cause of renal failure is tubular damage associated with the excretion of light-chain proteins. Not all these proteins are nephrotoxic, and some patients may excrete large amounts of them for years without developing renal failure. Patients excreting λ light chains are at greater risk than those excreting κ light chains.[354–356]

Multiple myeloma is usually a progressive disease. The doubling time of the abnormal plasma cells has been estimated to be 3–10 months. In rare cases, however, the preclinical stage may have a duration of years.[354–356]

The most frequent symptom of multiple myeloma is bone pain which occurs in about 70 percent of patients. Pain is often in the lower back or ribs and gradually increases in intensity. Sudden onset of pain often means that a vertebra has collapsed or there has been a spontaneous fracture through an involved area such as the shaft of a long bone, the pelvis, a rib, or a clavicle.

Systemic signs and symptoms include pallor, weakness, fatigue, dyspnea on exertion, and palpitations. These all result from the anemia present in about 70 percent of patients at the time of diagnosis. Signs of thrombocytopenia are common, such as ecchymoses, purpura, epistaxis, or excessive bleeding from trauma. Signs of infection also occur frequently as a result of neutropenia and immunoglobulin deficiency, and the patient may present with pneumonia, pyoderma, or pyelonephritis. Cold insensitivity and urticaria may result from cryoglobulinemia. Nephrotic syndrome is a rare presentation.

Hypercalcemia is very common in patients with destructive bone lesions and may result in anorexia, nausea, vomiting, polyuria, polydipsia, constipation, and dehydration. Particularly in elderly people, drowsiness, confusion, and coma can result from hypercalcemia.[354–356]

Acute renal failure may also develop in patients who have azotemia and who receive hypertonic contrast media during the performance of a diagnostic procedure. In patients with multiple myeloma, procedures such as intravenous or retrograde pyelograms or open bone biopsies should not be performed unless there is ample urine flow and hypercalcemia and hyperuricemia have been corrected.

Hyperviscosity syndrome occurs about 50 percent of the time if the monoclonal immunoglobulin is IgM (macroglobu-linemia). It is uncommon in multiple myeloma with another monoclonal protein. Purpura, ecchymoses, epistaxis, gastro-intestinal bleeding; blurred vision (associated with venous congestion, hemorrhages, and exudates), and ischemic neurological symptoms are common signs of hyperviscosity.[354–356]

Neurological signs and symptoms include mental confusion due to hypercalcemia, spinal cord and nerve root compression, myelomatous meningitis, carpal tunnel syndrome (due to deposition of amyloid), and sensorimotor polyneuropathy not due to amyloid or infiltration with plasma cells. Rarer CNS symptoms include intracerebral plasmacytomas, herpes zoster, and multifocal leukoencephalopathy.[354–356]

Laboratory data and diagnosis

If a monoclonal serum component is found in an otherwise asymptomatic patient, the skeleton should be X-rayed and a bone marrow aspiration should be performed. The absence of both lytic bone lesions and plasma cell infiltration makes a diagnosis of benign monoclonal gammopathy likely. Confirmatory tests for this diagnosis include absence of significant (less than 60 mg/24 h) amounts of a single type of light chain (Bence–Jones protein) in the urine and a serum monoclonal gammopathy of less than 2 g/dL. The presence in the bone marrow of more than 10 percent mature and immature plasma cells, osteolytic bone lesions, and a serum monoclonal protein is diagnostic of multiple myeloma. Excretion of light chains of more than 60 mg/24 h and of a monoclonal protein of greater than 2 g/dL (although it is usually greater than 3 g/dL) is very suggestive of multiple myeloma. If bone marrow plasmacytosis is not demonstrated, a repeat bone marrow aspiration and a search for an extraskeletal plasma cell tumor should be undertaken. Finally, one must keep in mind that idiopathic monoclonal components are sometimes seen with other cancers.[354–356] Patients should have a complete blood count, serum creatinine, uric acid, β2-microglobulin (β-2M), C-reactive protein, LDH and if possible a plasma cell labeling index (PCLI).

Prognosis

The only way to differentiate between some cases of early multiple myeloma and benign monoclonal gammopathy is observation over time. In a long-term follow-up study (median 22 years) in patients at the Mayo clinic with apparently benign monoclonal gammopathy, 19 percent had benign monoclonal gammopathy, 10 percent had a serum monoclonal protein value of 3 g/dL or more but did not require chemotherapy, 47 percent had died without evidence of myeloma, and 24 percent had multiple myeloma, systemic amyloidosis, macroglobulinemia, or malignant lymphoproliferative disease. In patients who developed multiple myeloma this was diag-

nosed a median of 10 years after the monoclonal protein was found, emphasizing the need for long-term follow-up.[385]

Once a diagnosis of multiple myeloma is made, the patient can be classified as a good or a poor risk. A good risk is defined as a hemoglobin of 9.0 g/dL or greater, a blood urea nitrogen of 30 mg/dL or less, and a serum calcium level of 12 mg/dL or less after hydration. The poor-risk group consists of patients who fail to meet these criteria.[354] With therapy, the good-risk group has a median survival of 42 months and the poor-risk group has only a 21-month survival. Both groups respond equally well to initial therapy. Besides clinical status, other important prognostic features are the β-2M level, which is an indicator of tumor mass,[386] PCLI, which measures the proliferative rate of the plasma cells,[386] and possibly the IL-6 level.[382,386] Patients with both a low PCLI and a low β-2M have a median survival of 6 years when treated with chemotherapy.

In some elderly people who fulfill the good-risk diagnostic criteria for multiple myeloma the disease progresses very slowly ("smoldering myeloma"). If the patient is asymptomatic or only mildly symptomatic and is not at risk of developing a complication, he can be followed over time to determine the pace of the illness.

Treatment

Since multiple myeloma is a neoplastic disorder, the mainstay of treatment is chemotherapy, with radiation reserved for localized painful lesions.[354–356]

All patients should be encouraged to keep active to prevent further bone demineralization. Lumbar corsets and braces may help to relieve pain and prevent further damage. Large osteolytic lesions should be irradiated before fractures occur. Actual fracture through a lytic lesion requires an intramedullary pin and radiation. Pamidronate, an intravenous bisphosphonate, administered monthly in stage III myeloma as an adjunct to chemotherapy has been shown to decrease skeletal events, reduce bone pain, and prolong survival.[387]

Patients must drink 2–3 L of fluid per day to maintain increased urine output to allow excretion of light chains, calcium, uric acid, and other metabolites. All infections must be treated promptly. Hyperuricemia should be treated with allopurinol. Hypercalcemia is usually treated with hydration and pamidronate.

Many chemotherapeutic regimens are currently in use for multiple myeloma. In elderly people with decreased bone marrow reserve, the most common regimen is intermittent melphalan and prednisone. The two drugs are given daily for 4 days, and treatment is repeated at intervals of 4–6 weeks for at least three courses before remission or resistance is confirmed.[387] In approximately 40 percent of patients remission is induced with the above therapy. The median duration of remission is about 2 years, and median survival about 3 years.[386] For patients who do not respond to the aforementioned regimen a wide variety of other options (e.g. vincristine, doxorubicin, and dexamethasone) are available.[355,386] Several maintenance therapies including continued melphalan and prednisone have been used,[386] and some success with increased remission duration has recently been reported with α-interferon.[388] Which maintenance therapies, if any (most studies do not show increased survival), to use are determined on an individual basis. Anemia can be palliated with erythropoietin administration. Hyperviscosity can be treated urgently with plasmapheresis.

Recently thalidomide was found to have substantial antitumor activity in patients with advanced myeloma who relapsed after high-dose chemotherapy.[388] Thalidomide is a known antiangiogenic agent and inhibits TNFα from monocytes among other effects. The role of thalidomide in first-line therapy and in combination with chemotherapy remain to be determined.

Lymphoma

Lymphomas are primary malignancies of the lymph nodes and include Hodgkin's disease and non-Hodgkin's lymphoma. They are distinct entities characterized by different patterns of spread, clinical behaviors, and cell of origin. Hodgkin's disease usually has a predictable pattern of spread to contiguous lymph node areas, while non-Hodgkin's lymphoma is usually widespread at diagnosis. Non-Hodgkin's lymphoma is more likely to have extranodal involvement. Both can be divided into subsets based on the histological appearance of the lymph nodes.[320,389,390]

The diagnosis of Hodgkin's disease depends on histological finding in the lymph node of the Reed–Sternberg cell, a giant cell with twin nuclei that give the cell the appearance of "owl's eyes." The Reed–Sternberg cell is probably the malignant cell, and the other cells surrounding it probably represent tissue reaction.[320,389,390]

Histologically, Hodgkin's disease is subdivided into the following four major types:

1. *Lymphocyte-rich*: mainly adult lymphocytes with few Reed–Sternberg cells.
2. *Mixed cellularity*: a cellular response of mature lymphoid cells, plasma cells, eosinophils, and Reed–Sternberg cells.
3. *Lymphocyte depletion*: a paucity of lymphoid cells with a majority of histiocytes, fibrotic reaction, and Reed–Sternberg cells.
4. *Nodular sclerosis*: effacement of lymphoid tissue by nodular aggregates of mature lymphoid cells and "lacunar" variants of Reed–Sternberg cells separated by bands of adult collagen.

Before modern therapies became available, it was noted that lymphocyte-rich and nodular sclerosis types carried a better prognosis.[320,389,390]

Systematic clinical staging is extremely important in the management of Hodgkin's disease. The currently accepted clinical stages are listed in Table 98-10.

Non-Hodgkin's lymphomas (NHL) are a heterogeneous group of lymphoid malignancies which have some common but many different features. The classification of non-Hodgkin's lymphomas has been a controversial subject and is undergoing revision. Table 98-11 shows the recent WHO classification that has been suggested by the International Lymphoma Study Group. It divides lymphoid neoplasms into B-cell neoplasms, T-cell neoplasms, and Hodgkin's disease and also lists classes not previously well defined such as mantle cell lymphoma and marginal zone B-cell lymphoma, which includes the mucosa-associated lymphoid tissue (MALT) type etc. (Table 98-11).[391]

Clinical staging is similar to that for Hodgkin's disease. However, over 90 percent of patients have stage III or IV disease at the time of presentation with NHL.

Incidence

The incidence of Hodgkin's disease is 2 per 100,000 per year in the United States, and there is a bimodal distribution as a function of age. There is an initial peak between 15 and 35 and a subsequent peak at age 50–80. At age 25, the incidence is approximately 5 per 100,000 per year, and at age 75 it is 7 per 100,000. The incidence is slightly greater for men.

The age-adjusted incidence of non-Hodgkin's lymphoma is 2.6–5.8 per 100,000 per year. There is a progressive increase in incidence with age similar to that seen in acute leukemia. At age 80, the incidence is approximately 40 per 100,000 per year.[320,389,390]

Etiology

The etiology of Hodgkin's disease remains unknown. However, based on seroepidemiological studies, there has been interest in the Epstein–Barr virus and other oncogenic viruses in relation to this disease. Patients with immunodeficiencies and autoimmune disease are at increased risk, which suggests that the immune system plays a role in the etiology. There are some suggestions that in the young, Hodgkin's disease may be an infectious disease, while in elderly people it is more likely a conventional malignancy.[392]

The etiology of most non-Hodgkin's lymphomas is also unknown. However, immunosuppressed patients (e.g. renal transplant recipients) and those with excessive function of the immune system (e.g. with Sjögren's syndrome) are at

Table 98-10 **Clinical staging of Hodgkin's disease**[a]	
Stage	**Definition**
I	Disease limited to one anatomical region
II	Disease in two or more anatomical regions on the same side of the diaphragm
III	Disease on both sides of the diaphragm but limited to lymph nodes, spleen, and/or Waldeyer's ring
III$_1$	Involvement limited to spleen, splenic nodes, and celiac and/or portal nodes
III$_2$	Involvement of para-aortic, pelvic, and iliac nodes
IV	Extranodal disease not directly contiguous with a nodal area (i.e., bone marrow, lung, pleura, liver)

[a]All stages are subclassified into A and B; A, no systematic symptoms; B, any one symptom of unexplained fever, or night sweats, or 10 percent or more loss of body weight.

Table 98-11 **WHO classification of lymphoid neoplasms**

B-cell neoplasms
Precursor B-cell neoplasm:
- Precursor B-lymphoblastic leukemia/lymphoma (precursor B-cell acute lymphoblastic leukemia)

Mature (peripheral) B-cell neoplasms:
- B-cell chronic lymphocytic leukemia/small lymphocytic lymphoma
- B-cell prolymphocytic leukemia
- Lymphoplasmacytic leukemia
- Splenic marginal B-cell lymphoma (± villous lymphocytes)
- Hairy cell leukemia
- Plasma cell myeloma/plasmacytoma
- Extranodal marginal sone B-cell lymphoma (±monocytoid B-cells)
- Follicular lymphoma
- Mantle cell lymphoma
- Diffuse large B-cell lymphoma
- Mediastinal B-cell lymphoma
- Primary effusion lymphoma
- Burkitt lymphoma/Burkitt cell leukemia

T and NK-cell neoplasms
Precursor T-cell neoplasm:
- Precursor T-lymphoblastic lymphoma–leukemia
- T-cell acute lymphoblastic leukemia

Mature peripheral T-cell neoplasms:
- T-cell prolymphocytic leukemia
- T-cell granular lymphocytic leukemia
- Aggressive NK-cell leukemia
- Adult T-cell lymphoma/leukemia (HTLV1+)
- Extranodal NK/T-cell lymphoma, nasal type
- Enteropathy-type T-cell lymphoma
- Hepatosplenic gamma-delta T-cell lymphoma
- Subcutaneous panniculitis-like T-cell lymphoma
- Mycosis fungoides/Sezary syndrome
- Anaplastic large cell lymphoma, T/null cell, primary cutaneous type
- Peripheral T-cell lymphoma, not otherwise characterized
- Angioimmunoblastic T-cell lymphoma
- Anaplastic large cell lymphoma, T/null cell, primary systemic type

Hodgkin's lymphoma
Nodular lymphocyte predominant Hodgkin's lymphoma
Classical Hodgkin's lymphoma:
- Nodular sclerosis Hodgkin's lymphoma (grades 1 and 2)
- Lymphocyte-rich classical Hodgkin's lymphoma
- Mixed cellularity Hodgkin's lymphoma
- Lymphocyte depletion Hodgkin's lymphoma

greater risk.[393] Viral etiologies are involved in at least some non-Hodgkin's lymphomas. African Burkitt's lymphoma is associated with Epstein–Barr virus infection,[393] and an aggressive T-cell leukemia or lymphoma is associated with HTLV-I infection in Japan and the Caribbean. Similarly, patients with human immunodeficiency virus (HIV) infection often develop aggressive non-Hodgkin's lymphoma and sometimes Hodgkin's disease.[394–397] It has been postulated that in acquired immunodeficiency syndrome (AIDS), lymphomas are secondary to Epstein–Barr virus activation of oncogene expression.[398] There is also some evidence that some early

MALT-type tumors are antigen responsive, and therapy directed against the antigen may result in regression of early lesions (*Helicobacter pylori* in gastric lymphoma).[399,400]

Chromosomal abnormalities are frequent in patients with lymphoma, and several abnormalities are often found simultaneously.[401] Translocations involving chromosomes 14 and 18 are the most common abnormalities found in non-Hodgkin's lymphoma. An oncogene *bcl-2* has been cloned from the region involved on chromosome 18 and has been shown to be activated through juxtaposition with the immunoglobulin heavy-chain locus.[401] The gene *bcl-2* produces a protein that helps block programmed cell death of B lymphocytes, possibly resulting in extended survival of cells carrying this translocation.[401]

Pathophysiology and signs and symptoms

In Hodgkin's disease normal lymphoid tissue is replaced by the malignant lymphoma, which can result in immunodeficiency and infections. The bone marrow may be replaced, resulting in pancytopenia and subsequent anemia, bleeding, and infection. The tumor bulk may obstruct vital organs and ultimately invade vital organs and cause death.

Patients with Hodgkin's disease usually have enlarged lymph nodes in the neck on presentation. Although any nodal group can be involved, the cervical or axillary lymph nodes are the most common. The patient may be asymptomatic, or the onset of symptoms may be marked by the B symptoms of fever, night sweats, or weight loss of greater than 10 percent of normal body weight. Pruritus may be present, but it is no longer considered diagnostic of a B classification. These constitutional symptoms are often associated with extensive disease. Patients may also present with advanced disease consisting of diffuse adenopathy and involvement of the spleen, liver, bone marrow, or lung. Elderly patients are more likely to present with B symptoms and advanced disease.[402]

Non-Hodgkin's lymphomas at all ages appear to be multi-centric in origin and have a tendency to spread widely during the course of the disease. A peripheral blood leukemic phase is not uncommon. Most patients seek medical care because of neck or inguinal node enlargement. However, skin, gastrointestinal tract, bone, liver, and CNS lymphomas make up about 10–20 percent of the primary sites at presentation. Splenomegaly, bone marrow failure, autoimmune hemolytic anemia, and autoimmune thrombocytopenia are occasional presenting features. Systemic B symptoms are not as common as in Hodgkin's disease. Waldeyer's ring involvement is strongly associated with gastrointestinal lesions. Hypercalcemia is a prominent feature in HTLV-I-related non-Hodgkin's lymphoma but it is rare in other lymphomas. Hypogammaglobulinemia may be present, but patients occasionally have a monoclonal serum M component.[320,389]

Laboratory data and diagnosis

The diagnosis is made based on biopsy and the histological picture of malignant lymphoma.

In Hodgkin's disease clinical staging is extremely important to determine treatment, and systemic staging includes the following:

1. Complete physical examination with careful attention to all lymph node areas.

2. Routine chemistry profile and CBC.
3. Computerized tomography scans of the abdomen, pelvis, and in some cases, the chest. Gallium scanning is also useful for follow-up if the tumor is gallium avid at presentation.
4. Lymphangiography via the pedal lymphatics to outline the femoral, inguinal, pelvic, and para-aortic nodes.
5. In cases in which the clinical stage may change the treatment modality, laparotomy (sometimes including splenectomy), liver biopsies, and sampling of suspicious nodes should be performed. A bone marrow biopsy is also required if it will change treatment. Up to 30 percent of patients have different clinical and pathological stages. In elderly patients, however, Hodgkin's disease is more likely to be manifested as advanced disease (stage III or IV). It has been suggested that patients past the age of 40, particularly those with mixed cellularity or lymphocyte depletion histologies, may not benefit from laparotomy.[320,389]

In non-Hodgkin's lymphoma systemic staging is rarely required. After a complete physical examination, CBC, chemistry profile, bone marrow aspirate and biopsy, chest X-ray or CT scan, and abdominal computerized tomography, about 90 percent of all patients are shown to have advanced-stage disease. Staging laparotomy is usually not required. Other studies such as serum protein electrophoresis, skeletal X-rays, and intravenous urography are sometimes useful.[320,389]

Prognosis

In Hodgkin's disease, elderly patients with advanced stages do not do as well as young people, since they are unable to tolerate maximal radiation and chemotherapy doses.[403] In non-Hodgkin's lymphoma, the prognosis relates to both age and factors that are intrinsic to the disease. Good prognostic indicators are nodular histology, limited stage, and young age. Marrow involvement is a poor prognostic sign in unfavorable histologies but not in favorable or intermediate histologies. Other poor prognostic signs are bulky abdominal disease, hemoglobin less than 12 g/dL, and serum LDH greater than 250 units/L.[393] Based on five clinical factors—age, tumor stage, serum LDH, performance status, and number of extranodal disease sites—some physicians categorize patients into four groups which help to predict complete response rates and survival.[404]

Treatment

In Hodgkin's disease, the primary therapeutic maneuver is the treatment of known disease and the next potential site of involvement. In general, limited radiation therapy is used for stages I and II (many institutions use chemotherapy and radiation therapy for stages IB and IIB), and combination chemotherapy with or without radiation is recommended for stages III and IV.[320,389] However, it must be kept in mind that regeneration of the bone marrow after radiation or chemotherapy is markedly diminished in patients past the age of 40, and gastrointestinal side-effects are much more severe. Thus, one must consider limiting the usual mantle field in elderly patients with early-stage disease. Similarly, it may be impossible to give optimal chemotherapy to elderly patients, even though the benefits of aggressive chemotherapy outweigh the risks. The survival of patients given palliative treatment rather than aggressive therapy is dramatically less. Many elderly patients can tolerate only 30–50 percent of the optimal dose of chemotherapy.[403] The duration of chemotherapy is 6–12 months or at least 2 months following attainment of complete remission. There is an increased incidence of a second malignancy in patients with Hodgkin's disease receiving therapy.[405,406] In a study at Stanford University, acute leukemia developed in about 4 percent of patients. However, the risk appeared to level off after 10 years.[406] and it was believed that risks were largely due to the chemotherapy. About 20 percent of patients developed solid tumors by 20 years after treatment, and these were believed to be primarily irradiation induced.[406] In the aforementioned study, by 18 years after treatment, about 5 percent of patients had developed non-Hodgkin's lymphoma.

In non-Hodgkin's lymphoma, there are marked differences in prognosis based on pathological classification. Very few cases are stage I, and therefore curative radiation is rarely possible. Most patients have advanced-stage disease and require chemotherapy. Chemotherapeutic "cures" in non-Hodgkin's lymphoma paradoxically tend to occur only in patients with intermediate and unfavorable prognosis histologies. In contrast, in lymphomas with a favorable prognosis, while they are extremely sensitive to chemotherapy, aggressive therapy does not seem to prolong survival. For these reasons, therapy is minimal in cases with a favorable prognosis and aggressive in those with unfavorable pathology.[320,389,393]

FAVORABLE PROGNOSIS HISTOLOGY IN NON-HODGKIN'S LYMPHOMA   Regional radiation is used in what appears to be disease of stage I or II, if any therapy is given. However, most patients relapse either because they were not truly in an early stage or because the disease is so indolent that recurrence may not occur for 5–10 years. Chemotherapy is rarely indicated in stage I or II and often no therapy is needed. Particularly in elderly patients close follow-up without treatment until problems develop is often a practical approach.[320,389]

In stages III and IV, the disease is still very indolent. Most patients respond to chemotherapy, but the relapse rate is 10–20 percent per year. Even though 80–90 percent with favorable prognosis histology achieve complete remission, at the 10-year mark only 10–20 percent will be without disease. Consequently, it is often wise to avoid both the serious systemic toxicity inherent in aggressive combination therapy and the potential risk of acute nonlymphocytic leukemia associated with chronic low-dose alkylating agents.[407] If treatment is necessary, chlorambucil is often used. Protocols involving different agents that have shown some promise in indolent lymphoma, such as fludarabine, are currently underway.[400] The most exciting recent developments are in the therapeutic use of monoclonal antibodies against CD20 (rituximab),[408] diphtheria toxin conjugated antibody against IL-2 receptor (denileukin difitox),[409] and new retinoids (bexarotene).[410] These are discussed in the biological therapy section.

INTERMEDIATE AND UNFAVORABLE PROGNOSIS HISTOLOGY IN NON-HODGKIN'S LYMPHOMA   These aggressive non-Hodgkin's lymphomas are rapidly growing tumors with a short natural history. For this reason, patients are generally treated with combination chemotherapy. Some patients with localized disease are, however, treated with combined limited-term chemotherapy and radiation therapy.[400] Regimens that might offer better tolerability in elderly people than older ones are being developed.[404] There have been advances in the treatment of lymphoma with high-dose therapy and allogeneic or autologous transplants but these aggressive treatments are usually reserved for patients <55 and <65 years old, respectively. There are studies ongoing combining immunotherapy with chemotherapy which include elderly patients (e.g. CHOP + rituximab).

Waldenstrom's macroglobulinemia

Waldenstrom's macroglobulinemia (WM) is a lymphoplasmacytoid lymphoma of elderly people associated with the production of monoclonal IgM greater than 2 g/L. The median survival of patients with WM averages 5 years but there is a 20 percent 10-year survival. The illness is insidious, with fatigue and weight loss being the predominant clinical findings. As the level of IgM monoclonal protein rises, hyperviscosity syndrome ensues with visual disturbances, lethargy, confusion, muscle weakness, neurological findings, congestive heart failure, cytopenias, and organomegaly. If the macroglobulins are cryoglobulins, Raynaud's phenomenon, cold agglutin disease, palpable purpura, or glomerulonephritis may occur. Tissue deposition of the macroglobulin may result in peripheral neuropathy which may be associated with demyelination if the IgM is a myelin-associated glycoprotein, renal disease (although this is less common and usually less severe than in multiple myeloma), or amyloidosis. Bleeding manifestations may occur as a result of interaction of the macroglobulin with platelets and coagulation factors. There is often anemia, but it may be artificially low because IgM causes expansion of the plasma volume. There is usually moderate lymphadenopathy and hepatosplenomegaly. Bence–Jones proteinuria may also be observed. Most patients die from progressive disease, although some develop treatment-related MDS or transform into large-cell lymphoma (Richter's transformation).[411]

Physical examination shows retinal changes with engorged veins, hemorrhages, exudates, and blurred disk margins. Moderate lymphadenopathy and hepatosplenomegaly may be present.

The diagnosis is made by demonstrating an IgM monoclonal spike in serum protein electrophoresis. Immunoelectrophoresis confirms that there is a monoclonal IgM and the other immunoglobulins may be depressed. Bone marrow examination reveals infiltration by lymphocytes, plasma cells, and plasmacytoid lymphocytes with immature forms. The peripheral blood smear often shows a mild lymphocytosis with plasmacytoid lymphocytes. Immunophenotypic analysis reveals CD19+, CD20+, CD5– and CD23–. Various cytogenic abnormalities have been described in 30 percent of bone marrow specimens studied and include abnormalities of chromosomes 10, 11, 12, 15, 20, and 21.[411]

In its early stages, Waldenstrom's disease does not require therapy. In a large series the combination of age >65 years, albumin < 4 g/dL, and presence of cytopenias (hemoglobin <12 g/dl, WBC <4×10^9/L and platelet <150 × 10^9/L) may help to select patients at high risk and in need of treatment. Treatment is necessary when there is anemia, bleeding, organomegaly, hyperviscosity, or severe B symptoms (weight loss, fever, night sweats). Treatment usually involves chemotherapy with an alkylating agent (traditionally chlorambucil), often together with prednisone if there is associated hemolysis, cold agglutins, or cryoglobin disease. Other therapies, involving agents such as α-interferon, nucleoside analogs (cladribine or fludarabine) and most recently anti-CD 20 MoAbs (rituximab) have been used. Nucleoside analogs may result in faster cytoreduction and disease control, although it is not yet clear if this translates into increased survival. There is a risk of opportunistic infections following treatment with nucleoside analogs because of the severe reduction of T-lymphocytes. Hyperviscosity is controlled with plasmapharesis.[411]

Hairy cell leukemia

Hairy cell leukemia (leukemic reticuloendotheliosis) is an uncommon chronic B-cell leukemia (occasionally T-cell) characterized by splenomegaly, pancytopenia, and sometimes lymphadenopathy. Characteristically here are lymphocytes with eccentric kidney-bean-shaped nuclei and filamentous cytoplasmic projections ("hairy" cells) in the blood and bone marrow ("fried egg" appearance). These hairy lymphocytes are unique in that they contain tartrate-resistant isozyme 5 of acid phosphatase (TRAP stain), ribosomal lamellar aggregates in the cytoplasm seen on electron microscopy, receptors for C3b, on their surface receptors for the Fc portion of IgG (Fc R), and frequent expression of monoclonal S IgG.[360,361]

Hairy cell leukemia usually appears at an earlier age, the median age being 53; the male/female ratio is more than 5:1 and this accounts for approximately 2 percent of the leukemias. Hairy cell leukemia is a chronic disease, with most patients surviving for more than 5 years. Initial presentation includes fatigue, weight loss, weakness, and infection. The most prominent clinical finding is splenomegaly. The massive splenomegaly is responsible for symptoms and for the hematological picture of hypersplenism.

At diagnosis, most patients are pancytopenic, and the characteristic hairy cells are seen on the peripheral blood smear. Bone marrow aspirate is usually unsuccessful, and a biopsy is necessary to demonstrate marrow infiltration. The malignant cells are CD19+, CD20+, CD11c+ and most specifically CD103+. Less common findings include osteolytic bone lesions, paraproteinemia, and skin involvement. Death is usually a result of infection and, less commonly, second malignancies.[412]

Therapy for hairy cell leukemia had included splenectomy or α-interferon prior to the development of the purine nucleoside analogs which target both resting and dividing lymphocytes. When treatment is required either deoxycoformycin (pento-statin) or 2-chlorodeoxyadenosine (cladribine) are the drugs of choice with 80–90 percent complete responses and more durable than with α-interferon.[413]

Angioimmunoblastic lymphadenopathy

Angioimmunoblastic lymphadenopathy is a systemic benign-appearing largely T-cell lymphoproliferative disorder with about a 20 percent predilection for transformation into lymphoma.[414] This is a disorder of late midlife (median age 60). Patients present with fever, night sweats, weight loss, pruritus, abdominal pain, painful cervical or generalized adenopathy, erythematous maculopapular rashes, and hepatosplenomegaly.[415] Frequently an anemia (often Coombs-positive) and polyclonal hyper-gammaglobulinemia are also found.[415] The clinical course is usually aggressive, with median survival of between 11 and 30 months, though some patients may experience spontaneous remission.[415] The major cause of mortality is infection or transformation into lymphoma, usually large-cell immunoblastic lymphoma, peripheral T-cell lymphoma, or Hodgkin's disease.[415] Treatment is usually combination chemotherapy that includes prednisone or more recently the purine nucleoside analog 2-chlorodeoxyadenosine (cladribine).[416]

Myeloproliferative diseases

Myeloproliferative disorders share a common origin in that they arise from monoclonal proliferation of the hematopoietic pluripotent precursor cell. In this respect, these illnesses can all be classified as malignancies. However, since in most myeloproliferative diseases the pluripotential precursor cells retain the ability to differentiate and mature into functional cells, they are usually fairly benign and chronic.[417,418]

Classification

Myeloproliferative diseases can be classified by their degree of maturation. Thus, they range from benign (hyperplastic) to dysplastic to malignant. The hyperplastic syndromes are polycythemia vera and essential thrombocythemia. Myeloid metaplasia is the dysplastic phase, and acute myelosclerosis, paroxysmal nocturnal hemoglobulinuria, aplastic anemia, and leukemia are malignant. This classification allows for the degree of overlap between the syndromes and the transition from one stage to the other (from more benign to more malignant). In these disorders, there is also a variable amount of fibrosis in the bone marrow.[417] Fibroblastic proliferation in myeloproliferative disease is of polyclonal origin and is a reactive phenomenon.[419]

The most benign proliferative states are characterized by panmyelosis of the central skeletal marrow with intact maturation of the red cells, white cells, and platelets (polycythemia vera and essential thrombocythemia). Dysplastic syndromes are characterized by reversion to a fetal distribution of the hematopoietic organ involving centrifugal expansion of the bone marrow from the axial skeleton to the long bones and reactivation of extramedullary hematopoiesis in the spleen and liver (myeloid metaplasia). This occurs in agnogenic myeloid metaplasia, polycythemia vera with myeloid metaplasia, and postpolycythemic myeloid metaplasia. Further malignant deterioration in myeloproliferative disease is characterized by ineffective erythropoiesis and a decrease in peripheral blood counts. Normal maturation is overcome by the production of abnormal cells. During this phase, hematopoiesis may develop into aplastic anemia, a myelodysplastic syndrome, or paroxysmal nocturnal hemoglobinuria. Final malignant deterioration is seen as acute nonlymphocytic or lymphocytic leukemia.[417]

Chronic myelogenous leukemia is also a clonal myeloproliferative disorder originating from a neoplastic transformation at the level of multipotential stem cells and is characterized by massive overproduction of slightly defective granulocytes. This illness does not arise from the other more benign myeloproliferative disorders but terminates with further deterioration to acute leukemia.[420–422]

Incidence

Accurate information on the incidence of myeloproliferative disorders is not available. These disorders are observed during the middle and later years of life and are rare in the young. Males are afflicted slightly more frequently than females. It has been suggested that there is an increased incidence in Ashkenazi Jews, but this is debatable.[417]

Etiology

Rare cases with a familial incidence or a history of exposure to mutagens or bone marrow toxins (benzene, radiation) suggest that there may be a chromosomal abnormality. However, this idea remains very speculative, except for chronic myelogenous leukemias.[422] At the present time, the etiology of these illnesses is still unknown.

Pathophysiology and signs and symptoms

Uncontrolled production of mature red blood cells is the predominant proliferative feature of polycythemia vera. This activity must be distinguished from other causes of erythrocytosis by the presence of an elevated red cell mass, normal oxygen saturation in the blood, normal p50 of the hemoglobin, and normal renal ultrasound (in selected patients abdominal and brain imaging studies to exclude certain specific diseases associated with erythrocytosis may also need to be performed). The erythropoietin level is low. A bone marrow biopsy shows hypercellularity, with most patients having trilinear hyperplasia. The leukocyte and platelet counts are usually elevated, and high leukocyte alkaline phosphatase and vitamin B_{12} levels are also often found. The increased blood volume and increased circulatory red cell mass lead to the complications of thrombosis and bleeding. Thrombosis may be arterial (coronary, cerebral, or peripheral vascular) or venous (peripheral, hepatic, or portal). Elderly patients are at increased risk for thrombotic events.[423,424] Small-vessel insufficiency produces cyanosis, erythromelalgia, or even frank gangrene of the fingers and toes. Mild hemorrhagic tendencies such as epistaxis, bruising, and gingival bleeding are common, while severe gastrointestinal, genitourinary, or pulmonary bleeding occurs in about 10 percent of patients. The major causes of mortality in untreated patients are thrombosis and hemorrhage.[417,418]

In essential thrombocythemia there is also hemorrhage and microvascular occlusions. However, there is generally a poor correlation between the occurrence of hemorrhagic phenomena and the platelet count or the presence of in-vitro platelet function abnormalities. It seems that the combination of erythrocytosis and thrombocytosis predisposes to large-vessel thrombosis. Thrombocythemia in the absence of an elevated red cell mass does not lead to large-vessel thrombosis. However, microvascular occlusion occurs very frequently, as does bleeding.[417,418]

In myeloid metaplasia, the degree of splenic involvement by extramedullary hematopoiesis is independent of the degree of marrow fibrosis. The dissociation invalidates the idea that myeloid metaplasia is compensatory to diminished bone marrow function.[417,418] The finding of increased numbers of granulocytic stem cells in the peripheral blood that show fetal characteristics suggests that it is possible that myeloid metaplasia arises from a homing of these cells to a favorable environment in the spleen and liver. When myeloid metaplasia occurs de novo, it is referred to as agnogenic myeloid metaplasia. The most common symptoms of agnogenic myeloid metaplasia are due to anemia or splenomegaly; half of patients have leukocytosis, and half have either thrombocytosis or thrombocytopenia.[425] In 12 percent of patients with polycythemia vera, about 10 years after diagnosis there is evolution into a picture indistinguishable from that of myeloid metaplasia. This may occur more frequently after ^{32}P treatment. Myeloid metaplasia may also occur early in the course of polycythemia vera. It is far less common to see myeloid metaplasia in the course of essential thrombocythemia.[417,418]

Patients with polycythemia and agnogenic myeloid metaplasia are at greater risk for developing acute leukemia. The leukemia may be acute lymphocytic, acute nonlymphocytic, or biphenotypic and is characteristically resistant to chemotherapy. Transformation into acute leukemia is an expression of myelodysplasia and occurs in both treated and untreated patients, even though it is more common in those who have received alkylating agents and radiation.

In chronic myelogenous leukemia over 90 percent of patients have the Ph[1] (Philadelphia) chromosome: this abnormality results from a T (9;22) translocation. The presence of this marker forecasts both a better prognosis and a better response to therapy.[422]

Patients with chronic myelogenous leukemia may present with almost identical physical and peripheral blood counts as myeloid metaplasia. However, in chronic myelogenous leukemia, leukocytosis is usually more prominent, teardrop cell forms are absent, and fibrosis of the bone marrow is uncommon. The differentiating features of chronic myelogenous leukemia are the presence of the Ph[1] chromosome, low or absent neutrophil alkaline phosphatase activity, and a high vitamin B_{12} serum level with a very high unsaturated binding capacity due to an increase in transcobalamin I.[417,418]

In other myeloproliferative disorders, the Ph[1] chromosome is not found, the neutrophil alkaline phosphate activity is normal or high, and serum vitamin B_{12} is only slightly elevated. In these other conditions, elevation is due to the elaboration of transcobalamin III. There is considerable elevation of the unsaturated B_{12} binding capacity.[417,418]

Early in the course of chronic myelogenous leukemia, the illness may be mistaken for another myeloproliferative disorder. It is important to distinguish it, as the prognosis and the treatment will be very different.

Prognosis

The median survival of patients with polycythemia vera who are treated is approximately 10–15 years.[426] In primary thrombocythemia, the median survival is about 5 years. Myeloid metaplasia patients have a 60 percent decrease in 5-year survival as compared to controls matched for age and gender.[420,421] Acute leukemias and myelosclerosis are usually rapidly fatal within months. Chronic myelocytic leukemia patients treated with conventional chemotherapy have a median survival of 47 months, and in rare cases patients survive for decades.

Treatment

In polycythemia, restoration of a normal blood volume and hematocrit markedly reduces the incidence of complications.[426]

At diagnosis the patient should undergo a series of phlebotomies of 250–500 mL every second or third day. If hydration is maintained, there is no need to readminister the patient's plasma. In patients with cardiovascular disease and in people over 75 years of age, it is usually prudent to phlebotomize only about 250–350 mL each time. Once the hematocrit is reduced to below 42 percent, the phlebotomy should be repeated as required to maintain the hematocrit at the desired level, at about 40–44 percent. Phlebotomy inevitably results in iron deficiency which serves to limit erythropoiesis. The phlebotomy requirement in iron deficiency should be less than 8 units per year. If an electronically derived hematocrit is used, it should be recognized that in the face of microcytosis the electronic cell counter underestimates the hematocrit up to 7 percent. Iron should not be given to correct the iron deficiency, as it will stimulate erythropoiesis.[426]

Occasionally a patient cannot tolerate phlebotomies or finds the symptoms of iron deficiency very troublesome. There are also certain subgroups of patients who are at especially high risk for thrombosis: patients older than 70 years of age, patients in whom erythropoiesis is so active that they have a high frequency of phlebotomy, and patients with a prior history of thrombosis.[424] In these individuals it is necessary to consider the use of myelosuppressive therapy. However, in patients treated with ^{32}P or chlorambucil, there is a danger of inducing leukemia or a second malignancy,[426] and the overall benefit of aggressive therapy has been questioned.[423] In a recent study in Italy four times as many patients who had previously received radiophosphorous alkylating or nonalkylating myelosuppressive agents died of cancer compared with patients who received phlebotomy or other pharmacological treatments.[423] At the present time, when myelosuppression is necessary, hydroxyurea is often used, although the previously believed safety of this agent in terms of mutagenicity has also recently been questioned.[424] Pruritus does not respond to phlebotomy and requires myelosuppression. Interferon is being used experimentally with some success in treating this disease.[424]

In essential thrombocythemia, myelosuppression is indicated in patients past the age of 60 who have marked thrombocythemia (platelet counts consistently over 1×10^6/mm^3) or a lower thrombocythemia with a past history of thrombosis or hemorrhage or a coexisting condition that places them at increased risk of these complications. Myelosuppression is usually achieved with hydroxyurea used in the same manner as in polycythemia vera.[427] The platelet count is usually reduced to a level of 500,000/mm^3. If surgery is necessary, the platelet count should be reduced to less than 500,000/mm^3. Postoperative bleeding should be managed with transfusion of normal platelets regardless of the platelet count. If a patient with thrombocythemia is bleeding or has active thrombosis, the platelet count should be reduced rapidly with plateletpheresis and hydroxyurea.[427] In any myeloproliferative disorder, the platelet count and red cell count must be normal before any surgery is performed. Newer approaches involving therapy with anagrelide, an agent believed to impair megakaryocytic maturation, is being evaluated with some success in patients with this disorder.[428]

In the asymptomatic phase of myeloid metaplasia no therapy is necessary unless the patient has thrombocythemia and is being prepared for surgery.[419] In myeloid metaplasia, splenomegaly is usually responsible for the major complications of the illness. Splenomegaly in myeloid metaplasia usually responds to myelosuppression. Hydroxyurea in doses of 1.0 g/d orally usually reduces the size of the spleen without achieving a significant decrease in marrow function. Anemia is not a contraindication to the use of myelosuppression, as transfusion may be given.[417]

Myelosuppressive therapy, however, cannot be used in the setting of neutropenia and thrombocytopenia because of hypoplasia or fibrosis of the bone marrow. Splenic irradiation has been tried, but even localized therapy is myelosuppressive. Therefore, splenic irradiation must be used sparingly and with extreme caution.[417–419] Splenectomy is used in some patients, but there is significant mortality and morbidity in elderly patients with myeloid metaplasia. Embolism via an arterial catheter has been proposed for use in elderly patients as an alternative safer method of infarcting the spleen.[419] Indications for splenectomy may include symptomatic splenomegaly, refractory thrombocytopenia, refractory hemolytic anemia, and portal hypertension due to splenomegaly.[425] Early splenectomy (at the point at which significant pancytopenia is present) in elderly patients has been advocated before cardiovascular complications occur.[417] Splenectomy is contraindicated if diffuse intravascular coagulation is found on laboratory testing (12 percent of patients have this condition without clinical bleeding). Thrombocythemia should be treated with hydroxyurea prior to splenectomy. Surgery is palliative therapy and usually should not be performed if there is high serum alkaline phosphatase, anemia with a spleen estimated to be greater than 3 kg, or anemia with a spleen estimated to be less than 1 kg.[417] Measurement of red cell production, survival, and splenic sequestration are not predictive of the effect of splenectomy on the anemia. The anemia should be evaluated to be sure that deficiencies are not present, such as iron, folate, or vitamin B_{12}. Hemolysis may respond to the use of corticosteroids and should be evaluated with chromium red blood survival. If ineffective erythropoiesis is present (shown by ferrokinetics), pyridoxine and androgens may be tried.[417–419,425]

The malignant phases of myeloproliferative disorders are notoriously resistant to therapy. However, treatment is similar to that described in previous sections.

In all myeloproliferative disorders hyperuricemia is treated with allopurinol. Hydration should be maintained, and hypertonic solutions for diagnostic purposes should be avoided as much as possible. Histamine symptoms (itching and pruritus after baths) may be relieved by use of the potent antihistamine agent cyproheptadine, 4 mg orally; other antihistaminics are usually not successful. Symptoms of gastrointestinal hyperacidity may be controlled with H2 blockers and/or antacids.[417]

Chronic myelocytic leukemia used to be controlled with oral busulfan or hydroxyurea. The current therapy for chronic myelocytic leukemia is evolving, however, and some studies have suggested that α-interferon prolongs survival and delays progression to the blastic phase when compared to therapy with hydroxyurea or busulfan.[429] Therefore, interferon-based regimens are being recommended more often. Bone marrow transplantation, which has met with some success in younger patients, is rarely used in the elderly because of the high mortality associated with this procedure.[429] Newer agents such as STI571, imatinib mesylate (Gleevec™), an oral protein kinase inhibitor that inhibits the constitutive abnormal Bcr-Abl tyrosine kinase has been shown to have efficacy in the chronic phase after interferon failure, and in the accelerated phase and the blast crisis of CML.[430,431] This new oral protein kinase inhibitor is discussed in the biological therapy section.

Myelodysplastic syndromes

Myelodysplastic syndromes (MDS) are a heterogeneous group of disorders in which the hematopoietic precursors are abundant but morphologically abnormal. There is ineffective hematopoiesis, and normal numbers of mature peripheral blood cells are not produced. If only the red cell line is affected, the term *refractory anemia* is used. There is often a progression from refractory anemia to a more serious myelodysplastic syndrome involving white cells and platelets.[432]

Morphological criteria are still the basis on which these myelodysplastic syndromes are classified (Table 98-8). If only the red cell line is involved and there are no ringed sideroblasts, the disorder is called refractory anemia. If there are more than 15 percent ringed sideroblasts, the diagnosis is refractory anemia with ringed sideroblasts. When there are excess blasts in the marrow but not in the peripheral blood, refractory anemia with excess blasts (RAEB) is the diagnosis. When RAEB is accompanied by peripheral blood monocytosis (1,000/mm^3 or greater), the illness is called chronic myelomonocytic leukemia. Finally, when there are 5 percent or more peripheral blood blasts, the illness is called RAEB in transformation. These terms have for the most part replaced the old term *preleukemia*, as only about 10–30 percent of patients with a myelodysplastic syndrome go on to develop acute leukemia.[320,432] A new classification system, the International Prognostic Scoring System (IPSS) for MDS is based scoring blast percentage, karyotype and cytopenias. This system allows stratification into low, intermediate-1, intermediate-2, and high-risk groups with predicted median survival of 5.7, 3.5, 1.2, and 0.4 years, respectively (Table 98-12).[433]

Incidence

The exact incidence is not known, but these syndromes are fairly common in elderly people. Ineffective erythropoiesis increases with the age of a population and in some studies on elderly people up to 20 percent had unexplained refractory anemia. These syndromes are more common in men than in women and are extremely rare under the age of 40. The older one gets, the more likely one is to develop these disorders (see the section on etiology). A history of exposure to radiation and/or chemical leukemogens is common.[434]

Etiology

While the etiology in most patients is unknown, it has become clear that treatment with prolonged courses of alkylating agents is associated with an increased risk of myelodysplastic syndromes and acute nonlymphocytic leukemia. Long courses of phenylalanine mustard for treatment of multiple myeloma or ovarian carcinoma, or of chlorambucil or nitrogen mustard plus radiation therapy for Hodgkin's disease, result in an incidence of acute nonlymphocytic leukemia of 2–7 percent. Anemia or pancytopenia associated with changes in the bone marrow and peripheral blood identical to those in

Table 98-12 WHO Classification—International Prognostic Scoring System (IPSS)

Overall IPSS risk score based on:
Marrow blast percentage

Blast (%)	IPSS score
<5	0
5–10	0.5
11–20	1.5
21–30	2.0

Cytogenic features[a]

Karyotype	IPSS score
Good prognosis (-Y, 5q-, 20q-)	0
Intermediated prognosis	0.5
Poor prognosis (abn. 7, complex)	1.0

Cytopenias[b]

Cytopenia	IPSS score
None or 1 type	0
2 or 3 types	0.5

Overall IPSS score and survival

Overall score	Median survival (yr)
Low (0)	5.7
Intermediate	
1 (0.5 or 1.0)	3.5
2 (1.5 or 2.0)	1.2
High (≥ 2.5)	0.4

[a]*PSS cytogenetic classification: Good prognosis: -Y only, del 5q only; del 20q only; Intermediate prognosis: +8, single (except -Y, 5q-, 20q-) or double abnormalities; Poor prognosis: complex (≥3) abnormalities; any chromosome 7 abnormality.*

[b]*IPSS cytopenias: hemoglobin <10g/dL; absolute neutrophil count <1,800/mm³; platelets <100,000/mm³.*

myelodysplastic syndromes develops 2–10 years after therapy.[435] The acute nonlymphocytic leukemia that may result is invariably fatal. It is very likely that this long-term complication of successful chemotherapy will become more prevalent, especially in an aging population, as the survival of patients with cancer continues to improve. Chemotherapeutic drugs that are not alkylating agents, such as methotrexate, do not seem to be associated with this danger.

Other etiological possibilities include RNA viruses, somatic mutations, radiation, and environmental toxins. Aging seems critical, and this has been interpreted as being related to the multihit theory of carcinogenesis.[436] Drugs and various illnesses can cause sideroblastic anemia. In these conditions, the inhibition of mitochondrial and heme synthesis and accumulation of the heme-controlled suppressor seems to be the pathogenic event.[15,67,74,85,437]

Pathophysiology and signs and symptoms

Most of these syndromes are thought to arise from a lesion in the pluripotential hematopoietic stem cell pool and to evolve from clonal expansion of a single stem cell or a very small number of such cells. Deletion of a major portion of the long arm of chromosome 5[59] is encountered in a wide spectrum of acquired hematological disease, including refractory anemias, acute nonlymphocytic leukemias, myeloproliferative diseases,

lymphomas, and occasional solid tumors.[438] About 50 percent of patients with myelodysplastic syndrome have chromosomal abnormalities, and abnormalities of chromosomes 7, 8, 11, 12, and 20 have also been described in addition to the abnormalities on chromosome 5.[439] The major specific pathophysiological mechanism is ineffective hematopoiesis, the defective maturation of marrow precursor cells. Proliferation of progenitor and early precursor cells is usually normal or enhanced, producing a hypercellular marrow, but there is a deficiency of the circulating fully mature cells. There is also a mild decrease in the cells' lifespan which contributes to the cytopenias.[320,432]

There are rare instances of such myelodysplastic syndromes in families. A protracted myelodysplastic syndrome lasting for 1–20 years occurs in about 5–10 percent of all cases of acute nonlymphatic leukemia.[320,432] The patient generally seeks medical care for symptoms of anemia, thrombocytopenia, or leukopenia. Thus, fatigue, decrease in exercise tolerance, purpura, fever, and infections are the common presenting problems. The male/female ratio is 2:1 and the patient is usually elderly. Hepatomegaly is present in about 5 percent of cases, while splenomegaly is present in about 10 percent. Pallor is found in about 50 percent of cases. Often the patient complains of arthralgias. Because development of the cytopenias is slow, many patients are asymptomatic and the diagnosis is made incidentally or the anemia is falsely attributed to aging.[432]

Laboratory data and diagnosis

The hallmark of the illness is anemia with reticulocytopenia, and red cell morphology is usually abnormal. A dimorphic population of red cells is usually present; some cells are microcytic and hypochromic, and others are normochromic and normocytic or macrocytic. Basophilic stippling, target cells, schistocytes, and nucleated red blood cells are often seen.[320]

Leukopenia is moderate in the white blood cell range of 1,000–4,000/mm³, with neutropenia being more pronounced than lymphopenia. Neutrophils are frequently poorly granulated, neutrophil alkaline phosphatase may be low, and acquired pseudo-Pelger–Huet anomaly (hypolobulation of the nuclei of the mature neutrophil) may be present. Granulocytes often have abnormal function, which further adds to the increased susceptibility to infection. Monocytosis is present in 30 percent of patients, and thus serum and urinary lysozyme may be elevated. Immature myeloid cells may seem to be present in the peripheral blood smear.[320]

Thrombocytopenia is common, even though patients occasionally have thrombocytosis. Platelets may have functional defects.

The bone marrow is diagnostic of myelodysplastic syndromes.[320] Erythroblasts may have double or fragmented nuclei or intranuclear bridging and budding. Ringed sideroblasts (excess iron in mitochondria) may be prominent and are usually found in patients with primarily abnormalities in red cell precursors. With mainly erythroid dysplasia, the ratio of myeloid to erythroid precursors (M/E ratio) is 1:1 to 1:10. There is an increase in reticuloendothelial iron, and serum iron and ferritin levels in plasma are elevated. Dyserythropoiesis results in moderate elevation of serum LDH and indirect bilirubin. Iron turnover studies reveal the ineffective erythropoiesis; there is an increase in the iron turnover rate but decreased incorporation of iron into circulating erythrocytes.[320]

Marrow myeloid cells may show poor maturation to mature neutrophils and have the acquired pseudo-Pelger–Huet anomaly. They are often poorly granulated. Eosinophils and basophils may also be dysplastic. In patients with mainly myeloid dysplasia, the M/E ratio is 3:1 to 10 to 20:1. Megakaryocytes may be immature and dysplastic as well.[320]

Most patients have increased iron stores, and many show clinical hemochromatosis with diabetes, cirrhosis, infiltrative heart disease, and pituitary dysfunction.[320]

Prognosis

Prognosis is variable, with survival of a few months to 10–15 years. Median survival ranges from 6 years for patients with refractory anemia with ringed sideroblasts to 5 months for those with refractory anemia with excess blasts in transformation.[433,439] The proportion of patients whose disease transforms into acute nonlymphocytic leukemia varies in the different subgroups, being about 50 percent in refractory anemia with excess blasts in transformation, 40 percent in refractory anemia with excess blasts, 35 percent in CMML, 15 percent in refractory anemia, and 5 percent in refractory anemia with ringed sideroblasts.[433,439] In a recent study from Australia on patients with myelodysplastic syndrome, the causes of death were infection (37 percent), acute leukemia (20 percent), bleeding (11 percent), and causes unrelated to myelodysplasia (37 percent). In 9 percent the cause of death was not recorded.[440]

Treatment

Transfusion of blood products is the mainstay of treatment;[320] however, this should be limited as much as possible. Transfusion of packed red cells entails the risk of iron overload, alloimmunization to red cell, white cell, and platelet antigens, and transmission of a variety of infections. The use of leukocyte depletion filters or washed red blood cells may slow the development of alloimmunization. Platelet transfusions should be used if the patient is thrombocytopenic and there is bleeding or if surgery is necessary. Granulocyte transfusions should be used only in neutropenic patients with documented Gram-negative infections who do not respond to antibiotics alone.[440] Colony-stimulating factors are often used to try to improve peripheral cell counts to avoid transfusions. Erythropoietin is frequently used to try to raise the hematocrit. About 20 percent of patients show a significant response[441,442] and there is some evidence that those with lower erythropoietin levels are more likely to respond.[442] GM-CSF and G-CSF regularly correct neutropenia but have not been shown to increase survival.[441]

Occasionally, patients with ringed sideroblasts respond to pharmacological doses of oral pyridoxine, 100–300 mg/d.[320] The response is only partial, and abnormal red cell morphology usually persists. Androgens and corticosteroids have usually been of little benefit.[440] Consideration should be given to the use of desferrioxamine when the total number of transfused units of red cells approaches 100.

Early treatment of myelodysplasia with excess blasts using chemotherapy has not shown any benefit on survival. The use of low-dose cytosine arabinoside to induce differentiation of blasts has been very controversial.[320,440] When the patient develops acute nonlymphocytic leukemia, the remission rate is even less than in cases of nonlymphocytic leukemia where

patients did not have prior myelodysplasia. Individuals with this secondary form of nonlymphocytic leukemia have prolonged marrow aplasia after chemotherapy. Recent approaches in elderly people have involved supportive care with blood products and an attempt to keep the white blood cell count below 50,000/mm³ with oral hydroxyurea.[320] Use of hematopoietic growth factors (GM-CSF, high doses of erythropoietin [EPO] and the combination of G-CSF + EPO) have been been used and in some cases there has been decreased infections and transfusion requirements. Treatment aproaches in younger patients have focused on bone marrow transplantation, which is seldom used in older adults because of poor tolerability and survival.

Newer approaches in clinical studies have focused on immunosupression and immunomodulation with amifostine, cyclosporin A, antithymocyte globulin, topotecan, melphalan, thalidomide, arsenic trioxide, and interleukins, all of which have shown benefit in some patients in small series and are reviewed in the literature.[440] Recently, the National Comprehensive Cancer Center (NCCN) proposed treatment guidelines for patients ≤60 and >60 years for management of low-risk intermediate-1, intermediate-2, and high-risk patients (www.NCCN.org). Management in elderly patients remains supportive care or low-intensity therapy at this time.

DISORDERS OF HEMOSTASIS

Hemostasis is maintained by a mechanism involving vascular, platelet, and coagulation components. A tendency to bleed may result from a disorder of one or more of these components. As a general rule, coagulation defects in elderly people may be treated as they are in other age groups. Purpura may occur with or without demonstrable platelet abnormalities. The most common purpura in elderly people are nonthrombocytopenic.

Nonthrombocytopenic purpuras

This condition has a different significance in elderly people than in the young. Anaphylactoid purpura is rare in old age, whereas senile purpura is very common.

Senile purpura

Senile purpura[443–445] occurs mainly on the extensor surfaces of the forearms and hands and may be seen in many otherwise normal old people. Loss of subcutaneous fat and changes in aging connective tissue permit undue mobility of an old person's skin, and the resulting shearing forces allow rupture of small vessels. The extravasated blood tracks widely, and the tissues' reaction to it is impaired. No history of trauma is usually obtained. In senile purpura individual lesions last longer than other types of purpura (from 1 to 3 weeks) and do not undergo the typical color changes as they resolve because of the poor phagocytic response to the extravasated blood. Senile purpura is more common in women. Platelets are normal both qualitatively and quantitatively in patients with senile purpura, and no correlation has been shown with ascorbic acid deficiency.

Scurvy

Scurvy is associated with purpura and more widespread bleeding from body surfaces, under the periosteum, or in the viscera. This hemorrhagic tendency has for a long time been attributed to disturbed collagen synthesis and an endothelial defect in the capillaries. In recent years, it has been demonstrated that impaired platelet function is also a feature of scurvy.[446] Dysproteinemias, infections, hypothermia, neoplasia, and drugs, have been implicated as causes of nonthrombocytopenic purpura.

Purpura due to platelet defects

Thrombocytopenia may occur as a primary (idiopathic) disorder or a secondary phenomenon (drug-induced or associated with other blood diseases, infections, neoplasia, or various other conditions). Occasionally thrombocythemia, thrombasthenia, or combined defects may be present.

Autoimmune (idiopathic) thrombocytopenic purpura

IgG autoantibodies against platelets can sensitize the platelets for destruction. Platelet autoantibodies may be a primary or secondary phenomenon. If they are secondary, they usually arise in the setting of systemic lupus erythematosus, immunodeficiency disorders, or B-cell lymphoproliferative syndromes (e.g. CLL).[447,448] Autoimmune thrombocytopenia may be the first sign of HIV infection and is found in about 10 percent of patients with AIDS. In children, acute autoimmune thrombocytopenia often follows a viral infection and remits spontaneously. In older people the onset is usually insidious and is not clearly related to another illness. The course is usually chronic and intermittent.[447,448]

Autoimmune platelet destruction results in thrombocytopenia and manifestations of hemorrhage in the patient. Unless severe acute or chronic bleeding has occurred or the patient has Evans syndrome (immune hemolytic anemia and thrombocytopenia), the red and white cell counts are normal. Few platelets are seen in the peripheral blood smear, and those that are present are large ("megathrombocytes").[447] The bone marrow shows an increase in megakaryocytes. There is usually no splenomegaly. In the serum, there are antibodies of the IgG class, and the few circulating platelets can be shown to be coated with antiplatelet IgG, C3, or both.[447,448] Testing for the presence of antibodies on platelet surfaces is, however, associated with many false positive results. Antibodies to specific platelet antigens (e.g. IIb/IIIa or Ib/IX complex) have been found in many patients with autoimmune thrombocytopenia, but tests for these are not available in most hospitals.[449] Treatment is usually initiated for bleeding or very low platelet counts (usually less than 30,000/μL) or prior to surgery. Therapy usually involves corticosteroids (prednisone 1–2 mg/kg per day). About 80 percent of patients respond in about 3–28 days after treatment is started.[449] Once a response has occurred, steroids should be tapered over 4–8 weeks. Splenectomy is often recommended for patients who relapse or who require high doses of prednisone to keep the platelet count acceptable. In life-threatening situations, high-dose methylprednisolone or intravenous γ-globulin is useful.[449] Other methods of treatment, if corticosteroids fail, are plasmapharesis,[449] more potent immunosuppressive drugs such as vinca alkaloids, danazol, or a monoclonal anti-FCR III antibody.[394,448]

Secondary thrombocytopenia

Drugs are a very important cause of thrombocytopenia. They may be direct marrow toxins or cause idiosyncratic or hypersensitivity reactions. Some drugs are known to cause selective thrombocytopenia only by decreasing megakaryocytes. They are all low-risk drugs and include sedormid, quinidine, sulfonamides, penicillin, tetracycline, chloramphenicol, salicylates, barbiturates, desipramine, chlorothiazide, digitoxin, insulin, cimetidine, and myelosuppressive drugs used as chemotherapeutic agents.[450]

Medication can also induce immune-mediated platelet destruction. Penicillin, quinidine, and quinine elicit antibodies that cause reactions similar to the hemolytic disorders produced by these drugs.[451] Antibodies against the anticoagulant heparin may produce thrombocytopenia, possibly because the heparin-antibody complexes bind to the platelets and activate them by binding to the platelet Fc receptor.[452] At the same time that the patient is at risk of bleeding from the thrombocytopenia, they are thus also subject to arterial thrombosis. When heparin-induced thrombocytopenia occurs, use of hirudin (Refludan™) is indicated. The initial use of low-molecular-weight heparins may reduce this problem.[452] Although the incidence of this complication is low, the widespread use of heparin in clinical practice makes it a familiar problem. Secondary thrombocytopenia is seen in acute and chronic leukemias, lymphomas, infections, myelodysplastic syndromes and myeloproliferative disorders, neoplasms, collagen vascular diseases, splenomegaly, paraproteinemia, cirrhosis of the liver, and hypersensitivity reactions. Ethanol use may also be associated with thrombocytopenia by direct suppression of platelet production, reduced survival, and secondary to the hypersplenism or folate deficiency that may be found in some alcoholics.

Transfusion thrombocytopenia

Antibodies directed against a platelet surface antigen (PL^AI), an epitope of platelet membrane glycoprotein IIb/IIIa, are very destructive to platelets.[450] PL^AI antigen is present on platelets of more than 98 percent of persons. Antibodies against PL^AI antigens only rarely are a problem in platelet transfusion therapy, but persons who lack the PL^AI antigen on their platelets and receive transfusions of PL^AI-bearing platelets may develop a condition called post-transfusion purpura. The platelets contained in whole blood transfusions are also sufficient to elicit this disorder. At some time following the transfusion, the patient generates anti-PL^AI antibodies. These antibodies are believed to bind PL^AI antigen released from the transfused platelets, and the antigen–antibody complex then binds to the patient's own PL^AI-negative platelets resulting in destruction of transfused and autologous platelets. The disorder has resulted in severe thrombocytopenia but is usually self-limited and remits completely.[450]

Thrombocytopenia caused by bone marrow failure is a common problem in hematology. It is treated with supportive care with platelet transfusions. However, anti-HLA antibodies arise in many transfused patients, limiting the effectiveness of platelet transfusions. Single donor infusions and HLA antigen matching of donors with recipients can eventually find platelets that can survive in such a sensitized recipient.[450] Thrombopoietin, the hormone thought to stimulate megakaryocytes, has recently been purified and cloned.[453] This molecule is in clinical trials.

Thrombotic thrombocytopenic purpura

Thrombotic thrombocytopenia purpura (TTP)[454] is a disseminated thrombotic microangiopathy first described in 1924 by Moschowitz. In some people the condition appears to be initiated by toxic endothelial damage: the toxin produced by *E. coli* 0157:H7 and various drugs including mitomycin C and cyclosporin A have been implicated in some cases.[449] The disorder known as the hemolytic–uremic syndrome (HUS) where renal failure is a prominent finding is similar to TTP but the pathophysiology may be different. TTP has a rapid onset, with widespread manifestations appearing over the course of a day or two. In the classic case, fever, thrombocytopenia with bleeding, traumatic hemolytic anemia, acute renal failure, and CNS disturbances are seen. Laboratory findings are very helpful in confirming the diagnosis and especially in making the sometimes difficult distinction between TTP and disseminated intravascular coagulation. The changes of traumatic anemia are present, including a low hematocrit and fragmented red cells on the blood smear. The platelet count is low, but there are many megakaryocytes in the marrow, indicating that the reduction in platelets is attributable to increased consumption rather than decreased production. Other clotting studies are usually normal, fibrinogen levels are normal or increased, and split products are usually absent. The diagnosis often has to be made on clinical grounds, but it can sometimes be made by biopsy, usually of the gum. The diagnostic finding is an arteriole containing a mass of fibrin. There is no evidence of inflammation, immunoglobulin, or complement to be found. The finding of an arteriole filled with a fibrin plug is pathognomonic for TTP in this clinical setting. The pathogenesis of this disorder has been debated but one unifying observation is of unusually large von Willebrand factor multimers (ULvWF) in remission plasma of relapsing patients. A protease was discovered in normal plasma that cleaves the UlvWF in normals and is absent in patients with TTP. This led to the hypothesis that this ULvWF under high shear in the microcirculation may be the cause of platelet aggregation as the inciting event. Most often the deficiency of the vWF-cleaving protease is acquired through an autoimmune mechanism with autoantibodies destroying activity but there are rare case reports of familial TTP with inherited deficiency. Assaying the vWF-cleaving protease may be useful in distinguishing TTP from HUS as the ULvWF multimers may be present in both due to endothelial cell damage but only in TTP is the protease deficient.[454]

TTP is usually treated by large-volume plasma exchanges. Cryodepleted (vWF poor) plasma can be used in combination with steroids. This form of therapy has decreased the mortality rate of TTP from 90 percent to less than 50 percent. In patients with TTP who do not respond to plasma exchange, a combination of steroids, antiplatelet agents, and emergency splenectomy has been used with some success. Eventually, if this new paradigm of TTP is confirmed, immunosuppressive therapy may be used in an attempt to restore the normal vWF-cleaving protease activity when patients are stable.

Thrombasthenia

This rare qualitative platelet defect affects platelet function and leads to a hemorrhagic tendency due to impaired platelet adhesiveness and a failure of clot retraction (despite a normal platelet count). Though mostly a hereditary disease, it is occasionally first diagnosed in older adults. It may also be secondary to scurvy, uremia, thrombocythemia, or macroglobulinemia.[451]

Drugs affecting platelet function

Many drugs have been shown to have effects on platelet behavior (adhesiveness, aggregation, and release phenomenon). Aspirin is the drug most commonly used and may be important in preventing thrombosis in older people.[455,456]

Defects of blood coagulation

Survival with congenital coagulation disorders in later life is possible, especially in von Willebrand's disease. Acquired disorders include vitamin K deficiency, which leads to a reduction in prothrombin (factor II) and in factors VII, IX, and X. This condition may occur in malabsorption syndromes, liver disease, prolonged obstructive jaundice, and biliary fistula and with oral broad-spectrum antibiotic therapy.[451,457] Renal failure, extracorporeal circuits, and acquired inhibitors may result in significant blood coagulation defects.[450]

Anticoagulant therapy with warfarin reduces hepatic synthesis of the same four factors. Chronic liver disease may lead to reduction in the above factors and also in fibrinogen (factor I) and factors V, XI, XII, and XIII. Factor X deficiency occurs in amyloidosis.[446,450]

Circulating anticoagulants

Circulating anticoagulants inhibit clotting factors. The most common, "lupus anticoagulant," is an antiphospholipid antibody and may be associated with thrombosis. This type of circulating anticoagulant usually proves to be the explanation for a prolonged partial thromboplastin time not corrected by normal plasma. The presence of this anticoagulant often means that the patient has lupus, but in elderly people it is often observed as an isolated entity.[458,459] Other acquired anticoagulants may be antibodies against the active site of the clotting factor and can result in a bleeding diathesis. Still others are seen when there is an elevation of fibrin, split products, and an anti-factor VIII antibody in hemophilia; when there are abnormal paraproteins; or if the patient is taking anticoagulant drugs.[450,451,457]

Fibrinogen deficiency

Fibrinogen deficiency may result from impaired formation (liver disease), intravascular clotting, or overactive fibrinolysis.[450,457]

Regulation of clotting

The clotting process is regulated by two general mechanisms: elimination of activated clotting factors and destruction of the fibrin clot (fibrinolysis). The activated clotting factors are removed by two circulating anticoagulant systems: the antithrombin III proteoglycan system and the protein C-protein S system.

Antithrombin III is a protease inhibitor which acts against all the proteolytic clotting factors except VIIa.[460–462] Antithrombin III binds to proteoglycans on the endothelial surfaces of blood vessels, thus layering them with an anticoagulant. Heparin works via its interaction with antithrombin III.

An inherited deficiency of this molecule leaves the individual highly suspectible to venous thrombosis.[460–462]

Protein C is a vitamin K-dependent protease that neutralizes factors V and VIII and must be activated by thrombin to work. Thrombin in turn must be modulated by thrombomodulin, before it can become an activator of protein C. Activated protein C then destroys the activity of factors V and VIII. Activated protein C requires Ca^{2+}, phospholipid, and another vitamin K-dependent protein, protein S (the accelerator). A deficiency in either protein C or S leads to a greatly increased risk of venous thrombosis.[462,463] Resistance to activated protein C has also been described as a major risk factor for thrombosis. In most cases it is the result of a single point mutation in the factor V gene, making factor V less sensitive to activated protein C-mediated inactivation.[464] Activated protein C resistance is found in about 4 percent of the population.[464] The presence of this abnormality may be especially important if the patient has other risk factors for thrombosis. High homocysteine levels have also been suggested as risk factors for thrombosis (see section on vitamin B_{12} deficiency). A recent study has suggested that patients with homocysteinemia and activated protein C resistance are at especially high risk for thrombosis.[465] These patients usually have a homozygous C677T mutation in the methylenetetrahydrofolate reductase or cystathionine β-synthase gene mutation resulting in elevated homocyteine plasma levels. Increased levels of factor VIII are a risk for thrombosis. Prothrombin mutations G20210A (heterozygotes or homozygotes) also are at risk for thrombosis and this mutation in combination with factor V Leiden or hyperhomocysteinemia increase the risk. The prothrombin mutation and the factor V Leiden mutation are the most common mutations in the Caucasian population.[466]

Fibrinolysis

Fibrinolysis is accomplished by a fibrin-splitting protease, plasmin. Plasmin is derived from its precursor, plasminogen.[467]

Disseminated intravascular coagulation

A syndrome of diffuse intravascular coagulation (DIC) may be seen in elderly people in an acute, subacute, or chronic form.[451–457] There is always a serious underlying disease process that leads to thromboplastic substances entering the circulation or direct endothelial cell damage from toxin or immune complexes.[451–457]

Criteria for diagnosis are not well defined; the most useful are a low platelet count, prolonged prothrombin time, and also often activated partial thromboplastin time, positive plasma protamine test for fibrin, monomer–fibrinogen complexes, D dimers, and levels of fibrinogen and fibrin degradation products related to the clinical condition. Therapy may include, under certain circumstances, restoration of depleted blood components with platelet concentrates, cryoprecipitate, and fresh frozen plasma in bleeding patients.[468] The most important therapy is to stop the underlying disease (e.g. infection, neoplasia, or tissue damage from trauma, burns, heatstroke, surgery, antigen–antibody reactions, drugs, incompatible transfusion, anaphylactic shock, and intravascular hemolysis). Aortic aneurysms have been associated with extensive coagulation disorders. Liver disease, acute pancreatitis, and nonbacterial thrombotic endocarditis have also been shown to cause DIC.[451–457]

The use of heparin in the treatment of DIC is controversial. In most cases of DIC (about 95 percent), heparin has not proved to be of value and may sometimes be harmful. Heparin may itself cause thrombocytopenia and thrombosis.[451–457] Even in complex situations such as promyelocytic leukemia the routine use of heparin remains controversial.[468]

Primary fibrinogenolysis (fibrinolysis)

Primary fibrinogenolysis occurs when active plasmin is generated in the circulation at a time when the clotting cascade is not operating. It is very rare and occurs only occasionally in severe liver disease, cancer of the prostate and lung, or heatstroke.[450] The illness is characterized by severe bleeding and must be differentiated from DIC by a normal platelet count, shortened euglobulin clot lysis time, fibrin degradation products present by immunological assay and absence of fibrin monomers and D-dimers.[446,450,451,468] It is important to make this distinction between DIC and fibrinogenolysis, as the latter can be treated with ε-aminocaproic acid, which inhibits both plasmin and plasminogen. If this drug is used in DIC, it will be very dangerous and thrombosis will be enhanced.

BIOLOGICAL THERAPY IN HEMATOLOGY

Biological materials derived from humans are being used to treat deficiencies of blood cells and hematological malignancies. The availability today of erythropoietin, granulocyte or granulyte–macrophage colony-stimulating factors (G-CSF and GM-CSF) and IL-11 (opreleukin) offer a potential for treating these specific anemia, leukopenias, and thrombocytopenias without resorting to transfusions.[469,470]

Biologicals are being developed to treat malignancies, including agents that boost host deficiencies, agents that kill tumors directly, and agents that alter tumor biology. The first class of agents (active immunotherapy) includes tumor-specific (tumor cell vaccines) and nonspecific agents (lymphokines, such as IL-2). The second category, immunotherapy, also includes tumor-specific (antitumor monoclonal antibodies) and nonspecific agents (tumor necrosis factor). Interferon has several modes of action in this category. The final category includes any agent that interferes with tumor biology and includes differentiating agents (retinoids), agents that block tumor growth (antibodies to growth receptors), and agents that alter the process of metastasis (laminine fragments). Ultimately, it may be possible to alter the DNA of the tumor cell and thereby cure malignancy.[471]

The following are some examples of recently developed products. Myelotarg®; gemtuzamab orgamycin, binds to the CD33 antigen on hematopoietic cells. The binding of this agent results in a complex which when internalized releases calicheamicin, which binds to DNA and causes strand breaks and cell deaths. Clinically this has been used to treat relapsed CD33+ AML and CML.[472,473] CAMPATH-1H® (alemtuzumab), a human immunoglobulin IgG1 anti-CD52 monoclonal antibody that binds to nearly all B- and T-cell leukemias has shown significant activity in patients with advanced and chemotherapy resistant CLL.[352] Rituxan® (rituximab), IDEC C_2–B_5, a monoclonal antibody against CD20 used in the treatment of follicular lymphoma, is under study for the treatment of intermediate grade lymphomas and CLL.[408] In a recently completed GELA trial using R-CHOP (rituximab plus CHOP [cytoxan, adriamycin, oncovin, prednisone]) vs CHOP alone in elderly patients with previously untreated diffuse large B-cell lymphoma, there was an increased complete response rate (CR) (R-CHOP 75 percent vs CHOP 60 percent). Bexxar® (tositumomab, iodine I[131] tositumomab), a radiolabeled anti-CD20 monoclonal antibody, has also been used in the treatment of low-grade NHL and targets the radioactivity to the CD20 positive cells.[474] Ontak™ (denileukin difitox) directs cytocidal action of the diphtheria toxin to cells expressing IL-2 receptors. These receptors are found in malignant cells of certain leukemias and lymphomas and have been effective in cutaneous T-cell lymphomas.[409] Bexarotene (Targretin®) is a novel oral synthetic retinoid analog that binds preferentially to RXR receptor subtypes and has been used to treat CD30+ cutaneous T-cell lymphomas.[410] STI 571, now known as imatinib mesylate (Gleevec™), is an oral protein kinase inhibitor that inhibits the constitutive abnormal Bcr-Abl tyrosine kinase created by the Philadelphia chromosome abnormality in CML. In clinical studies this agent has shown efficacy in chronic phase after α-interferon failure, accelerated phase, and myeloid blast crisis with complete hematological responses of 88, 63, and 26 percent, respectively.[430,431] In the clinical studies, approximately 40 percent of the patients were ≥60 years and 10–12 percent ≥ 70 years of age. Imatinib is not entirely selective for Bcr-Abl and has also been shown to inhibit the receptor tyrosine kinases for platelet-derived growth factor (PDGF), stem cell factor (SCF), and c-kit. Imatinib has also shown efficacy in gastrointestinal stroma tumors that express the c-kit tyrosine kinase.[475]

Multiple other agents are in varying stages of development. New agents include other tyrosine kinase inhibitors, retinoids, antiangiogenic agents, differentiation agents, metalloproteinase inhibitors, interferons, cytokines, antisense molecules, and ribozymes.[471]

At the present time, we have to combine biological therapy with traditional radiation and chemotherapy in treating hematological malignancies. Certain growth factors such as GM-CSF may make it possible to deliver higher levels of chemotherapy. Bone marrow transplantation (BMT) is invaluable in treating young people with hematological malignancy or aplastic anemia. The use of autologous BMT is now performed in patients up to age 70 with multiple myeloma and a good performance status. These new developments in biological therapy should prove to be invaluable resources in geriatric medicine. Specialized techniques of drug delivery with immunoconjugates, radioactive or toxin-loaded monoclonal antibodies, liposomal delivery systems, radiation by brachytherapy techniques, and special delivery systems for chemotherapeutics to affected organs will hopefully allow for more targeted treatment of malignancies in elderly people with reduction in systemic toxicity.[476]

Chemoprotectants

Special care must be taken in elderly, frail[477] patients, especially those being treated with chemotherapy. Hematapoietic growth factor support has resulted in reduction of anemia, transfusion requirements, and infections.[478] Newer antiemetics have markedly decreased emesis in patients on chemotherapy. Megesterol acetate has helped with cachexia. Guidelines for use have been published for growth factor and antiemetic use by the American Society of Clinical Oncology.[479,480]

Several reported chemoprotectants may help with quality of life and for dose escalation of chemotherapeutic agents.[481–483] Amifostine, glutathione, rosaxane, glutamate, and mesna have been used as cryoprotectants. Amifostine and glutathione decrease cisplatin-associated neurotoxicity and nephrotoxicity.[484,485] Amifostine also decreases radiotherapy toxicity, especially in head and neck radiation. Mesna decreases the urothelial toxicity from alkylating agents (e.g. ifosfamide).[485] Glutamate decreases cisplatin and paclitaxel neurotoxicity.[486] Rozoxane reduces the incidence of anthracycline-related cardiotoxicity.[487]

KEY POINTS   Blood disorders in old age

- Older patients with anemia require a diagnostic evaluation.

- Iron deficiency necessitates a gastrointestinal evaluation for sources of blood loss.

- B_{12} deficiency is common in elderly people.

- Acute leukemia in elderly people portends a poorer prognosis than in younger patients.

- Prognosis in myelodysplastic syndromes can be determined using the WHO Classification—International Prognostic Scoring System (IPSS).

REFERENCES

1. Department of Health, Education, and Welfare: The First Health and Nutrition Examination Survey. DHEW (HSM), Washington, DC, 1971–1972

2. Yip R, Johnson C, Dallman PR: Age-related changes in laboratory values in the diagnosis of an anemia and iron deficiency. Am J Clin Nutr 1984;39:427–436

3. World Health Organization: Iron Deficiency Anemia. Report of a Study Group. WHO Technical Reports Series 182. World Health Organization, Geneva, 1959:4

4. World Health Organization: Nutritional Anemias. Report of a WHO Scientific Group. WHO Technical Reports Series 405. World Health Organization, Geneva, 1968

5. Hill RD: The prevalence of anemia in the over 65s in a rural practice. Practitioner 1967;217:963–965

6. Myers MA, Saunders CRG, Chalmers DG: The hemoglobin level of fit elderly people. Lancet 1968;ii:261

7. Milner JS, Williamson J: Hemoglobin, hematocrit, leukocyte count and blood grouping in older people. Geriatrics 1972;27:118–126

8. Department of Health and Social Security: A nutritional survey of the elderly. Report on Health and Human Subjects 3. HMSO, London, 1972:57

9. Brocklehurst JC, Leeming JG, Carty MH, Robinson JM: Medical screening of old people accepted for residential care. Lancet 1978;ii:141–143

10. Htoo MS, Kofkoff RL, Freedman ML: Erythrocyte parameters in the elderly: an argument against new geriatric normal values. J Am Geriatr Soc 1978;27:547–555

11. Williams WJ: The effect of aging on the blood count. Compr Ther 1960;6:7–9

12. Lipshitz DA, Mitchell CO, Thompson C: The anemia of senescence. Am J Hematol 1981;11:47–54

13. Freedman ML, Marcus DL: Anemia and the elderly: is it physiology or pathology? Am J Med Sci 1980;280:81–85

14. Freedman ML: Anemias in the elderly. Compr Ther 1983;i:45–53

15. Babitz L, Freedman ML: Anemia and the elderly patient. Compr Ther 1988;14:55–64

16. Tibblin E, Bengtsson C, Hallberg L, Lennartsson J: Hemoglobin concentration and peripheral blood counts in women. Scand J Haematol 1979;22:5–16

17. Eisen ME, Hammond EC: The effect of smoking on packed cell volume, red cell counts, haemoglobin and platelet counts. Can Med Assoc J 1956;75:520–523

18. Isager H, Hagerup L: Relationship between cigarette smoking and high packed cell volumes and haemoglobin level. Scand J Haematol 1971;8:241–244

19. Sagone AL Jr, Bakcerzak SP: Smoking as a cause of erythrocytosis. Ann Intern Med 1975;82:512–515

20. Vaisrub S: On the fringes of smoke rings. JAMA 1976;234:520

21. Albert SN: Blood Volume. Charles C Thomas, Springfield, Il, 1963:24

22. Besa EC, Gorshein D, Gardner FH: Androgens and human blood volume changes. Arch Intern Med 1974;133:418–425

23. Besa EC: Physiological changes in blood volume. Crit Rev Clin Lab Sci 1975;6:67–79

24. Beaumont WV, Greenleaf JE, Juhos L: Disproportional changes in hematocrit, plasma volume and proteins during exercise and bed rest. J Appl Physiol 1972;33:55–61

25. Taylor HL, Ericson L, Hemschel A, Keys A: The effect of bed rest on the blood volume of normal men. Am J Physiol 1945;144:227–232

26. Fawcett JK, Wynn V: Effects of posture on plasma volume and some blood constituents. J Clin Pathol 1960;13:304–310

27. Rowe JW, Minaker KL, Sparrow D, Robertson GL: Age related failure of volume-pressure-mediated vasopressin release. J Clin Endocrinol Metab 1982;54:661–664

28. Sanchez C, Merino C, Figallo M: Simultaneous measurement of plasma volume and cell mass in polycythemia of high altitude. J Appl Physiol 1970;28:775–778

29. Purcell H, Brozovic B: Red cell 2,3-diphosphoglycerate concentration in man decreases with age. Nature 1974;251:511–512

30. Miller ME, Rorth M, Parving HH et al: pH effects on erythropoietin response to hypoxia. N Engl J Med 1973;288:706

31. Rorth M: Hypoxia, red cell oxygen affinity and erythropoietin production. Clin Haematol 1974;3:595–607

32. Besa EC: Approach to mild anemia in the elderly. Clin Geriatr 1988;4.1:43–55

33. Woo JE, Roy SB: The relationship of peripheral venomotor response to high altitude pulmonary edema in man. Am J Med Sci 1980;259:56–65

34. Dill BD, Horvath SM, Dahms TE et al: Hemoconcentration at altitude. J Appl Physiol 1969;27:514–518

35. Jung RC, Dill DB, Horton R, Hovarth SM: Effects of age on plasma aldosterone levels and hemoconcentration at altitude. J Appl Physiol 1971;31:593–597

36. Hartsock RJ, Smith EB, Petty CS: Normal variations with aging in the amount of hematopoietic tissue in bone marrow from the anterior iliac crest. J Am Clin Pathol 1965;43:326–331

37. Lipshitz DA, Udupa KB, Milton KY, Thompson CO: Effects of age on hematopoiesis in man. Blood 1984;63:502–509

38. Chen MG: Age related changes in hematopoietic stem cell populations of long lived hybrid mouse. J Cell Physiol 1971;78:225–232

39. Harrison DE: Normal function of transplanted marrow cell lines from aged mice. J Gerontol 1975;30:279–285

40. Freedman ML: Heme and iron metabolism in aging. Blood Cells 1987;13:234–241

41. Refino CJ, Dallman PR: Rate of repair of iron deficiency anemia and blood loss anemia in young and mature rats. Am J Clin Nutr 1983;37:904–909

42. Boggs DR, Patrene KD: Hematopoiesis and aging III: anemia and a blunted erythropoietic response to hemorrhage in aged mice. Am J Hematol 1985;19:327–328

43. Marx JJM: Normal iron absorption and decreased red cell iron uptake in the aged. Blood 1979;53:204–211

44. Piomelli S, Nathan DG, Cummins JF, Gardner F: The relationship of total red cell volume to total body water in octogenarian males. Blood 1962;19:89–98

45. Nathan DG, Piomelli S, Gardner F, Limauro AL: The effects of androgen on some aspects of body composition and erythropoiesis in octogenarian males. Ann NY Acad Sci 1967;110:965–977

46. Hurdle ADF, Rosin AJ: Red cell volume and red cell survival in normal aged people. J Clin Pathol 1962;15:343–345

47. Myers AM, Saunders CR, Chalmers DG: The haemoglobin level of fit elderly people. Lancet 1968;ii:261–263

48. Smith JS, Whitelaw DM: Hemoglobin values in aged men. Can Med Assoc J 1971;105:816–818

49. McLennan WJ, Andrews GR, Macleod C, Caird FI: Anemia in the elderly. Q J Med 1973;42:1–13

50. Jandl JH: Blood: Textbook of Hematology. Little Brown, Boston, 1987

51. Huehns ER: Control of red cell oxygen affinity by 2,3-DPG in disease. In Huntsman RG, Jenkins GC (eds): Advanced Haemotology, Butterworth, London, 1974:38–55

52. Huehns ER: The structure and function of haemoglobin: clinical disorders due to abnormal haemoglobin structure. In Hardisty RM, Weatherall DU (eds): Blood and Its Disorders. Blackwell, Oxford, 1974:526–629e

53. Brewer GJ: Red cell metabolism and function. In Surgenor DN (ed): The Red Blood Cell. 2nd Ed. Academic Press, New York, 1974:473–508

54. Thomas HM, Lefrak S, Irwin RS et al: The oxyhemoglobin disassociation curve in health and disease. Am J Med 1974;57:331–348

55. Weintraub NT, Freedman ML: Anemias. In Abrams WB, Berkow R (eds): The Merck Manual of Geriatrics. Merck, Sharp & Dohme, Whitehouse Station, NJ, 1990:643–684

56. Thompson W, Meola T, Lipkin M Jr, Freedman ML: The utility of the RDW, MCV and transferrin saturation in the diagnosis of iron deficiency anemia. Arch Intern Med 1988;148:2128–2130

57. Thompson WG, Cassino C, Babitz L et al: Hypersegmented neutrophils and vitamin B_{12} deficiency. Acta Haematol 1989;81:186–191

58. Coates CA: Routine testing in hematology. In Rodak BF (ed): Diagnostic Hematology. WB Saunders, Philadelphia, 1995:127–144

59. The Editors. Tenth Edition of the RDA. Nutr Rev 1990;48:28–29

60. Marcus DL, Freedman ML: Clinical disorders of iron metabolism in the elderly. Clin Geriatr Med 1985;1:729–745

61. Assessment of Iron Nutriture. In DHSS Publication 89–1255, National Center for Health Statistics:129–151

62. Schultz BM, Freedman ML: Iron deficiency in the elderly. Baillière's Clinical Haematology I:291–313

63. Guyatt GH, Patterson C, Ali M et al: Diagnosis of iron deficiency in the elderly. Am J Med 1990;88:205–209

64. Jacobs A: Non-haematologic effects of iron deficiency. Clin Haematol 1982;11:353–365

65. Marcus DL, Ibrahim NG, Gruenspecht N, Freedman ML: Iron requirement for isolated rat liver mitochondrial protein synthesis. Biochim Biophys Acta 1982;607:136–143

66. Marcus DL, Ibrahim NG, Freedman ML: Age-related decline in the biosynthesis of mitochondrial inner membrane proteins. Exp Gerontol 1980;17:333–341

67. Marcus DL, Freedman ML: Role of heme and iron metabolism in controlling protein synthesis. J Am Geriatr Soc 1986;34:593–600

68. Rabinovitz M, Freeman ML, Fisher JM, Maxwell CR: Translational control in hemoglobin synthesis. Symp Quant Biol 1969;34:567–568

69. Gross M, Rabinovitz M: Control of globin synthesis by hemin: factors influencing formation of an inhibitor of globin chain, initiation in reticulocyte lysates. Biochim Biophys Acta 1972;287:340–352

70. Rhoads RE, McNight GS, Schimke RT: Quantitative measurement of ovalbumin messenger ribonucleic activity: localization in polysomes, induction by estrogen, and effect of actinomycin D. J Biol Chem 1973;248:2031–2037

71. Freedman ML, Karpatkin S: Requirement of iron for platelet protein synthesis. Biochem Biophys Res Commun 1973;54:475–481

72. Lodish HF, Desalu O: Regulation of synthesis of nonglobin proteins in cell-free extracts of rabbit reticulocytes. J Biol Chem 1973;248:3420–3428

73. Lodish HF: Model for the regulation of mRNA translation applied to haemoglobin synthesis. Nature 1974;251:385–392

74. Freedman ML, Rosman J: A rabbit reticulocyte model for the role of hemin-controlled repressor in hypochromic anemias. J Clin Invest 1976;57:594–603

75. Freedman ML, Geraghty M, Rosman J: Hemin control of globin synthesis: isolation of a hemin-reversible translational repressor from human nature erythrocytes. J Biol Chem 1974;240:7290–7302

76. Freedman ML, Spieler PJ, Rosman J, Wildman J: Cyclic AMP maintenance of rabbit reticulocyte haem and protein synthesis in the presence of ethanol and benzene. Br J Haematol 1977;37:179–185

77. Ranu RS, London IM: Regulation of protein synthesis in rabbit reticulocyte lysates: purification and initial characterization of the cyclic 3':5'-AMP independent protein kinase of the hemeregulated translational inhibitor. Proc Natl Acad Sci USA 1976;73:4349–4355

78. Trachsel H, Staehelin T: Binding and release of eukaryotic initiation factor of eIF-2 and GTP during protein synthesis initiation. Proc Natl Acad Sci USA 1978;75:204–211

79. deHaro C, Datta A, Ochoa S: Mode of action of the hemin controlled inhibitor of protein synthesis. Proc Natl Acad Sci USA 1978;75:243–252

80. Ibrahim NG, Spieler PJ, Freedman ML: Ethanol inhibition of rabbit reticulocytes at the level of delta-aminolevulinic acid synthase. Br J Haematol 1979;41:235–241

81. Ibrahim NG, Gruenspecht NR, Freedman ML: Feedback inhibition rat reticulocyte delta at the level of delta aminolevulinic acid synthase. Biophys Res Commun 1978;80:722–730

82. Beuzard Y, Rodvien R, London IM: Effect of hemin on the synthesis of hemoglobin and other proteins in mammalian cells. Proc Natl Acad Sci USA 1973;70:1022–1031

83. Ibrahim NG, Marcus DL, Freedman ML: Maintenance of cytochrome P-450 content in old rat livers in spite of decreased mitochondrial protein synthesis. J Clin Exp Gerontol 1981;3:327–337

84. Ibrahim NG, Levere RD, Freedman ML: Effect of age on rat liver heme and drug metabolism. Exp Gerontol 1985;20:277–284

85. Freedman ML: Heme and iron metabolism in aging. Blood Cells 1987;13:234–241

86. Ibrahim NG, Hoffstein ST: Induction of liver cell haem oxygenase in iron overloaded rats. Biochem J 1979;180:257–263

87. Marcus DL, Lew G, Freedman ML: Increased inactivation of cytochrome P-450 in iron overloaded rats. J Clin Exp Gerontol 1985;7:257–270

88. Gubler CJ, Cartwright GE, Wintrobe MM: Studies on copper metabolism. XX. Enzyme activities and iron metabolism in copper and iron deficiencies. J Biol Chem 1957;224:533–546

89. Beutler E: Iron enzymes in iron deficiency. I. Cytochrome c. Am J Med Sci 1968;234:517–527

90. Beutler E: Iron enzymes in iron deficiency. IV. Cytochrome oxidase in rat kidney and heart. Acta Haematol 1959;21:371–377

91. Beutler E, Blaisdell RK: Iron enzymes in iron deficiency. V. Succinic dehydrogenase in rat liver, kidney and heart. Blood 1960;15:30–35

92. Masuya T: Pathophysiological studies in sideropenic symptoms: biochemical considerations. Isr J Med Sci 1965;1:733–734

93. Srivastava SK, Sanwal GG, Tewari KK: Biochemical alterations in rat tissue in iron deficiency and repletion. Indian J Biochem 1965;2:257–263

94. Dagg JH, Jackson JM, Curry B, Goldberg A: Cytochrome oxidase in latent iron deficiency (sideropenia). Br J Haematol 1966;12:331–333

95. Beveridge BR, Bannerman RM, Evanson JM, Witts L: Hypochromic anemia: a retrospective study and follow-up of 378 in-patients. Q J Med 1965;34:145–153

96. Jacobs A: Oral cornification in anaemic patients. J Clin Pathol 1959;12:235–241

97. Jacobs A: The buccal mucosa in anaemia. J Clin Pathol 1960;13:463–470

98. Paterson DR: A clinical type of dysphagia. J Laryngol Rhinol Otol 1919;34:289–295

99. Kelly AB: Spasm at the entrance to the oesophagus. J Laryngol Rhinol Otol 1919;34:285–289

100. Vinson PP: Hysterical dysphagia. Minnesota Med 1922;5:107–111

101. Entwistle CC, Jacobs A: Histological findings in the Patterson–Kelly syndrome. J Clin Pathol 1965;18:408–413

102. Ahlbom HE: Simple achlorhydric anemia, Plummer–Vinson syndrome and carcinoma of the mouth, pharynx, and esophagus in women. Br Med J 1936;ii:331–336

103. Wynder EL, Hultberg S, Jacobsson F, Bross IJ: Environmental factors in cancer of the upper alimentary tract. Cancer 1957;10:470–475

104. Dagg JH, Goldberg A, Anderson JM et al: Autoimmunity in iron deficiency anemia. Br Med J 1964;i:1349–1355

105. Chisholm M, Ardran GM, Callender ST, Wright R: A follow up study of patients with postcricoid webs. QJ Med 1971;40:409–420

106. Chisholm M, Ardran GM, Callender ST, Wright R: Iron deficiency and autoimmunity in postcricoid webs. Q J Med 1971;40:421–433

107. Coltman CA Jr: Pagophagia and iron lack. JAMA 1969;207:513–521

108. Sayers G, Lipschitz DA, Sayers M: The relationship between pica and iron nutrition in Johannesburg Bantu adults. South C J Nutr 1974;48:53–60

109. Markson JL, Moore JM: Autoimmunity in pernicious anaemia and iron deficiency anaemia. Lancet 1962;ii:1240

110. Jacobs A, Lawrie JH, Entwistle QC, Campbell H: Gastric acid secretion in chronic iron deficiency anaemia. Lancet 1966;ii:190–196

111. Stone WD: Gastric secretory response to iron therapy. Gut 1968;9:99–104

112. Jacobs A: Non-haematologic effects of iron deficiency. Clin Haematol 1982;ii:353–365

113. Judish JM, Naiman JL, Oski FA: The fallacy of the fat iron deficient child. Pediatrics 1965;37:987–993

114. Dallman PR: Tissue effects of iron deficiency. In Jacobs A, Worwood M (eds): Iron in Biochemistry and Medicine. Academic Press, London, 1974:437–475

115. Hood DA, Kelton R, Nishio ML: Mitochondrial adaptations to chronic muscle use: effect of iron deficiency. Comp Biochem Physiol 1992;101A:597–605

116. Holloszy JO: Biochemical adaptations in muscle: effects of exercise on mitochondrial oxygen uptake and respiratory enzyme activity in skeletal muscle. J Bio Chem 1967;242:2278–2282

117. Ekblom B, Goldbarg AN, Gullbring B: Response to exercise after blood loss and reinfusion. J Appl Physiol 1972;33:175–180

118. Viteri FE, Torun B: Anaemia and physical work capacity. Clin Haematol 1974;3:609–617

119. Finch CA, Miller LR, Inamdar AR et al: Iron deficiency in the rat: physiological and biochemical studies of muscle dysfunction. J Clin Invest 1976;58:447–453

120. Gardner GW, Edgarton VR, Senewiratne B et al: Physical work capacity and metabolic stress in subjects with iron deficiency anemia. Am J Clin Nutr 1977;30:910–917

121. Basta SS, Soekirman MS, Karydi D, Scrimshaw NS: Iron deficiency anemia and the productivity of adult males in Indonesia. Am J Nutr 1979;32:916–922

122. Edgerton VR, Gardner GW, Ohira Y et al: Iron deficiency anaemia and its effect on worker productivity and activity patterns. Br Med J 1979;2:1546–1549

123. Davies KJA, Packer L, Brooks GA: Biochemical adaptation of mitochondria muscle, and whole animal respiration to endurance training. Arch Biochem Biophys 1981;209:538–553

124. Dallman PR: Manifestations of iron deficiency. Semin Hematol 1982;19:19–30

125. Finch CA, Gollnick PD, Hlastala MP et al: Lactic acidosis as a result of iron deficiency. J Clin Invest 1979;64:129–137

126. Chandra RK, Saraya AK: Impaired immunocompetence associated with iron deficiency. J Pediatr 1975;86:899–909

127. Joynson DHM, Jacobs A, Walker DM, Dolby AE: Defect of cell mediated immunity in patients with iron deficiency anaemia. Lancet 1972;ii:1058–1059

128. Higgs JM, Wells RS: Chronic mucocutaneous candidiasis: associated abnormalities of iron metabolism. Br J Dermatol 1973;86(suppl 8):88–93

129. Macdougal LG, Anderson R, McNab GM, Katz J: The immune response in iron deficient children: impaired cellular defence mechanisms with altered humoral components. J Pediatr 1975;86:833–840

130. Cook JD, Lynch SR: The liabilities of iron deficiency. Blood 1986;68:803–809

131. Chandra RK: Reduced bacterial capacity of polymorphs in iron deficiency. Arch Dis Childhood 1973;48:864–870

132. Sagone AL, Balcerzak SP: Activity of iron containing enzymes in erythrocytes and granulocytes in thalassemia and iron deficiency. Am J Med Sci 1970;259:350–355

133. Sussman M: Iron and infection. In Jacobs A, Woorwood M (eds): Iron in Biochemistry and Medicine. Academic Press, London, 1974:664–679

134. Masawe AEJ, Muindi JM, Swai GRB: Infections in iron deficiency and other types of anaemia in the tropics. Lancet 1974;ii:314–320

135. Barry DMJ, Reeve AW: Increased incidence of gram negative sepsis with intramuscular iron administration. Pediatrics 1977;60:908–913

136. Murray MJ, Murray AB, Murray MB, Murray CJ: The adverse effect of iron repletion on the course of certain infections. Br Med J 1978;ii:1113–1121

137. Payne SM, Finkelstein RA: The critical role of iron in host-bacterial interactions. J Clin Invest 1978;61:1428–1435

138. Bullen JJ, Rogers HJ, Griffiths J: Role of iron in bacterial infection. Curr Topics Microbiol Immunol 1978;80:1–12

139. Fleming AF: Iron deficiency in the tropics. Clin Haematol 1982;11:365–371

140. Weinberg ED: Iron withholding: a defence against infection and neoplasia. Physiol Rev 1984;64:65–72

141. Glover J, Jacobs A: Activity pattern of iron deficient rats. Br Med J 1972;ii:627–633

142. Webb TE, Oski FA: Iron deficiency anemia and scholastic achievement in young adolescents. J Pediatr 1973;82:827–833

143. Webb TE, Oski FA: Behavioral status of young adolescents with iron deficiency status. J Spec Educ 1974;8:153–160

144. Pollitt E, Leibel RL: Iron deficiency and behavior. J Pediatr 1976;88:372–381

145. Tamir H, Klein A, Rapport MM: Serotonin-binding protein: enhancement of binding by Fe^{2+} and inhibition of binding by drugs. J Neurochem 1976;26:871–878

146. Youdim MBH, Green AR: Biogenic monoamine metabolism and functional activity in iron deficient rats: behavioral correlates. In Porter R, Fitzsimons DW (eds): Iron Metabolism. Elsevier/North Holland. Amsterdam, 1977:201–221

147. Oski FA, Honig AS: The effects of therapy on the developmental scores of iron-deficient infants. J Pediatr 1978;92:21–28

148. Bothwell TH, Carlton RW, Cook JD, Finch CA: Iron Metabolism in Man. Blackwell, Oxford, 1979

149. Weinberg J, Dallman PR, Levine S: Iron deficiency during early development in the rat: behavioral and physiological consequences. Pharmacol Biochem Behav 1980;12:493–502

150. Williamson AM, Ng KT: Activity and T-maze performance in iron deficient rats. Physiol Behav 1980;24:1157–1162

151. Youdim MBH, Green AR, Bloomfield MR: The effects of iron deficiency on brain biogenic monoamine biochemistry and function in rats. Neuropharmacology 1980;19:259–267

152. Deinard A, Gilbert A, Dodds M, Egeland B: Iron deficiency and behavioral defects. Pediatrics 1981;68:828–833

153. Sourkes TL: Transition elements and the nervous system. In Pollitt E, Leibel AL (eds): Iron Deficiency and Behavior. Raven Press, New York: 1–29

154. Youdim MBH, Yehuda S, Ben-Shachar D: Behavioral and brain biochemical changes in iron deficient rats: the involvement of iron in dopamine receptor function. In Pollit E, Leibel R (eds): Iron Deficiency: Brain Biochemistry and Behavior. Raven Press, New York, 1982:39–56

155. Lotzoff B, Brittenham GM, Viteri FE et al: Developmental deficits in iron-deficient infants: effects of age and severity of iron lack. J Pediatr 1982;101:948–956

156. Mackler B, Finch C: Iron in central nervous system oxidative metabolism. In Pollitt E, Leibel RL (eds): Iron Deficiency: Brain Biochemistry and Behavior. Raven Press, New York, 1982:31–38

157. Walter T, Kovalskys J, Stekel A: Effect of iron deficiency on infant mental development. J Pediatr 1983;10:519–525

158. Pollitt E, Leibel RL, Greenfield DB: Iron deficiency and cognitive test performance in preschool children. Nutr Behav 1983;1:137–142

159. Schoene RB, Escourrou P, Robertson HT et al: Iron depletion decreases maximal exercise lactate concentrations in female athletes with minimal iron deficiency anemia. J Lab Clin Med 1983;102:306–311

160. Vyas D, Chandra RK: Functional implications of iron deficiency. In Stekel A (ed): Iron Nutrition in Infancy and Childhood. Raven Press, New York, 1984:45–59

161. Tucker DH, Sanstead HH, Penland JG et al: Iron status and brain function: serum ferritin level associated with asymmetries of cortical electrophysiology and cognitive performance. Am J Clin Nutr 1984;39:105–112

162. Soemantri AG, Pollitt E, Kim I: Iron deficiency and education achievement. Am J Clin Nutr 1985;42:1221–1227

163. Symes AL, Missala K, Sourkes TL: Iron- and riboflavin dependent metabolism of a monoamine in the rat in vivo. Science 1981;74:153–155

164. Voorhess ML, Stuart MJ, Stockman JA, Oski FA: Iron deficiency anemia and increased urinary epinephrine excretion. J Pediatr 1975;86:542–547

165. Youdim MBH, Woods HF, Mitchell B, Boudin D: Human platelet monoamine oxidase activity in iron-deficiency anaemia. Clin Sci Mol Med 1976;48:289–295

166. Woods HF, Youdim MBH, Boudin D, Mitchell B: Monoamine metabolism and platelet function in iron-deficiency anaemia. Ciba Found Symp 1977;51:227–248

167. Dillman E, Johnson DG, Martin J et al: Catecholamine elevation in iron deficiency. Am J Physiol 1979;237:R297–R300

168. Dillman E, Mackler B, Johnson D et al: Effect of iron deficiency on catecholamine metabolism and body temperature regulation. In Pollitt E, Leibel RL (eds): Iron Deficiency: Brain Biochemistry and Behavior. Raven Press, New York. 1982:57–62

169. Davies DM, Smith A, Muller-Eberhard U, Margan WR: Hepatic-subcellular metabolism of heme from hemopexin: incorporation of iron into ferritin. Biochem Biophys Res Commun 1979;91:1504–1511

170. Callender ST, Mallet BJ, Smith MD: Absorption of hemoglobin iron. Br J Haematol 1957;3:186–192

171. Hussain R, Walker RB, Layrrise M et al: Nutritive value of food iron. Am J Clin Nutr 1965;16:464–471

172. Hallberg L, Solvell L: Absorption of hemoglobin iron in man. Acta Med Scand 1965;181:335–354

173. Conrad ME, Benjamin BI, Williams HL, Foy AL: Human absorption of hemoglobin iron. Gastroenterology 1967;53:5–10

174. Weintraub LR, Weinstein MB, Huser HJ, Rafal S: Absorption of hemoglobin iron: the role of a heme-splitting substance in the intestinal mucosa. J Clin Invest 1968;47:531–539

175. Raffin SB, Woo CH, Roost KT, Schmid R: Intestinal absorption of hemoglobin iron-heme cleavage by mucosal heme oxygenase. J Clin Invest 1974;54:1344–1352

176. Brown ER Jr, Justus BW: In vitro absorption of radioiron by everted pouches of rat intestine. Am J Physiol 1958;194:319–326

177. Beutler E, Kelly BM, Beutler F: The regulation of iron absorption. II. The relationship between iron dosage and iron absorption. Am J Clin Nutr 1962;11:559–567

178. Pollack S, Kaufman RM, Crosby WH: Iron absorption: effects of sugars and reducing agents. Blood 1964;24:577–581

179. Andrews NC: Disorders of iron metabolism. N Engl J Med 1999;341:1986–1995

180. Bendrich A, Cohen M: Ascorbic acid safety: analysis of factors affecting iron absorption. Toxicol Lett 1990;51:189–201

181. Lynch SR, Finch CA, Monsen ER, Cook JD: Iron status of elderly Americans. Am J Clin Nutr 1982;36:1032–1045

182. Rockey DC, Cello JP: Evaluation of the gastrointestinal tract in patients with iron-deficiency anemia. N Engl J Med 1993;329:1691–1695

183. Joosten E, Dereymaeker L, Perelmans W, Hiele M: Significance of a low serum ferritin level in elderly in-patients. Postgrad Med J 1993;69:397–400

184. Griffiths EK, Schapira DV: Serum ferritin and stool occult blood and colon cancer screening: cancer detection and prevention. 1991;15:303–305

185. Campbell NRC, Hasinoff BB: Iron supplements: a common cause of drug interactions. Br J Clin Pharmacol 1991;31:251–255

186. Campbell NRC, Hasinoff BB, Stalts H et al: Ferrous sulfate reduces thyroxine efficacy in patients with hypothyroidism. Ann Intern Med 1992;117:1010–1013

187. Cartwright GE, Lee GR: The anaemia of chronic disorders. Br J Haematol 1971;21:147–152

188. Frey R, Grimm J, Trachsler M, Rhyner K: Die wertigkeit von serum-ferritin, serumeisen and eisenbindungskapazitat in der differential diagnose der mikrozytarenhypochromen anamie. Schweiz Med Wochenschr 1982;112:13–17

189. Cartwright GE: The anaemia of chronic disorders. Semin Hematol 1996;3:351

190. Kluger MJ, Rothenburg BA: Fever and reduced iron: their interaction as a host defense response to bacterial infection. Science 1979;203:374–376

191. Pekarek RS: The effect of leukocytic endogenous mediator (LEM) on the tissue distribution of zinc and iron. Proc Soc Exp Biol Med 1972;140:684–686

192. Karle H, Hansen NE, Malmquist J et al: Turnover of human lactoferrin in the rabbit. Scand J Haematol 1979;23:303–312

193. Van Snick L, Masson PL: The binding of human lactoferrin to mouse peritoneal cells. J Exp Med 1976;144:1568–1580

194. Van Snick L: The ingestion and digestion of human lactoferrin by mouse peritoneal macrophages and the transfer of its iron into ferritin. J Exp Med 1977;146:817

195. Weinberg J: Iron and infection. Microbiol Rev 1978;42:45–66

196. Krantz SB: Pathogenesis and treatment of the anemia of chronic disease. Am J Med Sci 1994;307:353–359

197. Spivak JL: The blood in systemic disorders. Lancet 2000;355:1707–1713

198. Radtke HW, Claussner HW, Erbes PM et al: Serum erythropoietin concentration in chronic renal failure: relationship to degree in anemia and excretory renal function. Blood 1979;54:877–884

199. Van Dyke D, Keighley G, Lawrence J: Decreased responsiveness to erythropoietin in a patient with anemia secondary to chronic uremia. Blood 1963;22:838

200. Urabe A, Chiba S, Kosaka K, Takaku F: Response of uraemic bone marrow cells to erythropoietin in vitro. Scand J Haematol 1976;17:335–340

201. Wallner SF, Vautrin RM: The anemia of chronic renal failure: studies of the effect of organic solvent extraction of serum. J Lab Clin Med 1978;92:363–369

202. Pricto J, Barry M, Sherlock S: Serum ferritin in patients with iron overload and acute and chronic liver disease. Gastroenterology 1975;68:533–535

203. Larsson SD: Anemia and iron metabolism in hypothyroidism. Acta Med Scand 1967;157:349–363

204. Tudhope GR, Wilson GM: Anemia in hypothyroidism: incidence pathogenesis and response to treatment. J Med 1960;29:513–537

205. Freedman ML: Haemolytic disease. In Denham MJ, Chanorin I (eds): Blood Disorders in the Elderly. Churchill Livingstone, London, 1985:109–131

206. Dacie JV, Worlledge S: Autoimmune hemolytic anemias. Prog Hematol 1969;6:82–120

207. Worlledge S: Immune drug-induced hemolytic anemias. Semin Hematol 1969;6:181–200

208. Petz LD: Drug-induced immune hemolytic anemia. Clin Haematol 1980;4:181–197

209. Kirtland HH III, Mohler DN, Horowitz DA: Methyldopa inhibition of suppressor-lymphocyte function: a proposed cause of autoimmune hemolytic anemia. N Engl J Med 1980;30:825–832

210. Petz LD, Garratty G: Drug-induced haemolytic anaemia. Clin Haematol 1975;4:181–197

211. Pirofsky B: Autoimmunization and the Autoimmune Hemolytic Anemias. Churchill Livingstone, London, 1980

212. Madanes AE: Danazol. Ann Intern Med 1982;96:625–630

213. Ahn YS, Harrington WJ, Mylvaganam R: Danazol therapy in autoimmune hemolytic anemia. Blood 1983;62(suppl):102a

214. Jayid J: Immune hemolytic anemia in the aged. Clin Geriatr Med 1985;1:747–772

215. Allgood JW, Chaplin A Jr: Idiopathic acquired hemolytic anemia: a review of forty-seven cases treated from 1955 through 1965. Am J Med 1967;43:254–273

216. Kutti N, Wadenvik H, Safai-Kutti S et al: Successful treatment of refractory autoimmune hemolytic anaemia by plasmapheresis. Scand J Haematol 1984;32:149–152

217. Murphy S, LoBuglio AP: Drug therapy in autoimmune hemolytic anemia. Semin Hematol 1976;13:323–334

218. Heyssel RM, Bozian RC, Darby WJ, Bell MC: Vitamin B_{12} turnover in man: the assimilation of vitamin B_{12} from natural foodstuffs by man and estimates of minimal daily requirements. Am J Clin Nutr 1966;18:176–184

219. Hall CA: Long-term excretion of Co-57 B_{12} and turnover within the plasma. J Clin Nutr 1964;14:156–162

220. Adams JF: Considerations governing the maintenance treatment of patients with pernicious anemia. In Heinrich HC (ed): Vitamin B_{12} and Intrinsic Factor. Second European Symposium. Enke, Stuttgart, 1962

221. Grasbech R: Calculations on vitamin B_{12} turnover in man. Scand J Clin Lab Invest 1959;11:250–258

222. Beck WS: Metabolic aspects of vitamin B_{12} and folic acid. In Williams WJ, Beutler E, Erislev AJ, Lichtman MA (eds): McGraw-Hill, New York, 1983:311–331

223. Herbert V, Castle WB: Divalent cation and pH dependence of rat intrinsic factor action in everted sacs and mucosal homogenates of rat small intestine. J Clin Invest 1961;40:1978–1983

224. Grasbeck R: Soluble and membrane-bound vitamin B_{12} transport proteins. In Zagalak B, Freidrich W (ed): Vitamin B_{12}. Proceedings of the Third European Symposium on Vitamin B_{12}. and Intrinsic Factor. Walter de Gruyter, New York, 1979:743

225. Grasbeck R, Nyberg W, Reizenstein PG: Biliary and fecal vitamin B_{12} excretion in man: an isotope study. Proc Soc Exp Biol Med 1958;97:780–784

226. Reizenstein PG: Excretion of non-labelled vitamin B_{12} in man. Acta Med Scand 1959;165:313–319

227. Benson RE, Rappazzo ME, Hall CA: Late transport of vitamin B_{12} by transcobalamin II. J Lab Clin Med 1972;80:488–495

228. Gizis EJ, Arkun SN, Miller IF et al: Plasma clearance of transcobalamin I- and transcobalamin II-bound Co vitamin B_{12}. J Lab Clin Med 1969;74:574–580

229. Finkler AE, Hall CA: Nature of the relationship between vitamin B_{12} binding and cell uptake. Arch Biochem Biophys 1967;120:79–85

230. Carmel R, Herbert V: Deficiency of vitamin B_{12} binding alpha globulin in two brothers. Blood 1969;33:1–12

231. Hakami N, Neiman PE, Canellos GP, Lazerson: Neonatal megoblastic anemia due to inherited transcobalamin II deficiency in two siblings. N Engl J Med 1971;285:1163–1170

232. Herbert V: Megaloblastic anemias. Lab Invest 1985;52:3–19

233. Kuzminski AM, Del Giacco EJ, Allen RH, Stabler SP, Lindenbaum J: Effective treatment of cobalmin deficiency with oral cobalmin. Blood 1998;92:1191–1198

234. Lederle FA: Oral cobalamin for pernicious anemia: medicine's best kept secret. JAMA 1991;265:94–95

235. Hsing AW, Hansson L, McLaughlin JK et al: Pernicious anemia and subsequent cancer: a population based cohort study. Cancer 1993;71:745–750

236. Sjoblom SM, Sipponen P, Jarvinen H: Gastroscopic follow up of pernicious anemia patients. Gut 1993;34:28–32

237. Marcaurd SP, Albernaz L, Khazanie PG: Omeprazole therapy causes malabsorption of cyanocobalmin. Ann Intern Med 1994;120:211–215

238. Sumner AE, Chin MM, Abrahm JL et al: Elevated methymalonic acid and total homocysteine levels show high prevalence of vitamin B_{12} deficiency after gastric surgery. Ann Intern Med 1996;124:469–476

239. Bauman WA, Shaw S, Jayatilleke, Spungen AM, Herbert V: Increase intake of calcium reverses Vitamin B12 malabsorption induced by metformin. Diabetes Care 2000;23:1227–1231

240. Martin DC, Francis J, Protetch J, Huff JF: Time dependency of cognitive recovery with cobalamin replacement: report of a pilot study. J Am Geriatr Soc 1992;40:168–172

241. Stabler SP, Allen RH, Savage DG, Lindenbaum J: Clinical spectrum and diagnosis of cobalamin deficiency. Blood 1990;76:871–881

242. Thompson WG, Babitz L, Cassino C et al: Evaluation of current criteria used to order vitamin B_{12} levels. Am J Med 1987;82:291–294

243. Lindenbaum J, Healton EB, Savage DG et al: Neuropsychiatric disorders caused by cobalamin deficiency in the absence of anemia or macrocytosis. N Engl J Med 1988;318:1720–1728

244. Carmel R: Pernicious anemia: the expected findings of very low serum cobalamin levels, anemia, and macrocytosis are often lacking. Arch Intern Med 1988;148:1712–1714

245. Spivack JL: Masked megaloblastic anemia. Arch Intern Med 1982;142:2111–2114

246. Bessman JD, Gilmer PR Jr, Gardner FH: Improved classification of anemias by MCV and RDW. Am J Clin Pathol 1983;80:322–326

247. Bergia JJ: Evaluation of anemia. Postgrad Med 1985;77:253–269

248. Thompson WG, Cassino C, Babitz L et al: Hypersegmented neutrophils and vitamin B_{12} deficiency. Acta Haematol 1989;81:186–191

249. Cooper BA, Fehedy V, Blanshay P: Recognition of deficiency of vitamin B_{12} using measurement of serum concentration. J Clin Lab Med 1986;107:447–452

250. Karnaze DS, Carmel R: Low serum cobalamin levels in primary degenerative dementia: do some patients harbor atypical cobalamin deficiency states? Arch Intern Med 1987;147:429–431

251. Grinblat J, Marcus DL, Hernandez F, Freedman ML: Folate and vitamin B_{12} levels in an urban elderly population with chronic disease: assessment of two laboratory folate assays: microbiologic and radioassay. J Am Geriatr Soc 1986;34:627–632

252. Garry PJ, Goodwin JS, Hunt WC: Folate and vitamin B_{12} status in a healthy elderly population. J Am Geriatr Soc 1984;32:719–726

253. Marcus DL, Shadick N, Grantz J, Freedman ML: Low serum B_{12} levels in a hematologically normal elderly subpopulation. J Am Geriatr Soc 1987;35:635–638

254. Norman EJ: Gas chromatography mass spectrometry screening of urinary methylmalonic acid: early detection of vitamin B_{12} deficiency to prevent permanent neurologic disability. Gas Chromatogr Mass Spectrum News 1984;12:120–129

255. Weiland RG: Vitamin B_{12} deficiency in non-anemic elderly. J Am Geriatr Soc 1986;34:618

256. Kilpatrick GS, Withey JL: The serum vitamin B_{12} concentration in the general population. Scand J Haematol 1965;2:220–229

257. Elsborg L, Lund V, Bastrup MP: Serum vitamin B_{12} levels in the aged. Acta Med Scand 1976;200:309–314

258. Matchar DB, Feussner JR, Watson DJ et al: Significance of low serum B_{12} levels in the elderly. J Am Geriatr Soc 1985;34:680A–681A

259. Blundell EL, Matthews JH, Allen SM et al: Importance of low serum vitamin B_{12} and red cell folate concentrations in elderly hospital inpatients. J Clin Pathol 1985;38:1179–1184

260. Elwood PC, Shinton NK, Wilson CID et al: Haemoglobin, vitamin B_{12} and folate levels in the elderly. Br J Haematol 1971;21:557–563

261. Freedman ML: Status of vitamin B_{12} and folic acid in the elderly in the United States. In The Role of Folate and Vitamin B_{12} in Neurotransmitter Metabolism and Degenerative Neurological Changes Associated with Aging. NIA, NIDDKD Publication. Federation of American Societies for Experimental Biology, Bethesda, MD, 1989:25–31

262. Cole MG, Prichal JF: Low serum B_{12} in Alzheimer-type dementia. Age Ageing 1984;13:101–105

263. Carmel R, Karnaze DS: Physician response to low serum cobal-amin levels. Arch Intern Med 1986;146:1161–1165

264. Lindenbaum J: Status of laboratory testing in the diagnosis of megaloblastic anemia. Blood 1983;61:624–627

265. Carethers M: Diagnosing vitamin B$_{12}$ deficiency, a common geriatric disorder. Geriatrics 1988;43:89–112

266. Fairbanks VF: Test for pernicious anemia: the "Schilling test." Mayo Clin Proc 1983;58:541–544

267. Carmel R, Sinow RM, Siegel ME, Samloff M: Food cobalamin malabsorption occurs frequently in patients with unexplained low serum cobalamin levels. Arch Intern Med 1988;148:1715–1719

268. Savage DG, Lindenbaum J, Stabler SP, Allen RH: Sensitivity of serum methylmalonic acid and total homocysteine determinations for diagnosing cobalamin and folate deficiencies. Am J Med 1994;96:239–246

269. Stabler SP: Screening the older population for cobalamin deficiency. J Am Geriatr Soc 1995;43:1290–1297

270. Metz J, Kelly A, Swett VC et al: Deranged DNA synthesis by bone marrow from vitamin B$_{12}$-deficient humans. Br J Haematol 1968;14:575–592

271. Lindenbaum J: Status of laboratory testing in the diagnosis of megaloblastic anemia. Blood 1983;61:624–627

272. Metz J: The deoxyuridine suppression test: a review of its clinical and research applications. Crit Rev Lab Sci 1984;20:205–241

273. Wickramasinghe SN: The deoxyuridine suppression test: a review of its clinical and research applications. Clin Lab Haematol 1981;3:1–18

274. Wickramasinghe SN, Akinyanju OO, Grange A, Litwinczuk RAG: Folate levels and deoxyuridine levels in protein-energy malnutrition. Br J Haematol 1983;53:135–143

275. Fairbanks VF, Lennon VA, Kokmen E, Howard FM: Test for pernicious anemia: serum intrinsic factor blocking antibody. Mayo Clin Proc 1983;58:203–204

276. Herbert V: Don't ignore low serum cobalamin (vitamin B$_{12}$) levels. Arch Intern Med 1988;148:1705–1707

277. Herbert V, Herzlich B: A proposed model of sequential stages in the development of vitamin B$_{12}$ deficiency, abstracted. Blood 1985;66(suppl 1):54a

278. Herzlich B, Herbert V: Depletion of serum holotranscobalamin II: an early sign of negative vitamin B$_{12}$ balance. Lab Invest 1988;58:332–337

279. Perry IJ, Refsum H, Morris RW et al: Prospective study of serum total homocysteine concentration and risk of stroke in middle-aged British men. Lancet 1995;346:1395–1398

280. Fermo I, Vigano D'Angelo S, Paroni R et al: Prevalence of moderate hyperhomocysteinemia in patients with early onset venous and arterial occlusive disease. Ann Intern Med 1995;123:747–753

281. Stampfer MJ, Malinow R, Willet WC et al: Prospective study of plasma homocysteine and risk of myocardial infarction in U.S. Physicians. JAMA 1992;268:877–881

282. Den Heijer M, Koster T, Blom HK et al: Hyperhomocysteinemia as a risk factor for deep vein thrombosis. N Engl J Med 1996;334:759–762

283. Naurath HJ, Joosten E, Riezler R et al: Effect of vitamin B$_{12}$ folate, and vitamin B$_6$ supplements in elderly people with normal serum vitamin concentrations. Lancet 1995;346:85–89

284. Fata FT, Herzlich BC, Schiffman G, Ast AL: Impaired antibody responses to pneumococcal polysaccharide in elderly patients with low serum vitamin B$_{12}$ levels. Ann Intern Med 1996;124:299–304

285. Pennypacker LC, Allen RH, Kelly JP et al: High prevalence of cobalamin deficiency in elderly outpatients. J Am Geriatr Soc 1992;40:1197–1204

286. Read AE, Gough GH, Pardoe LJ, Nicholas A: Nutritional studies on the entrants to an old people's home with particular reference to folic acid deficiency. Br Med J 1965;ii:843–848

287. Batata M, Spray GH, Bottom FG et al: Blood and bone marrow changes in elderly patients with special reference to folic acid, vitamin B$_{12}$, iron and ascorbic acid. Br Med J 1967;ii:667–669

288. Girdwood RH, Thompson AD, Williamson J: Folate status in the elderly. Br Med J 1967;ii:670–672

289. Bailey LB, Wagner PA, Christakis GH et al: Folacin and iron status and hematological findings in predominately black persons from urban low-income households. Am J Clin Nutr 1979;32:2346–2353

290. Rosenberg IH, Bowman BB, Cooper BA et al: Folate nutrition in the elderly. Am J Clin Nutr 1982;16:1060–1066

291. Wagner PA, Bailey LB, Krista ML et al: Comparison of zinc and folacin status in elderly women from differing socioeconomic backgrounds. Nutr Res 1971;1:565–569

292. Baker H, Frank O, Thind IS et al: Vitamin profiles in elderly persons living at home or in nursing homes versus profile in healthy young subjects. J Am Geriatr Soc 1979;27:444–450

293. Hayes AN, Willans DJ, Skelton D: Vitamin B$_{12}$ (cobalamin) and folate blood levels in geriatric reference group as measured by two kits. Clin Biochem 1985;18:56–61

294. Garry PJ, Goodwin JS, Hunt WC: Folate and vitamin B$_{12}$ status in a healthy elderly population. J Am Geriatr Soc 1984;32:719–726

295. Grinblat J, Marcus DL, Hernandez F et al: Folate and vitamin B$_{12}$ levels in an urban elderly population with chronic diseases. J Am Geriatr Soc 1986;34:627–632

296. Marcus DL, Freedman ML: Folic acid deficiency in the elderly. J Am Geriatr Soc 1985;33:552–558

297. Botez MI, Young SN, Bachevalier J, Gauthier S: Effect of folic acid and vitamin B$_{12}$ deficiencies in 5-hydroxyindoleacetic acid in human cerebrospinal fluid. Ann Neurol 1982;12:479–484

298. Reynolds EH, Mattson RH, Gallagher BB: Relationships between serum cerebrospinal fluid anticonvulsant drug and concentrations in epileptic patients. Neurology 1972;22:841–844

299. Lanzkowsky P, Erlandson ME, Bezan AI: Isolated defects of folic acid absorption associated with mental retardation and cerebral calcification. Blood 1969;34:452–465

300. Coleman N: Folate deficiency in humans. In Draper HH (ed): Advances in Nutritional Research, Vol 1. Plenum, New York, 1977:80

301. Herbert V: Experimental nutritional folate deficiency in man. Trans Assoc Am Phys 1962;75:307–320

302. Reynolds FH, Rothfield P, Pincus JH: Neurological disease associated with folate deficiency. Br Med J 1973;ii:398–400

303. Runcie J: Folate deficiency in the elderly. In Boetz M, Reynolds EH (eds): Folic Acid in Neurology, Psychiatry and Internal Medicine. Raven Press, New York, 1979:493–595

304. Shulman R: An overview of folic acid deficiency and psychiatric illnesses. In Botez MI, Reynolds EH (eds): Folic Acid in Neurology, Psychiatry and Internal Medicine. Raven Press, New York, 1979:463–474

305. Carney MWP: Psychiatric aspects of folate deficiency. In Botez MI, Reynolds EH (eds): Folic Acid in Neurology, Psychiatry and Internal Medicine. Raven Press, New York, 1979:475–492

306. Botez MI, Botez T, Leville J et al: Neuropsychological correlates of folic acid deficiency: facts and hypotheses. In Folic Acid in Neurology, Psychiatry and Internal Medicine. Raven Press, New York, 1979:435–462

307. Rosenberg IH, Bowman BB, Cooper BA et al: Folate nutrition in the elderly. Am J Clin Nutr 1982;36:1060–1066

308. Reynolds EH: Neurological aspects of folate and vitamin B$_{12}$ metabolism. Clin Haematol 1976;5:661–696

309. Botez MI, Bachevalier J: The blood brain barrier and folate deficiency. Am J Clin Nutr 1981;34:1725–1730

310. Coleman N, Herbert V: Folate metabolism in brain. In Kumar E (ed): Biochemistry of the Brain. Pergamon Press, Oxford, 1979:103

311. Sneath RW, Chanarin I, Hodkinson HM et al: Folate status in a geriatric population and its relation to dementia. Age Ageing 1973;2:177–182

312. Melamed E, Reches A, Hershko C: Reversible central nervous system dysfunction in folate deficiency. J Neurol Sci 1975;25:93–98

313. Strachan RW, Henderson JG: Dementia and folate deficiency. J Med 1967;36:189–204

314. Hurdle ADF, Picton-Williams TC: Folic acid deficiency in elderly patients admitted to hospital. Br Med J 1966;ii:202–207

315. Shulman R: An overview of folic acid deficiency and psychiatric illness. In Botez MI, Reynolds EH (eds): Folic Acid in Neurology, Psychiatry and Internal Medicine. Raven Press, New York, 1979:463

316. Ten-State Nutrition Survey 1968–1970 (1970) IV DHEW Publication No. (HSM) US Department of Health, Education and Welfare, Communicable Disease Center IV: 72

317. Carney MWP: Serum folate values in 423 psychiatric patients. Br Med J 1967;4:512–516

318. Brigden ML: A systematic approach to macrocytosis: sorting out the causes. Postgrad Med 1995;97:171–186

319. Bennett JM, Catovsky D, Daniel MT: Proposals for the classification of the acute leukaemias. Br J Haematol 1976;33:451–458

320. Antin JH, Rosenthal DS: Acute leukemias, myeloplasia and lymphomas. Clin Geriatr Med 1985;1:795–826

321. Cohen HS, Freedman ML, Goldstein BD: The problem of benzene in our environment: critical and molecular considerations. Am J Med Sci 1978;275:124–136

322. Kyle RA: Second malignancies associated with chemotherapeutic agents. Semin Oncol 1982;9:131–142

323. Blayney W, Jaffe ES, Fisher RI et al: The human T-cell leukemia/lymphoma virus, lymphoma, lytic lesions and hypercalcemia. Ann Intern Med 1983;98:144–151

324. Chaganti RSK: The significance of chromosome change to hematopoietic neoplasms. Blood 1983;62:515–524

325. Bishop JM: The molecular genetics of cancer. Science 1987;235:305–311

326. Holt JT, Morton CC, Neinhuis AW, Leder P: Molecular mechanisms of hematological neoplasms. In Stamatoyannopoulos G, Neinhuis AW, Leder P, Majerus PW (eds): The Molecular Basis of Blood Diseases. WB Saunders, Philadelphia, 1987:347–376

327. Hayhoe FGJ, Rees J: The leukemias. In Denham MJM, Chanarin I (eds): Blood Disorders in the Elderly. Churchill Livingstone, London, 1985:188–207

328. Yunis JJ, Brunning RD, Howe RB, Lobell M: High-resolution chromosome as an independent prognostic indicator in adult acute non-lymphocytic leukemia. N Engl J Med 1984;311:812–818

329. Bloomfield CD: Acute myeloid leukemia. Semin Oncol 1987;14:357–471

330. Koeffler HP: Syndromes of acute non-lymphocytic leukemia. Ann Intern Med 1987;107:74–75

331. Devine SM, Larson RA: Acute leukemia in adults: recent developments in diagnosis and treatment. CA Cancer J Clin 1994;44:326–352

332. Hiddemann W, Kern W, Schoch C et al: Management of acute myeloid leukemia in elderly patients. J Clin Oncol 1999;17:3569–3576 (review, 48 refs)

333. Bodey GP, Bolivar R, Fainstein V: Infectious complications in leukemic patients. Semin Hematol 1982;19:193–236

334. Weiser B, Lange M, Fialk MA et al: Prophylactic trimethoprim sulfamethoxazole during consolidation chemotherapy for acute leukemia: a controlled trial. Ann Intern Med 1981;95:436–438

335. Mir MA, Delamore IW: Metabolic disorders in acute myeloid leukemia. Br J Haematol 1978;40:79–92

336. O'Regan S, Carson S, Chesney RW, Drummond KN: Electrolyte and acid base disturbances in the management of leukemia. Blood 1977;49:345–353

337. Grund FM, Armitage JO, Burns CP: Hydroxyurea in the prevention of the effects of leukostasis in acute leukemia. Arch Intern Med 1977;137:1246–1247

338. McKee I, Collins RD: Intravascular leukocyte thrombi and aggregates as a cause of morbidity and mortality in leukemia. Medicine 1974;53:462–478

339. Littman MA, Rowe JM: Hyperleukocytic leukemia: rheological, clinical and therapeutic considerations. Blood 1982;60:279–283

340. Stahl R, Silber R: Chronic lymphocytic leukemia. Clin Geriatr Med 1985;1:857–867

341. Mann DL, DeSantis PM, Mark G et al: HLTV-1 associated B-cell CLL: indirect role for retrovirus in leukemogenesis. Science 1987;236:1103–1106

342. Rozmin C, Montserrat E: Chronic lymphocytic leukemia. N Engl J Med 1995;333:1052–1057

343. Cheson BD, Bennett JM, Grever M et al.: National Cancer Institute-sponsored working group guidelines for chronic lymphocytic leukemia: revised guidelines for diagnosis and treatment. Blood 1996;87:4990–4997

344. Mangan KF, Chikkappa G, Farley PC: T gamma cells suppress growth of erythroid colony-forming units in vitro in the pure red cell aplasia of B-cell CLL. J Clin Invest 1982;70:1148–1156

345. Brouet JC, Flandrin G, Sasportes M et al: CLL of T cell origin: immunologic and clinical evaluation in 11 patients. Lancet 1975;ii:890–893

346. Carbone A, Santoro A, Pilotti S, Rilke F: Bone marrow patterns and clinical staging in CLL. Lancet 1978;i:606

347. Charron D, Dighiero G, Raphael M, Binet JL: Bone marrow patterns and clinical staging in CLL. Lancet 1977;ii:819

348. Ligler FS, Kettman JR, Smith G, Frenkel EP: Immunoglobin phenotype on B cells correlates with clinical stage CLL. Blood 1983;62:256–263

349. Dohner H, Stilgenbauer S, Benner A et al: Genomic aberrations and survival in chronic lymphocytic leukemia. N Engl J Med 2000;343:1910–1916

350. Lee JS, Dixon DO, Kantarjian HM et al: Prognosis of chronic lymphocytic leukemia: a multivariate regression analysis of 325 untreated patients. Blood 1987;69:929–936

351. Rai KR, Peterson L, Appelbaum FR et al: Fludarabine compared with chlorambucil as primary therapy for chronic lymphocytic leukemia. N Engl J Med 2000;343:1750–1757

352. Osterborg A, Dyer MJ, Bunges D et al: Phase II multicenter study of human CD52 antibody in previously treated chronic lymphocytic leukemia. European study group of CAMPATH-1H treatment in chronic lymphocytic leukemia. J Clin Oncol 1997;15:1567–1574

353. Weeks JC, Tierney MR, Weinstein MC: Cost effectiveness of prophylactic intravenous immune globulin in chronic lymphocytic leukemia. N Engl J Med 1991;325:81–86

354. Cohen HJ: Multiple myeloma in the elderly. Clin Geriatr Med 1985;1.4:827–855

355. Bataille R, Harousseau JL: Multiple myeloma. N Engl J Med 1997;1657–1664

356. Farhangi M (ed): Plasma cell myeloma and myeloma proteins. Semin Oncol 1986;13:1–382

357. Maldonado JE, Kyle RA: Familial myeloma: report of eight families and a study of serum proteins in their relatives. Am J Med 1976;57:875–884

358. McPhedran P, Health CW Jr, Garcia J: Multiple myeloma incidence in metropolitan Atlanta, Georgia: racial and seasonal variations. Blood 1972;39:866–873

359. Bertrams J, Kuwert E, Bohmeu U et al: HLA-antigens in Hodgkin's disease and multiple myeloma. Tissue Antigens 1972;2:41–46

360. Smith G, Wolford RL, Fishkin B et al: HLA phenotypes, immunoglobins and K and L chains in multiple myeloma. Tissue Antigens 1976;4:374–377

361. Ishimaru M, Ishimaru T, Mikamin M, Matsunaga M: Multiple myeloma among atomic bomb survivors, Hiroshima and Nagasaki, 1950–1976. Radiation Effects Research Foundation, Technical Report 9–79. Radiation Effects Research Foundation, Hiroshima, 1976

362. Isobe T, Osserman EF: Pathologic conditions associated with plasma cell dyscrasias: a study of 806 cases. Ann NY Acad Sci 1971;190:507–516

363. Frassanito MA, Cusmai A, Iodice G, Dammacco F: Autocrine interleukin-6 production and highly malignant multiple myeloma: relation with resistance to drug induced apoptosis. Blood 2001;97:483–489

364. Schafer AI, Miller JB: Association of IgA multiple myeloma with a preexisting disease. Br J Haematol 1979;41:19–24

365. Wohlenberg H: Osteomyelitis and plasmacytoma. N Engl J Med 1979;283:822–823

366. Penny R, Hughes S: Repeated stimulation of the reticuloendothelial system and the development of plasma cell dyscrasias. Lancet 1970;i:77–78

367. Rosenblatt J, Hall AC: Plasma-cell dyscrasias following prolonged stimulation of reticuloendothelial system. Lancet 1970;i:301–302

368. Goldenberg GJ, Paraskevas F, Israels LG: The association of rheumatoid arthritis with plasma cell and lymphocytic neoplasms. Arthritis Rheum 1969;12:569–579

369. Wegelius O, Skrifvars B: Rheumatoid arthritis terminating in plasmacytoma. Acta Med Scand 1970;187:133–138

370. Isomaki HA, Hakulmen T, Joustenlahti U: Excess risk of lymphomas, leukemias and myeloma in patients with rheumatoid arthritis. J Chron Dis 1978;31:691–696

371. Schaefer AI, Miller JB, Lester EP et al: Monoclonal gammopathy in heredity spherocytosis: a possible pathogenetic relation. Ann Intern Med 1978;88:45–46

372. Pratt PW, Estern S, Kochwa S: Immunoglobulin abnormalities in Gaucher's disease: report of 16 cases. Blood 1968;31:633–640

373. Wolf P: Monoclonal gammopathy in Gaucher's disease. Lab Med 1973;4:28

374. Turesson I, Rausing A: Gaucher's disease and benign monoclonal gammopathy. Acta Med Scand 1975;197:507–512

375. Macdonald M, McCathie M, Faed MJ: Gaucher's disease with biclonal gammopathy. J Clin Pathol 1975;28:757

376. Gerber MA: Asbestosis and neoplastic disorders of the hematopoietic system. Am J Clin Pathol 1970;53:204–208

377. Kagan E, Jacobson RJ, Yeung KY et al: Asbestos associated neoplasm of B cell lineage. Am J Med 1979;67:325–330

378. Porter DD, Dixon FJ, Larson AE: The development of a myeloma-like condition in mink with Aleutian disease. Blood 1965;25:736–742

379. Chapman I, Jimenez FA: Aleutian mink disease in man. N Engl J Med 1963;269:1171–1174

380. Helmboldt CR, Kenyon AJ, Dessel BH: The comparative aspects of Aleutian disease. In Slow, Latent and Temperate Virus Infections. NINBD Monograph 2. National Institute of Health. Bethesda, MD, 1964:315–319

381. Henry LW: Multiple myeloma in a mink handler following exposure to Aleutian disease. Cancer 1979;44:273–275

382. Klein B: Cytokine, cytokine receptors, transduction signals and oncogenes in human multiple myeloma. Semin Hematol 1995;32:4–19

383. Burger R, Neipel F, Fleckenstein B et al: Human herpesvirus type 8 interleukin-6 homologue is functionally active on human myeloma cells. Blood 1998;91:1858–1863

384. Durie BG, Salmon SE, Mundy GR: Relation of osteoclast activating factor production to extent of bone marrow disease in multiple myeloma. Br J Haematol 1981;47:21–30

385. Kyle RA: Benign monoclonal gammopathy—after 20 to 35 years of follow-up. Mayo Clin Proc 1993;68:26–36

386. Nordic Myeloma Study Group: Interferon-a2b added to melphalan-prednisone for initial and maintenance therapy in multiple myeloma. Ann Intern Med 1996;124:212–222

387. Berenson JR, Lichtenstein A, Porter L et al: Long-term pamidronate treatment of advanced multiple myeloma patients reduces skeletal events. Myeloma Aredia Study Group. J Clin Oncol 1998;16:593–602

388. Singhal S, Mehta J, Desikan R et al: Antitumor activity of thalidomide in refractory multiple myeloma. N Engl J Med 341;1999:1565–1571

389. Malpas JL: The lymphomas. In Denham MG, Chanarin I (eds): Blood Disorders in the Elderly. Churchill Livingstone, London, 1985:264–265

390. Koduru PR, Filippa DA, Richardson ME: Cytogenic and histological correlations in malignant lymphoma. Blood 1987;69:97–102

391. Harris NL, Jaffe ES, Diebold J et al: World Health Organization classification of neoplastic diseases of the hematopoietic and lymphoid tissues: report of the clinical advisory committee meeting, Airlie House, Virginia, November 1997. J Clin Oncol 1999;17:3835–3849

392. MacMahon B: Epidemiology of Hodgkin's disease. Cancer Res 1966;26:1189–1200

393. Jandl J: Non-Hodgkin's lymphoma. In Blood: Textbook of Hematology. Little Brown, Boston, 1964:891–964

394. Baer DM, Anderson ET, Wilkinson LS: Acquired immune deficiency syndrome in homosexual men with Hodgkin's disease: three case reports. Am J Med 1986;80:738–740

395. Ioachim HL, Cooper MC, Hellman GL: Lymphomas in men at high risk for acquired immune deficiency syndrome (AIDS): a study of 21 cases. Cancer 1985;56:2381–2842

396. Levine AM, Gill PS, Meyer PR et al: Retrovirus and malignant lymphomas in homosexual men. JAMA 1985;254:1921–1925

397. Ioachim HL, Cooper MC: Lymphomas of AIDS. Lancet 1986;i:96

398. Groopman JE, Sullivan JL, Mulder C et al: Pathogenesis of B cell lymphoma in a patient with AIDS. Blood 1986;67:612–625

399. Wotherspoon AC, Doglioni C, Diss TC et al: Regression of primary low grade B-cell gastric lymphoma of mucosa-associated lymphoid tissue type after eradication of *Helicobacter pylori*. Lancet 1993;342:575–577

400. Cavelli F: Recent advances in the management of lymphoma. Eur J Cancer 1995;31A:841–844

401. Mrozek K, Bloomfield CD: Cytogenetics of indolent lymphomas. Semin Oncol 1993;20(suppl 5):47–57

402. Lokich JJ, Pinkus CG, Moloney WC: Hodgkin's disease in the elderly. Oncology 1974;29:484–500

403. Eghbali H, Hoerni-Simon G, deMascarel I et al: Hodgkin's disease in the elderly: a series of 30 patients older than 70 years. Cancer 1984;53:2191–2193

404. Lichtman SM: Lymphoma in the older patient. Semin Oncol 1995;22(suppl 1):25–28

405. Boivin JF, Hutchinson GB: Second cancers after treatment for Hodgkin's disease: a review. In Boice JD, Fraumene JF Jr (eds): Radiation Carcinogens: Epidemiology and Biological Significance. Raven Press, New York, 1984

406. Rosenberg SA: The treatment of Hodgkin's disease. Ann Oncol 1994;5(suppl 2):17–21

407. Portlock CS: Management of the indolent non-Hodgkin's lymphomas. Semin Oncol 1980;3:292–301

408. Davis TA, Grillo-Lopez AJ, White CA et al: Rituximab anti-CD20 monoclonal antibody therapy in Non-Hodgkin's lymphoma: Safety and efficacy of retreatment. J Clin Oncol 2000;18:3135–3143

409. Saleh MN, Le Maistre CF, Kuzel TM et al: Antitumor activity of DAB389IL-2 fusion toxin in mycosis fungoides. J Am Acad Dermatol 1998;39:63–73

410. Abromowicz M (ed): Bexatotene (Targretin™) for cutaneous T cell lymphoma. Med Lett Drug Ther 2000;42:31–32

411. Dimopoulos MA, Panayiotis P, Maulopoulos LA, Sfikakis P, Dalakas M: Waldenstrom's macroglobulinemia: clinical features, complications and management. J Clin Oncol 2000;18:214–226

412. Westbrook CA, Groopman JE, Golde DW: Hairy cell leukemias: disease pattern and prognosis. Cancer 1984;59:500–506

413. Dearden CE, Matutes E, Hilditch BL, Swansbury GJ, Catovsky D: Long-term follow-up of patients with hairy cell leukemia after treatment with pentostatin or cladribine. Br J Haematol 1999;106:515–519

414. Weiss LM, Strickler JG, Dorfman RF et al: Clonal T-cell populations in angioimmunoblastic lymphadenopathy and angioimmunoblastic lymphadenopathy-like lymphoma. Am J Pathol 1986;122:392–397

415. Freter CE, Cossman J: Angioimmunoblastic lymphadenopathy with dysproteinemia. Semin Oncol 1993;20:627–635

416. Sabah S, Wehbie R, Lepera P, Sallah W, Bobzien W: The role of 2-chlorodeoxyadenosine in the treatment of patients with refractory angioimmunoblastic lymphadenopathy with dysproteinemia. Br J Haematol 1999;104:163–165

417. Gilbert HS: Myeloproliferative disorders. Clin Geriatr Med 1985;1:773–793

418. Middleton AM: Polycythemia and myelofibrosis. In Denham MJ, Chanarin I (eds): Blood Disorders in the Elderly. Churchill Livingstone, London, 1985:234–244

419. Gilbert HS: Myelofibrosis revisited: characterization and classification of myelofibrosis in the setting of myeloproliferative disease. In Berk PD, Castro-Malaspina H, Wasserman LR (eds): Myelofibrosis and the Biology of Connective Tissue. Alan R Liss, New York, 1984:3–18

420. Champlen RE, Golde DW: Chronic myelogenous leukemia: recent advances. Blood 1985;65:1039–1047

421. Sokol JE, Baccarani M, Russo D, Tura S: Staging and prognosis in chronic myelogenous leukemia. Semin Hematol 1988;25:49–61

422. Cannistraa SA: Chronic myelogenous leukemia as a model for the genetic basis of cancer. Hematol Oncol Clin North Am 1990;4:337–357

423. Gruppo Italiano Studio Policitemia: Polycythemia vera: the natural history of 1213 patients followed for 20 years. Ann Intern Med 1995;123:656–664

424. Bilgrami S, Greenberg BR: Polycythemia rubra vera. Semin Oncol 1995;22:307–326

425. Tefferi A, Silverstein MN, Noel P: Agnogenic myeloid metaplasia. Semin Oncol 1995;22:327–333

426. Berk PD, Goldberg JD, Donovan PD et al: Therapeutic recommendations in polycythemia vera based on Polycythemia Vera Study Group protocols. Semin Hematol 1986;23:132–143

427. Mitus AJ, Schafer AI: Thrombocytosis and thrombocythemia. Hematol Oncol Clin North Am 1990;4:157–178

428. Tefferi A, Silverstein MN, Hoagland CH: Primary thrombocythemia. Semin Oncol 1995;22:334–340

429. Giralt S, Kantarjian H, Talpazn M: Treatment of chronic myelogenous leukemia. Semin Oncol 1995;22:396–404

430. Druker BJ, Talpaz M, Resta DJ et al: Efficacy and safety of a specific inhibitor of the BCR-ABL tyrosine kinase in chronic myeloid leukemia. N Engl J Med 2001;344:1031–1037

431. Druker BJ, Sawyers CL, Kantarjian H et al: Activity of a specific inhibitor of the BCR-ABL tyrosine kinase in the blast crisis of chronic myeloid leukemia and acute lymphoblastic leukemia with the Philadelphia chromosome. N Engl J Med 2001;344:1038–1042

432. Griffin JD: Myelodysplasias. Clin Hematol 1986;15:909–1111

433. Greenberg P, Cox C, LeBeau MM et al: International scoring system for evaluating prognosis in myelodysplastic syndromes. Blood 1997;89:2079–2088 (erratum in Blood 1998;91:1100)

434. Brandt L: Environmental factors and leukemia. Med Oncol Tumor Pharmacother 1985;2:7–10

435. Zarrabi MH, Rosner F: Second neoplasms in Hodgkin's disease: current controversies. Hematol Oncol Clin North Am 1989;3:303–318

436. Jacobs A, Clark RE: Pathogenesis and clinical variations in the myelodysplastic syndromes. Clin Hematol 1986;15:925–951

437. Freedman ML: Hemoglobin synthesis in normal and abnormal states. In Gordon AS, Silber R, LoBue J (eds): The Year in Hematology 1977. Plenum, New York, 1977:47–101

438. Bunn HF: 5Q and disordered hematopoiesis. Clin Hematol 1986;15:1023–1035

439. Greenberg PL: Myelodysplastic syndrome. In Hoffman R, Benz E, Shattil S et al (eds): Hematology: Principles and Practice, 2nd Ed. Churchill Livingstone, New York, 1995;1098–1142

440. Saba HI: Myelodysplastic syndromes in the elderly. Cancer Control JMCC 2001;8:79–102

441. Estey EH: Treatment of acute myelogenous leukemia and myelodysplastic syndromes. Semin Hematol 1995;32:132–151

442. Hellstrom-Lindberg E: Efficacy of erythropoietin in the myelodysplastic syndromes: a meta-analysis of 205 patients from 17 studies. Br J Haematol 1994;89:67–71

443. Shuster S, Scarborough H: Senile pupura. QJ Med 1961;30:33–41

444. Shuster S, Black MM, McVitie E: The influence of age and sex on skin thickness, skin collagen, and density. Br J Dermatol 1975;93:639–643

445. Fritsch WC: Managing age-related vascular skin lesions. Geriatrics 1975;30:45–48

446. Grosset ABM, Rodgers GM: Acquired coagulation disorders. In Wintrobe's Clinical Hematology. Lippincott, Williams & Wilkins, 1999:1733–1780

447. Karpatkin S: Autoimmune thrombocytopenia purpura. Semin Hematol 1985;22:260–280

448. Bussel JB: Autoimmune thrombocytopenia purpura. Hematol Oncol Clin North Am 1990;4:179–191

449. Rutherford CJ, Frenkel EP: Thrombocytopenia issues in diagnosis and therapy. Med Clin North Am 1994;78:555–574

450. Joist JH, George JN, Francis CW et al: Acquired Hemorrhagic Disorders. In Hemostasis and Thrombosis. Lippincott, Williams & Wilkins, 2001;955–1070

451. Machin SJ: Bleeding and coagulation disorders. In Denham MJ, Chanarin I (eds): Blood Disorders in the Elderly. Churchill Livingstone, London 1985:132–156

452. Warkentin TE, Kelton JG: Temporal aspects of hepain induced thrombocytopenia. N Engl J Med 2001;344:1286–1292

453. Shick BP: Hope for treatment of thrombocytopenia. N Engl J Med 1994;331:875–876

454. Cines DB, Konkle BA, Furlan M: Thrombotic thrombocytopenia purpura: a paradigm shift? Thromb Hemost 2000;84:528–535

455. Webster MWI, Chesboro JH, Foster V: Platelet inhibitor therapy. Hematol Oncol Clin North Am 1990;4:265–289

456. Smith T, Viverette F, Adelman B: The use of antithrombotic therapy in the elderly. Clin Geriatr Med 1985;1:887–897

457. Stemerman MB: Coagulation in the elderly. Clin Geriatr Med 1985;1:869–885

458. Schleider MA, Nachman RL, Jaffe EA, Coleman M: A clinical study of the lupus anticoagulant. Blood 1976;48:499–509

459. Shapiro SS, Thiagarjian P: Lupus anticoagulants. Prog Hemost Thromb 1982;6:263–285

460. Chan TIC, Chan V: Antithrombin III, the major modulator of intravascular coagulation, is synthesized by human endothelial cells. Thromb Haemost 1981;46:504–506

461. Wunderwald P, Schrenk WJ, Port H: Antithrombin from human plasma: an antithrombin binding moderately to heparin. Thromb Res 1986;25:177–191

462. Furie B, Furie BC: The molecular basis of blood coagulation. Cell 1988;53:505–518

463. Clouse LH, Comp PC: The regulation of hemostasis: the protein C system. N Engl J Med 1986;314:1298–1304

464. Dahlback B: Inherited thrombophilia: resistance to activated protein C as a pathogenic factor of venous thromboembolism. Blood 1995;85:607–614

465. Mandel H, Brenner B, Berant M et al: Coexistence of hereditary homocysteinuria and factor Vleiden effect on thrombosis. N Engl J Med 1996;334:763–768

466. Seligsohn U, Lubetsky A: Genetic susceptibility to venous thrombosis. N Engl J Med 2001;344:1222–1231

467. Kaplan AP: Initiation of the intrinsic coagulation and fibrinolytic pathway of man. Prog Hemost Thromb 1978;4:127–175

468. Seligsohn U: Disseminated intravascular coagulation. In Hardin RI, Lux SE, Stossel TP (eds): Blood: Principles and Practice of Hematology. JB Lippincott, Philadelphia 1995:1289–1317

469. Golde DW (ed): Hematopoietic growth factors. Hematol Oncol Clin North Am 1989;3:369–554

470. Reynolds CH: Clinical efficacy of rhIL-11. Oncology 2000;14(9 suppl 8):32–40

471. Kirkwood J, Mier J, Atkins M et al: Pharmacology of cancer biotherapeutics. In DeVita VT, Hellman S, Rosenberg SA (eds): Cancer Principles and Practice of Oncology, 6th Ed. JB Lippincott, Williams & Wilkins, Philadelphia, 2001:461–548

472. van der velden VHJ, te Marvelde JG, Hoogeveen PG et al: Targeting of the CD33-calicheamycin immunoconjugate myelotarg® (CMA-676) in acute myeloid leukemia: in vivo and in vitro saturation and internalization by leukemic and normal myeloid cells. Blood 2000;96(11):481a

473. de Vetten MP, Jansen JH, van der Reijden BA et al: Molecular remission of Philadelphia/bcr-abl-positive acute myeloid leukaemia after treatment with anti-CD33 calicheamicin conjugate (gemtuzumab ozogamicin, CMA-676). Br J Haematol 2000;111:277–279

474. Kaminski MS, Estes J, Zasadny KR et al: Radioimmunotherapy with iodine (131)I tositumomab for relapsed or refractory B-cell non-Hodgkin lymphoma: updated results and long-term follow-up of the University of Michigan experience. Blood 2000;96:1259–1266

475. Joensuu H, Roberts PJ, Sarlomo-Rikala M et al: Brief report: Effect of the tyrosine kinase inhibitor STI571 in a patient with metastatic gastrointestinal stromal tumors. N Engl J Med 2001;344:1052–1056

476. Lefor A, Libutti S, Horne M III et al: Specialized Techniques in Cancer Management. In DeVita VT, Hellman S, Rosenberg SA (eds): Cancer Principles and Practice of Oncology, 6th Ed. JB Lippincott, Williams & Wilkins, Philadelphia, 2001:739–788

477. Hammerman S: Toward an understanding of frailty. Ann Intern Med 1999;130:945–950

478. Mertelsmann FS: Supportive care in hematologic malignancies: hematopoietic growth factors, infections, transfusion therapy. Curr Opin Hematol 2000;7:255–260 (review)

479. Ozer H. Armitage JO, Bennett CL et al: 2000 update of recommendations for the use of hematopoietic colony stimulating factors: evidence-based, clinical practice guidelines. J Clin Oncol 2000;18:3558–3585

480. Gralla RJ, Osoba D, Kris M et al: Recommendations for the use of antiemetics: evidence-based, clinical practice guidelines. J Clin Oncol 1999;17:2971–2994

481. Hensley ML, Schuchter LM, Lindley C et al: American Society of Clinical Oncology clinical practice guidelines for the use of chemotherapy and radiotherapy protectants, J Clin Oncol 1999;17:3333–3355

482. Awada A, Piccart M: Strategies offering protection from the toxic effects of anticancer treatments with a focus on chemoprotective agents. Curr Opin Oncol 2000;80:289–296

483. Links M, Lewis C: Chemoprotectants: a review of their clinical pharmacology and therapeutic efficacy. Drugs 1999;57:293–308

484. Hospers GA, Eisenhauer EA, de Vries EG: The sulfhydryl containing compounds WR-2721 and glutathione as radio- and chemoprotective agents. A review, indications for use and prospects. Br J Cancer 1999;80:629–638

485. Siu LL, Moore MJ: Use of mesna to prevent ifosfamide-induced urotoxicity. Support Care Cancer 1998;6:144–154

486. Boyle FM, Wheeler HR, Shenfield GM: Amelioration of experimental cisplatin and paclitaxel neuropathy with glutamate. J Neuro-Oncol 1999;41:107–116

487. Speyer J, Wasserheit C: Strategies for reduction of anthracycline cardiac toxicity. Semin Oncol 1998;25:525–537

Chapter 99

Aging of the skin

Rebecca C. C. Brooke and Christopher E. M. Griffiths

The cutaneous changes that occur with increasing age are universal and for the most part universally unwelcome. The immediate, and perhaps most telling, evidence of an individual's age is the appearance of their skin, hair, and nails. After all, the most that the outside world sees of us are our faces and hands, and as both of these are sun-exposed sites, this introduces a superimposed complexity almost unique to skin aging, namely the role of environmental factors, particularly sun exposure. It is only in the past 20 years that researchers have become aware of the distinction between intrinsic, chronological aging of the skin—which exists in its purest form in non-sun-exposed (photoprotected) body sites such as the buttocks—and extrinsic aging due to habitual sun exposure, most evident on face and hands. Extrinsic aging is never a pure phenomenon as it is inevitably superimposed on some degree of chronological aging—thus the term photoaging. However, as is elucidated in this chapter, the changes that sunlight wreaks upon the skin are more pronounced than those produced by longevity alone. Extrinsic aging seems to be influenced by outside elements, for example, wind, chemicals, cigarette smoke, and heat, of which by far the most influential is exposure to ultraviolet radiation. It is this inability to distinguish extrinsic from intrinsic skin aging that has eventuated in erroneous beliefs regarding wrinkles and age or liver spots: these clinical features, so often synonymous with old age, are merely the consequence of cumulative sun exposure. Proof of this is the paucity of wrinkling in black skin (markedly sun-protected by virtue of melanin) unless greatly sun-exposed. This confusion has led to the use of terms such as premature or accelerated aging to describe cutaneous changes resulting from chronic sun exposure. This chapter serves to help distinguish between intrinsic and extrinsic aging and photoaging (Table 99-1), and illustrates how relatively little is known about the processes that underlie intrinsic skin aging.

An anatomical approach to the epidermis and dermis and the cell types contained therein has been adopted and the clinical and histological features of intrinsic and photoaged skin compared and contrasted. The psychological effects of skin senescence probably outweigh the physiological and on these grounds alone there is an increasing need for prevention and/or treatment. On this basis, the chapter closes with a brief discussion of the nonsurgical approaches under investigation for treatment of aged skin.

EPIDERMIS

The epidermis is composed of a nonviable stratum corneum composed of enucleated squames and keratin and a viable cellular layer comprising keratinocytes, Langerhans cells, and melanocytes.

Stratum corneum

The stratum corneum supplies a barrier function to skin and it appears that this integral role is not appreciably affected by age.[1] Stratum corneal thickness is unchanged in elderly people[2] although its moisture content and cohesiveness are reduced, coupled with an increase in renewal time of damaged stratum corneum.[3] These changes are manifest clinically as dry, rough skin—so often the bane of elderly people—and enhanced susceptibility to irritants with consequent pruritus. Self-evidently such xerosis-induced pruritus is best treated with emollients as opposed to antihistamines and sedatives.

Keratinocytes

Epidermal thickness decreases slightly[4] with age—in men this is a gradual process beginning between 20 and 30 years old;[5] in women a reduction in epidermal thickness is apparent only after the menopause.[5] There is some evidence that estrogen replacement can slow or prevent this age-related epidermal atrophy in women. Photoaged epidermis is initially thickened but eventually atrophies.[6] Human epidermis is highly proliferative but in a steady-state condition dependent, as are other self-renewing structures, on slowly cycling, undifferentiated stem cells.[7] These stem cells are located within the basal compartment of the epidermis—the nonserrated keratinocytes at the tips of the epidermal rete ridges.[8] Loss of rete ridges and consequent flattening of the dermal–epidermal junction is a hallmark of intrinsically aged skin.[9] Such flattening results in a reduction in mean surface area of the dermal–epidermal junction. One study has estimated a reduction in mean area of dermal–epidermal junction/mm² from 2.6 at age 21–40 years to 1.9 at age 61–80 years.[10] These changes are accompanied by a reduction in microvilli[11]—cytoplasmic projections from basal keratinocytes into the dermis. There are also ultrastructural alterations in the dermal–epidermal junction that occur with

Table 99-1 Clinical features of intrinsic and extrinsic aging

Change with time	Intrinsic or chronological aging	Extrinsic or photoaging
Fine wrinkles	Yes	Yes
Skin laxity	Yes	Yes
Skin thinning	Yes	No
Xerosis (dryness)	Yes	Minimal
Coarse wrinkles	Minimal	Yes
Solar lentigines (age or liver spots)	No	Yes
Mottled dyspigmentation	No	Yes
Actinic keratoses	No	Yes

age. These include decreased reaction of hemidesmosomes from aged cells with β_4 integrin, a subunit essential for basal keratinocyte anchorage,[12] and a reduction in collagen IV, which is the main component of anchoring plaques.[12] In contrast, collagen VII containing anchoring fibrils are not known to vary with age but are reduced in photoaged skin.[13] Altogether, these alterations serve to reduce both the surface area of the dermal–epidermal junction and the anchoring of basal keratinocytes, possibly resulting in the susceptibility to shearing forces observed in elderly skin as evidenced by the ease of raising suction blisters on aged as opposed to young skin.[1] Photoaged skin has even greater fragility mainly because structures tethering epidermis to dermis, namely collagen-VII-containing anchoring fibrils[13] and fibrillin fibers[14] are greatly reduced in number in sun-exposed sites. The rate of epidermal renewal is reduced in the skin of individuals aged 60 years or greater.[15] Aging as a single factor reduces the ability of keratinocytes to proliferate in vitro.[16] This observation is in keeping with the Hayflick hypothesis of reduced numbers of cellular doublings with longevity.[17] Gilchrest has shown that the interleukin-1 receptor antagonist gene is increased in aged but decreased in photoaged epidermal keratinocytes.[18] Furthermore, levels of interleukin-1 in keratinocytes are not affected by intrinsic aging.[18] The ability of epidermal growth factor (EGF) to bind to its receptor is compromised in intrinsically aged skin and subsequently this may impair epidermal keratinocyte proliferation.

There is little difference in keratinocyte differentiation between photoaged, aged, and young epidermis, although there is marked heterogeneity of keratinocyte size and shape in intrinsically aged skin.[19] Melanin is uniformly distributed within aged keratinocytes but shows characteristic irregular clumping in photoaged epidermal keratinocytes.

Melanocytes

Melanocytes are decreased in number in intrinsically aged epidermis, although the estimates of this decrease vary from study to study according to the methodologies used to quantitate melanocyte numbers. This said, the reduction is in the order of 8–20 percent per decade compared to young adult skin.[20,21] By marked contrast, in chronically, sun-exposed, photoaged skin there is an increase in number of melanocytes.[21] In addition to a reduction in melanocyte number there is loss of melanocyte function eventuating in reduced tanning ability of intrinsically aged skin in response to ultraviolet radiation. The serious sequel to loss of melanocyte number and function in elderly skin is loss of photoprotection leading to an increased risk of skin cancer. Age or "liver" spots are more correctly known as actinic lentigines. These lesions are observed only on chronically sun-exposed sites, most particularly the dorsa of the hands. Their popular names, which include "autumn leaves" and "coffin spots" connote impending senility; however, they are commoner in the elderly only because cumulative sun exposure is necessarily greater in this group. Histologically, actinic lentigines are characterized by clusters of large, dendritic melanocytes within the basal layer of epidermis.

Langerhans' cells

The skin is the furthest outpost of the body's immune system, and is the largest immunologically active organ. Epidermal Langerhans' cells are bone marrow-derived and function as antigen-presenting cells integrally involved in immune surveillance. The number of Langerhans' cells is reduced in intrinsically aged epidermis[22]—a decrease that is compounded in photoaging.[23] Gilchrest demonstrated that subjects aged 62–86 years had a 42 percent reduction in number of Langerhans' cells in sun-protected, i.e., intrinsically aged skin as compared to young subjects aged 22–26 years.[22] A reduction in Langerhans' cell number equates to a loss of immune surveillance and a consequent increased risk of skin cancer; this may also explain the difficulty in sensitizing aged skin to contact allergens, e.g., 2,4-dinitrochlorobenzene[24] and the age-dependent decrease in the incidence of allergic contact dermatitis.[25]

DERMIS

Human dermis is divided into two components—a superficial, immediately subepidermal papillary dermis and the deeper reticular dermis. Although in comparison to epidermis the dermis is relatively hypocellular and has a longer cell turnover time, the changes wrought on it by chronological and photoaging are far more evident. Indeed it is dermal change that is responsible for some of the more characteristic features of cumulative sun exposure—namely wrinkles and elastosis (Fig. 99-1; see also Plate 99-1). Dermal changes also provide the most striking differences between the effects of chronological aging and photoaging—namely atrophy and hypertrophy respectively (Table 99.2). Sex differences are also apparent within the dermis in that it is generally thicker in males than in females—especially post-menopause.[1] The principal cells within the dermis are fibroblasts, although endothelial cells and mast cells are also affected by aging.

Fibroblasts

Numbers of dermal fibroblasts decrease with age associated with a reduction in fibroblast size and impaired capacity to produce extracellular matrix components—namely collagen, elastin, and glycosaminoglycans.[26] Collagen I is the predominant constituent of extracellular matrix, and collagen in total accounts for 70 percent dry weight of dermal tissue. Collagen provides skin with its tensile strength and structural integrity. Thus any loss in collagen imbues skin with a susceptibility to shearing force trauma. Age-related reduction in collagen is a subtle process, difficult to ascertain, whereas photoaging produces marked loss in collagen. Loss of collagen due to photoaging is a bipartite process resulting from decreased synthesis[27] coupled with increased breakdown by matrix metalloproteinases such as stromelysin and collagenase.[28] There is early evidence that intrinsically aged and photoaged skin share some molecular and biochemical features, especially in those over the age of 70 years.[29] In this age range non-sun-exposed skin also shows an increase in matrix metalloproteinases with concomitant reduction in collagens I and III.[29] Oxidative damage plays an important part in cellular aging, this process being mediated partly by mitogen-activated protein (MAP) kinases. In old skin (>70 years) extracellular-signal-regulated MAP-kinase activity is reduced, whereas stress-activated MAP-kinase activity is increased.[30] Ultraviolet irradiation of skin results in sustained elevation of matrix metalloproteinases[31] which

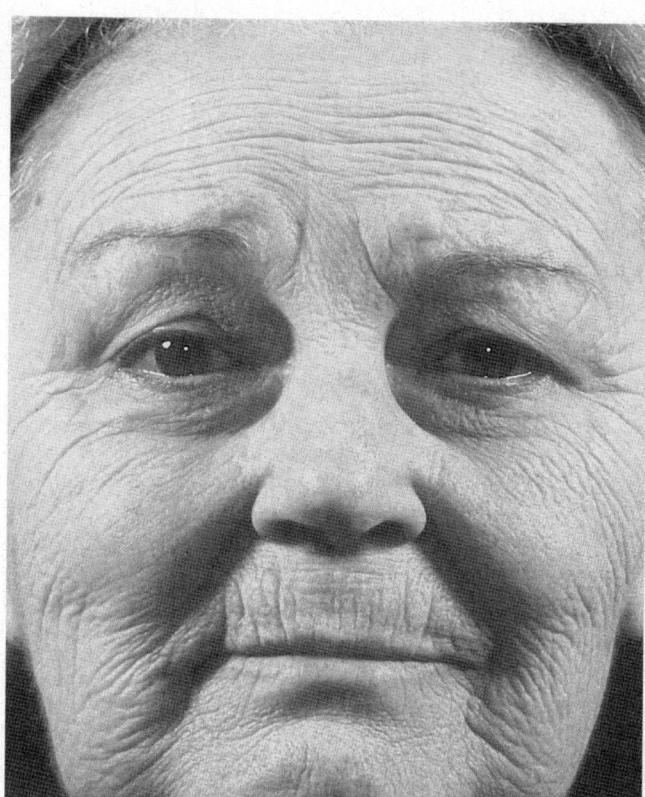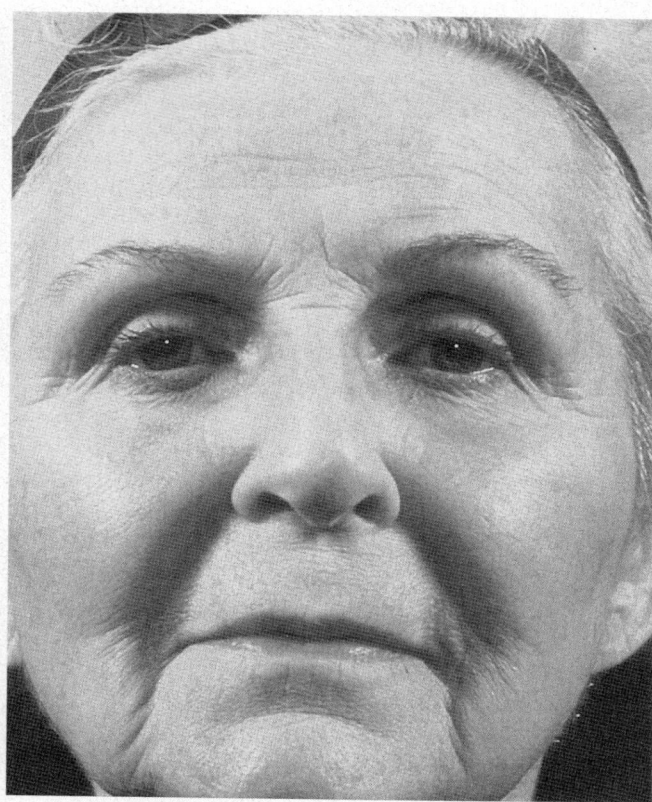

Figure 99-1 Faces of two 71-year-old women. The woman on the right has avoided sun exposure over most of her life and the changes are mostly those of intrinsic, chronological aging. The woman on the left has suffered a great deal of sun exposure and the wrinkles and thickened skin are evidence of photoaging. To the untrained observer the woman on the left appears older than her stated age.

break down collagen and may contribute to photoaging. In photoaged skin the papillary dermis is almost devoid of collagen synthesis,[32] and collagen-VII-containing anchoring fibrils, which tether epidermis to dermis, are significantly reduced in number.[13] Wound healing is impaired in intrinsically aged as compared to young skin in that rate of healing is appreciably slower, but paradoxically the resultant scar is usually more cosmetically acceptable. Loss of papillary dermal collagen and related structures most likely account for wrinkling due to photoaging. Sunlight is not the only extrinsic factor that causes skin wrinkling. Several studies[33,34] have confirmed that smoking is an independent causative factor of facial wrinkles, possibly as a result of metalloproteinase activation.[35]

There are many dermal glycosaminoglycans and proteoglycans (macromolecular conjugates of protein and carbohydrate), of which dermatan sulfate and hyaluronic acid diminish with age, as does versican[36] (large chondroitin sulfate proteoglycans) which may contribute to loss of dermal thickness and skin suppleness. This contrasts with decorin (small dermatan sulfate proteoglycans) which is increased.[36] In addition, another proteoglycan, smaller than decorin has been found in abundance in mature skin.[36] This has the same terminal amino-acid sequence and may be a catabolic fragment of decorin itself, which is known to influence collagen fibrillogenesis and fibril diameter, hence it may influence skin elasticity. By comparison, photoaging greatly increases the dermal content of glycosaminoglycans[37] and versican;[38] however, decorin is decreased.[38] The full range and influence of these

macromolecules is still being elucidated and their role in the aging process is not fully understood. Their importance perhaps lies in where they are deposited, for example decorin is associated with dermal collagen fibers,[39] whereas versican is found in the basal layer of the epidermis, around dermal elastic fibers and in hair follicle sheaths and sweat glands.[40]

One of the features of early, evolving photoaging is the presence of a periadnexal inflammatory infiltrate, consisting of macrophages and neutrophils.[41] It is postulated that enzymes and/or cytokines produced by this inflammatory infiltrate are responsible for the gross disruption of extracellular matrix observed in photoaged skin. No inflammation is seen in normal, intrinsically aged skin.

Fibroblasts also produce elastin—a protein that provides skin with its elasticity. The elastin content of intrinsically aged and photoaged skin is very different (Table 99-2 and Fig. 99-2; see also Plate 99-2). Intrinsically aged skin displays a reduction in elastic tissue. Elastin fibers deeper in the reticular dermis are disorganized, frayed, and contain cystic spaces.[11,42] These changes are most probably a combination of reduced synthesis and/or elastolysis. Photoaging markedly increases elastotic material within the dermis, so much so that the relatively subtle changes produced by intrinsic aging are overshadowed. Clumps of truncated, disorganized elastotic material are observed throughout the reticular dermis of photoaged skin. Chronic sun exposure has a hypertrophic effect on elastin, whereas fibrillin microfibrils, which provide the scaffolding on which elastin fibers are laid down, are markedly reduced

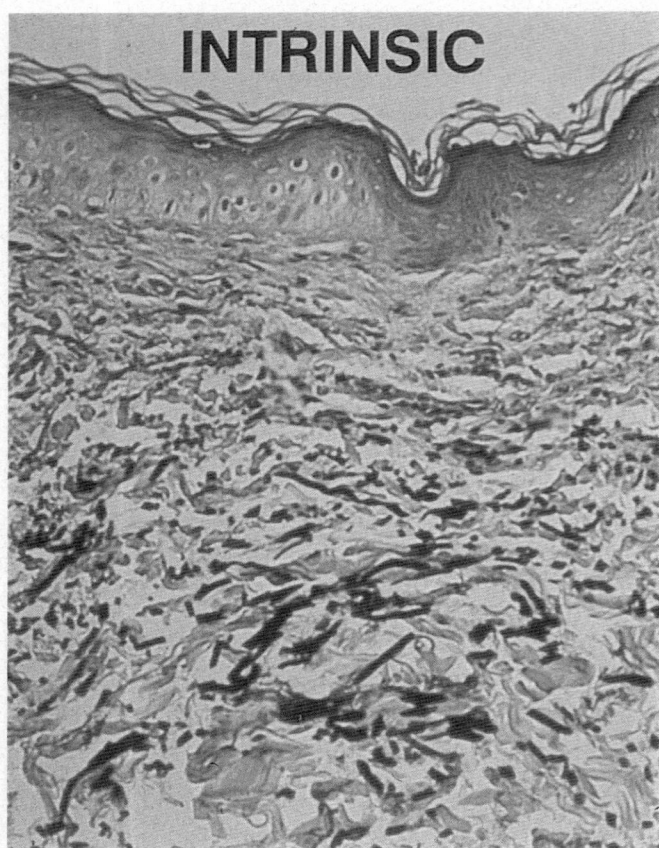
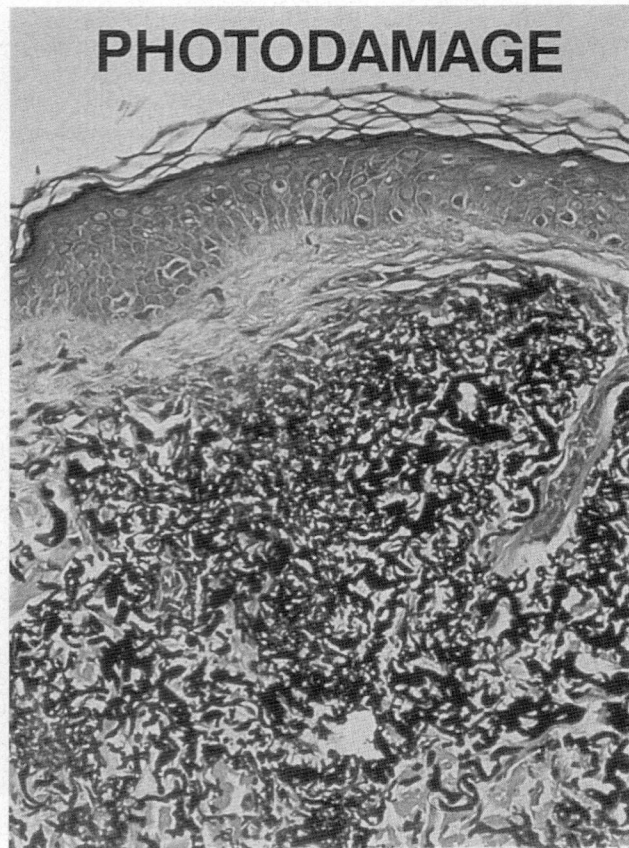

Figure 99-2 Photomicrographs of histological sections of intrinsic and extrinsically aged skin stained with Verhoeff van Giesen stain for elastin. The salient difference is the gross increase in black-staining, elastotic material in the reticular dermis of extrinsic, photoaged skin (×40).

Table 99-2 Intrinsic aging compared to extrinsic photoaging; structural protein changes within the extracellular matrix of the dermis

	Intrinsic aging	Extrinsic photoaging
Fibrillin	↓	↓↓
Elastin	↓	↑↑
Collagen I	↓	↓↓
Collagen III	↓	↓↓
Collagen IV	↓	Not known
Collagen VII	Not known	↓
Versican	↓	↑
Decorin	↑	↓
Hyaluronic acid	↓	↑

↑: increased.
↓: decreased.

in number in the papillary dermis of photoaged skin.[43] Indeed, fibrillin loss is an early and sensitive marker of photoaging. The mechanisms underlying this change are not fully understood. The elastotic material manifests clinically as yellow, pebbled, elastosis most easily observed on the temples of chronically sun-exposed individuals.

Endothelium

Aged skin is relatively hypovascular—particularly due to loss of small capillaries that run perpendicular to the dermal epidermal junction and form capillary loops.[44] This loss is concomitant with the loss of epidermal rete ridges.[45,46] Blood vessels within the reticular dermis are reduced in number and their walls are thinned. The consequent compromised blood flow is manifest physiologically as pale skin and an impaired capacity to thermoregulate[1,47]—possibly a contributing factor in the increased susceptibility of elderly individuals to hypo- and hyperthermia.

Likewise, photoaged skin is depleted of blood vessels but those remaining are tortuous, dilated, and telangiectatic[1,6,46]—resulting in venous lakes seen on the faces of photoaged individuals. The vessel walls are often thickened and rigid and this, coupled with loss of the buffer effect of perivascular collagen in sun damage, makes such blood vessels more susceptible to trauma, resulting in Bateman's or senile purpura at sun-exposed sites, particularly the extensor forearm—a feature exacerbated by systemic or topical glucocorticosteroids.

Mast cells

There is an approximate 50 percent reduction in numbers of mast cells in intrinsically aged skin.[48] Such a reduction may explain the relative rarity of urticaria in the elderly population.

APPENDAGES

Sweat glands

Eccrine glands are reduced in number and function in aged skin.[1,19] Impairment of sweating, as with loss of micro-circulation, disadvantages the thermoregulatory capacity of chronologically aged skin. Eccrine gland response to thermal and chemical (acetylcholine) stimuli is impaired. Apocrine gland activity is diminished, probably as a consequence of declining testosterone levels, leading to a reduction in both pheromone secretion and consequent body odor.[49] Both apocrine[19] and eccrine glands[50] in aged skin contain deposits of lipofuscin.

Sebaceous glands

Age does not alter the number of sebaceous glands, although they become hyperplastic and larger:[51] mean sebaceous gland size increases from 0.22 mm² in young adults to 0.4 mm² in elderly people. Although aged sebaceous glands are increased in size, they produce 50 percent less sebum than their younger counterparts.[52] The constituency of aged sebum is altered in that it contains less free cholesterol but more squalene.[53] Sebaceous gland hyperplasia may present clinically as giant comedones. Such hyperplasia is greatly exaggerated in photoaging, especially on the face. Some investigators believe that the reduction in sebum production that occurs with age, and contributes to xerosis of aged skin, is a reflection of reduced testosterone,[54] although this does not explain the hyperplasia.

Nerves

Skin is richly supplied by sensory receptors and free nerve endings which may permeate the epidermis and interact with Langerhans' cells.[55] Age probably reduces and disorganizes the nerve supply of skin; indeed there is an approximate two-thirds reduction in numbers of Pacinian and Meissner's corpuscles with age.[56] Partly as a consequence of these anatomical changes there is an increased threshold to pain in aged skin.[57]

Hair

A highly visible sign of age is the gradual loss of hair color to gray and in some individuals to white, this universal process begins around the temples and progresses.[58] Graying of the hair—canities—is due to a decreased number of active melanocytes in the hair follicle with associated decreased activity of remaining melanocytes. Purely white hair has an absence of α-melanocyte-stimulating hormone binding sites.[59]

Hair, particularly on the scalp, is lost with age in both sexes[60] and is associated with transition of terminal to vellus hairs. An Australian study reported that gray hair was found in only 22 percent of men aged 25–34 years as opposed to 95 percent of men over the age of 55 years.[1] Patterned, androgenetic alopecia is a genetically predetermined condition arising from increased sensitivity of hair follicles to the effects of dihydrotestosterone produced by breakdown of free testosterone by the enzyme 5α reductase. In some studies the prevalence of significant scalp hair loss approaches 70 percent in men over the age of 50 years.[61] The rate of hair growth decreases with age. Hair is not uniformly lost over the body as paradoxically men have an associated increase in hair growth in the nostrils, eyebrows and on the ears and elderly women often display conversion of vellus to terminal hairs on the chin and moustache areas.

Nails

Nails grow more slowly in elderly people and are characterized by brittleness and longitudinal, beaded ridging—so-called "sausage links." Nail-plate lipid composition varies with age at both extremes of life, apparently being influenced by sex-hormone status. After 60 years of age these changes seem to level out such that the proportion represented by more polar lipids (e.g. cholesterol sulfate) increase, while the amount of lipophilic sterols and free fatty acids declines,[62] possibly contributing to the characteristic brittleness of nails in elderly people.

PSYCHOLOGICAL EFFECTS

Although nobody has died as a result of cutaneous senescence (skin does not totally fail with age) the detrimental consequences of cutaneous aging, whether it be intrinsic or extrinsic, are not merely physiological. Skin represents our appearance to others and wrinkled, blemished, sagging skin is often as undesirable to elderly people as to the young. In modern day, youth-driven society the search for preservation of a youthful appearance has never been so important. Attractiveness induces feelings of self-worth and is strongly related to how favorably others perceive us. Furthermore, there is evidence that physically attractive individuals may live longer.[63] Men who looked "young for their age" lived longer than those who appeared older than their stated age.[63]

TREATMENT

Most of the cutaneous features erroneously ascribed to aging are merely a result of chronic sun exposure. One strategy, although very long term, is to prevent the ravages of excess sun exposure by educating young people about the dangers of ultraviolet irradiation and encouraging them to practice sun avoidance and use of sunblocks. It is estimated that 50 percent of sun exposure occurs before the age of 20 years—thus if you want to look good when you are a grandparent begin while your grandparents are still alive!

The "fountain of youth" is a mythical prize but nowadays may be more attainable than Ponce de Leon ever thought possible. Nonsurgical manipulation of aged and photoaged skin is feasible. In this regard, attention has been focused on the steroid hormone receptor superfamily[64] that contains the nuclear receptors for: retinoic acid; vitamin D; thyroid hormone; and glucocorticoids among others.[65] Topical retinoids—particularly all-*trans* retinoic acid, a metabolite of vitamin A—may improve clinical features of photoaged[65,66] and possibly intrinsically aged skin.[67,68] Retinoic acid effaces wrinkles by inducing synthesis of collagen I within the papillary dermis[32] both directly by stimulating fibroblasts[69] and indirectly by inducing transforming growth factor-β[70] which in turn stimulates fibroblast production of collagen. Topical retinoid use also increases anchoring fibril numbers at the dermal–epidermal junction of photoaged skin.[71] Recent work has demonstrated that topical retinoids may inhibit the induction of matrix metalloproteinases by ultraviolet irradiation[31,68] thereby preventing collagen breakdown. Alphahydroxy and glycolic acids may also have a reparative effect on photoaged and maybe aged skin,[72] but there are few data to support this.

Although the effects of topical retinoids on intrinsically aged skin are harder to address it appears that there may be an enhanced sensitivity of intrinsically aged skin to the reparative mechanisms of topical retinoids. Aged skin, as compared to young skin, appears to have less retinoid activity.[73] In-vitro evidence shows that adult skin from sun-exposed and sun-protected sites responds well to retinoic acid but neonatal skin is much less responsive, which would suggest that retinoids modulate skin repair mechanisms as a function of age per se rather than purely as a response to photodamage.[29] It may be that a feature of cutaneous aging is gradual loss of steroid superfamily activity: testosterone and estrogen are reduced, as is vitamin D synthesis.

CONCLUSIONS

Aging of the skin is, as with other organs, a highly complex process and intrinsic aging must be separated from the effects of environmental factors. The study of aging skin, particularly as a consequence of the ready accessibility of cutaneous tissue, is one that presents a paradigm for aging of other organs. With the exponential rise in numbers of old and very old individuals in the population coupled with the ever increasing emphasis on youth, the search for the "fountain of youth" will be redoubled as we begin the twenty-first century.

KEY POINTS   Aging of the skin

- Photoaging and intrinsic aging of skin are frequently confused.

- Photoaging (wrinkles and actinic lentigines) is mainly responsible for concerns about appearance.

- Wrinkles result from loss of extracellular matrix, e.g., collagen and fibrillin in the papillary dermis.

- Intrinsic aging, mainly responsible for functional changes in skin, e.g., reduction in number of epidermal Langerhans cells, leads to decreased incidence of allergic contact dermatitis.

- Intrinsic aging of skin is related to loss of extracellular matrix and increase in matrix metalloproteinase activity.

- Therapies for "aging skin," e.g., tretinoin, are mainly aimed at treatment of features of photoaged skin.

- Dermal blood vessels are depleted in aged skin.

- Number of dermal melanocytes are reduced in aged skin.

- There are fewer eccrine glands but no change in the number of sebaceous glands in aged skin.

- Advanced age is associated with graying and loss of hair.

REFERENCES

1. Balin AK, Pratt LA: Physiological consequences of human skin aging. Cutis 1989;43:431–436
2. Lavker RM: Structural alterations in exposed and unexposed aged skin. J Invest Dermatol 1979;73:59–66
3. Potts RO, Buras EM, Chrisman DA: Changes with age in the moisture content of human skin. J Invest Dermatol 1984;82:97–100
4. West MD: The cellular and molecular biology of skin aging. Arch Dermatol 1994;130:87–95
5. Branchet MC, Boisnic S, Frances C, Robert AM: Skin thickness changes in normal aging skin. Gerontology 1990;36:28–35
6. Lober CW, Finske NA: Photoaging and the skin: differentiation and clinical response. Geriatrics 1990;45:36–42
7. Miller SJ, Lavker RM, Sun TT: Keratinocyte stem cells of cornea, skin and hair follicle: common and distinguishing features. Dev Biol 1993;4:217–240
8. Lavker RM, Sun TT: Heterogenicity in epidermal basal keratinocytes: morphological and functional correlations. Science 1982;215:1239–1241
9. Hill WR, Montgomery H: Regional changes and changes caused by age in the normal skin. J Invest Dermatol 1940;3:321–345
10. Katzberg AA: The area of the dermal-epidermal junction in human skin. Anat Rec 1958;131:717–723
11. Lavker RM, Zheng PO, Dong G: Aged skin: a study by light transmission electron and scanning electron microscopy. J Invest Dermatol 1987;88:44s–51s
12. Le Varlet B, Chaudagne C, Saunois A et al: Age-related functional and structural changes in human dermo-epidermal junction components. J Invest Derm 1998;3:172–179
13. Craven NM, Watson REB, Jones C et al: Clinical features of photodamaged human skin are associated with a reduction in collagen VII. J Invest Dermatol 1997;137:344–350
14. Watson REB, Craven NM, Shuttleworth CA et al: Fibrillin in photoaged skin. Br J Dermatol 1996;134:573 (abstract).
15. Grove GL: Age-associated changes in human epidermal cell renewal and repair. In Balin AK, Kligman AM (eds): Aging and the Skin. Raven Press, New York, 1989;193–204
16. Gilchrest BA: In vitro assessment of keratinocyte aging. J Invest Dermatol 1983;81:184s–189s
17. Hayflick L: The cellular basis for biological ageing. In Finch CE, Hayflick L (eds): Handbook of the Biology of Aging. Van Nostrand Reinhold, New York, 1977
18. Gilchrest BA, Garmyn M, Yaar M: Aging and photoaging affect gene expression in cultured human keratinocytes. Arch Dermatol 1994;130:82–86
19. Montagna W: Morphology of the ageing skin: the cutaneous appendages. In Montagna W (ed): Advances in Biology of the Skin, Vol 6. Pergamon Press, Oxford, 1965;6:1–16
20. Quevedo WC, Szabo G, Virks J: Influence of age and UV on the populations of dopa-positive melanocytes in human skin. J Invest Dermatol 1969;52:287–290
21. Gilchrest BA, Blog F, Szabo G: Effecting of aging and chronic sun-exposure on melanocytes in human skin. J Invest Dermatol 1979;73:141–143
22. Gilchrest BA, Murphy GF, Soter NA: Effect of chronologic aging and ultraviolet irradiation on Langerhans' cells in human epidermis. J Invest Dermatol 1982;79:85–88
23. Gilchrest BA, Szabo G, Flynn E et al: Chronologic and actinically induced aging in human facial skin. J Invest Dermatol 1983;80:81s–85s
24. Kwngsukstith C, Maibach HI: Effect of age and sex on the induction and elicitation of allergic contact dermatitis. Contact Dermatitis 1995;33:289–298
25. Waldorf DS, Willkens RF, Decker JL: Impaired delayed hypersensitivity in an aging population: association with antinuclear reactivity and rheumatoid factor. JAMA 1968;203:831–834
26. Andrew W, Behnke R, Sato T: Changes with advancing age in the cell population of human dermis. Gerontologica 1964;10:1–19
27. Talwar HS, Griffiths CEM, Fisher GJ et al: Reduced type I and type III procollagens in photodamaged adult human skin. J Invest Dermatol 1995;105:285–290
28. Fisher GJ, Datta SC, Talwar HS et al: Molecular basis of sun-induced premature skin ageing and retinoid antagonism. Nature 1996;379:335–339
29. Varani J, Fisher GJ, Kang S, Voorhees JJ: Molecular mechanisms of intrinsic skin aging and retinoid induced repair and reversal. J Invest Dermatol Symp Proc 1998;3:57–60
30. Chung JH, Kang S, Varani J, Lin J, Fisher GJ, Voorhees JJ: Decreased extracellular-signal-regulated kinase and increased stress-activated MAP

kinase activities in aged human skin in vivo. J Invest Dermatol 2000;115:177–182

31. Fisher GJ, Wang ZQ, Datta SC et al: Pathophysiology of premature skin aging induced by ultraviolet light. N Engl J Med 1997;13:1463–1465

32. Griffiths CEM, Russman AN, Majmudar G et al: Restoration of collagen formation in photodamaged human skin by tretinoin (retinoic acid). N Engl J Med 1993;329:530–535

33. Daniell H: Smoker's wrinkles. A study in the epidemiology of "crow's feet". Ann Intern Med 1971;75:873–880

34. Kadunce DP, Burr R, Gress R et al: Cigarette smoking: a risk factor for premature facial wrinkling. Ann Intern Med 1991;114:840–844

35. Lahmann C, Bergemann, Harrison G, Young AR: Matrix metalloproteinase-1 and skin ageing in smokers. Lancet 2001;357:935–936

36. Carrino DA, Sorrell JM, Caplan AI: Age-related changes in the proteoglycans of human skin. Arch Biochem Biophys 2000;373:91–101

37. Smith JG, Davidson, EA, Sams WM et al: Alterations in human dermal connective tissue with age and chronic sun damage. J Invest Dermatol 1962;37:447–452

38. Bernstein EF, Fisher LW, Li K et al: Differential expression of the versican and decorin genes in photoaged and sun-protected skin: Comparison by immunohistochemical and northern analyses. Lab Invest 1995;72:662–669

39. Bianco P, Fisher LW, Young MF, Termine JD, Gehron Robey P: Expression and localisation of the two small proteoglycans biglycan and decorin in developing human skeletal and non-skeletal tissues. J Histochem Cytochem 1990;38:1549–1563

40. Zimmermann DR, Dours-Zimmerman MT, Schubert M, Bruckner-Tuderman L: Versican is expressed in the proliferating zone in the epidermis and in association with the elastic network of the dermis. J Cell Biol 1994;124:817–825

41. Lavker RM, Kligman AM: Chronic heliodermatitis: a morphologic evaluation of chronic actinic damage with emphasis on the role of mast cells. J Invest Dermatol 1988;90:325–330

42. Braverman IM, Fonferko E: Studies in cutaneous aging, I: the elastic fiber network. J Invest Dermatol 1982;78:434–443

43. Watson RE, Griffiths CE, Craven NM, Shuttleworth CA, Kielty CM: Fibrillin-rich microfibrils are reduced in photoaged skin. Distribution at the dermal-epidermal junction. J Invest Dermatol 1999;112:782–787

44. Montagna W, Carlisle K: Structural changes in aging human skin. J Invest Dermatol 1979;73:47–53

45. Braverman IM, Fonferko E: Studies in cutaneous ageing, II: the microvasculature. J Invest Dermatol 1982;78:444–448

46. Kligman AM: Perspectives and problems in cutaneous gerontology. J Invest Dermatol 1979;73:39–46

47. Howell TH: Skin temperature gradient in the lower limbs of old women. Exp Gerontol 1982;17:65–67

48. Gilchrest BA, Stoff J, Soter NA: Chronologic aging alters the response to ultraviolet-induced inflammation in human skin. J Invest Dermatol 1982; 79:47–53

49. Hurley JH, Shelley WB: The Apocrine Sweat Gland in Health and Disease. Charles C Thomas, Springfield, Illinois, 1960

50. Cawley E, Hsu YT, Sturgill BC, Harman LE: Lipofuscin (wear-and-tear pigment) in human sweat glands. J Invest Dermatol 1973;61:105–107

51. Plewig G, Kligman AM: Proliferative activity of the sebacous glands of the aged. J Invest Dermatol 1978;70:314–317

52. Pochi PE, Strauss JJ, Downing DT: Age-related changes in sebaceous gland activity. J Invest Dermatol 1979;73:108–111

53. Smith L: Histopathologic characteristics and ultrastructure of aging skin. Cutis 1989;43:414–424

54. Gilchrest BA: Aging. J Am Acad Dermatol 1984;11:955–997

55. Hosoi J, Murphy GF, Egan CL et al: Regulation of Langerhans cell function by nerves containing calcitonin gene-related peptide. Nature 1993;363:159–163

56. Schludermann E, Zubeck JP: Effects of age on pain sensibility. Percept Motor Skills Res Exchange 1962;14:295–301

57. Grove GL, Duncan S, Kligman AM: Effect of ageing on the blistering of human skin with ammonium hydroxide. Br J Dermatol 1982;107:393–400

58. Cline DJ: Changes in hair color. Dermatol Clin; 1998;6:295–303

59. Nanniaga PB, Ghanem GE, Lejeune FJ, Bos JD, Westerhof W: Evidence for alpha-MSH binding sites on human scalp hair follicles: preliminary results. Pigment Cell Res 1991;4:193–198

60. Barman JM, Astore I, Percorara V: The normal trichogram of the adult. J Invest Dermatol 1965;44:233–236

61. Burch PRJ, Murray JJ, Jackson D: The age prevalence of arcus senilis, greying of hair and baldness: etiological considerations. J Gerontol 1971;26:364–372

62. Helmdach M, Thielitz A, Röpke E-V, Gollnick H: Age and sex variation in lipid composition of human fingernail plates. Skin Pharmacol Appl Physiol 2000;13:111–119

63. Borkan GA, Norris AH: Assessment of biologic age using a profile of physical parameters. J Gerontol 1980;35:177–184

64. Evans RM: The steroid and thyroid hormone receptor superfamily. Science 1988;240:889–895

65. Kligman AM, Grove GL, Hirose R et al: Topical tretinoin for photoaged skin. J Am Acad Dermatol 1986;15:836–859

66. Weiss JS, Ellis CN, Headington JT et al: Topical tretinoin improves photoaged skin: a double-blind, vehicle-controlled study. JAMA 1988;259:527–532

67. Kligman AM, Dugadkina D, Lavker RM: Effects of topical tretinoin on non-sun-exposed skin of the elderly. J Am Acad Dermatol 1993;29:25–33

68. Varani J, Warner RL, Gharaee-Kermani M et al: Vitamin A antagonises decreased cell growth and elevated collagen-degrading matrix metalloproteinases and stimulates collagen accumulation in naturally aged human skin. J Invest Dermatol 2000;114(3):480–486

69. Federspiel SJ, DiMari SJ, Howe AM et al: Extracellular matrix biosynthesis by cultured fetal rat lung epithelial cells IV. Effects of chronic exposure to retinoic acid on growth, differentiation and collagen biosynthesis. Lab Invest 1991; 65:441–450

70. Glick AB, Flanders KC, Danielpour D et al: Retinoic acid induced transforming growth factor-β_2 in cultured keratinocytes and mouse epidermis. Cell Regul 1989;I:87–97

71. Woodley DT, Zelickson AS, Briggaman RA et al: Treatment of photoaged skin with topical tretinoin increases dermal-epidermal anchoring fibrils: a preliminary report. JAMA 1990;263:3057–3059

72. Ditre CM, Griffin TD, Murphy GF et al: Effects of α-hydroxy acids on photoaged skin: A pilot clinical, histologic and ultrastructural study. J Am Acad Dermatol 1996;34:187–195

73. Varani J, Perone P, Griffiths CEM et al: *All-trans* retinoic acid (RA) stimulates events in organ-cultured human skin that underlie repair. J Clin Invest 1994; 94:1747–1756

Chapter 100

Skin diseases and old age

W. Zoe D. Stitt and Barbara A. Gilchrest

DEMOGRAPHIC AND EPIDEMIOLOGICAL CONSIDERATIONS

Skin disease and symptoms referable to the skin are exceedingly common among elderly people. In the United States, nearly 20 percent of all outpatient visits to physicians by patients aged 65 years or older are motivated at least in part by a skin complaint,[1] approximately two-thirds of ambulatory older persons examined in survey studies have one or more dermatological disorders.[1-3] Including the cosmetically distressing and often anxiety-provoking benign neoplasms and other skin changes associated with aging, the percentage of the elderly population affected by abnormalities of the skin increases to 100 percent. Although these disorders are only rarely life threatening, they detract substantially from the quality of life and often lower self-esteem and psychosocial well-being.[4] The following sections seek to explain this high prevalence of skin disease and discuss the pathophysiology, diagnosis, and management of the more common disorders encountered in a geriatric practice.

Factors predisposing to skin disease in elderly people (see also Chapter 99)

Skin is the principal barrier between the body and its external environment. Thus, over many decades, the skin is modified not only by intrinsic aging processes, as are all tissues in the body, but also by cumulative environmental impacts. The relative contributions of these intrinsic and extrinsic processes on age-associated predisposition to injury and disease varies dramatically among individuals and from site to site on the skin surface. For most individuals, particularly fair-skinned Caucasians, the major lifelong environmental impact on skin is sun exposure. *Photoaging*, discussed separately below, is the term used to describe this superposition of cumulative sun damage on intrinsic aging. Another substantial environmental influence on skin aging is cigarette smoking, which exacerbates wrinkling and increases the risk of skin cancer.

Intrinsic aging processes have been shown to decrease maximum function and reserve capacity in skin as assessed in a variety of assays.[5,6] These age-associated functional decrements are widely and reasonably presumed to contribute to clinical skin disease, as well as to contribute to systemic health problems of elderly people. Of note, however, is that these decrements have relatively minor impact on the appearance of skin either clinically or histologically.[5,6] Photoaging exaggerates most of the functional losses observed in sun-protected old skin and greatly increases the risk of carcinogenesis.[7] In addition, photoaging is responsible for the great majority of age-associated changes in the skin's appearance.[7] Understanding this duality of aging processes in the skin is important not only in preventing and managing geriatric skin disease, but serves as well as an important reminder that the apparent aging of all organ systems is the combined result of innate aging and environmental influences.

APPROACH TO DERMATOLOGICAL DISEASE IN OLDER PATIENTS

Proper evaluation of a dermatological complaint entails at a minimum a pertinent medical history and skin examination. Full skin examination of all geriatric patients annually adds very little time to a standard physical examination and provides an excellent opportunity to counsel patients regarding sun protection, a highly effective measure to prevent skin cancers in high-risk individuals.[8] Skin cancer screenings by volunteer dermatologists throughout the USA have identified basal cell and squamous cell carcinomas in 7 percent of adults screened and biopsy proven melanomas in 0.2 percent of 140,038 self-selected Caucasians over 50 years of age, despite the fact that the great majority of these individuals had seen a primary care physician during the previous year.[9] This suggests an enormous opportunity for incidental diagnosis of skin cancer in older patients, for whom an earlier diagnosis implies reduced cost and morbidity associated with therapy and, at least in the case of melanoma, detection of thinner lesions with reduced risk of mortality.[10] Patients with evidence of sun damage, particularly those with actinic keratoses (see below) or a history of skin cancer or extensive past sun exposure should have a full skin examination at least annually. It is also important to inquire regarding topical and systemic treatments, either prescribed or self-determined. Over-the-counter topical remedies, cosmetics, bathing habits, and exposure to harsh detergents or inappropriate cleansers such as isopropyl alcohol, for example, often exacerbate skin conditions. The duration of a complaint, response to previous treatments, presence of similar condition in close contacts, and the patient's own opinions regarding etiology are among the information items to be elicited.

Often important physical findings are found in areas other than those mentioned by the patient. For example, the patient may not necessarily complain of genital lesions or may be unaware of cutaneous malignancies or other significant conditions unrelated to the chief complaint. At least cursory inspection of "hidden areas" (scalp, back, and buttocks for example) is warranted. Finally, age-associated blunting of vascular and immune responses may make skin findings more subtle in elderly patients than in younger patients with similar disorders, complicating diagnosis.

The older patient often has difficulty complying with topical treatment. He or she may not be able to reach the feet or back; may not be able to bathe, shower, or shampoo without assistance; and, as with oral medications, may become confused by complex regimens. Patient comprehension, mobility, and home situation should be carefully assessed initially and at the time of follow-up visits, particularly in the event of treatment failure. Written instructions that review the medications and skin care advised decrease the risk of error and are very helpful when more than one topical medication is given.

SELECTED SKIN DISEASES

Numerous skin diseases affect elderly people.[11] Those covered in the following sections are highly prevalent and/or highly symptomatic, mandating a geriatrician's familiarity with their pathogenesis, diagnosis, and treatment.

Summary of management algorithms

Herpes zoster
Acute outbreak
Presentation within 72 hours of onset:
- Immunocompetent elderly people
  - Topical management: Burow's solution or hypertonic saline, antibacterial wash, mupirocin ointment
  - Pain management
  - Oral antiviral: acyclovir 800 mg, 5× day, 7–10 days, famciclovir 500 mg, 3× day, 7 days, or valacyclovir 1,000 mg, 3× day, 7 days
- Immunocompromised elderly people, or disseminated disease
  - Topical management and pain management
  - Intravenous acyclovir 10 mg/kg q8 hr, 7 days (adjust for renal function)

Presentation after 72 hours of onset:
- As above, except oral antivirals may be of little help in immunocompetent patients

Post-herpetic neuralgia
Prevention:
- Incidence and degree of pain at 3 months lessened with early antiviral therapy
Treatment:
- Topical—capsasin, eutetic mixture of local anesthetics
- Analgesics—cautious use of narcotic analgesics
- Amitriptyline
- Carbamazepine, gabapentin
- Referral to pain clinic

Pruritus
Diagnosis
Presence of a rash:
- Diagnose and treat primary skin eruption
Absence of a rash:
- Symptoms attributable to systemic disease (fever, weight loss, nausea/vomit, cough/hemoptysis)
- History of new exposures—especially medication
- Physical examination—focus on thyroid, lymph node, liver, and spleen examination
- Laboratory evaluation
  - Liver function tests, complete blood count and differential, blood urea nitrogen and creatinine

- Chest X-ray
- Additional testing guided by history and physical
Treatment
- Treat systemic or local disease
- Topical—emollients, Sarna lotion
- Antihistamines
  - Sedating agents—with caution
  - Nonsedating
  - Cholestasis—consider cholestyramine
  - Opiate antagonists—experimental, with caution

Scabies
Noninstitutionalized, immunocompetent elderly people
- Permenthrin cream 5 percent
  - Neck to feet, overnight application
  - Treat household contact
  - Wash all bedding
  - May repeat in 1 week
- Antihistamines as needed
- Lindane, precipitated sulfur—second line

Institutionalized elderly people
- Permethrin cream 5 percent, treat all contacts
- Ivermectin 150–200 µg/kg—experimental
Hyperkeratotic scabies
- Keratolytic—12 percent lactic acid, 10 percent urea, 3–6 percent salicylic acid to decrease scale
- Permethrin cream 5 percent
  - Head to feet, overnight application
  - Repeat treatments—may require daily treatment
  - Treat contact, clean environment, antihistamines as needed
- Ivermectin—experimental

Herpes zoster

Herpes zoster (HZ), or "shingles," is due to reactivation of a latent varicella virus infection. Following a primary varicella infection, usually in childhood, the virus may remain dormant in dorsal sensory root ganglia and reactivate decades later at times of physical stress. Reactivation of varicella virus is thought to be due to waning immunity, specifically cell mediated immunity to the virus. The annual incidence of HZ in apparently healthy person ranges from approximately 1–2 cases per thousand in adolescents and young adults to 10 times this incidence in those aged 80 years and older.[12] The incidence of HZ in individuals with additional age-associated predisposing factors such as cancer, immunosuppressive therapy, and surgery is considerably higher. The lifetime risk of HZ is approximately 50 percent, with 10 percent of individuals experiencing at least two episodes,[12] making HZ a statistically likely event in the later decades of life.

HZ classically presents as paresthesia and/or dysesthesia affecting a single dermatome. These symptoms usually persist for several days, rarely more than a week, before skin lesions appear. The eruption of HZ is virtually pathognomonic. Clusters of vesicles, usually superimposed on erythematous plaques, erupt in a dermatomal distribution. In 98 percent of patients, the eruption is unilateral and lesions do not cross the midline, although occasional individual vesicles can be found outside the affected dermatome. Greater than 20 vesicles outside of the primary (or adjacent) dermatome is considered disseminated zoster, characteristic of severely immunocompromised patients.[13] The diagnosis of herpes virus infection may be confirmed by a Tzanck test of material scraped from the base of an intact vesicle. A positive test is indicated by the appearance of multinucleated giant cells indicative of herpetic infection, although this test cannot distinguish herpes simplex from herpes zoster. The initially clear vesicles may become pustular or, especially in the elderly, hemorrhagic within a few days. New lesions continue to appear for several days, often progressing distally along the dermatome. Widespread dissemination, if it is to occur, usually does so during this period. Pain and hyperesthesia are frequently prominent during the first days of the eruption. Vesicles usually begin to crust in the second week and resolve within 4 weeks in most patients; the eruption tends to persist longer and to be more severe in elderly patients than in younger adults. Permanent dyspigmentation or even hypertrophic scarring may occur in lesional skin.

Vesicle fluid is contagious, but the attack rate (cases of varicella) in susceptible household contacts is much less than for chickenpox (primary varicella infection). The course of HZ infection in young and old adults differs primarily in the incidence and severity of postherpetic neuralgia, variably defined as pain persisting after healing of skin lesions or pain of greater than 1–3, or 6 months duration. This problem occurs in approximately 10 percent of HZ cases overall, but although postherpetic neuralgia is uncommon in patients less than 40 years of age, it occurs in over one-half of patients aged 60 years and in over three-quarters of patients aged 70 years.[14] With age, the increase in severity and duration of postherpetic neuralgia is even more marked than the increase in incidence. Persistent pain is especially common in those patients with trigeminal involvement (10–15 percent of reported cases). The basis of the increased risk of postherpetic neuralgia in elderly people is unclear, but may be the consequence of less successful healing, with a greater tendency to perineural fibrosis and/or failure of involved neurons to re-establish normal signal transduction thresholds after the acute viral infection.

In 1995, the Food and Drug Administration (FDA) of the United States approved a live attenuated varicella virus vaccine. Currently, the vaccine is indicated for immunization of healthy infants, children, adolescents, and adults with a negative history of chicken pox, but vaccination trials in individuals over 60 years are underway with the rationale of enhancing cell-mediated immunity to varicella zoster virus in elderly people. At this time, however, there is no effective means of preventing varicella reactivation. Therapies are directed at reducing discomfort during the acute eruption and preventing or ameliorating postherpetic neuralgia.

During the acute phase of HZ infection, some patients require narcotic analgesics for adequate relief of pain. These agents should be prescribed cautiously in elderly people to avoid overmedication and adverse systemic effects. Early skin lesions are best treated with local compresses of Burow's solution (1:20 in cool water) or other hypertonic soaks for 10 minutes, three to four times daily, followed by gentle washing with Hibiclens or other antibacterial soap to hasten drying and prevent bacterial superinfection. A topical antibiotic alone, such as mupirocin ointment, should be applied two to three times daily to already crusted lesions. Systemic treatment is optional

in the immunocompetent host but studies have shown that patients who receive antiviral therapy experience faster healing, a shortened duration of viral shedding, decreased risk of dissemination, and a decrease in the severity and duration of acute pain.[15] Treatment should be started within 72 hours of the onset of symptoms to be effective. Currently there are three antiviral drugs approved for the treatment of HZ: acyclovir 800 mg five times a day for 7–10 days, its analog famciclovir 500 mg three times a day for 7 days, and its prodrug valacyclovir 1,000 mg three times a day for 7 days.[12] Severely immunosuppressed patients or patients with disseminated HZ require intravenous antiviral therapy with acyclovir.

Although antiviral therapy has definite proven benefit for the treatment of acute zoster, its role in the prevention of postherpetic neuralgia is less definite.[12] Review of placebo-controlled trials to date support the use of acyclovir 800 mg five times a day for 10 days to decrease the incidence of postherpetic neuralgia at 1–3 months.[16] In one study this regimen decreased the incidence of postherpetic neuralgia from 16.7 percent in the placebo group to 4.2 percent in the treated group during the first 3 months.[15] From 4 to 6 months, the groups did not differ statistically in neuralgia prevalence. These patient groups averaged 55 and 59 years of age, respectively, with more than 70 persons aged 50 years or older in each group, but data for the more elderly cohorts were not analyzed separately. However, no reduction in postherpetic neuralgia was detected in a second study of 364 patients aged 60 years or older,[17] using a very similar design in which acyclovir was administered for only 7 days. Neither study found medically significant side-effects of acyclovir. In a separate double-blind controlled study of HZ ophthalmicus, acyclovir 600 mg five times a day for 10 days was found to reduce the rate of ocular complications such as keratitis and uveitis when treatment was initiated as late as 7 days after the appearance of lesions.[18] Famciclovir at 500 mg and 750 mg three times a day for 7 days led to a significant decrease in duration of postherpetic neuralgia when compared to placebo, with a more marked decrease compared to placebo in patients over 50 years of age. Pain at six months was also less prevalent for the famciclovir-treated patients compared to control (15 percent compared to 23.8 percent).[19] Valacyclovir's effect on postherpetic neuralgia has not been studied in a placebo-controlled trial, but a study of valacyclovir 1,000 mg three times a day for 7 or 14 days compared to acyclovir 800 mg five times a day for 7 days, demonstrated persistent pain in 18.6 percent of the combined valacyclovir-treated patients compared to 25.7 percent of the acyclovir-treated patients.[20]

Treatment with systemic corticosteroids is likewise controversial. A randomized, controlled study of 349 subjects comparing 7- and 21-day treatments of acyclovir alone or in addition to prednisolone revealed that a longer course of acyclovir or the addition of steroids offered only minimal benefit, although an increase in adverse events was reported in the group treated with steroids.[21] These data contrast with earlier controlled trials examining the efficacy of oral corticosteroids in HZ management that reported a reduction in pain during the acute episode in all four of the five trials in which this variable was assessed.[12] All studies employed a dose of prednisone or its equivalent at a dose of 40–60 mg/day tapered over 21–28 days, and none found an increase in HZ complications or steroid-associated side-effects in treated patients. Two of the five trials found that corticosteroid therapy during the acute episode reduced the prevalence or severity of postherpetic neuralgia. Whether these discrepant results are the result of different selection criteria and patient age or borderline effectiveness of the intervention is unclear.

Treatment of already established postherpetic neuralgia can be frustrating. Often topical therapy is initiated as first-line treatment owing to its safety as compared with other modalities. Capsaicin, which exerts its effects via the local depletion of substance P and other neuropeptides, applied three to four times a day may decrease the pain of postherpetic neuralgia.[22] A 0.25 percent capsaicin cream is presently the only FDA-approved topical treatment for this neuralgia. However, transient stinging and burning at the time of application, incomplete pain relief, and the requirement for frequent, indefinite treatment greatly decrease patient satisfaction with this modality. Other topical treatments include topical anti-inflammatory agents, such as formulations containing aspirin or indomethacin, and topical anesthetics, such as EMLA (eutectic mixture of local anesthetics). This cream is most effective if applied under plastic wrap occlusion for a minimum of 1 hour, on a schedule dictated by patient symptoms. Data on the long-term efficacy of these agents are very limited.[14]

Despite trials and anecdotal use of numerous systemic agents for the treatment of postherpetic neuralgia, antidepressants such as amitriptyline remain the most consistently effective.[12,23] These drugs appear to act by blocking uptake of norepinephrine and serotonin by spinal neurons involved in pain perception, and often doses lower than those needed for antidepressant action are effective. Patients may begin with 12.5–25 mg at bedtime, increasing until the pain is controlled or unacceptable side-effects are encountered. Typical effective and well-tolerated doses are 75–150 mg/day. Particularly in patients with lancinating pain, carbamazepine 160 mg/day, increasing cautiously as necessary, may prove to be an effective alternative. A placebo-controlled trial of gabapentin, a structural analog of γ-aminobutyric acid, in patients with established postherpetic neuralgia demonstrated a reduction in average daily pain and in sleep interference but side-effects were frequent (somnolence, dizziness, ataxia, peripheral edema, and infection).[24] A variety of nonpharmaceutical therapies, such as acupuncture, nerve blocks, transcutaneous electrical nerve stimulation, and deep brain stimulation have also been employed.

Pruritus

Elderly people often experience localized or generalized pruritus. Depending on the population surveyed and the criteria employed, up to two-thirds report frequent bothersome itching.[1] For some, it is a minor annoyance; for others the pruritus leads to extensive, slow-healing excoriations or loss of sleep with associated irritability and impaired mental function.

Many patients presenting to the physician because of pruritus in fact have an eruption that is responsible for the symptom,[25] although its other manifestations may be so subtle that the patient or even the physician does not notice the rash. Because inflammatory responses may be muted in elderly people, a careful history and physical examination are necessary before excluding primary disorders of the skin such as eczema, early bullous pemphigoid, urticaria, scabies, or pediculosis. Proper identification of a causative dermatosis leads to effective treatment in most patients and enables the patient to avoid the hematological, radiographic, and other laboratory procedures that constitute the work-up for unexplained generalized pruritus.

Among all patients seeking medical attention for pruritus, the prevalence of underlying systemic disease has been reported as 10–50 percent,[26] the percentage depending on patient selection, diagnostic evaluation, and period of follow-up. Many authorities, however, believe the statistical association is far less strong among unselected older persons presenting to physicians with this symptom.

Numerically, perhaps the most important known cause of persistent generalized pruritus is chronic renal failure. However, the degree of renal failure necessary to cause pruritus is unknown, complicating interpretation of this symptom in the elderly patient with mild to moderate renal insufficiency. From a practical viewpoint, it is probably unwise to attribute pruritus to otherwise asymptomatic renal failure, or to renal insufficiency not requiring specific therapy for metabolic imbalance.

Pruritus is probably the most distressing and consistent symptom of chronic cholestasis, which underlies all the hepatic disorders associated with pruritus. Overall, pruritus occurs in approximately 20–25 percent of jaundiced patients, but it is rare in those with hepatic disease lacking cholestasis. Drugs that can cause pruritus by inducing cholestasis include phenothiazines, tolbutamide, erythromycin estolate, anabolic hormones, estrogens, and progestins. Opiates are perhaps the most common drugs to cause non-immunologically-mediated pruritus without cholestasis.

Approximately 30–50 percent of patients with polycythemia vera and up to 20 percent of patients with Hodgkin's disease experience pruritus. The incidence and significance of pruritus in other lymphomas and leukemias are unknown, but the occasional association cannot be disputed. Generalized pruritus has been reported as an initial symptom in patients with multiple myeloma, Waldenström's macroglobulinemia, and benign gammopathies. Iron deficiency anemia has been reported as the cause of generalized pruritus in more than 50 patients,[27] including 6 with polycythemia,[28] although this association is apparently rare. Pruritus attributable to endocrine or specific "miscellaneous" causes is rare.

Most elderly people experience extensive or generalized pruritus for which there is no apparent explanation. Hence, one must either accept a higher incidence of idiopathic pruritus with advancing age or infer the existence of "senile pruritus." Physiological factors that may contribute to this hypothetical entity include age-associated alterations in the skin, peripheral nerve endings, and dermal neuropeptide release.

Alterations in the barrier function of the skin, possibly facilitating low-grade irritant dermatitis, include decreased keratohyalin granule formation in the epidermis, decreased skin surface hydration, diminished stratum corneum lipids, and a slower rate of stratum corneum barrier repair.[29,30] In addition, altered sensory thresholds of C-fiber neurons as well as modifications in the synthesis, release, and clearance of dermal neuropeptides, such as substance P, histamine, neurokinin A, calcitonin gene-related peptide, and other mediators with opiate activity may also play a role.[30]

The appropriate laboratory evaluation for the patient with unexplained generalized pruritus remains a matter of opinion, as cost/benefit ratios for individual procedures have not been determined. Measurement of serum creatinine, blood urea nitrogen, bilirubin, hepatic enzymes, and a complete blood count seem to constitute a reasonable survey; a chest X-ray may also be justified as a screening for malignancy. Appropriate physical examination includes examination of the thyroid gland, lymph nodes, liver, and spleen. Additional tests may be suggested by history, review of systems, or physical examination.

The pathophysiology of pruritus associated with systemic disease is incompletely understood, and the optimal therapy is that for the underlying disease whenever possible. Specific approaches to the treatment of the pruritus itself are available in a few instances, but for most patients, nonspecific therapies must be employed.[30,31] Often it is worthwhile to prescribe an emollient, even in the absence of clinical xerosis, because minimal or intermittent "dryness," present in virtually all elderly individuals, may notably exacerbate pruritus of another cause. Patients should be cautioned specifically against topical application of alcohol or hot water (both of which may temporarily relieve but ultimately exacerbate pruritus) or excessive washing, especially with soap. Topical application of menthol and camphor in an emollient base, such as in Sarna lotion, may provide considerable temporary relief; other topical anesthetics can be used only at the risk of allergic sensitization. Oral antihistamines are widely prescribed for pruritus of all causes, although their efficacy is slight in most instances, even when combinations of H_1 and H_2 blockers are used. The use of antihistamines by elderly people may result in the additional problems of urinary retention, paradoxic restlessness, or significantly impaired psychomotor function. Newer nonsedating antihistamines have fewer neurological side-effects, but care must still be taken to avoid potential drug interactions. Pruritus associated with cholestasis may be best treated with the anion exchange resin, cholestyramine, given before and after meals (up to 16 g per day). Opiate receptor antagonists, including low-dose naltrexone (50 mg daily) and nalmetene, have shown promise in the treatment of pruritus due to systemic disease, pruritus associated with dermatological disease, and idiopathic pruritus.[32] Tolerance to these agents and recurrence of pruritus with discontinuation may occur. Side-effects to opiate receptor antagonists are minimal, but severe liver disease is a contraindication and their use in patients with milder cholestatic liver disease may be associated with an opiate-withdrawal syndrome due to increased endogenous opiates in these patients.[32]

Xerosis

Xerosis is the term used to describe the "dry" or rough quality of skin that is almost universal among elderly people. The condition may be generalized but is especially prominent on the lower legs and is exacerbated by low-humidity environments classically found in overheated rooms during cold weather. "Xerosis" is a misnomer; the initial assumption that the disorder resulted from a lack of water in the skin overall has been disproved.[33] In-vivo and in-vitro measurements demonstrate diminished hydration of the superficial portion of the stratum corneum only, with the deeper portion maintaining normal hydration.[34] The occasional classification of xerosis as a disorder of sebaceous (oil) glands is similarly without experimental basis. Xerosis probably reflects minor abnormalities in epidermal maturation that, in turn, result in an irregular surface and altered composition of the stratum corneum. These abnormalities that characterize xerotic skin histologically are similar in aged dry skin and young dry skin.[35] Xerotic skin in elderly people is often pruritic and may show evidence of inflammation, probably due to defects in the stratum corneum, with secondary entry of irritating substances into the dermis. Recovery to baseline after perturbation by irritants is delayed in aged skin compared to young skin.[36] The resulting inflammatory conditions, including *erythema craquele* or *winter eczema*, respond promptly to topical corticosteroid ointment and/or emollients, although these preparations do not correct the xerosis itself.

Frequent, regular use of a topical emollient makes dry skin more attractive and more comfortable and prevents the complications discussed previously. Emollients are most effective when applied to already moistened skin (e.g. immediately after the bath or shower). "Heavy," frankly greasy emollients are sometimes appealing to elderly people. They are often inexpensive and have the additional property of perceptibly coating the skin, producing a smooth surface film, and they are usually good barriers against evaporation. Preparations containing ammonium lactate or other α-hydroxy acids are more cosmetically elegant and often provide longer lasting improvements in skin barrier function and xerosis. Finally, it should be noted that emollients applied to the skin immediately after bathing retain water more effectively than gels or oils added to the bath water. Bath oils coat the bathtub as well as the skin, producing a dangerously slippery surface that is difficult to clean.

Seborrheic dermatitis

Seborrheic dermatitis is a very common dermatological condition in the geriatric population.[1,2] Clinically, it presents as erythema and greasy-appearing scales in what is referred to as a *seborrheic distribution*, namely the scalp; postauricular folds; central face, particularly the eyebrows, glabella, perinasal, nasolabial folds, and beard area; and the central chest and interscapular areas. On the scalp, it is referred to in lay terms as dandruff. Seborrheic dermatitis is found with greater frequency among patients with underlying neurological conditions, such as Parkinson's disease, facial nerve injury, spinal cord injury, poliomyelitis, and syringomyelia, as well as in patients taking neuroleptic medications with parkinsonian side-effects. Human immunodeficiency virus infection has also been associated with severe seborrheic dermatitis.

The role of resident lipophilic yeast, *Pityrosporum ovale*, is controversial, although studies have shown the organism to be present in greater numbers in patients with seborrheic dermatitis. Treatment is directed at either killing the yeast with topical antifungal preparations or directly suppressing inflammation via low-potency topical steroids. In a double-blind study comparing 2 percent ketoconazole cream to 1 percent hydrocortisone cream, therapeutic response was noted in 80.5 percent of subjects using ketoconazole and 94.4 percent of those using hydrocortisone, demonstrating a somewhat higher efficacy of hydrocortisone, although establishing keto-conazole as an effective, steroid-sparing alternative. For hair-bearing regions, shampoos containing ketoconazole, selenium sulfide, salicylic acid, zinc pyrithione, or tar are effective; for severe cases, a steroid-containing solution can be applied to the scalp after shampooing.

Rosacea

Also called acne rosacea, this is an idiopathic facial disorder of middle-aged and elderly fair-skinned persons consisting of inflammatory papules and pustules, telangiectasia, and easy sometimes florid flushing. The relative severity of these components varies markedly among patients; some, particularly men, may also develop marked coarsening and hypertrophy of the nasal skin, so-called rhinophyma.

The acneiform lesions usually respond dramatically to low-dose tetracycline (e.g. 250–500 mg twice daily) or other broad-spectrum antibiotics. Many patients can be maintained on even lower doses, and perhaps one-third have long-term remissions after a single 2–3-month antibiotic course. Good control can also be achieved with topical metronidazole.[37] Topical metronidazole is available as a gel, cream or lotion formulation for once daily (1 percent) or twice-daily (0.75 percent) use. Topical clindamycin and sulfacetamide preparations may also be effective. The mechanism of action of these agents is presumed to be dual anti-inflammatory and antimicrobial properties.

Management of the vascular component of rosacea is more difficult. The above antibiotics are claimed to reduce both telangiectasia and flushing, but the evidence for this benefit is slight. Patients should be advised to avoid known precipitants of flushing, such as alcohol, hot or spicy food, intense exercise, and emotional stress, but many are unable or unwilling to do so. Electrocautery and, more safely and reliably, pulsed dye laser therapy can eradicate individual dilated vessels; in extreme cases, laser treatment of the entire facial area subject to flushing can be performed and is reported to decrease the severity of vasodilation after challenge.

Reshaping of the rhinophymatous nose with removal of excess thickened skin can be accomplished by conventional surgery or use of the CO_2 laser.

Scabies

Scabies is a severely pruritic infestation by the *Sarcoptes scabiei* mite. Symptoms are due to a hypersensitivity reaction to the mite, explaining why pruritus can persist for days to weeks following adequate treatment and conversely why infested persons may be asymptomatic for days to weeks. While the male mite remains on the surface of the skin, the female burrows through the stratum corneum to lay her eggs. In an average infested host, only 10–12 live female mites are present at one time. Transmission is through person-to-person contact, and epidemics can arise among institutionalized or nursing home patients, necessitating widespread treatment of patients, staff, and visitors.

The hallmark lesion of scabies is the burrow, a linear ridge often ending with a tiny vesicle. Other cutaneous manifestations are due to the hypersensitivity reaction to the mite and include papules, vesicles, nodules, and excoriations. Lesions are concentrated in the interdigital web spaces, axillae, umbilicus, and on the volar wrists and genitalia. Diagnosis is confirmed by scraping the contents of the burrow onto a slide with mineral oil and examining it microscopically. The presence of a mite, eggs, or feces confirms the diagnosis, but this evidence is not essential to making the diagnosis if clinical suspicion is high. Immunocompromised patients or those who have an impaired ability to scratch may have an extensive hyperkeratotic and highly contagious eruption harboring thousands of mites.[38]

The two most widely used treatments are topical lindane and permethrin. Permethrin lacks the neurological toxicity sometimes seen with lindane, and it has the advantage of being able to kill the scabies eggs as well as mites; thus, in theory only one application is necessary. For successful treatment, all household members and other close contacts must be treated at the same time as the affected patient even if asymptomatic, because newly infested individuals develop pruritus only when allergically sensitized, often after a delay of 2 weeks or more. The medication is applied from the neck down, with particular attention to the subungual area and lesion-bearing sites including the genitalia, then washed off after 8 hours. At that time all clothing and linens should be washed in hot water and placed in a hot dryer, or dry cleaned. One week later, the entire process is repeated to kill any larvae that have hatched since the first treatment. It is essential to avoid application of lindane immediately following a hot bath, as increased absorption has been reported to cause seizures in some elderly individuals. Oral ivermectin has been reported to be as effective as topical lindane or permethrin in curing scabies,[39] but is not approved for this indication. Nevertheless, some advocate the use of ivermectin in a single dose of 150–200 µg/kg as first-line therapy for institutional scabies outbreaks, including nursing home outbreaks,[40] despite one report of unexplained deaths in such a nursing-home-treated population.[41] Treatment of hyperkeratotic scabies requires application of topical scabies lotions to the head and neck as well as neck down, and may require adjuvant keratolytic agents to remove scales and repeated treatments over several days to weeks. Residual pruritus can be managed with topical steroids or antihistamines. However, if pruritus continues beyond a few weeks or if new lesions appear, treatment failure, reinfestation, or misdiagnosis should be considered.

DRUG ERUPTIONS

Adverse cutaneous reactions to medications include expected, usually dose-related side-effects, such as an acneiform eruption following corticosteroid administration or xerosis from retinoids, and unexpected, immune-mediated, allergic reactions. These latter reactions typically occur within 3 days to 2 weeks of challenge and persist up to 2 weeks after the drug is discontinued. Rechallenge results in a more rapid onset of the eruption. Less commonly, a patient may have an adverse reaction to a medication after weeks, months, or rarely years of use.

Any medication can cause a drug eruption, but certain medications are statistically more likely to do so. In two separate survey studies of over 22,000 and 15,000 inpatients, respectively, the Boston Collaborative Drug Surveillance

Program[42] identified the following as most likely to cause a drug eruption: amoxicillin, ampicillin, penicillin, semisynthetic penicillins, trimethoprim-sulfamethoxazole, transfused blood, cephalosporins, gentamycin sulfate, acetylcysteine, allopurinol, quinidine, and dipyrone. Conversely, digoxin, antacids, meperidine, promethazine, and acetaminophen were among those medications administered to more than 1,000 patients with no reported cutaneous eruptions.

Central to management of a drug eruption is discontinuation of the culprit medication. In a patient ingesting multiple medications, it is prudent to discontinue or replace with a non-cross-reacting alternative all but those essential to his or her survival. This is particularly essential in the more serious and potentially life-threatening reactions. Failure to remove the immunological challenge may lead to a progressively more severe eruption. Midpotency topical steroids, antihistamines, and antipruritic lotions provide symptomatic relief during the period of resolution, after withdrawal of the suspected offending agent(s). Oral corticosteroids are not indicated in the management of drug eruptions, with the possible and controversial exception of those that are life threatening.

The most common form of drug eruption is the morbilliform or exanthematous eruption. Sometimes referred to as a "maculopapular" eruption, it is characterized by discrete and coalescing erythematous macules and papules symmetrically distributed on the trunk and extremities. The most common causative agents are those listed above. Morbilliform eruptions typically begin within 1 week of exposure, except in the case of penicillins when they may occur 2 weeks or longer after the initial exposure.[43]

Other forms of drug eruption include photosensitivity, as is seen with doxycycline, thiazides, and amiodarone; a lichenoid or lichen planus-like eruption, seen with gold and phenothiazines; and urticaria, often associated with penicillin or iodine-containing contrast media. Fixed drug eruption is manifest by one or few red to violaceous, round plaques that recur in the identical location if the patient is rechallenged. These lesions resolve with hyperpigmentation, which becomes more pronounced with each episode. Causes of fixed drug eruption include tetracyclines and nonsteroidal anti-inflammatory drugs.[44] Vasculitis, presenting as palpable purpura, can occur as the result of medication hypersensitivity, among many other possible causes. Immune complex formation can lead to a serum sickness reaction, characterized by an urticarial eruption, fever, arthritis, nephritis, and sometimes neurological symptoms. Penicillins, sulfonamides, and streptomycin are among the causative agents.[43]

Some uncommon drug reactions are important due to their life-threatening nature. These include hypersensitivity reaction, anaphylaxis/angioedema, exfoliative erythroderma, erythema multiforme major (Stevens–Johnson syndrome), and toxic epidermal necrolysis (TEN). These conditions often require hospitalization with intensive supportive care, as well as discontinuation of the causative agent.

Hypersensitivity reaction was first described with phenytoin, and is now recognized with drugs other than anticonvulsants, particularly sulfonamides. It is a multisystem response manifest by a cutaneous eruption, which may be of any type, in conjunction with fever, adenopathy, hematological abnormalities, and hepatitis.[45] It should be noted that phenytoin, carbamazepine, and phenobarbital cross-react with each other, so that all three agents are contraindicated in patients sensitive to any of them. Valproic acid is probably safe to use in these patients.

Anaphylaxis occurs on a spectrum of IgE-dependent reactions including urticaria, bronchospasm, laryngeal edema, and hypotension. Penicillins are the drugs most commonly associated with anaphylaxis, and the reaction is more likely to occur with intravenous administration.[43] Angioedema may occur with the use of angiotensin-converting enzyme inhibitors (ACE-I) and may not always be IgE mediated.[46] Exfoliative erythroderma presents as diffuse erythema and scaling. Temperature, fluids, electrolytes, and nutrition must be carefully monitored. Erythema multiforme is recognized by pathognomonic target lesions: a dusky center that sometimes progresses to a central blister or erosion, surrounded by pale edematous skin, with a macular erythematous perimeter. Most cases of erythema multiforme minor are due to infections, especially herpes simplex virus. When mucous membranes are involved the eruption is classified as Stevens–Johnson syndrome. The majority of Stevens–Johnson cases are due to medications. Large areas of sloughed skin are the hallmark of TEN characterized by skin tenderness and a positive Nikolsky sign, the shearing off of the epidermis with lateral force. TEN may appear de novo or may evolve from severe erythema multiforme. Again, fluid and electrolyte management and the avoidance of sepsis are crucial. Reported mortality rates for TEN are 30–50 percent and patients are best managed in a burns unit.[47]

Another adverse reaction to a medication may be the induction or worsening of a primary skin disease. For example, psoriasis may be triggered or worsened by lithium or beta-blocker administration and pemphigus has been associated with the use of penicillamine and captopril. Pseudolymphomas have been described with numerous medications and these drug-induced pseudolymphomas may also simulate cutaneous T-cell lymphoma.[48]

SKIN CANCER

Malignant neoplasms are strongly age-associated in most organ systems, including the skin. The most common cutaneous malignancies, basal cell carcinoma (BCC), squamous cell carcinoma (SCC), and malignant melanoma, account for perhaps one-half of all human malignancies and are rapidly increasing in incidence, to at least 1,200,000 cases per year as compared with half that number two decades ago.[49,50] Understandably, many authorities describe skin cancer as an epidemic, particularly affecting elderly people.

Ultraviolet irradiation, particularly ultraviolet B (290–320 nm, sunburn spectrum) is the major causative agent of skin cancer. The incidence of BCC and SCC rises with increased cumulative ultraviolet exposure, as assessed by lifelong geographic residence, employment, and recreational histories. Melanoma, with the exception of lentigo maligna melanoma (see below), is better correlated with intense intermittent exposures, such as those causing blistering sunburns.[51] Other risk factors include male gender and the interrelated features of fair skin, freckling, blue or light colored eyes, red or blond hair, and a tendency to sunburn rather than tan.[52]

A history of a previous BCC or SCC substantially increases an individual's risk for developing another skin cancer of that subtype; in one study the 1, 3, and 5 year risk of a subsequent malignancy developing was as high as 17, 35, and 50 percent respectively.[53] Cigarette smoking is also statistically associated with increased skin cancer risk.[53]

Unlike most malignancies, virtually all skin cancers can be recognized early in their course due to their visibility on the skin's surface. Cutaneous malignancies detected and treated at an early stage are nearly always curable, particularly in the case of nonmelanoma skin cancer, whereas malignancies left untreated have a greater risk of cosmetic disfigurement, functional impairment, metastasis, and fatal outcome.

Basal cell carcinomas

Approximately three-fourths of skin cancers are BCCs. Typical early lesions are asymptomatic, firm, opalescent or "pearly" papules, with fine surface telangiectases. Ninety percent occur on the face and neck, but unlike SCC, occurrence on the dorsal hands or forearms is uncommon. BCCs enlarge very slowly, and patients frequently insist that 4 mm lesions have been present for years. The classic, neglected "rodent ulcer" is uncommon today but can still be identified by its firm, opalescent, telangiectatic, rolled border. Differential diagnosis of BCC includes dermal nevi, which are flesh-colored but not as firm, and sebaceous hyperplasia, which is also less firm and is characterized by a slightly yellow color and a central punctum, the sebaceous orifice. Subtypes include nodular BCC, described above; superficial or multicentric BCC, which presents as a scaly red thin plaque often on the trunk, simulating dermatitis or psoriasis; morpheiform BCC, which appears waxy and scar-like and can often extend far beyond its clinically apparent borders; and pigmented BCC with black, brown, and gray pigmentation, often mistaken for a melanoma or seborrheic keratosis.[36]

BCCs have an extremely low incidence of metastasis, and thus mortality is low. However, if the lesion is untreated it may erode into adjacent structures and cause considerable local destruction.

A variety of treatment modalities exist. These include simple excision, micrographic surgery, electrodesiccation and curettage, cryotherapy, and X-irradiation, all of which have 5-year recurrence rates between 1 and 10 percent.[54] Medical therapy of BCCs is considered investigational, but agents that have shown promise include intralesional interferon, intralesional 5-fluorouracil, photodynamic therapy, and topical imiquimod (an immune modulator approved for the treatment of genital warts).[55,56] The appropriate treatment depends on numerous factors, such as the location, histological variant, size, and primary or recurrent status of the BCC, and the general health and cosmetic concerns of the patient.

Squamous cell carcinomas

SCCs occur in the same fair-skinned patient population, primarily in habitually sun-exposed areas, such as the head, neck, and upper extremities, but occasionally in sites of chronic ulceration or other skin damage. Early lesions are asymptomatic, firm red papules or plaques, usually with scale; more advanced lesions tend to ulcerate. Differential diagnosis includes premalignant actinic keratoses and, in the case of verrucous lesions, viral warts. Biopsy of suspect lesions is always indicated.

Like BCC, most SCCs are only locally invasive, but 2–10 percent metastasize.[52,57] Factors predisposing to metastasis are location on the lip or in areas of chronic inflammation, scarring or sites of prior ionizing irradiation, size greater than 1 cm in diameter and greater than 4 mm in thickness, and immunosuppression.[51] Treatment is usually simple excision or micrographic surgery.

Actinic keratoses

Actinic keratoses (AKs) are SCC precursor lesions. They occur in the same distribution, namely the head, neck, dorsal hands, and arms. Clinically, they appear as rough, scaly, pink-red, poorly circumscribed macules. Identification is sometimes easier by palpation than by visualization. Induration may be a sign of progression to invasive SCC or simply a manifestation of inflammation, and such lesions require biopsy to guide therapy. Multiple lesions are common. The rate of progression to invasive SCC for individual AKs is difficult to ascertain, and estimates range from less than 1 per 1,000 per year to 20 percent, although the true rate is probably closer to the former. An estimated 10–36 percent regress spontaneously,[58] particularly with sun avoidance.[59]

Initial treatment of individual AKs is usually cryotherapy.[60] Topical fluorouracil or masoprocol cream are often employed when numerous lesions are present, but unfortunately significant skin irritation is associated with their use and recurrences are common. Other destructive treatment modalities include curettage, dermabrasion and chemical peels; laser resurfacing has been associated with a high risk of recurrence of cutaneous malignancies.[61] Recently, topical photodynamic therapy for treatment of AKs has been FDA-approved for use in the United States. Regular application of a high sun-protection factor (SPF) sunscreen has been demonstrated to decrease the number of AKs.[59,62] Not all lesions require treatment, but all patients with multiple AKs should be monitored at least annually because of their high statistical risk of skin cancer of all types.

Malignant melanoma

Malignant melanoma is rare in comparison with nonmelanoma skin cancer, but in the United States it is now more common than Hodgkin's disease or thyroid carcinoma,[49] and incidence is increasing faster than for any other cancer.[63] Age-specific incidence increases throughout life, with statistically excess mortality among older men.[64] Even more than with other cutaneous malignancies, successful treatment depends on early recognition.

Clinical criteria for the diagnosis of melanoma have been extensively reviewed.[65] Signs include diameter greater than 6 mm, variation in color (red, white, and blue areas within a brown-black lesion), irregular border, and irregular surface topography. Bleeding and pain are late findings. The extremely common seborrheic or senile keratoses can usually be differentiated by their "stuck on" quality, even brown pigmentation, and "regularly irregular" surface. Any change or rapid growth of an existing nevus or new pigmented lesion arising in an elderly individual is suspect, however.

As is the case with BCCs, there are several clinical subtypes of melanoma. The most common type is superficial spreading melanoma, accounting for approximately 70 percent of cases. Lentigo maligna melanoma, arising from its slow-growing precursor, lentigo maligna, is often a large lesion with varied pigmentation, and occurs on sun-exposed surfaces, usually the face. It accounts for 10 percent of melanomas overall and occurs almost exclusively in elderly people. A lentigo maligna may be confused with a benign solar lentigo so that very large lesions, lesions with variegated color, or those reported as undergoing change, must be biopsied. Nodular melanomas are rapidly growing lesions that tend to invade deeply early in their course, with a resultant poor prognosis. Acrolentigenous melanoma, by definition a lesion of the hands and feet, often periungual, is the most common form of melanoma in blacks and Asians. A variant of this type of melanoma occurs on mucosal surfaces. Amelanotic melanoma accounts for less than 1 percent of all subtypes and poses a particular diagnostic challenge, owing to its lack of pigmentation.

The most important prognostic indicator in melanoma is the Breslow tumor thickness, the depth of malignant cell invasion as determined histologically. Five-year survival for lesions less than 0.76 mm thick is 96 percent, and for lesions between 0.76 and 1.49 mm, 87 percent, whereas survival falls to 75, 66, and 47 percent for lesions 1.5–2.49 mm, 2.5–3.99 mm, and greater than 4 mm thick, respectively. In general, older patients have a worse prognosis than younger ones.[65]

Surgical excision is the mainstay of treatment, and recommended margins of excision increase with tumor thickness. Sentinel lymph node biopsy utilizing dyes and radioactive tracers to track to the draining lymph node basin, and in particular the first (sentinel) draining lymph node, at the time of definitive melanoma excision is being used to select high-risk patients for adjuvant therapy with alpha-interferon or melanoma vaccine. Sentinel lymph node guided elective lymph node dissection also may improve survival of selected patients with intermediate thickness melanoma (1–2 mm).[66] As expected, sentinel lymph node metastasis has been shown to be a predictor of recurrence and death due to metastatic disease.[67,68] Patients diagnosed with melanoma must be closely monitored for local recurrence, metastasis, or development of a second primary melanoma, for which they are at increased risk. Such follow-up is best done by a physician with extensive experience in this field.

PHOTOAGING

Many older persons are distressed by the appearance of their skin. Treatment of the changes due to lifelong sun exposure is beneficial for many reasons. Medically, photodamaged skin demonstrates keratinocyte atypia and an increased rate of development of malignant skin lesions. Destruction of the photodamaged epidermis and subsequent re-epitheliazation, thus logically reduces this risk. Treatment may also provide a substantial morale boost; as well, participation in a comprehensive treatment regimen expected to improve their appearance may motivate otherwise noncompliant patients to avoid further sun exposure and thus reduce their skin cancer risk further (see above). Treatment of photoaging includes

medical therapies (below), chemical and physical resurfacing, injection of filler substances into skin folds, and denervation of motor nerves with botulinum toxin to erase expression lines.

It is now well established that sun avoidance and regular sunscreen use for periods as brief as 6–7 months can improve the skin's appearance[69–71] and permit regression of AKs.[59] Daily application of tretinoin 0.05–0.1 percent for 4–6 months in the context of such a regimen gives further improvement, with decreases in roughness, fine wrinkling, and mottled hyperpigmentation in 60–80 percent of patients[69–71] and an approximately 60 percent reduction in size and number of AKs.[72] Histological studies have established that tretinoin therapy reduces and redistributes epidermal melanin[73,74] and increases collagen deposition in the superficial dermis,[75] leading to lighter, more even skin color and decreased wrinkling, respectively. The mechanism of tretinoin's effect on AK regression is not known, but is presumably the same as for other retinoid compounds' antineoplastic effects.[76] In addition to treating pre-existing photoaging, topical tretinoin may prevent further damage via its inhibition of ultraviolet-induced collagen destruction.[77]

Tretinoin 0.05 percent, and more recently 0.02 percent, emollient cream are approved for the indication of photoaging in the United Kingdom as Retinova and in the United States as Renova, is customarily applied at bedtime to the face, dorsa of the hands, and other target areas. Moisturizer and sunscreen are applied in the morning. During the first weeks of treatment, nearly all patients experience retinoid dermatitis, consisting of erythema scaling, and itching or burning.[69–72] For most, symptoms are mild, peak at approximately 2 weeks, and then abate. Patients should be instructed to skip occasional days of application as necessary until their skin accommodates. As during other forms of topical chemotherapy, AKs may "light up," becoming more apparent during the early weeks of therapy. Treatment may be continued indefinitely, although improvement in appearance may plateau after 6–12 months. Less frequent tretinoin applications may then permit prior benefit to be retained in many patients.

Preparations containing α-hydroxyacids (AHAs) such as lactic acid or glycolic acid also improve the appearance of photodamaged skin when applied daily for several months[78,79] and may be less irritating than tretinoin, although in general less information is available regarding their effects. Preparations with up to 10 percent AHA are available over the counter, and higher concentrations are typically dispensed by or applied in dermatologists' offices. AHA-containing moisturizers are also highly effective in removing the hyperkeratosis (retained scale) often present on the extremities of older patients, as well as in areas of photodamage.

Systemic estrogen replacement may have a beneficial effect on skin aging, perhaps increasing skin thickness via its effects on collagen and elastic fibers. This beneficial effect has been debated; further studies are ongoing.[80,81]

BULLOUS PEMPHIGOID

Bullous pemphigoid (BP) is an idiopathic, antibody-mediated disease, which can be differentiated clinically, histologically, and immunologically from the much less common pemphigus vulgaris. Elderly people are affected far more commonly than young adults, and BP is the most common immune-mediated blistering disease affecting older patients. The disease is self-limited, lasting months to years, with recurrences following disease-free periods in a minority of patients.[82] Untreated, it ranges in severity from mild to disabling, and the resulting prolonged loss of an effective cutaneous barrier may be fatal. Certain medications, especially neuroleptics and diuretics may trigger or worsen BP.[83]

BP is characterized clinically by tense bullae arising on either erythematous or normal-appearing skin. Preceding or accompanying pruritus is common and may be intense. Crusted erosions and urticarial wheals may coexist with intact bullae, and hemorrhagic bullae are not unusual. Lesions occur most often on the trunk and proximal extremities, with a predilection for flexural surfaces. Approximately one-third of patients have oral blisters, although, unlike pemphigus vulgaris, the mouth is rarely the initial site of involvement. In some patients, bullae remain localized to one area for several months, and in a few, the lesions never become widespread.

Diagnosis is confirmed by skin biopsy. Immunofluorescent staining of perilesional skin is virtually, pathognomonic, showing linear deposition along the basement membrane zone of C_3 (third component of complement) in all patients and of IgG in most. Indirect immunofluorescent studies demonstrate anti-basement-membrane zone antibodies of the IgG class in approximately 70 percent of patients.[82] Recently developed, more sensitive, enzyme-linked immunosorbent assay (ELISA) techniques detect a higher number of circulating antibodies, but these tests, however, are not yet commercially available.[84]

The two recognized autoantibodies in BP are components of the hemidesmosome,[85] a structure that attaches the basal keratinocyte to the basement membrane. Immune-mediated disruption of this attachment leads to dermoepidermal separation and blister formation.

Corticosteroids are the first line of therapy. In mild or localized cases, topical or intralesional steroids may control the lesions, but almost all patients require systemic treatment at least initially. Patients with extensive or rapidly progressive disease should begin therapy with prednisone, 60–100 mg daily (some authors recommend two to three times this dose). Patients should be re-evaluated at weekly intervals and the prednisone dose slowly and progressively reduced once new blisters cease forming and clinical remission is achieved. If long-term prednisone use is anticipated, monitoring for side-effects and protection against osteoporosis (bone density testing, calcium and vitamin D supplementation; and if indicated, hormone replacement, bisphosphonate or calcitonin therapy) must be implemented.[86] An immunosuppressant such as azathioprine, low-dose methotrexate, or mycophenolate mofetil may be added to the regimen initially or at the time of remission in order to reduce the prednisone requirement.[82,87–89] Determination of thiopurine methyl transferase levels should be determined before azathioprine administration since patients with very low levels are at high risk of pancytopenia.[90] Six to 8 weeks are required for full expression of the steroid-sparing effect. Patients with less severe disease may initiate therapy with 40–60 mg of prednisone on alternate days and/or an immunosuppressant. More severe cases may require cyclophosphamide, chlorambucil, cyclosporin, pulse steroids, or plasmapheresis.[91] In all patients, drug dosages are decreased

gradually to zero over many months, provided the disease remains in remission. Recently, successful therapy with tetracycline (500 mg four times a day) and nicotinamide (500 mg three times a day) has been suggested as an alternative to prednisone.[92] Sulfapyridine or sulfones are also alternative therapies for patients with major contraindications to systemic steroids. Most patients achieve prolonged remissions and can ultimately discontinue treatment without recurrence of lesions. However, the possibility of disease exacerbation and the potential complications of therapy require close, expert monitoring of all patients throughout the course of their disease.

KEY POINTS   Skin diseases and old age

- Skin diseases and related symptoms are extremely common in elderly people.

- Skin disorders in elderly people are rarely life threatening, but detract substantially from the quality of life and often lower self-esteem and psychosocial well-being.

- Lifelong environmental impacts on skin, particularly sun exposure, account for the majority of age-associated changes in skin appearance and for skin cancer risk.

- Patients with herpes zoster benefit from antiviral therapy if begun within the first 3 days of the illness.

- Generalized pruritus may be due to occult systemic disease, although xerosis is often a contributing factor and may be the only identifiable factor.

- Skin cancer is the most common malignancy and its incidence increases exponentially with age.

REFERENCES

1. Fleischer Jr AB, McFarlane M, Hinds MA et al: Skin conditions and symptoms are common in the elderly: the prevalence of skin symptoms and conditions in an elderly population. J Geriatr Dermatol 1996;4:78–87
2. Beauregard S, Gilchrest BA: A survey of skin problems and skin care regimens in the elderly. Arch Dermatol 1987;123:1638–1643
3. Tindal JP: Skin changes and lesions in our senior citizens: incidences. Cutis 1976;18:359–362
4. Lutsky NS: Attitudes toward old age and elderly persons. In Eisdorfer C (ed): Annual Review of Gerontology and Geriatrics. Springer, New York, 1980:287–336
5. Gilchrest BA: Skin and Aging Processes. CRC Press, Boca Raton, FL, 1984
6. Gilchrest BA: Age-associated changes in the skin. J Am Geriatr Soc 1982;30:139–143
7. Gilchrest BA: Photodamage. Blackwell Science, Cambridge, MA, 1995
8. Dolan NC, Ng JS, Martin GJ et al: Effectiveness of a skin cancer control education intervention for internal medicine housestaff and attending physicians. J Geriatr Intern Med 1997;12(9):531–536
9. American Academy of Dermatology National Skin Cancer Screening Database 1986–99
10. Bruce AJ, Brodland DG: Overview of skin cancer detection and prevention for the primary care physician. Mayo Clin Proc 2000;75:491–500
11. Woodwell DA, Schappert SM: National Ambulatory Medical Care Survey: 1993 Summary. Advance Data from Vital and Health Statistics Number 40. National Center for Health Statistics, Hyattsville, 1995
12. Kost RG, Straus SE: Postherpetic neuralgia-pathogenesis, treatment, and prevention. N Engl J Med 1996;335:32–42
13. Liesegang TJ: Varicella zoster viral disease. Mayo Clin Proc 1999;74:983–998

14. Lee JJ, Gauci CAG: Postherpetic neuralgia: current concepts and management. Br J Hosp Med 1994;52:565–570
15. Huff JC, Bean B, Balfour HH et al: Therapy of herpes zoster with oral acyclovir. Am J Med 1988;85(suppl 2A):84–89
16. Alper BS, Lewis PR: Does treatment of acute herpes zoster prevent or shorten postherpetic neuralgia? A systemic review of the literature. J Fam Proc 2000;49(3):255–264
17. Wood MJ, Ogan PH, McKendrick MW et al: Efficacy of oral acyclovir treatment of acute herpes zoster. Am J Med 1988;85(suppl 2A):79–83
18. Cobo M: Reduction of the ocular complications of herpes zoster ophthalmicus by oral acyclovir. Am J Med 1988;85(suppl 2A):90–93
19. Tyring S, Barbarash RA, Nahlik JE et al: Famciclovir for the treatment of acute herpes zoster: effects on acute disease and postherpetic neuralgia, a randomized, double blind, placebo controlled trial. Ann Intern Med 1995;123:89–96
20. Beutner KR, Friedman DJ, Forszpaniak C et al: Valcyclovir compared with acyclovir for improved therapy for herpes zoster in immunocompetent adults. Antimicrob Agents Chemother 1995;39:1546–1553
21. Wood MJ, Johnson RW, McKendrick MW et al: A randomized trial of acyclovir for 7 days or 21 days with and without prednisolone for treatment of acute herpes zoster. N Engl J Med 1994;330:896–900
22. Bernstein JE, Korman NJ, Bickers DR et al: Topical capsaicin treatment of chronic postherpetic neuralgia. J Am Acad Dermatol 1989;21:265–270
23. Rowbotham MC: Treatment of postherpetic neuralgia. Semin Dermatol 1992;11:218–225
24. Rowbotham M, Harden N, Stacey B et al: Gabapentin for treatment of postherpetic neuralgia: a randomized controlled trial. JAMA 1998;280(21):1837–1842
25. Klecz RJ, Schwartz RA: Pruritus. Am Fam Physician 1992;45:2681–2686
26. Gilchrest BA: Pruritus: pathogenesis, therapy and significance in systemic disease states. Arch Intern Med 1982;142:101–105
27. Lewiecki MEM, Rahman F: Pruritus: a manifestation of iron deficiency. JAMA 1976;236:2319–2320
28. Salem HH, Van der Weyden MB, Young IF et al: Pruritus and severe iron deficiency in polycythemia vera. Br Med J 1982;285:91–92
29. Ghadially R, Brown BE, Sequeira-Martin SM et al: The aged epidermal permeability barrier: structural, functional, and lipid biochemical abnormalities in humans and a senescent murine model. J Clin Invest 1995;95:2281–2290
30. Gilchrest BA: Pruritus in the elderly. Semin Dermatol 1995;14:317–319
31. Fleischer AB: Pruritus in the elderly: management by senior dermatologists. J Am Acad Dermatol 1993;28:603–609
32. Metze D, Reimann S, Beissert S et al: Efficacy and safety of naltrexone, an oral opiate receptor antagonist, in the treatment of pruritus in internal and dermatologic disease. J Am Acad Dermatol 1999;41(4):533–539
33. Kligman AM: Perspectives and problems in cutaneous gerontology. J Invest Dermatol 1979;73:39–46
34. Tagami H: Quantitative measurements of water concentration of the stratum corneum in vivo by high-frequency current. Acta Derm Venereol 1994;185:29–33
35. Engelke M, Jensen J-M, Ekanayake-Mudiyanselage S et al: Effects of xerosis and aging on epidermal proliferation and differentiation. Br J Dermatol 1997;137:219–225
36. Schwindt D, Wilhelm K-P, Miller DL, Maibach HI: Cumulative irritation in older and younger skin: a comparison. Acta Derm Venereol (Stockh) 1998;78:279–283
37. Dahl M, Katz HI, Krueger GG et al: Topical metronidazole maintains remissions of rosacea. Arch Dermatol 1998;134(6):679–683
38. Estes SA, Estes J: Therapy of scabies: nursing homes, hospitals, and the homeless. Semin Dermatol 1993;12:26–33
39. Meinking TL, Taplin D, Herminda JL et al: The treatment of scabies with ivermectin. N Engl J Med 1995;333:26–30
40. Altman JS: Ivermectin for scabies. Arch Dermatol 1999;135:1550
41. Barkwell R, Shields S: Deaths associated with ivermectin treatment of scabies. Lancet 1997;349:1144–1145
42. Arndt KA, Jick H: Rates of cutaneous reactions to drugs: a report from the Boston Collaborative Drug Surveillance Program. JAMA 1976;235:918–922. Bigby M, Jick S, Jick H, Arndt K: Drug-induced cutaneous reactions: a report from the Boston Collaborative Drug Surveillance Program on 15,438 consecutive inpatients, 1975 to 1982. JAMA 1986;256:3358–3363
43. Wintroub BU, Stern R: Cutaneous drug reactions: pathogenesis and clinical classification. J Am Acad Dermatol 1985;13:167–179
44. Goldstein SM, Wintroub BU: A Physician's Guide-Adverse Cutaneous Reactions to Medication. CoMedia, New York, 1994
45. Shear NH, Spielberg SP: Anticonvulsant hypersensitivity syndrome: in vitro assessment of risk. J Clin Invest 1988;82:1826–1832
46. Daoud MS, Schanbacher CF, Dicken CH et al: Recognizing cutaneous drug eruptions. Postgrad Med 1998;104(1):101–115
47. Roujeau JC, Stern RS: Severe adverse cutaneous reactions to drugs. N Engl J Med 1994;331:1272–1285
48. Crowson AN, Margo CM: Recent advances in the pathology of cutaneous drug eruptions. Dermatol Clin 1999;17(3):537–560
49. Parker SL, Tong T, Bolden S et al: Cancer statistics, 1996. CA Cancer J Clin 1996;46:5–27
50. Miller DL, Weinstock MA: Nonmelanoma skin cancer in the United States: incidence. J Am Acad Dermatol 1994;30:774–778
51. Elmets CA, Mukhatar H: Ultraviolet radiation and skin cancer: progress in pathophysiologic mechanisms. Prog Dermatol 1995;30:1–16
52. Preston DS, Stern RS: Nonmelanoma cancers of the skin. N Engl J Med 1992;327:1649–1662
53. Karagas MR, Stukel TA, Greenberg ER et al: Risk of subsequent basal cell carcinoma and squamous cell carcinoma of the skin among patients with prior skin cancer. JAMA 1992;267:3305–3310
54. Rowe DE, Carroll RJ, Day CL et al: Long-term recurrence rates in previously untreated (primary) basal cell carcinoma: implications for patient follow-up. J Dermatol Surg Oncol 1989;15:315–328
55. Romagosa R, Saap L, Givens M et al: A pilot study to evaluate the treatment of basal cell carcinoma with 5-fluorouracil using phosphatidyl choline as a transepidermal carrier. Dermatol Surg 2000;26:338–340
56. Beutner KR, Geisse JK, Helman D et al: Therapeutic response of basal cell carcinoma to the immune response modifier imiquimod 5% cream. J Am Acad Dermatol 1999; 41(6):1002–1007
57. Salasche SJ, Cheney ML, Varvares MA et al: Recognition and management of the high-risk cutaneous squamous cell carcinoma. Curr Probl Dermatol 1993;5:141–192
58. Frost CA, Green AC: Epidemiology of solar keratoses. Br J Dermatol 1994;131:455–464
59. Thompson SC, Jolley D, Marks R et al: Reduction of solar keratoses by regular sunscreen use. N Engl J Med 1993;329:1147–1151
60. Feldman SR, Fleischer AB, Williford PM et al: Destructive procedures are the standard of care for treatment of actinic keratoses. J Am Acad Dermatol 1999;40(1):43–47
61. Fulton JE, Rahimi AD, Helton P et al: Disappointing results following resurfacing of facial skin with CO_2 lasers for prophylaxis of keratoses and cancers. Dermatol Surg 1999;25:729–732
62. Naylor MF, Boyd A, Smith DW et al: High sun protection sunscreens in the suppression of actinic neoplasia. Arch Dermatol 1995;131:170–175
63. Ries LAG, Miller BA, Hankey BF et al (eds): SEER Cancer Statistics Review, 1973–1991: Tables and Graphs, National Cancer Institute. NIH Pub. No. 94–2789. Bethesda, MD, 1994;287–299
64. Geller AC, Koh HK, Miller DR et al: Death rates of malignant melanoma among white men: United States, 1973–1988. MMWR 1992;41:20–21, 27
65. Koh HK: Cutaneous melanoma. N Engl J Med 1991;325:171–182
66. Balch CM, Seong SJ, Bartolucci AA et al: Efficacy of elective regional lymph node dissection of 1- to 4-mm thickness melanomas for patients 60 years of age or younger. Ann Surg 1996;224:255–263
67. Leong SP, Achtem TA, Steinmetz I et al: 1999 Am Soc Clin Oncol. Online. Available: http://www.asco.org
68. Essner R, Foshag LJ, Glass E et al: 1999 Am Soc Clin Oncol. Online. Available: http://www.asco.org
69. Weinstein GD, Nigra TP, Pochi PE et al: Topical tretinoin for treatment of photodamaged skin: a multicenter study. Arch Dermatol 1991;127:659–665
70. Olsen EA, Katz HI, Levine N et al: Tretinoin emollient cream: a new therapy for photodamaged skin. J Am Acad Dermatol 1992;26:215–224
71. Gilchrest BA: A review of skin ageing and its medical therapy. Br J Dermatol 1996;135:867–875
72. Kligman AM, Thorne EG: Topical therapy of actinic keratoses with tretinoin. In Marks R (ed): Retinoids in Cutaneous Malignancy. Blackwell Scientific, Oxford, 1991:66–73
73. Bhawan J, Gonzalez-Serva A, Nehal K et al: Effects of tretinoin on photodamaged skin: a histologic study. Arch Dermatol 1991;127:666–672
74. Rafal ES, Griffiths CEM, Ditre CM et al: Topical tretinoin (retinoic acid) treatment for liver spots associated with photodamage. N Engl J Med 1992;326:368–374
75. Griffiths CEM, Russman AN, Majmudar G et al: Restoration of collagen formation in photodamaged human skin by tretinoin (retinoic acid). N Engl J Med 1993;329:530–535

76. Moon RC, Itri LM: Retinoids and cancer. In Sporn MB, Roberts AB, Goodman DS (eds): The Retinoids, Vol 2. Academic Press, New York; 1984:327–372

77. Fisher GJ, Datta SC, Talwar HS et al: Molecular basis of sun-induced premature skin ageing and retinoid antagonism. Nature 1996;379:335–339

78. Ditre CM, Griffin TD, Murphy GF et al: Effects of alpha hydroxy acids on photoaged skin: a pilot clinical, histologic, and ultrastructural study. J Am Acad Dermatol 1996;34:187–195

79. Stiller MJ, Bartalone J, Stern R et al: Topical 8% glycolic acid and 8% L-lactic lactic acid creams for the treatment of photodamaged skin. Arch Dermatol 1996;132:631–636

80. Brincat MP: Hormone replacement therapy and the skin: beneficial effects: the case in favor of it. Acta Obstret Gynecol Scand 2000;79:244–249

81. Oikarinen A: Systemic estrogens have no conclusive effect on human skin connective tissue. Acta Obstret Gynecol Scand 2000;79:250–254

82. Mutasim DF: Bullous pemphigoid: review and update. J Geriatr Dermatol 1993;1:62–71

83. Bastuji-Garin S, Joly P, Picard-Dahan C et al: Drugs associated with bullous pemphigoid. Arch Dermatol 1996;132:272–276

84. Zillikens D, Mascaro JM, Rose RA et al: A highly sensitive enzyme-linked immunosorbent assay for detection of circulating anti BP 180 autoantibodies in patients with bullous pemphigoid. J Invest Dermatol 1997;109(5):679–683

85. Ishiko A, Shimizu H, Kikuchi A et al: Human autoantibodies against the 230-kD bullous pemphigoid antigen (BPAG1) bind only to the intracellular domain of the hemidesmosome, whereas those against the 180-kD bullous pemphigoid antigen (BPAG2) bind along the plasma membrane of the hemidesmosome in normal human and swine skin. J Clin Invest 1993;91:1608–1615

86. American College of Rheumatology Task Force on Osteoporosis Guidelines: Recommendations for the prevention and treatment of glucocorticoid-induced osteoporosis. Arthritis Rheum 1996; 39(11):1791–1801

87. Fine JD: Management of acquired bullous skin diseases. N Engl J Med 1995;333:1475–1484

88. Paul MA, Jorizzo JL, Fleischer AB et al: Low-dose methotrexate treatment in elderly patients with bullous pemphigoid. J Am Acad Dermatol 1994;31:620–625

89. Nousari HC, Griffin WA, Anhalt, GJ et al: Successful therapy for bullous pemphigoid with mycophenolate mofetil. J Am Acad Dermatol 1998;39(3):497–498

90. Snow JL, Gibson LE: The role of genetic variation in thiopurine methyltransferase activity and efficacy of azathioprine therapy in dermatologic patients. Arch Dermatol 1995;131:193–197

91. Scott JE, Ahmed AR: The blistering diseases. Med Clin North Am 1998;82(6):1239–1283

92. Fivenson DP, Breneman DL, Rosen GB et al: Nicotinamide and tetracycline therapy of bullous pemphigoid. Arch Dermatol 1994;130:753–758

Problem-based geriatric medicine

Chapter 101

Geriatric pharmacotherapy

*Joseph T. Hanlon, Catherine Lindblad,
Robert L. Maher, and Kenneth Schmader*

Pharmaceuticals are the most frequently used and misused form of therapy for the medical problems of elderly people. Geriatricians and their patients rely heavily on pharmacotherapy to palliate symptoms, improve functional status and quality of life, cure or manage diseases, and prolong survival. In the past 20 years there has been a major increase in our knowledge about the epidemiology and the clinical pharmacology of drugs in elderly people (see Chapter 14). The purpose of this chapter is to examine efficacy and problems of drug therapy in aged populations, measures to reduce drug-related problems in elderly people, and principles of optimal geriatric pharmacotherapy.

EFFICACY OF DRUG THERAPY FOR ELDERLY PATIENTS

The evidence for the efficacy of drug therapy in elderly patients has been bolstered in recent years by a number of seminal randomized controlled clinical trials for geriatric conditions (e.g. chronic pain) and diseases (e.g. isolated systolic hypertension).[1,2] Moreover, a number of new and improved therapeutic drug entities have come to market and improved the ability of healthcare professionals to treat certain conditions (e.g. cholinesterase inhibitors for Alzheimer's disease, alpha-blockers for prostatic hyperplasia, bisphosphonates for osteoporosis). In addition, the future seems bright for further drug discoveries that may benefit elderly people as nearly 700 new medicines are currently in Phase I to Phase III testing.[3]

Despite these optimistic trends, there are still major limitations in our knowledge regarding the efficacy of geriatric pharmacotherapy. Elderly patients are still under-represented in premarketing clinical drug trials.[4–6] While regulatory authorities have developed guidelines for pharmaceutical companies regarding new molecular entities that are likely to have significant use in elderly patients, the full impact of these guidelines has yet to be realized.[7] In addition, those trials that do include elders rarely include the "oldest-old" (i.e., 85+), those with multiple comorbidities, or those taking multiple medications.[4–6] These exclusions raise questions about the generalizability of the results to frail elderly people. Moreover, there are a paucity of post-marketing studies designed to compare the "effectiveness" of two drugs in the treatment of common conditions (e.g. desipramine vs gabapentin in management of postherpetic neuralgia). This makes it difficult for prescribers to choose the "best" drug therapy for their frail elderly patients. In part, these deficiencies in pre- and post-marketing evaluation of efficacy led to the development of Centers for Education and Research on Therapeutics in the USA (although none of the current centers focuses on elderly people).[8,9]

DRUG-RELATED PROBLEMS IN ELDERLY PATIENTS

The benefits of drug therapy in elderly patients are counterbalanced by the problems they pose. There are three major drug-related problems in elderly patients: (1) adverse drug reactions (ADRs), defined as "any response to a drug that is noxious and unintended and that occurs in doses in man for prophylaxis, diagnosis or therapy, excluding failure to accomplish the intended purpose"; (2) adverse drug withdrawal events (ADWEs), defined as a clinical set of symptoms or signs that are related to the removal of a drug; and (3) therapeutic failure, defined as a failure to accomplish the goals of treatment resulting from inadequate drug therapy and not related to the natural progression of disease.[10–12] Drug-related problems were cited in a recent Institute of Medicine report as a major patient-safety concern, especially in hospitals.[13] Two recent cost-of-illness analyses in the USA suggest that morbidity and mortality associated with drug-related problems cost an estimated $177.4 billion per year in ambulatory patients and an estimated $4 billion per year in nursing home residents.[14,15]

One potential source of information about drug-related problems in elderly patients is pre-marketing clinical trials but trials have a number of limitations. Pre-marketing clinical trials do not examine ADWEs and therapeutic failure so one must rely on clinical experience and published data in the post-marketing period to glean information about these problems. Pre-marketing clinical trial data on the adverse effects of pre-scription medications in elderly patients have been limited by the exclusion of elderly patients from trials of investigational drugs and by the small sample sizes of most Phase III trials.[4–6] In addition, a recent publication highlighted that researchers tend to under-report drug safety problems.[16] Formal post-marketing surveillance of drugs varies from country to country but usually it consists of case reports of potential ADRs by practitioners to medical journals or spontaneous reports by practitioners, patients, or pharmaceutical companies to regulatory agencies.[11] These methods are limited by under-reporting and the lack of denominator information about the population at risk. Thus, most ADR information must come from formal post-marketing observational studies of specific therapeutic classes or conditions. In part, these deficiencies in pre- and post-marketing evaluation of safety led to the development of the US Centers of Excellence for Patient Safety Research and Practice.[17]

Adverse drug reactions

Several authors have reviewed the epidemiology of ADRs.[11,18–20] The following paragraph summarizes data and highlights one or two major studies on the occurrence of ADRs leading to hospitalization, in hospital, in outpatient settings and in long-term care facilities, in that order.

One of the worst adverse consequences of drug therapy is hospitalization. The prevalence of ADR-related hospitalizations in studies of ambulatory elderly patients ranges from 3 to 17 percent. Mannesse et al. evaluated hospital admissions in patients over 70 years old during a 3-month period at a university teaching hospital in the Netherlands. Of 106 admissions, 13 patients (12 percent) were admitted probably because of an ADR.[21,22] Hallas et al. studied 1,999 admissions from six different types of medical wards that provide care to elderly persons in a defined region of Denmark and found a 7.9 percent incidence of ADRs leading to hospitalization.[23] Once hospitalized, the percentage of elderly patients experiencing ADRs range from 1.5 to 44 percent.[11] In the largest prospective study of ADRs in hospitalized patients, Carbonin et al. evaluated 9,148 patients over a 2-month period in 41 Italian hospitals.[24] Seven hundred eighty-eight (8.6 percent) patients experienced an ADR; 567 (6.2 percent) of the patient population was 60 years of age and older. Thomas et al. evaluated all types of adverse events in 15,000 hospitalized patients in Colorado and Utah, USA and discovered that elderly patients had significantly higher rates of preventable ADRs than the younger cohort (0.63 vs 0.17 percent, respectively).[25] Few investigators have studied ADRs in elderly outpatients and the prevalence rate of existing studies varies widely from 2.5 to 50.6 percent. In a carefully sampled, population-based study, Chrischilles et al. documented that 10 percent of 3,170 elderly residents of rural Iowa, USA, reported adverse drug events in the previous year.[26] In a group of outpatients taking five or more medications in North Carolina, USA, Hanlon et al. documented that 35 percent of 167 patients experienced an adverse drug event over a year, with 11 percent requiring hospitalization.[27] Studies of ADRs in the nursing home setting have revealed a prevalence ranging from 9.5 to 50.2 percent. Gurwitz et al. studied the occurrence of ADRs in 18 Massachusetts, USA, nursing homes.[28] Over a 1-year period, they found that 2,916 nursing home residents had 546 ADRs, an incidence rate of 1.89 ADRs per 100 patient-months. Nearly 44 percent of the ADRs were fatal, life-threatening or serious and 72 percent were preventable.[28] Collectively, these studies from a variety of settings document that ADRs are common phenomena in elderly patients.

ADR risk factors

Multiple medication use, multiple comorbidities and specific types of drugs increase the risk of ADRs in elderly patients.[11] Multiple medication use is an important factor because it is potentially modifiable. However, the reduction of number of medications in elderly patients with multiple diseases may be difficult because the diseases often require pharmacotherapy. It is also difficult to avoid the drug classes most associated with ADRs because these drug classes are essential to the management of older persons. While age and gender have previously been considered risk factors for ADRs in elderly patients, recent studies using multivariate analyses and controlling for known risk factors have found no association between age and gender and ADRs.[11,25]

Investigators have suspected that a previous history of an ADR, age-related alterations in pharmacokinetics and pharmacodynamics, fragmented medical care, suboptimal prescribing, and medication adherence influence the risk of ADRs, but study findings have been mixed. The latter two items are clinically important and will be discussed further below.

There are two major categories of suboptimal prescribing that may contribute to ADRs: (1) overuse or polypharmacy, and (2) inappropriate use.[29] While information is available about average drug use for elders by setting (see Chapter 14), there is limited information about polypharmacy defined as the administration of more medications than are clinically indicated.[29] In two separate ambulatory care studies in the USA, between 55 and 59 percent of elders were taking one or more potentially unnecessary drugs.[30,31] This problem is suspected to be higher in the nursing home setting; however, definitive studies are lacking.[32]

Inappropriate prescribing can be defined as prescribing that does not agree with accepted medical standards.[29] Epidemiological studies have found that 22 percent of community-dwelling elderly persons in the USA used medications that should be avoided in that age group.[33] Schmader et al. found that 74 percent of 1,644 drugs prescribed for 208 elderly ambulatory patients in the USA had one or more prescribing problems.[31] The most prevalent problem areas were incorrect and impractical directions, use of expensive drugs, and incorrect dosage. Of note is the lack of findings for clinically significant drug–drug interactions. Although commonly thought to be a major cause of drug-related problems in elderly patients, evidence-based data would suggest otherwise.[34] Recently, Osborne et al. evaluated prescribing for elderly inpatients in 19 hospitals in England and Wales using clinical review with explicit criteria.[35] Benzodiazepines prescribing was appropriate in only one-third of users. Other problems were noted with the coprescriptions of angiotensin-converting-enzyme inhibitor with a potassium-sparing diuretic or potassium supplement, and steroids with beta 2-adrenoceptor agonists. Finally, 40 percent of nursing home patients in the USA used medications that should be avoided in elderly patients.[36]

Medication adherence may also be a risk factor for ADRs. Approximately 50 percent of elderly patients are nonadherent with one or more of their medications, which is a rate similar to that in younger patients.[37,38] Intentional (some would say "intelligent") nonadherence may be more common in elderly than in younger individuals because of the presence of ADRs or the perception that they take too many medications.[38–41] Although nonadherence rates seem high, elderly patients may be compliant with up to 75 percent of their total number of medications, overall.[42] Overuse of medications is a type of medication adherence problem which could lead to ADRs and seems to be uncommon in elderly patients, although more data are needed.[41]

Adverse drug withdrawal events

ADWEs are a clinical set of symptoms or signs that are related to the removal of a drug.[11] The clinical manifestation of an ADWE may be either one of a physiological withdrawal reaction of the drug (e.g. beta-blocker withdrawal syndrome) or an exacerbation of the underlying disease itself.[43,44]

Clinicians and investigators have reported numerous cases of ADWEs but there have been few studies of this phenomenon in elderly patients. Gerety et al. investigated ADWEs in a single nursing home in Texas, USA, over an 18-month time period and found that 62 nursing home patients experienced a total of 94 ADWEs (mean 0.54 per patient), corresponding to an incidence of 0.32 reactions per patient-month.[45] Cardiovascular (37 percent), central nervous system (22 percent), and gastrointestinal drug classes were the most frequently associated with an ADWE. Over 27 percent of ADWEs were rated as severe. A study of ambulatory elderly patients by Graves et al. in the USA investigated ADWEs in 124 patients and discovered that out of 238 drugs stopped, 62 (26 percent) resulted in 72 ADWEs in 38 patients.[46] Cardiovascular (42 percent) and central nervous system (18 percent) drug classes were the most frequently associated with an ADWE. In 26 of the ADWEs (36 percent), patients required hospitalization, emergency room, or urgent care clinic visits. Most of the ADWEs were exacerbations of an underlying disease and some withdrawal events occurred up to 4 months after the medication was discontinued. Finally, in a more recent study, by Kennedy et al., ADWEs were investigated in the postoperative period in a single hospital.[47] Of 1,025 patients studied, 50 percent were over the age of 60 years. Thirty-four patients suffered post-surgical complications due to drug therapy withdrawal. Specific drug classes involved in ADWEs included antihypertensives (especially angiotensin-converting-enzyme inhibitors), antiparkinson medications (especially levodopa/carbidopa), benzodiazepines, and antidepressants.

ADWE risk factors

Little is known about the risk factors for ADWEs. In the study by Gerety et al., ADWEs were associated with multiple diagnoses, multiple medications, longer nursing home stays, and being hospitalized.[45] Graves et al. found that the number of medications stopped was a significant predictor of ADWEs.[46]

Analyses by Kennedy et al. revealed that the risk of an ADWE increased as the length of time off medication increased.[47]

Therapeutic failure

Therapeutic failure is defined by Grymonpre et al. as a failure to accomplish the goals of treatment resulting from inadequate or inappropriate drug therapy and not related to the natural progression of disease.[12] In addition to this definition, therapeutic failure can also be defined as a lack of therapeutic effect due to nonadherence, recent dose reduction/discontinuation, interaction, low prescribed dose or inadequate therapeutic monitoring.[23] Bootman et al. described treatment failure as a negative therapeutic outcome (not a new medical problem) that was due to a drug-related problem.[15] Despite taking on several meanings, the unfortunate similarity is that therapeutic failure may result in adverse outcomes in elderly patients including hospitalization, emergency department (ED) visits and nursing home admission. In a group of older Canadians, 19 percent of drug-associated hospital admissions were related to therapeutic failure.[12] Bero et al. found that 23 percent of drug-related problems leading to hospitalization in the USA were due to lack of a necessary drug therapy as well as under-dosage.[48] Other studies have reported rates of hospital admissions due to therapeutic failure around 2–3 percent.[23,49,50] Tamblyn and colleagues examined the impact of introducing drug cost-sharing on use of essential medications (defined as medications that prevent deterioration in health or prolong life) and the rates of ED visits. They found that increased cost-sharing for prescription drugs in elderly patients was followed by reductions in use of essential drugs and higher rates of ED visits.[51] Another study showed that limiting reimbursement of medications to Medicaid enrollees more than doubled the risk of admission of frail, low-income, elderly patients to a nursing home.[52]

Therapeutic failure risk factors

A major factor related to therapeutic failure is underuse of medications. Underuse is a problem of both suboptimal prescribing and patient nonadherence. The most common types of medication nonadherence in elderly patients are under- or erratic use.[41] Major and associates studied causes of therapeutic failure in children and adults, and found that 58 percent of the cases were attributable to nonadherence.[50] Nonadherence can also lead to a lack of disease control and hospital admissions or readmissions.[53] Sullivan and colleagues performed a meta-analysis of studies published before 1989, including patients of all age, and determined that the rate of hospital admissions due to nonadherence was 5.5 percent.[54] In 1990, one study evaluated 315 consecutive elderly hospital admissions and determined that 11.4 percent of those were due to nonadherence.[55]

From the standpoint of suboptimal prescribing, underutilization or underuse of medications can be defined as the omission of drug therapy that is indicated for the treatment or prevention of a disease or condition.[30] Lipton and colleagues developed a methodology to assess "omitted-but-necessary" drug therapies. They found that 55 percent of 236 ambulatory elderly patients had one or more necessary drug therapies omitted by lack of physician prescribing.[30] In 1998, Redelmeier et al., reported on the undertreatment of unrelated disorders in community-dwelling elders with chronic medical diseases.[56] They found that patients with diabetes mellitus were less likely to receive estrogen-replacement therapy and patients with pulmonary emphysema were less likely to receive lipid-lowering medications.[56] Clinical researchers have also detected underuse of medications in specific conditions. For example, several authors have investigated the underuse of angiotensin-converting-enzyme (ACE) inhibitors in patients with congestive heart failure with rates of use ranging from 33 to 75 percent.[57–62] Similarly, studies have shown that secondary preventive therapy (including aspirin, beta-blockers, and lipid lowering agents) is commonly omitted in older post acute myocardial infarction patients.[63–68]

MEASURES TO REDUCE DRUG-RELATED PROBLEMS IN ELDERLY PATIENTS

Given that drug-related problems are common, costly, and clinically important, how can they be reduced? The specific answer to this question is surprisingly difficult because there are few health services intervention clinical trials in elderly patients that examine measures to reduce ADRs, ADWEs, or therapeutic failure. Therefore, health policy makers and clinicians must look to reasonable, empiric approaches that are based on existing epidemiological and clinical information. These approaches include better systems design, improved health services, patient and family education, systematic medication review by pharmacists, and physician/provider education about optimal prescribing. Physician education will be discussed in the following section on the principles of geriatric pharmacotherapy.

Systems design

Several experts have suggested that faulty system design in the way that drugs are prescribed, dispensed, administered, and monitored induces errors that lead to ADRs or other drug-related problems.[20] The premise for reducing problems is improved system design. Most of the proposed solutions focus on computerized systems, such as computerized physician drug order entry with built-in screening for allergy, drug dosing errors or drug–drug interactions. Most work focuses on hospital patients but the concepts may be applicable to long-term care facilities and outpatient clinics and community pharmacies.

Health services approaches

Geriatric evaluation and management (GEM) units in hospitals or GEM clinics use an interdisciplinary approach to patient management. An important component of GEM is the assessment and management of medications. This attention to medications by GEM clinicians is thought to optimize prescribing and potentially reduce drug-related problems. However, how effectively GEM achieves a reduction in drug-related problems compared to usual care is unknown. Randomized controlled trials of GEM that included drug-related outcomes have shown improved prescribing and a reduction in the number of medications but these studies did not investigate the impact of

GEM on ADRs.[69–71] The GEM Drug Study, a substudy of the VA Cooperative Trial of GEM units and clinics, is investigating the impact of GEM vs usual care on ADRs in elderly patients and hopefully will provide results on the effectiveness of this health service.[72]

Patient education

Systematic education of patients and caregivers about ADRs may increase their ability to better report or avoid potential adverse drug events, thereby allowing clinicians to make medication changes before they become too serious. Likewise, education about ADWEs could prevent a patient or caregiver from stopping a drug abruptly that should be withdrawn slowly. Patient education and compliance aids can improve medication adherence which could potentially improve therapeutic failure due to a patient or caregiver's decision to stop a beneficial drug. The feasibility and effectiveness of more formal, systematic education efforts than what already occur in the course of usual care is unknown.

Systematic medication review

The objective of this type of formal systematic review of medications is to achieve the optimal drug regimen for a patient and hopefully reduce the occurrence of drug-related problems. Drug use evaluation (DUE) is one method where pharmacists use retrospective medication audits to assess drug use, usually in hospital and long-term care facilities. The reviewers develop explicit criteria (i.e., indication, contraindications, dosage, monitoring, outcomes) and apply the criteria to targeted drug classes (i.e., expensive, narrow therapeutic range, used frequently). The results of the review are communicated to the prescribing physician to improve prescribing. Explicit criteria can also be applied to drugs on a population level using large government or healthcare organization patient databases which some authors call drug utilization review (DUR).[29] DUE and DUR detect prescribing problems in elderly patients but whether they reduce drug-related problems is unknown.

PRINCIPLES OF GERIATRIC PHARMACOTHERAPY

Clinicians who care for elderly patients need to know and apply principles of geriatric pharmacotherapy in order to maximize the benefits of drugs in their elderly patients and minimize drug-related problems (Table 101-1). The first step in prescribing is to decide whether drug therapy is really necessary as many medical problems in elderly patients do not require a pharmacological solution. If the clinician decides that a drug is indicated and its benefits outweigh its risks, then the choice of the drug must factor in the drug's pharmacokinetics, the patient's renal and hepatic function, the drug's main potential adverse effects, and the patient's other drugs and diseases. The starting dose for most medications in elderly patients must be smaller, and the interval before modifying the dosage often must be extended. Cost and establishment of clear therapeutic endpoints are also important.

In the ongoing management of the patient and their medications, the clinician should monitor for potential ADRs via the

Table 101-1 Principles of geriatric pharmacotherapy

1. Consider whether drug therapy is necessary
2. Know the pharmacology of the drug in relation to age
3. Know the adverse effect profile of the drug in relation to the patient's other medication(s) and disease(s)
4. Choose initial dose, and adjust it carefully (doses will often need to be smaller in elderly people)
5. Select the least costly alternative
6. Establish clear, feasible therapeutic endpoints
7. Monitor for adverse drug reactions, an important cause of geriatric illness
8. Slowly taper medications to prevent/minimize adverse drug withdrawal events (if possible)
9. Regularly review the need for chronic medications and discontinue unnecessary ones
10. Assess whether there is omission of needed medication for established diagnosis/condition
11. Review compliance, simplify the medication regimen, if possible, and consider use of aids

history, physical examination, and, where appropriate, laboratory data.[11] The identification of ADRs can be a challenging task in elderly patients because their ADRs may present in a vague or atypical fashion and the causal link can be difficult to establish. The first step is to consider ADRs in the differential diagnosis of most geriatric syndromes. If the adverse event is a known side-effect of one or more of the patient's drugs, the clinician can further enhance their confidence in establishing ADR causality by considering the temporal relationship of onset of drug use to onset of event, competing causes, rechallenge, dechallenge, and other factors. Nonetheless, in some cases, the clinician may find it difficult, and sometimes impossible, to establish the ADR causal link between drug effect and illness in elderly patients.

In patients who have recently stopped a medication, it is important to consider the possibility of an ADWE. ADWEs in elderly patients can be overlooked when the withdrawal event is mistaken for a patient's disease state. Common events that may happen in the everyday care of an elderly patient such as discontinuation of unwanted medications, intentional noncompliance, stopping medications prior to a surgical procedure, and managed care practices of drug substitution within classes of medications may lead to an ADWE. Table 101-2 lists medications commonly used by elderly patients that may be associated with withdrawal syndromes or exacerbation of the underlying disease.[73-77] To prevent ADWEs, the clinician should take into account the dose of the medication, the length of therapy of the medication, and the pharmacokinetics of the medication. Risk can be minimized or eliminated by a slow, careful tapering of the drug over a period of time. This approach is similar to the time taken in the initiation and titration of a new drug. Unfortunately, precise tapering schedules have not been established for most drugs.

At every visit, it is necessary to review and, if possible, simplify the patient's medication regimen. This may be achieved by altering the dosing schedule and/or discontinuing medicines that are no longer needed. To conduct the review when faced with an elderly patient taking multiple medications, the clinician can utilize any of the standardized approaches such as the Medication Appropriateness Index (MAI) (Table 101-3).[78] The clinician should also consider whether there is omission of necessary medications. A standardized tool such as the Assessment of Underutilization of Medication (AOU) can be used, which requires having a health professional match the complete list of chronic medical conditions to the prescribed medications after reviewing the medical record.[79] In this manner, one can determine whether there was an omission of a needed drug for an established disease or condition based on the scientific literature. For each condition one of three ratings can be made: omission, marginal omission (e.g. have used appropriate nonpharmacological approach), or no omission.

The clinician should also consider providing adherence aids for their elderly patients. However, before providing the patient with methods to enhance adherence it is important to talk to the patient about how they take their medications so that an individualized plan can be developed. It is also important to identify risk factors for poor adherence (e.g. impaired hearing, vision, and cognition).[80] Healthcare professionals should also follow up with compliance recommendations by monitoring their patients.[81] Some general methods to enhance adherence in elderly patients include simplifying regimens, providing written instructions and considering generic formulations to reduce costs.[82] More specifically, pill boxes, increased font size on prescription labels, calendars, easy-to-swallow dosage forms, pill cutters, oral dosing syringes, insulin syringe magnification, tube spacer for inhalers, and easy-open caps may increase adherence in elderly patients.[41,81,83] There are also some highly technological devices available as compliance aids (e.g. alarm watches with messages, automated pill delivery systems, medication bottles with alarms).[84] These devices may prove to be beneficial, but probably not in the elderly "Luddite" population. Finally, active patient and family involvement should be encouraged.[41,81,83]

SUMMARY

Geriatric pharmacotherapy may greatly enhance the quality of life of elderly patients by effectively palliating, preventing, or treating many diseases and conditions in late life. The evidence for the efficacy of drugs in elderly patients has significantly increased over past decades by some clinical trials and many more potentially beneficial drugs are in development. However, clinical trial data may be limited by underrepresentation of older patients in many trials, the exclusion of frail elderly or oldest-old patients, and lack of post-marketing studies designed to assess the effectiveness of competing drugs. In addition, the benefits of drug therapy can be offset by ADRs, ADWEs, and therapeutic failure. Although variable in their estimates of the frequency of these drug-related problems, many epidemiological studies of drug-related problems agree that these are common, costly, and clinically important problems in elderly patients. Potential solutions to these problems include better systems design, health services approaches, patient and caregiver education, systematic medication review programs, and provider education. More research is needed to determine the feasibility and effectiveness of these approaches. Clinicians

Table 101-2 Drugs associated with medication withdrawal syndromes in the elderly [43–47,73–77]

Medications	Type of withdrawal[a]	Withdrawal syndrome
Alpha-antagonist antihypertensives	P	Hypertension, palpitations, headache, agitation
Angiotensin-converting-enzyme inhibitors	D,P	Hypertension, heart failure
Antianginal agents	D	Myocardial ischemia
Anticonvulsants	P,D	Seizures
Antidepressants	P,D	Akathisia, anxiety, irritability, gastrointestinal distress, malaise, myalgia, headache, coryza, chills, insomnia, recurrence of depression
Antiparkinson agents	P,D	Rigidity, tremor, pulmonary embolism, psychosis, hypotension
Antipsychotics	P	Nausea, restlessness, insomnia, dyskinesia
Baclofen	P	Hallucinations, paranoia, insomnia, nightmares, mania, depression, anxiety, agitation, confusion, seizures, hypertonia
Benzodiazepines	P	Agitation, confusion, delirium, seizures, insomnia
Beta-blockers	P	Angina, myocardial infarction, anxiety, tachycardia, hypertension
Corticosteroids	P	Weakness, anorexia, nausea, hypotension
Digoxin	D	Heart failure, palpitations
Diuretics	D	Hypertension, heart failure
Histamine-2 blockers	D	Recurrence of esophagitis and indigestion symptoms
Narcotic analgesics	P	Restlessness, anxiety, anger, insomnia, chills, abdominal cramping, diarrhea, diaphoresis
Nonsteroidal anti-inflammatory drugs	P	Recurrence of arthritis and gout symptoms
Sedative/hypnotics (e.g. barbiturates)	P	Anxiety, muscle twitches, tremor, dizziness

[a]P: Physiological withdrawal; D: exacerbation of underlying disease.

Table 101-3 Medication appropriateness index [78]

Questions to ask about each individual medication

1. Is there an indication for the drug?
2. Is the medication effective for the condition?
3. Is the dosage correct?
4. Are the directions correct?
5. Are the directions practical?
6. Are there clinically significant drug–drug interactions?
7. Are there clinically significant drug–disease/condition interactions?
8. Is there unnecessary duplication with other drug(s)?
9. Is the duration of therapy acceptable?
10. Is this drug the least expensive alternative compared to others of equal utility?

KEY POINTS Geriatric pharmacotherapy

- There are limitations in our knowledge about efficacy and safety of drugs in elderly people.

- Drug-related problems such as therapeutic failure, adverse drug withdrawal events and adverse drug reactions are common and result in considerable morbidity in elderly people.

- Strategies to modify or reduce drug-related problems will require that health systems design/institute new approaches to delivering care to elderly people.

- Clinicians should strive to conduct periodic systematic reviews of elderly patients' drug regimens as well as adhere to other principles to optimize geriatric pharmacotherapy.

who care for elderly patients need to know and apply principles of geriatric pharmacotherapy in order to maximize the benefits of drugs and minimize drug-related problems.

REFERENCES

1. Staessen JA, Gasowski J, Wang JG et al: Risks of untreated and treated isolated systolic hypertension in the elderly: meta-analysis of outcome trials. Lancet 2000;355:865–872
2. Weiner DK, Hanlon JT: Pain in nursing home residents: management strategies. Drugs Aging 2001;18:13–29
3. Pharmaceutical Research and Manufacturers of America: New medicines in development for older Americans. Washington, DC, 2002.
4. Avorn J: Including elderly people in clinical trials. Br Med J 1997;315:1033–1034
5. Schmucker DL, Vesell ES: Are the elderly underrepresented in clinical drug trials? J Clin Pharmacol 1999;39:1103–1108
6. Hutchins LF, Unger JM, Crowley JJ et al: Underrepresentation of patients 65 years of age or older in cancer-treatment trials. N Engl J Med 1999;341:2061–2067
7. US Food and Drug Administration: Guideline for industry: studies in support of special populations: geriatrics. ICH-E7 August 1994. http://www.fda.gov/cder/guidance/iche7.pdf
8. Agency for Healthcare Research and Quality (AHRQ) Centers for Education and Research on Therapeutics. http://certs.hhs.gov/.2000
9. Reidenberg MM: Centers for education and research in therapeutics. Clin Pharmacol Ther 2000;68:109–110
10. Karch FE, Lasagna L: Adverse drug reactions: a critical review. JAMA 1975;234:1236–1241
11. Hanlon JT, Schmader KE, Gray S: Adverse drug reactions. In Delafuente JC, Stewart RB (eds): Therapeutics in the Elderly, 3rd Ed. Harvey Whitney Books, Cincinnati, 2000;289–314
12. Grymonpre RE, Mitenko PA, Sitar DS et al: Drug-associated hospital admissions in older medical patients. J Am Geriatr Soc 1988;36:1092–1098
13. Kohn L, Corrigan J, Donaldson M: Committee on Quality of Health Care in America, Institute of Medicine. To Err Is Human: Building a Safer Health System. Washington, DC: National Academy of Sciences, 1999
14. Ernst FR, Grizzle AJ: Drug-related morbidity and mortality: updating the cost-of-illness model. J Am Pharm Assoc 2001;41:192–199
15. Bootman JL, Harrison DL, Cox E: The health care cost of drug-related morbidity and mortality in nursing facilities. Arch Intern Med 1997;157:2089–2096
16. Ioannidis JPA, Lau J: Completeness of safety reporting in randomized trials—an evaluation of 7 medical areas. JAMA 2001;285:437–443
17. Agency for Healthcare Research and Quality (AHRQ) of Centers of Excellence for Patient Safety Research and Practice. http://www.ahrq.gov, 2000
18. Atkin PA, Veitch PC, Veitch EM et al: The epidemiology of serious adverse drug reactions among the elderly. Drugs Aging 1999;14:141–152
19. Beyth RJ, Shorr RI: Epidemiology of adverse drug reactions in the elderly by drug class. Drugs Aging 1999;14:231–239
20. Rothschild JM, Bates DW, Leape LL: Preventable medical injuries in older patients. Arch Intern Med 2000;160:2717–2728
21. Mannesse CK, Derkx FH, de Ridder MA et al: Adverse drug reactions in elderly patients as contributing factor for hospital admission: cross sectional study. Br Med J 1997;315:1057–1058
22. Mannesse CK, Derkx FH, de Ridder MA et al: Contribution of adverse drug reactions to hospital admission of older patients. Age Ageing 2000;29:35–39
23. Hallas J, Gram LF, Grodum E et al: Drug related admissions to medical wards: a population based survey. Br J Clin Pharmacol 1992;33:61–68
24. Carbonin P, Pahor M, Bernabei R et al: Is age an independent risk factor for adverse drug reactions in hospitalized medical patients? J Am Geriatr Soc 1991;39:1093–1099
25. Thomas EJ, Brennan TA: Incidence and types of preventable adverse events in elderly patients: population based review of medical records. Br Med J 2000;320:741–744
26. Chrischilles EA, Segar ET, Wallace RB: Self-reported adverse drug reactions and related resource use: a study of community-dwelling persons 65 years of age and older. Ann Intern Med 1992;117:634–640

27. Hanlon JT, Schmader KE, Koronkowski MJ et al: Adverse drug events in high risk older outpatients. J Am Geriatr Soc 1997;45:945–948
28. Gurwitz JH, Field TS, Avorn J et al: Incidence and preventability of adverse drug events in nursing homes. Am J Med 2000;109:87–94
29. Hanlon JT, Schmader KE, Ruby CM et al: Suboptimal prescribing in elderly inpatients and outpatients. J Am Geriatr Soc 2001;49:200–209
30. Lipton HL, Bero LA, Bird JA et al: The impact of clinical pharmacists' consultations on physicians geriatric drug prescribing: a randomized controlled trial. Med Care 1992;30:646–658
31. Schmader K, Hanlon JT, Weinberger M et al: Appropriateness of medication prescribing in ambulatory elderly patients. J Am Geriatr Soc 1994;42:1241–1247
32. Montamat SC, Cusack B: Overcoming problems with polypharmacy and drug misuse. Clin Geriatr Med 1992;8:143–158
33. Hanlon JT, Fillenbaum GG, Schmader KE et al: Inappropriate medication use among community dwelling elderly residents. Pharmacotherapy 2000;20:575–582
34. Jankel CA, Fitterman LK: Epidemiology of drug-drug interactions as a cause of hospital admissions. Drug Safety 1993;9:51–59
35. Osborne CA, Batty GM, Maskrey V et al: Development of prescribing indicators for elderly medical inpatients. Br J Clin Pharmacol 1997;43:91–97
36. Beers MH, Ouslander JG, Fingold SF et al: Inappropriate medication prescribing in skilled nursing facilities. Ann Intern Med 1992;117:684–689
37. Stewart RB, Caranasos GJ: Medication compliance in the elderly. Med Clin North Am 1989;73:1551–1563
38. Weintraub M: Compliance in the elderly. Clin Geriatr Med 1990;6:445–452
39. Cooper JK, Love DW, Raffoul PR: Intentional prescription nonadherence (noncompliance) by the elderly. J Am Geriatr Soc 1982;30:329–333
40. Fincke BG, Miller DR, Spiro A 3rd: The interaction of patient perception of overmedication with drug compliance and side effects. J Gen Intern Med 1998;13:182–185
41. Murray MD, Darnell J, Weinberger M et al: Factors contributing to medication noncompliance in elderly public housing tenants. Drug Intell Clin Pharm 1986;20:146–152
42. Lipton HL, Bird JA: The impact of clinical pharmacists' consultations on geriatric patients' compliance and medical care use: a randomized controlled trial. Gerontologist 1994;34:307–315
43. Hodding GC, Jann M, Ackerman IP: Drug withdrawal syndromes: a literature review. West J Med 1980;133:383–391
44. Olmedo R, Hoffman RS: Withdrawal syndromes. Emerg Med Clin North Am 2000;18:273–288
45. Gerety M, Cornell JE, Plichta D et al: Adverse events related to drugs and drug withdrawal in nursing home residents. J Am Geriatr Soc 1993;41:1326–1332
46. Graves T, Hanlon JT, Schmader KE et al: Adverse events after discontinuing medications in elderly outpatients. Arch Intern Med 1997;157:2205–2210
47. Kennedy JM, van Rij AM, Spears RA et al: Polypharmacy in a general surgical unit and consequences of drug withdrawal. Br J Clin Pharmacol 2000;49:353–362
48. Bero LA, Lipton HL, Bird JA: Characterization of geriatric drug-related hospital readmissions. Med Care 1991;29:989–1003
49. Hallas J, Worm J, Beck-Nielsen J et al: Drug related events and drug utilization in patients admitted to a geriatric hospital department. Danish Med Bull 1991;38:417–420
50. Major S, Badr S, Bahlawan L et al: Drug-related hospitalization at a tertiary teaching center in Lebanon: incidence, associations, and relation to self-medicating behavior. Clin Pharmacol Ther 1998;64:450–461
51. Tamblyn R, Laprise R, Hanley JA et al: Adverse events associated with prescription drug cost-sharing among poor and elderly persons. JAMA 2001;285:421–429
52. Soumerai SB, Ross-Degnan D, Avorn J et al: Effects of Medicaid drug-payment limits on admission to hospitals and nursing homes. N Engl J Med 1991;325:1072–1077
53. Billups SJ, Malone DC, Carter BL: The relationship between drug therapy noncompliance and patient characteristics, health-related quality of life and health care costs. Pharmacotherapy 2000;20:941–949
54. Sullivan SD, Kreling DH, Hazlet TK: Noncompliance with medication regimens and subsequent hospitalizations: a literature analysis and cost of hospitalization estimate. J Res Pharm Econ 1990;2:19–33
55. Col N, Fanale JE, Kronholm P: The role of medication noncompliance and adverse drug reactions in hospitalizations of the elderly. Arch Intern Med 1990;150:841–845

56. Redelmeier DA, Tan SH, Booth GL: The treatment of unrelated disorders in patients with chronic medical diseases. N Engl J Med 1998;338:1516–1520

57. Havranek EP, Abrams F, Stevens E et al: Determinants of mortality in elderly patients with heart failure. Arch Intern Med 1998;158:2024–2028

58. Smith NL, Psaty BM, Pitt B et al: Temporal patterns in the medical treatment of congestive heart failure with angiotensin-converting enzyme inhibitors in older adults, 1989 through 1995. Arch Intern Med 1998;158:1074–1080

59. Gattis WA, Larsen RL, Hasselblad V et al: Is optimal angiotensin-converting enzyme inhibitor dosing neglected in elderly patients with heart failure? Am Heart J 1998;136:43–48

60. Croft JB, Giles WH, Roegner RH et al: Pharmacologic management of heart failure among older adults by office-based physicians in the United States. J Fam Pract 1997;44:382–390

61. Chin MH, Wang JC, Zhang JX et al: Utilization and dosing of angiotensin-converting enzyme inhibitors for heart failure. J Gen Intern Med 1997;12:563–566

62. Philbin EF: Factors determining angiotensin-converting enzyme inhibitor underutilization in heart failure in a community setting. Clin Cardiol 1998;21:103–108

63. Ganz DA, Lamas GA, Orav EJ et al: Age-related differences in management of heart disease: A study of cardiac medication use in an older cohort. J Am Geriatr Soc 1999;47:145–150

64. Mendelson G, Aronow WS: Underutilization of measurement of serum low-density lipoprotein cholesterol levels and of lipid-lowering therapy in older patients with manifest atherosclerotic disease. J Am Geriatr Soc 1998;46:1128–1131

65. Krumholz HM, Radford MJ, Ellerbeck EF et al: Aspirin for secondary prevention after acute myocardial infarction in the elderly: prescribed use and outcomes. Ann Intern Med 1996;124:292–298

66. Krumholz HM, Radford MJ, Wang Y et al: National use and effectiveness of β-blockers for the treatment of elderly patients after acute myocardial infarction. JAMA 1998;280:623–629

67. Hill JW, Roglieri JL, Warburton SW: Aspirin treatment after myocardial infarction: are health maintenance organization members, women, and the elderly undertreated. Am J Manag Care 1998;4:51–58

68. Aronow WS: Underutilization of aspirin in older patients with prior myocardial infarction at the time of admission to a nursing home. J Am Geriatr Soc 1998;46:615–616

69. Owens NJ, Sherburne NJ, Silliman RA et al: The Senior Care Study: the optimal use of medications in acutely ill older patients. J Am Geriatr Soc 1990;38:1082–1087

70. Burns R, Nichols LO, Graney MJ et al: Impact of continued geriatric outpatient management on health outcomes of older veterans. Arch Intern Med 1995;155:1313–1318

71. Toseland RW, O'Donnell MA, Engelhardt JB et al: Outpatient geriatric evaluation and management results of a randomized trial. Med Care 1996;34:624–640

72. Cohen HJ, Feussner JR, Weinberger M et al: Effect of Geriatric Evaluation and Management Units and Clinics on survival, health related quality of life and functional status: a VA cooperative trial. N Engl J Med 2002;346:905–912

73. Anon: Drugs that cause psychiatric symptoms. Med Lett 1998;40:21–24

74. Frishman WH: Beta-adrenergic blocker withdrawal. Am J Cardiol 1987;59:26F–32F

75. Packer M, Gheorghiade M, Young J et al: Withdrawal of digoxin from patients with chronic heart failure treated with angiotensin-converting-enzyme inhibitors. N Engl J Med 1993;329:1–7

76. Schatzberg AF, Haddad P, Kaplan EM et al: Serotonin reuptake inhibitor discontinuation syndrome. Discontinuation Consensus panel. J Clin Psychiatry 1997;58(suppl 7):5–10

77. Walma E, Hoes A, Van Dooren C et al: Withdrawal of long term diuretic medication in elderly patients: a double blind randomized trial. Br Med J 1997;315:464–468

78. Hanlon JT, Schmader KE, Samsa G et al: A method for assessing drug therapy appropriateness. J Clin Epidemiol 1992;45:1045–1051

79. Jeffery S, Ruby CM, Hanlon JT et al: The impact of an interdisciplinary team on suboptimal prescribing in a long-term care facility. Consult Pharm 1999;14:1386–1389

80. Ruscin JM, Semla TP: Assessment of medication management skills in older outpatients. Ann Pharmacother 1996;30:1083–1088

81. Cramer JA: Enhancing patient compliance in the elderly: role of packaging aids and monitoring. Drugs Aging 1998;12:7–15

82. Beers MH, Baran RW, Frenia K: Drugs and the elderly, part 2: strategies for improving prescribing in a managed care environment. Am J Manag Care 2001;7:69–72

83. Murray MD, Birt JA, Manatunga AK et al: Medication compliance in elderly outpatients using twice-daily dosing and unit-of-use packaging. Ann Pharmacother 1993;27:616–621

84. Durso SL: Technological advances for improving medication adherence in the elderly. Ann Long Term Care 2001;9:43–48

Chapter 102

Geriatric oncology

Margot Gosney

Cancer is a major cause of death and morbidity in elderly patients, with over 50 percent of new cases occurring in those aged 70 years or older. Within England and Wales there were 143,433 cancer deaths in 1999.[1] There are now more cancer-related deaths than those due to heart disease.[2] Cancer death rates in older people have increased by 17 percent despite a 23 percent decrease in the cancer death rate in those aged 65 years or less.[3] In the UK, 76 percent of cancer deaths occurred in people aged over 64 years and 47 percent in people over 74 years.[1] As the incidence and prevalence of cancer increases, coupled with improved diagnostic certainty and life expectancy, many doctors will be faced with caring for elderly patients with cancer. It is estimated that 6 percent of NHS expenditure is used in cancer care with elderly patients responsible for a large proportion of this expenditure. Although cancer was chosen as a key area in the "Health of the Nation" document,[4] elderly people were not specifically targeted and in the Department of Health document, "A Policy Framework for Commissioning Cancer Services"[5] which provides guidance for purchasers and providers of cancer services, there is no mention of involvement of geriatricians in the acute care or rehabilitation of elderly patients with cancer. Despite the recent publication in the United Kingdom of the National Service Framework for older people, cancer has not been highlighted as an area with clearly defined targets. The true impact of cancer in older people is unknown because of poor histological verification; often the first registration of cancer is at death certification. In the USA, in an attempt to focus attention on geriatric oncology, the American Cancer Society, the American Society of Clinical Oncology, and other research groups have formed subgroups specifically to deal with the problem of geriatric oncology. Within the USA, cancer mortality rates specific to older people (65 years or over) have increased over the past 10 years.[6] Similarly, in the Netherlands, age-specific cancer mortality rates have increased with increasing age for both males and females during 1991–1995.[7]

It is clear from work by Grulich et al.[8] that secular trends in cancer mortality are influenced by age. Between 1970 and 1990, for males and females aged 75–84 there has been a 16 and 18 percent increase, respectively, in cancer mortality. This is in contrast to males and females aged 45–54 who have had a 19 and 17 percent decrease in cancer mortality, respectively.

CANCER AND AGING

There is no doubt that older people are more likely to develop cancer and differences in tumor growth and spread occur as a result of aging. The relationship between cancer and aging is complex, and various factors including changes in host tumor defences, and exposure to carcinogens, have roles to play in the etiology of tumors. Although there are several distinct theories on cancer causation in older people, including decreased ability to repair DNA, oncogene activation or amplification, tumor suppressor gene loss, decreased immune surveillance, prolonged duration of carcinogenic exposure, or increase susceptibility of aged cells to carcinogens, no one theory has universal backing.[9]

There is debate as to whether carcinogenesis and aging are related phenomena. Many believe such a relationship exists[10,11] with some postulating that cancer develops due to normal processes occurring during aging[12] and others favoring a common etiological origin for both cancer and aging.[13] There is a relationship between chromosomal alterations and malignancy.[14] Several inherited disorders, featuring both chromosomal breakage and an increased frequency of malignant disease, show abnormalities of DNA repair or recombination[15] and many genetically determined syndromes have both an accelerated progression of biological aging and a high frequency of malignant disease.[16]

The increased incidence of cancer with age can be interpreted in accordance with two major theories of aging.[9,17] The first, the Damage or Error Theories, hold that over time there is an accumulation of damage to vital areas of cellular or organ function which culminates in the manifestations of the aging process. Mutations may occur in certain key genes or in many individual genes on a random basis. The multistep model of carcinogenesis fits with this theory as successive cancer-causing mutations accumulate during the aging process.[18] The Alternative or Program Theories, now largely discredited (see Chapter 4), consider aging as a latter stage of a program that proceeds through embryogenesis through growth development and maturation. During aging certain genes become expressed and others are shut down.

In 1858, Virchow[19] stated that each tissue present in the body has a limited response to injury. Since then, further work has described how various tissues of the body respond to damage. Those tissues having continuously mitotic cells, such as the gut and marrow, develop tumors, while those with intermittently mitotic cells, such as endothelial or smooth muscle, develop degenerative diseases such as atherosclerosis, but only rarely malignant change. Nonmitotic cells such as the neuron, virtually never develop tumors, but are associated with disorders such as Alzheimer's or Parkinson's disease, illustrating that frequent cell turnover is required for tumor development.[20]

A reduction in DNA methylation in some genes is more common in older subjects and results in an increase in cancer,[21,22] although this is not a consistent finding in all genes.[23] The formation of DNA adducts in a variety of tissues is seen in chemical carcinogenesis[24] and, in certain animal models, adduct-like compounds (I-compounds) accumulate with age.[25] Whether the I-compounds are responsible for tumor development or are merely markers of the aging process is debatable,[26] but they do have the capability to carry mutations, DNA chain breaks, and gene rearrangements.[25] Further evidence for the role of altered DNA repair in cancer causation is provided by the increased susceptibility of cells from older persons to chromosomal damage by ^{3}H-thymidine and to the toxic consequences of irradiation.[27]

In considering cancer in elderly people, the role of factors that increase lifespan (geroprotectors) and their effects on tumor development must be noted. Geroprotectors are of three types. First, those that decrease the mortality of a long-living subpopulation are effective in inhibiting carcinogenesis, prolong tumor latency, and decrease the incidence of cancers (e.g. calorie-restricted diet); second, those that increase the survival in a short-living subpopulation without a change in the maximum lifespan and may increase tumor incidence in an exposed population (e.g. tocopherol); finally, geroprotectors that prolong the lifespan equally in all members of the population, postpone the beginning of population aging, and in general do not influence the incidence of tumors, but do prolong tumor latency (e.g. 2-mecaptoethylamin).[28]

A large literature describes the gradual alteration of immune function that occurs with advancing age and that may contribute to the increase in malignancy. Many of these changes occur with the onset of thymic involution, which begins at puberty and results in only 10 percent of thymic function remaining by the age of 45. Although the total population of T-lymphocytes does not decline, the number of suppressor and killer cells decreases, the helper–suppressor ratio reverses, and there is an increase in the number of immature lymphocytes in the peripheral blood. Immune surveillance depends on the integrity of lymphocytes, and thymic function is critical for monitoring and disposing of cells that harbor replicative aggregations. Thymic hormones not only decline with age, but have also been shown to be significantly lower in age-matched patients with malignant disease.[29] Although reduction in immune surveillance may play a role in the development of cancer in older people, if it were to result in tumor development as seen in immunosuppressed patients, a lack of tumor diversity would be expected, which is not the case.[30]

Administration of L-argenine acts directly on the pituitary to increase thymulin levels and thus, the number of lymphocyte peripheral subsets.[29] However, there are no data on the use of L-argenine in immune activation in elderly patients with cancer.

There is conflicting opinion regarding the growth and spread of cancer in older patients, and although some evidence shows death to be earlier in older subjects, coexisting diseases have obvious effects on morbidity and mortality. Some experimental work has demonstrated slower tumor growth, fewer metastases, and longer survival in older rodents, and others have shown decreased tumor growth associated with impaired T-cell function.[31] Cultures from melanoma cell lines have demonstrated that T-cells from young, but not old, donors stimulate the growth of tumor cells, and T-cells from young, but not old, mice produce angiogenic factors resulting in a richer vascular supply that may be responsible for increased growth and metastases. The therapeutic implications of angiogenic factors produced by T-cells have yet to be explored. Additionally, a relationship between anergy and cancer

mortality, although not statistically significant, has been noted in older patients.[32]

Many elderly subjects have been exposed to carcinogenic agents as a result of their occupation (asbestos; inorganic chemicals such as arsenic or nickel; and plant products such as aflatoxin, polycyclic hydrocarbons, and dyes). Lifestyle and diet is dominated in older subjects by tobacco consumption and atmospheric pollution, and although studies have shown an increased incidence of cancer of the endometrium and breast associated with diet, other dietary factors such as fiber may protect against the development of carcinoma of the bowel.

The relationship between cancer and aging is clearly complex and various factors, including exposure to carcinogens and changes in the host defense, have roles to play in the etiology of tumors. With further understanding of normal aging its relationship to carcinogenesis should be further understood.[33]

CANCER PREVENTION

There are two main approaches to cancer prevention: *primary prevention*, which may be less applicable to older people, relates to changes in lifestyle, exercise, and diet to preclude the development of cancer; and *secondary prevention*, which involves screening tests and examinations to aid early detection of tumors, thereby decreasing morbidity and mortality, increasing the chance of cure, and prolonging disease-free interval following therapy.

Cancer becomes 100 times more common in men and 30 times more common in women between the ages of 25 and 75 years,[34] and therefore, secondary prevention should perhaps be targeted at older people rather than the young.[35]

Prevention strategies

Prevention has been classified into three types.[36] Primary prevention aims to prevent the onset of a disease and secondary prevention aims to halt progression of a disease once it has been established. By identifying the disease early, often while the patient is still asymptomatic, prompt and effective treatment may be given to stop the disease. Tertiary prevention aims to rehabilitate people with an established disease to minimize residual disabilities and complications.

The focus of many cancer studies is in both primary and secondary prevention. Approximately 80 percent of all cancers are potentially preventable and many public health strategies have been aimed at behavior modification such as smoking cessation, healthy diet, and protection from sunlight.[37]

Primary prevention and healthy promotion for older people are important issues not only for cancer but other common causes of morbidity and mortality. With regard to cancer, primary prevention may include elimination of environmental carcinogens through to chemoprevention, i.e., estrogen antagonists for breast cancer.[38]

It must be remembered that primary prevention, even at extreme old age, may result in decreased incidence of heart disease, colon cancer, and hypertension.[39]

For screening to be appropriate, a disease must be common, curable if diagnosed early, and the test involved must be highly sensitive. Screening in the UK is almost exclusively for tumors of the breast and cervix and is uncommonly performed in older people. The approach to screening varies: in the USA, screening tests are performed until studies show them to be ineffective, while in many areas of Europe screening is not carried out until shown to be effective. Older subjects are less likely than younger age groups to participate in screening and cancer detection behaviors[40,41] and this may be due to inadequate knowledge about cancer,[42] lower educational level, or being unaware of an increased risk.[43] Other factors such as fear of cancer and its treatment, difficulty differentiating between normal physiological changes and early symptoms or signs of cancer,[44] and fatalism[45] have also been implicated. Men participate less than women in screening procedures[46,47] and it has been found that elderly people who scored highly in a health perception questionnaire, which measured current health, prior health, health outlook, health worry/concern, resistance or susceptibility to illness, and rejection of the sick role, were also more likely to have participated in cancer screening programs.[47] This perception of health by older people playing an important role in cancer prevention has been reported by others.[48–51]

If screening in older subjects increases, the involvement of nurses will be important, although evidence suggests that patients perceive nurses not to focus on health promotion activities and to be more likely to perform examinations themselves, rather than teaching elderly women to examine their own breasts.[52]

In order to improve the early detection of cancer, several questions including the attitudes of older people towards screening, and the barriers perceived by the patient especially for skin, breast, and cervical cancer need to be explored.[53–55] Elderly people must be taught to differentiate symptoms and signs of aging from those of cancer, and the reasons for delay in seeking a medical opinion must be sought.

Breast cancer studies have shown a positive relationship between stage of disease and age at diagnosis.[40] However, older women are less likely to participate in screening programs for breast cancer than younger women.[41,56] In the UK the screening by mammography of women aged 50–64 on a triennial basis was recommended by the Forrest Report, and although women aged 65 years or older could attend for routine mammography, they were not invited to do so. However, the NHS Cancer Plan announced in September 2000 stated that by 2004, routine invitations would be extended to include women up to the age of 70 years.[57] Evidence from Hendry and Entwhistle,[58] in a study involving 1,500 women aged 65–69 years, which achieved a screening uptake of 74.6 percent and a cancer detection rate of 9.3/1,000, suggests that the NHS Cancer Plan will be both beneficial and cost-effective. Mammography reveals more tumors in older patients than in younger subjects,[59] increases the proportion of early cancers[60] and thereby reduces mortality.[61–65] Only 16 percent of all those performed are on women aged over 60 years.[43] Hobbs et al.[66] found that less women aged 65–79 (61 percent) than aged 50–64 years (77 percent) attended mammography after invitation, although the "pick up" rate was three times greater in the older group (11.6/1,000 vs 4.1/1,000). Factors that may reduce the number of elderly women attending for mammography are that they consider themselves less at risk for developing breast cancer than younger women[67] and consider self-examination

to be adequate. Older women are less likely to have breast examinations performed by their doctors,[68] despite this having been shown to result in less advanced disease at presentation[69] and physicians are less likely to send older people for screening.[70] Haigney et al.[71] assessed the views of both older women and hospital doctors on the performance of clinical breast examination. Despite older women stating they would accept clinical breast examination if it was offered by their doctor, only 7 percent of doctors said that they would routinely perform such an examination on women over 50 years of age. Previous assumptions that older women will not attend for routine screening have been inaccurate. An overall predicted uptake of previous nonattendees was found to be 50 percent and when studied by age group, 67 percent of patients aged 65–69 years, 53 percent of patients aged 70–99 years, and 27 percent of patients aged ≥85 years attended for mammographic screening.[72]

The American Cancer Society (ACS) recommends that women begin monthly breast self-examination at the age of 20 and between 20 and 39 years have a clinical breast examination every 3 years. They then recommend from age 40 onwards that women should have an annual mammogram and a clinical breast examination. Unlike the UK's National Screening Programme there is no upper age limit to ACS recommendations as long as women are in good health.[73,74]

If the percentage of older women who receive mammograms and breast examinations increased to 80 percent, mortality in this age group would fall by 30 percent[75] and data obtained from the SEER program showed a life extension of 178 days for those over 85 years and 617 days for those aged 65–69[76] if screening was extended. If quality of life is good following the diagnosis of cancer, the benefits of screening outweigh any anxiety generated by the procedures. There are no data to justify excluding women from breast cancer screening on an age basis alone.[77]

Colorectal screening using fecal occult blood, digital rectal examination, and sigmoidoscopy, although well-accepted in the USA, is not commonly performed in the UK.[78,79] Colon cancer is related to the presence of premalignant adenomas, which are more common in elderly people,[80,81] and although the life expectancy of many elderly patients with colorectal cancer is short, if early detection results in a reduction in the number of older people presenting with inoperable bowel obstruction secondary to advanced tumors, it should be considered. Although some studies have shown no increased survival following screening,[82] there is controversy surrounding patient numbers.[83] More recent studies however, suggest that population screening of people aged over 50 years can reduce mortality rates from bowel cancer.[84,85] Within the United Kingdom there are two pilot screening studies which are expected to be completed by 2002. However, the age band selected for screening by fecal occult blood testing is 50–69 years, not the upper age limit of 74 years as designated by Hardcastle et al.[84] and Kronborg et al.[85] The upper age screening limit may have been imposed because of a perceived lower acceptance of screening by patients aged 70 years or above, although the evidence for this is somewhat lacking.

In 1997 the UK Government accepted the advice of the National Screening Committee not to introduce a population screening program for prostate cancer because it would be neither cost-effective nor acceptable.[86] The main reasons against such an introduction were that prostate-specific antigen (PSA) has a low specificity and cannot reliably distinguish males with prostate cancer from males without the disease. In addition, there is no consensus on the treatment of prostate cancer and indeed many patients with the disease are unlikely to suffer any ill effects and the traumatic treatment of asymptomatic males because of a screening test could do more harm than good.

Screening for prostatic cancer using digital rectal examination is controversial,[77,87,88] as autopsy studies have shown that foci of adenocarcinoma in the prostate are almost universal in elderly men dying from unrelated causes. While PSA testing is widespread in the USA the impact of screening for prostate cancer remains controversial.[89] While the debate remains, it must be remembered that screening has not only an initial cost but also that of treatment of an often asymptomatic patient.[90]

Although lung cancer is common, survival is not improved by screening programs[77] and many physicians consider that older subjects have little or no benefit from smoking cessation despite a lack of evidence that ability to stop alters with age.[91] Immediately after cessation of smoking, a decline in the risk of developing lung cancer is seen such that 5–9 years after stopping, the risk is half, and by 15 years the risk is that of a lifelong nonsmoker.[92] Therefore, this, together with the life expectancy of patients aged 65 years being as great as 17 years, indicates that smoking cessation clearly has benefits. Indeed, Peto et al.[93] assessed the effects of smoking cessation and found that if people stopped smoking, even during middle age, the risk of developing lung cancer decreases.

Cervical screening has been aimed at young women, with over one-half the women aged 65 years or older not having had a Papanicolaou screen in the previous 3 years.[94] As the incidence of cervical cancer continues to increase in older women, a 63 percent improvement in mortality could result from routine screening of those over age 65.[95] Fahs et al.,[96] using a Markov computer model, found that the early detection of cervical cancer through screening programs may improve survival rates regardless of the patient's age. In addition, screening older women for cervical cancer remained cost-effective, although for women aged over 64 years with a history of regular negative smears, regular screening becomes inefficient and the cost increases. Various methods of improving participation in cervical screening, including the availability of testing in older person's accommodation, has been suggested.[97]

INCIDENCE

Overall cancer incidence rates are higher for males than for females, and males have a greater probability of dying from cancer compared with females.[98,99]

Malignant disease has a rising incidence with age, particularly for tumors of the prostate, stomach, colorectum, pancreas, and esophagus.[6–8,100,101] The most common cancer site for adult males (aged 25 years or above) is lung and for adult females is breast.[102] In the case of primary lung and breast tumors, although there is a similar rise in incidence with age, this falls away in the very old group, which may be due to poorer standards of diagnosis and certification or due to an increase in deaths from other causes. Smith[103] found that

although mortality rates increase with age, the relative frequency of cancer deaths declined. Almost 40 percent of all deaths between the ages of 50 and 69 years, but only 4 percent of deaths in those aged 100 years or older, were due to malignant disease. Of the 524 patients aged 100 years or older who died from malignant disease in the USA in 1990, the most common single site was the breast in 70 women, with 45 men dying of carcinoma of the prostate.[103] Similar studies in England and Wales looking at patients aged over 100 at the time of death showed a decreased mortality rate for males but a slow nonexponential increasing mortality rate in females.[104]

DIAGNOSIS

There is evidence that stage of disease varies in older subjects at presentation. In breast cancer, it has been found to be earlier in these subjects when screening is utilized,[59] and the number of cancer cases diagnosed and confirmed by mammography in older women appears to be increasing.[105] However, many older patients delay seeking medical advice and this may result in cancer being diagnosed at an advanced stage. The delay in diagnosis may have the same cause as the failure to participate in screening, namely a general lack of awareness of possible signs and symptoms of malignancy. Older people may still view cancer to be untreatable and to be invariably fatal. Some studies have found that elderly patients may have difficulty accessing diagnostic interventions.[106,107] Older people are significantly less likely to have their cancer verified histologically compared with younger patients.[108–110]

The diagnostic tests offered to older patients are influenced by the medical specialty to which they are referred. Fleming and Fleming[111] found that geriatricians were less likely to recommend mammography when compared to general physicians and older people with suspected lung cancer are less likely to be investigated by geriatricians than by chest physicians.[112] There is controversy as to whether the patient's age alone influences the method and the thoroughness of diagnostic investigations. Mulcahy et al.[113] concluded that the patient's age did not influence the method of detecting colorectal cancer. However, they did find that significantly more older patients with colorectal cancer were likely to present as emergency cases with advanced disease when compared with younger patients. These emergency cases are often referred to medicine or geriatric medicine rather than surgical units and this may be partly explained by atypical presentation and the general frailty of the patient.[114] The relative lack of investigations that are undertaken on an elderly person may be partly due to the oncologist's lack of understanding of normal aging. Geriatricians are experienced in assessing pre-existing disability and concurrent disease, understanding functional status, level of dependency, and psychological adjustment. This permits joint decisions with regard to further therapy prior to the rehabilitation and, hopefully, recovery of the elderly patient with cancer.[115]

STAGE OF DISEASE

Accurate cancer staging is an important component of appropriate management. If a cancer is detected at an early stage then curative treatment is likely to be attempted, whereas cancer at an advanced stage usually signals the need for palliative treatment. Early stage disease usually indicates a better prognosis than advanced cancer.[6]

When the stage of disease at diagnosis is considered, there is a clear relationship not only between age and stage at diagnosis, but also between age at diagnosis and treatment received by the patient with cancer.[116–118] In general, older patients are more likely to have advanced or unstaged disease when compared to younger patients,[119] and the stage of disease is determined by the cancer site. Havlik et al.[120] found, among patients aged over 74 years, 26.9 percent had unstaged stomach cancer, whereas only 2.4 percent had breast cancer that was unstaged. It is likely that these differences described are due to the type of available diagnostic techniques rather than chronological age alone. Older patients are also more likely to have "unknown" stage at diagnosis. Bergman et al.[121] and Martin et al.[122] found that older women with breast cancer were more likely to be diagnosed as stage unknown or stage 3 when compared with younger women. In contrast Busch et al.[123] found a lower proportion of older women (≥75 years) with breast cancer stage 2 or unknown when compared to younger women (13.7 vs 8.3 percent), although for stages 1, 3, and 4 there were comparable proportions for both age groups.

Older women with ovarian cancer have a higher proportion of advanced disease (stages 3 and 4) than younger women.[124,125] As with breast cancer there are reports that older women have the highest proportion of unstaged ovarian cancer.[6]

In contrast to other tumors the stage of colorectal cancer at diagnosis does not appear to correlate with the patient's age,[113,126] although over 10 percent of patients aged 75 years or above with colorectal cancer had an unknown stage recorded.[6]

TREATMENT

Elderly patients should receive therapy comparable to that received by their younger counterparts, although this is often not the case. Older patients with cancer are less likely to receive definitive treatment than younger people after the diagnosis of cancer.[117,125,127–129] When a comparison of the 1990 incidence data from the NCI Surveillance, Epidemiology and End Results (SEER) programme[130] was made to the National Cancer Institute (NCI) Treatment Trials, which included more than 8,000 elderly patients, a significant discrepancy between the incidence of cancer and participation in cancer treatment protocols was found. Only 39 percent of males and 25.9 percent of the women involved in the trials were 65 years or older, and as a result of this the USA, under the auspices of the NCI, have sponsored a number of trials specifically targeting older patients. Data published by Trimble et al.[131] showed the mean age of those receiving chemotherapy to be significantly younger than the mean age of those registered as incident cases of cancer by SEER. Mor et al.[116] showed that age was related inversely to subsequently receiving either chemotherapy or radiotherapy after controlling for the stage of disease and comorbidity. Patients with breast cancer aged 75 years or older were twice as likely as patients aged 45 years to undergo surgery as sole treatment and 60 percent of patients under 45 years with

regional node involvement received adjuvant chemotherapy compared to just 27 percent of those 65 years or older.[132]

The reasons behind the under-representation of older subjects in treatment figures are complex. The patient may not have full investigation and staging, and therefore not be eligible to enter into a trial. Some argue that older patients are more likely to suffer from toxicity with chemotherapy,[133] and although an increase in hematological toxicity with methotrexate and methyl-CCNU (lomustine) has been reported,[134] this may in part be due to aging changes present in the bone marrow and its response to growth factors.[135,136] Other authors[137] have found no increase in nephrotoxicity in elderly subjects despite clear pharmacological reasons why they may occur.

Data from chemotherapeutic studies have shown that attempts at curative cancer therapy decline in proportion to the age of the patient[117] and although the risk of adverse drug reactions may increase seven-fold in patients older than 70 years of age when compared with younger adults, most elderly patients benefit from anticancer therapy even when the therapeutic index is reduced.[138]

When side-effects of chemotherapeutic agents are considered, studies have documented that younger patients report more nausea, fatigue, and vomiting than their older counterparts,[139,140] and one possible explanation for the reduction in nausea and vomiting in older people is that younger patients have higher anxiety levels and greater expectation of being sick.[141]

Putative problems with compliance in older people has been cited as a reason for their nontreatment and elderly women with breast cancer have been found not to follow the prescribed adjuvant chemotherapy, although the reasons for this were not clear.[142] Further planning with regard to patient education is required as more elderly people undergo complex oral chemotherapeutic regimes at home. Other studies have shown, in contrast, that older patients are more compliant with therapeutic regimens than younger patients.[143]

Other reasons given for the nontreatment of elderly subjects with cancer have included the advanced stage of the disease at presentation, and although there is evidence that some patients over 55 years of age have more advanced disease, this is not universal.[40,116,118,132,144,145]

Some doctors caring for elderly patients with cancer consider that they are less likely to wish to receive treatment than their younger counterparts. This was not the finding of Yellen et al.,[146] who used structured scenarios to assess patients' willingness to accept toxic chemotherapy to enhance survival, and found that older patients were as willing to choose chemotherapy as younger patients, though the former required a greater survival advantage before they would choose a toxic regime over a less toxic alternative.

Myths about cancer may affect treatment. If older patients believe that cancer treatments are worse than the disease itself[147] or they have a greater fear of cancer than younger patients do[148] they may decline treatment. If adequate information is given to older patients they are likely to accept treatment in a similar fashion to younger patients[149,150] and indeed may experience less emotional distress following the diagnosis of cancer.[151]

Poor life expectancy in elderly subjects has been cited as a further reason for nontreatment; however, it must be remembered that a 90-year-old has a life expectancy of 5 years, an

80-year-old of 8 years, and a 70-year-old of 15 years. Age alone therefore should not be used to weigh against treatment.[152]

Greenfield et al.[127] found that the presence of comorbidity was associated with less treatment for breast cancer in older women, but even when controlled for comorbidity, there were substantial age effects on treatment decisions. Following an interview of 800 patients aged 65 years or older with newly diagnosed cancer of the breast, prostate, colon or rectum, logistic regression was used to assess factors potentially influencing the receipt of definitive treatment to each individual. The study showed that for breast and prostate cancer there was a clear increase in the percent of patients not receiving definitive treatment with increasing age,[153] and in colorectal cancer, men were more likely to receive definitive therapy than women.[153] This latter finding is in contrast to previous studies that have shown no effect of sex on treatment for colon cancer.[117] Other studies have found factors determining nontreatment with chemotherapy to include impaired ability to perform ADL (Activities of Daily Living), poor access to transportation, being unmarried, low income, and low educational achievement.[153] Surprisingly, the presence of other medical disorders, although reducing definitive treatment, was not statistically significant in the analysis. In contrast, advanced age, impaired access to transportation, and poor functional and cognitive status showed little influence on receipt of surgical therapy.

Coexisting diseases are well documented in older patients with cancer. Approximately 25 percent of patients over the age of 75 years with cancer have vascular disease and almost 10 percent have coexisting chronic obstructive pulmonary disease or diabetes mellitus.[154] It is important that such patients are included in clinical trials to determine the effect of comorbidity on treatment tolerance and survival.[155,156]

Surgery

Surgery is considered to be the treatment of choice for most cancers, and patients should not be denied on the basis of the patient's age.[157] Nonetheless, mortality and morbidity rates are often increased in older patients who undergo surgery for cancer. Consultation and teamwork can however, minimize mortality and morbidity.[158,159] In a review of 105 patients aged 75 years or above with a variety of recurrent solid tumors, postoperative mortality was 3.8 percent with a 5-year survival rate of over 40 percent for selected patients.[160]

Advanced age per se is often used by either the patient's family or the physician to justify not proceeding with surgery. However, there is no global rule to follow, and cases should therefore be assessed individually.[158]

Hebert-Croteau et al.[161] and Newschaffer et al.[162] after controlling various confounding factors, found that in older patients with breast cancer, age was independently and negatively associated with surgery being performed. The likelihood of women aged ≥85 years receiving surgery was less than one-third (OR 0.31, 95 percent CI 0.16–0.60) of that seen in women aged 66–74 years.

Surgery is the treatment of choice for patients with colorectal cancer. The patient's age should not be a reason to withhold surgery.[159,163–165] Unfortunately, older patients with colorectal cancer are more likely to present with advanced disease, twice as likely to have emergency surgery, and less likely to undergo curative surgery.[166] In addition, with increasing age the incidence of postoperative morbidity and mortality is also increased. While the proportion of older patients undergoing curative surgery for colorectal cancer has increased,[167] this may be because surgery is performed on most patients regardless of age.[168]

Drug therapy (see also Chapter 14)

The normal physiological changes of aging affect drug absorption, distribution, metabolism, and elimination and thus, when prescribing any drug for an elderly person, pharmacokinetics must be considered. Elderly patients with cancer may receive a wide range of drugs including chemotherapeutic agents, analgesics, antiemetics, antibiotics, and others, in addition to drug therapy that has previously been prescribed for coexisting medical disorders.[169]

While there is evidence that drug absorption is not greatly altered by age per se,[170] some normal changes of aging do affect drug absorption. Oral drugs are modified by gastric motility and emptying time, while the absorption of parenterally administered drugs is dependent on local blood flow in muscles and fatty tissue. Drug distribution is affected by the decrease in total body water and albumin and the change in the ratio of lean body weight to fat. The reduction in albumin results in a greater concentration of unbound drugs in the circulation able to exert their effects, such as the highly lipophilic agents, CCNU, and procarbazine.

Drug metabolism is affected by decreased liver mass and hepatic blood flow as well as decreased microsomal enzymatic activity in the liver and affects drugs such as adriamycin, which is degraded by a mixed-function oxidase system.[171] Elimination is affected by the reduction in glomerular filtration rate, decreased renal blood flow, and renal tubular function, and is particularly important with cyclophosphamide and methotrexate, which are both renally excreted.

Chemotherapy

Chemotherapy, often a primary systemic form of treatment for cancer, possesses either cytotoxic or cytocidal activity.[172] McKenna[158] found that adverse drug reactions from chemotherapy increased seven-fold for patients aged over 69 years when compared with younger patients. As already noted, however, not all studies confirm this;[139,140] see also below.

Older patients are less likely to receive chemotherapy, and if treated, it is more likely to be outside a clinical trial. This is due partly to age restrictions on trial entry, and partly to clinicians without clinical evidence, feeling the need to reduce drug dosages in such patients. All drug therapy in elderly people is affected by altered pharmacokinetics and pharmacodynamics and some chemotherapeutic agents pose special problems.[38,133,173–176] Reduction of chemotherapeutic drug dosages may reduce both toxicity and response rates,[177] lower response rate without effect on toxicity, or result in better tolerance, but provide no survival advantage.[144,178,179]

Other researchers have found that elderly subjects, when receiving drug dosages similar to their younger counterparts, have similar toxicity rates, although some trials do not clearly define how the patients aged over 70 years were selected.[133,134,180]

In order to avoid unnecessary toxicity, a decision regarding dose reduction should be made on the onset of treatment, because if dose reductions vary from cycle to cycle of therapy, although tailored for individual patients, little evidence is accrued with regard to toxicity and efficacy. While it is very difficult to establish general rules regarding administration of chemotherapy,[181] physicians must be aware of the diversity of the health of older people and tailor chemotherapy according to individual needs.[175]

Balducci and Beghe[176] set out guidelines on the administration of chemotherapeutic drugs for older people, which include:

- age 75 years defines older age for chemotherapeutic agents
- chemotherapeutic agents that are renally excreted should be dose adjusted according to the patient's glomerular filtration rate
- hemopoietic growth factors should be used in people receiving moderately toxic chemotherapy in order to reduce the duration and severity of neutropenia
- high-dose chemotherapeutic regimens should be avoided because the functional reserve of many older people (≥75 years) is decreased, and this population is more susceptible to complications of chemotherapy
- palliation for frail patients may include some mild form of chemotherapy.

There is an age-dependent decrease in bone marrow stem cells, which result in increased liability to neutropenic episodes. Both granulocyte macrophage-colony stimulating factor (GM-CSF) and granulocyte-colony stimulating factor (G-CSF) reduce the duration of severe neutropenia and accelerate neutrophil recovery following chemotherapy. There is no evidence that older people respond differently from younger patients to such agents,[182] and in patients aged between 60 and 70 years being treated with aggressive chemotherapy for non-Hodgkin's lymphoma, the addition of G-CSF reduced the number of chemotherapy courses that were delayed, the mean duration of delay, the incidence of severe infections, and hospitalization. Additionally, G-CSF was found to be cost-effective in this group of older people.[183]

The following are some of the drugs that are commonly used in older subjects with particular problems in this age group highlighted.

Cyclophosphamide is a stable inactive compound that is activated in the liver via the cytochrome-P450 system and is well-absorbed when taken orally. It is used in solid tumors such as small-cell lung cancer, lymphomas, and breast or ovarian cancer. The side-effect profile includes nausea and vomiting, hematological toxicity, pulmonary fibrosis, and hemorrhagic cystitis.

Chlorambucil is an oral-alkylating agent with a myelosuppressive effect that is gradual in onset. It is used in the palliative treatment of ovarian cancer and in low-grade lymphomas.

Methotrexate is a folic acid antagonist that can be administered orally, intravenously, or intrathecally. Toxicity is usually to the gastrointestinal tract, mucous membranes, and bone marrow, and if ascites or a pleural effusion is present, methotrexate may accumulate in these sites to be later released and result in toxicity. The drug is 50 percent bound to albumin and can be displaced by drugs such as salicylates and phenytoin.

Its excretion is mainly unchanged in the urine and is affected by glomerular and tubular alterations in older subjects. It is widely used in ovarian and breast carcinoma, as well as lymphomas and leukemia.

5-Fluorouracil is an agent that interferes with nucleic acid synthesis and is widely used for colorectal metastases, although also having activity in breast and ovarian tumors. It is well tolerated both orally and intravenously, but may cause nausea, diarrhea, myelosuppression, and cardiac disturbances.

Vincristine is an alkaloid that is administered intravenously in the treatment of lymphomas, small-cell carcinoma, and tumors of the breast. Its toxicity is mainly neurological with peripheral neuropathy occurring especially in older people and in those with hepatic impairment. The neuropathy is characterized by early loss of reflexes and paraesthesia, with motor weakness and peripheral sensory signs at a later stage. Although nerve conduction is usually preserved, the EMG shows denervation and in elderly patients an autonomic neuropathy may result in constipation and ileus.

Etoposide is one of the most widely used chemotherapeutic drugs in elderly patients and may be administered orally or intravenously. Its main role is in the palliative treatment of small-cell lung cancer, although it has been widely used in lymphomas in older patients. Its main toxic effects are nausea, vomiting, and neutropenia.

Cisplatin is a platinum complex used primarily in carcinoma of the ovary, although it has a role in the management of lymphomas and small cell carcinoma of the bronchus. It is highly nephrotoxic and a high urine flow must be obtained prior to drug administration. Even when there is adequate hydration and diuresis, renal function usually worsens during repeated cycles of therapy and repeated creatinine clearance estimations are mandatory. Nausea and vomiting, ototoxicity that may be irreversible, peripheral neuropathy, and biochemical abnormalities of potassium, magnesium, and calcium are common documented side-effects.

Adriamycin is an anthracycline antibiotic that is given intravenously and because of hepatic metabolization may result in toxicity in older patients with impaired liver function. Its main side-effects are bone marrow depression, nausea, vomiting, and alopecia. Cardiotoxicity may result in arrhythmias or cardiac failure and is related to the total dose administered. The main roles for adriamycin are in the management of lymphomas, small-cell carcinoma, and adenocarcinoma of the breast, ovary, and stomach.

Hormonal therapies

Hormonal therapies may provide a benefit to elderly patients with advanced cancer of the breast, prostate, and endometrium. In the management of metastatic breast cancer, the beneficial effects of estrogen therapy increase steadily with age in all postmenopausal women probably due to the increased incidence of estrogen–receptor positive tumors in older women that result in an increased response rate to such therapy.

Tamoxifen (an antiestrogen drug) prolongs survival of patients with breast cancer and also reduces recurrence rates. It is particularly useful if the tumor is estrogen–receptor positive as seen in many post-menopausal women. Tamoxifen, however, should not be used as an alternative to surgery in all but the frailest elderly patients who would not survive such treatment.[184–186] Some researchers have found that tamoxifen alone appears to delay definitive treatment and this should not be encouraged.[187–191] Although there is evidence that preoperative tamoxifen may be an appropriate approach before breast-conserving surgery,[150,192] its main role is in the prevention of recurrence of breast cancer in post-menopausal women. It should be administered daily for a maximum of 5 years as there is yet no evidence for a longer duration of therapy.[193,194]

Radiotherapy

If a tumor is radiosensitive radiotherapy may be appropriate and have positive results for older patients in good health.[158,168,195]

Little is known about organ-specific tolerance to radiation in relation to aging, although there is evidence that tolerance of normal tissues to radiation therapy is 10–15 percent less in the very old. Additionally, lymphocytes from both elderly experimental animals and man are more susceptible to damage induced by ionizing radiation. Because most radiotherapy in elderly patients is palliative in intent, it is important that minimal toxicity is experienced. However, radiotherapy can be highly effective with most patients completing the treatment with no serious complications. Zachariah and Balducci[196] found that 94 percent of patients aged 80 years or older diagnosed with cancer of the head and neck, lung, pelvis or breast tolerated and completed the planned course of radiotherapy, be it either curative or palliative, without serious complications. It must be remembered that unless the patient is severely debilitated there is no reason to modify a potentially curative approach.[197]

With regard to breast cancer, age unfortunately remains an independent factor which determines those patients who will receive postoperative radiotherapy even after adjusting for other variables, including stage.[198] While there is no evidence that older women tolerate postoperative radiotherapy following breast cancer less well than younger patients, fewer older women receive this therapy.[38,111,185,186,193,199]

Myelosuppression may be problematic as elderly patients have less functional bone marrow and a slower recovery of normal tissue. Fatigue may result in compliance problems and radiation may result in dry skin that is more susceptible to infection.[200] The normal aging of the gastrointestinal tract may result in increased susceptibility to anorexia and stomatitis following radiotherapy.[201]

The more commonly seen radiation side-effects that occur in elderly subjects are often added to pre-existing conditions; thus radiation to emphysematous lungs will increase dyspnea and irradiation of the mediastinum will impair declining left ventricular function. Compliance with radiotherapy in elderly subjects is additionally hampered by multiple visits and traveling. The use of split fractions does, however, reduce toxicity and is essential in the treatment of many tumors in older patients.

Patients with non-small-cell lung cancer who are unfit for or refuse surgery may receive radiotherapy as an alternative treatment. Patients who accept radiotherapy tolerate it well and consider it an acceptable treatment.[202]

Radiotherapy is a well-established and potentially curative treatment for small-volume prostate tumors. It is often the preferred treatment of choice because it carries fewer complications than surgery and in some series 15-year disease-free survival rates of up to 85 percent have been achieved.[203,204] Hanks et al.[205] found that the median age of patients with prostate cancer treated with radiotherapy has increased from 65 years in 1973 to 72 years in 1989.

NURSING CARE

Nursing research dealing with older subjects is limited, and where it does exist is most often related to the elderly people in nursing homes or long-term care. In 1986, Adams[206] reviewed 154 studies, and although the studies covered hypertension, medication, and chronic illness in older people, none dealt with cancer. In a similar fashion to medical papers on older people, most nursing research describes elderly subjects to be "65 years of age or over," which means that their findings may not be applicable to those patients usually seen in geriatric medicine practice who are frequently over 80 years.[53]

Agism is an important adverse influence on the prevention and diagnosis of cancer, but also in the nursing care of elderly patients with cancer, and nurses are just as likely as others to be biased by agism.[207] This may be due to the inadequate preparation of nurses[208] or to a perceived lack of attractiveness of a gerontological career.[209] The nurse may view cancer prevention to be unnecessary, may promote dependency and learned helplessness, and minimize the need for referral to clinicians or community resources.[208]

IMPACT ON THE FAMILY

The experience of cancer for both the patient and family is stressful, and although many treatments for cancer can be given on an outpatient basis, many require prolonged hospitalization. Upon discharge to the community, much of the physical and psychological care of the patients is placed on the family. This puts an enormous stress on elderly patients and their caregivers. Not surprisingly, there is a high correlation between severity of symptoms and impact on activities of daily living.[210] Additionally, there is evidence that many patients with cancer have depressive symptoms[211] and there is a positive correlation between patients' self-care needs and mood.[212] Kurtz et al.[213] assessed the mental health of patients and family members and found of the 208 patients in the study, of whom 83 were aged 65 years or older, the most common five symptoms were fatigue, pain, nausea, poor appetite, and constipation. In this study there was no relationship between age and level of symptoms, although older people tend to under-report and this may counteract a genuine age-related increase in symptoms. Caregivers are more likely to be wives than husbands, and to care single-handedly. Wives provide twice the hours of care that husbands provide, although this is compensated by female patients having more outside care than males.[214] When the patient was younger, the caregivers tended to be more depressed, and caring had a greater impact on the caregiver's schedule; friends did provide more support to the caregiver.

In 82 percent of cases, the caregivers were spouses of the patients and it is likely, therefore, that elderly spouses will be solitary caregivers and have little support from other friends and relatives.[212] Elderly caregivers require counseling, but this may present logistic difficulties. The use of telephone counseling is of potential value and removes the need for transport and alternative care arrangements.[215]

REHABILITATION

Where data are available on elderly patients following treatment for cancer, functional status is usually assessed via the Karnofsky performance status scale:

- The Karnofsky performance status is a 100-point scoring system.
- One hundred percent equates with normal ADL and no evidence of the disease.
- Seventy percent indicates a patient who cares for him/herself but is unable to carry on normal activity or do active work.
- Thirty percent indicates that the patient is severely disabled and although death is not imminent, hospitalization is indicated.

This however, is not specific to older subjects and ignores many of the more important activities of daily living that are included

in well-validated rating schemes used frequently by geriatricians. When geriatricians and oncologists work together in the assessment of elderly patients, a functional assessment that is familiar to both is mandatory.

SURVIVAL

Relative survival is lower among older people with cancer than among their younger counterparts. There are many possible explanations for these differences and these include tendency for cancer to be diagnosed at a later stage in older subjects, and differences in the treatments received by elderly patients. Other age-related factors, such as comorbidity, obviously alter outcome.[40,116,118,216,217] In women with breast cancer the overall survival rates are lower in those aged 74 years and above than those aged 55–64 years.[218] In contrast, Kant et al.[119] showed no significant difference in survival rates of breast cancer by age, which is in keeping with similar 5-year survival rates found for women with breast cancer once cancer stage had been taken into account.[186]

> ### KEY POINTS Geriatric oncology
>
> - Age-specific cancer mortality rates are increasing.
>
> - Patients aged 70 years or above account for more than half of all cancer diagnoses.
>
> - Aging and cancer may be accounted for by the same theories, especially when considering chromosomal mutation.
>
> - Primary prevention of cancer in older people will also affect other causes of morbidity and mortality.
>
> - Screening, especially for breast cancer, is cost-effective and research is ongoing into screening for colon cancer. In contrast, population screening for prostate cancer is not cost-effective.
>
> - Older patients with suspected cancer are less likely to be investigated aggressively, have histopathological confirmation, and be actively managed.
>
> - Older patients have more advanced or unstaged disease at presentation, are more likely to be treated with palliative intent and to have shorter survival.
>
> - Elderly patients with bowel cancer are more likely to present with advanced disease and have emergency surgery.
>
> - Patients over 75 years of age should be carefully assessed before administration of chemotherapeutic drugs.
>
> - Radiotherapy can be highly effective, especially for palliation of symptoms and many patients can have all their therapy as an outpatient.
>
> - Carers of older patients with cancer are often elderly themselves or may be siblings in full-time employment.

REFERENCES

1. Office for National Statistics: 1998 mortality statistics—1998 boundaries (registrations) England and Wales. London, HMSO, 1999
2. Mayor S: Cancer is the main cause of death in Britain. Br Med J 1998;316:576
3. Byrne A, Carney DN: Cancer in the elderly. Curr Prob Cancer 1993;17:145–218
4. Paine C: The Health of the Nation. HMSO, Department of Health, London, 1992
5. Calman K: A Policy Framework for Commissioning Cancer Services. HMSO, Department of Health, 1995
6. Yancik R, Ries LA: Cancer in older persons. Magnitude of the problem—how do we apply what we know? Cancer 1994;74:1995–2003
7. de Rijke JM, Schouten LJ, Hillen HF et al: Cancer in the very elderly Dutch population. Cancer 2000;89:1121–1133
8. Grulich AE, Swerdlow AJ, dos Santos Silva I, Beral V: Is the apparent rise in cancer mortality in the elderly real? Analysis of changes in certification and coding of cause of death in England and Wales 1970–1990. Int J Cancer 1995;63:164–168
9. Cohen HJ: Biology of aging as related to cancer. Cancer 1994;74(suppl 7):2092–2100
10. Dix D, Cohen P, Flannery J: On the role of aging in cancer incidence. J Theor Biol 1980;83:163–173
11. Ebbesen P: Cancer and normal aging. Mech Ageing Dev 1984;25:269–283
12. Dilman VM: Aging and cancer in the light of ontogenetic "model of medicine." In Likhachev A, Anisimov V, Montesano R (eds): Age Related Factors in Carcinogenesis. IARC Science, Lyons, 1985:21–23
13. Cutler RG, Semsei I: Development, cancer and ageing: possible common mechanisms of action and regulation. J Gerontol A: Biol Sci Med Sci 1989;44:25–34
14. Yunis JJ: The chromosomal basis of human neoplasia. Science 1983;221:227–236
15. Setlow RB: Repair deficient human disorders and cancer. Nature 1978;271:713–717
16. Goldstein S: Human genetic disorders which feature accelerated aging. In Schneider EL (ed): The Genetics of Aging. Plenum, New York, 1978:171–224
17. Afshari CA, Barrett JC: Molecular genetics of in vitro cellular senescence. In Holbrook NJ, Martin GR, Lockshin RA (eds): Cellular Ageing and Death. Wiley-Liss, New York, 1996:109–121
18. Kinzler KW, Vogelstein B: Lessons from hereditary colorectal cancer. Cell 1996;87:159–170
19. Virchow RLK: Cellular Pathology as Based Upon Physiological and Pathological Histology. A Hirschwald, Berlin, 1858

20. Lipschitz DA, Goldstein S, Reis R et al: Cancer in the elderly: basic science and clinical aspects. Ann Intern Med 1985;102:218–228

21. Ono T, Takahashi N, Okada S: Age-associated changes in DNA methylation and mRNA level of the c-myc gene in spleen and liver of mice. Mutat Res 1989;219:39–50

22. Mays-Hoopes LL: Age-related changes in DNA methylation: do they represent continued developmental changes? Int Rev Cytol 1989;114:181–220

23. Ono T: Changes of DNA methylation in aging and carcinogenesis. Cancer Res Clin Oncol 1990;116(suppl):1056

24. Singer B, Gruneberger D: Molecular Biology of Mutagens and Carcinogens. Plenum, New York, 1983

25. Randerath K, Liehr JG, Gladek A, Randerath E: Age-dependent covalent DNA alterations (I-compounds) in rodent tissues: species, tissue and sex specification. Mutat Res 1989;219:121–133

26. Warner HR, Price AR: Involvement of DNA repair in cancer and aging. J Gerontol A: Biol Sci Med Sci 1989;44:45–54

27. Staiano-Coico L, Darzynkiewicz Z, Melamed MR, Weksler ME: Changes in DNA content of human blood mononuclear cells with senescence. Cytometry 1982;3:79–83

28. Anisimov VN: Carcinogenesis and Aging. Vols 1 and 2. Boca CRC Press, Boca Raton, FL, 1987

29. Mocchegiani E, Cacciatore L, Talarico M et al: Recovery of low thymic hormone levels in cancer patients by lysine-arginine combination. Int J Immunopharmacol 1990;12:365–371

30. Ershler WB: Geriatric correlates of experimental tumor biology. Oncology Huntingt 1992;6(suppl 2):58–61

31. Weksler ME, Tsuda T, Kim YT, Siskind GW: Immunobiology of aging and cancer. Cancer Detect Prev 1990;14:609–611

32. Wayne SJ, Rhyne RL, Garry PJ, Goodwin JS: Cell-mediated immunity as a predictor of morbidity and mortality in subjects over 60. J Gerontol 1990;45:M45–M48

33. Dunn BK, Longo DL: Molecular biology and biological markers. In Hunter CP, Johnson KA, Muss HB (eds): Cancer in the Elderly. Marcel Dekker, New York, 2000:69–121

34. Brownson RC, Reif JS, Alavanja MCR, Bal DG: Cancer. In Brownson RC, Remington PW, Davis JR (eds): Chronic Disease, Epidemiology and Control. American Public Health Association, Washington, DC, 1993:137–167

35. Bal DG, Lloyd J: Advocacy and government action for cancer prevention in older persons. Cancer 1994;74:2067–2070

36. Donaldson L, Donaldson R: Promotion of health. In Donaldson L, Donaldson R (eds): Essential Public Health 2nd ed. Petroc Press, 2000:101–167

37. Gullatte M: Prevention, screening and detection. In Otto S (ed): Oncology Nursing, 3rd Ed. Mosby, 1997:30–48

38. Balducci L: Prevention strategies and treatment of cancer in the elderly. Oncol Issues 2000;15:26–28

39. Andrews GR: Promoting health and function in an ageing population. Br Med J 2001;322:728–729

40. Holmes F, Hearne E: Cancer stage-to-age relationship: implications of cancer screening in the elderly. J Am Geriatr Soc 1981;19:55–57

41. Costanza ME: The extent of breast cancer screening in older women. Cancer 1994;74(suppl 7):2046–2050

42. Weinrich SP, Weinrich MC: Cancer knowledge among elderly individuals. Cancer Nurs 1986;9:301–307

43. Robie PW: Cancer screening in the elderly. J Am Geriatr Soc 1989;37:888–893

44. Frank-Stromborg M: The role of the nurse in early detection of cancer: population sixty-six years of age and older. Oncol Nurs Forum 1986;13:66–74

45. Powe BD: Fatalism among elderly African Americans. Effects on colorectal cancer screening. Cancer Nurs 1995;18:385–392

46. Warren B, Pohl JM: Cancer screening practices of nursing practitioners. Cancer Nurs 1990;3:143–151

47. Zabalegui A: Secondary cancer prevention in the elderly. Cancer Nurs 1994;17:215–222

48. Yoder LE, Jones SC, Jones PK: The association between health care behaviors and attitudes. Health Values 1985;9:24–31

49. Speake DL: Health promotion and activity in the well elderly. Health Values 1987;11:25–30

50. Speake DL, Cowart ME, Pellet K: Health perceptions and lifestyles of the elderly. Res Nurs Health 1989;12:93–100

51. Barnes S, Thomas A: A modified cancer education program. Effect on cancer knowledge and beliefs of the elderly. Cancer Nurs 1990;13:48–55

52. Ludwick R: Registered nurses' knowledge and practices of teaching and performing breast exams among elderly women. Cancer Nurs 1992;15:61–67

53. Given B, Given CW: Cancer nursing for the elderly: a target for research. Cancer Nurs 1989;12:71–77

54. Rubenstein L: Strategies to overcome barriers to early detection of cancer among older adults. Cancer 1994;74(suppl 7):2190–2193

55. Roetzheim RG, Van-Durme DJ, Brownlee HJ et al: Barriers to screening among participants of a media-promoted breast cancer screening project. Cancer Detect Prev 1993;17:367–377

56. Foster RS, Long SP, Costanza MC et al: Breast self-examination practices and breast cancer stage. N Engl J Med 1978;299:265–270

57. Department of Health. The NHS Cancer Plan. HMSO, London, 2000

58. Hendry PJ, Entwistle C: Effect of issuing an invitation for breast cancer screening to women aged 65–69. J Med Screen 1996;3:88–89

59. Faulk RM, Sickles EA, Sollitto RA et al: Clinical efficacy of mammographic screening in the elderly. Radiology 1995;194:193–197

60. Tabar L, Fagerberg G, Day NE et al: Breast cancer treatment and natural history: new insights from results of screening. Lancet 1992;339:412–414

61. Collette DJA, Day NE, Rombach JJ, de Waard F: Evaluation of screening for breast cancer in a non-randomized study (the Dom project) by means of a case-control study. Lancet 1984;i:1224–1226

62. Morrow M: Breast disease in elderly women. Surg Clin North Am 1994;74:145–161

63. van Dijck JA, Holland R, Verbeek AL, Hendriks JH, Mravunac M: Efficacy of mammographic screening of the elderly: a case referent study in the Nijmegen program in the Netherlands. J Natl Cancer Inst 1994;86:934–938

64. Chen HH, Tabar L, Fagerberg G, Duffy SW: Effect of breast cancer screening after age 65. J Med Screen 1995;2:10–14

65. Blanks RG, Moss SM, McGahan CE, Quinn MJ, Babb PJ: Effect of NHS Breast Screening Programme on mortality from breast cancer in England and Wales 1990–98: comparison of observed with predicted mortality. Br Med J 2000;321:665–669

66. Hobbs P, Kay C, Friedman EHI et al: Response by women aged 65–79 to invitation for screening for breast cancer by mammography: a pilot study. Br Med J 1990;301:1314–1316

67. Harris RP, Fletcher SW, Gonzalez JJ et al: Mammography and age: are we targeting the wrong women? A community survey of women and physicians. Cancer 1991;67:2010–2014

68. King ES, Resch N, Rimer B et al: Breast cancer screening practices among retirement community women. Prev Med 1993;22:1–19

69. Samet JM, Hunt WC, Goodwin JS: Determinants of cancer stage. A population-based study of elderly New Mexicans. Cancer 1990;66:1302–1307

70. Weinberger M, Saunders AF, Samsa GP et al: Breast cancer screening in older women: practices and barriers reported by primary care physicians. J Am Geriatr Soc 1991;39:22–29

71. Haigney E, Morgan R, King D, Spencer B: Breast examination in older women: questionnaire survey of attitudes of patients and doctors. Br Med J 1997;315:1058–1059

72. Edwards NI, Jones DA: Uptake of breast cancer screening in older women. Age Ageing 2000;29:131–135

73. Costanza ME: Breast cancer screening in older women. Synopsis of a forum. Cancer 1992;69:1925–1931

74. American Cancer Society. Guidelines for the early detection of cancer. Cancer J Clinics 2000;50:34–49

75. Albert M: Health screening to promote health for the elderly. Nurse Pract 1987;12:42–58

76. Mandelblatt JS, Wheat ME, Monane M et al: Breast cancer screening for elderly women with and without comorbid conditions. A decision analysis model. Ann Intern Med 1992;116:722–730

77. Oddone EZ, Feussner JR, Cohen HJ: Can screening older patients for cancer save lives? Clin Geriatr Med 1992;8:51–67

78. Weinrich SP, Weinrich MC, Stromborg MF et al: Using elderly educators to increase colorectal cancer screening. Gerontologist 1993;33:491–496

79. Wagner JL, Herdman RC, Wadhwa S: Cost effectiveness of colorectal cancer screening in the elderly. Ann Intern Med 1991;115:807–817

80. Rex DK, Lehman GA, Ulbright TM et al: Colonic neoplasia in asymptomatic persons with negative fecal occult blood tests: influence of age, gender, and family history. Am J Gastroenterol 1993;88:825–831

81. DiSario JA, Foutch PG, Mai HD et al: Prevalence and malignant potential of colorectal polyps in asymptomatic, average-risk men. Am J Gastroenterol 1991;86:941–945

82. Kronborg O, Fenger C, Olsen J, Bech K, Sondergaard O: Repeated screening for colorectal cancer with faecal occult blood test. Scand J Gastroenterol 1989;24:599–606

83. Moss S, Draper GJ, Hardcastle JD, Chamberlain J: Calculation of sample size in trials for early diagnosis of disease. Int J Epidemiol 1987;16:104–110

84. Hardcastle J, Chamberlain J, Robinson M: Randomised controlled trial of faecal-occult-blood screening for colorectal cancer. Lancet 1996;348:1472–1477

85. Kronborg O, Fenger C, Olsen J, Jorgensen OD, Sondergaard O: Randomised study of screening for colorectal cancer with faecal-occult-blood test. Lancet 1996;348:1467–1471

86. National Screening Committee. Population screening for prostate cancer. Letter EL(97) 12. HMSO, London, 1997

87. Optenberg SA, Thompson IM: Economics of screening for carcinoma of the prostate. Urol Clin North Am 1990;17:719–737

88. Gerber FS, Chodak GW: Routine screening for cancer of the prostate. J Nat Cancer Inst 1991;83:329–335

89. Alexander F: Incidence and aetiology of prostate cancer. In Kirk D (ed): The International Handbook of Prostate Cancer. Rowe, London, 1999:1–12

90. Cookson MM: Prostate cancer: screening and early detection. Cancer Control 2001;8:133–140

91. Pederson LL: Compliance with physician advice to quit smoking. A review of the literature. Prev Med 1982;11:71–84

92. Holbrook J: Tobacco smoking. In Braunwald E, Fanci A, Kasper D, Mauser S et al (eds): Harrison's Principles of Internal Medicine, 15th Ed. McGraw-Hill, New York, 2001:1302–1305

93. Peto R, Darby S, Deo H et al: Smoking, smoking cessation, and lung cancer in the UK since 1950: combination of national statistics with two case-control studies. Br Med J 2000;321:323–329

94. Power EJ: Cervical cancer screening in elderly women: Congressional Office of Technology Assessment. JAMA 1990;263:2996

95. Fletcher A: Screening for cancer of the cervix in elderly women. Lancet 1990;335:97–99

96. Fahs MC, Mandelblatt J, Schechter C, Muller C: Cost effectiveness of cervical cancer screening for the elderly. Ann Intern Med 1992;117:520–527

97. White JE, Begg L, Fishman NW et al: Increasing cervical cancer screening among minority elderly. Education and on-site services increase screening. J Gerontol Nurs 1993;19:28–34

98. Monfardini S, Tirelli U, Serraino D, Fentiman I: After 65 years, cancer has a different impact on life expectancy in men and women. Eur J Cancer 1991;27:1065–1066

99. Yancik R, Ries LG: Cancer in the aged. An epidemiological perspective on treatment issues. Cancer 1991;68:2502–2510

100. Levi F, La Vecchia C, Lucchini F, Negri E: Worldwide trends in cancer mortality in the elderly 1955–1992. Eur J Cancer 1996;32A:652–672

101. Vercelli M, Capocaccia R, Quaglia A et al: EUROCARE Working Group: Relative survival in elderly European cancer patients: evidence for health care inequalities. Crit Rev Oncol Haematol 2000;35:161–179

102. Boyle P: Global burden of cancer. Lancet 1997;349(2):23–26

103. Smith EWE: Cancer mortality at very old ages. Cancer 1996;77:1367–1372

104. Barrett JC: The mortality of centenarians in England and Wales. Arch Gerontol Geriatr 1985;4:211–218

105. Cody HS: The impact of mammography on 1096 consecutive patients with breast cancer 1979–1993: equal value for patients younger and older than age 50 years. Cancer 1995;76:1579–1584

106. Mor V, Guadagnoli E, Weitberg A et al: Influence of old age, performance status medical, and psychosocial status on management of cancer patients. In Yancik R, Yates J (eds): Cancer in the Elderly. Springer Publishing, New York, 1989:127–146

107. Bennett C, Greenfield S, Avonow H et al: Patterns of care related to age of men with prostate cancer. Cancer 1991;67:2633–2641

108. Silcocks PB, Thornton-Jones H, Skeet RG: Making cancer statistics more informative: measures of the quality of recorded diagnosis in a population based registry. Eur J Cancer Clin Oncol 1989;25:1467–1473

109. Parkin DM, Chen V, Ferlay J et al: Comparability and quality control in cancer registration. International Association of Cancer Registries. IARC Technical Report No. 19, Leon 1994

110. Seddon E, Williams E: Data quality in population-based cancer registration: an assessment of the Merseyside and Cheshire Cancer Registry. Br J Cancer 1997;76:667–674

111. Fleming ID, Fleming MD: Breast cancer in elderly women. Cancer 1994;74:2160–2164

112. Muers MF, Howard RA: Management of lung cancer. Thorax 1996;51:557–560

113. Mulcahy HE, Patchett SE, Daly L, O'Donoghue DP: Prognosis of elderly patients with large bowel cancer. Br J Surg 1994;81:736–738

114. Curless R, French JM, Williams GV et al: Colorectal carcinoma: do elderly patients present differently? Age Ageing 1994;23:102–107

115. Corner J: Some reflections on frailty in elderly patients with cancer. Eur J Cancer Care 1993;2:5–9

116. Mor V, Masterson-Allen S, Goldberg R et al: Relationship between age diagnosis and treatments received by cancer patients. J Am Gerontol Soc 1985;33:585–589

117. Samet JM, Hunt WC, Key CR et al: Choice of cancer therapy varies with age of patient. JAMA 1986;255:3385–3390

118. Goodwin J, Sament J, Key C et al: Stage at diagnosis of cancer varies with age of the patient. J Am Geriatr Soc 1986;34:20–26

119. Kant AK, Glover C, Horm J, Schatzkin A, Harris TB: Does cancer survival differ for older patients? Cancer 1992;70:2734–2740

120. Havlik RJ, Yancik R, Long S, Ries L, Edwards B: The National Institute on Aging and the National Cancer Institute SEER collaborative study on comorbidity and early diagnosis of cancer in the elderly. Cancer 1994;74:2101–2106

121. Bergman L, Kluck HM, van Leeuwen FE et al: The influence of age on treatment choice and survival of elderly breast cancer patients in south-eastern Netherlands: a population-based study. Eur J Cancer 1992;28A:1475–1480

122. Martin LM, le Pechoux C, Calitchi E et al: Management of breast cancer in the elderly. Eur J Cancer 1994;30:590–596

123. Busch E, Kemeny M, Fremgen A et al: Patterns of breast cancer care in the elderly. Cancer 1996;78:101–111

124. Ries LA: Ovarian cancer. Survival and treatment differences by age. Cancer 1993;71:524–529

125. Markman M, Lewis JL Jr, Saigo P et al: Epithelial ovarian cancer in the elderly. The Memorial Sloan-Kettering Cancer Center experience. Cancer 1993;71:634–637

126. Doherty JG, Rufer A, Bartholomew P, Beaumont DM: The presentation, treatment and outcome of renal cell carcinoma of old age. Age Ageing 1999;28:359–362

127. Greenfield S, Blanco VM, Elashoff RM, Ganz PA: Patterns of care related to age of breast cancer patients. JAMA 1987;257:2766–2770

128. Silliman RA, Guadagnoli E, Weitgerg AB, Mor V: Age as a predictor of diagnostic and initial treatment intensity in newly diagnosed breast cancer patients. J Gerontol 1989;44:46–50

129. Bergman L, Dekker G, van Leeuwen FE et al: The effect of age on treatment choice and survival in elderly breast cancer patients. Cancer 1991;67:2227–2234

130. McBean AM, Warren JL, Babish JD: Measuring the incidence of cancer in elderly Americans using Medicare claims data. Cancer 1994;73:2417–2425

131. Trimble EL, Carter CL, Cain D et al: Representation of older patients in cancer treatment trials. Cancer 1994;74(suppl 7):2208–2214

132. Allen C, Cox E, Manton R, Cohen H: Breast cancer in the elderly. Current patterns of care. J Am Geriatr Soc 1986;34:637–642

133. Begg CB, Cohen JL, Ellerton J: Are the elderly predisposed to toxicity from cancer chemotherapy? An investigation using data from the Eastern Cooperative Oncology Group. Cancer Clin Trials 1980;3:369–374

134. Begg CB, Carbone PP: Clinical trials and drug toxicity in the elderly. Cancer 1983;52:1986–1992

135. Chatta GS, Andrews RG, Rodger E et al: Hematopoietic progenitors and aging: alterations in granulocytic precursors and responsiveness to recombinant human G-CSF, GM-CSF, and IL-3. J Gerontol 1993;48:M207–M212

136. Chatta GS, Price TH, Stratton JR, Dale DC: Aging and marrow neutrophil reserves. J Am Geriatr Soc 1994;42:77–81

137. Hrushesky WJM, Shimp W, Kennedy BJ: Lack of age-dependent cisplatin nephrotoxicity. Am J Med 1984;76:579–584

138. Balducci L, Mowry K: Pharmacology and organ toxicity of chemotherapy in older patients. Oncology 1992;6:62–68

139. Nerenz D, Leventhal H, Easterlin DV, Love RR: Psychosocial consequences of cancer chemotherapy for elderly patients. Health Serv Res 1986;20:961–976

140. Dodd MJ, Onishi K, Dibble SL, Larson PJ: Difference in nausea, vomiting and retching between younger and old out-patients receiving cancer chemotherapy. Cancer Nurs 1996;19:155–161

141. Fallowfield LJ: Behavioral interventions and psychological aspects of care during chemotherapy. Eur J Cancer 1992;28a:S39–S41

142. Bonnadonna G, Valagussa P: Dose-response effect of chemotherapy in breast cancer. N Engl J Med 1981;304:10

143. Holland JC, Massie MJ: Psychosocial aspects of cancer in the elderly. Clin Geriatr Med 1987;3:2766–2770

144. Cohen H, Silberman H, Forman W et al: Affect of age on response to treatment and survival of patients with multiple myeloma. J Am Geriatr Soc 1983;31:372–377

145. Warnecke RB: The elderly as a target group for prevention and early detection of cancer. In Yancik R, Yates JW (ed): Cancer in the Elderly: Approaches to Early Detection and Treatment. Springer Publishing, New York, 1989:3–14

146. Yellen SB, Cella DF, Leslie WT: Age and clinical decision making in oncology patients. J Natl Cancer Inst 1994;86:1766–1770

147. Sutton SM, Eisner EJ, Burklow J: Health communications to older Americans as a special population. The National Cancer Institute's consumer-based approach. Cancer 1994;74:2194–2199

148. Fratino L, Ferrario L, Redmond K, Audisio RA: Global health care: the role of geriatrician, general practitioner and oncology nurse. Crit Rev Oncol Hematol 1998;27:101–109

149. Sandison AJ, Gold DM, Wright P, Jones PA: Breast conservation or mastectomy: treatment choice of women aged 70 years and older. Br J Surg 1996;83:994–996

150. Silliman RA, Troyan SL, Guadagnoli E, Kaplan SH, Greenfield S: The impact of age, marital status, and physician-patient interactions on the care of older women with breast carcinoma. Cancer 1997;80:1326–1334

151. Ganz PA: Interaction between the physician and the older patient: the oncologist's perspective. Cancer 1997;80:1323–1325

152. Ganz PA: Does (or should) chronologic age influence the choice of cancer treatment? Oncology Huntingt 1992;6(suppl2):45–49

153. Goodwin JS, Hunt WC, Samet JM: Determinants of cancer therapy in elderly patients. Cancer 1993;72:594–601

154. Coebergh JW: Significant trends in cancer in the elderly. Eur J Cancer 1996;32A:569–571

155. Extermann M, Balducci L, Lyman GH: What threshold for adjuvant therapy in older breast cancer patients. J Clin Oncol 2000;18:1709–1717

156. Yancik R, Wesley MN, Ries LA et al: Effect of age and comorbidity in post-menopausal breast cancer patients aged 55 years and older. JAMA 2001;285:885–892

157. Walsh TH: Audit of outcome of major surgery in the elderly. Br J Surg 1996;83:92–97

158. McKenna RJ Sr: Clinical aspects of cancer in the elderly. Treatment decisions, treatment choices, and follow-up. Cancer 1994;74:2107–2117

159. Audisio RA, Geraghty JG: Signs, symptoms, early detection, staging and follow-up. Crit Rev Oncol Hematol 1998;27:119–120

160. Lehnert T, Pfitzenmaier J, Hinz U, Herfarth C: Surgery for local recurrence or distant metastases in patients aged 75 years or older. Eur J Surg Oncol 1998;24:418–422

161. Hebert-Croteau N, Brisson J, Latreille J, Blanchette C, Deschenes L: Compliance with consensus recommendations for the treatment of early stage breast carcinoma in elderly women. Cancer 1999;85:1104–1113

162. Newschaffer CJ, Penberthy LT, Desch CE, Tetchin SM, Whittemore M: The effect of age and comorbidity in the treatment of elderly women with nonmetastatic breast cancer. Arch Intern Med 1996;156:85–90

163. Shankar A, Taylor I: Treatment of colorectal cancer in patients aged over 75. Eur J Surg Oncol 1998;24:391–395

164. Marrelli D, Roviello F, De Stefano A et al: Surgical treatment of gastrointestinal carcinomas in octogenarians: risk factors for complications and long-term outcome. Eur J Surg Oncol 2000;26:371–376

165. Chiappa A, Zbar AP, Bertani E et al: Surgical outcomes for colorectal cancer patients including the elderly. Hepatogastroenterology 2001;48:440–444

166. Colorectal Cancer Collaborative Group. Surgery for colorectal cancer in elderly patients, a systematic review including aggregate data from 28 prospective surgical series. Lancet 2000;356:968–973

167. Arveux I, Boutron MC, El Mrini T et al: Colon cancer in the elderly: evidence for major improvements in health care and survival. Br J Cancer 1997;76:963–967

168. Turner NJ, Haward RA, Mulley GP, Selby PJ: Cancer in old age—is it inadequately investigated and treated? Br Med J 1999;319:309–312

169. Gosney M: Cancer. In Crome P, Ford G (eds): Drugs and the Older Population. Imperial College Press, London, 2000:601–651

170. Lamy P: Comparative pharmacokinetic changes and drug therapy in an older population. J Am Geriatr Soc 1982;30:S11–19

171. Robert J, Hoerni B: Age dependence of the early phase pharmacokinetics of doxorubicin. Cancer Res Clin Oncol 1983;43:4467–4469

172. Weiss G: Drugs in the treatment of cancer. In Weiss G (ed): Clinical Oncology. Prentice-Hall International, New York,1993:97–188

173. Hansen HH, Selawry OS, Holland JF, McCall CB: The variability of individual tolerance to methotrexate in cancer patients. Br J Cancer 1971;25:298–305

174. Haas CD, Coltman CA, Gottlieb AJ: Phase II evaluation of bleomycin: a Southwest Oncology Group study. Cancer 1976;38:8–12

175. Balducci L, Extermann M: Cancer chemotherapy in the older patient: what the medical oncologist needs to know. Cancer 1997;80:1317–1322

176. Balducci L, Beghe C: Pharmacology of chemotherapy in older cancer patient. Cancer Control 1999;6:466–470

177. Frei E, Canellos GP: Dose: a critical factor in cancer chemotherapy. Am J Med 1980;69:585–594

178. Bonadonna G, Valagussa P: Dose response effects of adjuvant chemotherapy in breast cancer. N Engl J Med 1981;304:10–15

179. Gelman R, Taylor SG: Cyclophosphamide, methotrexate and 5-fluorouracil chemotherapy in women more than 65 years old with advanced breast cancer: the elimination of age trends in toxicity by using doses based on creatinine clearance. J Clin Oncol 1984;2:1404–1413

180. Leslie WT: Chemotherapy in older cancer patients. Oncology Huntingt 1992;6(suppl 2):74–80

181. Zagonel V, Fratino L, Sacco C et al: Reducing chemotherapy-associated toxicity in elderly cancer patients. Cancer Treat Rev 1996;22:223–244

182. Shank W, Balducci L: Recombinant hemopoietic growth factors may protect older patients from chemotherapy myelodepression. Proc Am Soc Clin Oncol 1991;10:326

183. Kayahara M, Nagakawa T, Ueno K et al: Pancreatic resection for periampullary carcinoma in the elderly. Surg Today 1994;24:229–233

184. Gazet JC, Ford HT, Coombes RC et al: Prospective randomised trial of tamoxifen vs surgery in elderly patients with breast cancer. Eur J Surg Oncol 1994;20:207–214

185. Bellet M, Alonso C, Ojeda B: Breast cancer in the elderly. Postgrad Med J 1995;71:658–664

186. Ashkanani F, Eremin O, Heys SD: The management of cancer of the breast in the elderly. Eur J Surg Oncol 1998;24:396–402

187. Bates T, Riley DL, Houghton J, Fallowfield L, Baum M: Breast cancer in elderly women: a Cancer Research Campaign trial comparing treatment with tamoxifen and optimal surgery with tamoxifen alone. The Elderly Breast Cancer Working Party. Br J Surg 1991;78:591–594

188. Horobin JM, Preece PE, Dewar JA, Wood RA, Cushieri A: Long-term follow-up of elderly patients with locoregional breast cancer treated with tamoxifen only. Br J Surg 1991;78:213–217

189. Gaskell DJ, Hawkins RA, de Barteret S et al: Indications for primary tamoxifen therapy in elderly women with breast cancer. Br J Surg 1992;79:1317–1320

190. Bergmann L, van Dongen JA, van Ooijen B, van Leeuwen FE: Should tamoxifen be a primary treatment choice for elderly breast cancer patients with locoregional disease? Breast Cancer Res Treat 1995;34:77–83

191. Martelli G, DePalo G, Rossi N et al: Long-term follow-up of elderly patients with operable breast cancer treated with surgery without axillary dissection plus adjuvant tamoxifen. Br J Cancer 1995;72:1251–1255

192. Ellis MJ: Preoperative endocrine therapy for older women with breast cancer: renewed interest in an old idea. Cancer Control 2000;7:557–562

193. Silliman RA, Balducci L, Goodwin JS, Holmes FF, Leventhal EA: Breast cancer care in old age: what we know, don't know, and do. J Natl Cancer Inst 1993;85:190–199

194. Gottlieb S: Breast cancer patients can stop tamoxifen after 5 years. West J Med 2001;175:13

195. Pignon T, Scalliet P: Radiotherapy in the elderly. Eur J Surg Oncol 1998;24:407–411

196. Zachariah B, Balducci L, Venkattaramanabalaji GV et al: Radiotherapy for cancer patients aged 80 and older: a study of effectiveness and side effects. Int J Radiat Oncol Biol Phys 1997;39:1125–1129

197. Scalliet P: Radiotherapy in the elderly. Eur J Cancer 1991;27:3–5

198. Ballard-Barbash R, Potosky AL, Harlan LC, Nayfield SG, Kessler LG: Factors associated with surgical and radiation therapy for early stage breast cancer in older women. J Natl Cancer Inst 1996;88:701–703

199. de Graaf H, Willemse PH, Sleijfer DT: Review: breast cancer in elderly patients. Age Ageing 1994;23:427–434
200. Hilderley L: Clinical reviews: skin care in radiation therapy: a review of the literature. Oncol Nurs Forum 1983;10:51–56
201. Gunn W: Radiation therapy for the aging patient. Cancer 1980;30:337–347
202. Patterson CJ, Hocking M, Bond M, Teale C: Retrospective study of radiotherapy for lung cancer in patients aged 75 years and over. Age Ageing 1998;27:515–518
203. Dawson C, Whitfield H: ABC of urology. Urological malignancy—1: Prostate cancer. 1996;312:1032–1034
204. Kish JA: Neoadjuvant androgen ablation in localized carcinoma of the prostate. Cancer Control 2001;8:155–162
205. Hanks GE, Hanlon A, Owen JB, Schultheiss TE: Patterns of radiation treatment of elderly patients with prostate cancer. Cancer 1994;74:2174–2177
206. Adams M: Aging: gerontological nursing research. Annu Rev Nurs Res 1986;4:77–103
207. Chandler JT, Rachal JR, Kazelskis R: Attitudes of long term care nursing personnel towards the elderly. Gerontologist 1986;26:551–555
208. Boyle DM, Engelking C, Blesch KS et al: Oncology nursing society position paper on cancer and aging: the mandate for oncology nursing. Oncol Nurs Forum 1992;19:913–933
209. Siu AL: The quality of medical care received by older persons. J Am Geriatr Soc 1987;35:1084–1091
210. Holmes S, Dickerson J: The quality of life: design and evaluation of self-assessment instrument for use with cancer patients. Int J Nurs Stud 1987;24:15–24
211. Derogatis LR, Morrow G, Fettig J et al: The prevalence of psychiatric disorders among cancer patients. JAMA 1983;249:751–757
212. McCorkle R, Quint-Benoleil J: Symptoms distress, current concerns and mood disturbance after diagnosis of life-threatening illness. Soc Sci Med 1983;17:431–438
213. Kurtz ME, Given B, Kurtz JC, Given CW: The interaction of age, symptoms and survival status on physical and mental health of patients with cancer and their families. Cancer 1994;74:2071–2078
214. Allen SM: Gender differences in spousal caregiving and unmet need for care. J Gerontol 1994;49:S187–S195
215. Skipwith DH: Telephone counseling interventions with caregivers of elders. J Psychosoc Nurs Ment Health Serv 1994;32:7–12
216. Fentiman IS, Tirelli U, Monfardini S et al: Cancer in the elderly: why so badly treated? Lancet 1990;335:1020–1022
217. Vercelli M, Quaglia A, Casella C et al: Relative survival in elderly cancer patients in Europe. Eur J Cancer 1998;34:2264–2270
218. Bergman L, Dekker G, van Leeuwen FE et al: Dekker breast cancer survival rate. Cancer 1991;67:2227–2234

Constipation and fecal incontinence in old age

Danielle Harari

Material in this chapter contains contributions from the previous edition, and we are grateful to the previous author for the work done.

This chapter describes the epidemiology, pathogenesis, causes, diagnosis, and treatment of constipation and fecal incontinence in elderly people. Data sources were a computer-assisted search of the English language literature (1966 to present), reference lists from recent systematic reviews and book chapters, and expert committee reports and opinion. Strength of recommendations [A–D] are based on the following evidence levels: [A] meta-analysis of randomized controlled trials, or at least one randomized controlled trial; [B] at least one good-quality cohort or case-control study; [C] case series (and poor-quality cohort or case-control studies); [D] expert committee reports or opinion.[1]

CONSTIPATION IN THE OLDER ADULT

Constipation is a frequent health concern for elderly people and their healthcare providers. The number of physician visits for constipation increases markedly among people over 65 years,[2,3] as does regular laxative use.[4–6] The self-reported symptom of constipation has been associated with anxiety, depression, and poor health perception in older people, while clinical constipation in frail individuals may lead to complications such as fecal impaction, sigmoid volvulus, and urinary retention.

Definition of constipation

The feeling of being constipated will often mean different things to different individuals. Until 5 years ago, the nonspecific and subjective definition of "self-reported" constipation was used in epidemiological studies of older people. Based on the recommendations of an international workshop, constipation is now defined more symptom-specifically both in research and in clinical practice (see Table 103-1).[7] Objectively, however, the clinical definition of constipation relies on evidence of excessive stool retention in the rectum and/or colon.

Epidemiology of constipation in older people

The generally held belief that constipation is an inevitable consequence of aging stems partly from questionnaire-based studies showing a marked increase of self-reported constipation with age.[4–6] In the community, up to 34 percent of women and 26 percent of men over 65 report constipation;[4–6] the preponderance of women over men reporting the symptom attenuates in older cohorts aged 80 and over.[4,6,8] In contrast, the

Table 103-1 **Definitions of constipation**
Self-reported constipation
• Patient reports usual bowel habit as being constipated
Functional constipation

• Two or more of the following symptoms present for at least 12 months:
   • Two or fewer bowel movements per week
   • Straining on more than 1 in 4 occasions
   • Hard stools on more than 1 in 4 occasions
   • Feeling of incomplete evacuation on more than 1 in 4 occasions

Rectal outlet delay
• Feeling of anal blockage on more than 1 in 4 occasions *and*   • Prolonged defecation (>10 minutes to complete bowel movement); *or*   • Need for self-digitation (pressing in or around the anus to aid evacuation) on any occasion
Clinical constipation
• Large amount of feces in rectum on digital examination *and/or*   • Excessive fecal retention in the colon on abdominal radiograph

weekly frequency of bowel movements does not alter with aging, with only 1–7 percent of both young and older community-dwelling individuals reporting frequency below the normal range (≤ 2 bowel movements a week).[4,6,9] This consistent bowel pattern across age groups persists even after statistical adjustment for the greater amount of laxatives used by elderly people.[4] Even among older people complaining of constipation less than 10 percent report ≤ 2 weekly bowel movements, and over half move their bowels daily.[6,10] This suggests that bowel-related symptoms other than infrequent bowel movements drive self-reporting of constipation in elderly persons. These symptoms are in fact straining and passage of hard stools:[6,10] of older individuals who report constipation, 65 percent report persistent straining, and 39 percent report hard bowel movements.[10] Hence constipated older people tend to suffer primarily from difficulties with rectal evacuation, as shown by a prevalence rate of 21 percent for rectal outlet delay among community-dwelling people aged 65 and over.[7] A clear understanding of the specific bowel symptoms each individual has when reporting constipation is important in guiding the healthcare provider toward appropriate management of this common complaint [B].

Constipation is an even greater problem in the nursing home setting where 47 percent of individuals report constipation, 17 percent ≤ 2 bowel movements per week, and 30 percent persistent straining.[8] Over 40 percent of nursing home residents admitted to UK hospitals are already fecally impacted.[11] The high prevalence of constipation is all the more striking in that 50–58 percent of nursing home residents use one or more daily laxative.[8,12] This would imply that in the long-term care setting laxative prescribing may be ineffective, and that nonpharmacological approaches to treatment are currently underutilized. Periodic assessment for constipation in elderly nursing home residents should be incorporated into routine nursing and medical care [B].

Colonic function in healthy aging and in older patients with constipation

Colonic motility depends on the integrity of the central and autonomic nervous systems, gut wall innervation and receptors, circular smooth muscle and gastrointestinal hormones. Propagating motor complexes in the colon are stimulated by increased intraluminal pressure generated by bulky fecal content.

Studies of total gut transit time (passage of radio-opaque markers from mouth to anus) in healthy elderly people demonstrate no change with aging,[13,14] and motility studies show no effect of aging on colonic motor activity before or after meals.[15] In contrast, elderly people with constipation have prolonged total gut transit times of 4–9 days (normally <3 days).[13,16] Radiological markers pass especially slowly through the left colon with striking delay in evacuation from the rectosigmoid, suggesting that total transit time in elderly people with constipation is prolonged because of segmental dysmotility in the "hindgut."[17,18] Transit time is substantially slower in institutionalized or bedridden patients with constipation, ranging from 6 to more than 14 days.[19] Slower transit in frailer elderly people (often exacerbated by causes such as chronic illness, immobility, and drugs), creates a cycle of shrinking fecal bulk by reducing water content (normally 75 percent), hence diminishing intraluminal pressures and further inhibiting effective propagation through the colon.

Table 103-2 summarizes possible underlying mechanisms for colonic dysfunction in older persons with constipation. The aging rat model shows a 45 percent prolongation of transit time with senescence combined with a significant widening of the colon.[20] Colonic dilatation is seen in some elderly individuals with chronic constipation which could similarly prolong transit through a reduction in intraluminal pressures. Electrophysiological measurement of colonic motor activity in elderly constipated subjects has shown a reduced sigmoid

---

Table 103-2 Possible mechanisms for constipation in older people

Functional constipation
- Increased colonic diameter
- Myenteric plexus dysfunction
- Reduced inhibitory nerve input to circular muscle
- Increased binding of plasma endorphins to gut receptors

Rectal outlet delay
- Suppression or disregard of defecation urge
- Sacral cord dysfunction
- Pelvic floor descent
- Paradoxical contraction of pelvic floor muscles

---

motor response to intraluminal bisacodyl (a direct stimulant of the myenteric plexus), implying a degree of myenteric dysfunction.[18] This may contribute to primary gut pathology in constipated elderly people, independently of secondary causes such as heavy stimulant laxative use and diabetes. Myenteric plexus degeneration has been demonstrated in surgically removed colons of younger patients with severe idiopathic constipation,[21] but there are as yet no similar studies in elderly patients. In-vitro studies of colons from older persons show an age-related reduction in the amplitude of inhibitory junction potentials, but no decrease in the levels of inhibitory gut neuropeptides.[22] This age-related decrease in inhibitory nerve input to the circular smooth muscle occurs earlier in women as compared with men, and could result in segmental motor incoordination which may lengthen overall transit time. Individuals over 60 have higher plasma concentrations of beta-endorphin with increased binding to endogenous opiate receptors in the gut.[23] This may exacerbate the opiate effect of relaxing colonic tone, reducing motility, and inhibiting the gastrocolic reflex in older people receiving opiate analgesia. Parenthetically, it has been reported that naloxone, when given to nursing home residents with constipation, can result in an increase in stool output and a reduction in constipation symptoms.[23]

Anorectal function in healthy older adults

The internal anal sphincter is a continuation of the circular smooth muscle of the rectum which provides 75–80 percent of the anal closing pressure at rest.[24] The external sphincter is a striated muscle under voluntary control innervated by the pudendal nerve (as are the pelvic floor muscles). In normal defecation, stool enters and distends the rectal ampulla causing intrinsically mediated reflex relaxation of the internal anal sphincter (inhibitory reflex) followed promptly by reflex contraction of the external anal sphincter and pelvic floor muscles. The brain registers a desire to defecate, the external sphincter is voluntarily relaxed when appropriate, and the rectum evacuated with assistance from abdominal wall muscle contraction.

Anorectal function in healthy older persons is characterized by a tendency towards an age-related reduction in internal anal tone, and a more definite decline in external anal sphincter tone, especially in older women.[25,26] Rectal motility is well preserved,[15] though anorectal sensitivity appears to decline with age in women.[27] Aging alone however, appears to have little impact on anorectal function until later old age, from the seventh decade upwards in women and even later in men.[25,26]

Anorectal function in constipated older adults

Older persons with constipation may have one or more of four types of anorectal dysfunction. Most commonly seen in frail elderly people is *rectal dyschezia*, characterized by impaired rectal sensation (needing a larger-volume rectal balloon before feeling the urge to void), reduced rectal tone, increased rectal compliance, and impaired anal sensitivity.[11,18] Such patients are likely to have rectal impaction on digital examination of which they may be unaware, associated with fecal soiling due to locally secreted mucus from around the irritative fecal mass.[11] Rectal dyschezia may develop as a result of persistent disregard or suppression of the desire to defecate as occurs in patients with dementia, depression, immobility, or painful anorectal conditions (Table 103-2). The neuropathophysiology of the condition is also compatible with diminished parasympathetic outflow from the sacral plexus, which in elderly people may be due to local ischemia and spinal stenosis. *Pelvic dyssynergia* is failure to relax the puborectalis and external anal sphincter muscles during attempted defecation, resulting in paradoxical increases in anal pressure on straining.[28] This abnormal expulsion pattern is seen in some individuals with longstanding symptoms of rectal outlet delay, and in patients with Parkinson's disease.[29] The pelvic muscles show a decline in strength with aging women who have a history of childbirth,[30] which may result in *pelvic floor descent* with corresponding rectal evacuation difficulties.[11,18] Finally, some patients with a longstanding history of constipation will have increased rectal tone and reduced compliance indicative of *irritable bowel syndrome*; these patients often complain of difficult passage of small fecal pellets, and abdominal pain and distension relieved by defecation.[31] In summary, pathophysiological changes of colorectal dysmotility and anorectal dysfunction have been observed in elderly people who have constipation but not in healthy elderly people, and so cannot be considered inevitable consequences of aging [B]. Lower gut function is more influenced by chronic disease, immobility, and medications, than by aging itself.

Causes of constipation in older people

The identification of risk factors for constipation in elderly individuals is critical to achieve effective management of the condition [B]. In a prospective study, Robson et al. looked at baseline characteristics predictive of new-onset constipation in elderly nursing home patients, using the US Minimum Data Set instrument.[32] Seven percent ($n = 1,291$) developed constipation over a 3-month period. Independent predictors were white race, decreased fluid intake, Parkinson's disease, decreased mobility, arthritis, greater than five medications, and dementia. Table 103-3 summarizes predisposing causes of constipation.

Polypharmacy increases the risk of constipation in older patients,[6,32] particularly in nursing homes where each individual takes an average of six prescribed medications per day.[8] Certain classes of drugs are particularly implicated in promoting constipation. Drugs with strong anticholinergic properties reduce contractility of the smooth muscle of the gut via an antimuscarinic effect at acetyl-choline receptor sites, and in some cases, long-term use may induce chronic colonic dysmotility.[33,34] All types of iron supplements have the same propensity to cause constipation, though slow-release wax-matrix preparations may have a lesser impact on the large bowel.[35] Severe constipation has been reported in elderly patients taking calcium channel antagonists; nifedipine and verapamil are more potent inhibitors of gut motility than diltiazem and newer agents.[36] Nonsteroidal anti-inflammatory drugs increase the risk of constipation, most likely through prostaglandin inhibition.[37] Overall, constipation as a drug side-effect is likely to be substantially under-reported in elderly

Table 103-3 **Causes of constipation in older people**
Functional constipation
Medications:
• Anticholinergic drugs (tricyclics, antipsychotics, antihistamines, antiemetics, drugs for detrusor hyperactivity)
• Opiates
• Iron supplements
• Calcium channel antagonists
• Calcium supplements
• Nonsteroidal anti-inflammatory drugs
Immobility
Neurological conditions:
• Parkinson's disease
• Diabetes mellitus
• Stroke
• Spinal cord injury or disease
Dehydration
Low dietary fiber
Metabolic disturbances:
• Hypothyroidism
• Hypercalcemia
• Hypokalemia
Mechanical obstruction (e.g. tumor)
Rectal outlet delay
• Dementia
• Depression
• Lack of privacy or comfort
• Anorectal disease or prior surgery
• Weak pelvic and abdominal muscles
• Rectal dyschezia
Self-reported constipation
• Misperceptions regarding normal bowel habit
• Anxiety/depression

people. *Immobility* is a primary risk factor;[33] greater physical activity in elderly people reduces symptoms of constipation.[5,38] Exercise increases colonic propulsive activity, especially when measured post-prandially.[39] Patients with *Parkinson's disease* may be severely constipated because of dual pathologies of primary degeneration of dopaminergic neurons in the enteric nervous system resulting in prolonged transit throughout the entire gut, and pelvic dyssynergia resulting in rectal outlet delay and prolonged straining.[29,40] A survey of outpatients with *diabetes mellitus* showed that 60 percent complained of constipation.[41] Those with autonomic neuropathy are more likely to be affected due to markedly slowed transit throughout the colon.[42] Constipation is a significant clinical problem in the majority of people with *spinal cord disease or injury*.[43,44]

Low fluid intake in older adults has been related to slow colonic transit.[45] Withholding fluids over a 1-week period in young male volunteers significantly reduced stool output.[46] Elderly people are at greater risk of dehydration due to impaired thirst sensation, and less effective hormonal responses to hypertonicity, while those in nursing homes and hospitals may in addition have functional reasons for being unable to drink. *Dietary fiber* intake is often low in elderly people, but no clear association has been made with clinical constipation in this population. In younger healthy and constipated adults, low dietary fiber has been associated (through meta-analysis) with increased stool weight and decreased transit time.[47]

In elderly subjects, higher fiber intake correlated with lower laxative use among older women in one community study,[48] but in another, higher intake of bran was associated with no reduction in constipation symptoms and greater fecal loading in the colon on abdominal radiography.[5] *Dementia* predisposes individuals to rectal dyschezia,[11] possibly partly through ignoring the urge to defecate. A study in which young men deliberately suppressed defecation resulted in prolonged transit through the rectosigmoid with a marked reduction in frequency of bowel movements.[49] Psychological distress, *depression*, and anxiety are all associated with increased self-reporting of constipation in older persons.[50] In certain cases, the symptom of constipation is a somatic manifestation of psychiatric illness; a careful assessment is required to differentiate subjective complaints from clinical constipation in depressed or anxious patients. *Metabolic imbalances* of hypothyroidism, uremia, hypokalemia, and hypercalcemia should not be overlooked as remediable causes. Colorectal cancer is associated with both constipation and use of laxatives, though this risk association is likely to be confounded by the influence of underlying habits.[50a] As the prevalence of colorectal cancer increases with age, index of suspicion should be higher in older adults. Abdominal pain, rectal bleeding, recent change in bowel habit, and certainly any systemic features (weight loss, anaemia etc.) should prompt further investigations for underlying neoplasm.

Diagnosis of constipation in older people

Table 103-4 lists the important aspects of evaluating constipation in an elderly person. It is helpful to have patients keep a stool chart for at least 1 week to document frequency, consistency, and associated symptoms. Constipation can be underestimated in frailer elderly patients who do not report any bowel-related symptoms, and in those who may have regular bowel movements, despite significant impaction. This emphasizes the importance of a thorough bowel assessment in all elderly people at risk of clinical constipation, especially those in institutionalized settings [B]. An empty rectum on digital rectal examination does not exclude the diagnosis of constipation;[5] a plain abdominal radiograph is needed where clinical suspicion is present [C]. The abdominal radiograph will measure the extent and severity of fecal loading, identify impaction and evaluate the degree of associated bowel obstruction, and diagnose acute complications such as sigmoid volvulus (Fig. 103-1).[16,51] The presence of feces in the cecum on the abdominal radiograph (Fig. 103-2) is indicative of prolonged colonic transit.

Further investigation of constipated patients with colonoscopy or barium enemas is warranted if recently altered bowel habit, systemic illness, or laboratory abnormalities arouse suspicion of colorectal disease. In older patients, colonoscopy tends to provide more specific diagnoses with less patient discomfort than barium enemas. For both procedures, inadequate tests are not uncommon in elderly people due to poor bowel preparation,[52] and this is especially relevant in persons presenting with constipation. Polyethylene glycol may be better tolerated than sodium picosulfate in older people.[53,54] A pre-procedure plain abdominal X-ray for evaluation of fecal clearance is also helpful in predicting the adequacy of the test. Anorectal function tests may be useful in patients who report persistent and severe features of rectal outlet delay in order to diagnose pelvic dyssynergia, a condition amenable to biofeedback therapy.

Complications of constipation

The most important complication in older people is *overflow incontinence* (see below). In addition to overflow, features

Table 103-4 **Diagnosis of constipation in older people**
Bowel history
• Number of bowel movements per week
• Stool consistency
• Straining/symptoms of rectal outlet delay
• Duration of constipation
• Fecal/urinary incontinence
• Abdominal pain relieved by evacuation
• Rectal pain or bleeding
• Laxative use, prior and current
General history
• Mood/cognition
• Symptoms of systemic illness
• Diet
Specific physical examination
• Digital rectal examination including sphincter tone
• Perianal sensation/cutaneous anal reflex
• Abdominal palpation, auscultation
Tests
Indications for plain abdominal radiograph:
• Empty rectum with clinical suspicion of constipation
• Possible fecal impaction
• Fecal incontinence
• Evaluation for bowel dysmotility/redundant sigmoid loop/volvulus
Indications for colonscopy or barium enema:
• Systemic illness (weight loss, anaemia, etc.)
• New-onset fecal impaction without prior history of constipation
Indications for anorectal function tests:
• Severe or persistent symptoms of rectal outlet delay

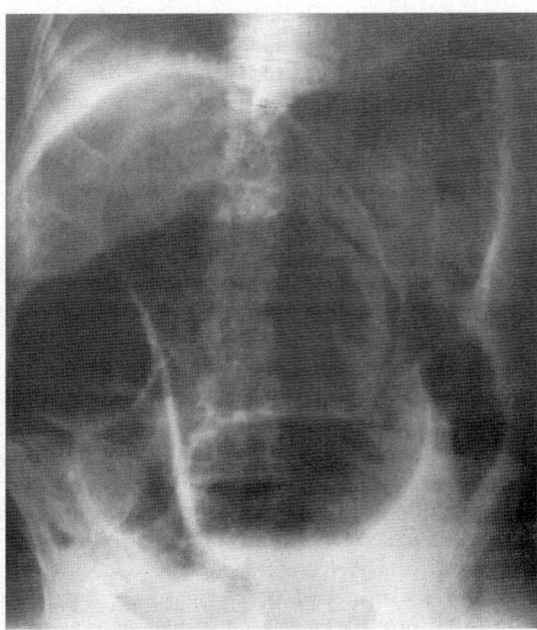

Figure 103-1 Anteroposterior radiographic view of sigmoid volvulus.

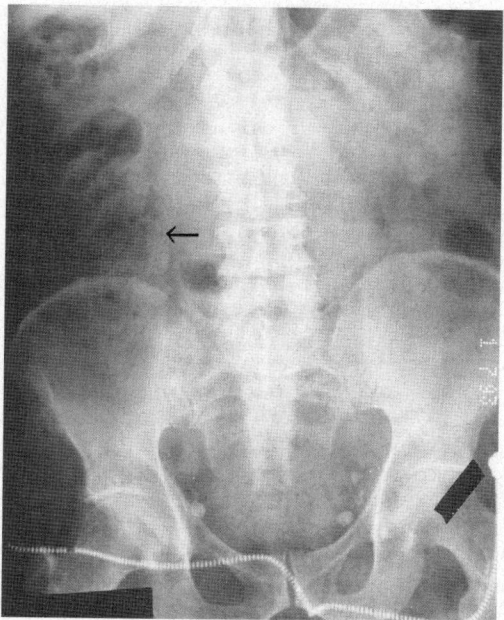

Figure 103-2 Plain abdominal radiograph showing fecal loading in the cecum (arrowed) and the presence of fecalomas in a 72-year-old patient with a long history of anticholinergic antipsychotic use.

of *fecal impaction* in older patients are anorexia, abdominal discomfort and distension, unexplained leukocytosis, delirium, and importantly, a nonspecific clinical deterioration. An abdominal radiograph will confirm the diagnosis of impaction; the closer the impacted stool is to the ileocecal valve, the more fluid levels are visible in the small bowel. *Stercoral perforation* of the colon can occur in chronically constipated persons (especially those with fecalomas), causing acute onset of abdominal pain, and high mortality. *Sigmoid volvulus* is the third commonest cause of large-bowel obstruction in the USA, and may require partial colectomy to prevent recurrences (Fig. 103-1).[55] Patients with redundant sigmoid loops loaded with stool (e.g. those with Parkinson's disease, or long-term users of anticholinergic psychotropic drugs) are at greatest risk of this complication.[56] A large rectal impaction can impinge on the bladder neck and cause significant *urinary retention*.

Nonpharmacological treatment

In mild constipation, elderly people should be treated initially with nonpharmacological measures, and these should remain the mainstay of treatment even when laxatives are necessary, both in community and institutionalized settings [C]. There are currently no rigorous clinical trial data evaluating the effectiveness of a nonpharmacological approach as compared to laxative therapy. The following measures are, however, likely to be clinically useful.

Education as to what constitutes normal bowel habit corrects patient misperceptions, and thereby may address self-reported constipation in some cases. In those with clinical constipation, *toileting habits* should be assessed with emphasis placed on comfort and privacy, particularly in institutional settings [B]. Individuals should be encouraged to attempt defecation within half an hour of breakfast to take

advantage of the gastrocolic reflex. Where straining is predominant and in patients with weak pelvic floor and abdominal muscles, leg elevation onto a *footstool* while on the toilet will promote effective use of the Valsalva maneuver [D]. Four small uncontrolled nursing home studies have suggested that daily bran *fiber* increases bowel movement frequency, reduces laxative intake and the need for nursing intervention.[57–60] Concomitant increased fluid intake may have contributed significantly to these positive results, however while the effectiveness of dietary fiber in treating constipation in elderly people remains to be established, current views are that fiber should be recommended to ambulant older people in the form of wholegrain bread, fresh fruit, seeded berries, vegetables, beans, lentils, etc. [C]. Coarse bran, although more effective than refined fiber in softening stool, is less palatable and may significantly reduce calcium and iron absorption due to its high phytic acid content. Daily *fluid intake* should be at least 1,500 mL (in the absence of medical restrictions) [C], and a program of regular *exercise* should be encouraged, within individual functional limitations [C]. Positioning immobile elderly patients out of bed and into a chair for up to 60-minute periods (with chairlifts at 15-minute intervals for prevention of pressure ulcers) may have similar beneficial effects. Daily exercise in bed and the use of abdominal massage have been shown to reduce laxative and enema use in chairfast geriatric long-stay patients, although transit time was unaffected.[61]

Laxative prescribing and pharmacological treatment

Currently the annual cost of laxative prescriptions in the UK is 43 million pounds, costing the National Health Service more than antihypertensive or diabetic drugs.[2] Osmotic laxatives are most frequently prescribed overall in the UK, followed closely by stimulant laxatives (most commonly senna). Prescription of bulk laxatives is actually declining.

A recent systematic review of effective laxative treatment in elderly persons found that the few published randomized controlled trials are potentially flawed due to small numbers and other methodological concerns.[2] The reviewers nevertheless commented that significant improvements in bowel movement frequency have been observed with a stimulant containing cascara and with lactulose, while bulk laxative psyllium and lactulose have individually been reported to improve stool consistency and related symptoms in placebo-controlled trials. The following summarizes available information on commonly used laxatives in elderly people. *Senna* works through direct stimulation of the myenteric plexus, and also has a prostaglandin-E-like effect which alters salt and water transportation; the result is an increase in transit and stool-softening effect. Animal studies have shown that senna does not cause myenteric plexus damage, and is therefore not implicated as a cause of "cathartic colon."[62] It is the preferred stimulant agent for treatment of functional constipation [C], oral *bisacodyl* having side-effects of inducing hypokalemia, and nausea and vomiting if taken with antacids. *Danthron* (the stimulant component of Codanthramer) causes unpleasant perineal skin burns in patients with fecal incontinence, and has recently been associated with increased risk of incontinence in nursing home residents.[12]

Bulk laxatives work by drawing in water, while being resistant to bacterial degradation. They hasten transit, soften and bulk stool, and have been shown to facilitate rectal evacuation in older people.[63] They may cause transient bloating and flatulence, and a good fluid intake is needed to avoid colonic retention, particularly in immobile patients. They can be considered a safe long-term laxative in treatment of chronic constipation or rectal outlet delay in ambulant elderly people [C].

Lactulose is a disaccharide which osmotically draws water into the gut lumen causing reflex contractions. It has been shown to reverse prolongation of transit time in frail nursing home residents,[64] and to treat chronic constipation effectively in ambulatory older patients [B].[65,66] *Polyethylene glycol* is a more potent osmolar laxative which in small studies appears to effectively treat fecal impaction in elderly patients.[54,64]

Docusate sodium (a stool softener) is the most frequently prescribed laxative in the USA, yet it has been demonstrated to have no effect on colonic motility, and hence no laxative action.[67] Widespread prescribing of docusate may be contributing to the high prevalence of constipation in elderly people in the USA.[8,67] Its use should be limited to situations where straining must be prevented in patients who are not constipated (such as unstable angina or painful anorectal conditions).

Prokinetic drugs are newly developed laxative agents which directly stimulate cellular release of acetyl choline in the myenteric plexus. Cisapride, a drug recently taken off the market because of cardiac side-effects, had been shown to be effective short-term in treating constipation associated with Parkinson's disease, diabetes, and spinal cord injury.[68] Safer alternative drugs within the same class are being developed and may have potential use as adjunctive therapy in constipated older patients with these neurological conditions.

Enemas are considered useful in the clinical setting for disimpaction, though there are no data examining effectiveness other than case reports. Phosphate enemas should be used cautiously in renal impairment,[69] and sodium citrate microl enemas may cause fluid retention in patients with cardiac failure. Tap water enemas are a suitable alternative. Bisacodyl suppositories are effective in treating severe constipation in patients with spinal cord injury.[70] Table 103-5 summarizes available information in the form of treatment protocols.

Conclusions

Constipation is not an inevitable consequence of aging, but may cause significant comorbidity and quality of life impairment in elderly people with risk factors. Straining and passage of hard stool are predominant symptoms in older individuals self-reporting constipation. More randomized controlled trials are needed to assess the impact of nonpharmacological interventions on constipation symptoms in older people, and to provide a more robust research evidence base for effective laxative prescribing in this population.

FECAL INCONTINENCE IN THE OLDER ADULT

Few medical symptoms are as distressing and social isolating for older people as fecal incontinence (FI), a condition which places them at greater risk of morbidity, dependency, hospital admissions, and institutionalization. Many older individuals

Table 103-5 Pharmacological treatment of constipation in older people

Functional constipation
- Bulk laxative 1–3 times daily with fluids in ambulant elderly persons
- In less mobile individuals, those with questionable fluid intake or those intolerant of bulk laxatives, give lactulose 30 mL daily titrating upwards to achieve regular (≥ 3 times a week) and comfortable evacuation
- In high-risk patients (e.g. immobile nursing home residents, patients with Parkinson's disease, etc.) or those with persistent constipation, *add* senna 1–3 tablets at bedtime

Rectal outlet delay
- Manual disimpaction where necessary, followed by enema for initial clearance
- Glycerine suppository once daily after breakfast for 2 weeks, then use as required to relieve symptoms. For recurrent rectal impaction or overflow fecal incontinence, use bisacodyl suppositories instead
- If stool is hard, add daily bulk laxative or lactulose

Colonic fecal impaction
- Daily arachis oil retention enema, or phosphate or enema with extension nozzle
- *When obstruction resolves*, give senna 3 tablets at bedtime and lactulose 30 mL 2 times daily with daily enemas until no further washout result
- Polyethylene glycol (Movicol) 1/2–1 sachet daily with fluids may be given instead of lactulose for rapid disimpaction (e.g. in hospital) or where stool retention is persistent. Provisions must be taken to manage the likely side-effect of fecal incontinence
- When impaction resolves, return to maintenance regimen for functional constipation

with FI will not volunteer the problem to their general practitioner, and regrettably, doctors and nurses do not routinely enquire about the symptom. This "hidden problem" therefore leads to social isolation and a downward spiral of psychological distress, dependency, and poor health. The condition takes its toll on carers also; FI surpasses even dementia as a leading reason for requesting nursing home placement.

Epidemiology of fecal incontinence in older people—prevalence and risk factors

The overall *prevalence* of fecal incontinence increases with age, particularly in the eighth decade and beyond.[71–73] Unlike younger populations, FI is as or more prevalent in older men than women.[12,72,74,75] The epidemiology of FI in older people varies according to the general health of the population and therefore study setting (community, hospital or nursing home) (Fig. 103-3). FI affects 9 percent of older *community-dwelling persons*, with 1 in 6 of these individuals experiencing daily incontinence.[71] Prevalence rates of 11 percent in men and 15 percent in women have been observed in a US community-based study,[72] with an age-related increase seen particularly in men (from 8 percent in their 50s to 18 percent in their 80s). The few studies of FI in *acutely hospitalized older patients* have shown rates of 14–22 percent.[76,77] The problem is greater still among *older institutionalized individuals* affecting 13 percent of those in residential homes, and on average 54 percent of those in

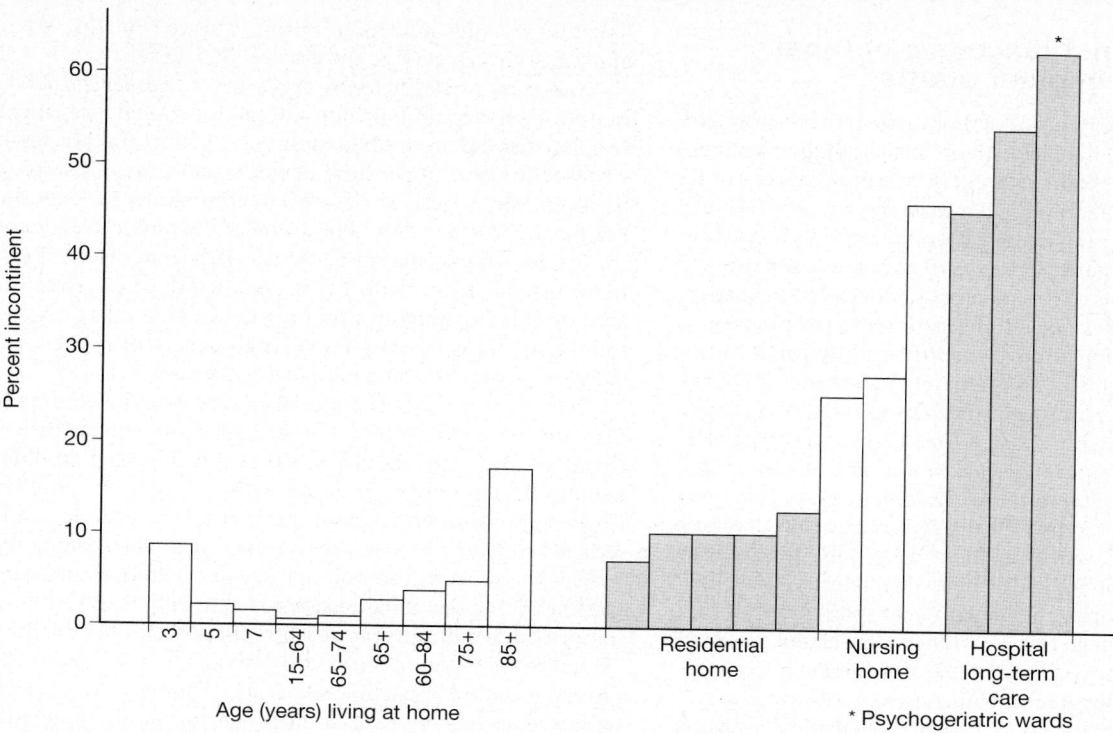

Figure 103-3 Prevalence of fecal incontinence in various settings. From Schultz et al. [77] Reprinted with permission of the publisher, the Society of Urologic Nurses and Associates, Inc., East Holly Avenue, Box 56, Pitman, NJ 08071-0056, USA.

nursing homes.[8,12,74–76] It is notable from these studies that the prevalence of FI varies widely from 17 to 95 percent between individual nursing homes. Even taking into consideration case-mix issues, this implies that different institutional standards of care can have an impact on the occurrence of the condition.

The *incidence* of new-onset FI over a 10-month period among elderly nursing home residents was shown to be 20 percent, with a mortality of 26 percent in those with persistent FI as compared with 6.7 percent in those who remained continent.[74] Independent baseline *risk factors* for new-onset FI in this study were age over 70, urinary incontinence, neurological disease, poor mobility, and impaired cognitive function. Retrospective studies in older adults have also shown restricted mobility to be a primary risk factor for FI,[12,73,75,76] particularly where help is needed to transfer from bed to chair. Other associated factors are loose stools, urinary incontinence, dementia, male gender, and poor general health perception.[72,73,75]

In summary, these findings indicate that bowel continence status should be identified by direct questioning and/or direct observation in community-dwellers in their 80s and beyond, nursing home residents, older hospital inpatients, and any older adult with impaired mobility, dementia, or urinary incontinence [B]. The high prevalence of FI in older men [B] should prompt exploration of etiologies other than childbirth in aging adults.

FI in older adults—the "hidden" problem

In a primary care study, only 50 percent of patients with FI or their carers had discussed the problem with a healthcare professional, and only 1 in 8 of those with daily FI had done

so.[71] Only 1 in 6 hospital inpatients reporting FI have the symptom documented by ward nursing staff,[77] while in the nursing home, nurses are aware of FI in only half of those residents self-reporting the condition.[8] Clearly these studies expose a low awareness of FI by physicians and nurses, and prompt the recommendation that general practitioners, community nurses, hospital ward staff, and nursing home staff should routinely enquire about FI in older patients [B]. Furthermore, one study showed that only 4 percent of nursing home residents with longstanding FI had been referred to their general practitioner for further assessment of this problem,[78] which may reflect a tendency toward unnecessarily conservative nursing management (e.g., use of pads and pants only). Older patients with FI should always be assessed for reversible causes, regardless of their institutionalization status [B].

Anorectal function in older adults with fecal incontinence

Studies of older people with FI suggest that age-related internal anal sphincter dysfunction is an important contributing factor,[79,80] as it lowers the threshold for balloon (stimulated stool) expulsion.[79] Childbearing is linked to later-life FI via structural damage to the external anal sphincter, and pelvic musculature.[81] Pudendal neuropathy is an age-related phenomenon in women with FI, but has an unclear role as a predisposing factor for incontinence.[80,82] Stool impaction predisposing to overflow is often related to rectal dyschezia in frail older adults.[11] Older adults with FI should therefore be clinically evaluated for anal sphincter dysfunction [B], and invariably undergo digital examination to identify rectal stool impaction [B].

Assessment and diagnosis of fecal incontinence in older adults

Current surveys indicate a lack of thoroughness by doctors and nurses in assessing FI in older patients in all healthcare settings, including failure to obtain an accurate symptom history or to perform rectal examinations.[83] For instance, a recent UK survey found that only 1 in 5 acutely hospitalized elderly patients with FI had undergone a physician rectal examination.[84] Table 103-6 highlights the essentials of standardized evaluation of FI in older people. The emphasis in older people is on a *structured clinical approach to identify multifactorial causes* of FI, including cognitive and functional assessments [B]. In most cases this approach will provide sufficient diagnostic information on which to base a feasible management plan without resorting to more specialized tests and assessments.

A careful *bowel symptom history* and assessment of *voiding pattern* by self-report,[85,86] proxy report or observation should form part of every assessment [B]. Constant leakage of loose stool or stool-stained mucus characterizes overflow around an impaction. Patients with anal sphincter dysfunction tend episodically to leak small amounts of stool preceded by a feeling of urgency where external anal sphincter weakness predominates, as compared with unconscious leakage seen with internal sphincter dysfunction.[87] Patients with dementia-related incontinence often pass complete bowel movements, especially after meals in response to the gastrocolic reflex.

Evaluation of *ability to use and access the toilet* should be multidisciplinary, and include a broad functional assessment (e.g. Barthel Index), mobility test (e.g. "get up and go" test), visual acuity test, upper limb dexterity assessment (undoing buttons), and cognitive measure. For community patients, the healthcare provider should be aware of the physical layout of the patient's home, and in particular bathroom details (location, distance from main living area, width of doorway for accommodating walking aids, presence of grab rails or raised toilet seat). Low lighting levels, high degree of clutter and hard-to-manage clothing may also be relevant.

Digital assessment of basal and squeeze tone can accurately discriminate sphincter function between continent and incontinent adults,[88] and should be a first-line approach in older people [B]. Easy finger insertion with gaping of the anus on finger removal indicates poor internal sphincter tone, while reduced squeeze pressure around the finger when asking the patient to "squeeze and pull up" suggests external sphincter weakness. Anorectal manometry is generally reserved for a minority in whom surgery or biofeedback seems feasible [D]. Digital rectal examination is also essential to assess anorectal disease and stool impaction. Older incontinent patients without evidence of stool retention per rectum should undergo a *plain abdominal radiograph* to rule out higher impaction and other problems [B].[5] Finally, observation of *pelvic floor descent* and rectal prolapse with straining, and of *sacral reflexes* should be included in every assessment.

Types of fecal incontinence in older people—causes and management

In many older individuals, methodical clinical assessment will identify multifactorial causes for FI leading to categorization into clinically meaningful types (below). There are very few randomized controlled trials of treatment of FI, so evidence presented is based largely on uncontrolled study data and expert opinion. An algorithmic management summary is provided on p. 1319.

Overflow incontinence secondary to constipation and stool impaction

Overflow incontinence is a treatable, preventable, and frequently overlooked condition in elderly patients, affecting 52 percent of nursing home residents with longstanding FI.[78] All too often untreated overflow leads to hospitalization of these frailer patients.[11] Patients with overflow should be carefully assessed for potentially modifiable causes, in particular immobility, medication side-effects, and low fluid and fiber intake [B]. A therapeutic intervention in frail nursing home residents with overflow (enemas until no further response followed by lactulose) achieved complete resolution of incontinence in 94 percent of those in whom full treatment compliance could be obtained.[78] Another nursing home study found that a regimen of daily lactulose and suppositories plus weekly enemas was effective in resolving overflow FI only when longlasting and complete rectal emptying was achieved.[89] An effective therapeutic program for overflow FI depends on monitoring of effect (by rectal examination and bowel chart),

---

Table 103-6 Clinical assessment of fecal incontinence in older people

Emphasis in older people is on a *structured clinical approach* to identify all contributing factors for fecal incontinence

History
- Duration of fecal incontinence
- Frequency of episodes
- Type (constant soiling, small amounts, complete bowel movement)
- Stool consistency (diarrhea, hard stool)
- Unconscious leakage or symptoms of urgency
- Constipation symptoms/current laxative use
- Systemic illness (confusion, depression, weight loss, anemia)
- Antibiotic use

General examination
- Cognitive and mood assessment
- Neurological profile (stroke, autonomic neuropathy, Parkinson's disease)

Toilet access
- Evaluate ability to use toilet based on muscle strength, coordination, vision, limb function, and cognition
- Place in context of current living environment

Specific examination
- Abdominal inspection for distension and tenderness
- Perineal inspection for skin breakdown, dermatitis, surgical scars
- Perianal sensation/cutaneous anal reflex
- Observe for excessive downward motion of the pelvic floor when asking patient to bear down in the lateral lying position
- Digital examination for stool impaction
- Digital examination for evaluation of impaired sphincter tone:
  - Anal gaping, and/or easy insertion of finger (internal sphincter)
  - Reduced squeeze pressure (external sphincter)
- Ask patient to strain while sitting on commode and observe for rectal prolapse

Summary of management algorithm

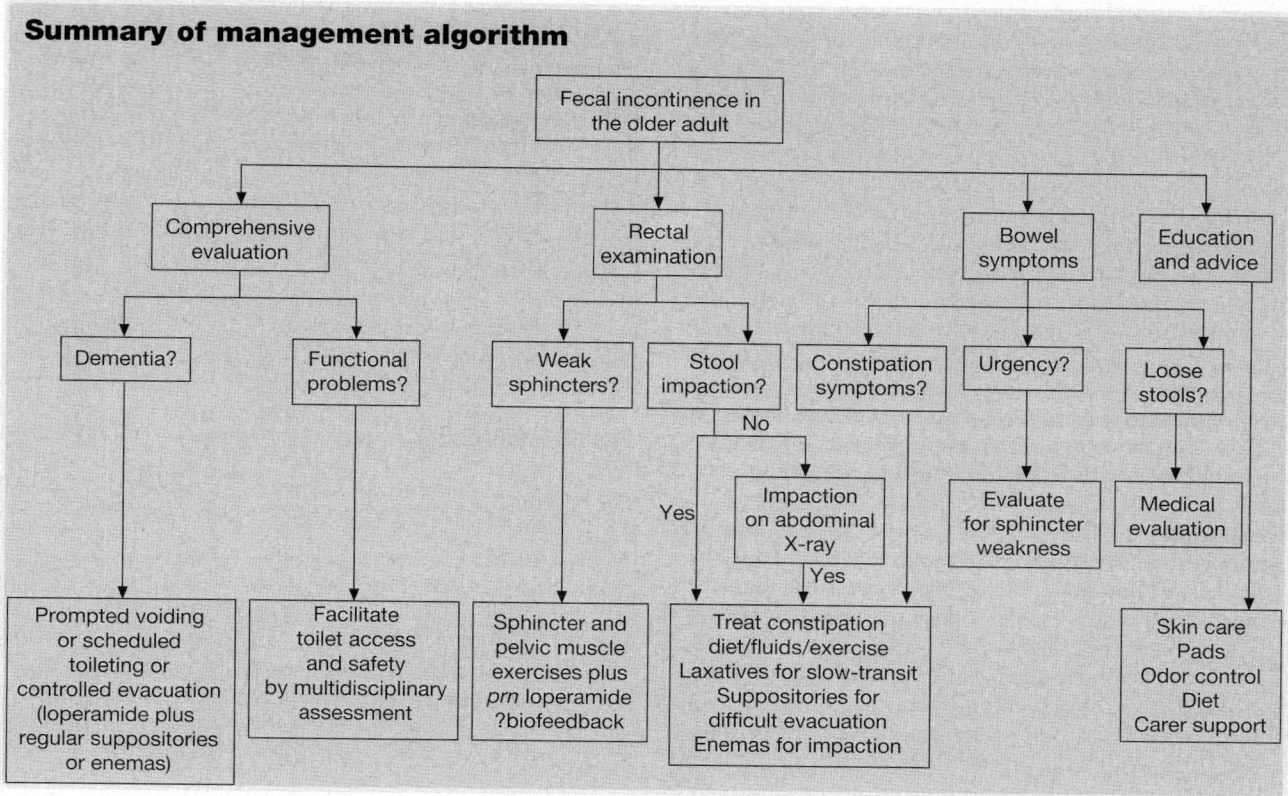

responsive stepwise drug and dosage changes, and a subsequent maintenance regimen to prevent recurrences [B]. Table 103-5 summarizes treatment recommendations for fecal impaction.

Functional incontinence

Functional incontinence occurs in individuals who are unable to access the toilet in time due to impairments in mobility, dexterity, or vision. These patients may even have normal lower gut function. Epidemiological studies of nursing home residents have repeatedly shown that poor mobility is a strong risk factor for FI after adjustment for confounding variables.[73–75] Functional FI should be identified early on in the assessment process [B], and management should be multidisciplinary.

Dementia-related incontinence

Advancing dementia may lead to a neurologically disinhibited rectum, associated with voiding of formed stool once or twice daily following mass peristaltic movements. Patients with dementia are more likely to exhibit multiple rectal contractions in response to rectal distension in physiological studies.[79,90] Dementia-related incontinence is the primary cause of FI in up to 46 percent of nursing home residents.[78] These individuals are very commonly incontinent of urine also. Treatment approaches to dementia-related FI include prompted or scheduled toileting, and controlled evacuation. Ouslander et al. showed that a 6-week prompted voiding program enabling incontinent nursing home patients with dementia to access a toilet more frequently, significantly increased their number of continent bowel movements.[91] This finding is relevant also for demented elderly patients in

hospital who may seldom be offered use of the toilet, especially if they have an indwelling urinary catheter. Tobin et al. evaluated a controlled evacuation program in 25 nursing home residents with dementia-related FI, consisting of daily codeine phosphate and twice-weekly enemas; continence was achieved in 75 percent of those fully treated.[78] The overall recommendation is for a stepwise approach to treatment where Step 1 is prompted voiding for those with mild to moderate dementia; Step 2 is scheduled toileting plus daily suppositories for those unresponsive to cues; and Step 3 for those with persistent and problematic FI is a controlled bowel program of stopping spontaneous evacuation with loperamide and administering suppositories or enema at a convenient time [C].

Comorbidity-related incontinence

Certain diseases that are more common in older people predispose individuals to FI. Immediately following acute *stroke* 40 percent of individuals are incontinent, and 10 percent remain so 3–6 months after the acute event.[92,93] One study found that FI in 3-month stroke survivors was more strongly associated with use of constipating medicines and functional problems with toilet access than with stroke severity or type.[93] This emphasizes the importance of assessing potentially reversible causes other than the primary diagnosis, in neurologically disabled patients [B]. FI may occur in people with longstanding *diabetes mellitus* through the dual mechanisms of bacterial overgrowth in a sluggish gut causing characteristic nocturnal diarrhea, and multilevel anorectal dysfunction (abnormal anorectal tone, reflexes, compliance, and sensation).[94,95]

Anorectal incontinence

Age-related as well as neurogenic anal sphincter dysfunction contribute to the increased prevalence of this type of FI in aging adults.[79,80] Loperamide is a useful drug treatment for anorectal FI in the absence of constipation [B], increasing basal tone and clinically reducing incontinent episodes and urgency.[96,97] In patients with external sphincter weakness, there is some evidence that biofeedback and sphincter and pelvic floor muscle strengthening exercises have a clinically beneficial effect [C].[98] However, this approach is unlikely to help more than a minority of highly selected older patients who have intact cognition, good motivation and preserved anorectal sensation.[99] Preliminary data suggest possible benefits from estrogen replacement therapy in post-menopausal women with anorectal FI,[100] but further research is required to substantiate this. In certain older incontinent patients extensive rectal prolapse or external sphincter damage are surgically treatable causes.[26]

Loose stools

Loose stool can cause FI in normally continent older adults by overwhelming a functional but age-compromised sphincter mechanism. Forty-four percent of cases of FI in a prospective nursing home study had diarrhea as a primary cause.[75] Certain causes of loose stools in older people are readily treatable. *Excessive use of laxatives* is an important one—one-third of community-dwelling people aged 65 and over regularly take laxatives, far exceeding the prevalence of constipation in this population.[4] Laxative use has been linked to FI in nursing home residents,[12] and potent laxatives such as sodium picosulfate and polyethylene glycol cause FI in a quarter of older users. Bulk laxatives may contribute to FI in some elderly patients who have greater difficulty retaining softer stool due to weak sphincters.[101] *Lactose malabsorption* is an age-related phenomenon,[102] leading in some cases to the clinical syndrome of loose stools, bloating, and cramps following ingestion of milk products. *Antibiotic-related diarrhea* and clostridium difficile colitis is particularly likely to affect older adults, especially women, and those resident in nursing homes.[103]

General measures

It is very important to provide patient and carer education to promote self-efficacy and other coping mechanisms. Where appropriate, self-management (e.g. reducing risk of constipation and impaction through dietary and lifestyle measures, advice on how to take loperamide) should be encouraged [D]. Advice on skin care, odor control, and continence aids should not be overlooked, though it is of note that very few products have specifically been designed for the problem of FI [D].

Conclusions

Greater emphasis needs to be placed on systematic and effective management of fecal incontinence in older people backed up by sound communications between doctors and nurses, in all healthcare settings [B]. There is a wide-open clinical research agenda in this area. As older adults with FI are not a homogenous group and causes are often multifactorial, randomized controlled trials need to be sufficiently large to permit subgroup analysis of targeted treatment protocols.

KEY POINTS Constipation and fecal incontinence in old age

- Constipation is not an inevitable consequence of aging, but may cause significant comorbidity and quality of life impairment in elderly people with risk factors.

- Straining and passage of hard stool are predominant symptoms in older individuals self-reporting constipation.

- Greater emphasis needs to be placed on systematic and effective management of fecal incontinence in older people, backed up by sound communications between doctors and nurses in all healthcare settings.

REFERENCES

1. Cook DJ, Guyatt GH, Laupacis A, Sackett DL, Goldberg RJ: Clinical recommendations using levels of evidence for thrombotic agents. Chest 1995;108(4 suppl):227S–230S
2. Petticrew M, Watt I, Sheldon T: Systematic review of the effectiveness of laxatives in the elderly. Health Technol Assess 1997;1(13):i–iv,1–52
3. Sonnenberg A, Koch TR: Physician visits in the United States for constipation: 1958 to 1986. Dig Dis Sci 1989;34:606–611
4. Harari D, Gurwitz JH, Avorn J, Bohn R, Minaker KL: Bowel habits in relation to age and gender: Findings from the National Health Interview Survey and clinical implications. Arch Intern Med 1996;156:315–320
5. Donald IP, Smith RG, Cruikshank JG, Elton RA, Stoddart ME: A study of constipation in the elderly living at home. Gerontology 1985;31:112–118
6. Whitehead WE, Drinkwater D, Cheskin LJ, Heller BR, Schuster MM: Constipation in the elderly living at home: Definition, prevalence and relationship to lifestyle and health status. J Am Geriatr Soc 1989;37:423–429
7. Talley NJ, O'Keefe E, Zinsmeister AR, Melton LJ: Prevalence of gastrointestinal symptoms in the elderly: A population-based study. Gastroenterology 1992;102:895–901
8. Harari D, Gurwitz JH, Choodnovskiy I, Avorn J, Minaker KL: Constipation: Assessment and management in an institutionalised population. J Am Geriatr Soc 1994;42:1–6
9. Everhart JE, Go VLW, Johannes RS et al: A longitudinal survey of self-reported bowel habits in the United States. Dig Dis Sci 1989;34:1153–1162
10. Harari D, Gurwitz JH, Avorn J, Bohn R, Minaker KL: How do older persons define constipation? J Gen Intern Med 1997;12:63–66
11. Read NW, Abouzekry L, Read MG et al: Anorectal function in elderly patients with fecal impaction. Gastroenterology 1985;89:959–966
12. Brocklehurst J, Dickinson E, Windsor J: Laxatives and faecal incontinence in long-term care. Nursing Standard 1999;52:32–36
13. Melkersson M, Andersson H, Bosaeus I, Falkheden T: Intestinal transit time in constipated and non-constipated geriatric patients. Scand J Gastroenterol 1983;18:593–597
14. Metcalf AM, Phillips SF, Zinsmeister AR et al: Simplified assessment of segmental colonic transit. Gastroenterology 1987;92:40–47
15. Loening-Baucke V, Anuras S: Sigmoidal and rectal motility in healthy elderly. J Am Geriatr Soc 1984;32:887–891
16. McKay LF, Smith RG, Eastwood MA et al: An investigation of colonic function in the elderly. Age Ageing 1983;12:105–110
17. Eastwood HDH: Bowel transit studies in the elderly; radio-opaque markers in the investigation of constipation. Geront clin 1972;14:154–159
18. Varma JS, Bradnock J, Smith RS, Smith AN: Constipation in the elderly. A physiologic study. Dis Colon Rectum 1988;31:111–115
19. Brocklehurst JC, Kirkland JL, Martin J: Constipation in long-stay elderly patients: its treatment and prevention by lactulose, poloxalkol-dihydroxyanthroquinolone and phosphate enemas. Gerontology 1983;29:181–184
20. McDougal JN, Miller MS, Burks TF et al: Age-related changes in colonic function in rats. Am J Physiol 1984;247:G542–G546
21. Krishnamurthy S, Schuffler MD, Rohrmann CA et al: Severe idiopathic constipation is associated with a distinctive abnormality of the colonic myenteric plexus. Gastroenterol 1985;88:26–34

22. Koch TR, Aiden Carvey J, Go VLW et al: Inhibitory neuropeptides and intrinsic inhibitory innervation of descending human colon. Dig Dis Sci 1991;36:712–718

23. Szurszewski JH, Holt PR, Schuster M: Proceedings of a workshop entitled "Neuromuscular function and dysfunction of the gastrointestinal tract in aging." Dig Dis Sci 34:1135–1146

24. Schweiger M: Method for determining individual contributions of voluntary and involuntary anal sphincters to resting tone. Dis Colon Rectum 1979;22:415–416

25. McHugh SM, Diamant NE: Effect of age, gender, and parity on anal canal pressures. Dig Dis Sci 1987;32:726–736

26. Matheson DM, Keighley MRB: Manometric evaluation of rectal prolapse and faecal incontinence. Gut 1981;22:126–129

27. Ryhammer AM, Laurberg S, Bek KM: Age and anorectal sensibility in normal women. Scand J Gastroenterol 1997;32:278–284

28. Bleijenberg G, Kuijpers HC: Treatment of spastic pelvic floor syndrome with biofeedback. Dis Colon Rectum 1987;30:108–111

29. Bassotti G, Maggio D, Battaglia E et al: Manometric investigation of anorectal function in early and late stage Parkinson's disease. J Neurol Neurosurg Psychiatry 2000;68:768–770

30. Bidmead J, Cardozo LD: Pelvic floor changes in the older woman. Br J Urology 1998;82(suppl 1):18–25

31. O'Keefe E, Talley NJ: Irritable bowel syndrome in the elderly. Clin Geriatr Med 1991;7:265–286

32. Robson KM, Kiely DK, Lembo T: Development of constipation in nursing home residents. Dis Colon Rectum 2000;43:940–943

33. Harari D, Gurwitz JH, Choodnovskiy I, Avorn J, Minaker KL: Correlates of regular laxative use in frail elderly persons. Am J Med 1995;99:513–518

34. Monane M, Avorn J, Beers MH, Everitt DE: Anticholinergic drug use and bowel function in nursing home patients. Arch Intern Med 1993;153:633–638

35. Brock C, Curry H, Hanna C, Knipfer M, Taylor L: Adverse effects of iron supplementation: A comparative trial of a wax-matrix iron preparation and conventional ferrous sulfate tablets. Clin Ther 1985;7:568–573

36. Traube M, McCallum RW and members of American College of Gastroenterology's Committee on FDA Related Matters: Calcium-channel blockers and the gastrointestinal tract. Am J Gastroenterol 1984;79:892–896

37. Jones RH, Tait CL: Gastrointestinal side-effects of NSAIDs in the community. Br J Clin Pract 1995;49:67–70

38. Kinnunen O: Study of constipation in a geriatric hospital, day hospital, old people's home and at home. Aging 1991;3:161–170

39. Dapoigny M, Sarna SK: Effects of physical exercise on colonic motor activity. Am J Physiol 1991;260:G646–G652

40. Edwards LL, Quigly EMM, Pfeiffer RF: Gastrointestinal dysfunction in Parkinson's disease. Neurology 1992;42:726–732

41. Feldman M, Schiller LR: Disorders of gastrointestinal motility associated with diabetes mellitus. Ann Intern Med 1983;98:378–384

42. Camilleri M: Gastrointestinal problems in diabetes. Endocrinol Metab Clin North Am 1996;25:361–378

43. Harari D, Gurwitz JH, Sarkarati M, McGlinchey-Berroth R, Minaker KL: Constipation: symptoms and management in persons with spinal cord injury. Spinal Cord 1997;35:394–401

44. Hinds JP, Eidelman BH, Wald A: Prevalence of bowel dysfunction in multiple sclerosis. Gastroenterology 1990;98:1538–1542

45. Towers AL, Burgio KL, Locher JL et al: Constipation in the elderly: Influence of dietary, psychological, and physiological factors. J Am Geriatr Soc 1994;42:701–706

46. Klauser AG, Schindlbeck NE, Muller-Lissner SA: Low fluid intake lowers stool output in healthy male volunteers. Z Gastroenterol 1990;28:606–609

47. Muller-Lissner SA: Effect of wheat bran on the weight of stool and gastrointestinal transit time: a meta analysis. Br Med J 1988;296:615–617

48. Johnson CK, Kolasa K, Chenoweth W et al: Health, laxation and food habit influences on fiber intake of older women. J Am Dietet Assoc 1980;77:551–557

49. Klauser AG, Voderholzer WA, Heinrich CA, Schindlbeck NE, Muller-Lissner SA: Behavioural modification of colonic function: can constipation be learned? Dig Dis Sci 1990;35:1271–1275

50. Garvey M, Noyes RJr., Yates W: Frequency of constipation in major depression; Relationship to other clinical variables. Psychosomatics 1009;3:204–206

50A. Sonnenberg A, Muller AD: Constipation and cathartics as risk factors of colorectal cancer: A meta-analysis. Pharmacology 1993;47 (suppl 1): 224–233

51. Starrveld JS, Pols JS, Van Wijk MA et al: The plain abdominal radiograph in the assessment of constipation. Z Gastroenterol 1990;28:335–338

52. Gurwitz JH, Noonan JP, Sanchez M, Lipsitz L: Barium enemas in the frail elderly. Am J Med 1992;92:41–44

53. Thomson A, Naidoo P, Crotty B: Bowel preparation for colonoscopy: a randomized prospective trial comparing sodium phosphate and polyethylene glycol in a predominantly elderly population. J Gastroenterol Hepatol 1996;11:103–107

54. Culbert P, Gillett H, Ferguson H: Highly effective oral therapy (polyethylene glycol electrolyte solution) for faecal impaction and severe constipation. Clin Drug Invest 1998;16:355–360

55. Morrissey TB, Deitch EA: Recurrence of sigmoid volvulus after surgical intervention. Am Surgeon 1994;5:329–331

56. Rosenthal MJ, Marshall CE: Sigmoid volvulus in association with parkinsonism. J Am Geriatr Soc 1987;35:683–684

57. Valle-Jones JC: An open study of oat bran meal biscuits ("Lejfibre") in the treatment of constipation in the elderly. Curr Med Opin 1985;9:716–720

58. Pringle R, Pennington MJ, Pennington CR: A study of the influence of a fibre biscuit on bowel function in the elderly. Age Ageing 1984;13:175–178

59. Hull C, Greco RS, Brooks DL: Alleviation of constipation in the elderly by dietary fiber supplementation. J Am Geriatr Soc 1985;28:410–414

60. Hope AK, Down EC: Dietary fibre and fluid in the control of constipation in a nursing home population. Med J Aust 1986;144:306–307

61. Resende TL, Brocklehurst JC, O'Neill PA: A pilot study on the effect of exercise and abdominal massage on bowel habit in continuing care patients. Clin Rehabil 1993;7:204–209

62. Dufour P, Gendre P: Ultrastructure of mouse intestinal mucosa and changes observed after long term anthraquinone administration. Gut 1984;25:1358–1363

63. Passmore AP, Wilson-Davies K, Stoker C et al: Chronic constipation in long stay elderly patients: a comparison of lactulose and a senna-fibre combination. Br Med J 1993;307:769–771

64. Puxty JA, Fox RA: Golytely: a new approach to faecal impaction in old age. Age Ageing 1986;15(3):182–184

65. Lederle FA, Busch DL, Mattox KM, West MJ, Aske DM: Cost-effective treatment of constipation in the elderly: A randomized double-blind comparison of sorbitol and lactulose. Am J Med 1990;89:597–601

66. Sanders JF: Lactulose syrup assessed in a double-blind study of elderly constipated patients. J Am Geriatr Soc 1978;26:236–239

67. Castle SC, Cantrell M, Israel DS, Samuelson MJ: Constipation prevention: empiric use of stool softeners questioned. Geriatrics 1991;46(11):84–86

68. Snape WJ: Role of colonic motility in guiding therapy in patients with constipation. Dig Dis 1997;15:104–111

69. Korzets A, Dicker D, Chaimoff C, Zevin D: Life-threatening hyperphosphatemia and hypocalcemic tetany following the use of Fleet enemas. J Am Geriatr Soc 1992;40:620–621

70. Steins SA: Reduction in bowel programme duration with polyethylene glycol based bisacodyl suppositories. Arch Phys Med Rehab 1995;76:674–677

71. Bradley W, Ferris W, Barr O: Continence promotion in adults with learning disabilities. Nursing Times 1995;91:38–39

72. Roberts RO, Jacobsen SJ, Reilly WT et al: Prevalence of combined faecal and urinary incontinence: a community-based study. J Am Geriatr Soc 1999;47(7):837–841

73. Nelson R, Norton N, Caulley E, Furner S: Community-based prevalence of anal incontinence. JAMA 1995;274:559–561

74. Chassagne P, Landrin I, Neveu C et al: Fecal incontinence in the institutionalized elderly: incidence, risk factors, and prognosis. Am J Med 1999;106(2):185–190

75. Johanson JF, Irizarry F, Doughty A: Risk factors for fecal incontinence in a nursing home population. J Clin Gastroenterol 1997;24:156–160

76. Peet SM, Castleden CM, McGrother CW: Prevalence of urinary and fecal incontinence in hospitals and residential and nursing homes for older people. Br Med J 1995;311:1063–1064

77. Schultz A, Dickey G, Skoner M: Urologic Nursing 1997;17:23–28

78. Tobin GW, Brocklehurst JC: Faecal incontinence in residential homes for the elderly: prevalence, aetiology and management. Age Ageing 1986;15:41–46

79. Barrett JA, Brocklehurst JC, Kiff ES, Ferguson G, Faragher EB: Rectal motility studies in faecally incontinent geriatric patients. Age Ageing 1990;19:311–317

80. Rasmussen OO, Christiansen J, Tetzschner T, Sorensen M: Pudendal nerve function in idiopathic fecal incontinence. Dis Colon Rectum 2000;43:633–636

81. Nygaard IE, Rao SSC, Dawson JD: Anal incontinence after anal sphincter disruption: a 30 year perspective. Obstet Gynecol 1997;89:896–901

82. Vaccaro CA, Cheong DM, Wexner SD et al: Pudendal neuropathy in evacuatory disorders. Dis Colon Rectum 1995;38:166–171

83. Incontinence. Causes, management and provision of services. Summary of a report of a working party of the Royal College of Physicians. J Royal Coll Phys London 1995;29:272–274

84. Morgan R, Spencer B, King D: Rectal examinations in elderly subjects: attitudes of patients and doctors. Age Ageing 1998;27:353–356

85. Osterberg A, Graf W, Karlbom U, Pahlman L: Evaluation of a questionnaire in the assessment of patients with faecal incontinence and constipation. Scand J Gastroenterol 1996;31:575–580

86. O'Keefe EA, Talley NJ, Tangalos EG, Zinsmeister AR: A bowel symptom questionnaire for the elderly. J Gerontol 1992;47:M116–M121

87. Engel AF, Kamm MA, Bartram CI, Nicholls RJ: Relationship of symptoms in faecal incontinence to specific sphincter abnormalities. Int J Colorect Dis 1995;10:152–155

88. Hallan RI, Marzouk DEMM, Waldron DJ, Womack NR, Williams NS: Comparison of digital and manometric assessment of anal sphincter function. Br J Surg 1989;76:973–975

89. Chassagne P, Jego A, Gloc P et al: Does treatment of constipation improve faecal incontinence in institutionalized patients. Age Ageing 2000;29:159–164

90. Barrett JA, Brocklehurst JC, Kiff ES: Anal function in geriatric patients with fecal incontinence. Gut 1989;30:1244–1251

91. Ouslander JG, Simmons S, Schnelle J, Uman G, Fingold S: Effects of prompted voiding on fecal continence among nursing home residents. J Am Geriatr Soc 1996;44:424–428

92. Nakayama H, Jorgenson HS, Pederson PM, Raaschou HO, Olsen TS: Prevalence and risk factors of incontinence after stroke. The Copenhagen Stroke Study. Stroke 1997;28:58–62

93. Harari D, Coshall C, Rudd AG, Wolfe CDA: New-onset faecal incontinence following stroke: Prevalence, natural history, risk factors and impact. Stroke 2002 (in press)

94. Wald A, Tunuguntla AK: Anorectal sensorimotor dysfunction in fecal incontinence and diabetes mellitus. N Engl J Med 1984;310:1282–1287

95. Sun WM, Katsinelos P, Horowitz M, Read NW: Disturbances in anorectal function in patients with diabetes mellitus and faecal incontinence. Euro J Gastroenterol Hepatol 1996;8:1007–1012

96. Kamm MA: Faecal incontinence. Br Med J 1998;316:528–532

97. Sun WM, Read NW, Verlinden M: Effects of loperamide oxide on gastrointestinal transit time and anorectal function in patients with chronic diarrhoea and faecal incontinence. Scand J Gastroenterol 1997;32:34–38

98. Norton C, Hosker G, Brazzelli M: Biofeedback and/or sphincter exercises for the treatment of faecal incontinence in adults. Cochrane Database Syst Rev 2000;2:CD002111

99. Whithead WE, Burgio KL, Engel BT: Biofeedback treatment of fecal incontinence in geriatric patients. J Am Geriatr Soc 1985;33:320–324

100. Donnelly V, O'Connell PR, O'Herlihy C: The influence of oestrogen replacement on faecal incontinence in postmenopausal women. Br J Obstet Gynaecol 1997;104:311–315

101. Ardron ME, Main ANH: Management of constipation. Br Med J 1990;300:1400

102. Goulding A, Taylor RW, Keil D et al: Lactose malabsorption and rate of bone loss in older women. Age Ageing 1999;28:175–180

103. Al-Eidan FA, McElnay JC, Scott MG, Kearney MP: Clostridium difficile-associated diarrhoea in hospitalised patients. J Clin Pharm Therapeutics 2000;25:101–109

Chapter 104

Urinary incontinence

James Malone-Lee

Nowadays the options available for the diagnosis and management of urinary incontinence reflect a transformation from earlier years. Incontinence is not a Cinderella subject and should be approached seriously, since therapeutic opportunities can be lost. There remains a paucity of centers which can provide training in the clinical skills needed for this subject and people new to the speciality of geriatrics are advised to arrange training attachments early on.

In the United Kingdom the prevalence of urinary incontinence increases from 2 percent in men and 9 percent in women aged 15–64 to 7 percent of men and 12 percent of women aged 65 and over.[1] A more recent survey has supported these observations.[2] The increased prevalence of incontinence in late life reflects functional deterioration and coincidental disability, the two working additively,[3] as would be expected intuitively. It is also now recognized that incontinence is not the only troublesome symptom; frequency, nocturia, urgency, and pain all rank similarly in their effects on life quality.[4–6]

ANATOMY AND PHYSIOLOGY

The smooth muscle fibers of the bladder, termed the detrusor, funnel at the bladder neck to be continued into the urethra as longitudinal fibers forming a tube. In the male these fibers are inserted into the verumontanum, but in the female they terminate in the distal urethra. The contraction of the detrusor results in a rise in bladder pressure associated with shortening of the urethra. The trigone forms a triangular baseplate with its apex at the bladder neck, and base running between both ureters. Contraction of the muscle of the trigone results in funneling of the bladder neck. There are some fibers which are inserted into the external surface of the trigone, distally. These pull the distal margins of the trigone apart, thus opening the bladder neck.

The detrusor has the ability to stretch considerably without developing an increase in tension: it is highly compliant. This means that it is normal for a bladder to be filled to 500 mL, and more, without an increase in intravesical pressure, other than the pressure head resulting from the height of the fluid in the bladder, which would be approximately 8 cm H_2O at 500 mL. If, during the filling phase of a urodynamic study, the detrusor contracts spontaneously, despite attempts to inhibit this, and thereby increases the pressure in the bladder, the detrusor is said to be "unstable." If the tension on the detrusor increases in association with filling, irrespective of any contractions, then the bladder is said to "lack compliance." "Low compliance" may result from fibrosis, detrusor hypertrophy or increased resting tone secondary to reduced neural inhibition.[7] The terminology is a little unsatisfactory. True compliance is a static measure obtained from a length/tension curve in which each pair of measures are taken at steady state. Many urodynamicists measure compliance from filling urodynamic studies during which the bladder volume is changing continuously. This means that the measurements are the sum of compliance and tissue viscosity, the latter dominating. The observation of unstable detrusor contractions and their quantification has been found to relate very weakly to symptoms.

The normal mechanism for activating contraction of the detrusor is the release of acetylcholine from parasympathetic nerves, stimulated by the spinobulbospinal micturition reflex, the main micturition reflex. Tension receptors in the detrusor activate afferents traveling in the pelvic nerves. These afferents pass through the lumbosacral dorsal roots to ascending tracts up to the pons. At this level the pontine micturition center provides the site where connections are made with descending motor tracts, destined for the sacral parasympathetic nuclei. The preganglionic, sacral parasympathetic axons originate in the sacral parasympathetic nuclei, leave the spinal cord through ventral roots, and travel in the pelvic nerves to ganglia in the pelvic plexus.[8,9]

While much of the functional neuroanatomy of the lower urinary tract has been explored by experiments conducted on cats, the advent of positron emission tomography has allowed some impressive studies on humans.[10] These have shown that humans and cats have remarkably similar arrangements. They show that micturition is associated with activity in the hypothalamus, periaqueductal gray matter, the right prefrontal cortex, anterior cingulate gyrus, and the dorsomedial pontine tegmentum.[11]

Since higher cerebral centers tend to inhibit the pontine micturition center, lesions above this are associated with detrusor hyper-reflexia. Subpontine lesions are more complex. There are some spinal micturition reflexes located below the pons which are weak in the adult and probably inactive in health. Therefore, lesions of the spinal cord below the pons, but rostral to the sacral nuclei, result in bladder areflexia initially. Subsequent to the injury, over weeks or months, reflex mechanisms in the spinal cord become active resulting in some uncoordinated and poorly sustained reflex bladder activity. However, if a spinal lesion involves complete destruction of the sacral nuclei, bladder areflexia will be permanent.[8,9]

The internal urethral sphincter is present only in the male, forming a circular collar continuous with the smooth muscle of the prostate. This sphincter is not part of the continence mechanism but contracts during ejaculation to prevent the retrograde flow of semen into the bladder. Failure of this sphincter leads to infertility, dry ejaculation, and seminuria. The internal sphincter is cut during transurethral resection of the prostate; however, continence is maintained.[8,9,12]

The external urethral sphincter is the principle mechanism for maintaining urethral continence in both sexes although the smooth muscle of urethra is important.[7] The circularly arranged muscle fibers are striated and predominantly slow twitch. The striated muscles of the pelvic floor and the external sphincter are supplied by somatic efferents originating in the anterior horns of the sacral cord segments S2–S4. The motor neurons are grouped in a specific region called Onuf's nucleus. This nucleus differs from other somatic motor nuclei with histochemical appearances similar to sacral parasympathetic nuclei along with evidence of adrenergic innervation. The axons, originating from Onuf's nucleus pass to the periphery through the pudendal nerve and the pelvic nerves. External sphincter activity is supported by the adrenergic smooth muscle of the urethra.[8,9,13]

The sympathetic innervation for the lower urinary tract comes from postganglionic nerves traveling in the hypogastric plexus, the pelvic nerves, and the pudendal nerves. The sympathetic innervation inhibits the detrusor and stimulates the urethral smooth muscle and the sphincters (Brading urethra). The stimulatory receptors on urethra, sphincter myocytes and prostatic smooth muscle are predominantly alpha-1A (sometimes termed alpha-1C) with some contribution from alpha-1L receptors.[13–16] The inhibitory noradrenergic receptors on detrusor cells are now recognized to be β_3 subtype and their significance is currently being invesigated.[17–21] The stimulatory action of noradrenaline on the smooth muscle of the prostate has precipitated an interest in selective alpha-1A receptor antagonists in the treatment of prostatism.[8,9,16]

Acetylcholine acts on muscarinic receptors, which when stimulated activate second messengers causing release of Ca^{2+} ions from intracellular stores in the sarcoplasmic reticulum. The rise in intracellular Ca^{2+} ion concentration activates actin and myosin, thereby promoting contraction. We know that the detrusor cell can depolarize with the inward current consisting of Ca^{2+} ions passing through L-type channels in sufficient magnitude to support depolarization.[22] The calcium influx may then trigger further intracellular Ca^{2+} ion release. However, acetylcholine does not cause depolarization and the role of detrusor depolarization is unexplained. Its limited influence may explain the lack of efficacy of calcium channel blockers in the treatment of detrusor overactivity.[22–24]

The muscarinic receptor is the focus of much current interest. Molecular biological studies have identified five subtypes of the muscarinic receptor (M1–M5). These are distributed throughout the central nervous system and in the periphery. Selective agonists and antagonists have identified five pharmacological subtypes (M1–M5) which correspond to the cloned M1–M5 receptors.[25] M1 activity is detected in the autonomic ganglia and central nervous system. M2 activity is found predominantly in the heart and M3 activity is found in glandular tissue and smooth muscle. mRNA activity for M4 receptors has been identified in rat striatum and rabbit lung. We know less about the role of M5 receptors limited because of the availability of specific agonists and antagonists.

Ligand studies of M2 and M3 receptors have shown that in the bladder the greater proportion (85 percent) are M2 receptors with only 20 percent being M3. It has been thought that the M2 receptors were largely redundant and all of the contractile activity could be attributed to the M3 receptor. However, recent studies suggest that the M2 receptor, may after all, be active.[26] In other smooth muscles the M2 receptor, on

stimulation, inhibits adenylate cyclase, which is stimulated by adrenoceptors. We do not know whether this system is active in the human bladder.[27,28] It has been found that some muscarinic antagonists prove selective for the bladder, and this tissue specificity has been claimed to be associated with either M2 selectivity or lack of M3 selectivity.[29,30] However, data from studies of the M3 selective agent darifenasin contradict these explanations.[31]

It is now known that acetylcholine and noradrenaline are not the only significant neurotransmitters in the lower urinary tract. Nonadrenergic noncholinergic (NANC) neurotransmitters are neuropeptides which modulate the actions of the classical transmitters and may act as transmitters themselves. Neuropeptide-Y (NPY) and vasoactive intestinal polypeptide (VIP) are important neuromodulators which are released at neuromuscular junctions so as to influence the release and uptake of acetylcholine and noradrenaline. Adenosine triphosphate (ATP) is thought to be an important neurotransmitter. It is known to cause depolarization of the detrusor. While in the normal human bladder ATP is not important, there is some evidence that in diseased states the activating mechanisms of the detrusor change and that NANC transmitters exert a much greater influence on the bladder.[29,30,32–34] There is also a growing interest in manipulating the activity of afferent pathway function, since inhibition of this might be an option in influencing bladder overactivity.[8,35]

PRESENTATION

It is frequently stated that the bladder is an unreliable witness and that the symptoms which a patient describes do not point to the true pathology.[36] This belief has arisen from the dubious assumption that patients can be fitted into distinct diagnostic categories and that meaningful symptoms should be unique to the diagnostic groups. In truth, it would seem that our diagnostic categories form intersecting continua which share some symptoms. This is important, because erroneous faith in diagnostic absolutes leads to dismissal of the significance of symptoms, which are the patients' experience of disease. It is my belief that the majority of symptoms can be explained by the physiological and mechanical principles which govern the lower urinary tract, and what the patients say usually makes sense. To date, our experimental data have supported this thesis, but rigor demands that we explore the subject much more.[37] However, I am going to discuss, critically, the nature of symptoms because expertise in this subject is important for patient relationships.

Frequency, urgency, urge incontinence, and nocturnal enuresis are symptoms associated with unstable contractions of the bladder and have been shown to be present during unstable bladder activity[38] and to reduce with documented resolution of the instability.[39,40] Frequency and urgency may be more noticeable when going out, and when opening the door on returning home, and to be subject to diurnal and seasonal variation. Intercurrent illness, particularly urinary infection will exacerbate instability. Urgency may vary as an experience between individuals. Some describe the idea of a growing potential for loss of bladder control, whereas others tell of a wholly physical sense of near incontinence.

Stress incontinence is incontinence associated with coughing, sneezing and other physical activity. It is associated with avoidance behavior prior to coughing. The term "genuine stress incontinence" is used to describe stress incontinence caused by an incompetent urethral sphincter. This terminology arose because it was noted that some women, with symptomatic stress incontinence were shown to have unstable bladders and it was believed that coughing induced unstable contractions which led to incontinence. It was proposed that instability could masquerade as stress incontinence. In fact, there are degrees of sphincter incompetence, which may coexist with degrees of detrusor instability and the two may interact.[41] We now know that the symptom of stress incontinence, with or without instability, is clearly associated with reduced sphincter function.[41,42] Where detrusor instability coexists, treatment of the instability may result in resolution in both symptom groups. This should be expected if the two pathologies work synergistically. Response to treatment of one pathology does not exclude the presence of the other.[43] On current evidence, if a woman describes stress incontinence, then there is a probability of some degree of sphincter dysfunction.

Sphincter dysfunction results in a reduction in the maximum closing pressure which can be generated in the urethra. This closing pressure must exceed the pressure of urine at the bladder neck for continence. As the bladder fills, a pressure will develop equal to the hydrostatic pressure of urine in the bladder plus the weight of any viscera pressing on the bladder. The hydrostatic pressure at 400 mL capacity is about 7 cm H_2O. If the maximum closure pressure is reduced below 10 cm H_2O then the woman will develop a sense of pending incontinence as the hydrostatic pressure rises towards the urethral threshold and minor positional changes may exacerbate this. The woman will be forced to maintain a bladder capacity with a hydrostatic pressure below the threshold. The symptoms of frequency, urgency and urge incontinence may all therefore be induced by an incompetent urethral sphincter. Additionally, rising during, or at the end of, the night, with a full bladder and suddenly applying an increased hydrostatic pressure to the faulty sphincter will lead to very severe urgency and precipitancy.

Hesitancy, a reduced stream, intermittency of stream, straining to void, manual abdominal compression during voiding, terminal dribbling, postmicturition dribbling and incomplete emptying are recognized symptoms of a voiding problem, be it obstructive or due to a failure of detrusor emptying function. Their presence correctly points to a requirement to check voiding efficiency. However, the physiology of micturition indicates that a high frequency will lead to similar symptoms. The bladder empties more efficiently from a higher capacity[44] when the hydrostatic pressure is greater, helping to open the urethra. Elongation of the detrusor fibers in response to filling promotes optimum contact between the actin and myosin so that a better contraction can be obtained.[45] Flow rates are well known to be related to the voiding bladder volume.[44] People with frequency therefore, commonly describe symptoms of poor voiding in the absence of detrusor underactivity or obstruction.

Dysuria is the experience of pain in association with micturition. The classical symptom of a burning in the urethra during voiding, caused by infection, is well known. Less appreciated is the external dysuria experienced by women with vaginitis when urine passes over the labia.[45] A persistent, low abdominal pain, partially relieved by micturition is a feature of chronic cystitis, particularly interstitial cystitis.[46,47] Instability may also cause poorly localized pains associated with unstable activity. This is particularly on rising in the morning. Very high frequencies may also result in lower urinary tract discomfort which tends to exacerbate frequency.

There are a variety of factors, unrelated to bladder physiology, which should be explored at the time of presentation. These commonly interact with a greater propensity for incontinence so as to cause it, such that correction will lead to continence. Adverse drug reactions, particularly caused by diuretics, sedatives, and alpha-receptor antagonists, should be identified. Diabetes may present as urinary incontinence. Toxic confusional states and intercurrent illness may precipitate the problem as can postoperative urinary retention, particularly on the orthopedic ward. It is often stated that fecal impaction causes urinary incontinence. While it certainly causes fecal incontinence, and may cause urinary retention, I am less certain of a valid relation with urinary incontinence. Physical problems around access to lavatory facilities also need to be considered.

URODYNAMICS

The urodynamic study has been the principal method used to explore the physiological changes particularly seen in elderly people. A urodynamic study is not necessary for the primary management of anyone presenting with urinary incontinence, be they young or old, and age should not influence the decision to use the investigation. However, an understanding of the test is certainly worthwhile.

A urodynamic study describes a number of aspects of lower urinary tract function extremely accurately,[48] particularly if proper attention is given to the laws of mechanics and the physiology governing the process. People err when they assume that their prior beliefs will be supported by results of the study. For example, a urodynamic study measures urinary outflow obstruction precisely.[48] It has been found, however, that urologists operate on the basis of symptoms rather than the physical demonstration of obstruction.[49] Because similar symptoms are found in urodynamically obstructed and unobstructed men it is inevitable that the clinical syndrome bearing the name "obstruction" is divorced from the urodynamic measure. Similarly, if you accept the definition of detrusor instability given in this chapter, you will find that patients with "urge incontinence" may prove to have "stable" bladders. This is not a problem with the measure, but with our theories about the nature of the clinical problem. With that said, I will describe the process of the test.[48,50]

On presentation, patients are asked to empty their bladders while urine flow rate is measured by means of a flow meter positioned in an adapted commode. A Jaques catheter (French gauge 10) and a nylon catheter (16G) are placed in the bladder via the urethra, which is anesthetized with 2 percent lignocaine gel. The postmicturition residual urine is drained off and measured. Another catheter (French gauge 10) tipped with a perforated latex sheath, to avoid fecal plugging, is introduced into the rectum. The smaller bladder catheter and the rectal catheter are filled with normal saline and then connected to force displacement transducers mounted at the level of the superior ramus of the pubic bone. This reference point is used to establish atmospheric pressure. The detrusor pressure, generated by the walls of the bladder, is calculated by subtracting the intra-abdominal pressure (measured via the rectal catheter) from the intravesical pressure (measured via the bladder catheter). The bladder is filled with a fluid (usually normal saline at 20°C) at a rate of between 50 and 100 mL min^{-1}. Unfortunately, filling rate, fluid temperature and content are not standardized and vary with department preference.

The analog data obtained from the transducers may be digitized and collected on magnetic disk. The bladder is filled until either a maximum of 500 mL has been infused, or unstable detrusor activity prohibits further filling, or the patient is found to be unable to tolerate any further infusion. On completion of the filling study the Jaques catheter, which was used for filling, is withdrawn from the bladder leaving the pressure measuring catheter in situ. The patient is then asked to void to completion. During voiding the bladder and rectal pressure and the flow rate are recorded simultaneously.

During normal filling to 500 mL the detrusor pressure rises to around 8 cm H$_2$O consequent on the pressure head of infused fluid and the relaxation of the detrusor in response to filling (Fig. 104-1). If the detrusor contracts whilst the patient is attempting to inhibit micturition an "unstable bladder" or "detrusor instability" is diagnosed. If this coexists with neurological disease, "detrusor hyper-reflexia" is diagnosed. As already emphasized, this nomenclature resulted from assumptions about pathophysiology and not observed differences in behavior,[51] although recent work supports such a differentiation.[52]

This basic test may be supplemented by fluoroscopic radiography and a number of other embellishments. There is no evidence for the value of these additional tests.

AGE-RELATED PATHOPHYSIOLOGY

Early studies of age-related urodynamic findings were conducted on samples of elderly people without younger comparisons.[53–56] In more recent studies, people with lower urinary tract symptoms have been compared across all age groups.[41,57–59] In 1995, data were published on normal, asymptomatic elderly people, but without comparative controls.[60]

Urge incontinence is the commonest cause of urinary incontinence in elderly people, this being due chiefly to detrusor instability. This is particularly the case in elderly people living in institutions.[61,62] Among outpatients presenting with lower urinary tract symptoms, between 75 and 85 percent of women aged 75 and over and 85 and 95 percent of similarly aged men will be found to have detrusor instability.[63]

Figures 104–2 and 104–3 are recordings obtained from women with detrusor instability and hyper-reflexia (detrusor instability with neurological disease). There are differences in the patterns of detrusor instability between the sexes. In addition, among women, contractions differ in relation to age and neuropathological state. Hyper-reflexic contractions occur on a background of poor compliance, caused by persistent muscle tone, and tend to summate. This differs from the pattern seen in detrusor instability where the contractions are less consistent on a background of persistent tone. With aging, in women, the detrusor instability is associated with increased excitability and similarly increased background tone.[59] Because of the similarities with detrusor hyper-reflexia, it is tempting to suspect that, in late life, detrusor instability is associated with age-related neurological degeneration. This has yet to be explored.

It is interesting to note that men with lower urinary tract symptoms do not demonstrate the age-related changes associated with women.[58] This probably relates to the higher urethral resistance caused by the prostate gland. The influence of this "obstructive" organ may dominate the evolution of bladder physiology. A recent publication, comparing obstructed and unobstructed elderly men supports this contention.[64]

Detrusor instability in both sexes is associated with lower bladder capacities in elderly people.[58] Contrary to expectations, lower bladder capacities, more aggressive detrusor instability,[59]

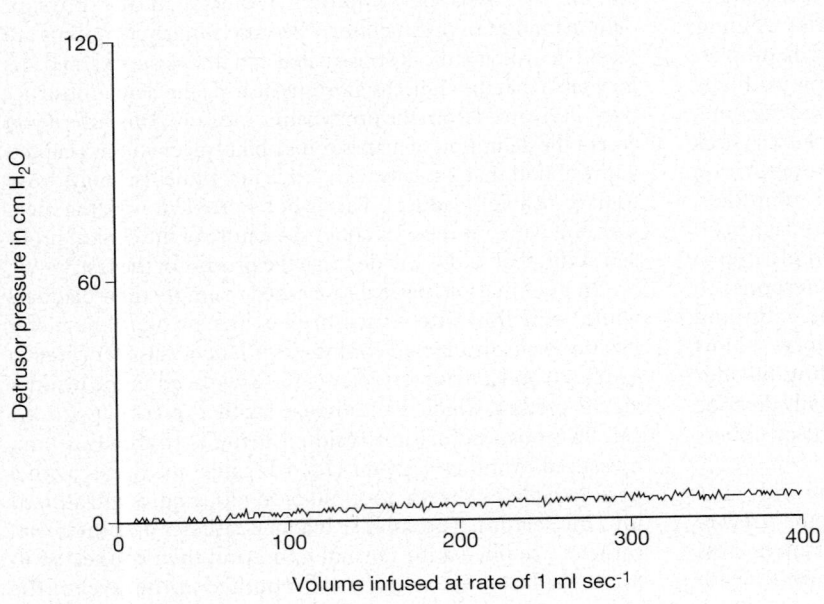

Figure 104-1 Detrusor pressure against infusion volume. Record obtained from a normal woman with a stable bladder.

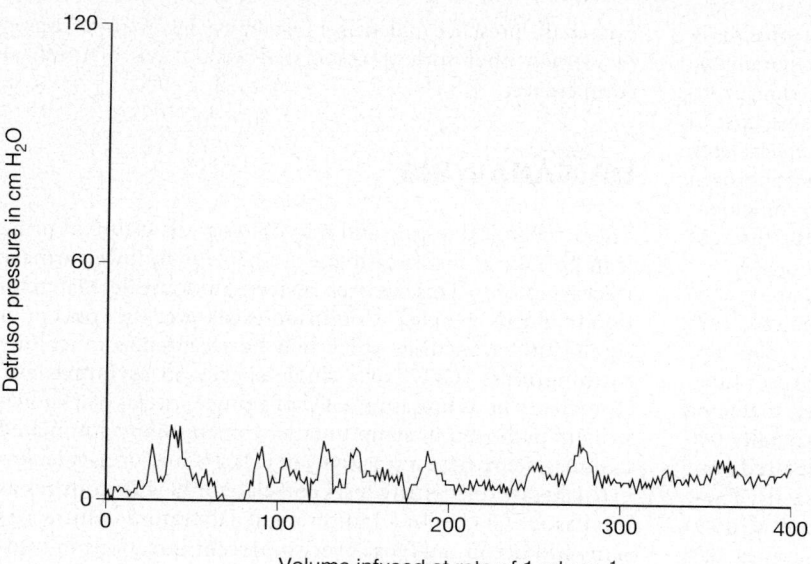

Figure 104-2 Detrusor pressure against infusion volume. Record obtained from a patient with instability.

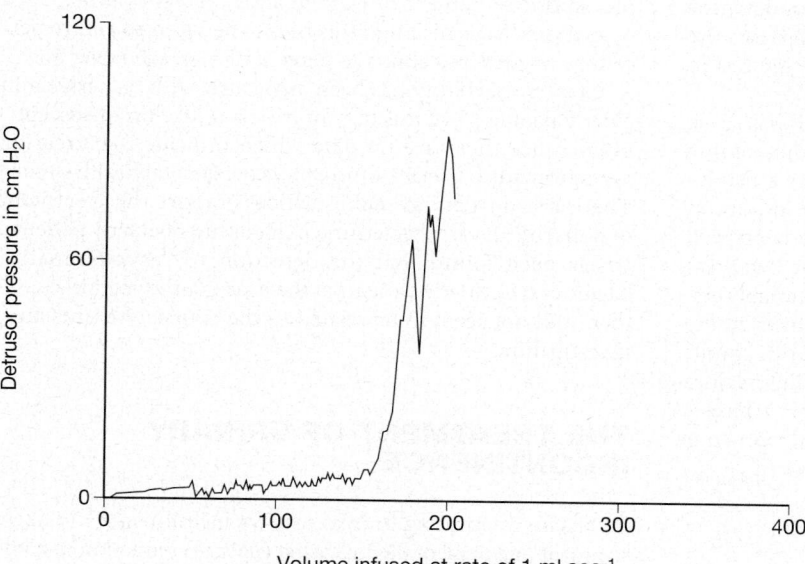

Figure 104-3 Detrusor pressure against infusion volume. Record obtained from a patient with multiple sclerosis. A hyper-reflexic bladder.

and older age do not appear to be associated with a poorer therapeutic prognosis.[63] In fact, there do not appear to be any urodynamic variables indicative of a poorer prognosis for the treatment of detrusor instability.[65] It is not appropriate therefore to talk of severity of detrusor instability.

Among women there are some interesting age-related changes involving bladder sensation. It has been found that the appreciation of bladder filling is reduced in association with age, and that this change in perception is very much more marked among women with detrusor instability and/or genuine stress incontinence.[57] This finding is unexpected, since the lower bladder capacities would seem to favor a contrary experience. Studies of bladder sensation combined with tests of cortical perfusion and cognition have shown that reduced bladder sensation in elderly people is associated with impaired cognition and reduced perfusion of specific parts of the cortex.[66,67]

Both sexes void less successfully in late life and voiding is associated with higher residual urine volumes and a higher proportion of patients with incomplete bladder emptying.[55,58,62] The explanations for this are probably complex. Obstruction will play a part in men but it is by no means the only explanation. There is evidence for a reduced speed of detrusor shortening in late life[58] as well as problems in sustaining adequate voiding contractions.[55,58,62]

The combination of detrusor instability and incomplete bladder emptying in elderly people raises the controversy of "Detrusor hyperactivity and impaired contractility" (DHIC).[55] This was described by Resnick and Yalla when reporting on 32 elderly nursing home residents in 1987.[55] They identified a specific physiological entity, being a subset of detrusor hyper-reflexia in elderly people. The characteristics were unstable detrusor contractions, a postmicturition residual urine volume, and reduced speed and amplitude of isometric detrusor contractions. In studying a much larger sample of elderly people, with younger comparators, my group have been unable to detect such a distinct physiological subgroup.[58] Voiding problems, detrusor instability, and contractility problems exist in elderly people but seem to be independent of each other. Derek Griffiths has also examined this issue, using a different approach to ours, and concluded that DHIC appeared to be a coincidental occurrence of two common conditions with different etiologies (Griffiths, D.J.; personal communication 1996).

However, Elbadawi et al.[68] have published data from electron microscopy studies of bladder biopsy specimens from elderly men ($n = 11$) and women ($n = 24$), which are in support of distinct pathophysiological subgroups of detrusor function. They reported four structural patterns precisely matching four urodynamic groups with no overlap. Additionally two subsets, "normal contractility" ($n = 11$) and "impaired contractility" ($n = 24$) matched histological subsets exactly. These findings have not been corroborated despite attempts to do so (Gosling, J.A., personal communication 1996). Carey et al.[69] have reported finding some of the defining histological characteristics described by Elbadawi et al.[68] evenly distributed between normal women ($n = 15$) and women with detrusor instability ($n = 22$).[69] This problem currently exercises the minds of many clinical and basic scientists with an interest in bladder function in elderly people.

There are changes in urethral function associated with aging in women. Figure 104-4 demonstrates a plot of the voiding detrusor pressure against flow rate recorded from a urodynamic study. The pressure–flow plot is extremely important in urodynamic analysis and its properties have been well reviewed elsewhere.[48,70] It has been shown that the two pressure intercepts shown, $p_{det.clos}$ and $p_{det.open}$, are invariably elevated in the presence of detrusor instability and lower in the presence of genuine stress incontinence. Where both conditions exist, the values take the middle ground. Highest values are seen in neurological diseases such as multiple sclerosis (Fig. 104-5). It has been shown that greater age in women is associated with lower values of both $p_{det.close}$ and $p_{det.open}$,

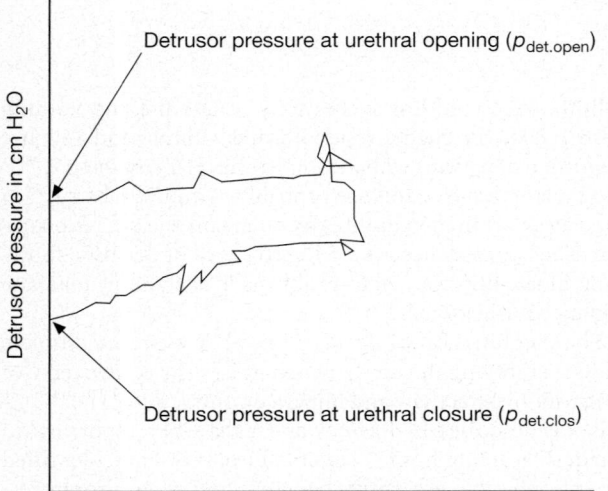

Figure 104-4 The pressure–flow plot.

even in the presence of detrusor instability (Fig. 104-6).[41] Aging in women, therefore, is associated with a loss of urethral competence.

URINANALYSIS

The biochemical testing and microbiological culture of urine is important in the assessment of people with lower urinary tract symptoms. This has been reviewed in some detail in relation to elderly people.[71] Confusion exists over the concept of significant bacteriuria, which may be accepted as 10^5 colony forming units (CFU) of a single species in asymptomatic women but be as low as 10^2 CFU of a single species of a known urinary pathogen in symptomatic women. Many automated culture systems have a sensitivity of 10^4 CFU and urinary leukocyte esterase and nitrite tests correlate only with cultures as high as 10^5 CFU.[72] In addition many laboratory culture systems will detect only just over 50 percent infections in midstream urine specimens from genuinely infected patients.[72,73] Asymptomatic bacteriuria is far more common in elderly people. About 20 percent of women and 3 percent of men aged 65–70 have bacteriuria and this rises to between 20 and 50 percent in women and about 20 percent of men aged over 80.[71]

Greater morbidity has been associated with bacteriuria in elderly people[74] but this may only be a reflection of susceptibility, since there are no data which indicate that treating asymptomatic bacteriuria influences the general health state.[74] There are no data available which support the treatment of nonacute dysuric bacteriuria in incontinent elderly patients. It has been found that the detection of "asymptomatic" bacteriuria in elderly patients at the time of urodynamic assessment did not seem to be related to the course of events after investigation.[75]

THE TREATMENT OF URINARY INCONTINENCE

Clinicians attempting to treat urinary incontinence are likely to aim at one or all of the following goals: (1) reduction of bladder sensitivity; (2) stabilization of the detrusor; (3) promotion of adequate bladder emptying during voiding; (4) competence of the urethral sphincter. Since a number of the therapeutic options will promote more than one of these objectives it is easier to consider treatment modalities individually.

Bladder retraining

This technique uses a protocol designed to encourage the patient to reduce the frequency of micturition. Several methods are proposed and none has been shown to be any better than others. There are a number of different bladder retraining charts, many of which are distributed by manufacturers of continence drugs or aids. The patient uses the chart to keep a record of episodes of micturition. During this time, efforts are made to delay micturition long after the urge to urinate is experienced. It has been found that while practicing the technique the frequencies of micturition tend to reduce.[76,77] In a recent randomized controlled trial[78] which included bladder

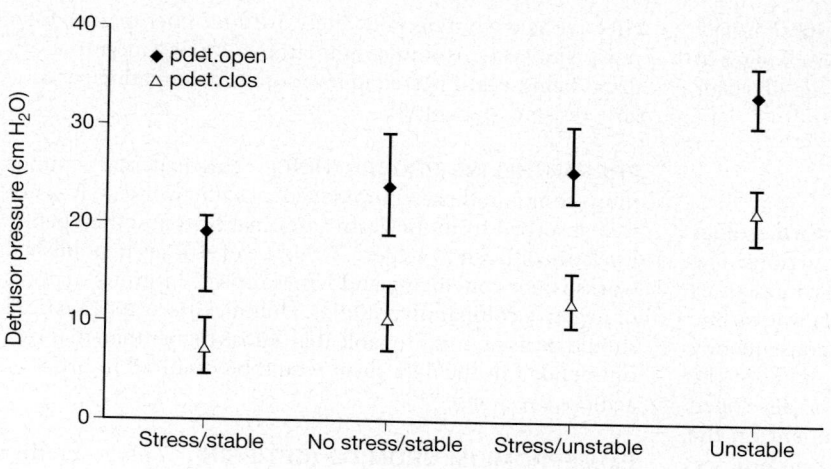

Figure 104-5 Detrusor pressures at urethral opening and closure for women with lower urinary tract symptoms.

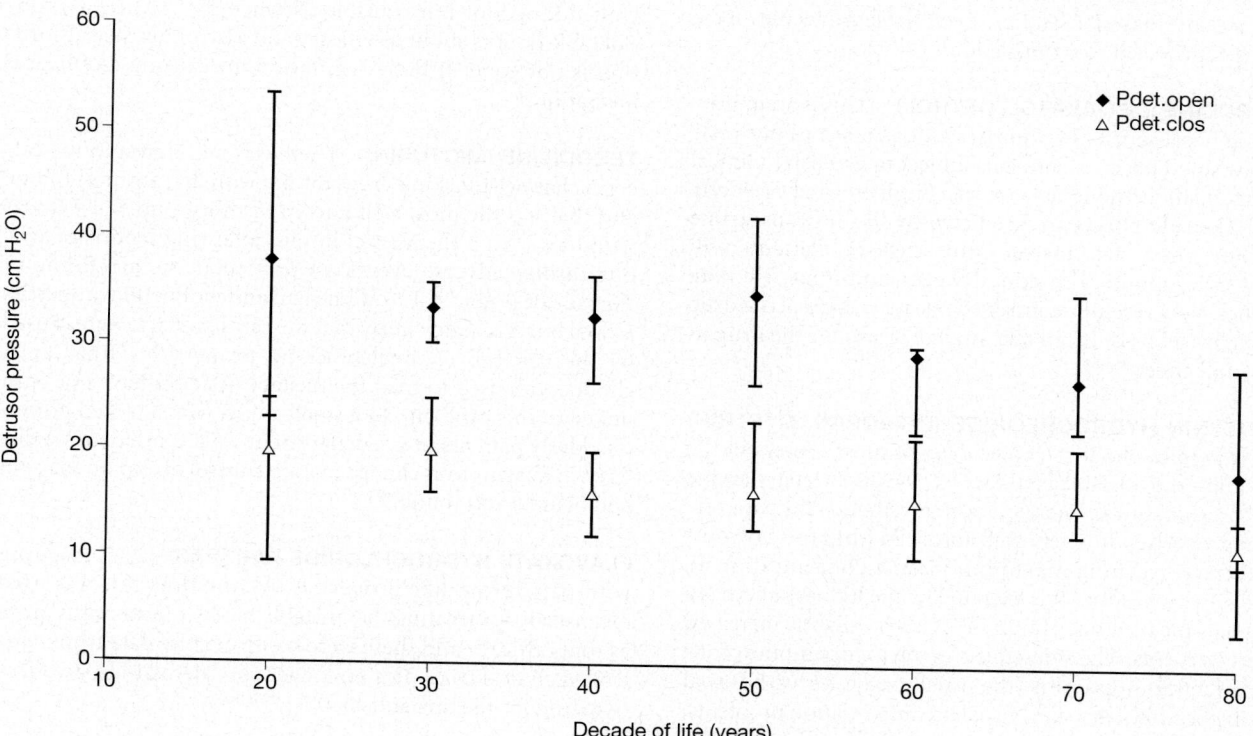

Figure 104-6 Detrusor pressures at urethral opening and closure for women with pure detrusor instability by decade of life.

retaining, we found that the period of change, in a patient who is responding, lasts about 3 weeks.

Patients with sensory urgency, who experience inappropriate desires to micturate at low bladder capacities in the absence of detrusor activity, may use this technique to reduce their frequency. However, it is not necessarily easy and the patient needs to be warned of this and persuaded of the great importance of compliance if there is to be any hope of recovery. An unstable bladder will tend to become less reactive if stretched by higher bladder volumes. This principle is used to treat detrusor instability where frequency predisposes to very low bladder capacities. Some patients with detrusor instability will experience pain while delaying micturition and there is a real possibility of urge incontinence while working with the regime.

Stretching the bladder can be augmented by encouraging higher fluid intakes while at home, and out of public scrutiny should an episode of incontinence occur.

As previously stated, if the urethral sphincter is incompetent, the greater pressure head applied to the bladder neck by larger bladder volumes will result in a strong sense of pending incontinence. This results in frequency being a feature of sphincter incompetence. For this reason it is appropriate to use a bladder retraining regime as part of the treatment of genuine stress incontinence, provided of course, that attention is also applied to the sphincter lesion.

Because a bladder will always empty more efficiently from a higher capacity, it is logical to use a bladder retraining regime to treat voiding problems secondary to detrusor muscle lesions.

Excessive delay, so that the bladder capacity rises substantially above 500 mL, should be avoided as there will be a danger of reducing detrusor power by overextension of the detrusor muscle fibers.

Stabilization of the bladder

To a very large extent the focus of much of our pharmacological effort is prevention of unstable bladder contractions. The most immediate precipitant of unstable detrusor contractions is probably the action of acetylcholine on the M3 muscarinic receptor on the detrusor membrane, which has consequently received much attention. Until very recently, none of the drugs available for treating detrusor instability was developed with the bladder in mind; we had been dependent on the accident of side-effects of drugs developed for other purposes. Tolterodine was recently introduced and darifenasin[26,40,79] is a subject of phase III studies. Both these molecules were developed specifically for the bladder.

TOLTERODINE (DETRUSITOL, DETROL)   This is an important drug because it has antimuscarinic properties but relatively few side-effects. It has been subject to extensive clinical trials that include a good data set specifically related to elderly people. The side-effects are predicted by the antimuscarinic properties which are not receptor-selective. Patients will describe a dry mouth, dry skin, dry eyes, and some will note headaches. Very recently, controlled release version of the drug has been introduced. It can take up to 8 weeks for the drug to exert its full effect.[80–85]

OXYBUTYNIN HYDROCHLORIDE (DITROPAN, CYSTRIN)   This seems to be the first-choice drug of most centers in the treatment of the unstable bladder.[78,86–89] It is a tertiary amine with powerful anticholinergic, local anesthetic and papaverine-like properties. It is very well absorbed from the gastrointestinal tract, reaching maximum plasma concentration 30 minutes after ingestion. It is excreted by the kidneys and has a plasma half-life of about 3 hours. This is very slightly increased in elderly patients. The side-effects involve a dry mouth, constipation, reflex esophagitis (the usual reason for withdrawal of this medication), dry skin, visual accommodation problems, and minor ankle swelling. Recent work has supported lower doses than those recommended in the data sheets for all age groups. We start all patients on 2.5 mg (or 3 mg) b.d. and titrate the dose in response to efficacy and side-effects.[89] It is probably best to wait for 4 weeks between dose alterations as the dynamics of the drug seem to be slower than the kinetics would suggest.[78,83] Oxybutynin's efficacy does seem to have been enhanced by the introduction of the new controlled-release preparation Ditropan XL.[90,91]

IMIPRAMINE (TOFRANIL)   This is a tricyclic antidepressant which has anticholinergic, alpha-agonistic, antihistaminic, and anti-5-HT properties.[92–95] Most patients respond to a single dose of between 10 mg and 25 mg at night. Some patients with troublesome daytime symptoms require an extra dose in the morning. The side-effects are similar to oxybutynin but milder; in addition, postural instability and drowsiness are problems experienced by elderly patients. Imipramine is probably not as effective as oxybutynin but there are a number of anecdotal reports of synergism in combination with oxybutynin, both drugs being administered in low dose, when treating particularly resistant patients.[94]

PROPANTHELINE (PROBANTHINE)   This quaternary ammonium compound is recommended by some workers. It is not well absorbed from the gastrointestinal tract and therapeutic levels are difficult to achieve. Evidence of efficacy in published works is not convincing and hangs on within-group analysis of negative comparative studies. Doubt exists as to what dose should be used. It is probable that a dose higher than that recommended in the data sheet would be required in order to achieve a response.[96–98]

EMMEPROMIUM BROMIDE (CETIPRIN)   This is another quaternary ammonium compound, no longer available in the United Kingdom, but available elsewhere.[99–101] There are considerable doubts about its efficacy and gastrointestinal absorption is not good. It has a reputation for causing esophageal ulceration.

TERODILINE (MICTURIN)   There was an interest in the calcium channel-blocking drugs for use with detrusor instability, and this was the most well known of this group.[102,103] It was withdrawn from the market in 1991 following reports of serious cardiac adverse events, in particular the arrythmia of Torsade de point.[104] Terodiline had anticholinergic properties as well but it is highly likely that the cardiac effects were caused by the calcium channel-blocking properties. Other anticholinergics used to treat the unstable bladder have not been linked to this problem. In a small study, which lacked power, on elderly patients in my department we did not detect a difference in symptom change from a control group on placebo and bladder retraining.[103]

FLAVOXATE HYDROCHLORIDE (URISPAS)   This is a drug with papaverine-like properties. At one time this was used extensively for treating the unstable bladder but doubts arose as to its efficacy and these were confirmed by data from controlled clinical trials. It is no longer considered to be an effective drug for the unstable bladder.[105–107]

Surgery for detrusor instability and hyper-reflexia

Three surgical procedures should be mentioned. Cystodistension, achieved by inflating a balloon in the bladder under anesthetic, produces a transient and unhelpful benefit.[108] Subtrigonal phenol injection was advocated for a while but has not stood the test of time.[109] The CLAM cystoplasty has proved to be a most important operative intervention for resistant patients.[46,110] There have to be some doubts about its applicability in late life, since the procedure makes voluntary bladder emptying ineffective and so voiding difficulties are inevitable. Patients therefore require clean intermittent self-catheterization to empty. This is particularly the case with detrusor hyper-reflexia.[111] Some elderly patients certainly can cope with intermittent self-catheterization, but the prevalence of multiple disabilities in late life demand some circumspection.

Correcting sphincter incompetence

PELVIC FLOOR EXERCISES These are a popular nonsurgical approach to urethral sphincter incompetence. The evidence for their efficacy is far from established and is based on data from open studies or within group analyses of comparative trial data.[112,113] Pelvic floor exercises have not been found to be superior to surgery. There is little consistency in the techniques which are adopted by different centers. While they have been advocated for the treatment of stress incontinence in older women, there is no evidence to support any specific efficacy in this group. It is regrettable that no large-scale studies of efficacy, which include age comparisons, have been conducted, so doubt hangs over their application.

SURGERY Until recently, the most widely accepted approach has been the colposuspension which seems to have achieved the most consistent successes across a wide variety of centers.[114-117] Some less invasive techniques have been promoted; in particular modifications of the Stamey endoscopic bladder neck suspension[118,119] and the use of injections into the paraurethral tissues.[120] We have to accept the fact that the results of these procedures are rather disappointing.

The most significant advance in surgery for stress incontinence for all age groups, but particularly elderly women, has been Ulmsten's work on "Tension free vaginal tape."[121] This new, simple and relatively noninvasive procedure is achieving very good results and is rapidly becoming the first surgical choice in many centers.[122,123]

THE AS ARTIFICIAL URINARY SPHINCTER This is an option for the management of urethral sphincter failure in both sexes. It is best suited to people who do not have unstable bladders. The operation involves the insertion of a cuff around the urethra. This cuff is passively inflated from a reservoir of fluid placed in the pelvis. The cuff can be deflated, so as to allow voiding, by activating a pump placed in the scrotum or labia major. After voiding, the cuff reinflates spontaneously. Complications include infection, displacement of the device, and mechanical failure. Some manual dexterity is required. These devices have been in use since 1972 and there is considerable experience and development favoring success. In correctly selected patients this prosthetic sphincter is highly effective.[12,124,125]

Treating voiding disorders

Intermittent self-catheterization has gained general acceptance in the management of voiding disorders associated with neurological disease.[126,127] We know that elderly people of both sexes have an increased tendency towards incomplete bladder emptying and this frequently coexists with detrusor instability. Voiding disorders in elderly people may occur in the absence of symptoms.[128] Treating detrusor instability in the presence of a voiding disorder may exacerbate the incomplete bladder emptying. The latter can be managed by intermittent catheterization. At this stage we do not know very much about the efficacy of this technique in elderly people. In addition, we are unclear as to which patients with voiding disorders can be safely left untreated.

Our policy is to identify patients with voiding disorders by including an assessment of the postmicturition residual urine volume as part of our standard assessment protocol. When we discover a significant problem, which we define as a residual of 150 mL or more, we institute a temporary, once daily intermittent catheterization program. If this results in a rapid and significant improvement in symptoms we then establish a more permanent regime, otherwise we take no further action.

The procedure may be difficult because of cognitive impairment and poor dexterity. It is more usual for us to enlist the services of a spouse or partner to administer the procedure, although a number of elderly people can self-catheterize. We have found that the fluid output in elderly people tends to be lower so that a less frequent regime of daily or twice daily catheterizations may prove adequate. Complications, in our selected elderly patients, do not seem to be greater than those among the young. Some older women, with delicate atrophic urethras, appear to be able to reduce urethral trauma by using estrogen replacement therapy.

Estrogen replacement therapy

The role of estrogen replacement therapy in the treatment of urinary incontinence remains unclear. Where this indication has been studied the results have not supported efficacy, despite widespread anecdotal advocacy.[129] It may, however, have a role in the management of recurrent urinary infection.[130] Estrogen withdrawal is associated with a fall in the levels of intravaginal glycogen on which lactobacilli depend. These bacteria cease to colonize the vagina, which is then occupied by colonic organisms that thrive in the higher pH associated with this change. The atrophy of the urethelium encourages colonization by Gram-negative fecal organisms and the urethelium becomes more adherent for these bacteria. There is some slim evidence that estrogen replacement therapy may reverse this process and give protection to elderly women with recurrent urinary tract infections.[129,131-133]

The primary concern in relation to hormone replacement therapy is the risk of triggering carcinoma of the uterus. This can be countered by using cyclical estrogen and progestogen therapy. There may be increased risk of breast cancer associated with the use of hormone replacement therapy over a long time but it reduces osteoporosis, stroke, and cardiac infarction.

A problem with cyclical combined therapy is the bleeding which will take place and this is not popular among elderly women. Estriol (Ovestin) may be useful here. Since there are no endometrial receptors, there is no risk of stimulating endometrial carcinoma and so it may be used continuously without progestogen in women who have not had a hysterectomy. The receptors for estriol are primarily in the vagina and lower urinary tract. Estriol does not effect bone so it is not possible to achieve an osteoporosis sparing effect with this drug.[134,135]

Treating urinary infection

In order to treat a urinary infection we need to choose a drug which is well absorbed from the gastrointestinal tract and therefore does not accumulate in the colon; is excreted in the urine rapidly; is not associated with high resistance rates; and is inexpensive. *Nitrofurantoin (Furadantin)* fits this bill. Some patients experience nausea with nitrofurantoin and in these circumstances the *macrocrystals (Macrodantin)* prove useful. *Trimethoprim (Monotrim)* is a useful urinary antibiotic provided there is not a great deal of local resistance. *Amoxycillin (Amoxil)* continues to be recommended for urinary infections and it is effective but particularly associated with the development of vaginal thrush infections. These occur in 25 percent of women prescribed amoxycillin. *Nalidixic acid (Negram)* is also a useful urinary antibiotic, is worth considering as a non-toxic first-line treatment. The quinolones such as *ciprofloxacin (Ciproxin)* should really be used as second-line therapies for resistant infections.[73,136–138]

The dose and duration should be designed to minimize the period of treatment. Clinical trials have shown that uncomplicated cystitis will respond usually to a 3-day course of trimethoprim, nitrofurantoin, or amoxycillin. Recurrent, postcoital cystitis usually responds to 100 mg nitrofurantoin immediately after intercourse. If the bladder is abnormal, 3-day courses may be less efficacious, and the recommendation is that antibiotic treatment be for 7 days at least. The published literature supports a 7-day course for elderly patients as a general rule. Nitrofurantoin does not penetrate the vagina. In theory this should be advantageous pre-menopausally when the vaginal lactobacilli need to be preserved. After the menopause, trimethoprim's ability to affect the vagina, which is likely to be colonized by the offending bacterium, may be a help.

If, in the rare circumstances of wishing to use prophylactic therapy in a patient experiencing recurrent urinary infections, then this is given as nitrofurantoin 100 mg nocte for 3 months. Long-term nitrofurantoin may, very rarely, cause peripheral neuropathy and pulmonary fibrosis. Since nitrofurantoin's action depends on rapid renal excretion, it is of no great use in renal impairment.[73,137,138] Cranberry juice is nowadays finding a role in prophylaxis against recurrent urinary infection.[139–141]

Devices

INCONTINENCE PADS These continue to play an important role in the management of uncontrolled urinary or fecal incontinence. They are best suited to patients with dementia and severe progressive disability. However, ambulant patients will need to use these devices while awaiting a permanent cure. The design, technology, function, and performance of incontinence pads have been reviewed with meticulous detail elsewhere.[142,143] Nowadays, there are some very effective products available, but care needs to be taken when choosing a suitable range. There are now considerable data on which to base an informed judgment of the most suitable products for a service. Too often decisions on the aids to provide for people are not given sufficient importance and tend to be hurried and ill-conceived. It is worth auditing the criteria adopted by local organizations when purchasing incontinence aids.[142–146]

PERMANENT INDWELLING CATHETERS These have a role in the management of some patients. They are not suitable in people with uncontrolled instability or hyper-reflexia, since they will cause pain and bypassing. They are best reserved for people with voiding problems, with or without controllable instability, who are unable to manage intermittent catheterization. A suprapubic catheter is by far the better option. It is easier to maintain and does not traumatize the urethra. Urethral catheters in women run the risk of inducing a vesico-vaginal fistula. If the bladder is impalpable the suprapubic catheter must be inserted under cystoscopic scrutiny.

Recurrent blocking and infections are complications of permanent catheterization. Anecdotal reports favor the use of vitamin C, 1 g q.d.s., and cranberry juice to combat blockage and infection but there are no clinical trial data to support this, although cranberry juice seems to have urinary antiseptic properties.[147] The former acidifies the urine and the latter reduces the tenacity of bacterial adhesion. Suby G bladder washouts do protect against blocking. A successful indwelling catheter need be changed only once every 3 months. Asymptomatic bacteriuria should be left untreated.[148]

EXTERNAL SHEATH DRAINAGE This is an option in some men. The old cumbersome latex contraptions have given way to penile sheaths, developed from the condom, which are fixed to the penis using adhesives specifically developed for this purpose. Urine drains from a tube connected at the apex of the sheath. The main problem is difficulty in fixation caused by penile retraction. Additionally, some patients have problems with displacement in response to the physical stresses of movement. There is an increased incidence of urinary infection from organisms ascending in the urinary column. Whilst skin ulceration has reduced with the advent of better adhesives, it remains a complication. A retractile penis can be splinted internally by implanting the Small Carrion prosthesis which is normally used for managing erectile failure.[149–151]

REFERENCES

1. Thomas TM, Flymat KR, Blannin J, Meade TW: The prevalence of urinary incontinence. Br Med J 1980;281:1243–1245
2. Brocklehurst JC: Urinary incontinence in the community—analysis of a MORI poll. Br Med J 1993; 306:832–834
3. Ding YY, Lieu PK, Choo PWJ, Tjia TTL: Urinary incontinence after ischaemic stroke—Predictive factors for its prevalence. Neurourol Urodyn 1996;15(4):262–264
4. Milsom I, Abrams P, Cardozo L et al: How widespread are the symptoms of an overactive bladder and how are they managed? A population-based prevalence study. BJU Int 2001;87(9):760–766
5. Milsom I, Stewart W, Thuroff J: The prevalence of overactive bladder. Am J Manag Care 2000;6(suppl 11):S565–S573
6. Simeonova Z, Milsom I, Kullendorff AM, Molander U, Bengtsson C: The prevalence of urinary incontinence and its influence on the quality of life in women from an urban Swedish population. Acta Obstet Gynecol Scand 1999;78(6):546–551
7. Brading AF, Turner WH: The unstable bladder: towards a common mechanism. Br J Urol 1994;73:3–8 (abstract)
8. Hoyle CHV, Lincoln J, Burnstock G: Neural control of pelvic organs. In Rushton DN (ed): Handbook of Neuro-Urology. Marcel Dekker, New York, 1994:1–54
9. De Groat WC: Neurophysiology of the pelvic organs. In Rushton DN (ed): Handbook of Neuro-Urology. Marcel Dekker, New York, 1995:55–93
10. Athwal BS, Berkley KJ, Hussain I et al: Brain responses to changes in bladder volume and urge to void in healthy men. Brain 2001;124 (Pt 2):369–377
11. Blok BFM, Holstege G: The human brain in the control of micturition and urine storage: A positron emission tomography study. Neurourol Urodyn 1996;15(4):261–262
12. Gousse AE, Madjar S, Lambert MM, Fishman IJ: Artificial urinary sphincter for post-radical prostatectomy urinary incontinence: long-term subjective results. J Urol 2001;166(5):1755–1758
13. Brading AF, McCoy R, Dass N: Alpha1-adrenoceptors in urethral function. Eur Urol 1999;36(suppl 1):74–79

14. Resnick NM, Yalla SV: Management of urinary incontinence in the elderly. N Engl J Med 1985; 313(13):800–805 (review)

15. Chapple CR: Alpha adrenoceptor antagonists in the year 2000: is there anything new? Curr Opin Urol 2001;11(1):9–16

16. Schwinn DA: Novel role for alpha 1-adrenergic receptor subtypes in lower urinary tract symptoms. Br J Urol Int 2000;86(suppl 2):11–20

17. Woods M, Carson N, Norton NW, Sheldon JH, Argentieri TM: Efficacy of the beta3-adrenergic receptor agonist CL-316243 on experimental bladder hyperreflexia and detrusor instability in the rat. J Urol 2001;166(3):1142–1147

18. Igawa Y, Yamazaki Y, Takeda H et al: Relaxant effects of isoproterenol and selective beta3-adrenoceptor agonists on normal, low compliant and hyperreflexic human bladders. J Urol 2001;165(1):240–244

19. Takeda M, Obara K, Mizusawa T et al: Evidence for beta3-adrenoceptor subtypes in relaxation of the human urinary bladder detrusor: analysis by molecular biological and pharmacological methods. J Pharmacol Exp Ther 1999;288(3):1367–1373

20. Fujimura T, Tamura K, Tsutsumi T et al: Expression and possible functional role of the beta3-adrenoceptor in human and rat detrusor muscle. J Urol 1999;161(2):680–685

21. Woods M, Carson N, Norton NW, Sheldon JH, Argentieri TM: Efficacy of the beta3-adrenergic receptor agonist CL-316243 on experimental bladder hyperreflexia and detrusor instability in the rat. J Urol 2001;166(3):1142–1147

22. Montgomery BSI, Fry C: The action potential and net membrane currents in isolated human detrusor smooth muscle cells. J Urol 1992;147:176–184

23. Palfrey ELH, Fry CH, Shuttleworth KED: A new *in vitro* perfusion technique for the investigation of human detrusor muscle. Br J Urol 1984;56:635–640

24. Wu CU, Kentish KJ, Fry CH: The effects of pH on Ca^{2+} activated force in α-toxin permealised detrusor smooth muscle isolated from guinea-pig bladder. J Physiol 1994;477:42

25. Eglen RM, Choppin A, Watson N: Therapeutic opportunities from muscarinic receptor research. Trends Pharmacol Sci 2001;22(8):409–414

26. Nilvebrant L, Sundquist S, Gillberg PG: Tolterodine is not subtype (m1-m5) selective but exhibits functional bladder selectivity in vivo. Neurourol Urodyn 1996;15(4):310–311

27. Shishido K, Yamaguchi O, Yokota T: Muscarinic receptor subtypes and their functional roles in rat detrusor muscle. Neurourol Urodyn 1996;15(4):313–314

28. Eglen RM: Muscarinic receptors and gastrointestinal tract smooth muscle function. Life Sci 2001;68(22–23):2573–2578

29. Jurgen W: Molecular basis of muscarinic acetylcholine receptor function. Trends Pharmacol Sci 1993;14:308–313

30. Eglen RM, Reddy H, Watson N, Challis JRA: Muscarinic acetylcholine receptor subtypes in smooth muscle. Trends. Pharmacol Sci 1994;15:114–119

31. Rosario DJ, Leaker BR, Smith DJ, Chapple CR: A pilot study of the effects of multiple doses of the M3 muscarinic receptor antagonist darifenasin on ambulatory parameters of detrusor activity in patients with detrusor instability. Neurourol Urodyn 1995;14(5):36–37

32. Bayliss M, Newgreen D, Fry CH: Changes to the functional properties of human detrusor smooth muscle and its innervation with disease. J Physiol 1998;507P:73

33. Wu C, Bayliss M, Newgreen D, Mundy AR, Fry CH: A comparison of the mode of action of ATP and carbachol on isolated human detrusor smooth muscle. J Urol 1999;162(5):1840–1847

34. Bayliss M, Wu C, Newgreen D, Mundy AR, Fry CH: A quantitative study of atropine-resistant contractile responses in human detrusor smooth muscle, from stable, unstable and obstructed bladders. J Urol 1999;162(5):1833–1839

35. De Groat WC, Kwatani M, Hisamitsu T: Neural control of micturition: the role of neuropeptides. J Auton Nerv Syst 1986;(suppl):369–387

36. Blaivas JG: The bladder as an unreliable witness. Neurourol Urodyn 1996;15:443–445

37. Wagg A, Bayliss M, Ingham NJ, Arnold K, Malone-Lee J: Urodynamic variables cannot be used to classify the severity of detrusor instability. Br J Urol 1998;82(4):499–502

38. van Waalwijk van Doorn ES, Remmers A, Janknegt RA: Extramural ambulatory urodynamic monitoring during natural filling and normal daily activities: evaluation of 100 patients. J Urol 1991;146:124–131

39. Tapp JS, Cardozo LD, Versi E, Cooper D: The treatment of detrusor instability in post-menopausal women with oxybutynin chloride: a double-blind placebo-controlled study. Br J Obstet Gynaecol 1990;97:521–526

40. Naerger H, Fry CH, Nilvebrant L: Effect of Tolterodine on electrically induced contractions of isolated human detrusor muscle from stable and unstable bladders. Neurourol Urodyn 1995;14(5):76–77

41. Wagg A, Lieu PK, Ding YY, Malone Lee JG: Age-related changes in female urethral function in association with detrusor instability. J Urol 1996;156:1984–1988

42. Lieu PK, Ng KJ, Malone-Lee JG: The voiding/pressure flow plot in the water cystometrogram is useful in inferring the possible existence of urethral sphincter incompetence in women. Neurourol Urodyn 1993;12:308–310

43. Wagg A, Malone Lee JG: Detrusor opening pressure and the prediction of outcome of treatment of instability in women with detrusor instability and stress incontinence. Neurourol Urodyn 1995;14:439–440

44. Haylen BT, Parys BT, Anyaegbunam WI, Ashby D, West CR: Urine flow rates in male and female urodynamic patients compared with the Liverpool nomograms. Br J Urol 1990;65:483–487

45. Hill AV: The heat of shortening and the dynamic constants of muscle. Proc Roy Soc 1938;126:136–195

46. Schaffer J, Fantl JA: Urogenital effects of the menopause. Baillière's Clin Obstet Gynaecol 1996; 10(3):401–417

47. Stamm WE, McKevitt M, Roberts PL, White NJ: Natural history of recurrent urinary tract infections in women. Rev Infect Dis 1991;13:77–84

48. Schafer W: Principles and clinical application of advanced urodynamic analysis of voiding function. Urol Clin North Am 1990;17:553–566

49. Cannon A, Chambers L, Bartlett E, Abrams P, Peters T: The natural history of bladder outlet obstruction and the longterm follow up of transurethral resection of the prostate. Neurourol Urodyn 1996;15(4):381–382

50. Griffiths DJ: Urodynamic assessment of bladder function. Br J Urol 1977;49:29–36

51. Abrams PH, Blaivas JG, Stanton SL, Andersen JT: Standardisation of terminology of lower urinary tract function. Neurourol Urodyn 1988;7:403–426

52. Malone-Lee JG, Wagg A, Mundy A et al: Science of urinary incontinence. Lancet 1994;344:311–315

53. Brocklehurst JC, Dillane JB: Studies of the female bladder in old age II. Cystometrograms on 100 incontinent women. Gerontol Clin 1966;8:306–319

54. Hilton P, Stanton SL: Algorithmic method of assessing urinary incontinence in elderly women. Br Med J 1981;282:940–942

55. Resnick NM, Yalla SV: Detrusor hyperactivity with impaired contractile function. An unrecognised but common cause of incontinence in elderly patients. JAMA 1987;257:3076–3081

56. Castleden CM, Duffin HM, Asher MJ: Clinical and urodynamic studies in 100 elderly incontinent patients. Br Med J Clin Res Ed 1981;282(6270):1103–1105

57. Collas DM, Malone-Lee JG: Age associated changes in detrusor sensory function in patients with lower urinary tract symptoms. Int Urogynecol J 1996;7:24–29

58. Malone-Lee JG, Wahedna I: Characterisation of detrusor contractile function in relation to old-age. Br J Urol 1993;72:873–880

59. Malone-Lee JG, Orugon O: A data reduction technique for describing and quantifying detrusor instability. Int Urogynecol J 1993;4:204–211

60. Resnick NM, Elbadawi A, Yalla SV: Age and the lower urinary tract: What is normal? Neurourol Urodyn 1995;14(5):577–579

61. Resnick NM, Yalla SV, Laurino E: The pathophysiology of urinary incontinence among institutionalized elderly persons. N Engl J Med 1989;320:1–7

62. Griffiths DJ, McCracken PN, Harrison GM, Gormley EA: Characteristics of urinary incontinence in elderly patients by 24-hour monitoring and urodynamic testing. Age Ageing 1992;21:194–201

63. Malone-Lee JG: Incontinence. Rev Clin Gerontol 1992;2:45–61

64. Lieu PK, Ding YY, Choo PWJ: Distinguishing unstable detrusor contractions of bladder outlet obstruction and cerebral disease. Neurourol Urodyn 1996;15(4):262–263

65. Wagg AS, Bayliss M, Arnold KG, Malone-Lee JG: Urodynamic prognosticators in detrusor instability. Neurourol Urodyn 1996;15(4):279–280

66. Griffiths DJ, McCracken PN, Harrison GM et al: Cerebral aetiology of urinary urge incontinence in elderly people. Age Ageing 1994;23:246–250

67. Griffiths DJ, McCracken PN, Harrison GM, Moore KN: Urinary incontinence in the elderly: the brain factor. Scand J Urol Nephrol 1994;157:83–88

68. Elbadawi A, Yalla SV, Resnick NM: Structural basis of geriatric voiding dysfunction, I. Methods of a prospective ultrastructural/urodynamic study and an overview of the findings. J Urol 1993;150:1650–1656

69. Carey M, Sapountzis K, Friedhuber A, Scurry J, Dwyer P: Electron microscopy study of detrusor muscle cell junctions in women with detrusor instability and controls. Neurourol Urodyn 1996;15(4):431–432

70. Griffiths DJ: Urodynamics: The mechanics and hydrodynamics of the lower urinary tract. Adam Hilger, Bristol, 1980

71. Gray RP, Malone-Lee JG: Review: Urinary tract infection in elderly people—Time to review management? Age Ageing 1995;24:341–345

72. Pappas PG: Laboratory in the diagnosis and management of urinary tract infections. Med Clin North Am 1991;75:313–325

73. Hooton TM, Stamm WE: Management of acute uncomplicated urinary tract infection in adults. Med Clin North Am 1991;75:339–357

74. Nicolle LE: Asymptomatic bacteriuria in the elderly. Infect Dis Clin North Am 1997;11(3):647–662

75. Harari D, Malone-Lee JG, Ridgway GL: An age related investigation of urinary tract symptoms and infection following urodynamic studies. Age Ageing 1994;23:62–64

76. Frewen WK: A reassessment of bladder training in detrusor dysfunction in the female. Br J Urol 1982; 54:372–373

77. Jarvis GJ, Millar DR: Controlled trial of bladder drill for detrusor instability. Br Med J 1980;281:1322–1323

78. Szonyi G, Collas DM, Ding YY, Malone-Lee JG: Oxybutynin with bladder retraining for detrusor instability in elderly people: a randomized controlled trial. Age Ageing 1995;24(4):287–291

79. Nilvebrant L, Stahl M, Andersson KE: Interaction of tolterodine with cholinergic muscarinic receptors in human detrusor. Neurourol Urodyn 1995;14(5):75–76

80. Van Kerrebroeck P: Tolterodine once-daily in treatment of the overactive bladder: Reply by the author. Urol 2001;58(5):831–832

81. Peters KM, Huang RR: Tolterodine once-daily in treatment of the overactive bladder. Urologia 2001; 58(5):829

82. Malone-Lee JG, Walsh JB, Maugourd MF: Tolterodine: a safe and effective treatment for older patients with overactive bladder. J Am Geriatr Soc 2001;49(6):700–705

83. Malone-Lee J, Shaffu B, Anand C, Powell C: Tolterodine: superior tolerability than and comparable efficacy to oxybutynin in individuals 50 years old or older with overactive bladder: a randomized controlled trial. J Urol 2001;165(5):1452–1456

84. Abrams P, Malone-Lee J, Jacquetin B et al: Twelve-month treatment of overactive bladder: efficacy and tolerability of tolterodine. Drugs Aging 2001;18(7):551–560

85. Kobelt G, Kirchberger I, Malone-Lee J: Review. Quality-of-life aspects of the overactive bladder and the effect of treatment with tolterodine. Br J Urol Int 1999;83(6):583–590

86. Malone-Lee JG: The clinical efficacy of oxybutynin. Rev Contemp Pharmacother 1995;5:195–202

87. Ouslander JG, Schnelle JF, Uman G et al: Does oxybutynin add to the effectiveness of prompted voiding for urinary incontinence among nursing home residents? A placebo-controlled trial. J Am Geriatr Soc 1995;43(6):610–617

88. Hughes KM, Lang JCT, Lazare R et al: The measurement of oxybutynin and its N-desethyl metabolite in plasma and its application to pharmacokinetic studies in young volunteers and elderly and frail elderly volunteers. Xenobiotica 1992;22:859–864

89. Malone-Lee JG, Lubel D, Szonyi G: Low dose oxybutynin for the unstable bladder. Br Med J 1992;304:1053

90. Hartnett NM, Saver BG: Is extended-release oxybutynin (Ditropan XL) or tolterodine (Detrol) more effective in the treatment of an overactive bladder? J Fam Pract 2001;50(7):571

91. Versi E, Appell R, Mobley D, Patton W, Saltzstein D: Dry mouth with conventional and controlled-release oxybutynin in urinary incontinence. The Ditropan XL Study Group. Obstet Gynecol 2000;95(5):718–721

92. Hindmarch I, Allford C, Barwell F, Kerr JS: Measuring the side effects of psychotropics: the behavioural toxicity of antidepressants. J Psychopharmacol 1992;6:167–173

93. Jarvis GJ: A controlled trial of bladder drill and drug therapy in the management of detrusor instability. Br J Urol 1981;53(6):565–566

94. Hunsballe JM, Djurhuus JC: Clinical options for imipramine in the management of urinary incontinence. Urol Res 2001;29(2):118–125

95. Andersson KE: Treatment of overactive bladder: other drug mechanisms. Urologia 2000;55(5A suppl):51–57

96. Holmes DM, Montz FJ, Stanton SL: Oxybutinin versus propantheline in the management of detrusor instability. A patient-regulated variable dose trial. Br J Obstet Gynaecol 1989;96:607–612

97. Thuroff JW, Bunke B, Ebner A et al: Randomized, double-blind, multicentre trial on treatment of frequency, urgency and incontinence related to detrusor hyperactivity: oxybutynin versus propantheline versus placebo. J Urol 1991;145:813–817

98. Zorzitto ML, Jewett MAS, Fernie GR, Holliday P, Bartlett S: Effectiveness of propantheline bromide in the management of geriatric patients with detrusor instability. Neurourol Urodyn 1986;5:133

99. Perera GL, Ritch AE, Hall MR: The lack of effect of intramuscular emepronium bromide for urinary incontinence. Br J Urol 1982;54(3):259–260

100. Walter S, Hansen J, Hansen L et al: Urinary incontinence in old age. A controlled clinical trial of emepronium bromide. Br J Urol 1982;54(3):249–251

101. Williams AJ, Prematalake JK, Palmer RL: A trial of emepronium bromide for the treatment of urinary incontinence in the elderly mentally ill. Pharmather 1981;2(8):539–542

102. Norton P, Karram M, Wall LL et al: Randomized double-blind trial of terodiline in the treatment of urge incontinence in women. Obstet Gynecol 1994;84(3):386–391

103. Wiseman PA, Malone-Lee J, Rai GS: Terodiline with bladder retraining for treating detrusor instability in elderly people. Br Med J 1991;302(6783):994–996

104. Thomas SH, Higham PD, Hartigan-Go K et al: Concentration dependent cardiotoxicity of terodiline in patients treated for urinary incontinence. Br Heart J 1995; 74(1):53–56

105. Chapple CR, Parkhouse H, Gardener C, Milroy EJ: Double-blind, placebo-controlled, cross-over study of flavoxate in the treatment of idiopathic detrusor instability. Br J Urol 1990;66(5):491–494

106. Milani R, Scalambrino S, Milia R et al: Double-blind cross-over comparison of flavoxate and oxybutynin in women affected by urinary urge syndrome. Int Urogynecol J 1993;4:3–8

107. Robinson JM, Brocklehurst JC: Emepronium bromide and flavoxate hydrochloride in the treatment of urinary incontinence associated with detrusor instability in elderly women. Br J Urol 1983;55(4):371–376

108. Lasanen LT, Tammela TL, Kallioinen M, Waris T: Effect of acute distension on cholinergic innervation of the rat urinary bladder. Urol Res 1992;20:59–62

109. Chapple CR, Hampson SJ, Turner Warwick RT, Worth PH: Subtrigonal phenol injection. How safe and effective is it? Br J Urol 1991;68:483–486

110. Flood HD, Malhotra SJ, O'Connell HE et al: Long-term results and complications using augmentation cystoplasty in reconstructive urology. Neurourol Urodyn 1995;14(4):297–309

111. Mast P, Hoebeke P, Wyndaele JJ, Oosterlinck W, Everaert K: Experience with augmentation cystoplasty. A review. Paraplegia 1995;33(10):560–564

112. Nilsson CG, Lukkari E, Haarala M et al: Comparison of a 10-mg controlled release oxybutynin tablet with a 5-mg oxybutynin tablet in urge incontinent patients. Neurourol Urodyn 1997;16(6):533–542

113. Bo K, Talseth T, Holme I: Single blind, randomised controlled trial of pelvic floor exercises, electrical stimulation, vaginal cones, and no treatment in management of genuine stress incontinence in women. Br Med J 1999;318(7182):487–493

114. Jarvis GJ: Surgery for genuine stress incontinence. Br J Obstet Gynaecol 1994;101:371–374

115. Hutchings A, Black NA: Surgery for stress incontinence: a non-randomised trial of colposuspension, needle suspension and anterior colporrhaphy. Eur Urol 2001;39(4):375–382

116. Fatthy H, El Hao M, Samaha I, Abdallah K: Modified Burch colposuspension: laparoscopy versus laparotomy. J Am Assoc Gynecol Laparosc 2001;8(1):99–106

117. Colombo M, Vitobello D, Proietti F, Milani R: Randomised comparison of Burch colposuspension versus anterior colporrhaphy in women with stress urinary incontinence and anterior vaginal wall prolapse. Br J Obstet Gynaecol 2000;107(4):544–551

118. Ganabathi K, Abrams P, Mundy AR, Dwyer PL, Glenning PP: Stamey-Martius procedure for severe genuine stress incontinence. Br J Urol 1992;69:34–37

119. Hilton P, Mayne CJ: The Stamey endoscopic bladder neck suspension: a clinical and urodynamic investigation, including actuarial follow-up over four years. Br J Obstet Gynaecol 1991;98:1141–1149

120. Radley SC, Chapple CR, Mitsogiannis IC, Glass KS: Transurethral implantation of macroplastique for the treatment of female stress urinary incontinence secondary to urethral sphincter deficiency. Eur Urol 2001;39(4):383–389

121. Ulmsten U, Falconer C, Johnson P et al: A multicenter study of tension-free vaginal tape (TVT) for surgical treatment of stress urinary incontinence. Int Urogynecol J Pelvic Floor Dysfunct 1998;9(4):210–213

122. Wang AC, Chen MC: Randomized comparison of local versus epidural anesthesia for tension-free vaginal tape operation. J Urol 2001;165(4):1177–1180

123. Ulmsten U, Johnson P, Rezapour M: A three-year follow up of tension free vaginal tape for surgical treatment of female stress urinary incontinence. Br J Obstet Gynaecol 1999;106(4):345–350

124. Mundy AR: Artificial sphincters. Br J Urol 1991;67:225–229

125. Montague DK, Angermeier KW, Paolone DR: Long-term continence and patient satisfaction after artificial sphincter implantation for urinary incontinence after prostatectomy. J Urol 2001;166(2):547–549

126. Michielsen DP, Wyndaele JJ: Management of false passages in patients practising clean intermittent self catheterisation. Spinal Cord 1999;37(3):201–203

127. Dowse J: Intermittent self-catheterisation: an option for all ages. Nurs Times 1999;95(6):67–68

128. Smith NKG, Morrant JD: Post-operative urinary retention in women: management of intermittent catheterization. Age Ageing 1990;19:337–340

129. Ouslander JG, Greendale GA, Uman G et al: Effects of oral estrogen and progestin on the lower urinary tract among female nursing home residents. J Am Geriatr Soc 2001;49(6):803–807

130. Hooton TM, Winter C, Tiu F, Stamm WE: Association of acute cystitis with the stage of the menstrual cycle in young women. Clin Infect Dis 1996;23(3):635–636

131. Messinger-Rapport BJ, Thacker HL: Prevention for the older woman. A practical guide to hormone replacement therapy and urogynecologic health. Geriatrics 2001;56(9):32–8,40

132. Mahavni V, Sood AK: Hormone replacement therapy and cancer risk. Curr Opin Oncol 2001;13(5):384–389

133. Cardozo L, Lose G, McClish D, Versi E, de Koning GH: A systematic review of estrogens for recurrent urinary tract infections: third report of the hormones and urogenital therapy (HUT) committee. Int Urogynecol J Pelvic Floor Dysfunct 2001;12(1):15–20

134. Raz R: Postmenopausal women with recurrent UTI. Int J Antimicrob Agents 2001;17(4):269–271

135. Lose G, Englev E: Oestradiol-releasing vaginal ring versus oestriol vaginal pessaries in the treatment of bothersome lower urinary tract symptoms. Br J Obstet Gynaecol 2000;107(8):1029–1034

136. Gupta K, Hooton TM, Roberts PL, Stamm WE: Patient-initiated treatment of uncomplicated recurrent urinary tract infections in young women. Ann Intern Med 2001;135(1):9–16

137. Hooton TM: Recurrent urinary tract infection in women. Int J Antimicrob Agents 2001;17(4):259–268

138. Hooton TM, Stamm WE: Diagnosis and treatment of uncomplicated urinary tract infection. Infect Dis Clin North Am 1997;11(3):551–581

139. Kontiokari T, Sundqvist K, Nuutinen M et al: Randomised trial of cranberry-lingonberry juice and Lactobacillus GG drink for the prevention of urinary tract infections in women. Br Med J 2001;322(7302):1571

140. Jepson RG, Mihaljevic L, Craig J: Cranberries for preventing urinary tract infections (Cochrane Review). Cochrane Database Syst Rev 2001;3:CD001321

141. Avorn J, Monane M, Gurwitz JJ et al: Reduction of bacteriuria and pyuria after ingestion of cranberry juice. J Am Med Assoc 1994;271(10):751–754

142. Cottenden AM, Fader MJ, Barnes KE, Jones TM, Malone-Lee JG: The clinical performance of incontinence products in relation to technical testing. Proc INSIGHT 1987;2:1–30

143. Cottenden AN, Malone-Lee JG, Butchers D: Technical testing and user requirements for adult incontinence products. Proc INSIGHT 1988;1:1–16

144. Cottenden AM, Fader MJ, Barnes KE, Jones TM, Malone-Lee JG: The clinical performance of incontinence pads in relation to their design and constituent materials. Proc TAPPI 1987;1:155–168

145. Fader M, Cottenden A, Brooks R: The CPE network: Creating an evidence base for continence product selection. J Wound Ostomy Continence Nurs 2001;28(2):106–112

146. Cottenden AM, Dean GE, Brooks RJ et al: Disposable bedpads for incontinence: predicting their clinical leakage properties using laboratory tests. Med Eng Phys 1998;20(5):347–359

147. Morris NS, Stickler DJ: Does drinking cranberry juice produce urine inhibitory to the development of crystalline, catheter-blocking Proteus mirabilis biofilms? Br J Urol Int 2001;88(3):192–197

148. Nicolle LE: The chronic indwelling catheter and urinary infection in long-term-care facility residents. Infect Control Hosp Epidemiol 2001;22(5):316–321

149. Pryor JP: Penile prostheses. In Gingell C, Abrams P (eds): Controversies and Innovations in Urological Surgery. Springer-Verlag, London, 1988:365–372

150. Fader M, Moore KN, Cottenden AM et al: Coated catheters for intermittent catheterization: smooth or sticky? Br J Urol Int 2001;88(4):373–377

151. Fader M, Pettersson L, Dean G et al: Sheaths for urinary incontinence: a randomized crossover trial. Br J Urol Int 2001;88(4):367–372

Chapter 105

Falls

Howard A. Fink, Jean F. Wyman, and Joseph T. Hanlon

Material in this chapter contains contributions from the previous edition, and we are grateful to the previous author for the work done.

Falls and their consequences are a well-recognized problem in elderly people. In adults, both falls and injurious falls increase with age. In addition to their association with injuries, falls may lead to future losses in function, increased fear of falling, and institutionalization. Moreover, falls are the most frequent cause of injury-related death in older adults. Well-designed epidemiological studies have estimated the incidence of falls and injurious falls in various elderly populations and have identified multiple risk factors. Knowledge of these risk factors may facilitate identification of individuals at risk for falls and associated injuries, and the presence of potentially modifiable risk factors provides targets for potential interventions to reduce risk of future falls. This chapter discusses the epidemiology of falls, assessment of falls, and interventions to prevent and reduce falls in geriatric patients.

EPIDEMIOLOGY OF FALLS

Definition

In epidemiological studies, a fall generally has been defined as an event that results in a person coming to rest inadvertently on the ground or other lower level.[1] Some studies have excluded events caused by a violent blow, loss of consciousness, or sudden onset of paralysis or seizure, circumstances that may still be relevant for clinical practice.[1] Ascertainment of falls in studies of community-dwelling elderly people has relied heavily on self-report, with ascertainment in studies of long-term care residents or hospitalized acute care patients often based on nurse or other incident reports. Though all these studies may use a narrower definition of falls than employed in clinical practice, and their ascertainment of falls may not be entirely complete, data from these studies provide the best information available in elderly people on the incidence of falls, their associated risk factors, and their sequelae.

Incidence of falls

Estimates from prospective observational studies indicate that approximately 25–50 percent of community-dwelling adults aged 65 years or older fall at least once annually, with roughly half of fallers falling multiple times.[2–5] In comparison, fall rates for residents in long-term care facilities range from 0.2 to 3.6 per bed per year (mean incidence of 1.5 falls per bed per year).[6] Among elderly in acute care hospitals, reported fall rates vary from 0.6 to 3.6 per 1,000 patient bed days.[7]

Circumstances of falls

COMMUNITY-DWELLERS   In community-dwelling elderly people, most falls occur during the daytime and at home or indoors.[2,3,8,9] Approximately half of falls involve a perturbation of the faller's base of support, such as occurs with a slip or trip, while more than one-quarter of falls occur during a moderate displacement of the faller's center of mass, such as occurs during bending over, reaching up, stepping up or down, or sitting or rising from a chair.[2,5]

LONG-TERM CARE RESIDENTS   In one long-term care facility consisting of residents of varying levels of dependency, most falls occurred during daytime and approximately half of falls occurred while ambulating.[10] Falls and injurious falls also frequently are associated with sitting or transferring from a chair, bed, or toilet, particularly in nonambulatory residents.[10–13]

ACUTE CARE PATIENTS   In acutely hospitalized patients, most falls occur during the waking activity hours, and many are associated with the changing of position or posture, notably in the course of using a wheelchair.[14]

Consequences of falls

DEATH   Complications related to falls have been considered the leading cause of death from injury in people older than 65.[15] In this population, deaths attributed to falls occur at a rate of approximately 2 per 1,000 persons per year, with the fall-related death rate increasing at older ages for all gender and ethnic categories.[16] While fractures have been considered to be the predominant mediating factor between falls and mortality, it appears that in most cases fractures, and by extension falls, do not directly lead to death but rather may be a marker of pre-existing frailty and heightened mortality risk.[17]

INJURY   Within community-dwelling elderly people, injuries occur commonly after falls, with 34–56 percent of falls leading to bruises, abrasions, or other minor soft-tissue injuries.[3,4,9,18] More serious injuries, such as dislocations, lacerations requiring suturing or other soft-tissue injuries requiring medical attention, occur after 1–10 percent of falls.[2–4,9,18] Further, 2–6 percent of falls result in a fracture(s), approximately one-fourth of which are hip fractures.[2–4,9,18] Within institutionalized elderly people, the rate of fall-related injuries is significantly higher than in those living independently in the community, even after accounting for differences in age and gender.[12]

Though most falls do not result in serious injury or fracture, falls still account for nearly 90 percent of all fractures in people aged 65 years and older, and each year approximately 5–8 percent of persons aged 70 years or older seek emergency care for one or more fall-related injuries.[16,19–21]

LONG LIE   After falling, 20–40 percent of elderly individuals are unable to get up without assistance.[3,9,18] Between 8 and 14 percent of fallers report an inability to rise without help for 5 minutes or greater, and 3 percent are unable to get up for more than 20 minutes.[3,18] Factors that increase the risk that a faller will be unable to get up without assistance after a fall include: age of 80 years or older, decreased strength, poor balance, arthritis, and dependency in activities of daily living (ADLs).[22] Within fallers, the inability to get up without help is a predictor of future loss of independence, institutionalization, and death.[22]

FEAR OF FALLING   Not surprisingly, many of those who have experienced a recent fall report a fear of future falls.[2,5,23–25] This fear of falling may be secondary to an individual's realistic perception of his or her functional impairment and resultant vulnerability to falls. Regardless, this fear may in turn increase the risk of falling, with possible mediating factors including the individual's avoidance of activity and resultant deconditioning, and his or her accentuated or ineffective reaction to postural disturbances.[26]

REDUCTION IN ACTIVITY AND INDEPENDENCE   Approximately 25 percent of recent fallers have been reported to restrict their activities at least temporarily after the fall, most often because of physical impairment resulting from a fall-related injury, but also frequently because of their fear of future falls.[2,3,18,25] As many as half of older people who are fearful of falling restrict or eliminate physical and social activities because of that fear.[2] In community-dwelling elderly people, falls, but in particular multiple falls, are associated with loss of independence in ADLs, increased risk of hospitalization and institutionalization, and increased risk of death.[2,27–30] Half of older adults hospitalized for a fall-related injury are unable to return home after their injury.[16] Nevertheless, analyses which account for other measures of chronic disease and disability suggest that multiple falls are not an independent predictor of these adverse outcomes but rather are a marker for other underlying factors that put older people at increased risk.[26,30]

Risk factors for falls

Numerous studies have examined factors for their possible association with falls in older adults. Within individual studies, multivariate analysis techniques have been utilized to determine whether specific factors are independently associated with falls after accounting for the presence or absence of other factors and their interactions. While some factors appear significant in one or more studies, a conclusive understanding about their relative importance in all older adults is limited by differences between studies with respect to populations enrolled, risk factors evaluated, and study-specific results. Associations between specific individual risk factors and falls appear stronger

when evaluated for multiple falls rather than for subjects with single falls.[3,8] This suggests that single falls may be more difficult to predict, and that there may be important differences between individuals who fall only once and those who fall repeatedly. Also, though some falls occur in individuals with no identified risk factors or only one risk factor, most take place in individuals with multiple, often interacting risk factors. The risk of falls appears to rise as the number of risk factors increases.[2,3]

ASSOCIATED INDEPENDENT RISK FACTORS   These independent risk factors are those identified in at least two prospective cohort studies.[2–4,8,9,31–35] These associated factors include older age, history of past falls, cognitive impairment, impairment in activities of daily living, lower extremity weakness or other disability, impaired balance or gait, dizziness, arthritis, history of stroke, increased number of medications, and psychotropic medication use (Table 105-1).

The association between psychotropic medications and falls was examined further in a recent meta-analysis that incorporated prospective cohort studies as well as studies of cross-sectional and retrospective design.[36] A statistically significant increase in risk of falls was evident with use of any psychotropic medication (odds ratio, OR = 1.7), as well as any sedative/hypnotic (OR = 1.7), benzodiazepine (OR = 1.5), antipsychotic (OR = 1.5), or antidepressant drug (OR = 1.5).[36] Fall risk appears similar for long vs short half-life benzodiazepines, and for tricyclic vs selective serotonin reuptake inhibitor antidepressants.[36,37] However, no data are available to date comparing the risk of falls with the new atypical antipsychotics to the risk with older agents.

SUSPECTED/CONTROVERSIAL FACTORS   A number of factors can be categorized as suspected or controversial risk factors for falls in elderly people.[9,38–43] Suspected or controversial risk factors are operationalized as such by their

---

Table 105-1 Evidence-based risk factors for falls[2–4,8,9,31–37]

Demographics:
- Advanced age (>80 years)

Medical conditions:
- Arthritis
- Cognitive impairment
- Dizziness
- History of stroke

Gait/balance/functional difficulties:
- Impaired activities of daily living
- Lower extremity weakness or disability
- Gait and/or balance deficit
- Previous fall history

Medication use
- Psychotropic medications
  - Antidepressants (both tricyclic and selective serotonin reuptake inhibitor antidepressants)
  - Antipsychotics
  - Benzodiazepines (both long and short half-life)
- Multiple medications (polypharmacy)

identification as being significantly associated with falls in some well conducted studies but not in others. These include certain medical conditions such as depression, visual impairment, glaucoma, urinary incontinence, lung disease, syncope, seizures, sleep problems, and cardiovascular conditions. Other suspected or controversial risk factors for falls include female gender, white race, use of an assistive device and environmental factors such as loose rugs, poor lighting, and slippery surfaces.[9,38–41]

Some other medications are considered suspected or controversial risk factors. A recent meta-analysis found that certain cardiac-related medications had relatively weak, but statistically significant associations with falls.[44] These include the use of type IA antiarrhythmics (OR = 1.6), digoxin (OR = 1.2) or diuretics (OR = 1.1). There was no increased risk of falls for other specific antihypertensive drug classes.[44] While this meta-analysis also found no association between falls and either narcotic or non-narcotic analgesic drugs, two previous studies reported an association between opioid analgesic use and an increased risk of hip fractures, including a possible dose–response relationship.[45,46] It also is possible that these studies have not identified all medications that increase fall risk. For example, it may be difficult to demonstrate associations for drugs that have a theoretical basis for an association with falls because of a low prevalence of use of these drugs (e.g. antiparkinson agents, those associated with myopathies/neuropathies, anticonvulsants).[47] However, a recent prospective cohort study by Ensrud et al., identified an increased risk of falls with anticonvulsant use (Adj OR = 1.7) in multivariate analyses that controlled for epilepsy as an indication.[48]

Risk factors for fall-related injuries

Risk factors for fall-related injuries are generally the same as those factors that predispose individuals to fall, but also include low bone mineral density (BMD), characteristics of the fall, and characteristics of the landing surface. For example, each standard deviation decrease in hip BMD is associated with a nearly three-fold increase in risk of hip fracture.[49] The risk of hip fracture also is greater for falls to the side or straight down on the hip, falls from standing height or more, and falls in which the faller lands on a hard surface.[18,24,50,51] The risk of wrist fracture appears to be greater when individuals have fallen backwards.[51]

ASSESSMENT OF FALLS
Screening

Assessment is the key to potential prevention of falls and their associated sequelae in elderly people. A recently released practice guideline by the American Geriatrics Society, British Geriatrics Society, and American Academy of Orthopedic Surgeons Panel on Fall Prevention recommends that all older adults should be screened annually for the occurrence of falls, with further evaluation in individuals who have experienced one or more falls (Fig. 105-1).[42]

It is important to note that even among older adults who experience one or more falls, many may fail to report fall events. Incomplete reporting may occur because individuals are embarrassed, or they may have forgotten about the fall(s), especially if the fall did not result in injury. Moreover, they

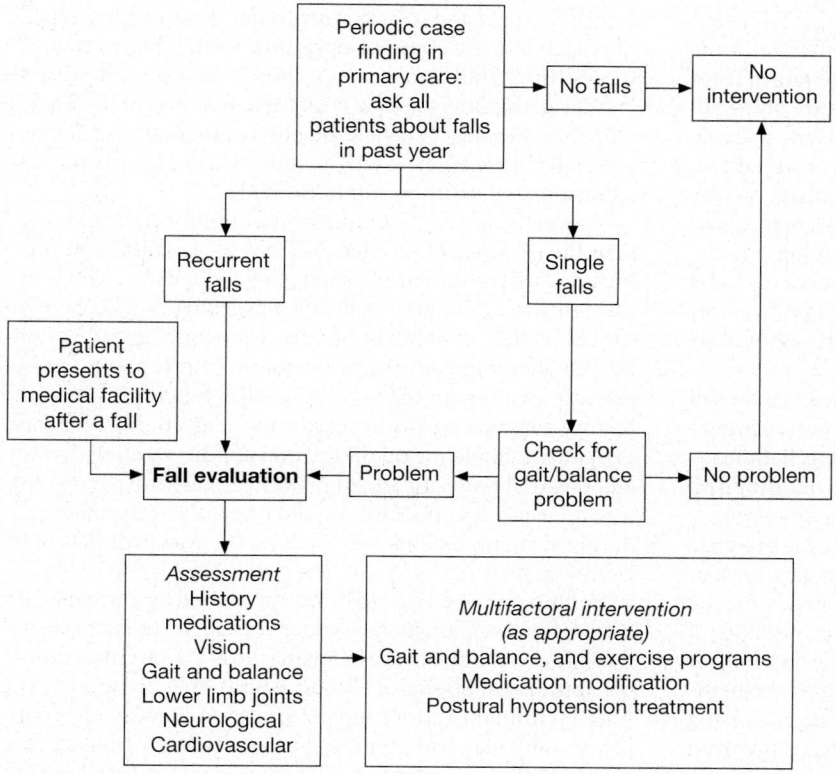

Figure 105-1 Algorithm summarizing the assessment and management of falls. (Reproduced from J Am Geriatr Soc 2001;49:664–672, with permission of Blackwell science, Inc.)

may minimize the significance of falls by attributing them to carelessness, or they may be fearful that in reporting falls that they might jeopardize their independence. In addition, patients will differ with respect to what they consider a fall event. When interviewing patients, clinicians should define a fall by asking whether the individual has experienced any episodes in which she/he accidentally came to rest on a lower level such as a chair or the floor.

There are a number of tests that can be used to assess gait and balance (Table 105-2).[52–56] It is recommended that the initial evaluation of individuals who report a single fall should consist of observation while they perform the "get-up and go" test.[54,55] This simple mobility test involves observation as an individual stands up from a chair without using his or her arms, walks a short distance, turns and walks back to the chair, and sits down (Table 105-2). A full fall assessment is then recommended only for those individuals who have difficulty or demonstrate unsteadiness on the get-up and go test, report recurrent falls over the past year, or present for medical attention because of a fall.[42]

Assessment

The goal of the fall assessment is to determine the mechanism(s) of the fall(s), to identify modifiable risk factors, and to characterize any impairment that may have resulted from a recent fall(s). The assessment should begin with a history to evaluate the circumstances surrounding the fall event(s), the individual's fear of falling, medication use and acute or chronic health problems that may have contributed to the fall. The history should be followed by a targeted physical examination, functional assessment, and, if indicated, diagnostic tests.

Evaluation of the circumstances surrounding a fall event often provides valuable clues as to the specific, often multiple factors that contributed to the fall. Information obtained from the history also may aid in characterizing the nature of the fall (e.g. whether it was syncopal or nonsyncopal), may provide guidance for what, if any, additional evaluation is warranted, and may identify situational and environmental risk factors that can be targeted for correction. Recurrent falls may follow a similar pattern that helps to reveal their etiology. If the individual is unable to recall the fall circumstances or had a loss of consciousness with the fall, the caregiver, family members, friends, or other witnesses to the fall event(s) should be questioned.

The mnemonic device SPLATT is useful in recalling the fall circumstances.[57] "S" stands for symptoms that occurred immediately prior to the fall or with the fall episode (e.g. lightheadedness, dizziness, vertigo, palpitations, chest pain, dyspnea, sudden focal neurological symptoms, aura, syncope, or urinary or fecal incontinence) that will help indicate the presence of new or exacerbated underlying illness. "P" stands for history of previous falls during the past year. "L" stands for the location of the fall. Did the fall occur indoors or outdoors; if indoors, in which room? "A" stands for the activity at the time of the fall. Was the individual rushing to the bathroom, getting out of the bathtub, descending stairs, arising from a chair or bed, reaching for a high object, or involved in some other physical activity where the center of gravity was displaced? "T" stands for the timing of the fall (e.g. falls

occurring soon after a meal may suggest postprandial hypotension as a possible cause) and the length of time on the ground. The second "T" stands for trauma or injury resulting from the fall.

The history may also include an assessment of the individual's fear of falling while performing specific daily activities (i.e., taking a bath or shower, getting dressed, walking outdoors or in stores), and should identify what activities the individual is now avoiding or limiting because of his or her fear of falling.[58] Several standardized instruments are available to assist in the assessment of fear of falling.[59–62]

The history also should focus on medications that can increase fall risk. The medication history should include a review of all drugs, including prescription, over-the-counter, herbal, and recreational drugs, including use of alcohol. Special attention should be given to newly started drugs or those for which the dose recently has been increased, as well as to key drug categories that have been associated with falls, such as psychotropic medications. Consideration also should be given to the individual's susceptibility for a future fall-related fracture, and to whether a bone strengthening agent(s) is indicated.

The history may identify numerous acute or chronic medical conditions possibly related to the fall(s), and the risk of falling is greater with an increased number of these conditions.[26] Acute conditions that may precipitate falls include metabolic imbalances, vertigo, delirium, postural hypotension, syncope, epileptic seizure, and alcohol intoxication. Some chronic conditions that may be associated with falls include sensory impairments, cognitive impairment, sleep problems, cardiovascular conditions, urinary incontinence, and musculoskeletal problems, and depression.[33,39,42,43] Because depression is frequently under-reported, it may be useful to incorporate a standardized instrument to screen for depression such as the Geriatric Depression Scale—short version.[63] In addition, functional status should be assessed with an instrument such as the Katz et al. basic activities of daily living (ADL).[64] Finally, a review of environmental risk factors, especially in areas where falls are most likely to occur (i.e., the bathroom and bedroom), may be helpful.

A targeted physical examination is useful to detect or confirm the presence of selected risk factors. Examination often includes an assessment of vision, gait and balance, and lower extremity joint function. A detailed neurological examination should include assessment of muscle strength, lower extremity peripheral nerves, proprioception, reflexes, and tests of cortical, extrapyramidal, and cerebellar function. When the history suggests a possible cardiovascular etiology for falls, assessment should include evaluation of heart rate and rhythm, and postural pulse and blood pressure.[42] Cognitive screening, if not previously completed, should be conducted using a standardized mental status test such as the Mini-Mental State Examination.[65]

Following the fall evaluation, specialized assessment may be indicated, especially for syncopal falls, injurious falls, and those for which the causes remain unclear. Determination of the appropriate specialized assessment should be based on the findings from the history and physical examination. For example, in the older adult with a syncopal fall, a formal cardiac work-up may be indicated. The emergency evaluation of an older adult who has had an injurious fall may warrant X-rays

Table 105-2 Tests to assist in the clinical assessment of gait and balance

Test	Description	Administration	Norms	
Functional reach[52]	Single item: scored in inches change while forward reaching using a fixed base of support. Extended arm is parallel to yardstick at shoulder level	3 minutes Yardstick, tape	*Age (yr)* 20–40 41–69 70–87	*Inches* 14–17 13–15 10–13
Berg balance test[53]	14-item categorical scale: sit to stand, stand to sit, transfer chair to chair, stand eyes open and closed, reach forward, pick object up from floor, single leg stance, tandem stance, look over shoulders, turn 360 degrees, alternate foot on stool	10–15 minutes Stopwatch, chair with armrest and bed or second chair with no arms, ruler, shoe, stool	Score <45 predicted multiple faller	
Timed get-up and go test[54,55]	Categorical scale and timed scoring Sit to stand from chair with armrests, walk 3 meters, turn, walk back to chair, sit down One trial run before timed test	1–2 minutes Measuring tape, arm chair, stopwatch	<10 seconds = freely mobile <20 seconds = mostly independent 20–29 seconds = variable mobility >29 seconds = impaired mobility	
Problem-oriented mobility assessment[56]	18 items with categorical scale and timed scoring *Balance subscale:* stand to sit, sitting, sit to stand, immediate standing, side-by-side standing, backward waist pull, single leg stance, semi-tandem stance, pick up object off floor, toe standing, heel standing *Gait subscale:* gait initiation, path deviation, missed step, turning while walking, stepping over obstacle	10 minutes Stopwatch, chair without arms, pen, two shoes, belt	≤19 = high risk of falling 20–25 = intermediate risk >25 = no unusual risk	

or other imaging studies. For falls that occur only at home for unclear reasons, a home safety evaluation could be considered.

Specialized assessment

Because falls are a multifactorial problem, fall evaluation may best be conducted by a multidisciplinary team, with the specific composition of the team varying depending on the healthcare setting and reimbursement factors. In the acute care or long-term care setting, referral may be made to a multidisciplinary falls consult team or to individual team members.

For elders with significant mobility and strength impairments, referral to a physical therapist may be indicated for a detailed assessment of gait, balance, and strength. Though some tests utilized by physical therapists to evaluate gait and balance impairments require specialized equipment, most frequently used measures may easily be administered in any setting with minimal equipment and time (Table 105–2). Further, in most fallers, a reasonable therapeutic plan may be developed with information obtained from simple observational tests. At present, there is no evidence that high-technology tests are essential in the evaluation of fallers.

For community-dwelling elders, referral to an occupational therapist or home health nurse may be indicated for evaluation of environmental risk factors and assessment of how the individual interacts with his/her environment when carrying out daily activities. A home safety evaluation should try to identify: possible tripping and slipping hazards, especially in the bathroom and in walkways within and outside the home; the presence of unsteady furniture such as chairs or tables; the site and preferred method for bathing; areas where lighting may be absent or inadequate; the state of repair of stairs, including whether handrails are present; and the height of the toilet, bed, and preferred sitting chairs, and the ability of the individual to easily negotiate getting on and off them. Referral to a pharmacist for a medication review, if not already included as part of the routine assessment, is valuable in determining whether specific drugs or combinations of drugs may be exposing the patient to an increased risk of falls, and whether any medications may be changed or discontinued.

INTERVENTIONS TO PREVENT/REDUCE FALLS

Because of the frequency of falls and their complications in older adults, the prevention of falls is an important clinical and public health issue. As described earlier, well-designed, prospective epidemiological studies have identified numerous factors that may predict falls, including some that potentially are modifiable. In turn, intervention studies have targeted one or more of these risk factors to determine whether falls may be prevented or reduced.

The strongest evidence regarding the efficacy of different interventions for prevention of falls should be available from well-designed, randomized controlled trials (RCTs) or systematic reviews and meta-analyses of such trials. While there are minimal RCT data on fall prevention interventions in hospitalized patients, and relatively limited data for elderly subjects living in long-term care settings, a great many RCTs

evaluating fall prevention interventions have been conducted in community-dwelling elderly populations.[66–92]

Intervention studies in community-dwelling or long-term care residents

Both falls prevention RCTs that enrolled participants who were community-dwelling and those that enrolled long-term care residents have generally evaluated the following types of interventions: identification and possible modification of falls hazards in the home environment, assessment and modification of medication regimens, and exercise to improve strength, balance, endurance and/or flexibility. In addition, trials involving community-dwelling subjects often have included subject education related to fall risk factors. Most trials involved a multifaceted intervention, incorporating a combination of these elements. The following summarizes the literature regarding these four approaches.

FALL-RELATED EDUCATION   There are limited data available from RCTs regarding the effectiveness of fall-related education alone for prevention of falls; nearly all trials that have evaluated fall-related education have included education as part of a multifaceted intervention. A single RCT by Reinsch and colleagues, conducted in 230 elderly adults recruited from community senior centers, compared a weekly fall-related curriculum with weekly discussions of health topics unrelated to falls.[85] Both intervention and follow-up were 1 year in duration. Fall-related education alone was not found to be beneficial for any measure of fall incidence.

ENVIRONMENTAL ASSESSMENT AND MODIFICATION   We are aware of no RCT data documenting the effectiveness of environmental assessment and modification alone for prevention of falls. However, environmental assessment and modification are incorporated in many multifaceted fall prevention RCTs, including one in which it was combined with only a very limited educational component.[75,77,79–81,86–88,90,91] In this latter RCT by Cumming and colleagues, 530 elderly subjects were randomized to receive usual care or an occupational therapist home safety assessment.[77] Subjects receiving the home visit were given individualized recommendations to reduce environmental fall hazards (e.g. removal of mats and rugs, installation of stair railing or night light) and to change personal behaviors that may increase their fall risk. Completion of recommended modifications was left to participants. Though the home visit was completed for only 67 percent of subjects in the intervention group and compliance with various specific recommendations ranged from 19 to 75 percent, subjects in the intervention group appeared to be nearly 20 percent less likely to experience a fall, with the benefit of intervention achieving borderline statistical significance.

MODIFICATION OF MEDICATION REGIMEN   RCT data are limited regarding the effectiveness of medication regimen modification as a sole intervention for falls prevention. In a double-blinded pilot study by Campbell and colleagues, 93 elderly men and women currently taking a benzodiazepine, other hypnotic, or any antidepressant or major tranquilizer, whose general practitioner thought might benefit from discontinuation, were randomly allocated to gradual withdrawal of psychotropic medication vs continued use.[73] In a multivariate analysis that adjusted for past history of falls and number of medications, subjects assigned to the medication withdrawal group were 66 percent less likely to experience a fall during the 44-week follow-up, a statistically significant reduction in falls compared with the control group. Perhaps not surprisingly, nearly half of subjects who successfully withdrew from their psychotropic medication during the study had restarted the medication within one month of study completion, often related to symptoms of stress or sleep disturbance. Additional studies incorporating nonpharmacological methods for supporting subjects discontinuing these medications and involving longer follow-up will be important for confirming and building on these promising results.

EXERCISE   Exercise modalities assessed in falls prevention RCTs have included: (1) strength/resistance exercise, (2) balance training, (3) aerobic/endurance training, (4) flexibility exercises, and (5) tai chi.[93] Based on data from RCTs that have incorporated an exercise component, the benefit of exercise for reducing falls is uncertain.[35,71–73,78,81–87,90–92] Among RCTs that evaluated exercise alone, one study found that subjects randomized to tai chi classes were significantly less likely to experience a fall during follow-up than those participating only in general health discussions.[92] No other single exercise modality has been shown to significantly reduce falls in isolation, or to consistently reduce falls as part of a multicomponent exercise-only intervention.

MULTIFACETED INTERVENTIONS   Results from RCTs that target multiple fall-related risk factors are mixed, with a nearly equal number of trials showing a significant reduction in falls in the intervention group compared to a control group as the number of trials showing no benefit. A meta-analysis of five RCTs by Gillespie and colleagues reported that subjects randomized to individualized assessment for falls risk factors by a health professional, with such findings made available for potential action, were significantly less likely to experience one or more falls during follow-up.[94] Of 10 additional RCTs involving multifaceted interventions to reduce falls that either were not mathematically pooled in the Gillespie meta-analysis or were reported after its publication, five showed a significant reduction in falls for the intervention group compared to the control group,[70,74,75,81,86] and five found no benefit with intervention.[68,76,80,85,88] These inconsistent results may be due to variability in the underlying falls risk of study participants, the type and number of component interventions included in each study, the intensity of each component intervention, and statistical issues such as the number of study participants, duration of follow-up and completeness of falls identification. The RCT by Tinetti and colleagues enrolled participants at high risk for falls, performed individualized assessments of fall risk factors, and individually targeted a multifaceted intervention that included education, environmental modification, medication changes if appropriate, and an exercise program incorporating strength, balance and flexibility.[87] Subjects in the intervention group were approximately 25 percent less likely to fall during the study, a significant protective effect compared to subjects in the control group. Though such a reduction in

falls should be clinically meaningful, and offers a possible intervention model, discrepant results in other trials are difficult to link to consistent differences in their respective study designs. Further research is needed to help determine which elements in interventions are most vital for their success.

Intervention studies in hospitalized patients

As noted above, few RCTs of falls prevention interventions have been conducted in hospitalized patients.[95] In one study, performed in 134 elderly inpatients in a rehabilitation unit who had at least one falls risk factor, assignment of patients to wear a bracelet designed to remind wearers to move about carefully did not reduce falls compared to falls observed in nonbracelet wearers.[66] A second RCT, carried out in 70 inpatients on an acute geriatric unit who were identified as being at high risk for falls from bed, found no significant reduction in bed falls with use of a pressure-sensitive alarm system designed to alert nursing staff when a patient was trying to get out of bed.[67]

A systematic review of hospital fall prevention programs included all studies that estimated fall rates before and after intervention, and in addition to the RCTs described above identified 18 nonrandomized, prospective studies that compared results in the intervention group with either parallel or historical controls.[96] Intervention strategies among included studies were heterogeneous, but tended to involve one or more of the following: (1) greater vigilance, (2) attention to equipment safety, and (3) proactive nursing assistance. While these nonrandomized studies appeared to demonstrate a statistically significant 24 percent reduction in the fall rate in the intervention group, limitations of these studies include their inability to account for changes in hospital unit or patient characteristics over time that may explain any observed reduction in falls. Oliver and colleagues rightly suggest that better-designed studies are needed before any firm conclusions can be made regarding the effectiveness of hospital fall prevention programs.[96]

Interventions studies to prevent fall-related injuries

Efforts to prevent falls, if successful, also may reduce fall-related injuries. However, in addition to falls, factors that contribute to fall-related injuries include the severity of the fall and the fragility of the faller. Given that no intervention will prevent all falls, in appropriately selected patients, strong consideration should be given to implementation of interventions that have been demonstrated to reduce clinical fractures through strengthening bone.[97–99] In addition, interventions to reduce clinical fractures by attenuating the impact transmitted to bone during a fall should be considered.[100–102]

SUMMARY

Falls and injurious falls occur frequently in community-dwelling elderly people, and appear to be an even greater problem in older adults who are hospitalized or who reside in a long-term care setting. Risk factors most rigorously associated with falls or recurrent falls in epidemiological studies include: older age, history of past falls, cognitive impairment, impairment in activities of daily living, lower extremity weakness or other disability, impaired balance or gait, dizziness, increased number of medications, psychotropic medication use, arthritis, and history of stroke. Results for all of the above risk factors appear to be heterogeneous between studies, and data suggest the possibility that many other factors also may be associated with falls. Primary fall prevention requires careful screening to determine those at increased risk of falling. In those who already have experienced a fall, the key to further fall prevention is a careful history and physical examination with judicious use of other health care professionals to help identify modifiable risk factors/causes. Evidence to date suggests that falls may be reduced or prevented by implementation of targeted, multifaceted interventions that include education, environmental modification, medication changes if appropriate, and an exercise program. Further research is needed to determine which aspects of multifaceted interventions may be responsible for a reduction in falls, as well as to evaluate the cost-effectiveness of interventions that demonstrate a significant clinical benefit.[103]

KEY POINTS Falls

- Falls occur frequently in elderly people and commonly result in morbidity.

- Risk factors most consistently associated with falls include: older age, history of past falls, cognitive impairment, impairment in activities of daily living, lower extremity weakness or other disability, impaired balance or gait, dizziness, increased number of medications, psychotropic medication use, arthritis and history of stroke.

- Careful history and physical with judicious use of other healthcare professionals is the key to fall prevention.

- Falls may be reduced or prevented by implementation of targeted, multifaceted interventions that include education, environmental modification, medication changes if appropriate, and an exercise program.

REFERENCES

1. Anonymous: The prevention of falls in later life: a report of the Kellogg International Work Group on the Prevention of Falls by the Elderly. Dan Med Bull 1987;34(suppl 4):1–24
2. Tinetti ME, Speechley M, Ginter SF: Risk factors for falls among elderly persons living in the community. N Engl J Med 1988;319:1701–1707
3. Nevitt MC, Cummings SR, Kidd S et al: Risk factors for recurrent nonsyncopal falls. JAMA 1989;261:2663–2668
4. O'Loughlin JL, Robitaille Y, Boivin JF et al: Incidence of and risk factors for falls and injurious falls among the community-dwelling elderly. Am J Epidemiol 1993;137:342–354
5. Maki BE, Holliday PJ, Topper AK: A prospective study of postural balance and risk of falling in an ambulatory and independent elderly population. J Gerontol A 1994;49:M72–M84
6. Rubenstein LZ, Josephson KR, Robbins AS: Falls in the nursing home. Ann Intern Med 1994;121:442–451
7. Tideiksaar R: Falling in Old Age: Prevention and Management, 2nd Ed. Springer, New York, 1997
8. Graafmans WC, Ooms ME, Hofstee HM et al: Falls in the elderly: a prospective study of risk factors and risk profiles. Am J Epidemiol 1996;143:1129–1136
9. Vellas BJ, Wayne SJ, Garry PJ et al: A two year longitudinal study of falls in 482 community dwelling elderly adults. J Gerontol A 1998;53:M264–M274
10. Gurwitz JH, Sanchez-Cross MT, Eckler MA et al: The epidemiology of adverse and unexpected events in the long-term care setting. J Am Geriatr Soc 1994;42:33–38
11. Thapa PB, Brockman KG, Gideon P et al: Injurious falls in nonambulatory nursing home residents: a comparative study of circumstances, incidence, and risk factors. J Am Geriatr Soc 1996;44:273–278
12. Luukinen H, Koski K, Honkanen R et al: Incidence of injury-causing falls among older adults by place of residence: a population-based study. J Am Geriatr Soc 1995;43:871–876
13. Ashley MJ, Gryfe CI, Amies A: A longitudinal study of falls in an elderly population: some circumstances of falling. Age Ageing 1977;6:211–220
14. Berry G, Fisher RH, Lang S: Detrimental incidents, including falls, in an elderly institutional population. J Am Geriatr Soc 1981;29:322–324
15. Sattin RW: Falls among older persons: a public health perspective. Ann Rev Public Health 1992;13:489–508
16. Sattin RW, Lambert Huber DA, Devito CA et al: The incidence of fall injury events among the elderly in a defined population. Am J Epidemiol 1990;131:1028–1037
17. Browner WS, Pressman AR, Nevitt MC et al: Mortality following fractures in older women: The Study of Osteoporotic Fractures. Arch Intern Med 1996;156:1521–1525
18. Nevitt MC, Cummings SR, Hudes ES: Risk factors for injurious falls: a prospective study. J Gerontol A 1991;46:M164–M170
19. Fife D, Barancik JI: Northeastern Ohio Trauma Study III: incidence of fractures. Ann Emer Med 1985;14:244–248
20. Fife D, Barancik JI, Chatterjee BF: Northeastern Ohio Trauma Study II: incidence rates by age, sex, and cause. Am J Pub Health 1984;74:473–478
21. Cummings SR, Kelsey JL, Nevitt MC et al: Epidemiology of osteoporosis and osteoporotic fractures. Epidemiol Rev 1985;7:178–208
22. Tinetti ME, Liu WL, Claus EB: Predictors and prognosis of inability to get up after falls among elderly persons. JAMA 1993;269:65–70
23. Walker JE, Howland J: Falls and fear of falling among elderly persons living in the community: occupational therapy interventions. Am J Occup Ther 1991;45:119–122
24. Grisso JA, Schwarz DF, Wolfson V et al: The impact of falls in an inner-city elderly African-American population. J Am Geriatr Soc 1992;40:673–678
25. Tinetti ME, Mendes de Leon CF, Doucette JT et al: Fear of falling and fall-related efficacy in relationship to functioning among community-living elders. J Gerontol A 1994;49:M140–M147
26. King MB, Tinetti ME: Falls in community-dwelling older persons. J Am Geriatr Soc 1995;43:1146–1154
27. Kiel DP, O'Sullivan P, Teno JM et al: Health care utilization and functional status in the aged following a fall. Med Care 1991;29:221–228
28. Wolinsky FD, Johnson RJ, Fitzgerald JF: Falling, health status, and the use of health services by older adults. Med Care 1992;30:587–597
29. Dunn JE, Furner SE, Miles TP: Do falls predict institutionalization in older persons? J Aging Health 1993;5:194–207
30. Dunn JE, Rudberg MA, Furner SE et al: Mortality, disability, and falls in older persons: the role of underlying disease and disability. Am J Pub Health 1992;82:395–400
31. Campbell AJ, Borrie MJ, Spears GF: Risk factors for falls in a community-based prospective study of people 70 years and older. J Gerontol A 1989;44:M112–M117
32. Davis JW, Ross PD, Nevitt MC et al: Risk factors for falls and for serious injuries on falling among older Japanese women in Hawaii. J Am Geriatr Soc 1999;47:792–798
33. Mahoney J, Sager M, Dunham NC et al: Risk of falls after hospital discharge. J Am Geriatr Soc 1994;42:269–274
34. Luukinen H, Koski K, Kivela SL et al: Social status, life changes, housing conditions, health, functional abilities and life-style as risk factors for recurrent falls among the home-dwelling elderly. Public Health 1996;110:115–118
35. Buchner DM, Larson EB: Falls and fractures in patients with Alzheimer-type dementia. JAMA 1987;257:1492–1495
36. Leipzig RM, Cumming RG, Tinetti ME: Drugs and falls in older people: a systematic review and meta-analysis: I. Psychotropic drugs. J Am Geriatr Soc 1999;47:30–39

37. Thapa PB, Gideon P, Cost TW et al: Antidepressants and risk of falls among nursing home residents. N Engl J Med 1998;339:875–882

38. Stone JK, Wyman JF: Falls. In Stone JK, Wyman JF, Salisbury (eds): Clinical Gerontological Nursing: A Guide to Advanced Practice, 2nd Ed. WB Saunders, Philadelphia, 2000

39. Brown JS, Vittinghoff E, Wyman JF et al: Urinary incontinence: does it increase risk for falls and fractures? Study of Osteoporotic Fractures Research Group. J Am Geriat Soc 2000;48:721–725

40. Kiely DK, Kiel DP, Burrows AB et al: Identifying nursing home residents at risk for falling. J Am Geriatr Soc 1998;46:551–555

41. Oliver D, Britton M, Seed P et al: Development and evaluation of evidence based risk assessment tool (STRATIFY) to predict which elderly inpatients will fall: case-control and cohort studies. Br Med J 1997;315:1049–1053

42. Anonymous: Guideline for the prevention of falls in older persons. J Am Geriatr Soc 2001;49:664–672

43. Brassington GS, King AC, Bliwise DL: Sleep problems as a risk factor for falls in a sample of community-dwelling adults aged 64–99 years. J Am Geriatr Soc 2000;48:1234–1240

44. Leipzig RM, Cumming RG, Tinetti ME: Drugs and falls in older people: a systematic review and meta-analysis: II. Cardiac and analgesic drugs. J Am Geriatr Soc 1999;47:40–50

45. Shorr RI, Griffen MR, Daugherty JR et al: Opioid analgesics and the risk of hip fracture in the elderly: codeine and propoxyphene. J Gerontol 1992;47:M111–M115

46. Guo Z, Wills P, Viitanen M et al: Cognitive impairment, drug use, and the risk of hip fracture in persons over 75 years old: a community-based prospective study. Am J Epidemiol 1998;148:887–892

47. Hanlon JT, Cutson T, Ruby CM: Drug-related falls in the elderly. Top Geriatr Rehabil 1996;11:38–54

48. Ensurd K, Blackwell T, Hanlon J et al: Central nervous system active medications and risk of falls and fractures in older women. J Bone Min Res 1999;14(suppl 1):S263 (abstract)

49. Cummings SR, Black DM, Nevitt MC et al: Bone density at various sites for prediction of hip fractures. The Study of Osteoporotic Fractures Research Group. Lancet 1993;341:72–75

50. Greenspan SL, Myers ER, Maitland LA et al: Fall severity and bone mineral density as risk factors for hip fracture in ambulatory elderly. JAMA 1994;271:128–133

51. Nevitt MC, Cummings SR: Study of Osteoporotic Fractures Research Group. Type of fall and risk of hip and wrist fractures: The Study of Osteoporotic Fractures. J Am Geriatr Soc 1993;41:1226–1234

52. Duncan PW, Weiner DK, Chandler J et al: Functional reach: a new clinical measure of balance. J Gerontol A 1990;45:M192–M197

53. Berg KO, Wood-Dauphinee SL, Williams JL et al: Measuring balance in the elderly: preliminary development of an instrument. Physiother Can 1989;41:304–311

54. Mathias S, Nayak US, Issacs B: Balance in elderly patients: the "get-up and go" test. Arch Phys Med Rehabil 1986;67:387–389

55. Podsiadlo D, Richardson S: The timed "up & go": a test of basic functional mobility for frail elderly persons. J Am Geriatr Soc 1991;39:142–148

56. Tinetti ME: Performance oriented assessment of mobility problems in elderly patients. J Am Geriatr Soc 1986;34:119–126

57. Tideiksaar R: Preventing falls: how to identify risk factors, reduce complications. Geriatrics 1996;51(2):43–46,49–53

58. Myers AM, Powell LE, Maki BE et al: Psychological indicators of balance confidence: relationship to actual and perceived abilities. J Gerontol A 1996;51:M37–M43

59. Tinetti ME, Richman D, Powell L: Falls efficacy as a measure of fear of falling. J Gerontol A 1990;45:M239–M243

60. Powell LE, Myers AM: The activities-specific balance confidence scale. J Gerontol A 1995;50:M28–M34

61. Rai GS, Kiniorns M, Wientjes H: Fall Handicap Inventory (FHI)—an instrument to measure handicaps associated with repeated falls. J Am Geriatr Soc 1995;43:723–724

62. Lachman ME, Howlan J, Tennstedt S et al: Fear of falling and activity restriction: the Survey of Activities and Fear of Falling in the Elderly (SAFE). J Gerontol B 1998;53:P43–P50

63. Yesavage JA, Brink TL, Rose TL et al: Development and validation of a geriatric depression rating scale: a preliminary report. J Psychiatr Res 1983;17:37–49

64. Katz S, Akpom CA: A measure of primary sociobiologic functions. Int J Health Serv 1976;6:493–507

65. Folstein MF, Folstein SE, McHugh PR: The mini-mental state: a practical method of grading the cognitive state of patients for the clinician. J Psychiatr Res 1975;12:189–198

66. Mayo NE, Gloutney L, Levy AR: A randomized trial of identification bracelets to prevent falls among patients in a rehabilitation hospital. Arch Phys Med Rehabil 1994;75:1302–1308

67. Tideiksaar R, Feiner CF, Maby J: Falls prevention: the efficacy of a bed alarm system in an acute-care setting. Mt Sinai J Med 1993;60:522–527

68. McMurdo ME, Millar AM, Daly F: A randomized controlled trial of fall prevention strategies in old peoples' homes. Gerontology 2000;46:83–87

69. Mulrow CD, Gerety MB, Kanten D et al: A randomized trial of physical rehabilitation for very frail nursing home residents. JAMA 1994;271:519–524

70. Ray WA, Taylor JA, Meador KG et al: A randomized trial of a consultation service to reduce falls in nursing homes. JAMA 1997;278:557–562

71. Buchner DM, Cress ME, de Lateur BJ et al: The effect of strength and endurance training on gait, balance, fall risk, and health services use in community-living older adults. J Gerontol A 1997;52:M218–M224

72. Campbell AJ, Robertson MC, Gardner MM et al: Randomised controlled trial of a general practice programme of home based exercise to prevent falls in elderly women. Br Med J 1997;315:1065–1069

73. Campbell AJ, Robertson MC, Gardner MM et al: Psychotropic medication withdrawal and a home-based exercise program to prevent falls: a randomized, controlled trial. J Am Geriatr Soc 1999;47:850–853

74. Carpenter GI, Demopoulos GR: Screening the elderly in the community: controlled trial of dependency surveillance using a questionnaire administered by volunteers. Br Med J 1990;300:1253–1256

75. Close J, Ellis M, Hooper R et al: Prevention of falls in the elderly trial (PROFET): a randomised controlled trial. Lancet 1999;353:93–97

76. Coleman EA, Grothaus LC, Sandhu N et al: Chronic care clinics: a randomized controlled trial of a new model of primary care for frail older adults. J Am Geriatr Soc 1999;47:775–783

77. Cumming RG, Thomas M, Szonyi G et al: Home visits by an occupational therapist for assessment and modification of environmental hazards: a randomized trial of falls prevention. J Am Geriatr Soc 1999;47:1397–1402

78. Ebrahim S, Thompson PW, Baskaran V et al: Randomized placebo-controlled trial of brisk walking in the prevention of postmenopausal osteoporosis. Age Ageing 1997;26:253–260

79. Fabacher D, Josephson K, Pietruszka F et al: An in-home preventive assessment program for independent older adults: a randomized controlled trial. J Am Geriatr Soc 1994;42:630–638

80. Gallagher EM, Brunt H: Head over heels: impact of a health promotion program to reduce falls in the elderly. Can J Aging 1996;15:84–96

81. Hornbrook MC, Stevens VJ, Wingfield DJ et al: Preventing falls among community-dwelling older persons: results from a randomized trial. Gerontologist 1994;34:16–23

82. Lord SR, Ward JA, Williams P et al: The effect of a 12-month exercise trial on balance, strength, and falls in older women: a randomized controlled trial. J Am Geriatr Soc 1995;43:1198–1206

83. McMurdo ME, Mole PA, Paterson CR: Controlled trial of weight bearing exercise in older women in relation to bone density and falls. Br Med J 1997;314:569

84. MacRae PG, Feltner ME, Reinsch S: A 1-year exercise program for older women: effects on falls, injuries, and physical performance. J Aging Phys Activity 1994;2:127–142

85. Reinsch S, MacRae P, Lachenbruch PA et al: Attempts to prevent falls and injury: a prospective community study. Gerontologist 1992;32:450–456

86. Steinberg M, Cartwright C, Peel N et al: A sustainable programme to prevent falls and near falls in community dwelling older people: results of a randomised trial. J Epidemiol Commun Health 2000;54:227–232

87. Tinetti ME, Baker DI, McAvay G et al: A multifactorial intervention to reduce the risk of falling among elderly people living in the community. N Engl J Med 1994;331:821–827

88. van Haastregt JC, Diederiks JP, van Rossum E et al: Effects of a programme of multifactorial home visits on falls and mobility impairments in elderly people at risk: randomised controlled trial. Br Med J 2000;321:994–998

89. van Rossum E, Frederiks CM, Philipsen H et al: Effects of preventive home visits to elderly people. Br Med J 1993;307:27–32

90. Vetter NJ, Lewis PA, Ford D: Can health visitors prevent fractures in elderly people? Br Med J 1992;304:888–890

91. Wagner EH, LaCroix AZ, Grothaus L et al: Preventing disability and falls in older adults: a population-based randomized trial. Am J Public Health 1994;84:1800–1806

92. Wolf SL, Barnhart HX, Kutner NG et al: Reducing frailty and falls in older persons: an investigation of Tai Chi and computerized balance training. Atlanta FICSIT Group. Frailty and Injuries: Cooperative Studies of Intervention Techniques. J Am Geriatr Soc 1996;44:489–497

93. Gregg EW, Pereira MA, Caspersen CJ: Physical activity, falls, and fractures among older adults: a review of the epidemiologic evidence. J Am Geriatr Soc 2000;48:883–893

94. Gillespie LD, Gillespie WJ, Cumming R et al: Interventions for preventing falls in the elderly. Cochrane Database Syst Rev 2000;CD000340

95. Feder G, Cryer C, Donovan S et al: Guidelines for the prevention of falls in people over 65. The Guidelines' Development Group. Br Med J 2000;321:1007–1111

96. Oliver D, Hopper A, Seed P: Do hospital fall prevention programs work? A systematic review. J Am Geriatr Soc 2000;48:1679–1689

97. Black DM, Cummings SR, Karpf DB et al: Randomised trial of effect of alendronate on risk of fracture in women with existing vertebral fractures. Fracture Intervention Trial Research Group. Lancet 1996;348:1535–1541

98. Cummings SR, Black DM, Thompson DE et al: Effect of alendronate on risk of fracture in women with low bone density but without vertebral fractures: results from the Fracture Intervention Trial. JAMA 1998;280:2077–2082

99. Harris ST, Watts NB, Genant HK et al: Effects of risedronate treatment on vertebral and nonvertebral fractures in women with postmenopausal osteoporosis: a randomized controlled trial. Vertebral Efficacy With Risedronate Therapy (VERT) Study Group. JAMA 1999;282:1344–1352

100. Lauritzen JB, Petersen MM, Laud B: Effect of external hip protectors on hip fractures. Lancet 1993;341:11–13

101. Kannus P, Parkkari J, Niemi S et al: Prevention of hip fracture in elderly people with use of a hip protector. N Engl J Med 2000;343:1506–1513

102. Harada A, Mizuno M, Takemura M et al: Hip fracture prevention trial using hip protectors in Japanese nursing homes. Osteoporosis Int 2001;12:215–221

103. Rizzo JA, Baker DI, McAvay G et al: The cost-effectiveness of a multifactorial targeted prevention program for falls among community elderly persons. Med Care 1996;34:954–969

Chapter 106

Pressure sores

Mary R. Bliss and Gerald C. J. Bennett

ETIOLOGY

The current renaissance across Europe in the scientific study of pressure sores has brought this important topic into the mainstream of clinical research for many healthcare professionals. However, pressure sores as a clinical problem and theories about their causation, management, and prevention have concerned doctors and nurses throughout history.

Peripheral tissue infarction

Pressure sores are areas of dead soft tissue caused by ischemia due to pressure which has cut off the blood supply for a critical length of time. They are acute, largely preventable medical injuries[1] which may occur within 1–2 hours,[2] causing pain and disability and sometimes death. The terms "sore" or "ulcer" are misleading in that they imply slow development and chronicity, whereas a pressure injury can occur almost as rapidly as a myocardial infarction with which it has much in common.[3,4] Both pressure injury and myocardial infarction affect patients with vascular disease who have abnormal microcirculatory reflexes[5] and impaired response to increased oxygen demand. Both may be worsened by reperfusion injury.[6,7] Both consist of circumscribed areas of dead tissue which results in scarring and functional loss.

Sites of sores

Pressure injuries typically occur over bony prominences where external pressures on the body are highest. The commonest sites are:

- *lying supine:* the sacrum, buttocks (Figs 106-1 and 106-2; see also Plates 106-1 and 106-2), and heels (Fig. 106-3; see also Plate 106-3)
- *lying in the lateral position:* the greater trochanters (Fig. 106–4; see also Plate 106-4)
- *sitting:* the ischial tuberosities (Fig. 106-5; see also Plate 106-5) and under surfaces of the thighs.

In a study of 2,526 sores in 1,455 patients being treated by home health agencies in the USA,[8] 79 percent of whom were aged over 65 years, 37 percent of sores were on the sacrum and buttocks, 5 percent on the trochanters, 4 percent on the ischia, and 14 percent on the heels. The mean number of sores per patient was 1.7.

Pressure injuries may, however, occur in any soft tissue which is subjected to prolonged external—or internal—pressure, for example, on the penis (Fig. 106-6; see also

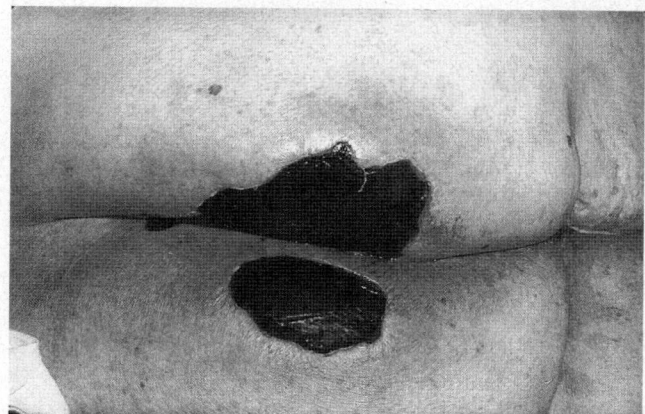

Figure 106-1 Acute pressure injury over the sacrum and buttocks in an elderly woman.

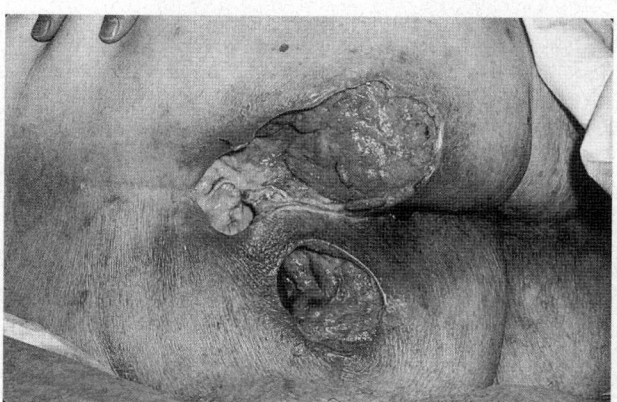

Figure 106-2 Natural debridement of the pressure injury shown in Figure 106-1 (see also Plate 106-1) at 2 weeks.

Plate 106-6) or the bladder trigone[9] due to a catheter. Pressure is the most likely cause of an isolated lesion on the skin of an elderly patient (Fig. 106-7).

Tissue distortion

Pressure injuries should be called "distortion injuries."[10] Pressure alone does not cause tissue ischemia. As recent deep sea exploration has shown, animals can thrive at pressures of over 191,000 mmHg.[11] Provided the pressure is evenly applied and has equal components inside and outside the body,[10] tissue distortion, and hence capillary closure, does not occur. In contrast, pressure by even a slight *localized* object which

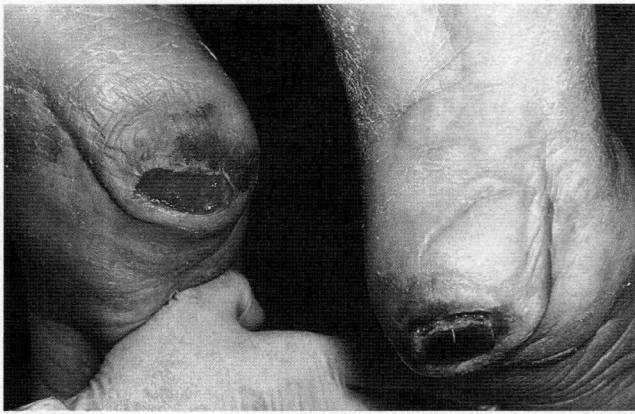

Figure 106-3 Pressure injuries of the heels.

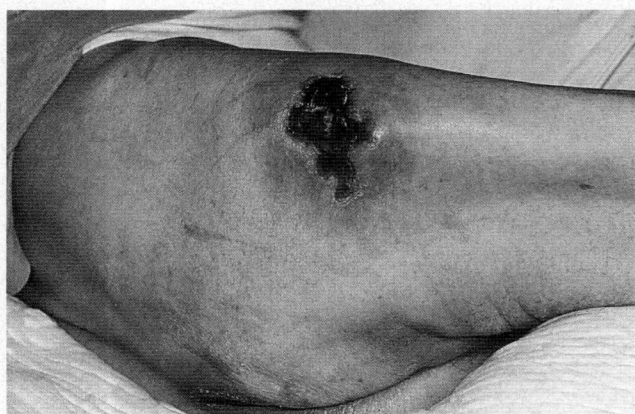

Figure 106-4 Pressure injury over the greater trochanter resulting from lateral turning on a hospital mattress.

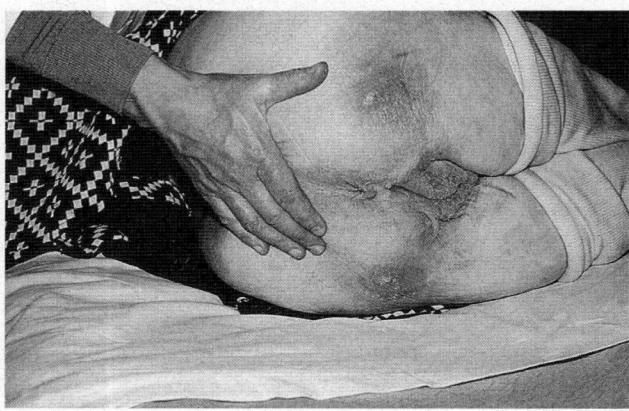

Figure 106-5 Pressure injuries over the ischial tuberosities caused by sitting in a chair.

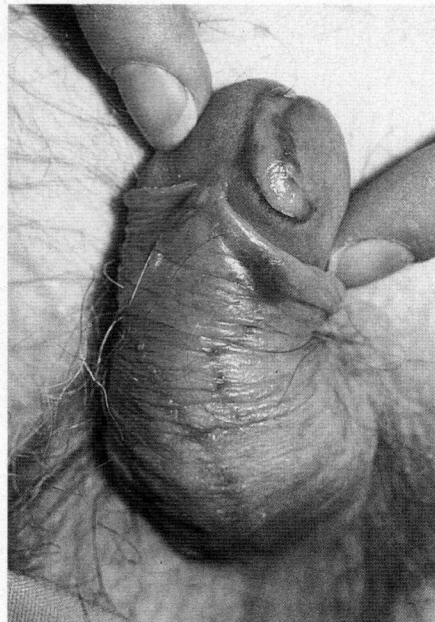

Figure 106-6 Pressure injury on the penis due to a catheter.

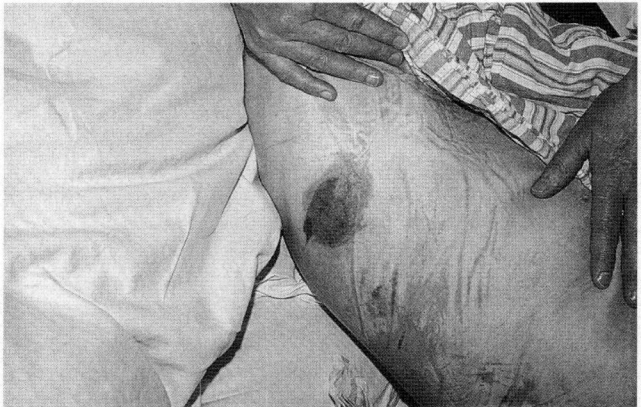

Figure 106-7 Early pressure sore over the inferior angle of the scapula.

indents soft tissue, e.g., a wrinkle in a sheet (Fig. 106-7; see also Plate 106-7),[12] causes shear stresses[13] which stretch and blanch the capillary beds. This will give rise to a pressure sore if it is maintained for too long. The higher the pressure, the shorter the time required to cause tissue damage.[14] However, the actual period depends on the health of the patient and low pressures for long periods can be as damaging as high pressures.[14,15]

Deep pressure

Internal bone itself can act as a localized source of pressure. Figure 106-8 shows how a bony prominence pressing down under the weight of the skeleton in a moderately obese patient lying on a soft mattress causes greater tissue distortion, and hence ischemia, in the periosteal tissues than in the skin. Animal experiments have shown that pressure and tissue damage is maximal in deep tissues.[16–20] Le et al.[19] found that the magnitude of an externally applied pressure increases with both lateral and vertical proximity of the pressure sensor to a bony prominence. Where bones are close to the surface, e.g., the heels, tissue damage will be full thickness from the start.[21] Flaccid muscles[10] and dehydrated skin and subcutaneous tissue which are easily deformed generate higher pressures than normal tissue.[22]

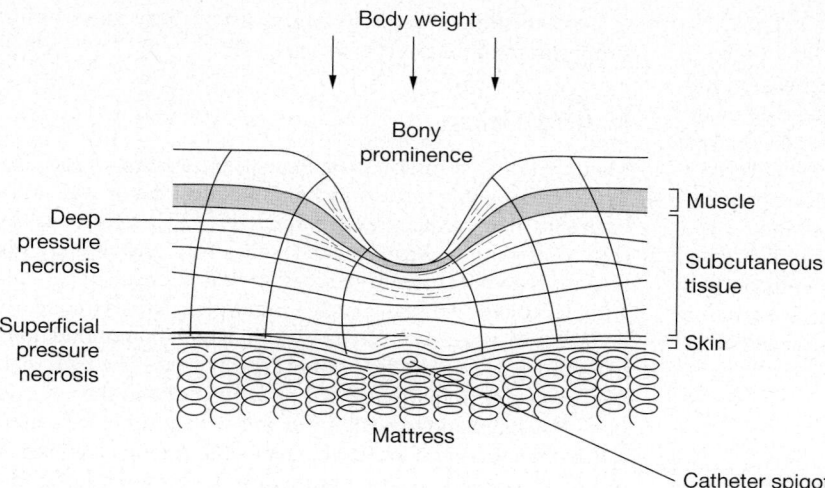

Figure 106-8 Diagram showing how tissue deformation under pressure may give rise to superficial and pressure sores. By permission of the Editor of the Lancet. (Bliss MR: Sir James Paget's legacy. Lancet 1992;339:221–223.)

Friction

Friction causes shear stresses in skin and subcutaneous tissues which disrupt capillary blood flow.[10,18] These may be exacerbated by reduced elasticity of aged skin[10] and maceration due to humidity or incontinence.[23] Friction may also be worsened by the sitting posture.[24]

Lymph drainage

Pressure and friction in immobile patients obstruct lymphatic drainage which is essential for healthy tissue.[25] Edema and accumulation of waste products increase the likelihood of cell death.

Immobility

In a normal person, ischemia due to pressure causes intolerable pain which prompts movement to ease it, thus relieving pressure and restoring the blood supply. However, in a patient with sensory loss, or who is unconscious, or too ill to move, or who cannot move because of restraints,[26] pressure injuries may occur. Impaired sensation is more important than immobility. Patients with purely motor diseases such as amyotrophic lateral sclerosis who have normal pain sensation, rarely develop sores.[27] In contrast, even mobile patients who cannot feel ischemic pain are at risk of pressure injury, as is shown by the prevalence of foot sores in people with diabetes.[28] Patients with sensory neglect due to strokes or Alzheimer's disease are very vulnerable. Reduced nocturnal movement has been shown to be correlated with the development of pressure sores.[29,30]

Reactive hyperemia

Relief of pressure on a tissue such as skin is normally instantly followed by reactive hyperemia.[31,32] Anoxia and accumulation of metabolites cause failure of cell processes and release of vasodilating substances.[33] The resulting increased blood flow restores tissue oxygen levels. Healthy microvessels have a continual rhythm of contraction and relaxation known as vasomotion,[34] the main component of which is controlled by the

vasomotor center in the brain.[33] Tonic sympathetic closure of arteriovenous shunts also regulates blood flow in the capillary network. Finally, the capillaries themselves are constantly opening and closing so that only about 5 percent are normally patent at any one time.[35] These mechanisms provide an enormous reserve circulation for activity such as exercise, and for responding to ischemic insults such as pressure.

Neurological disease

Impaired sympathetic control of the circulation increases susceptibility to pressure sores.[36] Reactive hyperemia and flow motion have been shown to be abnormal in patients with spinal cord injury,[3,36–38] especially in those with sensory loss,[36] and in elderly people.[38] Patients with neurological disorders[39,40] and older people[41] have the highest incidences of pressure injuries.

Vascular disease

Vascular disease also affects reactive hyperemia. Elderly patients,[38,42] patients with vascular disease,[43,44] hypertensives,[45] smokers,[45] and diabetics[46,47] all of whom have high incidences of pressure sores,[48] have abnormal hyperemic responses. Patients with vascular disease also have rheological disorders[49] which increase the likelihood of failure of reflow and thrombosis following occlusion.

Effects of pressure on tissue

Duration of reactive hyperemia is normally proportional to the duration of the ischemia.[31] However, prolonged ischemia damages endothelial cells and causes plateauing of the response, probably because of the release of inflammatory agents.[33] Adherence of platelets and leukocytes and the formation of microthrombi[50] prevent restoration of blood flow.[33] Endothelial damage caused by pressure itself may also play a part. Rendell and Wells[51] showed that reactive hyperemia in the finger in healthy volunteers was greater and lasted longer following application of pressure than when it was caused by occlusion of the circulation by means of a cuff.

Reperfusion injury

Reperfusion may also damage tissue.[16] Restoration of blood flow allows the formation of oxygen free radicals which may cause further injury to surviving cells.[33] Pierce et al.[6] showed that in rats, five ischemia reperfusion cycles which delivered a total of 10 hours compression caused more leukocyte extravasation and necrosis than one continuous compression for the same length of time. The effect may be worsened by disease. Bader[52] found that in normal people transcutaneous oxygen levels improved with repeated applications of pressure on the sacrum but that in patients with chronic neurological and other illnesses they deteriorated to dangerously low levels.

Illness

Acute illness is the precipitating factor in the development of a pressure injury. Even bedfast and chronically incontinent patients rarely develop sores while they are well but may do so very rapidly following an intercurrent infection or a fall. It is important to remember that illness in elderly patients is often manifest only by nonspecific symptoms such as decreased consciousness, loss of appetite, dehydration, incontinence, or constipation. Illness impairs mobility and sensation. Dehydration and muscle wasting increase tissue deformability. Pyrexia exacerbates humidity and friction. Pain inhibits movement and increases oxygen demand.[53] Incontinence and diarrhea excoriate skin and increase friction.[54] Confusion and agitation may occur which may be treated with restraints which are likely to cause pressure injury,[26] or with tranquilizers which cause drowsiness and hypotension. Profound hypotension has frequently been observed to precede the development of pressure injuries.[48,55,56] In shock, hypotension or vasoconstriction the vascular bed collapses.[57-59]

Microcirculatory failure

Reactive hyperemia microcirculatory reflexes are impaired in sick patients. Endothelial dysfunction[60] and reduced sympathetic vasomotor tone[61] cause vasodilatation and hypotension resulting in peripheral vascular failure.[62] With very severe infections or trauma maldistribution of blood flow to vital organs may cause multiorgan failure.[60] Patients with multiorgan failure[61] and patients with pressure sores[63] have been shown to have abnormal capillary vasomotion and reactive hyperemia. Meijer et al.[64] showed that elderly patients admitted to a nursing home who developed sores had delayed reactive hyperemia (measured by temperature responses) following experimentally applied pressure compared with similarly aged patients who did not. However, they were unable to study acutely ill or unconscious patients.

Age

Age changes in the skin[65] have not been shown to increase vulnerability to pressure.[66] The high incidence of pressure sores in elderly patients[48] is unlikely to be due to age itself, but to increased prevalence of illness. Old people often suffer from neurological and vascular disease and they have a greater incidences of severe infection, trauma,[67] and terminal illness than young patients. Lindholm[68] and Allman[69] found that 35 and 41 percent of older patients with pressure ulcers died within 3 months and 1 year, respectively.

Malnutrition

Malnutrition is common in patients with pressure sores,[70] and hypoalbuminemia is the only hematological factor which has been shown to predict pressure injury.[48,71,72] However, healthy thin old people with normal sensation and hyperemic responses do not suffer from sores,[73] while overweight patients with neurological diseases such as multiple sclerosis frequently do (Fig. 106-9; see also Plate 106-8). Piloian[74] did not find body mass index to be a predictor of pressure ulcers. The high incidence of sores in malnourished patients is due to the association of cachexia and hypoalbuminemia with advanced disease[75] rather than to weight loss itself. Hypoalbuminemia is a marker of illness as much as of malnutrition.[76] Malnourished individuals with immune deficiency are also more likely to suffer from acute illness than people of normal weight.[77]

Extrinsic causes of pressure injury

Pressures below the capillary closing pressure of 32 mmHg in a healthy person[78] are frequently cited as "safe."[24,79,80] However, in a hypotensive sick old person with deep tissue pressures over bony prominences and abnormal reactive hyperemia, critical ischemia may still occur.[54] Interface pressure itself is difficult to measure[24,81] and deep tissue pressure is almost impossible noninvasively except by imaging techniques[82-84] which are clinically impracticable. Laser Doppler flowmetry[38] or transcutaneous gas tensions[85] or temperature[64] may be more informative about the effect of pressure on oxygen levels and blood flow but need to be measured in acutely ill, not healthy people. Time must also be taken into account.[14,15] Rather than relying on physical measurements therefore, it is more important to *observe and document events which precede the development of pressure injuries*, including medical and nursing procedures.

LONG WAITING TIMES "Long lies" of patients in their homes, e.g., following a femoral neck fracture, usually cannot be avoided. However, these are often followed by many hours of waiting in accident and emergency and X-ray departments,

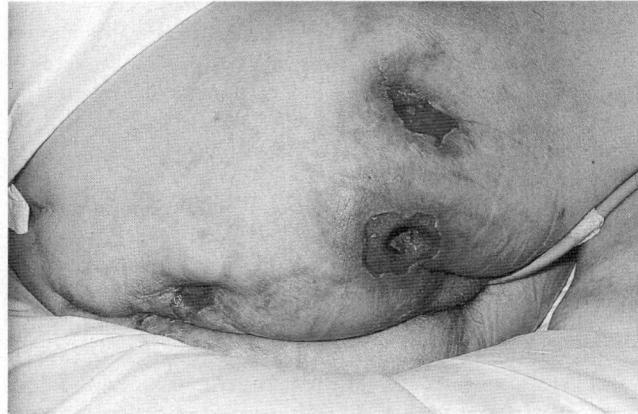

Figure 106-9 Deep pressure sore with sinuses in a patient with multiple sclerosis.

usually without pressure relief, oral fluids, food, or analgesics.[86,87] Up to 83 percent of sores have been shown to occur in the first 5 days following admission to hospital.[88]

"NIL BY MOUTH" Withholding oral fluids in patients awaiting operations[86,89] and with strokes[90] causes dehydration[89,90,91] which is likely to exacerbate pressure injury. Knowles[92] found that 27 percent of hospital patients with strokes awaiting long-term care had developed pressure sores since admission.

BEDS Hard hospital beds with worn mattresses[80,88,93] cause high pressures on the body. However, poorly designed pressure-relieving equipment[94] and broken-down powered supports[95] can also be damaging.

REGULAR REPOSITIONING "Side-to-side" turning on an ordinary hospital mattress causes high, repeated pressure on the hips[96] with the risk of reperfusion injury and the development of sores over the greater trochanters (Fig. 106-4; see also Plate 106-4). "Tilting" rather than turning causes less tissue hypoxemia,[96] but is badly tolerated by elderly patients. The use of pressure-reducing supports may provide a false sense of security which causes nurses to reduce the frequency of repositioning allowing tissue damage to occur.[97] In general, the ability to prevent sores by repositioning alone is limited by low staff–patient ratios.[67,98]

INTENSIVE CARE Preventing pressure injuries in intensive care patients may be difficult in spite of adequate staffing. Life support equipment may make repositioning difficult and cause additional pressure on soft tissues. Some patients cannot be moved for fear of dysrhythmias and other hazards.[24]

SURGERY AND ANESTHESIA Surgery is frequently associated with the development of sores, especially in elderly patients.[86] Versluysen[88] found that the highest incidence of pressure sores in patients with femoral neck fracture occurred on the day of operation. Elderly patients undergoing surgery are often already traumatized or ill and the operation adds to circulatory stress. Dehydration due to withholding oral fluids, and use of muscle relaxants, increases tissue deformability. Anesthetic drugs cause unconsciousness and hypotension.[48] Spinal anesthesia and analgesia may prolong sensory impairment and immobility.[99]

OPERATING TABLES Standard operating tables[88] and tables used for treating fractures[86] generate high pressures on the body. Kemp[48] noted that in 15 percent of surgical patients who developed postoperative sores, 70 percent were first observed when they were leaving the operating table. Bader and White[85] showed that in patients undergoing hip operations, applied pressures over the contralateral hip similar to those experienced on the operating table caused transcutaneous oxygen tensions to fall to levels which compromise tissue viability. Cardiovascular patients with extracorporeal circulation undergoing prolonged operations are at particularly high risk.[48] Diathermy plates can cause pressure injuries on the sacrum which have been mistaken for burns[100] (Fig. 106-10; see also Plate 106-9). Warming blankets may increase tissue damage.[101] In the USA, it has been estimated that a quarter of all pressure ulcers originate on the operating table.[102]

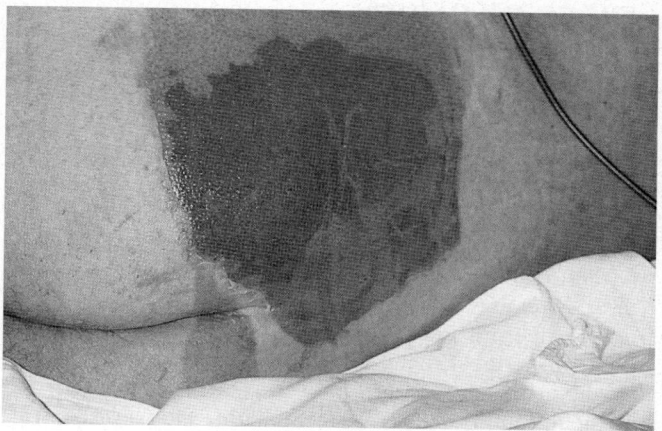

Figure 106-10 Pressure injury on the back caused by a diathermy plate. (Courtesy of Dr M. Lubbers, Academisch Medisch Centrum, Universiteit van Amsterdam.)

DRUGS Anesthetics, sedatives, and high doses of analgesics cause unconsciousness or drowsiness and hypotension.[55] Antipsychotic drugs which cause hypotension, Parkinsonism, and autonomic dysfunction are often associated with sores in elderly patients.[30] Beta-adrenoceptor blocking drugs cause hypotension and impair peripheral blood flow. Inotropes reverse hypotension at the expense of tissue perfusion.[103] Nonsteroidal anti-inflammatory drugs and high-dose steroids depress reactive hyperemia[104] and healing.[105] Cytotoxic drugs poison cells. Many drugs cause diarrhea in elderly patients, increasing the risk of superficial sores.

CHAIR NURSING Studies have shown that disabled[40] and postoperative[106] patients who are nursed in chairs for long periods tend to have more pressure sores than patients nursed in bed. Patients who cannot stand or move independently are unable to benefit from more than brief periods of physiotherapy[86] and become exhausted, hypotensive, and edematous if they have to remain upright for long periods.[106,107] Adequate rest and sleep are important for recovery and active patients usually spend frequent intervals lying on their beds.[106]

CUSHIONS Pressure-relieving cushions in chairs are relatively ineffective compared with pressure relieving mattresses.[12] Their use also encourages staff to sit patients out of bed for excessive periods. Footstools are not a substitute for bed rest and increase pressure on the heels.

BANDAGES AND COMPRESSION HOSIERY Doppler ankle/brachial pressure indices may be deceptive in patients with sclerosed arteries and are a poor indicator of the state of the microcirculation.[108] No attempt is usually made to assess the peripheral circulation before applying antiemboli stockings, which often cause sores in elderly patients[109] (Fig. 106-11; see also Plate 106-10).

OTHER CAUSES OF PRESSURE INJURY Wheelchairs, calipers, artificial limbs, trusses, dressings, spectacles, hearing aids, dentures, shoes, and tight clothing are common causes of pressure sores.

TYPES OF INJURY

The grading system recommended by the European Pressure Ulcer Advisory Panel[110] is shown in Table 106-1.

Sore grading

This classification has been mainly based on the studies of Shea.[111] Although he observed that "the elasticity of … tissues results in a force being distributed in a hammock … effect with the greatest pressure over the bone diminishing progressively towards the surface," he subsequently describes the injury as occurring in the skin and extending *inwards* toward the bone. He defined a Grade 4 sore as "penetration of the deep fascia by the infectious necrotic process eliminating the last barrier to extensive spread." This description has caused clinicians and manufacturers of pressure-relieving supports largely to ignore deep pressure as a cause of sores, and to exaggerate the importance of infection compared with ischemia in their etiology and development.

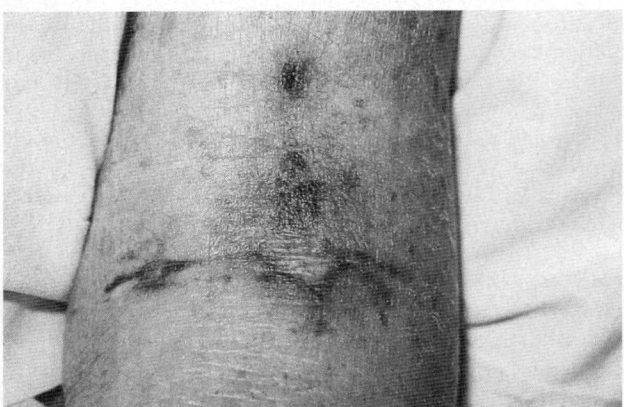

Figure 106-11 Pressure injury on the foot due to an antiemboli stocking.

Table 106-1 Pressure sore grades

Grade 1: Nonblanchable erythema of intact skin. Discoloration of the skin, warmth, edema, induration, or hardness may also be used as indicators, particularly on individuals with darker skin

Grade 2: Partial thickness skin loss involving epidermis, dermis or both. The ulcer is superficial and presents clinically as an abrasion or blister

Grade 3: Full thickness skin loss involving damage to or necrosis of subcutaneous tissue that may extend down to, but not through, underlying fascia

Grade 4: Extensive destruction, tissue necrosis or damage to muscle, bone or supporting structures with or without full thickness skin loss

Source: Pressure ulcer treatment and guidelines. European Pressure Ulcer Advisory Panel, EPUAP Business office, Department of Dermatology, Churchill Hospital, Oxford, UK.

Deep sores

As shown in Figure 106-8, a deep (Grade 4) sore *originates* in periosteal tissue and muscle. This can occur without any damage to the skin which only becomes secondarily involved following breakdown of the necrotic material and the formation of an abscess[17,50,55] (Fig. 106-9; see also Plate 106-8). Only when the dead tissue is discharged can the full extent of the original injury be seen (Figs 106-1 and 106-2). This causes apparent enlargement of the sore which is often mistaken for worsening. Because damage to the deep tissues is usually greater than in the skin, deep sores typically have overhanging edges (Fig. 106-2; see also Plate 106-2).

Infection

Pressure sores may enlarge due to repeated episodes of pressure and reperfusion injury causing new necrosis, but never due to infection. Cellulitis occurs in the skin and deep tissues surrounding a new pressure injury (Fig. 106-1; see also Plate 106-1) often accompanied by a leukocytosis and pyrexia. However, this is an inflammatory reaction caused by the presence of dead tissue, not infection.[67] It usually quickly subsides at the onset of natural debridement.

Superficial and deep sores

Groth[20] recognized only two types of sore: superficial "benign" and deep "malignant." In prevalence and incidence studies, undue emphasis has probably been placed on counting superficial sores, including persistent erythema, and not enough on their importance as a warning of the risk of deeper injury. Some superficial sores (Figs 106-5, 106-7; see also Plates 106-5 and 106-7) may be unavoidable in elderly patients.[112] Their appearance can be regarded as a physical sign equivalent to that of the doughy skin of dehydration. Like dehydration, they are an indication that the patient is seriously ill and that unless immediate measures are taken that his condition is likely to deteriorate. Hospitals cannot be held responsible for sores which are present on admission. However, they should be accountable for superficial sores which deteriorate, and for most new sores which develop, *particularly Grade 3 and 4 sores and heel sores.*[39] The incidence of Grade 3 and 4 sores would probably be a better measure of the success of clinical policies for prevention than counting all sores.

Dying patients

By far the majority of sores in dying patients can be prevented by the early provision of relatively simple measures for pressure relief.[98,113] However, occasionally the development of large or multiple gangrenous sores due to microcirculatory failure may be an inevitable part of the dying process.

PREVALENCE

A 1971 study in Denmark showed that 3 percent of hospital patients had a pressure sore, the minimum inclusion being "at least an epithelial defect."[114] In 1976 in the United Kingdom, two large prevalence surveys were performed in the greater

Glasgow[115] and Borders[116] Health Board Areas. They were carried out on a single day using a questionnaire completed by staff for hospital patients, excluding maternity, psychiatry, and learning disability but not psychiatry of old age. Patients in the community were included if they received a district nurse visit that day.

The greater Glasgow survey[115] contained data on 10,751 patients. The sore prevalence rate was 8.8, 1.5 percent of the patient population having a sore in the most severe category. Only established sores were included. The Borders survey covered a much smaller population in which the overall sore prevalence rate was 9.4 percent, with 2.1 percent having a severe sore. Subanalysis revealed a sore prevalence rate of 4.8 percent for patients nursed at home vs 11.7 percent for those nursed in a hospital. However, when patients of similar disability were compared, the difference disappeared.

More recently, prevalence rates in four European countries have been documented, including hospitals in the greater Paris region.[117,118] There are also data from Japan and Australia.[119,120] Prevalence studies in the United Kingdom indicate that between 8 and 20 percent of people in the hospital sector have pressure ulcers.[40,121] However, lower rates have been reported in units with a special interest.[122] O'Dea has analyzed the prevalence rates of pressure damage in acute care hospital patients.[123] Similar figures are found in the United States[124,125] where reports indicate that between 20 and 35 percent of elderly people have pressure ulcers at the time of admission to a nursing home.[126,127] Bergquist[128] investigated pressure ulcers in a community-based study involving older people receiving home care. There are few data on the nursing home population in the United Kingdom.

There is continuing confusion concerning the correct use of the terms prevalence and incidence.[129,130] A few countries have developed national survey models to provide accurate prevalence data[131] and reduce random variation in reported rates of pressure ulcer development.[132] However, interpretation of results is complicated by the use of a variety of populations in different settings, including continuing care.[133–136] Incidence rates have been reported as percentages of subjects[136] or as a number or range per 1,000 patient days.[137,138] In a 2-week prospective cohort study of elderly patients at risk, the incidence of pressure ulcers was 14 per 1,000 patient days.[139] Intergroup comparison within studies remains difficult.[140]

RISK ASSESSMENT
Prediction scores

A major difficulty in preventing pressure injuries is identifying patients at risk before tissue damage has occurred. The original risk assessment score, the Norton score, which was devised from observations of geriatric patients, is still widely used[141] (Table 106-2). Numerous more complicated risk calculators have been developed[142–144] but no score has been proven to be more effective than clinical judgment.[143] A summary of the predictive validity of the best-known risk assessment scores is given in *Effective Healthcare* 1995.[143] It is important to note that the same score may give different results depending on the type of patient being assessed, and that medical or nursing intervention not only may, but should, alter the expected outcome.[145]

Most risk calculators describe *disability* rather than acute illness. In a study of correlation matrices of the components of the Norton score, Goldstone and Goldstone[146] concluded that combining the categories "General condition" and "Incontinence" predicted pressure injuries as accurately as the complete score. Unfortunately, "General condition" has been omitted from many scales and replaced by "Nutrition" which, as we have seen, is not a good indicator. Acute loss of appetite which is a common presenting sign of illness is likely to be more important.[74]

Another problem is how often scores should be calculated. They are frequently documented only once or twice during a patient's hospital stay.[147] Scores assessed only on admission may convey a dangerous sense of security if the patient's health subsequently deteriorates or if he undergoes an operation.

Probably the most valuable use of risk assessment scores is to document the need for special care to prevent pressure injury, including that for pressure relieving supports. The score should be repeated when the support is removed. This is also important for medico-legal reasons.

Risk assessment scores may also be useful for identifying patients for clinical studies, or in surveys to assist with developing policies for prevention. However, care must be taken to ensure that they do not include only patients with chronic disabilities and ignore intercurrent illness.

Medical assessment

Instead of relying on scores, clinicians need to learn to recognize patients at risk of pressure injuries (Table 106-3) and to be prepared to provide pressure relief during acute illness. Deciding how ill a patient is requires the skills of a doctor as well as of the nurse.[148,149] However, doctors also find assessing severity of illness difficult.[150]

Examination

Peripheral tissue is easily accessible but compared with other organs is seldom examined. Firstly we need to know if the

Table 106-2 **Norton pressure sore prediction score**[a]				
Physical condition	**Mental state**	**Activity**	**Mobility**	**Incontinence**
4 Good	4 Alert	4 Ambulant	4 Full	4 Not
3 Fair	3 Confused	3 Walks with help	3 Limited	3 Occasional
2 Poor	2 Apathetic	2 Chairbound	2 Very limited	2 Usually urine
1 Bad	1 Stuporose	1 In bed	1 Immobile	1 Doubly incontinent

[a] *Patients with a score of 14 or lower are liable to develop pressure sores.*

Source: Norton D, McLaren R, Exton Smith AN: An Investigation of Geriatric Nursing Problems in Hospital. Churchill Livingstone, Edinburgh, 1975.

Table 106-3 Elderly patients at risk of pressure injury

- Patients with neurological injury or disease
- Patients with vascular disease
- Elderly patients newly admitted to hospital with acute illness or trauma
- Perioperative patients
- Normally stable disabled patients with intercurrent illness
- Dying patients

patient can turn over in bed, or stand unaided, because if he can, he is unlikely to be at risk. The pressure areas should then be examined, starting with the heels followed by the sacrum, trochanters, and ischial tuberosities. Dressings must be removed if necessary. Any part of the body complained about by the patient must also be inspected. This can be done as part of the general examination by the doctor or during toileting by the nurse. It should be routine during the visit of any professional to a sick or postoperative patient and is far more valuable than calculating complicated scores in the office. Persistent erythema, discoloration (Fig. 106-7; see also Plate 106-7), induration, blistering, or broken skin on any pressure area is evidence not only that the patient is at risk of an irreversible pressure injury, but also that he is seriously ill.

Assessment of the peripheral circulation

Many workers have tried to predict pressure injuries by measuring interface pressure,[12] transcutaneous gas tensions,[3,85] or skin blood flow[21] in the pressure areas, but this is difficult even in healthy volunteers[54] and still more so in patients.[151] In future, it may be possible to assess the state of the microcirculation in sick patients using pulse oximeters designed to detect poor peripheral perfusion,[108,152] or laser Doppler flowmeters in conjunction with challenge tests[153] in accessible areas such as the arms or legs.[42] Nevertheless, clinical examination is likely to remain of paramount importance.

PREVENTION
In the community

Once a patient is considered to be at risk of pressure injury, pressure must be relieved immediately. Supports therefore need to be *portable*, easy to install and to use, robust, not too expensive and readily available—in the community as well as in hospital. Healthcare workers visiting patients should be able to carry pressure-relieving supports in their cars as part of their emergency equipment. This may prevent hospital admission. If pressure sores can be avoided, families often feel more confident about looking after ill old people at home.

Treating acute illness

The patient's illness must be diagnosed and treatment begun as soon as possible.[67] The sooner he can be restored to health, the sooner the risk of pressure injury will diminish and existing sores begin to heal. Nonessential drugs should be stopped. With adequate bed rest, rehydration, treatment of infections or fractures, and vigorous care of the bowel and bladder (with a catheter if necessary)[67] most elderly patients will show improvement in their mental state, appetite and mobility within 1 or 2 days. With serious illnesses such as strokes, recovery may take longer, but the principles are the same. Only patients with irremediable illness are likely to need pressure relief indefinitely.

Nutrition

Although frequently advocated,[154] trying to improve the patient's nutritional state can play no part in the acute prevention of sores. Very ill patients may be either well or ill nourished, but nothing can be done about the latter in time to make any difference as to whether they will develop a pressure injury. Rehydration is very important, but attempts to force feed an anorexic, sick old person are merely likely to result in vomiting or diarrhea with a worsening of their general health[67] and to do nothing for their peripheral circulation. As the patient improves, his appetite usually improves also and nutritious meals, with assistance with feeding if necessary, will help to speed recovery and prevent further pressure injury. Supplements should rarely be necessary, but easily accessible drinks should be available at all times.

Chair nursing

Patients at risk of pressure injury should be nursed mainly in bed. The majority are too ill to be able to sit in a chair comfortably for more than short periods and pressure can be more effectively relieved in bed. Gebhardt and Bliss[106] found that elderly orthopedic patients who were allowed to be sat in chairs for not more than 2 hours per session had a lower incidence of sores (7% than those in whom chair nursing was unlimited (median 6 hours) (63% $P < 0.001$, 95% CI of the difference −77 to −36%). As their mobility improves, patients may sit out for longer but should be allowed to return to their beds if they request it. Muscle or mineral loss due to bed rest[155] during this short period is negligible and is more than outweighed by the patient's more rapid recovery and freedom from sores. Physical restraints should not be used.

Pressure relief

AT HOME Pillows can be positioned at the bottom of the bed in lieu of a bed cradle or placed under the calves to protect the heels. *It is important to note that pillows placed directly under pressure areas such as the heels do not give good pressure relief.* If there are signs of damage on the sacrum the patient should be tilted on to one side, and if on the ischial tuberosities, he should not be allowed to sit in a chair. Whatever position is adopted, instructions should be given for him to be moved every 1–2 hours. As this is seldom practicable for any length of time, an effective pressure relieving support should be procured as soon as possible, or admission to hospital arranged.

IN THE AMBULANCE AND ACCIDENT AND EMERGENCY DEPARTMENT Pressure-relieving supports should be available for at-risk patients. Alternatively, pillows can be used to relieve pressure on red or injured areas. Patients who cannot move their legs should always have the affected heel lifted off the mattress. They should be examined as soon as possible, and depending on the diagnosis and treatment plans, offered tea and sometimes a snack. Adequate analgesia must be given. If the patient is to be sent home, arrangements must be made for immediate continuing care, including pressure relief. Patients being admitted should reach the ward within 2 hours.[156]

IN THE WARD A pressure-relieving support should be placed on the bed before the patient is admitted. The next few days are likely to be when he is most ill and therefore at greatest risk. For this reason, the policy of providing "first line" *pressure-reducing* supports,[157] for patients with "low-risk" scores on admission and only changing these for more effective supports if their condition deteriorates is dangerous.[158] All too often, the reason for the change is because a pressure injury has developed. This is failure of care. *All patients deemed to be at any degree of risk should therefore be nursed on fully effective supports from the outset.* These should be used during the critical period of the patients' illness and removed when they are no longer necessary. Thereafter, most patients can safely be nursed on ordinary hospital mattresses.

Mechanical supports must never, however, be used as a substitute for nursing. Helping patients to sit up, or move, or to get in or out of bed is essential both to promote recovery and prevent sores. An adequate supply of pillows for making patients comfortable is as important as that of pressure-relieving mattresses.[159]

Skin care

The skin, including traumatized areas, should be kept as clean and dry as possible. Occlusive dressings may ease the pain of superficial sores but risk causing further skin trauma. Barrier creams have not been shown to prevent pressure sores.[160]

PRESSURE-RELIEVING SUPPORTS

Pressure-relieving mattresses for the prevention and treatment of pressure injuries should be used with the same care as other life support equipment, e.g., respirators. They fall into four main categories: *turning beds, profiling beds, constant low-pressure (LP) supports*, and *alternating-pressure (AP) mattresses.*

Turning beds

Turning beds which are used for spinal injury patients are unsuitable for elderly patients so will not be discussed here.

Profiling beds

Electrically operated profiling beds can improve pressure and friction and ease of positioning[161] but unless patients are capable of operating them themselves, restrict movement. Currently, they are mainly used for intensive care or very overweight patients.

Constant low-pressure supports

LP supports are soft or "flotation" mattresses or beds (Fig. 106-12) which aim to distribute body weight as widely as possible, thus reducing high pressure over bony prominences. They may be either static or powered.

Static supports

Deep flotation waterbeds have been in use since 1800[162] but are difficult to install and to nurse patients on. Instead, soft mattresses of *water, air, gel, foam, silicone beads, or fiber* etc. have been developed which it has been hoped might have a similar effect and be more practical.[80] Many show low interface pressures[54,163,164] and sustained oxygen tensions in healthy volunteers,[165] but their effect on deep pressure and in sick patients has not been assessed. In randomized controlled trials in elderly orthopedic and long-stay patients, Hofman et al.[166] and Bliss[98] found that slit and other designs of *foam mattresses* reduced sores compared with a standard hospital mattress, and water and fiberfill overlays respectively, but still allowed incidences of between 25 and 35 percent. Kemp[94] noted that patients on *convoluted foam overlays* developed significantly higher incidences of sores (45 percent) than on a solid foam overlay (39 percent). However, Gray,[167] in a study of younger medical and surgical patients at risk, found an incidence of only 7 percent on a *specialized foam mattress* compared with a hospital mattress (34 percent).

Static *air mattresses* may give good pressure relief[168] but are unreliable because of the difficulty of maintaining correct inflation. Lazzara and Buschmann,[79] who did not find any difference in the incidence of sores in elderly nursing home residents randomized to *air overlays* and gel mattresses (about 15 percent), noted that the air mattresses were often deflated and that the gel mattresses were heavy. In general, static LP supports cannot be relied on to prevent sores in sick patients without additional repositioning.

Powered low-pressure supports

Low air loss[169] and *air-fluidized bead beds*[170] have a similar floating action to a deep water bed but have the advantage that they can be switched to a static mode when required to facilitate patient care. However, they are cumbersome and very expensive.[169] Limited controlled trials have shown them to be effective in relieving pressure and healing sores in intensive care patients,[169,170] but they are unsuitable for prevention for elderly patients. Low air loss mattress overlays are available and a short trial has shown them to be as effective as low air loss

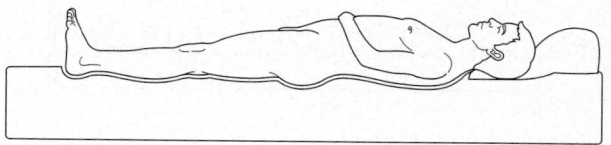

Figure 106-12 Diagram of a constant low-pressure support.

beds for healing.[171] They are mainly useful for patients who cannot tolerate alternating pressure.

Alternating-pressure supports

Unlike LP supports, AP supports (Fig. 106-13) do not aim solely to reduce pressure but to reproduce the alternation of high and low pressure in the weight-bearing areas which occurs in normal people as a result of postural changes in response to pressure pain.[172] They consist of two alternating systems of air cells powered by a pump which causes them to inflate and deflate reciprocally over a 5–10-minute cycle thus continually changing the supporting areas of pressure on the body.[168,172] (Reperfusion injury is avoided by the short timescale. Kosiak[17] showed that intermittent pressures of 5 minutes duration prevented tissue injury in rats exposed to pressures of 240 mmHg.) Studies of transcutaneous oxygen levels in the pressure areas in healthy volunteers have shown higher peak levels on AP mattresses than on low pressure supports,[173] probably because they stimulate reactive hyperemia.

Large-celled AP mattresses (cells >10 cm diameter) (Fig. 106-14; see also Plate 106-11) give better pressure relief and are more effective at preventing and healing sores[174] than small-celled mattresses (cells <5 cm) (Figs 106-15 and 106-16). In a variety of studies, only 13 percent of long-stay elderly patients,[98] 4 percent of newly admitted general hospital patients[175] and 0 percent of intensive care patients[113] deteriorated on large-celled overlays, compared with 25 percent of intensive care patients[24] and 54 percent of neurology patients[176] on small-celled mattresses.

Deeper AP mattress replacements (around 15 cm) with oval cells or a double layers of cells are marketed for overweight and "high-risk" patients.[177] However, large-celled mattress overlays which are less expensive and more portable are equally effective for the majority.[113,178,179]

Quality of manufacture of pressure-relieving supports is very important.[95] Early trials of AP supports are difficult to evaluate because demand was mainly for semi-disposable machines, which constantly broke down, permitting pressure sores to occur.[180] Following publication of a British Standard for AP air mattresses in 1989, stronger models became available. AP supports have since been widely used in the UK[181,182] with reduction in incidences of sores, particularly deep sores.[183]

Nursing

AP overlays are portable and easy to install in hospital or in the community. Patients can be nursed on them as on an ordinary mattress. In the absence of a profiling bed, a backrest can be placed over the support to allow patients to be sat up

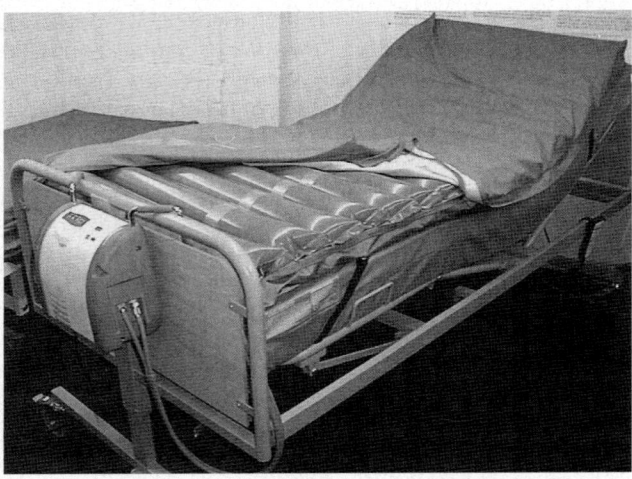

Figure 106-14 An alternating-pressure mattress overlay.

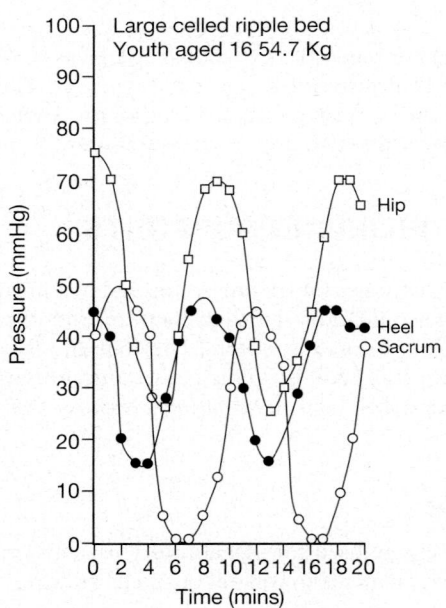

Figure 106-15 Changes in interface pressure over the sacrum, hip and heel measured by a Talley skin pressure evaluator (Talley Medical, Hants, UK) in a healthy youth lying on a large-celled alternating-pressure overlay (large-celled ripple bed).

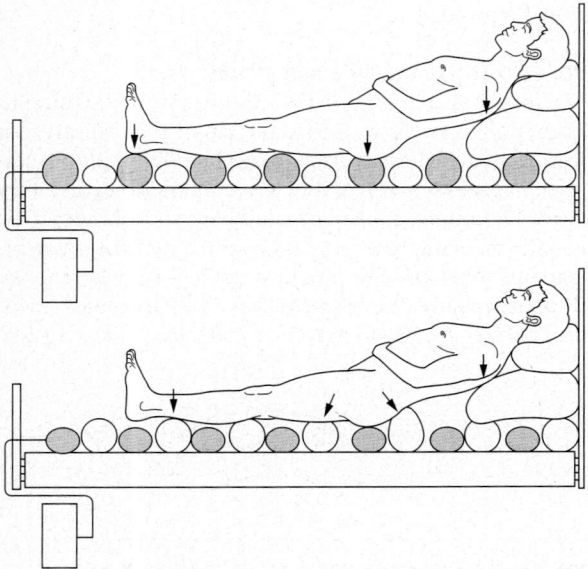

Figure 106-13 Diagram of an alternating-pressure support.

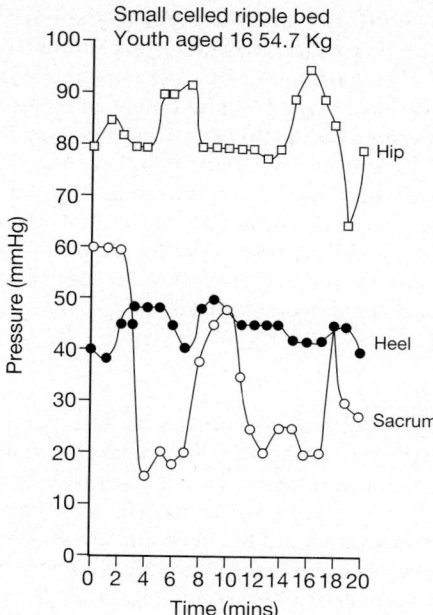

Figure 106-16 Changes in interface pressure in the same youth as in Figure 106-15 lying on a small-celled alternating-pressure mattress overlay (small-celled ripple bed).

adequately. Regular repositioning can be carried out but is not essential. Many supports can remain inflated during transport of the patient to theater. Most also have emergency deflation devices for cardiac resuscitation, although it is doubtful if these are necessary (J. Coakley, personal communication 1987) and they add to the hazards of misuse.[95]

Comfort

AP supports have a reputation for being uncomfortable. However, in a study of 115 patients of all ages, Gebhardt (personal communication 1996) found that at 65 percent of assessments patients were unaware of their support. Only eight patients asked to have their mattress removed. In a study of neurological patients, Pring[184] found that the Quattro mattress, which has a 1 in 4 sequential cycle, was more comfortable than the Pegasus Airwave or Nimbus II mattresses. Many patients who complain about discomfort are sufficiently alert and well not to need a special support. Alert patients who require pressure relief but cannot tolerate an AP support may be given a static air or flotation overlay.

Humidity

Humidity exacerbates discomfort and the risk of pressure injuries.[54] A fleece[185] or blanket placed over the mattress under the bottom sheet improves the comfort of AP supports and may help to prevent superficial sores by reducing temperature and friction.[21]

Covers

Covers on pressure-relieving supports are necessary for hygiene but should be as loose as possible to avoid hammocking under bony prominences such as the heel.[153] Even a flexible fitted cover impairs the pressure relief of a slit foam or AP mattress.[21,52]

Cleaning

Mattresses should be cleaned by sponging with hot water and antiseptic according to the manufacturer's instructions. Supports used for patients on barrier nursing (e.g. for methicillin-resistant *Staphylococcus aureus*) need to be cleaned by a gas cleaner or formalin spray (including the motor).

Servicing

Powered mattresses must be kept properly inflated and working throughout the 24 hours. In a survey of 53 AP overlays of six different types in use in a teaching hospital in 1 year, Gebhardt et al.[95] found 69 mechanical failures, 7 cases of physical damage and 56 errors in use (mainly units unplugged or not switched on). Simple, robust machines which are easy to understand and to operate and rigorous training of staff in both hospitals and the community are essential. Machines should be fitted with audible as well as visual alarms. A rapid replacement and repair service is essential. Static supports must also be regularly inspected and repaired or replaced when necessary. All pressure-relieving supports used in hospitals should be serviced and sterilized every 3 months. The employment of a technician with responsibility for ensuring that pressure-relieving supports in a hospital or community service are correctly installed and in working order would help to reduce pressure injuries resulting from malfunctioning equipment.

Cost

Excluding flotation beds which were found to be unnecessary, Gebhardt et al.[113] estimated that the overall costs per patient of LP and AP supports for preventing sores in intensive care patients were £86 and £44 (1995 prices) respectively.

Pressure-relieving cushions

Pressure-relieving cushions are seldom required for elderly patients. Patients at risk of pressure injuries should not sit out of bed for more than 2 hours, during which time they can safely sit in an ordinary armchair of the correct height. Immobile old people who insist on spending their days and nights in chairs may benefit from a pressure-relieving cushion. However, this is unlikely to prevent tissue breakdown during acute illness. Healthy wheelchair-bound patients should have cushions chosen for them with the help of an occupational therapist.[79] Comfort, stability, ease of transfer, cleaning and durability are as important as pressure relief.[186]

Footstools

Footstools increase pressure on the ischial tuberosities and heels. For patients who need to elevate their legs, rest on a bed is more comfortable and provides better circulation and pressure relief.

Trolleys

A good quality foam mattress, with a pillow under the calves if necessary, probably provides adequate pressure relief for a short period.

X-ray tables

If the patient has to spend any length of time on an X-ray table, it should be padded with a radiolucent material.

Operating tables

Pillows, bead,[187] gel,[188,189] foam,[48] liquid replacement,[190] and alternating pressure pads have been used to relieve pressure on the operating table, but none has proved wholly satisfactory. Stability, durability, ease of use and of cleaning and sterilizing, and antistatic properties are very important.[191] If no special support is available, high-risk patients can be positioned with pillows to relieve pressure on the sacrum and heels.[48] The patient may need to be lifted at intervals to restore circulation in the pressure areas. Alopecia following long operations has been shown to be prevented by anesthetists routinely repositioning patients' heads during surgery.[147]

Discontinuing pressure relief

As soon as patients can stand, or sit in a chair comfortably for 6 hours or more without developing pressure marks, bed supports can usually be removed. They should always be discontinued a few days before discharge to ensure that the patient is safe without a support. A few chronically ill patients may need a large-celled AP overlay indefinitely, in which case this must be arranged before discharge from hospital.

HEALING PRESSURE SORES

Pressure injuries are acute wounds which usually heal readily. Their reputation for chronicity is mainly due to continuing ischemia due to inadequate relief of pressure, or to injurious local treatment. Other causes of poor healing are peripheral vascular disease, poor nutrition or continuing illness. However, healing may occur even in dying patients.[98] Age slows healing but scar quality in old women may be better than in young women.[192]

Pressure relief

Pressure relief to heal sores is the same as for prevention except that it has to be continued for longer. Small superficial sores may heal within a week, but very extensive tissue loss may take up to 6 months, or may never heal satisfactorily without plastic surgery.

Bed rest

The importance of bed rest for healing sores in spinal injury patients is well recognized[193] but is often questioned in elderly people.[107] The belief that nursing patients in chairs is good for "bedsores" persists and is still taught to medical and nurse students. However, healing is inevitably delayed or prevented if a sore is deprived of a blood supply by sitting in chairs for long periods.[194] Pressure-relieving cushions do not allow adequate circulation to permit healing and risk causing new necrosis.[195] Patients should spend as much of their days as possible, when they are not walking about, on pressure-relieving mattresses on their beds. Sleep is also important for healing.[196] As the patient's condition and their sore improves, they may be dressed and allowed up for physiotherapy and for meals but should return to rest on their beds at other times.

Foot sores

Bed rest is also important for healing foot sores because it optimizes circulation in the legs. Sitting in a chair reduces venous and lymphatic flow and causes capillary stasis and edema which slow healing and encourage infection. Footstools increase pressure on the ischial tuberosities and the heels and are seldom tolerated for any length of time. Bed rest produces an immediate reduction in venocapillary pressure, resolution of edema, and beginning of healing, usually within 2 days. In elderly patients, the legs should not be raised above the horizontal because of the risk of arterial insufficiency.

Pressure-relieving supports

Five randomized trials of flotation beds for healing Grade 2–4 sores have been carried out in the USA, comparing air-fluidized[170,197,198] and low air loss beds,[143,199] respectively with "conventional therapy": turning 2 hourly on a hospital bed,[170] sheepskins,[197] gel pads,[197] convoluted foam mattresses,[199] and small-celled alternating pressure mattresses,[170,198] all of which are relatively ineffective methods of relieving pressure. Following these studies, flotation supports have been marketed for both prevention[67] and healing.[200] However, two trials of the air-fluidized bed were for less than 2 weeks because of the cost, and 50 percent of patients in the third were withdrawn over the 36-week trial period.[143] A low air loss bed for elderly nursing home residents was more satisfactory,[199] showing complete healing of 60 percent of superficial sores and a substantial decrease in the size of deep sores over a median follow-up period of 37.5 days. Caley[171] also found good healing rates over 24 days on less expensive and more practical low air loss overlays. However, flotation supports are complicated, expensive machines and are unsuitable for large numbers of elderly patients with sores which may take many months to heal. In relatively fit nursing home patients, Groen et al.[201] found healing rates of Grade 3–4 sores of 45 and 48 percent in one month on foam and water overlays.

No study comparing the effect of air flotation and large-celled AP supports on healing has been attempted.[200] In separate randomized trials, Devine[202] and Russell[203] showed similar good healing rates of Grade >2 sores on two deep AP mattress replacements. The effect of AP overlays on healing deep sores has not been evaluated. However, Keogh[204] noted that 19 elderly patients with sores, including Grade 4 sores, improved and 15 healed after being placed on large-celled Alpha X Cell overlays. In a randomized controlled study, Bliss[98] found that 45 percent of Grade 2 sores healed in 18 days on large-celled overlays compared with 37 percent on slit foam and 24 and 20 percent on water and fiberfill overlays respectively. AP overlays which permit an adequate circulation to prevent sores in acutely ill intensive care patients[113] are also likely to permit healing in convalescent patients.

Pain relief

Most pressure sores in elderly patients are very painful, limiting mobility and impairing sleep and healing. Pain relief should be started as soon as possible. For *superficial sores and heel sores*, positioning with pillows to avoid pressure on the injured area, a pressure-relieving mattress and an occlusive dressing if appropriate may be adequate. Analgesics such as paracetamol or coproxamol are ineffective. A patient with a *new deep sore* is usually toxic and shocked as well as in pain. He should be treated with bed rest, fluids, and analgesics. Nonsteroidal anti-inflammatory drugs may help traumatic pain but delay healing[105] and risk causing gastrointestinal bleeding. Diamorphine (2.5–5 mg), or morphine (5–10 mg) are usually necessary. They should be given 4 hourly subcutaneously or intramuscularly or via a subcutaneous pump until the slough has separated and the sore has begun to granulate, usually in 2–4 weeks. Long-acting oral preparations are less effective and more likely to cause drowsiness and confusion. Antiemetics are rarely required. The most important side-effect is constipation which must be treated with regular enemas and laxatives.

Nutrition

Good nutrition is important for optimal healing. However, decisions about artificial feeding for old people who cannot be fed orally should depend on their prognosis and the wishes of patients and their families. Tube feeding continuing-care patients has not been shown to prevent or heal pressure sores.[71]

In a young person, it has been calculated that twice the normal daily protein intake is required for healing a deep pressure sore.[205] Carbohydrate is also necessary to fuel cellular metabolism and vitamin C, zinc, iron, copper, manganese, and calcium for the synthesis of collagen.[206] However, supplements of vitamin C and zinc have not been shown to accelerate healing in nondeficient patients and hyperalimentation may cause metabolic disturbances.[77,207,208] Many nutritional parameters are altered by illness and age[76] and do not necessarily reflect intake or whole body balance. Hemoglobin and iron status should be checked and iron supplements given if necessary. Very debilitated patients may be helped by an initial blood transfusion. Anabolic steroids,[209] growth hormone,[209] and insulin[210] have been used to try to improve nutrition but with little success. In most patients, the improved appetite which occurs when pressure is relieved and pain and further tissue necrosis are prevented, makes nutritional supplements and drugs unnecessary.

Infection

Cellulitis, edema, pyrexia, and leukocytosis in a patient with a new pressure injury are normal inflammatory responses to the presence of dead tissue and do not indicate infection or the need for antibiotics. Similarly, discharge of foul-smelling necrotic material is the first stage of healing and not evidence of worsening infection. Pressure injuries are always colonized by bacteria, including pathogens, but these seldom cause clinically significant infection[211] and may even help to liquify the slough.[212] Osteomyelitis virtually never occurs in elderly patients, probably because those with deep sores do not survive long enough. Galpin et al.[213] found bacteremia in 76 percent of patients with deep sores, but half of these died despite being given antibiotics. Unnecessary antibiotics are merely likely to impair appetite and to cause diarrhea and encourage the growth of resistant organisms.

Pressure sores only need to be swabbed if the patient develops new signs of systemic toxicity after the initial inflammation has subsided or if the sore fails to improve despite adequate pressure relief. Infected sores are painful, red, and glistening with a discharge which often has a characteristic odor. Gram-negative organisms, coliforms, proteus, and pseudomonas predominate, but group A *streptococci* and *Staphylococcus aureus*, and anaerobes are common. Clinically significant infections are defined as those with more than 10^5 organisms per gram of tissue.[205] If required, antibiotics should be given systemically.

Methicillin-resistant *Staphylococcus aureus*

Many elderly patients are contaminated with methicillin-resistant *Staphylococcus aureus* (MRSA) and their sores soon become colonized. However, this rarely affects healing. The main danger is cross-infection in hospitals where isolation, barrier nursing, and eradication therapy are usually required. In the community, MRSA poses little threat and should not constitute a reason for refusing admission to a nursing home.[214] Patients should be given a single room if possible but should not be isolated from other residents. Where possible, wounds should be covered by impermeable dressings. Staff should use disposable gloves and aprons when dealing with wounds or bedding but thorough hand washing after other activities is sufficient. Clothes and bedding should be machine washed, preferably at a hot setting.

Local treatment

SURGICAL DEBRIDEMENT This is rarely necessary for pressure sores in elderly patients. Deep pressure sores almost never form abscesses or involve bone as in younger patients, and surgery merely causes additional stress in a sick old person. Providing pressure is relieved, the slough usually separates naturally within 1–4 weeks (Fig. 106-17; see also Plate 106-12). As it loosens, it can be snipped free with scissors and the cavity washed out twice daily with saline or tap water.[215] In rare cases in which the slough does not separate, the patient is usually dying so that surgery is inappropriate.

DEBRIDING AGENTS *Antiseptics* such as Eusol and povidone iodine which are toxic to granulation tissue[216] should not be used. *Topical antibiotics* which are likely to cause sensitivity reactions and encourage the growth of resistant organisms, should also be avoided. *Proteolytic enzymes* which are expensive and need to be applied twice daily are rarely necessary.

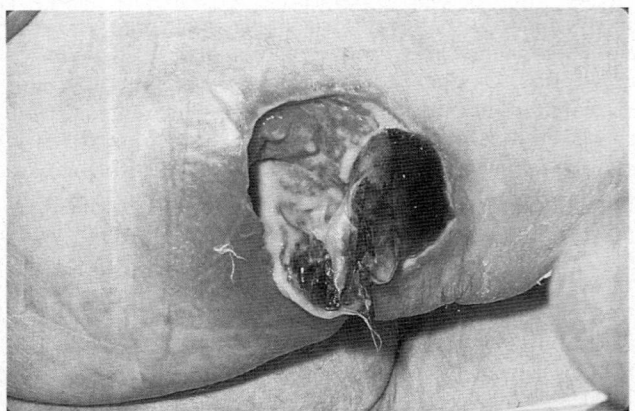

Figure 106-17 Naturally separating slough in a deep pressure sore.

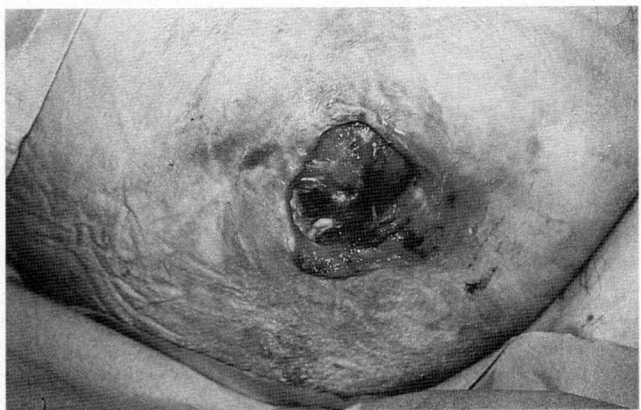

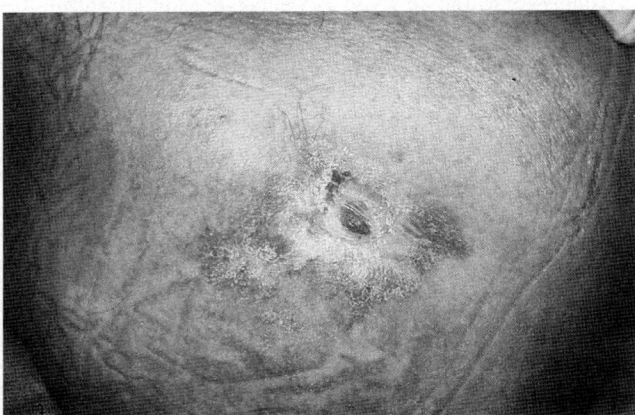

Figure 106-18 Deep pressure injury over the trochanter showing (top) contraction and (bottom) healing.

DRESSINGS Experimentally, healing has been shown to proceed faster in a moist environment,[217] but there have been few clinical trials and many workers prefer dry healing for some types of wound.[215] Dry dressings risk becoming incorporated into granulation tissue so that the wound may be retraumatized when they are changed.[215] Occlusive and semi-occlusive dressings reduce pain[218] and prevent scab formation and thus permit faster resolution of sloughs and epithelialization.[215] Hydrocolloid dressings may also reduce infection.[219] However, the presence of bacteria does not necessarily affect healing rates,[220] and different dressings may be needed in different situations. Bio-occlusive and hydrocolloid dressings are useful for treating sores on nonpressurized skin, but in areas such as the sacrum and heel they rumple and harden increasing tissue damage. They are also unsuitable for sores with a heavy exudate.

PACKING In elderly patients, packing deep sores to prevent loculation of infected material is unnecessary as this never occurs. Packing with gauze prevents discharge of necrotic material, damages granulation tissue and is very painful. It has been shown to slow healing compared with a hydrocolloid dressing.[221] Alginates and foam are less injurious, but all packing agents require a secondary dressing to keep them in place which risk causing dermatitis on the wound margins.[215] Nonirritant substances such as honey which has antibacterial properties,[222] or hydrogels which can be combined with metronidazole powder to reduce odor, can be placed in the cavity, but there is no evidence that they have any advantage over leaving it empty. Activated charcoal dressings should be avoided as they are costly, ineffective when saturated and may interfere with the growth of fibroblasts.[223] Once the slough has separated, myofibroblasts in healthy granulation tissue contract causing a rapid reduction in the size and depth of the wound (Fig. 106-18; see also Plate 106-13). This process may be delayed by inappropriate applications and dressings.

HEEL SORES Heel sores are best treated, at least initially, by exposing them and allowing them to dry. Attempts to keep the area moist increase maceration and pain and delay mobility. Superficial dried blisters can be ignored. Full-thickness eschars also often cause little inconvenience, but if, desired following demarcation, debridement can be expedited by a hydrogel or hydrocolloid dressing. Enzymes are seldom necessary and should never be injected underneath eschars in our experience as this is painful and injurious. Sharp debridement should also be avoided.

Healing agents

Wound therapy is nowadays big business and numerous physical, medical, and local treatments have been recommended for accelerating healing of pressure injuries. However, it cannot be emphasized too strongly that expenditure should be devoted to *prevention* rather than to *healing*,[200] and that pressure-relieving supports which are effective for prevention are also likely to be the most efficient aids for healing. Papers describing healing agents rarely include a description of the method of pressure relief being used, therefore their claims cannot be properly evaluated.

Electric currents influence the proliferation and migration of fibroblasts.[224] However, clinical studies of *electrical therapy*[225,226] have generally been poorly controlled or have included different types of wound, e.g., leg ulcers, diabetic foot sores. An uncontrolled trial of topical negative pressure showed possibly some improved healing in Grade >3 sores.[227] *Ultrasound*[228] and *hyperbaric oxygen*[229] have not been shown to be of benefit. *Platelet-derived growth factors* have been used in studies of healing pressure sores but with variable success.[230] *Cultured human skin equivalents* are being researched[231] but are extremely expensive and are unlikely to be required for pressure sores which usually heal readily once pressure is properly relieved.

Plastic surgery

Most pressure sores heal with relief of pressure and in the rare exceptions the patients are often too ill for surgery. Occasionally, however, an elderly patient may develop a deep sore during an acute illness which would normally take months to heal but who may be able to be discharged within 2 weeks following plastic surgery. He should be rendered as fit as possible preoperatively by physiotherapy, a high-protein diet and a blood transfusion or antibiotics if indicated. The wound is sterilized with antiseptics and is then completely excised and the tissue defect closed by skin flaps.[232] It is essential to maintain scrupulous pressure relief until the wound has healed and the patient has regained normal mobility.

EDUCATION
Clinical governance and pressure ulcers

Clinical governance has been defined as "a framework through which National Health Service (NHS) organisations are accountable for continuously improving the quality of their service and safeguarding high standards of care by creating an environment in which excellence in clinical care will flourish."[233] As in many other aspects of medicine, wound care is complex and a particular approach to the concept of governance is required.[234]

There are five components to the clinical governance framework: clinical audit, clinical effectiveness, risk management, quality assurance, and the development of staff and organizations.

Clinical audit is fully established in the NHS.[235] One large-scale chronic wound audit demonstrated that a large full-cycle clinical audit was feasible and that audit could lead to organizational changes and improvements in the quality of care.[236]

Clinical effectiveness is the process by which evidence-based healthcare is promoted.

Clinical risk management is defined as a means of reducing the risks of adverse events occurring in organizations by systematic assessment and review, and then seeking ways to prevent their occurrence. Pressure ulcers are not universally accepted as adverse events and hence are not routinely documented for this purpose. This lack of transparency by the medical and nursing profession raises fundamental questions concerning the rights of patients and the responsibilities of staff when damage occurs. This was not considered by the National Institute for Clinical Excellence when it published recommendations concerning pressure ulcer education initiatives for patients and carers.[237] Failure to accept responsibility has medico-legal implications. It is now accepted that, in some cases, pressure ulcer development constitutes neglect and legal redress with compensation is required.[238] What is not accepted is the contention that most pressure ulcers constitute neglect and that, except in specific defined circumstances, their occurrence is preventable. This would mean that all pressure ulcers became adverse events within a clinical governance framework

firmly linking quality assurance and clinical effectiveness to the individual patient. A culture of transparency would also ensure that patients and carers were part of the process by being made aware of the damage, its cause and management. Grade 1 and 2 pressure sores, which may not always be preventable and cause no lasting damage, would not constitute neglect in the legal sense but Grade 3 and 4 ulcers would lay the responsible organization open to claims for compensation in most circumstances. This process may, perversely, be more successful in encouraging the use of evidence-based local guidelines and protocols, audits, and standard setting, as well as patient pathway assessments, than the current clinical governance program. In a prospective post-mortem study of 10,222 corpses, 11.2 percent had a pressure ulcer (the majority deep and over the sacrum).[239] As the author states "… the prevalence of pressure sores in a defined population can be seen as a parameter for the quality of nursing and medical care. In bringing these fatalities to light, the field of legal medicine contributes to a general quality control of standards."

Medical education

The essential feature of pressure sore management is prevention, and to be successful, prevention must form part of the emergency care of susceptible patients. Doctors need to accept responsibility for maintaining the peripheral circulation as well as that of the heart or kidneys or any other organ. Preventing pressure necrosis requires an understanding of the etiology and pathology of peripheral circulatory failure and clinical judgment which should not be delegated to nurses alone. Patients at risk are found in almost every branch of medical practice. Doctors must be trained to recognize susceptible patients and know how to provide appropriate treatment. A survey of medical schools and colleges in the United Kingdom indicated that medical education in wound care was inadequate for their clinical and medico-legal needs.[240] A few centers are pioneering education for medical undergraduates in wound care, developing Study Guides (tutorials in print) available as hard copy and Intranet, and utilizing interactive CD-ROM computer-asssisted learning to promote interest and develop skills in trainee medical practitioners.[241]

Nurse education

Pressure care nurse specialists should be appointed in every health district. They should liaise with supplies officers and manufacturers to ensure that cost-effective, up-to-date pressure-relieving equipment is available in hospitals and in the community 24 hours a day[156] and should be responsible for servicing and redistribution. Innovative schemes include a mobile unit in Copenhagen, Denmark, which work out of a hospital base, but treat and teach in patients' own homes or nursing homes.[242] Specialists should also help to organize undergraduate and in-service training sessions on pressure care. Educational packages undertaken by nurses range from certificates (with no higher education validation) to diplomas, degrees, and postgraduate degrees. This situation will change with the implementation of the United Kingdom Central Council (UKCC)'s standards for postregistration nurse education.[243] However, although nurse specialists may give general advice about pressure relief, the decision to use pressure-relieving equipment should be a joint responsibility of the physician and nurse and form part of the general medical and nursing plan of treatment.[244]

KEY POINTS Pressure sores

■ Pressure injuries are caused by reduced mobility and peripheral circulatory failure in acutely ill patients.

■ They occur most commonly in patients with neurological and/or vascular disease.

■ Effective pressure relief for susceptible patients must be provided as early as possible following the onset of any acute illness or trauma, including surgery.

■ Patients at risk should not be nursed in chairs for more than a maximum of 2 hours per session.

■ Large-celled alternating-pressure mattress overlays prevent and heal most pressure injuries but must be robust, well serviced and correctly used.

REFERENCES

1. Rothschild JM, Bates DW, Leape LL: Preventable medical injuries in older patients. Ach Intern Med 2000;160:2717–2728

2. Gunnewicht BR: Prevention of pressure sores in acute spinal injury: outside the specialist unit. J Tiss Viabil 1997;7(4):124–129

3. Mawson AR, Siddiqui FH, Connolly BJ et al: Sacral transcutaneous oxygen tension levels in the spinal cord injured: risk factors for pressure ulcers? Arch Phys Med Rehab 1993;74:745–751

4. Creditor MC: Hazards of hospitalisation of the elderly. Ann Intern Med 1993;118:219–223

5. Shah AM: Vascular endothelium. Br J Hosp Med 1992;48: 540–549

6. Pierce SM, Skalak TC, Rodeheaver GT: Ischaemia-reperfusion injury in chronic pressure ulcer formation: a skin model in the rat. Wound Repair Regen 2000;8(1):68–76

7. Zhang JG, Ghosh S, Ockleford CD, Galinanes M: Characterisation of an in vitro model for the study of the short and prolonged effects of myocardial ischaemia and reperfusion in man. Clin Sci 2000;99:443–453

8. Meehan M, O'Hara L, Morrison YM: Report of the prevalence of skin ulcers in a Home Health Agency population. Adv Wound Care 1999;12(9):459–467

9. Lowthian P: Preventing pressure sores. Nurs Mirror 1985;160:18–20

10. Scales JT: Pathogenesis of pressure sores. In Bader DL (ed): Pressure: Sores. Clinical Practice and Scientific Approach. Macmillan Press, Basingstoke, 1990:15–26

11. Childress JJ, Felbeck H, Somero GN: Symbiosis in the deep sea. In Gould JL, Gould CG (eds): Life at the edge. Readings from Scientific American magazine. WH Freeman, New York, 1989:39–48

12. Bader DL, Hawken MB: Ischial pressure distribution under the seated person. In Bader DL (eds): Pressure Sores. Clinical Practice and Scientific Approach. Macmillan Press, Basingstoke, 1990:223–233

13. Bennett L, Lee BY: Pressure versus shear in pressure sore causation. In Lee BY (ed): Chronic Ulcers of the Skin. McGraw-Hill, New York, 1985:39–56

14. Kosiak M: Etiology and pathology of ischaemic ulcers. Arch Phys Med Rehab 1959;40:62–69

15. Reswick JB, Rogers JE: Experience at Rancho Los Amigos Hospital with devices and techniques for preventing pressure sores. In Kenedi RM, Cowden JM, Scales JT (eds): Bedsore Biomechanics. Macmillan Press, London, 1976:301–310

16. Salcido R, Donofrio JC, Fisher SB et al: Histopathology of pressure ulcers as a result of sequential computer controlled pressure sessions in a fuzzy rat model. Adv Wound Care 1994;7(5):23–40

17. Kosiak M: Etiology of pressure ulcers. Arch Phys Med Rehab 1961;42:19–29

18. Husain T: An experimental study of some pressure effects on tissues with reference to the bedsore problem. J Pathol Bacteriol 1953;66:347–358

19. Le KM, Madsen BL, Barth PW, Ksander GA, Angell JB, Vistnes LM: An in depth look at pressure sores using monolithic silicon pressure sensors. Plast Reconstr Surg 1984;74:745–754

20. Groth KE: Klinische Beobactungen und experimentelle Studien uber die Entstehung des Dekubitus. Acta Chirurgica Scand 1942;87 (suppl 76)

21. Ek AC, Gustavsson G, Lewis DH: Skin blood flow in relation to external pressure and temperature in the supine position on a standard hospital mattress. Scand J Rehab Med 1987;19:121–126

22. Bennett L, Kavner D, Lee BY, Trainer FS, Lewis JM: Skin stress and blood flow in sitting paraplegic patients. Arch Phys Med Rehab 1984;65:186–190

23. Cochran GVB: Measurements of pressure and other environmental factors at the patient-cushion interface. In Lee BY (ed): Chronic Ulcers of the Skin. McGraw-Hill, New York, 1985:23–37

24. Sideranko S, Quinn A, Burns K, Froman RD: Effects of position and mattress overlay on sacral and heel pressures in a clinical population. Res Nurs Health 1992;15:245–251

25. Ryan TJ: Cellular responses to tissue distortion. In Bader DL (ed): Pressure Sores. Clinical Practice and Scientific Approach. Macmillan Press, Basingstoke, 1990:141–152

26. Brandeis GH, Berlowitz DR, Hossain M, Morris JN: Pressure ulcers: the minimum data set and the resident assessment protocol. Adv Wound Care 1995;8(6):18–25

27. Raney JP: A comparison of the prevalence of pressure sores in hospitalised ALS and MS patients. Decubitus 1989;2(2):48–49

28. Uccioli L: Diabetic foot as a model of a pressure ulcer. EPUAP Rev 2001;3(1):14

29. Exton Smith AN, Sherwin RW: The prevention of pressure ulcers: significance of spontaneous bodily movements. Lancet 1961;2:1124–1126

30. Nicholson PW, Leeman AL, O'Neill CJA et al: Pressure sores: effect of Parkinson's disease and cognitive function on spontaneous movement in bed. Age Ageing 1988;17:111–115

31. Lewis T, Grant R: Observations upon reactive hyperaemia in man. Heart 1925–6;xii:75–120

32. Bliss MR: Hyperaemia. J Tiss Viabil 1998;8(4):4–13

33. Michel CC, Gillott H: Microvascular mechanisms in stasis and ischaemia. In Bader DL (ed): Pressure Sores. Clinical Practice and Scientific Approach. Macmillan Press, Basingstoke, 1990:153–163

34. Guyton AC: Capillary dynamics and exchange of fluid between blood and interstitial fluid. In Guyton AC. Medical Physiology. WB Saunders Company, Philadelphia, 1981:358–369

35. Lee BY, Thoden WR: Non invasive evaluation of the cutaneous circulation. In Lee BY (ed): Chronic Ulcers of the Skin. McGraw Hill, New York, 1985:77–89

36. Schubert V, Fagrell B: Post occlusive reactive hyperaemia and thermal response in the skin microcirculation of subjects with spinal cord injury. Scand J Rehab Med 1991;23:33–40

37. Teasell RW, Arnold MO, Krassioner A, Delaney GA: Cardiovascular consequences of loss of supra-spinal control of the sympathetic nervous system after spinal cord injury. Arch Phys Med Rehab 2000;81:506–516

38. Schubert V, Schubert P-A, Breit G, Intaglietta M: Analysis of arterial flow motion in spinal cord injured and elderly subjects in an area at risk for the development of pressure sores. Paraplegia 1995;33:387–397

39. Warner U, Hall D: Pressure sores: a policy for prevention. Nurs Times 1986;82(6):59–61

40. Barbenel JC, Jordan MM, Nicol SM, Clark ML: Incidence of pressure sores in the Greater Glasgow Health Board Area. Lancet 1977;ii:548–550

41. O'Dea K: Prevalence of pressure damage in hospital patients in the UK. J Wound Care 1993;2(4):221–225

42. Ardron ME, Helme RD, McKernan S: Microvascular skin responses in elderly people with varicose leg ulcers. Age Ageing 1991;20:124–128

43. Andersen TJ, Meredith IT, Yeung AC et al: The effect of cholesterol lowering and anti-oxidant therapy on endothelium-dependent coronary vasodilatation. N Engl J Med 1995;332:488–493

44. Struijker-Bondier HAJ, Crijns FRL, Stolte J, Van Essen H: Assessment of the microcirculation in cardio-vascular disease. Clin Sci 1996;91:131–139

45. Enggard E: Nitric oxide: mediator, murderer and medicine. Lancet 1994;343:1199–1206

46. Jaap AJ, Reza M, Leatherdale BA, Shore AC, Tooke JE: Impaired maximal hyperaemic response in the feet of non insulin dependent diabetic patients. Communications for the Winter Meeting of the Medical

Research Society, 5 and 6 November 1992. Royal College of Physicians, London, 46

47. Rayman G, Malik RA, Sharma AK, Day JL: Microvascular response to tissue injury and capillary ultrastructure in the foot of type 1 diabetic patients. Clin Sci 1995;89:467–474

48. Kemp MG: Factors which contribute to pressure sores in surgical patients. Res Nurse Health 1990;13(5):293–301

49. Lowe GDO: Rheology and arterial disease. Clin Sci 1986;71(2):137–146

50. Barton AA: Pressure sores. In Barbenel JC, Forbes CD, Lowe GDO (eds): Pressure Sores. Macmillan Press, London, 1983:53–57

51. Rendell MS, Wells JM: Ischemia and pressure induced hyperemia: a comparison. Arch Phys Med Rehab 1998;79:1451–1455

52. Bader DL: Effects of compressive loading regimens on tissue viability. In Bader DL (ed): Pressure Sores. Clinical Practice and Scientific Approach. Macmillan Press, Basingstoke, 1990:191–201

53. Anderson WG: Anaesthesia for patients with cardiac disease: post-operative care. Br J Hosp Med 1987;37:411–418

54. Krouscop JA, Garber SL: Pressure management and the recumbent person. In Bader DL (ed): Pressure Sores. Clinical Practice and Scientific Approach. Macmillan Press, Basingstoke, 1990:235–248

55. Vermillion C: Operating room acquired pressure ulcers. Decubitus 1990;3(1):26–30

56. Schubert V: Hypotension as a risk factor for the development of pressure ulcers. Age Ageing 1991;20:255–261

57. Severinghaus JW, Spellman MJ: Pulse oximeter failure thresholds in hypotension and vasoconstriction. Anaesthesiology 1990;73:532–587

58. Barton AA: The pathogenesis of skin wounds due to pressure. In Kenedi RM, Cowden JM, Scales JT (eds): Bedsore Biomechanics, Macmillan Press, London, 1983:55–62

59. de Bono DP: Cardiogenic shock. Hosp Update 1988;14(1):1083–1092

60. Evans TW, Smithies M: ABC of intensive care: organ dysfunction. Br Med J 1999;318:1606–1609

61. Young JD, Cameron EM: Dynamics of skin blood flow in human sepsis. Intens Care Med 1995;21:669–674

62. Hinds CJ, Watson D: ABC of intensive care; circulatory support. Br Med J 1999;318:1749–1752

63. Holloway GA, Tolentino G, De Latour BJ: Cutaneous blood flow responses to wheelchair cushion pressure loading measured by laser Doppler flowmetry. In Lee BY (ed): Chronic Ulcers of the Skin. McGraw Hill, New York, 1985

64. Meijer JH, Germs PH, Schneider H, Ribbe MW: Susceptability to decubitus ulcer formation. Arch Phys Med Rehab 1994;75:318–323

65. Desai H: Ageing and wounds. Part 2: healing in old age. J Wound Care 1997;6(5):237–239

66. Schubert V, Fagrell B: Local skin pressure and its effects on the skin microcirculation as evaluated by laser Doppler fluximetry. Clin Physiol 1989;9:535–545

67. Evans JM, Andrews KL, Chutka DS, Fleming KC, Garness SL: Pressure ulcers: prevention and management. Mayo Clin Proc 1995;70:789–799

68. Lindholm C: Chronic wounds and nursing care. J Wound Care 1999;8(1):5–10

69. Allman RM: The impact of pressure ulcers on healthcare costs and mortality. Adv Wound Care 1999;11(4) (suppl: OR acquired pressure ulcers): 2

70. Sparks S: Nurse validation of pressure ulcer risk factors for a nursing diagnosis. Decubitus 1992;5(1):26–35

71. Finucane JE: Malnutrition, tube feeding and pressure sores: data are incomplete. J Am Geriatr Soc 1995;43:447–451

72. Allman RM, Laprade CA, Noel LB et al: Pressure sores among hospitalised patients. Ann Intern Med 1986;105:337–342

73. Green SM, Franks PJ, Moffatt CJ, Eberhardie C, McLaren S: Nutritional intake in community patients with pressure ulcers. J Wound Care 1999;8(7):325–330

74. Piloian BB: Defining characteristics of the nursing diagnosis, 'High risk for impaired skin integrity'. Decubitus 1992;5(5):32–47

75. Kennedy KL: Involuntary weight loss: definition, diagnosis and documentation. Adv Skin Wound Care 2001;14 (suppl):4–6

76. Lehman AS: Nutrition in old age; an update and questions for future research. Rev Clin Gerontol 1991;1:135–145

77. Macallan D: Malnutrition and infection. Medicine 2001;29(1):17–19

78. Landis EM: Micro-injection studies of capillary blood pressure in human skin. Heart 1930;15:209–228

79. Lazzara D, Buschmann MBT: Prevention of pressure ulcers in elderly nursing home residents: are special support surfaces the answer? Decubitus 11991;4(4):42–48

80. Collier ME: Pressure reducing mattresses. J Wound Care 1996;5(5):207

81. Krouscop A, Garber SL: Interface pressure confusion. Decubitus 1989;2(3):8

82. Conner LM, Clack JW: In vivo (CT scan) comparison of vertical shear in human tissue caused by various support surfaces. Decubitus 1993;6(2):20–28

83. Reger SSI, McGovern TF, Chung KC: Biomechanics of tissue distortion and stiffness by electromagnetic resonance imaging. In Bader DL (ed): Pressure Sores. Clinical Practice and Scientific Approach. Macmillan Press, Basingstoke, 1990:177–190

84. Bosboom EMH, Nicolay K, Bouten CVC, Oomens CWJ, Baaijens FPT: Assessment of skeletal muscle damage after controlled compressive loading using high resolution MRI. In Prenergast PJ, Lee TC, Carr AJ (eds): Proceedings of the 12th Conference of the European Society of Biomechanics 2000, 28–30 August. Royal Academy of Medicine in Ireland, Dublini, 179

85. Bader DL, White SH: The viability of soft tissues in elderly subjects undergoing hip surgery. Age Ageing 1998;27:217–221

86. Bulstrode C: Orthopaedics. In Bader DL (ed): Pressure Sores. Clinical Practice and Scientific Approach. Macmillan Press, Basingstoke, 1990:55–64

87. Grewel PS, Sawant NH, Deaney CN et al: Pressure sore prevention in hospital patients: a clinical audit. J Wound Care 1999;8(3):129–131

88. Versluysen M: How elderly patients with femoral neck fracture develop pressure sores in hospital. Br Med J 1986;292:1311–1313

89. Wilson M-MG: The management of dehydration in the nursing home. J Nutr Health Ageing 1999;3(1):53–61

90. Li Pak Tong B, Langthorne P, Stott DDJ: Frequency and implications of dehydration in acute stroke. Age Ageing 2001;30(suppl 1):50

91. Bonn D: Ill health spiral in the elderly may be set off by poor hospital nutrition. Lancet 1999;353:1945

92. Knowles C: An audit of stroke patients referred to a special needs scheme. J Wound Care 1996;5(8):6(conference abstracts)

93. Santy J: Hospital mattresses and pressure sore prevention. J Wound Care 1995;4(7):329–332

94. Kemp MG, Kopanke D, Tordicilla L et al: The role of support surfaces and patient attributes in preventing pressure ulcers in elderly patients. Res Nurs Health 1993;16:89–96

95. Gebhardt KS, Hookway J, Bland JM: Evaluating alternating pressure mattress overlays. J Wound Care 1998;7(5):227–230

96. Colin D, Abraham P, Preault L, Bregeon C, Saumet J-L: Comparison of 90° and 30° laterally inclined positions in the prevention of pressure ulcers using transcutaneous oxygen and carbon dioxide pressures. Adv Wound Care 1996;9(3):35–38

97. Stoneberg C, Pitcock N, Myton C: Pressure sores in the homebound: one solution. Am J Nurs 1986;86:426–428

98. Bliss MR: Preventing pressure sores in elderly patients: a comparison of seven mattress overlays. Age Ageing 1995;24:297–302

99. Weiderman FJ, Wildsmith JAW, Duncan FM, Jury CS: Postoperative pressure sores after epidural anaesthesia. Br Med J 2001;322:732–734

100. Gendron F: Burns occurring during lengthy surgical procedures. J Clin Eng 1980;51(1):19–26

101. Grous CA, Reilly NJ, Gift AG: Skin integrity in patients undergoing prolonged operations. J Wound Ostomy Continence Nurse 1997;24:86–91

102. First annual OR acquired pressure ulcer symposium. Adv Wound Care 1998;11(suppl):8–9

103. Bliss MR, Simini B: When are the seeds of post operative pressure sores sown? Br Med J 1999;319:863–864

104. Larkin SW, Williams TJ: Evidence for sensory nerve involvement in cutaneous reactive hyperaemia in humans. Circul Res 1993;73:147–154

105. Barton A, Barton M: The Management and Prevention of Pressure Sores. Faber and Faber, London, 1981

106. Gebhardt KS, Bliss MR: Preventing pressure sores in orthopaedic patients—is prolonged chair nursing detrimental? J Tiss Viabil 1994;4(2):51–54

107. Gebhardt KS: The effect of limited and unlimited chair nursing on post operative recovery in elderly orthopaedic patients. University of Surrey: PhD Thesis, 1999

108. Joyce WP, Walsh K, Gough DB, Gorey TF, Fitzpatrick JM: Pulse oximetry: a new non invasive assessment of peripheral arterial occlusive disease. Br J Surg 1990;77:1115–1117

109. Bak-Christensen A, Dinio B, Samson D, Wille-Jorgensen P: Cutaneous reactions in relation to the use of TED stockings. Lancet 1989;ii:1346

110. Guidelines on treatment of pressure ulcers. EPUAP Rev 1999;1(2):31–33

111. Shea JD: Pressure sores. Classification and management. Clin Orthop Rel Res 1975;112:89–99

112. Barbenel JC: The limits of pressure sore prevention. J Roy Soc Med 1999;92(11):576–578

113. Gebhardt KS, Bliss MR, Winwright PL, Thomas J: Pressure relieving supports in an ICU. J Wound Care 1996;5(3):116–121

114. Peterson NC, Bittman S: The epidemiology of pressure sores. Scand J Reconstr Surg 1971;5:62

115. Jordan MM, Clark MO: Report on the Incidence of Pressure Sores in the Patient Community of the Greater Glasgow Health Board Area on Jan 1st 1976. University of Strathclyde, Glasgow, 1976

116. Jordan MM, Nichol SM, Melrose AL: Report on the Incidence of Pressure Sores in the Patient Community of the Borders Health Board Area on 13th October 1976. University of Strathclyde, Glasgow, 1976

117. O'Dea K: The prevalence of pressure sores in four European countries. J Wound Care 1995;4(5):234–236

118. Barrois B, Allaert FA, Colin D: A survey of pressure sore prevalence in hospitals in the greater Paris region. J Wound Care 1995;4:234–236

119. Saito E, Shirato M, Kanangwa K, Sagawa Y, Nakamura M: Incidence proportion estimation, prevalence and effective visiting nurse care of pressure ulcers. Nippon Koshu Eisei Zasshi (Jap J Pub Health) 1999;46(12):1084–1093

120. Pearson A, Francis K, Hodgkinson B, Curry G: Prevalence and treatment of pressure ulcers in northern New South Wales. Aust J Rural Health. 2000;8(2):103–110

121. Nyquist R, Hawthorn PJ: The prevalence of pressure sores within an Area Health Authority. Nursing 1987;12:183–187

122. Hibbs P: Pressure area care for the City and Hackney Health Authority. City and Hackney Health Authority, London, 1988

123. O'Dea K: The prevalence of pressure damage in acute care hospital patients in the UK. J Wound Care 1999;8(4):192–194

124. Allman RM: Pressure ulcers among the elderly. New Engl J Med 1989;320:850–853

125. Meehan M: National pressure ulcer prevalence survey. Adv Wound Care 1994;7:27–38

126. Shaughnessy PW, Kramer AM: Increased needs of patients in nursing homes and patients receiving home health care. N Engl J Med 1990;332:21–27

127. Sternberg J, Spector WD, Kapp MC, Tucker RJ: Decubitus ulcers on admission to nursing homes: prevalence and residents characteristics. Decubitus 1988;1:14–20

128. Bergquist S, Frantz R: Pressure ulcers in community-based older adults receiving home health care. Adv Wound Care 1999;12(7):339–351

129. Dealey C: Measuring the prevalence and incidence of pressure sores. Br J Nurs 1993;2:998–1000, 1002–1006

130. Baumgarten M: Designing prevalence and incidence studies. Adv Wound Care 1998;11(6):287–293

131. Bours GJ, Halfens RJ, Lubbers M, Haalboom JR: The development of a national registration form to measure the prevalence of pressure ulcers in The Netherlands. Ostomy Wound Manag 1999;45(11):28–33, 36–38, 40

132. Berlowitz DR, Anderson JJ, Ash AS et al: Reducing random variation in reported rates of pressure ulcer development. Med Care 1998;36(6):818–825

133. Dealey C: The size of the pressure-sore problem in a teaching hospital. J Adv Nurs 1991;16:663–670

134. Allcock N, Wharrad H, Nicolson A: Interpretation of pressure sore prevalence. J Adv Nurs 1994;20:37–45

135. Clark M, Watts S: The incidence of pressure sores within a National Health Services Trust hospital during 1994. J Adv Nurs 1994;20:33–36

136. Martin BJ: Incidence of pressure sores in geriatric long-term hospital care 1995. J Tiss Viabil 1995;5:83–87

137. Brandeis GH, Ooi WL, Hossain M et al: A longitudinal study of risk factors associated with the formation of pressure ulcers in nursing homes. J Am Geriatr Soc 1994;42:388–393

138. Rudman D, Mattson DE, Alvemo L et al: Comparison of clinical indicators in two nursing homes. J Am Geriatr Soc 1993;41:1317–1325

139. Bergstrom N, Braden B: A prospective study of pressure sore risk among institutional elderly. J Am Geriatr Soc 1992;40:747–758

140. Lake NO: Methodology. Measuring incidence and prevalence of pressure ulcers for intergroup comparison. Adv Wound Care 1999;12(1):31–34

141. Haalboom JRE: Risk assessment tools in the prevention of pressure ulcers. EPUAP Rev 1998;1(1):14

142. Hitch S: Prevention and management of pressure sores. A literature review. J Tiss Viabil 1995;5(1):3–24

143. Cullum N, Deeks J, Flethcher A et al: The prevention and treatment of pressure sores. Effect Healthcare 1995;2(1):1–16

144. Capobianco ML, Dillon McDonald D: Factors affecting the predictive value of the Braden Scale. Adv Wound Care 1996;9(6):32–36

145. Olshansky K: Pressure ulcer risk assessment scales—the missing link. Adv Wound Care 1996;11(2):90

146. Goldstone LA, Goldstone J: The Norton score: an early warning of pressure sores? J Adv Nurs 1982;7:419–426

147. Stotts N: Predicting pressure ulcer development in surgical patients. Heart Lung 1988;17(6):641–647

148. Francis J, Pica KJ: Pressure ulcers. Ann Intern Med 1996;125:421–422

149. Moody BL, Fanale JE, Thompson M et al: Impact of staff education on pressure sore development in hospitalised patients. Arch Intern Med 1988;148:2241–2243

150. Jandziol AK, Ridley SA: Validation of outcome prediction in elderly patients. Anaesthesia 2000;55:107–112

151. Baldwin KM: Transcutaneous oximetry and skin surface temperature as objective measures of pressure ulcer risk. Adv Wound Care 2001;14(1):26–31

152. Clayton DG, Webb RK, Ralston AC, Duthie D, Runciman WB: A comparison of the performance of 20 pulse oximeters under conditions of poor perfusion. Anaesthesia 1991;46:3–10

153. Abu-own A, Sommerville K, Scurr JH, Coleridge Smith PD: Effects of compression and type of bed surface on the microcirculation in the heel. Eur J Vasc Surg 1995;9:327–334

154. Hoffman DR: The False Claims Act as a remedy to the inadequate provision of nutrition and wound care to nursing home residents. Adv Wound Care 1996;9(5):25–29

155. Harper SM, Lyles YM: Physiology and complications of bedrest. J Am Geriatr Soc 1988;36:1047–1054

156. Hibbs P: Preventing an unnecessary evil. Nurs Stand 1987; 5th December

157. Torrance C: Pressure sore survey. Part 1. J Wound Care 1999;8(1):27–30

158. Smoot EC: Beware of the low-pressure bed substitute. Plast Reconstruct Surg 2000;105(5):1908

159. Hall C: People are just being written off by the system. Daily Telegraph 1999;6 Dec:11

160. Dealey C: Pressure sores and incontinence: a study evaluating the use of topical agents in skin care. J Wound Care 1995;4(3):103–105

161. Keogh A, Dealey C: Profiling beds versus standard hospital beds: effects on pressure ulcer incidence outcomes. J Wound Care 2001;10(2):15–19

162. Dr Arnott's hydrostatic bed for invalids. Lond Med Gazette 1832;10:712–714

163. Randorf-Klym LA, Langemo D: Relationships between body weight, body position, support surface and tissue interface pressure at the sacrum. Decubitus 1993;6(1):22–30

164. Medical Devices Agency. Evaluation of foam mattresses. No PS1. London, Department of Health 1993

165. Colin D, Loyant R, Abraham P, Saumet JL: Changes in sacral transcutaneous oxygen tension in the evaluation of different mattress in the prevention of pressure ulcers. Adv Wound Care 1996;9(1):25–28

166. Hofman A, Geelkarken RH, Wille J et al: Pressure sores and pressure decreasing mattresses: controlled clinical trial. Lancet 1994;343:568–571

167. Gray DG, Campbell MK: A randomised clinical trial of two foam mattresses. J Tiss Viabil 1994;4(4):128–131

168. Cooper PJ, Gray DG, Mollinson J: A randomised controlled trial of two pressure reducing surfaces. J Wound Care 1998;7(4):177–179

169. Inman KJ, Sibbald WJ, Rutledge FS, Clark BJ: Clinical utility and cost effectiveness of an air suspension bed in the preventing of pressure sores. JAMA 1993;269:1139–1143

170. Allman RM, Walker JM, Hart MK et al: Air fluidised beds or conventional therapy for pressure sores—a randomised controlled trial. Ann Intern Med 1987;107:641–648

171. Caley L, Jones S, Freer J, Miller JS: Randomised prospective trial of two types of low air loss therapy. In Anon (ed): 7th Symposium on Advanced Wound Care and 14th Annual Medical Research Forum on Wound Repair. Health Management Publications 1994

172. Clark M: Compare maximum and minimum pressures. Br Med J 1994;309:1436

173. Jakobsen J, Christensen KS: Transcutaneous oxygen tension over the sacrum on various anti-decubitus mattresses. Danish Med Bull 1987;34(6):330–331

174. Bliss M, McLaren R, Exton Smith AN: Mattresses for preventing pressure sores in geriatric patients. Med Bull Ministry Health 1966;25:238–267

175. Andersen KE, Jensen O, Kvorning SA, Bach E: Decubitus prophylaxis: a prospective trial of alternating pressure mattresses and water mattresses. Acta Dermatov (Stockholm) 1982;63:227–230

176. Conine JA, Daechsel D, Laus MS: The role of alternating air and silicone overlays in preventing decubitus ulcers. Int J Rehab Res 1990;13:57–65

177. Phillips L: Cost-effective strategy for managing pressure ulcers in critical care: a prospective non-randomised cohort study. J Tiss Viabil 2000;10(3):(suppl):22–26

178. Timmons JP: A randomised controlled trial of two alternating air pressure mattresses. Second European Pressure Ulcer Advisory Panel open meeting. Academic Centre, John Radcliffe Hospital, Oxford; 20–22 September 1998

179. Land L, Evans D, Geary A, Taylor C: A clinical evaluation of an alternating pressure mattress replacement system in hospital and residential care settings. J Tiss Viabil 2000;10(1):6–11

180. Bliss MR: The use of ripple beds in hospitals. Hosp Health Serv Rev 1979;74:190–193

181. Bethel E: Alternating pressure systems are useful. Br Med J 1994;309:1436

182. Bale S: Pressure sore prevention in a hospice. J Wound Care 1995;4:465–468

183. James HM, Fong A: Implementing and evaluating a pressure sore policy. J Tiss Viabil 1996;6:43–45

184. Pring J: Evaluating pressure relieving mattresses. J Wound Care 1998;7(4):177–179

185. Clark M: Pegasus Airwave and fleeces. J Tiss Viabil 1996;6(2):62

186. Wison J: Wheelchair cushioning. Spinal Injuries Assoc Newsl 1992;65:25

187. Goldstone LA, Norris M, O'Reilly M, White JA: Clinical trial of a bead bed system for the prevention of pressure sores in elderly orthopaedic patients. J Adv Nurs 1982;7:545–548

188. Defloor T, De Schuijmer JDS: Preventing pressure ulcers: an evaluation of four operating table mattresses. Appl Nurs Res 2000;13:134–141

189. Nixon J, McElvenny D, Mason S, Brown J, Bond S: A sequential randomised controlled trial comparing a dry viscoelastic polymer pad and standard operating table mattress in the prevention of post operative pressure sores. Int J Nurs Stud 1998;35:1932–1933

190. Moore E, Rithalia S, Gonsalkorale M: Assessment of the Charnwood operating table and hospital trolley mattresses. J Tiss Viabil 1992;2:71–72

191. Neander KD, Birkenfeld R: Decubitus prophylaxis in the operating theatre. J Tiss Viabil 1991;1:71–74

192. Ashcroft GS, Horan MA, Ferguson MWJ: The effects of ageing on cutaneous wound healing. Clin Sci 1995;89:43p–44p

193. Rogers MA: Pressure sores. In Rogers MA (ed): Living with Paraplegia. Faber and Faber, London, 1986:3–63

194. Bennett L, Lee BY: Pressure versus shear in pressure sore causation. In Lee BY (ed): Chronic Ulcers of the Skin. McGraw Hill, New York, 1985:39–56

195. Defloor T: The effect of sitting position and cushion on the development of pressure ulcers. First European Pressure Ulcer Advisory Panel open meeting. Academic Centre. John Radcliffe Hospital, Oxford, England, 21–23 September 1997:20

196. Adam K, Oswald I: Sleep helps healing. Br Med J 1984;289:1400–1401

197. Munro BH, Brown L, Heitman BB: Pressure ulcers: one bed or another. Geriatr Nurs 1989;10:190–192

198. Strauss MJ, Gong J, Gary BD et al: The cost of home air fluidised therapy for pressure sores. J Fam Pract 1991;33:52–57

199. Ferrell BA, Osterweil D, Christensen P: A randomised trial of low air loss beds for treatment of pressure sores. JAMA 1993;269:494–497

200. Stevenson A: Not doing RCTs. J Tiss Viabil 1999;9(1):36–37

201. Groen HW, Groenier KH, Schuling J: Comparative study of a foam mattress and a water mattress. J Wound Care 1999;8(7):333–335

202. Devine B: Alternating pressure air mattresses in the management of established pressure sores. J Tiss Viabil 1995;5:94–98

203. Russell L: Randomised comparative clinical trial of Pegasus Cairwave mattress and Proactive seating cushion and Huntleigh Nimbus 3 and Aura seating cushion. J Tiss Viabil 1999;9(3):103–104

204. Keogh A: An evaluation of alternating air mattresses. J Wound Care 1996; (Suppl abstracts from the 6th European Conference on Advances in Wound Management. RAI Conference Centre, Amsterdam 1–4 October):4

205. Constantian MB, Jackson HS: Biology and care of the pressure ulcer wound. In Constantian MB (ed): Pressure Ulcers: Principles and Techniques of Management. Little, Brown, Boston, 1980:69–100

206. Lewis BK, Harding KG: Nutritional intake and wound healing in elderly people. J Wound Care 1993;2:227–229

207. Tyrell DAJ: Vitamin C and the common cold. Prescrib J 1988;14:21–24

208. Lansdowne ABG: Zinc in the healing wound. Lancet 1996;347:706–709

209. Demling RH, De Santi: Involuntary weight loss and the non healing wound: the role of anabolic steroids. Adv Wound Care 1999;12(suppl 1):1–14

210. Joseph B: Insulin in the treatment of non diabetic bed sores. Ann Surg 1930;92:318

211. Bowler PG: The role of occlusive dressings in infection control. Wound Manag 1996;1:5–6

212. Hutchinson JJ, Lawrence JC: Wound infection under occlusive dressings. J Hosp Infect 1991;17:83–94

213. Galpin JE, Chow AW, Bayer AS, Guse LB: Sepsis associated with decubitus ulcers. Am J Med 1976;61:346–350

214. Working Party Report. Guidelines on the control of methicillin-resistant Staphylococcus aureus in the community. J Hosp Infect 1995;31:1–12

215. Miller M, Dyson M: Principles of Wound Care. Macmillan Press, London, 1996

216. Cameron S, Leaper D: Antiseptic toxicity in open wounds. Nurs Times 1988;84:77–78

217. Dyson M, Young S, Pendle CL et al: Comparison of the effects of moist and dry conditions on dermal repair. J Invest Dermatol 1988;91:434–449

218. Field FK, Kersein MD: Overview of wound healing in a moist environment. Am J Surg 1994;167:28–65

219. Mertz PM, Marshall PA, Eaglestein WH: Occlusive wound dressings to prevent bacterial invasion and wound infection. J Am Acad Dermatol 1985;12:662–668

220. Bowler PG: The role of occlusive dressings in infection control. Wound Manag 1996;1:5–6

221. Chang KW, Alsagoffs S, Ong KT, Sim PH: Pressure ulcers—randomised controlled trial comparing hydrocolloid and saline gauze dressings. Med J Malaysia 1998;53(4):428–431

222. Greenwood D: Honey for superficial wounds and ulcers. Lancet 1993;341:90–91

223. Thomas S: Wound Management and Dressings. Pharmaceutical Press, London, 1990

224. Anon: Adjunctive therapies in wound care. Adv Skin Wound Care 2001;14(1):24

225. Stefanovska A, Vodovnik L, Benko H, Turk R: Treatment of chronic wounds by electric and electromagnetic fields 2: value of FES parameters for pressure sore treatment. Med Biol Eng Comput 1993;31:213–220

226. Eason A, Lee MHM, Folk FS: Accelerated wound healing of pressure ulcers by high peak power electromagnetic energy (Diapulse). Decubitus 1991;4:24–34

227. Deva AK, Buckland GH, Fisher E et al: Topical negative pressure in wound management. Med J Aust 2000;173(3):128–131

228. Flemming K, Cullum N: Therapeutic ultrasound for pressure sores (Cochrane Review). Cochrane Data Base Syst Rev 2000;4:CDOO 1275

229. Upson AV: Topical hyperbaric oxygen in the treatment of recalcitrant open wounds. Practice 1986;66:1408–1412

230. Eaglstein WH, Falanga V: Tissue engineering and the development of Apligraf, a human skin equivalent. Adv Wound Care 1998;11(4):1–8

231. Pierce GF, Tarpley JE, Allman RA et al: Tissue repair processes in healing chronic pressure ulcers treated with recombinant platelet derived growth factor BB. Adv Wound Care 1995;8(5):9

232. Constantian MB: Pressure Ulcers. Principles and Techniques of Management. Little, Brown, Boston, 1980:249–289

233. Department of Health: A First Class Service. Quality in the new NHS. Health Services Circular 1998/113

234. North Thames paper on Clinical Governance, North Thames Office Department of Public Health, London June 1998

235. NHSE, Clinical audit in the NHS: using clinical audit in the NHS: a position statement. 1996

236. Bennett GCJ, Dickinson EJ, Thomas A: National Chronic Wound Audit (1995–1997) Proceedings 7th European Conference on Advances in Wound Management, Harrogate, UK, Nov 1997

237. National Institute for Clinical Excellence. Inherited clinical guidelines B. Pressure ulcer risk assessment and prevention. Department of Health (DOH), London, 2001

238. Bennett GCJ: Opinion: how we keep the truth from patients the NICE way. J Wound Care 2001;10(6):193

239. Tsokos M, Heinemann A, Puschel K: Pressure sores: epidemiology, medico-legal implications and forensic argumentation concerning causality. Int J Legal Med 2000;113(5):283–287

240. Bennett GCJ: Teaching of wound care to medical undergraduates (results from a UK national survey). J Tiss Viabil 1992;2:50–51

241. Hopkins A: Interactive CD-ROM (Wound Care). East London Wound Healing Centre. Presentation to the European Pressure Ulcer Advisory Panel Conference, Pisa, Italy, September 2000

242. Wahlers B, Zimmerdahl V, Muller K et al: Project "Out-patient Function—Prevention and Treatment of Pressure Sores:" Poster. European Wound Management Association Conference, Dublin, Ireland, May 2001

243. Flanagan M: Education and the development of specialist practice. J Wound Care 1998;7;6:304–305

244. Andrews J, Balai R: The prevention and treatment of pressure sores by use of pressure redistributing mattresses. Decubitus 1988;1:4–21

Chapter 107

Sleep, aging, and late-life insomnia

Kevin Morgan

Changes in the structure and quality of sleep have long been recognized as a feature of the aging process. Writing in *The Lancet* over 150 years ago, for example, Dr George Sigmond observed that "The duration of sleep should be, in manhood, about the fourth or the sixth of the 24 hours; children, the younger they are the more sleep they require; in advanced age there is more watchfulness."[1] Similar associations between "watchfulness" and age were noted by Herman Melville who, in his novel *Moby Dick*, commented that "Old age is always wakeful; as if, the longer linked with life, the less man has to do with aught that looks like death."[2] Developments in research methodology, particularly polysomnography, have since confirmed these changes in sleep structure which accompany advancing age,[3] while epidemiological studies have clearly described the age-related increase in complaints of insomnia.[4] Sleep disorders in later life are now an important focus for clinical[3] and economic[5,6] concern, and are widely regarded as a significant policy issue.[7,8] This chapter focuses mainly on insomnia, and aims to provide the background to this concern, and introduce the basis for clinical assessment and management. Since advances in sleep research have engendered an increasingly sophisticated taxonomy of sleep disorders, some familiarity with currently used diagnostic and classificatory systems are essential.

PRESENTATION AND CLASSIFICATION OF INSOMNIA

Broadly, complaints of disturbed sleep may be divided into sleep onset problems (trouble getting to sleep), sleep maintenance problems (trouble staying asleep), and early morning awakening (EMA). These symptoms may occur singly or in combination, and may be transient or long term. Disturbed sleep may also present, not as a complaint of sleeplessness, but rather as a report of excessive daytime sleepiness (hypersomnia). Building on these rather straightforward subjective reports, insomnia is now explicitly defined in three internationally recognized diagnostic systems: the ICD-10 Classification of Mental and Behavioral Disorders;[9] the Diagnostic and Statistical Manual of Mental Disorders (DSM-IV);[10] and the International Classification of Sleep Disorders (ICSD).[11] While all three classifications largely agree on the symptoms of insomnia, there are important differences both in terminology and emphasis.

Insomnia: ICD-10

ICD-10 broadly divides sleep disorders into organic and non-organic, with the latter category further subdivided into dyssomnias (disturbances of the amount, quality, or timing of sleep) and parasomnias (abnormal episodic events occurring during sleep, for example, sleepwalking, nightmares, etc.). In this system, "nonorganic insomnia" is a dyssomnia characterized by persistent (i.e., at least 3 times a week for at least 1 month) difficulty in getting to sleep or staying asleep (or poor quality sleep), which causes the individual concern, and markedly interferes with social or occupational functioning. ICD-10 does not explicitly discriminate between primary insomnia (where the sleep disturbance may be the *only* presenting condition) and secondary insomnia (where the sleep disturbance accompanies other physical or mental disorders).

Insomnia: DSM-IV

DSM-IV uses a broader classification which recognizes four main types of sleep disorder: sleep disorders related to another mental disorder; sleep disorders due to a general medical condition; substance-induced sleep disorders; and primary sleep disorders (i.e., those not associated with a psychiatric, medical, or pharmacological cause). *Primary sleep disorders* in DSM-IV are analogous to the *nonorganic sleep disorders* of ICD-10, and are similarly divided into dyssomnias and parasomnias, with insomnia (as "primary insomnia") again subsumed within the dyssomnias. In DSM-IV the diagnostic features of primary insomnia are also similar to those described in ICD-10 and include a persistent (i.e., for at least one month) complaint of difficulty initiating or maintaining sleep (or of nonrestorative sleep) which causes the individual "significant" distress and is associated with impaired social or occupational functioning. Unlike ICD-10, however, DSM-IV taxonomically separates primary insomnia from those secondary insomnias associated with other disorders. Nevertheless, the system does recognize that, under some circumstances, distinguishing *primary insomnia* from *insomnia related to another mental disorder* "can be especially difficult," and that *sleep disorders due to general medical conditions* are "characterized by symptoms similar to those in primary sleep disorders."

Insomnia: ICSD

The most detailed classification of sleep disorders is that provided by the ICSD, which defines 12 subtypes of "insomnia disorder" (i.e., disorders of initiating or maintaining sleep), and over 50 different insomnia syndromes. Since many of these diagnoses require specialized instrumental monitoring (often laboratory-based polysomnography) the value of the ICSD in everyday practice is probably limited.

The commonest forms of insomnia recognized by this classification (and those closest to the "nonorganic" and "primary" insomnias of ICD-10 and DSM-IV) include *psychophysiological insomnia* (characterized by psychosomatic arousal, excessive concern about sleep adequacy, and somatized tension) *inadequate sleep hygiene* (where the sleep problem appears to be caused or maintained by maladaptive practices), and so-called *sleep-state misperception* (where the chronic complaint of insomnia is not "corroborated" by polysomnographic findings). Though relatively rare, the ICSD diagnosis of *idiopathic insomnia* (a near lifelong constitutional predisposition to poor quality sleep) may also be regarded as a "classic" insomnia.

Overall, then, ICD-10, DSM-IV, and ICSD show widespread consensus as to what constitutes an insomnia, with many apparent differences being terminological rather than fundamental (in each system, for example, the same clinical presentation could attract the diagnosis of "organic insomnia," "primary insomnia," or "psychophysiological insomnia," respectively). In clinical field studies where all three systems have been used, diagnoses have been found to logically inter-relate.[12] In epidemiological studies, however, the strict application of diagnostic criteria possibly underestimates population levels of night-time sleep disturbance. For example, a survey of 12,778 adults in France[13] found that only 29 percent of those reporting "nocturnal sleep problems" met the frequency criteria for insomnia as defined by DSM IV (at least one problem occurring three times a week for at least 1 month), while only a further 19 percent reported sleep problems with "daytime consequences."

INSOMNIA AND AGING

While formal diagnostic classification is increasingly being used in epidemiological studies of insomnia, such categorization remains the exception. Nevertheless, since the seminal studies of McGhie and Russell[14] in the UK, and Karacan et al.[15] in the USA, and despite variations in methodology and criteria, community surveys have shown fairly consistent patterns in the prevalence and natural history of poor sleep quality.

Descriptive epidemiology

Prevalence
The prevalence of insomnia increases steadily with age, and is commonly reported by up to 1 in 3 people aged 65 and over (see Table 107-1). Epidemiological studies have also consistently shown that dissatisfaction with sleep is more common among elderly women than among elderly men (Table 107-1), and is higher among lower income and lower educational attainment groups.[14–18,23–25]

Incidence
In contrast to the abundance of prevalence data, information on the incidence of insomnia (i.e., the rate at which new cases come into existence) is scarce. Using conservative criteria to define cases (see Table 107-1) a modest age gradient in the 1-year incidence of insomnia was reported in the US National Institute for Mental Health (NIMH) catchment study, with incident complaints rising from 5.7 percent among those aged 18–25, to 7.3 percent among those aged 65 and over.[19] Lower estimates of incidence for the age group 65 years and over are reported by Morgan and Clarke,[31] who nevertheless found that incidence continued to show a clear age gradient after 65 years.

For each year at risk in a 4-year follow up, these researchers found incidence rates of 2.8, 3.2, and 3.5 percent for the age groups 65–69, 70–74, and 75–79, respectively.

In the largest study of insomnia incidence to date, Foley et al.[32] report older-age gradients among both men and women. Within the age groups 65–74, 75–84, and 85+, this study of 6,899 participants found 3-year insomnia incidence rates of 12.4, 15.1, and 20.5 percent for men and 14.4, 16.7, and 13.7 percent for women. Interestingly, the overall *annual* rate (unadjusted for mortality) in this US study was 5 percent which, as an overestimate of true person-years incidence, is very close to the 3.1 percent reported by Morgan and Clarke[31] in the UK.

Natural history
Increasing age is also associated with changes both in the nature, and the duration of sleep complaints. Table 107-2 shows the distribution of specific complaints among older people with insomnia (note that the categories are not mutually exclusive, and that a respondent may report more than one problem). Only two studies (Florida[15] and Nottingham[18]) report that, among older people with insomnia, onset problems predominate. The remaining studies all report a greater prevalence, within the insomnia grouping, of sleep maintenance problems, though in the case of the Liverpool[21] data, the differences are slight (73 vs 74 percent). Overall rates of EMA show considerable variation across studies, ranging from 4 percent in Florida[15] to 45 percent in Japan.[30]

Several epidemiological studies report data which indicate that symptoms of disturbed sleep are more persistent in older age groups. When asked to quantify the severity of insomnia, for example, older respondents are more likely to report that the problem occurs "often or all the time"[15] or "a lot."[16] In separate longitudinal follow-up studies conducted among random samples, persistent insomnia symptoms have been reported for 52 percent of older people with insomnia over 3 years,[32] and for 36 percent over 4 years.[31]

The extent to which reported dissatisfaction with sleep among elderly people (as measured in community surveys) translates into complaints of poor sleep (in primary care settings) has only recently attracted research attention. The evidence clearly shows, however, that insomnia remains both widely reported and widely treated in general practice settings.[23,28,33,34] In addition, those reporting sleep problems tend to show significantly higher primary care consultation rates than those who do not.[22,33]

STRUCTURAL CHANGES IN SLEEP

Since the discovery of rapid eye movement (REM) sleep,[35] and the subsequent upsurge of interest in all-night polysomnography, numerous EEG studies have reported age-related changes in the continuity, duration, and depth of sleep. Each of these changes has profound implications for subjective sleep quality as reported in population surveys, and each will be considered in turn.

Continuity of sleep

Relative to that of the young, the sleep of elderly people is characterized by more frequent "shifts" from one sleep stage to

Table 107-1 Prevalence of insomnia (variously defined) among older people living in the community

Location	Age	No. of older respondents	Prevalence (%) Overall	Women	Men
Florida, USA[15]	60–69	NR	20.9[a]	22.6[a]	18.3[a]
	70+	NR	25.9[a]	29.4[a]	20.0[a]
Los Angeles, USA[16]	51–80	336	39.8[b]	NR	NR
National Sample, USA[17]	65–79	798	25.0[c]	NR	NR
Nottingham, UK[18]	65+	1,023	22.5[d]	27.7[d]	14.6[d]
			16.0[e]	19.0[e]	11.6[e]
NIMH Catchment, USA[19]	65+	1,801	12.0[f]	NR	NR
London, UK[20]	60+ (women)			NR	—
		705	33.5[g]		
	65+ (men)			—	NR
Liverpool, UK[21]	65+	1,070	35.0[h]	40.7[h]	25.3[h]
Paris, France[22]	55+	758	31.0[i]	42.5[i]	22.5[i]
Mannheim, Germany[23]	66–92	330	23.0[j]	29.1[j]	7.9[j]
			17.0[k]	17.5[k]	16.9[k]
East Boston, USA[24]	65+	3,537	33.7[l]	36.4	29.4
New Haven, USA[24]	65+	2,717	27.5[l]	31.1[l]	21.2[l]
Iowa, USA[24]	65+	3,028	23.2[l]	25.4[l]	19.5[l]
National Sample, France[25]	65+	NR	NR	37.3[m]	28.7[m]
4 states,* USA[26]	65+	5,201	NR	30.0[n]	14.0[n]
4 states,* USA[26]	65+	5,201	NR	65.0[o]	65.0[o]
Veneto, Italy[27]	65+	2,398	NR	54.0[p]	35.6[p]
Montreal, Canada[28]	65+	227	15.1[q]	9.8[q]	18.7[q]
Lund, Sweden[29]	80+	212	19.0[r]	NR	NR
National Sample, Japan[30]	60+	766	29.5[s]	NR	NR

NR = data not reported.

* North Carolina, California, Maryland, and Pennsylvania.

Insomnia defined as: [a]trouble sleeping "often/all the time"; [b]current difficulty falling or staying asleep; [c]"had trouble and was bothered a lot" by "trouble falling asleep or staying asleep"; [d]problems sleeping "often/all the time"; [e]problems sleeping "sometimes"; [f]"... had trouble falling asleep, staying asleep, or waking too early" for a period of 2 weeks or more, and consulted a professional about it, took medication for it, or stated that it interfered with life a lot, and "... if it was not always the result of physical illness"; [g]having difficulty falling or staying asleep, waking early, or taking sleep medication (prevalence calculated from reported data); [h]"... trouble sleeping recently"; [i]reported "sleep disturbances"; [j]DSM-III-R criteria for severe insomnia; [k]DSM-III-R criteria for severe insomnia but without daytime impairment; [l]"trouble falling asleep and/or waking up too early and not being able to fall asleep again most of the time"; [m]"unsatisfied with sleep or taking medication for sleeping difficulties or anxiety with sleeping difficulties"; [n]sleep onset insomnia "difficulty falling asleep"; [o]sleep maintenance insomnia "frequent awakenings"; [p]compound sleep disturbance index; [q]"dissatisfied with quality of sleep with one or more indicators of insomnia"; [r]wakes 3+ times per night and describes usual sleep as "bad" or "very bad"; [s]"often" or "always" has trouble getting to sleep, staying asleep, or waking too early.

another, and more frequent episodes of intervening wakefulness during the night (see Fig. 107-1). Both events result in sleep which is more broken, and more likely to be rated as poor in quality.[36] Brief periods of EEG wakefulness (alpha activity) during the sleep period are normal at any age, but tend to become more frequent [37,38] in later life. Throughout adult life these "spontaneous" nocturnal awakenings tend to be more common among men, a finding possibly related to the disturbing effects of nocturnal penile tumescence (NPT) which occurs quite mechanically during REM sleep in sexually nondysfunctional men of all ages.[39–41]

In addition to the more conventionally recorded EEG awakenings (which can last for several minutes) "transient arousals" (2–15 second bursts of alpha activity) have also been observed in the sleeping EEG of elderly subjects.[42] While unrelated to behavioral awakenings, these brief episodes of alpha activity, indicative of sleep fragmentation, are positively related to daytime sleepiness (as measured by the Multiple Sleep Latency Test).[42]

Duration of sleep

As periods of intervening wakefulness increase with age in both frequency and duration, the total time spent asleep at night shows a reciprocal decrease. As a result, sleep efficiency (time spent asleep divided by time spent in bed) also tends to decrease. One of the most consistently reported age-related structural changes within NREM sleep is the progressive

Table 107-2 Distribution of specific complaints among older people with insomnia living in the community

Location	Age	Reported problems (%) among older people with insomnia[a]		
		Onset	Maintenance	EMA
Florida, USA[15]	60–69	58.1	20.2	4.0
	70+	53.8	20.9	3.3
Los Angeles, USA[16]	51+	39.9	47.8	41.8
London, UK[20]	65+	NR	NR	5.0
New York, USA[33]	65+	NR	NR	11.0[b]
Nottingham, UK[18]	65+	70.6	63.2	33.6
Uppsala, Sweden[34]	60–69[c]	21.8[d]	31.5[d]	NR
Liverpool, UK[21]	65+	73.0	74.0	23.0
4 states,*USA (men)[26]	65+	14.0	65.0	30.0
4 states,*USA (women)[26]	65+	30.0	65.0	34.0
Veneto, Italy (men)[27]	65+	20.3	60.8	24.5
Veneto, Italy (women)[27]	65+	38.9	59.8	33.3
National sample (Japan)[30]	60+	NR	77.0[e]	45.1[e]

*North Carolina, California, Maryland, and Pennsylvania.

Onset = problems getting to sleep; Maintenance = problems staying asleep;

EMA = early morning awakening; NR = data not reported.

[a]Categories not mutually exclusive.

[b]As defined in the CARE[7] schedule.

[c]Men only.

[d]At least "moderate" difficulty initiating or maintaining sleep.

[e]Calculated from reported data.

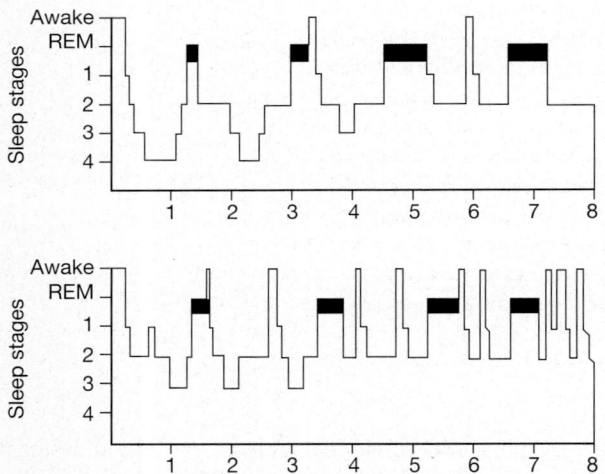

Figure 107-1 Sleep stage profiles for typical younger (above) and older (below) people. Note the decrease in stages 3 and 4, and the reciprocal increase in stages 1 and 2 with increasing age (for an 8-hour sleep period).

reduction in EEG slow waves (those associated with stages 3 and 4 or slow wave sleep)[e.g.,43] and, for many people, the virtual disappearance of stage 4 altogether (Fig. 107-1). These structural changes are particularly evident in spectral studies of the sleep EEG. Using appropriately transformed EEG data, advancing age is associated with significantly lower power densities for frequencies below 16 Hz (which includes stages 3 and 4 slow waves),[44–46] and significantly higher power densities for frequencies above 18 Hz.[44,45]

Depth of sleep

With advancing age depth of sleep is affected both quantitatively and qualitatively. Changes in the architecture of sleep so far considered result in a diminution of deeper slow wave sleep (SWS), and a reciprocal increase in stages 2 (light sleep) and 1 (drowsiness). Older sleep is therefore *structurally* lighter. In addition, studies of auditory awakening thresholds (the minimum amount of noise required to wake a sleeping person) show qualitative changes in the depth of individual sleep stages. It has been shown, for example, that during stages 2, 4, and REM, older people are more easily awakened by noise (i.e., have lower auditory awakening thresholds) than are younger people (this despite reductions in the hearing sensitivity of older subjects).[47] Age-related differences in auditory awakening thresholds have also been observed in comparisons of pre- and post-adolescent males (with older subjects again showing lower awakening thresholds).[48] Taken together, then, the evidence suggests a near lifelong modification of processes underlying arousal from sleep. It is relevant to note, however, that *outside* the laboratory auditory awakening thresholds may not be the best predictor of a given individual's response to nocturnal sound. In an extensive field study of the effects of aircraft noise on the sleep of people living near Heathrow Airport, London, Horne et al.[49] found that sleep disturbances did not increase with age. Rather, the behavior of bed partners and others living in the household appeared to be a more influential factor than aging in determining intrasleep arousals.

Gender differences in sleep quality

Collectively, then, these structural changes in sleep are broadly consistent with the subjective reports from community surveys. It is interesting to note, however, that while epidemiological studies tend to show that women are more likely to report sleep difficulties in later life, the EEG studies indicate that it is men who experience the greater deterioration in their sleep architecture.[50] The reasons for this discrepancy are not clearly understood, but possibly reflect cultural influences on the willingness of men and women to disclose symptoms and problems.

The aging circadian rhythm

In addition to changes in the architecture and depth of (usually night-time) sleep, the circadian rhythm itself also shows evidence of age-related decay, with sleep becoming desynchronized and more likely to encroach on daytime activities. Disturbances of the sleep–wake cycle which result from transmeridian travel[e.g.,51] (particularly where the sleep phase is advanced[52]), shift work,[53] or sleep deprivation[54] are also less well tolerated by older people.

Evidence that the strength of the circadian rhythm is strongly influenced by age-related changes in melatonin secretion has accumulated in recent years.[e.g.,55–57] In clinical trials among elderly people it has been shown that controlled-release melatonin replacement therapy can significantly improve both sleep efficiency[58,59] and sleep onset.[59] Nevertheless, negative associations between melatonin secretion and later-life sleep structure have been reported,[60] suggesting that relationships between this hormone and sleep disruption in older people are complex and, as yet, incompletely understood. Certainly, psychological contributions to circadian synchronization, such as the ability to perceive and respond to social zeitgebers (time cues), and the importance of maintaining regular social habits, should not be overlooked.[61,62]

Structural changes in sleep: normal or abnormal?

Ostensibly measured in healthy subjects, it has long been assumed that many of the age-related structural changes recorded in EEG laboratories reflected aspects of normal ontogenetic change. However, the possibility has now arisen that some of these apparently normal changes may be related to sleep-related respiratory disturbance (SRRD) or periodic leg movements (PLM), awareness of which has grown rapidly in the past 10 years.[3] Both SRRD and PLM are extremely prevalent in later life,[63,64] and are known to be disruptive of sleep continuity and quality. Whether, and to what extent, these conditions have "contaminated" earlier normative studies of human sleep, or whether structural changes in sleep predispose the individual to SRRD and PLM (or vice versa), remains unknown. Issues relating to SRRD are more fully discussed below.

THE ORIGINS OF INSOMNIA

Given that, in old age, structural changes in sleep are experienced by the majority, while complaints of unsatisfactory sleep quality are expressed by the minority, it is reasonable to conclude that age-related change per se is not a sufficient condition for the development of insomnia. Rather, the experimental and epidemiological evidence clearly points to the existence of health, situational, and psychological factors which are strongly associated with the onset and/or the maintenance of disturbed sleep. Since these factors may occur in combination, and are often superimposed upon sleep already compromised by ontogenetic change, it follows that sleep problems in later life are frequently multifactorial in origin. Some of the more important factors known to influence sleep quality in later life have been selected here for discussion (see Table 107-3).

Mental and physical health status

As a correlate of psychological well-being, insomnia continues to be regarded as a critical indicant of both mental health and quality of life; it appears as a prominent diagnostic feature in both ICD-10[9] and DSM-IV[10] (particularly in relation to depression and anxiety states) and is included in the most commonly used health-related quality of life outcome measures, including the Nottingham Health Profile[65] and the SF-36.[66] The symptom of disturbed sleep is also included in most of the available schedules for assessing the mental health of elderly people, including the Geriatric Mental State Schedule (GMS),[67] the Cambridge Mental Disorders of the Elderly Examination (CAMDEX),[68] and the Comprehensive Assessment and Referral Evaluation (CARE).[69] It is likely, however, that the specificity of insomnia as a symptom of mental ill-health is lowest in later life.

With advancing age, from early adulthood to at least the sixth or seventh decade of life, complaints of insomnia steadily increase[15–17,22,24,25,28,30] and are reported by approximately 5 percent of those aged 18–30, but by over 30 percent of those aged 65 years and over. In contrast, the prevalence of those psychiatric conditions most closely associated with insomnia, major depression and anxiety states, appears to peak in earlier adulthood, and decline thereafter.[e.g.,70–73] One result of these divergent patterns is that in later life, disturbed sleep and

Table 107-3 **Factors influencing sleep quality in later life**
• Antecedent history of insomnia
• Age-related changes in sleep structure
• Age-related changes in sleep depth
• Mental health status
• Depression
• Dementia
• Physical health status
• General symptoms
• Sleep related respiratory disturbance
• Periodic leg movements (nocturnal myoclonus)
• Institutionalization
• Poor sleep hygiene
• Personality factors
• Loss of stimulus control

insomnia appear to be far more common than the psychiatric conditions they are used to identify.

The relative contributions of mental and physical health factors to late-life insomnia can be directly assessed from the existing literature. Comparing the performance of various CARE indicator scales, Golden et al.[69] found high correlations not only between the sleep disorder and depression scales ($r = 0.55$), but also between sleep disorders and somatic symptoms ($r = 47$), arthritis (0.36), and leg swelling (0.36) scales. Similar associations are reported by Habte-Gabr et al.[74] for 3,097 elderly people living in rural Iowa, USA. In this extensive survey of health and disturbed sleep, recent hospitalization, limitations of physical function, self-perceptions of health, joint pain and stiffness, emphysema, a history of stroke or heart disease and depressive symptoms were all significantly associated with poor-quality, unrefreshing sleep.

Similarly, Gislason and Almqvist,[75] in their extensive postal survey among a random sample of Swedish men of all ages, conclude "Complaints of DMS [difficulty maintaining sleep] increased with increasing age ... multiple regression clarified that the increase was related to reporting of somatic diseases and overweight." From the same study it was also found that sleep complaints "were almost twice as common among men attending regular medical check-ups for somatic diseases ...." Mental health problems are, nevertheless, prevalent among older insomniacs. In a recent review of community studies, symptoms of depression and anxiety were associated with over 30 percent of later-life sleep complaints within random samples.[76] It is likely, however, that much higher levels of psychiatric comorbidity would be found among clinic populations and general practice attenders.[23]

Dementia

Dementia presents a special area of concern in late-life sleep disturbance, since many of the polygraphic sleep changes seen in normal aged individuals, and described above, are amplified in dementing illness.[77,78] Relative to age-matched controls, demented individuals take longer to get to sleep, wake up more frequently during the night, stay awake longer when disturbed, tend to be more active during periods of wakefulness, and in one study were found to be up to 20 times more likely to fall asleep during the day.[79,80] Changes in the circadian organization of *total* sleep have also been reported in patients with dementia. In a detailed comparison of demented and nondemented inpatients, Allen et al.[79] found that patients with dementia not only slept more during the day, but that some (10 percent) actually slept more during the day than during the night (so-called day–night reversal). These changes in the architecture and circadian timing of sleep, often accompanied by episodes of agitation and wandering (or "sundowning"),[3] contribute substantially to the demands of caring and are among the most frequently cited reasons for the breakdown of caregiving in the community.[e.g.,81]

Recent clinical studies indicate that the nature of a sleep disturbances may distinguish between dementia subtypes, with REM sleep behavior disorder (RBD, characterized by vigorous gross body movements and vocalizations during REM) indicative of dementia with Lewy bodies (DLB).[82,83] However, the existence of wide individual differences in the degree of sleep disturbance among similarly impaired individuals,[84,78] and the failure of sleep disturbance indicators reliably to discriminate between mildly demented patients and nondemented controls[85] suggest that etiological factors may not be alone in determining sleep disruptions in dementia. This conclusion is supported by the findings of Meguro et al.[86] who report that dementia severity (as indexed by the extent of white-matter lesions) and lowered activity levels (as measured by ADL scores) *interact* to increase sleep fragmentation.

Whatever the organic origin, it is likely that the disruption of sleep in dementia is exacerbated by behavioral and environmental factors which, as a result, provide targets for therapeutic interventions.[78] For example, the research evidence clearly indicates that regularizing daytime and night-time activities, optimizing daytime stimulation, minimizing daytime naps, and maximizing the psychological association between the bedroom and sleep all make significant contributions to the maintenance of satisfactory sleep–wake cycles in nondemented insomniacs.[87] In dementing illness, however, the influence of these and other factors may be greatly diminished or lost. For example, a demented patient with severely disturbed night-time sleep may be left to nap ad lib during the day by an exhausted relative. As a result the patient may be less tired and less likely to sleep during the night, which in turn can lead to sleepiness and excess napping the following day, and so on. Support for the general proposition that behavioral factors exacerbate sleep fragmentation in dementia can be found in the clinical literature. Hinchcliffe et al.,[88] for example, describe the successful management of dementia-related night-time sleeplessness and wandering through stimulating daytime "distractions" which prevented excessive napping.

Institutionalization

Relationships between institutionalization and disturbed sleep are strongly suggested by the high levels of hypnotic drug consumption that have consistently been found in hospitals, rest, residential, and nursing homes.[89–93] Within each of these settings, sleep disturbance can be related to the act of admission itself, the personal circumstances necessitating admission, or to the institutional environment. Each of these factors will be considered in turn.

The act of admission

It is well recognized in contemporary sleep research that environmental novelty (such as the first night in the EEG laboratory) results in sleep which is shorter, lighter, and more broken, a phenomenon originally described as the "first night effect,"[94,95] and observed in laboratory studies of older subjects.[38] After a brief period of adaptation (say, 1–2 nights), however, sleep returns to its more "normal" structure.[38] There is no reason to suppose that such phenomena do not accompany institutional admissions. It is possible, however, that such sleeplessness could be interpreted as a clinical event, and inappropriately treated with hypnotic drugs.

Reason for admission

Institutionalization is often accompanied by events which in themselves can be expected to disturb sleep—anxiety, discomfort, pain, bereavement, etc. In hospital settings it is also becoming increasingly apparent that many surgical and medical procedures have a quite detrimental effect on sleep continuity.[96,97]

The institutional environment

Undoubtedly one of the most significant environmental factors that has been shown to influence sleep quality in institutional settings is noise.[98,99] Thus, despite the theoretical importance of sleep in healing and tissue restoration,[100] hospitalization remains a major cause of insomnia.[101] A particularly interesting research finding which may help to explain this state of affairs concerns the discrepancy between sleep parameters as measured by the EEG, and sleep parameters as judged by observers. It was clearly shown in several early studies that, when compared with EEG measures recorded over the same period, nurse ratings consistently overestimate the sleep of hospital patients.[102,103] More recent studies indicate that, even in intensive care units where patients are continuously observed, nurses continue to overestimate the amount of time patients spend asleep.[96] Indeed, in a comparison of 26 studies in which the sleep of elderly people had been either observed or polygraphically recorded, direct observations were found to yield the highest estimates of total sleep time.[84]

The research evidence also suggests that institutional *regimes* can adversely affect sleep quality in old age. Again, while days lacking in structure and stimulation can disturb sleep at almost any age, elderly people do appear to be most at risk. In nursing home residents, for example, disturbed nighttime sleep has been associated with excessive periods in bed. Using wrist actigraphy[104] to monitor sleep and waking, Ancoli-Israel et al.[105] recorded up to five episodes of sleep during the day, and up to 32 episodes of wakefulness during the night in nursing home residents. These investigators concluded that residents had "very little sustained wakefulness and very little sustained sleep." Physical activity levels have also been implicated as a factor contributing to poor sleep in nursing home residents, though the evidence cautions against a simple cause–effect explanation. Thus, while lower activity levels have been significantly associated with sleep fragmentation in elderly nursing home residents,[86] structured activity programs appear to have little impact on the sleep quality of elderly people who are similarly institutionalized.[92]

Lifestyle

In recent years the clinical and research literature has established clear links between aspects of lifestyle (e.g. diet, exercise, sleeping habits, etc.) and sleep quality. Thus, degraded sleep quality in later life has been associated with tea consumption[106] and caffeine levels,[107] excessive daytime napping,[105] excessive time spent in bed,[105] and by unaccustomed night-time food-drinks.[108] Furthermore, in middle-aged people, body weight has also been shown to influence total and percentage REM sleep.[109] Improvements in "sleep hygiene," on the other hand, have been associated with significant and sustained improvements in sleep quality, particularly when combined with psychological therapies.[110] Certainly, regularizing daytime and night-time activities, optimizing daytime stimulation, minimizing daytime naps, and maximizing the psychological association between the bedroom and sleep all make a significant contribution to the maintenance of satisfactory sleep–wake cycles in both older and younger people with insomnia.

Personality factors

Studies comparing the personality profiles of otherwise healthy good and poor sleepers have found consistent differences in young,[111] middle-aged,[112] and elderly[106] subjects. In all cases poor sleepers have shown significantly elevated levels of anxiety and neuroticism as measured by the Minnesota Multiphasic Personality Inventory,[111] the Taylor Manifest Anxiety Inventory,[112] the Spielberger State-Trait Anxiety Inventory, and the Eysenck Personality Questionnaire.[106] Similar relationships between insomnia and anxiety/neuroticism have also been found in sleep clinic patients[113] and representative survey populations.[114] Given that many of these instruments reflect what are presumed to be enduring traits, such characteristics may act as risk factors for insomnia either directly, by contributing to levels of emotional arousal, or indirectly by lowering the threshold at which sleep is perceived to be a problem. That sleep quality is significantly influenced by constitutional factors is also strongly supported by evidence on hereditary predispositions. In a study of over 10,000 elderly people in Sweden, levels of insomnia were found to be significantly higher among those with parents who were both also poor sleepers.[115]

Learning and stimulus control

Stimulus control theory[116] presumes the influence of both operant and classical learning in the onset and maintenance of insomnia. As an operant behavior reinforced by sleep itself, sleep *onset* becomes associated with a number of factors (getting into bed, switching off the light, settling down to sleep) which ultimately become discriminative stimuli for reinforcement (in the presence of which sleep onset becomes more probable). In chronic insomnia, however (whatever the cause), where long periods in bed are increasingly associated with wakefulness, connections between these stimuli and sleep onset can be significantly weakened. Furthermore, through the repeated pairing of bedroom cues with the frustration of sleeplessness, these same stimuli can now, through the mechanisms of classical conditioning, become conditioned stimuli for negative emotional responses which antagonize and sustain episodes of insomnia. Thus factors which initiate insomnia may differ from those factors which maintain insomnia. Treatment, therefore, aims to maximize the stimulus control properties of the bedroom and recondition the environmental cues.[116]

Sleep-related respiratory disturbance

Classified within the ICSD[11] as a dyssomnia giving rise to either insomnia disorders or to disorders of excessive sleepiness, sleep-related respiratory disturbances (SRRD) refer to episodes of apnea and hypopnea which, in affected individuals, suppress the deeper stages of sleep. While criteria and terminology used to describe SRRD varied considerably in earlier studies,[117] the use of the respiratory disturbance index (RDI) has now been widely adopted for clinical and research purposes. Defined as the average number of apneic plus hypopneic episodes per hour of sleep, an RDI of ≥5 was originally considered pathogno-monic of sleep apnea syndrome (SAS).[118] In recent years, how-ever, higher RDI levels (e.g. RDI ≥15) have been found to offer a more realistic criterion for SAS.[119]

The prevalence of SRRD increases significantly with age,[120] with additional, risk factors including being male, snoring, and obesity.[121] Indeed, associations with daytime sleepiness and snoring have proved so robust that these two factors have been described as the "cardinal symptoms" of SAS.[3] The clinical rel-evance of SRRD in the absence of daytime symptoms, how-ever, remains unclear. Community-based studies have shown that low levels of SDB (RDI ≥5) are relatively common among noncomplaining older people, affecting approximately 24 per cent of asymptomatic Americans aged 65 and over.[120]

Using the more stringent criterion of RDI ≥15, however, there appears to be general agreement that SRRD is a major cause of reported sleep disturbance and excessive daytime som-nolence in older people.[122] Nevertheless, though associated with significant levels of morbidity in younger age groups, these higher RDI levels do not emerge as independent predictors of mortality (when chronological age and comorbidity are con-trolled) in elderly samples.[123,124]

While high in normal aged populations, levels of SRRD appear to be even higher among people with dementia,[125,126] particularly demented women.[127] Within small groups of women selected from an Australian retirement village, for example, 72 percent of the demented, compared with 46 per-cent of controls, were found to have RDIs of ≥5.[128] Again the precise clinical relevance of these events is uncertain. It seems reasonable to assume that respiratory disturbances which can be accompanied by prolonged oxygen desaturation and hypox-emia may further compromise neuropsychological functioning in dementing illness. In mildly and moderately demented peo-ple, however, Hoch et al.[129] found no consistent correlations between RDIs, apneic events/hour, lowest oxyhemoglobin desaturation, and psychometric test performance.

Periodic leg movements (PLM)

Also classified within the ICSD[11] as a cause of both insomnia and excessive daytime sleepiness, PLM are characterized by involuntary limb movements which can occur in all stages of sleep, but tend to predominate in the lighter stages (stages 1 and 2).[130] While movement and positional changes occur throughout normal sleep, four or more consecutive limb move-ments lasting 0.5–5 seconds (with an intermovement interval of 4–90 seconds) are regarded as PLM episodes.[131] More than five such episodes per night is considered pathological.[131] As with SRRD, PLM also increases with age, with an estimated prevalence among elderly people living at home of about 45 per cent.[63] Once again, however, not all those showing signs of PLM experience disturbed sleep. Thus, while undoubtedly a cause of disturbed sleep in later life, many of the links between PLM and sleep complaints remain to be explored.

MANAGING INSOMNIA

Advances in the understanding of factors which disturb sleep have, in recent years, been accompanied by substantial progress in the development of effective therapies and strategies for managing late-life insomnia.[87] These therapeutic options include health education, drug management, and psycholog-ical therapies, and their deployment places particular demands on clinical assessment and resource targeting. Combining empirical research findings,[132] authoritative clinical advice,[133] and current prescribing recommendations,[8] a schematic overview of management is presented in Fig. 107-2, and elab-orated below. The aim here is to describe the *structure* of man-agement, and introduce the appropriate therapeutic concepts. Issues of therapeutic practice are dealt with in greater detail in the literature cited.

Assessment

Assessment should aim to clarify the history and current dynamics of the presenting problem, and identify realistic tar-gets for clinical intervention. Since sleep problems occur over time, serial assessment of sleep patterns, using self-completed daily ratings (e.g. Fig. 107-3) or daily sleep diaries (e.g. Fig. 107-4), is extremely useful. Such ratings, continued throughout treatment and follow-up periods, also provide valuable outcome information, and can therefore be used to monitor and adjust management. Assessment should also cover relevant aspects of general health, the patient's sleep history and sleep hygiene, and their current expectations and under-standing of sleep.

While assessment methods can vary from formal question-naire procedures, to less structured clinical consultations, it is worth emphasizing here two assessment-related principles which emerge clearly from the scientific evidence reviewed above. First, since many patients enter middle and later life with pre-existing sleep problems, it should be recognized that sleep disturbances which are reported *in* old age are not nec-essarily due *to* old age. And second, given the operation of stim-ulus control influences, it should be remembered that factors which originally caused a sleep problem (e.g. acute trauma) may be less important than those behavioral factors which can *maintain* a sleep problem (e.g. the acquisition of maladaptive sleep habits).

Following assessment, onward referral may be considered depending on local resources (e.g. the existence of a special-ized service for insomnia or sleep apnea). If referral is not considered, then treatment may be delivered on the basis of triage, as shown in Fig. 107-2. Where insomnia is secondary (as, for example, in depression or arthritis) treatment, or a review of treatment, of the underlying cause may prove suffi-cient. Alternatively (or additionally), insomnia may be treated with one or more specific options as indicated in Fig. 107-2.

Treatment options

Having assessed the patient's understanding and management of their own sleep, information and sleep hygiene advice can be offered as appropriate. The remaining treatments can broadly be divided into drug management and psychological management (the latter including stimulus control approaches, relaxation-based approaches, and cognitive approaches). Detailed descriptions of treatment approaches can be found elsewhere.[87]

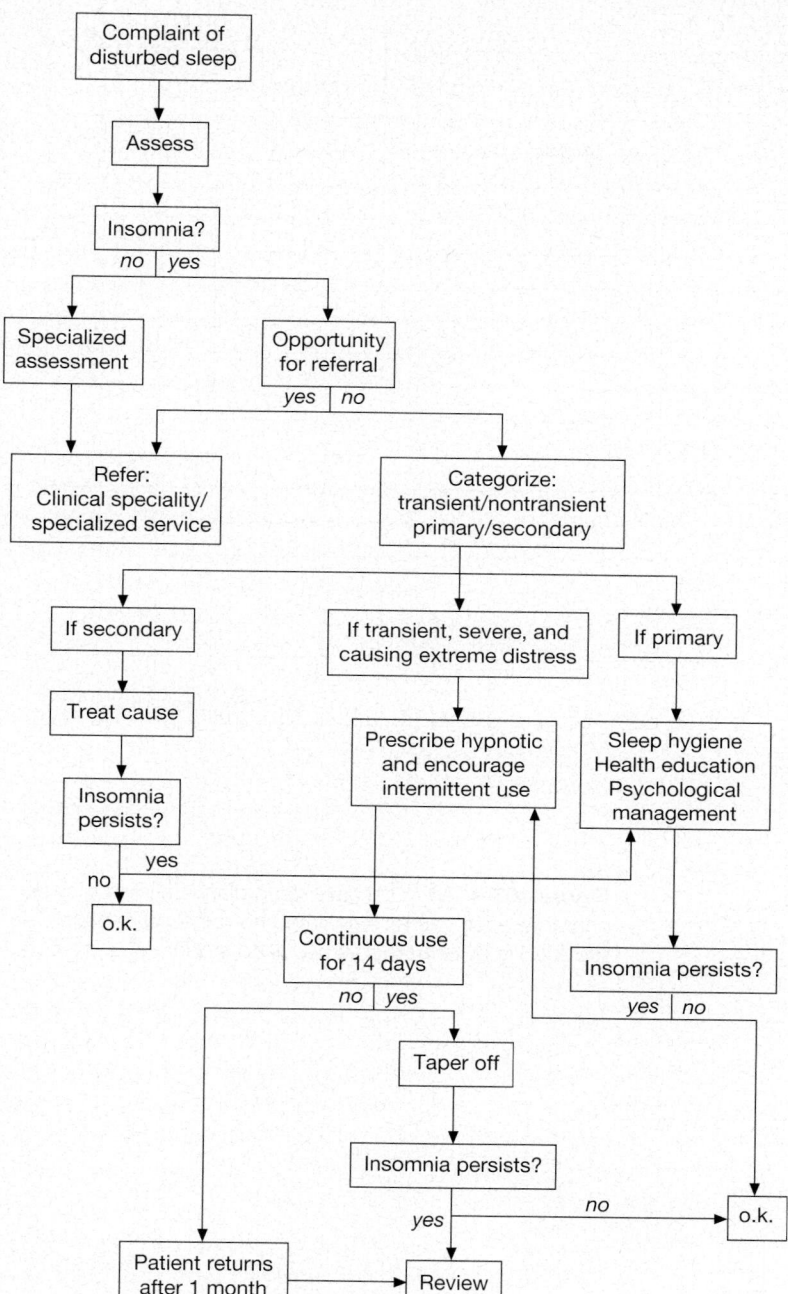

Figure 107-2 A proposed flow-chart for primary care insomnia management. Pathways and choice-points are informed by the literature reviewed in this chapter. (See particularly Refs 8, 133 and 134.)

Drug management

There is now widespread agreement that "hypnotic medication should not be the mainstay of management for most of the causes of disturbed sleep."[7] More recently, clinical guidelines in the UK have made it an explicit responsibility of primary care "to reduce the prescribing of long-term hypnotics for older people by asking older people if they would like to 'come off' long-term benzodiazepines and providing support for them to do so."[8] Nevertheless, hypnotics appear to have an important role in the management of *short-term* insomnias where the daytime consequences of such disturbance are "severe, disabling, or subjecting the individual to extreme distress."[134] From both a pharmacological and psychological perspective, great caution is required in the drug management of late-life insomnia, with hypnotics avoided if at all possible. Where drug management is unavoidable, shorter half-life drugs (at the lowest possible dose) are clearly preferable,[135] with intermittent use encouraged, and a limited "course" of drugs prescribed. Since even brief periods of hypnotic drug consumption may be accompanied by tolerance, products which minimize withdrawal effects should also be preferred, and abrupt discontinuation of the drug avoided.

Psychological management

Psychological approaches to the management of insomnia are now well established in specialized clinical practice,[132] have

Sleep latency (minutes)	120+															
	60															
	50															
	40															
	30															
	20															
	10															
Total sleep (hours)	8+															
	7															
	6															
	5															
	4															
	3															
	2															
	1															
Sleep quality	Very Good															
	Good															
	Average															
	Poor															
	Very poor															
Day		1	2	3	4	5	6	7	8	9	10	11	12	13	14	15
Start date																

Figure 107-3 A simple daily sleep log.

Name .... Date..................

1	At what time did you go to bed last night?
2	At what time did you settle down to sleep?
3	How long did it take you to fall asleep
4	How many times did you wake up?
5	What woke you up?
6	For how long do you think you were awake on each of these occasions?
7	At what time did you finally wake up?
8	How did you feel when you woke up this morning? (tick one) — Refreshed and alert ☐ / Alert but not at peak ☐ / Tired ☐ / Absolutely shattered ☐
9	At what time did you get up?
10	How would you rate last night's sleep? (tick one) — Very good ☐ / Good ☐ / Average ☐ / Poor ☐ / Very poor ☐
11	What medicines did you take yesterday?
12	How much alcohol did you drink yesterday?

Figure 107-4 A typical daily sleep diary. Estimated sleep characteristics can be calculated from the information provided (e.g. total sleep time, sleep efficiency).

been successfully deployed in primary care settings,[136] and are well tolerated and highly effective when used among elderly patients.[137]

STIMULUS CONTROL PROCEDURES One of the most successful psychological methods for treating insomnia,[132] stimulus control includes a variety of strategies for strengthening and maintaining associations between bedroom and sleep onset (see above). These include going to bed only when tired, using the bedroom only for sleep and sex, leaving the bedroom if sleep onset does not occur within 15–20 minutes (following either "lights-out," or a nocturnal awakening), and arising at a pre-set time irrespective of the amount slept. While shown to be effective in the management of late-life insomnias,[137] the standard stimulus control instructions (arising from bed in the night for example) may not be appropriate for all elderly patients.

RELAXATION-BASED TREATMENTS Progressive relaxation, autogenic training, and electromyographic feedback techniques for reducing somatic tension have all been found effective in the management of sleep-onset insomnia, with long-term benefits apparent at follow-up.[87] Evaluation studies among elderly people, however, remain rare. Nevertheless, it is reasonable to suggest that, under some circumstances (e.g. coexisting arthritis) progressive relaxation, with its emphasis on muscle tension, may be inappropriate.

COGNITIVE TREATMENTS Cognitive therapies have been found effective in the treatment of older insomniacs,[138] chronic insomniacs,[139] and clinically heterogeneous insomniac groups.[140] Aimed primarily at reducing cognitive arousal and focusing pre-sleep mentation, therapeutic strategies vary from imagery training to paradoxical intention (i.e. instructing the patient to remain awake, and thereby reducing anxieties about getting to sleep). While effective both alone, and in combination with relaxation therapies, the evidence does suggest that the benefits from some cognitive approaches may be less robust, and more variable than others.

Review

While the post-assessment triage in Fig. 107-2 suggests clear boundaries between diagnostic categories, the "Review" box acknowledges that not all the treatment options indicated will benefit all the patients. Review, therefore, presents an opportunity to consolidate experience gained, and consider remaining options. Persistent insomnias at first assumed to be transient, those who show poor compliance with psychological treatments, patients with complex sleep problems who may otherwise become chronic drug users, and secondary insomnias where the underlying condition, and hence the insomnia, vary in severity may all require reconsideration at this point.

CONCLUSIONS

In addition to senescent changes which directly influence the structure and quality of sleep, advancing age is also associated with an increasing number of events which can influence and disturb sleep indirectly. As a result, sleep problems in old age are both prevalent and complex. Academic and clinical sleep research has, in recent years, made considerable progress in identifying and clarifying some of the specific causes and correlates of disturbed sleep in later life. It is now clear that such problems, often multifactorial in origin, require a broad and flexible clinical response. Consonant with this growth in research knowledge, treatment approaches have become increasingly systematized in recent years, with due emphasis given to sleep assessments, health education and sleep hygiene, and the appropriate deployment of both pharmacological and psychological therapies. In this respect it is relevant to note that nonpharmacological treatments may often be more acceptable to patients.[141] The evidence also suggests, however, that there are many situations where, as elsewhere, prevention is better than cure.

KEY POINTS Sleep, aging, and late-life insomnia

- Insomnia increases steadily with age, affecting up to 30 percent of those aged 65 and over.

- Singly or in combination, physiological, clinical, situational, and personal factors can all influence sleep quality in later life.

- In addition to routine clinical examinations, assessments of sleep history, sleep hygiene, and patient expectations are essential for guiding insomnia treatment options.

- Evidence-based treatments for late-life insomnia include health education, improved sleep hygiene, psychological treatments, and hypnotic drugs.

- Treatment choice should be strongly influenced by the expected chronicity of the sleep complaint.

- The continuous, long-term use of hypnotics should be avoided.

REFERENCES

1. Sigmond GG: Lectures on materia medica and therapeutics. Lancet 1836; 37(1):214–220
2. Melville H: Moby Dick. Penguin, London, 1994 (original work published 1851)
3. Bliwise D: Sleep in normal aging and dementia. Sleep 1993;16:40–81
4. Partininen M: Epidemiology of sleep disorders. In Kryger MH, Roth T, Dement WC (eds): Principles and Practice of Sleep Medicine. Saunders, Philadelphia, 1994:437–452
5. Leger D: The cost of sleep related road accidents: a report for the National Commission on Sleep Disorders Research. Sleep 1994;17:84–93
6. Walsh JK, Engelhardt CL: The direct economic costs of insomnia in the United States for 1995. Sleep 1999;22:S386–S393
7. National Institutes of Health. Consensus development conference statement: the treatment of sleep disorders of older people. Sleep 1991;14:169–177
8. Department of Health: Medicines and older people: Implementing the medicines-related aspects of the NSF (National Service Framework) for older people. HMSO, London, 2001
9. World Health Organization: The ICD-10 Classification of Mental and Behavioral Disorders. World Health Organization, Geneva, 1993
10. American Psychiatric Association: Diagnostic and Statistical Manual of Mental Disorders: DSM-IV. American Psychiatric Association, Washington, DC, 1994
11. American Sleep Disorders Association. The International Classification of Sleep Disorders: Diagnostic and Coding Manual. American Sleep Disorders Association, Rochester, Minnesota, 1990

12. Buysse DJ, Reynolds CF, Kupfer DJ et al: Clinical diagnoses in 216 insomnia patients using the International Classification of Sleep Disorders (ICSD), DSM-IV and ICD-10 categories. A report from the APA/NIMH DSM-IV field trial. Sleep 1994;17:630–637

13. Leger D, Guilleminault C, Dreyfus JP et al: Prevalence of insomnia in a survey of 12778 adults in France. J Sleep Res 2000;9:35–42

14. McGhie A, Russell SM: The subjective assessment of normal sleep patterns. J Ment Sci 1962;108:642–654

15. Karacan I, Thornby JI, Anch H et al: The prevalence of sleep disturbance in a primarily urban Florida county. Soc Sci Med 1976;10:239–244

16. Bixler EO, Kales A, Soldatos CR et al: Prevalence of sleep disorders in the Los Angeles Metropolitan area. Am J Psychiatry 1979;10:1257–1262

17. Mellinger GD, Balter MB, Uhlenhuth EH: Insomnia and its treatment. Arch Gen Psychiatry 1985;42:225–232

18. Morgan K, Dallosso H, Ebrahim S et al: Characteristics of subjective insomnia among the elderly living at home. Age Ageing 1988;17:1–7

19. Ford DE, Kamerow DB: Epidemiologic study of sleep disturbances and psychiatric disturbances. JAMA 1989;262:1479–1484

20. Livingston G, Hawkins A, Graham N et al: The Gospel Oak study: prevalence rates of dementia, depression and activity limitation among elderly residents in Inner London. Psych Med 1990;20:137–146

21. Brabbins CJ, Dewey ME, Copeland JRM et al: Insomnia in the elderly: prevalence, gender differences, and relationships with morbidity and mortality. Int J Geriatr Psychiatry 1993;8:473–480

22. Jacquinet-Salord MC, Lang T, Fouriaud C et al: Sleeping tablet consumption, self reported quality of sleep, and working conditions. J Epidemiol Commun Health 1993;47:64–68

23. Hohagen F, Käppler C, Schramm E et al: Prevalence of insomnia in general practice attenders and the current treatment modalities. Acta Psychiatr Scand 1994;90:102–108

24. Foley DJ, Monjan AA, Brown SL et al: Sleep complaints among elderly persons: An epidemiologic study of three communities. Sleep 1995;18:425–432

25. Ohayon M: Epidemiologic-study on insomnia in the general-population. Sleep 1996;19:S7–S15

26. Newman AB, Enright PL, Manolio TA et al: Sleep disturbance, psychosocial correlates, and cardiovascular disease in 5201 older adults: the cardiovascular health study. JAGS 1997;45:1–7

27. Maggi S, Langlois JA, Minicuci N et al: Sleep complaints in community-dwelling older persons: prevalence, associated factors, and reported causes. JAGS 1998;46:161–168

28. Ohayon MM, Caulet M, Guilleminault C: How a general population perceives its sleep and how this relates to the complaint of insomnia. Sleep 1997;20:715–723

29. Jensen E, Dehlin O, Hagberg B et al: Insomnia in an 80-year-old population: relationship to medical, psychological and social factors. J Sleep Res 1988;7:183–189

30. Kim K, Uchiyama M, Okawa M et al: An epidemiological study of insomnia among the Japanese general population. Sleep 2000;23:41–47

31. Morgan K, Clarke D: Longitudinal trends in late-life insomnia: implications for prescribing. Age Ageing 1997;26:179–184

32. Foley DJ, Monjan A, Simonsick EM et al: Incidence and remission of insomnia among elderly adults: an epidemiologic study of 6,800 persons over 3 years. Sleep 1999;22(suppl 2):S366–S378

33. Weyerer S, Dilling H: Prevalence and treatment of insomnia in the community—results from the upper Bavarian field-study. Sleep 1991;14:392–398

34. Pharoah PDP, Melzer D: Variations in prescribing of hypnotics, anxiolytics and antidepressants between 61 general practices. Br J Gen Practice 1995;45:595–599

35. Aserinsky E, Kleitman N: Regularly occurring periods of eye motility, and concomitant phenomena during sleep. Science 1953;118:273–274

36. Oswald I: Sleep studies in clinical pharmacology. Br J Clin Pharmacol 1980;10:317–326

37. Webb WB: Sleep in older persons: sleep structures in 50-to 60-year-old men and women, J Gerontol 1982;37:581–586

38. Reynolds CF, Kupfer DJ, Taska LS et al: Sleep of healthy seniors: a revisit. Sleep 1985;8:20–29

39. Karacan I, Williams RL, Thornby JI et al: Sleep-related tumescence as a function of age. Am J Psychiatry 1975;132:932–937

40. Schiavi RC, Schreiner-Engel P: Nocturnal penile tumescence in healthy aging men. J Gerontol A 1988;43:M146–M150

41. Gheorghiu S, Mulligan T, Veldhuis JD: Lack of temporal association among REM sleep, LH secretion, testosterone secretion, and nocturnal penile tumescence (NPT) in healthy aged men. J Am Geriatr Soc 1995;43:SA81

42. Carskadon MA, Brown ED, Dement WC: Sleep fragmentation in the elderly: relationship to daytime sleep tendency. Neurobiol Aging 1982;3:321–327

43. Prinz PN, Vitaliano PP, Vitiello MV et al: Sleep, EEG and mental function changes in senile dementia of the Alzheimer's type. Neurobiol Aging 1982;3:361–370

44. Larsen LH, Moe KE, Vitiello MV, Prinz PN: Age trends in the sleep EEG of healthy older men and women. J Sleep Res 1995;4:160–172

45. Carrier J, Land S, Buysse DJ et al: The effects of age and gender on sleep EEG power spectral density in the middle years of life (ages 20–60 years old). Psychophysiology 2001;38:232–242

46. Landholt HP, Borbely AA: Age-dependent changes in sleep EEG topography. Clin Neurophys 2001;112:369–377

47. Zepelin H, McDonald CS, Zammit GK: Effects of age on auditory awakening thresholds. J Gerontol 1984;39:294–300

48. Busby KA, Mercier L, Pivik RT: Ontogenic variations in auditory arousal threshold during sleep. Psychophysiology 1994;31:182–188

49. Horne JA, Pankhurst FL, Reyner LA et al: A field study of sleep disturbance: effects of aircraft noise and other factors on 5,742 nights of actimetrically monitored sleep in a large subject sample. Sleep 1994;7:146–159

50. Rediehs MH, Reis JS, Creason NS: Sleep in old age: focus on gender differences. Sleep 1990;13:410–424

51. Dement WC, Seidel WF, Cohen SA et al: Sleep and wakefulness in aircrew before and after transoceanic flights. Aviat Space Environ Med (suppl 12) 1986:B14–B28

52. Monk TH, Buysse DJ, Carrier J, Kupfer DJ: Inducing jet-lag in older people: directional asymmetry. J Sleep Res 2000;9:101–116

53. Monk TH: Shift work. In Kryger MH, Roth T, Dement WC (eds): Principles and Practice of Sleep Medicine. WB Saunders, Philadelphia, 1994.

54. Webb WB: Sleep stage responses of older and younger subjects after sleep deprivation. Electroenceph Clin Neurophysiol 1981;52:368–371

55. Short RV: Melatonin: hormone of darkness. Br Med J 1993;307:952–953

56. Haimov I, Laudon M, Zisapel N et al: Sleep disorders and melotonin rhythms in elderly people. Br Med J 1994;309:167

57. Turek FW, Zee P, Reeth: Melatonin and aging. Adv Ex Med Biol 1999;460:435–440

58. Garfinkel D, Laudon M, Nof D, Zisapel N: Improvement of sleep quality in elderly people by controlled-release melatonin. Lancet 1995;346:541–544

59. Haimov I, Lavie P, Laudon M et al: Melatonin replacement therapy of elderly insomniacs. Sleep 1995;18:598–603

60. Youngstedt SD, Kripke DF, Elliott JA: Melatonin excretion is not related to sleep in the elderly. J Pineal Res 1998;24:142–145

61. Minors DS, Rabbitt PMA, Worthington H: Variation in meals and sleep-activity patterns in aged subjects—its relevance to circadian rhythm studies. Chronobiol Int 1989;6:139–146

62. Monk TH, Reynolds CF, Machen MA, Kupfer DJ: Daily social rhythms in the elderly and their relationship to objectively recorded sleep. Sleep 1992;15:322–329

63. Ancoli-Israel S, Kripke DF, Klauber MR et al: Sleep disordered breathing in community dwelling elderly. Sleep 1991;14:486–495

64. Ancoli-Israel, S, Kripke DF, Klauber MR et al: Periodic limb movements in sleep in community dwelling elderly. Sleep 1991;14:496–500

65. Hunt SM, McEwen J, McKenna SP: Perceived health—age and sex comparisons in a community. J Epidemiol Commun Health 1984;38:156–160

66. Brazier JE, Walters SJ, Nicholl JP et al: Using the SF-36 and Euroqol on an elderly population. Quality Life Res 1996;5:195–204

67. Copeland JRM, Kelleher MJ, Kellett JM et al: A semi-structured clinical interview for the assessment of diagnosis and mental state in the elderly. The Geriatric Mental State Schedule. 1. Development and reliability. Psychol Med 1976;6:439–447

68. Roth M, Tym E, Mountjoy CQ et al: CAMDEX: A standardised instrument for the diagnosis of mental disorder in the elderly with special reference to the early detection of dementia. Br J Psychiatry 1986;149:698–709

69. Golden RR, Teresi JA, Gurland BJ: Development of indicator scales for the Comprehensive Assessment and Referral Evaluation (CARE) interview schedule. J Gerontol 1984;39:138–146

70. Myers JK, Weissman MM, Tischler GL et al: Six-month prevalence of psychiatric disorders in three communities: 1980–1982. Arch Gen Psychiatry 1984;41:959–967

71. Kessler RC, McGonagle KA, Zhao S et al: Lifetime and 12-month prevalence of DSM-III-R psychiatric disorders in the United States. Arch Gen Psychiatry 1994;51:8–19

72. Weissman MM, Bland RC, Canino GJ et al: Cross-national epidemiology of major depression and bipolar disorder. JAMA 1996;276:293–299

73. Isometsä E, Aro S, Aro H: Depression in Finland: a computer assisted telephone, interview study. Acta Psychiatr Scand 1997;96:122–128

74. Habte-Gabr E, Wallace RB, Colsher PL et al: Sleep patterns in rural elders: demographic, health, and psychobehavioral correlates. J Clin Epidem 1991;44:5–13

75. Gislason T, Almqvist M: Somatic diseases and sleep complaints. Acta Med Scand 1987;221:475–481

76. Morgan K: Mental health factors in late-life insomnia. Rev Clin Gerontol 1996;6:75–83

77. Van Someren EJW, Hagebeuk EEO, Lijzenga C et al: Circadian rest-activity rhythm disturbances in Alzheimer's disease. Biol Psychiatry 1996;40:259–270

78. McCurry SM, Reynolds CF, Ancoli-Israel S, et al: Treatment of sleep disturbance in Alzheimer's disease. Sleep Med Rev 2000;4:603–628

79. Allen SR, Seiler WO, Stähelen HB, Speigel R: Seventy two hour polygraphic and behavioral recordings of wakefulness and sleep in a hospital geriatric unit: comparison between demented and nondemented patients. Sleep 1987;10:143–159

80. Prinz PN, Peskind ER, Vitaliano PP et al: Changes in the sleep and waking EEGs of nondemented and demented elderly subjects. J Am Geriatr Soc 1982;30:86–93

81. Pollak CP, Perlick D: Sleep problems and institutionalization of the elderly. J Geriatr Psychiatry Neurol 1991;15:123–135

82. Grace JB, Walker MP, McKeith IG: A comparison of sleep profiles in patients with dementia with Lewy bodies and Alzheimer's disease. Int J Geriatr Psychiatry 2000;15:1028–1033

83. Boeve BF, Silber MH, Ferman TJ et al: REM sleep behaviour disorder and degenerative dementia—An association likely reflecting Lewy body disease. Neurology 1998;51:363–370

84. Regestein QR, Morris J: Daily sleep patterns observed among institutionalized elderly residents. J Am Geriatr Soc 1987;35:767–772

85. Vitiello M, Prinz PN, Williams DE et al: Sleep disturbances in patients with mild-stage Alzheimer's disease. J Gerontol A 1990;45:M131–M138

86. Meguro K, Ueda M, Kobayashi I et al: Sleep disturbance in elderly patients with cognitive impairment, decreased daily activity and periventricular white matter lesions. Sleep 1995;18:109–114

87. Lichstein KL, Morin CM (eds): Treatment of Late-Life Insomnia. Sage Publications, Thousand Oaks, 1999:3–36

88. Hinchcliffe AC, Hyman I, Blizard B, Livingston G: The impact on carers of behavioural difficulties in dementia: a pilot study on management. Int J Geriatr Psychiatry 1991;7:579–583

89. Seppala M, Rajala T, Sourander L: Subjective evaluation of sleep and the use of hypnotics in nursing-homes. Aging Clin Exper Res 1993;5:199–205

90. Middelkoop HAM, Kerkhof GA, Smilde-Van Den Doel DA et al: Sleep and ageing: the effects of institutionalisation on subjective and objective characteristics of sleep. Age Ageing 1994;23:411–417

91. Snowdon J, Vaughan R, Miller R et al: Psychotropic-drug use in Sydney nursing-homes. Med J Aust 1995;163:70–72

92. Alessi CA, Schnelle JF, Traub S, Ouslander JG: Psychotropic medications in incontinent nursing home residents: Association with sleep and bed mobility. J Am Geriatr Soc 1995;43:789–792

93. Opedal K, Schjott J, Eide E: Use of hypnotics among patients in geriatric institutions. Int J Geriatr Psychiatry 1998;13:846–851

94. Agnew HW, Webb WB, Williams RL: The first night effect: an EEG study of sleep. Psychophysiology 1966;12:412–415

95. Scharf MB, Kales A, Bixler EO: Readaptation to the sleep laboratory in insomniac subjects. Psychophysiology 1975;12:412–415

96. Aureff J, Elmqvist D: Sleep in the surgical intensive care unit: continuous polygraphic recording of sleep in nine patients receiving postoperative care. Br Med J 1985;290:1029–1032

97. Meyer TJ, Eveloff SE, Bauer MS et al: Adverse environmental-conditions in the respiratory and medical ICU settings. Chest 1994;105:1211–1216

98. Soutar RL, Wilson JA: Does hospital noise disturb patients? Br Med J 1986;292:305

99. Yinnon AM, Ilan Y, Tadmor B et al: Quality of sleep in the medical department. Br J Clin Practice 1992;46:88–91

100. Adam K, Oswald I: Sleep helps healing. Br Med J 1984;289:1400–1410

101. Morgan K, Closs SJ: Sleep Management in Nursing Practice. Churchill Livingstone, Edinburgh, 1999:183–205

102. Kupfer DJ, Wyatt RJ, Snyder F: Comparison between electroencephalographic and systematic nursing observations of sleep in psychiatric patients. J Nerv Ment Dis 1970;151:361–368

103. Weiss BL, McPartland RL, Kupfer DL: Once more: the inaccuracy of non-EEG estimates of sleep. Am J Psychiatr 1973;130:1282–1285

104. Sadeh A, Hauri P, Kripke DF, Lavie P: The role of actigraphy in the evaluation of sleep disorders. Sleep 1995;18:288–302

105. Ancoli-Israel S, Parker L, Sinaee R et al: Sleep fragmentation in patients from a nursing home. J Gerontol A 1989;44:M18–M21

106. Morgan K, Healey DW, Healey P: Factors influencing persistent subjective insomnia in old age: a follow-up study of good and poor sleepers aged 65 to 74. Age Ageing 1989;18:117–122

107. Curless R, French JM, James OFW, Wynne HA: Is caffeine a factor in subjective insomnia of elderly people. Age Ageing 1993;22:41–45

108. Adam K: Dietary habits and sleep after food drinks. Sleep 1980;3:47–58

109. Adam K: Total and percentage REM sleep correlate with body weight in 36 middle-aged people. Sleep 1987;10:69–77

110. Schoicket SA, Bertelson AD, Lacks P: Is sleep hygiene a sufficient treatment for sleep-maintenance insomnia. Behav Therapy 1988;19:183–190

111. Monroe LJ: Psychological and physiological differences between good and poor sleepers. J Abnormal Psychol 1967;72:255–264

112. Adam K, Tomeny M, Oswald I: Physiological and Psychological differences between good and poor sleepers. J Psych Res 1986;20:301–316

113. Kales A, Caldwell AB, Soldatos CR et al: Biopsychobehavioral correlates of insomnia II: pattern specificity and consistency with MMPI. Psychosom Med 1983;45:341–356

114. Hyyppa MT, Kronholm E, Mattlar CE: Mental well-being of good sleepers in a random population sample. Br J Med Psychol 1991;64:25–34

115. Asplund R: Are sleep disorders hereditary? A questionnaire survey of persons about themselves and their parents. Arch Gerontol Geriatrics, 1995;21:231

116. Bootzin RR, Epstein D, Wood JM: Stimulus control instructions. In Hauri P (ed): Case Studies in Insomnia. Plenum Press, New York, 1991

117. Berry DTR, Phillips BA: Sleep disordered breathing in the elderly: review and methodological comment. Clin Psychol Rev 1988;8:101–120

118. Guilleminault C, van den Hoed J, Mitler M: Clinical overview of the sleep apnea syndromes. In Guilleminault C, Dement W (eds): Sleep Apnea Syndromes. Alan R Liss, New York, 1979:1–11

119. Gould GA, Whyte KF, Rhind GB et al: The sleep hypopnea syndrome. Am Rev Respirat Dis 1988;137:895–898

120. Ancoli-Israel S, Coy T: Are breathing disturbances in elderly equivalent to sleep apnea syndrome? Sleep 1994;17:77–83

121. Bliwise DL, Feldman DE, Bliwise NG et al: Risk factors for sleep disordered breathing in heterogeneous geriatric populations. J Am Geriatr Soc 1987;35:132–141

122. Ancoli-Israel S, Kripke DF, Mason WJ, Gabriel S, Kaplan D: Sleep apnea and PMS in a randomly selected elderly population: final prevalence results. Sleep Res 1986;15:101 (abstract)

123. Mant A, King M, Saunders NA et al: Four-year follow-up of mortality and sleep-related respiratory disturbance in non-demented seniors. Sleep 1995;18:433–438

124. Ancoli-Israel S, Kripke DF, Klauber MR et al: Morbidity, mortality and sleep-disordered breathing in community dwelling elderly. Sleep 1996;19:277–282

125. Erkinjuntti T, Partinen M, Sulkava R et al: Sleep apnea in multi-infarct dementia and Alzheimer's disease. Sleep 1987;10:419–425

126. Janssens JP, Pautex S, Hilleret H, Michel JP: Sleep disordered breathing in the elderly. Aging Clin Exp Res 2000;12:417–429

127. Frommlet M, Prinz P, Vitiello MV et al: Sleep hypoxemia and apnea are elevated in females with mild Alzheimer's disease. Sleep Res 1986;15:189 (abstract)

128. Mant A, Saunders NA, Eyland AE et al: Sleep-related respiratory disturbance and dementia in elderly females. J Gerontol A 1988;43:5:M140–M144

129. Hoch CC, Reynolds CF III, Nebes RD et al: Clinical significance of sleep-disordered breathing in Alzheimer's Disease: Preliminary Data. J Am Geriatr Soc 1989;37:138–144

130. Montplaisir J, Godbout R, Pelletier G, Warnes H: Restless legs syndrome and periodic movements during sleep. In Kryger MH, Roth T, Dement WC (eds): Principles and Practice of Sleep Medicine. WB Saunders, Philadelphia, 1994

131. Coleman RM: Periodic movements in sleep (nocturnal myoclonus) and restless legs syndrome. In Guilleminault C (ed): Sleeping and Waking

Disorders: Indications and Techniques. Addison-Wesley, Menlo Park, CA, 1982:265–295

132. Morin CM, Hauri PJ, Espie CA et al: Nonpharmacologic treatment of chronic insomnia. Sleep 1999;22:1134–1156

133. Sateia MJ, Doghramji K, Hauri PJ, Morin CM: Evaluation of chronic insomnia: An American Academy of Sleep Medicine Review. Sleep 2000;23:243–308

134. Committee on Safety of Medicines. Benzodiazepine dependence and withdrawal. Curr Problems 1988;21:1–2

135. Morgan K: Hypnotic drugs, psychomotor performance and ageing. J Sleep Res 1994;3:1–15

136. Espie CA, Inglis SJ, Tessier S, Harvey L: The clinical effectiveness of cognitive behaviour therapy for chronic insomnia: implementation and evaluation of a sleep clinic in general medical practice. Behav Res Ther 2001;39:45–60

137. Morin CM, Colecchi C, Stone J et al: Behavioral and pharmacological therapies for late-life insomnia—A randomized controlled trial. JAMA 1999;281:991–999

138. Morin CM, Azrin NH: Behavioral and cognitive treatments of geriatric insomnia. J Consult Clin Psychol 1988;56:748–753

139. Espie CA, Lindsay WR, Brooks DN et al: A controlled comparative investigation of psychological treatments for chronic sleep-onset insomnia. Behav Res Ther 1989;27:79–88

140. Morin CM, Culbert JP, Schwartz SM: Nonpharmacological interventions for insomnia: a meta analysis of treatment efficacy. Am J Psychiatry; 151:1172–1180

141. Morin CM, Gaulier B, Barry T, Kowatch RA: Patients' acceptance of psychological and pharmacological therapies for insomnia. Sleep 1992;15:302–305

Chapter 108

Eating disorders

Gerald Blandford

All living things must receive adequate nutrition to survive. In both animals and man the acts of food gathering and eating are innate and failure results in malnutrition, morbidity, and death. However, in man the acts and processes of food acquisition and preparation that precede eating are much more complicated than in other species. For elderly people, eating is a task that is not only complex, but often lonely and onerous, and hindered by multiple factors. These include the effects of aging, economic deprivation, poor social support, physical disability, acute and chronic disease states, and medication usage. As a consequence, the process of eating for elderly people is highly susceptible to failure, with subsequent inanition and its outcomes.[1] These consequences form the imperative for this chapter, which reviews the underlying causes, and diagnostic and management strategies for impaired eating in old age.

EPIDEMIOLOGY

The principal indicator for the presence of disordered eating in aging is malnutrition. The measurement of nutritional status is relatively imprecise and the prevalence of malnutrition varies based on the methods used and the population studied.[2–4] Undernutrition is the predominant problem and has been the subject of an excellent recent review.[5] Most geriatric studies have concentrated on protein calorie malnutrition. The prevalence of malnutrition in elderly people is variously estimated at 10–25 percent for those in the community over 65 years,[6,7] 30–61 percent for hospital patients,[6,8] and 17–85 percent for nursing home residents.[2,6,9] Any clinical condition with such serious consequences and such high prevalence must be taken seriously. Potential underlying causes require rigorous investigation.

AGING AND THE PROCESS OF EATING

The requirements for eating are listed in Table 108-1. Eating and drinking are driven by hunger or thirst, habit, or a deliberate wish to eat. Food must be acquired, prepared, and presented for eating, and the individual must be able to get the food from plate to mouth. There follows the complex neuromuscular processes of mastication, bolus preparation, bolus propulsion, airway closure, and swallowing. Every part of this process may be impacted by some of the losses and problems of aging, whether sociological, physiological, pathological, psychological, functional, or iatrogenic.

Motivation

The motivation to eat and drink may be voluntary or involuntary. Humans may eat because they wish to, whether hungry or not, or whether it is good for them or not. The choice

---

Table 108-1 The requirements for eating

Motivation
Involuntary drives:
- Hunger
- Thirst

Voluntary drives:
- Recognition of the need to eat or drink
- Acquired habits
- Eccentricity

Functional resources
Cognitive function:
- Prepare shopping list
- Obtain food
- Prepare a meal
- Recognize the need to eat

General physical function:
- Ability to shop (transportation, ambulation)
- Food preparation
- Ability to get food to mouth

Social support system:
- Family or other care provider
- Societal resources
- Economic resources
- Transportation
- Senior/community center
- Meals-on-wheels
- Home care

The act of eating
Voluntary phase:
- Oral
  - Open and close mouth
  - Moisten, chew, prepare bolus
  - Propel bolus to oropharyngeal junction
  - Start swallow

Involuntary phases:
- Pharyngeal
  - Stop breathing
  - Close airways
  - Propel bolus through pharynx
  - Open upper esophageal sphincter
- Esophageal
  - Peristalsis propels bolus to lower esophageal sphincter
  - Lower esophageal sphincter opens

---

is a cognitive process that may become a bad habit or idiosyncrasy carried into old age with resultant over- or undernutrition, and vitamin or mineral deficiencies. Because choice significantly affects dietary intake, cognitive impairment may also significantly alter the quality or quantity of what is eaten. In late Alzheimer's disease, however, and other progressive dementias, agnosias occur, such as failure to recognize the need to eat or the nature of food, and patients may therefore ignore food or eat nonedibles.[10–14] Further, when attempts are made to spoon-feed such patients they may exhibit resistive feeding behaviors such as biting, pushing away the hand that feeds, or striking out,[10–14] which further compromise food intake.

Appetite

Hunger is the involuntary drive to eat. It is regulated by various chemical mediators including hormones (e.g. insulin, corticosteroids, growth and thyroid hormones) and various cytokines (e.g. cholecystokinin,[15] serotonin.[16] interleukin-1-β (IL-1-β), tumor necrosis factor-α (TNF-α),[17] neuropeptide Y[18]), acting directly or indirectly through the hypothalamus and basal brain. Some increase in aging resulting in early satiety (e.g. cholecystokinin), some rise in response to stress or depression (e.g. serotonin), and others are produced in response to common disease processes in aging such as infection, inflammation, or cancer (e.g. TNF-α, IL-1-β). Endocrine diseases such as thyrotoxicosis or myxedema and diabetes produce their effects on nutritional status and eating by altering the body's metabolism. The metabolic rate is often reduced in aging because of an increasingly sedentary existence brought about by disease, disability, or various psychosocial factors. In addition, various chemical mediators, be they hormones, cytokines or drugs, may have their effects on appetite altered because of changes in receptor status that accompany old age (e.g. decreased opioid and insulin receptors).

Thirst

Body fluid homeostasis is frequently impaired in aging with potentially lethal consequences if the body is subject to certain stresses (e.g. increased ambient temperature, fever, vomiting). Changes occur in fluid ingestion in aging.[19] Thirst may be diminished by failure of osmotic regulation, by inappropriate antidiuretic hormone secretion or by changes in the basal brain. In addition, changes in renal function may impair the glomerular filtration rate, and electrolyte and water handling. In healthy elderly persons the nonstressed water deficits are generally made up by coingestion of water with solids.[19] However, this compensatory mechanism is not adequate if solid food ingestion is diminished from any cause, resulting in dehydration and its significant morbidity and mortality.

Many medications are anorexogenic or have a direct effect on fluid or electrolyte balance and may, therefore, contribute significantly to reduced nutritional intake, dehydration, or water overload. The multiple medications used in the management of various clinical problems of elderly people are a major cause of anorexia and impaired fluid homeostasis.

Food acquisition

Food gathering requires significant cognitive input—acknowledgment of the need to obtain food; ability to identify the food required; knowing where it can be acquired; having the necessary fiscal resources; and having the physical ability or the cognitive, financial, or social resources to acquire it and bring it home. Food then needs to be prepared, which requires cognitive input, a certain level of physical functioning (e.g. vision, upper extremity dexterity), and certain domestic resources (e.g. stove, microwave, a power supply). It is, therefore, apparent that depression, dementia, many different kinds of physical disability, poverty, lack of transportation, or an inadequate social support system, can all prejudice the food supply. Impaired vision and upper limb weakness, incoordination, or tremor may compromise the ability to get prepared food from table to mouth.

Chemosensory changes, oral health, and eating

The changes in taste and smell associated with aging, the effect these changes have on food intake, and the changes in mastication caused by dental problems, altered salivation, and oral motor performance in aging have been the subject of an excellent detailed review.[20]

Healthy older persons' ability to taste, food enjoyment, and salivary output are essentially unaffected, while chewing efficiency and swallowing are slightly diminished and smell is significantly diminished. In contrast, all are significantly diminished in medically compromised patients. The oral and systemic etiologies of gustatory and olfactory dysfunction, food selection, and chewing and swallowing problems in the geriatric population are summarized in Tables 108-2 and 108-3. They may lead to anorexia, oral pain, less enjoyment of eating, dysphagia and selective, though often unconscious, changes in food consistency or avoidance of certain foods. Smaller meals and smaller mouthfuls are taken, and the whole process of eating is slowed. These changes may also impair social interactions because of the particular food requirements and perceptions that certain changes in eating habits may be socially unacceptable.

THE ACT OF EATING

Eating begins as a voluntary act—a matter for serious consideration when confronted with patients with mid- to late-stage dementia—and the processes required to complete the task are highly sophisticated and delicately organized. The mechanical act of eating occurs in three phases.

The oral phase

The initial voluntary oral preparatory phase, consists of opening and closing the mouth, moistening food, chewing, bolus formation, passage of the bolus to oropharyngeal junction, and starting the swallow. This phase is entirely voluntary, controlled by the medial temporal lobes and limbic system. The tongue and neuromusculature of the oropharynx propel the bolus to the pharynx where the swallow is started.

Swallowing

The subsequent involuntary processes[21] and their changes in aging[22–24] have been well reviewed. The swallow includes pharyngeal and esophageal phases. Once started, the swallow may be partially interrupted by deliberately coughing or choking. The conscious awareness of eating stops when the automatic, reflex act of swallowing begins.

Table 108-2 Oral etiologies of gustatory and olfactory dysfunction, food selection, chewing, and swallowing problems

Etiology	Smell and taste problem	Food selection and chewing problem	Swallowing problem
Oral trauma:			
• Burns, lacerations, chemical damage	×	×	×
• Anesthetic, surgical	×	×	
• Removable prosthetic appliance	×	×	×
Oral diseases and problems:			
• Periodontal diseases	×	×	
• Dental-alveolar and other infections	×	×	
• Soft tissue lesions/oral tumors	×	×	×
• Candidiasis, denture stomatitis	×	×	
• Burning mouth syndrome	×	×	
• Salivary dysfunction	×	×	×
• Tooth loss		×	×
• Diminished activity of masticatory muscles		×	×
• Impaired chewing	×	×	×
• Velopharyngeal incompetence			×
Oral pain:			
• Treatment of oral diseases		×	
• Oral mouth rinses, gels, and dentifrices	×		
• Removable prosthetic appliances	×	×	×
• Drugs in saliva	×		
• Dental material interactions, galvanism	×		
• Poor dental restorations		×	
Chemosensory problems:			
• Dysosmia	×	×	
• Dysgeusia	×	×	
• Halitosis	×	×	

From Ship et al.,[20] with permission of Blackwell Science, inc.

Respiration ceases, and the following invariable sequence of events occurs. There is closure of the airways, velar elevation, laryngeal elevation, pharyngeal shortening, opening of the upper esophageal sphincter and pharyngeal contraction. This normally takes less than 1 second. The bolus is propelled into the esophagus where peristalsis carries it to the lower esophageal sphincter. When the bolus approaches the stomach, the lower esophageal sphincter relaxes and the bolus falls into the stomach. The process takes about 8 seconds for solids and 3 seconds for liquids. The swallowing reflex requires an intact medullary swallowing center, healthy striated and smooth muscle, sensory input from the cranial nerves V, X, and XI, and motor input from cranial nerves V, VII, IX, and XII.

Overall, the mechanics of eating require intact sensory and motor nerves, striated and smooth muscle, teeth, salivary glands, synovial joints (temperomandibular and cricothyroid), articular cartilage, the medial temporal lobes and limbic system of the cerebral cortex, and the swallowing center in the basal brain. Each stage or component may be affected by aging, disease, or by various therapeutic interventions.

Normal aging is associated with frequent, though clinically insignificant, delay in initiating the swallow. Increased laryngeal penetration has been reported in one study[25] but not in another.[26] However, the occurrence of aspiration in healthy old age has not been reported. Esophageal motility declines with age resulting in increased transit times and less efficient peristalsis[27] and gastroesophageal reflux occurs with greater frequency[28] but neither have been associated with dysphagia.[29]

Oropharyngeal and pharyngoesophageal dysphagia occur commonly (Table 108-4) after cerebrovascular accidents and in various neurological disorders, particularly Alzheimer's and Parkinson's diseases, in various systemic diseases, with cervical osteophytes, head and neck cancers, and following the surgical or radiation treatments used for these latter conditions. Chemotherapy may cause nausea and results in immunosuppression which may permit severe local candidiasis to occur. Dental problems and dentures may cause oral phase problems. In the latter case, impaired oral sensation, oral stereognosis, and taste are suggested causes although clinical significance has not been proven.[30] Salivary gland dysfunction and xerostomia caused by medications and Sjögren's syndrome may also cause delay in the initiation of swallowing and provoke complaints of dysphagia.[31,32]

Other functional impairments

The common end point of functional impairment is dependency for the task impaired. Thus, when a person has impaired vision, hearing, ambulation, toileting, bathing, or eating, they become more or less dependent for that task. We have seen that in the community, eating requires cognition, vision, ambulation and/or transportation, economic resources, social supports, manual

Table 108-3 Systemic etiologies of gustatory and olfactory dysfunction, food selection, chewing, and swallowing problems

Etiology	Smell and taste problem	Food selection and chewing problem	Swallowing problem
Upper respiratory tract problems:			
• Lesions of the nose/airways	×		
• Viral and bacterial infections	×		
• Exposure to toxic airborne contaminants	×		
Peripheral or central nervous system pathologies:			
• Head and neck trauma	×	×	×
• Tumors, lesions	×		×
• Neurological diseases (e.g. Alzheimer's)	×	×	×
Systemic diseases:			
• Systemic conditions			
• Cerebrovascular diseases	×	×	×
• Head and neck cancers	×	×	×
• Arthritides		×	×
• Psychiatric disorders	×	×	
• Endocrinopathies (e.g. diabetes)	×	×	×
• Pulmonary diseases			×
• Gastrointestinal disorders	×	×	×
• Swallowing disorders		×	×
• Sjögren's syndrome	×	×	
Treatment of systemic conditions			
• Prescription and nonprescription drugs	×		×
• Head and neck irradiation	×	×	×
• Chemotherapy	×	×	×
• Head and neck surgery	×	×	×
• Gastrointestinal surgery			×
Nutritional and dietary problems			
• Inappropriately restricted diet		×	
• Monotonous diet, poor texture and color		×	
• Insufficient smell/taste cues to initiate eating		×	
• Nutritional deficiencies	×	×	×
Psychosocial problems			
• Eating alone		×	
• Perceived chewing and eating problems		×	
• Low socioeconomic status		×	
Others			
• Aging	×	×	×
• Circadian variation	×		
• Functional problems (ADL, IADL)		×	

Modified from Ship et al.,[20] with permission of Blackwell Science, Inc.

dexterity, and the ability to eat safely. There are, therefore, many points at which an individual is potentially dependent and, if these dependencies are not adequately addressed then the food supply will be compromised and nutritional intake will decline resulting in potential morbidity and mortality. Eating dependency is a well recognized predictor of impending mortality in the geriatric population.[1] It is, therefore, essential when working up an elderly patient for undernutrition to complete a comprehensive multidimensional geriatric assessment (Chapter 26) which includes social, economic, medical, psychological, and functional data to ensure that all areas can be included in developing the subsequent care plan and in monitoring progress.

Sadly, even in professional care settings such as hospitals and nursing homes, where care for dependent persons should

be optimal, feeding patients is critically wanting. Butterworth[33] in 1974 declared that malnutrition was the skeleton in the acute care hospital closet. There is still inadequate flesh on those bones and nursing home closets contain the same skeletons.[9,10,34,35] The main causes for this problem have been known for more than 20 years,[36,37] yet the problem remains. The causes are itemized in the accompanying boxed list. As can be seen, the problems identified indicate that interdisciplinary care is required. The services of the dietitian, nursing staff, nursing attendants, physicians, and administration are needed to provide corrective action. Absent any other leader, the geriatrician should be the captain of this team and vigorously address all eating problems with the patient and the care team.

"FAILURE TO THRIVE"

The most frequent presentation of an eating problem in geriatrics is either an older person brought to the office for increasing dependency, unintended and often unrecognized weight loss, or an incidental finding of undernutrition in the office, at the hospital, or in the nursing home. Typical of geriatric medicine, this problem is a vague clinical syndrome without a single, potentially preventable, treatable, or identifiable cause. It is often termed "failure to thrive" (FTT), although many other terms have been applied.[38,39] Failure to thrive was given its own International Classification of Diseases, Ninth Revision (ICD-9) code in 1979, even though it does not fulfill the criteria for a specific disease entity. It has been defined by the National Institute on Aging as, "a syndrome of weight loss, decreased appetite, poor nutrition, and inactivity, often accompanied by dehydration, depressive symptoms, impaired immune function, and low cholesterol."[40] But this definition fails to include an important common association, namely cognitive impairment. All conditions associated with impaired eating cause FTT if present for long enough. An historic perspective, review of the syndrome, and a logical approach to its evaluation has been offered.[37] Evaluation begins with a nutritional assessment.

NUTRITIONAL ASSESSMENT

Many instruments have been developed to detect risk for malnutrition and nutritional screening methods, which could be used as a part of a multidimensional geriatric assessment in various settings, have been reviewed.[41] Unfortunately, the methodology remains suboptimal. The ability of the available instruments to detect risk varies between 36 and 93 percent for sensitivity and between 44 and 85 percent for specificity. Three instruments, designed for use in the hospital setting (Subjective Global Assessment,[42] Prognostic Nutritional Index [PNI],[43] and Nutritional Risk Index[42]), have been shown to be valid predictors for potential improvement with a nutritional intervention, and one of these (PNI) has been effective when used in ambulatory and nursing home patients. A new and promising internationally developed instrument, the Mini Nutritional Assessment (MNA), has been developed as a rapid and simple evaluation for at-risk elderly people and has been cross-validated in elderly populations from the very frail to the healthy.[44] The MNA includes the Body Mass Index (BMI),[45] which has often been used alone to estimate nutritional status and has the advantage of low cost, since it uses no laboratory data. An assessment instrument for classifying abnormal feeding behavior in dementia patients, the Aversive Feeding Behavior Inventory (AFBI) (Table 108-5)[46] has been developed and is currently being tested. It allows even lay persons to identify and distinguish behaviors due to agnosias and dyspraxias, physical resistance and oral and pharyngeal dysphagia.[13] It also is inexpensive, since it depends on bed or tableside observations only. The usefulness of these instruments in identifying problems which can be eased or reversed are subject to ongoing evaluation.

Low body weight, muscle wasting, absence of subcutaneous fat, sometimes clinical features of specific vitamin deficiencies (particularly vitamin C, thiamine, and B_{12}), various anthropomorphic measurements (BMI), a low white cell count, a low serum albumin, low cholesterol, low levels of vital nutrients (e.g. iron, zinc) and various vitamins can confirm the diagnosis of undernutrition and provide clinical parameters to follow progress.

Once a diagnosis of undernutrition has been made, then the usual diagnostic investigations are performed to identify

Table 108-4 Causes of oropharyngeal dysphagia

Neuromuscular:
- Stroke
- Parkinson's disease
- Brainstem tumors
- Multiple sclerosis
- Amytrophic lateral sclerosis
- Mononeuritis multiplex

Skeletal muscle disorders:
- Inflammatory myopathies
  - Polymyositis
  - Dermatomyositis
- Muscular dystrophies
  - Myotonic dystrophy
  - Oculopharyngeal dystrophy
- Myasthenia gravis
- Metabolic myopathies
  - Hyperthyroidism
  - Hypothyroidism
  - Steroid myopathy

Mechanical obstruction:
- Inflammatory conditions
- Extrinsic compression (thyromegaly, cervical hyperostosis, lymphadenopathy)
- Postsurgical changes
- Radiation scarring

Motility disorders:
- Zenker's diverticulum
- Cricopharyngeal bar

Salivary problems:
- Medications
- Sjögren's syndrome
- Postradiation

Cognitive dysfunction:
- Alzheimer's disease
- Parkinson's disease

specific treatable conditions (e.g. cancer, malabsorption, chronic inflammatory diseases, or endocrine abnormalities). At the same time, consideration must be given to the multiple functional and psychosocial factors that contribute to disordered eating outlined in Table 108-1.

DIAGNOSING EATING DISORDERS

After malnutrition and dental problems, the most frequent diagnosis made regarding eating disorders is that of "dysphagia." The word is derived from the Greek and means "difficulty eating." However, an important semantic problem has arisen. Specialists divide dysphagia symptomatically into oropharyngeal, pharyngoesophageal and esophageal types, but, common usage in medical practice has tended to limit "dysphagia" to describing only difficulty swallowing, the involuntary, pharyngoesophageal and esophageal phases of eating. Oral phase difficulties are frequently recognized by feeders but usually interpreted by nursing staff and reported to physicians, who rarely observe patients eating, as "dysphagia," and thus difficulty swallowing. It is suggested here that dysphagia should always be used with a defining adjective such as oral, pharyngeal or esophageal. In dementia the descriptors "oral dyspraxia" or "oral apraxia" would be even more accurate.

The symptoms of oral, pharyngeal, and esophageal dysphagia are usually well described by the cognitively intact and

Causes of esophageal dysphagia

- Achalasia
- Diffuse esophageal spasms
- Carcinoma
- Strictures
- Webs
- Rings
- Medication (chemical) injuries to gastric lining

physical examination frequently identifies the cause of the problem (e.g. oral infection, dental problems, arthritis, tumors, stroke, pseudobulbar palsy, Parkinson's disease, cranial nerve lesions, etc., Table 108-4).

In contrast, late-stage dementia patients, who all ultimately develop eating problems,[10,14] are unable to speak or express themselves. They tend to reside at home or in a nursing home and their problem is almost always described to the primary physician by feeders as "dysphagia," interpreted as difficulty swallowing or as "refusal" to eat or swallow. These patients are too cognitively impaired to rationally refuse anything. In the USA, dysphagia in dementia patients frequently results in tube feeding to prevent aspiration and to enhance or restore nutrition[47,48] so that in 1995 over 40,000 gastrostomy feeding tubes were inserted in dementia patients.[49] Systematic observation of such patients being fed or feeding themselves (Table 108-5) reveals a pattern of aversive behaviors that hinder or prevent effective oral feeding, most of which may be more appropriately managed without tube feeding.[10–14,47,48] Among them are a group of oral dyspraxias such as pursing of the lips instead of opening the mouth, failure to close the mouth, to chew, to

form or propel a bolus and failure to start the swallow. These behaviors occur almost exclusively in bedbound, incontinent, noncommunicative, end-stage patients incapable of any voluntary activity and may occur before and in the absence of pharyngeal dysphagia. In two different nursing home populations the presence of totally dependent feeding

---

Table 108-5 The Aversive Feeding Behavior Inventory (AFBI)

Feeding dependency scale
- Aversive self-feeder (displays one AFB, but self-feeds)
- Intermittently dependent feeder (occasionally requires feeding)
- Totally dependent feeder (will not eat unless fed)

Present

Resistive behaviors (RAFB):
- Turns head away from spoon
- Holds hands in front of mouth hindering or preventing access
- Pushes food or feeder away
- Grabs, hits, or bites feeder

Total

Global Dyspraxia/Agnosia (DA):
- Self-feeds with verbal coaxing or prompting
- Mixes and plays with food
- Uses fingers instead of utensils
- Unable to use utensils
- Throws food
- Continuous vocalization prevents food entry
- Eats nonedibles
- Ignores or fails to recognize food
- Wanders from the table

Total

Oral dyspraxia (oral dysphagia, OD)
- Fails to open mouth without physical prompting
- Puckers lips without opening mouth
- Closes mouth tightly on spoon preventing food entry
- Continuous mouth movements prevent food access
- Accepts food, forcibly expels it
- Accepts food, fails to swallow
- Accepts food, fails mouth closure, drools

Total

Pharyngeal dysphagia (PD)
- Coughing and choking on food
- Wet, gurgling voice

Total

Adapted from Blandford et al.[14]

Behaviors are observed while patient is feeding or being fed. The presence of one behavior from any group identifies the patient as displaying that type of behavior. Tube feeders who also receive oral nutrition may be similarly assessed. The total number of behaviors in each group may indicate severity and offer clinical parameters to follow progress. The Feeding Dependency is for aversive feeders only. Scale and its characteristics are mutually exclusive.

Each AFB group identifies a pattern of behaviors which suggest strategies which might enhance oral feeding. Preliminary data indicate that being a totally dependent aversive feeder and/or the presence of OD predict death within 1 year.

and unremitting oral dyspraxia were the best single predictors of death within 1 year.[14,50]

Barium radiographic studies are the most accurate tests for defining dysphagia. They should include anteroposterior and lateral projection videoradiography to properly elucidate mechanisms, and a solid bolus (cookie swallow) to identify obstructive lesions. An obstructive lesion may require endoscopy and biopsy. Motility disorders can be further elucidated with manometric studies. Sophisticated manometric studies help elucidate physiological mechanisms, but at present are of little practical help. In contrast, video-radiography can define strategies to improve feeding by identifying positional changes that may circumvent the hazards of pharyngeal penetration. Unfortunately, these techniques are expensive and very difficult to perform in late-stage dementia patients.

MANAGEMENT OF EATING DISORDERS

Throughout the foregoing, the need for an interdisciplinary approach has been emphasized. The social, economic, activities of daily living (ADL), instrumental activities of daily living (IADL), medical, psychological, and iatrogenic causes must be elucidated and comprehensively addressed. This requires a great deal of professional time and expertise, and substantial and varied resources. The expense is considerable and pragmatism is necessary in determining what is reasonable and what is not. In the latter regard the patient's life expectancy should not be ignored. Correctable medical problems should obviously be addressed, and reasonable achievable goals developed for restoring nutritional status and preventing and treating the complications of undernutrition.

A comprehensive and concise review of assessing and treating geriatric patients with undernutrition is available.[51] Treatment depends upon a correct diagnosis and finding reversible medical causes. The general approach is to eliminate conditions associated with anorexia, decreased food intake or increased energy usage. While these approaches are universal, their management in elderly people may be compromised by the patient's social circumstances, comorbidities and their individual treatment protocols, and not least, agreement and compliance with regimens suggested. It is equally important to recognize that elderly patients have a right to be properly informed regarding their diagnosis and the burdens and benefits of any and all potential treatment options, and to have their quality of life and their treatment choices respected.

Few causes of undernutrition in elderly people have been reversed successfully. Depression is one of these. Mood should always be evaluated with the Geriatric Depression Scale[52] and weight gain can almost invariably be obtained with antidepressant treatment even when there are significant debilitating underlying comorbidities.

Medications are another frequent cause of anorexia but may also cause undernutrition from nausea, diarrhea, constipation, cognitive disturbance, or an increase in metabolic rate. A comprehensive medication review is imperative and the emphasis should be on decreasing the number of medications and finding alternatives which will reduce or eliminate their negative effects on nutrition.

Many conditions respond poorly to attempts to restore nutritional status. These include undernutrition attributed to cancer, AIDS and congestive heart failure, and anorexia attributed to poor smell or taste. Unfortunately, the available data on replenishing and preventing nutritional deficits, with few exceptions, lack scientific support for their effectiveness.[2,39,41] Nevertheless, it is reasonable and humane to try to ensure that individuals receive adequate nutrition and social supports. This may at least improve the quality of life. Conditions in which maintenance nutrition therapy currently appears futile are presented in the accompanying boxed list.[5]

Summary of management algorithm

- Restrictive diets (e.g. salt, water, fats) should be used with caution in frail elderly patients. They are frequently unsavory or unpalatable, impairing quality of life, and may also compound pre-existing or imminent undernutrition or dehydration. They may also be too late to prevent pathology for which they have been shown to be beneficial in younger populations.

- Dietary supplements should be used with caution because of the cost to the individual and/or the health system and their propensity to cause gastrointestinal disturbances. The use of inexpensive balanced tasty (favorite) nutritious food should be constantly encouraged. A dietitian is a valuable resource in this regard.

- The effect of diet on the pharmacology and pharmacodynamics of the multiple medications commonly used by elderly individuals must be kept constantly in mind.

- Once identified the causes of malnutrition must be sought. This requires a comprehensive multidimensional geriatric assessment including assessments of social, economic, medical, psychological, and functional status.

- Therapeutic interventions to address malnutrition need to be equally multidimensional with the ultimate objective of defining a set of specific, reasonable and achievable goals for each problem identified.

- Current data fail to support the use of enteral feeding to treat failure to eat, correct weight loss, prevent aspiration, or prolong life in end-stage dementia patients. Burdens appear to outweigh benefits, suggesting that palliative care is the treatment of choice for this terminal condition.

Management of eating and swallowing difficulties

Appropriate treatment for malignancies and diseases such as polymyositis, Parkinson's disease, thyroid dysfunction, or myasthenia gravis, may result in significant improvement in eating and swallowing. The more permanent problems that follow a stroke, head and neck surgery, radiation or trauma, or degenerative neurological diseases, such as Alzheimer's disease or motor neuron disease, can be managed or improved to some extent by mechanical strategies and behavior modification.[53] Strategies that minimize laryngeal penetration include changes in food consistency and volume, frequent small feedings, postural modifications, instruction on certain physical maneuvers, and dental, prosthetic, or surgical interventions.[54] A speech therapist can be invaluable in assisting the care team

Conditions in which nutrition may never be regained or maintained

- Fasting
- Inability to accept oral nutrition (e.g. advanced dementia)
- Failure to accept alternative forms of nutrition (e.g. enteral or parenteral feeding)
- Prolonged nausea, vomiting, unrelieved diarrhea
- Increased energy consumption (e.g. open wounds, burns, fractures)
- Advanced disease, often preterminal (e.g. cancer, AIDS, malabsorption syndrome, congestive cardiac failure)
- Chronic renal failure
- Alcohol/drug abuse
- Chronic gastrointestinal blood loss
- Uncontrolled hyperthyroidism
- Gastrointestinal surgery
- Radiotherapy, chemotherapy

Complications of enteral tube feeding

- Discomfort
- Self-extubation
- Dislodgement
- Incorrect placement
- Tube trauma
- Erosions of nasal septum and passages
- Bleeding
- Tracheal perforation
- Pneumothorax
- Electrolyte disturbance
- Bloating
- Regurgitation
- Diarrhea
- Aspiration pneumonia
- Anxiety
- Imposition of chemical or mechanical restraints

Complications of gastrostomy and jejunostomy tube feeding

- All the complications of enteral tube feeding
- Peristomal discomfort
- Abdominal wall cellulitis
- Peritonitis
- Gastrointestinal bleeding
- Leakage
- Ileus
- Bowel obstruction
- Small bowel perforation and death
- Anesthetic problems (e.g. cardiopulmonary arrest)

identify the appropriate treatment. If these strategies are ineffective then enteral feeding should be considered.

Tube feeding

The principal mode of ensuring increased or sufficient nutritional intake in patients who are unable to eat is tube feeding. In this invasive procedure (which requires the patient's consent) a tube is inserted into the stomach through the nose (nasogastric [NG] tube), through an abdominal incision into the stomach (percutaneous endoscopic gastrostomy [PEG] or the jejunum (percutaneous endoscopic jejunostomy [PEJ]) through which nutrition, hydration, and medications can be passed. It is clearly indicated to provide nutrition and hydration to patients with serious acute illness where there is expectation of recovery of the ability to eat. It is also appropriate to supplement feeding in the short-term for patients unable to eat or drink sufficient amounts, to preserve or restore their fluid and nutritional balance while recovering from some temporary disability (e.g. transient ischemic attack [TIA], infections). In incurable illnesses tube feeding may be palliative, relieving hunger or thirst such as frequently occurs with head and neck tumors, postsurgery and/or radiation, or in treating the wasting syndromes of AIDS and cancer patients, if some improvement in their condition or function can reasonably be expected.

Four myths concerning tube feeding have been promulgated over time.[55] They are (1) that it is ordinary care analogous to spoon feeding, (2) that it prevents aspiration pneumonia, (3) that swallowing evaluations identify patients who should receive tube feeding, and (4) that withholding or withdrawing tube feeding leads to a painful death. All of these myths have been substantially refuted.

A recent excellent comprehensive review of the published findings of the outcome of tube feeding patients with progressive dementia has concluded that there are no published studies which show conclusively that tube feeding reduces the risk of aspiration pneumonia, prevents the complications of malnutrition, improves survival, or prevents or improves pressure ulcers.[47] Another current authoritative and thoughtful review of the same problem additionally found no legal or moral impediment to withholding or withdrawing tube feeding from such patients.[48] The medial temporal lobes and the limbic system are the main controlling sites for oral phase eating and also principle targets for Alzheimer's pathology. If it could be shown that end stage dementia patients with oral dyspraxia invariably had significant irreversible pathology at these sites, persistent oral dyspraxia could be designated a categorical terminal event since continued life would depend upon the provision of artificial nutrition and hydration. Palliative care could then become the treatment of choice, the most reasonable, appropriate, merciful and economical management for this dehumanizing and tragic condition.

It has been repeatedly confirmed that tube feeding brings many burdens to treated patients and that they may often outweigh the potential benefits.[47] Enteral feeding provides only chemical nutrition not food, and it is a potentially harmful and even a life-threatening procedure (see accompanying boxed lists on enteral tube feeding and gastrostomy and jejunostomy tube feeding). The literature on aspiration pneumonia is confounded by the inconsistent definitions of the syndrome, but the syndrome continues to occur in many tube-fed patients regardless of how it is defined or whether it is an NG, PEG, or PEJ. This may be due to aspiration of saliva or oral bacteria, by NG tubes causing incompetence of the gastroesophageal sphincter with consequent reflux, by PEG tubes increasing gastroesophageal reflux, or by regurgitation from an over-full stomach.

These problems may be minimized by keeping the patient at 30–35 degrees when in bed, by monitoring gastric residual before each feeding, and by ensuring that tube placement is correct.

The expensive diagnostic procedures for dysphagia, briefly described above, may clearly characterize abnormalities of the process of swallowing, but the clinical significance of the very subtle changes that can be identified are essentially unknown. Significant clinical judgment is required, taking into account both the severity of symptoms and the nature of the underlying disease. An abnormal result from a swallowing evaluation is not a categorical requirement to tube feed but very often will identify simple strategies for staff and cooperative patients to use to enhance safe oral food intake. Finally, the cruel and painful death by starvation claimed by some to occur when tube feeding is not provided has no scientific foundation.[56] Patients who are deprived of nutrition and hydration do not suffer from the discomfort of excessive respiratory secretions or the mechanical efforts to relieve it. Death occurs during a quiet coma, presumably the consequence of endorphin release.

SUMMARY

Undernutrition is common in aging and has multiple causes. Its presence indicates some disorder of eating. The common causes are failure to acquire or prepare food or to eat food provided, anorexia, depression, functional difficulties with eating, and an array of separate and distinct organ system problems and pathologies and the effects of polypharmacy. The great variety of causes for the syndrome is only exceeded by the heterogeneity of the elderly population.

The approaches to identifying causes and developing appropriate care plans include multidimensional geriatric assessment, nutritional status evaluation, and studies of the physiological processes of eating.

Management strategies focus first on treating underlying causes. In spite of the fact that supplemental feedings may not provide significant benefit in many circumstances, strategies to enhance and restore nutritional status should be developed and implemented.

In late-stage progressive dementia enteral feeding should not be used simply to sustain life. The presence of persistent oral dyspraxia (see the AFBI, Table 108-5) in these patients may define an absolute indication for a palliative care approach. This would permit a dignified, peaceful, symptom-free death for those who have been so sadly dehumanized by their irreversible disease and whose death is imminent. It would also significantly reduce the prolonged suffering and dying from co-morbid complications which frequently accompanies enteral feeding in end-stage dementia, substantially relieve care burden stress for the family and care providers, and significantly reduce the health care cost for this burgeoning population.

The fact that aged persons are frequently unaware of the benefits and burdens of modern diagnostic and treatment modalities and the fact that they have a right to know about such things and the right to choose or refuse such care modalities imparts a serious obligation to care providers. It is our obligation to try to ensure that patients are fully informed and able to make reasoned choices before proceeding. Where individuals have legally appointed decision makers for healthcare it is just as necessary that they be equally well informed and that they are instructed to make decisions based on what the patient would have wanted not on their own personal choice.

Further research into this common clinically problematic area of geriatric medicine is urgently needed. The elderly population in general, and of those who will suffer from disordered eating in particular, is growing faster than most other population groups in society. The methods for nutritional status evaluation and the results of nutritional interventions require further validation, and society will require that their respective cost/benefit ratios be favorable.

KEY POINTS   Eating disorders

- Qualitative and quantitative nutritional intake is often inadequate and sometimes inappropriate in individuals over 75.

- The consequences of malnutrition are symptomatically and clinically diverse, usually subtle and without specific complaints. The complications are potentially serious and may be irreversible. The diagnostic threshold should be low.

- Some degree of malnutrition is common in the elderly but methods to assess nutritional status are suboptimal. Unexplained weight loss over a defined period of time is the most objective and useful indicator.

- The best objective methods for detecting recent weight loss are changes in the way clothes fit, photographs taken over the preceding few months and physical changes observed by relatives and friends, including changes in eating patterns.

- In end-stage dementia, patients eventually fail to eat food provided and are unable to carry out the voluntary oral phase of the act of eating (oral dyspraxia). This includes opening and closing the mouth, mastication, bolus formation and propulsion, and starting the swallow. If oral dyspraxia fails to remit the patient may be considered terminal, since death is imminent unless artificial nutrition and hydration are provided.

REFERENCES

1. Sullivan DH: The role of nutrition in increased morbidity and mortality. Clin Geriatr Med 1995;11:661–673
2. Sullivan DH: Impact of nutritional status on health outcomes of nursing home residents. J Am Geriatr Soc 1995;43:195–196
3. Reuben DB, Greendale GA, Harrison GG: Nutrition screening in older persons. J Am Geriatr Soc 1995;43:415–425
4. Guigoz Y, Vellas B, Garry PJ: Assessing the nutritional status of the elderly: the mini nutritional assessment as a part of geriatric evaluation. Nutr Rev 1996;54:S59–S65
5. Sullivan DH: Undernutrition in older adults. Ann Long Term Care 2000;8:41–46
6. Verdery RB: Failure to thrive in the elderly. Clin Geriatr Med 1995;11:653–659
7. Wallace JI, Schwartz RS, LaCroix AZ et al: Involuntary weight loss in older outpatients: incidence and clinical significance. J Am Geriatr Soc 1995;43:329–337
8. Mowe M, Bohmer T: The prevalence of undiagnosed protein-calorie undernutrition in a population of hospitalized elderly patients. J Am Geriatr Soc 1993;41:283–296
9. Morley JE, Silver AJ: Nutritional issues in nursing home care. Ann Intern Med 1995;123:850–859
10. Siebens H, Trupe E, Siebens A et al: Correlates and consequences of eating dependency in institutionalized elderly. J Am Geriatr Soc 1986;34:192–198
11. Norberg A, Athlin E: Eating problems in severely demented patients. Issues and ethical dilemmas. Nurs Clin North Am 1989;24:781–787

12. Volicer L, Seltzer B, Rheaume Y et al: Eating difficulties in patients with probable dementia of the Alzheimer type. J Geriatr Psych Neurol 1989;2:188–194

13. Watkins LB, Blandford G: Aversive feeding behavior in dementia. J Am Geriatr Soc 1994;43:32

14. Blandford G, Watkins LB, Mulvihill MN et al: Assessing abnormal feeding behavior in dementia: a taxonomy and initial findings. In Vellas B, Riviere S (eds): Weight loss and eating behaviour disorders in Alzheimer's patients. Research and Practice in Alzheimer's Disease. Springer, New York, 1998:47–64

15. Morley JE, Silver AJ: Anorexia in the elderly. Neurobiol Aging 1984;9:9

16. Wallin MS, Rissanen AM: Food and mood: relationship between food, serotonin and affective disorders. Acta Psych Scand 1994;377(suppl):36–40

17. Martinez M, Arnalich F, Hernanz A: Alterations in anorectic cytokines levels from plasma and cerebrospinal fluid in idiopathic senile anorexia. Mech Aging Dev 1993;72:145–153

18. Leibowitz SF: Brain neuropeptide Y: an integrator of endocrine, metabolic and behavioral processes. Brain Res Bull 1991;27:333–337

19. de Castro JM: Age-related changes in natural spontaneous fluid ingestion and thirst in humans. J Gerontol B 1992;47:P321–P330

20. Ship JA, Duffry V, Jones JA, Langmore S: Geriatric oral health and its impact on eating. J Am Geriatr Soc 1996;44:456–464

21. Grohan ME: Dysphagia: Diagnosis and Management, 3rd Ed. Butterworth-Heinemann, Boston, 1997

22. Castell JA, Castell DO: Upper esophageal sphincter and pharyngeal function and oropharyngeal (transfer) dysphagia. Gastroenterol Clin North Am 1996;25:35–50

23. Sonies BC: Oropharyngeal dysphagia in the elderly. Clin Geriatr Med 1992;8:569–577

24. Schroeder PL, Richter JE: Swallowing disorders in the elderly. Semin Gastrointest Dis 1994;5:154–165

25. Robbins J, Hamilton JW, Lof GL, Kempster GB: Oropharyngeal swallowing in normal adults of different ages. Gastroenterology 1992;103:823–829

26. Tracy JF, Logemann JA, Kahrilas PJ et al: Preliminary observations on the effects of age on oropharyngeal deglutition. Dysphagia 1989;4:90–94

27. Mandelstam P, Lieber A: Cineradiographic evaluation of the esophagus in normal adults. Gastroenterology 1970;58:32–38

28. Dodds WJ, Hogan WJ, Helm JF, Dent J: Pathogenesis of reflux esophagitis. Gastroenterology 1981;81:376–394

29. Ergun GA, Miskovitz PF: Aging and the esophagus: common pathologic conditions and their effect upon swallowing in the geriatric population. Dysphagia 1992;7:58–63

30. Tallgren A, Tryde G: Chewing and swallowing activity of masticatory muscles in patients with complete upper and lower partial denture. J Oral Rehab 1991;18:285–299

31. Loesche WJ, Bromberg J, Terpenning MS et al: Xerostomia, xerogenic medications and food avoidances in selected geriatric populations. J Am Geriatr Soc 1995;43:401–407

32. Caruso AJ, Sonies BC, Atkinson JC, Fox PC: Objective measures of swallowing in patients with primary Sjogren's syndrome. Dysphagia 1989;4:101–105

33. Butterworth CE: The skeleton in the hospital closet. Nutrition Today 1974;March/April:4–8

34. Shaver HJ, Loper JA, Lutes N: Nutritional status of nursing home patients. J Parent Enteral Nutr 1980;4:367–370

35. Rudman D, Mattson DE, Nagmraj HS et al: Antecedents of death in men of a Veterans Administration nursing home. J Am Geriatr Soc 1987;35:496–502

36. MacLennan WJ, Martin P, Mason BJ: Causes for reduced dietary intake in a long-stay hospital. Age Ageing 1975;4:175–180

37. Edwards KA: Dining experience in the institutional setting. Nursing Homes 1979; March/April:6–17

38. Sarkisian CA, Lachs MS: "Failure to thrive" in older adults. Ann Intern Med 1996;124:1072–1078

39. Verdery RB: Failure to thrive in older people. J Am Geriatr Soc 1996;44:465–466

40. Lonergan ET (ed): Extending Life, Enhancing Life: A National Research Agenda. National Academy Press, Washington, DC, 1991

41. Reuben DB, Greendale GA, Harrison GG: Nutrition screening in older persons. J Am Geriatr Soc 1995;43:415–425

42. Veterans Affairs Total Parenteral Nutrition Cooperative Study Group: Perioperative total parenteral nutrition in surgical patients. N Engl J Med 1991;325:525–532

43. Dempsey DT, Mullen JL: Prognostic value of nutritional indices. JPEN 1987;11:109–114S

44. Guigoz Y, Vellas B, Garry PJ: Mini Nutritional assessment: a practical assessment tool for grading the nutritional state of elderly patients. Facts Res Gerontol 1994;(suppl. 2):15–59

45. Steen B: Body composition and aging. Nutrition Rev 1988;46:45–51

46. Blandford G, Watkins L, Mulvihill M, Taylor B: Feeding Alzheimer's patients. Facts Res Gerontol News 1995;4:5–8

47. Finucane TE, Christmas C, Travis K: Tube feeding in patients with advance dementia. JAMA 1999;282:1365–1370

48. Gillick MR: Rethinking the role of tube feeding in patients with advanced dementia. N Eng J Med 2000;342:206–210

49. Grant MD, Rudberg MA, Brody JA: Gastrostomy placement and mortality among hospital Medicare beneficiaries. JAMA 1998;279:1973–1976

50. Blandford G, Fann CF: Dementia, Abnormal feeding behavior and death. J Am Geriatr Soc 2000;48;S18, P27

51. Thomas DR, Morley JE: Assessing and Treating Undernutrition in Older Medical Outpatients. Part III. Clin Geriatr 2001; (suppl) March

52. Sheikh JI, Yesavage JA: Geriatric Depression Scale (GDS): Recent evidence and development of a shorter version. Clinical Gerontology: A Guide to Assessment and Intervention. The Haworth Press, New York, 1986;165–173

53. Linden P: Treatment strategies for adult neurogenic dysphagia. In Sonies B (ed): Seminars in Speech and Language. Thieme, New York, 1991:255

54. Logemann J: Evaluation and Treatment of Swallowing Disorders. College Hill Press, San Diego, 1993

55. Ahronheim JC: Nutrition and hydration in the terminal patient. Clin Geriatr Med 1996;12:379–391

56. Ahronheim JC, Gasner MR: The sloganism of starvation. Lancet 1990;1:278–279

Chapter 109

Pain in old age

Benny Katz and Robert D. Helme

Despite its increased prevalence in older individuals, pain should not be considered a normal consequence of aging. Pain is always due to pathology, either physical or psychological. Persistent pain interferes with enjoyment of life, and has deleterious effects on mood, social interaction, function, mobility, and independence. This chapter examines age-related changes in prevalence and perception of pain, and approaches to assessment and treatment. The focus is on pain and suffering, rather than the underlying causes of pain. The management of specific painful conditions is not discussed.

COMPONENTS OF PAIN

The pain experience is best understood by considering the influence of four determinants: nociception, pain perception, suffering, and pain behaviors.[1] *Nociception* is the detection of tissue damage by specialized transducers on primary afferent A delta and C nerve fibers in response to noxious stimuli. The subsequent *perception* of pain by the individual is effected by central processing of nociceptive input from the periphery, or from lesions in the peripheral and central nervous systems. Pain consequent upon nerve damage can occur with or without somatic nociceptive input. In the former case the perception of pain is altered from that which is usually reported following nociception. The intensity of pain under these circumstances bears little relationship to the extent and severity of pathology and tends to be less responsive to usual analgesic medications.

Suffering is a negative emotional response induced by pain, and also by fear, anxiety, loss, and other psychological states. Patients often use the language of pain to describe suffering, such as "heart ache," although not all suffering is caused by pain. *Pain behaviors* such as grimacing, lying down, limping, and avoidance of physical activity may result from pain perception and suffering. The clinician infers the existence of nociception, pain, and suffering from the patient's history, physical examination, and observation of pain behaviors.[1]

TYPES OF PAIN

Transient pain in response to nociceptor stimulation is ubiquitous in everyday life and is rarely a reason for seeking healthcare. It will not be discussed further. *Acute pain* usually has an identifiable temporal relationship with an injury or disease. In this setting pain may be seen to serve a useful role in drawing attention to injured tissues, altering behavior, and hence preventing further tissue damage. Autonomic overactivity such as diaphoresis and tachycardia may be present. Acute pain often leads the individual to seek medical attention. Pain often resolves before healing is complete.

Chronic pain persists beyond the normal duration of injury or tissue damage, or is associated with progressive disease. The time frame for the transition from acute to chronic pain is somewhat arbitrary, often determined by the underlying pathology, and not necessarily characterized by a change in quality or severity of symptoms. Chronic pain is often defined in arbitrary terms, such as pain persisting for longer than 3–6 months. There may be no identifiable pathology to account for the pain. Psychological and functional features often dominate but autonomic overactivity is not usually present. Once reversible factors have been excluded the pain rather than the pathology is considered the major problem. At this stage, the goal of treatment shifts from a disease focus to reduction of pain, suffering, and disability.

Prevalence studies

Older people have a higher burden of pathology, and consequently have more frequent hospitalizations and medical procedures, many of which are painful. Prevalence studies undertaken on individuals living in the community report similar rates of "temporary pain," or pain with "an onset in the last 3 months," across all age ranges.[2,3] The prevalence rates of chronic pain vary widely among studies, related to differences in population samples and survey methods.[3,4] Crook and colleagues[2] reported age-specific rates of persistent pain of 7.6 percent in subjects aged 18–30 years, increasing to 29 percent for those aged between 71 and 80 years. A similar age-associated increase in prevalence of chronic pain is a consistent finding up to age 60 years, although some studies have reported an attenuation in the prevalence of pain report in the over-85-year-old age group.[5–7] Reasons that might contribute to this include survivor effects, poor response rates in surveys, stoicism, reluctance to complain, the impact of other problems, inappropriate measurement tools and sequestration of the sickest in institutions. There is some consensus from epidemiological studies that pain affecting joints, feet, and legs is increased with age, that pain in the head, abdomen, and chest is reduced, but back pain frequency varies widely.[6–8] The high prevalence of degenerative joint disease overwhelms any contribution from other causes in all surveys. Studies undertaken in residential care settings for the elderly have shown prevalence rates of chronic pain between 66 and 80 percent[9–11] with low back pain reported in 40 percent, arthritis of appendicular joints 24 percent, followed by old fracture site pain and painful neuropathies.[10] Moss and colleagues[12] reported that during the last year of life 66 percent of individuals had frequent or continuous severe pain.

Most epidemiological studies indicate that women have a higher prevalence of pain compared with men at any given age,[5,6,8,13] although this is largely due to psychosocial issues such as living alone and widowhood. Lifestyle factors and preparedness to report pain may also be relevant.[13,14] As women represent a higher proportion of the older population the importance of this trend should not be underestimated.

Age-related changes in pain perception

Pain may not be the cardinal symptom of disease in older people. The incidence of silent myocardial infarction is strongly influenced by age with 47 percent being unrecognized between the ages of 75 and 79 years.[15] Similarly, in a retrospective study of elderly patients with peritonitis, abdominal pain was absent in nearly half of the cases[16] and several studies have suggested that older subjects report less postoperative pain. The physiological basis of these observations is uncertain. Clinicians should not underestimate the potential seriousness of underlying pathology in an older person because of the absence of severe pain.

There are widespread morphological, electrophysiological, neurochemical, and functional changes within the nociceptive pathways, as well as psychological factors which may alter pain experience in elderly people.[4] Most studies of experimental pain support the view that pain thresholds to short-duration noxious stimuli are increased in older people. Whether age also affects the level of discomfort and suffering associated with clinical pain is uncertain.[17] A recent study has identified reticence, self-doubt, and reluctance to label a stimulus as painful to underlie the perception that stoicism to pain increases with age. However, when pain is perceived the experience is the same, or under some circumstances, enhanced or prolonged.[18,19] Tolerance to severe pain may even be reduced in older people.

PATHOPHYSIOLOGICAL PERSPECTIVE

Inferences about the underlying pathophysiology of a painful condition assist the clinician in the selection of therapy and determining prognosis. Pain may be subdivided into three pathophysiological subtypes: nociceptive, neuropathic, and psychogenic. Pain that arises from noxious stimulation of specific peripheral or visceral nociceptors is termed *nociceptive pain*. Examples include pain arising from osteoarthritis, soft tissue injuries and visceral pathology. Pain arising from pathology of the peripheral nerves or within the central nervous system leading to aberrant somatosensory processing is termed *neuropathic pain*. This term encompasses a diverse range of conditions including painful peripheral neuropathies, phantom limb pains, post-herpetic neuralgia, trigeminal neuralgia and central post-stroke pain. Pain of neuropathic origin is often associated with abnormal and unpleasant sensations (dysasthesia) and may have a burning or shooting quality. Mild, normally non-noxious stimuli in the affected region may cause pain (allodynia), and repetitive stimulation results in summation and pain persisting longer than the stimulus (hyperpathia). There may be a delay between the precipitating injury and the onset of pain. The onset of central post-stroke pain syndrome occurs commonly between 1 and 3 months following the stroke, but may occur more than 1 year later.[20] Pain often persists in the absence of ongoing tissue damage.

When psychological or psychiatric factors are dominant, the pain is termed *psychogenic pain*. In the *Diagnostic and Statistical Manual of Mental Disorders*, 4th edition, of the American Psychiatric Association,[21] this entity is referred to as "Pain Disorder" and is diagnosed when psychological factors are judged to have the major role in the onset, severity, exacerbation, or maintenance of the pain. Pain Disorder is not diagnosed if pain is better accounted for by a mood, anxiety, or psychotic disorder. There may or may not be an associated medical condition. The absence of obvious pathology to account for the pain should not lead to the assumption that the pain is of psychological origin. The diagnosis should only be made in the setting of psychopathology. Previously this entity was called somatoform pain disorder.

It is not unusual for older individuals to have multiple mechanisms to account for their pain, or, indeed to have demonstrable local pathology unrelated to their pain. Pains associated with cancer often have features of acute and chronic pain, with different pathophysiological factors contributing to a variable extent at different times.

EVALUATION

Pain is inherently a subjective experience; the individual's self-report is the gold standard for assessment. The history should focus on the onset and temporal pattern of the symptoms, site and quality of the pain, the severity, aggravating and relieving factors, and the impact that pain is having on the patient's lifestyle. The assessment of a patient with a complex pain problem may need to take place over several consultations. The reliability of the history may be affected by the chronicity of the pain, past interventions, and age-related conditions that affect cognition. A collaborative history from a family member is often most helpful. Special emphasis should be placed on musculoskeletal and neurological examinations because of their importance in the genesis of pain in elderly people. The assessment should include functional and psychological aspects and where possible the individual should be assessed within their own environment. The open-ended question, "What would you do if you no longer had pain?" often reveals valuable information regarding mood state, attitudes, and disability. Part of the assessment needs to focus on the patient's comorbidities; how these affect function, their contribution to altered mood state, and their propensity to affect management with medications, and physical or psychological interventions. One must be vigilant not to falsely attribute drug side-effects to the underlying pathology.

Back pain will be used as an illustrative example. An estimated two-thirds of adults will experience back pain at some stage of their lives. Experimental studies reveal that pain may originate from any one of many structures. However, after clinical evaluation no precise patho-anatomical diagnosis can be established in 85 percent of cases.[22] Investigations are used to confirm a diagnosis and exclude more serious pathology. The diagnostic probabilities change with increasing age; cancers, compression fractures and spinal stenosis becoming more common. Plain radiology is not highly sensitive but findings on computerized tomography (CT) and magnetic resonance imaging (MRI) may be misleading. CT and MRI studies of asymptomatic individuals over 60 years of age reveal about 80 percent have abnormal findings such as disk prolapse and spinal canal stenosis. Therefore, the identification of pathology on diagnostic investigations does not necessarily indicate causality. Deyo and Weinstein[22] suggest that it is more helpful to address three questions during the assessment of a patient with low-back pain: Is a systemic disease causing the pain? Secondly, is there social or psychological distress that may amplify or prolong pain? And thirdly, is there neurological compromise that may require surgical evaluation? Under most circumstances, these questions can be answered from a careful history and physical examination without the need for further tests.

There are a number of validated psychometric instruments available to quantify and communicate the patient's pain experience. The McGill Pain Questionnaire[22] is a widely used measure appropriate for use in older people.[23] It consists of 78 adjectives describing emotional, sensory and evaluative dimensions of the pain experience. Words such as throbbing, sharp, cramping, burning, and aching describe a sensory dimension, whereas tiring, exhausting, cruel, punishing, fearful, and sickening describe an affective component. Among simpler instruments are the Visual Analogue Scale (VAS) for pain and the Present Pain Intensity Scale of the McGill Pain Questionnaire.

Psychological assessment

A comprehensive psychological assessment is not usually required in the setting of acute pain. However, chronic pain may have profound effects on mood, interpersonal relationships and activity level, and it may be difficult to ascertain which is cause and which is effect. Psychological evaluation is indicated when medical evaluation fails to adequately explain the severity of pain behaviors. Psychological evaluation can also be valuable when the pain causes severe distress, resulting in excessive health service utilization, or interference with normal activities or interpersonal relationships. Chronic pain patients are often resistant to psychological evaluation, considering this an inference that the pain is "in the head" rather than a physical problem. Patients often require careful explanation regarding the complex interaction between mind and body which often influences pain, suffering, and disability.[24] Acknowledging that the pain is real preserves the patient's sense of legitimacy and allows for a more complete evaluation of the psychological factors contributing to the maintenance of pain.

It is important to evaluate how the patient and their relatives conceptualize the pain and goals of treatment. They may believe that the pain has persisted because the medical assessment has been inadequate or specific interventions denied. Each time a new intervention is tried and fails the psychological distress is reinforced. Psychological strategies are not likely to be effective in teaching the patient how to manage with ongoing pain while the patient remains focused on seeking a cure. Pain behaviors such as limping, grimacing, inactivity, and verbalizing of pain complaints may be reinforced by social influences such as gaining attention, sympathy, or the ability to avoid unpleasant responsibilities. Fear of causing further pain or injury may lead to avoidance of activity. Attempts at management with medications and physical therapies, without addressing psychological factors, are often unsuccessful.

Assessment of pain in the presence of dementia

The prevalence of cognitive impairment rises sharply with advancing age with rates in excess of 30 percent after the age of 80 years. Dementia represents a major impediment to the evaluation and management of pain. Cognitive impairment may be aggravated by pain or medications used to treat the pain.[25] Bernabei and colleagues reported that low cognitive performance and age greater than 85 years were independent risk factors for lack of appropriate treatment of pain in cancer patients.[26] The report of pain in demented individuals may be affected by memory impairment or limited communication skills. A corroborative history from relatives or previous therapists is often required. There is no convincing evidence of enhancement of pain by dementia. In fact, Parmelee and colleagues[11] found a small negative relationship between pain intensity and cognitive impairment in a sample of 758 elderly institutionalized residents. Individuals with marked cognitive impairment were less likely to report pain in the back and joints. However, when pain was reported there was no difference in the presence or absence of a likely physical cause. In a sample of 325 nursing home residents, Ferrell and colleagues[27] reported that elderly subjects with mild to moderate cognitive impairment often require more time to assimilate and respond to questions regarding pain, but of the 62 percent reporting pain complaints, 83 percent were able to complete a unidimensional pain-intensity scale, with the Present Pain Intensity Scale of the McGill Pain Questionnaire having the highest completion rate of 65 percent. Pain report should therefore not be disregarded because the individual has cognitive impairment. Patients with dementia who are no longer able to verbally express their experience may manifest pain or other discomfort through nonverbal means including facial expressions, restlessness, agitation, hostility, aggression, body movements, postures, gestures, and vocalizations.[28]

Define the goals of therapy

Prior to embarking upon a treatment program the patient and the clinician should agree on the goals of therapy, particularly when pain eradication is not feasible. Involvement of family members often assists with ensuring compliance and successful outcomes. A frank discussion about the prognosis and therapeutic options is often accepted with gratitude, particularly in individuals who have had unsatisfactory experiences in the past. Even if the sensory component of pain cannot be eliminated, improved outcomes can be achieved by addressing factors such as disability and mood disturbance. Management of severe pain often requires establishing a balance between the severity of sensory symptoms, the level of disability, and medication side-effects. Disability may be more important to the patient than the pain. An improvement in the distance an individual is able to walk before being stopped by pain may be considered a positive outcome, although the intensity of maximum pain remains unaltered. Medication side-effects may be more troublesome than the condition for which they were prescribed. Pain management programs combine cognitive and rehabilitative approaches to enhance coping strategies and minimize the impact that persistent pain has on the individual.

MANAGEMENT

Medications

Pharmacological approaches with simple analgesics and non-steroidal anti-inflammatory drugs (NSAIDs) are the mainstay of most interventions for pain, whether self-initiated or prescribed by the doctor. This is often the most convenient and cost-effective approach. Selection of appropriate drug therapy for the older patient requires an understanding of age-related pharmacokinetic and pharmacodynamic changes, and needs to take into account any coexisting diseases and other medications, including those obtained without prescription. Selection of therapy needs to balance the potential efficacy with the potential for harm from the intervention. The timing of medication is very important. Analgesics may be prescribed on an "as required" basis for occasional pain or prophylactically for induced pain. However, for continuous pain, analgesics are best prescribed on a regular basis. Additional doses may be required prior to activities known to exacerbate pain or for breakthrough pain. Medications with long half-lives may be used to reduce the frequency of dosing. In general, medications should be commenced at low doses, titrating upwards and stopping at the lowest dose that achieves the desired outcome. Concern regarding potential adverse effects should not result in suboptimal treatment of pain. Although generally less effective when used for neuropathic pain, all analgesics can be reasonably trialed in that situation.

Simple analgesics

Paracetamol (acetaminophen) is the preferred analgesic for elderly people.[29] A trial of paracetamol is warranted as initial

therapy on the basis of cost, efficacy, and toxicity profile. For many patients paracetamol affords similar efficacy to that achieved with NSAIDs.[30] As a class, NSAIDs have been among the most frequently prescribed medications, particularly for pain associated with osteoarthritis and inflammatory arthropathies. Although effective in reducing signs and symptoms, they have no effect on the underlying musculoskeletal disease.[31] The side-effect and drug interaction profile of NSAIDs is of particular concern. At least 10–20 percent of patients taking NSAIDs will experience dyspepsia. Complications of ulcer disease such as hemorrhage and perforation occur far more often in patients taking NSAIDs. The overall risk for serious gastrointestinal events with NSAID use is about three times greater than that of controls, and in those over 60 years old, the risk rises to five times that of controls.[32] An estimated 16,500 deaths occurred from NSAID gastrointestinal toxic effects in the United States in 1997.[33] Renal toxicity is another concern with these agents. Risk factors for renal failure in patients with intrinsic renal disease treated with NSAIDs include age over 65 years, a history of hypertension, congestive cardiac failure, and concomitant use of diuretics or angiotensin-converting enzyme inhibitors. Most NSAIDs have a dose–response relationship with a ceiling effect. Increasing the dose above the recommended level or adding a second NSAID does not impart any greater analgesia, but increases the likelihood of drug toxicity.

The rate of NSAID-related serious gastrointestinal complications requiring hospitalization has decreased in recent years, in part due to extensive medical education campaigns and a move away from NSAIDs as first-line management of osteoarthritis.[33] Patients with inflammatory arthritides should preferentially be treated with disease modifying drugs. The options for management of patients with NSAIDs who are at high risk of serious upper gastrointestinal events are the use of a nonselective NSAID with gastroprotective therapy, or the use of a cyclo-oxygenase-2 (COX-2) specific inhibitor. Co-administration of misoprostol has been demonstrated to reduce the upper gastrointestinal complication rate of nonselective NSAIDs but is not well tolerated. Proton pump inhibitors are an acceptable alternative. H2 receptor antagonists have been shown to prevent duodenal ulceration only, and cannot be recommended.[32]

The two currently available COX-2 inhibitors, Celecoxib and Rofecoxib, have been shown to have significantly lower incidence of gastrointestinal toxicity than nonselective NSAIDs, similar to that of placebo.[34] This benefit appears to be attenuated by the co-administration of low-dose aspirin.[35] COX-2 inhibitors appear to affect renal function in a similar fashion to nonselective NSAIDs and particular care is required in patients with renal impairment, or those taking diuretics and angiotensin-converting enzyme inhibitors. COX-2 inhibitors may diminish the antihypertensive effects of ACE-inhibitors and diuretic effects of frusemide and thiazides. Celecoxib inhibits CP450 (CYP2C9) enzyme and thus may cause elevation of plasma concentrations of drugs metabolized by this enzyme, such as some beta-blockers, antidepressants and antipsychotics.[36]

Opioid analgesics

In the past, opioid analgesics have been divided into weak and strong categories according to their potency. This distinction

---

Summary of management algorithm

Paracetamol:
- First-line analgesic for older patients with chronic pain
- Often as effective as NSAIDs
- Best given regularly for persistent pain, rather than as required

NSAIDs:
- Increased risk of GI and renal complications in elderly
- Avoid if possible

Selective COX-2 inhibitors:
- Preferable to nonselective NSAIDs
- Similar nongastrointestinal side-effects to nonselective NSAIDs

Adjuvant analgesic (e.g. antidepressants and anticonvulsants):
- Proven role in neuropathic pain states
- Total pain eradication is unlikely
- Selection of medication is based on side-effect profile rather than comparative efficacy
- Start at low dose, increase slowly

Opioid analgesics:
- Have a role in chronic nonmalignant pain
- Treat constipation pre-emptively
- Drug dependence is uncommon in elderly people

Nonpharmacological approaches, e.g. physical and psychological therapies:
- Will reduce reliance on medications
- Failure to employ these strategies often accounts for treatment failure

has now become less distinct. All opioid analgesics have the potential to cause nausea, constipation, sedation, respiratory depression, and cognitive impairment. Increased cognitive impairment may itself lead to a diminished ability to cope with pain thus leading to a paradoxical increase in pain with increasing dose of opioid. Opioids are generally reserved for moderate or severe pain. Elderly patients tend to be more sensitive to equivalent doses and blood levels of opioids, receiving greater and more prolonged pain relief.[25,37] The analgesic effects of Codeine (methylmorphine) are mediated by its conversion to morphine via the cytochrome P450D6 (CYP2D6) system. About 8 percent of Caucasians and 2 percent of Asians are genetically deficient in CYP2D6 and obtain little pain relief with codeine. A number of medications frequently prescribed in elderly patients are capable of inhibiting CYP2D6 including cimetidine, quinidine, haloperidol, amitriptyline, and the selective serotonin reuptake inhibitors (SSRIs) including fluoxetine, paroxetine, and fluvoxamine. Side-effects of codeine are common, particularly constipation, nausea, and confusion. Other weak opioids include tramadol and propoxyphene. Tramadol is a centrally acting synthetic analgesic with opioid-like effects. Its mode of action is through binding to the mu-opioid receptor and inhibition of noradrenaline and serotonin reuptake. The efficacy of tramadol is comparable to ibuprofen in patients with hip and knee osteoarthritis. Dose reduction may be required in elderly patients. Propoxyphene should be used with caution in elderly patients because of the long half-life of its major metabolite and potential for central nervous system side-effects including hallucinations and seizures. Combinations of nonopioids with weak opioids, such as aspirin or paracetamol with codeine offer enhanced analgesia.[38] The combined medications may result in a lower incidence of side-effects as each analgesic can be used at a lower dose. The weak opioids have a ceiling effect for analgesia. If adequate pain relief is not obtained at optimal doses, change to a strong opioid should be considered.

Morphine is the prototypic opioid. The analgesic properties of morphine are not limited by a ceiling effect; however, side-effects are common. Tolerance to side-effects develops more rapidly than tolerance to analgesic effects, although constipation tends to persist. Once the daily opioid requirements have been established through the administration of a short-acting opioid on a regular basis, then the use of delayed-release opioid agents should be considered. Delayed-release morphine and oxycodone preparations may be used in elderly patients but care must be taken to prevent drug accumulation. Other strong opioids include methadone, pethidine (meperidine), and fentanyl. Pethidine is not appropriate for long-term use because of the risk of accumulation of its metabolite norpethidine, resulting in central nervous system excitation, tremors, and seizures. Methadone must be used with caution because it has a long half-life up to 2 or 3 days, resulting in accumulation in elderly patients.

Tolerance may develop with repeated administration of all opioids whereby higher doses are required to maintain equivalent analgesic effects. The rate of development of tolerance varies greatly. To overcome tolerance, the dose or frequency of dosing may be increased. Cross-tolerance with other opioids is not complete as they often act through different combinations of receptors. The problem may be overcome by changing to another oral opioid, commencing at one half of the equianalgesic dose. When a patient is unable to tolerate oral opioids, or has refractory pain, parenteral analgesia by the transdermal, subcutaneous, venous, epidural or intrathecal route should be considered. A transdermal fentanyl patch offers the advantage of one application every 72 hours. It has a similar side-effect profile to other opioids, although some subjects report less constipation than with other preparations. Fentanyl accumulates in skeletal muscle and fat and then is slowly released into the blood. Minimum effective concentrations are reached approximately 6 hours after application. Serum fentanyl concentrations fall by 50 percent approximately 17 hours after removing the patch. The clearance of fentanyl is delayed in elderly, cachectic, and debilitated patients. The 25 µg hour transdermal fentanyl patch is equivalent to about 90 mg of morphine per day. It is not recommended for opioid-naive patients.

Adjuvant analgesics

Adjuvant analgesics are drugs that have a primary indication other than pain but are analgesic in neuropathic pain syndromes. They include medications from heterogeneous therapeutic classes, including tricyclic antidepressants, anticonvulsants, oral antiarrhythmics, and neuroleptics.

Antidepressants and anticonvulsants have a proven role in the management of neuropathic pains that are often refractory to conventional analgesics. Pain relief is usually only partial, with 50 percent reduction in pain scores usually being classified as success in most studies. For every three patients treated with either an antidepressant or anticonvulsant for postherpetic neuralgia or diabetic neuropathy, one patient experiences 50 percent pain relief that they would not have received with placebo.[39] Empirically, antidepressants have been used for neuropathic pains with a burning quality and anticonvulsants for shooting pains, despite lack of evidence linking efficacy to the characteristics of pain. Tricyclic antidepressants also have a role in the management of non-neuropathic pain including tension and migraine headache, atypical facial pain, rheumatoid arthritis, chronic low-back pain, fibromyalgia, and cancer pain.[40] Tricyclic antidepressants have been widely used in older individuals despite their propensity for side-effects such as dry mouth, postural hypotension, falls, constipation, sedation, and urinary retention. The sedating side-effect may be used to advantage for some individuals with pain-related insomnia. The analgesic effects of tricyclic antidepressants are independent of antidepressant effects, occurring more rapidly and at a lower dose than used for depression. The median effective analgesic dose of agents such as amitriptyline or nortriptyline is in the order of 50–70 mg daily.[41] A low starting dose of around 10 mg is recommended. Newer antidepressant medications, such as SSRIs, have fewer side-effects but have not been demonstrated to be more effective than placebo in achieving analgesia, although there are insufficient data to draw a final conclusion.[39,42]

Anticonvulsants have been widely used for neuropathic pains despite surprisingly few trials of analgesic effectiveness.[43] Carbemazepine is the drug of choice for trigeminal neuralgia, with pain control achieved in about 75 percent of patients.[44] Anticonvulsants are considered second-line therapy following antidepressants for other neuropathic pain states.[43] Anticonvulsants shown to be of benefit for diabetic neuropathy and post-herpetic neuralgia are carbemazepine, phenytoin, and gabapentin.[43] Gabapentin has a lower incidence of side-effects than carbemazepine or phenytoin, but has not been proven to be more effective than the older anticonvulsants.[39,43] Other anticonvulsants that have been widely used to treat neuropathic pain without convincing evidence for benefit in clinical trials include valproate and lamotrigine.

The selection of an adjuvant analgesic agent for the management of neuropathic pain should be based on the side-effect profile, and the potential for drug interaction, rather than relative efficacy of different agents. There is considerable individual variation in the response to these agents. Failure to respond to one agent is not predictive of the response to another agent within the same therapeutic class.

Topical lignocaine (lidocaine) patches have been licensed for use in post-herpetic neuralgia in the United States. Extreme care must be used when using oral or parenteral local anesthetic agents, such as mexilitene and lignocaine to treat pain in older adults because of the potential for fatal arrhythmias. The use of neuroleptic medication for pain in older people is not indicated as side-effects outweigh benefits.

Nonpharmacological therapies

Nonpharmacological approaches, either alone or in combination with pharmacological approaches, should be an integral part of the care plan for older individuals with chronic pain.[29] Nonpharmacological approaches encompass a broad range of physical and other treatment modalities. They are widely used by patients, often without the knowledge of their healthcare provider. Few of these therapies have undergone formal evaluation.

Physical therapies

Simple adjustments in posture and daily routines, such as preparing meals in a seated position, breaking up the housework, or the provision of a walking aid can reduce the impact of pain on daily life. The use of a walking frame, which causes a mild degree of lumbar flexion, will often ease the pain of lumbar canal stenosis.

Exercise is a major component of most pain management programs, either alone or in conjunction with pharmacological and other nonpharmacological approaches. Even frail and institutionalized elderly people may benefit. Exercise can lead to decrease in pain, improvements in function and elevation of mood.[45] Hydrotherapy should be considered when weight-bearing exercises aggravate pain. The buoyancy effect of water reduces the weight of the body allowing joints to be moved with minimal friction through a full range of movements. The warmth of the water decreases pain and muscle spasm.

Transcutaneous electrical nerve stimulation (TENS) is a popular method of symptom relief for a wide range of painful conditions in elderly people such as low-back pain, osteoarthritis, and post-herpetic neuralgia. Other physical therapies used for a wide range of painful conditions include massage, cold and heat treatments, acupuncture, and electrotherapies such as ultrasound, infrared lamps, microwave, and shortwave diathermy.

Joint replacement surgery has had a major impact in alleviating the suffering of older people with degenerative joint disease who have experienced inadequate symptom control with conservative management.

Psychological approaches

Psychological factors may contribute to the maintenance of pain, or be causally related to the pain. Regardless of the pathophysiological basis of chronic pain, psychological strategies have a role in management. The essence of management is to establish appropriate pain coping strategies and discourage behaviors that may perpetuate the pain syndrome. Usually a combination of behavioral and cognitive strategies is employed. Cognitive strategies are aimed at modifying belief structures, attitudes and thoughts in order to modify the experience of pain and suffering. This approach also includes distraction therapy, relaxation, biofeedback, and hypnosis. The patient is encouraged to take an active role and accept responsibility for pain management, rather than being a passive victim.

Cognitive strategies are usually combined with a behavioral approach. Behavioral operant conditioning discourages pain behaviors such as limping, grimacing, inactivity, and verbalizing of pain complaints. Usually, in conjunction with the patient's relatives, positive reinforcement is provided for behavior unrelated to pain and for successfully achieving preset goals. All other pain behaviors such as moaning are ignored. A number of studies have demonstrated increased activity, reduced analgesic consumption and improved mood in middle-aged adults, with some reporting benefit for elderly patients with chronic pain.[46,47]

Pain and cancer

Half of all cancers occur in the population over 65 years of age.[48] In the advanced stages of cancer 70 percent experience pain, of which 80 percent is severe and persistent.[49] In up to 90 percent of cases cancer pain can be managed by relatively simple means.[50] The World Health Organization (WHO) has developed the Cancer Pain Relief Program to offer adequate pain relief to all cancer patients in the world, through the existing health system.[49]

The WHO method for relief of cancer pain is based on a three-step approach to the use of analgesia. The first step of the WHO analgesic ladder is the nonopioid analgesics including paracetamol and NSAIDs. The second step is the weak opioids and the third step is the strong opioid group. Nonopioid analgesics are usually combined with an opioid in steps two and three to give additive analgesia. At each stage, adjuvant analgesic drugs such as antidepressants and anticonvulsants should be added when there is a specific indication. Zech and colleagues[51] reported nearly 90 percent of 2,118 palliative care patients were able to obtain satisfactory pain control on this regimen up to the time of death. Patients with residual pain were often content with the balance of analgesic efficacy and troublesome side-effects. Emotional, spiritual, and functional aspects should not be neglected. Despite the widespread dissemination of the WHO ladder most cancer pain patients around the world still appear to have inadequate analgesia.[52]

The use of opioids in chronic noncancer pain

There is clear consensus about the use of opioids in severe acute and malignant pain; however, the role of opioid therapy in the management of chronic pain of nonmalignant origin remains controversial. Clinical experience demonstrates that selected patients obtain considerable benefit.[53] Exaggerated fear of adverse effects should not prevent a trial of opioid therapy in appropriately selected individuals who have not responded to other therapies. Maintenance opioid therapy for chronic pain of nonmalignant origin should only be considered after the patient has been thoroughly evaluated and has not responded to other conventional pharmacological and nonpharmacological therapies. There is an increased onus on the clinician to ensure the patient understands the risks and benefits of this therapy. The more serious the risk, the more important it is for the physician to outline such risk, even if the probability of it eventuating is small. To overcome anxiety about this form of therapy the clinician may need to explain to the patient the distinction between addiction, dependence, and tolerance. Physical dependence occurs with the prolonged use of all opioids. It is manifested by unpleasant symptoms following abrupt withdrawal, such as diaphoresis, abdominal cramps, malaise, and fear. Although the symptoms are similar to those experienced by opioid addicts, the normal person does not experience opioid craving. When there is a possibility of dependence, opioids should not be abruptly withdrawn. Addiction following the therapeutic administration of opioids is very rare, especially in older individuals. Opioid tolerance is manifested by reduced analgesic effect at the same dose. Its cause is unknown. Increased opioid dose requirements are more likely to be due to the progression of the underlying disease than the development of tolerance. With the relatively low doses of opioids used for the management of chronic nonmalignant pain in this population, the older individual is less likely to be troubled by these problems.[29]

The aims of treatment should be explicit, often aimed at easing the pain rather than total eradication. Total eradication of pain may occur at the expense of intolerable side-effects. Four factors should be regularly monitored; the dose of opioid, pain relief, side-effects, and overall functional status. The dose may be increased to obtain better pain control or functional status. If, however, the opioid dose is escalating at a time when pain control or functional status is declining, management should be reviewed. The physician must be familiar with and observe statutory requirements regarding the supply of opioids. Both parties must agree to close supervision for the duration of therapy.

CONCLUDING REMARKS

Advancing age is associated with an increased incidence of painful pathology. Anyone who has persistent pain despite what appears to be conventional treatment should be carefully reassessed to determine why there has been a failure of response to therapy. One should never conclude that it is the patient who has failed to respond to treatment; it is the treatment that has failed to achieve the desired result. Severe unrelieved pain has a profound impact on the individual. Various factors may preclude the older patient from the benefit of definitive therapy to eradicate pain and under these circumstances, symptom management is indicated. This must take into consideration the effect of comorbidities on the expression, assessment, diagnosis and treatment of the painful condition. Overemphasis on pharmacological approaches ignores the potential benefits of physical and cognitive–behavioral strategies. The persistence of pain despite apparently appropriate therapy raises the possibility of unrecognized mood disturbance, pain of neurogenic origin, or advancing pathology. Under these circumstances a multidisciplinary pain management approach involving medical, physical, and psychological therapeutic modalities is often more effective than a single disciplinary approach.[54] The proliferation of multidisciplinary pain management clinics over the past 30 years offers greater access to individuals with chronic pain, yet few have expertise or interest in geriatric medicine.[55] Age should not, however, be regarded as a barrier to successful outcomes from multidisciplinary management of pain problems. Even if pain cannot be eradicated, worthwhile improvements can often be achieved by addressing pain as a problem in a broader sense, not simply a sensory symptom.

KEY POINTS Pain in old age

Assessments:

- Contribution of nociceptive and neuropathic factors
- Impact of pain on function and mood state
- Comorbidities affecting assessment, function, and treatment selection

Investigations:

- Presence of radiological abnormalities does not prove causality
- Unexplained change in symptoms warrants reassessment to exclude serious pathology

---

REFERENCES

1. Loeser JD, Melzack R: Pain: an overview. Lancet 1999;353:1607–1609
2. Crook J, Rideout E, Browne G: The prevalence of pain complaints in a general population. Pain 1984;18:299–314
3. Helme RD, Gibson SJ: Pain in older people. In Crombie IK, Croft PR, Linton SJ, LeResche L, Von Korff M (eds): Epidemiology of Pain. IASP Press, Seattle, 1999:103–112
4. Gibson SJ, Helme RD: Age differences in pain perception and report: A review of physiological, psychological, laboratory and clinical studies. Pain Rev 1995;2:111–137
5. Mobily PR, Herr KA, Clark MK, Wallace RB: An epidemiologic analysis of pain in the elderly. J Ageing Health 1994;6:139–154
6. Andersson HI, Ejlertsson G, Leden I, Rosenberg C: Chronic pain in geographically defined general population: studies of different age, gender, social class, and pain localization. Clin J Pain 1993;9:174–182
7. Brattberg G, Thorslund M, Wilkman A: The prevalence of pain in a general population. The results of a postal survey in country Sweden. Pain 1989;37:215–222
8. Von Korff M, Dworkin SF, Resche L, Kruger A: An epidemiologic comparison of pain complaints. Pain 1988;32:173–183
9. Sengstaken EA, King SA: The problems of pain and its detection among geriatric nursing home residents. J Am Geriatr Soc 1993;41:541–544
10. Ferrell BA, Ferrell BR, Osterweil D: Pain in the nursing home. J Am Geriatr Soc 1990;38:409–414

11. Parmelee PA, Smith B, Katz IR: Pain complaints and cognitive status among elderly institution residents. J Am Geriatr Soc 1993;41:517–522
12. Moss MS, Lawton MP, Glicksman A: The role of pain in the last year of life of older persons. J Gerontol 1991:46:51–57
13. Tibblin G, Bengtsson C, Furunes B, Lapidus L: Symptoms by age and sex. Scand J Prim Health Care 1990;8:9–17
14. Ruda MA: Gender and pain. Pain 1993;53:1–2
15. Sigurdsson E, Thorgeirsson G, Sigvaldason H, Sigfusson N: Unrecognized myocardial infarction: epidemiology, clinical characteristics, and the prognostic role of angina pectoris. The Reykjavik Study. Ann Intern Med 1995;122:96–102
16. Wroblewski M, Mikulowski P: Peritonitis in geriatric inpatients. Age Ageing 1991;20:90–94
17. Harkins SW, Price DD, Bush FM, Small RE: Geriatric pain. In Wall PD, Melzack R (eds): Textbook of Pain, 3rd Ed. Churchill Livingstone, New York, 1994:769–784
18. Zheng Z, Gibson SJ, Khalil Z, Helme RD, McMeeken JM: Age related differences in the time course of capsaicin-induced hyperalgesia. Pain 2000;85:51–58
19. Washington LL, Gibson SJ, Helme RD: Age-related differences in the endogenous analgesic response to repeated cold water immersion in human volunteers. Pain 2000;89:89–96
20. Vestergaard K, Andersen G, Jensen TS: Central post-stroke pain. In Crombie IK, Croft PR, Linton SJ, LeResche L, Von Korff M (eds): Epidemiology of Pain. IASP Press, Seattle, 1999:155–158
21. American Psychiatric Association: Diagnostic and Statistical Manual of Mental Disorders, 4th Ed. American Psychiatric Association, Washington, DC, 1994
22. Deyo RA, Weinstein JN: Low Back Pain. N Engl J Med 2001;344:363–370
23. Gibson SJ, Farrell MJ, Katz B, Helme RD: Multidisciplinary management of chronic non-malignant pain in older adults. In Ferrell BR, Ferrell BA (eds): Pain in the Elderly. IASP Press, Seattle, 1996:91–99
24. Turner JA, Romano JM: Psychological and psychosocial evaluation. In Bonica JJ (ed): The Management of Pain, 2nd Ed. Lea and Febiger, Philadelphia, 1990
25. Montamat SC, Cusack BJ, Vestal RE: Management of drug therapy in the elderly. N Engl J Med 1989;321:303–309
26. Bernabei R, Gambassi G, Lapane K et al: Management of Pain in Elderly Patients with Cancer. JAMA 1998;279:1877–1882
27. Ferrell BA, Ferrell BR, Rivera L: Pain in cognitively impaired nursing home patients. J Pain Symptom Manag 1995;10:591–598
28. Hurley AC, Volicer BJ, Hanrahan PA, Houde S, Volicer L: Assessment of discomfort in advanced Alzheimer patients. Res Nurs Health 1992;15:369–377
29. AGS Panel on Chronic Pain in Older Persons: The management of chronic pain in older persons. J Am Geriatr Soc 1998;46:635–651
30. Bradley JD, Brandt MD, Katz BP, Kalasinski LA, Ryan SI: Comparison of an antiinflammatory dose of ibuprofen, and analgesic dose of ibuprofen, and acetaminophen in the treatment of patients with arthritis of the knee. N Engl J Med 1991;325:87–91
31. Gotzsche PC: Non-steroidal inflammatory drugs. Br Med J 2000;320:1058–1061
32. Lanza FL: A Guideline for the treatment and prevention of NSAID induced ulcers. Am J Gastroenterol 1998;93:2037–2046
33. Wolfe MM, Lichtenstein DR, Singh G: Gastrointestinal toxicity of nonsteroidal antiinflammatory drugs. N Engl J Med 1999;340:1888–1899
34. Hochberg MC, McAlindon T, Felson DT: Systemic and topical treatments. In Felson DT (conference chair): Osteoarthritis: new insights. Part 2. Treatment Approaches. Ann Intern Med 2000;133:726–729
35. Silverstein FE, Faich G, Goldstein JL et al: Gastrointestinal toxicity with celecoxib vs nonsteroidal anti-inflammatory drugs for osteoarthritis and rheumatoid arthritis. The CLASS study: A randomized controlled trial. JAMA 2000;284:1247–1255
36. Brooks PM, Day RO: COX-2 inhibitors. MJA 2000;173:433–436
37. Bellville JW, Forrest WH, Miller E, Brown BW: Influence of age on pain relief from analgesics. JAMA 1971;217:1835–1841
38. Moore A, Collins S, Carroll D, McQuay H: Paracetamol with and without codeine in acute pain: a quantitative systematic review. Pain 1997;70:193–201
39. Collins SL, Moore RA, McQuay HJ, Wiffen P: Antidepressants and anticonvulsants for diabetic neuropathy and post herpetic neuralgia: a quantitative systemic review. J Pain Symptom Manag 2000;20:449–458
40. Onghena P, Van Houdenhove B: Anti-depressant induced analgesia in chronic non-malignant pain: a meta-analysis of 39 placebo-controlled studies. Pain 1992;49:205–220
41. Watson CPN, Evans RJ, Watt VR, Birkett N: Post-herpetic neuralgia: 208 cases. Pain 1988;35:289–297
42. Sindrup SH, Jensen TS: Pharmacological treatment of pain in polyneuropathy. Neurology 2000;55:915–920
43. Wiffen P, Collins S, McQuay H et al: Anticonvulsant drugs for acute and chronic pain (Cochrane Review). In The Cochrane Library, 4. Update Software, Oxford, 2000
44. Fields HL: Treatment of trigeminal neuralgia. N Engl J Med 1996;334:1125–1126
45. Christmas C, Anderson RA: Exercise and older patients: guidelines for the clinician. J Am Geriatr Soc 2000;48:318–324
46. Gibson SJ, Katz B, Corran TM, Farrell MJ, Helme RD: Pain in older persons. Disab Rehab 1994;16:127–139
47. Puder RS: Age analysis of cognitive-behavioural group therapy for chronic pain outpatients. Psychol Ageing 1988;3:204–207
48. Cohen HJ: Oncology and aging: general principles of cancer in the elderly. In Hazzard WR, Bierman EL, Blass JP, Ettinger WH, Halter JB (eds): Principles of Geriatric Medicine and Gerontology, 3rd Ed. McGraw-Hill, New York, 1994:77–105
49. Tadeka F: WHO cancer pain relief programme. In Bond MR, Charlton JE, Woolf CJ, (eds): Proceedings of the VIth World Congress on Pain. Elsevier, Amsterdam, 1991:467–474
50. Jacox A, Carr DB, Payne R: New clinical-practice guidelines for the management of pain in patients with cancer. N Engl J Med 1994;302:651–655
51. Zech DFJ, Grond S, Lynch J, Hertel D, Lehman KA: Validation of World Health Organization guidelines for cancer pain relief: a 10 year prospective study. Pain 1995;63:65–76
52. Jadad AR, Browman GP: The WHO Analgesia Ladder for cancer pain management. JAMA 1995;274:1870–1878
53. Zenz M, Strumpf M, Tryba M: Long term oral opioid therapy in patients with chronic nonmalignant pain. J Pain Symptom Manag 1992;7:69–77
54. Flor H, Fydrich T, Turk DC: Efficacy of multidisciplinary pain treatment centres: a meta-analytic review. Pain 1992;49:221–230
55. Harkins SW, Price DD: Assessment of pain in the elderly. In Turk DC, Melzack R (eds): Handbook of Pain Assessment. The Guilford Press, New York, 1992:315–331

Chapter 110

Elder abuse

Claudine McCreadie and Anthea Tinker

While medical practitioners are generally aware and educated about the well-researched topic of child abuse, elder abuse has only recently been the subject of their attention.[1-5] In this chapter, we first examine the historical development of concern, definitions, prevalence, and risk factors. We then discuss ways in which elder abuse may be identified and consider prevention, treatment, and management. We write from the perspective of developments in the UK, themselves substantially influenced by experience and research in North America and elsewhere.[6-11] There is scope for continuing to draw lessons from cross-national perspectives on the problem, along with due recognition of differences in service provisions and the legal position between countries. Throughout we are concerned that, although there are lessons to be learned from child abuse, simplistic parallels might be drawn. For example, there are dangers in interventions focused on the *protection* of older people, if they are agist in philosophy, or undermine autonomy and rights in civil and criminal law. The European Convention on Human Rights, recently incorporated into UK domestic law, offers an important counter to these dangers.

HISTORICAL DEVELOPMENT

In the UK, early concerns about the problem of elder abuse were raised by doctors who saw a parallel with child abuse and placed the issue in the wider context of the care of older people both in their own homes and in institutions, emphasizing both the importance of awareness and of good geriatric practice.[12,13] Little was done to follow up this early recognition of the problem and, most crucially, virtually no research was undertaken in the UK until 1990.[14] In its absence, abuse was linked to concerns about family caregivers and the stress placed on them by the care of older people, particularly those with dementia.[15] There was concern with the appropriateness of applying contemporary law to situations involving older people with dementia and associated with risk of harm to all "vulnerable" adults, including those with learning disabilities and severe mental illness. This resulted in a major review of law involving extensive proposals for change.[16,17] Although changes in the law relating to incapacity have so far only taken place in Scotland, one response in England and Wales has been the development of guidance to establish multi-agency structures through which concerns about the abuse of "vulnerable adults" might be addressed.[18-20] This follows earlier policy and practice guidance on elder abuse, by the Department of Health's (DH) Social Services Inspectorate, the body responsible for professional and policy development in social care.[21]

In contrast, in both the USA and Canada, the role of government, at both state and federal level, has been more proactive and a significant benefit of this is that, unlike the UK, a substantial amount of research has taken place, much from a perspective of family violence.[22,23]

DEFINITION

Table 110-1 provides standard definitions and gives examples of both behavior and effect. Elder abuse refers to the ill-treatment

---

Table 110-1 Definitions of types of abuse, with examples of behavior and effects[8]

Physical abuse: Nonaccidental infliction of physical force that results in bodily injury, pain or impairment
- *Examples of behavior:* hitting, slapping, pushing, burning, physical restraint
- *Examples of effects:* bruises, fractures, burns, broken teeth, sprains, cuts, hair loss, bleeding from scalp, fear, anxiety, depression

Psychological abuse: The persistent use of threats, humiliation, bullying, swearing and other verbal conduct, and/or of any other form of mental cruelty, that results in mental or physical distress
- *Examples of behavior:* treating elder as a child, blaming, swearing, intimidating, name-calling, threatening violence, isolating elder
- *Examples of effects:* fear, depression, confusion, loss of sleep, loss of appetite

Financial abuse: Unauthorized and improper use of funds, property or any resources of an older person
- *Examples of behavior:* misappropriating money, valuables, or property; forcing changes to will; denying elder right to access personal funds
- *Examples of effects:* loss of money, etc., inability to pay bills, deterioration in health or standard of living, lack of amenities, unusual activity in bank accounts, signatures on documents uncertain, lack of solid arrangements for financial management, eviction or house sale notices

Sexual abuse: Direct or indirect involvement in sexual activity without consent
- *Examples of behavior*
- *Noncontact:* looking, photography, indecent exposure, harassment, serious teasing or innuendo, pornography
- *Contact:* touching breast, genitals, anus, mouth; masturbation of either or both persons; penetration or attempted penetration of vagina, anus, mouth, with or by penis, fingers, other objects
- *Examples of effects:* difficulty in walking or sitting, bruises, bleeding, venereal disease, psychological trauma

Neglect: Repeated deprivation of assistance needed by the older person for important activities of daily living
- *Examples of behavior:* failure to provide food, shelter, clothing, medical care, hygiene, personal care; inappropriate use of medication or over medication
- *Examples of effects:* malnutrition, pressure sores, oversedation; untreated medical problems, depression, confusion

of an older person (usually defined as over age 65) by commission or omission. Abuse may occur both in domestic settings (the older person's own home, a relative's home, in sheltered housing) and in institutions (day care, residential care, nursing homes, and hospitals). Some kinds of behavior defined as abuse are criminal acts, such as assault and theft; others, such as verbal abuse, or the restraint of someone who is aggressive, may seem more contingent upon particular circumstances. Definitions are important because they determine "who will be counted as abused and who will not."[23]

The importance of relationship to the concept of abuse

Where protection of the older person has dominated policy development, as in the USA, self-neglect is invariably included as part of the definition, and accounts for substantial numbers of reports of abuse.[24,25] However, there is a strong argument for treating self-neglect as a problem in its own right, because it will almost certainly have a different set of explanations from the problem of abuse by others and require different interventions.[9,26] In this chapter, therefore, abuse refers to behavior within a relationship connoting trust. This distinguishes actions by those closely linked to the older person, such as family members, or others in positions of responsibility (such as a member of staff) for their care, from actions by strangers.

Different types of abuse

A review of the research on elder abuse concludes that under the "umbrella" heading of elder abuse there is a diversity of problems and that it is of fundamental importance to distinguish these.[8] There is now widespread agreement about five categories of abuse: physical violence; psychological abuse, often measured by persistent verbal aggression; financial abuse; sexual abuse; and neglect.[23,27] Although sexual abuse is sometimes subsumed under physical abuse, it has been increasingly recognized as a form of abuse in its own right. There is still very limited information on how far these types of abuse occur together and how far they are separate phenomena, but the research suggests that they both occur singly *and* in combination, and that the explanations for the abuse, and therefore the factors relevant to risk, may vary accordingly.

Severity of abuse

The greater the violation of an individual, the more severe the harm to the person and the more distressed they may be.[28] Considering the degree of severity of effect of the abuse, its frequency, how long it has been going on, and the intentions of the abuser should help practitioners to judge the case for intervention and the kind of intervention that may be appropriate.[9]

Vulnerability of older people

In the context of elder abuse, vulnerability arises chiefly from the age-related conditions of physical and mental frailty, disability, and incapacity, but also from socio-economic factors: income, wealth, ethnic background, and social isolation. Older residents of nursing homes, or of any institution that provides them with personal social and healthcare, may be deemed vulnerable by virtue of living there. Service professionals are most likely to have contact with vulnerable older people, who because of their physical and/or mental impairments are least able to protect themselves.[22] This can be important in relation to financial exploitation.[29] The important national incidence study of elder abuse in the USA[30] found—not surprisingly—that reports to Adult Protective Services are much higher for older people who are unable to care for themselves and who have dementia. However, in itself, age is *not* a criterion of being vulnerable.

PREVALENCE AND INCIDENCE

Table 110-2 shows prevalence (in percentages) of elder abuse in North America, the UK, and The Netherlands. There have been two major studies of community prevalence in North America,[31,32] both based on telephone interviews, and one in The Netherlands.[33] Definitions were comparable, although the age range in the Dutch sample was more restricted. The only survey in Great Britain[34] employed broader definitions, and the different levels of abuse reported are more likely to reflect the questions asked rather than the actual levels of abuse in the community.

More recently, the US National Elder Abuse Incidence Study (NEAIS) was designed to obtain national estimates of both

---

Table 110–2 Prevalence of elder abuse in Boston USA, 1986,[31] Canada, 1990,[32] Great Britain, 1992,[34] and Amsterdam, The Netherlands, 1994[33]

Type of abuse	Boston, USA, 1986 (%)	Canada, 1990 (%)	Great Britain, 1992 (%)	Amsterdam, The Netherlands, 1994 (%)
Physical	2	0.5	1.5	1.2
Psychological[a]	1.1	1.1	5.4	3.2
Financial	Not in study	2.5	1.5	1.4
Neglect	0.4	0.4	Not in study	0.2
Multiple	Not in study	0.8	Not in study	Not in study
Base:	*2,020*	*2,008*	*593*	*1797*

[a] *Persistent verbal abuse.*

reported and unreported cases of elder abuse and neglect in 1996.[30] The NEAIS definitions included abandonment and defined psychological abuse in terms of effect, e.g. emotional upset or agitation, rather than behavior as in the prevalence studies, e.g., persistent verbal abuse. It was estimated that 450,000 older people in domestic settings in the United States were abused or neglected by other people in 1996. This constitutes 1.01 percent of people over the age of 60. Physical abuse accounted for only a small proportion of the total. The predominant forms of abuse by others were neglect and psychological abuse. In comparison with the prevalence studies, the overall rate was low and the incidence of neglect (after self-neglect was excluded) high.[35-37] These differences are likely in part to reflect differences between random community sampling in the prevalence research and reports by agencies and "sentinels"—agency staff not reporting cases officially—in the incidence study.

One particular difficulty for studies using the general population is that people who are highly dependent on another person, and particularly people who have significant mental impairment, are unable to participate, except by proxy. In the Dutch study, for example, nonresponse was relatively high for older women as well as for those with mental and physical incapacity.[33] Yet it is precisely these people whom practitioners would identify as most vulnerable.[38] Research in Australia, based on medical records (3 months retrospective study) and assessments (9 months prospective study) of all patients over the age of 65 referred to four Aged Care Assessment Teams in 1994 used similar definitions to the North American prevalence studies.[39] Overall prevalence was 1.2 percent, but varied between teams from 0.4 to 2.9 percent and retrospective rates were roughly twice as high as prospective rates. In smaller research studies, involving interviews with carers of older people with substantial disabilities including dementia, much higher rates of prevalence have been recorded.[12,40,41]

RISK FACTORS

The concept of risk refers to "the probability that a particular adverse event occurs during a stated period of time."[42] Current knowledge about elder abuse does not allow us to use the term in this precise sense, and we use it therefore to refer more generally to current understanding about the factors which appear to discriminate abusive from nonabusive situations. Because the term elder abuse is covering such a diversity of situations,[9] risk needs to be related both to the different types of abuse, and to the different settings in which it may occur. Some of these areas remain almost completely unresearched, so little can be said about them.

Physical and verbal abuse

Domestic settings

This has been the most thoroughly researched area of elder abuse. The key conclusions are:

1. Risk is higher for older people who live with someone.[23,31,32,43] Older people may be abused by their partners, and by other relations including their adult children. The gender differences that are so marked in younger age groups are much less striking among older people.[31,32,44] These probably relate to differences in coresidence patterns in old age. The majority of men of all ages in Great Britain live with a partner, but for women the pattern changes with age.[45] In Britain, two-thirds of women over the age of 80 live on their own.[45]

2. There is limited research linking abuse with socio-demographic variables such as income and education, although ethnic background has been the subject of more discussion.[23] An important exception is the only longitudinal study of its kind—in Connecticut—which was based on reported data from 2,182 adults over the age of 65 over a period of 9 years with sufficiently robust data for logistic regression techniques.[30] Being nonwhite roughly quadrupled the chance of reported abuse, while being poor (income under $5,000 a year) doubled it. However, the authors suggest that these factors are overemphasized by both reporting bias and the confounding of race and poverty.

3. Some abuse is longstanding—Homer and Gilleard[14] refer to the "elderly graduates of domestic violence." Lachs et al.[44] conclude as follows: "Clinicians should be particularly aware of high-risk situations in which functional and/or cognitive impairment are present, especially in circumstances where violent behavior has been known to exist previously."

4. Dependency in the abused person, measured in terms of their need for help with activities of daily living (ADLs), has not been found to be a significant risk factor in much of the research.[31,32,46,47] However, Lachs et al.[44] found that the number of ADL impairments approximately doubled the chance of reported abuse or neglect, and did not consider that reporting bias substantially influenced this particular finding.

5. There is little evidence that the stress of caring for a dependent elder is on its own a cause of abuse.[48-50] Large numbers of carers of are "under stress," but do not abuse their relative.[51] How carers react to the stresses associated with caring may, however, be important.[52]

6. Risk appears to depend more on problematic characteristics associated with the abuser—particularly their physical and mental health and notably, in many studies, their consumption of alcohol.[14,32,49,53-59] It is important to recognize that these problems may include aggressive behavior by an older person with dementia. In our research with general practitioners (GPs), we linked identification of abuse with knowledge of these kinds of factor in patients' households. GPs who identified five or more of 15 risk situations were seven times more likely (all other variables held constant) to have identified a case of abuse.[5]

7. The role of dementia as a risk factor is controversial. Lachs et al.,[44] using logistic regression techniques, found that cognitive impairment, particularly if it was new, was highly significant. Research specifically with dementia patients and their carers found that the factors distinguishing the abusive situations related to the "carers."[14,41] Aggressive and violent behavior by the patient may be associated with aggressive behavior in the person caring for them.[14,60-64]

Institutional settings

There is little research about abuse occurring in institutions.[65–67] Although the definitions used in the domestic setting apply to the communal one, methods of caring assume significance, particularly as the prevalence of physical and mental disability is generally so high among older people in communal settings.[68] Numerous inquiries in Britain into grave deficiencies in various areas of institutional care for all age groups have shown that abuse flourishes within a culture that allows it to be acceptable.[69,70] Research in 57 residential and nursing homes in the USA found that 10 percent of staff admitted to at least one act of physical abuse in the preceding year; excessive restraint was the most frequently recorded form.[71] Staff reported a very much higher rate of verbal than of physical abuse. Significant factors in explaining both kinds of abuse were staff burnout, patient aggression, and staff/patient conflict.[72] A recent research review about aggressive behavior toward staff by older people found substantial evidence that this is routine in many institutional settings, but can be significantly modified by a combination of factors to do with staffing, staff attitudes, environmental quality, and better understanding of the needs of the person with dementia.[73]

Sexual abuse

This type of abuse has been little researched, but such work as there is suggests that the victims are overwhelmingly female, and dependent on others for their care.[74,75] Their abusers may have problems themselves and need help.[74] Dementia increases vulnerability.[74] It has been suggested that greater attention should be paid to the potential for sexual abuse in residential and nursing home settings.[76]

Financial abuse

While nearly all definitions of elder abuse include financial abuse, there has been little research into financial abuse in its own right.[29] It has been stressed that there is a gray area between the financial mismanagement of people's affairs when they grow older and actual abuse.[77] The financial affairs of older people with dementia appear invariably to be incorrectly ordered, thus increasing the risk of financial abuse.[78,79] In contrast to physical and verbal abuse, the risk of abuse to older people in the community may be greater when they are living on their own.[32] This may in turn link to age, to gender (the substantially higher numbers of older women on their own), and to mental incapacity.[80,81] There is some evidence that financial abuse on its own is more likely to be perpetrated by not-so-close relations or paid carers.[29,32,46] When allied with physical and psychological abuse, the perpetrator is more likely to be a close adult relation (usually an adult child) with problems of their own, particularly relating to substance or alcohol abuse. Within institutional settings, very little is known. Again, there is an important issue over whether the appropriate arrangements for handling people's financial affairs are in place and whether there is someone responsible for seeing that these protect them from financial exploitation.[80,81]

Neglect

There are no clear messages from research about the distinguishing circumstances in which neglect occurs. Victims of neglect by others are more likely to be dependent on a caregiver, may be mentally frail, and—unsurprisingly—are in poor health.[32] Increasingly there is concern about neglect in nursing homes.[82–84]

IDENTIFICATION

The majority of cases, whether in domestic or institutional settings, are likely to arise in either primary or secondary care as part of some other presenting problem. Identification depends on a high index of suspicion.[9,85] Research in the USA suggests that there should be a high level of suspicion in accident and emergency departments.[86,87] Health professionals should not assume that health problems are due to age.[1] Two surveys in England showed that many GPs might not be recognizing abuse and would welcome training in both identification and management.[5] Abuse is frequently denied.[27,88] Physical symptoms may be common to frail older people suffering from chronic disease and be unreliable indicators.[7,14,89] When prevalence is relatively low, accurate diagnosis assumes great importance.[89–91] Incorrect diagnosis followed by misplaced interventions may damage all those concerned. Apart from increased sensitivity and awareness of the possibility of abuse, the first general principle, common to all good practice in geriatric medicine[92] and old age psychiatry[9] is that assessment must be holistic.[92] This may be time-consuming and it has been recognized that some doctors may, under pressures of time and shortage of resources, be particularly unwilling to address issues of family violence.[2] However, it is fundamental to view the patient in the context of their lifestyle and family or institutional environment.[8,89] The logic of current research findings is that the suspected perpetrator should be assessed as thoroughly as the victim of abuse.[5]

In the USA, where the law requires mandatory reporting of abuse cases, it is recommended that routine questioning should be built into daily practice and that in every clinical setting there should be a protocol for the detection and assessment of elder abuse.[93] Knowing what to look for is key.[94] There are benefits of a protocol or framework for questioning[1,27,93] and this can be useful in the context of possible financial abuse as well as physical and psychological abuse.[29] In Canada "tremendous energy has been invested in developing instruments to identify seniors at risk for abuse or neglect."[23] However, while recognizing that doctors need to be alert to the possibility of abuse, Canadian commentators have disagreed over whether there is currently sufficient evidence to justify including or excluding case findings for elder abuse as a matter of routine.[95,96]

Financial abuse is an issue that doctors may well encounter in various ways.[27] The *scope* for financial abuse among older people with dementia begins with the management of their finances, if they are no longer able to manage them themselves. Doctors may be approached to advise on this[78] and need to know to whom to refer people for appropriate guidance. However, they may also come across actual abuse in the course of patient contact and it is then necessary for them to know to whom the older person is most appropriately referred.

PREVENTION, TREATMENT, AND MANAGEMENT

The key objectives are the prevention of abuse and the promotion of the older person's autonomy.[12,18,22,23] At the level of policy and guidance, it is essential that the medical profession is properly represented where any professional or local initiatives are taking place to develop a response to abuse.[22,97] In the UK, government guidance has now been issued requiring multi-agency arrangements to protect vulnerable adults from abuse.[18] The appropriate involvement of medical practitioners in these structures is essential, but the experience from child abuse suggests that it will not be easy to achieve.[98]

In the context of patient care, doctors need to be sensitive to the appropriateness of arrangements for an older person's care—an issue raised directly in considering discharge arrangements—particularly from an accident or emergency department. The same considerations apply when considering the discharge of patients with challenging or aggressive behavior to an older person household: are those caring for them able and equipped to provide appropriate care? Two further general principles are "meticulous documentation"[22,89,93] and consultation with other professionals, both within and outside medicine.[22,89,97] Consultation takes time and the difficulties of this and the time it takes need to be taken into account.[22,99] The need to consult raises difficult ethical questions in terms of confidentiality of the doctor–patient relationship, should the older person request the doctor to "do nothing." The older person's rights to autonomy have to be balanced with the need for protection[80,95] and the need for legal intervention, and the possible danger in which they might be placed by misplaced intervention. The assessment of mental capacity, therefore, is of crucial importance and helps direct physicians to the options for intervention if the older person is unwilling to accept any help. Advocacy can be a particularly valuable service.[18]

Figure 110-1, interpreted in relation to the relevant type of abuse and to the legal and service provision context in which medical practitioners are working, gives general guidance. In the UK, the number of laws that potentially bear on abuse are considerable, and legal advice may be needed, because the issues around mental capacity are particularly difficult.[100] In the event of an emergency, the medical practitioner needs to make immediate contact with other responsible agencies, notably the police and social services in the UK, adult protection services in the USA, and act to protect the older person from any further harm. While safety of the victim is the first

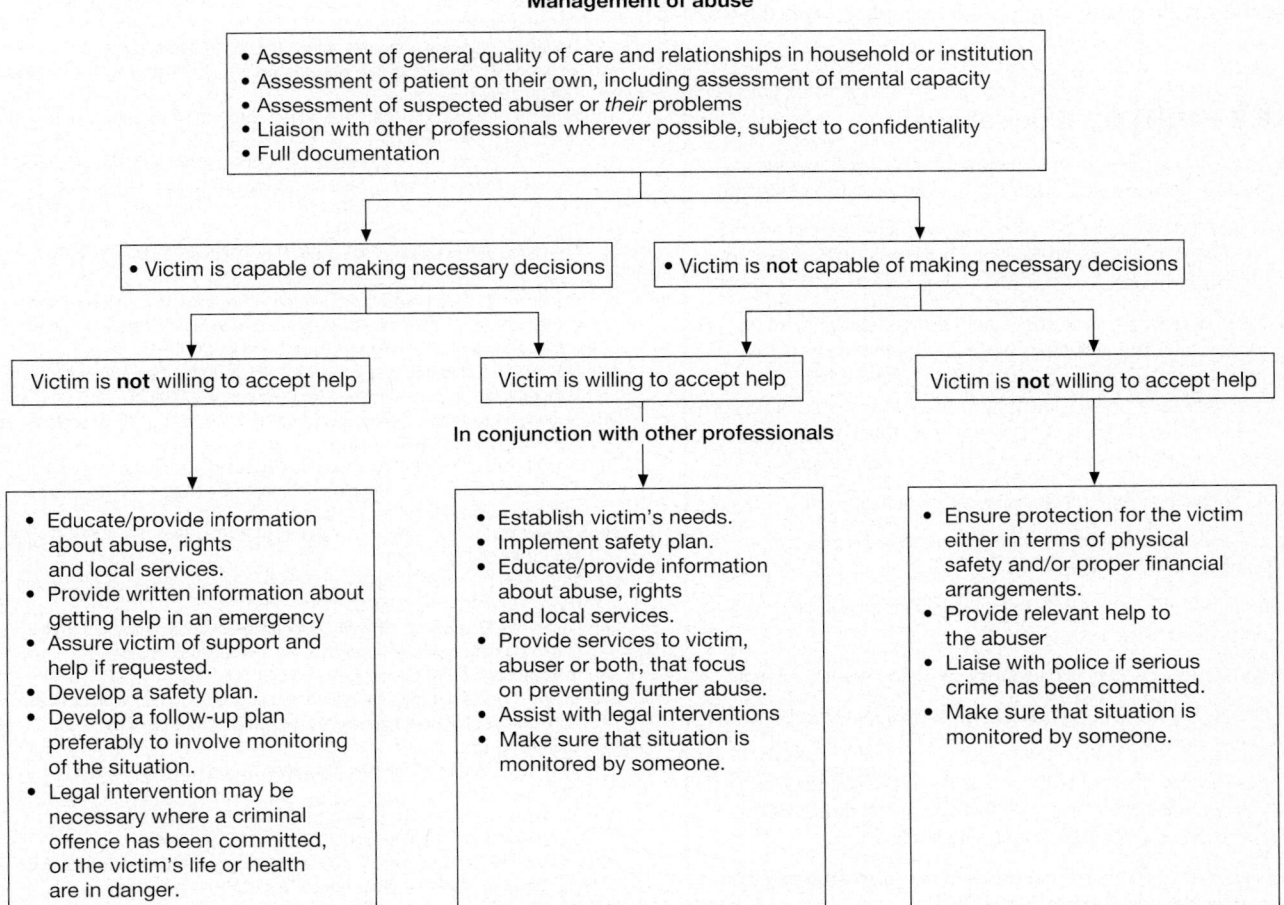

Figure 110-1 Management of abuse. (Data from Fisk,[9] Lachs and Pillemer,[22] Kurrle,[109] and American Medical Association.[93])

priority, situations arising are such that it is also essential to pay attention to the physical and psychological health of the suspected abuser, who themselves may be vulnerable.

CONCLUSION

Elder abuse "appears in many forms and for many reasons."[9] It encompasses domestic violence and harm inflicted on vulnerable adults. In some cases it is linked with shorter survival.[101] Overall, the primary aim should be to prevent abuse from occurring. There would appear to be at least four planks in prevention. The first is the provision of effective health and welfare services for older people, including pension and housing provision.[90,102,103] The second is awareness among a wide range of professionals, of whom the medical profession are crucial, that abuse can and does exist and requires a response, which is most effective when it is multidisciplinary.[1,18,97,104] This may involve training[5,23,105] and guidelines.[18,93] It also implies valid and reliable screening tools for detecting abuse.[27] Third, in the context of a policy emphasis on care in the community, is the need for recognition and action around caregivers, who may be both abuser and/or abused, older or younger themselves, and in their own right suffering from physical or mental illness.[106] Finally, in the context of institutional care, it is essential that all requirements within a nation for the monitoring or regulation of the quality of care are met, and that there is a general imperative to provide quality care to older people.[107] It is the worst of all possible worlds, as older people themselves are only too aware, to move an older victim to an institution only for them to suffer abuse there. In summary, "the challenge is to make sure that efforts on behalf of mistreated older persons do more good than harm and do not lead to the neglect of other societal needs."[108]

> ### KEY POINTS   Elder abuse
>
> ■ Elder abuse refers to the ill-treatment of an older person (usually defined as over age 65) by commission or omission.
>
> ■ Under the "umbrella" heading of elder abuse there is a diversity of problems and it is of fundamental importance to distinguish these.
>
> ■ Risk of physical/verbal abuse appears to depend more on problematic characteristics associated with the abuser—particularly their physical and mental health (including dementia) and notably, in many studies, their consumption of alcohol. There is little evidence that the stress of caring for a dependent elder is on its own a cause of such abuse.
>
> ■ Identification depends on a high index of suspicion.
>
> ■ Accurate diagnosis is particularly important because of relatively low prevalence.
>
> ■ Incorrect diagnosis followed by misplaced interventions may damage all those concerned.
>
> ■ Holistic assessment is necessary, including mental capacity.
>
> ■ Suspected perpetrators should be assessed as thoroughly as abuse victims.
>
> ■ The severity of effect of the abuse, its frequency, how long it has been going on, and the intentions of the abuser help practitioners judge the case for intervention.
>
> ■ Key objectives are the prevention of abuse and the promotion of the older person's autonomy.

REFERENCES

1. Bennett G, Kingston P, Penhale, B: The Dimensions of Elder Abuse: Perspectives for practitioners. Macmillan, London, 1997
2. Jones JS: Elder abuse and neglect: responding to a national problem. Ann Emerg Med 1994;23:845–848
3. Lachs MS: Preaching to the unconverted: educating physicians about elder abuse. J Elder Abuse Neglect 1995;4:1–12
4. Rosenblatt DE: Elder abuse. What can physicians do? Arch Fam Med 1996;5:88–90
5. McCreadie C, Bennett G, Gilthorpe MS, Houghton G, Tinker A: Elder abuse: do general practitioners know or care? J Roy Soc Med 2000;93:67–71
6. McCreadie C, Tinker A: Review: abuse of elderly people in the domestic setting: a UK perspective. Age Ageing 1993;22:65–69
7. Biggs S, Phillipson C, Kingston P: Elder Abuse in Perspective. Open University Press, 1995
8. McCreadie C: Elder Abuse: an Update on Research. Age Concern Institute of Gerontology. King's College, London, 1996
9. Fisk J: Abuse of the elderly. In Jacoby R, Oppenheimer C (eds): Psychiatry in the Elderly, 2nd ed. Oxford University Press, Oxford, 1997:736–748
10. Pritchard J (ed): Elder Abuse Work. Jessica Kingsley, London, 1999
11. Brogden M, Nijhar P: Crime, Abuse and the Elderly. Willan Publishing, Cullompton, Devon, UK, 2000
12. Baker AA: "Granny-battering". Mod Geriatr 1975;8:20–24
13. Burston GR: Do your elderly patients live in fear of being battered? Mod Geriatr 1977;5:54–55
14. Homer A, Gilleard CJ: Abuse of elderly people by their carers. Br Med J 1990;301:1359–1362
15. Tomlin S: Abuse of Elderly People: An Unnecessary and Preventable Problem. British Geriatrics Society, London, 1989
16. Law Commission: Mental Incapacity (Law Com. No. 231). Her Majesty's Stationery Office, London, 1995
17. Lord Chancellor: Making Decisions. The Stationery Office, London, 1999
18. Department of Health (DH): No Secrets: Guidance on developing and implementing multi-agency policies and procedures to protect vulnerable adults from abuse. DH/Home Office, London, 2000
19. McCreadie C: No Secrets: guidance in England for the protection of vulnerable adults from abuse. J Adult Protect 2000;2(3):5–16
20. National Assembly for Wales: In Safe Hands: Protection of Vulnerable Adults in Wales. Cardiff, 2000:6
21. Department of Health Social Services Inspectorate: No Longer Afraid: The Safeguard of Older People in Domestic Settings. Her Majesty's Stationery Office, London, 1993
22. Lachs MS, Pillemer KA: Abuse and neglect of elderly persons. N Engl J Med 1995;332:437–443
23. McDonald L, Collins A: Abuse and neglect of older adults: a discussion paper. Health Canada, 2000
24. Lachs MS, Berkman L, Fulmer T, Horwitz RI: A prospective community-based pilot study of risk factors for the investigation of elder mistreatment. J Am Geriatr Soc 1994;42:169–173
25. Tatara T: Understanding the nature and scope of domestic elder abuse with the use of state aggregate data. J Elder Abuse Neglect 1994;4:35–58
26. Cooney C, Hamid W: Review: Diogenes Syndrome. Age Ageing 1995;24:451–453
27. Silverman J, Hudson M: Elder mistreatment: A guide for medical professionals. N Carolina Med J 2000;61, 5, 291–296
28. Johns S, Hydle I, Aschjem O: The act of abuse: a two-headed monster of injury and offense. J Elder Abuse Neglect 1991;1:53–64
29. Tueth MJ: Exposing financial exploitation of impaired elderly persons. Am J Ger Psych 2000;8(2):104–111

30. Tatara T, Thomas C: National Elder Abuse Incidence Study. http://www.aoa.dhhs.gov/abuse/report/default.htm Accessed 30 March 2001

31. Pillemer KA, Finkelhor D: The prevalence of elder abuse: a random sample survey. Gerontologist 1988;28:51–57

32. Podnieks E: National Survey on Abuse of the Elderly in Canada. Ryerson Polytechnical Institute, Toronto, 1990

33. Comijs H: Elder Mistreatment: Prevalence, Risk Indicators and Consequences. Vrije Universsiteit, Amsterdam, 1999

34. Ogg J, Bennett GCJ: Elder abuse in Britain. Br Med J 1992;305:998–999

35. Thomas C: The first national study of elder abuse and neglect: contrast with results from other studies. J Elder Abuse Neglect 2000;12(1):1–14

36. Mixson P: Counterparts across time: comparing the national elder abuse incidence study and the national incidence study of child abuse. J Elder Abuse Neglect 2000;12(1):19–27

37. Callahan J: Elder abuse revisited. J Elder Abuse Neglect 2000;12(1):33–36

38. Decalmer P, Glendenning F: The Mistreatment of Older People, 2nd Ed. Sage, London, 1997

39. Kurrle S, Sadler P, Lockwood K, Cameron I: Elder abuse: prevalence, intervention and outcome in patients referred to four Aged Care Assessment Teams. Med J Aust 1997;166:119–122

40. Cooney C, Mortimer A: Elder abuse and dementia: a pilot study. Int J Soc Psych 1995;41:276–283

41. Compton SA, Flanigan P, Gregg W: Elder abuse in people with dementia in Northern Ireland: prevalence and predictors in cases referred to a psychiatry of old age service. Int J Ger Psych 1997;12:632–635

42. Royal Society, The Risk: analysis, perception and management, report of a Royal Society Study Group. The Royal Society, London, 1992

43. Penning MJ: Elder Abuse Resource Centre. Research component—Final Report. Centre on Aging. University of Manitoba, Winnipeg, 1992

44. Lachs MD, Williams C, O'Brien S, Hurst L, Horwitz R: Risk factors for reported elder abuse and neglect: a nine-year observational cohort study. Gerontologist 37(4):469–474

45. Askham J, Grundy E, Hancock R, Tinker A: Life after 60. A Report from the Gerontology Data Service of the Age Concern Institute of Gerontology, King's College, London, 1992

46. Wolf RS, Pillemer KA: Helping elderly victims: the reality of elder abuse. Columbia University Press, New York, 1989

47. Godkin MA, Wolf RS, Pillemer KA: A case-comparison analysis of elder abuse and neglect. Int J Aging Hum Dev 1989;288:207–225

48. Kurrle SE, Sadler PM, Cameron ID: Patterns of elder abuse. Med J Aust 1992;157:673–676

49. Pillemer KA, Finkelhor D: Causes of elder abuse: caregiver stress versus problem relatives. Am J Orthopsych 1989;59:179–187

50. Pittaway E, Gallagher E: Services for Abused Older Canadians. Centre on Aging, University of Victoria, Canada, 1995

51. Marin RS: The debate over dependency as a relevant predisposing factor in elder abuse and neglect. A research perspective. J Elder Abuse Neglect 1990;2:59–63

52. Steinmetz SK: The abused elderly are dependent: abuse is caused by the perception of stress associated with providing care. In RJ Gelles and DR Loseke (eds): Current Controversies on Family Violence. Sage, London, 1993

53. Anetzberger G, Korbin J, Austin C: Alcoholism and elder abuse. J Interpers Violence 1994;9:184–193

54. Greenberg J, McKibben M, Raymond J: Dependent adult children and elder abuse. J Elder Abuse Neglect 1990;2:73–86

55. Saveman B-I: Formal Careers in Health Care and the Social Services Witnessing Abuse of the Elderly in their Homes. Umea University Medical Dissertations, New Series no. 403, Umea, Sweden, 1994

56. Wolf RS: Spouse abuse and neglect in the aging family. In Wolf RS, Bergman S (eds): Stress, Conflict and Abuse of the Elderly. Brookdale Institute, Jerusalem, 1989

57. Bristowe E, Collins JB: Family mediated abuse of non-institutionalized frail elderly men and women living in British Columbia. J Elder Abuse Neglect 1989;1:45–64

58. Hwalek M, Neale A, Goodrich C, Quinn K: The association of elder abuse and substance abuse in the Illinois elder abuse system. Gerontologist 1996;36(5):694–700

59. McCreadie C, Claydon T, Denne C: Understanding elder abuse: the SAVE project. J Adult Protection 1999;1(1):23–30

60. Levin E, Sinclair I, Gorbach P: Families, Services and Confusion in Old Age. Gower Publishing Company, Avebury, Aldershot, 1989

61. Paveza GJ, Cohen D, Eisdorfer C et al: Severe family violence and Alzheimer's disease: prevalence and risk factors. Gerontologist 1992;32:493–497

62. Pillemer KA, Suitor JJ: Violence and violent feelings: what causes them among family caregivers? J Gerontol 1992;47:S165–S172

63. Coyne A, Reichman WE, Berbig LJ: The relationship between dementia and elder abuse. Am J Psych 1993;150:643–646

64. Cahill S, Shapiro M: "I think he might have hit me once": aggression towards caregivers in dementia care. Aust J Ageing 1993;4:10–15

65. Gilleard C: Physical abuse in homes and hospitals. In Eastman M (ed): Old Age Abuse. 2nd Ed. Age Concern England/Chapman and Hall, London, 1994:93–110

66. Glendenning F, Kingston P (eds): Elder Abuse and Neglect in Residential Settings: Different National Backgrounds and Similar Responses. The Haworth Press, New York, 1999

67. Stanley N, Manthorpe J, Penhale B (eds): Institutional Abuse: Perspectives Across the Life Course. Routledge, London, 1999

68. Martin J, Meltzer H, Elliot D: The Prevalence of Disability Among Adults. OPCS Surveys of Disability in Great Britain. Report 1. Her Majesty's Stationery Office, London, 1988

69. Clough R: Scandalous care: interpreting public enquiry reports of scandals in residential care. J Elder Abuse Neglect 1999;10(1/2):13–28

70. Camden and Islington Community Health Services NHS Trust: Beech House Inquiry. Camden and Islington CHS NHS Trust, London, 1999

71. Pillemer KA, Moore D: Abuse of patient in nursing homes: findings from a survey of staff. Gerontologist 1989;3:314–320

72. Pillemer KA, Bachman-Prehn R: Helping and hurting: predictors of maltreatment of patients in nursing homes. Res Aging 1991;1:74–95

73. McCreadie C: Review of research on violence towards social care staff with special reference to services for people with Alzheimer's disease. June 2001. www.doh.gov.uk/violencetaskforce/knowledge.htm Accessed 30 March 2001

74. Benbow SM, Haddad PM: Sexual abuse of the elderly mentally ill. Postgrad Med J 1993;69:803–807

75. Ramsey-Klawsnik H: Elder sexual abuse: preliminary findings. J Elder Abuse Neglect 1991;3:73–90

76. Sengstock M, McFarland MR, Hwalek M: Identification of elder abuse in institutional settings. J Elder Abuse Neglect 1991;1:31–50

77. Langan J, Means R: Financial management and elderly people with dementia in the UK: as much a question of confusion as abuse? Ageing Soc 1996;16:287–314

78. Rowe J, Davies KN, Baburaj V, Sinha RN: F.A.D.E. A.W.A.Y.: The Financial Affairs of Dementing Elders and Who Is the Attorney? J Elder Abuse Neglect 1993;2:73–79

79. Homer A: Abuse of elderly people. Br Med J 1992;305:1363 (letter)

80. Wilber KH, Reynolds SL: Introducing a framework for defining financial abuse of the elderly. J Elder Abuse Neglect 1996;2:61–80

81. Blunt AP: Financial exploitation of the incapacitated: investigation and remedies. J Elder Abuse Neglect 1993;1:19–32

82. Hirschel AE: Setting the stage: the advocates' struggle to address gross neglect in Philadelphia nursing homes. J Elder Abuse Neglect 1996;3:5–20

83. Age Concern New Zealand, Age Concern Elder Abuse and Neglect Services: Report of Statistics and Service Developments Covering the Three Years from July 1996 to June 1999. Age Concern New Zealand, 1999

84. Stevenson O: Elder Protection in Residential Care: What Can We Learn from Child Protection? DH, London, 1999

85. Kurrle S: Australian Society for Geriatric Medicine Position Statement on Elder Abuse. Aust J Ageing 1995;4:172–175

86. Lachs MS, Williams CS, O'Brien S et al: Emergency department use by older victims of family violence. Ann Emerg Med 1997;4:448–454

87. Kleinschmidt K: Elder abuse: a review. Ann Emerg Med 1997;4:463–472

88. Bennett G, Ogg J: Researching elder abuse. In McCreadie C (ed): Elder Abuse: New Findings and Policy Guidelines. Age Concern Institute of Gerontology, King's College, London, 1993

89. Lachs M, Fulmer T: Recognising elder abuse and neglect. Clin Geriatr Med 1993;3:665–679

90. McCallum J: Elder abuse: the "new" social problem? Mod Med Aust 1993;9:74–83

91. Duggan C: Introduction to risk assessment. Br J Psych 1997;170(suppl 32):1–3

92. Rubenstein LZ, Rubenstein LV: Multidimensional geriatric assessment. In Tallis RC, Fillit HM, Brocklehurst JC (eds): Brocklehurst's Textbook of

Geriatric Medicine and Gerontology, 5th Ed. Churchill Livingstone, New York, 1998:207–216

93. American Medical Association: Diagnostic and Treatment Guidelines on Elder Abuse and Neglect. American Medical Association, Chicago, 1992

94. Kruger RM, Moon CH: Can you spot the signs of elder mistreatment? Postgrad Med 1999;1106(2):353–358

95. Canadian Task Force on the Periodic Health Examination: Secondary prevention of elder abuse and mistreatment. Can Med Assoc J 1994;10:1413–1421

96. Kozak J: Difficulties in addressing abuse and neglect in elderly patients. Can Med Assoc J 1994;151(10):1401–1403

97. Anderson AJ: Elder Abuse; the Clinical Reality. In Pritchard J (ed): Elder abuse work. Jessica Kingsley, London, 1999

98. Birchall E, Hallett C: Working Together in Child Protection. A Survey of the Experience and Perceptions of Six Key Professions. Her Majesty's Stationery Office, London, 1995

99. O'Loughlin A, Duggan J: Abuse, neglect and mistreatment of older people: An exploratory study. National Council on Ageing and Older People, Dublin, 1998

100. British Medical Association: Assessment of Mental Capacity: Guidance for Doctors and Lawyers. Joint Report of the BMA and the Law Society. British Medical Association, London, 1996

101. Lachs MS, Williams CS, O'Brien S, Pillemer KA, Charlson ME: The mortality of elder mistreatment. JAMA 1998;5:428–432

102. Callahan JJ: Elder abuse: some questions for policymakers. Gerontologist 1988;4:453–458

103. Callahan JJ: Elder abuse revisited. J Elder Abuse Neglect 2000;1:33–36

104. Wolf RS: Testimony on behalf of the National Committee for the Prevention of Elder Abuse before the U.S. House Select Committee on Aging, Subcommittee on Human Services. J Elder Abuse Neglect 1991;4:87–99

105. Glendenning F: The abuse of older people in institutional settings. In Stanley N, Manthorpe J, Penhale B (eds): Institutional Abuse: Perspectives Across the Life Course. Routledge, London, 1999:173–190

106. Homer A: Prevalence and prevention of elder abuse. In Eastman M (ed): Old Age Abuse, 2nd Ed. Age Concern England/Chapman and Hall, London, 1994:31–50

107. Royal College of Physicians: High quality long-term care for elderly people: guidelines and audit measures. Report, Royal College of Physicians, British Geriatrics Society. Royal College of Physicians, London, 1992

108. Wolf RS: Making an issue of elder abuse. Gerontologist 1992;3:427–429

109. Kurrle S: Elder abuse: a hidden problem. Mod Med Aust 1993;9:58–72

Chapter 111

Sexuality in old age

Robert N. Butler and Myrna I. Lewis

MISINFORMATION, MYTHS, AND PREJUDICES

Older patients' sexuality is frequently overlooked by physicians during the typical medical examination and evaluation. As a result, physicians may miss the opportunity to offer their older patients reassurance about the normal changes in sexuality that may be troubling them; they may not advise these patients about the side-effects of medications that can impact adversely on continuing sexual activity; and they may fail to diagnose sexual dysfunction and recommend treatment possibilities.[1]

Lack of public and professional medical education is partially to blame for this neglect of late-life sexuality in the medical encounter. Centuries of myths about aging, as well as prudery and ignorance, have helped close the minds of laypeople and professionals alike to the fact that many older people wish to, and do, continue expressing their sexuality until the end of their life. Because few studies have been conducted on sexuality in general, and on late-life sexuality in particular, there have been scant data about the nature and frequency of sexual activity among older persons. However, self-reports from surveys of older people have demonstrated that, for many, sexual desire and satisfaction remain important aspects of their lives. The main barriers to sexual expression in late life are medical and psychological problems and social obstacles. A problematic marital relationship or lack of a partner due to the death of a spouse or companion may also interfere.[1]

With the discovery of the therapeutic effect in men of sildenafil citrate in erectile dysfunction (ED) and its introduction in 1998, the attitudes of physicians and that of the public have moved to more positive approaches and acceptance of sexuality for older persons. This includes a growing awareness of the need for further understanding of female sexuality, including better diagnosis and treatment for older women that parallels current breakthroughs for older men.

NORMAL AGING AND CHANGES IN SEXUALITY

Sexuality may be defined as the quality or state that comprises sexual desire (libido), arousal, function, and activity; physical satisfaction; and emotional intimacy. Many older people maintain desire (libido) and sexual capacity and satisfaction so long as they have their health, a healthy partner, and a good relationship with that partner. They experience the same four stages of the sexual act as younger people: desire, arousal, climax, and recovery. Sexual expression remains a highly complex process in old age, comprised of fantasy, the central nervous and peripheral nervous systems, the circulatory system, and all six senses. The capacity for fantasy may, however, decline for older men, according to the National Institute on Aging's Baltimore Longitudinal Study on Aging. We do not know if this is equally true for women because sexual fantasy in women was not documented in the study.

Normal change in sexual functioning is usually manifested as a gradual slowing; that is, more time is needed for arousal (erection in men; lubrication in women) and reaching a climax. Unlike women, healthy men can remain fertile until the end of life. There is no discrete climacteric for men, but rather, a gradual decline of testosterone levels after age 30 that usually do not fall below normal. Testosterone levels in 70 percent of healthy older men are in the same range as those of younger men. With aging, the testes may become smaller and penile flaccidity greater. More direct stimulation of the penis may be necessary to reach engorgement and erection. For some older men, orgasm may last a shorter time than it did when they were younger. The force of ejaculation and the volume of ejaculate decrease. A great concern for older men (and for younger men as well) is their ability to maintain sexual potency. Impotence and ED are often automatically and inaccurately attributed to increasing age. They can, in fact, occur at any age for a variety of reasons and, once properly diagnosed, are often treatable[1] (see ED below).

Owing to cultural emphasis on a youthful female body image, older women tend to be more concerned than men about physical appearance and their sexual desirability. However, those women who are healthy can usually continue earlier patterns of sexual functioning, which includes maintaining orgasmic capacity. For some women, sexual interest may increase after the menopause because they no longer experience concern about pregnancy. Nonetheless, reduced estrogen production due to the menopause may present both physical and emotional problems for a number of older women. Physical problems include a change in vaginal shape, vaginal dryness, and thinning of the vaginal walls, which may lead to pain and bleeding during coitus and a less well-protected bladder and urethra, with recurrent cystitis as a result. Less acidic vaginal secretions may lead to greater incidence of vaginal infections. Emotional problems accompanying menopause include increased irritability and lability, often due to sleep deprivation, which is itself a menopausal symptom. Although estrogen replacement therapy (ERT) helps relieve some symptoms, extensive studies by the National Institutes of Health's Women's Health Initiative (WHI) have implicated ERT in the development of gallbladder disease, and breast and uterine cancer. These studies also suggest that ERT may increase the risks of blood clots that can result in strokes and heart attacks. However, since the results of the WHI were based on estrogen derived from pregnant mares' urine (Premarin) that may be difficult to metabolize, further studies using other estrogen products are needed. In the meantime, to diet, exercise, as well as drugs that lower cholesterol and blood pressure can lower risk of heart disease, and nonhormonal drugs such as bisphosphonates may be effective in cutting the risk of fractures in women with osteoporosis. Women can often find relief for vaginal dryness and irritation during intercourse with off-prescription water-based vaginal lubricants.[2]

Women who wish to remain sexually active in later life may face barriers that have nothing to do with physical symptoms. Because women live nearly seven years longer than men and tend to marry men who are three or more years older, they have a much greater chance of surviving their male partners. About 60 percent of older women are without a spouse, as opposed to 20 percent of men, and many others may be living with a disabled spouse who cannot be a sexual partner. As they grow older, the ratio of women to men increases greatly, and the chances of finding another partner are greatly reduced. There are approximately 150 women to 100 men over the age of 65, and 250 women to 100 men over the age of 85.

It has been estimated that up to 10 percent of the general population is lesbian, gay, bisexual, or transgender (LGBT), although the exact number is unknown. Similar to the older heterosexual population, many LGBT individuals have long-term relationships and are emotionally stable, successful, and happy in their later years. When sexual difficulties occur for LGBT couples, they involve many of the same interpersonal, physical, social, and psychological problems faced by heterosexual couples. Physicians need to be sensitive to and accepting of alternative sexual expression.[2]

EXAMINATION AND EVALUATION OF THE PATIENT

The general medical evaluation of an older person should include a thorough sexual history, current sexual function, and a careful physical examination. The physician should initiate questions in these areas because older patients may not volunteer sexual information about themselves. Questions should be asked in an unintimidating and unembarrassing fashion. During the examination, the physician should pay special attention to the neurological, circulatory, and endocrine systems. Because some medical conditions, surgical procedures, and medications can affect sexual functioning, the physician should be sure to include a discussion of sexuality when treating disease or prescribing medication to patients for whom continuing sexual activity is important.

The physician should be aware of the fact that sexually transmitted diseases (STDs) occur in old as well as young persons. People of all ages should practice "safe sex." Ten percent of all AIDS patients in the USA are over 55 years of age, and not all of them contracted HIV through blood transfusions. Hepatitis B is the only sexually transmitted virus preventable by vaccine.[2]

EFFECTS OF MEDICAL PROBLEMS, SURGERY, AND MEDICATIONS

Sexual interest and capacity wane in the presence of illness, and some diseases have a much more powerful effect upon sexuality in the later years because of their frequency and character. Heart disease is three times more common in men than in women up to the age of 60, probably because of the protection afforded by estrogen, even postmenopausally. However, after the menopause the incidence of heart disease in women begins to rise and eventually reaches that of men in the early 60s. Heart disease is a source of considerable concern to sexually active older people because sexual activity increases the heart rate. Many who have had angina or a heart attack become anxious about future sexual encounters. The fear of dying during intercourse may also compound depression that is already present in response to the heart disease itself. Physicians should point out to their concerned patients that, in fact, oxygen usage or "debt" in a sexual encounter is the rough equivalent of walking up one or two flights of stairs. Physicians should reassure their patients that anyone who can carry out usual daily activities is able to engage in sexual activity. A study published in 1996 of over 800 men and women found that among individuals who had suffered a heart attack, the risk of a recurrent heart attack during sex was only two in one million.[3] An earlier large-scale study of more than 5,500 coronary deaths found that fewer than one percent were related to sex, with the majority of these involving extramarital relations (suggesting that stressful aspects associated with such affairs—guilt, anxiety, the need to hurry—may play a role).[4] Thus, sexual activity poses extraordinarily little risk.

Patients are often uneasy about recommencing their sex lives following coronary bypass surgery. Some 4 weeks or more of abstinence is recommended before resuming sexual activity, to allow full healing to occur.

Other medical conditions that can impact significantly on sexuality are stroke, diabetes, osteoarthritis and rheumatoid arthritis, backache, Parkinson's disease, chronic emphysema and bronchitis, chronic prostatitis in men, and stress incontinence in women. The effects on sexuality of these diseases and their treatment are summarized in Table 111-1.

Surgery can significantly impair sexual functioning as well. Common surgical procedures and their effects on sexuality are outlined in Table 111-2. Embarrassment or discomfiture from surgical procedures such as mastectomies or ostomies can inhibit sexual drive and performance. Prostate surgery is discussed in the section on ED below.

Medications are among the most common causes of sexual dysfunction. Commonly prescribed medications that adversely affect sexuality are listed in Table 111-3. Physicians should familiarize themselves with medications that have fewer toxic effects on sexual function and prescribe them whenever possible. For example, angiotensin-converting enzyme (ACE) inhibitors taken for hypertension are less apt to cause sexual dysfunction than methyldopa. Of the antidepressants, Wellbutrin is one of the least problematic. In addition, it is possible to reduce the dosage of some drugs to avoid adverse sexual and other effects without reducing the benefits of the drugs to the patient.[5] In certain cases, brief "drug holidays" may improve sexual function, but this requires discussion with one's physician.

Abuse of substances such as alcohol and tobacco also impairs sexuality (see Table 111-3). Alcohol may increase desire, but decrease performance. Tobacco adversely affects male sexuality and causes wrinkles in both men and women.

ERECTILE DYSFUNCTION

Causes and diagnosis

Because even occasional erectile dysfunction (ED) can have significant emotional consequences for many men, which can,

Table 111-1 **Effects of medical conditions on sexuality**

Medical condition	Effect on sexuality	Treatment
Arthritis	Sexual desire is usually unaffected, but disability due to osteoarthritis and rheumatoid arthritis may interfere with performance	Trying sexual positions that do not aggravate joint pain; planning sexual activity for times of day when pain and stiffness are diminished
Chronic emphysema and bronchitis	Shortness of breath hinders physical activity, including sex	Rest; supplemental oxygen
Chronic prostatitis	Pain may diminish sexual desire	Antibiotics; warm sitz baths, prostatic massage; Kegel exercises
Chronic renal disease	Impotence, possibly with anxiety and depression	Dialysis; psychotherapy for underlying emotional problems; kidney transplantation may restore sexual capacity
Diabetes mellitus	Impotence is common	Very tight control of diabetes may restore potency
Heart and vascular disease:		
Myocardial infarction	8–14 week recuperation period recommended before resuming sexual intercourse; depression and antidepressant drugs may reduce libido and capacity; fear of bringing on another heart attack if patient resumes sexual activity	Reassurance from the doctor about safety of sexual activity; exercise programs to improve cardiac function
Heart failure	Sexual dysfunction due to physical symptoms or medications; a 2–3 week recovery period is advised before resuming sex in cases of pulmonary edema	Reassurance from the doctor about safety of sexual activity for patients with effectively managed heart failure; exercise programs to improve cardiac function
Coronary bypass surgery	4 weeks or more of abstinence is recommended before resuming sexual intercourse	Alternatives such as self-stimulation or masturbation can usually be started earlier in the recovery period; exercise programs to improve cardiac function
Pelvic steal syndrome	Example of vascular impotence—male loses erection as soon as he enters his partner and begins pelvic thrusting due to gravity's redirecting blood supply away from the pelvis	Changing position may help (man should lie on his back or side)
Hypertension	Incidence of impotence in untreated male hypertensive patients is about 15%; effects on women not established	Choose hypertensive drugs that do not impair sexual response
Parkinson's disease	Lack of sexual desire in both men and women; impotence in men	Levodopa can improve sex drive and performance in some men for a limited period
Peyronie's disease	Intercourse is painful for many men with the disease; penetration may be difficult or impossible when penis is angled too sharply	Psychotherapy to help patient adjust to changes in the penis; symptoms occasionally disappear spontaneously; surgery helps in some cases
Stress incontinence	Sexual dysfunction has been reported in up to 50% of women with this condition	Solving the underlying problem may help; Kegel exercises to strengthen muscles supporting bladder; estrogen taken orally or locally to firm up vaginal lining; biofeedback training
Stroke	Sexual desire may not be impaired, but sexual performance likely to be affected (e.g. male erectile dysfunction either due to physical or psychological reasons, anesthetic areas, and/ or physical limitations due to paralysis)	Mechanical adjustments to assist positioning necessary for sexual activities; treatments for impotence

Data from Butler and Lewis.[1,2]

in turn, exacerbate physical problems, diagnosis should be made carefully. Erectile dysfunction should be diagnosed only when failure in sexual encounters occurs in at least a quarter of all attempts.

It is estimated that 10–20 million men in the USA experience some degree of erectile dysfunction. Although ED affects men of all ages, it tends to increase progressively with age because of the greater likelihood of accompanying medical conditions. The comprehensive Massachusetts Male Health Study found that 52 percent of men aged 40–70 experience some ED.[6]

It is estimated that 90 percent of erectile dysfunction cases are due to physical causes, including vascular disorders such as atherosclerosis and pelvic steal syndrome (Table 111-1); neurological disorders such as trauma (e.g. sports injuries) and diabetic neuropathy; and endocrine disorders, such as thyroid disease, diabetes, and low testosterone levels, although low testosterone affects only about 4 percent of men. Testosterone

Table 111-2 Effects of surgery on sexuality

Surgical procedure	Effect on sexuality
Hysterectomy	Need to refrain from sexual activity during healing (6–8 weeks after surgery); depression; possible reduction in sensation during orgasm
Mastectomy	Emotional reactions such as depression; loss of sexual desire due to emotional reactions of patient and partner
Prostatectomy	Need to refrain from sexual activity during healing (6 weeks); possible impotence due to surgery (nerve-sparing techniques help avoid this effect in some cases); possible psychogenic impotence
Orchiectomy	Impotence is common
Colostomy and ileostomy	Emotional reactions that can affect desire and potency (participation in ostomy clubs is recommended)
Rectal cancer surgery	Impotence is common

Data from Butler and Lewis.[1,2]

Table 111-3 Selected medications and substances that may adversely affect sexual functioning:

Psychotropics	Atenolol
Tricyclic antidepressants	Metoprolol
Clomipramine	Bisoprolol
Amitriptyline	Timolol
Doxepin	Betaxolol
Imipramine	α_1-blockers
Nortriptyline[a]	Prazosin[a]
Desipramine[a]	Doxazosin[a]
Monoamine oxidase inhibitors	α_2-agonists
Isocarboxazid	Clonidine
Phenelzine	Guanfacine
Tranylcypromine[a]	ACE inhibitors[c]
Serotonin reuptake inhibitors	Captopril[a]
Fluoxetine	Enalapril
Paroxetine	Calcium-channel blockers
Sertraline	Amlodipine
Fluvoxamine	Verapamil
Venlafaxine	Diltiazem
Mood stabilizers/anticonvulsants	Anticancer drugs
Lithium[b]	Vinblastine
Valproate[a]	5-fluorouracil
Carbamazepine	Tamoxifen
Phenytoin	Cold/allergy medications
Phenobarbitol	Chlorpheniramine
Antipsychotics/neuroleptics	Diphenhydramine hydrochloride
Phenothiazines	
Chlorpromazine	Pseudoephedrine
Fluphenazine[a]	Antiulcer medications
Perphenazine	Cimetidine
Thioridazine	Famotidine[a]
Other	Nizatidine[a]
Haloperidol	Ranitidine[a]
Thiothixene	Stimulants/anorectics
Risperidone	Phentermine
Antianxiety agents/tranquilizers	Fenfluramine
Benzodiazepines	Phenylpropanolamine
Diuretics	Diethylpropion
Thiazide-type	Mazindol
Chlorthalidone	Commonly abused substances
Hydrochlorothiazide	
Indapamide[a]	Alcohol
Loop diuretics	Barbiturates
Furosemide[a]	Cannabis
Potassium-sparing	Cocaine
Spironolactone	Opioids
Antihypertensives	Methylphenidate
Reserpine	Amphetamine
Methyldopa	Nicotine
Guanethidine	Hormones
β-blockers	Progesterone
Propanolol	Cortisol

[a]*Studies indicate that these drugs may have fewer sexual side-effects than others in their class.*

[b]*Direct sexual side-effects of lithium are only confirmed when taken in conjunction with benzodiazepines.*

[c]*ACE inhibitors have fewer sexual side-effects than other classes of antihypertensives.*

Data from Crenshaw and Goldberg.[5]

is more likely to be associated with decreased libido than with ED. Radiation and chemotherapy for cancer may destroy testicular function. In men with heart disease, fear that sex will cause a heart attack can cause sexual dysfunction.

Erectile dysfunction may also be caused by structural abnormalities such as Peyronie's disease (Table 111-1). Prostatectomies may create sexual problems. In some cases, a man who has had prostate surgery and has lost interest in sex may use the surgery as an excuse for avoiding sexual contact. ED may follow prostate surgery, but nerve-sparing surgical techniques, developed by Dr Patrick Walsh of Johns Hopkins University, are available and can help avoid ED in many cases.[7]

As described earlier, certain drugs may also cause sexual dysfunction, including antihypertensives, antidepressants, antipsychotics, and others (Table 111-3), as can overconsumption of alcohol.

Ten percent of cases of erectile dysfunction are due to psychological causes, including performance anxiety, stress, exhaustion, anger, bereavement, and depression. Sexual problems can be both the origin and symptom of depression. Losing one's partner may be followed by grief, sometimes complicated by depression. It may lead to a kind of "enshrinement" of the lost partner. In such cases, "widower's guilt" may block the development of new relationships and cause ED when the man tries to engage in sexual activity with a new partner.[2]

Proper diagnosis of erectile dysfunction depends on taking a thorough history; asking questions about changes in libido, nocturnal erections, and problems with relationships; and a review of diseases and medication and alcohol use. This should be followed by a physical examination and laboratory evaluation, including a testosterone level. ED during sleep can be checked by rigiscan, a means of measuring nocturnal tumescence associated with REM sleep. It should be noted, however, that this is an imperfect method for diagnosing ED.

Treatment

In general, the old adage "use it or lose it" appears to be true. Erections bring oxygen-rich blood to the penis, which contributes to continuing healthful functioning. Good health habits promote sexual capability. In addition to helping people stay healthy, a balanced diet, no tobacco, moderate consumption of alcohol, and exercise programs all help prevent sexual dysfunction.

Erectile dysfunction can often be treated successfully. For ED with a physical cause, the main treatment is of the underlying cause, such as diabetes or a reaction to medications. For psychogenic cases, psychotherapy, marital therapy, group therapy, and sex therapy—which is based on Masters and Johnson's use of "sensate focusing"—may be beneficial. These approaches are also useful when ED is physical in origin because there are often associated or concomitant emotional reactions to ED, and because such therapeutic approaches can help reassure the patient and his partner.

However, it should be noted that erectile dysfunction may be an early sign of heart disease, hypertension, or diabetes. It is a sign, not a diagnosis. Therefore, ED should prompt careful evaluation.

PHARMACOTHERAPY   Sildenafil has become widely used. In dosages of 25, 50, or 100 mg (in most cases starting with 25 mg) and taken one hour prior to a sexual encounter, sildenafil will produce an erection but only when the man is sexually stimulated. It is not an aphrodisiac, but a "mechanical" means to facilitate intercourse. Nor does it substitute for intimacy; indeed, it may reveal strains in relationships. Sildenafil blocks the action of an enzyme, phosphodiesterase type 5, so that nitric oxide dilates the penile blood vessels. It also increases clitoral blood flow and some women report its usefulness; however, comprehensive studies have not verified this. Although there are currently no reliable measurements of female sexual response, efforts are under way to develop such instruments.

Sildenafil can cause hypotension when nitrates are used concurrently, so it is contraindicated in patients who take nitrates to relieve angina. A patient who has had an adverse heart event and has taken sildenafil that day should not be given a nitrate. Sildenafil can also cause headaches, upset stomach, bluish vision, and nasal congestion. Rarely, priapism (4 hours of tumescence) occurs and must be treated to avoid damage to the penis.

Sildenafil has not been compared directly to other treatments for erectile dysfunction.[8] New oral drugs to treat erectile dysfunction are under study.

Other medications for erectile dysfunction include vasoactive compounds that are injected directly into the corpus cavernosum. Phentolamine, atropine, and prostaglandin-E have been shown to be effective given individually or together. Prostaglandin-E was the first FDA-approved prescription medication to treat ED. Erection should occur within 5–10 minutes after injection, and the erection can last 30 minutes or more. Injection with these substances should not be done more than once every 24 hours and not more than three times per week. Possible problems with this therapy include priapism

(4 percent), which can be reversed with epinephrine or ephedrine; mild to moderate pain at the site of injection; and some scarring. Contraindications include sickle-cell anemia, multiple myeloma, leukemia, anatomical deformities, and implants (see below). Treatment of men with ED with transurethral alprostadil (a synthetic compound identical to prostaglandin-E1) is effective in nearly 70 percent of cases, regardless of age. A major advantage of this treatment is that the drug is delivered transurethrally via an applicator, rather than through injection.[9]

VACUUM THERAPY   This involves placing a cylinder over an unerect penis, sucking out air to produce an erection, and applying a wide rubber band at the base to maintain the erection. One-third of individuals who try vacuum devices find them helpful. They should not be used by men taking anticoagulants or those who have low platelet counts.

IMPLANT   A permanent penile prosthesis may help a patient with an otherwise untreatable potency problem. Such a prosthesis is irreversible and therefore should be used only as a last resort. Penile implants can be noninflatable (positionable or semirigid rod prosthesis) and inflatable. Inflatable implants include an inflate/deflate pump with the cylinder in the penis or placed below the skin in the scrotum. There is a reservoir in the scrotum. Cylinders are placed behind the abdominal muscles. Contraindications to this treatment include psychiatric problems such as psychosis and untreated depression.[3] Complications include infection, mechanical failure, and penile fibrosis.

SURGERY   Revascularization surgery is still largely experimental. Some studies of the substance Yohimbine, which comes from the bark of an African tree, have shown that it has a positive effect on erection, probably because it acts on neurotransmitters such as acetylcholine and dopamine that are involved in the sexual response. However, undesirable side-effects have been noted.

THE "SECOND LANGUAGE OF SEX"

Some older people are not interested in sex because they were never interested in it, or their sexual desire has decreased, or their opportunities for sexual activity are significantly diminished, or other reasons. On the other hand, many older people are interested and want to continue to be sexually active. Whatever their point of view, each older person's wishes should be elicited and respected before treatment decisions are completed. There is a range of interest and degree of sexual activity among older people just as there is among other age groups, and treatment options can be as effective for them as for younger people.

The "first language" of sexuality, generally associated with youth, is biological and intense. The "second language" of sexuality, broader than the first, is learned by experience over a lifetime. Of course, some younger people are naturally adept at expressing the second language of sexuality and, conversely, some older people never quite learn it. But for many people, primary focus on genital contact gives way over time to a more encompassing definition of sexuality, which includes intimacy, mutuality, trust, love, romance, friendship, and caring.[2]

It is not known whether there is a clear association between sexual satisfaction and longevity, but there is evidence that love and sex enhance the quality of life. Some of the greatest obstacles to successful, intimate relationships in later life are the negative attitudes and practices toward older persons found among health professionals and the public at large. Health professionals must realize that their older patients have sexual interest, capacities, and pleasures, and that we have the means to repair many of the physical, emotional, and social impediments to continuing sexuality in late life through education and other interventions.

KEY POINTS Sexuality in old age

- Some medical conditions, surgical procedures, and medications can affect sexual functioning. The physician should include a discussion of sexuality when treating disease or prescribing medication to elderly patients for whom continuing sexual activity is important.

- It is estimated that 90 percent of cases of erectile dysfunction have a physical cause, while 10 percent are psychologically induced. Treatments for the latter include psychotherapy, marital therapy, group therapy, and sex therapy.

- Women who wish to remain sexually active in later life may face barriers that are unrelated to physical symptoms. For example, about 60 percent of elderly women are without a spouse, and many others live with a disabled spouse who cannot be a sexual partner.

- Medical conditions that can impact significantly on sexuality are coronary bypass surgery, stroke, diabetes, osteoarthritis and rheumatoid arthritis, backache, Parkinson's disease, chronic emphysema and bronchitis, chronic prostatitis in men, and stress incontinence in women.

- In men with heart disease, fear that sex will cause a heart attack can cause sexual dysfunction.

- With the discovery of the therapeutic effect in men of sildenafil citrate, the attitudes of physicians and the public have moved to more positive approaches towards the sexuality of older persons.

CONCLUSION

Physicians frequently fail to ask older patients about their sexual functioning during the typical medical examination and evaluation. Patients may be uncomfortable about revealing their sexual difficulties, and may not be aware that sexual dysfunction in both sexes can often be treated. In addition, erectile dysfunction may be an early sign of diseases such as heart disease, hypertension, or diabetes.

Normal change in sexual functioning is usually manifested as a gradual slowing; that is, more time is needed for arousal (erection in men, lubrication in women) and reaching a climax. Healthy older women can usually continue earlier patterns of sexual functioning, but reduced estrogen production due to the menopause may present physical and emotional problems. Studies at the National Institutes of Health are expected to help clarify indications, contraindications, and risks of hormone replacement therapy.

REFERENCES

1. Butler RN, Lewis MI: Sexuality. In: Merck Manual of Geriatrics, 3rd edn. Merck Research Laboratories, Whitehouse Station, NJ, 2000:1156–1164
2. Butler RN, Lewis MI: The New Love and Sex After 60. Ballantine Books, New York, 2000
3. Muller JE, Mittleman MA, Maclure M et al: Triggering myocardial infarction by sexual activity: low absolute risk and prevention by regular physical exertion. JAMA 1996;275:1405–1409
4. Ueno M: The so-called coital death. Jap J Legal Med 1963;7:330–340
5. Crenshaw TL, Goldberg JP: Sexual pharmacology: drugs that affect sexual functioning. WW Norton, New York, 1996
6. Carson C, Kirby R, Goldstein I (eds): Textbook of erectile dysfunction. Isis Medical Media, Oxford, 1999
7. Walsh PC: The preservation of sexual function in the surgical treatment of prostatic cancer: an anatomical surgical approach. In DeVit VT, Hellman S, Rosenberg SA (eds): Important advances in oncology. Lippincott–Raven, Philadelphia, 1988
8. Sadovsky R, Miller T, Moskowitz M et al: Three-year update of sildenafil citrate (Viagra) efficacy and safety. Int J Clin Pract 2001;55(2):115–128
9. Padma-Nathan H, Hellstrom WJG, Kaiser FE et al: Treatment of men with erectile dysfunction with transurethral alprostadil. N Engl J Med 1997;336:1–7

SECTION 4
Health systems and geriatric medicine

Chapter 112

The elderly in society: an international perspective

Robert N. Butler and Charlotte Muller

THE LONGEVITY REVOLUTION

The extraordinary growth in life expectancy at birth in nearly all countries of the world constitutes an ongoing revolution in longevity. This revolution encompasses both survival of individuals to older ages and changing age profiles of entire populations.

The impact of the longevity revolution has been pervasive and profound, and perhaps will prove to be as important as the Industrial Revolution was in the 1800s. In the earlier years of the last century, public health programs, better nutrition, and improved living standards worked to increase life expectancy; in the later years of the century, achievements in medical science applied to personal medical care decreased dramatically the death rates from heart disease, stroke, and some types of cancer after age 65 and significantly increased the numbers and proportions of persons aged over 65, over 75, and even over 90 years. In many countries men aged 65 can expect to live 13–16 more years, and women an extra 14–20 years. Today, however, demographic predictions are not secure because the spread of infectious diseases—notably AIDS—threatens the lives of younger populations in vulnerable countries: It can wipe out gains in longevity and hinder further advances.[1]

Women tend to live longer than men, and several explanations have been offered aside from possible gender differences in biological endowment and development. Women's lifestyles may be more healthful, with less smoking and alcohol use, and superior hygiene; while men, especially at younger ages, are more likely to pursue risky sports, to drive while under the influence of alcohol or other drugs, and to be in environments that promote violence. Women, as family healthcare representatives and users of reproductive healthcare, have tended to be more receptive to preventive services and more willing to accept help, which encourages early diagnosis. Yet in resource-scarce areas, tradition may favor allocation of household resources to the health of boys. Moreover, as women are more continuously exposed to workplace-related risks to health, the difference between the sexes may narrow. The strength of these diverse factors in different countries is likely to depend on cultural and economic patterns, including the degree of emancipation of women and the availability of modern health services.

Public concern with health and social services to maximize the personal and social benefits of increased longevity has spread. Furthermore, economic issues raised by such a rapid growth of older populations are now at the center of political debates in many developed and developing countries and on the agendas of international organizations. Much of the debate relates to the rising costs of pension and health programs.

Attention is also being directed to strengthening the quality of life of older persons, expanding their economic opportunities, and acknowledging their contributions to family and society. A major challenge has been meeting the needs of older men and women who can no longer manage daily functions because of physical or cognitive disabilities. Long-term care is beyond the financial and organizational capacities of most individual households, and countries with large older populations, such as Japan, Germany, and Sweden, have accepted public responsibility. This chapter reviews selected demographic aspects of the worldwide phenomenon of increased longevity and discusses the approaches used in different nations to provide economic security to their older residents.

A word of caution is applicable here: Nobody has a magic formula to resolve all the issues raised by an aging population. Given the long-term nature of demographic shifts and the difficulty of seeing far into the future, uncertainty is unavoidable. Birthrates and medical advances are surprisingly unpredictable, securities markets are immensely volatile, and even the most stable democracies may well experience sweeping transformations in politics and policy.[2]

Most censuses and surveys follow standard classifications and definitions of demographic and economic characteristics in creating national statistical systems, but some countries depart from these standards. Therefore, some readjustment in groupings was necessary in creating the accompanying tables, although national estimates were accepted as presented. The countries selected for inclusion here were chosen not only as representing different parts of the world but also as conforming to data quality standards.

AGE DISTRIBUTION AND LIFE EXPECTANCY

The United Nations regularly prepares mid-year estimates and projections of age and sex distributions of the populations of more than 200 countries and areas. Statistics in the first group of tables are based on the 1998 revision of these data.

In the period 1960–2000, the total population doubled in the world as a whole. Between 2000 and 2010, the rate of growth in Africa is expected to be three times as fast as the world rate, while the European population will actually decline. However, the prediction for vulnerable countries in Africa and elsewhere can be sound only if the threat to survival presented by the ravages of AIDS is brought under control.

For all age groups over 60 years, steady growth in numbers and proportions in their respective total populations occurred in all continents and countries, at a much more rapid rate than that of the global population. Older women in all countries tend to live longer than men and dominate numerically

in absolute numbers, proportion, and rates of increase. This trend will be maintained in the next decade. As early as 1960, at least 10 percent of the total population for each gender was aged 65 or over in Europe, North America, and Oceania. By 2000, females aged 70 or over had become a substantial proportion of all females in Europe and North America, and the trend towards a high age profile will continue in these continents.

Table 112-1 shows population aging in the period 1960–2000 in 56 selected countries that represent almost three-quarters of the world's population. It also shows the 19 countries with more than 3.5 million people over the age of 65 (both sexes) in 2000. By 2010 there will be 21 countries having more than 3.5 million older men and women. These countries contain three-quarters of the world population aged 65 and over. Table 112-2 shows gains in life expectancy at birth and at 65 in the period, 1900–2000. Countries with many older persons will need service development and implementation of social adjustments required to support health, living standards, and social integration.

In evaluating social progress, one must consider not only life expectancy but also quality of life, which has many dimensions, among them personal and family relations, adequacy of income, environmental safety, and opportunities for productive activity. Healthy life expectancy is an important spinoff as an indicator because it measures years free from disabilities that interfere with daily living, productivity, and enjoyment of leisure.

Table 112-1 Aging countries, census data, and mid-year estimates for 1960 and 2000 (percentages)

Country[a]	65 years of age and over (% of total)				65–79 years of age (% of total)				80 years of age and over (% of total)			
	1960		2000 (estimates)		1960		2000 (estimates)		1960		2000 (estimates)	
	M	F	M	F	M	F	M	F	M	F	M	F
Italy	7.9	10.3	15.3	20.9	6.8	8.8	12.6	15.6	1.1	1.4	2.6	5.3
Germany	9.9	12.9	12.7	19.8	8.6	11.2	10.8	14.6	1.4	1.7	1.9	5.2
Sweden	11.0	12.9	14.9	19.8	9.3	10.9	11.2	13.1	1.7	2.1	3.7	6.6
Greece	7.2	9.0	16.2	19.6	6.0	7.6	13.3	15.5	1.2	1.4	2.8	4.1
Belgium	10.3	13.5	13.7	19.5	8.9	11.3	11.6	14.6	1.4	2.2	2.1	5.0
Japan	5.1	6.4	14.6	19.4	4.6	5.4	12.2	14.6	0.4	0.9	2.4	4.8
Spain	7.0	9.4	14.5	19.4	6.1	7.9	12.0	14.5	0.9	1.5	2.6	4.9
France	8.9	14.2	13.2	18.5	7.5	11.6	10.8	13.4	1.3	2.6	2.4	5.1
UK	9.3	13.9	13.7	18.3	7.6	11.4	10.9	12.8	1.7	2.5	2.7	5.6
Portugal	6.6	9.2	13.2	18.1	5.8	7.9	11.1	14.1	0.8	1.3	2.2	4.0
Latvia	7.9	12.5	9.8	18.0	6.7	10.2	8.8	14.8	1.2	2.3	1.0	3.3
Austria	10.0	13.9	10.2	18.0	8.6	11.8	8.6	13.3	1.3	2.1	1.7	4.7
Finland	5.8	8.9	11.6	18.0	5.0	7.6	9.7	13.1	0.8	1.3	1.9	4.9
Norway	10.1	12.2	12.9	17.9	8.4	9.9	9.9	12.1	1.7	2.3	3.0	5.8
Hungary	7.8	10.0	11.6	17.7	6.8	8.8	9.9	14.4	0.9	1.2	1.6	3.4
Ukraine	5.7	9.0	10.1	17.7	5.0	7.5	9.0	14.3	0.8	1.6	1.1	3.3
Denmark	9.8	11.3	12.7	17.6	8.4	9.6	10.0	12.2	1.4	1.7	2.7	5.4
Estonia	7.3	12.9	9.6	17.3	6.4	11.0	8.5	14.2	0.9	1.9	1.1	3.1
Switzerland	8.7	11.7	12.1	17.3	7.3	9.7	9.6	12.1	1.4	2.0	2.5	5.1
Belarus	6.6	9.8	9.7	17.1	5.7	8.0	8.7	14.1	0.9	1.8	1.0	3.0
Luxembourg	9.6	11.9	11.8	16.9	8.3	10.2	10.4	13.2	1.3	1.8	1.4	3.7
Lithuania	6.1	9.1	9.6	16.6	5.3	7.5	8.4	13.4	0.8	1.7	1.3	3.2
The Netherlands	8.1	9.2	11.3	16.2	7.2	8.1	9.3	11.6	0.9	1.1	2.0	4.6
Russia	4.1	8.1	8.4	16.1	3.6	6.7	7.6	13.2	0.5	1.4	0.8	3.0
Poland	4.4	7.1	9.3	14.5	3.9	6.1	8.2	11.9	0.5	0.9	1.1	2.7

(continued)

Table 112-1 (continued)

Country[a]	65 years of age and over (% of total)				65–79 years of age (% of total)				80 years of age and over (% of total)			
	1960		2000 (estimates)		1960		2000 (estimates)		1960		2000 (estimates)	
	M	F	M	F	M	F	M	F	M	F	M	F
Canada	7.2	7.8	11.0	14.5	6.1	6.5	8.9	10.5	1.1	1.3	2.1	4.0
USA	8.5	10.0	10.5	14.4	7.3	8.3	8.3	10.1	1.2	1.6	2.2	4.3
Australia	7.2	9.7	10.7	13.5	6.3	8.3	8.6	9.9	0.9	1.5	2.0	3.6
New Zealand	7.6	9.7	10.2	13.0	6.4	8.0	8.3	9.3	1.2	1.7	1.9	3.7
Barbados	4.9	8.5	8.4	12.9	4.3	6.9	6.1	8.6	0.6	1.6	2.3	4.3
Ireland	10.5	11.8	9.7	12.8	9.6	9.6	8.0	9.4	1.0	2.2	1.7	3.4
Hong Kong	1.6	4.1	9.4	11.9	1.5	3.6	7.9	9.1	0.1	0.5	1.5	2.7
Puerto Rico	5.2	5.2	9.3	11.4	4.4	4.2	7.1	8.5	0.8	1.0	2.1	2.8
Argentina	5.4	5.9	8.1	11.2	4.8	5.1	6.9	9.0	0.6	0.8	1.2	2.3
Israel	4.6	5.2	8.4	11.2	4.0	4.4	6.6	8.6	0.6	0.8	1.7	2.6
Kazakhstan	5.2	6.2	5.0	9.0	4.5	3.3	4.5	7.4	0.6	2.9	0.5	1.6
Korea, Rep.	3.1	4.4	5.0	8.4	2.6	3.6	4.6	7.1	0.5	0.8	0.4	1.3
Singapore	1.6	2.6	6.5	8.0	1.4	2.2	5.5	6.3	0.2	0.4	1.0	1.7
Jamaica	3.7	4.9	6.4	7.6	3.0	3.8	4.9	5.6	0.7	1.2	1.5	2.0
China	4.3	5.4	6.1	7.6	4.0	4.9	5.5	6.4	0.3	0.5	0.6	1.2
Kyrgyzstan	6.7	7.4	4.5	7.4	5.9	6.2	4.1	6.2	0.8	1.1	0.4	1.2
Thailand	2.5	3.1	5.1	6.6	2.0	2.2	4.4	5.4	0.5	0.9	0.7	1.1
Turkey	2.7	4.3	5.3	6.3	2.3	3.6	4.8	5.5	0.4	0.8	0.5	0.8
Brazil	2.8	2.9	4.6	5.8	2.3	2.3	4.0	4.9	0.5	0.6	0.6	0.9
Panama	3.6	3.7	5.3	5.8	3.4	2.8	4.4	4.7	0.2	0.9	0.9	1.1
Cape Verde	2.9	5.7	3.0	5.7	2.7	5.2	2.5	4.8	0.2	0.6	0.5	0.9
Costa Rica	2.9	2.6	4.7	5.5	2.4	2.4	4.0	4.6	0.5	0.2	0.7	0.9
India	3.3	3.5	4.4	5.4	3.1	3.3	4.0	4.7	0.2	0.3	0.3	0.7
Mexico	3.3	3.5	4.3	5.1	2.6	2.7	3.6	4.2	0.7	0.8	0.7	1.0
Indonesia	3.2	3.5	4.3	5.1	2.9	3.2	3.8	4.5	0.3	0.3	0.4	0.6
Venezuela	2.4	2.7	4.0	4.9	2.2	2.4	3.5	4.1	0.2	0.2	0.5	0.8
Dominican Republic	3.0	2.9	4.3	4.7	2.4	2.3	3.7	4.0	0.6	0.7	0.6	0.7
Egypt	3.2	3.7	3.6	4.7	2.8	3.2	3.2	4.1	0.4	0.5	0.4	0.6
Philippines	2.7	2.8	3.3	4.0	2.2	2.4	2.9	3.4	0.5	0.3	0.4	0.6
Nigeria	2.2	2.7	2.8	3.3	2.0	2.4	2.5	2.9	0.2	0.2	0.3	0.4
Sierra Leone	2.7	3.4	2.6	3.3	2.6	3.2	2.4	2.8	0.2	0.2	0.2	0.5

[a] Countries with more than 3.5 million persons 65 years and over (both sexes) in 2000 are shown in bold. Countries are ranked by size of female population 65+ years of age in 2000.

Source: UN-1.

LABOR FORCE PARTICIPATION OF ELDERLY PEOPLE

In this section, "labor force" and "economically active persons," both men and women, are used interchangeably. Neither term is restricted to currently employed persons; that is, unemployed persons are considered to be part of the labor force.

Older people's participation in the labor force is a significant statistic for several reasons. It indicates receipt of income that supports a desired standard of living. Productive activity is a source of independence and self-esteem. Moreover, the potential for economic activity, if utilized, can reduce a nation's pension requirements. Historical evidence predicts that realization of this potential depends on resolution of controversies relating to competition for jobs with younger workers, employer costs based on customary higher wages for older employees, and age discrimination (see Chapter 18). In addition, health status and many older workers' own preference for retirement influence labor force participation rates.

The labor supply of older persons is promoted by the increase in disability-free years of life, the need for income to supplement their pensions, and perceived psychological and social benefits of work. But pension systems may discourage continued work through features such as early retirement options, absence of credits for work beyond the normal retirement age, and cessation of work as a requirement for award of pensions. One of the statistical measures presented is the percentage of the labor force that consists of older persons. This is influenced by the relative size of younger and older populations, the statutory retirement age, and the prevalence of work-limiting disability.

In examining labor force participation rates, we focus on age groups approaching and following the normal statutory ages of retirement: 50–59, 60–64, and 65+.

The world total of economically active persons doubled from 1960 to 2000, at an annual rate of 1.8 percent for men and 2.2 percent for women. Between 2000 and 2010, the rate of increase is expected to be 14.2 percent (an annual rate of 1.3 percent) for men and 16.8 percent (an annual rate

Table 112-2 Gains in life expectancy from 1900 to 2000 in selected countries (years)

Continent	No.	Country	Period	Males At birth	Males 65 yrs	Females At birth	Females 65 yrs	Period	Males At birth	Males 65 yrs	Females At birth	Females 65 yrs	Gain (at birth) Males	Gain (at birth) Females
Europe	1	England and Wales	1891–1900	44.1	10.3	47.8	11.3	1983–1985	71.8	13.4	77.7	17.5	27.7	29.9
Europe	2	Russian Fed.	1896–1897	29.4	…	31.7	…	1996	59.8	10.8	72.5	14.9	30.3	40.8
Europe	3	Spain	1900	33.9	9.0	35.7	9.2	1994–1995	74.3	16.1	81.6	20.0	40.5	45.9
Europe	4	Hungary	1900–1901	37.1	…	37.9	…	1997	66.4	12.2	75.1	15.9	29.3	37.2
N. Am.	5	USA	1900–1902	47.9	11.5	50.7	12.2	1997	73.6	15.8	79.2	19.0	25.7	28.5
Europe	6	Ireland	1900–1902	49.3	…	49.6	…	1990–1992	72.3	13.4	77.9	17.1	23.0	28.3
L. Amer. & Carib.	7	Trinidad & Tobago	1900–1903	36.7	8.5	38.8	9.8	1990 (PHC)	68.4	13.5	73.2	15.9	31.7	34.5
Europe	8	The Netherlands	1900–1909	51.0	11.6	53.4	12.3	1995–1996	74.5	14.6	80.2	18.9	23.5	26.8
Europe	9	Northern Ireland	1901	47.1	10.5	46.7	10.4	1983	69.3	12.4	75.7	16.1	22.2	29.0
Europe	10	Austria	1901–1905	39.1	10.1	41.1	10.2	1997	74.3	15.4	80.6	19.0	35.2	39.5
Europe	11	Denmark	1901–1905	52.9	11.9	56.2	13.0	1996–1997	73.3	14.5	78.4	17.9	20.4	22.2
Europe	12	Finland	1901–1910	45.3	10.8	48.1	11.9	1997	73.4	15.0	80.5	18.9	28.1	32.4
Europe	13	Germany	1901–1910	44.8	10.4	48.3	11.1	1994–1996	73.3	14.8	79.7	18.5	28.5	31.4
Europe	14	Iceland	1901–1910	48.3	11.7	53.1	13.4	1995–1996	76.2	16.2	80.6	19.1	27.9	27.5
Europe	15	Sweden	1901–1910	54.5	12.8	57.0	13.7	1996	76.5	16.1	81.5	19.7	22.0	24.5
Europe	16	Switzerland	1901–1910	49.3	10.1	52.2	10.7	1995–1996	75.7	16.3	81.9	20.3	26.5	29.8
Oceania	17	Australia	1901–1910	55.2	11.3	58.8	12.9	1994–1996	75.2	15.8	81.0	19.6	20.0	22.2
Asia	18	India	1901–1911	22.6	8.1	23.3	8.1	1991–1995	59.7	12.5	60.9	13.9	37.1	37.6
Europe	19	Italy	1901–1911	44.2	10.7	44.8	10.8	1995	74.6	15.5	81.0	19.4	30.4	36.2
Europe	20	Norway	1901–1919	54.8	13.5	57.7	14.4	1997	75.4	15.5	81.0	19.4	20.6	23.3
L. Amer. & Carib.	21	Puerto Rico	1902–1903	29.8	10.3	31.0	12.2	1990–1992	69.6	16.0	78.5	18.9	39.8	47.5
Europe	22	France	1908–1913	48.5	10.5	52.4	11.7	1996	74.2	16.1	82.0	20.7	25.7	29.6
Asia	23	Japan	1909–1913	44.3	10.6	44.7	12.0	1997	77.2	17.0	83.8	21.8	33.0	39.1
L. Amer. & Carib.	24	Jamaica	1910–1912	39.0	10.8	41.4	12.6	1995–2000	72.9	…	76.8	…	33.9	35.4
S. Am.	25	Guyana	1910–1912	29.9	7.8	32.4	9.6	1995–2000	61.1	…	67.9	…	31.2	35.5
S. Am.	26	Argentina	1914	45.2	10.9	47.5	12.4	1990–1992	68.4	13.5	75.6	17.3	23.2	28.1
Europe	27	Greece	1920	42.9	10.1	46.5	13.6	1997	75.3	16.2	80.6	18.7	32.4	34.1
Asia	28	Sri Lanka	1920–1922	32.7	8.9	30.7	8.2	1995–2000	70.9	…	75.4	…	38.2	44.7
Asia	30	Myanmar	1921–1931	30.6	8.7	31.0	9.2	1995–2000	58.5	…	61.8	…	27.9	30.8

Sources: United Nations Data Yearbooks, various issues. For Russia: Population of Russia, 1897–1997. Statistical Handbook, State Committee of the Russian Federation on Statistics, Moscow, 1998.

Table 112-3 **Distribution of the world total economically active male population in selected age groups (percentages)**

Continent	Year[a]	All ages	0–14 yrs	15–59 yrs	50–59 yrs	60+ yrs	60–64 yrs	65+ yrs
World	1960	100	5.1	87.4	12.2	7.4	3.6	3.9
	2000	100	2.1	91.4	11.6	6.5	3.4	3.0
	2010	100	1.3	92.1	14.2	6.5	3.4	3.1
Africa	1960	100	8.7	84.9	9.3	6.4	2.9	3.5
	2000	100	6.8	87.4	8.9	5.8	2.7	3.2
	2010	100	5.6	88.8	9.2	5.6	2.6	3.0
N. America	1960	100	0.4	89.2	16.5	10.4	5.5	4.9
	2000	100	0.0	95.3	16.5	4.7	3.4	2.4
	2010	100	0.0	93.3	20.4	6.7	4.4	2.3
Latin America +Caribbean	1960	100	5.1	87.3	10.6	7.5	3.3	4.2
	2000	100	1.9	92.1	10.3	5.9	2.9	3.0
	2010	100	0.9	92.7	12.2	6.4	3.3	3.1
Asia	1960	100	6.7	86.3	10.9	7.0	3.1	3.9
	2000	100	1.9	91.0	11.0	7.1	3.7	3.4
	2010	100	0.8	92.2	14.1	7.0	3.6	3.4
Europe	1960	100	0.6	91.1	16.3	8.2	4.6	3.7
	2000	100	0.0	95.2	16.3	4.8	3.1	1.7
	2010	100	0.0	95.3	19.6	4.7	3.1	1.6
Oceania	1960	100	1.6	90.7	14.5	7.7	4.4	3.3
	2000	100	0.8	94.5	14.9	4.7	2.9	1.7
	2010	100	0.6	94.0	16.3	5.4	3.7	1.8

[a] Mid-year estimates for 1960, 2000, and 2010.
Source: ILO-1.

Table 112-4 **Distribution of the world total economically active female population by selected age groups (percentages)**

Continent	Year[a]	All ages	0–14 yrs	15–59 yrs	50–59 yrs	60+ yrs	60–64 yrs	65+ yrs
World	1960	100	6.4	88.7	10.5	5.0	2.6	2.4
	2000	100	2.5	80.0	10.4	4.2	2.2	2.0
	2010	100	1.6	93.6	12.4	4.5	2.4	2.0
Africa	1960	100	10.4	83.6	9.6	6.1	2.9	3.2
	2000	100	8.0	86.8	8.7	5.2	2.4	2.8
	2010	100	6.8	88.5	8.4	4.7	2.2	2.4
N. America	1960	100	0.4	90.4	17.5	9.3	5.2	4.0
	2000	100	0.0	95.1	15.9	4.9	2.8	2.2
	2010	100	0.0	94.3	20.2	5.7	3.6	2.1
Latin America +Caribbean	1960	100	7.1	87.0	8.5	5.9	2.6	3.3
	2000	100	2.1	94.6	8.3	3.4	1.9	1.5
	2010	100	1.2	95.1	10.1	3.6	2.1	1.6
Asia	1960	100	8.2	87.7	8.8	4.1	2.1	2.0
	2000	100	2.4	72.1	9.5	4.2	2.2	2.0
	2010	100	1.0	94.3	11.8	4.6	2.5	2.1
Europe	1960	100	0.6	93.6	14.4	5.8	3.3	2.5
	2000	100	0.0	96.3	14.1	3.6	2.1	1.5
	2010	100	0.0	96.5	17.2	3.5	2.0	1.4
Oceania	1960	100	3.4	91.7	10.9	4.9	2.7	2.2
	2000	100	0.8	96.3	13.1	2.8	1.7	1.1
	2010	100	0.6	95.9	15.1	3.5	2.4	1.1

[a] Mid-year estimates for 1960, 2000, and 2010.
Source: ILO-1.

of 1.6 percent) for women. Europe's female labor force will have grown hardly at all: 1.8 percent in the decade. See Tables 112-3 and 112-4.

For the male labor force, the highest growth rate in 40 years was found in Africa (165 percent) with a 27.5 percent increase projected for the coming decade. For Europe, which had the lowest growth rates between 1960 and 2000, a decline in labor force activity rates is predicted by 2010.

Additional years of life gained during the past century did not result in larger labor force participation of older persons.

Reports from the International Labour Office on about 200 countries for decades from 1950 to 2010 show that, although the number of economically active older adults nearly doubled between 1960 and 2000 and will increase by about 15 percent in the next decade, their proportion of the labor force fell after 1960.

Overall, the number of men aged 60+ who are economically active grew from 65 million (1960) to 113.6 million (2000) and by 2010 will be 130.6 million. But their proportion of the total male labor force fell from 7.4 percent (1960) to 6.5 percent (2000) and will be about the same in 2010. Contrary to the general trend, Europe shows a decline in both numbers and proportions.

The worldwide trend for women aged 60 who are economically active is similar to that of men, except in Asia. The share of those 60+ in the total female labor force fell from 5.0 percent in 1960 to 4.2 percent in 2000; however, a slight increase is expected in the next decade. Although in Europe both the number of active female participants in this age category and their share of the female labor force have been dropping, in Asia the number of such women has risen at a striking pace and further growth to 40.2 million in the following decade is predicted. The share of these older women in the female labor force is also rising.

Overall, while the number of men aged 60–64 in the labor force almost doubled between 1960 and 2000 and is expected to reach 68.3 million in 2010, their share in the male labor force has stayed at 3–4 percent.

The trend for women aged 60–64 in the world labor force is similar to that of men. By 2010 one can expect 34.0 million such women, but their share in the total female labor force hovers at a little over 2 percent.

In Japan, where the standard retirement age was raised from 60 to 65 in 1996,[3] male workers aged 60+ more than doubled in number from 1960 to 2000, from 2.5 million (9.1 percent of all men in the labor force) to 5.6 million (14.1 percent), and an increase to 6.4 million (16.8 percent) is predicted. Their percentage of the entire male work force is, and will continue to be, the highest among all nations. In absolute numbers, however, the greatest growth took place in India, which added 12.3 million active men, 5.0 million of them aged 60–64 and 7.3 million 65+, over the course of 40 years; and in China, which added 10.6 million economically active men, 6.9 million aged 60–64 and 3.6 million 65+. However, these older men are not as large a proportion of the entire male labor force as in Jamaica and the Dominican Republic: 9.4 and 8.6 percent, respectively.

In contrast, significant declines in the number of economically active older men were reported by Hungary and the UK. The rates of change in both numbers and older workers' share in the total working population of each sex vary from country to country. In 1960, men aged 60+ accounted for 10 percent or more of the male labor force in 11 countries, but in the four ensuing decades these rates declined in 42 countries, while a drop in the numbers but not the rates occurred in 26 countries. Five countries, however, reported a substantial increase in the numbers of older men in the workforce, between 3.5 and 4.5 times their 1960 levels (China-Hong Kong, Nigeria, the Dominican Republic, Costa Rica, and Singapore).

There was a striking trend towards early retirement, shown by declines in the labor force participation rate of men aged 60–64 and 65+ in 52 countries, with two other countries showing the decrease for 60–64+ only and one other for 65+ only.

Steady growth in the numbers of older women in the labor force was reported by seven countries in Latin America and Asia, and the proportion of older women in the total female labor force also grew. This trend is seen for 60+, 60–64, and 65+ groups. In contrast, six European countries show a decrease in economically active older women. In Japan, where there will be 3.9 million women aged 60+ in the labor force in 2010, the proportion they represent of all women in the labor force is, and will continue to be, the highest among all nations. The greatest growth in numbers has occurred in China (5.4 million added in 40 years, 2.0 million of them 65+) and India (4.2 million added, 2.0 million of them 65+).

With increased life expectancy at age 65 including more disability-free years ahead, labor supply has the potential to increase. This will help keep the annual consumption expenditure (including health services) required to maintain daily living during the additional years of life in balance with annual incomes.

Paradoxically, recent history has shown a decline in the economic activity rate of men from age 50 onward in all continents, which is expected to continue in the years between 2000 and 2010. In 1960, work at older ages was relatively common in the world as a whole—of people aged 50–59, 92.8 percent were in the workforce, and the decline to 79.8 percent at ages 60–64 was relatively modest. Even at 65+, 48.3 percent of men were in the workforce. By 2000, there was a drop of about 7 percentage points at ages 50–59, but the economic activity rate for men aged 60–64 dropped by 12.9 percentage points, and at 65+, by 18.9 percentage points.

The economic activity rates are quite different for women. Globally, women's rate of economic activity for all ages has edged upwards since 1960 to about half of the adult female population, but this has not yet made itself felt in older age groups, and for older women an increase in the next decade is not expected.

The interpretation of the rates of economic activity for women is complex. Their retirement age may be adapted to that of a spouse who is retiring early. Women's activity in the informal sector usually is not reflected in official data, in the same way that nonmarket work of men is poorly represented by official data, and household work and family caregiving generally are not part of labor force statistics. In fact, statistics on women are more likely to be substantially affected by these practices because they are more often working in the informal sector. Furthermore, cultural attitudes towards women working outside the home often limit their participation in the labor markets of developing countries. Women's productive activities, whatever their form, generally support their consumption in old age. However, the scope of their activities is more limited and opportunities for mental stimulation would not be as extensive.

For men, the rate of labor force participation at age 60 and over declined between 1960 and 2000 in more than 40 of the 56 countries represented. While low rates are more typical in industrialized countries that have well-established retirement systems and greater longevity, declines are also occurring in less developed countries as urbanization increases and job structures change. Some of the decline in economic activity of men after age 65 is attributable to the emergence of disabling conditions with greater age, and to the higher age profile that appears within the 65+ population as longevity increases.

Gender differences in economic activity of older people are common. Labor force activity rates of women aged 60+ are above 20 percent in only 12 countries. After 65, only seven countries reported labor force participation of more than 20 percent, and in 40 countries under 10 percent of women 65+ were economically active, including 10 countries where under 2 percent were active.

In view of population aging, these statistics suggest major policy questions. Given older persons' low labor force activity, how can individuals and societies finance additional anticipated years of life? Nations are in the early stages of gearing retirement programs, employment practices, workplace culture, and other institutional features to the new age profiles. How can older women, now the majority, be relieved of fear of poverty and isolation, provided with more avenues of activity, and be equipped financially to attain a good quality of life? Healthcare professions and industries are involved as well in maintaining work-readiness, reducing the burden of chronic illnesses, protecting populations against threats to longevity, and promoting attitudes that will assist in personal and social adjustment to the new opportunities and responsibilities.

SOCIAL PROTECTION FOR OLD AGE
National resources

The standard of living of a country's older residents and the ability of the country to adjust smoothly to increased longevity are dependent on its overall resources and the commitment of the public sector to social expenditures. Important indicators of these factors include production per capita, government spending on consumption, and unemployment. In OECD countries, where population aging has been the most advanced, wide variation in these indicators can be observed.

Gross domestic product (GDP) per capita measures the annual total of national production available for all purposes, adjusted for population size. Government final consumption expenditure shows the extent to which household consumption of goods and services depends on public programs rather than private incomes. Sweden, with its tradition as a welfare state, leads with 26.2 percent of GDP. Social security and welfare programs account for as much as 6.7 percent of GDP in Denmark but less than 1 percent in several countries. These categories are important for older populations because they are likely to contain the programs intended to benefit older age groups.

The last of the selected indicators is unemployment. If the rate is high, the drain on unemployment insurance funds and social programs for supplementary income payments and job creation is likely to be substantial. Funds available for various services to older age groups will be more limited, and, furthermore, policymakers are less likely to be interested in expanding economic opportunities for older persons as an alternative to retirement.

Overview of pension systems

Income maintenance programs for old age were adopted throughout the world as market economies and industrialization spread along with institutions of political democracy. These programs varied widely in their coverage and specifications. The totality of the features vitally influences the standard of living of older populations, including ability to sustain healthful diets and living environments. While the systems came earlier and were generally more extensive in the developed countries, even developing countries tended to cover public employees and special groups and branched out in time to broader coverage.

The income programs for old age have been referred to by several different names, each with its own shade of meaning. The term "social insurance" stresses the concept of pooling of risk through either a nationwide governmental fund, or funds under national supervision maintained by industry, occupation groups, or geographical divisions. "Insurance" implies adherence to actuarial requirements—that is, expected probabilities regarding length of life and other contingencies—although important modifications of actuarial control have been numerous (such as a floor under benefits for low-wage workers). "Social security" has a rather similar meaning since it embraces statutory programs that insure against loss of earning power "as a result of old age" (which is not actually a determinant of lost earning power but represents the risks of unemployment and disability, when applied to an older population). Both social security and social insurance have been associated with a goal of averting destitution and deprivation caused by various occurrences throughout the life course, such as death of a parent of minor children. This inclusive approach most likely helps adults to prepare financially for old age. Risk pooling and a benefit structure that allows for alleviation of poverty distinguish social security from individual investment programs.

The term "social protection" has come into use to express a broader ambition—the use of public, private, and combined initiatives to mitigate income problems, aid the vulnerable, and secure minimum standards of well-being for all. At the same time, social protection as an umbrella concept acknowledges that priorities will vary with each country's circumstances. It also features a proactive dimension—averting risk through the delivery of targeted or population-wide services and providing programs to help people move out of poverty.

Old age benefit programs in the developing world tend to have narrow coverage and modest benefits. Owing to difficulties in compliance with respect to mandated contributions and in asset management, the ability to deliver benefits has not always been maintained. These problems have also afflicted countries which, despite universal pension systems, are in transition from state to private enterprise. Additionally, at least one international agency (the World Bank) and others interested in developing capital markets have favored privatized programs as a stimulus and an infrastructure for economic growth.

Social security systems use a variety of arrangements to deliver income in old age. Employment-related programs are mostly compulsory for defined categories of employees and employers, and sometimes permit self-employed persons to participate voluntarily. Length of employment and earning level determine benefit size. The government may contribute by subsidizing benefits for low-paid workers or meeting a fund deficit.

Universal or demogrant programs give a flat-rate cash benefit upon retirement, and are financed from general revenues.

Some length of residency is required, and they are often combined with an earnings-related tier. Contributions by employers and employees may be used even though major support comes from income taxes.

The publicly operated provident funds that are sometimes used in developing countries (such as Singapore) are based on employer and employee contributions but the distribution at retirement is received as a lump sum (one-time) rather than income over a period of years. While the lump sum, which reflects the accumulated amounts credited to each worker's account plus accrued interest, may help a retiree to start a small business or to acquire additional training, in this method retirement assets may be depleted by emergency use or the risks endemic to small enterprises.

Supplementing or replacing these program types, mandatory private insurance requires that either the employee alone or the employee and employer contribute to an employee's individual retirement account. Survivor benefits are not included and must be acquired by private purchase. Other countries require employers to provide a lump-sum refund of employer and employee contributions plus interest to an aged employee who leaves the firm. There is no pooling for risk across employers, although presumably in a large firm there is an implicit pool.

Complete or substantial retirement from the workforce is required for benefits in some countries (e.g. France, Finland, Egypt), but others start payments to all covered persons when they reach the specified retirement age. Some systems allow the individual to be credited for years out of the labor force for the purpose of childrearing. In some countries workers are allowed to accumulate wage credits after the normal retirement age, so as to entitle them to an adequate pension. Means-tested retirement pensions (as in Australia) may discourage labor force activity in the years preceding retirement by those who wish to reduce their earning record in order to qualify. This is a disincentive poorly adapted to the increased need for retirement savings created by greater life expectancy, as well as a divergence from the objective of relieving poverty in old age.

The usual age of retirement ranges between 60 and 65 but sometimes it is length of service that establishes eligibility. Lowering of the qualifying age in response to public pressure was sometimes reversed to cut costs. Usually the age for women is 5 years less than for men but the trend is towards equalization.

Many pension laws include an early retirement option when special conditions are met, such as an unhealthy occupation, unemployment near the normal retirement age, and many years in covered employment. The wage base used in calculating benefits is critical in determining retirement income. Depending on individual work history, it makes a difference whether the last years of coverage or the highest-earning years are used. Indexing benefits for price changes protects against inflation, and indexing for wage trends enables retirees to maintain the standard of living prevailing in the community. Such adjustments are subject to political trends and fiscal exigencies.[3,4]

Industrialized countries with extensive public pension systems have been facing fiscal and political problems as increasing longevity produces a growing number of pensioners. In some cases general unemployment and drains on unemployment insurance funds have been alleviated by shifting older unemployed workers to pensioner status. More generally, as macro-economies grew, workers became able to satisfy their desire to leave their long-term career jobs, especially physically demanding and psychologically stressful ones, for leisure or other uses of time, by early retirement.

This was made possible by provisions in social security laws that allowed benefits to start up to 5 years before the normal qualifying age when there were special circumstances and also without special circumstances but with actuarially reduced monthly pensions. The pronounced drop in labor force participation of older men that occurred after 1960 increased the annual obligations of public pension funds, while exits from the paid labor force reduced the productive resources of industrialized countries, in turn affecting (inter alia) the tax base supporting the pension system.

The trend of increased longevity and lower prevalence of disability in older age groups have led observers to question policies that tend to truncate the potentially active life years of aging persons. Specifically, provisions in pension laws that encourage early retirement are being scrutinized. If the normal retirement age is raised, economic support must be planned for those who can no longer work owing to impaired health; but disability insurance provides the community with the framework to handle this possibility.

A study of 11 industrialized countries measures the amount of wasted productive capacity implied by lowered economic activity rates. While at age 50 about 90 percent of men are in the labor force, by age 69 this rate has dropped, but the decline varies among countries. In Belgium, virtually no men aged 69 work and in fact most have left by age 65; in Japan, almost 50 percent still work at age 69. In the examples given, unused capacity is 61 percent of potential capacity of older workers in Belgium but much less (22 percent) in Japan. These measures are crude in that hours of work may vary among those who remain in the paid labor force, and much of their work may be at less productive tasks, while for many of those who leave, nonmarket activities, including caregiving, may contribute to society.[5]

Privatization experiences of three countries

Individual retirement accounts with tax deferment privileges as a vehicle for household saving for old age have now appeared in countries on several continents, sparking extensive debate as to the relative merits, risks, and costs involved. Proponents have stressed the opportunity to accumulate returns from investment in financial markets that funnel capital to corporate economies and thus participate in the gains from growth, as well as the wider range of options at the disposal of each active employee (compared, for example, with national funds restricted to buying government bonds). At the same time, the need for regulation of the investment and management companies that handle the placement of retirement savings into investment outlets and the administration of benefits is acknowledged. Regulations plus fees charged by the companies plus costs of competing for enrollees narrow the difference in returns to retirees compared with conventional social security. Since a long horizon for saving is necessary for sufficient accruals to occur, averaging good and bad periods, privatization programs would be more appropriate for younger workers than those nearing retirement.

The circumstances that led to privatization varied by country. For example, in Chile, there was dissatisfaction with the public program owing to mismanagement and political corruption, failure to keep up with inflation, and uneven coverage across occupations. Policymakers supported the opportunity to promote investment in the economy.[6,7] In China, pension cost allocation practices under the state system were obstructive to the transition to private enterprise, in which flexibility was important, and compliance with the state system was deficient. A potential problem is that low retirement ages were incorporated in the new legislation, limiting the amount that would be accrued in individual accounts, while the program was not fully geared to provide benefits for extended survival.[8]

The UK's privatized component was an outgrowth of an earnings-related tier that was added to the basic public pension system, and of allowing employers to offer their own plan as an alternative to the state system. Eventually, individuals were permitted to opt out of their employer's plan. When the economy declined, severe cuts in public pensions weakened support for the traditional system. The UK, like Chile, experienced problems under its new program, based on overselling, high charges, and limited utility of individual accounts to older workers that reduced overall net gains to participating workers.[9]

The privatization movement depends for success on a commitment of younger workers to save despite the stimulus of a consumerist economy, and has not had much to offer to those who could not afford to save much. Nor does "private security" provide accommodation, as can a state plan, for those whose work record is discontinuous because of childcare, illness, or unemployment. More experience will no doubt produce a more settled appraisal of the value of a substantial private investment component in the social planning for retirement security.[10]

Early retirement

Social security laws have the potential to influence both retirement before, and continued work after, the statutory pensionable age. In OECD countries, provisions for receipt of pension benefits vary considerably from country to country. Twenty have early-retirement options in their public pension programs, and among them 13 specify conditions under which early retirement is allowed. These provisions result in a difference between the standard retirement age stated in the law and the actual age at which pension benefits are awarded. The option allows older workers with sufficient credited years to change their time–use pattern. This could include self-employment as well as leisure pursuits and nonmarket services such as care of family members. Some countries, however, promoted early retirement as a response to high levels of unemployment, encouraging older workers receiving unemployment insurance benefits to leave the labor force. However, such a shift results in an increased social expenditure for pensions as well as loss of a productive resource to the labor market.

As pension systems mature over time, more workers have sufficient earnings to become eligible for benefit payments before reaching the statutory qualifying age. Provisions for early retirement generally allow such workers to start drawing their pension. Pensionable age is also reduced for women with dependent children or children with disabilities and for men and women employed in difficult or unhealthy work.

Partial retirement, legally available in some countries, has become an attractive option for many persons, but its utility to older workers depends on whether part-time jobs are available.

Labor force participation in OECD countries declines as people approach pensionable age under prevailing programs, but the trend differs by gender. The rate for men aged 60 and over is much greater than that for women, but the decrease in labor force participation among men aged 65 and over is quite dramatic, dropping from 3 to 12 percentage points in several countries.

In contrast, economic activity rates among older women in these OECD countries vary enormously. Rates are high in developing countries, where pension and retirement support systems are relatively infrequent, and are very low in the developed countries.

CONCLUSION: THE GERIATRICIAN'S ROLE

The demographic trend of an increased life expectancy has already changed the age profile of many countries and is continuing to be felt throughout the world, resulting in significant changes, both in private lives and public discourse.

Older persons will be affected by national economic resources, systems that are set in place to protect them from destitution, and their involvement in the paid labor force. These in turn will have an impact on the agendas and goals of healthcare professionals. The long-term variations in economic growth rates, pension policies, anticipated shortage of workers that will necessitate that older persons remain in the labor force longer, among other considerations, constrain long-range predictions and create difficulties in planning for the well-being of the aging population. For example, since nations are likely to raise the normal age of retirement in response to longevity changes, the interests of older persons whose disabilities preclude full-time work will need to be safeguarded.

The ongoing demographic changes increase the numbers of individuals who will be strongly affected by the availability, perspective, and content of geriatric services. The health professions must be prepared for this growing number of older persons (projecting from numbers of persons already born) and for a variety of life alterations. The changing social and economic environment in which the health and social care of older persons will be carried out will have an impact on important health service issues.

Geriatricians combine the application of medical science with a concern for the whole individual in responding to the challenge posed by demographic change. They must be prepared to make comprehensive assessments oriented (a) to preventive maintenance as well as restoration of function, and (b) not only to the seriously disabled but to the mostly well. Doctors who care for older patients should be cognizant of their economic and social resources, and of the setting in which they live, not only their biological parameters and organ integrity. The nature and stability of social support networks need to be understood, since changes in household composition, depletion of financial assets, and suitability of the housing environment can affect compliance with treatment, adherence to healthy regimens, and sources of morale and well-being. The death or disability of a spouse, migration of children, market fluctuations, and failures that affect the value of retirement savings are examples of risks embedded within the context of the individual's state of health. Thus, a patient's "fallback" options and the means of accessing them are important in effective care management.

Since most older persons are being treated for more than one ailment, the adoption of an integrated approach to care management can help doctors coordinate the stream of services that may be required. Geriatricians and other health-care professionals, who have an understanding of the resilience and determination of many older persons, can be effective advocates and facilitators for preventive behaviors and the delay of functional loss. This advocacy should extend to the specifics of long-term care, including its coordination with acute-care services that chronically ill persons may require and the particular needs associated with hospice care.

It is anticipated that the activity level of the aging population will continue to increase, along with their access to information as the Internet becomes more accessible worldwide. As the strengths and options of older persons increase and more and more of them remain highly functional for long periods of time, the outlook of doctors who treat them will change.

- Longevity creates economic problems because of the costs of retirement to individuals and society. Pension systems often contain counter-incentives to working, although use of the productive potential of older workers would help meet the costs of longevity to society as well as contribute to their morale and life quality.

- The labor force participation of older persons has not kept pace with the increase in their numbers and the control of late-life disability. Reports on about 200 countries show that although almost twice as many older adults were economically active in 2000 as in 1960, their proportion of the labor force had fallen.

- The spread of social security programs across the world means that both their built-in incentives to productive activity and their protective power against poverty are of wide interest at all levels of development. Indexing in benefit calculation, gender differences in the legal age of retirement, and incentives and disincentives relating to early retirement are among the features affecting whether the programs are compatible with the increased life expectancy and social goals of contemporary societies.

- Privatization of retirement programs has spread on several continents but is faced with many challenges. The problems include, among others, the level of fees charged by private companies administering the deposits, placement of investments, and payouts; the adequacy of retirement income afforded to older workers and low-wage workers, and the market risks encountered.

KEY POINTS The elderly in society

- The extraordinary growth in life expectancy at birth in nearly all countries of the world has changed both survival rates of individuals and age profiles of whole populations. Since 1950, scientific achievements applied to personal medical care decreased death rates from heart disease, stroke, and some types of cancer after age 65. In many countries, men aged 65 can expect to live 13–16 more years, and women an extra 14–20 years.

- Women's survival advantage may be due to a healthier lifestyle, more risk avoidance, and receptivity to prevention and early care of illness. The gender difference in longevity may vary between countries, depending on whether tradition favors allocation of household resources to boys' health, whether women are increasingly exposed to workplace risks, and whether modern health services are available.

REFERENCES

1. Rosenberg T: Look at Brazil. New York Times Magazine, 28 January 2001, Section 6:26–31,52,58,60–61
2. Butler RN, Grossman LK et al: Life in an older America. Century Foundation Press, New York, 1999:v
3. US Social Security Administration (SSA). Office of Policy, Office of Research, Evaluation and Statistics: Social Security Programs Throughout the World. SSA, Washington, DC, 1999
4. Remarks by John Langmore, Director, DSPD/DESA, United Nations, 39th Session of the Commission for Social Development, New York, 13 February 2001. SSA, Washington, DC, 1999
5. Gruber J, Wise D: Social security programs and retirement around the world: introduction and summary. National Bureau of Economic Research (NBER) working paper, 1998
6. Kritzer BE: Social security privatization in Latin America. Social Security Bull 2000;63(20):17–37
7. Williamson JB: Privatizing public pension systems: lessons for the United States from Latin America. CRR working paper 1999–03, November 1999
8. World Bank: Old age security: pension reform in China (China 2020 Series). World Bank, Washington, DC, 1997
9. Liu L: Retirement income security in the United Kingdom. Social Security Bull 1999;62(1):23–46
10. Liu L: Personal communication, February 2001

Chapter 113

Geriatric medicine: history and current practice in Europe

John C. Brocklehurst, Rebecca B. Dunn, and

Sijmen A. Duursma

For various historical reasons, specialist geriatric services developed as an integral part of the National Health Service in the UK earlier than in any other part of Europe. This chapter, therefore, deals principally with the evolution and present state of geriatric medicine in the UK. The second part deals more briefly with various aspects of geriatrics in a number of other European countries.

THE UNITED KINGDOM

Britain has been unique in as much as care of old people has been a state responsibility for about 400 years. In 1533, King Henry VIII divorced his first wife, Catherine of Aragon (who had produced no heir), and married Anne Boleyn. Because the Pope would not sanction the divorce, Henry broke with the church of Rome and established the Church of England. He dissolved the monasteries throughout the land that had until then provided refuge for the aged and chronic sick. As a result the "churches, streets and lanes of London became filled with sick and infirm poor men lying begging."[3] In 1552, a census—perhaps the first attempt ever to assess social need in England—was carried out by the citizens of London. It defined those in the city needing care as "fatherless children 350; sick and lame persons 200; aged and infirm 400; poor householders 600; idle vagabonds 200." Christ's Hospital was to take care of the children, while Bridewell took charge of the idle, and Bedlam the insane. St Bartholomew's and St Thomas' Hospitals between them cared for the remainder, "curable and incurable alike."[3] However, the problems remained, and in 1601 the responsibility for care was devolved to the local parishes under the Poor Relief Act. They were to provide for:

- the able bodied to work;
- children to be bound apprentice;
- the lame, impotent, old, and other persons unable to work to be relieved.

Relief could be in kind, but an Act of Parliament (the Knatchbull Act of 1723) permitted parishes to set up poor houses providing indoor relief. Parishes gradually ceased paying outdoor relief, poor houses gradually became "workhouses," also known as houses of industry and houses of correction. Gilbert's Act of 1782 was intended to promote humane houses for the old and indigent, but few were created. Gilbert's Act also empowered parishes to join together in unions to build workhouses that gradually included infirmaries

Geriatric medicine was established in Britain in the late 1930s by Margery Warren. Her message was the need for assessment and rehabilitation of elderly disabled people, education of medical students, and research into the problems of aging and old age.[1,2] This derived from her work in the workhouse infirmary associated with the West Middlesex Hospital in London: it is in the workhouse infirmary that the early history of elder care ended and the modern era began.

for the sick (the hospitals established at that time specifically excluding incurables). A Poor Law Commission was set up in 1832 and its report two years later (leading to the Poor Law Amendment Act of 1834) established the principle of less eligibility—that is life in the workhouse had to be less eligible (or more unpleasant) "than the situation of the independent labourer of the lowest class." The intention was to discourage all but the most desperate from entering the workhouse. Separation of the sexes was to be absolute, they were to "live, sleep and take their meals in totally different parts of the building each with its own enclosed yard." The work to be engaged in was "the hardest and most tedious labour human ingenuity could devise." Special treatment was to be provided for the "aged poor of good conduct," but this seldom occurred. As for those whose conduct was not regarded as good, the Minority Report had this to say: "For old men and women of this kind the general mixed workhouse with its stigma of pauperism, its dull routine, its exaction of such work as its inmates can perform and its deterrent regulations seems a fitting place in which to end a misspent life."

Because national old age pensions were not introduced until 1908, most people surviving into old age and having no savings and impoverished families had no alternative but to enter the generally hated workhouse.

The Metropolitan Asylums Board established provision in 1867 for Poor Law infirmaries separate from workhouses in London. "Chronic sick wards" were later provided in municipal hospitals set up under the Public Health Act of 1878. General hospitals established at that time specifically excluded "incurables."

THE EARLY TWENTIETH CENTURY

In 1929 the Local Government Act replaced the Boards of Guardians by local and county authorities and gradually there developed a series of general hospitals within whose walls many of the aged found refuge. A two-tiered hospital system resulted.

The newly created municipal hospitals retained responsibility for those with chronic diseases (predominantly elderly people) whom the long established voluntary hospitals (the seat of all medical training and research) would not admit. Huge waiting lists developed for admission to this chronic sick hospital accommodation. It was in the workhouse infirmary and municipal hospitals that geriatrics was born. In 1935, Margery Warren (a medical officer at the West Middlesex Hospital[4]), took over care of 858 chronic patients (including 144 mentally ill) in the adjoining workhouse infirmary. Following medical examination, 200 of these could be transferred elsewhere, beds were removed, wards improved physically, and gradually the numbers were reduced to 400 beds.[2] Her methods—careful medical and social assessment, medical treatment, and rehabilitation—were described in a series of publications.[1,2,4] Her general conclusion was that chronic sick patients should be treated in a special block in a general hospital because[1]

> Geriatrics is a significant subject for the teaching of medical students. It should comprise an essential part of the training of student nurses. General hospital facilities are necessary for correct diagnosis and treatment. Research on disease in old age can only be undertaken with the full facilities of a general hospital.

These were visionary proposals in 1943.

The coming of the National Health Service (NHS) in 1948 marked the end of the Poor Law. It firmly divided responsibility for elderly people between local authorities and the newly established Regional Hospital Boards. At first many of the former workhouses in which there were both dormitory and hospital accommodation became joint-user establishments between the NHS and the local authorities. However, Part III of the National Assistance Act of 1948 required the local authorities to provide care and attention for those who could not look after themselves, and many old people's homes were set up by these authorities as a result. Some were no more than old workhouses with slight modifications, others were large private houses or hotels that were especially adapted. Gradually the principle of purpose building of special residential accommodation for elderly people became established. There remained then under the Regional Hospital Boards a disparate collection of workhouse infirmaries, chronic sick wards in municipal hospitals and, as time went by, other hospitals whose use was changing (e.g. infectious diseases hospitals) into which elderly and infirm people were being admitted.

Throughout the 1940s a great deal of thought and discussion was given to the problems of the "chronic sick." Lord Amulree and Dr E. C. Sturdee—both at that time working in the Ministry of Health, and having been involved with chronically sick patients who were evacuated during World War II to sector hospitals under the emergency medical service—carried out surveys of hospitals in different parts of the country, and gave an overview to the Parliamentary Medical Group (PMG) as reported in the *British Medical Journal*.[5] They indicated that not all the chronically sick were old (data in 1943 showed 29 percent aged under 65), and many did not need to be in hospital. They clarified the reasons for the "chronically sick" status of these people. There were patients:

- with diseases that had become chronic and difficult to treat because they had not been treated early enough;
- with a disability who had been taken into hospital because their friends were unable to look after them;
- suffering from an illness which could have been prevented;
- admitted with a so-called chronic disease which under treatment had improved, but were still in hospital because they had nowhere to go.

These four categories encapsulated (perhaps unwittingly) the whole impetus for the emergence of geriatrics as a speciality.

Amulree and Sturdee suggested that 10–20 percent of beds in general hospitals should be allotted to this group of patients partly to counter the "present day tendency of giving priority to acute patients and leaving the others to shift for themselves" and to ensure accurate diagnosis and treatment. Their care should be "part of the duties of the more experienced medical staff."

They discussed accommodation for those no longer needing hospital care, recommending "hostels" run on the lines of boarding houses or hotels with special attention to the requirements of old people, some single rooms, and no more than four in any room. They should have good lighting (including over-bed lighting because "old people often like to read and knit in bed"), good heating, nonslip floors, chairs easy to get out of, and so on. In some cases, the hostel might be part of a group of "cottage homes." For long-stay patients requiring nursing care, small units with a homely atmosphere were required and "everything should be done to remove the institutional stigma."

Early followers of Margery Warren were Dr Lionel Cosin,[6] an orthopedic surgeon at Orsett Hospital, Essex, who promoted early rehabilitation, especially of fractured femur patients; Dr Eric Brooke at St Helier's Hospital, Carshalton, who had begun the practice of visiting waiting-list patients in their own homes by a "geriatric social worker;" and Dr Trevor Howell at the Royal Hospital, Chelsea (for retired servicemen).[7]

SURVEYS OF NEED

The dawning recognition of the needs of old people in an aging society led to a number of major surveys, producing data for the planning of services. In 1945, Curran and colleagues[8] published data on about 1,000 males aged 65 and females aged 60 and over living in poorer areas of Glasgow, all of whom were visited at home. A social and medical survey of people aged 65 and over in England was set up by the Nuffield Foundation in 1943, the results of which were published in two reports—*Old People* (1947)[9] and the *Social Medicine of Old Age* (1948).[10] The former covered several localities, while the latter was a random sample of the inhabitants of the town of Wolverhampton, yielding 143 males and 334 females aged 65 and over each visited at home by Dr Sheldon. Shortly afterward, a study of medical and social problems in old people in Northern Ireland was carried out by Adams and Cheeseman (1951).[11] This involved visits to 1,625 patients aged 60 and over in Northern Ireland hospitals, as well as a community survey in Belfast that included findings on medical examination. A further study in the UK was that of Hobson and Pemberton (1955).[12]

A more detailed study of disease and disability in 1,062 men aged 60–69 all on the lists of 11 general practitioners in Birmingham was reported by Brown et al.[13] in 1958. This showed a clear relationship between disease, disability, and social class. Nevertheless, 75 percent of men aged 66 and 50 percent aged 70 were still in full-time work.

In 1947, J. W. Affleck, a psychiatrist, published a survey of 788 chronic sick patients in five hospitals in Leeds[14] (all were cared for by general practitioners, 80 percent were over 65, and 35 percent suffered primarily from mental disorder). Affleck concluded: "the study of disease of the aged would be greatly assisted if, as suggested by Warren (1946), the 'geriatrics specialty' was developed in this country to the same extent as the pediatric to which it is analogous. It might develop into one of the most important services of the future anywhere."

In 1949, in his Lumleian Lectures to the Royal College of Physicians, A. P. Thompson[15] (Professor of Therapeutics at the University of Birmingham) described results of a survey of 50 institutions in Birmingham concerned with the reception of the aged and chronic sick—a total of 5,780 beds. These comprised 45 percent of all beds for general medicine and surgery in the region. In one hospital (Western Road Hospital) five full-time medical officers cared for 1,000 bedfast patients in addition to other responsibilities, including maternity beds and a venereal disease department. There was no attempt at rehabilitation, all day rooms were full of beds, and 97 percent of patients were bedfast, among whom one-half were incontinent. Thompson analyzed the reasons for this state of affairs in great detail. He concluded 100 days to be the critical period in hospital for elderly people; beyond that the expectation of discharge diminished, as did visiting by relatives. At that time also all the hazards of the bedfast state—contractures, decubitus ulcers, incontinence, apathy, and acceptance—became firmly established. Nevertheless, he did not support the concept of developing geriatrics as a specialty, but rather the establishment of wards in general hospitals, especially in teaching hospitals, where the aged and chronic sick would be cared for by general physicians.

In 1958 through 1959, a further study of hospital patients in all Birmingham general, special, and chronic hospitals was carried out by Thomas McKeown (Professor of Social Medicine) and his associates.[16] This involved 4,274 patients of whom in 4.7 percent it was considered that there were insufficient medical grounds for admission (11.8 percent in the chronic hospitals). The striking relationship of age with the type of hospital in which the patient was situated is shown in Figure 113-1. They concluded: "irrespective of their needs for care, physically ill patients are almost always in general and special hospitals if they are young and in chronic hospitals if they are old" and "the distribution of mentally disturbed patients who do not need the full services of a modern hospital between mental and chronic hospitals is sharply related to age."

The British Medical Association (BMA) set up a working group in 1947 to review care of the elderly and infirm and to make recommendations.[17] Of 21 members, four were active in the new specialty of geriatrics (Amulree, Brooke, Cousin, Warren). They noted that many elderly patients in institutions and hospitals for the chronic sick

... drift into "infirmary decubitus" with avoidable contractures and deformities fixed and immobile, unable to

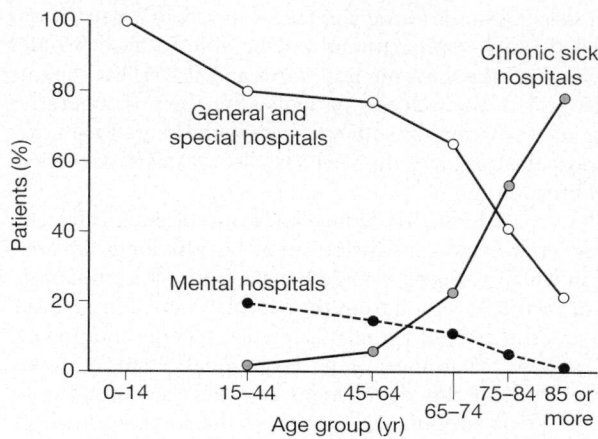

Figure 113-1 Age range of people treated in three different types of hospitals in Birmingham, UK, in 1960. From McKeown et al.,[16] with permission.

feed themselves or sit up in bed. An atmosphere of hopelessness is shared by staff and patients alike. The situation can lead to wasteful use of nurses and hamper recruitment to an already depleted profession."

The working group's report proposed a classification of the elderly population as follows:

1. *The elderly at home.*
2. *The elderly and infirm.* Their need was admission under guidance of the geriatric department to suitable homes or hostels providing domestic rather than continuous medical or nursing support, and looked after by general practitioners.
3. *The elderly sick*: (a) acute; (b) long-term sick (potentially remediable); and (c) irremediable, for whom long-stay annexes should be provided.
4. *Elderly psychiatric patients*: (a) those not requiring hospital treatment who could stay in their own homes; (b) those needing custodial care in long-stay annexes; and (c) those in need of active psychiatric care or treatment in a mental hospital.

They recommended the gradual establishment in general hospitals, including teaching hospitals, of special geriatric departments. A geriatric department was described as comprising wards reserved exclusively for elderly patients, all undergoing investigation or active treatment and rehabilitation so that in due course they could be discharged from such wards—either to their own homes or, after classification, to other appropriate accommodation. This included long-stay annexes which, under medical supervision of the geriatric department, would provide accommodation and nursing care for irremediable patients who, after full investigation and treatment in the geriatric department, showed no promise of further improvement. Residential homes would each provide, in close association with the geriatric department, accommodation for 20–40 elderly people in need of residential (but not nursing) care.

Admission to the geriatric department was to be directly from the patients' own homes, or in some cases transfer from other hospital wards for rehabilitation and resettlement. It was hoped that "this department will be able to absorb older patients from the acute medical wards and also relieve the surgical wards of their elderly patients after the post-operative phase and there must be sufficient beds in the long stay annexes to absorb the '20% residuum' which will be transferred to them from time to time."

The department should also have outpatient clinics, not only for consultation and investigation, but also for group exercises in which old people could benefit from the companionship of their fellows and from the stimulation of competition. Such an arrangement would "facilitate discharge and prevent readmission" (a harbinger of the day hospital). Vehicles should be provided for this department so that it was not wholly dependent on ambulance service of the local authorities. Liaison with local authorities and other bodies concerned with the problems of old age, public and voluntary, was regarded as of the highest importance.

This detailed account was published not only in the report of 1949—*The Care and Treatment of the Elderly and Infirm*—but also in a supplement to the report published in 1948, *The Right Patient in the Right Bed.*[17]

Regarding the fourth category—elderly psychiatric patients—the report proposed observation wards within the geriatric department that would be used for assessment by a psychiatric consultant as to whether the patient should be sent to a long-stay annex as irremediable or to a mental hospital as likely to benefit from the advice and from the active treatment. It emphasized the importance of avoiding the stigma (for the family) of mental hospital admission for the "mental debility associated with old age."

In 1972, the Royal College of Physicians of London set up a working party whose membership consisted of 13 geriatricians and some college officers.[18] It pointed out the varying admission procedures that were developing at different geriatric departments (e.g. participating in general medical rotas; admitting all patients aged 75 and over; admitting only patients referred from other clinicians). Regarding beds it reported: "most geriatric departments allot 30–40% of their beds for 'continuing care,' but it is obvious that the actual number of hospital beds for such patients with physical and mental infirmity must be increased during the next 30 years even if local authorities also expand their facility for the frail elderly." There were 40 vacancies for consultant geriatricians at that time, and the hope was expressed that the recently created academic departments would increase awareness of the role of geriatric medicine and the satisfaction this form of practice offers as a career. The need for specialist psychogeriatric services was also emphasized.

In 1976, yet another report of the British Medical Association was published.[19] Of a total working party membership of 17, six were consultant geriatricians (including three professors). A number of new developments were referred to, including assessment of unreported illness, good neighbor schemes, night sitters, soiled linen services, and admissions for respite care. Once again, staff shortages and inappropriate accommodation were emphasized. The importance of psychiatric assessment before the admission of mentally infirm elderly people to hospital; the involvement of health visitors in the early detection of unreported illness; and the recognition of one particular general practitioner as a visiting medical officer in a residential home with responsibility (in consultation with colleagues) for

contributing to medical policy within the home, were all emphasized, as was the importance of periodical review of medical and social needs of elderly people in residential homes and the possibilities for discharge.

THE STRUCTURE OF A GERIATRIC SERVICE

In 1948, the year the National Health Service began, the first new appointment of a consultant geriatrician was made in Cornwall, Dr Tom Wilson. This marked the recognition of a new specialty and one whose official status was the same as all other hospital specialties. By 1995, there were more than 600 consultant geriatricians in the UK. The first-generation geriatricians were each appointed to hospital management groups serving an average total population of between 200,000 and 250,000 people. The consultant was given responsibility for all the "chronic sick" beds usually in several hospitals and numbering between 200 and 400. There was generally a waiting list of similar proportions. The consultant's first clinical responsibility was to examine the patients occupying the beds, to make a diagnosis, and try to identify those who might respond to physical therapy and at least be able to be up and about and, in some cases, to move to residential homes or very occasionally, back home. At the same time, it was necessary to review those on the waiting list by visiting them at home or in the acute hospital beds they occupied, attempting to decide some alternative to long-term care and to allot some order of priority, having in mind again those likely to respond to treatment once properly assessed. It was then necessary to decide which of the hospital wards should be used for admission and assessment and which might appropriately be used for long-term care. A number of documented accounts for this process are available.

In 1949, Exton-Smith and Crockett[20] described the initiation of a service at a London County Council Hospital (St Pancras) after it had been taken over by a London teaching hospital (University College Hospital) under the care of a consultant, Lord Amulree. They described what they claimed was the first unit of its kind (being part of a teaching hospital) with facilities for investigation, treatment, and research. In 1949 also, Adams[21] described his work at the Belfast City Hospital, at one time the largest Poor Law Union Infirmary in the UK, but by then partly converted to a geriatric hospital with 500 to 600 of its 1,800 beds set aside for the chronic sick. Three hundred and fifty of these were in a "remote and antiquated brick building euphemistically named the 'convalescent buildings.'" They comprised 60 bedded wards with "no lifts, narrow stairs and poor light." Patients were kept in bed all day to avoid falls because staffing was minimal (at times, only one nurse and an orderly for 60 beds) and apathy was everywhere. This description echoes that of Marjory Warren and was repeated throughout the country where the first geriatric consultants were appointed— O. T. Brown in Glasgow, H. Droller in Leeds, J. Agate in Ipswich, T. Wilson in Truro, O. Olbrich in Sunderland, and so on.

The style of practice

Marjory Warren proposed that long-term care should be separate from other geriatric beds and most developments were along these lines.[22,23] Not all agreed however. Adams,[24] believed that all hospital wards should share the responsibility of care for long-stay patients, so in new wards for his unit in Belfast, each L-shaped 40-bed ward included 16 long-stay beds in a separate area, but integral to the ward and cared for by the ward staff. Because most first-generation geriatricians were given beds in more than one hospital, it became effective to designate those at different sites for different purposes. Wards in a general hospital were best used for acute admissions (often called "assessment wards") because of laboratory and radiological facilities and easy access to other specialists. Other beds were often in former tuberculosis sanatoria or infectious diseases hospitals and might adapt well to rehabilitation with space for physiotherapy and occupational therapy. Later, day hospitals developed in association with many of these. So a system of "progressive patient care" developed in many departments (reviewed by Irvine in 1963).[25] A national survey of style of practice was carried out in 1984 by Andrews and Brocklehurst.[26,27] Two hundred and thirteen geriatric departments provided information as follows: in 38 percent acute and rehabilitation patients shared the same wards and long-stay patients were separate; 24 percent practiced complete progressive patient care with separate acute, rehabilitation, and long-stay wards; and 21 percent combined all forms of care in all wards. In 8 percent the acute assessment wards were separate and rehabilitation and long-term care combined.

The department at Hull was a leading proponent of managing all types of patients in all wards.[28] The department consisted of 433 beds in three different hospitals. An age-related admissions policy was developed (all medical emergencies aged over 75 being admitted to these beds). By 6 years after the inception of this policy, long-stay beds had been reduced to 20 percent, and mean in-patient stay to under 30 days (including long-stay patients).

The advantages of progressive patient care include better use of medical staff time—consultant ward rounds being daily or at least two to three times weekly in acute wards, once weekly in rehabilitation wards, and less frequently in long-stay wards.[27] The ward structure and process also fit the different types of patients—technical medical procedures in acute wards, all staff involved in promoting independence in rehabilitation wards, and a homely atmosphere and provision of recreational activities in long-stay wards. The disadvantage of progressive patient care was the need for patients to move between different wards and different nurses, although medical staff usually maintained continuity; also the need to maintain available beds in a number of different locations. A profile of a geriatric rehabilitation ward in 1985 indicated an average length of stay of 31 days for patients being discharged home, but more than twice that for patients awaiting placements in nursing homes or long-stay wards.[29]

The concept of a "halfway house" for patients who had completed their medical care, but were not yet ready to live independently at home, was promoted by the National Corporation for the Care of Old People who set up a number of such units, usually in large houses outside hospital precincts.[30] In time, their short-stay function became lost and they added to long-stay beds.

Coordination of discharge

As the specialty developed, the need for coordination between the many agencies involved became apparent.[31] This applied not only within the hospital service, but also in the interface between primary care and hospital care and between geriatricians and psychiatrists.[32,33] While discharge planning was generally well-organized in departments of geriatric medicine, major problems remained in other hospital departments. In one study, 39 percent of the sample of people aged 65 and over were given less than 24 hours notice of discharge and less than 50 percent reported that a member of the hospital staff discussed their discharge with them while they were in hospital.[34] Lack of advice at the time of discharge was noted in 51 percent of elderly people readmitted within 28 days of discharge.[35] Another study[36] concluded that planned discharge for 650 patients aged 75 and over discharged over a period of 18 months from one hospital could have saved 6,700 bed-days by preventing readmissions.

Integrated services

An uneasy relationship between geriatric and general medicine was the constant background to the emergence of geriatrics as a specialty,[38,39] especially in two regards—the gatekeeper role of geriatrics for long-term care, which involved patients in general medical beds as well as the community; and increasing involvement of geriatricians in acute medicine of old age. Geriatricians relinquished care of patients aged under 65 with chronic illness as Young Disabled Units were established.[40] For those aged 65 and over, various admission policies were set up—some departments admitted according to need (i.e. those patients presenting with the "geriatric giants" or with mixed medical and social problems for which the geriatric department was specially adapted). Others were admitted on an age-related basis (varying from 65 and over to 85 and over).[41,42] These policies applied to emergency admissions while "cold" admissions referred by general practitioners through outpatients or domiciliary consultation usually included anyone aged 65 or over.[43,44] Gradually a reintegration with general medicine for emergency admissions gained impetus.[43] The move towards integration has been partially driven by the need to reduce junior hospital doctors' hours of work and the problem of "outliers"—patients of one consultant being admitted to many different wards of the hospital when their wards are full. Accommodation to these difficulties acquired more rational and economic use of beds and staff.

While most geriatricians are full-time specialists some have always had sessions in general (internal) medicine (joint appointments). These numbered 20 percent of geriatricians in 1988.[42] Half of these had five or more sessions devoted to general medicine (a full-time National Health Service consultant contract is for 10 sessions a week). Specialism on a part-time basis within geriatric practice also increased. In 1988, 26 percent of full-time geriatricians and 48 percent of those with joint appointments practiced special interests.[42] Gastroenterology was the most frequent (24 percent) followed by cardiology (20 percent) and diabetes (16 percent).

Domiciliary consultation

The practice of seeing the patients in their own homes was an essential part of geriatric practice in its early stages when consultants inherited large waiting lists. Such home visits were initiated by the hospital consultant, who usually carried out the visit, or sometimes by a social worker from the department.[45] Within the National Health Service they were part of the consultant's contract and called "assessment visits."[46,47]

Apart from deciding priority for admission, or whether some alternative form of care was more appropriate, these visits had the advantage of establishing a personal rapport between doctor and patient and affording the doctor an insight into the social circumstances of the patient (and of the geographic catchment area). They allowed discussion with patients and relatives of the proposed line of action and often allowed direct contact between consultant and general practitioner.[48] They also came to have a role in the teaching of medical students.[48] Now that most geriatric departments are able to admit patients immediately on referral, the need for assessment visits has diminished. However, a facility for consultants to offer advice to general practitioners on the diagnosis and management of patients at home remains and is allowed for within the National Health Service by a second type of home visit called a "domiciliary consultation." This is initiated by the general practitioner and attracts a fee to the specialist. While the intention of such consultations was that the specialist and general practitioner should both be present, in fact this happens only in a minority of cases.[48] The situation was reviewed in 1991.[49]

Special units

Stroke units and orthogeriatric units have been developed in a number of geriatric departments (by 1985 there were stroke units in 11 percent and orthogeriatric units in 20 percent of departments[26]). The number of stroke units has since risen sharply in the light of the evidence of the benefits of organized stroke care. These functioned in different ways—orthogeriatric wards having shared staffing with surgeons and geriatricians, stroke units usually being entirely staffed by geriatricians, but with specially trained physiotherapists, occupational therapists, and nurses. Early assessments of the effectiveness of some of these units was rather discouraging, but later reports were very positive.[50,51] (See also Chapter 50.)

Prevention in care

The extent of unreported illness among elderly people was investigated in Edinburgh in 1964 by Williamson and colleagues[52] who reported a considerable iceberg of morbidity. A clinic providing medical assessment associated with access to a health visitor (nurse), physiotherapist, chiropodist, and a voluntary welfare organizer was set up in 1952 in Rutherglen near Glasgow by Ferguson Anderson and Nairn Cowan.[53] Clients were referred by their general practitioners and findings on the first 500 were described in 1955.[52] Other schemes of screening or case finding have been published since then.[54,55] The responsibility for this service has been made a contractual obligation for general practitioners in the NHS and is now offered to all people aged 75 and over.

The geriatric day hospital

Geriatric day hospitals were preceded in the UK by some patients attending in the daytime only at geriatric wards or rehabilitation units, coming from their own homes.[56] The first day hospitals described in the literature were in Oxford[57] and Leeds.[58] In 1958 through 1959, James Farndale[59] visited nine geriatric day hospitals, describing them as small and experimental. The work of geriatric day hospitals was described in a number of publications in the early 1960s.[60–62] The first attempt to carry out a controlled trial of day hospital care was published by Woodford Williams and colleagues[63] in 1962. A government audit was published in 1994.[64,65]

Psychogeriatrics

The plight of mentally ill older people in general and chronic sick hospitals was highlighted in 1949 by Thompson[15] in his report—indicating 25 percent of the 1,000 patients in the Western Road Infirmary in Birmingham in 1948 as being certifiably insane. Twenty-two years later, a further study of patients in hospital in Birmingham[16] showed the switch in the number of patients requiring some supervision because of their mental state between mental hospital and chronic sick hospitals as a function of advancing age (Fig. 113-1). The widespread mixing of patients with mental illness and physical disability in mental hospitals, geriatric wards, and residential wards in Newcastle was highlighted by Kay and colleagues[66] in 1966. They advocated comprehensive psychogeriatric assessment units attached to general hospitals and staffed by geriatricians and psychiatrists. Developments in joint care between geriatrics and psychiatry by providing joint-assessment beds were demonstrated in Edinburgh in 1960,[67] and in Nottingham in 1968.[68] Joint-assessment wards received encouragement from the Department of Health in 1970.[69] Specialist consultant psychogeriatricians began to be appointed in the National Health Service through the 1970s, and the specialty received official recognition by the Department of Health in 1989.

Professional training

In the UK, registration as a medical practitioner requires 5 years' undergraduate study leading to the degree of Bachelor of Medicine and Bachelor of Surgery (MB, ChB) followed by 1-year internship as a House Officer (6 months in medicine and 6 months in surgery). Thereafter, specialist training involves at least a further 7 years. Geriatric specialization is usually by dual accreditation in geriatric medicine and general internal medicine. The diploma of membership of one of the Royal Colleges of Physicians in the UK (MRCP) by written or/and clinical examination is essential, and is usually obtained within the first 2 years of training. For those intending to specialize within academic geriatrics, a doctor's degree obtained by thesis (MD or PhD) is also generally required.

Early personalities

The British Geriatrics Society was formed as the Medical Society for the Care of the Elderly at a meeting convened by Dr Trevor Howell in 1947. Those present included Lord Amulree, Dr Sturdee, Dr Marjory Warren, Dr Eric Brooke, Mr Lionel Cousin, Dr Thomas Wilson, and Dr Alfred Mitchum who may be regarded as the founder members.[70]

In 1959, the name was changed to British Geriatrics Society, and since then there have been episodic discussions about changing the name once more because of the fairly widespread use of the word *geriatric* in a pejorative manner ("he's just an old geriatric"); but this is largely a UK phenomenon, relating probably to the workhouse origin of the specialty, and Nascher's word, *geriatric*, remains paramount worldwide. In the UK, many departments now call themselves Care of the Elderly or some similar title, but the Society's name persists. Membership is currently around 2,000.

MARJORY WARREN CBE (1897–1960)   In 1936, Marjory Warren became an Assistant Medical Officer at the West Middlesex County Hospital. Among her duties, she undertook more than 4,000 surgical operations. In 1935, the adjacent workhouse infirmary was annexed to the hospital and she took charge of it as described elsewhere. The reformed wards, with beds eventually diminished from 714 to 200, became a geriatric "Mecca" visited by physicians and others worldwide and inspiring the early pioneers to emulate her methods. She died prematurely in a car crash at the height of her career[71,72] (Fig. 113-2).

LORD AMULREE KBE (1900–1983)   Lord Amulree was recruited to the Ministry of Health in 1933 with responsibilities among others for the Poor Law. At the time, owing to wartime bombing of cities, many patients from chronic sick hospitals were transferred to temporary hospitals in the country, and Amulree, among others, became aware of the neglected state of these patients. Along with his senior colleague Sturdee, he brought this to the notice of the House of Lords[5] in 1946, and in 1949 he was appointed Consultant Physician in Geriatric Medicine at St Pancras' Hospital annexed to University College Hospital. This was the first teaching hospital appointment in geriatrics. He was president of the British Geriatrics Society from its inception in 1946 for 25 years[73] (Fig. 113-3).

A. L. STURDEE   After service in the Royal Navy in World War I, A. L. Sturdee joined the Ministry of Health with responsibilities for the administration of the Poor Law. He presented the case for geriatrics in the House of Lords (with Amulree as assistant).[5]

ERIC BROOKE (1896–1956)   Eric Brooke was Medical Superintendent of St Helier's Hospital in Surrey and was confronted with a large number of chronic sick beds and a considerable waiting list. He decided to visit the patients at home accompanied by a social worker—this was regarded as the beginning of domiciliary assessment visits. He is also credited with the origins of the day hospital, bringing patients up to hospital wards for physiotherapy and preventing the need for admission.[74]

LIONEL COSIN (1913–1994)   Lionel Cosin was an orthopedic surgeon who became Medical Superintendent of Orsett Hospital in Essex in 1937, and like Warren and Brooke, was confronted with the problem of the chronically sick. He developed a rehabilitation program, and when he moved to Cowley Road Hospital in Oxford he established an early-model geriatric unit, which became another focus for national and international visitors. He planned and developed the first purpose-built geriatric day hospital in 1958.[75]

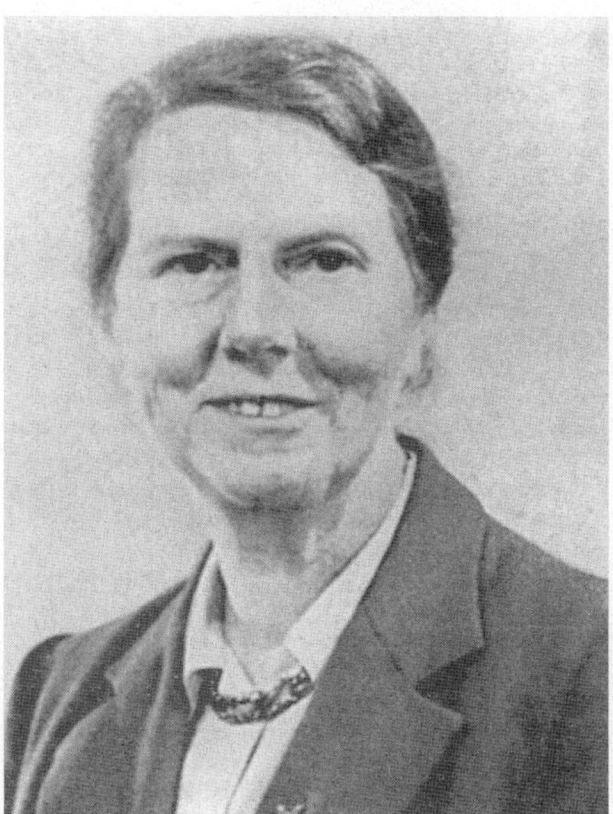

Figure 113-2 Dr Marjory Warren, founder of British geriatric medicine. From Adams,[71] with permission of Karger, Basel.

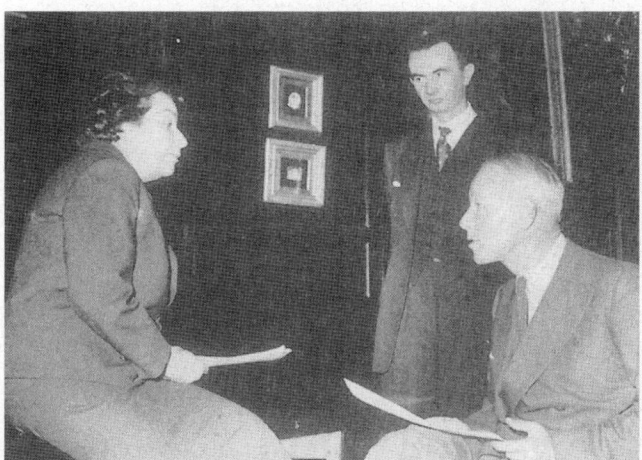

Figure 113-3 Lord Amulree (seated, right), first president and founding member of the Society for Care of the Elderly, later the British Geriatrics Society; Professor Norman Exton-Smith (standing), first joint editor of both *Gerontolgia Clinica* and *Age and Ageing*, and president of the British Geriatrics Society; and Professor Anna Aslan (left), director of the Institute of Gerontology, Bucharest, Romania.

TREVOR HOWELL (1908–1988) Trevor Howell, the prime mover in creating the Medical Society for Care of the Elderly, was its first secretary. After a period in general practice he was posted during World War II as a Medical Officer to the Royal Hospital Chelsea—a large hospital for retired military personnel. His interest in clinical aspects of aging led to a research fellowship after the war followed by consultant appointment as a Physician in Geriatric Medicine at St John's Hospital, Battersea, and subsequently at Queen's Hospital, Croydon.[76] He published widely in clinical medicine and medical history, including one of the early books (in 1946), *Old Age: Some Practical Points in Geriatrics*[77] (Fig. 113-4).

THOMAS WILSON (1918–) After wartime service in the RAF, Thomas Wilson joined Trevor Howell at St John's Hospital, and among other achievements, carried out the first series of cystometrograms in elderly people.[78] In 1948 he was appointed to the first advertised post of consultant geriatrician in the National Health Service, at Truro, Cornwall, where he developed early geriatric/psychogeriatric coordination.

J. A. SHELDON CBE (1893–1972) Dr Sheldon, whose survey of aging in Wolverhampton has been referred to already,[10] served as president of the Second International Congress of the International Association of Gerontology held in London in 1954. His researches included falls in old age, and he developed what was probably the first measurement of sway.[79]

SIR RONALD TONBRIDGE (1906–1954) Sir Ronald Tonbridge was appointed Professor of Medicine at the University of Leeds in 1944. He promoted the cause of geriatrics, being one of the two UK representatives at the formation of the International Association of Gerontology IAG (St Louis, 1951) and served as Chairman of the Second Congress of the IAG in 1954.

The individuals mentioned above were the early members of the British Geriatrics Society. Other early pioneers included Charles Andrews, who surveyed workhouses in Cornwall and recommended a countywide geriatric service headed by consultant geriatricians, which materialized in the appointment of Thomas Wilson. George Adams CBE, whose study of the aged in community and hospitals in Northern Ireland has already been referred to,[21] attended the first meeting of the Medical Society for Care of the Elderly in 1948 and became second president of the British Geriatrics Society. He became a consultant, and later Professor of Geriatric Medicine in Belfast. Sir Ferguson Anderson, appointed Coordinator of Geriatric Services in Glasgow, subsequently occupied the first chair of geriatric medicine in the UK. He became president of the Royal College of Physicians and Surgeons in Glasgow and the third president of the British Geriatrics Society (Fig. 113-5).

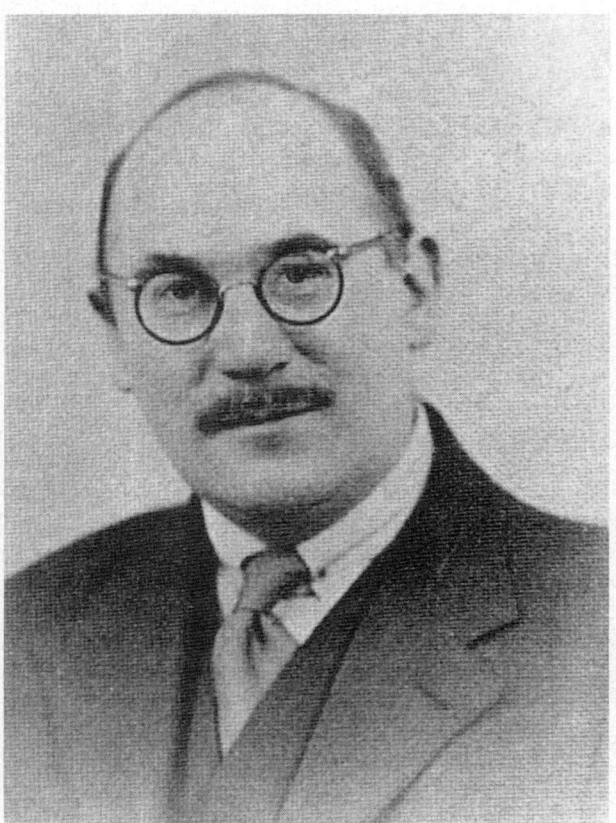

Figure 113-4 Dr Trevor Howell, first secretary and founding member of the Medical Society for Care of the Elderly, later the British Geriatrics Society.

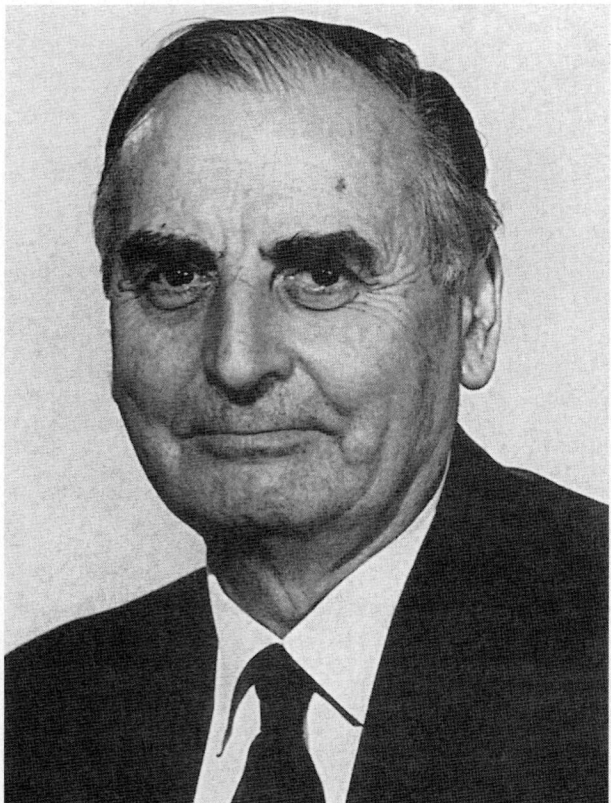

Figure 113-5 Professor Sir Ferguson Anderson, first professor of geriatric medicine in the UK, and president of the British Geriatrics Society.

Publications

Among early British publications concerned with old age were *Records of Longevity* by Thomas Bailey (1857)—an essay on the history of longevity followed by notes on hundreds of individuals reputed to have lived 100 years or longer—and Charcot's lectures to the New Sydenham Society in 1881. In 1922, Sir Humphrey Rolleston developed his Linacre lectures into *Aspects of Old Age*, a well-documented book. His definition of old age as the *period at which man ceases to adjust himself to his environment* is not far from a modern definition of aging as a failure of homeostasis.

Books describing aspects of geriatric practice include, *Old Age: Some Practical Points in Geriatrics* (Howell, 1946), *Adding Life to Years* (Amulree, 1957), *Medical Problems of Old Age* (Exton-Smith, 1955), *Modern Trends in Geriatrics* (Hobson, 1956), *Rehabilitation of the Elderly Invalid at Home* (Adams, 1957), and *Social and Medical Problems of the Elderly* (Hazel, 1960).

The first large textbook was the first edition of the present volume, *Geriatric Medicine and Gerontology*, edited by J. C. Brocklehurst (1973). It contained 760 pages contributed by 44 authors—modest numbers when compared with the present sixth edition.

Monographs include the two reports from the Nuffield Foundation already referred to—*Old People* (1947) and *Social Medicine of Old Age* (Sheldon, 1948); *Incontinence and Old People* (Brocklehurst, 1951), which described cystometry and anorectal manometry (using smoked drums and rubber tambours in the pretransducer era); and *Skill and Age* (Welford, 1951). Others were *The Biology of Senescence* (Comfort, 1956), *Family Life and Old People* (Townsend, 1957), *Physiological and Pathological Ageing* (Korenchevsky, 1958), and *Valvular Disease of the Heart in Old Age* (Bedford and Caird, 1960).

The first European journal, *Gerontologia Clinica*, edited by Woodford Williams and Exton-Smith and published by Karger, became the official publication of the British Geriatrics Society (first published in 1956) until its own journal, *Age and Ageing*, was produced in 1971, edited by Exton-Smith and Hodkinson. *Gerontologia Clinica* continues as the European journal, now entitled *Gerontology*.

CURRENT PRACTICE IN THE UNITED KINGDOM

During the 1980s and much of the 1990s, the trend in the UK was for geriatric practice to become more closely identified with acute general internal medicine and to be less involved with rehabilitation and long-term care. The improved access to acute diagnostic facilities for older people was welcome. In some departments, however, a concentration of resources at the acute end of care was at the expense of the other aspects of geriatric practice that had characterized a comprehensive geriatric service. This was largely a result of government policy and the need for greater consultant involvement with the increasing numbers of emergency medical admissions. It also reflected the interests of some of the physicians appointed as consultants with responsibility for geriatric services. Entering a new century, geriatric practice continues to evolve in response to changes in society and politically driven changes within the health and social services.

The patient as consumer

The rise in consumerism and desire for choice has resulted in the public having a higher expectation of all services. People are more questioning and critical of services and those who provide them. Inadequacies and inequalities in the healthcare of older people have had a major influence on current health policy.[80]

A campaign started by a Sunday newspaper led the government to commission an independent enquiry into the care of older people on acute wards in general hospitals. As a result of the findings, a National Service Framework containing standards of care for older people to be applied to the whole of the National Health Service (NHS) was to be implemented from 2001. The media and leading charities for older people have also drawn attention to age discrimination within the NHS. The identification and tackling of agism is being given high priority by the geriatrician who has been appointed the first National Director of Older People's Services in England.

Organizational change

The separation of the purchasing of healthcare from its provision has meant that the cost of healthcare has become more widely appreciated and has led to an acceptance of the need to provide value for money and therefore the need to measure and compare performance. Evidence-based practice has been boosted and quality has become a central tenet of the NHS (see also Chapter 119). A system for delivering improved quality is being implemented.[81] Standards of service are being set in so-called National Service Frameworks for the treatment of particular conditions or patient groups. A National Institute of Clinical Excellence is responsible for appraising new and existing treatments and disseminating advice on clinical and cost-effectiveness and drawing up guidelines. A system of clinical governance is being set up in hospitals and primary care whereby NHS organizations are accountable for local implementation of the national standards and continuously improving the quality of their services. A national body, the Commission for Health Improvement, is responsible for monitoring the quality of local clinical governance and clinical services.

Initially, providers, usually acute hospital trusts or community trusts, were expected to compete. This was a stimulus to service innovation but proved unpopular. Now government policy encourages cooperation.

The balance in terms of influencing resource allocation has shifted increasingly from hospital-based secondary care to the doctors and nurses in primary care. Since 1999 general practitioners (GPs) and community nurses have been part of primary care groups[81] each with a budget combining their population's share of the available resources for hospital and community health services with their general practice budget. They are being encouraged to take increasing responsibility for commissioning care and added responsibility for the provision of community services for their population. Freestanding Primary Care Trusts[81] bring primary and community health services within a single organization and are able to run community hospitals.

Health and social services are working more closely together, encouraged by changes in legislation which permit pooled budgets and resources, lead commissioning and integrated provision.[82] Eventually Primary Care Trusts may be able to merge with local social services to become Care Trusts.[80] This would mean that primary and community healthcare and social care were being commissioned and provided by a single organization. There is also greater scope for the public services to work with the private sector.[80] Joint working locally to develop services tailored to local needs is necessary, but the full implications of the latest partnership arrangements have yet to be realized.

Primary care trusts and care trusts will probably become responsible for providing most intermediate care[80] which, eventually, is likely to include geriatric services other than the acute inpatient work. The term "intermediate care" is firmly established but lacks a universally agreed definition. Most commonly it seems to encompass services that are an alternative to acute hospital admission and that expedite discharge from hospital, and includes rehabilitation. It is being promoted and funded by the government as part of its plan for investment and reform of the NHS but largely without evidence of effectiveness. This is reminiscent of the introduction of 75- and -over health checks into general practice a decade earlier when policy-making ran ahead of the evidence.[83] The challenge for geriatric practice is to ensure that geriatricians are part of the workforce to deliver intermediate care in community settings. Otherwise, rather than correcting the shortfall in rehabilitation and recuperation services for older people, providing appropriate alternatives to hospital admission and minimizing admission to long-term institutional care, intermediate care will deprive frail old people of specialist assessment and treatment.[84]

Health promotion in old age is also prominent in government policy.[80] A retirement health check is proposed. The first national campaign of vaccination against influenza for people 65 years or over was run in 2000.

Geriatric practice at the beginning of the twenty-first century

For the adequate provision of core services, the British Geriatrics Society recommends a minimum of one geriatrician for every 4,000 of the population aged 75 years or over.[85] This may, however, be insufficient given the increased time requirements for clinical governance and implementation of the National Service Framework and the current academic shortfall.

The core work is acute inpatient care, rehabilitation, and varieties of long-term care—although the nature of the workload can vary widely in content and intensity across the UK owing to variations in local supporting services, specialist activity, geographical sites to be covered, and the nature of the work. More than half of the geriatricians in England and Wales have some input to unselected acute general medical take. For some, this commitment plus the reduction in rehabilitation beds and loss of inpatient long-term care means that their geriatric work is predominantly acute inpatient care. They may also have another specialty interest.

The majority of acute hospitals in the UK have a medical admissions unit.[86] This is a ward to which patients presenting as acute medical emergencies are admitted, where immediate treatment and further assessment are instituted, and from which patients are either discharged or transferred to appropriate care within one or two days. Consultants carry out at least one round with the duty team in relation to each on-call period. Geriatricians may take their turn on the same on-call rota as the general physicians or work in parallel with responsibility for selected older patients. There are not usually enough consultants for a geriatrician and a general physician to do joint ward rounds seeing all new admissions. Systems are developed locally to ensure that old people who require acute admission and whose needs would best be met by geriatricians can be admitted directly by GPs or have immediate transfer following admission, to the care of a geriatric specialist. While the acute inpatient beds will be in the general hospital, the rehabilitation beds can be elsewhere—for example in a community hospital. In some acute hospitals geriatricians have developed liaison services to other surgical departments besides orthopedics.

The need to re-engage geriatricians in long-term care, now that it has been largely removed from hospitals, has been recognized.[87] The geriatrician can be a source of specialist opinion and advice to GPs in the management of nursing-home residents and act as educator, facilitator of good practice, and service developer. Specialist medical input is also needed to the planning, protocol development, and delivery of other aspects of community care such as acute-care schemes and rehabilitation. In the absence of evidence showing any advantage of day hospitals over alternative services,[88] resources have been diverted to expand domiciliary and outpatient therapy services and community outreach teams. The role of the day hospital has changed. It is often the setting for the interdisciplinary outpatient and domiciliary components of the specialized services for stroke and transient ischemic attack, movement disorders, and falls which geriatricians frequently lead. In addition it can be the base for the community teams that support discharge and provide a rapid response to assess and treat patients at home in order to prevent hospital admission. The day hospital can also be used for the assessment and rehabilitation of older people being considered for long-term institutional care.

GERIATRICS IN OTHER EUROPEAN COUNTRIES

The social, structural, and political systems across Europe vary considerably and this is reflected in the content and organization of geriatric services. The major differences lie between the countries of the European Union and those of eastern Europe. Their geriatric services will therefore be discussed separately.

THE EUROPEAN UNION (EU)

The proportion of the population of EU countries aged over 60 years in 1993, and the projected increase in this age group by 2020, is shown in Figure 113-6. The percentage increase varies from 9.4 in Finland to 3.9 in Sweden. Walker and Maltby[89] investigated 12 EU countries regarding personal care and healthcare. They showed that 28 percent of people aged over 60 received help or assistance with personal or household tasks, again with considerable variation from 24 percent in the UK to 47 percent in Portugal and 48 percent in Luxembourg. Consumer opinion is divided as to the method of funding personal and long-term care. Payment through taxation is favored by 60 percent in Denmark and the UK, but only by 20 percent in Germany and Luxembourg where a comprehensive public insurance system is favored.[89]

Geriatric services in EU countries

Medical care of elderly people involves many different practitioners and considerable variation in the content of the specialty of geriatric medicine is to be expected. Specialist geriatric services (acute, outpatient, day care) are universally available in Ireland, Norway, Sweden, and the UK; available in some areas in France, Denmark, Italy, Spain, Belgium, and the Netherlands; but in few or no areas in Austria, Greece, and Luxembourg.

In Portugal and Finland, long-term care is mainly in nursing homes staffed by general practitioners. The Netherlands is an interesting example, with specialists in nursing-home medicine as well as others in hospital-based geriatrics, psychogeriatrics, and social geriatrics (the last based on outpatient clinics and home visits).[90]

Undergraduate training in geriatric medicine

The development of academic departments of geriatric medicine with involvement of teaching undergraduates is shown in Table 113-1. The two countries with the largest number of medical faculties, France and Germany (73 medical faculties and only three professors of geriatric medicine), contrast with Sweden (six faculties and eight professors of geriatrics, all participating in undergraduate education) and the UK and Italy (48 medical faculties between them, 46 participating in undergraduate education in geriatrics with a total of 43 professors of geriatric medicine). These figures and Table 113-1 are derived from Stähelin et al.[91] and refer to the early 1990s. Further developments have been recorded (e.g. Denmark had three professors and Finland four in the 1998 publication of Michel et al.[92]).

A group of professors of medical gerontology established a European Academy of Medicine of Ageing to define and promote undergraduate and specialist training in geriatric

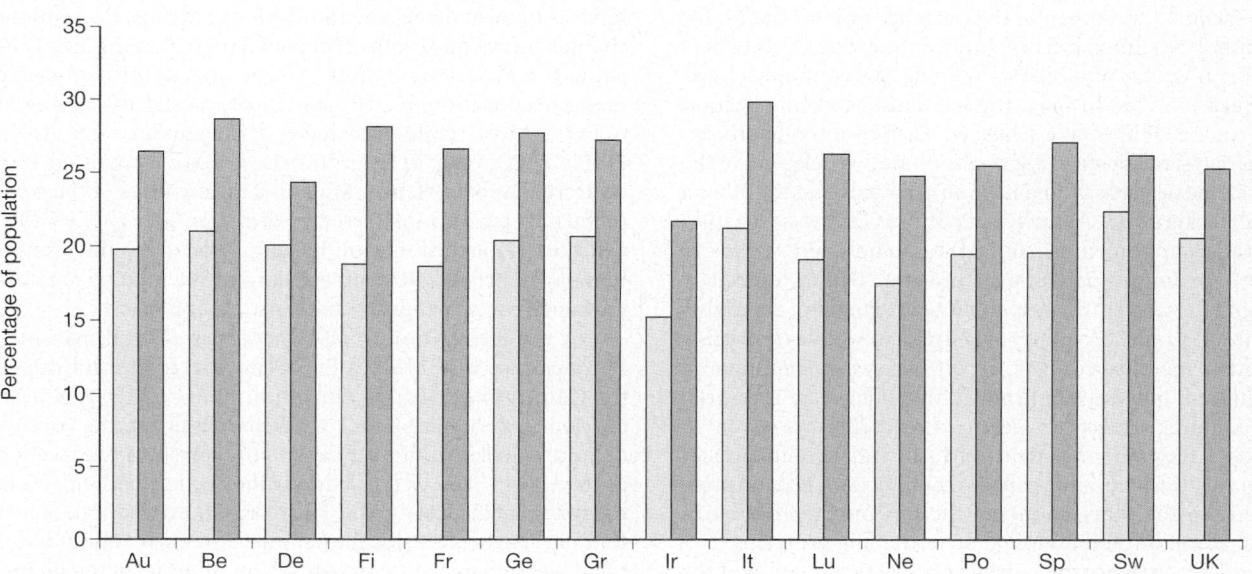

Figure 113-6 Changes in the percentage of people over 60 years of age between 1993 (plain bars) and 2020 (tinted bars) in the EU member countries. Au, Austria; Be, Belgium; De, Denmark; Fi, Finland; Fr, France; Ge, Germany; Gr, Greece; Ir, Ireland; It, Italy; Lu, Luxembourg; Ne, Netherlands; Po, Portugal; Sp, Spain; Sw, Sweden; UK, United Kingdom. From Walker and Maltby,[89] with permission.

Table 113-1 **Teaching facilities for geriatric medicine, psychogeriatrics, and gerontology at the universities in the EU member countries**

	Medical faculty	Professorial departments in:			Curriculum	
		Geriatrics	Psychogeriatrics	Gerontology	Undergraduate	Postgraduate
Austria	3	–	–	–	1	–
Belgium	11	2	–	1	5	Yes
Denmark	3	1	–	–	2	Yes
Finland	5	3	–	1	5	Yes
France	37	1	1	–	18	Yes
Germany	36	3	1	2	6	Yes
Greece	6	–	–	–	2	Yes
Ireland	2	1	–	–	1	Yes
Italy	22	22	–	22	22	Yes
Luxembourg	–	–	–	–	–	–
Netherlands	8	2	1	2	8	Yes
Portugal	5	1	–	–	1	–
Spain	23	–	–	1	1	Yes
Sweden	6	8	3	2	6	Yes
UK	26	21	4	1	24	Yes

Adapted from Stähelin et al.,[91] with permission of Oxford University Press.

medicine.[93] They set up 4-week courses for trainers (professors and senior staff members), three of which had been completed and the fourth started in 2001. The courses have received very positive evaluation.[94]

Specialist training in geriatric medicine

The recognition of geriatric medicine in the member countries made it possible to get the discipline accepted as a section of the European Union of Medical Specialists (UEMS). The UEMS was founded in 1958 and the goals are: to study, promote, and defend the free movement of specialists in the member countries; to collaborate with the Standing Committee of Doctors in Europe and with the European Union of General Practitioners; and to facilitate and organize the exchange of information for specialists.[95] Attention has been drawn towards aspects of harmonization, quality of specialists' training, and continuing medical education.[96,97] In 1997, the Geriatric Medicine Section (GMS) of the UEMS was established. Each country that recognizes geriatric medicine as a specialty sends two delegates to the section. One delegate should have an academic and the other a clinical background. An early aim of the GMS was to gather information from member countries as to how geriatric medicine was organized across the European Union, especially regarding the way in which specialists were trained. Specialists recognized in one EU country are eligible to work as specialists in another member country, so differences in training and accreditation may be significant. The results of an inventory about training aspects in geriatric medicine are given in Table 113-2. Luxembourg has no university and no training facilities. In Austria, Italy, and Spain the training is for general practitioners. In the other countries there is much variation in content, duration, and examination of training programs.

The GMS discusses the possible systematic visitation of the training institutes for geriatric medicine to enhance the quality and support harmonization. In the EU member countries the governments organize and regulate their national health care systems independently. To allow for free exchange for specialists and to guarantee the quality of services to patients, harmonization of the training programs is necessary. The GMS has developed guidelines for training in geriatric medicine in the European Union, which are accepted by the national societies.[98] However, such acceptance does not guarantee a rapid change at the national level, which requires intensive interaction with other medical specialties and the government. Financial consequences and the views of the society and of professionals in geriatric medicine are important in this discussion.

Continuing medical education in geriatric medicine

The main goal of geriatric medicine is to deliver high-quality services to meet the problems of elderly patients. Continuous changes in medical knowledge and the changing needs of patients and societies require a good system for continuing medical education (CME) and professional development (CPD). Most countries have arrangements for CME (Table 113-3). Only in five countries is CME formalized with an accreditation system. CME and CPD are parts of the goals of the European Union Geriatric Medicine Society (EUGMS) which was launched in 2001. Its main objective is the promotion of geriatric medicine in the European Union by organizing conferences, symposia, and personal contacts.

For the recognition of CME activities at local, national, European, or world level a European Accreditation Council for Continuing Medical Education (EAC-CME) has been developed. Recognition for accreditation is given after consent of the national scientific society and the corresponding section of the UEMS. The Geriatric Medicine Section participates in the system of the EAC-CME. The recognition of educational or training activities outside the national borders is a stimulus for the development and harmonization of geriatric medicine. Harmonization is necessary for the exchange of physicians; however, medical services, especially for geriatric patients, will always be adapted to national or local cultural and economic habits and possibilities.

Table 113-2 Aspects of training in geriatric medicine in the EU member countries

	Internal medicine (years)	Length of training (years)	Total training (years)	Number of trainees	Program[a]	Exam
Austria	No	_[b]	2	30–40/yr	T+C	Yes
Belgium	5	1	6	30	T+C	No
Denmark	4	2.5	6.5	36	C	No
Finland	2	3	5	25 approx	C	Yes
France	5	2	7	30–35	T+C	Yes
Germany	6	1.5	7.5	?	C	Yes
Greece	No[c]	2	2	20	T+C	No
Ireland	2	4	6	30 approx	T+C	No
Italy	No	4	4	220/yr	T+C	Yes
Netherlands	2	3	5	42	T+C	No
Spain	No	4	4	34/yr	T+C	No
Sweden	2	2	5	90 approx	T+C	No
UK	≥2	4	6	346	T+C	No

[a] T, theory; C, clinical.

[b] 8 weekends.

[c] The specialty has not been recognized in Greece, but the University of Thessaloniki organizes a course in geriatric medicine.

Adapted from Duursma.[90]

Table 113-3 Continuing medical education (CME) in the EU member countries

	CME	Type	National or local regulation	Accreditation
Austria	Yes	Formal	Medical Association of Austria	Yes
Belgium	Yes	Formal	National	Yes
Denmark	Yes	Informal	No	No
Finland	Yes	Informal	No	No
France	Yes	Informal	Regional Council	Yes
Germany	Yes	Informal	No	No
Greece	No	–	–	–
Ireland	Yes	Formal	Royal College of Physicians of Ireland	Yes
Italy	Yes	Informal	No	No
Netherlands	Yes	Formal	Dutch Society for Clinical Geriatrics	Yes
Spain	Yes	Informal	National Committee	No
Sweden	Yes	Informal	No	No
UK	Yes	Formal	Royal Colleges	Yes

Adapted from Hastie and Duursma.[90]

ICELAND, NORWAY, AND SWITZERLAND

These countries do not participate in the European Union, but their cultural, social, and medical structures are comparable to those of the EU countries, and they have a special relationship with the EU. All three recognize the specialty of geriatric medicine as part of internal medicine and participate in the activities of the GMS and the EUGMS. Iceland has one university but no chair in geriatric medicine. In Norway the four universities have three chairs,[91] and in Switzerland the five universities have six chairs—three for geriatric medicine, two for psychogeriatrics, and one for gerontology.[92,99]

EASTERN EUROPEAN COUNTRIES

Detailed information has not been published about the development of geriatric medicine in the Eastern European countries. Some data from 1991 are presented in Table 113-4. Poland, with four chairs, seems to be the best-equipped country regarding facilities for geriatric medicine. The former USSR, with

Table 113-4 Teaching facilities for geriatric medicine, psychogeriatrics, and gerontology at universities in eastern Europe. (med fac = medical faculty, psychoger = psychogeriatrics, gerontol = gerontology, undergrad = undergraduate and postgrad = postgraduate)

| | Medical faculties | Professorial departments in: | | | Curriculum | |
		Geriatrics	Psychogeriatrics	Gerontology	Undergraduate	Postgraduate
Slovakia	3	?	?	–	2	1
Hungary	4	–	–	–	2	Yes
Poland	11	4	–	1	5	3
Rumania	6	1	–	–	–	1
Ukraine	?	3	–	1	–	1

Data from Stähelin et al.[91] and Michel et al.[92]

87 universities, had only two chairs. The lack of information and the changed situation make a discussion about the development of geriatric medicine in this part of Europe uncertain.

CONCLUSION

The European Union is a well-developed part of the world with a high standard of living. Research and education have reached a high level of quality. Although differences exist between the member countries, geriatric medicine is well developed, despite many shortcomings. Over the last decade or so the EU-wide organization of geriatric medicine has been stimulated and has started promising activities for the future. It will take a high investment of energy, knowledge, and skills to build up a solid instrument to guarantee the services to meet elderly patients' needs. The professionals in the specialty in the EU also have the ethical duty to stimulate and support the development of geriatric medicine in other parts of the world, especially in the poor countries.

REFERENCES

1. Warren MW: Care of chronic sick: a case for treating chronic sick in blocks in a general hospital. BMJ 1943;ii:822–823
2. Warren MW: Care of the chronic aged sick. Lancet 1946;i:841–843
3. Ives AGL: Responsibility for the "chronic" sick: the historical perspective. Lancet 1946;ii:915–916
4. Warren MW: The role of a geriatric unit in a general hospital. Ulster Med J 1949;(May):3–12
5. Lord Amulree, Sturdee AL: Care of the chronic sick and of the aged. BMJ 1946;617–619
6. Cosin L: A statistical analysis of geriatric care. Proc R Soc Med 1948;XLI:333–336
7. Howell T: Aspects of the history of geriatric medicine. Proc R Soc Med 1976;69:445–449
8. Curran M, Hamilton J, Orr JS et al: The care of the aged: observations based on experience in Glasgow Outdoor Medical Service. Lancet 1945;i:149–152
9. Nuffield Foundation: Old People. Oxford University Press, Oxford, 1947
10. Sheldon JH: The Social Medicine of Old Age. Oxford University Press, Oxford, 1948
11. Adams GF, Cheeseman EA: Old people in Northern Ireland: A Report to the Northern Ireland Hospital Authority on Medical and Social Problems of Old Age, 1951
12. Hobson W, Pemberton JA: The Health of the Elderly at Home. Butterworth, London, 1955
13. Brown RG, McKeown T, Whitfield AGM: Observations on the medical condition of men in the seventh decade. BMJ 1958;555–562
14. Affleck JW: The chronic sick in hospital: a psychiatric approach. Lancet 1947;i:355–359
15. Thomson AP: Problems of ageing and chronic sickness. BMJ 1949;i:243–249,300–305
16. McKeown T, MacKintosh JM, Lowe CR: Influence of age on type of hospital to which patients are admitted. Lancet 1961;i:818–820
17. British Medical Association: (1) The Care and Treatment of the Elderly and Infirm (Report of a Special Committee of the British Medical Association). British Medical Association, London, 1949. (2) The Right Patient in the Right Bed (Supplement to a Report of the British Medical Association Committee on the Care and Treatment of the Elderly and Infirm). British Medical Association, London, 1947
18. Royal College of Physicians of London: A Report of the College Committee on Geriatric Medicine, London, 1972
19. British Medical Association Board of Education Science: Care of the Elderly. BMA, London, 1976
20. Exton-Smith AN, Crockett GS: The chronic sick under new management: experiences in starting a geriatric unit. Lancet 1949;i:1016–1018

KEY POINTS Geriatric medicine: history and current practice in Europe

- In the UK geriatric medicine is now a universally provided specialty in the National Health Service.

- The specialty was preceded by the gradual development of state care for old people following dissolution of the monasteries in the sixteenth century. This developed from outdoor relief to workhouses and chronic sick wards in municipal hospitals. Religious and private care was minimal.

- Early pioneers in the 1940s and 1950s realized that existing care had no basis in medical diagnosis and treatment.

- Advent of the National Health Service in 1948 allowed geriatric medicine to develop as a recognized medical specialty countrywide with a recognized academic basis.

- Developments in the 1990s with increased emphasis on acute medicine and less on long-term care have received a cautious welcome.

- Geriatric services in the European Union (EU) vary in content and training in different countries but specialist services are now established in all but three of the 15 member states.

- Within the EU there is a structure for the coordination of training and mutual recognition of specialist qualifications.

- Less information is currently available about non-EU countries in Europe, but numbers of university faculties provide undergraduate and postgraduate training in geriatric medicine.

21. Adams GF: Geriatrics in Northern Ireland. Lancet 1949;ii:1095–1097
22. Lord Amulree, Exton-Smith AN, Crockett, GS: Proper use of the hospital in treatment of the aged sick. Lancet 1951;i:123–126
23. Exton-Smith AN: Progressive patient care in geriatrics. Lancet 1962;i:260–262
24. Adams GF: The third phase in geriatric medicine: design and purpose of a hospital geriatric department. Lancet 1960;i:815–817
25. Irvine RE: Progressive patient care in the geriatric unit. Postgrad Med J 1963;39:401–407
26. Andrews K, Brocklehurst JC: Geriatric medicine: the style of practice. Age Ageing 1985;14:1–7
27. Andrews K, Brocklehurst JC: British Geriatric Medicine in the 1980s. King Edward's Hospital Fund for London. London, 1987
28. Bagnall WE, Datta SR, Knox J, Horrocks P: Geriatric medicine in Hull: a comprehensive service. BMJ 1977;ii:102–104
29. Andrews K, Brocklehurst JC: A profile of geriatric rehabilitation units. J R Coll Phys Lond 1985;19:240–243
30. Adams GF: Betwixt and between: a recovery home for the old. Lancet 1954;ii:486–488
31. Brocklehurst JC: Co-ordination of care of the elderly. Lancet 1966;i:1363–1366
32. Brocklehurst JC, Shergold M: What happens when geriatric patients leave hospital. Lancet 1968;ii:1133–1135
33. Brocklehurst JC, Shergold M: Old people leaving hospital. Gerontol Clin 1969;11:115–126
34. Victor VR, Vetter MJ: Preparing the elderly for discharge from hospital: a neglected aspect of patient care. Age Ageing 1988;17:155–163
35. Williams AEI, Fitton F: Factors affecting early unplanned re-admission of elderly patients to hospital. BMJ 1988;297:784–787
36. Townsend J, Piper M, Frank AO et al: Reduction in hospital in readmission stay of elderly patients by a community based hospital discharge scheme: a randomised control trial. BMJ 1988;297:544–547
37. British Geriatrics Society: The Discharge of Elderly Persons from Hospital for Community Care: A Compendium Document, Section 7. British Geriatrics Society, London, 1995
38. Leonard JC: Can geriatrics survive? BMJ 1976;i:1335–1336
39. O'Brien TD, Joshi DM, Warren EW: No apology for geriatrics. BMJ 1975;iv:277–280
40. Young Disabled Units: Chronically Sick and Disabled Persons Act 1970. HMSO, London, 1970
41. Kafetz K, O'Farrell J, Parry A et al: Age related geriatric medicine: relevance of special skills of geriatric medicine to elderly people admitted to hospital as medical emergencies. J R Soc Med 1995;88:629–633
42. Brocklehurst JC, Davidson C: Interface between geriatric and general medicine. Health Trends 1989;21:48–50
43. British Geriatrics Society: Acute Medical Care of Elderly People. British Geriatrics Society Compendium Document 12.2, Appendix 1. British Geriatrics Society, London, 1995
44. Grimley Evans J: Integration of geriatric with general medical services in Newcastle. Lancet 1983;i:1430–1433
45. Anonymous: Care of the old in their homes. Lancet 1949;i:462
46. Arcand M, Williamson J: An evaluation of home visiting of patients by physicians in geriatric medicine. BMJ 1981;283:718–720
47. British Geriatrics Society: Assessment Domiciliary Visits. British Geriatrics Society Compendium Document 22.1. British Geriatrics Society, London, 1995
48. Donaldson LJ, Hill PM: The domiciliary consultation service: time to take stock. BMJ 1991;302:449–451
49. Forsythe M: Domiciliary visits: we need to identify the ones worth doing. BMJ 1991;302:426–427
50. Gladman J, Barer D, Langhorne P: Specialist rehabilitation after stroke. BMJ 1996;312:1623–1624
51. Hempsall VJ, Robertson DRC, Campbell MJ, Briggs RS: Orthopaedic geriatric care: is it defective? J R Coll Phys 1990;24:47–50
52. Williamson J, Stokoe IH, Grey S et al: Old people at home: their unreported need. Lancet 1964;i:117–120
53. Anderson WF, Cowan NR: A consultative health centre for old people: the Rutherglen experiment. Lancet 1955;ii:239–240
54. Lowther CP, Macleod RDM, Williamson J: The evaluation of an early diagnostic service for the elderly. BMJ 1970;iii:275–277
55. Williams EI: A follow-up of geriatric patients: socio-medial assessments. J R Coll Gen Pract 1974;24:341–346
56. Brocklehurst JC: The Geriatric Day Hospital. King Edward's Hospital Fund, London, 1970
57. Cosin L: The place of the day hospital in the geriatric unit. Practitioner 1954:552–559
58. Droller H: A geriatric outpatient department. Lancet 1958;ii:739–741
59. Farndale J: The Day Hospital Movement in Great Britain. Pergamon Press, London, 1961
60. McComb SJ, Powell DJD: A geriatric day hospital. Gerontol Clin 1961;3:146–151
61. Fine W: Integration of a day hospital into a geriatric service. Geront Clin 1964;6:129–142
62. Brocklehurst JC: The work of a geriatric day hospital. Gerontol Clin 1964;6:151–166
63. Woodford Williams E, McKeown A, Trotter S: The day hospital in community care of the elderly. Gerontol Clin 1962;4:241–256
64. National Audit Office: National Health Service Day Hospitals for Elderly People in England. Report by Comptroller and Auditor General. HMSO, London, 1994
65. House of Commons Committee of Public Accounts: National Health Service Day Hospitals for Elderly People in England. HMSO, London, 1995
66. Kay DW, Roth M, Hall MRP: Special problems of the aged and the organisation of hospital services. BMJ 1966;ii:967–972
67. Fish F, Williamson J: A delirium unit in an acute geriatric hospital. Gerontol Clin 1964;6:71–80
68. Morton EVB, Barker ME, MacMillan D: The joint assessment and early treatment unit in psychogeriatric care. Gerontol Clin 1968;10:65–73
69. DHSS Psychogeriatric Assessment Unit: Circular HM (70) 11. HMSO, London, 1970
70. Howell T: Origins of the British Geriatrics Society. Age Ageing 1974;3:69–72
71. Adams GF: Margery Warren CBE, 1897–1960. Gerontol Clin 1961;3:1–4
72. Matthews DA: Dr Margery Warren and the origin of British geriatrics. J Am Geriatr Soc 1984;32:253–258
73. Lord Amulree: Obituary; Munks Roll, Vol VII. Royal College of Physicians, London, 1984;12–13
74. Brooke E: Obituary; Munks Roll, Vol V. Royal College of Physicians, London, 1968:52–53
75. Cosin L: Obituary. British Geriatrics Society Newsletter, London, May 1994
76. Howell JH: Obituary. British Geriatrics Society Newsletter, London, July 1988
77. Howell TH: Old Age: Some Practical Points of Geriatrics. Lewis, London, 1944
78. Wilson TS: Incontinence of urine in the aged. Lancet 1948;ii:374–377
79. Sheldon JH: Natural history of falls in old age. BMJ 1960;ii:1685–1690
80. Department of Health: The NHS Plan. Stationery Office, London, 2000
81. Department of Health: The New NHS. Stationery Office, London, 1997
82. The Health Act 1999. Stationery Office, London, 1999
83. Illiffe S, Gould M, Wallace P: Assessment of older people in the community: lessons from Britain's "75-and-over checks." Rev Clin Gerontol 1999;9:305–316
84. British Geriatrics Society: Intermediate Care: Guidance for Commissioners and Providers of Health and Social Care. Compendium Document D4. British Geriatrics Society, London, 2000
85. British Geriatrics Society: Workload of a Consultant. Compendium Document A5. British Geriatrics Society, London, 2000
86. Federation of Medical Royal Colleges: Acute Medicine: The Physician's Role. Royal College of Physicians, London, 2000
87. Royal College of Physicians, Royal College of Nursing, British Geriatrics Society: The Health and Care of Older People in Care Homes. Royal College of Physicians, London, 2000
88. Forster A, Young J, Langhorne P: Systematic review of day hospital care for elderly people. BMJ 1999;318:837–841
89. Walker A, Maltby T: Ageing Europe. Open University Press, Buckingham, 1997
90. Duursma SA: Teaching and training for geriatric medicine in the European Union. Europ J Geriatr 2002;4:59–67
91. Stähelin HB, Beregi E, Duursma SA et al: Teaching medical gerontology in Europe. Age Ageing 1994;23:179–181
92. Michel J-P, Rubinstein LZ, Vellas BJ, Albarede JL: Geriatric Programs and Departments Around the World. Serdi Publishers, Paris (and Springer), 1998
93. Verhaar HJJ, Becker C, Lindberg OIJ: European Academy for Medicine of Ageing: a new network for geriatricians in Europe. Age Ageing 1998;27:93–94

94. Michel JP, Stähelin H, Duursma SA et al: Un seignement innovant, une creation reussie: l'European Academy for Medicine of Ageing (EAMA): le point de vue des enseignemants et des etudiants. Rev Med Interne 1999; 20:531–535

95. Paul C: European Union of Medical Specialists. In: UEMS 1958–1998. Secretariat UEMS, Brussels, 1998;4–5

96. EUMS: Charter on training of medical specialists in the European Community. In: UEMS 1958–1998. Secretariat EUMS, Brussels, 1998:26–30

97. EUMS: Charter on continuing medical education of medical specialists in the European Union. In: UEMS 1958–1998. Secretariat EUMS, Brussels, 1998;31–34

98. Geriatric Medicine Section of EUMS: Training in Geriatric Medicine in the European Union. Department of Geriatric Medicine, St George's Hospital, London, 2001

99. Michel J-P, Proust J, Rapin CH, Stähelin H: The geriatrician in 1996: a viewpoint from Swizerland. Aging Clin Exp Res 1996;8:135–140

Chapter 114

Geriatrics in North America

William H. Barker

The present and future status of geriatric medicine in North America reflects national trends in demography and delivery and financing of health services, as well as academic and practice initiatives within the medical profession. This chapter reviews these several elements in the development of geriatrics in the USA and briefly considers and contrasts their counterparts in Canada.

THE UNITED STATES

TRENDS
Demography and disability trends

During the twentieth century, the US experienced a classic epidemiological and demographic transition, from a society characterized by mortality caused by short-lived acute infectious diseases and an average life expectancy of 47 years in 1900, to one characterized by mortality from protracted chronic diseases with average life expectancy of over 76 years in 2000.[1] While the increase in life expectancy during the first half of the century was almost entirely attributable to a dramatic decline in infant mortality, during the final quarter of the century an unprecedented additional increase in life expectancy occurred among persons after attaining 65 years of age. While life expectancy at age 65 increased by only 2 years (from 74 to 76 years) between 1900 and 1960, it increased by 3 more years (to 79 years) between 1960 and 1990.[2] As a consequence of this extended average life expectancy late in life, numerous studies have projected a disproportionately greater percentage growth in the population over 85 years of age in the first decades of the twenty-first century.[3]

Cross-sectional surveys conducted in the USA in the 1980s document strong correlations between increasing age, prevalence of chronic medical conditions, and need for assistance with activities of daily living. While 35 percent of men and 45 percent of women between 60 and 69 years of age report two or more chronic conditions, these figures rise to 53 and 70 percent, respectively, over the age of 80. Need for assistance increases from 9 to 10 percent between 65 and 75 years of age, to 45 percent at age 85 and above.[2] Recent studies of successive cohorts of aging persons in the USA reported lessening degrees of disability in general, and for specific conditions such as stroke among the black and nonblack population between 1982 and 1999.[4] In spite of such gratifying trends towards a healthier old age, the rapidly growing absolute numbers of very old persons portend a growing need for both acute and chronic care services.

Delivery systems trends

The evolution of financing and organization of acute and chronic care for older persons in the USA in the twentieth century has created dilemmas as well as opportunities for geriatric medicine. At the outset of the century, voluntary community hospitals, once equally open to young victims of accidents or infections and to aged persons with incurable and disabling chronic problems, began systematically to exclude the latter, leaving them to seek care in public almshouses or room and board homes. Despite compelling arguments in the pages of the forerunner of the *New England Journal of Medicine* and from the founder of Johns Hopkins Hospital, among others, exclusion of chronic care of older persons from the modern American hospital, and effectively from the study and practice of modern medicine, was a *fait accompli* in the USA by early in the century. Hardships of the Great Depression in the 1930s led to two important developments that further promoted the pattern of separate acute and chronic care sectors. First was the introduction of the Blue Cross and Blue Shield programs of voluntary private health insurance, whereby subscribers protected themselves against costs of acute hospitalization and physician services. This ushered in the now widely prevalent convention of private health insurance to pay for discrete episodes of hospital and physician care, but explicitly excluding coverage for continuing chronic care in the community or in institutions. Fueled by health insurance financing along with the rapid growth of medical science following World War II, the modern acute care hospital and hospital-oriented subspecialty medicine came to dominate healthcare in the USA.[5]

The second watershed event was the 1935 passage of the Social Security Act, which established a federally mandated payroll deduction to assure financial security in old age. Given the absence of dedicated funding or services for care of chronically ill older persons, the newly available pensions created a source of funds for privately operated rest homes. Thus was born the American private nursing home industry, which has flourished in parallel, but separately from, the acute care hospital industry.

The distinctly separate financing and development of the hospital and nursing home sectors, begun in the 1930s, was brought to fruition with passage of the landmark Medicare and Medicaid legislation in 1965. In this unprecedented legislation, the federal government expanded the Social Security payroll deduction to include a mandatory contribution to a trust fund (Medicare) to provide universal hospital insurance for retirees. Medicare includes limited coverage for posthospital, short-term skilled home care or nursing-home care. This "comprehensive health insurance" for the aged and disabled excludes coverage for chronic or long-term care, explicitly referred to as "custodial care." Enter Medicaid—this companion legislation is intended to provide comprehensive health insurance for the "medically indigent," primarily poor women and children; however, the program also covers the cost of custodial nursing-home care, a benefit largely used by elderly persons who divest themselves of their capital ("spend down") in order to qualify.

From comparatively modest beginnings, these two major financing programs have grown astronomically—Medicare from some 19 million beneficiaries and $4–5 billion expenditure in 1966 to 39 million beneficiaries and over $200 billion in 2000; and Medicaid from a "means-tested" recipient population of 18 million and annual expenditure of $12 billion in the early 1970s, to 36 million recipients and over $100 billion in the early 1990s. The pie charts in Figure 114-1 show proportionately how the Medicare and Medicaid dollars are spent among hospital, nursing-home, home health, physician, and other services. While Medicare dollars go primarily to hospital and physician services that meet the strict criterion of "medically indicated," the greatest single proportion of Medicaid dollars go to pay for chronic care for older persons in nursing facilities.[6] Conspicuously absent from Medicare is any coverage for prescription drugs, an increasingly large financial burden for older patients and the focus of much political attention in 2000–2001.

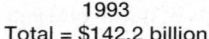
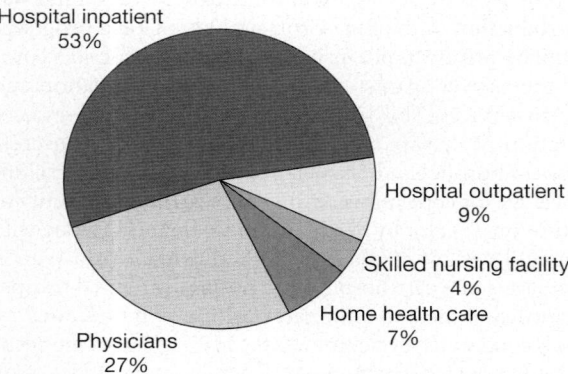

1993
Total = $142.2 billion

Hospital inpatient
53%

Hospital outpatient
9%

Skilled nursing facility
4%

Home health care
7%

Physicians
27%

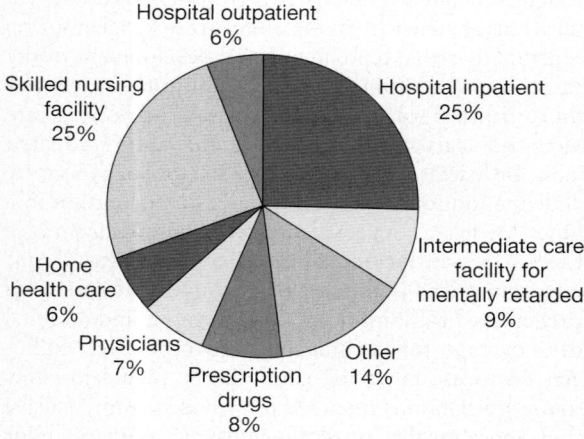

1993
Total = $101.7 billion

Hospital outpatient
6%

Skilled nursing facility
25%

Hospital inpatient
25%

Home health care
6%

Intermediate care facility for mentally retarded
9%

Physicians
7%

Prescription drugs
8%

Other
14%

Figure 114-1 Distribution of Medicare (top) and Medicaid (bottom) dollars (Health Care Financing Administration).

While both Medicare and Medicaid laws have been amended many times since inception, sometimes expanding coverage, often serving to constrain costs, the most profound changes respecting services for older Americans and their providers is embodied in the 1997 Balanced Budget Act.[7] In brief, this legislation on the one hand expands Medicare coverage for preventive screening tests and provides several novel ways for physicians and hospitals to form partnerships to care for older patients; on the other hand it substantially reduces Medicare payments for postacute home care and nursing-home care, two mainstays of geriatric services.

ACADEMIC EVOLUTION OF GERIATRIC MEDICINE

Study of the aging process and the characteristics and care for disease in old age have been of some identified interest to medical practitioners and investigators in the USA since the beginning of the twentieth century, long before the demographic transition to an "aging society." The seminal figure in this regard is Ignatz Leo Nascher (Fig. 114-2), a generalist physician, who devoted his career to studying, practicing, and promoting the medicine of old age—a field of work for which he first coined the now universal term, "geriatrics." Nascher vividly recalls an event that first kindled his lifelong interest during his medical school days in New York City in 1883.[8]

> A section of the class was taken to the Almshouse by one of the instructors. An old woman hobbled up to him with some complaint. The instructor said she was suffering from old age. "And what could be done for it?" "Nothing." Was old age, then, a painful, incurable disease from which those who reached advanced age must suffer and for which nothing could be done?

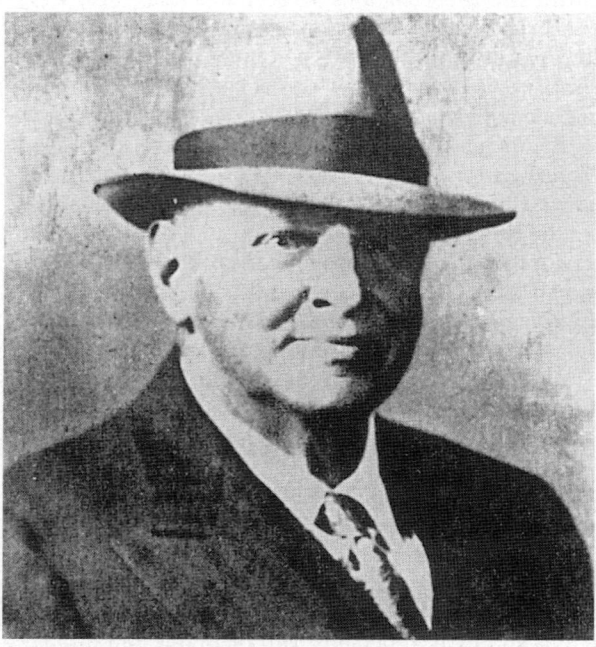

Figure 114-2 Ignatz Leo Nascher, MD (1863–1944).

Nascher thought otherwise, and devoted his career to refuting this conventional wisdom of the times. A prolific writer in professional and lay publications and author of a comprehensive text, *Geriatrics: The Diseases of Old Age and Their Treatment* (1914), he was convinced, partly through close collegial association with Dr Abraham Jacobi, founder of the specialty of pediatrics, that geriatrics would become a thriving speciality. "There are hopeful signs that such interest is spreading, that the cardinal principles of Geriatrics are becoming recognized, and that Geriatrics will soon be taught and practiced as one of the major specialties of medicine."[8] Nascher's "prophetic words" fell on deaf ears and little formal attention to geriatrics as a specialty was heard for decades to follow.

In spite of the failure of geriatrics to receive the formal recognition forecast by Nascher, the challenges to study and treat medical problems of aging, which he articulated so well, received growing organized attention in other important ways. Beginning in the 1930s, the Josiah Macey Jr Foundation sponsored a series of annual gerontology research conferences, each resulting in published proceedings, beginning with *The Problems of Aging* (1939), edited by the distinguished biologist, E. V. Cowdry. An outgrowth of the Macey Foundation's interest was establishment of the US Public Health Service Gerontology Research Center that has flourished to this day and has produced a formidable body of research on normal aging processes.[9] The 1940s saw the founding of the American Geriatrics Society (AGS) and the Gerontological Society of America (GSA), the former primarily representing practicing physicians, the latter primarily representing academicians from a number of disciplines concerned with biological, social, psychological, economic, and other dimensions of aging. At the public policy level, a series of White House Conferences on Aging, beginning in 1950, attended by scientists, consumers and policy-makers, have crystallized and advanced major national initiatives to address medical and related problems of old age. The 1961 conference was instrumental in promoting the subsequent 1965 enactment of the Medicare legislation, as well as the parallel Older Americans Act to support development of community social services.

The American Geriatrics Society

The AGS was founded in 1942, through the spirited leadership of Dr Malford Thewlis, a kindred spirit and longtime associate of Nascher. From its original 30 physician members, the Society has burgeoned to a membership of some 6,000.[10]

At its 1952 meeting, the members voted to establish a peer-reviewed journal, and in January 1953, the *Journal of the American Geriatrics Society* was launched. In an inaugural essay, "Aging Comes of Age—The Modern Concept of Geriatrics," journal editor Dr Willard Thompson laid out the broad philosophy that characterizes this field of medical work:[11]

> Geriatrics presents a great variety of problems and must be looked upon from the broadest possible point of view. The care of older people concerns physicians in practically every special field of medicine as well as the general practitioner who probably sees more older people than the specialist. ... Studies of the causes of aging and attempts to improve the medical care of older people must be correlated with developments in all other fields which contribute to the welfare of the aging population.

After Thompson's untimely death in 1954, Dr Edward Henderson assumed editorship for the next 18 years, during which he also served as executive director of the AGS. The society's highest lectureship award is named for Dr Henderson.

The AGS has taken active positions on national public policy since the early 1960s, when, ironically, along with most of organized medicine, it testified against the forerunner to the Medicare legislation, being wary of the effect of a government health insurance program on the practice of medicine. Issues of note on which the AGS has subsequently developed more progressive positions and testified before the US Congress include nursing-home standards and the concept of medical directors for nursing homes; patient and family rights to make decisions regarding life-sustaining interventions at the end of life; appropriate Medicare reimbursement for geriatric assessment, house calls, and nursing-home visits; and financing for a continuum of long-term care services as part of national healthcare reform. Medical education has been a principal concern of the AGS since its origin when one of two standing committees was established to aid medical societies in arranging geriatrics programs for practicing physicians. This focus has recently seen development of the "Geriatrics Review Syllabus," a self-administered core curriculum for physicians in training and in practice, coordination of a program sponsored by the Hartford Foundation to promote integration of geriatrics into surgical and medical specialties, and development and distribution to medical students of a handbook, *Geriatrics at Your Fingertips*, again funded by Hartford. Information on AGS policies, projects, products, affiliates, etc. may be accessed at its website, www.americangeriatrics.org.

Two AGS affiliated organizations, the Association of Directors of Academic Geriatric Programs (ADGAP) and the American Medical Directors Association (AMDA), serve respectively, to advance the interests of geriatric training and research and geriatric leaders in long-term care administration.

The National Institute on Aging

The principal legacy of the 1971 White House Conference on Aging was the 1974 founding of the National Institute on Aging (NIA) as a component of the National Institutes of Health. The leadership at the NIA during its first decades reflects several distinctive perspectives on solving medical problems of old age. The founding director, Dr Robert Butler (1974 to 1982), a psychiatrist, brought to the agency a broad background of teaching, research, and practice, with an emphasis on mental health. His Pulitzer prize-winning book, *Why Survive? Being Old in America*, published in 1975, brought to a wide professional and lay audience recognition of social and attitudinal ("agism") challenges as well as unmet chronic care needs. Following his tenure at the NIA, he joined the Mt Sinai Medical Center to be chairman of the first free-standing medical school geriatrics department in the USA. The institute's second director (1983 to 1991) was Dr T. Franklin Williams, an internist with a strong background in chronic metabolic diseases. Prior to his appointment, he served as medical director of a 600-bed former county poor farm in Rochester, New York, which was transformed under his leadership into a nationally renowned university affiliated center (Monroe Community Hospital) for treatment, teaching, and research related to chronic disease and disability of old age.[12] From this legacy he remains a tireless advocate for bringing geriatric assessment and rehabilitation to the mainstream of American medical education and practice. The third director of the NIA (1994 to the present), Dr Richard Hodes, comes from a background in molecular biology research at the National Cancer Institute, and signals increasing focus on basic science as related to aging, while retaining the institute's existing broad agenda of research.

In its first three decades, with an annual budget growing to almost $800 million, the NIA has sponsored research on a number of long-neglected specific health problems associated with aging as well as investigating fundamental biomedical, sociobehavioral, epidemiological, and health services problems. Exemplary large, multisite projects sponsored or cosponsored by the agency include:

- Established Populations for Epidemiologic Studies of the Elderly (EPESE): a longitudinal observational study of the natural history of many age-related problems, conducted in four different geographic sites and involving a combined cohort of some 10,000 subjects;
- The Teaching Nursing Home: a program devised to bridge the gap between acute medical and long-term care sectors by attracting medical school faculty and students to nursing homes for purposes of education, research, and practice;[13]
- Frailty and Injuries: Cooperative Studies of Intervention Techniques (FICSIT): a series of randomized clinical trials of various interventions to reduce musculoskeletal frailty and related injuries in later life, conducted at eight different sites;[14]
- Systolic Hypertension in the Elderly Program (SHEP): a randomized clinical trial of effectiveness of treating isolated systolic hypertension, conducted in collaboration with the National Heart, Lung, and Blood Institute, and involving some 4,800 subjects;[15]
- Claude Pepper Older American Independence Centers: named for a tireless congressional advocate in behalf of older people and based at a number of universities for the purpose of bringing together multidisciplinary research, training, and information dissemination on a variety of preventable or reversible causes of dependency;
- Alzheimer's Disease Centers: Based at 28 major medical institutions with the broad objective of conducting basic research on etiology, improving diagnosis and classification, evaluating clinical interventions, and disseminating information on Alzheimer's disease and related disorders;
- Nathan Schock Centers for basic biomedical science applied to aging;
- Study of Women's Health Across the Nation (SWAN). For further information: www.nia.n.ih.gov

Education and training

In spite of longstanding recognition that the health problems of old age are important, both for research and as a focus of national academic societies and journals, fully a decade following passage of the Medicare legislation there was a remarkable dearth of physician practice or educational commitment to the field. The American Medical Association (AMA) physician master file for 1977 revealed that only 0.2 percent of physicians listed geriatrics as a principal area of practice.[16] Surveys of medical students and practicing physicians in the 1970s revealed little formal training and a generally negative attitude toward care of elderly people. The failure of the field to develop as a medical specialty, analogous to pediatrics, is attributed to a lack of certain critical historic elements. The field clearly did not fit neatly into either of the two dominant trends in medical career development of the post-World War II era: biomedical subspecialities, dominant from 1945 to 1970; and primary care specialities from 1955 to 1980.

Facing this climate of medical noninvolvement, the USA has witnessed a spate of initiatives to redress the gap in medical education and training in geriatrics. Foremost among these has been a series of three major reports issued by the National Academy of Science's Institute of Medicine (IOM), which advises the federal government on health policy matters. The first report (1978) under the leadership of Dr Paul Beeson, a pre-eminent American professor of medicine and former Regius Professor of Medicine at Oxford, recommended that geriatrics be recognized as an academic discipline with a strong curricular presence in all medical schools. This would be accomplished by encouraging faculty to develop new courses or integrate pertinent material into existing courses. A variety of such undertakings ensued in response to state and federal grant support; however, relatively little substantial commitment to geriatrics was evident 5 years later. Re-evaluating the situation in 1985, Dr Beeson indicated his disappointment with "the half-way measures that we recommended" and cited certain more fundamental requirements for the success of geriatrics as a medical discipline. These included a tentative endorsement of the development of independent academic departments of geriatric medicine. Such departments would have their own faculty and required curriculum. He further pointed out the essential need for "a change in our system of health care payments whereby cognitive work and time spent in the care of people with chronic multiple disabilities is rewarded in a manner comparable to the rewards that come from carrying out procedures."[17]

The second IOM report (1987) recognized modest but clearly insufficient development of formal geriatrics undergraduate and postgraduate education. About 75 percent of medical schools reported offering elective courses, but fewer than 4 percent of students had enrolled. Only 40 percent of medical residencies offered geriatrics rotations and few residents took them. More than 60 small 1- or 2-year geriatrics fellowship programs had developed, but over 25 percent of the approximately 200 positions were unfilled. A fundamental problem in attracting candidates to the field was the absence of a well-defined career ladder, something which by contrast was noted to be well-developed in Great Britain. Two critical steps toward defining career standards were recognized and applauded by the report. The first was a set of Guidelines for Fellowship Training Programs in Geriatric Medicine, developed and published in 1987 by the AGS.[18] The second was the joint development by the American Boards of Internal Medicine (ABIM) and Family Practice (ABFP) of an examination to award a Certificate of Added Qualifications (CAQ) in geriatric medicine. Candidates qualified for the exam based on several educational and practice pathways indicative of expertise and commitment to care of elderly people. Of 4,282 candidates who sat the first exam in 1988, 2,398 (56 percent) passed and were awarded the CAQ.

With the forward-looking mission of defining and meeting needs for "Academic Geriatrics for the Year 2000," the 1987 IOM report focused upon current versus projected numbers of faculty. Compared to a projected need for up to 1,600 faculty members in geriatric medicine and 450 in geriatric psychiatry, as well as a complement of dedicated PhD investigators, by the end of the century, it was noted that only 250 to 300 of all medical school faculty members in the mid-1980s devoted substantial time to teaching aspects of geriatrics. To close this gap, the report emphasized the development of academic "centers of excellence" in geriatrics, analogous to cancer centers, which had greatly strengthened academic career development in the field of oncology. Each "center of excellence" would meet three central goals: (1) develop a geriatrics training program fulfilling the 1987 guidelines; (2) conduct a strong body of research and research training; and (3) provide clinical care in a variety of community and institutional settings. Existing Geriatric Research, Education and Clinical Centers (GRECCs) based at academically affiliated Veteran's Administration Hospitals were cited as models. It was recommended that funding for the proposed future "centers of excellence" come from a variety of sources, including the NIA, the National Institute for Mental Health, and other government agencies and private foundations.[19]

The third IOM report, published in 1994, took stock of the progress to date and focused on future potentials as well as obstacles.[20] A background document, drawing on extensive survey research conducted at UCLA and the RAND Corporation in the late 1980s and early 1990s, addressed the persisting modest progress in development of careers and education in geriatrics in the USA. As of 1992, 6,775 physicians from internal medicine, family medicine, and psychiatry, most of whom had not taken geriatric fellowships, had received certification in geriatrics. By 1993, there were 101 accredited geriatric medicine fellowship training programs with over 300 positions offered annually, but with fewer than 70 percent of positions filled. A high percentage of fellowship graduates were satisfied with their decision to pursue a career in geriatrics. A survey of residency programs found that 80 percent of family medicine programs, but only 36 percent of internal medicine programs required curriculum in geriatric medicine. Among 126 medical schools as of 1993, 14 taught geriatrics as a separate required course, while 102 taught geriatrics in the context of other required courses; only 2.9 percent of graduating students had taken an elective in geriatrics—essentially no change from 1987. With the exception of steady growth in the number and academic productivity of GRECCs in the VA system (a total of 16 sites with 284 completed traineeships and 617 total publications as of 1993), the development of centers of academic excellence was limited.

To explain the lack of greater progress, the 1993 IOM report noted the variable enthusiasm with which traditional leaders of academic medicine acknowledged the importance of geriatrics; the difficulty in finding stable funding to support both fellowships and centers of academic excellence; and, most fundamentally, the inadequate reimbursement provided by Medicare and other health insurers for the time-consuming, largely cognitive rather than procedure-governed work of those who would pursue a career in clinical geriatrics.

In an effort to awaken the academic establishment, the Association of Professors of Medicine convened a well-attended conference in 1993 on geriatrics curriculum. The conference was chaired by Dr William Hazerd, president of the AGS and chairman of internal medicine at the Bowman Gray School of Medicine. Among highlights were presentations on the extensive geriatric training programs of the VA and innovative mid-career geriatrics training programs for internists as well as for physicians in other specialities (e.g. gynecology, urology, orthopedics) sponsored by the John A. Hartford Foundation. Of particular interest was the strong recommendation that geriatrics as practiced in the USA should not be considered a subspecialty, but was rather more akin to primary care, a "supraspecialty" with added qualifications.[21] Bolstering this point of view was a survey of physicians who had taken the 1988 CAQ exam, which found that on average approximately 70 percent of their work represented primary care.[22] Others have made a persuasive argument, drawing comparisons to cardiology, rheumatology, and others, that the work pattern of the geriatrician more nearly fits that of a consulting subspecialty.[23] Depending on their work setting, geriatricians in the USA will de facto serve in some instances more like primary care practitioners, in other instances more like subspecialists.

National attention was most recently drawn to the serious shortage of physicians with geriatric training by a widely publicized report from the Alliance for Aging Research submitted to the US Senate Committee on Aging in May 1996.[24] Towards responding to this dilemma, a number of new national training and education initiatives were introduced in the late 1990s. Foremost was the joint decision by the governing boards of the AGS and the ABIM and ABFP to reduce eligibility requirements for the CAQ in Geriatric Medicine to one year of formal fellowship training in clinical geriatrics, while maintaining an additional two or more years of training for geriatric leadership careers in education, research, or administration.[25] A survey of physicians completing training between 1990 and 1998 documented increasing numbers of candidates completing fellowships of both 1 year and 2 or more years, with the latter generally pursuing academic careers.[26] Respecting medical education, two major programs funded between 1999 and 2001 by the Hartford Foundation (in collaboration with the American Association of Medical Colleges) and the Reynolds Foundation made awards to approximately half of the medical schools in the country to strengthen the integration of geriatric medicine across all 4 years of the undergraduate curriculum.

PRACTICE EVOLUTION OF GERIATRIC MEDICINE

By the mid-twentieth century as some members of the medical profession were becoming energized in Nascher's spirit, other professional and institutional associations were recognizing the implications of the trends in aging and chronic illness for organization and staffing of health services. In a joint report issued in 1947, addressed to the "general public as well as legislators and members of the health and welfare professions," the AMA, the American Hospital Association (AHA), the American Public Health Association (APHA), and the American Public Welfare Association made the following sweeping recommendations:[27]

- Care of the chronically ill should be inseparable from general medical care.
- Major emphasis should be placed on home and office care, with hospital care, convalescent care, and rehabilitation serving where possible to return the chronically ill to productive community life, and with nursing-home facilities providing for those whose medical condition is such that they cannot remain in their home environment.
- Major emphasis must be given to coordination and integration of services. Because the medical condition of the chronically ill person is not static, but changes with time, it is essential to develop smoothly operating mechanisms for referral from one type of care to another.

When Medicare was legislated in 1965, as pointed out earlier, insurance coverage was restricted to physician, hospital, and post-hospital services for discrete illness episodes, explicitly excluding chronic care. The long-term care sector accordingly grew up separately from mainstream health service financing and delivery. By the 1980s, in the absence of a system for managing both acute and chronic care interchangeably—to wit, "smoothly operating mechanisms for referral from one type of care to another"—a variety of inappropriate service utilization patterns emerged. Particularly conspicuous and costly among these were growing numbers of frail older patients "blocking beds" in acute care hospitals where restorative and health maintenance needs were neglected; and frequent disruptive transfers of nursing-home residents to hospitals because of the failure to provide timely onsite care for acute medical problems. Recognizing the dilemmas caused by the lack of integrated services for chronically ill aged persons, many groups called for national health policy reform to address the situation. Exemplary of such efforts was a position paper on "Long-term care of the elderly" issued by the American College of Physicians, which stated:[28]

> At present, there is not a comprehensive system of long-term care for the elderly in the United States. A confusing, fragmented, and expensive system exists that contains both gaps and duplication of services. ... Reimbursement procedures, both public and private, tacitly recognize the existence of two separate systems of health care: one for acute care and another for long-term care. ... A full array of services should be available through an integrated long-term care system. Such a continuum of care would better ensure that the elderly obtain appropriate services. The reimbursement system should foster, not impede, networking among hospitals and nursing homes.

In spite of a number of major healthcare reform proposals and legislative efforts in the late 1980s and early 1990s, most recently the thwarted effort of the Clinton Administration in 1994, national healthcare policy incorporating long-term care has not evolved and looks unlikely at the onset of the twenty-first century. Nonetheless, through public and privately funded demonstration projects, a variety of innovative healthcare strategies for meeting needs of frail older people have flourished during this time period. A selective review of such

projects across the spectrum of care sites reveals the unmistakable strong presence of principles of geriatric medicine and leadership by trained geriatric clinicians and academicians.

Hospitals

Largely emulating experiences pioneered in geriatric units in Great Britain, inpatient geriatric assessment services have been introduced in general hospitals in the USA in several distinctly different ways, as shown in Figure 114-3. These include, as labeled: geriatric consultation services (C), geriatric rehabilitation transfer units (T), and acute geriatric admission units (A).

Geriatric consultation services, being least obtrusive and demanding of hospital resources, represent the earliest and most widely implemented hospital-based geriatric strategy. Early observational studies of consultation services reported extensive findings of unaddressed problems among older patients, but only limited evidence of significant impact on patient functional status, length of stay, or level of care at discharge. Two later randomized trials failed to find measurable differences between patients receiving geriatric consultation and controls.[29,30] In thoughtful commentary, Winograd and colleagues,[29] as well as others, have drawn the general conclusion that such consultation services have little measurable impact because of lack of control over clinical management and resources for implementing their recommendations and indifferent attitudes of non-geriatric-trained hospital staff towards geriatric practices and patients.

Transfer units have been established and studied in a variety of hospital settings, including VA hospitals, academic medical centers, chronic disease hospitals, and rural community hospitals. The flagship example of this concept was the rigorously evaluated geriatric evaluation unit (GEU) developed at the Sepulveda VA Medical Center in Los Angeles. In a randomized clinical trial, Rubenstein and colleagues[31] reported that GEU patients, when compared with controls over a 1-year

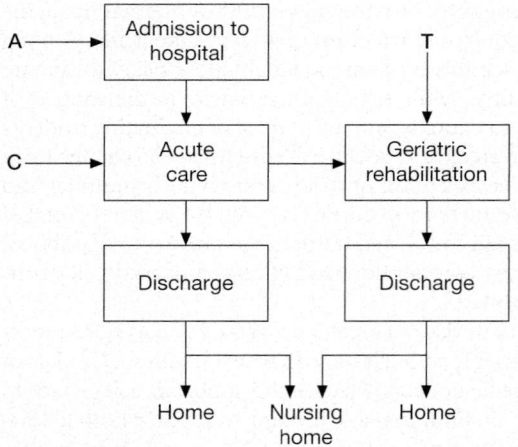

Figure 114-3 Potential intervention by special geriatric services in the course of acute hospital admission in the United States. A, admit to acute geriatric service; C, geriatric consultation on acute medical and surgical services; T, postacute transfer to special geriatric rehabilitation unit. From Barker.[5]

follow-up, experienced significantly lower mortality, reduced likelihood of nursing-home admission, fewer overall acute hospital or nursing-home days, greater improvement in functional status and morale, and lower average cost of care. A randomized trial of a unit developed and evaluated by Applegate and colleagues[32] in a large general hospital complex reported very similar findings.

Acute geriatric admission units have been introduced in relatively few US hospitals. One exemplary exception is the Acute Care for the Elderly (ACE) unit developed and carefully evaluated by Landefield and colleagues[33] at the Case Western Reserve Medical Center in Cleveland, Ohio, in the early 1990s. Designed to avoid the cascade of "hazards of hospitalization" for older patients,[34] the ACE unit incorporates a set of explicit geriatric care principles into routine acute care from the time of admission to hospital. These include environmental modification for safety and convenience; patient-centered care protocols dealing with potential problems with continence, mobility, skin integrity, mental health, etc.; and daily rounds by a multidisciplinary team led by medical and nursing directors. A randomized trial involving 651 patients showed significantly better functional status at discharge and lower rate of posthospital nursing home placement for the ACE unit patients, with comparable 7- to 8-day lengths of stay and hospital billing for intervention and control groups. Applying ACE unit principles in randomized trials to prevent delirium and its serious consequences in acute-care general medical patients and in post-hip fracture patients, Inouye and colleagues[35] and Marcantonio and colleagues,[36] respectively, both showed a more than 33 percent decrease in occurrence or severity of delirium and its costly consequences.

In recent years several well-planned programs of nurse-based geriatric interventions to improve outcomes of older patients hospitalized with congestive heart failure[37] and other high-risk conditions[38] have been shown to significantly reduce health decline and hospital readmission rate in the 3–6 months after discharge. Also emulating strategies developed in Great Britain, Australia, and Israel, the Geriatrics Center at Johns Hospital is exploring a "home hospital" alternative to hospitalization of acutely ill frail older patients.[39]

From their collective experience, hospital-based geriatric evaluation and management services (GEMs as they have come to be called) and related strategies, implemented in US general hospitals as inpatient and as outpatient modalities, appear to be both effective and efficient in influencing patient health status and health service utilization, particularly when they incorporate continuing care services.[40] However, the presence of such services is the exception rather than the rule in the vast majority of academic and community hospitals in the country.

Nursing homes

From the perspective of comprehensive medical services, perhaps the most costly and challenging problem among the 14,000 nursing homes in the USA is the high rate of transfer of acutely ill, frail residents to short-term hospitals in lieu of managing their medical problems onsite. Multiple national and regional surveys have documented rates of 20–30 such hospitalizations per 100 nursing-home beds per year, extrapolating to some 300 to 400 thousand in the country annually.[41]

A number of practical care strategies have been shown to significantly reduce hospital transfer from nursing homes.[42] The introduction of geriatric nurse practitioners to deal with intercurrent acute medical problems, as well as ongoing health promotion, has been most widely studied and consistently shown to reduce hospital use by nursing home residents.[43] This effect is attributable to both earlier identification and management of potentially serious illness (e.g. urinary tract infections, poor control of diabetes) and to the clinical management of frankly serious illness onsite (e.g. pneumonia, congestive heart failure). A second strategy that has received limited formal evaluation consists of providing financial incentives to physicians, nursing homes, and ancillary services (e.g. laboratory, radiology) to care for serious acute illness episodes within the facility. A further dimension of geriatric care that has the potential to reduce hospitalization of nursing-home residents is the growing use of advance directives to express patient or family preferences for receiving or withholding life-saving medical interventions, including hospitalizations. This ethical–legal strategy has been embodied in a variety of formal modalities, including "do not resuscitate" (DNR) orders, living wills, and healthcare proxies.[44,45]

Towards assuring quality care within nursing homes, ongoing monitoring with a uniform Resident Assessment Instrument was introduced in all US nursing homes in 1991 as a condition of participation in the Medicare and Medicaid programs. Details of this geriatric assessment and management strategy and its broadly positive effects in nursing homes are reported in the August 1997 issue of the *Journal of the American Geriatrics Society*.

Home and community

In the USA as elsewhere, more than 95 percent of persons over age 65, including most of those with chronic diseases and disabilities, live in the community. How best to anticipate and limit the impact of new intercurrent illness, prevent functional decline, and avoid admission to hospital and nursing homes among community-dwelling older persons has been the focus of extensive public policy experimentation in the past two decades and of targeted clinical geriatric strategies more recently.[46]

During the 1980s, more than two dozen largely government sponsored controlled studies of community-based long-term care (CBLTC) demonstrations, emphasizing home care and day care social support modalities, were conducted. In a careful synthesis of results it was found, with rare exception, that there was no improvement in functional status or survival, nor cost savings among those receiving the interventions. Among major concerns noted was the failure to include a strong clinical geriatric medicine component to complement the social component of these projects.[47]

While national policy for CBLTC or "home care" remains a quandary, there has been very active expansion of provision of "home healthcare" alternatives to hospital care, largely under sponsorship of the Medicare program. The focus has been to avoid or shorten hospitalizations by providing high-tech and acute and subacute care services in the home (e.g. parenteral nutrition and antibiotics, respirators, etc.).[48]

Often missing from both the chronic social support "home care" and acute hospital alternative "home healthcare" models are modalities to meet the ongoing medical and medically related needs of vulnerable community-dwelling older persons. Strategies, remarkably similar to ones long practiced in Great Britain, have recently been introduced in the USA. First, is provision of in-home geriatric assessment and follow-up by a geriatric nurse practitioner–geriatrician team. In a recently completed 3-year randomized trial,[49] those receiving this intervention experienced significantly less functional decline and permanent placement in nursing homes. In a variation on this strategy, a multisite demonstration supported by the Hartford Foundation has implemented practice models in which the ongoing care of frail older patients is shared by primary care physicians and geriatric nurse practitioners (GNPs). In this strategy, the patients are regularly seen at office visits by the physician and the GNP in tandem, while the GNP provides continuing care liaison. Geriatric nurse practitioner continuing care includes home visiting and telephone consultation with the objective of early detection and management of changes in mental or physical health as well as counsel on preventive health behaviors, etc. The current phase of this project focuses on developing techniques for training future physicians, nurses, and social workers to work effectively in such collaborative models (Donna Regenstreif, personal communication).

Managed care organizations

While, as evidenced above, there has been exciting progress with geriatric strategies at all levels of healthcare delivery, nonetheless, these specially funded "demonstrations" are the exception, not the rule, and will remain so as long as financing of healthcare is fragmented and fails to foster incorporation of such geriatric practices. Interestingly, as aspirations for comprehensive national healthcare reform have seriously waned since 1994, the dramatic surge of managed care organizations (MCOs) is providing, if not compelling, opportunities for the practice of geriatric medicine to flourish.[50] The role of managed care organizations in care of older persons

was the theme for special full-day workshops at the annual scientific meetings of both the AGS and the GSA in 1996 and 1997. The essence of MCOs is linking together a network of physician, hospital, home-care, nursing-home, and other service modalities to provide a defined scope of services for an enrolled population within a fixed budget, with considerable flexibility regarding the mix of service settings and personnel provided to meet the members' medical and related needs.

From the perspective of comprehensive services for older persons, three distinctly different variations on the MCO paradigm are briefly considered below: the Medicare Health Maintenance Organization (HMO), which provides a full complement of standard Medicare-coverable services as well as limited additional benefits, including vision and hearing services and prescription drugs; the Social Health Maintenance Organization (SHMO) and the On Lok/Program of All-Inclusive Care for the Elderly (PACE), both of which include chronic care services which are explicitly excluded from the standard Medicare program.

Medicare health maintenance organization

As a potential cost-saving policy, the Medicare program was amended in the 1980s to encourage HMOs to enroll large populations of Medicare beneficiaries and provide their full range of benefits under capitated payment, representing approximately 95 percent of the average fee-for-service cost per member. By 1999 some 15 percent of Medicare's beneficiaries were enrolled in HMOs. Surveys in the early 1990s found that over one-half of the Medicare HMOs employed geriatricians and were supporting some form of organized geriatric practices. Practices given priority in a sample of plans include geriatric assessment and targeted case management for high-risk patients, subacute geriatric rehabilitation services, and utilization of geriatric nurse practitioners.[51]

An exemplary Medicare HMO, the Health Partners Plan, located in the city of Minneapolis and caring for some 24,000 elderly persons (a subset of an all-ages HMO enrollment of 265,000) is illustrated in Figure 114-4. Those members of the older population who are identified as "frail" based on

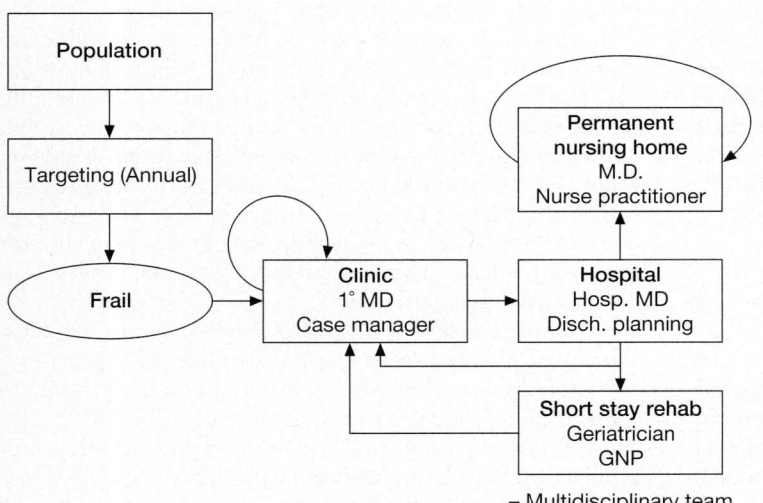

Figure 114-4 Network of services for Medicare patients enrolled in Health Partners health maintenance organization. Courtesy Thomas von Sternberg, MD.

– Multidisciplinary team

medical/functional/social assessment, are tracked by trained geriatricians who provide both consultative services to other physicians, as well as some direct patient care service. Geriatric services, involving nurse practitioners and full multidisciplinary team care under geriatrician leadership, are provided respectively in the ambulatory setting emphasizing case management in the community; in the acute hospital emphasizing expeditious and safe discharge; in short-stay geriatric rehabilitation units located in skilled nursing homes; and in long-stay nursing homes, managing intercurrent illness episodes on-site in lieu of transfer to a hospital.[52]

While conceptually attractive and initially growing at a steady pace, Medicare HMOs began to decline and disenroll members by the year 1999 as their private-sector sponsors found them to be difficult to implement and insufficiently profitable as investments.

Social Health Maintenance Organization (SHMO)

While Medicare HMOs do not typically provide ongoing chronic supportive care, a variant demonstration model sponsored by the Medicare program in the late 1980s, and known appropriately as the Social HMO, does in fact provide enrollees a limited amount of extended care service. The SHMO enrolls a relatively large population representing a cross-section of Medicare beneficiaries, all of whom agree to pay a supplemental premium into a fund that will finance a specified range of chronic social support services when and if needed. The chronic care benefits include case management, home nursing, homemaker services, day care, transportation, home-delivered meals, and limited amounts of skilled and custodial care in nursing homes.[53]

While successful in many respects, the initial SHMO demonstration sites encountered difficulties in efficiently

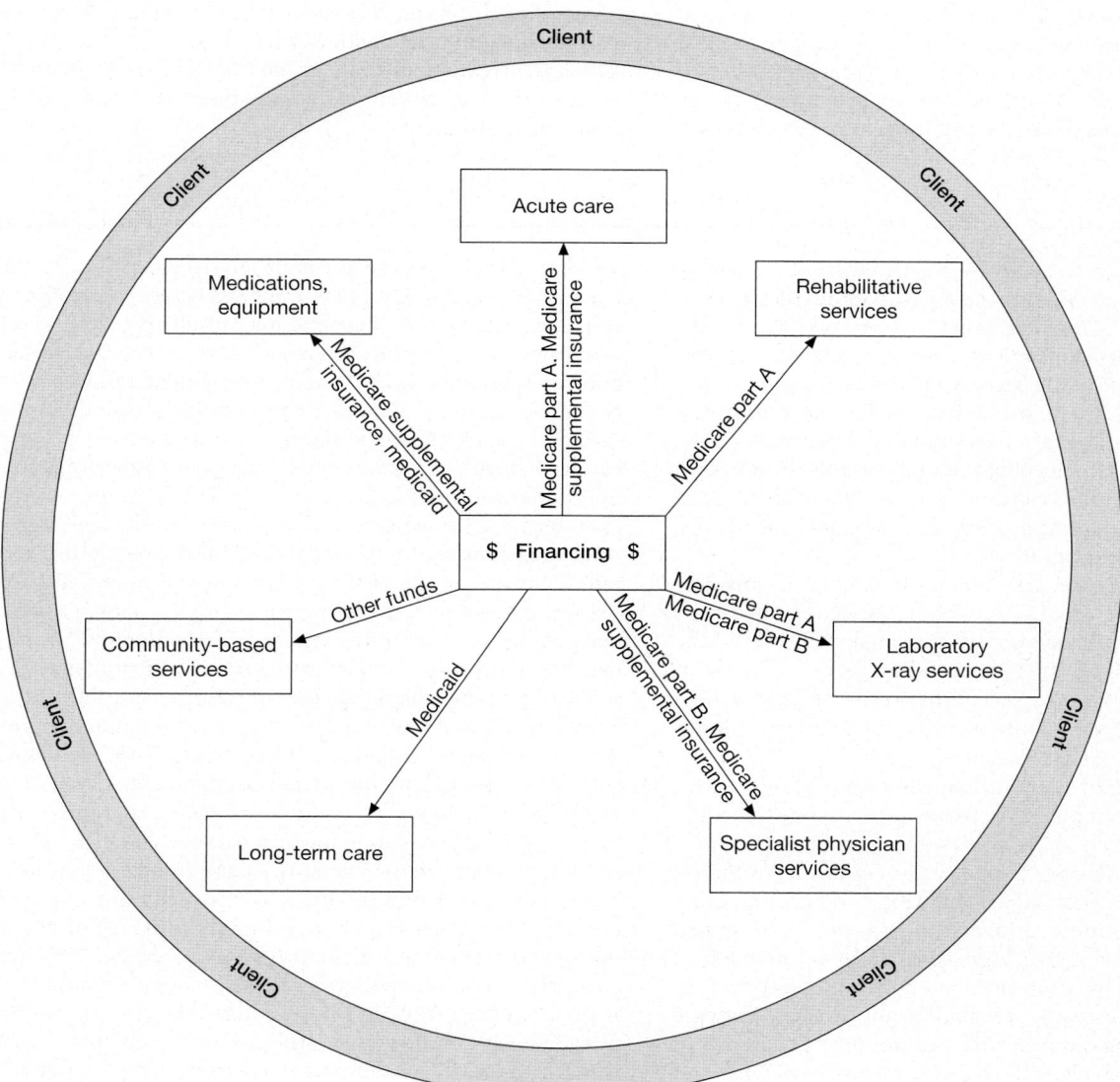

Figure 114-5 "Finance-oriented" system of care in which the patient/client must navigate a financially driven array of often disconnected services. From Calkins et al.,[57] used by permission of Springer Publishing Company, Inc., New York 10012.

integrating traditional medical services with the supplemental chronic care services and failed to achieve cost savings. In an effort to overcome these problems, a second-generation SHMO demonstration, initiated in 1996, was designed to more explicitly incorporate "a geriatric style of practice," emphasizing targeting high-risk patients, comprehensive assessment and rehabilitation, and including pivotal roles for geriatricians in coordination of services. As of 2001, only a single candidate site was fully operational under the SHMO II demonstration.[54]

On LOK/Program of All-inclusive Care for the Elderly (PACE)

The Program for All-Inclusive Care for the Elderly is a government-sponsored multisite service model designed to replicate the highly successful On Lok program, which integrates financing and delivery of a full range of acute and chronic care services for an enrolled population of several hundred nursing-home-eligible disabled older people. The prototype program evolved from its origins as a multipurpose day-care center in the Chinatown section of San Francisco to become a comprehensive system of medical and social services for functionally dependent elderly persons.[55] Combined Medicare–Medicaid funding provides coverage for all medical, rehabilitative, and long-term care services.

The resulting comprehensive delivery of care that is provided by a multidisciplinary geriatric team and emphasizes noninstitutional modalities, has been achieved at per capita costs substantially lower than would be incurred under the traditional fragmented provision of acute and long-term care services.[56] On Lok/PACE replications were conducted and evaluated in over 10 widely dispersed sites in the early 1990s, and based on a broad consensus of the model's success, the status of PACE was altered from a demonstration project to a certifiable Medicare provider under 1997 legislation. Currently over 40 PACE sites are operational nationwide; however, while commendable, these reach only some 10–12,000 total persons, a miniscule proportion of the frail older population in the country.

A thoughtful treatise entitled *New Ways to Care for Older People—Building Systems Based on Evidence*, published in 1999, contains excellent reviews of the many well-studied geriatric care strategies discussed here. In a pivitol chapter on "Integrating care," Boult points out the dilemma posed by the largely "finance-oriented" system of care, fraught with service gaps and discontinuities, with which frail elders and their physicians are currently confronted in the USA (Fig. 114-5). A model "client-oriented" system of care is presented as a desirable policy alternative.[57]

CANADA

Canada shares with the USA the twentieth-century demographic transition to an aging society with its attendant "geriatric imperative." Life expectancy at birth increased from 49 to 70 years between 1900 and 1965 in Canada, and had increased to over 76 at the century's end.

While sharing a common heritage of European conquest and colonization, Canada—in contrast to its breakaway neighbor to the south—remained formally linked with Great Britain well into the twentieth century and consequently retained certain distinctly European influences in both health service delivery and medical culture.

In the first instance, government financing of universal access to comprehensive health services, including substantial provision of chronic care, are fundamental principles of the Canada Health Act.[58] In the second instance, as in Great Britain, the roles of the medical profession are sharply divided between primary care and specialty medicine, the latter seeing patients on referral from the former.

Recognizing the need to address the health problems of increasing numbers of older Canadians, the Canadian Medical Association at its annual meeting in 1965 unanimously adopted a broad "Statement of Policy on Ageing."[59] Recommendations included placing greater emphasis on aging in medical school and resident training and in programs for practicing physicians; increasing numbers of medical and nonmedical professionals with primary interest in older people; increasing rehabilitation services, chronic hospitals, nursing homes, and community programs to serve frail older people; and targeting research on aging and chronic illness.

In 1978, following several years of debate, including serious misgivings expressed by the Specialty Committee in Internal

Medicine and the College of Family Physicians of Canada, the Canadian Royal College of Physicians and Surgeons established geriatric medicine as an academic and consultative subspecialty within internal medicine.[60] A set of requirements was developed to be used both for accrediting graduate training programs and for establishing eligibility of candidates to sit for the exam for the Certificate of Special Competence in Geriatric Medicine. Eligibility requirements included Royal College certification in internal medicine and completion of a 2-year program in geriatric medicine, which could be fulfilled through a variety of pathways. Importantly, in addition to acquiring attitudes, knowledge, and skills specific to medical problems of old age, trainees were to experience management of problems in inpatient and community settings, work with multidisciplinary healthcare teams, and learn to function primarily as a consultant, including planning for continuing care. In 1993, a revised specification of objectives for accredited training programs was issued by the Committee on Geriatric Medicine, again emphasizing the consultant role of the specialty.[61]

By the mid-1990s, accredited training programs were in place at 11 of Canada's 16 medical schools. The first certifying exam for specialists in geriatrics was administered in 1981. The number of certified geriatricians increased from 42 in 1987 to 130 in 1997. Their roles have primarily consisted of developing and staffing academic programs in medical schools and geriatric consultative services in major population centers. A Royal College study in 1987 predicted the country would need between 500 and 700 geriatricians by the year 2000, a goal which like its US counterpart is far from being attained.[61] The Canadian Society of Geriatric Medicine (now the Canadian Geriatrics Society) was established in 1981 to serve the professional interests of the new specialty.

The response to the call for dedicated geriatric content in medical school curricula has been well-documented through a series of surveys completed by geriatric medicine training program directors. Mandatory geriatric curriculum time increased from averages of 10 hours in 1982 (range of 0 to 50 hours) and 31 hours in 1987 to 65 hours (range of 3 to 205 hours) in 1992. In most schools, the majority of the teaching occurs during clinical training. Electives in geriatrics are taken by fewer than 2 percent of students.[62] At the graduate level, increasing numbers of family medicine and internal medicine residencies require a month or more of geriatric training, and the College of Family Physicians has established an optional 6- to 12-month add-on period of training in healthcare for elderly people.[60]

With regard to research in aging, attainments in geriatrics have been modest but steadily growing through efforts of the Canadian Geriatrics Society (CGS). While initial efforts were largely local clinical and health services studies focused on problems of frail older persons, the Canadian Study of Health and Aging launched in the early 1990s represents a large, multicenter, multidisciplinary cohort study involving over 10,000 subjects, designed much like the EPESE study in the USA to examine a wide range of questions regarding the natural history of aging and its attendant diseases and disabilities. A 1993 CGS review of research needs in geriatric medicine produced a "Blueprint for Discovery" which recommended that the Canadian Medical Research Council (MRC) establish an aging program. To date the MRC has declined to do so.[63]

Dedicated geriatrics services, while developed to varying degrees from province to province, are in principle fully covered as part of mainstream medical care under Canada's universal health system. As such, an older patient with acute and associated chronic care needs may be readily managed in a flexible continuing-care process under a global budget in Canada, in contrast to the fragmented approach to meeting (or possibly not meeting) the same care needs in mainstream medical services in the USA.[64] Given the status of geriatricians as a recognized part of the nation's health system, Canadian geriatricians have implemented a variety of strategies and systems of care within the institutional and community settings in which they work. In many instances they have emulated acute hospital-based units, day hospitals, and community outreach strategies developed in Great Britain or the USA.

Of particular note are several exemplary initiatives in which geriatricians have organized consultative and/or direct care systems that span the continuum of acute and chronic care services.

The Ottawa Regional Geriatric Assessment Program, implemented in the 1980s, comprises a model network of inpatient, day-hospital, and mobile geriatric assessment team services for meeting needs of community-dwelling frail older persons living within a defined area (William Dalziel, personal communication). The Regional Geriatric Program of Metropolitan Toronto serves primarily as a clearinghouse for facilitating efficient referrals of older patients from general practitioners to specialized geriatric services within a very large metropolitan healthcare system (Duncan Robertson, personal communication). The Baycrest Center for Geriatric Care, a microcosm of the Toronto metropolitan system, represents a model single institution providing a full spectrum of acute, short- and long-term rehabilitation, and chronic care services.[65] Seeking to provide similar comprehensive care services for community-dwelling populations of permanently disabled older persons, the Quebec Ministry of Health and Social Services has embarked on a well-funded demonstration of "Systems of Integrated Care for Frail Elderly," drawing on approaches used in the US PACE model (Howard Bergman, personal communication).

Development of the specialty of geriatric medicine in Canada has, from the beginning, received important contributions from British geriatricians, both as hosts to visitors in their home departments in Great Britain and as consultants on-site in Canada. Exemplary among these are Professor George Adams (Belfast) who, during a sabbatical in Manitoba, provided valued counsel on the decision in the 1970s to establish the specialty of geriatrics; Professor John Brocklehurst (Manchester) who planned and helped to implement Canada's first acute hospital-based geriatric service at the University of Saskatchewan; Professor James Williamson (Edinburgh) who consulted on geriatrics curriculum and service development at McMaster University and the University of British Columbia; and Dr John Dall (Glasgow) who provided extensive consultation on the development of regional geriatrics services in Ottawa.

CONCLUSION

The need for geriatric medicine, as one response to the aging of society, has been well-articulated in both the USA and Canada. With a legacy begun by Nascher, academic interest, particularly research in the medicine of old age, has flourished in the USA. Medical training and professional certification have evolved to accommodate both primary care and consultant geriatrician roles without formally recognizing geriatrics as a subspecialty. Many innovative geriatric service modalities, including managed care models with a chronic care component, have been introduced as demonstrations, but most of such services are not regularly covered, are often discouraged under prevailing healthcare financing programs, and have found limited implementation across the country. In Canada, geriatric medicine has evolved as a medical subspecialty, complementary to, but distinct from, primary care. Within the context of comprehensive national health services, regional geriatric consultation and delivery systems are in place, or planned in many, but not all, parts of the country. A vigorous aging research agenda was launched in the 1990s. Both countries enter the twenty-first century with a pressing challenge to overcome projected serious shortfalls in the supply of physicians trained in geriatrics to meet the needs of increasing numbers of older citizens.

Acknowledgments

A number of persons provided valuable resources and advice—in particular, Drs Chad Boult, Rebecca Elon, Bruce Leff, David Reuben, and T. Franklin Williams in the USA; and Drs Howard Bergman and William Dalziel in Canada.

KEY POINTS   Geriatrics in North America

In the United States

■ Separation of acute and chronic care delivery and financing has been detrimental to the development of geriatrics.

■ Aging-related research and academic developments flourished in the latter part of the twentieth century through organized government and professional efforts.

■ Need for medical education and postgraduate training in geriatrics has been repeatedly recognized and partially addressed, but remains seriously underdeveloped.

■ Effective geriatric health service strategies in hospital, nursing-home, community, and managed-care settings have been developed through demonstration projects. However, few have been incorporated into mainstream medical services.

■ Replacing the prevailing fragmented "finance-oriented" care system with integrated "client-oriented" services for older Americans is a central goal for the twentieth-first century.

In Canada

■ Geriatrics has been a recognized medical specialty, similar to the British model since the late 1970s; but as in the USA, there remains a serious shortage of geriatricians.

■ Dedicated geriatrics services are in principle included within the mainstream of the country's universal health system. However, developments have been highly variable across provinces and communities.

■ Research into aging has been modest, but expanding since the mid-1990s.

REFERENCES

1. Omran AR: Epidemiologic Transition in the United States: The Health Factor in Population Change. Population Bulletin Vol 32, No 2. Population Reference Bureau, Washington, DC, 1980
2. US Bureau of the Census: Current Population Reports, Special Studies, Sixty-Five Plus in America. US Government Printing Office, Washington, DC, 1992
3. Suzman RM, Willis DP, Manton KG: The Oldest Old. Oxford University Press, Oxford, 1992
4. Manton KG, Gu X: Changes in the prevalence of chronic disability in the United States black and non-black population above age 65 from 1982 to 1999. Proc Natl Acad Sci USA 2001;98:6354–6359
5. Barker WH: Health services for the elderly in the United States to 1980. In: Adding Life to Years: Organized Geriatrics Services in Great Britain and Implications for United States. Johns Hopkins University Press, Baltimore, 1987
6. DeLew N: The first 30 years of Medicare and Medicaid. JAMA 1995;274:262–267
7. Ettinger W: The Balanced Budget Act of 1997: implications for the practice of geriatric medicine. J Am Geriatr Soc 1998;46:530–533
8. Nascher IL: A history of geriatrics. Med Rev Rev 1926;32:281–284
9. Schock NW, Gruelich RC, Andres R et al: Normal Human Aging: The Baltimore Longitudinal Study of Aging. NIH Publication 84–2450. National Institutes of Health, Bethesda, 1984
10. Thewlis MW: History of the American Geriatrics Society. J Am Geriatr Soc 1953;1:3–8
11. Thompson WO: Aging comes of age. J Am Geriatr Soc 1953;1:1
12. Williams TF, Izzo AJ, Steel K: Innovations in teaching about chronic illness and aging in a chronic disease hospital. In Clark DW, Williams TF (eds): Teaching of Chronic Illness and Aging. DHEW Publication (NIH)75–876. National Institutes of Health, Bethesda, 1975
13. Schneider EL, Wendland CJ, Zimmer AW et al: The Teaching Nursing Home. Raven Press, New York, 1985
14. Ory MG, Schechtman KB, Miller JP et al: Frailty and Injuries in later life: the FICSIT trials. J Am Geriatr Soc 1993;41:283–343
15. SHEP Cooperative Research Group: Prevention of stroke by antihypertensive drug treatment in older persons with isolated systolic hypertension. JAMA 1991;265:3255–3264
16. Kane RL, Solomon D, Beck J et al: The future need for geriatric manpower in the United States. N Engl J Med 1980;302:1327–1332
17. Beeson, PB: The Institute of Medicine report in aging and medical education: 1984 update. Bull NY Acad Med 1985;61:478–483
18. Guidelines for fellowship training programs in geriatric medicine. J Am Geriatr Soc 1987;35:792–795
19. Report of the Institute of Medicine: Academic geriatrics for the year 2000. J Am Geriatr Soc 1987;35:773–791
20. Institute of Medicine: Training Physicians to Care for Older Americans: Progress, Obstacles, and Future Directions. National Academy Press, Washington, DC, 1993
21. Hazzard WR (ed): Geriatrics curriculum development conference and initiative. Am J Med 1994;97:4A1S–59S
22. Reuben DB, Zwanziger J, Bradley TB et al: Is geriatrics a primary care or subspecialty discipline? J Am Geriatr Soc 1994;42:363–367
23. Morley JE: Geriatric medicine: a true subspecialty. J Am Geriatr Soc 1993;41:1150–1154
24. Alliance for Aging Research: Will You Still Treat Me When I'm 65? The National Shortage of Geriatricians. Alliance for Aging Research, Washington, DC, 1996
25. AGS Education Committee: Guidelines for fellowship training in geriatrics. J Am Geriatr Soc 1998;46:1473–1477
26. Medina-Walpole A, Barker WH, Katz PR et al: The current state of geriatric medicine: a national survey of fellowship trained physicians 1990–98. J Am Geriatr Soc 2002;50:949–955
27. Special article: Planning for the chronically ill. JAMA 1947:343–347
28. American College of Physicians: Health and Public Policy Committee: long-term care of the elderly. Ann Intern Med 1984;100:760–763
29. Winograd CH, Gerety MB, Lai NA: A negative trial of inpatient geriatric consultation: lessons learned and recommendations for future research. Arch Intern Med 1993;153:2017–2023
30. Reuben DB, Borok GM, Wolde-Tsadik G et al: A randomized trial of comprehensive geriatric assessment in the care of hospitalized patients. N Engl J Med 1995;332:1345–1350
31. Rubenstein L, Josephson K, Wieland G et al: Effectiveness of a geriatric evaluation unit: a randomized clinical trial. N Engl J Med 1984;311:1664–1670
32. Applegate WB, Miller ST, Graney MJ et al: A randomized controlled trial of a geriatric assessment unit in a community rehabilitation hospital. N Engl J Med 1990;322:1572–1578
33. Landefield SC, Palmer RM, Kresevic DM et al: A randomized trial of care in a hospital medical unit especially designed to improve the functional outcomes of acutely ill older patients. N Engl J Med 1995;332:1338–1344
34. Creditor MC: Hazards of hospitalization of the elderly. Ann Intern Med 1993;118:219–223
35. Inouye SK, Bogardus ST, Charpentier PA et al: A multicomponent intervention to prevent delirium in hospitalized older patients. N Engl J Med 1999;340:669–676
36. Marcantonio E, Flacker J, Wright R et al: Reducing delerium after hip fracture: a randomized trial. J Am Geriatr Soc 2001;49:516–522
37. Rich MW, Beckham V, Wittenberg C et al: A multidisciplinary intervention to prevent the readmission of elderly patients with congestive heart failure. N Engl J Med 1995;333:1190–1195
38. Naylor MD, Brooten D, Campbell R et al: Comprehensive discharge planning and home follow-up of hospitalized elders: a randomized clinical trial. JAMA 1999;281:613–620
39. Leff B, Burton LC, Guido S: Home hospital program: a pilot study. J Am Geriatr Soc 1999;47:697–702
40. Stuck AE, Siu AL, Wieland D et al: Comprehensive geriatric assessment a meta-analysis of controlled trials. Lancet 1993;342:1032–1036
41. Barker WH, Zimmer JG, Hall WJ et al: Rates, patterns, causes, and costs of hospitalization of nursing home residents: a population-based study. Am J Pub Health 1994;84:1615–1620
42. Rubenstein LZ, Ouslander JG, Wieland D: Dynamics and clinical implications of the nursing home-hospital interface. Clin Geriatr Med 1988;4:471–491
43. Garrard J, Kane RL, Ratner ER, Buchanan JL: The impact of nurse practitioners on the care of nursing home residents. In Katz PR et al (eds): Advances in Long-Term Care I. Springer, New York, 1991

44. Miller TE: Advance directives: moving from theory to practice. In Katz PR et al (eds): Quality Care in Geriatric Settings. Springer, New York, 1995

45. Mott P, Barker WH: Hospital and medical care use by nursing home patients: The effect of care plans. J Am Geriatric Soc 1988;36:47–53

46. Campion EW: New hope for home care? N Engl J Med 1995;333:1213–1214

47. Weissert WG, Hedrick SC: Lesson learned from research on effects of community-based long-term care. J Am Geriatr Soc 1994;42:348–353

48. Vladeck BC, Miller NA: The Medicare home health initiative. Health Care Financ Rev 1994;16:7–16

49. Stuck A, Aronow HV, Steiner A et al: A trial of in-home comprehensive geriatric assessments for elderly people living in the community. N Engl J Med 1995;333:1184–1189

50. Wagner EH: The promise and performance of HMOs in improving outcomes in older adults. J Am Geriatr Soc 1996;44:1251–1257

51. Friedman B, Kane RL: HMO medical directors perceptions of geriatric practice in Medicare HMOs. J Am Geriatr Soc 1993;41:1144–1149

52. von Sternberg T: Geriatrics as a value-added service within an HMO. Clin Geriatr 1995;3:42–45

53. Leutz WN, Greenberg J, Abraham R et al: Changing Health Care for the Aging Society: Planning for the Social Health Maintenance Organization. DC Health, Lexington, 1985

54. Newcomer R, Harrington C, Kane R: Implementing the second generation social health maintenance organization. J Am Geriatr Soc 2000;829–834

55. Ansak M: The On Lok model: consolidating care and financing. Generations 1990;14:73–74

56. Eng C, Pedulla J, Eleazer GP et al: Program for All-Inclusive Care for the Elderly (PACE): an innovative model of integrated geriatric care and financing. J Am Geriatr Soc 1997;45:211–214

57. Calkins E, Boult C, Wagner E, Pacala J: New Ways to Care for Older People: Building Systems Based on Evidence. Springer, New York, 1999

58. Taylor MG: Insuring National Health Care: The Canadian Experience. University of North Carolina Press, Chapel Hill, 1990

59. Canadian Medical Association: Statement of policy on aging. Can Med Assoc J 1965;93:779

60. Hogan DB, Bergman H, McCracken P et al: The history of geriatric medicine in Canada. J Am Geriatr Soc 1997;45:1134–1139

61. Hogan DB, Patterson C, Boustcha E et al: Writing terminal educational objectives for the Royal College of Physicians and Surgeons of Canada accredited training programs in geriatric medicine. Ann R Coll Phys Surg Can 1995;28:291–296

62. Dalziel WB, Man-Son-Hing M: Survey of geriatric content in Canadian undergraduate medical school curricula. Ann R Coll Phys Surg Can 1994;27:476–478

63. Rockwood K, Bergman H, Hogan D et al: Aging-related clinical and health services research in Canada. J Am Geriatr Soc 1998;46:1469–1472

64. Bergman H, Clarfield AM, Ouslander J et al: Same patients, different systems: clinical implications for the care of the elderly. J Am Geriatr Soc 1992;40:1178–1182

65. Gordon M, Baycrest Centre for Geriatric Care: 75 years from clinical roots to academic present. Ann R Coll Phys Surg Can 1993;26:20–22

Chapter 115

Prospects for geriatric medicine in developing countries

Alexandre Kalache and Ingrid Keller

This chapter addresses the rapidity of the aging process in the developing world, discusses interrelated contributing demographic and socioeconomic factors, and examines the public health implications. There is a discussion on the need for appropriate policies within a conceptual framework of health promotion throughout the life course, and for the strengthening of the primary healthcare sector.

RAPID AGING IN DEVELOPING COUNTRIES

In 1950, the average life expectancy at birth in the developing world was around 40 years. By 2000 it had increased to 64 years, and is projected to reach 72 years by 2025.[1] With the exception of sub-Saharan countries hard hit by HIV/AIDS epidemics, life expectancy has constantly increased in all developing countries throughout the last few decades. In India, for example, life expectancy at birth for both sexes increased from 53 years in 1975 to 64 years in 2000, and is expected to increase further to 72 years in 2025. Respective figures for Pakistan are 53, 66, and 74 years, and for Brazil 60, 68, and 74 years.[1]

Such sharp increases reflect steep declines in mortality rates, particularly through the treatment and/or prevention of diseases associated with premature death. Thus, the advent of specific treatments for a range of infectious diseases (e.g. tuberculosis, respiratory infections, and gastroenteritis in childhood), along with immunization of many others (e.g. diphtheria, poliomyelitis, and measles), were the chief contributors to the survival of millions of children to adulthood throughout the developing world within the last 50 years. These adults are now aging. Already, most older people live in developing countries. These numbers will continue to rise at a far more rapid rate than in developed countries. It is estimated that by 2025, some 840 million people over the age of 65 will live in developing countries. This will represent 70 percent of all older people worldwide (Table 115-1).

However, rapid population aging is influenced also by the number of young people; in other words, in addition to a decline in mortality it is necessary that the population experiences a decline in the birth rate. Indeed, most of the developing world has experienced substantial decreases in fertility rates. For instance, in China, the total fertility rate (TFR; that is, the total number of children a woman in a given society expects to have had at the end of her reproductive life) declined from 3.2 in 1975 to 1.9 in 2000. In Brazil, respective figures are from 4.3 to 2.2, and in Thailand from 4.3 to 1.7. It is estimated that

Table 115-1 **Projected populations of the world (billions)**			
	2000	**2025**	**2050**
Total	6.0	7.8	8.9
More-developed countries	1.2	1.2	1.2
Less-developed countries	4.7	6.6	7.8
Population 65 years of age and over	0.4	0.8	1.5
More-developed countries	0.2	0.3	0.3
Less-developed countries	0.2	0.7	1.2

Source: United Nations.[1]

by 2020, 121 countries will have reached total fertility rates below replacement level (average fertility rate of 2.1 children per woman), a substantial increase compared to 1975, when just 22 countries had a total fertility rate below or equal to the replacement level—or the current figure of 68 countries.

As with the declines in mortality, fertility declines were made possible only through interventions based on medical technology. The availability of modern contraceptive methods has made it possible for such sharp declines in only a few years. In conclusion, in the same way as differences in life expectancy at birth in different regions of the world are rapidly disappearing, the large differentials between fertility rates are also decreasing (Figs 115-1 and 115-2). Population aging, then, is the effect of a combination of a shift from high to low mortality and high to low fertility (commonly referred to as the demographic transition): fewer children born and more individuals surviving into old age. A population pyramid shows the increases in the older age groups globally (Fig. 115-3).

The demographic transition can be illustrated clearly by the following data from Chile. Only 64 percent of the female children born in 1909 reached their fifth birthday, and only 13 percent of this birth cohort are living beyond their eighty-fifth birthday. In comparison, of the 1999 female cohort only 2 percent will have died before their fifth birthday, and virtually half are expected to live beyond 85 years.[2]

Contrast with already aged societies

In the developed world, population aging resulted also from the demographic transition, but the process took longer. For example, it took 114 years in France for the aged population to increase from 7 to 14 percent (from 1865 to 1979), and 82 years in Sweden (from 1890 to 1972). The same doubling will occur

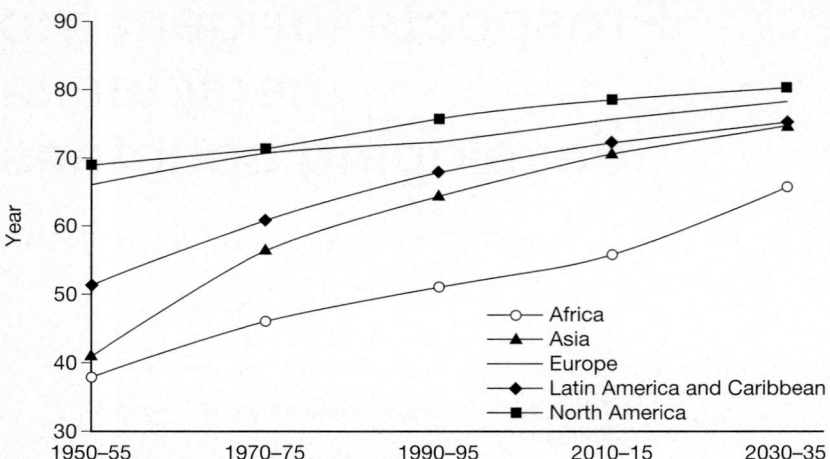

Figure 115-1 Life expectancy at birth in selected world regions (source: United Nations[1]).

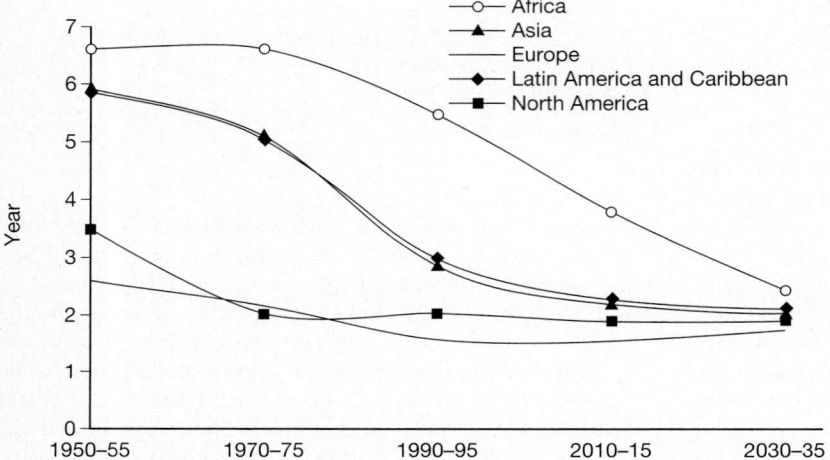

Figure 115-2 Total fertility rates in selected world regions (source: United Nations[1]).

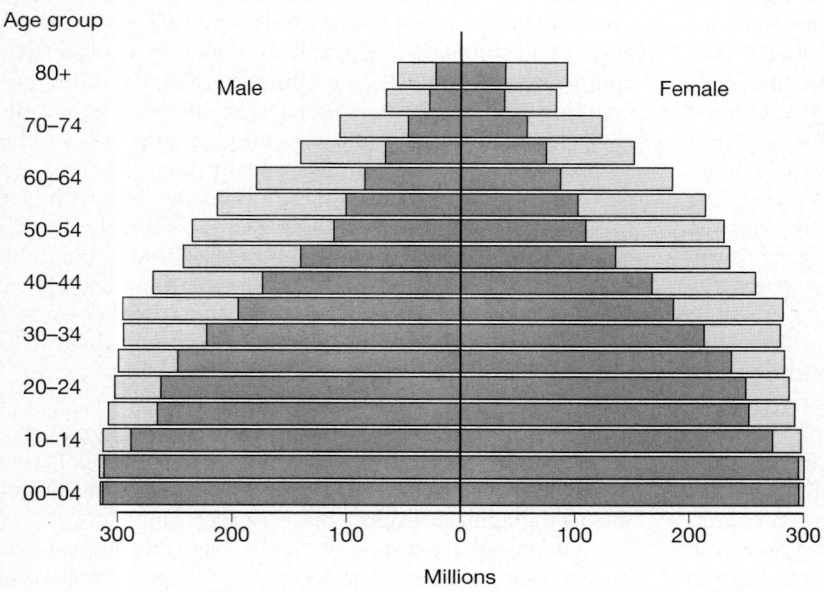

Figure 115-3 Population pyramid in 1995 ■ and 2025 □ (source: United Nations[1]).

in China in less than 30 years (from 2000 to 2027),[3] similar to the experiences in other developing countries—such as Malaysia and Brazil where a doubling will occur in 25 years (2000 to 2025).[2]

In developed countries, the demographic aging process followed the industrial revolution. Gradually, increasing segments of the population improved their living conditions by benefiting from rising socioeconomic standards. They were better housed, better nourished, and enjoyed healthier environments with improved working conditions. The contribution of advancing medical technology was minimal. For example, throughout the developed world diarrheal disease was virtually controlled as a cause of death in childhood well before the advent of antibiotic therapy. Tuberculosis was the leading cause of death in the USA by 1900; fifty years later (i.e. before the availability of specific treatment for the disease) mortality rates had declined to 10 percent of the 1900 level.

In contrast, the demographic transition in the developing world has been largely the result of medical interventions—effective treatments and vaccines for a wide range of infectious diseases. In spite of the poor, even miserable, conditions in which large numbers of the populations of developing countries still live, survival into adulthood (and from there to old age) is increasingly becoming the norm rather than the exception. Furthermore, in the past, a high educational level was a precondition for a woman to limit the size of her family; today, powerful contraceptive methods are effectively used throughout the world irrespective of women's literacy.

Beyond 2000, into the old-age era

Countries such as Indonesia, Kenya, Mexico, Taiwan, and Costa Rica will experience increases of 300 percent or more in their older populations from 1990 to 2025, far higher than the percentage increase in the total population within the same period.[3] Early in the twenty-first century, eight out of the eleven largest populations of older persons will be in the developing world: China, India, Brazil, Indonesia, Pakistan, Mexico, Bangladesh, and Nigeria—the others being in the USA, Japan, and the Russian Federation. By 2025 there will be 285 million people over the age of 60 years in China alone, more than the total present population of the USA; in India the total will be close to 150 million; while Brazil and Indonesia, with 32 million each, will have populations of older persons virtually as large as that of Japan.

PUBLIC HEALTH IMPLICATIONS OF AGING

Current WHO projections indicate that by the year 2020 over three-quarters of the burden of disease in the developing world will be attributable to noncommunicable diseases (NCDs)—a sizeable increase from current levels, as shown in Figure 115-4.

Risk factors for noncommunicable diseases—such as smoking, hypertension, obesity, or elevated cholesterol levels—are on the rise, especially in countries such as Chile and Mexico experiencing a rapid demographic and epidemiological transition. Table 115-2 shows the percentage of overweight and obese adults out of the total population in selected developing countries and countries in transition.

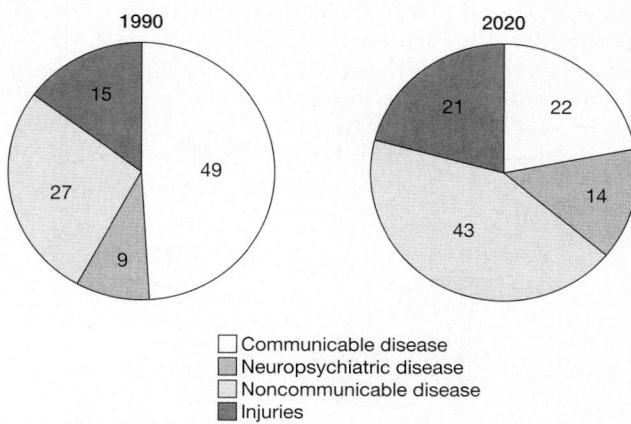

Figure 115-4 The global burden of disease 1990–2020, in developing and newly industrialized countries. From Murray and Lopez.[19]

Legend:
- □ Communicable disease
- ▨ Neuropsychiatric disease
- ▢ Noncommunicable disease
- ▧ Injuries

Table 115-2 Overweight and obese adults as a percentage of population in selected countries

Country (year)	Overweight men[a]	Overweight women[a]	Obese men[b]	Obese women[b]
Mexico (1995)	50	58	11	23
Philippines (1993)	11	12	2	3
Saudi Arabia (1996)	29	27	16	24
Tunisia (1990)	20	33	2	8
Russia (1996)	33	31	11	28

[a]Overweight: BMI > 25 kg/m^2. [b]Obese: BMI > 30 kg/m^2. BMI (body mass index) as person's bodyweight in kg/square of body height in meters.

Source: From Popkin and Doak.[20]

The contribution of communicable diseases to the disease burden will be reduced to around 22 percent by the year 2020—the same as for those caused by injuries. However, this reduction does not mean that communicable diseases will have become less important as public health threats. In order to keep them at bay it will be necessary to invest considerable resources towards their prevention (e.g. comprehensive vaccination and sanitation campaigns) and treatment (a challenge in the face of the re-emergence of epidemics from biopathogens increasingly resistant to available drugs). This double burden—continuing public health problems related to infectious diseases coupled to the emergence of noncommunicable diseases—is already affecting many developing nations. In all probability, it will become a standard feature in most of the developing world for the foreseeable future.

Figures 115-5 and 115-6 illustrate the share of noncommunicable diseases in the total causes of mortality presently in southeast Asian countries and in eastern Mediterranean countries.[4] In both regions, noncommunicable conditions already account for more than 50 percent of the causes of death.

The challenge for public health policy-makers is huge: scarce resources will be increasingly required to deal with NCDs while the old diseases will continue to be prevalent. This is an unprecedented phenomenon closely linked to the aging process.

Never before in the history of humankind has it been possible for societies to age—thus changing disease patterns—in the context of poverty. It is also a paradox: aging also makes it imperative for society to redefine itself.

The very nature of the health problems associated with aging—long-term, treatable but not curable, often requiring lifelong costly care, frequently disabling—highlight the impor-

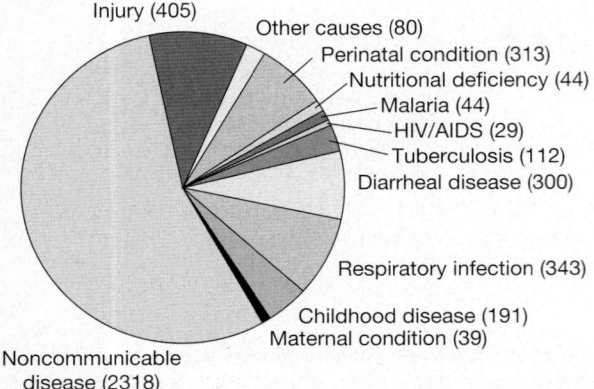

Figure 115-5 Distribution of causes of death in the eastern Mediterranean in 1999 (thousands) (source: WHO[4]).

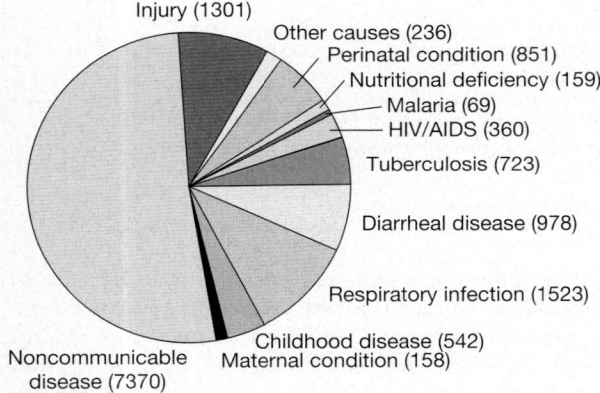

Figure 115-6 Distribution of causes of death in south-east Asia in 1999 (thousands) (source: WHO[4]).

tance of developing appropriate and cost-effective policies. In their absence, consequences for society could be devastating, eroding the very basis of overcoming underdevelopment.

Even the richest countries, which have taken much longer to age and to adapt to the new demographic order, are finding it difficult to find solutions. The perceived crisis of the "welfare state" throughout Europe is a clear example. Yet, World Bank figures indicate that in today's rich societies available resources are relatively much larger than those that will be at the disposal of developing countries by the time they become as old as the developed world is today. According to the World Bank,[5] in 1990 the per capita income in OECD countries was around US$18,000 (projected to reach US$ 44,000 by 2030); respective figures for Latin America are US$1,500 and US$6,000 (Fig. 115-7). That means that by 2030, when the Latin American demographic structure will be very similar to that of the OECD countries today, there will be merely one-third of the resources to be shared by competing problems. By then, South Asian countries are expected to reach the current US$1,500 current Latin American level, while Africa's GNP per capita will not change from the 1990s level of only US$300. In several countries with a large older population, the majority of the population lives with less than 2 dollars (purchasing power parity) per day (Table 115-3).[6]

The challenges will be compounded by the technological gap that will continue to grow, separating rich and poor nations. The US$44,000 GNP per capita in the OECD countries will be translated into a level of technological sophistication that is impossible to predict today. This will put extra pressure on developing countries, where the elites will continue to expect the same level of sophisticated healthcare that their counterparts will be enjoying in the rich world—thus exacerbating the challenges for the provision of equitable services and opportunities for all.

AGING AS A DEVELOPMENT ISSUE

A study of public spending on social programs in the mid-1980s in Brazil illustrates the dilemmas faced by developing nations as they age. By then, only 9 percent of the Brazilian population was aged 55 years or more, yet they absorbed 48 percent of the benefits provided by public money. The respective figures for

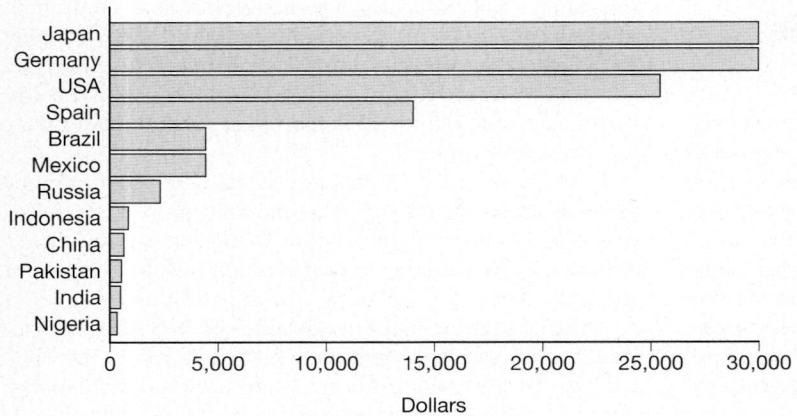

Figure 115-7 GNP per capita in 1999 (US dollars, atlas method) (source: World Bank[5]).

Table 115-3 Percentage of population below international poverty line in selected countries

	Population (millions)	<1 \$/day[a]	<2 \$/day[a]
China	1278	22	58
India	1014	53	89
Indonesia	212	12	59
Brazil	170	24	44
Nigeria	111	31	60
Ethiopia	63	46	89

[a]*Purchasing-power-parity dollars.*
Source: From World Bank.[6]

citizens aged under 15 years were 34 and 28 percent. Benefits for the aged were mostly related to pensions and healthcare, while for children education and healthcare generated the main costs. Underdevelopment will not be overcome unless tomorrow's adults grow in good health and attain high educational levels and are able to maintain themselves. Furthermore, the social fabric of any country requires intergenerational harmony. The tensions are clearly reflected in the Brazilian figures. However, they hide the lack of another basic prerequisite for harmonious development: equity. The same study indicated that the better-off 15 percent of the Brazilian population (with an average income higher than two minimum salaries) attracted seven times more publicly funded social benefits than the poorest fifth of the population (whose average income was less than half a minimum salary). All in all, the distribution of benefits in Brazil indicates that older rich individuals are receiving a disproportionate amount. These come in the shape of higher pensions and sophisticated healthcare. Meanwhile, the poor elderly population—and children in general—get very little in relative terms.

Aging-related policies in the developing world will have to take into account such inequities, since they could severely impair the capacity of societies to overcome underdevelopment. The models and practices from developed countries are of little relevance in this respect. Neither the resources they have available nor the pace of their aging process resemble what is now occurring in the developing world.

An aging policy framework, to be applicable worldwide, requires action on three basic pillars:

- *Health.* When the risk factors (both environmental and behavioral) for chronic diseases and functional decline are kept low and the protective factors are kept high, people enjoy both a longer quantity and higher quality of life. Older people will remain healthy and able to manage their own lives. Fewer older adults will need costly medical treatments and care services.
- *Participation.* Older people will continue to make a productive contribution to society in both paid and unpaid activities when the labor market, employment, education, health and social policies and programs support their full participation in socioeconomic, cultural, and spiritual activities, according to their capacities, needs, and preferences.
- *Security.* When policies and programs address the health, social, financial and physical security needs and rights of older people, older people are ensured of protection, dignity, and care in the event that they are no longer able to support and protect themselves. Families are supported in their efforts to care for older loved ones.

These three pillars are based on the UN Principles for older persons which focus on maintaining independence, participation, care, self-fulfillment and dignity of all older persons.

Key policy recommendations include reducing the prevalence of risk factors associated with most common chronic diseases, and increasing the prevalence of factors that protect health and well-being throughout the life course; developing health and social service systems that emphasize health promotion, disease prevention, and the provision of cost-effective, equitable and dignified long-term care; and preventing and reducing the burden of excess disabilities, especially in marginalized populations.[7]

Geriatric specialists have an important role to play as educators of future medical doctors—general practitioners with good knowledge of old-age care, as well as specialists in geriatrics. Old-age care cannot thrive if there are no centers of excellence and training.

THE CHANGING SOCIOCULTURAL CONTEXT

Population aging also modifies the demand for informal and formal long-term care. Although worldwide the bulk of care for frail elderly people is still provided by the family, changes in family structure and increasing participation of women in the paid workforce are gradually eroding the capacity of the family to provide care.[8] Accordingly, new models of home care, provided by professionals to support the family but avoiding costly stays in a nursing home, are being explored in most developed countries.

In the developing world, where healthcare systems are struggling with the double burden of diseases, the issues are more complex. There is a strong need to train primary healthcare personal in prevention and treatment of noncommunicable diseases, as well as to adapt healthcare systems in order to prepare them for an aged population. This is particularly important in areas where no health insurance or pension schemes exist. New and innovative schemes of community healthcare and long-term care for the aged are urgently required to counteract factors such as disrupted family ties due to, for example, the trend towards nuclear families, migration to cities of young people, increasing participation of women in the paid labor force and, particularly in sub-Saharan Africa, the HIV/AIDS epidemics leaving orphaned children to be looked after by their grandparents. This is a critical developmental issue for Africa and other similarly affected developing countries, with significant implications for future human capital. For the children, the trauma of losing one or both parents is often magnified by relocation, possibly from an urban to a rural living environment, within the extended family structure. The burden of care and support falls mostly on only slightly older brothers and sisters or on the grandparents. A clash of generations often ensues. Information and support for those older people providing care is essential to prevent an overextension of families' capacities to care for family members with AIDS, and subsequently for their orphans.

The World Health Organization has recently started to collaborate on projects that address the impact of this disease on older people in these countries. These projects, in association with HelpAge International, include for example interviews with grandparents caring for orphaned grandchildren in Zimbabwe. More collaborative efforts will be necessary to define and assess the scope of the problem, the subsequent implications for older individuals, their extended families, and society at large, and finally to strengthen the capacities of countries to develop solutions and policies to support their older populations.

The fast changes in demographic structure and in disease patterns are only part of the aging equation of the developing world. Table 115-4 shows the trends of urbanization. In many countries at a medium stage of development or in economic transition, the urbanization rate is already today as high as in fully industrialized countries; examples are Venezuela and Brazil. Today, 14 of the world's 19 largest cities, with more than 10 million inhabitants each, are in the developing world. By the year 2015 there will be 23 cities worldwide with over 10 million inhabitants, 19 of them in the developing world.[9]

Urbanization is but one mark of the modernization process. The trend towards the nuclear family is now becoming pronounced in many developing countries in the wake of urbanization. In Argentina, for example, in the early 1990s, more than half of older persons in urban districts were living alone or with their partner.[10] In São Paulo in the late 1980s, only 11 percent of older persons were living in multigenerational households; the majority were either living alone, with their spouse only, or in two-generation (nuclear-family) households.[11] This change in family structure—the social institution, which traditionally has cared for the aged—is not only in size but also in its capacity to provide fully for its aging members. Constraints include crowded housing, limited financial resources, and the increasing employment of women, the traditional carers for the frail and dependent in any society.

Urbanization also entails two further phenomena of great significance to population aging. On the one hand, throughout the world millions of earlier rural migrants are now aging without having been fully assimilated into the mainstream of their new home environment. On the other hand, those who migrate to urban areas are usually the young, who leave behind their elderly relatives without immediate support. Unless they succeed in the city (a prospect often denied to unskilled workers) they will not be in a position to assist financially their now distant relations, whatever their intentions were at the point of departure. For example, in Malaysia, about 80 percent of older persons living in urban areas live with their children, whereas only about half of the rural population of older persons lives with their children, about a quarter with the spouse only, and more than one in ten lives alone.[12] Policy-makers in developing countries are now starting to realize that unless family and community traditions of mutual aid are strengthened, a vast—yet unaffordable—service infrastructure will be required in coming decades to replace and expand previous informal care-giving.

Shifts from extended to nuclear families also imply the loss of older persons' roles as heads of families, and thus of their decision-making functions and financial responsibilities/privileges. Modernization undermines the status of older people by making their experience and attachment to tradition appear outmoded and irrelevant to technological progress. The socio-economic changes that are now taking place throughout the developing world often have the net effect of marginalizing the aged—that is, removing them from the mainstream of development, weakening their traditional sources of material support, and eliminating their purposeful social and economic role.

While the impact of urbanization has attracted intense research, rural aging has only recently been taken on by researchers and institutions. The International Rural Ageing Project (initiated in 1997 by the UN Programme on Ageing, the World Health Organization, and the International Association of Gerontology) is focusing on the needs of aging rural populations within the contexts of broad intersectoral policies and a life-course perspective. It aims at identifying policies and practices to address equitable distribution of resources to improve access to care and services for older persons in rural areas as well as education and training models in aspects of rural aging. The first global conference on rural aging took place in June 2000 (see www.ruralaging.org).

Common risk factors for noncommunicable diseases are often less frequent in older persons in rural areas than in urban areas; for example, the prevalence of diabetes type 2 is about 2.4 percent in rural India, while it is 11.6 percent in urban settings.[13] On the other hand, rural older adults in developing countries are much more prone to undernutrition. Studies from Malaysia, India, and Malawi have shown a high rate of undernutrition and micronutrient deficiency in older, rural persons, often living alone.[14–16] Health services, on the other hand, are often scarce in rural areas and may be impossible to reach, since adequate transportation for older people is not available. Also, primary healthcare workers often are neither trained nor equipped to detect and treat risk factors and/or diseases of older persons who need care. Thus, there is an urgent need to provide training in old-age care to primary healthcare workers, and to ensure access to healthcare services for older persons in rural areas.

GERIATRIC MEDICINE AT A CROSSROADS

By the year 2025 there will be more than 1.2 billion older people in the world, three-quarters of them in countries that are currently developing. The context in which this fast aging

Table 115-4 **Urban population as a percentage of the total, in selected countries**

Country	1975	1998	2015
Venezuela	75.8	86.8	90.4
Brazil	61.2	80.2	86.5
Turkey	41.6	73.1	84.5
Ukraine	58.3	71.6	78
Philippines	35.6	56.9	67.8
Malaysia	37.7	55.8	66.2
Indonesia	19.4	38.3	52.4
Pakistan	26.4	35.9	46.7
Zimbabwe	19.6	33.9	45.9
Thailand	15.1	20.9	29.3

Source: Human Development Report, UNDP.[21]

process is going to take place has been outlined above. However desirable, it is inconceivable that specialized geriatric care can be provided for such vast numbers of old individuals unless the speciality restructures itself.

Physicians in geriatric medicine will need to take the lead in disseminating their expertise and sharing their knowledge with other health professionals. This is easier said than done. Sharing knowledge is sharing power—an intrinsically difficult demand. Most of the problems presented by older people occur at community level where they will be expected to be solved—otherwise the costs will be prohibitive. Yet primary healthcare workers are mostly ill-equipped to deal with the problems of old age. The opportunities for geriatric medicine are immense. If the specialists seize these opportunities, adopting active roles as trainers, disseminators of knowledge, advocates of change, and policy developers, a revived discipline will emerge. Training of health and social service workers in enabling models of primary healthcare and long-term care that recognize the strengths and contributions of older people and reduce inequities in access to care in isolated and urban areas throughout the developing world will be an increasing imperative for the health sector. This will require the use of both high-tech solutions (e.g. telemedicine) and low-tech solutions (e.g. support to community-based outreach programs).

Geriatric medicine in the developing world should expand to encompass aging rather than just care of older people. The healthy aging message should increasingly be incorporated into the core of the speciality. After all, the future 1.2 billion older people are today's younger adults; the surest way to reduce their demand for services and their decline into disability is by investing on their health as they (we) age. Furthermore, an agenda for health and aging is an agenda for reducing the prevalence of noncommunicable diseases. In the developed as well as in the developing world, the diseases that most commonly affect older persons are noncommunicable diseases. Preventing them altogether—or postponing their onset—requires interventions much earlier in life when risk factors for these diseases are acquired or consolidated. In other words, it means bringing the "healthy aging" perspective to the entire life course.

HEALTH PROMOTION IN OLD AGE

Ultimately both individuals and societies share the same objective: successful aging. An indispensable prerequisite for that is health. Good health in older age is the major factor in ensuring that older people will continue to contribute to society and be providers of care, rather than recipients only. The body of knowledge developed by geriatric medicine over the last few decades can act as a foundation for the interventions to be widely implemented. That is why it is necessary to adopt a life-course perspective. Good health in older age depends largely on interventions and behavior changes that took place much earlier in life. However, it is never too late to promote health, as evidence presented elsewhere in this book demonstrates.

Older people continue to carry out activities for their daily living and therefore play an active part in their community. In this respect it is especially useful to examine the concept of functional capacity within a life-course perspective, as illustrated in Figure 115-8.

A person's capacity in relation to a number of functions (such as ventilatory capacity, muscular strength, cardiovascular output) increases in childhood and peaks in early adulthood. This peak is eventually followed by a decline. How fast the decline is, however, is determined largely by factors related to adult lifestyle often acquired in childhood or adolescence—such as smoking, alcohol consumption, and unhealthy diet. The natural decline in cardiac function, for example, can be accelerated by smoking, leaving the individual with a functional capacity lower than would normally be expected for his or her age. The gradient of decline may become so steep as to result in premature disability. However, the acceleration in decline may be reversible at any age. Smoking cessation and small increases in the level of physical fitness, for example, reduce the risk of developing coronary heart disease. Thus, the slope of the decline can be influenced in any stage through individual as well as policy measures. For example, smoking cessation at age 50 reduces the risk of dying within the next 15 years by 50 percent.[17]

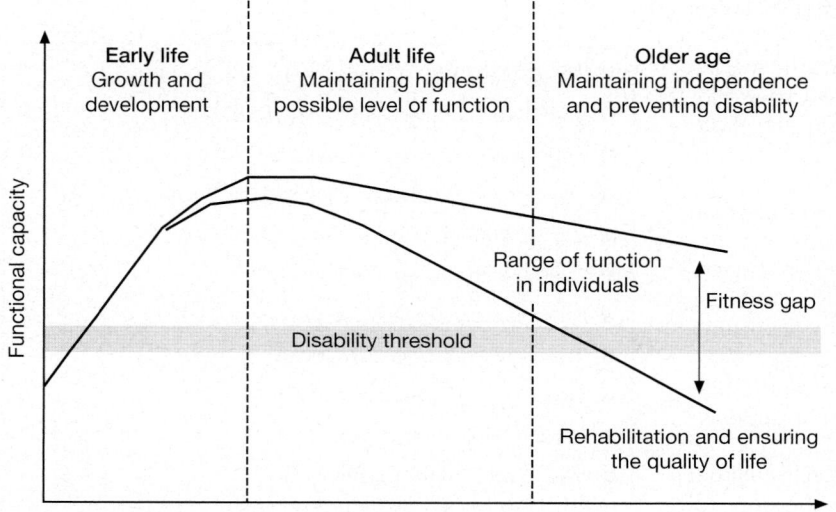

Figure 115-8 Life-course perspective for maintenance of the highest possible level of functional capacity (source: ref.[7]).

Other factors, conditioned by social class, also affect functional capacity. Poor education, poverty, and harmful living and working conditions all make reduced functional capacity more likely in later life. In those countries where people with poor functional ability are more likely to become institutionalized, this in itself can lead to or perpetuate dependence.

Finally, for those who become disabled, provision of rehabilitation and adaptations of the physical environment can greatly reduce the level of disability. Furthermore, specific interventions can improve functional capacity and thus quality of life. For example, cataract causes nearly 50 percent of all blindness worldwide, but it can be treated through a fairly simple surgical procedure, increasingly available in developing countries.[18]

Quality of life should be a major consideration throughout the life course, particularly for those whose functional capacity can no longer be maintained. For example, changes in the living environment can vastly improve quality of life. However, most of the gains are obtained by acting on the "care unit"—in most case the family and close friends. It is often by supporting the informed carer (frequently an older woman, in many cases in poor health herself) that the quality of life of the dependent older person can be most improved.

Within the model illustrated in Figure 115-8, consideration should also be paid to the disability threshold itself. Through appropriate environmental changes—such as adequate public transport in urban environments, the availability of lifts in apartment or office blocks, ramps, adapted kitchenware, or a toilet seat with rails—the disability threshold can be lowered. Such changes can ensure a more independent life well into very old age. One of the major challenges is to ensure access to them to all older persons, including the poor and those who live in remote areas.

THE WHO PROGRAM

If the main public health challenge of the last century was ensuring survival, that of the twenty-first century will be maintaining quality of life. With the steadily rising number of children who reach adulthood, and adults who reach old age, the most pressing concern becomes that of ensuring that all of them enjoy the highest attainable quality of life. For that, health comes first.

To help promote a global response to this major societal concern, the World Health Organization launched a new program on aging and health in 1995. Its perspectives can be summarized as follows.

- Approaching aging as part of the life course rather than compartmentalizing healthcare of elderly people.
- Promoting long-term health. There is increasing awareness of the need to focus on the process of healthy aging since, whether early or late in life, people have many opportunities to improve their health status as they age.
- Observing cultural influences. The settings in which individuals age play an important part in their health and well-being.
- Adopting community-oriented approaches. Throughout the world, even in the richest countries, the vast majority of

older people live in the community and it is at this level that most of their problems will have to be challenged—often outside the health sector but usually with implications for health.
- Recognizing gender differences. There are important differences in men's and women's health and ways of living, and they become more pronounced in later life.
- Strengthening intergenerational links. Emphasis is placed on strategies to maintain cohesion between generations and a common understanding of ethical issues. As populations age, vital issues must be considered such as undue hastening or delaying of death, human rights, long-term care, and abuse.

In conclusion, the appropriate model for the development of geriatric medicine in the developing world should encompass the perspectives laid down above. To this end, the WHO is strengthening its efforts—for instance through a workshop recently conducted with the aim of developing training modules on old-age care for primary healthcare workers in developing countries. The modules have been published.[22] They range from specific diseases and conditions to assessments of the nutritional and mental status of older persons.

Geriatric medicine in developing countries should avoid the limitations imposed by the adoption of a narrow disease-oriented model. Instead, it is health gains that should orient its development. This requires a combination of:

- clinical interventions, with emphasis on community-based interventions, informing and supporting effective primary healthcare;
- preventive interventions at primary, secondary, and tertiary levels;
- multisectoral actions.

Health, particularly in older age, depends on interventions from a wide range of sectors whose individual contributions and roles need to be defined. Geriatric medicine specialists could play a critical role in acting as catalysts, mediators, facilitators and advocates, as well as providers of services.

KEY POINTS Prospects for geriatric medicine in developing countries

- Rapid aging in developing countries.
- The contrast with already aged societies.
- Beyond 2000, into the old-age era.
- Public health implications of aging.
- Aging as a development issue.
- The changing sociocultural context.
- Geriatric medicine at a crossroads.
- Health promotion in old age.
- WHO's work on health and aging.

REFERENCES

1. United Nations (UN): World Population Prospects: The 1998 Revision (Medium Variant Projections), 1999
2. WHO: World Health Report, Geneva, 1999
3. Kinsella K, Taeuber C: An Aging World. II: International Population Reports P95/92–3, US Department of Commerce, Bureau of the Census, 1993
4. WHO: World Health Report, Geneva, 2000
5. World Bank: www.worldbank.org/data/databytopic/GNPPC.pdf, 2000
6. World Bank: World Development Report 1998/1999
7. WHO, Active Ageing, A Policy Framework, WHO/NMH/NPH/02.8, 2002
8. WHO/Millbank Memorial Fund: Towards an International Consensus on Policy for Long-Term Care of the Aging. WHO/HCS/AHE/00.1, 2000
9. World Bank: World Urban Prospects, 1999 Revision. www.un.org/esa/population/urbanization.pdf, 1999
10. Lloyd-Sherlock P: Living Arrangements of Older Persons and Poverty (UN/POP/AGE/2000/12) 2000.
11. Ramos et al: Profile of the elderly in a metropolitan area of Southeastern Brazil: results of a domiciliary survey (article in Portugese) Revista Saude Publica 1993;27(2):87–94
12. Chang TP, Tho NS, Peng TN, Awang H: Evaluating Programme Needs of Older Persons in Malaysia. Faculty of Economics and Administration, University of Malaya, Kuala Lumpur, 1999
13. Ramachandran A, Snehalatha C, Latha E, Manoharan M, Vijai V: Impacts of urbanization on the life style and on the prevalence of diabetes in native Asian Indian population. Diabetes Res Clin Pract 1999;44(3):207–213
14. Wadhwa A, Sabharwal M, Sharma S: Nutritional status of the elderly. Indian J Med Res 1997;106:340–348
15. Chilima DM, Ismail SJ: Anthropometric characteristics of older people in rural Malawi. Eur J Clin Nutr 1998;52:643–649
16. Shahar S, Earland J, Powers HJ, Rahman SA: Nutritional status of rural elderly Malays: dietary and biochemical findings. Int J Vitam Nutr Res 1999;Jul 69(4):277–284
17. WHO: Factsheet on Ageing and Tobacco (prepared by HSC/AHE for World Health Day), 1999,www.who.int/hpt/ageing
18. WHO: Factsheet on Ageing and Visual Disabilities (prepared by HSC/AHE for World Health Day), 1999,www.who.int/hpt/ageing
19. Murray C, Lopez A: Global Burden of Diseases. WHO, Harvard, 1996
20. Popkin BM, Doak CM: The obesity epidemic is a worldwide phenomenon. Nutr Rev 1998;56(4):106–114
21. United Nation's Development Program: Human Development Report, New York, 2000
22. CD-rom can be obtained from the Aging and Health Unit at the Pan American Health Organization, 525 23rd Street NW, Washington, DC 20037, USA, ENVEJECE @ PAHO.ORG

Chapter 116

Long-term care in the United Kingdom

Clive E. Bowman

OVERVIEW OF PRACTICE AND POLICY

The history of long-term care in the UK is a mixture of benevolence, denial, and pragmatism, driven more by social conscience and political pressure than by intelligent epidemiological understanding of needs and preferences. The key issue that *quality* of life rather than its length should be the guiding principle is widely accepted. Kirkwood[1] succinctly represents this widely held view. It is a curious phenomenon that, whilst strenuous medical endeavors to prolong life continue, the nature of life in long-term care remains inadequately described and understood.[2]

Poor Law policies of the nineteenth century sought to provide housing for the destitute unemployed, the sick, the blind, and people with epilepsy—as well as the elderly. The principle was to offer a standard of life below the lowest achievable by anyone in employment, the intention being to deter idleness! The advent of the National Health Service (NHS) in 1948 incorporated beds providing long-term care for elderly and disabled people into the service. The NHS inherited a motley collection of chronic sick wards in municipal hospitals, workhouse infirmaries, former infectious-disease hospitals and sanatoria. From this unpromising estate geriatric medicine emerged (see also Chapter 113). The principal objective of the management of the patients in these beds (and the many hundreds on lists waiting to occupy them) was to prevent long-term institutionalization through accurate diagnosis, where possible effective treatment, and the provision of physical and mental rehabilitation.[3] Through the 1950s and 1960s the management of long-term care remained the core of geriatric practice. The preoccupation with avoiding long-term care through comprehensive clinical and social assessment, treatment, and rehabilitation, together with increasing support at home, made the nature and issues of long-term care a secondary concern.

In 1962, Townsend published *The Last Refuge*, a landmark study of residential institutions and homes for the aged in England and Wales.[4] The study concluded that communal homes were not adequately meeting the physical, psychological, and social needs of the elderly people living in them, and that alternative services and living arrangements should quickly take their place. The number of geriatric beds in the NHS remained virtually unchanged from 1959 to 1985, with improved and new treatments, rehabilitation, and community care counterbalancing increasing numbers of older people. From 1986 to 1994, the number of these beds declined, while beds in private and voluntary nursing homes increased dramatically (Table 116-1). Similar trends were apparent in the local-authority residential home sector with an increase of 136 percent in private and voluntary homes. Hospitals for patients with mental illness also provided a good deal of long-term care for elderly people, but the psychogeriatric beds were separately counted and distinguished in official statistics only from 1988.[5]

Cochrane's seminal monograph[6] of 1971 foretold an inflation of acute healthcare and a widening gap in the standards between curative endeavor and caring. In 1972, Isaacs et al.[7] described the "hard core" of patients that a geriatric service traditionally looked after and emphasized that only well-coordinated health and care services could respond effectively to the needs of this group. In the early 1970s, such patients were still commonly the result of a neglect of the frail, isolated, sick and dispossessed old. Improvements in both living standards and aspects of health and care have considerably addressed the issues of "filth, hunger, cold and danger" confronting the frailest. However, Cochrane's concerns regarding the organization of care went unheeded.

In the early 1980s, social security payments were made available on demand, without comprehensive assessment, for residential and nursing-home care. This uncoordinated response to the aging population and the chronic underinvestment in buildings and services for chronically sick and disabled people resulted in a rapid development of an independent sector eager to satisfy a seemingly unending demand. The total scale of this expenditure escalated from £10,000,000 in England and Wales in 1979 to £190 million in 1983, £439 million in 1986, and £2.5 billion in 1992.[8] This rapid trend towards institutional care prompted a governmental review, and the

Table 116-1 Provision of residential care places in the UK				
	1980	**1985**	**1991/92**	**1994/95**
LA residential homes	134,500	137,100	117,400	86,400
Independent residential homes	80,000	130,400	203,100	218,200
Independent nursing homes	26,900	38,000	147,300	194,800
NHS geriatric/long-stay	46,100	46,300	44,300	34,700
Source: Department of Health.				

report *Caring for People* in 1989.[9] This resulted in a promotion of the development of domiciliary services to enable people to live in their own homes whenever feasible and sensible, with a renewed emphasis on proper assessments of need and case management.

The desirability of a flourishing independent sector along with good-quality public services and a new funding structure for social care were key elements of the report. The means to achieving this was to be through the transfer of the budget for long-term care to the social service departments of local municipalities, with a limitation on such expenditure. Social service departments became responsible for assessments of need, offering various choices, including (wherever possible) domiciliary support as an alternative to residential or nursing-home care. These recommendations were enshrined in the National Health Service Community Care Act 1990.[10]

Means testing, already an established feature of social services, was effectively extended to frail older people who were previously able to access free NHS care. Financial assessment frequently led to a requirement for self-funding until personal capital resources had dwindled to a very modest prescribed level. This was particularly discriminatory for nursing-home care in areas where a caucus of free NHS beds continued to exist side by side with private-sector provisions. Financial assessment took into account the value of a person's house, which had to be sold unless it was occupied also by an elderly spouse or other long-term relative.

Implemented in April 1993, these reforms brought marked and unintended inconsistencies in the level of care people experienced. Extraordinary packages of domiciliary care were sometimes provided, but the frailest entering institutional care were often placed in residential rather than nursing care because cost considerations displaced the broad awareness of the complexity and vulnerability of their clinical state. Social services funding for residential and nursing-care was not ring-fenced, financial settlements of local authorities tightened, and other competing statutory demands such as child protection services placed further pressures on funds for elderly care. Assessments became associated with rationing of placements into means-tested social care, with older people awaiting care acquiring the deplorable status of "hospital bed-blockers."

Some health authorities, particularly those with unsuitable outdated beds and a burgeoning independent provision, closed down their geriatric long-stay beds entirely, while others retained significant numbers. The anomaly of access to free NHS care for some and means-tested care for others, based more on geographic accident than need, was particularly unpopular among middle-class families—many of whom effectively became disinherited or resisted care in independent homes, insisting that it should be supplied free of charge by the health authority. Government guidance[11] required health authorities to provide some continuing NHS inpatient care, either in their own geriatric beds or in NHS-contracted beds in private nursing homes for people requiring long-term care in a number of categories detailed in the guidance. The processes and review procedures required to establish entitlement were labyrinthine, and in practice it seemed that if a similarly incapacitated person was being cared for in a nursing home there was no justification for NHS care. Unsurprisingly, this dogma made nursing-home care the norm for health authorities with

no long-term care beds, and the geographic lottery continued. This guidance also reaffirmed the rights of nursing-home residents to specialist care (whether placed there by social workers or self-financing) without payment. These services included stoma care, continence advice, diabetic advice, physiotherapy, speech therapy, and chiropody, as well as equipment not available on the general practitioner's prescription (with the exception of incontinence supplies).

Recently, care-home bed numbers have been declining. In the year 2000, of about 9,700 beds reported to have closed, 7,267 were in the private and voluntary sectors, and 2,481 were in local authority homes.[12] The balance of acute, rehabilitative, and long-term beds remains uncertain. However, the continuing problems that care homes experience in meeting escalating regulatory demands in the context of staff shortages and low fee levels undoubtedly have contributed to difficulties in the acute sector.

THE MEDICAL ROLE IN CARE

The medical supervision, leadership, and coordinated multidisciplinary care that had been the hallmark of traditional geriatric care in the UK did not follow the transfer and reclassification of NHS patients to care-home residents. General practitioners had new responsibilities thrust upon them, generally without contractual incentives to develop appropriate patterns of care and often in the absence of input from specialists.[13] The contrast with NHS care, where all long-stay patients remained under the nominal charge of a consultant physician in geriatric medicine, was stark. Discontinuities and inconsistencies of healthcare rapidly became evident.[14] Two surveys of consultant involvement in long-term care[15,16] produced similar findings, with 60–66 percent carrying out ward rounds once weekly or more often, although 15 percent visited the wards only monthly or less frequently. Consultants viewed their main role as providing expert medical advice and supporting nurses' morale. Day-to-day care was carried out by junior hospital doctors or general practitioners. Currently, the medical care provided by general practitioners in care homes is generally on a reactive episodic basis rather than planned, and the predictable medical needs of residents often remain unmet.[17] The largely empirically based model of British geriatric medicine featuring specialist assessment, treatment, and direction of rehabilitation are now seriously compromised.[18] Both primary and secondary healthcare are offering little more than a fire-fighting service to the most vulnerable.

Despite the official emphasis on the need for preadmission assessments, to avoid inappropriate institutionalization, evidence continues to indicate shortcomings. A multicenter audit in the late 1990s of nursing-home admissions revealed that only 40 percent had undergone specialist geriatric or psychogeriatric preadmission assessment.[19] A small single-center prospective study accepted older people referred by their general practitioners for long-term care for whom the responsible social workers had misgivings about the need for such care. Remarkably only 8 out of 33 were admitted to nursing-home care, with 13 being able to return home.[20] The trend for geriatric long-term care to be increasingly considered as part of primary care services, with regulation increasingly centered on style (process) rather than substance (outcomes), remains unsatisfactory.

QUALITY CONSIDERATIONS

For a long time there was no statutory mechanism for routine inspection of long-term care within the NHS. In 1969, a government agency—the Hospital Advisory Service, later renamed the Health Advisory Service (HAS)—was set up in response to a series of reports of patients mistreated in psychiatric hospitals. The HAS was charged with visiting geriatric and psychiatric departments of hospitals in rotation, the intention being to advise and encourage good practice rather than to admonish. A visiting team consisting of a consultant geriatrician, manager, nurse, and therapist would spend 1–2 weeks in a hospital and present a detailed report. Recommendations to the health authority would follow. For some time, HAS reporting had a limited circulation, although it did include the Secretary of State. Later reports became more generally available. The final report of the outgoing director of the HAS in 1987 stated: "The quality of long-term care offered to elderly people in hospital is still generally very poor. There is a growing contrast with the individual personal care offered in many local authority homes to elderly people with degrees of disability not significantly different from those seen in hospital."[21] The scope of the HAS inspection was restricted to hospitals, and proliferating nursing and residential care homes were outside its brief.

Many subsequent reports have encouraged positive attitudes for care, most notably *Home Life*, and its successor *A Better Home Life* which provides a code of good practice for residential and nursing-home care.[22] These reports espouse principles that should guide daily life in a continuing care setting (Table 116-2).

Clearly, maintenance of health at the best possible level is a prerequisite for care-home residents to be able to participate in a wide range of activities. In 1998, the Royal College of Physicians, the British Geriatrics Society, and the Royal Surgical Aid Society drew up clinical guidelines to enhance the health of older people in long-term care.[23] This report gave guidance on the management of dementia, depression, disability, autonomy, continence, medication, falls, and pressure care. Medication, particularly sedation, remains poorly managed[24] and has been the subject of explicit advice in a recent National Service Framework. This demands regular critical review of prescription charts,[25] and withdrawal of medicines likely to be unnecessary.

Table 116-2 Basic principles underpinning the rights accorded to all who find themselves in the care of others

- Respect for privacy and dignity
- Maintenance of self-esteem
- Fostering of independence
- Choice and control
- Recognition of diversity and individuality
- Expression of beliefs
- Safety
- Citizens' rights
- Sustaining relationships with relatives and friends
- Opportunities for leisure activities

Source: A Better Home, *Life Centre for Policy on Ageing, 1996.*

RECENT DEVELOPMENTS AND CONTEXT

Public and political uncertainty, particularly over the funding of care, prompted the establishment of a Royal Commission on long-term care.[26] The commission examined various funding options for the provision of housing and personal care. This authoritative review described the epidemiological uncertainties regarding future needs as the "funnel of doubt." This lack of knowledge regarding the illness and disability drivers that lead to care and the lack of intelligence regarding changing needs and expectations point to an urgent requirement for more epidemiological studies. Whilst it is unquestionably true that increasing numbers of older people are aging with greater success than ever, hopes that a compression of morbidity and dependency could render institutional care a transient historical phenomenon are perhaps overly optimistic (see Chapter 2). Stereotypes of a socially dispossessed elderly population are being replaced by a clinical reality of frail, very old people with complex physical and mental healthcare needs and an inherently unstable physiology.

Advances in healthcare techniques have resulted in the survival of many people who would previously have succumbed. This brings new and more complex clinical challenges in later life, with new patterns of disability and disease. It is paradoxical that, as levels of clinical need have increased, patients have been redesignated "residents and clients" with an illusory promise of increasing consumer rights, even though many care-home residents lack the ability to make informed choices. In reality their quality of life depends, as never before, on clinical care and health maintenance. Furthermore, the increasingly short lengths of stay in acute hospitals are leading to rapid discharge of older people who may not have received the personal health advocacy that traditionally was a feature of geriatric care. A typical instance would be a patient with a devastating stroke for whom enteral feeding is necessary to maintain hydration and nutrition in the period between acute stroke and time when a fully informed decision can be formulated regarding the need for and appropriateness of continued treatment. Such patients have traditionally remained in hospital with continuity of care being a positive contribution to difficult decision-making. Now it is not uncommon to see urgent insertion of feeding tubes and precipitant discharge, with scant regard to the planning of overall treatment objectives.

Currently there is an intense program of modernization of health and social care in the UK. A number of National Service Frameworks (NSFs), providing guidance in, and setting standards for, healthcare, have been established, including one for older people.[27] Care homes are destined to remain the focus of institutional long-term care. The government's response to the Royal Commission on long-term care has been to determine that, from October 2001, the separation of personal care and healthcare will be clarified through an eligibility assessment, with the professional nursing component of care being partly funded by the state and the remaining costs of care being met through a means-tested process. Real difficulties pervade the definition of "nursing care" as opposed to "personal care." The reality is that most requirements for professional nursing in care homes are dictated by regulation rather than evidence, and this underlines the need for a complete formulation of care. The NSF for older people includes a standard that "full multidisciplinary assessment should take place to identify and reduce inappropriate admission," and regulations surrounding the provision of monies for the nursing component of care demand regular reviews of needs. These developments may bring improvements, but another complicating factor is the prominence of Primary Care Trusts (PCTs) as principal commissioning agents in a revised NHS. PCTs are likely to serve similar populations as in social services departments. The establishment of Care Trusts that feature pooled budgets makes it possible that over the next decade such bodies could become the leading organizations for the provision of long-term care, in partnership with a variety of providers.

The Care Standards Act[28] presents an agenda that will reform the regulatory system for social care. National required standards for residential and nursing homes for older people were implemented from April 2002. The National Care Standards Commission (NCSC) is a single regulatory body replacing local authority registration and regulation of residential care and health authority regulation of nursing-home care. National consistency and a move away from a notion of adequacy to one of explicit standards are prime objectives of the new legislation; but the standards strongly emphasize the physical characteristics of the care institution, such as designating minimum room size and the fitness of care staff. The construct and outcomes management of care remain rather nebulous, and the NCSC has a structural bias to social care with attendant potential risk of clinical needs being overlooked. An expected collaborative involvement of the Commission for Health Improvement (CHI) with the NCSC may avoid this pitfall. Some reassurance may also be found in the NSF for older people through its requirement for the establishment of comprehensive assessment tools.

Nevertheless, a comprehensive strategy for long-term care in the UK remains elusive. A radical organizational proposal has been formulated by a working party of the Royal College of Physicians in partnership with the Royal College of Nursing and the British Geriatrics Society.[29] This features 10 recommendations that should collectively provide a comprehensive interdisciplinary approach to care (Table 116-3).

Several matters will greatly influence the future of long-term care in the UK beyond policy aspirations, expectations, and standard-setting. Improving packages of home care will bring increasing dependency in people being admitted to care homes, and cognitive impairment will grow as a principal determinant for institutionalization. There will be a predictable, continued increase in the complexity of individual and institutional management. The shortage of professional and general care support staff available for care is critical.[30] Low fee levels have meant poor levels of remuneration, dissuading some potential care staff and undermining staff retention, particularly in an economic climate of near full employment. An apparent widely held view was that the staff pool for the care sector was different, separate from that the NHS relied upon. The NHS faces a period where shortages of all professional staff are likely to constrain existing services, let alone allow development. An awareness that there is only one pool of staff may force the reformulation of long-term care in the spirit of the Royal College of Physicians' report of 2000. While long-term care in the UK remains inadequately defined and supported, to attention is likely to develop beyond the political difficulties of funding.

Table 116-3 Recommendations for a comprehensive interdisciplinary approach to the health and care of older people in care homes

- An agreed Comprehensive Assessment Tool should be adopted that records diagnoses along with disabilities to enable commissioning, inform care planning, and aid governance.
- Individual care planning should address clearly assessed needs and wishes of the individual. It should also identify expectations, responsibilities, and limitations of health and care. The care plan provides an individual benchmark from which an individual's care may be monitored.
- A population-based approach should be used for the planning and provision of services to residents in care homes. Integrating all the professions into an organization sized to address the care-home population needs is most likely to produce effective and efficient care.
- A specialist gerontological nurse should be the lead clinical practitioner for the identification and integration of healthcare support to the home in the care of its residents. Recognition, definition, development, and training within interdisciplinary care are required.
- General practitioners need their roles and responsibilities to be defined and supported in care homes. New ways of working should greatly improve patterns of care; training and qualifications should be encouraged and recognized.
- There is an urgent need to re-engage specialist geriatric medicine and old-age psychiatry in a structured manner with the care-home population.
- The management of medication and the role of the pharmacist may be enhanced through an institutional approach.
- The organization, application, and governance of all the professions allied to medicine may be enhanced through integration with other professionals and through core institutional-based care rather than individual contracting.
- A major investment in training, learning, and development is required for medical, nursing, social work, and paramedical professions. The concept of a "teaching nursing home" as a learning organization should be developed.
- Research is needed to inform further developments that aim to improve health and care outcomes through evidenced-based practice for care-home residents.

KEY POINTS UK long-term care

- Avoiding long-term care has been the priority of health and care services in the UK, with the consequence that long-term care itself is poorly developed.

- Inadequate epidemiological data regarding the population in long-term care has seriously undermined policy planning.

- Policy has centered on cost containment rather than needs, largely through ignorance.

- Regulation is being improved, but on its own will have limited effect in the improvement of care outcomes.

- A whole-system formulation (interdisciplinary and interorganizational) is required to provide integrated care for the emerging population in long-term care of clinically complex and unstable residents.

REFERENCES

1. Kirkwood T: The Time of Our Lives. Weidenfeld & Nicolson, London, 1999
2. Turrell AR, Castleton CM, Freestone B: Building on Sand: Long-stay care and the NHS—discontinuities between policy and practice. BMJ 1998;317:942–943
3. Warren M: Modern care of older people. Lancet 1947;i:761
4. Townsend P: The Last Refuge: A Survey of Residential Institutions and Homes for the Aged in England and Wales. Routledge & Kegan Paul, London, 1962
5. UK Department of Health: National Beds Inquiry. HMSO, London, 2000
6. Cochrane AL: Effectiveness and Efficiency: Random Reflections on Health Services. Nuffield Provincial Hospitals Trust, 1971
7. Isaacs B, Livingstone M, Neville Y: Survival of the Unfittest. Routledge & Kegan Paul, London, 1972
8. Care of Elderly People: Market Survey, 8th edn. Laing & Buisson, London, 1995
9. Secretary of State for Health and Social Services, Wales and Scotland: Caring for People: Community Care in the Next Decade and Beyond. HMSO, London, 1989
10. National Health Service and Community Care Act 1990: HMSO, London, 1990
11. UK Department of Health: NHS Responsibilities for Meeting Continuing Health Care Needs. Department of Health, London, 1995
12. Laing & Buisson: Community care. Market News 2001;8(1)
13. Black D, Bowman CE: Community institutional care for frail elderly: time to structure professional responsibility. BMJ 1997;315:441–442
14. Hepple J, Bowler I, Bowman CE: A study of private nursing home residents in Weston-super-Mare. Age Ageing 1989;18:61–63
15. Andrews K, Brocklehurst J: British Geriatric Medicine in the 1980s. King's Fund Publishing Office, London, 1987:46–48
16. Black JM, Knight PV: Continuing hospital care in Scotland: a survey of consultant geriatricians. Health Bull 1991;49(2):146–151
17. Pearson J, Challis L, Bowman CE: Problems of care in a private nursing home. BMJ 1990;301:371–372
18. Bowman C, Johnson M, Venables D, Foote C, Kane RL: Geriatric care in the United Kingdom: aligning services to needs. BMJ 1999;319:1119–1121
19. Millard PH: Nursing Home Placements for Older People in England and Wales. A National Audit 1995–1998. Department of Geriatric Medicine, St George's Hospital Medical School, London, 1999
20. Hutchinson SG, Tarrant J, Severs MP: An inpatient bed for acute nursing home admissions. Age Ageing 1998;27:95–98
21. Health Advisory Service: Annual Report. London, 1987
22. Centre for Policy on Ageing: A Better Home Life: A Code of Practice for Residential and Nursing Home Care. London, 1996
23. Royal College of Physicians, British Geriatrics Society, and Royal Surgical Aid Society: Enhancing the Health of Older People in Long-Term Care. Royal College of Physicians, London, 1998
24. McGrath AM, Jackson GA: Survey of neuroleptic prescribing in residents of nursing homes in Glasgow. BMJ 1996;312:611–612
25. UK Department of Health: Medicines and Older People: Implementing the Medicines-Related Aspects of the NSF for Older People. DoH, London, 2001
26. Royal Commission on Long Term Care: With Respect to Old Age. HMSO, London, 1999
27. UK Department of Health: National Service Framework for Older People. DoH, London, 2001
28. UK Department of Health: Care Standards Act 2001. HMSO, London, 2001
29. Royal College of Physicians: The Health and Care of Older People in Care Homes: A Comprehensive Interdisciplinary Approach. RCP, London, 2000
30. Henwood M for the King's Fund Care & Support Worker Inquiry: Future Imperfect. King's Fund, London, 2001

Chapter 117

Institutional long-term care services in the USA

Joseph G. Ouslander and Andrew D. Weinberg

The purpose of this chapter is to give non-American readers a brief perspective on the role of the nursing home and assisted living facilities (ALFs) in the care of the geriatric population in the USA. American nursing homes, also referred to as long-term care facilities (LTCs), are institutions that provide health, social, and recreational services to chronically ill people who, for a variety of reasons, cannot be managed in their own homes. There are several different types of LTC facilities, and the number of beds in each facility varies considerably, usually averaging 100–120 beds per facility. Because of the way that health and social services are funded, and the regulations imposed on LTC facilities by the federal and state governments, these facilities tend to follow a medical rather than a social model. Thus, most American LTC facilities look like and are administered in a manner similar to small acute-care hospitals, rather than residential homes in which skilled nursing, medical, and other services are available. Medical oversight of LTC facilities is provided by a physician medical director. This federally mandated position allows input by the medical director into policy and procedure development, and is a valuable liaison to the administrator and director of nursing. The medical director is also required to provide, or arrange for, emergency medical coverage when a resident's primary care physician-of-record cannot be reached.

At any one time about 5 percent, or 1.7 million, of America's population aged 65 years and older is in an LTC facility. But this is a deceiving statistic, for several reasons. First, the rate of LTC use varies considerably with age and sex. Among those 65–74 years of age, less than 3 percent are in an LTC facility; among those 85 years of age and older, about 15 percent of men and 25 percent of women are in an LTC facility, and close to one-half in this age group die there or shortly after discharge from an LTC setting to an acute-care hospital.[1] Second, a subgroup of LTC residents stay for only a short period. Thus, this lifetime risk of entering an LTC facility is underestimated by the prevalence data cited above. It is now estimated that Americans who were 65 years old in the year 1990 have a 43 percent chance of spending some time in an LTC facility; the chance is greater for women (about 50 percent) than for men (about 33 percent).[2] Third, for every elderly American in an LTC setting, there are two or three with a similar clinical and functional status living at home. The primary factors that determine whether an American enters an LTC setting include their medical and functional status, the availability and accessibility of noninstitutional community-based long-term care services, and economic factors.[1,3,4]

Despite the growth of community-based long-term care programs and the increasing number of assisted living facilities, the need for LTCs continues to grow. This is in large part due to the decreasing availability of children, especially daughters (who provide the most support to frail older Americans and who are increasingly joining the workforce, thus limiting their caregiving abilities) and to economic factors. Economic factors are critical, and are very different in the USA than in countries with a national health program. Thus, in order to understand the American LTC environment, one must understand how long-term care is financed in the USA.[1,5,6]

ECONOMIC CONSIDERATIONS

Healthcare for older Americans is funded in one of four basic ways: (1) private health insurance, (2) Medicare, (3) Medicaid, and (4) out-of-pocket expenditures. Although approximately 100 insurance companies are marketing long-term care policies, private insurance still plays a very small role in paying for LTCs at the present time. Medicare is a federally administered health insurance program for those aged 65 or older. The vast majority of older Americans qualify for basic Medicare coverage by contributions they or a spouse have made during their working years. Although most older Americans still incorrectly believe that Medicare will pay for LTC, it is not until they or a relative needs long-term care that reality sets in. Less than 5 percent of Medicare expenditures go to LTC settings, and overall less than 5 percent of long-term care is funded by Medicare.[3] Medicare will annually pay for up to 100 days of subacute long-term care after an acute illness, but only under specific circumstances. In order to qualify for Medicare reimbursement, subacute admission must follow a 3-day stay in an acute-care hospital, and the patient must require continuous "skilled" nursing care and/or active rehabilitation with carefully documented potential and progress to achieve the 100-day allocation.[7,8] Patients recovering from a hip fracture or stroke with good rehabilitation potential, and patients with unstable medical conditions (such as those requiring intravenous medications), will qualify for some Medicare coverage, usually for a few weeks. Patients with dementia and other chronic functional disabilities, on the other hand, are viewed as requiring "custodial" care, and do not qualify for Medicare coverage. Thus, the vast majority of funding for LTCs comes from Medicaid and out-of-pocket expenditures. Medicaid is a state-administered medical welfare program for the poor; one has to have very limited assets (for example, less than $2,000 monthly income, excluding a house) to qualify. This has created a phenomenon known as "spend down"; older Americans must spend down their assets to pay for long-term care until they become poor enough to qualify for Medicaid, which will then cover their LTC costs. Because private pay rates for most

LTC facilities are in the range of $4,000 to $5,000 per month, spend down occurs quickly for most older Americans who enter an LTC setting.[3]

The growth of managed, capitated systems of care is also substantially impacting the LTC industry in certain areas with a high penetration of managed care (e.g. California, Oregon, Arizona, Minnesota, Washington, Florida). In a capitated system of care, an insurance company (health maintenance organization) receives a fixed rate per Medicare beneficiary per month. One of the main ways of saving money in this system is to reduce the number of acute hospitals days. As a result, patients in these capitated health plans are being discharged very quickly from acute hospitals into nursing homes while still subacutely ill. In addition, because in capitated systems there is no 3-day acute hospital requirement for Medicare reimbursement of subacute days, some subacutely ill patients may completely bypass the acute hospital. For example, patients with deep vein thrombosis, or mild pneumonia or cellulitis requiring intravenous antibiotics, are commonly directly admitted to LTC facilities with subacute units without an acute hospital stay. These economic incentives are driving the growth of a new level of LTC called "subacute care" (discussed later in this chapter).

Home LTC facility care is presently a $60-plus billion industry, and the costs are expected to rise rapidly over the next several decades.[3,6] There are community-based long-term care services that may delay nursing-home admission for some older patients, but these services are still evolving, and some of them are rare (such as day hospitals). In most areas LTC services are poorly coordinated and difficult for older seniors and their families to locate, and they are generally not reimbursed by Medicare or private insurance. Care in assisted living facilities is not covered by Medicare or Medicaid, and can be a substantial out-of-pocket expenditure (as much or more than a nursing home, depending on the area and services provided). Thus, it is not surprising that the delivery and costs of long-term care have recently become major societal issues for US citizens as well as the politicians that govern the country.[6,9–11] Some states have attempted to decrease the rise in Medicaid LTC spending through the use of a waiver program. These programs allow older individuals eligible for Medicaid-covered long-term care to receive a range of community and home-based services (e.g. nursing assistants, nursing care, day care) to help prevent or delay the need for LTC placement.

ASSISTED LIVING FACILITIES

Assisted living facilities (ALFs) are a growing entity in the continuum of long-term care. In general, they are residential units that can provide additional services to residents, including meal preparation, laundry, housekeeping, incontinence care, and limited medication management. It is estimated by the American Health Care Association that there are at least 9,000 to 10,000 ALFs in operation with 500,000 to 1.1 million residents residing in these facilities.

Often costing 50 percent or less of the cost of care in an LTC facility, they cannot legally provide skilled nursing care, medical treatments, or direct administration of prescription medicines. The vast majority do not have medical oversight by a physician or licensed nurses present around the clock. Unlike skilled LTC facilities, physicians are not required to visit residents in these facilities.

The majority of ALFs are managed by a full-time care coordinator and a number of nursing assistants. Some ALFs may have licensed nurses present during daytime hours or are available on-call for emergencies. As ALFs do not receive Medicare funding, they are outside the purview and regulation of federal laws and are regulated in varying degrees on a state-by-state basis. Medical care is provided by a resident's own personal primary care physician, and most often families must arrange transportation to and from the doctor's office.

In summary, although ALF costs are, on average, less than institutional long-term care, this cost remains unaffordable to many low-and-moderate income seniors. Seniors needing skilled nursing care, intensive rehabilitation, and medication administration, will still generally require placement in an LTC facility.

CHARACTERISTICS OF NURSING HOMES

In the USA there are more nursing home/LTC beds than acute-care hospital beds. There are between 6,000 and 7,000 acute-care hospitals with a total of approximately 1 million beds, and there are over 17,000 nursing homes with over 1.6 million beds. Table 117-1 outlines selected characteristics of the nursing homes. Three-quarters are run for profit, and a large proportion of these are run by organizations that own several or a chain of nursing homes. Most LTC facilities average 100–120 beds. Thus, the typical American nursing home is a privately owned and operated free-standing facility of between 50 and 200 beds. A few nursing homes are hospital-based, occupying an unused ward in an acute-care hospital. Others are located on the campus of a multilevel long-term care community, such as a "life care" or "continuing care retirement" community. The federal and state governments also operate some nursing homes, including over 120 in the Veterans Administration system that serves veterans of US armed forces eligible for LTC placement.

Table 117-1 Selected characteristics of American long-term care facilities and assisted living facilities

Total number of nursing homes	16,706
Total number of residents	1.8 million
For-profit nursing homes	73%
Non-profit or church-related nursing homes	22%
Government-run nursing homes	4%
Nursing-home size (in number of licensed beds)	
50–100	48%
101–150	32%
151–200	13%
201+	7%
Assisted living facilities	11,472
Total number of residents	558,400

Data extracted from references 66, 67, and 68.

Nursing-home staff

The key staff in an American nursing home are the administrator, who is responsible for the day-to-day operation of the facility, and the director of nursing, who supervises the bulk of the facility's employees. Most nursing homes have very few registered and licensed nurses; staff ratios average about one registered nurse for each 50 beds and one licensed vocational nurse for each 25–30 beds. Over 90 percent of the hands-on care in American nursing homes is provided by certified nursing assistants (CNAs), who are generally poorly educated, may not speak English (especially in some areas), and are poorly paid (generally starting salaries under $7.00 per hour). CNA turnover rates exceed 90 percent a year in many facilities. In many, other members of the interdisciplinary team, including the rehabilitation therapists, social workers, activity therapists, and dietitians are part-time and work under contract, rather than as employees of the nursing home. Ancillary services, such as bioclinical laboratory, radiography, dentistry, and podiatry, are provided by outside contractors. Only in very large facilities will one find full-time multidisciplinary staff who provide the types of services mentioned above.

Nursing-home residents

Residents of American LTC facilities are generally characterized as predominantly older women with impaired mobility and dementia. It is true that close to three-quarters of LTC residents are women and older than 75 years, over one-half are nonambulatory and need assistance in transferring, and over one-half have some degree of dementia.[5] But this type of characterization masks the heterogeneity of the LTC population. Residents in American LTC facilities can be broadly characterized based on their length of stay: "short" (i.e. 1–6 months) versus "long." Short-stayers can be subdivided into two groups: patients who enter an LTC facility for short-term rehabilitation after an acute illness (e.g. hip fracture, stroke), and those who are medically unstable or terminally ill who are either quickly discharged to an acute hospital or will eventually die in an LTC setting. The proportion of LTC residents who are short-stayers is growing because patients are being rapidly discharged from acute hospitals, and, as mentioned earlier, some acutely ill patients in capitated systems of care are admitted directly to LTC facilities in order to avoid costly acute

hospital stays. Long-stayers can be subdivided into three groups: those with primarily cognitive impairment (e.g. the ambulatory, wandering resident with Alzheimer's disease or related dementia), those with primarily impairments of physical functioning (e.g. the resident with severe arthritis or end-stage heart or lung disease), and residents with both cognitive and physical impairments. Figure 117-1 illustrates this subgrouping of the LTC population. Obviously residents may move from one subgroup to another when acute illnesses intervene, chronic illness develops or progresses, or cognitive function declines.

Conceptualizing LTC residents in this manner has important implications for the goals of care, for quality assurance, and even for the structure of the LTC environment. The goals of caring for a previously healthy patient undergoing rehabilitation after a hip fracture are obviously very different from the goals of caring for an LTC resident with advanced dementia and related behavioral disorders, or the goals of caring for someone with a terminal malignancy. Similarly, from the perspective of quality assurance, processes and outcomes of care relevant for one subgroup of LTC residents may be inappropriate or irrelevant to another subgroup. From a structural standpoint, many American LTC facilities attempt to geographically separate different subgroups of patients. This approach offers many potential advantages when it is feasible: the physical environment can be modified for certain types of residents (e.g. wanderers), the staff can be trained and develop expertise in managing specific types of care (e.g. terminal or hospice type care, or rehabilitative care), and residents are often more comfortable when they are around others to whom they can relate. The latter is especially true for cognitively intact patients who are often very distressed by constant interaction, especially at mealtimes, with residents who have dementia and associated behavioral disorders.

MEDICAL CARE

The goals of medical care in American LTC facilities are listed in Table 117-2. Although these goals appropriately focus on several nonmedical aspects of care, the increasing acuity of medical conditions of residents in LTC facilities, and the influence

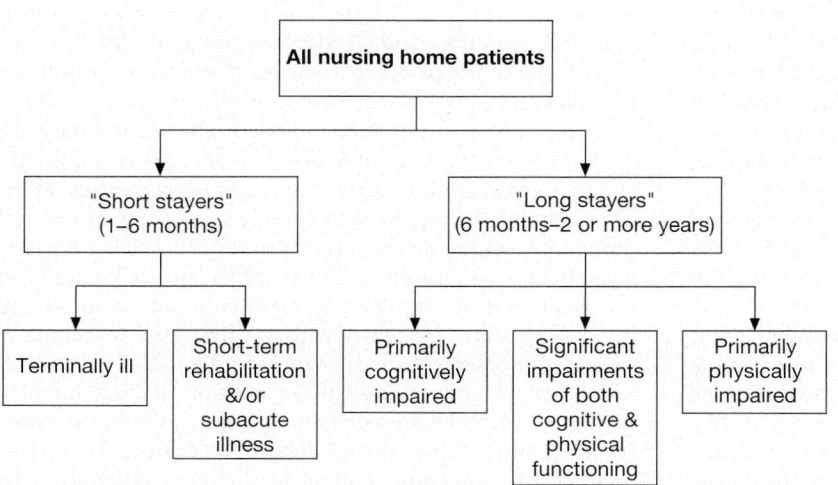

Figure 117-1 Types of patients in US long-term care (LTC) facilities. From Kane et al.,[1] with permission.

Table 117–2 Goals of care in American LTC facilities

- Provide a safe and supportive environment for chronically ill and dependent people.
- Restore and maintain the highest possible level of functional independence.
- Preserve individual autonomy.
- Maximize quality of life, perceived well-being, and life satisfaction.
- Provide comfort and dignity for terminally ill patients and their loved ones.
- Stabilize and delay progression, whenever possible, of chronic medical conditions.
- Prevent acute medical and iatrogenic illnesses, and identify and treat them rapidly when they do occur.
- Provide rehabilitation-oriented interdisciplinary care to subacutely ill patients

Source: Adapted from Ouslander et al.[5]

Table 117–3 Examples of admission criteria to subacute units

- Intravenous or central line administered antibiotics
- Physical therapy five times per week (minimum 90 min/d)
- Occupational therapy five times per week
- Weaning oxygen requirement with pulse oximetry
- Tracheal suctioning at least two times per shift
- Respiratory therapy treatment three times a day or more frequently
- Capillary blood glucose monitoring two times a day, with insulin coverage
- Injectable medications every 8 hours or twice a day
- Wound care (sterile) daily for pressure ulcers
- Tube feedings
- Laboratory monitoring required every 2–3 days
- Renal dialysis with monitoring
- Bladder/bladder training protocols
- Pain management (parenteral)
- Skilled nursing observation of congestive heart, liver, or renal failure

these conditions have on function and quality of life, demand that physicians be intimately involved in long-term care.[5,12]

Financial pressure to reduce the costs of care, especially acute hospital care, and the growth of capitated, managed care have led to the emergence of a new level of medical care in LTC facilities: "subacute care." Provided in designated units within free-standing LTC facilities and in acute hospital wards that have been designated as subacute or transitional care units, subacute care (post-acute care) has been defined by the Joint Commission on Accreditation of Health Care Organizations as comprehensive inpatient care designed for someone who has an acute illness, injury, or exacerbation of a disease process. It is goal-oriented treatment rendered immediately after, or instead of, acute hospitalization to treat one or more specific active complex medical conditions or to administer one or more technically complex treatments, in the context of a person's underlying long-term conditions and overall situation. Generally, the individual's condition is such that the care does not depend heavily on high-technology monitoring or complex diagnostic procedures. Subacute care requires the coordinated services of an interdisciplinary team including physicians, physician assistants, nurse practitioners, nurses, rehabilitation therapists, and other relevant professional disciplines, who are trained and knowledgeable to assess and manage these specific conditions and perform the necessary procedures. Subacute care is given as part of a specifically defined program, regardless of the site. It is generally more intensive than traditional nursing-home care and less than acute care. It requires frequent (daily or weekly) recurrent patient assessment and review of the clinical course and treatment plan for a limited period (several days to several months), until the condition is stabilized or a predetermined treatment course is completed. A maximum of 100 days' coverage per calendar year are allowed per Medicare Part A rules. Most patients, however, are not covered by Medicare for the full 100 days owing to current reimbursement rules.

Table 117-3 lists examples of conditions typically treated in subacute units. Subacute care poses a number of challenges for the American LTC facility. Nursing staff must become trained and experienced in the management of more acutely ill patients, and there is a more rapid turnover of patients, which requires more intensive discharge planning. Diagnostic testing (laboratory tests, X-rays, etc.) must be available with a rapid completion time. More comprehensive and integrated interdisciplinary involvement, especially by rehabilitative staff, is necessary, and structural changes in the facility may be required, such as in-room oxygen and larger therapy areas. The LTC facility administrative staff must be capable of accurately tracking costs of care, associated revenues, and patient outcomes. Finally, more intense involvement of medical staff than is typical in most American LTC facilities is essential.

The vast majority of American LTC facilities are too small to have a full-time medical staff or even a full-time medical director, although a small proportion of the larger facilities have both. Most facilities have a loosely organized medical staff supervised by a medical director who works part-time for the nursing home and is paid on an hourly, monthly, or annual basis.[13] Because most American LTC facilities are run for profit and have an open medical staff, numerous primary care physicians may be involved in a single facility. It is common for dozens of physicians to provide primary care for only a few residents in a small or medium-sized facility. This situation can make it difficult for nursing staff to develop effective communication and rapport with the medical staff, as well as making it more difficult for the medical director to monitor policies, procedures, and standards for medical care.

The role of the primary attending physician in American LTC facilities is to perform a comprehensive medical evaluation at the time of admission, to periodically reassess the resident's progress (visits at intervals of 30–60 days are required), and to assess acute and subacute changes when they occur.[5,14] Thus, physicians usually visit facilities only once or twice a month, depending on the number of residents they have in a given facility. Because physicians are generally not physically in the facility, various regulations and their interpretation result in nursing staff frequently calling physicians to report a variety of problems, such as changes in mental status, weight loss, laboratory values, and falls. In addition, acute changes in residents' conditions are generally reported by telephone, often resulting in transfer of the resident to the emergency department of an acute-care hospital for further evaluation.[15–19]

The lack of physician presence in American LTC facilities therefore results in many unnecessary phone calls and the overuse of acute-care hospital emergency departments for patient evaluation. One potential solution is the involvement of physicians' assistants (PAs) and/or nurse practitioners (NPs).[5,20–23] They are trained in basic patient care assessment techniques, and generally manage acute and subacute conditions using standard protocols under the supervision of a physician. They may be hired by a physician or a group of physicians and spend a substantial amount of their time in the facility. PAs and NPs are required to have clinical privileges granted at the nursing facility at which they work, and need ongoing supervision by the attending physician (either by telephone or in person). Currently they are reimbursed 85 percent of the physician's allowable scale.

A new model introduced during the mid-1990s, called EverCare, provides a nurse practitioner to cover a panel of nursing-home residents at no cost to the facility of the attending physicians.[24] This model, although funded as a pilot project by Medicare, is administered by a private insurance company and currently operates in 13 states.

QUALITY OF CARE

Unfortunately, the quality of medical care provided in most American LTC facilities is far from optimal.[10,25] Many treatable conditions, such as depression and urinary incontinence, are undiagnosed or misdiagnosed;[26–29] documentation in medical records is poor; many medications, especially psychotropic drugs and antimicrobials, are overused or misused;[29,30–33] and there is little if any input from psychiatrists or psychologists despite the high prevalence of mental morbidity among LTC patients.[27,28,34]

There are several factors that contribute to this less than optimal quality of care, including educational, attitudinal, and financial. Very few American physicians have had any formal training in geriatric medicine. Most medical schools have no required geriatric curriculum, and there are fewer than 2,000 physicians with postgraduate training in geriatric medicine.[35] Even among the latter, the majority do not spend a lot of time in LTC facilities and only a small proportion of practicing physicians attend at LTC facilities.[36] Currently there is a severe shortage of nurses and certified nursing assistants in the USA for several reasons, including work-related stress, understaffing issues, lower pay scales in the nursing-home setting, and heavy workloads with clinically difficult residents. Turnover rates for licensed nurses can exceed 45 percent a year and those of nursing assistants approach 100 percent a year. Many physicians have the same attitude as the American public: an LTC facility is the last stop on the way to death, and once in this setting there is little that can be done to improve the medical situation. To compound the educational and attitudinal barriers, caring for residents in LTC facilities is not often a rewarding activity. In addition to the financial disincentive, it is a logistical problem for physicians with busy office and hospital practices to go to such facilities frequently.[35] Thus, there are strong incentives for physicians to not visit residents in LTC facilities and to send these individuals to acute-care hospitals when their condition changes. Admission to an acute-care hospital is not only much more expensive than care in an LTC facility, the transfer can be physically and emotionally disruptive for residents and their families, and the acute-care hospital is fraught with iatrogenic hazards for this patient population (such as adverse drug reactions, falls, delirium, and pressure sores).[16,37]

New federal rules and regulations, implemented in 1991,[11] continue to help improve the quality of long-term care. They contain many provisions pertaining to resident's rights and quality of care, and require an active quality-assurance committee in each facility. The regulations also mandate a comprehensive, multidisciplinary assessment containing specific data (the Minimum Data Set or MDS). The MDS must be completed on admission, annually, and at the time of every major change in status; selected items on the MDS must be updated quarterly. The MDS is one component of the Resident Assessment Instrument, the other being the Resident Assessment Protocols (RAPs). The RAPs are "triggered" by specific items from the MDS, and basically represent clinical practice guidelines for 18 conditions common in the LTC population.[14] The American Medical Directors Association (AMDA) has introduced during the last five years a number of practice guidelines to help standardize the approach to a variety of clinical issues, including falls, incontinence, depression, dementia, altered mental status, pressure ulcers, chronic pain, and osteoporosis.[38] Although not yet widely implemented, these AMDA practice guidelines offer a rational and practical approach for nursing-home staff to utilize when addressing common clinical concerns.

ETHICAL ISSUES

Ethical issues arise on a daily basis in the care of LTC residents. Ethical considerations play an important role in decisions about the intensity of care provided to a very elderly and terminally ill LTC resident.[39–49] It is beyond the scope of this chapter to discuss these considerations in any detail; however, a few key issues will be mentioned briefly. One of the goals of long-term care is to preserve individual autonomy (see Table 117-2). The high prevalence of dementia among LTC residents makes this complicated as there are no validated methods of determining when patients with dementia are no longer capable of making healthcare decisions and no well-established standards for surrogate decision-makers.[50,51] Advance directives, such as a durable power of attorney for healthcare, offers a potential solution by enabling a person, while still capable, to designate a surrogate decision-maker and state his or her preferences in the event of serious illness.[51] The increased use of advance directives and their incorporation into nursing-home medical records will, it is hoped, preserve individual autonomy and at the same time guide physicians in managing serious illnesses that arise in their residents. Ethics committees may also play a role in approaching difficult clinical situations.[52]

FUTURE PERSPECTIVES

Although many American LTC facilities provide excellent care, the overall quality of care in this setting must be improved—especially given the projected enormous need for and costs of long-term care over the next several decades. At least three approaches will be required: changes in the way that LTC is financed, ongoing education and training, and research. The potential costs of LTC in the USA over the next several decades are staggering. At the present time many state governments are experimenting with a Medicaid payment system that would base reimbursement for custodial residents on the resources required to care for specific subgroups of residents, and the prevalence of the different subgroups in a particular facility (so-called RUGS or Resource Utilization Groups).[53] A prospective payment system based on RUGS is already in place for Medicare Part A subacute patient stays. The subgrouping will be based on assessment data that LTC facilities are required to collect as part of the MDS. In theory, RUGS will distribute reimbursement more equitably based on residents' needs. There is one caveat about this reimbursement scheme; it may create an incentive to keep residents sicker and more dependent to achieve higher reimbursement rates. Appropriate adjustments will have to be incorporated for rehabilitative approaches to care and new approaches to quality assurance are also being developed. Increasingly, principles of total quality management and continuous quality improvement are being applied in LTC facilities.[53,54] Quality indicators have also been developed that are derived from MDS data.[55] These and other quality indicators will be used by regulatory agencies to target more specific quality assurance activities on a state, regional, or national basis.

More than financial changes and regulations will be necessary to improve care in American LTC facilities. Education in geriatric medicine, gerontology, and long-term care must increase for physicians, nurses, and all other healthcare professionals who care for LTC residents.[56–58] The USA has made great strides in this regard over the last decade, but much more must be done to meet the tremendous needs for adequately trained health professionals over the next several decades. The LTC facility must increasingly become a research laboratory,[59–61] and a broad range of research is needed. Basic studies will help determine the causes, treatment, and prevention of conditions that lead to LTC admission, such as Alzheimer's disease, stroke, and osteoporosis. Clinical trials can also assist in identifying the most effective strategies for managing common conditions among LTC residents, such as urinary incontinence,[62,63] depression,[64] and behavioral disorders associated with dementia. There is some difficulty translating research into practical clinical practice in the nursing-home setting, and this remains an ongoing challenge. Nonbiomedical research is also needed to address issues of quality of life and ethics, which are so important in the LTC populations. Health services research will help identify methods of defining, measuring, and improving quality of care, and in determining the most cost-effective strategies for managing many aspects of long-term care. Only through this type of multifaceted research will we learn more about caring for the millions of people who will spend some time in an American LTC facility. Additionally, research can help identify methods of improving quality of care which may decrease the risk of litigation against LTC facilities seen during the last decade.[65]

KEY POINTS Long-term care in the USA

- At any one time, approximately 1.7 million Americans reside in a long-term care facility in the USA, with the majority being female and 85 years or older.

- The primary factors that determine admission to a nursing facility include an individual's underlying medical condition and functional status, and the availability of family support and community-based programs.

- Assisted living facilities are residential units that can provide meal preparation, laundry, housekeeping, incontinence care, and limited medication management but do not provide on-site medical or nursing services as do nursing facilities.

- Most US long-term care facilities are run for profit. Medicare (health insurance for the old) pays only for care for limited periods for those who meet specific criteria. Most care is an out-of-pocket expense for older individuals and their families, unless they are very poor and qualify for state medical assistance (Medicaid).

- In long-term care nursing facilities there are few registered nurses and often only one licensed practical (vocational) nurse for each 25–30 beds. Typically over 90 percent of the hands-on care in American nursing facilities is provided by certified nursing assistants who are generally poorly educated and paid low wages.

- Quality of care in nursing facilities remains a critical issue facing the long-term care industry. Many medical conditions, such as depression and urinary incontinence, remain misdiagnosed or untreated.

- Polypharmacy, including the overutilization of antipsychotics and antibiotics, remains an ongoing challenge to the healthcare provider in long-term care.

REFERENCES

1. Kane RA, Ouslander JG, Abrass IB: Essentials of Clinical Geriatrics, 4th edn. McGraw-Hill, New York, 1999

2. Kemper D, Murtaugh C: Lifetime use of nursing home care. N Engl J Med 1991;324:595–600

3. Kane RA, Kane RL: Long-Term Care: Principles, Programs and Policies. Springer-Verlag, New York, 1987

4. Mittleman M, Ferris S, Shulman E et al: A family intervention to delay nursing home placement of patients with Alzheimer disease. JAMA 1996;276:1725–1731

5. Ouslander JG, Osterweil D, Morley J: Medical Care in the Nursing Home, 2nd edn. McGraw-Hill, New York, 1996

6. Weiner J: Financing long-term care: a proposal by the American College of Physicians and the American Geriatrics Society. JAMA 1994;271:1525–1529

7. Loeser WD, Dickstein ES, Schiavone LD: Medicare coverage in nursing homes: a broken promise. N Engl J Med 1981;304:353–355

8. Smits HL, Feder J, Scanlon W: Medicare's nursing home benefit: variations in interpretation. N Engl J Med 1981;307:353–356

9. Harrington C, Cassel C, Estes CL et al: A national long-term care program for the United States: a caring vision. JAMA 1991;266:3023–3029

10. US Institute of Medicine: Improving the Quality of Care in Nursing Homes. National Academy Press, Washington, DC, 1986

11. Kane RL: Improving the quality of long-term care. JAMA 1995;273:1376–1380

12. US Department of Health and Human Services, Health Care Financing Administration: Medicare and Medicaid: Conditions of Participation for

Long-Term Care Facilities; Final Rule with Requests for Comments. Federal Register, 1989;54:5317–5373

13. Levenson S (ed): Medical Direction in Long-Term Care, 2nd edn. Carolina Academic Press, Durham, NC, 1993

14. Levenstein MR, Ouslander JG, Rubenstein LZ, Forsythe SB: Yield of routine annual laboratory tests in a skilled nursing home population. JAMA 1987;258:1909–1915

15. Kayser-Jones JS, Wiener CL, Barbaccia JC: Factors contributing to the hospitalization of nursing home residents. Gerontologist 1989;29:502–510

16. Rubenstein LZ, Ouslander JG, Wieland D: Dynamics and clinical implications of the nursing home: hospital interface. Clin Geriatr Med 1988;4:471–491

17. Weiner JM, Skaggs J: Current Approaches to Integrating Acute and Long-Term Care Financing and Services. American Association of Retired Persons Public Policy Institute, Publication 9516, Washington, DC, 1995

18. Ouslander J, Weinberg A, Phillips V: Inappropriate hospitalization of nursing facility residents: a symptom of a sick system of care for frail older people. J Am Geriatr Soc 2000;48:230–231

19. Saliba D, Kington R, Buchanan J et al: Appropriateness of the decision to transfer nursing facility residents to the hospital. J Am Geriatr Soc 2000;48:154–163

20. Martin SE, Turner CL, Mendelsohn S, Ouslander JG: Assessment and initial management of acute medical problems in a nursing home. In Bosker G (ed): Principles and Practice of Acute Geriatric Medicine. CV Mosby, St Louis, MO, 1989

21. Kane RA, Kane RL, Arnold S, Garrard J et al: Geriatric nurse practitioners as nursing home employees: implementing the role. Gerontologist 1988;28:469–477

22. Kane RA, Garrard J, Skay L et al: Effects of a geriatric nurse practitioner on process and outcome of nursing home care. Am J Pub Health 1989;79:1271–1277

23. Wieland D, Rubenstein LZ, Ouslander JG, Martin SE: Organizing an academic nursing home: impacts on institutionalized elderly. JAMA 1986;255:2622–2627

24. Kane R, Huck S: The implementation of the EverCare Demonstration Project. J Am Geriatr Soc 2000;48:218–223

25. Vladek B: Unloving Care: The Nursing Home Tragedy. Basic Books, New York, 1980

26. Ouslander JG, Kane RL, Abrass IB: Urinary incontinence in elderly nursing home patients. JAMA 1982;248:1194–1198

27. Borson S, Liptzin B, Nininger J et al: Psychiatry in the nursing home. Am J Psychiat 1987;144:1412–1418

28. Rovner B, German PS, Brant LJ et al: Depression and mortality in the nursing home. JAMA 1991;265:993–996

29. Zimmer JG, Bentley DW, Valenti WM et al: Systemic antibiotic use in nursing homes: a quality assessment. J Am Geriatr Soc 1986;34:703–710

30. Beers M, Avorn J, Soumerai B et al: Psychoactive medication use in intermediate-care facility residents. JAMA 1988;260:3016–3020

31. Ray WA, Federspeil CF, Schaffner W: A study of antipsychotic drug use in nursing homes: epidemiologic evidence suggesting misuse. Am J Pub Health 1980;70:485–491

32. Beers MH, Ouslander JG, Fingold SF et al: Inappropriate medication prescribing in skilled nursing facilities. Ann Intern Med 1992;117:684–689

33. Avorn J, Gurwitz JH: Drug use in the nursing home. Ann Intern Med 1995;123:195–204

34. Zimmer JG, Watson N, Treat A: Behavioral problems among patients in skilled nursing facilities. Am J Pub Health 1984;74:1118–1121

35. Rowe JW, Grossman E, Bond E: The institute of medicine committee on leadership for academic geriatric medicine: academic geriatrics for the year 2000. N Engl J Med 1984;316:1425–1428

36. Mitchell JB, Hewes HT: Why won't physicians make nursing home visits? Gerontologist 1986;26:650–654

37. Tresch DD, Simpson WM, Burton JR: Relationship of long-term and acute-care facilities: the problem of patient transfer and continuity of care. J Am Geriatr Soc 1985;33:819–826

38. American Medical Directors Association: Practice Guidelines. AHCPR Publications, Silver Spring, MD, 1996–1999

39. Besdine RW: Decisions to withhold treatment from nursing home residents. J Am Geriatr Soc 1983;30:602–606

40. Volicer L, Rheaume Y, Brown J et al: Hospice approach to the treatment of patients with advanced dementia of the Alzheimer's type. JAMA 1986;256:2210–2213

41. Lynn J (ed): No Extraordinary Means: The Choice to Forego Life-Sustaining Food and Water. University Press, Bloomington, IN, 1986

42. Uhlman RF, Clark H, Pearlman RA et al: Medical management decisions in nursing home patients: principles and policy recommendations. Ann Intern Med 1987;106:879–885

43. AGS Ethics Committee: The care of dying patients: a position statement from the American Geriatrics Society. J Am Geriatr Soc 1995;43:577–578

44. Steel K, Vitale C, Whang P: Annotated bibliography of palliative care and end-of-life care. J Am Geriatr Soc 2000;48:325–332

45. Zerzan J, Stearns S, Hanson L: Access to palliative care and hospice in nursing homes. JAMA 2000;284:2489–2494

46. Lynn J: Serving patients who may die soon and their families: the role of hospice and other services. JAMA 2001;285:925–932

47. O'Brien L, Grisso J, Maislin G et al: Nursing home residents' preferences for life-sustaining treatments. JAMA 1995;274:1775–1779

48. Molloy D, Guyatt G, Russo R et al: Systematic implementation of an advance directive program in nursing homes: a randomized controlled trial. JAMA 2000;283:1437–1444

49. Teno J: Advance directives for nursing home residents: achieving compassionate, competent, cost-effective care. JAMA 2000;283:1481–1482

50. Freedman M, Stuss DT, Gordon M: Assessment of competency: the role of neurobehavioral deficits. Ann Intern Med 1991;115:203–208

51. Emanuel EJ, Emanuel LL: Advance care planning as a process: structuring the discussions in practice. J Am Geriatr Soc 1995;43:440–446

52. Winn P, Cook J: Ethics committees in long-term care: a user's guide to getting started. Ann LTC 2000;8(1):35–42

53. Blumenthal D: Total quality management and physicians' clinical decisions. JAMA 1993;269:2775–2778

54. Schnelle JF, Ouslander JG, Osterweil D, Blumenthal S: Total quality management: administrative and clinical applications in nursing homes. J Am Geriatr Soc 1993;41:1259–1266

55. Zimmerman DR, Karon SL, Arling G et al: Development and testing of nursing home quality indicators. Health Care Financ Rev 1995;16:107–127

56. Aiken LH, Mezey MD, Lynaugh JE, Buck CR: Teaching nursing homes: prospects for improving long-term care. J Am Geriatr Soc 1985;33:196–201

57. Riesenberg D: The teaching nursing home: a golden annex to the ivory tower. JAMA 1987;257:3119–3120

58. Libow LS: The teaching nursing home: past, present and future. J Am Geriatr Soc 1984;32:598–603

59. Lipsitz LA, Pluchino FC, Wright SM: Biomedical research in the nursing home: methodological issues and subject recruitment results. J Am Geriatr Soc 1987;35:629–634

60. Rubenstein LZ, Wieland D (eds): Improving Care in the Nursing Home: Comprehensive Reviews of Clinical Research. Sage, London, 1993

61. Ouslander JG, Schnelle JF: Research in nursing homes: practical aspects. J Am Geriatr Soc 1993;41:182–187

62. Ouslander J, Schnelle J: Incontinence in the nursing home. Ann Intern Med 1995;122:438–449

63. Resnick N, Brandeis G, Baumann M et al: Evaluating a national assessment strategy for urinary incontinence in nursing home residents: reliability of the minimum data set and validity of the resident assessment protocol. Neurourol Urodynam 1996;15:583–598

64. The Medical Letter: Drugs for depression and anxiety. Med Lett Drugs Therapeut 1999;41(1050):33–38

65. Weinberg AD: Risk Management in Long-Term Care. Springer, New York, 1998

66. Marion Merrell Dow: Managed Care Digest, Long Term Care Edition. Marion Merrell Dow, Kansas City, MO, 1994

67. Stone RI: LTC for the Elderly with Disabilities: Current Policy, Emerging Trends and Implications for the 21st Century. Milbank Memorial Fund, New York, 2000

68. Hawes C, Rose M, Phillips CD et al: A National Study of Assisted Living for the Frail Elderly: Results of a National Telephone Survey of Facilities. Menorah Park Center for the Aging, Beachwood, OH, 1999

Chapter 118

Improving quality of care in the United Kingdom

David A. Black

Improving quality of care is difficult and controversial. Over the last 15 years in the UK there have been growing pressures from an increasing number of stakeholders to demonstrate and deliver quality improvement. From the inception of the National Health Service (NHS) politicians have been seen to be held responsible for a state-funded health service; patients are becoming increasingly knowledgeable and empowered to act and insist on improvements; healthcare purchasers have a particular interest in risk management processes owing to the influence of litigation; and finally the professions themselves have a growing interest in evidence-based medicine and delivering the best possible care. Yet the problems of improving care have recently been summarized by Brook who in a review states "in the last 30 years research has demonstrated that quality of care can be measured, the quality varies enormously, that where you go for care affects its quality far more than who you are, improving quality of care, while possible, is difficult, and in general has yet to be successfully accomplished."[1] Although this seems a pessimistic view, the gain from improving quality of care, when successful, can be spectacular. During the Crimea War, by enforcing improved standards of care and hygiene, Florence Nightingale reduced the mortality rates at the Scutari Military Hospital from 42.2 percent to 2 percent within 6 months.

Some may view the quality improvement movement as a management fashion. Yet the very success of geriatric medicine in the UK is a result of continuous improvements in the care of older people, starting in 1946 when Dr Marjory Warren identified the large numbers of older people confined in atrocious workhouse settings and denied effective healthcare. From those beginnings at the very onset of the NHS have evolved the comprehensive systems of assessment and care that are so different from the world of 1946. The development of geriatric medicine has been largely based on a persistent striving at local level for more and better services in the face of policy weakness, professional neglect, and resource starvation, coupled with poor training and a neglected research base. The healthcare of older people remains one of the major challenges for quality improvement within the health service particularly in the face of continual pressures to manage the growing number of the very old in the population.

The purpose of this chapter is to provide a theoretical understanding of the background to quality improvement by describing quality initiatives in the wider world of business and relating these to current health service policy with practical examples in geriatric medicine. A major problem for practitioners is the confusion of terminology and definitions. The experience of other areas, such as industry, has not been properly understood and the health service has been showered with initiatives, activities, jargon, and buzz words. The problems for clinicians have included failure to provide adequate commitment of time, significant problems with the information gathered, and difficulties implementing change when the needs have been identified. This chapter attempts to explain how the history of quality initiatives in business and the health service have led to the current government's approach, in particular the concept of clinical governance.

WHAT IS QUALITY?

At its very simplest, a basic working definition of highest quality care is "doing the right things well." In business, quality can be seen to have a number of dimensions:[2]

1. *Performance*—the primary operating characteristics or the product of services.
2. *Features*—add-ons or supplements.
3. *Reliability*.
4. *Conformance*—the degree to which a product's design and operating characteristics meet established standards.
5. *Durability*—measures of a product's life.
6. *Serviceability*—the speed and ease of repair.
7. *Esthetic*—the product's look, feel and taste.
8. *Perceived quality*—as viewed by a customer or client.

These dimensions do not map immediately to healthcare, and experts have struggled to find generally applicable definitions of the quality of healthcare.

The situation is especially complex as a service may have multiple customers, including the patient, the general practitioner (GP), and the local health authority. The World Health Organization divided quality into four aspects:[3]

- professional performance (technical quality);
- resource usage (efficiency);
- risk management (the risk of injury of illness associated with the services provided);
- patient satisfaction with the services provided.

Whatever definition is used, it must capture the complexity and variability of healthcare. One of the most widely used definitions was published by the Institute of Medicine in 1990 and states that quality consists of: *the degree to which health services for individual and populations increases the likelihood of desired health outcomes and are consistent with current professional knowledge.*[4]

Blumenthal has noted that healthcare professionals tend to define quality in terms of the attributes and results of care provided by practitioners.[5] This technical quality of care has two dimensions: the appropriateness of the services provided; and the skill with which appropriate care is performed. The biggest change for healthcare professionals has been to understand that care has also to be responsive to the preferences and values of consumers, particularly the individual patient.

A further view of quality, particularly in the UK, has been espoused by Maxwell.[6] This takes into account not just the individual patient but a wider population approach. Maxwell's six dimensions of quality are:

1. *Access* (issues such as physical accessibility and waiting times).
2. *Relevance to need* (appropriate to the assessed needs of the whole community).
3. *Effectiveness* (ability of the treatment or service to produce the desired result).
4. *Equity* (fair distribution of resources within the publicly funded system).
5. *Social acceptability* (including issues such as the environment and privacy).
6. *Efficiency and economy* (the best possible for the best possible price).

This model has been widely used for the purchasing or commissioning of services over the last decade in the UK.

MEASURING QUALITY OF CARE

Once the dimensions of quality have been identified, it should be possible to set standards and indicators of good practice (see later). However, we cannot start to improve the quality of care unless we are able to measure it. The real challenge is to find measures that are effective, that can be obtained inexpensively, and ideally that are part of the care process itself.

Quality of care may be assessed using measures of structure, process, or outcome. These three attributes were originally described by Donabedian.[7]

1. *Structure*—includes the building blocks and characteristics of healthcare, including buildings, equipment, and staff.
2. *Processes*—refers to all the activities forming the encounter between the healthcare professional and the patient, including diagnosis, tests, treatments, and record-keeping.
3. *Outcomes*—refers to the patient's subsequent health status as well as other effects of care, including knowledge and satisfaction.

These three attributes are interlinked, with both structure and process contributing to the outcome of care. There are implications:

- If quality-of-care criteria based on structural and process data are to be believed, it must be possible to show that variation in either process or structure leads to a difference in outcome.
- If outcome criteria are to be believable, it must be shown that differences in outcome will result if the processes under the control of the health professionals are altered.

Brook et al.[8] argue that, in healthcare, process measures are the most valid. Outcome measures which may seem at first to be the most obvious measure have also been widely used to assess quality but there are problems. Outcomes may be due, at least in part, to factors not related to the quality of care (e.g. a patient's physiological reserve or age). Also, some outcomes of care may become obvious only many years later; this will seriously limit their use as a tool for quality improvement. An example is the long-term outcome of good diabetic care in preventing vascular disease.

Measures of process are currently thought to be the tool of choice. An example is the management of stroke disease. The Cochrane Collaboration review of stroke units demonstrated that bringing together multidisciplinary teams and changing the process of care brought major benefits: patients managed within specialist stroke units are much more likely to be alive and at home a year after stroke than those managed on general medical wards.[9] Local measures of outcome would not have shown this as *individual* stroke units do not have enough patients to demonstrate improved survival. Process measures, however, are useful in enabling comparisons to be made with those processes shown in the Cochrane Collaboration.

Although there are exceptions to this rule (an example might be of the outcomes of carotid artery surgery in carotid artery stenosis), process measures then are most commonly used to assess quality. Several issues arise:

1. Which data should be used?
2. Are the data reliable? The problems of completeness and accuracy of data in the National Health Service are well described.
3. Are the data valid? Are we choosing the right measures to reflect changes in quality care?
4. Are the data sensitive enough?
5. Is the evidence generalizable? For example, are data about the management of incontinence applicable to both an acute hospital and a nursing home?
6. Does the importance of the quality data justify the cost of collecting them?
7. Are the measures understandable to all users, both professionals and patients? For example, are the patient surveys that are currently used as a measure of quality helpful and understandable by all parties?

RECENT QUALITY IMPROVEMENT INITIATIVES IN THE UK
Clinical audit

Audit was formally introduced into the NHS in 1989 and was the main quality improvement technique used by clinicians in the 1990s. Clinical audit can be described as "*systematically looking at processes used for diagnosis, care and treatment, examining how associated resources are used, and investigating the effect that care has on the outcome of quality of life for the patient.*"[10]

Clinical audit is usually described in the form of a cycle in which teams are encouraged to move through a process of setting standards, collecting and analyzing data, comparing the data with the standards set in a peer-review environment, and finally planning changes to improve the quality of care to meet the original standards set. The cycle is then repeated. In an environment of elderly care it is essential that audit is undertaken by multiprofessional teams and is focused on the needs of patients.

Clinical audit is not clinical research although, like research, it requires systematic collection of standardized data. Clinical audit is not simply counting but it is not necessarily complicated. It can be done just as effectively with a pencil and paper as with a computerized system. Clinical audit produced a great deal of activity among healthcare professionals, and by 1996 it was estimated that 20,000 projects had taken place with the majority of consultants (83 percent) and general practitioners (86 percent) participating. Major projects in geriatric medicine included the Royal College of Physicians' CARE scheme[11] and regional audits of hip fractures, for example in East Anglia.[12]

The criticism and challenges of clinical audit include:

- failure to use nationally set standards, and the use of resources on many small local projects with ill-defined standards and aims;
- failure to complete the audit cycle—projects demonstrate problems but changes are not made and no further re-audits are carried out to demonstrate improvement (or otherwise) in quality;
- a lack of patient-focused audits;
- a lack of links between audit and management, and between audit and education;
- far too few audits being multidisciplinary or multisectoral;
- constraints of time, staff shortages, and limitations of information technology—and the failure of some staff to participate at all.

Recently the General Medical Council has made it a requirement that all doctors in the UK take part in clinical audit, and it will be a requirement for revalidation.

The problems of single department or hospital audits being able to prove meaningful changes in quality have led to newer initiatives across networks of hospitals or even on a national basis. Examples include the Scottish Cancer Collaborative project, where surgeons in a clinical network are permitted to perform certain cancer operations only if they provide continuous audit data regularly discussed with their peers in other hospitals; and the national sentinel audit of stroke care by the Royal College of Physicians, a voluntary audit of stroke care involving over 70 percent of hospitals nationally, allowing all hospitals to measure their own performance against the national picture.[13]

Standards, guidelines, and protocols

To support clinical audit it is necessary to be clear about the standards that are being measured. During the 1990s many national and local organizations started to produce standard guidelines and protocols to inform the audit process, and to encourage a "clinical effectiveness" approach. Clinical effectiveness is seen as the extent to which the health status of patients can be expected to be enhanced by clinical interventions. Specific examples include the British Geriatrics Society's

compendium of guidelines,[14] and the work of the Royal College of Physicians' Clinical Effectiveness and Evaluation Unit.

Another major stimulus for assembling the evidence of effectiveness of interventions has been the Cochrane Collaboration launched in 1993. Cochrane reviews are systematic reviews of randomized control trials of healthcare carried out in a very precise way using the techniques of meta-analysis to pool the results of trials.[9] The six principles of the Cochrane Collaboration are: collaboration, building on people's enthusiasm and interest, minimizing duplication of effort, avoidance of bias, keeping up to date, and ensuring access.

NHS guideline production is now principally in the hands of the National Institute for Clinical Excellence (NICE: see later) and they have set out 10 key principles for NHS guideline production (Table 118-1). The Clinical Resource and Audit Group[15] defined standards, guidelines, and protocols as follows:

- *Standards*—specific statements relevant to particular criteria of care against which practice can be assessed.
- *Guidelines*—a systematically developed set of statements which assist in decision-making about appropriate healthcare for specific clinical conditions.
- *Protocols*—a fixed set of instructions to follow in the management of conditions, designed to reduce treatment variation and improve outcomes.

In practice, guidelines are seen as advisory and protocols as mandatory. The challenge for clinicians is to integrate guidelines or protocols into everyday care, usually in the form of integrated care pathways which aim to both ensure best care and allow easy audit to determine variation from the best pathway of care. This seems to be effective for single diseases, but becomes

---

Table 118-1 Principles for NHS guideline production

1. The objective of NHS clinical guidelines is to improve the quality of clinical care by making available to health professionals and patients well-founded advice on best practice.
2. Quality care is based on clinical effectiveness—the extent to which health status of patients can be expected to be enhanced by clinical interventions.
3. Quality of care in the NHS necessarily includes giving due attention to the cost-effectiveness of healthcare interventions.
4. NHS clinical guidelines are relevant to the care provided by the NHS throughout England and Wales.
5. NHS clinical guidelines are advisory.
6. NHS clinical guidelines are based on best possible research evidence, expert opinion, and professional consensus.
7. NHS clinical guidelines are developed using methods that command the respect of patients, the NHS, and NHS stakeholders.
8. Although NHS clinical guidelines are focused around clinical care provided by clinicians, patients are treated as full and equal partners along with relevant professional groups involved in a clinical guideline development.
9. All those who might be affected by NHS clinical guidelines deserve consideration within the clinical guideline development (usually including patients and their carers, service managers, the wider public, government, and healthcare industries).
10. NHS clinical guidelines should be both ambitious and realistic in nature. They should set out clinical care that might reasonably be expected throughout the NHS.

much more complex in the elderly-care environment even when there is a single primary defined problem such as stroke.[16]

The Health Advisory Service

In 1969, the Health Advisory Service (HAS) was established by the government to report on the management, organization, and standards of patient care for elderly and mentally ill patients predominantly in long-stay hospitals. This was in response to a series of critical reports. Over 20 years, multi-disciplinary review teams inspecting nationally all services for the care of the elderly reported to government ministers and health and local authorities about local services for older people. These services were reviewed every 5 years.

In 1991, the role of the HAS was changed to focus on thematic reviews to advise purchasers rather than reviewing services themselves. In 1997, the organization was reformed as a consortium of the Royal College of Psychiatrists, the British Geriatrics Society, the Royal College of Nursing Institute, and the Office for Public Management, to provide a proactive and advisory consultancy service for the National Health Service with the remit of improving delivery of services for mentally ill and older people. The approach taken was to develop evidence-based standards of clinical practice and organization, taking into account the views of users and carers, and to review services against these explicit standards. The organization has thrived and is currently the leading organization for detailed quality reviews and organizational development of mental health and older people services in England and Wales. It is working closely with the Commission for Health Improvement (see later).

The Audit Commission

The Audit Commission is an independent organization reporting to Parliament. It has a statutory role to report on value for money in both health services and local authorities. The auditors have a duty to examine the economy, efficiency, and effectiveness of use of public resources. Each year a small number of topics are chosen for detailed investigation, resulting in a report describing the issues and currently identified best practice. The following year all organizations in the NHS offering these features are reviewed by the commission. Those for whom indicators suggest problems have an in-depth review and detailed recommendations are produced for the Board of the organization. Follow-up to review progress against the objectives set usually occurs a year later.

Reports relating to older people include:[17] *Lying in Wait* (1992)—looking at the use of acute medical beds; *United They Stand* (update 1999)—reviewing the coordinated care of elderly people with hip fractures; *Fully Equipped* (2000)—the provision of equipment to older or disabled people by the NHS and social services in England and Wales; and *The Way To Go Home* (2000)—rehabilitation and remedial services for older people.

Accreditation

In the UK and elsewhere there are external inspection systems which may lead to accreditation. Both the Health Advisory Service and the Audit Commission provide external inspection but do not accredit. There are two inspecting bodies with

accreditation which may have some influence on services for elderly people:

- The Royal College of Physicians inspects all senior house officer posts in the UK and will accredit only those that meet their educational standards.
- The King's Fund, an independent healthcare advisory and organizational development organization, will provide accreditation of whole hospitals. It has a module for accrediting elderly-care services through the health quality service. Audit programs are usually based on self-audit against explicit standards based on processes and structures. Audit is completed with an inspection visit. There is no national requirement to participate and organizations usually use this accreditation process as a developmental tool.

Within industry, the British Standards Institution has accreditation standards BS5750 and ISO9000. These are voluntary schemes which identify organizations that have reached basic standard procedures to ensure that customer requirements are met. Accreditation depends upon documentation of procedures and policies, and assessment by an accrediting team visit. In the health services this has been used mostly in facilities departments, but clinical departments, including mental health services, have on occasion achieved these standards.

The Patient's Charter

The Patient's Charter was launched by the government in 1989 as an initiative to develop quality.[18] For the first time, users of the NHS were told what rights and standards they should expect. The original Patient's Charter was updated in 1995 and now includes standards on GP services, hospital services, community services, ambulance services, as well as dental, optical, pharmaceutical, and maternity services.

Some of the original rights included access to health records and a right to have a second opinion. The Charter also set out some very clear standards on waiting times for the ambulance service, waiting times for initial assessment in the accident and emergency department (A&E), as well as waiting times for outpatients and expectations after cancellation of operations. The Charter approach has certainly empowered patients who are now much more aware of their rights, as these rights are alluded to in complaints about services, and it appears to have provided a major impetus to change UK healthcare services towards a more patient-focused approach.

The Charter approach also demonstrated the problems that occur when setting and focusing on a very small number of standards. All efforts are made to achieve these without necessarily improving the performance of the whole organization. An example was the right to an immediate assessment in A&E. This led to the appointment of a large number of "hello nurses," who greeted the patient and performed a basic triage. This met statutory requirements without any demonstrable health gain benefit.

Charter Marks can be awarded to departments, or to whole organizations that can show an organizational-wide approach to quality and services, based on the Patient's Charter and patient involvement. A number of elderly-care departments have applied for a Charter Mark as an approach to quality.

The process of providing the evidence and inspection will often take up to 2 years, and then there is a reassessment process every 3 years to maintain the Charter Mark.

Complaints procedures

Complaints form another mechanism for monitoring the quality of healthcare delivery. In the UK, any complaint to a hospital must be acknowledged by the Chief Executive within 48 hours, and there is a national standard of the complainant receiving a reply following a completed investigation within 20 working days.

If a complainant is not satisfied and there is evidence that the complaint has not been dealt with in full, he or she may request an Independent Professional Review (IPR) of the whole complaint. This is decided by a convenor (a nonexecutive member of the hospital trust) and an independent lay chairman usually, with advice from the medical or nurse director of the hospital trust concerned. If an IPR is agreed, the convenor and lay chair set up and sit on the IPR panel, usually with two outside professional advisers whose clinical interests are relevant to the complaint. The panel produces a final report which goes to both the trust board and the health authority and is included in the final letter sent by the Chief Executive to the complainant. If the complainant is still dissatisfied, or issues remain outstanding, the person has the right to refer the matter to the National Health Service Ombudsman who may decide to investigate the complaint further. The Ombudsman produces an annual report to Parliament, which may "name and shame" publicly.

Since most complaints against doctors relate to poor communication, there may be particular challenges in elderly medicine both in avoiding complaints and in learning from them.[19] There are distinctive features which affect communication between older patients and physicians. For example, agism can occur in medical encounters, with physicians trivializing older people's problems. Physicians may spend less time with older people and may consider older patients to be more difficult to deal with than younger patients. Clinical discussion with older people is sometimes unusual in that a third person is often present, which complicates the communication process. These problems are additional to the generic problems of communication between doctor and patient.

The rise in the number of complaints about hospital-based elderly care was one of the main drivers that led to the setting up of the National Service Framework for Older People, an initiative from the Department of Health.

LESSONS FROM INDUSTRY ON QUALITY MANAGEMENT

The main advances in the business world in the field of quality improvement came during the 1970s and early 80s with the understanding that quality could not be improved simply by inspection, and problems corrected by removing those defective goods or poorly performing individuals found by the inspection. In healthcare this is called by Berwick "the bad-apple theory."[20] The bad-apple theory of improving healthcare suggests that, as there are increasingly sensitive and specific tools for identifying poor outlier performance (for example this might be the bottom performing 5 percent in a population of doctors, services, or hospitals), then by removing these outliers it is possible to improve quality. This is still the theory behind accreditation, revalidation, and purchasing to set standards.

The radical conceptual change to this was introduced by the management theorists William Deming and Joseph Duran who brought back from Japan to America the theory of continuous improvement. They found that problems in business were usually implicit in the complex production processes, and that problems with quality could only rarely be attributed to the lack of ability, will, or intention of the people involved with the processes. Thus removing the "bad apples" rarely worked. The problems were not of motivation or effort but of poor job design, failure of leadership, or unclear purpose. From this basic concept a number of models of quality improvement evolved in the business world which have subsequently been applied patchily to the healthcare environment. These include total quality management (TQM), re-engineering, benchmarking, and more recently the excellence model. Increasingly continuous quality improvement is influencing UK healthcare thinking.

Total quality management (TQM)

The most widely used quality intervention, certainly in business, is TQM. This has been defined as:[21]

> The management of activities involved in improving the quality of the organization's product or service. TQM is a philosophy and a set of guiding principles for continuous improvement. It applies human resources and analytical tools focused on meeting the customer's current and future needs and tries to integrate these into management's efforts.

There are several widely recognized key characteristics of TQM systems which must always involve the whole organization and focus on the customer.[21]

- TQM has to take into account all parts of the organization.
- The chief executive and all top managers must visibly support it.
- TQM is ingrained as a value in the organization and the culture. It is not an add-on, TQM is "how we do things around here."
- Partnerships with customers and suppliers are encouraged, and the aim is to exceed the customer's expectations.
- Everyone in an organization should be trying to exceed the expectations not just of external customers but of everyone with whom they interact within the organization who may equally be a customer.
- Cycle times can be reduced by focusing on doing the job faster.
- Statistical quality control and the use of self-managed work teams can improve processes.
- Do it right first time. Do not rely on inspection to identify defects, but correct the process to ensure that defects do not occur.

- There should be corporate citizenship. The organization values everyone, both those within it and those it serves—these are often called "stakeholders."
- No single formula works for everyone. Each organization is unique and must find its own way rather than taking an "off the shelf" approach.

Business process re-engineering (BPR)

Re-engineering, like TQM, is a system-wide change approach focusing on changing the basic processes of the organization.[22] BPR can be defined as the fundamental re-thinking and radical re-design of business processes to achieve dramatic improvements in performance. Re-engineering seeks to make all processes more efficient by combining, eliminating, or restructuring tasks, and the idea is to achieve large improvements in performance. Claims from the original studies suggested 100 percent improvement or more. Whereas TQM often looks at small continuous changes or improvements, re-engineering tries to take a radical approach to large-scale changes. Certainly in the business world re-engineering can be seen as a high-risk strategy. Its success rate is well under 50 percent and perhaps much less.

Benchmarking

Benchmarking, developed in the early 1990s, is the detailed study of productivity quality and value in different departments and activities in relation to performance elsewhere. The idea is basically simple. Find an organization that is good (ideally the best) at the particular process that you also carry out. Study carefully how it does well what it does, and then incorporate its technique into your own organization. This might involve looking at an organization in a completely different sector of the economy. An example in healthcare might be a hospital that looked at how a hotel managed its room booking processes in order to maximize the use of elective beds.

Outcomes in the health service

These three techniques for quality improvement and organizational development have been applied, some times indiscriminately,

in the healthcare environment. Pollitt noted how difficult it has been to implement them within the health service.[23]

Seventeen pilot total TQM projects were set up by the Department of Health in 1989, and the term "total quality management" has also been applied to other projects in the health service. A number of trusts also received considerable investment for pilot schemes of re-engineering. Leicester Royal Infirmary made a considerable name for itself for its one-stop neurology clinic, but demonstrable quality gains across a whole organization have not been found, at least in the NHS projects. Benchmarking as a specific project does not appear to have had an independent systematic evaluation in the health service.

Pollitt points out that these quality initiatives were difficult to implement within the health service.[23] In particular, they fail to take account of the professions and the complexity of standards and guidelines emanating from professional bodies. They all require considerable time and resources and yet specialist quality training is a resource that few healthcare organizations have been able to deliver. Moreover, a hospital environment is far more complex than the single-process environment of a manufacturing business. Hospitals fail to match many of the key elements that would be required to translate these business approaches into the NHS. Existing quality improvement activities reflect fragmented occupational structures and relationships within the organizations. In the NHS quality still remains, in large part, as a "bolt-on" extra.

The excellence model

The most recent model from the business world has been the excellence model (otherwise known as the business excellence model).[24] This derived from mainland Europe. It is currently espoused by the NHS Executive, the Cabinet Office, and the British Association of Medical Managers. The key premise is that "excellent results with respect to performance, customers, people and society are achieved through leadership driving policy and strategy, people, partnership and resources, and processes."

In essence this model is a development of TQM. It is used as a self-assessment approach to each of the elements set out in Figure 118-1. With self-assessment, organizations can measure their progress against the criteria and a scoring approach allows for a direct comparison with other organizations. Thus it can

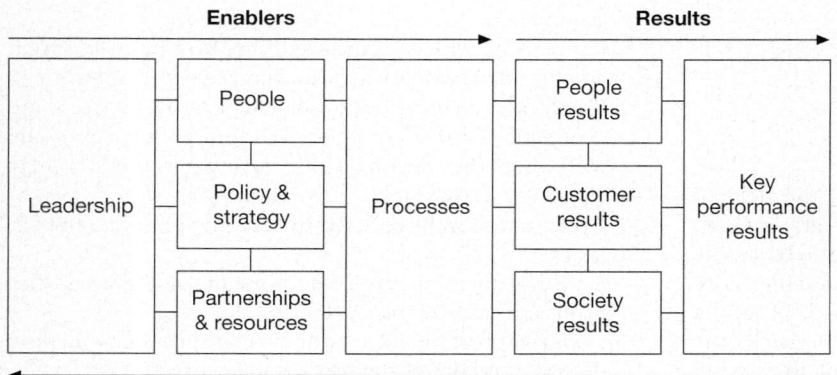

Figure 118-1 The EFQM model in diagrammatic form. The arrows emphasize the dynamic nature of the model. They show innovation and learning helping to improve enablers that in turn lead to improved results. The model's nine boxes represent the criteria against which to assess an organization's progress towards excellence. © 1999 EFQM. The model is a registered trade mark of the EFQM.

be used:

- for organizational self-assessment;
- as an integrative framework for organizational development and to incorporate previously adopted quality initiatives and practice;
- as a strategic and practical tool for performance management;
- as a means of addressing clinical governance agendas.

It is too early to say whether this will prove to be a more practical way of introducing total quality management into UK healthcare.

Continuous improvement

Despite the problems set out above, it is widely accepted that a continuous improvement model is most likely to succeed in achieving quality improvement in healthcare. It is clear that quality improvement is a painstaking and time-consuming business and that team working, team building, and leadership skills are all required for quality improvement.

One goal that has been suggested for healthcare is that the medical profession should move to so-called "six sigma quality."[25] The sixth-sigma goal aims for a rate of errors that lies six standard deviations outside of the normal distribution (i.e. fewer than 3.4 errors per one million events). Currently in anesthesia, using many techniques of quality improvement, deaths have been reduced to 5.4 per million, very close to the sixth-sigma goal. Yet 79 percent of eligible survivors after myocardial infarction do not receive beta-blockers, a rate equal to about one sigma.[25]

Berwick uses the term "continuous improvement" to mean "continuously improving systems."[26] He suggests a very simple model of system improvement, described by Langley et al.[27] This comprises three basic questions and a cycle for testing innovations (Fig. 118-2). The Plan–Do–Study–Act cycle describes the growth of knowledge through making changes and reflecting on the consequences. A simple model with clear leadership may be the best place to start quality improvement processes.

THE CURRENT NHS APPROACH

Service standards, delivery, and monitoring

Based on the 1997 NHS white paper[28] and the subsequent white paper, *A First Class Service*,[29] the government set out a new model for quality improvement within the health service. This has three main parts: clear standards of service; dependable local delivery; and monitored standards (Fig. 118-3).

Clear standards of service

Clear standards of service are being increasingly defined through two approaches. The first is the National Institute for Clinical Excellence (NICE). NICE promotes clinical and cost effectiveness through guidance and audit. It advises on best practice in existing treatment options, appraises new health interventions, and advises the health service on how they can

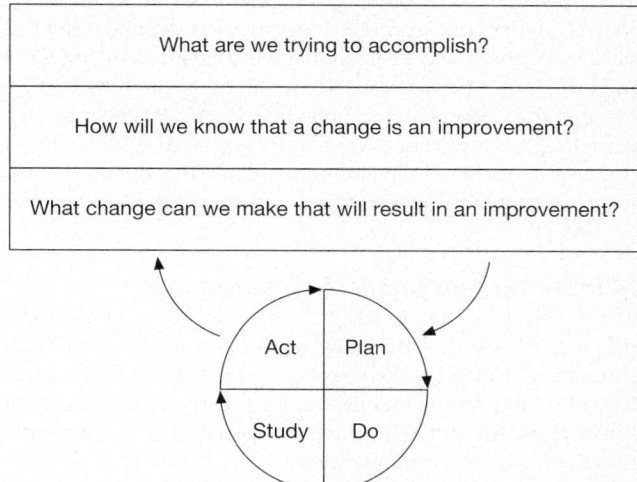

Model for improvement

What are we trying to accomplish?

How will we know that a change is an improvement?

What change can we make that will result in an improvement?

Act | Plan
Study | Do

Figure 118-2 A model of improvement adapted by Berwick from Langley et al.[27] Reproduced with permission from Berwick.[26]

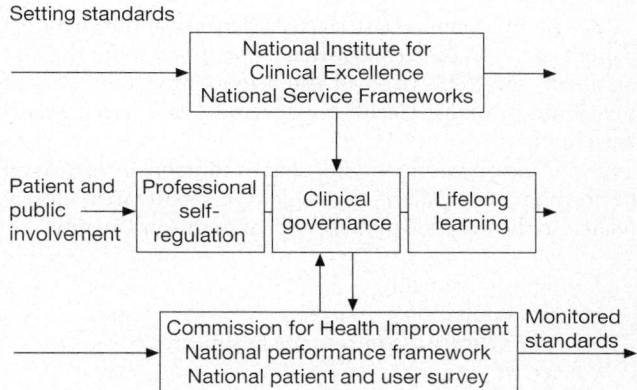

Setting standards

National Institute for Clinical Excellence National Service Frameworks

Patient and public involvement → Professional self-regulation | Clinical governance | Lifelong learning

Commission for Health Improvement National performance framework National patient and user survey

Monitored standards

Figure 118-3 A model for quality improvement in the NHS.

be implemented. One example has been the recent advice on the use of the new Alzheimer's disease drugs.[30]

The second approach to setting standards is through the National Service Frameworks (NSFs). These set national standards and define care models for specific services or care groups, put in place programs to support implementation, and establish performance measures against which the progress and timetable can be measured. A National Service Framework should bring together the best evidence of clinical and cost effectiveness with the views of the service users to determine the best ways of providing particular services. The National Service Framework in Elderly Care was published in April 2001. It contains guidelines on the management of specific conditions such as stroke and falls, on the organization of services with an emphasis on patient-centered care, and on the use of intermediate care facilities. It has policy statements about rooting out agism whereby older people are denied some treatments simply on account of their age.

Dependable local delivery

The second strand of *A First Class Service* is ensuring that arrangements are in place to support dependable local delivery of good care. Professional self-regulation includes the introduction of appraisal for all doctors and revalidation through the General Medical Council. It encourages programs of lifelong learning based on effective appraisal, and the introduction of personal development plans for all staff. It also involves the quality improvement tool of "clinical governance" (see later).

Monitoring and publicizing standards

Thirdly, the government has put in place plans to monitor and publicize standards. This includes the Commission for Health Improvement (CHI) which has been established as a new statutory body to provide independent scrutiny of local efforts to improve quality and help address serious problems. Currently the commission's core functions are:

- to inspect the clinical governance arrangements of all trusts (in both primary and secondary care) in the UK on a 4-year rolling cycle;
- to report on the implementation of the National Service Frameworks.

The government has also started a series of annual national patient surveys to determine what patients feel about the care offered by the NHS. This will also help to inform the work of the Commission for Health Improvement as it inspects each trust in turn.

Finally, the government has started to publish "high-level performance indicators" focusing on six main areas closely related to the Maxwell dimensions[6] of healthcare quality:

- health improvement;
- fair access to services;
- effective delivery of appropriate healthcare;
- efficiency;
- patient care experience;
- health outcomes of NHS care.

Some of the indicators currently published have direct relevance to services for elderly people—for example, inpatient mortality rate after stroke, inpatient mortality after fractured neck of femur, and the percentage of patients discharged home at 56 days after both of these conditions.

Clinical governance

Within the process of inspection, standard-setting, and attempts to measure quality, the main driver for quality improvement is the concept of "clinical governance."[31] Clinical governance is defined as: "a system through which NHS organizations are accountable for continuously improving the quality of their services and safeguarding high standards of care by creating an environment in which excellence in clinical care will flourish."

Clinical governance is seen as a process of continuous quality improvement in healthcare along the lines described by Berwick.[26] For the first time this is an attempt to put quality at the heart of what healthcare organizations do in the UK as opposed merely to bolting it on or "inspecting it in." Also for the first time, the chief executives of trusts are personally responsible for the quality of healthcare provided in their organizations.

For an organization to be able to turn this new concept into reality, change will have to occur in a number of ways. Quality improvement will need to be placed at the forefront, and this can be delivered only with clear leadership and using genuine multidisciplinary teams. Mechanisms will be required to put best evidence into practice in a systematic and guaranteed way. Poorly performing doctors need to be identified, and professional development beyond the simple remit of continuous medical education must become a priority. The quality and timeliness of data about activity and outcomes within the NHS will need to improve. Scally and Donaldson[31] point out the correspondence between corporate governance in the business world and clinical governance. They contend that if clinical governance is to be successful, it must have the same strengths as corporate governance: it must be rigorous in its application, have an organization-wide emphasis, and be accountable in its delivery, developmental in its thrust, and positive in its connotations. They assert that the emphasis of clinical governance is by far the most ambitious quality initiative that has ever been implemented in the NHS.

Clinical governance in geriatric medicine

The British Geriatrics Society and the Royal College of Physicians published a position paper in 1999 on interpreting clinical governance and its implications for geriatric medicine.[32] As well as recommending an integrated common scheme for clinical governance, the paper made specific recommendations for individual practitioners, and for services within an organization and the services crossing organizations. An integrated common scheme was based on the clinical governance cycle (Fig. 118-4). This requires practitioners or services to consider each aspect of the cycle.

- *Standards* include those set by NICE and the National Service Framework, as well as professional standards from the General Medical Council, Patient Charter standards, and legal standards.
- *Professional qualities* are based around the individual or the service needs for differing knowledge and skills. These may vary over time and are not exclusively clinical.
- *Service delivery and organization* includes the use of guidelines and protocols, and analysis of whether the structures available within the organization can deliver the care that is required.
- *Monitoring* includes systematic evaluation of clinical audit, both local and national; complaints; risk assessment; national performance indicators; critical incident reviews; Royal College visit reports; national patient surveys; and external body reviews such as the Health Advisory Service.
- *Change management* includes all those processes that can be used to improve the quality of care, such as the quality improvement tools discussed within this chapter.

The clinical governance cycle

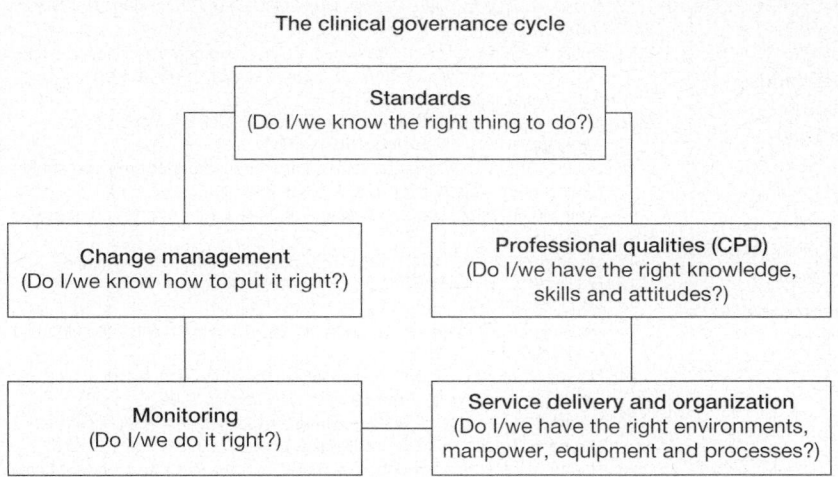

Figure 118-4 The clinical governance cycle. Reproduced with permission from reference 32.

The British Geriatrics Society has further considered guidelines for implementing clinical governance at the departmental level.[33] Key areas of implementation are:

1. Each department of geriatric medicine should have a nominated lead consultant in organizational service quality.
2. The appropriate participation of consultants in geriatric medicine in processes covering each element of the clinical governance cycle should be clearly demonstrable.

It is too early to say whether clinical governance will bring about the revolution in quality improvement that was promised at its launch. However, it can be seen how the various quality initiatives of the previous 20 years have been drawn together into an integrated common schema which is more closely in touch with the reality of the National Health Service rather than the business world.

Long-term care

Geriatric medicine in the UK grew out of long-term care with attempts to improve the quality of care of older people in that environment. As discussed earlier, the scandals that occurred in the 1960s led to the formation of the Health Advisory Service which continued to actively inspect NHS long-term care until 1991.

Changes in social security funding led to massive expansion of private sector provision, in particular nursing-home care in the 1980s and 1990s. The vast majority of long-term nursing-home and residential-home care is now in the private and "not-for-profit" sector. The main driver for standards is inspection. Health authorities are responsible for inspecting nursing homes, and local authorities for residential homes. These inspection processes are very much based on structure rather than process or outcome. The size of rooms, the facilities offered, and compliance with health, safety, and fire regulations are the main variables tested. Quality of care is not measured in any meaningful way.

In 1992, the Royal College of Physicians and the British Geriatrics Society produced a document on guidelines and audit measures in long-term care followed by a clinical audit

scheme called the CARE (Continuous Assessment Review and Evaluation) scheme.[11,34] This allowed users to audit seven main domains (Table 118-2) and encouraged a process of continuous review and reassessment. Although not widely used, where it has been used there is some evidence of improvement.[35] Yet the problems of improving quality in long-term care, particularly the medical aspects, remain, as a more recent publication from the Royal College of Physicians demonstrates.[36] Among the recommendations of this document are re-engagement of physicians in geriatric medicine in long-term care within the community, a whole-system approach to planning care, and the development of a new nursing role for the gerontological specialist.

Table 118-2 Key audit indicators for long-term care

Preserving autonomy
Promoting urinary continence
Promoting fecal continence
Optimizing drug usage
Managing falls and accidents
Preventing pressure sores
Environment and equipment
Aids and adaptations
The medical role in long-term care

KEY POINTS Improving quality of care in the UK

- Quality in healthcare has a number of dimensions, which makes definitions, standard setting, and measurement complex.

- Until recently the main approaches to improving quality involved inspection of services and encouragement for clinical audit.

(continued)

KEY POINTS (continued)

■ During the 1990s, new approaches from business introduced the ideas of continuous quality improvement, although implementation, in large part, has been haphazard and inadequately understood and resourced.

■ The UK government has introduced the concept of "clinical governance" which now places a responsibility on all professionals to be accountable for not only maintaining but also improving standards of care within the health service.

■ There is still huge room for improvement in our approaches to improving the quality of care of older people in the UK.

REFERENCES

1. Brook RH, McGlynn EA, Shekelle PG: Defining and measuring quality of care: a perspective from US researchers. Int J Qual Healthcare 2000;12:281–295
2. Bank J: The Essence of Total Quality Management. Prentice-Hall, Englewood Cliffs, 1992
3. World Health Organization: The Principles of Quality Assurance (report on a WHO meeting). WHO, Copenhagen, 1993
4. Lohr KN (ed): Medicare: a strategy for quality assurance. National Academy Press, Washington, 1990
5. Blumenthal D: Quality of health care. N Engl J Med 1996;335: 891–894
6. Maxwell RJ: Quality assessment in health. BMJ 1984;288:1470–1472
7. Donabedian A: Explorations in Quality Assessment and Monitoring. 1: The Definition of Quality and Approaches to its Assessment. Health Administration Press, Ann Arbor, 1990
8. Brook RH, McGlynn EA, Cleary PD: Measuring quality of care. N Engl J Med 1996;335:966–970
9. The Cochrane Library: Available at www.update.software.com/cochrane/cochrane-frame.html, 20 March 2001
10. UK Department of Health: Evolution of Clinical Audit. HMSO, London, 1994
11. Research Unit of the Royal College of Physicians: The CARE Scheme: Clinical Audit of Long-Term Care of Elderly People. Royal College of Physicians, London, 1992
12. Todd CJ, Freeman CJ, Camilleri-Ferrante C et al: Differences in mortality after fracture of hip: the East Anglian audit. BMJ 1995;310:904–908
13. Rudd A: The national sentinel audit for stroke and its lessons for clinical governance. In Potter J, Georgiou A, Pearson M (eds): Measuring the Quality of Care for Older People. Royal College of Physicians, London, 2000:61–73
14. British Geriatrics Society: Guidelines, Policy Statements and Statements of Good Practice. British Geriatrics Society, London, 1995. Available at www.bgs.org.uk, 20 March 2001
15. Clinical Resource and Audit Group: Clinical Guidelines: Report of a Working Party. Scottish Office, Edinburgh, 1993
16. Sulch D, Kalra L: Systematic review: integrated care pathways and stroke management. Age Ageing 2000;29:349–352
17. Audit Commission, London: Available at www.audit-commission.gov.uk, 20 March 2001
18. UK Department of Health: The Patient's Charter. DoH, London, 1991
19. Black DA: Complaints, Doctors and Older People. Age Ageing 2000;29:389–391
20. Berwick DM: Continuous improvement as an ideal in health care. N Engl J Med 1989;320:53–56
21. Harvey D, Brown DR: An Experiential Approach to Organizational Development, 5th edn. Prentice-Hall, New Jersey, 1996
22. Hammer M, Champy J: Reengineering the Corporation: A Manifesto for Business Revolution. Nicholas Brealey, London, 1993
23. Pollitt C: Business approaches to quality improvement: why they are hard for the NHS to swallow. Qual Healthcare 1996;5:104–110
24. Stahr H, Bulman B, Stead M: The Excellence Model in the Health Sector. Kingsham Press, Chichester, 2000
25. Chassin MR: Is health care ready for Six Sigma Quality? Milbank Quart 1998;76:565–591
26. Berwick DM: A primer on leading the improvement of systems. BMJ 1996;312:619–622
27. Langley GJ, Nolan KM, Nolan TW: The Foundation of Improvement. API Publishing, Silverspring, MD, 1992
28. UK Department of Health: The New NHS: Modern, Dependable. HMSO, London, 1997
29. UK Department of Health: A First Class Service: Quality in the New NHS. HMSO, London, 1998
30. National Institute for Clinical Excellence, London: Technology Appraisal Guidance 19: Guidance on the Use of Donepezil, Rivastigmine and Galantamine. Available at www.nice.org.uk, 20 March 2001
31. Scally G, Donaldson LJ: Clinical governance and the drive for quality improvement in the new NHS in England. BMJ 1998;327:61–65
32. British Geriatrics Society and Royal College of Physicians of London: Clinical Governance: A Position Paper. London, 1999
33. British Geriatrics Society: Guidelines for the Implementation of Clinical Governance in Geriatric Medicine. London, 2000
34. Royal College of Physicians and British Geriatrics Society: High-Quality Long-Term Care for Elderly People: Guidelines and Audit Measures. London: Royal College of Physicians, London, 1992
35. Dickinson E, Brocklehurst J: Improving the quality of long-term care for older people: lessons from the CARE scheme. Qual Healthcare 1997;6:160–164
36. Royal College of Nursing, Royal College of Physicians, and British Geriatrics Society: The Health Care of Older People in Care Homes: A Comprehensive Interdisciplinary Approach. London, 2000

Chapter 119

Quality improvement in the USA

Jerrold Hill, Samuel W. Warburton, and Randall K. Spoeri

Quality improvement in the USA has undergone substantial change in the last decade. The previous focus of quality improvement on audits of structure, process, and a limited number of outcomes has been transformed to an increasing focus on measuring outcomes and incorporating structured programs of continuous quality improvement. This transformation has occurred in response to mandates originating in both private and public sectors. In the private sector, the rapid growth of enrollment in managed care plans in the 1990s increased demands from employers and consumers that managed care plans demonstrate that restrictive provider networks and utilization management activities were not compromising quality of healthcare. In response, the National Committee for Quality Assurance (NCQA)[1] and similar organizations arose early in the 1990s to establish uniform measures of quality performance such as HEDIS (Health Plan Employer Data and Information Set)[2] and standards for the accreditation of managed care plans.[3] Surprisingly, public-sector organizations such as the Centers for Medicare and Medicaid (CMS, formerly the Health Care Financing Administration or HCFA) lagged behind the private sector, but later adopted similar requirements for quality performance measurement and quality improvement for Medicare and Medicaid managed care plans.[4]

Monitoring quality performance used to be focused primarily on inpatient hospital care and identifying "bad apples" or outliers of care.[5] In the 1990s, quality was monitored over a number of provider entities, indicating an increased scrutiny of physician and facility performance. The entire physician network of a managed care plan is monitored under HEDIS reporting. In addition, managed care plans often profile the quality and utilization performance of individual physicians and physician groups.[6,7] Several states have profiled surgical mortality rates for coronary artery bypass surgery (CABG) for individual hospitals and surgeons and have distributed profiles to the public.[8,9] Under the reporting requirements for the Resident Assessment Instrument (RAI)[10] mandated by Congress under the Omnibus Budget Resolution Act of 1987, nursing homes are required to monitor changes in medical conditions, functioning, and social interaction and respond to triggering conditions using standard Resident Assessment Protocols. Finally, quality of care in hospitals continues to be monitored by the Joint Committee for the Accreditation of Healthcare Organizations (JCAHO) and CMS's Peer Review Organizations (PROs).

Another profound change has been the dissemination of quality performance data to healthcare consumers, both through print media and more recently over the Internet. Sharing performance data is now accepted as a means of empowering consumers to make informed choices.[11]

The transformation of healthcare quality performance measurement and quality improvement initiatives represents a widespread endorsement of several principles. First, uniform measures of quality performance can be applied to a large segment of the healthcare industry. Second, the principles of continuous quality improvement should be applied to healthcare as has been done in other sectors of the economy. Third, it is possible to incorporate healthcare outcomes into quality performance measurement. Fourth, it is possible for healthcare consumers to use information on quality to make informed decisions.

Despite the widespread endorsement of these principles, the impact of increased measurement of, and interventions to improve, the quality of healthcare is not well-documented. Evidence from the 1999 Institute of Medicine (IoM) report of medical errors suggests that substantial problems with quality of care remain, despite the initiatives cited above.[12]

This chapter first presents the general principles of quality performance measurement and continuous quality improvement. Next, quality improvement initiatives are documented in several settings: commercial managed care plans, Medicare fee-for-service, Medicare managed care plans, and nursing homes. The methodological challenges to measuring quality, and the institutional challenges to implementing effective interventions to improve quality, are examined for each quality-improvement initiative.

PRINCIPLES OF QUALITY MEASUREMENT

Quality improvement initiatives are more likely to be successful if there is agreement among healthcare providers and consumers (including employers and government purchasers of healthcare) on how quality should be measured. Providers will be more committed to continuous quality improvement if they view the performance measures to be meaningful assessments of quality that are uniformly and fairly measured across providers.

Deciding what to measure

The necessity of measuring quality by structure, process, and outcomes as first suggested by Donabedian remains compelling[13,14] (Table 119-1). While healthcare outcomes are considered the best gauge of quality, they are often difficult to measure, or are not feasible for supporting quality improvement. For example, outcomes related to improved quality of periodic breast cancer screening, such as reduced mortality,

Table 119-1 **Measures of quality performance: structure, process, and outcomes**		
Structure: resources	**Process: activities**	**Outcomes: results**
Buildings	Technical care	Health status
Vehicles	Communication	Handicap
Equipment	Coordination	Disability
Staff and training	Teamwork	Impairment
Policies and procedures	Timeliness	Mortality
Intangibles: culture and philosophy		Satisfaction
Finance		Caregiver's views
Management systems		Avoidance of complications

will not be observed for many years, and the correlates of reduced mortality (e.g. a shift in the stage distribution toward earlier stage disease) are difficult and expensive to document. Similarly, outcomes associated with improved quality in the management of chronic diseases such as diabetes or conditions such as hypertension may not be realized for a number of years. Furthermore, random variations in outcomes, especially in low-incidence conditions, will not produce meaningful measurements in organizations with small patient populations (e.g. in healthcare plans or physician group practices with fewer than 10,000 members).

Process measures such as population-based rates of screening mammography and retinal and foot examinations for diabetics are not only reasonable measures of quality, but are often the most sensible since many quality-improvement interventions are focused on improving process. However, implicit in process measures of periodic screening is the assumption that all associated processes are being performed at acceptable levels of quality. The population rate of screening mammography, for example, is only a good indicator of secondary prevention of breast cancer if evaluations of mammography images by radiologists, pathology studies of tumors, and treatment of breast cancers are correctly performed. Intermediate outcomes, such as a lower hemoglobin A_{1c} level for diabetics achieved through changes in diet, exercise, or medication compliance, or lower blood pressure achieved through diet, behavior modification, or medication, are quality measures that will be acceptable to physicians and consumers.

Measures of structure such as physical characteristics of healthcare facilities and credentials of healthcare providers (e.g. the percentage of a managed-care organization's physician network that is board certified) are useful for determining whether the health plan or facility meets threshold standards of quality. Deficits on physical facilities or professional qualifications are credible indicators of poorer quality. In some instances, structural measures are the only data available (such as for a newly formed managed-care organization, or an MCO transformed by merger), and are the only source of information available to consumers and government agencies responsible for monitoring quality. Thus, structural measures of quality are essential for assessing the quality of new entities providing healthcare, and monitoring possible changes

for entities undergoing changes in physical facilities or provider networks. However, the weakness of using measures of structure as indicators of quality is that physicians, facilities, or health plans meeting threshold requirements on structure may perform poorly on process or outcome measures.

Uniform measurement

Uniform performance measures are essential when quality is compared across providers or health plans, especially when measures of quality are reported to consumers for the purpose of making decisions on the selection of provider or health plan.[15] Uniformity requires explicit specifications for measuring the quality indicator (e.g. explicit diagnosis codes for identifying diabetic patients from medical claims records), similar sources of data for the organizations or providers being compared, and a method for auditing the computed performance measures. While achieving uniformity seems simple, in practice it is often difficult to achieve given the heterogeneity of data systems for healthcare organizations under comparison.

Adjustments for case-mix and severity of illness

Healthcare providers are more likely to judge quality performance measurement as fair if the measurements incorporate adjustments for case-mix and severity of illness. For outcome measures such as mortality, prognosis is known to vary by number and type of comorbid conditions[16] and severity of illness by condition (e.g. stage of cancer). Failure to adjust for the variation in expected outcomes across healthcare providers due to differences in the prevalence of comorbid conditions and disease severity will produce unfair comparisons. Providers whose patients have a higher prevalence of comorbid conditions or a higher prevalence with more severe disease on specific comorbid conditions are likely to score lower on quality performance measures such as mortality.

Statistical methods for adjusting for case-mix and severity of illness have been applied to the measurement of hospital mortality,[17–19] mortality specific to CABG surgery,[8,9,20] consumers' satisfaction with their managed care plan,[21] and profiling of individual physician performance in a managed care setting. Typically, a three-step approach is used for adjustment.[22] In the first step, a regression model is estimated for the sample of patients under evaluation which has as the dependent variable the quality outcome of interest and as independent variables measures of case-mix and severity, such as presence of high-cost diagnoses, age, gender, and prior utilization. Logistic regression is typically used when the outcome variable of interest is a binary dependent variable such as whether the patient died during an inpatient hospital stay,[20] had an adverse outcome such as a surgical complication, or received a preventive examination. In the second step, the expected outcome for each patient is predicted from the regression model given his or her history with respect to medical conditions, severity of illness, and other patient-specific characteristics such as age and gender. The expected outcome for each patient is the average outcome across all providers for patients with the same medical conditions, severity of illness, and patient-specific characteristics. In step three, the provider's quality relative to others under evaluation is measured as the average difference between the actual and expected outcomes for the provider's patients. This difference yields the case-mix and severity adjusted measure of quality improvement.

In practice, case-mix and severity adjustments are difficult to implement. First, decisions on what should be included in the risk-adjustment model have to be made. Second, collecting data on the variables used for risk and severity adjustment can be costly, often requiring chart abstraction, supplementary data collection by provider, or supplementary data collection from a patient survey. Providers will be dissatisfied if they have to incur costs for data collection. In addition, while physicians want risk and severity adjustments for fair evaluation, they often do not understand the statistical methods used, and will object to being evaluated on a method they view as a "black box"—an arcane or propriety methodology not easily understood.

Population-based measurement for insured populations

For many measures of quality, such as rates of pediatric immunization or of immunization against pneumococcal influenza in the geriatric population, it is essential to know the population at risk. Because some members of the population at risk will not receive any healthcare in the time period over which quality performance is measured, quality measured from only patient records or administrative data such as health insurance claims will produce biased estimates of quality. Population-based measures of quality can be computed for members of managed care plans, because enrollment data are necessary for paying capitation to the managed care plan's providers. For other insured groups, such as persons insured under traditional indemnity coverage, enrollment data are often incomplete. Measuring quality from the public health perspective—that is, for the entire population including those not insured—presents special challenges. For example, to measure rates of pediatric immunization, the Centers for Disease Control and Prevention must rely on self-reported data from a survey of parents.

PRINCIPLES OF QUALITY IMPROVEMENT

Continuous quality improvement (CQI), or clinical quality improvement as it is sometimes called in healthcare, draws upon the principles originally proposed by Deming[23] and implemented by private corporations in the USA. CQI typically involves the following processes:[24]

- defining objectives;
- baseline measurement of performance;
- design and implementation of interventions to improve performance;
- follow-up measurement and assessment of performance;
- beginning the quality-improvement process again.

Each process is considered in more detail below.

Objectives for quality improvement in healthcare are often defined by evidence-based medicine; that is, scientific evidence on procedures, therapies, or processes found to be most efficacious in the diagnosis and treatment of specific illnesses. For example, a quality-improvement objective may be to improve care of patients after myocardial infarction.[25,26] Eliminating system failures such as medication errors in a hospital may also be an objective.[27]

Baseline measurement of performance involves assessment of the current state of affairs to identify possible problems and opportunities for improvement. It also involves identification of possible causes of problems or shortfalls in performance. These may include deficits in physician knowledge on the most efficacious procedures and therapies, patient compliance, barriers to receiving treatment (financial, socioeconomic, cultural—language and cultural orientation towards healthcare systems and specific therapies), and system failures (system too complex, no systematic checks for errors, provider fatigue increasing the likelihood of making errors, etc.).

Design and implementation of interventions to improve performance involves identifying successful models of quality improvement previously implemented. If multiple sources of failure were identified in the baseline evaluation, for example deficits in physician performance and patient compliance, then the design of intervention should address each source if feasible.

Follow-up measurement and assessment of performance (i.e. post-intervention performance compared to baseline) is necessary to determine whether interventions to improve performance were effective. This requires that performance measures and other analytic measures (e.g. measures of patient risk, case-mix, and other independent variables required for the evaluation) be clearly defined and that processes for data collection and analysis are in place. The data-collection plan may require specifications for selecting a sample of patients for measurement and evaluation if the costs of data collection are high (e.g. if data are obtained by survey or abstraction from medical records). For some CQI initiatives, it is important to measure the mean and variance of performance over time. Interventions to improve the performance of healthcare providers should not only improve mean performance, but also reduce variation as standards for treatment are adopted by providers. The literature on statistical process control provides a number of techniques for monitoring performance over time, and statistical software for computing and plotting performance measurement is now available.[28,29]

In addition to determining whether a CQI intervention was effective in the aggregate, evaluation of interventions should analyze whether effectiveness varies by characteristics of providers or patients. Evidence on the effectiveness of the individual components of a multifaceted intervention should be evaluated if possible. One would like to know, for example, whether a program to increase the use of beta-blockers in patients after myocardial infarction, through physician education to increase the rate of prescription and through patient reminders to increase compliance, was successful at increasing the rates of prescription and compliance. These additional analyses are useful for identifying opportunities for further improvement.

Even if quality improvements are achieved, the healthcare organization will begin the quality improvement process again, because opportunities for improvement will remain. As noted above, results from the evaluation of the intervention will be useful for identifying these opportunities.

MEASURING QUALITY PERFORMANCE IN MANAGED CARE

The case for monitoring quality performance in managed-care organizations (MCOs) is compelling. To control costs, MCOs selectively contract with a limited network of physicians willing to accept discounts on prevailing fee-for-service payments or willing to accept financial risk by receiving capitation payments to provide care to the MCO's members selecting or assigned to the physician. These contracting arrangements restrict the health-plan member's choice of physicians, and provide physicians with a financial incentive to provide less care. Furthermore, MCO members' access to specialists is restricted by requiring referrals from a member's primary care physician, and access to specific services, in particular inpatient services, is restricted by requiring pre-authorization from the MCO. These restrictions on choice of physicians and access to services raised concerns on whether members of MCOs receive poorer quality healthcare as a result.

HEDIS

In response to concerns that the restrictive policies on physician networks and access to care may adversely affect quality, initiatives to monitor quality performance in MCOs began in the early 1990s. The first of these was the development under the direction of the National Committee for Quality Assurance (NCQA) of the Health Plan Employer Data and Information Set (HEDIS). HEDIS is a set of uniformly defined measures of health-plan performance covering a number of domains including quality of care, consumer satisfaction, utilization and costs, geographic distribution of physicians across the MCO's service area, and financial indicators (Table 119-2).[2,30,31] The wide range of performance indicators which extends well beyond quality of care is in keeping with the original goal of providing employers with a set of uniform measures of performance to facilitate choice of MCOs on the basis of quality as well as cost.

Annual reporting of HEDIS is largely a voluntary activity (CMS requires HEDIS reporting for Medicare managed-care plans, and some states mandate HEDIS reporting). While voluntary, 51 million managed-care members covered under 466 health-plan products reported HEDIS data according to NCQA,[1] reflecting the demands of consumers for information on the healthcare quality of MCOs. NCQA facilitates access to HEDIS data by distributing detailed data by MCO on its Quality Compass website, making it easy for employers to compare MCOs when deciding which health plans should be offered to their employees.

HEDIS incorporates many of the desired attributes of quality performance measurement detailed above. Performance measures are based on a uniform set of detailed specifications. Many measures such as pediatric immunizations and periodic cancer screening are population-based. Many of the measures such as immunization rates, rates for screening examinations, care for patients with diabetes, care for patients with hypertension, and medication management for conditions such as asthma and depression are process measures for which evidence-based medicine predicts better outcomes with improved process.

Table 119-2 HEDIS performance measures: domains measured and specific measures of effectiveness of care

- Effectiveness of care:
  Childhood immunization status
  Adolescent immunization status
  Breast cancer screening
  Cervical cancer screening
  Chlamydia screening in women
  Controlling high blood pressure
  Beta-blocker treatment after a heart attack
  Cholesterol management after acute cardiovascular events
  Comprehensive diabetes care
  Use of appropriate medications for people with asthma
  Follow-up after hospitalization for mental illness
  Antidepressant medication management
  Advising smokers to quit
  Flu shots for older adults
  Pneumonia vaccination status in older adults
  The Medicare health outcomes survey

- Access/availability of care

- Satisfaction with the experience of care (CAHPS survey)

- Health plan stability

- Use of services

- Cost of care (currently no measure in this domain)

- Informed healthcare choices

- Health plan descriptive information

An important outcome measure, consumer satisfaction, is measured using a uniform instrument, the Consumer Assessment of Health Plans Survey (CAHPS), administered by survey specialists authorized by NCQA.[31] Thus, this important measure of performance cannot be manipulated in any way by the health plan. Furthermore, it provides uniform measures of satisfaction on how quickly members receive care, whether they get the care they need, their rating of healthcare received, whether their doctors communicate well, and their ease of getting referrals to a specialist.

The completeness and quality of health-plan data is a challenge to the validity of HEDIS measures of effectiveness of care. Many MCOs reimburse primary care physicians on a capitation basis (a fixed payment per month per health-plan member to cover all primary care services for the health-plan member). Unless the MCO requires primary care physicians reimbursed under capitation to submit a record for each health-care encounter, the MCO has no record of health-care services received by the health-plan member. (Even if the MCO requires the submission of encounter data, health-care encounters are under-reported by primary care physicians since they have little, and often no, financial incentive to submit these data.) This is in contrast to fee-for-service medicine, such as the traditional fee-for-service Medicare program, where claims are submitted to a third party payer for reimbursement and the concern is that some physicians will submit fraudulent claims. NCQA recognized this deficit in claims and encounter data. In recognition, it has permitted health plans to select a sample of health-plan members for each measure of effectiveness of care to review the sample's claims, encounters, or medical records data for evidence that the measure had been performed.[30] This methodology has several disadvantages. First, sampling reduces the precision of most estimates, meaning that comparisons of performance across health plans will be less precise. Second, reviewing medical records is costly, involving onsite review of one or more physicians providing care to the member over possibly a wide geographic area. The ability of the health plan to devote financial resources to medical records review will be positively correlated with the health plan's measured performance. That is, health plans with more resources or expertise for data collection will score higher on performance measures compared with health plans of equal quality, but with fewer resources or expertise for data collection. Thus, the possibility that performance as measured by HEDIS effectiveness of care may reflect quality of data collection rather than quality of care is a major weakness.

NCQA accreditation

NCQA is also the largest organization responsible for the accreditation of MCOs, and was the first organization to accredit health plans beginning in 1990.[3] NCQA is involved with the accreditation of half of all MCOs serving 75 percent of MCO members.[1] As Table 119-3 indicates, MCOs are evaluated in a number of its operations during the site visit by NCQA reviewers.[3] Many of the performance measures are process measures, such as whether the health plan has a written quality improvement plan which is updated annually, or whether it has written procedures for filing complaints or appeals that are distributed to its members. However, in recent years NCQA has given increased weight to clinical performance in its accreditation reviews. In particular, performance on HEDIS and CAHPS measures now accounts for 27.5 percent of the health plan's accreditation score.

Table 119-3 **Health-plan activities evaluated in an NCQA accreditation review**	
Processes and activities reviewed	**Content of review**
Quality improvement processes	Documentation of QI program and evidence of active QI committee; availability of providers; accessibility of services; member satisfaction; programs for chronic illness; continuity and coordination of care; measurement and evaluation of performance; evidence of meaningful improvements; oversight of QI activities in delegated providers
Processes for reviewing and authorizing medical care	Documented plan for managing care; criteria and procedures for approving or denying care; review of medical necessity by qualified health professional; timeliness of coverage decisions; communication of denial of coverage; process for reviewing coverage of new technologies; member satisfaction with authorization process; coverage of emergency services; procedures for drug coverage; monitoring over-use and under-use of medical services and corrective actions; triage and referral for behavioral healthcare; oversight of processes for coverage determination done by delegated providers
Quality of provider network	Procedures for assessing provider qualifications; committee to review decisions on credentials; validation of credentials; attestation of prior disciplinary actions and convictions and malpractice coverage; site visits of providers; re-evaluation of provider qualifications; process for dismissing providers with poor performance, including provider appeal; confirmation that healthcare facilities meet standards of state, federal, and private accreditation organizations; oversight of credentialing processes of delegated providers
Members' rights and responsibilities	Written statement of members' rights and responsibilities distributed to members and providers; policies for resolving complaints and appeals; handling of complaints and appeals; member information on coverage and the complaint and appeals process; insuring privacy of member information; oversight of processes for members' rights and responsibilities done by delegated providers
Preventive health activities	Guidelines for preventive healthcare and their distribution to providers; communication to members on guidelines and available preventive health programs; identification and referral of health-plan members with specific problems to available programs; oversight of processes on preventive health done by delegated providers
Medical records	Policies for keeping medical records confidential; standards for documenting in medical records and their distribution to providers; processes for assessing and improving the quality of medical records

NCQA accreditation reviews are comprehensive, involving on-site review of the health plan's documentation of compliance with the standards enumerated in Table 119-3. Accreditation decisions result in one of five possible determinations: denied, provisional, accredited, commendable, or excellent accreditation. MCOs undergo annual review of HEDIS and CAHPs data and on-site review every 3 years after receiving accreditation.

Physician profiling in MCOs

In addition to responding to external pressures to measure quality performance, some MCOs have taken the initiative to measure the quality performance of individual physicians or physician groups.[6,7] Typically, physician or physician group performance is compared to peers, adjusting for differences in case-mix. This profiling of physician performance relative to peers often includes comparisons on healthcare utilization and cost as well as measures of quality. The objective of the MCO is to compensate physicians on the basis of quality and utilization management.

In practice, producing credible physician profiles of quality are difficult for individual HMOs to do. The physician's contribution to healthcare utilization and costs is known to the health plan from administrative records (claims paid for services provided under fee-for-service, and capitation payments made for services provided under capitation). The physician's quality performance is more difficult to measure with the claims data typically used by health plans for this purpose. In particular, primary care physicians under capitation will generate limited claims for services assessed in process measures of quality. An exception is the fee-for-service reimbursement of immunizations to remove any disincentive to provide the preventive measure and to provide data to the health plan. Furthermore, some services of quality performance such as whether a diabetic in the health plan received a hemoglobin A_{1c} are not available on many MCO databases.

More importantly, since many physicians contract with several MCOs in their market area, only a portion of the physician's patients will be a member of a given MCO. A profile produced by any given MCO may be based on a small sample of the physician's patients. Furthermore, performance measures may differ on the profiles produced by the different MCOs for which the physician contracts. Because physicians are more likely to dismiss as flawed the results of profiles produced under these circumstances, their effectiveness in improving performance may be limited. Furthermore, some performance measures monitored by the MCO are population-based; however, a fraction of MCO members do not see their physicians regularly. Physicians have no opportunity or infrequent opportunities to demonstrate that they have provided quality care for this fraction of the MCO's members for which they are responsible. Again, physicians will not view such measures as credible gauges of performance.

Impact of quality improvement initiatives in managed care

Evaluation of the impact of HEDIS reporting and NCQA accreditation on clinical processes and outcomes has just begun. NCQA has reported improved performance over time for a number of measures of clinical performance for MCOs reporting HEDIS performance measures. For example, from 1998 to 1999, prescription rates for beta-blockers after acute myocardial infarction increased from 79.9 to 85.0 percent, rates for cholesterol screening from 59.1 to 68.9 percent, and rates for eye exams for diabetics from 41.4 to 45.3 percent. Performance was substantially better for accredited plans compared to nonaccredited plans. While HEDIS reporting is not universal, it measures quality of care for 51 million health-plan members. This would account for more than 60 percent of the 81 million enrolled in non-Medicare and Medicare MCOs.[32]

There is also some evidence that MCOs are using publicly reported performance measures for quality improvement and that consumers use these measures to choose their healthcare provider. A study of chief executive officers, medical directors, and quality-improvement directors from 24 MCOs reports that HEDIS and CAHPS measures were used to measure performance and target quality-improvement activities.[33] A study of 165 representatives from Medicare MCOs reports that CAHPS data enhanced awareness and knowledge of comparative performance of Medicare MCOs.[34] An evaluation of a community-based report card of quality performance for provider groups reports that 52 percent of subscribers with family coverage recalled seeing the report card during an open enrollment period for choosing their provider group, and of these 55 percent found the report card useful. Subscribers who actually changed provider groups were more likely to use the report cards and find them most useful, indicating that those "shopping" for a new provider group will use report cards on quality performance to make the decision.[35]

GOVERNMENT-SPONSORED PROVIDER PROFILING

In addition to provider profiling initiated by MCOs, the federal and several state governments have undertaken similar initiatives. The first and perhaps last initiative undertaken by CMS was its profile of mortality for Medicare beneficiaries in specific hospitals.[19] Using data on hospital discharges and mortality for Medicare beneficiaries and the regression-based case-mix methodology presented above, HCFA compared each hospital's annual mortality rate to the expected rate for hospitals with the same case-mix. The risk-adjustment methodology was further strengthened in the late 1980s.[18] The profiles were highly controversial among hospital providers and were abandoned by the 1990s. Their abandonment was most likely due to political pressures rather than methodological issues, since the statistical methods were endorsed by health services researchers.

Two states, New York and Pennsylvania, profiled hospital-specific mortality associated with coronary artery bypass graft surgery (CABG).[8,9,20,36] In New York, in-hospital mortality was initially profiled for 1989, and revealed that surgeons performing fewer than 50 procedures per year had a risk-adjusted mortality rate of 7.9 percent, more than double the 3.6 percent rate for surgeons performing 150 or more procedures.[8] Mortality rates specific to individual hospitals and surgeons were produced and distributed to hospitals and surgeons, and made available to the public. An evaluation of CABG mortality in New York based on profiles between 1989 and 1992 revealed several interesting trends. First, overall mortality for CABG declined by 41 percent between 1989 and 1992. Second, performance of low-volume surgeons improved substantially, with risk-adjusted mortality decreasing from 7.9 to 3.2 percent, but rates improved for higher-volume surgeons as well. Finally, improvement among low-volume performers was attributable in part to physicians with very high mortality rates in 1989 no longer performing CABG surgery in the subsequent years.

A similar program for profiling mortality for CABG surgery was initiated by the Pennsylvania Health Care Cost Containment Council (PH4C). As in New York, hospital-specific profiles were distributed to the public. However, in contrast to the New York program, Pennsylvania hospitals were required to collect data on a number of key clinical findings used in the computation of the Medisgroups severity scores (Admission Severity Grade and Morbidity), used in the risk-adjustment algorithm. Collection of these data cost hospitals (and ultimately healthcare consumers) a considerable amount. Furthermore, the weighting algorithm used to compute the Medisgroups severity scores is proprietary, meaning that one of the risk-adjustment variables was not public information to the provider. Data-collection costs and proprietary risk adjustment did not engender support among the provider support for the Pennsylvania profiles.

QUALITY PERFORMANCE MEASUREMENT AND QUALITY IMPROVEMENT IN THE MEDICARE PROGRAM

The Centers for Medicare and Medicaid Services (CMS, formerly HCFA) monitors quality for Medicare beneficiaries receiving services through fee-for-service providers and through MCOs contracting with CMS under the Medicare+Choice program. As in other sectors of the healthcare industry, quality initiatives in the Medicare program have increasingly emphasized the principles of continuous quality improvement.

Quality measurement and quality improvement in Medicare fee-for-service

Since the inception of the Medicare program in 1965, the quality of care received by beneficiaries has been monitored. The earliest organizations responsible for quality performance measurement were the Professional Services Review Organizations (PSROs), local review boards who reviewed care received by a limited number of beneficiaries during an inpatient hospital stay. The jurisdiction of PSROs was typically for one or several counties within a state, and had a primary focus on whether the healthcare received was medically necessary.[5]

In 1984, the PSROs were replaced by the Peer Review Organizations (PROs) with jurisdiction for an entire state (and for several of the 43 PROs, jurisdiction for more than one state).

Initially PROs monitored inpatient care by selecting random samples of inpatient admissions from computerized Medicare hospital claims records. Initial review of medical necessity and quality of care for the sampled admissions were performed by nurse reviewers. Admissions identified with problems were then reviewed by physician reviewers, who requested medical records for review if they concurred with the initial case review. Admissions judged to have problems after the review of medical records resulted in denial of payment for the admission.[5]

By the end of the 1980s, the PROs extended their review beyond inpatient care to include skilled nursing facilities, outpatient hospital departments, ambulatory surgery centers, and home health agencies. In addition, the reviews by the PROs increasingly focused on quality performance measures.

By the early 1990s, the effectiveness of the PROs in successfully monitoring quality performance and improving quality was questioned. The reliability of physician reviews done by the PROs was questioned in some influential studies. In particular, one study showed that the agreement between reviews of PRO reviewers compared with reviewers at Johns Hopkins were no better than what would be expected by chance.[37] The effectiveness of retrospective review in identifying the source of quality problems and preventing them was also questioned, given the elapse in time since specific cases were reviewed. Also, in contrast to provider profiling where quality performance is based on some or all of the provider's patients, a PRO's retrospective review of a random sample of cases will identify at most very few cases per provider subject to review and no cases for many providers. Under the PRO's system of review, this paucity of cases for any given provider invites attribution of quality problems for a specific case to random variation in outcomes rather than systemic problems with a physician or healthcare facility.

In light of this criticism of PROs, their activities were redefined under the Health Care Quality Improvement Program in 1993. Under this initiative, retrospective case review was replaced by collaborative initiatives with hospitals and physicians to improve quality that were closer to the model of CQI. While the aggregate impact of this new initiative is difficult to assess, case studies suggest success in specific settings. For example, results from one quality-improvement initiative for patients with congestive heart failure (CHF) showed that evaluation of left ventricular function improved from 53 to 65 percent and that appropriate use of ACE inhibitors improved from 54 to 74 percent.[38] Another initiative for CHF patients demonstrated improvements of left ventricular function, patient and caregiver education, and discharge planning, but no improvement in use of ACE inhibitors and calcium-channel blockers.[39]

Quality measurement and quality improvement in Medicare MCOs

Medicare beneficiaries began enrolling in Medicare MCOs in 1985 under provisions of the Tax Equity and Fiscal Responsibility Act (TEFRA). However, it would be more than a decade later that the Medicare program would begin ongoing review of healthcare quality in Medicare MCOs. This was because PROs had access to Medicare fee-for-service claims for random case selection, but did not have access to Medicare

MCO claims for the same purpose. In the interim, comprehensive evaluations of quality performance were conducted under contract with CMS by Mathematica Policy Research for both the Medicare HMO demonstrations and the Medicare MCOs contracting in the first 5 years of the TEFRA risk-contracting program.[40,41] The evaluations, which compared measures of process and outcomes for beneficiaries receiving care in Medicare MCOs to Medicare fee-for-service, reported that quality performance under MCOs and fee-for-service were quite similar. While comprehensive, these evaluations did not have the surveillance effect of the ongoing review of cases by the PROs. In addition, standards for quality performance and quality improvement measurement in commercial MCOs (i.e. MCOs other than Medicare and Medicaid) such as HEDIS and NCQA accreditation were in notable contrast to the lack of comparable quality performance standards for Medicare HMOs.

The lack of ongoing quality performance measurement in Medicare managed care ended in 1998, when CMS first required HEDIS reporting by Medicare MCOs. In addition, CMS required Medicare MCOs to submit for audit the beneficiary-level data used in the computation of the HEDIS measures. As part of the current HEDIS reporting set, CMS requires Medicare MCOs to conduct a longitudinal survey of health status for a random sample of the MCO's Medicare beneficiaries. Using the SF-36, the Health Outcomes Study compares the health status of beneficiaries surveyed in a baseline year with their health status measured two years later.

Under the 1997 Balanced Budget Act, the Quality Improvement System for Managed Care (QISMC) was established and became operational in 1999. QISMC applied many of the same principles of CQI adopted by the PROs in the Health Care Quality Improvement Program. More specifically, Medicare MCOs were required to measure clinical performance in the prevention or treatment of acute and chronic conditions, high-volume services, high-risk services, and continuity and coordination of care. Similarly, QISMC requires measurement of performance in nonclinical areas such as availability of and accessibility to care, quality of provider encounters, and resolution of appeals, grievances, and other complaints. For clinical and nonclinical areas selected by HCFA and the MCO, QISMC requires Medicare MCOs to develop and implement interventions for improving performance, and remeasure performance over time to demonstrate quality improvements. QISMC also imposes standards on methods of performance measurement; for example, they must be unambiguous, based on current clinical knowledge or health services research, and measure outcomes such as health status, functional status, beneficiary satisfaction, or valid proxies of these measures (ref. 4 QISMC standards). Performance must be measured over all relevant providers and beneficiaries at risk; and valid sampling methods must be used if performance is not measured for all beneficiaries at risk. A quality-improvement project under QISMC standards requires a minimum of 3 years: measurement of baseline performance in the first year, remeasurement of performance in the subsequent year when significant performance improvement is demonstrated, and continued measurement for a year beyond achieving significant improvement to demonstrate that higher performance has been sustained over time.[4]

MONITORING QUALITY PERFORMANCE IN NURSING HOMES

Under the Omnibus Budget Reconciliation Act (OBRA) of 1987, nursing homes participating in the Medicare and Medicaid programs are required to monitor nursing-home residents using the Resident Assessment Instrument (RAI). The RAI consists of the Minimum Data Set for Nursing Home Resident Assessment and Care Screening (MDS), which assesses functioning on activities of daily living (ADLs), cognition, continence, mood, behaviors, nutritional status, vision and communication, activities, and psychosocial well-being. Problems or risks for decline identified through the MDS assessment will trigger further assessment on one or more of the RAI's 18 Resident Assessment Protocols, that are used to identify treatable causes of problems common to nursing-home residents.[10] The OBRA 1987 requirements, which became federal law in 1990, were the result of widespread evidence of poor quality of care in nursing homes. Prior studies found prevalent use of physical restraints, inappropriate use of psychotropic medications, overuse of urinary catheters, and inadequate treatment of incontinence, pressure ulcers, nutritional problems, and behavioral problems.

Several studies compared process quality and patient outcomes prior to implementation of the RAI with the post-implementation period and found evidence of improvements. More specifically, in a study of 254 nursing homes in 10 states, accuracy of information in medical records, comprehensiveness of care plans, presence of advanced directives, participation in activities, and use of toileting programs for those with bowel incontinence improved after implementation of the RAI. Use of physical restraints declined by 25 percent and use of indwelling catheters declined by 29 percent.[42] Another study of 267 nursing homes showed that the rate of decline in ADLs, social engagement, and cognitive function was reduced after the introduction of the RAI.[43]

INITIATIVES TO REDUCE ADVERSE EVENTS ASSOCIATED WITH MEDICAL ERRORS

While the problem of medical errors has been known for some time, a concerted effort to address this problem has emerged only recently. The high likelihood of adverse events arising from medical errors was first documented in 1991 in the Harvard Medical Practice Study and in an evaluation of adverse events in Colorado and Utah.[12,44] The Harvard Medical Practice Study reports an adverse event in 3.7 percent of hospitalizations with 13.6 percent of these leading to death. The study of Colorado and Utah reports an adverse event in 2.9 percent of hospitalizations with 6.6 percent of these leading to death. Older patients (age greater than 64) face substantially higher risks than younger patients, 2.2 times higher for perioperative complications and 10 times higher for falling.[45] The 1999 Institute of Medicine (IoM) study projected the likely impact nationwide of medical errors and provided recommendations for addressing the problem. The IoM study estimates that between 44,000 and 98,000 patients in the USA die from adverse events occurring during a hospitalization;[12]

however, these estimates are likely to be biased upward since the study fails to adjust for expected mortality in the absence of medical errors.[46] Estimated annual mortality from medical errors exceeds mortality from motor vehicle accidents, breast cancer, or AIDs. The estimated financial costs associated with medical errors in the USA is immense—$17–29 billion annually.[12]

The IoM report cites many factors contributing to lack of action to address this important problem. These include: (1) limited attention by licensing and accreditation organizations to the problem of medical errors and the false sense of safety conveyed to the public by licensing or accrediting healthcare organizations without appropriate audit of medical errors; (2) the decentralized and fragmented nature of the healthcare system which does not share information across providers for patients receiving care from multiple providers, and makes implementation of systems for reducing medical errors more difficult to implement; and (3) the lack of demands from third-party payers of healthcare to improve safety and lack of incentives provided to providers to achieve this goal.

To address the problem of medical errors, the IoM report recommended a national commitment to the following objectives:

- The US Congress should create a Center for Patient Safety within the Agency for Healthcare Research and Quality (AHRQ) to set national goals for patient safety, track progress toward these goals, increase knowledge of medical errors, and establish a nationwide mandatory reporting system for medical errors.
- The performance standards imposed by government regulators, accreditation organizations, and healthcare purchasers on healthcare organizations should focus greater attention on patient safety.
- Performance standards and expectations for healthcare professionals from licensing bodies and professional societies should focus greater attention on patient safety.
- The Food and Drug Administration (FDA) should increase attention to the safe use of drugs in both the pre- and post-market phases of new drugs.
- Healthcare organizations and affiliated providers should make CQI inpatient safety a serious goal by establishing safety programs with defined executive responsibility.

There has been successful movement towards several of these goals. In particular, AHRQ has funded research on interventions to reduce medical errors; the JCAHO has instituted a policy of sanctions on healthcare organizations failing to disclose medical errors;[27] and there has been formation of the Leapfrog Group by the Business Roundtable to promote "leaps" in improved patient safety. The first three initiatives that have been endorsed by the Leapfrog Group are: (1) computer order entry system for hospital orders, (2) evidence-based referrals to hospitals for procedures such as coronary bypass surgery, carotid surgery, etc., and (3) full-time intensivists in the intensive-care units. These initiatives in metropolitan hospitals are expected to reduce death from medical error by more than 50 percent. This effort is in its infancy but is gaining momentum as the consumer begins to realize that not all hospitals are equal and that care in hospitals can be hazardous.

CONCLUSION

Quality improvement in the USA has changed dramatically since the 1980s, shifting from a focus on auditing of performance to a focus on continuous quality improvement and a greater emphasis on the measurement of outcomes. The geriatric population has been profoundly affected by several quality-improvement initiatives. These include NCQA's initiatives on annual quality-performance measurement (HEDIS) in MCOs and accreditation of MCOs; the adoption by HCFA of similar standards for Medicare managed care plans; the new emphasis on CQI initiatives by the PROs; and more comprehensive monitoring of nursing-home residents using the Resident Assessment Instrument.

These initiatives have had a positive impact on performance measures. NCQA reports improvements over time in several measures such as beta-blocker therapy after myocardial infarction and retinal examinations for diabetics. Similarly, the PROs have reported improvements in the treatment of Medicare patients with congestive heart failure. Other initiatives, such as QISMC and the Health Outcomes Study for Medicare MCOs, have just begun and have not been evaluated yet. Clearly, more evaluations of all of the initiatives of the past decade are needed to thoroughly assess their effectiveness, and to identify opportunities for improvement.

In spite of the optimism surrounding more comprehensive quality performance measurement and improvement, troubling signs of poor quality of healthcare remain. In particular, the incidence of medical errors resulting in death is astonishingly

---

KEY POINTS Quality Improvement in the USA

- Quality performance measurement and improvement have changed dramatically over the last decade with an increased focus on measuring outcomes and continuous quality improvement.

- Most managed care organization (MCOs) routinely measure and publicly report the clinical performance of their providers using HEDIS specifications and undergo accreditation review by NCQA.

- Quality measurement and improvement in the Medicare fee-for-service program is conducted by the Peer Review Organizations.

- Quality measurement and improvement activities in Medicare MCOs which are mandated by CMS include: HEDIS reporting, the Health Outcomes Survey, and the Quality Improvement System for Managed Care (QISMC) requirements.

- Quality of care in nursing homes is monitored by the Resident Assessment Instrument, a comprehensive assessment of health status, functioning, and behavioral problems.

- National initiatives to document medical errors and to redesign the health care delivery system to prevent them are now underway.

- While there is some evidence that quality improvement initiatives have been effective, further evaluation is needed.

high, and the quality of life of nursing-home patients remains poor by many objective standards in spite of increased monitoring of clinical conditions using the Resident Assessment Instrument. Actions by the JCAHO to improve the accuracy of reporting of medical errors, increased funding by the Agency for Healthcare Research and Quality (AHRQ) for research on methods for reducing medical errors, and the formation of the Leapfrog Group provide cautious optimism that the problem of medical errors is being addressed.

REFERENCES

1. NCQA: Overview. Available at www.ncqa.org/Communications/Publications/ncqaoverview.pdf, 24 August 2001
2. NCQA: HEDIS 2002. 1: Narrative—What's In It and Why It Matters. Washington, 2001
3. NCQA: Accreditation Programs. Available at www.ncqa.org/Programs/Accreditation/accreditation.htm,24 August 2001
4. HCFA: QISMC Standards. Available at www.hcfa.gov/Medicare/webquali.doc, 24 July 2001
5. Weinmann C: Quality improvement in health care: a brief history of the Medicare Peer Review Organization (PRO) initiative. Eval Health Profess 1998;21:413–418
6. Hanchak NA, Murray JF, Hirsch A, McDermott PD, Schlackman N: USQA health profile database as a tool for health plan quality improvement. Managed Care Q 1996;4(2):58–69
7. Hanchak NA: Using administrative data to evaluate the quality of care. Journal of Clinical Outcomes Management 1996;3(4):57–61
8. Hannan EL, Sui AL, Kumar D et al: The decline in coronary artery bypass graft surgery in New York State: the role of surgeon volume. JAMA 1995;273:209–213
9. Pennsylvania Health Care Cost Containment Council: Research Plan for Determining the Methodology and Reporting Issues for the 1990 Hospital and Physician Report for Coronary Artery Bypass Graft Surgery. Harrisburg, PA, 1992:1–18
10. Morris JN, Murphy K, Nonemaker S et al: Long-Term Care Facility Resident Assessment Instrument (RAI) User's Manual. Health Care Financing Administration, Baltimore, 1995
11. Fitzgerald ME, Molinari GF, Bausell RB: The empowering potential of quality improvement data. Eval Health Profess 1998;21:419–428
12. Kohn LT, Corrigan JM, Donaldson MS (eds) for the Committee on Quality Health Care in America: To Err Is Human: Building a Safer Health System. National Academy Press, Washington, 1999
13. Donabedian A: Evaluating the quality of medical care. Millbank Mem Fund Q 1966;44(3):166–206
14. Donabedian A: Quality assurance: structure, process and outcome. Nurs Stand 1992;7(11 suppl Qa):4–5
15. President's Advisory Commission on Consumer Protection and Quality in the Health Care Industry: Quality First: Better Health Care for All Americans. Final Report to the President of the United States. Government Printing Office, Washington, 1998
16. Charlson ME, Pompei P, Ales KI, MacKenzie CR: A new method of classifying prognostic comorbidity in longitudinal studies: development and validation. J Chronic Dis 1987;40:373–382
17. Health Care Financing Administration: Diabetes National Project Overview, 2000 (unpublished)
18. Health Care Financing Administration: Evaluation of the Adequacy of the Model Used for the Analyses of Mortality Rates Associated with Hospitalization. Office of Program Assessment and Information, Health Standards and Quality Bureau, Baltimore, 1989
19. Health Care Financing Administration: Medicare Hospital Mortality Information. US Government Printing Office, Washington, 1992
20. Smith DW: Analysis Plan for Coronary Artery Bypass Graft Surgery in Pennsylvania: Final Report. MediQual Systems Inc, 1993:1–11
21. Ullman R, Hill JW, Scheye EC, Spoeri RK: Satisfaction and choice: a view from the plans. Health Affairs 1997;16:209–217
22. Iezzoni LI (ed): Risk Adjustment for Measuring Health Care Outcomes, 2nd edn. Health Administration Press, Ann Arbor, 1997
23. Deming WE: Out of the Crisis. MIT Center for Advance Engineering Study, Cambridge, MA, 1986
24. King KM, Bungard TJ, McAlister FA et al: Quality improvement for CQI. Prev Med Managed Care 2000;1(3):129–137
25. Krumholz HM, Radford MJ, Ellerbeck EF et al: Aspirin for secondary prevention after acute myocardial infarction in the elderly: prescribed use and outcomes. Arch Intern Med 1996;124:292–298
26. McLaughlin TJ, Soumerai SB, Willison DJ et al: Adherence to national guidelines for drug treatment of suspected acute myocardial infarction: evidence for undertreatment in women and the elderly. Arch Intern Med 1996;156:799–805
27. Leape LL, Woods DD, Hatlie MJ et al: Promoting patient safety by preventing medical errors. JAMA 1998;280:1444–1447
28. Carey RG, Lloyd RC: Measuring Quality Improvement in Healthcare: A Guide to Statistical Process Control Applications. Quality Press, Miwankee, 2001
29. Montgomery DC: An Introduction to Statistical Quality Control. John Wiley, New York, 2001
30. NCQA: HEDIS 2002. 2: Technical Specifications. Washington, 2001
31. NCQA: HEDIS 2002. 3: Specifications for Survey Measures. Washington, 2001
32. Medicare 2000: 35 Years of Improving America's Health and Security. Available at www.hcfa.gov/stats/35chartbk. pdf, 12 September 2001
33. Scanlon DP, Darby C, Rolph E, Doty HE: The role of performance measures for improving quality in managed care organizations. Health Serv Res 2001;36:619–644
34. Smith F, Gerteis M, Downey N et al: The effects of disseminating performance data to health plans: results of qualitative research with the Medicare managed care plans. Health Serv Res 2001;36:643–663
35. Schultz J, Call KT, Feldman R, Christianson J: Do employees use report cards to assess health care provider systems? Health Serv Res 2001;36:509–530
36. Bentley JM, Nash DB: How Pennsylvania hospitals have responded to publicly released reports on coronary artery bypass graft surgery. J Qual Improv 1998;24(1):40–49
37. Rubin HR, Rogers WH, Kahn KL, Rubinstein LV, Brook RH: Watching the doctor-watchers. JAMA 1992;267:2349–2354
38. DeLong JF, Allman RM, Sherrill RG, Schiesz N: A congestive heart failure project with measured improvements in care. Eval Health Profess 1998;21:472–486
39. Caldwell GG, Berg P, Pritchard C, Lewis JN: Quality improvement in the diagnosis and treatment of heart failure by participating Indiana and Kentucky hospitals. Eval Health Profess 1998;21:461–471
40. Retchin SM, Brown RS, Cohen R et al: The Quality of Care in TEFRA HMOs/CMPs. Medical College of Virginia, Richmond, 1992
41. Brown R, Clement DG, Hill JW, Retchin SM, Bergeron J: Do health maintenance organizations work for Medicare? Health Care Finan Rev 1993;15(1):7–24
42. Hawes C, Mor V, Phillips CD et al: The OBRA-87 nursing home regulations and implementation of the Resident Assessment Instrument: effects on process quality. J Am Geriatr Soc 1997;45:977–985
43. Phillips CD, Morris JN, Hawes C et al: Association of the Resident Assessment Instrument (RAI) with changes in function, cognition, and psychosocial status. J Am Geriatr Soc 1997;45:986–993
44. Brennan TA, Leape LL et al: Incidence of adverse events and negligence in hospitalized patients: results of the Harvard Medical Practice Study I. N Engl J Med 1991;324:370–376
45. Rothschild JM, Bates DW, Leape LL: Preventable medical injuries in older patients. Arch Intern Med 2000;160:2717–2728
46. McDonald CJ, Weiner M, Hui SL: Deaths due to medical errors are exaggerated in the Institute of Medicine report. JAMA 2000;284:93–97

Chapter 120

Managed care for elderly people in the USA

Howard M. Fillit, Christine Himes, and Alan Lazaroff

Prepaid healthcare, in which individuals pay in advance for coverage of medical care, began in the USA with employers during the early part of the twentieth century.[1] Today, over 180 million Americans with health insurance are considered to be in some form of prepaid health insurance, or "managed care" through private or government insurance. The modern era of managed care was heralded by a new law enacted by the US Congress in 1973. The law allowed the establishment of health maintenance organizations (HMOs) whose purpose was to promote preventive healthcare for individuals enrolled in the prepaid health plan. For the elderly, HMOs receive government funds from the Health Care Financing Administration (HCFA) (now the Center for Medicare and Medicaid Services) through Medicare (the US program which pays for most aspects of healthcare for the elderly population) on a "capitated" or budgeted basis for each individual enrollee. These payments are based on a number of factors including age and geographic variations in healthcare costs. In return, the health plans are responsible for the costs of healthcare experienced by the individual enrollee. In addition, plans are held responsible for the quality of the medical care provided to the enrollee, as well as all other administrative aspects of the plans' business, such as marketing.

The Medicare managed-care program has expanded progressively, although growth has slowed recently. Revisions were enacted in the Medicare managed-care program by Congress in 1997 and 1999 which increased the administrative burden and reduced payments to health plans.[2] As a result, some Medicare health plans now called "Medicare+Choice" (M+C) plans exited the government program, resulting in recent declines in the number of Americans enrolled in Medicare managed-care plans. As of July 2001, about 5.5 million persons had enrolled in Medicare managed-care organizations (MCOs), or about 15 percent of Medicare eligible individuals.

Medicare managed-care plans have several potential advantages over the traditional Medicare fee-for-service program. M+C plans generally have lower deductibles and copayments. M+C plans may offer benefits that are not part of Medicare fee-for-service coverage, such as payments for preventive care including reimbursement for prescription drugs, eyeglasses, and hearing aids; health education and health-promotion programs such as case management and disease management; and discounts on or improved access to transportation, day care, respite care, or assisted living. Coverage for pharmaceutical costs has been a major reason why elderly Americans have joined the M+C plans. Recently, as many M+C plans have experienced financial difficulties, they have withdrawn or limited their coverage of pharmaceuticals, making them less attractive to elderly individuals.

The term "managed-care organization" refers to any healthcare organization which attempts to integrate the financing and delivery of healthcare in order to manage the quality and costs of care for an insured population. MCOs include payors such as health plans, as well as providers including independent practitioners associations (IPAs), medical groups, and hospital systems.

By integrating the financing of healthcare with its delivery, Medicare MCOs are in the difficult but important position of attempting to balance the needs of individual members of the MCO for "customized" healthcare with the quality, ethical, and cost concerns of the MCO population as a whole (population-based healthcare), essentially attempting to put into practice the principles of public health for large groups of individuals. In theory, the practice of population-based care should improve care for most individuals while reducing overall costs by reducing the variability in care and promoting "appropriate" care, reducing excess or unnecessary costs (such as unnecessary hospitalizations) while increasing utilization of interventions which promote health (such as the use of influenza vaccinations). In practice, MCOs have been criticized for prioritizing cost control at the expense of quality of care, for example by not allowing payment for procedures that may be necessary.

MODELS OF RELATIONSHIPS BETWEEN MCOS, PROVIDERS, AND INDIVIDUALS

There are several models of relationships between MCOs and insured individuals. These include health-maintenance organizations (HMOs) that restrict access to a limited panel of physicians, hospitals and other services that have agreed to provide care to health-plan members at a reduced price. Other less restrictive models such as point-of-service plans, preferred-provider plans, or managed indemnity plans allow members greater choice and access to a wider variety of providers. However, since larger networks of providers are more difficult to manage, these less restrictive plans are more costly to the individual through higher premiums, deductibles, and copayments.

There are also a variety of contractual relationships between MCOs and providers. These include the "staff model" in which the MCO is an insurer which also employs physicians and owns hospitals, clinics, and other facilities. The staff model is uncommon in the USA. Fewer than 5 percent of managed-care enrollees are in staff model plans. In the group model, MCOs have exclusive contracts with large multispecialty or primary care groups, but they do not own the providers.

The most common model is the independent practitioner association (IPA) model in which an insurer has contractual relationships with individual physicians or networks of physicians who generally retain ownership of their practices. The IPA to which the physician belongs may provide certain services to assist in managing care.

The method of physician payment can significantly affect the ability of an MCO to manage care through medical management programs.[3,4] Physician payment methodologies in managed care vary widely. Physicians may be paid for individual services (fee-for-service programs) or through various capitation models in which a budget is negotiated between payors and providers that covers healthcare costs for individuals or groups of individuals over a fixed time (usually a year). Full or global capitation refers to a contract in which a provider such as a physician group or health system is paid a budgeted amount and is responsible (or "at risk") for all medical costs of the insured population, including hospitalization. "Professional" or "primary care" capitation refers to a contract in which physicians are only "at risk" for their own services, but not other costs such as those of the hospital or home-care agency.

Capitation payment models involve considerable financial risk for providers, and many providers have gone bankrupt as a result of capitation.[4] Providers, such as hospital systems or physician groups, can lose money if patients are not well managed and medical costs exceed the budget. Providers can also lose money if the negotiated contract does not provide a reasonable rate to cover the costs of care. On the other hand, providers can profit if patients are well managed and preventive care is effective, resulting in care being delivered at less than budget.

Unburdened by traditional Medicare fee-for-service regulations and restrictions which can be considerable, capitation creates incentives for the redesign of health care in ways that are innovative and cost-effective (e.g. payments for geriatric assessment). However, in capitated arrangements, there are "perverse incentives" for under-utilization of needed services. For example, in an IPA with "global capitation" a physician may be reluctant to hospitalize a patient because of the expense involved. On the other hand, physicians have perverse incentives in fee-for-service to over-utilize and provide unnecessary care. The transition from fee-for-service to capitation is often difficult for physicians.

SERVICES PROVIDED BY MANAGED-CARE ORGANIZATIONS

Various services, many of which are mandated by the federal government, are provided by Medicare MCOs. Some of these functions are primarily related to the services of the insurer, such as marketing, sales, claims administration and payment, and member services. Network development attempts to create a coordinated continuum of care through contracting, insuring access to the most high-quality, cost-effective providers. Health plans must also ensure that all providers—including hospitals and physicians—meet credentialing standards. Quality oversight is an important mandated function of the health plan. In fee-for-service Medicare, there are few capabilities for quality oversight and other administrative services often provided by MCOs. The government now has regulated certain aspects of quality improvement that must be followed by Medicare+Choice, including accreditation by an independent organization, generally the National Committee for Quality Assurance (NCQA).

Medical management in MCOs

The process of managed care shares some common goals and processes with geriatric medicine.[5,6] Both emphasize preventive healthcare through risk screening. Similar to geriatric assessment, this process proactively identifies persons who may benefit from case management. Both also seek to provide healthcare to elderly individuals across a coordinated continuum of care employing the most cost-effective site (preferably the home) and avoiding hospitalization. This is often accomplished by effective contracting.

Medical management in Medicare MCOs has evolved in a fairly standard manner across the industry. These efforts are often led by a Medicare MCO medical director with experience in geriatric care. The lack of geriatricians in the USA limits their presence in the administration of Medicare MCOs.

Health risk screening is now mandated by HCFA for all new members enrolling in health plans. High-risk members identified by risk screening are referred to some form of follow-up through case management or disease management. Health risk appraisals (HRAs) are "screening instruments" used in managed care to initiate preventive population-based health care.[7,8] Managed-care health risk appraisals are provided to large populations and are implemented employing mailed surveys or telephonically. Telephone surveys are generally more expensive and time-consuming than mailed surveys, but they obtain more reliable information. HRAs are used to identify persons at risk of adverse health outcomes such as hospitalizations generating high healthcare utilization. Medicare fee-for-service does not employ risk screening in its programs.

Administrative data include data derived from insurance claims. Medical and pharmacy claims are used to evaluate the health status of individuals in MCOs. Administrative data are relatively inexpensive to obtain in most Medicare MCOs with sophisticated information systems. However, the quality, timeliness, and availability of such data can vary.[9–12]

In general, self-reported health risk data and administrative data equally predict healthcare use. However, because response rates to self-reported health surveys are generally only 50–60 percent, with nonresponders usually having higher health risk, administrative data have advantages because they can be obtained for all existing members of the MCO at a much lower cost.

Self-reported health surveys are more useful for persons who are newly enrolled in an MCO who do not have a claims history. Self-report surveys are also useful for identifying problems which cannot generally be identified by administrative data, such as smoking, alcohol use, cognitive impairment, falls, and nutritional problems. Self-reported health risk data are also useful for promoting well-being (e.g. exercise, stress reduction, smoking cessation) in the healthy elderly and for eliciting patient preferences, self-perceived health status, values, and the need for ancillary services (e.g. homemaker services, transportation).

It is illegal for an MCO to require health risk appraisals before individuals enroll in the MCO. This policy prevents MCOs from "cherry picking," the practice of enrolling only healthy persons. Under the payment system from the government at present, MCOs with many high-risk frail elderly members ("adverse selection") are more likely to lose money, whereas MCOs with few high-risk members ("favorable selection") may profit.[13] Responding to this situation, the Balanced Budget Act of 1997 required that the HCFA institute a health risk-adjusted payment system. This new system will attempt to pay Medicare+Choice health plans a capitated rate based on the relative illness burden of its members, decreasing payments to MCOs with favorable selection and increasing payments to MCOs with adverse selection. This payment system may increase the financial incentives of health plans to enroll, retain, and care for frail elderly patients.

Geriatric care management

Identification of high-risk members and triaging them to case management may reduce costs and improve the quality of care, although there are few data supporting this.[14–16] Frail elderly patients (generally those >75 years with multiple chronic health problems complicated by significant functional and psychosocial impairments) are generally classified as "high risk." Once identified, high-risk patients are assigned by triage to geriatric care management programs (Fig. 120-1).

Geriatric care management programs vary greatly. Most programs primarily use telephone communication, some may use home visits. Many geriatric care-management programs provided by MCOs promote patient self-management of chronic disease through education. Most attempt to improve access to the geriatric continuum of care and community resources to assist primary care physicians to provide better geriatric care.

An effective geriatric continuum of care enables the MCO to use the most cost-effective site of care while maintaining quality. Hospital admissions and prolonged hospital stays are the most expensive component of healthcare (generally accounting for about 40 percent of costs). Unnecessary hospitalizations can often be avoided through innovative use of subacute and home care (e.g. for community-acquired pneumonia). Shortening length of hospital stays (e.g. for hip fractures and strokes) is also a major emphasis of MCO medical-management programs.

Long-term care is covered by very few MCOs. Programs such as the Program of All-Inclusive Care for the Elderly (PACE) pool Medicaid and Medicare capitation to provide comprehensive geriatric care to those eligible for a nursing home.[17] Other models manage the Medicare portion of long-term custodial care; these models offer medical care primarily through extensive use of nurse practitioners.

Disease management

Disease management programs target high-prevalence, costly, chronic illnesses that may be effectively managed with a population-based approach (see Fig. 120-1). Management of chronic illness between physician visits is an important component of these programs, which typically use nonphysician providers to teach patients self-management and to coordinate care with physician providers.[18]

Disease-management programs are more difficult to implement in IPA models than in staff or group models. Physicians in an IPA model generally have too few patients from any one payor to attend to any individual payor's care-management program. However, contractual incentives such as capitation may create incentives for participation in disease-management programs.

Disease-management programs seek to improve the outcomes of patients with chronic diseases like diabetes and congestive heart failure by using an organized, often evidence-based approach to provide optimal treatment, preventing hospitalizations due to exacerbations and complications of these illnesses.[19,20] Improvements in care and control of costs may result from the same intervention. Many studies document the relatively poor performance of American medicine in providing treatments of proven effectiveness, such as angiotensin-converting enzyme (ACE) inhibitors for congestive heart failure or beta-blockers after myocardial infarction.[21] Disease-management programs attempt to improve care through proactive, preventive interventions such as patient education and disease-specific case management.

Disease-management programs may be operated by healthcare systems, physician organizations, or health plans. Typically, high-cost, high-volume conditions are targeted for disease management, especially when associated with potentially preventable events like hospitalization or emergency room usage. The availability of effective interventions and the likelihood of demonstrating clinical benefit and financial savings in a relatively short time frame are other desirable characteristics. Asthma, congestive heart failure, diabetes, and chronic obstructive pulmonary disease are among the most commonly addressed conditions.

Patients who are appropriate for disease-management programs may be identified through information systems, or referred by physicians or discharge planners, often according to

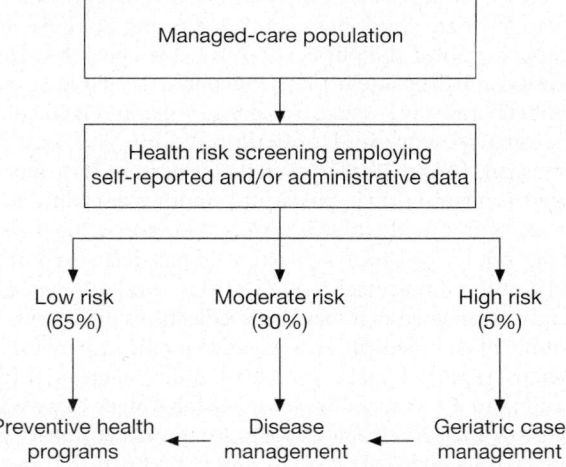

Figure 120-1 A population-based approach to geriatric care management. Patients are directed to appropriate programs on the basis of health risk appraisal. Adapted from Fillit HM et al.[103]

explicit eligibility criteria that include diagnosis, specific clinical characteristics such as disease stage, and heavy service and pharmaceutical use. Further assessment and risk stratification may be performed to identify the optimal group for the intervention. Since the benefits of preventive interventions may be difficult to discern in an individual patient, group outcomes will be the measure of success. This focus on the health of a population is consistent with the conceptual framework of managed care.

Disease-management programs use a variety of approaches, ranging from simple tracking and reminder systems, to telephone checks by a case manager, to comprehensive management by a multidisciplinary team. A program for congestive heart failure could be based on a CHF clinic housing a multidisciplinary team including cardiologist, nurse, physical therapist, health educator, social worker, and pharmacist. Alternately, increasing use of ACE inhibitors in patients with CHF may be the key goal of the program, with reminders mailed to physicians with patients not being so treated. Disease-management programs attempt to reduce variation in care by identifying and implementing best practices, often through the use of evidence-based clinical guidelines or protocols.

A well-designed study[22] of multidisciplinary team care after hospital discharge for congestive heart failure demonstrated a 56 percent decrease in readmission for CHF in the first 90 days after discharge, with an estimated saving of $460 per patient. A simpler, "home-based" intervention[23] produced a 43 percent decrease in CHF readmissions over a 6-month period. A protocol-driven, primary care-based program[24] achieved a 48 percent reduction in lower-extremity amputations among high-risk diabetic patients. Finally, the Arthritis Self-Management Program teaches patients the skills to live with their disease, and produces improvements in self-reported outcomes and a reduction in the demand for medical services.

Since disease-management programs segregate patients by diagnosis, problems may be encountered in serving the frail elderly patient with multiple chronic diseases. Fragmentation of care could result from the application of disease-management approaches for several conditions in a single patient. Frail geriatric patients may be served more effectively by care organized around function rather than diagnosis, such as geriatric care-management programs. Disease-management programs have been criticized for focusing too much on short-term financial outcomes, for giving inadequate attention to longer-term prevention opportunities, and for paying insufficient attention to psychosocial and other patient-specific issues.

Managing care for the geriatric syndromes

Expanding on programs that identify and manage health risk, the next generation of managed-care strategies for older adults will focus on building functional reserve and preventing unnecessary functional decline. This strategy is compelling because it both improves clinical outcomes and reduces the cost of caring for the expanding population of older persons with chronic illness and frail health. Functional decline and accompanying frailty is costly, with direct healthcare costs in the USA estimated at $24 billion and rising.[25]

Studies have shown that, compared with their counterparts whose functional status worsened over time, the direct cost of care among members who maintained high functional status despite comparable risks and chronic diseases was 62 percent lower.[26] Further, benefits with regard to both outcomes and costs can be realized in the relatively short time horizon of 6–12 months.[18] MCOs that invest in the management of geriatric syndromes with well-studied, effective interventions that improve function and quality of life are most likely to achieve greatest success.

"Functional reserve" refers to the capacity of individuals to withstand a threat to their health and functional status. Persons with limited functional reserve take longer to recover, or may not recover fully from their illness to the point where they can manage at home. Reduced functional reserve is frequently multifactorial, and different combinations of geriatric conditions and chronic diseases may contribute to decline in a given individual.

Although many conditions may potentially threaten functional reserve, six treatable geriatric syndromes have been well studied. They are becoming the focus for well-managed geriatric care because they represent common problems that adversely affect function and quality of life; they are frequently underdiagnosed and therefore undertreated; and effective evidence-based interventions are available (Table 120-1). These conditions cannot be viewed in isolation since they often occur concurrently and may interact with each other negatively or may confound treatment.[18,27,28]

An example of an MCO polypharmacy program included a direct-to-member and a physician component.[29] Members who were using five or more drugs were identified through administrative data obtained from electronic pharmacy records. These members were sent a brown bag together with an educational letter from the MCO medical director. The letter described the risks of taking multiple drugs and asked the members to place all their prescriptions and over-the-counter drugs in the bag and take them to their physician for a medication review. The physician was sent a drug-management report that listed all prescriptions filled by the member, including prescriptions prescribed by consultants that the primary care physician might be unaware of. The report enabled the physician to quickly check for drug duplication and drug interactions. Polypharmacy clinical practice guidelines or other educational information (e.g. recommendations on improved prescribing) were also sent to the physician. The program showed that 17 percent of members reported informing their physicians about prescription or nonprescription medicines they were taking that the physicians did not know about; 35 percent of physicians reported discontinuing unnecessary medications; and 20 percent of members reported that they had medications discontinued as a result of the medication review. Overall, 45 percent of physicians reported making at least one change in their prescribing to a member at risk for polypharmacy as a result of the program. Occasionally, such programs employ MCO pharmacists to review drug-management reports,[30] though this approach is considerably more expensive. Thus, polypharmacy programs can reduce unnecessary pharmacy costs, improve prescribing, and reduce the number of adverse drug interactions.

Table 120-1 Treatable geriatric syndromes in managed care

Geriatric syndrome	Prevalence and costs	Interventions
Physical inactivity	Principal risk factor for chronic health problems, loss of functional reserve and disability[26,31–34] Contributing factor for extended hospital stay and/or need for post acute care in skilled nursing facilities[35–37]	Programs that promote physical conditioning with a focus on muscle strengthening and flexibility exercises, for all members from healthy to frail[37–43]
Urinary incontinence	15–30% of community-dwelling older adults Direct cost of care in USA exceeds $11 billion[44–46] High impact on quality of life[47–51]	Behavioral therapy with nurse or physical therapist;[52–55] pelvic-floor exercises;[56] medications; surgery
Polypharmacy	14–24% of community-dwelling older adults take medications believed to be inappropriate[57–59] Medication-related complications account for 10–31% of all hospitalizations and 45% of hospital readmits[60,61]	Clinical pharmacist reviews; MD reviews; patient education[29,30,62–64]
Falls	30% community-dwelling older adults fall every year 50% of these fall repeatedly[65–68] 8% of people >70 will visit the ER as a result of falls every year, and 33% of these will be hospitalized[69]	Physical activity programs with emphasis on lower-extremity strengthening and balance; optimize vision; home safety evaluations; assistive devices; medication reviews[42,70–75]
Depression	5–10% of community-dwelling older adults; 30–40% of those recently hospitalized; 15–30% of nursing-home residents;[76,77] 47–61% higher costs of care for depressed patients 38% more visits[78–81]	Behavioral therapy including exercise and socialization; psychotherapy; medications[27,82–85]
Dementia	5–10% of adults over 65 years; 50% of adults over 85 years[86] Third most costly disease in the USA, with costs exceeding $100 billion Significant increase in hospital admissions and lengths of stay[86–91]	Caregiver support;[92–94] advanced planning;[95] management of comorbid diseases; medications; linkage to community resources[96–102]

KEY POINTS Managed care for elderly people in the USA

- Managed care is a continually evolving system that has great potential to improve the care of elderly people.

- Managed care attempts to combine the principles of population-based health with the needs of the individual.

- Managed care seeks to improve the quality and control the costs of care by a focus on preventive health.

- The principles of managed care are being adopted in many parts of the world outside the USA.

REFERENCES

1. Kongstvedt PR: The Managed Health Care Handbook, 3rd edn. Aspen, Gaithersburg, MD, 1996
2. Gold M: Medicare+Choice: an interim report card. Health Aff 2001;20:120–138
3. Boland P: The power and potential of capitation. Managed Care 1997;5:1–9
4. Robinson JC: Physician organization in California: crisis and opportunity. Health Aff 2001;20:81–96
5. The HMO Workgroup on Care Management: Identifying high-risk Medicare members. Case Manager 1997;8:57–61
6. The HMO Workgroup on Care Management: Essential components of geriatric care provided through health maintenance organizations. J Am Geriatr Soc 1998;46:303–308
7. Pacala JT, Boult C, Reed RL, Aliberti E: Predictive validity of the PRA instrument among older recipients of managed care. J Am Geriatr Soc 1997;45:614–617
8. Fillit HM, Picariello GP, Warburton SW: Health risk appraisals in the elderly: results from a survey of 70,000 Medicare HMO members. J Clin Outcomes Meas 1997;4:23–29
9. Iezzoni LI: Assessing quality using administrative data. Ann Intern Med 1997;127:666–674
10. Coleman EA, Wagner EH, Grothaus LC et al: Predicting hospitalization and functional decline in older health plan enrollees: are administrative data as accurate as self-report? J Am Geriatr Soc 1998;Apr;46(4):419–425
11. Mukamel DB, Chou C-C, Zimmer JG, Roethenberg BM: The effect of accurate patient screening on the cost-effectiveness of case management programs. Gerontologist 1997;37:777–784

12. Hornbrook MC, Goodman MJ, Fishman PA et al: Building health plan databases to risk adjust outcomes and payments. Int J Qual Health Care 1998;10:531–538

13. Brown RS, Clement DG, Hill JW, Retchin SM, Bergeron JW: Do health maintenance organizations work for Medicare? Health Care Fin Rev 1993;15:7–23

14. Boult C, Rassen J, Rassen A, Moore RJ, Robinson S: The effect of case management on the costs of health care for enrollees in Medicare Plus Choice plans: a randomized trial. J Am Geriatr Soc 2000;48:996–1001

15. Pacala JT, Boult C, Hepburn KW et al: Case management of older adults in health maintenance organizations. J Am Geriatr Soc 1995;43:538–542

16. Aliotta SL: Components of a successful case management program. Managed Care 1996;4:38–45

17. Branch LG, Coulam RF, Zimmerman YA: The Pace evaluation: initial findings. Gerontologist 1995;35:349–359

18. Leveille SG, Wagner EH, Davis C et al: Preventing disability and managing chronic illness in frail older adults: a randomized trial of a community-based partnership with primary care. J Am Geriatr Soc 1998;46:153–162

19. Rich MW: Heart failure disease management programs: efficacy and limitations. Am J Med 2001;110:410–412

20. Jedrey CM, Chaurette KA, Winn LB: Cooperative disease management programs. J Ambul Care Manage 2001;24:15–25

21. Roglieri JL, Futterman R, McDonough KL et al: Disease management interventions to improve outcomes in congestive heart failure. Am J Managed Care 1997;3:1831–1839

22. Rich M, Beckman V, Wittenberg C: A multi-disciplinary intervention to prevent the readmission of elderly patients with cognitive heart failure. N Engl J Med 1995;333:1190–1195

23. Stewart S, Pearson S, Horowitz J: Effects of a home-based intervention among patients with cognitive heart failure discharged from acute hospital care. Arch Intern Med 1998;158:1067–1072

24. Rith-Najarian S, Branchaud C, Beaulieu O: Reducing lower-extremity amputations due to diabetes: application of the staged diabetes management approach in a primary care setting. J Fam Pract 1998;47:127–132

25. National Institute on Aging: Physical Frailty. National Institutes of Health, 1991

26. Leveille SG, LaCroix A, Hecht JA, Grothaus L, Wagner EH: The cost of disability in older women and opportunities for prevention. J Womens Health 1992;1:53–61

27. Singh NA, Clements KM, Fiatarone MA: A randomized trial of progressive resistance training in depressed elders. J Gerontol A 1997;52:M27–M35

28. Dugan E, Cohen SJ, Bland DR et al: The association of depressed symptoms and urinary incontinence among older adults. J Am Geriatr Soc 2000;48:413–416

29. Fillit HM, Futterman R, Orland BI et al: Polypharmacy management in Medicare managed care: changes in prescribing by primary care physicians resulting from a program promoting medication review. Am J Managed Care 1999;5:8587–8594

30. Monane M, Matthias DM, Nagle BA, Kelly MA: Improving prescribing patterns for the elderly through an on-line drug utilization review intervention: a system linking the physician, pharmacist and the computer. JAMA 1998;280:1249–1252

31. Larson EB: Exercise, functional decline and frailty. J Am Geriatr Soc 1991;39:635–636

32. Berg RL, Cassells JS: The Second Fifty Years: Promoting Health and Preventing Disability. National Academy Press, Washington, 1990

33. Guralnick JM, LaCroix AZ, Abbott RD et al: Maintaining mobility late in life. I: Demographic characteristics and chronic conditions. Am J Epidemiol 1993;137:845–857

34. LaCroix AZ, Guralnick JM, Berkman LF, Wallace RB, Satterfield S: Maintaining mobility late in life. II: Smoking, alcohol consumption, physical activity and body mass index. Am J Epidemiol 1993;137:858–869

35. Kane RL, Finch M, Blewett L et al: Use of post-hospital care by Medicare patients. J Am Geriatr Soc 1996;44:242–250

36. Sager MA, Rudberg MA, Jalajuddin M et al: Hospital Admission Risk Profile (HARP): identifying older patients at risk for functional decline following acute medical illness and hospitalization. J Am Geriatr Soc 1996;44:251–257

37. Hoeing H, Nusbaum N, Brummel-Smith K: Geriatric rehabilitation: state of the art. J Am Geriatr Soc 1997;45:1371–1381

38. Wagner EH: Preventing decline in function: evidence from randomized trials around the world. West J Med 1997;167:295–298

39. Jette AM, Lachman M, Giorgetti MM et al: Exercise—it's never too late: the Strong for Life Program. Am J Pub Health 1999;89:66–72

40. Wallace JI, Buchner DM, Grothaus L, Leveille S, Tyll L, LaCroix AZ: Implementation and effectiveness of a community based health promotion program for older adults. J Gerontol A 1998;53:M301–M306

41. Fiatarone MA, Marks EC, Ryan ND et al: High-intensity strength training in nonagenarians: effects on skeletal muscle. JAMA 1990;263:3029–3034

42. Buchner DM, Cress ME, deLateur BJ et al: The effect of strength and endurance training on gait, balance, fall risk, and health services use in community living older adults. J Gerontol A 1997;52:M218–M224

43. National Institute on Aging: Exercise—A Guide from the National Institute on Aging. NIH99–4258, 1999

44. Hu TW: Impact of urinary incontinence on health-care costs. J Am Geriatr Soc 1990;38:292–295

45. Ruther M, Helbing C: Health care financing trends: use and costs of home care services under Medicare. Health Care Finan Rev 1988;10:105–108

46. Urinary Incontinence Guideline Panel: Urinary Incontinence in Adults: Clinical Practice Guideline. AHCPR No. 920038, Rockville, MD, 1992

47. Burgio KL, Ouslander JG: Effect of urge incontinence on quality of life in older people. J Am Geriatr Soc 1999;47:1033

48. Wyman JF: Quality of life in older adults with urinary incontinence. J Am Geriatr Soc 1998;46:779

49. Brown JS, Posner SF, Stewart S: Urge incontinence: new health related quality of life measures. J Am Geriatr Soc 1999;47:988

50. DuBeau CE, Kiely DK, Resnick NM: Quality of life impact of urge incontinence in older persons: a new measure and conceptual structure. J Am Geriatr Soc 1999;47:994

51. Johnson TMI, Kincaid JE, Bernard SL et al: The association of urinary incontinence with poor self-rated health. J Am Geriatr Soc 1990;38:282–288

52. Fantl JA, Wyman JF, McClish DK et al: Efficacy of bladder training in older women with urinary incontinence. JAMA 1991;265:609–613

53. Burgio KL, Locher JL, Goode PS: Combined behavioral and drug therapy for urge urinary incontinence in older women. J Am Geriatr Soc 2000;48:370–374

54. McDowell BJ, Enberg S, Sereika S et al: Effectiveness of behavioral therapy to treat incontinence in homebound older adults. J Am Geriatr Soc 1999;47:319

55. NIH Consensus Conference: Urinary incontinence in adults. JAMA 1989;261:2685–2690

56. Wells TJ, Brink CA, Diokno AC, Wolfe R, Gillis GL: Pelvic muscle exercise for stress urinary incontinence in elderly women. J Am Geriatr Soc 1991;39:791

57. Wilcox SM, Himmelstein DU, Woolhandler S: Inappropriate drug prescribing for the community dwelling elderly. JAMA 1994;272:292–296

58. Stuck A, Beers MH, Steiner A et al: Inappropriate medication use in community residing older persons. Arch Intern Med 1994;154:2195–2200

59. Hanlon JC, Schmader KE, Ruby CM, Weingerger M: Suboptimal prescribing in older inpatients and outpatients. J Am Geriatr Soc 2001;49:200–209

60. Bero LA, Lipton HL, Bird JA: Characterization of geriatric drug related hospital readmissions. Med Care 1991;29:989–1003

61. Bates DW, Spell N, Cullen DJ et al: The cost of adverse drug events in hospitalized patients. JAMA 1997;277:307–311

62. Hanlon JT, Weingerger M, Samsa GP et al: A randomized controlled trial of a clinical pharmacist intervention to improve inappropriate prescribing in elderly outpatients with polypharmacy. Am J Med 1996;100:428–437

63. Coleman EA, Grothaus LC, Sandhu N, Wagner EH: Chronic care clinics: a randomized, controlled trial of a new model of primary care for frail older adults. J Am Geriatr Soc 1999;47:775–783

64. McCombs JS, Liu G, Shi J et al: The Kaiser Permanente USC Patient Consultation Study: change in use and cost of health care services. Am J Health-sys Pharm 1998;55:2485–2499

65. Tinetti ME, Speechly M, Ginter SF: Risk factors for falls among elderly persons living in the community. N Engl J Med 1988;319:1701–1707

66. Sattin RW, Lambert HA, Devito CA: The incidence of fall injury among the elderly in a defined population. Am J Epidemiol 1990;131:1028–1036

67. King MB, Tinetti ME: Falls in community dwelling older persons. J Am Geriatr Soc 1995;43:1146–1154

68. Rubenstein LZ, Robbins AS, Josephson KR: The value of assessing falls in an elderly population. Ann Intern Med 1990;113:308–316

69. Campbell AJ, Borrie MJ, Spears GF: Risk factors for falls in a community-based prospective study of people 70 years and older. J Gerontol Med Sci 1989;44:M112–M117

70. Hauer K, Rost B, Rutchle K, Opitz H, Specht N: Exercise training for rehabilitation and secondary prevention of falls in geriatric patients with a history of injurious falls. J Am Geriatr Soc 2001;49:10–20

71. Lamb SE, Morse RE, Evans G: Mobility after proximal femoral fracture: the relevance of leg power, postural sway and other factors. Aging 1995;24:308–314

72. Fiaterone MA, O'Neill EF, Ryan ND: Exercise training and nutritional supplementation for physical frailty in very elderly people. N Engl J Med 1994;330:1170–1175

73. Tinetti ME, Baker DJ, McVay G: A multifactorial intervention to reduce the risk of falling among elderly people in the community. N Engl J Med 1994;331:821–827

74. Anonymous: The prevention of falls in later life. Dan Med Bull 1987;34(supp 4):1–24

75. Wolf ST, Barnhart H, Kutner NG: Reducing frailty and falls in older persons: an investigation of Tai Chi and computerized balance training. J Am Geriatr Soc 1996;44:489–497

76. Unutzer J, Patrick DL, Simon G et al: Depressive symptoms and the cost of health services in HMO patients aged 65 years and older: a four-year prospective study. JAMA 1997;277:1618–1623

77. Callahan CM, Hui SL, Nienaber NA: Longitudinal study of depression and health services use among elderly primary care patients. J Am Geriatr Soc 1994;42:833–838

78. Von KM, Ormel J, Katon W: Disability and depression among high utilizers of health care: a longitudinal analysis. Arch Gen Psychiat 1992;49:91–100

79. Harris R, Minion L, Patterson M: Severe illness in older patients: the association between depressive disorders and functional dependency during the recovery phase. J Am Geriatr Soc 1988;36:890–896

80. Kivela S, Pahkala K: Depressive disorder as a predictor of physical disability in old age. J Am Geriatr Soc 2001;49:290–296

81. Koenig H, George L: Depression and physical disability outcomes in depressed medically ill hospitalized older adults. Am J Geriatr Psychiat 1998;6:230–247

82. Djernes J, Gulmann N, Abelskov K: Psychopathologic and functional outcome in the treatment of elderly inpatients with depressive disorders, dementia, delirium and psychoses. Int Psychogeriatr 1998;10:71–83

83. Lebowitz B, Pearson J, Schneider L et al: Diagnosis and treatment of depression in late life. JAMA 1997; 278:1186–1190

84. Oslin D, Streim J, Katz I, Edell W, TenHave T: Change in disability follows inpatient for late life depression. J Am Geriatr Soc 2000;48:357–362

85. Simon G, Katon W, Rutter C: Impact of improved depression treatment in primary care on daily functioning and disability. Psychol Med 1998;28:693–701

86. US Government Accounting Office: Alzheimer's Disease: Estimates of Prevalence in the United States (HEHS-98-16). US Government Printing Office, Washington, 1998

87. Taylor D, Sloan F: How much do persons with Alzheimer's disease cost Medicare? J Am Geriatr Soc 2000;48:639–646

88. Ernst R, Hay JW, Fenn C, Tinklenberg J, Yesavage JA: Cognitive function and the cost of Alzheimer's disease. Arch Neurol 1997;54:687–693

89. Gutterman EM, Markowitz JS, Lewis B, Fillit H: Cost of Alzheimer's disease and related dementia in managed Medicare. J Am Geriatr Soc 1999;47:1065–1071

90. Fishman P, Von Korff M, Lozano P, Hecht J: Chronic care costs in managed care. Health Aff (Millwood) 1997;16:239–247

91. Weiner M, Powe NR, Weller WE, Schaffer TJ, Anderson GF: Alzheimer's disease under managed care: implications from Medicare utilization and expenditure patterns. J Am Geriatr Soc 1998;46:762–770

92. Wells DL, Dawson P, Sidani S, Craig D, Pringle D: Effects of an abilities focused program of morning care on residents who have dementia and on caregivers. J Am Geriatr Soc 2000;48:442–449

93. Max W, Webber P, Fox P: The unpaid burden of caring. J Aging Health 1995;43:179–199

94. Baumgarten M, Hanley J, Infante-Rivard C: Health of family members caring for elderly persons with dementia. Ann Intern Med 1994;120:126–132

95. Kinosian BP, Stallard E, Lee JH et al: Predicting 10-year care requirements for older people with suspected Alzheimer's disease. J Am Geriatr Soc 2000;48:631–638

96. Fillit H: Improving the quality of managed care for patients with mild to moderate Alzheimer's disease. Drug Benef Trends 1999;11 (11):BH6–BH11

97. Rojas-Fernandez CH, Lancotot KL, Allen DD, MacKnight C: Pharmacotherapy of behavioral and psychological symptoms of dementia: time for a different paradigm? Pharmacotherapy 2001;21(1):74–102

98. Van Dongen MCJM, Van Rossum E, Kessels AGH, Sielhorst HJG, Knipchild PG: The efficacy of Ginko for elderly people with dementia and age associated memory impairment: new results of a randomized clinical trial. J Am Geriatr Soc 2000;48:1183–1194

99. Sherwin B: Mild cognitive impairment: potential pharmacologic treatment options. J Am Geriatr Soc 2000;48:431–441

100. Mayeux R, Sano M: Treatment of Alzheimer's disease. N Eng J Med 1999;341:1670–1679

101. Galasko D: An integrated approach to the management of Alzheimer's disease: assessing cognition, function and behavior. Eur J Neurol 1998;5:S9–S17

102. Burke JR, Morgenlander JC: Promising advances in detection and treatment. Postgrad Med 1999;106:85–94

103. Fillit HM, Hill J, Picariello G, Warburton S: How the principles of geriatric assessment are shaping managed care. Geriatrics 1998;53:76

Index